Oxford Textbook of

Global Public Health

Oxford Textbook of
Global Public Health

SIXTH EDITION

Edited by

Roger Detels

Distinguished Professor of Epidemiology and Infectious Diseases,
Schools of Public Health and Medicine, University of California,
Los Angeles, CA, USA

Martin Gulliford

Professor of Public Health, Department of Primary Care and Public Health Sciences,
King's College London, UK

Quarraisha Abdool Karim

Associate Scientific Director, CAPRISA; Professor in Clinical Epidemiology,
Columbia University, USA; Adjunct Professor in Public Health,
University of KwaZulu-Natal, South Africa

and

Chorh Chuan Tan

President and Professor of Medicine, National University of Singapore, Singapore

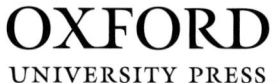

OXFORD

UNIVERSITY PRESS

OXFORD
UNIVERSITY PRESS

Great Clarendon Street, Oxford, OX2 6DP,
United Kingdom

Oxford University Press is a department of the University of Oxford.
It furthers the University's objective of excellence in research, scholarship,
and education by publishing worldwide. Oxford is a registered trade mark of
Oxford University Press in the UK and in certain other countries

First edition 1984
Second edition 1991
Third edition 1997
Fourth edition 2002 (reprinted in paperback 2004, 2005 twice)
Fifth edition 2009 (reprinted in paperback 2011)
Sixth edition 2015
First published in paperback 2017

Impression: 2

Published in the United States of America by Oxford University Press
198 Madison Avenue, New York, NY 10016, United States of America

British Library Cataloguing in Publication Data

Data available

Library of Congress Cataloging in Publication Data

Data available

ISBN 978–0–19–966175–6 (Set)
ISBN 978–0–19–871930–4 (Vol. 1)
ISBN 978–0–19–871931–1 (Vol. 2)
ISBN 978–0–19–871932–8 (Vol. 3)
ISBN 978–0–19–881013–1 (Combined pbk.)

Printed and bound in China by
C&C Offset Printing Co., Ltd

Preface to the sixth edition

There have been important developments in public health over the last decade, and these are reflected in the focus of this new edition of the *Oxford Textbook of Global Public Health*. There has been a dramatic decline in infant mortality and a commensurate increase in life expectancy, but at the same time, the disparities in health between rich and poor countries and between rich and poor within countries have increased. As life expectancy has increased in most regions of the world, so has the number of years individuals spend with significant disabilities from illnesses as reflected in higher disability-adjusted life years. The response to HIV/AIDS has forged new alliances between industry and public health and demonstrated the potential synergy between treatment and prevention approaches for control of infectious diseases. The speed of transmission of severe acute respiratory syndrome (SARS) in 2003 and the recent influenza epidemics which spread across continents within weeks have underscored the interdependency of nations, the need for international cooperation and the development of international and cross-border surveillance and control programs. The epidemic of chronic diseases has spread to middle- and low-income countries which now have the majority of cancer, diabetes, and heart disease occurring globally. Urbanization is occurring at an unprecedented rate and scale in rapidly emerging economies, bringing many new health and social challenges. These events, trends, and programs are rapidly changing the scope, reach, and character of public health.

Since the publication of the last edition it has become increasingly clear that public health must adopt a global perspective in assessing needs, developing interventions and ensuring good governance (Chapters 1.5, 11.13). This is underscored by the decision of the editors to change the title of the textbook to the *Oxford Textbook of Global Public Health* which better reflects the scope of the book and the issues covered in it. To capture this new perspective, we have updated all the chapters, added new chapters and recruited new authors with particular expertise in the rapidly changing scope and responsibilities of public health.

Global health problems of the 21st century

The development of real-time communication systems, rapid global travel and the pervasive use of the social media has had a huge impact on health and disease (Chapter 4.3). The outbreak of SARS, which began in Guangdong province in China in late 2002 and from Hong Kong, spread across the world in days to weeks underscores the rapidity with which epidemics can develop in the 21st century and the consequent challenges of controlling their rapid spread. The evolution of the internet while proving to be a useful tool in the control of disease through information sharing and dissemination of preventive and control strategies, has also greatly enabled activities that are detrimental to public health such as the sale of counterfeit drugs, propagation of misinformation about disease and strategies to control disease and spreading sexually transmitted diseases through websites facilitating sexual liaisons.

Chronic diseases have now overtaken infectious diseases as the major global health problem even in developing countries (Chapters 8.1–8.6). Developing countries must now face the dual challenge of rapidly increasing incidence of chronic diseases and the persistence of infectious diseases, many of which are becoming resistant to available drugs e.g. for tuberculosis, malaria, gonorrhea, etc. Many countries are now experiencing an epidemic of diabetes and obesity related to changing lifestyles associated with increasing prosperity.

As the physical health of the global population has generally improved, there has been growing awareness of the increasing prevalence of mental illness, especially depression, a leading cause of morbidity and non-productivity (Chapter 8.7). Concomitant with the increasing prevalence of mental illness, there has been an increase of overtreatment with anti-depressants and other drugs for mental illness which introduce drug-related problems. Overuse and abuse of anti-microbial drugs has also promoted the emergence of drug-resistant organisms. For a number of infectious diseases, there remains only one effective drug and in some cases, no effective drug leaving the population vulnerable to infections which had previously been considered to be under control.

Globalization has spurred internal migration of rural poor to urban centers, especially in developing countries, overwhelming the ability of cities to provide essential services such as clean water and safe disposal of waste (Chapters 1.5, 2.7, 6.2, 9.7, 10.1). Crowding in slums created by these migrants promotes the rapid spread of many infectious diseases, a hazard to all segments of the urban population. Internal migration also often leads to the break up of the family structure as it is the male who is more likely to migrate causing social disruption and the loss of the main social support system and social safety net in many developing countries.

Globalization has also been associated with the rapid development of industrialization and a steep increase in the number of vehicles, both of which have caused a severe increase in air and water pollution which in turn has increased the rate of climate change and its associated problems. The steep rise in water and air pollution and the impact of these on climate change transcend national boundaries and will require not only more comprehensive national responses but also greater international cooperation (Chapters 7.1–7.5).

Violence, only recently recognized as being in the sphere of public health, has been increasing in many parts of the world (Chapters 9.5, 9.6). The root causes of violence involve social inequality and the lack of access by much of the world's poor to basic social, economic and health resources. Thus, inequality, both between nations and within nations, a fundamental cause of the failure of many to attain the basic human right of good health, also affects the quality of life through promotion of violence. Although inequality is basically a political issue, public health must also play a role in reducing inequality (Chapters 2.2, 3.3). A component of this inequality affecting health is the lack of health professionals in both developing and developed countries (Chapter 11.9). Developing countries are effectively subsidizing the health of developed countries, as many of their citizens trained as healthcare professionals migrate to the more attractive positions offered in developed countries exacerbating the problem of health inequality suffered by developing countries.

Strategies to address public health problems in the 21st century

Traditionally public health professionals have relied on death rates, including infant mortality rates, to gauge the health status of a country. However, many diseases including mental illness and accidents impact the ability of individuals to function without necessarily increasing their probability of dying. The development of new metrics such as disability adjusted life years, years of healthy life lost and other strategies has provided important new ways to estimate the impact of these non-fatal diseases on health and the ability of individuals to function to their full potential (Chapter 5.17). The estimates developed from these strategies have contributed greatly to our ability to characterize health problems and to prioritize limited health resources to address key issues.

The 20th century also witnessed a rapid development of new technologies, including more sensitive approaches to identify genetic determinants of disease (Chapter 2.5). These technologies have been put in the service of public health and will play an increasingly role in the future. However, the development and application of these new technologies to assess health and to identify those at risk of disease also raise serious ethical issues (Chapter 3.2).

Surveillance has been an essential tool to monitor the magnitude and spread of disease in human and animal populations (Chapter 5.19). The increasing recognition that disease agents do not respect national boundaries and that emerging infectious diseases can spread between continents within days to weeks has highlighted the need to strengthen international surveillance strategies and cooperation to provide early warning of emerging and re-emerging health threats such as pandemic influenza so that more timely and effective strategies for containment can be implemented (Chapter 3.2).

The late 20th and early 21st centuries have witnessed the increasing commitment of some sections of the private sector to the health of the public as part of their corporate responsibility (Chapter 11.12). The private sector now plays a significant role in international public health through the contribution of pharmaceutical and other companies and foundations supported by the private sector such as the Ford Foundation, the Rockefeller Foundation and more recently the Gates Foundation. While it is clear that they can play a significant role in promoting health, it is crucial that they recognize the importance of working with developing countries in developing their health agendas so as to maximize their impact. The development of guidelines for health assistance such as those put forth in the Paris Declaration on Aid Effectiveness (2005), the Accra Agenda for Action (2008) and the International Health Partnership and Related Initiatives (2007) provide guidance for the private sector to maximize the contributions to international public health (Chapter 11.13).

The United Nations has spurred the contribution of developed countries to international health through the creation of the Global Fund to Fight AIDS, Tuberculosis and Malaria. This has been augmented by national bilateral and multilateral funds such as the US President's Emergency Plan for AIDS Relief and the programs of the European Union. These programs have made significant contributions to control of disease and promotion of global health.

The costs of drugs, protected by international trade and patent agreements, have been a major barrier to the control of such diseases as HIV/AIDS. Recently, however, pharmaceutical companies have been providing these drugs to developing countries at affordable prices and through outright donations (Chapter 8.3).

Public health challenges in the 21st century

The problems cited above persist in the 21st century, and will require international cooperation, research and public health action to address effectively. Many of the preventable infectious diseases have been brought under control through immunization programs although not eradicated (Chapters 8.11, 11.3, 11.4). Eradication of polio is within sight, but political issues in Pakistan and Nigeria have been associated with the killing of vaccinators, presenting a difficult problem not easily addressed by strategies available to public health.

Drug resistance will be an increasing problem that transcends national boundaries. New drugs need to be developed rapidly, but the issue of misuse of drugs, the cause of developing resistance to many drugs, needs to be urgently addressed as well (Chapters 8.12–8.15).

Although many infectious diseases have been brought under control, that control is very fragile and dependent on continued vigilance. Complacency is perhaps the worst enemy of vigilance undermining the considerable effort necessary to assure continued control of these preventable diseases (Chapter 11.13).

The epidemics of obesity and diabetes and the continuing problems of cardiovascular diseases and cancer need to be addressed in the 21st century (Chapters 8.1 and 8.2). This will be a particular challenge as it primarily involves changes in lifestyle from a sedentary existence requiring little effort to engaging in physical activities, changing eating habits and modifying many comfortable habits to which the public have become accustomed (Chapter 6.4). Prevention of chronic diseases requires taking personal responsibility for one's health. It is the job of public health to promote the assumption of that responsibility by the public (Chapter 8.4).

As rates of infant mortality have declined markedly in the late 20th century and duration of life has been extended, the population of the world is aging (Chapter 6.3). Thus the ratio of the productive age individuals to dependent age individuals has declined. Hence, a shrinking working age population will be responsible for supporting an increasing population of elderly. Increased worker productivity will be key to sustaining and improving the economic well-being of the global population. Increased health and the ability to function at full capacity will be key factors for increasing worker productivity and are the responsibility of public health (Chapters 3.1, 10.8). However, youth are increasingly vulnerable to drugs, violence, poverty, the changing make-up of the family, and mental health problems, exacerbated by increasing economic disparities between rich and poor globally and nationally (Chapters 8.7, 9.2, 9.5, 10.1, 10.4).

The world needs to ensure universal coverage of affordable health care and to increase the investment in the development and training of health professionals who will lead the essential public health initiatives of the 21st century. Distribution of this health workforce must be more equal and part of an effort to reduce health and social disparities (Chapters 2.2–2.4 and 11.3).

Recently there has been greater recognition of the need to scale up the effective implementation of strategies that have been demonstrated through research to improve health. Thus, the field of 'implementation science', which deals with issues of how to bring effective strategies to a scale which will impact the health of the public, has gained prominence as an important research thrust (Chapters 6.3, 6.4).

The sixth edition of the *Oxford Textbook of Global Public Health*

It is the intention of this 6th edition of the *Oxford Textbook of Global Public Health* to provide comprehensive insights into global health problems now and in the future, and to present strategies and initiatives to address these problems. Although public health professionals will agree on the problems that need to be addressed, there is a diversity of opinions on the optimal approaches to tackle them. It is also our intention to review the diversity of these opinions and to present our views and those of our expert contributors on the merits and shortcomings of these proposed strategies.

The 6th edition, as with previous editions, is targeted primarily at public health professionals, particularly those entering the field who wish to learn about the scope and diversity of global public health. Public health is an exciting field in which to work and has the ability and potential to substantially improve the health of millions of people all over the world. Above all, it is our intention to convey the excitement and the power of public health to promote 'health for all' through this 6th edition.

Introduction

The scope of public health

The scope of public health is vast and continues to evolve rapidly, seeking to address the daunting challenges to health in the twenty-first century while seizing new opportunities for advancing the well-being of the peoples of the world. From an earlier focus on population health, it has grown to encompass a greater emphasis on equity as encapsulated by the World Health Organization's goal of 'health for all' and, more recently, expanded into the concept of global health in recognition of the profound impact of globalization on health and its determinants. 'The scope of public health' traces the salient aspects of this evolution for countries at different stages of development, and provides in-depth overviews of long-standing as well as emerging issues of critical importance within the broad scope of public health.

'The scope of public health' maps the breadth of public health through three fully updated sections, namely, the history and development of public health; determinants of health and disease; and public health policies, law and ethics.

Section 1 sets the broad context and framework with Chapter 1.1 providing a high-level overview of contemporary health issues and the expanded functions of public health. The three chapters that follow describe how history, the phase of economic development and regional particularities have influenced the contours and directions of public health development in rich, low- and middle-income, and emerging economies respectively. All these countries, however, are experiencing the immense and growing impact of globalization on health and its determinants. Chapter 1.5 reviews the major forces and drivers associated with a much more globalized world, and the complex and varied influences that these are exerting on health and healthcare systems in different geographies. To respond adequately to these new challenges and dynamics, a much higher extent and depth of international coordination and cooperation across many sectors will be required.

These considerations set the essential backdrop for Section 2 which covers the determinants of health and disease, the thorough understanding of which is crucial to the development of effective and sustainable long-term interventions for public health problems. Chapter 2.1 provides a new overview of the determinants of health, emphasizing their complexity and inter-relatedness. A new chapter on poverty, justice and health (Chapter 2.2) discusses the meaning of justice as applied to health and focuses on factors that contribute to social inequities in health in both developed and resource-constrained countries. These issues are taken up in detail in the following chapters on socio-economic inequalities in health in high-income countries (Chapter 2.3), and reducing health inequalities in developing countries (Chapter 2.4).

Beyond the social determinants of health and disease, dramatic advances in genomics research are providing new insights into the causes and pathogenesis of diseases, and their genetic determinants. The application of genomics research techniques to public health and epidemiology, a topic covered in Chapter 2.5, also offers the potential for better designed public health programmes as well as more accurate stratification of sub-populations and individuals at significantly increased risk of specific diseases, raising the prospect for targeted public health interventions.

The chapters that follow provide updated reviews of long-standing public health concerns which remain critically important, namely water and sanitation; nutrition and food safety; and the environment with a strengthened focus on the public health impact of climate change. The high and rising prevalence of chronic non-communicable diseases throughout the world which have their roots in risk factors linked to lifestyles and behaviours, has led to heightened interest in the behavioural determinants of health and disease, an important subject covered in Chapter 2.9. The widespread adoption of health-promoting behaviours, at the level of individuals and societies, is arguably one of the most important challenges for public health in this century. Section 2, with its focus on social and health inequalities, is aptly rounded off with Chapter 2.10 which addresses key issues in access to healthcare, and the importance of universal coverage and equitable access to affordable and cost-effective health interventions.

The last section of 'The scope of public health' focuses on public health policies, law and ethics, builds on the issues and considerations discussed in the preceding sections. Section 3 starts with a discussion on the need for, and the changing forms of, leadership in public health. Chapter 3.2 considers key ethical issues in public health and the evolution of principles and guidelines for its practice and research, while Chapter 3.3 reaffirms the commitment of public health to work towards the highest attainable standard of health. These lead up to a new chapter on the role of law and legal instruments in achieving public health objectives at the local, national and global levels. A new Chapter, 3.5, reviews the complex but important issues of priority setting and rationing in public health and healthcare delivery. This is followed by discussion of the major drivers, forms and directions of health policy formulation and implementation in developing countries and developed countries, in Chapters 3.6 and 3.7 respectively. Given the high and growing interconnectedness of our world, and the powerful and pervasive impact of globalization on health and disease, Chapter 3.8 describes the importance of greater international collaboration and coordinated action, and the efforts jointly required and taken to promote public health in countries across the world.

The extensive responsibilities and the varied and changing scope of public health described in this book will require public health policy-makers and professionals to work closely together across a wide range of disciplines, to establish intersectoral partnerships and international coalitions that encompass the public, not-for-profit and private sectors, and, most importantly, to engage communities to achieve the goals of improving population health and promoting equity for all, so as to realise the full promise of public health for the 21st century.

The methods of public health

'The methods of public health' presents the methods which bring scientific rigour to the public health endeavour. With a firm and broad grounding in the methods of public health, students and practitioners will ensure that their research and practice is based on robust evidence; a critically important consideration in informing decision-making. The methodology utilized is key for assuring the strength and validity of evidence for decision-making. Randomized trials, systematic reviews, meta-analyses and economic evaluations are accepted methods for providing clinical evidence but there are difficulties in applying these in a public health context where there are large target populations and long timescales for the emergence of outcomes. Application of these techniques has become more common to inform public health decision-making but there is increasing appreciation of the complexity of public health interventions and the need to use a range of disciplinary approaches to develop and evaluate these.

The range and complexity of health problems facing populations is also increasing, and public health methodologies must evolve and expand to meet this challenge and ensure effective responses. With globalization of demographic, nutrition, and physical activity transitions, the methods of public health must be adapted to meet the new challenges. Since the 5th edition, the effects of globalization on health including the increasing importance of global environmental changes and notably climate change, have burgeoned. These new challenges are more difficult to study than the traditional concerns of infectious and non-infectious diseases and local environmental issues. The adaptation of old methods and the development of new ones are key to ensure the continued relevance and robustness of public health research. Public health practitioners have always had to face the dilemma of balancing delays in action emanating from concern for methodological rigor with the need to act expeditiously. This dilemma is becoming increasingly complex

and challenging as some of the new and emerging public health challenges are less amenable to traditional public health approaches and in some instances, are associated with ethical considerations that add to the complexity of the issue.

All the chapters in 'The methods of public health' have been extensively revised and updated, and several new chapters added. Organized into four sections: information systems and sources of intelligence; epidemiological and biostatistical approaches; social science techniques and environmental and occupational health sciences. Information systems are the foundation of all public health research and action. The lack of good information is still a barrier to effective action in much of the world. Basic information on births and deaths is not routinely available for most low-income and many middle-income countries. This gap remains a major impediment to tracking progress towards the Millennium Development Goals. Fortunately, a concerted effort is now being made to close the gap, especially for maternal and child statistics with the support of several philanthropic foundations. Three chapters in this section (Chapters 4.1–4.3) examine the contrasting challenges facing information systems in both high-income and low- and middle-income countries. Chapter 4.2 by Cherutich and Nduati captures the substantial advances being made in information systems and community diagnosis in low-and-middle income countries. Chapter 4.3 by Dutta, a new chapter in this section, provides an insightful overview of the impact of new communication streams on public health.

Epidemiology and biostatistics are the core sciences of public health. Public health practice requires a firm connection to the priority health needs of populations. Epidemiological research is almost always required to establish this connection, and exceptions are few; some major acute outbreaks or overwhelming catastrophes do not allow for serious epidemiological investigation before the response is required. However, epidemiological study is still needed to assess the scope of the problem and the effectiveness of the response. Public health methods to ensure the appropriateness of inferences (Chapter 5.14) drawn from public health investigations—perhaps the most difficult and certainly the most contentious aspect of public health science—are evolving. This process often requires a systematic approach to ensuring that all data from all studies—published and unpublished—are synthesized into a usable summary assessment (Chapter 5.15). A critical and expanding methodological area deals with interventions and their effectiveness (Chapters 5.7–5.10). Technological advances—computers and the Internet—are changing the scope of public health and opening new possibilities, from data collection and analysis for the early identification of disease outbreaks to the use of modelling of disease transmission to predict the future trends and needs (Chapters 5.4 and 5.18). The methods and special issues facing clinical epidemiology are discussed in Chapter 5.11. Chapter 5.19 stresses the essential importance of surveillance to monitor public health problems and the effectiveness of intervention programs. Increasingly a more systems-based approach is being utilized to understand disease and risk. Campbell and Bonell provide an excellent update on new developments in the implementation of multicomponent interventions (Chapter 6.5). The completion of the Human Genome Project is being translated to novel approaches to diseases including the use of gene therapy. Of note are two new contemporary chapters in Section 5, viz. genetic epidemiology (Young and Sandhu, Chapter 5.12) and life course epidemiology and analysis (Kuh et al., Chapter 5.20).

The methodologies for measuring burden of disease have been substantially revised (Vos and Murray, Chapter 5.17) and are particularly important as the implementation of these new methodologies is being used to provide the basis for both global and local rationing of resources and priority setting.

Social science techniques are assuming even greater importance to the practice of public health with the recognition that epidemiological information alone is not sufficient for the development and implementation of effective public health policies and programmes (Chapter 6.1). Demography is another underappreciated basic science of public health; the aging of all populations, especially in low- and middle-income countries, will be a critical public health issue for the economic survival of these countries in the 21st century (Chapter 6.3). Health economics and the use of cost-effectiveness analysis (Chapter 6.6) have expanded the audience for public health research to sectors outside health, especially the finance and development sectors, nationally and globally. Health promotion expands the focus of public health from a primary concern with disease prevention and control towards an understanding of the underlying determinants of health (Chapter 6.4). These and other social science tools, including management of the health programmes (Chapter 6.8), are key for the development and implementation of effective public health policy in all countries (Chapter 6.9). The HIV pandemic has brought renewed interest and focus on sexuality and health that Parker et al. cover eloquently in Chapter 6.2. A novel and increasingly used approach to programme and treatment adherence is incentivising and supporting desired behaviours which is captured in Chapter 6.7 on behavioural economics by Kessler and Zhang.

Environmental and occupational health sciences cover traditional public health issues, as well as the even more difficult global health challenges that are discussed in Volume 1. This section deals with both traditional and emerging environmental and occupational health hazards, many of which have been exacerbated by globalization (Chapters 7.1–7.4). The increasingly important issues of risk assessment and management, and risk perception and communication are covered in Chapters 7.5 and 7.6.

The importance of methodological advances in public health is illustrated by the way in which many chapters in this textbook consider methodological issues in considerable detail—for example, the chapters on measuring the global burden of diseases and responding to global environmental challenges. The chapters in this section illustrate the evolution and breadth of public health methods as its scope continues to expand. No doubt, this process will continue well into the future and remains a good marker of the growth and evolution of the public health sciences as sound and rigorous strategies to address emerging and ongoing public health challenges.

The practice of public health

Public health is what we, as a society, do collectively to assure the conditions for people to be healthy. This requires that continuing and emerging threats to the health of the public be successfully countered...through effective, organised and sustained efforts led by the public sector. Institute of Medicine (1988)[1]

---

[1] Institute of Medicine (1988). *The future of public health*. National Academies Press, Washington DC. Page 19.

'The practice of public health' provides an up-to-date account of the practice of public health through 48 chapters written by leading experts. The contents of 'The practice of public health' identify public health as a subject of local and national concern, and a key responsibility of governments and public agencies, with private industry also increasingly recognizing its responsibility to promote the health of the public. The contents also emphasize that public health is an international issue that must be addressed through good global governance. The focus is on the application of population science methods to the major challenges being addressed through public health intervention. The chapters in this edition reassess priorities, recognize the evolving burden of disease and recommend new strategies for intervention.

Beginning with a discussion of the major groups of non-communicable disorders, including cardiovascular and respiratory diseases and cancer (Section 8). This section now includes separate chapters on obesity, physical inactivity and diabetes, reflecting growing concern at the increasing prevalence and growing impact of these conditions on global health. This section continues with a series of chapters on communicable diseases, with chapters on tuberculosis, malaria, hepatitis and emerging and re-emerging infections. Together these conditions represent major priorities: tuberculosis accounts for an estimated 1.4 million deaths worldwide each year, with 8.7 million new cases; malaria accounts for 42.3 million disability-adjusted life years lost annually; while 500 million people are chronically infected with hepatitis viruses, with one million deaths annually. As well as outlining problems and their causes, each of these chapters discusses potential solutions, including national and international strategies for disease control and prevention.

The emphasis on intervention for prevention of disease and promotion of health is continued in 'The methods of public health' dealing with public health hazards including tobacco, alcohol, drug abuse, injuries and violence (Section 9). Proposed intervention strategies encompass both population-based approaches; including, for example, regulation, the use of deterrents and incentives, and public education; and strategies targeted at individuals at high risk through healthcare services. It remains clear, however, that the greatest risks are generally found among those groups for whom interventions are least accessible.

Section 10 considers the public health needs of different population groups paying particular attention to groups that for a range of reasons are vulnerable to public health hazards and disease risks. Separate chapters outline the needs of families, women, children, adolescents, older people, ethnic minorities, people with disabilities and forced migrants and displaced populations. New chapters are introduced on indigenous peoples and prisons and public health. Collectively, these chapters emphasize the importance of the public health role in analysing the health needs of these often marginalized populations, advocating for their rights to health, aiming to reduce inequalities in health.

Section 11 presents an analysis of the core public health skills required for improving population health and reducing inequalities in health. This section begins with a new chapter on the concept of need, which shows that technical assessments of the capacity to benefit from health intervention can rarely be separated from underlying assumptions concerning the justification and rationale for societal intervention. Involving several sectors is generally necessary and this is exemplified by chapters on current strategies for control of non-communicable diseases and infectious diseases. A series of chapters then outlines opportunities for intervention through the health sector including healthcare services, population screening, and environmental health practice. The section on the public health workforce is strengthened through the inclusion of new chapters on training of local health workers, and public health professionals, to meet public health needs. There are also chapters on planning and responding to public health emergencies, with a new chapter on chemical and radiological emergencies.

In the final section of the book, Quarraisha Abdool Karim and Roger Detels question the assumption that intervention on public health problems must be led by the public sector. They describe an enhanced role for powerful private sector advocates of public health intervention, while at the same time drawing attention to some of the challenges of this approach and the importance of the stewardship role of governments. The closing chapter, by Dr Margaret Chan and Mary Kay Kindhauser, comments on several key issues that have been raised in earlier chapters of the book, analysing the pressing challenges now facing the public health community globally, and emphasizing that public health is a powerful driver for positive change to dramatically improve the health and lives of all people.

Brief Contents

Contents

List of Contributors

Quarraisha Abdool Karim Associate Scientific Director, CAPRISA; Professor in Clinical Epidemiology, Columbia University, USA; Adjunct Professor in Public Health, University of KwaZulu-Natal, South Africa
Chapter 11.12 Private support of public health

Maia Ambegaokar Principal, Health Governance, Policy Planning Management consultancy, Sydney, Australia
Chapter 3.1 Leadership in public health

Anne-Emmanuelle Ambresin Senior Resident, Multidisciplinary Unit for Adolescent Health, University Hospital/CHUV, Lausanne, Switzerland
Chapter 10.4 Adolescent health

Ian Anderson Murrup Barak, Melbourne Institute for Indigenous Development, The University of Melbourne, Melbourne, VIC, Australia
Chapter 10.6 The health of indigenous peoples

Elena M. Andresen Interim Dean, Public Health, Oregon Health & Science University, and Portland State University, Portland, OR, USA
Chapter 10.7 People with disabilities

Tar-Ching Aw College of Medicine and Health Sciences, United Arab Emirates University, Al Ain, United Arab Emirates
Chapter 7.4 Occupational health
Chapter 7.5 Toxicology and risk assessment in the analysis and management of environmental risk

Gunilla Backman Swedish International Development Cooperation Agency, Stockholm, Sweden
Chapter 3.3 The right to the highest attainable standard of health

Rajiv Bahl World Health Organization, Geneva, Switzerland
Chapter 10.3 Child health

Lope H. Barrero Department of Industrial Engineering, Pontificia Universidad Javeriana, Bogotá, Colombia
Chapter 8.9 Musculoskeletal diseases

Natalie Bartle NHS Trust Development Authority, Midlands and East, UK
Chapter 11.1 Health needs assessment

Catherine R. Bateman Steel School of Social Sciences at the University of New South Wales, Sydney, NSW, Australia
Chapter 10.9 Forced migrants and other displaced populations

Frances Baum Director of the Southgate Institute of Health, Society and Equity at Flinders University, Adelaide, SA, Australia
Chapter 2.2 Poverty, justice, and health

Yoav Ben-Shlomo School of Social and Community Medicine, University of Bristol, Bristol, UK
Chapter 5.20 Life course epidemiology and analysis

Douglas Bettcher Director, Prevention of Noncommunicable Diseases, World Health Organization, Geneva, Switzerland
Chapter 3.8 International efforts to promote public health

Raj Bhopal Edinburgh Ethnicity and Health Research Group, University of Edinburgh, Edinburgh, UK
Chapter 10.5 Ethnicity, race, epidemiology, and public health

Zulfiqar A. Bhutta Robert Harding Chair in Global Child Health & Policy, Centre for Global Child Health, Hospital for Sick Children Toronto, Canada; Founding Director, Centre of Excellence in Women & Child Health, The Aga Khan University, Karachi, Pakistan
Chapter 8.11 Infectious diseases and prions

Marike Boezen University of Groningen, University Medical Center Groningen, Department of Epidemiology, Groningen, Netherlands
Chapter 8.3 Chronic obstructive pulmonary disease and asthma

Paolo Boffetta Director of the Institute for Translational Epidemiology at Mount Sinai Hospital, New York, NY, USA
Chapter 8.2 Cancer epidemiology and public health

Chris Bonell Department of Childhood, Families and Health, Institute of Education, University of London, UK
Chapter 6.5 Development and evaluation of complex multicomponent interventions in public health

Cynthia Boschi-Pinto World Health Organization, Geneva, Switzerland; and Universidade Federal Fluminense, Niterói, Brazil
Chapter 10.3 Child health

James Bowen Medical Director, Multiple Sclerosis Center, Swedish Neuroscience Institute, Seattle, WA, USA
Chapter 8.10 Neurological diseases, epidemiology, and public health

Naima Bradley Public Health England, Chilton, UK
Chapter 11.11 Principles of public health emergency response for acute environmental, chemical, and radiation incidents

Richard Brennan World Health Organization, Geneva, Switzerland
Chapter 11.10 Emergency public health and humanitarian assistance in the twenty-first century

Benjamin Bristow Mount Sinai Global Health, Icahn School of Medicine at Mount Sinai, New York, NY, USA
Chapter 8.15 Malaria

Collin Brooks Centre for Public Health Research, Massey University, Wellington, New Zealand
Chapter 8.3 Chronic obstructive pulmonary disease and asthma

James W. Buehler Health Management and Policy, School of Public Health, Drexel University, Philadelphia, PA, USA
Chapter 5.19 Public health surveillance

Wylie Burke Department of Bioethics and Humanities, University of Washington, Seattle, WA, USA
Chapter 2.5 Genomics and public health

Julie E. Byles Research Centre for Gender, Health and Ageing, at the University of Newcastle, Callaghan, NSW, Australia
Chapter 10.8 Health of older people

Alberto J. Caban-Martinez Department of Environmental Health, Harvard University School of Public Health, Boston, MA, USA
Chapter 8.9 Musculoskeletal diseases

Rona Campbell Director of the Centre for the Development and Evaluation of Complex Interventions for Public Health Improvement—DECIPHer, School for Social and Community Medicine, University of Bristol, UK
Chapter 6.5 Development and evaluation of complex multicomponent interventions in public health

Simon Carroll Community Health Promotion Research Centre, University of Victoria, BC, Canada
Chapter 6.4 Health promotion, health education, and the public's health

Richard F. Catalano Richard E. Chaisson, Johns Hopkins University School of Medicine and Bloomberg School of Public Health, Baltimore, MD, USA
Chapter 10.4 Adolescent health

Richard E. Chaisson Johns Hopkins University, School of Medicine and Bloomberg School of Public Health, Baltimore, MD, USA
Chapter 8.14 Tuberculosis

Margaret Chan World Health Organization, Geneva, Switzerland
Chapter 11.13 The future of international public health in an era of austerity

Leda Chatzi Department of Social Medicine, Medical School, University of Crete, Heraklion, Greece
Chapter 5.3 Cross-sectional studies

Chien-Jen Chen Graduate Institute of Epidemiology, National Taiwan University College of Public Health, Taipei, Taiwan
Chapter 7.1 Environmental health issues in public health

Peter Cherutich National AIDS & STI Control Programme–NASCOP, Kenyatta National Hospital Grounds, Nairobi, Kenya
Chapter 4.2 Information systems and community diagnosis in low- and middle-income countries

Gavin J. Churchyard Aurum Institute NPC, Johannesburg, Gauteng, South Africa
Chapter 8.14 Tuberculosis

Sarah Clark School of Public Policy at the Department of Political Science, University College London, London, UK
Chapter 3.5 Priority setting, social values, and public health

Mike Clarke Director of the MRC Hub for Trials Methodology Research at the Centre for Public Health, Queens University Belfast, Belfast, UK
Chapter 5.15 Systematic reviews and meta-analysis

Thomas Clasen Professor of Environmental Health, Rollins School of Public Health, Emory University, Atlanta, GA, USA; Reader in Water, Sanitation and Health, London School of Hygiene & Tropical Medicine, London, UK
Chapter 2.6 Water and sanitation

Hoosen Coovadia MatCH (Maternal Adolescent and Child Health) at the University of Witwatersrand, Nelson R. Mandela School of Medicine, Doris Duke Medical Research Institute, Durban, South Africa
Chapter 2.4 Reducing health inequalities in developing countries

Sue Crengle Senior Lecturer, Te Kupenga Hauora Maori, School of Population Health, University of Auckland, Auckland, New Zealand
Chapter 10.6 The health of indigenous peoples

Bernadette Daelmans World Health Organization, Geneva, Switzerland
Chapter 10.3 Child health

Julia Dalzell Program Director at the Center for Food Law and Policy, Los Angeles, CA, USA
Chapter 3.8 International efforts to promote public health

Manuel M. Dayrit Dean, Ateneo School of Medicine and Public Health, Ateneo de Manila University, Philippines
Chapter 3.1 Leadership in public health

Katherine DeLand World Health Organization, Geneva, Switzerland
Chapter 3.8 International efforts to promote public health

Don Des Jarlais The Baron Edmond de Rothschild Chemical Dependency Institute, Beth Israel Medical Center, New York City, NY, USA
Chapter 9.2 Public health aspects of illicit psychoactive drug use

Roger Detels Distinguished Professor of Epidemiology and Infectious Diseases, Schools of Public Health and Medicine, University of California, Los Angeles, CA, USA
Chapter 1.1 The scope and concerns of public health
Chapter 5.1 Epidemiology: the foundation of public health
Chapter 8.5 Physical activity and health
Chapter 11.8 Training of public health professionals in developing countries
Chapter 11.12 Private support of public health

Nancy Devlin Director of Research, Office of Health Economics, London, UK
Chapter 6.6 Economic appraisal in public healthcare: assessing efficiency and equity

Judith Diers Chief, Adolescent Development and Participation, UNICEF, New York, NY, USA
Chapter 10.4 Adolescent health

Ana V. Diez Roux Department of Epidemiology, University of Michigan School of Public Health, Ann Arbor, MI, USA
Chapter 5.2 Ecological variables, ecological studies, and multilevel studies in public health research

Allan Donner Department of Epidemiology and Biostatistics at the Schulich School of Medicine and Dentistry, University of Western Ontario, London, ON, Canada
Chapter 5.8 Methodological issues in the design and analysis of community intervention trials

Jeroen Douwes Centre for Public Health Research, Massey University, Wellington, New Zealand
Chapter 8.3 Chronic obstructive pulmonary disease and asthma

David W. Dowdy Department of Epidemiology, Johns Hopkins University, Baltimore, MD, USA
Chapter 8.14 Tuberculosis

Lesley Doyal Centre for Health and Social Care at the School for Policy Studies, University of Bristol, Bristol, UK
Chapter 10.2 Women, men, and health

Ernest Drucker Director of the Division of Public Health and Policy Research, Montefiore Medical Center, Albert Einstein College of Medicine, New York, NY, USA
Chapter 10.10 Prisons: from punishment to public health

Mohan J. Dutta Brian Lamb School of Communication, Purdue University, West Lafayette, IN, USA
Chapter 4.3 New communication technologies, social media, and public health

Lars Elhers Danish Center for Healthcare Improvements, Faculty of Social Science & Faculty of Health Science, Aalborg University, Aalborg, Denmark
Chapter 11.4 Population screening and public health

John W. Farquhar C.F. Rehnborg Professor in Disease Prevention and Professor of Medicine and Health Research and Policy, Stanford Prevention Research Center, Stanford University School of Medicine, Stanford, CA, USA
Chapter 5.9 Community intervention trials in high-income countries

Jonathan Feelemyer The Baron Edmond de Rothschild Chemical Dependency Institute, Beth Israel Medical Center, New York City, NY, USA
Chapter 9.2 Public health aspects of illicit psychoactive drug use

Louise Finer Her Majesty's Inspectorate of Prisons, London, UK
Chapter 3.3 The right to the highest attainable standard of health

Baruch Fischhoff Howard Heinz University Professor, Department of Social and Decision Sciences, Department of Engineering and Public Policy, Carnegie Mellon University, Pittsburgh, PA, USA
Chapter 7.6 Risk perception and communication

Dan W. Fitzgerald Weill Cornell Graduate School of Medical Sciences, Cornell University, New York, NY, USA
Chapter 6.9 Implementation science and translational public health

Julio Frenk Dean of the Faculty, T&G Angelopoulos Professor of Public Health and International Development, Harvard School of Public Health and Harvard Kennedy School, Harvard University, Boston, MA, USA
Chapter 3.6 Health policy in developing countries

Irwin Friedman The Health Programme of the SEED Trust, Durban, South Africa
Chapter 2.4 Reducing health inequalities in developing countries

Lawrence M. Friedman Independent Consultant, Rockville, MD, USA
Chapter 5.7 Methodology of intervention trials in individuals

Jonathan Garcia Center for the Study of Culture, Politics and Health, Department of Sociomedical Sciences, Mailman School of Public Health, Columbia University, New York City, NY, USA
Chapter 6.2 Sexuality and public health

Patricia J. Garcia Dean, School of Public Health and Administration (FASPA), Universidad Peruana Cayetano Heredia (UPCH), Lima, Peru
Chapter 8.12 Sexually transmitted infections

Bernard D. Goldstein Dean Emeritus, Graduate School of Public Health, University of Pittsburgh, Pittsburgh, PA, USA
Chapter 7.5 Toxicology and risk assessment in the analysis and management of environmental risk

Octavio Gómez-Dantés National Institute of Public Health, Cuernavaca, Mexico
Chapter 3.6 Health policy in developing countries

Miguel Angel González-Block National Institute of Public Health, Cuernavaca, Mexico
Chapter 3.6 Health policy in developing countries

Fernando Gonzalez-Martinez World Health Organization, Geneva, Switzerland
Chapter 3.8 International efforts to promote public health

Lawrence Gostin Faculty Director, O'Neill Institute for National and Global Health Law, Washington, DC; Director, WHO Collaborating Center on Public Health Law & Human Rights; Johns Hopkins University, Baltimore, MD; based at Georgetown Law, Washington, DC, USA
Chapter 3.4 Law and the public's health

Adele Green QIMR Berghofer Medical Research Institute, Brisbane, QLD; Cancer Research UK Manchester Institute, University of Manchester, Manchester, UK
Chapter 7.2 Radiation and public health

Lawrence W. Green Professor, Department of Epidemiology & Biostatistics at the University of California School of Medicine, San Francisco, CA, USA
Chapter 2.9 Behavioural determinants of health and disease
Chapter 5.9 Community intervention trials in high-income countries

Sander Greenland Department of Epidemiology, UCLA School of Public Health, Los Angeles, CA, USA
Chapter 5.13 Validity and bias in epidemiological research
Chapter 5.14 Causation and causal inference

Sian Griffiths Faculty of Medicine at the Chinese University of Hong Kong, Hong Kong
Chapter 11.6 Strategies and structures for public health intervention

Emily Grundy London School of Economics, London, UK
Chapter 6.3 Demography and public health

Martin Gulliford Department of Primary Care and Public Health Sciences, King's College London, London, UK
Chapter 2.10 Access to healthcare and population health

John Gulliver School of Public Health, Imperial College London, London, UK
Chapter 7.3 Environmental exposure assessment: modelling air pollution concentrations

Davidson H. Hamer Center for Global Health and Development, Boston University; Boston University Schools of Public Health and Medicine, Boston, MA; Tufts University Friedman School of Nutrition Science and Policy, Boston, MA, USA
Chapter 8.11 Infectious diseases and prions

Christopher Hamlin University of Notre Dame, Notre Dame, IN, USA
Chapter 1.2 The history and development of public health in developed countries

Piya Hanvoravongchai Faculty of Medicine, Chulalongkorn University, Bangkok, Thailand
Chapter 11.9 Training of local health workers to meet public health needs

Rebecca Hardy MRC National Survey of Health and Development at the MRC Unit for Lifelong Health and Ageing at UCL, London, UK
Chapter 5.20 Life course epidemiology and analysis

Deborah Hassin Columbia University, New York City, NY, USA
Chapter 9.2 Public health aspects of illicit psychoactive drug use

David L. Heymann Chairman, Health Protection Agency, London, UK
Chapter 8.17 Emerging and re-emerging infections

Robert A. Hiatt Professor and Chair, Department of Epidemiology & Biostatistics at the University of California School of Medicine, San Francisco, CA, USA
Chapter 2.9 Behavioural determinants of health and disease

Marcia Hills Community Health Promotion Research Centre, University of Victoria, BC, Canada
Chapter 6.4 Health promotion, health education, and the public's health

Gavin Hitchcock South African Centre for Epidemiological Modelling and Analysis (SACEMA), Stellenbosch, South Africa
Chapter 5.18 Mathematical models of transmission and control of infectious agents

Sai Yin Ho School of Public Health, The University of Hong Kong, Hong Kong
Chapter 9.1 Tobacco

Kristin S. Hoeft Department of Epidemiology & Biostatistics at the University of California School of Medicine, San Francisco, CA, USA
Chapter 2.9 Behavioural determinants of health and disease

Katherine J. Hoggatt Department of Epidemiology, UCLA School of Public Health, Los Angeles, CA, USA
Chapter 5.14 Causation and causal inference

San Hone Assistant Director, National Aids Control Program, Disease Control Complex, Department of Health, Nay Pyi Taw, Myanmar
Chapter 11.8 Training of public health professionals in developing countries

Kees de Hoogh School of Public Health, Imperial College London, London, UK
Chapter 7.3 Environmental exposure assessment: modelling air pollution concentrations

Paul Hunt School of Law, University of Essex, Colchester, UK
Chapter 3.3 The right to the highest attainable standard of health

Anne Huvos World Health Organization, Geneva, Switzerland
Chapter 3.8 International efforts to promote public health

Adnan Hyder Johns Hopkins University, Bloomberg School of Public Health, International Injury Research Unit, Baltimore, MD, USA
Chapter 9.4 Injury prevention and control: the public health approach

Sopon Iamsirithaworn Bureau of Epidemiology, Department of Disease Control, Ministry of Public Health, Thailand
Chapter 5.4 Principles of outbreak investigation

Richard J. Jackson Department of Environmental Health Sciences, Fielding School of Public Health, University of California, Los Angeles, CA, USA
Chapter 2.1 Determinants of health: overview

W. Philip T. James London School of Hygiene and Tropical Medicine, International Association for the Study of Obesity (IASO), London, UK
Chapter 8.4 Obesity

Rachel Jewkes Director, MRC Gender & Health Research Unit, South African Medical Research Council, Pretoria, South Africa
Chapter 9.5 Interpersonal violence: a recent public health mandate

Gavin W. Jones Director, J. Y. Pillay Comparative Asia Research Centre, Singapore
Chapter 10.1 The changing family

Mary L. Kamb Associate Director for Global Activities, Division of STD Prevention, National Center for HIV, Viral Hepatitis, STD and TB Prevention, US Centers for Disease Control and Prevention, Atlanta, GA, USA
Chapter 8.12 Sexually transmitted infections

Nancy Kass Johns Hopkins Berman Institute of Bioethics and Johns Hopkins Bloomberg School of Public Health, Baltimore, MD, USA
Chapter 3.2 Ethical principles and ethical issues in public health

Nicholas S. Kelley Center for Infectious Disease Research and Policy, University of Minnesota, Minneapolis, MN, USA
Chapter 8.18 Bioterrorism

Michael P. Kelly The Institute of Public Health, University of Cambridge, Cambridge, UK
Chapter 11.1 Health needs assessment

Judd B. Kessler Business Economics and Public Policy Department, The Wharton School, University of Pennsylvania, Philadelphia, PA, USA
Chapter 6.7 Behavioural economics and health

Leeka Kheifets Department of Epidemiology at UCLA School of Public Health, Los Angeles, CA, USA
Chapter 7.2 Radiation and public health

Rajat Khosla World Health Organization, Geneva, Switzerland
Chapter 3.3 The right to the highest attainable standard of health

Muin J. Khoury Office of Public Health Genomics, Centers for Disease Control and Prevention, Atlanta, GA, USA
Chapter 2.5 Genomics and public health

Ann Marie Kimball Bill and Melinda Gates Foundation, Seattle, WA, USA
Chapter 5.19 Public health surveillance

Robert J. Kim-Farley Director, Communicable Disease Control and Prevention, Los Angeles County Department of Public Health; Fielding School of Public Health, University of California, Los Angeles, CA, USA
Chapter 11.3 Principles of infectious disease control

Mary Kay Kindhauser World Health Organization, Geneva, Switzerland
Chapter 11.13 The future of international public health in an era of austerity

Bartha M. Knoppers Director, Centre of Genomics and Policy, Canada Research Chair in Law and Medicine, Faculty of Medicine, Department of Human Genetics, McGill University, Montreal, Quebec, Canada
Chapter 2.5 Genomics and public health

Manolis Kogevinas Centre for Research in Environmental Epidemiology (CREAL), Barcelona, Spain; IMIM (Hospital del Mar Medical Research Institute), Barcelona, Spain; CIBER Epidemiologia y Salud Pública (CIBERESP), Spain; and National School of Public Health, Athens, Greece
Chapter 5.3 Cross-sectional studies

David Koh Assistant Vice-Chancellor, Vice-President and Chair Professor, Universiti Brunei Darussalam, Brunei; Professor, Saw Swee Hock School of Public Health, National University of Singapore, Singapore
Chapter 7.4 Occupational health
Chapter 7.5 Toxicology and risk assessment in the analysis and management of environmental risk

Dragana Korljan UN Office of the High Commissioner for Human Rights, Geneva, Switzerland
Chapter 3.3 The right to the highest attainable standard of health

Diana Kuh MRC National Survey of Health and Development at the MRC Unit for Lifelong Health and Ageing at UCL, London, UK
Chapter 5.20 Life course epidemiology and analysis

Walter A. Kukull Director, National Alzheimer's Coordinating Center (NACC), Department of Epidemiology, University of Washington, Seattle, WA, USA
Chapter 8.10 Neurological diseases, epidemiology, and public health

Ronald Labonté Canada Research Chair and Globalization/ Health Equity; Faculty of Medicine, University of Ottawa, Ottawa, ON, Canada
Chapter 2.2 Poverty, justice, and health

Tai Hing Lam School of Public Health, The University of Hong Kong, Hong Kong
Chapter 9.1 Tobacco

Carlo La Vecchia Professor of Epidemiology, Department of Clinical Sciences and Community Health, University of Milan, Italy
Chapter 8.2 Cancer epidemiology and public health

Chien Earn Lee Chief Executive Officer, Changi General Hospital; Saw Swee Hock School of Public Health, Singapore
Chapter 11.7 Strategies for health services

Hin-Peng Lee Saw Swee Hock School of Public Health, National University of Singapore, Singapore
Chapter 1.4 Development of public health in economic transition: the middle-income countries

Kelley Lee Director of Global Health and Associate Dean, Research Faculty of Health Sciences, Simon Fraser University, Burnaby, BC, Canada
Chapter 1.5 Globalization

Vernon J. M. Lee Saw Swee Hock School of Public Health, National University of Singapore, Singapore
Chapter 8.17 Emerging and re-emerging infections

Tinne Lernout Centre for the Evaluation of Vaccination, Vaccine & Infectious Disease Institute, Faculty of Medicine and Health Sciences, University of Antwerp, Antwerp, Belgium
Chapter 8.16 Chronic hepatitis and other liver disease

Barry S. Levy Department of Public Health and Community Medicine at Tufts University School of Medicine, Boston, MA, USA
Chapter 9.6 Collective violence: war

Gemma Lien Public Health England, London, UK
Chapter 3.8 International efforts to promote public health

Peter Littlejohns Department of Primary Care & Public Health Sciences at King's College London, London, UK
Chapter 3.5 Priority setting, social values, and public health

Donald J. Lollar Professor, Public Health and Preventive Medicine, Oregon Health & Science University, Portland, OR, USA
Chapter 10.7 People with disabilities

Adetokunbo Lucas Department of Global Health and Population, Harvard School of Public Health, Harvard University, Boston, MA, USA
Chapter 3.6 Health policy in developing countries

Johan P. Mackenbach Department of Public Health, Erasmus MC, University Medical Center, Rotterdam, Netherlands
Chapter 2.3 Socioeconomic inequalities in health in high-income countries: the facts and the options

Alex Macmillan School of Population Health, University of Auckland, Auckland, New Zealand
Chapter 2.8 The environment and climate change

Rui T. Marinho Gastroenterology department, Hospital de Santa Maria, Portugal
Chapter 8.16 Chronic hepatitis and other liver disease

Tim Marsh UK Health Forum, London, UK
Chapter 8.4 Obesity

Zoe Marshman Dental Public Health, School of Clinical Dentistry, Sheffield University, Sheffield, UK
Chapter 8.8 Dental public health

Jose Martines Centre for Intervention Science in Maternal and Child Health, Centre for International Health, University of Bergen, Norway
Chapter 10.3 Child health

Elizabeth Mason Institute for Global Health, University College London, UK. Formerly World Health Organization, Geneva, Switzerland
Chapter 10.3 Child health

Kedar S. Mate Country Director, IHI South Africa Program at the Institute for Healthcare Improvement, Cambridge, MA; Department of Medicine, Division of Hospital Medicine, Cornell University, New York, NY, USA
Chapter 6.9 Implementation science and translational public health

Jill Meara Public Health England, Chilton, UK
Chapter 11.11 Principles of public health emergency response for acute environmental, chemical, and radiation incidents

Judith Bueno de Mesquita Human Rights Centre, School of Law, University of Essex, Colchester, UK
Chapter 3.3 The right to the highest attainable standard of health

Pierre-André Michaud Chief, Multidisciplinary Unit for Adolescent Health University Hospital/CHUV, Lausanne, Switzerland
Chapter 10.4 Adolescent health

Mark R. Montgomery Senior Associate of the Population Council, New York, NY; Professor of Economics, Stony Brook University, Stony Brook, NY, USA
Chapter 9.7 Urban health in low- and middle-income countries

Stephen Morris Chair of Health Economics, Epidemiology & Public Health, Institute of Epidemiology & Health, University College London, London, UK
Chapter 6.6 Economic appraisal in public healthcare: assessing efficiency and equity

Alvaro Muñoz Department of Epidemiology, Johns Hopkins Bloomberg School of Public Health, Baltimore, MD, USA
Chapter 5.6 Cohort studies

Miguel Muñoz-Laboy School of Social Work, College of Health Professions and Social Work, Temple University, Philadelphia, PA, USA
Chapter 6.2 Sexuality and public health

Michael Murphy London School of Economics, London, UK
Chapter 6.3 Demography and public health

Christopher J. L. Murray Director, Institute for Health Metrics and Evaluation, University of Washington, Seattle, WA, USA
Chapter 5.17 Measuring the health of populations: the Global Burden of Disease study methods

Virginia Murray Public Health England, London, UK
Chapter 11.11 Principles of public health emergency response for acute environmental, chemical, and radiation incidents

Ruth Nduati School of Medicine at the College of Health Sciences, University of Nairobi, Nairobi, Kenya
Chapter 4.2 Information systems and community diagnosis in low- and middle-income countries

Alfred I. Neugut Department of Epidemiology at the Mailman School of Public Health, Columbia University, New York, NY, USA
Chapter 8.2 Cancer epidemiology and public health

F. Javier Nieto Chair of the Department of Population Health Sciences, Helfaer Professor of Public Health, University of Wisconsin Medical School, Madison, WI, USA
Chapter 5.6 Cohort studies

Haik Nikogosian World Health Organization, Geneva, Switzerland
Chapter 3.8 International efforts to promote public health

Lisa Oldring UN Office of the High Commissioner for Human Rights, Geneva, Switzerland
Chapter 3.3 The right to the highest attainable standard of health

Michael T. Osterholm Center for Infectious Disease Research and Policy, Division of Environmental Health Sciences, School of Public Health; Medical School, University of Minnesota, Minneapolis, MN, USA
Chapter 8.18 Bioterrorism

Vural Özdemir School of Journalism, Faculty of Communications, Office of the Rector, Gaziantep University, Gaziantep, Turkey; School of Biotechnology, Amrita University, Kerala, India
Chapter 2.5 Genomics and public health

Tomás Pantoja Department of Family Medicine, School of Medicine, Pontificia Universidad Católica de Chile, Santiago, Chile
Chapter 5.11 Clinical epidemiology

Raymundo Paraná President of the Brazilian Society of Hepatology, Bahia, Brazil
Chapter 8.16 Chronic hepatitis and other liver disease

Richard Parker Center for the Study of Culture, Politics and Health, Department of Sociomedical Sciences, Mailman School of Public Health, Columbia University, New York City, NY, USA
Chapter 6.2 Sexuality and public health

David Parkin City University, London, UK
Chapter 6.6 Economic appraisal in public healthcare: assessing efficiency and equity

George C. Patton Centre for Adolescent Health, Murdoch Children's Research Institute, Melbourne, Australia
Chapter 10.4 Adolescent health

Amy Paul Johns Hopkins Berman Institute of Bioethics; Johns Hopkins Bloomberg School of Public Health, Baltimore, MD, USA
Chapter 3.2 Ethical principles and ethical issues in public health

Sarah Payne Centre for Health and Social Care, School for Policy Studies, University of Bristol, Bristol, UK
Chapter 10.2 Women, men, and health

Neil Pearce Centre for Public Health Research, Massey University, Wellington, New Zealand; Faculty of Epidemiology and Population Health, London School of Hygiene and Tropical Medicine, London, UK
Chapter 8.3 Chronic obstructive pulmonary disease and asthma

Corinne Peek-Asa University of Iowa, College of Public Health, Injury Prevention Research Center, Iowa City, IA, USA
Chapter 9.4 Injury prevention and control: the public health approach

Kai Hong Phua Lee Kuan Yew School of Public Policy, National University of Singapore, Singapore
Chapter 1.4 Development of public health in economic transition: the middle-income countries

Kevin Pottie Departments of Family Medicine and Epidemiology and Community Medicine, University of Ottawa, Ottawa, ON, Canada
Chapter 5.11 Clinical epidemiology

Jane E. Powell Professor of Public Health Economics, Department of Health and Social Science, University of the West of England, Bristol
Chapter 11.1 Health needs assessment

John Powles Department of Public Health and Primary Care, Institute of Public Health, University of Cambridge, Cambridge, UK
Chapter 3.7 Public health policy in developed countries

Stella R. Quah Duke-NUS Graduate Medical School, Singapore
Chapter 6.1 Sociology and psychology in public health

K. Srinath Reddy President of the Public Health Foundation of India, New Delhi, India
Chapter 11.2 Prevention and control of non-communicable diseases

Justin V. Remais Director, Graduate Program in Global Environmental Health, Department of Environmental Health, Rollins School of Public Health, Emory University, Atlanta, GA, USA
Chapter 2.1 Determinants of health: overview

Les Roberts Interim Director of the Program on Forced Migration and Health, Columbia University, New York City, NY, USA
Chapter 11.10 Emergency public health and humanitarian assistance in the twenty-first century

Peter G. Robinson Director of Research, School of Clinical Dentistry, Sheffield University, Sheffield, UK
Chapter 8.8 Dental public health

Nigel Rollins World Health Organization, Geneva, Switzerland
Chapter 10.3 Child health

Robin Room Melbourne School of Population and Global Health, University of Melbourne, Melbourne; Director of the Centre for Alcohol Policy Research (CAPR), Turning Point, Fitzroy, VIC, Australia; Centre for Social Research on Alcohol and Drugs, Stockholm University, Stockholm
Chapter 9.3 Alcohol

David Sanders People's Health Movement Director and Professor of the Public Health Programme, University of the Western Cape, Bellville, South Africa
Chapter 2.2 Poverty, justice, and health

Manjinder S. Sandhu Wellcome Trust Sanger Institute; Department of Public Health and Primary Care, University of Cambridge, Cambridge, UK
Chapter 5.12 Genetic epidemiology

Vonthanak Saphonn Vice Director of the University of Health Sciences and Head of Research Unit, National Center for HIV, AIDS, Dermatology and STDs, Phnom Penh, Cambodia
Chapter 11.8 Training of public health professionals in developing countries

Eleanor B. Schron Director of Clinical Applications at the National Eye Institute, Bethesda, MD, USA
Chapter 5.7 Methodology of intervention trials in individuals

Sara U. Schwanke Khilji Communicable Disease Policy Research Group, London School of Hygiene and Tropical Medicine, London, UK
Chapter 1.4 Development of public health in economic transition: the middle-income countries

Ulrike Schwerdtfeger World Health Organization, Geneva, Switzerland
Chapter 3.8 International efforts to promote public health

Than Sein President, People's Health Foundation, Yangon, Myanmar
Chapter 1.3 The history and development of public health in low- and middle-income countries

Shira Shafir Department of Epidemiology, School of Public Health, UCLA, Los Angeles, CA, USA
Chapter 8.15 Malaria

Jonathan Shaw Associate Director, Baker IDI Heart and Diabetes Institute, Melbourne, VIC, Australia
Chapter 8.6 Diabetes mellitus

Prakash S. Shetty Institute of Human Nutrition at the School of Medicine, University of Southampton, Southampton, UK; Hadassah Hebrew University Hospital, Jerusalem, Israel
Chapter 2.7 Food and nutrition

Daniel Shouval Chairman, Israel Foundation for Liver Diseases; Consultant of the World Health Organization; co-editor of the *Journal of Hepatology*
Chapter 8.16 Chronic hepatitis and other liver disease

Victor W. Sidel Montefiore Medical Center and Albert Einstein College of Medicine, Bronx, New York, NY, USA
Chapter 9.6 Collective violence: war

Andrew Siegel Johns Hopkins Berman Institute of Bioethics and Johns Hopkins Bloomberg School of Public Health, Baltimore, MD, USA
Chapter 3.2 Ethical principles and ethical issues in public health

Liam Smeeth London School of Hygiene & Tropical Medicine, London, UK
Chapter 4.1 Information systems in support of public health in high-income countries

Steven Solomon World Health Organization, Geneva, Switzerland
Chapter 3.8 International efforts to promote public health

Suniti Solomon Y. R. Gaitonde Center for AIDS Research and Education (YRG CARE), Chennai, Tamil Nadu, India
Chapter 8.13 HIV/acquired immunodeficiency syndrome

Marni Sommer Center for the Study of Culture, Politics and Health, Department of Sociomedical Sciences, Mailman School of Public Health, Columbia University, New York, NY, USA
Chapter 6.2 Sexuality and public health

Nasiha Soofie Centre for the Aids Programme of Research in South Africa (CAPRISA), Doris Duke Medical Research Institute, Nelson R. Mandela School of Medicine, University of KwaZulu-Natal, Congella, South Africa
Chapter 8.5 Physical activity and health

Frank Sorvillo Department of Epidemiology, School of Public Health, UCLA, Los Angeles, CA, USA
Chapter 8.15 Malaria

Allison Streetly Visiting Senior Lecturer, Division of Health and Social Care, King's College London, UK
Chapter 11.4 Population screening and public health

Sheena G. Sullivan WHO Collaborating Centre for Reference and Research on Influenza, Melbourne, Australia
Chapter 5.10 Community-based intervention trials in low- and middle-income countries

Theodore Svoronos Massachusetts Institute of Technology, Cambridge, MA, USA
Chapter 6.9 Implementation science and translational public health

Chorh Chuan Tan President and Professor of Medicine, National University of Singapore, Singapore
Chapter 1.1 The scope and concerns of public health

Meredith A. Tavener Research Centre for Gender, Health and Ageing, at the University of Newcastle, Callaghan, NSW, Australia
Chapter 10.8 Health of older people

Kate Tilling School of Social and Community Medicine, University of Bristol, Bristol, UK
Chapter 5.20 Life course epidemiology and analysis

Andrea C. Tricco Li Ka Shing Knowledge Institute, St Michael's Hospital, Toronto, ON, Canada
Chapter 5.11 Clinical epidemiology

Angelika Tritscher World Health Organization, Geneva, Switzerland
Chapter 3.8 International efforts to promote public health

Peter Tugwell University of Ottawa, Department of Medicine, Faculty of Medicine; Ottawa Hospital Research Institute, Clinical Epidemiology Program, University of Ottawa, Department of Epidemiology and Community Medicine, Faculty of Medicine; Institute of Population Health, University of Ottawa, Ottawa, Canada   *Chapter 5.11 Clinical epidemiology*

Kumnuan Ungchusak Bureau of Epidemiology, Department of Disease Control, Ministry of Public Health, Thailand
Chapter 5.4 Principles of outbreak investigation

Nigel Unwin Basic Medical Science Faculty of the University of the West Indies, Cave Hill, Barbados
Chapter 8.6 Diabetes mellitus

Pierre Van Damme Centre for the Evaluation of Vaccination, Vaccine & Infectious Disease Institute, Faculty of Medicine and Health Sciences, University of Antwerp, Antwerp, Belgium
Chapter 8.16 Chronic hepatitis and other liver disease

Tyler J. VanderWeele Department of Biostatistics, Harvard School of Public Health, Harvard University, Boston, MA, USA
Chapter 5.13 Validity and bias in epidemiological research
Chapter 5.14 Causation and causal inference

Koen Van Herck Centre for the Evaluation of Vaccination, Vaccine & Infectious Disease Institute, Faculty of Medicine and Health Sciences, University of Antwerp, Antwerp, Belgium
Chapter 8.16 Chronic hepatitis and other liver disease

Tjeerd-Pieter van Staa London School of Hygiene & Tropical Medicine, London, UK and Utrecht Institute for Pharmaceutical Sciences, Utrecht University, Utrecht, Netherlands
Chapter 4.1 Information systems in support of public health in high-income countries

Sten H. Vermund Institute for Global Health and Department of Pediatrics, Vanderbilt University School of Medicine, Nashville, TN, USA
Chapter 8.13 HIV/acquired immunodeficiency syndrome

Jimmy Volmink Centre for Evidence-based Health Care, Faculty of Medicine and Health Sciences, Stellenbosch University, Cape Town, South Africa; South African Cochrane Centre, South African Medical Research Council, Cape Town, South Africa
Chapter 5.15 Systematic reviews and meta-analysis

Yasmin E.R. von Schirnding The Mount Sinai Hospital, New York, NY, USA
Chapter 11.5 Environmental health practice

Theo Vos Institute for Health Metrics and Evaluation, University of Washington, Seattle, WA, USA
Chapter 5.17 Measuring the health of populations: the Global Burden of Disease study methods

Kristian Wahlbeck Finnish Association for Mental Health, Helsinki, Finland
Chapter 8.7 Public mental health and suicide

Richard Wakeford Dalton Nuclear Institute, University of Manchester, Manchester, UK
Chapter 7.2 Radiation and public health

Danuta Wasserman National Centre for Suicide Research and Prevention of Mental Ill-Health (NASP), Karolinska Institute, Stockholm, Sweden
Chapter 8.7 Public mental health and suicide

Albert Weale School of Public Policy at the Department of Political Science, University College London, London, UK
Chapter 3.5 Priority setting, social values, and public health

Noel S. Weiss Department of Epidemiology, School of Public Health, University of Washington, Seattle, WA, USA
Chapter 5.5 Case–control studies

Vivian A. Welch Bruyère Research Institute, Bruyère Continuing Care, Department of Epidemiology and Community Medicine, Faculty of Medicine, University of Ottawa, Ottawa, Canada
Chapter 5.11 Clinical epidemiology

Alex Welte South African Centre for Epidemiological Modelling and Analysis (SACEMA), Stellenbosch, South Africa
Chapter 5.18 Mathematical models of transmission and control of infectious agents

Suwit Wibulpolprasert Vice Chair, International Health Policy Program Foundation, Thailand
Chapter 11.9 Training of local health workers to meet public health needs

Brian Williams South African Centre for Epidemiological Modelling and Analysis (SACEMA), Stellenbosch, South Africa
Chapter 5.18 Mathematical models of transmission and control of infectious agents

Gail Williams School of Population Health, Faculty of Health Sciences, University of Queensland, Brisbane, QLD, Australia
Chapter 5.16 Statistical methods

Patrick Wilson Center for the Study of Culture, Politics and Health, Department of Sociomedical Sciences, Mailman School of Public Health, Columbia University, New York City, NY, USA
Chapter 6.2 Sexuality and public health

Nathan D. Wong Professor and Director, Heart Disease Prevention Program, Division of Cardiology, University of California, Irvine, USA; Adjunct Professor of Epidemiology (UC Irvine and UCLA) and Radiology (UC Irvine) USA; Past President, American Society for Preventive Cardiology
Chapter 8.1 Epidemiology and prevention of cardiovascular disease

Alistair Woodward Head of School, School of Population Health, University of Auckland, Auckland, New Zealand
Chapter 2.8 The environment and climate change

Zunyou Wu National Center for AIDS/STD Control and Prevention at the Chinese Center for Disease Control and Prevention, Beijing, China
Chapter 5.10 Community-based intervention trials in low- and middle-income countries

Mui-Teng Yap Institute of Policy Studies, Lee Kuan Yew School of Public Policy, National University of Singapore, Singapore
Chapter 1.4 Development of public health in economic transition: the middle-income countries

Eng-kiong Yeoh Faculty of Medicine, Chinese University of Hong Kong, Hong Kong
Chapter 6.8 Governance and management of public health programmes

Elizabeth H. Young Wellcome Trust Sanger Institute; Department of Public Health and Primary Care, University of Cambridge, UK
Chapter 5.12 Genetic epidemiology

C. Yiwei Zhang Business Economics and Public Policy Department, The Wharton School, University of Pennsylvania, Philadelphia, PA, USA
Chapter 6.7 Behavioural economics and health

Zuo-Feng Zhang Senior Professor of Epidemiology and Associate Dean for Research, Fielding School of Public Health, University of California, Los Angeles, CA, USA
Chapter 8.2 Cancer epidemiology and public health

Ron Zimmern Chairman, PHG Foundation, Cambridge, UK
Chapter 2.5 Genomics and public health

Anthony B. Zwi School of Public Health & Community Medicine at the University of New South Wales, Sydney, NSW, Australia
Chapter 10.9 Forced migrants and other displaced populations

SECTION 1

The development of the discipline of public health

The scope and concerns of public health

Roger Detels and Chorh Chuan Tan

Introduction to the scope and concerns of public health

There have been many definitions and elaborations of public health. The definition offered by the Acheson Report (Acheson 1988, p. 1) has been widely accepted:

> Public health is the science and art of preventing disease, prolonging life, and promoting health through the organized efforts of society.

This definition underscores the broad scope of public health and the fact that public health is the result of all of society's efforts viewed as a whole, rather than that of single individuals.

In 2003, Roger Detels defined the goal of public health as:

> The biologic, physical, and mental well-being of all members of society regardless of gender, wealth, ethnicity, sexual orientation, country, or political views. (cited in Detels 2009, p. 3)

This definition or goal emphasizes equity and the range of public health interests as encompassing not just the physical and biological, but also the mental well-being of society. The United Nation's Millennium Development Goals, the slogan of which is 'Health for All' (the Acheson report), and Detels' goals depict public health as being concerned with more than the mere elimination of disease and placing public health issues as a fundamental component of development.

To achieve the World Health Organization (WHO) goal of 'health for all', it is essential to bring to bear many diverse disciplines to the attainment of optimal health, including the physical, biological, and social sciences. The field of public health has adapted and applied these disciplines for the elimination and control of disease, and the promotion of health.

Functions of public health

Public health is concerned with the process of mobilizing local, state/provincial, national, and international resources to assure the conditions in which all people can be healthy (Detels and Breslow 2002). To successfully implement this process and to make health for all achievable, public health must perform the functions listed in Box 1.1.1.

Public health *identifies*, *measures*, and *monitors* health needs and trends at the community, national, and global levels through surveillance of disease and risk factor (e.g. smoking) trends. Analysis of these trends and the existence of a functioning health information system provides the essential information for predicting or anticipating future community health needs.

In order to ensure the health of the population, it is necessary to *formulate*, *promote*, and *enforce* sound health policies to prevent and control disease, and to reduce the prevalence of factors impairing the health of the community. These include policies requiring reporting of highly transmissible diseases and health threats to the community and control of environmental threats through the regulation of environmental hazards (e.g. water and

---

Box 1.1.1 Functions of public health

1. Prevent disease and its progression, and injuries.
2. Promote healthy lifestyles and good health habits.
3. Identify, measure, monitor, and anticipate community health needs (e.g. surveillance).
4. Investigate and diagnose health problems, including microbial and chemical hazards.
5. Formulate, promote, and enforce essential health policies.
6. Organize and ensure high-quality, cost-effective public health and healthcare services.
7. Reduce health disparities and ensure access to healthcare for all.
8. Promote and protect a healthy environment.
9. Disseminate health information and mobilize communities to take appropriate action.
10. Plan and prepare for natural and man-made disasters.
11. Reduce the impact of interpersonal violence and aggressive war.
12. Conduct research and evaluate health-promoting/disease-preventing strategies.
13. Develop new methodologies for research and evaluation.
14. Train and ensure a competent public health workforce.

Source: data from Office of the Director, National Public Health Performance Standards Program, *10 Essential Public Health Services*, Centers for Disease Control, 1994, available from www.cdc.gov/od/ocphp/nphpsp/EssentialPHServices.htm.

air quality standards and smoking). It is important to recognize that influencing politics and policies is an essential function of public health at the local, national, and global levels.

There are limited resources that can be devoted to public health and the assurance of high-quality health services. Thus, an essential function of public health is to effectively *plan, manage, coordinate*, and *administer cost-effective health services*, and to ensure their availability to all segments of society. In every society, there are *health inequalities* that limit the ability of some members to achieve their maximum ability to function. Although these disparities primarily affect the poor, minority, rural, and remote populations and the vulnerable, they also impact on society as a whole, particularly in regard to infectious and/or transmissible diseases. Thus, there is not only an ethical imperative to reduce health disparities, but also a pragmatic rationale.

Technological advances and increasing commerce have done much to improve quality of life, but these advances have often come at a high cost to the environment. In many cities of both the developed and developing world, the poor quality of air—contaminated by industry and commerce—has affected the respiratory health of the population, and has threatened to change the climate, with disastrous consequences locally and globally. We have only one world. If we do not take care of it, we will ultimately have difficulty living in it. Through education of the public, formulation of sound regulations, and influencing policy, public health can contribute much to the protection and monitoring of the environment to *ensure that it is conducive for the population to live healthily*.

To ensure that each individual in the population functions to his or her maximum capacity, public health needs to *educate the public, promote adoption of behaviours associated with good health outcomes*, and *stimulate the community* to take appropriate actions to ensure the optimal conditions for the health of the public. This is vital since many major public health problems are linked to human behaviour and lifestyles. Ultimately, public health cannot succeed without the support and active involvement of the community.

We cannot predict, and rarely can we prevent, the occurrence of natural and man-made disasters, but we can prepare for them to ensure that the resulting damage is minimized. Thus, *disaster preparedness* is an essential component of public health, whether the disaster is an epidemic such as influenza or the occurrence of typhoons and other natural disasters.

Unfortunately, in the modern world, interpersonal *violence* and *war* have become common. In some segments of society (particularly among adolescent and young adult minority males), violence has become the leading cause of death and productive years of life lost. Public health cannot ignore the fact that violence and wars are major factors dramatically reducing the quality of life for millions.

Many of the advances in public health have become possible through *research*. Research will continue to be essential for identifying and anticipating health problems and the optimal strategies for addressing them. Strategies that seem very logical may, in fact, not succeed for a variety of unforeseen reasons. Therefore, public health systems and programmes cannot be assumed to function cost-effectively without continuous monitoring and evaluation. Thus, it is essential that new public health strategies undergo rigorous evaluation before being scaled up, and once scaled up, are periodically reviewed to ensure their continuing effectiveness in diverse groups and populations.

Over the last century, the quality of research has been enhanced by the *development of new methodologies*, particularly in the fields of epidemiology, biostatistics, and laboratory sciences. Rapid advances in computational hardware and techniques have increased our ability to analyse massive amounts of data, and to use multiple strategies to aid in the interpretation of data. Despite this, it will be a major challenge to keep pace with the explosive growth in the volume and complexity of data being generated, driven by a range of factors from the pervasive use of the Internet, social media, and mobile phones, to the masses of data from molecular biology and sequencing studies. To glean valuable insights pertinent to public health from these huge datasets will require new approaches, strategies, and methodologies. It is essential that public health continues to use leading-edge technologies to develop more sophisticated research strategies to address public health issues.

A major problem in public health has been translating research advances into effective health practice and policy in a timely manner. A new area of research, *implementation science*, has been proposed to delineate barriers to and factors that facilitate rapid translation of scientific advances into improvements in health practice and development of more effective policies promoting health.

The quality of public health is dependent on the competence and vision of the public health *workforce*. Thus, it is an essential function of public health to *ensure the continuing availability of a well-trained, competent workforce* at all levels, including leaders with the vision essential to ensure the continued well-being of society and the implementation of innovative, effective public health measures.

Finally, a thread that runs through all these functions is the necessity for much greater international collaboration in data sharing, policy formulation and implementation, and the management of specific public health issues. With globalization, the rapid flow of information, people, goods, and services across national boundaries means that many public health concerns and issues are interconnected in complex ways. Effective solutions will therefore often depend on joint action between different countries. In addition, now more than ever, there are many opportunities for major public health attainments to be made through cooperative action at the global level, as has been demonstrated in the past by milestones such as the eradication of smallpox. The media can play an important role in educating the public and in facilitating public health interventions.

Contemporary health issues

Underlying the bulk of the public health problems of the world is the issue of poverty. More than half of the world's population lives below the internationally defined poverty line, and 22 per cent of the population in developing countries lives on less than US $1.25 per day (World Bank 2012). Although the majority of the world's poor live in developing countries, there are many poor living in the wealthiest countries of the world—underscoring the disparity of wealth between the poor and the rich in all countries. In the United States, 39.8 million Americans were living below the official poverty level in 2008. The proportion was highest among African Americans (24.7 per cent) and Hispanic Americans (23.2 per cent). Unfortunately, the disparity between the rich and the

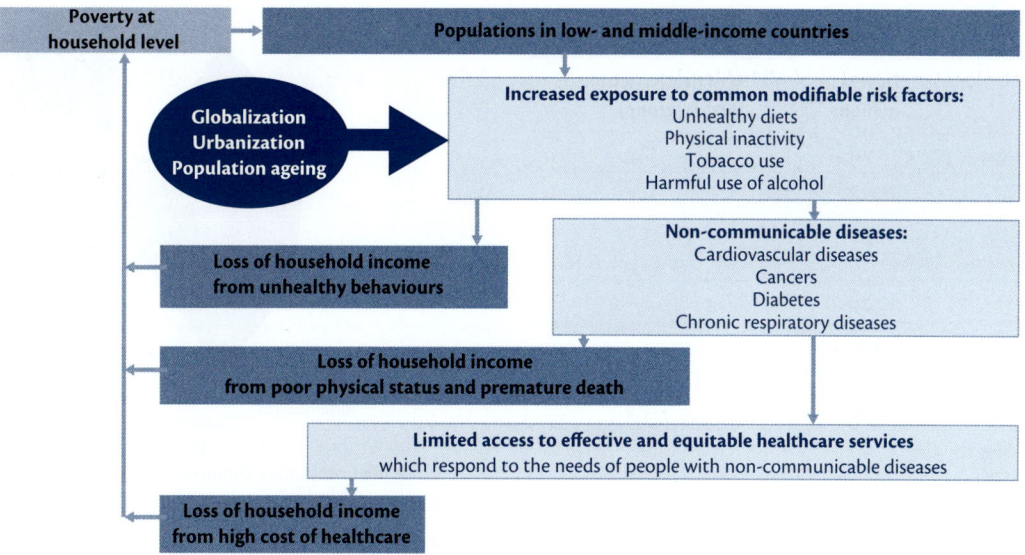

Fig. 1.1.1 From poverty to disease.

Reproduced with permission from World Health Organization, *Global Status Report on Noncommunicable Diseases 2010*, World Health Organization, Geneva, Switzerland, Copyright © 2011, available from http://www.who.int/nmh/publications/ncd_report_full_en.pdf.

poor is increasing within countries (US Census Bureau 2009). Poverty causes a cascade of problems leading to poor health (Fig. 1.1.1). It is incumbent on public health to work to reduce the impact of these disparities to ensure that all members of the global society share in a healthy quality of life.

The twentieth century witnessed the transition of major disease burdens, defined by death, from infectious and/or communicable diseases to non-communicable diseases (NCDs). In 1900, the leading cause of death in the United States and other developed countries was reported to be pneumonia and influenza. By the beginning of the twenty-first century, diseases of the heart and other chronic diseases were the leading causes of death, and pneumonia and influenza had dropped to seventh place, primarily affecting the elderly (Tables 1.1.1 and 1.1.2). Commensurately, the average lifespan increased significantly, compounding the problems introduced by population growth. The reduction in communicable diseases was not primarily due to the development of better treatments, although vaccines played an important role in the second half of the twentieth century; public efforts to reduce crowding and improve housing, enhance nutrition, and provide clean water and safe disposal of wastes were key to reducing communicable diseases.

By 1980, many leading public health figures felt that infectious diseases had been eliminated as a primary concern for public health; however, the discovery and expanding pandemic of acquired immunodeficiency syndrome (AIDS) caused by the human immunodeficiency virus (HIV) in the early 1980s, and subsequently, the severe acute respiratory syndrome (SARS) outbreaks in the early 2000s, demonstrated the fallacy of their thinking, as do the persisting high rates of infectious diseases, particularly in Africa.

Although communicable diseases persist as a major public health concern, globally chronic NCDs have become the major health problem, accounting for 70 per cent of deaths (Table 1.1.2). Even in poor, developing countries, NCDs are a dominant and growing challenge. Nearly 80 per cent of the deaths due to

Table 1.1.1 Leading causes of death in the United States (1900, 1950, 1990, 1997, 2001, 2011)

	1900	1950	1990	1997	2001	2011
Diseases of the heart	167	307	152	131	248	180
Malignant neoplasms	81	125	135	126	196	174
Cerebrovascular disease	134	89	28	26	58	39
Chronic obstructive lung diseases	—	4	20	13	44	42
Motor vehicle injuries	—	23	19	16	15	37
Diabetes mellitus	13	14	12	13	25	21
Pneumonia and influenza	210	26	14	13	22	16
HIV infection	—	—	10	6	5	3
Suicide	11	11	12	11	10	12
Homicide and legal intervention	1	5	10	8	7	6
Alzheimer's disease	—	—	—	—		23

Values expressed as rates per 100,000, age-adjusted.

Source: data from McGinnis, J.M. and Foege, W.H., Actual causes of death in the United States, *Journal of the American Medical Association*, Volume 270, Number 18, pp. 2007–12, Copyright © 1993 American Medical Association and Department of Health and Human Services, National Center for Health Statistics, *Health, United States, 1999*, US Centers for Disease Control and Prevention, Washington, DC, USA, 1999.

non-communicable or chronic diseases in 2008 occurred in developing countries, in part because many more people live in low- and middle-income countries than in high-income countries (World Health Organization 2011a). The age-standardized death rate due to NCDs among males in low- and middle-income countries was 65 per cent higher, and among females, 85 per cent higher than for men and women in high-income countries. This figure is particularly disturbing because low- and middle-income countries have

Table 1.1.2 Top ten causes of death worldwide, 2011

Causes of death	Deaths in millions	% of deaths (within income group)
Ischaemic heart disease	7.0	12.9
Stroke	6.2	11.4
Lower respiratory infections	3.2	5.9
Chronic obstructive pulmonary disease	3.0	5.4
Diarrhoeal diseases	1.9	3.5
HIV/AIDS	1.6	2.9
Trachea, bronchus, lung cancers	1.5	2.7
Diabetes mellitus	1.4	2.6
Road injury	1.3	2.3
Preterm birth complications	1.2	2.2

Reproduced with permission from World Health Organization, *The Top 10 Causes of Death*, Copyright © WHO 2013, available from: http://www.who.int/mediacentre/factsheets/fs310/en/index.html.

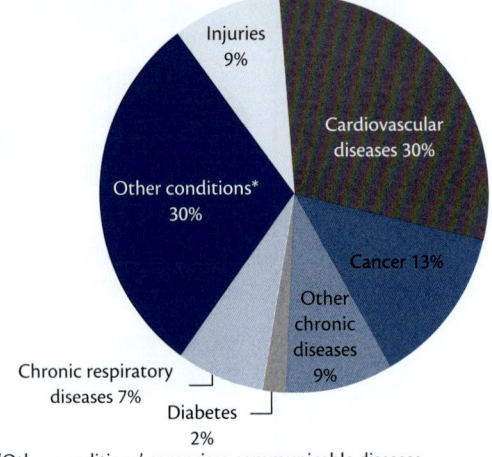

* 'Other conditions' comprises communicable diseases, maternal and perinatal conditions, and nutritional deficiencies.

Fig. 1.1.2 NCDs constitute more than 60 per cent of deaths worldwide. Reproduced with permission from World Health Organization, *Preventing Chronic Diseases: A Vital Investment*, World Health Organization, Geneva, Switzerland, Copyright © 2005, available from http://www.who.int/chp/chronic_disease_report/full_report.pdf

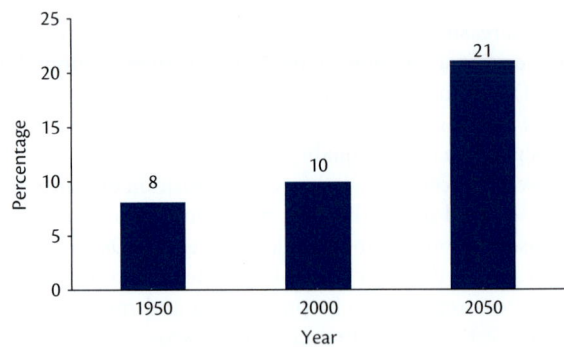

Fig. 1.1.3 Proportion of population 60 years or older: world, 1950–2050. Reproduced with the permission from Department of Economic And Social Affairs Population Division, *World Population Ageing: 1950–2050*, United Nations, New York, USA, Copyright © 2001, available from http://www.un.org/esa/population/publications/worldageing19502050/pdf/62executivesummary_english.pdf.

far fewer resources and capacity to address the epidemic of NCDs. Communicable diseases, however, still accounted for 30 per cent of the burden of disease worldwide (Fig. 1.1.2), but caused a majority of deaths only in Africa. The majority of communicable diseases are now preventable through vaccines, improved sanitation, behavioural interventions, and better standards of living.

Compounding the global shift to NCDs is the rapidly rising age of populations in many countries due to increased longevity and dramatically decreased birth rates (Fig. 1.1.3) (United Nations 2002). Population growth is already below replacement in many countries, both developed and developing. This demographic shift has widespread and profound implications. It will increase the burden of chronic disease in these countries, place increasing demands on healthcare and social support services, and strain public financing systems. This will occur even as the proportion of the population in the productive ages will decrease, which in turn will impact economic growth. The low- and middle-income countries in particular will be affected by the ageing of their populations.

Measuring disease occurrence

An essential step in defining health is to identify appropriate methods for measuring it. Traditionally, public health has defined disease in terms of mortality rates because they are relatively easy to obtain and death is indisputable. The use of mortality rates, however, places the greatest emphasis on diseases that end life, and tends to ignore those which compromise function and quality of life without causing death. Thus, the problems of mental illnesses, accidents, and disabling conditions are seriously underestimated if one uses only mortality to define health.

Two other strategies to measure health that evolved in the last half of the twentieth century have been 'years of productive life lost' (YPLL) (Lopez et al. 2007) and 'disability-adjusted life years' (DALYs) (Murray and Lopez 1995). The former emphasizes those

diseases that reduce the productive lifespan (currently arbitrarily defined as 75 years), whereas the latter emphasizes those diseases that compromise function but also includes a measure of premature mortality. Using either of these alternatives to define health results in very different orderings of diseases and/or health problems as public health priorities.

Using death to identify disease priorities, the leading cause is NCDs, which account for 70 per cent of diseases worldwide (Fig. 1.1.2). Among the chronic diseases, cardiovascular diseases account for half of the deaths. The proportion, however, varies markedly by regions of the world and level of affluence of the countries. Communicable diseases remain the major cause of death only in Africa, although they account for a significant proportion of deaths in South East Asia and the eastern Mediterranean. The major victims of these communicable diseases are infants and children under 5 years old. The persistence of communicable diseases in these areas represents a continuing major public health challenge.

DALYs and YPLL may be considered as better measures of the quality of life and functioning capacity of a country than mortality. Using DALYs to establish global disease priorities emphasizes communicable diseases and injuries, which tend to disproportionately affect the young, and reduces the relative importance of cardiovascular diseases and other chronic diseases that primarily affect the elderly. The WHO has projected that the ranking of total DALYs for neuropsychiatric disorders, injuries, and non-communicable and/or chronic diseases will increase by 2020, whereas the ranking for communicable diseases will decline. Communicable diseases, which currently account for 40 per cent of the DALYS, are expected to decline to 30 per cent by 2030 (Mathers and Loncar 2006).

On the other hand, according to projections by the WHO, while lower respiratory infections and diarrhoea remain the dominant communicable diseases, infections such as HIV, tuberculosis, and malaria will rise in terms of YPLL per 1000 population by 2030, even as other communicable diseases will yield to intervention efforts and account for progressively fewer YPLL (World Health Organization n.d.). The YPLL per 1000 population due to NCDs that tend to affect older people, however, is projected to remain constant, perhaps reflecting the optimism regarding the development of strategies for earlier diagnosis, better health habits, and better drugs to sustain life in patients with these conditions.

Communicable diseases

Many new vaccines against infectious agents have been and are being developed and many have become more affordable. The WHO's regional offices working with individual countries have conducted intensive immunization programmes against the major preventable infectious diseases of childhood, but there are significant barriers to complete coverage, including poverty, geographic obstacles, low levels of education affecting willingness to accept vaccination, logistical problems, civil unrest and wars, corruption, and mistrust of governments. Poverty, weak governments, and misuse of funds have also prevented the control of disease vectors that play a key role in diseases such as malaria and dengue, provision of clean water, and safe disposal of sanitation, all essential for the control of communicable diseases. (See Table 8.11.1 in Chapter 8.11.)

Another major factor in the rapid spread of communicable diseases has been the rapid growth in transportation. It is now possible for an individual with a communicable disease to circumnavigate the globe while still infectious and asymptomatic. Thus, cases of SARS were reported throughout South East Asia and as far as Canada within weeks of the recognition of the first cases in Hong Kong (Lee 2003). Similarly, due to the extensive global food supply chains, food-borne infections can spread rapidly within and across countries.

Another source of communicable diseases is the continuing emergence of new infectious agents, many of them adapting to humans from animal sources. Fig. 1.1.4 identifies new disease outbreaks from 1981 to 2003, including newly drug-resistant variants of new diseases occurring worldwide. Changes in food production, crowding of animals, mixing of live animal species in 'wet markets' (selling live animals for food) in Asia and elsewhere, and the introduction of hormones and antibiotics into animal feed have all contributed to the emergence of these new diseases.

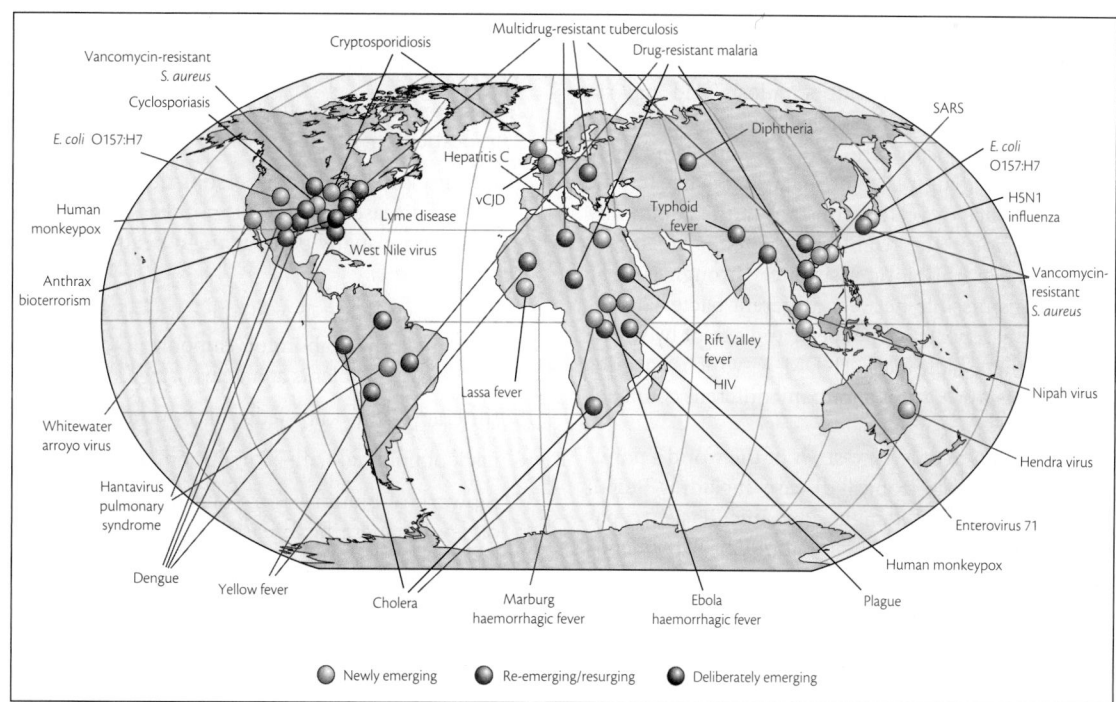

Fig. 1.1.4 Emerging and re-emerging disease worldwide, 1981–2003.

Adapted with permission from Morens D.M. et al., The challenge of emerging and re-emerging infectious diseases, *Nature*, Volume 430, Number 6996, pp. 242–9, Copyright © 2004, DOI:10.1038/nature02759.

Table 1.1.3 Newly identified infectious diseases and pathogens

Year	Disease/pathogen
2004	H1N1 avian influenza (human cases)
2003	SARS
1999	Nipah virus
1997	H5N1 (avian influenza A virus)
1996	New variant Creutzfeldt–Jakob disease; Australian bat lyssavirus
1995	Human herpes virus 8 (Kaposi's sarcoma virus)
1994	Savia virus; Hendra virus
1993	Hanta virus pulmonary syndrome (Sin Nombre virus)
1992	*Vibrio cholerae* O139
1991	Guanarito virus
1989	Hepatitis C
1988	Hepatitis E; human herpes virus 6
1983	HIV
1982	*Escherichia coli* O157:H7; Lyme borreliosis; human T-lymphotropic virus type 2
1980	Human T-lymphotropic virus

Reproduced from World Health Organization, Workshop presentation by David Heyman, World Health Organization, Geneva, Switzerland, Copyright © 1999, with permission of the author.

Table 1.1.3 lists many of the new diseases that have been recognized since 1980, and Box 1.1.2 lists the factors that contribute to the emergence of these new agents and disease threats.

In addition to the diseases listed in Table 1.1.3, antibiotic-resistant strains of known agents have emerged rapidly due, in part, to the widespread inappropriate use of antibiotics. Thus, resistant strains of gonorrhoea, *Staphylococcus*, tuberculosis, and malaria have become major problems. The latter two have now emerged as two of the three current major infectious disease problems globally. The development of drug-resistant malaria has been compounded by the emergence of vectors resistant to the commonly used chemical insecticides. The frightening potential for rapid and dangerous spread of antibiotic resistance through genetic elements that are transmissible between different bacterial species, was highlighted by reports of the speed and extent by which New Delhi metallo-beta-lactamase (NDM-1) which encodes multiple-antibiotic resistance, spread to many different countries (Moellering 2010).

Approximately 1 billion people, one-sixth of the world's population, suffer from one or more tropical disease, including Buruli ulcer, Chagas' disease, cholera, dengue, dracunculiasis, trypanosomiasis, leishmaniasis, leprosy, lymphatic filariasis, onchocerciasis, schistosomiasis, helminthiasis, and trachoma (WHO 2006). The functional ability of those so afflicted is severely compromised, in turn affecting the economic competitiveness of the poorest countries, which suffer the greatest burden of these tropical diseases. However, major strides have been achieved in reducing the burden of diseases such as leprosy, guinea worm disease, and lymphatic filariasis. Continuing efforts are needed to further reduce the burden of these and other tropical diseases.

Box 1.1.2 Factors contributing to the emergence or re-emergence of infectious diseases

1. Human 'demographic change' by which persons begin to live in previously uninhabited remote areas of the world and are exposed to new environmental sources of infectious agents, insects, and animals.
2. People living in close proximity to domestic animals, poor animal husbandry in many parts of the developing world leading to zoonotic infections.
3. Breakdowns of sanitary and other public health measures in overcrowded cities and in situations of civil unrest and war.
4. Economic development and changes in the use of land, including deforestation, reforestation, and urbanization.
5. Climate changes cause changes in geography of agents and vectors.
6. Changing human behaviours, such as increased use of child-care facilities, sexual and drug-use behaviours, and patterns of outdoor recreation.
7. Social inequality.
8. International travel and commerce that quickly transport people and goods vast distances.
9. Changes in food processing and handling, including foods prepared from many different animals and transported great distances.
10. Evolution of pathogenic infectious agents by which they may infect new hosts, produce toxins, or adapt by responding to changes in the host immunity (e.g. influenza, HIV).
11. Development of resistance of infectious agents such as *Mycobacterium tuberculosis* and *Neisseria gonorrhoeae* to chemoprophylactic or chemotherapeutic medicines.
12. Resistance of the vectors of vector-borne infectious diseases to pesticides.
13. Immunosuppression of persons due to medical treatments or new diseases that result in infectious diseases caused by agents not usually pathogenic in healthy hosts (e.g. leukaemia patients).
14. Deterioration in surveillance systems for infectious diseases, including laboratory support, to detect new or emerging disease problems at an early stage.
15. Illiteracy limits knowledge of prevention strategies.
16. Lack of political will—corruption, other priorities.
17. Biowarfare/bioterrorism—an unfortunate potential source of new or emerging disease threats (e.g. anthrax and letters).
18. War, civil unrest—creates refugees, food and housing shortages, increased density of living, etc.
19. Famine.

We now recognize that we will continue to see new human pathogens emerging in the future, and need to be prepared to contain them. Unless the world realizes the consequences of not protecting the environment in which we live, and acts on it, newly emerging diseases will continue to plague us.

Non-communicable diseases

With increasing control of communicable diseases and increasing lifespan, NCDs have emerged as the major global health problem in both developed and developing countries. Even in developing countries, NCDs have assumed greater importance. The prevalence of type 2 diabetes in rural India is 13.2 per cent (Chow and Raju 2006). Cardiovascular diseases have become a major cause of death in China. During 2000–2008, the incidence of stroke in low- and middle-income countries exceeded that in high-income countries by 20 per cent (Feigin et al. 2009).

The causes of NCDs are many and complex. Although the immediate causes are factors such as raised blood pressure, increased blood glucose, abnormal lipids and fat deposition, and diabetes, the underlying causes are behavioural and social. These behavioural factors include unhealthy diets that substitute pre-packaged and fast foods high in fats for a balanced diet, physical inactivity, and, especially, tobacco use; these in turn are the products of social change, including globalization, urbanization, and aging. WHO estimated that insufficient physical activity contributed to 3.2 million deaths and 32.1 million DALYs in 2008, and that obesity contributed to 2.1 million deaths and 35.8 DALYs globally (WHO 2011a). Some NCDs have been associated with infectious disease agents. For example, *Chlamydia pneumoniae* has been implicated in the development of atherosclerosis (Kuo and Campbell 2000), hepatitis C is a leading cause of hepatocellular (liver) cancer, and human papilloma virus (HPV), is a cause of cervical cancer. Recently, an effective vaccine has been developed, which protects against cervical cancer, but it is expensive and must be administered before sexual activity begins (i.e. early adolescence).

Fig. 1.1.5 shows the global distribution by gender of deaths from NCDs, demonstrating the higher rates of death from NCDs in developing countries, especially in Africa.

Another aspect of NCDs is the increasing survival of affected individuals who would not have survived as long previously. However, many of them are left with disabilities that require modified environments to experience a reasonable quality of life and to realize their full potential in order to contribute to society. Most NCDs can be reduced by a combination of healthy behaviours, including not smoking, moderate alcohol use, and exercise (Breslow and Breslow 1993). Many developed countries have been promoting healthy lifestyles, but there is a need for greater emphasis and development of these programmes in developing countries, where the major global burden of chronic diseases occurs.

Mental illness

Public health professionals have only relatively recently recognized the importance of addressing the mental health needs of society on a global scale, partly due to the difficulties in defining it. It is now estimated that 10 per cent of the world's population suffers from mental illness at any given time, and that mental illness accounts for 13 per cent of the global burden of disease (Collins et al. 2011) (Table 1.1.4). Mortality rates seriously underestimate the burden of mental health on society. The true extent of mental illness is probably greater—only 60 per cent of countries

report having a dedicated mental health policy and only 27 per cent report data on expenditures for mental health (WHO 2011b).

Global provisions for treatment of mental illness are still significantly below what is necessary to adequately address the problem. In developing countries, only US $0.25 is allocated per patient for mental health and there is less than one psychiatrist per 200,000 persons (WHO 2011b). Of those with mental illness in developing countries, 76–85 per cent do not have access to appropriate care (WHO 2001b). Although 87 per cent of the world's governments offer some mental health services at the primary care level, 30 per cent of them have no relevant programme, and 28 per cent have no budget specifically identified for mental health. Mental illness robs society of a significant number of potentially productive persons. With the diminishing proportion of productive people of working age and the increasing proportion of elderly dependants, it is important to assist those who are not productive because of mental illness to become healthy, productive members of society.

Population projections

Although the rate of growth of the world's population has slowed in the latter half of the twentieth century, the world's population, currently over 7 billion people, is still estimated to grow to 9 billion by 2050. The growth in the population will be mostly among the elderly and the old elderly (those over 80 years of age).

The well-being of society is dependent on the ratio of those who produce to those who are dependent. Improved technology and strategies will be required to increase worker productivity, because the majority of the population growth in the coming decades will be among the old and old elderly, not through increasing birth rates, and will result in a diminishing proportion of producers and an increasing proportion of dependants. It is also expected that more of the elderly will have to continue to be economically productive. In 2000, the proportion of the world's population who were 65 years and over was 8 per cent; by 2050, it will be at least 30 per cent (Index Mundi 2012). This will be further exacerbated because the majority of the oldest elderly will be single women who traditionally have more limited resources and lower levels of education, particularly in developing countries. The productivity and efficiency of those who produce must increase if we are to sustain and improve the quality of life for all.

The occurrence of disease in old age is directly correlated with unhealthy behaviours developed in early life. Unfortunately, concurrent with population growth, there has been a worldwide epidemic of obesity and decreased physical activity, which has increased the proportion of elderly who suffer from chronic debilitating diseases in both the developed and developing world. Thus, unless efforts to promote healthy lifestyles are successful, not only will there be an increase in the proportion of elderly, but also an increasing proportion of them will require assistive care, placing a further economic and social burden on families and society.

As the population grows, there is increasing pressure to provide food, water, and other necessities to maintain a high quality of life. Shifts in dietary preferences in developing countries towards greater meat consumption also puts additional strains on food production. Fertile farmlands are increasingly being converted to residential, commercial, or industrial use. Thus, more people will effectively need to be supported on less arable land. Food security will hence be a key issue for the future and this will be affected by a multitude of factors but most notably sufficiency of water

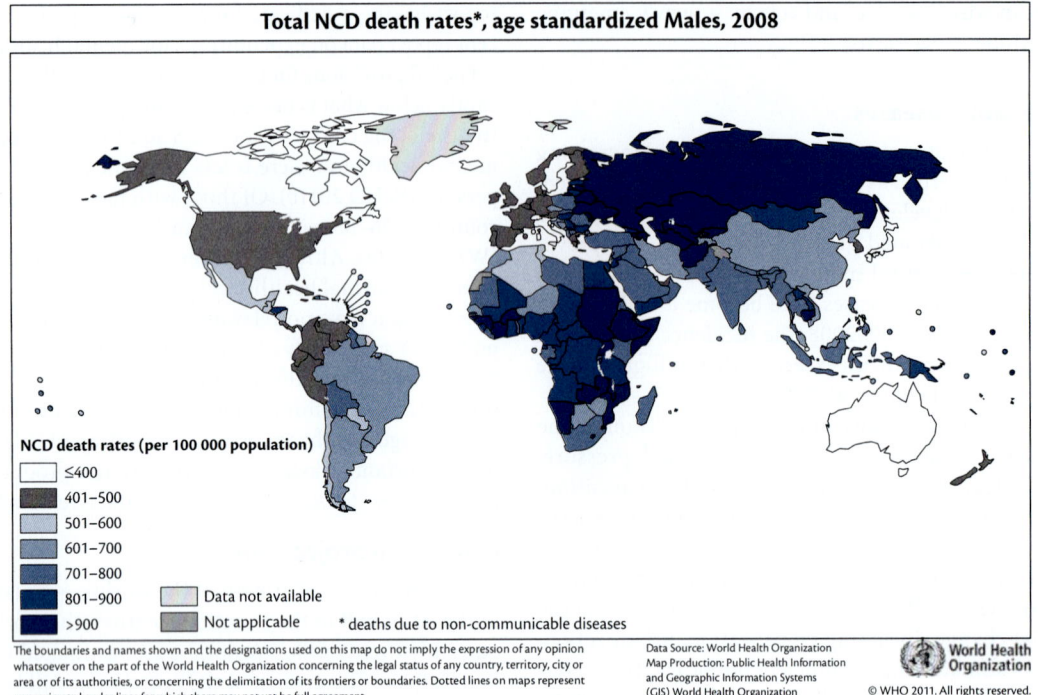

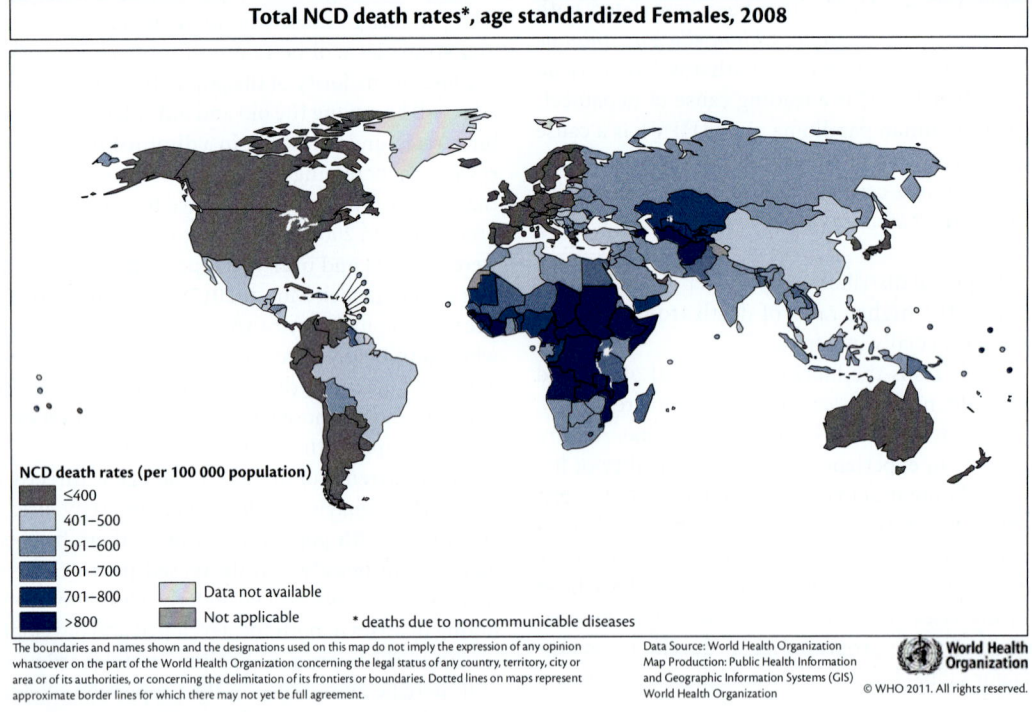

Fig. 1.1.5 Global distribution of non-communicable diseases (2008).

Reproduced with the permission from World Health Organization, *Global Status Report on Noncommunicable Diseases 2010*, World Health Organization, Geneva, Switzerland, Copyright © 2011, available from www.who.int/nmh/publications/ncd_report_full_en.pdf.

resources and whether there will be major increases in agricultural productivity.

Other public health issues

Nutrition

Appropriate nutrition is essential for health. In many developing countries (as well as among the poor and homeless in developed countries), undernutrition is a problem. Beyond access to nutritious and safe food, many of the poor have little knowledge about what constitutes a healthy diet, compounding the difficulties. At the same time, in developed and many rapidly developing countries such as China, overnutrition and obesity are a major problem. Some industry sectors have been more effective in promoting calorie-dense, salt-rich, and unhealthy diets than public health

Table 1.1.4 Global burden of mental, neurological, and substance-use (MNS) disorders

Rank	Worldwide		High-income countries[†]		Low- and middle-income countries	
	Cause	DALYs[‡] (millions)	Cause	DALYs (millions)	Cause	DALYs (millions)
1	Unipolar depressive disorders	65.5	Unipolar depressive disorders	10.0	Unipolar depressive disorders	55.5
2	Alcohol-use disorders	23.7	Alzheimer's and other dementias	4.4	Alcohol-use disorders	19.5
3	Schizophrenia	16.8	Alcohol-use disorders	4.2	Schizophrenia	15.2
4	Bipolar affective disorder	14.4	Drug-use disorders	1.9	Bipolar affective disorder	12.9
5	Alzheimer's and other dementias	11.2	Schizophrenia	1.6	Epilepsy	7.3
6	Drug-use disorders	8.4	Bipolar affective disorder	1.5	Alzheimer's and other dementias	6.8
7	Epilepsy	7.9	Migraine	1.4	Drug-use disorders	6.5
8	Migraine	7.8	Panic disorder	0.8	Migraine	6.3
9	Panic disorder	7.0	Insomnia (primary)	0.8	Panic disorder	6.2
10	Obsessive–compulsive disorder	5.1	Parkinson's disease	0.7	Obsessive–compulsive disorder	4.5
11	Insomnia (primary)	3.6	Obsessive–compulsive disorder	0.6	Post-traumatic stress disorder	3.0
12	Post-traumatic stress disorder	3.5	Epilepsy	0.5	Insomnia (primary)	2.9
13	Parkinson's disease	1.7	Post-traumatic stress disorder	0.5	Multiple sclerosis	1.2
14	Multiple sclerosis	1.5	Multiple sclerosis	0.3	Parkinson's disease	1.0

[†]World Bank criteria for income (2009 gross national income (GNI) per capita): low income is US $995 equivalent or less; middle income is $996–12,195; high income is $12,196 or more.

[‡] Disability-adjusted life years. Reproduced with permission from Pamela Y. Collins et al., Grand challenges in global mental health, *Nature*, Volume 475, Issue 7354, pp. 27–30, Copyright © 2011, DOI: 10.1038/475027a.

professionals have been in championing healthy food choices consumed in reasonable quantities. This has particularly been the case for the youth, and has contributed to rising childhood obesity in many countries, including the more affluent in developing countries.

Oral health

Good dental health is essential for maintaining adequate nutrition and a good quality of life. Worldwide, however, 60–90 per cent of school children and nearly 100 per cent of adults have dental cavities. About 30 per cent of adults aged 65–74 years have no natural teeth. It was also estimated in 2004, that globally, there was an average of 1.6 decayed, missing, or filled teeth (DMFT) among children aged 12 years old (WHO 2004). These high rates of dental problems reflect poor dental hygiene and preventive care (Pine and Harris 2007). Unfortunately, many people believe that dental care is an expendable luxury, and that visits to dentists are only necessary when there is a problem. Oral cancers are the sixth most common cause of cancer globally, with the 5-year prevalence estimated to be 6.8 per cent globally (WHO 2004). Poor dental hygiene is an important risk factor, together with smoking as well as the habit of betel nut chewing which is common in parts of Asia. Clearly the public health message regarding the importance of good dental hygiene, regular tooth-brushing, and regular dental check-ups is not reaching the majority of the people.

Injuries

Injuries and violence caused 5.8 million deaths in 2011, of which 1.6 million were due to global violence, 1.3 million to traffic accidents, and 844,000 to suicide. Deaths due to injuries are almost three times greater in developing than in developed countries. However, most of the injuries do not cause death, but may result in disability. Furthermore, they occur more commonly among younger persons and children. Injuries can be broadly categorized into the following groups: motor vehicle accidents, suicide, homicide, and unintentional injuries, including occupational injuries and falls. Motor vehicle accidents account for the largest proportion of deaths due to injury. The WHO projects that motor vehicle accidents will become the third highest cause of DALYs globally by 2020 (WHO 2013). Falls, particularly among the elderly, are a major cause of DALYs as well.

Unintentional injuries are largely preventable through community and governmental intervention. Thus, improved roads, separation of different modes of transportation, enactment and enforcement of seat belt and helmet laws, and improved designs of automobiles, ladders, and other equipment and tools have all been shown to significantly reduce injuries and deaths due to accidents.

Homicide, violence, and suicide

Homicide, violence, and suicide represent a growing problem, particularly among the young. Homicide and suicide are among the leading causes of death globally. In some minority groups in the United States, homicide and violence are the leading cause of death of youth, followed by suicide. In China, suicide remains the leading cause of death among women in rural areas. Globally, the WHO predicts that homicide and suicide will account for an increasing proportion of deaths. The WHO predicts that by 2020, war will become the eighth highest cause of DALYs, violence (including gender-based and personal) the twelfth, and self-inflicted injuries the fourteenth (Murray and Lopez 1997).

Vulnerable populations

Public health has always been concerned with the health and well-being of vulnerable groups who require special attention. The definition of a vulnerable population varies by time, situation, and culture, but the common characteristic across all vulnerable groups is their special susceptibility to adverse health and poor quality of life. The list of vulnerable groups includes the poor, minorities, women, children, the elderly, the handicapped, the illiterate, orphans and street children, immigrants, rural-to-urban migrants, refugees and displaced people, the homeless, and the mentally ill. In certain situations, other groups may be considered vulnerable. For example, in the face of epidemics such as HIV/AIDS, one should also consider adolescents to be a vulnerable group. Often vulnerable individuals live at the margins of society and have difficulty accomplishing the basic functions of living and accessing healthcare. Thus, they require assistance. In many societies, particularly in developing countries, the family acts as the safety net for these groups, but if the family itself is vulnerable or dysfunctional, this safety net is absent. Societies with ample resources have developed social support programmes that assist the vulnerable, but these programmes seldom cover the full range of vulnerable groups, and may not adequately support those whom they target. Universal access to healthcare is one component of assisting the vulnerable, but presently, even in rich, developed countries such as the United States, healthcare is not available to all, and strategies to fund universal healthcare are difficult to implement.

In almost every country, developed and developing, there are homeless people, many of whom suffer from multiple problems, including mental illness. The ability to function adequately and achieve good health among many vulnerable groups, including the homeless, mentally ill, alcoholics, and drug addicts, is adversely impacted by additional factors such as poverty, prejudice, and stigmatization by society. Thus, programmes to assist the vulnerable need to also encourage society to take supportive action, in order to be optimally effective. This is a particular challenge in respect to persons with handicaps. Many developed countries have adequate provision for persons with handicaps, but in poorer countries, those with handicaps face substantial difficulties to function in society, and many do not survive.

In designing programmes for vulnerable groups, a further complication is the fact that the specific problems and needs of each of these groups differ, and they thus require public health actions which are more tailored to their requirements. For some of these groups, such as mothers and children and the handicapped, there are well-established programmes, although coverage is far from complete and the quality of these programmes varies widely. For others, such as the illiterate and migrants, there are fewer established programmes. If we are to meet the public health goal of 'Health for All', we need to identify and assist the vulnerable groups within societies to achieve their maximum possible health and function.

The environment

> Environmental health comprises those aspects of human health, including quality of life, that are determined by physical, chemical, biological, social, and psychosocial processes in the environment.
> Draft definition developed at a WHO consultation in Sofia, Bulgaria, 1993 (WHO Regional Office for Europe 1994)

Currently, one of the major problems which the world faces is the deterioration of the environment caused by the increasing numbers of people and the accumulation of wastes produced by them, their vehicles, and the industries they support. Thus, the quality of the air that we breathe has declined, especially in developing countries where rapid economic growth has been achieved at the expense of the environment. The most polluted cities of the world are concentrated in developing countries, which often have the least capacity and political will to reduce pollutants. Pollution of the world's oceans, which receive massive amounts of biological and chemical wastes annually, affects not only the quality of the water but also the ability of the ocean to sustain marine life, an important source of food.

The number of known chemicals globally exceeds 14 million, of which over 60,000 are commonly used. All of these ultimately end up in the environment. They are the result of the huge proliferation of industry, technology, and automobiles in the twentieth century. The full health effects of many of these chemicals are still unclear and difficult to establish. Murray and Lopez (1995) estimated that 1,379,238 DALYs are caused annually by environmental pollutant exposures. As the twenty-first century progresses, the number of pollutants will continue to increase.

Problems of the environment occur at the personal level (at home and the workplace), the community level (e.g. air and water pollution), and globally (e.g. global warming, hazardous and radioactive waste). Although these problems may be viewed separately, they are in fact all global issues affecting both local and remote populations. Thus, slash-and-burn agricultural practices in Indonesia result in periodic, and sometimes severe, air pollution problems in neighbouring Singapore and Malaysia. Industrial pollutants released in the industrial states of northeastern United States cause acid rain, which adversely affects crops and people in the midwestern United States and southern Canada. Pollution of rivers upstream can adversely affect communities and countries downstream, as happened, for example, in 2005 when nitrobenzene was released into the Songhua River in Heilongjiang, China, contaminating drinking water downriver in both China and Siberia, Russia.

Air pollution

The rapid increase in automobiles and industry has caused widespread air pollution in most urban areas of the world, the worst occurring in the developing countries, which have rapidly industrialized at the expense of their environment. Now, in the early part of the twenty-first century, many of these countries are realizing the need to protect the environment. Unfortunately, reversal of decades of pollution is far more difficult and costly than prevention.

The harmful effects of air pollution extend beyond the environment. Many members of society, including asthmatics and persons with chronic respiratory disease, are vulnerable to even relatively low levels of pollutants. Studies of the urban air in Southern California have demonstrated that children chronically exposed to high levels of both primary pollutants and photochemical oxidants have decreased lung function (Detels et al. 1979). Studies have demonstrated that children living near freeways in Southern California also suffer long-term lung damage (Gauderman et al. 2007). Levels of pollutants observed in many developing countries, especially in China and India, are considerably higher than in developed countries. Studies have documented the serious health effects of long-term exposure to the levels of pollutants occurring in China (Chen et al. 2004; Wong et al. 2008). However, the true cost of uncontrolled industrialization and pollution in these countries is not known.

Indoor pollution is a particular problem in developing countries where cooking is traditionally carried out using coal or charcoal fires in poorly ventilated houses. However, it is also a problem in wealthier countries in which harmful chemicals are used for cleaning and household construction.

Water pollution

Those who live in developed countries take the provision of safe drinking water for granted, but 40 per cent of the world's population does not have access to clean drinking water, a basic necessity of life. As the world population expands, the production of waste increases, and the problem of protecting water supplies also rises. Approximately 60 per cent of the world does not have adequate facilities for waste disposal. Even in leading cities in developed countries, pollution of the water supply can occur, as happened in Milwaukee, Wisconsin, when cryptosporidia contaminated the water supply, causing severe illness and death, especially in vulnerable populations compromised by immune deficiency disorders (MacKenzie et al. 1994). The increased rate of upper respiratory infections and gastrointestinal disorders among surfers and others using the ocean for recreational purposes has been well documented. Beaches in most urban areas are frequently closed when the sewage disposal systems that drain into the vicinity become overwhelmed. Acid rain from industrialization has caused acidification of lakes, making them inhospitable for fish and other marine life, thus compromising the food supply. Recently there has been discussion about whether the benefits of omega-3 fatty acids found in fish outweigh the risk of mercury poisoning among those who eat large quantities of fish. Ensuring a safe, adequate water supply for people in both developed and developing countries must become a public health priority.

Other pollutants

As the population of the world rapidly increases and technology produces new substances and processes, not only the amount of pollutants, but also the varieties of pollutants increase. As new substances are developed, it would be ideal if their use is not permitted until plans and provisions have been developed and implemented for their safe disposal. However, this is often not the case in practice.

Biodegradable pollutants have a limited lifespan in the environment, but we are increasingly producing non-biodegradable substances such as plastics, which are now ubiquitous, and hazardous materials such as radioactive wastes that persist for generations. The problem of discarding these materials safely has become a major public health issue. In some cases, developed countries are paying developing countries to accept their hazardous waste products. This strategy does not solve the problem, but shifts it to those countries that have fewer resources with which to deal with the challenge.

In the last decade, nanoparticles (1 nanometre is 1 billionth of a metre) have been increasingly used in the production of foods, drugs, cosmetics, and other products used by humans. Particles of this small size become reactive in the body and, according to recent reports (Li et al. 2009), can cause serious damage to lung cells, the liver, and brain cells. Given this problem, it is important that the use of nanoparticles in products intended for human use be regulated.

Climate change

One of the most serious, long-term challenges of the twenty-first century is global warming due to the release of carbon dioxide and other 'greenhouse gases'. There is growing evidence that the consequential climate change will be associated with increased public health risks (Patz et al. 2005).

A major review by WHO to assess the public health impact of anthropogenic climate change to date, estimated that from the mid 1970s, climate change might already have contributed to 150,000 deaths and about 5 million DALYs per year. These are largely related to increased incidence of conditions such as malnutrition, diarrhoea, and malaria (WHO 2014). Mitigating the health impact of global warming and climate change at the regional level, will be a major public health issue for this century.

Rescuing the environment

To prevent further degradation of the environment and to tackle the threat of global climate change, strong political will is required of the countries of the world. For example, while the United States is one of the world's major producers of carbon dioxide and other greenhouse gases, it has yet to ratify the United Nations Framework Convention on Climate Change, an international treaty aimed at stabilizing global greenhouse gas at levels that would avoid dangerous climate change.

From a public health perspective, it is unrealistic to expect that the risks from environmental pollution and hazardous waste can be reduced to zero. Instead, the concept of 'acceptable risk' will continue to be a part of the process. Determining the level of acceptable risk will probably be arrived at through an interplay of the scientific data and evidence, with policy and political judgements. Public health professionals and researchers must endeavour to play a strong role in these determinations.

Occupational health

> Occupational diseases are different from other diseases, not biologically, but socially.
>
> Henry Sigerist, 1958 (Sigerist 1958–1961)

The International Labor Organization's Health and Safety Programme estimated that there were 2.3 million work-related deaths, 340 million work-related injuries, and more than 160 million cases of occupational disease annually worldwide (International Labor Organization 2011). In some developing countries, child labour is still the norm. Twelve million serious injuries occurred among young workers. This affects more people than those who have myocardial infarcts (heart attacks), strokes, or newly diagnosed malignancies annually. A significant proportion of these deaths and injuries are preventable by improving safety in the workplace. However, safeguarding the health of the worker often receives less priority than the need to produce goods cheaply, especially in developing countries.

The nature of the workplace is constantly changing, with increasing proportions of workers being involved in services industries rather than in manufacturing. Over the last decade particularly, the production of goods has shifted rapidly to developing countries, where labour costs are lower. The manufacturing industry in these countries is often subject to fewer and less comprehensive safety regulations, and in some cases, are associated with low salaries and few or low healthcare benefit provisions for workers, especially for migrant workers from rural areas. Increasingly, women are entering the workforce and must juggle work and family. Larger numbers of workers are being employed on an informal part-time basis. While this reduces labour costs for industry, these informal part-time workers do not usually receive work-related benefits. They now represent 50 per cent or more of the workforce globally. This segment of the workforce is particularly vulnerable to injury and limited access to healthcare.

As noted earlier, the population is ageing, and the proportion of the population that are economically active is diminishing. In response to this change, the age of eligibility for social security benefits in the United States is increasing, and mandatory retirement is being phased out. It is now projected that the proportion of workers over the age of 60 will increase to 20 per cent in Japan and 10 per cent in the United States by 2030 (Population Projections 2000). The needs of older workers are different from those of younger workers. Thus, the changing nature of the workforce will require corresponding changes in work safety regulations and health benefits to ensure a healthy, productive workforce.

Provision of and access to healthcare

Access to preventive and curative care is a requirement for health in every society, whether rich or poor. Access to affordable healthcare has long been a problem for the poor and for rural residents, especially in developing countries. However, in the United States, access to healthcare is even a problem for the middle class. Health insurance is prohibitively expensive and beyond the reach of many in the middle classes, unless it is subsidized by employers. Increasingly, employers are attempting to free themselves from the cost of health insurance for their employees through a variety of strategies. The elderly also have problems with healthcare; because healthcare costs increase with age, insurance companies are less willing to cover the elderly, and many governments, even in developed countries, do not provide adequate support for the elderly. Recently, President Obama and the US Congress implemented the Affordable Care Act, which will extend coverage significantly, but it is vigorously opposed by the Republican political party. In developing countries, the rural poor are particularly at risk. Few health professionals are willing to work in rural areas, and the cost of providing care in less populated areas is greater than in urban areas. Innovative strategies are needed to promote universal coverage and ensure that the rural poor and elderly have access to reasonable healthcare.

Bioterrorism and war

The history of use of biological weapons in war extends back for hundreds of years. In the Middle Ages, corpses of plague victims were catapulted into castles under siege. Recently, anthrax was used to contaminate the US postal system, resulting in several deaths. There has been a sharp increase in bioterrorist activities in this century. The WHO and public health agencies of individual countries have developed plans to quickly diagnose and control bioterrorist incidents. However, these threats to the health of the public will continue until we address the underlying causes of terrorism and bioterrorism.

Few actions can have the magnitude of negative impact on the health of the public that war has. Men, women, and children are killed, children are forced to serve as soldiers, homes are destroyed, major segments of the population become displaced refugees, and the social and/or economic fabric of the countries involved is destroyed. Recovery usually takes years to decades. The outside world, particularly those countries adjacent to warring nations, must cope with the huge influx of displaced persons, and action needs to be implemented to help those still in the country suffering from the impact of the war. The consequences of war are so severe and wide-ranging that it is imperative that better ways be reached to resolve international conflicts. The resources ploughed into armed conflict could be better deployed on humanitarian and public health support.

Ethics in public health

Although ethical issues are implicit in the delivery of public health, it was only after the Second World War and the recognition that 'scientific experiments' in Nazi Germany violated human rights that an emphasis was placed on recognizing the ethics of public health actions, particularly research. The Declaration of Helsinki (World Medical Association 2002), the Belmont Report (US National Commission for the Protection of Human Subjects of Biomedical and Behavioral Research 1979), and the Council for International Organizations of Medical Science (2002) have promulgated ethical guidelines for research and the establishment of institutional review boards worldwide to ensure that medical and/or public health research is conducted ethically and does not violate human rights. However, there are inherent ethical conflicts in many public health actions. For example, some consider that the human rights of 'typhoid Mary', a typhoid carrier who insisted on working as a cook in the early twentieth century, were violated when she was incarcerated to prevent her from continuing to prepare food that initiated epidemics. Protecting the human rights of a man to refuse testing for HIV may result in his unknowingly infecting his wife, yet-to-be-born children, and other sexual contacts. By protecting his human rights, the human rights of his wife or partner and future family will be violated.

Implementing public health programmes and research often results in ethical conflicts and the need to balance the good of society against potential harm to the individual. It is usually necessary to inform society, particularly those who will be involved in the public programme or research, about the nature of the ethical conflicts inherent in action. For example, a trial evaluating the effectiveness of prophylactic treatment to prevent HIV infection in sex workers in Cambodia was stopped by the prime minister, who felt that the prevention trial exploited Cambodian sex workers. A more intense effort on the part of the researchers to inform the public and politicians about the nature of the study and the potential benefit to sex workers, not only in Cambodia, but globally, might have averted this unfortunate outcome.

Public health interventions

One important task of public health professionals is to raise the level of anxiety of the public about public health problems to the level at which they will be willing to take an appropriate action. In this, an appropriate balance has to be struck since raising the level of anxiety too little will result in inadequate or no action, while raising the level too high may promote a fatalistic attitude and, as in the case of the recent HIV/AIDS epidemic, may promote stigmatization and isolation of affected individuals, seriously complicating the task of intervention. The difficulty for the public health professional is creating the level of anxiety that results in the required action while minimizing unintended consequences.

Public health interventions can be divided into four categories: social/biological/environmental, behavioural, political, and structural. The public health professional must use strategies in all four categories to achieve the maximum health of the public.

Social, biological, and/or environmental interventions

The strategy that has had the greatest impact on improving the health of the public has been an improved standard of living, including provision of clean water and safe disposal of wastes. Unfortunately, these interventions have not reached much of the world where crowding, unsafe and insufficient water, and accumulation of wastes, inadequate housing, and a lack of economic development persist.

The most cost-effective biological intervention strategy is immunization, in part because it requires minimal behavioural change and usually only a single series of actions. The WHO has taken the lead in promoting vaccine coverage worldwide through its Expanded Programme on Immunization. The appropriate use of vaccines has virtually eliminated the majority of childhood infections from the developed countries and significantly reduced them in most developing countries. Smallpox, a major infectious disease problem until the latter half of the twentieth century, has now been eliminated. We are well on our way to eliminating polio, but more challenges, such as hepatitis, tuberculosis, and measles, remain. However, it is important to realize that development and production of a vaccine is only the first step. An effective vaccine against smallpox was available for over 150 years before smallpox was eliminated. The key was the strategy of vaccine coverage, 'search and contain', together with adequate political will and funding that permitted global elimination of that disease. Thus, the strategy for utilizing the vaccine is perhaps equally important as the efficacy of the vaccine itself.

Another biological strategy is to eliminate the vectors of disease, the major approach currently in use for the control of dengue, arboviral diseases, and many of the parasitic diseases. However, overzealous use of pesticides can also create problems. For example, dichloro-diphenyl-trichloroethane (DDT), used widely in the twentieth century as an insecticide, still contaminates the food supply, creating other health problems, including the risk of malignancy.

Treatment can also be considered a biological intervention strategy. To confront tuberculosis, one of the major infectious diseases of the twenty-first century, directly observed treatment short course (DOTS) has been successfully implemented in countries where the disease persists, and reduces transmission and development of multidrug-resistant TB. Treatment of sexually transmitted infections and contacts is a major strategy for control of transmission, but has yet to prove effective in stopping the current epidemic. Recently there has been optimism that treatment as prevention can result in control of HIV (Cohen 2011).

Behavioural interventions

Most public health interventions depend ultimately on behaviour, whether it is personal or community behaviour. At the personal or individual level, promotion of good health habits and avoidance of smoking, excessive alcohol use, and other dependency disorders are important interventions that have a major impact on health. At the community level, attitudes towards acceptable sexual behaviour and persons with dependency disorders and stigmatizing diseases are key to establishing community 'norms' that promote a healthy lifestyle and include all segments of society. However, modifying individual behaviour and community norms is difficult; it is even more difficult to ensure persistence of the modified behaviour. Yet, the majority of the public health interventions will not be successful unless they are embraced and sustained by the community at the local, national, and international levels, and accompanied by appropriate regulations and policies. The success of the antismoking campaigns in the United States and Britain and population control in China (the one-child policy) affirm that it is possible to change community norms.

Many theories identifying strategies to modify behaviour have been proposed. One of the most interesting is the Popular Opinion Leader model (Kelly 2004), which utilizes the natural leaders found in any social group as agents of change. In the United States, this strategy has been demonstrated to change behaviour in groups of men who have sex with men, and is now being evaluated in other populations worldwide. Ultimately, if public health interventions are to be effective, they must be adopted by the community. The media can play an important role in facilitating these interventions and assuring that they become community norms.

Political interventions

Public health *is* politics. Any process that involves obtaining the support of the public will involve politics and differing points of view. For example, the campaign to stop smoking was strongly opposed by the tobacco industry, which spent millions of dollars trying to counter the many reports on the adverse health effects of smoking. Countering the efforts of the tobacco industry required obtaining the political support of the public in order to pass laws and regulations limiting smoking, placing health warnings on cigarette packages, and raising taxes on cigarettes. Many needed regulations transcend boundaries and require international cooperation (e.g. regulation of greenhouse gases).

If we are to succeed in safeguarding the oceans, inland waters, and the air we breathe, it will be through the political process requiring global coordination and joint action. This process has already begun in many of the developed countries, which have passed strong laws regulating the emissions from automobiles and factories. Now this process must be expanded to the developing countries, where the worst pollution is currently occurring.

One of the most urgent issues before the public today is the battle over emission of 'greenhouse gases', which are causing a rise in temperatures globally. This temperature rise will adversely affect the quality of life of our children, grandchildren, and their grandchildren. Unfortunately, we have not yet achieved the collective political will to take the necessary steps to arrest or reverse this detrimental warming trend.

It is important that the political process to put in place measures to improve the health of the public be based on sound scientific evidence. Pushing agendas not based on sound scientific evidence will undermine the credibility of public health professionals and our ability to accomplish our legitimate goals. Obtaining this evidence is not always easy. For example, accumulating evidence on the long-term (induction period of years to decades) impact of adverse exposures is not easily established, and often requires extrapolation from data on the impact of acute high-dose exposures to lower doses. This often requires relying on models, which are difficult for the public to understand, and are often subject to debate, even within the scientific community.

Structural interventions

An important end-point of the political process is the passage of laws and regulations. This action, if implemented, can have a very significant impact on the improvement of the health of the public. For example, the law reducing the maximum speed in California from 65 to 55 miles per hour had a significant impact on lowering the automobile fatality rate; unfortunately, this lower speed limit has been reversed. The passage and enforcement of helmet laws for motorcycles in Indonesia reduced the incidence of associated brain injuries and deaths. The incidence of lung cancer and heart disease among men has been significantly reduced, partly due to the laws regulating smoking in public spaces and the high taxes imposed on cigarettes. Many of the current public health problems of the world, particularly those involving protection of the environment, can be addressed best through structural changes requiring passage and implementation of laws and regulations. To accomplish this will require changing the attitudes and behaviour of the public and ensuring that public health regulations and laws are enforced.

Private support of public health

Private support has played an important role in the development of public health, especially in the twentieth century. The Rockefeller Foundation supported the first school of public health in the United States at Johns Hopkins University; set up the International Health Commission in 1913; established the China Medical Board in 1914, which established the first public health university in China, the Peking Union Medical College, in 1921; and has continued to contribute to global health since its founding in 1913 (Brown 1979; Berman 1983). Other foundations, including the Gates Foundation, the Ford Foundation, the Carnegie Foundation, and the Robert Wood Johnson Foundation, have made similar significant contributions to public health.

Private support of public health has been implemented through three strategies: establishment of charitable foundations by industry; development of international, national, and local non-governmental organizations (NGOs); and direct contributions by industry. Each makes and can continue to make a significant contribution to the health of the public.

Foundations have contributed enormously to the advancement of public health, but most identify their own priorities for funding. Usually they provide support for important public health needs, but foundations and public health leaders do not always agree on what the most important priorities are. Massive infusions of money into public health by organizations such as the Gates Foundation, which makes contributions to fight HIV, malaria, and tuberculosis, can have a significant positive impact, but they also tend to influence public health priorities. Some argue that developing strong public health infrastructures in developing countries will have a much greater impact on improving health than focusing funds on specific health issues (Garrett 2007).

NGOs tend to focus on specific health problems (e.g. American Cancer Society), specific health issues such as refugee health or medical care for the underserved (e.g. Doctors without Borders), and specific populations (e.g. drug users and sex workers). Often they can be more effective in reaching vulnerable populations and addressing specific health problems and issues because they are closer to the problem than health professionals who must handle a broad range of concerns. Public health programmes can increase their cost-effectiveness by cooperating with NGOs in addressing specific issues, health problems, and populations.

Industry is often viewed as part of the problem. Public health needs to convince industry to temper its profit motive to incorporate responsible citizenship at all levels. Certainly, industry is frequently a significant contributor to public health problems (e.g. air and water pollution). On the other hand, economic development can lead to an improved economic situation that reduces poverty and benefits all of society. However, industry, particularly the advertising industry, has clearly demonstrated that they are better at creating demand and influencing lifestyles than public health professionals. Thus, it behoves public health organizations to learn from industry and to work with industry to develop and implement healthy economic growth, while safeguarding the environment and benefiting the public.

Private support greatly benefited public health in the twentieth century. The challenge for the twenty-first century is for public health and private support to agree on the most effective use of private funds for achieving the greatest public health advances.

Social activism

Action by groups within society has led to improvements in the health of the public. Social activism by workers and others in the nineteenth and early twentieth century in England and the United States resulted in improved working conditions for workers in a variety of industries and to the development of the field of occupational health. More recently, social activism by social groups adversely affected by HIV/AIDS led to the policy to provide access to treatment for all with HIV infection and the need to recognize the human rights of marginalized groups in both developed and developing countries. Demands for better health conditions led by society itself are most likely to result in positive changes.

The future of public health

Public health does not lack challenges requiring solutions. Poverty is the major cause of poor health globally, yet income disparities in most countries of the world are growing. Developing countries must continue to cope with infectious diseases while confronting the epidemic of NCDs, further compounded by the threat of emerging diseases such as new variants of influenza. Rapid communications and transportation greatly increase the likelihood that local problems will quickly become global problems. This underscores the urgent need for much better international cooperation. An increasing proportion of the world's population will live longer. We have been successful at adding 'years to life', but chronic diseases such as Alzheimer's have reduced the quality of some of the years of life added. We must now concentrate on adding 'life to years', helping older people to continue to be healthy and productive.

We cannot afford to continue to ignore the quality of the environment. Continuing contamination of the air and water will not only cause and/or exacerbate chronic and infectious diseases, but will also compromise global food production. The world's population is still growing and together with increasing urbanization, will further exacerbate the problem of environmental degradation.

Despite the economic and health advances of the past century, disparities between the rich and the poor in many countries are widening. This gap needs to be narrowed, not at the expense of those who are better-off, but by improving the economic situation and health of the poor and disadvantaged. The rising cost of healthcare will make closing the gap in access to healthcare even more challenging.

Injuries and violence are robbing an increasing number of people of their ability to function and to enjoy a reasonable quality of life. Injuries can be easily prevented through a variety of preventive strategies, including better design of the workplace and tools, as well as behavioural and structural approaches.

Violence and war present a particularly great challenge, and will require new strategies not hitherto widely used in public health. Public health must contribute to strategies to resolve differences between countries by promoting cross-national and international cooperation in confronting global health problems, and contribute to strategies to implement successful conflict resolution.

Public health must convince people and provide the environment that allows them to adopt healthy lifestyles. The major strategies to combat the current epidemic of NCDs are regular exercise, a healthy diet, and development of good health habits.

Much is known about what needs to be done to significantly reduce the incidence of NCDs such as cardiovascular diseases, stroke, and cancer, but much more effective ways are needed to effect the necessary changes in personal and community behaviour, and to promote healthy lifestyles.

Tremendous strides have been made to improve the health of the public, but the challenge to do better remains. In subsequent chapters, public health experts discuss the challenges and potential solutions in detail.

References

Acheson, E.D. (1988). On the state of the public health. [The fourth Duncan lecture]. *Public Health*, 102(5), 431–7.

Berman, E.H. (1983). *The Ideology of Philanthropy: The Influence of the Carnegie, Ford, and Rockefeller Foundations on American Foreign Policy*. New York: University of New York Press.

Breslow, L. and Breslow, N. (1993). Health practices and disability: some evidence from Alameda County. *Preventive Medicine*, 22, 86–95.

Brown, E.R. (1979). *Rockefeller Medicine Men: Medicine and Capitalism in America*. Berkeley, CA: University of California Press.

Chen, B., Hong, C., and Kan, H. (2004). Exposures and health outcomes from outdoor air pollutants in China. *Toxicology*, 198(1–3), 291–300.

Chow, C.K. and Raju, R. (2006). The prevalence and management of type 2 diabetes in India. *Diabetes Care*, 29, 1717–18.

Cohen J. (2011). HIV treatment as prevention. *Science*, 334(6063), 1628.

Collins, P.Y., Patel, V., Joestl, S.S., et al. (2011). Grand challenges in global mental health. *Nature*, 475, 27–30.

Council for International Organizations of Medical Sciences (2002). *International Ethical Guidelines for Biomedical Research Involving Human Subjects*. Geneva: World Health Organization.

Detels, R. (2009). The scope and concerns of public health. In R. Detels, R. Beaglehole, M.A. Lansang, and M. Gulliford (eds.) *Oxford Textbook of Public Health* (Vol. 1, 5th ed.), pp. 3–19. Oxford: Oxford University Press.

Detels, R. and Breslow, L. (2002). Current scope and concerns in public health. In R. Detels, J. McEwen, R. Beaglehole, and H. Tanaka (eds.) *Oxford Textbook of Public Health* (Vol. 1, 4th ed.), pp. 3–20. Oxford: Oxford University Press.

Detels, R., Rokaw, S.N., Coulson, A.H., et al. (1979). The UCLA population studies of chronic obstructive respiratory disease: I. Methodology and comparison of lung function in areas of high and low pollution. *American Journal of Epidemiology*, 109(1), 33–58.

Feigin, V.L., Lawes, C.M., Bennett, D.A., Barker-Collo, S.L., and Parag, V. (2009). Worldwide stroke incidence and early case fatality reported in 56 population-based studies: a systematic review. *The Lancet Neurology*, 8(4), 355–69.

Garrett, L. (2007). The challenge of public health. *Foreign Affairs*, 86, 14–38.

Gauderman, W.J., Vora, H., McConnell, K., et al. (2007). Effect of exposure to traffic on lung development from 10 to 18 years of age: a cohort study. *The Lancet*, 369, 571–7.

Index Mundi (2012). *World Demographics Profile 2012*. [Online] Available at: http://www.index.mundi.com/world/demographics_profile.html.

International Labor Organization (2011). *World Statistics*. [Online] Available at: http://www.ilo.org/public/English.

Kelly, J.A. (2004). Popular opinion leaders and HIV prevention peer education: resolving discrepant findings, and implications for the development of effective community programmes. *AIDS Care*, 16(2), 139–50.

Kuo, C.C. and Campbell, L.A. Detection of *Chlamydia pneumoniae* in arterial tissues. *Journal of Infectious Diseases*, 181, S432–6.

Lee, S.H. (2003). The SARS epidemic in Hong Kong. *Journal of Epidemiology and Community Health*, 57(9), 652–4.

Li, C., Liu, H., Sun, Y., et al. (2009). PAMAM nonparticles promote acute lung injury by inducing autophagic cell death through the Akt-TSC2-m TOR signaling pathway. *Journal of Molecular and Cell Biology*, 1(1), 37–45.

Lopez, A., Mathers, C., Ezzati, M., Jamison, D., and Murray, C. (2007). Global and regional burden of disease and risk factors, 2001: a systematic analysis of population health data. *The Lancet*, 367, 1747–57.

MacKenzie, W.R., Hoxie, N.J., Proctor, M.E., et al. (1994). A massive outbreak in Milwaukee of cryptosporidium infection transmitted through the public water supply. *The New England Journal of Medicine*, 331, 161–7.

Mathers C.D. and Loncar D. (2006). Projections of global mortality and burden of disease from 2002 to 2030. *PLoS Medicine*, 3(11), e442.

Moellering, R.C. Jr (2010). NDM-1—a cause for worldwide concern. *The New England Journal of Medicine*, 363, 2377–9.

Murray, C.J.L. and Lopez A.D. (eds.) (1995). *The Global Burden of Disease: A Comprehensive Assessment of Mortality and Disability from*

Diseases, Injuries, and Risk Factors in 1990, and Projected to 2020. Cambridge, MA: Harvard University Press.

Murray, C.J.L. and Lopez A.D. (1997). Alternative projections of mortality and disability by cause 1990–2020: Global Burden of Disease Study. *The Lancet*, 349(9064), 1498–504.

Patz, J.A., Campbell-Lendrum, D., Holloway, T., and Foley, J.A. (2005). Impact of regional climate change on human health. *Nature*, 438, 310–17.

Pine, C. and Harris, R. (2007). *Community Oral Health*. London: Quintessence Books.

Population Projections (2000). Population projections. *Health Affairs*, 3, 191–203.

Sigerist, H.E. (1958–1961). *A History of Medicine*. Oxford: Oxford University Press.

United Nations (2002). *World Population Aging: 1950–2050*. New York: Population Division, Department of Economic and Social Affairs, United Nations.

US Census Bureau (2009). *International Database*. [Online]. Available at: http://www.census.gov/ipc/www/idbnew.html.

US National Commission for the Protection of Human Subjects of Biomedical and Behavioral Research (1979). *The Belmont Report: Ethical Principles and Guidelines for Protection of Human Subjects of Biomedical and Behavioral Research*. Washington, DC: US Department of Health & Human Services.

Wong, C.M., Vichit-Vadakan, N., Kan, H., and Qian, Z. (2008). Public Health and Air Pollution in Asia (PAPA): a multicity study of short-term effects of air pollution on mortality. *Environmental Health Perspectives*, 116(9), 1195–202.

World Bank (2012). *World Bank Sees Progress Against Extreme Poverty, But Flags Vulnerabilities*. [Online] Available at: http://www.worldbank.org/en/news/press-release/2012/02/29/world-bank-sees-progress-against-extreme-poverty-but-flags-vulnerabilities.

World Health Organization (2001a). *Mental Disorders Affect One in Four People*. Geneva: WHO. Available at: http://www.who.int/who/2001/media_centre/press_release/en/index.html.

World Health Organization (2001b). *Atlas Mental Health Resources in the World, 2001*. Geneva: WHO. Available at: http://whqlibdoc.who.int/whr/2001/WHR_2001.pdf.

World Health Organization (2002). *The World Health Report 2002*. Geneva: WHO.

World Health Organization (2004). *WHO Oral Health Program*. Sweden: Malmo University. Available at: http://www.whocollab.od.mah.se/index.html.

World Health Organization (2006). *Neglected Tropical Diseases—Hidden Successes, Emerging Opportunities*. Geneva: WHO. Available at: http://whqlibdoc.who.int/hq/2006/WHO_CDS_NTD_2006.2_eng.pdf.

World Health Organization (2011a). *Global Status Report on Non-Communicable Diseases, 2010*. Geneva: WHO.

World Health Organization (2011b). *Mental Health Atlas*. Geneva: WHO.

World Health Organization (2013). *Global Status Report on Road Safety*. Geneva: WHO.

World Health Organization (2014). *Fifth Assessment Report Climate Change 2014: Impacts, Adaptation and Vulnerability*. Geneva: WHO.

World Health Organization (n.d.). *Global Health Estimates*. [Online] Available at: http://www.who.int/healthinfo/global_burden_disease/en/index.html.

World Health Organization Regional Office for Europe (1994). *Action Plan for Environmental Health Services in Central and Eastern Europe and the Newly Independent States*. Report on a WHO Consultation, Sofia, Bulgaria, 19–22 October 1993 (Document EUR/ICP/CEH 123). Copenhagen: WHO. Available at: http://whqlibdoc.who.int/euro/1994-97/EUR_ICP_CEH_123_B.pdf.

World Medical Association (2002). *Declaration of Helsinki* (5th rev.). Washington, DC: World Medical Association.

1.2

The history and development of public health in developed countries

Christopher Hamlin

Introduction to history and development of public health in developed countries

Much more than is usually realized, public health is both a central and a problematic element of the history of the developed world—here conceived as Europe and the 'Neo Europes'; that is, the set of nations in broad latitude bands of the northern and southern hemispheres in which European institutions and biota have been particularly successful (Crosby 1986).

Over the last three centuries, health status has changed profoundly in these regions; arguably, it is in terms of health that our lives differ most strikingly from those of our ancestors. We live longer. Affluence and transportation mean most of us are no longer subject to periodic famines, and much less subject to epidemics of deadly infectious diseases, although we are less confident about that than we were two decades ago (Ward and Warren 2007). Most of us do not see life as a continuously painful experience and death as a merciful release, a view that is rather commonly found in books of theology from three centuries ago (Browne 1964).

Our health is adversely affected by aspects of the world we have built and the ways we choose to live individually and communally. A good deal is known about how to prevent those effects even if we do not always do so. Nonetheless, an expectation of health and a preoccupation with it are hallmarks of modernity. The freedom of action that ideally characterizes the lives of individuals in the developed world is predicated on health; so much of the agenda of development concerns health, that this transformation has some claim to be seen as one of the monumental changes in human history. It might be argued that economic and political progress are subordinate to securing health—they are means; health, which surely translates into life, liberty, and the pursuit of happiness, is the end.

Surprisingly, the history of public health is under-studied. There remain vast gaps in empirical knowledge, and relatively little comparative work (but see Baldwin 1999; Porter 1999; Kunitz 2007). Public health has sometimes seemed to historians a marginal and uncontroversial function of modern society. After all, we provide medicine, collect and evaluate demographic data, test water, and keep cities clean in roughly similar ways, according to the conventions of science, technology, and public administration that developed mainly in the nineteenth century. This view partly reflects a distortion of the history of public health by the modern professions and institutions of public health, which have often found it prudent to reduce the significance of the fact that they are necessarily political, even if their business is politics by medical means.

'Public health' is conceived broadly in this chapter. It is concerned with the general questions of how, why, and in what manners states came to take an interest in the peoples' health. The questions of what 'health' is, of what we mean by 'public', and of what we understand to be the proper domain of 'public health' remain contested matters. To define public health as that part of health that is the responsibility of the state does not help: what constitutes the state, and what are presumed to be state responsibilities vary in time and place. However broadly or narrowly we define 'health', it will be clear that many public actions affect the public's health, yet may not necessarily be seen as belonging to the domain of 'public health'.

An examination of actions taken in the name of protecting or improving the health of the public will illuminate the enigmatic relationship between that universal goal, the health of the public, and public health as an institution—as a profession, science, component of public administration. It will also address matters of moral and political philosophy (Rosen 1958; Fee 1993; Porter 1999), for, ultimately, a history of public health is necessarily part of an ongoing conversation about a programme of social change that is both rational and moral.

Themes and problems in the history of public health

It will help at the outset to recognize several of the most troublesome issues that face any historian of public health. Among these are the following:

1. The units of public health: states and publics:

   ◆ *The public and the state*: the state, concerned with population, may arrive at different health-related policies from a public sphere of groups of citizens, carrying out a rational and critical dialogue among equals (Sturdy 2002). Even when widely accepted agendas of state responsibility arose, not every state was in the position to act on them. Within the state, the focus of public health was quite often at the local rather than the central level, but responsibility and jurisdiction were often unclear or overlapping. Furthermore, the state may not be the optimal unit for addressing problems which are global such as epidemic infections.

 ◆ *Goals of the state:* although health is now thought of in terms of the biological well-being of individuals, in the past, the goals of programmes of public health have occasionally been directed at ensuring a good supply of labour or of soldiers, control of excess population, protection of elites, enhancement of the genetic stock of a population, or environmental stability.

2. The condition that is truly health:

 ◆ *The definition of health:* the combating of epidemic infectious diseases has often seemed to be the core of public health. Beyond these, questions arise as to the level and kind of physical and mental well-being the state should guarantee or require of its citizens, and of the status of health vis-à-vis other sources of imperatives such as the market, the environment, or individual liberty.

 ◆ *The problem of causation of disease:* in a broad sense, diseases have many causes—personal, social, cultural, political, and economic, as well as biological. Among the multiple antecedents that converge to produce an epidemic or endemic disease, there are numerous opportunities to intervene (MacMahon and Pugh 1970, chapter 2). Notions of rights that must be respected, or of political or technical practicality, narrow that list. Discussion of cause has often included notions of responsibility or preventability—of where in a social system there is flexibility, of who or what must change to prevent disease.

 ◆ *Equality and rights—race, class, gender:* the idea of 'health for all' disguises the fact that the interests of the so-called public have not always been the interests of all of its members. Public health actions have often reflected, and sometimes exacerbated, a view of the world in which some groups were seen primarily as perpetrators and others as victims. Often, views of the standards of health that were properly matters for the state varied with respect to different groups: key divisions were by sex, by age (infants, working adults, and the aged all had a different status), by wealth, and by race, religion, or historical heritage (indigenous people had a different status from colonial rulers). Whether the public's response to disease was to advise, aid, or condemn, or to imprison, banish, or kill, reflected the allocation of rights and the distribution of power more than the status of the biological threat.

3. The health that is truly public:

 ◆ *Health and public health:* most modern states have in principle distinguished aspects of health that are the business of the public from those that are for the individual to pursue in the medical marketplace, although the borders have been drawn in many different ways.

 ◆ *Medical and non-medical public health:* although public health has evolved into an ancillary medical science, with occasional involvement of engineering and the social sciences, the fact that health has been improved by many non-medical factors—prosperity, town planning, architecture, religious and humanitarian charity, the power of organized labour, and even the enlargement of political or economic rights—suggests that any comprehensive account of improved health must include these factors.

 ◆ *Health as authority:* given the amorphous nature of the concept of health and its status as the supreme good of human existence, it has been attractive as an imperative for political action. If other 'reasons of state' carry more immediacy, public health often has had better claim to the moral high ground because it is seen to be universal and apolitical.

These issues are too many to address fully, but they inform what follows. The history of public health in the developed world can be conceived in terms of three relatively distinct missions: public health as a reaction to epidemics, as a form of police, and as a means of human betterment. Public health was initially reactive; faced with epidemic disease, early modern European states closed borders and ports, instituted fumigation, shut down 'dangerous' trades, and isolated victims. Second, public health acted as a form of police. Wherever humans live in communities, customs arise for the regulation of behaviour and the maintenance of the communal environment. Gradually, much of the enforcement of community standards became medical. The control of food adulteration or prostitution, of the indigent and the transient, or concern over dung or smoke overlapped with the control of epidemics, but went well beyond it, and occurred in normal as well as in epidemic times.

Finally, public health became a proactive political vision for improvement of the health of all. Well into the nineteenth century, the view remained common that high urban or infant death rates were inevitable. A proactive public health involved the determination that *normal* conditions of health, if they could be improved, were not *acceptable* conditions of health. This shift was partly due to technical achievements—such as smallpox inoculation, and later, vaccination—and to better demographic information, but it rested on changed conceptions of human rights coupled with greater technical and economic optimism. Such visions sustained the building of comprehensive urban water and sewerage systems before there was wide acceptance that these needed to be universal features of cities. Such visions have periodically led public health to venture beyond traditional medical bounds, to recognize, for example, nuclear warfare or gun violence as public health problems.

The public health of epidemic crisis: reaction

Regardless of their virulence and pervasiveness, epidemic and, even more so, endemic diseases do not necessarily arouse comment or action—they may simply be acknowledged as part of life. For the public to decide to fight an epidemic, it must be sufficiently concerned and believe it can do something to mitigate the problem. While a belief in *the possibility of effective action* is a prerequisite for public health, an intriguing question in its history is the emergence of this belief. It does not coincide with the replacement of the supernatural by naturalistic explanations of disease causation. 'Will-of-God' explanations of disease have sometimes incited public action, but on other occasions implied abject resignation.

Similarly, naturalistic explanations—attributing epidemics to a mysterious element in the atmosphere or, as in the case of classical conceptions of smallpox, to a normal process of fermentation in the growing body—have on some occasions been taken as proof that we can do nothing beyond giving supportive care and on other occasions have sanctioned preventive public action. In each case, assessments of technical and political practicality are mixed with assessments of propriety: is taking such action part of our cultural destiny?

These issues are already evident in the first European account of a widely fatal epidemic, the unidentified plague that struck Athens in 430 bc. Athenians both recognized contagion and acknowledged a duty to aid the afflicted, as Thucydides informs us, but these recognitions did not translate into expectations of prevention, mitigation, or escape (Thucydides 1950; Longrigg 1992; Carmichael 1993; Nutton 2000). Few fled; on the contrary, the epidemic was exacerbated by an influx from the countryside. Although it was appreciated that those who survived the disease were unlikely to be affected again, the main response was to accept one's fate. The disease was attributed to the seasons as well as to the gods, and was said to have been prophesied. Such resignation would be central to the moral philosophies of the Roman world, Stoicism and Epicureanism, both of which taught one to accept what was fated or necessary (Veyne 1987). Later writers in the Christian world attributed the purported failure of Islam to take active steps against plague to such an outlook. Although classical Islamic doctors had developed a science of hygiene to a remarkable degree (Gori 2002), it did not follow that this had implications for intervention in an epidemic: if plague came, that was Allah's will. To fight it would be futile and impious; one's duty was to trust (Dols 1977; Conrad 1992; but see ibn Riḍwān 1984).

In contrast, the common response to epidemic disease in the late medieval Christian Latin countries would come to be activism. There was hope that one could prevent disease from taking hold in a community, extinguish it if it did, or at least avoid it personally. This activism had many sources. In the Old and New Testaments, disease had a multiplicity of significations. It represented the dispensation of God to an individual, perhaps as punishment or a test. To act against disease by intervening to help others stricken by a dangerous epidemic was an act of devotion. If one died in such a situation, it was a sign of grace; if one did not die, and helped to save others, this was equally a sign of grace. The laws of hygiene in the Pentateuch permitted a naturalistic interpretation of disease. Unclean acts or other transgressions, such as failing to isolate lepers from society, generated the retribution of disease through divinely appointed secondary or natural causes (Douglas 1966; Winslow 1943/1980; Amundsen and Ferngren 1986; Dorff 1986; Lieber 2000).

The two diseases that were most public in medieval Europe were leprosy and plague. Although it is difficult to assess the number of lepers in medieval Europe, the common view is of vast overreaction in terms of both investment in institutions—there were said to be several thousand leprosaria—and the detection and isolation of cases. In keeping with the prominence of leprosy in the Bible, the professionals who diagnosed it were churchmen, not medical men. The leprosy diagnosis was a loose one; it might be based on

skin blemishes alone. Often it led to the expulsion of the victim from ecclesiastical and civil society. Subsequently, no one was to touch or come near the leper or to touch what the leper touched. The theory of contagion provided the rationale for such action, but Skisnes (1973) has argued that the clinical characteristics of the disease itself—for example, its slow development, the visible disfigurement it produced—triggered such a reaction (Brody 1974; Richards 1977; Carmichael 1997; Touati 2000).

The prototypical institutional responses to epidemic disease, however, were those that arose in response to plague. The first wave of plague, the 'Black Death', spread across Europe from 1347–1353. Thereafter the disease returned to most areas about once every two decades for the next three centuries. Case-fatality rates appeared high, ranging from 30 to nearly 100 per cent depending on the strain of 'plague' (the identity of the microbe has been questioned) (Nutton 2008; Benedictow 2010; Cohn 2010), the means of transmission, and the immunological state of the population. Plague and accompanying diseases reduced the European population by a third or more in the fourteenth century and were responsible for the slowness of population growth during the following two centuries. As with leprosy, the aetiology of plague, and the associated means of prevention and mitigation of the disease were conceived in terms of divine will *and* natural processes (Nohl 1926; Ziegler 1969; Cohn 2010).

It is clear that in many communities plague could not be reconciled with the usual course of events, but indicated some fundamental violation of the cosmos. Boccaccio (1955), whose *Decameron* is a document on the Black Death, testifies to one form of activism—a discarding of social convention and religious duty, a devil-may-care indulgence in the present founded on the recognition that life was short and the future uncertain. Those with the means often fled plague-ridden places. Others, taking the view that the plague reflected God's just anger with hopelessly corrupt civil and ecclesiastical authority, saw a clear need to take charge of matters temporal and spiritual, to cleanse themselves, the state, and the church. Righteousness would end the plague.

Thus, the plague precipitated a social crisis, as would epidemics of other diseases in subsequent centuries. Beyond the massive disruption caused by high mortality and morbidity and an interruption of commerce and industry, the loss of faith in the conventions and institutions of society was a critical blow. Why respect property, family, or communal obligations, pay taxes, invest money, or tolerate rivals and others? Latent tensions within society had an excuse to become active.

When people acted precipitately and independently, civil and ecclesiastical institutions were threatened, and in their responses, we clearly see the emergence of public health as a form of public authority. For a state, to act in a crisis was to keep the state going; one maintained authority by acting authoritatively. If some state actions were rational in terms of the naturalistic aspects of theories of the plague, preserving the viability of civic authority itself was probably the key issue.

Unfortunately the source of hope, and mode of activism, was often blame. From the 'Black Death' onward, the fragility of pluralistic communities was overstrained as the epidemic was attributed to deliberate actions, accidental modes of being, or mere existence of some minority. The minorities might be foreigners, the poor, or Jews, and the actions against them included sequestration, expulsion, or even slaughter (Ziegler 1969). Such actions were often populist; they arose locally, and had often to be suppressed by national authorities. While it was easy to enlist conceptions of contagion as warrant for such actions, there were plenty of other explanatory options involving appeals to natural processes of disease transmission and generation as well as divine visitation.

Amidst episodes of civil disorder, there arose, particularly in the early modern Italian city-states, relatively successful approaches to plague prevention and control that were the forerunners of modern means of controlling epidemic outbreaks. They included the development of the 40-day hold on ships or other traffic coming from potentially infected places (quarantine), the isolation of victims (and families of victims), and numerous means of purifying the air and/or destroying contamination: bonfires, burning sulphur, burning clothes and bedding, washing surfaces with lime or vinegar, and killing or removing urban animals. Such actions were predicated on an understanding that the disease moved from place to place through some media, possibly involving person-to-person contact.

Although the eclecticism of this response reflected uncertainty about how plague spread, the actions do show a responsive civil authority (Cipolla 1979, 1992; Carmichael 1986; Cohn 2010). Indeed, in some ways plague prevention initiatives were themselves a means of state growth. Plague control required officials to oversee quarantine or isolation procedures. It required a staff to disinfect, and a structure to gather information on health conditions at remote ends of the state. An embassy, which in the high Middle Ages signified an official visit by one state to another, became the permanent presence of one state in the territory of another in the Italian city-states. Its initial purpose was to monitor the public health in the host country and to send word home if plague broke out (Cipolla 1981; Slack 1985).

Plague set the template for the mix of responses and reactions to other disease epidemics. These included flight, the exacerbation of social tensions, a heightening of religious seriousness, and pragmatic efforts to disinfect people, places, goods, or the environment, and to isolate victims or potentially contagious strangers. The theoretical frameworks to justify such actions included atmospheric factors ranging from hypothetical geophysical aberrations to local vitiation from decomposing matter, and various forms of interpersonal transmission. Before the nineteenth century, contagionist and environmental explanations were rarely mutually exclusive as factors implicated in disease (Pelling 2001; Kinzelbach 2006).

The patterns were repeated during the cholera pandemics which first reached Europe in the early 1830s. These brought forth accusations by the poor that the rich were poisoning them (and by the rich that the poor wantonly persisted in living in disease-nurturing squalor). They also engendered calls for public fasts, pure living, and declamations against sinful society, and a variety of attempts to disinfect, quarantine, and isolate (Briggs 1961; Rosenberg 1962; McGrew 1965; Durey 1979; Delaporte 1986; Richardson 1988; Evans 1990; Snowden 1995; Hamlin 2009). Often a key demarcator of class was the very possibility of flight. In nineteenth-century America, the response to yellow fever and malaria was the abandonment of cities during the summer by those who could afford to do so (Ellis 1992; Humphreys 1992). The summer home, in cooler, cleaner, and higher ground, became a mark of upper-middle-class life.

Significant alterations of that pattern came through efforts to control three other diseases: venereal diseases (particularly

syphilis), smallpox, and a mix of diseases including typhus, typhoid, relapsing fever, and ill-other defined conditions, collectively known as continued fever (or just 'fever').

Whether syphilis came to Europe from America or Africa, or had been present in Europe in a milder form has been much debated. What is clear is that a virulent epidemic often known as the French disease or pox began to spread quickly in the last years of the fifteenth century, and can be traced to the intercourse between Italian prostitutes and French and Spanish soldiers during the siege of Naples in 1494. The connection between the disease and sex was made quickly, partly because the initial signs and symptoms affected the external genitalia. In contrast to plague or leprosy, syphilis represented a serious epidemic disease that constituted a state, rather than a municipal, problem: it affected military strength, but was not susceptible to large-scale public action. It was further complicated by having variable symptoms and effects, a long often silent clinical course, and variability in contagiousness and virulence.

To control syphilis, states had to prevail on individuals to avoid behaviours that spread the disease. One might expect the moral opprobrium related to contracting a disease usually acquired through illicit sexual contact to have had some role in discouraging such practices, but it did not. For an adventurous young man, catching the pox was a cost of doing business, even a badge of achievement. The disease was deemed curable, chiefly through mercurial treatments. Although there are suggestions that by the eighteenth century syphilis had become something to hide, such was not the case during the sixteenth century, when the disease was spreading rapidly (Arrizabalaga 1993, 1997).

State attention shifted from cure to prevention only in the eighteenth century; partly because syphilis was becoming more clearly distinguished from other venereal conditions and as the varied manifestations of tertiary syphilis were becoming more evident. The priority European states placed on syphilis as a public problem differed but their approaches did not vary greatly: the disease was to be controlled by regulating prostitutes, who were regarded as the reservoir that maintained the contagion. While such approaches may have had a significant effect in controlling the disease, they exposed tensions between state and individual rights that have since become common in public health.

Such conflicts developed first in the United Kingdom following the first Contagious Diseases Act of 1862, even though its programme against venereal disease was much smaller than that of France, where regulation of prostitution was a central feature of public hygiene (Baldwin 1999). The British Act allowed the police in designated garrison towns to arrest and inspect women presumed to be prostitutes and to confine infected women in hospital. It led to a sustained campaign for repeal, which was ultimately successful in 1885. The repealers represented a broad coalition: some objected that the legislation was morally indefensible because it acquiesced in the immoral industry of prostitution, others that it singled out women whereas the men who used the services of prostitutes were equally responsible for the problem, while still others objected that the practice of arresting women was arbitrary and stigmatized working-class women who were not prostitutes (Walkowitz 1980; McHugh 1982).

The problem that the British parliament faced stemmed from liberal principles of human rights. Ironically, the Contagious Diseases Act had been touted as respecting rights—the rights of men: the state would inspect women because male soldiers and sailors would not put up with genital inspection. Nor should they be expected to in a state in which the male franchise was broadening and the public was becoming increasingly uneasy with declarations that part of its population existed as cannon fodder. But recognizing the rights of men thus highlighted the fact that the same were not accorded to women.

The issues that arose in combating venereal diseases surfaced in a more general way with smallpox. To the ninth-century doctor Al-Razi, smallpox had been a particularly dangerous stage of normal growth (Clendening 1942), but by the eighteenth century, it often accounted for 10–15 per cent of deaths. It was then widely recognized as a contagious disease of childhood. Many parents intentionally exposed their young children to it: sooner or later, one would be exposed, and the older child who died from it was a multi-year investment lost, while the younger one who survived was subsequently immune.

In many parts of the world, it was recognized that inducing smallpox by some means made it significantly less virulent. Mortality rates might drop from 25 per cent or more to a few per cent. Notwithstanding assertions that such practice defied providence and appeared counter-intuitive, such logic and experience had much to do with the relatively rapid acceptance of inoculation after 1721, when it was introduced into Western Europe by Lady Mary Wortley Montagu, a well-connected aristocrat who had observed the process in Turkey. It was first taken up in the British Isles; its subsequent spread resulted from the patronage of royalty and nobility, increases in the safety of the procedure, especially when carried out by the most highly skilled practitioners, and the acquiescence of at least a segment of the medical profession (Miller 1957; Razzell 1977; Hopkins 2002).

In 1798, the English practitioner Edward Jenner made immunization significantly safer by introducing the practice of vaccination with cowpox. Increasingly, smallpox prevention, hitherto a personal matter, became a state concern. Presumably, the institutions that orchestrated quarantines could also ensure universal vaccination. But here too there was ambiguity: in whose interests were vaccination programmes to be undertaken? England began offering free vaccination in 1840, made it compulsory in 1853, and instituted fines for non-compliance in 1873. The initial assumption that all would take advantage of this free medical service proved unfounded; as the authorities sought to give the vaccination laws more teeth, they encountered growing opposition and decreasing rates of compliance.

In 1898, anti-vaccinationists gained permission for conscientious objectors to forgo having their children vaccinated. The opposition was able to show that the dangerous procedure was not carried out everywhere with sufficient skill or care, and a real decline in smallpox meant decreasing risk to the unvaccinated. But mandatory vaccination also exposed underlying tension between the state and the public: in an atmosphere of distrust of the state, the more insistent the state became, the more convinced the public became that the state's actions were not in their interests (Porter and Porter 1988; Baldwin 1999; Durbach 2005; Brunton 2008).

It is important to emphasize that for most of the history of the West, efforts to combat epidemic disease were not reflective of a sense of obligation to the health of individuals. The welfare of individual subjects was incidental. Although states devoted substantial resources to enforcing quarantines and other health regulations (and absorbed considerable costs in lost commerce), it would be misleading to think of them acting in some quasi-contractual way as agents for groups of individuals who had recognized that public actions were necessary to secure their own health. Although many places had town or parish doctors, and there was often an expectation that the state take some steps to protect the welfare of its subjects (such as making food affordable in times of dearth), early modern political theorists recognized no general obligation of the state to protect the health of individuals. What was at risk in an epidemic was the state itself: the collection of taxes, the maintenance of defence, the continuance of commerce, and even the orderly transfer of property at a time of high mortality.

Perhaps nowhere was the tension between individual and state so great as in the combating of what was called 'continued fever'. Typhus, typhoid, relapsing fever, and yellow fever were among the several epidemic diseases that appeared or became increasingly prominent in the aftermath of the Black Death. This 'continued' fever (malaria was generally distinguished as 'intermittent' fever) was endemic as well as epidemic, and amidst vast disagreement about classification and cause, there was general agreement about its frequent association with social catastrophe and squalor—with war, jails, pestilence, famine, and overcrowded slums (Wilson 1978; Smith 1981; Hamlin 1998, 2006; Geary 2004). Although it was often associated with class, it did not limit itself to the poor. Many theorists believed the fever could spread from poor to rich, whether by person-to-person contact or by diffusion through some environmental medium from hovels and slums to mansions. But, as would later be the case with tuberculous diseases, it was not clear whether one could disentangle any single factor from the many conditions of poverty, nor did medical men necessarily think it made sense to try.

The public action that might have been taken was the comprehensive improvement of living conditions—the prevention of overcrowded dwellings; the insurance of sufficient food, fuel, and clothing; the provision of personal and environmental cleanliness, a safe work place, and a non-exhausting work day—in short, all the physical and social changes that would produce a sound human being. Yet, such far-reaching actions to defend the state also threatened to transform it and in essential ways—in its social distinctions, its institutions of property, even in the political rights it recognized. When the young Prussian radical doctors Rudolph Virchow and Sebastian Neumann investigated a typhus outbreak in Silesia in 1848, they argued that liberal political and economic reforms were the antidote to the squalor which caused the epidemic (Rosen 1947). Irish physicians made similar diagnoses in the pre-famine years, even proposing a 'political medicine' in which health outcomes would be a major consideration in public policy (Hamlin 2011).

The public health of communal life: police

Beyond the response to epidemics, Western societies had from early times taken steps to regulate their communities for the common good or public peace. By the eighteenth century, the term generally used for such efforts was 'police', but the control of crime was only a small part of it. It generally referred to matters of internal public order; that is, to all aspects of government other than military and diplomatic affairs, the raising of funds, import and export duties, matters of land tenure, and civil litigation. Box 1.2.1 lists common police functions.

Sometimes, doctors were involved in this enforcement, and some of these matters were overtly medical, but at least as often, doctors were part of the domain to be regulated.

The issues under the heading of police comprised problems at various levels: for individuals as town dwellers or as adjoining property owners within a neighbourhood, for towns as corporate entities, and for regional or national states. Public health, in the sense of a recognized obligation to protect the health of the people through public regulation, was only rarely the rationale for police, although improvement in the public's health was likely often a consequence of police action. In some cases, 'police' involved public means for the resolution of disputes between individuals as property owners, such as those that arose when drainage, smoke, or dung encroached on another's premises. At a municipal level, a widespread concern with the policing of commerce and manufacture reflected the town's dependence on its markets. The privileges of trade and industry within a town were rarely free; the concern with the quality of foods and drugs was less a matter of consumers' health than of fair competition, consumer satisfaction, and maintenance of the market's good reputation. Finally, at the state level, concern with midwifery, nutrition, or demographic statistics did not necessarily reflect concern with individuals' health. Early modern statecraft equated state strength with population.

The character of institutions of police varied considerably, although most medieval (and ancient) European towns had some kind of institution(s) to carry out the tasks listed earlier (Hope and Marshall 2000). Typically, these mirrored the political structure of the state. In medieval Islamic towns, a *muhtasib*, an appointee of the caliph oversaw public morals and commerce, but also regulated medical and veterinary practice, refuse disposal, water supply, the cleansing of the public baths, and the licensing of prostitutes (Karmi 1981; López-Piñero 1981; Palmer 1981). In England, where the state was weak and towns strong, police institutions were more community based; this bottom-up character of dispute resolution would evolve into common law. Among medieval English institutions of local government were the *leet* juries (groups of citizens who biannually perambulated through the town and 'presented' the nuisances they found to the magistrates, who would order abatement), and the courts of sewers, which acted similarly in trying to resolve conflicts about drainage. Whenever a landowner altered drainage patterns, others were affected, often deleteriously. The sewers court was a means of minimizing those adverse effects and compensating for damage when they were unavoidable. In a similar way, London's Assize of Nuisances managed disputes between neighbours about the location and cleansing of privies (Webb and Webb 1922; Redlich and Hirst 1970; Chew and Kellaway 1973; Leongard 1989; Novak 1996). The concept of 'nuisance', if not the term, underlay much of the work of public police. In the Anglo-French tradition, a 'nuisance' was an accusation, subsequently backed by a legal determination, that actions on one person's property or in the public domain annoyed and/or interfered with the enjoyment of another's rights (Blackstone 1892; Novak 1996; Hamlin 2002). Common forms of 'nuisance' included conditions offensive to health and sensibility, such as concentrations of pig manure or butchers' waste, as well as antisocial behaviour.

The business of the public police did affect health in many ways and also covered much of what would later belong to the domain of public health. The priority, however, was usually with amenity, morality, and conflict resolution. However, although the motives and contexts of police initiatives were broader than public health matters, there were overlaps in both practice and theory. The police institutions in late medieval Italian city-states evolved from means of plague response (Carmichael 1986; Cohn 2010), and almost always, a poorly administered town was looked upon as ripe for an epidemic. Moreover, within Hippocratic and Galenic frameworks, amenity was not clearly distinct from health: to feel well was to be well; unpleasant sights or smells, noises, or incidents, even if they did not lead to disease, constituted both a form of trespass and an assault on health (Carlin 2005). Concepts of specific diseases and vectors were far in the future. Notwithstanding the occasional speculation, such as that of the sixteenth-century Italian doctor Girolamo Fracastoro that each disease might be the product of an invisible living seed, most medical men were not thinking about individual diseases in a way that would encourage them to look for discrete agents. Because amenity, order, and health were so closely linked, a medical rationale could provide a basis for social action on behalf of a community.

Too little is known about the operation of these police institutions. What is known suggests that their performance varied enormously. It also suggests that the popular image of the pre-modern town as filthy and ungoverned is misleading. There may well have been filth on the streets, but clearly in some cases it was put there at prescribed hours prior to the rounds of the municipal street sweepers, who would collect it for manure or otherwise dispose of it. Many urban cottage industries—dyeing, soap making, the treating of leather or textiles—did use unpleasant

---

Box 1.2.1 Police functions

- The enforcement of basic rules of public behaviour.

- The enforcement of standards of building construction and use, with regard to noxious trades and basic sanitation.

- The care for the poor, the disabled, and for abandoned children or orphans.

- The regulation of hours and modes of work.

- The conduct of markets and the quality of the commodities sold in them.

- The regulation of marriage and midwifery.

- The supply of water to people and the treatment of cattle and other animals.

- The inspection and regulation of transients and prostitutes.

- The appropriate disposal of the dead, both human and animal.

- The prevention of fire and injury.

- The investigation of accidental deaths and other forensic matters.

- The maintenance of population statistics.

- The regulation of medical practice.

animal products; complaints about them often reflect the struggle between classes for control of the urban environment, with wealthy merchants or professionals appealing to supposedly universal standards of sensibility and health to enhance their status over those who worked in what Guillerme calls the fermentation industries (Guillerme 1988).

Two examples of the ongoing legacy of such institutions of police can be seen in the regulation of the food supply and the evolution of the concept of 'nuisances' in Anglo-American public health. The fight for pure food and drugs that developed in the later nineteenth century is often seen as an early manifestation of consumerism, and equally, the product of advances in chemistry, microscopy, and bacteriology as applied to foods. Currently, regulation of the food supply is one of the most common duties of public health departments—efficient inspection of meat- and milk-processing plants and institutional kitchens is seen as an essential component of a civilized society. There were changes in the late nineteenth century in the recognition of a wider range of food contaminants, and due to the need to grapple with a more ingenious group of food adulterers, whose doings were better hidden by an increasingly complicated system of food production and distribution. But the concerns of consumers with food safety and their view that food inspection was a duty of government was old and widely shared. The concern of many medieval food inspection officers was with honest weights and measures, but quality was always implicit—the just measure did not satisfy if the ale was diluted. Although there might not have always been objective ways of determining food quality, consumers knew and enforced a moral economy on transgressing vendors: The records of civil discord are packed with the trashing of shops and the thrashing of vendors (Thompson 1971).

Traditions of market regulation affected public health more broadly. Concern about water quality in metropolitan London, for example, reflected consumer outrage at high prices and poor quality and quantity of the water well before there was any epidemiological evidence of it causing cholera. Equally, public willingness to accept that epidemiological evidence was tied to anger at paying too much for an irregular and visibly dirty water supply (Hamlin 1990; Taylor and Trentmann 2005). It is also likely, although difficult to show, that the ready acceptance of the new scientific forms of food inspection in the late nineteenth century reflected consumer expectations that the service was necessary and appropriate for government to undertake (Waddington 2006).

In the case of environmental nuisances too, institutions of public health took over from long-standing institutions for settling civil disputes. Whereas in earlier centuries the concept had been very broad—including excessive noise, disturbances of the peace, the blocking of customary light—by the mid-nineteenth century, the quintessential nuisance had become urban dung, human and animal, and action against nuisances acquired a basis in statute law that supplemented its status in civil law. Beginning with the first English Nuisances Removal Act of 1846, passed in an expectation of the return of cholera, doctors, and later a new functionary called an inspector of nuisances (later a sanitary inspector), were charged with identifying nuisances and taking steps to have them removed (Wilson 1881; Hamlin 2005). The change from civil to criminal law reflects a recognition that a legal tradition built upon the power of property was ill-suited to a situation in which most property was not occupied by its owners, and equally to a situation in which most people's sensibilities were insufficiently

offended by the particular states of environment presumed to be associated with cholera.

Although this change was an emergency response, its effects were more far reaching. It represented the investing of community standards for health in a permanent institution with enforcement powers, rather than leaving them to be worked out incident-by-incident, through common law. The inspectors of nuisances did not restrict themselves to documented causes of disease, but continued to respond to community complaints, which sometimes were primarily aesthetic. They became the defenders of the ever-rising standards of middle-class life, and however far their activities might stray from any direct relation to disease control, they carried with them the authority of public health imperative (Hamlin 1988, 2005; Kearns 1991).

Towards the end of the nineteenth century, some epidemiologists, recognizing that the tracing of cases and contacts informed by the new science of bacteriology provided a more exact means of disease control, suggested that concern with general environmental quality was an unjustified expense that deflected the attention of public health departments from what really mattered (Cassedy 1962; Rosenkrantz 1974). In some cases, they were effective in severing sanitation and public works from public health, but often they found that the public, who tended to support clean streets and pleasant neighbourhoods, continued to use public health as justification. More common than the wholesale replacement of sanitation by bacteriology was the emergence of what has been called a 'sanitary–bacteriological synthesis' (Barnes 2006). Here too, medical science gave public action a legitimacy that would otherwise have been difficult to create.

The medicalization of public police that these examples suggest was clearly underway by the mid eighteenth century. The concept of medical police first arose in Germany and Austria, later in Scotland, Scandinavia, Italy, and Spain; in France the rough equivalent was *hygiene publique*. In America and in England, the term and concept never really caught on (Carroll 2002). Medicine's rise to prominence reflected an alliance between medical practitioners who sought state patronage and the 'enlightened despots'—rulers who, such as Austria's Joseph II, sought a science of good government that would significantly strengthen their states. Increasingly, rulers like Joseph felt obliged to test their policies against some tenets of rationality; health seemed to offer a well-defined arena of rational government, a set of means to improve the state and to measure the progress of that improvement (Rosen 1974, 2008). As the regulation of personal behaviour could improve the health of soldiers and sailors, why not practise the same techniques on the rest of society? The effect of this medicalization was to move matters of police further from the realm of local social relations and towards an all-encompassing scientific rationality.

The classic text of eighteenth-century medical police is medical professor and public health administrator Johann Peter Frank's six-volume *A System of Complete Medical Police*, which appeared between 1779 and 1819 (Frank 1976). The first two volumes discussed reproductive health, including suggestions for the regulation (and encouragement) of marriage, prenatal care, obstetrical matters, and infant feeding and care. The book then turned to diet, personal habits, public amusements, and healthy buildings. The fourth volume covered public safety from accident prevention to the injuries supposedly inflicted by witches, the fifth volume dealt with safe means of interment, and the sixth with the regulation of the medical profession. In Frank's cameralist view, anything that adversely affected health was a matter for public policy and an appropriate subject for regulation—rights, traditions, property, and freedom had no status if they interfered with the welfare of the population.

In its most far-reaching definitions, modern public health approaches the domain of a comprehensive police. It also recognizes that a wide range of factors is implicated in health conditions—current public health concerns include the effects of violent entertainment, the prevention of gun violence, and the conditions of the work place. But in modern liberal democracies, much of what Frank saw as the obvious business of the state is deeply problematic. For, in the nineteenth century, public health shifted radically in mission and constituency. It became less a means of maintaining the state, and more a means by which the state served its sovereign citizens with an (increasing) standard of health that they (increasingly) took as a right of citizenship.

The public health of human potential

We often think that health is a service that governments owe their citizens, that what separates past from present is not intent but simply sufficient knowledge of the means to provide that service—this is not so. A public health that is not merely reactive or regulative but which aims to reduce rates of preventable mortality and morbidity as its duty to its populace, is a product of the eighteenth century. It is also one of the most remarkable changes of sensibility in human history. Its causes are complex but poorly understood. Concepts of preventable mortality and excess morbidity required the ability to show that death and illness existed at much higher rates in some places than in others. It required also recognition of some ways to address these conditions.

Although there were a few attempts in seventeenth- and eighteenth-century Europe to determine local bills of mortality, they were too few to provide a basis for comparison. In contrast, by the late nineteenth century, annual mortality rates were an important focus of competition among English towns. The central government's public health officials, notably John Simon, chief medical officer of the Privy Council from 1857–1874, badgered towns with poor showings. Simon and his successors urged them to analyse the reasons for their excess mortality and to take appropriate action (Brand 1965; Lambert 1965; Eyler 1979; Wohl 1983). By the end of the century, and during the twentieth century, reliable morbidity statistics were available to provide a better understanding of the remediable causes of disease. The gathering of such data, and after about 1920 their analysis by modern means of statistical inference, has become a central part of modern public health (Desrosières 1998; Magnello 2002).

The mission of prevention was also tied to a very real growth in knowledge of the means of prevention. The widespread adoption of inoculation, and after 1800, of vaccination for smallpox, was the first clearly effective means to intervene decisively to prevent a deadly disease. Initially through the development of the numerical method and the cultivation of pathological anatomy in the Parisian hospitals in the first decades of the nineteenth century, and subsequently through bacteriological and later serological methods, infectious diseases were distinguished and their discrete causes and vectors identified (Ackerknecht 1967; Bynum 1994). Such recognition ultimately led not only to the 'magic bullet' thinking of vaccine development, but also underwrote campaigns to improve water quality and provide other means of sanitation,

and sometimes, as with tuberculosis and typhoid, programmes to identify, monitor, and regulate carriers.

Yet these factors alone cannot account for the widespread conviction that human health must be significantly improved—they are means, not ends. Despite the significance of effective action against smallpox, it did not imply that all infectious diseases could be controlled through a similar strategy. In most cases, the new medical knowledge did not precede the determination to improve the health of all, but was developed in the process of achieving that goal. A great deal of success was achieved despite quite erroneous conceptions of the nature of the diseases and their causes. The great sanitary campaign against urban filth (based on a vague concept of pathogenic miasms) is the best-known example (Barnes 2006).

Recognition of differential mortality was not new in the early 1800s, but it did not necessarily spur action. The mortality penalty associated with poverty, infancy, and urban living was regarded by some as a necessary corrective to the overfecundity of the countryside (Sadler 1830; Weyland 1816/1968). Even humane and optimistic writers saw infant mortality rates of 25 per cent or more as providential (Roberton 1827).

In contrast, the modern sensibility admits no justifiable reason (beyond, perhaps, the climatic factors that determine the range of some disease vectors) for differential mortality or morbidity. These changes in sensibilities towards state provision can be divided into three periods: an age of liberalism from 1790–1880; a golden age of public health to 1970; and a more confusing post-modern period in the last four decades, which may, at least in its most positive aspects, be seen as a return to liberalism.

The age of liberalism: health in the name of the people, 1790–1880

The social and intellectual movement known as liberalism, which began to prevail in the second half of the eighteenth century, included a wide range of philosophical, political, economic, and religious ideas, but at its heart were notions of individual freedom and responsibility, and usually, of equality in some form. In 1890, when John Simon, England's first chief medical officer and a pioneer of state medicine, surveyed progress in public health during the past two centuries in his *English Sanitary Institutions*, he included a lengthy chapter on the 'New Humanity'. In it, he covered the antislavery movement, the rise of Methodism, growing concern about cruelty to criminals and animals, legislation promoting religious freedom, the replacement of patronage by principle as the motor of parliamentary democracy, the introduction of free markets, the rationalization of criminal and civil law, and efforts towards international peace. Simon saw little need to explain how this concerned public health; he was sketching a fundamental change in 'feeling' that underlay changes in public health policy.

No longer were humans so much cannon fodder; the best policies were those which maximized 'human worth and welfare' (Simon 1890; compare with Pettenkofer 1941; Coleman 1974; Haskell 1985).

What Simon recognized was that with the granting of equal political and economic rights and responsibilities, it was no longer possible to see health status constrained by class, race, or sex. Nineteenth-century French and English liberals recognized that some—particularly women, children, and the poor—still suffered ill health disproportionately, but they saw such consequences as incidental, accidental, and increasingly, as unnecessary and objectionable: in principle, all had an equal claim to whatever human and health rights a society was prepared to recognize. This change in feeling was both the cause and effect of the widening distribution of political power.

And yet liberalism was no clear and compact doctrine, and its implications for public health were, and still are, by no means clear. Few of the pioneers of liberal political theory had bothered to translate human rights into terms of health. They wrote mainly with middle-class men in mind, and saw the threats to life, liberty, and property as political rather than biosocial. The expansion (or translation) of political rights into rights to health was gradual, piecemeal (it has never been the rallying cry of revolution), complicated, and even fundamentally conflictual—it was, and is, not always the case that the choices free individuals make will protect the public's health, or even their own. Concern with public health arose accidentally, and in different ways and at different times in the developed nations. At the beginning of the twenty-first century, an obligation to maintain and/or improve the health of all citizens exists only in varying degrees.

Many early liberals found health rights hard to recognize because so much of public health had been closely associated with the medical police functions of an overbearing state. In revolutionary France, the first instinct was to free the market in medical practice by abolishing medical licensing, a policy quickly recognized as disastrous for maintaining the armies of citizen-soldiers who were protecting the nation (Foucault 1975; Riley 1987; Weiner 1993; Brockliss and Jones 1997). Even after new, meritocratic, and science-based medical institutions had been established, the cadre of public health researchers that French medicine fostered—at the time, the world's leaders in epidemiology—found it difficult to conceive how their findings of the causes of disease could be translated into preventive legislation. Working and living conditions were dictated by the market; government mandates would induce dependence or simply shift the problem elsewhere. Thus, France was the scientific leader in public health for the first half of the nineteenth century without finding a viable political formula for translating that knowledge into prevention (Coleman 1982; LaBerge 1992).

In early-nineteenth-century Britain, the ideas of T.R. Malthus led a broad range of learned public opinion to similar conclusions. Disease was among the natural checks that kept population within the margins of survival. Successful prevention of disease would be temporary only; it would postpone an inevitable equilibration of the food–population balance that would then need to occur through some other form of catastrophe (Dean 1991; Hamlin 1998). Malthusian sentiment blocked attempts to establish foundling hospitals. Notwithstanding the fact that such institutions were notoriously deadly to their inmates, it was felt that their existence encouraged irresponsible procreation—faced with full economic responsibility for their actions, men would stifle their urges (McClure 1981). Malthusian views were prominent in British policy with regard to Ireland, Scotland, and India.

By 1850, in both France and England, it was no longer possible to maintain faith in the welfare-maximizing actions of a completely free society. A number of factors shattered this faith. First, no government ever adopted the programme of the early

nineteenth-century liberals in full. In Central, Eastern, and Southern Europe, the old concerns of state security continued to govern their public health. In Sweden and later France, concern about a state weakened by depopulation fostered attention to the health and welfare of individuals.

Second, working-class parties, although often generally sympathetic with political liberalism, saw no advantage in economic liberalism. Often, they demanded adherence to the moral economy of the old order, in which governments damped fluctuations in grain prices and enforced the working conditions that craft guilds had established. Most important is that many liberals themselves arrived at a biosocial vision, which recognized that it was impractical, inhumane, and injudicious to impose economic and political responsibilities on people who were biologically incapable of meeting those responsibilities: liberty had biological prerequisites.

These considerations were central to debates in France and Britain in the 1830s and 1840s. Governments in both countries were apprehensive of revolution and wary of an alienated underclass of people who could not be trusted with political rights and seemed immune to the incentives of the market. Such people represented a reservoir of disease, both literal physical disease and metaphorical social disease, that could infect those clinging precariously to the lower rungs of respectability. Reformers proposed to somehow transform these dangerous classes, usually with Bibles, schools, or experimental colonies. Such was the political background against which Edwin Chadwick (1800–1884), secretary of the English bureau charged with overseeing the administration of local poor relief, developed 'the sanitary idea' in the late 1830s (Finer 1952; Lewis 1952; Chadwick 1965; Richards 1980; Hamlin 1998).

Chadwick justified public investment in comprehensive systems of water and sewerage on the grounds that saving lives—particularly of male breadwinners—would be recompensed in lowered costs for the support of widows and orphans. But he also suggested that sanitation would remoralize the underclass, and for many supporters, this was its most attractive feature. Politically, sanitation was a brilliant idea, as every other general reform was deeply controversial: proposals for religion and education were plagued by sectarianism, calls to improve welfare by allowing free trade in grain (leading to lower food prices) ran afoul of powerful agricultural interests, proposals for regulating working conditions were unacceptable to powerful industrial interests. Notwithstanding complaints that towns should be allowed to reform in their own ways and their own good time rather than being forced to adopt Chadwick's technologies and deadlines, sanitation achieved remarkable popularity in nineteenth-century Britain.

In treating insanitation as the universal cause of disease, Chadwick hoped to establish a public health that was truly liberal. He sought to deflect attention from other causes of disease, such as malnutrition and overwork, for these were areas of great potential conflict between public health and liberal policy. For many political theorists, the liberty of the free adult to bargain in the market for labour without state intervention to limit hours or kinds of work was axiomatic. And the need for food was to be the spur for work and self-improvement. Interventions by a 'nanny state' seemed to imply an obligation to the state and to affirm the desirability of dependence and subjugation. There were grounds for such concern: the relations of political status to health were fraught with ambiguity. Frank had written passionately of misery as a cause of disease amongst the serfs of Austrian Italy, but had not advocated the elimination of serfdom. Virchow argued, in 1848, that liberal political rights were the answer to typhus in Silesia, while in Scotland, W.P. Alison argued the contrary, that too rigorous a liberal regime was the cause of poverty-induced typhus (Frank 1941; Rosen 1947; Weindling 1984; Hamlin 2006).

For about a generation, from 1850–1880, sanitation was unchallenged in Britain as the keystone of improved health. Chadwick's campaigns led to a series of legislative acts—beginning with the Public Health Act of 1848 and culminating with a comprehensive act in 1875—that established state standards for urban sanitation and a bureau of state medicine, staffed by medical officers in central and local units of government and charged with detecting, responding to, and preventing outbreaks of disease (Wohl 1983).

Outside Britain, although the ideals of sanitation might have had similar appeal, they did not warrant the same conclusions about state responsibility or sanitary technology. The English paradigm of a water-centred sanitary system was adopted only in the twentieth century (Simson 1978; Göckjan 1985; Goubert 1989; Labisch 1992; Münch 1993; Ramsey 1994; Melosi 2000; Hennock 2000). Often, the heritage of medical police was more prominent than that of sanitary engineering. Networks of local medical officers to control contagious disease transmission through the regulation of travel and prostitution were important.

Through the 1880s, the United States remained an exceptional case, coming closest to following a policy that an individual's health was a private matter alone. The national government maintained a system of marine hospitals along the coasts and navigable rivers, less for controlling the spread of epidemics than for relieving ports of the burden of caring for sick seamen. In the early 1880s, it established a National Board of Health to advance knowledge on key public health issues, but it was scrapped within a few years on the grounds that public health was the business of individual states and cities (Duffy 1990). Often dominated by rural interests, many state legislatures had little enthusiasm for public health. Louisiana, which established a state board of health to combat yellow fever, was an exception (Ellis 1992). Towns and cities were more active, but often only sporadically, taking steps when faced with epidemics. States that did establish boards of health usually focused on specific problems rather than on public health in general: in Massachusetts, the allotment of pure water resources was a key issue; elsewhere, it was food quality, care for the insane, vital statistics, or the threat of immigrants (Rosenkrantz 1972; Shattuck 1972; Kraut 1994). In Michigan, concern about kerosene quality (it was being adulterated with volatile and explosive petroleum fractions) and arsenical wallpaper dyes spurred the establishment of a state board of health in 1873 (Duffy 1990).

1880–1970: the golden age of public health?

By the 1880s, the liberalism of the first half of the century was giving way to a resurgent statism. The European nations, the United States, and later, Japan competed for colonies and international influence. If the newly liberated or enfranchised had claims to a right to health, they also had a *duty to the state* to be healthy. In most industrialized nations, there was renewed interest in monitoring social conditions.

Although the emerging techniques of empirical social research gave this inquiry the aura of quantitative precision, the surveys disclosed little that was distinctly new about the lives or health of the poor, the usual targets of public health and social reform. Much of it seemed new, however, because it now registered as problematic (Turner 2001). For example, the enormous contribution of infant deaths to total mortality had long been clear, but only towards the end of the century did persistently high infant mortality become a problem in itself as distinct from a general indicator of sanitary conditions. The health conditions of women and of workers began to command attention in a way that they had not done previously (Sellars 1997).

Although these newly recognized public health problems partly reflected the changing distribution of political power, they also reflected anxiety about the nation's vulnerability, and even the decadence of its population. Worried about the strengths of their armies, states such as Britain discovered in the 1890s that too few of those called up were competent to be mobilized, and this was attributed to causes ranging from poor nutrition (coupled with lack of sunlight in smoky cities), to bad sanitation, mothering, and heredity (Soloway 1982; Pick 1989; Porter 1991a, 1999; Stradling and Thorsheim 1999). Epidemics of smallpox following the Franco-Prussian War of 1870 and again in the 1890s disclosed the gaps in vaccination programmes (Baldwin 1999; Brunton 2008), resulting in states redoubling efforts to take responsibility for the immune status of their population (Brandt 1985; Baldwin 1999).

This led to an expanded public health, one highly successful in terms of reduced mortality and morbidity. It was undertaken jointly in the name of the state and the people, but it involved the regulation of an individual's life—home, work, family relations, recreation, sex—that went beyond the medical police of the previous century. From a later standpoint, such intimate regulation of the individual by the state may seem overbearing, but, with some notable exceptions, the populations of developed countries accepted it as legitimate and even desirable.

New diseases, or old diseases that were more prevalent or virulent, new public health institutions, and advances in medical and social science contributed to this new relation between states and people. During the 1860s, a long-standing analogy of disease with fermentation matured into the germ theory of disease as the research of Louis Pasteur and John Tyndall made clear the dependence of fermentation on some microscopic living ferment (Pelling 1978; Worboys 2000). During the 1880s, primarily through the work of emerging German and French schools of determinative bacteriology, it became possible to distinguish many separate microbe species, to ascertain the presence of particular species with some confidence, and therefore, to link individual species with particular diseases (Bulloch 1938). Through serological tests developed in the succeeding decades, the presence of a prior infection could be determined, regardless of the presence of symptoms.

Notwithstanding the increasing recognition of the many ways by which infectious microbes were transmitted from person to person, the effect of the rise of the germ theory was to focus attention on the body that housed and reproduced the germ—for example, the well-digger working through a mild case of typhoid—even when there were alternative strategies (water filtration or, by the second decade of the twentieth century, chlorination) that protected the public reasonably well most of the time (Hamlin 1990; Melosi 2000). The general interest in the human as germ-bearer and culture medium brought with it an emphasis on labour-intensive case-tracing, of keeping track of those with symptoms of the disease together with those with whom they had contact.

For key diseases like typhoid, syphilis, and tuberculosis, concern with the inspection and regulation of people was exacerbated by the recognition that not all who were infected were symptomatic. The case of 'Typhoid Mary' Mallon, the asymptomatic typhoid carrier who lived for 26 years as an island-bound 'guest' of the City of New York, is notorious, but it was also important in the working out of both legal limits and cultural sensibilities with regard to the trade-off between civil rights and public health (Leavitt 1996). Newly virulent forms of diphtheria and scarlet fever, deadly childhood diseases transmitted person to person or by common domestic media, also gave immediacy to decisive public health intervention.

Such monitoring could not have occurred without a large corpus of local public health officers. It was during the late nineteenth century that public health was identified as a distinct division of medicine and when most developed countries solidified a reasonably complete network of municipal and regional public health officers. Increasingly, these officers worked as part of hierarchical national health establishments to which they reported local health conditions and from which they received expert guidance.

Beginning in the mid 1870s, public doctors started to be specially trained and certified for public health work (Novak 1973; Watkin 1984; Acheson 1991; Porter 1991b). A commitment to public health was increasingly incompatible with ordinary medical practice, not because of its specialized knowledge, but because it was built upon a quite different ethic. There had long been economic tension between public and private medicine in areas of practice such as vaccination, in which public authorities either took over entirely or inadequately compensated private practitioners for services that had traditionally been part of the ordinary medical marketplace (White 1991; Brunton 2008).

But monitoring healthy carriers and those who might be susceptible to disease introduced a new regime of medicine—one which responded to an ethic of public good, even if there were no client-defined complaints. Effectively, bacteriology, epidemiology, and associated measures of immunological status redefined disease away from the patient complaint. The healthy carrier might see no need to seek medical care, but to the public health doctor that person was a social problem. On occasion, private doctors were appealed to for a diagnosis (bronchitis, pneumonia) that would protect one from the health officer's diagnosis of tuberculosis, which would bring loss of employment and social stigma (Smith 1988).

Rivalling the germ theory as the major motif of public health thinking from the 1890s to the 1950s was the application of the emerging science of heredity to the improvement of human populations—the science and practice of eugenics (Paul 1995; Kevles 1995). Whether or not eugenic concerns were the source of the greatest anxiety about the public's health is debatable, but they were the locus of the greatest hope for health progress. Even more than other forms of public health, eugenics exposed a class, and sometimes a racial, division that had long been a part of public health: much public health practice was predicated on a distinction between those, usually the poor, who were seen as the objects of public health efforts and those, often the well-to-do, who

authorized intervention, whether to improve the lot of the poor, to protect 'society', or perhaps even to block the physical or moral contagia that might infect their own class (Kraut 1994; Anderson 1995; Bashford and Hooker 2001; Carlin 2005). Eugenics appealed mainly to those with wealth and power: those others who were to be improved rarely identified heredity as the source of their problems.

Such an attitude is reflected in the most infamous application of the eugenic viewpoint, the attempt by Nazi Germany to exterminate Jews and other 'races' regarded as inferior and unfit to intermarry with so-called 'true Aryans', and even to exist. Although historians' views of the origins of the Holocaust differ, some of the immediate precedents for a state policy of negative eugenics—the prevention of the reproduction of those regarded as unfit—came from the sterilization laws that American states had begun to pass in the first decade of the century. The American laws focused on persistent immorality or criminality, and on what was called 'feeble-mindedness'.

In Germany, the acceptance of sterilization translated rather easily into the acceptance of euthanasia of the permanently institutionalized, and on to the extreme measures of the death camps, which were conceived of as facilities of state medicine. Even during the Holocaust, the prevailing rationality remained that of public health: the trade-off between individual rights and the state's welfare was a part of the working moral world of the public health officer. A campaign against Jews from Eastern Europe had already been rehearsed in typhus control efforts in the preceding generation (Weindling 1999). Just as an excision of cancerous matter might be necessary to maintain the body of the individual, so too an excision of a part of society might be necessary to maintain the health of the nation (Lifton 1986).

The horrors of the extreme version of eugenics practised in Nazi Germany have discredited eugenics to such a degree that it is difficult to recapture how central it seemed to reformers of the left as well as of the far right. It appealed for a number of reasons. First, it explained the failure of prior reforms, particularly sanitation, in effecting the physical and moral renewal of the lower classes.

Second, it seemed to be implied by Darwin's discoveries, which were themselves founded on deep familiarity with the remarkable transformations achieved by scientific agriculturalists in animal breeding. Those discoveries seemed particularly applicable within the utilitarian framework of the new statism: the task of governments was to reverse the trend towards decadence and produce uniform, reliable humans. Such concerns became powerful especially for nations that perceived themselves to be in demographic crisis, such as Sweden, which was experiencing depopulation and persistent tuberculosis, and the United States, where successive groups of immigrants found reasons to deplore the effects on the nation of the next immigrant group (Johannisson 1994; Kraut 1994; Broberg and Roll-Hansen 1996). Finally, it flattered those who held power and prominence by offering a simple explanation of all that was wrong, and a simple remedy for improvement based on an attractive sociological formula: more procreation for those who should breed and less for those regarded as inferior.

Eugenics sanctioned an enormous range of practices. Although eugenists focused attention on the human genotype and the inadequacy of public health programmes that ignored heredity, they were not uniformly dismissive of social and environmental reforms. These were needed to allow the better stock to fulfil its potential and because many believed that nurture *could* affect nature: heredity might be a limiting factor, but significant reforms were needed to fulfil hereditary potential. In almost every country in which eugenics was prominent—the United States, Britain, Japan, Germany, Russia, Brazil, and Argentina—it fitted into a comprehensive concept of social hygiene, albeit one that translated rather easily into racial hygiene (Schneider 1990; Porter 1991a; Stepan 1991; Gallagher 1999).

A third element of this phase of the development of public health was the rise of nutritional science. Although the effects of food on health had broadly been central to Western medicine throughout its history, apart from the linkage between scurvy and a lack of fresh vegetables, malnutrition and famine had remained outside public health. Remarkably, a science of nutrition that discriminated the particular effects of specific foods only began to take shape in the second half of the nineteenth century, chiefly in the new institutes of agricultural science where animal diets were being studied (Carpenter 1994). Most important was the link of several clinically distinct conditions with a deficit in trace substances in the diet. Particularly remarkable were Goldberger's association of pellagra in the American south with a too heavy reliance on maize, and the recognition of the roles of vitamin D and sunlight in the emergence of rickets. By the 1930s, public health included attention to a varied diet with adequate vitamins (Etheridge 1972; Apple 1996; Marks 2003; Kunitz 2007). Diet, like genes, loomed in the public imagination as the cause of all troubles, and a universal source of hope.

Thus, during this golden age of public health, people in the developed world learned to fear three malign entities: the invisible germs of disease, which might come through the most casual contact; the mysterious genes in their gonads; and the peculiar set of trace nutrients that their food might not contain. Their health and survival depended on all these, yet governments could control them only partially; successful control depended on their behaviour. Hence, a significant role of public health was to educate, advise, and admonish. The citizen, particularly the female citizen, was now being asked to uphold a new standard of cleanliness and to clean things that were not visibly dirty with new kinds of disinfectants. It became important to exercise new prudence in choosing a mate and controlling sexuality. A doctor was required to see whether the baby was being properly fed (Apple 1987; Hoy 1995; Tomes 1998).

Ignorance heightened these hygienic demands. It was clear from tuberculin tests, for example, that exposure to tuberculosis was widespread, in some places nearly universal, but far from clear what was required for exposure to evolve into pulmonary consumption: whether it was a matter of concentrated exposure, the victim's own constitution, or the diet and environment. All seemed plausible; the advice of public health authorities (who were concerned with infected cases and with their potential for infecting others) involved every aspect of life. It was not simply a matter of not spitting, but of disinfecting eating utensils, clothes, and bedclothes; transforming relations with a spouse, family, and co-workers; and changing diet, leisure activities, and the climate of dwellings (Newsholme 1935; Dubos and Dubos 1987; Smith 1988; Barnes 1995; Roberts 2009).

Some modern historians have been surprised that these long lists of seemingly exhausting and impossible hygienic expectations, each with no guarantee of health, did not trigger widespread

resentment, victim-blaming, and excessive violations of rights (Armstrong 1983). Four factors are important: first, this was an age stunned by scientific and technical achievement and lacking for the most part a critical vocabulary for mediating expert advice. Second, it was an age of mass aspiration to middle-class standards of living, which were manifested in health, behaviour, and cleanliness. Third, all this was taking place against the backdrop of falling mortality and morbidity, and increasing domestic comfort. Fourth, these efforts were redolent with the ethos of progressive development of the community and the state (Lewis 1986).

The return of liberalism, 1970 to the present day: lifestyle, environment, and welfare

The decades following the Second World War brought a marked shift in the focus of public health and the expectations of the public. In the developed world, the infectious diseases that had so long been the chief focus of public health receded, with effective immunizations, antibiotics, or epidemiological or environmental control (Rogers 1990). With the defeat of fascism and decline of communism, liberalism re-emerged. This was symbolized in the mission statement of the World Health Organization (WHO) that health and welfare were the birthright of all (WHO 1968). It was the obligation of states to deliver that right to their populations, who now, at least in the developed world, were made up of those who saw themselves as individual free agents, diverse perhaps in culture but equal in rights. In such a situation, the conflict between the imperatives of public health and civil rights re-emerged. It remains the most formidable issue that public health faces.

The retreat of infectious disease made clearer the failure of developed nations to grapple with chronic diseases, some of which were the price of longer lifespans (Fox 1993). Some of these could be prevented by changes in behaviour: epidemiological studies in the 1950s and 1960s showed the deadly effects of good living including smoking and a rich diet (Susser 1985; Marks 1997; Porter 1999). A new set of personal disciplines emerged to control lifestyle diseases and prevent accidents—apart from exercise and shedding weight, not smoking, avoiding fats, recreational drugs and alcohol, and using condoms, one was to use seat belts and child harnesses, cope with childproof caps on medicine bottles, and accept a fluoridated water supply. These measures often met with objections because they intruded into personal liberty or on culture, or were irksome or unpleasant.

Post-war, public health concerns also shifted from individual hygiene back to the environment (Hays 1987; Gottlieb 1993). To many, heart diseases and cancers, and other serious conditions such as birth defects and lowered sperm counts, had broader structural causes and could be prevented only by comprehensive changes in the physical and social environment (Epstein 1979; McNeill 2000). Thus, part of the liberal resistance to public health impositions was the argument that a focus on disciplining lifestyles detracted from attention to grander and more serious political issues (Tesh 1987; Turshen 1987; Levins and Lopez 1999).

While this new environmentalism harked back to nineteenth-century views of public health as environmental improvement, there were greater differences. The fear of insidious invisible radiation or toxic chemicals in consumer products mirrors the terror of germs or of invisible odourless miasmas; however, the blame was quite differently directed. The new problems of environmental public health were those in which individuals were victimized by corporate oligopolies and by the governments they influence.

Although Chadwick and his associates had warned of vested interests, such as those that perpetuated slum housing, nineteenth-century environmental health problems had a communal character that was missing from the twentieth. Everyone in a nineteenth-century town produced excrement, smoke, ash, and rubbish; the great problem was to find within the community the will and means to act collectively (Wohl 1977; Kearns 1988). Few in a twentieth-century community produced radiation or toxic chemical waste, and the reasons why nothing was done about these seemed clear. Public health had failed in its police function; an institution that had evolved to stop the selling of spoiled food by the individual grocer or restaurateur could not cope with the vast industry that sold goods whose harmful effects were less obvious and slower to appear but which might be much more widely distributed. Concern about the health effects of global climate change epitomized the problem: the scale and seriousness of the problem and attendant health problems often seem disproportionate to the heritage of environmental policing.

The growing gulf between potentially health-threatening factors and institutional responses has sometimes resulted in a fraught relationship between the people and public health. To the degree that governments were perceived as colluding with the proliferation of health-harming materials, public health institution as government departments were implicated too (Steneck 1984; Brown and Mikkelsen 1990; Edelstein 2004). Even the establishment of new departments of environmental protection to apply new expertise to environmental health problems, did not fundamentally alter the climate of distrust. Public health again became a matter for grassroots political agitation with the emergence of neo-populist Green parties, which gave prominent attention to health as part of environmental good. Public participation became increasingly important (Jasanoff 2005) as victims were not confident that the government would even recognize their disease unless a community of sufferers took it upon themselves to agitate for attention (Packard et al. 2004).

This focus on bad environmental policy even informed the response to AIDS and other infectious diseases like Ebola fever that appeared in the 1980s. Although it became clear that these diseases could be largely controlled through traditional approaches such as changes in personal behaviour and isolation or restriction of the activities of victims, it did not deflect demand for a vaccine, and investments to find a cure. These infections could be seen as diseases caused by environmental changes that allowed animal viruses to acquire secondary human hosts for whom they were highly virulent. Chief among these changes was the unwise exploitation of tropical forests by industries that put profit ahead of prudence (Garrett 1995).

Even lifestyle-related diseases could be attributed to the broader social environment. People smoked, drank, used drugs, ate too much or vastly too little, practised unsafe sex, spent hours immobilized before televisions absorbing images of violence, hit their spouses and children, or shot their co-workers or themselves because they could no longer cope. To expect disciplined personal behaviour from alienated people living in a stressful world was unrealistic, and public health institutions should recognize this.

However, critics were divided on the implications of such an analysis. Some felt the obvious response was to remake society with support structures more consistent with health behaviours it wished to promote. How absurd, for example, for a state to subsidize tobacco production while blaming its own citizens for smoking (Brandt 2006). For others, such a response sounded like an even more invidiously intrusive state. In this 'critical public health' view, the lifestyle agenda was suspicious. It was the public health agenda of an untrustworthy state, not one that its people would have chosen. It was not clear that the personal benefits of delayed or denied gratification were worth it: perhaps one should just enjoy life and rely on the miracles of modern medicine for redemption (Petersen and Lupton 1996).

This view, together with the emergence of cancers and other chronic illnesses for which there was no clear preventive strategy, including age-related debilitating conditions, raised the question of why supportive and curative medical care was not a public health concern or priority. It also highlighted the long-standing question of how far-reaching the health obligations of the liberal state to its citizens should be.

In socialist or social democratic politics, or where the legacy of medical police remained strong, there was often no clear boundary between public health and the public medical care most people demanded and received (Porter 1999). But elsewhere, the recognition that public health was bound up in the larger issue of human welfare, which in turn included the rest of medical care, was problematic. Many of the newly prominent diseases were not infectious; they could be experienced privately without disturbing community or state, hence the reactive and police rationales for public health did not apply. But they did disrupt the fulfilment of human potential, exacted great costs on productivity, increased the strains on publicly or risk-pooled funded health services for the treatment of advanced disease and their complications, and hence could justly take their place among the demands citizens could make of their governments.

In France, Germany, and Russia, public health services had emerged from, and had remained closely linked to, medical services for the poor (Labisch 1992; Ramsey 1994; Solomon 1994). In mid-nineteenth-century England, Edwin Chadwick, notwithstanding his own post as chief administrator of relief to the poor and the existence of a comprehensive national network of poor law medical officers, had deliberately severed public health (which he equated with sanitary engineering and saw as exclusively preventive) from medical care for the poor. Such medical care was second-rate, grudgingly made available because it was seen as a constitutional right. Expectations of effectiveness were low, however: it was hoped that the poor quality of public medical relief would spur the poor to pay for something better. While moderating the focus on sanitary engineering, Chadwick's English successors retained a distinction between public health medicine and social welfare, which seemed to them only marginally medical (Hamlin 1998). At the end of the nineteenth century, the Fabian socialists presented British parliament with a much expanded scheme of prevention, but which placed even greater impositions on personal and social behaviour in exchange for more guarantees from the state. The liberals, whose view prevailed, offered instead an insurance plan to pay for the medical care needed by stricken working men (Fox 1986; Eyler 1997). It was a policy acceptable to the rank and file of the medical profession and that retained and reinforced the split between public health and clinical medicine.

Subsequent efforts to expand state responsibility for health into matters of care and cure have generally worked when medical professions have seen them as advantageous (Starr 1982; Fox 1986; Levins and Lopez 1999; Epstein 2003). However, the kinds of objections that were made to Webb's scheme still arise: however laudable prevention as a goal, ironically, as we have seen with the concerns about lifestyles and the environment, the strategies and priorities of the preventive public health of the last two centuries have not always been those most desired by the masses of people. To many it has seemed that if the state was going to discipline behaviour for its own purposes, those who suffered that imposition deserved compensation for their trouble when things still went wrong.

Such logic was clearest in compensating war veterans. It underpinned the post-war establishment of Britain's National Health Service, which would provide 'health for heroes' and sustains the Veterans Administration medical system in the United States. Thus, what some have complained of as an unrealistic demand for risk-free living, in which people demand a political right to complete freedom of action without accepting responsibility for the consequences, may be better understood as a concern about the fairness of the basic social contract of modern societies.

In many respects, the political problem of the relationship between public health institutions and the citizenry for whom they claim to act, is the greatest challenge currently facing public health in the developed world—though it is an important issue elsewhere too. In the past decade, led by WHO, there has been much interest in an integrated approach to 'social determinants of health' and in particular to the impact of real or perceived social inequalities (Cook et al. 2009; Wilkinson and Marmot 2006; Wellcome Institution 2010). But the discoveries of increasingly sophisticated epidemiology do not quickly translate into political will or effective policy. Many diseases as well as poor health more generally result from many causes operating on many levels. Accordingly, there are numerous points where defensible preventive measures might be taken. But, almost all of them are likely to intrude on what are seen as rights or interests, and questions of fairness. Epidemiology therefore requires significant supplementation from a moral and political philosophy that must be acceptable to an increasingly diverse community. Without such a foundation, public health is forced to take refuge in science that is frequently challenged; but simultaneously, it is not clear whether the professional and educational institutions of public health, or the legal, political, and administrative structures that create and maintain it, will be able to initiate and implement a satisfactory approach to how these conflicting rights are to be adjudicated.

References

Acheson, R. (1991). The British diploma in public health: birth and adolescence. In E. Fee and R. Acheson (eds.) *A History of Education in Public Health: Health that Mocks the Doctors' Rules*, pp. 44–82. Oxford: Oxford University Press.

Ackerknecht, E. (1967). *Medicine at the Paris Hospital, 1794–1848*. Baltimore, MD: Johns Hopkins University Press.

Amundsen, D. and Ferngren, G. (1986). The early Christian tradition. In R. Numbers and D. Amundusen (eds.) *Caring and Curing: Health and Medicine in the Western Religious Traditions*, pp. 40–64. New York: Macmillan.

Anderson, W. (1995). Excremental colonialism: public health and the poetics of pollution. *Critical Inquiry*, 21, 640–69.

Apple, R. (1987). *Mothers and Medicine: A Social History of Infant Feeding, 1890–1950*. Madison, WI: University of Wisconsin Press.

Apple, R.D. (1996). *Vitamania: Vitamins in American Culture*. New Brunswick, NJ: Rutgers University Press.

Armstrong, D. (1983). *The Political Economy of the Body*. Cambridge: Cambridge University Press.

Arrizabalaga, J. (1993). Syphilis. In K. Kiple (ed.) *Cambridge World History of Human Disease*, pp. 1025–33. Cambridge: Cambridge University Press.

Arrizabalaga, J., Henderson, J., French, R. et al. (1997). *The Great Pox: The French Disease in Renaissance Europe*. New Haven, CT: Yale University Press.

Baldwin, P. (1999). *Contagion and the State in Europe, 1830–1930*. New York: Cambridge University Press.

Barnes, D. (1995). *The Making of a Social Disease: Tuberculosis in Nineteenth-Century France*. Berkeley, CA: University of California Press.

Barnes, D. (2006). *The Great Stink of Paris and the Nineteenth-Century Struggle Against Filth and Germs*. Baltimore, MD: Johns Hopkins University Press.

Bashford, A. and Hooker, C. (eds.) (2001). *Contagion: Historical and Cultural Studies*. London: Routledge.

Benedictow, O. (2010). *What Disease was Plague?: On the Controversy Over the Microbiological Identity of Plague Epidemics of the Past*. Leiden: Brill.

Blackstone, W. (1892). *Commentaries on the Laws of England*. New York: Strouse.

Boccaccio, G. (1955). *The Decameron*. London: Dutton.

Brand, J.L. (1965). *Doctors and the State: The British Medical Profession and Government Action in Public Health, 1870–1912*. Baltimore, MD: Johns Hopkins University Press.

Brandt, A. (1985). *No Magic Bullet: A Social History of Venereal Disease in the United States since 1880*. New York: Oxford University Press.

Brandt, A. (2006). *The Cigarette Century: The Rise, Fall and Deadly Persistence of the Product that Defined America*. New York: Basic Books.

Briggs, A. (1961). Cholera and society in the nineteenth century. *Past and Present*, 19, 76–96.

Broberg, G. and Roll-Hansen, N. (eds.) (1996). *Eugenics and the Welfare State: Sterilization Policy in Denmark, Sweden, Norway and Finland*. East Lansing, MI: Michigan State University Press.

Brockliss, L. and Jones, C. (1997). *The Medical World of Early Modern France*. Oxford: Clarendon Press.

Brody, S. (1974). *The Disease of the Soul: Leprosy in Medieval Literature*. Ithaca, NY: Cornell University Press.

Brown, P. and Mikkelsen, E. (1990). *No Safe Place: Toxic Waste, Leukemia, and Community Action*. Berkeley, CA: University of California Press.

Browne, T. (1964). Religio medici. In L.C. Martin (ed.) *Religio Medici and Other Works*, pp. 1–80. Oxford: Clarendon Press.

Brunton, D. (2008). *Political Medicine: The Construction of Vaccination Policy Across Britain, 1800–1871*. Rochester, NY: University of Rochester Press.

Bulloch, W. (1938). *The History of Bacteriology*. New York: Oxford University Press.

Bynum, W.F. (1994). *Science and the Practice of Medicine in the Nineteenth Century*. Cambridge: Cambridge University Press.

Carlin, C. (ed.) (2005). *Imagining Contagion in Early Modern Europe*. New York: Macmillan Palgrave.

Carmichael, A. (1986). *Plague and the Poor in Renaissance Florence*. Cambridge: Cambridge University Press.

Carmichael, A. (1993). Plague of Athens. In K. Kiple (ed.) *Cambridge World History of Human Disease*, pp. 934–7. Cambridge: Cambridge University Press.

Carmichael, A. (1997). Leprosy: larger than life. In K. Kiple (ed.) *Plague, Pox, and Pestilence*, pp. 50–7. New York: Barnes and Noble.

Carpenter, K. (1994). *Protein and Energy: A Study of Changing Ideas in Nutrition*. Cambridge: Cambridge University Press.

Carroll, P. (2002). Medical police and the history of public health. *Medical History*, 46, 461–4.

Cassedy, J. (1962). *Charles V: Chapin and the Public Health Movement*. Cambridge, MA: Harvard University Press.

Chadwick, E. (1965). *Report on the Sanitary Condition of the Labouring Population of Great Britain*. Edinburgh: Edinburgh University Press.

Chew, H. and Kellaway, W.E. (eds.) (1973). *London Assize of Nuisance, 1301–1431: A Calendar*. London: London Record Society.

Cipolla, C. (1979). *Faith, Reason, and the Plague in Seventeenth Century Tuscany*. New York: Norton.

Cipolla, C. (1981). *Fighting the Plague in Seventeenth-Century Italy*. Madison, WI: University of Wisconsin Press.

Cipolla, C. (1992). *Miasmas and Disease: Public Health and the Environment in the Pre-Industrial Age* (E. Potter, trans.). New Haven, CT: Yale University Press.

Clendening, L. (1942). *Source Book of Medical History*. New York: Dover Publications.

Cohn, S.K. (2010). *Cultures of Plague Medical Thinking at the End of the Renaissance*. Oxford: Oxford University Press.

Coleman, W. (1974). Health and hygiene in the *Encyclopedie*: a medical doctrine for the bourgeoisie. *Journal of the History of Medicine*, 29, 399–421.

Coleman, W. (1982). *Death is a Social Disease: Public Health and Political Economy in Early Industrial France*. Madison, WI: University of Wisconsin Press.

Conrad, L. (1992). Epidemic disease in formal and popular thought in early Islamic society. In T. Ranger and P. Slack (eds.) *Epidemics and Ideas: Essays on the Historical Perception of Pestilence*, pp. 77–99. Cambridge: Cambridge University Press.

Cook, H.J., Bhattacharya, S., and Hardy, A. (2009). *History of the Social Determinants of Health: Global Histories, Contemporary Debates*. Hyderabad: Orient BlackSwan.

Crosby, A. (1986). *Ecological Imperialism: The Biological Expansion of Europe, 900–1900*. Cambridge: Cambridge University Press.

Dean, M. (1991). *The Constitution of Poverty: Toward a Genealogy of Liberal Governance*. London: Routledge.

Delaporte, F. (1986). *Disease and Civilization: The Cholera in Paris, 1832*. Cambridge, MA: MIT Press.

Desrosières, A. (1998). *The Politics of Large Numbers: A History of Statistical Reasoning* (C. Naish, trans.). Cambridge, MA: Harvard University Press.

Dols, M. (1977). *The Black Death in the Middle East*. Princeton, NJ: Princeton University Press.

Dorff, E. (1986). The Jewish tradition. In R. Numbers and D. Amundusen (eds.) *Caring and Curing: Health and Medicine in the Western Religious Traditions*, pp. 5–39. New York: Macmillan.

Douglas, M. (1966). *Purity and Danger: An Analysis of the Concepts of Pollution and Taboo*. London: Routledge.

Dubos, R. and Dubos, J. (1987). *The White Plague: Tuberculosis, Man and Society*. New Brunswick, NJ: Rutgers University Press.

Duffy, J. (1990). *The Sanitarians: A History of American Public Health*. Urbana, IL: University of Illinois Press.

Durbach, N. (2005). *Bodily Matters: The Anti-Vaccination Movement in England, 1853–1907*. Durham, NC: Duke University Press.

Durey, M. (1979). *The Return of the Plague: British Society and Cholera, 1831–32*. Dublin: Gill and MacMillan.

Edelstein, M. (2004). *Contaminated Communities: Social and Psychological Impacts of Residential Toxic Exposure* (2nd ed.). Boulder, CO: Westview.

Ellis, J.H. (1992). *Yellow Fever and Public Health in the New South*. Lexington, KY: University Press of Kentucky.

Epstein, S. (1979). *The Politics of Cancer* (Rev. ed.). New York: Anchor.

Epstein, R. (2003). Let the shoemaker stick to his last: a defense of the 'old' public health. *Perspectives in Biology and Medicine*, 46, s138–59.

Etheridge, E. (1972). *The Butterfly Caste: A Social History of Pellagra in the South*. Westport, CT: Greenwood Press.

Evans, R.J. (1990). *Death in Hamburg: Society and Politics in the Cholera Years, 1830–1910*. London: Penguin Books.

Eyler, J.M. (1979). *Victorian Social Medicine: The Ideas and Methods of William Farr*. Baltimore, MD: Johns Hopkins University Press.

Eyler, J. (1997). *Sir Arthur Newsholme and State Medicine, 1885–1935*. Cambridge: Cambridge University Press.

Fee, E. (1993). Public health, past and present: a shared social vision. In G. Rosen (ed.) *A History of Public Health* (Expanded ed.), pp. ix–lxvii. Baltimore, MD: Johns Hopkins University Press.

Finer, S.E. (1952). *The Life and Times of Sir Edwin Chadwick*. London: Methuen.

Foucault, M. (1975). *The Birth of the Clinic*. New York: Vintage.

Fox, D. (1986). *Health Policies, Health Politics: British and American Experience, 1911–1965*. Princeton, NJ: Princeton University Press.

Fox, D. (1993). *Power and Illness: The Failure and Future of American Health Policy*. Berkeley, CA: University of California Press.

Frank, J.P. (1941). Academic address on the people's misery. *Bulletin of the History of Medicine*, 9, 88–100.

Frank, J.P. (1976). *A System of Complete Medical Police; Selections from Johann Peter Frank*. Baltimore, MD: Johns Hopkins University Press.

Gallagher, N. (1999). *Breeding Better Vermonters*. Hanover, NH: University Press of New England.

Garrett, L. (1995). *The Coming Plague: Newly Emerging Diseases in a World Out of Balance*. New York: Penguin.

Geary, L. (2004). *Medicine and Charity in Ireland, 1718–1851*. Dublin: University College Dublin Press.

Göckjan, G. (1985). *Kurieren und Staat Machen: Gesundheit und Medizin in der burgerlichen Welt*. Frankfurt am Main: Suhrkamp.

Gori, L. (2002). Arabic treatises on environmental pollution up to the end of the thirteenth century. *Environment and History*, 8, 475–88.

Gottlieb, R. (1993). *Forcing the Spring: The Transformation of the American Environmental Movement*. Washington, DC: Island Press.

Goubert, J.P. (1989). *The Conquest of Water* (A. Wilson, trans.). London: Polity Press.

Guillerme, A. (1988). *The Age of Water: the Urban Environment in the North of France, AD 300–1800*. College Station, TX: Texas A & M University Press.

Hamlin, C. (1988). Muddling in bumbledom: local governments and large sanitary improvements: the cases of four British towns, 1855–1885. *Victorian Studies*, 32, 55–83.

Hamlin, C. (1990). *A Science of Impurity: Water Analysis in Nineteenth Century Britain*. Berkeley, CA: Adam Hilger/University of California Press.

Hamlin, C. (1998). *Public Health and Social Justice in the Age of Chadwick: Britain 1800–1854*. Cambridge: Cambridge University Press.

Hamlin, C. (2002). Public sphere to public health: the transformation of 'nuisance'. In S. Sturdy (ed.) *Medicine, Health, and the Public Sphere in Britain, 1600–2000*, pp. 190–204. London: Routledge.

Hamlin, C. (2005). Sanitary policing and the local state, 1873–74: a statistical study of English and Welsh towns. *Social History of Medicine*, 18, 39–61.

Hamlin, C. (2006). William Pulteney Alison, the Scottish philosophy, and the making of a political medicine. *Journal of the History of Medicine and Allied Sciences*, 61, 547–66.

Hamlin, C. (2009). *Cholera: The Biography*. Oxford: Oxford University Press.

Hamlin, C. (2011). Environment and disease in Ireland. In V. Berridge and M. Gorsky (eds.) *Environment, Health, and History*, pp. 45–68. New York: Palgrave Macmillan.

Haskell, T. (1985). Capitalism and the origins of the humanitarian sensibility. *American Historical Review*, 90, 339–61.

Hays, S. (1987). *Beauty, Health, and Permanence: Environmental Politics in the United States, 1955–1985*. Cambridge: Cambridge University Press.

Hennock, E.P. (2000). The urban sanitary movement in England and Germany, 1838–1914: a comparison. *Continuity and Change*, 15, 269–96.

Hope, V. and Marshall, E. (eds.) (2000). *Death and Disease in the Ancient City*. London: Routledge.

Hopkins, D. (2002). *Princes and Peasants: Smallpox in History* (New ed.). Chicago, IL: University of Chicago Press.

Hoy, S. (1995). *Chasing Dirt: The American Pursuit of Cleanliness*. New York: Oxford University Press.

Humphreys, M. (1992). *Yellow Fever and the South*. New Brunswick, NJ: Rutgers University Press.

Ibn Riḍwān (1984). Medieval Islamic medicine: Ibn Riḍwān's treatise, 'On the Prevention of Bodily Ills in Egypt'. In M. Dols and J. Sulaymān (eds. and trans.), *Comparative Studies of Health Systems and Medical Care*, pp. 54–66. Berkeley, CA: University of California Press.

Jasanoff, S. (2005). *Designs on Nature: Science and Democracy in Europe and the United States*. Princeton, NJ: Princeton University Press.

Johannisson, K. (1994). The people's health: public health policies in Sweden. In D. Porter (ed.) *The History of Public Health and the Modern State*, pp. 165–82. Amsterdam: Rudopi.

Karmi, G. (1981). State control of the physician in the Middle Ages: an Islamic model. In A. Russell (ed.) *The Town and State Physician in Europe from the Middle Ages to the Enlightenment*, pp. 63–84. Wolfenbüttel: Herzog August Bibliothek.

Kearns, G. (1988). Private property and public health reform in England, 1830–1870. *Social Science & Medicine*, 26, 187–99.

Kearns, G. (1991). Cholera, nuisances, environmental management in Islington, 1830–1855. In W.F. Bynum and R. Porter (eds.) *Living and Dying in London*, pp. 94–125. London: Wellcome Institute for the History of Medicine.

Kevles, D. (1995). *In the Name of Eugenics: Genetics and the Uses of Human Heredity*. Cambridge, MA: Harvard University Press.

Kinzelbach, A. (2006). Infection, contagion, and public health in late Medieval and early modern German imperial towns. *Journal of the History of Medicine*, 61, 369–89.

Kraut, A. (1994). *Silent Travelers: Germs, Genes, and the 'Immigrant Menace'*. New York: Basic Books.

Kunitz, S. (2007). *The Health of Populations: General Theories and Particular Realities*. New York: Oxford University Press.

LaBerge, A. (1992). *Mission and Method: The Early-Nineteenth-Century French Public Health Movement*. Cambridge : Cambridge University Press.

Labisch, A. (1992). *Homo hygienicus: Gesundheit und Medizin in der Neuzeit*. New York: Campus.

Lambert, R. (1965). *Sir John Simon and English Social Administration*. London: McGibbon and Kee.

Leavitt, J. (1996). *Typhoid Mary: Captive to the Public's Health*. Boston, MA: Beacon Press.

Leongard, J. (ed.) (1989). *London Viewers and Their Certificates, 1508–1558: Certificates of the Sworn Viewers of the City of London*. London: London Record Society.

Levins, R. and Lopez, C. (1999). Toward an ecosocial view of health. *International Journal of Health Services*, 29, 261–93.

Lewis, J. (1986). *What Price Community Medicine? The Philosophy, Practice, and Politics of Public Health Since 1919*. Brighton: Wheatsheaf Books.

Lewis, R.A. (1952). *Edwin Chadwick and the Public Health Movement, 1832–1854*. London: Longmans Green.

Lieber, E. (2000). Old Testament 'leprosy', contagion and sin. In L.I. Conrad and K. Wujastyk (eds.) *Contagion: Perspectives From Pre-Modern Societies*, pp. 99–136. Aldershot: Ashgate.

Lifton, R. (1986). *The Nazi Doctors: Medical Killing and the Psychology of Genocide*. New York: Basic Books.

Longrig, J. (1992). Epidemic, ideas and classical Athenian society. In T. Ranger and P. Slack (eds.) *Epidemics and Ideas: Essays on the Historical Perception of Pestilence*, pp. 21–44. Cambridge: Cambridge University Press.

López-Piñero, J.M. (1981). The medical profession in sixteenth-century Spain. In A. Russell (ed.) *The Town and State Physician in Europe from the Middle Ages to the Enlightenment*, pp. 85–98. Wolfenbüttel: Herzog August Bibliothek.

MacMahon, B. and Pugh, T. (1970). *Epidemiology: Principles and Methods*. Boston, MA: Little, Brown.

Magnello, E. (2002). The introduction of mathematical statistics into medical research: the roles of Karl Pearson, Major Greenwood, and Austin Bradford Hill. In E. Magnello and A. Hardy (eds.) *The Road to Medical Statistics*, pp. 95–123. Amsterdam: Rodopi.

Marks, H. (1997). *The Progress of Experiment: Science and Therapeutic Reforming the United States, 1900–1990*. Cambridge: Cambridge University Press.

Marks, H. (2003). Epidemiologists explain pellagra: gender, race, and political economy in the work of Edgar Sydenstricker. *Journal of the History of Medicine and Allied Sciences*, 58, 34–55.

McClure, R. (1981). *Coram's Children: The London Foundling Hospital in the Eighteenth Century*. New Haven, CT: Yale University Press.

McGrew, R. (1965). *Russia and the Cholera, 1823–1832*. Madison, WI: University of Wisconsin Press.

McHugh, P. (1982). *Prostitution and Victorian Social Reform*. London: Croom Helm.

McNeill, J.R. (2000). *An Environmental History of the Twentieth-Century World*. New York: Norton.

Melosi, M. (2000). *The Sanitary City: Urban Infrastructure in America from Colonial Times to the Present*. Baltimore, MD: Johns Hopkins University Press.

Miller, G. (1957). *The Adoption of Inoculation for Smallpox in England and France*. Philadelphia, PA: University of Pennsylvania Press.

Münch, P. (1993). *Stadthygiene im 19 und 20 Jahrhundert*. Göttingen: Vandenhoeck und Ruprecht.

Newsholme, A. (1935). *Fifty Years in Public Health: A Personal Narrative with Comments. Volume 1: The Years Preceding 1909*. London: George Allen and Unwin.

Nohl, J. (1926). *The Black Death*. London: George Allen and Unwin.

Novak, S.J. (1973). Professionalism and bureaucracy: English doctors and the Victorian public health administration. *Journal of Social History*, 6, 440–62.

Novak, W.J. (1996). *The People's Welfare: Law and Regulation in Nineteenth-Century America*. Chapel Hill, NC: University of North Carolina Press.

Nutton, V. (2000). Did the Greeks have a name for it? Contagion and contagion theory in classical antiquity. In L.I. Conrad and K. Wujastyk (eds.) *Contagion: Perspectives From Pre-Modern Societies*, pp. 137–62. Aldershot: Ashgate.

Nutton, V. (ed.) (2008). *Pestilential Complexities: Understanding Medieval Plague*. London: Wellcome Trust Centre for the History of Medicine at UCL.

Packard, R.M., Brown, P.J., Berkelman, R.L., and H. Frumkin (2004). Introduction: emerging illnesses as social process. In R.M. Packard, P.J. Brown, R.L. Berkelman, and H. Frumkin (eds.) *Emerging Illnesses and Society: Negotiating the Agenda of Public Health*, pp. 1–36. Baltimore, MD: Johns Hopkins University Press.

Palmer, R. (1981). Physicians and the state in post-medieval Italy. In A. Russell (ed.) *The Town and State Physician in Europe from the Middle Ages to the Enlightenment*, pp. 47–62. Wolfenbüttel: Herzog August Bibliothek.

Paul, D.B. (1995). *Controlling Human Heredity: 1865 to the Present*. Atlantic Highlands, NJ: Humanities Press.

Pelling, M. (1978). *Cholera, Fever, and English Medicine, 1825–1865*. Oxford: Oxford University Press.

Pelling, M. (2001). The meaning of contagion: reproduction, medicine and metaphor. In A. Bashford and C. Hooker (eds.) *Contagion: Historical and Cultural Studies*, pp. 15–38. London: Routledge.

Petersen, A. and Lupton, D. (1996). *The New Public Health: Health and Self in the Age of Risk*. London: Sage.

Pettenkofer, M. (1941). *The Value of Health to a City* [translation, with an introduction by H.E. Sigerist]. Baltimore, MD: Johns Hopkins University Press.

Pick, D. (1989). *Faces of Degeneration: a European Disorder, c. 1848–1918*. Cambridge: Cambridge University Press.

Porter, D. (1991a). 'Enemies of the race': biologism, environmentalism, and public health in Edwardian England. *Victorian Studies*, 34, 159–78.

Porter, D. (1991b). Stratification and its discontents: professionalization and conflict in the British public health service, 1848–1914. In E. Fee and R Acheson (eds.) *A History of Education in Public Health: Health that Mocks the Doctor's Rules*, pp. 83–113. Oxford: Oxford University Press.

Porter, D. (1999). *Health, Civilization and the State*. London: Routledge.

Porter, D. and Porter, R. (1988). The politics of prevention: anti-vaccinationism and public health in nineteenth century England. *Medical History*, 32, 231–52.

Ramsey, M. (1994). Public health in France. In D. Porter (ed.) *The History of Public Health and the Modern State*, pp. 45–118. Amsterdam: Rudopi.

Razzell, P. (1977). *The Conquest of Smallpox: The Impact of Inoculation on Smallpox Mortality in Eighteenth Century England*. Firle: Caliban.

Redlich J. and Hirst F. (1970). *The History of Local Government in England* [reissue of Book I of *Local Government in England*] (2nd ed.). New York: Augustus Kelley.

Richards, P. (1977). *The Medieval Leper and his Northern Heirs*. Totowa, NJ: Rowman and Littlefield.

Richards, P. (1980). State formation and class struggle. In P. Corrigan (ed.) *Capitalism, State Formation, and Marxist Theory*, pp. 49–78. London: Quartet.

Richardson, R. (1988). *Death, Dissection, and the Destitute*. London: Penguin.

Riley, J.C. (1987). *The Eighteenth Century Campaign to Avoid Disease*. London: Macmillan.

Roberton, J. (1827). *Observations on the Mortality and Physical Management of Children*. London: Longman, Rees, Orme, Brown.

Roberts, S. (2009). *Infectious Fear: Politics, Disease, and the Health Effects of Segregation*. Chapel Hill, NC: University of North Carolina Press.

Rogers, N. (1990). *Dirt and Disease: Polio before FDR*. New Brunswick, NJ: Rutgers University Press.

Rosen, G. (1947). What is social medicine: a genetic analysis of the concept. *Bulletin of the History of Medicine*, 21, 674–733.

Rosen, G. (1958). *A History of Public Health*. New York: MD Publications.

Rosen, G. (1974). Cameralism and the concept of medical police. In G. Rosen (ed) *From Medical Police to Social Medicine: Essays on the History of Health Care*, pp. 120–41. New York: Science History.

Rosen, G. (2008). 'The fate of the concept of medical police, 1780–1890,' with commentaries by Christopher Hamlin and Michael Knipper. *Centaurus*, 50, 45–72.

Rosenberg, C. (1962). *The Cholera Years: the United States in 1832, 1849, and 1866*. Chicago, IL: University of Chicago Press.

Rosenkrantz, B. (1972). *Public Health and the State: Changing Views in Massachusetts, 1842–1936*. Cambridge, MA: Harvard University Press.

Rosenkrantz, B.G. (1974). Cart before horse: theory, practice and professional image in American public health, 1870–1920. *Journal of the History of Medicine*, 29, 55–73.

Sadler, M. (1830). *The Law of Population. A treatise in six books, in disproof of the superfecundity of human beings, and developing the real principle of their increase*. London: John Murray.

Schneider, W.H. (1990). *Quality and Quantity: The Quest for Biological Regeneration in 20th Century France*. Cambridge: Cambridge University Press.

Sellars, C. (1997). *Hazards of the Job: from Industrial Disease to Environmental Health science*. Chapel Hill, NC: University of North Carolina Press.

Shattuck, L. (1972). *Report of a General Plan for the Promotion of Public and Personal Health, Devised, Prepared, and Recommended by the Commissioners. . . Relating to a Sanitary Survey of the State*. New York: Arno.

Simon, J. (1890). *English Sanitary Institutions, Reviewed in their Course of Development, and in Some of Their Political and Social Relations*. London: Cassell.

Simson, J.V. (1978). Die Flussverungsreinigungsfrage im Jahrhundert. *Vierteljahrschrift für Sozial-und Wirtschaftgeschichte*, 65, 370–90.

Skisnes, O. (1973). Notes from the history of leprosy. *International Journal of Leprosy*, 41, 220–37.

Slack, P. (1985). *The Impact of the Plague in Tudor and Stuart England*. London: Routledge and Kegan Paul.

Smith, D.C. (1981). Medical science, medical practice, and the emerging concept of typhus. In W.F. Bynum and V. Nutton (eds.) *Theories of Fever from Antiquity to the Enlightenment*, pp. 121–34. London: Wellcome Institute for the History of Medicine.

Smith, F.B. (1988). *The Retreat of Tuberculosis, 1850–1950*. London: Croom Helm.

Snowden, F. (1995). *Naples in the Time of Cholera 1884–1911*. Cambridge: Cambridge University Press.

Solomon, S.G. (1994). The expert and the state in Russian public health: continuities and changes across the revolutionary divide. In D. Porter (ed.) *The History of Public Health and the Modern State*, pp. 183–223. Amsterdam: Rudopi.

Soloway, R.A. (1982). *Birth Control and the Population Question in England, 1877–1930*. Chapel Hill, NC: University of North Carolina Press.

Starr, P. (1984). *The Social Transformation of American Medicine*. New York: Basic Books.

Steneck, N. (1984). *The Microwave Debate*. Cambridge, MA: MIT Press.

Stepan, N. (1991). *The Hour of Eugenics: Race, Gender, and Nation in Latin America*. Ithaca, NY: Cornell University Press.

Stradling, D. and Thorsheim, P. (1999). The smoke of great cities: British and American efforts to control air pollution, 1860–1914. *Environmental History*, 4, 6–31.

Sturdy, S. (2002). Introduction: medicine, health, and the public sphere. In S. Sturdy (ed.) *Medicine, Health, and the Public Sphere in Britain, 1600–2000*, pp. 190–204. London: Routledge.

Susser, M. (1985). Epidemiology in the United States after World War II: the evolution of technique. *Epidemiologic Reviews*, 7, 147–77.

Taylor, V. and Trentmann, F. (2005). From users to consumers: water politics in nineteenth-century London. In F. Trentmann (ed.) *The Making of the Consumer: Knowledge, Power and Identity in the Modern World*, pp. 53–79. Oxford: Berg.

Tesh, S.N. (1987). *Hidden Arguments: Political Ideology and Disease Prevention*. New Brunswick, NJ: Rutgers University Press.

Thompson, E.P. (1971). The moral economy of the English crowd in the eighteenth century. *Past and Present*, 50, 76–136.

Thucydides (1950). *The History of the Peloponnesian War* (R. Crawley, trans.). New York: E.P. Dutton.

Tomes, N. (1998). *The Gospel of Germs: Men, Women, and the Microbe in American Life*. Cambridge, MA: Harvard University Press.

Touati, F.-O. (2000). Contagion and leprosy: myth, ideas and evolution in medieval minds and societies. In L.I. Conrad and K. Wujastyk (eds.) *Contagion: Perspectives from Pre-Modern Societies*, pp. 179–201. Aldershot: Ashgate.

Turner, S. (2001). What is the problem with experts? *Social Studies of Science*, 31, 123–49.

Turshen, M. (1987). *The Politics of Public Health*. New Brunswick, NJ: Rutgers University Press.

Veyne, P. (1987). The Roman empire. In P. Veyne (ed.) and A. Goldhammer (trans.) *A History of Private Life. Volume I: From Pagan Rome to Byzantium*, pp. 222–32. Cambridge, MA: Belknap Press of Harvard University Press.

Waddington, K. (2006). *The Bovine Scourge: Meat, Tuberculosis and Public Health, 1850–1914*. Woodbridge: Boydell.

Walkowitz, J. (1980). *Prostitution and Victorian Society: Women, Class and the State*. Cambridge: Cambridge University Press.

Ward J. and Warren, C. (2007). *Silent Victories: The History and Practice of Public Health in Twentieth-Century America*. Oxford: Oxford University Press.

Watkin, D. (1984). *The English revolution in social medicine, 1889–1911*. Unpublished PhD thesis, University of London.

Webb, S. and Webb, B. (1922). *English Local Government from the Revolution to the Municipal Corporations Act: Statutory Authorities for Special Purposes*. London: Longmans Green.

Weindling, P. (1984). Was social medicine revolutionary? Rudolph Virchow and the revolution of 1848. *Bulletin of the Society for the Social History of Medicine*, 34, 13–18.

Weindling, P. (1999). *Epidemics and Genocide in Eastern Europe, 1890–1945*. Oxford; New York: Oxford University Press.

Weiner, D. (1993). *The Citizen-Patient in Revolutionary and Imperial Paris*. Baltimore, MD: Johns Hopkins University Press.

Wellcome Trust (2010). *Social Determinants of Health: Assessing Theory, Policy and Practice*. New Delhi: Orient Blackswan.

Weyland, J. (1968). *The Principles of Population and Production as they are Affected by the Progress of Society with View to Moral and Political Consequences*. New York: Augustus Kelley. (Work originally published in 1816.)

White, K. (1991). *Healing the Schism: Epidemiology, Medicine and the Public's Health*. New York: Springer.

Wilkinson, R. and Marmot, M. (2006). *Social Determinants of Health* (2nd ed.). Oxford: Oxford University Press.

Wilson, F.R. (1881). *A Practical Guide for Inspectors of Nuisances*. London: Knight.

Wilson, L. (1978). Fevers and science in early nineteenth century medicine. *Journal of the History of Medicine*, 33, 386–407.

Winslow, C.A. (1980). *The Conquest of Epidemic Disease: A Chapter in the History of Ideas*. Madison, WI: University of Wisconsin Press. (Work originally published in 1943.)

Wohl, A. (1977). *The Eternal Slum: Housing and Social Policy in Victorian London*. London: Edward Arnold.

Wohl, A.S. (1983). *Endangered Lives: Public Health in Victorian Britain*. Cambridge, MA: Harvard University Press.

Worboys, M. (2000). *Spreading Germs: Disease Theories and Medical Practice in Britain, 1865–1900*. Cambridge: Cambridge University Press.

World Health Organization (1968). *Constitution of the* World Health Organization *in WHO Basic Documents* (19th ed.). Geneva: World Health Organization.

Ziegler, P. (1969). *The Black Death*. New York: Harper Torchbooks.

The history and development of public health in low- and middle-income countries

Than Sein

Introduction to the history and development of public health in low- and middle-income countries

The fundamental public health actions often have to take into account or to address social determinants of health, which fall outside the domain of the health sector and also beyond the individual's action. The socioeconomic, health, and other development status of the world have been changing rapidly and radically in recent decades. Nevertheless, the majority of people in many low- and middle-income countries (LMIC), which make up about 50 per cent of the world's population, are still living in poverty with very low health status. Based on the United Nations (UN) classification of countries by per capita gross national income (GNI), countries which have per capita GNI below US $1005 or less in 2011 are termed low-income countries (32 in total), those which have per capita GNI between US $1006 and $3985 are lower middle-income countries (38 in total), and those between US $3986 and $12,275 as upper middle-income countries (42 in total). Countries with per capita GNI above US $12,276 are categorized as high-income countries (UN 2012).

This chapter addresses the 112 countries which have been classified as the low-, lower middle, and upper middle-income countries, collectively referred to here as LMIC. The population of LMIC (excluding that of Brazil, China, and India) is around 3 billion (which is about half of the world's population), and, thus, the advancement of health in LMIC has a major impact on the health of the world. The present chapter highlights an updated review of the history and development of public health in LMIC, covering key factors and events during the transition period from the twentieth to twenty-first century.

The first section briefly traces public health development in LMIC from the colonial period to the present day, highlighting the importance of environmental promotion, prevention and control of old scourges like smallpox, cholera, plague and yellow fever (YF), and control of vaccine-preventable diseases with ultimate aim for elimination. The epidemiological, technical, political, and financing aspects of prevention and control of selected tropical diseases are highlighted. The emphasis on control of a few priority communicable diseases has often been associated

with less active attention to many other tropical diseases and chronic non-communicable diseases (NCDs). The subsequent section describes how the strengthening of health systems including human resources and health research has helped to shape the overall health development. The next section touches upon the influence of social determinants and health inequity which have led to conceptual changes on social medicine and public health. The last section covers the globalization, prevention, and control of emerging diseases. It ends with future challenges and opportunities for health development in LMIC.

Public health development

In LMIC which were colonial territories during the eighteenth and nineteenth centuries, both public health, including prevention and control of major tropical diseases like smallpox, cholera, plague, YF, etc., and health services for patients remained underdeveloped.

The initial foundations for public health were formally laid down through the intensification of international public health actions including international health diplomacy in the mid 1800s, when the United States and European countries applied protective legislative measures through international conventions. The World Health Organization (WHO) was born in 1946, as the first truly international and inter-governmental agency, whose two main functions were to direct and coordinate international health work, and to cooperate with Member States and partners in international health development.

Environmental health promotion

From the very beginning, the promotion of environmental health including public housing, public water supply, personal hygiene, and sanitation has been recognized as a key element for national public policies, legislative actions, and personal practices for effective health and social development in LMIC. Despite legislative measures supplemented by public health education campaigns, public subsidy support, and private donations, the progress in environmental health in LMIC has not been satisfactory. According to the *World Health Statistics 2012*, the population using improved drinking-water sources[1] in LMIC had increased from 70 per cent in 1990 to 87 per cent by 2010, while the population using improved sanitation[2] in the same group of countries in 2010 was still less than 50 per cent (WHO 2012a). By 2010, about 2.4 billion people around the world, mostly in Asia and Africa, were still lacking access to improved sanitation facilities, mainly due to the low priority given to the sector, inadequate financial resources, lack of sustainable water supply and sanitation services, and poor hygienic behaviours. The situation is exacerbated by inadequate provision of improved water supply and sanitation facilities in public places like wet-markets, movie theatres, schools, hospitals, health centres, and offices. Providing access to low-cost, adequate, and simple improved drinking water sources as well as improved facilities for sanitary disposal of excrement, and promoting sound hygienic behaviours amongst the general population in LMIC, are of critical importance in reducing the burden of communicable diseases (WHO/UNICEF 2012). Given the current economic growth prospects, LMIC have the challenge of getting additional financial support from external agencies, in order to achieve the Millennium Development Goal for environmental improvement.

Control of old scourges

Smallpox, cholera, plague, and yellow fever have been termed as scourges of the last centuries, since these diseases were major cripplers and killers during the eighteenth and nineteenth centuries. While effective prevention and control measures are available, a substantial portion of the world's population, especially in LMIC, has not been able to gain access to these preventative measures such as effective vaccination. As a consequence, mortality and morbidity associated with these infections remain unacceptably high.

The effective control of smallpox in LMIC in the early nineteenth century was hindered by a range of factors such as impurity and variable potency of the vaccine, poor vaccination techniques, low coverage among the general population, lack of commitment by the colonial administrations, insufficient quantities of heat-stable vaccine, and lack of confidence in vaccination amongst the local populace. Consequently, several thousands of people were infected and 30–50 per cent of affected people died. Those who survived were left disfigured by ugly pox-marks and blindness (Ko Ko 2005). With the assurance of adequate supplies of effective freeze-dried, heat-stable smallpox vaccine provided free-of-cost by major vaccine producers (United States and Soviet Russia) and with ample financial support for running the vaccination programmes, the worldwide control of smallpox with an ultimate aim of eradication was launched in 1958. Through mass smallpox vaccination campaigns, several LMIC were able to control smallpox outbreaks and cut the cycle of transmission. They all reported their last smallpox cases within the next 3–4 years. Nonetheless, as recently as 1967, some LMIC in Asia and Africa, especially those with weak health infrastructure, still experienced sporadic outbreaks of smallpox that killed 2–3 million people annually. However, continued global advocacy, and the provision of technical, financial, and human resources support, led to successful containment of the disease within a decade from 1967. A combination of strategies was used such as routine and mopping up mass vaccination, coupled with intensive case-detection, contact tracing, isolation of cases, and vaccination of individuals in the vicinity who could have been exposed to the infection. The last naturally-acquired human smallpox case in the world was reported in Somalia in October 1977. There was a laboratory accident which resulted in two human smallpox cases in the UK in 1978. By May 1980, the world was declared free from natural transmission of smallpox virus (Fenner et al. 1988). Although no further human case from natural infection by smallpox virus has been detected (zero case transmission) to date, a few vaccine-induced smallpox cases occurred in the United States, as recently as in 2010 (Centres for Disease Control and Prevention 2010). An international arrangement was made in 2011 to create an emergency stockpile of over 60 million doses of the first- and second-generation smallpox vaccines in safe and secure places, to be used for the effective control of any smallpox outbreak that might occur (WHO 2011a). The eradication of smallpox in 1980, however, stands out as the most successful public health intervention achieved globally in the twentieth century.

Cholera, one of the most devastating illnesses worldwide for many centuries due to its severity and quick and easy spread across borders, has thus been identified as a globally notifiable disease under the old version of International Health Regulations (IHR). It is still an international threat, since sporadic epidemics still occur in over 50 countries around the world (WHO 2011b). The last big-scale epidemic of cholera occurred in Haiti, in the aftermath of the massive earthquake in January 2010, which affected 230,000 people and caused more than 4500 deaths. Effective vaccines against cholera are still under development, and environmental health and good personal hygienic practices remain the only effective preventative and control measures. Properly administered rehydration therapy can also save thousands of lives who may otherwise die of dehydration and electrolyte imbalances.

Human plague, often regarded as a problem of the past or an ancient disease, resurfaced in the twenty-first century in 16 countries of Africa, Asia, and America, with around 12,500 cases of human plague (three-quarters of whom died). This clearly demonstrates the need for strengthening surveillance on rat falls (deaths of rats around human habitats) as well as human plague cases, improving preventative and control measures, and having early case finding and prompt treatment of human cases in endemic countries. All these require an effective public health and health systems infrastructure (WHO 2010a).

With the availability of an effective vaccine since 1940 together with vector control and the widespread adoption of personal protection measures, YF disease has been virtually wiped out in certain parts of Africa and Americas. As there is no effective specific treatment, immunization is the single most important means of protection against YF. However, due to inadequate health infrastructure and inadequate coverage of YF vaccination, the disease remains endemic in 34 African countries, with sporadic outbreaks occurring almost every year leading to an estimated 180,000 cases (WHO 2003). The ongoing circulation of wild YF virus, coupled with the low vaccination coverage and the presence of the vector mosquitoes around the world, means that YF will remain an important threat for international spread. Millions of lives could easily be lost, unless a substantially enhanced surveillance system and high coverage of YF vaccination in the countries at risk are sustained.

Elimination of vaccine-preventable diseases

With increasing availability and accessibility of improved vaccines for various infectious diseases which affect young children such as poliomyelitis, diphtheria, tetanus, measles, and tuberculosis, LMIC have initiated national immunization programmes, under the aegis of the global Expanded Programme of Immunization (EPI) in mid 1970. The EPI planned to control a few vaccine-preventable diseases with the ultimate aim of eliminating or eradicating them. With support from UN agencies and other development partners, all LMIC implemented the national EPI programme, by targeting universal child immunization (UCI), i.e. fully immunizing at least 80 per cent of all children at 2 years old, with essential vaccines. In reality, the majority of LMIC took more than two decades to improve their UCI coverage to the desired level for elimination of vaccine-preventable diseases. This was mainly due to the lack of human and financial resources to effectively deliver appropriate vaccines. In 2010, 130 countries (the majority from upper and lower middle-income groups) had achieved 90 per cent coverage for three doses of diphtheria–tetanus–pertussis (DTP3), and an estimated 85 per cent of infants worldwide (compared to 74 per cent in 2000) had received at least three doses of DTP vaccine. Despite this overall improvement in vaccination coverage, routine vaccination programmes need to be further strengthened nationally, especially in countries (the majority from least developed nations) with the greatest numbers of unvaccinated children. This situation highlights the need to address issues of limited national and community resources, competing health priorities, poor health systems management, and inadequate monitoring and supervision (Centres for Disease Control and Prevention 2011). Fig. 1.3.1 shows the immunization coverage of major childhood vaccine-preventable diseases by WHO Regions in 2010 (WHO 2011c).

Except for good coverage of BCG vaccination (at over 80 per cent), the coverage of all other vaccines is under 80 per cent in countries in Africa and South East Asia. Despite these challenges, the Global EPI initiative has been considered by many public health professionals as a silent revolution in public health in the late twentieth century.

Poliomyelitis is an acute potentially paralysing vaccine-preventable disease occurring in both tropical and temperate countries. When the initiative for Global Eradication of Poliomyelitis, within the EPI programme, was launched in 1988, many LMIC were faced with intense challenges since these countries had to improve and sustain the high coverage of routine immunization for all vaccines under the EPI programme, while improving their basic health infrastructure. At the start, the wild polio virus was circulating in more than 125 countries in five continents, disabling more than 1000 children every day. With concerted efforts, the average global coverage of polio immunization over two decades reached around 80 per cent, with Africa having the lowest coverage. Fig. 1.3.2 shows the trends for the coverage of poliomyelitis immunization (three doses) for infants by WHO regions, in 1980, and 1990 to 2009.

A campaign for national immunization day(s) (NID) was therefore launched globally in mid 1990, by assigning fixed date(s) of a year as special day(s) for polio immunization. Through NID campaigns in 2003, around 415 million children under 5 years old in the 55 LMIC were immunized with over 2.2 billion doses of oral polio vaccine. In addition, with support of the GAVI Alliance, 14 countries in Africa and Asia which had achieved the polio-free status could stop the spread in 2005 of wild polio virus imported from other countries. By the end of June 2009, infection due to indigenous wild polio virus existed in four countries only. Of the total of 440 new polio cases, ten cases were from Afghanistan, 30 from Pakistan, 89 from India, and 321 from Nigeria. A concerted effort to intensify polio eradication by interrupting transmission of wild polio viruses in all polio endemic countries was made by implementing multiple rounds of NIDs and other supplementary immunization activities, and by limiting the risk of reintroducing wild polio virus into other polio-free areas, especially neighbours. This was achieved through strong political will and support, community involvement, and national and international resources. India had reported no more internal transmission of all wild polio viruses for the whole year of 2011, and it had been removed from

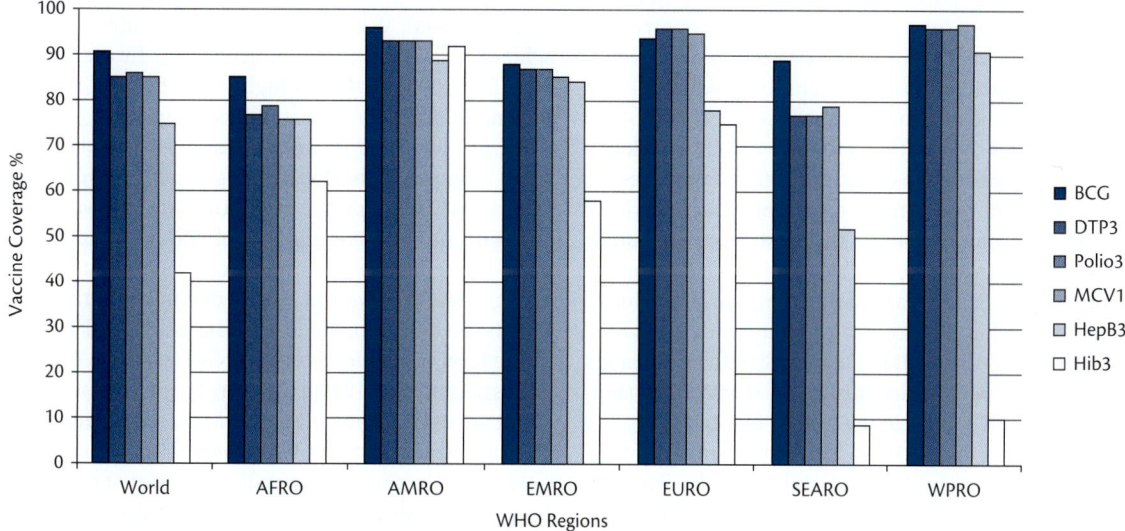

Fig. 1.3.1 Vaccination coverage of major vaccine-preventable diseases by WHO Regions in 2010. Abbreviations: BCG, Bacille Calmette–Guérin; DTP3, three doses of diphtheria–tetanus–pertussis vaccine; Polio3, three doses of polio vaccine; MCV1, one dose of measles-containing vaccine; HepB3, three doses of hepatitis B vaccine; Hib3, three doses of *Haemophilus influenza* type b vaccine.

Source: data from World Health Organization, Global Routine Vaccination Coverage, *Weekly epidemiological record*, Number 46, 2001, 86, pp. 509–20, Copyright © 2011, available from http:// www.who.int/wer/2011/wer8646.pdf.

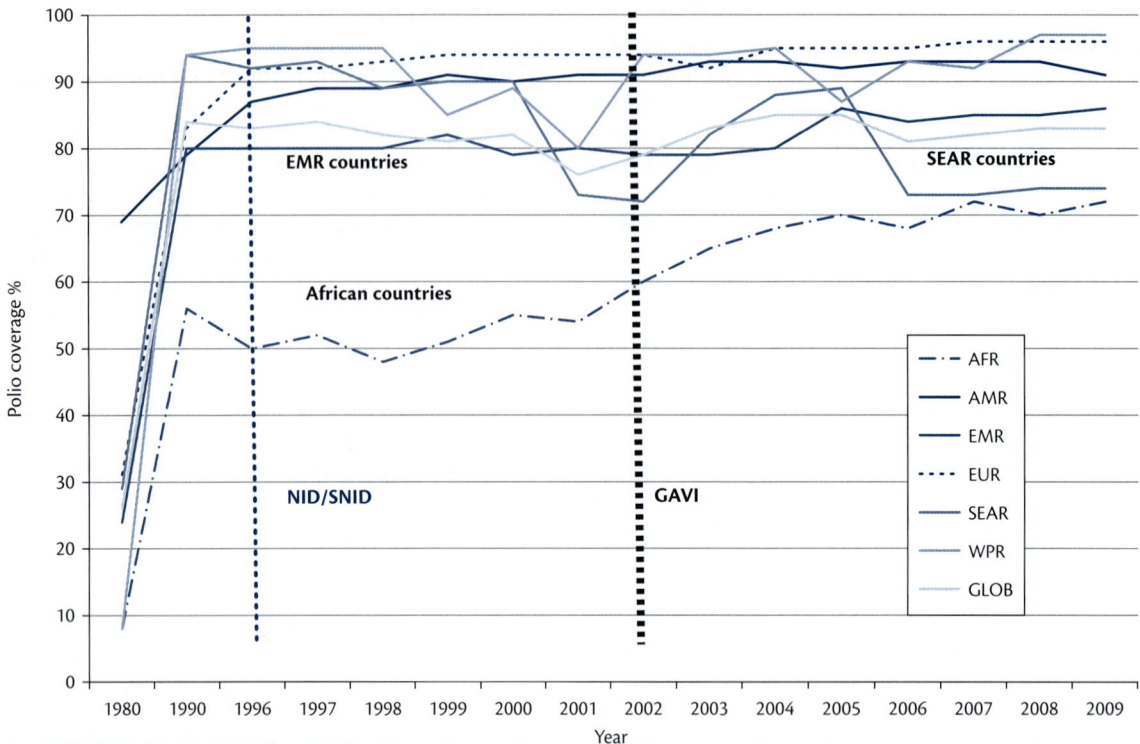

Fig. 1.3.2 Poliomyelitis immunization (three doses). Coverage for <1 year of age by WHO Regions, 1980 and 1990–2009.
Source: data from WHO Global Health Observatory Data Repository, Copyright © World Health Organization 2013, available from http://apps.who.int/gho/data/view.main.81605?lang=en.

the list of polio-endemic countries in February 2012. By mid 2012, only three countries, i.e. Afghanistan and Pakistan in Asia, and Nigeria in Africa, had endemic infections with indigenous transmission of wild polio viruses. These countries had accounted for 90 per cent of all new cases of polio in 2010 and 2011. Surveillance on new polio cases and acute flaccid paralysis cases with timely and prompt response for control is very crucial in these countries (WHO 2012b). The need for this was highlighted by outbreaks due to circulating vaccine-derived polio virus in nine countries in Asia and Africa, even in 2011. While the prize of achieving polio eradication is enormous with thousands of children spared paralysis or death every year, the continued transmission of wild polio virus in a few countries is the real threat to the possibility of global eradication. Failure of global polio eradication efforts, while seemingly unthinkable, would result in the return of polio infections around the world and would constitute the most expensive public health failure in history. In May 2012, the World Health Assembly called polio eradication a programmatic emergency for global public health, especially for those countries where wild polio virus transmissions still exist (WHO 2012c). If and when the world successfully eradicates wild polio virus, this would represent a major milestone of public health success in the twenty-first century.

Immunization against measles, an easily transmitted viral infection responsible for around 10 per cent of deaths from all causes among children aged under 5 years globally, was included as part of the routine EPI programme in all LMIC since mid 1970. By 2000, 72 per cent of the world's children received at least one dose of measles vaccine (against 16 per cent in 1980). The entire American continent had eliminated the measles infection (i.e. no indigenous case for more than 12 months) by 2002. This prompted

countries from other continents to launch the global measles initiative, aimed to boost routine coverage of measles vaccination (at least a single dose) to more than 90 per cent of children under 1 year in every district of the high-burden countries. Increased emphasis was placed on laboratory-backed surveillance of new measles cases, and continuous monitoring of vaccination coverage. The number of children dying from measles had dropped worldwide from an estimated 750,000 in 2000 to 197,000 in 2007 (WHO 2009a). While it may not be possible for many LMIC to achieve measles elimination in the near future, immunization of all infants is nevertheless highly beneficial in reducing sickness, lifelong disability, and deaths at early ages.

A high coverage of immunization with tetanus toxoid (TT) to all women of childbearing age and a high coverage of DPT (diphtheria, whooping cough, and tetanus) vaccine for infants and with boosters among school children, are the simplest and most cost-effective ways to reduce tetanus infection in women and neonates, as well as deaths due to neonatal tetanus (NNT). Efforts have been made to eliminate neonatal tetanus (reducing to the level of incidence of one NNT case per 1000 live-births in all districts) since 1989. However, by the end of 2010, around ten countries of the world, all from LMIC, remained tetanus endemic.

Immunization against hepatitis B (HepB) virus, another highly prevalent infection, was introduced as part of routine EPI vaccination in LMIC since early 1990. After two decades, almost all LMIC have used both plasma-derived and recombinant HepB vaccines, achieving over 70–80 per cent coverage. If the continuous vaccine supply can be ensured and the programme is properly managed, HepB infection could be under control and even eliminated within the next one to two decades.

A potent vaccine against infection by *Haemophilus influenzae* type b, or Hib has been available since mid 1980 in high-income countries. Large-scale studies in LMIC of Africa and Latin America, and recently in Asia showed a substantial reduction in the burden of pneumonia and meningitis among infants and young children (WHO 2006a). However, latest coverage data still showed that Hib vaccine coverage in Asia and the Pacific was lower than those of other regions.

Neglected tropical diseases

Neglected tropical diseases (NTD) are a group of infectious diseases of the tropical countries that cause illness and death of thousands of people living in the tropics worldwide. Leprosy, an age-old disease, but neglected for some decades, has been put under control by accelerated efforts in introducing multi-drug therapy and a call for its elimination. Extensive coverage of treatment of all registered leprosy cases with multidrug therapy (MDT) in endemic countries was pursued in early 1990. Within a decade, several millions of registered leprosy cases were put under supervised treatment, achieving cure of the disease within a year. By 2001, 107 of 122 endemic countries were able to achieve the global target of leprosy elimination, i.e. reducing the prevalence to a level below one case per 10,000 people. Globally, the number of new leprosy cases came down from a peak of 775,000 in 2001 to 299,000 in 2005, and by 2010, only 228,500 cases. The burden of leprosy continues to decline globally as a result of collaborative efforts carried out by national leprosy programmes along with continued support from both national and international partners. By the end of 2011, around 120 endemic countries achieved the global elimination target (WHO 2011d). If the current trend in disease reduction is well sustained with full support from the Global Alliance, the incidence and total burden of leprosy could be further reduced in all endemic countries in the near future. Leprosy elimination might become another public health landmark of the twenty-first century.

Visceral leishmaniasis or kala-azar, another NTD, has been put under control by using an oral medication, miltefosine. A new candidate vaccine is under trial in India in 2012. Until newer medicines and appropriate vaccine(s) are available at affordable prices, and made accessible to the mass population in the endemic countries, the misery and suffering of thousands of people from visceral leishmaniasis would continue.

Onchocerciasis also known as river blindness, another parasitic infection, is still endemic in 37 countries in Africa and Latin America. A million people are visually impaired and over 300,000 people are blind as a consequence of this disease. The Global Onchocerciasis Control Programme that was launched in 1974 tried to reduce severe pathological manifestations through community-based mass management with a microfilarial drug (ivermectin), combined with vector control. Although the disease is a preventable cause of blindness and its elimination goal is achievable, there is a great deal of work to be done in endemic countries (Diawara et al. 2009).

Dracunculiasis is a parasitic, vector-borne guinea worm infestation. Many endemic countries in Asia and Africa were able to achieve the global eradication target, set in 2004, by reducing the annual incidence from 3.5 million in 1986 to fewer than 1100 cases in 2011, with over 90 per cent of them in Sudan (WHO 2011e). If concerted efforts continued, eradication of dracunculiasis could be achieved in the near future without any use of vaccine and medicine.

Trachoma is a chronic repeated infection of the eyes by the bacterium *Chlamydia trachomatis*. It affects poor people and children living in the tropical countries of Asia and Africa, where unhygienic personal practices still prevail and people are not able to access adequate water supply. Surgical intervention, the grey-line split and splint technology to correct early cases of entropion and trichiasis of affected eyes, has saved millions of people from blindness (Wilfred 1979). Mass treatment with simple antibiotic (tetracycline) eye-ointment application daily for 6 months for both eyes, supplemented with field surgical treatment, and improvement of personal hygiene and sanitation, were effective strategies to reduce infection rate as well as cure the disease (Tun and Ko Ko 2007). Cost effectiveness of these multiple integrated strategies carried out in Myanmar has been documented (Evans et al. 1996). Many endemic countries implemented the WHO-advocated SAFE strategy (surgery, antibiotics, facial cleaning and environmental improvement) under the national integrated trachoma control programme, within the Vision 2020 strategy aiming for ultimate elimination of the disease.

The global eradication effort for yaws, another disabling NTD, through vaccination, has been launched in many countries around the world for the last five decades. However, sporadic epidemics and scattered foci of infection still persist in some parts of Latin America, the Pacific, and South and South East Asia. Extensive surveillance and case finding, use of newer antibiotics, and follow-up of treated cases and contacts, became important strategies for eradication of yaws from the remaining endemic countries.

Lymphatic filariasis (LF) is also a disabling NTD caused by blood-borne infection by microscopic thread-like parasitic worms—*microfilariae*. The global programme to eliminate LF was launched in 2000 and more than 3.4 billion doses of anti-microfilarial medicines were delivered to a targeted population of 897 million people. Vector control measures combined with mass drug administration can interrupt disease transmission and reduce the parasitic levels. Despite decades of such efforts, LF continues to be highly prevalent in many countries mainly in Asia, the Pacific, and Africa, with an estimated 120 million infected people in 72 countries in 2010 (WHO 2011f).

Chronic non-communicable diseases

While infectious diseases continue to be major public health problems in LMIC, chronic NCDs have become increasingly prevalent and important as a public health challenge. Recent estimates of the global burden of NCDs and their risk factors showed that over 36 million people died (almost 63 per cent of all deaths) in 2008, principally from cardiovascular diseases, diabetes, cancer, and chronic obstructive respiratory diseases. More than 60 per cent of the global burden of cardiovascular diseases is in LMIC. Many large-scale, well-designed clinical trials had shown that lowering the common risk factors like tobacco and alcohol use or unhealthy diets can reduce morbidity and death from NCDs. The dual approach of screening and mitigating risk factors in relatively high-risk groups and of promoting population-wide preventative activities to reduce health risks such as tobacco and alcohol use with policy and legislative measures is an appropriate strategy for LMIC.

Diabetes mellitus, either type 1 (insulin dependent) or type 2 (non-insulin dependent), has affected around 200 million people of above 20 years of age worldwide. Many patients with type 1 diabetes in LMIC still do not have adequate access to insulin. The number of patients with diabetes may increase to 370 million by 2030, if proper prevention and control strategies are not in place. With early screening and diagnosis, followed by effective management with diet, exercise, and essential medicines, diabetes and its complications can be potentially controlled.

Cancer is a well-known NCD and a leading cause of death worldwide with more than 70 per cent of all cancer deaths occurring in LMIC. Liver cancer affects approximately 5.5 million people, predominantly caused by viral hepatitides. Stomach cancer, caused by *Helicobacter pylori* infection, could be easily prevented by early prevention and control of infection with appropriate medicines. Early detection with proper screening and improved treatment of breast cancer has reduced mortality by 45 per cent in women above 50 years of age. Cancer of the uterine cervix, which is prevalent among women of childbearing age, is mainly due to chronic infection with sexually-transmitted human papilloma virus (HPV). Pap smear screening and early treatment has significantly reduced mortality from cervical cancer. Some high- and upper middle-income countries have introduced vaccination against HPV infection, with a view to reducing cervical cancer (WHO 2009b).

Strengthening health systems

For effective disease control, viable and efficient health systems are necessary. Many governments of LMIC at their independence tried to establish their public health facilities based on the model of their colonial masters. In general, the health systems in most countries were publicly funded, except in some African countries where basic healthcare was reliant on health facilities and staff supported by local and international nongovernmental organizations (NGOs). A number of medical schools and paramedical training institutes, public health training and research institutions, and health centres were established with technical assistance from the colonial rulers.

Up to the 1960s, many LMIC had weak health infrastructure for maternal and child health (MCH) care, despite the high mortality and morbidity from maternal and childhood diseases. Immunization coverage was very low and essential MCH care relied on poorly trained nurse-aids, midwives, or nurse-midwives at hospitals and hospital-based clinics, located mostly in urban areas. Even basic maternal and essential obstetric care services were not available. After a few decades, it was realized that the vertical approach of opening MCH centres and deploying MCH workers alone did not achieve the purpose of expanding MCH care. Various strategies were thus adopted to integrate and expand MCH services as part of essential healthcare packages. During 1960–1970, many LMIC started adopting comprehensive population policies, and family planning services as part of MCH care, to address both demographic challenges and maternal health problems. Even though simple and effective family planning techniques were available and within reach, only a fraction of women in LMIC could have access to these services.

Another critical challenge is making essential medicines available for needy patients. As many newer food supplements, medicines, and vaccines become available, the control of substandard, spurious, falsely-labelled, falsified, or counterfeit medical products must be closely monitored. LMIC have to continually strengthen their food and drug regulatory agencies to ensure effective implementation of their national policies. With the expansion of the private sector and health insurance, ensuring access to, and in particular affordability of, essential medicines and vaccines become more vital.

Health systems based on modern allopathic medicine intended to benefit the whole population barely existed a century ago in many LMIC. To date, healthcare provision in LMIC is by the publicly-financed health systems in conjunction with private healthcare providers, supported by NGOs. Development of infrastructure for public health, mainly for communicable disease prevention and control, was usually done as part of vertical campaign programmes. There are glaring contrasts between high-income countries and LMIC as well as among LMIC themselves in achieving a higher health status. The average life expectancy at birth in 1990, in low-income countries was around 52 years and that of lower- middle-income countries was 63 years, while the upper middle- and high-income countries range from 68 to 76 years, as estimated by WHO (WHO 2012a). Many low-income countries still have child mortality rates of above 100 per 1000 live births. During the 1980s and 1990s, many LMIC adopted the health-for-all (HFA) and primary healthcare (PHC) principles and approaches to restructuring their health systems, and formulated new health policies, strategies, and programmes on this basis (WHO 1998).

While some countries concentrated on vertical campaigns for expanding personal healthcare interventions like MCH, family planning, growth monitoring, breastfeeding and immunization, other countries tried to implement comprehensive health programmes, including health legislative and health finance reforms. This is important since lack of communication and a full understanding of the fundamental values, principles and policies of PHC and HFA applicable to national health development had resulted in limitations to access to essential healthcare. Also, there was inadequate coordination and collaboration between specific health intervention initiatives like immunization or specific disease campaigns, and the development of basic health systems infrastructure. This resulted in inadequate involvement of communities in their health development efforts, and also to the slow pace of integrating vertical disease control campaigns into the basic health services. It was compounded by weak planning and management of health development, especially at the operational levels at districts and below, and the imbalance and inappropriateness of some human resources for health (WHO 2008a).

Some health development programmes in LMIC showed that the conventional approach of merely expanding basic health services was inadequate, as the public sector could not bear the cost of expansion of basic healthcare services to the entire population, in the face of existing resource constraints. Thus, many countries sought partnerships with private healthcare providers, worked with community-based civil society organizations, and deployed a large number of community-level health volunteers, who were trained for short periods to serve as a third layer of human resources for health (Sein 2006). The increasing use of volunteers in health development proved successful for expanding essential healthcare coverage in many countries. With the involvement of private healthcare providers and community-based health volunteers, many essential public health interventions were enhanced especially in disease prevention and control including epidemic control and immunization, health promotion, maternal and child healthcare, information gathering and surveillance, treatment of minor ailments and environmental health promotion. A series of reforms in health systems such as improving the content of essential packages for health and the way these were financed were undertaken in many LMIC. The global trend in health systems development nowadays is towards the increasing role of both the for-profit and non-profit private sector.

Health planning and financing

The centrally directed planning framework using country health planning (CHP) or national planning process for health sector development, supported by WHO and UN agencies during 1970–1990, had moved many LMIC to a higher level of health attainment. It was highly successful when the health development projects based on selective healthcare interventions like immunization, malaria, or leprosy control, or selective maternal and child care, family planning, and growth monitoring were promoted on the national scale through centrally controlled, externally funded programmes. From mid 1990, external donors moved from planning multiple health development projects to an integrated sectoral planning of comprehensive health development programmes.

Around 2005, the UN introduced the principle of 'Delivering as One (DaO)', basically covering four areas: 'one leader, one budget, one programme, and one office', and later the Multi-donor Trust Fund (MDTF) mechanism to coordinate development resources and get more partners to support a single national strategy in selected LMIC (United Nations Development Group 2010). A group of development partners who share a common interest in improving health services and health outcomes for LMIC had launched, in 2007, another global initiative called IHP+ (International Health Partnership plus related initiatives). An inter-agency working group of IHP+ had developed a joint assessment tool for national health plans and strategies (JANs), and associated guidelines. In 2010, the JANs tool was applied in several LMIC as part of the national health policy development and planning process (IHP+ 2011). The national health planning processes cover now a comprehensive, balanced, and evidence-based assessment of the country's health and health system challenges. Many LMIC tried to strengthen their institutional capacity to harmonize and align donor programmes with their national policies, strategies, priorities, and plans (WHO 2011g).

The LMIC, while struggling to improve their health systems, increasingly realized the value of developing their own health systems to provide healthcare to all people, while financially protecting them in the fairest way possible. The key challenge of health financing reform, particularly the collection of revenue and pooling and use of financial resources, is to find a good balance between ensuring that the cost of care is affordable and fair for patients, while providing appropriate incentives to healthcare providers to motivate them to improve the health of the people by improving the responsiveness of care delivery. This is in keeping with the ideal for universal coverage, which means equity of access to key promotive, preventive, curative, and rehabilitative health interventions for all, at an affordable cost.

While high-income countries continued to increase public spending on health in response to growing expectations, LMIC were struggling with major problems in managing and financing their health systems. Total health expenditure as a proportion of GDP ranged from 1.9 per cent to 6 per cent in LMIC, while high-income countries spent more than 11 per cent. Per capita government expenditure on health varies from around US $30 in low-income, US $90 in lower middle-income, US $500 in upper middle-income, and more than US $2600 in high-income countries.[3] The relatively low public investment in health in LMIC has led to higher direct costs for healthcare in the form of out-of-pocket expenses for patients. In some LMIC, the local community organizes and manages their own community-based financing for healthcare, with government subsidies or technical support. While the coverage of social health insurance is high among LMIC in South and Central America, it is very low or almost non-existent in many LMIC of Asia and Africa. Where such social health insurance schemes are available, they usually cover formally employed workers as part of nation-wide social welfare schemes.

The degree of dependence on external resources for health as a percentage of the total health expenditure varied from country to country in 2009, ranging from 2–20 per cent for most LMIC in South- and South East Asia (WHO 2012a). Similarly, many LMIC in Africa had a range of 20–60 per cent, the highest being 80 per cent in Malawi. It is generally perceived that excessive dependence on external financial sources makes a country's health system vulnerable. External aid for health, especially through large international health partnerships, can create imbalances in the overall allocation of health resources and loss of a country's autonomy in making health decisions.

In addition to the support to health sector development by bilateral aid/grant programmes and multilateral financial institutions, there is an increasing investment in health by the national and international civil societies, and multinational pharmaceutical corporations through their foundations. The recent entry of private foundations set up by global entrepreneurs and private philanthropists in the health and social sectors, is an important trend with multibillion dollar contributions in specified funds and programmes for health development. The most recent study done by the Institute for Health Metrics and Evaluation (IHME), in its Financing Global Health Report 2011, stated that the development assistance in health (DAH) which is reaching US $27.73 billion, has more than doubled in size between 2001 and 2009 (IHME 2011). While the DAH is usually aligned with the health priorities of LMIC, some countries with high burden of diseases have been missed out for various reasons, mainly political ones. Similarly, the inputs from DAH may have benefited programmes which primarily target specific communicable diseases such as HIV/AIDS, tuberculosis, and malaria that may affect only a minority of people in the developing countries (see Chapter 11.12 for further discussion of these issues). The proliferation of bilateral and multilateral donors, multiple global initiatives, and international NGOs also generates the potential for weakening health systems, rather than strengthening them, allowing countries to avoid issues like long-term sustainability.

Human resources for health

One key factor for success in implementing healthcare, both for public health and health system development, is having a critical mass of competent human resources for health. As human resources consume as much as 60–70 per cent of the public health expenditure, they need to be fully developed and optimally utilized. The *World Health Report 2006* had provided a global analysis and identified effective strategies to strengthen the development of appropriate human resources for health (WHO 2006b). Despite concerted efforts to resolve imbalances and inequitable distribution, many LMIC are still confronted with basic human resources policy issues, such as the need for clear national policies on the development of an appropriate health workforce, inadequate norms and standards for health professionals resulting in inappropriate mix, inadequate mechanisms for exchange of information and insufficient standards for health professionals' education and training, and absence of quality control mechanisms for health professionals' practices. The development of human resources for health is crucial for improving health services coverage and for scaling up public health interventions. Major reasons for the health workforce shortage, while varying greatly among LMIC, include inadequate numbers due to underinvestment in basic undergraduate and graduate education and training; loss of existing workforce due to emigration to other countries; mismanagement and coordination (career structure and staff supervision); and inefficient planning.

Some of the impediments to the development of a relevant and adequately sized public health workforce are lack of incentives and career structure for public health professionals, public health training being seen as an extension of the biomedical model of clinical training, and the inclusion of many training courses and core curriculum which are either obsolete or irrelevant to the public health needs of the countries. Several networks, both formal and informal, among public health education institutions in Asia and Africa have been established to collaborate and support exchange programmes for faculty members and students, sharing of curriculum and training materials, and organizing joint research studies. The shortage of nurses and midwives in LMIC especially in Asia and Africa has been a chronic human resource issue for decades, and many countries have attempted to address this through expansion of nurse training institutions.

Health research development

While science and technology research and application have advanced rapidly in high-income countries, they have remained rudimentary in LMIC. While LMIC have to rely on the results of research and development on pharmaceuticals and vaccines from high-income countries, in practice, many breakthroughs have been contributed to by the experiences gained and the studies carried out in LMIC. In many LMIC, there are very few health research institutions and poor career prospects for researchers. Development of health research, both in biomedical and public health sciences, has been initiated in recent decades in LMIC, with respect to prevention and control of tropical diseases. Joint collaborative studies between LMIC, especially upper middle-income countries and high-income countries are carried out for development and use of medicines and vaccines for infectious diseases, promotion of human health and reproduction specifically on contraception and other fertility control measures, strengthening of health systems, promotion and protection of environmental health, and control of NCDs, and development of essential healthcare technologies. Considerable progress has been made in

capability strengthening for promoting health systems research, which has further paved the way for developing effective national health research systems. In recent years, the development of health research has been promoted through international exchanges of experience and expertise amongst the networks such as INCLEN Trust, Asia-Pacific Health Research System Network, and African Health Research System Network. A major issue faced by LMIC today is that while scientific advances and technological development of the high-income countries provide them with vast opportunities for their overall economic development, large numbers of people in LMIC are still suffering from neglected tropical diseases and undernutrition for which prevention or control interventions are already available (WHO 2010b).

Social determinants of health

The majority of LMIC are particularly susceptible to the negative impact of socially determined health inequities due to exposure to health risks, social exclusion, and other broader determinants associated with health risks including living conditions, work environment, unsafe sex, and changing consumption patterns of food, water, and information. After WHO released the report of the Commission on Social Determinants of Health in 2008 (WHO 2008b), LMIC considered the need to build up their national capacities to address advocacy, intersectoral action, evidence gathering of health inequity, and to address social determinants across sectors. They started establishing national mechanisms to coordinate and manage inter-sectoral actions for health and to bring into the mainstream consideration of social determinants of health, especially health inequities.

Tobacco is one of the common risk factors for many NCDs. Tobacco-related illnesses and deaths increased globally during the past decades with four million deaths every year, and if no proper control measures are instituted, the death toll may go up to 10 million. In South- and South East Asia, increasing use of the combination of betel-nut and tobacco as betel-quid has become a major issue, since it causes oral, laryngeal, and gastrointestinal cancer. After adoption in May 2003 of the WHO Framework Convention on Tobacco Control (WHO FCTC), LMIC have adopted or amended their tobacco control legislation. Several countries now have comprehensive national tobacco control legislation conforming to the provisions of the Convention (WHO 2011h).

Worldwide consumption of alcohol in 2008 was equivalent to 6 litres of pure alcohol consumed per person aged 15 or older, with a large portion of this—28.6 per cent or 1.76 litres per person—being homemade, illegally produced or sold outside normal government controls (WHO 2011i). Harmful use of alcohol is a major factor contributing to premature deaths and avoidable disease worldwide. A wide range of policy options and interventions for reducing public health problems caused by harmful use of alcohol was advocated for all countries (WHO 2010c).

Preventing injuries

Injuries, being caused intentionally and non-intentionally, have emerged as a major public health problem in the twenty-first century. The rapidly rising number of motor vehicles (48 per cent of the world's vehicles are registered in LMIC), and motorcycles (adding more than a million a day on the roads) has led to an equally rapid increase in traffic-related injuries and deaths. LMIC have a higher road-traffic related death rate of over 20 per 100,000 population, and accounted for over 90 per cent of the world's fatalities. Introduction and upgrading of safe public transport, improvement of road signs and pedestrian-crossings, compliance with traffic legislation like wearing helmets and seat-belts, and avoiding speeding and drink-driving, are important measures for reducing road-traffic injuries (WHO 2009c).

Social medicine and public health

The initial idea of social medicine or the social dimensions of public health had emerged in the early twentieth century. The concept of social medicine was developed as a new public health discipline in the late 1940s. At that time, leaders of both clinical medicine and public health questioned the perceived polarization of curative medicine and preventive medicine which included epidemiology and social medicine. The situation was exacerbated by continued specialization and the lack of cross-disciplinary interaction (Ko Ko 2011). However, the social and behavioural aspects that influenced illness and well-being are recognized and revisited in later decades, and many social and personal behavioural interventions are introduced as part of health promotion and disease prevention. Many universities and medical schools converted their departments, faculties, or schools of hygiene and public health into those of preventive and social medicine during the period 1960–1970. Instead of integrating curative and preventive medicine in the teaching of social medicine, educational institutions equated public health and hygiene with preventive and social medicine, and conventional public health teaching still has a primary focus on prevention and control of infectious diseases and hygiene. National health planners and public health specialists today need to have a better understanding about the integration of clinical medicine within its social context, and also to take into account political needs and demands of the community, widening gaps between personal and community health needs with available resources, and rising pressure of societal factors on healthcare. The general population is now becoming increasingly aware of the social and economic determinants impacting health. As a result, national debates on the linkages of health with social, environmental, economic, and political factors have started and there are more discussions at the global level to give a wider political and social dimension to international public health. Policymakers are increasingly concerned about finding equitable, realistic, and sustainable approaches to addressing social determinants of health with a view to improving health.

The history of public health development has shown the need for increasing cooperation between high-income countries and LMIC, in order to promote the health of the citizens of the world. Over the last 50 years, many international, intergovernmental, bilateral, and multilateral development agencies and organizations, as well as alliances have emerged out of necessity to deal with international developmental issues both in policy and programme terms. LMIC need to work in close collaboration with all development partners by focusing the global efforts to build healthy populations and communities by addressing the excess burden of sickness and suffering resulting from both communicable and non-communicable diseases especially in poor and marginalized populations. Partnerships could be established to sustain and support health system development so that equitable health outcomes are achieved and the needs of the people are met. More recently,

debates have intensified around global public health development and global governance of health (Dodgson et al. 2002; Kickbusch and Gleicher 2012).

Whither the new public health

In this century, many LMIC have moved from narrow, specific disease control interventions (vertical campaigns), to a wider perspective of integrated and comprehensive multi-sectoral interventions for health development. The approach of public health measures under full responsibility of the government has been supplemented with services provided by an increasing number of NGOs, foundations, and private sector agencies both at local and global levels. In addition to external financing and technical support by traditional international agencies like WHO and UN, bilateral aid agencies from high-income countries like the United States, United Kingdom, Australia, Japan or the Netherlands, and multilateral financial institutions such as the World Bank and Regional Development Banks, there are myriad international foundations and financing groups such as the GAVI Alliance and the Global Fund, as well as private foundations like the B&M Gates Foundation, that have transformed international health support and governance.

Globalization of public health

The UN launched the Joint United Nations Programme on HIV/AIDS (UNAIDS) in January 1996, with the UN-wide mission to lead, strengthen, and support an expanded response to HIV/AIDS. Another UN initiative was the organization of the UN Millennium Summit attended by 189 heads of states in 2000, where the UN Millennium Development Goals (UN MDG), of which the majority related to health, were adopted. The UN MDG targets for 2015 represented the world's commitment to deal with global poverty and health in several dimensions, with a global partnership that called for country-led strategies and support from developed countries in the areas of trade, official development assistance, debt sustainability, and access to medicine and technologies. The UN MDG became the aspirational goals for all countries, including LMIC, in reducing poverty and improving overall development, particularly health (UN 2011).

Analyses of the impact of rapid globalization on public health are available in much of the health and development literature (Drager and Beaglehole 2001) (see Chapter 1.5 on globalization in detail). Global trade, finance, information and people flows, governance, and security can all contribute to improving the health of people everywhere. The threats to and opportunities in public health, including cross-country control of infectious diseases and international governance, have been analysed extensively within the context of globalization (UN 2003; Fidler 2004). An updated version of the IHR, issued in 2008, is a guide for all countries to prevent, protect against, control, and provide a public health response to the international spread of a disease or diseases, in various ways that are commensurate with and restricted to public health risks, and that avoid unnecessary interference with international traffic and trade (WHO 2008c). There is a strong need for global collaboration to combat diseases of public health importance that are a significant threat to human health globally.

While many old scourges like tuberculosis, malaria, plague, cholera, and leprosy remain endemic or are re-emerging in some

LMIC, a few emerging infectious diseases of epidemic potential present a constant threat. These diseases include acquired immune deficiency syndrome (AIDS) and human immunodeficiency virus (HIV) infection, Ebola and other haemorrhagic diseases, severe acute respiratory syndrome (SARS), and avian influenza. A few old tropical diseases like cholera, dengue, and YF are also emerging in new geographical areas (see Chapter 8.17 on emerging and re-emerging infections in detail).

Healthy ageing

Many LMIC, which are experiencing an expansion of the proportion of people above 60 years of age, have started paying attention to the health of the elderly. These have focused on creating closer linkages between social welfare and health, providing care at home and in the community, promoting traditional family ties, optimizing the use of existing healthcare delivery systems, and setting up old-age homes. However, access to essential healthcare for the elderly is inadequate. Knowledge among basic health workers on specific needs of the elderly is also minimal. A few countries have organized research studies related to epidemiology, demography, and determinants of healthy ageing. Some countries have formulated comprehensive intersectoral national policies on ageing and health. The economic, social, and health status of the fast-growing elderly population in LMIC poses a great challenge to all sectors. The major difficulties in developing appropriate healthcare for the elderly include the lack of reliable data for programme planning, a virtual absence of national policies and strategies for the care and social welfare of the elderly, and inadequate infrastructure to cope with their rapidly increasing health needs.

Looking ahead

Many LMIC had undertaken a series of new, third-generation, health reforms, such as improving the content of essential packages for health and the way these were financed. Many models of health financing either at national or local levels were developed, including reforms in expanding social health insurance. Another global trend in health development is the increasing role of the private sector, both for-profit and non-profit. Fewer non-profit agencies were involved in public health development and medical care to under-served populations. It is not a simple solution of privatization, but a balanced mix of both public and private healthcare, that can fit within the existing socioeconomic, political, and health situation of the country, and the extent the national health plans would ensure that wider reforms would address the gaps in healthcare and create a pro-poor health system.

The linkages between social and economic development and health improvement were recognized by many LMIC in 1980–1990. There was a dramatic change in international public health development, especially global health governance and international cooperation. The centrality of health to human development is embedded in a wide range of national and international agreements and affirmed in action by a wide-ranging set of stakeholders. A multiplicity of new actors in national and international health had redefined the boundaries of health sector. Groups of individuals, united to a particular cause such as patient groups or civil society both at national and international levels, have become major players for policy and programme development in public health, by creating powerful lobbies and raising public awareness. Growing numbers and increasing involvement of NGOs in the direct delivery of healthcare had complemented the efforts of the publicly provided health systems. They have become influential players in policy development and decision-making in socioeconomic and health-related issues in many LMIC.

A new paradigm in health development in many LMIC, which have to rely heavily on external aid for health in earlier years and even now, has led to a complex relationship among traditional and new players in international health and health-related development, for guiding appropriate and effective planning and use for resources, and the need for delineation and harmonization of responsibilities. There are, however, a few concerns that the multiple international partnerships might widen the gaps by increasing fragmentation of international cooperation in health, overwhelming the national capacity to implement, distorting national priorities, diverting scarce human resources, and also marginalizing the UN system's agencies.

Conclusion

Health is a cause rather than an effect of economic development. The history of public health development in LMIC shows that important breakthroughs in public health interventions have led to great improvements in economic development. Health actually determines economic productivity and prosperity, and physical and emotional well-being of the people. The population afflicted with a high infant mortality rate usually lacks the secure knowledge of its children's longevity, witnesses higher rates of fertility, and experiences the quality–quantity trade-off in child rearing. The efforts of national and international communities should be aimed at promoting healthy living, reducing the double burden of disease, and making essential healthcare accessible to all. Ever since the health-for-all movement was initiated over three decades ago, health, equity, and social justice remain the main themes of social and health policy. It is essential for all public health professionals to sustain these values especially those in LMIC and the international community.

Notes

1. Improved drinking-water sources are those places where drinking-water is taken from: (1) piped water into dwelling, yard, or plot; (2) public tap or standpipe; (3) tube-well or bore-hole well; (4) protected spring; (5) protected dug well; and (6) rain-water collection (source: WHO/UNICEF 2012).
2. Improved sanitation means use of: (1) flush or pour-flush to piped sewage system, septic tank or pit-latrine; (2) ventilated improved pit (VIP) latrine; (3) pit latrine with slab; and (4) composting toilet (source: WHO/UNICEF 2012).
3. See details in Table 7, Annexure, *World Health Statistics 2012* (WHO 2012a).

References

Centres for Disease Control and Prevention (2010). Vaccinia virus infection after sexual contact with a military smallpox vaccine—Washington, 2010. *MMWR Morbidity and Mortality Weekly Report*, 59(25), 773–5.

Centres for Disease Control and Prevention (2011). Global routine vaccination coverage, 2010. *MMWR Morbidity and Mortality Weekly Report*, 60(44), 1520–2.

Diawara, L., Traoré, M.O., Badji, A., et al. (2009). Feasibility of onchocerciasis elimination with ivermectin treatment in endemic foci in Africa: first evidence from studies in Mali and Senegal. *PLoS Neglected Tropical Diseases*, 3(7), e497.

Dodgson, R., Lee, K., and Drager, N. (2002). *Global Health Governance: A Conceptual Review*. Geneva: WHO and London School of Hygiene and Tropical Medicine.

Drager, N. and Beaglehole, R. (2001). Globalization: changing the public health landscape. *Bulletin of World Health Organization*, 79(9), 803.

Evans, T.G., Ranson, M.K., Kyaw, T.A., and Ko, C.K. (1996). Cost effectiveness and cost utility of preventing trachomatous visual impairment lessons from 30 years of trachoma control in Burma. *British Journal of Ophthalmology*, 80, 850–9.

Fenner, F., Henderson, D.A., Arita, I., et al. (1988). *Smallpox and its Eradication*. Geneva: World Health Organization.

Fidler, D. (2004). *SARS, Governance, and the Globalization of Diseases*. London: Palgrave Macmillan.

Institute for Health Metrics and Evaluation (2011). *Financing Global Health 2011: Continued Growth as MDG Deadline Approaches*. Seattle: IHME.

International Health Partnership plus related initiatives (2011). *Combined Joint Assessment Tool and Guidelines*, Draft, Version 2, 2011, Geneva: IHP+. Available at: http://www.internationalhealthpartnership.net/en/home.

Kickbusch, I. and Gleicher, D. (2012). *Governance for Health in the 21st Century*. Copenhagen: WHO EURO.

Ko Ko, U. (2005). *The Eradication of Smallpox*. In U. Ko Ko, K. Lwin, and T.A. Kyaw (eds.) *Conquest of Scourges in Myanmar: An Update*, pp. 9–50, Yangon: Myanmar Academy of Medical Science.

Ko Ko, U. (2011). *Wither To—Preventive and Social Medicine?* Paper presented at the 57th Myanmar Medical Conference, 22 January 2011, Myanmar Medical Association, Yangon.

Sein, T. (2006). Health volunteers: third workforce for health-for-all movement. *Regional Health Forum*, 10(1), 38–48.

Tun A.K. and Ko Ko, U. (2007). A forty-year battle against blinding trachoma in Myanmar. *Regional Health Forum*, 11(2), 1–9.

United Nations (2003). *Human Security Now: Commission on Human Security*, pp. 95–112. New York: UN.

United Nations (2011). *Millennium Development Goals Report 2011*. New York: UN.

United Nations (2012). *World Economic Situation and Prospects 2012,* Table E, p. 137. New York: UN.

United Nations Development Group (2010). *UNDG Guidance Note on Establishing Multi-donor Trust Funds*. New York: UN.

Wilfred, W.N. (1979). Surgery for trachoma in Burma. *British Journal of Ophthalmology*, 63, 113–16.

World Health Organization (1998). *Health for All in the Twenty-First Century,* 51st World Health Assembly, May 1998, Document A51/15. Geneva: WHO.

World Health Organization (2003). Yellow fever vaccine. *Weekly Epidemiology Record*, 78(40), 349–60.

World Health Organization (2006a). WHO position paper on Haemophilus influenzae type b (Hib) conjugate vaccines. *Weekly Epidemiology Record*, 81(47), 445–52.

World Health Organization (2006b). *World Health Report 2006: Health Workforce*. Geneva: WHO.

World Health Organization (2008a). *World Health Report 2008, Primary Health Care: Now More Than Ever*. Geneva: WHO.

World Health Organization (2008b). *Closing the Gap in a Generation: Health Equity Through Action on the Social Determinants of Health: Final Report of the Commission on Social Determinants of Health*. Geneva: WHO.

World Health Organization (2008c). *International Health Regulations (2005), Second Edition*. Reprinted 2008. Geneva: WHO.

World Health Organization (2009a). *State of the World's Vaccines and Immunization* (3rd ed.). Geneva: WHO.

World Health Organization) (2009b). Human papillomavirus vaccines: WHO position paper. *Weekly Epidemiological Record*, 84(15), 118–31.

World Health Organization (2009c). *Global Status Report on Road Safety: Time For Action*. Geneva: WHO.

World Health Organization (2010a). Human plague: review of regional morbidity and mortality, 2004–2009. *Weekly Epidemiology Record*, 85(6), 37–48.

World Health Organization (2010b). *Research and the World Health Organization: A History of the Advisory Committee on Health Research, 1959–1999*. Geneva: WHO.

World Health Organization (2010c). *Global Strategy to Reduce Harmful Use of Alcohol*. Geneva: WHO.

World Health Organization (2011a). *Smallpox Eradication: Destruction of Variola Virus Stocks (A64/17)*. Geneva: WHO.

World Health Organization (2011b). *Cholera: Mechanism for Control and Prevention (A64/18)*. Geneva: WHO.

World Health Organization (2011c). Global routine vaccination coverage, 201. *Weekly Epidemiology Record*, 86(46), 509–13.

World Health Organization (2011d). Leprosy update, 2011. *Weekly Epidemiology Record*, 86 (36), 389–400.

World Health Organization (2011e). Dracunculiasis eradication: global surveillance summary, 2011. *Weekly Epidemiology Record*, 86(20), 189–204.

World Health Organization (2011f). Global programme to eliminate lymphatic filariasis: progress report on mass drug administration, 2010. *Weekly Epidemiology Record*, 86(35), 377–88.

World Health Organization (2011g). *Health Systems Strengthening: Improving Support to Policy Dialogues Around National Health Policies, Strategies and Plans (A64/12)*. Geneva: WHO.

World Health Organization (2011h). *WHO Report on the Global Tobacco Epidemic, 2011: Warning About the Dangers of Tobacco*. Geneva: WHO.

World Health Organization (2011i). *Global Status Report on Alcohol and Health*. Geneva: WHO.

World Health Organization (2012a). *World Health Statistics 2012*. Geneva: WHO.

World Health Organization (2012b). *Ten Months and Counting: Report of the Independent Monitoring Board of the Global Polio Eradication Initiative,* February, 2012. Geneva: WHO.

World Health Organization (2012c). *Poliomyelitis: Intensification of the Global Polio Eradication Initiative (A65/20)*. Geneva: WHO.

World Health Organization (2013). *WHO Global Health Observatory Data Repository: Immunization: Polio (Pol3) by WHO region*. Available at: http://apps.who.int/gho/data/view.main.81605?lang=en.

World Health Organization/UNICEF (2012). *Progress in Drinking Water and Sanitation: 2012 Update*. Geneva: WHO and UNICEF Joint Monitoring Programme for Water Supply and Sanitation.

1.4

Development of public health in economic transition: the middle-income countries

Kai Hong Phua, Mui-Teng Yap,
Sara U. Schwanke Khilji, and Hin-Peng Lee

Definitions of middle-income countries and emerging economies

The World Bank classifies economies according to gross national income (GNI) per capita, calculated using the World Bank Atlas method. The cut-off points are updated every year using purchasing power parities (PPP) at current international dollars. For 2011, the groups are: low income, $1025 or less; lower-middle income, $1026–4035; upper-middle income, $4036–12,475; and high income, $12,476 or more. The World Bank changed its terminology from the gross national product, or GNP, in previous publications to the GNI (World Bank 2012b). However, the definitions and groupings of 'transition economies' and 'emerging economies' in the literature have so far been hazy. The most comprehensive discussion on the terminology is by the *Centre d'Etudes Prospectives et d'Informations Internationales* (CEPII):

> The term 'emerging economies' corresponds to various and often blurred groupings. Sometimes it is used in relation to the four 'BRICs' (Brazil, Russia, India and China) or a group of 'fast growing economies', while on other occasions, it refers to all developing countries. (Gaulier, et al. 2009)

The term 'emerging economies' implies not only a rapid growth of gross domestic product (GDP) per capita or an increasing presence in world markets, but also entails several important ingredients of political economy. These countries have pursued a process of economic liberalization, promoted market orientation, and opened up to international flows of goods, services, and capital and this process has been associated with the building up of institutions and strong state regulation (Gaulier et al. 2009). Various classifications of 'emerging economies' include the countries which: (1) have a level of income below the threshold set by the World Bank (US $11,100 in 2006), and (2) have been able to increase their share in world markets of manufactured goods or services by at least 0.05 per cent points between 1995 and 2005. This group includes Brazil, India, Indonesia, China, South Africa, and Mexico. Similarly, the Organisation for Economic Co-operation and Development (OECD) describes Brazil, Russia, India, Indonesia, China, and South Africa, together known as the BRIICS, as the six largest non-OECD economies rapidly integrated into world markets during the past two decades (OECD 2009).

Tables 1.4.1–1.4.3, illustrate the rapidly rising trends in GNI per capita (in PPP at current international dollars) and corresponding improvements in the Human Development Index (HDI). The HDI is a composite index combining indicators of life expectancy at birth, educational attainment (mean years of schooling and expected years of schooling), and the gross national income per capita (PPP), to provide relative rankings among all countries. Despite the improving socioeconomic conditions, there are still vast inequalities in all middle-income countries, as reflected in the Gini Index and remaining high levels of poverty. The definition of middle-income countries is increasingly associated with the group of countries somewhere between the rich and poor countries, usually undergoing transition with their emerging economies.

Economic and health transitions in middle-income countries

The relationships between public health and rapid economic development can be illustrated by examples from the fastest emerging economies in East Asia in the past decades. The growth momentum was first propelled by the four 'tiger' economies of Hong Kong, Republic of Korea, Singapore, and Taiwan, which opened up their economies for export-led growth in the 1980s. Meanwhile, the opening up of the economies of China and India, countries which account for nearly one-third of the world's population, changed the dynamics of the regional and global economies. The average rate of economic growth among emerging countries in Asia at 7.5 per cent per annum during 1988–2005 was more than twice that of global economic growth over this period.

Income and health transition

The relationships between health and economic development can be examined by the correlations between national income and general health indicators. The relationship between per capita income and life expectancy among countries is non-linear. At low levels of income and development, there are discernible improvements

Table 1.4.1 Key macroeconomic indicators in middle-income countries

Country	GDP per capita PPP (int $) (2010)	Annual GDP growth % (2010)	GNI per capita PPP (int $) (2010)
Brazil	11,210.4	7.49	11,000
China	7598.8	10.40	7640
India	3425.4	8.81	3400
Indonesia	4325.3	6.10	4200
Jordan	5749.2	3.11	5800
Malaysia	14,730.9	7.19	14,220
Mexico	14,563.9	5.52	14,400
Russia	19,891.4	4.03	19,240
South Africa	10,565.2	2.85	10,360
Thailand	8553.8	7.81	8190
Tunisia	9549.8	3.70	9060

Note: GNI per capita of upper-middle-income group aggregate is 9971.85 (PPP int $).

Source: data from World Bank, *World Development Indicators and Global Development Finance*, 2012, Copyright © 2013 The World Bank Group, All Rights Reserved. Available from http://databank.worldbank.org/data/home.aspx.

Table 1.4.2 Human Development Index in middle-income countries

Country	HDI rank	HDI value	HDI group
Mexico	57	0.770	High
Malaysia	61	0.761	High
Russia	66	0.755	High
Brazil	84	0.718	High
Tunisia	94	0.698	High
Jordan	95	0.698	Medium
China	101	0.687	Medium
Thailand	103	0.682	Medium
South Africa	123	0.619	Medium
Indonesia	124	0.617	Medium
India	134	0.547	Medium

Source: data from United Nations, *Human Development Report 2011, Sustainability and Equity: A Better Future for All*, Copyright © 2011 by the United Nations Development Programme, available from http://hdr.undp.org/en/media/HDR_2011_EN_Complete.pdf.

in health with increases in income with a strong positive correlation up to a per capita income level of around US $4000 (current PPP terms). Beyond this threshold, the relationship becomes much weaker with rising income level but still remains positive. Similar to life expectancy, the relationship between income and infant mortality rate (IMR) is also non-linear. IMR declines faster with even small improvements in per capita income level at lower levels of development, but this correlation also becomes lower after the threshold level of around US $4000 (current PPP terms) is reached. Empirical econometric studies of global or country-specific data indicate a positive relationship between health and economic

growth. For example, a study in 2001 (Bhargava et al. 2001) shows strong correlations between average survival rate and economic growth. Conversely, there is also a positive impact of overall health conditions on economic growth, as shown in another study in 2004 (Jamison et al. 2004) that health improvements are correlated to a 0.2 per cent gain in annual growth rate of health expenditure.

Income and demographic transition

The demographic transition in middle-income economies is producing large changes in age structure that impact on economic growth and standards of living. For countries that are in the early stages of the transition, high fertility and declining infant and child mortality have led to a bulge in the population at younger ages. The middle range of the transition is marked by an increase in the share of the population at the working ages, as large cohorts of children reach adulthood and as the relative number of children is reduced by fertility decline. Towards the end of the transition, the share of the older population increases dramatically. This is a consequence of both the reductions in mortality rates, as well as low fertility rates.

Since the end of the Second World War, many emerging economies have undergone an unprecedented transition in the demographic patterns, from high fertility and high mortality to low fertility and low mortality. As the emerging countries experience positive economic growth, there is a corresponding demographic change in the distribution of population due to a reduction in fertility rate. This situation has come to be known as the 'demographic dividend'. The decrease in dependency due to the reduction in births could free up resources in the country for other investments leading to economic growth.

This is enhanced by a greater proportion of the adult, economically productive, population supporting the dependent population. This 'demographic bonus' where there is a higher proportion of working population groups with less economically dependent children and the elderly, can enable faster economic development. This phenomenon has been observed in many of the fastest growing emerging economies, creating the 'East Asian miracle' in Hong Kong, South Korea, Taiwan, and Singapore, which became newly industrialized economies in the recent past, and that of Thailand, Malaysia, Indonesia, and the Philippines currently. From 1975 to 2000, there has been a dramatic decrease in the dependency ratio in the region from 78 to 56 per cent (Asian Development Bank, 2011). The dependency ratio is projected to decrease further in Asia up to 46 per cent in 2025 as fertility rates continue to decline.

However, the 'demographic dividend' is not indefinite and newer public health issues will surface as the population ages. This will become one of the biggest challenges of the more developed middle-income countries where this window of opportunity might soon close. The economically active adult population will eventually mature into the elderly population 65 years and above, who will also have longer life expectancies, hence increasing the old-age dependency ratio. This situation will become more pronounced in middle-income countries with low fertility rates which result in a smaller number of the younger age group who will eventually replace the adult population engaged in productive employment.

Economic transition and global trade integration

With regard to transition economies, the International Monetary Fund has described the ingredients of the transition process to

Table 1.4.3 Indicators of income inequality and poverty in middle-income countries

Country	GINI index (%)	Income share held by lowest 20%	Poverty gap at $2 a day (PPP) (%)	Poverty head count ratio at $2 a day (PPP) (% population)	Poverty head count ratio at national poverty line (% population)
Brazil	54.69[c]	2.85[c]	5.4[c]	10.82[c]	21.4[c]
China	42.48[a]	4.99[a]	10.06[b]	29.79[b]	–
India	33.38[a]	8.64[a]	24.45[d]	68.72[d]	29.8[d]
Indonesia	34.01[a]	8.34[a]	14.29[d]	46.12[d]	12.5[e]
Jordan	35.43[d]	7.7[d]	0.24[d]	1.59[d]	13.3[b]
Malaysia	46.21[c]	4.54[c]	0.16[c]	2.27[c]	3.8[c]
Mexico	48.28[b]	4.73[b]	1.29[b]	5.19[b]	51.3[d]
Russia	40.11[c]	6.46[c]	0.01[c]	0.05[c]	11.1[f]
South Africa	63.14[c]	2.7[c]	10.16[c]	31.33[c]	23[f]
Thailand	40.02[c]	6.67[c]	0.77[c]	4.58[c]	8.1[c]
Tunisia	41.42[a]	5.92[a]	1.76[a]	8.06[a]	3.8[a]

Notes: [a]2005 data, [b]2008 data, [c]2009 data, [d]2010 data, [e]2011 data, [f]2006 data.

GINI index indicates inequality of income, with 'zero' expressing perfect equality and 100 per cent maximal inequality.

Poverty gap is the mean shortfall from the poverty line (counting the non-poor as having zero shortfall), expressed as a percentage of the poverty line. This measure reflects the depth of poverty as well as its incidence.

Source: data from World Bank, *World Development Indicators and Global Development Finance*, Copyright © 2013 The World Bank Group, All Rights Reserved. Available from http://databank.worldbank.org/data/home.aspx.

include liberalization, macroeconomic stabilization, restructuring and privatization, and legal and institutional reforms (International Monetary Fund 2000). As these economies develop, they are increasingly integrated into global trade and their roles evolve accordingly. This has brought along opportunities as well as challenges. There are many risks of increased trade for public health, including reduced access to medicines due to extended patent protection and restriction of national governments' abilities to regulate for public health (Labonte and Sanger 2006). On the other hand, there are opportunities including improved predictability in trading health-related goods and services, technology transfer, improved efficiency in allocating health resources, and better global coordination (Smith 2006).

The Trade-Related Intellectual Property Rights (TRIPS) Agreements, despite some flexibility, demand that World Trade Organization members protect intellectual property including medicines (Avafia and Narasimhan 2006). This can effectively restrict a country's ability to manufacture or import generic drugs (UNDP and UNAIDS 2012). Although the proponents of TRIPS argue that this would encourage innovation in healthcare, there are concerns over price escalation and affordability (Bettcher et al. 2000). For example, a study in Argentina estimated that the introduction of product patents would result in price increases of about 270 per cent, a reduction in consumption of medicines by 45.5 per cent, and an increased annual expenditure of US $194 million (Challu 1991). According to another analysis of the situation in Argentina, Brazil, Taiwan, India, Mexico, and South Korea, product patents would result in a minimum welfare loss of US $3500 million to US $10,800 million (Nogues 1993). One example is the effect of TRIPS on access to antiretroviral drugs (ARVs) in the fight against the AIDS pandemic in many emerging economies (Reich and Bery 2005; World Health Organization 2006).

TRIPS poses greater challenges to middle-income countries than to low-income ones. Least developed countries (LDCs) enjoy a general exemption from the TRIPS Agreement, but with a high proportion of the population still below the poverty line, middle-income countries bear the brunt of restrictions by such intellectual property enforcement. Another example is the General Agreement on Trade in Services (GATS) which can bring along opportunities, but also the risks of draining the public health workforce and misallocation of health resources (Drager and Fidler 2004).

Trade liberalization, particularly through the Uruguay Round of trade negotiation (Chaloupka and Corbett 1998), has also facilitated the penetration of tobacco industries into emerging markets. The expansion into transitional economies is a significant contributor to the increased risks of tobacco use and related diseases. As a response to declining sales in industrialized countries, major tobacco companies have targeted growing markets in Latin America in the 1960s and the newly industrialized economies of Asia (Taiwan, South Korea, and Thailand) in the 1980s (Connolly 1992).

Demography in middle-income economies

Population sizes in this group of countries vary widely. Four of the five most populous countries in the world—China, India, Indonesia, and Brazil (ranked 1st, 2nd, 4th, and 5th respectively)—that together account for nearly 3 billion persons of the world's 7 billion population in 2010, fall among this group. Two other countries, Russia and Mexico (ranked 9th and 11th respectively), together, make up in excess of another quarter billion. Countries with smaller populations account for another

164 million people, ranging from Jordan which has only six million persons to Thailand with 69 million persons.

The countries also vary in their stages of demographic development. For the majority, the transition from high to low death rate has already taken place such that in 2010, their crude death rates (CDRs) are below 10 per thousand population. Among these, Jordan has the lowest CDR (4.0 per thousand), followed by Malaysia and Mexico (4.7), Tunisia (5.6), Brazil (6.4), Indonesia (7.0), China (7.1), Thailand (7.4), and India (8.0). As the CDR is influenced by differences in population age structure, a comparison of life expectancy at birth in these countries is more reflective of their mortality transition. In 2010, the life expectancy for these countries ranged from 69 years for Indonesia to 77 years for Mexico.

South Africa and Russia are clearly outliers in this group, with crude death rates of 14.9 and 14.2 per thousand in 2010. Mortality levels in Russia have risen since the early 1990s following cataclysmic economic and political changes (Notzon et al. 1998; Men et al. 2003; Popov 2009). Life expectancy has declined as stress-related risk behaviour such as alcoholism rose and there was also an increase in violent deaths (suicides, homicides, unintentional alcohol poisoning, and traffic accidents). In the case of South Africa, there has been an increase in infectious and parasitic diseases related to AIDS. Life expectancy at birth in Russia is currently about the level in the 1960s, at nearly 69 years, after having risen to nearly 70 in the 1980s. South Africa's current life expectancy at birth, at 52 years, is well below the 61 years attained in the early 1990s.

Unlike the transition in the death rate, the transition from high to low birth rates has been less uniform, often lagging well behind the former. Thus while Jordan has the lowest CDR, its crude birth rate (CBR) is the highest, at 25 births per thousand population. With its rate of natural increase (RNI) of 21 per thousand, it is the most rapidly growing, and also the youngest, population among the group, with nearly 40 per cent aged below 15 years. Though further along in their transitions, Malaysia (CBR 20.3) and Mexico (CBR 19.5) also rank among the more rapidly growing, and youthful, countries among the group, due to lags in their fertility transition even as their death rates are among the lowest (CDRs of 4.7), bettered only by Jordan. At the other end of the spectrum, China, Thailand, and Russia are furthest along in their fertility transition, with CBRs of about 12 per thousand. Russia was the first to begin its fertility transition among this group of countries, although the transitions in China and Thailand were more rapid. All three countries are currently in the stage where they are reaping the demographic dividend, with more than 70 per cent of their populations in the working ages, 15–64 years. However, they are also furthest along in terms of the proportions of their population that are aged 65 years and older. China's and Thailand's fertility transitions appear to have been achieved at earlier stages of their demographic developments than Mexico and Tunisia: life expectancy at birth for China and Thailand, at 73 and 74 years respectively, are lower than Mexico's 77 and Tunisia's 75 years (with CBRs at 19.5 and 17.7 respectively). Russia appears to be in the post-transition stage only because of its anomalous mortality conditions.

Population density and urban agglomeration

While China is the most populous country in the world and among this group of countries, India is the most densely populated. With a population density of more than 400 persons per square kilometre, it is well ahead of the next band of countries comprising China, Thailand, and Indonesia (in rank order), with about half the density of India. The remaining countries form another band, led by Malaysia and rounded out by Russia.

Perhaps more important for its health and infrastructural implications than absolute density is the speed and level of urbanization. While cities and urban agglomerations perform useful economic functions in concentrating wealth and talent in a particular location:

> megacities are foci for risks because their unprecedented size magnifies the risks associated with any urban centre: natural disasters; infrastructure failures; pollution; poverty; shortages of food, water or fuel; crime and corruption; or social tensions. The human and economic loss potentials are much higher: not only are more people directly at risk but the repercussions of such an event will be felt by many, physically remote actors and systems, due to the interconnectedness of the megacity. (International Risk Governance Council 2010, p. 2)

Infectious diseases, non-communicable diseases (NCDs), and injuries resulting from accidents, violence, and crime are all potential health risks stemming from overcrowding, substandard housing, inadequate sanitation and waste disposal, and traffic congestion (WHO and UN-Habitat 2010).

In 2010, the level of urbanization was highest in Brazil and Jordan, with more than 80 per cent of their population living in urban areas (Fig. 1.4.1). Only Thailand and India have fewer than half of their population in urban areas, with China and Indonesia being the latest to achieve this milestone. In Thailand and India, only about one-third live in urban areas.

Concentration in agglomerations of more than 1 million persons is more likely to be found in the Latin American countries, Brazil and Mexico. While the Asian countries are generally concentrated at the lower levels along the scale of urban agglomeration (i.e. smaller proportions of their population live in cities of more than 1 million), there has been a sharp increase in China over the 1990–2010 period. Notably, there are currently more megacities in China and India than elsewhere.

Challenges and opportunities

The diverse demographic landscape among the emerging economies poses different health challenges and opportunities (see Tables 1.4.4 and 1.4.5). Rapid population growth and extremely young populations in countries that are still in the early stage of demographic transition (in Jordan, for example) present a different set of public health needs than those close to the final stages of the transition with slower growing, older populations. Rapid population growth, particularly if also highly concentrated in urban areas, is even more challenging as shown by megacities. However, there are also opportunities for those that are reaping the demographic dividend, where high fertility regimes have been followed by sharp fertility decline (as in the case of Brazil). Savings derived from having to provide for a less rapidly growing population may be better invested in higher quality of healthcare and other social infrastructure that could in turn lead to higher productivity and economic growth in a virtuous circle.

Rapid urbanization and internal migration also present critical health challenges in emerging economies. Between 1995 and 2005, the urban population of developing countries grew by an average of 1.2 million people per week (Population Division 2007). The

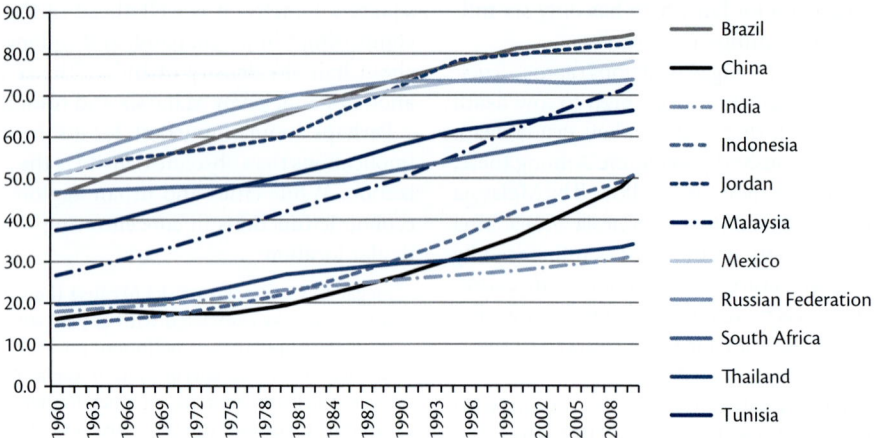

Fig. 1.4.1 Per cent urban population.

Source: data from World Bank, *World Development Indicators 2010*, Copyright © 2013 The World Bank Group, All Rights Reserved. Available from http://databank.worldbank.org/data/home. aspx.

Table 1.4.4 Demographic statistics in middle-income countries (2010)

Country	Population (millions)	Population age 65 and above (%)	Annual population growth (%)	Old-age dependency ratio	TFR	CBR per 1000
Brazil	194.9	7.00	0.88	10.37	1.8	15.49
China	1338.3	8.19	0.52	11.32	1.6	12.12
India	1224.6	4.92	1.39	7.63	2.6	22.17
Indonesia	239.9	5.55	1.03	8.24	2.1	18.22
Jordan	6.0	3.91	2.21	6.68	3.8	25.03
Malaysia	28.4	4.77	1.60	7.35	2.6	20.27
Mexico	113.4	6.35	1.23	9.84	2.3	19.55
Russia	141.7	12.80	−0.07	17.74	1.5	12.50
S. Africa	50	4.64	1.35	7.11	2.5	21.18
Thailand	69.1	8.89	0.60	12.59	1.6	12.14
Tunisia	10.5	6.95	1.04	9.99	2.0	17.70

Source: data from World Bank, *World Development Indicators and Global Development Finance*, 2012, Copyright © 2013 The World Bank Group, All Rights Reserved. Available from http://databank.worldbank.org/data/home.aspx.

number of megacities has grown from two in 1950 to 20 in 2005 (Population Division 2005). In 2011, 23 urban agglomerations qualified as megacities because they had at least 10 million inhabitants (Population Division 2011). By 2025 there will be 37 megacities globally, with about 13.6 per cent of the urban population of the world living in them, up from 9.9 per cent today (Population Division 2011). Thus the public health implications of this trend will be highly significant (International Risk Governance Council 2010).

Urban health is influenced by major factors such as standards of urban governance, population characteristics, natural and built environment, social and economic environment, food security and quality, services and health emergency management (WHO and UN-HABITAT 2010). WHO, through the Commission on Social Determinants of Health (2008), has urged policymakers to place health equity at the heart of urban governance and planning, as

'cities can also concentrate threats to health' (WHO 2010a). WHO highlighted urban health issues including substandard housing and crowded living conditions, problems with food and water safety, inadequate sanitation and solid waste disposal services, air pollution, and congested traffic (WHO and UN-HABITAT 2010). It was also stressed that chronic diseases and mental problems resulting from unhealthy lifestyles such as unhealthy diets, sedentary behaviours, smoking, alcohol, and other substance abuse are increasingly concentrated in the urban poor (Chan 2010). Public health risks and hazards can be concentrated in urban areas, as poverty has become heavily concentrated in cities (UN-HABITAT 2010). To summarize, cities face a triple threat: infectious diseases, NCDs, and injuries resulting from accidents, violence, and crime. These public health risks are aggravated in rapid, unplanned urbanization and with growing poverty in the urban slums of many middle-income countries. An estimated 828 million people,

Table 1.4.5 Urban population statistics in middle-income countries

Country	Population in largest city (million)	Urban population growth (annual %)	Urban population (% of total)	Megacities (2011)
Brazil	20.3	1.41	86.5	2
China	16.6	2.54	44.9	4
India	22.2	2.32	30.1	3
Indonesia	9.2	3.14	53.7	0
Jordan	1.1	2.26	78.5	0
Malaysia	1.5	2.89	72.2	0
Mexico	19.5	1.62	77.8	1
Russia	10.5	−0.10	72.8	1
South Africa	3.7	2.13	61.7	0
Thailand	7	1.61	34	0
Tunisia	0.8	1.64	67.3	0

Source: data from World Bank, *World Development Indicators and Global Development Finance*, 2012, Copyright © 2013 The World Bank Group, All Rights Reserved. Available from http://databank.worldbank.org/data/home.aspx.

one-third of the world's urban population, live in slum conditions, of which the vast majority of slums—more than 90 per cent—are located in the fastest growing cities of developing countries (Population Division 2007). It is of public health concern that slum dwellers experience different forms of deprivation (material, physical, social, and political) and poor access to health and other services (WHO and UN-HABITAT 2010).

The Millennium Development Goal (MDG) 7 includes a target of improving the lives of at least 100 million slum dwellers by 2020. This target has already been achieved earlier than expected and the proportion living in slums has apparently declined. According to UN-HABITAT, China and India had lifted at least 125 million people out of slum conditions between 2000 and 2010. They are the most successful countries in improving the lives of slum dwellers. Indonesia and Tunisia have also succeeded in lifting a large proportion of the population out of slum conditions (UN-HABITAT 2010). However, the absolute number of slum dwellers has risen since rapid urbanization continues to outpace slum improvements, and therefore, new and more realistic national and local targets might be required (United Nations 2011).

In addition to urbanization, internal migration is another public health challenge facing transitional countries. Some studies have pointed out inequality as a major factor driving both permanent and circular internal migration in Asian countries (Overseas Development Institute 2006). The report also highlights circular migration resulting from a lack of security in the country of destination which prevents people from settling down (Overseas Development Institute 2006). It also stressed the two-way relationship between migration and inequality, both within the poorer sending areas and between poor and rich regions (Overseas Development Institute 2006).

Recent studies on migration and health have pointed out the lack of policy coherence in addressing migration-related health issues. They revealed that most policies are narrowly focused although health intervention opportunities exist at each phase of the migratory process, including pre-departure, travel, destination, interception (temporary detention, interim residence by immigration control), and return (Zimmerman et al. 2011). Poor people continue to migrate despite restrictive policies, as in the case of China. Although these migrations can lead to higher productivity, higher income, and economic growth, migrants are usually excluded socially, economically, and politically. Their access to health, education, housing, sanitation, protection from exploitation, child care, and schooling are limited. Migrant children, adolescent girls, and women are particularly vulnerable to exploitation and infectious diseases (Overseas Development Institute 2006).

The International Organization for Migration has detailed many challenges, including health-related issues such as poor health status, environmental health and sanitation, lack of access to health services, and vulnerability to infectious diseases including HIV/AIDS, facing internal and cross-border migrants (International Organization for Migration 2008). All of these factors can have negative impacts, either direct or indirect, on migrants' health and their access to health services.

Health indicators in middle-income countries

From a cursory overview of health indicators in middle-income countries, there are discernible comparisons. Life expectancy at birth is generally between the 60s to 70s age range, except for South Africa which is in the low 50s and also has a very high maternal mortality ratio averaging 300. Similarly, countries including India and Indonesia with high maternal mortality also have high rates of infant, neonatal, and under-5 mortality. Conversely, countries with lower maternal mortality generally have lower child mortality and adolescent fertility rates (see Table 1.4.6).

Communicable diseases in middle-income countries

While it is true that, on the whole, the proportion of deaths from communicable disease in middle-income countries is decreasing

Table 1.4.6 Health indicators in middle-income countries

Country	Life expectancy at birth	Maternal mortality ratio[b]	Neonatal mortality rate[c]	Infant mortality rate[c]	Under 5 mortality rate[c]	Adolescent fertility rate[d]
Brazil	73.1	56 (36–85)	12	17.3	19.4	75.8
China	73.3	37 (23–58)	11	15.8	18.4	8.8
India	65.1	200 (140–310)	32	48.2	62.7	79.3
Indonesia	68.9	220 (130–350)	17	27.2	35.3	43.5
Jordan	73.3	63 (37–110)	13	18.4	21.7	24.8
Malaysia	74.0	29 (12–64)	3	5.4	6.3	11.6
Mexico	76.7	50 (44–56)	7	14.1	16.7	67.5
Russia	68.8	34 (26–42)	6	9.1	11.6	25.9
S. Africa	52.1	300 (150–500)	18	40.7	56.6	53.9
Thailand	73.9	48 (33–70)	8	11.2	13	39.5
Tunisia	74.6	56 (29–110)	9	13.8	16.1	4.9
UMI[a]	72.8	53.2	10.7	16.5	19.6	28.8

Notes:

[a] Upper-middle-income countries' group aggregate, World Bank 2010.

[b] Per 100,000 live births, Global Health Observatory Data Repository, 2010 estimates.

[c] Per 1000 live births, World Bank 2010.

[d] Births per 1000 women with age between 15 and 19, World Bank 2010.

Source: data from World Bank, *World Development Indicators and Global Development Finance,* 2012, Copyright © 2013 The World Bank Group, All Rights Reserved. Available from http://databank.worldbank.org/data/home.aspx.

as mortality due to NCDs rises (Heuveline et al. 2002; Miranda et al. 2008), communicable diseases remain a major public health challenge in these countries. Understanding communicable disease trends in middle-income countries is complex, because of the wide range of per capita incomes (O'Brien 2007) and differing health development challenges. Even within a given country, the health problems faced by the poorest 20 per cent are very different than those in the wealthiest 20 per cent. Because of this, it is possible for a single middle-income country to face a *double burden of disease*, with an increasing prevalence of NCDs despite the persistence of infectious diseases. This is particularly problematic for lower middle-income countries, where limited resources may be redirected to address the relative increase in NCDs and away from communicable disease control programmes. This would be a mistake, as the successes achieved in combating some of the most prominent communicable diseases, including tuberculosis, HIV/AIDS, and malaria can be quickly reversed.

Communicable diseases in decline in middle-income countries

The 1970s were a time of optimism that control of infectious diseases globally was at last within reach (WHO 2000). High rates of immunization against a number of childhood diseases, including diphtheria, measles, and tetanus, had had a significant impact on reducing child mortality; smallpox was at last on the verge of eradication; and a cocktail of effective antituberculosis medications made elimination seem a possibility. The emergence of the novel human immunodeficiency virus (HIV) in the 1980s, however, as well as growing resistance of tuberculosis to

available medications, provided a sombre reminder that the fight was far from over. The resurgence of previously contained infectious diseases and the increase in hospital-based antibiotic resistance provided further evidence that current containment and treatment strategies might not be sufficient for long-term control. Although the groundbreaking Global Burden of Disease (GBD) study, commissioned in 1990, proclaimed that the Group I causes of death (referring to the combination of communicable disease, maternal and perinatal disease, and nutritional deficiencies) were no longer responsible for the majority of deaths in developing regions (Murray and Lopez 1996), the World Health Report of 1996 reminded the global health community that communicable disease still played a very large role in morbidity and mortality, particularly in low- and middle-income countries (WHO 1996). This tension continues today: while the 2008 revision to the GBD, published in cooperation with the World Health Organization (WHO) and World Bank, reveals that the weight of communicable diseases among the top ten causes of death is relatively less in MICs than in low-income countries (see Tables 1.4.7 and 1.4.8), the fact remains that four of the ten leading causes of death in middle-income countries are due to an infectious cause.

A closer look at the three communicable diseases that have had the most significant health impacts worldwide helps to illustrate the overall decline of communicable disease in middle-income countries over the past decade.

HIV/AIDS

Since its identification in 1984, HIV/AIDS has caused more than 25 million deaths around the world. WHO estimates that

Table 1.4.7 Top ten causes of death in low-income countries

Cause	Deaths in millions	% of deaths
Lower respiratory infections	1.05	11.3
Diarrhoeal diseases	0.76	8.2
HIV/AIDS	0.72	7.8
Ischaemic heart disease	0.57	6.1
Malaria	0.48	5.2
Stroke and other cerebrovascular disease	0.45	4.9
Tuberculosis	0.4	4.3
Prematurity or low birth weight	0.3	3.2
Birth asphyxia and birth trauma	0.27	2.9
Neonatal infections	0.24	2.6

Reproduced with permission from World Health Organization, *The Top 10 Causes of Death*, Fact sheet No. 310, Copyright © WHO 2013, available from: www.who.int/mediacentre/factsheets/fs310/en/index.html.

Table 1.4.8 Top ten causes of death in middle-income countries

Cause	Deaths in millions	% of deaths
Ischaemic heart disease	5.27	13.7
Stroke and other cerebrovascular disease	4.91	12.8
Chronic obstructive pulmonary disease	2.79	7.2
Lower respiratory infections	2.07	5.4
Diarrhoeal diseases	1.68	4.4
HIV/AIDS	1.03	2.7
Road traffic accidents	0.94	2.4
Tuberculosis	0.93	2.4
Diabetes mellitus	0.87	2.3
Hypertensive heart disease	0.83	2.2

Reproduced with permission from World Health Organization, *The Top 10 Causes of Death*, Fact sheet No. 310, Copyright © WHO 2013, available from: www.who.int/mediacentre/factsheets/fs310/en/index.html.

approximately 34 million people are currently living with HIV. In low- and middle-income countries, more than 8 million people living with HIV were receiving life-saving antiretroviral therapy (ART), over half of those eligible (UNAIDS 2012a; WHO 2012a). Although still far below international goals, this has resulted in important achievements:

- A twentyfold increase in the number of people in developing countries receiving ART in less than a decade (2003–2011) (WHO 2012a).

- An overall decrease in global AIDS-related deaths from 2.3 million in 2005 to 1.7 million in 2011(UNAIDS 2012a).

- A more than 25 per cent decline in the rate of new HIV infections between 2001 and 2009, with above-average declines in

sub-Saharan Africa and South and South East Asia (UNAIDS 2012a).

HIV/AIDS disproportionately affects sub-Saharan Africa, the home to many low- and middle-income countries. In fact, the 20 countries with the highest HIV prevalence in 2009 were all in Africa. Of these, half were middle-income countries (UNAIDS 2012b). The top three countries with the highest absolute numbers of people living with HIV/AIDS are in South Africa, Nigeria, and India (Central Intelligence Agency 2012). The good news, however, is that of the ten middle-income countries amongst the top 20 countries for HIV prevalence rates, prevalence has decreased or remained stable in all but two since 2000 (UNAIDS 2012c). Outside Africa, middle-income countries are showing improvement as well. In India, estimated HIV prevalence decreased from 0.4 to 0.3 per cent between 2000 and 2009 (National AIDS Control Organisation 2011); it remained stable in Brazil at less than 0.1 per cent; and decreased significantly in Thailand, from 1.8 to 1.3 per cent (UNAIDS 2012d). Over that same period, however, the estimated prevalence of HIV increased from approximately 0.6 to 1.0 per cent in Russia, another highly populated middle-income country (UNAIDS 2012d); a reminder that the experience of middle-income countries in responding to infectious disease remains variable and heavily dependent on existing healthcare structures and systems.

Tuberculosis

Tuberculosis accounted for 1.4 million deaths in 2011, second only to HIV/AIDS for deaths due to communicable disease globally (WHO 2013a).The massive expansion worldwide of standardized tuberculosis diagnosis and treatment programmes (including directly observed therapy, short course, commonly referred to as DOTS) has resulted in a number of concrete successes:

- Worldwide incidence was estimated to peak in 2004, and has been gradually declining since, meeting MDG 6 (Lönnroth et al. 2010).

- Globally, more than 36 million people were cured between 1995 and 2008, with an estimated 6 million deaths avoided during that time (Lönnroth et al. 2010; Lawn and Zumla 2011).

- The case fatality rate during that period dropped by half, from 8 per cent to 4 per cent (Lönnroth et al. 2010).

It is important to recognize that the rapid increase in the world's population, particularly in middle-income countries such as China and India, means that the overall burden of tuberculosis in terms of incident cases and absolute number of deaths globally continues to increase, even though global incidence and per capita death rates have declined (Lönnroth et al. 2010). Additionally, low- and middle-income countries are disproportionately affected, accounting for 95 per cent of tuberculosis deaths. Of the 22 countries considered to have a high burden of tuberculosis, together claiming more than 80 per cent of cases worldwide, half are middle-income countries (Lönnroth et al. 2010).

The good news is that yearly incidence and estimated prevalence is stable or decreasing in nearly all of these 11 high-burden middle-income countries, with the notable exceptions of South African and Nigeria (Lönnroth et al. 2010), where tuberculosis control is complicated by very high prevalence of HIV/AIDS. The estimated death rate due to tuberculosis is generally decreasing, with significant declines noted in death rate between

1990 and 2008 in the following countries: Brazil, China, India, Indonesia, Pakistan, Russia, and Vietnam (Lönnroth et al. 2010). Similarly, the treatment success rate for new sputum-smear positive cases has met the MDG target of 85 per cent in most of these same countries, with the exception of Russia and Vietnam (Lönnroth et al. 2010). Russia's difficulty meeting the MDG target for treatment is due in large part to the very high rate of multi-drug-resistant tuberculosis (MDR-TB) there, the highest in the world at 13 per cent (Lönnroth et al. 2010). Of the 11 heavily burdened MICs, five suffer from MDR-TB rates greater than 2 per cent, with Russia, China, and India most heavily affected (Lönnroth et al. 2010).

Malaria

Malaria is the world's most deadly vector-borne disease and remains *endemic* in 106 countries as of 2010, of which 61 are middle-income countries (Roll Back Malaria 2010; WHO 2011a). Nearly half the world's population (approximately 3.3 billion) was estimated to be at risk for malaria in 2010, with an incidence rate of 219 million (WHO 2013b). Heavy investment of global development aid in highly cost-effective malaria interventions, including rapid diagnostic testing, insecticide treated nets (ITNs) and artemisinin-based combination therapies (ACTs), has resulted in substantial public health gains (WHO 2013b). Since 2000:

* malaria mortality rates have fallen more than 25 per cent globally (WHO 2011a)
* 43 of the 99 countries with ongoing malaria transmission reported greater than 50 per cent decreases in malaria incidence; an additional eight countries reported greater than 25 per cent decreases (WHO 2011a).

Where do the middle-income countries stand? On one end of the spectrum, the group of countries most heavily burdened by malaria and accounting for over 60 per cent of malaria deaths—Burkina Faso, Côte d'Ivoire, the Democratic Republic of Congo, Mali, Mozambique, and Nigeria—includes two middle-income countries (Nigeria and Côte d'Ivoire). At the other end, three of the four countries to become certified by WHO as free of malaria in the past 5 years were middle-income countries (Armenia, Morocco, and Turkmenistan) (WHO 2011a). As a group, the middle-income countries are showing significant progress in decreasing malaria incidence. While the majority of these countries remain in the control phase, one (Iraq) is in the prevention of re-introduction phase, four are in the elimination phase, and another nine are in the pre-elimination phase (WHO 2012b). Unsurprisingly, the countries in the elimination and pre-elimination phases have shown the most drastic reductions in malaria incidence since 2000; with the addition of successes in a number of countries still in the control phase, well over half the malaria-endemic middle-income countries reported decreases in malaria cases during that period. Indeed, even some middle-income countries in the control phase, such as Namibia and Nicaragua, reported decreases greater than 50 per cent (WHO 2012b).

As with tuberculosis, rising rates of drug resistance prove a significant challenge for global malaria control, including in middle-income countries. In fact, the origin of artemisinin-resistant *Plasmodium falciparum* malaria was on the border between Thailand, an upper-middle-income country, and Cambodia; this resistant form is now also suspected in Vietnam (another middle-income country) and Myanmar (WHO 2012c).

Emerging and re-emerging infectious diseases

An *emerging infectious disease* is a *pathogen* that is newly recognized as causing disease in humans. The term *re-emerging infectious disease* refers to an infectious disease already known to affect humans but which has expanded its potential range, whether by significantly increasing in incidence, re-entering a human population where it had previously been eliminated, infecting a geographic area not previously affected, or acquiring antimicrobial resistance (WHO n.d.). While any type of pathogen may infect humans, viruses are most likely to emerge as novel infectious diseases (Taylor et al. 2001; Woolhouse and Gowtage-Sequeria 2005) (see Chapter 8.17).

Factors leading to the emergence and re-emergence of infectious diseases

Several factors favour the development of emerging or re-emerging infectious diseases, of which human population growth and increasing density are two of the most important. Urbanization, characterized by large numbers of people living in close proximity and highly mobile populations, similarly poses risks for the emergence of new disease. Three-quarters of all emerging and re-emerging infectious diseases are thought to be *zoonotic* (Taylor et al. 2001), hence agriculture, animal husbandry and other food production, human encroachment on wild animal territories, deforestation, and water and sanitation all play a role in the potential for new zoonotic infections. Finally, healthcare practices at all levels, including global and national healthcare systems, pharmaceutical production, diagnosis, treatment, and patient behaviour, are important factors in the development of drug resistance.

Emerging and re-emerging infections in middle-income countries: the case of South East Asia

South East Asia, a geographic region made up of 11 countries, is a particular hotspot for emerging infectious diseases, as it acts as a melting pot for all of the factors that drive emergence. It is also the home of seven MICs: Indonesia, Philippines, Timor-Leste, Vietnam, Malaysia, Lao PDR, and Thailand. South East Asia as a whole, and Thailand and Indonesia (of the middle-income countries) in particular, were heavily impacted by the *SARS* (severe acute respiratory syndrome) epidemic in 2003 (Coker et al. 2011). When the *avian influenza A H5N1*, initially passed from birds to humans, broke out shortly after, there were concerns that it would similarly cause a pandemic; however, human-to-human transmission proved minimal so far. Although less publicized, the emergence of *Nipah virus* in Malaysia and Singapore in 1998 proved to be more deadly than SARS. The virus, which originated in pigs and causes severe febrile encephalitis with a case fatality rate of around 40 per cent, resulted in more than 100 deaths in these two countries (Lo and Rota 2008).

Middle-income countries in South East Asia are particularly vulnerable to the development of re-emerging infectious diseases, as well; indeed, South East Asia has been called the epicentre of antimalarial resistance. Artemisinin-resistant malaria emerged recently on the Thailand–Cambodia border, which was also the site of the emergence of chloroquine and sulphadoxine-pyrimethamine resistance in *P. falciparum* in the 1950s and 1960s (Coker et al. 2011).

All these underscore the need for stronger *surveillance systems*. These may take a variety of forms, including syndromic surveillance to identify both known and potentially novel infections;

surveillance for drug-resistance in known pathogens; and animal health surveillance. Since the emergence of SARS and H5N1, great attention has been paid toward strengthening communicable disease control in South East Asia. In Laos, for example, the government established multiple national institutions to strengthen infectious disease control, including a Centre for Laboratory and Epidemiology and a National Emerging Infectious Disease Control Office (Phommasack et al. 2012). Similarly, all the middle-income countries in South East Asia aside from Timor-Leste, are making concrete investments in strengthening their healthcare systems to more rapidly identify, contain, and control communicable diseases (Coker et al. 2011).

Challenges and possibilities for surveillance in middle-income countries

The surveillance strategies employed by middle-income countries are as varied as the group itself. Broadly, in the poorer middle-income countries, surveillance often comes behind more pressing health needs. The continuity required for a successful surveillance programme can be difficult to achieve in settings where resources are scarce and/or unpredictable. Inadequate or unevenly distributed laboratory services hinder active surveillance in some middle-income countries. Documentation of illness also varies greatly across and between countries, complicating attempts at passive surveillance.

Despite the concerns of its critics, syndromic surveillance holds potential for useful application in middle-income countries. The use of syndromic surveillance to strengthen existing measures globally was endorsed in the most recent revision of the *International Health Regulations* (IHR), internationally ratified guidelines for infectious disease notification. Specifically, the revised IHR recommend surveillance for acute respiratory syndrome, acute gastrointestinal syndrome, neurological syndrome, haemorrhagic fever, and novel severe infectious illness (World Health Assembly 2005). A number of middle-income countries have already successfully employed syndromic surveillance systems.

Non-communicable diseases in middle-income countries

With the exception of African region, the number of deaths from NCDs exceeds that from infectious diseases, maternal, perinatal conditions, and nutritional deficiencies combined. Of the estimated 57 million global deaths in 2008, 36 million (63 per cent) were due to NCDs. In 2008, around 80 per cent of all NCD deaths (29 million) occurred in low- and middle-income countries. In addition, a higher proportion (48 per cent) of all NCD deaths in low- and middle-income countries is estimated to occur in people under the age of 70 years—compared with an estimated 26 per cent in high-income countries and a global average of 44 per cent (WHO 2012d).

Top non-communicable diseases and risk factors

The leading causes of NCD deaths are cardiovascular disease, cancers, and chronic respiratory diseases. Over 80 per cent of cardiovascular and diabetes deaths, about 90 per cent of deaths from chronic obstructive pulmonary disease, and over two-thirds

of all cancer deaths occur in low- and middle-income countries (WHO 2010b). In low- and middle-income countries, 29 per cent of NCD deaths occur among people under the age of 60, compared to 13 per cent in high-income countries. The estimated percentage increase in cancer incidence by 2030, compared with 2008, will be greater in low- (82 per cent) and lower-middle-income countries (70 per cent) compared with the upper-middle- (58 per cent) and high-income countries (40 per cent) (WHO 2010b). Inadequate political commitment, insufficient engagement of non-health sectors, lack of resources, vested interests of critical constituencies, and limited engagement of key stakeholders have resulted in poor NCD prevention (WHO 2010b). WHO also pointed out that appropriate care for people with NCDs is lacking in low- and middle-income countries and populations (WHO 2010b).

Behavioural risk factors, including tobacco use, physical inactivity, unhealthy diet, and the harmful use of alcohol, are indicated to be responsible for about 80 per cent of coronary heart disease and cerebrovascular disease. Behavioural risk factors are associated with four key metabolic and/or physiological changes—raised blood pressure, increased weight leading to obesity, hyperglycaemia, and hyperlipidaemia. Every year, nearly 6 million people die from direct tobacco use and second-hand smoke. For the total population, smoking prevalence is highest among upper-middle-income countries (WHO 2010b). Tobacco use has declined in developed countries while it is rising rapidly in most developing countries, including middle-income countries. Studies from Brazil, China, India, South Africa, Vietnam, and Central America now show an inverse relationship: the prevalence of smoking is higher in low than high socioeconomic groups (WHO 2010c). Smoking rates are also rising rapidly among women, especially affluent urban young women in China, India, and Singapore (WHO 2010c). Approximately 2.3 million die each year from the harmful use of alcohol. While adult per capita consumption is highest in high-income countries, it is nearly as high in the populous upper-middle-income countries (WHO 2010b).

At least 2.8 million people die each year as a result of being overweight or obese which increase risks of heart disease, certain cancers, strokes, and diabetes (WHO 2010b). The prevalence of overweight is highest in upper-middle-income countries (WHO 2010b). Globalization and rapid urbanization have resulted in shifts towards diets high in sugar, fats, salt, and highly refined food. A recent review based on 14 surveys conducted between 1982 and 2003 in lower- to middle-income countries (Brazil, Chile, China, Cuba, India, Lithuania, Peru, Russian Federation, Samoa, and South Africa) showed the burden of obesity shifting towards individuals of lower socioeconomic status as a country's gross national product increased (Monteiro et al. 2004). This pattern is found at both individual and community level (WHO 2010c). Recent studies in Sri Lanka and India confirmed positive association, in both genders, between urbanicity and common modifiable risk factors for chronic diseases including smoking, low physical activity, low fruit and vegetable consumption, high body mass index, and high blood pressure (Allender et al. 2010, 2011).

Marketing activities for tobacco, alcohol, and junk food increasingly target people in developing countries and emerging economies (WHO 2010b). Many governments are not coping with this through policies, legislation, services, and infrastructure that could help protect their citizens from NCDs (WHO 2010b). One report estimated that losses in national income from heart disease, stroke, and diabetes in 2005 were US $18 billion in China, US $11 billion in the Russian Federation, US $9 billion in India, and US $3 billion in Brazil (WHO 2005). A macroeconomic analysis demonstrated that each 10 per cent rise in NCDs is associated with 0.5 per cent lower rate of annual economic growth (Stuckler 2008). From 2005–2015, China and India are projected to lose International $ (I$) 558 billion (0.93 per cent of the GDP) and I$ 237 billion (1.5 per cent of the GDP) respectively as a result of heart disease, strokes, and diabetes (WHO 2010b). Significant losses are also estimated for other countries. By 2025, the total direct and indirect costs from overweight and obesity alone among Chinese adults are projected to exceed 9 per cent of China's gross national product (Popkin et al. 2006). Infants and young children are getting more overweight in upper- and lower-middle-income countries than those in upper-income countries.

Selected country case: Thailand

In Thailand, according to a study by the Thai Ministry of Public Health comparing disease burden between 1999 and 2004, there was an increase in disability-adjusted life years (DALYs) due to NCDs (stroke, cancers, cardiovascular disease, chronic obstructive pulmonary disease, diabetes, cirrhosis) and mental health problems (alcohol dependence, depression) (Bundhamcharoen 2011). The study also reported a decrease in DALYs due to infectious diseases and maternal and nutritional deficiencies. Fig. 1.4.2 shows the dramatic increase in hospitalization for diabetes and heart diseases in Thailand over the last two decades (WHO 2011b).

Health systems development in middle-income countries

The pressures placed on national healthcare systems in many middle-income countries by recent demographic and epidemiological transitions are amplified by the growing demands of a more educated and affluent population for high-quality healthcare and the latest medical technologies. The demand from the expanding middle class in many higher-middle-income countries has fuelled a booming private healthcare sector. Rapid economic development is also requiring tremendous social, behavioural, and policy adjustments, and certain demographic, epidemiological,

and socioeconomic shifts are particularly accelerated for many middle-income countries. The delivery, financing, and regulatory functions of the public health system must adapt accordingly to such rapid societal changes. The need to restructure healthcare systems becomes even more critical for balancing such new demand and supply pressures (Phua and Chew 2002).

Most middle-income countries have built up capacity for basic health service delivery, according to the World Bank. They are now focusing more on the issues of universal health coverage, financial protection, and health system efficiency which face technical, institutional, and political challenges (Kremer and Besra 2002). They also face similar pressures of rising costs caused by demographic, epidemiological, and technological change; large out-of-pocket payments; inequitable and ineffective health financing systems; and inefficiencies in the healthcare system. The World Bank pointed out the need for improving equity and efficiency in tax-raising, resource mobilization, and risk pooling mechanisms to achieve universal coverage in middle-income countries. There are concerns over low-risk pooling and fragmentation which affects healthcare purchasing efficiency and equity. Fragmentation of health systems also hampers consistent policy focus and efficiency on both risk pooling and purchasing grounds. Improved pooling of out-of-pocket payments can provide middle-income countries with opportunities to mobilize substantial private resources in expanding in the risk pool. Health expenditure per capita has steadily increased in most of the middle-income countries (see Table 1.4.9).

The proportion of health expenditure by out-of-pocket payments (or direct payments) has declined in a few upper-middle-income countries, but such modes of payment still constitute a substantial proportion of health expenditure in middle-income countries. Direct payments can discourage early healthcare seeking, as many people who do seek treatment and have to pay for it at the point of delivery suffer severe financial difficulties as a consequence. The reduction in the incidence of financial hardship associated with direct payments is a key indicator of progress towards universal coverage (United Nations 2002; WHO 2002).

Examples of health system reforms in middle-income countries are discussed in World Bank publications (Gottret and Schieber 2006) and the World Health Report (WHO 2010d). Some success

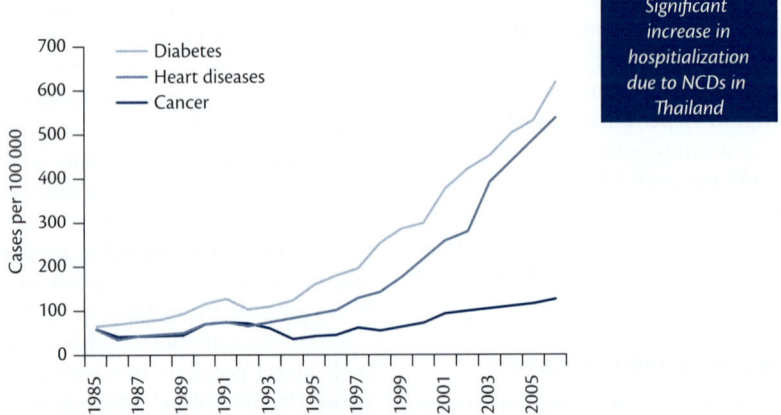

Fig. 1.4.2 Hospitalization rates for NCDs in Thailand.

Reproduced with permission from World Health Organization, *Non-communicable diseases in the South-East Asia Region: Situation and response 2011*, World Health Organization, Geneva, Switzerland, Copyright © 2011, available from http://apps.searo.who.int/pds_docs/B4793.pdf with data from Thai Health Profile, 2005–2007.

Table 1.4.9 Health expenditure in middle-income countries, 2010

Country	Health expenditure per capita (PPP constant 2005 Int $)	OOP[a] (% of total expenditure on health)	OOP[a] (% of private expenditure on health)	Health expenditure (% of government expenditure)	Public health expenditure (% of total health expenditure)
Brazil	1028.3	30.60	57.76	7.1	47.0
China	378.9	36.59	78.86	12.1	53.6
India	132.2	61.16	86.35	3.6	29.2
Indonesia	112.1	38.25	75.13	7.8	49.1
Jordan	448.4	25.11	77.64	18.6	67.7
Malaysia	641.1	34.17	76.81	9.2	55.5
Mexico	959.3	47.13	92.25	12.1	48.9
Russia	998.4	31.40	82.78	8.0	62.1
South Africa	934.9	16.57	29.64	11.9	44.1
Thailand	329.7	13.92	55.77	12.7	75.0
Tunisia	482.9	39.77	87.03	10.7	54.3
UMI[b]	594.2	33.38	76.38	NA	54.3

Notes:

[a]Out-of-pocket health expenditure (interchangeably used with the term 'direct payment' in WHO reports).

[b]Upper-middle-income group aggregate.

Source: data from World Bank, *World Development Indicators and Global Development Finance*, 2012, Copyright © 2013 The World Bank Group, All Rights Reserved. Available from http://databank.worldbank.org/data/home.aspx.

stories include those of Thailand, Brazil, Tunisia, Mexico, and Columbia (WHO 2002). China has embarked on ambitious plans to provide 'safe, effective, convenient and affordable health services' to all urban and rural residents by 2020. This is part of the reforms to address the high proportion of direct payments caused by earlier market-based approaches (WHO 2002). A series of reforms has included the New Cooperative Medical Schemes, initiated in 2003 to meet the needs of rural populations, and the Urban Residents Basic Medical Insurance scheme, piloted in 79 cities in 2007 (WHO 2002). While low-income countries are still struggling to raise sufficient resources to fund essential healthcare, countries in the middle-income group are focusing on a somewhat different set of priorities. With the ability to deliver basic health services, most middle-income countries are increasingly turning their attention to the issues of universal health coverage, financial protection, and health system efficiency. These objectives require an overhaul of the current financing structures—a prospect that raises technical, institutional, and political challenges (Peabody et al. 1999).

Conclusion: investing in cost-effective public health in middle-income countries

The economies of middle-income countries face significant health challenges in the decades ahead. While communicable diseases, including HIV/AIDS, remain a serious problem, the central health issue is that all countries face a rapid rise in chronic diseases such as cancer, diabetes, and cardiovascular diseases. The rise in chronic diseases will cause suffering and premature loss of life; they are also costly to diagnose and treat, and will impose new pressures

on health budgets. The combination of increasing chronic disease and rapid population changes creates an unprecedented challenge for many middle-income economies. An essential element in the response to this challenge to growth and financial sustainability will need to be substantial but well-planned investments in health systems, perhaps of a scale not previously contemplated (WHO 2005).

In some middle-income countries, inequality in access to health services has been exacerbated by the high reliance on private resources for health financing. This heavy reliance on meeting health costs from private incomes is common to many middle-income countries (e.g. China, Indonesia, Vietnam, and the Philippines, where less than 30 per cent of health costs are meet by the public sector). It contrasts sharply with the situation in developed countries and is the most notable difference in funding structure between the two groups of economies. A recent major review of studies investigating the performance of private and public sector delivery in low- and middle-income countries suggested that providers in the private sector more frequently violated medical standards of practice and had poorer patient outcomes, but had greater reported timeliness and hospitality to patients. Reported efficiency tended to be lower in the private than in the public sector, resulting in part from perverse incentives for unnecessary testing and treatment, whereas public sector services experienced more limited availability of equipment, medications, and trained healthcare workers. Competition for funding appeared between the two sectors, such that public funds and personnel were redirected to private sector development, followed by reductions in public sector service budgets and staff. The conclusions of the review do not support the claim that the private sector is more efficient, accountable, or medically effective than the public sector, but the public sector appears to frequently lack timeliness and hospitality towards patients (Basu et al. 2012).

Role of prevention, early detection, and early intervention

Given the human, economic, and financial costs of chronic diseases, there is a strong case for increased investment in prevention and early detection and intervention: preventive programmes, including lifestyle changes and health promotion based on known risk factors (such as smoking, alcohol use, obesity, and raised blood lipid levels) and systematic monitoring of such risk factors; expanded vaccination programmes, with older proven vaccines or new ones for the emerging infectious diseases; and screening to identify and treat early preconditions for NCDs. Middle-income countries face the challenges of growing domestic capability to be able to benefit from economic progress and biomedical science research innovations, and to meet the challenge of chronic diseases and rapidly ageing populations.

References

Allender, S., Lacey, B., Webster, P., et al. (2010). Level of urbanization and noncommunicable disease risk factors in Tamil Nadu, India. *Bulletin of the World Health Organization*, 88, 297–304.

Allender, S., Wickramasinghe, K., Goldacre, M., Matthews, D., and Katulanda, P. (2011). Quantifying urbanization as a risk factor for noncommunicable disease. *Journal of Urban Health*, 88, 906–18.

Asian Development Bank (2011). Asian Development Outlook 2011 Update: Preparing for Demographic Transition. Philippines: Asian Development Bank.

Avafia, T. and Narasimhan, S.M. (2006). *The TRIPS Agreement and Access to ARVs*. New York: United Nations Development Programme.

Basu, S., Andrews, J., Kishore, S., Panjabi, R., and Stuckler, D. (2012). Comparative performance of private and public healthcare systems in low- and middle-income countries: a systematic review. *PLoS Medicine*, 9(6), e1001244.

Bettcher, D.W., Yach, D., and Guindon, G.E. (2000). Global trade and health: key linkages and future challenges. *Bulletin of the World Health Organization*, 78, 521–34.

Bhargava, A., Jamison, D., Lau, L., and Murray, C. (2001). Modeling the effect of health on economic growth. *Journal of Health Economics*, 20(3), 423–40.

Bundhamcharoen, K., Odton, P., Phulkerd, S., and Tangcharoensathien, V. (2011). Burden of disease in Thailand: changes in health gap between 1999 and 2004. *BMC Public Health*, 11, 53.

Central Intelligence Agency (2012). *CIA World Factbook*. [Online] Available at: https://www.cia.gov/library/publications/the-world-factbook/.

Challu, P. (1991). Patenting pharmaceutical products: consequences. *World Competition (Law and Economics Review)*, 15(2), 65–126.

Chaloupka, F. and Corbett, M. (1998). Trade policy and tobacco: towards an optimal policy mix. In I. Abedian, R. van der Merwe, N. Wilkins, and P. Jha (eds.) *The Economics of Tobacco Control: Towards an Optimal Policy Mix*, pp. 129–45. Cape Town: University of Cape Town.

Chan, M. (2010). *Urban Health Threatened by Inequities*. [Online] Available at: http://www.who.int/dg/speeches/2010/urban_health_20100407/en/index.html.

Coker, R.J., Hunter, B.M., Rudge, J.W., Liverani, M., and Hanvoravongchai, P. (2011). Emerging infectious diseases in southeast Asia: regional challenges to control. *The Lancet*, 377, 599–609.

Commission on Social Determinants of Health (2008). *Closing the Gap in a Generation: Health Equity Through Action on the Social Determinants of Health*. Geneva: WHO.

Connolly, G.N. (1992). Worldwide expansion of transnational tobacco industry. *Journal of National Cancer Institute*, 12, 29–35.

Drager, N. and Fidler, D.P. (2004). *GATS and Health Related Services*. Geneva: WHO.

Gaulier, G., Lemoine, F., and Ünal, D. (2009). *EU15 Trade with Emerging Economies and Rentier States: Leveraging Geography*. Paris: Centre d'Etudes Prospectives et d'Informations Internationales.

Gottret, P. and Schieber, G. (2006). *Health Financing Revisited: A Practitioner's Guide*. New York: The World Bank.

Heuveline, P., Guillot, M., and Gwatkin, D. (2002). The uneven tides of the health transition. *Social Science & Medicine* 55, 313–22.

International Monetary Fund (2000). *Transition Economies: An IMF Perspective on Progress and Prospects*. [Online] Available at: http://www.imf.org/external/np/exr/ib/2000/110300.htm.

International Organization for Migration (2008). *World Migration Report 2008*. Geneva: International Organization for Migration.

International Risk Governance Council (2010). *Emerging Risks in Megacities*. [Online] Available at: http://www.irgc.org/IMG/pdf/Emerging_risks_Megacities.pdf.

Jamison, D., Lau, L., and Wang, J. (2004). *Health's Contribution to Economic Growth in an Environment of Partially Endogenous Technical Progress*. Disease control priorities project working paper No. 10. Bethesda, MD: Fogarty International Center. Available at: <http://www.fic.nih.gov/dcpp>.

Kremer, L. and Besra, G.S. (2002). Re-emergence of tuberculosis: strategies and treatment. *Expert Opinion on Investigational Drugs*, 11, 153–7.

Labonte, R. and Sanger, M. (2006). Glossary of the World Trade Organization and public health. *Journal of Epidemiology and Community Health*, 60, 655–61.

Lawn, S.D. and Zumla, A.I. (2011). Tuberculosis. *The Lancet*, 378, 57–72.

Lo, M.K. and Rota, P.A. (2008). The emergence of Nipah virus, a highly pathogenic paramyxovirus. *Journal of Clinical Virology*, 43, 396–400.

Lönnroth, K., Castro, K.G., Chakaya, J.M., et al. (2010). Tuberculosis control and elimination 2010–50: cure, care, and social development. *The Lancet*, 375, 1814–29.

Men, T., Brennan, P., Boffeta, P., and Zandze, D. (2003). Russian mortality trends for 1991–2001: analysis by cause and region. *BMJ* 327(7421): 964 (available online).

Miranda, J.J., Kinra, S., Casas, J.P., Davey Smith, G., and Ebrahim, S. (2008). Non-communicable diseases in low- and middle-income countries: context, determinants and health policy. *Tropical Medicine and International Health*, 13(10), 1225–34.

Monteiro, C.A, Moura, E.C., Conde, W.L., and Popkin, B.M. (2004). Socioeconomic status and obesity in adult populations of developing countries: a review. *Bulletin of the World Health Organization*, 82, 891–970.

Murray, C.J.L. and Lopez, A.D. (eds.) (1996). *The Global Burden of Disease: A Comprehensive Assessment of Mortality and Disability from Diseases, Injuries, and Risk Factors in 1990 and Projected to 2020*. Cambridge, MA: Harvard University Press.

National AIDS Control Organisation (2011). *Annual Report 2010–11*. New Delhi: National AIDS Control Organisation, Department of AIDS Control. Ministry of Health & Family Welfare, Government of India.

Nogues, J. (1993). Social costs and benefits of introducing patent protection to pharmaceutical drugs in developing countries. *The Developing Economies*, 31, 24–53.

Notzon, F.C., Komarov, Y.M., Ermakov, S.P., et al. (1998). Causes of declining life expectancy in Russia. *JAMA* (March), 279(10): 793–800 (available online).

O'Brien, T. (2007). *Development Results in Middle-Income Countries*. Washington, DC: World Bank.

Organisation for Economic Co-operation and Development (2009). *Policy Brief—Globalisation and Emerging Economies*. [Online] Available at: http://www.oecd.org/dataoecd/35/34/42324460.pdf.

Overseas Development Institute (2006). *Internal Migration, Poverty and Development in Asia*. Briefing Paper. London: Overseas Development Institute.

Peabody, J., Taguiwalo, M., Robalino, D., and Frenk, J. (1999). *Policy and Health: Implications for Development in Asia*. Cambridge: RAND Studies in Policy Analysis, Cambridge University Press.

Phommasack, B., Moen, A., Vongphrachanh, P., et al. (2012). Capacity building in response to pandemic influenza threats—Lao PDR case study. *American Journal of Tropical Medicine & Hygiene*, 87(6), 965–71.

Phua, K.H. and Chew, A.H. (2002). Towards a comparative analysis of health systems reforms in the Asia-Pacific region. *Asia-Pacific Journal of Public Health*, 14(1), 9–16.

Popkin, B.M., Kim, S., Rusev, E.R., Du, S., and Zizza, C. (2006). Measuring the full economic costs of diet, physical activity and obesity-related chronic diseases. *Obesity Reviews*, 7, 271–93.

Popov, V. (2009). *Mortality Crisis in Russia Revisited: Evidence from Cross-Regional Comparison*. Unpublished (available online).

Population Division (2005). *World Urbanization Prospects—The 2005 Revision*. New York: UN Department of Economic and Social Affairs.

Population Division (2007). *World Urbanization Prospects—The 2007 Revision*. New York: UN Department of Economic and Social Affairs.

Population Division (2011). *World Urbanization Prospects—The 2011 Revision—Highlights*. New York: UN Department of Economic and Social Affairs.

Reich, M.R. and Bery, P. (2005). Expanding global access to ARVs: the challenges of patents and prices. In K.H. Mayer and H.F. Pizer (eds.) *The AIDS Pandemic: Impacts on Science and Society*, pp. 324–50. New York: Academic Press.

Roll Back Malaria (2010). *Malaria Endemic Countries: 2010*. Roll Back Malaria: The Global Partnership for a Malaria-free World. [Online] Available at: http://www.rbm.who.int/endemiccountries.html.

Smith, R.D. (2006). Trade and public health: facing the challenges of globalisation. *Journal of Epidemiology and Community Health*, 60, 650–1.

Stuckler, D. (2008). Population causes and consequences of leading chronic diseases: a comparative analysis of prevailing explanations. *Milbank Quarterly*, 86, 273–326.

Taylor, L.H., Latham, S.M., and Woolhouse, M.E.J. (2001). Risk factors for human disease emergence. *Philosophical Transactions of the Royal Society: Biological Sciences*, 356, 983–9.

UNAIDS (2012a). *Global Report: UNAIDS Report on the Global AIDS Epidemic*. [Online] Available at: http://www.unaids.org/en/media/unaids/contentassets/documents/epidemiology/2012/gr2012/20121120_UNAIDS_Global_Report_2012_en.pdf.

UNAIDS (2012b). *AIDSinfo—Estimated HIV Prevalence 2011*. [Online] Available at: http://www.unaids.org/en/dataanalysis/datatools/aidsinfo/.

UNAIDS (2012c). *AIDSinfo—Estimated HIV Prevalence 2000*. [Online] Available at: http://www.unaids.org/en/dataanalysis/datatools/aidsinfo/.

UNAIDS (2012d). *AIDSinfo—Estimated HIV Prevalence 2000, 2009*. [Online] Available at: http://www.unaids.org/en/dataanalysis/datatools/aidsinfo/.

UNDP and UNAIDS (2012). *Potential Impact of Free Trade Agreements on Public Health*. New York: UNDP/UNAIDS.

UN-HABITAT. (2010). *State of the World's Cities 2010/2011—Bridging the Urban Divide*. Geneva: UN-HABITAT.

United Nations (2002). *Monterry Consensus on Financing for Development*. New York: United Nations.

United Nations (2011). *The Millennium Development Goals Report 2011*. New York: United Nations.

Woolhouse, M.E.J. and Gowtage-Sequeria, S. (2005). Host range and emerging and reemerging pathogens. *Emerging Infectious Disease*, 11(12), 1842–7.

World Bank (2012a). *World Development Indicators and Global Development Finance*. [Online] Available at: http://databank.worldbank.org/Data/Views/VariableSelection/SelectVariables.aspx?source=World%20 Development%20Indicators%20and%20Global%20Development%20 Finance#.

World Bank (2012b). *How we Classify Countries*. [Online] http://data.worldbank.org/about/country-classifications.

World Health Assembly (2005). *Revision of the International Health Regulations*. 58th World Health Assembly, Agenda item 13.1, WHA58.3. [Online] Available at: http://www.who.int/csr/ihr/IHRWHA58_3-en.pdf.

World Health Organization (1996). *The World Health Report 1996: Fighting Disease, Fostering Development*. Geneva: WHO.

World Health Organization (2000). *WHO Report on Global Surveillance of Epidemic-Prone Infectious Diseases*. WHO/CDS/CSR/ISR/2000.1. Geneva: World Health Organization Department of Communicable Disease Surveillance and Response. Available at: http://whqlibdoc.who.int/hq/2000/WHO_CDS_CSR_ISR_2000.1.pdf. See also http://whqlibdoc.who.int/hq/2000/WHO_CDS_CSR_ISR_2000.1.pdf. See also www.who.int/healthinfo/global_burden_disease/en/.

World Health Organization (2002). *The World Health Report—Health System Financing: The Path to Universal Coverage*. Geneva: WHO.

World Health Organization (2005). *Preventing Chronic Diseases: A Vital Investment*. Geneva: WHO.

World Health Organization (2006). Access to AIDS medicines stumbles on trade rules. *Bulletin of the World Health Organization*, 84, 5, 337–424.

World Health Organization (2010a). *News Release—Urban Planning Essential for Public Health*. [Online] Available at: http://www.who.int/mediacentre/news/releases/2010/urban_health_20100407/en/index.html.

World Health Organization (2010b). *Global Status Report on Non-communicable Diseases 2010*. Geneva: WHO.

World Health Organization (2010c). *Noncommunicable Disease Risk Factors and Socioeconomic Inequalities—What are the Links?: A Multicountry Analysis of Noncommunicable Disease Surveillance Data*. Geneva: WHO.

World Health Organization (2010d). *World Health Report 2010*. Geneva: WHO.

World Health Organization (2011a). *World Malaria Report 2011*. World Health Organization Global Malaria Programme. [Online] Available at: http://www.who.int/malaria/world_malaria_report_2011/WMR2011_noprofiles_lowres.pdf.

World Health Organization (2011b). *Non-Communicable Diseases in the South-East Asia Region: Situation and Response 2011*. Geneva: WHO.

World Health Organization (2012a). *HIV/AID: Fact Sheet No. 360*. World Health Organization Media Centre. [Online] Available at: http://www.who.int/mediacentre/factsheets/fs360/en/index.html.

World Health Organization (2012b). *Malaria: Country Profiles*. [Online] Available at: http://www.who.int/malaria/publications/country-profiles/en/index.html.

World Health Organization (2012c). *Update on Artemisinin Resistance—April 2012*. World Health Organization Global Malaria Programme. [Online] Available at: http://www.who.int/malaria/publications/atoz/arupdate042012.pdf.

World Health Organization (2012d). *World Health Statistics*. Geneva: WHO.

World Health Organization (2013a). *Tuberculosis: Fact Sheet No. 104*. World Health Organization Media Centre. [Online] Available at: http://www.who.int/mediacentre/factsheets/fs104/en/index.html.

World Health Organization (2013b). *Malaria: Fact Sheet No. 94*. World Health Organization Media Centre. [Online] Available at: http://www.who.int/mediacentre/factsheets/fs094/en/index.html.

World Health Organization (n.d.). *Zoonoses and Veterinary Public Health: Emerging Zoonoses*. [Online] Available: http://www.who.int/zoonoses/emerging_zoonoses/en/.

World Health Organization and UN-HABITAT (2010). *Hidden Cities—Unmasking and Overcoming Health Inequities in Urban Settings*. Geneva: WHO.

Zimmerman, C., Kiss, L., and Hossain, M. (2011). Migration and health: a framework for 21st century policy making. *PLoS Medicine*, 8, e1001034.

1.5

Globalization

Kelley Lee

Introduction to globalization

'Globalization' is a term associated with complex and varied changes to our world, and the costs and benefits of these changes to individuals and populations are still being debated. There is now a substantial body of scholarship on globalization and public health which seeks to explain how transboundary flows of people, other life forms, goods and services, capital, and knowledge are influencing health determinants and outcomes (Lee 2003b; Kawachi and Wamala 2006; Labonte et al. 2012). The greater scale and geographical reach of these flows pose three core challenges for the public health community: how can the evidence base on globalization and health continue to be strengthened; what effective policy responses are needed to optimize globalization's benefits, and minimize its costs, to population health; and how can these policy options be practically and effectively implemented?

This chapter is concerned with how globalization is influencing public health. It begins by defining globalization and its distinctive forms in the contemporary world. The key drivers of globalization are described, alongside their resultant changes and health impacts. The chapter then focuses on how public health practice is changing as a result of globalization. Many of the issues raised in this chapter are addressed in more detail elsewhere in this textbook, reflecting the importance of globalization across many aspects of public health. The chapter concludes by considering global health governance to strengthen collective action across societies to protect and promote population health. While the public health community has found itself at the frontline of many of globalization's impacts, it continues to play a limited role in managing and shaping its future trajectory. At the same time, greater attention to the public health impacts of globalization through effective collective action across all societies to tackle transboundary health determinants and outcomes will, in turn, contribute to more sustainable forms of globalization.

What is globalization?

The widespread use of the term 'globalization' has been accompanied by variation in its definition. In many cases, the term 'global' is used interchangeably with 'international' (subjects that concern two or more countries). At other times, globalization is used to refer to specific phenomena such as the spread of fast-food restaurants to far-flung locales, the worldwide popularity of American films, or the ease of information access through the Internet. Alongside definitional vagueness lie marked differences in how globalization is normatively assessed. Some writers see globalization as a unifying and progressive force, bringing unprecedented economic growth and prosperity to millions (Dollar and Kraay 2000). Others believe that globalization is a new form of colonialism which reinforces inequalities of wealth and power within and across countries (Cornea 2001). These different perspectives are reflected in the highly contested nature of policy analysis and scholarship in this field.

While it is beyond the scope of this chapter to review these debates in detail, it is an important starting point to approach the term critically. In the broadest sense, globalization has become widely understood as the closer integration or interconnectedness of human societies across geographical or political boundaries. While this has been the case for millennia, what is new in recent decades is the vast increase in the quantity and speed of transboundary flows, and their geographical reach. Held et al. (1999) write that it is this greater intensity and extensity of linkages across human societies that distinguish globalization today.

Three types of changes to social relations are occurring as a result of globalization (Lee 2003a). *Spatial change* refers to how people organize and interact across physical or territorial space. The familiar image of globalization as a 'global village' describes how social relations can increasingly happen on a worldwide scale. Long-haul flights, trade in foreign currencies, and the Internet are examples of social interaction across distant locations. This 'death of distance' has been driven largely by information and communication technologies of ever higher capacity, changing how we form and maintain social groups (Cairncross 2001). The creation of virtual communities, through social media such as Twitter, Facebook and YouTube, for example, allows individuals to communicate, and carry out social relations, irrespective of geographical location.

Temporal change concerns how we think about and experience time. The contemporary world is characterized by an acceleration of the timeframe in which many things can be, and are expected to be, done. For instance, global financial transactions such as foreign exchange, buying and selling equities (stocks and shares), and securing credit can take place in a matter of seconds. New modes of transportation have enabled larger numbers of people to travel greater distances in shorter amounts of time. Mechanization and scientific advances have sped manufacturing, agricultural, and construction processes.

Third, *cognitive change* concerns how we think about ourselves and the world around us. The dissemination and adoption of knowledge, ideas, values, and beliefs have become worldwide in scale through the global reach of the mass media (including the advertising industry), research and educational institutions, consultancy firms, religious organizations, and political parties. The ascendance of English, as the leading language for diplomacy, business, and science, is also a result of cognitive globalization. Some argue that this is leading to a dominant culture, largely of Western origin, threatening diversity and local cultures, languages, and belief systems (Barber 2003). Others believe it is allowing 'niche' communities to form or alternatively creating shared ideas and values such as human rights, gender equity, environmental and labour standards, and democracy (Gartzke and Li 2003). Overall, these three types of changes taking place as a result of globalization—spatial, temporal, and cognitive—are closely intertwined, and together are leading to a mixture of positive and negative impacts.

Another point of substantial debate surrounding globalization is an understanding of what is driving these change processes. Globalization is clearly enabled by technological advances which make flows across borders faster and cheaper, and hence much more pervasive. For example, the decline in freight cost per ton by sea and air freight has promoted the rapid growth of international trade (US Department of Transportation 2000; Teitel 2005) as well as the large-scale shift of manufacturing activities to low-cost countries. Not surprisingly, information and communication technologies have also been frequently cited as the major force behind globalization (Cairncross 2001; Hundley et al. 2003).

For some writers, however, technology is an enabler, but not the driver, of globalization. They argue that the real factors driving technological developments and their application are economic in nature. The global spread of capitalism has been spurred, on the one hand, by untold thousands of producers seeking access to cheaper inputs (i.e. raw materials, labour, research and development, transport and communications), most efficient (and greatest) economies of scale, and largest potential markets. Billions of consumers around the world, on the other hand, fuel this process by demanding the highest quality and quantity of goods and services at the lowest possible price. The economic transactions that result, what eighteenth-century economist Adam Smith called the 'invisible hand' of the market, are seen as the real force behind globalization (Dicken 1999; Schuh 2007).

A further perspective rejects globalization as an essentially technological or economically driven process which implies a degree of rationality and progress. Instead, current forms of globalization are seen as driven by particular ideologically based values and beliefs broadly referred to as neo-liberalism. It has been the global spread and dominance of this ideology from the 1980s, and its embedding within global institutional arrangements, that has, for instance, defined the industrial policies facilitating the development of such technologies (e.g. the promotion of an information economy through deregulation and privatization of the telecommunications sector), and their dissemination for particular purposes (e.g. deregulation of financial markets). It is argued that neo-liberalism has also defined economic policies which encourage trade liberalization, market-based competition, and foreign investment (e.g. tax incentives), while advocating a minimal role for the state at the expense of social welfare and environmental protections (Falk 1999). The global financial crisis from 2007 has led to a rethinking of neo-liberalism and calls for stronger global regulation (Brown and Sarkozy 2009).

Not surprisingly, differences in perspective about globalization's drivers reflect varying views about whether, on balance, it is beneficial or costly to human societies. 'Globalists' (supporters of contemporary globalization) predict a world of closer integration, shared identities, greater efficiency and productivity, rapid economic growth, and increased prosperity. While there may be bumps along the way, such as temporary inequalities in wealth within and across countries, it is believed that the globalization path is progressive in the longer term, bringing benefits for the greatest number of people. In sharp contrast, the opponents of contemporary globalization argue that there are fundamental flaws underpinning its logic in the form of stark imbalances in wealth and power which immutably divide the world into a few winners (those with access to technology, capital, knowledge, and gainful employment) and many losers. Although globalization may increase total wealth, critics challenge the assumption that this wealth will eventually 'trickle down' the global pecking order. Rather, it is argued that without strong commitment to redistributive policies, along with social and environmental protections, neo-liberal globalization will widen the gap between 'haves' and 'have-nots' (Mittelman 2002). In this sense, contemporary globalization is socially (Bacchetta and Jansen 2011) and environmentally unsustainable (Martens and Raza 2010).

From a public health perspective, there is strong evidence that globalization is leading to diverse and complex changes to health determinants, resulting in both positive and negative health outcomes for different populations. For the protection and promotion of population health, and as part of the longer-term sustainability of globalization, these changes must be actively managed to minimize the costs, and maximize the benefits, as well as ensuring that the costs and benefits to public health are equitably shared across societies. In order to develop effective responses to the public health implications raised by globalization, it is useful to consider in greater detail what changes are taking place and how they relate to public health.

Features of contemporary globalization

Globalization and the world economy

Current forms of globalization are characterized by the closer integration of systems of economic production, distribution, and consumption on a worldwide scale. While economists have varied opinions on the precise timing of these processes, most agree that the creation of the Bretton Woods Institutions—the World Bank, International Monetary Fund (IMF), and General Agreement on Tariffs and Trade (GATT)—after the Second World War laid its institutional and normative foundations. Each has played an important role in facilitating the emergence of a global economy defined by the liberalization of capital flows, and opening of national markets to trade and investment.

The first major pillar of a globalized world economy, the liberalization of capital flows, was introduced in the United States from the mid 1970s which, in turn, precipitated a complete restructuring of financial markets worldwide. Historically, banks, insurance companies, investment companies, and brokerage firms have been subject to heavy regulation. Deregulation of financial markets, such as the removal of restrictions on the types of securities that financial institutions could trade, levels of interest that could be paid on specific types of securities and bank accounts, and types of institution entitled to act as financial intermediaries, was introduced to increase competition and encourage capital flows within and across countries. Information and communication technologies enabled high-speed electronic-based transactions which eventually linked financial markets across countries. The result has been a globally integrated financial market capable of 24-hour trading in foreign exchange, commodities, capital, and other financial assets (Valdez 2006). The world's financial assets have correspondingly boomed, from US $136 trillion in 2005 to US $198 trillion in 2010. By 2020, this is expected to rise to US $371 trillion, with one-third accounted for by emerging economies (Roxburgh et al. 2011).

A second key pillar is the trade of goods and services. While trade has been the lifeblood of commerce for thousands of years, it is the global restructuring and integration of production, accompanied by the increased scale and scope of trade, which characterizes the world economy of recent decades. Historically, trade among countries has been dominated by raw materials and natural resources (e.g. oil, timber), commodities (e.g. grains, metals), or manufactured products (e.g. textiles and clothing, food products). In 1948, the GATT was established as an agreement under which signatories could negotiate reductions in tariffs on traded goods. Eight trade rounds were carried out between 1948 and 1994 by which thousands of tariff reductions were negotiated. During this period, membership grew from 23 countries in 1947 to 125 countries in 1994, thus establishing a worldwide trading system.

The growth of international trade led to renewed support for a permanent organization, resulting in the creation of the World Trade Organization (WTO) in 1995. As of 2012 there are 157 member states, with many more countries seeking accession. Moreover, the WTO's remit embraces trade in services, agriculture, intellectual property rights, government procurement, and other areas (Wilkinson 2006). The overall effect has been that world trade has grown faster than world output. In 2006, for example, world merchandise exports increased by 15 per cent to US $11.76 trillion, and commercial services exports grew by around 11 per cent (US $2.71 trillion), compared with global gross domestic production (GDP) growth of 3.7 per cent (WTO 2007). The global financial

crisis from 2008 has led to a significant downturn in trade volumes but the overall trend has been sharply upwards (WTO 2012).

The global restructuring of production and exchange processes has been an integral part of the boom in international trade over the past half century. In many sectors, transnational corporations (TNCs) have emerged which have relocated components of their business to different parts of the world. Thus, resource extraction may take place in one country, manufacturing in another, and research and marketing in still others (Dicken 1999). The targeted consumers have also changed, with TNCs seeking markets worldwide for global brands. According to the European Brand Institute (2012), the five most valuable global brands are Apple, Coca Cola, Microsoft, IBM, and Google.

Global economic restructuring can be observed in many sectors with direct or indirect impacts on public health. One important example is the pharmaceutical industry which is now dominated by a small number of large companies formed through mergers and acquisitions. The buying of domestic generic and manufacturing companies to access emerging markets, and the consolidation of the pharmaceutical and biotechnology industries, have been particular trends since 2008 (IMAP 2010). Table 1.5.1 describes the largest pharmaceutical companies in 2011 by revenue. In 1992, the ten largest companies accounted for one-third of world revenue (Tarabusi and Vickery 1998). By 2011, this had increased to 46 per cent. This trend towards consolidation has been driven by global competition. The cost of research and development (R&D), large-scale manufacturing, and worldwide marketing and distribution means that successful companies need to be of a certain size with considerable resources. For example, the reported cost of developing and bringing a new drug onto the market now averages US $4 billion, taking into account total R&D spend versus the number of actual new products (Herper 2012).

The tobacco industry offers another health-related example of the global restructuring of the world economy. As smoking prevalence has declined in the 'traditional markets' of North

Table 1.5.1 World's ten largest pharmaceutical companies (2011)

Company	HQ	Revenue (millions US$)	Growth (%)	Market share (%)
Pfizer	United States	57,747	−1	6.6
Novartis	Switzerland	47,935	10	6.0
Merck	United States	41,289	7	4.7
Sanofi Aventis	France	42,779	3	4.6
AstraZeneca	United Kingdom	32,981	3	4.3
Roche	Switzerland	34,900	6	4.0
GlaxoSmithKline	United Kingdom	35,594	1	4.0
Johnson & Johnson	United States	24,368	0	3.2
Abbott	United States	22,435	7	3.0
Teva	Israel	16,689	−2	2.8
Total				**43.2**

Adapted with permission from Roth, G.Y., Top 20 Pharma Report, *Contract Pharma*, 18 July 2011, Copyright © Rodman Media. All Rights Reserved. Available from http://www.contractpharma.com/issues/2012-07/view_features/top-20-pharma-report/#sthash.M9l1Gbei.dpuf and IMS, Top World Pharmaceutical Companies in *IMS Health World Review Analyst 2012*, Copyright © 2012, available from http://www.imshealth.com.

America, Europe, and Australia/New Zealand, the industry has focused on emerging markets in Asia, Middle East, Eastern Europe, Latin America, and Africa. Consequently, through mergers and acquisitions, the industry has become dominated by four transnational tobacco companies (TTCs)—Philip Morris, British American Tobacco, Japan Tobacco International, and Imperial Tobacco—controlling around 62 per cent of the world cigarette market by volume in 2008. This excludes the Chinese National Tobacco Corporation, a state monopoly, which accounts for 37 per cent of the world cigarette market, but concentrated on supplying 98 per cent of the 300 million smokers in China (WHO 2012b). Importantly, globalization has facilitated the tobacco industry's expansion into emerging markets through trade liberalization, foreign direct investment, increased economies of scale and marketing of global brands (McGrady 2012).

The public health consequences of economic globalization relate to the availability of health promoting or harming goods and services. In the pharmaceutical industry, consolidation can lead to improved efficiencies, R&D investments, distribution and safety of drug products. However, so-called 'Big Pharma' can also focus on the most profitable products and markets to recover high investment costs. The public health community has become concerned about the neglect of diseases and populations deemed to offer insufficient financial returns. For conditions where there are a relatively small number of sufferers, or the affected population is unlikely to afford cost-recovery level prices, companies may invest limited resources (Trouiller et al. 2002). For drugs reaching the market, affordability becomes a concern because patent-protected drugs are often too costly for patients in developing countries. The need to balance access to medicines with IPR protections led to the 2001 Doha Declaration on Intellectual Property Rights and Public Health, followed in 2003 by the WTO's Decision on Implementation of Paragraph 6, both intended to clarify flexibilities in the Agreement on Trade-Related Intellectual Property Rights permitting member states to take measures, such as compulsory licensing, that improves access to medicines (Kerry and Lee 2007). The formation of a WHO Commission on Intellectual Property Rights, Innovation and Public Health in 2003, investment by a few companies in 'rare disease' strategies and drug development for diseases in developing countries, and innovative financing schemes have sought to address the tension between industry interests and health equity goals.

The globalization of the food industry has raised widespread public health concerns about the rise in non-communicable diseases (NCDs) worldwide. Changing dietary patterns are one of multiple factors, notably physical inactivity, tobacco and alcohol use, and built environments, that must be better understood. The increased production and consumption of processed foods, for example, has increased salt intake and consequently hypertension among populations worldwide (Brown et al. 2009). The stark rise in adult and childhood obesity has been attributed to the availability and affordability of 'energy dense' foods (high fat and sugar) (Drewnoski 2007). Lang et al. (2006) assessed compliance by 25 of the world's largest food manufacturers and retailers to recommendations concerning ingredients, advertising, portion size, and labelling. Only a small proportion of companies are voluntarily reducing salt, sugar, and fats in their products. While the public health community has pushed for stronger regulation, governments to date have favoured industry initiatives such as voluntary codes. The 2004 WHO Global Strategy on Diet, Physical Activity and Health was also given no regulatory 'teeth' by member states, and the political declaration of the 2011 UN High Level Meeting on Non-Communicable Disease Prevention and Control has 'failed to generate the sustained popular attention and donor resources' (Johnson 2012).

Governments worldwide have committed to stronger tobacco control given 6 million deaths annually, rising to 8 million by 2030 (WHO 2012a). Of particular concern is the expansion of TTCs into the developing world where 70 per cent of tobacco deaths will occur in future. The WHO Framework Convention on Tobacco Control (FCTC) signed in 2003 sets out minimum measures that States Parties commit to. In addition, a Protocol to Eliminate Illicit Trade in Tobacco Products, representing 20–25 per cent of total consumption, was agreed in 2012.

Cigarette smuggling is part of a range of illicit activities, facilitated by globalization, which have direct implications for public health. Illegal psychoactive drugs, with a street value of US $322 billion in 2003, account for one in 100 adult deaths. Around 230 million people (or 5 per cent of the global population age 15–64) used illicit drugs at least once in 2010. In recent decades, the trade has become globalized in terms of producers and consumers, and the transboundary network of criminal organizations that connects them (United Nations Office on Drugs and Crime 2012). A related problem is counterfeit goods which comprise 5–7 per cent of world trade. Many counterfeits, notably medicines, food products, and cigarettes, are of dubious quality and content, and pose direct risks to public health. Counterfeit baby milk powder in rural China caused the deaths of 50 children and acute malnutrition in hundreds of others (Watts 2004). WHO estimates that counterfeit drugs account for 10 per cent of all pharmaceuticals, a figure much higher in some developing countries. For example, 80 per cent of drugs distributed by major pharmacies in Lagos, Nigeria were found to be counterfeit (WHO 2006a).

Population movements amid globalization

Globalization has been characterized by unprecedented levels of population movements in terms of frequency and distance travelled. Population movements are not new—humankind has been on the move since *Homo erectus* migrated out of Africa in about 1 million BC. What characterizes population mobility since the mid twentieth century has been its volume, geographical reach, speed, and frequency, resulting in what Castles and Miller (2009) call the 'age of migration'. International migration totals 214 million people per year (3.1 per cent of the world's population), an increase from 150 million in 2000 (UNDESA 2008). Two million people cross international borders daily, and 500 million people cross borders on commercial airlines annually. By 2012, 215 million people lived outside their country of birth, compared with 156 million in 1990 (UNCSD 2012).

The reasons why people migrate are diverse. For the relatively educated, highly skilled, and mobile, globalization offers new employment opportunities. For the poorly educated and low skilled, globalization has brought employment insecurity. In healthcare, this trend is evident in the migration of health workers. While health worker migration from poorer countries, notably sub-Saharan Africa, to the industrialized world has received much needed attention, migration patterns are complex. The decision to migrate is an individual one, based on personal circumstances and employment prospects, but broader forces shaped by globalization, affecting work and living conditions, are also at play (Bach 2003). The *World Health Report 2006* (WHO 2006c) estimated there are 59.2 million full-time paid health workers worldwide, with an estimated shortage of 4.3 million doctors, midwives, nurses, and support workers. This shortage is most critical in 57 countries, especially sub-Saharan Africa and South East Asia. The African region, for instance, has 24 per cent of the global health burden but only 3 per cent of health workers. This 'brain drain' of health workers from low- to high-income countries, has gravely worsened this problem. On average one in four doctors and one in 20 nurses trained in Africa is working in OECD countries.

The unprecedented speed and scale of urbanization worldwide over the past three decades raises profound challenges for public health. Globalization has accelerated the formation of mega-cities throughout the developing world, characterized by vast inequalities in income, living standards, environmental conditions, and life chances. In the Asia and the Pacific region over the last two decades, the urban population has risen by 29 per cent, and growing at 2 per cent per annum, reached 43 per cent in 2010. Africa is the least urbanized region but has the highest urban population growth in the world, at an average annual rate of 3.5 per cent (2005–2010). Latin America, in contrast, is the most urbanized at 80 per cent, a proportion predicted to rise to 90 per cent by 2050 (UN HABITAT 2012). In many countries, governments are struggling to provide appropriate infrastructure such as housing, water and sanitation, healthcare, transportation, security, and education that underpin health and well-being (Moore et al. 2003).

The implications of globalization for core public health functions

Public health is concerned with improving the health of whole populations within and across countries (Walley et al. 2001, p. 19).

As part of the review and renewal of public health systems worldwide since the late twentieth century, there has been much reflection on core public health functions. The Institute of Medicine (1988), for example, initiated a debate in the United States in its report, *The Future of Public Health*, later updated amid existing challenges such as 'obesity, toxic environments, a large uninsured population, and health disparities', with 'emerging threats' caused by rapid changes to the nation's social, cultural and global contexts, scientific and technological advances, and demographic shifts (Institute of Medicine 2002). The US Health and Human Services Public Health Service (1995) identifies ten core activities of public health such as preventing epidemic; protecting the environment, workplace, food and water; and promoting healthy behaviour. In the United Kingdom, the creation of a 'new public health system' in 2011 has led to reforms that delineate responsibilities between local authorities and Public Health England (UK Department of Health 2011). Similar reflection is being undertaken in a diverse range of countries including India (Planning Commission of India 2011), Brazil (Jerberg 2008), and China (2009). Fig. 1.5.1 illustrates the core functions for public health identified by the Ministry of Health for the Canadian province of British Columbia.

An important impetus for recent debate has been the need to adapt core public health functions to rapid globalization. As described earlier, spatial, temporal, and cognitive changes arising from globalization are having important impacts on population health determinants and outcomes. Globalization is not only leading to public health issues transcending national boundaries, but also to the need for collective efforts across countries to help shape more socially just and sustainable forms of globalization. Drawing on Fig. 1.5.1, the remainder of this chapter examines some of these core functions, how globalization may impact on their practice, and how the public health community might effectively respond to these impacts (Beaglehole and Bonita 2010).

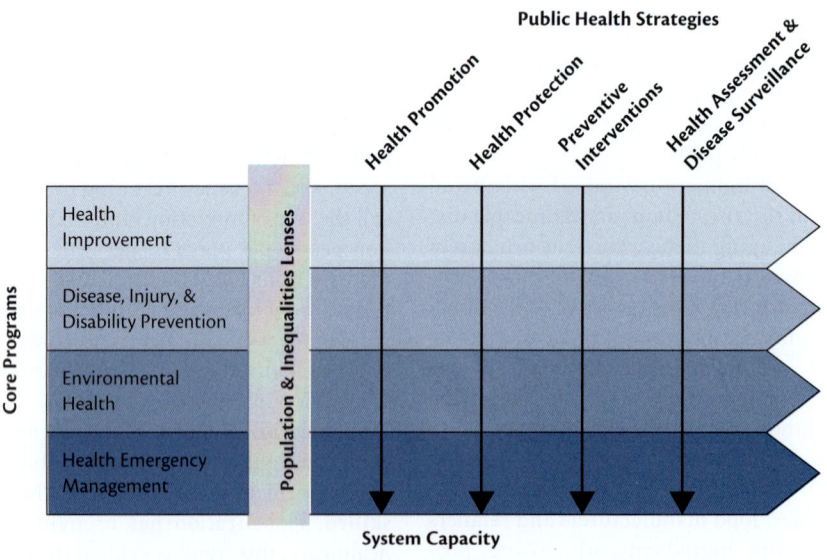

Fig. 1.5.1 Core functions framework.

Globalization and disease prevention and control

The prevention and control of disease is a core public health function. Historically, disease-causing microbes have travelled across vast distances for as long as human populations have come into contact with each other and other animal species. For example, the shift from hunting-gathering to agrarian societies and the domestication of animals, between 8000 and 3500 BC, led to the emergence and spread of new zoonotic diseases (Swabe 1999). The so-called 'Columbian exchange', following the arrival of Christopher Columbus in the Americas, is noted for the widespread exchange of plants, animals, foods, human populations (including slaves), and ideas that followed. Diseases, such as cholera, influenza, measles, malaria, smallpox, and tuberculosis, were also exchanged, resulting in the decimation of indigenous populations (Crosby 1972). Another notable example is the influenza pandemic of 1918–1919 which killed around 25 million people, demonstrating the capacity of infectious disease to spread worldwide amid large-scale human migration and weakened societies.

Contemporary globalization is creating new risks of disease outbreaks with a greater capacity to spread more rapidly and further afield. First, globalization may alter population size at risk of disease. Rapid urbanization, without sufficient attention to housing, clean water and sanitation, and access to healthcare, is creating large populations vulnerable to disease outbreaks. The world's urban population will almost double from 3.3 billion in 2007 to 6.3 billion in 2050, with most of this growth in cities within the developing world as hubs for the worldwide transmission of infectious diseases (Alirol et al. 2010). In cases where global population mobility comes together with local poverty, such as the arrival of UN soldiers from Nepal in 2010 to earthquake affected Haiti, diseases such as cholera have an opportunity to spread (Doyle 2012).

Importantly, globalization can also 'democratize' disease risks by making larger populations vulnerable. While tuberculosis and cholera are historically associated with the poor, other diseases do not discriminate by socioeconomic class. The rapid international response to the severe acute respiratory syndrome (SARS) outbreak in 2002–2003 was due to the recognized vulnerability of all populations, rich or poor, across the world (Woollacott 2003). The spread of SARS, from China to around 25 countries within weeks, illustrated how quickly infectious diseases can spread in a globalized world. There remain concerns about avian influenza (H5N1) causing a lethal human pandemic of unprecedented speed and reach (Lee and Fidler 2007). The 2009 H1N1 influenza pandemic had a lower case fatality rate than initially feared, but illustrated how such a pandemic could spread in a globalizing world.

Second, globalization may influence the *prevalence* (number of people with a disease within a given population) and *incidence* (number of new cases of a disease in a specified period of time per total population) of certain diseases. De Vogli and Birbeck (2005) argue that vulnerability to HIV/AIDS, tuberculosis, and malaria is closely linked to poverty, gender inequality, development policy, and health sector reforms that involve user fees and reduced access to care. Dorling et al. (2006) similarly argue that 'global inequality in wealth will have compounded the effects of AIDS on Africa', notably caused by globalization-related policies such as structural adjustment programmes. Changing employment patterns and conditions, as a result of economic globalization, have also had epidemiological consequences. Moody (2007) describes the globalization of the mining industry and its impact on local communities. Basu et al. (2009) observe how tuberculosis incidence among southern African miners is ten times greater than the general population, with migration to and from mines amplifying tuberculosis epidemics in the general population.

Third, globalization may increase the risks from emerging and re-emerging diseases. Environmental degradation, such as rainforest destruction and intense farming methods, can bring human and animal populations into closer contact. Sixty per cent of emerging infectious diseases that affect humans are zoonotic (originating in animals), and more than two-thirds of those originate in wildlife including HIV/AIDS, West Nile, Lyme disease, and Nipah virus. A 2012 study by the International Livestock Research Institute found that five countries—Bangladesh, China, Ethiopia, India, and Nigeria—are hotspots of poverty and zoonoses. The study also found that the northeastern United States, western Europe (especially the United Kingdom), Brazil, and parts of South East Asia may also be hotspots of 'emerging zoonoses'—those that are newly infecting humans, are newly virulent, or have newly become drug resistant (Grace et al. 2012).

The heightening of disease risks within a globalizing world has prompted efforts to develop more effective public health responses. Alongside risks, globalization brings opportunities to improve the capacity of public health institutions to respond more effectively to infectious disease outbreaks. Foremost is the advent of new information and communication technologies which, in principle, enable faster, cheaper, and more efficient gathering and sharing of knowledge. ProMED-mail (see Box 1.5.1) and regional disease

---

Box 1.5.1 Programme for Monitoring Emerging Diseases (ProMED-mail)

ProMED-mail—the Program for Monitoring Emerging Diseases—is an Internet-based reporting system dedicated to rapid global dissemination of information on outbreaks of infectious diseases and acute exposures to toxins that affect human health, including those in animals and in plants grown for food or animal feed. Electronic communications enable ProMED-mail to provide up-to-date and reliable news about threats to human, animal, and food plant health around the world, 7 days a week. By providing early warning of outbreaks of emerging and re-emerging diseases, public health precautions at all levels can be taken in a timely manner to prevent epidemic transmission and to save lives.

ProMED-mail is open to all sources and free of political constraints. Sources of information include media reports, official reports, online summaries, local observers, and others. Reports are often contributed by ProMED-mail subscribers. A team of expert human, plant, and animal disease moderators screen, review, and investigate reports before posting to the network. Reports are distributed by email to direct subscribers and posted immediately on the ProMED-mail web site. ProMED-mail currently reaches over 60,000 subscribers in at least 185 countries.

surveillance networks have facilitated the collection and reporting of epidemiological data. The lessons learned from SARS led to renewed efforts to revise the International Health Regulations (IHR), which came into effect in 2007, to harness a broader range of information sources. Another change is the expansion of the scope of the IHR beyond named diseases, notably plague, yellow fever, and cholera, to the broader term 'public health emergencies of international concern'. This may include human or natural disasters. Beyond surveillance, technological advances are also permitting faster development, such as drugs, vaccines, because of the capacity for more rapid development and testing, and potential dissemination of new knowledge within the medical research community (WHO 2005).

Protecting the natural and built environmental health in a global context

The discipline of environmental health concerns 'the theory and practice of assessing, correcting, controlling, and preventing those factors in the environment that can potentially affect adversely the health of present and future generations' (Pencheon et al. 2001, pp. 206–7). Environmental threats to public health range from local, small-scale factors (e.g. household exposures) to widespread exposures affecting whole populations. Protecting against a perceived environmental health threat involves identifying the hazard, determining the relationship between the hazard and the effect (dose–response assessment), exposure assessment, and risk characterization.

The possible impacts of globalization on environmental health are wide-ranging, potentially affecting populations at the global, regional, community, occupational, and household levels. These impacts can be direct, such as through the dumping of hazardous waste across borders, relocation of risky occupations (such as ship breaking or asbestos disposal in low-income countries), damage caused by acid rain, or a nuclear accident. Economic globalization, in which companies compete on a worldwide scale to increase returns, is raising concerns that profit-maximization motives can undermine environmental health. Governments, seeking to attract foreign direct investment to fuel economic growth and generate employment, are accused of engaging in a 'race to the bottom' by offering reduced taxation rates, lower wages, or weaker environmental, health and safety protections, although much depends on the domestic context and policies of neighbouring countries (Mosley and Uno 2007). As stated by the environmental organization, the Sierra Club (1999), 'By promoting economic growth without adequate environmental safeguards, trade increases the overall scale and pace of resource consumption; promotes adoption of high-consumption, high-polluting lifestyles; and prompts countries to seek international advantage by weakening, not raising, environmental protections'.

The World Bank (2000) argues that '[e]very society has to decide for itself on the relative value it places on economic output and the environment'. Others argue, however, that there are substantial inequities in terms of who bears the environmental costs. In addition, many of the environmental impacts can affect more than one country and can even be global in scope. More commitment is thus needed to better balance the trade-offs between economic growth and environmental protection, including a fuller understanding of environmental health risks.

In managing such trade-offs, the indirect effects of globalization on environmental health must also be recognized. A change in investment or lending policy by a global financial institution, such as the IMF, can have health consequences for local communities. For example, policy conditions set by the World Bank, or requirements to repay substantial sums of foreign debt, can restrict the public expenditure of borrowing countries on environmental protection or investment in basic infrastructure, such as water and sanitation. A cholera outbreak in South Africa in 2000–2001, which led to around 120,000 cases and 265 deaths, has been blamed on the introduction of user fees following the privatization of water utilities as part of the country's structural adjustment programme. As water supplies were cut to poor people unable to pay for the new charges, many resorted to using polluted river water (Anonymous 2006). Today, more than 2.6 billion people—over 40 per cent of the world's population—do not have access to basic sanitation, and more than 1 billion people still use unsafe sources of drinking water (WHO/UNICEF 2006). Predictions of the growing scarcity of fresh water supplies globally, and the continued trend towards the privatization of water utilities with ownership dominated by large TNCs, is likely to worsen this situation.

The capacity of the public health community to correct, control, and prevent environmental health risks can be affected by globalization. For example, globalization poses additional challenges for identifying a hazard and its causal relations. The tasks associated with identifying a hazard must take account of factors that extend far beyond national borders, a greater range of stakeholders, and jurisdictions that lie beyond the reach of public health authorities. A good example is the increase in reported outbreaks of food-borne illnesses involving more than one country which has been linked, in part, to the globalization of the food industry (Kaferstein et al. 1997; Hall et al. 2002). Tracing the source and cause of such an outbreak can be hindered by inadequate record-keeping in some countries, lack of timely sharing of information, inconsistency in labelling, or lack of access to production facilities abroad. The work of environmental health workers can be made even more difficult by hazards arising from illicit activities such as dumping, counterfeiting, or smuggling across borders (Kimball 2006).

The undertaking of risk assessment, defined as 'the process of estimating the potential impact of a chemical, physical, microbiological, or psycho-social hazard on a specified human population or ecological system under a specific set of conditions and for a certain timeframe' (Pencheon et al. 2001, p. 208), is also made more challenging by globalization. The population of interest may be widely dispersed, because of their mobility or transience, and identifying and measuring a suspected hazard requires large-scale analysis. Weiland et al. (2004) study 650,000 subjects as part of the International Study of Asthma and Allergies in Childhood. A collaboration among 155 participating centres worldwide, it is the first study 'to take a global view [of] . . . the relationship between asthma and eczema and climate' (Graham 2004).

Growing evidence suggesting that globalization is creating new environmental conditions, in which disease can emerge and spread more readily geographically and across species, has led to support for the so-called One Health approach. Ever growing human populations, reaching 7 billion in 2011 (UNFPA 2011), and the resulting environmental degradation from expanding land use, intensified agricultural and animal husbandry methods, and closer contact between humans and both domesticated and wild animal species, are recognized as key factors increasing shared risk across the animal–human-ecosystem interfaces (Ostfeld 2009; Sherman 2010). The concept of 'One Medicine' was coined in 1984 by the 'father of veterinary epidemiology' Calvin Schwabe (1984) who in his book *Veterinary Medicine and Human Health*, argued that 'the critical needs of man include the combating of diseases, ensuring enough food, adequate environmental quality, and a society in which humane values prevail'. Schwabe renewed the basic principle that a more holistic approach to human, animal, and environmental health was needed to better protect the health of all. Known as One Health, this approach has received growing attention over the past decade among policymakers, practitioners, and funders seeking more effective prevention, control and treatment responses in an increasingly populous and globalized world.

Harnessing new global information and communication technologies for public health

A key defining feature of contemporary globalization has been the spread of information and communication technologies (ICTs) worldwide, transforming almost every aspect of human life. Beginning with the advent of the personal computer in the 1980s, ever increasing processing speeds and storage capacity has led to the creation of new devices offering a wide range of mass applications at cheaper prices. Economic globalization has been enabled by the application of global networks of high-capacity computer systems which enable 24-hour financial systems and trading at an unprecedented scale and speed. Population mobility has been facilitated by online travel booking and the use of mobile technologies. How we work, shop, entertain and educate ourselves, and even form our individual and social identities, are all changing as a result of ICTs.

The global reach and application of ICTs are having profound impacts on health determinants and outcomes. The delivery of healthcare in many countries is being transformed by ICTs including research, diagnostics, patient care, planning and management, informatics, and health promotion. Often known as eHealth (or electronic health), technological change has been spurred by the increased complexity of health systems, need to manage ever larger and more complex datasets, rising cost of healthcare, need to provide longitudinal and comprehensive health records for individual patients, and increased mobility and/or geographically dispersal of many patient populations and healthcare providers. ICTs have been identified as particularly effective, for example, at reaching more individuals with effective health-related advice and information at a very low cost (Strecher 2007).

The use of mobile and wireless technologies in health (known as mHealth), in particular, has grown rapidly with advances in technologies and applications (or 'apps'), the declining cost of handsets and data transmission, and growth cellular network coverage. According to the International Telecommunication Union (ITU), there were over 5 billion wireless subscribers, over 70 per cent residing in low- and middle-income countries, in 2010 (ITU 2010). Commercial wireless signals cover over 85 per cent of the world's population, extending far beyond the reach of the electrical grid (WHO 2011). The potential for mHealth in low- and middle-income countries to improve healthcare, hindered in the past by a lack of infrastructure, is thus promising. Initiatives such as the mHealth Alliance (http://www.mhealthalliance.org/about) are seeking to catalyse the expanded use of such technologies in global health.

Social media, 'interactive platforms via which individuals and communities create and share user-generated content' (Kietzmann et al. 2011, p. 241), has also seen the blossoming of health-related applications. A systematic review of social media and public health messages finds that, as more consumers turn to the Internet for health-related information, health organizations have begun to use social media for connecting with the public (Newbold and Campos 2011). For example, health insurance companies are applying social media, health gaming apps, and other mobile apps to increase patient engagement in their own healthcare (Chilmark Research 2012). Evidence suggests considerable reach associated with social media applications, and the potential for engaging specific target audiences, although efficacy of public health messaging requires further investigation through controlled studies (Newbold and Campos 2011).

Overall, ICTs offer much promise for public health application. There has been substantial investment in such technologies by governments and the private sector, alongside promises to transform practice. However, a systematic review of eHealth technologies, and their impact on the quality and safety of healthcare delivery, found a lack of evidence about their benefits and cost-effectiveness (Black et al. 2011). Alongside their adoption by the public health community has been their use for commercial purposes to shape consumer choices and behaviour, many of which have impacts on the broad determinants of health. The online marketing and promotion of health-related goods and services has spread rapidly and, in many cases, been weakly regulated. The global reach of direct-to-consumer marketing of pharmaceuticals, authentic and counterfeit, via the Internet has been a particular source of regulatory concern. The challenge to national authorities of regulating Internet marketing and sales to ensure safety and efficacy of health-related goods arises from the transboundary nature of such transactions. How to strengthen regulatory mechanisms worldwide, notably in countries where such goods originate, has been the focus of growing policy debate (Institute of Medicine 2012). Greater scrutiny of such technologies and their uses remains much needed.

Globalization and health promotion

The rising burden from NCDs worldwide in recent decades (Beaglehole and Yach 2003; Matthews and Pramming 2003) has led to growing recognition of global approaches to health promotion (Lee 2007). NCDs are the leading causes of death and disability worldwide. Their prevalence rates are accelerating globally, in every region, and across all socioeconomic classes. Chronic diseases account for an estimated 60 per cent of all deaths worldwide (or 43 per cent of the global burden of disease), with 80 per cent occurring in low- and middle-income countries. By 2020, these figures are expected to rise to 73 per cent of all deaths and 60 per cent of the global burden of disease (Daar et al. 2007). Four chronic diseases—cardiovascular diseases (CVD), cancer, chronic obstructive pulmonary disease, and type 2 diabetes—are linked by common and preventable biological risk factors, notably high blood pressure, high blood cholesterol, and overweight, and by related major behavioural risk factors (unhealthy diet, physical inactivity, and tobacco use). Preventing these diseases should focus on controlling key risk factors in a well-integrated manner (WHO 2009b).

Health promotion is the process of enabling people to increase control over, and to improve, their health (WHO 1986). Interventions address three areas of activity in order to prevent disease and promote the health of a community: communication, service delivery, and structural (enabling factor) components (Walley et al. 2001, p. 147). A global approach to health promotion takes into account the ways in which globalization may be influencing the broad determinants of health, and health behaviours, as well as offering opportunities for providing appropriate interventions. The adoption of the Bangkok Charter for Health Promotion in a Globalized World in 2005 was in recognition of the major challenges, actions, and commitments needed to address the determinants of health in a globalized world by reaching out to people, groups, and organizations that are critical to the achievement of health. How this might be achieved can be understood in relation to two key issues—obesity and tobacco control.

The rapid increase in overnutrition and obesity, among both adults and children, has attracted substantial public health concern in recent years. According to WHO (2012a), around 500 million people worldwide are obese (body mass index (BMI) >30), with levels rising rapidly in the twenty-first century. At least 200 million school-age children are overweight or obese, with 40–50 million classified as obese (International Association for the Study of Obesity 2010). Importantly, these upward trends are not limited to high-income countries. Changes in diet, levels of physical activity, and nutrition have led to sharp increases in obesity rates in such wide-ranging countries as India, Thailand, Brazil, and China. Drewnoski and Popkin (1997, p. 32) write:

> Whereas high-fat diets and Western eating habits were once restricted to the rich industrialized nations…the nutrition transition now occurs in nations with much lower levels of gross national product (GNP) than previously…. First, fat consumption is less dependent on GNP than ever before. Second, rapid urbanization has a major influence in accelerating the nutrition transition.

Similarly, Prentice (2006, p. 93) links the trend to globalization of food production and lifestyles:

> The pandemic is transmitted through the vectors of subsidized agriculture and multinational companies providing cheap, highly refined fats, oils, and carbohydrates, labour-saving mechanized devices, affordable motorized transport, and the seductions of sedentary pastimes such as television. This trend has been linked to the globalisation of sedentary lifestyles alongside changes in food production and consumption.

Many interventions to address the obesity epidemic have focused on the modification of individual behaviours, such as healthy eating initiatives and the promotion of physical activity. Global health promotion, however, would also seek to tackle the structural factors that constrain or enable lifestyle choices. This includes what and how food is produced and marketed by a globalized food industry. For example, the Institute of Medicine (2005) report, *Food Marketing to Children and Youth: Threat or Opportunity?*, recognizes that dietary patterns begin in childhood and are shaped by the interplay of genetics and biology, culture and values, economics, physical and social environments, and commercial media environments. Importantly, the report provides a comprehensive review of the scientific evidence on the influence of food marketing on diets and diet-related health of children and youth. It argues that environments supportive of good health require leadership and action from the food, beverage, and restaurant industries; food retailers and trade associations; the entertainment industry and the media; parents and caregivers; schools; and governments.

Global-level regulation of food-related industries, however, remains problematic. The process of adopting the WHO Global Strategy on Diet, Physical Activity and Health was hindered by the food industry's opposition to explicit recommendations on healthy levels of salt, sugar, and fats intake (Lang et al. 2006). In the United States, the powerful food industry has instead succeeded in promoting voluntary and self-regulation. As Kelly (2005) writes:

> So far the U.S. government has declined to regulate the aggressive ways in which food producers market high-energy, low-nutrition foods to young people. That public-health responsibility has been left to an industry-created scheme of self-regulation that is deeply flawed; there is a compelling need for government involvement.

Lessons for global health promotion can be drawn from efforts to strengthen tobacco control worldwide. As described earlier, the globalization of the tobacco industry has led to a rise in tobacco consumption, facilitated by the industry's consolidation, greater economies of scale, and aggressive marketing strategies to gain access to emerging markets (Bettcher and Yach 2000). WHO initiated the FCTC in the mid 1990s in recognition of the need to globalize tobacco control policies (Reid 2005). WHO Director-General Gro Harlem Brundtland (2000, p. 2) stated:

> [O]ver the past fifteen years, we have seen that modern technology, has limited the effectiveness of national action. Tobacco advertising is beamed into every country via satellite and cable. Developing countries are the subject of massive marketing campaigns by international tobacco companies. In the slipstream of increasing global trade, new markets are opened to international tobacco companies which see these emerging markets as their main opportunity to compensate for stagnant or dwindling markets in many industrialized countries.

The FCTC negotiation process encompassed regional consultations, public hearings, contributions by civil society organizations (CSOs), and old-fashioned diplomacy among member states. The process also faced extensive efforts by the tobacco industry to undermine negotiations through participating on some national delegations, lobbying of tobacco leaf-producing countries and farmers, orchestrating criticism of WHO, and even challenging the science on tobacco and health (Weishaar et al. 2012).

Despite industry opposition, the treaty was signed in 2003 and came into effect in 2005. As of 2012, 176 countries are parties to the treaty. Importantly, the FCTC represents a collective effort across WHO member states to address a clear global public health challenge. The involvement of a broad spectrum of stakeholders, notably CSOs, was critical to raising public awareness and support at the regional, national, and local levels. The mobilization of public health advocates, led by the Framework Convention Alliance, was greatly facilitated by the use of the Internet (focused on the Globalink network) which enabled groups to follow negotiations, organize advocacy activities, and share experiences (Collin et al. 2004). While weaker on some aspects of globalization, such as international trade, than initially hoped, protocols could address

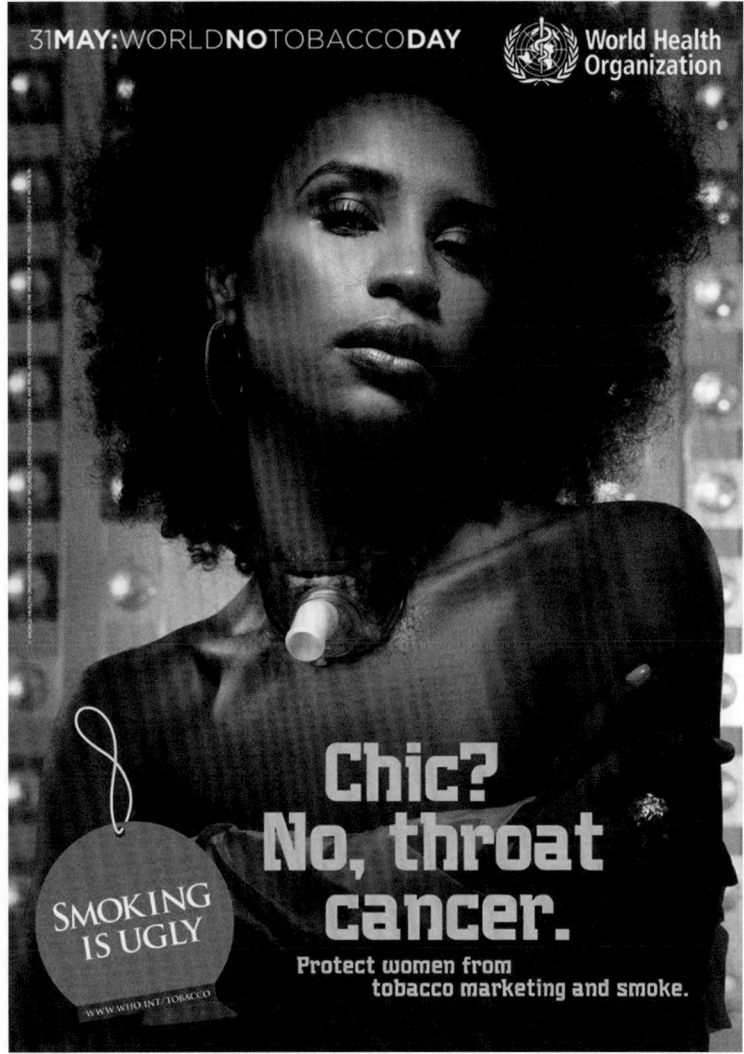

Fig. 1.5.2 Campaign poster for World No Tobacco Day.

Reproduced with permission from the Tobacco Free Initiative, World Health Organization, Geneva, Switzerland, Copyright © 2011, available at: http://www.who.int/tobacco/wntd/2010/en_wntd_2010_chic_no_throat_cancer.pdf.

other transboundary issues such as smuggling and marketing (e.g. sports sponsorship, Internet sales).

Initiating policies, such as the Global Strategy on Diet, Physical Activity and Health and the FCTC, can raise the profile of health promotion and be effective vehicles for addressing global challenges. The experiences of established campaigns, such as the WHO/UNICEF International Code on the Marketing of Breastmilk Substitutes and Healthy Cities Initiative, and initiatives such as the Public–Private Partnership for Handwashing, show that signing agreements is only a starting point. Implementation requires longer term mobilization of political will, resources, and technical capacity to translate commitments into effective action. Globalization can also be harnessed for health promotion purposes. For example, the tobacco control community has developed campaigns to challenge advertising imagery associating cigarette smoking with glamour and excitement in emerging markets (Fig. 1.5.2). Worldwide consumer boycotts of TNCs, such as Nestlé and McDonalds, have been organized via social media to pressure companies to change

their marketing practices or unhealthy product ranges (Yach and Beaglehole 2003).

In summary, the global spread of unhealthy lifestyles and behaviours pose new challenges for health promotion. In many cases, powerful vested interests within key sectors of the global economy have facilitated this process through foreign investment, production, trade, and marketing practices. There is substantial evidence that these practices are resulting in a sharp increase in NCDs. The public health community faces major challenges in influencing these practices, as well as opportunities to harness aspects of globalization to promote healthier lifestyles and behaviours. Collective action across societies to appropriately regulate the harmful aspects of the global economy remains urgently needed.

Measuring and monitoring the health status of populations

Assessing the health of a given population is the starting point for a wide range of public health activities such as policy reviews, programme development, goal setting, and resource allocation. There are well-recognized steps for assessing population health status:

◆ Define the purpose of the assessment.

◆ Define the population concerned and any comparator population.

◆ Define the aspects of health to be considered.

◆ Identify and review existing data sources.

◆ Select the most appropriate existing data (Gentle 2001).

In assessing the linkages between globalization and population health status, two challenges are presented. First, there is variable capacity within and across countries to collect and manage basic health data. Data remains of poor quality or limited availability for many populations as a result. According to WHO (2006b):

> A country health information system comprises the multiple sub-systems and data sources that together contribute to generating health information, including vital registration, censuses and surveys, disease surveillance and response, service statistics and health management information, financial data, and resource tracking. The absence of consensus on the relative strengths, usefulness, feasibility, and cost-efficiency of different data collection approaches has resulted in a plethora of separate and often overlapping systems.

To address this problem, the WHO Health Metrics Network (HMN) was formed as a global partnership to strengthen and align health information systems around the world. The partnership is comprised of countries, multilateral and bilateral development agencies, foundations, global health initiatives, and technical experts that aim to increase the availability and use of timely, reliable health information by catalysing the funding and development of core health information systems in developing countries.

A second challenge is the limitations of existing data sources in capturing health needs that cut across the national level. For each country, health data is collected and managed by a department of health and associated institutions. The WHO Statistical Information System (WHOSIS), in turn, collects and coordinates data on core health indicators, mortality and health status, disease statistics, health system statistics, risk factors and health service coverage, and inequities in health from its 194 member states. This is compiled in the *World Health Statistics*. By definition, globalization is eroding, and even transcending, national borders so that health and disease patterns may be emerging that do not conform to such delineations. As a result, national level data may need to be aggregated and disaggregated in novel ways to reveal these new patterns.

A good example is the earlier discussed increase in obesity rates. Improving data on trends in different countries reveal a complex picture. In high-income countries, obesity is rising rapidly across all social classes but is particularly associated with social deprivation. In the United Kingdom, for example:

> Obesity is linked to social class, being more common among those in the routine or semi-routine occupational groups than the managerial and professional groups. The link is stronger among women. In 2001, 30 per cent of women in routine occupations were classified as obese compared with 16 per cent in higher managerial and professional occupations. (UK Office of National Statistics Office 2004, pp. 111–12)

In France, Romon et al. (2005) found that genetic predisposition influences the prevalence of obesity and changes in BMI among children from the higher social class. For children within the lowest social class, which has seen an increase in BMI across the whole population, environmental factors appear to have played a more important role. In contrast, in low- and middle-income countries, the total number of obese or overweight people is projected to grow by 50 per cent by 2015 alongside the persistence of undernutrition (Fig. 1.5.3). Social class is one factor. In such diverse countries as Kenya, China, India, and Brazil, obesity among an increasingly affluent middle class has been observed (McLellan 2002). A high BMI may even be considered socially desirable as a sign of affluence. At the same time, some populations within the lower social classes are also experiencing rising rates of overweight and obesity. For example, Monteiro et al. (2004) find that a country's level of wealth is an important factor, with obesity starting to fuel health inequities in the developing world when the GNP reaches a value of about US \$2500 per capita. Trends in over/undernutrition, in other words, are complex and changing over time, and require sufficiently detailed and comparable data across population groups defined along additional variables (e.g. gender, socioeconomic status, occupation).

The need to improve available data on the health of populations affected by globalization is illustrated by a wide range of other examples. The outsourcing of manufacturing to the developing world by TNCs, for example, has led to the employment of hundreds of thousands of workers. What public health needs do these workers have and are they addressed by local occupational health policies? Similarly, the greater movement of people across national borders may require increased attention to the health needs of different types of migrants. Alternatively, what public health issues arise for populations from global environmental change? All of these examples suggest the need to redefine new population groups within a global context, and to develop data sources that measure population health patterns which do not conform to national borders.

The governance of global public health

Governance broadly concerns the agreed actions, rules, and means adopted by a society to promote collective action and solutions in pursuit of common goals. Governance takes place whenever people seek to organize themselves to achieve a shared end through agreed rules, procedures, and institutions. This can take place at different levels of decision-making and action. In public health, if a local community decides to initiate a campaign to slow traffic speed and improve road safety, this requires some form of governance to organize the effort. If a national policy is adopted to improve food labelling and increase the taxation of unhealthy foods, governance is needed to set the agreed labelling standards and rates of taxation, as well as enforce compliance. If a global campaign is initiated to strengthen tuberculosis control, an agreed form of governance is needed to take decisions, for example, on agreed treatment, resource mobilization, and implementation of agreed actions across countries. To what extent is there need for more effective governance to protect and promote public health within an increasingly globalized context?

The existing institutional arrangements for global health cooperation have historical roots dating from the International Sanitary Conferences of the nineteenth century. This series of

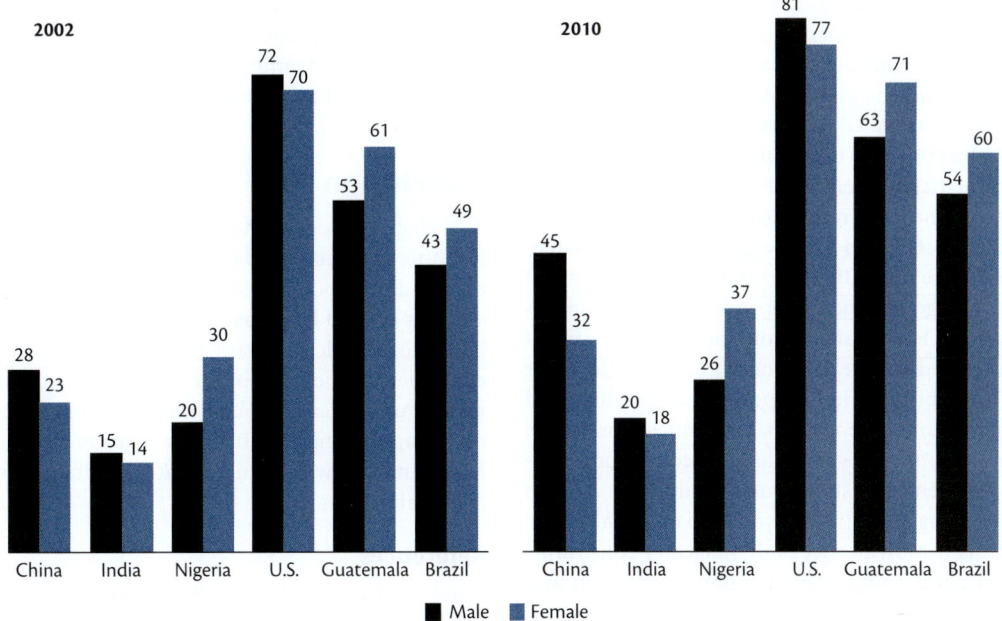

Fig. 1.5.3 Per cent of population that is overweight, selected countries, 2002 and 2010 (projected).

Note: 'overweight' is defined as having a body mass index (weight in kilograms divided by height in metres squared) of between 25 and 30. 'Obese' is defined as having a body mass index of 30 or more.

Reproduced with permission from Nugent, R., *Obesity Creeping up on Less Developed Countries*, Population Reference Bureau, Copyright © 2005, available from http://www.prb.org/Articles/2005/ObesityCreepingUponLessDevelopedCountries.aspx.

meetings, largely dominated by European countries, focused on protecting trading interests from epidemic diseases such as cholera and plague. The institutions eventually created, such as the *Office International d'Hygiène Publique*, were primarily concerned with collecting and disseminating epidemiological data on these diseases (Fidler 2001). The creation of the WHO as a specialized agency of the United Nations in 1948 was intended to universalize membership, and broaden the scope of, international health cooperation. Its objective, 'the attainment by all peoples of the highest possible level of health', was reflected in the vast array of programmes initiated under WHO's auspices (Lee 2008).

Recent decades have seen challenges to WHO's designated role as 'the directing and co-ordinating authority on international health work' (WHO Constitution, Article 2(a)). In part, this has arisen from differences in perspective on whether WHO should be biomedically (disease) focused, or whether the organization should address the broad social determinants of 'health for all'. These debates have been accompanied by rapid changes in WHO's operating environment, with the ascendance of new institutional players with often competing resources, technical expertise and normative perspectives (McInnes and Lee 2012). From the 1980s, the World Bank became a major influence as the biggest source of financing for health development (Buse 1994), while other UN bodies such as the UN Children's Fund and UN Development Programme (UNDP) expanded their health portfolios. The 1990s saw the creation of numerous global public–private partnerships for health which attracted additional resources, but rendered the policy environment far more complex and crowded (Buse and Walt 2000). In recent years, charitable foundations led by the Bill and Melinda Gates Foundation, have become perhaps the biggest players in the funding of health development (McCoy et al.

2009). This influx of institutions and resources has, on the one hand, reflected the higher priority to health development given by governments, corporations, and CSOs. On the other hand, there is substantial evidence of overlapping mandates, duplication of effort, and, above all, a lack of consensus about how to effectively tackle the collective public health challenges posed by globalization.

The governance of global public health can thus be seen as undergoing a period of transition. In principle, the existing institutions formally responsible for governing public health remain governmental. Public health authority lies within the ministries of health of each WHO member state, and collaboration across countries and regions is expected to take place on a wide range of functions through governmental bodies. However, as described in this chapter, intensified flows of people, other life forms, goods and services, capital, and knowledge are creating transboundary health determinants and outcomes that can transcend state capacity to manage them. This is due, in part, to differences in perspective about what priority goals and actions should be pursued, the capacity of governments to act, and even a willingness to act collectively. Where governments cannot or will not assume a global health governance role, non-state actors in the form of CSOs, charitable foundations, and even corporations have been looked to as potentially filling this governance gap. Many scholars of global governance point to the need for new institutional arrangements to enable more effective action in the face of urgent need. Examples described in this chapter—such as tobacco control, obesity, and infectious disease outbreaks—demonstrate the need for innovation but also the political challenges posed.

What can the public health community do to foster such innovation? Globalization is now an established subject of discussion and debate at public health meetings around the world, and there has been no shortage of commitments to addressing its impacts. Processes of globalization continue apace and show little signs of reversal. At the same time, the global financial crisis of the early twenty-first century has revealed many weaknesses—the availability of easy credit, incentives to undertake high-risk lending and borrowing, poor fiscal management by governments, and rampant speculative investing. The deep reflection that has accompanied this crisis has included efforts to 'fix' the global financial system by creating more effective institutional arrangements that support better global economic governance. There are also opportunities to draw broader lessons. Foremost is a profound understanding of how globalization has tied the fate of billions more closely together than ever before. The debt crises in Europe, for example, have had direct and prolonged consequences for economies worldwide. Problems in the global financial system have profound local consequences for employment, investment, and production. And an ailing world economy has impacts far beyond the financial sector. Public health systems worldwide face both budgetary constraints and increased need amid rising economic hardship within and across countries (WHO 2009). Low- and middle-income countries, especially those dependent on health sector aid, face particular challenges. Since 2009, health sector aid has grown by 4 per cent annually after growing 13 per cent between 2002 and 2008 (Institute of Health Metrics and Evaluation 2011). There are reports that this trend is having direct effects on the ground where aid is used to provide life-saving drugs and treatments not otherwise available (Bennett 2012).

As heads of state, ministers of finance and banking executives ponder over the future of economic globalization, and the need for better checks and balances, how can the public health community play a part in the improved global governance? Public health representation in policy debates on trade and finance to date has been limited yet, for the earlier given reasons, increasingly critical. WHO and other public health institutions have remained marginal observers in the WTO and other key decision-making forums. The controversy surrounding intellectual property rights and access to medicines, the substantial concern by consumers about the social and environmental harms of globalization, the looming economic time bomb of NCDs, and the potential costs to the world economy of a lethal infectious disease pandemic demonstrate the scope for greater collaboration across sectors. The global public goods for health approach, for example, addresses globalization and health from an economic perspective. The concept identifies where a good or service (such as knowledge of an infectious disease outbreak), which would be of benefit globally, will not be produced or disseminated if left to the market because no one can be excluded from accessing the good, and thus no charge can be levied for its use and no costs recouped. There may even be economic disincentives to produce certain goods, such as outbreak reports, because of resultant negative economic consequences. At the national level, the production of these goods is usually ensured by government intervention, but at the global level there remains no 'global government' to undertake this role. Certain functions of public health may be classed as global public goods (e.g. immunization programmes, disease surveillance), which require collective action to overcome market failures (Smith et al. 2005). The concept might thus be an appealing rationale to non-health policymakers shaping global change. The potential role of health

impact assessment for informing non-health policy proposals is another such approach (Lee et al. 2007). Most importantly, the long-term sustainability of globalization requires public health to be a core part of any efforts to build better global governance.

Conclusion

This chapter has described key ways in which globalization is relevant to the theory and practice of public health. There are both threats and opportunities arising from the complex and diverse changes created by globalization, although current forms of globalization are clearly characterized by an inequitable distribution of winners and losers. For the public health community, there is a need to understand and contribute to more effective management of the rapid changes taking place. Greater attention to these public health impacts will, in turn, contribute to more sustainable forms of globalization.

References

Alirol, E., Laurent, G., Stoll, B., Chappuis, F., and Loutan L. (2010). Urbanisation and infectious diseases in a globalised world. *The Lancet*, 10, 131–41.

Anonymous (2006). Report: water problems remain in rural areas. *Mail & Guardian*, 12 July.

Bacchetta, M. and Jansen, M. (2011). *Making Globalization Socially Sustainable*. WTO/ILO, Geneva. Available at: http://www.wto.org/english/res_e/booksp_e/glob_soc_sus_e.pdf.

Bach, S. (2003). *International Migration of Health Workers: Labour and Social Issues*. Working Paper, Sectoral Activities Programme. Geneva: ILO. Available at: http://www.ilo.org/public/english/dialogue/sector/papers/health/wp209.pdf (accessed 26 March 2007).

Barber, B. (2003). Jihad vs McWorld. In H. Lechner and J. Boli (eds.) *The Globalization Reader*, pp. 21–6. London: Blackwell Publishing.

Basu, S., Stuckler, D., Gonsalves, G., and Lurie, M. (2009). The production of consumption: addressing the impact of mineral mining on tuberculosis in southern Africa. *Globalization and Health*, 5(11), 1–8.

Beaglehole, R. and Bonita, R. (2010). What is global health? *Global Health Action*, 3, 5142. Available at: http://www.ncbi.nlm.nih.gov/pmc/articles/PMC2852240/pdf/GHA-3-5142.pdf (accessed 30 September 2012).

Beaglehole, R., and Yach, D. (2003). Globalisation and the prevention and control of non-communicable disease: the neglected chronic diseases of adults. *The Lancet*, 362, 903–6.

Bennett, S. (2012). Financial crisis may kill in Congo as global health aid stalls. *Bloomberg News*, 18 January. Available at: http://www.businessweek.com/news/2012-01-18/financial-crisis-may-kill-in-congo-as-global-health-aid-stalls.html (accessed 24 October 2012).

Bettcher, D. and Yach, D. (2000). Globalisation of tobacco industry influence and new global responses. *Tobacco Control*, 9(2), 206–16.

Black, A., Car, J., Pagliari, C., et al. (2011). The impact of eHealth on the quality and safety of health care: a systematic overview. *PLoS Medicine*, 8(1), e 1000387.

Brown, G. and Sarkozy, N. (2009). For global finance, global regulation. *Wall Street Journal*, 9 December. Available at: http://online.wsj.com/article/SB10001424052748704240504574585894254931438.html.

Brown, I., Tzoulaki, I., Candeias V., and Elliot, P. (2009). Salt intakes around the world: implications for public health. *International Journal of Epidemiology*, 38(3), 791–813.

Brundtland, G.H. (2000). *Opening Statement*. First meeting of Intergovernmental Negotiating Body, Framework Convention on Tobacco Control, Geneva, 16 October. Available at: http://www.who.int/director-general/speeches/2000/english/20001016_tobacco_control.html (accessed 27 March 2007).

Buse, K. (1994). Spotlight on international organizations: the World Bank. *Health Policy and Planning*, 9, 95–9.

Buse, K., and Walt, G. (2000). Global public–private partnerships: part I—a new development in health? *Bulletin of the World Health Organization*, 78(4), 549–61.

Cairncross, F. (2001). *The Death of Distance: How the Communications Revolution Is Changing Our Lives*. Cambridge, MA: Harvard Business Press.

Castles, S., and Miller, M. (2009). *The Age of Migration, International Population Movements in the Modern World* (4th ed.). London: Macmillan.

Chilmark Research (2012). *Benchmark Report: Payer Adoption of Emerging Consumer Tech*. Press release, August 2012. Available at: http://www.informationweek.com/healthcare/mobile-wireless/health-insurers-ramp-up-social-media-mhe/240006028 (accessed 16 October 2012).

China (2009). *Deepening the Reform of Health-care System*. Beijing, Central Committee of the Communist Party of China and the State Council.

Collin, J., Lee, K., and Bissell, K. (2004). Negotiating the framework convention on tobacco control: the politics of global health governance. In R. Wilkinson and C. Murphy (eds.) *The Global Governance Reader*, pp. 254–73. London: Routledge.

Cornea, G.A. (2001). Globalization and health: results and options. *Bulletin of the World Health Organization*, 79(9), 834–41.

Crosby, A. (1972). *The Columbian Exchange: Biological and Cultural Consequences of 1492*. Westport, CT: Greenwood Press.

Daar, A., Singer, P., and Persad D. (2007). Grand challenges in chronic non-communicable diseases. *Nature* 450, 494–6.

De Vogli, R. and Birbeck, G.L. (2005). Potential impact of adjustment policies on vulnerability of women and children to HIV/AIDS in Sub-Saharan Africa. *Journal of Health Population and Nutrition*, 23, 105–20.

Dicken, P. (1999). *Global Shift, Transforming the World Economy*. London: Paul Chapman Publishing.

Dollar, D. and Kraay, A. (2000). *Growth is Good for the Poor*. Research Paper. Washington, DC: World Bank.

Dorling, D., Shaw, M., and Davey Smith, G. (2006). Global inequality of life expectancy due to AIDS. *BMJ*, 332, 662–4.

Doyle M. (2012). Haiti cholera epidemic 'most likely' started at UN camp—top scientist. *BBC News*, 22 October. Available at: http://www.bbc.co.uk/news/world-latin-america-20024400 (accessed 23 October 2012).

Drewnoski, A. (2007). The real contribution of added sugars and fats to obesity. *Epidemiologic Reviews*, 29(1), 160–71.

Drewnoski, A. and Popkin, B. (1997). The nutrition transition: new trends in the global diet. *Nutrition Reviews*, 55(2), 31–43.

European Brand Institute (2012). *Top 100 Brand Corporations Worldwide*. Vienna: European Brand Institute. Available at: http://www.eurobrand.cc/studien-rankings/eurobrand-2012/.

Falk, R. (1999). *Predatory Globalization: A Critique*. London: Polity Press.

Fidler, D. (2001). The globalization of public health: the first 100 years of international health diplomacy. *Bulletin of the World Health Organization*, 79(9), 842–9.

Gartzke, E. and Li, Q. (2003). War, peace, and the invisible hand: positive political externalities of economic globalization. *International Studies Quarterly*, 47(4), 561–86.

Gentle, P. (2001). Assessing health status. In D. Pencheon, C. Guest, D. Melzer, and J.A. Muir Gray (eds.) *Oxford Handbook of Public Health Practice*, pp. 28–30. Oxford: Oxford University Press.

Grace, D., Mutua, F., Ochungo, P., et al. (2012). *Mapping of Poverty and Likely Zoonoses Hotspots*. Nairobi: International Livestock Research Institute.

Graham, S. (2004). Global study links climate to rates of childhood asthma. *Scientific American*, 21 June. Available at: http://scientificamerican.com/article.cfm?chanID=sa003andarticleI

D=000624A7-66A2-10D3-A6A283414B7F0000 (accessed 27 March 2007).

Hall, G., D'Souza, R.M., and Kirk, M. (2002). Foodborne disease in the new millennium: out of the frying pan into the fire? *The Medical Journal of Australia*, 177(1112), 614–18.

Held, D., McGrew, A., Goldblatt, D., and Perraton, J. (1999). *Global Transformations*. Stanford, CA: Stanford University Press.

Herper, M. (2012). The truly staggering cost of inventing new drugs. *Forbes*. 10 February. Available at: http://www.forbes.com/sites/matthewherper/2012/02/10/the-truly-staggering-cost-of-inventing-new-drugs/ (accessed 28 September 2012).

Hundley, R.O., Anderson, R.H., Bikson, T.K., and Neu, C.R. (2003). *The Global Course of the Information Revolution, Recurring Themes and Regional Variations*. Washington, DC: National Defense Research Institute, RAND.

IMAP (2010). *Pharmaceuticals and Biotech Industry Global Report—2011*. Available at: http://www.imap.com/imap/media/resources/IMAP_PharmaReport_8_272B8752E0FB3.pdf (accessed 28 September 2012).

Institute of Health Metrics and Evaluation-IHME (2011). *Financing Global Health 2011: Continued Growth as MDG Deadline Approaches*. Available at: http://www.healthmetricsandevaluation.org/publications/policy-report/financing-global-health-2011-continued-growth-mdg-deadline-approaches.

Institute of Medicine (1988). *The Future of Public Health*. Washington, DC: IOM.

Institute of Medicine (2002). *The Future of the Public's Health in the 21st Century*. Washington, DC: National Academy of Sciences.

Institute of Medicine (2005). *Food Marketing to Children and Youth: Threat or Opportunity?* Washington, DC: National Academy of Sciences.

Institute of Medicine (2012). *Ensuring Safe Foods and Medical Products Through Stronger Regulatory Systems Abroad*. Washington, DC: National Academy of Sciences.

International Association for the Study of Obesity (2010). *Obesity: Understanding and Challenging the Global Epidemic*. London: International Association for the Study of Obesity.

ITU (2010). *Mobile eHealth Solutions for Developing Countries*. Geneva: International Telecommunication Union. Available at: http://www.itu.int/dms_pub/itu-d/opb/stg/D-STG-SG02.14.2-2010-PDF-E.pdf (accessed 16 October 2012).

Jerberg, C. (2008). Flawed but fair: Brazil's health system reaches out to the poor. *Bulletin of the World Health Organization*, 86(4), 248–9.

Johnson, T. (2012). *UN High-Level Meeting on NCDs: One Year Later, Interview with Thomas Bollyky, Council on Foreign Relations*, 19 September. Available at: http://www.cfr.org/global-health/un-high-level-meeting-ncds-one-year-later/p29090 (accessed 28 September 2012).

Kaferstein, F.K., Motarjemi, Y., and Bettcher, D.W. (1997). Foodborne disease control: a transnational challenge. *Emerging Infectious Diseases*, 3(4), 503–10.

Kawachi, I. and Wamala, S. (eds.) (2006). *Globalization and Health*. Oxford: Oxford University Press.

Kelly, D. (2005). To quell obesity, who should regulate food marketing to children? *Globalization and Health*, 1(9). Available at: http://www.globalizationandhealth.com/content/1/1/9.

Kerry, V.B. and Lee, K. (2007). TRIPS, the Doha declaration and paragraph 6 decision: what are the remaining steps for protecting access to medicines? *Globalization and Health*, 3(3), 1–12.

Kietzmann, J.H., Hermkens, K., McCarthy, I.P., and Silvestre, B.S. (2011). Social media? Get serious! Understanding the functional building blocks of social media. *Business Horizons*, 54(3), 241–51.

Kimball, A.M. (2006). *Risky Trade Infectious Disease in the Era of Global Trade*. London: Ashgate.

Labonte, R., Schrecker, T., Packer, C., and Runnels, V. (2012). *Globalization and Health: Pathways, Evidence and Policy*. London: Routledge.

Lang, T., Rayner, G., and Kaelin, E. (2006). *The Food Industry, Diet, Physical Activity and Health: a Review of Reported Commitments and Practice of 25 of the World's Largest Food Companies*. London: Centre for Food Policy, City University. Available at: http://www.city.ac.uk/news/press/The%20Food%20Industry%20Diet%20Physical%20Activity%20and%20Health.pdf (accessed 13 June 2007).

Lee, K. (2003a). *Globalization and Health: An Introduction*. London: Palgrave Macmillan.

Lee K. (ed.) (2003b). *Health Impacts of Globalization: Towards Global Governance*. London: Palgrave Macmillan.

Lee, K. (2007). Global health promotion: how can we strengthen governance and build effective strategies? *Health Promotion International*, 21(1), 42–50.

Lee, K. (2008). *The World Health Organization*. London: Routledge.

Lee, K. and Fidler, D. (2007). Avian and pandemic influenza: progress and problems for global governance. *Global Public Health*, 2(3), 215–34.

Lee, K., Ingram, A., Lock, K., and McInnes, C. (2007). Bridging health and foreign policy: the role of health impact assessment? *Bulletin of the World Health Organization*, 85(3), 207–11.

Martens, P. and Raza, M. (2010). Is globalization sustainable? *Sustainability*, 2, 280–93.

Matthews, D. and Pramming, S. (2003). Diabetes and the global burden of non-communicable disease. *The Lancet*, 362(9397), 1763–4.

McCoy, D., Kembhavi, G., Patel, J., and Luintel, A. (2009). The Bill and Melinda Gates Foundation's grant-making programme for global health. *The Lancet*, 373, 1645–53.

McGrady B. (2012). *Confronting the Tobacco Epidemic in a New Era of Trade and Investment Liberalization*. Geneva: WHO Tobacco Free Initiative. Available at: http://whqlibdoc.who.int/publications/2012/9789241503723_eng.pdf (accessed 28 September 2012).

McInnes, C. and Lee, K. (2012). *Global Health and International Relations*. Oxford: Polity.

McLellan, F. (2002). Obesity rising to alarming levels around the world. *The Lancet*, 359(315), 1412.

Ministry of Health (2005). *A Framework for Core Functions in Public Health*. Resource Document. Victoria: Government of British Columbia. http://www.health.gov.bc.ca/public-health/pdf/core_functions.pdf (accessed 11 October 2012).

Mittelman, J.H. (2002). Making globalization work for the have nots. *International Journal on World Peace*, 19(2), 3–25.

Monteiro, C.A., Conde, W.L., Lu, B., and Popkin, B.M. (2004). Obesity and inequities in health in the developing world. *International Journal of Obesity*, 28(9), 1181–6.

Moody, R. (2007). *Rocks and Hard Places: The Globalization of Mining*. New York: Zed Books Ltd.

Moore, M., Gould, P., and Keary, B. (2003). Global urbanization and impact on health. *International Journal of Hygiene and Environmental Health*, 206(4/5), 269–78.

Mosley, L. and Uno, S. (2007). Racing to the bottom or climbing to the top? Economic globalization and collective labor rights. *Comparative Political Studies*, 40(8), 923–48.

Newbold, K.B. and Campos, S. (2011). *Media and Social Media in Public Health Messages: A Systematic Review*. Hamilton: McMaster Institute of Environment and Health. Available at: http://www.mcmaster.ca/mieh/documents/publications/Social%20Media%20Report.pdf (accessed 16 October 2012).

Ostfeld, R.J. (2009). Biodiversity loss and the rise of zoonotic pathogens. *Clinical Microbiology and Infection*, 15(Suppl. 1), 40–3.

Pencheon, D., Guest, C., Melzer, D., and Muir Gray, J.A. (2001). *Oxford Handbook of Public Health Practice*. Oxford: Oxford University Press.

Planning Commission of India (2011). *High Level Expert Group Report on Universal Health Coverage for India*. New Delhi. Available at: http://planningcommission.nic.in/reports/genrep/rep_uhc0812.pdf.

Prentice, A. (2006). The emerging epidemic of obesity in developing countries. *International Journal of Epidemiology*, 35(1), 93–9.

Reid, R. (2005). *Globalizing Tobacco Control, Anti-smoking Campaigns in California, France, and Japan*. Bloomington, IN: Indiana University Press.

Romon, M., Duhamel, A., Collinet, N., and Weill, J. (2005). Influence of social class on time trends in BMI distribution in 5-year-old French children from 1989 to 1999. *International Journal of Obesity*, 29, 54–9.

Roxburgh, C., Lund, S., Dobbs, R., Manyika, J., and Wu, H.H. (2011). *The Emerging Equity Gap: Growth and Stability in the New Investor Landscape*. McKinsey Global Institute. Available at: http://www.mckinsey.com/insights/global_capital_markets/emerging_equity_gap.

Schuh, A. (2007). Brand strategies of Western MNCs as drivers of globalization in Central and Eastern Europe. *European Journal of Marketing*, 41(3/4), 274–91.

Schwabe, C. (1984). *Veterinary Medicine and Human Health* (3rd rev. ed.). Philadelphia, PA: Lippincott Williams and Wilkins.

Sherman, D.M. (2010). A global veterinary medical perspective on the concept of One Health: focus on livestock. *ILAR Journal*, 51, 281–7.

Sierra Club (1999). *Comments to the Trade Policy Staff Committee, United States Trade Representative*, 20 May, Washington, DC: Sierra Club.

Smith, R., Beaglehole, R., Woodward, D., and Drager, N. (eds.) (2005). *Global Public Goods for Health, Health Economic and Public Health Perspectives*. Oxford: Oxford University Press.

Strecher, V. (2007). Internet methods for delivering behavioral and health-related interventions (eHealth). *Annual Review of Clinical Psychology*, 3, 53–76.

Swabe, J. (1999). *Animals, Disease, and Human Society: Human-Animal Relations and the Rise of Veterinary Medicine*. London: Routledge.

Tarabusi, C. and Vickery, G. (1998). Globalization in the pharmaceutical industry. *International Journal of Health Services*, 28(1), 67–105.

Teitel, S. (2005). Globalization and its disconnects. *Journal of Socio-Economics*, 34(4), 444–70.

Trouiller, P., Olliaro, P., Torreele, E., Orbinski, J., Laing, R., and Ford, N. (2002). Drug development for neglected diseases: a deficient market and a public-health policy failure. *The Lancet*, 359(9324), 2188–94.

UK Department of Health (2011). *The New Public Health System: Summary*. London: Department of Health. Available at: http://www.dh.gov.uk/prod_consum_dh/groups/dh_digitalassets/documents/digitalasset/dh_131897.pdf.

UK Office for National Statistics (2004). Health. In *Social Trends 34: 2004 Edition*, pp. 105–117. London: Office for National Statistics.

UNCSD (2012). *Migration and Sustainable Development*. Rio 2012 issues briefs No. 15. Available at: http://www.uncsd2012.org/content/documents/443Migration%20Issues%20Brief_final_June%208.pdf.

UNDESA (2008). *Trends in International Migrant Stock: The 2008 Revision*. New York: United Nations Department of Economic and Social Affairs. Available at: http://esa.un.org/migration/index.asp?panel=1 (accessed 27 September 2012).

UNFPA (2011). *The World at 7 Billion*. Available at: http://www.unfpa.org/public/home/7Billion (accessed December 2011).

UN HABITAT (2012). *State of Latin America and Caribbean Cities 2012: Towards a New Urban Transition*. Nairobi: UN Human Settlements Programme.

UN Office on Drugs and Crime (2012). *World Drug Report 2012*. New York: UN Office on Drugs and Crime.

US Department of Transportation (2000). *The Changing Face of Transportation*. BTS00-007. Washington, DC: Bureau of Transportation Statistics. Available at: http://www.rita.dot.gov/bts/sites/rita.dot.gov.bts/files/publications/the_changing_face_of_transportation/index.html (accessed 30 September 2012).

US Health and Human Services Public Health Service (1995). *For a Healthy Nation: Returns on Investment in Public Health*. Washington, DC: US Government Printing Office.

Valdez, S. (2006). *An Introduction to Global Financial Markets*. London: Palgrave Macmillan.

Walley, J., Wright, J., and Hubley, J. (2001). *Public Health: An Action Guide to Improving Health in Developing Countries*. Oxford: Oxford University Press.

Watts, J. (2004). Chinese baby milk blamed for 50 deaths. *The Guardian*, 21 April. Available at: http://www.guardian.co.uk/china/story/0,7369,1196996,00.html (accessed 13 June 2007).

Weiland, S.K., Hüsing, A., Strachan, D. P., Rzehak, P., Pearce, N., and the ISAAC Phase One Study Group (2004). Climate and the prevalence of symptoms of asthma, allergic rhinitis and atopic eczema in children. *Occupational and Environmental Medicine*, 61(7), 609–15.

Weishaar H., Collin, J., Smith, K., Gruning, T., and Gilmore, AB. (2012). Global health governance and the commercial sector: a documentary analysis of tobacco company strategies to influence the WHO Framework Convention on Tobacco Control. *PLoS Medicine*, 9(6), e1001249.

Wilkinson, R. (2006). *The WTO, Crisis and the Governance of Global Trade*. London: Routledge.

World Bank (2000). *Is Globalization Causing a 'Race to the Bottom' in Environmental Standards?* Briefing Papers, April. Washington DC: PREM Economic Policy Group and Development Economics Group. Available at: http://www1.worldbank.org/economicpolicy/globalization/documents/AssessingGlobalizationP4.pdf (accessed 27 March 2007).

WHO (1986). *The Ottawa Charter for Health Promotion*. First International Conference on Health Promotion, Ottawa, 21 November 1986.

WHO (2005). *The World Health Assembly adopts resolution WHA59.2 on application of the International Health Regulations (2005) to strengthen pandemic preparedness and response. Epidemic and Pandemic Alert and Response*. Geneva: WHO. Available at: http://www.who.int/csr/ihr/wharesolution2006/en/index.html (accessed 20 June 2007).

WHO (2006a). *Counterfeit Medicines. Fact Sheet No. 275*, 14 November. Geneva: WHO. Available at: http://www.who.int/mediacentre/factsheets/fs275/en/print.html (accessed 13 June 2007).

WHO (2006b). *Health Metric Network (HMN) Workshop—better health information systems*. Geneva: Health Metrics Network. Available at: http://www.who.int/healthmetrics/news/20061027/en/index.html (accessed 20 June 2007).

WHO (2006c). *World Health Report 2006—Working Together for Health*. Geneva: WHO.

WHO (2009a). *The Financial Crisis and Global Health, Report of a High-Level Consultation*, 19 January. Geneva: WHO. Available at: http://www.who.int/topics/financial_crisis/financialcrisis_report_200902.pdf (accessed 24 October 2012).

WHO (2009b). *Global Health Risks: Mortality and Burden of Disease Attributable to Selected Major Risks*. Geneva: WHO.

WHO (2011). *mHealth: New Horizons for Health Through Mobile Technologies*. Global Observatory for eHealth Series, Volume 3. Geneva: WHO.

WHO (2012a). *Obesity and Overweight. Fact Sheet No. 311*, May. Geneva: WHO.

WHO (2012b). *Tobacco. Fact Sheet No. 339*, May. Geneva: WHO. Available at: http://www.who.int/mediacentre/factsheets/fs339/en/index.html (accessed 28 September 2012).

WHO/UNICEF (2006). *Meeting the MDG Drinking-Water and Sanitation Target: The Urban and Rural Challenge of the Decade*. Geneva: WHO. Available at: http://www.who.int/water_sanitation_health/monitoring/jmpfinal.pdf (accessed 27 March 2007).

Woollacott, M. (2003). The new killer threatening rich and poor alike. *The Guardian*, 25 April. Available at: http://www.guardian.co.uk/comment/story/0,,943179,00.html (accessed 20 June 2007).

World Tourism Organization (2011). *UNWTO Tourism Highlights 2011 Edition*. Madrid: World Tourism Organization. Available at: http://mkt.unwto.org/sites/all/files/docpdf/unwtohighlights11enlr.pdf (accessed 28 September 2012).

WTO (2007). *Risks Lie Ahead Following Stronger Trade in 2006*. Press Release, 472. Geneva: WHO. Available at: http://www.wto.org/english/news_e/pres07_e/pr472_e.htm (accessed 13 June 2007).

WTO (2012). *Trade Growth to Slow in 2012 After Strong Deceleration in 2011*. Press Release, 12 April. Geneva: WHO. Available at: http://www.wto.org/english/news_e/pres12_e/pr658_e.htm (accessed 24 October 2012).

Yach, D. and Beaglehole, R. (2003). Globalization of risks for chronic diseases demands global solutions. *Perspectives on Global Development and Technology*, 3(1–2), 1–21.

SECTION 2

Determinants of health and disease

Determinants of health: overview

Justin V. Remais and Richard J. Jackson

Introduction to determinants of health

The determinants of health are classically categorized into behavioural factors, impacts of the natural environment, genetic determinants, and social determinants, but these overarching categories mask the complexity and diversity of, and interaction between, the drivers of health and disease. These fundamental determinants have acted, and interacted, within populations in complex ways throughout history. For example, the European conquest of the Americas in the sixteenth century decimated native American populations not just through subjugation (social determinants), but also through land confiscation and associated food insecurity (social and environmental determinants), and the spread of infectious diseases— smallpox, measles and plague among them—that Europeans had developed moderate resistance to over generations (biological determinants) (Brooks 1993; Eyler 2003). More nuanced views of the determinants of population health include disease prevention efforts and medical interventions, as well as genetic predispositions to disease and immunological naiveté. Spanning the fundamental determinants are the additional issues of population dynamics, and political and cultural factors, which can have a wide range of impacts both health promoting and health damaging.

Specific cultural practices, for instance, can make a population more or less susceptible to disease. The wiping of an infant's umbilical cord with dung can raise the risk of tetanus and other infections (World Health Organization 1999), while use of lead-containing pigments in cosmetics and medicaments can lead to anaemia, nerve damage, and other disorders (Al-Saleh et al. 2009). Conversely, breastfeeding is a cultural practice that is health protective, reducing the risk of diarrhoeal infections and death among infants in particular (Smith et al. 1973). Meanwhile, tobacco use and tobacco restriction are other examples where cultural practices exert strong influences on population health and well-being, and an improved cultural understanding of tobacco use can provide new opportunities for changing smoking behaviour and approaches to tobacco control (Nichter 2003; Unger et al. 2003).

Similarly, economic conditions are major determinants of health. Countries that experienced increasing prosperity during the twentieth century achieved better housing, reduced crowding, improved water and food quality, and reduced dangerous working conditions (Kangas 2010). These improvements have contributed to reduced rates of a multitude of diseases—e.g.

diarrhoea, tuberculosis (TB), occupational respiratory diseases—and have led to dramatically increased lifespan and better health (Kjellstrom and Mercado 2008). Yet as the twentieth century progressed, certain aspects of increased affluence led to new population health risks, such as increased consumption of calories and salt. The abundance of relatively inexpensive processed foods high in sugar, fat, and salt has been associated with epidemics of obesity, diabetes, and other chronic diseases across most of the wealthier nations, as well as in the rising middle class in certain low- and middle-income countries (LMICs) (McLellan 2002; Remais et al. 2013). At the other end of the economic spectrum, poverty and resource limitations are associated with unhealthy housing, deficient infrastructure, malnutrition, and dangerous sweatshop working conditions.

As economic conditions improve, opportunities arise to invest in relatively inexpensive and widely distributed public health interventions. Examples include the provision and disinfection of water supplies, or the fortification of foodstuffs—flour and other grain products being most common—with micronutrients (Backstrand 2002; Thompson et al. 2003). Similarly, reduction in unventilated cooking with solid fuels in the home can reduce the risk of severe respiratory disease (Smith et al. 2011), while chemicals can be regulated to reduce exposures, and vehicular and building safety codes enacted and enforced. The impact of such basic measures to protect health can be tremendous: a magnitude 7.0 earthquake in 2010 in Haiti resulted in over 200,000 deaths, while a much larger earthquake in Chile that same year resulted in the loss of 700 lives (Harrell 2010). While there is a range of economic, social, political, and resource differences between the two countries, the fundamental importance of the establishment and enforcement of building codes was made apparent in these two tragic disaster contexts.

As our understanding of the determinants of health has expanded, the catalogue of determinants has grown as well, as has appreciation for their interaction at individual and population levels. Distal, far-reaching drivers of health and disease have recently been acknowledged as central determinants of public health. Globalization, climate change, and urbanization, for example, are receiving increasing attention as complex socioenvironmental phenomena—linked to health though rapidly shifting pathways—that fit poorly into the classical categorizations (McMichael 2000; McMichael and Campbell-Lendrum 2003; Gong et al. 2012). To address the key public health challenges and capacities of the twenty-first century, the catalogue of determinants will need to expand further, but their interactions must also be understood and acted upon. For instance, the convergence of infectious and non-communicable diseases in rapidly changing settings like India reflects the dynamic interplay between diverse heath determinants (Remais et al. 2013), requiring a synthetic and comprehensive approach to health determinants, as well as new approaches to research and public health response. In this chapter, we discuss several such complicating features of the determinants of health, addressing the challenges they raise for public health institutions, professionals, and the policies and interventions they develop and deploy.

We describe how the temporal characteristics of health determinants—their dynamism—introduces complex delays and feedbacks, issues related to cumulative exposures, and raises the need for a life-course perspective and a lasting commitment to longitudinal studies, and long time-horizons for policy analysis. We explore the how the multiple scales of health determinants—from molecular to global, distal to proximal—will require cross-sector and cross-disciplinary science, and new technologies for studying, interpreting, and acting on multi-scale health challenges. The cross-boundary nature of the determinants of health are discussed, including the movement of people, policies, capital, and pollutants inherent in global migration, trade, finance, and the transport of transboundary pollutants. Finally, we discuss the influence of abrupt state changes, such as those brought about by conflict or disasters, on health, addressing the need for leadership that is robust to, and prepared for, change, as well as policies that enhance resilience.

Complicating features of determinants

Dynamism

The determinants of health are complicated by their dynamism. The common practice of expressing the relationship between exposure and disease as a relative risk does little to convey the complexities of the temporal relationship between exposure and disease. An abrupt change in exposure, for instance, may not lead to a sudden change in the associated disease response. Time lags between exposure and disease, or disease responses for which cumulative exposures are required, have posed significant challenges to improving our understanding of important health risks, such as indoor air pollution and cancer risk assessment. Health-damaging exposures themselves have complex temporal characteristics, with specific time-scales relevant to particular health outcomes—i.e. cumulative long-term levels are most relevant to some exposures, peak levels most relevant to others.

These exposures are experienced over a series of life stages, and factors influencing growth and development early in life can have dramatic consequences for health in adulthood. A life-course perspective highlights the importance of considering the dynamic nature of health outcomes, as insults during fetal, infant, and childhood development—such as those stemming from maternal and childhood undernutrition, childhood infections, and certain environmental exposures—can lead to susceptibility to multiple health outcomes later in life (Cohen et al. 2004; Gluckman et al. 2008; Chan et al. 2009; Dowd et al. 2009; Winans et al. 2011). Inadequate development of the human body early in life, which is prevalent in LMICs, can impede vitality and

ultimately longevity. There is increasing evidence that certain *in utero* and early-life conditions individuals and populations can lead to both infectious and non-communicable chronic diseases later in life (Gluckman et al. 2008; Rinaudo and Wang 2012; Remais et al. 2013).

The dynamism of the determinants of health raises methodological challenges when carrying out research to clarify the relationship between time-varying exposures and outcomes. Methods are needed to contend with dynamism, for instance by accounting for the timing of exposure and resulting disease, and applying analytical approaches to adjust for effects experienced in the future, such as discounting. Such approaches must reconcile tricky issues related to the relative importance of current versus future conditions when little consensus exists as to which discount rates are best used in such analyses (Weitzman 2001). This poses special challenges for assessing the health impacts of exposures that extend far into the future (e.g. those associated with global climate change), as well as policies and interventions that are phased in over decades (e.g. smoking cessation campaigns). Indeed, dynamism introduces major policy challenges weighing the relative importance of experiencing a given outcome in the present versus the future, forcing the public health community to strike an explicit balance between the interests of current and future generations.

Addressing the dynamic characteristics of the determinants of health will require a commitment to addressing these difficult estimation, valuation, and policy issues, including longitudinal studies with tailored designs that capture the time-course of complex exposures and outcomes. Research designs that span the life-course are one example, as are approaches to account for the diverse time-course of health interventions. Likewise, long time horizons for policy analysis are needed in order to account for long-term impacts that may be overlooked in near-term analyses, such as those that stem from changes to diet and nutrition. These temporal issues, which complicate the timing of exposure and disease as well as our ability to study and respond to them, combine with the challenges associated with health determinants that are multi-scale.

Multi-scale

The determinants of health are not only dynamic and changing, they operate at various scales. Persons who are charged with promoting health—both directly and indirectly—typically operate at the scale of their training. Physicians and nurses work at a personal scale, hospital administrators and health product manufacturers at a more derivative scale, ministers of health at a focused governance level, and at the top level, elected (or arrogating) officials develop and execute military, industrial, agricultural or other policies with sweeping and sometimes global consequences for health. Indeed, at this level national and international leaders frequently make decisions that have great influence on health with limited awareness or consideration of impacts on health. It is the role of health officials to assure that political and institutional leaders at all levels understand health determinants, which themselves span a wide range of scales and domains. Solutions to interconnected challenges, for example, prevention of waste or contamination of drinking water, can offer benefits across not just health domains, but benefits for food and industrial production, cost, and environmental savings (Hanjra et al. 2012).

Virtually all health challenges span scales ranging from the molecular to the microscopic to the global. For example, transmission of *Plasmodium* spp. malaria parasites is regulated by host factors (e.g. immunological, nutritional, etc.), by the local population prevalence and dynamics of mosquito vectors, and by global factors such as climate change that can influence the parasite's spread across regions and continents (Pascual and Bouma 2009; Moore et al. 2012; Dhingra et al. 2013). These scales are not equally valued by health practitioners, who may, for instance, consult with immunologists and microbiologists about the first and second scales, and neglect the latter. Management of multi-scale issues requires that practitioners understand the range of parameters, from microbiological to climatological, that drive such health threats, often requiring them to identify the limits of their expertise, and to articulate the need to abate large-scale determinants, not merely the narrow ones. The spread of malaria is influenced by actions at the personal, community, and governmental levels, which together determine housing infrastructure, availability of bednets, types of livestock, degree and extent of mosquito abatement, insecticide resistance, heat island effects, cost of diagnosis and treatment, and other factors. Managing multi-scale challenges requires cross-domain awareness, technical training, analytical skills, and practical experience.

Cross-boundary

Many key public health threats pose risks that transcend international borders, such as risks resulting from mobile atmospheric or aquatic environmental pollutants, and those that stem from global socioeconomic integration (e.g. increases in global air transport, trade, and migration). In the former category, air pollutants, for instance, are transported internationally and intercontinentally (Zhang et al. 2008; J. Liu et al. 2009), and the consequences for public health thus extend far from the site of emissions. Dust from sources in Asia traverses the Pacific and has reached surface locations in the United States in a matter of days (Husar et al. 2001), and mercury emitted mainly from coal combustion remains in the atmosphere for about a year and poses a serious cross-boundary threat (Selin 2005). Likewise, greenhouse gases (e.g. carbon dioxide and methane) lead to global climate change no matter where emissions occur, and thus the health and economic consequences, such as loss of life and property resulting from increased frequency of extreme temperature events, are widely dispersed across national and continental boundaries (Zhang et al. 2010).

Meanwhile, tighter global economic integration has important public health consequences that are in the early stages of comprehension. For instance, biofuel energy policies in established market economies can have a nutritional impact in developing countries when a portion of global agricultural production is switched to biofuel feedstocks. The macroeconomic effects of such a switch can yield rapid changes in prices of global food staples (Chakravorty et al. 2009), such as occurred in 2007 when average global grain prices rapidly increased in part as a consequence of the expansion of biofuels to meet national blending targets in the European Union, United States, and other countries (Mitchell 2008; Rosegrant 2008). Increases in food prices, and other economic shocks, can have major consequences for undernutrition (Friel et al. 2009; Bloem et al. 2010), yet large uncertainties remain in our understanding of the complex factors that link global economic integration and public health, such as those that drive global food prices (Mitchell 2008) and determine regional resilience to price spikes (Webb 2010) in this example.

Responding to these and other transboundary risks requires coordination of policy goals and regulations between diverse governments, increasingly involving a range of public and private actors at various policy levels (Winter 2006). The World Health Organization and other multilateral institutions can play a key role in coordinating policies to confront transboundary risks, and in facilitating uptake of interventions that are tailored to national and regional needs. International scientific collaboration has been essential to the characterization of the health risks of global climate change and stratospheric ozone depletion, and policy measures that sustain such interactions are needed, such as open-access publication and data sharing requirements, coupled with open-government transparency initiatives that make essential data public. Besides transcending boundaries, certain health determinants are characterized by abrupt shifts, raising additional challenges.

State changes

Large, abrupt changes at societal or planetary levels can drive patterns of health and illness, often for generations. Conflicts between nation states often originate from resource competition, although camouflaged as moral, religious, or ethnic disputes, and can affect health not just for years but for generations (Klare et al. 2011). Wars fought over land and water rights, for instance, can exact heavy and rapid health and economic tolls, and can arise even among seemingly similar religious or ethnic groups, such as Protestants and Catholics in Europe, or the Tutsi and Hutus in Africa. National conflicts can cause abrupt tears in the social fabric, including scores of civilian casualties, the loss of homes and community support systems, sudden depletion or loss of food, water, and other essential resources, and large, rapid unplanned migrations of populations under dangerous conditions. Mental health consequences invariably accompany these abrupt changes to systems that support health (Murthy and Lakshminarayana 2006), and when a new stable state is achieved, it can often be far inferior in its support of population health, such as the establishment of long-term refugee camps, forced repatriation, or loss of nationhood accompanied by ongoing social unrest.

Strategies, diplomatic and technological, to mitigate the flash points for conflict will be necessary, and such strategies must be included in the domain of the health professions. While it may seem a truism that state conflict is a powerful determinant of ill health, health leaders have often shied away from confronting and addressing such threats. In 1985, the Nobel Committee awarded its Peace Prize to International Physicians for the Prevention of Nuclear War, validating the work of health professionals confronting the threats of nuclear war, and elevating the role of health leaders in preventing abrupt state changes to the systems that support health, and minimizing the devastation, health and otherwise, that follows conflict. When conflicts do occur, the important roles of the Red Cross, Red Crescent, and other voluntary health organizations are critical. Large-scale movements of displaced persons give rise to highly vulnerable populations—for example, children and the elderly—placed in circumstances directly hazardous to health and prone to epidemics. Provision of fundamental public health services in such settings is essential, yet as in most circumstances, never as effective as prevention of the conditions that brought on displacement in the first place.

Besides being a source of conflict, resource depletion can itself directly cause abrupt state changes to key earth systems that support health (Tong 2000). These can be brought on by increasing population, emissions of greenhouse gases, and depletion of fresh water, arable land, and other essential resources. A major challenge is that climate change and other global shifts with large consequences for health are often seen as slow moving threats, perhaps best dealt with at some later date. Evolving threats, such as the gradual increase in surface temperatures across the planet, are punctuated by abrupt state changes as well, for example, increased frequency of extreme weather events, which can generate immediate and large health crises. Perhaps the most dramatic example of this is the 2005 heat wave in Europe that caused over 40,000 deaths as a consequence of lasting, dangerous heat conditions that transpired more rapidly than the public health response could mitigate. Such weather extremes, stemming from steady changes in climate, are an inevitable consequence of unmitigated emissions of greenhouse gases, though impacts are difficult to precisely attribute. Avoiding large, irreversible negative health outcomes from abrupt state changes brought on by poor energy, agricultural, and other national policies demands rigorous analysis and leadership from the health sector.

Examples of determinants exhibiting such complexity

Interactions between migration, healthcare delivery, and immunization: an example in China

A range of determinants illustrates the complications described earlier, and among them global urbanization serves as an especially illuminating example. Urbanization is proceeding at rapid pace globally, presenting substantial health risks, such as the challenges of meeting the healthcare needs of large, migrating populations. Urbanization impacts health through complex and multifactorial pathways, involving a number of the complications already described. In China, for instance, the health risks of urbanization are not borne equally: the major healthcare delivery challenges that arise from rapid rural-to-urban migration have diverse impacts on migrant populations. Provision of childhood immunization services to the children of migrants, for example, has been significantly complicated by urbanization (Gong et al. 2012). The country established extensive programmes in the early 1970s to provide basic childhood vaccines—e.g. TB, diphtheria, pertussis, tetanus, polio, measles, and more recently hepatitis B (HBV)—and since 2005 has offered nine vaccines to all neonates and infants nationwide without regard to ability to pay. Coverage has increased dramatically in rural areas, e.g. for HBV from less than 50 per cent in 1993 to greater than 80 per cent by 2006 (Zeng et al. 1998; Cui et al. 2007).

Having dramatically reduced the urban–rural gap in coverage is a major accomplishment for China, yet the country's mass rural-to-urban migration phenomenon has generated a new trend: immunization coverage among the children of migrants is now lower than that of both urban and rural children (Zeng et al. 1998; Cui et al. 2007; Lin et al. 2007, 2011; Liu et al. 2007;

Qin et al. 2007; Zhou et al. 2008). Thus, an urban–rural gap in immunization coverage has given way to a gap between migrant and non-migrant populations, and this problem has been compounded by the unprecedented, dynamic timeline of the country's migration phenomenon. The country's migrant population has risen to more than 260 million, up from 98 million in 2004 (NBSC 2011), and urbanization equivalent to the scale of China's experience over the past few decades was accomplished over hundreds of years in the West. The extraordinary pace of change has produced complex interactions between migration, healthcare delivery, and immunization, but has also driven trends in other key health determinants for migrant populations, such as dangerous working and living conditions, income inequality, and psychological stressors (Gong et al. 2012). Strengthening health programmes to reach migrant populations must be made a high priority for rapidly urbanizing countries, yet a better understanding of the complex pathways linking urbanization to health is urgently needed. Characterizing the causal web will require a multidisciplinary research approach, as well as a commitment to longitudinal studies capable of quantifying the long-term impacts of the transition from rural to urban living in a way that captures both health opportunities and risks (Gong et al. 2012).

Interactions between determinants of infectious disease and of non-communicable chronic disease

Another key example where the determinants of health are interacting in novel ways is the convergence of non-communicable disease (NCD) and infectious disease (ID) in LMICs—a convergence that existing health systems and public health approaches must grapple with. Prevention and control programmes for NCDs—like cardiovascular disease and diabetes mellitus—and IDs—such as TB, HIV/AIDS, and certain parasitic diseases—rarely interact, even though NCDs and IDs share important common features. There are common risk factors for NCDs and IDs, and key interactions between NCDs and IDs lead some individuals with NCDs to be more susceptible to IDs. For example, diabetes increases susceptibility to various communicable diseases, such as TB and malaria. As a result, LMICs are experiencing a large, simultaneous burden of disease from NCDs and IDs (Remais et al. 2013). Diabetes in India, for instance, is estimated to be responsible for more than 10 per cent of the country's 2 million annual TB cases (Ruslami et al. 2010). Diabetes prevalence is projected to increase in India, and as a result the proportion of TB cases attributable to diabetes is projected to increase as well (Ruslami et al. 2010). These interactions between two categories of diseases historically separated by deep professional divides will necessitate new collaborations between NCD and ID researchers and between NCD and ID programme leadership (Remais et al. 2013).

Fundamental data on ID and NCD co-morbidity in LMIC populations must be collected to understand their overlap in populations (Ebrahim et al. 2013), and public health services must be targeted to reach populations found to be exposed to common ID and NCD risk factors, and provide for their healthcare needs. Importantly, the presentation of comorbid NCDs will likely pose new complications to treating IDs, and vice versa, in ways not yet fully explored (Remais et al. 2013). Clinical vigilance will be called for, and as new information emerges, screening and treatment programmes will have to efficiently adapt. Although the convergence of NCD and ID stems from a well-understood risk overlap that drives epidemiological transitions (Smith and Ezzati 2005), the phenomenon presents challenges to the historic divisions in the public health professions, such as the partitioning of chronic and infectious disease epidemiology (Barrett-Connor 1979; Remais et al. 2013). These will need to be overcome if the necessary changes in policy and research are to be enacted, and new approaches to prevention that acknowledge common determinants of NCD and ID, particularly those outside the health sector, will be crucial to doing so (Yang et al. 2008; Gong et al. 2012; Remais and Eisenberg 2012).

Environmental health versus economic development and inequality

Historically, the early stages of national economic development begin with resource extraction and resource-rich developing countries are often courted by industrial countries and their multinationals for access to their raw materials, along with their inexpensive labour, weak environmental regulations, and sites for hazardous waste disposal. These industries can generate rapid wealth, and the political and financial conditions that accompany extraction economies run the risk of becoming repressive toward labour rights, and indifferent and hostile to environmental protections (Reed 2002). What is more, extraction and commodity industries are often subject to 'boom and bust' cycles, which can be detrimental to social stability and health. Maintaining good governance in the face of an influx of new wealth, generated by a small number of industrial agents, can be challenging, and political processes have been observed to be manipulated by vested interests (Hilson and Maconachie 2008). Weak governance during boom-bust cycles can render public services such as schools, transportation, and healthcare ineffective and at times non-existent.

Understanding and addressing issues of environmental health and economic development is essential for ensuring that cycles of resource extraction, political corruption, environmental pollution, and occupational illness are avoided, and examples of successful and environmentally sustainable industrial development are broadly adopted. For example, while extraction of precious metals can present grave risks for miners and smelter workers—for example, gold miners exposed to toxic cyanide or mercury, or diamond miners working in extremely hazardous pits—mining practices have been developed that protect worker health, reduce environmental pollution and are economically viable (Amezaga et al. 2011). Historically, the health sector has argued persuasively for expansive policies to address industrial pollution, urging that societal response should extend beyond the clinical setting (e.g. treating an individual poisoned by metals pollution) into the environment where exposures were taking place (e.g. preventing exposures before they occur) (Remais and Eisenberg 2012). Public health leaders will need to resuscitate this historical role, insisting that funding priorities, research, and policies ensure that sustainable industrial development be implemented based on the best evidence and experience to date.

Ageing and urbanization

Ageing and urbanization are occurring simultaneously in many settings, raising unique public health challenges and illustrating the dynamic, multi-scale nature of the global determinants of health. China, for instance, is experiencing a demographic age shift as a result of declining fertility and increasing life expectancies (Lutz et al. 2008). Fertility has declined nearly 70 per cent since 1950 (Chen and Liu 2009) and life expectancy reached 73 years in 2005 (Zeng 2009). Accordingly, the proportion of China's population 65 years of age and above is projected to reach 25 per cent by 2050, up from 7.6 per cent in 2005 (Flaherty et al. 2007; Chen and Liu 2009). The health determinants unique to ageing populations are interacting with those that accompany the urbanization experience described earlier. China's urban populations have lower fertility and longer life expectancy on balance (Zeng and Vaupel 1989; Li and Tan 2011), which thus tends to yield rapidly ageing urban populations. At the same time, however, tens of millions of migrants, most of whom are young (Wang 2008; Yeh et al. 2011), have flowed into urban areas in China, counterbalancing the tendency of ageing in urban settings. Meanwhile, as a result of the same flux of youth into urban centres, rural areas are ageing very rapidly, raising unique public health issues in these settings (Gong et al. 2012).

For instance, the children left behind when working-age adults leave rural areas—20 million such children are estimated throughout China (Duan and Zhou 2005)—may be at greater risk of injury in part because of reduced supervision of young children under the care of a single parent (Shen et al. 2009). Deleterious mental health effects have also been observed in this so-called 'left-behind' population (Z. Liu et al. 2009). At the same time, the rural elderly population is becoming increasingly dependent on familial support, rather than pensions or social security, for their income (Wang 2006), and mass migration has had the dual effect of both increasing the geographic distance between adult children and their parents (Joseph and Phillips 1999; Chen and Liu 2009) and also providing job opportunities in cities that can increase financial transfers from adult children to their parents (Giles et al. 2010). Addressing the public health effects of these complex interactions between urbanization and population ageing will require approaches and policies that differ from traditional modes of strengthening social security. Expanding support networks for rural elders in the absence of familial ties may be one such approach, as well as injury prevention programmes aimed specifically at reducing accidents among children under the care of single parents, or grandparents, in rural areas. Development of such initiatives will require interaction between a range of social programmes, healthcare systems, and pension schemes, and such efforts are steadily gaining support in China and elsewhere (Gong et al. 2012).

Health risks and benefits of urbanization

No major social, environmental, or behavioural change is without health impacts, both positive and negative, and examining the benefits, alongside health risks, is essential. Returning to urbanization, the phenomenon in LMICs is frequently characterized as essential to future prosperity, while at the same time a threat to health and, in the case of unplanned urban expansion and sprawl, harmful to local and global environmental quality. Globally, migrant flows are continuing into cities at a rapid pace, and important adverse health effects that have long been associated with living in urban areas have been extensively reviewed (e.g. Whiting and Unwin 2009; Gong et al. 2012), some of which have already been discussed.

Notable adverse health impacts include transmission of infectious diseases, such as TB and HIV, facilitated by increased density and mobility of populations, especially within urban slums (Alirol et al. 2011); obesity and diabetes linked to sedentary urban lifestyles and greater access to fatty and sweetened processed foods in urban areas (Ford and Mokdad 2008; Townshend and Lake 2009); and malaria, dengue, and other diseases carried by vectors that capitalize on urban landscapes with poor management of water resources and high host population densities (Keiser et al. 2004). Urban environments are associated with a breakdown of traditional support networks, decreasing social capital and increasing susceptibility to stress, mental illness, and violent crime (Galea et al. 2011). These adverse health effects have been found to vary between countries, among cities in the same country, and within cities (Ompad et al. 2007), and the urban poor disproportionately experience the burden of these ill effects (Kjellstrom and Mercado 2008). In fact, in some instances the urban poor can suffer greater morbidity and mortality from infectious diseases than the rural poor, an indication of the substandard living conditions and poor services in some urban areas, such as a near-complete lack of sanitation facilities and a wide variety of barriers to accessing health services in cities (Satterthwaite 2011).

Conversely, a number of possible health benefits accrue to urban populations, many of which may be unique to urban areas. Greater access to improved water and sanitation facilities, healthcare infrastructure, and nutritional opportunities are examples (Bissonnette et al. 2012), and with decades of rapid urbanization ahead for most LMICs, a comprehensive characterization of the health benefits is needed, alongside extensive research on adverse effects. An analysis of both the health risks and benefits of urbanization can help in the development of strategies to alleviate the ills of urban living, while maximizing the health benefits urban settings offer. Importantly, examining the mechanisms by which urban areas may lead to health gains will be essential, including those that flow from the main distinguishing characteristics of urban areas: high population density, concentration of infrastructure, and rapid social and environmental change. In a future public health environment where political leaders need access to the best evidence to inform policies ranging from industrial to banking, agricultural to social, transportation to health, it will be essential to fully characterize health benefits of policies alongside their adverse impacts.

Conclusion

Addressing the public health challenges of the twenty-first century will require new approaches to understanding, quantifying, and responding to complex, dynamic health determinants. Interactions between health determinants at multiple scales will need to be understood and acted upon, departing from traditions among healthcare providers to consider, and act at, only scales within their training. The cross-boundary nature of health determinants, highlighted by rapid trends in the international movement of people, policies, capital, and pollutants, must be addressed through new global policy mechanisms. There will be a need for global leadership from the health sector to address these major challenges, both from within public health institutions, as well as within other private and public sector institutions setting a range of global policies that influence health through both direct and indirect pathways.

References

Alirol, E., Getaz, L., Stoll, B., Chappuis, F., and Loutan, L. (2011). Urbanisation and infectious diseases in a globalised world. *The Lancet Infectious Diseases*, 11, 131–41.

Al-Saleh, I., Al-Enazi, S., and Shinwari, N. (2009). Assessment of lead in cosmetic products. *Regulatory Toxicology and Pharmacology*, 54, 105–13.

Amezaga, J.M., Rotting, T.S., Younger, P.L., et al. (2011). A rich vein? Mining and the pursuit of sustainability. *Environmental Science & Technology*, 45, 21–6.

Backstrand, J.R. (2002). The history and future of food fortification in the United States: a public health perspective. *Nutrition Reviews*, 60, 15–26.

Barrett-Connor, E. (1979). Infectious and chronic disease epidemiology: separate and unequal? *American Journal of Epidemiology*, 109, 245–9.

Bissonnette, L., Wilson, K., Bell, S., and Shah, T.I. (2012). Neighbourhoods and potential access to health care: the role of spatial and aspatial factors. *Health & Place*, 18, 841–53.

Bloem, M.W., Semba, R.D., and Kraemer, K. (2010). Castel Gandolfo workshop: an introduction to the impact of climate change, the economic crisis, and the increase in the food prices on malnutrition. *Journal of Nutrition*, 140, 132S–5S.

Brooks, F.J. (1993). Revising the conquest of Mexico: smallpox, sources, and populations. *Journal of Interdisciplinary History*, 24, 1.

Chakravorty, U., Hubert, M.H., and Nostbakken, L. (2009). Fuel versus food. *Annual Review of Resource Economics*, 1, 645–63.

Chan, J.C., Malik, V., Jia, W., et al. (2009). Diabetes in Asia: epidemiology, risk factors, and pathophysiology. *JAMA*, 301, 2129–40.

Chen, F. and Liu, G. (2009). Population aging in China. In P. Uhlenberg (ed.) *International Handbook of Population Aging*, pp. 157–72. New York: Springer.

Cohen, S., Doyle, W.J., Turner, R.B., Alper, C.M., and Skoner, D.P. (2004). Childhood socioeconomic status and host resistance to infectious illness in adulthood. *Psychosomatic Medicine*, 66, 553–8.

Cui, F., Purha, T., Hadler, S., and Liang, X. (2007). Analysis on newborn hepatitis B immunization coverage and pregnant women hospital delivery rate in different regions. *Chinese Journal of Vaccine and Immunization*, 13, 1–3.

Dhingra, R., Jimenez, V., Chang, H., et al. (2013). Spatially-explicit simulation modeling of ecological response to climate change: methodological considerations in predicting shifting population dynamics of infectious disease vectors. *ISPRS International Journal of Geo-Information*, 2, 645–64.

Dowd, J.B., Zajacova, A., and Aiello, A. (2009). Early origins of health disparities: burden of infection, health, and socioeconomic status in U.S. children. *Social Science & Medicine*, 68, 699–707.

Duan, C. and Zhou, F. (2005). Studies on left behind children in China. *Population Research*, 25, 29–36.

Ebrahim, S., Pearce, N., Smeeth, L., Casas, J.P., Jaffar, S., and Piot, P. (2013). Tackling non-communicable diseases in low- and middle-income countries: is the evidence from high-income countries all we need? *PLoS Medicine*, 10, e1001377.

Eyler, J.M. (2003). Smallpox in history: the birth, death, and impact of a dread disease. *Journal of Laboratory and Clinical Medicine*, 142, 216–20.

Flaherty, J.H., Liu, M.L., Ding, L., et al. (2007). China: the aging giant. *Journal of the American Geriatrics Society*, 55, 1295–300.

Ford, E.S. and Mokdad, A.H. (2008). Epidemiology of obesity in the Western Hemisphere. *The Journal of Clinical Endocrinology & Metabolism*, 93, S1–8.

Friel, S., Dangour, A. D., Garnett, T., et al. (2009). Public health benefits of strategies to reduce greenhouse-gas emissions: food and agriculture. *The Lancet*, 374, 2016–25.

Galea, S., Uddin, M., and Koenen, K. (2011). The urban environment and mental disorders: epigenetic links. *Epigenetics*, 6, 400–4.

Giles, J., Wang, D., and Zhao, C. (2010). Can China's rural elderly count on support from adult children? Implications of rural-to-urban migration. *Journal of Population Ageing*, 3, 183–204.

Gluckman, P.D., Hanson, M.A., Cooper, C., and Thornburg, K.L. (2008). Effect of in utero and early-life conditions on adult health and disease. *The New England Journal of Medicine*, 359, 61–73.

Gong, P., Liang, S., Carlton, E.J., et al. (2012). Urbanisation and health in China. *The Lancet*, 379, 843–52.

Hanjra, M.A., Blackwell, J., Carr, G., Zhang, F., and Jackson, T.M. (2012). Wastewater irrigation and environmental health: implications for water governance and public policy. *International Journal of Hygiene and Environmental Health*, 215, 255–69.

Harrell, E. (2010). When the earth moves. *Time*, 175, 22–5.

Hilson, G. and Maconachie, R. (2008). 'Good governance' and the extractive industries in sub-Saharan Africa. *Mineral Processing and Extractive Metallurgy Review*, 30, 52–100.

Husar, R.B., Tratt, D.M., Schichtel, B.A., et al. (2001). Asian dust events of April 1998. *Journal of Geophysical Research – Atmospheres*, 106, 18317–30.

Joseph, A.E. and Phillips, D.R. (1999). Ageing in rural China: impacts of increasing diversity in family and community resources. *Journal of Cross-Cultural Gerontology*, 14, 153–68.

Kangas, O. (2010). One hundred years of money, welfare and death: mortality, economic growth and the development of the welfare state in 17 OECD countries 1900–2000. *International Journal of Social Welfare*, 19, S42–59.

Keiser, J., Utzinger, J., Caldas De Castro, M., Smith, T.A., Tanner, M., and Singer, B.H. (2004). Urbanization in sub-Saharan Africa and implication for malaria control. *American Journal of Tropical Medicine and Hygiene*, 71, 118–27.

Kjellstrom, T. and Mercado, S. (2008). Towards action on social determinants for health equity in urban settings. *Environment and Urbanization*, 20, 551–74.

Klare, M.T., Levy, B.S., and Sidel, V.W. (2011). The public health implications of resource wars. *American Journal of Public Health*, 101, 1615–19.

Li, G.-P. and Tan, Y.-G. (2011). China's urbanization: characteristics, regional differences, and influencing factors. *Social Science Journal*, 106–10.

Lin, X.-D., Chen, L.-P., Zheng, X.-C., Li, W.-C., Wang, Z.-G., and Deng, Z.-J. (2011). Analyses of factors influencing the coverage of national immunization program in migrant children in Wenzhou. *Chinese Journal of Child Health Care*, 59–61.

Lin, Y.-J., Lei, R.-Y., Luo, Y.-X., et al. (2007). Analysis of immunization coverage rate and its influencing factor of floating children in Zhujiang Delta River Area of Guangdong Province. *Chinese Journal of Vaccine and Immunization*, 13, 87–90.

Liu, D.-W., Sun, M.-P., Liu, W.-X., et al. (2007). Comparative study on immunization coverage rates of nine vaccines between local and floating children in Beijing. *Chinese Journal of Vaccine and Immunization*, 13, 165–9.

Liu, J., Mauzerall, D.L., Horowitz, L.W., Ginoux, P., and Fiore, A.M. (2009a). Evaluating inter-continental transport of fine aerosols: (1) methodology, global aerosol distribution and optical depth. *Atmospheric Environment*, 43, 4327–38.

Liu, Z., Li, X., and Ge, X. (2009). Left too early: the effects of age at separation from parents on Chinese rural children's symptoms of anxiety and depression. *American Journal of Public Health*, 99, 2049–54.

Lutz, W., Sanderson, W., and Scherbov, S. (2008). The coming acceleration of global population ageing. *Nature*, 451, 716–19.

McLellan, F. (2002). Obesity rising to alarming levels around the world. *The Lancet*, 359, 1412.

McMichael, A.J. (2000). The urban environment and health in a world of increasing globalization: issues for developing countries. *Bulletin of the World Health Organization*, 78, 1117–26.

McMichael, A.J., and Campbell-Lendrum, D.H. (2003). *Climate Change and Human Health: Risks and Responses*. Geneva: World Health Organization.

Mitchell, D. (2008). *A Note on Rising Food Prices*. Washington, DC: The World Bank, Development Prospects Group.

Moore, J.L., Liang, S., Akullian, A., and Remais, J.V. (2012). Cautioning the use of degree-day models for climate change projections in the presence of parametric uncertainty. *Ecological Applications*, 22, 2237–47.

Murthy, R.S., and Lakshminarayana, R. (2006). Mental health consequences of war: a brief review of research findings. *World Psychiatry*, 5, 25–30.

NBSC (2011). *Bulletin of Main Statistics of the Sixth National Census*. Beijing: National Bureau of Statistics.

Nichter, M. (2003). Smoking: what does culture have to do with it? *Addiction*, 98(Suppl. 1), 139–45.

Ompad, D.C., Galea, S., Caiaffa, W.T., and Vlahov, D. (2007). Social determinants of the health of urban populations: methodologic considerations. *Journal of Urban Health*, 84, i42–53.

Pascual, M. and Bouma, M.J. (2009). Do rising temperatures matter? *Ecology*, 90, 906–12.

Qin, X.-L., Li, J.-L., and Qin, C.-W. (2007). Immunization of floating children in clustered areas of migrant workers and the influencing factors. *Journal of Applied Preventive Medicine*, 31–2.

Reed, D. (2002). Resource extraction industries in developing countries. *Journal of Business Ethics*, 39, 199–226.

Remais, J.V., and Eisenberg, J.N.S. (2012). Balance between clinical and environmental responses to infectious diseases. *The Lancet*, 379, 1457–9.

Remais, J.V., Zeng, G., Li, G., Tian, L., and Engelgau, M.M. (2013). Convergence of non-communicable and infectious diseases in low- and middle-income countries. *International Journal of Epidemiology*, 42, 221–7.

Rinaudo, P. and Wang, E. (2012). Fetal programming and metabolic syndrome. *Annual Review of Physiology*, 74, 107–30.

Rosegrant, M. (2008). *Biofuels and Grain Prices: Impacts and Policy Responses*. Testimony for the U.S. Senate Committee on Homeland Security and Governmental Affairs, 7 May. Washington, DC: International Food Policy Research Institute.

Ruslami, R., Aarnoutse, R.E., Alisjahbana, B., Van Der Ven, A.J., and Van Crevel, R. (2010). Implications of the global increase of diabetes for tuberculosis control and patient care. *Tropical Medicine and International Health*, 15, 1289–99.

Satterthwaite, D. (2011). Editorial: why is urban health so poor even in many successful cities? *Environment and Urbanization*, 23, 5–11.

Selin, N.E. (2005). Mercury rising: is global action needed to protect human health and the environment? *Environment*, 47, 22–35.

Shen, M., Yang, S., Han, J., et al. (2009). Non-fatal injury rates among the 'left-behind children' of rural China. *Injury Prevention*, 15, 244–7.

Smith, K.R. and Ezzati, M. (2005). How environmental health risks change with development: the epidemiologic and environmental risk transitions revisited. *Annual Review of Environment and Resources*, 30, 291–8.

Smith, K.R., McCracken, J.P., Weber, M.W., et al. (2011). Effect of reduction in household air pollution on childhood pneumonia in Guatemala (RESPIRE): a randomised controlled trial. *The Lancet*, 378, 1717–26.

Smith, L.E., Jr., Sitton, G.D., and Vincent, C.K. (1973). Limited injections of follicle stimulating hormone for multiple births in beef cattle. *Journal of Animal Science*, 37, 523–7.

Thompson, T., Sobsey, M., and Bartram, J. (2003). Providing clean water, keeping water clean: an integrated approach. *International Journal of Environmental Health Research*, 13(Suppl. 1), S89–94.

Tong, S. (2000). The potential impact of global environmental change on population health. *Australian & New Zealand Journal of Medicine*, 30, 618–25.

Townshend, T. and Lake, A.A. (2009). Obesogenic urban form: theory, policy and practice. *Health & Place*, 15, 909–16.

Unger, J.B., Cruz, T., Shakib, S., et al. (2003). Exploring the cultural context of tobacco use: a transdisciplinary framework. *Nicotine & Tobacco Research*, 5(Suppl. 1), S101–17.

Wang, D.W. (2006). China's urban and rural old age security system: challenges and options. *China & World Economy*, 14, 102–16.

Wang, D.W. (2008). *Rural-Urban Migration and Policy Responses in China: Challenges and Options*. Bangkok: International Labour Office; ILO Regional Office for Asia and the Pacific, Asian Regional Programming on Governance of Labour Migration.

Webb, P. (2010). Medium- to long-run implications of high food prices for global nutrition. *Journal of Nutrition*, 140, 143S–7S.

Weitzman, M.L. (2001). Gamma discounting. *American Economic Review*, 91, 260–71.

Whiting, D. and Unwin, N. (2009). Cities, urbanization and health. *International Journal of Epidemiology*, 38, 1737–8.

Winans, B., Humble, M.C., and Lawrence, B.P. (2011). Environmental toxicants and the developing immune system: a missing link in the global battle against infectious disease? *Reproductive Toxicology*, 31, 327–36.

Winter, G. (2006). *Multilevel Governance of Global Environmental Change: Perspectives from Science, Sociology and the Law*. Cambridge: Cambridge University Press.

World Health Organization (1999). *Care of the Umbilical Cord: A Review of the Evidence*. Geneva: World Health Organization.

Yang, G., Kong, L., Zhao, W., et al. (2008). Emergence of chronic non-communicable diseases in China. *The Lancet*, 372, 1697–705.

Yeh, A., Xu, J., and Liu, K. (2011). China's post-reform urbanization: retrospect, policies and trends. New York: United Nations Population Fund (UNFPA) and the International Institute for Environment and Development (IIED).

Zeng, X.J., Yang, H.G., Miao, S., Chen, A., Tan, J., and Huang, Z. (1998). A study on the coverage, strategies and cost of hepatitis B vaccination in China, 1996. *Chinese Journal of Epidemiology*, 277–81.

Zeng, Y. (2009). Challenges of population aging in China. *China Economic Journal*, 2, 277–83.

Zeng, Y. and Vaupel, J.W. (1989). The impact of urbanization and delayed childbearing on population-growth and aging in China. *Population and Development Review*, 15, 425–45.

Zhang, J., Mauzerall, D.L., Zhu, T., Liang, S., Ezzati, M., and Remais, J.V. (2010). Environmental health in China: progress towards clean air and safe water. *The Lancet*, 375, 1110–19.

Zhang, L., Jacob, D.J., Boersma, K.F., et al. (2008). Transpacific transport of ozone pollution and the effect of recent Asian emission increases on air quality in North America: an integrated analysis using satellite, aircraft, ozonesonde, and surface observations. *Atmospheric Chemistry and Physics*, 8, 6117–36.

Zhou, Y.-H., Wu, C., and Zhuang, H. (2008). Vaccination against hepatitis B: the Chinese experience. *Chinese Medical Journal*, 121, 98–102.

Poverty, justice, and health

Ronald Labonté, Frances Baum,
and David Sanders

Introduction to poverty, justice, and health

> Poverty has to be understood not just as a disadvantaged and inse-
> cure economic *condition*, but also as a shameful and corrosive social
> *relation*. (p. 7, emphasis in original)
> Reproduced from Lister, R., *Poverty*, Polity Press, Copyright © 2004.

Poverty has long been a concern in public health. Not only do the poor generally suffer higher burdens of disease, but during periods of infectious epidemics or pandemics they are perceived as posing a risk to the non-poor as well. Recent studies even suggest that high poverty and disease rates together can contribute to social unrest and 'failed' (or failing) states (Cheek 2001; Hotez 2002; Singer 2002; Peterson and Shellman 2006). Apart from these more 'public' (or population) health risks, the persistence of poverty has also led many public health theorists and practitioners to ask why poverty continues to exist in times of great global wealth, and to argue that a socially just society would seek to eliminate poverty. The reasons for the persistence of poverty lie in how societies' economic and political systems allocate the opportunities and resources people need to be 'non-poor' and healthy, or intervene to reduce inequities (avoidable inequalities) in their access to services and resources. Thus, any discussion of poverty, and of its impacts on health, unavoidably intersects with understanding how inequalities arise in the distribution of income and wealth, and of the material and psychosocial resources these socioeconomic privileges accord. As the British economist-cum-philosopher, Adam Smith, known best for his writings extolling the virtues of free markets, noted:

> Wherever there is great property, there is great inequality. For one
> very rich man, there must be at least five hundred poor, and the afflu-
> ence of the few supposes the indigence of the many. (Smith 1776,
> p. 419)

But what exactly is poverty? How is it affecting health, and ill health affecting poverty? And what theories or practices of justice should guide public health interventions based on poverty's persisting health risks? These three questions form the basis of the chapter that follows.

What is poverty?

At first glance, it may seem simple to define poverty: the inability of people to provide for the basic necessities of life. But there are actually many forms of poverty, all of them important to public health and to public policy; and the concept of poverty itself is 'highly contested' (Alcock 1993, p. x). Its contestation is not simply theoretical (what does it mean?) or empirical (how do we measure it?) but also political, since it is the same sociopolitical structures and economic arrangements that give rise to both poverty and affluence.

Absolute poverty

Absolute poverty is foundational to an understanding of the concept, and is commonly considered to be the lack of a minimum income necessary for simple survival based upon the price of a basket of 'essential' goods and services (Masters and Wickstrom 2006; Saunders et al. 2008). The World Bank has standardized poverty measures globally through its 'dollar a day' and 'two dollars a day' poverty rates. The dollar-a-day level, close to the national poverty line in India, has since been raised to $1.25/day as a more common metric, a figure that represents the average national poverty line of the poorest 10–20 countries (Chen and Ravallion 2012). The two-dollar-a-day level is the median national poverty line for all developing countries. Dollar-a-day poverty describes subsistence consumption at a level that is minimally life-supporting and 'exceptionally frugal . . . even by the standards of the world's poorest countries' (Chen and Ravallion 2012, p. 1). Raising this to $1.25/day does little to improve the material circumstances of those who live on it. Two-dollar-a-day poverty describes consumption that accommodates other essential basic needs such as land, agricultural tools, and some access to education and healthcare, although it remains associated with comparatively low life expectancies and high infant and maternal mortality rates. (We discuss the relationship between poverty and health later in this chapter.)

Global poverty rates at all three levels ($1, $1.25, and $2/day) have continued to fall since the baseline year of 1981 (Table 2.2.1), often attributed to globalization-associated economic growth (Santarelli and Figini 2002; World Bank 2002). The absolute number of people worldwide who are living below these levels has also fallen, but there are important regional variations. Poverty rates and absolute numbers fell most dramatically in East Asia and China. Poverty rates and absolute numbers rose in Latin America and the Caribbean during the 1980s and 1990s—the 'lost decades' that many attribute to structural adjustment programmes imposed by the World Bank and International Monetary Fund (Grindle 1996)—before beginning to

Table 2.2.1 Percentage and number of people in the developing world living below World Bank poverty levels, 1981 and 2008

Poverty level	1981 percentage	1981 number	2008 percentage	2008 number
$1/day	42	1.54 billion	14	801 million
$1.25/day	52	1.94 billion	22	1.29 billion
$2/day	70	2.59 billion	43	2.47 billion

Source: data from Shaohua Chen and Martin Ravallion, *An update to the World Bank's estimates of consumption poverty in the developing world*, Briefing Note 03-01-12, Development Research Group, World Bank, Copyright © 2012.

fall in the 2000s. The recent decline in poverty in this region is a result of economic growth combined with redistributive social policies and programmes (Birdsall et al. 2011). Poverty rates in sub-Saharan Africa fell only very slightly over this 30-year period, and failed completely to keep pace with population growth as the continuing rise in number of poor indicates (Fig. 2.2.1). Globally, there were only modest gains in decreasing poverty at the two-dollar-a-day level, and a substantial rise in the number subsisting between the $1.25 and $2/day rates, which 'points to the fact that a great many people remain vulnerable' (Chen and Ravallion 2012, p. 3).

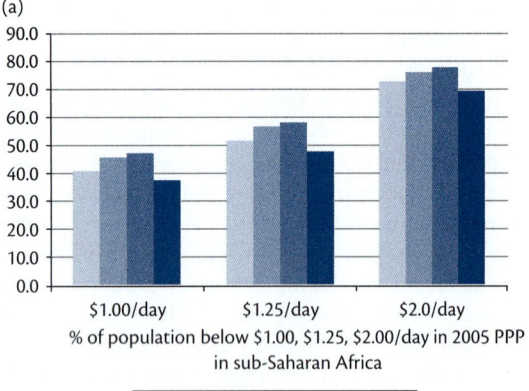

(a)

% of population below $1.00, $1.25, $2.00/day in 2005 PPP in sub-Saharan Africa

1981   1990   1999   2008

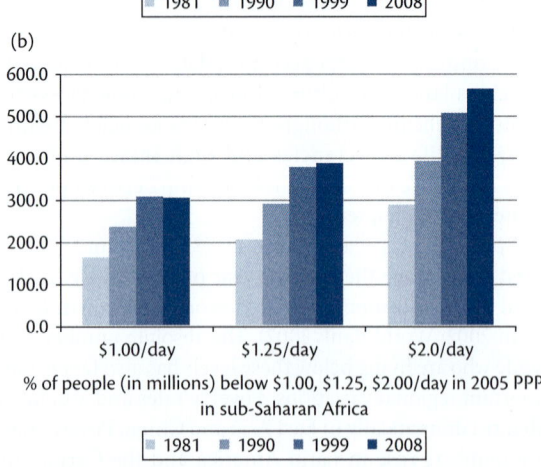

(b)

% of people (in millions) below $1.00, $1.25, $2.00/day in 2005 PPP in sub-Saharan Africa

1981   1990   1999   2008

Fig. 2.2.1 Proportion of population and number of people living in poverty in sub-Saharan Africa between 1981 and 2008.
Source: data from Shaohua Chen and Martin Ravallion, *An update to the World Bank's estimates of consumption poverty in the developing world*, Briefing Note 03-01-12, Development Research Group, World Bank, Copyright © 2012.

These data mean that the not very ambitious Millennium Development Goal of halving the number of people living in extreme poverty ($1 or $1.25/day) between 1990 and 2015 has been achieved. Of comparative significance is that the value of the global economy more than quadrupled during this same time period—from US $18 trillion in 1980 (De Long 1998) to US $80 trillion in 2011 (Central Intelligence Agency 2013), indicative that very little 'trickle down' of the benefits of that growth reached the 'bottom billion' (Collier 2007). Neither does halving these rates say anything of the adequacy of the poverty lines themselves, to which other analysts have responded with estimates of an 'ethical poverty line'. The ethical poverty line was established by working backwards from countries with an average life expectancy at birth of 74 years (considered an ethical minimum) to the average level of consumption associated with such a life expectancy (around $3/day) (Edward 2006). Using this $3/day poverty line increases the number of global poor by 1.3 billion to around 3.7 billion, or roughly half the planet's total population. By one estimate, which assumes a continuation of global economic growth and poverty reduction rates of the past two decades, cutting 'ethical poverty' by half would take between 116 and 209 years (Woodward and Simms 2006), would still leave half the world behind, would achieve life expectancies for those above the ethical poverty line a decade less than that enjoyed by wealthier people in high-income countries, and would almost certainly destroy the ecological resources required for life long before achieving this effect.

Finally, the World Bank's estimates of people living in absolute poverty are generally based on what people report consuming. Since many of the world's poor consume healthcare for which they have to pay, this can result in *medical poverty*, when catastrophic illness forces people to sell their assets and exhaust their savings to pay for treatment. These people may lift themselves out of 'consumption' poverty (since they are consuming healthcare at a high level) but leave themselves in income poverty (since they no longer have money for other goods or services). In 2005, the World Health Organization (WHO) estimated that:

> Each year 100 million people slide into poverty as a result of medical care payments. Another 150 million people are forced to spend nearly half their incomes on medical expenses. That is because in many countries people have no access to social health protection — affordable health insurance or government-funded health services. (WHO 2005)

Recognizing the seriousness of medical poverty, in December 2012, the United Nations General Assembly passed a resolution calling on Member States to develop universal health coverage systems to prevent significant payments at the point of delivery and to pool risks to avoid catastrophic healthcare spending and impoverishment (United Nations General Assembly 2012).

Absolute poverty informs public health by way of a presumption that people living at or below such poverty lines lack access to sufficient material resources to develop or maintain their health. Apart from the ethical poverty line, this level of poverty represents a form more commonly associated with poor groups in low-income and middle-income countries than with poor groups in high-income countries. This poverty concept nonetheless applies to high-income countries where some households live in 'deep poverty', where income levels are 75 per cent or less of nationally established poverty lines and are considered inadequate to meet even basic needs of food, shelter, and clothing (Beiser et al. 2002).

Conservative think-tanks in high-income countries have sometimes argued that absolute poverty, which is indifferent to measures of income or wealth distribution, should be the only policy concern. Not all agree. Apart from growth-related poverty reduction being much less under conditions of high income-inequality (Bourguignon 2004), most of the world's absolute poor now live in middle-income countries such as India and China, making governance, taxation, and redistribution of paramount importance in reducing levels of absolute poverty (Sumner 2010).

Relative poverty

Poverty means going short materially, socially and emotionally. It means spending less on food, on heating and on clothing than someone on an average income—above all, poverty takes away the tools to build the blocks for the future. It steals away the opportunity to have a life unmarked by sickness, a decent education, a secure home. (p. 3)
> Reproduced with permission from Oppenheim C. and Harker L., Poverty: the facts, Child Poverty Action Group, London, UK, Copyright © 1990.

Relative poverty introduces the idea that it is not enough simply to be able to meet the material necessities of life. One is poor if one lacks the resources required to engage in some meaningful ways in society and its sundry activities (social, economic, political, cultural, and recreational). That is, relative poverty is concerned with *living standards*—which vary by place and over time, but which convey the notion of comparatively full social functioning. This concept of relative poverty as the inability to function socially to

some normative standard can be traced in Western thought as far back as Aristotle (Sen 2000). Peter Townsend was one of the first of the recent theorists to criticize the policy use of absolute poverty:

> He, and others since, argued for a concept of 'relative poverty' based less on minimal needs for survival and more on needs conditioned by societal expectations—that is, on what people require to participate fully in society (Nunes 2008; Eurostat 2010). This concept of relative poverty is actually reasonably old even in liberal economic thought, having been famously proposed by Adam Smith in his statement that 'a creditable day-labourer would be ashamed to appear in public without a linen shirt, the want of which would be supposed to denote that disgraceful degree of poverty' (cited in Ravallion 2011). (Labonté et al. 2012, p. 15)

As Martin Ravallion, the World Bank's expert on global poverty and lead analyst for the absolute measures discussed earlier, points out, this passage from Smith implies that 'certain socially-specific expenditures are essential for social inclusion, on top of basic needs for nutrition and physical survival' and that 'the way this idea is implemented in practice is to set a 'relative poverty line' that is a constant proportion of average income for the country' (Ravallion 2011). The common relative poverty measure is having a net household income (one that takes into account government cash transfers and taxes, and that is adjusted for family size and often also for urban or rural location) that is below 50 per cent of the country median. This measure is commonly used for comparative studies within or across high-income countries, i.e. those belonging to the Organization for Economic Cooperation and Development (OECD). Fig. 2.2.2 provides an example using

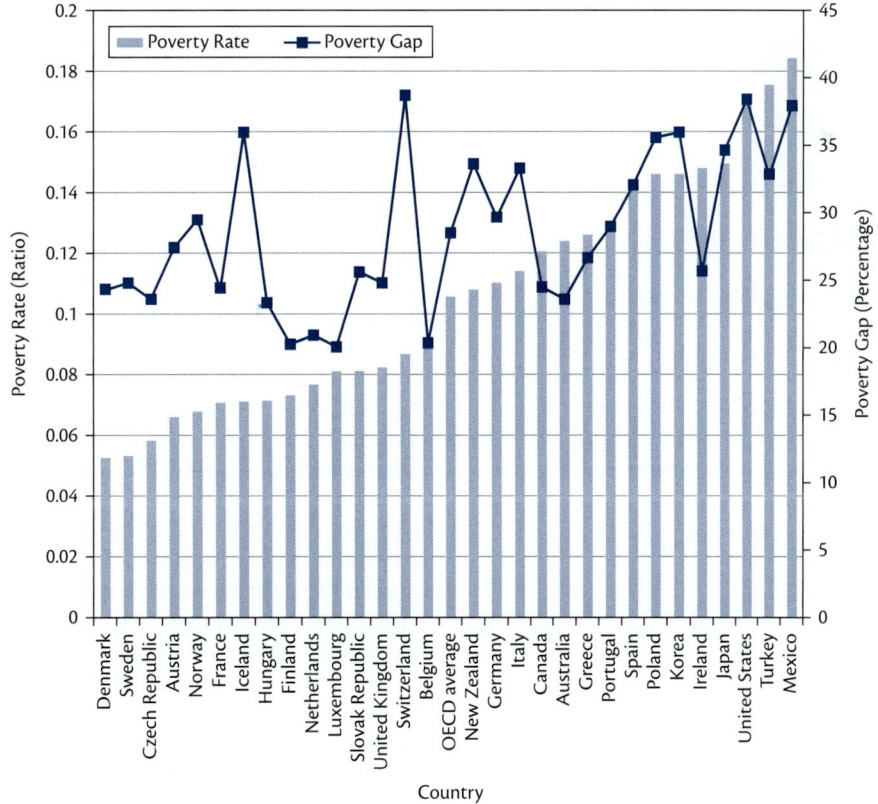

Fig. 2.2.2 Poverty rate and poverty gap, selected OECD countries.

Adapted with permission from Organisation for Economic Co-operation and Development (PECD), *OECD Factbook 2010: Economic, Environmental and Social Statistics*, OECD Publishing, p.237, Copyright © 2010, DOI: 10.1787/factbook-2010-en.

OECD countries, which includes the 'poverty gap'—the median of how far below the relative poverty line a household falls and a measure of 'deep poverty' (OECD 2010). Fig. 2.2.3 focuses on child poverty in economically advanced countries (UNICEF Innocenti Research Centre 2012). A relative concept of poverty informs public health by expanding the range of goods and services that members of a household should be able to access to experience, in Ravallion's terms, social inclusion, and the mental and physical health benefits such inclusion might garner. At the same time, the monetization of the concept (pegging it to a percentage of average or median income) has been criticized since it represents a form of poverty that will never disappear. As average or median incomes rise in a population, there will always be some who will fall below these cut-offs. It is possible for absolute poverty to fall within a country or region, while relative poverty rises; since the relative

poverty cut-offs can be affected by disproportionate increases in income amongst a minority of the population, even if the material conditions of those at the bottom of the income gradient improve. As the UNICEF Innocenti Research Centre (2012) warns, relative poverty is not a good metric for comparison across countries except for those wealthier nations where falling below 50 per cent of the median income does risk social exclusion (a concept we define later in this chapter).

Poverty as lack of capabilities

> The capability approach...builds a bridge between absolute and relative concepts of poverty. It is absolute in identifying the capabilities or functionings that people should experience, but relative in the income or resources that may be required.
>
> Reproduced from Labonté, R. et al., *Indicators of Social Exclusion and Inclusion: A Critical and Comparative Analysis of the Literature*, E/Exchange Working Paper Series, PHIRN, University of Ottawa, Canada © 2012, with permission from the author.

While relative poverty presents a more nuanced understanding of 'being poor' than does absolute poverty, it still relies upon indicators of income. Amartya Sen (1985), in his pioneering capability approach to poverty, focused attention on the infrastructural enabling conditions ('capabilities') that allow people to attain desirable states ('functionings'), without which a minimally dignified human existence is not possible. This has brought in different kinds of indicators that are much more transparent and direct reflections of people's actually achieved levels of well-being and ability 'to accomplish what [they] value' (Alkire 2002, p. 6, cited in Nunes 2008). Income is simply a means to a valued and socially purposeful end. Sen considered indicators such as life expectancy, literacy, and infant mortality to be important proxies for capabilities (at least at a population level) and more useful than income alone to identify poor from non-poor groups or countries. He proposed that indicators of these other characteristics should be aggregated into a more complex poverty measure (Nunes 2008). This approach became the basis of the *Human Development Index* (HDI), first released in 1990 and issued annually by the United Nations Development Program (UNDP), and which combines data on health, education, and living standards (this last dimension using the income indicator of log gross domestic product (GDP)/capita) (see Table 2.2.2) (UNDP 2011). The capability approach from which the HDI arose has since been considerably elaborated (Ranis et al. 2007), including the UNDP's creation of a *multidimensional poverty index* (MPI) in which additional weighted measures have been added to its HDI (Box 2.2.1).

The key contribution the capability approach makes to public health is that it de-couples meaningful social participation (the concern of relative poverty) and, in broader conceptual terms, the notion of 'development' itself, from a purely or primarily economic growth/income growth model. It identifies a range of goods and services for which social (state) provision is important due to their cost or to market failures in ensuring equitable access. The capability approach arose, in part, to challenge the dominance in public policy of the GDP measure, which critics argued was a deeply flawed indicator of how well countries were doing in providing for the general health or welfare of their citizens.

While Sen (1999) argued effectively for the obligations on states to provide a minimum basket of resources allowing people to

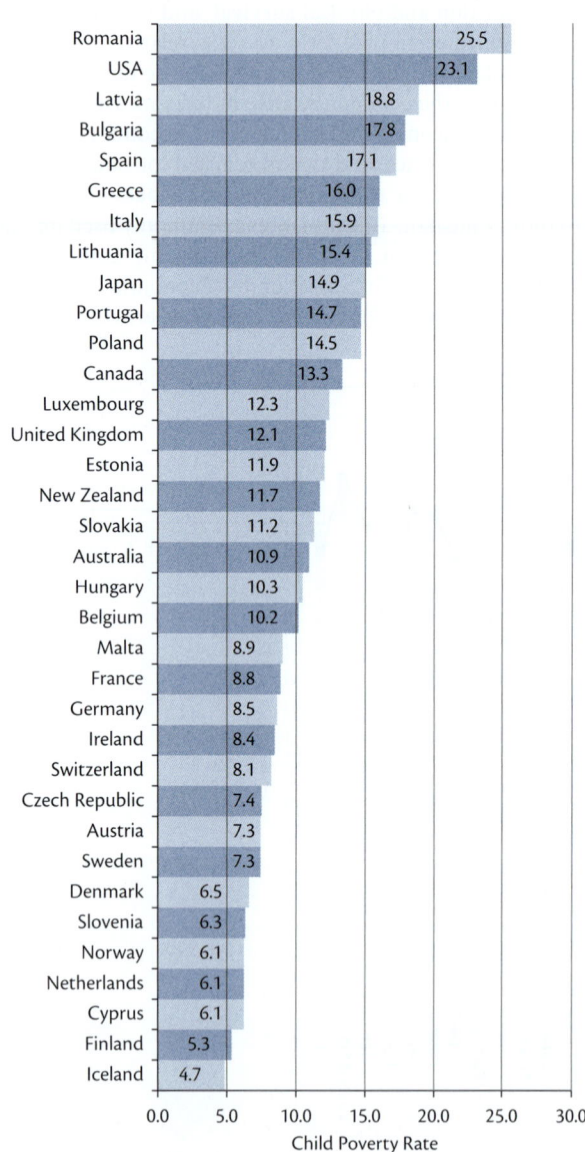

Fig. 2.2.3 Child poverty rate (%) in selected countries. Data generally for 2009.
Adapted with permission from UNICEF Innocenti Research Centre, *Measuring Child Poverty: New league tables of child poverty in the world's rich countries*, p.3, UNICEF Innocenti Research Centre, Innocenti Report Card 10, Florence, Italy, Copyright © 2012.

Table 2.2.2 Human Development Index (HDI) 1980 and 2011, selected countries

HDI rank	Country	HDI value	
		1980	2011
Very high human development			
1	Norway	0.796	0.943
2	Australia	0.850	0.929
3	Netherlands	0.792	0.910
4	United States	0.837	0.910
5	New Zealand	0.800	0.908
6	Canada	0.817	0.908
7	Ireland	0.735	0.908
High human development			
48	Uruguay	0.658	0.783
49	Palau	–	0.782
50	Romania	–	0.781
51	Cuba	–	0.776
52	Seychelles	–	0.773
53	Bahamas	–	0.771
54	Montenegro	–	0.771
Medium human development			
95	Jordan	0.541	0.698
96	Algeria	0.454	0.698
97	Sri Lanka	0.539	0.691
98	Dominican Republic	0.532	0.689
99	Samoa	–	0.688
100	Fiji	0.566	0.688
101	China	0.404	0.687
Low human development			
183	Chad	–	0.328
184	Mozambique	–	0.322
185	Burundi	0.200	0.316
186	Niger	0.177	0.295
187	Congo (Democratic Republic of the)	0.282	0.286
Very high human development		0.766	0.889
High human development		0.614	0.741
Medium human development		0.420	0.630
Low human development		0.316	0.456
Regions			
Arab States		0.444	0.641
East Asia and the Pacific		0.428	0.671
Europe and Central Asia		0.644	0.751
Latin America and the Caribbean		0.582	0.731

HDI rank	Country	HDI value	
		1980	2011
South Asia		0.356	0.548
Sub-Saharan Africa		0.365	0.463
World		**0.558**	**0.682**

Note: the top five countries in each of the first three categories (very high, high and medium) are shown, while for contrast purposes the bottom five countries for the fourth category (low) is shown.

Adapted with permission from United Nations Development Programme (UNDP), *Human Development Report 2011: Sustainability and Equity: A Better Future for All*, Copyright © 2011by the United Nations Development Programme, available from http://hdr.undp.org/en/media/HDR_2011_EN_Complete.pdf.

develop their capabilities (hence their choice of 'functionings', including choices concerning their health), his collaborator in developing this theory, Martha Nussbaum, attempted to identify the contents of that basket:

1. Life: being able to live to the end of a human life of normal length; not dying prematurely, or before one's life is so reduced as to be not worth living.

Box 2.2.1 Multidimensional poverty index

1. *Education* (each indicator is weighted equally at 1/6):
   ◆ Years of schooling: no household member has completed 5 years of schooling.
   ◆ School attendance: no school attendance in years 1–8.

2. *Health* (each indicator is weighted equally at 1/6):
   ◆ Child mortality: if any child has died in the family.
   ◆ Nutrition: if any adult or child for whom there is nutritional information is malnourished.

3. *Standard of living* (each indicator is weighted equally at 1/18):
   ◆ Electricity: the household has no electricity.
   ◆ Drinking water: the household lacks access to clean drinking water within a 30-minute walk from home.
   ◆ Sanitation: the household has no adequate sanitation or only a shared toilet.
   ◆ Flooring: the household has a dirt, sand, or dung floor.
   ◆ Cooking fuel: the household cooks with wood, charcoal, or dung.
   ◆ Assets: the household does not own more than one of: radio, TV, telephone, bike, motorbike, or refrigerator and does not own a car or tractor.

Reproduced with permission from Alkire, S. and Santos, M.E., *Measuring acute poverty in the developing world: Robustness and scope of the Multidimensional Poverty Index*, OPHI Working Paper 59, Oxford, UK, Oxford Poverty and Human Development Initiative, Copyright © 2013, also available from http://www.ophi.org.uk/measuring-acute-poverty-in-the-developing-world-robustness-and-scope-of-the-multidimensional-poverty-index-2/

2. Bodily health: being able to have good health, including reproductive health, to be adequately nourished; to have adequate shelter.

3. Bodily integrity: being able to move freely from place to place; being able to be secure against assault, including sexual assault, having opportunities for sexual satisfaction and for choice in matters of reproduction.

4. Senses, imagination, and thought: being able to use the senses, to imagine, think, and reason—and to do these things in a way informed and cultivated by an adequate education, including but not limited to literacy and basic mathematical and scientific training. Being able to use one's mind in ways protected by guarantees of freedom of expression with respect to both political and artistic speech. Being able to search for ultimate meaning of life in one's own way.

5. Emotion: being able to have attachments to things and people outside ourselves.

6. Practical reason: being able to form a conception of the good and to engage in critical reflection about planning one's life; Nussbaum recognizes that this entails protection for the liberty of conscience and religious observance.

7. Affiliation: being able to live with and toward others; to engage in various forms of social interaction; having the social bases of self-respect and non-humiliation; being able to be treated as a dignified being including protection against discrimination on the basis of race, sex, sexual orientation, religion, caste, ethnicity, or national origin.

8. Other species: being able to live with concern for and in relationship to the world of nature.

9. Play: being able to laugh, or play, to enjoy recreational activities.

10. Control over one's environment both politically and materially, including having the right to political participation and having property rights on an equal basis with others, having the right to seek employment on an equal basis with others (Nussbaum 2000, pp. 77–80).

Defining poverty as capability-failure, especially given the long list of positively stated attributes of 'flourishing' that Nussbaum provides, nonetheless risks taking policy attention away from income poverty. In commodified, wage-based market systems, income (and its quantity) represents both choice (capabilities) and power (Lister 2004). Money may not be everything, but adequate income (however adequacy is determined) remains basic to any understanding of poverty. We note that in some low-income countries market systems are less entrenched and access to the capabilities through subsistence farming and strong cohesive communities remain important protections against absolute poverty.

Poverty as deprivation

> Deprivation…exists when people lack or are denied resources to participate in social and economic activities in the society in which they live.
>
> Reproduced from Labonté, R. et al., *Indicators of Social Exclusion and Inclusion: A Critical and Comparative Analysis of the Literature*, E/Exchange Working Paper Series, PHIRN, University of Ottawa, Canada © 2012, with permission from the author.

Deprivation entered the poverty literature in the late 1960s (Yitzhaki 1979). Like poverty, deprivation has both absolute and relative conceptualizations. As an absolute condition, deprivation is an undesired state that arises when people are unable to access necessary goods and services due to a lack of resources (Hallerod 1996); much depends here on where one draws a line under 'necessary' which immediately takes us into the terrain of relative deprivation. As a relative condition, deprivation exists when people lack or are denied resources to participate in social and economic activities in the society in which they live (Bailey 2004). One example is the UNICEF Innocenti Research Centre's measure of 'child deprivation' based upon the percentage of children aged 1–16 lacking two or more items from a list of 14 considered essential to acceptable child functionings in economically advanced countries (Fig. 2.2.4) (UNICEF Innocenti Research Centre 2012). Like relative poverty, the emphasis of relative deprivation is on *social participation*. The notion of being 'denied' resources for such participation is captured evocatively in deprivation as an 'enforced lack of socially perceived essentials' (Saunders et al. 2008, p. 175). Deprivation, like multidimensional poverty, can be multiple, when people lack access to sufficient levels of several attributes important to social participation, such as income, housing, healthcare, and education. Moreover, deprivation is an *enforced* state; that is, its origins can be traced directly to certain political, economic, or policy choices made by governments and which are entrenched in economic systems such as capitalism.

While emerging from the poverty literature, there are important conceptual differences between deprivation and poverty. A person may be poor in terms of income but not deprived in terms of, for example, housing, healthcare, education, or transportation, to the extent these are publicly subsidized or provided. Conversely, a person could experience deprivation in multiple dimensions while

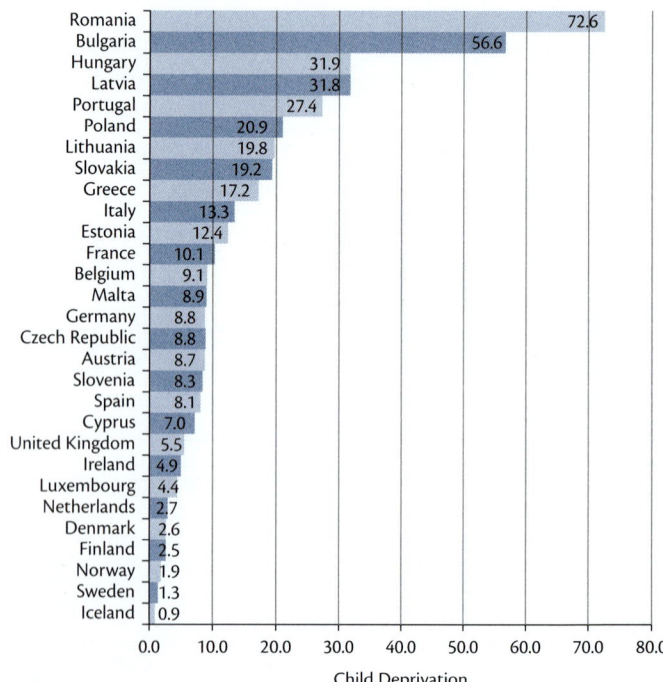

Fig. 2.2.4 Child deprivation in selected countries. Data for 2009.

Adapted with permission from UNICEF Innocenti Research Centre, *Measuring Child Poverty: New league tables of child poverty in the world's rich countries*, p. 2, UNICEF Innocenti Research Centre, Innocenti Report Card 10, Florence, Italy, Copyright © 2012.

not being income poor, such as experiencing discrimination by virtue of one's gender, ethnicity, or sexual orientation (Saunders et al. 2008). This 'intersectionality' of social identity and health risk has become increasingly invoked as a way of incorporating a broader understanding of poverty and inequality, by exploring 'simultaneous intersections between aspects of social difference and identity (e.g. as related to meanings of race/ethnicity, indigeneity, gender, class, sexuality, geography, age, disability/ability, migration status, religion) and forms of systemic oppression (e.g. racism, classism, sexism, ableism, homophobia)' (Springer et al. 2012, p. 1661). It shifts an understanding of poverty well away from matters of simple material goods and physical functioning, which some critics argue deflects attention away from the financial needs of the many who live in absolute or relative poverty (Nolan and Whelan 1996), to a much broader concern with multiple forms of what has been termed *social exclusion.*

Poverty as social exclusion

Poverty and social exclusion refer to when people are prevented from participating fully in economic, social and civil life and/or when their access to income and other resources (personal, family, social and cultural) is so inadequate as to exclude them from enjoying a standard of living and quality of life that is regarded as acceptable by the society in which they live. In such situations people often are unable to fully access their fundamental rights. (p. 11)

Reproduced from European Commission, *Draft Joint Report on Social Exclusion*, European Commission, Brussels, Copyright © 2001.

Social exclusion extends beyond poverty and deprivation concepts by incorporating a broader understanding of social processes and their consequences (Bailey et al. 2004). Both poverty and deprivation are components of social exclusion but, as Berger-Schmitt and Noll (Berger-Schmitt and Noll 2000) point out, income-poverty can be both a cause and a consequence of social exclusion. But income-poverty is only one possible cause or consequence. As with deprivation, one can be wealthy (not poor) and still experience social exclusion, as has been the case with gay and lesbian people in many of the world's countries (Estivill 2003). Social exclusion, although sharing much in common with Townsend's concept of relative deprivation, differs in the emphasis it places on non-material aspects, from 'prospects and networks' (which work to reduce exclusion) to prejudice and discrimination (which work to increase it) (Saunders and Wong 2009).

Social exclusion first arose in research and policy discourse in France in the early 1970s, and was used both to explain the effects of extreme economic restructuring on social solidarity beyond what poverty and deprivation alone could describe, and to assist in developing policies to promote social cohesion within the European Union (Gore and Figueiredo 1997; Aasland and Flotten 2001; Rawal 2008). Rene Lenoir in 1974 was the first to coin the term as a way to define the condition of a large portion of the population that included the poor, handicapped, vulnerable, aged, abused children, substance abusers and other marginalized groups or 'social misfits' (de Haan 1999; Sen 2000). A broader conceptualization was later proposed to incorporate the 'social, economic, political and cultural systems which determine the integration of a person in society' (Walker 1997, cited in Lessof and Jowell 2000, p. 5)—that is, the social processes of exclusion.

Economic exclusion is a term frequently used synonymously with social exclusion. Dertwinkel (Dertwinkel 2008, p. 4) argues that the 'meaning of social exclusion has always been an economic and less a political or cultural one' and defines economic exclusion as a state of 'non-participation in or blocked access to the labor market, public services, finance, housing, educational and health sector, among other possibilities'. (Labonté et al. 2012, pp. 19–20)

This emphasis on labour market attachment is most often encountered in European writing on social exclusion, even when other dimensions of exclusion are considered. Part of the reasoning behind this emphasis is that it creates greater social cohesion and reduces social conflict, given evidence that high levels of youth unemployment and poverty are associated in many countries with gang participation or rebel group involvement, motivated primarily by a desire to earn income (World Bank 2011). Other theorists, however, give greater attention to the *relational* aspects of social exclusion, linking exclusion to inadequate social participation, lack of social integration and lack of power (Room 1995, p. 5). As Sen (2000, p. 6) puts it, social exclusion (unlike poverty or deprivation) gives 'a central role to relational connections'. Work, like the income it generates, is simply one of the means of making such connections. This emphasis was echoed in the final report of the Social Exclusion Knowledge Network of the WHO Commission on Social Determinants of Health which distinguished between 'social exclusion as a state experienced by particular groups (common in policy discourse) as opposed to the relational approach ... [in which] exclusion is viewed as a dynamic, multi-dimensional process driven by unequal power relations' (Popay et al. 2008, p. 7). This process results in unequal resources, reduced capabilities, and fewer claims on human rights leading to inequalities in access to entitled services. This perspective on social exclusion also points the policy spotlight at unfair economic and social structures rather than on deficiencies of individuals.

Gough et al. (2006) discuss social exclusion in terms of the ways in which it is an inevitability of neo-liberal capitalism. They acknowledge that it is a highly ambiguous concept (Gough et al. 2006, p. 49), and one that can be used to support a neo-liberal status quo by regarding as unproblematic the 'inclusion' of elite and wealthy groups whose privileges and practices contribute to the exclusion of others. They maintain that a broad notion of social exclusion should be centrally concerned with social oppression in particularly those of 'race', gender, sexuality, disability, and age. Crucially for the discussion in this chapter they note that the discourse of inclusion avoids confronting the question of justice and that 'one can be included in any social arrangement in an unjust fashion' (Gough et al. 2006, p. 4). As Levitas noted:

The term social exclusion is intrinsically problematic. It represents the primary ... division in society as one between an included majority and an excluded minority. ... The solution ... is a ... transition across the boundary to become an insider rather than an outsider in a society whose structural inequalities remain largely uninterrogated. (Levitas 2005, p. 7)

Poverty summarized

Taking account of these various attempts to define and understand poverty, the concept might usefully be summarized as an absolute and comparative lack of resources and capabilities, comprised principally of the following:

1. Adequate material resources (food, shelter, clothing, and other normatively defined social necessities).

2. Income to acquire such necessities (generated through employment or government subsidies and transfers).

3. Access to formal labour markets or post-retirement or child-rearing income support (to provide adequacy and security of income, as well as access to social relations).

4. Access to adequate and affordable housing (extending beyond basic shelter to incorporate aspects of overcrowding, disrepair, insecure tenancy), and to services basic to health (e.g. sanitation, water).

5. Access to educational and healthcare opportunities (to improve access to formal labour markets and reduce barriers to broader forms of social participation).

6. Socially conditioned and structured forms of discrimination (which reduce access to formal labour markets, educational and healthcare opportunities, and broader forms of social participation).

7. Power or voice to influence the policy choices of governments affecting all of the above conditions (which extends to lack of political freedoms or human rights) (Labonté et al. 2012, p. 15).

There are finally three cautions about poverty that need issuing. The first is that poverty mobility can be dynamic, with people moving in and out of income- or consumption-based poverty (whether absolute or relative) even within short time periods. The chronic poor are those who 'remain trapped in situations and relationships which produce deprivation and capability losses over long periods' (Policy Analysis Discussion Group 2012, p. 6). The second is that people living in poverty, however conceptualized or measured, may not view themselves as poor, deprived, or without capabilities. 'Subjective' poverty differs from its objective measure, and may reflect people's perception of their agency, their rejection of the stigmatizing label of being one of 'the poor', or an internalized resignation to the inevitability of their circumstances. The third is that, just as poverty is now regarded as multidimensional, people's identities and capabilities are multiple. A focus only on people's relative deprivation without appreciating their relative capabilities risks creating or reinforcing resignation to their circumstances, rather than mobilization to change them.

How does poverty affect health and ill health affect poverty?

> Whatever is going round, people in lower social positions tend to get more of it, and to die earlier even after adjustment for the effects of specific individual or environmental hazards. (p. 1355)
> Reproduced with permission from *Social Science & Medicine*, Volume 31, Issue 12, Evans R. and Stoddart G., Producing Health, Consuming Health Care, pp. 1347–63, Copyright © 1990.

On average, the lower the socioeconomic position, the lower one's health status. Socioeconomic status (SES) is usually measured by income, occupation, or education, but also includes stratification by social class, gender, and race/ethnicity—examples of the intersectionality of different deprivations discussed earlier. One of the key findings in recent years has been that differences between social position and health status follow a gradient, a step-wise pattern between where one sits in a SES hierarchy and most health outcomes. Although not all health conditions follow a socioeconomic gradient (a few diseases are more common in higher than in lower SES groups) the pattern is robust, observed in many countries, persists over time, and is evident for all age groups and

for both men and women. Recent research has also shown that health inequities accumulate over a lifetime and that disadvantage at each stage of the life course affects health (Lynch et al. 1997; Smith et al. 1997, 1998). Adverse social and economic conditions in the early years of life are increasingly being shown to have a lifelong impact on health (Lynch and Smith 2005; Hertzman and Boyce 2010; Power et al. 2012). Much of this textbook is concerned with the determinants of the gradient in health; here, we recount briefly the three major explanatory models for this gradient: natural or social selection, cultural/behavioural, and materialist or structural (Baum 2008).

Natural or social selection

The social selection argument suggests that healthier people become wealthier people, enjoying greater social mobility than their poorer fellows. There is some evidence that better health is associated with social mobility, especially at younger ages; but this accounts for only a small portion of health differences between social groups (Whitehead 1992; Power et al. 1996). The social selection and mobility argument comes with its inverse: people are poor because they are unhealthy. Again, there is some evidence for this, particularly in low-income countries. We have already noted the problem of medical poverty, where the absence of affordable healthcare pushes sick people into poverty. There is also evidence that people living in countries with high burdens of particular diseases (such as HIV/AIDS, tuberculosis, or malaria) and with poor social protection safety nets (such as income transfers or sickness and unemployment benefits) can suffer greater poverty due to their illness reducing their ability to earn income. Poor health also contributes to poverty through its debilitating effects of inadequate nutrition on individual development and later economic productivity (Horton and Ross 2003; Sanders et al. 2007; Baum 2008). Early insults to the growth and brain development of children, even with intensive interventions later in life, are partially irreversible. In many cases, the damage is done even before the child is born. Undernutrition among mothers is a major reason why babies are born with a low birth weight, a result of small maternal size at conception and low pregnancy weight gain or inadequate food and energy intake during pregnancy (Kramer 1987). Malnutrition among infant girls is therefore one of the main routes for the intergenerational transmission of poverty (Horton and Ross 2003).

That sick people become poor, in other words, reflects the same dynamics of social stratification and material circumstances that explain why poor people are more likely to become ill in the first place. This accounts for why some wealthy but highly unequal countries with limited social protection can have poorer population health outcomes than poorer but more equal countries with high levels of social programme spending (notably for primary healthcare, education, women's literacy, land reforms, and physical infrastructure) (Balabanova et al. 2011). Sen (1999, pp. 335–6) showed this very clearly when he compared the life expectancies in the early 1990s of US whites with US African Americans, and with Indians in Kerala and the Chinese. While African Americans are very many times richer in income terms than the people in China and Kerala (even after correcting for cost of living differences) they are less likely to live as long. Sen explains this by reference to 'the social arrangements and community relations such as medical coverage, public healthcare, elementary education, law and order, and prevalence of violence'. In other words: there is nothing 'natural' about 'social selection'; such selection arises as an effect of how the political and economic systems of countries are structured.

Cultural/behavioural explanations

A more commonly encountered reason for the SES gradient in health is that poorer people make unhealthier lifestyle choices. This is not a new argument. During the early decades of the nineteenth century Industrial Revolution in Europe, with its dislocating impacts on rural agricultural livelihoods and explosion of ghettoes in rapidly expanding cities (a phenomenon now characteristic of many developing countries in late twentieth- and early twenty-first-century globalization) the poor were seen as a palpable disease threat to the rich. Their poverty, in turn, was not regarded as an effect of their economic dislocations, but as 'the interaction of the twin problems of indolence and vice' (Alcock 1993, p. 12). The British 'father' of public health, Sir Edwin Chadwick, in his reforms of the poor laws requiring urban paupers to earn their minimal allowance in workhouses, and so to become 'deserving poor', argued that:

> The population so exposed is less susceptible to moral influences, and the effects of education are more transient than with a healthy population; these adverse circumstances tend to produce an adult population short-lived, improvident, reckless and intemperate, and with habitual avidity for sensual gratifications. (Chadwick 1930)

Even while acknowledging the 'adverse circumstances' of the poor, Chadwick posits that the poor health of the poor results primarily from their lack of the proper behaviours and morality of the healthier and wealthier. A more socially critical observer of the same era, Friedrich Engels, agreed with Chadwick that alcohol was fairly prevalent amongst the poor labouring classes, but that 'it was almost their only source of pleasure':

> The working man comes home from his work tired, exhausted, finds his home comfortless, damp, dirty, repulsive; he has urgent need of recreation, he must have something to make…the prospect of the next day endurable. (Engels 1845/1999, p. 113)

The same dichotomy between a behavioural and a socially critical account of the poverty/health relationship persists today. Many (although not all) unhealthy behaviours do tend to be more prevalent as one moves down the social gradient. Even in developing countries undergoing nutritional transitions (where traditional diets are being replaced by increased consumption of high-fat, energy-dense, low-nutrient food commodities), what might begin as a status choice amongst a rising middle class quickly becomes a necessity choice (due to availability and cost) for poorer social classes (Drieskens et al. 2009; Monteiro et al. 2010; Stuckler and Nestle 2012). The same is true for smoking, originally more common amongst elite social classes, and, to lesser degrees, alcohol and other drug use (Drieskens et al. 2009). But explaining these behaviours as 'cultural' effects of poorer groups (their improvident or reckless 'lifestyle'), or as their lack of knowledge or motivation to adopt healthier patterns, ignores the social contexts that condition and constrain individual choice (Layte and Whelan 2009). It also fails to account for the excess disease burden faced by many poorer groups, even after accounting for all of the individual/behavioural risk factors (Lynch and Smith 2005).

Materialist or structural explanations

The limitation of a narrowly behavioural understanding of the poverty/health relationship draws attention to how the material conditions of poverty affect health. Here the enumeration of, and evidence for, the health determining effects of these conditions is plentiful, reflecting many of the material circumstances identified in this chapter's discussion of poverty and deprivation: access to income, housing, employment, nutritious food, safe water and sanitation, unemployment protection, health services, education services, and other socially provided resources that allow for the development of capabilities. These structural factors (so named because they reflect embedded economic and power relations within societies) are also related to what have been called psychosocial risk factors: the isolation, low social support, poor social networks, high self-blame, and low perceived power that are more frequent among poorer and less educated groups (Najman 1994; Lynch and Smith 2005; Kawachi et al. 2008). Racism has also been shown to have a powerful effect on health status (Krieger 2000; Paradies 2006; Ziersch et al. 2011), psychosocial and material risks cluster together, and poorer groups (those lower along the SES gradient) are more likely to experience all three. In countries where material inequalities have been significantly reduced through welfare measures, for example, health inequalities experienced by poorer groups are more likely to be a result of greater behavioural and psychosocial risks; although, as Johan Mackenbach, whose work is the topic of Chapter 2.3, suggests, 'the persistence of health inequalities in modern European welfare states can partly be seen as a failure of these states to implement more radical redistribution measures' (Mackenbach 2012, p. 761). Behavioural, psychosocial, and material risks matter and interact with each other (Krieger 2000; Paradies 2006; Ziersch et al. 2011).

What theories of justice should guide our interventions?

The public health concern with justice, poverty, and health enjoys a rich history. Over 150 years ago the young Prussian physician, Rudolf Virchow, hired by the government to recommend how to control a typhoid epidemic amongst poor coal miners, famously called for massive social reforms that ranged from progressive taxation and organized food cooperatives, to improved wages and working conditions, strong local government, improved education, and an end to church interference urging the poor to suffer now and to reap their rewards in heaven. Friedrich Engels, writing around the same time as Virchow, published his lengthy analysis of *The Condition of the Working Class in England*, leading to his co-authorship with Karl Marx of the influential *Communist Manifesto* with its call for a revolutionary social justice. Some of this early concern with poverty and its social and physical ills continued into the late nineteenth and into the twentieth century, although it became muted by the rise of 'scientific medicine' and its promise of a cure for most diseases. Supported by industrialist philanthropies (notably in the Americas, by The Rockefeller Foundation), scientific medicine's emphasis on cure rather than prevention deflected much public health attention away from the social roots of disease (Brown 1979; Tesh 1988). Poverty as a public health issue occasionally surfaced, especially during times of economic recession or depression when high poverty rates were associated with the spread of diseases such as tuberculosis and cholera. But it was in Latin America that the radicalism of nineteenth-century public health activism became institutionalized in the practice of what has been called 'social medicine' (Waitzkin 2005). One of its major proponents was the Chilean physician (and later socialist President) Salvador Allende who, as health minister in the late 1930s and 1940s, approached health inequities in Chile as a direct result of historic underdevelopment, international economic dependency, and foreign debt. He argued that the 'medico-social problems of the country…require precisely the solution of the economic problems' (Waitzkin 2005, p. 740). Allende's reforms, echoing those of Virchow, included wage improvements, wealth redistribution, land reforms, improved food security measures, and publicly supported housing development.

More recently, the WHO Commission on the Social Determinants of Health (2008) took a clear stand that inequities in health (avoidable inequalities) were unacceptable and the goal of policy should be to eliminate these and so argued for closing the life expectancy gap in a generation.

These are bold public health proposals, generally framed in broadly stated concerns with justice (fairness). But how should we determine when poverty's health risks become unacceptable? What theories of social justice might guide our public health interventions or advocacy?

Equality of opportunity or equality of outcome?

Social justice theory is generally associated with European societies and particularly with struggles during the industrial revolution and the emergence of socialist, social democratic or other models of redistributive welfare states: 'Social justice is not possible without strong and coherent redistributive policies conceived and implemented by public agencies' (United Nations Division for Social Policy 2006, p. 6). Social justice theory is essentially concerned with equity, or fairness. On this basis, it is argued that social justice (equity) is a universal concern, since all social arrangements, to be legitimate and to function at all, must attend to issues of equality (Sen 1992). But there are subtleties to how equity is conceived with two main dimensions: equality of opportunity, achieved through procedural justice or 'horizontal equity' in which equals are treated the same; and equality of outcome, achieved through substantive justice or 'vertical equity' in which people are treated differently according to their initial endowments, resources, privileges or rights. Both equalities (opportunity, outcome) are ideal types; neither exists in 'true' form. They represent aspirational ideals of what societies strive to create for their members (fairness in outcomes) and how they believe this should be accomplished (fairness in opportunity). (Labonté 2010, p. 84)

There is a political, as well as philosophical, difference in these two broad social justice streams. (Labonté 2010, p. 84).

Recent decades of global market integration and the collapse of Soviet-style 'socialism' have been accompanied by the increasing dominance of neo-liberal ideology which has supplanted concerns with social justice by an exclusive focus on economic growth which, it is suggested, will result in greater and better-distributed wealth—the trickle-down theory.

In turn, proponents of more open markets and conventional approaches to growth and development emphasize equality of opportunity, with only residual attention to equality of outcome. This was the position taken by the World Bank's 2006 *World Development*

Report on the theme of equity and development, which was less supportive of post-market income redistribution to achieve greater equality, instead favouring greater individual equality of opportunity through *inter alia* 'equality before the law, equal enforcement of personal and property rights, non-discriminatory institutions, and equal access to public services and infrastructure' (World Bank 2006, pp. 18–19). The slight nod to a concern with outcomes was reference to avoidance of absolute deprivation. (Labonté 2010, p. 84)

Theories of justice

Moral defense for some mitigation of health and social inequalities arising from poverty is a recurrent theme in much contemporary Western philosophy. Peter Singer (1972) posits 'a Greater Moral Evil Principle,' that it is both just and of collective benefit to act to relieve poverty and deprivation if, in doing so, we do not sacrifice something of comparable moral significance. Around the same time John Rawls published his highly influential *Theory of Justice*. Standing behind a 'veil of ignorance' as to their social standing at birth, Rawls argues that people would choose a justice that guaranteed a minimum of primary goods that any rational person would choose as basic to their needs. This justice theory builds upon two principles. The first principle is the 'priority of the equal' (basic liberties), which roughly equates with individuals having civil and political rights that protect them against excess authoritarian rule by the state. The second principle is based on legal equality of opportunity, which roughly equates with individuals having economic, cultural and social rights that obligate states to provide certain goods or services (the minimum resources or capabilities required to exercise one's functionings). His second principle also invokes the 'difference principle': that inequality in the distribution of social and economic goods ('primary goods') are allowable only to the extent that they also improve the lot of the least advantaged. The difference principle obliges a degree of state interventions of redistribution and regulation, although Rawls did not believe that the extreme differences in wealth and power that markets create was of moral concern provided the conditions of the least advantaged improved. He also emphasized the centrality of better procedural justice (Schaefer 2007). (Labonté 2010, p. 85)

Rawls' justice theory is located within the social contract school, which views nation states as the primary actors in international relations. He held that poverty in low-income countries was primarily an effect of domestic policies and practices with little international or global causality. Pogge (2002), drawing on cosmopolitan arguments, challenges Rawls on this conclusion, as well as on evidence that poverty cannot be de-linked from global economic institutions and actors. In doing so, he extends Rawls' basic justice theory to a global level, contending that there are not simply 'positive duties' to assist those in need, but moral obligations (negative duties) to prevent harm (Pogge 2004).

Pogge's theory of relational justice (Pogge 2002) is based on three lines of argument:

1. The radical inequalities observed between peoples and nations today are partly an effect of a violent history in which some gained at the expense of others. While we individually cannot be held responsible for the actions of our forebears in this 'conquest,' as moral persons we can be held accountable for rectifying the vast disparities in initial conditions that this history has created.

2. Not only does procedural justice by itself fail to account for these vast disparities in initial conditions; it is impossible to conceive of these disparities existing on the scale that they do without 'an organized state of civilization' (Pogge 2005) to uphold them. Both procedural and substantive injustices thus endure.

3. There is evidence that economic institutions operating on an international scale (the 'organized state of civilization') have been complicit in upholding these injustices. There are also feasible alternatives to these economic institutions that would reduce the "radical inequality" of persisting poverty. Persons involved in upholding these institutions are thus implicated in creating subsequent ill health, even though they may be half-way around the world (Pogge 2004).

Pogge concludes that: 'we are *harming* the global poor if and insofar as we collaborate in imposing an *unjust* global institutional order on them;' and proceeds to offer an evidence-informed argument to establish that present global institutional rules and procedures are unjust (Pogge 2005, emphasis in original). The justice implication is one of immediately engaging in 'rectification' through strengthened human rights and more progressive systems of global resource redistribution; but also an obligation to change the very rules of economic governance in order to overcome the historic and radical inequalities in initial conditions. (Labonté 2010, pp. 85–6)

A similar theory of social justice has been argued by Iris Marion Young. Accepting that there are demonstrable 'structural injustices' that 'put large categories of persons under a systematic threat of domination or deprivation of the means to develop and exercise their capacities, at the same time as these social processes enable others to dominate' (Young 2006, p. 114), Young argues that 'all agents who contribute by their actions to the structural processes that produce injustice have responsibilities to work to remedy these injustices' (Young 2006, pp. 102–3). Her 'social connection model' of responsibility extends these moral obligations beyond those more directly (causally) liable to a larger body of people who may be only indirectly connected. An example she offers is responsibility for retaining developing country 'sweatshops', which includes those who shop at retailers sourcing their goods from such shops as well as the retailers and factory owners themselves. The limitation of this model is that its extensive diffusion of responsibility may limit the ability to enforce changes in practice.

The role of human rights

Several justice theories make reference to human rights. Not only do human rights conventions, ratified by most of the world's states, represent a consensus on citizen rights and state obligations (Mack 2009), but there is widespread agreement that 'poverty is the principal cause of human rights violations in the world' (Office of the High Commissioner for Human Rights 1999, para. 9) and that 'poverty constitutes a denial of human rights' (Office of the High Commissioner for Human Rights 1999, para. 1). First established after the Second World War with the UN Declaration on Human Rights, several subsequent conventions have been agreed upon that detail specific citizen rights and state duties. These include the Covenant on Civil and Political Rights (intended to protect individuals against abuses of state authority) and the Covenant on Economic, Social and Cultural Rights (intended to guarantee individuals certain entitlements from the state); as well as specific treaties on the rights of children and women, racial minorities, indigenous peoples and numerous other facets of social justice. Together these treaties comprise an 'International Human Rights Framework' which, although lacking enforcement measures, empowers different UN committees and 'special rapporteurs' to review countries' compliance with their legally binding

obligations. Central to concerns with the poverty/health relationship is Article 12 of Covenant on Economic, Social and Cultural Rights (technically known as the Right to the Highest Attainable Standard of Physical and Mental Health, see Chapter 3.3) and its General Comment 14, which identifies a broad range of actions required for the progressive realization of this right. Health is considered a basic right, since it is foundational to the enjoyment of most other human rights.

The right to health, when adopted in countries' own constitutions or laws, however, can be and has been interpreted in legal decisions or national policy as an individual right only. Individual rights to treatment have been used to force public payment of costly medicines with opportunity costs to other facets of public health access of greater importance to the poor (Hogerzeil et al. 2006; Gianella-Malcam et al. 2009; Yamin and Parra-Vera 2009). International legal scholars argue that human rights emphasis, instead, should be placed on poorer and more vulnerable populations. This requires greater attention to collective rights. Collective rights are implied in General Comment 14 on the right to health (Committee on Economic Social and Cultural Rights 2000), and are explicit in the Declaration on the Right to Development (Office of the High Commissioner for Human Rights 1986). Though the right to development is not a binding treaty, it is considered to have some standing in international human rights law (Aguirre 2008) and has strong normative support through UN agencies especially in the context of the Millennium Development Goals.

Some activist scholars and civil society organizations argue against the present international emphasis on human rights for their lack of class and political economy analysis. Others contend that human rights, with their individualistic and legalistic focus, 'are not sufficient to serve as ethical criteria in solving the fundamental problems of the absolute poor' partly because within these static statements, the 'poor are not invited…to articulate their moral needs and rights for themselves' (Mack 2009, p. 11). At the same time, human rights are considered the most globalized social justice statements of our era; and human rights treaties are being used to advance policies to improve health and to assist the poor (Dasgupta 1995; Schrecker et al. 2010).

Inequalities in initial conditions

Confronting inequalities in initial conditions (the lives people are born into) is vital especially given the evidence cited earlier on the lifetime impact of adverse living circumstances in early life. A focus on initial conditions begins to blur the earlier distinctions between equality of opportunity (procedural justice) and equality of outcome (substantive justice). Equality of opportunity, to be just, requires vertical equity: a disproportionate provision of public goods and capability resources for those whom history's conquests, and today's political institutions, place in highly unequal initial conditions. Departing from the redistributive minimalism of the World Bank's 2006 World Development Report, a later report of the Bank's Latin American Development Forum argues that:

A better understanding of the importance of inequality of opportunity in the determination of inequality of outcomes may change attitudes towards redistribution. People dislike and consider unfair inequalities associated with differences in circumstances, which many argue should be compensated for by society. By highlighting that component of inequality attributable to circumstances, this type of analysis can help build a social and political consensus on…the best means for addressing inequality of opportunity. (p. 50)

What remains at issue is the extent of moral (or legal) obligation for amelioration of gross inequalities in initial conditions that create 'shortfall inequalities in central health capabilities' (Ruger 2008, p. 440). Is there an ethically defensible scale of rectification?

There is no answer to this question, apart from the imperative to seek one. In this quest, norms of procedural justice re-assume importance. Boggio (2009), in an argument for why international organizations and those within them have an ethical obligation to act to redress systematic health inequalities arising from poverty, addresses *how* such policy decisions can be made in a just manner. He identifies three basic principles for an 'ethically-informed deliberative process': publicity (transparency in process, a comprehensible rationale, and public argument and evidence); relevance (trust in actors/institutions by recipients, opportunity for wide participation, and interventions based on recipients' needs, values and aspirations); and revisability (policies and programmes can be challenged over time and improved, and individuals and institutions can be held accountable to purpose) (Boggio 2009). Several of these conditions are similar to principles of good governance widely held by governments and multilateral organizations; that is, they can be considered as having a broad normative base.

What public policies will reduce poverty?

The last decade of research on the causes of chronic poverty has shown that *a key factor in keeping certain categories or social groups in a state of chronic poverty* (transmitted through the generations) *is the operation of power relations* which stigmatise the people involved, undermine their confidence, and systematically close off options for individual or collective advancement…A stronger focus on structural inequalities, on systematic obstacles to redistributive processes and on social groups and interactions between them is part of this. (p. 6, emphasis in original)

The first issue public health confronts in grappling with the poverty, health, and justice relationship is simply this: if it is possible to improve the health of the poor without necessarily reducing income inequalities or relative poverty, is this sufficient? Some of the justice theories cited earlier might be content with saying yes to this, as their emphasis was more on absolute than on relative poverty. More recent poverty theories (capabilities, social exclusion/inclusion), however, give greater emphasis to the core value of ensuring human dignity or 'flourishing'. There is no justice if one simply survives; one must be able to live with purpose and meaning. Public health concern with poverty, then, extends beyond simply the specific disease risks poverty creates (both for the poor, and for the non-poor), to the existence of poverty itself—both absolute and relative.

The existence of poverty is inherently political, and there are different political theories for how poverty might be reduced. Alcock

(1993) distils these to four dominant models: neo-liberalism, conservatism, social democratic, and socialist, to which Gough et al. (2006) add a fifth: the associational.

The *neo-liberal model* is associated with policy responses to the declining profit rates, economic recessions, and developing world debt problems that arose in the 1970s and 1980s. Promoted by conservative governments in the United Kingdom, United States, and Germany (in the 1970s, the major economic powers in the world), neo-liberalism is based on a belief that free markets, sovereign individuals, free trade, strong property rights, and minimal government interference is the best means to enhance human well-being. Its policy platform rested on what became known in later years as the 'Washington Consensus': privatization, deregulation, tax reform (lower corporate and marginal rates), deficit reduction, and trade and financial liberalization. In general, the neo-liberal view is that governments should avoid poverty reduction as a policy matter, and instead rely upon economic growth through stronger free markets and economic liberalization to 'trickle down' and lift the poor out of their condition. Extreme neo-liberals have argued that the state should not interfere at all with conditions of poverty (Murray 1984), although this was rarely pursued as a policy option. Instead, neo-liberal-dominated governments tend towards a 'welfare minimalism', with benefits or entitlements at a level that prevents the worst forms of deprivation, but that is rarely sufficient for 'flourishing' or 'health capabilities'.

The *conservative model* overlaps with the neo-liberal, although it holds to the importance of some state intervention to ameliorate the worst inequities arising from markets, and specifically market failures (Alcock 1993). Persisting chronic poverty is symptomatic of market failures, implying that free markets and economic growth are unable, by themselves, to create equal opportunities for all. Conservative policies are not aimed at preventing poverty, which would require strong regulation of markets, but with relieving the worst of its effects. The approach is selective (means-tested benefits), often punitive (distinguishing between the 'deserving' and the 'undeserving' poor, the latter being people who could work even if their employment kept them in relative poverty), and minimalist (offering supports well below the minimum wage that could be earned in work, thus creating an incentive to 'labour market attachment').

The *social democratic model*, historically associated most with northern European countries, but also found in other parts of the world, emphasizes universalism in its poverty reduction policies. Social democracies are often highly interventionist in markets to prevent poverty in the first instance, as well as using high taxation and social spending to reduce residual levels of poverty. As with the previous two models, there is still an emphasis on labour market participation and an expectation that those who can engage in work will do so. But there is also greater emphasis on extending positive incentives to people entering lower-waged positions to overcome what has been called the 'welfare wall', a term that describes the loss of non-income benefits when moving off social assistance to minimum waged positions. Although universalism in benefits and entitlements helps to build cross-class solidarity, the non-income benefits of social spending (e.g. in healthcare, education, transportation services, and the like) can be disproportionately 'captured' by wealthier social groups. This has led to calls for 'proportional universalism' in which policies are constructed such that those in greater need enjoy disproportionate levels of benefits (Marmot 2010); and for some degree of targeting of benefits to maximize their poverty reducing efficiencies (OECD 2008).

The *associational model* also reflects opposition to neo-liberalism and is based on the need to involve people in economic models and reduce the extent to which they are alienated by them (Gough et al. 2006). Building strong social capital, voluntary organizations, and civil society are considered to be the key poverty-reducing components. Micro credit banks such as the Grameen Bank are an example in low-income countries where (mainly) women can obtain loans to set up their own business. A further example is the Indian Self-Employed Women's Association, which organizes millions of women to provide their own banks, workers' cooperatives, child care, and health and unemployment insurance. In rich countries, examples would be locally based bartering systems, food and worker cooperatives. These initiatives are based on self-help, are democratically run, have a local focus, and depend on forms of collectivity that can be plural, multiple, and diverse. Gough et al. (2006) indicate that the expectation is that states should be subordinate to these myriad local organizations and that political democracy should grow out of the practical economic and social democracy. They go on to note that asssociationalist projects are usually hemmed in by disciplinarian capital and the localist strategies leave the power structures that create poverty in the first place untouched.

The *socialist model*, though less prominent in recent decades since the collapse and failure of the Eastern Bloc countries, holds that capitalist market systems inevitably create poverty and that the only enduring means to reduce poverty is to replace capitalism with a socialist system of governance. This implied a radical transformation of capitalist labour markets, which inevitably create unemployment and poverty, to socialist (collective) forms of production and ownership. In the absence of a political revolution, the entrenchment of neo-liberal politics and ideology means that a process of transition to a socialist society needs to be envisaged. Moves towards greater egalitarianism include: protection of workers' conditions and rights; progressive taxation and tax enforcement measures for the wealthy and corporations; combating the multiple forms of discrimination in jobs, housing, and public services; withdrawal of public support for private education and health; public provision of good quality education and health services; provision of universal lifelong social security for all citizens; and maintaining public spaces for community use. Many of the critiques of market economics made by socialism are finding more policy and media traction in the wake of the 2007 global financial and employment crises; accompanied by civil society calls for progressive taxation, stronger market regulations, and enforceable citizen rights to hold government to account (Labonté and Schrecker 2009).

The role of policy initiatives and civil society mobilization for poverty reduction and fairer societies

Most countries have organized civil society groups, including labour organizations, campaigning for policy actions to reduce poverty. These groups generally blend the broad approaches of the social democratic and revolutionary socialist models. They often provide detailed policy analyses and briefs, and collaborate with some academic researchers to ensure the empirical and theoretical integrity of their work. Some groups focus on reducing poverty while others argue that poverty reduction will only result from a broader reform of the economic system and the inequities to which it gives rise. There are several examples in history of social and labour movement mobilization forcing changes in government and social policies, including those directly related to poverty reduction and health improvement (Szreter 2003). We offer two here, one a governmental example and the other capturing civil society activism.

Brazil's governmental reforms

Significant gains in poverty reduction, health system development, and health outcomes have been achieved in several countries through progressive social policies, resulting ultimately from political mobilization. Brazil's progress over the past 20 years provides a contemporary example of progressive change within a market economy. Infant mortality, for example, fell from 114 per 1000 live births in 1970 to just 19.3 per 1000 live births in 2007, while life expectancy at birth increased by almost 40 per cent, reaching 72.8 years in 2008. It is not possible (or even likely) to attribute these impressive advances to health sector activities alone, since these activities were part of several large-scale social reforms initiated in the country. These reforms led to steep increases in school attendance and decreases in illiteracy rates, both of which are pathways to better health. As well, Brazil's gross domestic product doubled between 1981 and 2008, potentially lifting more families out of income poverty; and its high levels of income inequality fell substantially as a result of such social policies as the Bolsa Família conditional cash transfer programme, which covers 10.5 million families, and increases in the legal minimum wage. Other social determinants of health were also improved substantially, including increases in provision to households of indoor water, sewage disposal and electricity (Paim et al. 2011). Sustained and significant investment in the creation of a universal health system, the centrepiece of which is the Family Health Programme, is mostly directed at providing more accessible and equitable health services, particularly at the primary level, but also engages community health workers who identify in their localities social factors that negatively affect socioeconomic and health status and enrol other sectors in addressing them (Macinko et al. 2007; People's Health Movement et al. 2011).

The political context of Brazil's reforms dates back to the late 1980s when popular mobilization challenged a conservative government with strong pro-market policies. This mobilization against a military dictatorship brought together oppositional political parties (at the time, illegal), grassroots groups, progressive academics and researchers, and trade unions. This movement catalysed the institution of many progressive health policies. With the election of the Workers' Party in 1989, popular mobilization waned as progressive social policies were introduced, although 'social participation' in local government continues through such bodies as the National Health Council, which plays an ongoing role in democratizing policy development (Paim et al. 2011). In 2013, 'middle-class' protests began once again in Brazil, which some attribute to the country's targeting of many of its social reforms to the poorest sectors of the population. The challenge now is to universalize the benefits of these reforms, building the cross-class solidarity that remains important in sustaining support for redistributive social protection programmes (People's Health Movement et al. 2011).

Civil society challenges to unhealthy globalization

Another important recent example of civil society activism that catalysed far-reaching policy change that indirectly impacts on health equity is the campaign against the Multilateral Agreement on Investment (MAI). The Association for the Taxation of Financial Transaction for the Aid of Citizens (ATTAC) was founded in France in 1998 to mobilize support for the Tobin tax on currency transactions as part of a broader movement against inequitable globalization arising from cross-border speculative finance. ATTAC, which has now established itself in many countries, played a leading role in France's decision to withdraw from OECD talks on the MAI, resulting in the failure of the talks (Waters 2004).

The People's Health Movement (PHM), another global civil society group, is a grassroots organization linking health activists around the world. It was formed following the First People's Health Assembly in 2000 and its political position is outlined in the People's Charter for Health (People's Health Movement 2009) and summarized in the Preamble as:

> Health is a social, economic and political issue and above all a fundamental human right. Inequality, poverty, exploitation, violence and injustice are at the root of ill-health and the deaths of poor and marginalised people. Health for all means that powerful interests have to be challenged, that globalisation has to be opposed, and that political and economic priorities have to be drastically changed.
>
> Reproduced with permission from People's Health Movement, The People's Charter for Health, Copyright © 2009.

The Charter goes on to call for much broader political, economic, and social participation from poor people. Since 2000 the PHM has grown to encompass around 70 national circles which are organized into regional networks. A Right to Health campaign, whose parameters have been defined at a global level but whose country-level activities vary according to context and conjuncture, has placed the responsibility for poverty reduction and the reduction of health inequities firmly on the shoulders of national states and international organizations. PHM has also collaborated with other organizations to produce three editions of a publication, 'Global Health Watch' (http://www.ghwatch.org), which present alternative and more progressive versions of the World Health Reports produced by the World Health Organization. The GHWs provide a critical 'watch' on international organizations including the World Bank and the World Health Organization; offer evidence-informed critiques of neoliberal globalization; and argue strongly for its replacement by a more just and equitable system of global governance and economic system to achieve poverty eradication and health equity.

Conclusion

This chapter has analysed the various definitions of poverty and considered their philosophical and political implications. We have examined a variety of explanations for why poverty affects health adversely. On the basis of this examination we concluded that poverty reflects structural features of global and national economic and social systems and, in particular, that unequal societies give rise to greater poverty. We examined the norms of justice that can guide policy interventions to reduce poverty and its causes. We argued that both equality of opportunity and outcome are essential considerations in public policy and that confronting

inequalities in initial conditions is vital. Political responses to poverty reflect philosophical and ideological positions. Social democratic and socialist responses place emphasis on tackling the underlying structural causes of poverty and seek to provide non-stigmatizing supports to those living in poverty. Socialism also seeks to replace capitalist modes of production with those that socialize both production and profits and argues that a transition to such an economy would result in a significant reduction in poverty. Despite the efforts of many civil society groups around the world, poverty or near poverty, and its health consequences, although showing recent decline, are still the reality for about half of the world's population. This fact, together with growing economic inequities, does suggest that a new world economic and social order are required to dramatically reduce or eliminate poverty and the adverse health outcomes to which it gives rise.

Acknowledgements

Text extracts from Labonté, R. et al., *Indicators of Social Exclusion and Inclusion: A Critical and Comparative Analysis of the Literature*, E/Exchange Working Paper Series, PHIRN, University of Ottawa, Canada © 2012, reproduced with permission from the author.

Text extracts from Labonté, R., *Global Health Policy: Exploring the Rationale for Health in Foreign Policy*, Globalization and Health Equity Working Papers, University of Ottawa, Canada, Copyright ©2010, reproduced with permission from the author.

References

Aasland, A. and Flotten, T. (2001). Ethnicity and social exclusion in Estonia and Latvia. *Europe-Asia Studies*, 53(7), 1023–49.

Aguirre, D. (2008). *The Human Right to Development in a Globalized World*. Aldershot: Ashgate Publishing Company.

Alcock, P. (1993). *Understanding Poverty*. London: Macmillan.

Bailey, N., Spratt, J., Pickering, J., Goodlad, R., and Shucksmith, M. (2004). *Deprivation and Social Exclusion in Argyll and Bute: Report to the Scottish Centre for Research on Social Justice*. Glasgow: Scottish Centre for Research on Social Justice, Universities of Glasgow and Aberdeen.

Balabanova, D., McKee, M., and Mills, A. (2011). *'Good Health at Low Cost' 25 Years On: What Makes a Successful Health System?* London: London School of Hygiene & Tropical Medicine.

Baum, F. (2008). The commission on the social determinants of health: reinventing health promotion for the twenty-first century? *Critical Public Health*, 18(4), 457–66.

Beiser, M., Hou, F., Hyman, I., and Tousignant, M. (2002). Poverty, family process, and the mental health of immigrant children in Canada. *American Journal of Public Health*, 92(2), 220–7.

Berger-Schmitt, R. and Noll, H.H. (2000). *Conceptual Framework and Structure of a European System of Social Indicators*. Report No.: 9. Mannheim: Centre for Survey Research and Methodology ZUMA.

Birdsall, N., Lusting, N., and McLeod, D. (2011). *Declining Inequality in Latin America: Some Economics, Some Politics*. Washington, DC: Center for Global Development.

Boggio, A. (2009). Health and development: an ethics perspective. In A. Gatti and A. Boggio (eds.) *Health and Development: Towards a Matrix Approach*, pp. 140–52. Houndmills: Palgrave Macmillan.

Bourguignon, F. (2004). *The Poverty-Growth-Inequality Triangle*. Paper presented at the Indian Council for Research on International Economic Relations, New Delhi, 4 February.

Brown, R. (1979). Exporting medical education: professionalism, modernization and imperialism. *Social Science & Medicine*, 13(A), 585–95.

Central Intelligence Agency (2013). *The World Fact Book*. [Online] Available at: https://www.cia.gov/library/publications/the-world-factbook/geos/xx.html.

Chadwick, E. (1930). Edwin Chadwick, Report of Poor Law Commissioner to the British Parliament on Sanitary Conditions, 1842. In J.F. Scott and A. Baltzly (eds.) *Readings in European History Since 1814*. New York: Appelton Century-Crofts Inc.

Cheek, R.B. (2001). Playing God with HIV. *African Security Review*, 10(4), 19–28.

Chen, S. and Ravallion, M. (2012). *An Update to the World Bank's Estimates of Consumption Poverty in the Developing World*. Briefing Note 03-01-12. Washington, DC: World Bank.

Collier P. (2007). *The Bottom Billion: Why the Poorest Countries are Failing and What Can Be Done About It*. New York: Oxford University Press.

Commission on Social Determinants of Health (2008). *Closing the Gap in a Generation: Health Equity Through Action on the Social Determinants of Health (Final Report)*. Geneva: World Health Organization.

Committee on Economic Social and Cultural Rights (2000). *Substantive Issues Arising in the Implementation of the International Covenant of Economic, Social and Cultural Rights: General Comment No. 14*. Report No.: E/C.12/2000/4. Geneva: United Nations Economic and Social Council.

Committee on Economic Social and Cultural Rights (2001). *Substantive Issues Arising in the Implementation of the Interantional Covenant on Economic, Social and Cultural Rights: Poverty and the International Covenant on Economic, Social and Cultural Rights*. Report No.: E/C 12/2001/10. New York: UN Economic and Social Council.

Dasgupta, P. (1995). *An Inquiry into Well-Being and Destitution*. Oxford: Oxford University Press.

De Barros, R.P. and Ferreira, F.H.G. (2009). *Measuring Inequality of Opportunities in Latin America and the Caribbean*. Washington, DC: World Bank Publications.

De Haan, A. (1999). *Social Exclusion: Towards an Holistic Understanding of Deprivation*. London: Department for International Development.

De Long, B. (1998). *Estimates of World GDP, One Million B.C. Present*. [Online] Available at: http://delong.typepad.com/print/20061012_LRWGDP.pdf.

Dertwinkel, T. (2008). *Economic Exclusion of Ethnic Minorities: On the Importance of Concept Specification*. Flensburg: European Centre for Minority Issues.

Drieskens, S., Van Oyen, H., Demarest, S., Van der Heyden, J., Gisle, L., and Tafforeau, J. (2009). Multiple risk behaviour: increasing socio-economic gap over time? *The European Journal of Public Health*, 20(6), 634–9.

Edward, P. (2006). The ethical poverty line: a moral quantification of absolute poverty. *Third World Quarterly*, 27(2), 377–93.

Engels, F. (1999). *The Condition of the Working Classes in England in 1844*. Oxford: Oxford University Press. (Originally published in 1845.)

Estivill, J. (2003). *Concepts and Strategies for Combating Social Exclusion: An Overview*. Portugal: International Labour Office.

European Commission (2001). *Draft Joint Report on Social Exclusion*. Brussels: European Commission.

Eurostat (2010). *Combating Poverty and Social Exclusion. A Statistical Portrait of the European Union*. Luxembourg: Eurostat.

Evans, R. and Stoddart, G. (1990). Producing health, consuming health care. *Social Science & Medicine*, 31(12), 1347–63.

Gianella-Malcam, C., Parra-Vera, O., Eli Yamin, A., and Torres-Tovar, M. (2009). Democratic deliberation or social marketing? The dilemmas of a public definition of health in the context of the implementation of Judgment T-760/08. *Health and Human Rights*, 11(1).

Gore, C. and Figueiredo, J.B. (1997). *Social Exclusion and Anti-Poverty Policy: A Debate*. Geneva: International Labour Organization.

Gough, J., Eisenschitz, A., and McCulloch, A. (2006). *Spaces of Social Exclusion*. Abingdon: Routledge.

Grindle, M.S. (1996). *Challenging the State: Crisis and Innovation in Latin America and Africa*. Cambridge: Cambridge University Press.

Hallerod, B. (1996). Deprivation and poverty: a comparative analysis of Sweden and Great Britain. *Acta Sociologica*, 39(2), 141–68.

Hertzman, C. and Boyce, T. (2010). How experience gets under the skin to create gradients in developmental health. *Annual Review of Public Health*, 31, 329–47.

Hogerzeil, H.V., Samson, M., Casanovas, J.V., and Rahmani-Ocora, L. (2006). Is access to essential medicines as part of the fulfilment of the right to health enforceable through the courts? *The Lancet*, 368, 305–11.

Horton, S. and Ross, J. (2003). The economics of iron deficiency. *Food Policy*, 28(1), 51–75.

Hotez, P.J. (2002). *Appeasing Wilson's Ghost: The Expanded Role of the New Vaccines in International Diplomacy*. Washington, DC: Chemical and Biological Arms Control Institute.

Kawachi, I., Subramanian, S.V., and Kim, D. (2008). *Social Capital and Health: A Decade of Progress and Beyond*. New York: Springer.

Kramer, M. (1987). Determinants of low birth weight: methodological assessment and meta-analysis. *Bulletin of the World Health Organization*, 65(5), 663–737.

Krieger, N. (2000). Discrimination and health. In L.F. Berkman and I. Kawachi (eds.) *Social Epidemiology*, pp. 36–75. Oxford: Oxford University Press.

Labonté, R. (2010). *Global Health Policy: Exploring the Rationale for Health in Foreign Policy*. University of Ottawa: Globalization and Health Equity Working Papers.

Labonté, R., Hadi, A., and Kaufmann, X. (2012). *Indicators of Social Exclusion and Inclusion: A Critical and Comparative Analysis of the Literature*. University of Ottawa: E/Exchange Working Paper Series, PHIRN.

Labonté, R. and Schrecker, T. (2009). Rights, redistribution and regulation. In R. Labonté, T. Schrecker, C. Packer, and V. Runnels (eds.) *Globalization and Health: Pathways, Evidence and Policy*, pp. 317–33. New York: Routledge.

Layte, R. and Whelan, C.T. (2009). Explaining social class inequalities in smoking: the role of education, self-efficacy, and deprivation. *European Sociological Review*, 25(4), 399–410.

Lessof, C. and Jowell, R. (2000). *Measuring Social Exclusion*. Oxford: University of Oxford.

Levitas, R. (2005). *The Inclusive Society?: Social Exclusion and New Labour* (2nd ed.). Basingstoke: Palgrave Macmillan.

Lister, R. (2004). *Poverty*. London: Polity Press.

Lynch, J., Kaplan, G., and Shema, S. (1997). Cumulative impact of sustained economic hardship on physical, cognitive, psychological, and social functioning. *The New England Journal of Medicine*, 337(26), 1889–95.

Lynch, J. and Smith, G.D. (2005). A life course approach to chronic disease epidemiology. *Annual Review of Public Health*, 26, 1–35.

Macinko, J., de Fa'tima Marinho de Souza, M., Guanais, F., and da Silva Simoes, C. (2007). Going to scale with community-based primary care: an analysis of the family health program and infant mortality in Brazil, 1999–2004. *Social Science & Medicine*, 65(10), 2070–80.

Mack, E. (2009). Introduction. In E. Mack, M. Schramm, S. Klasen, and T. Pogge (eds.) *Absolute Poverty and Global Justice*, pp. 1–18. Burlington, VT: Ashgate.

Mackenbach, J.P. (2012). The persistence of health inequalities in modern welfare states: the explanation of a paradox. *Social Science & Medicine*, 75(4), 761–69.

Marmot, M. (2010). *Fair Society, Healthy Lives: The Marmot Review*. London: The Marmot Review.

Masters, J. and Wickstrom, T. (2006). *Defining and Measuring Poverty: Challenges and Opportunities*. Berkeley, CA: Center for Community Futures.

Monteiro, C.A., Levy, R.B., Claro, R.M., de Castro, I.R.R., and Cannon, G. (2010). Increasing consumption of ultra-processed foods and likely impact on human health: evidence from Brazil. *Public Health Nutrition*, 14(1), 5.

Murray, C. (1984). *Losing Ground: American Social Policy, 1950–1980*. New York: Basic Books.

Najman, J.M. (1994). Class inequalities in health and lifestyle. In C. Waddell and A.R. Petersen (eds.) *Just Health: Inequalities in Illness, Care and Prevention*, pp. 27–46. Melbourne: Churchill Livingston.

Nolan, B. and Whelan, C.T. (1996). *Resources, Deprivation, and Poverty*. Oxford: Clarendon Press.

Nunes, C. (2008). *Poverty Measurement: The Development of Different Approaches and Its Techniques*. Report No.: ECINEQ WP 2008–93. Portugal: Society for the Study of Economic Inequality.

Nussbaum, M.C. (2000). *Women and Human Development: The Capabilities Approach*. Cambridge: Cambridge University Press.

Office of the High Commissioner for Human Rights (1986). *Declaration on the Right to Development*, 41/128. New York: Office of the High Commissioner for Human Rights.

Office of the High Commissioner for Human Rights (1999). *Human Rights and Extreme Poverty. Report of the Independent Expert on Human Rights Submitted to Commission on Human Rights*. 55th Session. Report No.: E/CN 4/1999/48. New York: UN Economic and Social Council.

OPHI and UNDP (2010). *Multidimensional Poverty Index*. Oxford Poverty and Human Development Initiative. University of California, Berkeley, Department of Economics. Available at: http://www.ophi.org.uk/wp-content/uploads/MPI_One_Page_final_updated.pdf?cda6c1.

Oppenheim, C. and Harker, L. (1990). *Poverty: The Facts*. London: Child Poverty Action Group.

Organisation for Economic Co-operation and Development (2008). *Growing Unequal? Income Distribution and Poverty in OECD Countries*. Paris: OECD.

Organisation for Economic Co-operation and Development (2010). Poverty rates and gaps. In OECD (ed.) *OECD Factbook 2010: Economic, Environmental and Social Statistics*, pp. 236–7. Paris: OECD Publishing.

Paim, J., Travassos, C., Almeida, C., Bahia, L., and Macinko, J. (2011). The Brazilian health system: history, advances, and challenges. *The Lancet*, 377, 1778–97.

Paradies, Y. (2006). A systematic review of empirical research on self-reported racism and health. *International Journal of Epidemiology*, 35(4), 888–901.

People's Health Movement (2009). *The People's Charter for Health*. Available at: http://www.phmovement.org/en/resources/charters/peopleshealth.

People's Health Movement, Medact, Health Action International, Medico International and Third World Network (2011). Primary health care: a review and critical appraisal of its 'revitalisation'. In *Global Health Watch 3: An Alternative World Health Report*, pp. 45–61. London: Zed Books.

Peterson, S. and Shellman, S. (2006). *AIDS and Violent Conflict: The Indirect Effects of Disease on National Security*. Working Paper. Williamsburg, VA: College of William and Mary.

Pogge, T. (2002). *World Poverty and Human Rights*. Cambridge: Polity.

Pogge, T. (2004). Relational conceptions of justice: responsibilities for health outcomes. In S. Anand, P. Fabienne, and A. Sen (eds.) *Public Health, Ethics and Equity*, pp. 135–61. Oxford: Clarendon Press.

Pogge, T. (2005). World poverty and human rights. *Ethics & International Affairs*, 9(1), 1–7.

Policy Analysis Discussion Group (2012). *Understanding Poverty and Well-Being: A Note with Implications for Research and Policy*. London: Overseas Development Institute.

Popay, J., Escorel, S., Hernández, M., Johnston, H., Mathieson, J., and Rispel, L. (2008). *Understanding and Tackling Social Exclusion*. Final Report to the WHO Commission on Social Determinants of Health From the Social Exclusion Knowledge Network, SEKN. Geneva: SEKN.

Power, C., Matthews, S., and Manor, O. (1996). Inequalities in self rated health in the 1958 birth cohort: lifetime social circumstances or social mobility? *British Medical Journal*, 313, 449–53.

Power, C., Thomas, C., Li, L., and Hertzman, C. (2012). Childhood psychosocial adversity and adult cortisol patterns. *British Journal of Psychiatry*, 201(3), 199–206.

Ranis, G., Stewart, F., and Samman, E. (2007). Human development: beyond the human development index. *Journal of Human Development*, 7(3), 323–58.

Ravallion, M. (2011). *What Does Adam Smith's Linen Shirt Have to do with Global Poverty? Let's Talk Development*. A blog hosted by the World Bank's Chief Economist. [Online] Available at: http://blogs.worldbank.org/developmenttalk/node/616.

Rawal, N. (2008). Social inclusion and exclusion: a review. *Dhaulagiri Journal of Sociology and Anthropology*, 2, 161–80.

Room, G. (1995). *Beyond the Threshold: The Measurement and Analysis of Social Exclusion*. Bristol: The Policy Press.

Ruger, J. (2008). Normative foundations of global health law. *Georgetown Law Journal*, 96, 423–43.

Sanders, D. and Chopra, M. (2007). Poverty, social inequity, and child health. In M. Kibel, H. Saloojee, and T. Westwood (eds.) *Child Health for All* (4th ed.), pp. 22–30. Oxford University Press Southern Africa Ltd.

Santarelli, E. and Figini, P. (2002). *Does Globalization Reduce Poverty? Some Empirical Evidence for the Developing Countries*. Working Paper. Bologna: Dipartimeto Scienze Economiche, Università di Bologna.

Saunders, P., Naidoo, Y., and Griffiths, M. (2008). Towards new indicators of disadvantage: deprivation and social exclusion in Australia. *Australian Journal of Social Issues*, 43(2), 175.

Saunders, P. and Wong, M. (2009). *Still Doing it Tough: An Update on Deprivation and Social Exclusion Among Welfare Service Clients*. Sydney: Social Policy Research Centre, University of New South Wales.

Schaefer, D.L. (2007). Procedural versus substantive justice: Rawls and Nozick. *Social Philosophy and Policy*, 24(1), 164–86.

Schrecker, T., Chapman, A.R., Labonté, R., and De Vogli, R. (2010). Advancing health equity in the global marketplace: how human rights can help. *Social Science & Medicine*, 71(8), 1520–6.

Sen, A. (1985). *Commodities and Capabilities*. Amsterdam: North-Holland.

Sen, A. (1992). *Inequality Re-examined*. Boston, MA: Harvard University Press.

Sen, A. (1999). *Development as Freedom*. Oxford: Oxford University Press.

Sen, A. (2000). *Social Exclusion: Concept, Application and Scrutiny*. Manila: Office of Environment and Social Development, Asian Development Bank.

Singer, P. (1972). Famine, affluence, and morality. *Philosophy & Public Affairs*, 1(1), 229–43.

Singer, P.W. (2002). AIDS and international security. *Survival*, 44(1), 145–58.

Smith, A. (1776). *An Inquiry into the Nature and Causes of the Wealth of Nations*. London: A. and C. Black.

Smith, G.D., Hart, C., Blane, D., Gillis, C., and Hawthorne, V. (1997). Lifetime socioeconomic position and mortality: prospective observational study. *British Medical Journal*, 314, 547.

Smith, G.D., Hart, C., Blane, D., and Hole, D. (1998). Adverse socio-economic conditions in childhood and cause specific adult mortality: prospective observational study. *British Medical Journal*, 316, 1635.

Springer, K.W., Hankivsky, O., and Bates, L.M. (2012). Introduction to special issue on gender and health: relational, intersectional, and biosocial approaches to gender and health. *Social Science & Medicine*, 74(11), 1661–6.

Stuckler, D. and Nestle, M. (2012). Big food, food systems, and global health. *PLoS Medicine*, 9(6), e1001242.

Sumner, A. (2010). Global poverty and the new bottom billion: what if three-quarters of the world's poor live in middle-income countries? *IDS Working Papers*, 2010(349), 1–43.

Szreter, S. (2003). The population health approach in historical perspective. *American Journal of Public Health*, 93(3), 424.

Tesh, S. (1988). *Hidden Arguments: Political Ideology and Disease Prevention Policy*. New Brunswick, NJ: Rutgers University Press.

UNDP (2011). *Human Development Report 2011: Sustainability and Equity: A Better Future for All*. New York: Palgrave Macmillan.

UNICEF Innocenti Research Centre (2012). *Measuring Child Poverty: New League Tables of Child Poverty in the World's Rich Countries*. Innocenti Report Card 10. Florence: UNICEF Innocenti Research Centre.

United Nations Division for Social Policy (2006). *Social Justice in an Open World: The Role of the United Nations*. New York: United Nations Publications.

United Nations General Assembly (2012). *Global Health and Foreign Policy*. Report No.: A/67/L.36. New York: United Nations.

Waitzkin, H. (2005). Commentary: Salvador Allende and the birth of Latin American social medicine. *International Journal of Epidemiology*, 34(4), 739–41.

Waters, S. (2004). Mobilising against globalisation: Attac and the French intellectuals. *European Politics*, 27(5), 854–74.

Whitehead, M. (1992). The concepts and principles of equity in health. *International Journal of Health Services*, 22, 429–45.

Woodward, D. and Simms, A. (2006). *Growth Isn't Working: The Unbalanced Distribution of Benefits and Costs from Economic Growth*. London: New Economics Foundation.

World Bank (2002). *Globalization, Growth, and Poverty: Building an Inclusive World Economy*. New York: Oxford University Press.

World Bank (2006). *World Development Report 2006: Equity and Development*. New York: Oxford University Press for the World Bank.

World Bank (2011). *World Development Report 2011: Conflict, Security, and Development*. Washington, DC: World Bank.

World Health Organization (2005). *Medical Costs Push Millions of People into Poverty Across the Globe*. Geneva: WHO. Available at: http://www. who.int/mediacentre/news/releases/2005/pr65/en/index.html.

Yamin, A.E. and Parra-Vera, O. (2009). How do courts set health policy? The case of the Colombian Constitutional Court. *PLoS Medicine*, 6(2), 147–50.

Yitzhaki, S. (1979). Relative deprivation and the Gini coefficient. *The Quarterly Journal of Economics*, 93, 321–4.

Young, I.M. (2006). Responsibility and global justice: a social connection model. *Social Philosophy and Policy*, 23(1), 102–30.

Ziersch, A.M., Gallaher, G., Baum, F., and Bentley, M. (2011). Responding to racism: insights on how racism can damage health from an urban study of Australian Aboriginal people. *Social Science & Medicine*, 73(7), 1045–53.

2.3

Socioeconomic inequalities in health in high-income countries: the facts and the options

Johan P. Mackenbach

Introduction to socioeconomic inequalities in health in high-income countries

At the start of the twenty-first century, all high-income countries are faced with substantial inequalities in health within their populations. People with a lower level of education, a lower occupational class, or a lower level of income tend to die at a younger age, and to have, within their shorter lives, a higher prevalence of all kinds of health problems. This leads to large differences between socioeconomic groups in the number of years that people can expect to live in good health ('health expectancy').

Socioeconomic inequalities in health currently represent one of the greatest challenges for public health worldwide. This chapter aims to review the available evidence on the magnitude and explanation of these health inequalities (the 'facts'), and to present the available evidence on what we can do to reduce health inequalities (the 'options'). Socioeconomic inequalities in health will be defined as systematic differences in morbidity or mortality rates between people of higher and lower socioeconomic status, as indicated by, for example, level of education, occupational class, or income level.

This chapter only deals with the situation in high-income countries. Wherever possible, we will draw upon international overviews, such as comparative studies, in order to avoid biases related to the selective experiences of single countries. Most of the illustrations will be drawn upon the European experience, which has become very well documented in the past three decades.

Historical notes

Historical evidence suggests that socioeconomic inequalities in health are not a recent phenomenon. However, it was only during the nineteenth century that socioeconomic inequalities in health were 'discovered'. Before that time, health inequalities simply went unrecognized because of lack of information. In the nineteenth century, great figures in public health, such as Villermé in France, Chadwick in England, and Virchow in Germany, devoted a large part of their scientific work to this issue (Ackerknecht 1953; Coleman 1982; Chave 1984). This was facilitated by national population statistics, which permitted the calculation of mortality rates by occupation or by city district. Louis René Villermé (1782–1863), for example, analysed inequalities in mortality between 'arrondissements' in Paris in 1817–1821. He showed that districts with a lower socioeconomic level, as indicated by the proportion of houses for which no tax was levied over the rents, tended to have systematically higher mortality rates than more well-to-do neighbourhoods. He concluded that life and death are not primarily biological phenomena, but are closely linked to social circumstances (Coleman 1982). Rudolf Virchow (1821–1902) went even further in his famous statement that 'medicine is a social science, and politics nothing but medicine at a larger scale' (Mackenbach 2009).

Since the nineteenth century, there has been a marked decline in mortality in all current high-income countries, leading to a doubling of average life expectancy at birth. As a result, some inequalities in mortality have declined as well, but this is far from a generalized phenomenon. For example, in England and Wales, the only European country where long time-series about occupational class differences in mortality are available, inequalities in infant mortality declined substantially between the 1920s and 1970s, but over the same period inequalities in adult mortality remained largely stable in absolute terms, and even increased in relative terms (Pamuk 1985). Since then, further increases have been observed in many high-income countries (Mackenbach et al. 2003), and these have contributed to a heightened awareness of health inequalities, and of the challenge they pose to public health policy, around the world.

The start of the resurgence of an active interest in health inequalities in Europe can be linked to the publication of the Black Report in England in 1980 (Department of Health and Social Services 1980), which has been followed by an enormous rise of descriptive studies in many other countries, testifying to the existence of substantial inequalities in health in all countries with available data. Gradually the emphasis of academic research in this area has shifted from description to explanation, not only to satisfy scientific curiosities but also to find entry-points for policies and interventions to reduce health inequalities (Mackenbach and Bakker 2002; Marmot and Wilkinson 2006). This was greatly facilitated by increased research funding, both from national research programmes (e.g. in England, the Netherlands, and Finland), and by international agencies (e.g. the European Commission and the European Science Foundation) (Siegrist and Marmot 2006).

As a result, our understanding of the causes of socioeconomic inequalities in health has expanded tremendously, and has allowed interested policymakers to start searching for strategies to reduce these inequalities. While countries are in different stages of policy development in this area (Whitehead 1998), the World Health Organization has actively promoted the issue of health inequalities by creating a Commission on Social Determinants of Health that has issued a major report urging policy action to 'close the gap in a generation' (Commission on Social Determinants of Health 2008). In some countries (e.g. England) political windows of opportunity have arisen which have led to national programmes to tackle health inequalities, the results of which are gradually becoming clear (Department of Health 2010), pointing to a need to double our efforts to find effective interventions and policies that can be implemented on a sufficiently large scale to achieve population-wide impacts (Mackenbach 2011).

The facts: description

Socioeconomic position should be measured by individual-level indicators like education (e.g. highest completed level of education), occupation (e.g. occupational class), or income (e.g. household income adjusted for household size), but can sometimes only be measured by area-level indicators (e.g. neighbourhood deprivation). Usually, all these indicators point in the same direction, with health being worse for those in lower socioeconomic positions, but there is often substantial variation between indicators in the strength of the association, suggesting that the underlying aetiological mechanisms are different as well (Galobardes et al. 2007).

The magnitude of socioeconomic inequalities in health can be measured in different ways, ranging from simple measures like rate ratios and rate differences (indicating relative and absolute differences in morbidity or mortality rates between two contrasting groups), to more complex measures like the relative index of inequality and the slope index of inequality (indicating relative and absolute differences in rates between those with the lowest and highest socioeconomic position, taking all groups into account and calibrating the social position of each group to its relative size) (Mackenbach and Kunst 1997). Although the choice of measure will partly depend on technical considerations, each emphasizes different aspects of health inequalities, often at the expense of others, and it may therefore be important to combine different measures (Harper et al. 2010).

Socioeconomic inequalities in health usually present themselves as a gradient, in the sense that there is a stepwise increase of rates of morbidity and mortality with every step down the social ladder, implying that social inequality affects the health of nearly everybody, not only the worst-off. This suggests that explanations should be sought in factors operating across society (Marmot 2003, 2004), and that policies to reduce health inequalities should do more than closing the gap between the worst- and best-off (Graham 2004).

Mortality

Total mortality

In all high-income countries with available data, mortality rates are higher among those in less advantaged socioeconomic positions (Mackenbach 2006; Commission on Social Determinants of Health 2008). Fig. 2.3.1 shows that the relative index of inequality is greater than 1 for both men and women in all countries, indicating that, throughout Europe, mortality is higher among those with less education (Mackenbach et al. 2008). Relative inequalities in mortality are seen at all ages, and are often largest in early middle age, but because of the higher average mortality rates at older ages, absolute inequalities tend to rise with age (Huisman et al. 2004).

The magnitude of these inequalities varies substantially among European countries. For example, in Sweden, the relative index of inequality for men is less than 2, indicating that mortality among those with the least education is less than twice that among those with the most education; on the other hand, in Hungary, the Czech Republic, and Poland, the relative index of inequality for men is 4 or higher, indicating that mortality differs by a factor of more than 4 between the lower and upper ends of the education scale. The smallest inequalities for both men and women are found in the Basque country of Spain, whereas the largest inequalities are found in the Czech Republic and Lithuania. Education-related inequalities in mortality are smaller than the European average in all southern European populations and larger than average in most countries in the eastern and Baltic regions. Similar patterns are seen for occupation-related inequalities in mortality among middle-aged men (Mackenbach et al. 2008).

Within Europe, the international pattern observed for relative inequalities in mortality also applies to absolute inequalities in mortality, as indicated by the slope index of inequality. This is because countries with larger relative inequalities in mortality, i.e. those in the eastern and Baltic regions, also tend to have higher average rates of mortality. As a result, the range of variation of absolute inequalities in mortality is even larger than that seen for relative inequalities. The magnitude of absolute inequalities in mortality varies more than sixfold among men and more than 20-fold among women, suggesting that there is an enormous scope for reducing inequalities in mortality (Mackenbach et al. 2008).

While the mortality rates of the higher educated are rather similar in different countries, the mortality rates of the lower educated are much more variable, and higher in countries with larger inequalities in mortality. In other words, the mortality rates among the lower educated drive the magnitude of inequalities in mortality in a country. It is as if the higher educated manage to keep their mortality levels low, regardless of national conditions, whereas the lower educated are more vulnerable to unfavourable national conditions (van Raalte et al. 2011).

Cause-specific mortality

Countries do not only differ in the magnitude of their inequalities in total mortality, but also in the causes of death contributing to higher mortality in lower socioeconomic groups (Table 2.3.1). Within Europe we observe three different 'regimes' of inequalities in cause-specific mortality: a North-western regime with large inequalities in mortality from cardiovascular disease (men and women) and cancer (men only); a Southern regime with small

(a) Education, men

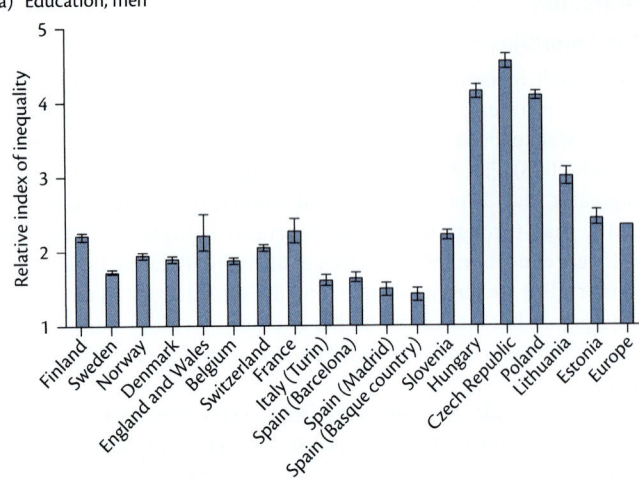

(b) Education, women

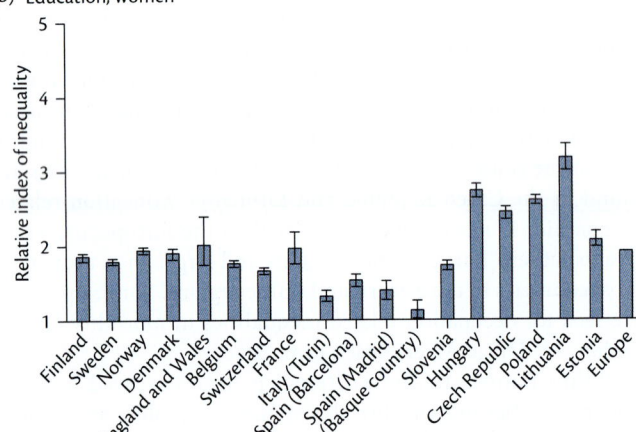

Fig. 2.3.1 Relative inequalities in mortality by level of education in 16 European countries, 1990s. Note: the graph shows the relative index of inequality, indicating the rate ratio of mortality between those with the lowest and the highest socioeconomic position. This is a regression-based measure that takes into account all socioeconomic groups and calibrates the social position of each group to its proportion in the total population.
From the *New England Journal of Medicine*, Mackenbach, J.P. et al., Socioeconomic inequalities in health in 22 European countries, Volume 358, Issue 23, pp. 2468–81, Copyright ©2008 Massachusetts Medical Society. Reprinted with permission from Massachusetts Medical Society.

inequalities in mortality from cardiovascular disease (men and women) and large inequalities in mortality from cancer (men only); and an Eastern regime with huge inequalities in mortality from cardiovascular disease, cancer and injuries (men and women) (Table 2.3.1) (Huisman et al. 2005a; Mackenbach et al. 2008).

Whereas mortality from stroke is always higher in the lower socioeconomic groups, this is not the case for ischaemic heart disease (IHD) (Avendano et al. 2004). For IHD, a North–South gradient within Europe has been found, with relative and absolute inequalities being larger in the North of Europe (e.g. the Nordic countries and the United Kingdom) than in the South (e.g. Portugal, Spain, and Italy) (Kunst et al. 1999; Mackenbach et al. 2000; Avendano et al. 2006).

This international pattern for IHD results from differences between countries in how the 'epidemic' of IHD has developed over time. In many countries, particularly in the North of Europe, mortality from IHD increased substantially after the Second World War, probably as a result of changes in health-related behaviours, such as smoking, diet, and physical exercise. During the 1970s, however, a decline set in, and is still continuing. During this epidemiological development, important changes occurred in the association between socioeconomic position and IHD mortality. In the North of Europe, during the 1950s and 1960s IHD mortality was higher in the higher socioeconomic groups, leading to the notion of IHD being a 'manager's disease'.

It was only during the 1970s, coinciding with the start of the decline of IHD mortality in the population as a whole, that a reversal occurred, and the current association emerged (Marmot and McDowall 1986; Gonzalez et al. 1998). This is due to differences between socioeconomic groups in both the timing and the speed of decline of IHD mortality. In the South of Europe, however, a similar 'epidemic' of IHD mortality has not occurred, and similar inequalities in IHD mortality have not arisen, partly as a result of the protection of traditional Mediterranean living habits against IHD (Avendano et al. 2006). These smaller inequalities in IHD explain much of the smaller inequalities in total mortality in Southern Europe, and suggest that the latter do not result from effective policies to reduce inequalities.

Inequalities in mortality from cancer are often large among men, partly because of the excess lung cancer mortality in lower socioeconomic groups (Menvielle et al. 2007; Menvielle et al. 2008; Van der Heyden et al. 2009). Among women, inequalities in cancer mortality are often smaller than among men. Sometimes they are really small or even have a 'reverse' direction, with higher mortality among the higher educated, particularly in Southern Europe (Mackenbach et al. 2008). This is because lung cancer mortality does not (yet) have the same negative association with socioeconomic status among women as it has among men, and because the most important cause of cancer mortality among women, breast cancer, often has a 'reverse' association with socioeconomic position (Strand et al. 2007). Both reflect the diffusion of 'modern' patterns of behaviour (i.e. smoking and delayed age of child-bearing) among women, with women in the North-western part of Europe and women in higher socioeconomic groups adopting these behaviours first (Cavelaars et al. 2000).

Unfortunately, the favourable situation in women, with small or absent socioeconomic inequalities in total cancer mortality, is likely to be a temporary phenomenon. In some countries in Western Europe, it has been found that in younger birth cohorts rates of breast cancer mortality now tend to be higher in lower socioeconomic groups than in higher socioeconomic groups. For lung cancer, there are similar indications for a future change in gradient among women (Mackenbach et al. 2004; Van der Heyden et al. 2009).

External causes of injury (road traffic accidents, other accidents, and suicides) are another important contributor to socioeconomic inequalities in mortality, particularly (but not exclusively) in Eastern Europe. Mortality from road traffic accidents, from suicides and from homicides is higher in lower socioeconomic groups among men, but not or less clearly so among women (Borrell et al. 2005; Lorant et al. 2005; Stickley et al. 2012). The larger inequalities in injury mortality in Eastern Europe are likely to be related to

Table 2.3.1 Absolute inequalities in cause-specific mortality by level of education in 16 European countries, 1990s[a]

Country	Average rate of death from any cause[a]	Slope index of inequality according to cause of death (deaths/100,000 person-years)											
		All causes	All cancer-related causes	Breast cancer[b]	Lung cancer	All cardiovascular disease	Ischaemic heart disease	Cerebrovascular disease	Injuries	All other diseases	Alcohol-related causes[c]	Smoking-related causes[d]	Causes amenable to medical intervention[e]
Men													
Finland	1673	1255	213		135	533	393	94	143	347	101	215	88
Sweden	1188	625	90		37	309	229	50	52	175	50	71	26
Norway	1529	980	169		95	434	307	78	70	305	62	166	49
Denmark	1344	828	126		75	235	157	39	89	363	23	60	44
United Kingdom (England and Wales)	1124	862	225		141	401	284	67	19	157	28	241	NA
Belgium	1510	915	274		179	233	99	55	64	340	36	302	28
Switzerland	1475	1012	283		136	401	132	61	91	348	117	260	61
France	1241	1044	333		71	232	67	68	109	357	196	204	114
Italy (Turin)	1377	639	232		107	140	57	52	23	243	63	177	24
Spain (Barcelona)	1370	662	230		90	88	26	40	38	304	77	218	36
Spain (Madrid)	1355	530	181		56	38	−16	11	26	278	75	170	34
Spain (Basque country)	1108	384	107		39	16	−6	3	63	177	46	107	24
Slovenia	1902	1439	303		124	405	67	219	203	482	224	327	83
Hungary	2110	2580	666		260	1003	482	385	222	671	420	508	66
Czech Republic	1664	2130	676		247	825	472	259	138	489	146	364	73
Poland	1804	2192	589		260	750	295	223	187	637	145	408	75
Lithuania	2531	2536	383		197	807	505	159	643	677	304	424	195
Estonia	2799	2349	355		191	929	610	263	436	618	286	323	162
Europe total	1635	1333	328		153	451	233	131	147	425	141	288	72
Women													
Finland	811	483	49	−8	14	262	168	72	25	161	31	28	42
Sweden	673	381	73	−6	20	172	104	44	8	128	15	39	18
Norway	811	518	103	−14	44	239	141	62	5	169	16	79	30
Denmark	830	511	103	−12	63	160	90	42	22	230	9	70	27

(Continued)

Table 2.3.1 Continued

Country	Average rate of death from any cause[a]	Slope index of inequality according to cause of death (deaths/100,000 person-years)											
		All causes	All cancer-related causes	Breast cancer[b]	Lung cancer	All cardiovascular disease	Ischaemic heart disease	Cerebrovascular disease	Injuries	All other diseases	Alcohol-related causes[c]	Smoking-related causes[d]	Causes amenable to medical intervention[e]
United Kingdom (England and Wales)	672	462	111	−22	59	236	154	31	1	96	7	103	NA
Belgium	761	417	47	−11	11	195	77	55	11	163	6	29	10
Switzerland	676	337	53	−3	10	158	74	46	5	120	10	21	22
France	536	375	50	35	6	130	33	44	36	163	30	17	82
Italy (Turin)	721	197	15	−17	−9	94	34	34	−3	94	8	−4	11
Spain (Barcelona)	569	236	7	−12	−14	103	36	34	5	126	7	−14	12
Spain (Madrid)	543	175	−12	−29	−17	96	30	29	−1	94	−3	−17	9
Spain (Basque country)	422	51	−76	−19	−20	56	23	17	7	74	3	−24	2
Slovenia	853	459	−13	−21	−18	263	62	127	28	180	44	−3	33
Hungary	1023	948	120	−17	20	511	237	216	51	258	82	61	26
Czech Republic	868	726	144	10	17	356	112	134	26	203	23	33	32
Poland	840	750	139	6	10	356	117	142	29	222	23	28	27
Lithuania	1053	1099	130	7	7	535	297	162	178	251	87	39	51
Estonia	1213	851	7	−5	4	493	273	187	109	252	101	16	48
Europe total	778	492	55	−9	10	251	120	85	30	172	30	28	27

Code numbers of the causes of death according to the 9th and 10th revisions of the *International Classification of Diseases, Clinical Modification* (ICD-9-CM and ICD-10-CM) are given in table 1 of the supplementary appendix in Mackenbach et al. (2008). The slope index of inequality is a regression-based measure of absolute differences in mortality rates between the lowest and the highest ends of the socioeconomic scale. NA denotes not available.

[a] Age-standardized rates of death for all educational groups are given.

[b] Rates of death from breast cancer among men are not given.

[c] Alcohol-related causes are accidental poisoning by alcohol and alcoholic psychosis, dependence, abuse, cardiomyopathy, and cirrhosis of the liver and pancreas.

[d] Smoking-related causes are chronic obstructive pulmonary disease and cancer of the buccal cavity, pharynx, oesophagus, larynx, trachea, bronchus, and lung.

[e] Causes amenable to medical intervention are tuberculosis and other infectious and parasitic diseases, cervical cancer, breast cancer, Hodgkin's disease, leukaemia, hypertension, cerebrovascular disease, pneumonia or influenza, appendicitis, hernia, peptic ulcer, cholelithiasis and cholecystitis, and complications of childbirth.

Note: the slope index of inequality indicates the mortality rate difference between those with the lowest and the highest socioeconomic position. It is a regression-based measure that takes all socioeconomic groups into account and calibrates the social position of each group to its proportion in the total population.

From the *New England Journal of Medicine*, Mackenbach, J.P. et al., Socioeconomic inequalities in health in 22 European countries, Volume 358, Issue 23, pp. 2468–81, Copyright ©2008 Massachusetts Medical Society. Reprinted with permission from Massachusetts Medical Society.

higher rates of excessive alcohol consumption (Mackenbach et al. 2008).

As is clear from Fig. 2.3.1, inequalities in mortality tend to be smaller among women than among men. This is partly because of a different cause-of-death pattern among women (with, e.g. high mortality rates from breast cancer, which as noted earlier happens to have 'reverse' inequalities), partly because of smaller inequalities among women (e.g. no clear socioeconomic gradients for road traffic and suicide mortality among women) (Mackenbach et al. 1999).

Trends

Mortality differences between socioeconomic groups have widened considerably in many European countries during the last three decades of the twentieth century. For relative inequalities this widening has been seen in all countries with available data; absolute inequalities, on the other hand, have remained stable in some countries and increased in others (Mackenbach et al. 2003; Wamala et al. 2006; Krieger et al. 2008; Strand et al. 2010; Shkolnikov et al. 2012).

The explanation of this disturbing phenomenon is only partly known. One aspect which should certainly be taken into account, however, is that this widening is generally the result of a difference between socioeconomic groups in the speed of mortality decline. While mortality declined in all socioeconomic groups, the decline has been faster in the higher socioeconomic groups than in the lower. The faster mortality declines in higher socioeconomic groups were in their turn mostly due to faster mortality declines for cardiovascular diseases (Mackenbach et al. 2003).

In many developed countries, the 1980s and 1990s have been decades with substantial improvements in cardiovascular disease mortality. These have been due to improvements in health-related behaviours (less smoking, modest improvements in diet, more physical exercise, etc.), and to the introduction of effective healthcare interventions (hypertension detection and treatment, surgical interventions, thrombolytic therapy, etc.) (Unal et al. 2005). While these improvements have to some extent been taken up by all socioeconomic groups, the higher socioeconomic groups have tended to benefit more.

The widening of the gap in death rates has been particularly strong in Eastern Europe, probably as a result of economic and social developments following the political changes around 1990 (Leinsalu et al. 2009). Since these transitions, mortality rates have changed dramatically in many countries in Eastern Europe, with increases followed by declines in many countries. The temporary increases in mortality were due to a combination of (interlinked) factors: a rise in economic insecurity and poverty; a breakdown of protective social, public health, and healthcare institutions; and a rise in excessive drinking and other risk factors for premature mortality (McKee 2009).

The evidence clearly shows that these changes in mortality have not been equally shared between socioeconomic groups: in the countries with available data, mortality rates have generally increased more, or declined less, in the lower socioeconomic groups. Apparently, people with higher levels of education have been able to protect themselves better against increased health risks, and/or have been able to benefit more from new opportunities for health gains. Evidence from several Eastern European countries (Estonia, Hungary, Russia) suggests a much larger widening of the gap in death rates than in Western European countries (Shkolnikov et al. 2006; Leinsalu et al. 2009).

Life expectancy is shorter in lower socioeconomic groups

As a result of these differences in the risk of dying, people from lower socioeconomic groups live considerably shorter lives than those with more advantaged social positions. Differences in life expectancy at birth between the lowest and highest socioeconomic groups (e.g. manual versus professional occupations, or primary school versus postsecondary education) are typically in the order of 4–6 years among men, and 2–4 years among women, but sometimes larger differences have been observed (Mackenbach 2006). In England and Wales, for example, inequalities in life expectancy at birth among men have increased from 5.4 years in the 1970s to more than 8 years in the 1990s, and remained stable at this high level in the early 2000s (2010). Increases have also been observed in several other countries (Deboosere et al. 2009; Palosuo et al. 2009; Bronnum-Hansen and Baadsgaard 2012; Steingrimsdottir et al. 2012).

Morbidity

Many countries have nationally representative surveys with questions on both socioeconomic status and self-reported morbidity (e.g. self-assessed health, chronic conditions, disability). Inequalities in the latter are substantial everywhere, and practically always in the same direction: persons with a lower socioeconomic status have higher morbidity rates.

Inequalities in generic health indicators

For one indicator, self-assessed health (measured with a single question on an individual's perception of his or her own health), the availability of these data is almost as great as that for inequalities in mortality (Fig. 2.3.2). The overall pattern is clear again: prevalence rates of less than 'good' self-assessed health are higher in lower socioeconomic groups. No clear patterns have emerged in the magnitude of socioeconomic inequalities in self-assessed health between European countries (Cavelaars et al. 1998a, 1998b; Eikemo et al. 2008; Mackenbach et al. 2008).

Beyond early adulthood, socioeconomic differences in self-reported morbidity have been found in all European countries where this has been examined (Cavelaars et al. 1998a, 1998b; Dalstra et al. 2005). For children and adolescents, however, the picture is more mixed. Some studies have suggested that in adolescence, the period between childhood and adulthood, there is a genuine narrowing of health inequalities, perhaps as a result of the transition between socioeconomic position of family of origin and own socioeconomic position. Among children the picture is more consistent: many studies find that parents in lower socioeconomic groups report more ill health for their children than parents in higher socioeconomic groups (Halldorsson et al. 1999).

Inequalities in diseases and disabilities

Socioeconomic inequalities have not only been found for general health indicators, which are usually measured on the basis of self-reports, but can also be found for many specific indicators, including objective measurements of the incidence or prevalence of diseases and disabilities. In the large majority of these studies, higher incidences or prevalences of health problems have been found in the lower socioeconomic groups (Dalstra et al. 2005).

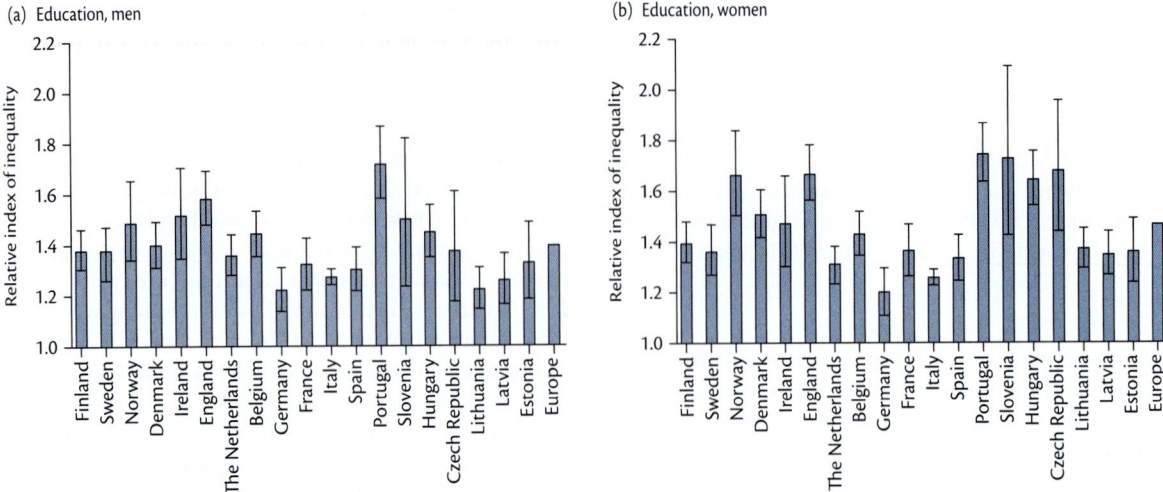

Fig. 2.3.2 Inequalities in self-assessed health in 19 European countries. Note: the graph shows the relative index of inequality, indicating the rate ratio of less-than-good self-assessed health between those with the lowest and the highest socioeconomic position. This is a regression-based measure that takes into account all socioeconomic groups and calibrates the social position of each group to its proportion in the total population.

From the *New England Journal of Medicine*, Mackenbach, J.P. et al., Socioeconomic inequalities in health in 22 European countries, Volume 358, Issue 23, pp. 2468–81, Copyright ©2008 Massachusetts Medical Society. Reprinted with permission from Massachusetts Medical Society.

Since the start of the decline of IHD mortality in the 1970s and 1980s, it has been observed that the timing and magnitude of the decline have been different between socioeconomic groups. The decline generally started earlier and has proceeded more rapidly in higher socioeconomic groups, and as a result, people with a lower socioeconomic position currently experience a higher IHD mortality in most industrialized countries (Avendano et al. 2006). In many countries, these inequalities are due to both inequalities in IHD incidence and inequalities in case fatality after myocardial infarction (Salomaa et al. 2000; Stirbu et al. 2012).

Similarly, inequalities in cancer mortality reflect inequalities in both incidence and survival.

Many cancers, particularly those associated with smoking, excessive alcohol consumption, and other lifestyle factors, such as cancers of the respiratory and upper digestive tract, have a higher incidence in the lower socioeconomic groups, whereas risks of cancer of the prostate, breast, ovary, and colon and malignant melanoma are often reduced (Faggiano et al. 1997; Aarts et al. 2010). By contrast, cancer prevalence tends not to be different between socioeconomic groups (Dalstra et al. 2005), perhaps because longer survival of higher socioeconomic status patients 'compensates' their lower incidence. Most studies show a survival advantage for patients with a higher socioeconomic position (Kogevinas and Porta 1997), which is at least partly explained by more favourable prognostic factors (e.g. less co-morbidity, more favourable stage at presentation, etc.) (Louwman et al. 2010).

As suggested by data on mortality from suicide (see earlier), mental ill health tends to be more prevalent in lower socioeconomic groups (Fryers et al. 2005; Lorant et al. 2007). The higher prevalence of mental illness in lower socioeconomic groups is likely to have a complex explanation. In psychiatric epidemiology, there is a long tradition of looking at the possible effects of mental health problems on downward social mobility. This 'drift hypothesis' has indeed found some support, for example, in the case of schizophrenia, whose onset usually occurs in adolescence and young adulthood, and which may consequently interfere with school and early work careers. On the other hand, incidence studies have also found higher rates of many mental health problems among those who are currently in a lower socioeconomic position. It seems likely that this at least partly reflects a causal effect, perhaps through a higher exposure to psychosocial stressors and/or a lack of coping resources (Lorant et al. 2007).

As a result of the higher frequency of physical and mental health problems in lower socioeconomic groups, the prevalence of limitations in functioning and various forms of disability also tends to be higher. This applies to many aspects of functioning (mobility, sensory functioning, grip strength, walking speed, etc.) and is particularly evident among the elderly (Avendano et al. 2005). These inequalities in functioning translate into inequalities in limitations with activities of daily living such as dressing and bathing, and limitations with instrumental activities of daily living such as preparing hot meals and making telephone calls. This illustrates the high burden of physical limitations among those with a lower socioeconomic position, and is likely to contribute to substantially higher professional care needs, including institutionalized care (e.g. nursing homes). As suggested by the results for objective measures of grip strength and walking speed, inequalities in self-reported disability are real, and not a matter of reporting bias (Mohd Hairi et al. 2010).

'Healthy life expectancy' is shorter in lower socioeconomic groups

We have seen in earlier sections that the higher mortality rates in lower socioeconomic groups lead to substantial inequalities in life expectancy: people in lower socioeconomic groups tend to live between 2 and 8 years less than people in higher socioeconomic groups. The fact that morbidity rates (among those who are still alive) are higher too, contributes to even larger inequalities in 'healthy life expectancy' (the number of years which people can expect to live in good health). Inequalities in the number of years lived in good health are often seen of more than 10 years (Sihvonen et al. 1998; Majer et al. 2011).

Costs of health inequalities

Health inequalities do not only represent an enormous loss of human well-being, but also generate economic costs, for example, through excess use of healthcare and social security benefits and through lost labour productivity. Currently, there is no established methodology to estimate these economic costs, but the few studies that have explored this issue have concluded that the economic costs may well be substantial. One study found that the higher rates of health problems among those in the lower half of the socioeconomic distribution account for 20 per cent of the total costs of healthcare, and 15 per cent of the total costs of social security benefits in the European Union (EU), and that the associated losses to labour productivity take 1.4 per cent off gross domestic product each year (Mackenbach et al. 2011). Largely similar findings, interpreted as 'the costs of inaction', were reported from a British study (2010).

The facts: explanation

During the past decade, great progress has been made in unravelling the determinants of health inequalities in high-income countries, and here we will summarize the evidence under three headings: '"selection" versus "causation"', 'specific causal pathways', and 'overarching ideas'. While we present these explanatory insights for general use, it is important to note that the contribution of each of these factors and pathways differs between countries, even within this relatively homogeneous group. This has been shown decisively for smoking, which is much more important as a determinant of health inequalities in the North of Europe than in the South, but is likely to be true for many other factors and pathways. This is due to the 'distal' nature of socioeconomic status: unlike more 'proximal' determinants of health like smoking, socioeconomic status exerts its effects indirectly, which leaves a lot of room for interaction with national circumstances.

'Selection' versus 'causation'

Early debates

Early debates about the explanation of socioeconomic inequalities in health focused on the question of whether 'causation' or 'selection' was the more important mechanism (Macintyre 1980, 1997). Selection explanations imply that health determines socioeconomic position, instead of socioeconomic position determining health. Because of the occurrence of 'social mobility' (changes in socioeconomic position during a person's lifetime) there is ample scope for selection processes: health problems may lead to downward social mobility, and upward mobility may be more likely for those with above-average health. The unspoken assumption in these debates was that selection would be less of a problem for public policy than causation. This assumption was incorrect, however, because limiting the social consequences of health problems is one of the classical objectives of social security and public health policies in many developed countries (Burstrom et al. 2000).

The occurrence of health-related selection is undisputed: during social mobility, some degree of selection on (ill) health does indeed occur, with people who are in poor physical or mental health being more likely to be downwardly mobile (e.g. get a lower status job, or lose income) and less likely to be upwardly mobile (e.g. finish a high level education, or obtain a highly-paid job),

than people who are in good health. Research has shown, however, that the contribution of health-related selection to the explanation of socioeconomic inequalities in health is small, at least when occupational class or education is used as an indicator of socioeconomic status (Bartley and Plewis 1997; van de Mheen et al. 1999). The main reason is that most health problems occur in late middle or old age, after people have reached their final level of education and main occupational status. This is consistent with the fact that longitudinal studies in which education or occupational class have been measured before health problems are present, and in which the incidence of health problems has been measured during follow-up, show clearly higher risks of developing health problems in the lower socioeconomic groups (Marmot et al. 1991; Marmot and Wilkinson 2006).

The conclusion is, however, different for income and wealth as indicators of socioeconomic status. Studies from the United States have found that 'health shocks' lead to wealth depletion, partly through medical care costs, partly through income losses due to reduced labour supply, suggesting that these 'reverse' effects are actually stronger than the effect of income on health (Smith 1999). Income appears to be much more sensitive to health status than education or occupational class, and in contrast to education and occupational class longitudinal studies that relate income to health outcomes at a later stage have produced inconsistent results (Cutler et al. 2006).

Recent extensions

While the impact of such 'direct selection'—that is, selection on health or ill health—is likely to be small, particularly when educational level or occupational class is used as an indicator of socioeconomic status, there is more scope for an impact of what has been called 'indirect selection'—that is, selection on determinants of health. For example, there is some evidence that behavioural risk factors such as obesity affect social mobility, perhaps because of discrimination during recruitment for jobs or promotion (Karnehed et al. 2008; Heraclides and Brunner 2010).

Potentially more important is selection on the basis of personal attributes such as cognitive ability, coping styles, control beliefs, personality, and bodily and mental fitness (Mackenbach 2010). These may influence educational and occupational achievement, and at the same time determine later health, either directly or through health-related behaviours such as consumption and exercise patterns and use of health services. Empirical studies have found associations between many of these personal attributes and social mobility (Atkinson et al. 1993; Judge et al. 1999; Lounsbury et al. 2003), and some multivariate analyses suggest that factors like personality and cognitive ability do indeed contribute to the explanation of health inequalities (Singh-Manoux et al. 2005; Batty et al. 2006; Nabi et al. 2008; Chapman et al. 2010).

This perspective also suggests ways for genetic factors to contribute to health inequalities. Genetic factors do not easily fit into 'causation'-type explanations, because temporally a person's genotype precedes his/her socioeconomic status, and a causal effect of the latter on the first is therefore logically impossible. Genetic factors can more easily be seen to operate within a 'selection' framework (Mackenbach 2005). An association between socioeconomic status and a certain genotype will arise when the genotype is a determinant of social mobility, for example, through an effect on personal attributes related to social mobility. To the extent that personal attributes that influence social mobility (cognitive ability, coping styles, control beliefs, personality, bodily and mental fitness, etc.) are genetically co-determined, the underlying genotypes will tend to be more common in the upper or lower social classes (Mackenbach 2005).

Evidence suggests that intelligence and personality profiles are indeed genetically co-determined (Bouchard 1998; Plomin and Spinath 2004), and although their specific genetic determinants have not yet been definitively identified, some role of the genetic determinants of social mobility in the explanation of health inequalities seems plausible. Because of the same social mobility, however, a more direct role of genetic determinants of disease in the explanation of health inequalities is less likely. Research has so far been limited but has not found differences between socioeconomic groups in the prevalence of genetic determinants of disease (Holzapfel et al. 2011).

Disentangling causal effects

Confounding by personal attributes is difficult to get rid of in observational studies, and because experimentation (with random allocation of individuals to higher and lower socioeconomic positions) is impossible, situations have been sought that mimic such experimental manipulation. Lotteries are an example: in lotteries large amounts of money are allocated randomly, and studies have found that the recipients of lottery prizes experience positive changes in self-reported health. These positive effects are particularly seen for mental health and less so for physical health, perhaps because winning a lottery also tends to increase smoking and social drinking (Lindahl 2005; Apouey and Clark 2010).

Similarly, historical changes in the age of compulsory education have been used to study the causal effect of education on mortality. In the United States, between 1915 and 1939, at least 30 states changed their compulsory schooling laws. A comparison

of later-life mortality of children attending school just before and just after the changes took effect showed that 1 year of extra schooling reduced mortality substantially (Lleras-Muney 2002). Such results have also been reported for several other countries (Kippersluis et al. 2011; Lager and Torssander 2012).

Specific causal pathways

The findings summarized in the previous paragraph suggest that socioeconomic inequalities in health at least partly reflect a causal effect of socioeconomic position on health, but the debate on the relative contribution of such causal mechanisms is far from closed. That also applies to the exact nature of these causal mechanisms, which are likely to be largely indirect, by raising the prevalence of specific determinants of morbidity or mortality in lower socioeconomic groups.

Many risk factors for morbidity and mortality are more prevalent in lower socioeconomic groups. Three groups of explanatory factors are likely to explain the bulk of health inequalities in high-income countries: material, psychosocial, and behavioural risk factors. Healthcare may also play a role. Fig. 2.3.3 provides a schematic representation of these mechanisms.

Material factors

There is no doubt that financial resources are very unevenly distributed between people with lower and higher socioeconomic positions, even in high-income countries with strong egalitarian traditions. For example, according to Eurostat, the statistics office of the EU, the 20 per cent of the population with the highest income in the EU-25 received 4.9 times more than the 20 per cent of the population with the lowest income in 2005. The proportion of the population who is at risk of poverty (defined as having an income less than 60 per cent of the national median income) was 16 per cent in the EU as a whole.

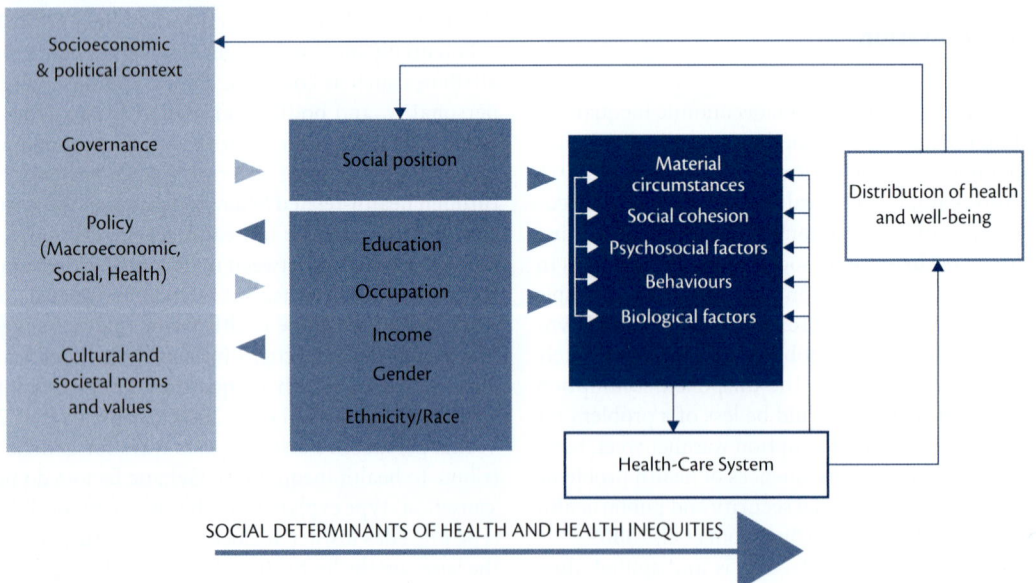

Fig. 2.3.3 A possible model for the explanation of health inequalities.

Income inequality and poverty rates differ substantially between countries, partly as a result of differences in income taxation and social security schemes. For example, within the EU-25 the ratio of income going to the upper as compared to the lower 20 per cent of the population varied from 3.3 to 8.2 in 2005, and the proportion of the population having an income less than 60 per cent of the national average varied between 9 per cent and more than 20 per cent. Nevertheless, it is quite likely that inequalities in financial disadvantage play an important role in the explanation of health inequalities in all high-income countries.

Financial disadvantage may affect health through various mechanisms: psychosocial stress and subsequent risk-taking behaviours (smoking, excessive alcohol consumption, etc.), reduced access to health-promoting facilities and products (fruits and vegetables, sports, preventive healthcare services, etc.), and so on. Research on the role of the specific contribution of financial disadvantage to inequalities in health is scarce, but as the lowest possible costs for healthy living (as defined by health-based needs for nutrition, physical activity, housing, medical care, social needs, hygiene, and transport) tend to exceed minimum benefit levels (Morris et al. 2007), this role is likely to be substantial.

Variations between countries in income inequality have also been linked to variations in average health: countries and other territorial units with larger income inequalities tend to have lower life expectancy (Wilkinson 1992) and higher rates of mortality and self-reported ill health, even in studies controlling for individual income levels (Kondo et al. 2009). This has been interpreted as indicating a 'contextual effect' of income inequality, which may increase health risks for everyone, perhaps through social comparisons and the resulting psychosocial stress (Wilkinson and Pickett 2009), or through erosion of social capital (Kawachi et al. 1997). It is unclear, however, whether larger income inequalities also go together with larger health inequalities within populations, and the relevance of these findings for explaining health inequalities therefore remains unclear.

Other 'material' risk factors that tend to be more prevalent in lower socioeconomic groups include occupational health risks (exposure to chemicals, accident risks, physically strenuous work, etc.) (Costa and D'Errico 2006), health risks related to housing (crowding, dampness, accident risks, etc.) (Dunn and Hayes 1999), and environmental health risks (air pollution, traffic noise, etc.) (Kruize et al. 2007). Some of these have been shown to make important contributions to the explanation of health inequalities (Marmot and Wilkinson 2006; Siegrist and Marmot 2006).

Psychosocial factors

The second group of specific determinants which contribute to the explanation of health inequalities are psychosocial factors. Those who are in a low socioeconomic position on average are exposed to more psychosocial stressors, in the form of negative life events (loss of beloved ones, financial difficulties, etc.), daily hassles, 'effort–reward imbalance' (high levels of effort without appropriate material and immaterial rewards), and a combination of high demands and low control both in the workplace and beyond (Siegrist and Marmot 2004).

At the same time, they also tend to have smaller social networks, and to have lower levels of social support (Stansfeld 2006), as well as less effective coping styles (Kristenson 2006) and a weaker sense of control over their life and living conditions (Bosma et al. 1999).

This combination of a higher exposure to psychosocial stressors and less capacity to remove or buffer these exposures may explain part of the higher frequency of health problems in the lower socioeconomic groups. This has been best documented for psychosocial factors related to work organization, such as job strain, which have been shown to play a role in the explanation of socioeconomic inequalities in cardiovascular health (Marmot et al. 2006).

Two possible pathways may be involved. The first is a behavioural pathway: psychosocial stress and other unfavourable psychosocial factors increase the likelihood of unhealthy behaviours in lower socioeconomic groups, such as smoking (Droomers et al. 2002), excessive alcohol consumption (Droomers et al. 1999, 2004), and lack of physical exercise (Droomers et al. 1998, 2001). The second is a biological pathway. The experience of stress affects the neural, endocrine, and immune systems of the body, and chronic stress may lead to maladaptive responses in the form of, for example, high blood pressure, a prolonged high level of cortisol, higher blood viscosity, or a suppression of the immune response, which may in their turn increase the susceptibility to a range of diseases (Brunner 1997; Brunner and Marmot 2006; Steptoe, 2006).

Health-related behaviours

The third group of contributory factors are health-related behaviours, such as smoking, inadequate diet, excessive alcohol consumption, and lack of physical exercise. In many developed countries one or more of these 'lifestyle' factors are more prevalent in the lower socioeconomic groups. As we have already seen, many of the disease-specific patterns of health inequalities also suggest a substantial contribution of health-related behaviours to inequalities in mortality.

By far the most widely available data on a specific determinant of health inequalities relate to smoking. In many European countries, particularly in the North of Western Europe, cigarette smoking is the number one determinant of health problems. This is not only because of its role in lung cancer and some other specific diseases, for which it is the main cause. It is also because of its role in (premature) mortality in general, in less than 'good' self-assessed health and in disability, for which smoking is an important contributory factor. The prevalence of smoking differs strongly between socioeconomic groups in many European countries, so one can safely assume that it plays an important role in generating health inequalities (Fig. 2.3.4) (Cavelaars et al. 2000; Huisman et al. 2005b).

In general, the prevalence of smoking is higher in the lower socioeconomic groups, but there are important differences between countries in the magnitude, and sometimes even the direction, of these inequalities. A number of comparative studies within Europe have demonstrated a North–South gradient, with larger inequalities in current smoking in the North of Europe and smaller (sometimes even 'reverse') gradients in the South (Fig. 2.3.4) (Cavelaars et al. 2000; Huisman et al. 2005b). This is particularly clear in the case of women: higher educated women smoke less in the North of Europe (represented by the Nordic countries, Great Britain, the Netherlands, Belgium, etc.), but they smoke more than lower educated women in the South of Europe (represented by Italy, Spain, Greece, Portugal, etc.).

Current rates of smoking are the result of trends which have played out over the past decades: the habit of cigarette smoking started early in the twentieth century with the advent of industrially produced cigarettes, and in many European countries it was

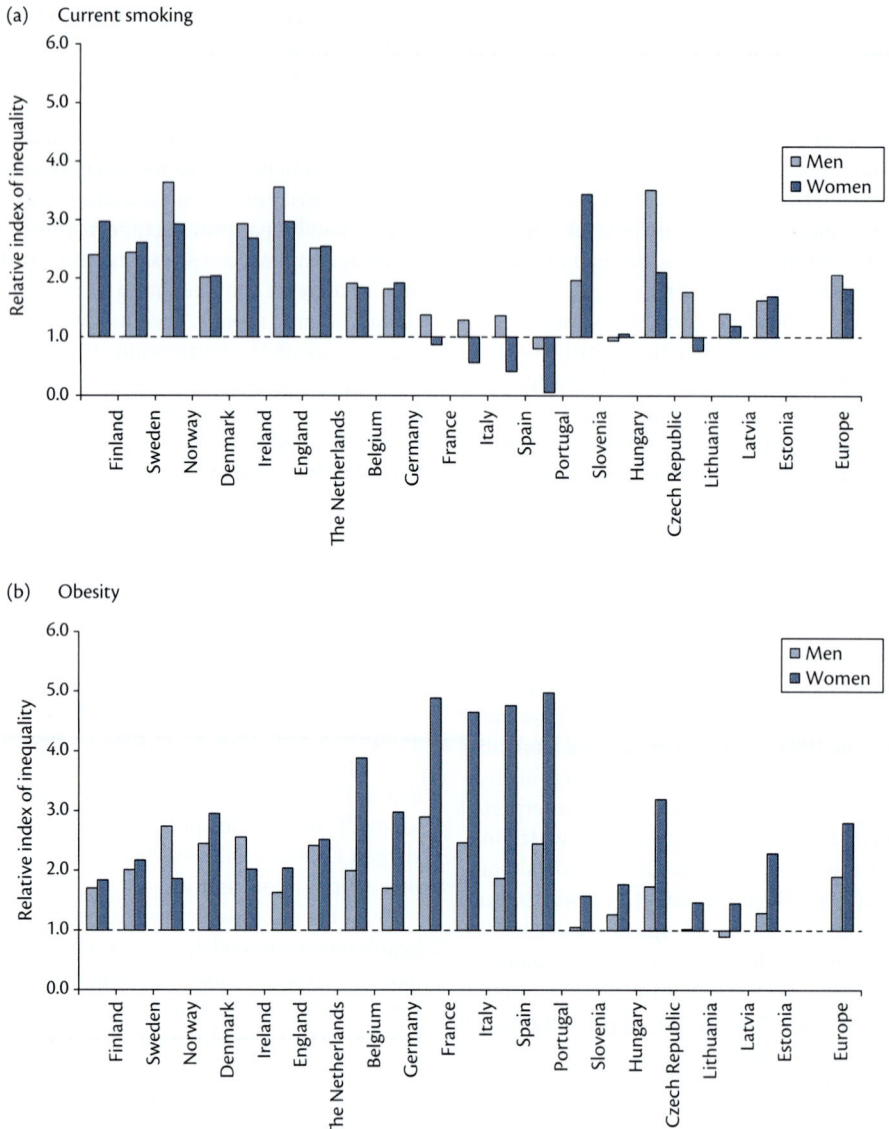

Fig. 2.3.4 Inequalities in smoking and overweight in 19 European countries. Note: the graph shows the relative index of inequality, indicating the rate ratio of current smoking or being obese between those with the lowest and the highest socioeconomic position. This is a regression-based measure that takes into account all socioeconomic groups and calibrates the social position of each group to its proportion in the total population.

From the *New England Journal of Medicine*, Mackenbach, J.P. et al., Socioeconomic inequalities in health in 22 European countries, Volume 358, Issue 23, pp. 2468–81, Copyright ©2008 Massachusetts Medical Society. Reprinted with permission from Massachusetts Medical Society.

only after the Second World War that smoking became highly prevalent, first among men (with rates of up to 90 per cent smokers), then among women. In many countries, smoking prevalence has declined over the past decades, at least among men, as a result of health education efforts and other anti-tobacco measures such as raising excise taxes and bans on smoking in public places. This decline in smoking is still continuing, but there have been, and still are, clear socioeconomic differences in this decline (Giskes et al. 2005; Schaap et al. 2008).

While smoking is clearly bad for health, alcohol is a more complex risk factor: both abstinence and excessive alcohol consumption are bad for health (as compared to moderate drinking). Abstinence usually is more common in the lower socioeconomic groups, both among men and among women; however, the pattern

for excessive alcohol consumption is more variable. Many studies report a higher prevalence in lower socioeconomic groups, particularly among men, but the results for women are far from consistent (Droomers et al. 1999, 2004). These inconsistencies may well be due to real differences between countries in the social patterning of excessive alcohol consumption.

In some countries, such as the Nordic countries (e.g. Finland) and several Eastern European countries, 'binge drinking' (drinking more than, say, 8 units on a single occasion) is a more serious source of health problems than regular overconsumption of alcohol. In these countries, binge drinking tends to be more common in lower socioeconomic groups, and is likely to contribute to the explanation of health inequalities, e.g. through a higher rate of IHD, stroke, and injury mortality (Makela et al. 1997).

Comparable data on dietary behaviour by socioeconomic status are even more difficult to obtain. The measurement of diet is notoriously difficult, and collecting nationally representative data on diet by socioeconomic position from a range of countries is a costly exercise. Only a few comparative studies have been conducted, and these show that men and women in lower socioeconomic groups tend to less frequently eat fresh vegetables, particularly in the North of Europe. Differences in fresh vegetable consumption are smallest in the South of Europe, perhaps because of the larger availability and affordability of fruits and vegetables in Mediterranean countries. A similar North–South gradient has been found for the consumption of fruits (Cavelaars et al. 1997). Literature reviews have shown that it is likely that many other aspects of diet, such as consumption of meat, dairy products, and various fats and oils, also are socially patterned in many European countries, and that these social patterns differ between countries (Lopez-Azpiazu et al. 2003; Prattala et al. 2003).

Lack of leisure-time physical activity tends to be more common in the lower socioeconomic groups, and so do overweight and obesity. Interestingly, this is one of the very few health aspects where patterns of social variation are clearer for women than for men. Among women, overweight and obesity are more prevalent in lower socioeconomic groups in all countries with available data, with clearly large inequalities in overweight and obesity in Southern Europe (Fig. 2.3.4) (Sobal and Stunkard 1989; Roskam et al. 2010).

The systematic nature of these differences in health-related behaviour clearly demonstrates that these are not a matter of free choice, but must be determined by conditions which are at least partly beyond the control of the individual. Some psychosocial factors that could play a role in generating these behaviour patterns were mentioned earlier. Another possibility is neighbourhood conditions: people with a lower socioeconomic position tend to live in less well-to-do neighbourhoods which may have limited opportunities for physical exercise and purchase of healthy foods (Giskes et al. 2007, 2009; Kamphuis et al. 2007, 2009).

Healthcare

Unequal access to effective healthcare could theoretically also play a role in the explanation of health inequalities. Most high-income countries, however, have healthcare financing systems that have reduced inequalities in access to rather low levels. This is clear from studies of healthcare utilization, which typically show that lower socioeconomic groups tend to use more care than higher socioeconomic groups in accordance with their higher levels of need, and that relatively low use of specialist care in lower socioeconomic groups goes together with relatively high use of primary care (van Doorslaer et al. 2006; Lemstra et al. 2009).

Studies of variations in healthcare outcomes do suggest that there may be inequalities in quality of care that are not captured by studies of global indicators of healthcare utilization. As was mentioned earlier, survival after a cardiovascular event or after a diagnosis of cancer is often shorter for patients in lower socioeconomic groups. Some studies have found higher rates of utilization of surgical and non-surgical interventions among hospitalized patients with a higher socioeconomic position (Hetemaa et al. 2004; Stirbu et al. 2012). Like inequalities in survival after myocardial infarction, inequalities in survival of cancer patients are likely to be partly determined by inequalities in co-morbidity or

other risk factors for mortality independent of care received, but there is some emerging evidence that inequalities in treatment may also play a role, for example, in the case of breast cancer (Aarts et al. 2012).

At the population level, mortality from causes of death that have become amenable to medical intervention also is higher in lower socioeconomic groups. One recent study of educational variations in mortality from amenable conditions in 16 European populations showed that inequalities in mortality from these conditions are often substantial, and contribute between 11 and 24 per cent to inequalities in partial life expectancy between the ages of 30 and 64 (Stirbu et al. 2010). To what extent these inequalities really reflect inequalities in healthcare access or quality is, however, uncertain. Countries with larger inequalities in healthcare utilization have not been found to also have larger inequalities in amenable mortality (Plug et al. 2012).

Overarching ideas

What has emerged from recent research efforts is a rather complex picture of how individuals in the lower socioeconomic strata are exposed over their lifetime to a wide variety of unfavourable and interacting material, cultural, and psychological conditions, and how these exposures lead to ill health—either directly, or indirectly through unhealthy behaviours or psychosocial stress. Various attempts have been made to combine these factors and pathways into overarching theories. We discuss some of these attempts in the following sections.

Life-course perspective

A life-course perspective, which sees the higher rates of illness and premature death among adults and older persons in lower socioeconomic groups as the result of socially patterned exposures acting at different stages of the life course, has proven to be a very useful way of integrating different pieces of evidence. The simplest conceptual model for life course influences is that of 'accumulation of risk'. Different forms of material and immaterial disadvantage tend to cluster in the same persons, with one disadvantage increasing the likelihood of another one at a later point in time, and studies have found dose–response relationships between measures of cumulative disadvantage and health outcomes (Power and Matthews 1997; Smith et al. 1997).

Such accumulation models can be refined to take into account chains of events reinforcing each other. Interestingly, this also resolves the 'selection' versus 'causation' debate, because a low socioeconomic position in one stage of the life course may translate into a health disadvantage in the next, which may then lead to a still lower socioeconomic position some years later, and so on. Health-induced downward social mobility then becomes just another form of accumulation of disadvantage (Mheen et al. 1998).

Another type of life-course model focuses on 'critical periods', time windows of exposure that are particularly important for health at later ages. One example of such a 'critical period' model is the 'fetal origins of adult disease' hypothesis. This hypothesis arose when it was seen that low birth weight is not only associated with infant health, but surprisingly also with adult health, e.g. coronary heart disease, stroke, hypertension, and diabetes, probably due to 'fetal programming' of growth patterns and related metabolic and endocrine processes (Barker and Robinson 1992). This hypothesis would imply that inequalities in adult cardiovascular disease may partly be attributable to differences in prevalence of low birth weight and other aspects of early growth, but so far the evidence on this life-course pathway is inconclusive (Power and Kuh 2006).

However, early life influences on inequalities in adult health are not limited to fetal programming of growth patterns. The child's physical, cognitive, and emotional development is strongly influenced by socioeconomic circumstances, and in its turn influences adult health in many ways. Childhood socioeconomic position has an independent effect on adult obesity and smoking, probably because it has a lasting influence on attitudes (Power et al. 2005). Cognitive ability is also shaped by childhood socioeconomic circumstances, and has been shown to mediate the association between childhood socioeconomic position and adult mortality (Hart et al. 2003). Circumstances in early life also set up a pattern of social learning, which may generate a sense of powerlessness reinforced by others in the social network who have been similarly disadvantaged and socially excluded, sometimes over generations (Keating and Hertzman 1999).

Fundamental causes

The theory of 'fundamental causes' stipulates that it is the social forces underlying social stratification which ultimately cause health inequalities, and not exposure to the proximal risk factors which are usually studied by social epidemiologists (like smoking, psychosocial stress, working conditions, etc.). According to this theory, the persistence of health inequalities in different time-periods and different national conditions is due to the fact that a person's socioeconomic status provides him or her with 'flexible resources'. These include 'knowledge, money, power, prestige, and beneficial social connections' which can be used 'to avoid disease risks or to minimize the consequences of disease once it occurs' regardless of the prevailing circumstances. The association between socioeconomic status and health 'is reproduced over time via the replacement of intervening mechanisms', and as opportunities for avoiding disease continue to expand so will health inequalities continue to exist (Link and Phelan 1995; Phelan et al. 2010).

This theory provides an elegant summary of all the more specific explanations, which fail to explain why health inequalities are seen in all countries with available data, and persist over time, regardless of variations in the proximal determinants of health. Although it does not help us to identify the mechanisms underlying health inequalities, it is a useful reminder that in the end the existence of health inequalities depends on the existence of socioeconomic inequalities.

Health inequalities and the welfare state

The persistence of socioeconomic inequalities in health is one of the great disappointments of public health. All countries, including those ranking high on indices of economic prosperity and human development, have systematic inequalities in mortality and morbidity between citizens with a higher and a lower socioeconomic position, as indicated by education, occupation, income, or wealth. This also applies to the highly developed 'welfare states' of Western Europe. All Western European countries have created extensive arrangements aiming to reduce socioeconomic inequality and its various consequences. With notable variations all these 'welfare regimes' include measures to redistribute income (e.g. by progressive taxation and social security)

and a range of collectively financed provisions (e.g. public housing, education, healthcare, access to culture and leisure facilities) (Esping-Andersen 1990).

There is good evidence that welfare policies have contributed to a reduction of inequalities in income, housing quality, healthcare access, and other social and economic outcomes (Esping-Andersen 1990; Kautto et al. 2001), but they have apparently been insufficient to eliminate health inequalities. The explanation of this paradox has puzzled many observers (Huijts and Eikemo 2009; Bambra 2011), and several hypotheses have emerged. Three circumstances may help to explain the persistence of health inequalities despite attenuation of inequalities in material conditions by the welfare state: (1) inequalities in access to material and immaterial resources have not been eliminated by the welfare state, and are still substantial; (2) due to greater intergenerational mobility, the composition of lower socioeconomic groups has become more homogeneous with regard to personal characteristics associated with ill health; and (3) due to a change in epidemiological regime, in which consumption behaviour became the most important determinant of ill health, the marginal benefits of the immaterial resources to which a higher social position gives access have increased (Mackenbach 2012).

The options: how to build a strategy to reduce inequalities in health?

With all these advances in our understanding of health inequalities, we are now in a much better position than, say, in 1980 when the Black Report appeared (Department of Health and Social Services 1980), to develop rational strategies to tackle them. Several European countries have taken steps to develop such strategies, by commissioning evaluation studies of policies and interventions, and by drawing on expert advice to create comprehensive programmes to reduce health inequalities. Bringing together evidence from around the world, the World Health Organization has even called upon all countries to 'close the gap in a generation' (Commission on Social Determinants of Health 2008).

Normative assessment of health inequalities

Reducing inequalities in health, by levelling up the health status of those in lower socioeconomic positions, has thus become an important policy goal in many high-income countries. One reason is technical: potential health gains are larger in lower socioeconomic groups, and raising their health status may therefore be a very effective way to improve average population health. Another reason is normative: health inequalities are widely perceived to be 'unjust'. One particularly striking illustration of this perception can be found in the report of the WHO Commission on Social Determinants of Health, which stated that '[p]utting right these inequities is a matter of social justice. Reducing health inequities is an ethical imperative. Social injustice is killing people on a grand scale' (Commission on Social Determinants of Health 2008).

It is important, however, to first outline the reasoning behind this move from 'inequalities' (a term with ethically neutral connotations, like 'disparities' or 'variations') to 'inequities' (a term which implies that these variations are 'unjust'). This was first done by Whitehead in a simple but effective scheme consisting of two criteria: 'avoidability' (are health inequalities caused by changeable social conditions, and therefore unnecessary?) and 'unfairness' (do health inequalities result from conditions out of people's direct control, not from free choice?) (Whitehead 1992).

According to these criteria, health inequalities caused by exposure to health hazards in the environment, or by restricted access to healthcare, would be considered unjust, as would health inequalities caused by health-damaging behaviour restricted by socioeconomic factors. On the other hand, health inequalities caused by natural biological variation (e.g. genetic factors) or freely chosen health-damaging behaviour would not (Whitehead 1992). Application of this scheme thus requires empirical evidence on the determinants of health inequalities, and on the role of free choice versus 'conditions out of people's direct control'—evidence that is actually hard to obtain, although it is hard to imagine that systematic differences in behaviour between socioeconomic groups are based on truly free choice.

Attempts to further formalize the normative assessment of health inequalities have tried to use Rawls's influential 'theory of justice' (Daniels et al. 1999) or Sen's capability theory (Venkatapuram 2011). The latter theory has become especially popular among social epidemiologists because, in contrast to other theories of justice, it gives a central place to health. It argues that all human beings are entitled to a certain set of 'capabilities', such as the ability to live a life of normal length, to have good health, to have emotional attachments to others, and to participate effectively in political decisions. From this perspective, tackling health inequalities should be a central objective of all governments pursuing justice (Venkatapuram 2011).

Policy development vis-à-vis health inequalities

In reality, different countries are in widely different phases of awareness of, and willingness to take action on, socioeconomic inequalities in health. Common milestones in policy development are: high-profile independent reports recommending research or policy on health inequalities; national research programmes on health inequalities; government advisory committees recommending policies to reduce health inequalities; and coordinated government action to reduce health inequalities (Mackenbach and Bakker 2003).

Whitehead has proposed a schematic 'action spectrum' to characterize the stage of diffusion of ideas on socioeconomic inequalities in health (Fig. 2.3.5). Starting with a primordial stage in which socioeconomic inequalities in health are not even measured, the spectrum covers the stages of 'measurement', 'recognition', 'awareness', 'denial/indifference', 'concern', 'will to take action', 'isolated initiatives', 'more structured developments', and 'comprehensive coordinated policy' (Whitehead 1998).

Even among high-income countries there are several that find themselves still in a pre-measurement stage. In a country like Greece, for example, data on socioeconomic inequalities in health are almost completely lacking, and awareness of the issue is limited to a small number of academics who do not have structural research funding for studies in this area. Other countries, such as Spain, after a period with heightened awareness due to the publication of high-profile reports, find themselves in a 'denial/indifference' stage. Still others, such as France and Italy, are in a 'concern' stage: important reports on socioeconomic inequalities in health have been published, and policymakers are increasingly paying attention to the issue, but real

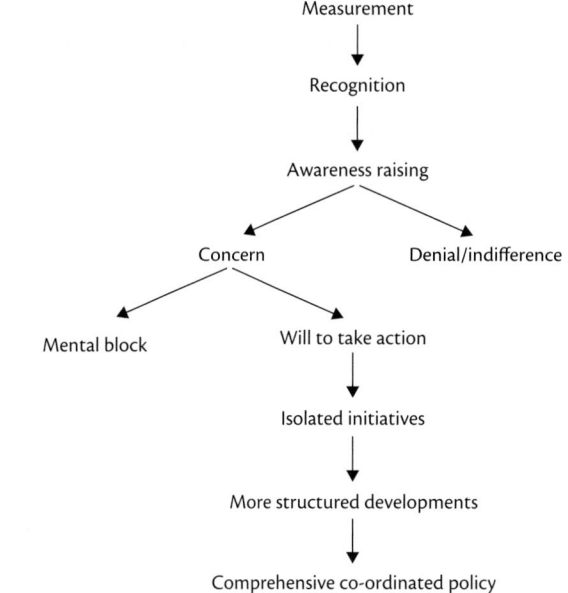

Fig. 2.3.5 Whitehead's action spectrum.
Reproduced from Whitehead, M., Diffusion of ideas on social inequalities in health: a European perspective, *Milbank Quarterly*, Volume 76, Issue 3, pp. 469–92, Copyright © 1998 Milbank Memorial Fund, with permission from John Wiley & Sons, Inc.

action has not yet been taken. Only a few countries have entered a 'more structured developments' stage, with national research programmes as well as high-level advisory committees that have issued comprehensive policy advice on how to reduce socioeconomic inequalities in health, and still fewer have started 'comprehensive coordinated policy' (Whitehead 1998; Mackenbach and Bakker 2003).

A rational approach to tackling health inequalities should be based on logical reasoning: dependent on the causes of the problem, and on what is known about possible ways to address these causes, interventions and policies should be developed and tested for effectiveness, and then implemented systematically on the scale required to have population-wide impacts (Whitehead 2007). A possible typology of actions to tackle health inequalities is: (1) strengthening individuals (e.g. improving individuals' abilities to make healthy lifestyle choices), (2) strengthening communities (e.g. community development initiatives to create healthier conditions in neighbourhoods), (3) improving living and working conditions (e.g. improve access to adequate housing and eliminate work-related health risks), and (4) promoting healthy macro-policies (e.g. reduce income inequalities) (Whitehead 2007).

Within high-income countries, there is considerable diversity in the way scientific evidence is being used to underpin policies to reduce health inequalities. Often, most of the evidence used relates to the contribution of specific factors to the explanation of health inequalities, not to the effectiveness of policies and interventions tackling them (Macintyre et al. 2001). It is only rarely that strategies are developed primarily on the basis of evaluation studies of various intervention options (Mackenbach and Stronks 2004). As we will see in the next section the evidence base is still very limited, and opinion differs on what type of evidence is needed to underpin policies and interventions in this field.

There are those who argue that in view of the urgency of starting to tackle health inequalities ('doing nothing is not an option') (Petticrew et al. 2004), one should be prepared to start intervening on the basis of plausibility. Political 'windows of opportunity' are usually short, for example, 4 years at most, and they may be closed before careful evaluation studies have been conducted (Whitehead et al. 2004). A parallel has been drawn with nineteenth-century public health interventions for which controlled intervention studies have never been done, but which were implemented on the basis of plausibility and have proven to be highly successful (Davey Smith et al. 2001). Under the pressure of politicians wanting to see rapid results, the best that can be achieved in terms of scientific evaluation may then be large-scale implementation accompanied by a 'real-time' evaluation study of the intervention, concurrent with its implementation, using some quasi-experimental design (before–after study, interrupted time-series study, and so on) (Macintyre 2003).

On the other hand, there are those who argue that this is a strategy with serious risks. Like in other areas of social and health policy, the actual results of policies and interventions to reduce health inequalities could easily be counterintuitive. There are many historical examples of 'plausible' interventions and policies that did not work, or actually had adverse effects (Macintyre et al. 2001). In addition to that, one could argue that any investment in reducing health inequalities should be justified on the basis of a comparison of its cost-effectiveness with that of other possible investments in health and well-being, and that producing credible evidence is therefore essential (Oliver 2010).

Another issue for debate is what types of evidence are best suited to underpin policy decisions in this area. Clearly, randomized controlled trials will not always be feasible, particularly for the evaluation of policies and interventions that are applied on a population-wide scale. Sometimes, community intervention trials, in which groups of people (school classes, neighbourhoods, etc.) instead of individuals are allocated to the intervention and control condition, will then be a good alternative. But in many circumstances one will have to rely on quasi-experimental or even observational designs to inform policymakers on the effectiveness of new approaches. Controlled before–after studies or interrupted time-series designs could then be used, or observational studies of 'natural experiments', for example, by making comparisons between countries (Thomson et al. 2004). Useful guidance has been developed to support further research in this area (Craig et al. 2008, 2011). Also, a Cochrane and Campbell Equity Methods group has been set up to ensure that research about differential effectiveness of health interventions is available worldwide (http://equity.cochrane.org/).

A complicating factor in evaluating the effectiveness of policies and interventions to reduce health inequalities is that this effectiveness should be measured in terms of favourably changing the distribution of health problems in the population, not of reducing the rate of health problems in a particular group. A 'full' study design therefore requires the measurement, in one or more experimental populations and one or more control populations, of changes over time in the magnitude of health inequalities. Any other design, such as an experimental study of changes over time in the rate of health problems in lower socioeconomic groups only, requires rather strong assumptions to be made, in this case on the absence of health effects in higher socioeconomic groups (Mackenbach and Gunning-Schepers 1997).

Innovative approaches

A number of innovative approaches to reduce health inequalities have been developed, for which there is at least some empirical evidence suggesting that they can help to reduce health inequalities (Mackenbach and Bakker 2002). A few examples are discussed here.

Health inequalities are partly due to labour market and working conditions. Swedish labour market policies enforce strong employment protection and active promotion of labour market participation for citizens with chronic illness. A comparison with England suggests that these policies have been effective in protecting vulnerable groups from labour market exclusion during the recession of the 1990s (Burstrom et al. 2000). In France, occupational health services are mandatory and include an annual health check for every employee. This provides a good setting for introducing preventive activities for those who otherwise have few medical contacts, particularly those in manual occupations. Randomized controlled trials within this setting have shown that interventions aimed at detection and treatment of hypertension and smoking cessation were successful (Lang et al. 1995, 2000). Improvements of working conditions have made important contributions to reducing health inequalities in the past, but a lot remains to be done. In the Netherlands a recent intervention study suggests that task rotation among garbage collectors reduces sickness absenteeism. Rotation of tasks (truck driving and minicontainer loading) reduces physical load and possibly also increases job control (Kuijer et al. 1999).

Health-related behaviours like food consumption, smoking, and physical exercise also contribute to socioeconomic inequalities in health. Finnish nutrition policies have followed the Nordic welfare ideology where universalism has been the general principle. School children, students, and employees in Finland receive free or subsidized meals at school or workplace, and special dietary guidelines have been implemented ensuring the use of low-fat food products. This has probably contributed to the favourable trend of narrowing socioeconomic inequalities in use of butter and high-fat milk in Finland (Prattala et al. 1992). In many countries, smoking is increasingly concentrated in lower socioeconomic groups, and reviews show that a variety of policies and interventions is effective in reducing smoking in these groups. Whereas the price weapon (raising excise taxes) is very effective, its regressive impact on the poorest smokers who cannot stop should be counteracted by active promotion of the use of nicotine replacement therapy and other cessation support. A national programme which created smoking cessation services in disadvantaged areas in England has effectively reached disadvantaged smokers and reduced the gap in smoking somewhat (Bauld et al. 2007).

Despite these and many other advances, however, the evidence base for tackling inequalities in health remains thin. An 'umbrella review' of social interventions covering housing, work, transport, unemployment, food, and education showed that differential impact on socioeconomic groups was only occasionally studied. Only in the case of work interventions did the authors see some evidence for an effect on reducing inequalities (Bambra et al. 2010). A similar 'umbrella review' of smoking interventions covering price increases, access restrictions, and smoking bans only found evidence for an inequalities-reducing effect of price increases (Main et al. 2008). Evidence-based policymaking to reduce health inequalities therefore remains a great challenge.

Comprehensive strategies

As it is unlikely that any single policy or intervention will significantly reduce socioeconomic inequalities in health, 'packages' of policies and interventions of a more comprehensive nature have been devised by government advisory committees in Britain, Sweden, the Netherlands, Norway, and Finland.

Britain

The Black Report, commissioned by a Labour government to investigate the causes and possible remedies for Britain's undiminished social class inequalities in mortality, had proposed a radical change in social and healthcare policies but had disappeared in a desk drawer after the Conservatives won the 1979 elections (Department of Health and Social Services 1980). However, research continued and when Labour came back into power almost 20 years later, it again commissioned an expert report to bring together all the evidence—the Independent Inquiry into Inequalities in Health (Department of Health 1998)—and developed a comprehensive programme to tackle health inequalities.

This programme consisted of a range of new government policies including the introduction of a national minimum wage, higher benefits and pensions, and substantially increased spending on education, housing, urban regeneration, and healthcare. It also announced a number of specific initiatives including the 'Sure Start' programme (free child care, early education, and parent support for low-income families), 'Health Action Zones' (local strategies to improve health in deprived areas), and a series

of anti-tobacco policies (including free nicotine replacement therapy for low-income smokers) (Department of Health 1999). In a further evolution of the programme two quantitative targets (to narrow the socioeconomic gap in life expectancy and that in infant mortality by 10 per cent in 2010) were added, and priority was given to key interventions expected to contribute to closing the life expectancy gap, such as reducing smoking in manual social groups, managing risks for coronary heart disease and cancer (poor diet and obesity, physical inactivity, hypertension), and reducing accidents at home and on the road (Department of Health 2003). The total budget exceeded £20 billion (Table 2.3.2).

The strategy came to an end with the 2010 parliamentary elections and the formation of a Conservative/Liberal Democrat coalition government. An extensive review of the achievements of the programme showed that it had been a mixed success: despite positive effects in some areas (e.g. reduction of child poverty, improvements in housing, better uptake of influenza vaccination) most indicators showed a widening instead of a narrowing of health inequalities, and the programme missed its targets (Department of Health 2010). Further analyses showed that the failure to achieve the targets was due to the fact that the strategy had not sufficiently focused on the most relevant entry-points, that effective policies were unavailable at that point in time, and that the scale of implementation had not been sufficient for achieving population-wide impacts (Mackenbach 2011).

Other European countries

Despite its partial failure, the British programme has set an extremely valuable example that deserves to be followed elsewhere. Its combination of an evidence-based approach (choosing entry-points on the basis of scientific evidence, and regular monitoring to keep track of progress) with a strong implementation

Table 2.3.2 The English programme to tackle health inequalities: commitments and their achievement

'Departmental commitments'	Examples	Budget (2004–2007)[a]	Direct relevance for life-expectancy target	Direct relevance for infant-mortality target	Commitments mostly met (2007)[b]
Maternal and child health	Sure Start, chikcare, Welfare Food Scheme	>£2 billion	No	Yes	Yes
Improving life chances for children	Mental health, sports facilities, education	>£2 billion	No	No	Yes
Reducing teenage pregnancy	Sex education, care access	Not specified	No	Yes	Yes
Engaging communities	Neighbourhood Renewal, homelessness reduction	>£1.5 billion	No	No	Yes
Prevention	Smoking cessation, 5 A Day, injury prevention	Not specified	Yes	No	Yes
Primary care	Facilities, breast cancer screening, flu immunization	>£1 billion	Yes	No	Yes
Effective treatment	Access to cancer services, access to coronary-heart-disease services	>£0.5 billion	No	No	Yes
Underlying determinants	Child poverty, fuel poverty, Pathways to Work	>£15.5 billion	No	No	Yes

Source: *Tackling Health Inequalities: A Program for Action.*

[a] A '>' sign indicates that amounts exclude commitments for which no budget was specified.

[b] Source: *Tackling Health Inequalities: 2007 States Report of the Program for Action.*

plan (clear commitments shared between government sectors, and supported by serious budget allocations) has so far not been matched elsewhere.

In the Netherlands a national 'Program Committee on Socioeconomic Inequalities in Health' issued a set of 26 specific recommendations in 2001. The recommendations were partly based on a series of intervention studies in which 12 different interventions addressing specific inequalities in health were evaluated. Examples of recommendations include 'no further increase in income inequality', 'no cuts in disability benefits', 'increase labour participation of the chronically ill', 'reduce physically demanding work', 'increase tobacco taxation', 'implement school health policies' and 'strengthen primary care in deprived areas' (Mackenbach and Stronks 2002). Due to changes and instability in the composition of national governments in the Netherlands, the recommendations have so far not been followed. At the local and regional level, however, many new initiatives have been taken to tackle health inequalities (Mackenbach and Stronks 2004).

Several of the Nordic countries have also developed comprehensive strategies to reduce health inequalities. In Sweden the National Public Health Commission, a committee consisting of representatives of all political parties, scientific experts, and advisers from governmental and non-governmental organizations, has developed a new national health policy with a strong focus on reducing health inequalities. It further involved extensive consultation of numerous organizations, and the proposal itself includes action by a wide range of actors in society. The commission formulated 18 health policy objectives grouped in six large areas: strengthening social capital, growing up in a satisfactory environment, improving conditions at work, creating a satisfactory physical environment, stimulating health-promoting life habits, and developing a satisfactory infrastructure for health (Swedish National Institute of Public Health 2005). So far, the results of national programmes to tackle health inequalities in Sweden and the other Nordic countries have not been systematically assessed.

Conclusion

Whether it will actually be possible to substantially reduce socioeconomic inequalities in health remains an open question. The good news, however, is that there has been enormous progress in explanatory research, and that this has identified a large number of targets for policies and interventions to tackle health inequalities. There has also been a beginning of research and development for effective interventions and policies to tackle health inequalities. While this is still a modest beginning, it does put us in a better position to reduce socioeconomic inequalities in health in the coming decades. A number of innovative approaches have been developed for which there is at least some evidence of effectiveness. Comprehensive packages have been developed in several countries that have a sound theoretical basis and clear inspirational value.

Developing effective strategies to reduce health inequalities is a daunting task. No single country has the capacity to contribute more than a fraction of the necessary knowledge. This is a matter not only of restricted manpower or financial resources for research, but also of restricted opportunities for implementing and evaluating policies and interventions. Some policies can be implemented and evaluated in some countries and not in others, either because they have already been implemented or because

they are politically infeasible. International exchange is therefore necessary to increase learning speed.

References

Aarts, M.J., Hamelinck, V.C., Bastiaannet, E., et al. (2012). Small but significant socioeconomic inequalities in axillary staging and treatment of breast cancer in the Netherlands. *British Journal of Cancer*, 107, 12–17.

Aarts, M.J., Van Der Aa, M.A., Coebergh, J.W., and Louwman, W.J. (2010). Reduction of socioeconomic inequality in cancer incidence in the South of the Netherlands during 1996–2008. *European Journal of Cancer*, 46, 2633–46.

Ackerknecht, E.H. (1953). *Rudolf Virchow. Doctor, Statesman, Anthropologist*. Madison. WI: University of Wisconsin Press.

Apouey, B. and Clark, A.E. (2010). *Winning Big but Feeling No Better? The Effect of Lottery Prizes on Physical and Mental Health*. IZA Discussion Papers. Bonn: Institute for the Study of Labor (IZA).

Atkinson, R.L., Atkinson, R.C., Smith, E.E., and Bemm, D.J. (1993). *Introduction to Psychology*. Fort Worth: Harcourt Brace Jovanovich College Publishers.

Avendano, M., Aro, A.R., and Mackenbach, J.P. (2005). Socio-economic disparities in physical health in 10 European countries. In A. Boersch-Supan, A. Brugiavini, H. Juerges, J.P. Mackenbach, J. Siegrist, and G. Weber (eds.) *Health, Ageing and Retirement in Europe. First Results of the Survey of Health, Ageing and Retirement in Europe*, pp. 102–7. Morlenbach: Strauss.

Avendano, M., Kunst, A.E., Huisman, M., et al. (2004). Educational level and stroke mortality: a comparison of 10 European populations during the 1990s. *Stroke*, 35, 432–7.

Avendano, M., Kunst, A.E., Huisman, M., et al. (2006). Socioeconomic status and ischaemic heart disease mortality in 10 western European populations during the 1990s. *Heart*, 92, 461–7.

Bambra, C. (2011). Health inequalities and welfare state regimes: theoretical insights on a public health 'puzzle'. *Journal of Epidemiology and Community Health*, 65, 740–5.

Bambra, C., Gibson, M., Sowden, A., Wright, K., Whitehead, M., and Petticrew, M. (2010). Tackling the wider social determinants of health and health inequalities: evidence from systematic reviews. *Journal of Epidemiology and Community Health*, 64, 284–91.

Barker, D.J.P. and Robinson, R.J. (eds.) (1992). *Fetal and Infant Origins of Adult Disease*. London: British Medical Journal.

Bartley, M. and Plewis, I. (1997). Does health-selective mobility account for socioeconomic differences in health? Evidence from England and Wales, 1971 to 1991. *Journal of Health and Social Behaviour*, 38, 376–86.

Batty, G.D., Der, G., Macintyre, S., and Deary, I.J. (2006). Does IQ explain socioeconomic inequalities in health? Evidence from a population based cohort study in the west of Scotland. *BMJ*, 332, 580–4.

Bauld, L., Judge, K., and Platt, S. (2007). Assessing the impact of smoking cessation services on reducing health inequalities in England: observational study. *Tobacco Control*, 16, 400–4.

Borrell, C., Plasencia, A., Huisman, M., et al. (2005). Education level inequalities and transportation injury mortality in the middle aged and elderly in European settings. *Injury Prevention*, 11, 138–42.

Bosma, H., Schrijvers, C., and Mackenbach, J.P. (1999). Socioeconomic inequalities in mortality and importance of perceived control: cohort study. *BMJ*, 319, 1469–70.

Bouchard, T.J., Jr. (1998). Genetic and environmental influences on adult intelligence and special mental abilities. *Human Biology*, 70, 257–79.

Bronnum-Hansen, H. and Baadsgaard, M. (2012). Widening social inequality in life expectancy in Denmark. A register-based study on social composition and mortality trends for the Danish population. *BMC Public Health*, 12, 994.

Brunner, E. (1997). Stress and the biology of inequality. *BMJ*, 314, 1472–6.

Brunner, E. and Marmot M. (2006). Social organization, stress, and health. In M. Marmot and R.G. Wilkinson (eds.) *Social Determinants of Health* (2nd ed.), pp. 6–30. Oxford: Oxford University Press.

Burstrom, B., Whitehead, M., Lindholm, C., and Diderichsen, F. (2000). Inequality in the social consequences of illness: how well do people with long-term illness fare in the British and Swedish labor markets? *International Journal of Health Services*, 30, 435–51.

Cavelaars, A.E., Kunst, A.E., Geurts, J.J., et al. (1998a). Differences in self reported morbidity by educational level: a comparison of 11 western European countries. *Journal of Epidemiology and Community Health*, 52, 219–27.

Cavelaars, A.E., Kunst, A.E., Geurts, J. J., et al. (1998b). Morbidity differences by occupational class among men in seven European countries: an application of the Erikson-Goldthorpe social class scheme. *International Journal of Epidemiology*, 27, 222–30.

Cavelaars, A.E., Kunst, A.E., Geurts, J.J., et al. (2000). Educational differences in smoking: international comparison. *BMJ*, 320, 1102–7.

Cavelaars, A.E., Kunst, A.E., and Mackenbach, J.P. (1997). Socio-economic differences in risk factors for morbidity and mortality in the European Community: an international comparison. *Journal of Health Psychology*, 2, 353–72.

Chapman, B.P., Fiscella, K., Kawachi, I., and Duberstein, P.R. (2010). Personality, socioeconomic status, and all-cause mortality in the United States. *American Journal of Epidemiology*, 171, 83–92.

Chave, S.P.W. (1984). The origins and development of public health. In W.W. Holland, R. Detels, and E.G. Knox (eds.) *Oxford Textbook of Public Health*, pp. 1–20. Oxford: Oxford University Press.

Coleman, W. (1982). *Death is a Social Disease; Public Health and Political Economy in Early Industrial France*. Madison, WI: University of Wisconsin Press.

Commission on Social Determinants of Health (2008). *Closing the Gap in a Generation. Health Equity Through the Social Determinants of Health*. Geneva: World Health Organization.

Costa, G. and D'Errico, A. (2006). Inequalities in health: do occupational risks matter? *European Journal of Public Health*, 16, 340–1.

Craig, P., Cooper, C., Gunnell, D., et al. (2011). *Using Natural Experiments to Evaluate Population Health Interventions: Guidance for Producers and Users of Evidence*. Glasgow: Medical Research Council.

Craig, P., Dieppe, P., Macintyre, S., Michie, S., Nazareth, I., and Petticrew, M. (2008). *Developing and Evaluating Complex Interventions: New Guidance*. London: Medical Research Council.

Cutler, D.M., Deaton, A., and Lleras-Muney, A. (2006). The determinants of mortality. *Journal of Economic Perspectives*, 20, 97–120.

Dalstra, J.A., Kunst, A.E., Borrell, C., et al. (2005). Socioeconomic differences in the prevalence of common chronic diseases: an overview of eight European countries. *International Journal of Epidemiology*, 34, 316–26.

Daniels, N., Kennedy, B.P., and Kawachi, I. (1999). Why justice is good for our health: the social determinants of health inequalities. *Daedalus*, 128, 215–51.

Davey Smith, G., Ebrahim, S., and Frankel, S. (2001). How policy informs the evidence. *BMJ*, 322, 184–5.

Deboosere, P., Gadeyne, S., and Van Oyen, H. (2009). The 1991–2004 evolution in life expectancy by educational level in Belgium based on linked census and population register data. *European Journal of Population*, 25, 175–96.

Department of Health (1998). *Independent Inquiry into Inequalities in Health (Acheson Report)*. London: Department of Health.

Department of Health (1999). *Reducing Health Inequalities: An Action Report*. London: Department of Health.

Department of Health (2003). *Tackling Health Inequalities: A Program for Action*. London: Department of Health.

Department of Health (2010). *Fair Society, Healthy Lives (Marmot Review)*. London: Department of Health.

Department of Health and Social Services (1980). *Inequalities in Health: Report of a Research Working Group (Black Report)*. London: Department of Health and Social Services.

Droomers, M., Schrijvers, C.T., and Mackenbach, J.P. (2001). Educational level and decreases in leisure time physical activity: predictors from the longitudinal GLOBE study. *Journal of Epidemiology and Community Health*, 55, 562–8.

Droomers, M., Schrijvers, C.T., and Mackenbach, J.P. (2002). Why do lower educated people continue smoking? Explanations from the longitudinal GLOBE study. *Health Psychology*, 21, 263–72.

Droomers, M., Schrijvers, C.T., and Mackenbach, J.P. (2004). Educational differences in starting excessive alcohol consumption: explanations from the longitudinal GLOBE study. *Social Science & Medicine*, 58, 2023–33.

Droomers, M., Schrijvers, C.T., Stronks, K., Van De Mheen, D., and Mackenbach, J.P. (1999). Educational differences in excessive alcohol consumption: the role of psychosocial and material stressors. *Preventive Medicine*, 29, 1–10.

Droomers, M., Schrijvers, C.T., Van De Mheen, H., and Mackenbach, J.P. (1998). Educational differences in leisure-time physical inactivity: a descriptive and explanatory study. *Social Science & Medicine*, 47, 1665–76.

Dunn, J.R. and Hayes, M.V. (1999). Identifying social pathways for health inequalities. The role of housing. *Annals of the New York Academy of Sciences*, 896, 399–402.

Eikemo, T.A., Kunst, A.E., Judge, K., and Mackenbach, J.P. (2008). Class-related health inequalities are not larger in the East: a comparison of four European regions using the new European socioeconomic classification. *Journal of Epidemiology and Community Health*, 62, 1072–8.

Esping-Andersen, G. (1990). *The Three Worlds of Welfare Capitalism*. Cambridge: Polity.

Faggiano, F., Partanen, T., Kogevinas, M., and Boffetta, P. (1997). Socioeconomic differences in cancer incidence and mortality. *IARC Sci Publ*, 65–176.

Fryers, T., Melzer, D., Jenkins, R., and Brugha, T. (2005). The distribution of the common mental disorders: social inequalities in Europe. *Clinical Practice & Epidemiology in Mental Health*, 1, 14.

Galobardes, B., Lynch, J., and Smith, G.D. (2007). Measuring socioeconomic position in health research. *British Medical Bulletin*, 81–2, 21–37.

Giskes, K., Kunst, A.E., Benach, J., et al. (2005). Trends in smoking behaviour between 1985 and 2000 in nine European countries by education. *Journal of Epidemiology and Community Health*, 59, 395–401.

Giskes, K., Van Lenthe, F.J., Brug, J., Mackenbach, J.P., and Turrell, G. (2007). Socioeconomic inequalities in food purchasing: the contribution of respondent-perceived and actual (objectively measured) price and availability of foods. *Preventive Medicine*, 45, 41–8.

Giskes, K., Van Lenthe, F.J., Kamphuis, C.B., Huisman, M., Brug, J., and Mackenbach, J.P. (2009). Household and food shopping environments: do they play a role in socioeconomic inequalities in fruit and vegetable consumption? A multilevel study among Dutch adults. *Journal of Epidemiology and Community Health*, 63, 113–20.

Gonzalez, M.A., Rodriguez Artalejo, F., and Calero, J.R. (1998). Relationship between socioeconomic status and ischaemic heart disease in cohort and case-control studies: 1960–1993. *International Journal of Epidemiology*, 27, 350–8.

Graham, H. (2004). Tackling inequalities in health in England: remedying health disadvantages, narrowing health gaps or reducing health gradients? *Journal of Social Policy*, 33, 115–31.

Halldorsson, M., Cavelaars, A.E., Kunst, A.E., and Mackenbach, J.P. (1999). Socioeconomic differences in health and well-being of children and adolescents in Iceland. *Scandinavian Journal of Public Health*, 27, 43–7.

Harper, S., King, N.B., Meersman, S.C., Reichman, M.E., Breen, N., and Lynch, J. (2010). Implicit value judgments in the measurement of health inequalities. *Milbank Quarterly*, 88, 4–29.

Hart, C.L., Taylor, M.D., Davey Smith, G., et al. (2003). Childhood IQ, social class, deprivation, and their relationships with mortality and morbidity risk in later life: prospective observational study linking the Scottish Mental Survey 1932 and the Midspan studies. *Psychosomatic Medicine*, 65, 877–83.

Heraclides, A. and Brunner, E. (2010). Social mobility and social accumulation across the life course in relation to adult overweight and obesity: the Whitehall II study. *Journal of Epidemiology and Community Health*, 64, 714–19.

Hetemaa, T., Keskimaki, I., Salomaa, V., Mahonen, M., Manderbacka, K., and Koskinen, S. (2004). Socioeconomic inequities in invasive cardiac procedures after first myocardial infarction in Finland in 1995. *Journal of Clinical Epidemiology*, 57, 301–8.

Holzapfel, C., Grallert, H., Baumert, J., et al. (2011). First investigation of two obesity-related loci (TMEM18, FTO) concerning their association with educational level as well as income: the MONICA/KORA study. *Journal of Epidemiology and Community Health*, 65, 174–6.

Huijts, T. and Eikemo, T.A. (2009). Causality, social selectivity or artefacts? Why socioeconomic inequalities in health are not smallest in the Nordic countries. *European Journal of Public Health*, 19, 452–3.

Huisman, M., Kunst, A.E., Andersen, O., et al. (2004). Socioeconomic inequalities in mortality among elderly people in 11 European populations. *Journal of Epidemiology and Community Health*, 58, 468–75.

Huisman, M., Kunst, A.E., Bopp, M., et al. (2005a). Educational inequalities in cause-specific mortality in middle-aged and older men and women in eight western European populations. *Lancet*, 365, 493–500.

Huisman, M., Kunst, A.E., and Mackenbach, J.P. (2005b). Educational inequalities in smoking among men and women aged 16 years and older in 11 European countries. *Tobacco Control*, 14, 106–13.

Judge, T.A., Higgins, C.A., Thoreson, C.J., and Barrick, M.R. (1999). The big five personality traits, general mental ability, and career success across the lifespan. *Personnel Psychology*, 52, 621–52.

Kamphuis, C.B., Van Lenthe, F.J., Giskes, K., Brug, J., and Mackenbach, J.P. (2007). Perceived environmental determinants of physical activity and fruit and vegetable consumption among high and low socioeconomic groups in the Netherlands. *Health & Place*, 13, 493–503.

Kamphuis, C.B., Van Lenthe, F.J., Giskes, K., Huisman, M., Brug, J., and Mackenbach, J.P. (2009). Socioeconomic differences in lack of recreational walking among older adults: the role of neighbourhood and individual factors. *International Journal of Behavioral Nutrition and Physical Activity*, 6, 1.

Karnehed, N.E., Rasmussen, F., Hemmingsson, T., and Tynelius, P. (2008). Obesity in young adulthood is related to social mobility among Swedish men. *Obesity (Silver Spring)*, 16, 654–8.

Kautto, M., Fritzell, J., Hvinden, B., Kvist, J., and Uusitalo, H. (eds.) (2001). *Nordic Welfare States in the European Context*. New York: Routledge.

Kawachi, I., Kennedy, B.P., Lochner, K., and Prothrow-Stith, D. (1997). Social capital, income inequality, and mortality. *American Journal of Public Health*, 87, 1491–8.

Keating, D.P. and Hertzman, C. (eds.) (1999). *Developmental Health and the Wealth of Nations: Social, Biological and Educational Dynamics*. New York: Guildford.

Kippersluis, H.V., O'Donnell, O., and Doorslaer, E.V. (2011). Long run returns to education: does schooling lead to an extended old age? *Journal of Human Resources*, 46, 695–721.

Kogevinas, M. and Porta, M. (1997). Socioeconomic differences in cancer survival: a review of the evidence. *IARC Scientific Publications*, 177–206.

Kondo, N., Sembajwe, G., Kawachi, I., Van Dam, R.M., Subramanian, S.V., and Yamagata, Z. (2009). Income inequality, mortality, and self rated health: meta-analysis of multilevel studies. *BMJ*, 339, b4471.

Krieger, N., Rehkopf, D.H., Chen, J.T., Waterman, P.D., Marcelli, E., and Kennedy, M. (2008). The fall and rise of US inequities in premature mortality: 1960–2002. *PLoS Medicine*, 5, e46.

Kristenson, M. (2006). Socio-economic position and health: the role of coping. In J. Siegrist and M. Marmot (eds.) *Social Inequalities in Health. New Evidence and Policy Implications*, pp. 127–52. Oxford: Oxford University Press.

Kruize, H., Driessen, P.P., Glasbergen, P., and Van Egmond, K.N. (2007). Environmental equity and the role of public policy: experiences in the Rijnmond region. *Environmental Management*, 40, 578–95.

Kuijer, P.P., Visser, B., and Kemper, H.C. (1999). Job rotation as a factor in reducing physical workload. *Ergonomics*, 42, 1167–78.

Kunst, A.E., Groenhof, F., Andersen, O., et al. (1999). Occupational class and ischemic heart disease mortality in the United States and 11 European countries. *American Journal of Public Health*, 89, 47–53.

Lager, A.C. and Torssander, J. (2012). Causal effect of education on mortality in a quasi-experiment on 1.2 million Swedes. *Proceedings of the National Academy of Sciences of the United States of America*, 109, 8461–6.

Lang, T., Nicaud, V., Darne, B., and Rueff, B. (1995). Improving hypertension control among excessive alcohol drinkers: a randomised controlled trial in France. The WALPA Group. *Journal of Epidemiology and Community Health*, 49, 610–16.

Lang, T., Nicaud, V., Slama, K., et al. (2000). Smoking cessation at the workplace. Results of a randomised controlled intervention study. Worksite physicians from the AIREL group. *Journal of Epidemiology and Community Health*, 54, 349–54.

Leinsalu, M., Stirbu, I., Vagero, D., et al. (2009). Educational inequalities in mortality in four Eastern European countries: divergence in trends during the post-communist transition from 1990 to 2000. *International Journal of Epidemiology*, 38, 512–25.

Lemstra, M., Mackenbach, J., Neudorf, C., and Nannapaneni, U. (2009). High health care utilization and costs associated with lower socio-economic status: results from a linked dataset. *Canadian Journal of Public Health*, 100, 180–3.

Lindahl, M. (2005). Estimating the effect of income on health using lottery prizes as exogenous source of variation in income. *Journal of Human Resources*, 40, 144–68.

Link, B.G. and Phelan, J. (1995). Social conditions as fundamental causes of disease. *Journal of Health and Social Behaviour*, Spec No, 80–94.

Lleras-Muney, A. (2002). *The Relationship Between Education and Adult Mortality in the United States*. NBER Working Paper Series. Cambridge: National Bureau of Economic Research.

Lopez-Azpiazu, I., Sanchez-Villegas, A., Johansson, L., et al. (2003). Disparities in food habits in Europe: systematic review of educational and occupational differences in the intake of fat. *Journal of Human Nutrition and Dietetics*, 16, 349–64.

Lorant, V., Croux, C., Weich, S., Deliege, D., Mackenbach, J., and Ansseau, M. (2007). Depression and socio-economic risk factors: 7-year longitudinal population study. *British Journal of Psychiatry*, 190, 293–8.

Lorant, V., Kunst, A.E., Huisman, M., Costa, G., and Mackenbach, J. (2005). Socio-economic inequalities in suicide: a European comparative study. *British Journal of Psychiatry*, 187, 49–54.

Lounsbury, J.W., Sundstrom, E., Loveland, J.M., and Gibson, L.W. (2003). Intelligence, "big five" personality traits, and work drive as predictors of course grade. *Personality and Individual Differences*, 35, 1231–9.

Louwman, W.J., Aarts, M.J., Houterman, S., et al. (2010). A 50% higher prevalence of life-shortening chronic conditions among cancer patients with low socioeconomic status. *British Journal of Cancer*, 103, 1742–8.

Macintyre, S. (1997). The Black Report and beyond: what are the issues? *Social Science & Medicine*, 44, 723–45.

Macintyre, S. (2003). Evidence based policy making. *BMJ*, 326, 5–6.

Macintyre, S., Chalmers, I., Horton, R., and Smith, R. (2001). Using evidence to inform health policy: case study. *BMJ*, 322, 222–5.

Mackenbach, J.P. (2005). Genetics and health inequalities: hypotheses and controversies. *Journal of Epidemiology and Community Health*, 59, 268–73.

Mackenbach, J.P. (2006). *Health inequalities. Europe in profile*. London: Department of Health.

Mackenbach, J.P. (2009). Politics is nothing but medicine at a larger scale: reflections on public health's biggest idea. *Journal of Epidemiology and Community Health*, 63, 181–4.

Mackenbach, J.P. (2010). New trends in health inequalities research: now it's personal. *Lancet*, 376, 854–5.

Mackenbach, J.P. (2011). Can we reduce health inequalities? An analysis of the English strategy (1997–2010). *Journal of Epidemiology and Community Health*, 65, 568–75.

Mackenbach, J.P. (2012). The persistence of health inequalities in modern welfare states: the explanation of a paradox. *Social Science & Medicine*, 75, 761–9.

Mackenbach, J.P. and Bakker, M. (eds.) (2002). *Reducing Inequalities in Health: A European Perspective*, London: Routledge.

Mackenbach, J.P. and Bakker, M.J. (2003). Tackling socioeconomic inequalities in health: analysis of European experiences. *Lancet*, 362, 1409–14.

Mackenbach, J.P., Bos, V., Andersen, O., et al. (2003). Widening socioeconomic inequalities in mortality in six Western European countries. *International Journal of Epidemiology*, 32, 830–7.

Mackenbach, J.P., Cavelaars, A.E., Kunst, A.E., and Groenhof, F. (2000). Socioeconomic inequalities in cardiovascular disease mortality; an international study. *European Heart Journal*, 21, 1141–51.

Mackenbach, J.P. and Gunning-Schepers, L.J. (1997). How should interventions to reduce inequalities in health be evaluated? *Journal of Epidemiology and Community Health*, 51, 359–64.

Mackenbach, J.P., Huisman, M., Andersen, O., et al. (2004). Inequalities in lung cancer mortality by the educational level in 10 European populations. *European Journal of Cancer*, 40, 126–35.

Mackenbach, J.P. and Kunst, A.E. (1997). Measuring the magnitude of socio-economic inequalities in health: an overview of available measures illustrated with two examples from Europe. *Social Science & Medicine*, 44, 757–71.

Mackenbach, J.P., Kunst, A.E., Groenhof, F., et al. (1999). Socioeconomic inequalities in mortality among women and among men: an international study. *American Journal of Public Health*, 89, 1800–6.

Mackenbach, J.P., Meerding, W.J., and Kunst, A.E. (2011). Economic costs of health inequalities in the European Union. *Journal of Epidemiology and Community Health*, 65, 412–19.

Mackenbach, J.P., Stirbu, I., Roskam, A.J., et al. (2008). Socioeconomic inequalities in health in 22 European countries. *New England Journal of Medicine*, 358, 2468–81.

Mackenbach, J.P. and Stronks, K. (2002). A strategy for tackling health inequalities in the Netherlands. *BMJ*, 325, 1029–32.

Mackenbach, J.P. and Stronks, K. (2004). The development of a strategy for tackling health inequalities in the Netherlands. *International Journal for Equity in Health*, 3, 11.

Main, C., Thomas, S., Ogilvie, D., et al. (2008). Population tobacco control interventions and their effects on social inequalities in smoking: placing an equity lens on existing systematic reviews. *BMC Public Health*, 8, 178.

Majer, I.M., Nusselder, W.J., Mackenbach, J.P., and Kunst, A.E. (2011). Socioeconomic inequalities in life and health expectancies around official retirement age in 10 Western-European countries. *Journal of Epidemiology and Community Health*, 65, 972–9.

Makela, P., Valkonen, T., and Martelin, T. (1997). Contribution of deaths related to alcohol use to socioeconomic variation in mortality: register based follow up study. *BMJ*, 315, 211–16.

Marmot, M., Siegrist, J., and Theorell, T. (2006). Health and the psychosocial environment at work. In M. Marmot and R.G. Wilkinson (eds.) *Social Determinants of Health* (2nd ed.), pp. 97–130. Oxford: Oxford University Press.

Marmot, M. and Wilkinson, R.G. (eds.) (2006). *Social Determinants of Health*. Oxford: Oxford University Press.

Marmot, M.G. (2003). Understanding social inequalities in health. *Perspectives in Biology and Medicine*, 46, S9–23.

Marmot, M.G. (2004). *Status Syndrome. How Your Social Standing Directly Affects Your Health and Life Expectancy*. London: Bloomsbury.

Marmot, M.G. and McDowall, M.E. (1986). Mortality decline and widening social inequalities. *Lancet*, 2, 274–6.

Marmot, M.G., Smith, G.D., Stansfeld, S., et al. (1991). Health inequalities among British civil servants: the Whitehall II study. *Lancet*, 337, 1387–93.

Mckee, M. (2009). Public health in Central and Eastern Europe and the former Soviet Union. In R. Beaglehole and R. Bonita (eds.) *Global Public Health. A New Era*, pp. 101–22. Oxford etc.: Oxford University Press.

Menvielle, G., Kunst, A.E., Stirbu, I., et al. (2007). Socioeconomic inequalities in alcohol related cancer mortality among men: to what extent do they differ between Western European populations? *International Journal of Cancer*, 121, 649–55.

Menvielle, G., Kunst, A.E., Stirbu, I., et al. (2008). Educational differences in cancer mortality among women and men: a gender pattern that differs across Europe. *British Journal of Cancer*, 98, 1012–19.

Mheen, H.V.D., Stronks, K., and Mackenbach, J.P. (1998). A lifecourse perspective on socioeconomic inequalities in health: the influence of childhood socioeconomic position and selection processes. *Sociology of Health and Illness*, 20, 754–77.

Mohd Hairi, F., Mackenbach, J.P., Andersen-Ranberg, K., and Avendano, M. (2010). Does socio-economic status predict grip strength in older Europeans? Results from the SHARE study in non-institutionalised men and women aged 50+. *Journal of Epidemiology and Community Health*, 64, 829–37.

Morris, J.N., Wilkinson, P., Dangour, A.D., Deeming, C., and Fletcher, A. (2007). Defining a minimum income for healthy living (MIHL): older age, England. *International Journal of Epidemiology*, 36, 1300–7.

Nabi, H., Kivimaki, M., Marmot, M.G., et al. (2008). Does personality explain social inequalities in mortality? The French GAZEL cohort study. *International Journal of Epidemiology*, 37, 591–602.

Oliver, A. (2010). Reflections on the development of health inequalities policy in England. *Health Care Analysis*, 18, 402–20.

Palosuo, H., Koskinen, S., Lahelma, E., et al. (eds.) (2009). *Trends in Socioeconomic Health Differences 1980–2005*. Helsinki: Ministry of Social Affairs and Health.

Pamuk, E.R. (1985). Social class inequality in mortality from 1921 to 1972 in England and Wales. *Population Studies (Cambridge)*, 39, 17–31.

Petticrew, M., Whitehead, M., Macintyre, S.J., Graham, H., and Egan, M. (2004). Evidence for public health policy on inequalities: 1: the reality according to policymakers. *Journal of Epidemiology and Community Health*, 58, 811–16.

Phelan, J.C., Link, B.G., and Tehranifar, P. (2010). Social conditions as fundamental causes of health inequalities: theory, evidence, and policy implications. *Journal of Health and Social Behaviour*, 51(Suppl.), S28–40.

Plomin, R. and Spinath, F.M. (2004). Intelligence: genetics, genes, and genomics. *Journal of Personality and Social Psychology*, 86, 112–29.

Plug, I., Hoffmann, R., Artnik, B., et al. (2012). Socioeconomic inequalities in mortality from conditions amenable to medical interventions: do they reflect inequalities in access or quality of health care? *BMC Public Health*, 12, 346.

Power, C., Graham, H., Due, P., et al. (2005). The contribution of childhood and adult socioeconomic position to adult obesity and smoking behaviour: an international comparison. *International Journal of Epidemiology*, 34, 335–44.

Power, C. and Kuh, D. (2006). Lifecourse development of unequal health. In J. Siegrist and M.G. Marmot (eds.) *Social Inequalities in Health. New Evidence And Policy Implications*, pp. 27–54. Oxford: Oxford University Press.

Power, C. and Matthews, S. (1997). Origins of health inequalities in a national population sample. *Lancet*, 350, 1584–9.

Prattala, R., Berg, M.A., and Puska, P. (1992). Diminishing or increasing contrasts? Social class variation in Finnish food consumption patterns, 1979–1990. *European Journal of Clinical Nutrition*, 46, 279–87.

Prattala, R.S., Groth, M.V., Oltersdorf, U.S., Roos, G.M., Sekula, W., and Tuomainen, H.M. (2003). Use of butter and cheese in 10 European countries: a case of contrasting educational differences. *European Journal of Public Health*, 13, 124–32.

Roskam, A.J., Kunst, A.E., Van Oyen, H., et al. (2010). Comparative appraisal of educational inequalities in overweight and obesity among adults in 19 European countries. *International Journal of Epidemiology*, 39, 392–404.

Salomaa, V., Niemela, M., Miettinen, H., et al. (2000). Relationship of socioeconomic status to the incidence and prehospital, 28-day, and 1-year mortality rates of acute coronary events in the FINMONICA myocardial infarction register study. *Circulation*, 101, 1913–18.

Schaap, M.M., Kunst, A.E., Leinsalu, M., et al. (2008). Effect of nationwide tobacco control policies on smoking cessation in high and low educated groups in 18 European countries. *Tobacco Control*, 17, 248–55.

Shkolnikov, V.M., Andreev, E.M., Jasilionis, D., Leinsalu, M., Antonova, O.I., and McKee, M. (2006). The changing relation between education and life expectancy in central and eastern Europe in the 1990s. *Journal of Epidemiology and Community Health*, 60, 875–81.

Shkolnikov, V.M., Andreev, E.M., Jdanov, D.A., et al. (2012). Increasing absolute mortality disparities by education in Finland, Norway and Sweden, 1971-2000. *Journal of Epidemiology and Community Health*, 66, 372–8.

Siegrist, J. and Marmot, M. (2004). Health inequalities and the psychosocial environment—two scientific challenges. *Social Science & Medicine*, 58, 1463–73.

Siegrist, J. and Marmot, M. (eds.) (2006). *Social Inequalities in Health. New Evidence and Policy Implications*. Oxford: Oxford University Press.

Sihvonen, A.P., Kunst, A.E., Lahelma, E., Valkonen, T., and Mackenbach, J.P. (1998). Socioeconomic inequalities in health expectancy in Finland and Norway in the late 1980s. *Social Science & Medicine*, 47, 303–15.

Singh-Manoux, A., Ferrie, J.E., Lynch, J.W., and Marmot, M. (2005). The role of cognitive ability (intelligence) in explaining the association between socioeconomic position and health: evidence from the Whitehall II prospective cohort study. *American Journal of Epidemiology*, 161, 831–9.

Smith, G.D., Hart, C., Blane, D., Gillis, C., and Hawthorne, V. (1997). Lifetime socioeconomic position and mortality: prospective observational study. *BMJ*, 314, 547–52.

Smith, J.P. (1999). Healthy bodies and thick wallets: the dual relation between health and economic status. *Journal of Economic Perspectives*, 13, 144–66.

Sobal, J. and Stunkard, A.J. (1989). Socioeconomic status and obesity: a review of the literature. *Psychological Bulletin*, 105, 260–75.

Stansfeld, S.A. (2006). Social support and social cohesion. In M. Marmot and R.G. Wilkinson (eds.) *Social Determinants of Health* (2nd ed.), pp. 148–71. Oxford: Oxford University Press.

Steingrimsdottir, O.A., Naess, O., Moe, J.O., et al. (2012). Trends in life expectancy by education in Norway 1961–2009. *European Journal of Epidemiology*, 27, 163–71.

Steptoe, A. (2006). Psychobiological processes linking socio-economic position to health. In J. Siegrist and M. Marmot (eds.) *Social Inequalities in Health. New Evidence and Policy Implications*, pp. 101–26. Oxford: Oxford University Press.

Stickley, A., Leinsalu, M., Kunst, A.E., et al. (2012). Socioeconomic inequalities in homicide mortality: a population-based comparative study of 12 European countries. *European Journal of Epidemiology*, 27, 877–84.

Stirbu, I., Kunst, A.E., Bopp, M., et al. (2010). Educational inequalities in avoidable mortality in Europe. *Journal of Epidemiology and Community Health*, 64, 913–20.

Stirbu, I., Looman, C., Nijhof, G.J., Reulings, P.G., and Mackenbach, J. P. (2012). Income inequalities in case death of ischaemic heart disease in the Netherlands: a national record-linked study. *Journal of Epidemiology and Community Health*, 66, 1159–66.

Strand, B.H., Groholt, E.K., Steingrimsdottir, O.A., Blakely, T., Graff-Iversen, S., and Naess, O. (2010). Educational inequalities in mortality over four decades in Norway: prospective study of middle aged men and women followed for cause specific mortality, 1960–2000. *BMJ*, 340, c654.

Strand, B.H., Kunst, A., Huisman, M., et al. (2007). The reversed social gradient: higher breast cancer mortality in the higher educated compared to lower educated. A comparison of 11 European populations during the 1990s. *European Journal of Cancer*, 43, 1200–7.

Swedish National Institute of Public Health (2005). *The 2005 Public Health Policy Report*. Stockholm: Swedish National Institute of Public Health.

Thomson, H., Hoskins, R., Petticrew, M., et al. (2004). Evaluating the health effects of social interventions. *BMJ*, 328, 282–5.

Unal, B., Critchley, J.A., and Capewell, S. (2005). Modelling the decline in coronary heart disease deaths in England and Wales, 1981–2000: comparing contributions from primary prevention and secondary prevention. *BMJ*, 331, 614.

Van de Mheen, H., Stronks, K., Schrijvers, C.T., and Mackenbach, J.P. (1999). The influence of adult ill health on occupational class mobility and mobility out of and into employment in the Netherlands. *Social Science & Medicine*, 49, 509–18.

Van der Heyden, J.H., Schaap, M.M., Kunst, A.E., et al. (2009). Socioeconomic inequalities in lung cancer mortality in 16 European populations. *Lung Cancer*, 63, 322–30.

Van Doorslaer, E., Masseria, C., and Koolman, X. (2006). Inequalities in access to medical care by income in developed countries. *Canadian Medical Association Journal*, 174, 177–83.

Van Raalte, A.A., Kunst, A.E., Deboosere, P., et al. (2011). More variation in lifespan in lower educated groups: evidence from 10 European countries. *International Journal of Epidemiology*, 40, 1703–14.

Venkatapuram, S. (2011). *Health Justice. An Argument from the Capabilities Approach*. Cambridge: Polity Press.

Wamala, S., Blakely, T., and Atkinson, J. (2006). Trends in absolute socioeconomic inequalities in mortality in Sweden and New Zealand. A 20-year gender perspective. *BMC Public Health*, 6, 164.

Whitehead, M. (1992). The concepts and principles of equity and health. *International Journal of Health Services*, 22, 429–45.

Whitehead, M. (1998). Diffusion of ideas on social inequalities in health: a European perspective. *Milbank Quarterly*, 76, 469–92, 306.

Whitehead, M. (2007). A typology of actions to tackle social inequalities in health. *Journal of Epidemiology and Community Health*, 61, 473–8.

Whitehead, M., Petticrew, M., Graham, H., MacIntyre, S.J., Bambra, C., and Egan, M. (2004). Evidence for public health policy on inequalities: 2: assembling the evidence jigsaw. *Journal of Epidemiology and Community Health*, 58, 817–21.

Wilkinson, R.G. (1992). Income distribution and life expectancy. *BMJ*, 304, 165–8.

Wilkinson, R.G. and Pickett, K. (2009). *The Spirit Level: Why More Equal Societies Almost Always Do Better*. London: Allen Lane.

2.4

Reducing health inequalities in developing countries

Hoosen Coovadia and Irwin Friedman

Introduction: why is health inequity an issue?

Well-being is profoundly impacted by many social and economic determinants. Clearly, access to basic needs such as food, water, shelter, education, decent employment, safe working conditions, and so on are crucial to health. But even many higher-order needs such as social inclusion, involvement in governance issues such as policy development (e.g. on human rights and gender equity), the right to critique unfair administration, or participate in the exercise of political power are also important. Indeed, well-being is so tightly linked to the broad ecology of social determinants, it has become increasingly evident that the health of a population is fundamentally dependent on fair access to social goods and processes within the society. Health equity and social justice are interlinked. Well-being depends on fairness (McKeown 1976; Acheson 2000; Deaton 2003; Wilkinson and Marmot 2005). While the insight may not be new, what is of contemporary relevance is that the causes of health inequity, once thought to be beyond the realms of intervention, are now routinely being considered for inclusion within the parameters of progressive health programming. Close examination of the evidence by expert groups has indeed shown that effective interventions to address injustices in the socioeconomic conditions underpinning health are not only possible, but warranted. Where avoidable systematic disparities in health occur in situations which could be avoided by reasonable, timeous action, then they can be judged as unfair. This unfairness can be labelled as health inequity. These insights formed the basis for the conclusions and recommendations of the Commission for Social Determinants of Health (CSDH) (CSDH 2008), which are discussed in some detail in the following sections.

Definition

Health equity relates to the fairness in distribution of health resources and outcomes. This applies both to equity between citizens in specific countries (intra-country) as well as between countries (inter-country) or regions (inter-regional). The World Health Organization (WHO) defines health inequalities as 'differences in health status or in the distribution of health determinants between different population groups' (Quigley et al. 2006; WHO n.d.). Putting right these inequities—the huge and remediable differences in health between and within countries—is a matter of social justice, founded on the linked concepts of fairness, justice,

and freedom. These ideas echoed the sentiments of strong equity advocates such as Amartya Sen (Sen 1999), who for many years had argued that freedom from poverty, social deprivation, political tyranny, and cultural authoritarianism was crucial if the social and economic development to which all countries aspire was to be achieved. Inequity was anathema for socioeconomic well-being. Development was therefore dependent on social justice, founded on a system of supportive institutions and all citizens having access to basic education and essential health. For John Rawls (Rawls 1958), justice is fairness.

Absolute and relative health inequalities and socioeconomic status

There are health inequities everywhere, but they are more pronounced in certain settings. Rather than viewing this in terms of absolute differences between rich and poor they should be understood as comprising relative social gradients. It follows that where societal resources are maldistributed by elements such as income, class, spatial location, race, and gender, population health will correspondingly be unequally distributed. Interventions to deal with these are discussed in the section entitled 'Tackle the inequitable distribution of resource and power'.

Improving health inequalities by addressing social determinants

One of the earliest attempts to understand health inequity dates back to the work of Edwin Chadwick, a leading figure in the effort to investigate and combat the considerable differences in health that existed in nineteenth-century Britain. Documented in his famous report on *Enquiry into the Sanitary Condition of the Labouring Population of Great Britain and the Means of its Improvement* (Chadwick 1843) was a description of the awful living conditions endured by the poorest in society compared to those that were relatively well off (Table 2.4.1). The findings of his report helped pave the way for the introduction of the Public Health Act of 1848 in Britain.

Despite progress in public health for more than a century and a half, even in developed countries such as Britain, health inequalities continue to persist. Unsurprisingly they present among the biggest of global health challenges.

One of the most significant efforts to counter health inequalities was the 'Health for All' (HFA) programme of the WHO, which

Table 2.4.1 Key finding of Edwin Chadwick's report

	Average age of deceased
Liverpool 1840	
Gentry and professional persons	35 years
Tradesmen and their families	22 years
Labourers, mechanics, and servants	15 years
Bath 1840	
Gentry and professional persons	55 years
Tradesmen and their families	37 years
Labourers, mechanics, and servants	25 years

Reproduced from Edwin Chadwick, *Report on the Sanitary Condition of the Labouring Population of Great Britain: A Supplementary Report on the results of a Special Inquiry into The Practice of Internment in Towns*, printed by R. Clowes and Sons, for Her Majesty's Stationery Office, London, UK, 1843.

was based on the 1978 Alma Ata Declaration, which set out the principles of primary healthcare (PHC). This approach introduced a radically new equitable approach to the provision of health services which was of particular relevance to developing countries. During the 1980s this approach became the impetus for health activities based on addressing the range of factors impacting on well-being. Increasingly the social and economic determinants of health became a focal point of HFA programmes (WHO 2003). There were setbacks, however, when a downturn in global economic conditions, accompanied by adverse conditions in developing countries, slowed and in some cases, reversed progress. Sadly, despite growing attention, increased global funding as well as innovative programming, the problem of inequity in health systems is little better. In fact, despite the considerable efforts to achieve the Millennium Development Goals (MDGs), the prospects of achieving these by 2015 is unlikely. A new paradigm is needed to deal with the powerful forces that have shaped and will continue to shape the world health scene. Without such a change, inequity and health injustice will persist (Gostin 2012).

Quite what a new post-MDG framework focused on global health justice will look like is not yet clear, despite the attention that the issue is receiving from many groups. One example of a promising approach, however, is that being pursued by the Joint Action and Learning Initiative on National and Global Responsibilities for Health (JALI). As a global coalition of civil society and academics, JALI is championing an international campaign of advocacy for a Framework Convention on Global Health (FCGH). Its approach includes novel ideas such as defining both national and international responsibilities to improve health equity by setting global health priorities and arguing for reliable, sustainable funding; overcoming fragmented activities; reshaping global health governance; and providing strong global health leadership through the WHO (UN Millennium Project 2005).

The WHO Commission on Social Determinants of Health

In an effort to address the social, economic, and environmental conditions that impact on health and cause health inequity, in 2005, the WHO established the Commission on Social

Determinants of Health[1] (CSDH) to provide context-specific advice for regions, countries and global health partners (Gostin 2012; The Commission on Social Determinants of Health Knowledge Networks 2011).

Some novel WHO activities have grown out of the insights of the CSDH and several are now global initiatives. The three focal areas of the CSDH findings are to: (1) improve daily living conditions, (2) tackle inequality in the distribution of resources and power, (3) understand and measure the extent of health inequity and take action.

These three focal areas have become the pillars for reducing health inequities, which may require attention in several dimensions such as equality of rights and opportunities as well as equity in living conditions to achieve fairness in distribution.

Improve daily living conditions

Promote equity from conception

Child development begins with the health of the mother during pregnancy. Once born, many factors may affect the child in its physical, social, emotional, linguistic, and cognitive milieu. All of these critically influence the growth, development, and health of the child. Any may influence the child's life chances and affect well-being, education, and occupational opportunities. In turn, such factors affect diverse risks of individual propensity to obesity, malnutrition, mental health disorders, cardiovascular diseases, and criminality.

The evidence suggests that pre- and postnatal interventions reduce health inequalities and improve maternal and child health outcomes, particularly if these are aimed at the poorest quintiles in low- and middle-income countries (Carrera et al. 2012; Chopra et al. 2012; Countdown 2012 Report Writing Group 2012).

Provide a more equitable start in early life

A comprehensive approach to early life, built on the experience of existing child survival programmes, but including also early learning activities to stimulate social/emotional and language/cognitive development is important. Increased coverage of high-impact child survival interventions such as skilled birth attendants, measles vaccination, treatment of childhood diarrhoea and pneumonia, provision of insecticide-treated bednets for children, offering nutrition support, and introducing appropriate socioeconomic measures can all have these effects. The outcomes may reduce neonatal morbidity as well as longer-term reductions in stunting and underweight (Amouzou et al. 2012; Victora et al. 2012).

Create healthy places for people

The environments where people live and work profoundly affect their lives and well-being. Taking action to promote fair planning and improving habitats in both rural and informal urban areas through proactive town planning is essential for long-term health equity. Sustained investment in rural development, removing exclusionary policies and processes that lead to rural poverty, dealing with landlessness, and reducing the displacement of people from their homes are all measures that improve the settings in which people live and work. Climate change and other policies or programmes to prevent environmental degradation should also take health equity into account.

Meaningful employment and decent work

Unemployment is one of the major determinants of health inequity.

Meaningful employment and work opportunities for disadvantaged populations profoundly affects health equity. When people have jobs they value the opportunity for work as this boosts their self-esteem and provides financial security. This in itself may be a prerequisite to self-development, enhancement in social standing, and better relationships both within the family and society. Working people are less vulnerable to physical dangers and societal hazards such as alcohol dependency. Unemployment, precarious employment, indecent work, or poor working conditions can result in the opposite with damage to self-esteem, and exposure to a variety of social ills including the need to engage in transactional sex, sell or use drugs, or resort to crime.

Actions to make full and fair employment, as well as decent work, the cornerstones of national and international social and economic policymaking are crucial to achieving health equity. Improving working conditions for all workers reduces accidents, minimizes harmful exposures to material hazards, decreases work-related stress, and diminishes health-damaging behaviours. If health equity is to be achieved, safe, secure, fairly paid, all-year-round work opportunities, and a sound work–life balance are basic needs for all citizens.

Social protection throughout the full life cycle

People of all ages, whether they are infants, toddlers, children, adolescents, young people, working adults, or older persons, need social protection. Everyone is at all times vulnerable to adverse life events which can strike even those who are well endowed. Especially during periods of grave disturbances in their lives such as catastrophic diseases, disabilities, and unemployment, social protection is important.

All governments should be proactive in creating social protection policies that mitigate the impacts of life-disturbing events that may affect individuals.

Comprehensive social protection should include the public provision of basic utilities such as free or low-cost water, sanitation, electricity, housing services, as well as education, health, and welfare services. Provision of such public goods and services, also known as the social wage, comprises the building blocks of a fair and just society.

Universal healthcare

The health system itself can be considered a social determinant of health. While a good system with a well-trained, capable, and motivated workforce can improve health equity, a poor system may make things worse by imposing costs through out-of-pocket expenses without offering sufficiently good care. This can delay or deny health services and may also aggravate poverty. To deal with this, the action that is necessary is for governments to strive to provide universal health coverage of sound quality based on the principles of PHC. This would include the provision of equitable, accessible, appropriate, affordable services focused on health promotion, disease prevention, and multi-sectoral social development in which citizens are active participants.

Tackle the inequitable distribution of resources and power

Health equity in policies and programmes

All dimensions of societal activity, the economy and finance, education, sanitation, housing, transport, employment creation, and so on, have the potential for affecting health and well-being of the population and individuals. Socioeconomic status (SES) and health are associated across a continuous gradient at all levels (Alder et al. 1994), and not just at the extremes of wealth and poverty. This relationship is true whether measured as income, employment, education, residential environment, social status, occupation, or other stratifications. Action requires placing responsibility for action-on-health and health equity at the highest level of government, to ensure its coherent implementation across all policies. This requires that ministries of health adopt a social determinants approach and develop a framework across all of its policy and programmatic functions. Indeed, ministries of health should become champions advocating adoption of the social determinants approach across government. Where such attempts at coherence are being made in developing countries, as described later under 'National health insurance and universal coverage', there has been opposition from many vested interests, such as the private sector, pharmaceutical companies, international corporations with investments in developing countries, and right-wing social groups. The lack of will by governments in the developing world, often buttressed by demands of their elites, exacerbates the implementation of socially just public health programmes.

Many health indicators such as standard mortality ratios, annual death rates, and infant mortality are strongly correlated with SES, even though the full explanation underlying the environmental, biological, psychosocial, and behavioural mechanisms that explain this association are not fully understood (Alder et al. 1994) (Fig. 2.4.1).

In the past researchers usually simply controlled for SES rather than attempting to change it. And even today, only the effects on lower, poverty-level SES are generally examined. Excessive wealth, for example, is not considered a problem. There might, however, in the light of recent findings, be good reasons to undertake wealth studies to supplement those on poverty and to demonstrate that greater equity is beneficial for all, even the wealthy (Wilkinson and Pickett 2010). This observation requires that fresh thinking and novel approaches about the domains through which SES may exert its health effects are needed.

Adopting the health equity paradigm requires rephrasing of commonly asked questions which challenge the structural issues underpinning inequity to shift the burden away from its 'victims': 'How can we promote healthy behaviour?' by 'How can we target dangerous conditions and reorganize resource use and public policies to ensure healthy spaces and places?'. Instead of 'How can we reduce disparities in the distribution of disease and illness?' ask instead, 'How can we eliminate differentials in the distribution of power and resources that shape health outcomes?'. Similarly, we could ask 'What types of institutional and social changes are necessary to tackle health inequities?' and 'What kinds of alliance building and community organizing are necessary to mobilize and protect communities?'. This different paradigm recognizes that structural social, economic, historical, and ideological factors play a fundamental role shaping health outcomes and in the increasing health inequities that characterize many aspects of the global landscape.

There is considerable empirical evidence that health inequities are growing between the advantaged and marginalized, wealthy and poor, both within and between different countries (Dahl et al. 2002) as well as global regions (Kahn et al. 2000; Lochner et al. 2001; Deaton 2003; UC Atlas of Global Inequality 2007).

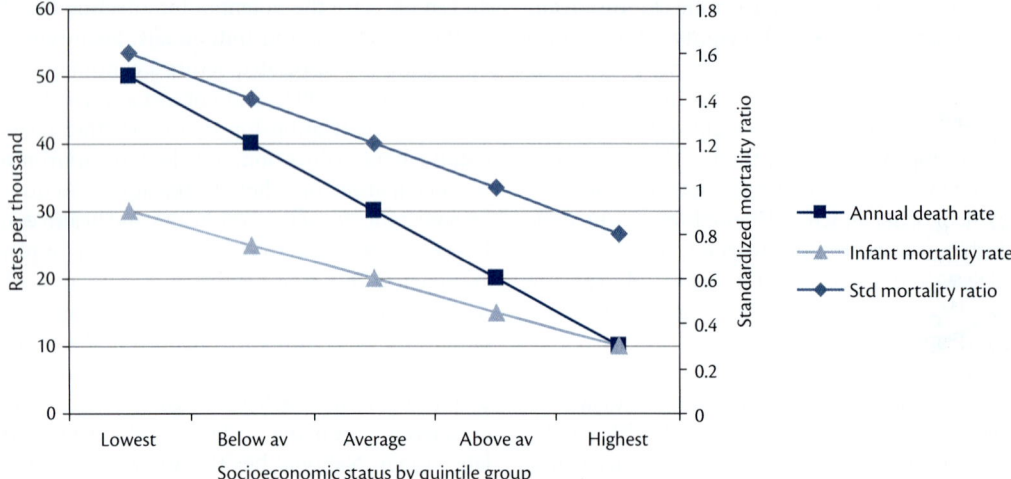

Fig. 2.4.1 The negative association between socioeconomic status (horizontal axis) and mortality indicators (vertical axis) (Alder et al. 1994).
Source: data from Alder NE et al., Socioeconomic status and health: The challenge of the gradient, *American Psychologist*, Volume 49, Issue 1, pp. 15–24, Copyright ©1994.

The greater the differences in health between social groups within a society or between countries the steeper the gradient or the greater the inequity (WHO 2003). This relationship between an Index of Health and Social Problems and Income Inequality has been extensively documented (Wilkinson and Pickett 2006, 2010, figure 13.1; Inequality.org 2012).

The relationship between longevity and healthcare spending in the public sector, in selected countries, at varying levels of development, is shown in Fig 2.4.2 (UC Atlas of Global Inequality 2007). Levels of development are clearly linked, unsurprisingly, to life expectancy. As important, is the group of countries (ringed) which gain years of longevity similar to those reached by the upper income countries but at much lower cost. Similar graphs with a wider spread of countries are available from the UC Atlas of Global Inequality (2007).

It is clear that above a certain threshold of health expenditure there is no commensurate benefit in life expectancy, as dramatically illustrated by the differences between high expenditures in the United States and far lesser expenditures in Singapore and Cuba. There are also discrepancies if one considers only averages. One reason for the discrepancy is that these averages mask inequalities. Nevertheless, it is clear that disparities within countries explain the outliers as shown in the comparison of the following Gini[2] coefficients (Central Intelligence Agency 2009). South Africa (Gini 65 per cent in 2005), for example, which has very high levels of inequity, has low levels of life expectancy (Weissman 1999). In comparison, Cuba (Gini 30 per cent) and Singapore (Gini 47 per cent), which have a much lower level of inequity, correspondingly have life expectancies that are as high as the wealthiest countries. And extreme wealth does not guarantee equity. For example, in the United States (Gini 45 per cent), despite the clinical excellence of its private health services, millions of Americans lack basic health insurance, and are therefore less likely to receive preventive care. In contrast, Cuba, despite its limited resources, and many economic problems, has achieved a similar longevity in its population by prioritizing the provision of universal health. It has, despite its evident lack of resources, even created very high doctor-to-patient ratios.

Fair financing

Public financing for the social determinants of health is fundamental to the promotion of health and prevention of disease. Public financing and the progressive achievement of universal coverage in the developed world has historically led to socioeconomic progress. Accepting that there is market failure (as, for example, in the United States), in the delivery of equitable health services and the prevention of certain diseases (public goods), public finance is therefore necessary to ensure universal access to health. As a result, strong public sector leadership and adequate budgets are the foundations of an equitable health system. Action is required to strengthen public finance for action on the social determinants of health. It means that national governments fairly allocate tax resources for implementation of the social determinants of health. A national health insurance, as one of the components of social spending, funded from progressive taxation and from other sources, should become the cornerstone of redistributive policies aimed at counteracting health inequity and reducing poverty. This is necessary at country level, but important also globally. Increased international finance for health equity, coordinated through a 'social determinants of health action framework', is as important as redistribution at a national or regional level. The United Kingdom, Australia, Canada, Italy, New Zealand, and Sweden are examples of developed countries in which general taxes are the main source of public funds for health services (National Audit Office 2003). In middle- and low-income countries there are several examples as well. Thailand (Evans et al. 2012), Israel (Cohen 2012), Taiwan (Chiang 1997; Cheng 2003; Lu and Hsiao 2003), Mexico (Anonymous 2012), Trinidad and Tobago (Tsountal 2009), and Chile (Government of Chile 2005) also have publicy funded schemes that provide universal access.

Market regulation

Using an unfettered market-orientated approach to health development is a double-edged sword. While it may assist with introducing new technologies and services which provide some benefit, it is as likely to cause unintended consequences in creating unnecessary or unhealthy goods and services, exacerbating unhealthy

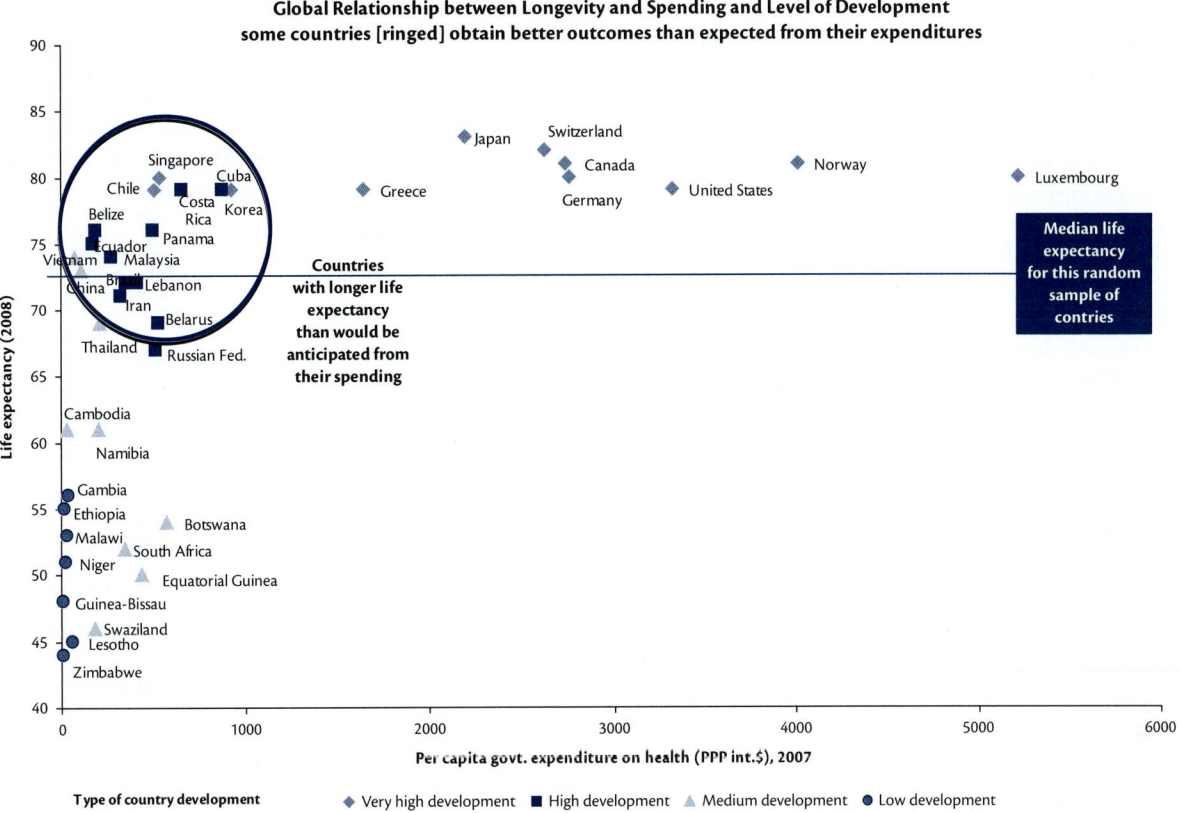

Fig. 2.4.2 The parabolic relationship between per capita healthcare spending (horizontal axis) and life expectancy (vertical axis) showing a plateau at about US $500 per capita.

Data reproduced with permission from Save the Children, Connecticut, USA from *The State of the World`s Children, Special Edition; State of the World`s Mothers; Champions for Children;* Save the Children, World Health Statistics, Copyright © May 2011.

working conditions, and increasing health inequity by serving mainly those with financial resources.

At the international level, the World Trade Organization's Agreement on Trade-Related Aspects of Intellectual Property Rights (TRIPS) provides a case in point. While efforts to protect the intellectual property rights of innovating companies has encouraged investment in drug discovery, the creation of the 20-year patent for new drugs has meant that many poor people have not been able to afford them and therefore access to novel medicines in poor countries has been limited. This contradiction was brought to the fore in the late 1990s when life-saving antiretroviral drugs were initially denied to those in developing countries because of the unreasonably high costs of the drugs. This led to an intense struggle against injustice. Although vigorous global advocacy eventually forced concessions from patent holders, TRIPS remains. Health equity in respect of access and availability to medicines will be severely challenged until there is greater flexibility or elimination of this restriction (Gwatkin and Ergo 2011; Latko et al. 2011).

Responsible governments should take steps to introduce some degree of market regulation to enable the realization of the benefits of free enterprise, while limiting the damage that could exist in a free-for-all situation. It remains important for governments to continue to play an active role in the provision of basic services essential to health (such as water, sanitation, housing, and education) and the regulation of goods and services with a major impact on health (such as medicines, medical devices, alcohol, tobacco, and food).

Gender equity

Gender inequities, characterized by harmful masculine norms, pervasive in almost all societies, impact significantly on child health and survival. The uneven power relationships, resources, entitlements, norms and values, as well as the way in which organizations are structured, and programmes are run, although they impact mostly on girls and women also have serious consequences for boys and men. There are innumerable ways that gender impacts on inequity whether as a result of unfair feeding patterns, violence against women, unfair divisions of work, leisure, and opportunities to improve life as well as inequitable decision-making. This ultimately leads to poor access to health resources. Profound as these gender inequities are, they are socially generated and therefore can be changed. Interventions to counter this require that the gender biases in the structures of society be challenged and new norms established in the formulation of laws and their enforcement. Also important is to reorganize the way institutions are run. Creative rethinking is necessary in regard to the development of national economic policies to close the gaps in education and skills development such that they are supportive of female economic participation. Greater spending on sexual and reproductive health services and programmes as part of universal coverage and rights are very important.

Political empowerment

Democratic participation in a full and unrestricted manner is a very important aspect in creating an equitable society which is free of material and psychosocial deprivation. Exclusion from participatory processes is one of the key dimensions that adversely affect well-being. People's movements and community empowerment initiatives can mitigate exclusionary social practices. Ultimately, however, although civil society and the private sector can support policies which advocate for active social inclusion, it is the government that has to adopt legislation that will guarantee citizen rights to participation. Action steps to improve this require that all groups in society be empowered to participate in democratic, participatory processes. Inclusive social practices enable civil society organizations to promote political and social rights in a way that improves health equity.

Good global governance

The huge disparities between the lives and health of people in different parts of the world are a reflection of the unequal distribution of power and wealth of different countries. While there are benefits to globalization, there are also severe consequences for the poor and this has highlighted the need for the WHO's efforts to strengthen multi-sectoral action for development and improve global leadership to take proactive steps to tackle the social determinants of health and to institutionalize these efforts as a guiding principle.

Measure and understand the problem and assess the impact of action

The social determinants of health: monitoring, research, and training

Reliable data are essential to identify health problems and devise solutions to factors impacting the social determinants of health. This requires: ensuring that routine monitoring systems for health equity and the social determinants of health are in place, locally, nationally, and internationally; investing in generating and sharing new evidence on the ways in which social determinants influence population health equity; and on evaluating the effectiveness of measures to reduce health inequities through action on social determinants.

Differences of SES can be measured in two main ways: individual household measures and geographic/area based measures, each with advantages and disadvantages.

Individual measures use indicators such as income (personal or individual), educational levels, or occupation. Although the value of these is their specificity, often such information is not generally available. Within countries the income inequities between the top 20 per cent and the bottom 20 per cent of the population can be used for this purpose.

Geographic-based information relates to areas and although not applicable to all individuals can be applied to a group of people.

South Africa—an example measuring extreme inequality

Measuring changes in such inequalities is of great importance in monitoring and evaluating programmes designed to ameliorate this.

South Africa has the worst global indicators of inequality. One example of an approach to measure this is charting the relative deprivation of populations across districts within the country as developed by a South African non-governmental organization, the Health Systems Trust (Day et al. 2011). It ranks districts in relation to a Deprivation Index (DI) derived from a set of demographic and socioeconomic variables (see list) obtained from national General Household and Community Surveys, which are generally available in the country. These surveys provide measurements of various indicators of vulnerability:

◆ Under-5 population.

◆ Black Africans as a proportion of the total population.

◆ Female-headed households.

◆ Household heads with no formal education.

◆ Working-age population that is unemployed (not working, whether looking for work or not—the official definition of unemployment in South Africa).

◆ People living in a traditional dwelling, informal shack, or tent.

◆ Households with no piped water in their house or on site.

◆ Households with a pit or bucket toilet or no form of toilet.

◆ Households which do not have access to electricity, gas, or solar power for lighting, heating, or cooking.

A technique called principal component analysis (PCA) was then used to produce a composite index of deprivation. The objective of the PCA was to create an index of composite measurements that reflects social and material deprivation from a set of variables that are indicators of deprivation. Using the DI, the 52 districts in South Africa were then ranked into socioeconomic quintiles. Those districts that fell into the lowest quintile (the bottom 20 per cent) were the most deprived districts.

In the final part of the analysis various health problems and indicators could be correlated with the DI to provide an understanding of the impact that deprivation contributes to health inequalities. The result is displayed in a bar chart showing the districts ranked by district and grouped by quintile with unique colours for each of the nine provinces in which the districts fall. This provides a simple graphic way of illustrating the districts needing intervention.

National health insurance and universal coverage

The terms national health insurance (NHI) and universal coverage (UC) have been used interchangeably, to indicate the two essential components of an equitable health system, universal access to services at health facilities and elimination of financial barriers to care. For example, the World Health Report 2011, endorsed by the World Health Assembly, urged member states to 'aim for affordable universal coverage and access for all citizens on the basis of equity and solidarity' (World Health Assembly 2011). Several countries have lately developed policy proposals to pursue this goal. NHI and UC are rooted in a human rights philosophy: the right to health and the right to social security, which could, at a stretch, be extended to the rights to life and freedom. These policy tools aim at achieving social justice through establishing equity in health. These systems, common and effective in richer countries, have been introduced recently in countries at different levels of development: Brazil, Thailand, China, Mexico, Ghana, and

Tanzania. Before we describe a few of the most striking examples, we dwell on the substantial difficulties in the early stages of implementation, and use South Africa, the most extreme example of inequity, as a case in point

South Africa—the legacy of colonialism and systematic oppression

South Africa, with its population of about 51 million people, has a nominal gross domestic product (GDP) per capita of US $8066 and Human Development Index (HDI) of 0.619[3] and is a middle-income country. Despite almost a century-long positive engagement with the idea of a NHI and more recently a willing political leadership with a receptive population, the country illustrates the numerous hurdles to achieving UC to healthcare. South Africa, although the largest economy in Africa, has a high rate of poverty and low GDP per capita with an unemployment rate of about 25 per cent and among the top ten countries globally for income inequality as measured by the Gini coefficient. The Lancet South Africa Series in 2009 (Abdool Karim et al. 2009; Chopra et al. 2009; Coovadia et al. 2009; Mayosi et al. 2009; Seedat et al. 2009) showed clearly the residual imprint of the colonial and apartheid eras, an inequitable and inefficient health system, feeling the weight of multiple health burdens, and a backdrop of pervasive racial disparities in socioeconomic indicators, with high levels of poverty and unemployment, despite progressive policies.

The solutions proposed in the Series dealt primarily with recommendations on health systems strengthening. It was believed that these actions could be implemented from 2009 when a new administration took office, by an established and more capable Health Ministry working with functioning provincial counterparts, and a receptive population willing to participate in public health programmes.

Leadership has indeed been a critical element of change in South Africa's recent history. Within the health management bureaucracy there has been stasis for more than 10 years (Abdool Karim et al. 2009). Weakness in the supervision and leadership of the public sector has resulted in falling performance of public servants which is a major factor in poor government delivery of health, educational, and other services. The public sector faced a shortage of staff and specialized skills, and corruption undermined state legitimacy and service delivery. Leadership flaws cause tensions in the political–administrative interface in the public service with an erosion of accountability and authority, a lack of effective organizational design, inappropriate staffing, and low staff morale (Coovadia et al. 2009).

At the highest levels, the Health Minister and his senior staff have made radical policy changes and vigorously engaged leadership and civil society. The role of managers has been identified as crucial for transformation. Some of the other major forces envisaged likely to influence change in the health system were relative stability, growth of the economy, intersectoral engagement (government, civil society, business, funders and global initiatives), high-quality research, and a clear programme of action.

The outcomes from these programmes may be realized if the policy proposals by the government of South Africa, especially on 'universal coverage' (Republic of South Africa 2011; Mills et al. 2012), are successfully implemented. Recent policies envisage that the NHI will be phased in over a period of 14 years and it will gradually transform the existing health system distorted currently by both race and class into a new NHI providing universal coverage based on principles such as social cohesion, equity, social solidarity, fairness, affordability, appropriateness, and effectiveness.

Recent progress on the NHI following release of a Green Paper described later in this section has been regularly reported in the media (South Africa Council for Medical Schemes 2009; KPMG 2011; National Planning Commission 2011). Over 75 per cent of all public health facilities have been audited, but few facilities yet comply with standards and norms.

The new policy aims, in particular, to overcome the inequities and inefficiencies of the current two-tier system between a well-resourced private sector and poorly resourced public sector (Shisana 2010). The inequities are worsening: over the past decade, private hospital costs and specialist costs have increased above the Consumer Price Index (South Africa Council for Medical Schemes 2009), and there is further maldistribution of specific skilled human resources to the advantage of the private sector. The arguments in favour of an NHI, and comparisons with other countries, have been provided in the 'Green paper' (Republic of South Africa 2011) and shown in recent studies (South Africa Council for Medical Schemes 2009; Mills et al. 2012).

A 're-engineered PHC' will realign the dominance of a curative and hospital-centred service. Quality control and regulation will be implemented through the Office of Health Standards Compliance. The NHI will be funded from a number of sources: a mandatory tax, the fiscus, and from a payroll tax (South Africa Minister of Finance 2012); 'sin taxes' have also been raised unofficially in public discussions by state officials. A fundamental criticism is that there is very little chance of successful implementation of the NHI in the present situation of a debilitated, inefficient, ineffective, and dysfunctional state.

We have shown that it is not simply a lack of funds or even facilities which are the central factors to explain the poor health and development returns under the current system (Coovadia et al. 2009). There is, as pointed out earlier, a national unevenness in the capabilities of the civil service (Chopra et al. 2009). A recent publication comes to similar conclusions on the central problem of implementation and capability of the state (National Planning Commission 2011). The costing of the NHI has been both supported (Shisana 2010) and criticized by local economists (van den Heever n.d.). The 2012 Budget anticipates that the real GDP growth will stabilize to 4.2 per cent per annum by 2014 (South Africa Minister of Finance 2012). KPMG's recent report is much more optimistic and indicates the benefits of externalities (KPMG 2011). It is evident that much more operational and implementation research will be required given the complexity and scale of the transformation necessary to establish the NHI.

In a recent comparison of financing of health services in Ghana and Tanzania in comparison to South Africa (Republic of South Africa, 2011):

> overall health-care financing was progressive in all three countries, as were direct taxes. Indirect taxes were regressive in South Africa but progressive in Ghana and Tanzania. Out-of-pocket payments were regressive in all three countries. Health-insurance contributions by those outside the formal sector were regressive in both Ghana and Tanzania. The overall distribution of service benefits in all three countries favoured richer people, although the burden of illness was greater for lower-income groups. Access to needed, appropriate services was the biggest challenge to universal coverage in all three countries.

Syria—the subtle impacts of neo-liberalism

Syria has a population of 20.8 million people and a nominal GDP per capita of US $2802 and HDI of 0.632. For many years, joblessness, food riots, and hunger have become commonplace, and like many lower- and middle-income countries much of this being related to structural reforms and austerity measures promoted in the past by the International Monetary Fund and World Bank.

More recently, the volatility and uprisings of several countries in the Arab world, typified by Syria, have often been oversimplified as simply being viewed as an expression of the popular clamour for democracy. What is often less understood is that the situation is a manifestation of underlying economic dysfunction which has been fuelled, inter alia, by misplaced development efforts of Western countries keen to promote market reforms. Kasturi Sen and Waleed al Faisal (Sen and Faisal 2012) investigated the neo-liberal economic policies implemented in Syria and showed that it is leading to rising health inequity in the country. Although health indicators have been improving in Syria over the last 30 years, infant mortality rate (132 in 1970 to 14 in 2010); under-5 mortality (164 in 1970 to 16 in 2010); and maternal mortality rate (482 per 100,000 registered live births in 1970 to 45 in 2010), the introduction of neo-liberal market reform policies from 2003, several years before the current volatility, have begun to reverse these gains. Supported by the European Union and German Technical Cooperation agency, the Syrian State included in its 10th Five-Year Plan (2006–2010) a package of economic liberalization policies. Changes made to the operation of the health sector and the labour environment included: new health insurance schemes to replace universal coverage, fee-for-service charges introduced at public hospitals, which also led to numerous job losses. The impact was felt mainly at primary healthcare level where the increases of user fees have increased out-of-pocket expenses with the net result that the people can no longer afford the service, and rising disparity and inequity.

There is now evidence (Sen and Faisal 2012) that the economic liberalization measures are playing a significant role in reversing the gains previously made, reinforcing the rich–poor divide, fostering inequality, suffering, social divisions, and creating discontent, consequences which have often been overlooked by Western observers. In Syria, previously providing a top-down centrally managed state with a command and control structure and a strong emphasis on public health, primary care, health promotion, and disease prevention which, while being directive, had led to important health gains. The new measures, however, introduced to liberalize and commercialize the health system, despite benevolent intentions, have produced the opposite effect. While the West views discontent in Syria as largely political, the fact that it had been behind the promotion of liberalizing economic reforms is either discounted or dismissed (Sen and Faisal 2012).

Thailand—transforming towards universal access to health

Thailand has a population of 70 million, a nominal GDP per capita of US $5394 and HDI of 0.682. After improving health infrastructure for 30 years and implementing a range of different financial risk protection schemes over 40 years, Thailand was finally able to achieve universal health coverage in 2002 (Evans et al. 2012). This provides health insurance for all Thai citizens which guaranteed them access to a comprehensive package of health services.

Although this achievement was the result of many factors, the most significant intervention was an inspiring health reform scheme known as the Universal Coverage Scheme (UCS).

The intervention included policy formulation and implementation to provide an equitable entitlement to healthcare for all Thais in the form of a universal coverage system with three main features: (1) a tax-financed scheme providing services at the point of delivery free of charge. Although a small co-payment or fee of 30 baht or US$ 0.70 was charged per visit or admission, this was later abandoned in 2006. (2) A comprehensive benefits package with a primary care focus, including disease prevention and health promotion. (3) A fixed budget with caps on provider payments to control costs. In addition to this several mechanisms were set up to protect UCS beneficiaries. This included more stringent hospital accreditation requirements, an information hotline, a patient complaints service, and a no-fault compensation fund.

By the end of 2001 the UCS provided coverage to 75 per cent (47 million) of the Thai population. This was an especially impressive achievement given that 18 million people had previously been uninsured. Furthermore the 25 per cent of the population (18 million people) not covered in the UCS were either civil servants, retired people and dependants, covered by the Civil Servant Medical Benefit Scheme (CSBMS), or participants of the contributory Social Security Scheme (SSS) which covered private-sector employees.

Achieving the establishment of the UCS was remarkable. Not only was it achieved in the aftermath of the 1997 Asian financial crisis when the per capita gross national income was very modest (US $1900), but it went against the advice of external experts sceptical of its financial viability and was implemented with unprecedented speed.

In a recent 2011 assessment, which, a decade after its implementation, aimed to review the scheme's performance, the results show the impressive extent to which health inequities have been addressed, teasing out also what worked well and what did not; the reasons for these outcomes in equity were also elucidated (Evans et al. 2012). It was found that between 2003 and 2010 the number of outpatient visits rose from 2.45 to 3.22 per member per year and the number of hospital admissions rose from 0.094 to 0.116 per member per year. This improved access has led to much greater service equity and reduced medical impoverishment, which are indicators of the additional number of non-poor households falling below the national poverty line caused by the out-of-pocket costs of medicines and/or health services. This decreased significantly from 2.71 per cent in 2000 before the UCS was introduced to 0.49 per cent in 2009. It is not surprising that there is now a very low level of unmet need for health services in Thailand.

The UCS has led to a situation where there has been a marked decrease of out-of-pocket expenditure, which has been compensated for by an increase of government health sector spending through public subsidy. This progressive pro-poor spending has eliminated the rich–poor gap in out-of-pocket expenditure.

In addition to the described outcomes the scheme's success has proved to be resoundingly popular. The high percentage of UCS members who express satisfaction has grown from 83 per cent in 2003 to 90 per cent in 2010. Encouragingly also for the private sector, was that although many contracted healthcare providers were initially unhappy with the UCS, their own satisfaction rose from 39 per cent in 2004 to 79 per cent in 2010.

Although there has been much impressive improvement as already described, some other important areas that were part of the ambitious UCS reform did not make the same gains. There was very little strengthening of the primary healthcare system, primary prevention was not effective, and the reliability of the referral system is still weak. Furthermore there has not been much progress towards rationalizing the three insurance schemes; this revealed that further challenges were related to the political influences and power dynamics of institutional reform.

It is important to note that politicians, civil society, and technocrats all played major roles in pushing for the UCS reform. It required securing parliament's commitment to universal health coverage and advocacy through the policy, design, implementation, and evaluation processes. Prior experience gained from existing health insurance schemes was both positive and negative, and the lessons learned proved helpful in designing the UCS. The rapidity with which the plan was rolled out was because, even in 2001, Thailand already had a firm foundation upon which to implement the scheme. There was an extensive network of government-owned district health facilities, well-established health policy and systems, research institutions, public health administration capacities, and a computerized civil registration system.

One of the important innovations in the creation of the UCS was the creation of the National Health Security Office (NHSO) which acted as the purchaser on behalf of UCS beneficiaries. This meant that the Ministry of Public Health (MOPH) no longer wielded control over government spending on healthcare services and was able to focus on improving the quality of service provision. Throughout the process, research was vital in building up a supportive body of evidence. This was essential in countering fierce resistance to change from some stakeholder groups and establishing a critical mass of support.

There are important lessons in establishing universal coverage including extension of access to services, containment of costs, and strategic purchasing. Financing reform must go hand in hand with improving physical access to services.

India—shifting towards NHI at scale

India, the second largest country by population (with over 1.2 billion people), is the most populous democracy in the world. It has a nominal GDP per capita US $1388 and HDI of 0.547. Despite enormous recent development strides, the Indian economy is still, however, only the world's tenth-largest by nominal GDP. From 1991 the country began to adopt market-based economic reforms and has since become one of the fastest-growing major global economies, even though it is still a newly industrializing country. India faces many challenges. These include poverty, illiteracy, malnutrition, poor healthcare, and corruption. Indeed, though planning for a UC has begun, there remain deep flaws in the Indian Health System (High Level Expert Group 2011). *The Lancet* ran a series of seven papers on India with the final article (Reddy et al. 2011) concluding on one of the points of major relevance to this paper: the creation of an integrated national health system through universal health insurance. It is recognized that for this to work it will have to offer good quality healthcare provided by well-trained health staff. Given the current organization of healthcare this will mean restructuring of health governance. It will also be necessary to develop greater engagement with the community and being proactive in developing the necessary legislation that would enshrine the important

health entitlements that the Indian people need and deserve. The current public health system which is the primary provider of promotive, preventive, and curative health services to most of the people in India, has to be greatly improved, and the other providers in the health system (including the private sector) need to be steered towards integration. A call is made in *The Lancet* series for India to achieve universal healthcare for all by 2020. Given the massive scale and need for reorganization, this call appears to be unrealistic. Sengupta and Prasada (2011) point out that the economic growth path of India is dominated by a powerful corporate private sector, whose actions exacerbate rather than ameliorate inequities. Hence the de facto planning process does not concern itself with the health burdens of the majority nor indeed deal with the persistent, widespread, and crippling poverty, and the need for a public sector response, but tends rather to drift towards a laissez-faire, free-market approach. Although India desperately needs an efficiently managed and well-resourced public health system based on the principles of UC, the markedly dysfunctional health system requires a paradigm shift in making the transition.

Mexico—a labour-based approach

Mexico, with a population of 115 million people (13th largest in the world), a nominal GDP of US $10,153 per capita, and an HDI of 0.770, has a tragic history of colonization, dictatorship, rebellion, civil conflict, territorial wars, and economic instability. Against this background and despite great challenges, there has been surprising progress in implementing a UC scheme based on the principle of broadening coverage of workers (Knaul et al. 2012). In 2003, the country introduced *Seguro Popular*, an NHI scheme, which by 2012 had virtually become a UC which provided healthcare access to more than 50 million Mexicans previously excluded from insurance. The programme is based on three principles of protection: insurance against health risks, providing quality healthcare assurance, and insurance against the financial consequences of disease and injury. *Seguro Popular* has been successful in improving access to health services, providing financial protection, and reducing the prevalence of catastrophic health expenditures, which further impoverish the poor. *Seguro Popular* provides access to a package of universally comprehensive health services, which in Mexico is synonymous with social protection of health. Initially the system was a labour-based social security system but has progressed from then to become a vehicle for the universal social protection of health. The ethical basis for the reform is that access to effective healthcare is seen as a universal right based on citizenship. Each year the effects and impacts of the reform initiative are published and made available in the public domain through the scientific literature and release of new data. Despite the progress, the struggle to shift the health system so that it becomes an increasingly effective, equitable, and responsive health service remains a challenge. Further reforms will be required before the health system has been reorganized to function correctly. Nevertheless this carefully recorded documentation of the process to establish UC has considerable relevance for low- and middle-income countries.

Brazil—promoting equity through health and human rights

Brazil, the largest country in South America and the world's 5th largest country, both by geographical area and by population with over 193 million people (with a nominal GDP per capita of US $12,788 and HDI of 0.718), provides a striking example of how a country steeped in a long tradition of inequity can rapidly transform. It also shows that this can be achieved in a manner that is compatible with economic growth. Indeed with an impressive economic growth rate of 7.5 per cent (2010) Brazil has made formidable health achievements in recent years in fulfilment of the goal of universal, equitable, and sustainable healthcare and the right to health enshrined in its 1988 constitution (Kleinert and Horton 2011).

The historical development of the current health system has several unique features. Public health, created at the end of the nineteenth century has always featured as an important aspect of the health system. For example, two of Brazil's greatest scientific leaders, Oswaldo Cruz and Carlos Chagas, acted decisively against public health threats of the time. These included tropical diseases such as yellow fever, bubonic plague, and smallpox. In the process these public health interventions laid the foundation for the internationally renowned Oswaldo Cruz Foundation (FIOCRUZ) which continues these efforts and now employs over 7500 people across the country. It remains an institution which specializes in education, research, pharmaceutical, and vaccine production. Regrettably the health system was not always so progressive. Until 1985 a hospicentric, biomedical approach backed by a military dictatorship dominated the approach. Although it suppressed moves towards social and health equity, it nevertheless created the conditions for a strong civil-society movement that still flourishes today. With a change in government, that movement mounted a powerful drive for health reform, that ultimately resulted in the Unified Health System (SUS). These reforms broadened the definition of health beyond the biomedical paradigm. They incorporated stewardship into the thinking of the social determinants of health, education, poverty reduction, and preventive measures within the broader context of health as a human right. Especially interesting was the promotion of community participation at all administrative levels.

In 1989, Brazil was one of the most unequal countries. In the two decades since then, much progress has been made, which has significantly reduced regional and socioeconomic inequalities and poverty. According to the World Bank, poverty (at purchasing power parity of US $2 per day) has fallen from 20 per cent of the 190 million citizens in 2004 to 7 per cent in 2009. In the health sector the SUS has vastly improved access to primary and emergency care, notably enabling Brazil to have already achieved one target of MDG 1, to reduce by half the number of underweight children. Brazil is also on track to meet MDG 4 and realize a reduction in the mortality rate of children younger than 5 years by two-thirds. Brazil's HIV/AIDS policies and achievements have also been widely praised.

Comparisons

There are different approaches to the incorporation of private healthcare into national systems of UC. There are seven countries which finance more than 20 per cent of their healthcare through private health insurance: Brazil, Chile, Namibia, South Africa, the United States, Uruguay, and Zimbabwe. In South Africa, where privatized health services comprise the largest financial proportion of the total health system, there are many barriers.

The dominance of the private sector places constraints on achieving a fair, just, and equitable health system (Sekhri and Savedoff 2005).

A recent study (Lagomarsino et al. 2012) examined the structure of NHI reforms in nine countries: Ghana, Indonesia, the Philippines, Rwanda, and Vietnam are five countries which are at intermediate stages of reform. Four (India, Kenya, Mali, and Nigeria) are at a very early stage. On the whole, progress is unsatisfactory. Although the authors report some progress towards UC, citing increasing enrolment in government health insurance, enlarging the benefits packages, and reducing out-of-pocket spending with an increasing of the share of government in health spending, it is suggested that it would be helpful if there was one set of common, comparable indicators of progress towards UC.

Important as UC is as a strategy, some key observers (Gwatkin and Ergo 2011; Latkoet al. 2011) have warned about over-optimism in the provision of UC through NHI.

Intersectoral action for health

Given the wide range of social determinants of health, it is clear that interventions are required in many sectors of society, hence the importance of intersectoral action.

In a systematic review of intersectoral actions to promote the socioeconomic determinants of health it was found that few studies have been able to assess their extremely complex and context-specific nature. In one such study, an expedited, systematic 3-month review critically appraised some 10,000 selected articles against review criteria and found only 17 which met the inclusion criteria (Ndumbe-Eyoh and Moffatt 2012): a few of these studies reported on interventions which deal with structural determinants of health. The evaluation of the impact of intersectoral action was mixed, showing that it had either a moderate effect or no effect on the social determinants of health, and consequently a limited effect on health equity.

Overall these findings (Ndumbe-Eyoh and Moffatt 2012) suggest that much of the literature on the social determinants of health to advance health equity is mainly descriptive. There has been up until this time little emphasis on undertaking interventions. There has been even less concern with the types of measurements required to evaluate these. The earlier cited study emphasized the lack of available high-quality, rigorously evaluated evidence.

Global initiatives to address health inequality

A book produced by the WHO (Blas and Kurup 2010), *Equity, Social Determinants and Public Health Programmes* and edited by Erik Blas and Anand Sivasankara Kurup, stemming from the recommendations of the CSDH, offers a collection of different approaches and analyses of the social determinants of health that impact on specific health conditions.

There has been a number of recent global initiatives aimed at reducing health inequities. One notable example of this is that at the conclusion of the 13th World Congress on Public Health, held 22–27 April 2012 in Addis Ababa (Ethiopia), the World Federation of Public Health Associations (WFPHA) produced the *Addis Ababa Declaration on Global Health Equity* (World Congress on Public Health 2012), which was 'a call to act on closing some of the critical gaps in global health and well-being'. An article about the 13th World Congress on Public Health and the Addis Ababa Declaration by Dr Peter Byass, a Professor and Director of the Umea Centre for Global Health Research (Sweden), also appeared in the *Huffington Post* (Byass 2012).

A second example is the Global Health Corps. Founded in 2009, Global Health Corps (GHC) is developing a health equity movement by energizing a global community of emerging leaders. The programme had grown to 68 fellows, by 2012, serving in Burundi, Malawi, Rwanda, Uganda, and the United States (Global Health Corps 2012).

A third example is the Training for Health Equity Network (THEnet) (THEnet n.d.). THEnet is a consortium of health professional education institutions committed to achieving health equity. Responding to the priority needs of communities, it works by reforming medical education, research, and service. THEnet schools are consistent with this vision, demonstrating their social accountability by committing themselves to measure their own success by how well they meet the needs of people they serve.

A final example, the Global Action for Health Equity Network (Global Action for Health Equity Network n.d.) (HealthGAEN), is a global movement for health equity. It develops a programme of action to deal with the social and environmental determinants of health. It was established to build on the momentum, expertise, and partnerships that arose following the establishment of the WHO CSDH.

Global endorsement towards a new great transition

At the 67th meeting of the UN's General Assembly on 12 December 2012, the assembly unanimously adopted a resolution on global health and foreign policy. It urged governments to begin to move towards providing universal access to affordable and quality healthcare services (UN General Assembly 2012).

The Assembly also recognized that improving social protection was a necessary step towards UC. It saw social protection as empowering investment in people. It could assist people to adjust to changes in the labour market and economy. This was a necessary step to support a transition to a more inclusive, sustainable, and equitable economy. While planning or pursuing the development of UC, Member States were encouraged to continue investing in health-delivery systems. This was to be done to increase and safeguard the range and quality of services. It could also help meet population health needs.

Member States were also encouraged to recognize the interrelationships between the promotion of UC and other international policy issues, such as the social dimension of globalization, which includes inclusive policies, equitable growth, and sustainable development.

These global reforms, like those of demography and sanitation movements of the eighteenth and nineteenth centuries, and the continuing public health improvements in the twentieth century, including the expansion of immunization, promise another great transition—the provision of universal care by altering how the mechanisms of healthcare are financed and how health systems are organized (Forum on Universal Health Coverage 2012; Prince Mahidol Award Conference 2012; World Health Assembly 2011).

Acknowledgements

Text extracts from Republic of South Africa, National Department of Health, *National Health Insurance in South Africa*, Policy Paper, Government Gazette No. 34523, Government Notice No. 65712, Copyright © 2011, reproduced with permission from the South African Department of Health.

Notes

1. For more information about the WHO Commission on Social Determinants of Health, visit http://www.who.int/social_determinants/en.
2. Gini coefficient: this index measures the degree of inequality in the distribution of family income in a country. The index is calculated from the Lorenz curve, in which cumulative family income is plotted against the number of families arranged from the poorest to the richest. If income were distributed with perfect equality, the Lorenz curve would coincide with the 45-degree line and the Gini index would be zero; if income were distributed with perfect inequality, the Lorenz curve would coincide with the horizontal axis and the right vertical axis and the index would be 100 (Central Intelligence Agency 2012; World Bank 2012).
3. The Human Development Index (HDI) is a composite statistic of life expectancy, education, and income indices to rank countries into four tiers of human development. It was created by economist Mahbub ul Haq, followed by economist Amartya Sen in 1990, and published by the United Nations Development Programme. Its range is between 0 and 1 with higher indices being more desirable.

References

Abdool Karim, S.S., Churchyard, G.J., Abdool Karim, Q., and Lawn, S.D. (2009). HIV infection and tuberculosis in South Africa: an urgent need to escalate the public health response. *The Lancet*, 374, 921–33.

Acheson, D. (2000). Health inequalities impact assessment. *Bulletin of the World Health Organization*, 78(1), 75–6.

Alder, N.E., Boyce, T., Chesney, M.A., et al. (1994). Socioeconomic status and health. The challenge of the gradient. *American Psychologist*, 49(1), 15–24.

Amouzou, A., Habi, O., Bensaid, K., and Niger Countdown Case Study Working Group (2012). Reduction in child mortality in Niger: a countdown to 2015 country case study. *The Lancet*, 380, 1169–78.

Anonymous (2012). Mexico: celebrating universal health coverage. *The Lancet*, 380, 622.

Blas, E. and Kurup, A.S. (eds.) (2010). *Equity, Social Determinants and Public Health Programmes*. Geneva: World Health Organization.

Byas, P. (2012). Mind the gap ...*Huffington Post*, 28 April.

Carrera, C., Azrack, A., Begkoyian, G., et al. (2012). Equity in Child Survival, Health and Nutrition Analysis Team. The comparative cost-effectiveness of an equity-focused approach to child survival, health and nutrition: a modelling approach. *The Lancet*, 380, 1341–51.

Central Intelligence Agency (2009). *The World Factbook 2009*. Washington, DC: Central Intelligence Agency. Available at: https://www.cia.gov/library/publications/the-world-factbook/index.html.

Chadwick, E. (1843). *Report on the Sanitary Condition of the Labouring Population of Great Britain. A Supplementary Report on the Results of a Special Inquiry into the Practice of Internment in Towns*. London: Printed by R. Clowes & Sons, for Her Majesty's Stationery Office.

Cheng, T.-M. (2003). Taiwan's new national health insurance program: genesis and experience so far. *Health Affairs*, 22(3), 61–76.

Chiang, T.-L. (1997). Taiwan's 1995 health care reform. *Health Policy*, 39, 225–39.

Chopra, M., Daviaud, E., Panninson, R., Fonn, S., and Lawn, J.E. (2009). Saving the lives of South Africa's mothers, babies and children: can the health system deliver? *The Lancet*, 374, 835–46.

Chopra, M., Lawn, J.E., Sanders, D., et al. (2009). Achieving the health Millennium Development Goals for South Africa: challenges and priorities. *The Lancet*, 374, 1023–31.

Chopra, M., Sharkey, A., Dalmiya, N., Anthony, D., Binkin, N., on behalf of the UNICEP. (2012). Equity in Child Survival, Health and Nutrition Analysis Team. Strategies to improve health coverage and narrow the equity gap in child survival, health and nutrition. *The Lancet*, 380, 1331–40.

Cohen, N. (2012). Policy entrepreneurs and the design of public policy: conceptual framework and the case of the National Health Insurance Law in Israel. *Journal of Social Research & Policy*, 3 (1), 5–26.

Commission on Social Determinants of Health (2008). *Closing the Gap in a Generation, Health Equity Through Action on the Social Determinants of Health. Final Report of the Commission on Social Determinants of Health*. Geneva: Commission on Social Determinants of Health.

Coovadia, H., Jewkes, R., Barron, P., Sanders, D., and McIntyre, D. (2009). The health and health system of South Africa: historical roots of current public health challenges. *The Lancet*, 374, 817–34.

Countdown 2012 Report Writing Group (2012). Building a future for women and children. *The Lancet*, 379, 2121–2.

Dahl, E. (2002). Health inequalities and health policy: the Norwegian case. *Norsk Epidemiologi*, 12(1), 69–75.

Day, C., Barron, P., Massyn, N., Padarath, A., and English, R. (eds.) (2011). *District Health Barometer 2010/2011*. South Africa, Durban: Health Systems Trust.

Deaton, A. (2003). Health, inequality, and economic development. *Journal of Economic Literature, American Economic Association*, 41(1), 113–58.

Evans, T.G., Chowdhury, A.M.R., Evans, D.B., et al. (2012). *Thailand's Universal Coverage Scheme: Achievements and Challenges. An Independent Assessment of the First 10 Years (2001–2010)*. Nonthaburi, Thailand: Health Insurance System Research Office.

Forum on Universal Health Coverage (2012). *Mexico City Political Declaration on Universal Health Coverage: Sustaining Universal Health Coverage, Sharing Experiences and Promoting Progress*. Available at: http://www.who.int/healthsystems/topics/financing/MexicoCityPoliticalDeclarationUniversalHealthCoverage.pdf.

Global Action for Health Equity Network (n.d.). *Asia Pacific Health GAEN* [Online] Available at: http://www.hapi.org.uk/about-us/partners/healthgaen/.

Global Health Corps (2012). *History. Why We're Here*. [Online] Available at: http://ghcorps.org/why-were-here/history/.

Gostin, L.O. (2012). A framework convention on global health: health for all, justice for all. *Journal of the American Medical Association*, 307(19), 2087–209.

Government of Chile (2005). *The General Regime on Explicit Guarantees was established by Law 19.966. A list of 40 diseases and health conditions, and guaranteed services relating to those conditions, was established by Supreme Decree 228, issued by the Ministry of Health and the Treasury in 2005*. Government of Chile.

Gwatkin, D.R. and Ergo, A. (2011). Universal health coverage: friend or foe of health equity? *The Lancet*, 377, 2160–1.

High Level Expert Group (2011). *Report on Universal Health Coverage for India*: submitted to Planning Commission of India. New Delhi: Planning Commission of India.

Inequality.org (2011). *Cross-National Comparisons: Inequality and Health. Resource and Data Pack*. Inequality.org. Available at: http://inequality.org/inequality-health/.

Kahn, R.S., Wise, P.H., Kennedy, B.P., and Kawachi, I. (2000). State income inequality, household income, and maternal mental and physical health: cross sectional national survey. *British Medical Journal*, 321, 1311–15.

Kleinert, S. and Horton, R. (2011). Brazil: towards sustainability and equity in health. *The Lancet*, 377, 1721–2.

Knaul, F.M., González-Pier, E., Gómez-Dantés, O., et al. (2012). The quest for universal health coverage: achieving social protection for all in Mexico. *The Lancet*, 380, 1259–79.

KPMG (2011). *Funding NHI: A Spoonful of Sugar? An Economic Analysis of the NHI*. South Africa: KPMG.

Lagomarsino, G., Garabrant, A., Adyas, A., Muga, R., and Otoo, N. (2012). Moving towards universal health coverage: health insurance reforms in nine developing countries in Africa and Asia. *The Lancet*, 377, 933–43.

Latko, B., Temporão, J.G., Frenk, J., et al. (2011). The growing movement for universal health coverage. *The Lancet*, 377, 2161–3.

Lochner, K., Pamuk, E., Makuc, D., Kennedy, B.P., and Kawachi, I. (2001). State-level income inequality and individual mortality risk: a prospective, multilevel study. *American Journal of Public Health*, 91, 385–91.

Lu, J.-F.R. and Hsiao, W.C. (2003). Does universal health insurance make health care affordable? Lessons from Taiwan. *Health Affairs*, 22(3), 77–88.

Mayosi, B.M., Flisher, A.J., Lalloo, U.G., Sitas, F., Tollman, S.M., and Bradshaw, D. (2009). The burden of non-communicable diseases in South Africa. *The Lancet*, 374, 934–47.

McKeown, T. (1976). *The Modern Rise of Population*. London: Edward Arnold.

Mills, A., Ataguba, J.E., Akazili, J., et al. (2012). Equity in financing and use of health care in Ghana, South Africa and Tanzania: implications for paths to universal coverage. *The Lancet*, 380(9837), 126–33.

National Audit Office (2003). *International Health Comparisons. A compendium of published information on healthcare systems, the provision of healthcare and health achievement in 10 countries*. London: National Audit Office. Available at: http://www.nao.org.uk/idoc.ashx?docId=e902d344-ab56-4808-ab63-399241d33484&version=-1.

National Planning Commission (2011). Building a Capable State. In *National Development Plan. Vision for 2030*, pp. 363–99. Republic of South Africa: The Presidency.

Ndumbe-Eyoh, S. and Moffatt, H. (2012). *Assessing the Impact and Effectiveness of Intersectoral Action on the Social Determinants of Health and Health Equity: An Expedited Systematic Review*. Antigonish, Nova Scotia: National Collaborating Centre for Determinants of Health, St. Francis Xavier University.

Prince Mahidol Award Conference (2012). *Bangkok Statement on Universal Health Coverage*. Bangkok, Thailand, 24–25 January 2012. Available at: http://www.pmaconference.mahidol.ac.th/index.php?option=com_content&view=article&id=525:2012-bkk-statement-final&catid=981:cat-2012-conference.

Quigley, R., den Broeder, L., Furu, P., Bond, A., Cave, B., and Bos, R. (2006). *Health Impact Assessment International Best Practice Principles*. Special Publication Series No. 5. Fargo, USA: International Association for Impact Assessment.

Rawls, J. (1958). Justice as fairness. *The Philosophical Review*, 67, 164–94.

Reddy, K.S., Patel, V., Jha, P., et al. (2011). Towards achievement of universal health care in India by 2020: a call to action. *The Lancet*, 377, 760–8.

Republic of South Africa. National Department of Health (2011). *National Health Insurance in South Africa, Policy Paper*. Government Gazette No. 34523. Government Notice No. 657. Pretoria: National Department of Health.

Seedat, M., Van Niekerk, A., Jewkes, R., Suffla, S., and Ratele, K. (2009). Violence and injuries in South Africa: prioritising an agenda for prevention. *The Lancet*, 374, 1011–22.

Sekhri, N. and Savedoff, W. (2005). Private health insurance: implications for developing countries. *Bulletin of the World Health Organization*, 83(2), 81–160.

Sen, A. (1999). *Development as Freedom*. Oxford: Oxford University Press.

Sen, K. and Faisal, W. (2012). Syria neoliberal reforms in health sector financing: embedding in unequal access? *Social Medicine*, 6(3).

Sengupta, A. and Prasada, V. (2011). Towards a truly universal Indian health system. *The Lancet*, 377, 702–3.

Shisana, O. (2010). NHI consensus: fix the existing system or risk failure. *South African Medical Journal*, 100, 791–3.

South Africa Council for Medical Schemes (2009). *Annual Report 2008–09*. Pretoria: South Africa Council for Medical Schemes.

South Africa Minister of Finance (2012). *2012 Budget Speech by Minister of Finance, Pravin Gordhan*. Pretoria: National Treasury.

The Commission on Social Determinants of Health Knowledge Networks, Lee, J.H., and Sadana, R. (eds.) (2011). *Improving Equity in Health by Addressing Social Determinants*. Geneva: World Health Organization.

THEnet (n.d.). *Social Accountability in Action. What we do. Evaluation framework*. [Online] Available at: http://www.thenetcommunity.org./what-we-do.html.

Tsountal, E. (2009). *Universal Health Care 101: Lessons for the Eastern Caribbean and Beyond*. IMF Working Paper. New York: Western Hemisphere Department.

UC Atlas of Global Inequality (2007). *Health Care Spending*. Santa Cruz, CA: Institute for the Future and Centre for Global and Regional Studies, University of California. Available at: http://ucatlas.ucsc.edu/spend.php.

UN Millennium Project (2005). *Investing in Development: A Practical Plan to Achieve the Millennium Development Goals. Overview*. New York: UN Millennium Project. Available at: http://www.unmillenniumproject.org/documents/overviewEngLowRes.pdf.

United Nations General Assembly (2012). *Sixty-seventh General Assembly. 53rd Meeting, Plenary. Adopting Consensus Text, General Assembly Encourages Member States to Plan, Pursue and Transition of National Health Care Systems towards Universal Coverage*. 12 December 2012. New York: UN General Assembly.

van den Heever, A. (n.d.). *Evaluation of the Green Paper on National Health Insurance. Old Mutual Chair of Social Security Policy Management and Administration*. Graduate School of Public and Development Management. University of Witwatersrand, Johannesburg, South Africa. Unpublished paper.

Victora, C.G., Barros, A.J., Axelson, H., et al. (2012). How changes in coverage affect equity in maternal and child health interventions in 35 Countdown to 2015 countries: an analysis of national surveys. *The Lancet*, 380, 1149–56.

Weissman, R. (1999). *AIDS and Developing Countries: Democratizing Access*. Washington, DC: Foreign Policy In Focus.

Wilkinson, R. and Pickett, K. (2010). *The Spirit Level. Why Equality is Better for Everyone*. London: Penguin Books Ltd.

Wilkinson, R.G. and Marmot, M.G. (2003). *Social Determinants of Health: The Solid Facts*. Geneva: World Health Organization.

Wilkinson, R.G. and Pickett, K.E. (2006). Income inequality and population health: a review and explanation of the evidence. *Social Science & Medicine*, 62(7), 1768–84.

World Bank (2012). *Development Research Group. Gini Index*. Washington, DC: The World Bank. Available at: http://data.worldbank.org/indicator/SI.POV.GINI.

World Congress on Public Health (2012). *The Addis Ababa Declaration on Global Health Equity: A Call to Action*. Geneva: World Federation of Public Health Associations. Available at: http://bit.ly/JMP6oS.

World Health Assembly (2011). *Sustainable Health Financing Structures and Universal Coverage*. Geneva: World Health Organization. Available at: http://apps.who.int/gb/ebwha/pdf_files/WHA64/A64_R9-en.pdf.

World Health Organization (2003). *Overview of the World Health Report 2003: Shaping the Future*. Geneva: WHO.

World Health Organization (n.d.). *Health Impact Assessment. Glossary of Terms Used*. Geneva: WHO. Available at: http://www.who.int/hia/about/glos/en/index1.html.

2.5

Genomics and public health

Vural Özdemir, Wylie Burke, Muin J. Khoury, Bartha M. Knoppers, and Ron Zimmern

Introduction and historical perspectives of genomics and public health

A grand challenge for twenty-first-century medicine is to understand how knowledge about human genomic variation and its interaction with the environment can be used, across the lifespan, to improve health and prevent disease. Some genomic applications are already well embedded in health systems; for example, many countries have newborn screening programmes that aim to reduce morbidity, mortality, and disability in people affected by hereditary conditions. The scope and context of genomic applications have evolved, however, since the completion of the Human Genome Project a decade ago. A growing number of candidate applications are currently in transition from basic science to public health practice, in the face of an increasingly global science (Rajan 2006; Bernstein et al. 2011; Hotez 2011; Lancet editors 2011; Suresh 2011; Dandara et al. 2012). Between 2009 and November 2012, more than 450 new genomic tests were identified from horizon scanning by the US Centers for Disease Control and Prevention (GAPP Finder 2012).

Until recently, genomics and public health rarely came together except in the context of population screening programmes for certain rare single-gene disorders (Burke et al. 2010; Zimmern 2011; Zimmern and Khoury 2012; Ozdemir 2014). The first of these was newborn screening for the inherited metabolic disease phenylketonuria (PKU), for which biochemical screening and diagnostic tests became available during the 1960s (Botkin 2005). Although this genetic disease was rare, screening was recognized as a public health responsibility because early diagnosis and treatment of affected infants could prevent serious mental and physical disability in the population.

As new interventions such as antenatal diagnosis for genetic disorders were developed during the next few decades, geneticists and some public health professionals became involved in assessing population needs for services offering these interventions (Royal College of Physicians of London 1991) and, in countries such as the United Kingdom where public health has a role in healthcare service organization and delivery, in commissioning and allocating resources for them. Enthusiasm for population screening broadened after the success of the early newborn screening programmes, to include screening adult populations for certain genetic conditions. However, a general distrust of public health motives for population screening, together with the malign legacy of the eugenics movement of the early to mid twentieth century, resulted during the late 1970s and 1980s in the distancing of medical genetics from mainstream public health.

The impact of the Human Genome Project: from medical genetics to genomic medicine

In 1990, the Human Genome Project began. This ambitious enterprise aimed to sequence the entire 3 billion DNA base pairs of the human genome within a 15-year time frame, providing the raw material for discovering the sequences of the complete set of human genes and, eventually, discerning their functions and how they contribute both to normal physiology and initiation and progression of disease. As it turned out, the sequencing project was finished ahead of schedule: a 'reference sequence' for the genome, including the almost complete sequences for its complement of around 25,000 genes, was published in 2003 (Collins et al. 2003).

The Human Genome Project accelerated progress in finding the genes that, when mutated, cause heritable diseases such as cystic fibrosis, Duchenne muscular dystrophy, and Huntington's disease. By the early years of the twenty-first century, the genes implicated in some 1800 of these genetic diseases (most of them very rare) had been identified and catalogued in the Online Mendelian Inheritance in Man database (Online Mendelian Inheritance in Man, OMIM® n.d.). The availability of molecular diagnosis for many of these conditions began to transform the practice of medical genetics and spurred attempts to find effective treatments.

The Human Genome Project also generated data and tools for a new wave of genetic epidemiology projects to search for gene–disease associations. In an effort to provide tools for such studies, research consortia, largely funded by public funding sources, instigated first the single nucleotide polymorphism (SNP) project and then the HapMap, 1000 Genome Project, the Encyclopedia of DNA Elements (ENCODE), and the Human Variome Project (Guttmacher and Collins 2005; ENCODE Project Consortium 2012; Patrinos et al. 2012). These initiatives collectively provided a map of common structural and functional variation across the genome in different populations. These resources are beginning to bear fruit in whole-genome association studies, where markers distributed across the entire genome are scanned for putative associations with the environment, a disease, or other phenotypes such as drug effectiveness and safety (Nuzhdin et al. 2012; Ritchie 2012). These studies, often carried out by large international consortia and involving many thousands of study participants, have also signalled the rise of 'infrastructure science' such as population biobanks, consortia and networks, and cloud computing that coexists with, and sustains, the classic discovery science (Knoppers and Hudson 2011; Shanker 2012; Knoppers and Özdemir 2014). The introduction of genomic infrastructure science has successfully led to discovery of common genomic variants associated with conditions including type 2 diabetes, coronary artery disease, and breast cancer (see, for example, The Wellcome Trust Case Control Consortium 2007; Nuzhdin et al. 2012).

During the same period, attention has also turned towards the subject of 'normal' human genetic variation and the opportunity of using data-intensive 'omics' technology platforms (genomics, proteomics, metabolomics) developed as a result of the Human Genome Project to identify biomarkers for common human diseases. A biomarker, as noted by the US National Institutes of Health (NIH) Biomarkers Definitions Working Group, is 'a characteristic that is objectively measured and evaluated as an indicator of normal biological processes, pathogenic processes, or pharmacological responses to a therapeutic intervention' (Biomarkers Definitions Working Group 2001). Seen in this light, a biomarker can be genetic, biochemical, or any other clinical measure, provided that it meets the definition as an indicator (Collins and McKusick 2001; Guttmacher et al. 2001; Burke and Trinidad, 2011; Khoury et al. 2012a; Özdemir et al. 2012).

Public health genomics

The population-level goals of the Human Genome Project, and the expectation that it will have a major impact on clinical health services and disease prevention, make the evaluation of genomics as a component of public health practice an essential part of the current life sciences agenda (Burke et al. 2010; Khoury et al. 2012a, 2012b). Genomics may assist public health practitioners to address heterogeneity of risks and stratified interventions. Genomic factors may also contribute to the assessment and management of important public health issues such as environmental health, nutrition, vaccines and infectious disease (Zimmern 2011). The growing understanding of genomic contributors to disease need not detract from efforts to address disease modifiable risk factors such as environmental exposures, social structure, and lifestyle. Rather, the unproductive debate about nature versus nurture can now be replaced with an integrated and synergistic approach of nature *and* nurture in public health practice (Burke et al. 2010; Zimmern 2011; Zimmern and Khoury 2012).

As with other emerging technologies, the challenge is to devise an efficient strategy to strike the right balance between 'premature translation' of genomics discoveries to public health practice versus the 'lost in translation syndrome' where genuine innovations fail to be recognized or used in practice, be it in clinical medicine or public health. A related challenge is to weigh the potential benefits and harms of genomics applications. The recognition of these challenges and opportunities and the need for an overarching integrative strategy to address them have led over the last decade to the emergence of the new field of public health genomics (Khoury 2003; Khoury et al. 2000, 2012a; Stewart et al. 2007).

This chapter outlines the theoretical underpinnings of public health genomics and its applications in practice. We then look in detail at important areas where public health and genomics intersect, underscoring populations as heterogeneous and dynamic structures: the use and evaluation of genetic and genomic tests, the criteria for population screening programmes involving genomic factors, and the use of genomics in disease prevention. We provide a three-tiered approach to group public health genomics applications based on their readiness for practice (Khoury et al. 2011). This is essential because we now have reached a stage in the field where claims for genomics tests are rapidly proliferating well beyond newborn screening. An evidence-based approach to public health genomics practice equips researchers, practitioners, patients, and policy makers with tools for informed decision-making. We note that new and innovative ways to evaluate evidence on new genomics applications are needed (Evans and Khoury 2013). Indeed, we will likely never have sufficient resources or time to conduct randomized controlled trials for each candidate genomics test. Of particular concern is the ascertainment of clinical and real-life utility of new genomics tests that will vary in different contexts. These analyses are followed by horizon-scanning on 'big data'-driven public health science, using the intersection of vaccine science and genomics (vaccinomics) as an example. We conclude by a consideration of the ethical principles for the application of genomics in public health practice and the challenges and prospects for public health genomics.

We assume that readers have an understanding of the basic principles of genetics. A glossary of important terms and their definitions is provided in Box 2.5.1.

Genes as determinants of health

The new era of genomics recognizes genes as one of the determinants of health (Fig. 2.5.1). An important feature of this model is that it emphasizes the interplay between genomic and environmental factors (an 'environmental' factor in this context is anything that is not genomic).

DNA sequence variation is not the only source of variation in gene function. In multicellular organisms, different types of cells acquire their functional characteristics by expressing different subsets of their genome in a specific temporal pattern. Differential gene expression is associated with chemical modifications to the DNA (such as methylation) that do not change the primary DNA sequence and are termed epigenetic. As cells of a specific type multiply, they stably transmit these epigenetic modifications to the cells they give rise to. Epigenetic mechanisms are likely to play a role in mediating changes in gene expression in response to environmental signals (Slomko et al. 2012). Epigenetic mechanisms are emerging as an important consideration in many common complex diseases, including diabetes and cancer (Sandoval et al. 2012; Slomko et al. 2012). Epigenetic changes are not generally thought to be heritable by the organism's offspring but there is evidence that trans-generational effects may occur (Richards 2006; Bohacek et al. 2012). More significantly, clarification of the role of epigenetics in disease aetiology may have important implications for public health action, related to the environmental factors associated with epigenetic change.

As discussed in Chapter 5.12 on genetic epidemiology, genetic components of human traits are dynamic, be they disease or drug exposure related, and fluctuate depending on the environmental context (Kalow et al. 1999; Özdemir et al. 2005; Begum et al. 2012). A book by Tobias et al. (2011) provides additional, practical background to all aspects of medical genetics and its clinical practice.

Box 2.5.1 Glossary of basic terms in genetics and genomics

Alleles	Variant forms of the same gene
Autosomes	Chromosomes that are not concerned with sex determination. Humans have 22 pairs of autosomes and two sex chromosomes
Biomarker	A factor used to indicate or measure a static or dynamic biological process (for example, a specific protein or genetic polymorphism)
Carrier	Usually refers to an individual who is heterozygous for a recessive disease-causing allele
Chromosomes	The structures within cells that carry the genetic information in the form of DNA
Dominant	A characteristic that is expressed even when the relevant gene is present in only one copy
Epigenetic	A factor or mechanism that changes the expression of a gene without affecting its DNA sequence, and is stably transmitted during cell division
Genome	The complete set of genetic information of an organism
Genotype	The specific genetic constitution of an individual
Germline	Relating to the sex cells, which transmit genetic information from one generation to the next
Haplotype	A specific set of alleles located on the same chromosome
Heterozygous	Carrying two different alleles of a gene
Homozygous	Carrying two identical alleles of a gene
Karyotype	A description of the number and structure of chromosomes in an individual
Locus	The location of a gene or DNA marker on a chromosome
Marker	A gene or other segment of DNA whose chromosomal position is known
Meiosis	The specialized cell division that takes place when sex cells (sperm or eggs) are produced. The members of each chromosome pair separate so each sex cell receives only one copy of each gene
Mendelian	Relating to the laws of inheritance discovered by Gregor Mendel
Mutation	A change in the sequence of DNA
Nucleotide	The molecular units that make up DNA and RNA. A nucleotide of DNA consists of a base (A, C, G, or T) linked to the sugar deoxyribose and a phosphate group
Penetrance	The likelihood that an individual carrying a specific genetic variant will show the characteristic determined by that variant
Phenotype	The observable traits of an organism such as eye colour and disease characteristics or response to a health intervention (e.g. drug side effects)
Polymorphism	A common genetic variant or allele (present in at least 1 per cent of the population)
Recessive	A characteristic that is only expressed when two copies of the relevant gene are present
SNP	Single nucleotide polymorphism: a DNA sequence variation that involves a change in a single nucleotide
Somatic	Relating to the cells of the body other than the germline (sex) cells and their precursors

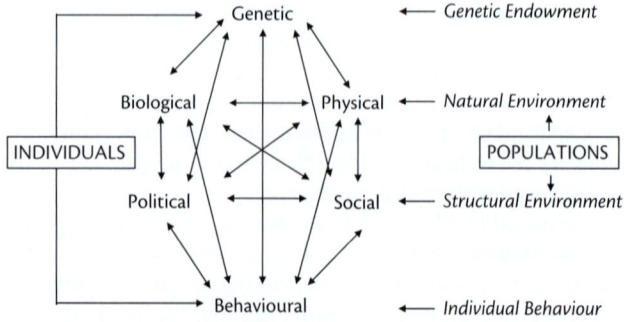

Fig. 2.5.1 Determinants of health.

Genomics and improving health

In this section, we discuss the range of use of genetic and genomic tests for improving population health. Some uses, such as newborn screening programmes, represent public health interventions. Others represent the use of genetic tests and knowledge in clinical care.

Newborn screening

Most highly penetrant genetic diseases are incurable, but clinical management of many of these conditions has improved in recent years, and for some conditions, life expectancy has increased significantly. In some cases, early detection of the disease, and early initiation of treatment, can significantly reduce mortality and morbidity. The classic example is the disease PKU, which is caused by deficiency of the enzyme phenylalanine hydroxylase (Kaye et al. 2006). If the disease is untreated, build-up of phenylalanine causes irreversible brain damage soon after birth. Early detection and initiation of a phenylalanine-free diet enables near-normal development. Sickle cell disease and cystic fibrosis also respond to early diagnosis and initiation of treatment in the newborn period, though the benefits are less dramatic than for PKU (Kaye et al. 2006). Newborn screening programmes may have other less direct benefits, such as in sparing parents of an affected child the often prolonged process of obtaining a diagnosis, and in counselling parents about the risk to subsequent pregnancies.

Newborn screening programmes for various conditions are in place in many Western countries. In some jurisdictions, including the United States, newborn screening programmes are state-mandated. In others, for example the United Kingdom, parental consent is sought. The apparent success of newborn screening for PKU, the development of new diagnostic technologies such as tandem mass spectrometry, and powerful advocacy by patient groups have led to pressure for widening newborn-screening programmes to include an increasing number of conditions. The Secretary's Advisory Committee on Heritable Disorders in Newborns and Children recommends screening for 31 core disorders and 26 secondary disorders (US Secretary's Advisory Committee on Heritable Diseases of Newborns and Children 2011).

There is ongoing debate about the scope of newborn screening (see Chapter 11.4). Serious concerns have been expressed about pressures to expand newborn screening panels (Botkin et al. 2006; Grosse et al. 2006; Elliman 2012). A major criticism is that many of the additional conditions depart from the key criteria identified (Wilson and Jungner 1968) for ensuring that population screening programmes deliver public health benefits. These criteria include the need to demonstrate that the natural history of the disorder is understood, that the characteristics of the screening test have been thoroughly evaluated, that an effective preventive intervention is available, and that screening is necessary to prevent death or serious disability. Some have called for a clear distinction between screening tests that meet the original goals of newborn screening, focused on improved health outcomes for infants, while others have called for expanding the purpose of newborn screening, to include other benefits, such as providing information to parents about reproductive risk or creating opportunities for research on rare diseases (Bailey et al. 2005; Alexander and van Dyck 2006; Baily and Murray 2008; President's Council on Bioethics 2008; Cody 2009).

The approach to the assessment of potential population screening programmes varies in different countries. In the United Kingdom, a National Screening Committee considers the evidence base for all proposed screening programmes, including those for genetic conditions. The Health Technology Assessment research programme has carried out reviews of newborn screening for some conditions (see, for example, Pandor et al. 2004), and most proposed programmes are piloted on a regional basis before being rolled out nationally. For example, a national newborn screening programme for medium-chain acyl-CoA dehydrogenase deficiency (MCADD) was introduced following a successful pilot study (National Screening Committee 2007). Ideally, research and clinical trials of new screening technologies should be funded promptly and adequately so that evidence to inform decisions about proposed screening programmes can be obtained as efficiently as possible.

Using genomics in risk assessment and disease prevention

An ultimate objective for those wishing to apply genomics in public health would be the ability to use genotypic information to identify groups of individuals who are at increased risk of disease and who could be offered opportunities to reduce their risk by means of interventions aimed at modifiable environmental factors such as diet. However, this is by no means a simple goal to attain.

The predictive value of genotypic information

The first problem in using genotypic information for prevention is the low penetrance of most of the alleles implicated in susceptibility to common disease. Individually, such alleles are typically associated with odds ratios of around 1.1 to 2.0, though rarer alleles may confer higher risks. For this reason, the positive and negative predictive values of tests for single alleles are likely to be low (see Fig. 2.5.2): most individuals who tested positive would gain no benefit from a preventive intervention because they would not have developed the disease in any case. Those who tested negative might be falsely reassured.

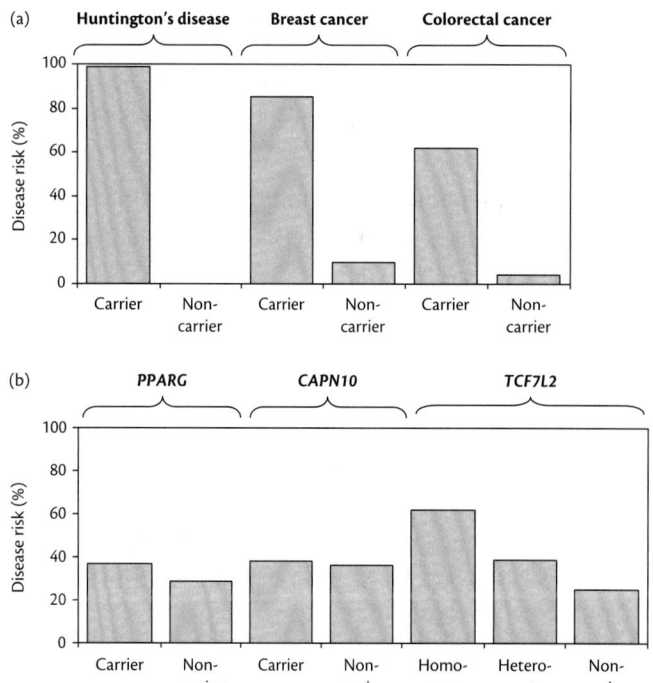

Fig. 2.5.2 Disease risks of carriers and non-carriers in genetic testing. In monogenic (Mendelian) disorders (a), carriers have a substantially increased risk of disease; non-carriers have a disease risk that approximates the population average. In the case of common disease (b), because risk alleles are generally common (population frequency 1 per cent or higher), carriers and non-carriers have disease risks that are only slightly higher or slightly lower, respectively, than the population average.

Reproduced with permission from Janssens and Khoury, Predictive value of testing for multiple genetic variants in multifactorial diseases: Implications for the discourse on ethical, legal and social issues, *Italian Journal of Public Health*, Year 4, Volume 3, Number 3–4, pp. 35–41, Copyright © 2006.

Some premature applications of genotypic information in prevention have been advocated. For example, since the discovery of the *HFE* gene, which is mutated in the iron-overload disease hereditary haemochromatosis, population screening for hereditary haemochromatosis has been proposed, based on *HFE* genotype. The rationale is that serious disease (liver cirrhosis, fibrosis, or diabetes) may be prevented by the simple procedure of frequent phlebotomy. However, although about 25–50 per cent of people with a predisposing *HFE* genotype have evidence of iron overload, it is not known how many of these people would, if untreated, progress to symptomatic disease; the penetrance of overt liver disease may be as low as 1–10 per cent. Public health has played an important role in the evidence-based evaluation of population screening for hereditary haemochromatosis.

It has been suggested that the predictive power of genotypic information would be increased if more alleles were considered together. This approach is called genomic profiling (Yang et al. 2003). Although individuals who carry multiple risk alleles will have a very high risk of disease, these individuals constitute a very small percentage of the population (Janssens et al. 2004). For the bulk of the population, genomic profiling will be extremely complex, depending on the number of risk genotypes tested for, the spectrum of risk alleles an individual carries, and the odds ratios associated with each of them (Janssens and Khoury 2006).

Pleiotropic effects of susceptibility genes must also be taken into account. For example, the *APOE4* variant increases risk for both Alzheimer's dementia and coronary heart disease but reduces risk for macular degeneration. Interventions aimed at preventing the negative effects of a gene variant might increase risk for another disease.

Behavioural responses to genomic risk information

The second problem is whether risk information based on genetic factors is likely to be effective in motivating the *sustained* behavioural change that would be needed to achieve health benefits. Current evidence on this issue is limited and more research is needed. The availability of an effective intervention is also important, as is the individual's assessment of his or her ability to achieve behavioural change; this assessment, in turn, is strongly dependent on the person's familial and social environment. There is some evidence that reactions to genetic risk information may differ from those to other types of risk information. For example, a recent study of individuals recently diagnosed with familial hypercholesterolamia through DNA testing found that perceived risk, and perceived efficacy of medication were higher than the 'no genetic predisposition' control sample (Claassen et al. 2012). This points to the need to present genetic risk information in such a way that it does not undermine the individual's belief in the efficacy of behavioural change.

There could also be a danger that information indicating an average or reduced genetic risk might be falsely reassuring, leading people to underestimate their risk and ignore advice about a healthy lifestyle. To date there is little evidence that false reassurance is a significant concern, though some more subtle effects of negative genetic test results have been observed. For example, among people with a family history of Alzheimer's disease (and therefore at increased risk),

those whose risk estimate included a negative test result for the *APOE4* polymorphism perceived their risk as lower than those with the same risk estimate based only on family history information (LaRusse et al. 2005).

A further relevant factor is the likelihood that people will take up an offer of genetic testing to indicate their risk. The public health impact of genetic susceptibility testing is likely to be low if few are motivated to take advantage of it. Those who have poor motivation to improve their health through behavioural and lifestyle change, or perceive a test result as a threat to their well-being rather than an opportunity to improve their health, are unlikely to perceive benefits from genetic susceptibility testing.

High-risk versus population approaches to prevention

The fundamental rationale for using genomics in the primary prevention of common diseases with environmental causes has also been questioned (see, for example, Merikangas and Risch 2003). One argument is based on Rose's (1985) observation that a greater reduction in overall disease incidence can be achieved by a small reduction in disease risk over a whole population, whereas targeting an intervention at a high-risk group results in a larger absolute reduction in risk for those individuals.

A further issue is the need for caution in applying population-derived risk estimates to decisions about individual patients (Rockhill et al. 2000). For example, Elmore and Fletcher (2006) have calculated that, although the Gail model for breast cancer risk prediction performs well at a population level, with a concordance of 0.96 between the expected and actual number of women in a population who develop breast cancer, at an individual level the concordance is only about 0.6. This problem is, of course, not unique to risk estimates based on genetics. Population-based risk estimates may best be used to stratify risk (so that, for example, an individual falls into a specific quintile) rather than to attempt to pinpoint individual risk. Population-based data will generate hypotheses about preventive action but these hypotheses must be tested rigorously in prospective outcome studies. Scientifically validated genotypic risk information is best used to enhance the predictive value of a 'package' of risk information that also incorporates measures of lifestyle and behavioural factors as well as relevant phenotypic biomarkers (Haga et al. 2003). Another approach is the Boadicea (Breast and Ovarian Analysis of Disease Incidence and Carrier Estimation Algorithm) that is used as a risk model to compute *BRCA1* and *BRCA2* mutation carrier probabilities and age-specific risks for breast and ovarian cancer (Antoniou et al. 2008). Further research is needed to determine the best way to communicate genetic risk information in order to achieve beneficial health outcomes.

Using family history in disease prevention

It is likely to be many years, perhaps decades, before it will be possible to use genotypic information routinely in the assessment of risk for common chronic diseases. It has been suggested that, in the meantime, family history information represents a useful surrogate that could be used more effectively and systematically in preventive healthcare than is currently the case (Yoon et al. 2002; Khoury et al. 2010b).

Family history is a risk factor for almost all diseases of public health significance, including most chronic diseases. Family history reflects the consequences of shared genetic variation at multiple loci (first-degree relatives such as siblings share 50 per cent of their genes), shared exposures to environmental factors, and shared behaviours.

Methods have been proposed for quantifying the risk associated with family history based on the number of family members affected, the degree of closeness of their biological relationship to the individual under consideration, and their ages at onset of disease (Yoon et al. 2002). From this information about their relatives, it is suggested that people can be stratified into average-risk, moderate-risk, and high-risk groups, and given appropriate preventive advice (Khoury et al. 2005). Those at average risk would be encouraged to adhere to standard public health prevention recommendations. Those at moderate or high risk would be given personalized recommendations including, for example, assessment and modification of risk factors, lifestyle changes, alternative early detection strategies, and perhaps chemoprevention. Those at high risk would also be referred to the specialist clinical genetics service to investigate the possibility of a high-penetrance genetic disorder. Although only a few people are expected to fall into the high-risk group, a much larger number will be assessed as being at moderate risk, offering the possibility of augmenting and improving the standard population approach to prevention.

Risk stratification based on family history is already in clinical practice as a form of triage for individuals concerned about a family history of some common cancers, such as breast/ovarian and colorectal cancer (see, for example, guidelines of the United Kingdom's National Institute for Health and Clinical Excellence (2006) for management of women with a family history of breast cancer and Doerr and Teng (2012) for primary care applications). This approach is not, however, used proactively as a screening programme.

The added value of the proactive use of family history risk-stratification as an adjunct to population-level prevention activities needs rigorous evaluation (Khoury et al. 2005, 2010b). Issues that must be addressed include the degree of accuracy of family history reporting, the optimum algorithm for stratifying risk, and the value of family history as a motivator for behavioural change. Particularly rigorous evaluation will be needed if a positive family history is used as an indication for any preventive intervention that carries risk, such as chemoprevention. Health service providers, particularly family practitioners, will need education and training in taking and assessing family histories, and provision must be in place for effective follow-up of individuals who fall into higher-risk groups. Health economic analysis should also form part of the overall assessment of the family history approach.

Genetic and genomic tests in clinical practice

Genetic and genomic tests may be used in clinical care for various purposes, including diagnosis of a disease, prognosis, assessment of disease risk, and prediction of response to a therapeutic (e.g. drugs) or preventive (e.g. vaccines) intervention (Burke et al. 2007; Teutsch et al. 2009).

Diagnostic genetic tests

Diagnostic genetic tests may be used to detect a DNA or chromosomal variant (or variants), or pathognomonic metabolic changes, associated with a disease. For example, in an infant with ambulatory problems, a DNA test may confirm a diagnosis of Duchenne muscular dystrophy. Often a diagnosis of a genetic disease provides important prognostic information as well. Where specific treatments are available, diagnosis may provide an essential guide to treatment. For example, a diagnosis of haemochromatosis provides information about the need to manage iron stores to prevent diseases associated with iron overload.

Risk assessment

Risk assessment is also an important tool in clinical practice: family history, as discussed earlier, provides an important risk assessment tool, and when family history suggests increased risk, genetic testing may offer an opportunity to identify specific individuals at high risk who would benefit from aggressive prevention efforts— e.g. BRCA testing to identify women with a high risk of breast and ovarian cancer.

Predictive genetic tests

Because an individual's germline DNA remains largely unchanged throughout life, DNA testing can in some circumstances be used in an asymptomatic individual to predict the risk of a specific genetic disease occurring in the future. The classic example is Huntington's disease, which may be predicted with almost 100 per cent certainty by a DNA test even before birth. A positive test result for a pathogenic mutation in the *APC* gene associated with familial adenomatous polyposis, an inherited form of bowel cancer, predicts future disease with 90–100 per cent certainty. In the context of highly penetrant Mendelian conditions, predictive testing is sometimes termed *presymptomatic testing*. However, this high degree of predictive value is rare. Huntington's disease has a population prevalence of about 1 in 20,000–40,000, and fewer than 0.5 per cent of bowel cancer cases are thought to be due to inherited mutations in the *APC* gene. In relation to common disease, the predictive value of DNA test information is much lower; such tests may be better described as susceptibility or predispositional tests.

Pharmacogenetic tests

Heritable genetic factors are known to result in marked person-to-person and population variability in drug effectiveness and safety. With origins in advances in biochemical genetics in the first half of the twentieth century, the field of pharmacogenetics examines these variable responses to drugs. For example, variants of genes encoding members of the cytochrome P450 family of drug metabolizing enzymes affect dosage requirements for a wide range of drugs including warfarin, codeine, clozapine, timolol and abacavir (Sim and Ingelman-Sundberg 2011; Warnich et al. 2011). The concept underlying pharmacogenetics is that it may be possible to use DNA testing, be it genotyping or gene expression analysis, to tailor drug prescribing to an individual's genetic make-up, thereby optimizing response and minimizing adverse reactions. The path from discovery of a validated polymorphism influencing drug response to a clinically useful pharmacogenetic test is a complex one. The anticoagulant drug warfarin provides an instructive example. Warfarin dose requirement is affected by variation in both the *CYP2C9* gene through effects on its pharmacokinetics, and in the *VKORC1* gene through effects on its molecular targets (Sanderson et al. 2005; Eriksson and Wadelius 2012). However, other factors such as age, sex, other genes, gene–gene and drug–drug interactions also affect warfarin response (and response to most other drugs). Further prospective studies in real-life clinical settings will help discern the extent to which *CYP2C9* and *VKORC1* testing might offer appreciable advantages over current best practice in warfarin prescribing, which includes careful clinical evaluation of the patient and post-prescription therapeutic drug monitoring.

Proposed pharmacogenetic tests need careful consideration based on intended clinical scenarios, including determination of diagnostic performance indicators such as sensitivity, specificity, positive and negative predictive values, and cost-effectiveness. The optimal parameters for a pharmacogenetic test will vary for different test indications. Pharmacogenetic tests for heritable variants remain mostly at the research stage but some somatic pharmacogenetic tests are already in clinical use, particularly in oncology. An example is the typing of *HER2* gene expression in breast tumours to test for responsiveness to the drug Herceptin® (trastuzumab), an antibody drug that targets the HER2 protein on the surface of tumour cells.

Gene expression profiling is under investigation as a tool to guide optimal treatment. For example, patients whose tumour gene expression profile, together with standard clinical criteria, indicates a good prognosis and a low probability of metastasis may be spared debilitating aggressive treatment with adjuvant chemotherapy. Gene expression profiling needs further evaluation before adoption for mainstream use in clinical pharmacology and therapeutics. In all, pharmacogenetic tests signal an expansion in the scope of genetic testing to address inter-individual differences in outcomes of health interventions such as drug therapy, in addition to disease susceptibility and prognosis. As we discuss later in the chapter, the emerging subspecialty of vaccinomics is yet another example of application of knowledge on human genomic variation to optimize health interventions.

Diagnostic genomic biomarkers

Genomic biomarkers such as gene expression, proteomic, or metabolomic profiles convey information about the molecular-genetic characteristics of somatic cells that may be correlated with clinical parameters such as disease staging, prognosis, and response to therapy. A hallmark of these data-intensive 'omics' biomarkers is that they offer a systems perspective on the informational value of a test, over and above the biological redundancies (e.g. overlapping metabolic pathways) preserved throughout the course of human evolution (Haring and Wallaschofski 2012). By contrast, biomarkers that target a singular pathway may incorrectly over- or underestimate their attendant predictive value. Gene expression and proteomic profiling remain an active area of clinical research, particularly in oncology, in part owing to ready availability of tumour biopsy specimens required for gene and protein expression analysis. Data on differences in regulation of gene expression is emerging as an important factor in health outcomes (Osman 2012), and this approach is postulated as an important avenue for identification of clinically useful biomarkers and, ultimately, new therapeutic approaches (Tian et al. 2012). Difficulties that need to be overcome include inadequate reproducibility, lack of standardization, failure to demonstrate improved outcomes as compared with current clinical practice, and poor positive predictive values, especially when used as screening tests in a population setting. Systematic approaches to ensure adequate validation of new tests have been proposed (Institute of Medicine 2012).

Reproductive genetic testing

Genetic testing also offers options for the assessment and management of reproductive risk. Diagnostic DNA tests carried out before birth (preimplantation or antenatal genetic diagnosis) may be used by couples at risk of transmitting a specific genetic disease to determine whether the embryo or fetus is affected by the disease. The purpose of testing is to enable the couple to exercise reproductive choice by either preparing for the birth of an affected child, opting to terminate a pregnancy, or, in the case of preimplantation diagnosis, choosing unaffected embryos to establish a pregnancy.

A special category of reproductive genetic test is a carrier test, which is used to detect a carrier of a Mendelian autosomal recessive or sex-linked disease. Individuals in families or populations affected by such diseases may wish to know whether they are carriers and therefore, although not themselves affected, at risk of transmitting the disease to their children.

Because decisions based on genetic information about reproductive risk are determined by personal values, these tests should not be recommended by health professionals. Rather, they are offered as an option, and the primary role of the health provider is to provide information and counselling so that prospective parents can make decisions about testing and follow-up that are most consistent with their goals and values. This testing therefore differs in its scope from testing intended to improve the health of the individual undergoing testing. Medical genetics has developed a supportive approach to counselling, focused on the educational and emotional needs of the individual or family seeking care (sometimes referred to as 'non-directive counselling') to address this practice need.

Evaluation of genetic and genomic tests

A US Task Force on Genetic Testing has defined a genetic test as 'the analysis of human DNA, RNA, chromosomes, proteins, and certain metabolites in order to detect heritable disease-related genotypes, mutations, phenotypes, or karyotypes for clinical purposes' (Holtzman and Watson 1997; see also definitions in Box 2.5.1). This definition implies that a genetic test is a test that enables a direct inference about the state of the germline genetic material. Any diagnostic test for a Mendelian disease or chromosomal disorder qualifies as a genetic test because it allows such an inference. For example, a renal ultrasound test for autosomal dominant polycystic kidney disease may be considered a genetic test because it enables the inference that there is or is not a lesion in one of the genes causally implicated in this disease. A biochemical analysis to detect haemoglobin variants causing sickle cell disease is also a genetic test. Any direct DNA test is a genetic test, whether it relates to a single-gene or chromosomal disorder, or to a low-penetrance genetic factor implicated in a common disease. However, a blood pressure test, for example, is not a genetic test by this definition because it does not enable any direct inference about the sequence or properties of a specific gene or genes.

The nature and implications of a genetic test can vary widely, depending largely on the penetrance of the condition or the genotype in question. It is important, when using the term genetic test, to be clear about whether it is being used to denote a test for a genetic (highly penetrant heritable) disease, or simply to mean a test of the genetic material (Zimmern 2001, 2014). A test for a genetic condition may have serious implications both for the person tested and for his or her blood relatives. In contrast, a test for a common DNA polymorphism associated with susceptibility to, say, coronary heart disease will probably have no more serious implications for health than analysis of blood lipids, and no greater consequences for other family members.

The 1997 US Task Force's definition cited earlier, specifically excludes somatic genetic tests, such as tests of the genetic material in tumour cells or gene expression profiles in different tissues or organs. However, the development, use, and evaluation of somatic genetic tests—perhaps better termed 'genomic tests'—also pose both opportunities and challenges for public health. Somatic genomic tests may also include tests for other complex genomic biomarkers such as proteomic or metabolomic profiles.

Evaluation of genetic and genomic tests

Public health programmes have an important role in ensuring that any diagnostic, predictive, or pharmacogenetic tests used in health practice are properly evaluated in order to protect the public's health and assure validated health services. A genetic test (or any other clinical test) encompasses more than a laboratory assay. Rather, it is a complex process that is part of an overall regime of disease prevention or management for a specific individual in an intended clinical scenario (Kroese et al. 2004). A test is best conceived of as the application of an assay for a particular disease, in a particular population, and for a particular purpose (Kroese et al. 2004; Zimmern 2014). An assay may be deemed highly effective in one set of circumstances but not in another.

The first attempt to devise an evaluation framework for genetic tests was the ACCE evidentiary framework (Haddow and Palomaki 2004), using criteria originally proposed by the 1997 Task Force on Genetic Testing (Holtzman and Watson 1997). ACCE is an abbreviation standing for **A**nalytical validity, **C**linical validity, **C**linical utility, and **E**thical, legal, and social implications. It has been acknowledged that ethical, legal, and social implications such as potential discrimination, stigmatization, and psychosocial consequences form part of the assessment of the overall utility of a test (Grosse and Khoury 2006; Burke et al. 2010), and there has been a trend away from regarding them as a separable set of issues. Additionally, the scope of ethics is presently expanding beyond classic issues such as informed consent and protection of research subjects to examine the issues related to genomics evidence: which evidence, generated, synthesized and funded by whom, should be employed to adopt or reject genetic tests? (Özdemir et al. 2013a, 2013b).

Analytical validity

The analytical validity is the means by which an assay is evaluated. It is defined as the assay's ability to measure accurately (in the case of a genetic test) the genotype of interest. It is important to define the genotype precisely. A test to detect 24 specific mutations in the *CFTR* gene is not the same test as one designed to detect only four mutations, for example. The test characteristics will differ in these two circumstances because the reference standard will be different. A distinction can also be made between open-ended assays such as karyotyping (microscopic examination of the chromosomes) or mutation scanning across a gene, in which any abnormality is sought, and closed assays, which specify in advance the spectrum of mutations or abnormalities the assay is designed to test (Burke and Zimmern 2007).

Clinical validity

Clinical validity is the ability of a test to diagnose or predict a specific phenotype (usually, a specific disease); here, the reference standard is a clinical one. The clinical validity of a test encompasses more than a demonstration of good epidemiological association between a test result (the presence of a genetic variant) and the disease. There must additionally be a formal evaluation of test performance in practice.

For closed assays, parameters such as sensitivity, specificity, positive and negative predictive values, likelihood ratios, and the receiver operating characteristic (ROC) curve can be measured as diagnostic test performance. Even if there is a strong association between a genetic variant and a disease, as has been shown for the *TCF7L2* polymorphism and type 2 diabetes, a clinical test for this polymorphism may have very limited predictive value and thus poor clinical validity (Janssens et al. 2006).

Assessment of clinical validity is more difficult for open-ended assays because the sought after variants or their proxies are not known in advance, thereby raising challenges to estimate the clinical performance of an open-ended test. Microarray comparative genomic hybridization (CGH) offers an example (Subramonia-Iyer et al. 2007). CGH is a new technique for detecting submicroscopic chromosomal abnormalities, including some never detected before, and some that are unlikely to be of clinical significance. In this setting, measures based on biological plausibility can be used to estimate the likelihood that a detected abnormality is clinically significant (e.g. nature and location of the abnormality; whether similar chromosomal abnormalities have been described in normal populations). With the use of these parameters, the test can be evaluated for its estimated diagnostic yield (proportion of those tested with a positive result) and false positive yield.

Clinical utility

Clinical utility refers to the likelihood that a test will lead to an improved health outcome, by way of reduced mortality or morbidity or improved healthcare. Factors that may be considered include the clinical risks and benefits of testing, such as the availability of an effective intervention and the risks associated with any interventions (Burke 2002; Burke et al. 2002; Burke and Zimmern 2007), and health economic assessment.

Clinical utility may be poor if, for example, available interventions are not genotype-specific. Carriers of the Factor V Leiden or *G20210A* prothrombin variants have an increased risk for venous thromboembolism (VT). However, genetic testing of VT patients does not aid clinical management, as current evidence suggests that these genetic variants do not significantly increase the recurrence risk for VT.

Clinical utility has proved very difficult to assess in practice. Burke and Zimmern (2007), using criteria based on Donabedian's work (Donabedian 1978, 2005) on the quality of medical care, suggest that the main dimensions of clinical utility relate to the purpose for which a test is used (legitimacy, efficacy, effectiveness, and appropriateness), and the feasibility of test delivery (acceptability, efficiency, and the economic dimensions of optimality and equity) (Table 2.5.1). This approach has merit when looking at a utility from an objective population health perspective. However, one may also conceptualize utility as being primarily a subjective parameter, and that presented with the same data and evidence, individual citizens may interpret those data differently and take a different view as to the appropriate action for them as individuals.

Table 2.5.1 Key questions in genetic test evaluation

Domain	Questions
Assay	*How accurate is the assay?*
Analytical validity	What are the analytical sensitivity, specificity, PPV, and NPV of the assay, as compared to a gold standard?
Reliability and reproducibility	How reproducible are the test results under normal laboratory conditions?
Clinical validity	*What is the predictive value of the test in a defined population, for the specified disease?*
Gene–disease association	What is the strength of the association between genotype and disease?
	Is the genotype a minimally sufficient cause of disease?
	Is the genotype necessary for disease to occur?
Clinical test performance	What are the sensitivity, specificity, PPV, NPV, LR+, LR–, and ROC of the test, compared to a gold standard?
	If these measurements are not possible, what is the basis for proposing clinical validity for the test?
Clinical utility	
Test purpose	*What is the purpose of the test?*
Legitimacy	Is the proposed test in keeping with societal values, norms, and ethical principles?
	Is test delivery in compliance with laws and regulations?
Efficacy	Can the test and associated services achieve the intended purpose under ideal circumstances?
Appropriateness	What are the benefits and negative consequences of testing?
	Do the benefits sufficiently outweigh the negative consequences?
Feasibility of test delivery	*Can the test and associated services be delivered equitably, and in an acceptable manner, for a reasonable cost?*
Acceptability	Is the test delivered in conformity to the wishes, desires, and expectations of patients and their families?
Efficiency	Can the cost of the test and associated services be lowered without diminishing benefits? If there is an alternative for achieving the same purpose, is the test more or less efficient?
Optimality	What are the costs of the test relative to the benefits? Is a formal analysis of cost-effectiveness needed?
Equity	Can the test and associated services be provided equitably among different members of the population?

We note that the acceptable answers to the questions are context sensitive, and do vary across different tests, persons, countries and technology governance frameworks.

Reproduced from Burke, W. and Zimmern, R., *Moving beyond ACCE: An expanded framework for genetic test evaluation*, Paper prepared for the UK Genetic Testing Network, Copyright © 2007, with permission of the authors.

The full evaluation of a genetic test is a complex process that requires significant resources. Because it is not possible to apply the full process to all tests, different levels of evaluation may be applied, depending on the nature of the test, its purpose, and the population in which it is to be carried out. For example, most tests for rare disorders require a less stringent programme of evaluation than tests for common disorders or population screening. This is because, when penetrance is high, the association between a positive test and ultimate outcome is more predictable, and the rarity of the condition means that the number of tests will be small.

In the United States, an ongoing model initiative of the Centers for Disease Control and Prevention, the Evaluation of Genomic Applications in Practice and Prevention (EGAPP n.d.), is spearheading the integration of various models of genetic test evaluations including in-depth assessments and fast-track evaluation.

Evidence-based classification of recommendations on use of genomic tests in practice

As the number of genetic tests increases, the task to evaluate the available evidence has become ever more challenging and data- and labour-intensive, suggesting a need for a system to classify genomics applications with a view to their readiness for public health action. Those who produce evidence (e.g. genomics test providers, scientists) and those who evaluate evidence (e.g. public health practitioners, regulatory scientists, social scientists) need to maintain an analytical distance for credibility and impartiality of decisions to transition (or not) candidate genomics applications to practice. The range of evidence taken into consideration may include prospective randomized controlled trials (RCTs) but often extend beyond so as to include observational and user-driven qualitative evidence, particularly on clinical utility of genomics tests. In addition, the existing binary (up or down) evidence-based recommendation for use of genomics tests often returns 'insufficient evidence' of clinical validity and utility for their use in clinical practice. The problem of insufficient evidence is not unique to genomics tests but is exacerbated by the lack of comparative effectiveness research (Khoury et al. 2010a). Binary or insufficient evidence recommendations do not permit refined decision-making, especially for clinicians who need to provide advice in the face of insufficient evidence. Khoury et al. (2011) have recently suggested a three-tier evidence-based classification of recommendations for use of genomic tests:

◆ Tier 1: 'use in practice'.

◆ Tier 2: 'promote informed decision-making'.

◆ Tier 3: 'discourage use'.

The intermediate category of promoting informed decision-making is particularly notable because it provides interim guidance for clinical and public health practice. The framework for assigning genomics applications to one of the three tiers requires consideration, in the context of intended use, of the analytic validity, clinical validity and clinical utility of the test, and the existence of an evidence-based recommendation.

Tier 1 applications demonstrate analytic validity, clinical validity, clinical utility, and there are evidence-based guidelines encouraging their use.

Tier 2 applications demonstrate analytic and clinical validity, display potential for clinical utility (e.g. well-designed trials with appropriately selected endpoints are known to be in progress), but there are no evidence-based guidelines recommending clinical use.

Tier 3 applications have not yet demonstrated adequate analytic validity, clinical validity or clinical utility, or have demonstrated evidence of harms. The use of such applications is discouraged.

The CDC Office of Public Health Genomics provides a list of genomic tests and family health history in practice according to the three levels of evidence to researchers, providers, public health programmes, and others. As this list of applications is updated dynamically on an ongoing basis, we encourage the reader to consult with the attendant online source (Centers for Disease Control and Prevention n.d.).

Integrating genomics into public health practice

We are moving from an era in which genetics has been a small specialist clinical service dealing with patients and families affected by rare heritable diseases, to one in which genomic information and technologies may become a normal part of mainstream clinical and public health practice (Khoury et al. 2011; Zimmern 2011). During the past 10 years, public health professionals have begun to realize that this transformation must be rationally managed and to put in place organizations and steering strategies for achieving this aim. Introduction of genomics to public health practice requires multilayered evidentiary frames integrated across stakeholders, and from analytical validity to clinical utility and public health ethics dimensions.

The emergence of public health genomics

During the 1990s, some public health professionals in the United States and the United Kingdom began to realize that public health practice must take account of developments in genomics. In the decade since 1997, public health genomics has increased in strength and influence. A growing body of academic literature has established the intellectual foundations of the discipline. Groups focused on public health genomics have been set up within both government organizations (for example, the Office of Public Health Genomics, US Centers for Disease Control and Prevention, and the Office of Population Health Genomics in the Western Australian Department of Health) and academia (for example, centres at the Universities of Washington and Michigan and at Maastricht University).

Translation of genomics to public health practice is at the epicentre of the current life sciences R&D agenda, and can be expected to remain in focus for at least the next decade. The recent US National Institutes of Health initiative to establish the National Center for Advancing Translational Sciences (NCATS) to pursue opportunities for disruptive translational innovation (Collins 2011) attests to the urgency of supporting translation science to move genomics to public health action. As we move towards an increasingly global science, public health genomics research and practice programmes with a similar mission and ethos need to be established in resource-limited settings in different countries. Conceivably, the existing genomics medicine networks can be scaled up so as to cultivate public health genomics in hitherto underrepresented global locales (e.g. Asia-Pacific, the Middle-East, Africa, etc.) and to ensure responsible integration of genomics to population health beyond a narrow technology-driven framework. Global expansion of public health genomics to developing countries and resource-limited settings is more than essential, to prevent a narrow technology lens in evaluation and implementation of genetic and genomic tests (Dandara et al. 2012; Özdemir and Knoppers 2013).

The Bellagio model for public health genomics

A multidisciplinary workshop convened in Bellagio, Italy proposed the following definition for public health genomics: 'Public health genomics is the responsible and effective translation of genome-based knowledge and technologies for the benefit of population health' (Bellagio Group 2005; Burke et al. 2006). This definition of public health genomics takes a population perspective to applications of new genome-based technologies to improve health. It focuses on prevention, evidence-based multidisciplinary science, and ethical, legal, and social implications, including addressing health disparities. The use of the term 'genomics' rather than 'genetics' signals that the subject matter is not confined to rare heritable diseases, and that much of the effort going forward will be directed at determining the contribution of genomic variants to disease pathogenesis using new genome-based technologies.

Building on this consensus definition, the Bellagio workshop developed a visual representation of the 'enterprise' of public health genomics (Fig. 2.5.3). The functions and activities shown in dark grey define the scope of the field. Several key features emerge from this representation:

1. The input to the enterprise is knowledge generated by genome-based science and technology, together with knowledge derived from academic research in the population sciences and practice on the ground, as well as the humanities and social sciences.

2. The driving force of public health genomics is knowledge integration. This term encompasses the activity of selecting, storing, collating, analysing, integrating, and disseminating knowledge, both within and across disciplines. It is the means by which genomics knowledge is transformed into 'situated' innovation that is contextualized for a given application, attuned to societal norms and hence, robust and sustainable (Ommer et al. 2011).

3. The integrated and interdisciplinary knowledge base is used to underpin four core sets of activities:

   (a) Communication and stakeholder engagement (including, for example, public dialogue and involvement, and engagement with a broad range of genomics stakeholders for an

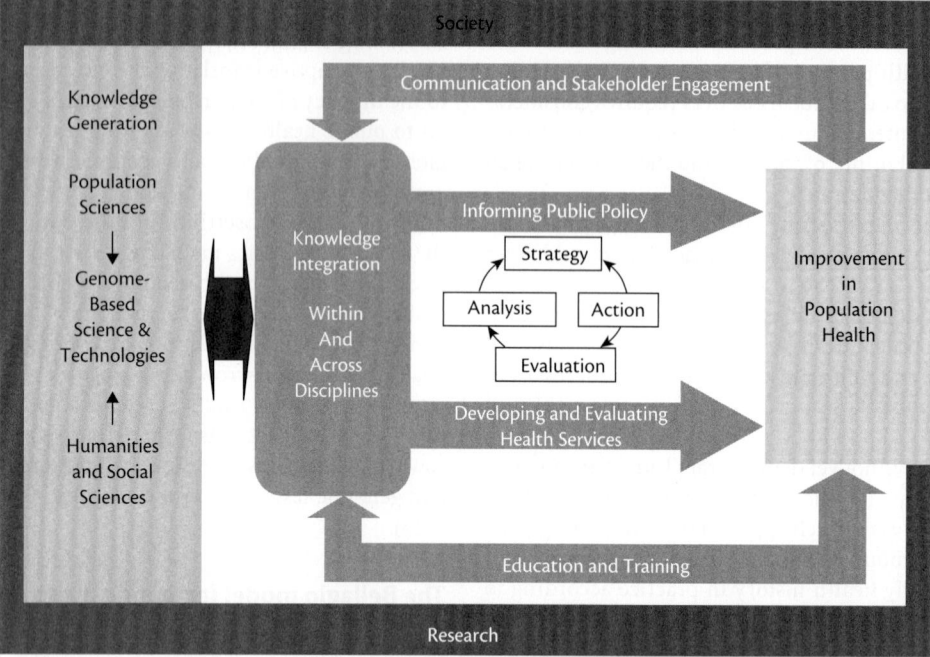

Fig. 2.5.3 The 'enterprise' of public health genomics. The scope of public health genomics is defined by the areas shown in dark grey.

'extended peer review' of genomics innovations in public health) (Özdemir and Knoppers 2013).

(b) Informing public policy (including applied legal and policy analysis, engagement in the policy-making process, seeking international comparisons, and working with governments and other innovation stakeholders).

(c) Developing and evaluating health services (including strategic planning, manpower planning, and capacity building; service review and evaluation; and development of new programmes and services).

(d) Education and training (including programmes of genetic literacy for health professionals and generally within society, specific training for public health genomics specialists, and development of courses and materials).

4. The mode of working of public health genomics is described by the recursive cycle of analysis–strategy–action–evaluation–calibration/adjustment, which is a widely recognized representation of public health practice, and one that allows mutual dynamic learning among the innovation stakeholders.

5. Public health genomics does include a research component defined in a classic sense, shown at the bottom of the diagram. This component is not generally basic research; rather, it is programmes of applied and translational research that contribute directly to the goal of improving population health and also identify gaps in the knowledge base that need to be addressed by further basic research. Hence, public health genomics is presently expanding the boundaries of classic notions of 'research' in that knowledge integration and bringing about 'change on the ground' are included. Ultimately, this is an invitation to rethink what is meant with 'research' and that the earlier mentioned hitherto underappreciated components are also *legitimate* building blocks of a research activity in twenty-first-century science.

6. Public health genomics does not operate in a vacuum. It is embedded within a social and political context and is informed by societal priorities. In other words, public health genomics recognizes that scientific knowledge is 'socio-technical' in nature, and a co-product of both technology and the social/political systems whose boundaries are highly porous. For robust knowledge-based innovations, public health genomics advocates tackling the socio-technical systems attendant to knowledge co-production, not to mention the provenance of the trajectory from data to knowledge to action.

7. Double-headed arrows throughout the diagram indicate the dynamic, bi-directional, and interactive nature of the enterprise: it generates knowledge as well as using it, and it is reflexively governed by the effects of its own outputs and activities.

An international network, the Genome-based Research and Population Health International Network (GRaPH Int n.d.) has been established to support the development of public health genomics and the sharing of resources worldwide (Stewart et al. 2006). The administrative hub of the network was based in Montreal and funded by the Public Health Agency of Canada. Today, it is located at the University of Maastricht, the Netherlands.

More recently, an international public health genomics meeting was held at Ickworth House, Suffolk, United Kingdom (Burke et al. 2010). The latter meeting has further endorsed the basis for public health genomics as the entire set of information stemming from the Human Genome Project and related environmental factors and data-intensive 'omics' sciences: not only gene sequences and gene–disease associations, but also information about the spectrum of gene expression activity, gene products and metabolites in different tissue types, and in normal and disease states (functional genomics, proteomics, and metabolomics) are taken into account.

'Big data' and vaccinomics for twenty-first-century vaccines

Twenty-first-century public health: data-intensive and collective innovation driven

'Big data' are now being sought to address the complex challenges we face in biology and other scientific fields such as global warming, climate change, and astronomy (Raddick and Szalay 2010). In the case of public health and biomedicine, the transition from genetics to genomics and other omics fields (proteomics, metabolomics, theranostics, etc.), new sensor and imaging systems to capture human phenotypic and biological variation, and attendant data-intensive simulation and computing have collectively resulted in a 'data deluge' in the twenty-first century (Smith et al. 2011; DaSilva et al. 2012; Özdemir and Cho 2012). Public health practitioners and life scientists increasingly have to deal with massive amounts of data in the order of petabytes (10^{15} = 1 million gigabytes = 1 thousand terabytes).

We are confronted with immense, globally distributed and heterogeneous datasets. Direct to consumer personal genomics tests that rely on big data (e.g. whole genome or exome sequencing for prediction of individual health risks) are bypassing the classic physician-centred health services and thus challenging the extant public health systems. Citizen-scientists also contribute to big data R&D, for example, in collection of high-granularity observations for ecosystem epidemiology where geographically distributed real-time science is crucial for human health. No longer are scientists forced to wait to generate data about human biological variation; instead, entire sets of scientific projects can be accomplished with online data sources. Moreover, social media analyses generate copious volumes of data that reveal insights on spread of infectious diseases and other emergency-preparedness measures to be taken in support of population health (Merchant et al. 2011). For example, after the 2010 earthquake in Haiti, crowd-sourced information on an open-source Web platform has served well to link healthcare providers requiring supplies to those who had them (Ushahidi-Haiti at Tufts University 2010). In the 2009 influenza pandemic, health departments have tweeted and texted to direct the public to sites where vaccine against H1N1 influenza was available (Merchant et al. 2011).

With declining cost of genome sequencing and the current age of big data science, genomics has also breached *Moore's law*: the concept that the number of transistors (and by extension, computation and data storage and analysis capacity) on a computer chip doubles every 24 months, allowing 'chip scale' to be reduced proportionately. Consequently, the bottleneck in data-intensive fields such as public health genomics has shifted to that of addressing the issues pertaining to *data analysis and storage* instead of the past emphasis on *sequencing* or data generation alone (Figure 2.5.4).

A very recent exemplary application of the big data and collective innovation driven science that is currently impacting twenty-first-century public health is the ENCODE, the Encyclopedia Of DNA Elements Project. ENCODE aimed to describe all functional elements encoded in the human genome and announced its results on 6 September 2012, 9 years after its inception (ENCODE Project Consortium et al. 2012). While the Human Genome Project completed a decade ago provided the code for human genetic make-up, ENCODE provides deeper insights

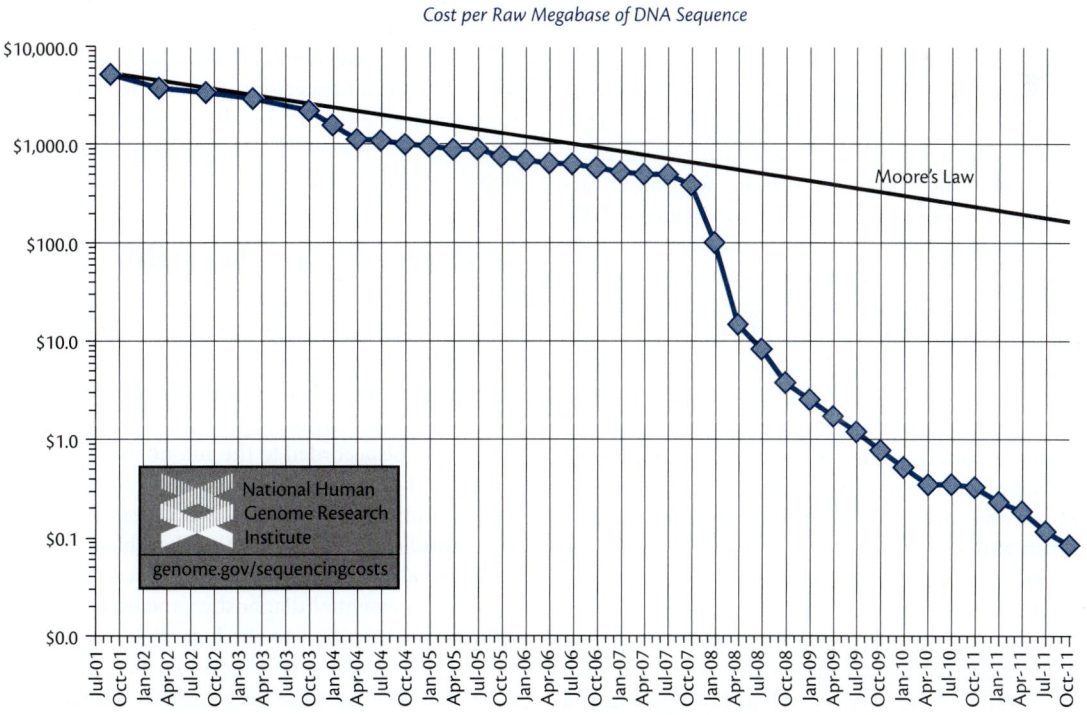

Fig. 2.5.4 Declining cost of sequencing a human genome. Moore's law is the concept that the number of transistors (and by extension, computation and data storage and analysis capacity) on a computer chip doubles every 24 months, allowing 'chip scale' to be reduced proportionately. However, in the years from 2007–2011, the rate of reduction in human genome sequencing cost has far exceeded the data analysis and storage capacity defined by Moore's law.

on the *functional architecture* of the human genomics variation. Most importantly, ENCODE has now assigned more than 80 per cent of the human genome's components to at least one biochemical function (ENCODE Project Consortium et al. 2012). ENCODE has ramifications not only for modern biology and public health in the decades to come, it also firmly attests to massively collaborative science, collective innovation and dizzying volumes of data that increasingly define and shape twenty-first-century scientific practice.

No doubt, striking the right balance between data collection and analysis is the next grand challenge, as we move towards genomics applications for public health practice in the age of ENCODE and other similar big science projects.

Vaccinomics: designing the next generation of vaccines

The collective innovation and big data driven science is being exemplified in new subspecialties emerging within the field of public health genomics. Vaccinomics is one such prototype example. Vaccinomics represents the entry of data-intensive 'omics' health technologies such as genomics to the practice of vaccine science. Vaccinomics is a rapidly emerging frontier in genomics medicine and twenty-first-century public health. Much like pharmacogenetics, discussed earlier, it is based on the premise that genomic differences at the individual and population levels can be used to develop safe and effective pharmacological treatments targeted to subgroups in the population, the development of vaccinomics is based on genomic (as well as integrated proteomic and metabolomic) variations which regulate the host immune response and host–pathogen interactions to develop safer and more effective personalized vaccine strategies.

In a recent analysis of the new field of vaccinomics, Bernstein et al. (2011) noted 'despite the historic successes of vaccines, or perhaps because of these successes, vaccinology has evolved to rely almost entirely on an empirical, trial-and-error process, in which the pathways to protective immunity remain largely unknown'. Enabled with systems-oriented omics health technologies, vaccinomics offers unprecedented promise to transform vaccine R&D and health promotion in the twenty-first century, with novel vaccines for common infectious pathogens (e.g. tuberculosis, HIV, malaria) as well as therapeutic vaccines for NCDs (Fig. 2.5.5). By virtue of broad applications in both preventive and therapeutic contexts, vaccinomics brings about a broadening in the scope and ethos of vaccine-based health interventions. The US NIH Clinical Trials registry identifies over 20 clinical trials at Phase III stage for therapeutic cancer vaccines (O'Meara and Disis 2011). The first therapeutic cancer vaccine (Sipuleucel-T) for castration-resistant prostate cancer was approved by the US Food and Drug administration. The US National Comprehensive Cancer Network recognized this agent as a Category 1 (highest recommendation) in 2010 (O'Meara and Disis 2011).

Vaccinomics can be anticipated to grow as a new strand of public health genomics scholarship in the next decade. On the other hand, for big data-driven fields such as vaccinomics to have a concrete and compelling impact on population health, the entire data to analysis to innovation trajectory, as well as both people and technology, need to be connected in order to achieve a form of knowledge ecosystem and 'collective intelligence' that is far more effective than any individual or singular group of people and

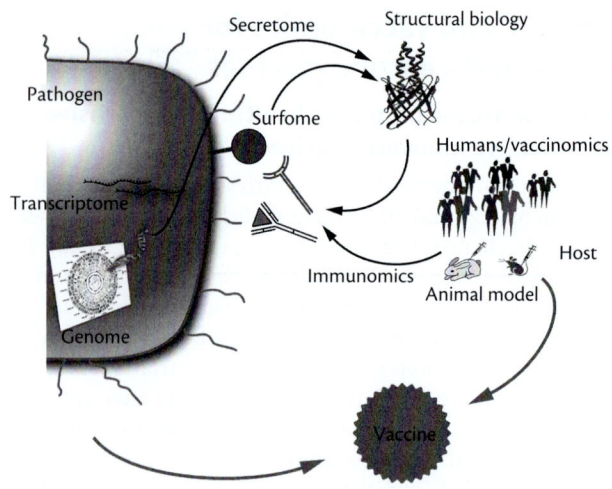

Fig. 2.5.5 Vaccinomics guided design of the new generation of vaccines. Vaccine candidates can be identified by analysis of the pathogen's genome and/or pan-genome (the complete genetic content of the organism/species), transcriptome (the complete set of RNA transcripts), surfome (the complete set of expressed surface proteins), or secretome (the complete set of expressed secreted proteins), immunomics (the set of antigens that are recognized by the human or animal host), and vaccinomics (human responses to a vaccine). Finally, structural biology is expected to provide the first information to build prediction methods to identify protective epitopes.

Reproduced with permission from Bagnoli, F., et al., Designing the next generation of vaccines for global public health, *OMICS: A Journal of Integrative Biology*, Volume 15, Issue 9, pp. 545–66, Copyright © 2011, doi:10.1089/omi.2010.0127.

computers. This seems essential given that vaccines and genomics have been met with both hope and pressures from funders and citizens to demonstrate their impacts for population health. Conflation of genomics and vaccine science in the form of vaccinomics offers much potential to engage with it at this early stage of the innovation trajectory, so as to steer it towards responsible innovation, one that is socially contextualized and subjected to 'extended peer review', as indicated earlier by the Bellagio model for public health genomics.

Genomics and public health ethics

The combination of genetics and public health has had an uneasy history, largely because of the legacy of the eugenics movement. Even today, there are still concerns about the potential tension between the population-level objectives of public health, the sensitive and personal nature of genomic information, and the priority that should be accorded to the autonomy of the individual citizen and the utility that he or she assigns to such information.

The traditional population-level approach of public health also raises another, more subtle, ethical problem in the era of genomic medicine: a reliance on the ethos of 'access' and 'provision'—for example, to essential diagnostics, medicines, and nutrition—but without due attention to the heterogeneity of the population to which these health-related services and goods are offered. It is important to allay these fears, which in many cases arise from framing of populations as a homogenous construct that may in turn compromise the ethical imperative to achieve optimum benefit from these interventions.

The legacy of eugenics

The term 'eugenics', literally meaning 'well born', was coined by Francis Galton in 1883. Its central philosophy was that the human gene pool could be 'improved' by selective breeding (Kevles 1995). Individuals judged to have a 'good' genetic constitution would be encouraged to have children, while those with 'poor' genes would be discouraged. The idea gained ground both in a number of European countries (including the United Kingdom and Sweden) and in the United States, despite ultimately discredited scientific backing. Some eugenic programmes involved the involuntary sterilization of large numbers of people deemed genetically 'unfit' because they were poor, homeless, or 'morally degenerate'. In Nazi Germany, eugenic principles were invoked to justify the murder of millions of people.

Beyond the human rights abuses, an important lesson of the eugenics movement is that efforts to define 'good' or 'bad' genetic heritage are deeply flawed and problematic. Moreover, definitions of allegedly good and bad human characteristics falsely assume that they are merely a result of an individual's genetics or autonomous moral agency; the acts and behaviours of human kinds are also co-produced by the 'habitus' wherein they reside, and the embedded power structures that interact with human agency (Bourdieu and Wacquant 1992; Rajan 2006; Özdemir et al. 2012). Even if 'good' and 'bad' traits could be defined, it would be impossible to select simultaneously for multiple 'good' traits and against multiple 'bad' traits. The eugenics movement has been rightly condemned, and repudiated in most countries of the world.

Use of genomic information: balancing the rights of individuals and society

Revulsion against eugenics has led to an insistence that genomic information is the property of the individual and his or her family. Individual autonomy, informed consent, and the privacy and confidentiality of genomic information have been paramount concerns. Numerous authors have warned about the dangers of stigmatization and discrimination against individuals on the basis of genetic characteristics.

Recently there have been attempts to re-balance the ethical debate and to move away from the concept that genetic information necessarily has a power and significance beyond that of other types of personal medical information—a concept known as 'genetic exceptionalism' (Murray 1997).

The development of applications for genomics to improve health will depend on the willingness of individuals to allow their genomic information to be used in population-based research projects designed to investigate low-penetrance genomic variants and genome–environment interactions that affect disease susceptibility. Concerns have been raised about the privacy and confidentiality of the genetic information of individuals participating in such projects. For example, full anonymization of samples and data may not be possible because the research may depend on the ability to link data to individuals. Moreover, the prospective nature of some epidemiological projects can mean that informed consent is difficult to implement fully: individuals may be asked to consent now to future uses of their samples and data that are currently unknown with additional data security and ethical oversight.

On the other hand, the ethical problems of large population studies may have been over-played. With appropriate protections in place, genomic studies are not likely to pose risks different from those people experience in their usual contact with the healthcare system and other entities that collect personal information. Although individual rights must be upheld, and genetic information must be protected just like any other personal data, community-centred ethical values such as solidarity, altruism, and citizenry must also be given due weight (Knoppers and Chadwick 2005). In this view, biobanks and population genomic research are seen as global public goods to be used for the benefit of current society and future generations (Knoppers 2005; Knoppers and Özdemir 2014).

These arguments do not deny the importance of high ethical standards for population-based projects and biobanking initiatives, in order to maintain the degree of public confidence that will be essential for the success of these long-term projects. Iceland's deCODE project attracted criticism as a result of the Icelandic Government's decision to assume that every individual in the country would be a participant in the project unless they specifically opted out, and to grant a commercial monopoly on any results from the project to the deCODE company. Other large-scale population biobanking projects have been more careful to avoid ethical controversy, for example, by establishing mechanisms for independent ethical oversight, paying careful regard to procedures for seeking informed consent from participants, and carrying out public consultations on project plans. Such measures appear to command broad approval although some disquiet persists, for example, over issues such as feedback of results to individuals, and terms for commercial access to samples and data. For the current biobanks initiatives around the world, the reader is referred to the international Public Population Project in Genomics (P3G) and Society (http://www.p3gconsortium.org). The P3G is also providing a platform for sharing best practice in ethical standards for biobanking initiatives.

Although procedures and norms for protection of individual research participants are well established, the potential for group harm from genomic research has received little attention, and represents an important area for both empirical and conceptual investigation. A qualitative study of stakeholder views related to genomic research in Africa identified a potential for group harm if the research involves populations already subject to stigmatization or addresses questions that have important ethical corollaries (de Vries et al. 2012). This concern points to the need for careful consideration of governance structures for data repositories, and, in particular, that the appeal to solidarity, altruism, and communal benefit is supported by vigorous oversight that ensures the use of data for societal benefit.

Population biobanks and databases are public goods; they are conceptualized as an unprecedented new configuration in twenty-first-century science—'infrastructure science'—in contrast to the long-standing, single scientist-driven entrepreneurship frames on 'discovery science' (Schofield et al. 2010). Infrastructure science represents an invaluable resource for subsequent discovery-oriented science. Hence, we are presently witnessing a new dual reconfiguration of twenty-first-century data-intensive public health science exemplified by the coexistence of infrastructure science and discovery science (Rajan 2006; Ozdemir et al. 2014).

Challenges and prospects for public health genomics

Integrating genomics into public health and behavioural research

Research is needed to strengthen the evidence base for applications of genomics in public health, particularly with respect to major public health problems such as obesity, outbreaks of infectious disease, or effects of exposure to environmental toxins and pollutants (Khoury et al. 2004, 2005; Evans and Khoury 2013).

Toxicogenomics and nutrigenomics

Toxicogenomics (sometimes referred to as 'ecogenomics') and nutrigenomics are important evolving areas of research that are attempting to unravel interactions between genomic variants and responses to toxic environmental agents and dietary constituents, respectively. There is good evidence that genomic variants do affect responses to these exposures but as with alleles associated with susceptibility to common disease, the predictive value of the individual risk alleles is generally low. For example, a polymorphism in the *DPB1* gene (part of the major histocompatibility complex, which encodes components of the immune system) increases risk of sensitization to inhaled beryllium dust, encountered by workers in the nuclear industry. However, although the relative risk conferred by the sensitizing *DPB1* allele is high (odds ratio ~10), the specificity of the *DPB1* marker is low, thus limiting its utility.

Many reported associations and gene–environment interactions in toxicogenomics and nutrigenomics have not been independently confirmed. For example, different studies have found opposite effects of the Pro12Ala variant of the PPAR-γ gene on the association between the dietary P:S (polyunsaturated:saturated fat) ratio and body mass index. Although non-replication can be due to poor study design, under-powered studies, and type 1 errors, these differences could also reflect true differences between the populations studied, as well as the known biological complexity of the role of PPAR-γ.

The fields of toxicogenomics and nutrigenomics are in their infancy, and it is likely that many years of research will be needed before validated evidence will be available to inform public health action. It is also important to ensure that this evidence, when it does become available, is used responsibly. Genetic effects on responses to environmental toxins or dietary components may identify some individuals or populations at high risk for whom specific preventive advice may be appropriate. Toxicogenomic and nutrigenomic research will also reveal important aspects of the biological mechanisms of interaction between environmental exposures and the human body. Such information could lead, for example, to better definition of the lowest tolerable dose for a toxin, based on the most susceptible genotype.

In terms of prevention, however, genomics is unlikely to supersede the value of standard public health advice for the bulk of the population. Public health practitioners must ensure that the benefits and risks of any proposed interventions or programmes based on toxicogenomics or nutrigenomics are carefully weighed, and that people are not misled by unsupported claims made by companies selling direct-to-consumer genetic test kits.

Infectious disease

The complete genomes of many important human pathogens have been sequenced, including those of the organisms implicated in tuberculosis, malaria, plague, leprosy, diphtheria, cholera, and typhoid. Genomic information is being used to develop new diagnostics, vaccines, and drug treatments (Warnich et al. 2011). For example, genomic technology and data-intensive omics sciences have provided important new leads for diagnosis of dengue fever in resource-limited countries (Ray et al. 2012). Research on the genome of the malaria parasite *Plasmodium falciparum* identified an unusual biochemical pathway for steroid synthesis and suggested that a drug (fosmidomycin) known to inhibit a crucial step in a similar pathway operating in bacteria and plants might be useful in treating malaria. Enabled by genomics, discovery of fosmidomycin is interesting because it is directed uniquely against *Plasmodium falciparum* malaria by inhibiting 1-deoxy-D-xylulose 5-phosphate reductoisomerase, an enzyme which is absent in humans (Umeda et al. 2011).

The process of infection involves not just the pathogen genome but also that of the host organism. The genomes of human populations have co-evolved with those of the pathogens that infect them, and resistance or susceptibility to infection has been a strong selective pressure in human evolution. A wide range of human genes, including the highly polymorphic genes of the immune system, are involved in human responses to pathogens. In some cases a single genetic variant appears to be significantly associated with susceptibility or resistance to a disease. For example, a specific polymorphism in the gene encoding the cell-surface receptor molecule CCR5 is associated with resistance to infection by human immunodeficiency virus (HIV). This candidate gene is of interest because the encoded receptor was known to be involved in entry of the virus into specific cells of the immune system. Analysis of genomic variants in resistant individuals may suggest new mechanisms and targets for drug development, or strategies for enhancing protective immunity in exposed populations.

Behavioural research

Public health programmes of disease prevention depend to a large extent on promoting behavioural change, but genomics has so far had little impact on behavioural research. It is particularly important, for example, that individuals who believe genetic testing has revealed they are at reduced risk from, for example, bladder cancer due to smoking, or coronary heart disease due to a high-fat diet, do not interpret 'reduced risk' as 'no risk'.

In addition, the role of genomic factors in health-related behaviours must be more fully explored. For example, genomic factors are known to affect the likelihood that smokers will develop lung cancer, but the picture is incomplete without an understanding of the genomic factors that affect risk-taking behaviour and nicotine addiction. A fuller understanding of the role of genomics in human behaviour may suggest new strategies to promote public health and prevent avoidable death and disease.

The impact of genomics on epidemiology

Genomics offers new opportunities for epidemiological research. In time, the familiar 2×2 table correlating disease status (for example, in a case–control study) with the presence or absence of an exposure or risk factor may routinely be replaced by a 2×4

table in which the underlying genotype at a particular locus or groups of loci will be measured and evidence sought for interaction with the risk factor.

New tools and resources are being developed for epidemiological studies involving genomics. For example, as mentioned earlier in this chapter, genomics is inspiring the establishment of large population cohorts and 'biobanks' to provide resources for the discovery and characterization of genes associated with common diseases. In addition to promoting gene discovery, biobanks will help epidemiologists to quantify the occurrence of diseases in different populations and to understand their natural histories and risk factors, including gene–environment interactions. Large cohorts may also be used for nested case–control studies or case-only studies as an initial screening method. These studies will produce a large amount of data on disease risk factors, lifestyles, and environmental exposures, and they will provide opportunities for data standardization, data sharing, and joint analyses (Khoury et al. 2004; Davey Smith et al. 2005).

Genomic research may also help to identify unknown environmental risk factors for disease or confirm suspected environmental risk factors, through the approach of Mendelian randomization (Davey Smith et al. 2005). The reasoning behind this approach is that if a genetic polymorphism affects the level of a biological intermediate in a way that mirrors the effect of an environmental exposure on the same intermediate, and if the biological intermediate in turn affects disease risk, then an association between the polymorphism and disease risk can act as a proxy for the relationship between the environmental exposure and disease risk. Mendel's law of random assortment of traits during transmission from parents to offspring means that this proxy relationship can be viewed as protected from the various confounding factors that affect observational studies of exposures.

The concept of Mendelian randomization can be illustrated by the example of the C677T polymorphism of the methylenetetrahydrofolate reductase (*MTHFR*) gene, which is needed for conversion of homocysteine to methionine (Khoury et al. 2005). The C677T polymorphism reduces MTHFR enzyme activity and increases levels of homocysteine, thereby mimicking the effects of low dietary folate intake. Thus a confirmed association between the C677T polymorphism and neural tube defects enhances causal inferences about the role of folate in neural tube defects. Although Mendelian randomization can potentially help epidemiologists derive better causal inferences about environmental exposures and disease, its application is currently limited by the paucity of confirmed genotype–disease associations, and incomplete understanding of the gene functions and biological pathways involved in the pathogenesis of common diseases.

Human genome epidemiology

Although thousands of gene–disease associations have been reported, only a small fraction of these have been independently replicated and fewer still can be considered fully validated (Khoury et al. 2007). Problems include publication bias, confounding by population stratification, faulty selection of control subjects, genotyping errors, deviations from Hardy–Weinberg equilibrium, linkage disequilibrium issues, misclassification of exposures and outcomes, inadequate statistical power, and type 1 errors (false positive associations). These problems point to a need for systematic evaluation and meta-analysis of studies to identify validated associations, question unsubstantiated claims, and flag promising candidates for further investigation.

The Human Genome Epidemiology Network, HuGENet, is a global collaboration of individuals and organizations that develops methods and guidance for integrating and disseminating knowledge on the prevalence of genomic variants in different populations, genotype–disease associations, gene–gene and gene–environment interactions, as well as evaluating genetic tests for screening and prevention (Khoury 1999; Little et al. 2003).

HuGENet's Web-accessible knowledge base captures ongoing publications in human genome epidemiology and is searchable by disease, gene, and disease risk factors. In collaboration with several journals, HuGENet also sponsors systematic reviews of the evidence on genotype–disease associations, using specific published guidelines for this work (the HuGENet handbook) as well as applying quantitative methods for evidence synthesis. Over 50 HuGENet reviews have been published on various diseases ranging from single-gene conditions to common complex diseases.

In 2005, HuGENet formed a network of investigator networks; these are mostly disease-specific research consortia that share knowledge, experience, and resources for human genome epidemiology investigations. The HuGENet Network of Networks has published a 'road map' for using consortia-driven pooled data and meta-analyses to augment the knowledge base on gene–disease associations (Ioannidis et al. 2006a, 2006b) and guidelines on the assessment of cumulative evidence on genetic associations (Ioannidis et al. 2008). HuGENet is also working on ways of integrating genetic epidemiological evidence on gene–disease associations with biological evidence.

Genomics in the developing world

Genomics and genomic technology will not replace traditional public health measures such as combating malnutrition, providing clean water and access to sanitation, alleviating poverty, and promoting sexual health. However, genomics offers potential benefits to the developing world, for example, in more rapid and accurate diagnosis of infectious disease (as discussed earlier in this chapter), enhancing the nutritional value of staple foods, bioremediation to reverse environmental degradation, and prevention of widespread human suffering by better recognition and management of genetic disease (Genomics Working Group of the Science and Technology Task Force of the United Nations Millennium Project 2004; Dandara et al. 2012).

It will be appropriate for different countries to adopt different strategies depending on the nature of their health problems, their economic situation, their social and political climate, their clinical and public health infrastructure, and the availability of trained medical and public health personnel. It is important to ensure that applications of genetics and genomic technology are thoroughly evaluated in pilot studies; that local expertise is fully engaged at all stages of the research, development, and implementation pathway; and that international aid is focused appropriately on developing local capacity, networks, and partnerships to cascade expertise and promote best practice. The appropriate targeting of global genomics research, in a manner that reflects the local and regional public health priorities, will remain an important challenge in the coming years. For example, in an analysis based on a PubMed-based systematic review of all the studies on human genetics that used Cameroonian DNA from 1989 to 2009, very few studies dealt with public health-related genetic issues: only 10 per cent of the reports were related to haemoglobinopathies such as sickle cell anaemia despite its pressing public health importance (Wonkam et al. 2011).

Management and prevention of genetic disease

As mentioned earlier in this chapter, the developing world carries the heaviest burden of genetic disease, contributing to a birth defects prevalence that is 50–100 per cent higher than in the developed world (Christianson et al. 2006). The most prevalent genetic disorders in the developing world are the haemoglobin disorders (sickle cell disease and thalassaemia) and glucose-6-phosphate deficiency. Approximately 7 per cent of the world's population are carriers of a haemoglobin disorder, and 300,000–400,000 babies with severe forms of these diseases are born every year, mostly in tropical regions (Weatherall and Clegg 2001). The public health impact of haemoglobin disorders is substantial and in some regions is increasing, as falling rates of childhood mortality due to malnutrition and infection mean that more individuals survive to present for diagnosis and treatment. Demographic changes such as migration are also increasing the prevalence of haemoglobin disorders in the developed world.

Chromosomal disorders and multifactorial conditions with a strong genetic component also have a significant impact on the developing world. For example, lack of effective family planning, leading to high birth rates for older mothers, contributes to a significant birth prevalence for Down syndrome. Congenital heart defects and neural tube defects make a substantial contribution to childhood mortality and morbidity. High rates of consanguineous marriages in some societies may increase the birth frequency of rare recessive diseases.

As a first step towards improving management and prevention of genetic conditions, both low-income and middle-income countries should seek to educate their communities and health professionals about these conditions, promote family planning, improve maternal health and nutrition, and establish child health services (Christianson et al. 2006). If economic and political circumstances allow, it may be possible to establish a medical genetics service, including training appropriate health professionals in clinical diagnosis of genetic conditions and basic genetic counselling, and considering implementation of appropriate neonatal and antenatal screening programmes.

For sickle cell disease, the most cost-effective approach is likely to be the development of national centres with expertise in screening, DNA diagnosis, education, counselling, and management of the conditions (World Health Organization Advisory Committee on Health Research 2002). Ideally, such centres would support and train personnel for a network of peripheral screening clinics focusing on neonatal screening and administration of oral antibiotic prophylaxis in childhood, and taking the lead in programmes of public education.

The thalassaemias present a different range of problems. Simple and cheap diagnostic techniques are available to diagnose the condition and detect carriers. However, disease management is more complex and costly than for sickle cell disease because the severe forms require lifelong blood transfusion (using blood that has been screened to prevent transmission of pathogens) and expensive drug treatment to remove the excess iron introduced by multiple transfusions. In some countries, programmes of antenatal carrier screening are considered acceptable to reduce the birth prevalence of disease. Once again, the model of centralized diagnostic laboratories and a network of peripheral screening clinics (in this case, for antenatal screening) may be appropriate. Antenatal carrier screening programmes have been in operation for many years in some Mediterranean countries, where as a result the birth frequency of beta thalassaemia has fallen by over 80 per cent (Cao et al. 2002).

In some middle-income, developing countries, such as the countries of South East Asia, changing lifestyles are leading to an increasing burden of disease from multifactorial conditions such as heart disease and diabetes, which may before long overtake communicable diseases as the major public health scourge in these countries. Although, as in the developed world, preventive strategies will be aimed at altering diet and lifestyle, some of the genetic variants underlying susceptibility to these conditions are likely to be population-specific. Genomic research in developing-world populations will be needed for a full understanding of the aetiology of disease and may point to a need for therapies and preventive interventions that are tailored for different population groups.

Genomic technologies in the developing world

In the wider sphere of genomic biotechnology, too, different strategies are appropriate for different countries (Genomics Working Group of the Science and Technology Task Force of the United Nations Millennium Project 2004). For some of the poorest countries, cheap genomics-based diagnostics may be cost-effective in programmes of infectious disease monitoring and control. International collaborations between the developed and developing world can help scientists in developing countries to gain access to appropriate technology, and to adapt this technology to a low-resource setting and a specific set of local conditions. Ongoing evaluation of any applications is also essential.

Some middle-income countries such as Cuba, Brazil, and Thailand are in a position to be able to develop their own biotechnology capacity. Governments in such countries need to create a favourable policy environment for genomic technology by investing in appropriate research, instituting transparent legal and regulatory frameworks and protection for intellectual property rights, stimulating their own biotechnology and pharmaceutical industries, and fostering public–private partnerships that are accountable to the public interest (World Health Organization Advisory Committee on Health Research 2002). Policies for applications of genomics and genetics must be sensitive to the ethical and cultural values of the country.

Training partnerships between industrialized and developing countries can help to develop human resources, and in some cases joint academic or clinical appointments can prevent the 'brain drain' of highly trained scientists and clinicians to more lucrative jobs in the developed world.

Education and training

In both the developed and the developing world, public health professionals must be prepared for the impact genomics will have on their practice (Austin et al. 2000; Burton 2003; Rajan 2006; Hotez 2011). As well as a working knowledge of basic genetics,

Box 2.5.2 Examples of some current initiatives in public health genomics

Centres

Office of Public Health Genomics, US Centers for Disease Control and Prevention

http://www.cdc.gov/genomics

Carries out research on how human genomic discoveries can be used to improve health and prevent disease. Established and coordinates the HuGENet (Human Genome Epidemiology Network) initiative.

Foundation for Genomics and Population Health (formerly the Public Health Genetics Unit)

http://www.phgfoundation.org

Multidisciplinary group that assesses advances in genetic science and their impact on health services and healthcare policy.

Centers for Genomics and Public Health

http://www.sph.umich.edu/genomics/
http://depts.washington.edu/cgph/

Established by collaboration between the US Centers for Disease Control and Prevention and the Association of Schools of Public Health, and located at the Universities of Michigan and Washington. The Centers contribute to the knowledge base, provide technical assistance to local, state, and regional public health organizations and develop and deliver training to the public health workforce.

Genomics, Health, and Society

http://genopole-toulouse.prd.fr/index.php?id=57

A multidisciplinary research centre located at the Toulouse Genopole, University of Toulouse, France, and including biologists, clinicians, geneticists, lawyers, sociologists, and economists.

Office of Population Health Genomics, Western Australian Department of Health

http://www.genomics.health.wa.gov.au/home/index.cfm

Aims to facilitate the integration of genomics into all aspects of public health, policy, and programmes.

Resources

HumGen

http://www.humgen.umontreal.ca

An international database on the legal, ethical, and social aspects of human genetics, developed as a collaboration between academia, government, and industry located at Faculty of Medicine, McGill University, Canada.

GDPinfo

http://apps.nccd.cdc.gov/genomics/GDPQueryTool/default.asp

A searchable database of all the documents available on the Office of Genomics and Disease Prevention Website, including the HuGENet database.

PHGU Genomics Policy Database

http://www.phgfoundation.org/policydb

A searchable web-based database of literature on policy development for genomics in health services and healthcare.

Projects

Evaluation of Genomic Applications in Practice and Prevention (EGAPP)

http://www.cdc.gov/genomics/gtesting/egapp.htm

The project aims to develop a coordinate process for evaluating genetic tests and other genomic applications that are in transition from research to clinical and public health practice.

P3G Consortium—Public Population Project in Genomics

http://www.p3gconsortium.org/

An international consortium to provide the international population genomics community with the resources, tools, and know-how to facilitate data management for improved methods of knowledge transfer and sharing.

Canadian Programme on Genomics and Global Health

http://www.utoronto.ca/jcb/genomics/index.html

Promotes the use of genomics and biotechnologies to improve health in developing countries.

HuGENet

http://www.cdc.gov/genomics/hugenet/default.htm

A global collaboration of individuals and organizations committed to the assessment of the impact of human genome variation on population health and how genetic information can be used to improve health and prevent disease.

they will need an understanding of human genome epidemiology and the criteria for evaluation of genetic tests, and an appreciation of the ethical, legal, psychosocial, and policy dimensions of applications of genomics and genomic technologies.

A set of competencies in genomics for the US public health workforce has been developed (US National Office of Public Health Genomics 2001). Competencies are documented for the workforce as a whole and for specific groups including leaders/administrators, clinicians, epidemiologists, health educationalists, laboratory staff, and environmental health workers.

In addition, some individuals will require an in-depth knowledge of public health genomics, for example, those involved in screening and other preventive programmes, health service development and evaluation, public health education, and policy analysis and development. Educational programmes in public health genomics are already underway at some centres.

Conclusion

While the full benefits of genomics for public health practice are likely to take many years to materialize, new technologies such as next-generation sequencing (NGS) have markedly reduced the cost and time (e.g. from 10 years to 1 week) required to sequence a genome (Raffan and Semple 2011). Moreover, NGS and other emerging high-throughput genomics technologies present an invitation to better understand the molecular basis of 'missing heritability' for traits that otherwise display a strong hereditary component. In particular the 'common trait, rare variants' hypothesis—an alternative (or complementary) to the hitherto prevailed 'common trait, common variant' hypothesis is now amenable for testing in clinical studies as we can more readily identify rare genetic variants with NGS. In the case of the 'the common trait, rare variants' hypothesis, multiple rare variants with moderate to high penetrances are assumed to collectively influence disease susceptibilities. Together with direct to consumer availability of NGS-driven personal genomics tests, this enhanced ability to characterize human genomics variation is blurring the boundaries between research and clinical practice (Dove and Ozdemir 2013, 2014a, 2014b; Petersen 2013), and creating a demand for more innovative frameworks to approach and evaluate clinical utility (Evans and Khoury 2013; Özdemir et al. 2013b).

In the course of these important changes brought upon by new genomics technologies and conceptual frameworks, public health genomics must take on the 'steering' role for the long-haul as knowledge strands converge and coalesce from public health and data-intensive genomics sciences (Halliday et al. 2004; Davey Smith et al. 2005; Zimmern and Khoury 2012). However, there is a need now to establish integrated and inter-generational capacity for both discovery and infrastructure science for the decades ahead. Leadership, sharing of resources (Box 2.5.2), and knowledge through international networks such as GRaPH Int and the Public Health Genomics European Network (PHGEN n.d.), programmes of professional education and training, and engagement with public policy development for genomics will all contribute to timely progress.

Ultimately, we need to rethink public health genomics as an effort to bring modern biology and science to public health to address population heterogeneity in disease and health intervention outcomes. In the absence of such knowledge, we risk a public

health practice that delivers inadequate and suboptimal responses to the extant disease burden in the population, not to mention health interventions such as drugs and vaccines with poor safety and effectiveness (Ozdemir 2014).

References

Alexander, D. and van Dyck, P.C. (2006). A vision of the future of newborn screening. *Pediatrics*, 117, S350–4.

Antoniou, A.C., Cunningham, A.P., Peto, J., et al. (2008). The BOADICEA model of genetic susceptibility to breast and ovarian cancers: updates and extensions. *British Journal of Cancer*, 98, 1457–66.

Austin, M.A., Peyser, P.J., and Khoury, M.J. (2000). The interface of genetics and public health: research and educational challenges. *Annual Review of Public Health*, 21, 81–9.

Bagnoli, F., Baudner, B., Mishra, R.P., et al. (2011). Designing the next generation of vaccines for global public health. *OMICS*, 15(9), 545–66.

Bailey, D.B., Jr., Skinner, D., and Warren, S.F. (2005). Newborn screening for developmental disabilities: reframing presumptive benefit. *American Journal of Public Health*, 95, 1889–93.

Baily, M.A. and Murray, T.H. (2008). Ethics, evidence, and cost in newborn screening. *The Hastings Centre Report*, 38, 23–31.

Begum, F., Ghosh, D., Tseng, G.C., et al. (2012). Comprehensive literature review and statistical considerations for GWAS meta-analysis. *Nucleic Acids Research*, 40(9), 3777–84.

Bellagio Group (2005). *Genome-Based Research and Population Health*. Report of an international workshop held at the Rockefeller Foundation Study and Conference Center, Bellagio, Italy, 14–20 April 2005. Available at: http://www.graphint.org/docs/BellagioReport230106.pdf.

Bernstein, A., Pulendran, B., and Rappuoli, R. (2011). Systems vaccinomics: the road ahead for vaccinology. *OMICS*, 15(9), 529–31.

Biomarkers Definitions Working Group (2001). Biomarkers and surrogate endpoints: preferred definitions and conceptual framework. *Clinical Pharmacology & Therapeutics*, 69(3), 89–95.

Bohacek, J., Gapp, K., Saab, B.J., et al. (2012). Transgenerational epigenetic effects on brain functions. *Biological Psychiatry*, 73(4), 313–20.

Botkin, J.R. (2005). Research for newborn screening: developing a national framework. *Pediatrics*, 116, 862–71.

Botkin, J.R., Clayton, E.W., Fost, N.C., et al. (2006). Newborn screening technology: proceed with caution. *Pediatrics*, 117, 1800–5.

Bourdieu, P. and Wacquant, L. (1992). *An Invitation to Reflexive Sociology*. Chicago, IL: University of Chicago Press.

Burke, W. (2002). Genetic testing. *The New England Journal of Medicine*, 347, 1867–75.

Burke, W., Atkins, D., Gwinn, M., et al. (2002). Genetic test evaluation: information needs of clinicians, policy makers, and the public. *American Journal of Epidemiology*, 256, 311–18.

Burke, W., Burton, H., Hall, A.E., et al. (2010). Extending the reach of public health genomics: what should be the agenda for public health in an era of genome-based and 'personalized' medicine? *Genetics in Medicine*, 12(12), 785–91.

Burke, W., Khoury, M.J., Stewart, A., et al. (2006). Bellagio working group. The path from genome-based research to population health: development of an international public health genomics network. *Genetics in Medicine*, 8, 451–8.

Burke, W. and Trinidad, S.B. (2011). Systems medicine and the public's health. *Genome Medicine*, 3(7), 47.

Burke, W. and Zimmern, R. (2007). *Moving Beyond ACCE: An Expanded Framework for Genetic Test Evaluation*. Paper prepared for the UK Genetic Testing Network.

Burke, W., Zimmern, R.L., and Kroese, M. (2007). Defining purpose: a key step in genetic test evaluation. *Genetics in Medicine*, 9, 675–81.

Burton, H. (2003). *Addressing Genetics, Delivering Health*. Cambridge: Public Health Genetics Unit.

Cao, A., Rosatelli, M.C., Monni, G., et al. (2002). Screening for thalassae-mia: a model of success. *Obstetrics and Gynecology Clinics of North America*, 29, 305–28.

Centers for Disease Control and Prevention (n.d.). *Genetic Testing: Genomic Tests and Family History by Levels of Evidence.* [Online]. Available at: http://www.cdc.gov/genomics/gtesting/tier.htm.

Christianson, A., Howson, C.P., and Modell, B. (2006). *March of Dimes Global Report on Birth Defects. The Hidden Toll of Dying and Disabled Children.* White Plains, NY: March of Dimes Birth Defects Foundation.

Claassen, L., Henneman, L., van der Weijden, T., Marteau, T.M., and Timmermans, D.R. (2012). Being at risk for cardiovascular dis-ease: perceptions and preventive behavior in people with and without a known genetic predisposition. *Psychology, Health & Medicine*, 17, 511–21.

Cody, J.D. (2009). An advocate's perspective on newborn screening policy. In M.A. Baily and T.H. Murray (eds.) *Ethics and Newborn Genetic Screening*, pp. 89–105. Baltimore, MD: Johns Hopkins University.

Collins, F.S. (2011). Reengineering translational science: the time is right. *Science Translational Medicine*, 3, 90cm17.

Collins, F.S. and McKusick, V.A. (2001). Implications of the human genome project for medical science. *JAMA*, 285, 540–4.

Collins, F.S., Morgan, M., and Patrinos, A. (2003). The human genome pro-ject: lessons from large-scale biology. *Science*, 300, 286–90.

Dandara, C., Adebamowo, C., de Vries, J., et al. (2012). An idea whose time has come? An African foresight observatory on genomics medicine and data-intensive global science. *Current Pharmacogenomics and Personalized Medicine*, 10, 7–15.

Dasilva, N., Díez, P., Matarraz, S., et al. (2012). Biomarker discovery by novel sensors based on nanoproteomics approaches. *Sensors (Basel)*, 12, 2284–308.

Davey Smith, G., Ebrahim, S., Lewis, S., et al. (2005). Genetic epidemiology and public health: hope, hype, and future prospects. *The Lancet*, 366, 1484–98.

de Vries, J., Jallow, M., Williams, T.N., et al. (2012). Investigating the potential for ethnic group harm in collaborative genomics research in Africa: is ethnic stigmatisation likely? *Social Science & Medicine*, 75(8), 1400–7.

Doerr, M. and Teng, K. (2012). Family history: still relevant in the genomics era. *Cleveland Clinic Journal of Medicine*, 79, 331–6.

Donabedian, A. (1978). The quality of medical care. *Science*, 200, 856–64.

Donabedian, A. (2005). Evaluating the quality of medical care. *Milbank Quarterly*, 83, 691–729.

Dove, E.S. and Ozdemir, V. (2013). All the post-genomic world is a stage: the actors and narrators required for translating pharmacogenomics into public health. *Personalized Medicine*, 10(3), 213–16.

Dove, E.S. and Ozdemir, V. (2014a). Glocal bioethics: when international IRB collaboration confronts local politics. *American Journal of Bioethics*, 14(5), 20–3.

Dove, E.S. and Ozdemir, V. (2014b). The epiknowledge of socially responsi-ble innovation. *EMBO Reports*, 15(5), 462–3.

Elliman, D. (2012). Ethical aspects of the expansion of neonatal screen-ing programme due to technological advances. *Clinical Chemistry and Laboratory Medicine*, 50, 999–1002.

Elmore, J.G. and Fletcher, S.W. (2006). The risk of cancer risk predic-tion: 'What is my risk of getting breast cancer?' *Journal of the National Cancer Institute*, 98, 1673–5.

ENCODE Project Consortium, Dunham, I., Kundaje, A., et al. (2012). An integrated encyclopedia of DNA elements in the human genome. *Nature*, 489(7414), 57–74.

Eriksson, N. and Wadelius, M. (2012). Prediction of warfarin dose: why, when and how? *Pharmacogenomics*, 13, 429–40.

Evaluation of Genomic Applications in Practice and Prevention (EGAPP) (n.d.). Website. Available at: http://www.egappreviews.org/default.htm.

Evans, J.P. and Khoury, M.J. (2013). The arrival of genomic medicine to the clinic is only the beginning of the journey. *Genetics in Medicine*, 15(4), 268–9.

GAPP Finder (2012). *Genomic Applications in Practice and Prevention (GAPP) Finder*. Atlanta, GA: Office of Public Health Genomics, Centers for Disease Control and Prevention (GAPP). Available at: http://www.hugenavigator.net/GAPPKB/topicStartPage.do (accessed 5 November 2012).

Genome-based Research and Population Health International Network (GRaPH Int) (n.d.). Website. Available at: http://www.graphint.org.

Genomics Working Group of the Science and Technology Task Force of the United Nations Millennium Project (2004). *Genomics and Global Health*. Toronto: University of Toronto Joint Centre for Bioethics.

Grosse, S.D., Boyle, C.A., Kenneson, A., et al. (2006). From public health emergency to public health service: the implications of evolving crite-ria for newborn screening panels. *Pediatrics*, 117, 923–9.

Grosse, S.D. and Khoury, M.J. (2006). What is the clinical utility of genetic testing? *Genetics in Medicine*, 8, 448–50.

Guttmacher, A.E. and Collins, F.S. (2005). Realizing the promise of genom-ics in biomedical research. *JAMA*, 294, 1399–402.

Guttmacher, A.E., Jenkins, J., and Uhlmann, W.R. (2001). Genomic medi-cine: who will practice it? A call to open arms. *American Journal of Medical Genetics*, 106, 216–22.

Haddow, J. and Palomaki, G. (2004). ACCE: a model process for evaluating data on emerging genetic tests. In M. Khoury, J. Little, and W. Burke (eds.) *Human Genome Epidemiology*, pp. 217–33. Oxford: Oxford University Press.

Haga, S.B., Khoury, M.J., and Burke, W. (2003). Genomic profiling to pro-mote a healthy lifestyle: not ready for prime time. *Nature Genetics*, 34, 347–50.

Halliday, J.L., Collins, V.R., Aitken, M.A., et al. (2004). Genetics and pub-lic health—evolution, or revolution? *Journal of Epidemiology and Community Health*, 58, 894–9.

Haring, R. and Wallaschofski, H. (2012). Diving through the '-omics': the case for deep phenotyping and systems epidemiology. *OMICS*, 16(5), 231–4.

Holtzman, N.A. and Watson, M.S. (eds.) (1997). *Promoting Safe and Effective Genetic Testing in the United States*. Final report of the Task Force on Genetic Testing. Available at: http://www.genome.gov/10001733.

Hotez, P.J. (2011). New antipoverty drugs, vaccines, and diagnostics: a research agenda for the US President's Global Health Initiative (GHI). *PLoS Neglected Tropical Diseases*, 5 (5), e1133.

Institute of Medicine (2012). *Evolution of Translational Omics: Lessons Learned and the Path Forward*. Washington, DC: National Academy Press.

Ioannidis, J.P.A., Boffetta, P., Little, J., et al. (2008). Assessment of cumula-tive evidence on genetic associations: interim guidelines. *International Journal of Epidemiology* 37, 120–32.

Ioannidis, J.P.A., Gwinn, M., Little, J., et al. (2006a). A road map for effi-cient and reliable human genome epidemiology. *Nature Genetics*, 38, 3–5.

Ioannidis, J.P.A., Trikalinos, T.A., and Khoury, M.J. (2006b). Implications of small effect sizes of individual genetic variants on the design and interpretation of genetic association studies of complex diseases. *American Journal of Epidemiology*, 164, 609–14.

Janssens, A.C.J.W., and Khoury, M.J. (2006). Predictive value of testing for multiple genetic variants in multifactorial diseases: implications for the discourse on ethical, legal and social issues. *Italian Journal of Public Health*, 4, 35–41.

Janssens, A.C.J.W., Pardo, M.C., Steyerberg, E.W., et al. (2004). Revisiting the clinical validity of multiplex genetic testing in complex disease. *American Journal of Human Genetics*, 74, 585–8.

Janssens, A.C., Gwinn, M., Valdez, R., et al. (2006). Predictive genetic test-ing for type 2 diabetes. *BMJ*, 333, 509–10.

Kalow, W., Özdemir, V., Tang, B.K., et al. (1999). The science of pharmacological variability: an essay. *Clinical Pharmacology & Therapeutics*, 66, 445–7.

Kaye, C.I., Committee on Genetics, Accurso, F., et al. (2006). Newborn screening fact sheets. *Pediatrics* 118, e934–63.

Kevles, D.J. (1995). *In the Name of Eugenics: Genetics and the Uses of Human Heredity*. Cambridge, MA: Harvard University Press.

Khoury, M.J. (1999). Human genome epidemiology (HuGE): translating advances in human genetics into population-based data for medicine and public health. *Genetics in Medicine*, 1, 71–3.

Khoury, M.J. (2003). Genetics and genomics in practice: the continuum from genetic disease to genetic information in health and disease. *Genetics in Medicine*, 5, 261–8.

Khoury, M.J., Bowen, M.S., Burke, W., et al. (2011). Current priorities for public health practice in addressing the role of human genomics in improving population health. *American Journal of Preventive Medicine*, 40(4), 486–93.

Khoury, M.J., Burke, W., and Thomson, E.J. (2000). *Genetics and Public Health in the 21st Century*. New York: Oxford University Press.

Khoury, M.J., Coates, R.J., and Evans, J.P. (2010a). Evidence-based classification of recommendations on use of genomic tests in clinical practice: dealing with insufficient evidence. *Genetics in Medicine*, 12(11), 680–3.

Khoury, M.J., Davis, R., Gwinn, M., et al. (2005). Do we need genomic research for the prevention of common diseases with environmental causes? *American Journal of Epidemiology*, 161, 799–805.

Khoury, M.J., Feero, W.G., and Valdez, R. (2010b). Family history and personal genomics as tools for improving health in an era of evidence-based medicine. *American Journal of Preventive Medicine*, 39(2), 184–8.

Khoury, M.J., Gwinn, M.L., Glasgow, R.E., et al. (2012b). A population approach to precision medicine. *American Journal of Preventive Medicine*, 42(6), 639–45.

Khoury, M.J., Gwinn, M.L., Khoury, M.J., Coates, R.J., Fennell, M.L., et al. (2012a). Multilevel research and the challenges of implementing genomic medicine. *Journal of the National Cancer Institute*, 2012(44), 112–20.

Khoury, M.J., Little, J., Gwinn, M. et al. (2007). On the synthesis and interpretation of consistent but weak gene-disease associations in the era of genome-wide association studies. *International Journal of Epidemiology*, 36, 439–45.

Khoury, M.J., Millikan, R., Little, J., et al. (2004). The emergence of epidemiology in the genomics age. *International Journal of Epidemiology*, 33, 936–44.

Knoppers, B.M. (2005). Of genomics and public health: building public 'goods'. *Canadian Medical Association Journal*, 173, 1185–6.

Knoppers, B.M. and Chadwick, R. (2005). Human genetic research: emerging trends in ethics. *Nature Reviews Genetics*, 6, 75–9.

Knoppers, B.M. and Hudson, T.J. (2011). The art and science of biobanking. *Human Genetics*, 130(3), 329–32.

Knoppers, B.M. and Özdemir, V. (2014). Biogenetics and the concept of humanity. In B.B. Van Beers (ed.) *Research Project in Humanity*. Cambridge: Cambridge University Press.

Kroese, M., Zimmern, R.L., and Sanderson, S. (2004). Genetic tests and their evaluation: can we answer the key questions? *Genetics in Medicine*, 6, 475–80.

Lancet editors. [No authors listed] (2011). Two days in New York: reflections on the UN NCD summit. *Lancet Oncology*, 12(11), 981.

LaRusse, S., Roberts, J.S., Marteau, T.M., et al. (2005). Genetic susceptibility testing versus family history-based risk assessment: impact on perceived risk of Alzheimer disease. *Genetics in Medicine*, 7, 48–53.

Little, J., Khoury, M.J., Bradley, L., et al. (2003). The human genome project is complete. How do we develop a handle for the pump? *American Journal of Epidemiology*, 157, 667–73.

Merchant, R.M., Elmer, S., and Lurie, N. (2011). Integrating social media into emergency-preparedness efforts. *The New England Journal of Medicine*, 365(4), 289–91.

Merikangas, K.R. and Risch, N. (2003). Genomic priorities and public health. *Science*, 302, 599–601.

Murray, T. (1997). Genetic exceptionalism and 'future diaries': is genetic information different from other medical information? In M.A. Rothstein (ed.) *Genetic Secrets: Protecting Privacy and Confidentiality in the Genetic Era*, pp. 60–73. New Haven, CT: Yale University Press.

National Institute for Health and Clinical Excellence (2006). *Familial Breast Cancer: The Classification and Care of Women at Risk of Familial Breast Cancer in Primary, Secondary and Tertiary Care*. London: NICE. Available at: http://www.nice.org.uk/guidance/CG41.

National Office of Public Health Genomics (2001). *Genomic Competencies for the Public Health Workforce*. Available at: http://www.cdc.gov/genomics/training/competencies/default.htm.

National Screening Committee (2007). *National Screening Committee Policy—Medium Chain Acyl CoA Dehydrogenase Deficiency Screening*. Available at: http://www.library.nhs.uk/guidelinesfinder/ViewResource.aspx?resID=57173.

Nuzhdin, S.V., Friesen, M.L., and McIntyre, L.M. (2012). Genotype phenotype mapping in a post-GWAS world. *Trends in Genetics*, 28(9), 421–6.

O'Meara, M.M. and Disis, M.L. (2011). Therapeutic cancer vaccines and translating vaccinomics science to the global health clinic: emerging applications toward proof of concept. *OMICS*, 15(9), 579–88.

Ommer, R., Wynne, B., Downey, R., et al. (2011). *Pathways to Integration*. Vancouver: Genome British Columbia GSEAC Subcommittee on Pathways to Integration.

Online Mendelian Inheritance in Man, OMIM® (n.d.). McKusick-Nathans Institute of Genetic Medicine, Johns Hopkins University (Baltimore, MD). Available at: http://omim.org/.

Osman, A. (2012). MicroRNAs in health and disease—basic science and clinical applications. *Clinical Laboratory*, 58, 393–402.

Özdemir, V. (2014) Personalized medicine across disciplines and without borders. *Personalized Medicine* 11(7), 687–691. Available from: http://www.futuremedicine.com/doi/pdfplus/10.2217/pme.14.70

Özdemir, V., Joly, Y., Kirby, E., et al. (2013a). Beyond ELSIs—where to from here? from 'regulator' to anticipating and shaping the innovation trajectory in personalized medicine. In Y.W.F. Lam and L. Cavallari (eds.) *Pharmacogenomics: Challenges and Opportunities in Therapeutic Implementation*, pp. 406–28. Amsterdam: Elsevier.

Özdemir, V., Badr, K.F., Dove, E.S., et al. (2013b). Crowd-funded micro-grants for genomics and 'big data': an actionable idea connecting small (artisan) science, infrastructure science and citizen philanthropy. *OMICS*, 17(4), 161–72.

Özdemir, V. and Cho, C.W. (2012). Theranostics: rethinking postgenomics diagnostics. *Expert Review of Molecular Diagnostics*, 12(8), 783–5.

Özdemir, V., Fisher, E., Dove, E.S., et al. (2012). End of the beginning and public health pharmacogenomics: knowledge in 'mode 2' and P5 medicine. *Current Pharmacogenomics and Personalized Medicine*, 10(1), 1–6.

Özdemir, V., Kalow, W., Tothfalusi, L., et al. (2005). Multigenic control of drug response and regulatory decision-making in pharmacogenomics: the need for an upper-bound estimate of genetic contributions. *Current Pharmacogenomics and Personalized Medicine*, 3, 53–71.

Özdemir, V. and Knoppers, B.M. (2013). From government to anticipatory governance: responding to challenges set by emerging technologies and innovation. In I. Kickbusch (ed.) *Governance for Health in the 21st Century*. New York: Springer.

Özdemir, V., Kolker, E., Hotez, P.J., et al. (2014). Ready to put metadata on the post-2015 development agenda? Linking data publications to responsible innovation and science diplomacy. *OMICS*, 18(1), 1–9.

Pandor, A., Eastham, J., Beverley, C., et al. (2004). Clinical effectiveness and cost effectiveness of neonatal screening for inborn errors of metabolism using tandem mass spectrometry. *Health Technology Assessment*, 8(12), iii, 1–121.

Patrinos, G.P., Smith, T.D., Howard, H., et al. (2012). Human variome project country nodes: documenting genetic information within a country. *Human Mutation*, 33, 1513–19.

Petersen, A. (2013). From bioethics to a sociology of bio-knowledge. *Social Science & Medicine*, 98, 264–70.

President's Council on Bioethics (2008). *The Changing Moral Focus of Newborn Screening*. Washington, DC: President's Council on Bioethics.

Public Health Genomics European Network (PHGEN) (n.d.). Website. Available at: http://www.phgen.eu/typo3/index.php.

Raddick, M.J. and Szalay, A.S. (2010). The universe online. *Science*, 329(5995), 1028–9.

Raffan, E. and Semple, R.K. (2011). Next generation sequencing—implications for clinical practice. *British Medical Bulletin*, 99, 53–71.

Rajan, K.S. (2006). *Biocapital: The Constitution of Postgenomic Life*. Durham, NC: Duke University Press.

Ray, S., Srivastava, R., Tripathi, K., et al. (2012). Serum proteome changes in dengue virus-infected patients from a dengue-endemic area of India: towards new molecular targets? *OMICS*, 16, 527–36.

Richards, E.J. (2006). Inherited epigenetic variation—revisiting soft inheritance. *Nature Reviews Genetics*, 7, 395–401.

Ritchie, M.D. (2012). The success of pharmacogenomics in moving genetic association studies from bench to bedside: study design and implementation of precision medicine in the post-GWAS era. *Human Genetics*, 131(10), 1615–26.

Rockhill, B., Kawachi, I., and Colditz, G.A. (2000). Individual risk prediction and population-wide disease prevention. *Epidemiological Reviews*, 22, 176–80.

Rose, G. (1985). Sick individuals and sick populations. *International Journal of Epidemiology*, 14, 32–8.

Royal College of Physicians of London (1991). *Purchasers' Guide to Genetic Services in the NHS*. London: Royal College of Physicians.

Sanderson, S., Emery, J., and Higgins, J. (2005). CYP2C9 variants, drug dose, and bleeding risk in warfarin-treated patients: a HuGENet systematic review and meta-analysis. *Genetics in Medicine*, 7, 97–104.

Sandoval, J. and Esteller, M. (2012). Cancer epigenomics: beyond genomics. *Current Opinion in Genetics and Development*, 22, 50–5.

Schofield, P.N., Eppig, J., Huala, E., et al. (2010). Sustaining the data and bioresource commons. *Science*, 330 (6004), 592–3.

Shanker, A. (2012). Genome research in the cloud. *OMICS*, 16(7–8), 422–8.

Sim, S.C. and Ingelman-Sundberg, M. (2011). Pharmacogenomic biomarkers: new tools in current and future drug therapy. *Trends in Pharmacological Sciences*, 32, 72–81.

Slomko, H., Heo, H.J., and Einstein, F.H. (2012). Minireview: epigenetics of obesity and diabetes in humans. *Endocrinology*, 153, 1025–30.

Smith, A., Balazinska, M., Baru, C., et al. (2011). Biology and data-intensive scientific discovery in the beginning of the 21st century. *OMICS*, 15(4), 209–12.

Stewart, A., Brice, P., Burton, H., et al. (2007). *Genetics, Health Care and Public Policy*. Cambridge: Cambridge University Press.

Stewart, A., Karmali, M., and Zimmern, R. (2006). GRaPH Int: an international network for public health genomics. In B.M. Knoppers (ed.) *Genomics and Public Health. Legal and Socio-Economic Perspectives*, pp. 257–71. The Netherlands: Martinus Nijhoff Publishers.

Subramonia-Iyer, S., Sanderson, S., Sagoo, G., et al. (2007). Array-based comparative genomic hybridization for investigating chromosomal abnormalities in patients with learning disability: systematic review and meta-analysis of diagnostic and false-positive yield. *Genetics in Medicine*, 9, 74–9.

Suresh, S. (2011). Moving toward global science. *Science*, 333(6044), 802.

Teutsch, S.M., Bradley, L.A., Palomaki, G.E., et al. (2009). The Evaluation of Genomic Applications in Practice and Prevention (EGAPP) Initiative: methods of the EGAPP Working Group. *Genetics in Medicine*, 11(1), 3–14.

The Wellcome Trust Case Control Consortium (2007). Genome-wide association study of 14,000 cases of seven common diseases and 3,000 shared controls. *Nature*, 447, 661–78.

Tian, Q., Price, N.D., and Hood, L. (2012). Systems cancer medicine: towards realization of predictive, preventive, personalized and participatory (P4) medicine. *Journal of Internal Medicine*, 271, 111–21.

Tobias, E.S., Connor, M., and Ferguson Smith, M. (2011). *Essential Medical Genetics*. Oxford: Wiley-Blackwell.

Umeda, T., Tanaka, N., Kusakabe, Y., et al. (2011). Molecular basis of fosmidomycin's action on the human malaria parasite Plasmodium falciparum. *Scientific Reports*, 1, 9.

Ushahidi-Haiti at Tufts University (2010). *Haiti: The 2010 Earthquake in Haiti*. Available at: http://haiti.ushahidi.com.

US Secretary's Advisory Committee on Heritable Diseases of Newborns and Children (2011). Available at: http://www.hrsa.gov/advisory committees/mchbadvisory/heritabledisorders/ (accessed 30 October 2012).

Warnich, L., Drögemöller, B.I., Pepper, M.S., Dandara, C., and Wright, G.E. (2011). Pharmacogenomic research in South Africa: lessons learned and future opportunities in the Rainbow Nation. *Current Pharmacogenomics and Personalized Medicine*, 9, 191–207.

Weatherall, D.J. and Clegg, J.B. (2001). Inherited haemoglobin disorders: an increasing global health problem. *Bulletin of the World Health Organization*, 79, 704–12.

Wilson, J.M.G. and Jungner, G. (1968). *Principles and Practice of Screening for Disease*. Public health paper no. 34. Geneva: World Health Organization.

Wonkam, A., Kenfack, M.A., Muna, W.F., et al. (2011). Ethics of human genetic studies in sub-Saharan Africa: the case of Cameroon through a bibliometric analysis. *Developing World Bioethics*, 11(3), 120–7.

World Health Organization Advisory Committee on Health Research (2002). *Genomics and World Health*. Geneva: World Health Organization.

Yang, Q., Khoury, M.J., Botto, L., Friedman, J.M., and Flanders, W.D. (2003). Improving the prediction of complex diseases by testing for multiple disease susceptibility genes. *American Journal of Human Genetics*, 72, 636–49.

Yoon, P.W., Scheuner, M.T., Peterson-Oehlke, K.L., et al. (2002). Can family history be used as a tool for public health and preventive medicine? *Genetics in Medicine*, 4, 304–10.

Zimmern, R. (2001). What is genetic information: whose hands on your genes? *Genetics Law Monitor*, 1, 9–13.

Zimmern, R.L. (2011). Genomics and individuals in public health practice: are we luddites or can we meet the challenge? *Journal of Public Health (Oxford)*, 33(4), 477–82.

Zimmern, R.L. (2012). Issues concerning the evaluation and regulation of predictive genetic testing. *Journal of Community Genetics*, 5(1), 49–57.

Zimmern, R.L. and Khoury, M.J. (2012). The impact of genomics on public health practice: the case for change. *Public Health Genomics*, 15(3–4), 118–24.

2.6

Water and sanitation

Thomas Clasen

Introduction to water and sanitation

Background

Safe drinking water and sanitary waste disposal are among the most fundamental of public health interventions. When readers of the *British Medical Journal* were asked in 2006 to name the 'greatest medical advance' since 1840, their top choice was clean drinking water and waste disposal, beating antibiotics, anaesthesia, vaccines, and germ theory (Ferriman 2007). Deaths from diarrhoeal diseases and typhoid fever showed dramatic declines in Europe and North America when cities and towns began filtering and chlorinating their water and safely disposing of human and animal excreta (Cutler and Miller 2005). The field of epidemiology arguably has its origins in John Snow's nineteenth-century mapping of cholera cases and the eventual intervention at London's Broad Street pump that demonstrated waterborne transmission of the disease.

While diseases associated with poor water and sanitation are now comparatively unknown in higher-income countries, they still impose a heavy burden elsewhere, especially among young children, the infirm, the poor, the immunocompromised, and the displaced. The World Health Organization (WHO) estimates that diarrhoeal diseases alone are responsible for 1.5 million deaths annually, including 760,000 among children under 5 years (WHO 2013). Diarrhoea is the third leading cause of deaths of children <5 years in low-income countries, accounting for 11% of the overall disease burden in this population. Improvements in water, sanitation, and hygiene have the potential to reduce this disease burden by an estimated 58% (Prüss-Ustün et al. 2014). As discussed below, poor water and sanitation is also associated with a heavy disease burden from malnutrition, parasite and worm infection, trachoma, and environmental enteropathy. Water and sanitation are not only a matter of public health, but also of poverty, equity, and justice (United Nations Development Programme 2007). Because they are less likely to have access to safe water and sanitation, the poor bear most of the burden of water-related diseases, driving them further into poverty through lost productivity and expenditure on treatment (Blakley et al. 2005). Time spent in collecting water from distant sources and the inability to procure sufficient quantities of water for irrigating crops, watering animals, and carrying out other productive activities aggravates poverty. While urban-rural disparities in water and sanitation coverage are well documented (WHO and UNICEF 2014), a recent analysis of sub-Saharan Africa also demonstrated important geographic inequalities in use of water and sanitation previously hidden within national statistics (Pullan et al. 2014). These results confirm the need for targeted policies and metrics that reach these marginalized populations.

(Pickering and Davis 2012). Inadequate water and sanitation are also associated with poor school attendance (Hutton et al. 2007). For these and other reasons, water and sanitation have been recognized as a fundamental human right (United Nations 2010).

Nevertheless, basic water security and sanitation still elude much of the world's population living in low-income countries. An estimated 748 million people lack improved access to water supplies; hundreds of millions more rely on water that is unsafe for drinking (WHO and UNICEF 2014). An estimated 2.5 billion people—40 per cent of the world's population—lack access to improved sanitation; more than 1 billion of those still practise open defecation. Coverage is lowest in developing regions, where people are most vulnerable to infection and disease. In sub-Saharan Africa, improved water and sanitation coverage is just 63 per cent and 30 per cent, respectively. Rural areas also lag behind their urban counterparts. By the end of 2011, 83 per cent of the population without access to an improved drinking-water source lived in rural areas. If current trends continue, more than half of the rural population will still be without sanitation coverage in 2015, and more than 700 million mainly poor rural dwellers will still lack improved water (WHO and UNICEF 2014).

The shortfall in water and sanitation coverage is not the result of a failure to recognize the need or declare goals at the highest international levels. The 1977 Mar del Plata Declaration by the United Nations (UN) expressed the goal of providing safe water and sanitation for all by 1990, launching the Water and Sanitation Decade (1981–1990) (Cairncross 1992). In 1990, the UN renewed the call and extended the deadline to the end of the century. The UN Millennium Development Goals (MDGs) call for halving, by 2015, the portion of the population without sustainable access to safe drinking water or basic sanitation (United Nations 2000). As the research described in this chapter suggests, such coverage would not only advance the environmental security targets under MDG 7, but also make contributions to reducing poverty (MDG 1), increasing primary education (MDG 2), promoting gender equality (MDG 3), reducing child mortality (MDG 4), and combating major diseases (MDG 6). In a further effort to attract attention to this deficit and additional priority to the sector, the UN General Assembly declared 2005–2015 as the Decade for Action, Water for Life (WHO and UNICEF 2005), and 2008 as the International Year of Sanitation. Proposals for post-2015 goals call for universal access to drinking water at home, schools, and clinics, greater progress on sanitation coverage, and improved equity in access (WHO and UNICEF 2014).

Traditionally, much of the work in water and sanitation has been undertaken by engineers and has consisted of infrastructural improvements. Low-cost community- and household-based interventions, such as protected wells, boreholes, and communal stand pipes for improved water supplies, and various types of latrines, septic tanks, and composting systems for improved sanitation, have been largely conceived by and constructed with the assistance of engineers. There are numerous books, manuals, and other resources that describe these systems in detail, including Cairncross and Feachem (1993), the UK Department of International Development (1998), Davis and Lambert (2002), the quarterly *Waterlines*, and the World Bank Water and Sanitation Programme (WSP) 'Field Notes' (World Bank n.d.). Readers are encouraged to refer to such sources for details on the design, installation, and operation of such systems, technology innovations, and the programmatic challenges associated with achieving widespread use on a sustained basis.

This chapter focuses solely on the public health issues concerning water and sanitation. After introducing some basic terminology, it begins by describing the diseases associated with inadequate water and sanitation and their contribution to the overall burden of disease. It then presents evidence of the effectiveness of water and sanitation interventions to prevent such diseases, the economic implications (especially cost-effectiveness and cost–benefits) of such interventions, and some of the other non-health benefits associated therewith. Recent and emerging developments in water, sanitation, and health are then discussed, along with some issues relevant to water and sanitation interventions. The chapter closes with a discussion of some of the continuing challenges in water and sanitation.

Terminology

At the outset, it is useful to understand some of the terminology used in describing the diseases, transmission routes, and interventions associated with the water and sanitation sectors. Water-related diseases are sometimes classified according to their disease transmission routes as *waterborne* (ingested in drinking water), *water-washed* (associated with inadequate supplies of water for proper personal hygiene), *water-based* (transmitted through an aquatic invertebrate host), or linked to a *water-related vector* (involving an insect vector breeding in or near water) (White et al. 1972). Most waterborne organisms that are human pathogens colonize the gut of humans and certain other mammals and are transmitted through the *faecal–oral* route. The transmission of common waterborne diseases can thus be interrupted by improvements in sanitation (*excreta disposal*), personal hygiene (especially *hand washing with soap*), and microbiological *water quality*, while those that are water-washed are impacted by improvements in *water supplies* (quantity and access) for personal hygiene. Improving water supplies can also help prevent water-based diseases (such as schistosomiasis and dracunculiasis) by reducing the need to enter infected water bodies.

The term 'sanitation' is vague and has multiple meanings. Within the public health sector two definitions are used. Under the broader definition, sanitation extends to the process whereby people demand, effect, and sustain a hygienic and healthy environment for themselves. This definition could include safe food production, solid waste management, industrial waste, animal waste, control of chemicals, environmental pollution, storm water drainage, wastewater disposal, human settlements, personal and domestic hygiene, vector and vermin control, occupational health and safety, mining and quarrying, port health, and disposal of the dead. A second definition is more specific, extending only to the process of separating humans from their excreta. This chapter uses this second, more specific definition and regards sanitation as a system in which excreta is: (1) collected safely and with dignity, (2) transported to a suitable location, (3) treated or contained to eliminate pathogenicity, and (4) reused and/or discharged to the environment.

The MDG targets for water and sanitation are expressed in terms of *sustainable access to safe drinking water* and of *basic sanitation*. The water target has been interpreted as 'sufficient drinking water of acceptable quality as well as sufficient quantity of water for hygienic purposes' (UN Millennium Project 2005). Basic sanitation, in turn, has been defined as 'the lowest-cost option for securing sustainable access to safe, hygienic, and convenient facilities and services for excreta and sewage disposal that provide privacy and dignity, while at the same time ensuring a clean and healthy living environment both at home and in the neighbourhood of users' (UN Millennium Project 2005). Progress toward the MDGs, however, is measured with reference to the Joint Monitoring Programme (JMP) that adopts an indicator approach based on facilities or level of service. For water supplies, the JMP distinguishes only between *improved water supplies* (piped-in tap water, public tap/standpipe, borehole/tubewell, protected well/spring, rainwater harvesting), and *unimproved water supplies* (surface water, unprotected well/spring, tankered water, bottled water) (WHO and UNICEF 2013). *Improved sanitation* includes a private flush or pour-flush toilet or latrine connected to a piped sewer system or septic system, simple pit latrine with slab, ventilated improved pit (VIP) latrine, or composting toilet; *unimproved sanitation* includes any other flush or pour-flush latrine, open pit latrine, bucket latrine, hanging latrine, any public or shared facility, or open defecation (WHO and UNICEF 2014). Some of these definitions are being reconsidered in the context of developing a set of post-MDG water and sanitation targets (WHO and UNICEF 2014).

Burden of disease

General

Poor water and sanitation are associated with a variety of infectious diseases transmitted through various pathways by helminths, protozoa, bacteria, and viruses. Table 2.6.1 summarizes the most important of these diseases, their transmission routes, aetiological agents, and epidemiological significance. Some of these diseases also contribute to malnutrition, a separate cause of substantial morbidity and mortality that is not reflected in the direct burden of disease figures cited in this chapter (Black et al. 2003).

Certain diseases associated with water are not addressed in this chapter. First, in addition to microbial agents, water is a medium for the transmission of chemical pathogens, including arsenic and other metals, fluoride, nitrates, and volatile organic compounds (including pesticides and herbicides). Accordingly, WHO guidelines and many national water standards establish maximum allowable limits for such chemicals (WHO 2012). However, except for arsenicosis and fluoridosis, which are especially serious in focal areas in Asia and parts of Africa, most of these contaminants represent hazards to health only over the longer term. Second, although improvements in water supplies (to discourage contact

Table 2.6.1 Principal infectious diseases, disease agents, transmission routes, and annual morbidity and mortality related to poor water and sanitation

Disease	Aetiological agent	Transmission	Infected[1] (millions)	Mortality[1] (thousands)
Diarrhoea (dysentery, cholera)	**Virus** *Rotavirus*	Faecal–oral	4000 (annual morbidity)	1400–1800
	Bacteria *Escherichia coli* (ETEC) *Shigella* spp. *Salmonella* spp. *Vibrio* spp. *Campylobacter* sp.	Faecal–oral		
	Protozoa *Giardia lambia* *Cryptosporidium parvum* *Entamoeba histolytica*	Faecal–oral		
Schistosomiasis	*Schistosoma haematobium* *S. mansoni* *S. japonicum*	Penetration through skin exposed to contaminated freshwater	207	15–280
Ascariasis	*Ascaris lumbricoides*	Faecal–oral	1221–1472	3–60
Trichuriasis	*Trichuris trichuria*	Faecal–oral	759–1050	3–10
Hookworm infection	*Necator americanus* *Ancylostoma duodenale*	Penetration through skin exposed to faecally-contaminated soil Faecal–oral	740–1300	3–65
Typhoid and paratyphoid fever	*Salmonella* spp.	Faecal–oral	26	216
Trachoma	*Chlamydia trachomatis*	Fingers Clothing Eye-seeking flies (*Musca sorbens*) Coughing/sneezing	Blind from trachoma: 1.3 Active trachoma: 40 Trachiasis: 8.2	

Note: [1] estimates vary according to method.

Morbidity and mortality estimates for diarrhoeal disease: data from World Health Organization and UNICEF, *Progress on Sanitation and Drinking Water: 2013 Update*, World Health Organization and UNICEF Joint Monitoring Programme on Water and Sanitation, New York, USA, Copyright © 2013.

Schistosomiasis and soil-transmitted helminth infections (STH) (ascariasis, trichuriasis, hookworm): data from Lustigman et al., A research agenda for helminth diseases of humans: the problem of helminthiases, *PLoS Neglected Tropical Diseases*, Volume 6, Issue 4, e1582, Copyright © 2012 Lustigman et al.

Typhoid and paratyphoid: data from Crump et al., The global burden of typhoid fever, *Bulletin of the World Health Organization*, Volume 82, Number 5, pp. 346–53, Copyright © 2004.

Trachoma figures: data from Burton MJ and Mabey DC, The global burden of trachoma: a review, *PLoS Neglected Tropical Diseases*, Volume 3, Issue 10, e460, Copyright © 2009 Burton, Mabey.

with water) and point-of-use water treatment (with filters) are important interventions in preventing dracunculiasis (Cairncross et al. 2002), efforts to control Guinea worm infection have been largely successful and the disease is now of public health interest in limited areas. Finally, this chapter does not address a variety of diseases associated with waterborne pathogens, such as poliomyelitis and hepatitis A and E, which are controlled mainly by vaccines and other non-environmental measures (Leclerc et al. 2002).

Diarrhoeal diseases

Diarrhoeal diseases represent the leading cause of mortality and morbidity associated with unsafe drinking water and poor sanitation. For those infected with the human immunodeficiency virus (HIV) or who have developed acquired immune deficiency syndrome (AIDS), diarrhoea can be prolonged, severe, and life-threatening (Hayes et al. 2003). Diarrhoea is characterized by stools of decreased consistency and increased number. The clinical symptoms and course of the disease vary greatly with the age, nutritional and immune status, and the pathogen (Black and Lanata 1995). Most cases resolve within a week, though a small percentage continue for 2 weeks or more and are characterized as 'persistent' diarrhoea. Dysentery is a diarrhoeal disease defined by the presence of blood in the liquid stools. Though epidemic diarrhoea such as cholera and shigellosis (bacillary dysentery) are well-known risks, particularly in emergency settings, their global health significance is small compared to endemic diarrhoea (Hunter 1997). The immediate threat from diarrhoea is dehydration, a loss of fluids and electrolytes. Thus, the widespread

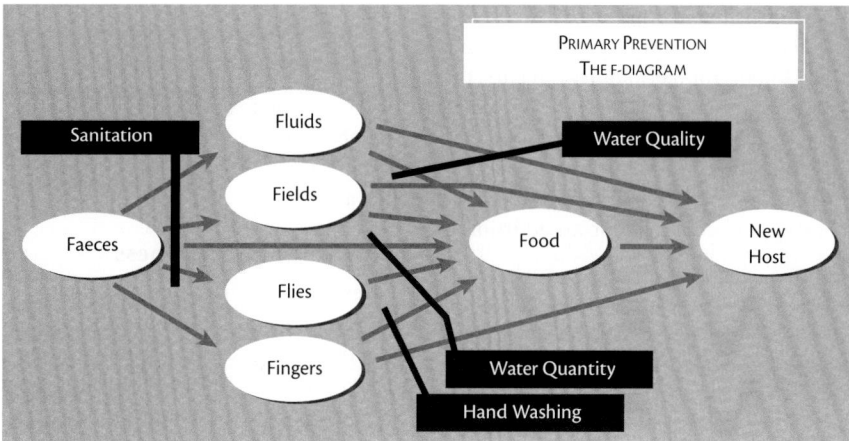

Fig. 2.6.1 The F-diagram.
Reproduced with permission from Wagner, EG and Lanois, JN, *Excreta disposal for rural areas and small communities.* WHO monograph series No.39, World Health Organization, Geneva, Switzerland, Copyright © 1958.

promotion of oral rehydration therapy (ORT) has significantly reduced the case-fatality rate associated with the disease. Such improvements in case management, however, have not reduced morbidity, which is estimated at 4 billion cases annually (Kosek et al. 2003). And since diarrhoeal diseases inhibit normal ingestion of foods and adsorption of nutrients, continued high morbidity is an important cause of malnutrition, leading to impaired physical growth and cognitive function, reduced resistance to infection, and potentially long-term gastrointestinal disorders.

The infectious agents associated with diarrhoeal disease are transmitted chiefly through the faecal–oral route (Leclerc et al. 2002). Safe excreta disposal thus represents a primary barrier that should contribute to the prevention of indirect transmission via food, water, hands, fomites, and mechanical vectors (flies) (Fig. 2.6.1). A wide variety of bacterial, viral, and protozoan pathogens excreted in the faeces of humans and animals are known to cause diarrhoea. While the importance of individual pathogens varies among settings, seasons, and conditions, a recent multicountry study has shed important light on the principal aetiological agents responsible for much of the disease burden in Africa and South Asia (Kotloff et al. 2013). Investigators found that most attributable cases of moderate-to-severe diarrhoea were due to four pathogens: rotavirus, *Cryptosporidium*, enterotoxigenic *Escherichia coli* producing heat-stable toxin (ST-ETEC) and *Shigella. Aeromonas, Vibrio cholerae* O1, and *Campylobacter jejuni* were also important in selected sites. They reported that the odds of dying during follow-up were 8.5 times higher in patients with moderate-to-severe diarrhoea than in controls (odd ratio (OR) 8.5; 95 per cent confidence interval (CI) 5.8–12.5, p < 0.0001) and that 88 per cent of deaths occurred during the first 2 years of life. Pathogens associated with increased risk of case death were ST-ETEC (hazard ratio (HR) 1.9; 95 per cent CI: 0.99–3.5) and typical enteropathogenic *E. coli* (HR 2.6; 95 per cent CI: 1.6–4.1) in infants aged 0–11 months, and *Cryptosporidium* (HR 2.3; 95 per cent CI: 1.3–4.3) in toddlers aged 12–23 months. Although diarrhoea is also associated with the ingestion of metals, nitrates, organics, and other chemicals, the burden of disease arising from such exposure is small relative to infectious diarrhoea (Hunter 1997).

Schistosomiasis

Schistosomiasis affects 200 million people all over the world, with *Schistosoma haematobium* and *S. mansoni* being the most common species. The schistosomiasis life cycle involves contamination of freshwater by eggs carrying excreta and urine and an intermediate host, a freshwater snail. Larvae released in the water infect humans by penetrating through the skin. Parasites develop and migrate to the intestines and bladder where thousands of eggs are produced. Like other intestinal helminths, schistosomes are associated with impaired physical and mental development and anaemia. Furthermore, schistosomiasis may cause serious damage to the bladder and intestine walls as a result of parasite egg entrapment within tissues. Chronic infection with *S. haematobium* has been associated with increased risk of bladder cancer in adulthood (Gryssels et al. 2006).

Soil-transmitted helminth infection

More than 2 billion of the world's population are infected with soil-transmitted helminths. A disproportionate burden of helminthiasis occurs in marginalized, low-income, and resource-constrained regions of the world, largely in developing areas of sub-Saharan Africa, Asia, and the Americas (Lustigman et al. 2012). About 300 million people suffer from heavy worm load and related severe morbidity (deSilva et al. 2003). *Ascaris lumbricoides, Trichuris trichuria*, and hookworm (*Ancylostoma duodenale* and *Necator americanus*) are the most prevalent intestinal helminths. Transmission occurs via ingestion of eggs present in faecally contaminated soil, or via penetration of the larvae through the skin. Children are particularly vulnerable to chronic and heavy infections, which result in malnutrition, stunted growth, reduced physical fitness, and impaired cognitive development (Stephenson et al. 2000). Hookworm infection is an important cause of anaemia, not only in children, but also among women of reproductive age and pregnant women leading to premature birth and low birth weight (Hotez et al. 2004).

Typhoid and paratyphoid fevers

While enteric fevers such as typhoid and paratyphoid were leading causes of waterborne disease in previous centuries, morbidity and mortality diminished dramatically with the provisions of disinfected water supplies and improved sanitary facilities (Cutler and Miller 2005). The aetiological agents for typhoid and paratyphoid fevers are *Salmonella enterica* serovar Typhi (formerly *S. typhi*) and *S. enterica* serovar Paratyphi A and B (formerly *S. paratyphi*). There are an estimated 21 million cases of typhoid annually, causing 216,000 deaths (Crump et al. 2004). The milder paratyphoid accounts for an additional 5 million cases each year.

Trachoma

Trachoma accounts for 15 per cent of world blindness, with 6 million people affected and 150 million at risk of visual impairment (Kumaresan and Mecaskey 2003). Trachoma is caused by repeated eye infection with *Chlamydia trachomatis*. Children are the main reservoir for infection, with high prevalence of active trachoma (Mabey et al. 2003). Repeated infections result in deformation of the upper eye lid, abrasion of the cornea, and progressive loss of vision in later life. *C. trachomatis* is transmitted from the discharge of an infected eye via contaminated fingers, clothing, and eye-seeking flies (*Musca sorbens*) (Hu et al. 2010). Although the role of flies in the transmission of infection remains unclear, studies have shown that *M. sorbens* breed mainly in solid human faeces present in the environment and not in latrines (Emerson et al. 2000). Thus, safe excreta disposal may play an important role in reducing trachoma transmission. Improving water supplies and sanitation is part of the WHO-backed SAFE (surgery, antibiotics, facial hygiene, environmental improvement) strategy for controlling and preventing the disease.

Malnutrition

Water and sanitation are also linked to malnutrition, a separate source of significant morbidity and mortality. An estimated 165 million children under 5 are stunted (i.e. have a height-for-age Z score of less than −2); 55 million children are wasted (i.e. have a weight-for-height Z score of less than −2), of whom 19 million have severe wasting (weight-for-height Z score of less than −3) or severe acute malnutrition (weight-for-height Z score of −3 or lower or associated oedema) (Bhutta et al. 2013). Child underweight or stunting causes about 20 per cent of all mortality of children younger than 5 years of age; it also contributes to long-term cognitive impairment, poorer performance in school, fewer years of completed schooling, and lower adult economic productivity.

Effectiveness of water and sanitation in preventing disease

Barriers to transmission of faecal–oral diseases

As illustrated by the so-called 'F-diagram' (Fig. 2.6.1), the safe disposal of human faeces is the primary barrier in preventing faecal–oral transmitted diseases. Without removing excreta from potential contact with humans, animals, and insects, pathogens may be carried on unwashed hands, in contaminated water or food, or via flies and other insects on to further human hosts. Whether or not sanitation is adequate, hands can become contaminated with faeces, especially during anal cleansing following defecation or in cleaning a child after defecation. This may result in further transmission, either directly or indirectly through food, water, or other beverages, or fomites. Accordingly, hand washing is an important secondary barrier to faecal–oral disease

transmission (Curtis and Cairncross 2003). Other secondary barriers include: (1) water quality interventions (e.g. safe distribution and storage or use of boiling or other point of use water treatment), (2) water supply interventions to increase the quantity and availability of water for personal and domestic hygiene, (3) proper cooking and food handling, and (4) control of mechanical vectors such as flies.

Evidence of effectiveness

Scores of studies have been conducted and published on the effectiveness of water, sanitation, and hygiene interventions to prevent infection and disease. Systematic reviews (Chapter 5.15) are a means of identifying, summarizing, synthesizing, explaining, and assessing the methodological quality of evidence of the effectiveness of health interventions with a variety of studies relating to a particular health intervention. In some cases, such reviews also employ meta-analyses or other statistical methods to estimate the pooled effect of the intervention across the studies included in the review. A number of such reviews have examined the evidence of effectiveness of water, sanitation, and hygiene interventions to prevent disease and infection.

Diarrhoeal diseases

Table 2.6.2 summarizes the results of five different systematic reviews of water and sanitation interventions to prevent diarrhoeal diseases published over the last 25 years. While there is conflicting evidence on the impact of water supply (quantity and access), there is consistent evidence that improvements in water and sanitation can make substantial contributions to the prevention of diarrhoeal diseases.

Soil-transmitted helminth infection

A more recent review assessed not only the impact of sanitation interventions on soil-transmitted helminth infections but also water and hygiene (Strunz 2014). The review covers 94 studies, though only 5 were randomized controlled trials. Use of treated water was associated with lower odds of infection from any soil-transmitted helminth (OR 0.46, 95% CI 0.36–0.60). Piped water access was associated with lower odds of *A. lumbricoides* (OR 0.40, 95% CI 0.39–0.41) and *T. trichiura* infection (OR 0.57, 95% CI 0.45–0.72), but not any STH infection (OR 0.93, 95% CI 0.28–3.11). Access to sanitation was associated with decreased likelihood of infection with any soil-transmitted helminth (OR 0.66, 95% CI 0.57–0.76), *T. trichiura* (OR 0.61, 95% CI 0.50–0.74), and *A. lumbricoides* (OR 0.62, 95% CI 0.44–0.88), but not with hookworm infection (OR 0.80, 95% CI 0.61–1.06).

In one systematic review, the authors reported larger protective effect of sanitation interventions to prevent soil-transmitted helminth infection despite acknowledging significant imitations (most studies used a cross-sectional design and were of low quality, with potential biases and considerable heterogeneity) (Ziegelbauer et al. 2012). Availability of sanitation facilities was associated with significant protection against infection with soil-transmitted helminths, with ORs ranging from 0.46–0.58 depending on the type of helminth. Pooling studies reporting on latrine use yielded ORs of 0.54 (95 per cent CI: 0.28–1.02), 0.63 (95 per cent CI: 0.37–1.05), and 0.78 (95 per cent CI: 0.60–1.00) for *Trichuris trichiura*, hookworm, and *Ascaris lumbricoides*, respectively. The overall ORs, combining sanitation availability and use, were 0.51 (95 per cent CI: 0.44–0.61) for the three soil-transmitted helminths combined,

Table 2.6.2 Estimate of effect[1] (and number of studies in square brackets) of systematic reviews of water and sanitation interventions to prevent diarrhoeal diseases

Intervention (Improvement)	Esrey et al. (1985) (range)	Esrey et al. (1991)	Fewtrell et al. (2005) (95% CI) (No. studies)	Clasen et al. (2006) (95% CI) (No. studies)	Waddington et al. (2009) (95% CI) (No. studies)	Wolf et al. (2014) (95% CI)[2]
Water quantity	25% (0–100%) (17)	27% (7)				
Water quality			0.69 (0.53–0.89) (15)	0.57 (0.46–0.70) (38)	0.58 (0.50–0.67) (31)	
Source	16% (0–90%) (9)	17% (7)	0.89 (0.42–1.90) (3)	0.73 (0.53–1.01) (6)	0.79 (0.62–1.02) (3)	0.89 (0.78–1.01)
Household (point-of-use)			0.65 (0.48–0.88) (12)	0.53 (0.39–0.73) (32)	0.56 (0.45–0.65) (28)	
Chlorination				0.63 (0.52–0.75) (16)		0.63 (0.55–0.72)
Filtration				0.37 (0.28–0.49) (6)		0.41 (0.33–0.50)
Solar disinfection				0.69 (0.63–0.74) (2)		0.63 (0.55–0.72)
Floc-disinfection				0.69 (0.58–0.82) (6)		
Water supply (point-of-distribution)	37% (0–82%) (8)	16% (22)	0.75 (0.62–0.91) (6)	0.73 (0.53–1.01) (6)	0.98 (0.89–1.06) (8)	0.89 (0.78–1.01)
Water supply and sanitation/hygiene		20% (7)			0.43 (0.33–0.55) (3)	
Sanitation	22% (0–48%) (10)	22% (11)	0.68 (0.53–0.87) (2)		0.63 (0.43–0.93) (6)	0.84 (0.77–0.91)

Note: [1] for studies by Esrey and colleagues, estimate of effect is the median reduction in diarrhoeal disease from the reported studies; for other studies, estimate of effect is the pooled risk ratio from meta-analysis using random effects model. To compare results, the percentage reduction is 1 − RR (e.g. RR of 0.69 implies a 31 per cent reduction in risk).
[2] Pooled estimates of effect in settings with unimproved water supply and prior to adjustment for non-blinding. For household interventions, estimates are for studies that combine treatment with safe storage.

0.54 (95 per cent CI: 0.43–0.69) for *A. lumbricoides*, 0.58 (95 per cent CI: 0.45–0.75) for *T. trichiura*, and 0.60 (95 per cent CI: 0.48–0.75) for hookworm.

Schistosomiasis

Esrey and colleagues (1991) reported a median reduction in the prevalence of schistosomiasis of 73 per cent (range 59–87 per cent) from four water and sanitation interventions; the reduction was 77 per cent among the three studies they deemed rigorous. Piped-in water supplies and community washing and bathing facilities that reduced contact with surface waters were especially protective, leading to reductions in both prevalence and severity (Esrey et al. 1991). The reviewers noted that in Kenya, the installation of boreholes without laundry or shower facilities failed to reduce infection.

Two quasi-randomized, controlled interventional studies from China also suggest that improved excreta disposal is protective against schistosomiasis. In a 3-year quasi-randomized controlled trial (RCT), Chen et al. (2004) recorded a 43 per cent reduction from combined water, sanitation, and hygiene interventions that also included a snail control component. Zhang et al. (2005) reported a 45 per cent reduction in a 2-year quasi-RCT that included water, sanitation, and hygiene. Once again, these trials did not include sufficient clusters to reliably calculate confidence intervals around the point estimates of effect.

Typhoid and paratyphoid

No RCTs of water or sanitation interventions to prevent typhoid or paratyphoid have been reported. A recent review of global trends in these enteric fevers identified little direct evidence of the potential contribution of water or sanitation interventions (Crump and Mintz 2010). Nevertheless, there is evidence suggesting the

effectiveness of water quality interventions. Cutler and Miller (2005) have shown the historical evidence on reductions in mortality associated with the introduction of clean water and sanitation in the United States. Case–control studies do suggest that the diseases are still associated with unsafe water and sanitation. In a study in Uzbekistan where typhoid remains endemic, cases were more likely to drink unboiled surface water outside the home (OR 3.0; 95 per cent CI: 1.1–8.20) (Srikantiah et al. 2007). In a similar case–control study in Bangladesh, drinking unboiled water at home was a significant risk factor (OR 12.1; 95 per cent CI: 2.2–65.6) (Ram et al. 2007). Among the risk factors for typhoid and paratyphoid in an urban setting in Indonesia were lack of a toilet in the household (OR 2.20; 95 per cent CI: 1.06–4.55) and use of ice cubes (OR 2.27; 95 per cent CI: 1.31–3.93). Enteric fevers are also a risk among travellers to endemic area, but effective vaccines are usually recommended against the risk of waterborne or foodborne transmission.

Trachoma

The evidence of the effectiveness of environmental interventions (including water and sanitation) alone to prevent active trachoma is not clear (Rabiu et al. 2012). Reviews of the WHO-backed SAFE strategy for trachoma control conclude that there is comparatively weak evidence of the effectiveness of the 'F' (facial cleanliness) and 'E' (environmental improvement) components that encompass improved access to water and better sanitation (Emerson et al. 2000a; Kuper et al. 2003). In a 6-month cluster RCT of 21 villages in the Gambia, Emerson and colleagues (Emerson et al. 2004) reported a reduction in fly catches among study clusters receiving latrines. However, the prevalence of active trachoma associated with the intervention was not statistically lower than among seven control clusters (RR 0.81; 95 per cent CI: 0.54–1.22). The study has not been repeated. In another review, access to sanitation was associated with lower trachoma as measured by the presence of trachomatous inflammation-follicular or trachomatous inflammation-intense (TF/TI) (OR 0.85, 95% CI 0.75–0.95) and *C. trachomatis* infection (OR 0.67, 95% CI 0.55–0.78) (Stocks et al. 2013). Hygiene practices that require adequate supplies of water, such as facial cleansing, were also protective against trachoma. However, living within 1 km of a water source and the use of sanitation facilities was not found to be significantly associated with TF/TI.

Malnutrition

Malnutrition is linked to water and sanitation, both through food production (irrigation and safe use of waste for fertilizer) and by preventing diarrhoea and enteric infections that interfere with normal adsorption of nutrients (Fewtrell et al. 2007). An association of malnutrition with diarrhoea has been well established, but the impact of interventions is less clear. In a pooled analysis of nine studies with diarrhoea and growth data for 1393 children, the probability of stunting at 24 months of age increased by 2.5 per cent per episode of diarrhoea, and 25 per cent of all stunting in 24-month-old children was attributable to having five or more episodes of diarrhoea in the first 2 years of life (Checkley et al. 2008). The Maternal and Child Undernutrition Series in *The Lancet* estimated that sanitation and hygiene interventions implemented with 99 per cent coverage would reduce diarrhoea incidence by 30 per cent, which would in turn decrease the prevalence of stunting by only 2.4 per cent (Bhutta et al. 2013). A report for the World Bank suggests that open defecation explained 54 per cent of international variation in child height by contrast with gross domestic product, which only explained 29 per cent (Spears 2013). However, a recent systematic review and meta-analysis of water, sanitation, and hygiene interventions on nutritional status found no evidence on impact on weight-for-age Z-scores and only a small benefit on height-for-age Z-scores in children under 5 years of age (Dangour et al. 2013).

Economic implications of water and sanitation interventions

Cost-effectiveness and cost–benefit analyses

Hutton and colleagues (Hutton et al. 2007) assessed the cost–benefit ratios in 17 WHO epidemiological subregions of five categories of water and sanitation interventions based on the MDG water and sanitation targets and additional steps to minimize environmental exposure. The interventions included: (1) improvements required to meet the MDGs for water supply, (2) interventions to meet the water and sanitation MDG, (3) increasing access to improved water and sanitation for everyone, (4) providing disinfection at point-of-use over and above increasing access to improved water supply and sanitation, and (5) providing regulated piped water supply in house and sewage connection with partial sewerage for everyone. The study found that all water and sanitation improvements were cost-beneficial in all developing world subregions. The main contributor to economic benefits was timesaving associated with better access to water and sanitation services, contributing at least 80 per cent to overall economic benefits. A more recent analysis confirmed these results, concluding that the global return per dollar invested was $5.50 for

sanitation, $2.0 for water supply, and $4.30 for combined sanitation and water supply (Hutton 2013). It estimated the global costs of universal access amount over the 5-year period 2010–2015 to US$ 35 billion per year for sanitation and US$ 17.5 billion for drinking-water.

A more recent economic analysis estimated the cost–benefit ratios of water quality (point-of-use filtration or chlorination) and sanitation (community-led total sanitation) interventions and placed them in the context of other comparable interventions (long-lasting insecticide treated nets and cholera vaccination (Whittington et al. 2012)). The study also found the water and sanitation interventions to be cost-beneficial. Most of the benefits, however, arose from improved health outcomes, principally reductions in mortality. Significantly, the study found substantial heterogeneity among the results; it also emphasized the sensitivity of the findings to assumptions about benefits, uptake, and usage. It cautions against generalizing the results to settings where the underlying assumptions about the population and the intervention can vary dramatically. It recommends decentralized decision-making and priority setting of water and sanitations in contrast to setting targets and subsidies by international organizations and large donors.

Willingness to pay; pricing strategies

Despite fairly consistent evidence that water and sanitation interventions are cost-effective and cost-beneficial, consumer demand varies with the type of products and services offered. Demand for piped water services in developing countries is especially inelastic (Nauges and Whittington 2009), even though their corresponding health benefits are not well established as noted earlier. This is likely to be due to the perceived value of timesaving. On the other hand, point-of-use water chlorination, though potentially among the most cost-effective of WASH interventions, has achieved only limited market penetration despite large-scale social marketing campaigns (Clasen 2009).

There is also continuing debate over user fees and subsidies to support the dissemination of interventions such as water and sanitation. Public health officials generally support free or heavily subsidized services, citing positive externalities, price elasticity, and the need to reach the lowest income households with services. On the other hand, water and sanitation officials as well as governments often insist on the need for user fees, noting the need for cost recovery strategies to ensure expansion and maintenance of services.

Cost-effectiveness analyses and cost–benefit analyses suggest that improvements in water and sanitation yield both health and other valuable benefits, not only to those who receive the intervention but also to the public sector. Inadequate water and sanitation services also have significant negative externalities (costs imposed on others), such as the costs of over-extraction from water supplies, pollution of water sources, and environmental degradation. Even those who promote water as a basic right accept that some value must be attached to water to reduce waste, encourage conservation, and promote higher value uses. Infrastructural improvements in water and sanitation often fail to be initiated or sustained because of a reluctance to charge fully for the cost of delivering the services, inefficiency in collecting such charges, or diversion of the fees away from operation and maintenance. Understanding who benefits from improvements in water and sanitation can help justify the allocation of costs and secure financing.

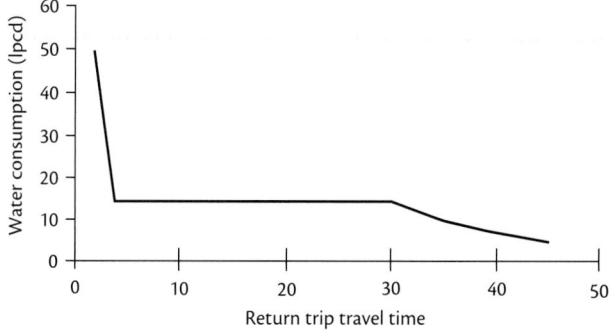

Fig. 2.6.2 Time travel (in minutes) versus consumption (in litres per capita per day).

Reproduced from Cairncross, S. and Feachem, R., Environmental health engineering in the tropics: An introductory text, Second Edition, John Wiley and Sons Ltd., Chichester, West Sussex, UK, Copyright © 1993, by permission of John Wiley and Sons Ltd.

Other benefits of water and sanitation interventions

Improving water availability (quantity and access)

As the section 'Evidence of effectiveness' suggests, improving water availability—even without a corresponding improvement in water quality—is associated with reductions of diseases transmitted through waterborne, water-washed, and water-based routes. This is partly due to the well-established relationship between the amount of water that people use and the time required to collect it (Cairncross and Feachem 1993). Fig. 2.6.2 shows the L-shaped curve that characterizes water consumption patterns based on service levels. While significant quantities of water are used if delivered directly to the home, the quantity used is fairly constant when the collection time is 5–30 minutes and further diminishes for longer collection times. In lower-income settings, average daily per capita consumption is about 150 L for those with household connections, 50 L for yard taps, and just 15 L for communal sources such as stand posts, wells, and springs. Thus, assessments of water availability are expressed in terms of distance: normally 1 km or round trip collection time (normally 30 minutes) (WHO and UNICEF 2013) but 0.5 km in disaster response (Sphere Project 2004).

A WHO report concluded that a minimum quantity of water for basic health protection is 20 L/person/day (Hutton and Bartram 2003). Of this, 7.5 L is for consumption (hydration and food preparation) and therefore must be of a quality to present minimal health risk; the balance is for basic personal and domestic hygiene. The report recognizes, however, that in addition to the direct health benefits associated with improving water supplies, there are indirect health and other benefits. Indirect health benefits may accrue from reducing the amount of time collecting water which can then be used more effectively at home caring for children or engaging in other productive activities (Cairncross 1987). Services at clinics, medical posts, and other healthcare facilities also benefit from improved water supplies. Sufficient water for irrigating gardens and crops can improve nutrition and generate income (Thompson et al. 2001). Vending water and making and selling beverages can also impact poverty. Finally, to the extent that people are paying for water, improved water supplies may result in savings that can be used for food and other necessities that may impact health outcomes.

Ecological sanitation

Within the sanitation sector there is an active group of advocates who promote the use of ecological sanitation (Winblad and Simpson-Hébert 2004). Ecological sanitation (EcoSan) works on the principle that urine and faeces are not just waste products, but assets that if properly managed, can contribute to better health and food production and reduce pollution. Managing such assets includes reducing pathogen loading to a safe level which is achieved by a combination of drying the faeces, increasing the pH, and storage for at least 12 months. Without good latrine management, pathogens can survive and create a risk to public health. The pathogen that causes greatest concern is *Ascaris*, which has a long persistence in the environment and a low infective dose (Cairncross and Feachem 1993). Public health risks need to be balanced against the potential benefits. In areas where land fertility is low, artificial fertilizer is expensive, and livelihoods are dependent on subsistence farming, the benefits of using excreta as a fertilizer/soil amendment could be considerable. Even when potential benefits can be demonstrated, local beliefs and taboos may limit acceptability or prevent adoption of the practice (Jackson 2005).

Improved school attendance

Although weaker than often asserted, there is some evidence that water and sanitation interventions at schools can improve school attendance, at least among girls (Freeman et al. 2012). This may be due to reduced incidence of disease resulting in fewer days of school missed as a result of illness. In Africa alone, Hutton et al. (2007) estimated that meeting the MDGs for water and sanitation would increase school attendance by 99 million days annually; full access to basic water and sanitation for all would increase school attendance by 140 million days each year. The sanitary needs of girls and the negative impact of lack of sanitation adversely impacts their attendance levels. In a recent trial in Kenya, schools with poor water access during the dry season that received combined water supply, hygiene promotion and water treatment together with improvements in sanitation experienced an increase in average attendance equal to 26 additional pupils per school on average (Garn et al. 2013). The proportion of girls enrolled in school also increased by 4%. In Uganda, 94 per cent of girls reported problems at school during menstruation and 61 per cent reported staying away from school (IRC International Water and Sanitation Centre 2006). Cultural and religious constraints in many settings make menstruation a taboo. If menstruation lasts over a week, there is a tendency for girls to skip the entire school year (Bharadwaj and Patkar 2004). Sanitation can play an important role in improving educational access for children with disabilities, through the improvement of paths, latrine floors, and installation of handrails (Bannister et al. 2005).

Security and gender equality

Improved sanitation and water supplies advance security and gender equality for women and girls. Household sanitation can increase their safety by avoiding the dangers of sexual assault and harassment faced when practising open defecation or using latrines away from their homes. Safe, private, and proximate latrines are now considered a basic human right (United Nations 2010); they are a particular issue for women in emergencies and conflicts (Sphere

Project 2004). Research in Kenya revealed that women would defecate into plastic bags and throw them into streets ('flying toilets') because they feared being raped when using latrines shared with men (Maili Saba Research Report 2005). They were also afraid of being seen to be using latrines too regularly and preferred to bathe within their own homes after dark where they felt safer. Young children often prefer open defecation due to fear of falling into pits in poorly-designed or unsuitably-adapted latrines.

HIV/AIDS

It is well known that access to safe drinking water and sanitation prolongs the lives of people living with HIV/AIDS (PLWHA) by reducing the risk of opportunistic infections, including diarrhoeal diseases (Peletz et al. 2013). Household-based water treatment has been shown to be an effective intervention in preventing mortality and morbidity in a population with one or more persons infected with HIV (Colford et al. 2005; Lule et al. 2005; Peletz et al. 2012). There is also evidence that household-based water filters and insecticide treated bednets for malaria slow the progression of HIV (Walson et al. 2012). Water and sanitation are now recognized as particular priorities in home-based care of PLWHA (WHO 2008). Point-of-use water treatment products are now included in health kits for people living with HIV/AIDS (Colindres et al. 2007). Efforts are also encouraged to ensure that mothers infected with HIV have safe drinking water (or point-of-use water treatment products) to prepare infant formula for use as an alternative to breastfeeding in order to minimize mother–child transmission.

Recent and emerging developments in water and sanitation

Post-2015 goals in water and sanitation

The MDG water and sanitation targets—to halve the proportion of the 1990 population without sustainable access to safe drinking water and basic sanitation—have been a major factor in mobilizing efforts to expand water and sanitation coverage. While there is still some controversy about JMP claims on the water target and overall disappointment on progress to the sanitation target, efforts are now underway to establish successor goals. As this chapter goes to press, it is still unclear what form these goals and the corresponding targets will take. However, recent proposals have included four possible targets: (1) by 2025, no one practises open defecation; (2) by 2030, everyone uses a basic drinking-water supply and handwashing facilities when at home, all schools and health centres provide all users with basic drinking-water supply and adequate sanitation, handwashing facilities, and menstrual hygiene facilities; (3) by 2040, everyone uses adequate sanitation when at home, the proportion of the population not using an intermediate drinking-water supply service at home has been reduced by half, the excreta from at least half of schools, health centres, and households with adequate sanitation are safely managed; and (iv) all drinking-water supply, sanitation, and hygiene services are delivered in a progressively affordable, accountable, and financially and environmentally sustainable manner (WHO and UNICEF 2014). In addition, there are proposals to change certain definitions used in monitoring these targets. A 'basic drinking-water supply' would include the JMP's current 'improved' water supplies (excluding protected wells or springs in urban areas) provided the time for collection/return does not exceed 30 minutes. An 'intermediate' water supply would mean an improved drinking-water source on premises that delivers acceptable quantities at least 12 of the past 14 days of water with <10 cfu (colony-forming units) of *Escherichia coli* per 100mL. 'Adequate' sanitation would mean use of an 'improved' sanitation facility at home, and shared sanitation would be treated as 'improved' if it otherwise meets the required service level and was shared by no more than five households or 30 people. Future developments on the post-2015 water and sanitation targets can be followed by consulting the JMP website: http://www.wssinfo.org/post-2015-monitoring/overview.

Systems approach to understanding enteric pathogen transmission

Much of the research described in previous sections regarding the health impact of water and sanitation interventions has focused on assessing the impact of interrupting particular transmission pathways. Increasingly, epidemiologists are recognizing the interaction and interdependencies that characterize the transmission of enteric pathogens. This is leading to calls for a systems approach that not only acknowledges the multiple transmission pathways and varied aetiological agents involved in diarrhoea and other enteric diseases but also their dynamism and the community level impact of interventions (Eisenberg et al. 2012). Examples of this community effect are the health benefits that inure to non-adopters who live adjacent to households with latrines or who practise effective household water treatment. Interventions that interrupt transmission of one or more pathways can also impact transmission through other pathways of one or more pathogens. It is important that studies endeavour to capture externalities and the wider impact of an intervention at the community level, both to understand and design interventions that that optimize this larger effect and to correctly assess the impact (and cost-effectiveness) of the interventions.

Water safety plans and microbial risk assessment

Traditionally, the water sector relied on compliance with end-product standards to ensure the safety of drinking water. Most drinking water standards are based on WHO guidelines that establish maximum limits for known or suspected microbial and chemical pathogens as well as physical/aesthetic characteristics. Under this approach, drinking water is to be free of pathogens at the point of delivery as demonstrated by the absence of a prescribed indicator of faecal contamination, such as *Escherichia coli* or thermotolerant coliforms (TTCs). However, the WHO adopted a risk assessment and risk management approach for improving drinking water quality (WHO 2012). The approach calls on water providers to develop and implement water safety plans similar to the hazard assessment critical control point (HACCP) approach used in the food industry to identify and control potential threats to safety. This latest rolling revision to the GDWQ also encourages greater surveillance to verify compliance.

This risk-based approach uses health-based targets for water quality. This is based on quantitative microbial risk assessment (QMRA), an approach developed for calculating the burden of disease from potential pathogens. QMRA sets pathogen limits based on the evidence concerning exposure assessment, dose–response analysis, and risk characterization (Haas et al. 1999). Risk assessment and acceptable levels of risk are expressed in terms of DALYs. Reference pathogens are defined for each category of microbes. Significantly, these do not necessarily coincide with long-standing indicator organisms and may require capacity building in new laboratory techniques. Limited country-specific data and other resources may also delay full implementation of this approach in many countries.

Need for consistency/adherence in safe water consumption

Epidemiological modelling using QMRA has also been used to estimate the impact of sporadic exposure to contaminated drinking water, either as a result of interruptions in water supplies (Hunter et al. 2009) or from inconsistent use of point-of-use water treatment (Brown and Clasen 2012; Enger et al. 2013). The models show that in settings with moderately contaminated water supplies, much of the health benefit from improved drinking water quality is vitiated by even occasional consumption of untreated water. These results raise questions about the health benefits that can be gained from unreliable water supplies. Moreover, insofar as point-of-use water treatment campaigns often fail to achieve high levels of adherence, these models raise questions about the potential health benefits from household-based water treatment.

Wastewater reuse

QMRA is also used in the second edition of the WHO's *Guidelines for the Safe Use of Wastewater, Excreta and Greywater* for agriculture and aquaculture (WHO 2006). As an estimated 70 per cent of water withdrawals from surface and subsurface sources are used for agricultural purposes (Water Resources Institute 2007), the agricultural sector is particularly eager to develop safe, economical, and effective water sources for crop irrigation. Wastewater can be high in plant nutrients (nitrogen, phosphorus, and potassium), minimizing the need for chemical fertilizers and producing higher incomes for farmers (Ensink and van der Hoek 2007). As municipalities in lower-income settings struggle to treat even drinking water, however, few are able to remove potential pathogens from wastewater, leaving an estimated 80 per cent of sewage untreated. The WHO *Guidelines* attempt to balance the benefits of wastewater reuse with the need for food security. As treated wastewater is also being increasingly viewed as a potential source of drinking water in water stressed regions, additional guidance based on public health evidence will be necessary.

Household-based water treatment

For the hundreds of millions who lack household water connections that provide drinking water on a 24/7 basis, water is often collected and stored in the home until needed. It is well known that even water that is safe at the point of collection undergoes frequent and extensive re-contamination during collection (or compromised distribution), storage, and use in the home (Wright et al. 2004). While providing safe, piped in, disinfected water to each household is an important goal, even the purported achievement of the MDG water target leaves more than three-quarters of a billion people without access to improved water and hundreds of millions more without safe drinking water (Clasen 2012). Accordingly, the WHO and others have called for other approaches

that will accelerate the heath and economic gains associated with safe water while progress is made in improving infrastructure.

Household water treatment and safe storage (HWTS) represent one such alternative (Sobsey 2002). Boiling, filtering, and chemically disinfecting water in the home are already in use, with more than 1 billion people reportedly treating their water at home before drinking it (Rosa and Clasen 2009). In many settings, both rural and urban, populations have access to sufficient quantities of water, but that water is unsafe. Because point-of-use interventions can improve the microbiological integrity of the water at the point of ingestion, they can reduce exposure if used correctly and consistently (exclusively) by a vulnerable population. Recent systematic reviews have shown household-based interventions (home-based boiling, chlorination, filtration, solar disinfection, and flocculation/disinfection) to be significantly more effective than traditional, non-reticulated source-based interventions (protected wells and springs, boreholes, communal tap stands) in improving microbiological water quality and reducing diarrhoeal disease (Fewtrell et al. 2005; Clasen et al. 2006; Waddington et al. 2009). The up-front cost of treating such water at the point-of-use can be dramatically less than the cost of conventional water treatment and distribution systems. Point-of-use water treatment, such as household-based chlorination, is the most cost-effective intervention to prevent diarrhoeal disease across a wide range of countries and settings (WHO and UNICEF 2002; Clasen et al. 2007). It is also among the most cost-beneficial (Hutton et al. 2007).

In 2003, the WHO helped organize the International Network for the Promotion of Safe Household Water Treatment and Storage, a global collaboration of UN and bilateral agencies, non-governmental organizations, research institutions, and the private sector committed to improved household water management as a component in water, sanitation, and hygiene programmes. The Network's website contains a considerable amount of information on household water management (http://www.who.int/household_water/en).

There is evidence, however, that the health impact from HWTS intervention trials may be exaggerated due to placebo effect and reporting bias. While more than three dozen studies of HWTS interventions reported a protective effect, none of the blinded studies that attempted to blind the intervention with a placebo found the effect to be statistically significant (Clasen et al. 2006). A large-scale double blind trial of chlorine tablets in India reported no impact of the intervention on diarrhoea or weight-for-height Z-scores in children under 5 years old (Boisson et al. 2013). This and other evidence of the lack of successful strategies for achieving adoption of HWTS interventions at scale has led some investigators to conclude that further efforts to scale up the intervention are not supported by the evidence (Schmidt and Cairncross 2009). Other investigators have noted, however, that if the estimates of effect of HWTS interventions are discounted by the exaggerated effect associated with open trials of reported outcomes (like self-reported diarrhoea), the interventions are still protective, particularly for those HWTS methods whose sustainability can be maintained (Hunter 2009; Wolf et al. 2014).

There is a need for additional assessments of HWTS interventions using placebos and objective outcomes in order to determine the actual protective effect of HWTS interventions to prevent diarrhoea. Even so, the size of the effect, if any, is likely to depend largely on the level of exposure, principal aetiological agent, other potential sources of exposure, the efficacy of the HWTS method, the consistency of its use, and other factors that research may not yet have identified.

Shared and public sanitation

An estimated 450 million people—including a fifth of the population of sub-Saharan Africa and Eastern Asia—rely on public or other shared sanitation facilities (WHO and UNICEF 2013). Historically, such shared facilities are excluded from the definition of 'improved' sanitation for purposes of monitoring progress toward the MDG sanitation target, regardless of the level of service or number of people sharing them, because they are deemed unacceptable, unhygienic, and inaccessible. The JMP is currently considering a revision to this policy that would allow shared latrines to be considered 'improved' if they otherwise meet the required service level and are shared by no more than five households or 30 persons. However, there is little evidence to support this change. A systematic review and meta-analysis of 11 studies reporting on diarrhoea found increased odds of disease associated with reliance on shared sanitation (OR 1.39; 95 per cent CI: 1.14–1.70) (Heijnen et al. 2014). While there was some evidence of increased risk with the number of households sharing, there was an elevated risk at any level of sharing. An analysis of JMP data also found evidence of increased risk of diarrhoea associated with sharing latrines, even after adjusting for likely confounders (Fuller et al. 2014).

There are various reasons why observational studies might find shared sanitation to be associated with adverse health outcomes. These include differences in the underlying risk profile of people who rely on shared sanitation rather than individual household latrines, differences in latrine maintenance and use, increased exposure to pathogens circulating in the public domain, and differences in sludge management that increase community exposure. Shared sanitation is likely a necessity, particularly in high-density urban settings. It represents an increasing proportion of the types of sanitation on which populations in low-income settings rely. It is therefore necessary for research to determine whether shared sanitation actually increases risk, and if so, the reasons therefor and the interventions that can be implemented to mitigate any such increased risk.

Safe disposal of child faeces

While there are few published studies, the evidence suggests that in many low-income settings, nappies and potties are rarely available or used, making the hygienic collection of early child faeces difficult; if collected, such faeces are often disposed of in a manner that does not prevent further exposure (Gil et al. 2004). In fact, the unsanitary disposal of child faeces may present a greater health risk than that of adults. First, young children represent the highest incidence of enteric infections, and their faeces are most likely to contain agents. Second, young children tend to defecate in areas where susceptible children could be exposed. Third, young children who are also most at risk of mortality and the serious sequelae associated with enteric infection are most likely to be exposed to these ambient agents due to the time they spend on the ground, their tendency to put fingers and fomites in their mouths, and common behaviours such as geophagia. In a meta-analysis of ten observational studies published between 1987 and 2001, Gil et al. (2004) found that child faeces disposal behaviours considered risky (open defecation, stool disposal in the open, stools not removed from soil, stools seen in household soil, and children

seen eating faeces) were significantly associated with an increased risk of diarrhoeal diseases (relative risk (RR) 1.23; 95 per cent CI: 1.15–1.32); behaviours considered safe (use of latrines, nappies, potties, toilets, washing diapers) was borderline protective (RR 0.93; 95 per cent CI: 0.85–1.00).

There is evidence that even households with latrines often fail to disposal of child faeces safely; more commonly, they are either not collected or are disposed of with the household's other solid waste (Majorin 2012). By definition, this renders the practice 'open defecation' even though these households are usually counted as having 'improved sanitation' due to the presence of the latrine (WHO and UNICEF 2013). Efforts to end open defecation will not be successful unless they include interventions to ensure the safe disposal of child faeces.

Technological and programmatic innovations

Steps to improve water supplies and sanitation, particularly in rural and remote locations, have proved especially challenging. Despite concerted efforts over past decades, vast numbers in Africa and South/South East Asia still lack improved water and sanitation (WHO and UNICEF 2014). While a variety of communal and household-level options have been promoted as alternatives to customary approaches in order to improve water quality, quantity, and proximity, some of these have been found wanting in terms of technological suitability, cost, and sustainability. New challenges include natural or man-made chemical contamination, saline intrusion, increasing urbanization, falling water tables, threats associated with climate change, and increasing demand for agricultural and industrial uses of water. High upfront costs, lack of financing, uncertain land tenure, inadequate skilled masons for construction, pit-emptying, longer-term waste disposal, and urbanization are major challenges in sanitation.

Public health professionals, donors, programme implementers, social entrepreneurs, and the private sector have responded to these challenges by developing and promoting a variety of technological and programmatic innovations for improving water supplies and sanitation, especially among low-income populations. In water, these include developments in rainwater harvesting, water locating, borehole drilling, well digging, locally-fabricated pumps and other water lifting devices, self-supply strategies, small community water treatment and/or distribution systems, water filling stations/kiosks, and a variety of point-of-use water treatment technologies. In sanitation, much of the effort in low-income settings focuses on improved on-site solutions in rural settings and alternatives to conventional sewerage in urban settings. Communal private latrines have been promoted widely in India and elsewhere. New technologies include cheaper, lightweight squatting slabs, composting toilets, digestion chemicals, multichamber pits, pit-emptying, and improved separation of liquid and solid excreta. Sludge is increasingly being viewed as a useful product rather than waste, with innovations in collection and processing. Many of these innovations are accompanied by entrepreneurial initiatives and public–private partnerships; others through micro-finance and base-of-the-pyramid marketing. While some of these innovations appear promising, lessons from the past suggest that understanding and responding to the particular circumstances present in a given setting—and especially what the target population itself wants and is willing to pay for—are especially important in achieving large-scale sustainable improvements that will also impact public health. Technical innovations in water and sanitation that do not address the need for behaviour change are also unlikely to achieve optimal uptake and impact.

Water and wastewater testing and microbiology

American Public Health Association (APHA), the American Water Works Association (AWWA), and the Water Environment Federation (WEF) jointly publish *Standard Methods for the Examination of Water and Wastewater*, the definitive guide for water quality testing. The 22nd edition published in 2012 and available online (APHA et al. 2012) contains methods for assessing physical properties, metals, inorganic non-metallic constituents, aggregate organic constituents, individual organic compounds, radioactivity, toxicity, microbiological examination, and biological examination (APHA et al. 2012). Nevertheless, there are continuing debates about even fundamental issues, such as the use of indicators of faecal contamination such as coliforms, thermotolerant coliforms (TTC), and *Escherichia coli* (Gleeson and Gray 1997). The International Water Association's Health Related Water Microbiology Specialist Group is a rich source of research and new developments in the microbiology of water and waste, including water and wastewater treatment and its effects on health and the environment (including chlorinated by-products), methods in microbiology, microbe tracking and behaviour in water systems and the environment, rapid testing and monitoring, issues presented by bioterrorism, epidemiology and microbial risk assessment, and treatment processes.

Community-led total sanitation

First developed in Bangladesh in 1999 and expanding widely elsewhere, community-led total sanitation (CLTS) is an approach that empowers local communities to stop open defecation and to build and use latrines without the support of external hardware subsidies. Through the use of participatory techniques, community members analyse their own sanitation situation, including the extent of open defecation and the possibilities of faecal–oral contamination. This is designed to ignite a personal sense of disgust and shame that translates into collective action to reduce the impact of open defecation (Kar 2003). By triggering collective behaviour change, CLTS places the community, rather than the household, at the centre of the decision-making process. Peer pressure and civic pride are important motivating factors. The particular design of a latrine is secondary to the emphasis on 100 per cent coverage. The results can be impressive, with whole communities changing from open defecation to latrine use in a matter of months (Kar 2003). The approach has since been rolled out in Africa and Asia, and there is some evidence of its sustainability (Kar and Bongartz 2006). Nevertheless, the use of shaming and other social pressure to encourage latrine ownership is controversial (Bartram et al. 2012). Recent reconsideration of various aspects of the approach has resulted in proposed changes that are now promoted under the moniker 'CLST+'.

Sanitation marketing

Sanitation marketing uses a commercial approach to the production and delivery of sanitation technologies and engages the private sector for production and delivery in a financially and institutionally sustainable manner (Jenkins and Sugden 2006). Such a marketing approach has been recommended over typical public-sector promotion of sanitation since it helps ensure that people choose to receive what they want and are willing to pay for, is financially sustainable, is cost-effective, and can be taken to scale (Cairncross 2004). Sanitation marketing adopts a consumer perspective, starting with an understanding of which products and services the target population wants, will pay for, will maintain, and are appropriate to the local context. It seeks to develop a sustainable sanitation industry, which is not dependent on external donors for hardware subsidies or long-term support for its continuation (Water and Sanitation Program n.d.). It recognizes the household as the key decision-maker regarding their defecation practice and the importance of effective public private partnerships. The extent to which the approach is capable of reaching the base of the economic pyramid has not yet been shown.

Scaling up sanitation; subsidies

Research has begun to explore the drivers and constraints toward latrine adoption (Jenkins and Curtis 2005; Jenkins and Scott 2007). Results demonstrate that while public health and economic benefits are the main societal reasons for investing in sanitation, householders have different reasons for wanting a latrine (Table 2.6.3). Research has shown that the rate of uptake of sanitation interventions increases as information spreads from one household to another, much like the adoption curves that characterize many new innovations (Cairncross 2004; Jenkins and Curtis 2005). Householder-perceived advantages of using a latrine become apparent as housing density starts to increase and when the need for privacy, convenience, and maintaining dignity become more important.

Subsidizing latrine construction is a controversial issue within the sanitation sector. Public incentives to private individuals are justified in an economic sense when there are externalities—social benefits that go beyond the private benefits associated with a given private action. As the public health benefits of limiting open defecation are greater than the private benefits an individual gains by choosing use of latrines over open defecation, sanitation may constitute a public good, thus justifying subsidies. However, for scaling up of sanitation to be successful, subsidies must be used to encourage householders to build and use latrines and help them overcome the constraints rather than to cover the actual costs of construction. Moreover, the public service priority needs to focus on safely and efficiently managing excreta within the larger community, especially in dense urban slums, after it has left the private domain of households (Evans et al. 2004; Methra and Knapp 2005). Inappropriately applied subsidies also have the negative effects of creating dependency, distorting the behaviour of the private supply market, and perhaps most importantly, not reaching the poor.

Enteropathy

Beyond the impact of diarrhoea on malnutrition, researchers have postulated that repeated exposure to faecal pathogens may be a significant cause of environmental (tropical) enteropathy, a subclinical condition characterized by malabsorption, villus atrophy, crypt hyperplasia, T-cell infiltration, and general inflammation of the jejunum (Humphrey 2009). Enteropathy is caused by faecal bacteria ingested in large quantities by young children living in conditions of poor sanitation and hygiene. Humphrey has suggested that that the primary causal pathway from poor sanitation

Table 2.6.3 Inventory of stated benefits of improved sanitation from the private vs. public perspectives

Household perspective[1]	Society–public perspective[2]

• Increased comfort
• Increased privacy
• Increased convenience
• Increased safety, for women, especially at night, and for children
• Dignity and social status
• Being modern or more urbanized
• Cleanliness
• Lack of smell and flies
• Less embarrassment with visitors
• Reduced illness and accidents
• Reduced conflict with neighbours
• Good health in a very broad cultural sense, often linked to disgust and avoidance of faeces
• Increased property value
• Increased rental income
• Eased restricted mobility due to illness, old age
• Reduced fertilizer costs (ecological sanitation)
• Manure for crop production (ecological sanitation)
	• Reduced excreta-related disease burden (morbidity and mortality) leading to:
	  • Reduced public healthcare costs
	  • Increased economic productivity
	• Increased attendance by girls at school (for school sanitation) leading to broad development gains associated with female education
	• Reduced contamination of ground water and surface water resources
	• Reduced environmental damage to ecosystems
	• Increased safety of agricultural and food products leading to more exports
	• Increased nutrient recovery and reduced waste generation and disposal costs (for ecological sanitation)
	• Cleaner neighbourhoods
	• Less smell and flies in public places
	• More tourism
	• National or community pride

Notes:

[1] Source: data from Jenkins (2004); Jenkins and Curtis (2005); Obika et al. (2002); Mukherjee (2000); Allan (2003); and Water and Sanitation Program (2002).

[2] Reasons for public action stated in studies and documents but rarely quantified or ranked, see Evans et al. (2004); Jenkins and Sugden (2006).

and hygiene to undernutrition is tropical enteropathy and not diarrhoea. If so, current estimates may have substantially underestimated the contribution of sanitation and hygiene to growth because the effect is modelled entirely through diarrhoea. A recent study in Bangladesh found that markers of enteropathy linked to unhygienic environments (Lin et al. 2013). Further research is underway to assess the impact of water and sanitation interventions on this condition (Arnold et al. 2013).

Challenges in water and sanitation

Failure to treat diarrhoea as a serious disease

One of the threshold constraints to scaling up water and sanitation is the belief that diarrhoea—the main health threat associated with poor water and sanitation coverage—is not a disease. Figueroa and Kincaid (2010) cite numerous studies from various countries in which participants reported diarrhoea to be a natural and even desirable condition, especially in young children, not worthy of special preventative measures. Although health benefits often lack significant motivational impetus for driving preventative measures, the fact that diarrhoea is not even considered a disease by many of the most vulnerable populations further limits this strategy. Among policymakers and health officials faced with a variety of life-threatening diseases, diarrhoea may not receive the commitment of resources that its status as the third leading cause of morbidity and mortality from infectious disease would suggest it deserves.

Lack of public-sector coordination

In most countries, a variety of agencies and authorities are responsible for some part of water and sanitation. These typically include the ministries of water, health, water resources, environment, local government, rural development, and education. In many cases, there are also federal, regional, district, and local levels of government. Rarely do any of these ministries take full responsibility for all aspects of water or of sanitation. The result is often a patchwork effort that lacks funding and coordination. There are important examples of successful coordinated public sector efforts. In South Africa, strides in sanitation are occurring because of a national decision and plan which set out targets, clear strategies, significant resources, and accountability (Muller 2002). Ethiopia has also achieved considerable success in improving water and sanitation coverage, particularly in the Southern Nations, Nationalities and Peoples Region, where a commitment at the senior levels translated into coordinated and sustained action (Bibby and Knapp 2007).

Bias toward large, infrastructural solutions

Public-sector advocacy, funding, and support has been shown to be an important factor in the successful scaling up of oral rehydration salts, insecticide-treated nets, and other interventions directed at environmental health. To date, however, governmental support for community and household-based water and sanitation interventions programmes has not been extensive in most countries. This is due in part to the engineering orientation of the applicable ministries, and their emphasis on larger-scale, infrastructural improvements, especially in urban and peri-urban settings. Nearly all populations who do not enjoy piped-in water on a 24/7 basis express priority for increasing the quantity and access to water over improving its quality. Governments respond accordingly, aware not only of the political value from these popular projects (and the particularly photogenic value of water emerging from massive new pipes), but also the economic gains that are available from reducing the time people spend collecting and transporting water to their homes and from the productive use of water in agricultural activities. Multilateral and bilateral funding also tends to focus on such infrastructural water projects, despite compelling evidence that HWTS is more cost beneficial and highly cost-effective (Clasen et al. 2007; Hutton et al. 2007).

Uncertainty about the role of the private sector

Water and sanitation have traditionally been supplied by the public sector, particularly in Europe and North America where coverage, service levels, and costs are optimal. As governments, particularly in lower-income settings, have been unable to deliver services such as power, transportation, and even health and education to much of the population, they are increasingly relying on the private sector to provide such services. There are some apparent success stories where the private sector, through concessions, public–private partnerships, or other vehicles, enhances the coverage and service level of water and sanitation through increased investment and improved management of fee collection and delivery. At the same time, there are at least some notorious cases, such as Cochabamba, Bolivia, where a concession was opposed due to the perception at least that the private-sector partners were putting profits ahead of performance. There is certainly a need for regulation, as these services are usually a natural monopoly and market forces, if left unchecked, will favour delivery to higher-density and higher-income areas where paybacks are faster and costs/risks lower. The United Nations Development Programme (UNDP), World Bank, and others have examined the constructive role that the private sector can play in helping scale up the delivery of water and sanitation services (UNDP 2007). Balancing the potential contribution of the private sector against the needs of the target population will continue to represent a significant challenge for policymakers.

Decoupling sanitation from water

Since the 1990s, there has been an effort to always integrate water supply, sanitation, and hygiene promotion in developing countries within the same project. As a result, sanitation and hygiene have piggybacked on the political and community demand for improved water supplies. However, many effective interventions to improve excreta disposal do not require improvements in water supplies. While the water supply sector is dominated by engineers who lean towards technical solutions, sanitation, and hygiene promotion rely more heavily on understanding and changing behaviour, a different set of skills. As a result, staff in integrated projects naturally concentrate on water supplies, whilst excreta disposal fails to receive the resources it requires. The sanitation element is usually built around the process of providing the water supply; in fact, sanitation differs in that it requires a household rather than a community decision, requires more time, and is more complex from a behaviour change perspective. By decoupling sanitation from water, it may be possible to increase coverage more rapidly, particularly in remote areas in which water interventions are unlikely to reach in the near future.

Excreta disposal in urban unplanned areas

While urban areas generally have higher rates of sanitation than rural areas, the rapid growth of informal settlements and urban slums presents a particular challenge for sanitation (WHO and UNICEF 2014). The lack of planning controls can result in ever increasing housing densities as plots are divided and subdivided either to house expanding extended families or to increase rental income. Eventually the area becomes saturated. This complicates excreta management in two ways: (1) streets and passages become very narrow making it impassable for latrine- and septic-emptying vehicles, and (2) the space available in each compound is insufficient to build initial or replacement latrines.

Another important and sensitive question with urban sanitation is the divide between public and private responsibility. Public funds are used to install, manage, and maintain public sewers and tariffs or taxation used to recover costs. No such publicly funded services are provided for the poor living in the unplanned high-density areas, and excreta disposal is regarded as being the sole responsibility of the household. It is arguable that the public health benefits from providing an appropriate pit emptying service could be so great that it warrants total public funding and provided free of charge to the poor.

Conflicting objectives in sanitation

Sanitation projects usually aim for a combination of four often-conflicting objectives. The first is to build a large number of latrines in a relatively short time, driven in part by the MDGs or national targets. In such cases, projects often use a supply-driven approach that coerces, entices, or persuades householders to build latrines by providing a generous subsidy, normally in the form of free hardware and/or labour. But when funding ends, the delivery and support mechanisms dissolve and the community members are left, as they started, with a lack of latrine component supply chains and nowhere to turn to for support. The second objective is to develop a sustainable sanitation industry that can continue providing latrines for many generations to come. This requires a good understanding of demand, the motivations and constraints of households in building and using latrines, and the use of marketing techniques to develop, promote, and supply better latrine components. This is a longer-term process which will not result in a large number of latrines being built in a short period of time and is therefore not attractive to politicians, donors, government officials, and implementers wanting instant MDG-driven solutions and to be seen to be doing something. The third objective driving sanitation is to enhance sustainable livelihoods and environmental improvements. This can be achieved by taking an ecological sanitation approach to latrine building which ensures that the nutrients in the excreta are reused to grow crops. The fourth objective is organizational insistence that their work must be targeted at the poorest of the poor. These are the most risk adverse, hardest to reach, price-sensitive members of the population who are also likely to be the least well educated and socially or politically connected. This makes them the least likely people to benefit from either a supply- or a demand-driven approach. While a targeted, sustainable, demand-driven, livelihood-enhancing latrine building programme that builds a large number of latrines in a short period of time is the ideal, decision-makers need to understand the weaknesses of each approach and prioritize their expectations accordingly.

Conclusion

Unlike many of the other challenges in public health, the solutions for eliminating most of the disease burden associated with poor water and sanitation are well known. All but the poor have enjoyed the health, economic, and other benefits associated with safe drinking water and basic sanitation for decades. The fact that hundreds of millions still lack access to these fundamental resources is a scandal that generations have allowed to persist simply as a matter of misguided priorities. And as the 'haves' continue to make rapid gains, they are not only increasing the gap over the 'have-nots' but also using up larger amounts of the world's limited water supplies and capacity for waste disposal, making it more difficult and costly for others to join their privileged club.

The need to extend water and sanitation coverage is acknowledged at the highest international levels, and progress is being made. Whether these efforts will be any more successful than those expressed in previous international declarations and goals is not yet clear. As the poor continue to wait for the piped-in water supplies and sanitary disposal that they deserve, however, it is incumbent on the public health community to develop, assess, and promote effective, low-cost, and sustainable alternatives and creative delivery strategies in order to accelerate access to the health gains associated with safe drinking water and basic sanitation.

Key points

◆ While safe drinking water and sanitation are widely recognized as fundamental public health interventions, more than a sixth of the world's population still lack improved water supplies and 40 per cent lack basic sanitation.

◆ The infectious diseases associated with unsafe drinking water and poor sanitation impose a heavy burden, especially on the poor, the very young, and the immunocompromised; they also aggravate poverty, education, and economic development.

◆ There is strong evidence that interventions to improve water supplies or sanitation can be effective in preventing diarrhoea, soil-transmitted helminth infections, schistosomiasis, and typhoid fevers.

◆ Water and sanitation interventions have also been shown to be cost-effective and cost-beneficial, with significant savings to the public sector from reduced healthcare costs; there is also evidence of other economic and developmental benefits from improved access to water and sanitation.

◆ A variety of recent and emerging developments, including new methods for assessing and monitoring the risk of diseases associated with water and sanitation as well as alternative technologies, programmatic approaches, and implementation strategies, may contribute to improved targeting, coverage, uptake, and sustainability.

◆ Nevertheless, significant political, social, economic, and developmental challenges must be addressed in order to successfully scale up some of these interventions on a sustainable basis and thus provide the most vulnerable populations with the health and other benefits of safe drinking water and sanitation.

Acknowledgements

The author acknowledges the contributions of Steven Sugden to a previous version of this chapter.

References

Allan, S.C. (2003). *The WaterAid Bangladesh/VERC 100% Sanitation Approach: Bangladesh*. IDS Working Paper 194. Brighton: Institute of Development Studies, Brighton.

American Public Health Association, American Water Works Association, and the Water Environment Federation (2012). *Standard Methods for the Examination of Water and Wastewater* (22nd ed.). Washington, DC: American Public Health Association, the American Water Works Association, and the Water Environment Federation. Available at: http://www.standardmethods.org.

Arnold, B., Null, C., Luby, S., et al. (2013) Cluster-randomized controlled trials of individual and combined water, sanitation, hygiene, and nutritional interventions in rural Bangladesh and Kenya: The WASH Benefits Study design and rationale. *BMC Open*, 3(8), e003476.

Bannister, M., Hannan, M.D., Jones, H., et al. (2005). *Water and Sanitation for All: Practical Ways to Improve Accessibility for Disabled People*. 31st WEDC Conference, Maximising the benefits from water and environmental sanitation, Kampala, Uganda.

Bartram, J., Charles, K., Evans, B., O'Hanlon, L., and Pedley, S. (2012). Commentary on community-led total sanitation and human rights: should the right to community-wide health be won at the cost of individual rights? *Journal of Water and Health*, 10(4), 499–503.

Bharadwaj, S. and Patkar, A. (2004). *Menstrual Hygiene and Management in Developing Countries: Taking Stock*. Mumbai: Junction Social, Social Development Consultants.

Bhutta, Z.A., Das, J.K., Rizvi, A., et al. (2013). The Lancet Nutrition Interventions Review Group, and the Maternal and Child Nutrition Study Group. Evidence-based interventions for improvement of maternal and child nutrition: what can be done and at what cost? *The Lancet*, 382, 452–77.

Bibby, S. and Knapp, A. (2007). *From Burden to Communal Responsibility: A Sanitation Success Story from Southern Region in Ethiopia*. Field Note. Washington, DC: World Bank Water and Sanitation Programme.

Black, R.E. and Lanata, C.F. (1995). Epidemiology of diarrhoeal diseases in developing countries. In M.J. Blaser, P.D. Smith, J.I. Ravdin, H.B. Greenberg, and R.L. Guerrant (eds.) *Infections of the Gastrointestinal Tract*, pp. 11–29. New York: Raven Press.

Black, R.E., Morris, S.S., and Bryce, J. (2003). Where and why are 10 million children dying every year? *The Lancet*, 361, 2226–34.

Blakely, T., Hales, S., Kieft, C., Wilson, N., and Woodward, A. (2005). The global distribution of risk factors by poverty level. *Bull World Health Organ*, 83(2), 118–26.

Boisson, S., Stevenson, M., Shapiro, L., et al. (2013). Effect of household-based drinking water chlorination on diarrhoea among children under five in Orissa, India: a double-blind randomised placebo-controlled trial. *PLOS Medicine*, 10(8), e1001497.

Brown, J. and Clasen, T. (2012). High adherence is necessary to realize health gains from water quality interventions. *PLoS One*, 7(5), e36735.

Burton, M.J. and Mabey, D.C. (2009). The global burden of trachoma: a review. *PLOS Neglected Tropical Diseases*, 3(10), e460.

Cairncross, S. (1987). The benefits of water supply. In J. Pickford (ed.) *Developing World Water*, pp. 30–4. London: Grosvenor Press.

Cairncross, S. (1992). *Sanitation and Water Supply: Practical Lessons from the Decade*. Washington, DC: World Bank.

Cairncross, S. (2004). *The Case for Marketing Sanitation*. Field Note. Nairobi: Water and Sanitation Programme Africa.

Cairncross, S. and Feachem, R. (1993). *Environmental Health Engineering in the Tropics: An Introductory Text* (2nd ed.). Chichester: John Wiley and Sons Ltd.

Cairncross, S., Muller, R., and Zagaria, N. (2002). Dracunculiasis (Guinea worm disease) and the eradication initiative. *Clinical Microbiology Reviews*, 15, 223–46.

Checkley, W., Buckley, G., Gilman, R.H., et al. (2008). The Childhood Malnutrition and Infection Network. Multi-country analysis of the effects of diarrhoea on childhood stunting. *International Journal of Epidemiology*, 37, 816–30.

Chen, G., Wang, M.H.S., Ou, N., et al. (2004). Observation on the effect of the comprehensive measures of replacing cattle with machine and reconstructing water supply and lavatory to control the transmission of schistosomiasis. *Journal of Tropical Disease and Parasitology*, 2, 219–22.

Clasen, T. (2009). *Scaling Up Household Water Treatment in Low-Income Settings*. Geneva: World Health Organization. Available at: http://whqlibdoc.who.int/hq/2009/WHO_HSE_WSH_09.02_eng.pdf.

Clasen, T. (2012). MDG water target claim exaggerates achievement. *Tropical Medicine & International Health*, 17(10), 1178–80.

Clasen. T., Haller, L., Walker, D., et al. (2007). Cost-effectiveness analysis of water quality interventions for preventing diarrhoeal disease in developing countries. *Journal of Water and Health*, 5 (4), 599–608.

Clasen, T., Roberts, I., Rabie, T., et al., (2006). Interventions to improve water quality for preventing diarrhoea. *Cochrane Database of Systematic Reviews*, 3, CD004794.

Colford, J.M. Jr, Saha, S.R., Wade, T.J., et al. (2005). A pilot randomized, controlled trial of an in-home drinking water intervention among HIV + persons. *Journal of Water and Health*, 3(2), 173–84.

Colindres, R., Mermin, J., Ezati, E., et al. (2007). Utilization of a basic care and prevention package by HIV-infected persons in Uganda. *AIDS Care*, 24, 1–7.

Crump, J.A., Luby, S.P., and Mintz, E.D. (2004). The global burden of typhoid fever. *Bulletin of the World Health Organization*, 82, 346–53.

Crump, J.A. and Mintz, E.D. (2010). Global trends in typhoid and paratyphoid fever. *Clinical Infectious Diseases*, 50, 241–6.

Curtis, V. and Cairncross, S. (2003). Effect of washing hands with soap on diarrhoea risk in the community: a systematic review. *The Lancet Infectious Diseases*, 3, 275–81.

Cutler, D. and Miller, G. (2005). The role of public health improvements in health advances: the twentieth-century United States. *Demography*, 42 (1), 1–22.

Dangour, A.D., Watson, L., Cumming, O., et al. (2013). Interventions to improve water quality and supply, sanitation and hygiene practices, and their effects on the nutritional status of children. *Cochrane Database of Systematic Reviews*, 8, CD009382.

Davis, J. and Lambert, R. (2002). *Engineering in Emergencies*. London: Intermediate Technology Publications, Ltd.

Department of International Development (1998). *Guidance Manual on Water Supply and Sanitation Programmes*. London: Department of International Development.

Desilva, N.R., Brooker, S., Hotez, P.J., et al. (2003). Soil-transmitted helminth infections: updating the global picture. *Trends in Parasitology*, 19, 547–51.

Eisenberg, J.N., Trostel J., Sorensen R.J., and Shields K.F. (2012). Toward a systems approach to enteric pathogen transmission: from individual independence to community interdependence. *Annual Review of Public Health*, 33, 239–57.

Emerson, P.M., Bailey, R.L., and Mahdi, O.S. (2000). Transmission ecology of the fly *Musoca sorbens*, a putative vector of trachoma. *Transactions of the Royal Society of Tropical Medicine and Hygiene*, 94, 1–5.

Emerson, P.M., Cairncross, S., Bailey, R.L., et al. (2000a). Review of the evidence base for the 'F' and 'E' component of the SAFE strategy for trachoma control. *Tropical Medicine and International Health*, 5(8), 515–27.

Emerson, P.M., Lindsay, S.W., Alexander, N., et al. (2004). Role of flies and provision of latrines in trachoma control: cluster-randomised controlled trial. *The Lancet*, 363, 1093–8.

Enger, K.S., Nelson, K.L., Rose, J.B., and Eisenberg, J.N. (2013). The joint effects of efficacy and compliance: a study of household water treatment effectiveness against childhood diarrhea. *Water Research*, 47(3), 1181–90.

Ensink, J.H. and van der Hoek, W. (2007). New international guidelines for wastewater use in agriculture. *Tropical Medicine and International Health*, 12(5), 575–7.

Esrey, S.A., Feachem, R.G., and Hughes, J.M. (1985). Interventions for the control of diarrhoeal diseases among young children: improving water supplies and excreta disposal facilities. *Bulletin of the World Health Organization*, 63, 757–72.

Esrey, S.A., Potash, J.B., Roberts, L., et al. (1991). Effects of improved water supply and sanitation on ascariasis, diarrhoea, dracunculiasis, hookworm infection, schistosomiasis, and trachoma. *Bulletin of the World Health Organization*, 69, 609–21.

Evans, B., Hutton, G., and Haller, L. (2004). *Closing the Sanitation Gap—The Case for Better Public Funding of Sanitation and Hygiene*. Oslo: Commission on Sustainable Development.

Ferriman, A. (2007). BMJ readers choose the 'sanitary revolution' as greatest medical advance since 1840. *British Medical Journal*, 334, 111.

Fewtrell, L., Kaufmann, R., Kay, D., et al. (2005). Water, sanitation, and hygiene interventions to reduce diarrhoea in less developed countries: a systematic review and meta-analysis. *The Lancet Infectious Diseases*, 5, 42–52.

Fewtrell, L., Pruss-Ustun, A. Bos, R., et al. (2007). *Water, Sanitation and Hygiene—Quantifying the Health Impact at National and Local Levels in Countries with Incomplete Water Supply and Sanitation Coverage*. Environmental Burden of Disease series No. 15. Geneva: World Health Organization.

Figueroa, M.E. and Kincaid, D.L. (2010). *Social, Cultural and Behavioral Correlates of Household Water Treatment and Storage*. Center Publication HCI 2010-1: Health Communication Insights. Baltimore, MD: Johns Hopkins Bloomberg School of Public Health, Center for Communication Programs.

Freeman, M.C., Greene, L.E., Dreibelbis, R., et al. (2012). Assessing the impact of a school-based water treatment, hygiene and sanitation programme on pupil absence in Nyanza Province, Kenya: a cluster-randomized trial. *Tropical Medicine & International Health*, 17(3), 380–91.

Fuller, J.A., Clasen, T., Heijnen, M., and Eisenberg, J.N. (2014). Shared sanitation and the prevalence of diarrhea in young children: evidence from 51 countries, 2001–2011. *American Journal of Tropical Medicine and Hygiene*, 91(1), 173–80. doi: 10.4269/ajtmh.13-0503

Garn, J.V., Greene, L.E., Dreibelbis, R., Saboori, S., Rheingans, R.D., and Freeman, M.C. (2013). A cluster-randomized trial assessing the impact of school water, sanitation, and hygiene improvements on pupil enrollment and gender parity in enrollment. *J Water Sanit Hyg Dev*, 3(4).

Gleeson, C. and Gray, N. (1997). *The Coliform Index and Waterborne Disease*. London: E and FN Spon.

Gil, A., Lanata, C., Kleinau, E., and Penny, M. (2004). *Children's Feces Disposal Practices in Developing Countries and Interventions to Prevent Diarrheal Diseases*. Environmental Health Project. New York: USAID.

Gryssels, B., Polman, K., Clerinx, J., et al. (2006). Human schistosomiasis. *The Lancet*, 368, 1106–18.

Haas, C.N., Rose, J.B., and Gerba, C.P. (1999). *Quantitative Microbial Risk Assessment*. New York: John Wiley and Sons.

Hayes, C., Elliot, E., Krales, E., et al. (2003). Food and water safety for persons infected with human immunodeficiency virus. *Clinical Infectious Diseases*, 36(Suppl 2), S106–109.

Heijnen, M., Cumming, O., Peletz, R., Chan, G.K., Brown, J., Baker, K., and Clasen, T. (2014). Shared sanitation versus individual household latrines: a systematic review of healthoutcomes. *PLoS One*, 2014 Apr 17;9(4):e93300. doi: 10.1371/journal.pone.0093300.

Hotez, P., Brooker, S., Bethony, J., et al. (2004). Hookworm infection. *The New England Journal of Medicine*, 351, 799–807.

Hu, V.H., Harding-Esch, E.M., Burton, M.J., Bailey, R.L., Kadimpeul, J., and Mabey, D.C. (2010). Epidemiology and control of trachoma: systematic review. *Tropical Medicine & International Health*, 15(6), 673–91.

Humphrey, J.H. (2009). Child undernutrition, tropical enteropathy, toilets, and handwashing. *The Lancet*, 374, 1032–5.

Hunter, P.R. (1997). *Waterborne Disease Epidemiology and Ecology.* Chichester: John Wiley and Sons.

Hunter, P.R. (2009). Household water treatment in developing countries: comparing different intervention types using meta-regression. *Environmental Science & Technology*, 43(23), 8991–7.

Hunter, P.R., Zmirou-Navier, D., and Hartemann, P. (2009). Estimating the impact on health of poor reliability of drinking water interventions in developing countries. *Science of the Total Environment*, 407(8), 2621–4.

Hutton, G. (2013). Global costs and benefits of reaching universal coverage of sanitation and drinking-water supply. *Journal of Water and Health*, 11(1), 1–12.

Hutton, G. and Bartram, J. (2003). *Domestic Water Quantity, Service Level and Health.* Geneva: World Health Organization.

Hutton, G., Haller, L., and Bartram, J. (2007). Global cost-benefit analysis of water supply and sanitation interventions. *Journal of Water and Health*, 5(4), 481–502.

IRC International Water and Sanitation Centre (2006). *Girl Friendly Toilets for School Girls.* [Online] Available at: http://www.washinschools.info/page/319.

Jackson, B. (2005). *A Review of EcoSan Experience in Eastern and Southern Africa.* Field Note. Washington, DC: World Bank Water and Sanitation Programme.

Jenkins, M.W. and Curtis, V. (2005). Achieving the 'good life'; why some people want latrines in rural Benin. *Social Science & Medicine*, 61, 2446–59.

Jenkins, M.W. and Scott, B. (2007). Behavioral indicators of household decision-making and demand for sanitation and potential gains from social marketing in Ghana. *Social Science & Medicine*, 64(12), 2427–42.

Jenkins, M.W. and Sugden, S. (2006). *Rethinking Sanitation—Lessons and Innovation for Sustainability and Success in the New Millennium.* UNDP HDR, Sanitation Thematic Paper. London: London School of Hygiene and Tropical Medicine.

Kar, K. (2003). *Subsidy or Self-Respect? Participatory Total Community Sanitation in Bangladesh.* IDS Working Paper 184. Brighton: Institute of Development Studies, Brighton.

Kar, K. and Bongartz, J. (2006). *Update on Some Recent Developments in Community-Led Total Sanitation.* Brighton: Institute of Development Studies, Brighton.

Kosek, M., Bern, C., and Guerrant, R.L. (2003). The global burden of diarrhoeal disease, as estimated from studies published between 1992 and 2000. *Bulletin of the World Health Organization*, 81, 197–204.

Kotloff, K.L., Nataro, J.P., Blackwelder, W.C., et al. (2013). Burden and aetiology of diarrhoeal disease in infants and young children in developing countries (the Global Enteric Multicenter Study, GEMS): a prospective, case-control study. *The Lancet*, 382, 209–22.

Kumaresan, J. and Mecaskey, J. (2003). The global elimination of blinding trachoma: progress and promise. *The American Journal of Tropical Medicine and Hygiene*, 69, 24–8.

Kuper, H., Solomon, A.W., Buchan, J., et al. (2003). A critical review of the SAFE strategy for the prevention of blinding trachoma. *The Lancet Infectious Diseases*, 3(6), 372–81.

Leclerc, H., Schwartzbrod, L., and Dei-Cas, E. (2002). Microbial agents associated with waterborne diseases. *Critical Reviews in Microbiology*, 28(4), 371–409.

Lin, A., Arnold, B.F., Afreen, S., et al. (2013). Household environmental conditions are associated with enteropathy and impaired growth in rural Bangladesh. *The American Journal of Tropical Medicine and Hygiene*, 89(1), 130–7.

Lule, J.R., Mermin, J., Ekwaru, J.P., et al. (2005). Effect of home-based chlorination and safe storage on diarrhea among persons with HIV in Uganda. *Tropical Medicine and International Health*, 73, 926–33.

Lustigman, S., Prichard, R.K., Gazzinelli, A., et al. (2012). A research agenda for helminth diseases of humans: the problem of helminthiases. *PLoS Neglected Tropical Diseases*, 6(4), e1582.

Mabey, D.C., Solomon, A.W., and Foster, A. (2003). Trachoma. *The Lancet*, 362, 223–9.

Maili Saba Research Report (2005). *Livelihood and Gender in Sanitation And Hygiene Water Services Among Urban Poor.* London: Overseas Development Institute.

Majorin, F. (2012). *Child Faeces Disposal Practices in Rural Orissa: A Cross Sectional Study.* MSc Thesis, London School of Hygiene and Tropical Medicine.

Methra, M. and Knapp, A. (2005). *The Challenge of Financing Sanitation for Meeting the Millennium Development Goals.* Commissioned by the Norwegian Ministry of the Environment for the Commission on Sustainable Development. Water and Sanitation Program—Africa. Nairobi: World Bank.

Mukherjee, N. (2000). *Myth vs. Reality In Sanitation and Hygiene Promotion.* Field Note, Jakarta: World Bank Water and Sanitation Programme—East Asia and the Pacific.

Muller, M. (2002). *The National Water and Sanitation Programme in South Africa.* Field Note, Water and Sanitation Program—Africa. Nairobi: World Bank.

Nauges, C. and Whittington, D. (2009). Estimation of water demand in developing countries: an overview. The World Bank Research Observer, 25, 263–94.

Obika, A., Jenkins, M., Howard, G., et al. (2002). *Social Marketing for Urban Sanitation, Inception Report.* DFID KAR Project R7982. Loughborough: WEDC.

Peletz, R.L., Mahin, T., Elliot, M., et al. (2013). Water, sanitation and hygiene interventions to improve health among people living with HIV/AIDS: a systematic review. AIDS, 27(16), 2593–601.

Peletz, R., Simunyama, M., Sarenje, K., et al. (2012). Assessing water filtration and safe storage in households with young children of HIV-positive mothers: a randomized, controlled trial in Zambia. *PLoS One*, 7(10), e46548.

Pickering, A.J. and Davis, J. (2012). Freshwater availability and water fetching distance affect child health in sub-Saharan Africa. *Environmental Science & Technology*, 46(4), 2391–7.

Pullan, R.L., Freeman, M.C., Gething, P.W., and Brooker, S.J. (2014). Geographical inequalities in use of improved drinking water supply and sanitation across Sub-Saharan Africa: mapping and spatial analysis of cross-sectional survey data. *PLoS Med*, 11(4):e1001626. doi: 10.1371/journal.pmed.100162.

Prüss-Üstün, A., Bartram, J., Clasen, T., et al. (2014). Burden of disease from inadequate water, sanitation and hygiene in low- and middle-income settings: a retrospective analysis of data from 145 countries. *Tropical Medicine & International Health*, 19(8), 894–905.

Rabiu, M., Alhassan, M.B., Ejere, H.O., and Evans, J.R. (2012). Environmental sanitary interventions for preventing active trachoma. *Cochrane Database of Systematic Reviews*, 2, CD004003.

Ram, P.K., Naheed, A., Brooks, W.A., et al. (2007). Risk factors for typhoid fever in a slum in Dhaka, Bangladesh. *Epidemiology and Infection*, 135(3), 458–65.

Rosa, G. and Clasen, T. (2010). Estimating the scope of household water treatment in low- and medium-income countries. *The American Journal of Tropical Medicine and Hygiene*, 82(2), 289–300.

Schmidt, W.P. and Cairncross, S. (2009). Household water treatment in poor populations: is there enough evidence for scaling up now? *Environmental Science & Technology*, 43(4), 986–92.

Sobsey, M.D. (2002). *Managing Water in the Home: Accelerated Health Gains from Improved Water Supply.* WHO/SDE/WSH/02.07. Geneva: World Health Organization.

Spears, D. (2013). *How Much International Variation in Child Height can Sanitation Explain?* World Bank policy research working paper, no. WPS 6351. Available at: http://go.worldbank.org/SZE5WUJBI0.

Sphere Project (2004). *Humanitarian Charter and Minimum Standards in Disaster Response.* Geneva: The Sphere Project.

Srikantiah, P., Vafokulov, S., Luby, S.P., et al. (2007). Epidemiology and risk factors for endemic typhoid fever in Uzbekistan. *Tropical Medicine and International Health*, 12(7), 838–47.

Stocks, M.E., Ogden, S., Haddad, D., Addiss, D.G., McGuire, C., and Freeman, M.C. (2014). Effect of water, sanitation, and hygiene on the prevention of trachoma: a systematic review and meta-analysis. *PLoS Med*, 11(2):e1001605. doi:10.1371/journal.pmed.1001605.

Strunz, E.C., Addiss, D.G., Stocks, M.E., Ogden, S., Utzinger, J., and Freeman, M.C. (2014). Water, sanitation, hygiene, and soil-transmitted helminth infection: a systematic review and meta-analysis. *PLoS Med*, 11(3):e1001620. doi: 10.1371/journal.pmed.1001620.

Stephenson, L.S., Latham, M.S., and Ottensen, E.A. (2000). Malnutrition and parasitic helminth infections. *Parasitology*, 121, S23–38.

Thompson, J., Porras, I.T., Tumwine, J.K., et al. (2001). *Drawers of Water II: 30 Years of Change in Domestic Water Use and Environmental Health in East Africa*. London: IIED.

UN Millennium Project (2005). *UN Millennium Project Task Force on Water and Sanitation—Health, Dignity and Development: What Will it Take?* London: Earthscan.

United Nations (2000). *United Nations Millennial Declaration*. General Assembly Res. 55/2, 18 September 2000. New York: United Nations.

United Nations (2010). *The Human Right to Water and Sanitation*. United Nations General Assembly Res. 64/292, 3 August 2010. New York: United Nations.

United Nations Development Programme (2007). *Beyond Scarcity: Power, Poverty and the Global Water Crisis*. Human Development Report 2006. New York United Nations Development Programme.

Waddington, H., Snilstveit, B., White, H., and Fewtrell, L. (2009). *Water, Sanitation and Hygiene Interventions to Combat Childhood Diarrhoea in Developing Countries*. New Delhi: 3ie.

Wagner, E.G. and Lanois, J.N. (1958). *Excreta Disposal for Rural Areas and Small Communities*. WHO monograph series no. 39. Geneva: WHO.

Walson, J.L., Sangaré, L.R., Singa, B.O., et al. (2013). Evaluation of impact of long-lasting insecticide-treated bed nets and point-of-use water filters on HIV-1 disease progression in Kenya. *AIDS*, 27(9), 1493–501.

Water and Sanitation Program (2002). *Selling Sanitation in Vietnam: What works?* Jakarta: World Bank Water and Sanitation Program—East Asia and the Pacific.

Water and Sanitation Program (n.d.). *Sanitation Marketing Toolkit*. World Bank. Available at: http://www.wsp.org/toolkit/toolkit-home.

Water Resources Institute (2007). *Water Resources Institute. EarthTrends Environmental Resource Portal*. Available at: http://earthtrends.wri.org/text/water-resources/variable-10.html.

White, G.F., Bradley, D.J., and White, A.U. (1972). *Drawers of Water: Domestic Water Use in East Africa*. Chicago, IL: University of Chicago Press.

Whittington, D., Jeuland, M., Barker, K., and Yuen Y (2012). Setting priorities, targeting subsidies among water, sanitation, and preventive health interventions in developing countries. *World Development*, 40(8), 1546–68.

Winblad, U. and Simpson-Hébert, M. (eds.) (2004). *Ecological Sanitation*. Stockholm: Stockholm Environmental Institute.

Wolf, J., Prüss-Ustün, A., Cumming, O., et al. (2014). Assessing the impact of drinking water and sanitation on diarrhoeal disease inlow- and middle-income settings: systematic review and meta-regression. *Trop Med Int Health*, 19(8):928–42.

World Bank (n.d.). *Water and Sanitation Program*. Available at: http://www.wsp.org/.

World Health Organization (2006). *Guidelines for the Safe Use of Wastewater, Excreta and Greywater*, Vols. 1–4. Geneva: WHO.

World Health Organization (2008). *Essential Prevention and Care Interventions for Adults and Adolescents Living with HIV in Resource-Limited Settings*. Geneva: WHO.

World Health Organization (2012). *Guidelines for Drinking-Water Quality* (Vol. 1, 4th ed.). Geneva: WHO.

World Health Organization (2013). *Global Health Observatory*. [Online] Available at: http://www.who.int/gho/en/.

World Health Organization and the United Nations Children's Fund (2002). *Global Water Supply and Sanitation Assessment*. Geneva: WHO and UNICEF.

World Health Organization and the United Nations Children's Fund (2005). *Water for Life: Decade for Action 2005–2015*. Geneva: WHO and UNICEF.

World Health Organization and the United Nations Children's Fund (2014). *Progress on Sanitation and Drinking Water: 2014 Update*. New York: WHO and UNICEF Joint Monitoring Programme on Water and Sanitation.

Wright, J., Gundry, S., Conroy (2004). Household drinking water in developing countries: a systematic review of microbiological contamination between source and point-of-use. *Tropical Medicine and International Health*, 9 (1), 106–17.

Ziegelbauer, K., Speich, B., Mäusezahl, D., Bos, R., Keiser, J., and Utzinger, J. (2012). Effect of sanitation on soil-transmitted helminth infection: systematic review and meta-analysis. *PLoS Medicine*, 9(1), e1001162.

Zhang, S.-Q., Wang, T.-P., Tao, C.-G., et al. (2005). [Observation on comprehensive measures of safe treatment of night-soil and water supply, replacement of bovine with machine for schistosomiasis control]. *Zhongguo Xue Xi Chong Bing Fang Ji Za Zhi* [*Chinese Journal of Schistosomiasis Control*], 17(6), 437–42.

Food and nutrition

Prakash S. Shetty

Introduction to food and nutrition

Food and the nutrients in it, habitually consumed by individuals, are important determinants of the health of populations worldwide. Nutrition and health interactions are complex and their determinants include: the social, economic, and cultural issues related to making the right food choices; purchasing and eating the 'correct' types of food in 'appropriate' quantities; as well as the daily human activity and behaviour related to food. Just as the acquisition of the knowledge of microbiology influenced our understanding of infectious diseases which in turn led to preventive measures for the population, so the historical advances in nutrition have led to a more coherent understanding of the patterns of and the prevention of diet-related diseases of public health importance.

Environmental determinants of variations in disease rates include food and nutrition as one of the primary determinants. In the developing world, numerous nutrient deficiency diseases persist and now coexist with the increasing incidence of diet-related chronic diseases. Developing societies now bear the 'double burden' of malnutrition with the emergence of the so-called 'diseases of affluence' amidst persisting undernutrition in their populations. Changes in the rates and patterns of nutritional disease and their contribution to premature death within a population depend largely on the environmental factors, which include changes in social and economic conditions, the implementation of immunization programmes, improvements in women's social and educational status within the society, and changes in agriculture and food systems and in the availability of food. These changes have been influenced in recent times by globalization and the increasing global trade and the remarkable advances and changes in agricultural practices and the food systems that affect individual diets and lifestyles. National policies that seek to promote economic activity and international trade to boost foreign exchange earnings ignore the impact of these measures on the health of the populations. Economic development is normally accompanied by improvements in the quantity and quality of a nation's food supply and improvements in the immediate environment and living standards of the community. Beneficial environmental influences operate through changes in the provision of and access to hygienic and nutritious food; the availability of potable water, clean housing, and sanitary surroundings; and lack of exposure to environmental toxins. These changes contribute to a food and nutrition-mediated improvement in the body's resistance to infections and better health. The mutual interdependence of the immune and nutritional status of the population probably explains at least some of the gains in public health in Britain in the last century (McKeown 1976).

The quantitative and qualitative changes in our food patterns that lead to such dramatic changes in life expectancy also result in the problems of diet-related chronic diseases. Diet-related chronic diseases occur typically in middle and later adult life and can, by increasing the incidence of premature mortality, undermine the gains in life expectancy. More importantly they lead to morbidity and the resultant disability-adjusted life years (DALYs) lost as well as contributing to economic losses and reducing the quality of life. These diet-related chronic diseases are traditionally regarded as manifestations of overconsumption and self-indulgence in an affluent society. In practice, some of these chronic diseases may be compounded by relatively deficient intakes of some nutrients, thus emphasizing the need for a diversified and balanced daily diet for good health.

Nutrition has re-emerged as being fundamental to public health. Nutritional issues were seen in industrialized, developed societies as relating to deficiency diseases, which were conquered in the early part of the twentieth century while continuing to persist in the relatively poor, developing countries. Now, food and nutrition are recognized as one of the principal environmental determinants of a wide range of diseases of public health importance globally. These diseases reflect the cumulative impact of a variety of pathophysiological processes over a lifetime and the interactions are often seen as reflecting individual genetic susceptibility, but the different disease patterns of groups living on different diets being manifestly a societal reflection of the impact of dietary factors. The display of nutrient–gene interactions is evident, for example, in obesity, alcoholism, cardiovascular disease, type 2 diabetes mellitus, many gastrointestinal disorders, neural tube defects, and the most prevalent cancers. Molecular epidemiology unravels the basis for genetic susceptibility to some of these disorders while the gene inducers or repressors often prove to be of dietary or environmental origin. Societal features, which determine human behaviour and economic well-being as well as climate, tradition, and culture, all affect food consumption patterns and dietary practices. These are features which need to be considered in public health rather than simply the epidemiological or aetiological aspects of diet-related diseases.

This chapter seeks to take a global view of food and nutrition as determinants of public health. This is particularly important because deficiency diseases are widespread in several parts of the world and yet coexist in the same country with chronic diet-related diseases in adults. Vitamin deficiencies, both clinical and subclinical, continue to manifest in poor communities as well as in apparently healthy populations. Threat of hunger and starvation and severe dietary inadequacy resulting in malnutrition often emerges during conflict and other emergencies. This chapter is structured in such a way that it deals with both sides of the 'mal' nutrition in humans as relevant to public health.

Food and nutrition security

The pre-eminent determinant of 'hunger' (household food insecurity) is poverty in societies. The recognition that poverty and hunger go hand in hand is manifest in the United Nations (UN) Millennium Development Goals (MDGs), which specify targets for the reduction of both global poverty and hunger by the year 2015 (MDG 1). Improving household food security is one of the objectives of all democratic societies and constitutes an important element of the human right to adequate food. *Food security* is defined as 'the access by all people at all times to the food they need for an active and healthy life'. The inclusion of the term 'household' ensures that the dietary needs of all the members of the household are met throughout the year. According to the UN Food and Agricultural Organization (FAO) food insecurity is thus, 'a situation that exists when people lack secure access to sufficient amounts of safe and nutritious food for normal growth and development and an active and healthy life' (FAO 2000). Food insecurity may be caused by the unavailability of food, insufficient purchasing power, inappropriate distribution, or inadequate use of food at the household level. Hence current definitions of food security emphasize the 'availability', 'accessibility', 'stability', and 'utilization' of food.

The achievement of household food security requires an adequate supply of food to all members of the household, ensuring stability of supply all year round, and the access, both physical and economic, which underlines the importance of the entitlement to produce and procure food. Food insecurity may be a result of the unavailability of food, inadequate purchasing power, or inappropriate utilization of food at the household or individual level. Thus, food security at the household level is a complex phenomenon attributable to a range of factors that vary in importance across regions, countries, and social groups, as well as over time (Shetty 2006). It is described in terms of the availability and stability of good quality, safe, and nutritious food supplies, and the access to, and utilization of, this food. All these criteria must be met for the consumption of a healthy diet and the achievement of nutritional well-being.

Availability relates to the adequacy of a varied and nutritious food supply and is influenced principally by factors that promote agricultural production and trade. Factors that influence this include policies and incentives, access to natural resources, and the availability of agricultural inputs, skills, and technologies including biotechnology. Stability of the level and types of foods available for consumption is subject to seasonality and by the sustainability of production and farming systems in practice. These in turn depend on the efficiency of market systems, including pricing mechanisms and infrastructure such as transport and warehousing, which influences the storage, distribution, and flow of food. While reduction of food losses through improvements in food storage and processing also affects stability, the nature of the farming system adopted and its effect on the environment and on sustainability is also a key determinant of the stability of food supplies in the medium to long term.

Access that a community, household, or individual has to food is a reflection of the ability to either grow and retain the food grown for consumption, to purchase the food from the market, or to acquire it by a combination of strategies that are described as representing 'entitlements' to food (Sen 1981). This system depends on a range of factors such as: access to resources such as land, water, agricultural inputs, and improved technologies; the nature of the food marketing system and the infrastructure to support it; purchasing power and food prices; and consumer perceptions, behaviour, and preferences. Utilization is more concerned with the biological availability of the food after it has been ingested. While age, body size, and physical activity levels are important determinants, the absence of disease and parasitic infestations also influence the utilization of nutrients by the body. As a consequence, the biological utilization of food is largely influenced by environmental factors such as clean water and good sanitation.

The necessity to include nutrition into food security evolved over time as nutrition security in principle is more than food security (Shetty 2009). The nutrition focus adds physiological requirements for different nutrients and the determinants of their bioavailability and bioutilization as well as aspects of caring practices and health services and healthy environments that influence it. *Nutrition security* can be defined as 'adequate nutritional status in terms of protein, energy, vitamins, and minerals for all household members at all times' (Quisumbing et al. 1995, p. 12). While this definition illustrates the consideration of the need for food to ensure optimal supply of nutrients in the diet, i.e. physiological needs, other definitions of nutrition security focus on the vulnerable individual and their needs related to non-food factors. While pointing out the need for a paradigm shift in policy formulation from attention to food security at the aggregate level to nutrition security at the level of each individual, Swaminathan (2008) defines nutrition security as, 'physical, economic and social access to balanced diet, safe drinking water, environmental hygiene, primary health care and primary education'. This definition of nutrition security involves both food and non-food factors and consequently food and nutrition security integrates both conceptual frameworks. The recognition that food, which includes water, is a substance that people eat and drink to achieve an adequate nutritional status, i.e. maintain life and physical, cognitive, and social development, and that it has to meet physiological requirements in terms of quantity, quality, and safety and be socially and culturally acceptable, influenced and amended the definition further. Accordingly, '*food and nutrition security* is achieved, if adequate food (quantity, quality, safety, socio-cultural acceptability) is available and accessible for and satisfactorily utilized by all individuals at all times to achieve good nutrition for a healthy and happy life' (Weingartner 2005, p. 5).

Undernutrition in children and adults

The causes of undernutrition are multidimensional and its determinants include both food- and non-food-related factors such as socioeconomic, cultural, and environmental deprivations. Although establishing a relationship between these variables, and the indicators of undernutrition do not necessarily imply causality, they demonstrate that in addition to food availability many social, cultural, health, and environmental factors influence its prevalence. People faced with inadequacy of food are generally poor, but not all the poor are undernourished. Even in households that are food secure, some members may be undernourished. Income fluctuations, seasonal disparities in food availability, demand for high levels of physical activity, and proximity and access to marketing facilities may singly or in combination influence the nutritional status of an individual or a household. Transition from subsistence farming to commercial agriculture and cash crops may help improve nutrition in the long run; however, over the short term they may have negative impacts unless accompanied by improvements in access to health services, environmental sanitation, and other social investments. Rapid urbanization and rural to urban migration may lead to nutritional deprivation and alter cultural attitudes in food preferences and practices, and women's time constraints including that available for child-rearing practices, and thus influence the health of the vulnerable in societies. Inadequate housing and over-crowding, poor sanitation, and lack of access to a protected water supply, through links with infectious diseases, are potent environmental factors that influence biological food utilization and nutrition. Inadequate access to food, limited access to healthcare, and clean environments and insufficient access to educational opportunities are in turn determined by the economic and institutional structures as well as the political and ideological superstructures within society. Thus the presence of undernutrition is not only causally related to food insecurity at the household or individual level, but is also determined by other health-related factors such as access to safe water, good sanitation, healthcare, and appropriate care practices and ensuring fair intra-household food distribution.

Poor nutritional status of populations affects physical growth, cognitive development, intelligence, behaviour, and learning abilities of children and adolescents. It impacts on their physical and work performance and has been linked to impaired economic work productivity during adulthood. Inadequate nutrition predisposes them to infections and contributes to the negative downward spiral of malnutrition and infection. Good nutritional status, on the other hand, promotes optimal growth and development of children and adolescents. It contributes to better physiological work performance, enhances adult economic productivity, increases levels of socially desirable activities, and promotes better maternal birth outcomes. Good nutrition of a population manifested in the nutritional status of the individual in the community contributes to an upward positive spiral and reflects the improvement in the resources and human capital of society.

Low birth weight

Intrauterine growth retardation (IUGR) resulting in low birth weights constitutes a major public health problem in developing countries. A World Health Organization (WHO) Technical Report (WHO 1995) recommended that the 10th percentile of a sex-specific, birth weight-for-gestational-age distribution be designated for the classification of small-for-gestational-age (SGA) infants. While it is difficult to establish with certainty whether the reduced birth weight is the result of *in utero* growth restriction; in developing-country populations the high incidence of SGA infants is largely the result of IUGR.

The definition of IUGR is an infant born at term (>37 weeks of gestation) with a low birth weight (<2500 g). The causes of IUGR are multiple and the most important determinant is maternal environment of which nutrition is the most important factor. Poor maternal nutritional status at conception and inadequate maternal nutrition during pregnancy can result in IUGR. Short maternal stature, low maternal body weight and body mass index at conception, and inadequate weight gain during pregnancy are all associated with IUGR. Thus IUGR is closely related to conditions of poverty and chronic undernutrition of economically disadvantaged mothers.

More than 96 per cent of low-birth-weight (LBW) infants are born in the developing world and over 20 million children are born each year with LBW accounting for 15 per cent of all births—more than double the level in the developed world (UNICEF 2012). The incidence of low birth weight varies across regions, but South Asia has the highest incidence, at 27 per cent (with India at 28 per cent and Pakistan at 32 per cent).

LBWs due to IUGR are associated with increased morbidity and mortality in infancy. It is estimated that term infants weighing less than 2500 g at birth have a four times increased risk of neonatal death as compared to infants weighing between 2500 and 3000 g and ten times higher than those weighing between 3000 and 3500 g. The risk of morbidity and mortality in later infancy is also considerably higher in these LBW infants and is largely due to increased risk of diarrhoeal diseases and respiratory infections. Barker's studies have consistently demonstrated a relationship between LBW and later adult disease and provide an important aetiological role for fetal undernutrition in amplifying the effect of risk factors in later life thereby increasing the risk of developing diabetes, hypertension, dyslipidaemia, cardiovascular disease, and obesity in adult life (Barker 2004).

Childhood undernutrition

The clinical conditions of childhood undernutrition like kwashiorkor and marasmus are severe forms of malnutrition. They are the tip of an iceberg of widespread mild-to-moderate childhood undernutrition within the community that is relevant from a public health perspective.

The determinants of child undernutrition can be considered as operating at three levels of causality: immediate, underlying, and basic. The immediate determinants are dietary intakes and health status which are in turn influenced by three underlying determinants—household food and nutrition insecurity, care for children and their mothers, and the health environment which includes access to safe water, sanitation, and health services. Care encompasses such variables as breastfeeding and proper and timely introduction of complementary feeding, and the education of women—the primary caregiver, their status, their autonomy, and their access to resources. A poor health environment can result in frequent episodes of infection. A vicious cycle may be established and children in poor communities fail to thrive once they have succumbed to an infectious disease and they then languish, responding poorly to therapy and failing to grow even when presented with apparently adequate amounts of food.

Undernutrition in childhood is characterized by growth failure and hence, in children, assessment of growth has been the single most important measurement that best defines their nutritional status. Measures of height and weight are the commonly used indicators of the nutritional status of the child and classification of childhood undernutrition based on height, weight and age continues to be the backbone of nutritional assessment of both populations and individuals (WHO 1995) when compared against international growth reference standards developed by WHO (2006).

Children throughout the world when well fed and free of infection tend to grow at similar rates irrespective of their ethnic or racial origin, and healthy children everywhere can, when fed appropriately, be expected to grow on average along the 50th centile of a reference population's weight and height for age. By expressing both height and weight as standard deviations or Z-scores from the median reference value for the child's age, the normal range will correspond to the 3rd and 97th centile, (i.e. ±2 SDs or ±2 Z-scores). By expressing data in this way, it is possible to express the weight and height data for all children across a wide age range in similar Z-score units and thereby produce a readily understandable comparison of the extent of growth retardation at different ages and in different countries.

A deficit in height is referred to as 'stunting' whereas a deficit in weight-for-height is considered as 'wasting'. These two measures are subsumed in the designation of a child's failure to grow in terms of weight-for-age when the deficit is termed 'underweight'. Wasting can occur on a short-term basis in response to illness with anorexia or malabsorption or because the child goes hungry for several weeks. Changes in weight-for-height therefore reflect the impact of short-term changes in nutritional status. Growth in height, however, is much more a cumulative index of long-term health because growth in length or height stops when a child develops an infection and the subsequent growth may be slow during the recovery period. Children normally grow in spurts and intermittently. Energy intake is not a crucial determinant of height and the energy cost of growth and weight gain is only 2–5 per cent of total energy intake once the child is 1 year of age. Impairment of growth in height occurs in many communities at the time of weaning and up to about 2 years of age. Once the children have failed to maintain their proper growth trajectory for stature they tend to remain on the lower centiles and 'track' at this low level for many years.

While the MDGs targeted underweight in children, more recently the emphasis has shifted from underweight to stunting. The damage caused by lack of good nutrition in the first 5 years of life is largely irreversible and stunted children achieve less in school, are paid less when they enter the workforce, and are at greater risk of becoming overweight and developing chronic diseases later in life. There is now a better appreciation of the crucial importance of nutrition during the critical 1000-day period covering pregnancy and the first 2 years of a child's life, that stunting reflects deficiencies during this period and that health and nutrition interventions need to focus on this crucial period.

Global estimates of the main forms of child undernutrition are summarized in Table 2.7.1. Comparisons from earlier estimates indicate that the prevalence of underweight and stunting remain high despite substantial progress (Black et al. 2013). In most parts of Africa the numbers of underweight and stunting increased during this period while the dramatic progress in Asia is outweighed by the persisting high prevalence and numbers of children affected. Stunting is a serious problem reflecting poor nutrition and frequent infections during the early growth period. Stunting in South Asia seems also to be related to the high incidence in LBW in this region.

Underweight in children is being used as an indicator for monitoring progress towards the MDGs. Overall current analyses demonstrate some progress in reducing child undernutrition—but progress is uneven and in some countries has even deteriorated.

Table 2.7.1 Current estimates and progress since 1990 in the prevalence and numbers of child undernutrition globally and in developing countries of Africa, Asia, and Latin America

	Underweight		Stunting	
	1990	2011	1990	2011
Global				
Prevalence (%)	26.5	15.7	33.5	25.7
Numbers ($\times 10^6$)	163.4	100.7	206.5	164.8
Africa				
Prevalence (%)	23.6	17.7	36.9	35.6
Numbers ($\times 10^6$)	25.3	27.9	39.6	56.3
Asia				
Prevalence (%)	35.1	19.3	41.1	26.8
Numbers ($\times 10^6$)	131.9	69.1	154.6	95.8
Latin America				
Prevalence (%)	8.7	3.4	18.3	13.4
Numbers ($\times 10^6$)	4.8	1.8	10.0	7.1

Prevalence expressed as percentage below −2 SD of WHO International reference value.

Global estimates are predominantly developing countries in the three regions. Latin America includes the Caribbean.

Source: data from *The Lancet*, Volume 382, Issue 9890, Black RE et al., Maternal and child undernutrition and overweight in low-income and middle-income countries, pp. 427–451, Copyright © 2013 Elsevier Ltd. All rights reserved.

To achieve the MDGs more concerted effort is needed, especially in those regions with stagnating or increasing trends in child undernutrition. Well-nourished children have a better chance of surviving and growing into healthy adults. Improving child nutrition requires attention to all three components, i.e. access to adequate and safe food, freedom from illness, and appropriate care. Ensuring optimal child health and growth can contribute to a healthy adult population and accelerate economic growth of countries.

Adult undernutrition

Undernutrition among adults has been neglected and this may have profound significance for the economic growth of developing countries. One simple measure of adult nutritional status is the *body mass index* (BMI), (i.e. body weight in kilograms divided by the square of the height in metres); the most suitable index for both under- and overnutrition in adults (Shetty and James 1994). Adults with a BMI less than 18.5 are considered chronically undernourished while those with a BMI greater than 25.0 or greater than 30.0 are overweight or obese respectively (WHO 2000); the same BMI cut-offs apply to both males and females. Undernourished adults show impairment of physical well-being and exercise capacity and susceptibility to illness and the ability to sustain economic productivity. Hence, it is important to examine adult undernutrition.

Anthropometric measures of adult undernutrition provide objective estimates of the prevalence of undernutrition worldwide. In practice, children and adults may adapt to a shortage of food by reducing their physical activity without changing their body weight. Thus, measures of the prevalence of low weight-for-height provide only a limited index of food insecurity as physical activity is fundamental and desirable for physiological well-being and for limiting the development of chronic disease while promoting societies to prosper through physically demanding economic activity.

For many years the FAO has attempted to assess the global prevalence of food insecurity by relating complex measures of food supply and its variable distribution between households with estimates of the population's energy needs. The numbers of undernourished estimated most recently by FAO are 870 million of which 850 million are in developing countries (FAO 2012). Since reducing by half the proportion of the food insecure by 2015 is one of the targets set in MDG 1, monitoring progress is essential. While there has been progress in this direction since the 1990s, most of the progress has been achieved before 2007/2008, and since then progress has stalled. While the prospect of meeting the MDG 1 target is good, progress has been variable with some regions showing a worsening of the situation. Reliable global estimates of adult undernutrition based on BMI are not available since nutritional surveys rarely include adult men and the issue of adult undernutrition has also largely been ignored. With awareness of the increasing problem of overweight and obesity, more information based on anthropometric surveys of adults is being generated which will provide global data on adult undernutrition.

The basic causes of undernutrition are clearly political and socioeconomic. Agricultural revolutions such as the green revolution have increased food availability and helped meet the food needs of the population. Agricultural productivity has increased worldwide and developing countries are increasingly producing more food even when expressed on a per capita basis. Food prices for most commodities, particularly for cereals, had also fallen to their lowest until the food price crisis in 2007/2008. However, poverty is often the basis of a failure to have access to food even when food is available in plenty; and is aggravated by the rise in food prices. Accelerated food production will alleviate hunger only to the extent that the resources used in the process reduce poverty more than they would if used in other ways. Thus food entitlement decline is a more important force in sustaining poverty and undernutrition than a decline in the availability of food in developing societies.

Micronutrient malnutrition

Micronutrient malnutrition, also referred to as 'hidden hunger', is caused by lack of adequate micronutrients (vitamins and minerals) in the habitual diet. Diets deficient in micronutrients are characterized by high intakes of staple food and cereal crops, but low consumption of foods rich in bioavailable micronutrients such as fruits, vegetables, and animal and marine products, i.e. the lack of a diversified diet. Micronutrient deficiencies are important from a public health perspective as they affect several billion people worldwide (Table 2.7.2) and can impair cognitive development and lower resistance to disease in children and adults. They increase the risk to both mothers and infants during childbirth and impair the physical ability and economic productivity of men. The costs of these deficiencies in terms of lives lost and reduced quality of life are enormous, not to mention the economic costs to society.

Strategies to combat micronutrient deficiencies in communities have included: (1) *supplementation* of specific nutrients to meet

Table 2.7.2 Estimated global impact of micronutrient malnutrition

Micronutrient malnutrition	Estimated impact
Vitamin A deficiency	140 million preschool children affected with VAD[1]
	Contributes to 1.15 million deaths in children every year[2]
	4.4 million children suffer from xerophthalmia[1]
	6.2 million women suffer from xerophthalmia[1]
Iron deficiency	2.0 billion women (96 million of them pregnant)[2]
	67,500 maternal deaths per year from severe anaemia[2]
Iodine deficiency	1.98 billion at risk with insufficient or low iodine intakes[3]
	15.8% of population worldwide have goitre[3]
	17.6 million infants born mentally impaired every year[2]
Folate deficiency	Responsible for 200,000 severe birth defects every year[2]

Source: data from [1] Standing Committee on Nutrition, *Fifth report on the world nutrition situation: Nutrition for improved development*, World Health Organization, Geneva, Switzerland, Copyright © 2004; [2] UNICEF/Micronutrient Initiative, *Vitamin and Mineral deficiency: A World progress report* UNICEF/Micronutrient, Canada, Copyright © 2004; and [3] World Health Organization, *Iodine status worldwide*, World Health Organization, Geneva, Switzerland, Copyright © 2004.

the immediate deficits; (2) *fortification* of staple food items in the daily diet—another successful strategy that has been adopted to deal with specific nutrient deficiencies like iodine; (3) *food-based approaches* which include promoting kitchen gardens to enable families to produce and consume a diversified diet and improve the nutrition of households—promoted to reduce vitamin A deficiency in developing countries; (4) a potential strategy that is showing signs of great promise is to improve the nutrient quality of commonly consumed staples by agricultural biotechnology—a process referred to as *biofortification*. The micronutrient deficiencies that will be addressed in this chapter include only the significant ones from a public health viewpoint.

Iron deficiency and anaemia

Iron deficiency is probably the most common nutritional deficiency disorder in the world and it is estimated that globally about 1.62 billion people suffer from anaemia (de Benoist et al. 2008). Hence anaemia and iron deficiency are major public health problems with adverse consequences especially for women of reproductive age and for young children. The predominant cause of iron deficiency is nutritional, the diet failing to provide for the body's requirements of iron. Intestinal helminthic infestations exacerbate iron deficiency by loss of blood from the gut and malaria also contributes to anaemia in tropical countries. A low intake of iron and/or its poor absorption then fails to meet the enhanced demands for iron and anaemia results. Low intakes of folic acid and vitamin B_{12} also contribute to anaemia.

The consequences of iron deficiency are numerous as iron plays a central role in the transport of oxygen in the body and is also essential in many enzyme systems. Iron deficiency leads to changes in behaviour, such as attention, memory, and learning in infants and children, and negatively influences the normal defence systems against infection. T-lymphocyte function, phagocytosis, and the killing of bacteria by neutrophilic leucocytes are affected. In pregnant women, iron deficiency contributes to maternal morbidity and mortality, and increases risk of fetal morbidity, mortalitym, and LBWs (Viteri 1997). Iron deficiency results in a reduction in physical working capacity and productivity of adults both in agricultural and industrial work situations. These functional impairments are economically important as it is estimated that median value of productivity losses is about 0.9 per cent gross domestic product (GDP) and the economic impact of iron deficiency can vary from 2 per cent GDP in the case of Honduras to 7.9 per cent in Bangladesh (Horton and Ross 2003).

Iron deficiency disorders encompass a range of body iron depletion states. The least severe is *diminished iron stores* diagnosed by decreased serum ferritin levels and not usually associated with adverse physiological consequences. The intermediate, *iron deficiency without anaemia* on the other hand, is severe enough to affect production of haemoglobin without haemoglobin levels falling below clinical criteria indicative of anaemia and characterized by decreased transferrin saturation levels and increased erythrocyte protoporphyrin. The severe form with clinical manifestation is *iron deficiency anaemia* (IDA).

IDA is a serious problem worldwide and the dominant cause in all cases is nutritional iron deficiency (Table 2.7.3). The highest prevalence figures for IDA are seen in developing countries. Global estimates are 18.1 per cent for children under 5 years and 19.2 per cent among pregnant women (Black et al. 2013). Even in developed countries the prevalence of IDA is significant. Based on the estimates of IDA as a risk factor for mortality, the total attributed global burden is estimated at 841,000 deaths and over 35 million DALYs (Stoltzfus et al. 2004).

In Africa, Asia, and South America, the availability of iron in diets has been deteriorating and IDA continues to be a serious public health problem. The availability of iron in the diet for absorption is affected by both the form of iron and the nature of foods concurrently ingested. Iron exists in the diet in two forms: (1) as 'haem iron', found only in animal source foods, readily absorbable and not influenced by other dietary constituents; and (2) as 'inorganic iron', not readily available and strongly influenced by foods ingested at the same time. Both animal foods and ascorbic acid promote the absorption of inorganic iron. Diets which are primarily cereal- and legume-based may contain much iron but, in the absence of co-factors such as ascorbic acid or presence of phytates,

they provide only low levels of bioavailable iron. Concern about iron deficiency is an important reason for recommending the consumption of some animal source foods as well as foods with ascorbic acid for populations who rely predominantly on a cereal-based diet.

The strategies to combat iron deficiency include: (1) iron *supplementation*; (2) iron *fortification* of certain foods; (3) *dietary modification* to improve the bioavailability of dietary iron by modifying the composition of meals; and (4) *parasitic disease control*. Iron and folate supplementation for pregnant women are currently widely implemented in several countries; and many countries have a universal preventive supplementation programme during pregnancy. Iron supplementation of preschool- or school-aged children is also carried out in several countries. Fortification of foods with iron is a preventive measure for improving and sustaining adequate iron nutrition over a longer term. Many countries like Canada and the United States have fortified foods with iron and studies in developing countries have demonstrated the effectiveness of iron fortification of foods and salt provided these programmes are based on careful planning and follow well-established guidelines (Viteri 1997). Improvement in the supply, consumption, and the bioavailability of iron in food is an important strategy to improve iron status of populations. Food-based approaches such as diversification and modification of the diet and the inclusion of animal source foods have been tried successfully to improve iron intakes. The bioavailability of iron is influenced by the composition of the meal and food preparation methods. The consumption of ascorbate-rich foods enhances iron absorption while limiting the content of phytate will improve iron bioavailability. All of these barriers can be addressed by diversification and modification of the diets at the household or community level. Sustainable and successful strategies include the promotion of homestead gardening, small livestock production, and investment in community level technologies for preservation and storage of seasonal fruits and vegetables that are rich in micronutrients like iron (Thompson and Amoroso 2011). The introduction of biofortified cereal crops with higher content of minerals like iron and zinc is also undergoing trials to address this huge public health problem.

Table 2.7.3 Numbers of people (in millions) affected with iron deficiency anaemia based on blood haemoglobin concentration in different regions of the world

	Children		Women (15–49 years)		Men (15–59 years)	Elderly
	Preschool (millions)	School age (millions)	Pregnant (millions)	Non-pregnant (millions)	(millions)	(millions)
Global	293.1	305	56.4	468.4	260	164
Africa	83.5		17.2	69.9		
Americas	23.1		3.9	39.0		
South East Asia	115.3		18.1	182.0		
Europe	11.1		2.6	40.8		
East Mediterranean	0.8		7.1	39.8		
Western Pacific	27.4		7.6	97.0		

Source: data from Bruno de Benoist et al. (eds), *Worldwide prevalence of Anaemia 1993–2005: WHO global database on anaemia*, World Health Organization, Geneva, Switzerland, Copyright © 2008.

Malaria and intestinal parasites are important contributors to IDA in endemic areas. In populations where hookworm is prevalent, effective treatment of this infection has reduced IDA in school-age children (Stoltzfus et al. 1997). Thus strategies that address iron nutrition whether food based, or by supplementation or fortification, must be integrated with programmes such as malaria prophylaxis, helminth control, environmental health, and control of other micronutrient deficiencies to maximize effectiveness (WHO/UNICEF/UNU 2001).

Iodine deficiency disorders

The term 'iodine deficiency disorder' (IDD) refers to a complex of effects arising from deficient intakes of iodine. The mountainous areas of the world are likely to be iodine deficient because rain leaches iodine from the rocks and soils. Severely deficient areas are the Himalayas, the Andes, the European Alps, and the vast mountainous regions of China. It also occurs in flooded river valleys of Eastern India, Bangladesh, and Burma. The Great Lake basins of North America are also iodine deficient. Excessive intakes of goitrogens in food (excessive consumption of *cassava* or *brassica* group of vegetables) and water, as well as the deficiency of certain trace elements in the soil or food chain (e.g. selenium) may interfere with iodine uptake and metabolism and can cause or amplify the effects of iodine deficiency.

The prevalence of manifest IDD in the form of goitre varies globally and at present is confined to developing countries, largely because public health initiatives such as mandated or permitted iodization of salt have been in force in the developed world. Iodine deficiency and goitre is still prevalent in Central and Eastern Europe. According to recent estimates, goitre prevalence in developing countries is 15.8 per cent (WHO 2004). However, this figure masks the enormous numbers who are at risk of IDD based on urinary iodine status that reflects the insufficiency of iodine intake in the diet (Table 2.7.4). Iodine deficiency is also responsible for over 200,000 severe birth defects worldwide while also contributing to lower the intellectual capacity by as much as 10–15 percentage points (UNICEF and Micronutrient Initiative 2004).

IDD in humans is due to deficiency of iodine in the diet. Both water and foods are sources of iodine with marine fish being the richest source of iodine. Milk and meat are rich sources of iodine and fruits, legumes, vegetables, and freshwater fish are also important sources. Goitrogens in the diet are of secondary importance as aetiological factors in IDD. It has been shown that staple foods consumed largely by poor rural populations, such as cassava, maize, sweet potatoes, and lima beans contain cyanogenic glucosides which release a goitrogen thiocyanate. Cassava is now implicated as an important contributor to the endemic goitre and cretinism in non-mountainous Zaire and in Sarawak in Malaysia. Selenium deficiency in the soil can result in manifestations of IDD in the presence of modest iodine deficiency and is considered relevant in several regions of China.

Iodine is readily absorbed from the diet and is essential for the synthesis of thyroid hormones which are essential for normal growth and development. Failure to synthesize sufficient triiodothyronine as a result of iodine deficiency may be a factor in the stillbirths that occur as a part of the spectrum of IDD. Thyroid hormone deficiency leads to severe retardation of growth and maturation of all organs and the brain is particularly susceptible to damage during the fetal and early postnatal periods. The

Table 2.7.4 Proportion of population and number of individuals with insufficient iodine intake in school-age children (6–12 years) and the general population and total goitre prevalence in the same UN regions

UN region	Insufficient iodine intake (urinary iodine <100 micrograms/L)		Total goitre prevalence
	School-age children	General population	
Africa	42.7% (59.7 millions)	43.0% (324.2 millions)	26.8%
Asia	38.3% (187.0 millions)	35.6% (1239.3 millions)	14.5%
Europe	53.1% (26.7 millions)	52.7% (330.8 millions)	16.3%
Latin America and The Caribbean	10.3% (7.1 million)	10.0% (47.4 millions)	4.7%
North America	9.5% (2.1 millions)	64.5% (19.2 millions)	–
Oceania	59.4% (2.1 million)	64.5% (19.2 million)	12.9%
Total	**36.5% (285.4 millions)**	**35.2% (1988.7 millions)**	**15.8%**

Figures in parentheses are numbers of individuals at risk estimated from UN Population estimates for 2002.

Adapted with permission from World Health Organization, *Iodine status worldwide*, World Health Organization, Geneva, Switzerland, Copyright © 2004.

spectrum of IDDs in humans, from the fetus to the adult, has been outlined by Hetzel (1987).

The public health initiatives for correcting iodine deficiency include the following: *iodization* of salt has been the most favoured method and has greatly reduced the prevalence of IDDs in Switzerland, the United States, and New Zealand. Since its first successful introduction in the 1920s in Switzerland (Bürgi et al. 1990) successful programmes have been reported in Central and South America, in Europe, and in Asia. However, several developing countries have encountered problems with salt iodization programmes because it is difficult to produce and maintain enough high-quality iodized salt for large populations such as in India and Bangladesh. The costs of iodized salt and its availability and distribution to remote regions can also be a problem and may be compounded by cultural prejudices about the use of iodized salt and the loss of iodine with cooking if salt is not added after cooking. *Iodized oil* injections have been used to prevent goitre and cretinism in New Guinea (Pharoah and Connolly 1987). Iodized oil is suitable for mass programmes and can be carried out alongside mass immunization programmes. These methods have been successful in China, Indonesia, and Nepal. The major problems with iodized oil are the cost, the initial discomfort, and the likely potential risk of the transmission of hepatitis B and HIV. The need for trained personnel to inject iodized oil can be a further disadvantage. Iodized oil by mouth may be an alternative and oral iodized oil has been shown to be as effective in a single oral dose as an intramuscular injection (Phillips et al. 1988).

Although the effects of oral iodized oil seem to last for only half as long as a similar dose of injected iodized oil, oral iodized oil does not suffer from the disadvantages of iodized oil injections and so is a preferred method for use in remote areas. IDDs are excellent examples of nutritional deficiency disorders of public health importance which can readily be addressed if mass community programmes are undertaken.

Zinc deficiency

Zinc deficiency is the result of inadequate intake or absorption of zinc from the diet. Excess losses of zinc during episodes of diarrhoea also contribute to deficiency. The composition of the diet can influence zinc bioavailability as high levels of phytates in the diet may result in poor absorption while animal source foods increase availability. Based on inadequate intakes in the diet it has been estimated that globally 31.3 per cent of the population have inadequacy of zinc in the diet (Caulfield and Black 2004) while zinc deficiency has been estimated globally at 17.3 per cent (Black et al. 2013).

Worldwide, zinc deficiency is responsible for approximately 16 per cent of lower respiratory tract infections, 18 per cent of malaria, and 10 per cent of diarrhoeal disease and 1.4 per cent (0.8 million) of deaths worldwide. Attributable DALYs were higher, with zinc deficiency accounting for about 2.9 per cent of worldwide loss of healthy life years. Dietary diversification and the addition of animal source foods in the diet have helped reduce zinc deficiency and agricultural technologies such as addition of zinc enriched fertilizer to the soil (Gibson et al. 2007) and the use of biofortified crops with higher zinc and iron content have also been successfully tried to reduce the burden of zinc deficiency as a public health problem.

Vitamin A deficiency

Vitamin A deficiency (VAD) is a major public health problem in many developing countries. VAD leads to night blindness and xerosis of the conjunctiva and cornea and disrupts the integrity of their surface and causes corneal clouding and ulceration and may lead to blindness in children. Xerophthalmia continues to be a major cause of childhood blindness despite the intensive prevention programmes worldwide. The parts of the world most seriously affected include South and South East Asia, and many countries in Africa, Central America, and the Near East. Extrapolations from the best available data suggest that 140 million preschool children and more than 7 million pregnant women suffer from VAD every year (Standing Committee on Nutrition 2004). This report also states that another 4.4 million children and 6.2 million women suffer from xerophthalmia. Nearly half the cases of VAD and xerophthalmia occur in South and South East Asia.

VAD manifests as night blindness and it is estimated that globally 5.17 million preschool age children and 9.75 million pregnant women suffer from night blindness—the highest prevalence in pregnant women in Africa and South and South East Asia (WHO 2009). Global estimates are 0.9 per cent for preschool children and 7.8 per cent for pregnant women (Black et al. 2013). Based on low serum retinol levels the estimates globally are much higher at 190 million preschool children and 19.1 million pregnant women with Africa and South and South East Asia having the highest prevalence. Global estimates are 33.3 per cent for preschoolers and 15.3 per cent for pregnant women (Black et al. 2013). About

20–40 million suffer from subclinical deficiency of vitamin A which has serious consequences for child survival since VAD decreases resistance to infections and increases risk of mortality and estimates suggest this to be between 1.2 to 3.0 million children. VAD may also be associated with increased maternal morbidity and mortality.

Vitamin A belongs to a class of compounds called retinoids. Pro-vitamin A carotenoids, chiefly β-carotene, is also included. Preformed vitamin A is chiefly found in dairy products, egg yolk, in some fatty fish, and in the livers of farm animals and fish. Carotenes are generally abundant in yellow fruits (papayas, mangoes, apricots, peaches) and vegetables (carrots). Absorption of vitamin A is about 80 per cent complete in the presence of an adequate fat intake, while the absorption of carotenoids is highly bile salt dependent. Vitamin A (retinol and retinoic acid) plays a very important role in the body in cellular development and differentiation. Retinol also has a vital role in normal vision, particularly by the rods in the retina. Thus, one of the earliest manifestations of VAD is night blindness.

There is now increasing evidence that vitamin A supplements in deficient populations can reduce morbidity, mortality, and blindness although there is emerging evidence that this is not always the case (Awasti et al. 2013). Xerophthalmia has become less prevalent in hyperendemic areas in recent years and intervention strategies with periodic megadose vitamin A supplementation may have contributed to this. It is now the practice to provide vitamin supplements with immunization programmes in many countries with the aim of providing at least one dose of vitamin A per year for all children aged 6 months to 5 years. The fortification of dietary items which are universally consumed, e.g. sugar in Central America (Arroyave et al. 1981) and monosodium glutamate in Indonesia (Muhilal et al. 1988), have also had a favourable impact on the vitamin A status of the population. Triple fortification (iodine, iron, and vitamin A) of salt using microcapsules has been shown to be effective (Zimmerman et al. 2004). Following on the success of sugar fortification in Central America it has been successfully tried in Zambia and South Africa and the Philippines have successfully implemented fortification of cereals (wheat and maize flour) with vitamin A (UNICEF and Micronutrient Initiative 2004).

The problems with food fortification are essentially logistical and technological and many developing countries are beginning the process of fortifying staple foods and condiments, including margarine, cooking oil, and soya sauce, with vitamins (and minerals). Food intakes from different regions of the world show limited vitamin A availability, and the problem is exacerbated by withholding vegetables and fruits from children and pregnant and lactating women for cultural reasons in some parts of the world. Nutrition education is the only approach when VAD develops despite fruit and vegetable sources of the vitamin being in plentiful supply. These foods are not incorporated into the diets of young children and mothers, due either to lack of knowledge or cultural biases. Nutrition education together with practical advice and help with growing cheap, nutritious vegetables in home kitchen gardens may help eradicate VAD. Horticultural approaches are effective and potentially sustainable in improving vitamin A status and micronutrient status generally. Economic development and poverty reduction programmes are likely to improve socioeconomic status and may indirectly contribute to reducing the problem of VAD.

Folate deficiency

Folate enables cell division and tissue growth. Adequate folate in the diet helps prevent malformations that affect the neural tube and spinal cord such as anencephaly and spina bifida as well as birth defects like cleft lip and palate. Without adequate folate in the diet, two in every 1000 pregnancies may end up with a serious birth defect. Folate deficiency is also associated with increased risk of preterm delivery and LBW (Scholl and Johnson 2000) and may also contribute to anaemia, especially in pregnant and lactating mothers (Dugdale 2001). It may thus contribute indirectly to increased maternal illness and mortality. With the increasing awareness of the role of folate in reducing the risk of heart disease and stroke, a case is being made for folate fortification of flour, a strategy already adopted in the United States and Canada.

Addressing the challenge of micronutrient malnutrition

It is important to acknowledge the contribution of several non-government organizations (NGOs), many of them specialized in addressing specific micronutrient deficiencies (e.g. International Council for the Control of Iodine Deficiency Disorders (ICCIDD) with the objective of the sustainable elimination of IDD) while many others such as Micronutrient Initiative tackle all major micronutrient deficiencies of public health significance and the important role they play in addressing the problem of 'hidden hunger' worldwide. They closely work in partnership with governments, aid agencies, and with the UN agencies and the community to further this laudable objective.

This section has hitherto dealt with only some of the more important nutritionally determined deficiency disorders of public health importance. It is important to know that segments of populations in the world suffer from other nutritional disorders such as the deficiency of fluoride, zinc, selenium, B group vitamins, and ascorbic acid. Some of these seem to occur during seasonal deficiencies in their availability and accompany famine and conflict situations when they are seen in refugee camps. In all regions of the world there are still populations affected by one or more of these deficiencies despite the significant advances that have been made in controlling nutritional deficiency disorders. In some regions of the world, largely the result of increasing population size, the numbers of undernourished are increasing even if the population prevalence is declining. In many there is a shift in the severity of the deficiency diseases with decreasing numbers with severe deficiency and increasing numbers with mild-to-moderate deficiencies. For a majority of these countries there is still the need to pursue vigorous policies and targeted action to combat the various nutritional deficiency disorders as a part of the comprehensive health-oriented national food and nutrition policies.

Consequences of undernutrition and micronutrient deficiencies

An issue that that deserves attention is to ask the question: humanitarian considerations apart, does widespread undernutrition and micronutrient malnutrition matter? And is there a case for investing in better nutrition? According to UNICEF, approximately half the economic growth achieved by developed countries of Western Europe since 1790 until 1980 can be attributed to better nutrition

and improved health and sanitation (UNICEF 1997). The social and economic costs, apart from costs to the individual due to poor nutrition, are huge. Improving nutrition of communities reduces healthcare costs. More than half of child mortality in developing countries is attributable to underweight and the increased risk of infectious diseases. Underweight is the leading risk factor in the global burden of disease, and among developing countries with high mortality it contributes to nearly 15 per cent of the attributable DALYs (WHO 2002). Preventing LBW and stunting also reduces childhood mortality and morbidity. The intimate links between undernutrition in early life, including LBW and the increasing risk of chronic disease in later adult life, are well established. Diagnosis and treatment of chronic diseases like heart disease, diabetes, and cancer are expensive and will distort the limited public health budgets of developing countries.

Undernourished children become smaller adults and demonstrate lower physiological performance and reduced physical and work capacity. Employment prospects and productivity of short-statured and undernourished individuals are impaired (Spurr 1987). It shortens productive lives and increases absence due to illness; impacting in turn on economic productivity of countries. Micronutrient deficiencies such as iron deficiency impair physical capacity and work productivity and contribute to economic losses.

Poor nutrition impairs cognitive development and learning in undernourished children in developing societies. Grantham-McGregor (1995) has demonstrated that children who are stunted and live in deprived circumstances have major deficits in intellectual and cognitive development and social behaviour. Children's scholastic ability in their teens can be strongly influenced by interventions in the second and third year of life. Iodine deficiency and the syndrome of cretinism is another example of the role of nutrition in brain development and function. Even postnatal iodine deficiency can lead to slowing of mental processing that results in permanent impairment of mental development because of the need for adequate nutrition during critical periods of brain development. Similarly, Pollitt (1991a, 1991b) has demonstrated that iron deficiency anaemia can permanently handicap children at a crucial time in their development even though iron deficiency per se is not enough to produce demonstrable clinical deficiency. Grantham-McGregor's (1995) studies show that food that stimulates longitudinal bone growth also stimulates brain development, thus implying a more generic demand for a range of nutrients if mental function is to improve. All of these have significant relevance to the fact that children's education is the cornerstone to social and economic development of nations and is now an important component of the MDGs (MDG 2). The benefits of sustained mental and physical development from childhood into adult life ensure that healthy adults with the physical capacity to maintain high work outputs and with the intellectual ability to flexibly adapt to new technologies in this rapidly globalizing world will be a national asset. The importance of food and nutrition in the development of human capital in developing societies can never be underestimated.

Strategies to address the problem of undernutrition in developing societies

Reduction of poverty and hunger are high up among MDGs since achieving MDG 1—halving poverty and hunger by 2015—is central to achieving the other health-related MDGs. Economic growth and development should reduce the burden of undernutrition, but the reduction is slow and many people continue to suffer needlessly. There is thus a need for well-conceived policies for sustainable economic growth and social development that will benefit the poor and the undernourished. Given the complexity of factors that determine malnutrition of all forms, it is important that appropriate food and agricultural policies are developed to ensure household food security and that nutritional objectives are incorporated into development policies and programmes at national and local levels in developing countries. The deleterious consequences of rapid growth and development need to be guarded against and policies need to be in place to prevent one problem of malnutrition replacing another in these societies.

The pre-eminent determinant of household food insecurity is poverty in societies. Several policy measures undertaken by governments in developing countries are aimed at ensuring food supply and household food security. Good governance and democracy and well-targeted aid and the implementation of policies and relevant programmes will reduce the burden of hunger and undernutrition in developing countries. The adoption of the MDGs by the world's leaders at the Millennium Summit of the UN and the declaration to 'free all men, women, and children from the abject and dehumanizing conditions of extreme poverty' contributed a sense of urgency to address issues of nutrition and public health. Several programmes to address the problem of nutrition worldwide have been initiated; significant among them has been the Scaling Up Nutrition (or SUN) Initiative. The SUN movement is built through the engagement of nations affected by undernutrition and is a country-led movement that brings organizations together across sectors to support national plans to scale up nutrition and focuses attention on the 1000-day window of opportunity for impact. The SUN movement promotes the implementation of evidence-based nutrition interventions, as well as integrating nutrition goals into broader efforts in critical sectors such as health, social protection, development, and agriculture. The latter has resulted in the recent focus on agricultural strategies to sustainably reduce undernutrition just as this approach in the past addressed the challenge of food insecurity.

Diet, nutrition, and chronic non-communicable diseases

The evidence relating food and nutrition to chronic non-communicable diseases (NCDs) such as cardiovascular disease, type 2 diabetes mellitus, and cancers comes from population-based epidemiological investigations and trials. Descriptive population-based epidemiological investigations yield valuable data that lead to important hypotheses, but cannot be used alone to establish the causal links between diet and disease. The most consistent correlation between diet and chronic diseases has emerged from comparisons of populations or segments of population with substantially different dietary habits. Epidemiological studies, such as cohort studies and case–control studies, that compare information from groups of individuals within a population usually provide more accurate estimates of associations. Examining population-based epidemiological data relating diet to disease recognizes that every population consists of individuals who vary in their susceptibility to each disease and

part of this difference in susceptibility is genetic. As the diet within a population changes in the direction that measures the risk of the specific disease, an increasing proportion of individuals, particularly those most susceptible to the risk, develop the disease. As a result of this interindividual variability in the interaction of diet with an individual's genetic make-up and the individual's susceptibility to disease, some diet–disease relationships are difficult to identify within a single population. In experimental clinical studies and randomized and controlled trials, long exposures may be required for the effect of diet as a risk factor to be manifest. Strict inclusion criteria for participants need to be adhered to, to show the effect with small numbers in a reasonable length of time. These in turn may restrict the study to homogenous samples and thus limit the applicability of results to the population at large. Despite these limitations, when carefully designed studies show consistent findings of an association between specific dietary factors and a chronic disease, they generally indicate a cause and effect relationship.

Diet and cardiovascular diseases

The commonest cardiovascular diseases that are diet-related are coronary heart disease (CHD) and hypertension.

Coronary heart disease

CHD emerged as a burgeoning public health problem in Europe and North America after the Second World War and by the end of the 1950s had become the single major cause of adult death. The rates of CHD showed marked international differences with overall rates being higher among men than women. Mortality rates were sevenfold higher in some Eastern European countries while threefold differences were evident between Scotland and Spain or Portugal. Migration can contribute to either an increase, as in the case of Japanese moving to the United States, or decrease when Finns move to Sweden—migrants tending to approach the rates in their host countries. In the case of migrants from South Asia to the United Kingdom, however, the rates exceed the hosts implying some genetic susceptibility increasing risk in the host environment. The nearly fivefold difference in CHD rates among different countries and the intrapopulation variations in rates, by socioeconomic class, ethnicity, and geographical location, have revealed the dietary basis of CHD. The marked changes in CHD rates in migrant populations that moved across a geographical gradient in CHD risk provided evidence of the environmental nature of the causative factor.

Several prospective population studies have documented the relationship between habitual diets and the risk of CHD. These longitudinal studies have shown that several foods in the diet like wholegrain cereals, fish, fruits and vegetables, nuts, and moderate intakes of red wine are protective and reduce risk of CHD while others such as dietary saturated fat, trans fatty acids, and increased consumption of coffee may increase the risk of CHD. On the basis of the evidence, the WHO Expert Committee on Prevention of CHD (WHO 1982) concluded that the relationship of lipids in the diet and blood met the criteria for an epidemiological association to be termed causal. These data were backed by other evidence from intervention trials and animal experiments demonstrating the effects of diet on coronary artery atherosclerosis.

This relationship between dietary factors and CHD was supported by the results of the Seven Country Study (Keys 1980). The *saturated fat intake* varied between 3 per cent total energy in Japan and 22 per cent in Finland while the 15-year CHD incidence rates varied between 144 per 10,000 in Japan and 1202 per 10,000 in Finland. The annual incidence of CHD among 40–59-year-old men initially free of CHD was 15 per 100,000 in Japan and 198 per 100,000 in Finland. Evidence from 16 well-defined cohorts in seven countries and its correlation to the 10-year incidence rate of CHD deaths provided further support for this causal association. The strongest correlation was noted between CHD and percentage of energy derived from saturated fat, while total fat was not significantly correlated with CHD.

In the Seven Country Study, the *serum total cholesterol* values were 165 mg/dL in Japan and 270 mg/dL in Finland, and the variation in serum total cholesterol levels between populations could largely be explained by differences in saturated fat intake. The risk of CHD seemed to rise progressively within the same population with increases in plasma total cholesterol. Observational studies suggest that one population with an average total cholesterol level 10 per cent lower than another will have one-third less CHD and a 30 per cent difference in total cholesterol predicts a fourfold difference in CHD (WHO 1990). The Seven Country Study showed a strong positive relationship between saturated fat intake and total cholesterol level; populations with an average saturated fat intake between 3 per cent and 10 per cent of the energy intake were characterized by serum total cholesterol levels below 200 mg/dL and by low mortality rates from CHD. As saturated fat intakes increased to greater than 10 per cent of energy intake a marked and progressive increase in CHD mortality was noticed. Saturated fats raise total and *low-density lipoprotein* (LDL) cholesterol; and of these fatty acids myristic and palmitic acids abundant in diets rich in dairy and meat products have the greatest effects (Table 2.7.5).

Several prospective studies have shown an inverse relation between *high-density lipoprotein* (HDL) cholesterol and CHD incidence. However, HDL cholesterol levels are influenced by several non-dietary factors and HDL levels do not explain differences in CHD mortality between populations. HDL levels are increased by alcohol, weight loss, and by physical activity. Populations who have high intakes of mono-unsaturated fatty acids (from olive oil) or have diets rich in n-3 polyunsaturates of marine origin (like Eskimos) also have low CHD rates. Both *mono-unsaturated* and n-3 and n-6 *polyunsaturated fatty acids* (PUFAs) lower plasma total and LDL cholesterol; PUFAs are more effective than monounsaturates (Kris-Etherton 1999; Mori and Beilin 2001). There is good evidence that some isomers of fatty acids, such as *trans fatty acids*, increase the incidence of CHD by increasing LDL cholesterol levels and decreasing the HDL levels, by interfering with essential fatty acid metabolism and by enhancing the concentrations of the lipoprotein Lp(a) which, in genetically susceptible people, seems to be an additional risk factor through mechanisms which include an antiplasminogen effect to limit fibrinolysis.

Other dietary components, for example, *dietary fibre or complex carbohydrates*, seem to influence serum cholesterol levels and the incidence of CHD. Populations consuming diets rich in plant foods high in complex carbohydrates have lower rates of CHD; vegetarians have a 30 per cent lower rate of CHD mortality than non-vegetarians and their serum cholesterol levels are significantly lower than that of lacto-ovo-vegetarians and non-vegetarians. *Alcohol* consumption also reduces the incidence of CHD. A number of observational studies suggest that light-to-moderate drinkers

Table 2.7.5 Summary of strength of evidence of dietary and lifestyle factors and risk of developing cardiovascular disease

Evidence	Decreased risk	No relationship	Increased risk
Convincing	Regular physical activity	Vitamin E supplements	Myristic and palmitic acids
	Linoleic acid		Trans fatty acids
	Fish and fish oils[1]		High sodium intake
	Vegetables and fruits		Overweight
	Potassium		High alcohol intake[4]
	Alcohol intake (low to moderate)[2]		
Probable	α Linolenic acid	Stearic acid	Dietary cholesterol
	Oleic acid		Unfiltered boiled coffee
	NSP[3]		
	Wholegrain cereals		
	Nuts (unsalted)		
	Plant sterols/stanols		
	Folate		

Notes:
[1] Eicosapentaenoic acid and docosapentaenoic acid.
[2] For CHD risk.
[3] NSP, non-starch polysaccharide.
[4] For risk of stroke.

Adapted with permission from World Health Organization/FAO, *Diet, nutrition and the prevention of chronic diseases*, WHO Technical Report Series 916, World Health Organization, Geneva, Switzerland, Copyright © 2003, available from http://whqlibdoc.who.int/trs/who_trs_916.pdf.

have a slightly lower risk of CHD than abstainers. However, the relationship between alcohol intake and CHD is complicated by changes in blood pressure and also the nature of the alcoholic drink. The presence of phenolic compounds in red wine may contribute to the benefits of drinking red wine as compared to alcohol consumption per se in reducing the risk.

The risk of CHD in individuals is dominated by three major factors: (1) high serum total cholesterol, (2) high blood pressure, and (3) cigarette smoking (WHO 1982). There is also a synergism between risk factors, with the Japanese notable for their high smoking rates and hypertension but very low cholesterol levels: smoking and hypertension are particularly harmful to individuals with high cholesterol levels. Body weight changes induced by diet and levels of physical activity, are strongly related to changes in serum total cholesterol, blood pressure, and obesity. Obesity in turn, particularly when associated with high waist circumference or waist/hip ratio, is strongly related to diabetes mellitus, both of which are risk factors for CHD.

Hypertension and stroke

The risk of CHD and that of cerebrovascular disease presenting clinically as stroke, increases progressively throughout the observed range of blood pressure, in a number of different countries (MacMohan et al. 1990). From the combined data it appears that there is a fivefold difference in CHD and a tenfold risk of stroke over a range of diastolic blood pressure of only 40 mmHg. Analysis indicates that a sustained difference of only 7.5 mmHg in diastolic pressure confers a 28 per cent difference in risk of CHD and a 44 per cent difference in risk of stroke.

Nutritional determinants of hypertension are contributory and are causally linked to stroke. Obesity and alcohol intake are related to hypertension since weight reduction and restricting alcohol intake can lower blood pressures. The dietary factors that are implicated (in addition to alcohol and caffeine intakes) are excessive sodium and saturated fat intake and low potassium and calcium intake. The Intersalt Study (1988) compared blood pressure measurements with 24-hour urinary sodium excretion in 10,000 individuals aged 20–59 years in 32 countries and showed that populations with very low sodium excretion and intakes had low median blood pressures, a low prevalence of hypertension, and no increase in blood pressure with age. Although sodium intake was related to blood pressure levels and also influenced the extent to which blood pressures increased with age, the overall association between sodium, median blood pressure, and the prevalence of hypertension was less than significant. A number of explanations have been put forward to explain why studies such as the Intersalt Study underestimate the relationship between dietary sodium and blood pressure. These include among others: unreliability of assessing dietary intake of sodium accurately, genetic variability, and the contribution of other factors such as obesity or alcohol intake.

Reviews based on meta-analysis correlated blood pressure recordings in individuals with measurements of their 24-hour sodium intake (Law et al. 1991); an association increasing with age and the initial blood pressure. The results of intervention trials of sodium restriction support this relationship. Aggregation of the results of 68 cross-over trials and ten randomized control trials of dietary salt reduction have shown that moderate dietary salt reduction over a few weeks lowers systolic and diastolic pressure in those individuals with high blood pressure (Law et al. 1991). It was estimated that such reductions in salt intake by population would reduce the incidence of stroke by 26 per cent and that of CHD by 15 per cent in Western countries. Reduction of salt in processed food would lower blood pressure even further and would prevent as many as 70,000 deaths per year in the UK. Results of therapeutic trials of drug therapy also support the fact that the incidence of stroke can be reduced if blood pressure is lowered, although the beneficial effect of lowering the incidence of CHD is lower than expected. A recent Cochrane review of 34 clinical trials (He et al. 2013) showed that a modest reduction in salt intake for 4 or more weeks causes significant and important falls in blood pressure in both hypertensive and normotensive individuals, irrespective of sex and ethnic group. The review supports the view that a long-term reduction in population salt intake will lower population blood pressure and thereby reduce cardiovascular disease. The observed significant association between the reduction in 24-hour urinary sodium and the fall in systolic pressure indicates that larger reductions in salt intake will lead to larger falls in systolic blood pressure. The current recommendation is to reduce salt intake to 5–6 g/day and this will have a major effect on blood pressure. This review indicates that further reductions to 3 g/day will have a greater effect and should become the long-term target for population salt intake.

The other dietary component that has been investigated by the Intersalt Study (1988) is potassium. Urinary potassium excretion, an assumed indicator of intake, was negatively related to blood pressure as was the urinary sodium/potassium concentration ratio. It has also been observed that potassium supplementation reduces blood pressure in both normotensive and hypertensive subjects (Cappucio and MacGregor 1991). A recent systematic review of 22 randomized control trials (Aburto et al. 2013) supports the view that increased potassium intake reduces blood pressure in people with hypertension and has no adverse effect on blood lipid or catecholamine concentrations, or renal function. The higher potassium intake was associated with a 24 per cent lower risk of stroke. These results suggest that increased potassium intake is potentially beneficial to most people for the prevention and control of elevated blood pressure and stroke.

Some, but not all, cross-sectional and intervention studies suggest a beneficial effect of calcium intake on blood pressure. Epidemiological studies also consistently suggest lower blood pressures among vegetarians independent of age and body weight. These studies may also support the role of other dietary components because vegetarian diets rich in complex carbohydrates are also rich in potassium and other minerals.

Nutritional intervention is likely to reduce the occurrence of hypertension and the complications of stroke and CHD in the community, demonstrated in Finland where the average blood pressure has fallen by nearly 10 mmHg and the prevalence of hypertension is only a quarter of what it was prior to the intervention. Along with the falls in average cholesterol levels, CHD and stroke rates in Finland have fallen dramatically as the population's diet was transformed to change its fat content and to more than double the average vegetable and fruit intakes. The decline in CHD and stroke rates was predominantly dependent on the fall in cholesterol and blood pressure levels respectively and these changes occurred despite increasing obesity rates (Puska et al. 1995).

A summary of the strength of evidence (convincing and probable) on diet and lifestyle factors and risk of developing cardiovascular diseases (CHD and stroke) based on the recent Joint WHO/FAO Expert Consultation is provided in Table 2.7.5 (WHO/FAO 2003). There is now general agreement on the population strategies that need to be adopted to reduce both the frequency and extent of the risk factors of cardiovascular disease based on this report. The nutritional approach including increasing physical activity is aimed at reducing obesity, lowering blood pressure, lowering total and LDL cholesterol and increasing HDL cholesterol, and lowering sodium intakes. Current recommendations take into consideration both the entire spectrum of cardiovascular risks including effects on thrombosis as well as providing a holistic approach to recommending a healthy diet that will reduce all chronic NCDs including cancers. These recommendations include lowering total fat intake to between 30 to 35 per cent of total calories, restricting saturated fat intake to a maximum of 10 per cent of total calories, and increasing contribution from monounsaturated and polyunsaturated fatty acids (n-3 and n-6 PUFAs) and to increase intakes of complex carbohydrates or dietary fibre. Translated into food components this would mean reducing in particular intake from animal fat, hydrogenated and hardened vegetable oils, and increasing the consumption of cereals, vegetables, and fruits. Dietary advice appears to be effective in bringing about modest beneficial changes in diet and cardiovascular risk factors over approximately a year (Rees et al. 2013).

Diet nutrition and cancers

It is now widely accepted that one-third of human cancers could relate directly to some dietary component (Doll and Peto 1981) and it is probable that diet plays an important role in influencing the permissive role of carcinogens on the development of many cancers. Thus up to 80 per cent of all cancers may have a link with nutrition.

Evidence that diet is a determinant of cancer risk comes from several sources. These include correlation between food consumption data and the incidence of cancers in the population. Studies on the changing rates of cancer in populations as they migrate from a region or country of one dietary culture to another have contributed to many important hypotheses. Case–control studies of the dietary habits of individuals with and without a cancer and prospective studies as well as intervention trials have provided evidence for the effects of diet on cancer. Only those human cancers where the role of diet or a nutrient is reasonably well established (summarized in Table 2.7.6) are discussed here.

Cancers of the gastrointestinal tract may be influenced by the diet. The intake of alcohol appears to be an independent risk factor for oral, laryngeal, and pharyngeal cancers as well as for oesophagus, liver, and breast cancers. Consumption of salted fish (Cantonese style), preserved, and fermented foods containing nitrosamines as weaning foods or from early childhood may introduce a substantial risk of *nasopharyngeal cancer*. *Stomach cancer* is also associated with diets comprising large amounts of salted and salty foods and low levels of fresh fruit and vegetables which may contain nutrients that possibly inhibit the formation of nitrosamines. Non-starchy vegetables, allium vegetables (onion, garlic, etc.), and fruits probably decrease risk of stomach cancer.

Cancers of the colon and rectum are the third commonest form of cancer and the incidence rates are high in Western Europe and North America while they are low in sub-Saharan Africa (Boyle et al. 1985). International comparisons indicate that diets low in dietary fibre and high in animal fat and animal protein increase the risk of colon cancer. The epidemiological data relating dietary fibre to colorectal cancer generally support the existence of an inverse relationship between the intake of foods rich in dietary fibre and colon cancer risk and meta-analysis indicates a 10 per cent decreased risk per 10 g fibre per day. Diets rich in fibre are also rich sources of antioxidant vitamins and minerals with potential cancer inhibiting properties. Vegetarian diets seem to provide a protective effect from the risk of colon cancer. There is now convincing evidence that red meat and processed meat in the diet increases the risk of colon and colorectal cancers while physical activity decreases risk. Alcohol intake in men and women as well as obesity and abdominal fatness increase risk of this cancer (World Cancer Research Fund and American Institute for Cancer Research 2007; Vargas and Thompson 2012).

Primary *liver cancers* have been correlated with mycotoxin (aflatoxin) contamination of foodstuffs.

The primary causal factor for *lung cancer*, a leading cause of death among men, is cigarette smoking. Several studies have shown an interactive effect between cigarette smoking and low frequency of intake of green and yellow vegetables rich in β-carotene. In prospective studies, the frequency of the consumption of foods

Table 2.7.6 Associations between nutritional factors and some common cancers

Cancer	Decreasing risk of cancer	Increasing risk of cancer
Breast	Lactation Physical activity	Alcohol Obesity
Colorectal	Physical activity NSP[1]/dietary fibre Milk, calcium	Processed red meat Alcohol Obesity
Endometrium, and kidney	Physical activity	Obesity
Liver		Aflatoxin Alcohol
Lung	Fruits Physical activity	High-dose supplements of β-carotene
Mouth, larynx, pharynx	Vegetables and fruits	Alcohol
Nasopharynx		Salted fish[2]
Oesophagus	Fruits and vegetables	Alcohol Obesity
Pancreas	Folate rich foods	Obesity
Prostate	Lycopene and selenium rich foods	High calcium diets
Stomach	Fruits and vegetables	High salt intake

Notes:
Both convincing and probable evidence for decreasing and increasing risk combined.
[1] NSP, non starch polysaccharide/dietary fibre
[2] Specifically Cantonese style salted fish

Source: data from World Cancer Research Fund / American Institute for Cancer Research, *Food, Nutrition, Physical Activity, and the Prevention of Cancer: a Global Perspective*, American Institute for Cancer Research, Washington, USA, Copyright © 2007 World Cancer Research Fund International All rights reserved.

rich in β-carotene has been inversely associated with lung cancer risk. However, high intakes of β-carotene as supplements increase risk significantly; and so does arsenic in drinking water.

Breast cancer is a common cause of death among women both in the United States and in the United Kingdom. The most convincing evidence is that lactation protects against risk of breast cancer in both pre- and postmenopausal women. Physical activity probably also decreases risk while increases in body fatness after menopause increases risk. While other nutritional factors such as greater birth weight, attained adult stature, and weight gain increase risk, consumption of alcoholic drinks also convincingly increases risk of breast cancer both pre- and post-menopause.

Dietary factors are important in the causation of cancers of many sites and dietary modifications may reduce cancer risk. In general diets high in plant foods, especially vegetables and fruits, are strongly associated with a lower incidence of a wide range of cancers. Such diets tend to be low in saturated fat, high in complex carbohydrate and fibre, and rich in several antioxidant vitamins. Sustained and consistent intake of alcohol, physical inactivity, and obesity and body fatness are also associated with several cancers. On the basis of the evidence, a recent report (World Cancer Research Fund and American Institute for Cancer Research 2007) makes the following recommendations: (1) be within the normal range of body weight for height and be physically active; (2) eat mostly foods of plant origin and limit intake of red meat and avoid processed meat; (3) limit consumption of energy dense foods and avoid sugary drinks; (4) limit alcohol intake; (5) limit consumption of salt, and avoid mouldy food; (6) mothers must be encouraged and supported to breastfeed their children.

Diet, lifestyles, and obesity

Obesity is one of the most important public health problems and the prevalence of obesity is increasing worldwide. In developing countries undergoing rapid economic growth, relatively affluent and urbanized communities are showing an increasing prevalence of obesity among adults and children.

Overweight and obesity is normally assumed to indicate an excess of body fat. Like adult undernutrition, BMI is used as an indicator of choice for obesity and Table 2.7.7 outlines the diagnostic criteria for overweight and obesity in infants and children, adolescents and adults (WHO 1995, 2000). Recent recommendations are that a BMI of between 18.5 and 24.9 in adults be considered appropriate weight-for-height; BMI between 25 and 29.9 be indicative of overweight and possibly a pre-obese state; while obesity is diagnosed at a BMI greater than 30.0.

The main health risk of obesity is premature death due to heart disease and hypertension and other chronic diseases. In the presence of other risk factors (both dietary and non-dietary), obesity increases the risk of CHD, hypertension, and stroke. In women, obesity seems to be one of the best predictors of cardiovascular disease. Longitudinal studies have demonstrated that weight gain, both in men and women, is significantly related to increases in

cardiovascular risk factors. Weight gain was strongly associated with increased blood pressure, elevated plasma cholesterol and triglycerides, and hyperglycaemia. The distribution of fat in the body in obesity may also contribute to increased risk; high waist–hip ratios (i.e. fat predominantly in abdomen and not subcutaneous) increase the risk of heart disease and type 2 diabetes. The coexistence of diabetes is also an important contributor to morbidity and mortality in obese individuals. Obesity also carries increased risk of gall bladder stones, breast and uterine cancer in females, and possibly of prostate and renal cancer in males, as well as osteoarthritis of weight-bearing joints and obstructive sleep apnoea. While obesity contributes to social problems such as low self-esteem and reduced employability it is also associated with increasing mortality both in smokers and non-smokers.

Several environmental factors, both dietary and lifestyle related, contribute to increased obesity. Social and environmental factors that either increase energy intake and/or reduce physical activity are of primary interest. Changes in the environment that affect the levels of physical activity and changes both in the food consumed and in the patterns of eating behaviour may contribute to increase energy intakes beyond one's requirement, thus causing obesity. Increased intake of dietary fat as energy-dense food may result in poor regulation of appetite and food intake while fibre-rich complex carbohydrates tend to bulk the meal and limit intakes.

International comparisons reveal that obesity increases as the fat percentage of calories in the diet increases (Lissner and Heitmann 1995). A recent systematic review indicates that increased intake of sugars was associated with increase in body weight while iso-energetic exchange of dietary sugars with other carbohydrates showed no change in body weight (Morenga et al. 2013). Patterns of eating, particularly snacking between meals, may contribute to increased intakes. However, evidence supports the view that much of the energy imbalance in modern societies is largely the result of dramatic reductions in physical activity levels (both occupational and leisure time) when food availability is more than adequate.

Tackling overweight and obesity that is approaching epidemic proportions worldwide is of crucial importance since it is associated with several co-morbidities and the consequent increased healthcare costs. It has been estimated that the direct costs of obesity for healthcare in the United States in 1995 were US$ 70 billion and those of physical inactivity another US$ 24 billion (Colditz 1999). These are enormous costs and a huge drain on healthcare budgets of countries.

Preventive measures to tackle the increasing obesity worldwide are reliant on the strength of evidence related to the factors that increase or reduce the risk of weight gain. The WHO report (WHO and FAO 2003) and a more recent review of the evidence is provided in Table 2.7.8 (World Cancer Research Fund and American Institute for Cancer Research 2007). Preventive measures have to start very early and primary prevention may have to be aimed at young children. This includes nutrition education of children and parents and dealing with problems of school meals, snacking, levels of physical activity, and other related issues. Public health initiatives need to address all social and environmental issues that contribute to the increasing energy and fat intakes and reductions in physical activity. Since the issues are complex, attempts have to be made to interact with a wide range of stakeholders and address issues relevant to work sites, schools, supermarkets, and deal with marketing, advertising, and promoting activity, etc., and

Table 2.7.7 Diagnostic criteria for overweight and obesity in infants and children, adolescents and adults

Infants and children (all ages)	Weight-for-height	>+ 2 Z scores
Adolescents		
Overweight	BMI-for-age	>85th percentile
Obese	BMI-for-age	>85th percentile of BMI plus
	Triceps-for-age	>90th percentile of TSKF
	Subscapular-for-age	>90th percentile of SSSKF
Adults		
Normal weight range	BMI	18.5–24.9
Overweight or pre-obese	BMI	25.0–29.9
Obese—Grade I	BMI	30.0–35.9
Grade II	BMI	35.0–39.9
Grade III	BMI	> 40.0

SSSKF, supraspinal skinfold thickness; TSKF, triceps skinfold thickness.
Adapted with permission from World Health Organization, *Physical status: the use and interpretation of anthropometry*, WHO Technical Report Series 854, World Health Organization, Geneva, Switzerland, Copyright © 1995 and World Health Organization, *Obesity: preventing and managing the global epidemic*, World Health Organization, Geneva, Switzerland, Copyright © 2000.

Table 2.7.8 Summary of factors that decrease risk (i.e. promote appropriate energy intake relative to energy expenditure) and those that increase risk (i.e. promote excess energy intake relative to energy expenditure) of weight gain and obesity

Evidence	Decreased risk	Increased risk
Convincing	Physical activity	Sedentary living
Probable	Low energy-dense foods[1]	Energy-dense foods[2]
	Being breast fed	Sugary drinks[3]
		'Fast foods'
		Television viewing

Notes:
[1] Low energy-dense food, wholegrain cereals, cereal products, non-starchy vegetables, and dietary fibre.
[2] Energy-dense foods are mostly from animal fat and fast foods.
[3] Sugary drinks have sucrose or high fructose corn syrup.

This material has been adapted with permission from the 2007 WCRF/AICR Report Food, *Nutrition, Physical Activity and the Prevention of Cancer: a Global Perspective*.

not merely expect the health sector to provide solutions. A recent high-level exercise in the UK is a good example of such an integrated approach to the problem (Foresight 2007).

Type 2 diabetes mellitus

Type 2 diabetes mellitus (formerly non-insulin dependent diabetes mellitus) is a chronic metabolic disorder which occurs in adulthood and is strongly associated with an increased risk of CHD. Type 2 diabetes mellitus has to be distinguished from type 1 diabetes mellitus (formerly insulin dependent diabetes mellitus) and from gestational diabetes of pregnancy. Obesity is a major risk factor for the occurrence of type 2 diabetes mellitus; the risk being related both to the duration and the degree of obesity. The occurrence of type 2 diabetes mellitus appears to be triggered by environmental factors such as sedentary lifestyle, dietary factors, stress, urbanization, and socioeconomic factors. Certain ethnic or racial groups seem to have a higher incidence of type 2 diabetes mellitus; these include Pima Indians, Nauruans, and South Asians (i.e. Indians, Pakistanis, and Bangladeshis). Type 2 diabetes mellitus also seems to occur when the food ecosystem rapidly changes, for example, urbanization of Australian aborigines or adoption of Western dietary patterns by Pima Indians.

The cause of type 2 diabetes mellitus is unclear, but it seems to involve both an impaired pancreatic secretion of insulin and the development of tissue resistance to insulin. Overweight and obesity, particularly the central or truncal distribution of fat accompanied by a high waist–hip ratio and a high waist circumference, seems to be invariably present with type 2 diabetes mellitus. Hence the most rational approach to preventing type 2 diabetes mellitus is to prevent obesity. Weight control and increasing physical activity levels are fundamental both as a population strategy for the primary prevention of this disorder but also to tackle high-risk individuals. Physical activity improves glucose tolerance by weight reduction and by its beneficial effects on insulin resistance. Diets high in plant foods are associated with a lower incidence of type 2 diabetes mellitus and vegetarians have a lower risk.

Expert groups have provided dietary recommendations for both the primary prevention of type 2 diabetes mellitus, the management of diabetes, and the reduction of secondary complications which include CHD risk and renal, ocular, and neurological complications of diabetes. Prevention of weight gain and reduction of obesity is the key, as is increasing levels of physical activity. The specific dietary recommendations include providing diets with carbohydrates contributing 55–60 per cent of energy, maximizing content of complex carbohydrates and dietary fibre, and reduction of simple sugar intakes. In addition the general recommendations for fat (saturated fat to <10 per cent of calories) are emphasized due to the associated high risk of CHD. Maintaining a desirable body weight and preventing weight gain is most important.

Diet and osteoporosis

The increase in numbers of the elderly in the developed world has seen an increase in their health problems, which affects their quality of life. Fracture of the hip is an important health problem, particularly among postmenopausal women. Fractures occur in the elderly following a relatively trivial fall when there is osteoporosis and the density of the bone is reduced. Bone density increases in childhood and adolescence and reaches a peak at about 20 years of age. Bone density falls from menopause in women and from about the age of 55 years in men. The variation in bone density between individuals and different racial groups is large and of the order of ± 20 per cent. Since bone density declines with increasing age, those that attain high levels of peak bone mass at the end of adolescence and retain higher levels of bone density during adulthood become osteoporotic with advancing age much more slowly than those with lower bone densities to start with. Hence factors that influence the attainment of peak bone density may play a crucial role in the development of osteoporosis and the occurrence of fractures with ageing.

Several factors influence the onset of osteoporosis and include the lack of oestrogen in postmenopausal women, degree of mobility, smoking, and alcohol intake. Calcium intake may influence the onset and degree of osteoporosis. Evidence from some countries indicates that osteoporosis may be diet related since the fracture rate is halved among individuals in the higher calcium intake range. However, there are regions where the lower rates of fracture and osteoporosis are associated with lower calcium intakes. The rates are lower in Singapore compared to the United States, although the calcium intakes are lower than the United States. The traditional emphasis on calcium intakes possibly reflects the recognition of its importance in contributing to the density of bone during growth and the need for attaining dense bones at the peak of adult life. High protein and high salt diets are known to increase bone loss while calcium supplements, well above what may be considered physiological, in postmenopausal women, may reduce the rate of bone loss and slow down osteoporosis. Adequate levels of vitamin D are important factors that diminish risk of osteoporosis. Poor vitamin D status has been linked with age-related bone loss and osteoporotic fractures in the elderly.

Other nutrients may be important for long-term bone health and the prevention of osteoporosis. Consumption of dairy products, fruits, and vegetables are important modifiable protective factors for bone health, and nutrients like magnesium, potassium, vitamins C, K, and B, and carotenoids have been shown to be more important than previously realized (Tucker 2009). Current research on diet and bone status supports encouragement of balanced diets with plenty of fruit and vegetables, adequate dairy and other protein foods, and limitation of foods with low nutrient density. Moderate alcohol intake shows positive effects on bone, particularly in older women, while high intakes of alcohol increase risk of osteoporosis. Convincing evidence indicates that physical activity is an important determinant of bone health.

It is generally believed that populations in developing countries are at less risk of developing osteoporosis in spite of low calcium intakes. This may be related to the fact that they do more physical work, smoke less, drink less alcohol, and have diets which are generally not high in protein or salt content. However, osteoporosis is seen in developing countries in regions where low intakes of dietary calcium are associated with high fluoride intakes. No osteoporosis occurs if high intakes of fluoride are accompanied by dietary intakes of calcium which are also high.

Diet and dental caries

Dental caries is a common disease of the teeth, which results in decay of the tooth surface, usually beginning in the enamel. An essential feature in the causation of dental caries is dental plaque which is largely made up of microorganisms. Dietary sugars diffuse into the dental plaque where they are metabolized by the microorganisms to acids which can dissolve the mineral phase of the enamel causing dental decay. The process is, however, much more complex and is related to the quantity and quality of saliva produced in the mouth among other factors.

The evidence relating diet to dental caries has been well reviewed and overwhelming evidence indicates that sugars are cariogenic. Good correlations exist between the sugar supply and the occurrence of dental caries in children and adults (WHO and FAO 2003). The consumption of refined sugar in many parts of the world seems to be accompanied by an increase in dental caries in communities which were hitherto free of the problem. Cross-sectional studies demonstrate good correlations between sugar consumption and incidence of dental caries, particularly among young children. Consumption of sugars between meals is associated with a marked increase in caries compared to consumption of sugars with meals. Sucrose is the predominant dietary cariogenic agent, although the current emphasis is on the consumption of all free sugars, particularly between meals. Analysis of epidemiological data from several countries suggests that a much closer relationship exists between dental caries and free sugars than between caries and starchy cereal foods. Fresh fruit, although it contains intrinsic sugars, has a lower cariogenic potential while fruit juices are cariogenic, which may be related to the added sugars in fruit juices or from the lack of adequate salivary stimulation. Food may also contain protective factors that prevent the occurrence of dental caries. This includes fluoride and inorganic phosphates in the diet which protect against dental caries.

Prevention of dental caries can be achieved by health education aimed at the individual beginning in infancy. Avoidance of the addition of free sugars to bottle feeds and milk and fruit drinks are a must. An adequate intake of fluoride is desirable quite early in life. During childhood and adolescence, the restriction of the three major sources that contribute to two-thirds of our intake of sugars, i.e. confectionery, table sugar, and soft drinks, will help reduce the increment of caries in childhood. At local and national level, the main interventions should include fluoridation of water supply, labelling of foods, and possible changes in policies that promote the production and marketing of free sugars.

Population nutrient intake goals in the prevention of chronic diseases

The distribution and determinants of risk factors in a population have direct implications for population-based prevention strategies. Risk typically increases across the spectrum of the risk factor and is a continuum. Thus, individuals at increased risk are not a distinct group or deviant minority, but a part of the risk continuum. Hence population-based strategies must seek to shift the whole distribution of risk factors downwards and thus reduce population incidence of the disease.

Population nutrient intake goals represent the mean population intake of the nutrient that is judged to be consistent with the maintenance of good health, i.e. a low prevalence of diet-related diseases in the population. There is no single best value and the safe range of intakes that constitute the nutrient goals would be consistent with maintenance of health. If the existing population averages move outside the recommended ranges, health concerns are likely to arise. Thus population nutrient intake goals are useful signposts for population-based strategies to help shift the risk distribution in a population downwards and thus reduce risk of the disease. The recommended population nutrient goals based on critical examination of the evidence from an Expert Consultation (WHO/FAO, 2003) are summarized in Table 2.7.9.

Emerging food and nutrition issues of public health concern

Over the last decade several issues of public health concern related to food and nutrition have emerged globally. These include

Table 2.7.9 Ranges of the population nutrient intake goals

Dietary factor/nutrient	PNI goal[1]
Total fat	15–30%
Saturated fat	< 10%
Polyunsaturated fatty acids (PUFAs)	6–10%
n-6 PUFAs	5–8%
n-3 PUFAs	1–2%
Trans fatty acids	< 1%
Monounsaturated fats (MUFAs)	By difference
Total carbohydrate	55–75%
Free sugars	<10 %
Protein	10–15%
Cholesterol	< 300 mg per day
Sodium chloride	<5 g per day
Fruits and vegetables	> 400 g per day

Note: [1] expressed as per cent of energy.

Adapted with permission from World Health Organization/FAO, *Diet, nutrition and the prevention of chronic diseases*, WHO Technical Report Series 916, World Health Organization, Geneva, Switzerland, Copyright © 2003, available from http://whqlibdoc. who.int/trs/who_trs_916.pdf.

problems related to microbiological safety of foods, concerns related to genetically modified foods, issues of labelling of processed foods, and the emerging epidemic of diet-related chronic diseases and obesity.

Food safety

Food safety refers to whether food is safe for human consumption and hence lacking in biological and chemical contaminants that have the potential to cause illness. The increasing concern over the safety of foods in the West is a paradox in that the epidemiological evidence on the safety of foods is quite contrary to the perceptions of the public and the media that the food available now is less safe than it used to be. The improvements in public health have virtually eradicated primarily food-borne infections that were associated with morbidity and mortality. The common food-borne diseases currently encountered in the West are usually associated with mild self-limiting gastroenteritis. Studies of risk perception suggest that the public becomes alarmed by health threats which are disproportionate to the actual risk associated with the disease and that this public concern is fuelled by the media which make health issues into media health scares depending on the newsworthiness of the incidents.

There have been several food-borne epidemics that have raised concerns about food safety in recent years. These include for instance the *Salmonella enteritidis pt4 (Se4)* epidemic. This was attributed to the ability of *Se4* to invade the oviduct of poultry and get deposited in the albumin of the egg. At the consumer level the outbreak of the infection was linked to the use of raw egg in recipes or cross-contamination from raw to cooked foods. *Campylobacter* infection is the commonest food-borne disease in the UK and the increase in its incidence may partly be explained by the better ascertainment and reporting of cases with this infection. The more recent food scare was the emergence of *Escherichia coli* O157 in Scotland which caused several deaths and was attributable to changes in husbandry and the movement of livestock and the rapid growth of the fast food industry. *Listeria* is another cause of food-borne disease exemplifying of the role of globalization and international trade in the spread of food-borne diseases.

In the developing world the issues of food safety are related to microbiological agents that contaminate food and water and spread disease rapidly in the warm humid environments aided by the improper or poor food hygiene practices, poor environmental sanitation, and inadequate regulation of food-related commerce. The safety of foods in the developing world is also compromised by the presence of toxins like aflatoxins due to poor food storage practices or due to cyanogens in the diet due to inadequate preparation of foods such as cassava. Aflatoxins are linked to hepatocellular cancer and the risk appears to be higher among those who are likely to be hepatitis B positive. In addition, the food chain in poor countries is contaminated by pesticide and chemical residues compromising the safety of the food consumed by populations in these countries.

Genetically modified foods

Another issue that has created a considerable degree of controversy is the use of biotechnology to produce genetically modified (GM) foods. Genetic modification of food crops can be used to reduce food losses by increasing resistance to drought, frost, diseases, and pests and help control weeds and reduce post-harvest losses. Biotechnology can improve the nutritional value of foods, for example, by increasing protein or micronutrient content or by reducing saturated fat content. They could help slow down ripening so that foods retain their quality much longer. Biotechnology can increase both the yield and the quality of crops grown on existing farmland and thereby reduces pressure on wildlife habitats. In the West, particularly in the United Kingdom and Europe, the opposition to GM foods is based largely on arguments that raise concerns with ecological damage that may follow large-scale use of GM crops.

In developing countries the concerns are more related to the use of the 'terminator gene' technology and the dependence on the large multinationals for seeds and chemicals that the small farmers will inherit. At the heart of this controversy and the raging debate is the gulf between plant breeders, seed and agrochemical industries who promote biotechnology, and the campaigners who argue that GM technology may have hazardous consequences on the environment. This is a debate replete with numerous paradoxes and the climate of mistrust, some of it associated with the bovine spongiform encephalopathy and new variant Creutzfeldt–Jakob disease scare, and is obscuring the real issues and clouding objective decisions from being made with regard to the production and consumption of GM foods (Dixon 1999).

Agricultural biotechnology is essential to increase food production to an increasing global population that is increasingly diverting food from human use to biofuels and animal feed; the latter the consequence of increased meat consumption with economic growth, as seen in China. It has the potential to improve the quality and the nutrient content of the food to address both nutritional needs that pose public health challenges (such as iron, zinc, and vitamin A deficiencies) as well as consumer demands. It is interesting to note that the perception and acceptance of GM foods in developing societies is at variance to the concerns in developed countries (FAO 2004). Agricultural biotechnology will have an important role to play if emphasis is placed on agriculture and farming systems as a means to sustainably improve nutrition.

Food labelling

An important source of information for the consumer about the food on the supermarket shelf is the label on a food product. Food labels provide information that may be of interest to the consumer, especially with regard to the added chemicals (additives, pesticide residues, colouring and flavouring agents, and preservatives), fats, sugars, and energy content. Although about two-thirds of shoppers claim to read the information on the labels of new or unfamiliar food products to check their contents, this interest in labels does not mean that consumers always understand the information in the labels. Consumers are even more confused by the nutrition information panel which appears on many food labels.

Food label information is usually designed by experts. A prototype label was produced by the *Codex Alimentarius Commission* of the FAO and WHO, which is the organization charged with advising on international food standards, and this prototype is followed by Food Standards Committees around the world. According to this prototype the nutrients—energy, carbohydrate, protein and fats—are listed according to their amounts per serving and per 100 g. Most consumers, however, have hardly any idea of what a 100 g serving is, or for that matter what a normal or average serving is. A further problem is that these labels designed by experts are also beset with problems with terminology. Health benefits or nutritional claims are not meant to be part of the food labels and they also do not provide information to cover ecological and ethical issues which may be of concern for some consumers. More recently the need to highlight the source or origin of foods and in particular the labelling of GM sources of the food product has been a serious concern of consumers. In January 2007, the Food Standards Agency in the United Kingdom agreed on the nutritional criteria for a 'traffic light' labelling of food products to identify products high in fat, sugar, and/or salt. Consumer organizations supported this move while some of the major food companies and supermarkets initially opposed the scheme. In recent years there is generally more acceptance of this simple labelling scheme. Food labelling is an important issue of public health concern and despite the considerable progress made so far there is much to be achieved.

Functional foods

New food products are being marketed as health-enhancing or illness-preventing foods. These are called functional foods or otherwise 'pharmafoods', 'nutriceuticals', or novel foods. Functional foods are generally defined as food products that deliver a health benefit beyond providing nutrients. The health benefits of functional foods may be conferred by a variety of production and processing techniques which include: fortification of certain food products with specific nutrients, using phytochemicals and active microorganisms, and by genetic modification of foods. The topic of functional foods is complex and controversial. An assumption implicit in the functional foods and health benefit claims is that the food supply needs to be fixed or doctored (or medicalized) on public health grounds. The assumption therefore is that the current food supply is in some way deficient, that the habitual diets are inadequate, and a technological fix will solve the problem. Thus the emerging debate viewed from the perspective of the proponents of functional foods is that these novel foods may reduce healthcare expenditure by promoting good health and that functional foods are a legitimate nutrition education tool, which will help inform consumers of the health benefits of certain food products. The opponents on the other hand rightly state that it is the total diet that is important for health. They believe that the functional foods are a 'magic bullet' approach which enables manufacturers to indulge in marketing hyperbole, exploit consumer anxiety, and essentially blur the distinction between food and drugs. Ironically the production and marketing of functional foods is on the rise in most developed countries. Regulatory bodies in developed societies have a huge and uphill task ahead to ensure that health claims made for these novel foods is evidence based.

Emerging epidemic of obesity and diet-related chronic diseases and the 'double burden' of malnutrition in developing societies

A critical examination of the principal causes of mortality and morbidity worldwide indicates that malnutrition and infectious diseases continue to be significant contributors to the health burden in the developing world. Although reductions in the prevalence of undernutrition are evident, the numbers of individuals affected remain much the same or have even increased, largely due to increases in the population. What is striking, however, is

that the health burden due to NCDs is dramatically increasing in some of these developing countries with modest per capita GNPs, particularly among countries in rapid developmental transition. Even the modest increases in prosperity that accompany economic development seem to be associated with marked increases in the mortality and morbidity attributable to these diet-related NCDs. These transitions in the disease burden of the population are mediated by changes in the dietary patterns and lifestyles that typify the acquisition of urbanized lifestyles.

Most developing countries, particularly those in rapid developmental transition, are in the midst of a demographic and epidemiological transition. Economic development, industrialization, and globalization are accompanied by rapid urbanization. These developmental forces are bringing about changes in the social capital of these societies as well as increasing availability of food and changing lifestyles. The changes in food and nutrition are both quantitative and qualitative; there is not only access to more than adequate food among some sections of the population, but also a qualitative change in the habitual diet. Lifestyle changes contribute to a reduction in physical activity levels. The essence of these changes is captured by the term 'nutrition transition' (Popkin 1994) which accompanies the demographic and epidemiologic transition in these countries. The poor consumer resistance and inadequate regulation compromises food safety and increases contaminants in the food chain. In addition the deterioration of the physical environment, particularly the increase in levels of environmental pollution, contributes to the health burden. Developing societies suffer a 'double burden'—an unfinished agenda of pre-existing widespread undernutrition superimposed by the emerging burden of obesity and NCDs.

Food and nutrition in the prevention of diseases of public health importance

The public health approach to the prevention of nutrition-related diseases requires the adoption of health-oriented nutrition and food policies for the whole population. In most developing countries, the first priority must be ensuring the production or procurement of adequate food supply and its equitable distribution and availability to the whole population along with the elimination of the various forms of nutritional deficiencies. Efforts must also be made to improve the quality of the food which includes ensuring food safety while reducing spoilage and contamination of foods as well as diversifying the availability and use of foods. In agrarian societies, consideration must be given to the short- and long-term effects of agricultural policies which affect the income and buying power of the small producers. Particular attention needs to be paid to the impact the promotion of cash and export crops has on the availability and ability to procure the principal staples in the diet. Special attention needs to be paid to the feasibility of fortification of foods to deal with localized or widespread deficiencies of iodine, iron, and vitamin A as a mass intervention measure.

In developed countries, the burgeoning costs of tertiary healthcare related to the diagnosis and management of the increasing burden of obesity and NCDs have had an impact. There is increasing recognition of the need for prevention-oriented health and nutrition policies and changes in behaviour and lifestyle to reduce the occurrence of these diseases. Some developed countries have been active in the field of public education using national dietary guidelines as a major stimulus. It is important to remember that nutrition education of the public operates in the area where advice is given on a balance of probabilities, rather than irrefutable evidence or any degree of certainty. There is bound to be information that does not fit in with the consensus view since the consensus is based on the balance of the available evidence. It is important to recognize that the causes of these chronic diseases are complex and dietary factors are only a part of the explanation. Individuals differ in their susceptibility to the adverse health effects of specific dietary factors or deficiencies of others. Within the context of public health the focus is the health of the whole population and interventions are aimed at lowering the average level of risk.

Changes in consumer preferences have emerged, initially among the upper socioeconomic and educated masses. The media attention, along with the behavioural changes in food preferences and food choices, are in turn influencing the industry to modify the systems for food production and processing. However, progress in changing consumer behaviour and preferences is by its nature intrinsically rather slow and has until recently largely occurred without support from public policies in any but the health sector. The process of changing unsatisfactory dietary practices and thus promoting health is not easy to achieve. Despite these limitations the occurrence of and mortality associated with some NCDs such as heart disease have declined, reflecting changes in lifestyles of populations.

The dynamic relationship between changes in a population's diet and changes in its health is reflected well in two critical situations. One is the changes in disease and mortality profiles of migrant populations moving from a low-risk to a high-risk environment. An example is the change in disease pattern of Japanese migrants to the United States. The other is the rapid change seen within a country as rural to urban migration occurs or more frequently as a developing country undergoes rapid industrialization and economic development and in the process acquires a dietary change and the consequent morbidity and premature mortality profile characteristic of developed countries. Several developing countries have urban pockets of affluent diet and lifestyles and related disease burdens in the midst of problems typical of a poor country. Such countries in transition, like India and Brazil, bear the dual burdens of diseases of affluence and the widespread health problems of a poor country. Developing countries can benefit by learning from the experience of dietary change and adverse health effects of the developed world. By recognizing this problem, governments of developing countries can gain for their people the health benefits of avoiding nutritional deficiencies without encouraging at the same time the development of NCDs that invariably accompany economic development.

It is thus possible for a country to achieve a reduction in infant and childhood mortality and an increase in life expectancy by the pursuance of health and nutrition policies that aim to provide adequate and equitable access to safe and nutritious food and to minimize at the same time the occurrence of diet-related chronic diseases. This in turn will help avoid the social and economic costs of morbidity and premature death in middle age—a period of highest economic activity and productivity to the nation and to society at large. If such a socially and economically desirable goal is to be achieved, then national governments worldwide must aim towards achieving a population-based dietary change (WHO 1990). In the pursuance of this objective UN agencies established

the scientific basis for Food Based Dietary Guidelines (FBDGs) (FAO and WHO 1996).

The development of food-based dietary guidelines

FBDGs are developed and used in order to improve the food consumption patterns and nutritional well-being of individuals and populations. FBDGs can address specific health issues without the need to fully understand the biological mechanisms that link constituents of food and diet with disease. FBDGs do take into account the considerable epidemiological data linking specific food consumption patterns with a low or high incidence of certain diet-related diseases.

Disseminating information and educating the public through FBDGs is a 'user friendly' approach since consumers think in terms of foods rather than nutrients. They provide a means for nutrition education and are intended for use by individual members of the general public, are written in ordinary language, and as far as possible avoid the use of technical terms in nutritional science. FBDGs will vary with the population group and have to take into account the local or regional dietary patterns, practices, and culture. It is important to underline that more than one dietary pattern is consistent with good health. FBDGs can serve as an instrument of nutrition policies and programmes. Since they are based directly on diet and health relationships of particular relevance to the individual country or region, they can help address those issues of public health concern, either dietary insufficiency or dietary excess. Food and diet are not the only components of a healthy lifestyle and it is important that other relevant messages related to health promotion are integrated into dietary guidelines.

Global strategies to reduce the burden of nutritional disorders

The prevalence of chronic diseases is increasing dramatically, with the majority occurring in developing countries. According to estimates made by WHO, 36 million people die annually from NCDs, 63 per cent of all global deaths are due to NCDs, and 9 million people die too young from NCDs, i.e. before the age of 60. WHO and the FAO earlier proposed an integrated global strategy for the prevention and control of NCDs entitled, 'Diet, physical activity and health' in 2003 and highlighted the fact that chronic diseases are the leading cause of disease and disability, but are neglected elements of the global health agenda (Beaglehole et al. 2007). They proposed a global goal for the prevention and control of chronic diseases to complement the MDGs. The goal is to reduce by 2 per cent per year the age-specific rates of death attributable to chronic diseases, achievement of which would avert 36 million deaths by 2015. Because most of the deaths averted would be in low- and middle-income countries and would mainly affect people less than 70 years, it would bring major economic benefits and reduce the health burden of these nations.

These efforts were followed up by a UN Summit on Non Communicable Diseases in 2011 that recognized 'the urgent need for greater measures at the global, regional and national levels to prevent and control non-communicable diseases'. Unfortunately, much of the emphasis of this summit was focused more on meeting the challenges to the health systems and health services than to prevention apart from tobacco. Dietary interventions to promote population health and reduce risk of NCDs received less attention.

Strategies that are developed to tackle global nutritional problems need to be joined up to deal simultaneously with both ends of the spectrum of nutritional disorders and need to encompass a wide range of stakeholders in an integrated manner to be effective.

References

Aburto, N.J., Hanson, S., Gutierrez, H., et al. (2013). Effect of increased potassium intake on cardiovascular risk factors and disease: systematic review and meta-analyses. *British Medical Journal*, 346, 1378.

Arroyave, G., Mejia, L.A., and Aguilar, J.R. (1981). The effect of vitamin A fortification of sugar on serum vitamin A levels of pre-school Guatemalan children: a longitudinal evaluation. *American Journal of Clinical Nutrition*, 34, 41–9.

Awasti, S., Peto, R., Read, S., et al. (2013). Vitamin A supplementation every 6 months with retinol in 1 million pre-school children in north India: DEVTA, a cluster-randomised trial. *The Lancet*, 381, 1469–77.

Barker D.J.P. (2004). Fetal origins of adult disease. In R.A. Polin, W.W. Fox, and S.H. Abman (eds.) *Fetal and Neonatal Physiology* (3rd ed.), pp. 160–4. Philadelphia, PA: W.B. Saunders,

Beaglehole, R., Ebrahim, S., Reddy, S., et al. (2007). Prevention of chronic diseases: a call to action. *The Lancet*, 370, 2152–7.

Black, R.E., Victora, C.G., Walker, S.P., et al. (2013). Maternal and child undernutrition and overweight in low-income and middle-income countries. *The Lancet*, 382, 427–51.

Boyle, P., Earidze, D.G., and Simans, M. (1985). Descriptive epidemiology of colo-rectal cancer. *International Journal of Cancer*, 36, 9–18.

Bürgi, H., Supersaxo, Z., and Selz, B. (1990). Iodine deficiency diseases in Switzerland one hundred years after Theodor Kocher's survey: a historical review with some new goiter prevalence data. *Acta Endocrinologica (Copenhagen)*, 123, 577–90.

Cappucio, F.P. and MacGregor, G.A. (1991). Does potassium supplementation lower blood pressure? A meta-analysis of published trials. *Journal of Hypertension*, 9, 465–73.

Caulfield, L.E. and Black, R.E. (2004). Zinc deficiency. In M. Ezzati, A.D. Lopez, A. Rodgers, and C.J.L. Murray (eds.) *Comparative Quantification of Health Risks: Global and Regional Burden of Disease Attributable to Selected Major Risk Factors* (Vol. 1), pp. 257–9. Geneva: World Health Organization.

Colditz, G. (1999). Economic costs of obesity and inactivity. *Medicine and Science in Sport and Exercise*, 31, S663–67.

De Benoist, B., McLean, E., Egli, I., et al. (2008). *Worldwide Prevalence of Anaemia 1993-2005. WHO Global Database on Anaemia.* Geneva: World Health Organization.

Dixon, B. (1999). The paradoxes of genetically modified foods. *British Medical Journal*, 318, 547–8.

Doll, R. and Peto, R. (1981). *The Causes of Cancer*. Oxford: Oxford University Press.

Dugdale, M. (2001). Anemia. *Obstetrics and Gynaecology Clinics of North America*, 28, 363–81.

Food and Agricultural Organization (2000). *State of Food Insecurity in the World 2000.* Rome: FAO.

Food and Agricultural Organization (2004). *Agricultural Biotechnology: Meeting the Needs of the Poor?* Rome: FAO.

Food and Agricultural Organization (2012). *State of Food Insecurity in the World 2012.* Rome: FAO.

Food and Agricultural Organization and World Health Organization (1996). *Preparation and Use of Food-Based Dietary Guidelines.* Geneva: World Health Organization.

Foresight (2007). *Tackling Obesity: Future Choices – Project Report.* London: The Stationery Office

Gibson, R.S., Winichagoon, P., Pongcharoen, T., et al. (2007). The feasibility of using zinc fertilizers to improve adequacy of zinc intakes of children consuming rice based diets in North-East Thailand. Paper presented at *Zinc Crops 2007: Improving Crop Production and Human Health*, 24–26 May, Istanbul, Turkey. Available at: http://zinc-crops.ionainteractive.com/ZnCrops2007/PDF/2007_zinccrops2007_gibson.pdf.

Grantham-McGregor, S. (1995). A review of the studies of the effect of severe malnutrition on mental development. *Journal of Nutrition*, 125, 2232S–8S.

He, F.J., Li, J., and Macgregor, G.A. (2013). Effect of longer term modest salt reduction on blood pressure: Cochrane systematic review and meta-analysis of randomised trials. *British Medical Journal*, 346, 1325.

Hetzel, B.S. (1987). An overview of the prevention and control of iodine deficiency disorders. In B.S. Hetzel, J.T. Dunn, and J.B. Stanbury (eds.) *The Prevention and Control of Iodine Deficiency Disorders*, pp. 7–31. Amsterdam: Elsevier.

Horton, S. and Ross, J. (2003). The economics of iron deficiency. *Food Policy*, 28, 51–75.

Intersalt Cooperative Research Group (1988). Intersalt: an international study of electrolyte excretion and blood pressure. *British Medical Journal*, 298, 920–4.

Keys, A. (1980). *Seven Countries: A Multivariate Analysis of Death and Coronary Heart Disease.* Cambridge, MA: Harvard University Press.

Kris-Etherton, P.M. (1999). Monounsaturated fatty acids and risk of cardiovascular disease. *Circulation*, 100, 1253–8.

Law, M.R., Frost, C.D., and Wald, N.J. (1991). By how much does dietary salt reduction lower blood pressure? *British Medical Journal*, 302, 811–24.

Lissner, L. and Heitmann, B.L. (1995). Dietary fat and obesity: evidence from epidemiology. *European Journal of Clinical Nutrition*, 49, 969–81.

MacMohan, S., Peto, R., Cutler, J., et al. (1990). Blood pressure, stroke and coronary heart disease. *The Lancet*, 335, 765–74.

McKeown, T. (1976). *The Modern Rise of Population.* London: Edward Arnold.

Mori, T.A. and Beilin, L.J. (2001). Long-chain omega 3 fatty acids, blood lipids and cardiovascular risk reduction. *Current Opinion in Lipidology*, 12, 11–17.

Muhilal, P.D. Idjrodinata, Y.R., and Karyadi, D. (1988). Vitamin A fortified monosodium glutamate and health, growth and survival of children: a controlled field trial. *American Journal of Clinical Nutrition*, 48, 1271–6.

Pharoah, P.O.D. and Connolly, D.C. (1987). A controlled trial of iodinated oil for the prevention of endemic cretinism: a long-term follow-up. *International Journal of Epidemiology*, 16, 68–73.

Phillips, D.I.W., Lusty, T.D., Osmond, C., et al. (1988). Iodine supplementation: comparison of oral or intramuscular iodized oil with potassium iodide. A controlled trial in Zaire. *International Journal of Epidemiology*, 17, 142–7.

Pollitt, E. (1991a). Effects of diet deficient in iron on the growth and development of preschool children. *Food and Nutrition Bulletin*, 13, 521–37.

Pollitt, E. (1991b). Iron deficiency and cognitive function. *Annual Review of Nutrition*, 13, 521–37.

Popkin, B. (1994). The nutrition transition in low-income countries: an emerging crisis. *Nutrition Reviews*, 52, 285–98.

Puska, P., Tuomilehto, J., Nissinen, A., et al. (1995). *The North Karelia Project. 20 year results and experiences.* Helsinki: Helsinki University Press.

Quisumbing, A.R., Brown, L.R., Feldstein, H.S., Haddad, L., and Peña, C. (1995). *Women: The Key to Food Security.* Washington, DC: Food Policy Report, IFPRI.

Rees, K., Dyakova, M., Ward, K., et al. (2013). Dietary advice for reducing cardiovascular risk. *Cochrane Database Systematic Reviews*, 3, CD002128.

Scholl, T.O. and Johnson, W.G. (2000). Folic acid: influence on the outcome of pregnancy. *American Journal of Clinical Nutrition*, 71, 1295S–303S.

Sen, A. (1981). *Poverty and Famines: An Essay on Entitlement and Deprivation.* Oxford: Clarendon Press.

Shetty, P. (2006). The Boyd Orr lecture: achieving the goal of halving global hunger by 2015. *Proceedings of the Nutrition Society*, 65, 7–18.

Shetty, P. (2009). Incorporating nutritional considerations when addressing food insecurity. *Food Security*, 1, 431–40.

Shetty, P.S. and James, W.P.T. (1994). *Body Mass Index: An Objective Measure for the Estimation of Chronic Energy Deficiency in Adults.* FAO Food and Nutrition Paper. Rome: FAO.

Standing Committee on Nutrition (2004). *Fifth Report on the World Nutrition Situation: Nutrition for Improved Development* Standing Committee on Nutrition. Geneva: WHO.

Stoltzfus, R.J., Chwaya, H.M., Tielsch, J.M., et al. (1997). Epidemiology of iron deficiency anaemia in Zanzibari schoolchildren: the importance of hookworms. *American Journal of Clinical Nutrition*, 65, 153–9.

Stoltzfus, R.J., Mullany, L., and Black R.E. (2004). Iron deficiency anemia. In M. Ezzati, A. Rodgers, and C.J.L. Murray (eds.) *Comparative Quantification of Health Risks: The Global and Regional Burden of Disease Attributable to Selected Major Risk Factors*, pp. 163–209. Geneva: WHO.

Swaminathan, M.S. (2008). *Achieving Sustainable Nutrition Security for All and Forever.* International Union of Food Science and Technology (IUFOST) Congress. Available at: http://www.iufost.org/world_congress/documents/IUF.Food.Security.Swami.2.pdf.

Te Morenga, L., Mallard, S., and Mann, J. (2013). Dietary sugars and body weight: systematic review and meta-analyses of randomised controlled trials and cohort studies. *British Medical Journal*, 346, 7492.

Thompson, B. and Amoroso, L. (2011). *Combating Micronutrient Deficiencies: Food Based Approaches.* Wallingford: CABI.

Tucker, K.L. (2009). Osteoporosis prevention and nutrition. *Current Osteoporosis Reports*, 7, 111–17.

UNICEF (1997). *The State of the World's Children 1997.* Oxford: Oxford University Press.

UNICEF (2012). *The State of the World's Children 2012: Children in an Urban World.* New York: UNICEF.

UNICEF and Micronutrient Initiative (2004). *Vitamin and Mineral Deficiency: A World Progress Report.* Ottawa: Micronutrient Initiative.

Vargas, A.J. and Thompson, P.A. (2012). Diet and nutrient factors in colorectal cancer risk. *Nutrition in Clinical Practice*, 27, 613–23.

Viteri, F.E. (1997). Prevention of iron deficiency. In Institute of Medicine (ed.) *Prevention of Micronutrient Deficiencies. Tools for Policy-makers and Public Health Workers*, pp. 45–102. Washington, DC: National Academy Press.

Weingartner, L. (2005). The concept of food and nutrition security. In K. Klennert (ed.) *Achieving Food and Nutrition Security: Actions to Meet the Global Challenge*, pp. 1–28. Bonn: InWEnt (Internationale Weiterbildung und Entwicklung gGmbH).

World Cancer Research Fund and American Institute for Cancer Research (2007). *Food, Nutrition, Physical Activity and the Prevention of Cancer: A Global Perspective.* Washington, DC: American Institute for Cancer Research.

World Health Organization (1982). *Prevention of Coronary Heart Disease.* Technical Report Series. Geneva: WHO.

World Health Organization (1990). *Diet, Nutrition and the Prevention of Chronic Disease.* WHO Technical Report Series 797. Geneva: WHO.

World Health Organization (1995). *Physical Status: The Use and Interpretation of Anthropometry.* Geneva: WHO.

World Health Organization (2000). *Obesity: Preventing and Managing the Global Epidemic.* Geneva: WHO.

World Health Organization (2002). *The World Health Report: Reducing Risks, Promoting Healthy Life.* Geneva: WHO.

World Health Organization (2004). *Iodine Status Worldwide.* Geneva: WHO.

World Health Organization (2006). *WHO Child Growth Standards.* Geneva: WHO.

World Health Organization (2008). *Worldwide Prevalence of Anaemia 1993–2005.* WHO global database on anaemia. Geneva: WHO.

World Health Organization (2009). Global Prevalence of Night Blindness and Number of Individuals Affected in Populations of Countries at Risk of Vitamin A Deficiency 1995–2005. WHO Global Database on Vitamin A Deficiency. Geneva: WHO.

World Health Organization and Food and Agricultural Organization (2003). *Diet, Nutrition and the Prevention of Chronic Diseases.* Technical Report Series 916. Geneva: WHO.

World Health Organization, UNICEF, and UNU (2001). *Iron Deficiency Anemia: Assessment, Prevention and Control.* Geneva: WHO.

Zimmerman, M.B., Wegmueller, R., Zeder, C., et al. (2004). Triple fortification of salt with microcapsules of iodine, iron, and vitamin A. *American Journal of Clinical Nutrition*, 80, 1283–90.

2.8

The environment and climate change

Alistair Woodward and Alex Macmillan

Introduction to the environment and climate change

In 2006, George Pell, Archbishop of Sydney, compared those who seek cuts in greenhouse gas emissions with pagans who seek to pacify the gods by animal and human sacrifice. In both cases, he argued, spiritual emptiness and fears about the natural world lead to extreme and unreasonable behaviours (Pell 2006).

Cardinal Pell is not alone. Climate change attracts a lot of attention, and many people are prepared to express an opinion, often strongly worded and frequently poorly informed. This chapter aims to introduce readers to the basic science underlying climate change, so they are better placed to judge extreme claims of all kinds. We will explore the links between climate change and health, and examine the implications of this knowledge for public health policy and practice.

As a start, readers are invited to check their understanding of the field against the multiple-choice questions in Box 2.8.1. (The answers are shown at the end of the chapter in Box 2.8.4.) This is not a comprehensive test but a starting point and a guide to what is contained in the chapter.

The Earth has an average surface temperature suitable for life that is the product of a number of natural influences on the balance of radiation (radiative 'forcing' at the top of the atmosphere). These include solar activity (the amount of energy produced by the sun), the tilt and orbit of the planet, volcanic activity that injects gases and ash into the upper atmosphere, other dusts and aerosols that block incoming solar radiation, and the amount of reflection ('albedo') by clouds, ice, and snow. Also important is the concentration of so-called 'greenhouse' gases. These gases are transparent to relatively high-frequency incoming solar radiation in the visible spectrum. However, when this radiation is absorbed on the surface of the earth it is re-emitted in the infra-red range, which is trapped by the greenhouse gases. This action is similar to the effect of a pane of glass in a greenhouse (or the window of a car sitting in the sun). Without the blanket for the planet that is provided by the greenhouse gases, the Earth would be approximately 30 degrees centigrade (C) colder than it is at present. Carbon dioxide (CO_2) is the most abundant of these heat-trapping gases.

CO_2 levels in the atmosphere vary over long timescales due to transfers from the atmosphere to the biosphere and the oceans, and from the oceans carbon is eventually sequestered in sedimentary rocks. In the very long term, carbon from the earth's crust is ejected by volcanic eruptions into the atmosphere, and the cycle begins again.

What has changed in the last 200 years or so is the large-scale emission of CO_2 (and other heat-trapping gases) as a result of human activities, such as clearing of forests and burning of fossil fuels. This process began in pre-industrial times as a relatively minor addition of carbon to the atmosphere but has escalated rapidly in the last 50 years. In the early 2000s, roughly 27 giga-tonnes (Gt) of CO_2 were released into the atmosphere each year. (This equates to the mass of 3 million Eiffel Towers.) CO_2 is a long lived greenhouse gas: about half of the carbon that is emitted into the atmosphere is taken up by natural sinks within 30 years, but about 30 per cent will persist in the atmosphere for centuries.

The concentration of CO_2 in the atmosphere has risen steadily from about 280 parts per million (ppm) in pre-industrial times, to 315 ppm in 1960 when direct measurements were first made, and exceeded 400 ppm in 2014. Indirect measures, using ice cores and other indications of historic conditions, tell us that the present levels are higher than at any time in the last 400,000 years. Concentrations of other, shorter-lived but more potent greenhouse gases, such as methane and nitrous oxide, have also increased acutely in the last 50 years (Solomon et al. 2007).

Consequences of these changes in atmospheric chemistry are evident in the recent temperature record at or close to the earth's surface, and are expressed also in sea level rise, reduced snow and ice cover, and a variety of impacts on physical and biological systems. The year-to-year variability in average global temperatures is dominated by natural factors such as the El Niño Southern Oscillation (ENSO), so the effect of persistent, external forcing such as steadily rising greenhouse concentrations is seen most clearly on longer timescales. Indeed each of the last three decades has been warmer than all earlier decades, and the warmest years on record have occurred in the 2000s, according to NASA (Arndt et al. 2010). This rise in global average temperatures has occurred in every region, over both land and ocean, and cannot be explained by time trends in solar activity and other natural forcings. On the other hand, climate simulations that include anthropogenic contributions (i.e. the increase in CO_2 and other greenhouse gases) match well with the last 40 years of temperature records (Fig. 2.8.1).

Other evidence of global warming includes the predominance of highest ever temperatures in the record of temperature extremes (in the western United States, record high temperatures

Box 2.8.1 Carbon IQ quiz

Indicate which of the following, A to E, is the best answer for each question.

1. If the planet's atmosphere consisted of oxygen and nitrogen, the global average temperature would change by:

   A. −30 degrees C

   B. −10 degrees C

   C. +10 degrees C

   D. +30 degrees C

   E. 0 degrees C

2. Climate is 'average weather'. Over what period?

   A. At least a week

   B. >2 years

   C. >20 years

   D. A century at least

   E. Millennia

3. One-third of the CO_2 emitted today will still be in the atmosphere in:

   A. 1 year

   B. 10 years

   C. 100 years

   D. 1000 years

   E. 10,000 years

4. Combustion of biomass releases black carbon, other particulates, and aerosols. The effect is to:

   A. Warm

   B. Cool

   C. Affect regional climate, mostly

   D. Accelerate ice melt

   E. All of the above

5. In the last 50 years, what proportion of the warming due to greenhouse emissions has been absorbed by the ocean?

   A. 5 per cent

   B. 80 per cent

   C. 0 per cent

   D. 20 per cent

   E. 100 per cent

6. Globally, the warmest year on record was:

   A. 2010

   B. 1998

   C. 1992

   D. 1980

   E. 1260

7. How many return flights, Singapore to Rome, are required to generate the annual average emissions of CO_2 per capita for Laos?

   A. 200

   B. 20

   C. 1

   D. 0.2

   E. 0.02

8. If there was a food with the energy intensity of oil, how many litres would be required to cycle 100 km?

   A. 200

   B. 20

   C. 1

   D. 0.2

   E. 0.02

9. Which US President gave a commitment to translate the UN Framework Convention on Climate Change into 'concrete action to protect the planet'?

   A. George H.W. Bush

   B. Bill Clinton

   C. George W. Bush

   D. Jimmy Carter

   E. Richard Nixon

10. Take the number of deaths in New Orleans caused by Hurricane Katrina, and make the numerator the average number of fatalities resulting from storms of a similar severity in Cuba in the preceding 5 years. The fraction is:

    A. 0.1

    B. 0.5

    C. 2.0

    D. 0.05

    E. 1.0

now outnumber record low measurements each year by about three to one) (Meehl et al. 2009), and increasing temperatures in the upper layers of the ocean (which absorbs more than 80 per cent of the solar energy that is trapped by greenhouse gases) (von Schuckmann et al. 2009). Summertime Arctic sea ice is reducing year on year, more rapidly than was forecast in the Intergovernmental Panel on Climate Change (IPCC) Fourth Assessment Report and global average sea level is rising at about 3.0 mm/year (twice the rate observed before 1990) (Australian Academy of Sciences 2010).

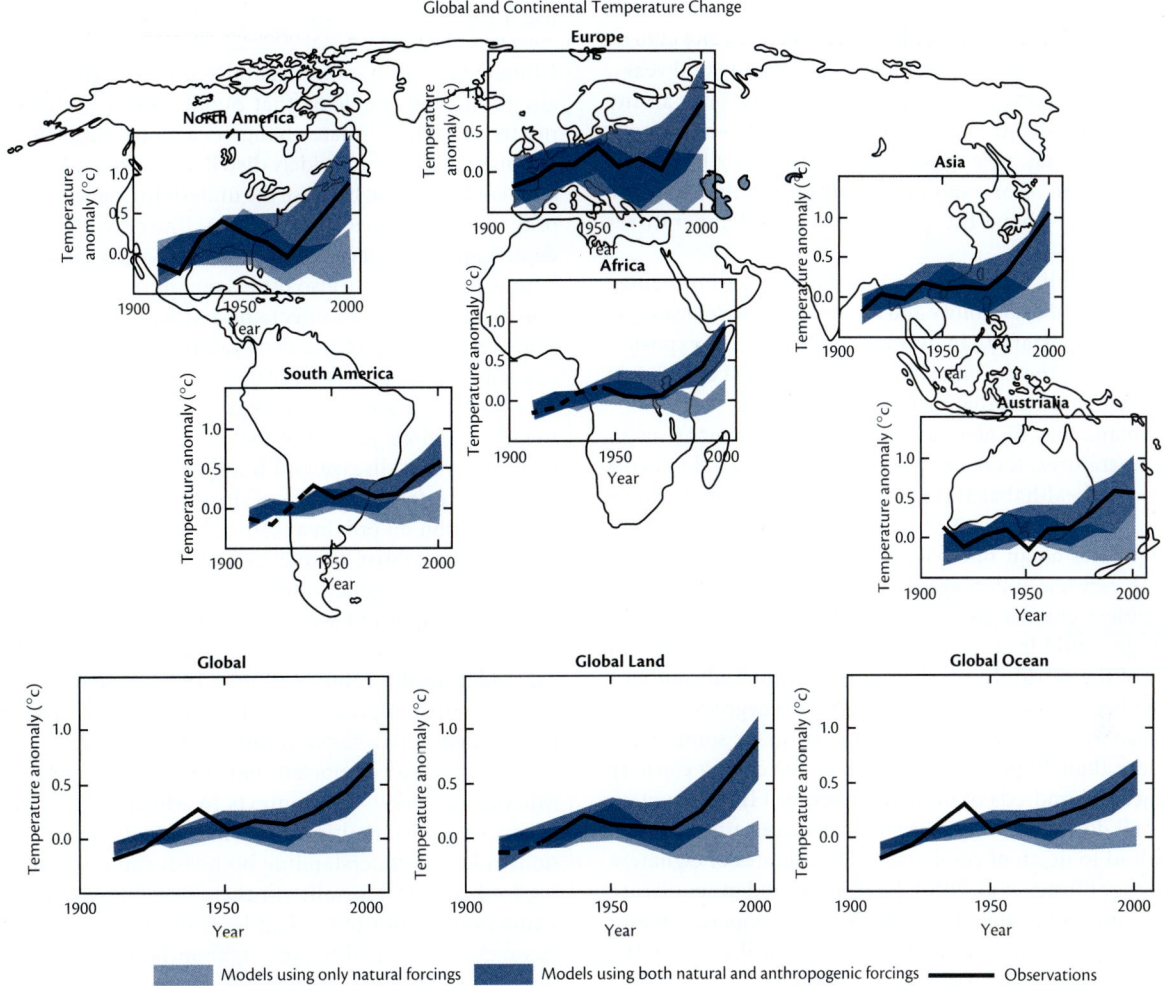

Fig. 2.8.1 Observed and modelled temperatures, 1906–2005. Decadal averages, observed (black lines), modelled using only natural forcings (lower shaded areas), and modelled using natural and anthropogenic forcings (upper shaded areas).

Reproduced with permission from *Climate Change 2007: The Physical Science Basis. Working Group I Contribution to the Fourth Assessment Report of the Intergovernmental Panel on Climate Change*, Figure 2.5. Cambridge University Press.

Since the 1960s, emissions of greenhouse gases have tracked upwards, the rise halted only briefly by major economic disturbances, such as the Asian financial crisis of the late 1990s (Peters et al. 2011). Emissions in the first decade of the twenty-first century have matched, or exceeded, the figures forecast by the most extreme of the climate scenarios (A1FL) reported in the Third Assessment Report in 2001.

What about the future? The IPCC in AR4 forecast that the 'business as usual' trajectory would result in atmospheric CO_2 doubling pre-industrial levels sometime between 2050 and 2100, and global average temperatures rising as a result by between 2 and 4.5 degrees C by 2100 (Solomon et al. 2007).

A global average temperature rise reflects a shift of the whole temperature distribution to the right, but there will also be an increase in the variability of the distribution. This combination of distribution shift and increased variability translates a 2–4 degrees C increase (which may sound small) into a very marked increase in the frequency of very high temperatures that are presently experienced rarely. It is projected that 'mega-heatwaves' of the kind that caused more than 50,000 excess deaths in Russia in 2010 may increase by a factor of 5–10 in Europe, within the next 40 years (Barriopedro et al. 2011). As average temperatures rise, the incidence of cold events is likely to fall, all else being equal, although there may be unexpected effects in some regions. In one example, melting of the Arctic ice has affected the high level jet stream over Europe and North America, and there is evidence of more severe winters occurring in these regions as a consequence (Liu et al. 2012).

The effects of warming and changes in rainfall will be unevenly distributed, geographically. For instance, a global average of 4 degrees C of warming may be associated with an increase in temperatures in the Arctic of 10 degrees C or more, a decline in rainfall by 40–50 per cent in North Africa, droughts threatening the viability of rain-fed agriculture in many parts of sub-Saharan Africa by the end of the century, and much of south-eastern Australia experiencing extreme fire risks as often as every second summer (4 degrees & beyond 2009).

In summary, the greenhouse effect is long known and well described. The rate at which greenhouse gas levels in the atmosphere are increasing is unprecedented in the last 400,000 years, and absolute concentrations are presently higher than at any time in the same period. In association with these changes, the world is warming, in a manner that carries a discernible human 'finger print'. For example, heating is confined to the lower atmosphere—above the greenhouse layer temperatures are falling.

Why is this a public health issue? It is important to recognize that for human health, variability and frequency of extreme events are often more important than average conditions. On exposure to heat or cold, it is the deviation from usual or most commonly experienced temperatures that carry the greatest risk.

While humans may be able to cope with modest increases in baseline temperatures, there are physical and ecological systems of importance to health that are exposed to environmental change and may be exquisitely sensitive to temperature rise. Agriculture generally operates as an open system, directly exposed to the weather, with very few buffers against extreme events or long-term shifts in ambient conditions. Warming of 2–4 degrees C in the global average would lead to substantial falls in productivity in some parts of the world. In much of sub-Saharan and southern Africa, it has been projected that an increase of 5 degrees C in the global average would reduce the growing period for some staple crops by more than 20 per cent, threatening the coping capacity and resilience of hundreds of millions of people (Thornton et al. 2010). A small degree of ocean warming above certain threshold limits may lead to death of coral and increased rates of ciguatera (fish poisoning) (Tester et al. 2010). Mosquitoes and other disease vectors also respond acutely to small shifts in temperature and rainfall, and increases in average temperatures will increase the potential for disease transmission in some populations (Wandiga et al. 2009). (Conversely, disease risks may be reduced in areas where conditions are presently close to the upper limits of vector survival (Gething et al. 2010).)

Another mechanism by which an extra degree or two (or four) of global warming may affect human health is through displacement of populations. Projected effects of climate change include sea level rise, increased intensity of storms and floods, prolonged droughts and crop failure, all of which may cause large numbers of people to move, bringing heightened risks of poverty, conflict, and violence (see Box 2.8.2) (McMichael et al. 2012).

Observational studies of weather, climate, and health

A great deal has been written about variations in weather (day-to-day conditions) and climate (average weather over a period of decades) to health outcomes. One of the exposures most closely studied is temperature, which may be expressed in many ways, commonly as the daily average or maximum temperature, with or without an adjustment for humidity. Fig. 2.8.2 shows a pattern that is frequently observed—a U- or J-shaped relation between temperature and health outcomes (in this case, mortality excluding accidental deaths). The optimal temperature (the point at which mortality is lowest) differs from one setting to another. In the case of Haerbin, a city located in the far north of China, the number of deaths is at its lowest when the average temperature

---

Box 2.8.2 Too big? Or too big to ignore? The challenge of scale

Climate change is fundamentally different from most other environmental problems that public health has faced. It is a matter of scale. Climate change is a global problem, not only because the effects are widely distributed, like acid rain, or influenza epidemics, but because the underlying cause is a disruption of the planet's homeostatic systems. The only forerunner is the depletion of high-level atmospheric ozone by chlorofluorocarbons. Climate change also moves on unprecedented timescales. For instance, the full effects of a spike in greenhouse emissions on warming of the deep ocean and associated sea-level rise may not be apparent for 5000 years or more (Stouffer 2012). This provides a serious challenge to public health scientists. In the last hundred years, the focus has shifted to finer-grained explanations of disease and injury, assisted by new technologies and greater knowledge of the mechanisms of disease. The concentration on proximal causes has brought many successes (such as the control of infectious diseases, and opportunities for specific nutritional interventions). Some have argued that there is an important lesson here, that engaging with upstream causes may be a distraction, and is unlikely to provide significant public health gains (Rothman 1998). Others maintain that a fine-grained approach, in which the unit of observation is increasingly microscopic (individual, organ, genes, and molecules) misses an important part of the public health picture (McMichael 1999). The contexts in which chemical reactions occur, microbes multiply, and individuals make their decisions is key to understanding both risk and resilience, according to this view. Mortality in the 1995 Chicago heatwave was a function of both individual-level variables (such as age and income), and the qualities of neighbourhoods. The poor and the elderly were at much greater risk during the heatwave if they lived in areas with rundown businesses, abandoned housing, and degraded public spaces (Klinenberg 2003). Climate change represents a particularly stark example of a big-picture problem, featuring extended timescales, ubiquitous exposures, and the confounding effects of human adaptation. If public health intends to grapple with the most important health problems, some contend there is no choice but to move upstream, to move from studies of the variations between individuals to studying causes on a larger scale, and to embrace and overcome the difficulties that will, inevitably, be encountered (Pearce 2011). This will very likely require refinement of established methods of public health inquiry (such as time series analysis, and ecological research designs); an understanding of climate science and meteorology; the creative use of analogues; and the application of relevant modelling methods from other disciplines (e.g. systems dynamic modelling) (Woodward 2002).

---

is close to 0 degrees C (Yang et al. 2007). In cities located closer to the equator, the optimal temperature tends to be higher (Fig. 2.8.2). The overall shape of the curve relating temperature to mortality remains similar, but the point of inflection on the curve moves towards the right in cities in which high temperatures are more commonly experienced (McMichael et al. 2008). This is a reminder that populations do adapt to their ecological context, physiologically and socially. What is less clear is how quickly this

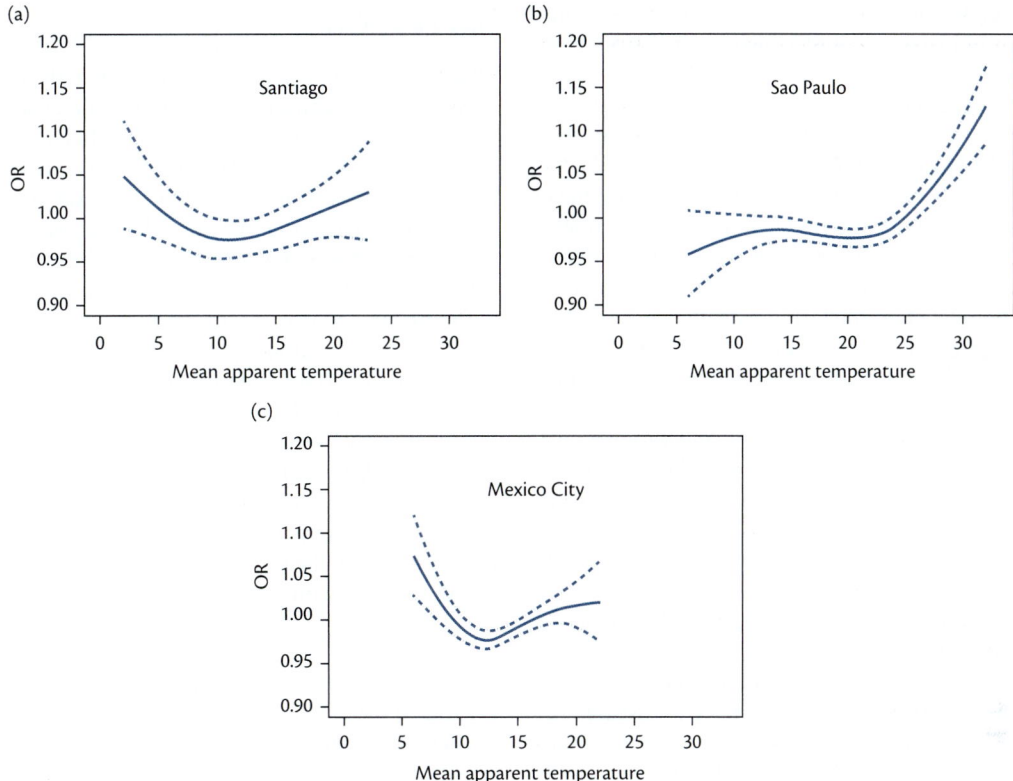

Fig. 2.8.2 Average daily apparent temperature and total mortality: Santiago (33 degrees S), Sao Paulo (24 degrees S), and Mexico City (19 degrees N). Solid lines show central estimate, dashed lines the 95 per cent confidence intervals. Adjusted for particulate pollution and ozone levels.
Reproduced from Bell ML et al., Vulnerability to heat-related mortality in Latin America: a case-crossover study in Sao Paulo, Brazil, Santiago, Chile and Mexico City, Mexico, *International Journal of Epidemiology*, Volume 37, Issue 4, pp. 796–804, Copyright © The Author 2008, with permission from Oxford University Press.

adaptation can occur, if people move, or the climate changes, and what are the limits of adaptation—how much heat is tolerable?

Higher temperatures have been linked with a range of health outcomes including deaths and hospital admissions for respiratory and cardiovascular diseases. In heatwaves, which may be defined as prolonged exposure to temperatures in the top 5–10 per cent of the range for that location, the effects appear to be greater than would be expected by simply extrapolating the temperature–health outcome relationship (Anderson and Bell 2011; Rocklöv et al. 2012). Duration of heat, frequency of heatwaves, and timing (early or late in the season) all appear to modify the effects of high temperatures. It is unclear how much of the elevated mortality risk associated with low temperatures is explained by seasonal factors other than cold weather, such as outbreaks of influenza and other infections that may be linked to winter crowding, as well as conditions attributed to decreased exposure to sunlight and reduced vitamin D levels (Goldstein et al. 2011). Mortality from cardiovascular conditions, the most common cause of death in many countries, is only weakly associated with low temperatures (Ebi and Mills 2013).

There is considerable variation within populations in vulnerability to heat. Older people (70 years and over) and children are generally at greater risk. There is no consistent pattern with gender. Men were found to be at greater risk in Sao Paulo and Santiago (Bell et al. 2008); whereas a study in Brisbane, Australia reported a more marked increase in mortality risk for women than men (Huang et al. 2012). In many countries, low socioeconomic

status (SES) has been associated with increased risk of heat- and cold-related poor health, but again, this is not universal. There is, for example a greater variation by SES in heat mortality in the United States than in England, perhaps because the use of air conditioning is distributed differentially in the US but not so much in the United Kingdom (where few houses have artificial cooling and there is much less social variation) (Armstrong et al. 2011). Vulnerability is also expressed spatially (Uejio et al. 2011) reflecting the geographical distribution of individual and household characteristics (such as prevalence of chronic diseases, housing design, and poverty) and also district-level variables (urban form, quality of services). It is not just the maximum or average temperatures that affect health. Variability is important as well. In 135 United States cities, for example, the standard deviation of summer temperatures was associated with mortality of older people suffering from chronic disease, after adjustment for a wide range of risk factors including average temperature (Zanobetti et al. 2012).

As with many climate change impacts, more is known about the effects of high temperatures in high-income countries than in the developing world, although the problem is likely to be more severe in the latter, given the high temperatures that already apply in many low-latitude countries, the very large populations, often with multiple health problems, that are exposed, and the low quality of housing and urban environments. Given climate change projections, there is renewed interest in the effects of heat on the health of workers. This is especially significant in equatorial countries where high temperatures already place severe restraints on the duration and intensity of outdoor work (Kjellstrom et al. 2013).

In 2003, Europe experienced a particularly severe heatwave, affecting France most notably. In July, a spike in temperature of 5–8 degrees C resulted in about 100 extra deaths in Paris. The following month Paris experienced almost 2 weeks of daily mean temperatures that were 10–12 degrees C above the normal level for the season. The heatwave caused about 1000 extra deaths in Paris in July, and altogether more than 30,000 deaths across the whole of Europe (Fouillet et al. 2008). These deaths were not simply events brought forward by a few days or weeks, since mortality rates after the heatwave did not fall below the long-term average until the following year.

In addition to the direct effects of extreme and variable temperatures on mortality, the effects of climate on infectious disease have long been known (see Box 2.8.3). The first textbook of tropical medicine, by Patrick Manson, was published in 1900, and was called *A Manual of the Diseases of Warm Climates* (Manson 1900). Manson wrote principally of infectious diseases but he recognized that few conditions were peculiar to the tropics. In other words, he understood that climate variables such as temperature and precipitation play an important part in, but are seldom the entire explanation for, the distribution and occurrence of disease. The mosquito-borne diseases are good examples. In warmer conditions, vectors such as *Aedes aegypti* (responsible most commonly for the transmission of dengue fever) develop more quickly from the immature stage (Tun Lin et al. 2000). In tropical countries in which temperatures vary little through the year, the transition from a time of low rainfall to the rainy season may act as a powerful climatic trigger for outbreaks of dengue (Schreiber 2001). However, other factors, such as the degree of urbanization and the quality of housing, commonly have a strong role in modifying the effect of climate on dengue risk (Wu et al. 2009).

The sensitivity of dengue to climate variations has been demonstrated on a regional scale from investigations of the ENSO in the Pacific. Every 4–6 years, approximately, the prevailing east-to-west flow of the trade winds across the Pacific weakens, ocean currents are affected, and warm water spreads from the west Pacific to the east. In the southern Pacific (including Fiji, Samoa, Tonga, the Cook Islands) the La Nina stage of ENSO, which brings warmer

> **Box 2.8.3** Plague and climate
>
> Plague is caused by infection of humans with *Yersinia pestis*. The organism is established in rodent populations in parts of Asia, Africa, and the Americas, and periodically causes outbreaks of disease in local populations. The prevalence of *Yersinia* in animal hosts is climate sensitive. For example, a study of gerbils in Kazakhstan found the risk of disease was increased by warmer springs and wetter summers (Stenseth et al. 2006). An increase of 1 degree C in spring was associated with an increase of more than 50 per cent in the prevalence of animals infected with *Yersinia*. Climate also affects the abundance of rodent hosts and flea vectors, as well as the chances of humans coming into contact with the pathogen. Consequently, it is not surprising that many historical studies have shown a link between climate and plague epidemics. As one example: a study of plague in China between 1850 and 1960 found the number of cases per year was positively related to rainfall, although extremely high precipitation in the wetter parts of the country led to lower than expected plague intensity (Xu et al. 2011).

and wetter conditions to that part of the world, has been strongly associated with the number of dengue outbreaks (Fig. 2.8.3).

There are many other examples of health conditions that are sensitive to variations in climate or weather. In the south-western part of Australia, the prevalence of depression has been related to the severity of long-term drought (measured as dry-land salinity) (Speldewinde 2009). In Bangladesh the dry season is marked by increasing salinity and rising temperatures of the ground water, and it is thought these changes are linked to marked seasonal variations in the incidence of high blood pressure and eclampsia in pregnancy (precipitated by increases in sodium loading), and cholera (Xun et al. 2010).

In summary, humans have evolved to experience minimal mortality in narrow temperature ranges that are context specific. The connection between extremes of cold and heat on mortality is well established through our understanding of excess winter mortality and deaths resulting from heatwaves. In addition there are studies of specific infectious and non-infectious diseases demonstrating variation with both climate and weather.

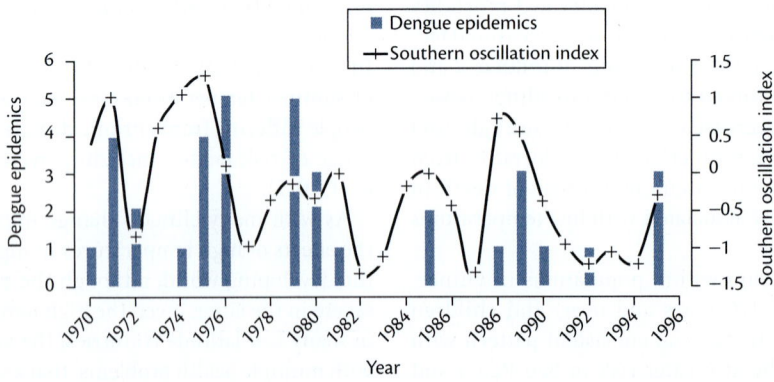

Fig. 2.8.3 Dengue and the El Niño Southern Oscillation.

Reprinted from *The Lancet*, Volume 348, Issue 9042, S Hales, P Weinstein, A Woodward, Dengue fever epidemics in the South Pacific: driven by El Niño Southern Oscillation?, p1664–1665, Copyright © 1996, with permission from Elsevier, http://www.sciencedirect.com/science/journal/01406736.

Attribution—present impacts of climate change

In its Fourth Assessment Report, published in 2007, the IPCC concluded that 'warming of the climate system is unequivocal' and 'most of the observed increase in temperatures since the mid-twentieth century is very likely due to the increase in anthropogenic greenhouse gases' (Solomon et al. 2007). The Fifth Assessment Report confirms that we are extremely likely to be experiencing the early stages of human-induced climate change (reference to 5th assessment report WG1). In other words, according to the IPCC, we are (very likely) seeing the early stages of human-induced climate change.

As well as temperatures increasing beyond the bounds of what are regarded as natural variability, the IPCC assessment documented numerous changes in physical and biological systems that are consistent with global warming. For example, nearly two-thirds of fish species in the North Sea have shifted in latitude or depth or both, over the space of 25 years, in accord with warming of the ocean (Perry 2005). In the Alsace region of France, in association with higher summer temperatures, the potential alcohol content of Riesling grapes, at harvest, has climbed by almost 1 per cent per year (Duchene and Schneider 2005). These changes in physical and biological systems are clearly attributable to climate change. It is more difficult to attribute effects of climate change on the frequency of injury or disease, or other measures of human ill health, than on measures such as the location of fish stocks or levels of sugar in grapes. There are three reasons. The phenomenon of adaptation has been mentioned already—most human societies are well buffered against the effects of climate variability and extremes. Second, it is often difficult to distinguish effects of climate from other co-temporaneous causes of ill health (for example, the disruptive effects of migration or expanding settlements in disaster-prone locations). Third, because climate change takes place over decades, we need outcome data for the same length of time. But it is unusual, especially in the most vulnerable parts of the world, to have accurate and reliable information on health status over such long periods.

Finding early evidence of health effects attributable to climate change requires data extending over many years, in areas where the relationship between climate and health is strongest, where adaptive capacity is weak, and where there are few competing explanations (Woodward and McMichael 2001). It is a challenge to identify conditions and settings that meet all these criteria.

The story of tick-borne encephalitis (TBE) illustrates well these complexities of attribution. In the last decade of the twentieth century the vector for TBE moved northward across the Baltic and Scandinavia, in association with warming that has been most marked in winter and early spring (Lindgren 2001). The incidence of TBE surged in the early 1990s in the Baltic states, but disease trends do not fit neatly with the change in climate. There were considerable variations within the Baltic in TBE rates, and although warming has continued, TBE rates have diminished since 2000 (Sumilo et al. 2007). Clearly there are other factors that are important besides the arrival of a climate that was more favourable for transmission of the TBE virus. When the Soviet Union broke up in 1989, many collective farms ceased to operate, areas that had been used for pasture and agriculture were left untended, and these provided new habitat for rodents and deer. At the same time, during a period of economic disruption and transition, people were more dependent than before on wild food sources, including mushrooms and small game, and as a result spent more time in the countryside. In combination these changes, climatic and non-climatic, may have increased tick abundance and boosted, for a short time, the exposure of humans to tick-borne diseases (Sumilo et al. 2007).

In public health, the accepted way around this difficulty of attribution is a risk-based approach which estimates the increase in the probability of an event occurring due to a particular exposure. No one would think inability to attribute a particular instance of lung cancer to cigarette smoking is inconsistent with a firm conviction that smoking causes the majority of such cancers in populations in which tobacco use is common. But such an approach to detection and attribution is less frequently applied in the natural and biological sciences—the disciplines that by and large are responsible for the production and assessment of much of the evidence on climate change (Parmesan et al. 2011).

Here are two examples of risk-based approaches to attribution. A study of the 2003 European heatwave concluded it was very likely (probability greater than 90 per cent) that human influences on climate had more than doubled the risk of such an extreme event (Stott 2004). Note that a relative risk of more than 2.0 means it is more likely than not that the outcome is attributable to the exposure, and this is the standard of proof that is applied in some jurisdictions to establish liability (in, for example, disputes over diseases related to exposures in the workplace). This raises the tantalizing question of who or what should be held liable, globally, for warming that raises the risk of damaging heatwaves more than twofold.

As part of the 2002 Global Burden of Disease project, the contribution of climate change up to the year 2000 was estimated, providing an overall assessment of present impacts. This followed the steps that are usually taken in a health risk assessment: choose the conditions that are thought to be sensitive to the exposure; quantify the dose–response relationship; define alternative exposure scenarios; and calculate the burden of disease attributable to the difference in exposure between what is observed and what would have applied in the counterfactual situation. The increase in average temperatures across the globe between 1961–1990 and 2000 was calculated, and applied to the population distribution worldwide in 2000. Included as outcomes were heatwave deaths from cardiovascular causes, episodes of diarrhoea (in countries with gross domestic product (GDP) per capita less than US $6000), clinical cases of malaria and dengue, fatal injuries due to natural disasters, and the prevalence of malnutrition (Campbell-Lendrum et al. 2006). The findings are shown in Fig. 2.8.4, along with future impacts which will be discussed in the next section. Note that the direct effects (fatalities due to floods), and the impacts on vector-borne diseases, are much less than what is estimated to be the additional mortality and ill health attributable to climate-induced malnutrition.

This work rests on assumptions that are critical to the calculations and appear plausible but remain uncertain. The assumptions include: the effect of warming on disease and injury is independent of the original temperature; there are no interactions between the outcomes of climate change (e.g. malnutrition and incidence of diarrhoea); risk coefficients are valid (unconfounded) and precise, and can be generalized to all populations; climate sensitivity declines as countries become richer; and the extent of warming assigned to climate change is accurate.

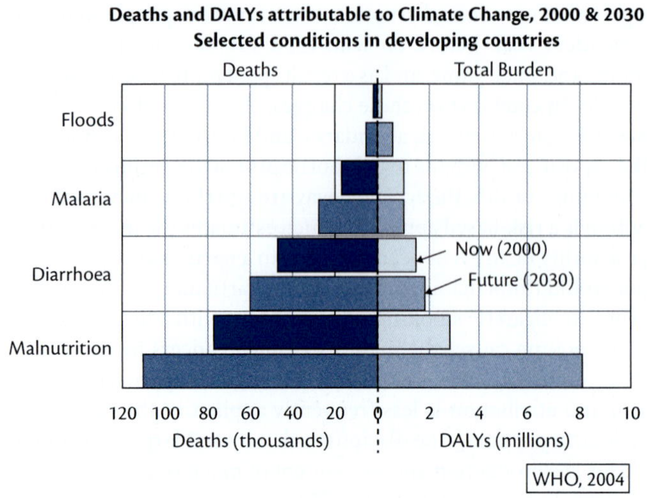

Fig. 2.8.4 The burden of disease attributable to climate change in 2000 and 2030. DALYs, disability-adjusted life years.
Source: data from World Health Organization, The Global Burden of Disease 2004 Update, World Health Organization, Geneva, Switzerland, Copyright © World Health Organization 2008.

Forecasting

We have demonstrated how difficult it is to attribute past and present morbidity and mortality to climate change, but future attribution presents even greater difficulties. There is no certainty about how much the climate will change in the future, or what the consequences will be, but it does seem clear that the most important risks lie ahead of us. Present-day effects of climate change on health may be miniature versions of future effects, or perhaps not: future challenges may be threshold-crossing novelties. For this reason, a great deal of effort has been applied to attempts to project future climates and the consequent impacts through modelling studies. One approach is to attempt to isolate the effect of an altered climate on specific diseases by holding all other independent variables constant. We will look at examples of this approach using several diseases known to be highly climate sensitive: diarrhoeal disease, malaria, schistosomiasis, and urinary stones. Since climate change acts as a multiplier of disadvantage, ideally studies would go further and ask: how are the 'baseline' risks likely to change in the short to medium term? This is a difficult undertaking but could, potentially, provide a more accurate description of future impacts of climate change on human health. Modelling studies that have taken this approach are less common and require methods less familiar to epidemiologists—methods that can deal with significant levels of complexity, non-linear interactions and feedback dynamically over time.

In addition to estimating the present burden of disease from climate change, the 2002 Global Burden of Disease project included estimates of deaths and disability-adjusted life years attributable to climate change in 2030 (Fig. 2.8.4). In the case of diarrhoeal disease, this was done by estimating average temperatures across the globe in 2030, at a very fine geographic scale, overlaid on an estimate of the world population distribution in 2030 (Campbell-Lendrum et al. 2006). It was assumed that the relation between temperature and incidence would not change, and that vulnerability to warming-related diarrhoeal disease would also

remain as it is currently. (Countries with a GDP per capita less than US $6000 were treated as susceptible: countries with higher levels of GDP were assumed to be unaffected.) It was assumed also that the effect of rising temperatures is independent of the starting temperature, and that there are no effects of changes in rainfall.

In a similar vein, a study of future impacts of climate change on the 'potential transmission' of malaria in Zimbabwe attempted to isolate the effects of climate between 2000 and 2050, by assuming there would be no other changes (Ebi et al. 2005). The suitability of the climate for stable transmission of *Plasmodium falciparum* malaria was related to mean temperatures, winter minimum temperatures, and monthly rainfall, based on outputs from the MARA (Mapping Malaria Risk in Africa) project. On this basis the researchers reported that within 50 years malaria could be established in the densely populated and presently malaria-free highlands of Zimbabwe. The model used in this study was risk based (suitability varied from 0 to 1), was explicitly projecting the potential for disease, rather than predictions of disease occurrence, and set aside the question of how other influences on malaria, apart from climate, might differ in 2050 from the present day.

In China, it has been observed that the snail that harbours the parasite responsible for schistosomiasis is restricted to areas in which the average January temperatures are above freezing, and on the basis of this, and other parameters, climate change models have been applied to estimate that an additional 8 per cent of the land area of the country may be suitable for transmission of the disease in 2030 (Zhou et al. 2008). No allowance was made in this study for future changes in land use, healthcare, housing conditions, or other factors that are known to affect susceptibility to schistosomiasis.

Finally, in a less common non-communicable disease example, a study in the United States modelled the current relation between mean annual temperature and hospital admissions for stones in the urinary tract in the United States. In general, nephrolithiasis is more common in populations living in warm climates, and this trend is apparent in the United States. The authors applied projections of mean annual temperatures in the future and calculated the potential increase in hospital admissions and associated costs (Brikowski et al. 2008). Since both linear and non-linear relationships between temperature and risk fitted the present data, both forms were modelled. Projections were based on one of the IPCC's intermediate severity climate change scenarios (SRES A1B). Fig. 2.8.5 shows the projected increase in risk by 2050, using the linear model to relate prevalence to temperature. The authors calculated that the increase attributed to climate amounts to approximately 2 million additional lifetime cases.

There has been much interest in projections for dengue fever, given the rapid spread of the disease in the last 50 years, and the lack of a vaccine or effective treatment (Degallier et al. 2009). Outbreaks of dengue fever have been related to monthly average vapour pressure. Assuming no change in population susceptibility, it is therefore possible to map the potential extension of dengue in a warmer and wetter world (Hales et al. 2002). However, the relation between climate and dengue transmission is complex (Russell et al. 2009). Increasing temperatures may reduce virus incubation, extend the transmission season, and increase vector feeding rates. But mosquito mortality also increases (especially if the humidity falls). Heatwaves may increase the risk of explosive outbreaks through increased mosquito breeding, but

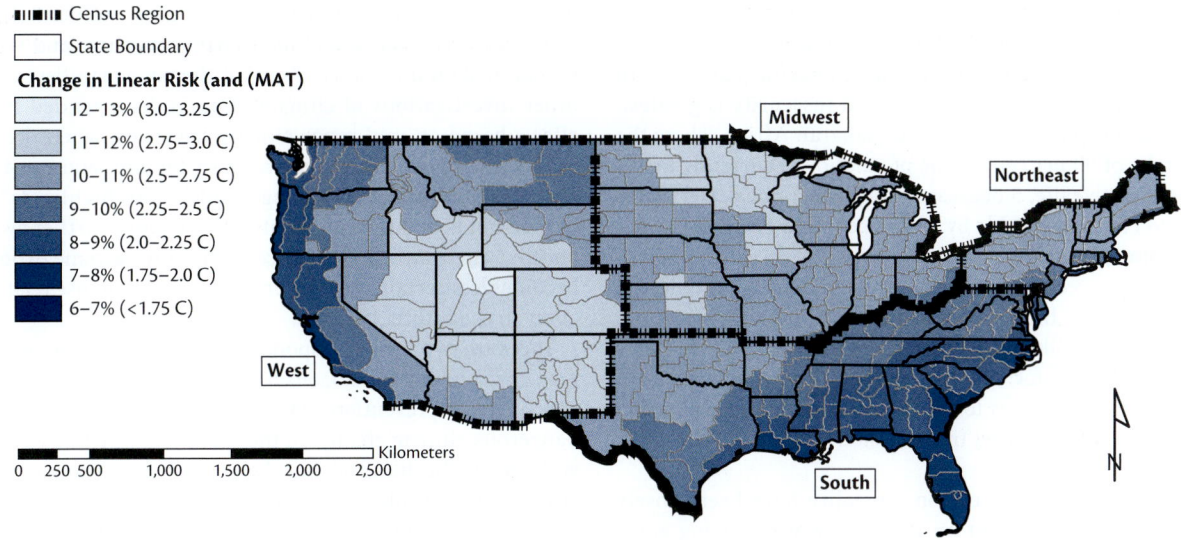

Fig. 2.8.5 Increase in mean annual temperature and risk of nephrolithiasis with the SRES A1B scenario, United States, 2050.
Reproduced with permission from Brikowski TH et al., Climate-related increase in the prevalence of urolithiasis in the United States, *Proceedings of the National Academy of* Sciences, Volume 105, Number 28, pp. 9841–6, Copyright © 2008 National Academy of Sciences, USA.

if populations have access to air conditioning, and spend more time indoors, there will be less exposure to the disease vector, and transmission of dengue may be inhibited. Droughts may reduce vector numbers if there are fewer free-standing and accessible bodies of water for mosquito breeding, but if instead there is widespread use of unscreened water storage, vector numbers will rise. A New Zealand study modelled future high-risk areas for dengue transmission by adding population growth, travel, and freight imports to changes in temperature and rainfall projections (De Wet et al. 2001). New Zealand is presently free of the disease and also does not host competent mosquito vectors. So projections included factors such as container traffic that might influence the risk of importing the most likely vector, *Aedes albopictus*.

Demographic projections are important, since climate change impacts will depend on the size, structure, and health status of world populations. The mid-range estimate is for the world population to increase from about 7 billion presently to around 9.5 billion by 2050, with most of the growth occurring in developing countries (Stephenson et al. 2010). The proportion of the population in older age groups is likely to increase, almost everywhere, although the average years of life remaining will change much less (Lutz et al. 2008). Mortality is projected to decline, in most countries, leading to increases in life expectancy at birth of around 5–6 years by the mid-century (World Health Organization 2011). Assuming that present trends of social and economic development continue, illness rates will also decline, and it has been estimated that the overall burden of disease (measured in disability-adjusted life years) will be reduced by about 30 per cent by 2030 (World Health Organization 2008). Child mortality is falling, worldwide, with no sign of a reduction in the rate of improvement (Rajaratnam et al. 2010). However, there are still very large differences between countries, and some countries, especially in sub-Saharan Africa, are improving slowly, if at all (World Health Organization 2011).

The emission scenarios adopted by the IPCC in its Third Assessment Report assumed that per capita incomes in developing countries would grow by about 4 per cent per year throughout the first half of this century, considerably more than the rate observed over the last 50 years. A similar bias is apparent in the World Health Organization's (WHO) projections, in which GDP growth continues in all countries, even the worst-case scenarios (Mathers and Loncar 2006). Whether social and economic development does continue on present trajectories is of course uncertain, but is fundamental to projections of climate change (because current patterns of economic growth increase greenhouse gas emissions) and vulnerability to its effects. In turn, uncertainty about the pace of social and economic development stems, in part, from the possible effects of climate change on societies and economies. Overall, one would say, the IPCC and WHO assumptions are optimistic.

Furthermore, health is sensitive to the manner in which economic growth occurs. If development is not inclusive, then vulnerability to the effects of climate change may not improve. India, for instance, has taken great strides, economically, in the last 20 years, but the health problems of poverty persist for many people. The prevalence of child underweight and stunting fell modestly between 1992 and 2005 (from 49 per cent to 40 per cent underweight, for instance), but there was no relation, at the state level, with income growth (Subramanyam et al. 2011). Child health measured in this way advanced no faster in the richest states than the poorest.

Finally, will there be positive effects of climate change, and if so, how will they balance the negative impacts? This is not a straightforward question to answer. It is likely there will be some positive effects in the short term, but it is difficult to judge their magnitude. For instance, it is likely that modest warming will boost agricultural yields in temperate parts of the world, increasing food production in these regions. Moreover, food crops such as wheat, rice, barley, and oats, tend to grow more quickly in higher levels of CO_2. Together, these effects may reduce the risk of food shortages and under-nutrition caused by lower production in hot, low-latitude countries (Gornall et al. 2010). The balance of gains and losses will depend on whether populations at risk of food shortages can in fact get access to the climate dividend, and the relief may be temporary: the increase in crop yields in temperate zones will almost certainly diminish as warming continues (Teixeira et al. 2011). In tropical developing countries, where food insecurity is greatest, the impact will be most severe. In sub-Saharan Africa, where the caloric intake of 60 per cent of the population is currently insufficient for an active life, 5 degrees of warming (global average) is projected to cut maize yields by 19 per cent and beans by 68 per cent (Thornton et al. 2010).

Where disease vectors and pathogens are already close to the upper temperature limit for reproduction and transmission, further warming is likely to reduce the risk of disease. In parts of equatorial Africa, for example, projected temperatures will exceed the optimal settings for both the vector and the parasite, and the potential for malaria transmission will rapidly diminish (Mordecai et al. 2012).

The effects of cold and heat on mortality have been closely studied, and shed some light on the matter of balancing gains and losses with global warming (Ebi and Mills 2013). The U- or J-shaped relation between ambient temperature and mortality suggests that warming will lead to fewer cold-related deaths, and greater heat-related mortality. But as noted already, it is unclear how many of the deaths that occur at colder times of the year are in fact due to low temperatures, rather than other phenomena that vary with season (such as infectious disease epidemics). Also, the U- or J-shaped curve is rarely symmetrical—in cooler locations, the right-hand arm of the curve (associated with heat) tends to rise more rapidly, and the opposite is true for populations living in relatively warm conditions. This means that if there is a trade-off of gains and losses with warming, the balance will depend on the initial conditions. But it is more complicated still—it is not clear whether cool-location populations will retain their (relatively greater) tolerance for cold as temperatures rise, or whether the shape of the temperature–mortality curve will change. Finally there is evidence that many populations in colder parts of the world, where the most affluent and best buffered populations in the world are located, have adapted to a large extent to cold, and the impacts of both cold spells and ambient low temperatures have much reduced over time. Consequently, the added benefits of global warming in these locations may be modest and are outweighed by the additional burden of heat-related ill health in the much larger and more vulnerable populations living in low latitudes (Kinney et al. 2012).

It is also necessary to consider the most important sources of uncertainty in projections of this kind. An analysis of the projections for diarrhoeal disease attempted to distinguish the effects of uncertainties in temperature changes and the exposure–response function (change in disease incidence per unit warming) (Kolstad and Johansson 2010). The focus in future-oriented studies tends to be on the climate modelling, given the many assumptions that have to be incorporated. However in this case it was evident that uncertainty associated with the risk coefficient (which varied almost fourfold between studies) caused more variation in the outcome than the choice of climate change model. Another study in the United States examined the effects of modelling choices on national mortality attributable to low-level ozone, in the presence of climate change (Post et al. 2012). Results varied from about 600 deaths per year avoided as a result of climate change to 2500 deaths attributable to climate change (although most models

projected increases in mortality). The most influential analytic steps were the choices of climate change scenario and air quality model. It should be noted also that the ozone studies, and many other investigations of climate impacts, have tended to project effects based on mid-range climate scenarios, when the globe is in fact tracking on a steeper trajectory for emissions, one that fits more closely with the high-range models. This highlights the issue of thresholds and tipping points—as we move further away from familiar environments and encounter more extreme exposures, it becomes less certain that present exposure–response relations will apply in the future.

There are two ways of responding to climate change: adapt to the new environment (analogous to secondary prevention), and mitigate (primary prevention—take whatever steps are needed to avoid dangerous climate change in the first place). Primary prevention is the public health ideal, but there are strong arguments for now also investing in adaptation: in particular, we are committed to the warming that will occur as a result of greenhouse gases already emitted, due to the long time-course of global carbon cycles and heat transfers. This is regardless of future emission trajectories.

Adaptation to expected climate change

The importance of adaptation is proportional to the momentum of climate change—when there are very long lag times in the climate system then interventions to reduce emissions will take a very long time to have their full effect, and in the meantime, steps must be taken to cope with changes that are, in effect, unavoidable. It has been estimated that warming of about 0.7 degrees C is already committed by the greenhouses gases that are now in the atmosphere. Also in the atmosphere are airborne particulates that have a cooling effect, and are tending to dampen down the global warming signal. It is difficult to determine the size of this effect, but it may be as much as 0.6 degrees C of warming will result when particulate levels fall (Stern 2007). Then there is the question of future emissions, and how rapidly these will be reduced. At present, global emissions are close to 50 Gt CO_2 equivalent per year, about 14 per cent higher than the level required to hold warming to around 2 degrees C, the amount of warming that has been adopted (controversially) in international negotiations as the threshold for 'dangerous climate change'. Moreover, total emissions continue to increase by about 2 per cent per annum (United Nations Environment Programme 2012). If emissions peaked in 2025, which would seem a relatively optimistic scenario, and then reduced by 3 per cent per year, global average surface temperatures would rise by as much as 4 degrees C by the end of this century (Parry et al. 2009). We have already discussed the way extremes of temperature are hidden within such average rises.

Given current forces driving emissions upwards, it is becoming less and less likely the world can keep to the 2-degree C target. These drivers include the population pressures identified earlier (a 50 per cent increase projected worldwide in the next 50 years) and economic development 'catch up': 90 per cent of the growth in emissions this century will come from states that are presently in the low- and middle-income categories. Perhaps most importantly, there continues to be a lack of leadership from the governments of most high-income countries which are responsible for 90 per cent of the emissions currently in the atmosphere.

The already locked-in climate change and the risk of mitigation failure are both compelling reasons to find options for coping with climate change impacts, particularly adaptation to increasing average and extreme temperatures, as well as resilience to storms, flooding, sea level rise, and disruption to agricultural production and distribution. Here we will examine some of the opportunities for adaptation, ranging from individual behaviours to neighbourhood interventions, to sector-wide changes. Some of the available options for adapting to climate change can also assist with climate change mitigation, or have other co-benefits for health and equity, while others may hamper efforts in these areas. We cover some examples relating to heat and storm events.

At an individual level, improving the body's physiological response to temperature extremes can assist with adaptation. Increasing physical activity and reducing obesity both have many benefits to health, including enhanced capacity to deal with heat. Clinical trials have shown that short-term endurance training increases sweat rate and peripheral blood flow and leads to more effective control of body temperature during exercise (Ichinoseet al. 2009). Overweight military recruits in the United States were found to be seven times more likely to suffer heat illnesses during training than their colleagues (Bedno et al. 2010). Work of this kind indicates that public health programmes to promote physical activity, prevent unhealthy weight gain, and reduce the prevalence of obesity are likely to reduce vulnerability to heat.

Community-oriented interventions have promise, since risk factors for heat-attributable deaths tend to cluster spatially. For instance, a study in Chicago found that poverty, social isolation, lack of access to air conditioning, age, and the prevalence of diabetes were concentrated in a relatively small number of neighbourhoods (Reid et al. 2009).

Although air conditioning is an important measure for coping with high temperatures (Ostro et al. 2010), it brings vulnerability, as well as consuming large amounts of (potentially carbon-generating) electricity, and transferring heat outdoors. Artificial cooling relies on a consistent power supply, and heatwaves may trigger electricity outages due to overload (largely driven by the demands of air conditioning plants) (Anderson and Bell 2011). In these circumstances, populations accustomed to living with air conditioning may be at increased risk of ill health due to high temperatures. Cities that are built for air conditioning are often poorly designed in other ways to deal with heat (with large, exposed surfaces of glass, and minimal natural shade, for instance). Also, physiological adaptation requires some exposure to heat strain, that is, an increase in body temperature (Maloney and Forbes 2010). Populations with around-the-clock access to air conditioning are effectively isolated from heat, and therefore are less likely to develop the capacity to respond to extreme temperatures, when and if this occurs.

Cities are significantly warmer than their surrounding rural areas (the urban heat island effect) due to darkly paved surfaces and dense anthropogenic heat generation (for example, from vehicles and buildings). City-level interventions to reduce the health risks due to high temperatures will therefore be important. Designing cities to reduce the heat-island effect can also make them safer during times of high temperature. A study in Phoenix, Arizona estimated the reduction that could be made in heat-related emergency calls by an urban re-design package (Silva et al. 2010). This included changes in building and road materials to increase heat flows, more urban green spaces, rooftop treatments, and widespread application of reflective paints. In combination, the authors estimate, these interventions could reduce inner-city temperatures sufficiently to almost halve the number of annual heat-related emergency calls. Measures at a city-level to manage high temperatures when they do occur include heat-health early warning systems, better cooling of at-risk environments (such as residential care facilities for the elderly), identifying the isolated and most vulnerable citizens, and improving the preparedness of the healthcare sector.

The contrast between more aggressive air conditioning and greater provision of green space in cities is an example of how 'business as usual' approaches can miss important opportunities (Hess 2012). On the one hand, enhancing air conditioning of all health facilities helps to protect some of the most vulnerable individuals from high temperatures, though it carries a heavy cost in power consumption. On the other hand, a radical expansion in urban green spaces may bring a range of benefits (in addition to cooling), including carbon sequestration and health benefits due to reduced air pollution, better mental health, and more opportunities for physical activity (Groenewegen et al. 2006). But these 'win win' interventions are seldom straightforward: green spaces on their own may not be sufficient to achieve health gains. A study of the 49 largest cities in the United States (Richardson et al. 2011) compared the extent of green space with all-cause mortality, adjusting for important social and demographic differences, but not for measures of urban density. The result, against expectations, was that health appeared to be worse in greener cities. The explanation is that other elements of urban renovation are critical, in combination with greening. Transport policy and land use regulation are particularly important. Otherwise, at least in the US context, the undesirable effects of urban sprawl predominate.

In France, many changes to heatwave responsiveness were made following the severe heatwave in 2003. These included public education, better emergency preparedness, and healthcare improvements. When another heatwave occurred in July 2006, the question asked was: did the country cope better this time than it did in 2003? In July 2003, the increase in daily temperatures was theoretically sufficient to increase daily mortality by about 230 per cent, according to the long-run (1975–1999) relation between temperatures and daily deaths (Fouillet et al. 2008). But a 290 per cent increase was observed, an excess of more than 15,000 deaths. In 2006, the heatwave temperatures were not as high as 3 years earlier, and it was theoretically projected to raise mortality by about 60 per cent. In fact the death rate increased by only 14 per cent (2065 excess deaths observed of about 6400 predicted). One possible explanation is that the 2003 disaster brought forward so many deaths in relatively frail individuals that the pool of susceptibles was much reduced in 2006. However, the mortality trends indicate the 4600 fewer-than-expected deaths in July 2006 were indeed evidence of effective adaptation.

Another important area for adaptation is in preparedness and resilience to severe storms and flooding. Most climate change models project an increase in the intensity of tropical storms, though it is less clear whether the frequency of storms will change. These extreme events already cause substantial loss of life and economic damage. For example, in Burma in 2008, Cyclone Nargis caused approximately 138,000 deaths and US $10 billion damage (Fritz et al. 2009); in the United States, Hurricane Katrina in 2005 was responsible for about a thousand deaths (Brunkard et al. 2008) and direct losses of over US $130 billion (Field and Barros 2012). But there are also examples of countries managing the health risks of storms and cyclones. In Cuba, for example, between 1998 and 2002 the island was struck by four destructive hurricanes (category 2 or greater). Tens of thousands of homes were damaged, and hundreds of thousands of people were evacuated, but there were very few deaths (12 in all) (Thompson and Gaviria 2004).

Cuba invests heavily in traditional civil defence activities, including stockpiles of equipment, clothing, fuel, and food. There are effective storm warning systems, and good means of communicating information to the public. Other factors that contribute to resilience are high levels of literacy, provision of basic facilities in all rural areas, and a comprehensive and accessible primary healthcare system. An Oxfam analysis of disaster preparedness in Cuba found there was strong community engagement, so that populations that are threatened can be mobilized rapidly, and protection extends to all social groups, not just those with personal resources (Thompson and Gaviria 2006). In contrast, the large number of deaths associated with Hurricane Katrina was a result of serious deficiencies in the public health system, and lack of protection for the poorest and most marginalized social groups in the city (Brunkard et al. 2008).

There are other opportunities to learn from the variability in past experience of coping with climate-related health problems. For instance, enteric infections such as that caused by *Salmonella* tend to be more common at higher temperatures, but the size of the increase in disease rates for a given amount of warming varies from one site to another. A study of the five largest Australian cities found that all showed an increase in *Salmonella* notifications with monthly mean temperature, but one city stood out as following a much steeper trajectory than the others (D'Souza et al. 2004). Perhaps aspects of the food safety programmes present elsewhere are missing in this apparently particularly temperature-sensitive city.

There is no doubt that climate change acts principally as a risk multiplier. The greatest impact will occur in populations that, for other reasons, already have the worst health statistics. The World Bank, in its 2010 World Development Report concluded that 'baseline health status is the single most important determinant of both future losses, and the cost of adaptation' (World Bank 2009). It follows that adaptation must include improvements in the social determinants of health, as well as essential public health services. But is it true that this is all that is needed? In other words, is business as usual development, the package of improvements that we would want to be making anyway, sufficient preparation for climate change?

We argue that business as usual development will not be sufficient. Climate change is a special problem, and requires special responses, in addition to improvements in baseline health. To begin with, climate change is unique because of the scale on which it operates. This is a global phenomenon, and adaptation has to take account of distant as well as local effects. There is a time dimension also. Climate change accumulates and progresses, with such long lag times (apparent, for instance, in projected sea level rise) that the process must be regarded as irreversible, to a large extent. The force of change must be noted. This is not a one-off event, but a new environmental dynamic, with enormous momentum. We

are likely to be pushed to the edge of what is familiar, and beyond, leading potentially to abrupt and radical changes in Earth systems (McNeall et al. 2011). In epidemiological terms, even if the trends in exposures (rising temperatures, changing patterns of precipitation) remain the same, it may be difficult to anticipate the dose–response relationships that apply in the future, due to unforeseen tipping points, thresholds, and non-linearities. The much greater than expected impact of the 2003 European heatwave is one example of non-linear effects; another is the damage caused by unprecedentedly intense bushfires in Victoria, Australia in 2009 (Teague et al. 2010).

Climate change does not *only* multiply existing risks. It may contribute to new risks where ecosystems are pressed beyond significant thresholds. This may happen on the edges of areas affected by climate-sensitive diseases. One example is the acute illness that occurs after eating sea-foods contaminated with *Vibrio parahemolyticus*. The organism is temperature sensitive, and until 2004 no instances of this particular food poisoning had been reported in North America above the US/Canada border. In that year there was an outbreak of cases on a cruise ship in Alaska, linked to shell-fish from a local oyster farm in Prince William Sound. On investigation, it was found that water temperatures at the farm (and the surrounding ocean) had been rising steadily for a decade, and presumably had crossed a critical boundary beyond which the organism could be sustained in local shell-fish (McLaughlin et al. 2005).

In summary, given the extent of committed warming, and the difficulty of achieving substantial reductions in emissions, the world almost certainly faces large changes in the next century. Improving baseline health status is fundamental to adaptation, but not sufficient—there are distinctive features of climate change that have to be taken into account.

Mitigation: scale, possible co-benefits, and unintended harms

There is debate about how far greenhouse gas levels in the atmosphere must fall to avoid dangerous climate change, but it is absolutely clear that big changes will be required to lower risks to a level that most governments believe is acceptable. In the past, energy revolutions have been disruptive. They have caused serious environmental damage, increased social inequalities, and shortened life expectancy. Are there paths to a low-carbon future that can achieve the opposite result—simultaneous improvements in the quality of the environment and public health? We will review the evidence for common solutions and discuss ways in which 'co-benefits' might influence policy settings for climate change.

In 2009 the World Bank reported that if the increase in emissions that has been seen in the first decade of this century continues unchecked, annual emissions of CO_2 in 2050 will be around 62 Gt, more than twice the present levels (and not counting other greenhouse gases) (World Bank 2009). If warming by the end of the century is to be contained to around 2 degrees C, then CO_2 emissions must be reduced to around 14 Gt per year in 2050, less than a quarter of business as usual projections. The later the world turns the corner on emissions, the steeper the subsequent decline will need to be. If CO_2 emissions peak in 2020, and it is assumed that climate safety amounts to a global cap of 750 Gt of carbon released between 2000 and 2050, then CO_2 emissions will need to fall by about 9 per cent per year, a radical change in the shape of trends—from accelerating growth to steep decline (Anderson and Bows 2008). This is a tall order, and if reductions of this order of magnitude are going to be achieved, there will need to be radical changes in the way humans use energy. It will require deeper social changes than merely identifying and bringing forward renewable technologies—over the last 50 years each added unit of energy from wind, hydro, and other renewables has displaced only a quarter of a unit of energy from fossil fuel sources and has had an even smaller impact on electricity generation (York 2012). In order to meet greenhouse targets, there will need to be serious deterrents to fossil fuel use, including prices that reflect the full environmental cost.

The 2010 World Development Report talked about changes that are so large they constitute 'an energy revolution'. Revolutions may re-orient society in a way that is beneficial, in the long run, but they tend to be disruptive and harmful, in the short term. The last energy revolution began in England in the nineteenth century and ushered in what has been in many respects a golden age of industrialization. But England, and every other country that went through the process, also experienced the 'four Ds'—disruption, deprivation, disease, and death (Szreter 2004). In the large English cities in the 1840s, crowding, pollution, and social upheaval affected everyone, but particularly those at the bottom of the social hierarchy. For instance, life expectancy at birth fell to medieval levels, less than 30 years among the working classes (Szreter and Mooney 1998).

The challenge with climate change mitigation will be to disrupt present patterns of energy use, while avoiding the very high and inequitable social and health costs that were carried by nineteenth-century cities like Birmingham and Manchester. Early experience with alternative energy sources has not been altogether reassuring. One stark example is the encouragement of biofuels. There have been large-scale moves to use food crops for bioethanol and biodiesel, often with substantial government subsidies. (In 2009 about a quarter of all US corn was diverted to biofuel production as a result of federal intervention.) This has reduced the demand for petroleum products, but has increased competition for food staples such as soybeans, maize, and cereals—according to one analysis, increasing biofuel demand accounted for about 30 per cent of the increase in world grain prices between 2000 and 2007 (Rosegrant 2008). It remains to be seen whether second-generation biofuels, extracted from non-edible plants such as jatropha that are grown on marginal lands and don't compete directly with food production, will bring the same energy benefits without the health risks.

It is possible to identify a low-risk climate path that can enhance rather than worsen health and equity. One easy example is provided by the link between short-lived climate pollutants and air quality. Emissions of black carbon particles, the precursors of low-level ozone, and methane, all of which have stronger heat-trapping properties than CO_2 on a weight-for-weight basis, have local toxic effects, and pass through the atmosphere relatively quickly. Black carbon or soot is the second most important greenhouse forcing agent, after CO_2. It acts by absorbing sunlight and darkening ice and snow, and remains in the atmosphere for about 7–10 days, on average (Kerr 2013). Typically black carbon is emitted as part of a complex mixture, including other particles that tend to be cooling (as a result of reflecting sunlight). The ratio

of black carbon to other organic material (and hence the warming potential) varies depending on the source (tending to be high in diesel fumes and smoke from cook stoves; low with forest fires).

The United Nations Environment Programme estimated what could be achieved by widespread application of measures that are proven to reduce black carbon and methane (United Nations Environment Programme 2011). These measures include particle filters for disease engines, clean burning biomass cook stoves, and bans on the open field burning of agricultural waste. Assuming full implementation by 2030, the effects compared with 'business as usual' emissions amounted to saving 0.5 degrees C of warming in 2050, while the reduction in local pollution would save about 50 million tons per year of lost crop yields, and avoid about 2.5 million premature deaths worldwide.

Transport and housing are two sectors where health co-benefits can be achieved, but there might also be adverse consequences for health if interventions are not carefully thought through. One example is the health and energy efficiency benefits of home insulation and efficient heating. In New Zealand, although the climate is moderate, many homes are relatively cold and damp owing to a lack of insulation, ineffective heating, and poor building design. A randomized community trial tested the effect of home insulation on indoor temperatures, energy consumption, and respiratory health (Howden-Chapman et al. 2007). Insulated homes were found to be warmer, drier, used 20 per cent less electricity than the control homes, and children in them were sick less frequently (Table 2.8.1). The findings led subsequently to a national roll-out of insulation subsidies and installation.

However, alterations to improve energy efficiency may increase health risks. For example, there is a balance in houses between airtightness and ventilation that provides for efficient warming while allowing for adequate air flow to reduce indoor air pollution, and prevent moisture from reaching levels conducive to mould growth (Davies and Oreszczyn 2011).

In many countries, emissions from the transport sector are growing more rapidly than those from any other sector. Yet there are many opportunities in transport policy to simultaneously cut carbon and improve health. This is particularly so in cities that are currently highly car-dependent. For example, in New Zealand about 80 per cent of travel is by private car, and yet many vehicle trips, in

Table 2.8.1 Outcomes of a randomized trial of insulation in 1350 New Zealand households. All households included one or more children with asthma

	Outcome
Average bedroom temperature in winter	Warmer by 0.5 degrees
Relative humidity in bedroom	Reduced by 2.3%
Energy consumption	81% of controls
Self-reported wheeze	OR 0.57 (0.47–0.70)
Days off school	OR 0.49 (0.31–0.80)
Visits to general practitioner	OR 0.73 (0.52–0.87)

OR, odds ratio.

Source: data from Howden-Chapman P et al., Effect of insulating existing houses on health inequality: cluster randomised study in the community, *British Medical Journal*, Volume 3, Issue 334, pp. 460, Copyright © 2007, DOI: 10.1136/bmj.39070.573032.80.

the city, cover very short distances. In the New Zealand Household Travel Survey 2003–2006, it was reported that about three-quarters of car trips in urban areas were 7 km or less, and almost a third (31 per cent) were 2 km or less (Lindsay et al. 2011). Shifting 5 per cent of those short trips (7 km or less) from cars to bicycles would, it was estimated, save 22 million litres of fuel per year, avoid six deaths a year from air pollution, and as a result of promoting physical activity, postpone a further 116 deaths a year from chronic diseases such as stroke, diabetes, and heart disease (Lindsay et al. 2011). If no changes were made to the road system, the additional cycle traffic might lead to an extra five deaths from crash injuries, but overall, it was estimated that the health benefits of a 5 per cent mode shift would outweigh the costs of injury by more than ten to one.

A similar modelling exercise was undertaken in Delhi, India, comparing the health effects of different mitigation strategies (Woodcock et al. 2009). The city has set targets for greenhouse gas emission reduction, and this could be achieved by increasing the numbers of low-carbon vehicles, encouraging more active transport (walking and cycling), or a combination. The low-carbon vehicle option would avoid premature deaths and illness, mainly as a result of reduced air pollution in the city, but it was estimated these co-benefits were roughly ten times less than what could be achieved by the 'active transport' or 'combined' strategies.

In summary, global greenhouse gas emissions need to be reduced by about 60 per cent by 2050 to provide a reasonable chance of holding warming by the end of the century to 2 degrees C or less. Radical mitigation of this kind might be seriously health damaging. But there are opportunities for co-benefits: well-chosen interventions could produce health gains (early), as well as long-term climate security. See Box 2.8.4.

Box 2.8.4 Answers to the carbon IQ quiz

1. Without greenhouse gases, the temperature at the Earth's surface would be below freezing (about −15 degrees C). The global average is instead about +15 degrees C. The answer is A.

2. Climate is long-range weather, over a timescale of decades. The British Meteorological Office, for example, uses 30 years as the averaging period, though in some recent assessments 20 years of weather has been considered long enough to define a climate. The answer is C.

3. C is closest to the mark: today's choices about the level of emissions will have long-term consequences (Stouffer 2012). AR4 says 'about 50 per cent of a CO_2 increase will be removed from the atmosphere within 30 years, and a further 30 per cent will be removed within a few centuries. The remaining 20 per cent may stay in the atmosphere for many thousands of years' (Solomon et al. 2007). There are many caveats, because the various processes that soak up carbon work at different speeds, and on a large scale, the lifetime of CO_2 depends on the amount emitted, and the rate of emission. But as a rough guide, about 40 per cent is likely to be still in the atmosphere after 100 years, and just over 20 per cent after 1000 years.

4. Combustion of biomass releases a complex soup of pollutants, and reactions in the atmosphere generate 'secondary' agents such as ozone and other photochemical oxidants. The effects on climate are complex. Black carbon absorbs heat; sulphur aerosols have a reflective (cooling) effect. Because these agents are short-lived (remaining in the atmosphere for days or weeks), the impact is local/regional. Deposition of soot on ice causes increased absorption of solar energy, and accelerated melt. The answer is E.

5. The oceans absorb 80–90 per cent of the solar energy that is trapped by greenhouse gases. Additional amounts of heat go toward melting glaciers and sea ice, as well as warming the land and parts of the atmosphere. Only a tiny fraction warms the air at the planet's surface.

6. According to the British Meteorological Office, 1998 still holds the record, and 2010 was the second warmest. In the United States, NASA report that 2010 was equal warmest (tied with 2005): the answer varies a little depending on which weather stations are included. Some have argued that the answer is 1260 (the period of the medieval warming)—this is definitely not true (NASA n.d.).

7. Laos emits about 0.2 tons CO_2 per head (Carbon Dioxide Information Analysis Center n.d.). A 747 jet emits about 100 g of CO_2 per passenger kilometre (Carbon Independent n.d.). Singapore to Rome return is roughly 10,000 km, which amounts to about 1 ton CO_2 per passenger, based solely on the fuel consumed during the flight. Note that this does not allow for the greater warming effect of CO_2 released high in the atmosphere, nor the embedded fossil fuel costs of aviation, which include those incurred in building jets, running airports and training staff. But on this basis the solution is 0.2 and the best answer is D.

8. A cyclist would travel 570 km on a litre of comparably energy dense food, which is 0.2 L/100 km (Wilson 2004). But this refers to a racing cyclist moving at 30 kph. Note that wind resistance falls away rapidly as speed drops—less than half the energy would be required for travel at an average of 20 kph (which means no more than 100 mL of oil-equivalent per 100 km).

9. George H.W. Bush, made this commitment at the Rio Summit in 1992, after signing the UN Framework Convention on Climate Change. In the subsequent 20 years Republican leaders have shifted their ground, and increasingly they have denied that climate change is a serious threat (Oreskes and Conway 2010).

10. There were about a thousand deaths caused by Katrina: there were typically four or five deaths in Cuba from hurricanes of similar severity (categories 2–4) between 1998 and 2002 (Thompson and Gaviria 2004). On the whole, wealthy countries are less seriously affected by climate extremes, but this is not always the case, which points to some lessons, possibly, for adaptation to climate change.

Conclusion

Climate change is a new kind of environmental problem—the scale of the phenomenon dwarfs the issues that public health workers have encountered previously. Its effects on health will result, mainly, from exacerbating disease and injury from familiar causes. Understanding how multiple variables will interact in the future to diminish or magnify the effects of climate change on health requires methods not currently familiar in public health. Complex models are needed that can incorporate non-linear interactions, feedbacks and tipping points dynamically over time.

Climate change is undoubtedly an issue of health and social equity—those at greatest risk already carry a heavy load of disadvantage, and have contributed little to the CO_2 that now sits in the atmosphere. This means that many of the impacts can be avoided, or reduced in magnitude, by providing basic health improvements to the world's poor populations.

Targeted adaptation efforts, such as early warning systems and good disaster management, are necessary also: there is plenty of evidence that high-income countries are not immune from the effects on health of climate variability. But the world is not making rapid progress on either poverty reduction or targeted adaptation, so we expect the public health dimensions of climate change to become more prominent in the next few decades. In the medium to longer term (2050 and beyond), unless there are radical reductions in emissions beforehand, it is possible the average temperature of the globe will rise by more than 4 degrees C over the pre-industrial baseline. If this happens, impacts of climate change may overwhelm all efforts at adaptation. For this reason, the response to climate change must be two-pronged—coping with adverse effects of rising temperatures and changing patterns of rainfall, and at the same time, finding ways of slashing emissions and reducing levels of climate active pollutants in the atmosphere. On the positive side, well-chosen adaptation and mitigation measures may achieve substantial health gains. Strengthening the place of public health in multidisciplinary decision-making about climate change can assist with identifying low-risk climate paths that enhance rather than worsen health and equity.

References

4 degrees & beyond (2009). *Implications of a Global Climate Change of 4+ Degrees for People, Ecosystems and the Earth-System.* Abstract book. International Climate Conference, 28–30 September 2009, Oxford, UK.

Anderson, G. and Bell, M. (2011). Heat waves in the United States: mortality risk during heat waves and effect modification by heat wave characteristics in 43 US communities. *Environmental Health Perspectives,* 119(2), 210–18.

Anderson, K. and Bows, A. (2008). Reframing the climate change challenge in light of post-2000 emission trends. *Philosophical Transactions. Series A, Mathematical, Physical, and Engineering Sciences,* 366, 3863–82.

Armstrong, B.G., Chalabi, Z., Fenn, B., et al. (2011). Association of mortality with high temperatures in a temperate climate: England and Wales. *Journal of Epidemiology and Community Health,* 65(4), 340–5.

Arndt, D., Baringer, M.O., and Johnson, M.R. (2010). State of the climate in 2009. *Bulletin of the American Meteorological Society,* 91(6), S1–224.

Australian Academy of Sciences (2010). *The Science of Climate Change. Questions and Answers.* Canberra: Australian Academy of Sciences.

Barriopedro, D., Fischer, E.M., Luterbacher, J., Trigo, R.M., and García-Herrera, R. (2011). The hot summer of 2010: redrawing the temperature record map of Europe. *Science,* 332, 220–4.

Bedno, S.A., Li, Y., Han, W., et al. (2010). Exertional heat illness among overweight U.S. army recruits in basic training. *Aviation, Space, and Environmental Medicine,* 81(2), 107–11.

Bell, M.L., O'Neill, M.S., Ranjit, N., Borja-Aburto, V.H., Cifuentes, L.A., and Gouveia, N.C. (2008). Vulnerability to heat-related mortality in Latin America: a case-crossover study in Sao Paulo, Brazil, Santiago, Chile and Mexico City, Mexico. *International Journal of Epidemiology,* 37(4), 796–804.

Brikowski, T.H., Lotan, Y., and Pearle, M.S. (2008). Climate-related increase in the prevalence of urolithiasis in the United States. *Proceedings of the National Academy of Sciences of the United States of America,* 105(28), 9841–6.

Brunkard, J., Namulanda, G., and Ratard, R. (2008). Hurricane Katrina deaths, Louisiana, 2005. *Disaster Medicine and Public Health Preparedness,* 2(4), 215–23.

Campbell-Lendrum, D. and Woodruff, R. (2006). Comparative risk assessment of the burden of disease from climate change. *Environmental Health Sciences,* 114(12), 1935–41.

Carbon Dioxide Information Analysis Center (n.d.). *Ranking of the World's Countries by 2008 Per Capita Fossil-Fuel CO_2 Emission Rates.* [Online] Available at: http://cdiac.ornl.gov/trends/emis/top2008.cap.

Carbon Independent (n.d.). *Aviation Sources.* [Online] Available at: http://www.carbonindependent.org/sources_aviation.htm.

Davies, M. and Oreszczyn, T. (2011). The unintended consequences of decarbonising the built environment: a UK case study. *Energy and Buildings,* 46, 80–5.

Degallier, N., Favier, C., Menkes, C., et al. (2009). Toward an early warning system for dengue prevention: modeling climate impact on dengue transmission. *Climatic Change,* 98(3–4), 581–92.

De Wet, N., Ye, W., Hales, S., Warrick, R., Woodward, A., and Weinstein, P. (2001). Use of a computer model to identify potential hotspots for dengue fever in New Zealand. *The New Zealand Medical Journal,* 114(1140), 420–2.

D'Souza, R.M., Becker, N.G., Hall, G., and Moodie, K.B.A. (2004). Does ambient temperature affect foodborne disease? *Epidemiology,* 15(1), 86–92.

Duchene, E. and Schneider, C. (2005). Grapevine and climatic changes: a glance at the situation in Alsace. *Agronomy for Sustainable Development,* 25(1), 93–9.

Ebi, K.L., Hartman, J., Chan, N., McConnell, J., Schlesinger, M., Weyant, J. (2005). Climate suitability for stable malaria transmission in Zimbabwe under different climate change scenarios. *Climatic Change,* 73(3), 375–93.

Ebi, K.L. and Mills, D. (2013). Winter mortality in a warming world: a re-assessment. *WIREs Climate Change,* 4, 203–12.

Field, C. and Barros, V. (eds.) (2012). *Managing the Risks of Extreme Events and Disasters to Advance Climate Change Adaptation.* New York: Cambridge University Press.

Fouillet, A., Rey, G., Wagner, V., et al. (2008). Has the impact of heat waves on mortality changed in France since the European heat wave of summer 2003? A study of the 2006 heat wave. *International Journal of Epidemiology,* 37(2), 309–17.

Fritz, H.M., Blount, C.D., Thwin, S., Thu, M.K., and Chan, N. (2009). Cyclone Nargis storm surge in Myanmar. *Nature Geoscience,* 2(7), 448–9.

Gething, P.W., Smith, D.L., Patil, A.P., Tatem, A.J., Snow, R.W., and Hay, S.I. (2010). Climate change and the global malaria recession. *Nature,* 465, 342–5.

Goldstein, M.R., Mascitelli, L., and Grant, W.B. (2011). Might vitamin D explain the seasonal variation of cardiovascular disease in Tromso? *European Journal of Cardiovascular Prevention & Rehabilitation,* 18(4), 678–9.

Gornall, J., Betts, R., Burke, E., et al. (2010). Implications of climate change for agricultural productivity in the early twenty-first century. *Philosophical Transactions of the Royal Society of London. Series B, Biological Sciences,* 365(1554), 2973–89.

Groenewegen, P.P., van den Berg, A.E., de Vries, S., and Verheij, R.A. (2006). Vitamin G: effects of green space on health, well-being, and social safety. *BMC Public Health*, 6, 149.

Hales, S., de Wet, N., Maindonald, J., and Woodward, A. (2002). Potential effect of population and climate changes on global distribution of dengue fever: an empirical model. *The Lancet*, 360(9336), 830–4.

Hales, S., Weinstein, P., and Woodward, A. (1996). Dengue fever epidemics in the South Pacific: driven by El Nino Southern Oscillation? *The Lancet*, 348, 1664–5.

Hess, J.J. (2012). Integrating climate change adaptation into public health practice: using adaptive management to increase adaptive capacity and build resilience. *Environmental Health Sciences*, 120(2), 171–9.

Howden-Chapman, P., Matheson, A., Crane, J., et al. (2007). Effect of insulating existing houses on health inequality: cluster randomised study in the community. *British Medical Journal*, 334, 460.

Huang, C., Barnett, A.G., Wang, X., and Tong, S. (2012). The impact of temperature on years of life lost in Brisbane, Australia. *Nature Climate Change*, 2(4), 265–70.

Ichinose, T.K., Inoue, Y., Hirata, M., Shamsuddin, A.K.M., and Kondo, N. (2009). Enhanced heat loss responses induced by short-term endurance training in exercising women. *Experimental Physiology*, 94, 90–102.

Kerr, R. (2013). Soot is warming the world even more than thought. *Science*, 339, 382.

Kinney, P.L., Pascal, M., Vautard, R., and Laaidi, K. (2012). La mortalité hivernale va-t-elle diminuer avec le changement climatique? [Winter mortality in a changing climate: will it go down?]. *Bulletin Epidémiologique Hebdomadaire*, 12–13, 149–51.

Kjellstrom, T., Lemke, B., and Otto, M. (2013). Mapping occupational heat exposure and effects in South-East Asia: ongoing time trends 1980–2011 and future estimates to 2050. *Industrial Health*, 51, 56–67.

Klinenberg, E. (2003). *Heat Wave: A Social Autopsy of Disaster in Chicago.* Chicago, IL: University of Chicago Press.

Kolstad, E.W. and Johansson K.A. (2010). Uncertainties associated with quantifying climate change impacts on human health: a case study for diarrhea. *Environmental Health Sciences*, 119(3), 299–305.

Lindgren, E. (2001). Tick-borne encephalitis in Sweden and climate change. *The Lancet*, 358, 16–18.

Lindsay, G., Macmillan, A., and Woodward, A. (2011). Moving urban trips from cars to bicycles: impact on health and emissions. *Australian and New Zealand Journal of Public Health*, 35(1), 54–60.

Liu, J., Curry, J.A., Wang, H., Song, M., and Horton, R.M. (2012). Impact of declining Arctic sea ice on winter snowfall. *Proceedings of the National Academy of Sciences of the United States of America*, 109(11), 4074–9.

Lutz, W., Sanderson, W., and Scherbov, S. (2008). The coming acceleration of global population ageing. *Nature*, 451, 716–19.

Maloney, S.K. and Forbes, C.F. (2010). What effect will a few degrees of climate change have on human heat balance? Implications for human activity. *International Journal of Biometeorology*, 55(2), 147–60.

Manson, P. (1900). *Tropical Diseases. A Manual of the Diseases of Warm Climates.* London: Cassell.

Mathers, C. and Loncar, D. (2006). Projections of global mortality and burden of disease from 2002 to 2030. *PLoS Medicine*, 3(11), e442.

McLaughlin, J., DePaola, A., Bopp, C., et al. (2005). Outbreak of Vibrio parahaemolyticus gastroenteritis associated with Alaskan oysters. *The New England Journal of Medicine*, 353(14), 1463–70.

McMichael, A. (1999). Prisoners of the proximate: loosening the constraints on epidemiology in an age of change. *American Journal of Epidemiology*, 149(10), 887–97.

McMichael, A.J., Wilkinson, P., Kovats, R.S., et al. (2008). International study of temperature, heat and urban mortality: the 'ISOTHURM' project. *International Journal of Epidemiology*, 37(5), 1121–31.

McMichael, C., Barnett, J., and McMichael, A.J. (2012). An ill wind? Climate change, migration, and health. *Environmental Health Sciences*, 120(5), 646–54.

McNeall, D., Halloran, P.R., and Good, P. (2011). Analyzing abrupt and nonlinear climate changes and their impacts. *WIREs Climate Change*, 2, 663–86.

Meehl, G.A., Tebaldi, C., Walton, G., Easterling, D., and McDaniel, L. (2009). Relative increase of record high maximum temperatures compared to record low minimum temperatures in the U.S. *Geophysical Research Letters*, 36(23), L23701.

Mordecai, E.A., Paaijmans, K.P., Johnson, L.R., et al. (2012). Optimal temperature for malaria transmission is dramatically lower than previously predicted. *Ecology Letters*, 16(1), 22–30.

NASA (n.d.). *Piecing Together the Temperature Puzzle.* [Online] Available at: http://climate.nasa.gov/warming_world.

Oreskes, N. and Conway, E.M. (2010). *Merchants of Doubt.* New York: Bloomsbury Press.

Ostro, B., Rauch, S., Green, R., Malig, B., and Basu, R. (2010). The effects of temperature and use of air conditioning on hospitalizations. *American Journal of Epidemiology*, 172(9), 1053–61.

Parmesan, C., Duarte, C., Poloczanska, E., Richardson, A.J., and Singer, M.C. (2011). Overstretching attribution. *Nature Climate Change*, 1(1), 1–3.

Parry, M., Lowe, J., and Hanson, C. (2009). Overshoot, adapt and recover. *Nature*, 458, 1102–3.

Pearce, N. (2011). Epidemiology in a changing world: variation, causation and ubiquitous risk factors. *International Journal of Epidemiology*, 40(2), 503–12.

Pell, G. (2006). *Islam and Western Democracies: An Address from the Legatus Summit*, Naples, Florida, USA, 4 February. Available at: http://web.archive.org/web/20060605154745/http://www.sydney.catholic.org.au/Archbishop/Addresses/200627_681.shtml.

Perry, A.L. (2005). Climate change and distribution shifts in marine fishes. *Science*, 308, 1912–15.

Peters, G.P., Marland, G., Le Quéré, C., Boden, T., Canadell, J.G., and Raupach, M.R. (2011). Rapid growth in CO_2 emissions after the 2008–2009 global financial crisis. *Nature Climate Change*, 2(1), 1–3.

Post, E.S., Grambsch, A., Weaver, C., et al. (2012). Variation in estimated ozone-related health impacts of climate change due to modeling choices and assumptions. *Environmental Health Sciences*, 120(11), 1559–64.

Rajaratnam, J.K., Marcus, J.R., Flaxman, A.D., et al. (2010). Neonatal, postneonatal, childhood, and under-5 mortality for 187 countries, 1970–2010: a systematic analysis of progress towards Millennium Development Goal 4. *The Lancet*, 375, 1988–2008.

Reid, C.E., O'Neill, M.S., Gronlund, C.J., et al. (2009). Mapping community determinants of heat vulnerability. *Environmental Health Sciences*, 117(11), 1730–6.

Richardson, E.A., Pearce, J., and Kingham, S. (2011). Is particulate air pollution associated with health and health inequalities in New Zealand? *Health & Place*, 17(5), 1137–43.

Rocklöv, J., Barnett, A.G., and Woodward, A. (2012). On the estimation of heat-intensity and heat-duration effects in time series models of temperature-related mortality in Stockholm, Sweden. *Environmental Health*, 11(1), 23.

Rosegrant, M. (2008). *Biofuels and Grain Prices: Impacts and Policy Responses.* Washington, DC: International Food Policy Research Institute.

Rothman, K.J. (1998). Should the mission of epidemiology include the eradication of poverty? *The Lancet*, 352, 810–13.

Russell, R., Currie, B., Lindsay, M., Mackenzie, J., Ritchie, S., and Whelan, P. (2009). Dengue and climate change in Australia: predictions for the future should incorporate knowledge from the past. *Medical Journal of Australia*, 190(5), 265–8.

Schreiber, K. (2001). An investigation of relationships between climate and dengue using a water budgeting technique. *International Journal of Biometeorology*, 45(2), 81–9.

Schuckmann, K von., Gaillard, F., and Le Traon, P.Y. (2009). Global hydrographic variability patterns during 2003–2008. *Journal of Geophysical Research*, 114(C9), C09007.

Silva, H.R., Phelan, P.E., and Golden, J.S. (2010). Modeling effects of urban heat island mitigation strategies on heat-related morbidity: a case study for Phoenix, Arizona, USA. *International Journal of Biometeorology*, 54(1), 13–22.

Solomon, S., Qin, H., Manning, M.R., et al. (eds.) (2007). *Climate Change 2007: The Physical Science Basis. Contribution of Working Group I to the Fourth Assessment Report of the Intergovernmental Panel on Climate Change. IPCC. Summary for Policymakers*. New York: Cambridge University Press.

Speldewinde, P. (2009). A relationship between environmental degradation and mental health in rural Western Australia. *Health & Place*, 15, 880–7.

Stenseth, N., Samia, N., Viljugrein, H., et al. (2006). Plague dynamics are driven by climate variation. *Proceedings of the National Academy of Sciences of the United States of America*, 103(35), 13110–15.

Stephenson, J., Newman, K., and Mayhew, S. (2010). Population dynamics and climate change: what are the links? *Journal of Public Health*, 32(2), 150–6.

Stern, N. (2007). *The Economics of Climate Change: The Stern Review*. Cambridge: Cambridge University Press.

Stott, P. (2004). Human contribution to the European heatwave of 2003. *Nature*, 432, 610–12.

Stouffer, R.J. (2012). Oceanography: future impact of today's choices. *Nature Climate Change*, 2(6), 397–8.

Subramanyam, M.A., Kawachi, I., Berkman, L.F., and Subramanian, S.V. (2011). Is economic growth associated with reduction in child undernutrition in India? *PLoS Medicine*, 8(3), e1000424.

Sumilo, D., Asokliene, L., Bormane, A., Vasilenko, V., Golovljova, I., and Randolph, S. (2007). Climate change cannot explain the upsurge of tick-borne encephalitis in the Baltics. *PLoS ONE*, 2(6), e500.

Szreter, S. (2004). Industrialization and health. *British Medical Bulletin*, 69(1), 75–86.

Szreter, S. and Mooney, G. (1998). Urbanization, mortality, and the standard of living debate: new estimates of the expectation of life at birth in nineteenth-century British cities. *The Economic History Review*, 51(1), 84–112.

Teague, B., McLeod, R., and Pascoe, S. (2010). *Victorian Bushfires Royal Commission. Parliament of Victoria*. [Online] Available at: http://www.royalcommission.vic.gov.au/Commission-Reports/Final-Report/Volume-1/High-Resolution-Version.

Teixeira, E.I., Fischer, G., and van Velthuizen, H. (1970). Global hot-spots of heat stress on agricultural crops due to climate change. Agricultural and forest. *Agricultural and Forest Meteorology*, 170, 206–15.

Tester, P.A., Feldman, R.L., Nau, A.W., Kibler, S.R., and Litaker, R.W. (2010). Ciguatera fish poisoning and sea surface temperatures in the Caribbean Sea and the West Indies. *Toxicon*, 56(5), 698–710.

Thompson, M. and Gaviria, I. (2004). *Weathering the Storm: Lessons in Risk Reduction from Cuba. An Oxfam America Report*. Boston, MA: Oxfam America.

Thornton, P.K., Jones, P.G., Ericksen, P.J., and Challinor, A.J. (2010). Agriculture and food systems in sub-Saharan Africa in a 4 C+ world. *Philosophical Transactions of the Royal Society A: Mathematical, Physical and Engineering Sciences*, 369, 117–36.

Tun Lin, W., Burkot, T., and Kay, B. (2000). Effects of temperature and larval diet on development rates and survival of the dengue vector Aedes aegypti in north Queensland, Australia. *Medical and Veterinary Entomology*, 14(1), 31–7.

Uejio, C.K., Wilhelmi, O.V., Golden, J.S., Mills, D.M., Gulino, S.P., and Samenow, J.P. (2011). Intra-urban societal vulnerability to extreme heat. The role of heat exposure and the built environment, socioeconomics, and neighborhood stability. *Health & Place*, 17(2), 498–507.

United Nations Environment Programme (2011). *Integrated Assessment of Black Carbon and Tropospheric Ozone. Summary for Decision Makers*. New York: UNEP.

United Nations Environment Programme (2012). *The Emissions Gap Report 2012*. Nairobi: UNEP.

Wandiga, S.O., Opondo, M., Olago, D., et al. (2009). Vulnerability to epidemic malaria in the highlands of Lake Victoria basin: the role of climate change/variability, hydrology and socio-economic factors. *Climatic Change*, 99(3–4), 473–97.

Wilson, D.G. (2004). *Bicycling Science*. Cambridge, MA: MIT Press.

Woodcock, J., Edwards, P., Tonne, C., et al. (2009). Public health benefits of strategies to reduce greenhouse-gas emissions: urban land transport. *The Lancet*, 374, 1930–43.

Woodward, A. (2002). Epidemiology, environmental health and global change. In P. Martens and A.J. McMichael (eds.) *Environmental Change, Climate and Health. Issues and Research Methods*, pp. 290–310. Cambridge: Cambridge University Press.

Woodward, A. and McMichael, T. (2001). Climate change: what's new? *Australasian Epidemiologist*, 8(1), 10–12.

World Bank (2009). *World Development Report 2010. Development and Climate Change*. Washington, DC: World Bank.

World Health Organization (2008). *The Global Burden of Disease*. Geneva: WHO.

World Health Organization (2011). *World Health Statistics 2011*. Geneva: WHO.

Wu, P.-C., Lay, J.-G., Guo, H.-R., Lin, C.-Y., Lung, S.-C., and Su, H.-J. (2009). Higher temperature and urbanization affect the spatial patterns of dengue fever transmission in subtropical Taiwan. *The Science of the Total Environment*, 407(7), 2224–33.

Xu, L., Liu, Q., Stige, L.C., et al. (2011). Nonlinear effect of climate on plague during the third pandemic in China. *Proceedings of the National Academy of Sciences of the United States of America*, 108(25), 10214–19.

Xun, W.W., Khan, A.E., Michael, E., and Vineis, P. (2010). Climate change epidemiology: methodological challenges. *International Journal of Public Health*, 55(2), 85–96.

Yang, C., Cai, T., and Zhou, H. (2007). Impact of low temperature on population death in a typical city of North China. *Chinese Journal of Public Health Engineering*, 2, 77–9.

York, R. (2012). Do alternative energy sources displace fossil fuels? *Nature Climate Change*, 2(6), 441–3.

Zanobetti, A., O'Neill, M.S., Gronlund, C.J., and Schwartz, J.D (2012). Summer temperature variability and long-term survival among elderly people with chronic disease. *Proceedings of the National Academy of Sciences of the United States of America*, 109(17), 6608–13.

Zhou, X., Yang, G., Yang, K., et al. (2008). Potential impact of climate change on schistosomiasis transmission in China. *The American Journal of Tropical Medicine and Hygiene*, 78(2), 188–94.

Behavioural determinants of health and disease

Lawrence W. Green, Robert A. Hiatt, and Kristin S. Hoeft

Introduction to behavioural determinants of health and disease

Lifestyle is widely implicated in disease incidence and prevalence. That behaviour is associated with health and disease has never been in doubt. Indeed, the tendency to blame sinful, negligent, indulgent, ignorant, reckless, slothful, or selfish behaviour for health problems has too often placed undue emphasis on individual responsibility and culpability when the solution to health problems of populations demanded attention to the social and physical environment. But no matter how behaviour is framed or moralized in relation to its causes, it remains an inescapable variable in the pathway between ultimate upstream aetiologies and the incidence or prevalence of most diseases and health conditions downstream. Approaches to public health have sought throughout the history of civilization to: (1) control or cajole the health-related behaviour of individuals, (2) protect individuals from the behaviour of others, and (3) mobilize the behaviour of groups to influence health-related policies, organizations, and social or physical environments.

This chapter reviews ways in which behaviour relates to the spectrum of health and disease determinants, from environmental to genetic, in shaping health outcomes. It builds on the previous chapters in recognizing the powerful influence of socioeconomic and cultural factors, especially poverty and discrimination, in influencing both behaviour and health. Many commentaries in the past four decades have attempted to correct the overemphasis on behavioural determinants of health by discounting and sometimes disparaging any focus on individual behaviour or personal responsibility in disease prevention and health promotion, often referring to it as 'victim blaming' (e.g. Crawford 1977), and on another side, 'scapegoating' people with health problems as the cause of rising costs of healthcare (e.g. Minkler 1983). This chapter seeks a middle ground, building on the growing understanding of the ecological and cultural context of the behaviour–health relationship. It seeks to integrate that knowledge in an approach to public health that acknowledges the reciprocal determinism of behavioural, environmental, and biological determinants rather than minimizing the importance of behaviour in these complex interactions. This is consistent with a concept of 'behavioural justice' that Adler and Stewart (2009, p. 49) refer to as a 'principle that individuals are responsible for engaging in health-promoting behaviors but should be held accountable only when they have adequate resources to do so. This perspective maintains both individuals' control and accountability for behaviors and society's responsibility to provide health-promoting environments'.

The shifting role of behaviour as a determinant of health and disease

Simple, discrete behaviours account for many of the infections and injuries of the past. Today's growing chronic disease burden relates more to complex behaviours, sometimes referred to as 'lifestyle'. We use the term 'complex behaviour' to refer to combinations of interrelated practices and their environmental contexts, reflecting patterns of living influenced by the family and social history of individuals and communities, their environmental and socioeconomic circumstances, and their exposure to cultures and communications. We know that discrete behaviours can be influenced directly by health education targeted at individuals and groups. Complex behaviour, however, changes more slowly and usually requires some combination of educational, organizational, economic, and environmental interventions in support of changes in both behaviour and conditions of living. This combination of strategies has defined health promotion and public health programmes addressing complex behaviour change through combined efforts to predispose, enable, and reinforce the behaviours (Green and Kreuter 2005; Smith et al. 2006; Swan et al. 2012). The predisposing interventions are directed particularly at the individual, but the enabling and reinforcing interventions are directed at policies in support of, and environments in which, predisposed individuals would seek to enact and maintain the behaviour.

Obesity and HIV/AIDS present two obvious contemporary examples of health-related conditions and diseases awaiting technological solutions, for which behaviour, in the meantime, is a necessary route of intervention and change. Virtually every public health breakthrough has had a behavioural change process that served the public until the technology was at hand. Then, behavioural change processes were needed to diffuse, adapt, and apply the new technology to varying cultural and social circumstances.

For example, unless and until an obesity prevention vaccine or HIV vaccine is developed, society must depend on behavioural preventive measures to curb the spread of obesity and AIDS. These include, of course, policies, environmental changes, and health educational programmes that support behavioural changes.

Much of the early success in controlling HIV infections through change in sexual practices (especially use of condoms) among men in urban gay communities appears to have been in response to health education programmes (Petrow 1990). Reviews also show increases in the use of clean needles for at least 15 years among intravenous drug users (e.g. Wodak 2006), which has required a combination of policy and educational interventions to make clean needles accessible and more acceptable than the culture of needle sharing. Evidence that health education leads to the regular use of condoms among sexually active adolescents, however, has not held up consistently (Cervantes et al. 2011; Klein et al. 2011). The parallel lessons from the success of tobacco control programmes also point to the need for combined policy, regulatory, organizational, environmental, and educational interventions to influence population changes in tobacco consumption (Institute of Medicine 2003; Eriksen et al. 2007). Many of the same types of interventions are under consideration and evaluation for obesity control (Mercer et al. 2005; Institute of Medicine 2010, 2012).

Specific behaviours and health—the causal links

Some behaviour clearly increases the risk of developing disease and can be considered a proximal cause of disease, such as hygienic practices that expose one to infections. Other behaviours correlate with and precede better health, increased longevity, and decreased disease risk, but their causal link is more tenuous, variable, delayed, cumulative, or indirect, warranting their inclusion with more distal determinants, such as development of dietary and physical activity patterns. Examining the correlations between specific behavioural and social patterns and indicators of health and disease status provides the foundation for assessing behavioural factors as population health determinants (Evans et al. 1994). Examining the covariation of these relationships with other characteristics of the populations and their environmental circumstances helps put behaviour into its ecological, social, and cultural context (Institute of Medicine 2010, 2012).

The causal link is relatively easy to establish for single-agent communicable or infectious diseases. Evidence from observational epidemiological studies, human experimental trials, and animal models, together with clear mechanisms of biological action, lead one to conclude that many behaviours are, in fact, contributing causes (causal risk factors) of specific diseases. Again, the easiest examples of clear causal linkages are those established for single-action behaviours such as ingesting a contaminated food, getting an immunization that confers lifetime immunity, or taking a one-dose medication that leads to rapidly improved symptoms. As the number of booster shots required for immunization or doses required for cure increases, for example, the behaviour becomes more complex, requiring repetition or timing, and the causal linkage more difficult to unravel among the biomedical agent, the behaviour, and all the other events and circumstances that might have intervened and influenced the person's exposure, susceptibility, and outcome along the way.

Complex behaviours and health—the synergistic causal pathways

More difficult still are causal attributions and allocations for long-term behavioural patterns that are not under medical supervision and relate to multiple-cause chronic diseases and conditions (Glass and McAtee 2006; Krieger 1984). We present three examples of evidence supporting causal links between behaviours and coronary heart disease: smoking, diet, and physical inactivity. These three examples illustrate that even in the absence of direct experimental evidence in human beings, strong evidence of other types can be combined for the steps in a causal chain from behaviour through physiological effects to disease or health. In addition, the synergistic effects of two or more behaviours on health outcomes have been established.

A plausible biological model of the relationship between smoking behaviour and coronary heart disease has been available for decades (Dawber 1960). Observational epidemiological studies—including within- and between-population designs, case–control, and prospective designs—produced strong and consistent measures of association, the hypothesized temporal sequence, and dose–response relationships in subsequent decades (Stamler 2005). Additional randomized trials have included smoking cessation programmes that provide experimental evidence for smoking as a cause of coronary heart disease. Although the overall results of the Multiple Risk Factor Intervention Trial (MRFIT) in the United States were disappointing, in both MRFIT (Ockene et al. 1990) and the British trial on the effect of smoking reduction (Rose and Colwell 1992), cessation interventions showed decreases in coronary heart disease mortality respectively of 13 per cent after 20 years and 12 per cent after 10.5 years. In addition, when smokers at baseline from the experimental and control groups were pooled, quitters had a significant decrease in their risk of mortality from coronary heart disease compared with non-quitters (Ockene et al. 1990).

On the dietary front, evidence that saturated fat and cholesterol consumption behaviour contributes to coronary heart disease came first from ecological studies showing a correlation between dietary patterns and serum cholesterol levels (Keys et al. 1958), and later dietary fat consumption levels, and the corresponding geographical coronary heart disease incidence rates and mortality (Keys 1970). A 30-year follow-up of the Framingham cohort samples showed that high levels of serum cholesterol predicted the risk of coronary heart disease development (Anderson et al. 1987). In a meta-analysis of 27 trials, Mensink and Katan (1992) found that changes in dietary saturated fat and cholesterol led to changes in serum cholesterol. In the Helsinki Heart Study, Frick et al. (1987) showed that interventions to lower serum cholesterol levels decreased the occurrence of coronary heart disease. A definitive demonstration of the diet–heart hypothesis by a true experimental study might never occur because of the large sample size required, the sustained differential changes needed between intervention and control groups, and the long-term follow-up required for such a trial. The strong evidence for each step in a causal chain from diet to coronary heart disease and mortality, however, led to major national and international recommendations that diet be a first-line approach to reduce blood cholesterol to prevent disease, and more urgently today in the face of the global obesity epidemic (e.g. WHO 1990, 2000; Health Canada 2003; National Heart,

Lung, and Blood Institute 2004; Institute of Medicine 2005, 2012; US Department of Health and Human Services 2011).

Physical inactivity as a risk factor for coronary heart disease is the third example. Evidence that physical inactivity contributes to coronary heart disease came from studies of the biological effects of exercise on cardiovascular physiology, observational epidemiological studies, and randomized controlled trials of physical activity and physiological coronary heart disease risk factors, such as high blood pressure, obesity, and diabetes. The biological effects of exercise training to enhance cardiovascular health were well established by the 1980s (McArdle et al. 1986). Epidemiological evidence continues to show consistent and relatively strong associations, the hypothesized temporal sequence, and a dose–response relationship between physical activity and coronary heart disease (Ahmed et al. 2012). Observational epidemiological and randomized controlled trials demonstrated the beneficial effects of physical activity on blood pressure (Arroll and Beaglehole 1992) and on blood lipids and lipoproteins (Lokey and Tran 1989), which have, in turn, been causally linked with subsequent coronary heart disease. The combination of these sources of evidence for each of the steps in a causal chain provides a plausible model for the sequence.

Some of the immediate causal risk factors are not themselves behaviours, but have determinants that are behaviours. In these cases, the behavioural determinants can be regarded as indirect risk factors that act earlier in the causal pathway. For example, a combination of overeating and sedentary behaviour produce high caloric intake and low energy output, which together mediate the behavioural determinants of obesity. Obesity, in turn, is a physiological risk factor for cardiovascular diseases (CVD) and type 2 diabetes (Institute of Medicine 2005).

Behaviour also contributes to the prognosis of diseases at each stage where the screening, diagnosis, or the compliance with prescribed regimens of treatment or self-care affects outcomes. For example, the prognosis of breast cancer depends on the stage of disease at which the person obtains screening, diagnosis, and medical care. The prognosis for type 1 (insulin-dependent) diabetes depends on the patient's compliance with his or her insulin prescriptions. Because behaviour is so central to disease outcomes, a large literature on patient education and patient compliance with medical regimens has been catalogued and subjected to meta-analyses with regularity (e.g. Mullen et al. 1985; US Preventive Services Task Force 1989 and continuously updated on http://www.ahrq.gov/clinic/uspstfix.htm).

Behavioural risk factors in population health

The causal pathways by which behaviour can influence health (or its negative manifestations) can be broadly classified as direct (as shown by arrow 1 in Fig. 2.9.1) and indirect, where the indirect pathways (arrows 2 and 3 in Fig. 2.9.1) are largely mediated through the environment or through healthcare organization and personnel. These three determinants of health—behaviour, environment, and healthcare organization—in addition to human biology, were cast as the 'Health Field Concept' as part of the Lalonde Report on the Health of Canadians (Canada 1974), which many credit with having launched or at least facilitated the health promotion, health determinants and population health movements in public health (cf. Green and Allegrante 2011). The third indirect pathway

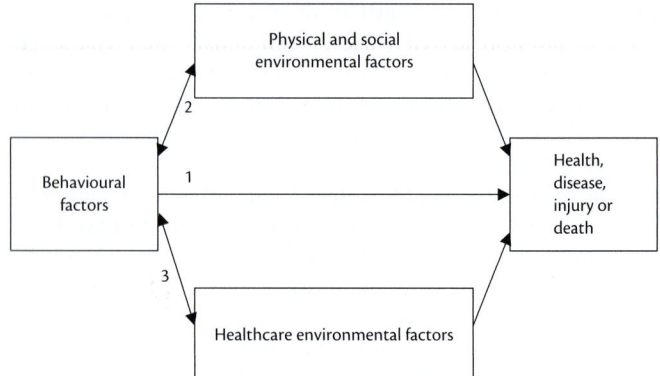

Fig. 2.9.1 Three pathways for behavioural influence on health, disease, injury, or death.

could be drawn through genetics, the main pathway by which individuals can make some reproductive decisions independent of the medical care system, but such non-medically mediated decisions are largely mediated by the social environment. Fig. 2.9.1 is hardly a full representation of the three sets of variables (behaviour, environment, healthcare organization), much less the genetic interactions, insofar as there is much reciprocal determinism between behaviour and each of the various environments, as well as with genetics. These environmental influences on behaviour will be examined in the next section, and behaviour's influence on the environment in a later section.

Behaviour itself as a risk factor for disease

The direct pathway suggested by arrow 1 in Fig. 2.9.1 includes the broad array of actions people take, consciously or unconsciously, that can have an immediate or cumulative effect on their health status. The effect on health may be intended (health-directed) or unintended (health-related), but the behaviour is nevertheless direct in its effect. The most dramatic of these are the violent injury-causing actions people may take behind the wheel of an automobile, with weapons, or unintentionally with the careless use of tools or toxic substances or merely walking absent-mindly on a slippery or cluttered surface. Less dramatic, but no less lethal, are the cumulative little actions people take each time they light a cigarette, imbibe or inject an addictive or mind-altering substance, or neglect physical activity or healthful foods.

Table 2.9.1 lists the nine leading causes of death in most of the more developed countries, as reflected here by the United States, and relates those to the risk factors for each in column 2, which McGinnis and Foege (1993, 2004) and Mokdad et al. (2004) refer to as the 'actual causes of death'. Colditz (2001) has noted that more than half of all cancer is a consequence of behaviour, much of which is embedded in culture. Most of the risk factors in Table 2.9.1 are themselves behaviours. Those that are not behaviours themselves—such as high serum cholesterol, obesity, hypertension, and diabetes mellitus—are the physiological consequence, in large part, of behaviours. The behavioural determinants of risk factors in column 3 present some of the most challenging targets for public health intervention, because they require decreasing behaviours that are perceived as pleasurable (e.g. types of food, sedentary entertainment, casual or spontaneous sexual encounters) and increasing behaviours perceived as boring, painful, or inconvenient (e.g. less sugary or salty foods, more strenuous or frequent physical activity, use of condoms). Their challenges are compounded by the fact that most of the instances of these behavioural determinants of risk can be carried out very privately with limited opportunity for monitoring, enforcement or social influence.

Tobacco consumption alone accounts for a large proportion of deaths in developed countries, implicated as a direct risk factor in all five of the leading causes of death shown in Table 2.9.1. At least one of the three main behavioural risk factors—smoking, dietary practices, and alcohol use—is causally related to each of the nine leading causes of death shown in Table 2.9.1. Active smoking has been established as a risk factor for coronary heart disease, diabetes, stroke, and adverse pregnancy outcomes, such as low birth weight, premature rupture of membranes, and abruption placentae (US Department of Health and Human Services 2004). As examples of how the behaviour of some individuals can influence the health of others, passive smoking (i.e. exposure to environmental

tobacco smoke) has been related to lung cancer and other respiratory diseases, as an independent risk factor for coronary heart disease, and exposure to environmental tobacco smoke in the home has been associated with asthma, other respiratory conditions, and with ear infections in infants and children (US Department of Health and Human Services 2006). Although still controversial, the California Environmental Protection Agency (2005) has concluded from its reviews that passive smoking is also a risk factor for breast cancer. This has been supported in a review of studies in Japan (Iwasaki and Tsugane 2011) and by the Canadian Expert Panel on Tobacco Smoke and Breast Cancer (Johnson et al. 2011).

As noted in previous chapters, the causes of death in developing countries differ markedly from the patterns reflected in Table 2.9.1, although the demographic profiles are converging. World Health Organization (WHO) estimates of the four leading causes of death for the developing countries have been respiratory diseases, infectious and parasitic diseases, CVD, and perinatal mortality. As tobacco use has increased and problems of macro-nutrients have

Table 2.9.1 Nine leading causes of death (United States 2003), their generally accepted risk factors, and their behavioural determinants

Causes of death (age-adjusted death rates in the United States per 100,000 population)	Selected risk factors	Behavioural determinants of risk factors
Diseases of the heart (232.3)	Tobacco smoke	Smoking
	Sedentary living	Physical inactivity
	High serum cholesterol	High-fat diet
	Obesity, diabetes mellitus	High-calorie diet, physical inactivity
	Hypertension	High-salt diet
Malignant neoplasms (190.1)	Smoking	Smoking
	Low-fibre diet	Low-fibre diet
	Physical inactivity	Physical inactivity
	Sexually transmitted diseases	Sexual behaviours
Cerebrovascular diseases (53.5)	Hypertension	High-salt diet
	Atherosclerosis	High-fat diet
	Smoking	Smoking
Chronic obstructive pulmonary disease (43.3)	Smoking	Smoking
Unintentional injuries, traffic-related (37.3)	Alcohol abuse	Alcohol use before or while driving
	No seat belt engaged	Seat belt non-use
	Unsafe driving	Behavioural distractions (e.g. smoking, texting) while driving; speeding
	Drug abuse	Drug use before or while driving
Diabetes mellitus (25.3)	Obesity	High-calorie diet, physical inactivity
Pneumonia and influenza (22.0)	Immunization status	Failure to obtain immunization
	Malnutrition	Diet
Suicide (10.8)	High blood-alcohol abuse	Alcohol use
	Handgun use	Handgun possession
	Drug abuse	Drug use
Chronic liver disease and cirrhosis (9.3)	Alcohol abuse	Alcohol use

Source: data from National Center for Health Statistics, *Health, United States, 2006 with Chartbook on Trends in the Health of Americans, Center for Disease Control*, p. 179, 2006, available from http://www.cdc.gov/nchs/data/hus/hus06.pdf. Death data from Mokdad et al., Actual causes of death in the United States, 2000, *Journal of the American Medical Association*, Volume 291, Number 1238, Copyright © 2000 American Medical Association.

replaced some of the micro-nutrient problems in those countries, other chronic diseases, in addition to CVD, have increased. By 2020, according to WHO (1998) estimates, the tobacco epidemic is expected to kill more people than any single disease. Because it is a known probable determinant of at least 25 diseases, and the most important determinant of some of the leading causes of death, tobacco use will cause nearly 18 per cent of all deaths in developed countries and 11 per cent in developing countries. This alone warrants the concerted global attention to this behaviour that has been proposed by the Framework Convention on Tobacco Control.

Behaviour as a determinant of other risk factors

Besides the cumulative effect of behaviours on physiological risk factors, such as the energy balance between calorie intake and physical activity producing weight gain, obesity, and hypertension, many of the health consequences of behaviour are secondary to their impact on the immediate environment. Individuals are not merely the passive victims of the environments they inhabit or traverse. They are agents of change in those environments, and their ability to alter or control environmental threats to their own health increases with technological innovations. The growing capacity of individuals and groups to alter their environments through technological means, such as transport, also produces negative consequences for their health. Hence, health promotion and health protection have emphasized mobilizing individuals and groups to undertake personal conservation behaviours and collective actions to support policy changes and regulatory initiatives in support of more healthful environments.

Among the most striking differences in health between the developed and the developing countries are the perinatal–juvenile mortality rates. In their analysis of 66 countries, Hertz et al. (1994) found the three most important predictors of infant mortality rates to be percentage of households without sanitation, illiteracy rate, and the percentage of households without safe water. The major public health goals in developing nations have related to the provision of immunization, access to a sufficient supply of clean water, and the installation of proper sanitation facilities (WHO 1981). But the more recent Millennium Development Goals (MDGs) aimed to cut global poverty by half by the year 2015, with three goals focused directly on health, covering maternal mortality, infant mortality, HIV/AIDS, malaria, and tuberculosis.

These environmental and age-specific or disease-specific health measures, however, achieve their intended health goals only to the extent that an informed population accepts and uses them properly. A report by the World Bank (1993) suggested that the single most important public health policy for developing countries lies in the improvement of the education of young girls. Better educated women have fewer children, who tend to be healthier and, in turn, better educated and able to respond to the technological advances offered by such environmental measures. They also become a better informed electorate to demand and support healthful policies for the installation of such facilities. In short, behaviour remains a critical mediator of the relationships between environmental measures and health outcomes, as well as the relationship between the health needs and the political actions to create the environmental changes.

The behaviour–policy link in the causal chains becomes more important as the chronic diseases creep into the developing

countries. Inspection of the recent trends in the richest of the developing countries provides evidence that improvement of the socioeconomic condition is accompanied by a shift in mortality towards the chronic diseases and their behavioural risk factors reviewed earlier. In Mexico, for example, as early as 1991, infectious and parasitic diseases were only the fourth leading cause of death, following diseases of the heart, malignant neoplasms, and unintentional injuries. Developing countries are now the primary target for market expansion for the multinational tobacco companies, with convenience food companies close behind them. Behaviour will be an issue both in personally resisting the temptations offered by these industries and in collective action to restrain their advertising, promotion, ingredients, and location.

Behaviour as a consequence of cognitions, environments, and genetics

Notwithstanding the implied simplicity of identifying a few behaviours that account for the majority of deaths in developed countries, those and other behaviours are highly complex, value-laden, and over-determined. Most behavioural risk factors and healthcare behaviours as well, are the product of a variety of component behaviours, tasks, skills, or actions. For example, food consumption confronts most people with a chain of related behaviours that includes procuring and selecting food, planning menus or selecting from a menu, preparing or ordering foods, and eating with literally hundreds of food-related choices, including where to shop or eat, what to purchase or prepare, how to season food, and with whom to eat (Simons-Morton et al. 1986). One can identify similar chains of component behavioural choices for each of the other health behaviours identified in Table 2.9.1.

Not only are the behaviours complex, but each behaviour has numerous influences or determinants. Factors that influence behaviours can be grouped into three major categories (Green and Kreuter 2005; with adaptation from Andersen 1969): predisposing, enabling, and reinforcing, as shown in Fig. 2.9.2. Both positive and negative behaviours are predisposed, enabled, and reinforced by forces in the culture and the environment. This broad categorization has proved useful in public health programme planning (with more than 1000 published applications, see http://lgreen.net/bibliog.htm for bibliography) because it groups the determinants of behaviour according to the major strategies used in public health to influence them. *Direct communications* through mass media, schools, worksites, other organizations, and through patient counselling in health clinics are used to influence the predisposing factors. *Indirect communications* through parents, teachers, clergy, community leaders, employers, peers, and others are used to strengthen the reinforcing factors with organizational rewards or social-normative influence. *Community organization*, *political activation*, and *training* strengthen the enabling factors by mobilizing and moving resources, policies, and building skills and capacities.

Predisposing factors

Predisposing factors reside in the individual and include attitudes, values, beliefs, and perceptions of need, but these are shaped over time by cultural and social exposures, which produce reinforcing factors (see later). Predisposing factors are those antecedents to behaviour that provide the rationale, motivation, or drive for an

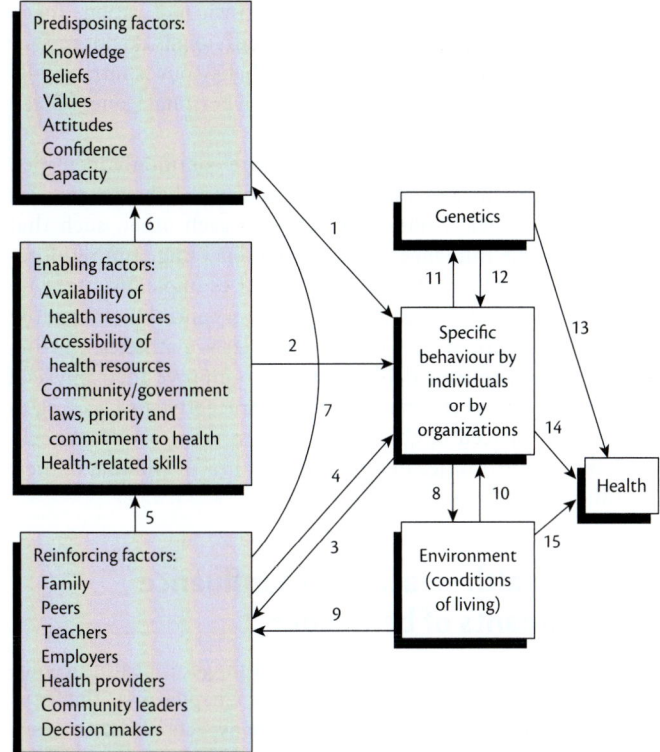

Fig. 2.9.2 This portion of the Precede–Proceed Model includes additional lines and arrows to outline a theory of causal relationships and order of causation and feedback loops for the three sets of factors influencing behaviour. In addition to the lines shown, an arrow from 'enabling factors' to 'environment' would elaborate the ecological aspect of factors that influence behaviour indirectly through changes in the environment.
Reproduced from Green, L.W. and Kreuter, M., *Health Program Planning: An Educational and Ecological Approach*, Fourth edition, McGraw-Hill Higher Education, New York, USA, Copyright © 2005, with permission from McGraw-Hill Education.

individual's or group's behaviour. They mostly fall in the psychological domain of determinants, though genetics and environment shape them across the life span. They include the cognitive and affective dimensions of knowing, feeling, believing, valuing, and having self-confidence or a sense of self-efficacy.

Because these determinants of behaviour reside in individuals, public health must seek to influence behaviour by assessing the prevalence and distribution of key predisposing factors and look for opportunities to communicate differentially with various segments of the populations, according to an educational diagnosis or 'social marketing' assessment of their knowledge, attitudes, values, beliefs, and perceptions. The behavioural science literature, especially in health psychology, is replete with competing theories of the relative importance of particular predisposing factors and how they interact with each other (e.g. Glanz et al. 2008). Some of these theories, such as the Health Belief Model (Becker 1974), Social Cognitive Theory (Bandura 2004), and the Transtheoretical Model of Stages of Change (Prochaska et al. 2002), have become mainstays of the intervention literature on health education and behaviour change. These frequent uses of selected models have produced sufficient numbers of comparable studies or programme evaluations to permit meta-analyses of their applications across different health behaviours (e.g. Spencer et al. 2005; Tuah et al.

2011). These applications of theory, in turn, have led to enough consistency in the construction of interventions and programmes that these have lent themselves to systematic reviews, notably by national panels such as the Task Force on Community Preventive Services (www.thecommunityguide.gov) and the UK's National Institute for Health and Care Excellence (http://www.nice. org.uk).

Enabling factors

Underplayed in most psychological studies of health behaviour, but critical to the role of public health as a complement to the roles of parents, schools, and mass media in the development of a healthy population, are the enabling factors influencing behaviour. These are often conditions of the environment that facilitate (or impede) the performance of a predisposition or motivated action by individuals or groups. Included are the availability, accessibility, and affordability of healthcare and community resources. Also included are conditions of living that act as facilitators or barriers to action, such as availability of transportation or child care to release a parent from that responsibility long enough to participate in a health programme, clinic, or service. It also includes features of the built environment, such as bicycle lanes, sidewalks, proximity of housing to workplaces, and other physical conditions of the environment that make physical activity more or less convenient and inviting (e.g. Taylor et al. 2007). Enabling factors also include new skills that a person needs—or new capacities that a group, organization, or community needs— to be able to accomplish health goals.

Public health addresses the enabling factors for behavioural change through policy changes and resource allocations at the national, regional, and local level, community organization for such policy and resource allocation at the local level when government programmes and services are insufficient or inappropriate to local perceptions of need. Training in the skills needed to take certain complicated actions is the other behavioural intervention used by public health to address the enabling factors.

In an era of constrained public health resources, many communities have resorted to more intensive community organization to build coalitions of multiple agencies including government and non-governmental organizations, and intersectoral collaboration between the health agencies and the community's schools, worksites, transportation, and other such sectors. Public–private collaboration on issues of enabling a more healthful food supply in school lunches, for example, or less accessibility of children to vending machines with cigarettes or 'junk food', have become increasingly common strategies for addressing the behaviour–environment interaction issues at the heart of most enabling factors (e.g. Institute of Medicine 2012).

Reinforcing factors

Before chronic diseases became the prevailing concern of public health in developed countries, behaviour was perceived as less important than today. The types of behaviour required to implement many of the most important public health interventions such as immunization and fluoridation of water supplies were less complex. Immunizations, for example, could confer long-term immunity for an individual with a single act. Fluoridation or chlorination of water supplies could be implemented in many communities with no engagement of the public, although when water fluoridation did become a local political issue requiring a local vote, the behaviour in question for most people was, again, a single action. As chronic diseases became more prevalent, the behaviours in question were largely ones that had to be repeated frequently, some for a lifetime, such as dietary practices, hypertension medication regimens, smoking cessation, and physical activity. For these behaviours, the predisposing and enabling factors remain important, but reinforcing factors take on increased importance because maintaining a behaviour requires strong or repeated extrinsic reinforcement in the form of rewards or incentives, or highly internalized intrinsic reinforcements in the form of values and personal commitments.

Reinforcing factors are those consequences of action that determine whether the actor receives positive (or negative) feedback and is supported socially or financially after it occurs. Reinforcing factors thus include social support, peer influences, and advice and feedback by healthcare providers, as well as a sense that the benefits of the action outweigh the costs. In consideration of the benefits (and costs), they also include physical consequences of behaviour, which may be separate from the social context. Examples include the feeling of well-being (or pain) caused by physical exercise and the alleviation of respiratory symptoms (or the experience of side effects) following the use of asthma medication, or gaining weight while quitting cigarettes.

Public health uses reinforcing factors such as denormalizing smoking in public places, social reinforcement with encouraging words in personal counselling, small-group health education sessions in which behaviour is publicly endorsed and praised, or mass media images of attractive role models with whom people wish to be associated by their own behaviour. No matter how effective these extrinsic reinforcements might be in the short term in strengthening a behavioural tendency, they must be internalized over time to become intrinsic motivation. Token rewards lead to token behaviour if the individuals do not replace them over time with the belief that the behaviour is intrinsically valuable because it accords with their own personal values (Green et al. 1986).

Table 2.9.2 gives examples of the more commonly identified influences on each of four most important behavioural risk factors. These behaviours interact with each other, such that changes in one influence predisposing, enabling, and reinforcing factors for others. Young women, for example, may take up smoking in the belief that it will help them control their appetite and thereby their weight. Other examples are athletes quitting smoking and limiting alcohol intake to improve their physical activity or sport performance; and contraceptive use leading to fewer, more spaced births, which lead in turn to women seeking other opportunities to improve their health and that of their families.

Public health strategies to influence determinants of behaviour

Another chapter will deal with the full range of health promotion and health education strategies (see Chapter 6.4). The focus of this section is specifically on how the aspects of the environment discussed in the previous sections that shape health-related behaviour can be targeted for strategic intervention for public health purposes. Three types of strategies are used in public health to accomplish health promotion and disease prevention goals through behaviour change:

◆ *Educational strategies* inform and educate the public about issues of concern, such as the dangers of drug misuse, the benefits of automobile restraints, or the relationship of maternal alcohol consumption to fetal alcohol syndrome.

Table 2.9.2 Some known and suspected predisposing (a), enabling (b), and reinforcing (c) influences on four major behavioural risk factors

Cigarette smoking	Dietary practices	Alcohol use/abuse	Physical inactivity
Knowledge of adverse health effects of smoking (a)	Personal food preferences (a)	Expectations of alcohol effects (a)	Beliefs in physical activity benefits (a)
Attitudes about smoking (a)	Cultural food preferences (a)	Child of alcoholic (a)	Attitudes toward physical activity (a)
Skills in smoking cessation/prevention (b)	Perceived social acceptance of foods (a and c)	Alternatives to alcohol (a and b)	Self-efficacy (a)
Cigarette cost (b and c)	Social context of eating (b and c)	Psychological stress (a, b and c)	Resources, facilities for exercise (b)
Availability of cigarettes (b)	Availability and convenience of healthful foods (b)	Low self-esteem (a)	Cost of exercise facilities (b)
Cigarette advertising (a)	Skills in menu planning (b)	Early drinking experience (c)	Skills in relapse prevention (b)
Peer influences to smoke (c)	Skills in food preparation (b)	Heavy social drinking (c)	Skills in goal setting (b)
Social support for non-smoking (c)	Skills in food selection (b)	Parent and peer influences (c)	Enjoyability of physical activity (c)
Smoke-free policies in worksite (b and c)	Food advertising (a and c)	Alcohol advertising (a, c)	Family support (c)
Access to cessation services (b)	Healthful options in vending machines (b)	Cost of alcohol (b)	Design of the built environment (b and c)
Attitude toward tobacco industry practices (a)	Belief in personal susceptibility to risk factors (a)	Availability of alcohol (b)	Belief in benefits of physical activity

- *Automatic-protective strategies* are directed at controlling environmental variables, that minimize the need for individual decisions in structuring each behaviour, such as public health measures providing for milk pasteurization, water fluoridation, infant immunizations, and the burning or chemical killing of marijuana crops, but these often involve individual and group decisions and actions about which policies to support, since they limit degrees of freedom in choice of behavioural options.

- *Coercive strategies* employ legal and other formal sanctions to control individual behaviour, such as required immunizations for school entry, mandatory tuberculosis testing of hospital employees, compulsory use of automobile restraints, and arrests for drug possession or use or for drunk driving.

Illustrative of successful public health measures reflecting this range of strategies directed at influencing health-related behaviours are the efforts to control tobacco consumption. Influencing tobacco-related knowledge and attitudes has been declared one of the great public health achievements of the twentieth century, at least in the United States (Centers for Disease Control 1999) and several other countries. Considering that these successes, as measured by the reductions in tobacco consumption behaviour, were achieved largely in the last third of the century, they represent both a remarkable turn-around of an epidemic of smoking behaviour that had increased inexorably through the first two-thirds of the century, and an inspiration for public health approaches to other health-related behaviours that now show similar epidemic trends. The application of the lessons from tobacco control to reversing, for example, the obesity epidemic through similar influences on dietary and physical activity behaviours has become a point of major public health debate in the early years of the new millennium (Mercer et al. 2005; Green et al. 2006; Eriksen et al. 2007; Institute of Medicine 2012).

Influences on smoking initiation and cessation are numerous, and many of them are also intertwined with diet, alcohol, and physical activity. Predisposing factors include attitudes about smoking and beliefs about and knowledge of the health effects of smoking. Enabling factors of access to tobacco products and price are influential. The price elasticity has been documented at a 3 per cent decrease in tobacco consumption for every 10 per cent increase in the price, and a greater relative decrease in youth, for whom disposable income is less (Ranson et al. 2002; Wilson et al. 2012). The influence of raising taxes on cigarettes, then, has been a major public health strategy with known effects on consumption. With the dedication of part of the tax revenues to the funding of comprehensive tobacco control programmes, some jurisdictions have achieved a doubling and even tripling of the rate of decline in per capita consumption compared with other jurisdictions in the same country (Mercer et al. 2005). But more powerful still are the cumulative reinforcing factors of growing social support and pressure for smoke-free environments as smoking becomes denormalized with the decline in prevalence rates and the legal restrictions on smoking in public places (Eriksen et al. 2007; Wilson et al. 2012).

Cigarette advertising and promotions by the tobacco industry have proved to be powerful negative predisposing and reinforcing influences on smoking behaviour that are highly adaptable to changing regulatory attempts to control their content and channels. Initial restrictions on US tobacco advertising in the broadcast media in the mid 1960s, for example, resulted in the tobacco industry voluntarily withdrawing from radio and television advertising, but adroitly using those resources from mass media to expand its advertising vastly on more targeted print media in magazines, billboards, and youth-oriented outlets. Sponsorship of sports and arts events and clubs, for example, provided a more targeted venue for reaching youth and other susceptible markets. Response of some jurisdictions in restricting these sponsorships has produced reductions in youth uptake of tobacco products (Hagmann 2002; Perez et al. 2012). Diversification of advertising to youth-oriented media and point-of-purchase settings such as stores near schools has resulted in increased restrictions in many jurisdictions. The restrictions have been largely disappointing, which is attributed to the agility of the industry in finding loopholes and ways to circumvent the new legal restrictions.

Attempts to control the determinants of tobacco consumption also illustrate an essential public health lesson in the importance of comprehensive programmes to affect the complex behaviours associated with chronic diseases (Centers for Disease Control and Prevention 1999, 2007). Comprehensive approaches have proved critical because:

- No single intervention reaches all segments of susceptible people in a population (Green and Glasgow 2006).

- No single intervention reaches different segments with the same degree of effectiveness (Warner 2011).

- Different interventions are differentially effective in the different phases of change (Prochaska et al. 2002).

- Different interventions variously influence the predisposing, enabling, and reinforcing determinants of behaviour in a population (Green and Kreuter 2005).

- This comprehensiveness lesson has been carried forward to public health efforts in diet, alcohol, and physical activity insofar as they have increasingly engaged multiple organizations in community coalitions and multiple sectors and national programmes to address the various determinants that extend beyond the purview of the medical and public health sectors at the local level. The complexity of these organizational and ecological layers and intersections of influence on both physical activity and food consumption have driven a concerted effort in the rush to find remedies for the obesity epidemic to include ecological models and systems models (Institute of Medicine 2005, 2010, 2012).

The promotion of physical activity or active living illustrates the lessons of comprehensiveness and multi-sector involvement in public health strategies to influence a complex behaviour. Increasing attention has been given in recent years to the built environment, including the density of housing, mixed-use neighbourhoods, and sidewalks that encourage walking to and from home for shopping, work, and recreation; provision of mass transit that also supports walking the distance to and from transit stops rather than driving to work and other destinations (Frank 2000; Sallis et al. 2012).

The recent growth of the active living field is an extension and integration of traditional public health approaches with more collaborative approaches involving sectors such as housing, parks and recreation, and transportation. It responds to the increasing recognition of the complexity of health-risk behaviours related to chronic diseases and their numerous determinants. The performance of each behaviour is interwoven with or ecologically embedded in other behaviours, organizations, and ecologies (Ottoson et al. 2009).

Behaviour as determinant of environmental and genetic predispositions

Population behavioural and educational diagnoses enable public health to intervene strategically on the behaviour of populations. But health problems have other determinants in the environment and in genetics. Behaviour also can play a role in influencing those determinants.

The reciprocal influence of individual behaviour on environments

A fundamental precept of human ecology is the reciprocal determinism of behaviour and the environment (Green et al. 1996; Sallis et al. 2012). The literature on health promotion took a sharp turn away from behaviour in the 1980s to give attention to the policy and environmental determinants of health. This was partly in response to a period in which public health was perceived to have taken too much of a psychological approach to the determinants of health (Green 2006). As early as 1968, Edward S. Rogers had appealed to sociology for the assistance public health needed from the social sciences to address the ecological issues (Rogers 1968). Psychologists, however, were more available, at least in the United States, to step into the perceived social science void of public health and to take up the new professorships in public health. They brought an emphasis on testing theories of individual behavioural change. As the ecological imperative of multi-level interventions (individual, family, organizational, community, regional, national, and global) gained growing emphasis in public health (e.g. Kickbusch 1989; Green et al. 1996), a gradual turn to the study of behaviour-in-context gave reciprocal determinism a new lease on life in public health (Stoto et al. 1997; Institute of Medicine 2001, 2003) in the decade bridging the millennium. One theory of behavioural change that gained particular public health prominence in this era was Albert Bandura's social cognitive theory, with its emphasis on self-efficacy and individual agency in changing one's environment at the same time that it gave prominence to the social environment in shaping behaviour (Bandura 2004).

Some of the environmental determinants of health beyond the behavioural control of individuals nevertheless lend themselves to group political behaviour or collective action through community intervention. Communities, neighbourhoods, or special-interest (self-help) groups can organize, vote, lobby, boycott, and otherwise support or prevent some environmental changes. To varying degrees, individuals can avoid or limit their exposure to environmental risks such as solar radiation, lead paint, and ambient smoke. In short, individual behaviour can be mobilized to influence the environment, so that individuals need not be seen only as passive objects of environmental influence.

The projected but still limited mobilization of behaviour to influence genetics

The Human Genome Project and the explosion of research on human genetics have raised very hopeful scenarios of 'personalized medicine', in which individuals could know more precisely their genetic risk of certain diseases or causes of death. The usual assumptions are that such information could be made readily available to individuals, and that having such information would be considerably more compelling in motivating behaviour than the usual statistical risk of groups of people without the personalized association with the individual in question.

The first assumption remains to be supported by true evidence of effectiveness. For example, in about 30 per cent of women with breast cancer, overexpression of a protein called HER2/neu is associated with a worse prognosis and in such women the drug trastuzumab is especially effective. The US Food and Drug Administration approved the drug and a test for HER2/neu for use in women with metastatic breast cancer in 1998 and more recently for women with early stage breast cancer (Hortobagyi 2005; Braga et al. 2006). The co-development and approval of the drug and test is considered one of the real successes of the application of genetics to modern medical practice and among the best examples of 'personalized medicine'. One might think the story is complete. However, although this information about the efficacy and availability of the test and the drug was published and promulgated by commercial backers, the behaviour of clinicians and their patients has been a more complicated matter. There is little known about how many women have access to testing and treatment. The costs of both are high and cost-effectiveness issues have not been resolved. Also how best to administer the test has not been resolved (e.g. timing) and there are reports of an increased risk of heart failure, the effect of which on acceptance is not known.

The second assumption, that having such information would motivate more concerted effort to change one's behaviour, is only partially supported by: (1) the logic and evidence from other areas of health counselling and communications that more personally tailored health information based on the individual's own family history or biological risk information adds motivational value to the experience with health advice that is based on more generic information (Kreuter and Wray 2003; Kreuter et al. 2005); (2) limited direct evidence from the few instances in which such genetic information has been used to counsel individual behavioural choices of action. The latter is illustrated by the examples in the previous paragraph and those from prenatal testing and counselling for birth defects. However, a meta-analysis of 21 controlled trials showed that while genetic counselling improved knowledge of cancer genetics, it did not increase the level of perceived risk and few studies examined cancer surveillance behaviours (Braithwaite et al. 2006).

Public health faces two major limiting factors in pursuing this pathway of behaviour influencing health through genetic determinants: (1) the limited influence of the genes so far implicated in specific mortality or morbidity outcomes, and their interactions with the environment, and (2) the ethics of offering such information to the individual with anything more than a cautionary note of possible relevance to their reproductive decisions or their behavioural choices. The first is a limit that could be partially overcome with further breakthroughs in the human genomics research. But apart from some prenatal tests for genetic defects in the fetus, most of the other genetic markers associated with predispositions to illnesses or premature mortality are highly interactive with other genes and the environment. Therefore, any course of action recommended to the individual remains probabilistic in its assurance of a health benefit. In combination with the other risk factors that can be more readily identified, the addition of personalized genetic information might raise the probabilities sufficiently to help the individual reach a tipping point in motivation to take action on complex health-related behaviours. But whether it really adds motivational value to what could be similarly known from a good family history has yet to be demonstrated.

The other limiting factors for this behaviour–genetic pathway as a public health consideration are the ethical complications that arise with the technology and the information. The concern, as in other screening technologies, with false-positive results can be multiplied in their ethical considerations for genetic information on individuals. The usual issues of protecting the privacy of such information and the potential discrimination in hiring, placement, retention, and promotion of individuals with known genetic predispositions will continue to be debated before the 'personalized medicine' potential of expanding the behaviour–genetic pathway can be pursued as public health policy. Meanwhile, private medicine is opening opportunities for individuals to explore this option in structuring their behavioural response to personal genetic information, as research on the behavioural implications mounts with three priorities: '(1) improving the public's genetic literacy in order to enhance consumer skills; (2) gauging whether genomic information improves risk communication and adoption of healthier behaviors more than current approaches; and (3) exploring whether genomic discovery in concert with emerging technologies can elucidate new behavioral intervention targets' (McBride et al. 2010). Other chapters in this volume addresses human genetics more thoroughly (see Chapters 2.5 and 5.12).

One still speculative pathway for social-behavioural influence on genetics is probed by a review of evidence for developmental and epigenetic pathways linking early life (perinatal) environments with CVD, and critically evaluates their possible role in the origins of African-American racial health disparities in CVD (Kuzawa and Sweet 2009). They observed, 'extensive evidence for a social origin to prematurity and low birth weight in African Americans, reflecting pathways such as the effects of discrimination on maternal stress physiology' (p. 2). They concluded 'environmentally responsive phenotypic plasticity, in combination with the better-studied acute and chronic effects of social-environmental exposures, provides a more parsimonious explanation than genetics for the persistence of CVD disparities between members of socially imposed racial categories' (p. 2). The prospects for finding ways for behaviour to influence DNA methylation are tantalizing.

The interaction of socioeconomic status, environments, and behaviour

Of all the interactions in the association of behaviour and health, none is more pervasive, consistent, and robust than that of socioeconomic status (SES). The relationship between SES and measures of health or mortality is shown in other chapters to be a gradient rather than a threshold effect, though threshold effects (or points of diminishing returns) are sometimes found beyond which income or other SES indicators have no further beneficial effects (e.g. Finch 2003). Those at the top of the SES hierarchy usually have better health and lower mortality rates than those just below them who are themselves better off than the others below them, and so on down to those in poverty at the very bottom. The

gradient adheres whether the SES measure is education, income, occupational status, or place of residence. The gradient globally is anchored at the lowest end by the poorest developing countries. Some 1.2 billion people globally in 2008 lived in extreme poverty on an income of just US $1.25 a day, of whom 70 per cent were in Asian and Pacific countries (World Bank 2012). Many of the poor lack access to basic health services and are at exaggerated risks for many of the leading causes of death in those countries. The gradients are complicated by the varied statistical interactions of gender, racial and ethnic discrimination with income, education, and occupation—the usual metrics of SES—in different countries.

The question here is how the mortality and morbidity gradients with socioeconomic status might operate through health-related behaviours, cultures, and environments to suggest mechanisms by which the pervasive SES gradient influences health, and ways in which the behavioural pathway can be made more protective or preventive.

SES as a predisposing determinant of behaviour

The ecological perspective on SES as a determinant of behaviour related to health would suggest first that environments shape behaviour from early childhood onward. Shaping behaviour in the first instance (rather than enabling it in the second or reinforcing it in the third) qualifies this environmental influence as a predisposing factor. Homes, neighbourhoods, towns, cities, regions, and whole countries with their variable physical, social, economic, and cultural environments differ in relation to SES measured at individual, family, neighbourhood, and other geographic levels. Once the measures of SES and health or mortality are aggregated above the individual level, their relationships constitute ecological correlations. Studies have examined the ecological relationship between mortality rates and various indicators of social inequalities in geographical areas varying in size from metropolitan areas (Lynch et al. 1998) to whole countries (Wilkinson and Marmot 1998). These studies showed that those areas where inequalities between those at the top of the hierarchy and those at the bottom were the largest were also those in which the mortality gradient was the strongest (Wilkinson 1996). Similar findings were found with other indicators of social inequities such as differences in social capital (Kawachi et al. 1997). Health disparities between socioeconomic groups appear from Canadian data to increase with age across the lifespan, which supports the notion of a cumulative effect over time of the health- and mortality–SES gradient (e.g. Prus 2007).

One implication of this relative deprivation dimension of the SES–health gradient is that perception of one's status relative to others de-motivates or discourages one's efforts to take greater control over the behavioural and environmental determinants of one's health. Whether consciously discouraged or unconsciously conditioned by repeated confrontations with inequalities and inequities that conspire against one's efforts, the hypothesis is that disparities make those exposed to relative deprivation less predisposed or motivated to take preventive and healthcare actions. Two specific mechanisms have been suggested for this de-motivation or lack of predisposition to undertake behaviour. One is a chronic pessimism that has been found in adolescent children of lower SES parents, and that pessimism was associated with stress (Finkelstein et al. 2007). The other possibly related mechanism is the theoretical construct of 'self-efficacy', widely measured in association with social cognitive theory applications in health behaviour research (Bandura 2004; Jang and Yoo 2012).

SES as an enabling determinant of behaviour

Socioeconomic standing also confers capabilities and resources that enable the predisposed behaviours to be carried out, for better or for worse. With higher standing come more resources and the associated education and training that endow individuals, families, groups, and communities with enabling judgements, resources, and skills. No matter how motivated people may be by their predisposing factors, they may not have the income and other resources, including accessible and affordable services within reach of their residences or workplaces, to be able to carry out the behaviour without great sacrifice and inconvenience. But environmental variables of accessible fruit and vegetable outlets in local neighbourhoods, for example, only partially explain or mediate the relationship between SES and fruit or vegetable consumption (Ball et al. 2006). The 'food deserts' of poor access to fruits and vegetables in neighbourhood stores of poor areas are compounded by the high accessibility of the 'food swamps' of fast food restaurants with their calorie-dense menus (Fielding and Simon 2011).

The educational enabling influence of SES on behaviour

Among the SES indicators, education has for decades demonstrated the strongest association with most health-behaviour measures (Green 1970a, 1970b; Metcalf et al. 2007), and this association has been found to have a major part of its essence in health literacy (e.g. Curtis et al. 2012). It also stands out among the indicators of inequities in confirming the relative deprivation hypothesis (Kunst and Mackenbach 1994). Education can be viewed as a proxy for a variety of predisposing and enabling factors in explaining the causes of behavioural determinants as mediators of at least part of the SES–health gradient. Prominent among these are optimism (a predisposing factor) and education as an enabling or coping resource (Finkelstein et al. 2007), with the knowledge, attitudes, and skills that come with years of schooling.

The Canadian Health Promotion Survey (Adams 1993) showed that men and women with a higher level of education self-rated their health as excellent or good in a much higher proportion than individuals with lower education (noting that self-rated health is a well-established proxy for objective measures of general health). The proportion of people in Canada who are smokers is double in people with elementary or lower education, compared with people with university degrees (Health and Welfare Canada et al. 1993). This spread in proportions of smokers was greater for the highest and lowest education categories than for the highest and lowest income or occupational status categories (Pederson 1993). Data from the major US community trials in cardiovascular disease prevention showed that the dramatic drop in smoking prevalence over the 1980s was more pronounced for people with higher education compared with people with less education (Winkleby et al. 1992a; Luepker et al. 1993). The same trend was observed in Canada for the period 1985–1991 (Millar and Stephens 1993).

These historical associations between health behaviours and SES have been confounded in the more recent tracking of obesity, physical activity, and food consumption. The more sedentary work and modes of travel of a majority of white collar workers blur the educational, income, and occupational correlations with physical activity (e.g. Tjepkema 2005; Canadian Institute for Health Information 2006). In Canada, for example, 'of the demographic variables examined, income, occupation, and employment status were unrelated to obesity, while education was negatively associated with the prevalence of obesity' (Raine 2004, p. 6).

The cultural–environmental predisposing influence of SES

The strong relationships between education and smoking and other health behaviours are only slightly less so when adjusted for age, sex, and ethnicity or race (Winkleby et al. 1992b; Shea et al. 1991). Culture and gender do appear to play important roles, but these are highly intertwined with SES and acculturation. The early ecological studies remain some of the most compelling in establishing and explaining the role of culture in health. The studies of Japanese men who had lived in Japan and emigrated to California showed clear dietary changes and increased heart disease and stroke rates only in their offspring, i.e. the second generation. Those who immigrated to Hawaii had intermediate rates of dietary change and coronary and stroke rates (Keys 1970; Kato et al. 1973). As the Japanese became acculturated, they assumed both the dietary and cardiovascular patterns of their new country.

Another classic study providing evidence of the effects of culture on health was the series on the Roseto community. Early observations showed that this ethnically homogeneous Pennsylvania community experienced a significantly lower mortality from myocardial infarction than the nearby community of Bangor despite a higher prevalence of hypertension and obesity and a similar proportion of smokers (Lynn et al. 1967). These results were attributed to the apparent protective effect of a unique social, ethnic, and family cohesion in the community (Bruhn et al. 1982). More recent analyses show that Rosetans lost that relative protection over subsequent decades (Egolf et al. 1992). This loss was accompanied by an increase in the number of intermarriages of Rosetans with people of non-Italian decent, a decrease in social participation in Roseto, and an increase in the general wealth of the community, as the original Italian-born generation was gradually replaced by their ageing American-born offspring (Lasker et al. 1994).

In short, to the extent that minority cultures can remain sheltered from the pervasive influences of the majority culture, they can have powerful predisposing influences on health-related behaviour. With acculturation, however, comes the displacement of minority cultural influence with the majority culture. Culture, nevertheless, remains a conceptually useful construct for understanding both the minority and majority processes of socially transmitted beliefs and values that predispose people to one choice of behaviour over another.

SES as a reinforcing determinant of behaviour

A behaviour that is predisposed and enabled might still fail to persist beyond a trial stage of acting if it fails to produce satisfying results. Satisfaction comes from various sources that can have the effect of reinforcing behaviour. SES can contribute to the availability of reinforcements by putting people into association with other people and environments that are more likely to produce satisfaction with behaviours. Two examples follow.

The 'status identity factor' and social norms

The social-normative theory underlying the notion of SES functioning like a reinforcing factor would predict that people will identify with a place in the social hierarchy that they can justify on the basis of their highest achievement. Unlike the usual measure of SES produced by averaging standardized or weighted measures of education, income, and occupation, one hypothesis derived from social reinforcement theory was that people will aspire to and adhere to that norm of a particular behaviour associated with their highest measure on the gradient of SES. For example, a person who is relatively high on education, but of moderate income and occupational status, would tend to adhere to the behavioural norms of the highest, rather than the average, of the person's three status scores. The hypothesis was tested in a California state-wide sample of mothers of children under 5 years, demonstrating that the immunization status of the children and five other measures of early childhood care followed a gradient with SES, but that the best predictor of the mother's behaviour on these five measures was her highest standardized SES among income, education, and occupation, not the average. This inferred 'status identity' of the mothers provided a basis for linking the psychological phenomena of identification and role modelling with the sociological concept of normative influence (Green 1970a).

Denormalizing behaviour

In retrospect, one of the most important elements of the tobacco control success of the last third of the twentieth century in the United States and Canada was the 'denormalization' of smoking behaviour in public places (Eriksen et al. 2007; Rogers 2010). What had been a normative behaviour of smoking in the workplace and in restaurants, meeting rooms, and other public places became increasingly unacceptable, first by legal restrictions, then by social norms, by which the growing majority of non-smokers expected and even insisted on smoke-free environments. The combination of new smoke-free or 'clean air' ordinances and by-laws with mass media emphasizing the carcinogenic properties of second-hand smoke and the rights of non-smokers to be spared the exposure to this carcinogen resulted in a dramatic drop in this public behaviour. It was during this period of the 30-year decline in smoking that the rate of decline accelerated most dramatically. One reason for the importance of this element of the tobacco control campaigns was that the passage and enforcement of policies restricting a personal behaviour faced strong opposition as long as it was perceived by the public to be a matter of individual rights and the threat to be only to the person's own health. When the threat is seen to be to other people's health, especially to the health of children, the support of passage and enforcement of the laws and regulations grows. Other public health campaigns are attempting to model this experience, which builds on the social responsibility notions associated with communicable diseases of the past, but with most of the chronic disease-related behaviours, such as overeating and sedentary living, it has been more complicated to relate the normative behaviour of individuals to the health of others.

The interaction of socioeconomic status, gender, and behaviour

Men's and women's relative risk of disease or death in relation to specific behavioural risk factors such as smoking are generally similar (e.g. Oliveira et al. 2007), but their experiences with health differ markedly (Chapman Walsh et al. 1995). These differences cannot be attributed solely to biological determinants related to sexual differentiation (Krieger et al. 1993). The social construct of gender, as opposed to the biological categories of sex, was conceptualized to refer to cultural and social conventions, roles, and behaviours assigned to men and women (Krieger 1996). These in turn shape the social, political, cultural, and economic circumstances experienced by men and women. Gender thus attempts to capture this differential experience that men and women have with their environment and the possibilities and constraints associated with these differences (Potvin and Frohlich 1998). Some of these constraints and possibilities are interacting with the living conditions associated with SES to shape the health of people (Wilkinson and Pickett 2008).

The correlation of SES with health appears stronger for men than for women; the SES–health gradient is steeper for men (Arber and Cooper 1999), except in their twenties and thirties when the gradients are similar (Matthews et al. 1999). The gender interactions with SES and health have been variously attributed to differential occupational experiences (e.g. Ross and Bird 1994), marital experiences (Koskinen and Martelin 1994), and degree of emancipation of women (Kawachi et al. 1999). These and other possible explanations generally require assumptions of behavioural mediators. Such mediators are as likely to be 'health-related' behaviour (e.g. sedentary living or food consumption patterns) as 'health-directed' behaviour (e.g. exercise or high-fibre diet). This distinction (Green and Kreuter 2005) recognizes the centrality of behaviour in the causal chains even when (perhaps especially when) it is not consciously health-*directed* behaviour.

Relationships among health-related behaviours

The interplay among habitual behavioural patterns and the socioeconomic and cultural conditions reviewed in the last half of this chapter leads one to put into a broader context the reductionist examinations, presented in the first half, of specific behaviours as they relate to health, disease, and mortality. The dynamic relationships among the specific measures create a complex system of social, economic, cultural, and behavioural factors, interwoven with disease risk factors and health status, and influenced by the healthcare and physical environments.

Early studies of the relationships among health behaviours showed weak correlations, typically below $r = 0.20$ (Green 1970b; Steele and McBroom 1972). Those in subsequent studies that maintained correlations in the 0.20 range were smoking with alcohol use, alcohol use and exercise (Calnan 1989), and smoking and diet (Blaxter 1990). With the decline in smoking, less variation in smoking produces less co-variation with other behavioural variables. Given these low correlations, there is little evidence supporting a one-dimensional concept of health-related behaviours (Calnan 1994) or a uniform 'healthy lifestyle'. It supports, instead, the reciprocal and ecological system of relationships laid out in the various sections of this paper, showing behaviour as both a product and an active ingredient in the mix of culture, socioeconomic and environmental conditions affecting individual and population health.

Conclusion

Behaviour is an inescapable link in the chain of causation between most environmental and genetic determinants and the health outcomes in which they are implicated. Some toxins and infectious environmental agents can affect health directly without behaviour as a mediator, but even these *can* be mediated by individual action to avoid exposures, and collective behaviour of groups or communities to protect themselves.

The *social* environment presents a further complexity in the mediating and moderating of behaviour and environment in their determination of population health. Most health-related behaviour occurs in the context of the social environment, so it involves the behaviour of other people as well as that of the person whose health is in question. The individuals are acting upon, and in reaction to, each other as their health outcomes are being shaped by their actions. This reciprocal determinism of behaviour and the social environment applies as well to the physical environment and the genetic determinants of health. These interactions make up the ecology of health, and call upon public health to take an ecological approach to the management of population health.

One way to structure the ecological approach to the planning of public health programmes in which behaviour change has a role is to examine the factors that influence behaviour in three categories of determinants: predisposing factors, enabling factors, and reinforcing factors. These roughly correspond to strategies, respectively, that would use: (1) direct communications to influence the knowledge, attitudes, beliefs, and perceptions of the population concerning the behaviour–health relationship; (2) legal, engineering, financial, organizational levers, and resource development that would enable, restrain, or prohibit the behaviour; and (3) indirect communications through social organizations, parents, peers, employers, and others who control rewards and approval that would reinforce behaviour. By combining public health strategies directed at these three categories of determinants (predisposing, enabling, and reinforcing factors) the strategies will be comprehensive in their coverage and impact.

All of what has been understood as determinants of the health behaviour of individuals applies with some variation to the behaviour of health professionals, other practitioners and policymakers who could serve as channels through which to reach individuals, groups, and whole populations to influence their health behaviour. The actions of all of these categories of individuals, as well as their organizations, can be analysed in relation to the factors that predispose, enable, and reinforce their actions, and these analyses can point, in turn, to the development of strategies to change those behaviours.

Acknowledgements

We are indebted to Denise Simons-Morton, MD, PhD, and Louise Potvin, PhD, co-authors of this chapter respectively in its first and second editions, for remnants of their earlier contributions that remain in this fourth revision.

References

Adams, O. (1993). Health status. In T. Stephens and D. Fowler Graham (eds.) *Health and Welfare Canada. Canada's Health Promotion Survey 1990: Technical Report*, p. 23. Ottawa: Ministry of Supply and Services.

Adler, N.E., and Stewart, J. (2009). Reducing obesity: motivating action while not blaming the victim. *Milbank Memorial Fund Quarterly*, 87(1), 49–70.

Ahmed, H.M., Blaha, M.J., Nasir, K., et al. (2012). Effects of physical activity on cardiovascular disease. *American Journal of Cardiology*, 109, 288–95.

Andersen, R.M. (1969). *A Behavioral Model of Families' Use of Health Services*. University of Chicago Center for Health Administration Studies, Research Series No. 25. Chicago, IL: University of Chicago Press.

Anderson, K.M., Castelli, W.P., and Levy, D. (1987). Cholesterol and mortality: 30 years of follow-up from the Framingham Study. *Journal of the American Medical Association*, 257, 2176–80.

Arber, S. and Cooper, H. (1999). Gender differences in health in later life: the new paradox? *Social Science & Medicine*, 48, 61.

Arroll, B. and Beaglehole, R. (1992). Does physical activity lower blood pressure: a critical review of the clinical trials. *Journal of Clinical Epidemiology*, 45, 439–47.

Ball, K., Crawford, D., and Mishra, G. (2006). Socio-economic inequalities in women's fruit and vegetable intakes: a multilevel study of individual, social and environmental mediators. *Public Health Nutrition*, 9, 623–30.

Bandura, A. (2004). Health promotion by social cognitive means. *Health Education and Behavior*, 31, 143.

Becker, M.H. (1974). The Health Belief Model and personal health behaviour. *Health Education Monographs*, 2, 324.

Blaxter, M. (1990). *Health and Lifestyles*. London: Routledge.

Braga, S., dal Lago, L., Bernard, C., et al. (2006). Use of trastuzumab for the treatment of early stage breast cancer. *Expert Review of Anticancer Therapy*, 6, 1153–64.

Braithwaite, D., Emery, J., Walter, F., et al. (2006). Psychological impact of genetic counseling for familial cancer: a systematic review and meta-analysis. *Familial Cancer*, 5, 66–75.

Bruhn, J.G., Philips, B.U., and Wolf, S. (1982). Lessons from Roseto 20 years later: a community study of heart disease. *Southern Medical Journal*, 75, 575.

Calnan, M. (1989). Control over health and patterns of health-related behavior. *Social Science & Medicine*, 26, 435.

Calnan, M. (1994). Lifestyle and its social meaning. *Advances in Medical Sociology*, 4, 69.

Canada (1974). *A New Perspective on the Health of Canadians (Lalonde Report)*. Ottawa: Department of National Health and Welfare.

Canadian Institute for Health Information (2006). *Improving the Health of Canadians: Promoting Healthy Weights*. Ottawa: Canadian Institute for Health Information.

Centers for Disease Control and Prevention (1999). Achievements in public health 1900–1999: tobacco use—United States, 1900–1999. *MMWR Morbidity and Mortality Weekly Reports*, 48, 986–93.

Centers for Disease Control and Prevention (2007). *Best Practices for Comprehensive Tobacco Control Programs* (2nd ed.). Atlanta, GA: Centers for Disease Control and Prevention, Office on Smoking and Health.

Cervantes, R., Goldbach, J., and Santos, S.M. (2011). Familia adelante: a multi-risk prevention intervention for Latino families. *Journal of Primary Prevention*, 32, 225–34.

Chapman Walsh, D., Sorensen, G., and Leanord, L. (1995). Gender, health and cigarette smoking. In B.C. Amick III, S. Levine, A.R. Tarlov, and D. Chapman Walsh (eds.) *Society and Health*, p. 131–71. New York: Oxford University Press.

Colditz, G.A. (2001). Cancer culture: epidemics, human behavior, and the dubious search for new risk factors. *American Journal of Public Health*, 91, 357.

Crawford, R. (1977). You are dangerous to your health: the ideology and politics of victim blaming. *International Journal of Health Services*, 7, 663.

Curtis, L.M., Wolf, M.S., Weiss, K.B., and Grammer, L.C. (2012). The impact of health literacy and socioeconomic status on asthma disparities. *Journal of Asthma*, 49(2), 178–83.

Dawber, T.R. (1960). Summary of recent literature regarding cigarette smoking and coronary heart disease. *Circulation*, 22, 164.

Egolf, B., Lasker, J., Wolf, S., et al. (1992). The Roseto effect: a 50-year comparison of mortality rates. *American Journal of Public Health*, 82, 1089.

Eriksen, M.P., Green, L.W., Husten, C.G., et al. (2007). Thank you for not smoking: the public response to tobacco-related mortality in the United States. In J.W. Ward and C. Warren (eds.) *Silent Victories: The History and Practice of Public Health in Twentieth-Century America*, pp. 423–36. New York: Oxford University Press.

Evans, R.G., Barer, M.L., and Marmor, T.R. (eds.) (1994). *Why Are Some People Healthy and Others Not? The Determinants of Health of Populations*. New York: Aldine de Gruyter.

Fielding, J.E. and Simon, P.A. (2011). Food deserts or food swamps?: comment on 'Fast food restaurants and food stores'. *Archives of Internal Medicine*, 171(13), 1171–2.

Finch, B.K. (2003). Socioeconomic gradients and low birth-weight: empirical and policy considerations. *Health Services Research*, 38, 1819.

Finkelstein, D.M., Kubzansky, D.M., Capitman, J., et al. (2007). Socioeconomic differences in adolescent stress: the role of psychological resources. *Journal of Adolescent Health*, 40, 127–34.

Frank, L.D. (2000). Land use and transportation interaction: implications on the public health and quality of life. *Journal of Planning Education and Research*, 20, 6–22.

Frick, M.H., Elo, M.O., Happa, K., et al. (1987). Helsinki Heart Study: primary-prevention trial with gemfibrozil in middle-aged men with dyslipidemia. Safety of treatment, changes in risk factors, and incidence of coronary heart disease. *The New England Journal of Medicine*, 137, 1237–45.

Glanz, K., Rimer, B.K., and Viswanath, K. (2008). *Health Behavior and Health Education: Theory, Research, and Practice* (4th ed.). San Francisco, CA: Jossey Bass.

Glass, T.A. and McAtee, M.J. (2006). Behavioral science at the crossroads in public health: extending horizons, envisioning the future. *Social Science & Medicine*, 62, 1650.

Green, L.W. (1970a). Manual for scoring socioeconomic status for research on health behavior. *Public Health Reports*, 85, 185.

Green, L.W. (1970b). *Status Identity and Preventive Health Behavior*. Pacific Health Education Reports, No. 1. Berkeley, CA: University of California School of Public Health.

Green, L.W. (2006). Public health asks of systems science: to advance our evidence-based practice, can you help us get more practice-based evidence? *American Journal of Public Health*, 96, 406.

Green, L.W. and Allegrante J.P. (2011). Healthy people 1980–2020: raising the ante decennially, or just the name from health education to health promotion to social determinants? *Health Education and Behavior*, 38(6), 558.

Green, L.W. and Glasgow, R. (2006). Evaluating the relevance, generalization, and applicability of research: issues in external validation and translation methodology. *Evaluation and the Health Professions*, 29, 126.

Green, L.W. and Kreuter, M. (2005). *Health Program Planning: An Educational and Ecological Approach* (4th ed.). New York: McGraw-Hill Higher Education.

Green, L.W., Orleans, C.T., Ottoson, J.M., et al. (2006). Inferring strategies for disseminating physical activity policies, programs, and practices from the successes of tobacco control. *American Journal of Preventive Medicine*, 31(Suppl. 4), S66.

Green, L.W., Richard, L., and Potvin, L. (1996). Ecological foundations of health promotion. *American Journal of Health Promotion*, 10, 270–81.

Green, L.W., Wilson, A., and Lovato, C.Y. (1986). What changes can health promotion produce and how long will they last? Trade-offs between expediency and durability. *Preventive Medicine*, 15, 508–21.

Hagmann, M. (2002). WHO attacks tobacco sponsorship of sports. *Bulletin of the World Health Organization*, 80, 80.

Health and Welfare Canada, Stephens, T., and Fowler Graham, D. (eds.) (1993). *Canada's Health Promotion Survey 1990: Technical Report*. Ottawa: Minister of Supply and Services.

Health Canada (2003). *Canadian Guidelines for Body Weight Classification in Adults*. Ottawa: Health Canada.

Hertz, E., Hebert, J.R., and Landon, J. (1994). Social and environmental factors and life expectancy, infant mortality, and maternal mortality rates: results of a cross-national comparison. *Social Science & Medicine*, 39, 105.

Hortobagyi, G.N. (2005). Trastuzumab in the treatment of breast cancer. *The New England Journal of Medicine*, 353, 1734.

Institute of Medicine (2001). *Health and Behavior: The Interplay of Biological, Behavioral, and Societal Influences*. Washington, DC: National Academies Press.

Institute of Medicine (2003). *The Future of Public Health in the 21st Century*. Washington, DC: National Academies Press.

Institute of Medicine (2005). *Preventing Childhood Obesity: Health in the Balance*. Washington, DC: National Academies Press.

Institute of Medicine (2010). *Bridging the Evidence Gap in Obesity Prevention: A Framework to Inform Decision Making*. Washington, DC: National Academies Press.

Institute of Medicine (2012). *Accelerating Progress in Obesity Prevention: Solving the Weight of the Nation*. Washington, DC: National Academies Press.

Iwasaki, M. and Tsugane, S. (2011). Risk factors for breast cancer: epidemiological evidence from Japanese studies. *Cancer Science*, 102(9), 1607–14.

Jang, Y. and Yoo, H. (2012). Self-management programs based on the social cognitive theory for Koreans with chronic disease: a systematic review. *Contemporary Nurse*, 40(2), 147–59.

Johnson, K.C., Miller, A.B., Collishaw, N.E., et al. (2011). Active smoking and secondhand smoke increase breast cancer risk: the report of the Canadian Expert Panel on Tobacco Smoke and Breast Cancer Risk (2009). *Tobacco Control*, 20(1), e2.

Kato, H., Tillotson, J., Nichaman, M.Z., et al. (1973). Epidemiological studies of coronary heart disease and stroke in Japanese men living in Japan, Hawaii, and California. Serum lipids and diet. *American Journal of Epidemiology*, 97, 372–85.

Kawachi, I., Kennedy, B.P., Gupta, V., et al. (1999). Women's status and the health of women and men: a view from the States. *Social Science & Medicine*, 48, 21–32.

Kawachi, I., Kennedy, B.P., Lochner, K., et al. (1997). Social capital, income inequality, and mortality. *American Journal of Public Health*, 87, 1491–8.

Keys, A. (ed.) (1970). Coronary heart disease in seven countries. *Circulation*, 41(Suppl. 1), 1–200.

Keys, A., Kimura, N., Kusukawa, A., et al. (1958). Lessons from serum cholesterol studies in Japan, Hawaii, and Los Angeles. *Annals of Internal Medicine*, 48, 83.

Kickbusch, I. (1989). Approaches to an ecological base for public health. *Health Promotion*, 4, 265–8.

Klein, C.H. and Card, J.J. (2011). Preliminary efficacy of a computer-delivered HIV prevention intervention for African American teenage females. *AIDS Education and Prevention*, 23(6), 564–76.

Koskinen, S. and Martelin, T. (1994). Why are socioeconomic mortality differences smaller among women than among men? *Social Science & Medicine*, 38, 1385–96.

Kreuter, M.W. and Wray R.J. (2003). Tailored and targeted health communication: strategies for enhancing information relevance. *American Journal of Health Behavior*, 27 (Suppl. 3), S227–32.

Kreuter, M.W., Sugg-Skinner, C., Holt, C.L., et al. (2005). Cultural tailoring for mammography and fruit and vegetable intake among low-income African-American women in urban public health centers. *Preventive Medicine*, 41, 53–62.

Krieger, N. (1984). Epidemiology and the web of causation. Has anyone seen the spider? *Social Science & Medicine*, 39, 887–903.

Krieger, N. (1996). Inequality, diversity, and health: thoughts on 'race/ethnicity' and 'gender'. *Journal of American Medical Women's Association*, 51, 133–6.

Krieger, N., Rowley, D.L., Herman, A.A., et al. (1993). Racism, sexism, and social class: implications for study of health, disease, and well being. *American Journal of Preventive Medicine*, 9 (Suppl.), 82–122.

Kunst, A.E. and Mackenbach, J.P. (1994). The size of mortality differences associated with educational level in nine industrialized countries. *American Journal of Public Health*, 84, 932–7.

Kuzawa, C.W. and Sweet, E. (2009). Epigenetics and the embodiment of race: developmental origins of US racial disparities in cardiovascular health. *American Journal of Human Biology*, 21, 2–15.

Lasker, J.N., Egolf, B.P., and Wolf, S. (1994). Community social change and mortality. *Social Science & Medicine*, 39, 53.

Lokey, E.A. and Tran, Z.V. (1989). Effects of exercise training on serum lipid and lipoprotein concentrations in women: a meta-analysis. *International Journal of Sports Medicine*, 10, 424–9.

Luepker, R.V., Rosamond, W.D., Murphy, R., et al. (1993). Socioeconomic status and coronary heart disease risk factor trends: the Minnesota Heart Health Survey. *Circulation*, 88, 2172–9.

Lynch, J.W., Kaplan, G.A., Pamuk, E.R., et al. (1998). Income inequality and mortality in metropolitan areas of the United States. *American Journal of Public Health*, 88, 1074–80.

Lynn, T.N., Duncan, R., Naughton, J.P., et al. (1967). Prevalence of evidence of prior myocardial infarction, hypertension, diabetes, and obesity in three neighboring communities in Pennsylvania. *American Journal of Medical Services*, 254, 385–91.

McArdle, W.D., Katch, F.L., and Katch, V.L. (1986). *Exercise Physiology: Energy, Nutrition, and Human Performance* (2nd ed.). Philadephia, PA: Lea and Febiger.

McBride, C.M., Bowen, D., Brody, L.C., et al. (2010). Future health applications of genomics: priorities for communication, behavioral, and social sciences research. *American Journal of Preventive Medicine*, 38(5), 556–65.

McGinnis, J.M. and Foege, W.H. (1993). Actual causes of death in the United States. *Journal of the American Medical Association*, 270, 2207–12.

McGinnis, J.M., and Foege, W. (2004). The immediate vs the important. *Journal of the American Medical Association*, 291(10), 1263–4.

Matthews, S., Manor, O., and Power, C. (1999). Social inequalities in health: are there gender differences? *Social Science & Medicine*, 48, 49–60.

Mensink, R.P. and Katan, M.G. (1992). Effect of dietary fatty acids on serum lipids and lipoproteins: a meta-analysis of 27 trials. *Arteriosclerosis and Thrombosis*, 12, 911–19.

Mercer, S.L., Kahn, L.K., Green, L.W., et al. (2005). Drawing possible lessons for obesity prevention and control from the tobacco control experience. In D. Crawford and R.W. Jeffrey (eds.) *Obesity Prevention and Public Health*, pp. 231–64. New York: Oxford University Press.

Metcalf, P., Scragg, R., and Davis, P. (2007). Relationship of different measures of socioeconomic status with cardiovascular disease risk factors and lifestyle in a New Zealand workforce survey. *New Zealand Medical Journal*, 120(1248), U2392.

Millar, W.T. and Stephens, T. (1993). Social status and health risk in Canadian adults: 1985–1991. *Health Reports*, 5, 143–56.

Minkler, M. (1983). Blaming the aged victim: the politics of scapegoating in times of fiscal conservatism. *International Journal of Health Services*, 13(1), 155–68.

Mokdad, A.H., Marks, J.S., Stroup, D.F., et al. (2004). Actual causes of death in the United States, 2000. *Journal of the American Medical Association*, 291, 1238–45. Erratum, *Journal of the American Medical Association*, 293, 293.

Mullen, P.D., Green, L.W., and Persinger, G.S. (1985). Clinical trials of patient education for chronic conditions: a comparative meta-analysis of intervention types. *Preventive Medicine*, 14, 753–81.

National Center for Health Statistics (2006). *Health, United States, 2006*. Hiattsville, MD: US Department of Health and Human Services, Centers for Disease Control.

National Heart, Lung, and Blood Institute (2004). *Detection, Evaluation and Treatment of High Blood Cholesterol in Adults*, NIH Publication 93 updated. Bethesda, MD: National Institutes of Health.

Ockene, J.K., Kuller, L.H., Svendsen, K.H., and Meilahn, E. (1990). The relationship of smoking cessation to coronary heart disease and lung cancer in the Multiple Risk Factor Intervention Trial (MRFIT). *American Journal of Public Health*, 80, 954–8.

Oliveira, A., Buros, H., Maciel, M.J., et al. (2007). Tobacco smoking and acute myocardial infarction in young adults: a population-based case-control study. *Preventive Medicine*, 44, 311–16.

Ottoson, J.M., Green, L.W., Beery, W.L., et al. (2009). Policy-contribution assessment and field-building analysis of the Robert Wood Johnson Foundation's Active Living Research Program. *American Journal of Preventive Medicine*, 36(2, Suppl. 1), S34–S43.

Pederson, L. (1993). Tobacco use. In Health and Welfare Canada, T. Stephens, and D. Fowler Graham (eds.) *Canada's Health Promotion Survey 1990: Technical Report*, pp. 97–108. Ottawa: Minister of Supply and Services Canada.

Perez, D.A., Grunseit, A.C., Rissel, C., et al. (2012). Tobacco promotion 'below-the-line': exposure among adolescents and young adults in NSW, Australia. *BMC Public Health*, 12(12), 429.

Petrow, S. (1990). *Ending the HIV Epidemic*. Santa Cruz, CA: Network Publications.

Potvin, L. and Frohlich, K.L. (1998). L'utilité de la notion de genre pour comprendre les inégalités de santé entre les homes et les femmes. *Ruptures, Revue Transdisciplinaire en Santé*, 5, 142.

Prochaska, J.O., Redding, C.A., and Evers, K.E. (2002). The Transtheoretical model and stages of change. In K. Glanz, B.K. Rimer, and F.M. Lewis (eds.) *Health Behavior and Health Education: Theory, Research, and Practice* (3rd ed.), pp. 99–120. San Francisco, CA: Jossey-Bass.

Prus, S.G. (2007). Age, SES, and health: a population level analysis of health inequalities over the life course. *Sociology, Health and Illness*, 29, 275–96.

Raine, K.D. (2004). *Overweight and Obesity in Canada: A Population Health Perspective*. Ottawa: Canadian Institute for Health Information.

Ranson, M.K., Jha, P., Chaloupka, F.J., et al. (2002). Global and regional estimates of the effectiveness and cost-effectiveness of price increases and other tobacco control policies. *Nicotine and Tobacco Research*, 4, 311–19.

Rogers, E.S. (1968). Public health asks of sociology…Can the health sciences resolve society's problems in the absence of a science of human values and goals. *Science*, 159, 506–8.

Rogers, T. (2010). The California Tobacco Control Program: introduction to the 20-year retrospective. *Tobacco Control*, 19(2), i1–i2.

Rose, G. and Colwell, L. (1992). Randomized controlled trial of anti-smoking advice: final (20-year) results. *Journal of Epidemiology and Community Health*, 46, 75–7.

Ross, C.E. and Bird, C.E. (1994). Sex stratification and health lifestyle: consequences for men's and women's perceived health. *Journal of Health and Social Behavior*, 35, 161–78.

Sallis, J.F., Floyd, M.F., Rodríguez, D.A., and Saelens, B.E. (2012). Role of built environments in physical activity, obesity, and cardiovascular disease. *Circulation*, 125(5), 729–37.

Shea, S., Stein, A.D., Basch, C.E., et al. (1991). Independent associations of educational attainment and ethnicity with behavioral risk factors for cardiovascular disease. *American Journal of Epidemiology*, 134, 567–82.

Simons-Morton, B.G., O'Hara, N.M., and Simons-Morton, D.G. (1986). Promoting healthful diet and exercise behaviors in communities, schools, and families. *Family and Community Health*, 9, 1–13.

Smith, B.J., Tang, K. C., and Nutbeam, D. (2006). WHO Health Promotion Glossary: new terms. *Health Promotion International*, 21, 340–5.

Spencer, L., Pagell, F., and Adams, T. (2005). Applying the transtheoretical model to cancer screening behavior. *American Journal of Health Behavior*, 29, 36–56.

Stamler, J. (2005). Established major coronary risk factors: historical overview. In M. Marmot and P. Elliott (eds.) *Coronary Heart Disease Epidemiology* (2nd ed.), pp. 18–31. Oxford: Oxford University Press.

Steele, J. and McBroom, W. (1972). Conceptual and empirical dimensions of health behavior. *Journal of Health and Social Behavior*, 13, 382–92.

Stoto, M.A., Green, L.W., and Bailey, L.A. (eds.) (1997). *Linking Research and Public Health Practice: A Review of CDC's Program of Centers for Research and Demonstration of Health Promotion and Disease Prevention*. Washington, DC: National Academy Press. Available at: http://books.nap.edu/catalog/5564.html.

Swan E., Bouwman L., de Roos, N., and Koelen, M. (2012). How science thinks and practice acts: bridging the gap in weight management interventions for adolescents. *Family Practice*, 29(Suppl.), i117–125.

Taylor, W.C., Sallis, J.F., Lees, E., et al. (2007). Changing social and built environments to promote physical activity: recommendations from low income, urban women. *Journal of Physical Activity and Health*, 4, 54–65.

Tjepkema, M. (2005). *Nutrition: Findings from the Canadian Community Health Survey. Issue No. 1 Measured Obesity: Adult Obesity in Canada*. Ottawa: Statistics Canada.

Tuah, N.A., Amiel, C., Qureshi, S., et al. (2011). Transtheoretical model for dietary and physical exercise modification in weight loss management for overweight and obese adults. *Cochrane Database of Systematic Review*, 5(10), CD008066.

US Department of Health and Human Services (2004). *The Health Consequences of Smoking: A Report of the Surgeon General*. Washington, DC: U.S. Department of Health and Human Services, Centers for Disease Control and Prevention, Coordinating Center for Health Promotion, National Center for Chronic Disease Prevention and Health Promotion, Office on Smoking and Health, Atlanta.

US Department of Health and Human Services (2006). *The Health Consequences of Involuntary Exposure to Tobacco Smoke: A Report of the Surgeon General—Executive Summary*. Atlanta, GA: U.S. Department of Health and Human Services, Centers for Disease Control and Prevention, Coordinating Center for Health Promotion, National Center for Chronic Disease Prevention and Health Promotion, Office on Smoking and Health.

US Department of Health and Human Services (2011). *Healthy People 2020: National Health Promotion and Disease Prevention Objectives*. Washington, DC: US Government Printing Office.

US Preventive Services Task Force (1989). *Guide to Clinical Preventive Services: An Assessment of the Effectiveness of 169 Interventions*. Baltimore, MD: Williams & Wilkins.

Warner, K.E. (2011). Disparities in smoking are complicated and consequential. What to do about them? *American Journal of Health Promotion*, 25, S5–S7.

Wilkinson, R.G. (1996). *Unhealthy Society. The Afflictions of Inequality*. London: Routledge.

Wilkinson, R.G. and Marmot, M. (1998). *The Solid Facts*. Geneva: World Health Organization.

Wilkinson, R.G. and Pickett, K.E. (2008). Income inequality and socioeconomic gradients in mortality. *American Journal of Public Health*, 98, 699–704.

Wilson, L.M., Avila Tang, E., Chander G., et al. (2012). Impact of tobacco control interventions on smoking initiation, cessation, and prevalence: a systematic review. *Journal of Environmental and Public Health*, 2012, 961724

Winkleby, M.A., Fortman, S.P., and Rockhill, B. (1992a). Trends in cardiovascular risk factors by educational level: the Stanford Five City Project. *Preventive Medicine*, 21, 592–601.

Winkleby, M.A., Jatulis, D.E., Franck, E., et al. (1992b). Socio-economic status and health: how education, income, and occupation contribute to risk factors for cardiovascular disease. *American Journal of Public Health*, 82, 816–20.

Wodak, A. (2006). Controlling HIV among injecting drug users: the current status of harm reduction. *HIV AIDS Policy and Law Review*, 11, 77–80.

World Bank (1993). *World Development Report 1993. Investing in Health*. New York: Oxford University Press.

World Bank (2012). *Poverty*. [Online] Available at: http://www.worldbank.org/en/topic/poverty.

World Health Organization (1981). *Global Strategy for Health for All by the Year 2000*. Geneva: WHO.

World Health Organization (1990). *Prevention in Childhood and Youth Adult Cardiovascular Diseases: Time for Action*. WHO technical report 792. Geneva: WHO.

World Health Organization (1998). *Tobacco Epidemic: Health Dimensions*. Fact Sheet No. 154, revised. Geneva: WHO.

World Health Organization (2000). *Obesity: Preventing and Managing the Global Epidemic*. WHO technical report series no. 894. Geneva: WHO.

Access to healthcare and population health

Martin Gulliford

Introduction to access to healthcare and population health

Facilitating access to healthcare should address the health needs of populations, but the role of health services in improving population health is disputed. Earlier commentators argued that access to healthcare could not be considered as one of the determinants of population health because interventions were generally ineffective at prolonging life and even caused premature mortality through iatrogenic disease (Illich 1976). A more recent consensus is that health services play an important role in delivering clinical interventions for the treatment and cure of disease, as well as population interventions for the prevention of disease and promotion of health. Health services represent one of three key areas of public health activity alongside health protection and health improvement. Public health specialists often play an important role in planning and managing health services. This chapter evaluates the relationship between healthcare and public health; it asks 'What is the role of health services in improving population health?'.

Concepts and values in healthcare

Purpose and value of health services

The boundaries of health services and health systems are difficult to define (Table 2.10.1). Broader definitions encompass 'all the activities whose primary purpose is to improve or maintain health' (Murray and Frenk 2000, p. 718). This definition includes interventions that are not implemented through healthcare services but such multisectoral interventions are generally considered to contribute to health improvement and not healthcare.

Health services serve several objectives. Health services can improve health by preventing or delaying the onset of disability or death; they contribute to relieving pain and suffering; healthcare is also valued for providing information concerning diagnosis and prognosis. Through its influence on individuals' health status, access to healthcare may determine what opportunities individuals will have in life, and how their lives will begin and end (President's Commission for the Study of Ethical Problems in Medicine and Biomedical and Behavioural Research 1983). Facilitating access to healthcare represents a tangible expression of the value that communities place on life and health.

For individuals, as well as for private providers and commercial interests, healthcare is valued as a private good that can be utilized to preserve or improve health. Markets generally fail to provide a satisfactory distribution of healthcare because the risk of illness is unpredictable, the costs of healthcare can be extremely high, and consumers may have limited information on which to base choices. For these reasons, communities and national governments are usually involved in arrangements for the delivery of healthcare in order to pool risks and regulate healthcare markets. Healthcare also yields benefits that extend beyond individual recipients. The treatment of pulmonary tuberculosis has value in controlling the spread of disease to others. Such positive externalities may be more important to communities than to individuals. Societies may facilitate access to these benefits, as merit goods, which would otherwise be under-produced if individuals only valued their own personal benefits. Extending this argument, it may be desirable to organize healthcare so as to generate public goods that benefit all. Objectives such as the eradication of an infectious disease, or the control of antimicrobial drug resistance, offer benefits that are freely accessible to the global population, with a value that extends beyond national boundaries (Smith et al. 2003).

Guiding principles

Obtaining needed healthcare is sometimes regarded as the responsibility of individuals and families. This is often the case in low-income countries where government or externally funded health services may not be available and families necessarily make out-of-pocket payments to private providers or do not obtain healthcare (van Doorslaer et al. 2006b). In high-income countries, obtaining needed care is sometimes also viewed primarily as an individual responsibility with the government, representing the organized efforts of society, having a minimal role in the regulation of the healthcare market. This libertarian view is often advocated in the United States. One proposed justification is that taxation to provide healthcare for others infringes against individuals' freedom of choice. From this perspective, fairness only concerns basic opportunities to compete for health resources and does not require that a fair distribution of healthcare is realized. A more moderate position is that individual responsibility may be promoted through the use of co-payments, or user charges, that discourage over-consumption of healthcare and reduce moral hazard. However, such charges generally impact disproportionately on the poor, who generally have

Table 2.10.1 Aspects of health and healthcare

Term	Meaning
Healthcare need	Capacity to benefit from healthcare (Stevens et al. 2004)
Health improvement	Population health benefit associated with intervention on the determinants of health
Health gain	Individual or population health benefit associated with healthcare intervention
Health outcome	Change in individual or population health status associated with utilization of needed healthcare
Health system	(1) All the activities whose primary purpose is to improve or maintain health (Murray and Frenk 2000)
	(2) The economic, fiscal, and political management method that nations use to run the national healthcare services (Last 2007)
	(3) A local or regional group of organized health services (Last 2007)
Healthcare	Services provided to individuals or communities by agents of the health services or professions to promote, maintain, monitor, or restore health. Healthcare is not limited to medical care, which implies therapeutic action by or under the supervision of a physician. The term is sometimes extended to include self-care (Last 2001)
Health services	Services that are performed by healthcare professionals, or by others under their direction, for the purpose of promoting, maintaining, or restoring health. In addition to personal healthcare, health services include measures for health protection, health promotion, and disease prevention (Last 2001)

worse health, and can lead to their exclusion from healthcare (Sachs 2012). Many high-income countries have adopted a more egalitarian approach, with the ideal of universal eligibility to services and the objective of equity of access to healthcare (Mossialos and Thomson 2003). This ideal has now been adopted more widely, with a resolution supporting the objective of universal coverage being passed by the United Nations (UN) General Assembly in 2012 (United Nations General Assembly 2012)

The distribution of the outputs of healthcare is also an important concern. From a utilitarian perspective, health services should maximize the health gains obtained across all individuals. This idea is summed up by the slogan 'the greatest good for the greatest number'. This is sometimes regarded as 'the guiding principle for many of the decisions and actions of public health professionals' (Last 2007, p. 385). The objective of maximizing the health gain to be achieved from the available resources is closely related to the economic principle of efficiency. Resources for health will be used most efficiently when health gain is maximized (Table 2.10.2).

The utilitarian approach is problematic because it only requires that the sum of health gains in a population should be maximized, it does not require that all individuals receive a fair distribution of potential benefits from healthcare. In contrast, approaches based on concepts of human rights and social justice view each individual as having a right to health. All individuals are considered to be entitled to healthcare even when the contribution this makes to

the aggregate benefit of the wider community does not require that they receive it (Dworkin 1977). The rights to health and medical care are recognized in the Universal Declaration of Human Rights (United Nations 2007). The International Covenant on Economic, Social and Cultural Rights goes further and requires that governments create 'conditions which would assure all medical services and medical attention in the event of sickness' (Office of the High Commissioner for Human 2007). These international statements do not guarantee that access to needed services will be possible for every individual but they are important in offering a degree of protection to marginalized and vulnerable groups (see Chapter 3.5). An approach based on human rights favours a just or equitable distribution of healthcare over the maximization of potential health gains across the population. The pursuit of equity is also justified in terms of Rawls' theory of justice as fairness, which proposed that a just society will be arranged so as to achieve fair equality of opportunity (Rawls 2007). Daniels (2008) observed that health is an important determinant of the extent of an individual's opportunities and therefore requires special consideration in a fair society. Based on the concepts of human rights and social justice, equity may be regarded as a moral value which health services should strive to promote (Braveman et al. 2001). Equity and efficiency are often viewed as conflicting objectives. For example, delivering equitable access to specialist services in sparsely populated rural areas may compromise efficiency.

Table 2.10.2 Dimensions for evaluation of health services

Dimension	Description
Effectiveness	Extent to which a healthcare intervention achieves the intended outcome (Last 2007)
Efficiency	Outcome achieved in relation to expenditure of resources (Last 2007)
Equity	Fairness, or justice, in respect of treatment of different individuals or groups (Last 2007)
Access	Extent to which services are available, can be utilized, deliver needed services and achieve appropriate outcomes
Appropriateness	Relevance to need (Maxwell 1984)
Responsiveness	Social acceptability (Maxwell 1984)

However, where health services are both inefficient and inequitable, with costly services delivering suboptimal population health outcomes, widening access to cost-effective services may enhance both equity and efficiency.

The conflicting principles underlying the financing and delivery of healthcare outlined in this section are apparent in the differing approaches to facilitating access to health services in different countries. Existing health systems result from compromises that are made through the policy process. In the healthcare systems of high-income countries, collective healthcare provision based on universal eligibility is favoured but individuals may not be prevented from purchasing healthcare privately. Equity of access is an objective, but this is only to the extent to which it is considered acceptable to compromise efficiency. In other systems, such as in the United States or in middle-income countries, private financing of healthcare through insurance or out-of-pocket payments may predominate, but governments may facilitate access to basic health services for vulnerable groups such as the poor and elderly.

Dimensions for evaluation

The diverse objectives, and the complex organization and delivery of healthcare, require evaluation on several different conceptual dimensions. Maxwell (1984) suggested a framework of six dimensions (Table 2.10.2). Each dimension represents a complex, multifaceted concept that is not easily defined. Maxwell's dimensions are reflected in the 'National Scorecard' approach used by the US Commonwealth Fund in its 2011 report (The Commonwealth Fund 2011). This used multiple indicators to evaluate five dimensions of health service performance:

◆ *Access* including the ability to participate in affordable care.

◆ *Efficiency* including appropriate use of resources to deliver cost-effective interventions at appropriate levels of care.

◆ *Equity* including the extent of inequalities in health status and eligibility for, and receipt of care.

◆ *Quality* including the provision of safe, well-coordinated, patient-centred care.

◆ *Healthy lives* including life-expectancy, mortality, activity limitations, and risk factors such as smoking.

Definition of 'access to healthcare'

In general terms, 'access to healthcare' is said to exist when individuals or families can mobilize the resources they need to preserve or improve their health (Gulliford et al. 2002). At the simplest level, having access to healthcare may be judged in terms of the availability of services (Table 2.10.3). This may include the geographical proximity or physical accessibility of services. Availability may also encompass the supply of services in terms of the numbers of doctors, nurses, or hospital beds per 1000 population. At the next level, gaining access to healthcare means that services are utilized when they are needed. There may be considerable barriers to the uptake of services even when these are available. Obstacles to utilization include *affordability* with financial barriers, such as the costs to individuals or households of utilizing care; physical barriers, including distance or difficulties of travel; personal barriers leading to problems of *acceptability*, as when services are not viewed as culturally appropriate, socially acceptable, or consistent with personal beliefs; or organizational barriers, as when there are difficulties obtaining a consultation, or delays in receiving needed treatment, because of waiting lists or limited capacity of services (Aday and Anderson 1981; Pechansky and Thomas 1981). Utilization of services only offers benefit when care provided is relevant to need and effective in addressing people's health problems (Table 2.10.3). Finally, access to healthcare should deliver effective care that meets people's health needs and achieves the intended health outcome.

This traditional, structured approach to the concept of access has been the subject of recent reappraisal. Dixon-Woods et al. (2006) suggested that access should be understood in terms of individuals' *candidacy*, that is their eligibility for healthcare. Candidacy is defined both by individuals' perceptions of their own interests and concerns, as well as by health providers' views of the appropriate roles and spheres of activity for health services. Mooney (2009) argued that access should be understood in terms of the *empowerment* of individuals and communities to gain access to needed health resources. This idea draws attention to the importance of the inequality in power between service providers and more vulnerable service users, in determining who gains access to care, and what services they receive.

Table 2.10.3 Dimensions of access to healthcare

Dimension of access	Meaning	Potential indicators
Availability	Whether there is an adequate supply of health services in an area	• Number of physicians or nurses per 1000 population • Number of hospital beds per 1000 population • Distance to nearest primary care provider • Distance to nearest hospital
Utilization	Whether health services are utilized	• Primary care consultations for 1000 population • Hospital admissions per 1000 population
Relevance to need	Whether appropriate services are received by people who need them	• Proportion of births attended by trained healthcare professional • Proportion of subjects with elevated blood pressure who receive antihypertensive therapy
Outcomes	Whether achievable health outcomes are realized	• Maternal mortality rate • Mortality rate from appendicitis

Definition of equity

Equity in healthcare can be evaluated in several different ways (Table 2.10.4). An important distinction, which is attributed to Aristotle, is the one between horizontal as compared to vertical equity (Gillon 2005). Horizontal equity requires that equals should be treated in proportion to their equality, while vertical equity requires that unequals should be treated in proportion to their inequality. It is generally easier to evaluate horizontal equity, as this requires that all people with the same needs have access to the same services, 'equal access for equal need'. Horizontal inequity in access to healthcare, like inequality in income or health, is often measured using Gini-like metrics known as concentration indices (Mackenbach and Kunst 1997). In reality, different groups in a population often have different needs and require appropriately differentiated services. This is evident, for example, in the healthcare needs of indigenous peoples in Australia whose life expectancy at birth is some 17 years shorter than that of the general population. Mooney posed the question, what would amount to a fair distribution of health resources, given this large difference in health status? (Mooney 1996). There is little consensus on how questions concerning this vertical dimension of equity should be answered. Marginalized groups such as indigenous populations, new migrants, homeless people, or prisoners may be regarded as 'hard to reach' or at least 'underserved' by standard services and there may sometimes be a case for developing targeted services. There is a concern that such targeted services may become 'poor services for poor people'. More generally, there is increasing emphasis on designing local services to meet locally expressed needs, leading to greater variation in the organization and delivery of services, in contrast to the uniform approach implied by the pursuit of horizontal equity. In the United Kingdom, the tension between these two dimensions of equity has been addressed by introducing national level service specifications, while accommodating local discretion in organizing their implementation.

In the following sections, approaches to the relationship between access to health services and population health are divided into those that are predominantly motivated by the pursuit of efficiency and those driven by the goal of greater equity. Two specific questions are addressed: 'How do health services aim to optimize health gains?' and 'How do health services ensure an optimal distribution of health gains?'.

Efficiency-oriented approaches

Underlying problems

Lack of effectiveness

Illich claimed that 'a vast amount of contemporary clinical care is incidental to the curing of disease, but the damage done by medicine to the health of individuals and populations is very significant' (Illich 1976, p. 23). Illich acknowledged that medicine has some effect in preventing and curing infectious diseases through the use of vaccinations and antimicrobial drugs, but he argued that the historical reductions in mortality from infectious diseases in high-income countries occurred before these technologies became available. In his opinion, treatment of non-communicable diseases such as cancer and cardiovascular disease was of negligible benefit and might cause considerable harm (Illich 1976).

Illich's interpretation was supported by McKeown's (1979) analysis of historical trends in mortality in Britain. This analysis was important in identifying the limited role of medicine as a determinant of health in the historical era. For example, relative reductions in mortality between 1881 and 1950 ranged from 30-fold for tuberculosis, 20-fold for digestive diseases, and 15-fold for respiratory disease (Office for National Statistics 1998). Most of these reductions occurred before the widespread use of specific antimicrobial treatment after 1945. These trends support the interpretation that environmental influences, particularly improved nutrition, clean water supplies, and better housing and sanitation, were largely responsible for historical reductions in mortality from infectious diseases in high-income countries with limited gains from health service interventions (McKeown 1979). Wooton (2006) argued that in the historical era, progress in medicine was largely confined to the development of a body of scientific knowledge concerning health and disease. This knowledge was not translated into practical applications and consequently medicine did not develop as a technology for improving health until more recent decades.

A similar argument was developed by Cochrane in his book *Effectiveness and Efficiency* (Cochrane 1972). Cochrane commented on the rising costs of medical care and the dominance of treatment of established disease over preventive medicine. He showed that in many instances there was little evidence available concerning whether medical interventions were beneficial, ineffective, or harmful. When randomized controlled trials (RCTs) were conducted, they often showed that benefits of intervention

Table 2.10.4 Aspects of equity in health and healthcare

Term	Meaning
Equity	Fairness, or justice, in respect of treatment of different individuals or groups (Last 2007)
Horizontal equity	The extent to which equals are treated in proportion to their equality
Vertical equity	The extent to which unequals are treated in proportion to their inequality
Equity in financial contribution	The extent to which individual or household contributions are consistent with their capacity to pay
Equity in access to healthcare	The extent to which there is a fair distribution of access to healthcare in relation to need
Equity in health	The extent to which there is a fair or just distribution of health among individuals and groups in a population
Effective coverage	The proportion of the population in need of an intervention that has received an effective intervention (Shengelia et al. 2005)

were smaller than anticipated and unexpected adverse effects of treatment were not uncommon. Cochrane advocated a now generally accepted view that all healthcare interventions should be tested in RCTs, and the results of all such trials should be systematically collected, analysed, and implemented in clinical practice.

Tradition and professional opinion were, for a long time, the main drivers of clinical practice and the organization and delivery of medical care. However, tradition came under attack through research from epidemiologists and social scientists that questioned the effectiveness of widely used procedures, demonstrated inexplicable variations in clinical practice, widespread problems with medical errors and poor quality of care, and showed that methods for organizing and delivering care were not consistent with patients' wants and needs.

Quality of care and variations in practice

'Quality of care' is a wide-ranging concept that includes departures from optimal standards of healthcare judged on any of Maxwell's dimensions (Maxwell 1984). In Donabedian's framework (Donabedian 2003), quality may be assessed in terms of the organizational structures for care, the processes of care that are delivered, or the health outcomes of care. Problems with quality of care are often revealed through variations in the organization and delivery of care. For example, in Brazil, 72 per cent of women giving birth in private clinics had Caesarean sections, compared with 31 per cent in public hospitals; yet 70–80 per cent of women in either setting expressed a preference for vaginal delivery (Potter et al. 2001). In Pakistan, 68 per cent of subjects in a household survey had received one or more injections for treatment of acute symptoms in the preceding 3 months, with an average of 13.6 injections per person per year. A new needle was reportedly used in only 53 per cent of instances (Janjua et al. 2005). In the United Kingdom, 36 per cent of patients with common colds and upper respiratory infections are prescribed antibiotics (Gulliford et al. 2009). At different family practices the proportion prescribed antibiotics ranged from 0–97 per cent for influenza and 0–84 per cent for common colds (Ashworth et al. 2005).

Variations such as these may originate in uncertainty concerning the optimal use of specific medical interventions. This uncertainty permits the outcome of clinical decisions to be influenced by factors such as the supply of medical services, financial incentives to providers, or practitioner and patient preferences, leading to wide and often idiosyncratic variations in practice. Variations in practice may result in health resources being used inefficiently; in patients being treated in ways that are contrary to their expressed preferences; in the widespread use of potentially harmful procedures; or patients being denied the potential benefits of effective therapy.

Iatrogenic illness and patient safety

Iatrogenic illness and problems with patient safety represent a particular set of concerns with quality of care. Errors in medical care have been shown to be common, especially in hospital settings. In the US Harvard Medical Practice Study of 30,121 subjects from 51 acute hospitals in 1984 (Brennan et al. 1991), injuries caused by medical management occurred in 3.7 per cent of hospital admissions. A quarter of these adverse events were judged to be caused by negligence, 2.6 per cent were permanently disabling, and 13.6 per cent led to death. Based on these results, it was estimated that there may be between 44,000 and 88,000 deaths in the United States annually from errors in medical care (Kohn et al. 2000). In primary care, there may be significant errors in 0.1–1 per 100 consultations (Bhasale et al. 1998). These include delays in diagnosis, wrong diagnoses, errors in prescribing, failure to prescribe needed treatment, and difficulties with communication and referral (Burgess et al. 2012).

Healthcare-associated infections are an increasing problem. A meta-analysis of 220 reports worldwide suggested that about 15 patients per 100 admitted will experience a healthcare-associated infection, with much higher rates in middle- and low-income countries than in Europe and the United States (Allegranzi et al. 2011).

Misallocation of resources and problems in service organization and delivery

The World Health Organization (WHO) has estimated that between 20 and 40 per cent of all health spending is wasted (WHO 2010). A common problem is over-allocation of resources to hospitals. In high-income countries about 70 per cent of health services expenditure is on hospital services, a pattern of expenditure that has been exported to middle- and low-income countries. Hospital-based services generally deliver interventions of low cost-effectiveness compared with those delivered in primary care (World Bank 1993). Other problems concern the relationship between public and private sectors with doctors employed in the public sector often 'moonlighting' in private clinics, or charging for services provided in public clinics (WHO 2000). The private sector may be inadequately regulated. There is often a lack of respect for the comfort, dignity, and concerns of patients (Phillips 1996; Burgess et al. 2012).

Proposed solutions

Clinical effectiveness and health technology assessment

Cochrane's book *Effectiveness and Efficiency* (Cochrane 1972) was influential in leading to the development of strategies for improving clinical effectiveness, including the promotion of 'evidence-based medicine' grounded in the belief that clinical decision-making should be informed as far as possible by the results of well conducted RCTs that provide evidence for the effectiveness of interventions (Sehon and Stanley 2003). This requires that the results of all available RCTs should be analysed in systematic reviews and meta-analyses such as those produced by the Cochrane collaboration. This approach has been extended to cover not just therapeutic interventions but diagnostic techniques, screening strategies, and methods for delivering care under the more general heading of health technology assessment.

Health technology 'includes any method used to promote health, prevent and treat disease and improve rehabilitation or long-term care' (The NHS Health Technology Assessment Programme 2007). Health technology assessment includes evaluation of both the effectiveness and resource use associated with new medical technologies. Cost-effectiveness analysis is now commonly integrated into the implementation of RCTs so that the cost per unit benefit from an intervention may be estimated. Cost–utility analysis allows the health benefits from different interventions to be compared using a common metric such as the quality-adjusted life year (QALY). This permits more explicit comparison of the benefits obtained, and the resources used by different interventions, thus informing choices made in resource allocation decisions.

Processes for assessing population health needs have also been made more explicit, based on the incidence and prevalence of disease and the effectiveness of interventions, so that health services can be designed to deliver services that are relevant to the population's health problems (Stevens et al. 2004).

Quality improvement, implementation research, and patient safety

The increasing availability of objective evidence concerning effective treatment for different conditions has been associated with increased evaluation of medical care against agreed standards. It is clear that there is widespread failure to achieve standards of good clinical practice or to implement fully interventions that have been shown to be effective in RCTs. For example, the technique of cumulative meta-analysis showed a delay of many years between evidence of efficacy and implementation of thrombolytic therapy in myocardial infarction (Lau et al. 1992). These problems have given rise to a new area of research known as 'implementation research' that aims to evaluate and identify methods to encourage health professionals to practice in accordance with evidence-based guidelines (Eccles et al. 2005). Studies in implementation research typically combine a range of interventions such as the provision of guidelines, invitations to educational meetings, provision of advice from respected peers, or the inclusion of prompts in the medical record. Such combinations of interventions commonly offer modest benefits in terms of promoting evidence-based practice (Oxman et al. 1995). In the United Kingdom, the government introduced a system of financial incentives to encourage family doctors to deliver specified processes of care and designated intermediate outcome targets in their patients, with a main emphasis on chronic illness management (Roland 2004). Initial results appear to be favourable (Doran et al. 2011).

Alongside quality improvement initiatives, and requiring similar techniques for implementation, there have been specific initiatives to increase patient safety. In some countries, special organizations have been set up with the brief of improving patient safety through surveillance of critical events, identifying risks, and feeding back information to improve services. The WHO launched a World Alliance for Patient Safety with a headline campaign of 'Clean Care is Safer Care' focusing on safe blood transfusion, injection and immunization, safer clinical procedures, clean water, sanitation and hand hygiene (World Alliance for Patient Safety 2007).

There has also been increasing recognition of the importance of good governance in health services. This includes both *clinical governance*, to ensure that services deliver safe and effective care that is acceptable to users, as well as *organizational governance*, to ensure that organizational objectives are achieved through effective leadership, accountability, and monitoring, with a specific focus on the use of resources.

Systems redesign and service organization and delivery research

The organizational context in which care is delivered is increasingly viewed as important in influencing the effectiveness and efficiency of care (Sheldon 2001). Whether services are delivered in primary or secondary care, by physicians or nurses, by specialist teams or generalists, the financial arrangements, including the payment and reimbursement methods used, may be important in influencing the costs and outcomes of care. The size and workload of an organization, its staffing levels, the management strategies, and organizational culture may also influence the quality and safety of services (Mannion et al. 2005). Consequently there has been an expansion of social science-based research into organization and delivery of health services. This includes investigation of the nature of patient and carer interactions with the health system, the roles of the healthcare workforce, or the impact of organizational change on the various dimensions of quality of care (Fulop et al. 2003). At the same time, there has been a much greater interest in experimentation with different models of organizing care including transferring care from hospital to primary and community settings, utilizing staff with different types of training, integrating specialist skills into primary care service delivery, and making use of new information and communication technologies in delivering services. Such changes have sometimes been facilitated by health sector reforms that remove commissioning and service planning functions from the hands of service providers.

Redesign and modernization of service delivery have been particularly important in the management of chronic conditions. Health services have been designed traditionally to deal with acute episodes of illness but most contacts with health services are now for chronic conditions (Bodenheimer et al. 2002). More than two-thirds of adults in high-income countries have one or more chronic conditions, and chronic conditions account for 80 per cent of primary care consultations and 60 per cent of hospital bed days. The management of chronic conditions requires ongoing surveillance of the patient's condition, management of risk factors, early detection of complications, and education of patients so that they can actively manage their own illness and reduce risk through appropriate lifestyle and behavioural changes. Traditionally designed health services are often very ineffective at delivering services that can achieve these outcomes. The US Institute of Medicine referred to a 'quality chasm' representing the discrepancy between the potential for delivering effective care and the reality of chronic illness management (Institute of Medicine and Committee on Quality of Health Care in America 2005). This has led to the development of new models of service delivery in chronic illness care with a focus on developing care in primary settings, linking appropriately trained staff skilled in education and promoting self-care, with easy access to specialist advice, supported by reliable and easy to use clinical information systems (Bodenheimer et al. 2002).

Investing in Health and essential packages of care

The World Bank's World Development Report for 1993 (World Bank 1993) applied the tools of needs assessment, health technology assessment, and cost-effectiveness analysis to model potential solutions to a range of health problems in middle- and low-income countries. The motivation behind the report was summarized in its title, *Investing in Health*. A healthy population is a major resource that can contribute to stronger economic growth and improving standards of living (Bloom et al. 2004). On average each 10 per cent increase in life expectancy at birth in a country is associated with an increase in economic growth of 0.3–0.4 per cent per year (Commission on Macroeconomics and Health 2001). Improved health can lead to greater productivity because there are more economically active adults, fewer dependent adults affected by illness, children who are better able to participate in education enhancing their productivity as adults, and rising expectations of longevity providing a motivation to save for later life.

The 1993 World Bank Report, and the follow-on second edition of the *Disease Control Priorities* project (Jamison 2007), argued that existing resources for healthcare were utilized extremely inefficiently and that major health gains could be achieved through focused investment in limited packages of highly effective but low-cost clinical interventions and public health measures delivered through health and other services. This investment could be justified in economic terms through the benefits it could bring to productivity and economic growth.

The Global Burden of Disease study and the Disease Control Priorities project were influential in identifying, quantifying, and prioritizing needs for healthcare intervention in countries at different levels of development (Lopez et al. 2006). Using information about the burden of disease and the cost-effectiveness of different interventions it was possible to model the health gain, measured in terms of disability-adjusted life years (DALYs), that could result from different interventions and identify priorities for investment (Table 2.10.5). The World Development Report estimated that a gain of DALYs equivalent to about 25 per cent of the burden of disease in middle- and low-income countries could be achieved through implementation of programmes of low-cost public health interventions, partly delivered through health services, as well as essential cost-effective clinical services (World Bank 1993). A recommended package of essential measures included extended and increased uptake of immunization, improved nutrition education and micronutrient supplementation, treatment of sick children, and reproductive health interventions including prevention and treatment of sexually transmitted diseases and safe motherhood. It was estimated that significant health gains could be achieved with little additional overall cost to governments, through disinvestment from public spending on what it termed 'discretionary clinical services' including interventions of low cost-effectiveness delivered in hospital settings.

The World Development Report contributed to an important shift in thinking in several respects. Providing health services to the poor in middle- and low-income countries was no longer to be regarded as a weak form of buffering against the consequences of poverty. Instead, delivering health interventions to the poor was viewed as attacking the causes of poverty and contributing towards establishing conditions that could lead to economic growth, providing households with a route out of a continuing cycle of poverty and illness. Following on from the publication of the report, the WHO established a Commission on Macroeconomics and Health (2001) whose report endorsed the importance of preventing and treating disease as a means of promoting wealth as well as health. This facilitated the mobilization of resources for health in middle- and low-income countries. A Global Fund was established to attract funds to be directed towards programmes for the prevention and treatment of AIDS, tuberculosis, and malaria (The Global Fund 2007). The GAVI Alliance (formerly the Global Alliance on Vaccines and Immunisation) was set up to promote immunization programmes in the poorest countries through both public and private sector funding (GAVI Alliance 2007).

The World Development Report was also important in encouraging a more explicit approach to rationing of services and priority setting for health investment, justified by the extent of health gains that could be achieved through this approach. For example, it is estimated that for a cost of US $1 million the loss of 50,000–500,000 DALYs could be averted through extended vaccine coverage, the loss of 50,000–125,000 DALYs could be averted through improved malaria treatment programmes. Estimates such as these encouraged governments to promote the notion of universal access to essential services. Updated estimates were published for the global burden of disease and risk factors (Lopez et al. 2006) and revised estimates for the costs and effectiveness of different packages of intervention were published (Laxminarayan et al. 2006; Jamison 2007). These included a growing appreciation of the present and likely future impact of chronic non-communicable diseases affecting adults in middle- and low-income countries, together with a recognition that selected interventions for these conditions could be very cost-effective. The WHO has developed the concept of 'effective coverage' (Table 2.10.4) as a measure of the extent to which health services deliver appropriate interventions to those groups of people who need them. Effective coverage is defined as the proportion of the population in need of an intervention that receives an effective intervention (Shengelia et al. 2005).

The thinking in *Investing in Health* was also influential in high-income countries. For these countries, a major implication is that appropriate healthcare as well as population strategies to promote health are important for containing the costs associated with an ageing population and a high prevalence of chronic illness. In the United Kingdom, the Treasury commissioned a former chief executive of a leading bank to examine the case for increasing investment in health services (Wanless 2004). His

Table 2.10.5 Selected cost-effectiveness estimates from the *Disease Control Priorities Project* (2nd ed.)

Service or intervention	Cost per DALY (US $)	Estimated DALYs averted per million US $ spent
Care of infants under 28 days old	10–400	2500–100,000
Expanding immunization coverage with standard childhood vaccines	2–20	50,000–500,000
Treating sexually transmitted infections to interrupt HIV transmission	50–200	5000–20,000
Using antiretroviral therapy that achieves high adherence for a high proportion of patients	350–500	2000–3000
Treating myocardial infarction with an inexpensive set of drugs	10–25	40,000–100,000
Performing coronary artery bypass grafting for high-risk cases (e.g. disease of left main coronary artery)	>25,000	<40

report recognized the increasing costs associated with chronic conditions and argued for the need 'to invest in reducing demand by enhancing the promotion of good health and disease prevention' (p. 3) with 'health services evolving from dealing with acute problems through more effective control of chronic conditions to promoting the maintenance of good health' (Wanless 2004, p. 10).

Criticisms of the essential package of care approach

The essential package of care concept represents a rational, utilitarian approach to addressing urgent health needs in the context of scarcity of resources. However, the projected benefits of the essential package of care approach have rarely been realized through successful implementation (WHO 2013). In reality, the elements of the package must be determined through negotiation, both at the planning stage and during implementation. Pressure from stakeholders, including patients and professionals, may cause the package to be expanded to address other health needs or different elements of care. Proposed disinvestment from specialist services of low-cost effectiveness is unlikely to prove politically acceptable (Gwatkin et al. 2004). Cost-effectiveness analysis is useful in defining the set of interventions that should be delivered by health services but has a more limited role in defining the systems that should be organized to deliver them. A study in Malawi found that although there was an agreed essential package of care, there were important barriers to implementation including insufficient trained healthcare workers and inadequate supplies of essential drugs and equipment (Mueller et al. 2011). The appropriateness of disease-focused intervention strategies has been debated (Taylor et al. 1997; Hopkins 2013). The resources allocated to intensified intervention against a single disease might arguably be invested in long-term efforts to strengthen health systems that can deliver interventions for a range of priority conditions (Taylor et al. 1997). These arguments point to the need for the development of health systems that offer access to affordable care to everyone.

Equity-oriented approaches

Equity in healthcare may be evaluated in terms of the availability and use of health services, as well as in terms of health outcomes (Table 2.10.6).

Availability of services

Table 2.10.6 provides illustrative data for indicators of health services availability for several countries at different levels of economic development (World Bank 2006). It is clear that the countries with the lowest incomes and worst health also have the smallest share of resources committed to health services. In the high-income countries, per capita expenditure on health is some 200 times greater than in the low-income countries and health conditions, measured in terms of life expectancy at birth, are substantially better. These variations among countries illustrate enormous inequality in distribution of healthcare resources, and access to healthcare, at the global level.

Table 2.10.6 also illustrates considerable variation among countries in the same income category. There is variation in the overall level of resources devoted to the health sector; in the relative proportions of public and private sector spending and out-of-pocket expenditure; as well as variation among countries in health outcomes at a given level of expenditure on health. For example, among middle-income countries, Costa Rica has been successful at mobilizing resources for health and life expectancy is higher than expected. Among the high-income countries, the United States is unusual in having exceptionally high health expenditure but life expectancy is lower than expected. These variations reflect societal views of the purpose of health services and the nature of policies, institutions, and community responses to questions of health and healthcare, in addition to the availability of resources.

Health services in middle- and low-income countries do not often provide universal population coverage. Gwatkin characterized health systems in middle- and low-income countries as

Table 2.10.6 Health expenditures, healthcare resources, and life expectancy at different levels of economic development (2010)

	Gross national income per capita (2010 $)	Health expenditure (per cent GDP)	Public expenditure (% total)	Out of pocket (% total)	Health expenditure per capita (dollars)	Doctors per 1000 population	Hospital beds per 1000 population	Life expectancy at birth (years)
Low income								
Kenya	790	4.8	44.3	42.7	37	–	1.4	56
Pakistan	1050	2.2	38.5	50.5	22	0.8	0.6	65
Middle income								
Albania	3960	6.5	39.0	60.8	241	1.2	2.8	77
Costa Rica	6810	10.9	68.1	27.8	811	–	1.2	79
Indonesia	2500	2.6	49.1	38.3	77	0.3	0.6	69
High income								
Japan	41,850	9.5	82.5	14.3	4065	2.1	13.7	83
United Kingdom	38,200	9.6	83.9	10.0	3503	2.7	3.3	80
United States	47,340	17.9	53.1	11.8	8362	2.4	3.0	78

Source: data from World Bank, *World Development Indicators 2012*, World Bank Washington, DC, USA, Copyright © 2012. Data for 2010.

'consistently inequitable, providing more and higher quality services to the well-off, who need them less, than to the poor, who are unable to obtain them' (Gwatkin et al. 2004, p. 1273). In some of the more affluent middle-income countries, such as the small islands of the Caribbean, government services offer access to primary care services that are mainly used by the poor, while private practitioners' services are utilized by the better off. However, as national income decreases, government expenditure on healthcare as a percentage of gross domestic product (GDP) declines and population coverage by government services diminishes (Table 2.10.6). Services tend to be concentrated close to urban areas, where they may be more readily utilized by better-off groups leading to a markedly pro-rich distribution of expenditure on government health services. The distribution of expenditure on primary healthcare services generally shows a lesser degree of inequity than all healthcare spending (Fig. 2.10.1). In rural areas, access to government health services may be extremely limited, with non-governmental organizations such as religious bodies and charities sometimes offering alternative sources of provision. Geographical barriers to accessing services are important not only in terms of distance but also in terms of the difficulty and costs of travelling long distances to access services. In some regions, the rapid pace of urbanization may lead to situations in which large populations of urban poor may have limited access to any health services.

In China, the lack of availability of rural health services was addressed between 1965 and the early 1980s by the development of 'barefoot doctors'. These were rural farm workers who were given basic health training over several months in order to provide a combination of traditional Chinese and Western medicines to rural communities. The 'barefoot doctor' approach was regarded as a model for the development of community health workers in other countries and provided an important inspiration for the 1978 Alma Ata Declaration that initiated the 'Health for All' strategy. The Alma Ata Declaration promoted access to primary care, with an emphasis on community participation and universality, as a means of facilitating equity in health. The importance of the concept of primary healthcare was restated in the 2008 World Health Report (WHO 2008) which advocated primary care as a route to reducing inequalities in health outcomes.

Definition of primary healthcare

There are several definitions of primary healthcare. The WHO makes a distinction between primary healthcare, which encompasses public health activities directed at environmental determinants of health, and primary medical care, including first point of contact care in the community. The English Department of Health defines primary healthcare simply as care provided outside hospitals by family health services (including family physicians, dentists, pharmacists, and opticians) and community health services (including community doctors, dentists, nurses, midwives and health visitors, and other allied professions). Other definitions characterize primary healthcare according to key attributes (Table 2.10.7). Primary care providers are community based, easily accessible, and offer population coverage. Primary care provides the first point of contact with the health system and is comprehensive in its scope, addressing all potential health problems. Primary care also provides ongoing care over time

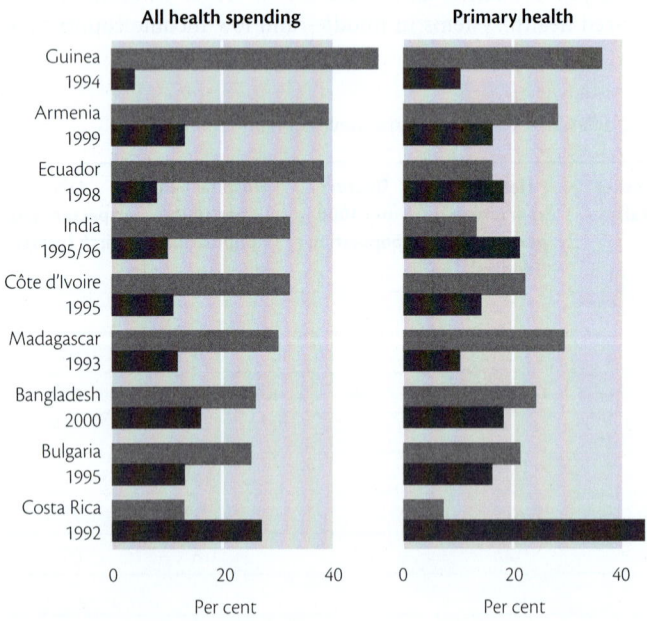

Fig. 2.10.1 Share of public spending that accrues to the richest (top bar) and poorest fifths (bottom bar) of the population.

Reproduced with permission from World Bank, *World Development Report 2004: Making services work for poor people*, World Bank, Washington DC, USA, Copyright © 2004 The World Bank Group, All Rights Reserved.

Table 2.10.7 Primary medical care: definition and key elements

Definition of primary medical care
Care which provides integrated, accessible health care services by clinicians who are accountable for addressing a large majority of personal healthcare needs, developing a sustained partnership with patients, and practising in the context of family and community (Institute of Medicine 1994)

Characteristics of primary medical care

Attribute	Meaning
Universal	Population-based, open to everyone
Accessible	Enabling people to use services when they are needed
Community-based	Placing the patient within the wider familial or social context necessary for addressing multiple causes of illness
First point of contact	Providing entry into the health system
Comprehensive	Addressing most personal care needs including preventive, curative and rehabilitative
Continuity	Providing care that is patient-focused over time
Coordination	Coordinating and regulating use of other levels of care
Affordable	Consistent with capacity to pay

Source: data from Macinko J et al., *The contribution of primary care systems to health outcomes within Organization for Economic Cooperation and Development (OECD) countries, 1970–1998*, Health Services Research, Volume 38, Issue 3, pp. 831–65, Copyright © 2003 John Wiley & Sons, Inc. All Rights Reserved.

with continuity or longitudinality representing a key element in most definitions. Primary care services are generally less costly and more affordable than specialist services. In high-income countries, primary medical care practitioners generally have a gatekeeper role in which they regulate and coordinate access to specialist care (Starfield 1992). However, specialist expertise is increasingly being embedded in primary care teams in order to improve the quality of chronic illness management (Bodenheimer et al. 2002).

Through its emphasis on universality, accessibility, and affordability, primary medical care generally promotes equity of access to healthcare. Through its community orientation and emphasis on out-of hospital care, primary medical care generally enhances efficiency through the application of more cost-effective and appropriate health technologies. The gatekeeper role of the primary care practitioner generally has the consequence of promoting more efficient utilization of resources compared with systems where individual patients can gain direct access to specialists.

Inverse care law

Inequality in the availability of health services is a concern for all countries. Without regulation, the supply of healthcare resources is distributed towards more affluent areas with fewer health needs. This situation was described by the British general practitioner Julian Tudor Hart as an 'inverse care law' with 'the availability of good medical care tending to vary inversely with the need for it in the population served' (Tudor Hart 1971, p. 405).

In countries which, like the United Kingdom, have a dominant national health service funded from general taxation, this situation has been addressed through the development and application of explicit formulae linking the allocation of resources for hospital and community services in different areas to measures of population size and health needs. The number of primary care doctors in an area is also regulated. Nevertheless, historical patterns of the supply of services have been resistant to change and socioeconomically deprived areas continue to have fewer doctors and less well-developed primary care facilities. Similar resource allocation methods have been recommended for application to public services in middle- and low-income countries (Laxminarayan et al. 2006.) In countries, with more pluralistic systems of providing care, or where fee-for-service payment is dominant, greater inequities in the supply of services develop. For example, in US cities the poor are significantly 'underserved' by health services both because of inequalities of supply and because of financial barriers to accessing care (National Research Council 2003). In most countries, the rural poor are significantly disadvantaged by relative or absolute lack of availability of services.

Availability of primary care and population health

Does the availability of primary healthcare contribute to improved population health? In general, those countries that have followed policies emphasizing universal primary healthcare coverage have achieved more favourable health outcomes. The Cuban health system is frequently cited as one that has successfully adopted the primary care approach. In 2009, life expectancy at birth in Cuba was 76 years in men and 80 years in women, compared with 77.4 years in the United States, and the infant mortality rate was 7.2 per 1000 in both countries in spite of the great disparity in economic conditions (Pan American Health Organization 2007). In Costa Rica, commitment to the development of public health

services and primary care has been associated with favourable health outcomes and the second highest life expectancy in the Americas (Table 2.10.6) (Unger et al. 2007).

Evidence is also provided by ecological analyses from high-income countries. In the United States, states with a greater supply of family physicians have lower mortality rates after adjusting for income inequality and smoking (Shi et al. 1999). In the United Kingdom, districts with higher supply of family physicians have lower mortality from all causes but this association is sensitive to adjustment for several measures of healthcare needs. Hospital utilization shows a strong negative association with the supply of primary care physicians (Gulliford 2002). In an analysis of data for 18 Organisation for Economic Cooperation and Development (OECD) countries, Macinko and colleagues (Macinko et al. 2003) suggested that the strength of a country's primary healthcare system is associated with lower all-cause mortality and reduced premature years of life lost from all causes and from respiratory and cardiac disease.

Utilization of services

Donabedian (2003) argued that utilization of services represented proof of access to healthcare. The availability of services does not ensure that those who need them will use them and there may be important personal, financial, or organizational barriers to the uptake of services. Patterns of utilization may not be consistent with medically defined need, as when people do not take up preventive services, delay in presenting with serious conditions, or utilize services for apparently trivial conditions. In many health systems, the financial cost of utilizing healthcare may present a very significant barrier to utilization. McIntyre and colleagues (McIntyre et al. 2009) identified *affordability* and *acceptability* as important dimensions of access, alongside service *availability*.

Financial barriers to access

Fees paid by service users as out-of-pocket expenditures are important in funding healthcare in middle- and low-income countries (Table 2.10.6). This impacts disproportionately on those who are poor or sick (WHO 2010). This has the consequence that poor people may be unable to obtain needed healthcare, or may find it necessary to utilize less costly and less appropriate forms of care such as private drugs vendors. People may delay accessing care until their illness becomes more severe, requiring more costly treatment. Health expenditures for serious illness may then be catastrophic leading to impoverishment of households. Xu and colleagues (Xu et al. 2003) reported a study of catastrophic health expenditures, defined as health expenditure exceeding 40 per cent of household income after subsistence needs were met. More than 2 per cent of households in 17 out of 59 countries experienced catastrophic expenditures. Based on between-country comparisons, high healthcare expenditures were more likely if health services require direct out-of-pocket payment, if households have limited capacity to pay, and if methods to pool risks were lacking. In Asia, illness is one of the principal, reasons for households falling into poverty. Across eleven Asian countries, if household expenditures on healthcare are taken into account, then an additional 2.7 per cent of the population (78 million people) live in absolute poverty with household incomes of less than US $1 per person per day when compared with conventional estimates (van Doorslaer et al. 2006b). Frenk observed a paradox that while healthcare should be an important factor in reducing poverty, expenditure on healthcare is itself a cause of poverty (Frenk 2006).

The 2010 World Health Report (WHO 2010) analysed these issues and advanced the principle that there should be reduced reliance on direct, out-of-pocket, payments for healthcare, with greater use of 'pre-payment' through taxation or insurance to finance healthcare. These approaches should provide a mechanism for increasing population coverage, with the risk of illness pooled across the population, so that healthcare for the sick is under-written by the healthy, and for the poor by the wealthy (WHO 2010, p. 5). This approach was subsequently endorsed by a UN resolution in 2012. Recent Mexican health reforms provide an example from a middle-income country, with the introduction of a new form of health insurance that extended coverage of the poor and provided access to a set of basic medical interventions (Frenk et al. 2006).

Sachs (2012) suggested that, in low-income settings, 'universal coverage' should be understood in terms of coverage with a minimum package of low-cost interventions to meet basic health needs. This should initially focus on maternal and child health needs, communicable disease control, and nutrition, with a more selective approach for non-communicable diseases and injuries. However, universal access to even a minimum package might cost considerably more than the maximum available revenues in a typical low-income country indicating a requirement for substantial additional external resources to achieve universal coverage (Sachs 2012).

Healthcare utilization in high-income countries

Many studies have evaluated the overall impact of barriers to the utilization of medical care in high-income countries that, with the exception of the United States, generally offer universal healthcare coverage. In a recent study, the utilization of physician services was evaluated in relation to respondents' self-rated needs for care (van Doorslaer et al. 2006a). Gini-like indices of horizontal inequity were estimated to summarize the utilization of care in relation to household income level. The results showed that utilization of primary care visits was generally either equitably distributed among income groups, or showed a pro-poor distribution. However, utilization of specialists' services generally showed some degree of pro-rich inequity, that is higher-income groups utilized more specialist care than lower-income groups at a given level of need. This is a consistent finding from a number of studies and suggests that higher socioeconomic position, including higher income or education, may facilitate access to specialist care through increased ability to negotiate financial or organizational barriers. These results from a range of countries suggest that in many instances a degree of equity of access to primary care has been achieved, but inequity persists in the utilization of specialist care.

Socioeconomic groups differ not only with respect to the volume of care consumed but also with respect to the type of care utilized. There is a considerable body of evidence to show that preventive medical interventions are taken up less by lower socioeconomic groups, with a risk of increasing inequalities in health. In Belgium, for example, overall utilization of family physician services showed substantial pro-poor inequity, but there was marked pro-rich inequity in the uptake of influenza vaccination, cholesterol testing, mammography, and cervical cancer screening (Lorant et al. 2002). Problems of poor quality care typically vary between socioeconomic groups with disadvantaged groups receiving lower quality care. The US Institute of Medicine has reviewed a large and consistent body of evidence to show that US black and ethnic minority populations are less likely to receive needed care even after allowing for socioeconomic variables including insurance status, income, age, and severity of condition (National Research Council 2003). For example, there are lower rates of utilization of appropriate cardiac treatment including coronary artery bypass surgery, lower rates of renal dialysis, or transplantation, but higher rates of unfavourable events such as diabetes-related lower limb amputations.

Healthcare and population health

Perceptions of the role of health services as a determinant of population health have evolved. Historically, medical care was of limited importance as a determinant of health; medical care was often ineffective and had a considerable capacity for causing harm. In the twentieth century, however, the pace of technological innovation accelerated and from 1948 onwards the application of RCTs to evaluate the effectiveness of health technologies was increasingly accepted. Effective interventions came to be widely used. These included vaccination and immunization against infectious disease, screening for early stages of cancer, treatment of risk factors for cardiovascular disease, or treatment services for the major causes of mortality. The impact of the widespread implementation of such interventions on population health is difficult to evaluate because of the contribution of wider and more powerful determinants of population health cannot be readily controlled as they might be in a randomized trial. Three main approaches have been used to evaluate the impact of healthcare on population health indicators.

The 'sentinel indicator' approach supposes that if a given condition is amenable to medical intervention, then there should be few or no deaths from the condition. Mortality rates may be used as sentinel indicators of the effectiveness of healthcare services. For example, if surgical services are effective then there should be few deaths from acute appendicitis, cholecystitis, or abdominal hernia. This method was developed and implemented extensively by Holland (1991) who mapped the distribution of 'avoidable' deaths in Europe.

If a health service intervention is implemented across a population over a short space of time, changes in trends in mortality or morbidity may be used to evaluate the effectiveness of the intervention. There have been well-documented reductions in the incidence of infectious diseases following the implementation of new vaccination programmes. There have also been changes in mortality from cancer following the implementation of screening programmes. This approach is complicated by underlying secular trends in disease incidence as well as by changes over time in the effectiveness of case management.

Modelling approaches to the evaluation of health service effectiveness vary in their sophistication but all utilize evidence concerning the incidence and prevalence of disease, the effectiveness of clinical interventions, and the expected coverage and quality of services in the population at risk. This information is used to estimate the contribution of medical care to real or projected changes in mortality or other health outcomes in populations of interest.

Healthcare and population health: high-income countries

Bunker and colleagues (Bunker et al. 1994) modelled the contribution of medical care to life expectancy in the US population.

Their report concluded that medical care, including preventive and treatment services, contributed about 5 years additional life expectancy in the United States with potential for gain of an additional 1.5–2 years if effective interventions were implemented more completely, with improved population coverage, and higher standards of care. In a more recent study, Cutler et al. (2006) estimated changes in life expectancy at birth in the United States between 1960 and 2000. The cumulative increase in life expectancy during this period was 6.97 years with reduced mortality from cardiovascular disease accounting for 4.88 years (70 per cent) and reduced rates of infant deaths accounting for 1.35 years (19 per cent). Based on Bunker's estimates, as well as analyses of the decline in mortality from cardiovascular disease (Unal et al. 2004), Cutler et al. (2006) attributed half of this increased life expectancy to more effective medical intervention. Several examples illustrate the substantial benefits to be obtained from effective medical care.

Survival with human immunodeficiency virus

The first illustration concerns the survival of people who are infected with the human immunodeficiency virus (HIV). Lohse et al. (2007) compared the survival of HIV-infected individuals in Denmark with that of controls matched for age, sex, and place of residence drawn from the general population. The estimated median survival of incident HIV cases after 25 years of age was 7.6 years in 1995–1996, 22.5 years in 1997–1999, and 32.5 years in the period 2000–2005. This dramatic improvement in survival following diagnosis was attributed to the introduction of highly active antiretroviral therapy (HAART). This improvement is all the more remarkable when it is remembered that HIV was first identified in 1984. This example illustrates the capability of medical care to change the clinical course of a condition. In this case HIV became a chronic disease requiring active medical therapy over many years, with a prognosis similar to that of insulin-treated type 1 diabetes mellitus. Indeed, before insulin treatment became available, the prognosis of type 1 diabetes was similar to, or worse than, that of HIV infection in the pre-HAART era.

Breast cancer mortality

Another example concerns mortality from breast cancer, the most frequent cancer among women in high-income countries. In the United Kingdom, population-based mammographic screening was introduced for women aged 50–64 years after 1988. The decision to introduce screening was based on strong, but disputed, evidence from RCTs (Gotzsche and Olsen 2000; Nystrom et al. 2002). Around this time, there was also accumulating evidence for increasing survival following clinical diagnosis through more effective use of specific therapies, including the oestrogen receptor antagonist tamoxifen as well as other newer drugs. An analysis of breast cancer mortality for women aged 55–69 years in England and Wales, showed an estimated 21.3 per cent reduction in breast cancer mortality between 1990 and 1998 compared with the predicted trend (Blanks et al. 2000). The authors estimated that approximately one-third of this decrease could be attributed to breast cancer screening with two-thirds of the reduction attributed to improved treatment. Allgood et al. (2008) compared women who died of breast cancer with control women who did not die and found that attending for breast screening was associated with between a 35 per cent and 65 per cent reduction in odds of mortality depending on assumptions. Cancer Research UK

(2007) reported that 5-year survival of women diagnosed with breast cancer increased from 52 per cent in 1971–1973 to 85 per cent in 2005–2009. The example of breast cancer illustrates the difficulty of analysing longer-term outcomes of health service interventions. Analysis required estimation of the secular trend, in this case increasing, as well as separate effects of a population screening intervention and the outcomes of improved clinical treatment.

Coronary heart disease mortality

These same difficulties are also evident in the third example, which concerns the impact of healthcare on declining mortality from coronary heart disease (CHD). In Finland, as in a number of other high-income countries, CHD mortality has been declining since the 1960s. During the 1980s and 1990s a number of new therapies were introduced, whose effectiveness had been demonstrated in large RCTs. These included more effective drug therapy for patients with myocardial infarction, angina, or heart failure as well as coronary artery bypass surgery for patients with angina. There were also declining trends in the major risk factors for CHD including elevated cholesterol and blood pressure levels and cigarette smoking. Based on observed trends in risk factors and uptake of specific therapies, Laatikainen and colleagues (Laatikainen et al. 2005) estimated that about 53 per cent of the reduction in CHD mortality in Finland between 1982 and 1997 could be attributed to changes in risk factor levels, while 23 per cent could be attributed to more effective medical care, including secondary prevention, in those affected by the condition. In England and Wales, CHD mortality declined by 62 per cent in men and 45 per cent in women between 1981 and 2000, and about 42 per cent of the decline was attributed to medical intervention (Unal et al. 2004).

These analyses of CHD trends and their determinants raise important questions concerning the priority to be given to prevention efforts through population strategies as compared to healthcare intervention, contributing 'high-risk' approaches to primary prevention and to secondary and tertiary prevention in those with established disease. Comparison of the potential costs and outcomes of population strategies for primary prevention, as compared to medical care intervention, should generally favour the former. However, the dominant epidemiological approach to evaluation, the RCT, lends itself most readily to the evaluation of medical care interventions. The application of epidemiological designs to the evaluation of population-wide prevention strategies has generally given disappointing results (Ebrahim and Smith 2001). This may have encouraged epidemiologists to give undue priority to medical care interventions with less attention given to the implementation and evaluation of population strategies. For example, Wald and Law (2003) used the results of meta-analyses of clinical trials to support the concept that a 'polypill' containing a number of effective but low-cost pharmaceuticals (a statin, three blood pressure-lowering drugs, as well as aspirin and folic acid) may have the potential to prevent up to 80 per cent of stroke and CHD deaths. However, a pill is not a panacea for a lifetime of exposure to unhealthy risks and a strategy grounded in the high-risk approach may not be appropriate for population-wide implementation.

Access to care and inequalities in health

In high-income countries, the consequences of inequities in healthcare access may not be easy to discern because problems resulting from inadequate healthcare are not easily distinguished from the consequences of inequalities in the wider determinants of health, often sustained over generations. Here, promoting a greater degree of equity of access to healthcare than already exists is not usually viewed as a major strategy for reducing inequalities in health. Instead, inequalities in the wider determinants must be addressed more directly. This does not mean, however, that it is not important to ensure that all groups have equal access to the benefits offered by effective healthcare interventions, with access to preventive medical interventions over the life-course being key to reducing inequalities in healthy life expectancy (Acheson 1998).

Some indirect evidence suggests that inequity in access to specialist care may contribute to inequalities in health in high-income countries. In England and Wales, there are substantial socioeconomic inequalities in survival with cancer that have been increasing over time and are greater for treatable cancers (Coleman et al. 2004). For example, the difference in 5-year survival between the highest and lowest quintiles of deprivation in women is 5.8 per cent for breast cancer, 8.3 per cent for rectal cancer, and 7.3 per cent for colon cancer, compared with 0.2 per cent for oesophageal cancer, a less treatable condition. Evidence such as this has been used to advocate the routine implementation of 'equity audit' as part of routine service evaluation. In the United States, there are significant black–white inequalities in mortality, with life expectancy for black men being 6.3 years lower, and for women 4.5 years less, than for white people. Cardiovascular disease and diabetes account for 35 per cent of this difference in men and 52 per cent in women (Harper et al. 2007). Differential access to healthcare may contribute to these differences (National Research Council 2003).

In order to promote equity in health, new policies and services have sometimes been implemented on the basis of their potential to reduce inequalities in health. In England, following a White Paper on cigarette smoking, smoking cessation services were developed in deprived areas, providing nicotine replacement therapy free of charge (Chambers 1999). Universal antenatal and newborn screening programmes for sickle cell disease and thalassaemia were implemented with specific recognition of their potential to reduce health inequalities associated with black and ethnic minority status (Sassi et al. 2001). At local level, outreach services have been developed to target specific groups such as homeless people with serious mental illness.

Healthcare and population health: middle- and low-income countries

Millennium Development Goals

While sentinel events, such as maternal and child deaths, are an infrequent occurrence in high-income countries, this is not so in middle- and low-income countries. The health-related Millennium Development Goals (MDGs) were designed to reduce maternal and child mortality, as well as reducing deaths from tuberculosis, malaria, and other diseases. Focused strategies for intervention have been advocated to achieve these objectives. There are four main strands to the strategy to reduce child mortality, including better treatment of complications for newborn infants, integrated management for childhood illnesses, expanded programmes for immunization, and improved nutrition for infants and young children. In the context of a 2015 target for the achievement of the MDGs, reports have evaluated progress towards these targets. Rates of maternal and child deaths have been declining overall, but

the rate of decline is generally lower in those regions with highest mortality rates (Lozano et al. 2011). At present rates of progress, it is unlikely that the targets for health outcomes will be achieved until considerably later than intended, reflecting continuing difficulties in accessing healthcare. At the same time, the growing prevalence of chronic non-communicable diseases coming on top of an existing high burden of infectious diseases, is contributing to a 'double burden' of disease in middle- and low-income countries. The importance of universal health coverage has therefore received increasing attention as a key route to addressing these problems (WHO 2010) and was advocated by a resolution of the UN General Assembly in 2012 (United Nations General Assembly 2012). There are many obstacles to achieving universal coverage, including the absolute shortage of resources in the poorest countries, weak governance in public services, and problems in the relationship with the private sector (Moreno-Serra and Smith 2012; Sachs 2012). However, recent empirical analyses suggest that there are substantial population health benefits associated with increasing access to health services by increasing government health expenditures and reducing the share of out-of-pocket health expenditure (Moreno-Serra and Smith 2012).

Conclusion

This chapter started by asking 'What is the role of health services in improving population health?'. It went on to distinguish two separate questions: 'How can health gains be maximized?' and 'How should health gains be distributed?'. The negative argument that health services have little impact on population health is untenable. Modern healthcare offers a wide range of interventions of proven effectiveness that when implemented widely can be shown, at least indirectly, to contribute to improving trends in population health status in countries at different levels of economic development. Population health gains can be increased by investing resources in the most cost-effective interventions, by increasing effective coverage of the population, increasing quality of care, and optimizing systems for organizing and delivering care. Inequalities in health continue to be sustained by the inequalities in distribution of the determinants of health both within and between countries. While a degree of equity of access to primary care has been achieved in high-income countries, this is generally far from being the case in middle- and low-income countries. The challenge now is to ensure that all groups obtain a fair share of the benefits of healthcare intervention. Public health specialists should advocate principles of efficiency and universal coverage and contribute to realizing these through participation in processes of needs assessment, health technology assessment, quality improvement, and facilitating access to needed healthcare for all groups.

References

Acheson, E.D. (1998). *Independent Inquiry into Inequalities in Health.* London: The Stationery Office.

Aday, L.A. and Anderson, R.M. (1981). Equity of access to medical care: a conceptual and empirical overview. *Medical Care*, 19(Suppl.), 4–27.

Allegranzi, B., Nejad, S.B., Combescure, C., et al. (2011). Burden of endemic health-care-associated infection in developing countries: systematic review and meta-analysis. *The Lancet*, 377, 228–41.

Allgood, P.C., Warwick, J., Warren, R.M., Day, N.E., and Duffy, S.W. (2008). A case-control study of the impact of the East Anglian breast screening programme on breast cancer mortality. *British Journal of Cancer*, 98, 206–9.

Ashworth, M., Charlton, J., Ballard, K., Latinovic, R., and Gulliford, M. (2005). Variations in antibiotic prescribing and consultation rates for acute respiratory infection in UK general practices 1995–2000. *British Journal of General Practice*, 55, 603–8.

Bhasale, A.L., Miller, G.C., Reid, S.E., and Britt, H.C. (1998). Analysing potential harm in Australian general practice: an incident-monitoring study. *Medical Journal of Australia*, 169, 73–6.

Blanks, R.G., Moss, S.M., McGahan, C.E., Quinn, M.J., and Babb, P.J. (2000). Effect of NHS breast cancer screening programme on mortality from breast cancer in England and Wales, 1990–8: comparison of observed with predicted mortality. *British Medical Journal*, 321, 665–9.

Bloom, D.E., Canning, D., and Jamison, D.T. (2004). Health, wealth and welfare. *Finance and Development*, 41, 10–15.

Bodenheimer, T., Wagner, E.H., and Grumbach, K. (2002). Improving primary care for patients with chronic illness: the chronic care model, part 2. *JAMA: The Journal of the American Medical Association*, 288, 1909–14.

Braveman, P., Starfield, B., Geiger, H.J., and Murray, C.J.L. (2001). World Health Report 2000: how it removes equity from the agenda for public health monitoring and policy. Commentary: comprehensive approaches are needed for full understanding. *British Medical Journal*, 323, 678–81.

Brennan, T.A., Leape, L.L., Laird, N.M., et al. (1991). Incidence of adverse events and negligence in hospitalized patients. Results of the Harvard Medical Practice Study I. *The New England Journal of Medicine*, 324, 370–6.

Bunker, J.P., Frazier, H.S., and Mosteller, F. (1994). Improving health: measuring effects of medical care. *Milbank Quarterly*, 72, 225–58.

Burgess, C., Cowie, L., and Gulliford, M. (2012). Patients' perceptions of error in long-term illness care: qualitative study. *Journal of Health Services Research & Policy*, 17, 181–7.

Cancer Research UK (2007). *Breast Cancer Survival Statistics*. London: Cancer Research UK.

Chambers, J. (1999). Being strategic about smoking. *British Medical Journal*, 318, 1–2.

Cochrane, A.L. (1972). *Effectiveness and Efficiency. Random Reflections on Health Services*. London: Nuffield Provincial Hospitals Trust.

Coleman, M.P., Rachet, B., Woods, L.M., et al. (2004). Trends and socio-economic inequalities in cancer survival in England and Wales up to 2001. *British Journal of Cancer*, 90, 1367–73.

Commission on Macroeconomics and Health (2001). *Macroeconomics and Health: Investing in Health for Economic Development. Report of the Commission on Macroeconomics and Health*. Geneva: World Health Organization.

Cutler, D.M., Rosen, A.B., and Vijan, S. (2006). The value of medical spending in the United States, 1960–2000. *The New England Journal of Medicine*, 355, 920–7.

Daniels, N. (2008). *Just Health*. Cambridge: Cambridge University Press.

Dixon-Woods, M., Cavers, D., Agarwal, S., et al. (2006). Conducting a critical interpretive synthesis of the literature on access to healthcare by vulnerable groups. *BMC Medical Research Methodology*, 6, 35.

Donabedian, A. (2003). *An Introduction to Quality Assurance in Health Care*. Oxford: Oxford University Press.

Doran, T., Kontopantelis, E., Valderas, J.M., et al. (2011). Effect of financial incentives on incentivised and non-incentivised clinical activities: longitudinal analysis of data from the UK Quality and Outcomes Framework. *British Medical Journal*, 342, d3590.

Dworkin, R. (1977). *Taking Rights Seriously*. London: Duckworth.

Ebrahim, S. and Smith, G.D. (2001). Exporting failure? Coronary heart disease and stroke in developing countries. *International Journal of Epidemiology*, 30, 201–5.

Eccles, M., Grimshaw, J., Walker, A., Johnston, M., and Pitts, N. (2005). Changing the behavior of healthcare professionals: the use of theory

in promoting the uptake of research findings. *Journal of Clinical Epidemiology*, 58, 107–12.

Frenk, J. (2006). Bridging the divide: global lessons from evidence-based health policy in Mexico. *The Lancet*, 368, 954–61.

Frenk, J., Gonzalez-Pier, E., Gomez-Dantes, O., Lezana, M.A., and Knaul, F.M. (2006). Comprehensive reform to improve health system performance in Mexico. *The Lancet*, 368, 1524–34.

Fulop, N., Allen, P., Clarke, A., and Black, N. (2003). From health technology assessment to research on the organisation and delivery of health services: addressing the balance. *Health Policy*, 63, 155–65.

GAVI Alliance, G. (2007). *GAVI Alliance*. [Website] Available at: http://www.gavialliance.org/.

Gillon, R. (2005). *Philosophical Medical Ethics*. Chichester: John Wiley.

Gotzsche, P.C. and Olsen, O. (2000). Is screening for breast cancer with mammography justifiable? *The Lancet*, 355, 129–34.

Gulliford, M., Figueroa-Munoz, J., Morgan, M., et al. (2002). What does 'access to health care' mean? *Journal of Health Services Research & Policy*, 7, 186–8.

Gulliford, M., Latinovic, R., Charlton, J., Little, P., van Staa, T., and Ashworth, M. (2009). Selective decrease in consultations and antibiotic prescribing for acute respiratory tract infections in UK primary care up to 2006. *Journal of Public Health*, 31, 512–20.

Gulliford, M.C. (2002). Availability of primary care doctors and population health in England: is there an association? *Journal of Public Health Medicine*, 24, 252–4.

Gwatkin, D.R., Bhuiya, A., and Victora, C.G. (2004). Making health systems more equitable. *The Lancet*, 364, 1273–80.

Harper, S., Lynch, J., Burris, S., and vey Smith, G. (2007). Trends in the black–white life expectancy gap in the United States, 1983–2003. *JAMA: The Journal of the American Medical Association*, 297, 1224–32.

Holland, W.W. (1991). *European Community Atlas of 'Avoidable Death'* (2nd ed.). Oxford: Oxford Medical Publications.

Hopkins, D.R. (2013). Disease eradication. *The New England Journal of Medicine*, 368, 54–63.

Illich, I. (1976). *Limits to Medicine. Medical Nemesis: The Expropriation of Health*. Harmondsworth: Penguin Books.

Institute of Medicine (1994). *Defining Primary Care. An Interim Report*. Washington, DC: National Academies Press.

Institute of Medicine and Committee on Quality of Health Care in America (2005). *Crossing the Quality Chasm: A New Health System for the 21st Century*. Washington, DC: National Academy Press.

Jamison, D.T. (2007). Investing in health. In D.T. Jamison, J.G. Breman, A.R. Measham, et al. (eds.) *Disease Control Priorities in Developing Countries*, pp. 3–34. Washington, DC: World Bank.

Janjua, N.Z., Akhtar, S., and Hutin, Y.J.F. (2005). Injection use in two districts of Pakistan: implications for disease prevention. *International Journal for Quality in Health Care*, 17, 401–8.

Kohn, L.T., Corrigan, J.M., and Donaldson, M.S. (2000). *To Err is Human*. Washington, DC: National Academy Press.

Laatikainen, T., Critchley, J., Vartiainen, E., Salomaa, V., Ketonen, M., and Capewell, S. (2005). Explaining the decline in coronary heart disease mortality in Finland between 1982 and 1997. *American Journal of Epidemiology*, 162, 764–73.

Last, J.M. (2001). *Dictionary of Epidemiology*. Oxford: Oxford University Press.

Last, J.M. (2007). *A Dictionary of Public Health*. Oxford: Oxford University Press.

Lau, J., Antman, E.M., Jimenez-Silva, J., Kupelnick, B., Mosteller, F., and Chalmers, T.C. (1992). Cumulative meta-analysis of therapeutic trials for myocardial infarction. *The New England Journal of Medicine*, 327, 248–54.

Laxminarayan, R., Mills, A.J., Breman, J.G., et al. (2006). Advancement of global health: key messages from the Disease Control Priorities Project. *The Lancet*, 367, 1193–208.

Lohse, N., Hansen, A.B., Pedersen, G., et al. (2007). Survival of persons with and without HIV infection in Denmark, 1995 to 2005. *Annals of Internal Medicine*, 146, 87–95.

Lopez, A.D., Mathers, C.D., Ezzati, M., Jamison, D.T., and Murray, C.J.L. (2006). Global and regional burden of disease and risk factors, 2001: systematic analysis of population health data. *The Lancet*, 367, 1747–57.

Lorant, V., Boland, B., Humblet, P., and Deliege, D. (2002). Equity in prevention and health care. *Journal of Epidemiology and Community Health*, 56, 510–16.

Lozano, R., Wang, H., Foreman, K.J., et al. (2011). Progress towards Millennium Development Goals 4 and 5 on maternal and child mortality: an updated systematic analysis. *The Lancet*, 378, 1139–65.

Macinko, J., Starfield, B., and Shi, L. (2003). The contribution of primary care systems to health outcomes within Organization for Economic Cooperation and Development (OECD) countries, 1970–1998. *Health Services Research*, 38, 831–65.

Mackenbach, J.P. and Kunst, A.E. (1997). Measuring the magnitude of socio-economic inequalities in health: an overview of available measures illustrated with two examples from Europe. *Social Science & Medicine*, 44, 757–71.

Mannion, R., Davies, H.T., and Marshall, M.N. (2005). Cultural characteristics of 'high' and 'low' performing hospitals. *Journal of Health Organization and Management*, 19, 431–9.

Maxwell, R.J. (1984). Quality assessment in health. *British Medical Journal*, 288, 1470–2.

McIntyre, D., Thiede M., and Birch S. (2009). Access as a policy relevant concept in low- and middle-income countries. *Health Economics Policy and Law*, 4, 179–93.

McKeown, T. (1979). *The Role of Medicine*. Oxford: Blackwell.

Mooney, G. (1996). And now for vertical equity? Some concerns arising from aboriginal health in Australia. *Health Economics*, 5, 99–103.

Mooney, G. (2009). Is it not time for health economists to rethink access and equity? *Health Economics Policy and Law*, 4, 209–21.

Moreno-Serra, R. and Smith, P.C. (2012). Does progress towards universal health coverage improve population health? *The Lancet*, 380, 917–23.

Mossialos, E. and Thomson, S. (2003). Access to health care in the European Union: the impact of user charges and voluntary health insurance. In M.C. Gulliford and M. Morgan (eds.) *Access to Health Care*, pp. 143–73. London: Routledge.

Mueller, D.H., Lungu, D., Acharya, A., and Palmer, N. (2011). Constraints to implementing the Essential Health Package in Malawi. *PLoS One*, 6, e20741.

Murray, C.J. and Frenk, J. (2000). A framework for assessing the performance of health systems. *Bulletin of the World Health Organization*, 78, 717–31.

National Research Council (2003). *Unequal Treatment: Confronting Racial and Ethnic Disparities in Health Care (2003)*. Washington, DC: National Academies Press.

Nystrom, L., Andersson, I., Bjurstam, N., Frisell, J., Nordenskjold, B., and Rutqvist, L.E. (2002). Long-term effects of mammography screening: updated overview of the Swedish randomised trials. *The Lancet*, 359, 909–19.

Office for National Statistics (1998). *Mortality Statistics: Cause, England and Wales*. Series DH2. Number 25. London: Office for National Statistics.

Office of the High Commissioner for Human Rights (2007). *International Covenant on Economic, Social and Cultural Rights*. Geneva: Office of the High Commissioner for Human Rights.

Oxman, A.D., Thomson, M.A., Davis, D.A., and Haynes, R.B. (1995). No magic bullets: a systematic review of 102 trials of interventions to improve professional practice. *Canadian Medical Association Journal*, 153, 1423–31.

Pan American Health Organization (2007). *Regional Core Health Data System. Country Profile: Cuba*. Data updated for 2001. Available at: http://www.paho.org/.

Pechansky, R. and Thomas, W. (1981). The concept of access. *Medical Care*, 19, 127–40.

Phillips, D. (1996). Medical professional dominance and client dissatisfaction: a study of doctor–patient interaction and reported dissatisfaction with medical care among female patients at four hospitals in Trinidad and Tobago. *Social Science & Medicine*, 42, 1419–25.

Potter, J.E., Berquo, E., Perpetuo, I.H.O., et al. (2001). Unwanted caesarean sections among public and private patients in Brazil: prospective study. *British Medical Journal*, 323, 1155–8.

President's Commission for the Study of Ethical Problems in Medicine and Biomedical and Behavioural Research (1983). *Securing Access to Health Care*. Washington, DC: US Government Printing Office.

Rawls, J. (2007). *Theory of Justice*. Cambridge, MA: Harvard University Press.

Roland, M. (2004). Linking physicians' pay to the quality of care—a major experiment in the United Kingdom. *The New England Journal of Medicine*, 351, 1448–54.

Sachs, J.D. (2012). Achieving universal health coverage in low-income settings. *The Lancet*, 380, 944–7.

Sassi, F., Archard, L., and Le Grand, J. (2001). Equity and the economic evaluation of healthcare. *Health Technology Assessment*, 5, 1–138.

Sehon, S.R. and Stanley, D.E. (2003). A philosophical analysis of the evidence-based medicine debate. *BMC Health Services Research*, 3, 14.

Sheldon, T.A. (2001). It ain't what you do but the way that you do it. *Journal of Health Services Research & Policy*, 6, 3–5.

Shengelia, B., Tandon, A., Adams, O.B., and Murray, C.J.L. (2005). Access, utilization, quality, and effective coverage: an integrated conceptual framework and measurement strategy. *Social Science & Medicine*, 61, 97–109.

Shi, L., Starfield, B., Kennedy, B., and Kawachi, I. (1999). Income inequality, primary care, and health indicators. *Journal of Family Practice*, 48, 275–84.

Smith, R., Beaglehole, R., Woodward, D., and Drager, N. (2003). *Global Public Goods for Health. Health Economic and Public Health Perspectives*. Oxford: Oxford University Press.

Starfield, B. (1992). *Primary Care: Concept, Evaluation and Policy*. New York: Oxford University Press.

Stevens, A., Raftery, J., and Mant, J. (2004). The epidemiological approach to health care needs assessment. In A. Stevens, J. Raftery, J. Mant, and S. Simpson (eds.) *Health Care Needs Assessment: The Epidemiologically Based Needs Assessment Reviews*, pp. 1–15. Oxford: Radcliffe Medical Press.

Taylor, C.E., Cutts, F., and Taylor, M.E. (1997). Ethical dilemmas in current planning for polio eradication. *American Journal of Public Health*, 87, 922–5.

The Commonwealth Fund (2011). *Why Not the Best? Results from the National Scorecard on US Health System Performance, 2011*. Washington, DC: The Commonwealth Fund.

The Global Fund (2007). The Global Fund to Fight AIDS, Tuberculosis and Malaria. [Website] Available at: http://www.theglobalfund.org.

The NHS Health Technology Assessment Programme (2007). *Health Technology Assessment*. Available at: http://www.nets.nihr.ac.uk/programmes/hta.

Tudor Hart, J. (1971). The inverse care law. *The Lancet*, i, 405–12.

Unal, B., Critchley, J.A., and Capewell, S. (2004). Explaining the decline in coronary heart disease mortality in England and Wales between 1981 and 2000. *Circulation*, 109, 1101–7.

Unger, J.P., De Paepe, P., Buitron, R., and Soors, W. (2007). Costa Rica: achievements of a heterodox health policy. *American Journal of Public Health*, 98, 636–43.

United Nations (2007). *Universal Declaration of Human Rights*. New York: United Nations.

United Nations General Assembly (2012). *Resolution on Universal Health Coverage*. New York: United Nations General Assembly.

van Doorslaer, E., Masseria, C., Koolman, X., for the OECD Health Equity Research Group (2006a). Inequalities in access to medical care by income in developed countries. *Canadian Medical Association Journal*, 174, 177–83.

van Doorslaer, E., O'Donnell, O., Rannan-Eliya, R.P., et al. (2006b). Effect of payments for health care on poverty estimates in 11 countries in Asia: an analysis of household survey data. *The Lancet*, 368, 1357–64.

Wald, N.J. and Law, M.R. (2003). A strategy to reduce cardiovascular disease by more than 80%. *British Medical Journal*, 326, 1419.

Wanless, D. (2004). *Securing Good Health for the Whole Population. Final Report*. London: HMSO.

Wooton, D. (2006). *Bad Medicine: Doctors Doing Harm Since Hippocrates*. Oxford: Oxford University Press.

World Alliance for Patient Safety (2007). *Clean Care is Safer Care*. Geneva: World Health Organization.

World Bank (1993). *World Development Report 1993*. New York: World Bank and Oxford University Press.

World Bank (2006). *World Development Indicators 2006*. Washington, DC: World Bank.

World Health Organization (2000). *The World Health Report 2000*. Geneva: WHO.

World Health Organization (2008). *Primary Health Care. Now More Than Ever. The World Health Report 2008*. Geneva: WHO.

World Health Organization (2010). *Health Systems Financing. The Path to Universal Coverage*. Geneva: WHO.

World Health Organization (2013). *Essential Health Service Packages*. Geneva: WHO.

Xu, K., Evans, D.B., Kawabata, K., Zeramdini, R., Klavus, J., and Murray, C.J.L. (2003). Household catastrophic health expenditure: a multi-country analysis. *The Lancet*, 362, 111–17.

SECTION 3

Public health policies, law, and ethics

3.1

Leadership in public health

Manuel M. Dayrit and Maia Ambegaokar

Introduction to leadership in public health

Imagine that tomorrow you were suddenly appointed into a prominent health leader position in your country—as a Director of Department or perhaps even Minister of Health. Upon taking office, you are presented with the following urgent dilemmas by your chief advisers:

◆ We are suffering perennial outbreaks of water-borne diarrhoea in the urban slums of our largest city, caused by the illegal tapping of water lines. How can we prevent this in both the short and long terms?

◆ Other departments are preventing us enacting any measures to stop smoking in public places. How can we convince them to collaborate on this critical health issue?

◆ How can we take steps to provide antiretrovirals for the tens of thousands of our citizens suffering from HIV/AIDS?

◆ Our government is in moral opposition to abortion, despite scientific evidence showing that decriminalizing abortion prevents maternal deaths from sepsis. Illegal abortion is high in our country. What action should we take?

How would you proceed to address these issues? Would you be able to think on your feet and respond promptly and effectively to the health needs of your populace? In other words, are you capable of being a public health leader?

Think about these questions as we explore the nature of leadership and the possibility of learning it.

Overview of leadership in public health

There is growing recognition of the importance of leadership in public health. This is reflected in recent domestic and international initiatives to train or 'develop' leaders in the health sector (Wright et al. 2001; Cardenas et al. 2002; Saleh et al. 2004; Umble et al. 2005), to identify the skills and personal qualities of leaders (Wright et al. 2000; NHS Leadership Centre 2006), and to assess the effect of different types of leadership on outcomes (Firth-Cozens and Mowbray 2001; Xirasagar et al. 2005). In this chapter, we examine what is involved in public health leadership. We set four tasks: to define the difference between management and leadership; to describe the core competencies and personal

characteristics of leaders; to discuss whether leadership can be taught; and to demonstrate why leadership is so important in public health. We argue that it is the complex, multiorganizational, and team-based nature of health work that necessitates leadership at many levels in order to result in success.

There is an urgent need around the world for strong public health leaders to promote the health of populations, particularly the poor and vulnerable. Unfortunately, calls for stronger and better leadership are often taken as imprecise and unachievable demands. In this chapter, we attempt to circumvent that accusation by demonstrating that effective leaders have existed and continue to exist in health, and that strong leadership can be encouraged and developed. In addition, we have built the chapter on findings from interviews with individual health sector leaders.

At the end of the chapter, we turn to the targeted reader of this book—an early-to-mid-career public health worker—and suggest ways to develop his or her own 'path to leadership'. We urge the aspiring health leader not to forget the inseparable link between what is needed for leadership to occur and the kind of principled leadership most required in global health today.

Among the chapter's most important points:

◆ There is a distinction between leadership and management. Leadership has to do with the visionary activities of setting direction, while management has to do with the controlling tasks associated with implementation.

◆ Leadership is fundamentally about influence. Academic thinking about leadership has evolved from a focus on the characteristics of the individual leader to a more complex understanding of the dynamic interaction between leaders and followers in specific contexts. But there is no established 'science of leadership', as there is in medicine.

◆ Public health leaders need to be able to imagine and create evidence-based change. They need to be able to influence and lobby key actors for support of their public health agenda. They must operate across disciplinary and organizational boundaries, and they must be skilled at developing and working through diverse teams.

◆ Leaders are not simply born. Public health leaders can be developed by means of team-based training, mentoring, and repeated practice of leadership skills at all levels and all types of public health organizations. The aspiring health leader can create her or his path to leadership.

◆ Public health challenges are often politically and procedurally complex and do not lend themselves to simple medical or technical solutions. A set of guiding principles will help the leader to define appropriate actions.

Leadership is not the same as management

Much literature and research conflate leadership and management, but the two are not identical:

> 'Management' derives from the Latin word 'manus' (meaning hand) and the subsequent Italian word 'maneggiare' (to control, often horses)...'Leadership', however, is from the Old German word 'Lidan' and the Old English derivation 'lithan' (to travel, to show the way, to guide). (Grint 2002, p. 248)

This distinction between the controlling tasks associated with implementation and the visionary activities associated with setting a direction is a useful, if simplified, way of defining management as compared to leadership. In practice, the two are often linked, in a single individual or in a particular job description. As a result, separating the characteristics of good leadership from those of good management is not straightforward.

To a certain extent, the confusion arises because historical reviews of research on leadership often begin with the early research on what makes a good manager. For example, Stone and Patterson (2005) begin with Max Weber's interest in bureaucratic hierarchies as an efficient solution to getting things done in the workplace. This led to classical management theory, with its emphasis on using the bureaucracy to achieve objectives, and scientific management theories with their focus on 'control, ruthless efficiency, quantification, predictability, and de-skilled jobs' (Stone and Patterson 2005, p. 2). In this context, managers who could organize and direct workers below them in the hierarchy were crucial. There was little emphasis, during this period in the early part of the twentieth century, on the behavioural aspects of organizations. Instead, workers were seen as machine-like, and managers needed only to establish and oversee the correct procedures. By the middle of the twentieth century, management theorists shifted their focus to the factors that motivate people at work and the ways in which managers could harness motivation to achieve results. 'A new theory of organizations and leadership began to emerge based on the idea that individuals operate most effectively when their needs are satisfied' (Stone and Patterson 2005, p. 3). In this context, good managers were perceived as those who could do more than structure the work and give orders. They also needed to inspire their workers to lead them.

The tendency to link the characteristics of good managers with those of leaders is thus partly the result of changes in the understanding of the role of a manager. Still, the distinction between the leadership role and the managerial role is widely perceived as the difference between vision and implementation.

These distinctions between leaders and managers apply as well in the health sector. For example, the director of a health district might choose to have an operations director who manages the finances and daily implementation, thus allowing her/ himself the freedom to develop strategies and engage diverse actors in a shared vision of the district's health goals. A hospital, to give another example, needs a manager who with limited finances can organize and implement a detailed schedule of surgeries involving people, equipment, and other resources. However, a hospital also needs a leader who can motivate staff to provide high-quality work in the context of budget restrictions. Sometimes these skills and job responsibilities may exist in the same person, but the nature of management tasks differ from leadership tasks.

In this chapter, we are particularly interested in leadership, rather than management. We do not mean to imply that competent management is not important. On the contrary, the ability to take care of the controlling tasks associated with implementation is crucial to the delivery of programmes and services in public health, and certainly research and funding are needed to improve management in order to strengthen the functioning of health systems (see, for example, Egger et al. 2005). However, the current interest in public health leadership is in itself worth exploring. Public health requires people who can move the agenda in a world dominated by the politics of vested interest groups. It requires individuals who can take scientific evidence and use it to change the direction of policy. This calls for 'big picture' skills and the ability to influence people both inside and outside the public health field.

If we are not mainly interested here in management, we are also not only concerned with leadership within organizations. 'Leadership deals with interpersonal influence, and management deals with acquiring and allocating resources to achieve work, unit or organisational goals' (Campbell 2013, p. 412). Leadership is, therefore, broader than the leading of employees within organizations. Leadership takes place in all social and political contexts. In public health, leaders are needed not only in hospitals and department divisions, but also in local, regional, and national government, in other related sectors like education and in large- and small-scale settings. For a broader understanding of leadership, we turn next to a review of academic thinking about leadership.

Evolution of thinking about leadership

Research on leadership, like that on management, has evolved over time (Van Wart 2003). More than a century ago, thinking about leadership focused on the inherent personality of the individual leader: 'This 'Great Man Theory' approached leadership capacities as innate, fixed and cross-contextual...the leader as solitary actor' (Turning Point 2001, p. 14).

This 'great leader' theory was deepened, in the first part of the twentieth century, by attempts to identify the key 'traits' or 'attributes' of successful leaders. Leadership attribute research was still focused on the individual, not the context. This research has continued into the present day and has generated many lists of leader traits (Zaccaro et al. 2013), including some specific to the health sector, as we show in the next section.

The 'special individual' has certainly been invoked in the health sector. For example, Halfdan Mahler, a former head of the World Health Organization (WHO), and James Grant, a former head of UNICEF, were widely thought to have innate leadership qualities that largely explained the success of their agendas. When we interviewed people who had risen to public health leadership positions within their countries and internationally (for an earlier version of this chapter), we noted that leaders are often people who are willing to take risks and to do things that defy convention. However, research and thinking on the question of leadership moved on in the middle of the twentieth century to a 'contingency' approach (Van Wart 2003), taking into account the attributes not only of the leader, but also of the followers and the context in which he or she leads, for a more nuanced understanding of leadership success. While acknowledging that 'the essence of leadership is influence', this approach accepts that 'no single leader trait…or style explains leadership in all circumstances' and focuses instead on 'the dynamics of leadership—the coming together of leader and follower behaviour in a social and/or organisational context' (Rumsey 2013a, pp. 1, 2, and 6).

One corollary of the contingency approach is the use of parables or stories to illustrate types of leadership. Stories serve the purpose of simplifying the underlying psychology, sociology, political economy, etc., that might provide theoretical explanations of leadership success. Box 3.1.1 provides some examples, and many others can be imagined. The author argues not only that such stories are explanatory but also that successful leaders use their 'wisdom, intelligence and creativity to synthesize stories' that suit their own traits, the context and the followers (Sternberg 2013).

This method of understanding leadership through simplified parables has the value of demonstrating that many different personality types and various character traits may be suited to leadership roles. It also shows that context matters—the level of the leader in the organization, the type and number of followers, the stability of the setting all interact with the leader's traits (Rumsey 2013b). Among the many variables that may play a role in explaining leadership success are the interpersonal situation, emotional situation, and psychological situation of the leader and followers, as well as the organizational or cultural system of norms and practices and the economic setting (Klimoski 2013).

> Simply stated, context presents the leader with any number of situations…; it offers opportunities and constraints. Yet it also should be clear that our current theories or models do not do an adequate job in capturing the various ways that context can, and especially will play out. (Klimoski 2013, p. 283)

Thinking about leadership has thus evolved to acknowledge the great complexity involved in achieving or understanding leadership success. This is a striking change from the earliest 'great man' theories:

> [C]omplexity leadership [thinking] challenges traditional leadership [thinking] at almost every turn: It challenges the assumptions that individuals are independently responsible for their own failures and successes, or that successful organisations need foster only their human capital (largely ignoring their social capital). It debunks the heroic leader and top-down coordination strategies so central to leadership studies in the 20th century. (Marion 2013, pp. 198–9)

Box 3.1.1 Leadership stories

- The carpenter—the leader who can build a new organization or society.
- The CEO—the leader who can 'get things done'.
- The communicator—the leader who can communicate with diverse followers.
- The conqueror—the leader who is going to conquer all enemies.
- The conserver—the leader who will make sure things stay the wonderful way they are.
- The cook—the leader who has the recipe to improve the life of his or her followers.
- The deep thinker—the leader who will make sense out of what is going on.
- The defender—the leader who will save all followers from harm.
- The deity—the leader who presents him or herself as saviour.
- The diplomat—the leader who can get everyone to work together.
- The doctor—the leader who can cure what is wrong with the organization.
- The ethicist—the leader who pledges to clean up the place.
- The lifesaver—the leader who will rescue followers from otherwise certain death.
- The organizer—the leader who can create order out of chaos.
- The plumber—the leader who can fix all the leaks.
- The politician—the leader who understands how 'the system' works.
- The replicator—the leader who is going to be like some past individual.
- The scout—the leader who can lead followers to new and uncharted territory.
- The ship captain—the captain of a ship navigating through turbulent times.
- The turn-around specialist—the leader who can turn around a failing organization.
- The warrior chieftain—the leader who will lead followers to fight, defensively or offensively, enemies, seen or unseen.

Reproduced from Robert J. Sternberg, 'The WICS Model of Leadership' pp. 47– 62 in Michael G. Rumsey (ed.), *Oxford Handbook of Leadership*, Oxford University Press, New York, USA, Copyright © 2013, by permission from Oxford University Press USA.

In addition, many contemporary settings have seen developments 'such as team emphasis, delegation, participative decision-making, flatter organisational structures, self-managed work teams and telecommuting, [that] have rendered leader-centred approaches obsolete' (Hollander 2013, p. 139). For a leader, achieving results in such a context requires not just the use of skills that will enable individuals to get things done, but also the ability to facilitate disparate group efforts by collaborating and sharing the leadership task: 'we have shifted from a view of leader as sole or unitary actor to a team or community centred view of leadership...from a hierarchical model of leadership into collaborative models' (Turning Point 2001, p. 15). In public health, the collaborative approach may be a necessity, as we illustrate in later sections of this chapter dealing with the complexity inherent in public health practice.

This shift in the way of thinking about leadership—from a top–down model to a participatory one— does not alter the ongoing interest in understanding the competencies and attributes of good leaders. Next we consider these, with an emphasis on health sector contexts.

Leadership competencies, personal qualities, and behaviours

The literature on leadership is replete with definitions and lists of leadership characteristics. In this section, we present two that are particularly thorough and intuitively useful in public health. However, we do so with a couple of caveats. First, research on leadership has not yet presented definitive descriptions, much less definitive prescriptions. As Grint (2002, p. 249) says: 'a science of leadership...has proved incredibly elusive...[and yet] there are indeed plenty of leadership recipes on the market'. In the health sector, this is as true as in other sectors.

Second, there is reason to be concerned that some of the elements of these lists may be 'culture-bound' and thus more accurate in the North American and European settings in which they were developed. Some research has identified culture-specific differences in observed leadership traits and 'many scholars have argued that the effectiveness of a given leadership style varies across cultures in important ways' (Kumar and Chhokar 2013, p. 238). For example, 'participatory' working behaviour may be more relevant in some cultural contexts than others (Flahault and Roemer 1986). In addition, 'directive [as opposed to supportive] leadership seems to be more problematic in individualistic cultures' (Kumar and Chhokar 2013, p. 234). Having said this, there is no harm in advocating the leadership behaviours presented in the two lists in the following sections—such as acting with high ethical integrity, developing an evidence-based vision of the future, and empowering others to work towards public health goals—whatever the cultural context.

Competencies of leaders in health

What do we expect leaders in public health to be able to do? One comprehensive list (Wright et al. 2000) defines the following core competencies of public health leaders:

1. *Transformation*—public health needs and priorities require leaders to engage in systems thinking, including analytical and critical thinking processes, envisioning of potential futures, strategic and tactical assessment, and communication and change dynamics.

2. *Legislation and politics*—the field of public health requires leaders to have the competence to facilitate, negotiate, and collaborate in an increasingly competitive and contentious political environment.

3. *Transorganization*—the complexity of major public health problems extends beyond the scope of any single stakeholder group, community unit, profession or discipline, organization, or government unit, thus requiring leaders with the skills to be effective beyond their organizational boundaries.

4. *Team and group dynamics*—effective communication and practice are accomplished by leaders through building team and work group capacity and capability (Wright et al. 2000, p. 1204).

In other words, public health leaders need to be able to imagine and create evidence-based change; they need to be able to influence and lobby politicians for support of their public health agenda; they must operate across disciplinary and organizational boundaries; and they must be skilled at developing and working through diverse teams. The authors go on to give more detail about each competency area (Wright et al. 2000). We present a summary in Table 3.1.1. In a practical way, the information in this table answers the question: what do public health leaders do?

Interviews with public health leaders suggest that this is an appropriate list of the types of skills public health leaders need and use in varying degrees. All the leaders we interviewed for an earlier version of this chapter had some vision of an alternate future to which they are committed. Whether it was to improve the health services in a remote location of a country, strengthen the performance of an international public health bureaucracy, or lead research towards better understanding of breast cancer, each had a vision of contributing towards improving the people's health and well-being. Interviewees acknowledged the necessity of working in the political arena, although the extent of political engagement much depended on whether their job allowed them the opportunity to do so. The frustration of not being able to exert influence effectively beyond the health sector was a frequent observation. This confirmed the importance of working trans-organizationally as well as trans-sectorally. Working with ministries of finance was a frequently cited example of doing so. The interviewees acknowledged the critical importance of collaborative work, of building and working in teams. However, it was also suggested by some interviewees that the conventional way in which medical doctors were trained did not necessarily provide them with the skills to work collaboratively in public health teams.

Personal characteristics of leaders

The ability to conduct the change-related, trans-organizational, political, and team-building activities associated with public health leadership seems to rely on a core set of personal qualities. One particularly useful summary argues for a framework of 15 qualities important in a public health leader, broken down into three groups: *personal*, *cognitive*, and *social* qualities (NHS Leadership Centre 2006).

As Fig. 3.1.1 demonstrates, at the core are the five personal qualities of *self-belief*, *self-awareness*, *self-management*, *drive for improvement*, and *personal integrity*. The five cognitive qualities at the top make possible the necessary analytical and procedural skills: *seizing the future*, *intellectual flexibility*, *broad scanning*, *political astuteness*, and *drive for results*. These are then rounded off by five social qualities at the bottom: *leading change through*

Table 3.1.1 Competencies needed by leaders in public health

Creating change	Influencing politics	Working trans-organizationally	Building teams
Visionary leadership Be able to articulate an evidence-based vision of the future and incorporate it into strategy	*Political processes* Determine appropriate actions on policy and political issues, organize key actors to cooperate for regulatory and legislative changes, and translate policies into programmes and services	*Understanding of organizational dynamics* Assess and develop systems structures based on an understanding of culture and organizational behaviour	*Develop team-oriented structures and systems* Change system infrastructure to encourage innovative, learning teams
Sense of mission Facilitate the development of a mission, communicate it, and 'model' it through personal behaviour	*Negotiation* Mediate potential crises, bargain, and coordinate with key stakeholders	*Inter-organizational collaborating mechanisms* Involve key actors and networks across a broad range of organizations and groups in collaborative coalitions	*Facilitate development of teams* Empower, motivate, and reward teams *Serve in facilitation and mediation roles* Negotiate and intervene to help teams function
Effective change agent Think creatively and analytically about systems and change strategies, and facilitate dialogue and empowerment of others to take action	*Ethics and power* Identify and use alliances based on ethical principles *Marketing and education* Use social marketing and health education to influence key audiences	*Social forecasting* Analyse trends and communicate predictions to consortium partners	*Serve as an effective team member* Through own behaviour, 'model' the key characteristics of listening, encouraging and motivating while displaying integrity, commitment, and honesty

Source: data from Wright, K. et al., Competency development in public health leadership, *American Journal of Public Health*, Volume 90, Issue 8, pp. 1202–7, Copyright © 2000 American Public Health Association.

people, holding to account, empowering others, effective and strategic influencing, and *collaborative working.*

The ten qualities associated with 'setting direction' and 'delivering the service' shown as the outer ring of the doughnut in Fig. 3.1.1 can be viewed as another way of presenting the same basic material we have illustrated in Table 3.1.2. But the core personal qualities presented at the centre of the doughnut are worth emphasizing because they represent the personal behaviour of a leader. These core personal characteristics explain *how* leaders are able to do what they do. Self-belief, for example, is a 'positive "can do" sense of confidence which enables [outstanding leaders] to be shapers rather than followers, even in the face of opposition' (NHS Leadership Centre 2006, p. 4). Leaders are also self-aware. They know their own emotions and learn from mistakes (NHS Leadership Centre 2006, p. 13). Leaders demonstrate self-management. They are 'tenacious and resilient' in complex and difficult working environments (NHS Leadership Centre 2006, p. 5). They do not lose control, but manage their emotions (NHS Leadership Centre 2006, p. 14). Public health leaders have a vocation that feeds a 'drive for improvement': 'Outstanding leaders are motivated by wanting to make a real difference to people's health...[by] investing their energy in bringing about health improvements—even to the extent of wanting to leave a legacy which is about effective partnerships, inter-agency working and community involvement [rather than their own reputation]' (NHS Leadership Centre 2006, p. 5). And finally, leaders demonstrate personal integrity: 'a strongly held sense of commitment to openness, honesty, inclusiveness and high [ethical and performance] standards' (NHS Leadership Centre 2006, p. 16).

This NHS Leadership Centre framework of the personal characteristics of leaders is reinforced by consideration of one recent academic review summarizing leader attributes cited in scholarly reviews of leadership (not specifically in health) over many decades (Zaccaro et al. 2013). Among the domains identified are the following (excerpts):

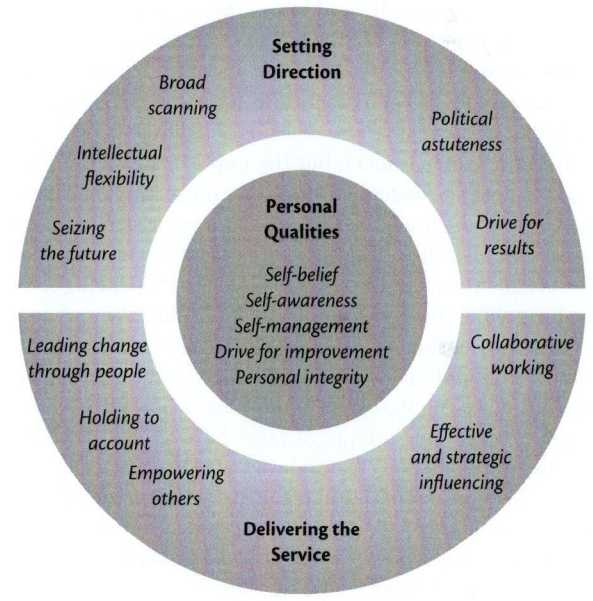

Fig. 3.1.1 NHS leadership qualities framework.

- *Cognitive capacities*: general intelligence, judgement/decision-making skills, organizing skills
- *Social capacities*: social intelligence/sensitivity, communication skills
- *Personality*: extraversion, conscientiousness, openness, agreeableness, neuroticism/emotional stability
- *Motives*: dominance, drive/purpose, energy, tenacity/persistence
- *Core beliefs/self-evaluation*: self-confidence, self-efficacy
- *Knowledge*: knowledge of the business/sector
- *Other*: honesty/integrity.

Transactional, transformational, and servant leadership behaviours

In addition to their personal qualities, leaders tend to behave in one of two ways when seeking to accomplish something: They may be 'transactional' or 'transformational' in their approach (Avolio and Bass 1999). Transactional leadership behaviour uses rewards and punishments deliberately. In contrast, transformational behaviour is more likely to mean presenting a vision of how things could be done differently:

> Thus, transactional leadership is based on exchange; for example, in business, this is often financial rewards for productivity, whereas transformational leadership is a process of inspiring people to achieve shared goals through recognizing individuals' needs, stimulating creative thinking and aligning values between individuals and groups. (Walumbwa and Wernsing 2013, p. 393)

These two ways of behaving are not mutually exclusive. Indeed, in the past two decades, leadership theory and research has focused on a 'multifaceted' approach to understanding leadership success, integrating transactional and transformational elements (Van Wart 2003).

Research on leaders in the public sector (including health workers) suggests they are more likely to be transformational in their approach (Alban-Metcalfe and Alimo-Metcalfe 2000). Research on the leadership styles of doctors also indicates that those with transformational behaviours are perceived as more effective leaders and are able to deliver better healthcare results (Xirasagar et al. 2005, 2006). Some may argue that this is likely to be true generally of health sector leaders, but the importance of the distinction could depend on context. Perhaps transactional leaders are needed in certain urgent settings (such as emergency epidemic responses or operating theatres) while transformational leaders are needed in more complex domains (such as influencing changes in health policy). Both transformational leadership and contingent reward leadership have been shown to have positive effects on performance in different contexts, although research does provide 'evidence suggesting that transformational-leadership behaviour does indeed add some unique variance beyond that provided by transactional leadership' (Walumbwa and Wernsing 2013, p. 393). However, '[c]ross-cultural studies [of] transformational leadership suggest that there are similarities as well as differences about the nature and impact of transformational leadership across cultures' (Kumar and Chhokar 2013, p. 239).

Finally, leadership research has recently also identified behaviours of the 'servant leader'—one who takes on an ethical responsibility to his or her followers, to all relevant stakeholders, even to society as a whole (Van Wart 2003). These behaviours include acting with humility, integrity, altruism, and trust while collaborating with and empowering followers (Dennis and Bocarnea 2005; Sendjaya et al. 2008). These behaviours may be particularly relevant in public health. As we discuss later in this chapter, public health leadership is by its very nature about service to people.

Emphasizing the special qualities of public health leaders, as we have done in this section, seems to imply that leaders are somehow born exceptional. But the personal qualities and competencies cited earlier, such as self-knowledge and political skill, might also result from a maturity of experience. Similarly, people may pick up transformational or transactional behaviour as they progress through their careers. Thus, it seems likely that leadership can be learned, at least in part. But can it be taught? We turn next to that question.

Training leaders

Around the world, isolated initiatives to train health sector leaders have been developed and implemented, often focused on enhancing technical skills or improving workplace interactions. But '[p]ublic health has only recently begun to explore the potential of formal leadership education and training' (Koh and Jacobson 2009, p. 201).

Many training efforts are focused on the traditional attempt to ensure that public health leaders have the epidemiological and statistical skills to understand research and evaluation of interventions and outcomes. The curriculum in most schools of public health is focused on such technical areas and the phrase 'public health training' is often used as shorthand for education in epidemiology and its related domains of statistics, demography, etc. In light of the importance of such skills, the Training Programmes in Epidemiology and Public Health Interventions Network (TEPHINET) was established in association with the WHO, the US Centers for Disease Control and Prevention, and the Fondation Mérieux to train public health personnel around the world. 'These programmes are becoming increasingly recognized as catalysts for strengthening the scientific basis of policy-making through the continuous examination of data' (Cardenas et al. 2002, p. 196). Now part of the Task Force for Global Health, TEPHINET 'is a professional alliance of more than 55 Field Epidemiology (and Laboratory) Training Programs with participants from over 80 countries' (TEPHINET 2012).

In order to be able to analyse trends and articulate a vision of the future, public health leaders clearly need to be able to assess and use the available research evidence. This skill is conventionally believed to be one that can be taught. But what about skills like trans-organizational work and team-building? Can these be conferred on a potential leader by means of a training programme? Some interesting evaluations suggest they can.

Saleh et al. (2004) evaluated training provided by the Northeast Public Health Leadership Institute (NEPHLI) in the United States. Issues covered in the year-long programme include such slightly nebulous topics as building collaborative relationships, group problem-solving, and dealing with cultural diversity. The evaluation results show that the participants clearly believe their abilities were enhanced in the 15 competency areas assessed. In addition, those who had reason to use certain particular skills as part of their work were more likely to perceive an improvement in their competence as a result of training. A key aspect of this training was, thus, the relevance of the topics to the participants' daily work. There may be, of course, a distinction between the participants' perception that the training improved their skills and the reality when they apply these skills. Nevertheless, it seems reasonable that those (such as doctors and nurses) whose basic training and earlier work skills are technical medical ones would benefit from training that emphasizes a very different set of procedural skills. For example, in this case, the '[t]opics covered included influencing others, measuring and improving public health performance, developing collaborative relationships and partnerships, risk communication, team building, group problem solving, responding to the needs for cultural diversity and competence, and emergency preparedness training' (Saleh et al. 2004, p. 1245).

Another training programme evaluation sheds some light on the mechanism by which these behavioural skills are transferred to the participants. Umble et al. (2005, 2011a, 2011b) assessed a leadership training programme in which all the members of a public health team participated together in the training. In addition, the training was based on the participants' real work and on typical projects. The results showed improved outcomes with regard to collaborating and networking, key aspects of leadership.

This team training approach seems to have improved the participants' confidence to work collaboratively and to lead a team, as well as improving their practice of these behaviours. The authors conclude from this evaluation that 'networks and collaborative leaders can be developed through education, and that groups thus created can improve services and programmes' (Umble et al. 2005, p. 642). This approach to bringing together, as a team, leaders who will have to work together to solve public health problems has the potential to work elsewhere. See, for example, a story from the Philippines presented in Box 3.1.2 which shows that training medical, political, and community leaders together fosters the networking skills and builds the very communication links

needed to address public health priorities. The evidence suggests that this is an approach that might reasonably be tried elsewhere.

In addition to formal training programmes, the development of leaders has also been promoted by means of 'mentoring', 'shadowing', or 'coaching' (Turning Point 2001, p. 51). Mentoring is the process by which a more experienced person guides a more junior person with regard to various work- and career-related decisions. It may involve helping the junior person solve problems at work by empathetic listening and feedback. Mentoring may also involve the experienced person giving career advice to the junior.

Shadowing can work with a more senior person either being shadowed or doing the shadowing. In the former approach, a more junior person follows the senior one in his or her job over several months. In this way, learning takes place by observing and participating in the work of an established leader. The latter approach involves a more experienced person shadowing a junior over a shorter period of a day or few days, and then giving constructive feedback on the junior's behaviour and activities at work.

Coaching does not necessarily involve a senior and junior person. A coach may be a specialist psychologist or counsellor who can provide assessment and feedback about skills and practice to a leader or someone wishing to develop leadership skills. Coaches may set goals and tasks for the subject, followed by discussion

---

Box 3.1.2 Training local teams to be health leaders in poor communities: a case from the Philippines

The Philippines provides an innovative approach to leadership for the health needs of the most deprived and vulnerable populations. Begun in 2002, the Leaders for Health Program (LHP) was predicated on the understanding that health professionals must work in concert with political and community actors if basic health problems are to be addressed in low-income communities. This 'Tri-Leader' approach brought together the community doctor, the mayor, and a local community leader and trained them, both individually and as a team.

To address the need that medical leaders understand and are able to use evidence to inform policy, doctors received postgraduate training resulting in a Master in Community Health Management. Recognizing that the local political and community leaders often did not have an advanced level of education, the programme created a certificate course in community health management tailored to them, but paralleling the master's training provided to doctors. Joint workshops and training sessions were also held for the tri-leaders together. In addition, all three benefited from coaching and mentoring from a more experienced leader of their own category from another part of the country. Once this team began to identify priorities in its locality, the LHP provided assistance in identifying donors for specific interventions. For example, some communities invested in sanitation and clean water systems. One community established a local pharmacy; another invested in a boat for emergency transport of patients.

By taking this innovative approach to leadership—one that recognizes the importance of joint leadership in the medical, political, and local communities in order to address public health needs—the LHP has been able to demonstrate greater success than other initiatives that focus only on placing trained doctors in low-income areas. Its success would seem to be due to the programme's understanding of the complexity of health systems. For example, addressing water-borne diseases properly requires sanitation systems, and sanitation systems cannot be built without political support. In addition, the programme's training of doctors together with mayors and community leaders helps doctors to see beyond the narrow biomedical domain to the broader political and sociological setting in which public health problems must be tackled. One mayor reported that earlier attempts to post doctors to his village were unsuccessful because the doctor was perceived to be making demands arrogantly of a resource-poor community, rather than working with the community to reach a common understanding.

A cost analysis of the programme found that the cost per person for the close to 1 million beneficiaries in the 36 towns that participated in the LHP over its initial 4-year period was Philippine pesos 60 or USD 1.50 per year. Furthermore, for every peso invested in the programme as grant, the local government and other national government partners were able to raise a counterpart share of Philippine pesos 1.27. LHP therefore stimulated the mobilization of local resources for health system development. Most of the graduates of the LHP have continued to work in their posts. Some joined various units of the Department of Health, the US Agency for International Development and Médecins Sans Frontières, showing a remarkable record for retaining health professionals in places of need. As a result of the LHP's success, its expansion to other local government units is now being considered as part of the national effort to strengthen local health systems.

Source: data from Baquiran et al., *Leaders for Health Program 2005*, Copyright 2006 and R. Baquiran, personal communication, 2013.

sessions designed to help him or her learn from the experience. Peers may sometimes coach one another, although this may be more successful when the peers are not in direct competition with one another (Turning Point 2001, p. 52).

Among the leaders we interviewed, mentoring and shadowing experiences occupied a prominent place in their development. Many cited their mentors with great fondness and appreciation. And there were instances when more than one mentor was acknowledged by a leader.

It appears, then, that the training and development of leaders is possible: 'You cannot transform a person with no talent into a successful collaborative leader, but you can take a rough diamond and polish it. You can hone the skills of those who have some aptitude for it' (De Meyer 2011, p. 59). The old assumption that leaders are born with innate skills that cannot be taught, no longer seems true. Waiting for great leaders to emerge is not necessary. Instead, the health sector can seek to train, develop, and promote leaders. Although 'we have only barely scratched the surface in our efforts to build a science of leadership development', there is now evidence that training can build specific leadership skills (Day 2013, p. 76). And, equally importantly, it is clear that 'the role of leader identity construction is emerging as a central process in the effective development of leaders' (Day 2013, p. 87). That is, as a person begins to think of him/herself as a leader, he/she is motivated to learn more about what to do and how to act as a leader.

In this chapter so far, we have reviewed the concepts behind leadership studies and research and considered the matter of training and developing leaders. But, beyond this, how does leadership work in the gritty, very real world of day-to-day public health work? In the next section, we reflect on the practice of public health leadership, using real examples.

Leadership in health today

Acknowledging and addressing complexity— putting theory into practice

Health systems are complex. In all countries, health systems are broad and multisectoral. They involve complicated interactions among politics and policy-making, financing, training and education, and public and private organizations. It is not easy to define where public health activities end: a large manufacturing company may employ someone to conduct health education with its staff, just as the government might engage outreach workers to do the same with villagers. In the context of a very complex system that extends far beyond the boundaries of any one organization, it is not possible to 'manage' things in a mechanical way (Plsek and Wilson 2001). Imposing simple managerial or technical–medical solutions on a public health problem will not solve it. Indeed, if technical and mechanistic solutions were all that were needed to address public health problems, we would not need leaders. Instead, the complex, multi-organizational, and team-based nature of public health work requires people who can inspire others to achieve results working through the complexity.

The leaders we interviewed voiced both enthusiasm and frustration with the work they were engaged in. While they spoke of positive gains in their work, they also spoke of conditions beyond their sphere of influence, and of existing economic and political forces far beyond their personal or their organization's capacities to change. Despite these difficulties, hardly any interviewee suggested

that they should give up. Instead they seemed to understand that their mission of service will come up against problems and dilemmas inherent to this complex world. As Binney et al. (2005) note:

> [L]eaders are able to use all their intelligence, senses and experience to connect with others and make sense of the context…They are able to tolerate the complexity of events and people and not rush to simple-minded solutions that don't make sense. Their focus is on both long- and short-term issues. (Binney et al. 2005, p. 93)

Let us look at four examples of complexity faced by public health leaders.

First, consider the relationship between disease and poverty manifest in epidemics. In Manila, there are perennial outbreaks of diarrhoea in the urban slums because residents illegally tap water lines causing contamination of water. When such a water-borne outbreak occurs, the water company needs to step in. It removes the illegal connections, repairs leaks, flushes out the contamination, and increases the chlorination levels in the affected water lines. Public health authorities undertake epidemic investigations and related measures to treat the sick and prevent the infection from spreading in households.

While appearing to be a local issue, this phenomenon is a microcosm of a global problem described in the text of a WHO poster that reads: 'For the first time in history, more than half of the world's population lives in urban settings. Three billion people live in cities. One billion people live without access to safe drinking water' (WHO n.d.).

What can be done to prevent perennial outbreaks of water-borne diarrhoea in urban slums caused by the illegal tapping of water lines? How could a public health leader deal with this situation in order to find a longer-term answer to it?

Second, consider the relationship between disease and people's lifestyles. The association between smoking cigarettes and cancer is now well established. In 2003, the World Health Assembly ratified the Framework Convention on Tobacco Control, which urged member states to undertake a variety of actions in order to reduce smoking among their populations (WHO 2003). Despite scientific advances leading to a better understanding of the ill effects of smoking and the aforementioned landmark global agreement, the prevalence of smoking among youth and women is on the rise in many countries. And while some countries now have legislation to ban smoking in public places, governments in many countries seem not to be doing enough to discourage and reduce smoking among their citizens.

How could the public health leader, such as a city health officer, deal with the situation if the city mayor or the city council have not enacted any measures to stop smoking in public places?

Third, consider the relationship between a disease, the necessary medicines for its treatment, and the commercial interests involved in making those medicines accessible to the people who need them. HIV/AIDS has become a drag on social and economic development. Life expectancies have been shortened drastically in many countries because thousands of people succumb to AIDS at an early age. Large numbers of AIDS orphans are overwhelming the capacities of families and societies to provide and care for them. Antiretrovirals exist, but they are expensive and still inaccessible to millions of infected people.

How could a public health leader, such as a Minister of Health in a country with a large burden of HIV/AIDS, take steps to provide antiretrovirals for thousands of citizens with the disease?

Fourth, consider the relationship between people's reproductive choices and the prevailing traditions, moral views and teachings of religious institutions. Faced with unwanted pregnancies, women may seek abortions. Often, these abortions are conducted under surreptitious and illegal conditions, placing women at high risk of life-threatening bleeding and infection. Legalizing abortions will result in better regulation of the practice of abortion, thereby making the procedure less risky.

How does a public health leader deal with a situation where the scientific evidence shows that decriminalizing abortion prevents maternal deaths from sepsis, but his moral beliefs run counter to implementing such a change?

These four examples are only a few of the many complex issues that public health leaders face. As they bring themselves to lead under these challenging circumstances, their personal qualities, technical, and social competencies will be tested. It can be overwhelming to lead in such complex situations, and leaders must be realistic about what they and their organizations can accomplish.

Principled leadership

In the face of such challenges, leaders need more than the attributes described earlier to help them succeed. Also vitally important is a set of principles that can serve as a guide to thought and action. Where would public health leaders find such a set of principles? We offer five principles derived from the WHO Constitution (WHO 1946; see Box 3.1.3):

1. Commitment to the vision of total human development.

2. Commitment to empowering the poor and the vulnerable with knowledge and opportunity.

3. Pursuit of evidence and truth.

4. Commitment to fairness and equity in the provision of adequate health and social measures.

5. Trustworthiness and public accountability.

Applied singly or in varying combinations, we submit that these principles provide the foundation and inspiration for public health work.

Let us examine how these five principles might help a public health leader address the four complex challenges set out previously. In the first challenge discussed earlier, public health leaders are asked to find a longer-term solution to control water-borne outbreaks of diarrhoea in urban slums. Principle 1, which calls for commitment to total human development, urges these leaders to think beyond epidemic control. It challenges them to address the problem of urban slums to tackle the social determinants of water-borne outbreaks. This is exceedingly complex and difficult. However, where Principle 1 is combined with Principle 2, more durable solutions have been found. The experience of Gawad Kalinga in the Philippines demonstrates how a movement to eradicate urban slums has improved the health of people in such communities and in the process has prevented the perennial occurrence of outbreaks there (see Box 3.1.4). By addressing the land and housing issues at the root of urban slum communities, Gawad Kalinga was able to build low-cost houses and proper water supplies for the families previously dwelling in slums.

Principle 5, trustworthiness and public accountability, is applicable to the second challenge. Big business interests protect and

---

Box 3.1.3 WHO Constitution

THE STATES Parties to this Constitution declare, in conformity with the Charter of the United Nations, that the following principles are basic to the happiness, harmonious relations and security of all peoples:

- Health is a state of complete physical, mental, and social well-being and not merely the absence of disease or infirmity.

- The enjoyment of the highest attainable standard of health is one of the fundamental rights of every human being without distinction of race, religion, political belief, economic or social condition.

- The health of all peoples is fundamental to the attainment of peace and security and is dependent upon the fullest co-operation of individuals and States.

- The achievement of any State in the promotion and protection of health is of value to all.

- Unequal development in different countries in the promotion of health and control of disease, especially communicable disease, is a common danger.

- Healthy development of the child is of basic importance; the ability to live harmoniously in a changing total environment is essential to such development.

- The extension to all peoples of the benefits of medical, psychological and related knowledge is essential to the fullest attainment of health.

- Informed opinion and active co-operation on the part of the public are of the utmost importance in the improvement of the health of the people.

- Governments have a responsibility for the health of their peoples, which can be fulfilled only by the provision of adequate health and social measures.

ACCEPTING THESE PRINCIPLES, and for the purpose of co-operation among themselves and with others to promote and protect the health of all peoples, the Contracting Parties agree to the present Constitution and hereby establish the World Health Organization as a specialized agency within the terms of Article 57 of the Charter of the United Nations.

Reproduced with permission from World Health Organization, *WHO Constitution, adopted by the International Health Conference held in New York from 19 June to 22 July 1946*, Copyright © 1946, available from http://apps.who.int/gb/bd/PDF/bd47/EN/constitution-en.pdf.

---

promote the sale of cigarettes. Some of these business interests may even have philanthropic projects which benefit the public, such as grants to educational institutions or youth scholarships. It can be convenient for public health leaders to take the path of least resistance and not call for a ban on cigarettes in public places. Principle 5 calls on public health leaders to be faithful to their calling of safeguarding public health despite the odds against them. In this respect, they are trustworthy and accountable to the public for their actions, even if some of their actions may be politically unpopular. There are public health leaders who have unstintingly used the built-up scientific evidence on the ill effects of smoking

Box 3.1.4 Gawad Kalinga: improving well-being by empowering the poor

Gawad Kalinga (GK) means to 'give care.' GK is a non-profit foundation whose vision for the Philippines is a slum-free, squatter-free nation achieved through a strategy of providing land for the landless, homes for the homeless, and food for the hungry in order to attain dignity and peace in poor Filipino communities.

What started in 1995 as a daring initiative by a faith-based organization to rehabilitate juvenile gang members and help out-of-school youth in a large squatters' relocation area in Metro Manila, has evolved into a multisectoral movement supported by local and multinational corporations.

GK works actively in the poorest urban areas and concentrates on providing decent homes and the resources necessary for self-sufficiency. It seeks a holistic approach to poverty alleviation that includes various components: the provision of basic healthcare, community organization, livelihood programmes, and values formation. Even before a GK house is built in a slum community, issues of land ownership, capital for house materials, participation of the residents in the construction of the houses, eventual ownership of the built houses, and community building are considered and dealt with. Complex social dynamics are involved in dealing with these varied issues.

Part of the current success of GK is attributed to this stewardship component which integrates leadership building into the GK communities. Every GK village has a Caretaker Team comprised mainly of resident volunteers who undertake specific responsibilities like assisting in resolving conflicts, ensuring the proper management of the resources for constructing the houses, and seeing to it that the GK standards for a well-organized community are maintained.

GK was given the Ramon Magsaysay Awardee in 2006 and the Skoll Award for Social Entrepreneurship in 2012.

Source: data Habaradas, R.B., *The Economic and Artistic Flows of Gawad Kalinga*, Paper presented at the Arts Congress of De La Salle University, Manila, Philippines, Copyright © 2010. Available from http://www.academia.edu/735064/ The_economic_and_artistic_flows_of_Gawad_Kalinga.

to persist in the campaign to fight against cigarette smoking. The recent implementation in Australia, for example, of plain cigarette packaging with antismoking messages and photographs showing the ugly effects of cigarette smoking are a breakthrough in the fight against the tobacco industry (BBC News Asia 2012).

Principle 4, commitment to fairness and equity, may be applicable in the third challenge. In the face of the complex issues concerning the way in which pharmaceuticals are produced, sold, and distributed, answers must be found to address the lack of access to medicines by millions of people. The solutions to these imbalances are not straightforward. They involve the dynamics of the domestic and international market for medicines. Where patents for new medicines are involved, there are international agreements that govern the production and marketing of generic copies during the patent term. In addition, negotiations with pharmaceutical companies have resulted in agreements to sell critical drugs at reduced prices in developing countries. There are concerns that pharmaceutical companies may stop investing in research and development of drugs that might benefit the poorest countries, leading to calls for a new model for funding research into new drugs. Notwithstanding these complexities, public health leaders, seeking to broaden their populations' access to medicines, are persevering with the global and domestic politics needed to accomplish this goal.

The application of Principle 3—the pursuit of evidence and truth—is relevant to the fourth challenge and may guide a public health leader to advocate for the legalization of abortion, explaining that this policy significantly decreases maternal deaths. But those against abortion will resist this evidence, taking the view that no law can justify terminating the fetus in early pregnancy. The leader may persist, providing other evidence, namely that limiting access to legal abortion is not associated with lower abortion rates. But people's beliefs and values vary, and these beliefs may dominate evidence in policymaking. In the Philippines, while a reproductive health bill was recently signed into law mandating government funding for contraceptives, legalization of abortion remains politically unacceptable as public policy (Sandique-Carlos 2012). So, even as public health leaders pursue the evidence to justify health interventions, there may be historical and social considerations that override it. Public health leaders, whatever their moral beliefs, will have to confront those realities as they continue to present the evidence and promote equity for women.

These four complex challenges illustrate the broad range of skills required by successful public health leaders. As we showed in Table 3.1.2, the competencies needed extend far beyond medical and epidemiological skills to incorporate the systems thinking and political skills needed to influence change.

The path to leadership

You too can become a public health leader—but how can you develop the personal qualities and competencies needed to do so?

There are many paths to leadership. The public health leaders we interviewed first entered the profession with a strong desire to serve. Through the course of their careers, they were exposed to circumstances that deepened their commitment. Frequently, they sought out challenging circumstances in which to gain much needed experience. They travelled, engaged in development work, often involving poor countries and communities. In the course of this exposure, they took up more advanced public health studies, perhaps did some research, wrote articles in scientific journals, or managed a healthcare facility. Some had long periods of service in their own country before being exposed to international work. For others, international exposure came early, usually through some clinical or public health training abroad.

Some of our interviewees moved into public health after years of working in the clinics, practising a speciality like paediatrics, obstetrics, or surgery. Others came into positions of leadership through the field services, rising through a public health organization, or a non-governmental organization. Others were involved in academia, teaching and research, consulting, or working with a development agency. Public health leaders could also have been involved in politics. Or they could once have been cause-oriented activists, involved in issues such as HIV prevention and primary healthcare.

Mentors play a significant role in the development of the public health leader. Nearly everyone we interviewed cited people significant to their career at various stages. One public health leader we spoke to for this chapter put it this way: 'A leader creates a path for others to succeed'. Another interviewee mentioned how his boss and mentor encouraged him and other young people in the organization to think up and explore new ideas.

Central to the growth and development of the public health leader are the years when he/she developed the personal qualities of self-awareness, self-belief, and self-management. In those we spoke to, there was the strong conviction that their involvement in public health was imbued with higher purpose and even that they were instruments of a higher power to do good work. Certainly, the sense of 'other-orientedness' was quite a major motivation infusing the leaders' sense of service. Among those interviewed, none said that money was a strong motivating factor for the choice of a public health career. A desire to continue learning new things was often mentioned as a source of great satisfaction. One public health leader emphasized the necessity to listen and learn from others before making decisions.

We encourage potential health leaders of tomorrow to forge their 'path to leadership' on three fronts:

1. Know your guiding principles.

2. Seek mentors and aim to learn from every situation you face.

3. Pursue leadership, not the leadership position.

Know your guiding principles

The WHO Constitution—drawn up in a fertile climate of unprecedented hope by international leaders in every field—can be distilled into fundamental guiding principles that are central to a public health leader's work. In reality, individual context, culture, and background dictate that each leader will interpret these principles slightly differently and will complement them with additional principles derived from their personal philosophy of life. Together, this collection of principles will serve to give focus and meaning to the health leader's work.

These principles must be embedded firmly in the mind. Leaders need to think and act on their feet. Unless one is sure of one's principles, in a time of crisis—with perhaps many lives at stake—panic and uncertainty might take over. There will not be time to think about remembering your principles when the need to make a decision is immediate. For this reason, taking the time to understand what guides you—to 'know thyself'—is invaluable. Take time to think about what it is that guides you, or what you would like to guide you.

Seek mentors and aim to learn from every situation you face

Both the literature on leadership and the practical experience of today's health leaders underline the crucial importance of mentorship in the development of the complete public health leader. To achieve self-improvement, being prepared to learn from superiors, fellow colleagues, friends, and public figures is essential. But how does one 'obtain' a mentor?

There is no fixed prescription for mentorship. By its very nature, it is a personal arrangement between two parties. Some programmes encourage their participants to go out and seek a mentor other than their direct supervisor—someone they admire, probably working in their vicinity—and to invite them to act as a mentor. Following this, an arrangement can be struck that is convenient and suitable to the mentor and the mentee. The mentoring relationship could be formal and structured, with regular meetings and log book entries; or it could be more informal and sporadic, with the occasional chat over coffee or e-mail correspondence.

The opportunity should be taken for the mentor to impart advice, the mentee to report on recent events, and for both to share thoughts on work and even wider aspects of life, particularly if relevant to a career in health and leadership. Ideally, a mentoring relationship should be mutually beneficial, with both parties learning from one another, enriching their understanding of their work and purpose.

Pursue leadership, not the leadership position

Looking back to the beginning of this chapter, at the distinction between leadership and management, it is clear that whereas to exercise management it is necessary to be in a management position, the skills, characteristics, and competencies of leadership can be practised regardless of one's position in a hierarchy. One pursues leadership by steadily inculcating in oneself the personal qualities, competencies, and principles that make up a true leader. One does not acquire these necessary attributes and skills simply by ascending to a leadership position, often via political patronage, especially if one lacks adequate preparation. Study, training, reflection, exposure, and experience are all elements of this preparation. Thus, as one's leadership traits flourish, the time will come when one is ready to assume a leadership position. Leadership should be sought in this way from day one of any career and hence, any strong public health organization should encourage leadership development at all levels.

When does one know that he/she is ready to take up a position of leadership? The trajectory of an individual's path to leadership can rise steeply or gently. It is one's willingness to step forward, given one's self-awareness and knowledge of the prospective job, however incomplete, which might mark a person's readiness to lead. A potential leader will almost always be selected by having already demonstrated leadership and by showing readiness to lead. In deciding if one is ready to assume the responsibility of a public health leader, it of course helps to discuss the opportunity with mentors, co-workers, and family members.

Once in a leadership position, the leader must keep learning. Mistakes will be made, disappointments and conflicts will occur. The strong face of leadership is well observed, but how do top health leaders deal with themselves during the dark hours, when the tasks seem overwhelming and when results fall short of expectations? It is often said that in these situations, leaders dig deep into themselves to find internal resources of strength. The capacity to affirm self-belief and overcome self-doubt is an important ingredient in surviving the difficult times; but it is also true that the leader turns outward to others for strength. One leader whom we interviewed emphasized that she turned to her community for rejuvenation and inspiration. 'We hold on to each other', she said. Others turn to family members or colleagues for support. And there are many who through prayer and meditation, turn to their faith or guiding principles to find inner strength.

How can a leader know how he/she is doing? A leader can listen closely to what the boss, spouse, colleagues, friends, constituencies, or even opinion surveys say. Or a leader may listen inwardly reflecting on thoughts, actions and lived experience in the midst of complexity, adversity, and uncertainty. Sometimes, institutional awards and honours may bestow recognition. By learning to be truly honest with oneself and seeking objective, constructive, and critical feedback from others, a leader can begin to find an answer to this question and sustain self-improvement. We find that the unsolicited compliment like 'Thank you for your fine example' or the gentle rebuke 'Perhaps if you had done it this way…' provide invaluable inputs to a leader's self-awareness.

We hope that the reflections presented here will help to direct the interested and motivated reader in tracing his/her own 'path to leadership'. Before bringing this chapter to a close, and as a final pointer for those wishing to serve the needy through public health leadership, we might look at things from another perspective. Instead of asking 'What do I need in order to become a health leader?' perhaps we should ask 'What kind of leader does the world need?'

Getting the public health leaders the world needs

We need public health leaders everywhere and at every level of the health system. However, good leaders are most needed in places where people are poor and suffering simply because there is such a scarcity of them there. Committed and effective leaders often provide the vision and impetus to mobilize people and resources in needy areas. How can the international health community help developing countries develop the needed leaders? A good starting point is to aim at strengthening educational institutions, which can provide relevant, team-based training. Schools of public health have an important role to play (Colgrove et al. 2010). Helping governments and their partners to improve public health working conditions, including financial and non-financial incentives, will also help to attract and retain talented people. From an international perspective we can work towards empowering nations to do this self-sufficiently, strengthening their own frameworks for leadership. Health leaders have used the term 'capacity release' in reference to this kind of endeavour (Chan 2007). It must be stressed that training programmes are only one component of a comprehensive approach that should include strategies to retain promising public health workers and sustain the idealism of leaders who are prepared to venture forth to places of hardship. We must encourage and support them to stay where they are most needed. Examples of work being done on this include the WHO framework on training leaders and managers (Egger et al. 2005) and related work to strengthen leadership at all levels of the health system.

The challenge now is particularly great. We have not yet established systematic ways to develop public health leaders, while the context is becoming ever more complex. To address the social determinants of health, confront the ongoing communicable disease burden as well as the rising burden of non-communicable diseases, and truly ensure 'health in all policies' will require devoted and determined public health leaders at all levels of society and in all sectors.

Conclusion

As we reach the end of this chapter, here are some key points for the aspiring leader:

- Leadership is displayed in a complex interaction between the leader, the followers, and the context. Parables about different types of leadership illustrate the diversity of contexts and behaviours that may be associated with successful leadership.

- In the face of ever-increasing complexity, public health leaders are needed to prevent, treat, and eliminate disease and promote the health and well-being of all people. Such leadership can be developed by local, national, and international actors.

- Public health leaders demonstrate personal qualities and skills, underpinned by fundamental principles, which enable them to influence actions and results. The constant manifestation and practice of these attributes and beliefs is a continuing challenge in a leader's job and career.

- Each 'path to leadership' is unique and very personal. However, exposure, training, mentors, and guiding principles all help in the development of leadership qualities in individuals who aspire to lead. These should be sought by anyone interested in serving as a public health leader.

The pursuit of leadership should ennoble the mind and the heart of those who aspire to it. It is a dignified and never-ending quest. We bid the reader all success.

Acknowledgements

The authors would like to thank Amimo Agola, Anand Kurup, Chadia Wannous, Christine Lamoureux, Claudia Vivas, Delanyo Dovlo, Dick Chamla, Francis Omaswa, Guangyuan Liu, Helen Robinson, Lealou Reballos, Maria Eufemia Yap, and Miriam Were, among others, for their insights into the issues of leadership in public health. The authors would also like to acknowledge the contributions of Carmen Dolea, Daniel Shaw, and Joanne McManus to an earlier version of this chapter.

References

Alban-Metcalfe, R.J. and Alimo-Metcalfe, B. (2000). An analysis of the convergent and discriminant validity of the transformational leadership questionnaire. *International Journal of Selection and Assessment*, 8(3), 158–75.

Avolio, B.J. and Bass, B.M. (1999). Re-examining the components of transformational and transactional leadership using the multifactor leadership questionnaire. *Journal of Occupational and Organizational Psychology*, 72(4), 441–62.

Baquiran, R., Yap, M.E., and Bengzon, A.R.A. (2006). *Terminal Grant Report: Leaders for Health Program 2002–2006*. Manila: Pfizer Philippines Foundation Inc.

BBC News Asia (2012). *Australia Smokers Given Plain Packs*. 1 December 2012. Available at: http://www.bbc.co.uk/news/world-asia-20559585.

Binney, G., Wilke, G., and Williams, C. (2005). *Living Leadership: A Practical Guide for Ordinary Heroes*. London: Pearson Education Limited.

Campbell, J.P. (2013). Leadership, the old, the new, and the timeless: a commentary. In M.G. Rumsey (ed.) *The Oxford Handbook of Leadership*, pp. 401–19. New York: Oxford University Press.

Cardenas, V.M., Roces, M.C., Wattanasri, S., et al. (2002). Improving global public health leadership through training in epidemiology and public health: the experience of TEPHINET. Training Programs in Epidemiology and Public Health Interventions Network. *American Journal of Public Health*, 92(2), 196–7.

Chan, M. (2007). Address to WHO staff. 4 January 2007. Geneva: World Health Organization.

Colgrove, J., Fried, L.P., Northridge, M.E., and Rosner, D. (2010). Schools of public health: essential infrastructure of a responsible society and a 21st-century health system. *Public Health Reports*, 125(1), 8.

Day, D.V. (2013). Training and developing leaders: theory and research. In M.G. Rumsey (ed.) *The Oxford Handbook of Leadership*, pp. 76–93. New York: Oxford University Press.

De Meyer, A. (2011). Collaborative leadership: new perspectives in leadership development. In J. Canals (ed.) *The Future of Leadership Development*, pp. 44–63. Basingstoke: Palgrave Macmillan.

Dennis, R.S. and Bocarnea, M. (2005). Development of the servant leadership assessment instrument. *Leadership and Organization Development Journal*, 26(8), 600–15.

Egger, D., Travis, P., Dovlo, D., et al. (2005). *Strengthening Management in Low-Income Countries*. Making Health Systems Work: Working Paper Series Number 1. Geneva: World Health Organization.

Firth-Cozens, J. and Mowbray, D. (2001). Leadership and the quality of care. *Quality in Health Care*, 10 (Suppl. 2), ii3–7.

Flahault, D. and Roemer, M.I. (1986). *Leadership for Primary Health Care*. Geneva: World Health Organization.

Gawad Kalinga (2012). *Skoll award to Gawad Kalinga: freedom to serve*. Available at: http://gk1world.com/skoll-world-forum-2012 (accessed 8 January 2013).

Grint, K. (2002). Management or leadership? *Journal of Health Services Research and Policy*, 7(4), 248–51.

Habaradas, R.B. (2010). *The Economic and Artistic Flows of Gawad Kalinga*. Paper presented at the Arts Congress of De La Salle University, Manila, Philippines. Available at: http://www.academia.edu/735064/The_economic_and_artistic_flows_of_Gawad_Kalinga.

Hollander, E.P. (2013). Inclusive leadership and idiosyncrasy credit in leader–follower relations. In M.G. Rumsey (ed.) *The Oxford Handbook of Leadership*, pp. 122–43. New York: Oxford University Press.

Klimoski, R. (2013). Commentary: when it comes to leadership, context matters. In M.G. Rumsey (ed.) *The Oxford Handbook of Leadership*, pp. 267–87. New York: Oxford University Press.

Koh, H.K and Jacobson, M. (2009). Fostering public health leadership. *Journal of Public Health*, 31(2), 199–201.

Kotter, J.P. (2008). *Force for Change: How Leadership Differs From Management*. [eBook] New York: Free Press.

Kumar, R. and Chhokar, J.S. (2013). Cross-cultural leadership. In M.G. Rumsey (ed.) *The Oxford Handbook of Leadership*, pp. 225–40. New York: Oxford University Press.

Leaders for Health Program (2005). *The LHP Experience: 5 Stories of Hope and Transformation in Municipal Health Practices (Program Document)*. Makati, Philippines: Ateneo Professional Schools. Available at: http://www.leadersforhealth.ph.

Marion, R. (2013). Organizational leadership and complexity mechanisms. In M.G. Rumsey (ed.) *The Oxford Handbook of Leadership*, pp. 184–202. New York: Oxford University Press.

NHS Leadership Centre (2006). *NHS Leadership Qualities Framework*. London: National Health Service Institute for Innovation and Improvement.

Plsek, P.E. and Wilson, T. (2001). Complexity, leadership, and management in healthcare organisations. *British Medical Journal*, 323(7315), 746–9.

Rumsey, M.G. (2013a). Introduction: leadership in five parts. In M.G. Rumsey (ed.) *The Oxford Handbook of Leadership*, pp. 1–7. New York: Oxford University Press.

Rumsey, M.G. (2013b). Commentary: a way ahead. In M.G. Rumsey (ed.) *The Oxford Handbook of Leadership*, pp. 94–100. New York: Oxford University Press.

Saleh, S.S., Williams, D., and Balougan, M. (2004). Evaluating the effectiveness of public health leadership training: the NEPHLI experience. *American Journal of Public Health*, 94(7), 1245–9.

Sandique-Carlos, R. (2012). Philippines adopts contraception law. *The Wall Street Journal* (Europe edition), 29 December 2012. Available at: http://online.wsj.com/article/SB10001424127887324669104578208889139000 6944.html.

Sendjaya, S., Sarros, J.C., and Santora, J.C. (2008). Defining and measuring servant leadership behaviour in organizations. *Journal of Management Studies*, 45(2), 402–24.

Sternberg, R.J. (2013). The WICS model of leadership. In M.G. Rumsey (ed.) *The Oxford Handbook of Leadership*, pp. 47–62. New York: Oxford University Press.

Stone, A.G. and Patterson, K. (2005). *The History of Leadership Focus*. Servant Leadership Research Roundtable—August 2005. School of Leadership Studies, Regent University.

TEPHINET (2012). *15th Anniversary Report 1997–2012*. Decatur, GA: The Task Force for Global Health, Inc.

Turning Point Program (2001). *Collaborative Leadership and Health: A Review of the Literature*. Seattle, WA: Leadership Development National Excellence Collaborative, Turning Point Program.

Umble, K., Baker, E., Diehl, S., et al. (2011a). An evaluation of the National Public Health Leadership Institute–1991–2006: Part II. Strengthening public health leadership networks, systems, and infrastructure. *Journal of Public Health Management and Practice*, 17 (3), 214–24.

Umble, K., Baker, E., and Woltring, C. (2011b). An evaluation of the National Public Health Leadership Institute—1991–2006: Part I. Developing individual leaders. *Journal of Public Health Management and Practice*, 17 (3), 202–13.

Umble, K., Steffen, D., Porter, J., et al. (2005). The National Public Health Leadership Institute: evaluation of a team-based approach to developing collaborative public health leaders. *American Journal of Public Health*, 95(4), 641–4.

Van Wart, M. (2003). Public sector leadership theory: an assessment. *Public Administration Review*, 63(2), 214–28.

Walumbwa, F.O. and Wernsing, T. (2013). From transactional and transformational leadership to authentic leadership. In M.G. Rumsey (ed.) *The Oxford Handbook of Leadership*, pp. 392–400. New York: Oxford University Press.

World Health Organization (1946). *WHO Constitution, adopted by the International Health Conference held in New York from 19 June to 22 July 1946*. Available at: http://apps.who.int/gb/bd/PDF/bd47/EN/constitution-en.pdf.

World Health Organization (2003). *WHO Framework Convention on Tobacco Control*. Geneva: World Health Organization. Available at: http://www.who.int/fctc/text_download/en/index.html Accessed on 9 January 2013.

World Health Organization (n.d.). *Knowledge Network On Urban Settings*. [Poster] Kobe, Japan: WHO Commission on Social Determinants of Health, WHO Centre for Health Development.

Wright, K., Rowitz, L., and Merkle, A. (2001). A conceptual model for leadership development. *Journal of Public Health Management and Practice*, 7(4), 60–6.

Wright, K., Rowitz, L., Merkle, A., et al. (2000). Competency development in public health leadership. *American Journal of Public Health*, 90(8), 1202–7.

Xirasagar, S., Samuels, M.E., and Curtin, T.F. (2006). Management training of physician executives, their leadership style, and care management performance: an empirical study. *The American Journal of Managed Care*, 12(2), 101–8.

Xirasagar, S., Samuels, M.E., and Stoskopf, C.H. (2005). Physician leadership styles and effectiveness: an empirical study. *Medical Care Research and Review*, 62(6), 720–40.

Zaccaro, S.J., LaPort, K., and Irwin, J. (2013). The attributes of successful leaders: a performance requirements approach. In M.G. Rumsey (ed.) *The Oxford Handbook of Leadership*, pp. 11–36. New York: Oxford University Press.

Ethical principles and ethical issues in public health

Nancy Kass, Amy Paul, and Andrew Siegel

Medical ethics, bioethics, and the emergence of public health ethics

While some cite the Hippocratic Oath as the first articulation of moral duties of physicians, and others cite John Gregory or Thomas Percival as giving birth to medical ethics, codes and teachings about moral duties of physicians have existed for hundreds, if not thousands, of years (Percival 1985; McCullough 1998). Medical ethics focuses primarily on physicians' interactions with individual patients and is the focus of significant scholarship. The American Medical Association has longstanding codes of medical ethics, and instruction on medical professionalism is nearly universal in US and Canadian medical schools (Kao et al. 2003). The American Association of Medical Colleges requires that principles related to medical ethics should be taught in medical core curricula (Allen 2007); the UK General Medical Council requires medical schools to teach medical ethics; and the Medical Council of India requires students to 'observe medical ethics' as part of exemplary behaviour (Ravindran 2008).

Bioethics emerged more recently, with a broader focus. 'Bioethics' as a field arose in the 1960s and 1970s (Walter and Klein 2003) arising from questions of resource allocation, moral questions raised by new reproductive and genetic technologies, a growing patients' rights movement, and a lack of oversight in human subject research. Important scholarship grew, and a national commission was convened in the 1970s to examine questions of human research ethics. The National Commission drafted the Belmont Report (National Commission for the Protection of Human Subjects of Biomedical and Behavioral Research 1979) delineating three ethics principles for human research—beneficence, respect for persons, and justice. This early work in bioethics not only went beyond the individual doctor–patient dyad but also informed public policy.

Bioethics ignited. Centres were created, journals started, meetings convened, and professionals from various disciplines started calling themselves 'bioethicists'. The three 'Belmont principles' became the foundation for a widely used bioethics text (Beauchamp and Childress 1979). While some suggested alternative approaches, 'principlism' remains a widely used framework for healthcare and research ethics (Clouser 1995; Jonsen 1995; Pellegrino 1995), and Belmont principles were adopted for the Council for International Organizations of Medical Sciences (CIOMS) international ethics guidelines (CIOMS 2002).

Early framers of these principles suggested no principle, a priori, should have moral superiority over any other (Beauchamp and Childress 1979). Nonetheless, issues animating bioethics early on—the need to tell patients and research participants the truth and the right to refuse medical care or research participation—were ones where respect for autonomy, perhaps given too little moral attention previously, was given pre-eminent moral status (Callahan 1984; Pellegrino and Thomasma 1988; Steinbock 1996). Informed consent, an application of the autonomy principle, became a hallmark of the new bioethics. Codes of ethics for clinical practice, which previously focused on not harming patients, added requirements to respect patients' right to decide about their own care (American Medical Association 1990).

The subfield of *public health ethics*, articulated as such, did not appear significantly in the literature until the 1990s, although Marc Lappe had a chapter 'Ethics and Public Health' in the 1986 Maxcy-Rosenau text *Public Health and Preventive Medicine* (Lappe 1986).[1] This chapter outlined core public health ethics challenges: fair distribution of resources, rights of individuals versus groups, and promoting efficiency while recognizing the 'special standing of those who are disadvantaged in terms of their health status' (Lappe 1986, p. 1875). Moreover, Lappe asserted that whereas medical ethics is more concerned with individual autonomy and duties of single health professionals, public health ethics focuses more on equity and efficiency. Lappe suggested individual rights can be compromised for community interests, but only with proportionality—an intervention's benefit must outweigh its harm, and the absolute level of infringement must be minimal. Related, since many public health programmes do not grant individuals right of refusal, there must be evidence that programmes will provide the good promised. He suggested an inevitable tension between utilitarianism and justice with an ethic of public health capturing the urgency for efficiency, while recognizing the special standing of those in greatest need.

An additional exception from this early history is Dan E. Beauchamp's work, suggesting social justice and communitarian traditions should drive public health (Beauchamp 1976b). While public health practitioners had recognized, for more than a century, the relationship between social conditions and health (see Fee 1977),[2] Beauchamp's work suggested a new idea *within bioethics* that exclusive attention to individual interests, particularly through market justice, will hinder protecting the public's health. Rather, public health should 'require thinking about and reacting to the problems of disability and premature death as collective problems of the entire society' (Beauchamp 1976b, p. 9).

Furthermore, Beauchamp challenged bioethics to see public health as furthering community interests in terms of shared commitments we have to one another. Through collective actions in health and safety, for example, we share commitments to the common life (Beauchamp 1985, p. 34). While Beauchamp did not use the words 'public health ethics', his work is foundational in putting forward the idea that public health has its own set of moral priorities.

By the early 2000s a need for a more structured way to examine ethics issues in public health surfaced, and literature examined how public health ethics issues differed from those in medicine or other areas of bioethics. In 2001 and 2002, four articles were published defining the territory of public health ethics and/or offering tools and frameworks for its analysis (Kass 2001; Callahan and Jennings 2002; Childress et al. 2002; Roberts and Reich 2002), suggesting public health ethics requires identifying programme goals, determining effectiveness, minimizing burdens, proportionality, furthering social justice, and ensuring procedural justice. Publication of the first code of ethics by the American Public Health Association, an organization that had existed since 1832, followed in 2002 (*APHA Code of Ethics*; American Public Health Association 2002).

Ethics and health promotion

In the 1970s, several scholars began addressing the degree to which governments should regulate personal behaviour to promote public health. While many of the discussions were influenced by John Stuart Mill's view that government restrictions on an individual's liberty are justified only to prevent harm to others (Mill 1869), debates ensued over whether interventions to improve the health of the person targeted could be morally acceptable. Daniel Wikler suggested that promoting certain lifestyles conveyed a set of moral values when 'It is not self-evident that this vision of a safe society, with its lack of immoderation, stress, and risk-taking, is to be favoured over others whose constitutive elements have incidental adverse effects upon health' (Wikler 1978a, p. 231).

Edmund Pellegrino, one of the 'fathers of bioethics', described an ethics of prevention (Pellegrino 1981). Preventive interventions, he suggested, ranged from more voluntary approaches like health education to increasingly less voluntary ones like opinion manipulation through mass media, tax and insurance incentives and disincentives, and legal prohibitions in the name of what some consider to be 'the good life', highlighting that we are forced to make decisions about what constraints we will accept to further the common good.

Faden and Faden, similarly, described interventions ranging from facilitation to persuasion to manipulation to coercion, arguing the acceptability of different approaches rests on how rational and resistible they are (Faden and Faden 1978). Described here, to be cited frequently throughout future public health ethics writings, was the concept of *proportionality*: the burden posed by (particularly non-voluntary) interventions should be low and benefits high. As such, incentives should be favoured over disincentives, education favoured over manipulative messages, and government intervention ought not occur without considerable evidence about effectiveness.

The Society of Public Health Educators' code of professional ethics went further, calling voluntariness the *only* acceptable approach, suggesting health educators should 'empower individuals to adopt healthy lifestyles through informed choice rather than by coercion (Society for Public Health Education n.d.).

Purely voluntary interventions do not always work, however (Glanz et al. 1997; Roter et al. 1998), and the question for ethics scholars became whether or under what conditions more controlling interventions were acceptable. Furthermore, since governments would be implementing stricter measures, how could one ensure their agenda related to public health rather than politics? (Faden 1987). Involuntary measures also assume 'a benign, wise, and responsive government, something history finds singularly rare' (Pellegrino 1981, p. 375).

Dan Beauchamp suggested shifting focus from the degree to which governments can regulate individual behaviour to, instead, the legal authority of public health to regulate behaviour of those marketing and distributing harmful products (Beauchamp 1976a). Wikler similarly suggested that if outside influences encourage an individual to alter his or her preferences unknowingly, this diminishes the autonomy with which those choices are made (Wikler 1978b). Coercive measures may be needed to control the manipulation of messages that run counter to the interests of public health.

The rise of chronic disease has more recently shifted the focus of public health ethics back to the acceptability of different types of behavioural interventions or public policies designed to influence behaviour. The high burdens of tobacco-related illness, injury, obesity, and diabetes have prompted interventions that target environmental, behavioural, and lifestyle determinants. In obesity prevention, for example, public health ethics must consider the justifiability of government action to restrict access to unhealthy products such as sugar sweetened beverages in various programmes or institutions as well as the effects such proposals would have on morally relevant values such as liberty, privacy, and fairness. Ethics debate surrounds whether all consumer choices constitute protected liberties, and when, if ever, restrictive policies are justifiable absent direct threats to others.

Infectious disease and public health ethics: HIV and pandemic preparedness

HIV/AIDS

Few challenges have forced examination of ethics and public health as much as HIV/AIDS. Multiple public health ethics tensions surfaced, from societal rights versus individual liberties to justice and healthcare access, and arose in core functions of public health: surveillance, disease reporting, containment, and resource allocation. As policymakers navigated tough decisions, much bioethics literature emerged, influencing what would soon be called public health ethics. Arguably, it was HIV that introduced many bioethics scholars to the world of public health.

In 1983, the Public Health Service (PHS) recommended that gay men be discouraged from donating blood (Centers for Disease Control (CDC) 1983), and soon policy documents and individual scholars examined ethics in HIV policy (Bayer 1983; Institute of Medicine 1986; Presidential Commission on the Human

Immunodeficiency Virus Epidemic 1988). Fear and uncertainty precipitated proposals from tattooing infected persons to full quarantine that were highly restrictive while having little evidence of efficacy. Despite almost uniform rejection from bioethics and legal communities (Gostin and Curran 1986; Koop 1986; Macklin 1986; Musto 1986; Porter 1986), policy proposals continued to recommend exclusion of HIV-infected persons from employment, housing, insurance, and school. Bioethicists jumped into the fray to help articulate appropriate public health response and put forward ethical requirements for new screening programmes (Bayer et al. 1986; Childress 1987; Gostin and Curran 1987; Gostin et al. 1987; Hunter 1987; Bayer 1989), cognizant of the tension between potential public health benefits and concerns of exposing at-risk individuals to stigma with no treatment in return.

HIV renewed interest in the ethics of other tools of public health with calls for mandatory HIV reporting, contact tracing, and partner notification. Proponents suggested mandatory reporting would improve understanding of the disease and target education and potential treatments. Critics argued education and treatments could be provided without reporting, which was an unjustified invasion of privacy, particularly when strong antidiscrimination laws did not exist; concerns existed that at-risk individuals would avoid testing, fearing consequences. Support for mandatory reporting increased when treatments became available. HIV stimulated ethics debate in almost every area of public health including health education, duty to treat, resource allocation, access, and financing. While the phrase 'public health ethics' was not yet used, the foundation of the field had been laid.

Pandemic preparedness

The re-emergence of pandemic disease in the 2000s pushed public health ethics thinking to modify frameworks for the pandemic context. While the infectious nature of pandemic flu raised familiar tensions between individual interests and population health, the urgency and potential for insufficient resources highlighted additional challenges. Avian flu and severe acute respiratory syndrome outbreaks, for example, were met with insufficient healthcare workforce, vaccine shortages, and complex global governance challenges when pandemics crossed borders, raising questions of healthcare worker obligations, fair resource allocation, and justifications for restricting liberty interests (Gostin 2004; Kotalik 2005). Resulting ethical guidance (University of Toronto 2005; Thompson et al. 2006; CDC 2007, 2011) offered principles for a response while acknowledging the importance of procedural values including reasonable and evidence based decision-making, inclusivity, transparency, and accountability.

Pandemic influenza also renewed focus within public health ethics on resource allocation as questions arose concerning how best to allocate scarce vaccines, hospital beds, ventilators and everyday supplies. The US National Vaccine Advisory Committee and Advisory Committee on Immunization Practices recommended giving priority to those in greatest medical need (US Department of Health and Human Services 2005), some asserted priority be given to those in whom we have invested some societal resources, yet who have not had opportunity to experience multiple life-stages, meaning young adults would be prioritized above infants (Emanuel and Wertheimer 2006), others underscored the importance of considering vulnerable populations in allocation (Uscher-Pines et al. 2007; Rosoff and DeCamp 2011; DeBruin et al.

2012), and some emphasized the importance of securing access for those with important roles in maintaining societal functioning and infrastructure (Kass 2001). Questions of resource allocation in a pandemic prompted procedural interests in public engagement as a strategy to incorporate public input into policy decisions (Bailey et al. 2011; Vawter et al. 2011).

Public health and social justice

Until recently, the more theoretical literature on justice and health focused almost exclusively on issues of access to healthcare and the allocation of scarce healthcare resources. While these remain important and contested areas of inquiry, the epidemiological evidence indicates that healthcare plays a relatively limited role in determining health status (Wilkinson and Marmot 2003). It has long been understood in public health that socioeconomic status (SES) (viz. status as defined by income, education, and occupation) is a major determinant of health, giving rise to significant health inequalities between social groups. Some health disparities are due to material conditions related to poverty, such as poor nutrition and crowded and unsanitary living conditions. But studies over the past two decades suggest that poverty alone does not explain the effects of SES on health. There is a gradient in life expectancy, mortality, and morbidity across all levels of the SES hierarchy (Marmot et al. 1991; Marmot and Shipley 1996). Health inequalities in the gradient that exist in the absence of material deprivations appear to be best explained by psychosocial factors, such as levels of social support and integration, control in the workplace, and hostility (Marmot 2004). There are also studies that, while controversial, suggest that an individual's health is influenced by the level of income inequality in society as a whole, and not just by her own level of income (Kawachi et al. 1999). Increasing attention to the social determinants of health has given rise to a heightened focus on social justice in public health.

The central social justice issue in the context of public health concerns when health inequalities between social groups are unjust. There are several approaches in the literature to addressing this question, all of which are developed from more general theoretical accounts of distributive justice. Theories of distributive justice identify a metric specifying the good that is sought and a principle for the distribution of that good. The primary metrics include welfare, resources, and capabilities, while the competing principles of distribution appeal to equality, priority, and sufficiency.

Metrics of justice vary, with some viewing health as purely instrumental to the good justice seeks and others viewing health as intrinsic to that good. Instrumentalist accounts include Norman Daniels' view that the value of health lies in its serving to secure equality of opportunity to pursue life plans (Daniels 1985, 2008) and the welfare egalitarian and contemporary utilitarian view that health is valuable insofar as it fulfils individual preferences. Each account is subject to the objection that health has value even when failing to promote these ends. Health seems important even for those near the end of life who have completed their life plans (Brock 1989; Segall 2010); health further can have value where one has a weak preference for it, particularly where the preference is due to an adaptation to conditions under which one has been persistently deprived of health (Sen 2009).

An alternative to the instrumentalist perspective conceives of health as partly constitutive of the ends of justice. Various capabilities theorists have argued that a person's ability to achieve good health is a fundamental capability inasmuch as health is essential to human life and flourishing (Sen 2002; Nussbaum 2006; Ruger 2009; Venkatapuram 2011). Madison Powers and Ruth Faden offer a related but distinct conception, viewing health as one of several dimensions of well-being (which also include personal security, respect, attachment, self-determination, and reasoning) that justice aims to secure. But they privilege the achievement of positive health outcomes over capabilities to achieve health, both because some individuals (children, in particular) are not well positioned to make free and informed choices about their health and because there are threats to health that may not be within an individual's ability to control (e.g., exposure to environmental harms) (Powers and Faden 2006, 2011).

In assessing whether a given health disparity is unjust, one must turn to distributive principles. On a strict egalitarian account, everyone should, as far as possible, have equal health status. This account has been widely dismissed as it would permit 'levelling down' the health status of some without improving the health of others as a means to achieve equality (Parfit 1998). Alternatively, the prioritarian account permits inequalities where they benefit those who are worst off. John Rawls' Difference Principle, which allows inequalities in income and wealth (among other goods) only where they benefit the worst off, is a prominent example of prioritarianism (Rawls 1971). Daniels has applied this view to health, suggesting that distributing social goods in accordance with the Difference Principle would substantially reduce the steepness of the health gradient (2008). Another prioritarian account gives weight to personal responsibility for health differentials, positing that those who do more to promote their health should be given priority (Segall 2010). Sufficientarians, like prioritarians, are concerned with how persons fare in absolute terms; but they hold that justice should ensure that everyone has enough of the goods essential to living a decent life, without regard to inequalities beyond the sufficiency threshold (Frankfurt 1987). Powers and Faden, for example, maintain that justice demands that everyone have a sufficient amount of health, and that the most pressing health inequalities are those that are systematically accompanied by inadequately met needs in other core dimensions of well-being (Powers and Faden 2006).

Given how many people lack adequate health and how little of the vast social and economic gains to the well-off have been accompanied by gains to the worst-off, following either the prioritarian or sufficientarian views of justice likely would lead to profound improvements in population health. While public health practitioners do not bear primary responsibility for addressing the full range of the social determinants of health, some argue that public health should more explicitly incorporate a social justice orientation. Strategies to do so are of course more challenging, and include monitoring social indicators related to health inequalities to engaging in community organization and collaborative practices that help promote the structural changes necessary to address the material and psychosocial causes of health disparities (Plough 2005).

Public health research

Literature in ethics and public health research falls into two categories. First, there is literature exploring how public health research can be distinguished, conceptually and operationally, from public health practice (CDC 1999; Casarett et al. 2000; Bellin and Dubler 2001; Amoroso and Middaugh 2003). This literature outlines criteria for when an activity is quality assurance, surveillance, or evaluation versus when it is research requiring regulatory oversight (US Department of Health and Human Services 2009). This growing body of literature recognizes the blurry lines between research and practice in many arenas, including public health, and increasingly questions whether distinguishing research from practice is the most salient approach for ensuring ethical protection (Faden et al. 2013). As more data are available electronically, and with greater emphasis on learning healthcare systems and evidence-based practice (Institute of Medicine 2007; Kass et al. 2013), blurriness between research and practice will only grow larger.

Second, there is literature examining activities that unquestionably are research, but exploring whether public health research is different from clinical research, such that it should be exempt from certain regulatory requirements; literature also has addressed whether ethical challenges differ when entire populations are targeted for research.

Distinguishing public health research from non-research activities of public health

In 1999, the Centers for Disease Control and Prevention (CDC) issued what has become a widely cited document aimed at distinguishing public health research from non-research (CDC 1999). These guidelines were written in response to queries from outsiders whether certain data gathering activities conducted by CDC or by state health departments for public health practice should be categorized as research (Burris et al. 2003). While the guidelines were written to guide CDC employees in their own work, they have been used more broadly. The document asserts that public health practice can be distinguished from research based on what the primary intent of the activity is. If an activity is designed, primarily, to help a public health department do its job furthering the health interests of a particular community, even if it *also* produces data of more generalizable interest, the activity should be called non-research. Research, the guidance continued, is intended to produce generalizable knowledge, to have relevance beyond the population or programme from which data were collected. Surveillance, then, would be considered non-research when conducted in response to 'lawful state disease reporting or monitoring' activities. In 2001, the National Bioethics Advisory Commission echoed CDC guidance stating that projects *intended* to produce generalizable knowledge must be subject to the oversight provided by the Common Rule (National Bioethics Advisory Commission 2001).

The scholarly literature has echoed many of these concepts, especially that intention to produce generalizable knowledge characterizes research requiring federal oversight. Casarett et al. (2000), by contrast, suggest that activities should be regulated as research if: (1) the majority of patients involved are not expected to benefit directly from the knowledge to be gained and (2) additional risks and burdens exist as a result of wanting findings to be generalizable. Participants in a CDC workshop on practice versus research recommended research oversight to be determined by level of risk, rather than distinguishing based on primary intent (MacQueen and Buehler 2004). Bellin and Dubler suggested activities can be considered non-research if there is a commitment to modify programs based on collected data (Bellin and Dubler 2001), and a recent framework suggests that the degree to which learning and collecting data increase risks or threaten important interests or well-being should dictate the degree of ethical oversight required, regardless of whether an activity is called research or practice (Faden et al. 2013).

Burris et al. contend that collection of data by government agencies fulfils their mandated functions and should be exempt from federal research regulations specifically because they are conducted by public health departments. They suggest an alternative, internal oversight system be created to ensure that 'human beings who become involved in activities that increase our knowledge (whether defined as research or not) should be protected' and ensure that data collection activities are conducted in the least harmful, least restrictive, and most respectful way possible (Burris et al. 2003).

Fairchild and Bayer, however, suggest *all* data collection by federal or state governments should be subject to ethical review. While not suggesting institutional review boards (IRBs) necessarily perform this review, they advocate for universal review of these activities (Fairchild and Bayer 2004). With so much non-health data widely used and shared through social media, and through the Internet more broadly, questions are emerging going forwards about whether views about health privacy will change as the sharing of health data likely also becomes more widespread (Voyena et al. 2012).

Ethical issues raised by public health research

Other literature explores whether ethics issues in *public health research* differ from those of clinical research. Papers from the 1970s and 1980s suggested that certain types of epidemiological studies using identifiable records should be exempt from informed consent requirements (Gordis et al. 1977; Kelsey 1981; Waters 1985). Gordis et al. provide dozens of examples, from identifying the link between cigarette smoking and lung cancer, to the link between high concentrations of oxygen for premature infants and blindness, to the link between oral contraceptives and stroke, illustrating the contributions that epidemiological record review has made to public health and suggesting such methods would be nearly impossible if consent were required (Gordis et al. 1977). More recent literature examines whether and how population-based or prevention research differs in ethically relevant ways from clinical research (Taylor and Johnson 2007). Population-based research may not allow individual participants the opportunity to refuse participation, for example, when studies investigate community-wide interventions, like the impact of health promotion media campaigns in some communities and not others. In such cases, IRBs must confirm that risk to individuals is minimal and public health benefit from the research outweighs concerns imposed by individuals' inability to refuse. Data are generally collected at the population level without individual identifiers.

Population-based research has the potential to stigmatize identifiable groups if the research targets specific geographic, religious, or ethnic communities, or groups defined by a risk behaviour such as injection drug use or sexual orientation. The potential for stigma and social harms was a prominent concern of genetic research and the launch of the Human Genome Diversity Project in 1991, as entire races and indigenous communities were the unit of interest. Social harms animated a recent case, *Havasupai Tribe v. Arizona Board of Regents*. Stored genetic samples for research ultimately undermined traditional understandings of the tribe's ancestral origin, indicated high levels of inbreeding within the tribal community, and assessed associations with schizophrenia, a highly stigmatized condition within the tribe (*Havasupai Tribe v. Arizona Board of Regents* 2008). While research ethics has traditionally allowed analysis of samples that are not individually identifiable, this case demonstrated that population-based research carries the risk that outsiders might think differently about an entire social group as a result of research findings.

It is then not surprising that population-based research is the origin of both community advisory boards (Strauss et al. 2001; Morin et al. 2003; Quinn 2004) and community-based participatory methods (Israel et al. 1998; Macaulay et al. 1999), strategies designed to include community input into planned research methods and dissemination plans. Challenges remain regarding what is meant by 'community' and 'engagement' in the context of research (Hillery 1955; CDC 1997; MacQueen et al. 2001; Sharp and Foster 2007), as well as determining when community input must be sought, when a community has been fully represented, and how to resolve disputes within communities (Sharp and Foster 2007).

Research in resource-poor settings raises additional ethical challenges, both globally and domestically, and points to why the CIOMS guidelines include sections that other research ethics guidelines do not on incentives, responsibilities when studies are over, and justice. A major controversy erupted in 1997 after US-funded HIV trials in low-income countries tested the efficacy of drugs to prevent vertical transmission of HIV. Studies were placebo-controlled even when an effective, albeit expensive and complex, treatment protocol existed. While some scholars and human rights activists asserted that use of placebo was in clear violation of ethical guidelines, causing millions of infants to contract HIV (see Lurie and Wolfe 1997), others argued that women in the trials were no worse off by participating in trials, and placebo-controlled designs more validly tested whether locally relevant interventions were effective, to then be implemented in the field more quickly (Varmus and Satcher 1997). The controversy resulted in multiple revisions of the Declaration of Helsinki and CIOMS guidelines on the use of placebos, yet consensus on this question has not been reached.

Finally, similar to clinical trials, population-based trials—particularly those conducted in resource-poor settings—increasingly must consider what, if anything, will be made available to study communities when the research is completed. Several national and international bodies have suggested that successful research interventions should be made reasonably available to host country communities (CIOMS 2002; National Bioethics Advisory Commission 2001)—or at least justify why such availability is impossible if that is the case (Nuffield Council of Bioethics 2002), while others argued that many donor or government commitments never could have been secured until study results were in hand. An alternative approach suggested that 'fair benefits' should be provided to communities, regardless of whether those benefits are directly related to the study intervention being tested (Conference on Ethical Aspects of Research in Developing Countries 2004). Recent HIV Prevention Trial Network (HPTN) ethics guidance acknowledges that although conclusive definitions of post-study access agreements may not be possible prior to testing the intervention, the development of a detailed, preliminary plan of post-study access is nonetheless necessary (HPTN 2009).

Important in the evolution of thinking about public health research ethics was a controversial legal case of 2001 related to a lead abatement trial conducted in the 1990s in Baltimore (*Ericka Grimes v. Kennedy Krieger Institute, Inc.* 2001). This trial targeted low-income housing units in old neighbourhoods that had significant lead paint in units and where units often were in disrepair; that is, where children would be at risk of lead poisoning due to the existing poor conditions (Farfel and Chisolm 1990, 1991, 1994; Pollak 2002). Despite evidence existing for decades documenting the danger of lead paint to children, no laws existed requiring that houses be safe or abated before they could be rented to families. In the trial, households were randomized to one of several different lead abatement strategies to see the effect on both household lead dust and children's own blood lead levels of the different abatement strategies. Two families later brought lawsuits, charging that researchers failed to warn them in a timely manner that children might still be at risk of lead poisoning. This case was paradigmatic of certain types of public health research, in that it targeted a particular community, it dealt with prevention of a major public health problem, and, significantly, it was designed to respond to a series of baseline conditions that were harmful to public health. There remains no consensus regarding whether research is exploitive when situated in settings of neglect and when testing interventions that may improve conditions, but will not improve them as much as other, existing, but clearly unavailable interventions. Scholars have questioned whether conducting research on 'partial solutions' condones the idea that partial solutions are adequate for the disadvantaged (Farmer and Campos 2004; Spriggs 2004; Buchanan and Miller 2006; Kass 2008). Miller and Buchanan suggest that rejecting all research on partial solutions out of a 'presumption that a particular conception of justice will eventually prevail'—sacrifices the welfare of 'literally millions' of (in this case) children who could benefit from the results of the partial solutions tested through public health prevention research. Related, they assert that it is inappropriate to blame researchers for 'the lack of social consensus' on the right to better social conditions and that doing so is 'misplaced indignation' (Buchanan and Miller 2006). Others, however, suggest that even the perception of exploitation raised through this case is harmful for the research enterprise and suggests a need for 'true partnership in the research enterprise, particularly when proposed research involves vulnerable communities' (Mastroianni and Kahn 2002).

Ethical issues raised by genetic research

The rapid advancement of genetic research over the past two decades has presented new challenges for public health research, including issues of consent for storage of genetic material, return of genetic test results, and assignment of ownership of genetic material.

Because biospecimens used in genetic research are frequently collected and stored in a 'biobank' from which they are accessed for a wide range of future studies, it is not always possible to know how specimens may be used in the future. Re-contacting participants each time their sample will be used has been viewed as impractical and overly burdensome to both researchers and participants, yet 'blanket consent,' in which participants agree to any future use of their samples, has been criticized as an insufficient means of respecting participant autonomy (McGuire and Beskow 2010). While empirical work shows most participants support data-sharing initiatives that enable widespread use of their samples, participants expressed lingering concerns about the capacity of data-sharing initiatives to fully protect participant data, suggesting initiatives should be transparent to maintain trust with participant populations (Trinidad et al. 2010). At the same time, there is increasing opportunity for individuals to upload their own genetic data into private non-profit and commercial databases for use by a wide network of researchers, for example, through online initiatives such as 'Consent to Research' (http://weconsent.us/) and the 'Personal Genome Project' (www.personalgenomes.org). As biobanks have sprung up across the globe and information is increasingly available electronically, the potential for global data sharing is quickly becoming a reality (Kaye 2011). While such interconnectedness leverages the resources available to researchers and opens new opportunities for research, it amplifies the potential for uncontrolled use of specimens well beyond original and anticipated uses. Consent procedures for biobanking and the ethics of global data sharing is in its infancy, and ethicists are grappling with the challenges of developing controls and accountability mechanisms (Gottweiss and Lauss 2010; O'Doherty et al. 2011).

Disclosure of results from genetic tests performed during research also raises controversy. Some argue results should be returned as a way to respect autonomy and allow participants to find meaning in results even without clinical implications; returning results may also demonstrate reciprocity for having participated in research (Ravitsky and Wilfond 2006). Others counter that supplying genetic results that are often complex and offer limited clinical value would be misleading and potentially harmful (Beskow 2006). Even when results are readily interpretable and have clinical implications, informing participants of results requires retaining linkages to individual samples. The National Bioethics Advisory Commission and the National Cancer Institute's Best Practices for Biospecimen Resources state merely that the informed consent document contain a statement explaining whether, which, and to whom individual results would be released (National Bioethics Advisory Commission 1999; National Cancer Institute 2011). Taking a stronger stance, the National Heart, Lung and Blood Institute convened working groups in 2004 and 2009 that drafted recommendations outlining conditions under which results ethically should be returned, circumstances in which research may but should not be expected to return results, and that emphasized the importance of community engagement when working with identifiable communities (Fabsitz et al. 2010).

Finally, genetic research has given rise to questions of identity, ownership, and property in ways not seen in other types of public health research. Law suits filed in the early 1990s and 2000s addressed ownership of biological material used in genetic research (*Moore v. Regents of the University of California* 1990; *Greenberg v. Miami Children's Hospital Research Institute* 2003; *Washington University v. Catalona* 2007) and plaintiffs claimed a property right to the materials developed from their genetic samples. Defendants argued that samples were 'donated' and individuals relinquished ownership rights when samples were collected. Case law to date has favoured the research enterprise in rulings that do not recognize participant ownership of biospecimens collected for research, yet questions remain, ethically, as to whether viewing biospecimens as property is appropriate. McGuire and Beskow outline numerous approaches to informed consent in genetic research, (McGuire and Beskow 2010), and the National Human Genome Research Institute maintains a comprehensive web resource for conducting informed consent in genetic research. In addition, new initiatives seek to address these challenges through participant engagement (Kaye et al. 2012). Finally, emerging participatory models propose the use of social media as a way to form relationships between participants and researchers. As a means of ongoing communication, these initiatives empower participants to make informed choices over the use of their samples and provide a mechanism to communicate findings as their interpretation changes over time.

Conclusion

Public health has been given significant attention in the bioethics literature only in the last three decades. Public health must balance furthering the health of communities through education, surveillance, interventions, and regulations with needing to restrict the freedoms or privacy of individuals affected to the minimum degree possible while also addressing core commitments to social justice. Public health is granted statutory authority to protect the public's health and, indeed extraordinary public health improvement has been achieved through sanitary measures, restaurant inspections, immunizations, and health education. At the same time, it is expressly because of this authority that ethics has such a critical role to play. Clear frameworks of ethics that outline a need for data, minimizing of harms, fair procedures, and clear principles to follow, including transparency, reciprocity, and equity, can help public health fulfil its duty to improve health on behalf of all of us, while allowing individuals to feel confident that any restrictions are appropriate and fairly defined. Public health research requires some new considerations for research ethics including the need to be more cognizant of the implications of research for populations as a whole, for finding creative ways to seek community-wide input, and to begin to consider how to ensure that communities, as well as individuals, realize research benefit.

Notes

1. Note that the 11th edition of the same textbook (1980) had a chapter entitled 'Legal and Ethical Issues in Public Health' by Sidney Shindell. The bulk of this chapter is devoted to legal issues in public health, however, rather than ethics issues, and thus is not discussed here.
2. Note that this article describes the work of Edward Chadwick in England in the early 1800s demonstrating that differences in social conditions led to a more than twofold difference in life expectancy between upper and lower classes. Also in the 1800s, governments began conducting investigations of housing conditions and garbage heaps and mapping them in relation to outbreaks of disease, and by the end of the nineteenth century, state and local boards of health were being created to enforce sanitary regulations.

References

Allen, R. (2007). *Fostering Professionalism During Medical School and Residency Training. CME Report 3-A-01. Report of the Council on Medical Education.* Chicago, IL: American Medical Association.

American Medical Association. Council on Ethical and Judicial Affairs (1990). Fundamental elements of the physician–patient relationship. *Journal of the American Medical Association*, 264, 3133.

American Public Health Association (2002). *APHA Code of Ethics.* Washington, DC: American Public Health Association.

Amoroso, P.J. and Middaugh, J.P. (2003). Research vs. public health practice: when does a study require IRB review? *Preventive Medicine*, 36, 250–3.

Bailey, T., Haines, C., Rosychuk, R.J., et al. (2011). Public engagement on ethical principles in allocating scare resources during an influenza pandemic. *Vaccine*, 29, 3111–17.

Bayer, R. (1983). Gays and the stigma of bad blood. *Hastings Center Report*, 13, 5–7.

Bayer, R. (1989). Ethical and social policy issues raised by HIV screening: the epidemic evolves and so do the challenges. *AIDS*, 3, 119–24.

Bayer, R., Levine, C., and Wolf, S.M. (1986). HIV antibody screening: an ethical framework for evaluating proposed programs. *Journal of the American Medical Association*, 256, 1768–74.

Beauchamp, D.E. (1976a). Alcoholism as blaming the alcoholic. *International Journal of Addiction*, 11, 41–52.

Beauchamp, D.E. (1985). Community: the neglected tradition of public health. *The Hastings Center Report*, 15, 28–36.

Beauchamp, D.E. (1976b). Public health as social justice. *Inquiry*, 13, 1–14.

Beauchamp, T.L. and Childress, J.L. (1979). *Principles of Biomedical Ethics.* Oxford: Oxford University Press.

Bellin, E. and Dubler, N.N. (2001). The quality improvement–research divide and the need for external oversight. *American Journal of Public Health*, 91, 1512–17.

Beskow, L. (2006). Considering the nature of individual research results. *American Journal of Bioethics*, 6, 38–40.

Brock, D. (1989). Justice, health care, and the elderly. *Philosophy and Public Affairs*, 18, 297–312.

Buchanan, D.R. and Miller, F.G. (2006). Justice and fairness in the Kennedy Krieger Institute lead paint study: the ethics of public health research on less expensive, less effective interventions. *American Journal of Public Health*, 96, 781–7.

Burris, S, Buehler, J., and Lazzarini, Z. (2003). Applying the Common Rule to public health agencies: questions and tentative answers about a separate regulatory regime. *Journal of Law and Medical Ethics*, 31, 638–53.

Callahan, D. (1984). Autonomy: a moral good, not a moral obsession. *The Hastings Center Report*, 14, 40–2.

Callahan, D. and Jennings, B. (2002). Ethics and public health: forging a strong relationship. *American Journal of Public Health*, 92, 169–76.

Casarett, D., Karlawish, J.H.T., and Sugarman, J. (2000). Determining when quality improvement initiatives should be considered research: proposed criteria and potential implications. *Journal of the American Medical Association*, 283, 2275–80.

Centers for Disease Control (1983). Current trends prevention of acquired immune deficiency syndrome: report of inter-agency recommendations. *Morbidity and Mortality Weekly Report*, 32, 101–3.

Centers for Disease Control (1997). *Community Engagement: Definitions and Organizing Concepts from the Literature, Part 1. Principles of Community Engagement: CDC/ATSDR Committee on Community Engagement.* Atlanta, GA: CDC.

Centers for Disease Control (1999). *Guidelines for Defining Public Health Research and Public Health Non-Research.* Atlanta, GA: CDC.

Centers for Disease Control (2007). *Ethical Guidelines in Pandemic Influenza*. Atlanta, GA: CDC.

Centers for Disease Control (2011). *Ethical Consideration for Decision Making Regarding Allocation of Mechanical Ventilators during a Severe Influenza Pandemic or Other Public Health Emergency*. Atlanta, GA: CDC.

Childress, J.F. (1987). An ethical framework for assessing policies to screen for antibodies for HIV. *AIDS Public Policy Journal*, 2, 28–31.

Childress, J.F., Faden, R.R., Gaare, R.D., et al. (2002). Public health ethics: mapping the terrain. *Journal of Law and Medical Ethics*, 30, 170–8.

Clouser, K.D. (1995). Common morality as an alternative to principlism. *Kennedy Institute of Ethics Journal*, 5, 219–36.

Conference on Ethical Aspects of Research in Developing Countries (2004). Moral standards for research in developing countries: from 'reasonable availability' to 'fair benefits'. *The Hastings Center Report*, 34, 17–27.

Council for International Organizations of Medical Sciences (2002). *International Ethical Guidelines for Biomedical Research Involving Human Subjects*. Geneva: World Health Organization.

Daniels, N. (1985). *Just Health Care*. New York: Cambridge University Press.

Daniels, N. (2008). *Just Health: Meeting Health Needs Fairly*. New York: Cambridge University Press.

DeBruin, D., Laischenko, J., and Marshall, M. (2012). Social justice in pandemic preparedness. *American Journal of Public Health*, 102, 586–91.

Emanuel, E. and Wertheimer, A. (2006). Public health: who should get influenza vaccine when not all can? *Science*, 312, 854–5.

Ericka Grimes, v. Kennedy Krieger Institute, Inc. (2001). *West's Atlantic Reporter*, 782, 807–62.

Fabsitz, R.R., McGuire, A., Sharp, R.R., et al. (2010). Ethical and practical guidelines for reporting genetic research results to study participants: updated guidelines from an NHLBI working group. *Circulation: Cardiovascular Genetics*, 3, 574–80.

Faden, R.R. (1987). Ethical issues in government sponsored public health campaigns. *Health Education Quarterly*, 14, 27–37.

Faden, R.R. and Faden, A.I. (1978). The ethics of health education as public policy. *Health Education Monographs*, 6, 180–97.

Faden, R., Kass, N., Goodman, S., et al. (2013). An ethics framework for learning healthcare systems. *The Hastings Center Report*, 43, S16–27.

Fairchild, A.L. and Bayer, R. (2004). Public health: ethics and the conduct of public health surveillance. *Science*, 303, 631–2.

Farfel, M.R. and Chisolm, J.J. (1990). Health and environmental outcomes of traditional and modified practices for abatement of residential lead-based paint. *American Journal of Public Health*, 80, 1240–5.

Farfel, M.R. and Chisolm, J.J. (1991). An evaluation of experimental practices for abatement of residential lead-based paint: report on a pilot project. *Environmental Research*, 55, 199–212.

Farfel, M.R. and Chisolm, J.J. (1994). The longer-term effectiveness of residential lead paint abatement. *Environmental Research*, 66, 217–21.

Farmer, P. and Campos, N.G. (2004). New malaise: bioethics and human rights in the global era. *Journal of Law and Medical Ethics*, 32, 243–51.

Fee, E. (1977). History and development of public health. In F.D. Scutchfield and C.W. Keck (eds.) *Principles of Public Health Practice*, pp. 10–30. Boston, MA: Delmar Publishers.

Frankfurt, H. (1987). Equality as a moral ideal. *Ethics*, 98, 21–43.

Glanz, K., Lewis, F.M., and Rimer, B.K. (1997). *Health Behavior and Health Education: Theory, Research and Practice* (2nd ed.). San Francisco, CA: Jossey-Bass.

Gordis, L., Gold, E., and Seltser, R. (1977). Privacy protection in epidemiologic and medical research: a challenge and a responsibility. *American Journal of Epidemiology*, 105, 163–8.

Gostin, L. (2004). Pandemic influenza: public health preparedness for the next global emergency. *Journal of Law, Medicine, and Ethics*, 32, 565–73.

Gostin, L. and Curran, W.J. (1986). The limit of compulsion on controlling AIDS. *Hastings Center Report*, 16, 24–9.

Gostin, L. and Curran, W.J. (1987). Legal control measures for AIDS: reporting requirements, surveillance, quarantine, and regulation of public meeting places. *American Journal of Public Health*, 77, 214–18.

Gostin, L., Curran, W.J., and Clark, M.E. (1987). The case against compulsory casefinding in controlling AIDS—testing, screening and reporting. *American Journal of Law and Medicine*, 12, 7–53.

Gottweiss, H. and Lauss, G. (2010). Biobank governance in the post-genomic age. *Personalized Medicine*, 7, 187–95.

Greenberg v. Miami Children's Hospital Research Institute (2003). 264 F.Supp.2d 1064 (S.D. Fla. 2003).

Havasupai Tribe v. Arizona State University Board of Regents (2008). 204 P.3d 1063 (9th Cir. 2008).

Hillery, G. (1955). Definitions of community: areas of agreement. *Rural Sociology*, 20, 111–24.

HIV Prevention Trials Network Ethics Working Group (2009). *HIV Prevention Trials Network Ethics Guidance for Research*. New York: HPTN.

Hunter, N.D. (1987). AIDS prevention and civil liberties: the false security of mandatory testing. *AIDS Public Policy Journal*, 2, 1–10.

Institute of Medicine (1986). *Confronting AIDS: Directions for Public Health, Health Care, and Research*. Washington, DC: National Academies Press.

Institute of Medicine (2007). *IOM Roundtable on Evidence-Based Medicine, The Learning Healthcare System: Workshop Summary*, L. Olsen, D. Aisner, and J.M. McGinnis (eds.). Washington, DC: National Academies Press.

Israel, B.A., Schulz, A.J., Parker, E.A., et al. (1998). Review of community-based research: assessing partnership approaches to improve public health. *Annual Review of Public Health*, 19, 173–202.

Jonsen, A.R. (1995). Casuistry: an alternative or complement to principles? *Kennedy Institute of Ethics Journal*, 5, 237–51.

Kao, A., Lim, M., Spevick, J., et al. (2003). Teaching and evaluating students' professionalism in US medical schools, 2002–2003. *Journal of the American Medical Association*, 290, 1151–2.

Kass, N. (2001). An ethics framework for public health. *American Journal of Public Health*, 91, 1776–82.

Kass, N. (2008). Just research in an unjust world: can harm reduction be an acceptable tool for public health prevention research? In R.M. Green, A. Donovan, and S.A. Jauss (eds.) *Global Bioethics*, pp. 89–116. Oxford: Oxford University Press.

Kass, N., Faden, R., Goodman, S., et al. (2013). The research–treatment distinction: a problematic approach for determining which activities should have ethical oversight. *The Hastings Center Report*, 43, S4–15.

Kawachi, I., Kennedy, B.P., and Wilkinson, R.G. (1999). *The Society and Population Health Reader, Vol. I: Income Inequality and Health*. New York: The New Press.

Kaye, J. (2011). From single biobanks to international networks: developing e-governance. *Human Genetics*, 130, 377–82.

Kaye, J., Curren, L., Anderson, L., et al. (2012). From patients to partners: participant-centric initiatives in biomedical research. *Nature Reviews Genetics*, 13, 371–6.

Kelsey, J.L. (1981). Privacy and confidentiality in epidemiological research involving patients. *IRB*, 3, 1–4.

Koop, C.E. (1986). Surgeon General's report on acquired immune deficiency syndrome. *Journal of the American Medical Association*, 256, 278–89.

Kotalik, J. (2005). Preparing for an influenza pandemic: ethical issues. *Bioethics*, 19, 422–31.

Lappe, M. (1986). Ethics and public health. In J.M. Last (ed.) *Maxcy-Rosenau Public Health and Preventive Medicine* (12th ed.), pp. 1867–77. Norwalk, CT: Appleton-Century-Crofts.

Lurie, P. and Wolfe, S. (1997). Unethical trials of interventions to reduce perinatal transmission of the human immunodeficiency virus in developing countries. *New England Journal of Medicine*, 337, 853–6.

Macaulay, A.C., Commanda, L.E., Freeman, W.L., et al. (1999). Participatory research maximizes community and lay involvement. *British Medical Journal*, 319, 774–8.

Macklin, R. (1986). Predicting dangerousness and public health response to AIDS. *The Hastings Center Report*, 16, 16–23.

MacQueen, K.M. and Buehler, J.W. (2004). Ethics, practice, and research in public health. *American Journal of Public Health*, 94, 928–31.

MacQueen, K.M., McLellan, E., Metzger, D.S., et al. (2001). What is community? An evidence-based definition for participatory public health. *American Journal of Public Health*, 91, 1929–38.

Marmot, M. (2004). Social causes of social inequalities in health. In A.Sudhir and F. Peter (eds.) *Public Health, Ethics, and Equity*, pp. 37–62. Oxford: Oxford University Press.

Marmot, M., Davey Smith, G., Stansfeld S., et al. (1991). Health inequalities among British social servants: the Whitehall II Study. *Lancet*, 337, 1387–93.

Marmot, M. and Shipley, M. (1996). Do socio-economic differences in mortality persist after retirement? 25 year follow up of civil servants from the first Whitehall Study. *British Medical Journal*, 33, 1177–80.

Mastroianni, A.C. and Kahn, J.P. (2002). Risk and responsibility: ethics, Grimes v Kennedy Krieger, and public health research involving children. *American Journal of Public Health*, 92, 1073–6.

McCullough, L.B. (ed.) (1998). *John Gregory's Writings on Medical Ethics and Philosophy of Medicine*. Dordrecht: Kluwer Academic Publishers.

McGuire, A. and Beskow, L. (2010). Informed consent in genomics and genetic research. *Annual Review Genomics and Human Genetics*, 11, 361–81.

Mill, J.S. (1869). *On Liberty*. In J. Gray (ed.) (1998) *On Liberty and Other Essays* (2nd ed.), pp. 1–129. New York: Oxford University Press.

Moore v. Regents of the University of California (1990). 793 P.2d 479 (Cal. 1990).

Morin, S.F., Maiorana, A., Koester, K.A., et al. (2003). Community consultation in HIV prevention research: a study of community advisory boards at 6 research sites. *Journal of Acquired Immune Deficiency Syndromes*, 33, 513–20.

Musto, D.F. (1986). Quarantine and the problem of AIDS. *Milbank Memorial Fund Quarterly*, 64, 113.

National Bioethics Advisory Commission (NBAC) (1999). *Research Involving Human Biological Materials: Ethical Issues and Policy Guidance*. Vol. 1. Rockville, MD: NBAC.

National Bioethics Advisory Commission (NBAC) (2001). *Ethical and Policy Issues in International Research Clinical Trials in Developing Countries*. Vol. 1. Rockville, MD: NBAC.

National Cancer Institute (2011). Best Practices for Biospecimen Resources). Available at: http://biospecimens.cancer.gov/bestprac tices/2011-NCIBestPractices.pdf (aAccessed 25 April 25, 2013).

National Commission for the Protection of Human Subjects of Biomedical and Behavioral Research (1979). *The Belmont Report: Ethical Principles and Guidelines for the Protection of Human Subjects of Research*. Washington, DC: Government Printing Office.

Nuffield Council of Bioethics (2002). *The Ethics of Research Related to Healthcare in Developing Countries*. Available at: http://www.nuffield bioethics.org/research-developing-countries (accessed 25 April 2013).

Nussbaum, M. (2006). *Frontiers of Justice: Disability, Nationality, Species Membership*. Cambridge, MA: The Belknap Press of Harvard University Press.

O'Doherty, K., Burgess, M., Edwards, K., et al. (2011). From consent to institutions: designing adaptive governance for genomic biobanks. *Social Science and Medicine*, 73, 367–74.

Parfit, D. (1998). Equality and priority. In A. Mason (ed.) *Ideals of Equality*, pp. 21–36. Oxford: Blackwell Publishers.

Pellegrino, E.D. (1981). Health promotion as public policy: the need for moral groundings. *Preventive Medicine*, 10, 371–8.

Pellegrino, E.D. (1995). Toward a virtue-based normative ethics for health professions. *Kennedy Institute of Ethics Journal*, 5, 253–77.

Pellegrino, E. and Thomasma, D.C. (1988). *For the Patient's Good: The Restoration of Beneficence in Health Care*. New York: Oxford University Press.

Percival, T. (1985). *Medical Ethics; or a Code of Institutes and Precepts, adapted to the Professional Conduct of Physicians and Surgeons…together with an Introduction by Edmund D. Pellegrino*. Birmingham, AL: Classics of Medicine Library.

Plough, A. (2005). Promoting social justice through public health policies, programs, and services. In B.S. Levy and V.W. Sidel (eds.) *Social Justice and Public Health*, pp. 418–31. Oxford: Oxford University Press.

Pollak, J. (2002). The lead-based paint abatement repair and maintenance study in Baltimore: historic framework and study design. *Journal of Health Care Law and Policy*, 6, 89–108.

Porter, R. (1986). History says no to the policeman's response to AIDS. *British Medical Journal*, 293, 1589–90.

Powers, M. and Faden, R. (2006). *Social Justice: The Moral Foundations of Public Health and Health Policy*. New York: Oxford University Press.

Powers, M. and Faden, R. (2011). Health capabilities, outcomes, and the political ends of justice. *Journal of Human Development and Capabilities*, 12, 565–70.

Presidential Commission on the Human Immunodeficiency Virus Epidemic (1988). *Final Report*. Washington, DC: Government Printing Office.

Quinn, S.C. (2004). Ethics in public health research: protecting human subjects: the role of Community Advisory Boards. *American Journal of Public Health*, 94, 918–22.

Ravindran, G.D. (2008). Medical ethics education in India. *Indian Journal of Medical Ethics*, 5, 18–19.

Ravitsky, V. and Wilfond, B. (2006). Disclosing individual genetic results to participants. *American Journal of Bioethics*, 6, 8–17.

Rawls, J. (1971). *A Theory of Justice*. Cambridge, MA: The Belknap Press of Harvard University Press.

Roberts, M.J. and Reich, M.R. (2002). Ethical analysis in public health. *The Lancet*, 359, 1055–9.

Rosoff, P. and DeCamp, M. (2011). Preparing for pandemic influenza: are some people more equal than others? *Journal of Health Care for the Poor and Underserved*, 3S: 19–35.

Roter, D.L., Hall, J.A., Merisca, R., et al. (1998). Effectiveness of interventions to improve patient compliance: a meta-analysis. *Medical Care*, 36, 1138–61.

Ruger, J. (2009). *Health and Social Justice*. Oxford: Clarendon Press of Oxford University Press.

Segall, S. (2010). *Health, Luck, and Justice*. Princeton, NJ: Princeton University Press.

Sen, A. (2002). Why health equity? *Health Economics*, 11, 659–66.

Sen, A. (2009). *The Idea of Justice*. Cambridge, MA: The Belknap Press of Harvard University Press.

Sharp, R. and Foster, M. (2007). Grappling with groups: protecting collective interests in biomedical research. *Journal of Medicine and Philosophy*, 32, 321–37.

Society for Public Health Education (n.d.). *Code of Ethics for the Health Education Profession*. Section 4. Available at: http://www.sophe.org/Ethics.cfm (accessed 25 April 2013).

Spriggs, M. (2004). Canaries in the mines: children, risk, non-therapeutic research, and justice. *Journal of Medical Ethics*, 30, 176–81.

Steinbock, B. (1996). Liberty, responsibility, and the common good. *The Hastings Center Report*, 26, 45–7.

Strauss, R.P., Sengupta, S. Quinn, S.C., et al. (2001). The role of community advisory boards: involving communities in the informed consent process. *American Journal of Public Health*, 91, 1938–43.

Taylor, H.A. and Johnson, S. (2007). Ethics of population-based research. *Journal of Law, Medicine and Ethics*, 35, 295–9.

Thompson, A., Faith, K., Gibson, J., et al. (2006). Pandemic influenza preparedness: an ethical framework to guide decision-making. *BMC Medical Ethics*. 7, 12.

Trinidad S., Fullerton, S., Ludman, E., et al. (2010). Genomic research and wide data-sharing: views of prospective participants. *Genetics and Medicine*, 12, 486–95.

University of Toronto Joint Centre on Bioethics (2005). *Stand on Guard for Thee: Ethical Consideration in Preparedness Planning for Pandemic Influenza.* Toronto: University of Toronto Joint Centre on Bioethics.

Uscher-Pines, L. Duggan, P.S., Garoon, J.P., et al. (2007). Social justice and disadvantaged groups. *The Hastings Center Report,* 37, 32–9.

US Department of Health and Human Services (HHS) (2005). *HHS Pandemic Influenza Plan. Appendix D.* Washington, DC: HHS. Available at: http://www.flu.gov/planning-preparedness/federal/hhspandemicinfluenzaplan.pdf (accessed 25 April 2013).

US Department of Health and Human Services (HHS) (2009). *Protection of Human Subjects, 45 CFR 46.* Washington, DC: HHS.

Varmus, H., and Satcher, D. (1997). Ethical complexities of conducting research in developing countries. *New England Journal of Medicine,* 337, 1003–5.

Vawter, D.E., Garret, J.E., Gervais, K.G., et al. (2011). Attending to social vulnerability when rationing pandemic resources. *Journal of Clinical Ethics,* 22, 42–53.

Venkatapuram, S. (2011). *Health Justice.* Cambridge: Polity Press.

Voyena, E., Mastroianni, A., and Kahn, J. (2012). Ethical issues in health research with novel online sources. *American Journal of Public Health,* 102, 2225–30.

Walter, J. and Klein, E. (2003). *The Story of Bioethics: from Seminal Works to Contemporary Explanations.* Washington, DC: Georgetown University Press.

Washington University v. Catalona (2007). 490 F.3d 667, 675 (8th Cir. 2007).

Waters, W.E. (1985). Ethics and epidemiological research. *International Journal of Epidemiology,* 14, 48–51.

Wikler, D.I. (1978a). Coercive measures in health promotion: can they be justified? *Health Education Monographs,* 6, 223–41.

Wikler, D.I. (1978b). Persuasion and coercion for health. *Milbank Memorial Fund Quarterly/Health and Society,* 56, 303–33.

Wilkinson, R.G. and Marmot, M. (2003). *Social Determinants of Health: The Solid Facts* (2nd ed.). Geneva: WHO.

3.3

The right to the highest attainable standard of health

Paul Hunt, Gunilla Backman, Judith Bueno de Mesquita, Louise Finer, Rajat Khosla, Dragana Korljan, and Lisa Oldring

Human rights

What are human rights?

Human rights are freedoms and entitlements concerned with the protection of the inherent well-being, dignity, and equality of every human being. They include civil, political, economic, social, and cultural rights. The international community has accepted the position that all human rights are universal, indivisible, interdependent, and interrelated (United Nations (UN) 1993).

Although inspired by moral values, such as dignity and equality, human rights are more than moral entitlements: They are legally guaranteed through national and international legal obligations on duty bearers. They are enshrined, for example, in various international treaties and declarations.

International human rights treaties (often called covenants or conventions), such as the International Covenant on Economic, Social and Cultural Rights (ICESCR), are legally binding on the States that ratify them ('States parties'). In contrast, human rights declarations, such as the Universal Declaration of Human Rights, are non-binding, although many of them do include norms and principles that reflect obligations that are binding under customary international law.

Human rights have traditionally been concerned with the relationship between the State, on one hand, and individuals and groups on the other. By ratifying international human rights treaties, States assume binding legal obligations to give effect to the human rights enumerated within them.

Additionally, all States have national laws that protect some human rights. Moreover, some States have enshrined human rights—civil, political, economic, social, and cultural—in their constitutions.

Historic neglect of economic, social, and cultural rights, such as the rights to health and shelter, is gradually being overcome, thanks in part to civil society organizations across the world that have campaigned for their equal representation and advocated for specific mechanisms for their enforcement.

Who has human rights duties?

Although only States are parties to international and regional human rights treaties, and are thus fully accountable for compliance with their provisions, all members of society have responsibilities regarding the realization of human rights, including the right to the highest attainable standard of health (UN 1948, preamble; UNCESCR 2000, para. 42). This includes health workers, families, communities, inter- and non-governmental organizations, civil society groups, as well as the private business sector: these so-called 'non-State actors' all have responsibilities regarding the realization of the right to health. States, as parties to international treaties, have a duty to provide an environment in which all of these individuals and groups can discharge their human rights responsibilities.

Approaches to human rights

One approach to the vindication of human rights is via the courts, tribunals, and other judicial and quasi-judicial processes (the 'judicial' approach). Another approach, however, brings human rights to bear upon policymaking processes so that policies and programmes that promote and protect human rights are put in place (the 'policy' approach). Although the two approaches are intimately related and mutually reinforcing, the distinction between them is important because the 'policy' approach opens up challenging new interdisciplinary possibilities for the operationalization of human rights.

Lawyers have played an indispensable role in developing the norms and standards that today constitute international human rights law. Naturally, when it comes to the 'judicial' and 'policy' approaches, some lawyers are professionally drawn to the former. Indeed, in the context of the right to health, despite some suggestions to the contrary, this approach has a vital role to play and many courts have demonstrated that they have a crucial contribution to make (UNHRC, 2007; Gauri and Brinks 2008; Yamin and Gloppen 2011). It is important that this judicial contribution deepens and becomes more widespread.

In addition to this approach, however, it is vital that the right to health is brought to bear upon all relevant local, national and international policymaking processes This 'policy' approach depends upon techniques and tools—indicators, benchmarks, impact assessments, and so on—that demand close cooperation across a range of disciplines. Given its historic role and traditional expertise, public health has an indispensable contribution to make to the 'policy' approach. The later section 'New tools and techniques' briefly introduces some of these techniques and tools in the specific context of the right to the highest attainable standard of health.

What is the right to health?

Sources of the right to health

The origins of the international right to the highest attainable standard of health can be traced back over 60 years. Adopted in 1946, the World Health Organization's (WHO) Constitution states: 'The enjoyment of the highest attainable standard of health is one of the fundamental rights of every human being without distinction of race, religion, political belief, economic or social condition'. Two years later, article 25(1) of the Universal Declaration of Human Rights laid the foundations for the international legal framework for the right to health. Since then, the right to health has been codified in numerous legally binding international and regional human rights treaties, and enshrined in many national laws, some of which are signalled in the following paragraphs. This gives rise to one of the most important and distinctive characteristics of human rights, including the right to the highest attainable standard of health. Human rights place legally binding obligations on States.

International human rights law

Concrete legal duties are conferred upon States when they ratify international treaties; they must ensure that all individuals within their jurisdiction can enjoy the rights envisaged within them. The cornerstone protection of the right to health in international law is found in Article 12 of ICESCR. Over 155 States have legally bound themselves, through ratification of this treaty, to its implementation.

Additional right to health protections are contained in international treaties that address issues specific to marginalized groups, such as the International Convention for the Elimination of All Forms of Racial Discrimination (CERD, Article 5(e)(iv)); the International Convention on the Elimination of All Forms of Discrimination Against Women (CEDAW, Articles 11(1)f, 12, and 14(2)b); the Convention on the Rights of the Child (CRC, Articles 3(3), 17, 23, 24, 25, 28, and 32); and the Convention on the Rights of Persons with Disabilities (CRPD, Articles 25 and 26).

Authoritative and interpretive guiding principles of several of these treaty provisions on the right to health—called General Comments or General Recommendations—shed further light on the parameters and content of the right to health generally, and in relation to the application of the right to specific groups. In 2000, for example, the UN treaty-body responsible for monitoring ICESCR adopted General Comment 14 on the right to the highest attainable standard of health.

Moreover, some UN treaty-bodies have decided cases that shed light on the scope of health-related rights. Recently, for example, the Human Rights Committee considered the case of a 17-year-old Peruvian who was denied a therapeutic abortion. When K.L. was 14 weeks pregnant, doctors at a public hospital in Lima diagnosed the fetus with an abnormality that would endanger K.L.'s health if pregnancy continued. However, K.L. was denied a therapeutic abortion by the hospital's director. In *K.L. v. Peru*, the Human Rights Committee decided that by denying the young woman's request to undergo an abortion in accordance with Peruvian law, the Government was in breach of its right-to-life obligations under the International Covenant on Civil and Political Rights (UNHRCttee 2003).

Further standards relating to specific groups are set out in non-binding legal instruments, such as the Declaration on the Elimination of Violence against Women. Additional international human rights instruments contain protections relevant to the right to health in various situations, environments and processes, including armed conflict, development, the workplace, and detention (UNCHR 2003a, Annex I).

Significantly, resolutions of the UN Commission on Human Rights, including those on disabilities and access to medication (UNCHR 2002a, 2002b), have articulated the right to the highest attainable standard of health; while other important resolutions contain provisions that bear closely upon the right (UNCHR 2003a, Annex II).

Far-reaching commitments relating to the right to health have been made in the outcome documents of numerous UN world conferences, such as the International Conference on Population and Development (UN 1994), the Fourth World Conference on Women (UN 1995), and the Millennium Declaration (UNGA 2000). These conferences have helped to place international problems, including health issues such as HIV/AIDS, at the top of the global agenda and their outcome documents influence international and national policymaking. Several refer to the right to health and health-related rights.

Regional human rights law

The right to health is recognized in human rights treaties drafted and monitored by the different regional human rights systems. These have effect only in their respective regions and include: the African Charter on Human and Peoples' Rights (Article 16); the African Charter on the Rights and Welfare of the Child (Article 14); the Additional Protocol to the American Convention on Human Rights in the Area of Economic, Social and Cultural Rights, known as the 'Protocol of San Salvador' (Article 10); and the European Social Charter (Article 11). Other regional instruments, such as the American Convention on Human Rights (OAS 1969) and European Convention for the Protection of Human Rights and Fundamental Freedoms (Council of Europe 1950), provide, through health-related rights, indirect protection of the right to health.

At regional level there are also judicial and other mechanisms that adjudicate cases involving the right to health. A notable case in 2002 was the finding by the African Commission on Human and Peoples' Rights of a violation of the right to health by the Federal Republic of Nigeria, on account of violations against the Ogoni people in relation to the activities of oil companies in the Niger Delta (ACHPR 2001).

Significantly, regional mechanisms have also found breaches of other health-related rights, including the violation of the right to a home and family and private life, arising from environmental harm to human health in *López Ostra v. Spain* (ECtHR 1994), as well as the negative consequences on children's health stemming from the occurrence of child labour in *ICJ v. Portugal* (ECSR 1998).

Another important development has come from the Inter-American Commission on Human Rights, which expressed its willingness to 'take into account' provisions of the regional treaty (the Protocol of San Salvador) related to the right to health when analysing the merits of a case, even though it lacked competence to determine violations under them (IACHR 2000).

National law

A study has shown that 67.5 per cent of the constitutions of all nations have provisions regarding health and healthcare (Kinney and Clark 2004). In addition, a large number of constitutions set out States' duties in relation to health, such as the duty to develop health services, from which it is possible to infer health entitlements.

In some jurisdictions these constitutional provisions have generated significant jurisprudence, such as the decision of the Constitutional Court of South Africa in *Minister for Health v. Treatment Action Campaign*. In this case, the Court held that the Constitution required the Government 'to devise and implement a comprehensive and coordinated programme to realize progressively the right of pregnant women and their newborn children to have access to health services to combat mother-to-child transmission of HIV' (CCSA 2002, para. 135 (2) (a)). This case—and numerous other laws and decisions at the international, regional, and national levels—confirms that the courts have an important role to play in the protection of the right to the highest attainable standard of health.

Right to health in the context of other human rights

As already indicated, the right to health is closely related to and dependent upon the realization of other fundamental human rights contained within international law. These include the rights to life, food, housing, work, and education, as well as rights based on the freedom not to be tortured or discriminated against. Similarly, the rights to privacy, equality, access to information, and freedom of association, as well as other rights and freedoms, relate to and address integral components of the right to health.

The right to health—like other economic, social, and cultural rights—does not escape controversy and ideological objections. Some States are still reluctant to see it as a right of similar weight to others, such as the right to a fair trial. However, under international law, the right to the highest attainable standard of health is an integral part of the international code of human rights and must be given equal treatment and attention. Importantly, the interdependence and equal footing of all human rights was reaffirmed in the Vienna Declaration (UN 1993, para. 5). Furthermore, jurisprudence and international standards are gradually clarifying the mutually reinforcing relationship between the right to health and other health-related rights, such as the right to life (UNCESCR 2000, para. 3).

The complementary relationship between public health and the right to health

With a few exceptions, the relationship between health and human rights was not subject to close examination until the 1990s. Of course, the Constitution of WHO (WHO 1946) affirms the right to health and so does the Declaration of Alma Ata (WHO 1978a). Also, some of those who were struggling against HIV/AIDS in the 1980s recognized the crucial importance of human rights.

But, for the most part, these important developments were not accompanied by a detailed examination of the substantive relationship between health and human rights. That had to wait until the early 1990s. A great debt is owed to the late Jonathan Mann and his colleagues at the Harvard School of Public Health and the Francois-Xavier Bagnoud Center for Health and Human Rights for their pioneering work on the relationship between health and human rights, especially in the context of HIV/AIDS (Grodin et al. 2013).

In the 1990s, however, Dr Mann and others suffered from a serious limitation that does not apply today. At that time, although there was a widespread and detailed understanding of many human rights, there was no comparable understanding of the right to the highest attainable standard of health, even though this human right is the cornerstone of the relationship between health and human rights.

Today, however, the situation is significantly different. In 2000, an authoritative understanding of the right to health emerged when the UN Committee on Economic, Social and Cultural Rights, working in close collaboration with WHO and many others, adopted General Comment 14 (UNCESCR 2000). Also, some international bodies like WHO, UNFPA, UNICEF, and UNAIDS, as well as civil society organizations, have begun to give more careful attention to health-related rights, including the right to the highest attainable standard of health. These and other developments have deepened understanding of the right to health, enabling linkages to be made between public health and human rights, a process that continues to accelerate through good practice, the academic literature and widening jurisprudence.

Although in some quarters there is a presumption that the right to health relates to medical care, such a narrow definition is in fact inconsistent with international human rights law, which encompasses both medicine and public health, as confirmed by Article 12 of ICESCR and Article 24 of CRC. As well as access to medical care, the right to health encompasses the social, cultural, economic, political, and other conditions that make people need medical care in the first place (WHO 1946, preamble; Beaglehole 2002), as well as other determinants of health such as access to water, sanitation, nutrition, housing, and education. This wider perspective underscores the very extensive common ground between public health and the right to the highest attainable standard of health.

The right to the highest attainable standard of health depends upon public health measures, such as immunization programmes, the provision of adequate sanitation systems and clean drinking water, health promotion (e.g. regarding domestic violence, healthy eating, and taking exercise), road safety campaigns, nutrition programmes, the promotion of indoor stoves that reduce respiratory diseases, and so on. Also, however, the classic, long-established public health objectives can benefit from the newer, dynamic discipline of human rights. In other words, just as public health programmes are essential to the realization of the right to health, so too can human rights help to reinforce existing, good, health programmes and identify new, equitable, health policies. This chapter focuses on the relevance of the right to the highest attainable standard of health to public health. However, the indispensable contribution of public health to the right to the highest attainable standard of health also deserves careful study.

Both public health and human rights advocates wish to establish effective, integrated, responsive health systems that are accessible to all. Both stress the importance not only of access to healthcare, but also to water, sanitation, health information, and education. Both understand that good health is not the sole responsibility of the Ministry of Health, but belongs to a wide range of public and private actors. Both prioritize the struggle against discrimination and disadvantage, and both stress cultural respect. At root, those working in health and human rights are both animated by a similar concern: the well-being of individuals and populations.

Health workers—defined in the World Health Report of 2006 (WHO 2006a) as 'all people engaged in actions whose primary intent is to enhance health'—can use health-related rights to help them devise more equitable policies and programmes; to place important health issues higher up national and international agendas; to secure better coordination across health-related sectors, as well as between services within the health sector; to raise more funds from the treasury; to leverage more funds from developed countries to developing countries; in some countries, to improve the terms and conditions of those working in the health sector; and so on. The right to the highest attainable standard of health is not just a rhetorical device, but also a tool that can save lives and reduce suffering, especially among the most disadvantaged.

The following sections provide examples that illustrate the resonance between public health and the right to the highest attainable standard of health.

Although these two disciplines are, in many ways, complementary, in practice public health has been used by some States as a ground for limiting the exercise of some human rights. Indeed, under international law, States are allowed to impose some limitations on human rights, in some circumstances, for the protection of public health, an issue briefly revisited in the following section.

The contours and content of the right to health

The right to health is not a right to be healthy. It is a right to facilities, goods, services, and conditions that are conducive to the realization of the highest attainable standard of physical and mental health. Understanding of the content of the right has evolved considerably over the last 60 years, with jurisprudence, international standards, and practical implementation of the right all contributing to this process.

As we have seen, an inclusive approach to implementing the right to the highest attainable standard of health calls for its reach to extend not only to timely and appropriate medical care, but also to the underlying determinants of health, such as access to safe and potable water and adequate sanitation, healthy occupational and environmental conditions, and access to health-related education and information (UNCESCR 2000, para. 8).

The right to health can also be broken down into more specific entitlements, such as the rights to: maternal, child, and reproductive health; healthy workplace and natural environments; the prevention, treatment, and control of diseases, including access to essential medicines; and access to safe and potable water.

In times of emergency, States have a joint and individual responsibility to cooperate in providing disaster relief and humanitarian assistance, including medical aid and potable water as well as assistance to refugees and internally displaced persons (UNCESCR 2000, para. 40).

Certain limitations on the right to health do exist, as issues of public health are sometimes used by States as grounds for limiting the exercise of other fundamental rights. For such limitations to be implemented legitimately, they must be in accordance with the law and international human rights standards. In particular, they should be strictly necessary for the promotion of the general welfare in a democratic society, proportional, subject to review, and of limited duration (UN ECOSOC 1985, Annex; UNCESCR 2000, paras. 28–9).

The right to health analytical framework

In recent years, the Committee on Economic, Social and Cultural Rights, WHO, the first Special Rapporteur on the right of everyone to the enjoyment of the highest attainable standard of physical and mental health, civil society organizations, academics, and many others, have developed a way of 'unpacking' or analysing the right to health with a view to making it easier to understand and apply to health-related policies, programmes, and projects in practice. The analytical framework that has been developed is made up of ten key elements and has general application to all aspects of the right to health, including the underlying determinants of health: this has been demonstrated by the first Special Rapporteur in his use of the framework throughout his work (Hunt and Leader 2010).

National and international human rights laws, norms, and standards

The relevant laws, norms, and standards relevant to the particular issue, programme, or policy must be identified. These will include both general provisions and standards relating to the right to health, in addition to international instruments that relate to specific groups and contexts (see the section 'What is the right to health?') (UNCHR 2003a, Annex 1).

Resource constraints and progressive realization

International human rights law recognizes that the realization of the right to health is subject to resource availability. Thus, what is required of a developed State today is of a higher standard than what is required of a developing State. However, a State is obliged—whatever its resource constraints and level of economic development—to realize progressively the right to the highest attainable standard of health (UN 1966b, Art. 2(1)). In essence, this means that a State is required to be doing better in 2 years' time than it is doing today. In order to measure progress (or the lack of it) over time, indicators and benchmarks must be identified (see the section 'New tools and techniques').

Obligations of immediate effect

Despite resource constraints and progressive realization, the right to health also gives rise to some obligations of immediate effect, such as the duty to avoid discrimination (UNCESCR 2000, para. 43). These are obligations without which the right would be deprived of its *raison d'être* and as such they are not subject to progressive realization, even in the presence of resource constraints (UNCESCR 1990, para. 10). The precise scope of these immediate obligations has not yet been clearly defined; for the health and human rights communities, this remains important work-in-progress.

Freedoms and entitlements

The right to health includes both freedoms (for example, the freedom from discrimination or non-consensual medical treatment and experimentation) and entitlements (for example, the provision of a system of health protection that includes minimum essential levels of water and sanitation). For the most part, freedoms do not have budgetary implications, while entitlements do.

Available, accessible, acceptable, and good quality

All health services, goods, and facilities should comply with each of these four requirements. An essential medicine, for example, should be *available* within the country. Additionally, the medicine should be *accessible*. Accessibility has four dimensions: accessible without discrimination, physically accessible, economically accessible (i.e. affordable), and accessible health-related information. As well as being available and accessible, health services should be provided in a culturally *acceptable* manner. This requires, for example, effective coordination and referral with traditional health systems. Lastly, all health services, goods, and services should be of *good quality*; a medicine, for example, must not be beyond its expiry date. These four requirements are further explored and applied in the section 'Right to health issues through the analytical framework'.

Note the similarity between these requirements and the four 'As' of public healthcare envisaged since the 1978 Alma Ata Declaration: geographical accessibility, financial accessibility, cultural accessibility, and functional accessibility (WHO 1978b).

Respect, protect, fulfil

This subsidiary framework relates to the tripartite obligations of States to respect, protect, and fulfil the right to the highest attainable standard of health, as explained and used by CESCR, the Committee on the Elimination of Discrimination Against Women (CEDAW) and the Sub-Commission on the Promotion and Protection of Human Rights. A version of this subsidiary framework is also enshrined in the Constitution of South Africa.

For example, the obligation to *respect* places a duty on States to refrain from interfering directly or indirectly with the enjoyment of the right to health. The obligation to *protect* means that States must prevent third parties from interfering with the enjoyment of the right to health. The obligation to *fulfil* requires States to adopt necessary measures, including legislative, administrative and budgetary measures, to ensure the full realization of human rights, including the right to the highest attainable standard of health.

Non-discrimination, equality, and vulnerability

Because of their crucial importance, the analytical framework demands that special attention be given to issues of non-discrimination, equality, and vulnerability in relation to all elements of the right to the highest attainable standard of health.

Active and informed participation

Participation is grounded in internationally recognized human rights, such as the rights to participate in the formulation and implementation of government policy (CEDAW, Article 7(b)), to take part in the conduct of public affairs (ICCPR, Article 25(a); UN 1966a), and to freedom of expression and association (ICCPR, Articles 19 and 22). The right to health requires that there be an opportunity for individuals and groups to participate actively and in an informed manner in health policymaking processes that affect them (UNCESCR 2000, para. 54).

International assistance and cooperation

In line with obligations envisaged in the UN Charter and some human rights treaties, such as the ICESCR (Article 2) and the CRC (Article 4), developing countries have a responsibility to seek international assistance and cooperation, while developed States have some responsibilities towards the realization of the right to health in developing countries (Hunt et al. 2010; Maastricht Principles on Extraterritorial Obligations of States in the Area of Economic, Social and Cultural Rights 2011).

Monitoring and accountability

The right to health introduces globally legitimized norms or standards from which obligations or responsibilities arise. These obligations have to be monitored and those responsible held to account. Without monitoring and accountability, the norms and obligations are likely to become empty promises. Accountability mechanisms provide rights-holders (e.g. individuals and groups) with an opportunity to understand how duty-bearers have discharged their obligations, and it also provides duty-bearers (e.g. ministers and officials) with an opportunity to explain their conduct. In this way, accountability mechanisms help to identify when—and what—policy adjustments are necessary. Accountability tends to encourage the most effective use of limited resources, as well as a shared responsibility among all parties. Transparent, effective, and accessible accountability mechanisms are among the most crucial characteristics of the right to the highest attainable standard of health.

These ten key elements of the right-to-health analytical framework underscore what the right to health contributes to public health. For example, the preoccupation with non-discrimination, equality, and vulnerability requires a State to take effective measures to address the health inequities that characterize some populations. The focus on active and informed participation requires a State to adopt, so far as possible, a 'bottom–up' participatory approach in health-related sectors. The requirement of monitoring and accountability can help to ensure that health policies, programmes, and practices are meaningful to those living in poverty.

Crucially, the key elements of the right-to-health analytical framework are not merely to be followed because they accord with sound management, ethics, social justice, or humanitarianism. States are required to conform to the key features *as a matter of binding law*. Moreover, they are to be held to account for the discharge of their right-to-health responsibilities arising from these legal obligations.

Right to health issues through the analytical framework

In this section, elements of the analytical framework signalled in the section 'The contours and content of the right to health' are applied to a selection of health issues. While space does not permit all of the elements to be applied to all of the selected issues, each element is applied to at least one of them.

The selected health issues are: neglected diseases; mental disabilities; sexual and reproductive health, including maternal mortality; and water and sanitation. The right to health is among the most extensive and complex in the international lexicon of human rights. As already signalled, it extends much further than these four issues which are simply provided as an illustration of how the right-to-health analytical framework applies to this selection of important health issues.

Neglected diseases

Although there is no standard global definition of 'neglected diseases', nor are they homogenous, they tend to share some common features. For example, they typically affect neglected populations, those least able to demand services. They are a symptom of poverty and disadvantage. Fear and stigma are attached to some neglected diseases, leading to delays in seeking treatment and to discrimination against those afflicted.

Neglected diseases include lymphatic filariasis, schistosomiasis, onchocerciasis (river blindness), trachoma, Buruli ulcer, soil-transmitted helminths, leishmaniasis, leprosy, and human African trypanosomiasis (sleeping sickness). According to WHO, 'the health impact of…neglected diseases is measured by severe and permanent disabilities and deformities in almost 1 billion people' (WHO 2002, p. 96).

Where curative interventions for neglected diseases exist, they have generally failed to reach populations early enough to prevent impairment. Furthermore, the development of new tools to diagnose and treat them has been underfunded, largely because there has been little or no market incentive (WHO 2004a, p. 22).

Non-discrimination, equality, and vulnerability

Discrimination and social stigma can be both causes and consequences of certain neglected diseases. As non-discrimination and equal treatment are cornerstone principles in international human rights law, a rights-based approach to neglected diseases pays particular attention to policies, programmes, and projects that impair the equal enjoyment of the human rights of people suffering from these diseases (WHO and TDR 2007).

Stigmatization and discrimination heighten people's vulnerability to ill health. Often, stigmatization is based on myths, misconceptions, and fears, including those related to certain diseases or health conditions. In turn, fear of stigmatization can lead people living with neglected diseases to avoid diagnosis, delay seeking treatment and hide the diseases from family, employers, and the community at large.

Discrimination involves acts or omissions which may be directed towards stigmatized individuals on account of their health status and/or related disabilities. For example, leprosy, lymphatic filariasis and leishmaniasis may cause severe physical disabilities, including deformities and scarring, giving rise to discrimination in the workplace, and limiting access to healthcare and education.

The socioeconomic consequences of stigmatization and discrimination associated with neglected diseases can have devastating consequences for individuals and groups that are already marginalized, leading to further vulnerability to neglected diseases. For example, stigma related to tuberculosis can be greater for women: it may lead to ostracism, rejection, and abandonment by family and friends, as well as loss of social and economic support and other problems (WHO 2001a, p. 12). Social and behavioural research on stigma and neglected diseases suggests that women also may experience more social disadvantages than men, in particular from physically disfiguring conditions like lymphatic filariasis (Coreil et al. 2003, p. 42).

The guarantee of non-discrimination and equal treatment enshrined under national and international human rights law requires the government to adopt wide-ranging measures, including through the implementation of health-related laws and policies, which confront discrimination in the public and private sector.

Active and informed participation

A human rights approach not only attaches importance to reducing the incidence and burden of neglected diseases, but also to the democratic and inclusive processes by which these objectives are achieved. Such processes require the active, informed, and meaningful participation of communities affected by neglected diseases.

Affected communities have sometimes participated in aspects of prevention, treatment, and control of neglected diseases. For example, they are sometimes involved in vector control programmes, such as bednet impregnation to combat malaria, or housing improvements to combat Chagas disease, which is caused by parasites living in cracks in housing. Communities have also been involved in treatment strategies, for example, through community health workers who have been selected and trained to administer vaccinations and treatment (Espino et al. 2004).

However, the human rights approach means that affected communities should participate in a range of contexts, not just in implementing programmes. They should be actively involved in setting local, national, and international public health agendas; decision-making processes; identifying disease control strategies and other relevant policies; and holding duty bearers to account. While it is not suggested that affected communities should participate in all the technical deliberations that underlie policy formulation, their participation can help to avoid some of the top–down, technocratic tendencies often associated with old-style development plans and policy implementation.

Although effective participation is not straightforward, and takes time to generate, it is nonetheless an important means by which to empower and build capacity in affected communities, enhance accountability, and improve the effectiveness of interventions. Therefore, as demonstrated in the following examples, participation has a positive impact on the enjoyment of the right to health.

In Peru in the 1980s, patients' associations, spontaneously set up in response to the government's failure to provide drugs and financial compensation for people who had suffered from leishmaniasis, were eventually successful in securing support from the regional and national health authorities. They became forums for discussions of wide-ranging social and political issues. This movement, which became more structured and organized over time, provided local institutions with detailed knowledge and made links with local populations so that it became possible to determine the best control and intervention strategies, and implement them successfully (Guthman et al. 1997, p. 17).

In Uganda, Village Health Teams are able to help dispel the neglect that characterizes certain diseases and populations, ensuring that local needs are clearly identified, understood, and addressed. Moreover, the Teams can provide the crucial grassroots delivery mechanisms for community interventions in relation to neglected diseases, and health protection generally (UNCHR 2006a).

Vehicles for community participation such as these require adequate resources, training, and support. They must be listened to and used strategically as delivery mechanisms in relation to neglected diseases, with smooth and effective coordination, cooperation, and collaboration between them and the local political structure and health centres. For this reason, government, development actors, and others should sustain and foster vital community-based initiatives to ensure that full and effective participation can support the realization of the right to health.

Monitoring and accountability

In practice, few accountability mechanisms give sufficient attention to neglected diseases, and often prove inaccessible to impoverished members of neglected communities. Within a national jurisdiction, parliamentarians might hold the Minister of Health to account in relation to the discharge of his or her responsibilities, yet the ability of these and other general mechanisms (such as judicial processes) to provide adequate accountability in relation to neglected diseases and the right to health is doubtful.

The right to the highest attainable standard of health demands accessible, transparent, and effective monitoring and accountability mechanisms that are meaningful to neglected communities. These could include independent national human rights institutions that monitor the incidence of neglected diseases and the initiatives taken to address them. Adopting an evidence-based approach, the institution could scrutinize who is doing what and whether or not they are doing all that can reasonably be expected of them to realize the right to health of those concerned. Whenever possible, the institution should identify realistic and practical recommendations for all those involved.

International human rights machinery can also draw attention to the issue of neglected diseases and neglected populations. For example, when a relevant State presents its periodic reports to CESCR, both the Government's reports and the human rights body's examination of them should give careful attention to the issue of neglected diseases and neglected populations, in accordance with the national and international right to health standards to which the Government is bound.

International assistance and cooperation

This feature of the right to health requires that donors and the international community pay particular attention to the health problems of the most vulnerable and disadvantaged individuals and communities in developing countries. For example, donors and the international community have a duty to help developing countries enhance their capacity so they can determine their own national and local health research and development priorities, such as neglected diseases.

Mental disabilities

Too often, disability issues do not attract the attention they demand and deserve. This is especially true in the context of mental disabilities, which include all major and minor mental illness and psychiatric disorders, as well as intellectual disabilities. The right to the highest attainable standard of health demands that due attention is given to both physical and mental disabilities.

A significant development in the field of disability was achieved with the adoption of a new international human rights treaty in 2006, the Convention on the Rights of Persons with Disabilities. Alongside this important new treaty, there are many important provisions contained in non-binding principles that have profound connections to the right to health, such as the *UN Principles for the Protection of Persons with Mental Illness and the Improvement of Mental Health Care*, even if some elements are inadequate and need revisiting (UNGA 1991). Where appropriate, these specialized instruments should be used as interpretive guides in relation to the right to health as it is enshrined in international law.

International human rights treaties and specialized international instruments relating to mental disabilities are mutually reinforcing, even if, as the UN Secretary General recently put it, 'a more detailed analysis of the implementation of State human rights obligations in the context of mental health institutions would be desirable' (UNGA 2003, para. 43). Inadequate attention has been given to the implementation of these obligations to date. It is hoped that the new UN Convention will help to remedy this situation.

Freedoms and entitlements
Freedoms

Freedoms of particular relevance to the experience of individuals with mental disabilities include the right to control one's health and body. Forced sterilizations, rape, and other forms of sexual violence, to which women with mental disabilities are particularly vulnerable, are inherently inconsistent with their sexual and reproductive health rights and freedoms, are psychologically and physically traumatic, and thus jeopardize mental health even further.

Several international human rights instruments allow for exceptional circumstances in which persons with mental disabilities can be involuntarily admitted to a hospital or another designated institution (ECHR, Article 5 (1) (e); UN Mental Illness Principles, Principle 16). However, because involuntary detention is an extremely serious interference with the freedom of persons with disabilities, in particular their right to liberty and security, international and national human rights law attaches numerous procedural safeguards to involuntary detention cases. Moreover, these safeguards are generating a significant jurisprudence, most notably in regional human rights commissions and courts (ECtHR 1979; Gostin 2000; Lewis 2002; Gostin and Gable 2004).

Entitlements

The right to health includes an entitlement to a system of health protection which provides equality of opportunity for all people to enjoy the highest attainable standard of health through access to both healthcare and the underlying determinants of health, all of which play a vital role in ensuring the health and dignity of persons with mental disabilities (UNGA 1993, Rules 2–4).

States are required to take steps to ensure a full package of community-based mental healthcare and support services conducive to health, dignity, and inclusion. These should include medication, psychotherapy, ambulatory services, hospital care for acute admissions, residential facilities, rehabilitation for persons with psychiatric disabilities, programmes to maximize the independence and skills of persons with intellectual disabilities, supported housing and employment, income support, inclusive and appropriate education for children with intellectual disabilities, and respite care for families looking after a person with a mental disability 24 hours a day. In this way, unnecessary institutionalization can be avoided.

Scaling up interventions to ensure equality of opportunity for the enjoyment of the right to health requires that adequate numbers of appropriate professionals be trained. Similarly, primary care providers should be provided with essential mental healthcare and disability sensitization training to enable them to provide front-line mental and physical healthcare to persons with mental disabilities.

Underlying determinants of health that are particularly relevant to persons with mental disabilities, who are disproportionately affected by poverty and as such often deprived of important entitlements, include adequate sanitation, safe water, and adequate food and shelter (UNCESCR 2000, para. 4). The conditions in psychiatric hospitals, as well as other institutions used by persons with mental disabilities, are often grossly inadequate from this point of view.

Obligations of immediate effect and progressive realization

It is reasonable to expect that countries, even those with very limited resources, undertake to implement certain measures towards realization of the right to health for people with disabilities. For example they can be expected to: include the recognition, care, and treatment of mental disabilities in training curricula of all health personnel; promote public campaigns against stigma and discrimination of persons with mental disabilities; support the formation of civil society groups that are representative of mental healthcare users and their families; formulate modern policies and programmes on mental disabilities; downsize psychiatric hospitals and, as far as possible, extend community care; in relation to persons with mental disabilities, actively seek assistance and cooperation from donors and international organizations (WHO 2001b, pp. 112–15).

Respect, protect, fulfil

Specifically in relation to mental disabilities, the obligation to *respect* requires States to refrain from denying or limiting equal access to healthcare services and underlying determinants of health, for persons with mental disabilities. They are also required to ensure that persons with mental disabilities in public institutions are not denied access to healthcare and related support services, or underlying determinants of health, including water and sanitation (IACHR 1997).

The obligation to *protect* means that States are required to take actions to ensure that third parties do not harm the right to health of persons with mental disabilities. For example, States should take measures to protect persons with mental disabilities from violence and other right to health-related abuses occurring in private healthcare or support services.

The obligation to *fulfil* requires States to recognize the right to health, including the right to health of persons with mental disabilities, in national political and legal systems, with a view to ensuring its implementation. States should adopt appropriate legislative, administrative, budgetary, judicial, promotional, and other measures towards this end (ICESCR Article 2(1); UNCESCR 2000, para. 36). For example, States should ensure that the right to health of persons with mental disabilities is adequately reflected in their national health strategy and plan of action, as well as other relevant policies, such as national poverty reduction strategies, and the national budget (WHO 2004B). Mental health laws, policies, programmes, and projects should embody human rights and empower people with mental disabilities to make choices about

their lives; give legal protections relating to the establishment of (and access to) quality mental health facilities, as well as care and support services; establish robust procedural mechanisms for the protection of those with mental disabilities; ensure the integration of persons with mental disabilities into the community; and promote mental health throughout society (WHO 2005). Patients' rights charters should encompass the human rights of persons with mental disabilities. States should also ensure that access to information about their human rights is provided to persons with mental disabilities and their guardians, as well as others who may be institutionalized in psychiatric hospitals.

International assistance and cooperation

The record shows that mental healthcare and support services are not a priority health area for donors. Furthermore, donors have sometimes supported inappropriate programmes, such as the rebuilding of a damaged psychiatric institution constructed many years ago on the basis of conceptions of mental disability that have since been discredited. In so doing, the donor inadvertently prolongs, for many years, seriously inappropriate approaches to mental disability.

It is unacceptable for a donor to fund a programme that, in moving a psychiatric institution to an isolated location, makes it impossible for its users to sustain or develop their links with the community (MDRI 2002). If a donor wishes to assist children with intellectual disabilities, it might wish to fund community-based services to support children and their parents, enabling the children to remain at home, instead of funding new facilities in a remote institution that the parents can only afford to visit once a month, if at all (Rosenthal et al. 2000).

Donors have a right to health duty to consider more—and better quality—support in the area of mental disability. In accordance with their responsibility of international assistance and cooperation, they are required to consider adopting measures such as: supporting the development of appropriate community-based care and support services; supporting advocacy by persons with mental disabilities, their families and representative organizations; and providing policy and technical expertise. Furthermore, donors should ensure that all their programmes promote equality and non-discrimination for persons with mental disabilities, while international agencies fulfil the role that corresponds to them by providing technical support.

Monitoring and accountability

The right to health requires that States have in place effective, transparent, and accessible monitoring and accountability mechanisms in relation to the health of persons with mental disabilities.

In many countries, there is an absence of sustained and independent monitoring of mental healthcare, resulting in frequent abuses in large psychiatric hospitals and community-based settings going unnoticed. The Mental Illness Principles emphasize the importance of inspecting mental health facilities, as well as investigating and resolving complaints where an alleged violation of the rights of a patient is concerned (UN Mental Illness Principle 22).

Lack of surveillance is doubly problematic because persons with mental disabilities, especially those who are institutionalized, are often unable to access independent and effective accountability mechanisms when their human rights have been violated. Where accountability mechanisms do exist, the severity of their condition may render them unable to protect their interests independently through legal proceedings, to demand effective procedural safeguards where these may be lacking, or to access legal aid.

For example, the right to health requires that an independent review body must be made accessible to persons with mental disabilities, or other appropriate persons, to review cases of involuntary admission and treatment periodically (UN Mental Illness Principle 17).

Although there is a range of detailed international standards concerning the human rights of persons with mental disabilities, and procedural safeguards to protect them (UN Mental Illness Principles 11, 18), their lack of implementation poses a real challenge. The new Convention on the Rights of Persons with Disabilities will be crucial to international monitoring and accountability, especially if its Optional Protocol, which introduces a procedure under which individuals and groups can lodge complaints, were to come into force. Significantly, this mechanism strengthens the existing standards relating to the right to health of persons with mental disabilities that do not establish specific monitoring or accountability mechanisms.

Alongside this Convention, other international human rights treaties (including ICESCR, CRC, CEDAW and CERD, and ICCPR) extend protections to persons with mental disabilities. For this reason, States should pay greater attention to them in their State party reports, and examination of these reports by the human rights treaty bodies should, in turn, give a greater focus to these issues through their discussions with States parties, concluding observations, and general comments or recommendations. Relevant civil society organizations, including representatives of persons with mental disabilities, play an important role by engaging with UN treaty bodies and special procedures.

Sexual and reproductive health, including maternal mortality

The Commission on Human Rights confirmed in 2003 that 'sexual and reproductive health are integral elements of the right of everyone to the enjoyment of the highest attainable standard of physical and mental health' (UNCHR 2003b, preamble and para. 6). The outcomes of world conferences, in particular the International Conference on Population and Development (UN 1994), the Fourth World Conference on Women (UN 1995), and their respective 5-year reviews, confirm that human rights have an indispensable role to play in relation to sexual and reproductive health issues.

More recently, there has been a deepening conceptual and operational understanding of maternal mortality as a human rights issue (Freedman 2003; Ministry for Foreign Affairs 2006; UNHRC 2010a; Kaur 2012; Kismodi et al. 2012; UNOHCHR 2012b; Hunt and Gray 2013). Although the issue is connected to a number of human rights, the right to the highest attainable standard of health is of particular relevance, and is the focus of the following remarks.

Monitoring and accountability
Freedoms
In the context of sexual and reproductive health, freedoms include a right to control one's health and body. Rape and other forms of sexual violence, including forced pregnancy, non-consensual contraceptive methods (e.g. forced sterilization and forced abortion),

female genital mutilation/cutting (FGM/C), and forced marriage all represent serious breaches of sexual and reproductive freedoms, and are therefore fundamentally and inherently inconsistent with the right to health. In the specific context of maternal mortality, relevant freedoms include freedom from discrimination; harmful traditional practices, such as early marriage; and violence.

For example, some cultural practices, including FGM/C, carry a high risk of disability and death. This means that where the practice exists, States should take appropriate and effective measures to eradicate it, in accordance with their obligations under the Convention on the Rights of the Child. Early marriage, which disproportionately affects girls, is predominantly found in South Asia and sub-Saharan Africa, where over 50 per cent of girls are married by the age of 18. Among other problems, early marriage is linked to health risks including those arising from premature pregnancy. Finally, in the context of adolescent health, States are obliged to set minimum ages for sexual consent and marriage (UNCRC 2003, paras. 9, 19).

Entitlements
Entitlements that form part of the rights to reproductive and sexual health include equal access, in law and fact, to reproductive and child health services, as well as information about sexual and reproductive health issues.

Specifically, States are required to provide a wide range of appropriate and, where necessary, free sexual and reproductive health services, including access to family planning, pre- and post-natal care, emergency obstetric services, and access to information (Cottingham et al. 2012). They should also ensure access to such essential health services as voluntary testing, counselling, and treatment for sexually transmitted infections, including HIV/AIDS, and breast and reproductive system cancers, as well as infertility treatment.

Unsafe abortions kill some 68,000 women each year, and thus constitute a right to life and right to health issue of enormous proportions. They also give rise to high rates of morbidity. Women with unwanted pregnancies should be offered reliable information and compassionate counselling, including information on where and when a pregnancy may be terminated legally. Where abortions are legal, they must be safe: public health systems should train and equip health service providers and take other measures to ensure that such abortions are not only safe but accessible (WHO 2003). In all cases, women should have access to quality services for the management of complications arising from abortion. Punitive provisions against women who undergo abortions are inconsistent with the right to the highest attainable standard of health (UNGA 2011; Kismodi et al. 2012).

Certain entitlements envisaged in international law are directly relevant to reducing maternal mortality (CEDAW Article 12 (2); UNCESCR 2000, para. 14) and, if fulfilled, would reduce its incidence. For example, an equitable, well-resourced, accessible, and integrated health system—a crucial entitlement arising from the right to health—is widely accepted as a vital pre-condition for guaranteeing women's access to the interventions that can prevent or treat the causes of maternal deaths (Freedman 2005). Other entitlements include education and information on sexual and reproductive health (UNCEDAW 1999, para. 18), safe abortion services where not against the law, and primary healthcare services (UN 1994, para. 8.25; UNCEDAW 1999, para. 27; UNCESCR

2000, paras. 14, 21), especially universal access to reproductive healthcare (UNMP 2005b).

The entitlement to specific underlying determinants of health relevant to maternal mortality must also be guaranteed. The failure to safeguard women's rights is often manifested in low status of women, poor access to information and care, early age of marriage, and restricted mobility, among other problems (DFID 2005). Specifically, gender equality has an important role to play in preventing maternal mortality as alongside empowerment it can lead to greater demand by women for family planning services, antenatal care, and safe delivery. Another relevant determinant of health and element of the right to health that must be ensured in order to address problems of maternal mortality is water and sanitation, which are vital to the provision of prenatal care and emergency obstetric care.

Available, accessible, acceptable, and good quality

In many countries, information on sexual and reproductive health is not readily available and, if it is, it is not accessible to all, in particular women and adolescents. Sexual and reproductive health services are often geographically inaccessible to communities living in rural areas, or provided in a form that is not culturally acceptable to indigenous peoples and other non-dominant groups. Similarly, services, and relevant underlying determinants of health, such as education, are often of substandard quality.

In order to address the problem of maternal mortality, the concept of availability calls for collective action to enhance care and improve human resource strategies, including increasing the number and quality of health professionals and improving terms and conditions (UNMP 2005c). Accessibility considers whether physical access and the cost of health services influence women's ability to seek care (UNMP 2005c). Furthermore, discriminatory laws, policies, practices, and gender inequalities prevent women and adolescents from accessing good quality services or information on sexual and reproductive health, and have a direct impact on maternal mortality (Cook et al. 2006). To prevent maternal mortality, scaling up technical interventions, or making the interventions affordable is insufficient: strategies ensuring the *acceptability* of services through their sensitivity to the rights, cultures and needs of pregnant women, including those from indigenous peoples and other minority groups, are also vital (Shiffman 2006). Quality of care will influence both a woman's decision whether or not to seek care, as well as the outcome of interventions, and so is key to tackling maternal mortality through the provision of maternal healthcare services.

Discrimination, vulnerability, and stigma

Discrimination and stigma continue to pose a serious threat to sexual and reproductive health for many groups, including women, sexual minorities, refugees, people with disabilities, rural communities, indigenous persons, people living with HIV/AIDS, sex workers, and people held in detention. Some individuals suffer discrimination on several grounds, e.g. gender, race, poverty, and health status (UNCHR 2003a, para. 62).

Discrimination based on gender hinders the ability of many women to protect themselves from HIV infection and to respond to the consequences of HIV infection. Women and girls' vulnerability to HIV and AIDS is compounded by other human rights issues including inadequate access to information, education, and services necessary to ensure sexual health; sexual violence;

harmful traditional or customary practices affecting the health of women and children (such as early and forced marriage); and lack of legal capacity and equality in areas such as marriage and divorce.

Stigma and discrimination associated with HIV/AIDS may also reinforce other prejudices, discrimination, and inequalities related to gender and sexuality. The result is that those affected may be reluctant to seek health and social services, information, education, and counselling, even when those services are available. This, in turn, will contribute to the vulnerability of others to HIV infection.

Vulnerability in the context of sexual and reproductive health is particularly relevant to adolescents and young people, who find themselves lacking access to relevant information and services during a period characterized by sexual and reproductive maturation. Important protections for adolescents are enshrined in CRC, which includes a number of cross-cutting principles which have an important bearing on adolescents' sexual and reproductive health, namely: the survival and development of the child, the best interests of the child, non-discrimination, and respect for the views of the child (CRC Articles 2, 3, 5, 6, and 12; UNCRC 2003, para. 12).

Discrimination on the grounds of sexual orientation is impermissible under international human rights law. The legal prohibition of same-sex relations in many countries, in conjunction with a widespread lack of support or protection for sexual minorities against violence and discrimination, impedes the enjoyment of sexual and reproductive health by many people with lesbian, gay, bisexual, and transgender identities or conduct (UNCHR 2001, paras. 48–50; UNGA 2001, paras. 17–25; UNHRC 2010c, para. 6–26). Similarly, criminalization can impede programmes which are essential to promoting the right to health and other human rights (UNHRCttee 1994, para. 8.5).

Arising from their obligations to combat discrimination, States have a duty to ensure that health information and services are made available to vulnerable groups. For example, they must take steps to empower women to make decisions in relation to their sexual and reproductive health, free of coercion, violence, and discrimination. They must take action to redress gender-based violence and ensure that there are sensitive and compassionate services available for the survivors of gender-based violence, including rape and incest. States should ensure that adolescents are able to receive information, including on family planning and contraceptives, the dangers of early pregnancy, and the prevention of sexually transmitted infections including HIV/AIDS, as well as appropriate services for sexual and reproductive health. Consistent with *Toonen v. Australia* and numerous other international and national decisions, they should ensure that sexual and other health services are available for men who have sex with men, lesbians, and transsexual and bisexual people. It is also important to ensure that voluntary counselling, testing, and treatment of sexually transmitted infections are available for sex workers (UNHRCttee 1994).

Finally, in the context of sexual and reproductive health, breaches of medical confidentiality may occur. Sometimes these breaches, when accompanied by stigmatization, lead to unlawful dismissal from employment, expulsion from families and communities, physical assault, and other abuse. Also, a lack of confidentiality may deter individuals from seeking advice and treatment, thereby jeopardizing their health and well-being. States are obliged to take effective measures to ensure medical confidentiality and privacy.

Water and sanitation

Healthcare attracts a disproportionate amount of attention and resources. Yet access to water and sanitation, as well as other underlying determinants of health, are integral features of the right to the highest attainable standard of health.

Available, accessible, acceptable, and quality
Available
The right to health requires a State to do all it can to ensure that safe water and adequate sanitation are available to everyone in its jurisdiction. The quantity of water available for each person should correspond to the quantity specified by WHO (Howard and Bartram 2002), though some individuals and groups may require additional water due to health, climate, and work conditions, and the State should therefore ensure that this is also available. The right to health stipulates that States must ensure the availability of safe water for personal and domestic uses such as 'drinking, personal sanitation, washing of clothes, food preparation, personal and household hygiene' (UNCESCR 2003 para. 12 (a)).

Accessible
The right to health also requires that water and sanitation be accessible to everyone without discrimination. In this context, accessibility has four dimensions.

First, water and sanitation must be within safe physical reach for all sections of the population, in all parts of the country. Water and sanitation therefore should be *physically accessible* within, or in the immediate vicinity of, the household, educational institution, workplace, and health or other institution (UN 2005, guideline 1.3). The inaccessibility of water within safe physical reach can seriously impair health, including the health of women and children responsible for carrying water. Carrying heavy water containers for long distances can cause fatigue, pain, and spinal and pelvic injuries, which may lead to problems during pregnancy and childbirth. Similarly, the absence of safe, private sanitation facilities subjects women to a humiliating, stressful, and uncomfortable daily routine that can damage their health (UNMP 2005a, pp. 23–5). When designing water and sanitation facilities in camps for refugees and internally displaced persons, special attention should be given to prevent gender-based violence. For example, facilities should be provided in safe areas near dwellings (UNHCR 2005).

Second, water and sanitation should be *economically accessible*, including to those living in poverty. Poverty is associated with inequitable access to health services, safe water, and sanitation. If those living in poverty are not enjoying access to safe water and adequate sanitation, the State has a duty to take reasonable measures that ensure access to all.

Third, water and sanitation should be *accessible* to all *without discrimination* on any of the grounds prohibited under human rights law, such as sex, race, ethnicity, disability, and socioeconomic status.

Finally, reliable *information* about water and sanitation must be *accessible* to all so that they can make well-informed decisions.

Acceptable
The right to health requires that water and sanitation facilities be respectful of gender and life-cycle requirements and be culturally *acceptable*. For example, measures should ensure that sanitation facilities are mindful of the privacy of women, men, and children.

Quality
Both water services and sanitation facilities must be of good *quality*: this reduces susceptibility to anaemia, diarrhoea, and other conditions that cause maternal and infant mortality and morbidity (UNMP 2005a, p. 18). Water required for personal and domestic use should be safe and free from 'micro-organisms, chemical substances and radiological hazards which constitute a threat to a person's health' (UNCESCR 2003, para. 12(b)). States should establish water quality regulations and standards on the basis of the *WHO Guidelines for Drinking Water Quality* (WHO 2006b).

Similarly, each person should have affordable access to sanitation services, facilities, and installations adequate for the promotion and protection of their human health and dignity. Good health requires the protection of the environment from human waste; this can only be achieved if everyone has access to, and utilizes, adequate sanitation (UNCHR 2004, para. 44).

In 2008, the UN Human Rights Council appointed a Special Rapporteur on the human right to safe drinking water and sanitation whose reports shed light on the contours and content of this important human right (UNHRC 2010b).

New tools and techniques

The 'Human rights' section introduced the idea, which is increasingly recognized, that one way of vindicating the right to the highest attainable standard of health is by way of the 'policy approach' i.e. the integration of the right to health in national and international policymaking approaches. For this approach to prosper, the traditional human rights techniques—taking test cases in the courts, 'naming and shaming', letter-writing campaigns, slogans, and so on—will not be sufficient. The 'policy approach' demands the development of new right-to-health skills and tools, such as budgetary analysis, indicators, benchmarks, and impact assessments. In recent years, the health and human rights community has made significant progress towards the development of these new methodologies. Here, by way of illustration, indicators, benchmarks, and impact assessments are briefly introduced in the context of the right to the highest attainable standard of health.

A human rights-based approach to health indicators

The international right to the highest attainable standard of health is subject to progressive realization. Inescapably, this means that what is expected of a State will vary over time. With a view to monitoring its progress, a State needs a device to measure this variable dimension of the right to health. The most appropriate device is the combined application of indicators and benchmarks. Thus, a State selects appropriate indicators that will help it monitor different dimensions of the right to health. These indicators might include, for example, maternal mortality ratios and child mortality rates. Most indicators will require disaggregation, such as on the grounds of sex, race, ethnicity, rural/urban, and socioeconomic status. Then the State sets appropriate national targets or benchmarks in relation to each disaggregated indicator.

In this way, indicators and benchmarks fulfil two important functions. *First*, they can help the State to monitor its progress over time, enabling the authorities to recognize when policy adjustments are required. *Second*, they can help to hold the State to account in relation to the discharge of its responsibilities arising from the right to health, although deteriorating indicators do not necessarily mean that the State is in breach of its international right to health obligations (UNCHR 2006b, para. 35). Of course, indicators also have other important roles. For example, by highlighting issues such as disaggregation, participation, and accountability, indicators can enhance the effectiveness of policies and programmes.

Health professionals and policy makers constantly use a very large number of health indicators, such as the HIV prevalence rate. Is it possible to simply appropriate these health indicators and call them 'human rights indicators' or 'right to health indicators'? Or do indicators that are to be used for monitoring human rights and the right to health require some special features? If so, what are these special attributes?

The considered view is that some of these health indictors may be used to monitor aspects of the progressive realization of the right to health, provided the following conditions are met (UNGA 2004):

1. They correspond, with some precision, to a right to health norm.

2. They are disaggregated by at least sex, race, ethnicity, rural/urban, and socioeconomic status.

3. They are supplemented by additional indicators—rarely found among classic health indicators—that monitor five essential and inter-related features of the right to health:

  ◆ A national strategy and plan of action that includes the right to health.

  ◆ The participation of individuals and groups, especially the most vulnerable and disadvantaged, in relation to the formulation of health policies and programmes.

  ◆ Access to health information, as well as confidentiality of personal health data.

  ◆ International assistance and cooperation of donors in relation to the enjoyment of the right to health in developing countries.

  ◆ Accessible and effective monitoring and accountability mechanisms.

In this way, many existing health indicators, such as the maternal mortality ratio and HIV prevalence rate, have an important potential role to play in measuring and monitoring the progressive realization of the right to health, provided that they conform to these conditions (Hunt and MacNaughton 2007; UNOHCHR 2012a).

Impact assessments and the right to the highest attainable standard of health

A further tool that can be employed to monitor the fulfilment of the right to health and hold duty-bearers to account is through impact assessments. They are an aid to equitable, inclusive, robust, and sustainable policymaking, and have the objective of informing decision-makers and the people likely to be affected by a new policy, programme, or project so that the proposal can be improved to reduce potential negative effects and increase positive ones. They are one way of ensuring that the right to health—especially

of marginalized groups, including the poor—is given due weight in all national and international policymaking processes. From the right to health perspective, an impact assessment methodology is a key feature of a health system and an essential means by which a government can gauge whether or not it is on target to realize progressively the right to health.

At least two distinct methodological approaches are available: to develop a self-standing methodology for human rights impact assessments such as has been done in other fields, such as environmental and social policy; or to integrate human rights into *existing* types of impact assessments. The second approach is consistent with the call on governments to mainstream human rights into all government processes and requires interdisciplinary collaboration (MacNaughton and Hunt 2009).

In order that an impact assessment uphold rights-based principles, it must: (1) use an explicit human rights framework, (2) aim for progressive realization of human rights, (3) promote equality and non-discrimination in process and policy, (4) ensure meaningful participation by all stakeholders, (5) provide information and protect the right to freely express ideas, (6) establish mechanisms to hold the State accountable, and (7) recognize the interdependence of all human rights (MacNaughton and Hunt 2011).

If the second approach is adopted, there are six steps that should be followed to ensure that the right to health is integrated into existing impact assessments: (1) perform a preliminary check on the proposed policy to determine whether or not a full-scale right-to-health impact assessment is necessary; (2) prepare an assessment plan and distribute information on the policy and the plan to all stakeholders; (3) collect information on potential right-to-health impacts of the proposed policy; (4) prepare a draft report comparing the potential impacts with the State's legal obligations arising from the right to health; (5) distribute the draft report and engage stakeholders in evaluating the options; and (6) prepare the final report detailing the final decision, the rationale for the choices made, and a framework for implementation and evaluation.

Overall, the human rights framework for impact assessment adds value because human rights: (1) are based on legal obligations to which governments have agreed to abide; (2) apply to all parts of the government, encouraging coherence to policymaking and ensuring that policies reinforce each other; (3) require participation in policymaking by the people affected, enhancing legitimacy and ownership of policy choices; (4) enhance effectiveness by demanding data disaggregation, participation, and transparency; and (5) demand mechanisms through which policy makers can be held accountable.

Conclusion: key features of a health system from a right to health perspective

The right to the highest attainable standard of health can be understood as a right to an effective and integrated health system, encompassing healthcare and the underlying determinants of health, which is responsive to national and local priorities, and accessible to all.

At the heart of this understanding of the right to health is a package of health services, facilities, and goods, extending to healthcare and the underlying determinants of health, such as access to safe water, adequate sanitation, and health-related information. This package must be available, accessible, and of good quality. Also, it must be sensitive to different cultures. While this package will have many features that are common to all countries, there will also be differences between one country and another, reflective of different disease burdens, cultural contexts, resource availability, and so on. This chapter has signalled some elements of this package in relation to neglected diseases, mental disability, sexual and reproductive health, and water and sanitation.

However, besides this essential package of health services, facilities, and goods, a health system must have some additional features if it is to reflect the right to the highest attainable standard of health (Backman et al. 2008). These additional features derive from international norms, including CESCR's General Comment 14 on the right to the highest attainable standard of health. While some of these additional features have been described in the preceding paragraphs, they include the following:

1. Formal legal recognition of the right to health in either a national Constitution, or bill of rights, or other statute.

2. An elaboration of what the right to health means, for both the public and private sectors, for example by way of regulations, guidelines, and codes of conduct.

3. Research and development for national and local health priorities.

4. A comprehensive situational analysis identifying, *inter alia*, the health needs of the population, upon which (5) is based.

5. A comprehensive national health plan, including objectives, timeframes, who is responsible for what, reporting procedures, indicators and benchmarks (to measure progressive realization), and a detailed budget.

6. A health financing system that is equitable and evidence-informed.

7. An ex-ante right to health impact assessment methodology that permits the Government to foreshadow the likely impact of a draft law, policy, or programme on the enjoyment of the right to the highest attainable standard of health, thereby enabling it, when necessary, to revise the projected initiative.

8. As much 'bottom–up' participation as possible, in relation to policymaking, implementation, and accountability.

9. Access to health-related information and data; data will have to be disaggregated so that the health situation of disadvantaged populations is properly understood, enabling the authorities to devise measures that address health inequities and disadvantage; at the same time, however, arrangements must be in place to ensure that personal medical data remains confidential.

10. As well as effective mechanisms for coordination within the health sector, there must also be effective mechanisms for inter-sectoral coordination in health, because the right to health extends beyond the health sector; moreover, where relevant, there must be effective coordination and referral with traditional health systems.

11. A sufficient number of domestically trained health workers enjoying good terms and conditions of employment; they should be reflective of the country's cultural diversity, including language, and strike a balance between men and women; health workers' training should include human rights.

12. An international dimension, for example, low-income countries should seek international assistance and cooperation in health and high-income countries should provide it.

13. Educational campaigns and other arrangements so that the public knows about its right to health entitlements and how to vindicate them.

14. Effective, transparent, and accessible monitoring and accountability mechanisms, including redress, for both the public and private health sectors.

States have a legal obligation to ensure that their health systems not only include an appropriate package of health services, facilities, and goods, but also the additional features briefly summarized in points 1–14.

A key challenge for the future is to conduct multidisciplinary and multimethod research on the evidence of impact of human rights on health (Bustreo et al. 2013).

Key points

◆ The right to the highest attainable standard of health is enshrined in several international treaties and numerous national constitutions.

◆ It gives rise to legally binding obligations on States.

◆ There is a complementary relationship between public health and the right to the highest attainable standard of health.

◆ The right to health analytical framework deepens understanding of contemporary public health issues and can help to identify appropriate responses to them.

◆ The right to the highest attainable standard of health can be understood as a right to an effective and integrated health system, encompassing healthcare and the underlying determinants of health, which is responsive to national and local priorities, and accessible to all.

Acknowledgements

Thanks are due to Genevieve Sander, Senior Research Officer, Human Rights Centre, University of Essex, for her assistance in preparing this chapter for the 6th edition.

References

ACHPR (African Commission on Human and Peoples' Rights) (2001). *Communication No. 155/96: The Social and Economic Rights Action Center for Economic and Social Rights v. Nigeria*. Fifteenth Annual Activity Report of ACHPR, 2001–2002, Annex V.

Backman, G., Hunt, P., Khosla, R., et al. (2008). Health systems and the right to health: an assessment of 194 countries. *Lancet*, 372 (9655), 2047–85.

Beaglehole, R. (2002). Overview and framework. In R. Detels, J. McEwen, R. Beaglehole, and H. Tanaka (eds.) *Oxford Textbook of Public Health* (4th ed.), pp. 83–7. Oxford: Oxford University Press.

Bustreo, F., Hunt, P., Gruskin, S., et al. (2013). *Women's and Children's Health: Evidence of Impact of Human Rights*. Geneva: WHO.

CCSA (Constitutional Court of South Africa) (2002). *Minister of Health et al v. Treatment Action Campaign* et al. Case CCT 8/02, decided on 5 July 2002.

Coreil, J., Mayard, G., and Addiss, D. (2003). *Support Groups for Women with Lymphatic Filariasis in Haiti*. Report Series No. 2, Social, Economic and Behavioural Research, Special Programme for Research and Training in Tropical Diseases (TDR), p. 42.

Cottingham, J., Germaine, A., and Hunt, P. (2012). Use of human rights to meet the unmet need for family planning. *Lancet*, 380, 172–80.

Council of Europe (1950). *Convention for the Protection of Human Rights and Fundamental Freedoms*. ETS No. 5. Strasbourg: Council of Europe.

DFID (Department for International Development) (2005). *How to Reduce Maternal Deaths: Rights and Responsibilities*. London: DFID.

ECSR (European Committee on Social Rights) (1998). *International Commission of Jurists v. Portugal*. Case No. 1/1998.

ECtHR (European Court of Human Rights) (1979). *Winterwerp v. The Netherlands, Judgement 24 October 1979*. Application No. 6301/73. Reported at 2 EHRR 387.

ECtHR (European Court of Human Rights) (1990). *E. v. Norway, Judgement of 29 August 1990*. Application No. 11701/85, Series A, No. 181–A.

ECtHR (European Court of Human Rights) (1994). *Lopez Ostra v. Spain, Judgement of December 9, 1994*. Case No. 41/1993/436/515.

Espino, F., Coops, V., and Manderson, L. (2004). *Community Participation and Tropical Disease Control in Resource-poor Settings*. Geneva: UNICEF/UNDP/World Bank/WHO Special Programme for Research and Training in Tropical Diseases.

Freedman, L. (2003). Human rights, constructive accountability and maternal mortality in the Dominican Republic: a commentary. *International Journal of Gynecology and Obstetrics*, 82, 111–14.

Freedman, L. (2005). Achieving the MDGs: health systems as core social institutions. *Development*, 48(1), 19–24.

Gauri, V. and Brinks, D. (2008). *Courting Social Justice: Judicial Enforcement of Social and Economic Rights*. Cambridge: Cambridge University Press.

Gostin, L.O. (2000). Human rights of persons with mental disabilities: the European Convention of Human Rights. *International Journal of Law and Psychiatry*, 23, 125–59.

Gostin, L.O. and Gable, L. (2004). The human rights of persons with mental disabilities: a global perspective on the application of human rights principles to mental health. *Maryland Law Review*, 63, 20–121.

Grodin, M., Tantola, D., Annas, G., and Gruskin, S. (eds.) (2013). *Health and Human Rights in a Changing World* (3rd ed.). New York: Routledge.

Guthman, J., Calmet, J., Rosales, E., Cruz, M., Chang, J., and Dedet, J.P. (1997). Patients' associations and the control of leishmaniasis in Peru. *Bulletin of the World Health Organization*, 75, 6–13.

Howard, G. and Bartram, J. (2002). *Domestic Water Quantity: Service Level and Health*. Geneva: WHO.

Hunt, P., and Gray, T. (eds.) (2013). *Maternal Mortality, Human Rights and Accountability*. New York: Routledge.

Hunt, P. and Leader, S. (2010). Developing and applying the right to the highest attainable standard of health: the role of the UN Special Rapporteur. In J. Harrington and M. Stuttaford (eds.) *Global Health and Human Rights: Philosophical and Legal Perspectives*, pp. 28–61. New York: Routledge.

Hunt, P. and MacNaughton, G. (2007). A human rights-based approach to health indicators. In M. Baderin and R. Mccorquodale (eds.) *Economic, Social and Cultural Rights in Action*, pp. 303–30. Oxford: Oxford University Press.

Hunt, P., Mesquita, J., and Khosla, R. (2010). The human rights responsibilities of international assistance and cooperation in health. In M. Gibney and S. Skogly (eds.) *Universal Rights and Extraterritorial Obligations*, pp. 104–29. Pennsylvania Studies in Human Rights. Pennsylvania, PA: University of Pennsylvania Press.

IACHR (Inter-American Commission on Human Rights) (1997). *Victor Rosario Congo v. Ecuador*. Case 11.427, Report No. 12/97, OEA/Ser.L/V/II.95 Doc. 7 rev at 257 (1997).

IACHR (Inter-American Commission on Human Rights) (2000). *Jorge Odir Miranda Cortez et al v. El Salvador*. Case 12.249, Report No. 29/01, OEA/Ser.L/V/II.111 Doc. 20 rev. at 282 (2000).

ICJ (International Court of Justice) (1996). *Advisory Opinion: Legality of the Threat or Use of Nuclear Weapons*, ICJ Reports 1996. Vol. I. The Hague: ICJ.

Kaur, J. (2012). The role of litigation in ensuring women's reproductive rights: an analysis of the Shanti Devi judgment in India. *Reproductive Health Matters*, 20(39), 21–30.

Kinney, E. and Clark, B.A. (2004). Provisions for health and health care in the constitutions of the countries of the world, *Cornell International Law Journal*, 37, 285.

Kismodi, E., Bueno de Mesquita, J., Andión Ibañez, X., Khosla, R., and Sepúlveda, L. (2012). Human rights accountability for maternal death and the failure to provide safe, legal abortion: the significance of two ground-breaking CEDAW decisions. *Reproductive Health Matters*, 20(39), 31–9.

Lewis, O. (2002). Protecting the rights of people with mental disabilities: the ECHR. *European Journal of Health Law*, 9(4), 293–320.

Maastricht Principles on Extraterritorial Obligations of States in the Area of Economic, Social and Cultural Rights (2011). Maastricht: International Commission of Jurists, Maastricht University.

MacNaughton, G. and Hunt, P. (2009). Health impact assessment: the contribution of the right to the highest attainable standard of health. *Public Health*, 123(4), 302–5.

MacNaughton, G. and Hunt, P. (2011). A human rights based approach to social impact assessment. In F. Vanclay and A.M. Esteves (eds.) *New Directions in Social Impact Assessment: Conceptual and Methodological Advances*, pp. 355–68. Cheltenham: Edward Elgar.

MDRI (Mental Disability Rights International) (2002). *Not on the Agenda: Human Rights of People with Mental Disabilities in Kosovo*. Washington, DC: MDRI.

Ministry for Foreign Affairs (2006). *International Policy on Sexual and Reproductive Health and Rights*. Stockholm: Swedish International Development Cooperation Agency.

OAS (Organization of American States) (1969). *American Convention on Human Rights*. OAS Treaty Series No. 36, 1144 U.N.T.S. 123. Adopted at the Inter-American Specialized Conference on Human Rights, San Jose, Costa Rica, 22 November 1969. Washington DC: OAS.

Rosenthal, E., Bauer, E., Hayden, M.F., and Holley, A. (2000). Implementing the right to community integration for children with disabilities in Russia: a human rights framework for international action. *Health and Human Rights: An International Journal*, 4, 82–113.

Shiffman, J. and Garces del Valle, A. (2006). Political histories and disparities in safe motherhood between Guatemala and Honduras. *Population and Development Review*, 32(1), 53–80.

UN (United Nations) (1948). *Universal Declaration of Human Rights*. GA Resolution 217A (III), UN GAOR, Resolution 71, UN Document A/810. New York: UN.

UN (United Nations) (1965). *Convention on the Elimination of All Forms of Racial Discrimination*, (ICERD). UN GA Resolution 2106A (XX). New York: UN.

UN (United Nations) (1966a). *International Covenant on Civil and Political Rights* (ICCPR). UN GA Resolution 2200A (XXI), 16 December 1966. New York: UN.

UN (United Nations) (1966b). *International Covenant on Economic, Social and Cultural Rights* (ICESCR). UN GA Resolution 2200A (XXI), 16 December 1966. New York: UN.

UN (United Nations) (1979). *Convention on the Elimination of All Forms of Discrimination Against Women* (CEDAW). GA Resolution 34/180, UN GAOR, 34th Session, Supplement No. 46 at 193, UN Document A/34/46. New York: UN.

UN (United Nations) (1989). *Convention on the Rights of the Child* (CRC). UN GA Resolution 44/25, 20 November 1989. New York: UN.

UN (United Nations) (1990). *International Convention on the Protection of the Rights of All Migrant Workers and Members of Their Families* (ICRMW). GA Resolution 45/158, 18 December 1990. New York: UN.

UN (United Nations) (1991). *Principles for the Protection of Persons with Mental Illness and the Improvement of Mental Health Care*, GA Resolution 46/119, 17 December 1991. New York: UN.

UN (United Nations) (1993). United Nations General Assembly. *Vienna Declaration and Programme of Action. World Conference on Human Rights*, Vienna 14–25 June 1993, UN Document A/CONF.157/23. New York: UN.

UN (United Nations) (1994). *International Conference on Population and Development*. 5–13 September 1994, Cairo, Egypt.

UN (United Nations) (1995). *Report of the Fourth World Conference on Women*. Beijing, China 4–15 September 1995. UN Document A/CONF.177.20.

UN (United Nations) (2005). *Sub-Commission Draft Guidelines for the Realisation of the Right to Drinking Water and Sanitation*. Adopted by the Sub-Commission in Resolution 2006/10. UN Document A/HRC/Sub.1/58/L11.

UNCEDAW (United Nations Committee on the Elimination of Discrimination Against Women) (1999). *General Recommendation No. 24 on Women and Health*, EDAW/C/1999/1/WGII/WP2/Rev.1. Geneva: UN.

UNCESCR (United Nations Committee on Economic, Social and Cultural Rights) (1990). *General Comment No. 3 (Fifth Session). The Nature of States Parties Obligations (Art.2, par.1)*. UN Document E/1991/23. Geneva: UN.

UNCESCR (United Nations Committee on Economic, Social and Cultural Rights) (1994). *General Comment No. 5 (Eleventh Session). Persons with Disabilities*. UN Document E/C.12/1194/13. Geneva: UN.

UNCESCR (United Nations Committee on Economic, Social and Cultural Rights) (2000). *General Comment No. 14 (Twenty Second Session). The Right to the Highest Attainable Standard of Health*. UN Document E/C.12/2000/4. Geneva: UN.

UNCESCR (United Nations Committee on Economic, Social and Cultural Rights) (2003). *General Comment No. 15 (Twenty Ninth Session). The Right to Water*. UN Document E/C.12/2002/11. Geneva: UN.

UNCHR (United Nations Commission on Human Rights) (2001). *Civil and Political Rights, Including the Question of Disappearances and Summary Executions: Report of the Special Rapporteur*, 11 January 2001, UN Document E/CN.4/2001/9). Geneva: UN.

UNCHR (United Nations Commission on Human Rights) (2002a). *Access to Medication in the Context of Pandemics such as HIV/AIDS*, Resolution 2002/32, 22 April 2002. Geneva: UN.

UNCHR (United Nations Commission on Human Rights) (2002b). *Human Rights of Persons with Disabilities*, Resolution 2002/61, 25 April 2002. Geneva: UN.

UNCHR (United Nations Commission on Human Rights) (2003a). *The Right of Everyone to the Enjoyment of the Highest Attainable Standard of Physical and Mental Health, Report of the Special Rapporteur*, 13 February 2003, UN Document E/CN.4/2003/58). Geneva: UN.

UNCHR (United Nations Commission on Human Rights) (2003b). *The Right of Everyone to the Enjoyment of the Highest Attainable Standard of Physical and Mental Health*. 22 April 2003, Resolution 2003/28. Geneva: UN.

UNCHR (United Nations Commission on Human Rights) (2004). *Relationship Between the Enjoyment of Economic, Social and Cultural Rights and the Promotion of the Realization of the Right to Drinking Water Supply and Sanitation: Final Report of the UN Sub-commission Special Rapporteur*. 14 July 2004. UN Document E/CN.4/Sub.2/2004/20. Geneva: UN.

UNCHR (United Nations Commission on Human Rights) (2006a). Mission to Uganda, *Report of the Special Rapporteur on the Right of Everyone to the Enjoyment of the Highest Attainable Standard of Health*, 19 January 2006. UN Document E/CN.4/2006/48/Add.2. Geneva: UN.

UNCHR (United Nations Commission on Human Rights) (2006b). *The Right of Everyone to the Enjoyment of the Highest Attainable Standard of Physical and Mental Health, Report of the Special Rapporteur*, 3 March 2006, UN Document E/CN.4/2006/48). Geneva: UN.

UNCRC (United Nations Committee on the Rights of the Child) (2003). *General Comment No. 4. Adolescent Health and Development in the Context of the Convention on the Rights of the Child*. UN Document CRC/GC/2003/4. Geneva: UN. paras 9 and 19.

UN ECOSOC (United Nations Economic and Social Council) (1985). *Siracusa Principles on the Limitation and Derogation Provisions in the International Covenant on Civil and Political Rights*. UN Document E/CN.4/1985/4, Annex.

UNGA (United Nations General Assembly) (1991). *Principles for the Protection of Persons with Mental Illness and the Improvement of Mental Health Care*. Adopted by Resolution 46/119, 17 December 1991.

UNGA (United Nations General Assembly) (1993). *Standard Rules on the Equalization of Opportunities for Persons with Disabilities*. Adopted by Resolution 48/96, 20 December 1993. New York: UN.

UNGA (United Nations General Assembly) (2000). *United Nations Millennium Declaration*. Adopted by Resolution 55/2, 8 September 2000.

UNGA (United Nations General Assembly) (2001). *Question of Torture and Other Cruel, Inhuman or Degrading Treatment or Punishment, Note by the Secretary-General*. 3 July 2001, UN Document A/56/156. paras 17–25.

UNGA (United Nations General Assembly) (2003). *Progress of Efforts to Ensure the Full Recognition and Enjoyment of the Human Rights of Persons with Disabilities: Report of the Secretary General*. 24 July 2003, UN Document A/58/181. New York: UN. para 43.

UNGA (United Nations General Assembly) (2004). *Report of the Special Rapporteur on the Right of Everyone to the Enjoyment of the Highest Attainable Standard of Physical and Mental Health*. 8 October 2004, UN Document A/59/422. New York: UN.

UNGA (United Nations General Assembly) (2011). *Report of the Special Rapporteur on the Right of Everyone to the Enjoyment of the Highest Attainable Standard of Health*. 3 August 2011. UN Document A/66/254. Geneva: UN.

UNHCR (United Nations High Commissioner for Refugees) (2005). *Access to Water in Refugee Situations: Survival, Health and Dignity for Refugees*. Geneva: UNHCR.

UNHRC (United Nations Human Rights Council) (2010a). Mission to India, *Report of the Special Rapporteur on the Right of Everyone to the Enjoyment of the Highest Attainable Standard of Physical and Mental Health*. 15 April 2010. UN Document A/HRC/14/20/Add.2. Geneva: UN.

UNHRC (United Nations Human Rights Council) (2010b). *Report of the Independent Expert on the Issue of Human Rights Obligations Related to Access to Safe Drinking Water and Sanitation, Catarina de Albuquerque*. 29 June 2010, UN Document A/HRC/15/31. Geneva: UN.

UNHRC (United Nations Human Rights Council) (2010c). *Report of the Special Rapporteur on the Right of Everyone to the Enjoyment of the Highest Attainable Standard of Physical and Mental Health, Anand Grover*. 27 April 2010. UN Document A/HRC/14/20. Geneva: UN.

UNHRC (United Nations Human Rights Council) (2007). *Report of the Special Rapporteur on the Right of Everyone to the Enjoyment of the Highest Attainable Standard of Physical and Mental Health, Paul Hunt*. 17 January 2007, UN Document A/HRC/4/28. New York: UN.

UNHRCttee (UN Human Rights Committee) (1994). *Toonen v. Australia*. 4 April 1994, UN Document CCPR/C/50/D/488/1992. New York: UN. para 8.5.

UNHRCttee (UN Human Rights Committee) (2003). *Karen Noelia Llantoy Huaman v. Peru (K.L. v. Peru)*. UN Document CPR/C/85/D/1153/2003. New York: UN.

UNMP (United Nations Millennium Project) (2005a). *Health, Dignity and Development: What Will it Take?* Report of the Task Force on Water and Sanitation. New York: UN.

UNMP (United Nations Millennium Project) (2005b). *Taking Action: Achieving Gender Equality and Empowering Women*. Report of the Taskforce on Education and Gender Equality. London: Earthscan.

UNMP (United Nations Millennium Project) (2005c). *Who's Got The Power?* Report of the Task Force on Child Health and Maternal Health. New York: UN.

UNOHCHR (United Nations Office of the High Commissioner for Human Rights) (2012a). *Human Rights Indicators: A Guide to Measurement and Implementation*. HR/PUB/12/5. Geneva: UN.

UNOHCHR (United Nations Office of the High Commissioner for Human Rights) (2012b). *Technical Guidance on the Application of a Human Rights-based Approach to the Implementation of Policies and Programmes to Reduce Preventable Maternal Morbidity and Mortality.* UN Document A/HRC/21/22. Geneva: UN.

WHO (World Health Organization) (1946). *Constitution of the* World Health Organization, adopted by the International Health Conference, New York, 19 June–22 July 1946, and signed on 22 July 1946. Geneva: WHO.

WHO (World Health Organization) (1978a). *Declaration of Alma-Ata: International Conference on Primary Health Care.* 6–12 September, USSR.

WHO (World Health Organization) (1978b). *A Joint Report by the Director-General of the WHO and the Executive Director of UNICEF Presented at the International Conference on Primary Health Care, 1978, Alma-Ata.* Geneva: WHO.

WHO (World Health Organization) (2001a). *A Human Rights Approach to Tuberculosis.* Geneva: WHO.

WHO (World Health Organization) (2001b). *World Health Report 2001. Mental Health: New Understanding, New Hope.* pp. 112–15. Geneva: WHO.

WHO (World Health Organization) (2002). *Global Defence Against the Infectious Disease Threat.* Geneva: WHO.

WHO (World Health Organization) (2003). *Safe Abortion: Technical and Policy Guidance for Health Systems.* Geneva: WHO.

WHO (World Health Organization) (2004a). *Intensified Control of Neglected Diseases: Report of an International Workshop, Berlin, 10–12 December 2003.* WHO/CDS/CPE/CEE/2004.45. Geneva: WHO. p22.

WHO (World Health Organization) (2004b). *Mental Health Policy, Plans and Programmes.* Geneva: WHO.

WHO (World Health Organization) (2005). *Resource Book on Mental Health, Human Rights and Legislation.* Geneva: WHO.

WHO (World Health Organization) (2006a). *World Health Report 2006, Working Together for Health.* Geneva: WHO.

WHO (World Health Organization) (2006b). *Guidelines for Drinking Water Quality.* Geneva: WHO.

WHO (World Health Organization) and TDR (Special Programme for Research and Training in Tropical Diseases) (2007). *Neglected Diseases: A Human Rights Analysis.* Document reference TDR/SDR/SEB/ST/07.2. Geneva: WHO.

Yamin, A.E. and Gloppen, S. (eds.) (2011). *Litigating Health Rights: Can Courts Bring More Justice to Health?* Cambridge, MA: Human Rights Program, Harvard Law School.

Law and the public's health

Lawrence Gostin

Introduction to law and the public's health

Public health law can be defined as the legal powers and duties of government, in collaboration with multiple partners (e.g. healthcare, business, the community, the media, and academe), to assure the conditions for people to be healthy and safe (to identify, prevent, and ameliorate risks to health in the population). The prime objective of public health law is to pursue the highest possible level of physical and mental health in the population, consistent with the values of social justice (Gostin 2008).

Although government needs adequate power to safeguard the public's health, it should not interfere with the civil rights and liberties of individuals without adequate justification. Government therefore has limitations—both legal and ethical—in exercising power that constrains the autonomy, privacy, liberty, proprietary, or other legally protected interests of individuals. Some of the most challenging, and enduring, debates in public health law are the conflicts between individual liberties and the common good.

Public health laws have deep roots in social history, ranging from the ancient use of quarantines at land and at sea, to sanitary laws in the wake of the Industrial Revolution, through to injury prevention, and non-communicable disease (NCD) control in the late twentieth century. Domestic public health laws operate at the local (e.g. municipal codes) and national level. Often, federalist states such as Brazil, Canada, India, and the United States have complex constitutional arrangements between local, regional, and national public health laws.

Domestic public health laws and regulations also intersect with international health law (e.g. the International Health Regulations and Framework Convention on Tobacco Control), 'soft' law (e.g. World Health Organization (WHO) codes of practice and global strategies), and wider international regimes that impact on health (e.g. trade, migration, human rights, and the environment). The complex intersections between local, national, and international law to protect the public's health cannot be overemphasized.

This chapter first examines the powers and duties of government to protect the public's health and safety, together with the limits on its authority to protect a sphere of individual rights and liberties. Second, it explores the central value of public health law—social justice, with particular attention to unconscionable inequalities in health based on socioeconomic status. Third, the chapter examines the statutes and regulations that create public health agencies—defining their mission, powers, funding, and scope. Fourth, the chapter categorizes seven legal 'tools' at the state's disposal to promote the health, safety, and well-being of the population: taxing and spending, the informational environment, the built environment, the socioeconomic environment, direct regulation, indirect regulation, and deregulation. Finally, the chapter turns to how legal interventions can be used to prevent or ameliorate three major health hazards: infectious diseases, NCDs, and injuries (both unintentional and intentional).

Public health: powers, duties, and limits

Governments have the power and duty to safeguard the public's health and safety. The international human right to health, which virtually all countries accept as part of treaty obligations, imposes on governments the primary responsibility for the public's health. In many newer democracies (for example, in Africa and Latin America), national constitutions also guarantee the right to health, as well as other socioeconomic rights such as the right to life and to a safe environment (Friedman and Gostin 2012). Emerging economic powers such as Brazil, India, and South Africa have had robust 'right to health' litigation in their judicial systems. Whether through international law or national constitutions, the state's highest obligation is the defence of the social and economic well-being of the population, with health and security being among the most vital. In most theories of democracy health and security are seen as quintessential aspects of the social contract between individuals and their governments (Walzer 1983).

Beyond socioeconomic rights, virtually all states around the world—older constitutions such as in the United States, newer ones such as in South Africa, and even those without written constitutions such as the United Kingdom—protect civil and political rights—for example, bodily integrity, privacy, liberty, and non-discrimination. At the same time, national constitutions, as well as public health laws, also usually afford individuals civil and political rights, which can constrain the power of ministries to use compulsion. Provided that agencies act for an important public health purpose, and use means that are proportionate to the ends, they can require conformance with publicly established standards of conduct.

Protecting and preserving the public's health and safety is often not possible without constraining a range of private activities that pose unacceptable risks. Private actors can profit by engaging in practices that damage the rest of society: individuals can spread infectious disease; industry has a profit motive, which can result in unsafe workplaces, environmental pollution, or unhealthy products. Some industries are inherently dangerous (e.g. tobacco), while others can have harmful effects (e.g. alcoholic beverages). In each instance, individuals or organizations act in their own interests, but their actions may adversely affect communal health and safety. In the absence of governmental authority and willingness to coerce, such threats to the public's health could not easily be reduced.

Although regulation in the name of public health is intended to safeguard the health and safety of whole populations, it often benefits those most at risk of injury and disease. Everyone gains value from public health regulations, such as food and water standards, but some regulations protect the most vulnerable. For instance, eliminating a toxic waste site, enforcing a building code in a crowded tenement, or closing an unhygienic restaurant holds particular significance for those at immediate risk. Frequently, those at increased risk are particularly vulnerable due to their race, gender, or socioeconomic status.

Individuals and businesses often oppose government regulation. Resistance is sometimes based on philosophical grounds of autonomy, choice, or freedom from government interference. Citizens, and the groups that represent them, claim that regulating self-regarding behaviour, such as the use of seat belts or motorcycle helmets, is not the business of government. Or they harbour suspicions about government's intent, such as fluoridation of drinking water. Public health agencies sometimes have to defend charges of paternalism, or the 'Nanny State,' such as with Mayor Bloomberg's decision to limit portion size of sugary drinks in New York City (Gostin and Gostin 2009).

Public health has historically constrained the rights of individuals and businesses to protect community interests in health. Reporting and surveillance diminish privacy; mandatory testing, vaccination, and treatment invade bodily integrity; environmental standards reduce property values; industrial regulation impedes economic freedom; and isolation and quarantine deprive individuals of liberty. In each of these cases, and more, public health has not shied from regulating individuals and businesses for the common good.

Public health powers can legitimately be used to restrict human freedoms and rights, but they must be exercised consistent with constitutional and statutory constraints on state action. Governments cannot over-reach, such as constraining liberty without sufficient evidence of public benefit. When agencies coerce they must do so proportionately, such as by using the least restrictive measure needed to avert the health threat. And they must always act fairly, without discrimination on grounds such as race, gender, or disability. Achieving a just balance between the powers and duties of the state to advance the public's health and constitutionally protected rights poses an enduring challenge for public health law.

Social justice

Social justice is viewed as so central to the mission of public health that it has been described as the field's core value: 'The historic dream of public health . . . is a dream of social justice' (Beauchamp 1999, p. 105). Among the most basic and commonly understood meanings of justice is fair, equitable, and appropriate treatment in light of what is due or owed to individuals and groups (Rawls 1971).

Social justice captures the twin moral impulses that animate public health: to advance human well-being by improving health and to do so particularly by focusing on the needs of the most disadvantaged (Gostin and Powers 2006). This account of justice has the aim of bringing about the human good of health for all members of the population. An integral part of that aim is the task of identifying and ameliorating patterns of systematic disadvantage that profoundly and pervasively undermine prospects for well-being of oppressed and subordinated groups—people whose prospects for good health are so limited that their life choices are not even remotely like those of others (Powers and Faden 2006). These two aspects of justice—health improvement for the population and fair treatment of the disadvantaged—create a richer understanding of public health law and ethics. Seen through the lens of social justice, the central mission of the public health system is to engage in systematic action to assure the conditions for improved health for all members of the population, and to redress persistent patterns of systematic disadvantage.

Imagine a government policy designed to reduce tobacco consumption in the population. If the government were to lower the smoking prevalence from, say, 30 per cent to 15 per cent, would that be acceptable if marginalized groups such as institutionalized populations (e.g. prisoners and mental patients) continue to have high smoking prevalence? What if the government explicitly targets smoking prevention messages to the well-off but not in poor neighbourhoods? Is that acceptable as a matter of social justice?

These are the quintessential values of public health law—government power and duty, coercion and limits on state power, and the value of social justice. To achieve the goals of population health under the rule of law requires sound legal foundations. Statutes and regulations—as interpreted by the judicial system—establish the infrastructure for public health agencies ranging from their mission, functions, and powers, to their organization and funding.

Public health statutes: legal foundations of public health agencies

The field of public health is typically regarded as a scientific endeavour, and undoubtedly our understanding of the aetiology and response to disease is heavily influenced by technical inquiry. Less well understood is the role of law in public health. Law defines the jurisdiction of public health officials and specifies the manner in which they may exercise their authority. Public health statutes create public health agencies, designate their mission and core functions, appropriate their funds, grant their power, and limit their actions to protect a sphere of freedom. They authorize the collection of health information and enable monitoring and regulation of dangerous activities. The most important public health debates take place in legal forums—legislatures, courts, and administrative agencies—and in the law's language of rights, duties, and justice (Grad 2004).

The quality and modernity of public health laws around the world are highly variable (Institute of Medicine 2011). Some states have relatively recent and comprehensive public health laws; others have older statutes, while still others have virtually no public health laws. Overall, public health statutes often have a number of deficiencies. They may be quite old, reflecting an era when infectious and sexually transmitted infections were the major health hazards. They can be highly fragmented, built up in layers over time, for example, beginning with tuberculosis and sexually transmitted diseases (e.g. syphilis and gonorrhoea), through to polio and then AIDS, and more recently traffic safety and diet and physical activity. These laws may not afford the state sufficient authority to protect the public's health and safety and they may fail to adequately protect individual rights and freedoms. For example, many older statutes do not ensure natural justice or procedural due process before the exercise of compulsory powers.

Given the importance of sound, modern public health laws, many (if not most) states should examine the corpus of their public health laws and regulations. Low- and middle-income countries may need the capacity and knowledge to reform their laws. The influential Institute of Medicine in the United States issued a major report on public health law reform in 2011, urging states to adopt the 'Turning Point' Model Public Health Act (Hodge et al. 2006). That model act could provide a template for other countries. Additionally, the WHO and International Development Law Organization are planning to release a 'Public Health Law Manual' that would provide law reform guidance particularly in low- and middle-income countries.

The WHO Constitution requires member states to notify the Organization of its major public health statutes and regulations, even though few states actually comply. The WHO publishes a *Health Law Digest*, but the Organization has drastically cut back resources for the *Digest*. The Director-General's reorganization several years ago removed 'law' from the title of the department charged with publishing the *Digest*. Today, the *Digest* is solely in electronic form and has lost its utility to provide a systematic account of national public health laws.

The lawmaking process: building constituencies and forming partnerships

The methods and goals of public health are often misunderstood and undervalued within government and society. Public health needs opportunities to draw attention to its resource requirements and its achievements so that it can develop constituencies for programmes. The lawmaking process provides such an opportunity. A bill is the first step towards a coalition. It is an occasion for contact with interest groups and affected communities, some of whom may be motivated to act in support of the bill. Contacts and collaborative efforts also help to establish long-term ties and identify important sources of support for other programmes. Moreover, the process of negotiating for support can be a useful and concrete way for health agencies to incorporate the views of persons who receive public health services or are subject to regulation.

Legal reform also has the potential to enhance health agencies' relationships with the legislature. Positive lawmaking offers a different sort of contact with legislators than tends to occur in the appropriations process. Public health law reform may offer an occasion to deal with a far greater range of legislators outside the context of contentious budget discussions. The drafting, negotiating, and hearing processes provide a variety of forums for educating lawmakers and their staffs about public health needs and methods and also provide health planners with better information about legislative views and priorities.

Law reform, of course, cannot guarantee better public health. However, by crafting a consistent and uniform approach, carefully delineating the mission and functions of public health agencies,

designating a range of flexible powers, and specifying the criteria and procedures for using those powers, the law can become a catalyst, rather than an impediment, to reinvigorating the public health system.

Models of legal interventions: law as a tool for the public's health

Law can be empowering, providing innovative solutions to the most implacable health problems. Many of the great public health achievements in the twentieth century were realized, at least in part, through law reform or litigation, including vaccinations, safer workplaces, safer and healthier foods, motor vehicle safety, control of infectious diseases, tobacco control, and fluoridation of drinking water (Centers for Disease Control and Prevention 2000).

The study of public health law, therefore, requires a detailed understanding of the various legal tools available to prevent injury and disease and to promote the health of the populace. There are a number of models for using law as a tool for the public's health and safety, including: taxation and spending, the informational environment, the built environment, the socioeconomic environment, direct regulation, indirect regulation through the tort system, and deregulation. Although in each case the law can be a powerful agent for change, the interventions can also raise critical social, ethical, or constitutional concerns (Gostin 2008).

Model 1: the power to tax and spend

The power to tax and spend—the quintessential governmental function found everywhere—provides government with an important regulatory technique. Most governments invest in a broad array of services to promote public health ranging from surveillance to education and research. Although funding is far too limited, many governments spend to establish and maintain a public health infrastructure consisting of: a trained workforce, electronic information and communications systems, rapid disease surveillance, laboratory capacity, and response capability. In some states, governments can attach 'conditions' to public spending that are intended to be health promoting. For example, in the United States, the federal government requires states to have a drinking age of 21 years as a condition of the receipt of highway funds.

The power to tax is primarily designed to raise revenue, but it also can provide significant inducements to engage in beneficial behaviour and disincentives to engage in risk activities. Tax relief can be offered for health-producing activities such as healthcare services, childcare, and charitable contributions. At the same time, tax burdens can be placed on the sale of hazardous products such as cigarettes, alcoholic beverages, and firearms. Of course, taxation can create perverse incentives such as tax relief for the purchase of unsafe and fuel-inefficient motor vehicles. A carbon tax offers a good example of an economic vehicle that would be beneficial to the public's health and the environment.

Model 2: the power to alter the informational environment

The public is constantly exposed to images and information that influence their life choices, and this undoubtedly affects health and behaviour. The reliability and usefulness of information is variable. Some messages are educational, such as child nutrition campaigns. Other information can be biased—either inaccurate or misleading. For example, the corporate profit motive can result in advertisement of harmful products, such as foods with excess sugar and salt. Messages such as 'low fat,' 'low calorie,' or 'light' can be confusing or deceptive.

Regulating the flow in information can be challenging. In practical terms, governments do not have the available resources to compete with large advertising budgets that market unhealthy foods, alcoholic beverages, or tobacco. In constitutional terms, there can be questions about whether advertising restrictions violate the corporation's right to free expression.

Governments have several tools at their disposal to alter the informational environment thereby encouraging people to make more healthful choices about diet, physical activity, tobacco, and alcohol. First, government, as a health educator, can use communication campaigns that warn consumers of high risks (e.g. smoking or driving while intoxicated) or encourage safer activities (e.g. wearing seat belts or motorcycle helmets). Second, government can require businesses to label their products to inform consumers: instructions on safe product use, disclosure of contents or ingredients, or warnings about hazards. Third, government can regulate advertising and promotions for potentially harmful products such as cigarettes and firearms. They can also limit marketing certain products to vulnerable populations, such as children and adolescents.

Regulating tobacco packaging and advertising offers a good illustration. The WHO's Framework Convention on Tobacco Control (WHO 2005a) requires states to adopt supply and demand reduction strategies, including advertising restrictions. Yet, the tobacco industry has challenged advertising restrictions and packet labels in countries as diverse as Australia, Uruguay, and the United States. Australia was the first country to introduce plain packaging legislation with graphic images of the harms of tobacco. Although Australia's highest court upheld the legislation, the government is defending its law both in an Investment Treaty dispute and at the World Trade Organization (*British American Tobacco Australia Limited v. The Commonwealth* 2012). Uruguay's tobacco control legislation is also being challenged in a separate Investment Treaty case (*FTR Holding v. Oriental Republic of Uruguay* 2010). 'Big Tobacco' is claiming that the state is unfairly 'taking' their property or diminishing the value of their private investments. Although this may seem to be an outrageous claim, it is expensive for states to defend their public health laws.

In the United States, the Food and Drug Administration's requirement of graphic warning labels is going to be decided by the Supreme Court. Tobacco companies are claiming that the graphic image requirement violates their rights to free expression (*R.J. Reynolds Tobacco Company v. Food and Drug Administration* 2012). The United States is one of the world's outliers in that its highest court ardently defends the right of corporations to free expression, thus thwarting public health restraints on advertising hazardous products.

Model 3: the power to alter the built environment

The design of the 'built' or 'physical' environment can hold great potential for creating healthier and safer communities. Public health has a long history of altering the built environment to reduce injuries (e.g. workplace safety, traffic calming, consumer protection, and fire codes), infectious diseases (e.g. sanitation, nuisance abatement, and housing codes), and environmentally associated harms (e.g. lead paint and toxic emissions). Sanitary laws go back hundreds of years, designed to ensure more hygienic conditions in growing cities; occupational health and safety became prominent following the Industrial Revolution, which exposed workers to toxins and unsafe working conditions; and more modern laws provide patients and consumers with protection against unsafe products.

The epidemiological transition from infectious to chronic diseases raises new challenges in the design of neighbourhoods. For example, urban design can encourage more active lifestyles (walking lanes, bicycle paths, parks, green fields, and playgrounds); improve nutrition (zoning to limit fast food); discourage the use of hazardous products ('tobacco-free' indoor spaces); reduce violence (well-lit streets, safe storage of firearms); and increase social interactions (helping neighbours and building social capital) (Perdue et al. 2003).

Many zoning laws in the mid and late twentieth century were unfavourable to healthy lifestyles, such as those giving preference to motor vehicles over pedestrians and bicycle riders, or preferring commercial development over playgrounds. Municipalities often facilitated the expansion of unhealthy fast foods, forming 'food deserts' in poor neighbourhoods. These are political choices, and debates still rage over whether government should use health as a major factor in designing living spaces, rather than, say, economic development. What seems certain is that it is within the power of government to structure the environment in ways that are more conducive to a healthy diet and physical activity.

Model 4: the power to alter the socioeconomic environment

A strong and consistent finding of epidemiological research is that socioeconomic status (SES) is correlated with morbidity, mortality, and functioning (Marmot 2005). SES is a complex phenomenon based on income, education, and occupation. The relationship between SES and health often is referred to as a 'gradient' because of the graded and continuous nature of the association; health differences are observed well into the middle ranges of SES. These empirical findings have persisted across time and cultures and remain viable today.

Some researchers go further, concluding the overall level of economic inequality in a society correlates with (and adversely affects) population health. That is, societies with wide disparities between rich and poor tend to have worse health status than societies with smaller disparities, after controlling for per capita income. These researchers hypothesize that societies with higher degrees of inequality provide less social support and cohesion, making life more stressful and pathogenic. Drawing upon this line of argument, some ethicists contend, 'social justice is good for our health' (Daniels et al. 2000).

The WHO issued a report on social determinants of health, urging more attention to the underlying factors in influencing health outcomes (WHO 2008b). However, the WHO never put significant resources into social determinants and did not follow the Commission Report with international law or softer norms. From government's perspective, ensuring a healthy population that is fair and equitable requires an 'all of government,' indeed 'all of society' approach that transcends the health sector.

Although social determinants powerfully affect health, they can require redistribution of wealth and hence are often hotly contested. Opponents of redistributive policies argue such policies punish personal accomplishment, thereby discouraging economic growth. Still, it is impossible to make significant inroads into health disparities without careful attention to the deeper social and economic determinants of health.

Model 5: direct regulation of persons, professionals, and businesses

Government has the power to directly regulate individuals, professionals, and businesses. In a well-regulated society, public health authorities set clear, enforceable rules to protect the health and safety of workers, consumers, and the population at large.

Regulation has long been a staple of injury control. In most Western countries, for example, the rate of motor vehicle-related injuries and deaths has plummeted due to law reform. Governments required individuals to engage in safer behaviour, such as by using seat belts and motorcycle helmets. The law also compelled manufacturers to design and sell safer vehicles, such as cars with airbags and with the ability to better withstand crashes. The law also set standards for governmental and commercial development such as safer roads and traffic calming. Yet, with the explosion of motorized vehicles in newly emerging states, the injury and death rates from motor vehicles are alarming. The streets of Bangkok, Delhi, and Hanoi (among many others) are teeming with unsafe vehicles, chaotic roads, and motorcycle drivers and passengers without helmets.

Perhaps the most ancient use of direct public health regulation is in the control of infectious diseases. Governments often mandate vaccination, screening, partner notification, directly observed therapy, and isolation or quarantine. Originating from the ancient scourges such as leprosy, malaria, and tuberculosis, through to syphilis and herpes, and to the modern AIDS pandemic, states—for good or bad—have enacted civil and criminal laws to deter or punish perceived risk behaviours. Early in the AIDS pandemic, for example, many states enacted laws to require testing (e.g. prisoners), travel and immigration restrictions, and even quarantine (e.g. Cuba). Criminal laws were altered to punish behaviours conducive to transmitting HIV, and to targeting risk populations such as injecting drug users and commercial sex workers.

Direct regulation also plays a major role in ensuring that professionals and businesses operate safely and with the requisite level of skill and knowledge. Licences and permits enable government to monitor and control the standards and practices of healthcare professionals, hospitals, and nursing homes. By licensing and accrediting health professionals, public health agencies can help ensure safe, competent, and well-qualified practitioners. Finally, inspection and regulation of businesses helps to assure humane conditions at work, reduced toxic emissions, and improved consumer product safety.

The control of chronic diseases is becoming the new battleground over the wisdom of direct regulation. Some jurisdictions have banned harmful ingredients such as trans fatty acids; others have reduced harmful additives, such as excess sugar or sodium; while still others have regulated portion size, such as the size of a sugary soft drink. Recent research suggests, 'sugar is toxic', which may require public health agencies to set or recommend safer levels of sugar intake (Basu et al 2013).

When regulating what people eat or their physical activity, governments often face the stinging criticism that they are acting paternalistically, with the charge of running a 'Nanny State'. To public health advocates, these are all necessary measures to make health the 'easier' or 'default' choice. But to many in society, it restricts their freedoms to make their own decisions about their health and well-being (Gostin and Gostin 2009).

Model 6: indirect regulation through the tort system

Ministries of justice and health, as well as private citizens, possess a powerful means of indirect regulation through the tort system. Civil litigation can redress many different kinds of public health harms: environmental damage (e.g. air pollution or groundwater contamination), exposure to toxic substances (e.g. pesticides, radiation, or chemicals), hazardous products (e.g. tobacco or firearms), and defective consumer products (e.g. children's toys, recreational equipment, or household goods).

The most prominent illustration of using judicial remedies for a public health purpose is tobacco litigation. Tort litigation against the tobacco industry began in the United States. This litigation had multiple benefits. It resulted in a 'Master Agreement' between states and tobacco companies, with large sums given to states. It uncovered highly damaging evidence about the deceptive behaviour of the industry, such as raising the nicotine level of cigarettes, hiding information about the hazards of smoking, and targeting young girls, racial minorities, and minors with cigarette advertisements and promotions.

More modern litigation has been waged under the constitutional right to health in places such as India and Latin America. Public health advocates in these and other countries have sued tobacco companies for knowingly misleading the public. They have also sued their own governments to force them to adopt more rigorous tobacco control measures, such as clean air acts (Cabrera and Gostin 2011).

Perhaps it would be predictable for Big Tobacco to use the law as a sword against government regulation. Increasingly, the industry is using the constitutional right to property or commercial speech, bilateral investment treaties to safeguard their investments, or World Trade Organization treaties to stall or block tobacco control (Mitchell and Studdert 2012).

Using tobacco litigation as a model, public health advocates have sought to use tort law to attack the deceptive and harmful practices of other powerful industries. This litigation ranges from lawsuits against the food industry (e.g. marketing unhealthy products to minors), the firearms industry (e.g. trafficking in dangerous weapons), and the alcohol industry (e.g. glamorizing underage or excessive drinking). Thus far, many of these lawsuits have not been successful. One difference is that food, firearms, and alcoholic beverages when used responsibly are not harmful, while tobacco use is always hazardous.

To what extent should the harmful activities of these and other industries be immune from tort litigation on the theory that autonomous consumers are free to make their own decisions—whether healthful or harmful? Given that individuals are embedded in communities and societies that profoundly affect their personal choices, laws should enable consumers to litigate if the private sector has exposed them to unnecessary and serious risks.

Model 7: deregulation: law as a barrier to health

Sometimes laws are harmful to the public's health and stand as an obstacle to effective action. In such cases, the best remedy is deregulation. Politicians may urge superficially popular policies that have unintended health consequences. Consider laws that prohibit or penalize needle exchange programmes and pharmacy sales of sterile syringes. Even though access to sterile injection equipment significantly reduces the risk of needle-borne infections (e.g. HIV and hepatitis B or C) and does not encourage illicit drug use, many governments discourage or ban the distribution of these products, including by public health agencies.

A further illustration is the decision to close bathhouses, making it more difficult to reach gay men with condoms and safe sex literature. Rather than banning these activities, government could use them as venues for education and harm reduction.

Finally, but perhaps even more importantly, governments throughout the world criminalize high-risk activities. They punish sex workers, drug users, and even those who engage in same-sex sexual activities. Criminal laws that punish activities that risk transmission of HIV, for example, do not appear to reduce unsafe behaviour, but rather drive the epidemic underground.

Criminal law is usually a blunt, ineffective, and unfair tool when used for an allegedly public health purpose. Deregulation, however, can be controversial because it often involves a direct conflict between public health and other values that society may favour, such as crime prevention or morality. Drug laws, the closure of bathhouses, and HIV-specific criminal penalties represent society's disapproval of disfavoured behaviours. Deregulation becomes a symbol of weakness that is often politically unpopular. Public health advocates may believe passionately in harm-reduction strategies, but the political community may want to use the law to demonstrate social disapproval of certain activities such as illicit drug use, commercial sex, or unprotected sex.

The government, then, has many legal 'levers' designed to prevent injury and disease and promote the public's health—taxing and spending, the informational environment, the built environment, the socioeconomic environment, direct regulation, indirect regulation, and deregulation. Legal interventions can be highly effective and need to be part of the public health officer's arsenal. However, legal interventions can also be controversial, raising vital ethical, social, constitutional, and political concerns.

Case studies of four major health hazards

The previous sections often used major health hazards as illustrations of the use of public health law. This chapter concludes with four brief case studies: infectious diseases, NCDs, unintentional injuries, and violence to self or others. This final section shows how the intersection between public health law at the local, national, and international levels can influence health outcomes.

Infectious disease law

As mentioned earlier, infectious disease law has ancient origins (Markel 2005). Epidemic disease has historically had profound implications, not only for animal and human health, but also for security, trade, tourism, and social relationships. Infectious diseases often bring out the worst in people and societies, provoking stigma and discrimination against disfavoured groups such as immigrants and ethnic or religious minorities. Rapidly emerging diseases (such as novel influenzas) often provoke unjustified trade or travel restrictions. At the same time, governments are likely to spend disproportionate public health resources on highly transmissible or novel infections—disproportionate at least insofar as infectious pathogens receive so much more attention than equally destructive health hazards, such as NCDs, injuries, and mental illness.

This dynamic can be seen in the emphasis in domestic and international laws on infectious diseases. The oldest international health law—dating from mid-nineteenth-century sanitary conferences in Europe—is the International Health Regulations, which are devoted almost exclusively to health security. The one and only time the International Health Regulations (WHO 2005b) were used was in relation to the influenza A (H1N1) pandemic. Before that, governments were planning and spending large resources on novel influenzas, in response to H5N1.

The emphasis on epidemic diseases can also be seen in domestic law, where most public health statutes are devoted to infectious disease powers, such as testing, screening, partner notification, directly observed therapy, and isolation or quarantine. During the SARS outbreaks, states—particularly in North America and Asia—exercised public health powers extensively including travel restrictions, trade barriers, border security, and quarantine (Fidler 2004).

Even in the realm of international relations, infectious diseases have dominated funding and political attention. The AIDS pandemic fundamentally changed the political and funding calculus for global health. The United States launched the greatest effort by a single country against a single disease—PEPFAR. The United Nations (UN) formed a new agency to coordinate work on AIDS—UNAIDS. And powerful new public/private partnerships emerged to provide unprecedented funding for work on AIDS, tuberculosis, and malaria, such as the Global Fund and UNITAID, while the GAVI Alliance supports another infectious disease initiative—immunizations. Most impressively, the international community has vastly ramped up research, funding, and access to antiretroviral treatment for HIV/AIDS.

Non-communicable disease law

Four NCDs—cardiovascular disease, cancer, respiratory disease, and diabetes—account for 63 per cent of global deaths annually. The conventional wisdom, which conceives of NCDs as a 'First World' problem, is starkly belied by data: 80 per cent of the 35 million people who die annually from NCDs live in low- and middle-income countries. The death toll is projected to rise by 17 per cent over the next decade, unless meaningful steps are taken urgently. With the exception of sub-Saharan Africa, NCD mortality now exceeds that of infectious, maternal, perinatal, and nutritional conditions combined (WHO 2011).

The suffering and early deaths from NCDs, and the disproportionate burden in lower-income countries, will only grow. And they will interact with existing health challenges in poorer countries, creating the 'double burden' of hunger alongside obesity. Although longer lifespans partly explain the increased burden of NCDs, human behaviour plays a central role: unhealthy diets, sedentary lifestyles, smoking, and excessive alcohol consumption account for more than two-thirds of all new NCD cases.

The moral tragedy lies in the fact that much of this suffering and early death is preventable, and many of the solutions are to be found in law—at both the domestic and international levels. Local and national governments have all the public health law tools at their disposal in fighting the NCD epidemic. They can tax unhealthy products such as tobacco, alcoholic beverages, sugary drinks, and sodium-laden processed foods. Equally, rich states could cease subsidizing unhealthy foods, such as high-fructose corn syrup, cane sugar, and even red meat and dairy, while subsidizing healthy fruits and vegetables.

Governments can also alter the informational environment, counteracting incessant commercial messages—for example by package labelling, health warnings on cigarettes and alcohol, and comprehensible nutritional information on food packages and restaurant menus. The United Kingdom Food Standards Agency developed a voluntary system 'traffic light' system that is visible and simple to follow. By putting a series of bright red lights on food packages with excessive saturated or trans fats, sodium, sugar, and calories, it incentivizes food companies to be more responsible, while clearly informing consumers. The state can restrict advertising unhealthy products, particularly when aimed at minors (Hawkes 2007).

Individual choices are not made in isolation, but reflect the environment in which people live. Government could use its powers to plan cities and zones to facilitate healthy lifestyles, including supermarkets and farmers' markets. It can build bike and walking paths, designate pedestrian areas, subsidize mass transit, and discourage motor vehicle use—such as the 'congestion tax' instituted by the city of London in the United Kingdom. Government could require 'health impact assessments' as a condition of new government or commercial development.

Although incentives and voluntary approaches are often more politically palatable, there is also a role for direct regulation. Some products, such as trans fatty acids, are so hazardous to health that they should be removed from the market, as Denmark has done (see Table 3.4.1).

It is equally important to marshal a transnational response. The impact of globalization—globalized food and tobacco markets and the homogenization of cultures and behaviours—means that no country can effectively tackle NCDs without the support and cooperation of the international community. Global governance for health requires a multifaceted approach (Gostin 2014). The international community could set norms for healthy activities, such as the Framework Convention on Tobacco Control (WHO 2005a). The WHO has also developed 'Global Strategies' covering: NCD prevention and control (2000); diet, physical activity, and health (2008); and the harmful use of alcohol (2010). In 2008, the Assembly adopted the 2008–2013 Action Plan for its Global Strategy on NCDs, and in 2010, it adopted recommendations on the marketing of foods and non-alcoholic beverages to children (WHO 2008a, 2010).

The decade of WHO governance on NCDs failed to raise NCDs to the same high profile and impact as HIV/AIDS. But the UN General Assembly (2011) hosted a high-level meeting on NCDs in September 2011, adopting a *Political Declaration on the Prevention and Control of Non-Communicable Diseases*—a 65-point document, cataloguing many of the global challenges, and calling for a whole-of-government/whole-of-society response. Broadly speaking, the Declaration recommends preventative measures, health system strengthening, international cooperation, research and development, and monitoring and evaluation of progress. Sadly, however, the UN failed to set clear targets, a tangible road-map to meet those targets, and the resources needed to tackle the global NCD pandemic.

Just as domestic governments need to adopt an 'all-of-government/all-of-society' approach, so too must global institutions look beyond WHO to a more expansive view of governance. In short, there is a need for 'total global engagement,' encompassing trade, investment, development, intellectual property, and human rights—all international law regimes in their own right. The private sector is a vital part of the solution, but the major companies operate all over the world, so corporate governance must also operate at the global, as well as the national, level.

Injury control law

Injuries are often portrayed as 'accidents' or 'random events' that are unpredictable and therefore unpreventable, as opposed to a serious public health concern, which explains the field's historical neglect. However, injuries are a leading cause of death and disability worldwide, resulting in nearly 6 million deaths annually and representing 17 per cent of the global burden of disease; by 2020 the global burden of injuries is projected to increase to 20 per cent (WHO 2011). The injury epidemic has been compounded by rapid unplanned urbanization, increased motorization, and dramatic changes in the built environment in low- and middle-income countries (Lozano et al. 2012; Murray et al. 2012; Salomon et al. 2012).

There are marked inequalities in the global distribution of injuries, with >90 per cent of all deaths and disability-adjusted life years occurring in low- and middle-income countries, mostly among young people. The economic burdens for those countries are staggering: traffic incidents alone cost $65 billion or 1–1.5 per cent of GDP annually (Norton et al. 2006).

The WHO differentiates between unintentional injuries (no predetermined intent such as road traffic incidents, poisonings, falls, fires, and drowning) and intentional injuries (self-directed such as suicide or self-mutilation, interpersonal such as domestic violence or murder, or collective violence such as war-related injuries). Law reform can help prevent both of these.

The UN Convention on the Rights of the Child (UN 1989) guarantees all children the right to a safe environment and to protection from injury and violence. Yet, injuries are the single greatest cause of death and disability among children in low- and middle-income countries. Drowning is a leading cause of morbidity and premature mortality in children under 5 years of age. With increasing age, mortality resulting from road traffic crashes surpasses that from drowning, with traffic deaths being the greatest overall killer of children aged 15–19.

Men often suffer injuries in the course of paid labour or occupational pursuits, while women suffer burns as a result of their customary domestic role—in the kitchen, from fires or scalding water, and as a result of cooking on open fires. The home use of kerosene or paraffin lamps, which are easily knocked over and ignited, is also a large contributor. Above all, underlying gross poverty heavily influences many of these injuries, irrespective of age and gender.

Table 3.4.1 Domestic strategies to address NCD risk factors

Domain	Goal	Intervention	Example
Healthy lifestyles	Optimal nutrition	Agricultural production	Incentives to produce healthier foods
		Food manufacturing, processing, and distribution	Regulation of food industry and retailers
		Disincentives for buying and selling unhealthy food	'Fat tax'
		Marketing unhealthy foods	Restricting advertisements targeting children
		Nutritional information disclosure and education	Providing government nutritional guidelines; improving package labelling; menu labelling
		Direct regulation	Banning unhealthy ingredients (such as trans fats)
		Public–private partnership	Voluntary targets for nutritional values
	Physical activity	Incentives for exercise	Subsidies for physical exercise and organized activities
		Flexible spending accounts	Corporate allowances for fitness activities
		Monitor community physical activity	Public health surveillance of monitoring prevalence of NCDs
Healthy places	Places to buy and eat food	Access to affordable, healthy foods	Farmers' markets; zoning of unhealthy fast foods
		Healthy foods in schools, workplaces, etc.	Vending machines, snacks, meals
		School/childcare curricula and programmes	Body mass index (BMI) surveillance; nutrition education
	Places to walk, recreate, and play	Workplace/education settings and programmes	Organized activities; fitness memberships
		Urban land use and planning	Attractive, accessible, safe public places and paths
		Tax incentives for building design	Businesses incorporating building designs that promote physical activity
		Transportation	Mass transit and safe routes
		Health impact assessments	Consultation with affected communities; public health evaluations
Healthy societies	Social justice	Antidiscrimination laws	Proscribe medical condition-related discrimination
	Access to services	Services to support life functions of ill individuals	At-home support services
		Encourage prevention and treatment	Metabolic screening; counselling
		Monitoring disease in the community	Surveillance through BMI reporting

National public health laws are perhaps the single most potent interventions to prevent injuries. Developed countries have used a multitude of regulations to vastly curtail traffic injuries and deaths—e.g. driving licences, speed limits, vehicle safety, motorcycle helmets, and road design. Yet, in many low- and middle-income countries, the roads are chaotic and very dangerous, with vehicles unfit for travel and roads poorly planned. The mix of pedestrians, bicycles, and motorized vehicles on unsafe roads that do not separate the types of traffic is lethal. To further compound the problem, roadways are usually designed with the convenience of the drivers in mind and little thought for the safety of pedestrians. In Nairobi, residents of Kibera, one of the largest urban slums in the world, suffer inordinate road traffic injuries and deaths, as they have to run across dangerous roads to get to work, school, or shops to buy food and clothing.

Work-related injuries are ubiquitous in low-resourced countries. The rise in industrial development and the lack of attention to safety will ensure that occupational injuries double by 2025. Again, this situation is very different in the developed world, which has steadily decreased occupational injury rates over the years. Most industrial work in low-resourced countries such as

agriculture, manufacturing, and mining is already associated with high rates of injury from electrical, mechanical, and physical hazards. Now, the steady expansion of chemical and biotechnology industries has introduced new injury risks.

Yet, occupational health and safety laws cover only 10 per cent of the population in low-resourced countries. Without adequate regulations, businesses do not invest in quality equipment or train workers to ensure safety. Companies often expect workers to take inordinate risks because labour is cheap and plentiful. If developing countries do not soon implement effective safety standards, the health costs to workers in high-risk jobs will outweigh the financial benefits of industrial development.

Intentional injuries are also a vast and growing problem, particularly in low- and middle-income countries. Rates of robberies, assaults, rapes, and homicides can be devastating in major cities such as Johannesburg. India has experienced an epidemic of gender-related violence, which also occurs in many other parts of the world. In some African countries, gay men are subjected to brutal assaults and murders. Yet, it is possible to prevent most injuries through technological innovation, safety regulation, and law enforcement. However, the same ingenuity and resources that make the home, workplace, and the streets safer in richer countries have not been applied in low-resourced countries. The WHO devotes <1 per cent of its budget to injuries and violence.

Developed countries, of course, are not immune from violence, which could be dramatically lowered with sound firearm regulation and enforcement. In the United States, for example, firearm-related deaths are roughly equal to road traffic deaths, with few checks on gun buyers or the lethality of weapons and bullets.

If the public health community wishes to close the 'injury gap' between rich and poor, it will have to devise evidence-based solutions, demonstrate their effectiveness, engage the private sector, gain the cooperation of police and the courts, devote the resources, and advocate for strong occupational health and safety laws throughout the developed world.

Conclusion: the future of public health law reform

This chapter has sought to demonstrate the powerful potential of law to prevent injuries and disease. Law can build the infrastructure of public health agencies, ensuring a broad mission and adequate powers. It can protect individuals from excessive or unjustified coercion or discrimination. It can promote social justice by narrowing health disparities. At the same time, government has multiple legal tools available to improve the public's health and safety, ranging from its economic power to tax and spend, to its authority to alter the environments in which people live (e.g. informational, built, and socioeconomic), through to direct and indirect regulation, including, where necessary, deregulation.

With the potential for rapid dissemination of pathogens, products, services, and marketing throughout the world, the need for global governance cannot be overstated. No country acting alone can stem the tide of injuries and disease. Global health leadership could establish health-promoting norms, set benchmarks, monitor progress, and encourage compliance by state and non-state actors. Global leadership, moreover, must act beyond the health sector, engaging legal regimes such as trade, intellectual property, food, migration, and the environment.

When law is used in a systematic and coordinated way at the local, national, and international levels, it can go a long way towards preventing infectious diseases, NCDs, and injuries (both unintentional and violence-related). For public health practitioners, the lesson is to effectively use the battery of legal tools at their disposal. And when those tools are inadequate, public health agencies must work with civil society and communities to raise the level of political awareness. In a complex and globalized world, public health is a deeply legal and political pursuit—well beyond purely science and technology.

References

Basu, S., Yoffe, P., Hills, N., and Lustig, R.H. (2013). The relationship of sugar to population-level diabetes prevalence: an econometric analysis of repeated cross-sectional data. *PLoS One*, 8(2), e57873.

Beauchamp, D.E. (1999). Public health as social justice. In D.E. Beauchamp and B. Steinbock (eds.) *New Ethics for the Public's Health*, pp. 105–14. New York: Oxford University Press.

British American Tobacco Australia Limited v. The Commonwealth (2012). HCA 43.

Cabrera, O.A. and Gostin, L.O. (2011). Human rights and the Framework Convention on Tobacco Control: mutually reinforcing systems. *International Journal of Law in Context*, 7(3), 285–303.

Centers for Disease Control and Prevention (2000). *Ten Great Public Health Achievements in the 20th Century*. [Online] Available at: http://www.cdc.gov/about/history/tengpha.htm.

Daniels, N., Kennedy, B., and Kawachi, I. (2000). Justice is good for our health. *Boston Review*, 25, 6–15.

Fidler, D.P. (2004). *SARS, Governance and the Globalization of Disease*. Houndmills: Palgrave Macmillan.

FTR Holding v. Oriental Republic of Uruguay (2010). ICSID, Request for Arbitration, 3–5, 77.

Friedman, E.A. and Gostin, L.O. (2012). Pillars for progress on the right to health: harnessing the potential of human rights through a framework convention on global health. *Health and Human Rights: An International Journal*, 14(1), 1–16. Available at: http://ssrn.com/abstract=2086456.

Gostin, L.O. (2008). *Public Health Law: Power, Duty, Restraint* (2nd ed.). Berkeley, CA: University of California Press.

Gostin, L.O. (2014). *Global Health Law: International Law, Global Institutions, and World Health*. Cambridge, MA: Harvard University Press.

Gostin, L.O. and Gostin, G.G. (2009). A broader liberty: JS Mill, paternalism, and the public's health. *Public Health*, 123, 214–22. Available at: http://dx.doi.org/10.1016/j.puhe.2008.12.024.

Gostin, L.O. and Powers, M. (2006). What does justice require for the public's health? Public health ethics and policy imperatives of social justice. *Health Affairs*, 25, 1053–60.

Grad, F.P. (2004). *The Public Health Law Manual* (3rd ed.). Washington, DC: American Public Health Association.

Hawkes, C. (2007). Regulating food marketing to young people worldwide: trends and policy drivers. *American Journal of Public Health*, 97, 1962–73.

Hodge, Jr. J.G., Gostin, L.O., Gebbie, K., and Erickson, D.L. (2006). Transforming public health law: the Turning Point Model State Public Health Act. *Journal of Law, Medicine and Ethics*, 33(4).

Institute of Medicine (2011). *For the Public's Health: Revitalizing Law and Policy to Meet New Challenges*. Washington, DC: National Academy Press.

Lozano, R., Naghavi, M., Foreman, K., et al. (2012). Global and regional mortality from 235 causes of death for 20 age groups in 1990 and 2010: a systematic analysis for the Global Burden of Disease Study 2010. *Lancet*, 380, 2095–128.

Markel, H. (2005). *When Germs Travel: Six Major Epidemics that Have Invaded America and the Fears They Have Unleashed*. New York: Vintage.

Marmot, M. (2005). Social determinants of health inequalities. *Lancet*, 365, 1099–104.

Mitchell, A.D. and Studdert, D.M. (2012). Plain packaging of tobacco products in Australia: a novel regulation faces legal challenge. *JAMA*, 307, 261–2.

Murray, C., Vos, T., Lozano, R., et al. (2012). Disability-adjusted life years (DALYs) for 291 diseases and injuries in 21 regions, 1990–2010: a systematic analysis for the Global Burden of Disease Study 2010. *Lancet*, 380, 2197–223.

Norton, R., Hyder, A.A., Bishai, D., and Peden, M. (2006) Unintentional injuries. In D.T. Jamison, J.G. Breman, A.R. Measham, et al. (eds.) *Disease Control Priorities in Developing Countries*, pp. 737–54. New York: Oxford University Press.

Powers, M. and Faden, R. (2006). *Social Justice: The Moral Foundations of Public Health and Health Policy*. New York: Oxford University Press.

Perdue, W.C., Stone, L.A., and Gostin, L.O. (2003). The built environment and its relationship to the public's health: the legal framework. *American Journal of Public Health*, 93, 1390–4.

Rawls, J. (1971). *A Theory of Justice*. Cambridge, MA: Harvard University Press.

R.J. Reynolds Tobacco Company v. Food and Drug Administration (2012). US Court of Appeals for the District of Columbia. Available at: http://www.cadc.uscourts.gov/internet/opinions.nsf/4C0311C78EB11C5785 257A64004EBFB5/$file/11-5332-1391191.pdf.

Salomon, J.A., Wang, H., Feeman, M.K., et al. (2012). Healthy life expectancy for 187 countries, 1990—2010: a systematic analysis for the Global Burden Disease Study 2010. *Lancet*, 380, 2144–62.

United Nations (1989). *Convention on the Rights of the Child*. UN GA resolution 44/25, UN Doc. A/RES/44/25, 20 November 1989. New York: United Nations.

United Nations (2011). *Political Declaration of the High-Level Meeting of the General Assembly on the Prevention and Control of Non-Communicable Diseases*. New York: United Nations.

Walzer, M. (1983). *Spheres of Justice: A Defense of Pluralism and Equality*. New York: Basic Books.

World Health Organization (2005a). *Framework Convention on Tobacco Control*. Geneva: World Health Organization. Available at: http://www.who.int.

World Health Organization (2005b). *International Health Regulations*. Geneva: World Health Organization.

World Health Organization (2008a). *2008–2013 Action Plan for the Global Strategy for the Prevention and Control of Noncommunicable Diseases*. Geneva: World Health Organization.

World Health Organization (2008b). *Commission on Social Determinants of Health. Closing the Gap in a Generation: Health Equity Through Action on the Social Determinants of Health*. Geneva: World Health Organization.

World Health Organization (2010). *Set of Recommendations on the Marketing of Foods and Non-Alcoholic Beverages to Children*. Geneva: World Health Organization.

World Health Organization (2011). *Global Status Report on Noncommunicable Diseases 2010*. Geneva: World Health Organization.

3.5

Priority setting, social values, and public health

Peter Littlejohns, Sarah Clark, and Albert Weale

Introduction to priority setting, social values, and public health

Around the world, policymakers are facing the dilemma of how to allocate resources to healthcare in ways that are both effective and that can be justified to their citizens in terms of fairness and appropriateness. In the United Kingdom, the National Institute for Clinical Excellence (NICE, currently the National Institute for Health and Care Excellence) was created in 1999 in order to provide recommendations for medical care based on appraisals of cost-effectiveness evidence. NICE recommendations include explicit advice on which medical interventions should, and which should not, be offered to patients in a predominantly public healthcare system. Similar bodies now exist in France, Germany, Thailand, and South Korea. In Latin America, constitutional courts have been used by plaintiffs denied access to care as a means to enforce a right to health included in the constitutions of Columbia and Brazil. Even in the United States, which has long been a country hostile to explicit priority setting, the Affordable Care Act, passed by the Obama administration in 2011, established the Patient-Centered Outcomes Research Institute to provide evidence about the effectiveness of medical interventions in the context of the long-standing and persistent concerns about lack of cost-control in US health spending. The proposed institutional solutions vary from country to country; but the underlying problem of how best to allocate healthcare resources to good effect and in ways that can be publicly justified is common and pervasive.

Cost pressures on healthcare resources arise from a number of causes that are well understood in general terms, although the relative contribution of each is subject to dispute. People are living longer, not only increasing population size but also creating populations that are older. Citizens have rising expectations of health services and the quality of life that those services should deliver. Innovation in healthcare technology means that some very expensive pharmaceutical interventions, like NovoSeven®, a second-order treatment for haemophilia, are made available for relatively small groups of patients whose treatment may be very costly on a 'per case' basis. Alternatively, some pharmaceuticals, like statins, turn out to be relevant to a wider group of patients, contributing a large total increase in spending. As a result of these pressures, rising expenditure means that healthcare needs are in competition with one another and healthcare itself is in competition with other potential uses of the same resources. In 1980 a typical west European state would spend 6–8 per cent of its national income on healthcare; in 2009 the equivalent figure was between 10 and 12 per cent of national income. In the same period, expenditure in the United States rose from approximately 9 per cent of national income to over 16 per cent. In virtually all developed societies, workers take half a day a week of their working life just to pay for healthcare, and in the United States it is closer to a day a week.

Public health has traditionally been concerned with such matters as the protection of populations from widespread communicable diseases or the promotion of healthy living as a means of prevention. It is sometimes contrasted with medical care, understood as the provision of diagnostic and therapeutic treatments to individuals in need. Public health is targeted at populations; medical care is targeted at individuals. This difference matches the distinction that economists make between public goods and private goods. Pure public goods, like clean air or water, are non-competitive, because they are available to everybody who falls within their scope. No one can be excluded from the benefit they supply, and their provision raises general social well-being. By contrast, private goods, like hip operations or cataract surgery, necessarily involve a competitive element. Resources made available for some individuals mean that there are fewer resources for other individuals. Priority setting in health policy is a problem of allocating healthcare resources, thought of as private goods, in a fair and efficient way. The typical issues that fall under the heading of priority setting include such questions as to whether to pay for highly expensive pharmaceutical products that provide only a few extra weeks or months of low-quality life, or whether to prioritize a small number of people in great need compared to a larger number of people in modest need.

The contrast between public goods, which have traditionally been the focus of public health, and medical interventions, which should be thought of as private goods, might suggest that problems of priority setting for medical care are not relevant for the study of public health. Because medical care inevitably involves allocating resources among patients according to an order of priority, much of the work of policymaking concerns the process of priority setting. By contrast, implementation of public health measures makes it possible to secure a gain for all, since members of a population are not in competition with one another for the same resource, and individual interventions may benefit others through externalities or 'spill-over' effects. A vaccination pro-gramme will benefit all members of a population by reducing the risk of contagion. Clean water supplies will benefit all those who have access to them. Better road design will reduce the risk of acci-dents for all, just as good building standards will protect against the effects of disasters.

However, although there is a contrast between the competitive character of resource allocation in medicine on the one hand and the non-competitive measures aimed at improving public health on the other, the principles and practices of priority setting are nonetheless relevant to public health for a number of reasons. Firstly, public health measures involve spending resources, and so raise exactly the same questions about their priority as does provision for sickness. For example, vaccination programmes cost money as do public health education campaigns on such matters as smoking, obesity, and sexual health. Medicines stocked for pre-ventive health reasons are a call on the budget in the same way that therapeutic medicines are a call on the budget. A concern for priorities inevitably raises the question of whether the money spent on these programmes provides better value than the alter-native uses to which it could be put.

There is often perceived to be a potentially large gain for health budgets if effective public health measures can be undertaken. Effective control of tobacco, or reductions in the number of peo-ple who are obese, would save the medical services money, it is sometimes asserted, because it would reduce the number of peo-ple who would have to be treated. The evaluation of this claim is not straightforward, because if effective public health measures prolong life, their consequence may simply be to postpone costs onto the treatment and care of the degenerative diseases of old age. However, this point offers a good illustration of the way in which traditional public health concerns and priority setting concerns interact.

Since no country can afford to provide all its residents with every possible medical or public health intervention, all health systems face the problem of how to set priorities in the allocation of resources. These decisions cannot be made simply by appealing to technical tests of 'what works' because measuring what works inevitably involves a set of value judgements. Even something as seemingly technical as a satisfactory clinical outcome presup-poses that quality of life is satisfactory and such a judgement is not purely technical. Moreover, priority setting decisions can be politically controversial. When NICE decided in 1999 not to rec-ommend Relenza® within the National Health Service, its manu-facturers, then Glaxo Wellcome, even spoke about relocating its production facilities outside of the United Kingdom in retaliation. Priority setting in healthcare inevitably means looks at the social values that are part of the civic and political cultures of different societies.

'Social values' is a term with no agreed precise definition. In this chapter we use it to designate the reasons that are used in policy deliberation that involve reference to those features of the content and processes of decision-making to which the members of a society attach importance. Such features may concern the decision-making process itself, for example, its transparency, or the content of the decision that is made, for example, whether it meets the entitlements to care that people are thought to have. In relation to these values, we can ask both how such considerations are taken into account in priority-setting processes and whether there are some values that ought to be given greater weight in decision-making.

How are values in play?

Setting priorities is undertaken at many different levels of decision-making, ranging from the highest level of policy, where governments allocate overall national budgets or decide on reim-bursement schemes for intervention, through the local level, as administrations balance delivering public health and clinical ser-vices to their communities, to the individual bed-side level where practitioners make decisions affecting individuals. Priority set-ting in healthcare is also not unique to governments. It is always apparent in commercial insurers' decisions about the limits of coverage. It is also implicit in the priorities that non-governmental organizations and philanthropic foundations give to some inter-ventions over others. In every case, we can ask what are the social values implicated in the decisions that are made.

The most important development in recent years is that a num-ber of countries have developed specific institutions or agencies to advise on cost-effectiveness and priority setting and to provide the evidence upon which they aim to assess value for money in healthcare. These agencies include: the National Evidence-Based Healthcare Collaborating Agency (NECA) in Korea; the Health Improvement and Technology Assessment Programme (HITAP) in Thailand; the new Instituto de Evaluación Tecnológica en Salud (IETS) in Columbia, established in September 2012; the National Institute for Health and Care Excellence (NICE) in the United Kingdom; the recently established Patient-Centered Outcomes Research Institute in the United States; the Haute Autorité de Santé (HAS) in France; and the Institut für Qualität und Wirtschaftlichkeit im Gesundheitswesen (IQWiG) in Germany (Littlejohns et al. 2012a).

All agencies such as these face the problem of how to integrate social values into their decision-making on health priority setting. For example, in Thailand HITAP has confronted difficult ques-tions about what should be included in its basic package of care. In particular, in a case of diapers for adult incontinence, a decision was required that paid attention to income distribution considera-tions, since the cost of diapers was absorbing a high proportion of the budget for poor households (see case study in Table 3.5.1).

Along with other systems, the Korean National Health Insurance system is facing the challenges of increased expendi-ture associated with an ageing population. In one example, the Korean health technology assessment (HTA) agency, NECA, had to deal with the case of glucosamine for osteoarthritis in the elderly, which raised questions about how to assess the value of a product for which there was little evidence of effectiveness, but which occupied a special position in the gift culture of the society. Ahn et al. have described the way in which pharmaceuticals, med-ical devices, diagnostics, and procedures are assessed in South Korea and shown how issues of accountability are of concern to stakeholders (Ahn et al. 2012).

HTA agencies in Europe are similarly challenged by how to take into account social values in their policymaking. Even for a well-established agency such as NICE in the United Kingdom, which has sophisticated decision protocols and a formalized approach to cost-effectiveness, unforeseen social values conse-quences of 'technical' decisions can challenge those decisions

Table 3.5.1 Social values and health priority setting case study

Title of case study	Absorbent Products for Adult Disabled and Elderly Incontinence in Thailand
Author	Dr Sarah Clark, School of Public Policy, UCL
	Dr Utsana Tomayakul, Health Intervention and Technology Assessment Programme (HITAP), Thailand
Author contact	s.l.clark@ucl.ac.uk
Date of Submission	11 July 2012
Case summary (approx. 350 words) Please include information here about why the case is of particular interest	This case concerns 'adult diapers' on which many elderly and disabled people in Thailand rely to enable them to cope with the problem of incontinence. Currently these products must be purchased by individuals or by households at some cost (an estimated $1200 per year). The imposition of such costs on groups who are already vulnerable and socially disadvantaged raises issues of equity and solidarity. Despite being proven to be well below the Thai cost-effectiveness threshold and decision-makers recognizing the important solidarity values implied in the case, the products were not ultimately included in the Universal Coverage package on the grounds of the large numbers of those eligible for coverage, leading to a budget impact which was considered unacceptably high.
Facts of the case Please include information on as many of the following as are relevant to the case: • At what condition is the intervention, programme, or service aimed? • What are its effects? E.g. Is it curative, preventative, palliative, life-prolonging, rehabilitative? • Is there a relevant comparator? If so how does this intervention, service or program compare to the alternative? Include ICER estimates/QALY costs if relevant. • What are the significant features about the condition and/or about the patient population in this case? E.g. patient population is very young, very old, condition is rare, life-threatening, life-limiting, etc. • How are the benefits of the intervention distributed across the patient population and/or across time? • What is the cost or budget impact of the intervention/service/programme?	The use of absorbent products—'diapers'—is necessary on a daily basis for those with incontinence, often occurring as a result of age or disability. Without these products, the quality of life of people with incontinence is impaired, and normal life hindered in a significant way. Catheterization is an alternative approach to incontinence but carries the risk of complications. Currently in Thailand, absorbent products are purchased privately. However given the daily, ongoing use of these products, their cost can be considerable for the elderly or disabled and for the families who support them. It has been estimated by a HITAP (Health Intervention and Assessment Program) assessment that on average families spend around $1200 (37,000 Thai Baht) per year on these products and that around 360,000 people need to use them (Tantivess et al. 2012). To put these costs in perspective and to give an indication of affordability, in Thailand the average teacher annual net income is 192,000 THB, that of a dentist/GP is 375,000 THB, and that of a bus driver is 96,000 THB. The cost of these absorbent products, at least for lower-income families, is therefore likely to form a significant portion of household expenditure. A HITAP assessment estimated that provision of adult diapers to disabled people with incontinence produced a positive and statistically significant 32 per cent improvement in quality of life scores of over 10 weeks. The cost-effectiveness of including provision of adult diapers for the disabled within the Universal Coverage package was estimated at $1200 per QALY or 37,000 Thai Baht.

and provide cause for revising and modifying policy. For example, NICE has modified its technical guidance in respect of the threshold ICER to deal with considerations around treatments for patients at the end of their life and for children.

Similarly, the Haute Autorité de Santé in France, an established HTA agency, had to determine the value of a growth hormone, both in terms of how to assesses 'normal' height and how to balance risks against benefits, leaving them with a decision involving issues of social values as profound as how to define 'normal'. In Germany, IQWiG has to make its decisions against the background of the German Constitutional Court decision in the 2005 *Nikolaus* case, according to which the individual judgement of a treating physician concerning the effectiveness of a treatment has to be respected and the health insurance system cannot deny reimbursement, thus demonstrating a deep commitment to the principle of clinical need which may on occasion conflict radically with considerations of cost-effectiveness (Bundesverfassungsgerichts 6, 2005).

In other parts of the world, the challenges of social values are worked out in very different ways. Recent developments in Latin America have seen the growth of a rights-based approach to health and, in particular, an increase in the use of the courts to press for accountability in cases where individuals believe they have been denied equitable access to healthcare and their 'right' to health thereby violated. Cases brought to court on the basis of the right to health in countries such as Columbia and Brazil, have become known as 'tutelas' and have arisen as a consequence of a legal procedure known as a writ of protection, in the context of the constitutional changes that followed democratization in such countries (Cubillos et al. 2012). However, while court decisions in 'tutelas' may provide accountability in individual cases, this does not mean that the cumulative effect of such decisions is necessarily to move towards a more equitable system of care for the population as a whole. How social values are played out when national bodies decide on individual cases can thus be very different and not indicative of how they are played out at the level of policymaking as it affects the wider population.

These brief examples show that there are many common challenges faced by different decision-making systems but the ways in which social values are brought into play, and the ways in which their challenges are dealt with, varies considerably. One example of this is the contrasting decision processes of the United Kingdom and Germany in respect of high-cost health interventions: in the United Kingdom, NICE explicitly uses quality-adjusted life years (QALYs) in determining priorities, whereas German HTA regards their use as incompatible with Germany's Basic Law. Social values thus help define the policy paradigm of different countries. A policy paradigm is defined by the basic concepts that are used in policy deliberation and such paradigms are embodied in institutional processes of decision in different countries (see Weale 2010 for a recent summary). Policy paradigms shape the way in which problems are understood, and the definition of what counts as success for a policy.

Despite the need for prioritization, formal approaches to addressing the challenge have so far not been as successful as hoped. There are a number of reasons:

1. More emphasis has been placed on the technical assessment of efficiency as manifested by the increasing number of national HTA programmes and less attention directed to issues of equity.

2. Compared to the amount of effort put into creating the evidence base for making prioritization decisions, little effort has been targeted at understanding the relationship between the outputs of HTA organizations and the political process of translating this evidence into national policy and then implementing that policy. Priority setting should aim to produce an allocation of healthcare resources that can be ethically justified, especially to those who lose out as a result of resource allocation decisions. Such an ethical justification requires articulation of social value judgements, both in terms of the process of decision-making, on which allocation decisions rest, and in terms of the content of those decisions. Such a justification is a vital element in any public legitimation of how priorities are set. Yet there are legitimate disagreements about which social value should dominate as they can be contradictory. To date, most attempts of adding dimensions other than efficiency have relied on creating lists of values with little emphasis on how these could actively inform real decisions (Culyer and Bombard 2012; Johri and Norheim 2012).

3. Prioritization means that de-prioritization has also to occur which results in exclusions of cover for some programmes. The dynamics of removing well-established health interventions are very different from those of introducing new ones and have received little attention although this is beginning to be rectified (Elshaug et al. 2007; Garner et al. 2013). The process of limiting access to interventions (either stopping old or restricting new) makes the process a political one with all that that implies.

4. There is a tendency to separate out components of healthcare; for example, emerging technologies are assessed separately from chronic disease management which is separate from primary and community care and all are separate from public health initiatives. This separation not only occurs in the context of planning and delivering services but also most importantly in budgetary management making prioritization complex with the result that often no one has overall responsibility for a coherent approach to priority setting.

So, although many of the challenges are common, healthcare systems in various national settings will make different decisions about priorities, differences based on the distinctive balance of social values in each country, as well as their particular methods for capturing and incorporating values in decision-making. These differences will also reflect the level of economic development of each country, its institutional arrangements for deciding on healthcare priorities, the balance of power between competing social groups within the decision-making system, and the distinctive civic culture that prevails. It is this combination of common challenges, encompassing both management challenges and ethical challenges, and distinct institutional and cultural differences, that makes the cross-national comparative study of social values and health priority setting so important to understand. Before systems can learn lessons or even exchange experiences with one another, they first need to locate the social value challenges in their specific circumstances.

A new approach: 'values-based' prioritization

We have suggested so far that all healthcare systems face common problems of priority setting, and that more attention needs to be paid to the way in which the social values of different societies condition the way in which those priority-setting decisions are made. If we are to go beyond this generalization, we need to identify more systematically what the key social values are that are relevant to priority setting. Identifying such values is potentially a large data-gathering task. However, as a way of seeking to answer this question, we convened, in February 2011, participants from seven countries in London, United Kingdom, with a follow-up meeting in Rio de Janeiro, Brazil, in June 2011 to discuss the issues. The starting point for the discussion was the creation of a draft template (see Table 3.5.2) for assessing the role of social values in healthcare priority setting in each country, the object of the template being to detail the logical pattern of such values (Clark and Weale 2012).

What emerged from the workshops was a view that procedural values like transparency, accountability, and participation play an important role in policy deliberation in different contexts alongside substantive values like clinical effectiveness, cost-effectiveness, justice (also sometimes called equity), solidarity, and autonomy.

There are potentially a large number of content values, but five seem to dominate the current approaches to priority setting—clinical effectiveness, cost-effectiveness, justice/equity, solidarity, and autonomy. That list draws upon a reading of statements of social values from NICE (Rawlins and Culyer 2004; NICE 2008) and from the wider bioethics literature (Cookson and Dolan 2000; Hoedemaekers and Dekkers 2003; Oliver 2003; Powers and Faden 2008; Chalkidou et al. 2009; Persad et al. 2009).

The process values selected—transparency, accountability, and participation—are those commonly associated with processes of public reasoning and legitimacy in democratic decision-making (for example, see Gutmann and Thompson 2004). They also draw on the values inherent in what has become the leading framework for procedural justice—Daniels' accountability for reasonableness model (Daniels 2000)—and on the values adhered to by NICE in its decision-making processes (NICE 2012).

Table 3.5.2 Description of content and process social values

Content values	Meaning, purpose, and values-based questions
Clinical effectiveness	• *Meaning*: the ability of a procedure to accomplish a given clinical purpose. Commonly considered to imply that a given treatment is better than existing alternatives because it provides greater health benefits. • *Purpose*: to secure patient safety and to ensure that resources are not wasted on ineffective or harmful interventions. • *Values-based questions*: how *much* benefit has to be achieved for an intervention to be classed as clinically effective? This can be a matter of value judgement, rather than scientific evidence.
Cost-effectiveness	• *Meaning*: an intervention is cost-effective if the difference in costs between it and alternative interventions can be justified in terms of the health benefits it produces. • *Purpose*: to secure value for money in terms of ensuring that the *most* health benefits are obtained from available resources—does this by assessing opportunity costs. • *Values-based questions*: QALYs might be impartial, but can health states and health benefits produced by different treatments be valued objectively in this way? Does cost-effectiveness focus too much on capacity to *benefit* from interventions rather than on the *need* which exists for them?
Justice/equity	• *Meaning*: there are many conceptions of justice, but one meaning common to all is that like cases should be treated as like and unlike cases as unlike. In the case of healthcare, likeness will be that of patients' conditions. • *Purpose*: seeks to ensure an equitable distribution of resources wherein only those factors which are morally relevant to healthcare are taken into account, and that morally *ir*relevant considerations are excluded. • *Values-based questions*: determining what counts as a 'morally relevant factor' is highly arguable—to what extent are, for example, age, personal responsibility, economic, or health inequality morally relevant or morally irrelevant factors when determining priorities in the allocation of healthcare resources?
Solidarity	• *Meaning*: all members of society will stand together and will support those who are worst off either in health or in financial terms, depending on the particular form of solidarity espoused. • *Purpose*: to ensure that no member of society is denied healthcare because of financial barriers to access, and to improve the lot of the worst off (either the sickest or the poorest) in society. • *Values-based questions*: given the pressures of demography and high-cost pharmaceuticals on available resources, how far do the limits of solidarity stretch?
Autonomy	• *Meaning*: many conceptions, but one meaning common to all is the ability of individuals to be self-directing and to make decisions for themselves about important matters, including healthcare. • *Purpose*: to secure certain freedoms for the individual to choose the form of healthcare they might prefer and, in some conceptions, to confer responsibility upon the individual for those choices. • *Values-based questions*: to what extent is it desirable—or possible—to foster individual autonomy in circumstances of limited budgets, where doing so can have negative consequences for justice and for collective healthcare choices?
Process values	
Transparency	• *Meaning*: making both the content and the process of decision-making visible and comprehensible to all relevant parties. • *Purpose*: making decision arrangements as transparent as possible allows stakeholders—from patients to politicians to clinicians—to evaluate how decisions have been arrived at and thereby increases the chances of decisions being viewed as legitimate, especially by those who lose out. • *Values-based questions*: what does genuine transparency require, given that the mere transfer of information will not necessarily enable stakeholders to comprehend or evaluate decisions?
Accountability	• *Meaning*: one party justifies and takes responsibility for its activities to another party. Being accountable in priority setting means having the obligation to answer questions regarding decisions about which interventions are prioritized and why. • *Purpose*: at one level, to ensure that those who are responsible for decisions are able to provide justifiable reasons for priority setting to those affected—especially to those who lose out—and to taxpayers or insurance payers for how their money is spent. • *Values-based questions*: how to secure meaningful accountability? How much accountability might be too much?
Participation	• *Meaning/purpose*: to allow different interests to contribute and have their voices and experiences heard—thereby contributing to the quality, legitimacy and democratic validity of decisions. • *Values-based questions*: how best can we capture what is morally and politically important about engaging the public and other stakeholders in priority setting decisions? Who should be involved? And by what methods is genuine, democratic participation best secured?

The content of decision-making

Clinical effectiveness

The clinical effectiveness of a health intervention refers simply to the quality of the benefits it provides for patients. As such, clinical effectiveness is a fundamental value in priority-setting decisions, given that it is clearly undesirable to waste limited resources on procedures that provide low levels, or indeed no benefits to patients or, worse still, that may actually do harm. The positive aim of the principle, then, is to ensure that health benefits are achieved. One way of measuring effectiveness is in terms of the advantage an intervention has over the relevant alternatives, so the benefit or effect of a treatment is the difference it makes to the health state of patients over and above the benefits provided by alternative treatments.

There are some practical issues concerning the principle of clinical effectiveness. There may be different attitudes towards testing of established interventions and innovative ones, with the latter often being subject to much more rigorous standards of effectiveness than the former. Problems can also arise around lack of evidence of effectiveness of new treatments: while it seems entirely proper that clinical effectiveness should be assessed according to the highest scientific standards, this may mean waiting for long periods of time before the effectiveness of a treatment is fully proven. Therefore, questions about how much benefit is required for a treatment to be classed as 'clinically effective' often turn on value—rather than purely technical—judgements. Where there is unmet need and no other clinical developments have been available to a particular patient group over recent years, a lower level of benefit might be thought acceptable on grounds that such patients should be offered 'something', even if the clinical effectiveness of that 'something' is lower than might ideally be sought. The simple fact that 'something is being done', even if it only provides a small or uncertain benefit, may be very important (Clark and Weale 2012).

Cost-effectiveness

The aim of cost-effectiveness analysis is to ensure that the *most* health benefits are obtained from limited resources. Cost-effectiveness seeks to establish whether differences in costs between alternative interventions can be justified in terms of the health benefits they respectively produce. As such, opportunity costs are the central concern: comparison between health gained and health forgone is at the heart of the rationale for cost-effectiveness analysis, such that the benefits provided by a treatment for one set of patients must be more than the benefits forgone by not providing a treatment to another set of patients. Further, by using estimates of health benefits and economic costs that are equivalent across treatments, cost-effectiveness evaluation can, in principle, compare the relative worth of healthcare interventions even if those interventions are quite different. QALYs provide a means of doing this (➲ see Chapter 6.6).

Supporters of QALYs point to impartiality as a strength of the approach since a year of life has the same value regardless of whose year of life it is—someone old or young, rich or poor, etc. However, questions arise around the subjectivity of how people value health states. The valuation of health states which inform QALYs can be thought to be problematic because there is no reason to expect that different people, different groups of people, or even the same people at different points in their lives, will value health states in

the same way. Also, it is important to consider *whose* quality of life is judged—just the person with the illness, or that of her family too, given that ill health can have a detrimental effect on the well-being of carers and other family members. Another issue of value judgement in relation to QALYs is their reliance on the conception of need as capacity to benefit. This conception values the *outcomes* of health interventions, rather than the 'inputs' to which they respond, and logically entails that the more one can benefit from a treatment, the more one needs it.

As the earlier contrast between the United Kingdom and Germany illustrated, the use of QALYs can be controversial. Some object to the use of QALYs because using them seems to imply that the sole purpose of a healthcare system is to maximize benefit, that is to secure the largest gain in health improvement aggregated over a given population. Taken in this way, the use of QALYs would not accord with important social values. As the example of priority setting in Oregon showed, a simple maximizing approach would mean that a small benefit for a large number of people would outweigh a significant benefit for a small number of people: tooth-capping could be given higher priority than appendectomies. However, using QALYs is not logically tied to a maximizing approach. A QALY is simply a measure of benefit, akin to the disability-adjusted life year (DALY). How those benefits are given priority for any one population depends upon the social values that are relevant to that population.

A second concern in connection with the value of cost-effectiveness is that it is incompatible with asserting a universal right to health (see Chapter 3.3). The idea of the right to health has been an important element in the 'health for all' movement and the idea also plays an important role in arguments for universal coverage. To say that cost-effectiveness is important seems to suggest that the right to health should be curtailed when there are insufficient resources—or worse still when governments decide that there are insufficient resources, even though wasteful expenditures may be taking place elsewhere in the public or private sectors. However, this conflict between cost-effectiveness and the right to health is more apparent than real. The right to health has always been recognized as the right to the 'highest attainable' level of health, and in this respect resource and cost concerns have always been accepted through the idea of the 'progressive realization' of the right to health. Moreover, the principle of cost-effectiveness applies even when universal access to good healthcare has been secured. Indeed, it can be argued that cost-effectiveness is highly important within systems that secure universal coverage, since avoiding the distorting effects of low value interventions enables more to be done for everyone.

Justice

The value of justice or fairness is fundamental to priority-setting decisions and, in terms of its inclusion in the list, perhaps the least controversial. It is, however, one of the most contested values not only in priority setting but in bioethics and indeed political philosophy more widely, with multiple models available (see Hoedemaekers and Dekkers (2003) for a summary of dominant conceptions of justice and their application to healthcare). One notion is common across very many of these models however: this is the principle that like cases should be treated as like and unlike as unlike. In decisions about healthcare, the most obvious condition of likeness of patients is likeness of their illness: so it is equitable for two people who have cancer to be treated similarly—the relevant characteristic here is having cancer. Irrelevant characteristics to take into account in this situation might be the gender or ethnicity or sexual orientation of the patients: to base priority-setting decisions on these considerations would be unjust because they make distinctions between persons which are irrelevant to their health condition. However, it is not always easy to distinguish which characteristics of persons are relevant and which are irrelevant: some have argued that the 'merit' of individuals based on judgements about their contribution to society can be taken into account (Mooney 1987; McIntyre and Gilson 2000); others argue that it is fair to provide greater benefits to the young or middle aged rather than to the elderly on grounds that the old have already had a 'fair innings' (Williams 1997), or that if people were to prudently allocate resources to themselves, they may do so in a way which favours their young and middle-aged selves who have projects to fulfil or dependants to care for (Daniels 1988). Arguments of principle also abound as to whether personal responsibility for health states should influence resource allocations (see Cappelen and Norheim 2005). Further questions arise over the justifiability of according special priority to particular health needs—for example, to different kinds of diseases, to care at the end of life or to curative over preventive interventions.

Some conceptions of justice can justify weighting some considerations more heavily than others if they are concerned with redressing health inequalities. A concern with these inequalities may lead to according public health interventions greater priority—for example, to targeting interventions at those with co-morbidity factors, or focusing resources on preventive rather than curative interventions in order to tackle health inequalities at the outset, where they are related to socioeconomic background. Further, the idea of justice also applies to how healthcare is financed—notably, the effect that different systems of financing have on social or health-related inequalities, for example, the potentially catastrophic levels of expenditure incurred in countries where health-related costs have to be met by individuals paying direct, out-of-pocket charges for treatment.

Overall, how fairness in healthcare is conceived in different systems will naturally be shaped by wider conceptions of social justice, which may in turn be affected, for example, by levels of social inequality and attitudes to discrimination, as well as by social institutions such as written constitutions or bills of rights. Which conception of justice or fairness is in operation will also be substantially informed by the balance of the other social values in the list.

Solidarity

Solidarity is a value which can be particularly influential in shaping conceptions of justice. The principle of solidarity implies a commitment to the idea that all members of society will stand together and will not leave anyone behind, no matter how needy or disadvantaged. However, solidarity can take different forms: it can take a contractual form, such as membership of a welfare state or of a basic healthcare package, where it is primarily expressed through a willingness to share the financial risks of ill health, or a more generalized humanitarian form which is expressed in decisions which give priority to those who are worst-off in health terms. As such, the principle can be manifested either in concern about the negative effects of healthcare financing overall or in the process

of priority setting. The two forms of solidarity converge on the issue of cost-sharing or co-payment, particularly in systems which are mainly publicly financed: given the limits of funding in these systems, some element of cost-sharing is often present so that the state pays for some aspects of healthcare, and the individual for others. In privately financed systems, decisions have to be made as to what interventions will be funded by insurance premiums, and what levels of 'excess' individuals are left to pay themselves. The effect of a decision to make a certain intervention the subject of a co-payment—that is, a private payment by the individual—is to put that intervention beyond both the bounds of financial solidarity and health solidarity (Weale and Clark 2010). The relevant intervention may be either so expensive (whether clinically effective or not) as to impose an unjustified burden on the pool of risk-sharers, or its benefits may be either sufficiently uncertain and/or trivial for it to be justified in terms of health solidarity. The value of solidarity is also highlighted in responses to the tension between the principles of medical need and cost-effectiveness, and in how those principles are ordered. Where humanitarian solidarity is valued particularly highly, medical need may be prioritized over all other considerations, including cost-effectiveness. This has been the case in Sweden where, although scarce resources have called for cost-effectiveness considerations to be taken into account in priority setting, such is the social and political commitment to solidarity in the form of meeting medical need that issues of cost-effectiveness are sidelined.

However, the way in which demography, the increase in chronic diseases, and the high cost of pharmaceuticals are combining in many countries is increasingly putting strains on solidaristic healthcare arrangements, and raising questions as to where the reasonable limits of solidarity might lie. In such circumstances, attention may turn to the value of individual autonomy as decision-makers reflect on the possibilities for increasing personal responsibility either for health states or for healthcare financing, in order to ease pressure on the public purse.

Autonomy

The value of autonomy has a varied set of meanings (see Feinberg 1986) but it is often used to refer to the ability of individuals to be self-directing and to make decisions for themselves about important matters. Indeed, it is often taken to be one of the fundamental principles in medico-moral decisions, along with requirements of beneficence, non-maleficence, and justice (Beauchamp and Childress 1989). However, autonomy can be instrumental not only at the clinical level but also at the macro level of policy decisions about priority setting, both in terms of questions about individual responsibility for one's own health and in terms of questions about individual freedoms, perhaps most notably the freedom to choose the form of healthcare one prefers—and the responsibility that goes with that freedom to pay for those choices with one's own money (see Richards (2008) and Weale and Clark (2010) for examples of this conception of autonomy). Market-based approaches to healthcare tend to value autonomy more highly than other, notably solidarity-based, approaches. This might affect how priorities are set in a number of ways: it might be thought best that individuals are left to decide individually about how they spend their money and what healthcare goods and services they choose to purchase, and so perhaps only the most severe and urgent medical needs will be prioritized for public funding, with the rest being met either by insurance premiums or ad hoc out-of-pocket expenses. As we have already seen, there will likely be negative implications for justice from such an approach. When health-care priorities are set collectively, decisions may perhaps ignore what matters to some individuals with regard to their own medical need and treatment preferences. Where a healthcare budget is limited, giving full scope to individual self-determination will lead either back to collective healthcare choices in order to secure economies of scale or to long waiting lists—and there is arguably little self-determination to be pursued while one sits on a waiting list. However, it is possible to conceive of ways in which greater individual autonomy could be secured without necessarily leading to negative effects on justice. Priorities could be set so that aspects of care which are not central to clinical effectiveness are left to the individual to select and make the appropriate 'top-up' payment—for example, around different standards of accommodation in hospitals or around medically 'unnecessary' treatments. However, this runs into problems of defining what is medically necessary, and how apparently marginal factors like different standards of hospital accommodation can affect patients' over-all levels of well-being and their recovery from interventions. So, while they might be 'strictly' irrelevant from the perspective of the values of justice and effectiveness, it is not clear that this can be guaranteed in practice with real human individuals.

The process of decision-making

There has been increasing emphasis over recent years on the importance of procedural values in priority setting, partly in recognition of the significance of the quality of policy processes to the public legitimacy of decisions. As norms of democratic legitimacy are diffused around the world, so the values of transparency and accountability become more important. However, given that the content values are themselves subject to dispute, some way has to be found procedurally of dealing with the plurality of perspectives that this implies. As Daniels has commented, 'establishing a fair process for priority setting is easier than agreeing on principles' (Daniels 2000). In this context, three values are particularly important: transparency, accountability, and participation.

Transparency

The value of transparency has both normative and practical purposes (Clark and Weale 2012). Where people lose out as a result of priority-setting decisions it may be thought important, as a matter of principle, that they are able to see that both the reasons upon which such a decision is based, and the processes involved in reaching it, are fair. The instrumental value of transparency is also related to this ability of all interested parties to see the fairness of decisions: in this way, trust in decision-makers is increased, and clinicians, patients, and the public are left in a better position to accept priority-setting decisions as fair even (and especially) for those who may lose out—if they can see that those decisions are based on appropriate and relevant reasons.

Transparency in decision-making is often associated with explicit priority setting, where reasons and criteria are openly stated, and where it is clear who makes the decisions and how they do so. Contrary to this, implicit priority setting, where decision-makers, decision protocols, and criteria are not openly stated, tends to obscure decision processes from public and patient scrutiny: what is not known cannot be challenged or criticized,

and those who do what is not known are themselves not known, and so cannot be held responsible. As such, implicit priority setting may hinder public understanding and acknowledgement of the real limitations that exist with regard to resources in healthcare. While the demand for transparency might arise most in the context of publicly funded systems where it is necessary as an element of democratic accountability, it is also relevant in privately funded systems: that is, when private providers claim to be providing a benefit for which they should be fairly recompensed by funders of either a public or private nature, that claim should be capable of being openly demonstrated to all interested parties.

Biron et al. (2012) drawing upon O'Neill (2002) and Rid (2009), have argued that the mere disclosure of information will unlikely be sufficient for transparency. Simple disclosure does not ensure that information will be intelligible to the public but may instead simply provide a 'flood of information', causing a great deal of uncertainty in the public mind. However, in many societies the problem is more likely to be too little information rather than too much. In the People's Republic of China, for example, where the World Bank estimates that there are some 750,000 premature deaths through pollution, levels of soil pollution are not made publicly available (Hook 2013). Just as there should be transparency in respect of public health risks, so there should be transparency in respect of priority setting decisions, no matter how demanding the task may seem.

Accountability

Accountability occurs when one party to the decision-making process justifies and takes responsibility for its activities to another. Being accountable in health priority setting means having the obligation to answer questions regarding decisions about which interventions are prioritized and why. We can think of accountability in terms of three questions: 'Who?', 'What?', and 'How?' (Clark and Weale 2012). The answers to each of these questions will vary considerably depending on the nature of the health system in question.

In terms of 'Who?' we can ask both who is held accountable, and who does the holding to account—who should answer the accountability questions and who should ask them. Those who should answer the questions will be those who make the decisions: for example, central or local government, civil servants, health professionals, medical institutions, or insurers. Pharmaceutical companies may also have an important role in influencing decisions and there may be good grounds for holding them to account too. There is a range of possibilities as to who asks accountability questions: patients, the public, and health professionals most obviously, although the courts have also become important actors in holding decision-makers to account in some countries, and in privately financed systems, employers and individual payers will likely be those who ask questions of insurers.

The 'What?' question, we might phrase as 'Accountability for what?'. The main answer to this in publicly funded systems has traditionally been the spending of taxpayers' money. In privately funded systems, financial accountability is also primary: private and corporate payers will want to ensure that their money is being used responsibly. However because decisions about priority setting involve value judgements as well as purely economic ones, so financial accountability alone does not provide a comprehensive answer to accountability questions. Accountability around value judgements can be difficult to assign however, since even where priority setting is explicit in economic terms, it may not be so in respect of social values.

With regard to the 'How?' question, two general types of accountability can be identified. The first type is simply about providing information on decisions and implies a one-way transmission of information from decision-makers to, for example, the public. The second type of accountability moves beyond simple reporting of decisions and attends not just to what was decided but to the reasons for decisions, often in the form of a two-way dialogue. This can help build trust in decision-makers by signalling that they are interested in the views and well-being of patients and the public. In this way, the value of accountability is complemented by the value of participation.

As even this brief discussion suggests, discharging the obligation of accountability can be complex and demanding. It requires decision-makers to assemble the relevant information and provide a chain of reasoning from evidence to policy that a variety of audiences can follow. Concerns have also been raised that an emphasis upon accountability can descend into mere formal compliance in the form of a 'box-ticking' culture rather than a commitment to communicating the reasons for decisions (O'Neill 2002). Of course, this is always a possibility, and where top-down (and often poorly thought out) performance targets are used, the risk is increased. However, there is no reason to believe that this sort of distortion is intrinsic to the practice of accountability, which is a value that plays an important role in the public justification of priority-setting decisions.

Participation

Participation refers to the opportunity that those affected by public decisions have to contributing towards the formation of those decisions. One primary reason why participation is a value is because it can allow different interests to contribute and have their voices heard. This is important for several reasons. Firstly, because prioritization decisions are fundamentally value judgements—and value judgements inevitably vary between individuals and groups within society—having those individuals and groups participate in decision-making is likely to help make both the process and the outcome more legitimate and more likely to be accepted, especially by those who lose out. However, including different viewpoints in the decision-making process can also improve the quality of decisions, given that it widens the range of information taken into consideration: for example, patients can make important contributions to the technical quality of decisions via their direct experience of pharmaceuticals. Participation in the decision-making process is also a mechanism for engaging powerful constituencies in a constructive manner—for example, leaders of the medical profession—as well as for improving the transparency and sharing accountability for decisions. However, within democracies, there is a deeper reason for participation: it is commonly thought that citizens should be able to participate in decision-making about issues that affect their vital interests—and access to appropriate healthcare is clearly one of the most important of such interests. Healthcare priority setting, then, is an obvious candidate for a democratic mandate.

The most obvious answer to the question of who should participate is 'patients'—the people directly affected by priority-setting decisions. However, the patient perspective is not the only relevant one: it has been argued that the perspective of the citizen should also be engaged in order to gain a wider and more inclusive view of the issues. Engaging only patient groups can exclude those who are not current users but who may use the services in the future, and the narrow perspective of a patient who has a particular personal interest in a service may conflict with the broader, longer-term interest of a citizen who is a taxpayer, a voter, and a member of any number of communities. There is an increasing tension in some healthcare services between the push to increase individual rights and 'consumer interests' in healthcare and the need to make collective decisions which are in the interests of the citizen and the wider community (Montgomery 1996).

Process and content

How do these process and content values relate to one another? Although transparent and accountable processes are necessary to make resource allocation decisions in ways that are justifiable, we should not assume that process alone will be sufficient (Powers and Faden 2008). This in turn raises the question of whether there is a cultural bias in supposing that some content values are always relevant to ethically justified priority setting. Does justice in China, Thailand, Korea, Colombia, Germany, or the United Kingdom mean the same thing? The short answer is that we do not know until we see their priority-setting processes develop and decisions are made. However, it is striking that as countries like China, Korea, and Thailand develop, they have moved towards policies based on the principle of universal access, in that respect at least following the European model.

A similar question can be raised about process values. Can fair priority-setting decisions be reached in contexts where procedural values are not considered to be particularly important or necessary? Again, the answer to this question must remain open. However, we should always bear in mind that those who say that certain process values associated with transparency and accountability are culturally specific risk underestimating the extent to which there is a willingness to protest where standards of openness are not met. As our earlier example of pollution in China showed, the demand for greater transparency is widespread where there is a threat to human health.

One special case where we might observe difference in social values is in the importance attached to public participation as compared to expert judgement.

A recent study of priority setting in eight different countries notes that many countries without widespread public involvement in decision-making have achieved priority-setting objectives that are largely accepted by the public. In Norway, for example, 'the recommendation was that this process [of decision-making] should be expert-driven, and not involve much public debate' (Sabik and Lie 2008). Yet, there is also a complex interplay between the value and technical components of health priority-setting decisions as well as between the values themselves. Different conceptions of the values of justice and solidarity in particular are significant in how technical judgements are worked out and how the various reasons within decisions are weighted. The degree to which a society values solidarity will have a large impact on how it weighs justice considerations in decisions, and what form those considerations take, particularly in determining which characteristics of persons are relevant—and therefore legitimate—to take into account in priority-setting decisions and which are not. As such, a purely technical approach to quality of life measures that does not acknowledge the values it assumes will likely be lacking in some way—and it will make accountability for, transparency and participation in those value judgements difficult if not impossible. The Oregon priority setting experiment where a ranked list of interventions was produced on the basis of cost-effectiveness alone, produced considerable counter-intuitive effects (Hadorn 1991) and further, there is evidence to suggest that the public in some countries at least wish for both accountability and participation in relation to value judgements.

Important values underlie both the 'process' and 'content' elements of decision-making in health priority setting. The 'process' values of transparency, accountability, and participation are closely linked: transparency forces governance to be more careful so as to stand up to public scrutiny. In this way, it is the instrument of accountability and justifiability: if transparency is lacking, it will be difficult for decision-makers to be held accountable in any meaningful way since those who wish to hold them to account will not have the relevant knowledge with which to do so. One way to advance transparency may be to increase participation, especially in an area like health where citizens (as well as patients) are directly affected by decisions and where they may have much to contribute to governance. In turn, increasing participation may be a pre-condition to increasing transparency. In terms of 'content', value judgements are often hidden in technical criteria such as clinical and cost-effectiveness measures.

A research programmme

If almost all decisions in health priority setting involve complicated issues of social values, they are nonetheless often only implicit and unrecognized by policymakers. There is often a sense of 'muddling through' when it comes to social values. The challenge of values is demanding, but the capacity to address it when there are many other challenges may be limited, given the complexity of the values-based issues and the unfamiliarity of policymakers with them. This practical need for greater understanding of the role and significance of social values in health priority setting became apparent to the authors and all of those present at the international conference held in London in early 2011. A new research programme was finally launched at the HTAi conference in Bilbao in 2012.

This new research programme (see http://www.ucl.ac.uk/socialvalues for further details) (Littlejohns et al. 2012b) has as its central focus an international comparison of the role that social values play in the setting of healthcare priorities in Thailand, Korea, Columbia, the United Kingdom and the United States. It requires the collection of complex data from a variety of agencies in the different countries. The research will be carried out through a network of policymakers and researchers, and will involve a cross-national comparative empirical analysis of priority setting together with policy evaluation informed by recent developments in normative political theory, culminating in the production of a decision tool aimed to help policymakers integrate social values considerations more easily and effectively into their decision-making processes.

Two main questions are at the heart of the research programme. What role *do* social values play in decisions about health priority setting and how are they currently taken into account by policymakers? And what role *should* social values play and how *should* they be taken into account by policymakers?

One distinctive approach to these questions is the use of case studies to provide insight into the challenges of priority setting and into the role that social values play in priority setting decisions. As an 'inductive' research tool, they offer a focus for gathering rich information about particular instances of social values issues in 'real life' priority setting and, as such, they facilitate comparative research. And for policymakers, case studies offer a means of accessing the experiences of others facing similar problems and provide an opportunity for shared learning. An online 'catalogue' of case studies is currently in development as part of the research programme, and uses a standardized reporting template to enable comparison.

However, the ultimate aim of our research programme is not only to improve understanding of the role that social values do and should play in health priority setting, but to translate our findings into a usable tool for policymakers as they confront questions of value choice. The challenge here is to develop a comprehensive, easily usable, and policy-relevant tool which provides a way for policymakers systematically to identify and consider the social values which are involved in their decisions. This is a question of translational research involving the validation of the tool through developmental work with policymakers and other stakeholders. Improving decision-making in the light of important social values is a collective enterprise, and we are sure that many others will be involved in the challenges that are set us all.

References

Ahn, J., Kim, G., Suh, H., and Lee, S.M. (2012). Social values and health care priority setting in Korea. *Journal of Health Organization and Management*, 26(3), 343–50.

Beauchamp, T.L. and Childress, J.F. (1989). *Principles of Biomedical Ethics* (3rd ed). New York: Oxford University Press.

Biron, L., Rumbold, B., and Faden, R. (2012). Social value judgements in health care. *Journal of Health Organization and Management*, 26(3), 317–30.

Bundesverfassungsgerichts 6 (December 2005). 1 BvR 347/98. [Judgement of *Nikolaus* case.]

Cappelen, A. and Norheim, O. (2005). Responsibility in health care: a liberal egalitarian approach. *Journal of Medical Ethics*, 31, 476–80.

Chalkidou, K., Tunis, S., Lopert, R., et al. (2009). Comparative effectiveness research and evidence-based health policy: experience from four countries. *The Milbank Quarterly*, 87(2), 339–67.

Clark, S. and Weale, A. (2012). Social values in health priority setting: a conceptual framework. *Journal of Health Management and Organisation*, 26(3), 293–316.

Cookson, R. and Dolan, P. (2000). Principles of justice in health care rationing. *Journal of Medical Ethics*, 26, 323–9.

Cubillos, L., Escobar, M.L., Pavlovic, S., and Lunes, R. (2012). Universal health coverage and litigation in Latin America. *Journal of Health Organization and Management*, 26(3), 388–404.

Culyer, A. and Bombard, Y. (2012). An equity framework for health technology assessments. *Medical Decision Making*, 32(3), 428–41.

Daniels, N. (1988). *Am I My Parents' Keeper?* Oxford: Oxford University Press.

Daniels, N. (2000). Accountability for reasonableness in private and public health insurance. In A. Coulter and C. Ham (eds.) *The Global Challenge of Health Care Rationing*, pp. 89–106. Buckingham: Open University Press.

Elshaug, A., Hiller, J., Tunis, S., and Moss, J. (2007). Challenges in Australian policy processes for disinvestment from existing, ineffective health care practices. *Australia and New Zealand Health Policy*, 4, 23.

Feinberg, J. (1986). *The Moral Limits of the Criminal Law: Harm to Self*, Vol. 3. Oxford: Oxford University Press.

Garner, S., Docherty, M., Somner, J., et al. (2013). Reducing ineffective practice: challenges in identifying low-value health care using Cochrane systematic reviews. *Journal of Health Services Research and Policy*, 18(1), 6–12.

Gutmann, A. and Thompson, D. (2004). *Why Deliberative Democracy?* Princeton, NJ: Princeton University Press.

Hadorn, D. (1991). Setting healthcare priorities in Oregon: cost effectiveness meets the rule of rescue. *Journal of the American Medical Association*, 265(17), 2218–25.

Hoedemaekers, R. and Dekkers, W. (2003). Key concepts in health care priority setting. *Health Care Analysis*, 11(4), 309–23.

Hook, L. (2013). Weibo alters China's environmental debate. *The Financial Times*, 4 March.

Johri, M. and Norheim, O. (2012). Can cost-effectiveness analysis integrate concerns for equity? Systematic review. *International Journal of Technology Assessment in Health Care*, 28(2), 125–32.

Littlejohns, P., Weale, A., Chalkidou, K., Faden, R., and Teerawattananon, Y. (eds.) (2012a). Social values and healthcare priority-setting, special issue. *Journal of Health Organization and Management*, 26(3), 285–421.

Littlejohns, P., Weale, A., Chalkidou, K., Faden, R., and Teerawattananon, Y. (2012b). Social values and health policy: a new international research programme. *Journal of Health Organization and Management*, 26(3), 285–92.

McIntyre, D. and Gilson, L. (2000). Redressing disadvantage: promoting vertical equity within South Africa. *Health Care Analysis*, 8, 235–58.

Montgomery, J. (1996). Patients first: the role of rights. In K. Fulford, F. Erssen, and T. Hope (eds.) *Essential Practice in Primary Care*, pp. 142–51. Oxford: Blackwell Science.

Mooney, G. (1987). What does equity in health mean? *World Health Statistics Quarterly*, 40(4), 296–303.

NICE (2008). *Social Value Judgements: Principles for the Development of NICE Guidance* (2nd ed.). London: National Institute for Health and Clinical Excellence. Available at: http://www.nice.org.

NICE (2012). *How We Work*. London: London: National Institute for Health and Clinical Excellence. Available at: http://www.nice.org.uk/aboutnice/howwework/how_we_work.jsp.

Oliver, A. (ed.) (2003). *Equity in Health and Healthcare*. London: Nuffield Trust.

O'Neill, O. (2002). *Lecture 3: Called to Account*. Reith lecture. Available at: http://www.bbc.co.uk/radio4/features/the-reith-lectures/transcripts/2000/.

Persad, G., Wertheimer, A., and Emanuel, E. (2009). Principles for allocation of scarce medical interventions. *Lancet*, 373, 423–31.

Powers, M. and Faden, R. (2008). *Social Justice: The Moral Foundations of Public Health and Health Policy*. New York: Oxford University Press.

Rawlins, M.D. and Culyer, A.J. (2004). National Institute for Clinical Excellence and its value judgements. *British Medical Journal*, 329, 224–7.

Richards, M. (2008). *Improving Access to Medicines for NHS Patients: A Report to the Secretary of State for Health*. Available at: http://www.dh.gov.uk/en/Publicationsandstatistics/Publications/PublicationsPolicyAndGuidance/DH_089927.

Rid, A. (2009). Justice and procedure: how does accountability for reasonableness result in fair limit-setting decisions? *Journal of Medical Ethics*, 35(1), 12–16.

Sabik, L. and Lie, R. (2008). Priority setting in health care: lessons from the experiences of eight countries. *International Journal for Equity in Health*, 7(4), 4–17.

Tantivess, S., Perez Velasco, R., Yothasamut, J., Mohara, A., Limprayoonyong, H., and Teerawattananon, Y. (2012). Efficiency or equity: value judgments in coverage decisions in Thailand. *Journal of Health Organization and Management*, 26, 3.

Weale, A. (2010). Political theory and practical public reasoning. *Political Studies*, 58(2), 266–81.

Weale, A. and Clark, S. (2010). Co-payments in the NHS: an analysis of the normative arguments. *Health Economics, Policy and Law*, 5(2), 225–46.

Williams, A. (1997). Intergenerational equity: an exploration of the fair innings argument. *Health Economics*, 6, 117–32.

3.6

Health policy in developing countries

Miguel Angel González-Block, Adetokunbo Lucas, Octavio Gómez-Dantés, and Julio Frenk

Introduction to health policy in developing countries

Most developing nations are making important strides towards better health and universal health service coverage through policies that are increasingly influenced by international experience. The flow of financial resources is also expanding rapidly thanks to the role that health investments are playing in the wider strategy towards democracy, economic growth, and global security (Brown et al. 2001; Hecht and Shah 2006; Frenk and Gómez-Dantés 2007). Health policy in the South is thus increasingly being influenced by globalization, both by responding to global threats and by doing so through extensive use of the pool of global experiences.

Health policy has been critical for the diffusion of life-saving technologies and knowledge that are behind the drop in disparities in life expectancy across rich and poor countries at least since the middle of the last century. Taken as a group, the poorer countries have seen gains of about 5 years on average per decade since 1960, against half this much by the better-off. Critically, the pace of technology diffusion has been more influential for health than changes in the levels of income. Increased access to knowledge and technology thanks to appropriate health policies has accounted for perhaps as much as two-thirds of the 2 per cent per year rate of decline in under-5 mortality rates (Jamison 2006).

However, health policy still has important challenges in a world saddled with conflict, poverty, and the pandemic of HIV/AIDS. In some African countries, the trend in the mortality rate for children under 5 has been reversed. While, between 1960 and 1990, African countries made substantial progress in reducing this rate, in many countries this effort was slowed down considerably, and in some others mortality even rose between 1990 and 2002 (United Nations Children's Fund (UNICEF) 2004).

In this chapter we review the context in which health policies are being developed in low- and middle-income countries. We discuss several key concepts associated with health policy, and describe some of the tools available for policymaking. In the first part, we discuss the role of health policy as a stewardship instrument and the general context in which health policies are being designed and implemented in developing nations. In the second part, we describe some of the novel tools available for policymaking, including burden of disease, national health accounts, and

health system performance assessment. We discuss the increasing international financing for healthcare and the alternatives for achieving universal health coverage (UHC) with financial protection against catastrophic costs of healthcare. We then analyse the search for equity in health and discuss the role of international agencies and health research in the design and implementation of health policies.

The main messages of the chapter are the following:

1. Sound health policies balancing the best evidence, ethical principles, and political realities are needed in developing countries not only to address the pressing needs of infectious diseases and malnutrition and the rapidly emerging problems of non-communicable diseases and injuries, but also the new challenges related to globalization, including pandemics and the health consequences of climate change.

2. Sound health policymaking can contribute to the consolidation of democracy, to economic growth, and to global security. The broad consensus generated around this issue has helped to mobilize *more money for health* in developing nations.

3. Policy-making should be evidence-based, and also results-oriented. Careful planning and skilled management can achieve good results and allow developing countries to deliver *more health for the money*.

Health policy as stewardship

Health policymaking in developing countries is seeking a new model of action to increase health and welfare, largely based on the separation of health system stewardship from service delivery through various forms of decentralization (Bossert 1998; Murray and Frenk 2000). Policymaking is increasingly being envisaged as a stewardship process concerned with attaining trust and legitimacy between a government and its people towards the improvement of the welfare of populations (Londoño and Frenk 1997; Gilson 2003; Bankauskaite et al. 2007; Garret 2007). The *World Health Report 2000* defined stewardship of the health system by national governments as a critical function to realign incentives and to mobilize and allocate resources to achieve the final goals of health gain, financial protection, and responsiveness. Stewardship has also been defined as a function of international agencies to enable coordination of health systems at the global level (WHO 2000).

Stewardship is an ethically-based, outcome-oriented policy approach and as such it is more interventionist than the economically driven agency approach to state regulation (Table 3.6.1). The notion of stewardship, if properly developed, is also consistent with an evidence-based health policy framework (Saltman and Ferroussier-Davis 2000). A national health strategy based on stewardship can marshal the available evidence to support population-based measures that can improve overall health status. Stewardship capacity is synonymous with the quality of governing institutions within countries, and with the trust that societies place in their governments. In a global climate of increased support for public investments in health, greater attention is being paid to differentiate countries with 'good' and 'stressed' governance in order to marshal international aid support for policymaking.

The process of policymaking for the health sector has become increasingly intricate. Health practitioners, policymakers, planners, and resource providers have to contend with three main issues: *diversity, complexity,* and *change.*

There is often great *diversity* within developing countries, as well as between and within different geographical areas. Ecological and geographical factors are recognized as important determinants of health conditions. Economic, social, and cultural determinants also contribute to diversity. The association of poverty, exclusion, and discrimination with poor health status is a consistent finding in both developed and developing countries and has a long research tradition (Evans et al. 1994). In general, policymaking fails to systematically recognize and act on these determinants. The World Health Organization (WHO) Commission on Social Determinants of Health attempted to redress this shortcoming by creating awareness of such determinants among political leaders and stakeholders, and helping countries adopt comprehensive health and development policies oriented towards them (Irwin et al. 2006).

Complexity in health needs of populations is another challenge. In contrast with rich countries that experienced a substitution of old for new patterns of disease, developing nations are facing a triple burden of ill health: first, the unfinished agenda of infections, malnutrition, and reproductive health problems; second, the emerging challenges represented by non-communicable diseases and injuries; third, the health risks associated with globalization, including the threat of pandemics like AIDS and influenza, the trade in harmful products like tobacco, and other drugs, the health consequences of climate change, and the dissemination of harmful lifestyles. A recent study of risk factors at global and regional levels based on the measurement of burden of disease for 2010 attests to a major shift in risk factors to disease burden, moving away from risks for communicable diseases in children and towards those for non-communicable diseases in adults. According to this study, in much of sub-Saharan Africa the leading risks are still poverty related and affect children (Lim et al. 2012).

Annual changes in mortality projections between 2002 and 2020 suggest decreases in tuberculosis (TB) of over 5 per cent yet increases of between 2.1 and 3 per cent for HIV/AIDS. Diabetes mellitus and road traffic mortality are projected to increase over 1 per cent per year, an alarming rate. In projections to 2030, cardiovascular disease will account for 13.4 per cent of the total world mortality and will rank as the first or second cause of mortality in all income regions (Mathers and Loncar 2006). Tobacco consumption is largely responsible for many disease trends, and particularly ischaemic heart disease. This is a product of relentless push of industry into new, unregulated contexts susceptible to lifestyle changes.

While knowledge and innovative health technologies have been critical in healthcare in developing countries, the explosion of new technologies designed for rich countries as well as innovations of critical importance to the South such as antiretrovirals and Integrated Management of Childhood Illness (IMCI) have markedly increased the *complexity of healthcare*. The expanding scope of prophylactic, diagnostic, and therapeutic options demands an increasing range of specific programmes with the associated need for specialist personnel, new categories of support staff, high-technology equipment, and infrastructure. Fig. 3.6.1 illustrates the complex interaction of medical and non-medical factors that are involved in perpetuating the high maternal mortality rates occurring in the developing world. It also offers clues as to the package of interventions that are required to reduce maternal mortality (McCarthy and Maine 1992). A particular challenge is a renewed tendency to deliver new technologies through vertical programmes that may fail to support the health system while weakening existing programmes (Unger et al. 2003; Molineux and Nantulya 2004; Garret 2007). New approaches to integrate disease control programmes with the health system as to obtain reciprocal benefits are now being proposed and evaluated (González-Block et al. 2012).

Table 3.6.1 Comparison of agency theory and stewardship theory

Characteristic	Agency theory	Stewardship theory
1. Model man	Economic man	Self-actualizing man
Behaviour	Self-serving	Collective serving
2. Psychological mechanisms	Lower order/economic needs (physiological, security, economic)	Higher-order needs (growth achievement, self-actualization)
Motivation	Extrinsic	Intrinsic
Social comparison	Other managers	Stakeholders
Identification	Low-value commitment	High-value commitment
Power	Institutional (legitimate, coercive, reward)	Personal (expert, referent)
3. Situation mechanisms	Control-oriented	Involvement-oriented
4. Management philosophy	Control mechanisms	Trust
Risk orientation	Short term	Long term
Time frame	Cost control	Performance enhancement
Objective	Individualism	Collectivism
5. Cultural differences	High-power distance	Low-power distance

Adapted with permission from Davis, J. et al., Towards a stewardship theory of management, *Academy of Management Review*, Volume 22, Issue 1, pp. 20–47, Copyright © 1997 Academy of Management Review.

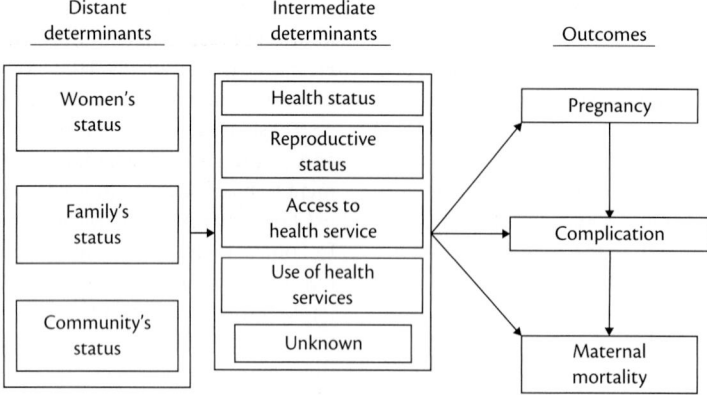

Fig. 3.6.1 Interaction of factors involved in the epidemiology of maternal mortality.
Reproduced with permission from McCarthy, J. and Maine, D., A framework for analyzing the determinants of maternal mortality, *Studies in Family Planning*, Volume 24, pp. 23–33, Copyright © 1992.

The interaction of medical and non-medical factors in the dynamics of health and disease calls for a critical analysis of needs and opportunities as a basis of designing and managing health programmes. Due to the important influence of non-medical factors on health, it is also necessary to mobilize intersectoral action to complement inputs from the health sector. In this process, policymakers in developing countries should measure their capacity and ensure they first reap their benefits of interventions they can directly control within their health systems (Jamison 2006).

Policymaking in developing countries also has to be fluid and dynamic to adapt strategies and programmes to the many *changes* that are occurring in the environment. Two critical changes are accountability and socioeconomic change.

Global as well as national influences are leading towards greater *accountability* of policymakers to parliaments, provincial stakeholders, as well as to donors, clients, and populations. Decentralization has continued its pace giving provincial authorities and local officials greater autonomy for innovations but also increased responsibility (Hutton 2002; Bossert 1998). Policymaking in the health sector is thus moving from a technical and highly hierarchical approach towards recognizing the role of new actors and processes set in a political and participatory environment.

Changes in the economic and social situation in countries may have a profound effect on the health sector. Health policies have had to be modified in the light of rapid development in some countries and economic recession in others. In the immediate post-Second World War era, macroeconomic policies emphasizing central planning and welfare programmes gained popularity. During the 1980s and 1990s, this trend was reversed, with national policies increasingly favouring free market economy in place of welfare programmes and central control. These changes brought about a slowdown in public health sector investments and the introduction of user fees, without visible improvements (Alliance HPSR 2004). Today, international agencies such as the International Monetary Fund (IMF) and the World Bank have reversed their policies (World Bank IMF Development Committee 2003), and funding has been substantially increased aiming to double the level of international aid to support the Millennium Development Goals (MDGs). Government capacity is being revamped to ensure efficiency and equity in investments.

Countries face different degrees of resource development, of government control, and of private sector participation. These dimensions define a spectrum of country situations that goes from the accumulated conditions of poverty and underdevelopment seen in low-income countries, to the emerging conditions most notably seen in middle-income countries (Table 3.6.2). This chapter focuses on eight critical issues along this spectrum:

1. Health reform with special emphasis on structural reform and decentralization

2. Tools for policymaking—burden of disease, national health accounts, and performance assessment

3. Financing healthcare—sector-wide approaches (SWAps), health insurance and UHC

4. Human resources for health

5. Public–private contracting

6. Equity in health

7. International agencies and public–private partnerships

8. Health research.

Health reform

The rapid rise of non-communicable diseases, the advances in health technologies, the escalating cost of healthcare, and the increasing demands and expectations of populations are leading governments, both in developed and developing countries, to undertake reforms of the health sector.

Structural reform

Health sector reform has been defined as the sustained and purposeful change to improve efficiency, equity, and effectiveness of the health sector (Berman and Bossert 2000; Roberts et al. 2003). Reforms have also been equated with comprehensive and integral change at the systemic, programmatic, organizational, and instrumental levels of the health system (Frenk 1994; González-Block 1997).

At the *systemic* level, changes such as the universalization of access to services, new financing arrangements, and the separation of stewardship and delivery functions have been critical. In turn, reforms at the *programmatic* level may include the definition of specific service

Table 3.6.2 Challenges facing health systems in developing countries, by population and institutional components

Component	Type of challenge	
	Accumulated	**Emerging**
Population	• Epidemiological backlog:	• New pressure:
	• Common infections	• Non-communicable diseases
	• Malnutrition	• Injuries
	• Reproductive health problems	• Emerging infections
	• Health gap	• Changes in demand patterns
	• Inequity	• Political pressures
Institutions	• Insufficient coverage	• Cost escalation
	• Poor technical quality	• Inadequate incentives
	• Allocational inefficiency	• Financial insecurity
	• Inadequate patient referral	• Patient dissatisfaction
	• Deficient management of institutions	• Deficient management of the system

Reproduced from *Health Policy*, Volume 41, Issue 1, Londoño, J. and Frenk, J., Structured pluralism: Towards an innovative model for health system reform in Latin America, pp. 1–36, Copyright © 1997, with permission from Elsevier, http://www.sciencedirect.com/science/journal/01688510.

rights and predefined packages of interventions through explicit choices based on a calculus of benefits and costs. Changes at the *organizational* level may involve introducing quality improvement strategies, increasing provider choice, and implementing provider payment mechanisms to promote quality, safety, and efficiency. At the *instrumental* level, reforms may imply increasing reliance on research, evaluation, and monitoring mechanisms, as well as incentives for human resource and technology development.

Health reforms require the development of monitoring mechanisms to ensure the attainment of objectives within different time spans. Such mechanisms should pay attention both to the technical and the ethical components of health reforms. A number of technical areas for monitoring and decision-making have been identified. These areas include effective coverage, general

level and distribution of health conditions, general level and distribution of responsiveness, and fair financing (see later in 'Health system performance assessment') (WHO 2000). This framework was successfully used for monitoring and evaluation purposes at the subnational level in the reform of the Mexican health system aiming towards UHC (Frenk et al. 2006).

The ethical monitoring of health sector reforms has been enabled through a set of benchmarks of fairness (Daniels et al. 1996). These benchmarks identify and measure the degree of fairness of health systems and of the different objectives pursued by health reforms and has been tested in several developing countries with some success (Daniels et al. 2005).

Decentralization

The decentralization of the planning and management of health services from national authorities to provincial governments is a common feature of structural reforms. However, we are witnessing new trends towards recentralizing services, due both to an assessment of past strategies but more importantly as a result of scaling-up efforts for disease control.

Especially in large countries with dispersed populations, governments cannot efficiently manage the delivery of healthcare from their central offices. In a decentralized system, the central Ministry of Health can set national goals and targets, establish performance-based incentives and monitor their attainment, while devolving the responsibility for detailed management of programmes and services to local authorities. Such arrangements promise improved allocative and technical efficiency, organizational innovation to meet local needs, improved service quality as well as greater equity, together with transparency, accountability, and legitimacy for the health sector as a whole. Three questions are critical to assess the effectiveness of decentralization: (1) the amount of choice that is transferred from central institutions to institutions at the periphery of health systems, (2) what choices local officials make with their increased discretion, and (3) what effect these choices have on the performance of the health system; see Fig. 3.6.2 and Table 3.6.3 (Bossert 1998).

Decentralization entails the establishment of principal–agent relationships, whereby the principal transfers responsibilities but tries to maintain overall control, for example, on the kind of services provided, their quality, and the equity attained (Bossert 1998). Information, assessment, and monitoring instruments are therefore critical for the success of decentralization reforms.

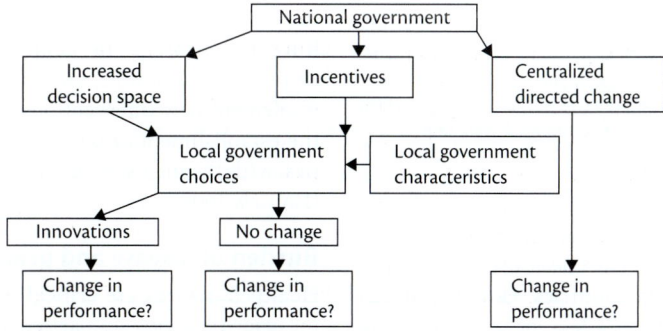

Fig. 3.6.2 Decision space and changes in performance in a decentralized healthcare system.
Reproduced from *Social Science and Medicine*, Volume 47, Issue 10, Bossert, T., Analyzing the decentralization of health systems in developing countries: Decision space, innovation and performance, pp. 1513–27, Copyright © 1998, with permission from Elsevier, http://www.sciencedirect.com/science/journal/02779536.

Table 3.6.3 Comparing the decision space in Ghana, Philippines, Uganda, and Zambia

Functions	Range of choice		
	Narrow	Moderate	Wide
Financing			
Source of revenue	Zambia	Ghana, Uganda	Philippines
Expenditures		All four	
Income from fees		Ghana, Zambia, Uganda	Philippines
Service organization			
Hospital autonomy	Ghana, Zambia	Uganda	Philippines
Insurance plans	Ghana, Uganda		Zambia, Philippines
Payment mechanisms	Ghana, Uganda	Philippines	Zambia
Contracts with private providers		Ghana, Zambia, Philippines	Uganda
Human resources			
Salaries	All four		
Contracts	Ghana,	Philippines	Zambia, Uganda
Civil service	Ghana	Zambia, Uganda, Philippines	
Access rules	Ghana	Zambia, Uganda, Philippines	
Governance			
Local government	Ghana, Zambia		Uganda, Philippines
Facility boards	All four		
Health offices	Ghana, Philippines	Zambia, Uganda	
Community participation	Ghana, Uganda	Zambia Philippines	
Country totals			
Ghana	11	4	0
Zambia	5	7	3
Uganda	5	7	3
Philippines	3	7	5

Reproduced from Thomas J. Bossert and Joel C. Beauvais, Decentralization of health systems in Ghana, Zambia, Uganda and the Philippines: a comparative analysis of decision space, *Health Policy and Planning*, Volume 17, pp. 14–31, Copyright © 2002, with permission from Oxford University Press.

Economic theories based on the choice that consumers have on the consumption of public resources have been useful to understand decentralization in developed countries. However, under conditions of meagre resources there is less local political and economic competition. More important perhaps is the reliance on trusted institutions at the local level and the strengthening of their capacity to ensure common interests across the multiple actors and often multiple principals that exert influence on health service providers (Gilson 2003).

Decentralization has not been without its critics, arguing that it has been often imposed upon local governments as a means of reducing central government obligations (Ugalde and Homedes 2006). The assessment of the effects of decentralization is now leading to recentralize a number of health functions such as public health surveillance in Mexico. Of greater significance for recentralization, however, is the increased funding by national governments as part of efforts towards UHC as well as by global health initiatives for disease control programmes such as malaria and HIV/AIDS.

Tools for policymaking

Policymaking in developing countries has not always been guided by the best available evidence. In the immediate post-independence period, some developing countries copied models of health services in developed countries with particular emphasis on specialized curative care and the construction of large tertiary hospitals. The high cost of maintaining such establishments often distorted the national health budget, leaving very little resources for supporting less expensive but highly effective community-based services. Because of severe resource constraints, developing countries should set clear priorities and adopt policies that help achieve maximum improvement in health in return for minimum expenditure. This is particularly the case as governments strive to attain UHC of a package of cost-effective interventions.

The establishment of priority lists of disease conditions and interventions was relatively easy in the traditional epidemiological situation where a few major conditions, mainly acute infectious diseases, accounted for a high proportion of deaths. In such situations one could rank priorities by considering the mortality rates from specific acute infectious diseases or the prevalence of chronic disabling diseases like onchocerciasis, a blinding disease. The process of priority setting has become more complex with the epidemiological transition, the increasing differentiation of health systems—including community participation—and the rising demands for equitable coverage.

Efficient decision-making for the allocation of scarce resources for health interventions requires setting priorities in terms of a wide range of considerations (Musgrove 1999; Gericke et al. 2005), to include: (1) the potential health impact and cost of interventions, (2) the 'public good' character of interventions as well as their externalities and their consequence for catastrophic expenditure in the absence of public interventions, (3) anti-poverty and equity considerations, and (4) the capacity of health systems to implement new interventions. This process should also consider the establishment of fair procedures for the definition of priorities, with the inclusion of the voice of patients and the community (Daniels 2008).

Burden of disease and priority setting

Health measures are critical for policymaking, in general, and for priority setting, in particular. One of the most widely applied indexes used to measure health needs is disability-adjusted life years (DALYs), which combines losses from premature death and from disability (Murray 1994a, 1994c).

The most common use of the DALY is simply to rank diseases and conditions by the burden of disease (the sum of healthy life years lost and years lived with disability) that they contribute, thus highlighting their relative importance for population health. The DALY is also being used to measure the burden of disease attributable to specific risk factors such as tobacco and obesity. On the basis of such measures, DALYs have been used to assess the contribution of specific risks and risk factors to the disease burden and the impact of major control programmes as well as to estimate cost-effectiveness of interventions by comparing the cost of averting a DALY across them. In its *World Health Report 2000*, the WHO published data on healthy life expectancy (HALE), which is defined as the average number of years that a person can expect to live in 'full health' by taking into account years lived in less than full health due to disease and/or injury. The most recent global measurement of disease burden was undertaken in 2010 by the Institute of Health Metrics and Evaluation, demonstrating the global rise in non-communicable diseases from 43 per cent of total DALYs for 1990 to 54 per cent for 2010 (Murray et al. 2012).

The DALY approach has been critiqued by several authors with respect to technical, methodological, and conceptual issues (Schneider 2001). The data required to estimate the DALY is extensive and is not always available to the extent necessary or with the required quality in developing countries. This has led to the use of questionable assumptions, such as the use of data for non-representative population segments. Another difficulty with the DALY is the combination of death and disability measures under the assumption that these phenomena lie on the same continuum along time (Anand and Hanson 1997).

Most critique of the DALY has centred on the large number of value-based judgements necessary to assign unequal age weights, to estimate the discounting of future health years, as well as to establish the disability weights (Anand and Hanson 1997). Furthermore, disability is quantified with respect to the limitation that diseases impose on individual functionality and does not consider pain and suffering.

The DALY is proving a useful tool but more work is required to refine and simplify it. Under the guidance of WHO, low- and middle-income countries are striving to improve the quality of data collection so as to improve the accuracy of national estimates of burden of disease. Some middle-income countries like Sri Lanka, Mexico, and Brazil are already making effective use of these tools (Morrow and Bryant 1995; Hyder et al. 1998). In Tanzania, the burden of disease approach was adapted to prioritize interventions in the rural districts of Morogoro and Rufiji. After a 5-year period of offering a package of essential health services, under-5 mortality rates had declined by 40 per cent, to less than 100 deaths per 1000 live births, in contrast with the child mortality rate for the country as a whole which remained in 160 deaths during the period of the intervention (de Savigny et al. 2004).

The public good character of interventions offers another criterion for priority setting. Public investment will be justified if the interventions do not have sufficient supply or demand. Such is the case for vector control or environmental risk surveillance. However, even if there is some private supply and demand, the public intervention would be justified if it can be demonstrated that enlarging services would benefit an even wider population beyond that which is consuming the service directly. Such is the case of immunizations, where individual consumption offers herd immunity to populations at large.

The risk by the poor or the near-poor of incurring catastrophic expenditures when seeking healthcare or as a result of disability to work is in itself a reason to invest public resources. Indeed, in Mexico, around 3 million households suffered impoverishing or catastrophic health expenditures annually in the early 2000s, a situation that led the government to implement the programme *Seguro Popular* (Popular Health Insurance) as a means of achieving UHC with financial protection, a goal that was achieved in 2012 (Knaul et al. 2012).

The condition of poverty of specific population groups is in itself an important criterion to consider for allocating resources on a priority basis. However, poverty in itself is not a reason to provide services indiscriminately, as scarce resources would not be used efficiently in the fight against poverty. This is why it is ethically acceptable to provide a package of highly cost-effective services for the poor, so long as the package is also acceptable to the poor themselves.

The criteria thus far considered for prioritizing public investments in health interventions can be summarized in Fig. 3.6.3, which suggests that investments should be spent on public goods only when they are cost-effective and when they have inadequate private supply and demand. Interventions that particularly benefit the poor should also be prioritized, as should those threatening with catastrophic health expenditure. Vertical and horizontal equity will not always be compatible with cost-effectiveness, leaving decision-making open to political criteria (Musgrove 1999).

The setting of priorities to invest in specific interventions should also consider the capacity of the health systems to formulate appropriate programmes and to deliver on the ground. Assessing health system capacity is today paramount, as new interventions are being scaled-up for the control of malaria, TB, and HIV/AIDS, among other diseases. These interventions require human, technical, and material resources that are often lacking. Four dimensions have been proposed for the assessment of the organizational and economic context (Gericke et al. 2005): (1) technical characteristics of interventions, (2) the logistical and delivery requirements, (3) the requirements stemming from governmental regulation, and (4) the characteristics of demand and utilization.

Technical characteristics of interventions include the basic design of products and technologies, such as stability and shelf-life. Product standardization is critical as similar interventions will be more easily implemented. Costs that are incurred during implementation but that may not have been considered in cost-effectiveness analysis include safety monitoring, supervision, storage, and regular, on-time delivery. Regulatory costs can be considerable, such as accreditation of health providers and facilities to ensure service quality as well as measures to curb corruption. Often the costs necessary to ensure compliance and coercion are not considered when formulating new programmes, leading to low enforcement of measures to increase quality and efficiency. Finally, priority setting should consider the ease of use of technologies by the population at large, including the extent to which health education is required to ensure demand and compliance. Ease of use may also be related to the proliferation of black markets and forgery for which countermeasures should be implemented.

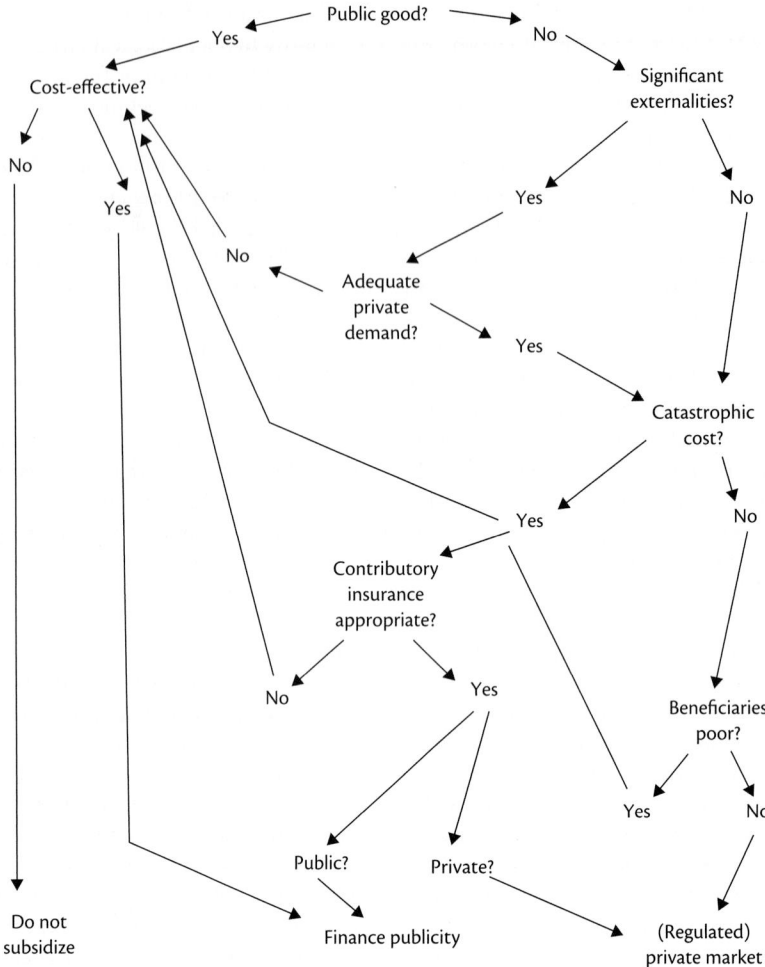

Fig. 3.6.3 Decision tree for assessing public investments in health.

Reproduced from *Health Policy*, Volume 47, Issue 3, Musgrove, P., Public spending on health care: How are different criteria related?, pp. 207–23, Copyright © 1999, with permission from Elsevier, http://www.sciencedirect.com/science/journal/01688510.

National health accounts

In the past, policymakers concentrated mainly on spending within the public sector, ignoring private spending through insurance, corporate arrangements, and employees' schemes, and out-of-pocket spending. Furthermore, spending within the public sector lacked clear indicators on resource flows, thus contributing to growing inequity and inefficiency. Policymakers now obtain a more comprehensive view of health expenditures thanks to the use of national health accounts developed through a uniform methodology. These analyses integrate health spending from all sources—public and private, corporate, and personal, national and international—within comprehensive accounts. National health accounts can affect the choices made within the public sector but also influence the role of public agencies in providing guidelines to the private sector and to communities regarding the most cost-effective uses of their investments and expenditures.

Health accounts consist of a basic matrix, where the columns list all sources of health spending—public (taxation and national social insurance), and private sources including employment-based schemes, privately financed insurance, and out-of-pocket expenditure. The rows of the matrix show the distribution of expenditure

for personal healthcare, public health, and environmental sanitation services, and administration. Disaggregating the items in the columns and rows generates more elaborate analyses, providing more detailed information about sources and spending. Thus, the analyses could show variations over time, by geography, by population subgroups, or any other variable that is relevant to policymaking (Berman 1997; WHO 2003). Today, health accounts are being prepared not only at the national level but also by specific programmes such as HIV/AIDS and reproductive health.

Health system performance assessment

The *World Health Report 2000* offered a comprehensive methodology and reported results to assess the overall performance of health systems in terms of health gain, responsiveness to the legitimate expectations of the population, and fairness of financing (WHO 2000). The degree to which these outcomes are achieved depends on how well the basic health system functions of stewardship, financing, resource generation, and service provision are carried out (Fig. 3.6.4). The three health system outcomes were assessed in terms of equity and efficiency, except financial fairness for which only equity is appropriate. Health gain was measured through

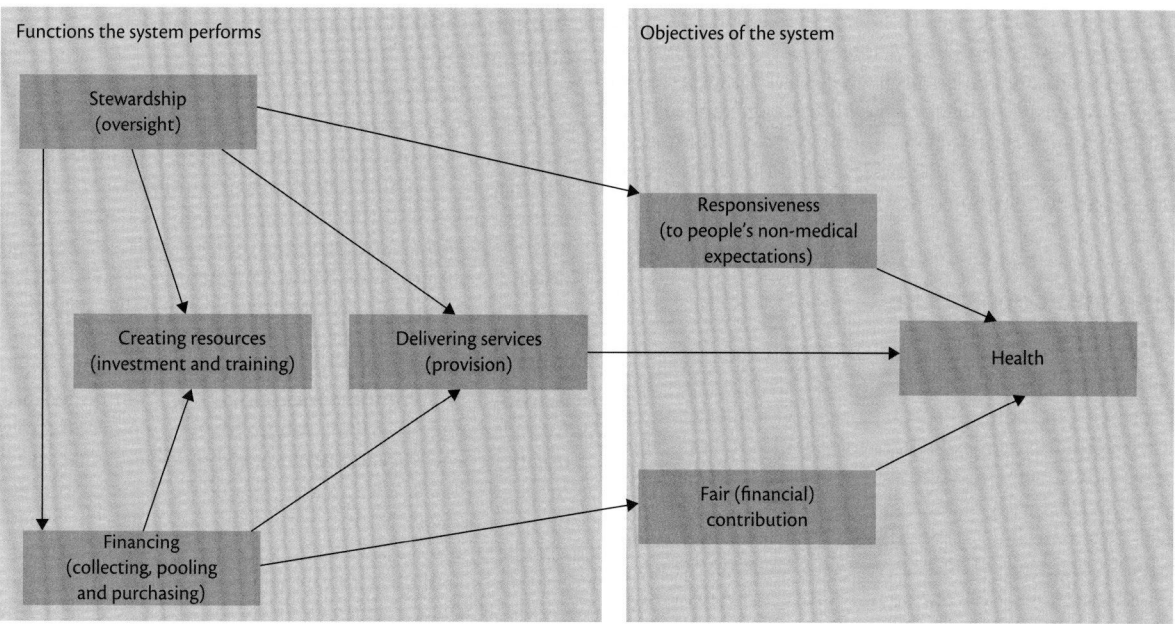

Fig. 3.6.4 Functions and objectives for the measurement of health system performance.
Reproduced with permission from World Health Organization, *The World Health Report 2000, Health Systems: Improving Performance*, World Health Organization, Geneva, Switzerland, Copyright © 2000, available from http://www.who.int/whr/2000/en/whr00_en.pdf.

healthy life expectancy, already described under the priority setting section above. The methodology enabled the measurement of each health system goal separately as well as through a combined indicator. All WHO member countries were then ranked as a means of highlighting the benefits and limitations of health system designs as well as to promote analysis and improvements.

Performance assessment can support policymaking in monitoring and evaluating attainment of critical outcomes and the efficiency of the health system in a way that allows comparison over time and across systems. Performance assessment enables the measurement of the relationship between design of health systems and outcomes and the dissemination of evidence on the benefits of diverse health system designs and reforms. The use of a widely accepted, comparative method was intended to feedback the policy debate as well as to empower the public with information relevant to their well-being (Murray and Evans 2003).

The methodology for performance assessment was widely debated by academics and governments and the Executive Board of WHO called for the establishment of a Scientific Peer Review Group (107th Session, EB107.R8, 15–22 January 2001). It was argued that intersectoral action for health was not subject to monitoring, focusing only on those functions and outcomes that are more directly under the control of ministries of health. Given that health sector policymaking may be the result of actions taken in an indefinite past, it will not be clear whose actions are being assessed at any given point in time.

Perhaps most controversial was the lack of consensus on the weighting that was given to each of the three separate dimensions of performance, where following a Web survey, health gain was assigned 50 per cent and responsiveness and financial protection 25 per cent each. Data used for the 2000 report was also faulted for excessive use and lack of clarity of the estimations that were necessary, given poor data quality and availability in many countries.

Performance assessment has been widely endorsed as a tool for policymaking for developing countries and, as mentioned earlier, was the basis for the monitoring of health sector reform in Mexico. WHO has called for improvements (WHO 2007), among them paying more attention to the broader health system as well as to the relationship between measured outcomes and health system functions. The Expanded Chronic Care Model could point towards new approaches to measure the contribution of the community, health policy and health systems towards more performing health strategies that take into account critical actors and multilevel chains of causation (Barr et al. 2003). Inequality should be more broadly measured, to include both health as well as socioeconomic inequality. In this respect, the Commission on Social Determinants for Health provided ample evidence and methods on how to integrate equity in health policy (Irwin et al. 2006). Subnational analyses should be carried out to identify success and limitations that can be more easily disseminated at the national level. Implementation research is being increasingly funded as a way to identify process bottlenecks and access barriers hampering the performance of policies and programmes (WHO 2011).

WHO also called to strengthen national health information systems as tools for performance assessment through the development of a broad range of health metrics. Mexico demonstrates how middle-income countries with reasonably developed information systems can make use of data for health system performance assessment. From 2000 to 2006, a set of health conditions and service benchmarks were systematically measured at state level and disseminated at yearly intervals. Evidence indicates that state authorities agreed on the quality and relevance of these measures and have accepted on this basis to be systematically monitored by federal health authorities and interested actors. Systematic monitoring has also led to the development of effective coverage measures, defined as the proportion of potential health gain that could be delivered by the health system to that which is actually delivered (Lozano et al. 2006). A total of 14 health interventions have been monitored and overall effective coverage assessed through a comprehensive indicator. Overall coverage ranged from 54 per cent in Chiapas, a poor state, to 65.1 per cent in Mexico's capital. These findings suggest that basic health interventions are much more equitably distributed in Mexico with respect to other health indicators.

Financing and contracting for healthcare

During the 1980s, international financing agencies restrained public investments in health as part of structural adjustment programmes with negative consequences for health systems. These policies have now been reversed as the United Nations (UN) enshrined the MDGs with important health targets for maternal and child health as well as HIV/AIDS, TB, and malaria among other epidemic diseases. MDGs served as a basis on which to mobilize national and international resources (World Bank IMF Development Committee 2003). Also, the Commission on Macroeconomics and Health, convened by WHO under the leadership of Jeffrey Sachs, produced analytical data advocating massive investments in health as a means of spurring economic growth (Commission on Macroeconomics and Health 2001). The Monterrey Consensus agreed at the 2002 UN Financing for Development Conference intends to double the level of international aid through an additional US$20 billion per annum to enable poor countries to achieve the MDGs (Sachs 2004).

Scaling up health financing in poor countries

Government capacity is now being revamped in many countries to ensure that massive scaling-up of health interventions can be undertaken under conditions of efficiency and equity. However, before interventions can be scaled up, low-income countries under stress—essentially countries with low governance—will have to strengthen their institutional capacity to ensure efficient and equitable resource allocation. It has also been recommended that resources be allocated to interventions whose delivery is least covered by the market so as to increase the impact of government services (Filmer et al. 2000).

The IMF and World Bank estimate that large increases in aid (a doubling or more of current flows) could be used effectively in countries with good governance such as Bangladesh, India, Indonesia, Pakistan, and Vietnam, and in some sub-Saharan African countries, such as Ethiopia. These countries have a combination of good policies and prospects for further improvement, large unmet needs relative to the MDG targets, and relatively low levels of aid dependence. Sub-Saharan African countries considered to have good governance such as Burkina Faso, Mozambique, Tanzania, and Uganda could also use additional aid productively to supplement the sizable flows they already receive—an increase of about 60 per cent on average in the medium term.

Evidence suggests that international short-term health aid is indeed supporting economic growth, regardless of the strength of governments (Clemens et al. 2004). Effective low-cost health interventions have also been effectively put in place and sustained in countries with weak governments or even under conflict situations (Medlin et al. 2006; Center for Global Development 2007).

Aid harmonization and sector-wide approaches

Donors and recipient countries have achieved a high degree of consensus regarding the provision of international aid. The Paris Aid Harmonization Declaration and Principles commits partners to recognize developing country ownership of development policies, and the alignment of donors with country strategies, institutions, and procedures. This implies a commitment by donors to support capacity strengthening of government procedures, rather than supporting specific aid delivery mechanisms. In terms of harmonization, the Paris declarations commit donors to a more harmonized, transparent, and collectively effective giving through common arrangements and simplified procedures. Complementarity is to be sought through a more effective division of labour while greater attention should be paid to aid provision in fragile states. Aid policies should be devised so that they can be managed by results, furthering collaborative behaviour and through mutual accountability (Paris Declaration 2005).

Donor harmonization in health has also been pursued through sector-wide approaches (SWAps), a process whereby funding for the sector—whether internal or from donors—supports a single policy and expenditure programme, under government leadership, and adopting common approaches across the sector. It is generally accompanied by efforts to strengthen government procedures for disbursement and accountability. A SWAp should ideally involve broad stakeholder consultation in the design of a coherent sector programme at micro, meso, and macro levels, and strong coordination among donors and between donors and government (Brown et al. 2001).

Universal health coverage

Health system financing has proven to be double-edged, mobilizing increasing amounts of resources for health but also driving millions of families into hardship or poverty when resource mobilization forces families to pay excessive amounts through out-of-pocket payments, chiefly for essential medicines and curative care. WHO proposed governments in its 2005 report *Health Systems Financing. The Path to Universal Coverage* to critically analyse how the health system is financed, how to protect people from the financial consequences of ill health, and how to encourage the optimum use of available resources (WHO 2005). Today, many developing countries are proposing to achieve UHC in the short to medium term, broadly understood as fair financing of essential healthcare through prepayment of health services and broad-based resource pooling. Two criteria are key to assess if a health system is offering UHC: financial protection for all from the costs of healthcare and effective access to needed healthcare for all citizens (McIntyre and Mills 2012). To attain this, UHC requires effective resource mobilization as well as reducing out-of-pocket payments in the context of more efficient health services. For health systems to function equitably towards UHC, financing should balance the depth, breadth, and proportion of health costs covered (Chua and Cheah 2012).

Community health insurance has been proposed to improve access by rural and informal sector workers to needed healthcare. Macro-level cross-country analyses give empirical support to the hypothesis that risk-sharing in health financing matters in terms of its impact on both the level and distribution of health, financial fairness, and responsiveness indicators (Preker et al. 2003; Alliance HPSR 2004).

Five key policies are available to governments to improve the effectiveness and sustainability of community financing schemes:

◆ Increased and well-targeted subsidies to pay for the premiums of low-income populations.

◆ Insurance to protect against expenditure fluctuations and re-insurance to enlarge the effective size of small risk pools.

◆ Effective prevention and case management techniques to limit expenditure fluctuations.

◆ Technical support to strengthen the management capacity of local schemes.

◆ Establishment and strengthening of links with the formal financing and provider networks.

Middle-income countries with segmented health systems face particular challenges to extend insurance coverage to a rising population employed in the informal sector. China has made impressive progress towards UHC as it increased coverage to health insurance schemes for its population from 29.7 per cent in 2003 to 90 per cent at the end of 2010. Behind this rapid expansion are two insurance schemes: the New Cooperative Medical Scheme for the Rural Population (NCMS) and the Urban Resident Basic Health Insurance (URBMI) (Tang et al. 2012). However, it is of concern that this rapid expansion has also been accompanied by cost explosion at an annual rate of 17 per cent in the past two decades. The total health expenditure increased from 74.7 billion Chinese Yuan in 1990 to 1998 billion Yuan in 2010, while average health expenditure per capital reached 1490.1 Yuan per person in 2010, rising from only 65.4 Yuan per person in 1990 (Tang et al. 2012).

New schemes have been implemented aiming at universal access to care through voluntary, government-subsidized schemes such as *Seguro Popular* in Mexico. Short-term assessments point to success in improving access to health services and reducing the prevalence of catastrophic and impoverishing health expenditures, especially for the poor, as well as improvements in access to priority interventions (Gakidoue et al. 2006; King et al. 2009). However, research also points to opportunities to diversify the health provider network and to encourage more effective, equitable and responsive health services (Knaul et al. 2012).

The effects of voluntary insurance schemes upon formal sector employment need to be addressed to ensure that morally just and cost-effective schemes also fuel the economy and are a step towards fully integrated, equitable publicly financed health systems. Using a robust database, Wagstaff and colleagues were able to establish for Thailand that universal coverage had a mixed effect, encouraging employment generally but discouraging formal sector employment among married men, yet not in other groups (Wagstaff and Wanwiphang 2012a). UHC had a positive impact on economic development through reducing the likelihood of people reporting themselves to be too sick to work (Wagstaff and Wanwiphang 2012b). These findings point to the importance of envisioning UHC schemes as transitory arrangements towards universal health systems.

Human resources for health

The WHO has estimated that, to meet the ambitious targets of the MDGs, health services in Africa will need to train and retain an extra 1 million health workers by 2010, chiefly nurses and other classes of health workers who constitute the bulk of the workforce. Health systems in poor countries face a very low-density health workforce, compounded by poor skill mix and inadequate investment. In addition, migration of trained human resources to more developed countries is becoming an ever more important issue.

Mass migration of health personnel is often a symptom of the 'sick system syndrome', in which many essential components of healthcare services are malfunctioning and mismanaged. Policies on migration must tackle the 'pull factors', which induce trained personnel to seek better living conditions abroad, as well as the 'push factors', which make disaffected and frustrated health workers seek employment elsewhere. Health challenges, such as the HIV/AIDS epidemic, impose additional pressures on health workers in their workplaces and at home, exposing them to contagious hazards, which adversely affect the morbidity and mortality of the workforce. The 'anchor factors' which encourage workers to remain in public service are important too. These should include financial incentives as well as well-designed training programmes that increase workers' skill and competence, boost their morale, increase their job satisfaction, and improve the performance of services (Lucas 2005).

Effective policymaking for human resources has to overcome the low attention that is given by both national governments and international agencies. Fiscal discipline depends on restriction of staff numbers and compensation levels, with staff salaries now consuming 60–80 per cent of diminished public budgets in the health sector. There is also a lack of coherent and integrated investment strategies to strengthen the workforce, resulting in an overemphasis on workshops and training sessions that have an unclear effect. Such constraints operate in a context of health-sector and civil-service reforms that have altered the work environment through expansion of the private sector, downsizing, and decentralization in the public sector. Public–private contracting has thus been increasingly sought after as a means of addressing multiple constraints.

An informal global network of health leaders supported by the Rockefeller Foundation's Joint Learning Initiative has proposed four immediate steps towards a reinvigorated human resources for health policy (Joint Learning Initiative 2004):

◆ Large-scale advocacy to achieve heightened political awareness within countries and globally, leading to a social mobilization to respond to the crisis in the short term.

◆ Improve information and develop a commonly accepted framework of ideas, terms, and relations to guide analysis for policy formulation, particularly on the mobility of health professionals and the relations between health equity and human resources.

◆ Learn from history and identify success stories demonstrating the goodwill and commitment of health workers in spite of adverse conditions. Lessons from BRAC in Bangladesh are highlighted, employing over 30,000 village health workers to raise awareness of health issues among the rural poor.

◆ Address the supply, demand, and mobility of personnel, linking across training and education, health systems, and labour markets to develop a system that ensures continuity of policies over time. This includes a process of addressing low wages, as well as creating an incentive structure that supports providers over the course of their working lives.

International debate around the responsibilities of all actors has also produced an interesting range of proposals, including ethical recruitment guidelines and financial compensation for exporting countries (Brush et al. 2004). Diagnostic approaches are required to inform evidence-based action: identify signs and causes of the 'sick system syndrome'. These should lead to the development and adoption of policies on human resources which are relevant, affordable, and sustainable, and are realistic about migration of trained staff (Lucas 2005).

Policymaking and the public–private mix

The private health sector may be defined as comprising all providers who exist outside the public sector, whether their orientation is philanthropic or commercial, and whose aim is to treat illness or prevent disease (Mills et al. 2002). However, the public and private sectors are highly related as public sector workers often have a private practice and many public facilities offer private wards or services or operate in such a manner that they are indistinguishable from profit-seeking private providers (Meng et al. 2004).

As stated previously, even in developing countries with a widespread public system such as Mexico, catastrophic or impoverishing out-of-pocket health expenditures, which imply an extensive use of private medical services, affect a large proportion of the population (Knaul and Frenk 2005). In these contexts, it is vital to support consumers in their use of health services. Such efforts could stimulate appropriate demand through improving consumer information or could make services or products more affordable. Efforts can also influence the supply of services through creating institutions that give consumers greater authority to challenge care of poor quality (Mills et al. 2002, Söderlund et al. 2003).

Social marketing is an approach to stimulate demand of cost-effective interventions by increasing consumer information and subsidizing access to services. This approach has been particularly used to demand services within the private sector for reproductive health and basic sanitation. Limitations have been identified with regard to the extent to which social marketing stimulates or rather limits the private sector, the targeting of the poor, and leakage of benefits to the better-off who could afford to pay full price for health services and commodities.

The use of vouchers has been tested on a limited scale as a means of targeting the poor without having to provide a generic subsidy. Protection of patients has also been pursued through the establishment of specialized government agencies to facilitate the settlement of malpractice and negligence, attempting to reduce the costs and negative consequences of litigation (Tena and Sotelo 2005).

Efforts on the supply side to improve the quality and value of private providers have included the promotion of professional training and accreditation as well as giving access to their patients to a limited range of public goods or services as for the treatment of TB (Marek et al. 1999). However, the most important efforts have been in the area of purchasing or contracting of a full range of primary or hospital services for specific population groups. These functions involve the separation of purchasing and provision at the government level and exercising stewardship functions, as already noted at the beginning of this chapter. The main challenge with these approaches lies in the capacity by government to develop contracts, set prices, and monitor and supervise private providers (Slack and Savedoff 2001; Palmer et al. 2003).

Equity in health

Policymakers in most developing countries are aware that poverty and ill health are intertwined and that important differences in health exist both across countries and provinces and across socioeconomic groups (Figs 3.6.5 and 3.6.6). It is now accepted that poverty breeds ill health and that ill health keeps poor people poor (Fig. 3.6.5). The concept of equity in health is based on a fundamental principle: that differences in health that are the result either of the exposure to unhealthy life or working conditions or

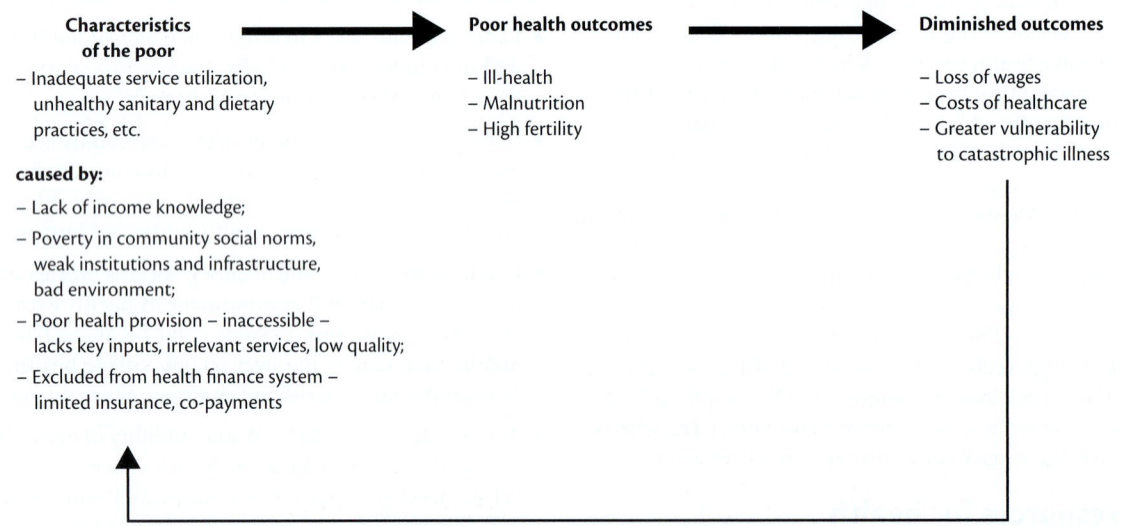

Fig. 3.6.5 The cycle of health and poverty.

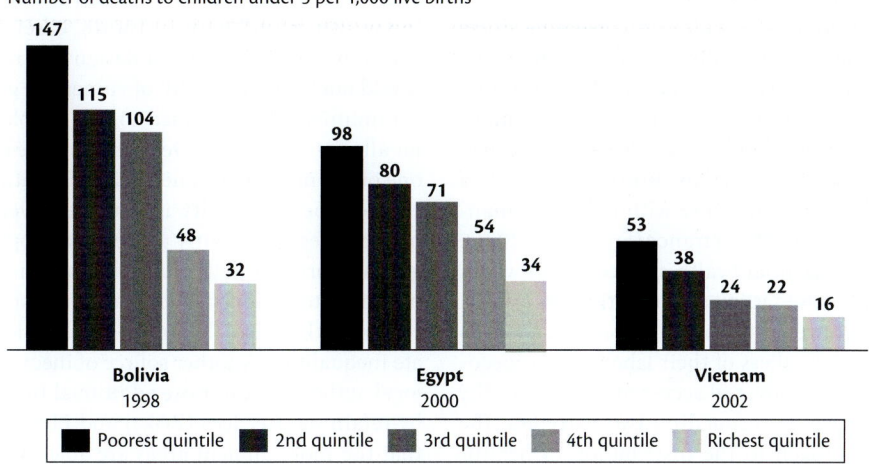

Number of deaths to children under 5 per 1,000 live births

Fig. 3.6.6 Inequalities in under-5 mortality rates within socioeconomic groups of selected developing countries, 1998–2002.
Reproduced from *The Lancet*, Volume 361, Issue 9357, Gwatkin, D.R., How well do health programmes reach the poor?, pp. 540–1, Copyright © 2003, with permission from Elsevier, http://www.sciencedirect.com/science/journal/01406736.

limited access to essential health services are morally unacceptable (Whitehead 1990; Dahlgren and Whitehead 1991).

Inequality in the health status of individuals and communities is a global phenomenon. Such disparities have been observed even in the most affluent countries but are most striking in developing countries where the poorest citizens often lack access to the most basic healthcare. Efforts to reduce such disparities have only been partially successful and too little is known on the reasons behind failure (Wagstaff 2002).

Equity can be assessed in three complementary dimensions: in health status of families, communities, and population groups; in allocation of financial, technical, and material resources; and in access to, and utilization of, high-quality services. Attention must be paid to political commitment towards equity and to equitable policy formulation. To this end, information, monitoring, and evaluation for equity should be in place. Each of these dimensions of equity and of their political and policy dimensions are now considered.

The basic dimensions of health equity

Gross inequality in health status is regarded as prima facie evidence of inequities in the healthcare system. Significant inequalities in health status are found even in the most affluent developed countries, with long traditions of national health services that are designed to provide universal coverage (Black et al. 1998; Pollock 1999). A consistent finding is the strong association between poverty and poor health as defined by such indicators as the expectation of life, the incidence of acute diseases and injuries, the prevalence of chronic diseases and disabilities, and low access to services (Gwatkin 2000; Wagstaff 2002).

This consistent association of poverty with ill health makes it necessary for health systems to address the needs of the poor, and it strengthens the case in favour of programmes for the alleviation of poverty as important strategies for health promotion. It also draws attention to the influence of factors outside the health sector on health development: the levels of education and especially of girls, which has proven to be among the most powerful factors in reducing infant mortality; access to adequate quantity of safe water and environmental sanitation; as well as food and nutrition. Lifestyle and human behaviour, including such personal choices like smoking, use of alcohol, sexual behaviour, and physical exercise, also have important effects on health outcomes (Gwatkin 2003).

Equity is also examined in terms of the allocation of resources to different sections of the population. On moral and ethical grounds, the objective of allocative equity is for public resources to be shared out in a fair manner (Taipale 1999). The simplest formula would be a uniform per capita allocation. However, if large differences in health status already exist, an equal allocation would tend to perpetuate the inequalities. It can be argued that it is the responsibility of governments to perform a re-distributive function by allocating resources from the more affluent sector of society to meet the needs of lower-income individuals and families, the so-called vertical equity already mentioned when addressing priority setting.

Another view of equity is that everyone should have an equal opportunity of receiving care. This so-called horizontal equity proposes that individuals in like situations should be treated in like manner. Access is often defined in terms of the availability of services and its geographical coverage but experience has shown that the potential access, i.e. the services are within geographical range, does not necessarily correspond to real access as measured by the utilization of services (Jacobs and Price 2006).

Marked disparities are often found in the geographical distribution of health facilities: between regions, between urban and rural areas, between rural areas and within urban areas (Phillips 1990). The differential ratios of persons per facility—hospital beds, nurses, and doctors—are used to measure the disparities. The distribution of health centres and other institutions in relation to the population—how far people have to travel to reach such facilities—are also used to indicate the uneven distribution of resources.

Political commitment for equity and equitable policy formulation

The political commitment of the government is the essential basis for promoting equity in health (Feacham 2000). The objective of equity in health fits well with the political philosophy in welfare states that have the clear goal of providing universal coverage of comprehensive healthcare for the entire population 'from the womb to the tomb'. In such countries, the question is not whether the State should embrace equity in health but how to achieve this goal in practice. Many developing countries have adopted more limited but realistic goals of providing universal access to a cost-effective package of services, together with universal financial protection through social health insurance (Frenk et al. 2006). In Mexico, the package of essential health services upon which *Seguro Popular* relied was devised using cost-effectiveness criteria as a priority-setting tool. However, the package was also a means to ensure that all citizens, regardless of their labour or socioeconomic status, have the right to universal access to healthcare. The Mexican model may be seen as reconciling two extremes: the selective, technocratic approach to the distribution of healthcare, which provides practical alternatives but is usually morally neutral, and the rights-based approach, which has a strong value foundation but has lacked operational support (Frenk and Gómez-Dantés 2007).

UHC efforts need to place health equity in the forefront, making it an end in itself and ensuring the most efficient systems are put in place to make cost-effective services available (Reidpath et al. 2012). Furthermore, UHC policy has to be rolled-out with a clear equity goal in mind so as to avoid 'regressive universalization', a paradoxical condition where the better-off would benefit first and could capture a greater proportion of benefits (Gwatkin and Ergo 2011). Research suggests that some countries manage to implement UHC equitably. Thailand implemented a universal coverage for its 47 million uninsured and was able to do so through a resource allocation scheme with strong pro-poor features that ensured equity (Limwattananon et al. 2012). However, effective access to essential health services has to be ensured through culturally appropriate models that ensure that the needs of diverse groups of population are fully met. Political commitment for equity is also required to correct the inequities that result from discrimination on the basis of gender, race, ethnic group, and religion. Often, inequalities in health status reflect the marginalization of disadvantaged groups (Brockerhoff and Hewett 2000). The plight of indigenous populations in the Americas and Australasia is a special case.

In weighing policy options, a good guideline would be to examine critically the expected impact of the selected option on equity. The formulation of health policies has to contend with a variety of pressures including the increasing demands of populations for more services, the desire to achieve maximal improvement in health of the populations served, and the need to contain costs. Reforms of the health sector aim at improving efficiency, effectiveness, cost-effectiveness, and equity. It is not always easy to reconcile these goals. For example, the delivery of care to the populations in remote areas is relatively expensive and less cost-effective than services to dense urban areas. However, in the interest of equity, health services should reach the underserved populations even in remote settings.

The impact of macroeconomic policies on health also deserves attention. For example, under pressure from the international finance agencies, some developing countries undertook Structural Adjustment Programmes (SAP) and markedly reduced public investment in health and other social sectors. UNICEF (2004) and other agencies drew attention to negative impact of SAP on the health of children. In future, careful analysis and relevant research would be used to design macroeconomic policies that would not harm the health of vulnerable groups. The international community has responded to this problem by adopting policies for alleviating poverty. Debt relief for the poorest nations has been one of the major mechanisms for alleviating poverty.

One aspect of equity is that the government should allocate financial resources fairly to the entire population. A simple demographic formula that allocates funds simply on population size may need to be adjusted to take note of special needs of particular regions; otherwise, the uniform allocation may tend to perpetuate inequalities. Another source of inequity is the degree to which local authorities can raise additional funds through taxation and by retaining user fees (Brikci and Phillips 2007). Again, the fact that the more affluent areas are able to raise much larger funds than the poorer areas may tend to widen the gap in the quantity and quality of healthcare.

Within the health budget, there is the difficult task of allocating resources to the needs of the various groups within the community (Castro-Leal et al. 2000; Makinen et al. 2000). With finite resources, even the most affluent nations have to accept limits to the services that the public sector can provide. Hence, rationing is an inevitable feature of health planning. In the interests of equity and social justice, if economies have to be made, the burden should be fairly shared among various sectors of the community. Quantitative estimates of burden of disease and of the cost-effectiveness of various interventions help to rationalize the selection of priorities (Murray 1994a, 1994b, 1994c; Hyder et al. 1998). But a point is reached at which hard choices cannot be made solely on the basis of objective measurements. At this stage, the debate must include philosophical and ethical considerations about the value of human life (Morrow and Bryant 1995).

The Poverty Reduction Strategy Papers (PRSPs) are a promising avenue to focus policymaking on the poor, although much needs to be done to influence health policymaking through this strategy (Laterveer et al. 2003). The majority of PRSPs lack country-specific data on the distribution and composition of the burden of disease, a clear identification of health system constraints and an assessment of the impact of health services on the population. More importantly, they make little effort to analyse these issues in relation to the poor. Furthermore, only a small group explicitly includes the interests of the poor in health policy design. Attention to policies aiming at enhancing equity in public health spending is even more limited. Few papers that include expenditure proposals also show pro-poor focused health budgets.

Tools are available to trace the extent to which investments at national levels benefit the poor and needy, taking into consideration the effects on income and health and considering the relative size of benefits given the levels of health and income (Gwatkin 2000 and 2003). The better-off in Africa and in India benefit far more than the poor from public spending (Castro Leal et al. 2000). Recent analyses in Mexico suggest that the incidence of health benefits is improving for the poor thanks to financial reforms, although still inequitable (Frenk et al. 2006). However, analysis of a wide range of evidence suggests that tax-based funding distributes health benefits more evenly and targets the poor more effectively than social health insurance (Wagstaff 2007).

New tools are also being developed to forecast demand for global health funding of programmes benefiting the poor (Sekhri 2006). These efforts stem from the realization that the lack of accurate and credible information about the demand for essential health products costs lives. Gaps and weaknesses in demand forecasting result in a mismatch between supply and demand—which in turn leads to both unnecessarily high prices and supply shortages.

Equity information, monitoring, and evaluation

In order to design services that are equitable and to monitor performance of health services, each health authority needs an appropriate management information system which must include measuring inequalities in health status and inequities in access to healthcare. The data collecting instruments must be designed to take note of groups and subgroups especially vulnerable groups whose access to services is restricted by geographical, economic, social, and cultural factors. It should include the usual demographic indicators—age, sex, and marital status, as well as socioeconomic indicators—race, ethnic origin, occupation, residence, and other social variables (Rosen 1999).

The health system should include mechanisms for monitoring equity objectively. Interest in measuring equity has generated some useful tools and some valuable experience is accumulating. In the first instance, monitoring equity is the responsibility of health authorities at each level of care. They must build into their service, sensitive indicators that would inform them of their performance with regard to equity and access to care.

In addition to such internal processes, it would be valuable to commission independent reviews of equity within the health system by groups outside the health departments. Another option would be to assign responsibility for a national equity watch to a local non-governmental organization.

International organizations

International organizations, bilateral and multilateral, are influential in developing country policy under many circumstances. A new breed of agencies, development banks, global health programmes (GHPs), and public–private partnerships (PPPs) are also increasing their presence in policy design, implementation and evaluation in low- and middle-income countries, particularly through financing health interventions. Global philanthropic organizations are also playing a major role in the definition of the global health agenda and in the mobilization of financial resources for health. Salient among them is the Bill and Melinda Gates Foundation (*The Lancet* 2009).

UN agencies

WHO is the lead agency for health within the UN system. In recent years, other international agencies have increased their involvement in the health sector. The United Nations Children's Fund (UNICEF) through its child survival programme, provides massive input into the health sector often in collaboration with WHO. With the leadership of James Grant in the 1980s, UNICEF was key in substantially increasing immunization coverage in poor countries. This support flattened out after Grant's period, but was boosted again when UN and private agencies established the innovative Global Alliance for Vaccines and Immunizations (GAVI).

Other UN agencies like the United Nations Fund for Population Action (UNFPA), the International Labor Organisation (ILO), and the Food and Agriculture Organization (FAO) have relevant programmes involving specific aspects of the health sector. The United Nations Development Programme (UNDP) issues a highly influential annual report that includes the Human Development Index, a composite of indicators including key health measures. The International Monetary Fund (IMF) plays a key role in national financing policies. Its Structural Adjustment Programme in the 1980s was widely critiqued—starting with UNICEF—for restraining key public health programmes in poor countries. Through its lending programme, the World Bank represents an important source of external finance for the health sector and has stimulated countries to develop more efficient and cost-effective health programmes.

Generally, these external agencies operate independently of each other at country level but there have been some attempts at coordination and collaboration. UNICEF and WHO have established mechanisms of collaboration including such formal mechanisms as the Task Force for Child Survival. WHO also sometimes executes health programmes on behalf of other external agencies. A more ambitious attempt at interagency collaboration is the UNAIDS programme; six UN agencies jointly manage this programme for the global control of HIV/AIDS epidemic.

Global health programmes and public–private partnerships

There has been a proliferation of GHPs and public–private partnerships, with more than 70 in existence. They account for close to 20 per cent of international aid for health. Examples include Roll Back Malaria (RBM), the Global Alliance for Vaccines and Immunization (GAVI), the International AIDS Vaccine Initiative (IAVI), and the Global Fund for AIDS, TB and Malaria (GFATM). The vast majority focus on communicable diseases—60 per cent of identified GHPs target the big three diseases—HIV/AIDS, TB, and malaria—with HIV/AIDS attracting the most GHPs by some margin. However, almost all the 'most neglected' diseases (such as lymphatic filariasis and leishmaniasis) are now supported by at least one GHP, many of which have been established in recent years. No GHPs address non-communicable diseases or health systems per se.

Africa has the highest number of GHPs per country, followed by Asia (East, South East, and Central). GHPs vary substantially in scale, cost, operational structure, and impact on systems at country level, including research and development as well as technical assistance and service support. GHPs which support improved service access may provide discounted or donated drugs, and give technical assistance. Some GHPs are dedicated to advocacy for increased international and/or national response and resource mobilization. The Global Fund is dedicated to financing for specific disease programmes.

GHPs are generally considered to deliver positive results in the following areas: leverage of additional funds (including from private sector); promotion of global public goods, raising profile of neglected issues, more inclusive governance, enhanced aid effectiveness through pooling of resources, and reduced commodity prices. On the other hand, common criticisms levelled at GHPs are the creation of additional complexity in an international aid system that is already overloaded. For certain GHPs, poorer countries do not meet eligibility criteria or have the capacity to frame successful proposals. Other limitations include the distortion of national priorities, the provision of international aid made ad hoc and less predictable, dysfunctional national coordination mechanisms, the establishment of parallel structures or additional burden on existing national systems, displacement of existing government services, disproportionate demands on time of Ministers and senior officials, national strategic planning and budgeting processes undermined, and diminished political accountability (Buse and Waxman 2001; Widdus 2003).

Health research

In many respects, health policy in developing countries is all about the encouragement of innovation and the scaling-up of life-saving technologies and system processes. As highlighted previously, increased access to knowledge and technology has accounted for perhaps as much as two-thirds of the 2 per cent per year rate of decline in under-5 mortality rate (Jamison 2006). Furthermore, there is increasing realization that research and evaluation can play a valuable role for shared learning from health sector reforms (González-Block 1997).

The case has been made that it is as unethical to introduce health reforms that have not been previously validated or thoroughly analysed as it is to introduce untested medical technology into healthcare. Indeed, both can have important health consequences, even more so population interventions that are adopted on a massive scale (Daniels 2006). WHO has recognized that 'Ignoring research evidence is harmful to individuals and populations, and wastes resources' (WHO 2004).

Health research—including health policy and systems research—thus plays a double role in policymaking. As a core function of health systems, research contributes knowledge as one of the most critical resources for healthcare. Formulating and implementing health research policy is therefore a key component of health policy overall. On the other hand, research on health policy and systems contributes knowledge and applications to improve the way that societies organize themselves to respond to health problems and challenges (Alliance HPSR 2004). Such knowledge is today one of the scarce resources limiting health system performance.

Health research systems and policy

WHO together with the Council on Health Research for Development and the Global Forum for Health Research advocate health research policy through the development of health research systems at national level and through a well-structured international architecture (Pang et al. 2003). Health research systems should be strengthened by building relevant capacity, developing capable leadership, providing essential monitoring and evaluation tools, improving capacity for ethical review of research, and putting in place necessary ethical standards and regulations for population health, health services, and clinical research. Health systems should further promote access to reliable, relevant, and up-to-date evidence on the effects of interventions, based on systematic reviews of the totality of available research findings (WHO 2004).

Health research systems provide a promising opportunity to link knowledge generation with practical concerns to improve health and health equity. Pioneer health research systems from Canada and the UK show that academic centres and service agencies can be related in ways that encourage the utilization of research (Lomas 2000; Kogan et al. 2006), such as networking between existing stakeholders (Department of Health 2006). A key issue is the balance between funding research through independent research councils that have science-led priorities and funding research in response to the priorities of healthcare systems.

New science frameworks are solving these dilemmas through positing a move from the traditional discipline-centred mode of knowledge production (characterized as Mode 1), towards a broader conception (Mode 2) where knowledge is generated through a context of application and thus addresses problems identified through continual negotiation between actors from a variety of settings (Gibbons et al. 1994). Another conceptualization, Pasteur's Quadrant, suggests how types of research can be considered according to two dimensions, a quest for understanding and considerations of use. This gives rise to three categories of research depending on the extent to which general understanding arises in the process of solving specific problems, or whether only pure knowledge or pure application is generated (Stokes 1997).

Evidence-based policymaking

New science frameworks are being applied to policymaking though novel strategies such as the interfaces and receptor model (Hanney et al. 2003) or the 'linkage and exchange' model proposed by the Canadian Health Services Research Foundation (Lomas 2000). Such strategies are promoting collaborative approaches to organizing health research systems. They have also promoted the use of knowledge brokers between researchers and policymakers. In the end, demonstrating the benefits of research for policymaking and for population health and national well-being will be critical (Hanney and González-Block 2006).

Evidence-based policymaking can be made a reality if research and analysis is carefully introduced along the critical steps of issue identification, policy development, implementation, monitoring, evaluation, and feedback. Evidence can provide the rationale for an initial policy direction; it can set out the nature and extent of the problem, suggest possible solutions, look to the likely impacts in the future, and evidence from piloting and evaluation can provide motivation for adjustments to a policy or the way it is to be implemented (Campbell et al. 2007).

Conclusion

Policymaking for the design, implementation, and management of effective, efficient, and equitable health systems is today more critical than ever to address the developing country health challenges. Health policy is being called not only to address the pressing needs of infectious diseases and malnutrition and the emerging problems of violence, lesions, tobacco, and obesity. New challenges are being addressed, including the fight against poverty and the increasing global threats. The belief that sound health policymaking can contribute to democracy, economic growth, and global security has influenced the availability of greater financial resources for health. However, relaxing this constraint has now brought much greater awareness to needs in key areas such as human resources and health system strengthening and research.

The information now being produced can provide valuable guidance to policymakers, although it also threatens to overpower capacities in poor countries. Not only must policymaking be knowledge-based—it must also be result-oriented. Careful planning and skilled management can achieve good results even where financial resources are limited. The countries that have achieved good health at low cost challenge other countries to adapt and adopt relevant aspects of their policies.

Policymakers must give high priority to strategies that will eliminate the major items of the unfinished agenda that still plague many developing countries. Many lives can be saved and much disability prevented by measures like boosting immunization programmes, ensuring access to adequate supplies of safe water and good sanitation, providing effective treatment for common childhood ailments, and ensuring skilled care during childbirth including emergency obstetric care (Center for Global Development 2007). More daunting tasks include the pandemic of HIV/AIDS and the emerging non-communicable challenges, which may require complex and expensive care. Evidence has shown that progress can be made through the application of social and behavioural interventions, which can act on those risks that are responsible for the increasing burden of disease associated to chronic ailments and injuries in the developing world. In addition, developing nations must invest in health system strengthening so they can better respond to the increasingly complex challenges that will define the global and national agendas in the decades ahead.

Key points

◆ Health policymaking in developing countries is intricately related to global health policies and actors.

◆ Health financing has been increasing, thanks to policy advocacy, but more resources and improved governance are required to meet the MDGs.

◆ Policy tools are available to support decision-making at national and global levels.

◆ Equity and efficiency trade-offs should be addressed on the basis of sound research.

References

Alliance AHPSR (2004). *Strengthening Health Systems: The Role and Promise of Policy and Systems Research*. Geneva: Alliance AHPSR.

Anand, S. and Hanson, K. (1997). Disability-adjusted life years: a critical review. *Journal of Health Economics*, 16(6), 685–702.

Bankauskaite, V., Dubois, H.F.W., and Saltman, R. (2007). Patterns of decentralization across European health systems. In R. Saltman, R. Busse and E. Mossialos (eds.) *Decentralization in Health Care*, pp. 22–43. Maidenhead: Open University Press.

Barr, V.J., Robinson, S., Marin-Link, B., et al. (2003). The expanded chronic care model. An integration of concepts and strategies from population health promotion and the chronic care model. *Hospital Quarterly*, 7(1), 73–82.

Berman, P.A. (1997). National health accounts in developing countries: appropriate methods and recent applications. *Health Economics*, 6, 11–30.

Berman, T.J. and Bossert, T. (2000). *A Decade of Health Sector Reform in Developing Countries: What Have We Learned?* Data for Decision Making Project. Cambridge, MA: IHSG, Harvard School of Public Health.

Black, D., Morris, J.N., Smith, C., et al. (1998). Better benefits for health: plan to implement the central recommendation of the Acheson report. *British Medical Journal*, 318, 724–7. Available at: http://otpubh.oxfordmedicine.com/cgi/external_ref?access_num=000079495700032&link_type=ISI.

Bossert, T. (1998). Analyzing the decentralization of health systems in developing countries: decision space, innovation and performance. *Social Science & Medicine*, 47, 1513–27.

Bossert, T. and Beauvais, J.C. (2002). Decentralization of health systems in Ghana, Zambia, Uganda and the Philippines: a comparative analysis of decision space. *Health Policy and Planning*, 17, 14–31.

Brikci, N. and Philips, M. (2007). User fees or equity funds in low-income countries. *The Lancet*, 369(9555), 10–11.

Brockerhoff, M. and Hewett, P.C. (2000). Inequality of child mortality among ethnic groups in sub-Saharan Africa. *Bulletin of the World Health Organization*, 78, 30–41.

Brown, A.M., Foster, A., Norton, A., et al. (2001). *The Status of Sector-Wide Approaches*. Working Paper 142. London: ODI.

Brush, B., Sochalski, J., and Berger, A. (2004). Imported care: recruiting foreign nurses to US health care facilities. *Health Affairs*, 23(5), 78–87.

Buse, K. and Waxman, A. (2001). Public–private health partnerships: a strategy for WHO. *Bulletin of the World Health Organization*, 79(8), 748–54.

Campbell, S., Benita, S., Coates, E., et al. (2007). *Analysis for Policy: Evidence-Based Policy in Practice*. London: Government Social Research Unit, HM Treasury.

Castro-Leal, F., Dayton, J., Demery, L., et al. (2000). Public spending on health care in Africa: do the poor benefit? *Bulletin of the World Health Organization*, 78(1), 66–74.

Center for Global Development (2007). *Millions Saved: Proven Successes in Global Health. 2007 Edition*. Washington, DC: CGD.

Clemens, M., Radelet, S., and Bhavnani, R. (2004). *Counting Chickens When They Hatch: The Short-Term Effect of Aid on Growth*. Working Paper 44. Washington, DC: Center for Global Development.

Commission on Macroeconomics and Health (2001). *Macroeconomics and Health: Investing in Health for Economic Development—Report of the Commission on Macroeconomics and Health*. Geneva: World Health Organization.

Chua, H.T. and Cheah, J.C.H. (2012). Financing Universal Coverage in Malaysia: a case study. *BMC Public Health*, 12(Suppl 1), S7. Available at: http://www.biomedcentral.com/content/pdf/1471-2458-12-S1-S7.pdf.

Dahlgren, G. and Whitehead, M. (1991). *Policies and Strategies to Promote Equity in Health*. Copenhagen: WHO Regional Office.

Daniels, N. (2006). Toward ethical review of health system transformations. *American Journal of Public Health*, 96, 3.

Daniels, N. (2008). *Just Health. Meeting Health Needs Fairly*. Cambridge: Cambridge University Press.

Daniels, N., Flores, W., Pannarunotha, S., et al. (2005). An evidence-based approach to benchmarking the fairness of health-sector reform in developing countries. *Bulletin of the World Health Organization*, 83(7), 534–9.

Daniels, N., Light, D.W., and Caplan, R.L. (1996). *Benchmarks of Fairness for Health Care Reform*. New York: Oxford University Press.

Davis, J., Donaldson, L., and Schoorman, D. (1997). Towards a stewardship theory of management. *Academy of Management Review*, 22(1), 20–47.

De Savigny, D., Kasale, H., Mbuya, C., et al. (2004). *Fixing Health Systems*. Ottawa: IDRC.

Department of Health (2006). *Best Research for Best Health: A New National Health Research Strategy*. London: Department of Health.

Evans, R., Barer, M., and Marmor, T. (1994). *Why Are Some People Healthy and Others Not? The Determinants of Health of Populations*. New York: Aldine de Gruyter, Hawthome.

Feacham, R.G.A. (2000). Poverty and inequity: a proper focus for the new century. *Bulletin of the World Health Organization*, 78(1), 1.

Filmer, D., Hammer, J.S., and Pritchett, L.S. (2000). Weak links in the chain: a diagnosis of health policy in poor countries. *World Bank Research Observer*, 15(2), 199–224.

Frenk, J. (1994). Dimensions of health system reform. *Health Policy*, 27(1), 19–34.

Frenk, J. and Gómez-Dantés, O. (2007). La globalización y la nueva salud pública. *Salud Publica de Mexico*, 49(2), 156–64.

Frenk, J., Gonzalez-Pier, E., Gómez-Dantes, O., et al. (2006). Comprehensive reform to improve health system performance in Mexico. *The Lancet*, 368, 1524–34.

Gakidou, E., Lozano, R., González-Pier, E., et al. (2006). Assessing the effect of the 2001–06 Mexican health reform: an interim report card. *The Lancet*, 368(9550), 1920–35.

Garret, L. (2007). The challenge of global health. *Foreign Affairs*, 86, 14–38.

Gericke, C.A., Kurowski, C., Ranson, M.K., et al. (2005). Intervention complexity—a conceptual framework to inform priority-setting in health. *Bulletin of the World Health Organization*, 83, 285–93.

Gibbons, M., Limoges, C., Nowotny, H., et al. (1994). *The New Production of Knowledge: The Dynamics of Science and Research in Contemporary Societies*. London: Sage.

Gilson, L. (2003). Trust and the development of health care as a social institution. *Social Science & Medicine*, 56, 1453–68.

González-Block, M.A. (1997). Comparative research and analysis methods for shared learning from health system reforms. *Health Policy*, 42, 187–209.

González-Block, M.A., Akisa, A.B., and Chowdhury, A. (2012). Health systems research and infectious diseases of poverty: from the margins to the mainstream. In WHO (ed.) *Global Report for Research on Infectious Diseases of Poverty*, 67–93. Geneva: WHO.

Gwatkin, D.R. (2000). Critical reflection: health inequalities and the health of the poor: what do we know? What can we do? *Bulletin of the World Health Organization*, 78(1), 3–18.

Gwatkin, D.R. (2003). How well do health programmes reach the poor? *The Lancet*, 361, 540–1.

Gwatkin, D.R. and Ergo, A. (2011). Universal health coverage: friend or foe of health equity? *The Lancet*, 377, 2160–1.

Hanney, S. and González-Block, M.A. (2006). Building health research systems to achieve better health. *Health Research Policy and Systems*, 4, 1–6. Available at: http://www.health-policy-systems.com/content/4/1/10.

Hanney, S.R., González-Block, M.A., Buxton, M.J., et al. (2003). The utilisation of health research in policy-making: concepts, examples and methods of assessment. *Health Research Policy and Systems*, 1, 2.

Hecht, R.M. and Shah, R. (2006). Recent trends and innovations in development assistance for health. In D.T. Jamison, J.G. Breman, A.R. Measham, et al. (eds.) *Disease Control Priorities in Developing Countries* (2nd ed.), pp. 243–58. Washington, DC: Oxford University Press for The World Bank.

Hutton, G. (2002). *Decentralization and the Sector-Wide Approach in the Health Sector*. Basel: SDS.

Hyder, A.A., Rotllant, G., and Morrow, R.H. (1998). Measuring the burden of disease: healthy life-years. *American Journal of Public Health*, 88, 196–202.

Irwin, A., Valentine, N., Brown, C., et al. (2006). The Commission on Social Determinants of Health: tackling the social roots of health inequities. *PLoS Medicine*, 3(6), e106.

Jacobs, B. and Price, N. (2006). Improving access for the poorest to public sector health services: insights from Kirivong Operational Health District in Cambodia. *Health Policy Plan*, 21(1), 27–39.

Jamison, D.T. (2006). Investing in health. In D.T. Jamison, J.G. Breman, A.R. Measham, et al. (eds.) *Disease Control Priorities in Developing Countries* (2nd ed.), pp. 3–34. Washington, DC: Oxford University Press for The World Bank.

Joint Learning Initiative (2004). *Human Resources for Health. Overcoming the Crisis*. Cambridge, MA: Harvard University Press.

King, G., Gakidou, E., Imami, K., et al. (2009). Public policy for the poor? A randomized assessment of the Mexican universal health insurance programme. *The Lancet*, 373, 1447–54.

Knaul, F.M. and Frenk, J. (2005). Health insurance in Mexico: achieving universal coverage through structural reform. *Health Affairs (Project Hope)*, 24(6), 1467–76.

Knaul, F.M., Gonzalez-Pier, E., Gomez Dantes, O., et al. (2012). The quest for universal health coverage: achieving social protection for all in Mexico. *The Lancet*, 380, 1259–79.

Kogan, M., Henkel, M., and Hanney, S. (2006). *Government and Research: Thirty Years of Evolution* (2nd ed.). Dordrecht: Springer.

Laterveer, L., Niessen, L.W., and Yazbeck, A.S. (2003). Pro-poor health policies in poverty reduction strategies. *Health Policy Plan*, 18, 138–45.

Lim, S.S., Vos, T., Flaxman, G., et al. (2012) A comparative risk assessment of burden of disease and injury attributable to 67 risk factors and risk factor clusters in 21 regions, 1990–2010: a systematic analysis for the Global Burden of Disease Study 2010. *The Lancet*, 380, 2224–60.

Limwattananon, S., Tangcharoensathien, V., Tisayaticom, K., Boonyapaisarncharoen, T., and Prakongsai, P. (2012), Why has the Universal Coverage Scheme in Thailand achieved a pro-poor public subsidy for health care? *BMC Public Health*, 12(Suppl. 1), S6. Available at: http://www.biomedcentral.com/content/pdf/1471-2458-12-S1-S6.pdf.

Lomas, J. (2000). Using 'linkage and exchange' to move research into policy at a Canadian Foundation. *Health Affairs*, 19, 236–40.

Londoño, J. and Frenk, J. (1997). Structured pluralism: towards an innovative model for health system reform in Latin America. *Health Policy*, 41(1), 1–36.

Lozano, R., Soliz, P., Gakidou, E., et al. (2006). Benchmarking of performance of Mexican states with effective coverage. *The Lancet*, 368(9548), 1729–41.

Lucas, A.O. (2005). Human resources for health in Africa. Better training and firm national policies might manage the brain drain. *British Medical Journal*, 331, 1037–8.

Makinen, M., Waters, H., Rauch, M., et al. (2000). Inequalities in health care use and expenditures: empirical data from eight developing countries and countries in transition. *Bulletin of the World Health Organization*, 78, 55–65.

Marek, T., Diallo, I., Ndiaye, B., et al. (1999). Successful contracting of prevention services: fighting malnutrition in Senegal and Madagascar. *Health Policy and Planning*, 14(4), 382–9.

Mathers, C.D. and Loncar, D. (2006). Projections of global mortality and burden of disease from 2002 to 2030. *PLoS Medicine*, 3(11), e442.

McCarthy, J. and Maine, D. (1992). A framework for analyzing the determinants of maternal mortality. *Studies in Family Planning*, 23, 23–33.

McIntyre, D. and Mills, A. (2012). Research to support universal coverage reforms in Africa: the SHIELD project. *Health Policy and Planning*, 27, i1–i3

Medlin, C.A., Chowdhury, M., Jamison, D.T., et al. (2006). Improving the health of populations: lessons of experience. In D.T. Jamison, J.G. Breman, A.R. Measham, et al. (eds.) *Disease Control Priorities in Developing Countries* (2nd ed.), pp. 165–80. Washington, DC: Oxford University Press for The World Bank.

Meng, Q., Shi, G., Yang, H., et al. (2004). *Health Policy and Systems Research in China*. Geneva: UNICEF/UNDP/World Bank/WHO. Special Programme for Research and Training in Tropical Diseases (TDR).

Mills, A., Brugha, R., Hanson, K., et al. (2002). What can be done about the private health sector in low-income countries? *Bulletin of the World Health Organization*, 80, 325–30.

Molineux, D. and Nantulya, V. (2004). Linking disease control programmes in rural Africa: a pro-poor strategy to reach Abuja targets and Millennium Development Goals. *British Medical Journal*, 328(7448), 1129–32.

Morrow, R.H. and Bryant, J. (1995). Health policy approaches to measuring and valuing human life: conceptual and ethical issues. *American Journal of Public Health*, 85, 1356–60.

Murray, C.J. (1994a). Quantifying the burden of disease: the technical basis for disability-adjusted life years. *Bulletin of the World Health Organization*, 72, 429–45.

Murray, C.J. (1994b). National health expenditures: a global analysis. *Bulletin of the World Health Organization*, 72, 623–37.

Murray, C.J. (1994c). Cost-effectiveness analysis and policy choices: investing in health systems. *Bulletin of the World Health Organization*, 72, 663–74.

Murray, C.J.L. and Evans, D.B. (eds.) (2003). *Health Systems Performance Assessment: Debates, Methods and Empiricism*. Geneva: WHO.

Murray, C.J. and Frenk, J. (2000). A framework for assessing the performance of health systems. *Bulletin of the World Health Organization*, 78(6), 717–31.

Murray, C.J.L., Vos, T., Lozano, R., et al. (2012). Disability-adjusted life years (DALYs) for 291 diseases and injuries in 21 regions, 1990–2010: a systematic analysis for the Global Burden of Disease Study 2010. *The Lancet*, 380, 2197–223.

Musgrove, P. (1999). Public spending on health care: how are different criteria related? *Health Policy*, 47, 207–23.

Palmer, N., Mills, A., Wadee, H., et al. (2003). A new face for private providers in developing countries: what implications for public health? *Bulletin of the World Health Organization*, 81(4), 292–7.

Pang, T., Sadana, R., Hanney, S., et al. (2003). Knowledge for better health—a conceptual framework and foundation for health research systems. *Bulletin of the World Health Organization*, 81(11), 815–20.

Paris Declaration on AID effectiveness Ownership, Harmonisation Alignment Results and Mutual Accountability Paris, 2 March 2005.

Phillips, D.R. (1990). *Health and Health Care in the Third World*. Chapter 4. London: Longmans.

Pollock, A.M. (1999). Devolution and health: challenges to Scotland and Wales. *British Medical Journal*, 319, 94–8.

Preker, A.S., Suzuki, E., Bustero, F., et al. (2003). *Costing the Millennium Development Goals*. Background paper to The Millennium Development Goals for Health: Rising to the Challenges. Washington, DC: World Bank.

Reidpath, D., Olafsdottir, A.E., Pokhrel, S., and Allotey, P. (2012). The fallacy of the equity–efficiency trade off: rethinking the efficient health system. *BMC Public Health*, 12(Suppl 1), S3. Available at: http://www.biomedcentral.com/content/pdf/1471-2458-12-S1S3.pdf.

Roberts, M.J., Hsiao, W., Berman, P., and Reich, M.R. (2003). *Getting Health Reform Right: A Guide to Improving Performance and Equity*. New York: Oxford University Press.

Rosen, M. (1999). Data needs in studies on equity in health and access to care—ethical considerations. *Acta Oncologica*, 38, 71–5.

Sachs, J. (2004). Health in the developing world: achieving the Millennium Development Goals. *Bulletin of the World Health Organization*, 82(12), 947–52.

Saltman, B. and Ferroussier-Davis, O. (2000). On the concept of stewardship in health policy. *Bulletin of the World Health Organization*, 78(6), 732–9.

Schneider, M. (2001). *The Setting of Health Research Priorities in South Africa*. Johannesburg: South African Medical Research Council, Burden of Disease Research Unit.

Sekhri, N. (2006). *Forecasting for Global Health: New Money, New Products & New Markets*. Background Paper for the Forecasting Working Group. Washington, DC: Center for Global Development.

Slack, K. and Savedoff, W.D. (2001). *Public Purchaser-Private Provider Contracting for Health Services: Examples from Latin America and the Caribbean*. Sustainable Development Department Technical Paper 111. Washington, DC: Inter-American Development Bank.

Söderlund, N., Mendoza-Arana, P., and Goudge, J. (2003). *The New Public/Private Mix in Health: Exploring the Changing Landscape*. Geneva: Alliance for Health Policy and Systems Research.

Stokes, D.E. (1997). *Pasteur's Quadrant: Basic Science and Technological Innovation*. Washington, DC: Brookings Institute.

Taipale, V. (1999). Ethics and allocation of health resources—the influence of poverty on health. *Acta Oncologica*, 38(1), 51–5.

Tang, S., Tao, J., and Bekedam, H. (2012). Controlling cost escalation of healthcare: making universal health coverage sustainable in China. *BMC Public Health*, 12(Suppl. 1), S8.

Tena-Tamayo, C. and Sotelo, J. (2005). Malpractice in Mexico: arbitration not litigation. *British Medical Journal*, 331, 448–51.

The Lancet (2009). What has the Gates Foundation done for health? *The Lancet*, 373, 1577.

Ugalde, A. and Homedes, N. (2006). Decentralization: the long road from theory to practice. In A. Ugalde and N. Homedes (eds.) *Health Services Decentralization in Mexico. A Case Study in State Reform*, pp. 3–44. La Jolla: Center for US-Mexico Studies.

Unger, J.P., De Paepe, P., and Green, A. (2003). A code of best practice for disease control programmes to avoid damaging health care services in developing countries. *International Journal of Health Planning and Management*, 18, S27–S39.

UNICEF (2004). *Progress for Children. A Child Survival Report Card: Number 1*. New York: UNICEF.

Wagstaff, A. (2002). Poverty and health sector inequalities. *Bulletin of the World Health Organization*, 80(2), 97–105.

Wagstaff, A. (2007). *Social Health Insurance Reexamined*. World Bank Policy Research Working Paper 4111. Washington, DC: World Bank.

Wagstaff, A. and Wanwiphang, M. (2012a). *Universal Health Care and Informal Labor Markets: The Case of Thailand*. Washington, DC: World Bank.

Wagstaff, A. and Wanwiphang, M. (2012b). *The Health Effects of Universal Health Care: Evidence from Thailand*. Washington, DC: World Bank.

Whitehead, M. (1990). *The Concepts and Principles of Equity and Health*. Copenhagen: WHO Regional Office.

Widdus, R. (2003). Public–private partnerships for health require thoughtful evaluation. *Bulletin of the* World Health Organization, 81(4), 235.

World Bank–IMF Development Committee (2003). *Supporting Sound Policies with Adequate and Appropriate Financing*. Discussion paper. Washington, DC: World Bank.

World Health Organization (2000). *Health Systems: Improving Performance. World Health Report 2000*. Geneva: WHO.

World Health Organization (2003). *Guide to Producing National Health Accounts with Special Applications for Low-Income and Middle-Income Countries*. Geneva: WHO.

World Health Organization (2004). *Ministerial Summit (Web)*. World Health Organization. *World Health Report 2004. Changing History*. Ginebra: WHO.

World Health Organization (2005). *Health Systems Financing. The Path to Universal Coverage*. Geneva: WHO. Available at: http://www.who.int/whr/2010/overview.pdf.

World Health Organization (2007). *Health Metrics Network Biennial Report 2005/2006*. Geneva: WHO.

World Health Organization (2011). *Implementation Research for the Control of Infectious Diseases of Poverty. Strengthening the Evidence Base for the Access and Delivery of New and Improved Tools, Strategies and Interventions*. Geneva: WHO. Available at: http://www.who.int/tdr/publications/documents/access_report.pdf.

3.7

Public health policy in developed countries

John Powles

Introduction: scope of public health policy

>...wise consumption is a far more difficult art than wise production
>
> John Ruskin, 1862 (Ruskin 1985)

The scope and purpose of public health policy may be seen as implicit in widely used definitions of public health. Winslow's definition, as adapted by the Acheson Report in England, is: 'The science and art of preventing disease, prolonging life and promoting health through organised efforts of society' (Secretary of State for Social Services 1988).

Public health policies might thus be thought of as the policies that guide these 'organized efforts' to protect and improve health. The scope of such policies depends a good deal, however, on what is considered to be entailed by 'organized efforts', and on how centrally 'organized efforts' are understood to be related to efforts that are more decentralized, more informal, less organized, perhaps even 'spontaneous'. The relative importance and legitimacy of centralized versus decentralized uses of knowledge in protecting and enhancing health is a central and controversial underlying theme in discussion of public health policy.

We need first to define our scope by deciding which countries are currently classifiable as 'developed'. Many answers are clearly possible, but for the purposes of this chapter the boundary will be drawn as follows: the 31 high-income members of the Organisation for Economic Cooperation and Development (OECD) plus six member states of the European Union (EU) that are not included in the OECD list (these six are indicated with '(EU)' in the following). European developed countries divide into western and 'post-communist' groups: western—Austria, Belgium, Cyprus (EU), Denmark, Finland, France, Germany, Greece, Iceland, Ireland, Italy, Luxembourg, Malta (EU), Netherlands, Norway, Portugal, Spain, Sweden, Switzerland, United Kingdom; post-communist—Bulgaria (EU), Czech Republic, Estonia, Hungary, Latvia (EU), Lithuania (EU), Poland, Romania (EU), Slovakia, Slovenia. OECD members elsewhere include two countries each in East Asia—Japan and South Korea; North America—Canada and the United States; and Oceania—Australia and New Zealand. In addition there is Israel which will be grouped with Western Europe in this discussion.

Discussion of public health policy can be pursued from either end of an epistemological/disciplinary polarity—or from somewhere in between. At one pole are sociological and political science analyses of how 'health problems make it onto the political agenda' and studies of the social and political processes by which policies come to be articulated, adopted, and implemented. Such investigations may be pursued without formally connecting policies to actual health trends. Oliver's discussion of 'the politics of public health policy' in the United States (Oliver 2006) illustrates this approach. At the other, 'objectivist' or 'scientific' pole are works concerned above all, to assess the effects of policy on health trends. *Successes and Failures of Health Policy in Europe* by Mackenbach and McKee (2013) illustrates this approach. This chapter will begin from this second viewpoint.

The unit of analysis for policy is typically the nation state. The diversity of health experience in developed countries over recent decades provides extremely rich raw material for exploring connections between political and economic institutions and policies on the one hand and health trends on the other. The experience of individual countries will be noted according to what it might be telling us about the variety of experience among developed countries. The chapter will focus on the relationship of policy to average levels of population health, not on relationships with inequalities in health levels within countries. This is dealt with in Chapter 2.3. The topics considered will be deliberately restricted to those most closely linked to the main theme. Specialized topics receive attention elsewhere in this textbook.

The remainder of the chapter will be organized as follows: the second section surveys trends in survival over the last four decades. The third section explores, through case studies of road traffic injuries, tobacco and circulatory diseases, the apparent sources of success in reducing non-communicable diseases (NCDs) and injuries in adults. The fourth section notes two public health failures—obesity and habitat degradation—and the fifth considers wider determinants of average levels of population health. The sixth concludes with a tentative vindication of pluralism—ideological, methodological, and institutional.

Success and failure among developed countries

For the 37 developed countries, proportional changes between 1970 and 2010 in the probability of dying before the 5th birthday (child mortality) and the probability of 15-year-olds dying before their 60th birthday (adult mortality) are shown in Fig. 3.7.1. The

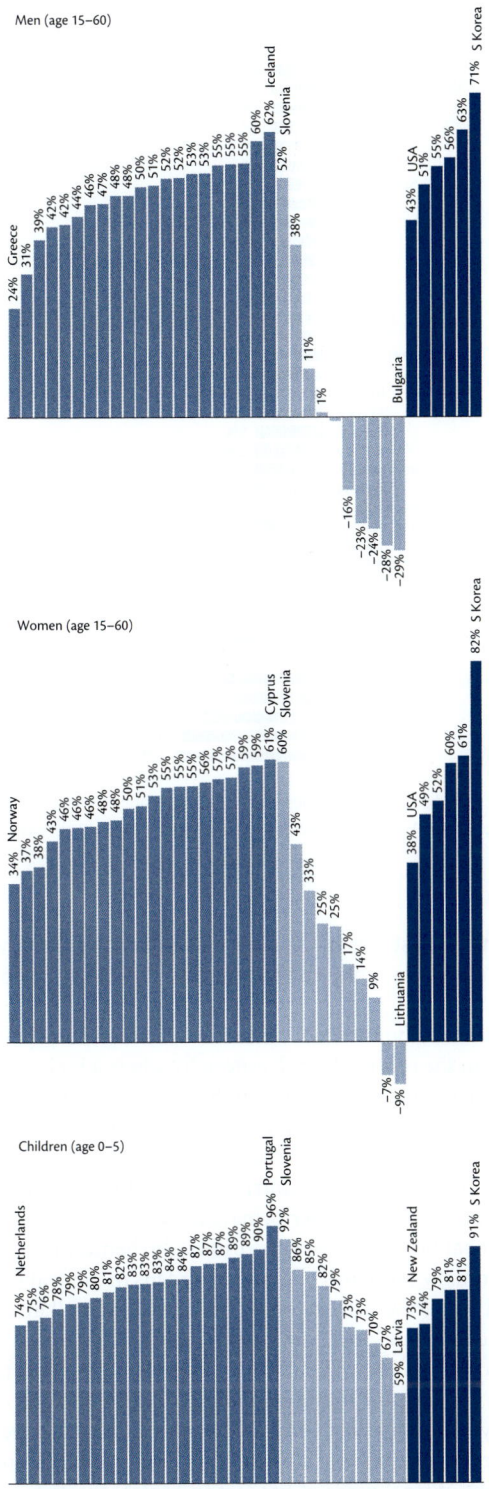

Fig. 3.7.1 Proportional reductions, between 1970 and 2010, in risks* of dying before the 5th birthday and of dying between 15th and 60th birthdays in 37 developed countries, grouped into 21 western European countries (medium blue), ten central and eastern European countries (light blue) and six countries from north America, Australasia, and Asia (dark blue). They are ranked successively in ascending, descending and ascending order to illustrate the extent of variation within and between the groups of countries. (*The calculated risks would apply if mortality rates for each reference year were sustained indefinitely.) Source: data from *The Lancet*, Volume 380, Issue Wang, H. et al., Age-specific and sex-specific mortality in 187 countries, 1970–2010: a systematic analysis for the Global Burden of Disease Study 2010, pp. 2071–94, Online appendix, Copyright © 2012.

absolute adult mortality risks at the end of this period are given in Fig. 3.7.2.

First, a guide to the layout: countries are placed in three groups—West European countries (in medium blue and on the left) are sorted from worst, left to best, right; next are the post-communist countries (light blue), sorted from best to worst; the third group includes North America, Australasia, and east Asia (dark blue), sorted from worst to best.

This figure reveals broad similarities and stark contrasts. Reductions in child mortality (bottom panel) have been universal and substantial, reaching a remarkable 96 per cent in Portugal (from a 7.4 per cent risk of death before the 5th birthday in 1970 down to a 0.3 per cent risk in 2010). The median reduction in the post-communist countries (76 per cent) was below that for countries of Western Europe (83 per cent), but also slightly better than that for the United States (74 per cent).

As attention moves from changes in the risks of death in childhood to changes in the risks of premature adult death in women and men, the variation within and between country groups increases markedly. Within the Western European group, reductions in the risks of premature adult death were around twice as great for men in Italy, Malta, and Iceland as for men in Greece and Denmark. Far more striking were the disparate performances among the post-communist states—ranging from a halving of risks in Slovenian men to an almost 30 per cent increase in Bulgarian men. (The values for Slovenia for 1970 have been imputed and are more uncertain; however, the documented Slovenian trend was strongly downward through the 1980s, differing from the other countries then under communist rule.) For six of the ten post-communist countries, risks of premature death in men were higher in 2010 than they had been 40 years earlier. The biggest reductions in adult male mortality over this period were in South Korea (71 per cent), followed by Australia (63 per cent). The reduction in the United States (43 per cent) was below the median for Western Europe (50 per cent).

For women outside of post-communist Europe, proportional reductions were broadly comparable to those for men but the rank ordering of countries differed somewhat. Within the post-communist group, heterogeneity was again marked, with Slovenia equalling the best performing Western countries while Latvia and Lithuania failed, in 2010, to regain the level of adult female survival they had achieved 40 years earlier.

The absolute risks of premature adult mortality attained by 2010 (Fig. 3.7.2) also reveal a marked heterogeneity. For males, levels were more than three times higher in Hungary and Estonia (both now classified by the World Bank as high income (World Bank 2013)) than they were in the most favoured countries such as Australia, Switzerland, Netherlands, Malta, Sweden, and Iceland. For females, the range was somewhat less but still exceeded twofold. The poor ranking of US women was notable, with their mortality risks exceeded only by some (but not all) of the post-communist countries.

These data present powerful challenges for those wishing to link attained levels of health to differences in political and economic histories and health policies. The contrast between the relative homogeneity in the reduction in child mortality and the diversity of trends in adults calls for explanation. On the provisional assumption that knowledge-based processes are of primary

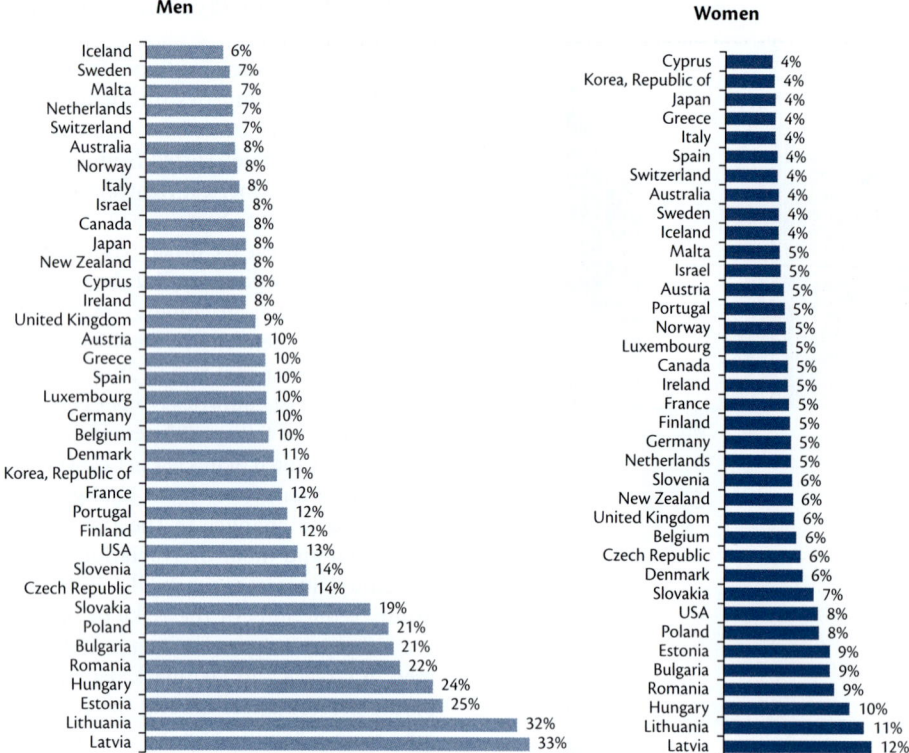

Fig. 3.7.2 Risks of dying between the 15th and 60th birthdays based on the age-specific mortality risks of 2010. Countries are ranked separately by sex.
Source: data from *The Lancet*, Volume 380, Issue Wang, H. et al., Age-specific and sex-specific mortality in 187 countries, 1970–2010: a systematic analysis for the Global Burden of Disease Study 2010, pp. 2071–94, Online appendix, Copyright © 2012.

importance in the explanation of health trends, this relative homogeneity could be consistent with:

1. Advances in knowledge of how to protect and enhance child health being widely diffused among professional medical staff and general publics in all developed countries.

2. Action to protect child health, based on that knowledge, being seen as both desirable and legitimate across diverse political settings.

3. Much of this action being amenable to central (state) initiation, coordination or support, resulting in widespread realization of the gains promised by the advances of knowledge (immunization providing an obvious example).

For adults, one question compels attention before all others: why was communist rule in Europe so destructive of adult health in most—but not all—countries? Why was this more so for males than females? And why was this public health failure so specific? It did not, as already noted, apply to child health. Nor was it manifest in adults before around 1970. The public health system developed in the Soviet Union in the 1920s (based on a network of 'sanitary-epidemiological stations' and often referred to as the Shemashko system after the first People's Commissar of Public Health), dealt effectively with the problems, predominantly of communicable disease, that it was designed to address (Field 1967; Riley 2008). The countries of central Europe that implemented this system in the first two decades of communist rule achieved rapid declines in adult mortality: Poland almost closed its life expectancy gap with West Germany by the mid 1960s (Zatonski

1996), and in East Germany adult male mortality was lower than in West Germany until the late 1970s (Fig. 3.7.3) (Anonymous 2013c).

Discussion of the even more extreme trends in Russia has directed attention to the role to alcohol, especially where a high average volume of consumption has been combined with the binge drinking pattern. However, among the developed countries in our sample, the binge drinking pattern is mainly limited to the Baltic states and Poland; it is not typical of countries such as Hungary and Bulgaria, whose poor public health performance also needs explanation.

The Global Burden of Disease 2010 study (henceforth GBD) provides summary estimates of disease burdens in 'central Europe' in 1990 and 2010 (this GBD category includes some Balkan countries not included in our 'post-communist' group) (Anonymous 2013a). These show that cardiovascular diseases were the dominant contributors to the continuing gap with Western Europe. In 2010, rates of years of life lost from cardiovascular causes were more than twice as high in central as in Western Europe, accounting for 43 per cent of total years of life lost in central Europe, compared to 29 per cent in Western Europe. Estimates from the GBD 2010 study of the contributions of leading risk factors to rates of years of life lost in 1990 and 2010 show substantial contributions from the following risk factors (and risk factor clusters) to the central/west Europe gap in years of life lost in males in both 1990 and 2010:

1. Physiological risk factors (blood pressure, blood cholesterol levels, raised BMI, raised plasma glucose)

2. Diet and physical activity (including intakes of fruit and vegetables, sodium, dietary fats)

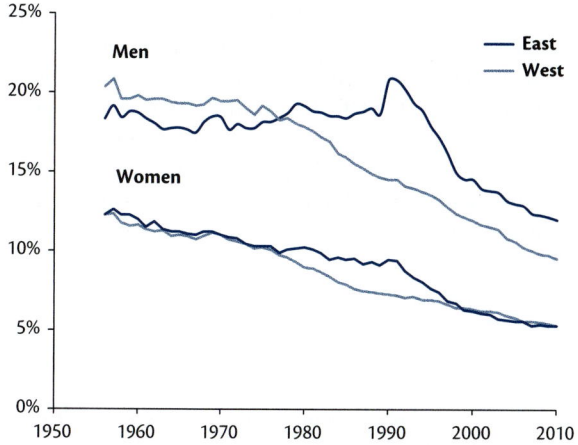

Fig. 3.7.3 East and West Germany (former boundaries): trends in the risk of dying between the 15th and 60th birthdays, 1956 to 2010*. (* The calculated risks would apply if mortality rates for each calendar year were sustained indefinitely.) Source: data from *Human Mortality Database*, University of California, Berkeley, USA, and Max Planck Institute for Demographic Research, Germany, available at http://www.mortality.org.

3. Tobacco

4. Alcohol.

The gap in the contributions of these risk factors did not generally reduce over this period (which corresponds to the period since the end of communist rule). For females, tobacco and alcohol made smaller contributions to the central/west differences than did the physiological risk factors and diet. The lack of convergence of the burdens attributable to these risk factors between 1990 and 2010 may appear surprising given that the mortality trajectories of most of the post-communist countries changed abruptly in the early years of the post-communist period (Wang et al. 2012). However, the declines in adult mortality risks tended to be of comparable magnitude, proportionally, in the central and the western groups (30–40 per cent over the 20-year period) so while there was consistency in the direction of change, there was little overall convergence in absolute levels by 2010.

The GBD 2010 data also cover the other developed regions. Years of life lost attributable to these leading risk factors tended to be lower in 'high-income East Asia' (mainly Japan and South Korea) in both time periods. Trends for Australasia were more favourable than those for North America, consistent with their divergent mortality trends. However, the GBD comparative risk assessments generally fail to illuminate the reasons for the increasing divergence in mortality risks between North America and Western Europe. (Some cautions are in order in interpreting these GBD estimates: sources for risk factor levels were scarce for many countries and gaps were filled using Bayesian imputation (with typical 95 per cent uncertainty ranges of the order of plus or minus 6 per cent). Also aggregation of specific risk factors (especially in the physiological and diet groups) involves some double counting, e.g. the effects of adiposity are partially mediated by effects on blood pressure—so the true combined effects of these aggregates will be smaller than their sums (Lim et al. 2012).)

The poor performance of the United States in terms of population health measures deserves note. This has occurred in spite of an extraordinarily high level of expenditure on professional medicine and of major investment in the creation of new knowledge in medicine and public health. Comparisons with Australia and with Western Europe for the period since 1970 show that the US disadvantage has extended across a wide range of causes. Trends over time show adult mortality decline slowing in the United States since the 1980s, resulting in increasing the gap with other developed countries; mortality levels reached in the United States by 2010 were comparable to those achieved more than 20 years earlier in the leading countries.

In summary:

1. The sample of 37 countries classified as developed on the basis of recent characteristics has diverse cultural, political, and economic histories.

2. Since 1970 there has been substantial and relatively uniform success in reducing mortality risks in children which contrasts with dramatically unequal achievements in reducing adult mortality risks, especially in men. From around 1970 most central European countries experienced serious institutional failures in responding to these adult mortality risks. Although adult male mortality has declined substantially since the end of communism, in six of the ten post-communist countries the gains in this period have been insufficient to offset the losses of the preceding 20 years.

3. The performance of the United States in reducing adult mortality risks has lagged increasingly behind that of the most successful countries. This lag now exceeds 20 years.

4. Differences in adult mortality risks are mainly due to differences in NCDs, especially cardiovascular diseases, and to injuries. These, in turn, are related to differences in a broad range of NCD and injury risk factors—physiological risk factors, dietary composition, tobacco and alcohol use, and risks associated with motor vehicle use.

These major variations in achieving reductions in adult mortality risks remain poorly explained. The next section considers advances in reducing road traffic injuries, tobacco-related disease, and cardiovascular diseases in the hope of throwing light on the institutional origins of success in reducing risks of these kinds.

Case studies of public health success
Road traffic injuries

Deaths from traffic injury per unit of exposure (e.g. per 10,000 vehicles per year) have fallen around tenfold in many developed countries over the past half century. Despite this outstanding public health success, traffic injuries still ranked 8th in their contribution to the burden of disease and injury in developed countries in 2010 (Anonymous 2013a). Because of the short time lags between control measures and their effects, traffic injury control provides a sensitive field in which to explore the relationship between policy adoption, programme implementation, and health effects.

First, it is appropriate to note that success has not flowed exclusively from centrally initiated policies, especially in the early decades of motorization. Smeed writing in the early 1970s showed that deaths from traffic crashes in relation to the number of registered vehicles had followed a general, and pronounced, downward trend as the number of motor vehicles increased in relation to population (Smeed's law: deaths/vehicle = 0.0003 (vehicles/population)$^{-0.66}$) (Smeed 1972). In the mid 1960s, two-thirds of 70 populations analysed by Smeed had rates within 40 per cent of his prediction. This implies that, up until then, societies had generally learnt how to use motor vehicles more safely as familiarity with them and the resources available for safety measures both increased. Because the overall tendency was general, it is unlikely to have depended on the specifics of policies variably adopted. However, over the last four or five decades organized policy responses have clearly made a bigger contribution. The Australian state of Victoria has been a pioneer in traffic injury control and its experience will be briefly reviewed here.

Consistent with Smeed's prediction, deaths per 10,000 vehicle years fell in Victoria as the number of vehicles increased in relation to population—from over 20 in the 1930s to about 9 in the early 1960s. During these early decades, Victoria generally had rates in excess of Smeed's prediction and from the late 1940s onwards, the 'road toll' was increasingly seen to be unacceptable. Early policy responses relied on exhortation—for example, encouraging motorists to sign a pledge to abstain from 'careless and discourteous behaviour' on the roads. This approach was not successful. A campaigning young police surgeon engaged journalists in the cause by taking them to the scenes of alcohol-related accidents on Friday and Saturday nights. A committee of the Royal Australasian College of Surgeons made a case before the parliamentary committee on road safety for more rigorous surveillance and for compulsion. In 1970, these submissions convinced the main political parties to support legislation, the first in the world, compelling Victorians to fit and wear seat belts. Compliance with the new law was high and road deaths fell (Fig. 3.7.4). In 1976, the Victorian parliament was the first in the world to legislate for random breath alcohol testing, responding again to advice from professionals. Deaths declined over the following decade. In 1986, a Transport Accident Commission was established, with secure funding from a levy on motorists. It paid no-fault compensation to those injured, which gave it a financial incentive to reduce injuries. A specified proportion of its spending on injury prevention was required to be spent on programme evaluation—thus supporting the development of an independent accident research institution. In late 1989, after traffic deaths had begun to rise again, it launched one of the most intensive mass media campaigns ever run in Australia—combined with intensified police enforcement (Davison and Yelland 2004). This combination of intensive mass communication, enforcement and evaluative research has continued. For example, in 2009 police performed 1.24 million random breath tests in a total population of 5.4 million persons (Transport Accident Commission 2013a). A local historian commented in 2004:

> Probably nowhere else in the world was the conduct of the individual motorist more closely monitored or more rigorously controlled. Yet, with only occasional grumblings, motorists overwhelmingly accepted these measures. (Davison and Yelland 2004, p. 167)

These strategies of education and enforcement were combined with those of engineering. In 1965, Ralph Nader denounced US cars as 'unsafe at any speed' (Nader 1965). In Australia, the national government negotiated against the resistance of the international automobile industry for 'design rules' to make cars safer—e.g. collapsible steering columns, shatter-proof windshield glass, and the removal of dangerous protrusions from the passenger cabin (T. Ryan, personal communication). For the United States, Robertson has documented the continuing resistance of the motor industry to manufacturing safer cars (Robertson 2010).

By 2010, across developed countries as a whole, transport fatality rates varied more than fivefold from less than 0.6 per 10,000 vehicle years in Switzerland, Sweden, Finland, Malta, and Iceland to more than 3.0 in Latvia, South Korea, and Romania (calculated from data in Anonymous (2013b)). Interestingly, Slovenia (1.06) and the Czech Republic (1.10) outperformed other post-communist states as well as the United States (1.37).

Globally, the success of traffic injury control has depended on institutional evolution over several decades. Pioneer jurisdictions moved from considering traffic injury as a moral issue to a public health one and acted on the advice of professionals—whose knowledge at that time typically reflected its early stage of development.

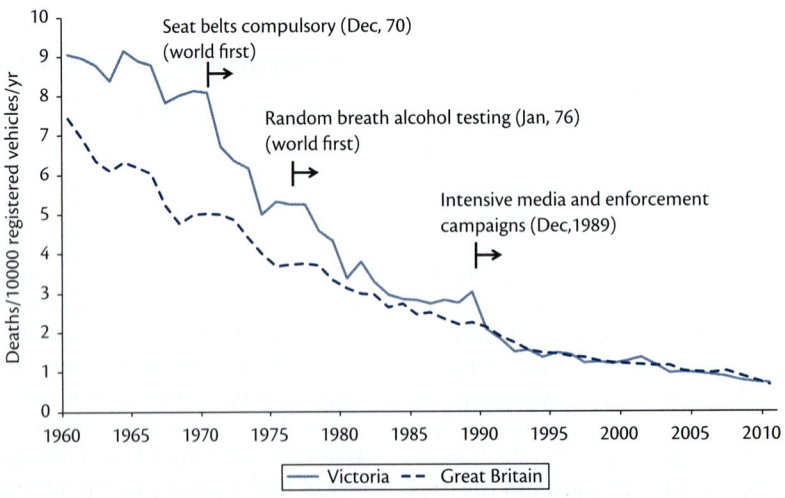

Fig. 3.7.4 Decline in traffic fatalities per 10,000 vehicles per year, 1960–2010, State of Victoria, Australia and Great Britain.

Source: data from Victoria Transport Accident Commission, Road safety statistical summary (yearly), Transport Accident Commission, Victoria, Australia, Copyright © 2013; and World Health Organization, *Global Status Report on Road Safety 2013: Supporting A Decade of Action*, World Health Organization, Geneva, Switzerland, Copyright © 2013.

Emergent control measures have been multifaceted, extending from modifying driver behaviour (including drink driving and speeding) to the redesign of cars and roads. Sustained reduction of injury rates has depended on the concurrent discovery of what to do — by programme supported research bodies such as the Monash University Accident Research Centre (in Victoria), the Insurance Institute for Highway Safety (in the United States), and the Transport Research Laboratory (in the United Kingdom). A body of experience now exists to guide the intensification of control measures. The United Nations has declared 2011 to 2020 as a Decade of Action for Road Safety resting on five pillars: (1) road safety management, (2) safer roads and mobility, (3) safer vehicles, (4) safer road users, and (5) improved post-crash responses. Illustrating the potential for rapid gains from the application of knowledge built up over previous decades, Spain managed to halve fatality rates in just 5 years (from 1.61 per 10,000 vehicle years in 2005 to 0.80 in 2010 (Dirección General de Tráfico, Spain 2013).

In addition to the measures considered here for reducing injury risks per unit exposure to car usage, there are other powerful health and environmental considerations favouring a reduction in car use itself and a switch to more active forms of commuting (Woodcock et al. 2009).

Tobacco

The first English-language demonstrations of the quantitative relationships between smoking and lung cancer risk were reported in 1950. By 2010, all of the 37 developed countries except the United States and Switzerland had ratified an international treaty on tobacco control, committing themselves to a full repertoire of evidence-based measures to reduce tobacco smoking (World Health Organization 2013). Over a 60-year interval, the currently established set of measures for tobacco control was invented, tried, and tested—ultimately gaining political support at the highest level.

The early 1950s to the 1970s was a period of gradual clarification at a scientific, professional, political, and public level of the nature and meaning of the health risks arising from tobacco use. The epistemology of professional medicine was still prequantitative. As reports from epidemiological studies accumulated, high-level policy debates continued to revolve around a largely illusory search for 'proof of causation' (Pollock 1999). Many physicians remained unconvinced of the hazards. In the United States a 1960 poll found that only one-third of physicians were convinced that smoking was a 'major cause' of lung cancer and 43 per cent were still regular smokers (Proctor 2011). Physicians who appreciated the magnitude of the risks and who were in a position to do something about it struggled to find a way forward.

In the late 1950s, George Godber was Deputy Chief Medical Officer in Britain and was very keen to help reduce harm from cigarette smoking. But his superior, the Chief Medical Officer, did not want to take the matter forward with the Minister of Health who was known to be unenthusiastic about taking on the Chancellor of the Exchequer (Treasurer). The Treasury was keen to protect the 15 or so per cent of central government revenue provided by tobacco tax (Berridge 2007). Godber visited Charles Fletcher, a respiratory physician, at a London teaching hospital and invited him to his club for lunch so that they could discuss strategies. They decided on working through the Royal College of Physicians in order to by-pass the Chief Medical Officer. The College took up

the matter energetically and decided to produce a report aimed at a large audience. In 1962, *Smoking and Health* appeared and quickly sold out (Pollock 1999; Lock et al. 1998). The United States followed suit and in 1964 the Surgeon General's report on *The Health Effects of Smoking* appeared. The mass media covered these reports extensively and Pierce and colleagues have shown that smoking cessation rates in US middle-aged adults were, in turn, responsive to the extent of news coverage (Pierce and Gilpin 2001). Coverage of the Surgeon-General's report was not the beginning of mass media coverage of smoking and health in the United States—as early as 1946 a news magazine story 'Cigarettes cause cancer?', based on experimental work on the carcinogenicity of cigarette tar, was 'widely read' (Proctor 2011)—but there is good reason to see it as a turning point in increasing public awareness of the hazards of smoking.

A major difficulty, in the 1950s, was that public health authorities were reluctant to tell adult men how they should behave. Reluctance of this kind had not previously inhibited anti-spitting campaigns to reduce risks of transmitting a communicable disease (tuberculosis). Nor had it inhibited strong and detailed directions to mothers, early in the twentieth century on how they should care for their children (Lewis 1980). But advising adult men to abandon a widely accepted habit was seen as different. Crossing this frontier would ultimately change 'the discourse of public health' in Britain and legitimize government activity to promote health favouring lifestyles (Berridge 2007).

Early tobacco control activists set out to build political constituencies in support of action by parliament. This turned out to be a slow process. In the United Kingdom, Kenneth Robinson who was health minister through the mid-1960s said that lack of public support had prevented him acting (Berridge 2007, p. 102). In 1971, the Royal College of Physicians established a pressure group—Action on Smoking and Health—'to make non-smoking the norm in society and to inform and educate the public about the death and disease caused by smoking' (Action on Smoking and Health 2013). Most of the early office holders were activist physicians. Major breakthroughs in mobilizing public support came in the mid to late 1980s in Victoria, Australia and in California. The 1987 Victorian Tobacco Act was the first to secure a hypothecated tax to be allocated to health promotion—in this case to the Victorian Health Promotion Foundation (Vichealth). Vichealth then used this money (AU $23 million per year—about US $7 per person per year) to buy out tobacco sponsorship of sporting and arts events and to fund health promotion programmes. The close passage of this Act was the outcome of careful planning, initially conducted in strict secrecy in order to catch the tobacco industry off-guard and prevent it deploying its enormous resources against the Act. Once the campaign was public, the large contributor base of the Anti-Cancer Council of Victoria was mobilized. Newspaper coverage was sympathetic—the main morning paper reported more correspondence on the topic than any other in the paper's history (Borland et al. 2009). Over 150 000 letters of support were sent to state politicians and church leaders were engaged in the campaign. The idea of an hypothecated tax was taken to California and included in Proposition 99 which won voter approval in November 1988—a victory gained by a largely volunteer workforce of canvassers against massive industry spending (Glanz and Balbach 2000). Twenty per cent of the 25 cents per pack hypothecated tax was to be allocated to education and prevention. Secure funding enabled the California Tobacco Program to achieve bigger reductions in tobacco consumption than happened elsewhere in the United States (Pierce et al. 2011).

From the 1990s onwards, the tobacco industry has suffered further losses of legitimacy and support in the developed world. In the United States, the 1998 Tobacco Master Settlement Agreement between 46 states and the largest cigarette manufacturers resulted in the industry agreeing to restrict some marketing practices, to dissolve its three main front organizations and to pay the states US $206 billion (sic) over 25 years to compensate for the extra state medical expenditures attributable to cigarette smoking. Interpretation of the potential effects on the Settlement on tobacco control have been mixed (Schroeder 2004) but the public release of previously secret industry documents disclosed during the discovery phase of the litigation has led to further damage to the industry. Proctor used these documents to show how the industry deliberately and secretly modified the composition of cigarettes to make the smoke more inhalable and the smoker more dependent (Proctor 2011).

In 2006, Philip Morris was convicted by a US federal court under legislation designed to counter organized crime (the Racketeer Influenced and Corrupt Organizations Act) for having: falsely denied that they market to youth, falsely denied that they manipulated cigarette design, falsely represented that light and low-tar cigarettes deliver less nicotine and tar, falsely denied that ETS (second-hand smoke) causes disease and suppressed documents, information, and research (Proctor 2011). In November 2012 they were ordered to make public statements admitting that they had lied to the public (Associated Press 2012). Elsewhere, the closing off of marketing opportunities in high-income countries was taken one step further when, in December 2012, Australia enacted a law requiring that all cigarettes be sold in plain standardized packaging.

In 2008, the World Health Organization (WHO) summarized current 'best practice' in anti-tobacco policy under the abbreviation MPOWER:

> **M**onitor tobacco use and prevention policies
>   **P**rotect people from tobacco use
>   **O**ffer help to quit tobacco use
>   **W**arn about the dangers of tobacco
>   **E**nforce bans on tobacco advertising, promotion and sponsorship
>   **R**aise taxes on tobacco. (WHO 2008)

Detailed country profiles are available on the WHO website tracking implementation within this framework (Anonymous 2013e). The most robust indicator of success in reducing cumulative tobacco exposure is lung cancer mortality—preferably at younger ages so as to reflect the recent experience of young adults (Fig. 3.7.5). For males, lung cancer mortality under the age of 50 peaked in nearly all developed countries before the year 2000, implying a peaking of smoking uptake in adolescents before about 1980. The epidemic in females has lagged relative to that in males, with six of the 37 countries (Portugal, Spain, Italy, Greece, Ireland, and Germany) showing rates still rising between 2005 and 2010.

Despite these shifts towards declining deaths from smoking, tobacco was still ranked third, after dietary composition and high blood pressure, as a cause of health loss in developed countries in 2010 (Anonymous 2013a). The century-long epidemics of cigarette smoking and its consequent disease burdens illustrate well

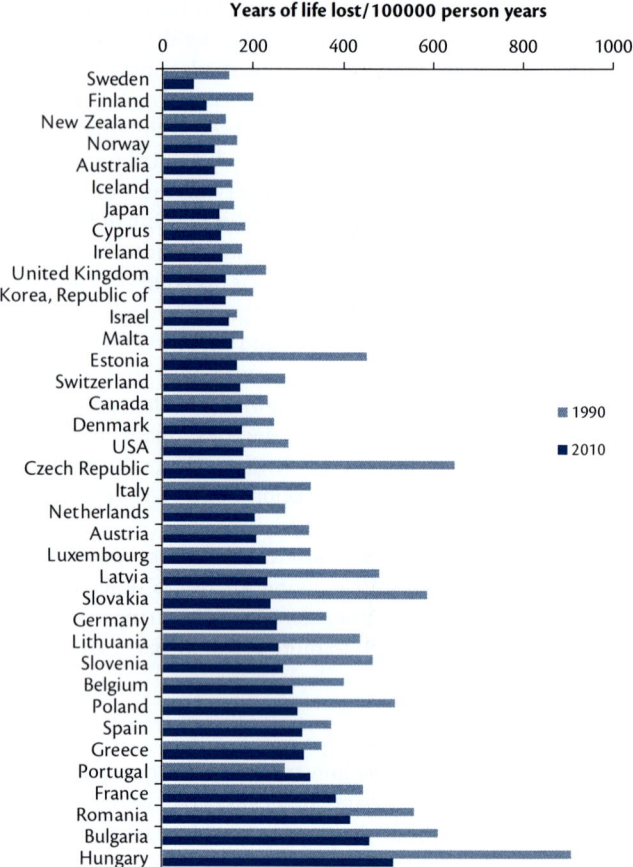

Fig. 3.7.5 Years of life lost from lung cancer deaths in males aged 15–49, rates per 100,000 person years for 1990 and 2010, countries ranked by level in 2010*. (*Years of life lost have been calculated by the Global Burden of Disease Project using a model life table with a life expectancy at birth of 86 years.)

Source: data from *Global Burden of Disease Visualizations*, Institute for Health Metrics and Evaluation, University of Washington, Seattle, USA, Copyright © 2013, available from http://www.healthmetricsandevaluation.org/gbd/visualizations/country.

the long time frame over which chronic disease determinants may rise and fall, making campaigns to reduce them into long wars of attrition. Tobacco control also illustrates how the development of quantitative methods has supported appropriate policy responses. With increased acceptance of epidemiological reasoning and its transmission to political and wider publics (for example, Peto et al. 2013), quantitative assessments have become more central to policy deliberations, facilitating effective institutional responses, nationally and globally.

Circulatory diseases

Despite the marked reductions of the last two decades, circulatory diseases, mainly ischaemic heart disease and stroke, remain the leading causes of lost life years in developed countries. The overall change from 1990 to 2010 in the level of lost life years from these diseases is shown in Fig. 3.7.6. There is a clear bi-modality of the mortality levels in 1990 (once Slovenia is transferred out of the post-communist group). On average, mortality halved over this interval. Levels became more similar among the 'other' group of countries; for example, reductions were less in France and Japan which began with the lowest levels in 1990. Among the

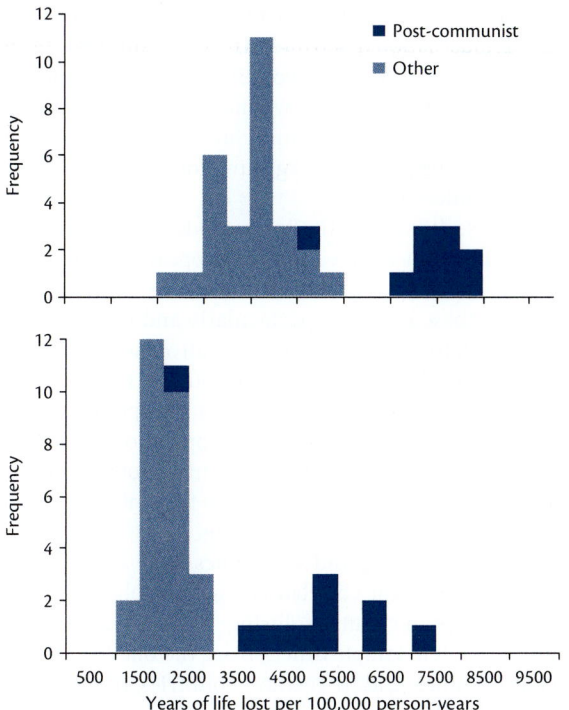

Fig. 3.7.6 Distribution of 37 developed countries by rates of life years lost to circulatory diseases in 1990 and 2010.

Source: data from *Global Burden of Disease Visualizations*, Institute for Health Metrics and Evaluation, University of Washington, Seattle, USA, Copyright © 2013, available from http://www.healthmetricsandevaluation.org/gbd/visualizations/country.

post-communist group, however, levels became less similar—a reduction of 52 per cent in the Czech Republic contrasted with a reduction of just 15 per cent in Bulgaria. Overall there was no 'catch-up' by the post-communist group. The United States performed poorly with a reduction of 39 per cent, compared, for example, to a 53 per cent reduction in the United Kingdom.

These trends prompt three policy-related questions:

1. What have been the main contributors to progress over recent decades?

2. Why have the trends since 1990 in the post-communist group been so diverse?

3. Why has the United States been less successful?

Changes contributing to the decline in circulatory diseases

As with road traffic injuries and tobacco-caused disease, endeavours to control circulatory diseases have been pursued in conjunction with determined attempts to better understand their causes. In the United States, President Harry Truman signed the National Heart Act in June 1948. Between 1950 and 2012 the budget of what was to become the National Heart Lung and Blood Institute rose from US $10 million to US $3100 million (National Institutes of Health 2012). The deliberate rapid expansion of research into the causes of ischaemic heart disease contributed strongly to the development of modern epidemiology, including the concept of 'risk factors'. The causation of these diseases has turned out to be complex. In GBD 2010, 11 dietary, five physiological, and three environmental risk factors plus alcohol and tobacco use were modelled as influencing vascular risk.

Notwithstanding this increasing complexity of the acknowledged determinants of vascular risk, much of its variation, at individual and population levels, continues to be explicable by the three classic risk factors—blood pressure, blood cholesterol concentration, and cigarette smoking—whose quantitative relationship to risk is now well understood. Trends in smoking have already been discussed, including the peaking of the smoking epidemic in young adult males before 1980 in most of the developed countries. Less data is available on trends in blood pressure and blood cholesterol concentrations. Where documented, trends in both sexes in developed countries have tended to follow a broadly similar time course to those of cigarette smoking in males—that is, to have been generally favourable, especially since around 1990 (Danaei et al. 2011; Farzadfar et al. 2011). The development of drugs that are effective in lowering blood pressure and blood cholesterol concentrations has enabled clinicians to also make an important contribution to the prevention of these diseases. More effective treatments for heart attacks and for precursor coronary artery disease also mean that the trends in mortality from heart attack reflect not only the extent of success in preventing disease onset but also in reducing the risk of death after onset.

In seeking to characterize societal responses to heart disease and stroke one might start with a hypothetical chain from the advance of scientific knowledge to increased professional and public knowledge, constituency building by activists, enactment of policy, programme implementation, changes in risk factors, and finally changes in disease incidence. However such sequences cannot be easily documented or established in a convincing way. Early phases of development were often marked by the formation of physician-led voluntary organizations which sought to mobilize public support for research, prevention, and treatment in many countries: the American Heart Association (founded 1924), the National Heart Foundation in Australia (founded 1959), and the British Heart Foundation (founded 1961). The European Heart Network now unites 31 member organizations from 24 European countries. In Australia, the National Heart Foundation, with extensive public support, was rich enough to actually lead in establishing national risk factor surveys during the 1980s. In Finland, the local government of North Karelia, a district with extremely high risks of premature death from vascular disease, petitioned the national government for support in reducing their disease burden. From this emerged the North Karelia project which spanned epidemiological investigation and mass mobilization to promote dietary change. Finland became an exemplar in the implementation of science-based policies to reduce vascular risk (Puska 2005).

Few countries have long time-series of surveillance data for levels of public knowledge of risk factors or of risk factor levels. For the United States, data from the National Health and Nutrition Examination Survey is available from the early 1960s. These show substantial reductions in the prevalence of hypertension—from 31 per cent in 1960–1962 to 17 per cent in 1999–2000 (Gregg et al. 2005) with no further reduction to 2007–2008 (Yoon et al. 2010). The prevalence of raised blood cholesterol fell from 34 per cent in the early 1960s to 17 per cent at the end of the 1990s (Gregg et al. 2005), with little further improvement since (CDC 2011).

Capewell and colleagues have shown, in a series of studies, that favourable shifts in risk factors contributed much more than clinical measures (pharmacoprevention plus treatment) to the reductions in years of life lost from ischaemic heart disease in Scotland (1975–1994), United States (1980–2000), Ireland (1985–2000), and England and Wales (1981–2000) (Gouda et al. 2012).

To all of these activities intended to reduce disease risk must be added other background factors. As early as the 1960s, results from the study of 'Coronary Heart Disease in Seven Countries' confirmed that local food cultures varied markedly in their effects on coronary risk—protective in the Mediterranean area and in Japan and adverse, for example, in northern Europe (Keys 1980). Favourable trajectories in mortality from circulatory diseases in countries such as France and Japan may owe as much to protective material cultures as to deliberate efforts to reduce risk. While the effects of rising incomes on animal fat and cigarette consumption may have been adverse in the early decades of the twentieth century, once the associated risks were understood, rising incomes will have brought benefits, for example, via the ability to support further scientific research and by the diversification of food supplies—reduced fat dairy products, margarines with low trans-fat content, year-round supplies of fresh fruit and vegetables, etc. Richer populations can also afford the relatively expensive strategy of controlling blood pressure and high cholesterol by long-term medication. These changing patterns of association between vascular risk factors and national income levels have recently been described (Danaei et al. 2013).

The diverse trends of the post-communist countries

The constellation of institutional responses and background trends just noted was associated with marked declines in vascular diseases in Western countries that were not matched by comparable declines in the European communist countries. In the case of males, the gap was widened by actual increases in incidence in the communist world. But even in the case of females, declines in the West were not matched by declines in the East: for example, rates of vascular mortality in middle-aged women were 1.5 times higher in Hungary than in Spain in the 1950s but a remarkable 4.5 times higher in the 1990s. All of the increase in the difference was due to favourable changes in Spain that failed to occur in Hungary (author's analyses using data from Anonymous (2013f)).

The communist countries failed to build the scientific foundations for responding to these diseases: they did not invest in the relevant science and they failed to make good use of international findings. The early years of the Soviet regime had been characterized by an enthusiasm for science but subsequent developments were not favourable to population-based aetiological research in medicine. The policy of Nikolai Semashko, first People's Commissar of Public Health, of integrating prevention and treatment led, in practice, to the domination of Soviet medicine by clinicians rather than by public health experts (Terris 1988); legacies of the 'Lysenko affair' weakened all biological sciences (Krementsov 1997), the control of science through hierarchical systems of research institutes limited innovation, while Soviet political economy saw the route to human betterment through the physical domination of nature, not by attending to the biological bases of human well-being—hence the physical sciences and engineering were valued and rewarded more than medicine (Field 1967). These adverse internal characteristics were augmented by the isolation of the cold war years; as late as 1988, Terris observed that there were no Soviet members of the International Epidemiological Association (Terris 1988). The transformative potential of the quantitative revolution in medicine and, in particular, of the randomized trial, was never realized. Finally, empty shelves in the shops and continuing consumer frustration may not have provided a propitious background for programmes promoting dietary prudence.

Despite these difficulties, the Soviet model of medicine and public health, as broadly adopted in the European communist states, had been initially successful—until it met its nemesis: NCDs of adults. With these it failed, spectacularly and tragically. Twenty years after the fall of communism, nearly all of the post-communist states in our sample continue on less favourable adult survival trajectories than their Western counterparts. Exceptions are Slovenia and the Czech Republic, whose female populations had overtaken the United States by 2010, and East German women, who caught up to their Western counterparts, within the ambiance of a reunified Germany, around the year 2000 (Fig. 3.7.3).

Mackenbach, McKee, and colleagues have made a detailed empirical analysis of the correlates of 'health policy performance' among 42 European countries during the first decade of the new millennium. (Their sample differs from the one for this chapter in including more middle-income countries from the former USSR and the Balkans and in not including North America, Australasia, Japan, and South Korea.) Their composite 'health policy performance score' combined information on a maximum of 27 indicators across ten policy areas. They explored the association of this score with income per person, score on the survival/self-realization scale from the World Values Survey, 'democracy', government effectiveness, political orientation (proportion of cabinet seats held by left-wing parties between 1990 and 2009), and ethnic fractionalization. They did not include an indicator of economic inequality. Political composition of governments was not associated with the outcome. In a multivariate analysis only the survival/self-expression score ($r^2 = 87$ per cent) and ethnic fractionalization (combined $r^2 = 90$ per cent) were significant. They conclude:

> These findings indicate that performance on health policy is driven substantially by the dominant values in the population, for example because a popular demand to do something is communicated to politicians. (Mackenbach and McKee 2013, p. 338)

Higher average scores on the self-expression scale correspond to greater satisfaction with levels of personal autonomy and with levels of creativity at work. However it is interpreted, average scores on this scale clearly separate the three higher-income members of the post-communist group with divergent health outcomes—Slovenia and the Czech Republic each had mean scores of 0.38 on the self-expression scale in the 2006 wave of the World Values Survey and also the most favourable survival trends in contrast to Hungary with a score of −1.22 and less favourable survival trends.

For three of the main mortality indicators for 2010 used in this chapter—traffic deaths per 10,000 vehicle years, years of life lost from male lung cancer deaths before age 50, and years of life lost from circulatory diseases—the ratio of the median level in the post-communist group to the median of west European group exceeds 2.5. This suggests a persisting lag in developing cultures of prudent consumption across motor cars, tobacco, and diet. Countries in the post-communist group tend to show consistent rankings across these and related variables.

Why has the United States been less successful?

The experience of the United States may be compared with the medians for the 26 other developed countries excluding the post-communist group. Such comparisons show the United States to have a mean income 30 per cent above the reference and a strong orientation towards self-expression in the World Values Survey (mean score 1.76, reference 1.13) (James et al. 2012; Anonymous 2013d). To these advantages must be added the relative strength of knowledge infrastructures in medicine and public health and the remarkably high levels of expenditure on professional medicine. Despite these multiple advantages, mortality risks between the ages of 15 and 60 are around 50 per cent higher in each sex than in the reference and the United States has been falling further behind over time. These observations suggest that opportunities for health improvement in the United States are being restricted by other societal characteristics.

These developments have not passed unnoticed in the United States, with a major report (*Shorter Lives, Poorer Health*) from the National Research Council and the Institute of Medicine in 2013 (Woolf and Aron 2013a). The authors show that factors influencing the distribution of health levels, while important in themselves and the subject of much attention in the literature, are not at the heart of the problem: privileged groups in the United States are similarly disadvantaged relative to their counterparts in other countries. The US disadvantage extends across a range of major health outcomes. Traffic fatalities per 10,000 vehicle years are 65 per cent higher than the developed country reference; years of life lost from lung cancer under age 50 is 9 per cent higher for males but 65 per cent higher for females and years of life lost from circulatory diseases are 34 per cent higher. As with the post-communist group of countries, patterns of commodity use unfavourable to health appear to underlie the US disadvantage. In order ' to make sense of why Americans are more likely to engage in certain unhealthy behaviors or injurious practices…, the role of societal values in enacting or resisting countermeasures cannot be ignored' (Woolf and Aron 2013a, p. 222).

The report cites approvingly another National Academies report on traffic injuries which shows how jurisdictions in the United States resist the application of measures proven effective elsewhere for reducing drink driving, increasing seat belt and motorcycle helmet use and controlling speed (Woolf and Aron 2013a, pp. 227–31). The main report concludes that it will be 'important for Americans to engage in a thoughtful discussion about what investments and compromises they are willing to make to keep pace with health advances other countries are achieving' (Woolf and Aron 2013a, p. 6).

Public health failures

Energy intake, energy expenditure, and obesity

In contrast to the preceding areas of success, this is an area of generalized failure. In developed countries there has been an almost universal tendency for obesity prevalences to rise over recent decades, with this tendency accelerating over the past decade or so (Stevens et al. 2012). Prevalences in males and females in the United States and in males in the Czech Republic now exceed 30 per cent, while prevalences in South Korea and Japan are still below 10 per cent. Surprisingly, trends in attributable

disease burdens from GBD 2010 show little increase through the last decade (Anonymous 2013a) suggesting that favourable trends in background risks for circulatory diseases may have been offsetting much of the potential harm from rising obesity—i.e. an increasing obesity multiplier may have been applied to a shrinking background vascular risk level (Powles et al. 2010).

The UK Foresight Report on 'Tackling obesities' sought to understand and respond to the societal determinants of rising obesity prevalence. 'The technological revolution of the twentieth century has left in its wake an 'obesogenic environment' that serves to expose the biological vulnerability of human beings' (Butland et al. 2007, p. 8). Adequate responses will require 'changes in the environment and organizational behaviour, as well as changes in group, family and individual behaviour' (p. 15), that will need to span generations (p. 131). Parallels with the challenges posed by climate change are noted. So far, however, the authors are able to find few international examples of success.

Habitat degradation and public health

In the early phases of industrialization 'point source' pollution damaged health by contaminating local (or regional) air, water, and soil. Over recent decades, the cumulative effects of global industrialization have been found to be disturbing the large-scale natural processes on which the stability of our human habitat and the long-term health and survival of human populations depend (McMichael 2013) (see also Chapter 2.8). Human-induced climate change is part of a larger pattern of systemic environmental and ecological changes due to the now excessive and widespread human pressures on the biosphere (Rockstrom et al. 2009). These include stratospheric ozone depletion, ocean acidification, soil losses and groundwater depletion, disruption of global nitrogen and phosphorus cycles, and rapid loss of biodiversity. The WHO, through its Director General, noted in 2008 that 'climate change endangers health in fundamental ways': disruption of food production, increased storms and floods, water shortage and excess, heatwaves and changes in the distribution of insect vectors of disease (Chan 2008).

Lagged, large-scale adverse effects of these kinds differ qualitatively, and very significantly, from other connections between productive activity and health—their main threats to health lie ahead of us, as current trends continue, they are global or regional in scope, they are mainly predicted rather than currently manifest, and their specific manifestation in a given time and place is highly uncertain—as are the final pathways by which the health of individuals will be harmed. Despite these differences, there are common threads with the epidemics of NCD. Both arise from attending exclusively to human wants rather than also attending to the biological requirements for human well-being. Adequate responses cannot be built on approaches that respond only to demand. The rewards of economic development, so highly valued by economic liberals, can now only be protected by attending to the objective requirements for their sustainability—by means which economic liberals mostly oppose.

Governments and public health professionals in developed countries have responded to the challenge of climate change in three main ways:

1. First, by securing the participation of public health experts in national and global expert panels assessing climate change, notably the 6 yearly Intergovernmental Panel on Climate

Change (IPCC) Assessments, the fifth of which was published in 2013–14. Such participation is especially important for the Health chapter (Working Group II), but is not limited to it.

2. Second, by identifying and elaborating strategies that promise 'double dividends'—that is, changes that both favour health and mitigate climate change. Examples include transport policies that both increase physical activity and reduce carbon emissions (Woodcock et al. 2009) and reductions in red and processed meat consumption that reduce both risks of NCDs and the major greenhouse gas emissions produced by livestock production (Aston et al. 2012).

3. Third, by ensuring that the medical care sector, itself a major industry in developed countries, acts as an exemplar in moving towards sustainability. For example the English National Health Service has a Sustainable Development Unit 'to ensure that the health and care system fulfils its potential as a leading sustainable and low carbon service' (NHS Sustainable Development Unit 2013). The English unit is a founding member of the Global Green and Healthy Hospitals network (Global Green and Healthy Hospitals n.d.).

Wider determinants of the public health

The marked increase over the past two decades or so in discussion of the 'social' or 'wider' determinants of health has been associated with the belief that distributional considerations are central to understanding these phenomena. The final report of the WHO Commission on the Social Determinants of Health, for example, was titled: *Closing the Gap in a Generation: Health Equity Through Action on the Social Determinants of Health* (Commission on the Social Determinants of Health 2008). Evidence presented in this chapter, consistent with that marshalled by Mackenbach and McKee for Europe (Mackenbach and McKee 2013) and with the US National Academies report (Woolf and Aron 2013a), suggests that it may instead be helpful to distinguish between the wider determinants of average levels of population health and the wider determinants of the dispersion (or inequality) of health levels within populations.

A pragmatic reason for doing so is the availability of evidence on variation in the dependent variable. We have seen that multiple indicators are available, showing variation in average levels across developed countries that are often greater than twofold. Variation in dispersion, as measured, for example, by the relative index of inequality, may in some cases be of comparable magnitude, but tends to be available in comparable form for fewer populations and time periods (Mackenbach et al. 2008). Investigation of the causes of variation in average levels of population health may therefore be more empirically tractable than explanation of variations in levels of inequality within populations.

A second reason for this distinction is that variation in levels of economic or social equality may not be central to the explanation of variation in average levels of health. For example, the communist states of Europe had both more equal distribution of incomes and much less favourable average levels of adult health. The US report discussed earlier also notes that differences in levels of inequality do not account for poorer outcomes in the United States because the US disadvantage is experienced across all social strata.

A third reason is that when considering wider determinants of average levels of health it is possible to give due recognition to the institutional and ideological determinants of the consumption habits underlying variation in health levels. By contrast, much discussion of the wider determinants of health inequalities considers consumption habits to be characteristic of individuals—as in the oxymoron 'individual lifestyle'. (The concept of a style is intrinsically social (Cockerham et al. 1997).) The much cited Dahlgren/Whitehead model places 'individual lifestyle factors' in the zone closest to individuals (Bambra et al. 2010).

I will briefly consider the following as 'wider determinants' of average levels of population health (henceforward just public health):

1. Knowledge

2. Income

3. Values

4. Corporate power

5. Political economy.

Knowledge

Avoidable weaknesses in the knowledge infrastructure for public health prevented the European communist countries from responding effectively to the challenge of NCD in adults. Outcomes for these countries in the post-communist period were noted to be variable, with Slovenia and the Czech Republic showing the biggest gains. There is little evidence, however, of these countries making determined efforts in the post-communist period—via research funding, attractive scholarships tenable internationally, etc.—to build scientific capacities supportive of modern responses to NCD. A bibliometric index of research papers published in 2001–2010 and indexed in PubMed with MESH terms relating to the epidemiology and control of heart disease and stroke shows that the median for the post-communist group of countries was only 15 per million mid-period population, compared with five times that rate in the United States and the United Kingdom and more than ten times that rate in Sweden, Denmark, and Israel (personal analyses).

It is likely that relevant national research strengths are much more important in the early developmental phases of responses to public health challenges. Knowledgeable experts were seen to have played important roles in the early development of measures to control traffic injury, to reduce tobacco use and to control cardiovascular risk—even though relevant knowledge was, at those early stages, often tentative and incomplete. As control measures against these challenges have been developed, tested and achieved international acceptance, countries are able to make use of them, to some extent independent of their local research strengths in these areas. In the long run, knowing what to do has been powerfully permissive of it (eventually) being done.

Income

Other things being equal, higher incomes should facilitate health protective patterns of living: for example, safer cars and roads will be more affordable, as will a wider variety of foods associated with lower circulatory disease risk. The median income level among the post-communist group of countries remains 50 per cent below the reference group and this could be constraining the implementation of public health programmes in those countries. Mackenbach and McKee found that gross domestic product per person (in 2000) was a strong correlate of their 'health policy performance score' across European countries (Mackenbach and McKee 2013). However, discordant national experiences reviewed here indicate that income per se has been unable to over-ride the effects of unfavourable institutional circumstances: between 1970 and 1990, real income per person is estimated to have almost doubled in Hungary and to have more than doubled in Bulgaria but over these intervals the risks of dying between ages 15 and 60 rose from 20 per cent to 30 per cent in Hungarian men and from 16 per cent to 22 per cent in Bulgarian men. In 2010, the United States ranked third out of 37 in real income per person (using purchasing power adjusted estimates (James et al. 2012)) but 30th out of 37 for adult female survival and 27th out of 37 for adult male survival. A high level of command over resources has not automatically led to patterns of resource use favourable to health. Other circumstances need also to be favourable.

Values

As noted earlier, Mackenbach and McKee found that the 'self-realization' score from the World Values Survey was even more strongly associated with 'policy performance' than was income (Mackenbach and McKee 2013, p. 338). It is hypothesized that the attainment of material security enables more attention to be paid to self-realization—including a greater interest in reducing longer term health risks. Part of the limited catch up of the post-communist states could plausibly be associated with the extent of their other preoccupations. However, evidence on this topic is limited. The United States scores highly on 'self-expression'. Its deviance in the World Values Survey is in the strength of 'traditional/religious values'; on this dimension it sits with Latin American and Islamic states.

Corporate power

Large corporations are a salient feature of the contemporary capitalist world. In 2000, of the 100 largest economic entities in the world (ranked by value added), 63 were countries and 37 were corporations (De Grauwe and Camerman 2002). Adverse effects of corporations on health are claimed via three channels: (1) illegal behaviour, (2) disreputable behaviour, and (3) normal behaviour.

As already noted, the cigarette industry illustrates the first: by making cigarette smoke more inhalable and cigarettes more dependence creating and therefore more deadly while conspiring to conceal the fact. Claimed disreputable actions include the behaviour of the 'big food' companies, for example, in marketing directed to children (Brownell and Warner 2009).

The third claim is that corporations, in their legal obligation to give priority to returns to shareholders, will automatically devalue ends that are not monetized and not relevant to their profitability (Wiist 2010). In this view it is inappropriate to regard corporations as good or bad. Corporations in the cigarette, alcohol, motor vehicle, pharmaceutical, and food industries damage health as a consequence of the objectives they are required to pursue. The appropriate response, for public health advocates, is to seek to limit corporate power by 'redesigning or restructuring the corporation as an institution'—for example, by banning all corporate political activity, by removing the right to legal personhood,

and by eliminating or reducing limited liability (Wiist 2010, pp. 47–48). This analysis is largely based on US sources. The volume cited does not explain how the health disadvantage of the United States compared to other developed capitalist countries is attributable to differences in the legal privileges of corporations.

Prevailing ideas on political economy

Theories of political economy lie close to the surface of many discussions of policies to change consumption habits in order to prevent disease. In the United States, liberal/libertarian political economy exerts pervasive influence. Both the neo-classical ('Chicago') and 'Austrian' schools seek to minimize state coercion and emphasize the virtues of markets in regulating economic activity and individual behaviours.

Many public health policies to reduce chronic disease and injury do indeed include coercive elements e.g. traffic law, bans on indoor smoking etc. The liberal criticism of them as coercive is, however, weakened by its abstraction from social and historical contexts. As was noted in the case of measures to reduce traffic injury in Victoria, high levels of surveillance and coercion may achieve wide public support because of the perceived benefits in safer car travel produced. In practice, for public health policies to be enacted in democratic polities, the case for any coercive elements has to be made in the light of the health benefits expected. They cannot be introduced behind the public's back.

A more fundamental liberal/libertarian criticism is that even where public health policies are effective in improving health, this will not constitute an improvement in well-being (utility) if it is achieved by violating existing consumer preferences. This is because, in the liberal/libertarian perspective, value arises solely from meeting the subjective preferences of consumers—by fulfilling their demands, not by meeting their needs. This perspective is consistent with neo-classical economic approaches which Hodgson characterizes as those that:

1. Assume rational, utility-maximizing behaviour by agents with given and stable preferences.

2. Focus on attained equilibrium states or movements towards them.

3. Are marked by an absence of chronic information problems (Hodgson 2013a).

Gary Becker's elaboration of 'rational choice theory' illustrates a neo-classical approach to consumption and its connections to well-being. For Becker, the household is the locus of production of final commodities such as health, social standing, and 'pleasures of the senses', using inputs such as market goods, time, and consumer and social capital (Becker 1996b). As societies become richer, time becomes relatively scarcer and market goods less so. The capacity to gain utility using time and market goods is enhanced by education and 'social' resources (the latter conceived in a restricted sense). Within this framework, Becker is able to interpret opiate, alcohol and nicotine addiction as 'rational' (Becker 1996a). Given this, the case for public policies to reduce them loses legitimacy.

The Austrian school of liberal political economy differs in important respects from the neo-classical school (Aranzadi del Cerro 2006). It is exemplified in works such as Friedrich Hayek's *Constitution of Liberty* (Hayek 1960) (acknowledged by Margaret

Thatcher as a key influence on her programme to revive economic liberalism in 1980s Britain) and Ludwig von Mises' *Human Action* (von Mises and Greaves 2007). Although no less determined to minimize state coercion and to extol the virtues of markets, the Austrian approach provides a richer account of the way in which the decentralized exchange of knowledge through markets creates stable social orders (catallaxis). Gamble sees Hayek's approach as rooted in 'epistemological pessimism', regarding as a 'fatal conceit' 'the belief that in the modern era human beings were able to throw off the chains of tradition, superstition, convention, and precedent and design institutions, choose morals, invent values, and plan societies as though they were starting from a blank sheet' (Gamble 2006). Hayek preferred instead 'the tacit knowledge encoded in the traditions, conventions, and rules which had been inherited, and were the fruit of human action over millennia'. Hayek was inclined to oppose all centralized uses of knowledge—not just by governments seeking to regulate economic life but also by elite groups of scientists seeking disproportionate influence on public affairs (variously referred to as scientism or 'constructivism'). The suspicion among US liberal/libertarian groups of bodies such as the Intergovernmental Panel on Climate Change, to the extent that it is not based on irrational 'denialism' (Diethelm and McKee 2009), likely owes a good deal to this sentiment.

Gamble notes how Hayek's logic could be turned in the opposite direction: the way in which he 'approaches the social world is paralleled in the way in which environmentalists approach the natural world. Both are conceived as extremely delicate, living organisms…whose operations are imperfectly understood'. But Hayek 'never extended to natural science and technology his critique of constructivist rationalism in social science'.

Alternatives to liberal/libertarian political economy are provided by heterodox approaches. In Europe, the best established of these is that of evolutionary political economy (European Association for Evolutionary Political Economy n.d.). These typically depart from the neo-classical approach by:

1. Abandoning exclusive reliance on a subjective theory of value by also valuing the meeting of objective needs.

2. Seeking greater consistency with the substantive findings of the natural sciences.

3. Attending to human capacities for creativity, morality and institutional evolution.

Hodgson's *From Pleasure Machines to Moral Communities: An Evolutionary Economics Without Homo Economicus* (Hodgson 2013) illustrates an approach likely to be more congenial to public health professionals. Hodgson embraces a pluralist theory of value—'health is an objective, universal need, irrespective of whether it is also a want' (Hodgson 2013, p. 174; Woolf and Aron 2013a)—and notes the consequent difficulties in arbitrating needs:

> Some middle ground must be found between the propositions that the consumer always knows best and the state or the experts always know best: neither extreme is defensible…The problem is to design institutions that set up a creative dialogue between individual preferences and expert advice, embody mechanisms to scrutinize the skills and claims of experts, and facilitate the creation and distribution of relevant knowledge. (Hodgson 2013, p. 192)

Hodgson does not evade the fact that '[S]cience is unavoidably elitist. It depends on the interactions and evaluations of a selected group of highly trained experts and specialists' (Hodgson 2013, p. 223). He also considers many forms of collective action to be well founded because our evolution has left us 'biologically and culturally primed to be sensitive to such issues as fairness, care for the needs of others and an unspoiled environment' (p. 204). By contrast it is a fatal weakness of neo-classical welfare economics that it can provide no useful guidance when confronted with the challenge of climate change (p. 197).

Clarifying theoretical viewpoints held in good faith is one thing, but in real political contests, propositions may be advanced for the purpose of defending vested interests in ways that bear little connection to the actual beliefs of those advancing them—as has been documented in the behaviour of the cigarette manufacturers. Especially in the United States, liberal/libertarian anti-state arguments are heavily promoted by those who stand to gain from them (Cohen et al. 2000). But such beliefs also have strong historical and constitutional foundations in that country. Individual autonomy and freedom of choice are valued, rather than fairness and social solidarity, leading to hostility to regulation that is seen to infringe choice, for example, firearms control. Whatever their origins, the strength of 'anti-government' viewpoints makes it difficult for the United States to implement public health policies found effective elsewhere (Woolf and Aron 2013b).

Conclusion

For this chapter, a sample of 37 developed countries was identified based on their recent status as high-income members of the OECD or membership of the EU. They are heterogeneous in culture and in their political and economic histories. When examining changes in survival patterns over the last 40 years, it was found that gains in child survival were substantial and broadly similar across all 37 countries. By contrast, trends in adult survival between ages 15 and 60 differed dramatically. These differences mainly arose from a relatively small group of diseases and injuries related to patterns of commodity consumption. Attention was therefore focused on how differing experience of these conditions might have been related to those differences in political histories and public health policies most likely to influence relevant consumption habits.

Although the wider determinants of inequalities in health is an important topic, for the purpose of this chapter it was found to be more useful to concentrate on wider determinants of average levels of population health. In relation to broad systems of political economy, poorer outcomes were associated with the extremes of the state-centred systems of the European communist countries (and their institutional legacies in the post-communist period) and the United States, where ideas of liberal/libertarian political economy and associated 'anti-government' sentiments are most dominant. Health trends in countries lying between these two poles have not shown any straightforward association with the political alignment of their governments. European countries tend to have a wider range of political opinion represented both inside and outside their parliaments. In many, the influence of non-liberal Catholic social teaching on right-of-centre parties has been important, and has moderated the linkage between right-of-centre politics and economic liberalism. These countries have generally pursued more pragmatic or pluralist approaches to protecting adult health—consistent with Popper's idea of 'piecemeal social engineering' (Popper 1957). It is thus the capacity of the dominant liberal/libertarian political economy in the United States to restrict more pluralist approaches that appears to have been important. Notwithstanding these obstructions there have been strong state or city level programmes for NCD control within the United States—for example, the California Tobacco Control Programme and the more recent programmes of the New York City Health Department (New York City Health Department 2014). As awareness within the US that it is falling behind other developed countries increases, ways may be found to further develop and replicate public health programmes that are acceptable and effective within the US context.

Some recent trends in developed countries have not been favourable. Without effective responses to the rise in obesity, the substantial health gains of the last couple of decades may erode. The medium- to longer-term future is clouded by potential large-scale harms from climate change. Meeting these challenges will require the renovation and transformation of economic, social and public health institutions—complex processes, that are presenting difficult challenges to public health professionals as to others. The recent run of success may not last.

Key points

◆ Over the last four decades, developed countries have achieved broadly similar success in reducing risks of death in childhood but have varied markedly in their success in reducing adult mortality.

◆ Most variation in adult mortality risks is accounted for by circulatory diseases and a limited number of other conditions related to patterns of commodity consumption.

◆ The European communist countries failed tragically to control adult mortality risks; improvements since the fall of communism have been variable.

◆ The United States has also performed poorly, especially in the light of its financial and scientific resources; it now lags more than 20 years behind its comparators.

◆ Effective counter-measures for traffic injuries, tobacco-caused disease, and circulatory disease evolved over time; early leadership came mostly from informed professionals, then broadened as supportive constituencies were built, knowledge advanced, and effective measures were identified and given international sanction.

◆ The rising prevalence of obesity and habitat degradation by greenhouse gas emissions are current policy failures.

◆ Theories of political economy that have little respect for biologically based needs may, where dominant, restrict societal responses to NCD and habitat degradation.

◆ Prospects for further sustainable health gains are now uncertain, but are likely to improve under conditions of pluralism.

Acknowledgements

Tony McMichael, Paul Lincoln, and Adela Sanz provided helpful advice and Ildiko Varga provided research assistance.

References

Action on Smoking and Health (2013). *Key Dates in the History of Anti-Tobacco Campaigning.* London: Action on Smoking and Health.

Anonymous (2010). *Global Burden of Disease 2010.* Data downloads. Seattle, WA: Institute of Health Metrics and Evaluation, University of Washington.

Anonymous (2013a). *Global Burden of Disease Visualizations.* Seattle, WA: Institute of Health Metrics and Evaluation, University of Washington.

Anonymous (2013b). *Global Status Report on Road Safety 2013: Supporting a Decade of Action.* Geneva: World Health Organization.

Anonymous (2013c). *Human Mortality Database.* University of California, Berkeley (USA), and Max Planck Institute for Demographic Research (Germany). Available at: http://www.mortality.org.

Anonymous (2013d). *Nation-Level Mean Scores on Traditional/ Secular-rational and Survival/Self-Expression Values Dimensions, 1981–2007.* Stockholm: World Values Survey Association.

Anonymous (2013e). *Tobacco Free Initiative, Tobacco Control Country Profiles.* Geneva: World Health Organization.

Anonymous (2013f). *WHO Mortality Database.* Geneva: World Health Organization.

Aranzadi del Cerro, J. (2006). *Liberalism Against Liberalism.* New York: Routledge.

Associated Press (2012). Tobacco companies are told to correct lies about smoking. *New York Times,* 27 November, B8.

Aston, L.M., Smith, J.N., and Powles, J.W. (2012). Impact of a reduced red and processed meat dietary pattern on disease risks and greenhouse gas emissions in the UK: a modelling study. *BMJ Open,* 2, e001072.

Bambra, C., Gibson, M., Sowden, A., Wright, K., Whitehead, M., and Petticrew, M. (2010). Tackling the wider social determinants of health and health inequalities: evidence from systematic reviews. *Journal of Epidemiology and Community Health,* 64, 284–91.

Becker, G.S. (1996a). A theory of rational addiction. In G.S. Becker *Accounting for Tastes,* pp. 50–76. Cambridge, MA: Harvard University Press.

Becker, G.S. (1996b). *Accounting for Tastes.* Cambridge, MA: Harvard University Press.

Berridge, V. (2007b). *Marketing Health: Smoking and the Discourse of Public Health in Britain, 1945–2000.* Oxford: Oxford University Press.

Borland, R., Winstanley, M., and Reading, D. (2009). Legislation to institutionalize resources for tobacco control: the 1987 Victorian Tobacco Act. *Addiction,* 104, 1623–9.

Brownell, K.D. and Warner, K.E. (2009). The perils of ignoring history: Big Tobacco played dirty and millions died. How similar is Big Food? *Milbank Quarterly,* 87, 259–94.

Butland, B., Jebb, S., Kopelman, P., et al. (2007). *Foresight: Tackling Obesities: Future Choices—Project Report.* London: Foresight Programme, Government Office for Science.

CDC (2011). Vital signs: prevalence, treatment, and control of high levels of low-density lipoprotein cholesterol—United States, 1999–2002 and 2005–2008. *MMWR,* 60, 109–14.

Chan, M. (2008). *The Impact of Climate Change on Human Health: Statement by WHO Director-General Dr Margaret Chan, 7 April 2008.* Geneva: World Health Organization.

Cockerham, W.C., Ruetten, A., and Abel, T. (1997). Conceptualizing contemporary health lifestyles: moving beyond Weber. *The Sociological Quarterly,* 38, 321–42.

Cohen, J.E., Milio, N., Rozier, R.G., Ferrence, R., Ashley, M.J., and Goldstein, A.O. (2000). Political ideology and tobacco control. *Tobacco Control,* 9, 263–7.

Commission on the Social Determinants of Health (2008). *Closing the Gap in a Generation: Health Equity Through Action on the Social Determinants of Health. Final Report of the Commission on Social Determinants of Health.* Geneva: World Health Organization.

Danaei, G., Finucane, M.M., Lin, J.K., et al. (2011). National, regional, and global trends in systolic blood pressure since 1980: systematic analysis of health examination surveys and epidemiological studies with 786 country-years and 5.4 million participants. *The Lancet*, 377, 568–77.

Danaei, G., Singh, G.M., Paciorek, C.J., et al. (2013). The global cardiovascular risk transition: associations of four metabolic risk factors with national income, urbanization, and Western diet in 1980 and 2008. *Circulation*, 127, 1493–502.

Davison, G. and Yelland, S. (2004). Blood on the bitumen. In *Car Wars: How the Car Won Our Hearts and Conquered Our Cities*, pp. 143–67. Crows Nest, Australia: Allen & Unwin.

De Grauwe, P. and Camerman, F. (2002). *How Big are the Big Multinational Companies?* Leuven: University of Leuven.

Diethelm, P. and McKee, M. (2009). Denialism: what is it and how should scientists respond? *European Journal of Public Health*, 19, 2–4.

Dirección General de Tráfico, Spain (2013). *Series Estadísticas Sobre Accidentes y Víctimas I (Annual)*. Madrid: Dirección General de Tráfico.

European Association for Evolutionary Political Economy (EAEPE) (n.d.). Website. Available at: http://eaepe.org/.

Farzadfar, F., Finucane, M.M., and Danaei, G., et al. (2011). National, regional, and global trends in serum total cholesterol since 1980: systematic analysis of health examination surveys and epidemiological studies with 321 country-years and 3.0 million participants. *The Lancet*, 377, 578–86.

Field, M.G. (1967). *Soviet Socialized Medicine: An Introduction*. New York: Free Press.

Gamble, A. (2006). Hayek on knowledge, economics and society. In E. Feser (ed.) *The Cambridge Companion to Hayek*, pp. 111–31. Cambridge, MA: Cambridge University Press.

Glanz, S.A. and Balbach, E.D. (2000). *Tobacco War: Inside the California Battles*. Berkeley, CA: University of California Press.

Global Green and Healthy Hospitals (n.d.). Website. Available at: http://greenhospitals.net/.

Gouda, H.N., Critchley, J., Powles, J., and Capewell, S. (2012). Why choice of metric matters in public health analyses: a case study of the attribution of credit for the decline in coronary heart disease mortality in the US and other populations. *BMC Public Health*, 12, 88.

Gregg, E.W., Cheng, Y.J., Cadwell, B.L., et al. (2005). Secular trends in cardiovascular disease risk factors according to body mass index in US adults. *JAMA: The Journal of the American Medical Association*, 293, 1868–74.

Hayek, F.A. (1960). *The Constitution of Liberty*. Chicago, IL: University of Chicago Press.

Hodgson, G.M. (2013). *From Pleasure Machines to Moral Communities: An Evolutionary Economics Without Homo Economicus*. Chicago, IL: University of Chicago Press.

James, S.L., Gubbins, P., Murray, C.J., and Gakidou, E. (2012). Developing a comprehensive time series of GDP per capita for 210 countries from 1950 to 2015. *Population Health Metrics*, 10, 12.

Keys, A. (1980). *Seven Countries: A Multivariate Analysis of Death and Coronary Heart Disease*. Cambridge, MA: Harvard University Press.

Krementsov, N.L. (1997). *Stalinist Science*. Princeton, NJ: Princeton University Press.

Lewis, J. (1980). *The Politics of Motherhood. Child and Maternal Welfare in England, 1900–1939*. London: Croom Helm.

Lim, S.S., Vos, T., Flaxman, A.D., et al. (2012). A comparative risk assessment of burden of disease and injury attributable to 67 risk factors and risk factor clusters in 21 regions, 1990–2010: a systematic analysis for the Global Burden of Disease Study 2010. *The Lancet*, 380, 2224–60.

Lock, S., Reynolds, L.A., and Tansey, E.M. (1998). *Ashes to Ashes: The History of Smoking and Health Symposium and Witness Seminar Organized by the Wellcome Institute for the History of Medicine and the History of Twentieth Century Medicine Group on 26–27 April 1995*. Amsterdam: Rodopi.

Mackenbach, J. and McKee, M. (2013). *Successes and Failures of Health Policy in Europe: Four Decades of Divergent Trends and Converging Challenges*. Maidenhead: Open University Press.

Mackenbach, J.P., Stirbu, I., Roskam, A.J., et al. (2008). Socioeconomic inequalities in health in 22 European countries. *The New England Journal of Medicine*, 358, 2468–81.

McMichael, A.J. (2013). Globalization, climate change, and human health. *The New England Journal of Medicine*, 368, 1335–43.

Nader, R. (1965). *Unsafe at Any Speed*. New York: Grossman Publishers.

National Institutes of Health (2012). *The NIH Almanac. Appropriations (Section 1)*. Available at: http://www.nih.gov/about/almanac/appropriations/index.htm.

New York City Health Department (2014). *Smoking Legislation*. [Online] Available at: http://www.nyc.gov/html/doh/html/environmental/smoke-law.shtml.

NHS Sustainable Development Unit (2013). *Sustainable Development Strategy for the Health, Public Health and Social Care System: Consultation Jan–May, 2013*. London: NHS Sustainable Development Unit.

Oliver, T.L. (2006). The politics of public health policy. *Annual Review of Public Health*, 27, 195–233.

Peto, R., Watt, J., and Boreham, J. (2013). *Deaths from Smoking*. [Online] International Union Against Cancer. Available at: http://www.ctsu.ox.ac.uk/deathsfromsmoking/.

Pierce, J.P. and Gilpin, E.A. (2001). News media coverage of smoking and health is associated with changes in population rates of smoking cessation but not initiation. *Tobacco Control*, 10, 145–53.

Pierce, J.P., Messer, K., White, M.M., Cowling, D.W., and Thomas, D.P. (2011). Prevalence of heavy smoking in California and the United States, 1965–2007. *JAMA: The Journal of the American Medical Association*, 305, 1106–12.

Pollock, D. (1999). *Denial and Delay: The Political History of Smoking and Health, 1951–1964*. London: Action on Smoking and Health.

Popper, K. (1957). *The Open Society and Its Enemies: Volume 1: The Spell of Plato*. London: Routledge and Kegan Paul.

Powles, J., Shroufi, A., Mathers, C., Zatonski, W., Vecchia, C.L., and Ezzati, M. (2010). National cardiovascular prevention should be based on absolute disease risks, not levels of risk factors. *European Journal of Public Health*, 20, 103–6.

Proctor, R. (2011). *Golden Holocaust: Origins of the Cigarette Catastrophe and the Case for Abolition*. Berkeley, CA: University of California Press.

Puska, P. (2005). Community change and the role of public health. In M. Marmot and P. Elliott (eds.) *Coronary Heart Disease Epidemiology: From Aetiology to Public Health* (2nd ed.), pp. 893–907. Oxford: Oxford University Press,

Riley, J. (2008). *Low Income, Social Growth, and Good Health: A History of Twelve Countries*. Berkeley, CA: University of California Press.

Robertson, L.S. (2010). Motor vehicle industry. In W.H. Wiist (ed.) *The Bottom Line on Public Health: Tactics Corporations Use to Influence Health and Health Policy and What We Can Do to Counter Them*, pp. 225–48. Oxford: Oxford University Press.

Rockstrom, J., Steffen, W., Noone, K., et al. (2009). A safe operating space for humanity. *Nature*, 461, 472–5.

Ruskin, J. (1985). Unto this last: four essays on the first principles of political economy [originally published 1862]. In C. Wilmer (ed.) *John Ruskin: Unto this Last, and Other Writings*, p. 217. London: Penguin Books.

Schroeder, S.A. (2004). Tobacco control in the wake of the 1998 master settlement agreement. *The New England Journal of Medicine*, 350, 293–301.

Smeed, R.J. (1972). The usefulness of formulae in traffic engineering and road safety. *Accident Analysis and Prevention*, 4, 303–12.

Stevens, G.A., Singh, G.M., Lu, Y., et al. (2012). National, regional, and global trends in adult overweight and obesity prevalences. *Population Health Metrics*, 10, 22.

Terris, M. (1988). Restructuring and accelerating the development of the Soviet health service: preliminary observations and recommendations. *Journal of Public Health Policy*, 9, 537–43.

Transport Accident Commission (2013a). *Drink Driving Statistics*. Victoria: Transport Accident Commission.

Transport Accident Commission (2013b). *Road Safety Statistical Summary (Yearly)*. Victoria: Transport Accident Commission.

United Kingdom and Secretary of State for Social Services (1988). *Public Health in England: The Report of the Committee of Inquiry into the Future Development of the Public Health Function (D. Acheson, Chairman)*. London: HMSO.

von Mises, L.A. and Greaves, B.B.E. (2007). *Human Action: A Treatise on Economics,* Liberty Fund, Indianapolis.

Wang, H., Dwyer-Lindgren, L., Lofgren, K.T., et al. (2012). Age-specific and sex-specific mortality in 187 countries, 1970–2010: a systematic analysis for the Global Burden of Disease Study 2010 (online appendix). *The Lancet*, 380, 2071–94.

Wiist, W.H. (2010). The corporation: an overview of what it is, its tactics, and what public health can do. In W.H. Wiist (ed.) *The Bottom Line on Public Health: Tactics Corporations Use to Influence Health and Health Policy and What We Can Do to Counter Them*, pp. 3–72. Oxford: Oxford University Press.

Woodcock, J., Edwards, P., Tonne, C., et al. (5-12-2009). Public health benefits of strategies to reduce greenhouse-gas emissions: urban land transport. *The Lancet*, 374, 1930–43.

Woolf, S.H. and Aron, L. (eds.) (2013a). *U.S. Health in International Perspective: Shorter Lives, Poorer Health*. Washington, DC: National Research Council and Institute of Medicine, National Academies Press.

Woolf, S.H. and Aron, L. (2013b). Policies and social values. In S.H. Woolf and L. Aron (eds.) *U.S. Health in International Perspective: Shorter Lives, Poorer Health*, pp. 207–38. Washington, DC: National Research Council and Institute of Medicine, National Academies Press.

World Bank (2013). *World Development Report Online*. Washington, DC: World Bank.

World Health Organization (2008). *WHO Report On The Global Tobacco Epidemic*. Geneva: World Health Organization. Available online: http://whqlibdoc.who.int/publications/2008/9789241596282_eng.pdf.

World Health Organization (2013). *WHO Framework Convention on Tobacco Control*. Geneva: World Health Organization.

Yoon, S.S., Ostchega, Y., and Louis, T. (2010). Recent trends in the prevalence of high blood pressure and its treatment and control, 1999–2008. *NCHS Data Brief*, 48.

Zatonski, W. (1996). *Evolution of Health in Poland Since 1988*. Warsaw: Maria Sklodowska-Curie Cancer Center and Institute of Oncology.

3.8

International efforts to promote public health

Douglas Bettcher,[1] Katherine DeLand, Gemma Lien, Fernando Gonzalez-Martinez, Anne Huvos, Steven Solomon, Ulrike Schwerdtfeger, Haik Nikogosian, Angelika Tritscher, and Julia Dalzell

Introduction: global health governance, international health instruments, and global public goods

As detailed in Chapter 1.5 on globalization, the world today is becoming less recognizable as a system of independent states and is instead increasingly viewed as a complex network of interdependent states and non-state actors, linked in multifaceted ways. Globalization forces such as migration, trade, food production and movement, insect/microbe resistance to drugs, and environmental change increase the speed and geographical scope of cross-border health risks and directly challenge the existing system of international health governance defined by national borders (Dodgson et al. 2002). In light of these shifts in the broad global landscapes, the notion of global health governance (GHG) should also shift and be recast to reflect the new realities. This chapter continues the examination of GHG begun in Chapter 1.5, expanding the discussion to address international legal instruments and global public goods as key elements of GHG.

GHG has been defined as 'the use of formal and informal institutions, rules and processes by states, intergovernmental organizations, and non-state actors to deal with challenges to health that require cross-border collective action to address effectively' (Fidler and Calamaras 2010, p. 3). The fundamental idea underpinning GHG is that the world has assets capable of improving population health and these should be deployed and distributed more equitably and effectively (WHO 2013a).

The essential functions of GHG 'are generally agreed upon and include convening, defining shared values, ensuring coherence, establishing standards and regulatory frameworks, providing direction (e.g. setting priorities), mobilizing and aligning resources, and promoting research' (Sridhar et al. 2008/2009, p. 2).

International governmental cooperation in the governance of health issues resulted in the establishment of the World Health Organization (WHO) in 1948, arguably one of the greatest achievements of GHG to date. Since then, various forms and mechanisms of health governance have been developed under the auspices of WHO, in accord with the provisions of the WHO Constitution: formal decision-making forums (for example, the World Health Assembly), legally binding instruments (for example, the International Health Regulations (2005) and the WHO Framework Convention on Tobacco Control (WHO FCTC)), voluntary agreements (such as the Pandemic Influenza Preparedness (PIP) Framework), and shared goals or strategies (such as the health objectives contained in the Millennium Development Goals). As a formalized, intergovernmental agency, WHO has provided and continues to provide a robust platform for state-to-state negotiations on agreed approaches towards global health aims.

However, as globalization has progressed and our understanding of the complexity of global health, health interventions, and health systems has become more sophisticated, it is clear that GHG is no longer solely a matter of intergovernmental concern, nor is there always the necessary political will or mandate to address all transborder public health issues through governmental mechanisms. As noted in Chapter 1.5, often civil society and foundations seek to fill these gaps. More and more commonly, the public health community is also creating public–private partnerships, like the Global Fund to Fight AIDS, Tuberculosis and Malaria (Global Fund), the Global Alliance for Vaccines and Immunization (GAVI Alliance), and Roll Back Malaria. It is worth noting that, while these partnerships involve WHO and other United Nations (UN) agencies, all are outside of the purely intergovernmental context, to allow for adequate flexibility for the formal participation and contribution of key non-state actors.

Global public–private partnerships (GPPPs) represent a qualitatively new hybrid form of governance, bringing together in a partnership bodies such as intergovernmental organizations, states, non-governmental organizations, development banks, philanthropic foundations, and multinational corporations to achieve a shared health-creating goal. The Global Polio Eradication Initiative is one such example of a GPPP, bringing together WHO, the UN Children's Fund (UNICEF), the United States Centers for Disease Control and Prevention, and Rotary International in the effort to eradicate polio.

Critics of these new approaches are concerned that public and private goals are not mutually compatible and argue that the new initiatives may be susceptible to undue influence of private interests. The increase in the number of GPPPs in the health sector may have 'significant implications for the exercise of governance of health through the multilateral UN regime' and may ultimately 'undermine the ability of WHO to effectively contribute to health governance at the global level' (Buse and Walt 2002). These new initiatives may increase competition for scarce resources and influence and have the potential to cause verticalization within health policymaking. To be most effective, GHG must include both vertical and horizontal approaches, particularly with regard to complicated issues like those identified in Chapter 1.5 (i.e. tobacco, obesity and infectious disease outbreaks or public health emergencies). The harmonization of efforts by the traditional entities, like WHO, and the new contributors, like the GPPPs, is key to the longer-term success of GHG in addressing major health concerns.

Two distinct concepts have begun to emerge in the field of GHG: governance *of* health and governance *for* health. Governance of health entails coordinating and directing public health efforts (for example, through resolutions of the World Health Assembly). Governance for health, however, is an advocacy and policy function seeking to influence the governance of other sectors (for example, agriculture, trade, and environment) to include and benefit health efforts (WHO 2013a).

Governance for health recognizes that a broad range of social, economic, political, and environmental determinants impact population health and that public health solutions must be found to address issues such as poverty, access to affordable healthcare and medicines, climate change, and food security. States are beginning to recognize that health is important not just for population well-being, but also for national and international security, economic well-being, and the economic and social development of developing countries (Fidler and Calamaras 2010). Approaching these issues from a 'health-in-all-policies' perspective enables governments to factor health impact into law and norm development.

However, it is also essential to consider the role of non-state actors. As the global health policy landscape responds to globalization, non-state actors like multinational corporations and philanthropic foundations become more and more involved. While interest in and support for public health are critical, it is worth noting that the substantial financial influence these non-state actors can wield may lead to a shift not only in how global health is funded, but in what is funded (Smith 2010).

It has been argued that the biggest obstacle for GHG 'might not be unstructured plurality but the plurality of incapacity', given that despite large donors and the increased profile of GHG, 'the political and financial responsibility for public health infrastructure and capacity' still falls on governments (Fidler 2007). More needs to be done to build and sustain public health systems and capabilities within states. Whether hard (i.e. binding) or soft (i.e. non-binding) law is developed through GHG, the fact remains that states still need the national capacity to implement and enforce those laws.

To remedy the 'unstructured plurality' of the current fractured global landscape, it has been suggested that a new global agreement or a treaty on global health may be the answer (Kickbusch 2006; Gostin 2007). Other suggestions include adding a 'Committee C'

to the World Health Assembly with the aim of providing a forum for non-state actors (Silberscmidt et al. 2008). As part of its recently initiated reform process, WHO's Executive Board and the World Health Assembly have both considered next steps in developing a policy on engagement with non-governmental organizations (WHO 2013a, 2013b). Regardless of the approach taken, WHO's Constitution mandates it to act as 'the directing and coordinating authority on international health work' (WHO 1946).

Global public goods

Economists have used the term *public good* for centuries to think about and analyse national governance. A public good is a good that has two characteristics: (1) it is non-rival in consumption—that is, its consumption by an individual does not impede someone else from consuming it—and (2) it is non-excludable, which means that one cannot prevent someone else from consuming it. One example of a public good is street lighting. As a person walks down a street at night, the light illuminates the sidewalk. Using the light does not impede other people from using that same light as they walk. While often tangible, like the street light, public goods can also be intangibles, like security or education. Since public goods tend to be underprovided in the absence of government intervention, due to the 'free-rider problem' (i.e. taking advantage of a public good without providing for its existence or maintenance), it is often the role of governments to provide them.

The interconnectedness of states as a result of globalization naturally leads to an increase in domestic public goods common to the interacting states. Correlatively, the singular nature of some of what were once solely domestic public goods has progressively declined as the creation and maintenance of those public goods became shared enterprises. This has led to the emergence of the concept of the global public good (GPG). Kaul et al. define GPG as a public good having three characteristics (Box 3.8.1).

Based on these criteria, health is arguably a GPG. As a public good, health is a positive sum: one person's good health does not detract from another's (characteristic 1). Indeed, better individual health usually has positive effects on entire populations—for example, through reduced disease transmission. As health is not only an end in itself but is also inseparable from social and economic welfare, health is also a key element for economic and social growth. An improvement in individual health can improve

---

Box 3.8.1 Global public goods

1. Covers more than one group of countries.

2. Its benefits [...] reach [...] a broad spectrum of the global population (which means that access to them must not be limited to certain economic classes, gender, religious groups, or any other discrete community).

3. It meets the needs of present generations without jeopardizing those of future generations (Kaul et al. 1999).

Source: data from Kaul, I. et al., 'Defining global public goods', in Kaul, I. et al. (Eds), *Global Public Goods: International Cooperation in the 21st Century*, pp. 2–19, Oxford University Press, New York, USA, Copyright © 1999 by the United Nations Development Programme.

the community-level economy and social fabric (characteristics 2 and 3). Furthermore, although the onus of providing health remains primarily on national governments, globalization means that the determinants of health, as well as the requisite means to deliver health, are increasingly global (characteristic 1) (Jamison et al. 1998).

Two forces are moving health progressively toward the centre of the stage in the discussion of GPGs. First, as already noted, enhanced international linkages in trade, migration and information flows have accelerated the cross-border transmission of disease and the international transfer of non-communicable behavioural health risks. Second, intensified pressure on common-pool global resources, such as air and water, has generated shared, transnational environmental threats. However, the notion of health as a GPG is not uncontested. It has been argued that an individual's health—or even an entire country's health status—primarily benefits only the individual or country and that the resources necessary to provide better health are indeed 'predominantly rival and exclusive' (Woodward and Smith 2003). This school of thought agrees that some aspects of health, including control of globally threatening communicable disease like HIV/AIDS and tuberculosis, may be GPGs, but there is some concern that 'relaxing' the interpretation of GPG to include health may dilute the usefulness of GPGs as means to secure funding (Smith and Woodward 2003). Perhaps most importantly, if health as a GPG is limited to very prescribed circumstances like control of an infectious disease, then it loses its capacity as an organizing principle for global health priorities (Smith et al. 2004).

Nonetheless, even among those who maintain that health is not a GPG, there is a strong sense that collective action and coordination, as the core notion of GPGs, can be used to great and measurable effect to promote and improve global health, through, for instance, the development of international public health legal instruments.

As well as being the means to a GPG end (in this case, health), international instruments *themselves* could also be considered within the rubric of GPGs, insofar as they provide a shared platform for the process of improving social and economic welfare. However, the agreement to coordinate and to act in concert, while critical for reaching a GPG, is part of the process rather than an outcome in and of itself. This conceptualization allows us to introduce a typology that distinguishes two different types of GPGs: final GPGs and intermediate GPGs:

1. Final global public goods are outcomes rather than 'goods' in the standard sense. They may be tangible (such as the environment or the common heritage of mankind) or intangible (such as peace or financial stability).

2. Intermediate global public goods, such as international regimes, contribute towards the provision of final global public goods (Kaul et al. 1999).

As there is no supranational authority that can ensure the provision of GPGs, the implications of globalization include the need for increased transnational cooperation and partnerships, as well as greater intersectoral action. Intermediate GPGs (see Box 3.8.2), like international norms, agreements and regulations, play an important role in this dynamic (Kaul et al. 2003; Fidler 2002; Taylor et al. 2003). The WHO FCTC provides an example of an intermediate GPG. As an intermediate GPG, the WHO FCTC establishes a basis

---

Box 3.8.2 Intermediate global public goods

Instruments that contribute to the provision of final global public goods.

Box 3.8.3 Final global public goods

Outcomes that can be tangible (such as the environment or the common heritage of mankind) or intangible (such as peace or financial stability).

---

for coordinated action among states, which will bring about a significant health improvement not otherwise efficiently obtainable by states acting on their own (Taylor et al. 2003).

Using the intermediate GPG of international law to achieve the final GPG of health

Using international law to produce health, the goal and final GPG (see Box 3.8.3) of international health instruments, comprises four essential aspects. First, states use international law to establish formal institutions empowered to work on global public health problems. The modern classic example of this is, of course, WHO itself, but it is reasonable to also include certain others, such as the United Nations Environment Programme (UNEP) and the International Labor Organization (ILO), that also, if somewhat indirectly, promote and foster health.

Second, states use international law to establish procedures through which states and non-state actors can tackle specific global public health problems. For example, to effectively address the transnationalization of health risks and diseases, instruments like the WHO FCTC and the International Health Regulations (IHR) provide frameworks for efficient multilateral information and surveillance systems. Implementation and ongoing evolution and improvement of these systems are critical, and the complexity inherent in this kind of information gathering is exemplified by WHO's strengthening global monitoring and alert systems, which link together, *inter alia*, specialized laboratories, disease surveillance systems, sources of relevant expertise, and state governments via electronic and printed media.

Third, states use international law to craft substantive duties in connection with particular global public health challenges. The IHR, for example, obligate WHO Member States to notify the Organization of specific public health events. The WHO FCTC requires Parties to implement specific obligations like adhering to a discrete tobacco product labelling and warning regime, as well as to incorporate the general obligations and objectives of the Convention into their approaches to providing health.

Fourth, states use international law to create mechanisms to enforce substantive legal duties undertaken by states that have agreed to be bound by international instruments. Enforcement mechanisms come in many forms, from states self-reporting on progress made in connection with certain goals articulated in a treaty, as is common in multilateral environmental agreements like the Basel Convention on the Control of Transboundary Movements of Hazardous Wastes and their Disposal (1992), to formal adjudication of state-to-state disputes by an international tribunal, as seen in the WTO's dispute-settlement mechanism.

While various instruments can be intermediate GPGs for health, international legal agreements are among the most important. International legal agreements provide a foundation for many other intermediate products with global public benefits, including institutionalized forums for global cooperation, research, surveillance, technical assistance programmes, and information clearing-houses. Global agreements are negotiated to secure global cooperation, and that cooperation, in turn, leads to the sustained creation and promotion of health and related GPGs.

Case studies

The intermediate GPGs that comprise health-related international normative agreements, strategies, and instruments will improve public health, reduce the burden of disease, and lead to reductions in poverty and increases in economic development. Globalization has been a cardinal factor triggering the expansion of international health law and has compelled the international community to think creatively and to develop new models of cooperation, including the expanded use of international health law, to protect and promote the health of populations worldwide. The five case studies that follow illustrate the relevance of norms, standards, agreements, and regulations in transnational disease control and discuss the impact of such instruments now and in the future.

Case study: the WHO Framework Convention on Tobacco Control

The WHO FCTC is a carefully balanced legal instrument, adopted following vigorous negotiations, which took into account scientific, economic, social, and political considerations. The launch of WHO's first treaty negotiation was catalysed by a unique convergence of a number of factors, including the accumulation of scientific evidence demonstrating the causal links between tobacco use and more than 20 major categories of disease (Doll 1998), and evidence pointing to the global toll of tobacco-related diseases, the release as a result of litigation in the United States of over 35 million pages of previously secret tobacco industry documents, which provided a unique opportunity to better understand the strategies and tactics of the tobacco industry and, in doing so, to advance the public health agenda (Yach and Bettcher 2000), the establishment of a WHO cabinet project, the Tobacco Free Initiative, and the support of civil society in the form of public pressure on governments for strengthened tobacco regulations as the public became more aware of the dangers of tobacco (Da Costa e Silva and Nikogosian 2003).

The WHO FCTC is the first treaty negotiated under the auspices of WHO. As such, it is a milestone in public health and it provides new legal dimensions in international health cooperation. This case study explores the status of the WHO FCTC, demonstrates how the provisions of the Convention promote evidence-based interventions that have been proven to be effective, and finally discusses how the WHO FCTC is an intermediate GPG for health.

Fast-paced ratification

The WHO FCTC entered into force on 27 February 2005 when it had 40 Parties, only about one and a half years after it had been opened for signature (WHO 2003c). Those 40 rapidly grew to 177 in 2013. The WHO FCTC now covers about 90 per cent of the world's population (see Fig. 3.8.1).

Key provisions of the WHO FCTC

The Convention includes a number of provisions regarding demand- as well as supply-reduction measures. Key provisions also include obligations to establish or reinforce a national coordinating mechanism for tobacco control, to protect public health policies with respect to tobacco control from interests of the tobacco industry and to consider taking legislative action to address liability, including compensation. In addition, the Convention addresses international cooperation as well as reporting and the exchange of information.

Demand-reduction measures
Price measures
Price and tax measures are an important and effective means of reducing tobacco consumption—a fact recognized in Article 6. It is estimated that a 10 per cent increase in the price of cigarettes will reduce consumption by approximately 4 per cent in a high-income country and by approximately 8 per cent in a low- or middle-income country (World Bank 1999). Furthermore, it has been shown that tax increases have a stronger impact on young people, which is particularly important, as the risk of lung cancer increases exponentially with the duration of smoking. Lastly, increases in tobacco taxes increase government revenue.

Non-price measures
Protection from exposure to tobacco smoke. Article 8 of the WHO FCTC requires Parties to provide 'for protection from exposure to tobacco smoke in indoor workplaces, public transport, indoor public places and, as appropriate, other places' (WHO 2003c).

Packaging and labelling of tobacco products. When warning labels contain large, graphic, thought provoking, and factual information, they are effective in deterring tobacco use. Article 11 obliges Parties to appropriately label packages of tobacco products. Tobacco product label warnings are unique in prevention because the consumer receives the warning at the time of use.

Education, communication, training, and public awareness. In Article 12, Parties are required to adopt legislative or other measures that promote public awareness and access to information on the dangers of tobacco.

Tobacco advertising, promotion, and sponsorship. Article 13 requires each Party to undertake comprehensive bans of all tobacco advertising, promotion and sponsorship, as far as constitutionally possible for each Party.

Article 14 requires Parties, for example, to create cessation programmes, including in workplaces, educational institutions, and other settings; and to include diagnosis and treatment of nicotine dependence in national health programmes.

Supply-reduction measures

In Article 15, the WHO FCTC recognizes that the elimination of smuggling and all forms of illicit trade in tobacco products is an essential component of tobacco control. The first Protocol to the WHO FCTC builds upon and complements Article 15.

Further supply-reduction measures in the WHO FCTC include measures to protect minors (Article 16) and to provide support for economically viable alternatives to tobacco growing (Article 17).

Treaty bodies

The Convention's main treaty bodies, the Conference of the Parties (COP) and the Convention Secretariat, have been established and

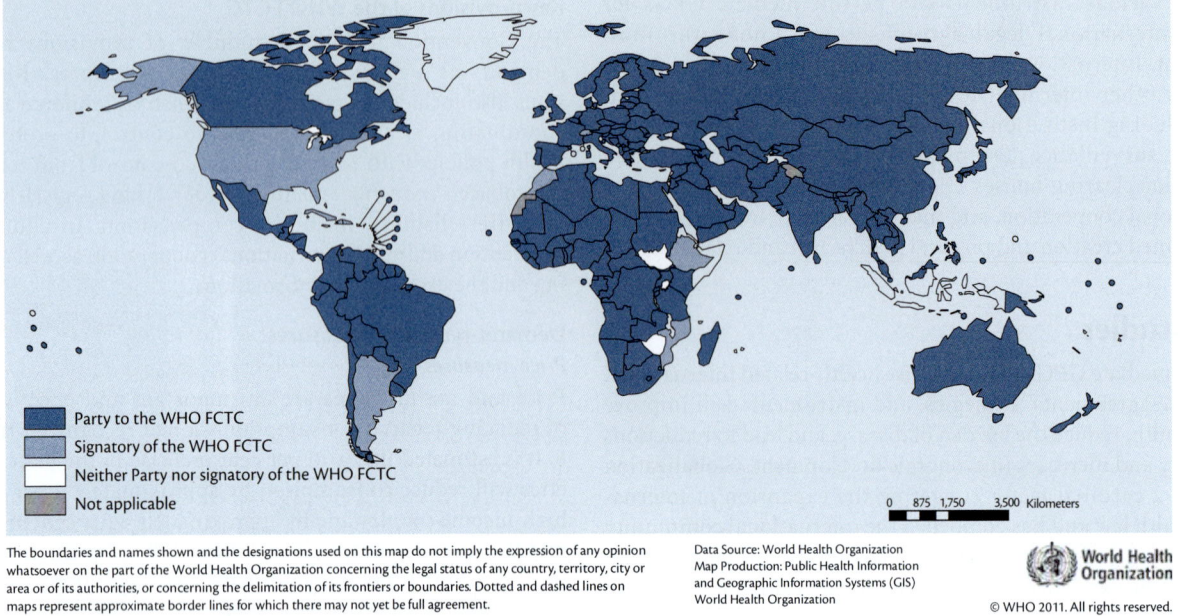

Party to the WHO FCTC
Signatory of the WHO FCTC
Neither Party nor signatory of the WHO FCTC
Not applicable

The boundaries and names shown and the designations used on this map do not imply the expression of any opinion whatsoever on the part of the World Health Organization concerning the legal status of any country, territory, city or area or of its authorities, or concerning the delimitation of its frontiers or boundaries. Dotted and dashed lines on maps represent approximate border lines for which there may not yet be full agreement.

Data Source: World Health Organization
Map Production: Public Health Information
and Geographic Information Systems (GIS)
World Health Organization

World Health Organization

© WHO 2011. All rights reserved.

Fig. 3.8.1 Parties to the WHO Framework Convention on Tobacco Control (FCTC).
Reproduced with permission of the World Health Organization, Copyright © 2011

are fully functional (Nikogosian 2010). The governing body of the WHO FCTC, the COP, now meets every 2 years. Starting from its second session, Parties have been hosting this global public health event. The first COP (COP1) was held in 2006 in Geneva, and subsequent sessions were hosted by Thailand, South Africa, Uruguay, and the Republic of Korea (COP 2007, 2008, 2010, 2012). The sixth session of the Conference was hosted by the Russian Federation (COP 2014).

Treaty instruments

One notable development is the rapid development of treaty instruments, namely implementation guidelines and the first Protocol.

Article 7 of the WHO FCTC obliges the COP to propose 'appropriate guidelines for the implementation...of' the non-price measures to reduce the demand for tobacco products. The COP has met this obligation by adopting guidelines for Articles 8 (COP 2007), 11, 12, and 13 (COP 2008 and 2010). Partial guidelines for Articles 9 and 10 have been adopted and remain work in progress (COP 2006, 2007, 2008, 2010, 2012). Although not directly referred to in Article 7, the Parties also adopted guidelines for Articles 5.3 and 14 (COP 2008 and 2012). The COP's initiative to elaborate guidelines on Article 5.3 corresponds with the large extent of interference of the tobacco industry experienced by Parties while implementing the WHO FCTC (COP 2012; WHO 2012a).

In addition, guidelines and policy options are being developed for Articles 6, 17, and 18 (COP 2012) and the COP also established an intergovernmental working group on sustainable measures to strengthen the implementation of the WHO FCTC (COP 2012). Therefore, the COP adopted guidelines and established processes for further instruments for the majority of substantive articles of the WHO FCTC in the brief period between 2006 and 2012.

Reporting system

Under Article 21, Parties have an obligation to submit periodic reports on the status of implementation to the COP. The reporting system was established and refined quickly; it is now functional and synchronized with the biennial cycle of the COP. More than 90 per cent of Parties submitted at least one implementation report after the entry into force of the Convention (WHO 2012a). The Secretariat regularly issues global progress reports based on the reports submitted by Parties. The latest report was issued in 2012, with plans to publish new reports every 2 years.

International cooperation and assistance

The importance of implementation assistance to Parties has risen steadily. Constraints and barriers encountered by Parties are manifold (WHO 2012a) and require adequate assistance. A range of mechanisms of assistance and international cooperation modes were systematized and promoted by the COP and in the UN system. Based on Article 26, a database of resources available to support the implementation of the Convention was created. Needs assessment exercises are carried out in many Parties jointly between the government and the Convention Secretariat, also involving the respective WHO office and relevant UN agencies and other international partners. The integration of the WHO FCTC in national health and development programmes has emerged as a central mechanism in implementation assistance. The role of the WHO FCTC has also been highly recognized in the action against the growing burden of non-communicable diseases (NCDs) as stated in the 'Political Declaration of the High-level Meeting of the General Assembly on the Prevention and Control of NCDs' (United Nations 2012).

In a recent decision, the United Nations Economic and Social Council (ECOSOC) called for UN system-wide coherence on tobacco control. In particular, it encouraged the members of the

Ad Hoc Inter-Agency Task Force on Tobacco Control to promote effective tobacco control policies and assistance mechanisms at the national level, including by integrating WHO FCTC implementation within the United Nations Development Assistance Frameworks (ECOSOC 2012).

Newly adopted treaty: Protocol to Eliminate Illicit Trade in Tobacco Products

The COP recognized that 'cooperative action is necessary to eliminate all forms of illicit trade in tobacco products' and established the Intergovernmental Negotiating Body (INB), mandated with negotiating a protocol (COP 2007).

The INB held five sessions between 2008 and 2012. The absolute majority of WHO FCTC Parties participated in the negotiating sessions. At its fifth session, the INB agreed on a draft text of a protocol to eliminate illicit trade in tobacco products. The Protocol was adopted on 12 November 2012 at the fifth session of the COP in Seoul (COP 2012).

The Protocol comprises a variety of obligations, namely the Supply Chain Control, including the establishment of a licensing system, an international tracking and tracing regime, due diligence, provisions for free zones, duty free sales, and the sale by Internet. In addition, the Protocol aims to protect personal data and addresses unlawful conduct including criminal offences, 'seizure payments', the disposal of confiscated products, information sharing, assistance and cooperation, mutual legal assistance and reporting.

One of the lessons learned during the negotiations was that one way to reach consensus on a controversial matter is to refer it to the governing body. For example, the Protocol refers two technical matters to its governing body, the Meeting of the Parties (MOP): whether key inputs exist and the extent of illicit trade related to duty free sales (WHO 2013b).

The Protocol includes time-bound provisions. Within 5 years of entry into force, Parties have to establish a global tracking and tracing regime (WHO 2013b). Each Party has to ensure that 'unique identification markings' are affixed to packets and outside packaging of cigarettes within 5 years and other tobacco products within 10 years of entry into force of the Protocol for that Party (WHO 2013b). Regarding free zones, Parties have to control the manufacture and transactions in tobacco and tobacco products within 3 years of entry into force (WHO 2013b).

The infrastructure established under the WHO FCTC is used for the Protocol—this concerns the rules of procedure and financial rules of the COP, the reporting being incorporated into the COP reporting, and the sessions of the MOP to be held back-to-back with those of the COP (WHO 2013b).

Impact of WHO FCTC

The implementation of the Convention already demonstrated its impact on national legislation. One key conclusion of Parties' reports is that following ratification, 80 per cent of Parties either adopted new tobacco control legislation or strengthened existing legislation (Fig. 3.8.2). The COP decided at its fifth session that an impact assessment, linked to the tenth anniversary of the entry into force of the Convention in 2015, should be carried out.

Empirically, increasing the price of tobacco products is a strong measure to curb consumption. The potency of this measure is clear in economic terms: a 33 per cent increase in the price of tobacco would yield a cost-effectiveness ratio of US $3 to $42 for every disability-adjusted life year (DALY) averted in low- and middle-income countries, and of US $85 to $1773 in high-income countries (Jamison et al. 2006). An averted DALY has sizeable financial implications, with less public and private expenditure on healthcare for tobacco-attributed illnesses. And contrary to critics' fears, taxation on tobacco products actually raises government revenues because consumption usually falls at a slower rate than price increases (Frank et al. 2000).

The implementation of price and other strong measures are linked with public health and broader economic gains, with positive implications for long-term development. The treaty also serves as a legal resource and catalysed strong movement to address the growing burden of NCDs worldwide.

The WHO FCTC as an intermediate global public good for health

The WHO FCTC and the process of negotiating the WHO FCTC both have important intermediate GPG characteristics. The Convention and its negotiation are intermediate GPGs in that both have facilitated the development of tobacco control policies globally (Taylor et al. 2003). The WHO FCTC facilitates the flow of information about tobacco control and serves as a mechanism to coordinate various transnational aspects of tobacco control, including smuggling, advertising, packaging, and labelling. It enhances global surveillance, information exchange, and international technical, legal, and financial cooperation in tobacco control. The WHO FCTC process continues to provide a global instrument for public health professionals to distribute their evidence to governments and to get this evidence incorporated into binding agreements including future protocols to the Convention. Overall, it provides new legal dimensions for international health cooperation.

Conclusion: the WHO Framework Convention on Tobacco Control

The strength of the WHO FCTC resides in several elements. First, it is an evidence-based treaty. All the tobacco control measures required by the WHO FCTC have been proven to be effective and are based on numerous experiences and facts. Second, it is a comprehensive tool that addresses all the effective tobacco control policies that can be implemented to reduce tobacco consumption; its effect will exceed the sum of the results of each measure taken separately because some measures increase the effectiveness of others. Third, the process of developing the Convention showed how the growing role of transnational factors in health can be addressed through a legally binding instrument, a new direction in international health. Fourth, the Convention demonstrated its attractiveness as a new type of global public health instrument— more than half of States ratified it within less than three years of entry into force, and the absolute majority had done so by 2012. Fifth, Parties displayed high commitment in the implementation of the Convention, including by promptly establishing the principal treaty instruments, such as guidelines, the reporting system, the mechanisms of assistance and the first protocol to the WHO FCTC. Finally, the years after the entry into force have shown growing political recognition of the role of the WHO FCTC on the global health and development agenda, including in the UN system.

The WHO FCTC provides a legal framework for improving the health of all people. It is a model for an effective global response

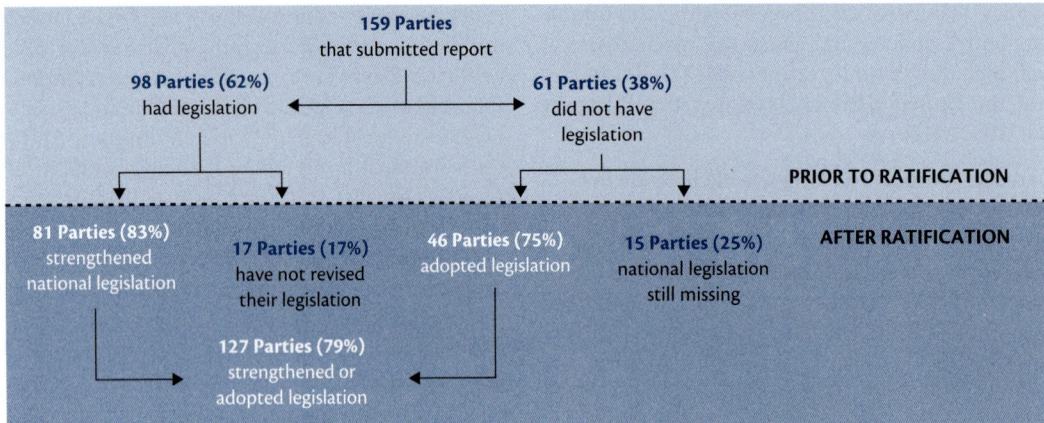

Fig. 3.8.2 Adoption of legislative, executive, administrative, and other measures in relation of ratification of the WHO FCTC.
Reproduced from World Health Organization, xxx, World Health Organization, Geneva, Switzerland, Copyright © 2013, available from xxx. Reproduced with permission from World Health Organization, *2012 global progress report on implementation of the WHO Framework Convention on Tobacco Control*, p. 11, Copyright © World Health Organization 2012, available from http://apps.who.int/iris/bitstream/10665/79170/1/9789241504652_eng.pdf?ua=1

to the negative effects of globalization on health. However, the Convention remains a tool and its success depends on governments' dedication to making the best use of it (Nikogosian 2010).

Case study: the International Health Regulations (2005)

The International Health Regulations (2005) (hereinafter 'IHR' or 'the Regulations') are an instrument of international law adopted by the World Health Assembly, WHO's supreme decision-making body,[2] on 23 May 2005 under Article 21 of the WHO Constitution. They entered into force, generally, on 15 June 2007 and are legally binding on 196 States Parties, including all WHO Member States. The Regulations apply to emerging infectious diseases like SARS and pandemic influenza, as well as to those cross-border threats that arise as a result of public health risks and emergencies whose origin may be biological, chemical or radiological in nature. The 2011 nuclear accident in Fukushima, Japan, is an illustration of how the IHR may apply to an event which is not biological in nature. The stated purpose and scope of the Regulations are to prevent, protect against, control, and provide a public health response to the international spread of disease in ways that are commensurate with and restricted to public health risks, and which avoid unnecessary interference with international traffic and trade. In order to fully appreciate their broad scope, however, it is necessary to refer to key terms, which are defined in the IHR, including event, disease, public health risk, public health emergency of international concern and international traffic (WHO 2005). This case study describes experiences and progress in implementing the IHR in States Parties with the support of the WHO Secretariat with a view to showing how the Regulations may, in part, be considered an intermediate GPG for health.

The IHR as an intermediate global public good for health

The concept of public goods and what makes them global have been defined and discussed elsewhere in this chapter. Relevant to the examination of the IHR, disease control at the national level through the adoption of regulatory measures can be seen as a public good for health. That is, such a public good is non-excludable because it benefits those who are not even aware that there is a risk (of disease) and non-rivalrous due to the fact that one person benefiting from disease control does not prevent another from also benefiting. With regard to the global nature of the public good of infectious disease control it is clearly the intent of the IHR to be a transboundary, globally inclusive instrument. Article 3 (Principles) of the 2005 IHR provides that the implementation of the new rules 'shall be guided by the goal of their universal application for the protection of all people of the world from the international spread of disease' (WHO 2005).

In terms of the IHR as an intermediate GPG for health, the freedom from epidemics (or epidemic control) is a final GPG for health, while the surveillance and control mechanisms required to attain this goal are an intermediate GPG for health. A functioning IHR provides the set of rules that establish administrative and legislative structures in support of these intermediate GPGs for health. Therefore, inasmuch as they deal with epidemic control, the IHR may constitute an intermediate GPG for health. Although it remains difficult to assess the extent to which the IHR will be an effective tool to curb epidemics, it is clear that its purpose and scope continue to make it a strong candidate as an intermediate GPG for health.

As is shown by the monitoring framework developed by WHO (see later) to assess progress in implementing the IHR, the Regulations' coverage is considered broad enough to encompass relevant public health risks involving biological, chemical, or radiological agents (WHO 2007b). It is also important to reiterate that the IHR are designed to contain the international spread of disease while at the same time ensuring that the international movement of people and goods is not unnecessarily restricted. This nexus between public health and international traffic, as well as between the law of infectious disease and trade law, continues to be an important and defining aspect of the Regulations.

Strengthening capacities for IHR implementation

A major focus of IHR implementation has been to support States Parties to strengthen existing surveillance and response capacities. Indeed, according to Article 5 and 13 of the Regulations, IHR States Parties have 5 years from entry into force (i.e. 15 June

2007) 'to develop, strengthen and maintain the capacities to detect, assess, notify and report events' (to WHO) and 'to respond promptly and effectively to public health risks and public health emergencies of international concern', as set out in Annex 1. The 5-year period for developing, strengthening or maintaining these capacities expired for most IHR States Parties on 15 June 2012. It is important to highlight that under the IHR, States Parties that have not met their capacity requirements may apply for and obtain a further 2-year period to establish them (i.e. through 15 June 2014) based on a justified need and upon presentation of an implementation plan. To date, more than one-half of IHR States Parties have obtained such an extension.

A key issue in applying for extensions is the progress States Parties have made to implement the Regulations and how this progress has been measured. Moreover, under Article 54 of the IHR and World Health Assembly resolution WHA61.2 (WHO 2008), States Parties must report to the Assembly, WHO's supreme governing body, on progress made in implementing the Regulations. To assist countries to assess this progress and meet this reporting requirement, WHO has developed a monitoring framework with eight core capacities for tracking IHR implementation: (1) national legislation, policy, and financing; (2) coordination at national level and the communication of National IHR Focal Points,[3] both globally and nationally; (3) surveillance; (4) response; (5) preparedness; (6) appropriate communication of risks; (7) human resources; and (8) adequate laboratory services. The framework also defines five relevant hazard types: (1) infectious, (2) zoonotic, (3) food safety-related, (4) chemical, and (5) radionuclear (WHO 2011a). In line with this framework, States Parties are annually requested to complete a self-assessment questionnaire. The latest questionnaire from 2012 has garnered the following summary results based on 127 (of 195) responses (WHO 2013c): progress has been made with respect to surveillance (with a global average score of 81 per cent), response (78 per cent), and zoonotic events (80 per cent). Low capacities were reported for human resources (with a global average of 53 per cent), chemical events (51 per cent), and radiological events (53 per cent). In addition to the self-assessment questionnaire, a number of IHR States Parties have requested WHO to conduct assessment missions and conduct desk audits to, *inter alia*, identify gaps and develop action plans for IHR implementation through 2014 (WHO 2013c).

Evaluating the functioning of the IHR and pandemic influenza (H1N1) 2009

On 25 April 2009, the WHO Director-General determined that the ongoing human influenza event in Mexico and the United States of America constituted a public health emergency of international concern[4] (WHO 2009). This was the first time (and the only time to date) since the entry into force of the Regulations that such an international emergency had been declared by the WHO Director-General.[5] This determination was an important step because until that date a host of IHR provisions had not been tested since PHEICs are (almost by definition) rare occasions and in 'peace time' the Regulations are applied on a daily basis to other types of public health events, risks and emergencies that do not reach the 'PHEIC' threshold, as determined by the Director-General. The significance of this event as relates to the IHR as GPG for health is that, in the aftermath of the pandemic,

concerns were raised that the IHR, the WHO and the world community had not met up to their expectations and that there was a need to draw lessons from this unique experience. In addition to this, under Article 54 of the IHR, the Health Assembly is required to review the *functioning* of the IHR and this review must take place 'no later than five years after the entry into force of these Regulations'. The timing of this review was further decided by the Health Assembly in resolution WHA61.2. Article 54 also provides that this review may be conducted with the advice of a Review Committee to be convened by the Director-General. In 2010, WHO's Executive Board[6] welcomed the proposal of the WHO Director-General to establish such a Committee whose objectives were to: (1) assess the functioning of the IHR, (2) assess the ongoing global response to pandemic (H1N1) 2009, and (3) identify lessons learned important for strengthening preparedness and response for future pandemics and public-health emergencies (WHO 2011b). With regard to the first objective, a major conclusion of the Review Committee was that the IHR had 'helped make the world better prepared to cope with public-health emergencies'. This optimistic finding, however, was immediately followed by this statement: 'The core national and local capacities called for in the IHR are not yet fully operational and are not now on a path to timely implementation worldwide.' Judging from the number of States Parties seeking and obtaining extensions to establish these capacities by 2014 the Review Committee's conclusion on this point still holds true.

Conclusion: the International Health Regulations (2005)

The IHR have shown their potential to become an intermediate GPG for health. Their purpose of preventing and protecting against the international spread of disease, including epidemic control, while avoiding unnecessary interference with world traffic, continues to fall within the definition of a public good. Moreover, the global nature of this public good is clear, given the Regulations' textual intent of universal application. Regarding the IHR's enabling role as an intermediate GPG for health, implementation of the Regulations has met with mixed results. Although States Parties are highly committed to implementing the IHR (WHO 2012b), the necessary resources to achieve this have been hampered by the current economic and financial climate. This has resulted in an intensified effort by WHO to galvanize States Parties and to match their needs with the priorities of partners and stakeholders, including the donor community, the common goal being to lend their support to ensure that the number of countries that have obtained extensions to the 2012 deadline will be significantly reduced by June 2014. Finally, although not within the scope of this case study, a recurring debate surrounding IHR implementation is the question of its contribution to the at times nebulous concept of global (public) health security (WHO 2007b), which could itself be seen as a potential GPG for health candidate.

Case study: food safety—the Codex Alimentarius Commission and the International Food Safety Authorities Network

Food safety and food control have been recognized as important issues for decades. The rapid globalization of food production and trade has increased the potential for international incidents involving contaminated food. As a result, international monitoring and control as well as rapid exchange of information in case of emergencies need to be improved. Many major initiatives both in safe food production and in monitoring and control have contributed to improving food production systems and to the prevention of food-borne disease in most developed countries. But serious outbreaks of food-borne disease have been documented on every continent in the past decade, illustrating the public health implications and social significance of unsafe food. Additionally, recent incidences have shaken the consumers' trust in food safety systems. Bovine spongiform encephalopathy (BSE), dioxin, melamine, *Escherichia coli* O157, *Salmonella*—all food-borne hazards that were virtually unknown 10–15 years ago—are now household names in most families.

Food-borne diseases not only significantly affect people's health and well-being, they also have economic consequences for individuals, families, communities, businesses, and countries. These diseases impose a substantial burden on healthcare systems and markedly reduce economic productivity. The loss of income due to food-borne disease perpetuates the cycle of poverty. Estimating direct as well as indirect costs of food-borne disease is difficult. An estimate in the United States places the medical costs and productivity losses in a population of approximately 250 million in the range of US $6.6–37.1 billion (Buzby and Roberts 1997).

Global improvement to assure a safe and sufficient food supply requires a strategic approach, in strengthening national food safety systems, fostering and formalizing a strong cross-sectoral approach linking the agriculture, veterinary, and public health sectors, and implementing evidence-based measures along the food chain to reduce food-borne health risks. One of the primary multilateral responses to the need for internationally harmonized food safety management is the Codex Alimentarius Commission (CAC), an intergovernmental body formed in 1963 that operates under the joint auspices of the Food and Agriculture Organization of the United Nations (FAO) and WHO. The objective of the CAC is to protect the health of consumers and to ensure fair practices in the food trade, while promoting coordination of all food standards work undertaken by intergovernmental and non-governmental organizations (FAO and WHO 2006, 2007). The international food standards and related texts adopted by CAC constitute the Codex Alimentarius (Codex). All food standards and related texts in the Codex are voluntary and become binding only when they are converted into national legislation or regulation. Membership in the CAC is open to all member nations and associate member nations of FAO and WHO, and currently covers more than 99 per cent of the world population.

Despite improved food safety systems in many parts of the world, the occurrence of food contamination events cannot be avoided. In response to the 2000 WHA resolution on food safety and to address the need for rapid access and exchange of information in case of a food contamination event of international concern, the International Food Safety Authorities Network (INFOSAN) was established. INFOSAN provides tools and support to increase Member States' capacity to respond to health emergencies posed by natural, accidental, and intentional contamination of food.

This case study examines the global burden of food-borne disease and provides overviews of CAC and INFOSAN, the most salient international responses to food safety concerns. As part of the review of these mechanisms, the question of the CAC and INFOSAN providing intermediate GPGs for health is considered.

Food-borne disease burden

Food-borne and water-borne diarrhoeal diseases kill an estimated 2.2 million people annually, most of whom are children. While diarrhoea is the most common immediate symptom of food-borne illness, other serious consequences include kidney and liver failure, and brain and neural disorders. Food contamination also contributes to the burden of NCDs, in particular cancer and cardiovascular diseases, and can also affect reproductive health and the immune system.

Further, diarrhoeal diseases only constitute a fraction of disease caused by food. Microorganisms transmitted through food can cause many other types of disease, including very serious long-term infections. Even more important, the disease burden caused by chemical hazards in food is largely unknown. Therefore, determinations of the impact of food-borne disease have always relied heavily on estimates and assumptions. To address this lack of knowledge, WHO has started to estimate the global burden of food-borne disease, taking enteric, parasitic and chemical hazards into account, and it is expected to have a broader knowledge base on the global burden of food-borne illness in the near future.

The risk of spread of food-borne diseases is greatly increased with increasing global trade of feed, food ingredients, partially processed food, and final food products. International travel also represents a significant source of food-borne disease for some countries. For example, in 2005, Sweden reported that 80.2 per cent and the Netherlands reported 87 per cent of their salmonellosis cases acquired their infection while overseas (EFSA 2007). It has become imperative to address the matters related to food safety and quality at the international level—to complement and assist the actions taken by national governments that carry the primary responsibility to ensure food safety for their population.

The Codex Alimentarius Commission
Legal basis and organizational structure

The CAC was established as a joint commission, to be the executive organ of the Joint FAO/WHO Food Standards Programme. The CAC enjoys certain autonomy on procedural and programmatic matters, whereas the strategic direction of the Joint Programme is laid out by the Member States in the respective governing bodies of the two parent organizations. The highest governing body of the Codex is the Commission. The CAC Secretariat is located at FAO headquarters in Rome and supports the work of the CAC and its subsidiary bodies.

The preparatory work of the Codex (i.e. development of draft international standards and related texts), is undertaken by the subsidiary bodies of the CAC; namely, Codex committees and task forces. They are classified into two categories: (1) general subject committees that address horizontal aspects of food standards (additives, contaminants, pesticide and veterinary drug residues, labelling, hygiene, nutrition, methods of analysis and sampling, etc.); and (2) commodity committees that address specific groups of commodities (fish and fishery products, milk and milk products, fats and oils, etc.).

Codex Standards, in particular safety standards, are based on independent scientific advice provided through international expert committees convened by FAO and WHO, including: Joint FAO/WHO Expert Committee on Food Additives (JECFA),

Joint FAO/WHO Meetings on Pesticide Residues (JMPR) and Joint FAO/WHO Expert Meetings on Microbiological Risk Assessment (JEMRA). Ad hoc expert meetings are convened to address emerging and emergency issues, such as the 2008 melamine contamination of the global food supply.

Operations and procedure

The operation of the Codex system is guided by the Rules of Procedure, adopted by the Commission and endorsed by the Directors-General of FAO and WHO. The process of elaboration and adoption of international standards and related texts follows a procedure consisting of eight steps.

- Step 1: a proposal for new work is reviewed and a decision on whether or not to undertake new work is taken by the Commission.

- Steps 2, 3, and 4: a draft text is prepared and circulated to governments and all interested parties for comment, followed by review by the relevant Committee.

- Step 5: the Commission reviews the progress made and agrees that the draft should go to finalization.

- Steps 6 and 7: the approved draft is sent again to governments and interested parties for comment and is finalized by the relevant Committee.

- Step 8: following a final round of comments, the Commission adopts the draft as a formal Codex text.

An accelerated procedure whereby the elaboration of a text is concluded by adoption at Step 5/8 can be used, thereby skipping steps 6 through 8. Increasing application of this accelerated procedure has led to a significant increase of adoption of standards, particularly in the area of pesticide and veterinary drug residues in food.

International importance

The Codex system has become the global reference point for consumers, food producers and processors, national food control agencies, and the international food trade. Codex standards are recognized in the World Trade Organization's (WTO) Agreement on the Application of Sanitary and Phytosanitary Measures (SPS Agreement) and the Agreement on Technical Barriers to Trade (TBT Agreement), and have become the benchmarks against which national food measures and regulations are evaluated within the legal parameters of the WTO Agreements.

In particular, the SPS Agreement specifically designates Codex standards, guidelines, and recommendations as the international benchmark in food safety, with which WTO members are encouraged to harmonize their sanitary measures. The SPS Agreement acknowledges that governments have the right to take sanitary measures necessary for the protection of human health. WTO members applying measures that deviate from Codex standards are allowed to do so but are required to provide scientific justification based on risk assessment for such measures.

The International Food Safety Authorities Network

In collaboration with FAO, WHO initiated the International Food Safety Authorities Network (INFOSAN) in 2004. Recognizing the continuous increase in global food trade and travel, INFOSAN was developed to share food safety information and experience, as well as to promote collaboration between food safety authorities at national and international levels. An integral part of the INFOSAN network is the rapid exchange of emergency information between such authorities relative to food safety events or emergencies. This is known as INFOSAN Emergency.

As of May 2013, INFOSAN has 181 member countries and is advised on its strategic functions by an external advisory group. Non-emergency related activities include sharing experience and best practices between members and the publication of INFOSAN Information Notes, describing the latest food safety knowledge. Multilateral communication is also encouraged as a means of countries learning from each other's experiences, facilitated through a closed, web-based communication platform.

INFOSAN Emergency operates within the International Health Regulations (2005) (WHO 2005) and oversees all food safety related events in close cooperation with IHR focal points, inclusive of food contamination and food-borne disease. On average, 200 food safety events per month are investigated to determine their public health impact, including events of unusual or unexpected natures, distribution, and possible trade restrictions. The network actively shares information about one or two such events per month deemed of international public health significance. For example, when two shigellosis outbreaks occurred in two countries both implicating baby corn from a third country, INFOSAN Emergency sought information from the exporting country. Through this process it was determined that a further three countries were at risk since they had imported the affected baby corn. INFOSAN Emergency alerted all three countries, enabling a process where these countries could determine the risk for their population and implement their own appropriate risk management options.

Membership in INFOSAN is voluntary. However, the legal obligation with regard to INFOSAN Emergency is a mix of both hard and soft law: the 2005 IHR (hard law) and the instruction to WHO to maintain a list of primary contacts from the CAC (soft law). FAO and WHO encourage the rapid notification of food safety events or emergencies associated with traded foods to international bodies and to the INFOSAN network.

The Codex and INFOSAN as intermediate GPGs for health

Both the Codex and INFOSAN have proven capacity to improve health and health systems, the predicate for an intermediate GPG for health. The success of CAC as the multilateral framework for global food safety is the result of the global scale and scope of a large number of commodity standards and safety standards covering the farm-to-table approach. In addition many consider the Codex a successful UN initiative because of a high level of transparency and inclusiveness ensured by the participation of a large number of governmental and non-governmental observer organizations in the eight-step rule-based standards-setting process, and the fact that the safety standards are evidence-based.

In 2012, the CAC adopted close to 500 standards based on scientific assessments:

- 27 maximum residue limits (MRLs) for veterinary drug residues.

- 270 MRLs for pesticide residues in specified crops.

- 165 maximum use levels for food additives in specified food categories.

◆ Two maximum limits for containments (melamine and aflatoxins).

◆ Two food hygiene standards.

Contributing to the success of Codex is the FAO/WHO Project and Fund for Enhanced Participation in Codex (known as the Codex Trust Fund). The Codex Trust Fund was established to enhance participation in Codex by developing and transition economy countries by: (1) providing support to allow delegates of eligible countries to attend Codex meetings, (2) supporting Codex training courses and workshops to build capacity for more effective participation in Codex, and (3) supporting scientific and technical input from eligible countries into the Codex process.

INFOSAN has demonstrated its function as an intermediate GPG for health, strengthening international as well as national food safety systems and providing a platform for the development of the GPG of health, itself. The provision of INFOSAN Information Notes provides technical support for national food regulators when considering the impact and management of evolving food safety issues. INFOSAN Emergency activities enable rapid alerts to countries about food safety events or emergencies that may impact both the health and the economy of these countries. INFOSAN also assists national governments with the necessary public health response as required.

Conclusion: food safety

The ability of national governments to regulate food safety as they simultaneously move to increase food security presents many challenges. Food production systems need to be improved and these improvements should be informed by the lessons learned through food safety mistakes. When confronted with growing levels of international food trade, cross-border competition, increasing corporate and supplier power, and rapid consolidation of global agrifood markets and industries, governments recognize that the domestic food systems cannot be regulated unilaterally. Consequently, there is increased interest in and support for collective policy action at the multilateral level to protect citizens and to achieve the collective good.

Case study: Pandemic Influenza Preparedness Framework

Humanity has confronted infectious pathogens that cause epidemic or pandemic disease since its origins. Of all the microorganisms that have resulted in outbreaks of deadly disease, among the most deadly in human history is the Orthomyxoviridae family of viruses, known commonly as influenza. This family of viruses is characterized by its capacity to change into new, sustainably transmissible viruses to which humanity has little or no pre-existing immunity. Those new viruses are called pandemic influenza viruses.

One of the most lethal influenza viruses in the recent past was the 1918 A(H1N1) virus which, according to epidemiological estimates, caused 20–50 million deaths worldwide. While the advent of post-Second World War medicine, including improvements in vaccine production and technology, may have allowed the fear of pandemic flu to recede in the public mind, apprehension among public health experts about another 1918-like flu event has never waned. Indeed, concern over the continued threat posed by

influenza prompted WHO, very soon after its creation in 1947, to establish the first truly global network of laboratories to gather and monitor flu viruses, assess attendant risks and, eventually, coordinate the selection of strains for vaccines.

That network, which has since become known as the Global Influenza Surveillance and Response System (GISRS), operated for decades receiving little, if any, attention outside of public health circles. However, the appearance of the severe acute respiratory syndrome (SARS) coronavirus—a virulent viral pathogen—around 2003, and a spike of concern about the A(H5N1) influenza virus, known commonly as bird flu, in 2005, renewed awareness of the potentially devastating health, economic and social impacts of infectious, pandemic diseases. Suddenly, the existing public health system to address those threats became of intense political interest. And as scrutiny increased, so did interest in improving it.

SARS was extinguished less than 6 months after its detection, and H5N1 has so far not mutated to a form easily and sustainably transmissible among people, but their public health legacies are numerous (Heymann 2012). Among their most direct and potentially far reaching is the 2011 global arrangement known as the PIP Framework, short for the 'Pandemic Influenza Preparedness Framework for the sharing of influenza viruses and access to vaccines and other benefits'.

The PIP Framework represents the culmination of a 5-year, global effort in public health diplomacy to improve pandemic preparedness and response so that all countries, irrespective of wealth, could access the technologies and products needed to prepare for and protect their populations from flu pandemics.

Influenza-related burden of disease

The WHO-coordinated, international network of laboratories, or GISRS, operates for two principal purposes: (1) to gather representative samples of circulating influenza viruses to conduct detailed risk assessment, including pandemic risk, and (2) to develop candidate vaccine viruses and provide them to influenza vaccine manufacturers for vaccine production.

Influenza is normally a seasonal disease that is well understood in industrialized countries, where awareness of its health and economic impact has prompted governments to develop a vaccination policy that is supported by a well-established and resourced flu-vaccine manufacturing industry. The disease and its burdens, however, are far less well assessed in resource-poor developing states.

The emergence of H5N1 and its potential to trigger a pandemic brought new focus on GISRS and pandemic flu. As the perceived threat of an H5N1 pandemic increased, influenza vaccine manufacturers started to develop and test H5N1 vaccines. Rich and poor countries alike took measures to ensure their future access to vaccines. In a world of limited resources, however, where total pandemic flu vaccine demand far outstrips global production capacity, developing countries found themselves at a significant disadvantage. The precipitating cause of the PIP Framework negotiations was the difficulty for many of these developing countries to secure H5N1 vaccine at affordable prices, or even at all. In a measure that drew attention to this inequitable situation, some developing countries decided to withhold or delay sharing A(H5N1) viruses with GISRS laboratories, denying GISRS access to biological materials that were needed for risk assessment, preparedness, and response. In a number of developing countries, the question, in effect, was asked: why share the virus if the vaccine produced from it is out of reach?

The need for a more transparent, fair, and equitable system for the sharing of viruses as well as the access to the benefits derived from such virus sharing, namely vaccines and other medical necessities, became pressing. As a result, in May 2007 the 60th World Health Assembly adopted Resolution WHA60.28 requesting the WHO Director-General to, *inter alia*, convene an Intergovernmental Meeting with a view to reforming many of the practices and processes of GISRS and the pandemic influenza preparedness system it supports.

Over the next four years, Member States, with WHO support, worked through the intergovernmental process to develop the PIP Framework.

Overview of the PIP Framework

The PIP Framework has an intentionally narrow scope, covering only the sharing of influenza viruses with pandemic potential (under the Framework, these are known as 'PIP biological materials') and the fair and equitable access to benefits derived from such virus sharing. Legally speaking, the PIP Framework is a unique document: although adopted as a resolution of the World Health Assembly, and therefore technically a 'recommendation' of that body,[7] it includes several novelties, including a 'Partnership Contribution' mechanism addressed to certain manufacturers, as well as a system to conclude legally binding contracts designed to ensure benefit sharing commitments from both public and private entities.

The structure of the Framework is straightforward: it opens with several Principles that are central to the rest of the text. Following this, after succinct sections on objective, scope and definitions, the Framework addresses three core elements: virus sharing, benefit sharing, and governance. Additionally, annexed to the Framework are five additional and critical instruments: two Standard Material Transfer Agreements; Terms of Reference for the Director-General's Advisory Group; and Terms of Reference, including a set of Guiding Principles, for the four categories of laboratories in the WHO network.

Principles

The nineteen statements in this section reflect the intensity and breadth of Member States discussions during the 4 years of negotiations. Two principles in particular lend the Framework its distinctive, pioneering aspect. The first places both virus sharing and benefit sharing on an 'equal footing', underscoring that they are 'equally important parts of the collective action for global public health' (WHO 2011c). Reaching consensus on this provision in December 2008 was the catalyst for breaking 2 years of gridlock over the framing of virus sharing in relation to benefit sharing. It allowed the negotiation of other parts of the Framework to move ahead. Second, benefits are to be made available on the basis of public health risk and need rather than in relation to the level of virus sharing (WHO 2011c). Early in the negotiations, Member States rejected a direct link between virus sharing and access to benefits: benefits were to be made available to countries in need regardless of their contribution of materials to the system. This was considered a critical, ethical principle.

Virus sharing

Responsibility for this activity, which is at the core of the PIP Framework, rests with WHO Member States. Through their duly authorized or designated 'National Influenza Centres' Member States undertake to share with the WHO network material from all cases of infection due to influenza viruses with pandemic potential. Through this, the global scientific community is assured of access to biological materials that are critical for conducting pandemic risk assessment, and that may also be useful in developing vaccines or other medicines to respond to pandemic influenza.

Benefit sharing

Under the PIP Framework, WHO Member States, working with WHO, established a benefit sharing system, which operates to, *inter alia*, prioritize important benefits, such as vaccines, antiviral medicines and diagnostic tools, as high priorities for developing countries, and to secure binding commitments and resources to provide such benefits. The benefit sharing system also operates to build capacity over time, through technical assistance and transfer of technology, skills and know-how to countries in need.

Two innovative tools were developed by Member States to facilitate the successful achievement of the benefit sharing goals of the PIP Framework: an annual cash Partnership Contribution from influenza vaccine, diagnostic and pharmaceutical manufacturers using the WHO network (WHO 2011c) and a legally binding 'Standard Material Transfer Agreement-2' ('SMTA-2') to be concluded by WHO with all recipients of PIP biological materials outside the WHO network (WHO 2011c).

The Partnership Contribution is one of the most groundbreaking features of the PIP Framework. Addressed directly to manufacturers, this mechanism establishes a link between their use of the WHO GISRS network and a financial contribution to WHO. Each manufacturer's contribution is based on its individual nature and capacity (WHO 2011c), in accordance with a fully transparent and equitable formula developed with the input of industry and other stakeholders. The resources collected through this mechanism will be used by WHO to improve pandemic preparedness and response (WHO 2011c). It is a novel mechanism for public health and should allow measurable progress in many areas where preparedness is weakest: laboratory and surveillance capacities in developing countries.

The SMTA-2 is another cutting-edge, tailor-made mechanism that addresses the need for real-time access to specific pandemic products—notably vaccines, diagnostic materials and antiviral medicines—at the time of a pandemic. On the one hand, it is a classic contract, binding WHO and the recipient of 'PIP biological materials'. With respect to the benefit-sharing commitments that may be selected by recipients, however, the SMTA-2 is atypical in its prescriptiveness. The instrument was carefully constructed by Member States to ensure that at the time of a pandemic, countries in need would have real-time access to products necessary for a response. For this reason, the generic SMTA2 which is found in Annex 2 of the Framework provides only six benefit-sharing options from which influenza vaccine and antiviral manufacturers may choose: four of these concern real-time provision of pandemic vaccines and antivirals, and two concern licences to technology relevant to the production of vaccines, adjuvants, antivirals or diagnostics (WHO 2011c). Again, there is no direct, one-for-one link between receipt of PIP biological materials by the recipient and performance of the commitments selected. As long as such materials are received, the selected commitments must be performed. Thus, for example, a vaccine manufacturer that receives PIP biological materials must provide pandemic vaccines even if a particular production run is not based on those materials. Further, since all recipients of PIP biological materials must conclude an SMTA2, even research and academic institutions are covered, although the benefit sharing requirements addressed to them are far more flexible.

The PIP Framework benefit sharing system, however, is not limited to these two mechanisms. It also promotes more traditional benefit sharing by Member States to, among other things, strengthen laboratory and surveillance capacity, support regulatory authorities, promote technology transfer, and close the gap in the understanding of influenza disease burden in the developing world. This last element is a critical piece of the WHO-led effort to extend seasonal influenza vaccination programmes in the developing world, where epidemiologically warranted. Such seasonal flu programmes are essential to the sustainable functioning of flu vaccine manufacturing capacity, and, consequently, to increasing the global capacity to produce vaccines in the event of a flu pandemic.

Governance

The Framework, given its many novel elements, needed a robust system to advance and monitor its implementation. Its drafters therefore established a three-pillared oversight mechanism, involving the World Health Assembly, the WHO Director-General and a PIP 'Advisory Group'. The overall objective of the oversight mechanism is to ensure effective, efficient, transparent and accountable progress on implementation of the PIP Framework and the achievement of its objectives, both in the short and long terms.

The PIP Framework as an intermediate GPG

As with the other international instruments showcased in this chapter, the PIP Framework and the negotiating process that lead to the Framework can both be viewed as intermediate GPGs, in that they 'contribute towards the provision of final global public goods' (Kaul et al. 1999). The PIP Framework increases global and national capacities to address influenza and improves information flow and financial cooperation on matters relevant to pandemic influenza. Additionally, the PIP Framework demonstrably has the capacity to improve health systems and, very like the IHR (2005), at its core is designed to prevent and control the spread of infectious disease. These characteristics, as well as the laboratory, surveillance, and monitoring strengthening that spring from the PIP Framework, allow for a characterization of the Framework as an intermediate GPG for health.

Conclusion: overview of the PIP Framework

The PIP Framework is a unique, forward-looking instrument that provides pragmatic approaches and solutions to address specific public health problems. Its adoption was a landmark achievement, marking a departure from ad hoc pandemic response to a more structured, equitable, predictable, and efficient system for both preparedness and response. Its successful implementation and evolution will depend on many factors, particularly the trust of its many stakeholders in WHO as the body charged with its operationalization. By forging a new modus operandi between countries, both developed and developing, and stakeholders, in the public and private sectors, it has strengthened the global community's collective effort to protect all people from the international spread of disease.

Case study: the Minamata Convention: a cross-cutting approach to intermediate GPGs for health

Traditionally, subject areas like international environmental law, trade law, and humanitarian law have been treated as isolated areas of work (Sands 1999). As a result, instruments have often been developed in discrete fora and from discrete vantage points. However, as argued in this and other chapters, there are very few areas that can be conclusively categorized as 'health' or as 'non-health'. Infectious disease control can affect trade and commerce; environmental protection can affect NCD prevalence; and economic or trade decisions can have profound health and environmental impacts. In 2010 the Director-General of WHO addressed the need for cross cutting, multi-sector approaches: 'Policy spheres are no longer distinct. Lines of responsibility are blurred. A policy that makes perfect sense for one sector can have a highly negative impact on others, including health…The lesson is obvious. If policies that serve economic goals want to improve the human condition, they must include health as an explicit policy objective' (WHO 2010). In the same ethos, WHO's *Health in all Policies* approach encourages health to be integrated UN- and government-wide.

Concepts like governance *for* health move actors from working in separate silos to embracing multidisciplinary approaches. Allowing for specialized input from other sectors can encourage the integration of valuable perspective and expertise, and prevent duplication of efforts or adoption of contradicting policies. A recent example of a successful multisectoral collaboration on an international instrument is the Minamata Convention.

Mercury: the Minamata Convention

Mercury is a naturally occurring element found in air, water, and soil. Exposure to mercury generally occurs through consumption of fish and shellfish that have been contaminated with methyl mercury, though people can also be exposed through inhaling mercury vapours from fossil fuel combustion, industrial processes, and small-scale gold mining operations. Mercury can also be found in electrical and electronic devices, energy efficient fluorescent light bulbs, and batteries. However, at sufficient levels of exposure, mercury can be toxic. Mercury poisoning, to which children are particularly susceptible, can negatively affect the nervous, digestive, and immune systems and, in severe cases, can be fatal.

The continued release of mercury into the environment from human activity, the presence of mercury in the food chain and the demonstrated adverse effects on humans were of such concern that in 2009 governments agreed on the need to develop a global, legally binding instrument on mercury. Environment Ministers at the 2009 session of the United Nations Environmental Protection (UNEP) Governing Council took the decision to launch the negotiations; in 2013, the Minamata Convention, as it was named, was finalized. More than 140 nations negotiated and agreed on the language contained in the Minamata Convention and the document will open for signature in October 2013. The treaty will enter into force once it has been ratified by 50 parties.

Highlights of the Minamata Convention are as follows:

- Production, export, and import of a range of mercury-containing products will be banned by 2020.

◆ Parties are required to develop strategies to reduce the amount of mercury used by small-scale miners.

◆ Parties with artisanal and small-scale gold mining operations are required to develop national plans to reduce and, if possible, eliminate the use of mercury in such operations within 3 years of the treaty entering into force.

◆ Mercury emissions and releases from various large industrial facilities ranging from coal-fired power stations and industrial boilers to certain kinds of smelters will be controlled.

◆ Best available technologies will be used on new power plants and facilities, with plans to be developed to bring emission levels down from current rates.

The results of the UNEP-led negotiations could have been a treaty that addresses only the environmental impact of mercury. However, recognizing that mercury has serious health impact, the negotiating states invited WHO to provide its expertise to inform the development of relevant provisions. WHO provided background materials highlighting where the greatest health gains could be made and provided evidence regarding the use of mercury in medical instruments. The results of the WHO and UNEP joint work can most concretely be seen in the Objectives of the Convention which include clear reference to the protection of the environment *and* human health. Further, Article 16 of the Convention centres on health, encouraging Parties to implement health education and prevention programmes in vulnerable communities and indicating that the Conference of the Parties should consult, collaborate, and promote cooperation and information exchange with WHO, ILO, and other relevant intergovernmental organizations (UNEP 2013). The Minamata Convention, though not a specifically international health instrument, clearly contributes to improving health and, as an international instrument, is an intermediate GPG for health.

International legal paradigms, enforcement, and intermediate global public goods for health

As noted earlier in this chapter, the production of GPGs for health is most effective when states create international legal instruments that contain four essential aspects:

1. The establishment of formal institutions empowered to work on global public health problems.

2. The establishment of procedures through which states and non-state actors can tackle specific global public health problems.

3. The enumeration of substantive duties in connection with particular global public health challenges.

4. The creation of mechanisms to enforce substantive legal duties undertaken by states that have agreed to be bound by international instruments.

The WHO FCTC and the 2005 IHR both integrate all four aspects, as they address institutional, procedural, substantive, and enforcement aspects of the regulation of tobacco products and disease spread, respectively. As binding instruments, these instruments are often called 'hard law'. However, as demonstrated

by the non-binding Codex Alimentarius and INFOSAN and PIP Framework, which are voluntary, it is not only binding multilateral legal instruments that make up the landscape of intermediate GPGs for health. Those agreements and arrangements that are non-binding, and sometimes identified as 'soft law', can play a critical role in establishing the foundations required to produce the ultimate GPG—in this case, health.

The following section provides a brief review of health as a GPG in the context of international law and the spectrum of agreements between nations. The contrasts and similarities between hard and soft international law are presented and the institutional capacity, responsibility, and role of WHO in the creation of intermediate GPGs for health is examined.

Law and non-law: binding and non-binding international instruments and GPGs for health

The ideas and characteristics of soft law and hard law, and their relationship and usefulness, are common themes among international legal scholars and practitioners. With regard to the GPG of health, a very cogent and useful set of articles on this area was presented in the Bulletin of the WHO in December 2002, a special edition focusing on international law and public health (WHO 2002).

As exemplified by the case studies in this chapter, public health concerns are becoming increasingly complex as globalization progresses; so, too then, must and have the international responses been. In overcoming the Westphalian notion of single-nation solutions, 'the complex network of global health governance structures that are emerging indicates the need for an inclusive approach to engagement with new global health actors', including civil society, private actors, and public organizations (Taylor 2002; Taylor and Bettcher 2002). It is perhaps reasonable, then, to assert that the first step to producing the GPG of health is to examine the entire spectrum of stakeholders and create processes that are inclusive, to ensure that the intermediate GPG international legal instruments are as effective and efficient as possible.

Among the intermediate GPG legal instruments, traditional legal instruments—namely, treaties—provide the strongest, most effective tools for improving health (Taylor 2002), though they are commensurately difficult to negotiate because they bind parties to discrete, identifiable obligations. Although treaties have variable success in being implemented and enforced, the gestalt created by a negotiation, adoption, and entry into force can be tremendous (Taylor 2002). This certainly was the case for the WHO FCTC process, during which 'the power of the process' was often noted as one of the key ingredients to its success.

Perhaps because of the substantial challenges inherent in successfully negotiating a treaty on a topic as multifaceted as health, non-binding instruments have become increasingly utilized as nations seek to reach agreement and move a number of multilateral agendas forward (Chopra et al. 2002). Non-binding agreements provide the kind of flexibility that allows nations to act cooperatively and in concert without limiting their own autonomy (Chopra et al. 2002). However, the position and essential nature of non-binding instruments like resolutions and codes, sometimes called soft law and sometimes called 'non-law', remain unsettled in the rubric of international law (Taylor and Bettcher 2002). In terms of intermediate GPGs for health, non-binding arrangements like the Codex and INFOSAN and the PIP Framework certainly have demonstrated their usefulness, even in the face of not having the more robust implementation and enforcement opportunities that come with traditional international legal instruments.

Global health and GHG is a dynamic, exciting arena with an increasingly complex landscape being painted with each new transboundary health challenge that emerges or is identified. The relationship between hard and soft law has and will continue to adapt to best respond to the needs of global communities, which will in turn look to the WHO FCTC, IHR (2005), the Codex, INFOSAN and the PIP Framework and the Minamata Convention as models of intermediate GPGs on which to build.

WHO and institutional roles and responsibilities in the creation of intermediate GPGs for health

In a review of the nature and usefulness of international instruments for health, it would be remiss not to consider the role of WHO, as the UN specialized agency for health, in the creation of these intermediate GPGs for health. As the institutional umbrella home of four of the five instruments considered in this chapter, it plays a key and central role in fostering and providing a forum for its Member States to create agreements. Notwithstanding this, though, the question of what it can do and what it should do remain topics worth considering.

According to its Constitution, WHO is not simply an institutional home for multilateral health programmes and technical expertise; WHO is vested with substantial normative functions as well, including the Articles 19 and 21 powers to adopt conventions and regulations on matters within its competence (WHO 2007a). Though, with the exception of regulations, these powers are only 'quasi-legislative' in that Member States are not automatically bound to provisions of a given negotiated text, this is nonetheless one of the Organization's most important functions (Burci and Vignes 2004).

By design of its founding Member States, WHO does not, and perhaps should not, have full legislative capacity (Burci and Vignes 2004). It does have substantial comparative advantage, though, in being the primary agent for actualizing international agreements on health. The Organization has the capacity to coordinate its Member States, promote dialogue, and set the global health agenda and provide a platform for negotiations (Taylor 2002), provided it maintains adequate supporting political will and consensus among its constituency (Taylor 2002; Burci and Vignes 2004). WHO is one of, if not the, most potent sources of intermediate GPGs for health.

Conclusion

As intermediate GPGs for health, international legal instruments take on an additional layer of importance in GHG. In providing a robust framework for improving and occasionally even creating health, these instruments are important not only for what they are already doing, but for the potential good new instruments might be able to deliver. As WHO continues to grow into its normative role, it is likely that additional opportunities to exercise its Constitutional quasi-legislative powers will present themselves. The five examples of intermediate GPGs examined in this chapter, the WHO FCTC, the 2005 IHR, and the Codex and INFOSAN, the PIP Framework and the Minamata Convention, have laid a solid foundation on which WHO and its Member States may build to continue to work toward achieving the GPG of health.

Notes

1. The authors alone are responsible for the views expressed in this publication and they do not necessarily represent the decisions, policy or views of the World Health Organization.
2. The work of the World Health Organizations is carried out by three organs: the World Health Assembly, the Executive Board, and the Secretariat. See chapter IV of the WHO Constitution available at http://apps.who.int/gb/bd/PDF/bd47/EN/constitution-en.pdf.
3. A National IHR Focal Point is defined in Article 1 of the Regulations as 'the national centre, designated by each State Party, which shall be accessible at all times with WHO IHR Contact Points'.
4. Defined in Article 1 of the IHR as an 'extraordinary event which is determined (by the WHO Director-General) [...]: (i) to constitute a public health risk to other States through the international spread of disease and (ii) to potentially require a coordinated international response'.
5. It should be noted that under Annex 2 of the IHR, States Parties are required to notify WHO of cases of human influenza caused by a new subtype.
6. The WHO Executive Board's main function is to give effect to the decisions and policies of the World Health Assembly (see Article 28 of the WHO Constitution).
7. The document was adopted by the 64th World Health Assembly under Article 23 of the WHO Constitution.

References

Burci, G.L. and Vignes, C.-H. (2004). Normative functions. In G.L. Burci and C.-H. Vignes, *World Health Organization*, pp. 124–53. The Hague: Kluwer Law International.

Buse, K. and Walt, G. (2002). Globalisation and multilateral public–private partnerships: issues for health policy. In K. Lee, K. Buse, and S. Fustukian (eds.) *Health Policy in a Globalising World*, pp. 41–62. Cambridge: Cambridge University Press.

Buzby, J.C. and Roberts, T. (1997). Economic costs and trade impacts of microbial foodborne illness. *World Health Statistics Quarterly*, 50(1/2), 57–66.

Chopra, M., Galbraith, S., and Darnton-Hill, I. (2002). A global response to a global problem: the epidemic of overnutrition. *Bulletin of the World Health Organization*, 80 (12), 952–8.

Conference of the Parties to the WHO Framework Convention on Tobacco Control (2006). *Decisions*. Document A/FCTC/COP/1/DIV/8. Available at: http://apps.who.int/gb/fctc/PDF/cop1/FCTC_COP1_DIV8-en.pdf.

Conference of the Parties to the WHO Framework Convention on Tobacco Control (2007). *Decisions*. Document A/FCTC/COP/2/DIV/9. Available at: http://apps.who.int/gb/fctc/PDF/cop2/FCTC_COP2_DIV9-en.pdf.

Conference of the Parties to the WHO Framework Convention on Tobacco Control (2008). *Decisions*. Document FCTC/COP/3/DIV/3. Available at: http://apps.who.int/gb/fctc/PDF/cop3/FCTC_COP3_DIV3-en.pdf.

Conference of the Parties to the WHO Framework Convention on Tobacco Control (2010). *Decisions*. Document FCTC/COP/4/DIV/4. Available at: http://apps.who.int/gb/fctc/PDF/cop4/FCTC_COP4_DIV6-en.pdf.

Conference of the Parties to the WHO Framework Convention on Tobacco Control (2012). *List of Decisions*. FCTC/COP/5/DIV/5. Available at: http://apps.who.int/gb/fctc/PDF/cop5/FCTC_COP5_DIV5-en.pdf.

Da Costa e Silva, V.L. and Nikogosian, H. (2003). Convenio marco de la OMS para el control del tabaco: la globalizacion de la salud publica. [WHO Framework Convention on Tobacco Control: the globalization of public health. *Prevencion del Tabaquismo* [Prevention of tobacco addiction], 5(2), 71–5.

Dodgson, R., Lee, K., and Drager, N. (2002). *Global Health Governance: A Conceptual Review*. Key Issues in Global Health Governance Discussion Paper No. 1. Geneva: Centre on Global Change & Health and World Health Organization. Available at: http://whqlibdoc.who.int/publications/2002/a85727_eng.pdf.

Doll, R. (1998). Uncovering the effects of smoking: historical perspective. *Statistical Methods in Medical Research*, 7, 87–117.

European Food Safety Authority (EFSA) (2007). *The Community Summary Report on Trends and Sources of Zoonoses, Zoonotic Agents, Antimicrobial Resistance and Foodborne Outbreaks in the European Union in 2005*. Brussels: EFSA.

Food and Agriculture Organization of the United Nations and World Health Organization (2006). *Understanding the Codex Alimentarius* (3rd ed.). Rome: FAO. Available at: ftp://ftp.fao.org/codex/Publications/understanding/Understanding_EN.pdf.

Food and Agriculture Organization of the United Nations and World Health Organization (2007). *Codex Alimentarius Commission. Procedural Manual* (17th ed.). Rome: FAO. Available at: ftp://ftp.fao.org/codex/Publications/ProcManuals/Manual_17e.pdf.

Fidler, D. (2002). *Global Health Governance: Overview of the Role of International Law in Protecting and Promoting Global Public Health* (Key issues in Global Health Governance Discussion Paper 3). Geneva: World Health Organization and London School of Hygiene and Tropical Medicine. Available at: http://www.lshtm.ac.uk/cgch/ghg3.pdf.

Fidler D. (2007). Architecture amidst anarchy: global health's quest for governance. *Global Health Governance*, 1(1), 1–17.

Fidler, D. and Calamaras, J. (2010). *The Challenges of Global Health Governance*. New York: Council on Foreign Relations Press.

Frank, J., Chaloupka, F.J., Hu, T., et al. (2000). The taxation of tobacco products. In Jha P. and F. Chaloupka (eds.) *Tobacco Control in Developing Countries*, pp. 237–72. Oxford: Oxford University Press.

Gostin, L.O. (2007). A proposal for a framework convention on global health. *Journal of International Economic Law*, 10, 989–1008.

Heymann, D.L. (2012). *The Legacy of SARS Ten Years On*. Chatham House Centre on Global Health Security. Available at: http://www.chathamhouse.org/media/comment/view/187187.

Jamison, D.T., Breman, J.G., Measham, A.R., et al. (2006). Cost-effective strategies for noncommunicable diseases, risk factors, and behaviors. In D.T. Jamison, J.G. Breman, A.R. Measham, et al. (eds.) *Priorities in Health*, pp. 97–128. New York: Oxford University Press.

Jamison, D.T., Frenk, J., and Knaul, F.I. (1998). International collective action in health: objectives, functions, and rationale. *The Lancet*, 351, 514–17.

Kaul, I., Conceição, P., Le Goulven, K., and Mendoza, R.U. (2003). *Providing Global Public Goods: Managing Globalization*. New York: Oxford University Press.

Kaul, I., Grunberg, I., and Stern, M.A. (1999). Defining global public goods. In I. Kaul, I. Grunberg, and M.A. Stern (eds.) *Global Public Goods, International Cooperation in the 21st Century*, pp. 2–19. Oxford: Oxford University Press.

Kickbusch I. (2006). Mapping the future of public health: action on global health. *Canadian Journal of Public Health*, 97(1), 6–8.

Nikogosian, H. (2010). WHO Framework Convention on Tobacco Control: a key milestone. *Bulletin of the World Health Organization*, 88, 83–3.

Sands, P. (1999). Sustainable development: treaty, customs and the cross-fertilization of international law. In A. Boyle and D. Freestone

(eds.) *Sustainable Development and International Law*, pp. 39–60. Oxford: Oxford University Press.

Silberscmidt, G., Matheson, D., and Kickbusch, I. (2008). Creating a Committee C of the World Health Assembly. *The Lancet*, 371, 1483–6.

Smith, R. (2010). The role of economic power in influencing the development of global health governance. *Global Health Governance*, 3(2), 1–12.

Smith, R. and Woodward, D. (2003). Global public goods for health: use and limitations. In R. Smith, R. Beaglehole, D. Woodward, and N. Drager (eds.) *Global Public Goods for Health: Health Economic and Public Health Perspectives*. Geneva: World Health Organization. Available at: http://www.who.int/trade/distance_learning/gpgh/gpgh9/en/index.html.

Smith, R., Woodward, D., Acharya, A., et al. (2004). Communicable disease control: a 'global public good' perspective. *Health Policy and Planning*, 19, 271–8.

Sridhar, D., Khagram, S., and Pang, T. (2008/2009). Are existing governance structures quipped to deal with today's global health challenges—towards systematic coherence in scaling up. *Global Health Governance*, 2(2), 1–25.

Taylor, A.L. (2002). International health law and the WHO. *Bulletin of the World Health Organization*, 80, 975–80.

Taylor, A.L. and Bettcher, D.W. (2002). WHO framework convention on tobacco control: a global 'good' for public health. *Bulletin of the World Health Organization*, 78, 920–9.

Taylor, A.L., Bettcher, D.W., and Peck, R. (2003). International law and the international legislative process: the WHO Framework Convention on Tobacco Control. In R. Smith, R. Beaglehole, D. Woodward, and N. Drager (eds.) *Global Public Goods for Health: Health Economic and Public Health Perspectives*, pp. 212–32. Oxford: Oxford University Press.

United Nations (2012). *Political Declaration of the High-level Meeting of the General Assembly on the Prevention and Control of Non-communicable Diseases*. Document A/RES/66/2 Available at: http://www.un.org/ga/search/view_doc.asp?symbol=%20A/RES/66/2.

United Nations Economic and Social Council (ECOSOC) (2012). *United Nations System-Wide Coherence on Tobacco Control*. Document E/RES/2012/4. Available at: http://www.un.org/ga/search/view_doc.asp?symbol=E/RES/2012/4.

United Nations Environment Programme (UNEP) (2013). *Annex to the Report of the Intergovernmental Negotiating Committee to Prepare a Global Legally Binding Instrument on Mercury on the Work of its Fifth Session—Draft Minamata Convention on Mercury*. Document UNEP(DTIE)/Hg/INC.5/7. Available at: http://www.unep.org/hazardoussubstances/Mercury/Negotiations/INC5/INC5Report/tabid/3496/Default.aspx.

Woodward, D. and Smith, R.D. (2003). Global public goods and health: concepts and issues. In R. Smith, R. Beaglehole, D. Woodward, and N. Drager (eds.) *Global Public Goods for Health: Health Economic and Public Health Perspectives*, pp. 3–29. Geneva: World Health Organization. Available at: http://www.who.int/trade/distance_learning/gpgh/gpgh1/en/index.html.

World Bank (1999). *Curbing the Epidemic: Governments and the Economics of Tobacco Control*. Washington, DC: World Bank.

World Health Organization (1946). *Constitution of the World Health Organization*. New York: World Health Organization.

World Health Organization (1963). *Article 18 of the WHO 16th World Health Assembly Resolution WHA16*

World Health Organization (2002). Special the and international law. *Bulletin of th* 923–1000.

World Health Organization Cessation and Trea

World Health Organi Regulations. Worl at: http://www.wh

World Health Organization (2003c). *WHO Framework Convention on Tobacco Control*. Geneva: WHO Press.

World Health Organization (2005). *Revision of the International Health Regulations*. World Health Assembly resolution WHA58.3. Available at: http://www. who.int/gb/ebwha/pdf_files/WHA58/WHA58_3-en.pdf.

World Health Organization (2007a). *Basic Documents* (46th ed.), pp. 1–18. Geneva: WHO Press.

World Health Organization (2007b). *The World Health Report 2007: A Safer Future: Global Public Health Security in the 21st Century*, p. 5. Geneva: WHO Press.

World Health Organization (2008). *Implementation of the International Health Regulations (2005)*. Resolution WHA61.2. Available at: http://apps.who. int/gb/ebwha/pdf_files/WHA61-REC1/A61_Rec1-part2-en.pdf.

World Health Organization (2009). *Swine Influenza*. Statement by the WHO Director-General. Available at: http://www.who.int/mediacen tre/news/statements/2009/h1n1_20090425/en/index.html.

World Health Organization (2010). *Policies in Non-Health Sectors Can Have a Profound Impact on Health*. Bangkok, Thailand, 8 September 2010. The WHO Director-General's address to the Regional Committee for South-East Asia. Available at: http://www.who.int/dg/speeches/2010/searo_regcom_20100908/en/index.html.

World Health Organization (2011a). *Implementation of the International Health Regulations (2005): Report by the Director-General*. Document A64/9. Available at: http://apps.who.int/gb/ebwha/pdf_files/WHA64/A64_9-en.pdf.

World Health Organization (2011b). *Implementation of the International Health Regulations (2005): Report of the Review Committee on the Functioning of the International Health Regulations (2005) in relation to Pandemic (H1N1) 2009*. Document A64/10. Available at: http://apps. who.int/gb/ebwha/pdf_files/WHA64/A64_10-en.pdf.

World Health Organization (2011c). *Pandemic Influenza Preparedness Framework for the Sharing of Influenza Viruses and Access to Vaccines and Other Benefits*. Geneva: WHO Press. Available at: http://whqlib doc.who.int/publications/2011/9789241503082_eng.pdf.

World Health Organization (2012a). *Global Progress Report on Implementation of the WHO Framework Convention on Tobacco Control*. Geneva: WHO Press. Available from: http://www.who.int/fctc/reporting/2012_global_progress_report_en.pdf.

World Health Organization (2012b). *Implementation of the International Health Regulations (2005)*. Resolution WHA65.23 Available at: http://apps.who.int/gb/ebwha/pdf_files/WHA65-REC1/A65_REC1-en.pdf#page=25.

World Health Organization (2013a). *WHO's Role in Global Health Governance*. Document EB132/5 Add.5. Available at: http://apps.who.int/gb/ebwha/pdf_files/EB132/B132_5Add5-en.pdf.

World Health Organization (2013b). *Protocol to Eliminate Illicit Trade in Tobacco Products*. Geneva: WHO Press. Available at: http://apps.who.int/iris/bitstream/10665/80873/1/9789241505246_eng.pdf.

World Health Organization (2013c). *Implementation of the International Health Regulations (2005): Report by the Director-General*. Document A66/16. Available at: http://apps.who.int/gb/ebwha/pdf_files/WHA66/A66_16-en.pdf.

Yach, D. and Bettcher, D. (2000). Globalisation of tobacco industry influence and new global responses. *Tobacco Control*, 9, 206–16.

SECTION 4

Information systems and sources of intelligence

4.1

Information systems in support of public health in high-income countries

Tjeerd-Pieter van Staa and Liam Smeeth

Introduction to information systems

Public health sciences have been described by a Wellcome Trust working group as follows: 'effective public health actions are based on scientifically derived information about factors influencing health and disease and about effective interventions to change behaviour at the level of the individual, the family, the community or wider society' (Public Health Sciences Working Group et al. 2004, p. 5). This field of science has made major contributions to the improvement of health such as the effects of sanitary reforms on infant mortality and, more recently, the reductions in cardiovascular disease incidence due to lipid lowering and blood pressure control. However, many challenges remain, such as how to tackle the increased prevalence of obesity and diabetes and how to relate the costs of interventions to their benefits (Public Health Sciences Working Group et al. 2004). This chapter will describe how information systems containing healthcare data can support public health research. We will first describe examples of public health information systems, followed by a description of various developments in these systems, including increased public health use of routinely collected electronic healthcare records (EHRs). More and more clinicians and healthcare professionals are using computers to store information: indeed the 'meaningful use' of electronic health records for patient care has recently been mandated in the United States (Blumenthal et al. 2010). These data sources provide opportunities, among others, to test the effectiveness and impact of public health interventions. We discuss the role of randomization in public health research and conclude this chapter by highlighting the importance of an impact assessment of public health interventions.

Sources of public health information

Vital statistics

Death certificates are routinely collected in many countries in order to report on specific causes of death including, for example, alcohol-related deaths, suicides, and drug-related deaths, deaths involving methicillin-resistant *Staphylococcus aureus* (MRSA) and *Clostridium difficile*, and estimates of excess winter mortality. Trends in, for example, all-age all-cause mortality, deaths from cancer, circulatory diseases, suicide and injury of undetermined

intent, and accidents are reviewed periodically as are the association of mortality rates with socioeconomic deprivation. Live and stillbirth figures are also routinely collected in many countries. The birth counts may be stratified by occurrence within or outside marriage, multiple births, mother's area of residence and country of birth, place of confinement, and father's social class (examples are given at http://www.statistics.gov.uk).

Population surveys

Population surveys are frequently used information resources. One example is the US National Health Interview Survey, which targets annually an interview with 40,000 households. Questions include health status and health services utilization and activity limitations due to ill health. The Behavioural Risk Surveillance System is a telephone survey in the US involving 150,000 people. Data are collected on health risks and behaviours, exercise, and diet. The National Health and Nutrition Examination Survey examines diet, nutrition, health behaviours, and risk factors in 5000 randomly selected persons.

A population census provides information about the characteristics of the population and facilitates understanding of the similarities and differences in populations locally, regionally, and nationally. The results are then used to allocate public money for services including healthcare services. They are also used to identify areas with the greatest public health needs. As an example, national census data from the Strasbourg metropolitan area in eastern France were used to develop a small-area index of socioeconomic deprivation. It showed an association between increased rates of myocardial infarction and worse neighbourhood deprivation (Havard et al. 2008).

Disease surveillance

In many countries, there are systems for reporting and notification of cases of certain diseases to the public health authorities. Infectious diseases such yellow fever and diphtheria are notifiable on diagnosis of a suspected case and should not wait for laboratory confirmation. All notifiable cases are then reviewed and appropriate action may be taken. Analyses of local and national trends are typically published on a regular basis. Despite legal requirements to report certain infectious diseases, reporting rates for these conditions are not always optimal. To address this, for example, a New York public health institute facilitated public health reporting by creating alerts within EHRs to remind clinicians at the point of care that a particular diagnosis is reportable and providing a link to the reporting form. Patient demographics are automatically populated in the form (Calman et al. 2012).

Administrative databases

There are many administrative databases that contain information recorded for the purposes of managing the healthcare system. Several of these systems can be used for public health research. The Hospital Episode Statistics is a data warehouse containing details of all admissions to National Health Service hospitals in England. It contains clinical information about diagnoses and operations on individual patients, demographic information such as age, gender, and ethnicity, administrative information such as time waited and date of admission, and geographical information on where the patient was treated and the area in which they lived. Main procedures (such as surgical operations) are also recorded. It contains admitted patient care data from 1989 onwards, with more than 12 million new records added each year, and outpatient attendance data from 2003 onwards, with more than 40 million new records added each year (Health and Social Care Information System n.d.).

Registries

A registry is an organized system that uses observational study methods to collect uniform data (clinical and other) to evaluate specified outcomes for a population defined by a particular disease, condition, or exposure. There are many different types of registries. An example of a product registry is the UK national registry of patients on biological therapy: patients starting such therapy are registered and followed, for example, for long-term safety issues. Healthcare service registries include patient-based individual clinical encounters, such as office visits or hospitalizations, and procedures. Examples include registries enrolling patients undergoing a procedure (e.g. carotid endarterectomy, appendectomy, or primary coronary intervention) or admitted to a hospital for a particular diagnosis (e.g. community-acquired pneumonia). These registries may be used to evaluate the processes and outcomes of care for quality measurement purposes. Disease registries use the state of a particular disease or condition as the inclusion criterion. These registries typically enrol the patient at the time of diagnosis at a routine healthcare service. Examples include cancer registries which are widely used for research (Edwards and Bell 2000).

Immunization registries have been created in order to assemble in one site a record of all immunizations and to provide reminder and recall notices when an immunization is due or late. Vaccination schedules are becoming complex due to the number of different vaccinations a child should receive. These may be further complicated by frequent changes of healthcare provider or insurance company. Immunization registries can provide a central repository of all the vaccinations given to children (Linkins 2001).

Electronic health records databases

EHRs are increasingly being used for research and public health purposes. There are currently over 300 EHR databases in 45 countries (http://www.ispor.org/intl_databases). This section describes a few examples of EHR databases that have been widely used for research. The Clinical Practice Research Datalink, previously known as the General Practice Research Database, collates the anonymized EHR information for over 5 million patients currently registered at participating general practices. General Practitioners (GPs) play a key role in the UK healthcare system, as they are responsible for primary healthcare and specialist referrals. If a patient is treated in secondary care or by a specialist, the GP is informed about major clinical outcomes, and long-term treatments are frequently handed back to the GP. Almost all GPs in the UK use computers for maintaining health records, and communications between different health providers are increasingly sent electronically (Williams et al. 2012). The Dutch PHARMO Record Linkage System collects information on patient demographics, drug dispensings, hospital morbidity, clinical laboratory and pathology results, and GP information for more than 3 million community-dwelling inhabitants of 48 geographic areas in the Netherlands (Herings et al. 2012). A recent development in the Netherlands is the Mondriaan project that has developed an IT and governance infrastructure for enrichment and linkage of EHR. Privacy enhancing technology such as linkage through a trusted third party (TTP) is applied and currently data from GPs (one million), community pharmacists (12 million), and various other EHR sources are retrieved for research purposes and as feedback information to healthcare providers (www.projectmondriaan.nl). In Denmark and Sweden, each national healthcare system provides universal coverage to all residents (5.5 million inhabitants in Denmark and 9.2 million inhabitants in Sweden). Healthcare coverage includes visits to GPs, specialists, hospital admissions, and outpatient visits; drug costs are either partially or completely covered. A centralized civil registration system has been in place in each country for many years, allowing for personal identification of each person in the entire population and for the possibility of linkage to all national registries containing civil registration numbers, for example, patient registry, cancer registry, prescription databases, and registry of causes of death (Furu et al. 2010). The Rochester Epidemiology Project medical records-linkage system captures healthcare information for the entire population of Olmsted County in the United States. It includes a dynamic cohort of over half a million patients who received healthcare for any reason. The data available electronically include demographic characteristics, medical diagnostic codes, surgical procedure codes and death information (including causes of death). The system covers residents of all ages and both sexes, regardless of socioeconomic status, ethnicity, or insurance status (St Sauver et al. 2012).

Recent developments in information systems

The electronic information systems in the healthcare system are evolving and increasing (Table 4.1.1). Initial use of electronic healthcare data mostly consisted of aggregate analyses of administrative data such as hospital admission data. When clinicians started to use computers for record keeping, the first research databases collating anonymized EHRs were created. One of the first of these was the VAMP research database that

Table 4.1.1 Stages in the development of EHR databases

Time period (approximate)	Development of EHR databases
1980s onwards	Data collected for administrative purposes (such as hospital admission data and death certificates); mainly used for aggregate analyses
1990s onwards	Clinicians starting to use computers for record keeping (replacing paper records) and data collated into research database. These data initially mainly used for drug safety monitoring
2000s onwards	Monitoring of clinic encounters for symptoms that may represent infectious diseases and other conditions of public health concern
2000s onwards	Linkages between various EHR databases; mainly used to obtain complementary information or to validate outcomes
2010s onwards	Enrichment of routinely collected data by prospective data collection within EHR databases (e.g. collection of blood samples for genetic analyses or patient questionnaires)
2010s onwards	Development and implementation of triage tools to guide clinicians in hospital referral of patients with, e.g. influenza; electronic alerts for eligible patients
2010s onwards	Introduction of randomization at the point of care using the EHR database to identify potentially eligible patients and for follow-up collection of major clinical outcomes (i.e. pragmatic and cluster trials); mainly used to evaluate the effects of medicines in routine clinical practice

started in 1987. This database eventually developed into the Clinical Practice Research Datalink. The richness and completeness of many EHR databases have been increasing over time as more information is being shared electronically between different parts of the healthcare system. Laboratory data provide an example in which test results are increasingly being communicated electronically and loaded automatically into the patient's EHR.

An important development is the increased linkage between different healthcare databases. Typically, linkages are done by a TTP that collects from each data source the patient's identifiers (such as registration number in the healthcare system, patient's date of birth, gender, and postcode) and research numbers. The TTP then matches the records of the various databases retaining the linked records with the various research numbers without any patient identifiers. This approach allows the combination of different healthcare databases. Linkages between different EHR datasets are being done more frequently, benefiting both the quality and completeness of the EHR data. The UK Clinical Practice Research Datalink has been linked individually and anonymously to other healthcare datasets, including the national registry of hospital admissions, the national death certificates (with primary and secondary cause of death), and prospective disease registries,

such as the cancer and cardiovascular disease registries (Williams et al. 2012).

Comparisons of the information in linked EHR databases can highlight incomplete data records and inform efforts to improve data recording in the healthcare system. In a cohort study, primary care records were linked with those from cancer registries in the UK National Cancer Data Repository. Comparison of the two datasets showed a concordance rate of 83.3 per cent, which varied by cancer type. Cancer registries recorded larger numbers of patients with lung, colorectal, and pancreatic cancers, whereas GPs recorded more haematological cancers and melanomas (Boggon et al. 2013).

Anonymized linkages between local air pollution data, records from primary care, hospital admissions and death certificates have been used recently to evaluate the relationships between ambient outdoor air pollution and incident myocardial infarction, stroke, arrhythmia, and heart failure. While evidence was weak for relationships with myocardial infarction, stroke, or arrhythmia, consistent associations between pollutant concentrations and incident cases of heart failure were found (Atkinson et al. 2013).

An example of a public health resource that uses linked healthcare databases is the CALIBER programme. It is linking multiple data sources including the longitudinal primary care data from the Clinical Practice Research Datalink, the national disease registry of acute coronary syndrome, hospitalization and procedure data from hospital admission records, cause-specific mortality from death certificates, and postcode-based social deprivation. Current cohort analyses involve a million people in initially healthy populations and disease registries (Denaxas et al. 2012). A recent study that used this resource was an analysis of the effect of influenza and influenza-like illnesses on triggering acute myocardial infarction (AMI). A self-controlled case series (i.e. only cases were evaluated) identified cases of myocardial infarction from the national registry of acute coronary syndromes and looked for associations with exposure to influenza from the consultation records of GPs. It found that influenza and other acute respiratory infections can act as a trigger for AMI (Warren-Gash et al. 2012).

The Massachusetts Department of Public Health in the United States has developed a system that loads EHRs every 24 hours from clinicians' proprietary software systems. These extracts are organized into separate databases for patient demographics, vital signs, diagnosis codes, test orders and results, medication prescriptions, allergies, social histories, and provider contact details. These data provide clinically detailed surveillance data. Sensitive and specific disease-detection algorithms have been developed to overcome the limited accuracy of code diagnostic data by considering all available data. Diabetes surveillance is done using these algorithms and can provide information on, for example, the frequency of referrals for medical nutrition counselling stratified by race and locality. A comparison of this system and conventional reporting by clinicians showed a significant increase in the quantity and quality of case reports of notifiable conditions (Klompas et al. 2012).

The minimization of risk of preventable harm to patients is a priority for many healthcare organizations. In Scotland, a system has been implemented in routine primary care that provides a rapid audit method of screening electronic patient records to detect patient harm. The objective of this tool is to support clinical improvement efforts (De Wet and Bowie 2011).

The combination of routinely collected EHRs with prospectively collected data is an important development in improving the quality of information resources. An ongoing study in the Clinical Practice Research Datalink is recruiting 6000 persons aged 50–64 year for a survey about working life. Study participants will complete questionnaires about their work and home circumstances and their EHRs will be reviewed anonymously. The inter-relationship between changes in employment (with reasons) and changes in health (e.g. major new illnesses, new treatments, mortality) will be examined. This study will contribute to the evidence-base as to whether working beyond the traditional retirement age is feasible for those with major health problems associated with ageing and the effect of occupational and personal circumstances (e.g. savings, retirement intentions, domestic responsibilities, whether work is arduous or rewarding) (K. Palmer, personal communication 2012).

Syndromic surveillance is the practice of monitoring clinic encounters for symptoms that may represent infectious diseases and other conditions of public health concern. There are several examples in which EHRs are used to conduct this surveillance. An example is QSurveillance which provides weekly information on the consultation rates of flu-like illness in general practices covering a total population of almost 22 million patients (QSurveillance n.d.). A comparable system has been developed in New York State, United States, in which routinely collected EHRs from health centres are transferred daily to the research database. Respiratory illness, fever, diarrhoea, and vomiting are the key symptoms monitored, with analysis to determine when the incidence of these syndromes exceeds expected thresholds (Calman et al. 2012).

Research in EHR databases is now being carried out to refine and validate triage tools to guide clinicians in hospital referral of patients with influenza-like illness during a pandemic. In the first phase of this study (called FLU-CATS), clinicians will record their assessment and management of patients with influenza-like illness. They will be prompted by a pop-up box to provide this information when a diagnosis of influenza-like illness is being entered into the EHR. There will be an automated daily transfer of the anonymized EHRs to the research database (the Clinical Practice Research Datalink). The EHRs will be linked periodically to hospital admission records and data from a regional microbiology network which includes laboratory results on investigations for respiratory pathogens. The collected data will be used to refine and update the triage tools. If the pilot phase is successful, this system could be rolled out to a much larger group of clinics. Such a system is also potentially adaptive, since with ongoing data collection, triage tools can be regularly adapted to changes in virus, human behaviour, and models of healthcare provision in the community (M.G. Semple, personal communication 2012)

Pandemic preparedness is a major public health activity in many countries, including the United Kingdom. The major objectives of the UK strategy are, in case of an influenza pandemic, to identify key clinical, epidemiological, and virological features of the new influenza virus, to count severe cases and identify risk groups affected, to describe the evolving pandemic and its impact at the population level (e.g. by age-group) particularly in relation to hospitalizations and mortality, and to measure the uptake and safety of various pharmaceutical countermeasures. Several information systems would be used to collect the data to be used for this, including primary care consultations, records of calls to telephone help-lines and web-based advisory services relating to influenza-like illness, virological 'sentinel' surveillance schemes in primary care, laboratory analysis of a sample of cases to identify the genetic features of the virus and analysis of death records (Department of Health 2011).

Future developments in information systems

There is an increasing need to perform studies across different EHR systems and across different countries mainly because of the need for a larger sample size. The healthcare systems in most countries consist of multiple healthcare providers who often use different systems to store data, either on paper or electronically. Furthermore, physicians often record data differently and inconsistently, both on paper and electronically. Various international initiatives are currently ongoing which use different approaches to combine heterogeneous EHR databases. One approach focuses on IT aspects with the aim to develop EHR systems that are interoperable and allow seamless transfer of data (http://www.transform project.eu/; http://www.ehr4cr.eu/). All the information in the various databases is mapped together with a detailed understanding of the content of each of the data elements and use of a single coding dictionary across the different databases. An alternative approach is to maintain the EHR data structure as collected by the participating health professionals but to develop a common protocol across the different databases. The operational definitions of how the data are classified will vary by individual EHR database but the research questions will be kept similar. This model is currently used by the Innovative Medicines Initiative PROTECT project (http://www.imi-protect.eu/). The third approach is used by the OMOP initiative in the USA: all EHR data from the different databases are integrated into a central research database according to a common data model (http://omop.fnih.org/). A distributed network model where basic analyses are run on federated datasets generating common input data and subsequent local aggregation and central pooling of results, constitutes the fourth approach to dealing with heterogeneous EHR databases. The EU-ADR project uses this approach. In one of their studies, data from eight European healthcare databases (administrative claims, medical records) were combined. This dataset included over 1.9 million individuals (59,594,132 person-years follow-up) who used 2289 different drugs. It found for a frequent event such as AMI, there were 531 drugs (23 per cent of total) for which an association with relative risk ≥ 2, if present, can be investigated. For a rare event such as rhabdomyolysis, there are 19 drugs (1 per cent) for which an association of same magnitude can be investigated. It concluded that even larger databases would be required to detect signals for less frequent exposures and outcomes (Coloma et al. 2012).

A recent development is the use of EHRs to measure the quality of clinical care and provide financial incentives through 'pay-for-performance' programmes (Campbell et al. 2009). EHRs are used to evaluate clinician and system performance with the goal of making healthcare safer and more efficient. The adoption of computerized clinical records itself may be associated with improved care and outcomes (Cebul et al. 2011) although some doubts remain (Classen and Bates 2011). There are several different dimensions in which quality of healthcare can be measured.

Examples of different quality measures include the number of patients with diabetes seeing an ophthalmologist, clinical outcomes in patients with hypertension, percentage of clinicians reviewing out-of-range laboratory results with a certain number of hours, and the percentage of patients receiving incorrect medications (Weiner et al. 2012). The quality and completeness of the EHRs are of course critical in achieving the goals of the 'pay-for-performance' programmes.

Internet postings, blogs, and social media postings may provide another source of information for the early detection of new infectious disease epidemics. A recent study analysed the queries to online search engines, which are used by millions of people around the world each day. It concluded that this approach accurately estimated the level of weekly influenza activity in each region of the United States, with a reporting lag of about 1 day. The use of search queries could detect influenza epidemics in areas with a large population of web search users (Ginsberg et al. 2009). This potential use of Internet searches was tested in a US study that compared Internet searches with rates of outpatient visits for influenza-like illness and of confirmed laboratory tests. It was found that Internet searches were highly correlated with rates of outpatient visits for influenza-like illness but less correlated with rates of laboratory-confirmed influenza (Ortiz et al. 2011). The main limitation of these analyses of unstructured Internet data is that it may be difficult to separate activities by concerned healthy people from those with the disease of interest. Healthcare seeking behaviour, physician testing practices, and Internet search behaviour can be influenced by high levels of media coverage (Ortiz et al. 2011).

The information on the Internet can also be evaluated for the monitoring of side effects of medicines. A study evaluated the text on Internet message boards dedicated to drug abuse in order to compare different prescription opioids. Over 48,000 posts were analysed and the unstructured text was coded. It was found that the number of posts on these drug abuse message boards varied between the different opioids (Butler et al. 2007). While this approach is interesting, one cannot conclude that these differences in drug abuse messages were caused by the pharmacological differences between the opioids. Different levels of information provision by, for example, the clinicians or in the information sheet or prescribing to different patient populations could also lead to different levels of Internet activities.

Randomization in public health research

The present allocation of healthcare interventions is often inconsistent. Clinicians will be influenced in their prescribing behaviour, not only by clinical considerations, but also by other issues including drug preferences, exposure to marketing materials, and guidance from the local healthcare funders, which will vary considerably between practices and clinicians (Adamson et al. 2012). Clinicians will respond differently to uncertainties in the evidence base. The prescribing of antibiotics to patients with mild to moderate exacerbations of chronic obstructive pulmonary disease provides an example of this. A review of EHRs found major differences in the rate of antibiotics prescribing to these patients. Very few patients received an antibiotic in some clinics while antibiotics were routinely prescribed in other clinics. This variability in care (due to a lack of randomized trials conducted in these patient

groups) produces a potentially unfair lottery for the receipt of healthcare interventions. Treating patients in this inconsistent manner generates no new evidence to improve clinical practice. On the other hand, randomization with structured data collection would provide the evidence to guide clinicians in selecting treatments. A possible model would be to offer randomization to all willing patients as part of routine clinical care in every situation where there is genuine uncertainty about which of two or more widely accepted treatments is best. The EHRs could be used to measure major clinical outcome and follow progress (van Staa et al. 2012). An analysis of the trial evidence for medicines used by millions of patients and with blockbuster sales showed that only one of the 24 top blockbusters in 2011 had a randomized trial including more than 10,000 participants and only few of the blockbusters had evidence of beneficial effects on mortality (Ioannidis 2013). A mega-trial with mortality as an outcome could address concerns about side effects and also provide evidence of effectiveness of medicines in routine clinical practice.

EHR databases could offer an ideal platform to undertake large pragmatic trials, with randomization at the point of care and collection of follow-up data using the EHR (van Staa et al. 2012). Such an approach would allow the assessment of effectiveness of healthcare interventions in everyday clinical practice among representative populations. An example of an ongoing study is the RETROPRO trial, in which patients with high cardiovascular risk are randomized between simvastatin and atorvastatin (van Staa et al. 2012). After confirmation of trial eligibility by the patient's clinician and after informed consent, a patient is then randomized between simvastatin and atorvastatin. Heart attacks are measured using the routinely collected data from primary care, linked data from hospital admissions, from a prospective disease registry, and from death certificates. The patient's clinician can also be asked to confirm and validate the occurrence of a heart attack. The outcome of death can be measured using the primary care data and linked death certificates; this outcome is generally well recorded as the payments to primary care clinics will depend on the number of live patients and notification of death certificates is well established. Discontinuation and non-compliance with statin treatment over time is also an important outcome measurement in this pragmatic trial. For example, if patients preferentially use atorvastatin for a longer period of time, this could mean a substantially lower number of patients suffering a heart attack. In most trials, study participants are regularly monitored and instructed how to take their medicines. But the rates of persistence are often considerably lower in routine clinical practice, as stringent monitoring procedures do not apply. Pragmatic trials that collect follow-up information unobtrusively (e.g. from EHR databases) would provide the answers that decision makers need: that is, will this intervention make a difference in routine clinical practice compared to alternative strategies (Tunis et al. 2003).

Cluster trials randomly allocate entire areas or health service organizational units to intervention or control groups, with outcomes evaluated for individuals within each cluster. They facilitate pragmatic evaluation of the effectiveness of interventions delivered in routine practice settings. Public health interventions could be tested in cluster trials as one can, for example, implement the novel intervention in one set of randomly selected clinics and the old intervention in the remaining clinics. The effectiveness of screening programmes could also be tested in cluster trials, with half of the clinics conducting the screening and the other half not. An example of a study that used EHR data is a study that tested the effectiveness of providing clinicians with the guideline recommendations on antibiotic prescribing in respiratory illness. Electronic prompts are activated during a patient's consultation for upper respiratory illness. The EHRs are used to measure the outcomes of interest, which include the rate of antibiotic prescribing (Gulliford et al. 2011).

Phased access to new interventions has been proposed as a method to measure effectiveness and safety. Practices or regions would be randomized to early or late access and the EHR data would be used to measure the outcomes of interest. Because practices are randomly chosen for each new intervention, a practice will have access to some of the new interventions (Adamson et al. 2012).

Impact assessment of public health interventions

The measurement of outcomes of public health interventions in routine clinical practice should be considered a major public health activity. This impact assessment can inform the extent of uptake but also identify any issues with the implementation of the public health activity. However, this impact assessment is not consistently done. For example, measurements of outcomes are lacking in a major UK programme that targeted the use of statins in patients with high cardiovascular risk. Following a detailed review of evidence, the UK National Health Service introduced a population-wide vascular risk assessment programme. This consists of a systematic approach to assessing risk of vascular diseases for everyone between 40 and 74 years who is not yet diagnosed with cardiovascular disease or treated for risk factors. Statin treatment should be initiated if a patient has a high risk (20 per cent or greater 10-year risk) of cardiovascular disease (National Health Service Health Check Programme 2008). However, a recent analysis of the EHRs found that many healthy patients were prescribed a statin despite having a below-threshold cardiovascular risk and that there was wide variation between practices in the extent of statin prescribing to patients at high risk.

Another example of the difference between intended use according to guidelines and actual use in clinical practice concerns the selective cyclooxygenase-2 inhibitors (coxibs). These drugs ranked, before September 2004, among the most commonly used medications in the world. They were developed to minimize the upper gastrointestinal side effects of conventional non-steroidal anti-inflammatory drugs. A large number of cost-effectiveness analyses were conducted in order to provide clinicians with guidance on which patient groups should be treated with coxibs. These analyses were based on mathematical models that took into account the higher prescription costs and lower incidence of gastrointestinal side effects of coxibs. The assumptions that were used in these models were obtained from the main coxibs randomized trials. However, an analysis of EHRs found that the vast majority of coxib users in routine clinical practice would not have been eligible for the main coxibs randomized trials, as they did not have osteoarthritis or rheumatoid arthritis and only used coxibs intermittently or short term. Thus, the many cost-effectiveness analyses that were conducted for coxibs lacked external validity and were of limited value in guiding clinicians on how to treat

patients in routine clinical practice. The authors of the EHR analyses concluded that the field of health technology assessments should move from evaluating cost-*efficacy* in ideal (hypothetical) populations with ideal interventions, to cost-*effectiveness* in real populations with pragmatic interventions (van Staa et al. 2009). The clinicians were not provided with any guidance on how to use coxibs in the vast majority of patients who could be treated with coxibs. Public health interventions should be developed with a focus on who could be targeted in routine clinical practice rather than on who had been included into randomized trials. It has been proposed that public health programmes should be preceded by a systematic review of the research evidence assessing the likely effects of these programmes followed by an impact evaluation after launch (Oxman et al. 2010).

Scientific challenges in research with electronic healthcare data

Data quality is of course very important for research that uses EHR data. There are several dimensions of data quality. The accuracy and validity of the information in EHR databases will depend on the level and specificity of the coding of medical data at the clinics. A clinic that mostly records data using unstructured free-text or using non-specific codes will provide data that are less useful for research. Data quality also depends on the completeness of information. A clinic that is not routinely informed about, for example, hospitalizations of their patients will not provide complete data, even if the clinic codes the medical data to highest standards. Reliability of information includes the level of changes in data collection over time. As an example of secular changes, the Quality and Outcomes Framework introduced in England in 2004 resulted in a substantive increase of the data included in this framework. Relevance of the collected data for the desired use is another component of data quality. An EHR database that is based on records from GPs may not contain all the data considered relevant by a specialist for making a diagnosis. Timeliness of information processing is also critical for data quality (Audit Commission 2007). Studies that use EHR data for public health research will need to consider these different aspects of data quality.

There are many different EHR systems and similar information may be recorded and stored differently, making it difficult to extract information in a standardized manner or to share information between different partners. Complex systems may need to be built in order to make computer systems interoperable and to exchange EHR data with public health agencies. An example of such a system is the US National Electronic Disease Surveillance System. This is a web-based infrastructure for public health surveillance data exchange between the Centers of Disease Control and the 50 US states. Forty-seven states had in 2010 fully operational general communicable disease electronic surveillance systems, of which 39 states had systems that were interoperable and 42 states had the capacity to receive electronic laboratory reports (Centers for Disease Control and Prevention 2011).

Ethical aspects of research with electronic healthcare data

Healthcare data contain sensitive information about individuals. Adequate protection of individuals' privacy and data security are very important requirements for researchers to adhere to. EHR databases typically remove patients' identifiers (such as name, address, and postcode) from the research database. In some databases, researchers will never be able to contact the clinician or patient; these data are considered fully anonymized. In other databases, researchers will not know the patients' identifiers but they are able to contact the clinician or patients through a gatekeeper; these data are considered pseudo-anonymized. In the Clinical Practice Research Datalink, the patient's clinician can be contacted (following approval by an ethics committee), who can then review the request and contact the patient, if appropriate.

There is considerable debate about whether (pseudo)anonymized healthcare data should be made available for research. In an opt-in system, data can only be made available to researchers dependent on their informed consent. In an opt-out system, patients can refuse to have their data used for research. In other systems, anonymized data are considered exempt from consent or dissent requirements and can be used for research as long as the data do not contain patient identifiers. A recent discussion in the European parliament proposed that 'processing of sensitive data for historical, statistical and scientific research purposes is not as urgent or compelling as public health or social protection.' Identifiable health data about an individual could never be used without their consent (such as cancer registries). Pseudo-anonymized data could be used without consent, but only in cases of 'exceptionally high public interest' such as bioterrorism (European Parliament 2012). At the time of this writing, the discussions around European data privacy regulations are still ongoing.

The critical question is whether the right of data privacy trumps all other rights and duties or whether there is a balance between different considerations. There is the right of patients to receive proper treatments and the duty of the healthcare to, for example, monitor treatments for effectiveness and safety and be cost-effective. A healthcare system that generates and applies the best evidence for collaborative healthcare choices of each patient and provider has been defined as a learning healthcare system (McGinnis 2010). Such a system would continuously test interventions and collect data on the outcomes and then use the results to inform and improve clinical practice. Scientific research including public health requires high-quality data, and a learning healthcare system that aims to continuously improve cannot be achieved without such data. It has been proposed that data governance should be viewed as a matter of weighing up the value accruing to individuals, such as privacy and consent, against the value that the research may generate for the public (Rumbold et al. 2011).

The discussion about rights of data privacy and the research use of EHRs should not be restricted to abstract legal notions but also consider the likelihood of data privacy breaches and how these can be minimized. Staff training and standard procedures are essential, but the skills and attitudes of staff are also very important to ensure that data are treated with appropriate care. Regular audits of data security by external experts can also help to maintain a culture of continuous improvement (MacKenzie et al. 2011). With appropriate data security procedures, the risk of breaches of data privacy could be minimized. Also, the standards and quality of research are important considerations in the balancing of rights of data privacy and the research use of EHRs. Registration of the study prior to the start of the analyses and external access to protocols after completion of the analyses have been advocated

strongly for randomized trials (Chan et al. 2006). External access to protocols and the possibility for independent researchers to replicate the study findings could help to improve research standards. A public health system that uses EHRs for high-quality and transparent research and with minimal risk of privacy breaches is clearly ethically superior to a system that applies few standards.

Conclusion

Information systems are critical for public health activities with information being exchanged between public health agencies, clinicians/healthcare providers, individuals, and communities. The EHRs can provide information on diseases and healthcare activities and electronic alerts within the EHRs can be used to remind clinicians of necessary or required public health activities. The effectiveness of some public health interventions can be monitored and also tested using the EHRs. Better data on risks and benefits of healthcare interventions can also help to improve decision-making and informed consent by individuals (Calman et al. 2012). The increasing computerization of the healthcare system will offer many important opportunities to improve public health activities.

References

Adamson, J., van Staa, T., and Torgerson, D. (2012). Assuring the safety and effectiveness of new drugs: rigorous phase IV trials randomizing general practices to delayed access to new drugs. *Journal of Health Services Research & Policy*, 17(1), 56–69.

Atkinson, R.W., Carey, I.M., Kent, A.J., van Staa, T.P., Anderson, H.R., and Cook, D.G. (2013). Long-term exposure to outdoor air pollution and incidence of cardiovascular diseases. *Epidemiology*, 24(1), 44–53.

Audit Commission (2007). *Improving Information to Support Decision Making: Standards for Better Quality Data*. Report. London: Audit Commission.

Blumenthal, D. and Tavenner, M. (2010). The 'meaningful use' regulation for electronic health records. *The New England Journal of Medicine*, 363(6), 501–4.

Boggon, R., van Staa, T.P., Chapman, M., Gallagher, A.M., Hammad, T.A., and Richards, M.A. (2013). Cancer recording and mortality in the General Practice Research Database and linked cancer registries. *Pharmacoepidemiology and Drug Safety*, 22(2), 168–75.

Butler, S.F., Venuti, S.W., Benoit, C., Beaulaurier, R.L., Houle, B., and Katz, N. (2007). Internet surveillance: content analysis and monitoring of product-specific internet prescription opioid abuse-related postings. *The Clinical Journal of Pain*, 23(7), 619–28.

Calman, N., Hauser, D., Lurio, J., Wu, W.Y., and Pichardo, M. (2012). Strengthening public health and primary care collaboration through electronic health records. *American Journal of Public Health*, 102(11), e13–18.

Campbell, S.M., Reeves, D., Kontopantelis, E., Sibbald, B., and Roland, M. (2009). Effects of pay for performance on the quality of primary care in England. *The New England Journal of Medicine*, 361(4), 368–78.

Cebul, R.D., Love, T.E., Jain, A.K., and Hebert, C.J. (2011). Electronic health records and quality of diabetes care. *The New England Journal of Medicine*, 365(9), 825–33.

Centers for Disease Control and Prevention (CDC) (2011). State electronic disease surveillance systems—United States, 2007 and 2010. *MMWR Morbidity and Mortality Weekly Report*, 60(41), 1421–3.

Chan, A.W., Upshur, R., Singh, J.A., Ghersi, D., Chapuis, F., and Altman, D.G. (2006). Research protocols: waiving confidentiality for the greater good. *BMJ*, 332(7549), 1086–9.

Classen, D.C. and Bates, D.W. (2011). Finding the meaning in meaningful use. *The New England Journal of Medicine*, 365(9), 855–8.

Coloma, P.M., Trifirò, G., Schuemie, M.J., et al. (2012). Electronic healthcare databases for active drug safety surveillance: is there enough leverage? *Pharmacoepidemiology and Drug Safety*, 21(6), 611–21.

Denaxas, S.C., George, J., Herrett, E., et al. (2012). Data resource profile: cardiovascular disease research using linked bespoke studies and electronic health records (CALIBER). *International Journal of Epidemiology*, 41(6), 1625–38.

Department of Health (2011). *UK Influenza Pandemic Preparedness Strategy 2011*. London: Department of Health. Available at: https://www.gov.uk/government/uploads/system/uploads/attachment_data/file/213717/dh_131040.pdf.

De Wet, C. and Bowie, P. (2011). Screening electronic patient records to detect preventable harm: a trigger tool for primary care. *Quality in Primary Care*, 19(2), 115–25.

Edwards, D. and Bell, J. (2000). Cancer registries—future development and uses in Britain. *Journal of Public Health Medicine*, 22(2), 216–19.

European Parliament. Committee on Civil Liberties, Justice and Home Affairs (2012). *Draft report on the proposal for a regulation of the European Parliament and of the Council on the protection of individual with regard to the processing of personal data and on the free movement of such data (General Data Protection Regulation) (COM(2012)0011 – C7-0025/2012 – 2012/0011(COD))*. Available at: http://www.europarl.europa.eu/meetdocs/2009_2014/documents/libe/pr/922/922387/922387en.pdf.

Furu, K., Wettermark, B., Andersen, M., Martikainen, J.E., Almarsdottir, A.B., and Sørensen, H.T. (2010). The Nordic countries as a cohort for pharmacoepidemiological research. *Basic & Clinical Pharmacology & Toxicology*, 106(2), 86–94.

Ginsberg, J., Mohebbi, M.H., Patel, R.S., Brammer, L., Smolinski, M.S., and Brilliant, L. (2009). Detecting influenza epidemics using search engine query data. *Nature*, 457(7232), 1012–14.

Gulliford M.C., van Staa T., McDermott L., et al. (2011). Cluster randomised trial in the General Practice Research Database: 1. Electronic decision support to reduce antibiotic prescribing in primary care (eCRT study). *Trials*, 12, 115.

Havard, S., Deguen, S., Bodin, J., Louis, K., Laurent, O., and Bard, D. (2008). A small-area index of socioeconomic deprivation to capture health inequalities in France. *Social Science & Medicine*, 67(12), 2007–16.

Health and Social Care Information System (n.d.). *Hospital Episode Statistics*. [Online] Available at: http://www.hscic.gov.uk/hes.

Herings, R.C. and Pedersen, L. (2012). Pharmacy-based medical record linkage systems. In: B.L. Strom, S.E. Kimmel, and S. Hennessy (eds.) *Pharmacoepidemiology* (5th ed.), pp. 270–86. New York: Wiley-Blackwell.

Ioannidis, J.P.A. (2013). Mega-trials for blockbusters. *JAMA*, 309(3), 239–40.

Klompas, M., McVetta, J., Lazarus, R., et al. (2012). Integrating clinical practice and public health surveillance using electronic medical record systems. *American Journal of Preventive Medicine*, 42(6 Suppl. 2), S154–62.

Linkins, R.W. (2001). Immunization registries: progress and challenges in reaching the 2010 national objective. *Journal of Public Health Management and Practice*, 7(6), 67–74.

Mackenzie, I.S., Mantay, B.J., McDonnell, P.G., Wei, L., and MacDonald, T.M. (2011). Managing security and privacy concerns over data storage in healthcare research. *Pharmacoepidemiology and Drug Safety*, 20(8), 885–93.

McGinnis, J.M. (2010). Evidence-based medicine—engineering the Learning Healthcare System. *Studies in Health Technology and Informatics*, 153, 145–57.

National Health Service Health Check Programme (2008). *Putting Prevention First—Vascular Checks: Risk Assessment and Management*. London: Department of Health. Available at: http://www.healthcheck.nhs.uk/Library/F26E1C01d01.pdf.

Ortiz, J.R., Zhou, H., Shay, D.K., Neuzil, K.M., Fowlkes, A.L., and Goss, C.H. (2011). Monitoring influenza activity in the United States: a comparison of traditional surveillance systems with Google Flu Trends. *PLoS One*, 6(4), e18687.

Oxman, A.D., Bjørndal, A., Becerra-Posada, F., et al. (2010). A framework for mandatory impact evaluation to ensure well informed public policy decisions. *The Lancet*, 375(9712), 427–31.

Public Health Sciences Working Group convened by the Wellcome Trust (2004). *Public Health Sciences: Challenges and Opportunities*. London: The Wellcome Trust. Available at: http://www.wellcome.ac.uk/stellent/groups/corporatesite/@policy_communications/documents/web_document/wtd003191.pdf.

QSurveillance (n.d.). Website. [Online] Available at: http://www.qsurveillance.org.

Rumbold, B., Lewis, G., and Bardsley, M. (2011). *Access to Person-Level Data in Health Care: Understanding Information Governance*. London: Nuffield Trust. Available at: http://www.nuffieldtrust.org.uk/publications/access-person-level-data-health-care-understanding-information-governance.

St Sauver, J.L., Grossardt, B.R., Yawn, B.P., et al. (2012). Data Resource Profile: The Rochester Epidemiology Project (REP) medical records-linkage system. *International Journal of Epidemiology*, 41(6), 1614–24.

Tunis, S.R., Stryer, D.B., and Clancy, C.M. (2003). Practical clinical trials: increasing the value of clinical research for decision making in clinical and health policy. *JAMA*, 290(12), 1624–32.

Van Staa, T.P., Leufkens, H.G., Zhang, B., and Smeeth, L. (2009). A comparison of cost effectiveness using data from randomized trials or actual clinical practice: selective cox-2 inhibitors as an example. *PLoS Medicine*, 6(12), e1000194.

Van Staa, T.P., Goldacre, B., Gulliford, M., et al. (2012). Randomised Evaluations of Accepted Choices in Treatment (REACT) trials: large-scale pragmatic trials within databases of routinely collected electronic healthcare records. *BMJ*, 344, e55.

Warren-Gash, C., Hayward, A.C., Hemingway, H., et al. (2012). Influenza infection and risk of acute myocardial infarction in England and Wales: a CALIBER self-controlled case series study. *The Journal of Infectious Diseases*, 206(11), 1652–9.

Weiner, J.P., Fowles, J.B., and Chan, K.S. (2012). New paradigms for measuring clinical performance using electronic health records. *International Journal for Quality in Health Care*, 24(3), 200–5.

Williams, T., van Staa, T.P., Puri, S., and Eaton, S. (2012). Recent advances in the utility and use of the General Practice Research Database as an example of a UK Primary Care Data resource. *Therapeutic Advances in Drug Safety*, 3, 89–99.

Information systems and community diagnosis in low- and middle-income countries

Peter Cherutich and Ruth Nduati

Introduction to information systems and community diagnosis in low- and middle-income countries

Individuals, local communities, governments, and national and international bodies are heavily investing in health as a key pillar for development. The International Covenant on Economic, Social and Cultural rights of the United Nations Assembly of 1966 and the WHO Constitution affirm that all human beings have inalienable rights that include 'the enjoyment of the highest attainable standard of health' (UN General Assembly 1966). And in Ottawa in 1998, the World Medical Association declared that 'children need to grow up in a place where they can thrive—spiritually, emotionally, mentally, physically and intellectually' (World Medical Association 1998) with access to health services when needed. The global community has further shaped the global health landscape over the last few decades through political declarations, research, and increased funding. The Declaration of Alma Ata, Health for All by the year 2000, the UN charter on human rights, the Abuja Declaration, and the G8 summits have created a momentum for global health. Health is therefore part of a global social and human rights imperative. The overarching international global health aspirations are captured in the commitments made to achieve the Millennium Development Goals (MDGs) (UN General Assembly 2000) by the year 2015.

Three of these MDGs—4, 5, and 6—are directly health related while the others have an indirect but nevertheless significant effect on health and quality of life. Each of the MDGs has a defined set of targets whose attainment has galvanized the international community. Following these declarations of commitment to the promotion of health globally, significant resources have been made available through the President's Emergency Plan for AIDS Relief (PEPFAR), the GAVI Alliance, The Bill and Melinda Gates Foundation, The Global Fund for AIDS, TB and Malaria, and others to support these objectives. Countries and communities are obligated to ensure these resources are utilized accountably in terms of outcomes and impact and information systems and community diagnosis are tools for evaluating accountability.

One major drawback to the attainment of the MDGs is that many MDG-related health indicators cannot attract major international attention or investments and that in low- and middle-income countries data availability on these indicators is limited (Murray 2007). Monitoring the flow of resources as well as the potential impact of those resources on health outcomes especially in low- and middle-income countries where the burden of disease is high constitute a major goal of community diagnosis.

Overview of community diagnosis

Community diagnosis is a composite mechanism that informs priorities and tracks the progress of health metrics. Community diagnosis, in contrast with clinical diagnosis which is a patient–clinician interaction, refers to the identification and quantification of health problems at the population level. Information systems and community diagnosis in low- and middle-income countries fundamentally builds on the core of epidemiological surveillance and includes the following:

1. Systems to monitor magnitude and temporal trends of disease/health.

2. Identifying risk factors driving continued trends.

3. Targeting/prioritizing interventions or planning services and/or rationing limited resources (human and financial) for maximum impact.

4. Assessing impact of intervention on desired outcome.

The World Health Organization (WHO) defines community diagnosis as a quantitative and qualitative description of the health of citizens and the factors which influence their health including the population's perception of their own health. It identifies problems, proposes areas for improvement, and stimulates action. Community diagnosis provides data reference for the region and provides an overall picture of the local community and the residents' concerns.

For the purposes of public health, a community is defined as a cluster of people with at least one common characteristic (geographic location, occupation, ethnicity, housing condition, exposure to similar risk factor, etc.). For example, mine workers constitute a community since their occupation exposes them to high risk for HIV transmission and acquisition as well as other occupational hazards (respiratory illnesses, injury, etc.).

Process of community diagnosis

There are four steps in carrying out a community diagnosis:

Initiation of a community diagnosis: a community diagnosis begins with the determination of the scope of areas to be studied. The study may include health status, lifestyles, living conditions, socioeconomic conditions, physical and social infrastructure, inequalities, as well as public health services and policies. The scope of the community diagnosis depends on the client, the purpose and the resources that are available for the exercise.

Data collection: tools for community diagnosis include primary and secondary data collection techniques. The primary data collecting techniques include key informant interviews, mapping, questionnaires, observations, focus group discussions, anthropometric surveys, and participatory rapid appraisals. Secondary data collection techniques generally involve review of records.

A community diagnosis should be well designed to ensure adequate representation of different members of the community. Typically, community diagnosis is cross-sectional but repeated measurements enable determination of trends in the population and may be used to monitor the impact of an intervention.

Data analysis: the raw data then needs to be organized and statistical tests and inferences made. The statistical information is best presented as rates or ratios such as mortality and morbidity rates which can be further analysed to determine their correlates for the purpose of defining those at risk or those in need of healthcare. Trends and projections are useful for monitoring changes over a time period for future planning, for example, mortality trends as presented in demographic health surveys or monitoring of the progress on the implementation of health interventions as well as community perceptions regarding health. Local district data can be compared with other districts or the whole population and help identify the priority areas of hot spots for immediate intervention.

Diagnosis: the diagnosis of the community is based on evaluation of the analysed data. Ideally the community diagnosis should be arranged around the following themes:

◆ Health status of the community—measures of disease occurrence are used to describe the status of health of the community such as incidence and prevalence.

◆ Determinants of health in the community—measures of disease association such as odds ratios, population attributable risks.

◆ Potential for health interventions.

Community engagement

Community diagnosis is a dynamic process. Applying the methods of community diagnosis requires meticulous planning and community mobilization. Large-scale household surveys like the Demographic and Health Surveys (DHS) and community-based studies (Joint United Nations Programme on HIV/AIDS 2011) typically involve the community in the planning, implementation, and feedback. The opportunity cost of not engaging survey participants and the relevant communities is very high since surveys are expensive. In order to achieve high participation rates, community leaders and other opinion shapers may aid in convincing reluctant survey participants and dispel myths, especially around blood draws. A further example is in the conduct of verbal autopsies. To achieve a balance between recall bias and sensitivities around grieving, administrators of verbal autopsy require skill to

interact with the community but also to ensure that they engage respondent families after a reasonable duration (usually 3 weeks) following the death of a member.

Key steps of community entry are outlined as follows:

◆ Set up a coordinating committee at national and regional level. Designate one of the subcommittees to spearhead community engagement:
  • Provide advance notice to the local community about the survey.
  • Identify regional or local coordinators of the survey.

◆ Develop key messages with details of the goal, the process, and outcome of the survey.

◆ Map out key community leaders and identify local structures for engagement:
  • Identify community needs though structured process.
  • Identify community champions.
  • Align community expectations (e.g. for recruitment as survey personnel) with survey realities and possibilities.

◆ Sensitize the media and launch media campaign if necessary.

◆ High-profile launch of survey by key political leaders may be appropriate in some settings.

◆ Regular feedback on the progress of survey—clarify any misconceptions that may continue to arise.

◆ Final feedback on the findings of the survey and return of any biomarker results if appropriate.

Community involvement further assures that the knowledge derived from any domain of community diagnosis can be repackaged in a manner relevant to the beneficiaries (Madhavan et al. 2007). Health programme managers and policymakers should also make sure that they consult with frontline healthcare workers before they introduce any new health information system. A comprehensive review of existing solutions must be done before decisions on high-technology investments are made (Detels et al. 2005). Failure to do this will result in resentment and rejection of the new system.

There are numerous examples of questions that are well addressed by conducting a community diagnosis. Are trends in mortality and nutritional status moving in the right direction? Is the country on track to achieve the health MDGs? How high is coverage for each intervention? Are trends moving in the right direction towards universal coverage? Are there gaps in coverage for specific interventions? How equitable is coverage? Are certain interventions particularly inaccessible for the poorest segment of the population?

Community diagnosis and information systems are useful in determining the Global Burden of Disease (GBD) (Murray et al. 2011), populations at risk, generating denominators for coverage, unit costs, etc. The data generated from community diagnosis may inform mathematical modelling aimed at prioritizing interventions with the highest public health impact (Hallett et al. 2008; Njeuhmeli et al. 2011).

Community diagnosis, if appropriately done and well disseminated, has the potential to:

◆ Improve national and subnational delivery of health services through properly costed national health plans that emphasize service integration and include programmes for reproductive, maternal, newborn, and child health.

◆ Strengthen health information systems, including vital registration systems and national health accounts, so that timely, accurate data can inform policies and programmes.

◆ Increase domestic funding allocations for and expenditures on health.

◆ Build the numbers, motivation, and skill mix of the health workforce.

◆ Analyse subnational data to identify gaps and inequities and to monitor and evaluate programmes and policies.

◆ Develop strategies to reduce the burden of disease and improve efficiency of health programmes.

Priority health metrics for community diagnosis in low- and middle-income countries

Depending on specific health priorities of countries, the burden of disease and risk factor profile, the data required may include demographic characteristics, educational infrastructure (schools) and educational attainment, waste disposal, housing conditions, vector control, nutritional status of the population, and the social environment, etc. (MacQueen et al. 2011).

Outlined in the following sections are the key health metrics relevant to low- and middle-income countries, and which are of interest to the global health community.

Demographic: life expectancy at birth

The number of years that a person born today (or at any other designated point in time) is expected to live, given the mortality patterns for the country in which he or she lives at the time of birth. This metric is modelled based on the age-specific death rates obtained from a combination of sources including vital registration systems and household surveys and censuses. Advances in public health and improvement in quality of life are accompanied by increased life expectancy.

Mortality

The vital events necessary for measurement of mortality are live births, deaths, and still births. A complete vital registration (VR) is the best source of mortality data. However, most low- and many middle-income countries have incomplete VR systems, especially data pertaining to perinatal deaths (stillbirth and early neonatal deaths) and therefore information collected through this system is often non-representative. In settings where VR is incomplete, reliance on interviews from relatives to ascertain probable cause of death is essential. This is called verbal autopsy (VA). The mortality questions frequently asked include household deaths in the last 12 months, and about parental, spousal, and sibling survival (Gakidou et al. 2004). Although these surveys are subject to recall bias, they nevertheless provide a robust source of mortality data for resource limited settings.

Maternal mortality ratio

Maternal death is defined as the death of a woman as a result of pregnancy or childbirth, during pregnancy, or within 42 days after delivery. Classification of a death as a maternal death is highly dependent on a recorded diagnosis or the conduct of a VA to ascertain the cause of death. Pregnancy-related deaths in early gestation may be under-reported. Secrecy and stigma surrounding pregnancy may also impede reporting of a maternal death. Standardized interview tools to document maternal deaths to be used during surveys have been developed. The maternal mortality ratio (MMR) is expressed as the number of maternal deaths per 100,000 live births over a specified period.

Child mortality

Age-specific mortality rates are categorized and defined as follows:

◆ Neonatal mortality: the probability of dying within the 1st month of life.

◆ Post-neonatal mortality: the difference between infant and neonatal mortality.

◆ Infant mortality: the probability of dying before the first birthday.

◆ Child mortality: the probability of dying between the first and fifth birthday (the sum of the probabilities of dying in the 2nd, 3rd, 4th, and 5th years of life).

◆ Under-5 mortality: the probability of dying between birth and the 5th birthday.

All rates are expressed per 1000 live births, except for child mortality, which is expressed per 1000 children surviving to 12 months of age. The other important measure is perinatal death rate which is total stillbirths plus 1st-week deaths as a ratio of the total live births.

Calculation of the probability of dying for each year of life usually relies on data from a survey or registry of all birth and death histories. When such data are not available, child mortality would be estimated for any given calendar year by summing all reported deaths of children 1–4 years of age that occurred in a given year and dividing that number by the number of live births in the same year or the estimated number of children aged 1–4 years. When VR is incomplete, periodic surveys (Demographic Surveys and Census) data is used to determine the estimates of infant and child mortality.

Cause of death

VR is the gold standard for obtaining cause of death information. The quality of information collected determines the extent to which deaths can be attributed to different causes. The ICD-10 provides standard disease classification although its utility in the context of community diagnosis is diminished by incomplete medical records and failure of the clinician to commit to a specific diagnosis. VA is increasingly being used to supplement incomplete VR systems. Abbreviated verbal autopsies have also been used in refugee camps and in emergency situations. Accuracy of the verbal autopsies requires careful development of the case definition to be used in the survey. Community members may use medical jargon with a completely different meaning from the health worker and therefore formative research is required to anchor the VA in the local context (Irimu et al. 2008). VA reports are used to trigger important health action. For example, a recorded increase in mortality from measles should trigger a vaccination campaign in the affected area.

Morbidity

Morbidity estimates the relative prevalence (new and old cases) of a particular disease. In developing countries, most morbidity data is obtained from hospital records. Health facility data is almost always available in low-resource settings. Aside from the fact that these data are rarely collated and disseminated, health facility records including hospital discharge records are frequently biased since it is usually the most severe cases that are admitted to hospital. Additionally, those who are poorer and live further from health facilities are unlikely to utilize them. One innovative way of obtaining morbidity data is through demographic surveillance systems (DSSs), which are typically community-based systems in defined geographical areas that integrate regular household surveys and health examinations.

Composite measures of death and morbidity

The disability-adjusted life year (DALY) combines years of life lost (YLL) due to premature mortality and time spent with reduced health that is years lived with disability (YLD) into one measure. This is the metric employed by WHO to estimate the global burden of disease. The GBD 2010 shows a decrease in DALYs by 23 per cent in the period 1990–2010 with contribution of deaths by children aged less than 5 years declining from 41 per cent in 1990 to 25 per cent in 2010 (Murray et al. 2012). However, estimation of DALYs is not without controversy although recent iteration of DALY estimations is more robust (Box 4.2.1). Additionally the GBD 2010 highlighted significant disparities in burden of disease across countries and within regions (Fig. 4.2.1). Low- and middle-income countries should utilize the information available through the GBD for priority setting and allocation of resources.

Risk factors

The determination of risk factors for major health outcomes is vital if countries are to improve health outcomes. The assessment of population exposure of these risk factors through surveys has been widely used (Ministry of Health, Kenya 2007; Cherutich et al. 2012). When applied correctly, surveys produce valid trend data and can be used to plan interventions and project future health needs. Health examination surveys are rarer and more expensive. National censuses, although appropriate, are less often used to elicit risk factor assessment mainly because of the tremendous cost that would be involved. Cross-sectional surveys are not able to explain causal relationships since exposure (risk) and outcome are measured at the same time.

Functional health status

Functional health status of communities is important so that prevention of harm and improvement of quality of life can be prioritized (Institute of Health Metrics and Evaluation 2009). Information regarding vision, hearing, cognition, and pain can be collected through community surveys although in many developing countries it can be expensive. However, simpler tools such as MOS short form 36 (SF-36) (http://www.sf-36.org) and the Euroquol EQ-5D (http://www.euroquol.org) are available and can be utilized in low-resource settings to capture self-reported critical information on physical functioning, mental/emotional function, pain, mobility, cognition, etc.

Box 4.2.1 Case study: the Global Burden of Disease

Disability-adjusted life years (DALYs) account for both premature mortality and time spent with reduced health, that is years lived with disability (YLDs) whether short or long term. In order to determine the impact of disease or injury at population level there is a need to have valid measurements of health which are replicable across different populations. Furthermore, there is a need to determine the severity of one outcome relative to the other and therefore a weighting system-disability weight was used where 0 = minimal or no disability and 1 = severe disability equivalent to death.

Since the GBD work was published in 1990 there has been debate on the validity of the disability weights used in the original study especially since these weights were now being used on a much wider scale and in different settings. The discussions have revolved around: (1) how do you define the construct being measured, (2) what methods should be used to measure the construct to elicit responses from individuals or groups, (3) whose responses should be elicited, and (4) how universal are the resulting weights?

The GBD 2010 study teams have conducted a multi-country study to validate the disability weights (Murray 2012). The consensus was that the construct would be health outcome and not welfare outcome since the latter varies considerably with the social and environmental context. Method of trade-offs was used with a series of paired questions associated with the 220 unique health outcomes that described the non-fatal outcomes of the GBD study. The comparisons were based on a lay description of each of the conditions that emphasized the major functional symptoms associated with each health state using non-clinical vocabulary. The responses from the general public were adopted in formulating disability weights unlike the past where disability weights were derived from the judgements of a small group of health professionals. Individuals with the various conditions were not interviewed since this would introduce an adaptation bias. Finally to address the question of their applicability in different global locations, the study was carried out in five countries: the United States, Bangladesh, Indonesia, Peru, and Tanzania. At household level an individual aged 18 years or more was randomly selected to respond to the questions. Within these countries rural and urban populations were surveyed across different socioeconomic strata. In addition, an open-access web-based survey was carried out. The study demonstrated that disability assessments are consistent across diverse populations and different cultural environments. There was a pattern of agreement in the disability weights derived in this 2010 study compared to the 1990 study; however, in the mild range, many disabilities had lower weights.

The refinement of these disability weights means that countries can use data from the GBD to plan healthcare or even in the clinical setting improve communication regarding long-term outcomes. The study also illustrates the importance of collaboration between public health departments and research institutes/universities. The authors of this paper rightfully highlight the need to do further work to refine the lay description of the health outcomes of the different conditions.

Communicable, maternal, neonatal, and nutritional disorders
Both sexes, All ages, 2010
DALYs per 100,000

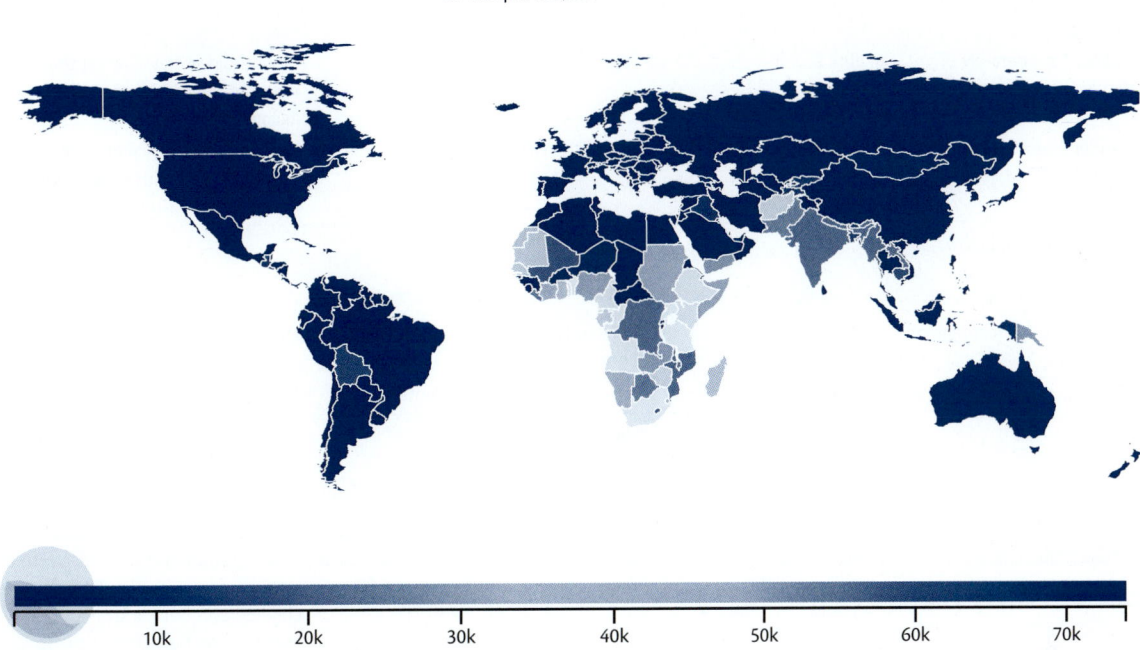

Fig. 4.2.1 Heterogeneity of global disease burden, GBD 2010.
Reproduced with permission from Institute for Health Metrics and Evaluation, University of Washington, Copyright © 2013, http://viz.healthmetricsandevaluation.org/gbd-compare/.

Health expenditure per capita

Healthcare providers, managers, and policymakers are accountable to communities, governments, and donors for the utilization of financial resources. Conversely donors and governments require financial information in order to allocate resources more equitably and efficiently. Many developing countries have now set up systems to produce National Health Accounts (http://www.who.int; http://www.phrplus.org/Pubs/prim1.pdf). National Health Accounts (NHA) is an internationally accepted tool for summarizing, describing, and analysing the financing of national health systems. The NHA is derived from data on disbursements, budgetary allocations, and expenditures by different entities within the healthcare system. In order to inform the NHA, household surveys as well as facility surveys are used. Household surveys among others, provide information on the balance of payments between out-of-pocket and institutional expenditures. Health facility surveys provide information on the costs of services to both the user and supplier and these surveys may include inventory recording, equipment audit, infrastructure assessments, etc.

Human resource inputs

Human resources data in terms of numbers, geographical distribution, type and level of skills, as well as repartition across the public and private sectors, is rarely available. The International Health Facility Assessment Network (IHFAN) supported by USAID and MEASURE Evaluation is one such mechanism for obtaining relevant data in the health workforce in developing countries. With slight modifications, countries can integrate these measurements into the country health information system. Key aspects for this metric include training, specialty or cadre, education levels, skills, and whether they work in the private or public settings.

Effective coverage

Effective coverage measures the proportion of health gain realized through delivering quality interventions (Shengelia et al. 2005). To calculate effective coverage, one requires information on the population in need, the utilization of the particular intervention, and the quality of the delivery of the intervention. Surveys provide the best information regarding the burden of disease in a community and the denominator population. Utilization rates can be collected from health facilitates and community surveys. For example, effective coverage for childhood immunization is defined as children having received BCG (Bacille Calmette–Guérin), three doses of DPT+P (diphtheria, pertussis, tetanus, and polio) vaccines, and measles vaccine by 12 months of age.

Cost-effectiveness

Cost-effectiveness analysis (CEA) is a tool that is used to compare the cost of a health intervention with the expected health gains. To impute CEA several pieces of information are required including costs of inputs (such as human resources, medical supplies, etc.) and outputs (such as number of caesarean sections done). NHA, where available, and health facility surveys are important sources of information for input and output data. Using the CEA approach it is possible to identify a minimum package of interventions that may impact a certain health outcome, for example, neonatal survival (Darmstadt et al. 2005).

Measurement strategies for key health metrics

Disease-specific indicators of global health importance have been integrated into information systems of many countries. However, as outlined in Table 4.2.1, some of these indicators are minimally

Table 4.2.1 Measurement of selected indicators for the Millennium Development Goals

Indicator	Type of indicator	Public health importance	Measurement strategy
4. Prevalence of underweight children under 5 years of age			
4a. Children under 5 moderately or severely underweight, percentage	Risk factor	High	Household surveys with anthropometric measurements with some inconsistency across age groups measured
4b. Children under 5 severely underweight, percentage	Risk factor	Adds little value to 4a	Household surveys with anthropometric measurements with some inconsistency across age groups measured
5. Proportion of population below minimum level of dietary energy consumption.			
5a. Undernourished as a percentage of total population	Risk factor	Low, adds little value to prevalence of underweight	Details not available
5b. Undernourished, number of people	Risk factor	Low, same information content as 5a	Details not available
13. Under-5 mortality rate	Health outcome	High	Vital registration in countries with completer systems, complete with birth histories, or children ever born and children surviving questions on household surveys
14. Infant mortality rate	Health outcome	Low; redundant, correlation coefficient with under-5 mortality rate in 0.99	Vital registration in countries with completer systems, complete with birth histories, or children ever born and children surviving questions on household surveys
15. Proportion of 1 year-old children immunized against measles	Intervention coverage	Medium/low; represents less than 10 per cent of the package for child survival	Health service provider registries in the public sector; household surveys
16. Maternal mortality ratio	Health outcome	High	Vital registration in countries with complete systems, sibling histories collected in household surveys
17. Proportion of births attended by skilled health personnel	Intervention coverage	High; but not the only intervention needed to reduce maternal mortality	Household surveys, definition of skilled health personnel varies across countries
18. HIV prevalence among women aged 15–24			
18a. AIDS estimated deaths	Health outcome	High	Vital registration in countries with complete systems, modelling of mortality based on estimated sero-prevalence in other countries.
18b. HIV prevalence rate, aged 15–49, percentage	Health outcome	High	ANC clinic sero-surveillance in sentinel sites, household sero-surveys; ANC sentinel surveillance overestimates national population prevalence
18c. HIV/AIDS prevalence rate for pregnant women 15–24 attending antenatal care in clinics in capital city	Health outcome	Low; represents only a partial fraction of the national prevalence, but has been used to estimate incidence of HIV	Capital city ANC sero-surveillance, because of variability in representativeness of sentinel clinics and demographic significance of capital city, comparability limited
18d. HIV/AIDS prevalence rates, men, estimated from national population surveys	Health outcome	Subset of 18b	Household sero-surveys
18e. HIV/AIDS prevalence rates, women, estimated from national population surveys	Health outcome	Subset of 18b	Household sero-surveys
19. Condom use to overall contraceptive use among currently married women, aged 15–49	Intervention coverage	Low; not a good measure of condom use in high-risk sexual intercourse	Household surveys
19a. Condom use, men aged 15–24 years at last high-risk sex	Intervention coverage	Medium; condom use for any age group for high-risk sex would be of public health interest	Household surveys but validity of reported rates of high-risk sex not established
19b. Condom use, women aged 15–24 years at last high-risk sex	Intervention coverage	Correlation coefficient with 19a in 2000 is 0.85	Household surveys but validity of reported rates of high-risk sex not established

(Continued)

Table 4.2.1 Continued

Indicator	Type of indicator	Public health importance	Measurement strategy
21. Prevalence and death associated with malaria			
21a. Malaria deaths rate per 100,000, ages 0–4	Health outcome	High	Vital registration in countries with complete systems, in nearly all endemic countries, based on verbal autopsy data for demographic surveillance sites, or epidemiological models
21b. Malaria deaths rate per 100,000, all ages	Health outcome	Low; death rates over the age 0–4 very low	Vital registration in countries with complete systems, in nearly all endemic countries, based on verbal autopsy data for demographic surveillance sites, or epidemiological models
21c. Malaria prevalence, notified cases per 100,000 population	Health outcome	Low; notified cases are not a measure of prevalence	Administrative data collected at health facilities
22. Proportion of population in malaria-risk areas using effective malaria prevention and treatment measures			
22a. Malaria prevention, use of insecticide treated bednets in population <5, percentage	Intervention coverage	High	Household surveys
22b. Malaria treatment, percentage of population <5 with fever being treated with antimalarial drugs	Intervention coverage	Moderate; resistance makes effective antimalarial drugs a better indicator	Household surveys, validity not established
23. Prevalence and death rates associated with tuberculosis			
23a. Tuberculosis death rate per 100,000	Health outcome	High	Vital registration in countries with complete VR, modelled for all other countries
23b. Tuberculosis prevalence rate per 100,000 population	Health outcome	High	No measurement strategy, modelled estimates based on case notifications
24. Proportion of tuberculosis cases detected and cured under directly observed therapy (DOTS)			
24a. Tuberculosis, DOTS detection rate, percentage	Intervention coverage	High	Health service provider registers for detected cases, no measurement strategy for denominator
24b. Tuberculosis, DOTS treatment success, percentage	Intervention coverage	High	Health service registers
31. Proportion of the population with access to improved sanitation, urban and rural			
31a. Water, percentage of population with access to improved sanitation, rural	Risk factor	Moderate; not clear whether separate indicators for rural and urban necessary	Household surveys
31b. Water, percentage of population with access to improved sanitation, total	Risk factor	High	Household surveys
31c. Water, percentage of population with access to improved sanitation, urban	Risk factor	Moderate; not clear whether separate indicators for rural and urban necessary	Household surveys
46. Proportion of population with access to affordable essential drugs on a sustainable basis	Intervention coverage	High	No measurement strategy

Adapted from *The Lancet*, Volume 369, Issue 9564, Murray C., Towards good practice for health statistics: lessons from the Millennium Development Goal health indicators, pp. 863–73, Copyright © 2007 with permission from Elsevier, http://www.sciencedirect.com/science/journal/01406736.

informative; and still others cannot be estimated at all or are subject to measurement errors and poor validation. For a health indicator to be measured successfully, public health specialists, information system experts, advocates, implementers, and funders need to concur.

Methods for community diagnosis

Health information systems

A *health information system* includes procedures to collect, store, analyse, transfer, and retrieve data or health metrics for decision-making. The data may be stored in paper and/or electronic form, and the collection, analysis, transfer, and retrieval may be performed by human beings or electronic information technology, but usually by some combination of both. Advances in information technology, and the increase in the penetration of cellular mobile phones, offer opportunities to revolutionize information systems in low- and middle-income countries.

A combination of data from community and facility-based systems are used for community diagnosis. An ideal health information system is driven by community needs and provides sufficient feedback to district and local health planners for the purposes of decision-making, quality improvement, and planning. We shall describe these key data sources outlining their potential in low- and middle-income countries.

Household surveys

Household surveys are some of the most commonly used methods for documenting burden of disease, risk factor surveillance, and health expenditures. Often they are nationally representative and utilize a two-stage stratified sampling design. There are several resources on how to conduct health surveys (Institute for Health Metrics and Evaluation n.d.; The DHS Program n.d.).

Countries such as Kenya, Uganda, Swaziland, Thailand, Mexico, Brazil, Chile, and Columbia have incorporated biomarkers such as dry blood spots for HIV and other infections, into their household surveys (Central Statistical Office (CSO) and Macro International Incorporated 2008) at marginally higher costs.

Implementing surveys requires several considerations. Designing the questionnaire is the single most critical stage in the survey development process. As such, key questions to tackle include, but are not limited to: What is the question that the survey aims to answer? How do I design my survey instrument to capture information that will allow me to answer that question? Who is the target population? They are there a need to stratify the population? What is the sample size that is required to reach a scientifically sound conclusion? Is the sample representative?

In conducting surveys, communities must be active participants and must be engaged very early in the process. Inappropriate consultation with the community may lead to failure or may compromise the validity of the survey. However, when properly done, community mobilization and engagement can yield participation rates of up to 98 per cent (Central Statistical Authority (Ethiopia) and ORC MACRO 2001). Return of biomarker results and dissemination of results to survey participants is increasingly becoming an ethical requirement and needs to be considered.

The Multiple Indicator Cluster Surveys (MICS) are special surveys developed by the United Nations Children's Fund to provide internationally comparable, statistically rigorous data on the situation of children and women. They are particularly tailored to track progress towards the attainment of the MDGs. Using this method, it has been documented that 9 per cent of children under the age of 15 in sub-Saharan Africa have lost at least one parent (Monasch et al. 2004).

Where two-stage cluster sampling is not feasible, a single-stage cluster sampling may provide a reasonable alternative. With single-stage cluster sampling, an area is divided into non-overlapping units, called clusters. A limited number of clusters are randomly sampled for inclusion into the study, and then all units within the selected clusters are sampled. This has the advantage of avoiding costs of developing a sampling frame and

further enhances efficiency since it ensures that survey areas are limited geographically. One further advantage of cluster sampling is that it can be integrated with lot quality assurance sampling (LQAS) (Hoshaw-Woodard 2001).

Lot quality assurance sampling

In some instances, household surveys are either expensive or impractical. LQAS provides an alternative to identify priority areas or indicators that are not reaching average coverage at subnational level. LQAS can provide an accurate measure of coverage or health system quality at a more aggregate level (e.g. programme catchment area or district or refugee camp), typically caller 'supervision area' and at a lesser cost. It can be used for quality assurance using a 'minimal sample', 'maximal security' principle. A typical sample size is five to six supervision areas each comprising 19 facilities. In Uganda, it has been used to assess the performance of HIV/AIDS control programmes at the district and subdistrict levels as well as at the national level. There are now several examples applying LQAS for ongoing supervision, and the most well-documented example is from a maternal and child health project in rural Nepal (Valadez and Devkota 2002).

A detailed description of the methodology and its application is available (Lemeshow and Stroh 1988; Myatt et al. 2003).

Vital registration

VR—the systematic recording of births and deaths—has both legal and health significance. Specifically, as an integral part of community diagnosis, VR enables countries to track health related targets of the MDGs (Liu et al. 2012). Specifically VR has been used, in combination with VA, to monitor stillbirth rates (Cousens et al. 2011) and adult mortality (Rajaratnam et al. 2010) and the overall impact of the Millennium Villages Project (Ohemeng-Dapaah et al. 2010). In HIV clinics, linking to VR systems can provide more accurate assessments of programme effectiveness and target lost patients most at risk for mortality (Foxet al. 2010).

VR systems are now fairly well established around the world with about 115 countries reporting death statistics to the World Health Organization in 2003 (Matherset al. 2005). Although it is the ideal method for mortality estimation, many low- and middle-income countries have incomplete VR systems. In one study in Great Accra, the rate of under-registration of maternal mortality was 28 per cent, mainly due to misclassification (Zakariah et al. 2006). Nonetheless, interest in establishing sample VR, in which a subset of VR is studied, is rapidly growing in Africa and Asia.

Limitations

VR systems are expensive to set up and require close collaboration between Ministries of Health, and sectors responsible for registration of persons, immigration, and the judiciary. Misclassification of cause of death is a major drawback for VR. Adjusting for this can improve death registration data and provide empirical estimates of mortality (Birnbaumet al. 2011). Furthermore, statistical modelling can be used to estimate the causes of child mortality for settings with incomplete VR (Murray et al. 2010). Another means of improving measures of adult mortality is using sibling survival (Obermeyer et al. 2010).

Verbal autopsy

Cause-of-death data derived from VA are increasingly used for health planning, priority setting, monitoring, and evaluation in countries with incomplete or no VR systems. Currently, the VA method is routinely used at over 35 sites, mainly in Africa and Asia. In Kenya, between August 2002 and December 2008, a total of 1823 VA interviews were reviewed by physicians. The patterns of mortality as determined by both methods showed a high burden of infectious diseases, including HIV/AIDS, tuberculosis, and pneumonia (Oti and Kyobutungi 2010).

However, since VA procedures vary from setting to setting and may include physician reviews and/or computer automated methods, these instruments must be standardized and assessed with rigour in order to make accurate national and international comparisons of VA data. Traditional means of comparing VA methods include specificity, sensitivity, and cause-specific mortality fraction (CSMF). At the Institute of Health Metrics and Evaluation at the University of Washington, Seattle, a further refinement of the assessment of VA methods has been done (Murray et al. 2011).

Fig. 4.2.2 outlines the process of conducting and interpreting VA, assigning cause of death, and calculating CSMFs (Soleman et al. 2006).

Limitations

Although it has challenges relating to level of subjectivity associated with physician reviews, and is time and resource intensive, VA may be useful in generating probable disease mortality trends in a community, particularly when applied over time and integrated in routine DSSs.

Demographic surveillance systems

Demographic surveillance—the process of monitoring births, deaths, causes of deaths, and migration in a population over time—is one of the cornerstones of public health research and community diagnosis. DSSs involve continuous longitudinal recording of demographic data usually within small geographically defined populations and on a regular basis. The periodicity of follow-up varies somewhere between monthly household visits (Indepth NETWORK n.d.) to about yearly visits (Collinson et al. 2002; Razzaque and Streatfield 2002; Indepth NETWORK n.d.). However, for most of the DSSs the average visitation cycle is about three times a year. DSSs start with an initial census to define the baseline denominator population and thereafter continuously monitor this population at well-defined periods of time in order to observe changes or events that occur within the initial population. During the routine visits, vital events such as births, deaths, and migrations and, in some areas like Kisumu, Kenya, pregnancies and new HIV and tuberculosis infections are registered and monitored. DSSs may yield critical information regarding magnitude and determinants of mortality and since they collect more detailed information on risk factors for disease, DSSs may inform morbidity patterns in the community.

DSS sites have provided platforms for research on pneumococcal vaccines in Basse (Gambia), maternal mortality in Matlab (Bangladesh), non-communicable disease in Filabavi (Vietnam), and HIV/STIs (sexually transmitted infections) in Rakai (Uganda), insecticide-treated nets in Navrongo, Farafeni (Gambia), Ifakara (United Republic of Tanzania), Kisumu (Kenya), and Oubritenga (Burkina Faso). DSSs are critical for measuring impact of health interventions, for example, malaria (Alba et al. 2011), track mortality and morbidity patterns of internally displaced persons (Feikin et al. 2010), and through initiatives of pooling together DSS information (Indepth NETWORK n.d.) it is possible to generate new standardized mortality rates and life-tables (Sankoh et al. 2006).

Limitations

DSSs like many other surveys rely on self-report; this limitation can be overcome by supplementing self-reported with actual physical exam. Whether data from DSSs can be generalized is a matter of debate. In South Africa, maternal recall of vaccination through DSSs has been found to be comparable to information retrieved from the vaccination (Ndirangu et al. 2011) and from demographic health surveys (Hammer et al. 2006).

Routine information systems

Practically every country in resource-limited settings maintains some form of health facility information system albeit with varying degrees of complexity. Typically these systems are paper-based registers but if applied well, health facility records yield information on patient load, service utilization, and health system infrastructure. The number of indicators that health information systems can collect through health facilities is finite and limited by the information system infrastructure and availability of human resources. The determination of the extent of information that can be accommodated through facility registers requires delicate balance between the necessity of the information and the burden to healthcare providers.

Routine systems can be integrated in surveillance systems particularly for communicable diseases like polio, measles, or malaria. A sharp increase in facility reported cases for malaria may point towards an impending outbreak, and facilitate a prompt public health response.

Limitations

One major limitation for routine records is the selection bias where those with severe illness and those with resources are more likely to seek care. Moreover, since the population at risk cannot be determined through facility records, rates of disease and injuries cannot be calculated.

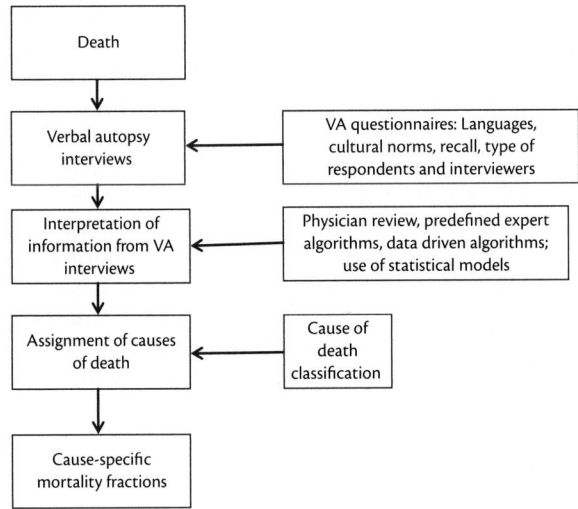

Fig. 4.2.2 Verbal autopsy process.
Adapted with permission from Soleman, N. et al., Verbal autopsy: current practices and challenges, *Bulletin of the World Health Organization*, Volume 84, Number 3, pp. 239–45, Copyright © 2006 World Health Organization, http://www.who.int/bulletin/en/.

Opportunities for improving community diagnosis

Electronic medical records

In response to major global health challenges such as HIV and malaria, the years 2002–2012 witnessed unprecedented development assistance for health mainly driven by PEPFAR, the President's Malaria Initiative, the Global Fund for AIDS, TB and Malaria, and GAVI Alliance as well as the Bill and Melinda Gates Foundation. In order to document the attainment of ambitious targets by these agencies, innovative methods including electronic medical records (EMRs) have been devised to complement the traditional health information systems. EMR platforms can be expensive to install and implement in developing countries. However, open-source systems which are cost-effective and flexible are available, for example, Open Medical Record System (OpenMRS). OpenMRS has been implemented in several African countries, including South Africa, Kenya, Rwanda, Lesotho, Zimbabwe, Mozambique, Uganda, and Tanzania.

Box 4.2.2 Case studies of various initiatives to enhance utilization of electronic medical records in low- and middle-income countries

Stand-alone databases

The AMPATH in Kenya supports HIV treatment at Moi University and utilizes EMR. In a review of the system a comparison of the clinic before and after adoption of the EMR showed patient visits were 22 per cent shorter, provider time per patient was reduced by 58 per cent (P <0.001), and patients spent 38 per cent less time waiting in the clinic (P <0.06); clinic personnel spent 50 per cent less time interacting with patients, two-thirds less time interacting with each other, and more time in personal activities (Cherutich et al. 2012). The EMR has also vastly simplified the generation of mandatory reports to the Ministry of Health.

Internet-based medical record systems

The PIH-EMR system was created to support the management of drug-resistant tuberculosis in Peru. This system was built using the Linux operating system, Apache web server, Tomcat Java Servlet engine, and Oracle database. It supports clinical care, logistics such as assessment of drug requirements, and research studies.

Web-based collaboration and telemedicine systems (not specifically for HIV)

Satellife are using the cell phone network in Uganda to transfer data to a central site. Local healthcare workers collect data on Palm Pilots and then connect to a local, battery-powered server called a Wide Ray Jack. This server allows data to be sent to and from a central database via a cell phone modem. More information is at http://pda.healthnet.org/.

Adapted by permission from BMJ Publishing Group Limited. *British Medical Journal*, Fraser, H. et al., An information system and medical record to support HIV treatment in rural Haiti, Volume 329, pp. 1142–6, Copyright © 2004 BMJ Publishing Group Ltd.

Box 4.2.2 provides case studies of application of EMRs in low- and middle-income countries (Fraser et al. 2004).

Advances in information technology and communications

Rapid developments in information technology have greatly reduced the costs of setting up information systems. Plans were announced to develop a laptop PC for US $100 (Bray 2005). At the same time, Internet access is now relatively widely available in many developing countries (Peru, Ghana, Kenya, etc.) and there exists a broad range of robust and flexible devices to manage data, including personal digital assistants (PDAs) and smartphones. Indeed in Africa and the rest of the developing nations, mobile phone subscription penetration ranges from 53–79 per cent. There exist tremendous opportunities to improve health information systems and inject efficiencies in the methods and tools of community diagnosis. These include geographical information systems (GIS) and electronic medical records.

Geographic information systems

GIS are a combination of computer hardware and software used to store, manipulate, analyse, and display spatial or geographic data. GIS had been widely used in many disciplines such as agriculture, forestry, environmental engineering, and urban planning prior to its applications in public health. Today, more public health professionals are aware of the usefulness of GIS; spatial data in small areas are more readily available and technology is more easily accessible. GIS is an appropriate and practical tool for governments and other agencies to use in identifying regional disparities and for priority setting. It has been used to track spatial distribution of human resources, health services and diseases (Rutto and Karuga 2009; Simoonga et al. 2009; Cooke et al. 2010; Massey 2011), ongoing disease transmission (Murray et al. 2009), and inform the design of emergency obstetric services (Bailey et al. 2011). In Kenya, for example, the entire Northern Corridor highway was studied to characterize the 'hotspots' where transactional sex is concentrated and to provide estimates of numbers of truckers and sex workers and the volumes of transactional sex taking place on the highway (Ferguson and Morris 2007). An average of 2400 trucks parked overnight at the 39 hotspots were identified and mapped using GIS. As a consequence, the Kenya National AIDS/STD Programme in Kenya has instituted HIV prevention and treatment services along these 'hotspots'. In the Greater Mekong area, a hotspot mapping was able to determine the need for more comprehensive programming for the key population groups (sex workers, males who have sex with males, intravenous drug users, and people living with HIV/AIDS (USAID 2006).

By layering different types of HIV/AIDS-related information such as prevalence rates and behavioural surveillance, GIS technology allows this information to be integrated into a choropleth map (Fig. 4.2.3) and visually compared with other information, such as the programme response in a given area (Larmarange et al. 2011).

Conclusion

Community diagnosis and information systems are key ingredients for improving public health outcomes. Without appropriate tools and methods for community diagnosis, stakeholders may

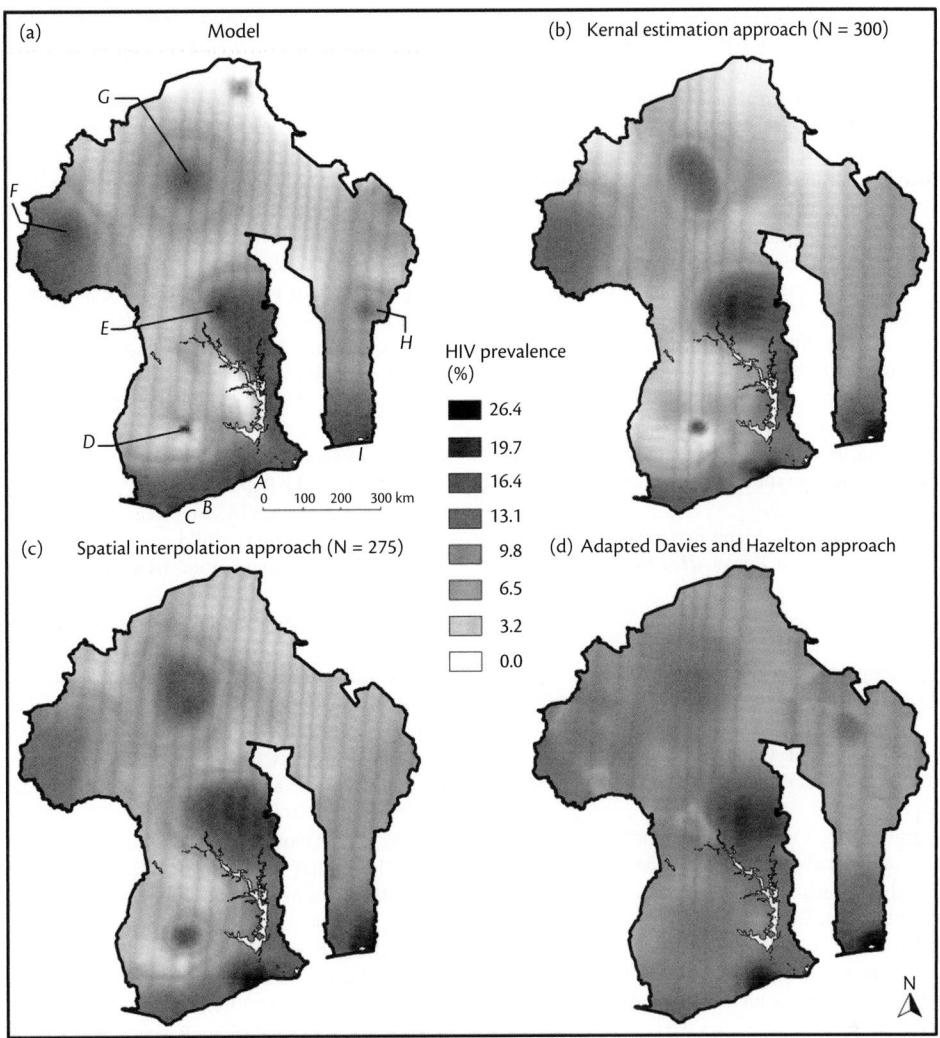

Fig. 4.2.3 Model prevalence surface and estimated prevalence surfaces using three different approaches based on the same DHS simulation.
Reproduced with permission from Joseph Larmarange et al., Methods for mapping regional trends of HIV prevalence from Demographic and Health Surveys (DHS), *European Journal of Geography*, Document 558, Copyright © 2001 CNRS-UMR Géographie-cités 8504, DOI: 10.4000/cybergeo.24606.

not have the means to document the burden of disease, identify risk factors for adverse health outcomes, and prioritize health interventions. However, none of the methods are reliable on their own and each should be validated and complemented by other methods to yield robust estimates of key health metrics. As the countdown to the MDGs for 2015 begins and as the international community prepares to set new targets beyond the MDGs, developing countries have to demonstrate, through robust methods and tools, that the burden of disease in their regions warrants further global attention. Therefore, low- and middle-income countries need to invest in these information systems and seize opportunities offered by increasing access to technology and the Internet to strengthen community diagnosis.

References

Alba, S., Hetzel, M., Nathan, R., Alexander, M., and Lengeler, C. (2011). Assessing the impact of malaria interventions on morbidity through a community-based surveillance system. *International Journal of Epidemiology*, 40(2), 405–16.

Bailey, P.E., Keyes, E.B., Parker, C., Abdullah, M., Kebede, H., and Freedman, L. (2011). Using a GIS to model interventions to strengthen the emergency referral system for maternal and newborn health in Ethiopia. *International Journal of Gynecology and Obstetrics*, 115(3), 300–9.

Birnbaum, J., Murray, C., and Lozano, R. (2011). Exposing misclassified HIV/AIDS deaths in South Africa. *Bulletin of the World Health Organization*, 89, 278–85.

Bray, H. (2005). A $100 laptop to change the world. *Boston Globe*, 7 February.

Central Statistical Authority (Ethiopia) and ORC MACRO (2001). *Ethiopia Demographic and Health Survey*. Addis Ababa, Ethiopia, and Calverton, MD: Central Statistical Authority and ORC MACRO.

Central Statistical Office (CSO) and Macro International Incorporated (2088). *Swaziland Demographic and Health Survey 2006–2007*. Mbabane, Swaziland: Central Statistical Office.

Cherutich, P., Kaiser, R., Galbraith, J., et al. (2012). Lack of knowledge of HIV status a major barrier to HIV prevention, care and treatment efforts in Kenya: results from a nationally representative study. *PLoS ONE*, 7(5), e36797.

Collinson, M., Mokoena, O., Mgiba, N., et al. (2002). Demographic surveillance system (Agincourt DSS). In O.A. Sankoh, K. Kahn, E. Mwageni,

P. Ngom, and P. Nyarko (eds.) *Population and Health in Developing Countries* (Vol. 1), pp. 197–205. Ottawa: IDRC & INDEPTH.

Cooke, G.S., Tanser, F.C., Bärnighausen, T.W., and Newell, M.L. (2010). Population uptake of antiretroviral treatment through primary care in rural South Africa. *BMC Public Health*, 10, 585.

Cousens, S., Blencowe, H., Stanton, C., et al. (2011). National, regional, and worldwide estimates of stillbirth rates in 2009 with trends since 1995: a systematic analysis. *The Lancet*, 377, 1319–30.

Darmstadt, G., Bhutta, Z., Cousens, S., Adam, T., Walker, N., Bernis, L., for the Lancet Neonatal Survival Steering Team (2005). Evidence-based, cost-effective interventions: how many newborn babies can we save? *The Lancet*, 365, 977–88.

Detels, R., Beaglehole, R., Lansang, M., and Gulliford, M. (eds.) (2009). *Oxford Textbook of Public Health* (5th ed.). Oxford: Oxford University Press.

Feikin, D.R., Adazu, K., Obor, D., et al. (2010). Mortality and health among internally displaced persons in western Kenya following post-election violence, 2008: novel use of demographic surveillance. *Bulletin of the World Health Organization*, 88, 601–8.

Ferguson, A.G. and Morris, C.N. (2007). Mapping transactional sex on the Northern Corridor highway in Kenya. *Health & Place*, 13(2), 504–19.

Fox, M.P., Brennan, A., Maskew, M., MacPhail, P., and Sanne, I. (2010). Using vital registration data to update mortality among patients lost to follow-up from ART programmes: evidence from the Themba Lethu Clinic, South Africa. *Tropical Medicine & International Health*, 15, 405–13.

Fraser, H., Jazayeri, D., Nevil, P., et al. (2004). An information system and medical record to support HIV treatment in rural Haiti. *British Medical Journal*, 329, 1142–6.

Gakidou, E., Hogan, M., and Lopez, A. (2004). Adult mortality: time for a reappraisal. *International Journal of Epidemiology*, 33(4), 710–17.

Hallett, T.B., Singh, K., Smith, J.A., et al. (2008). Understanding the impact of male circumcision interventions on the spread of HIV in Southern Africa. *PLoS ONE*, 3(5), e2212.

Hammer, G., Somé, F., and Becher, H. (2006). Pattern of cause-specific childhood mortality in a malaria endemic area of Burkina Faso. *Malaria Journal*, 5, 47.

Hoshaw-Woodard, S. (2001). *Description and Comparison of the Methods of Cluster Sampling and Lot Quality Assurance Sampling to Assess Immunization Coverage*. Geneva: World Health Organization, Department of Vaccines and Biologicals.

Indepth NETWORK (n.d.). *International Network of Field Sites with Continuous Demographic Evaluation of Populations and Their Health in Developing Countries*. [Online] Available at: http://www.indepth-network.org/.

Institute for Health Metrics and Evaluation (2009). *Role of Health Surveys in National Health Information Sytems: Best Use Scenarios*. Working Paper Series No. 6. Seattle, WA: University of Washington.

Institute for Health Metrics and Evaluation (n.d.). Website. Available at: http://www.healthmetricsandevaluation.org/.

Irimu, G., Nduati, R.W., Wafula, E., and Lenja, J. (2008). Community understanding of pneumonia in Kenya. *African Health Sciences*, 8(2), 103–7.

Joint United Nations Programme on HIV/AIDS (UNAIDS) (2011). *Good Participatory Practice: Guidelines for Biomedical HIV Prevention Trials*. Geneva: UNAIDS.

Larmarange, J., Vallo, R., Yaro, S., Msellati, P., and Méda, N. (2011). Methods for mapping regional trends of HIV prevalence from Demographic and Health Surveys (DHS). *European Journal of Geography*, 2011, 558.

Lemeshow, S. and Stroh, G. (1988). *Sampling Techniques for Evaluating Health Parameters in Developing Countries*. Washington, DC: National Academy Press.

Liu, L., Johnson, H., Cousens, S., et al., for the Child Health Epidemiology Reference Group of WHO and UNICEF (2012). Global, regional, and national causes of child mortality: an updated systematic analysis for 2010 with time trends since 2000. *The Lancet*, 379, 2151–61.

MacQueen, K., McLellan, E., Metzger, D., et al. (2001). What is community? An evidence-based definition for participatory public health. *American Journal of Public Health*, 91(12), 1929–38.

Madhavan, S., Collinson, M., Townsend, N.W., Kahn, K., and Tollman, S.M. (2007). The implications of long term community involvement for the production and circulation of population knowledge. *Demographic Research*, 17(13), 369–88.

Massey, P. (2011). Reducing maternal mortality in Senegal: using GIS to identify priority regions for the expansion of human resources for health. *World Health & Population*, 13(2), 13–22.

Mathers, D., Fat, D.M., Inoue, M., Rao, C., and Lopez, A.D. (2005). Counting the dead and what they died from: an assessment of the global status of cause of death data. *Bulletin of the World Health Organization*, 83, 171–7.

Ministry of Health, Kenya (2007). *Kenya AIDS Indicator Survey (KAIS, 2007)*. Nairobi: Republic of Kenya.

Monasch, R., Reinisch, A., Steketee, R., Korenromp, E., Alnwick, D., and Bergevin, Y. (2004). Child coverage with mosquito nets and malaria treatment from population-based surveys in African countries: a baseline for monitoring progress in Roll Back Malaria. *The American Society of Tropical Medicine and Hygiene*, 71(2 Suppl.), 232–8.

Murray, C. (2007). Towards good practice for health statistics: lessons from the Millennium Development Goal health indicators. *The Lancet*, 369, 862–73.

Murray, C., Lozano, R., Flaxman, A., Vahdatpour, A., and Lopez, A. (2011). Robust metrics for assessing the performance of different verbal autopsy cause assignment methods in validation studies. *Population Health Metrics*, 9, 28.

Murray, C.J., Rajaratnam, J.K., Marcus, J., Laakso, T., and Lopez, A.D. (2010). What can we conclude from death registration? Improved methods for evaluating completeness. *PLoS Medicine*, 7(4), e1000262.

Murray, E.J., Marais, B.J., Mans, G., et al. (2009). A multidisciplinary method to map potential tuberculosis transmission hot spots in high-burden communities. *The International Journal of Tuberculosis and Lung Disease*, 13(6), 767–74.

Murray, J.L., Vos, T., Lozano, R., et al. (2012). Disability-adjusted life years (DALYs) for 291 diseases and injuries in 21 regions, 1990–2010: a systematic analysis for the Global Burden of Disease Study 2010. *The Lancet*, 380, 2197–223.

Myatt, M., Limburg, H., Minaissan, D., and Katyola, D. (2003). Field trial of applicability of lot quality assurance sampling survey method for rapid assessment of prevalence of active trachoma. *Bulletin of the World Health Organization*, 81, 877–85.

Ndirangu, J., Bland, B., Bärnighausen, T., and Newell, M. (2011). Validating child vaccination status in a demographic surveillance system using data from a clinical cohort study: evidence from rural South Africa. *BMC Public Health*, 11, 372.

Njeuhmeli, E., Forsythe, S., Reed, J., et al. (2011). Voluntary medical male circumcision: modeling the impact and cost of expanding male circumcision for HIV prevention in Eastern and Southern Africa. *PLoS Medicine*, 8(11), e1001132.

Obermeyer, Z., Rajaratnam, J.K., Park, C.H., et al. (2010). Measuring adult mortality using sibling survival: a new analytical method and new results for 44 countries, 1974–2006. *PLoS Medicine*, 7(4), e1000260.

Ohemeng-Dapaah, S., Pronyk, P., Akosa, E., Nemser, B., and Kanter, A.S. (2010). Combining vital events registration, verbal autopsy and electronic medical records in rural Ghana for improved health services delivery. *Studies in Health Technology and Informatics*, 160(Pt 1), 416–20.

Oti, S.O. and Kyobutungi, C. (2010). Verbal autopsy interpretation: a comparative analysis of the InterVA model versus physician review in determining causes of death in the Nairobi DSS. *Population Health Metrics*, 8, 21.

Rajaratnam, J.K., Marcus, J.R., Flaxman, A.D., et al. (2010). Neonatal, postneonatal, childhood, and under-5 mortality for 187 countries, 1970–2010: a systematic analysis of progress towards Millennium Development Goal 4. *The Lancet*, 375, 1988–2008.

Razzaque, A. and Streatfield, P.K. (2002). Matlab demographic surveillance system, Bangladesh. In O.A. Sankoh, K. Kahn, E. Mwageni, P. Ngom, and P. Nyarko (eds.) *Population and Health in Developing Countries* (Vol. 1), pp. 287–95. Ottawa: IDRC & INDEPTH.

Rutto, J.J. and Karuga, J.W. (2009). Temporal and spatial epidemiology of sleeping sickness and use of geographical information system (GIS) in Kenya. *Journal of Vector Borne Diseases*, 46(1), 18–25.

Sankoh, O.A., Ngom, P., Clarks, J., de Savigny, D., and Binka, F. (2006). Levels and patterns of mortality at INDEPTH demographic surveillance systems. In D.T. Jamison, R.G. Feachem, M.W. Makgoba, et al. (eds.) *Disease and Mortality in Sub-Saharan Africa*, pp. 75–86. Washington, DC: World Bank.

Shengelia, B., Tandon, A., Adams, O.B., and Murray, C.J. (2005). Access, utilization, quality, and effective coverage: an integrated conceptual framework and measurement strategy. *Social Science & Medicine*, 61(1), 97–109.

Simoonga, C., Utzinger, J., Brooker, S., et al. (2009). Remote sensing, geographical information system and spatial analysis for schistosomiasis epidemiology and ecology in Africa. *Parasitology*, 136(13), 1683–93.

Soleman, N., Chandramohan, D., and Shibuya, K. (2006). Verbal autopsy: current practices and challenges. *Bulletin of the World Health Organization*, 84, 239–45.

The Demographic and Health Surveys (DHS) Program (n.d.). Website. Available at: http://dhsprogram.com/.

UN General Assembly (1966). *International Covenant on Economic, Social and Cultural Rights, 16 December 1966*. Available at: http://www.ohchr.org/EN/ProfessionalInterest/Pages/CESCR.aspx.

UN General Assembly (2009). *United Nations Millennium Declaration. Resolution Adopted by the General Assembly*, 18 September 2000. A/RES/55/2. New York: UN General Assembly.

USAID (2006). *Mapping HIV/AIDS Service Provision for Most At Risk and Vulnerable Populations in the Greater Mekong Sub-Region*. Core Initiative, USAID funded project. Available at: http://www.unaids.org.vn/facts/docs/MappingHIVAIDS.pdf.

Valadez, J. and Devkota, B. (2002). Decentralized supervision of community health programs: using LQAS in two districts of Southern Nepal. In J. Rohde and J. Wyon (eds.) *Community Health Care: Lessons from Bangladesh to Boston*, pp. 169–200. Boston, MA: Management Sciences for Health.

World Medical Association (1998). *Declaration of Ottawa on Child Health*, adopted by the 50th World Medical Assembly, Ottawa, Canada, October 1998. Available at: http://www.wma.net/en/30publications/10policies/c4/.

Zakariah, Y., Alexander, S., van Roosmalen, J., and Kwawukume, E.Y. (2006). Maternal mortality in the Greater Accra region in Ghana: assessing completeness of registration and data quality. *Acta Obstetricia et Gynecologica Scandinavica*, 85(12), 1436–41.

New communication technologies, social media, and public health

Mohan J. Dutta

Introduction to new communication technologies

New communication technologies play vital roles in the realm of public health, both in terms of contributing towards positive health outcomes as well as possibly generating a variety of adverse health effects. In recent years, the advent of web 2.0 technology has fundamentally shifted the terrain of how users and communities engage with technologies in communicating about health. As opposed to the earlier web 1.0 technology that sends out one-way communication through static pages, web 2.0 technology allows for users to both produce and distribute content (Thackeray et al. 2008, 2013). These new communication technologies have also been referred to as social media because of their fundamental nature of usage that is grounded in social and community networks, shifting traditional forms of sender-driven media uses towards more two-way forms of communication (McNab 2009). Social media, descriptive of participative media applications on the Internet, utilize the next generation of web 2.0 technologies to enable users to share, collaborate, link, and include user-generated content (Thackeray et al. 2008). The current repository of new technologies enables collaborative writing (blogs, wikis, etc.), sharing of content (Facebook, text, YouTube, Flickr), social networking (Facebook, Twitter), social bookmarking (ratings, tagging, etc.), and syndication (blogs, RSS feeds, etc.) (Thackeray et al. 2008). Essential then to the functioning of social media are the networks and ties within which they are embedded, in addition to their participatory characteristics that enable user active engagement, co-scripting, and active dissemination of content.

The important role of these new communication technologies in redefining the landscape of communication is often acknowledged in coining the term 'revolution' to depict the shifts in the nature of communication (Della et al. 2008). The powerful role of these new communication technologies has been acknowledged by public health and health communication scholars, attending to the broader connectivity in communities leveraged by the various forms of social media (Della et al. 2008; McNab 2008; Thackeray et al. 2008; Taubenheim et al. 2012). Health scholars have noted that new communication technologies democratize the landscape of health information processing by creating multiple loci of health information dissemination, and by shifting the very nature of health information dissemination into the hands of publics.

However, simplistic depictions of the growth of these new communication technologies as cyber-revolution need to be tempered with nuanced attention to the complexities of social, cultural, political, and economic contexts that shape the penetration of, access to, and usage of these technologies globally. Also, discussions of the public health implications of these new communication technologies need to be based on detailed analyses of the complex social, economic, and political fabrics within which they are constituted. Geographically, for instance, there exist differential patterns in the penetration of new communication technologies that are similar to patterns witnessed in the diffusion of traditional media. In addition, within nation states, there exist differential patterns of uses of new communication technologies, mapping out along the lines of differentials in access by socioeconomic status (SES), age, and race.

The patterns of access to and usage of new communication technologies continue to mirror the inequities in patterns of media usage that are seen in the context of traditional media, thus risking the perpetuation of similar inequities in knowledge and behaviour often generated by health campaigns in the case of the traditional media. The growing body of research on the 'digital divide' points towards the differential patterns of access to new communication technologies. How then to conceptualize the broader public health implications of the growth of social media? In this chapter, attention will be drawn to the positive uses of social media for health promoting goals, followed by discussion of the adverse public health outcomes of social media.

Trends in social media

The trends in social media reflect growing user participation in creating, curating, and sharing content through the uses of new communication technologies. Globally, there has been an increase in social media usage among Internet users and this is particularly the case in low- and middle-income countries. Further, there has been a global growth in mobile technologies and the uses of these technologies for accessing information, posting content, tagging and sharing content, collaborating, etc. According to a Pew Global

Attitudes Survey conducted in 2011 across 21 countries, a median of 75 per cent of mobile phone owners say they text. Among the mobile phone owners, 50 per cent report that they take pictures/video and 23 per cent report that they use the Internet on their mobile phones (Pew Research Center 2011). The report also notes that social networking usage typically tends to be higher in higher-income countries as compared to lower-income countries. However, taking into account the obvious differences in Internet access between higher- and lower-income countries, people in lower-income countries that have online access are equally or more likely to use social networking sites as compared to people in higher-income countries (Pew Research Center 2011).

Texting is most common among mobile phone owners in Indonesia (96 per cent), Kenya (89 per cent), and Lebanon (87 per cent). Also in Poland, Mexico, Japan, and China, 80 per cent or more mobile phone users say that they regularly text. Regarding the usage of their mobile devices to access the Internet, at least 30 per cent in six countries, namely Israel, Japan, United States, Britain, China and Poland, go online using their phone. In 15 countries among the 21 countries polled, at least 25 per cent of those polled note having visited a social networking site. Social networking usage is highest among the respondents in Israel and the United States, with more than 50 per cent of respondents stating that they use a social networking site. In Britain, Russia, and Spain, more than 40 per cent of the respondents note that they use a social networking site. Growth of social networking was highest in Egypt and Russia, two countries that experienced a great deal of political participation through social media, and was approximately 10 per cent, growing from 18 per cent in 2010 to 28 per cent in 2011 in Egypt, and growing from 33 per cent in 2010 to 43 per cent in 2011 in Russia.

Globally, there is increasing participation of Internet users in social media. On the basis of a US-wide survey conducted in August 2012, Rainie et al. (2012) observed that 46 per cent of Internet users post original photos and videos that they themselves have created, and 41 per cent of adult Internet users repost photos and videos that they have found online. These creators and curators comprise a major segment of the US population of Internet users, playing an active role in constituting online content. Currently, approximately one-third of adults utilize health-related social media (Taubenheim et al. 2012). Furthermore, individuals who seek out health information online are also likely to use a wide variety of social media such as blogging, using Facebook and using other status update services (Fox and Jones 2009; Hughes 2010).

Online support groups

The earliest forms of social networking platforms that became vital health communication tools were online social support groups. These online support groups emerged as communities in the virtual space where patients and their family members could interact, exchange information about diseases and their treatments, and seek out solutions through participation.

Facebook

Facebook is a social networking site that enables users to post information, share information, tag and rate resources, and form groups based on interests. In the United States, in a survey conducted nationwide between 2 and 5 August 2012, 66 per cent of all Internet users used Facebook (Rainie et al. 2012). Along the lines of gender, 63 per cent of Internet users among men and 70 per cent Internet users among women reported having used Facebook. The highest percentage of Facebook users was in the 18–29 age group (83 per cent) compared to 40 per cent of Internet users in the 65+ category, suggesting that Facebook is more likely to have a younger audience.

Twitter

Twitter is a social messaging service that allows the instant dissemination of information between publics across the world. Users can post their own 'tweets' as well as follow health information, developing health stories, health conferences, etc. They can also search for health information on Twitter, resulting in new information, contacts, and networks. In the same survey in the United States reported earlier, 16 per cent of Internet users in the US reported using Twitter (Rainie et al. 2012). The Singapore Health Promotion Board uses Twitter to reach out to its audiences with health information and has 2266 followers. The World Health Organization utilizes Twitter to disseminate information to a wide net of globally distributed audiences.

Podcasts

Podcasts are voice-recorded information resources that can be downloaded from the web. Multiple health agencies and institutions such as the US Centers for Disease Control and Prevention (CDC), Mayo Clinic, Harvard's School of Medicine, the World Health Organization, the Public Broadcasting Service, and HealthBeat utilize podcasts to reach out to their audiences. Many of these health information podcasts are available for free from iTunes or can be downloaded directly from the respective websites. According to the study published by Della et al. (2008), CDC had published over 250 podcasts by 2008, and the podcasts had been downloaded more than 180,000 times.

YouTube

YouTube is a video networking and video-sharing website, where users can upload, view, and share videos. Video materials posted on YouTube include movie clips, TV clips, music videos as well as video blogging (vlogging) and short original videos. On 3 October 2012, 29.39 per cent of Internet users globally used YouTube, with an Alexa Traffic Rank of third globally and in the US (Alexa n.d.). According to the same report, roughly 20 per cent of visitors to YouTube come from the United States. The Singapore Health Promotion Board utilizes YouTube to post its video content of health promotion campaigns. For instance, The Bepositiveproject campaign has a YouTube page that posts the video materials of the campaign, with 299 subscribers and 137,556 video views (TheBepositiveproject n.d.). The campaign page has 15 videos, and audience members post comments on the YouTube videos. Similarly, the 'Let's Stop HIV Together' campaign in the United States targeting Americans with the message of HIV prevention ran multiple YouTube videos (Centers for Disease Control and Prevention (CDC) n.d.). The videos generated a great deal of viewership, resulting in over 130,000 views. The CDCStreamingHealth YouTube page has over 14,000 subscribers and more than 25 million video views, posting health information and prevention-based resources on the page (viewing data from 5 November 2013).

Blogs

Blogs are user-driven informational and discussion sites where users design and craft content, organized as distinct entries in reverse chronological order. Blogs can be single authored or multi-authored, and are considered a form of social media because most posters not only provide content on the blog but also share this content in a social network, engaging with their readers as well as other bloggers. According to a Nielsen report published in 2011, there were 156 million public blogs in existence by February 2011 (Nielsen 2011a). In the United States, in May 2011, Blogger reported over 50 million unique visitors and Wordpress reported over 22 million unique visitors (Nielsen 2011b). In 2006, the CDC launched the *Health Marketing Musings* blog on its Health Marketing website, fostering a space for health marketing professionals to publicly discuss relevant communication and marketing strategies (Della et al. 2008). The CDC website provides a listing of all the blogs posted by CDC, now adding up to 13 blogs on various topics. For instance, the *Global Voices* blog provides information on health initiatives from across the globe. In the United States, among 41 per cent of users of Blogger, household income is greater than $75,000, and 25 per cent of visitors to Wordpress have a Bachelor's degree.

mHealth

mHealth is the delivery of health related services via mobile communications technologies such as mobile phones and PDAs (United Nations Foundation 2009). In nations where shortage of workers continues to be a key problem and the penetration of mobile communication technologies is high, mobile health services offer important avenues for reaching out to underserved audiences, especially in hard-to-reach and resource-poor environments. In areas where access to medical services is the key challenge, mobile technologies offer health workers means for providing diagnoses as well as real-time health information. Health clinics, home providers, and health workers can rely on these technologies to secure quality health information in their delivery of care. mHealth programmes can also serve as resources for digitizing patient health records into national health systems, thus standardizing these health records and creating a national-level inventory. The United Nations Foundation report cited earlier documents 51 mHealth programmes in 26 different countries including India, South Africa, Uganda, Peru, and Rwanda, offering the following functions: (1) education and awareness, (2) remote data collection, (3) remote monitoring, (4) communication and training of healthcare workers, (5) disease and epidemic outbreak tracking, and (6) diagnostic and treatment support. In the backdrop of the digital divide, these mobile communications technologies also serve as avenues for reaching out to resource-poor audiences through mobile devices that are accessible. For example, Project Masiluleke and Text to Change utilize SMS message campaigns to provide HIV/AIDS education in South Africa and Uganda, respectively. In Georgia, a film on HIV/AIDS created by Save the Children and UNICEF with the goal of educating the youth was disseminated via mobile phones, encouraging the youth to pass it on to others. Similarly, the Freedom HIV/AIDS games launched in India in December, 2005 run on mobile phones and have been created with the goal of fostering HIV/AIDS awareness through the 'play-and-learn' method. Within 4 months, 10 million games

had been downloaded, many of them having been downloaded in cities and towns where the vulnerability is higher.

Social media as health resources

Social media usage is constituted amid various forms of functions offered by social media as resources. These forms of user-driven collaborative media on the Internet have shifted the ways in which traditional mediated communication takes place, turning mediated communication into a two-way process where users have an active role to play (Thackeray et al. 2008; McNab 2009). A resource-based approach to social media examines the communicative functions played by social media, drawing upon the argument that social media play different functions in different contexts, and the specific uses of social media are driven by the needs felt by the user at a given point of time. Social media as resources for health operate across a wide variety of functions, meeting a wide variety of health needs of users. Whereas social media differ substantively from traditional forms of media in terms of audience participation, in other ways, social media are very similar to traditional media in their information dissemination functions. In the United States, the use of social network sites has multiplied over the last decade (Jones and Fox 2009; Pew Internet and American Life Project 2012). Also, in other parts of the globe, increasingly Internet users have become social media users, with a large percentage of Internet users from low-economic development countries being social media users.

Social media as social capital resources

Broadly, social media are defined as the category of Internet-driven media platforms that involve collaboration and sharing. On social media, audience members participate actively in posting content, in commenting upon content posted by others, in sharing information-based resources, and in having conversations about ideas or causes that are of interest to them (Chou et al. 2009; Hughes 2010). As opposed to traditional media that are typically static in content encoded by a sender to be decoded by a receiver, social media are dynamic and context-driven, creating opportunities for co-creation of communication. Co-creation refers to a partnership among multiple participants, where they come together to engage in mutually meaningful communicating. As a result, communication emerges through interactions on social media, taking on varying interpretive frames based on social interactions among participants on the media platform.

The capacity of social media to catalyse communication within and across social networks is critical to the role of social media in generating social capital, referred to as the collective participatory strands and networks of trust within communities. Social media enable the formation of social capital through the specific linkages that it fosters among community members. It enables the formation of communities in virtual spaces that are not restricted by geographic boundaries and other structural features. For instance, a specific community formed on a social medium develops into a resource for the community, enabling participation and collaboration virtually among community members. Online health communities for example have emerged as vital resources for social support for acute as well as chronic disease patients and their families. The American Cancer Society operates multiple community forums that are disease specific, and that emerge as resources for community members, sharing information, guiding each other, offering emotional support, providing guidance in the context of decision-making, mobilizing resources collectively, etc.

Also, in the realm of health campaigns, the social capital generated on social media emerges as a channel for disseminating health information as well as for building communication networks for the dissemination of preventive health information resources. The trust and credibility of health communication messages increase when the messages are embedded within interpersonal and community networks. The Heart Truth campaign launched by the National Heart, Lung, and Blood Institute utilizes a variety of social media in order to connect with audience members, leveraging the strong social networks and social support resources of women to empower women and to educate them about heart disease, their number one killer.

Launched in 2008, The Heart Truth Facebook fan page (The Heart Truth n.d.) gained over 3500 fans by early 2011. By November 2013, the page had over 38,000 'likes'. Fans participate in conversation with the materials posted by the team, and interact with the content through 'likes', through the posting of their own comments in response to the materials posted by the campaign team, and sharing the information posted on the Facebook page on their own Facebook pages. Pieces of information shared by the campaign team become the basis for additional sharing of resources among community members on the Facebook page, this leading to the widespread dissemination of the information. Along these lines, tweets offer ways of connecting user communities through key pieces of scientific and/or health information, and blogs also serve as important social capital resources by connecting individuals and communities into networks.

Social media as information resources

Social media have high levels of reach, and therefore, serve as important tools for the dissemination of information, leveraging the multiplicative reach of social networks to disseminate information. One of the key elements of contemporary health communication is the need for health information capacity building, developing resources that enable participation in healthcare decision-making. Social media such as Facebook and Twitter can play important roles in building the information capacities of publics, making science and scientific decision-making processes more widely accessible to the public, and enabling public participation in the utilization of science. For example, comparative effectiveness information on effects, side effects, risks, and costs of various preventive and treatment options can be disseminated widely through the leveraging of social media. The emphasis on comparative effectiveness information seeks to democratize the nature of health decision-making, driving decision-making on the basis of systematic evidence on effectiveness, risks, side effects, costs etc.

Take the example of the World Health Organization (WHO). The WHO uses tweets to reach out to global publics with health information, reaching over 900,000 'followers' (World Health Organization n.d., viewing data from 5 November 2013). During the H1N1 pandemic, the WHO leveraged the social networking function of Twitter to disseminate information to geographically spread audiences. Information posted on Twitter is then followed by audiences, thus embedding the information within social

networks. In addition, the 'retweet' function allows interested audience members to share the information with others, thus disseminating the information further through social networks.

Similarly, the Health Promotion Board in Singapore, a government agency that works on dissemination of health information and promotion of healthy behaviours, runs a Facebook page (Health Promotion Board, Singapore n.d.). As of November 2013, the Facebook page of the Health Promotion Board had over 97,000 likes. The Board utilizes the Facebook page to disseminate health information. For instance, it offers information on breast cancer detection in the month of October, synergizing with the Breast Cancer Awareness Month. One of the Facebook postings notes that breast cancer is the most common cause of cancer among Singapore women and early detection can save life. The posting then provides a detailed image of breast self-examination and walks the participant in depth through the various steps of self-examination. It connects to a webpage posted by the Health Promotion Board on its website, discussing the risk factors, the importance of breast self-exams and mammograms, and the basics of treatment.

Social media as channels of persuasion

A growing body of research suggests that social media are important channels of persuasion, based on the argument that involved audiences that participate in co-creating the persuasive messages are more likely to be persuaded by those messages as compared to audiences that receive top–down persuasion messages (Thackeray et al. 2008; Taubenheim et al. 2012). Social media are therefore being used as vital resources in health campaigns on a variety of topics ranging from suicide prevention to heart health promotion, and also for the purposes of promoting dialogues among campaign planners and the broader public health community (Hughes 2010; Taubenheim et al. 2012). Strategic uses of social media for health campaigns involve the deliberate consideration of digital goals and objectives, segmenting and prioritizing audiences, and optimizing the content of the strategic communication effort by listening to and engaging audiences in bidirectional conversation (Taubenheim et al. 2012).

The Think HIV: This Is Me campaign was launched by MTV and the Kaiser Family Foundation in the United States, encouraging youth aged 15–25 to become video bloggers by developing video content on the impact of HIV on their lives. Based on about 200 hours of video footage submitted by nearly 100 audience members in the target segment, the show *Think HIV* was created and aired four times by MTV, receiving more than 3 million viewings (Hoff et al. 2008). In the United States, The Heart Truth campaign launched by the National Heart, Lung, and Blood Institute in collaboration with Ogilvy Public Relations Worldwide utilized social media to: (1) increase women's awareness that heart disease is a leading cause of death; and (2) encourage women to find their personal risks, talk to their doctors, and take action to lower heart disease. The digital component of the campaign sought to: (1) connect women to create an online community, (2) motivate women to take action through online tools, and (3) promote partnerships for amplifying the campaign message through content integration and online engagement. Outreach to bloggers, launching a Twitter handle, developing a Facebook fan page, creating a Bit.ly account, utilizing Flickr, developing a YouTube presence, and developing Widgets and Badges were all components of the social media strategy of the campaign. The campaign has been successful in fostering a women's health community, and in generating greater awareness of The Heart Truth campaign. After considering the possible influences of extraneous variables and secular trends, Taubenheim et al. (2012) report the increase in awareness regarding heart disease among women throughout the campaign period, along with increases in preventive action and decreases in heart disease deaths among women.

In New Zealand, the Txt2Quit campaign utilized text messaging along with an interactive web-based intervention to target people trying to quit smoking. Audience members could receive automated messages on quitting and text 'crave' and 'slip up' to receive instant messages with tips. Similarly, the Health Promotion Board in Singapore launched social media components of its 'Beat the Blues' campaign, posting campaign messages on Facebook and driving user-generated discussion, tagging, sharing, and participation.

Social media as resources for listening

Not only are social media important in reaching out to audiences with relevant and necessary health information, but they are also vital tools for listening. The difference between social media and traditional media lie in the specific ways in which social media are actively used by audience members, emerging as content-generating and content-sharing tools in communities. Given the active participation of individuals, families, and communities on social media platforms, media such as Facebook and Twitter also become vital avenues for listening to the voices of the people, creating active contexts for content to be co-produced. The traditional top–down nature of public health programming can be countered by the active role of social media in tapping into the voices of people and communities, and in fostering communicative avenues for them to participate in. The National Library of Medicine (NLM) utilizes its Facebook page as a platform not only to disseminate information, but also to listen to community members and to engage in dialogue. For health organizations that typically serve as repository of health information and perform the traditional function of information dissemination, social media open up opportunities for listening to communities, for engaging them in dialogue, and for co-constructing solutions. The NLM not only posts information on the Facebook site, but also responds to comments posted by users, thus creating a thread of dialogue.

Social media as avenues of expression and performance

Because of the content generating role of social media, they also emerge as communicative avenues for expression and performance, thus connecting biomedical narratives of health with lived experiences, stories, and frameworks of meanings among users. Social media enable authorship and participation by audiences. For instance, patients undergoing treatment utilize blogs and Facebook to communicate about their health, to interpret health information, to connect such information with their lived experiences, to make sense of their lived experiences in the backdrop of the information, to make a variety of health-related decisions, and to share this information with others.

Social media as advocacy and activist resources

Social media are not only critical in the dissemination of information guiding individual behaviour and lifestyle choices, but they are also pivotal to the organizing of advocacy and activist efforts directed at bringing about transformations in unhealthy policies. In the backdrop of contemporary globalization politics, it is particularly relevant to draw attention to the inequalities produced by economic liberalization, and the health consequences of these inequalities. For example, large-scale disparities in health outcomes are observed between the haves and have-nots in the global South. Similar discrepancies are witnessed in the global North as well. Even in nation states where growth rates are high, high Gini coefficients draw attention to the landscape of inequalities. Of particular importance for public health are the negative consequences of large-scale liberalization based on the principles of trickle-down economics.

Challenging the taken-for-granted assumptions around trickle-down, global activist movements draw attention to the increasing inequalities that have been produced by trade liberalization and opening up of markets. With the global rise in inequalities accompanied by rising unemployment, rising food prices, and rising displacements of the poorer and middle classes, the social media have emerged as sites of organizing, creating innovative avenues for connecting multiple stakeholders, drawing attention to information that is typically absent from mainstream media, and organizing resistance in opposition to inequitable structures. The interactive storytelling feature of social media has emerged as a key resource in the sharing of stories of adversity and economic hardship, co-creating a story of inequality that becomes the organizing feature for social change processes globally. For example, the Occupy Wall Street movement emerged in the United States and globally in response to the rising inequalities, the growing unemployment, the impoverishment of the middle class, and fundamental lack of basic resources (Dutta 2012).

Public health implications of social media

Social media also need to be examined in the context of their public health implications, especially as they relate to the adverse health implications of social media usage. For instance, with the absence of adequate regulatory processes that evaluate the quality of health information being circulated on social media, it is important to consider the health implications of circulating information that is not grounded in the evidence base. Another domain of interest to public health is the prevalence of unhealthy branding tactics on social media, especially in avenues that are directed towards children. Also, given the multiplicity of authors of health information in social media spaces, it is critical to consider the role of quality of health information in guiding health decision-making by publics. Along similar lines, given the variety of interpersonal communications that are generated on social media, it is important to consider the health implications on negative interpersonal communication such as cyberbullying and sexting.

Food marketing on social media

The food and beverage industry has adopted social media on a large scale to reach out to their target audiences. The strong food industry in the United States, for instance, spends US $1.6 billion every year targeting young people (Richardson and Harris 2011; Yale Rudd Center for Food Policy and Obesity n.d.). Facebook and Twitter have emerged as key channels for reaching out to large segments of consumers, especially in the youth segment (Richardson and Harris 2011). Richardson and Harris (2011), in their content analysis of Facebook campaigns launched by the food and beverage industry, noted that Coca-Cola is the most popular Facebook brand and Starbucks is the third-most popular Facebook brand. Also, the brands Red Bull, Monster, Dr. Pepper, Oreo (#4), Skittles (#8), Pringles (#11), Ferrero Rocher (#14), and Nutella (#16) ranked among the top 20 most popular brands on Facebook.

Especially given the high penetration of the Internet and social media among the younger segment of the population, one of the key strategies in food and beverage marketing is the strategic utilization of social media such as Facebook. For example, Cheerios runs a Facebook page that is targeted at children. The Facebook page depicts imagery of children, and utilizes the tagline 'Your moments. Our timeline. The story of Cheerios, as told by you' (Cheerios n.d.). Interactive storytelling, a key feature of social media, is strategically utilized to promote Cheerios. Audience ownership of storytelling is utilized in order to embed the brand Cheerios into the everyday lives of children. The Cheerios campaign utilizes language such as 'community building' and 'participation' in order to market the product.

On a similar note, the Facebook campaign of Coca-Cola has over 75 million 'likes' and uses localized storytelling to narrate the stories of users, sharing their stories about consuming Coke (Coca-Cola n.d., viewing data from 5 November 2013). Consumers post their stories of drinking Coke along with their images. These stories and images are embedded within images of Coke logos on the Facebook site of Coke. The images then serve as spaces for co-constructive storytelling, with users sharing the images, posting their comments, posting additional stories in response in the 'Comments' section etc.

Also, social media such as Facebook emerge as interactive storytelling sites for global brands, targeting the campaign to the local culture, and simultaneously drawing upon culturally specific strategies through participation of communities in country-specific campaigns. For example, the Facebook McDonald's Malaysia page has over 1.7 million 'likes,' as recorded in November 2013 (McDonald's Malaysia n.d.). The site emerges as a space for organizing contests, getting consumers to take pictures of trying out products, and sharing stories that are shared by consumers. The McDonald's brand is reinforced among consumers through the various Facebook stories and participatory tools that are utilized by consumers. Pictures of winners of different contests such as the Egg McMuffin Photo Contest on Instagram are then posted on the Facebook site.

Social media and existing disparities

Because social media are much more likely to be used among audience segments with higher levels of education and income, what are the consequences of developing social media-based messaging systems and strategies that don't attend to the inequities in access and usage (Chou et al. 2009; Lustria et al. 2011)? Furthermore, as reported in a series of health communication studies on health information seeking, extant research documents that more health-oriented segments of the population are also more likely to seek out health-based information resources on the Internet and utilize more information-heavy resources (Dutta-Bergman 2003). Given the active focus of social media, the relationship between health-orientation and health-based social media usage is critical

to examine, with attention paid to the role of social media in the context of health disparities. This is especially important in the light of the existing disparities in the penetration of social media globally and within countries.

In sum, without the critical consideration of the specific patterns of usage of social media, especially among hard-to-reach segments of the population, a one-size-fits-all approach is unlikely to reach out to the underserved and hard-to-reach segments of the population. A celebratory and uncritical stance towards social media as a resource for public health is likely to exacerbate health disparities rather than ameliorate them. What is the role of social media in the context of existing structural disparities within social systems? How are social media situated in relationship to the broader structures of social systems?

Social media and health

With the increasing participation of the public in social media platforms for health-related functions, attention needs to be drawn to questions of privacy and confidentiality (Pinnock et al. 2007). To what extent do social media participants understand the issues of privacy when sharing health information and the consequences associated with the various levels of privacy? What are the norms of privacy in the context of health information that are shared in social media platforms? Similarly, the increasing use of mobile technologies for health-related purposes raises concerns about health data security and confidentiality (Patrick et al. 2008).

The sharing of health information at multiple interfaces ranging from uploading of the information from a mobile device, linking it to a server, transmitting it to some form of electronic medical record, use and interpretation of the data by care providers, and the delivery of health information back to the patient involve multiple levels of information sharing, each with its corresponding issues of confidentiality. Noting the lack of guidance for professionals on the safe use of mobile phone technology for the delivery of healthcare, Pinnock et al. (2007) outline the need for national and international policies that guide and regulate mobile technology use, transfer of health-related data, and the status of health consultations that are offered through mobile technologies.

In addition to issues of privacy and confidentiality, it is also worthwhile to consider the quality of health information shared on social media and in peer-to-peer networks. For example, Syed-Abdul et al. (2013) noted that a large number of YouTube videos promote misleading information about anorexia nervosa, and that pro-anorexia videos are more highly favoured and rated by viewers as compared to informative videos. The widespread use of social media also increases the likelihood of dissemination of non-credible and potentially erroneous information (Kortum et al. 2008; Habel et al. 2009). Use of mobile health devices is also related with repetitive strain injury, a painful condition that can result in disability because of repeated movements (Karim 2009). 'BlackBerry thumb', for instance, results from the repeated use of the thumbs to type on the small keyboards that accompany many mobile devices.

Social media and interpersonal communication

A growing body of research is starting to document the negative interpersonal and social consequences of social media, especially in the context of bullying, clique-forming, and sexual experimentation, manifesting in the forms of issues of cyberbullying, privacy management, and sexting (Patchin and Hinduja 2006; Hinduja and Patchin 2007; Lenhart 2009; MTV 2009; O'Keefe et al. 2011). In a 2009 survey conducted among 1247 respondents in the 14–24 age range, 50 per cent of young people reported having experienced some form of digital abuse (MTV 2009). The social networking capacities of social media can also become tools for bullying, perpetuating forms of exclusion and harassment. The anonymity on social media can contribute to cyberbullying, with important health consequences. Moessner (2007) defined cyberbullying as 'the use of the Internet, cell phones or other technologies to send or post text or images intended to hurt or embarrass another person' (p. 1).

A study analysing the 'Growing Up with Media' survey reported by Ybarra et al. (2007) observed that youth who were targets of rude and nasty comments or rumours being spread about them online as well as offline were more likely to experience distress by the incident as compared to youth who were targeted only in the online environment. The study also reported that 64 per cent of youth who were harassed online did not report being bullied at school. Most importantly, youth who were harassed online were also more likely to ditch or skip school as well as carry weapons to school. Youth who reported being harassed online were eight times more likely as compared to all other youth to concurrently report carrying a weapon to school in the past 30 days.

Wolak et al. (2007) reported that nine per cent of the 1499 youth surveyed were harassed online in the past year, and in this group, whereas 43 per cent were harassed by known peers, 57 per cent reported being harassed by online-only contacts. For targets of online-only harassments, the extent of distress experienced is much more likely to be higher when the harassment is repeated, when the harasser was 18 years or older, and when the harasser asked for pictures. In the opening commentary in the *Journal of Adolescent Health*, guest editors David-Ferdon and Hertz (2007) note that new media technologies are increasingly becoming sites of harassment and aggression, and therefore electronic aggression is becoming a public health problem, calling for additional prevalence and aetiological research to guide the development of interventions.

Theories of new media

The communication literature has developed a range of theories for understanding the uses and distributions of media, ranging from small-scale micro-level theories to large-scale macro-level theories. Whereas some of these theories focus on individual-level explanations for the usage of particular media types, other theories offer societal-level descriptions of uses of media.

Selective processing theories

Based on the notion that publics are inundated with media messages around them, selective process theories suggest that individuals attend to, cognitively process, and retrieve mass media messages that are consistent with their own attitudes and beliefs (Dutta-Bergman 2004a, 2004b; Della et al. 2008). Drawing upon the principles of selective processing, existing scholarship documents systematic within-population differences in audience interest in health issues. This body of research empirically documents

intrinsic differences in interest in health issues, captured in the concept of health orientation. Health-oriented individuals are more likely to search for online health information, and make decisions on the basis of this information. Reflecting the functional approach to media use, selective processing theories suggest that individuals orient their attention to specific stimuli in their environment, selecting and processing information that is consistent with existing attitudes and beliefs, and avoiding information that is discrepant with their existing dispositions (Atkin 1985; Zillman and Bryant 1985).

Selective processing of media messages plays out in the context of selective exposure, interpretation, and memory (Oliver 2002). Selective exposure theory suggests that audiences select media messages that match their existing attitudes and beliefs based on the notion that individuals seek consistency in their cognitions (Webster and Wakshlag 1985; Oliver 2002). Selective perception theory suggests that readers and viewers ascribe meanings to and judgements of media messages that are consistent with their existing values and beliefs. Also, pre-existing beliefs and attitudes influence what is remembered by audience members (Oliver 2002). In the context of health information processing, Dutta-Bergman (2004a, 2004b) demonstrated that health-active individuals that are highly engaged in health-related issues are more likely to seek out health specialized media content as compared to the individuals who are not involved in issues of health. In other words, an intrinsic interest in health issues is tied to the active seeking out of health information resources.

In the context of social media then, it may be argued that health-oriented individuals who are intrinsically interested in health issues are also the ones that attend to health-related social media. Furthermore, healthcare consumers selectively orient their attention to specific health-based social media resources that match their existing interest in health issues. This is particularly the case with the social media where the choices of social media as well as the specific groups selected are driven by an active interest in specific issues and topical areas. The two-way communication enabled by web 2.0 facilitates selective processing of information such that the participation in specific Facebook sites and interactions is driven by an intrinsic interest in the topical area. Health-motivated public who are intrinsically interested in health issues are also likely to seek out health-related social media such as specific Facebook sites and blogs, remember specific aspects of health messages aligned with their intrinsic interest, and then act on the knowledge gained through this process.

Uses and gratifications theory

Founded on the principles of an actively engaged audience, the uses and gratifications perspective conceptualizes media consumption in terms of the specific functions served by the media (Katz et al. 1974; Rubin 1994). This line of research suggests that media serve a wide variety of functions for different segments of the population, and the consumption of media is driven by the choice patterns of receivers (Rubin 1994, 2002). Beginning with developing a framework for understanding the felt needs of the audience, the uses and gratifications framework argues that these felt needs drive specific forms of media consumption.

According to Katz et al. (1974), the uses and gratifications framework seeks to: (1) explain how people use media to satisfy their needs, (2) understand motives underlying media behaviour, and

(3) identify functions or consequences that emerge from the intersection of needs, motives, and behaviours. Rubin (1994) suggests five core elements of uses and gratifications research: (1) communication behaviour is goal-directed, (2) individuals select and use communication channels to satisfy felt needs, (3) individual communication behaviour is mediated by a plethora of social and psychological factors, (4) media compete with other forms of communication, and (5) although individuals are typically more influential than the media in the relationship, this is not always the case. Audience members systematically differ in their motives for information, surveillance, entertainment, habit, social interaction, escape, pass time, and relaxation from the consumption of specific media, and they satisfy these motives by building a repertoire of media they consume.

Extant research demonstrates systematic differences in motives for consuming new communication technologies (Palmgreen and Rayburn 1982; Becker and Schoenbach 1989). In a national random-digit-dialling telephone survey conducted in 1994, Perse and Dunn (1998) reported that home computers were typically associated with ritualistic uses such as keeping busy and passing time. In addition, such ritualistic use was positively related with greater computer use. On a similar note, Parker and Plank (2000) reported that university students were primarily using on-line sources for relaxation and escape. Ferguson and Perse (2000) observed the salience of entertainment as a motive for visiting the World Wide Web among college students. The most visited web sites were sports and entertainment websites. Also, another important motive for using the web in the college sample was acquisition of information. Kargaonkar and Wolin (1999) reported that web usage was positively correlated with social escapism, information, interactive control, and socialization motivations. Papacharissi and Rubin (2000) similarly demonstrated that information seeking and entertainment were the most salient motives for using the Internet.

Theory of channel complementarity

What is the relationship between traditional and new media? The theory of channel complementarity suggests that new media consumption patterns mirror consumption patterns of traditional media, thus reiterating the existing forms of access and usage (Dutta-Bergman 2004c, 2004d, 2004e). Media consumption is driven by intrinsic interest in a specific content type, and therefore, consumption of traditional media is complementary to consumption of new media, grounded in notions of active participation. Therefore, there exists a positive relationship among the usage of different communication channel types that share similar functions and serve similar needs for their audiences (Stempel et al. 2000; Dutta-Bergman 2004c, 2004e). Channel types that offer similar functions for the consumer exist in complementary relationships, such that the usage of one channel type is reinforced by the usage of another channel type. These complementary patterns are reported by Stempel et al. (2000), who noted that Internet users were also more likely to be newspaper readers and radio news listeners. Also, LaRose and Atkin (1992) observed that the use of local audiotext information services was complementary with the use of similar information technologies such as videotexts, ATMs, 800 numbers, and telephone answering services that shared the function of providing information on demand to the user.

Channel complementarity in content areas is observed because of high consumer involvement in the content area (Dutta-Bergman 2004c, 2004d; Rice 1993). People using one particular medium to gather information in one particular area are also likely to use other media to gather information in that area. In the domain of health, the health-motivated consumer who is intrinsically interested in issues of health is not only likely to read health magazines and health-related sections of news, but is also likely to watch health television, surf health-related websites to gather health information, and participate in health-related social media. Underlying the consumption of health content across these various channels is an enduring consumer interest in health (Dutta-Bergman 2004c, 2004d). Dutta-Bergman (2004c) observed that use of the Internet for science and health information was congruent with the use of traditional media for science and health information.

In this sense then, new media extend traditional media consumption patterns, thus replicating existing disparities in knowledge as well as health outcomes. Tian and Robinson (2008) observed that cancer patients and non-patients utilize traditional media, the Internet, and face-to-face communication to gather health information. Complementary patterns therefore extend beyond the media context to interpersonal and community contexts, such that health information seekers in online media are also more likely to seek out health information from interpersonal contexts. Similarly, participation in offline communities is likely to be correlated positively with participation in online communities.

Diffusion of innovations

The diffusion of innovations framework offers an organizing lens for understanding the ways in which a new technology spreads within a population (Rogers 1995). The framework lends itself especially well to the study of social media because of the community-driven and network-based nature of social media. Rogers (1995) outlined specific characteristics of an innovation such as relative advantage, compatibility, trialability, and observability as pivotal in shaping the diffusion process. Furthermore, the innovation gets adopted differentially among different segments of the population, ultimately spreading across the population. The earliest users of the innovation are called adopters, individuals who are eager to try out new products and have strong social networks. These adopters play key roles in the dissemination of the innovation across the population. In the case of social media, early adopters link others in their network to social media platforms, thus driving the diffusion of these platforms.

The culture-centred approach

The culture-centred approach (CCA) attends to the role of communication in enabling the active participation of individuals, families, and communities in health-related decision-making. It notes that communication is an active meaning-making process that is constituted in relationship with organizational and societal structures. Structures refer to the ways in which resources are organized in societies and in the institutions and organizations within them. Access to communication avenues mirrors patterns of access to other structural resources such that those segments of society that are historically disenfranchised in their access to health resources also have minimal or no access to communicative infrastructures. Acknowledging the role of structural features in organizing communication access and usage, the CCA suggests the important role of addressing the underlying structural features of communication even as policies and programmes are driven towards building communication infrastructures such as information communication technologies (Dutta 2008, 2011).

Individuals, families, and communities respond to structures by enacting their agency. Agency refers to the choices and decisions enacted by individuals, families, and communities in order to negotiate structures. From a communicative standpoint, agency is enacted in the everyday forms of communication that emerge as avenues for expression. Therefore, CCA attends to the role of communication resources as enablers of participation. In the context of new communication technologies and social media, individuals and communities utilize these resources in variety of ways in order to fulfil their needs. Efforts that are grounded in an understanding of local cultures emphasize the role of culture in shaping the technological spaces that are created and fostered through social media (Ali 2011).

In the CCA, structure and agency find meaning in their interaction with culture. Culture refers to the dynamic framework of meanings that offers a guiding framework of actions. Structural features in the environment are understood through the cultural artefacts and symbols that are available to communities. In the backdrop of the existing patterns of disparities in public health outcomes, the interactions among culture, structure, and agency offer avenues for understanding the role of new communication technologies in addressing unequal structures. Furthermore, the CCA offers a framework for understanding the role of scientific information capacity building within grassroots community networks as avenues for facilitating community-involved decision-making. Health communication processes grounded in the CCA underscore the importance of social networks in building health information capacity grounded in scientific information.

Directions for consideration: social media and health

In the conclusion of this chapter, considering the relationship between social media and health raises key questions regarding the role of social media in public health. The directions for consideration include: (1) dynamism, (2) access and usage, (3) participation, (4) literacy, (5) global research on social media, and (6) social media openness and regulation.

Dynamism

New technologies are continually emerging, always shifting, and evolving to address a variety of user needs and motives. For example, new platforms such as Klout have emerged as avenues for integrating Twitter, Facebook, and LinkedIn, offering a Klout rating of a user on the basis of the network strength of the user. Pinterest, Instagram, and Tumblr have emerged as additional social media sites for user participation and collaboration. Also, the rise of YouTube and the newer services such as Pinterest, Instagram, and Tumblr have enabled curating activities as they are organized for image and video sharing.

Access and usage

The Pew Report on Global Technology Uses documents the positive relationship between gross domestic product (GDP) per capita (PPP) and the level of social networking (Pew Research Center 2011). In the Pew Research Center list of countries surveyed, the United States has the highest GDP per capita and also has the highest percentage of adults using social networking sites. Pakistan and India have the lowest GDP per capita and also have the lowest percentage of adults using social networking sites. Education is a key factor in usage of social networking sites (Pew Research Center 2011). Therefore, access and patterns of usage are key components in considering the role of social media in the context of public health. In determining how social media are strategically leveraged in public health campaigns and advocacy efforts, attention needs to be paid to the structural differentials in access to as well as usage of social media (Dutta et al. 2007). Specifically, in interventions with information dissemination components, attention needs to be paid to the potential knowledge gaps that are likely to be generated with the widespread uses of social media without the appropriate consideration of the consequences of these gaps. Across the globe, the widespread diffusion of mobile phones is being leveraged to deliver web-driven content through phones. The fastest growth in mobile phone adoption is taking place in many low-income countries, thus offering opportunities for leveraging mobile phones for delivering web-based resources. Multiple 'mHealth' or mobile health information resources have been launched globally with the goals of reaching out to underserved populations (McNab 2009; United Nations Foundation 2009). Also, specific training programmes have been created with the goal of developing mobile media use capacities for health.

Participation

The user-driven technology of platforms such as Facebook and Twitter enables the participation of community members in the posting and sharing of stories (Thackeray et al. 2008). Users as participants engage in collaborative writing, in the creation of stories and in the sharing of these stories in their social networks. Therefore, essential to social media is their grassroots-driven nature, lending to the social networking technologies that enable user-driven communication within their networks (Thackeray et al. 2013). However, the nature of participation on platforms such as Facebook and Twitter can also be shaped by the broader agendas of public health agencies, marketing departments, policymakers, etc., thus raising important questions about the very nature of participation. To what extent did the solutions originate from within the community of participants as opposed to being imposed by external actors? To what extent is communication in social media contexts truly participatory as opposed to being co-opted within marketing strategies as channels for disseminating top-down information? Future scholarship on social media and public health needs to engage in theoretically understanding the nature of participation on social media and develop appropriate metrics for delineating the various types of participation on social media. Nuanced understandings of participation need to consider the dialogic potential of social media in the backdrop of the co-optive potential of social media as channels for top–down management of health issues. An emphasis on the participatory elements of social media is central to greater citizen participation in scientific and health-based decision-making processes, turning information into the hands of users and collectives as resources for decision-making through engagement with policymakers and a variety of health services providers.

Literacy

As depicted in the various sections of this chapter, it is not adequate to conceptualize technologies for public health simply in terms of problems of access. Creating access to computers and the Internet is the first step, although there remain multiple additional barriers to the uses of technology (Dutta et al. 2007). These barriers are embedded at the intersections of structure and culture, suggesting that the local cultural needs of underserved communities are often ignored by structures of information communication technologies. As elucidated by the Heart Health Indiana project that was grounded in community-based culturally-centred processes, underserved African American community members resisted the use of technology as a platform for collaboration and instead preferred face-to-face meetings. In spite of specific training programmes and workshops that were directed at building capacities of community members in using technology as a means of collaboration, the community–academic partnership team observed limited uses of technology, especially among low SES community members, resulting in reliance on face-to-face meetings as platforms for collaboration.

Global research on social media

Much of the published research discussed in this chapter suffers from the ethnocentrism of being driven by US-specific research or research available in high-income contexts. What are the ramifications and utilities of social media that fall outside the realm of the typically young, higher-income, educated, English-speaking users of various social media? Whereas much of the digital divide research documents the non-users of specific technologies, more attention needs to be paid to understanding the broader communicative environment of marginalized groups that remain on the outskirts of the landscape of new communication technologies, both in terms of access and also in terms of the variety of communicative barriers that minimize opportunities for participation.

Social media openness and regulation

On the one hand, social media are one of the earliest forms of media that allow two-way participation, bringing two-way dialogue into a mediated context and creating opportunities for wider public participation in shaping policies and programmes. On the other hand, as depicted through the growing research on the public health implications of social media, questions arise regarding the role of policy-based interventions that regulate the usage of social media. Similarly, what are the implications of social-media driven food and sugary drink advertising campaigns that leverage the social media to reach out to the youth? Future research and theorizing needs to engage with questions of values in the context of the regulation of social media with regard to its possible effects on public health.

Conclusion

In conclusion, new communication technologies, specifically social media, intersect with public health issues in complex and dynamic ways. The changing landscape of media consumption opens up new avenues for audience participation in health-related issues. These various forms of participation constitute a range of functions from information gathering to offering social support to participating in health advocacy. Furthermore, in areas such as food advertising on social media as well as online harassment, attention needs to be paid to the policy-based and intervention frameworks around social media. Finally, public health considerations of social media not only need to attend to the individual level uses of these media forms but also to the broader social and structural patterns within which social media uses are constituted. The emphasis of this chapter was specifically on social media; however, attention also needs to be paid to other forms of technological innovations in healthcare such as electronic health records that may not fall directly under the heading of social media.

References

Alexa (n.d.). *How Popular is youtube.com?* [Online] Available at: http://www.alexa.com/siteinfo/YouTube.com.

Ali, A.H. (2011). The power of social media in developing nations. *Harvard Human Rights Journal*, 24, 185–219.

Becker, L.B. and Schönbach, K. (1989). When media content diversifies: anticipating audience behaviors. *Audience Responses to Media Diversification: Coping with Plenty*, S.1–28.

Centers for Disease Control and Prevention (CDC) (n.d.). In *YouTube*. [Online] Available at: https://www.youtube.com/user/cdcstreaminghealth?feature=results_main.

Cheerios (n.d.). In *Facebook*. [Online] Available at: https://www.facebook.com/Cheerios.

Chou, W.S., Hunt, Y.M., Beckjord, E.M., Moser, R.P., and Hesse, B. (2009). Social media use in the United States: implications for health communication. *Journal of Medical Internet Research*, 11, e48.

Coca-Cola (n.d.). In *Facebook*. [Online] Available at: https://www.facebook.com/cocacola.

David-Ferdon, C. and Hertz, M.F. (2007). Electronic media, violence, and adolescents: an emerging public health problem. *Journal of Adolescent Health*, 41, S1–5.

Della, L.J., Eroglu, D., Bernhardt, J., Edgerton, E., and Nall, J. (2008). Looking to the future of new media in health marketing: drawing propositions based on traditional theories. *Health Marketing Quarterly*, 25, 147–74.

Dutta, M.J. (2008). *Communicating Health: A Culture-Centered Approach*. London: Polity Press.

Dutta, M.J. (2011). *Communicating Social Change: Structure, Culture, Agency*. New York: Routledge.

Dutta, M.J. (2012). *Voices of Resistance: Communication for Social Change*. West Lafayette, IN: Purdue University Press.

Dutta, M.J., Bodie, G.D., and Basu, A. (2007). Health disparity and the racial divide among the nation's youth: Internet as an equalizer? In A. Everett (ed.) *Learning Race and Ethnicity: Youth and Digital Media*, pp. 175–97. Cambridge, MA: MIT Press.

Dutta-Bergman, M.J. (2003). A descriptive narrative of healthy eating: a social marketing approach using psychographics in conjunction with interpersonal, mass media and new media activities. *Health Marketing Quarterly*, 20, 81–101.

Dutta-Bergman, M. (2004a). Developing a profile of consumer intention to seek out health information beyond the doctor. *Health Marketing Quarterly*, 21, 91–112.

Dutta-Bergman, M. (2004b). Primary sources of health information: comparison in the domain of health attitudes, health cognitions, and health behaviors. *Health Communication*, 16, 273–88.

Dutta-Bergman, M.J. (2004c). Complementarity in consumption of news types across traditional and new media. *Journal of Broadcasting and Electronic Media*, 48, 41–60.

Dutta-Bergman, M.J. (2004d). Interpersonal communication after 9/11 via telephone and internet: a theory of channel complementarity. *Journal of Computer-Mediated Communication*, 11, 469–84.

Dutta-Bergman, M. (2004e). A descriptive narrative of healthy eating: a social marketing approach using psychographics. *Health Marketing Quarterly*, 20, 81–101.

Ferguson, D.A. and Perse, E.M. (2000). The World Wide Web as a functional alternative to television. *Journal of Broadcasting & Electronic Media*, 44(2), 155–74.

Fox, S., and Jones, S. (2009). *The Social Life of Health Information*. Pew Internet and American Life Project. Available at: http://www.pewinternet.org/Reports/2009/8-The-Social-Life-of-Health-Information.aspx.

Habel, M.A., Liddon, N., and Stryker, J.E. (2009). The HPV vaccine: a content analysis of online news stories. *Journal of Womens Health*, 18, 401–7.

Health Promotion Board, Singapore (n.d.). In *Facebook*. [Online] Available at: https://www.facebook.com/hpbsg.

Hinduja, S. and Patchin, J. (2007). Offline consequences of online victimization: school violence and delinquency. *Journal of School Violence*, 6, 89–112.

Hoff, T., Mishel, M., and Rowe, I. (2008). Using new media to make HIV personal: a partnership of MTV and the Kaiser Family Foundation. *Cases in Public Health Communication and Marketing*, 2, 190–7.

Hughes, A. (2010). *Using Social Media Platforms to Amplify Public Health Messages: An Examination of Principles and Best Practices*. Ogilvy Washington and the Center for Social Impact Communication at Georgetown University. Available at: http://smexchange.ogilvypr.com/wp-content/uploads/2010/11/OW_SM_WhitePaper.pdf.

Jones, S. and Fox, S. (2009). *Generations Online in 2009*. Washington, DC: Pew Internet and American Life Project.

Karim, S.A. (2009). From 'playstation thumb' to 'cellphone thumb': the new epidemic in teenagers. *South African Medical Journal*, 99, 161–2.

Katz, E., Blumler, J.G., and Gurevitch, M. (1974). Utilization of mass communication by the individual. In J.G. Blumler and E. Katz (eds.) *The Uses of Mass Communications: Current Perspectives on Gratifications Research*, pp. 19–32. Beverly Hills, CA: Sage.

Korgaonkar, P.K. and Wolin, L.D. (1999). A multivariate analysis of web usage. *Journal of Advertising Research*, 39, 53–68.

Kortum, P., Edwards, C., and Richards-Kortum, R. (2008). The impact of inaccurate health information in a secondary school learning environment. *Journal of Medical Internet Research*, 10, e7.

LaRose, R. and Atkin, D. (1992). Audiotext and the reinvention of the telephone as a mass medium. *Journalism Quarterly*, 69(2), 413–21.

Lenhart, A. (2009). *Teens and Sexting*. Washington, DC: Pew Research Center. Available at: http://pewinternet.org/Reports/2009/Teens-and-Sexting.aspx.

Lustria, M.L., Smith, S.A., and Hinnant, C.C. (2011). Exploring digital divides: an examination of e-health technology use in health information seeking, communication and personal health information management in the USA. *Health Informatics Journal*, 17, 224–43.

McDonald's Malaysia (n.d.). In *Facebook*. [Online] Available at: https://www.facebook.com/My.McDonalds.

McNab, C. (2009). What social media offers to health professionals and citizens. *Bulletin of the World Health Organization*, 87, 566.

Moessner, C. (2007). Cyberbullying. *Trends & Tudes*, 6, 1–4.

MTV (2009). *A Thin Line: 2009 AP-MTV Digital Abuse Study*. [Online] Available at: http://www.athinline.org/MTV-AP_Digital_Abuse_Study_Executive_Summary.pdf.

Nielsen (2011a). *Blogpulse*. New York: The Nielsen Company.

Nielsen (2011b). *State of the Media: The Social Media Report*. New York: The Nielsen Company. Available at: http://nmincite.com/wp-content/uploads/2012/09/State-of-the-Media-The-Social-Media-Report.pdf.

O'Keefe, G.S., Clarke-Pearson, K., and Council on Communications and Media (2011). The impact of social media on children, adolescents, and families. *Pediatrics*, 127, 800–5.

Oliver M.B. (2002). Individual differences in media effects. In J. Bryant and D. Zillman (eds.) *Media Effects: Advances in Theory and Research*, pp. 507–24. Mahwah, NJ: Lawrence Erlbaum.

Palmgreen, P. and Rayburn, J.D. (1982). Gratifications sought and media exposure: an expectancy value model. *Communication Research, 9*(4), 561–80.

Papacharissi, Z. and Rubin, A.M. (2000). Predictors of Internet use. *Journal of Broadcasting & Electronic Media*, 44(2), 175–96.

Parker, B.J. and Plank, R.E. (2000). A uses and gratifications perspective on the Internet as a new information source. *American Business Review*, 18, 43–9.

Patchin, J.W. and Hinduja, S. (2006). Bullies move beyond the schoolyard: a preliminary look at cyberbullying. *Youth Violence and Juvenile Justice*, 4, 148–69.

Patrick, K., Griswold, W.G., Raab, F., and Intille, S.S. (2008). Health and the mobile phone. *American Journal of Preventive Medicine*, 35, 177–81.

Perse, E.M. and Dunn, D.G. (1998). The utility of home computers and media use: implications of multimedia and connectivity. *Journal of Broadcasting and Electronic Media, 42*, 435–56.

Pew Research Center. (2011). *Global Digital Communication: Texting, Social Networking Popular Worldwide*. Washington, DC: Pew Research Center.

Pinnock, H., Slack, R., and Sheikh, A. (2007). Misconnecting for health: (lack of) advice for professionals on the safe use of mobile phone technology. *Quality & Safety in Health Care*, 16, 162–3.

Rainie, L., Brenner, J., and Purcell, K. (2012). *Photos and Videos as Social Currency Online*. Washington, DC: Pew Research Center's Internet & American Life Project.

Rice, R.E. (1993). Media appropriateness: using social presence theory to compare traditional and new organizational media. *Human Communication Research*, 19(4), 451–84.

Richardson, J. and Harris, J.L. (2011). Food marketing and social media: findings from fast food facts and sugary drinks facts. Presented at American University Digital Food Marketing Conference on 5 November 2011.

Rogers, E.M. (1995). *Diffusion of Innovations*. New York: Free Press.

Rubin, A. (1994). Media uses and effects: a uses and gratifications perspective. In J. Bryant and D. Zillman (eds.) *Media Effects: Advances in Theory and Research*, pp. 417–36. Mahwah, NJ: Lawrence Erlbaum.

Rubin, A. (2002). The uses and gratifications perspective of media effects. In J. Bryant and D. Zillman (eds.) *Media Effects: Advances in Theory and Research*, pp. 525–48. Mahwah, NJ: Lawrence Erlbaum.

Stempel, G.H., Hargrove, T., and Bernt, J.P. (2000). Relation of growth of use of the Internet to changes in media use from 1995 to 1999. *Journalism and Mass Communication Quarterly*, 77(1), 71–9.

Syed-Abdul, S., Fernandez-Luque, L., Jian, W., et al. (2013). Misleading health-related information promoted through video-based social media: anorexia on YouTube. *Journal of Medical Internet Research*, 15, e30.

Taubenheim, A.M., Long, T., Wayman, J., Temple, S., McDonough, S., and Duncan, A. (2012). Using social media to enhance health communication campaigns. In S.M. Noar and N. Harrington (eds.) *eHealth Applications: Promising Strategies for Behavior Change*, pp. 218–34. Hoboken, NJ: Routledge.

Thackeray, R., Crookston, B.T., and West, J.H. (2013). Correlates of health-related social media use among adults. *Journal of Medical Internet Research*, 1, e21.

Thackeray, R., Neiger, B., Hanson, C., and McKenzie, J. (2008). Enhancing promotional strategies within social marketing programs: using web 2.0 social media. *Health Promotion Practice*, 9, 338–43.

The BePositiveproject (n.d.). In *YouTube*. [Online] Available at: http://www.YouTube.com/user/TheBepositiveproject.

The Heart Truth (n.d.). In *Facebook*. [Online] Available at: https://www.facebook.com/hearttruth.

Tian, Y. and Robinson, J.D. (2008). Media use and health information seeking: an empirical test of complementarity theory. *Health Communication*, 23, 184–90.

United Nations Foundation (2009). *mHealth for Development: The Opportunity for Mobile Technology for the Developing World*. Washington, DC: United Nations Foundation. Available at: http://www.unfoundation.org/news-and-media/publications-and-speeches/mhealth-for-development-1.html.

Webster, J.G. and Wakshlag, J. (1985). Measuring program choice. In D. Zillman and J. Bryant (eds.) *Selective Exposure to Communication*, pp. 35–62. Hillsdale, NJ: Lawrence Erlbaum Associates.

Wolak, J., Mitchell, K., and Finkelhor, D. (2007). Does online harassment constitute bullying? An exploration of online harassment by known peers and online-only contacts. *Journal of Adolescent Health*, 41, S51–8.

World Health Organization (n.d.). In *Twitter*. [Online] Available at: https://twitter.com/WHO.

Yale Rudd Center for Food Policy and Obesity (n.d.). Website. [Online]. Available at: http://www.yaleruddcenter.org/.

Ybarra, M.L., Diener-West, M., and Leaf, P. (2007). Examining the overlap in Internet harassment and school bullying: implications for school intervention. *Journal of Adolescent Health*, 41, S42–50.

Zillman, D. and Bryant, J. (1985). *Selective Exposure to Communication*. Hillsdale, NJ: Lawrence Erlbaum Associates.

SECTION 5

Epidemiological and biostatistical approaches

5.1

Epidemiology: the foundation of public health

Roger Detels

Introduction to epidemiology

Epidemiology is the basic science of public health, because it is the science that describes the relationship of health and/or disease with other health-related factors in human populations, such as human pathogens. Furthermore, epidemiology has been used to generate much of the information required by public health professionals to develop, implement, and evaluate effective intervention programmes for the prevention of disease and promotion of health, such as the eradication of smallpox, the anticipated eradication of polio and guinea worm disease, and the prevention of heart disease and cancer. Unlike pathology, which constitutes a basic area of knowledge, and cardiology, which is the study of a specific organ, epidemiology is a philosophy and methodology that can be applied to learning about and resolving a very broad range of health problems. It is not enough to know what the various study designs and statistical methodologies are. The 'art' of epidemiology is knowing when and how to apply the various epidemiological strategies creatively to answer specific health questions.

The uses and limitations of the various epidemiological study designs are presented in this chapter to illustrate and underscore the fact that the successful application of epidemiology requires more than a knowledge of study designs and epidemiological methods. These designs and methods must be applied appropriately, creatively, and innovatively if they are to yield the desired information. The field of epidemiology has been expanding dramatically over the last three decades, as epidemiologists have demonstrated new uses and variations of traditional study designs and methods (Pearce 2012). We can anticipate that the scope of epidemiology will expand even more in the future as increasing numbers of creative epidemiologists develop innovative new strategies and techniques.

The chapters in this section present detailed discussions of the principles and methods of epidemiology. In this introductory chapter, I will attempt to define epidemiology, to present ways in which epidemiology is used in the advancement of public health, and finally, to discuss the range of applications of epidemiological methodologies.

What is epidemiology?

There are many definitions of epidemiology, but every epidemiologist will know exactly what it is that he or she does. Defining epidemiology is difficult primarily because it does not represent a body of knowledge, as does, for example, anatomy, nor does it target a specific organ system, as does cardiology. Epidemiology is a scientific strategy/method for studying a health problem that can be applied to a wide range of problems, from transmission of an infectious disease agent to the design of a new strategy for healthcare delivery. Furthermore, this methodology is continually changing as it is adapted to a greater range of health problems and more techniques are borrowed and adapted from other disciplines such as mathematics and statistics.

Maxcy, one of the pioneer epidemiologists of the past century, offered the following definition:

> Epidemiology is that field of medical science which is concerned with the relationship of various factors and conditions which determine the frequencies and distributions of an infectious process, a disease, or a physiologic state in a human community. (Lilienfeld 1978, p. 88)

The word itself comes from the Greek *epi, demos*, and *logos*; literally translated, it means the study (*logos*) of what is upon (*epi*) the people (*demos*). John Last, in the *Dictionary of Epidemiology* (Last 2001), has defined epidemiology as follows:

> The study of the distribution and determinants of health-related states or events in specified populations, and the application of this study to the control of health problems.

Last's definition underscores that epidemiologists are concerned not only with disease but also with 'health-related events', and that ultimately epidemiology is committed to control of disease. All epidemiologists, however, will agree that epidemiology concerns itself with populations rather than individuals, thereby separating it from the rest of medicine and constituting the basic science of public health. Following from this, therefore, is the need to describe health and disease in terms of frequencies and distributions in the population. The epidemiologist relates these frequencies and distributions of specific health parameters to the frequencies of other factors to which populations are exposed in order to identify those that may be causes of ill health or promoters of good health. Inherent in the philosophy of epidemiology is the idea that ill health is not randomly distributed in populations, and that elucidating the reasons for this non-random distribution will provide clues regarding the risk factors for disease and the biological mechanisms that result in loss of health.

Because epidemiology usually focuses on health in *human* populations, it is rarely able to provide experimental proof in the sense of Koch's postulates, as can often be done in the laboratory sciences. Epidemiology more often provides an accumulation of increasingly convincing indirect evidence of a relationship between health or disease and other factors. This process, referred to as causal inference (see Chapter 5.14), includes considering an observed relationship in terms of its strength, consistency, specificity, temporality, biological gradient, plausibility, coherence, and experimental evidence (Hill 1965).

Although they will differ on the exact definitions of epidemiology, most epidemiologists will agree that they try to characterize the relationships among the *agent*, the *environment*, and the *host* (usually human). The epidemiologist considers health to represent a balance among these three forces, as shown in Fig. 5.1.1.

Changes in any one of these three factors may result in loss of health. For example, the host may be compromised as a result of treatment with steroids, making him or her more susceptible to agents that do not ordinarily cause disease. On the other hand, a breakdown in the water supply system may result in an increased exposure of people to agents such as cryptosporidium, as happened in 1993 in Milwaukee, Wisconsin (MacKenzie et al. 1994). Finally, some agents may become more or less virulent over time—often because of the promiscuous use of antibiotics—thereby disturbing the dynamic balance among agent, host, and environment. Two examples are the cases of acute necrotizing fasciitis caused by group A streptococcus (Communicable Disease Surveillance Centre 1994) and the development of multidrug-resistant tuberculosis (Chapman and Henderson 1994).

The epidemiologist uses another triad to study the relationship of agent, host, and environment: *time–place–person*. Using various epidemiological techniques, described in subsequent chapters, the epidemiologist describes disease or disease factors occurring in the population in terms of the characteristics of time (e.g. trends, outbreaks, etc.), place (the geographic area in which the disease is occurring), and person (the characteristics of the affected individuals; e.g. age, gender, etc.) to elucidate the causative agent, the natural history of the disease, and the environmental factors that increase the likelihood of the host acquiring the disease. With this information, the epidemiologist is able to suggest ways to intervene in the disease process to prevent either disease or death.

Epidemiology has been described as the 'art of the possible'. Because epidemiologists work with human populations, they are rarely able to manipulate events or the environment as can the laboratory scientist. They must, therefore, exploit situations as they exist naturally to advance knowledge. They must be both pragmatic and realistic; they must realize both the capabilities and limitations of the discipline. Morris has said that the 'epidemiologic method is the only way to ask some questions. . ., one way of asking others and no way at all to ask many' (Morris 1975, p. 96). The art of epidemiology is to know both when epidemiology is the method of choice and when it is not, and how to use it to answer the question.

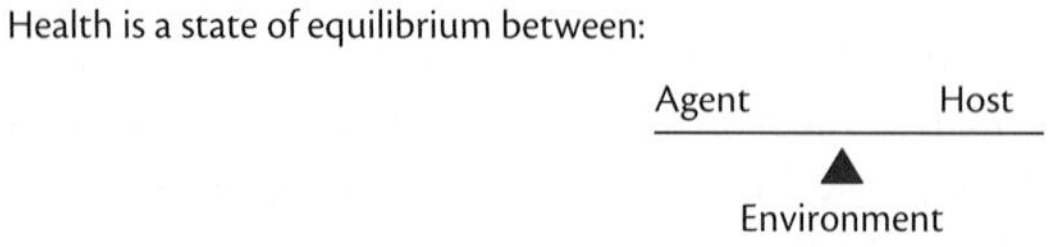

Health is a state of equilibrium between:

Agent   Host

Environment

Fig. 5.1.1 The dynamic relationship between agent, host, and environment in epidemiology.

Applying the epidemiological method to resolve a health question successfully can be compared to constructing a memorable Chinese banquet. It is not enough to have the best ingredients and to know the various Chinese cooking methods. The truly great chefs must be able to select the appropriate ingredients and cooking methods to bring out the flavours of each dish, and further, must know how to construct the correct sequence of dishes to excite the palate without overwhelming it. They create a memorable banquet by adding their creative genius to the raw ingredients and the established cooking methods. Similarly, it is not enough for the epidemiologist to know the various strategies and methods of epidemiology; the innovative epidemiologist must be able to apply them creatively to obtain the information needed to understand the natural history of the disease. It is not enough to know what a cohort study is; the epidemiologist must know when the cohort design is the appropriate design for the question at hand, and then must apply that design appropriately and creatively. These skills make epidemiology more than a methodology. It is this opportunity for creativity and innovation that provides excitement for the practitioner and makes the successful practice of epidemiology an art.

For example, Imagawa et al. (1989) identified probable transient HIV-1 infection in men, implying clearance of the virus by the immune system of the men, by focusing their viral isolation studies on the relatively few HIV-1-antibody-negative homosexual men who had many different sexual partners; a simple cohort study of antibody-negative individuals would have required a cohort of thousands of men rather than the 133 studied. the effects of passive smoking were demonstrated by cohort studies of non-smoking family members of smokers and in nursing students by comparing the reported symptoms in room-mates of smokers and non-smokers who kept diaries of their symptoms: the room-mates of the smokers had a 1.8 greater risk of episodes of phlegm than room-mates of non-smokers (Colley et al. 1974; Tager et al. 1979; Schwartz and Zeger 1990). Tashkin et al. (1984) demonstrated that children of smokers had lower levels of lung function than children of non-smokers. All of these investigators used traditional study designs, but demonstrated their creativity by applying that design to those specific populations which were most likely to reveal a relationship if it existed.

Epidemiological studies rarely provide 'proof' of a causal relationship. Thus, there is continuing debate among epidemiologists about what constitutes adequate criteria for inferring a causal relationship from epidemiological studies (Rothman 1988). Hill (1965) suggested the following minimum criteria for establishing a causal relationship between exposure and consequence/outcome: strength of association (statistical probability and risk ratio), consistency of findings across multiple studies, specificity of the relationship, temporality (outcome follows causation not heuristic), biological gradient (a dose–response relationship), plausibility, coherence (consistency with prior knowledge), experimental evidence, and analogy (relationship hypothesized is similar to that in known relationships). Susser has added to these criteria the ability of the observed relationship to correctly predict other relationships (Rothman 1988). Rothman and Greenland define a cause as 'an event, condition or characteristic that preceded the disease onset and that, if the event, condition or characteristic has been different in a specified way, the disease would not have occurred at all or would not have occurred until sometime later' (Rothman and Greenland 1998, p. 8). The sufficient component cause model defined a sufficient cause as 'a complete causal mechanism' that inevitably produces disease (Rothman and Greenland 1998, p. 8). A minimal set of factors results in an outcome, that is, each factor in a sufficient cause is a component cause and most 'causes' that are the 'causes of interest' in studies are component causes of a sufficient cause, for example, HIV infection can only occur following exposure to the HIV virus (sufficient cause). The exposure to the virus occurs through component causes (unprotected heterosexual intercourse, intravenous drug use). Therefore, a sufficient cause is a minimal set of factors that will cause the outcome. The debate goes on, but the principle is the same: epidemiological studies seldom provide 'proof' of a causal relationship in the sense of Koch's postulates, but may be used to reveal a possible relationship and build a convincing case that this relationship is causal. However, the presence of a relationship does not imply a causal relationship and the 'art' of causal inference assists in distinguishing causal from non-causal relationships (Aschengrau and Seage 2008).

More recently there is increased recognition that disease is not a product of individual circumstances at a given point of time, but rather a product of circumstances over a life course, possibly beginning *in utero* and continuing during a life course (Galea et al. 2010). This includes the complex interactions over time that result in a dynamic up- or down-regulation of different factors that closely approximates the temporal nature of causality (Galea et al. 2010).

Uses of epidemiology in support of public health

Epidemiology is the basic science of public health because it is the health science that describes health and disease associations in *populations* rather than in individuals, information essential for the formulation of effective public health initiatives to prevent disease and promote health in the community. I have taken the liberty of updating the 'Functions of Epidemiology', first expounded by Morris (1957) and Holland et al. (2007). They are as follows:

1. *Describe the spectrum of the disease*: disease represents the end point of a process of alteration of the host's biological systems. Although many disease agents are limited in the range of alterations they can initiate, others, such as measles, can cause a variety of disease end points. For example, the majority of infections with rubeola (measles) virus result in the classical febrile, blotchy-rash disease, but the rubeola virus can also cause generalized haemorrhagic rash and acute encephalitis. Years after initial infection, rubeola can also cause subacute sclerosing panencephalitis (SSPE), a fatal disease of the central nervous system.

    Various types of epidemiological studies have been used to elucidate the spectrum of disease resulting from many agents and conditions; for example, cohort studies have been used to document the role of high blood pressure as a major cause of stroke, myocardial infarct, and chronic kidney disease. For rare diseases such as SSPE and multiple sclerosis, case–control studies have been useful to identify the role of the rubeola virus (Detels et al. 1973; Alter 1976). Knowing the spectrum of disease that can result from specific infections and conditions allows the public health professional to design more effective intervention strategies; for example, education, screening, and treatment programmes to reduce the prevalence of high blood pressure will also reduce the incidence of myocardial infarct, stroke, and chronic kidney disease (Hypertension Detection and Follow-up Program Cooperative Group 1979).

2. *Describe the natural history of disease*: epidemiological studies can be used to describe the natural history of disease, to elucidate the specific alterations in the biological system in the host, and to improve diagnostic accuracy. For example, cohort studies of individuals who were infected with HIV, the 'AIDS virus', revealed that a drop in the level of T lymphocytes having the CD4 marker was associated with being infected with HIV (Polk et al. 1987), and that a further decline in CD4 cells was associated with developing clinical symptoms and AIDS (Detels et al. 1987). This observation stimulated immunologists to focus their research on the interaction of the immune system and HIV. From a clinical perspective, clinicians can target HIV-antibody-positive individuals who have declining CD4 cells for viral suppressive or antiretroviral treatment when it is clinically indicated. Epidemiology can also be used to describe the impact of treatment on the natural history of disease. For example, a cohort study design was used to demonstrate the public health effectiveness of combined highly active antiretroviral therapy on reducing the incidence of AIDS and extending survival of those who already had the disease (Detels et al. 1998). Thus, describing the natural history of AIDS among both treated and untreated individuals has assisted researchers to focus their studies and clinicians to use the limited treatment modalities available more effectively (Phair et al. 1992). The field of 'clinical epidemiology' applies research on the natural history of disease to improving the diagnostic accuracy of physicians in their clinical practice (Sackett et al. 1991).

3. *Community diagnosis*: epidemiological surveys are often used to establish the morbidity and mortality from specific diseases, allowing efficient use of limited public health funds for control of those diseases having the greatest negative impact on the health of the community. For example, an epidemiological survey in one area of China identified the epidemic of HIV due to plasma donations in villages (Wu and Detels 1995; Wu et al. 2001; Ji et al. 2006). The use of disability-adjusted life years (DALYs) has allowed quantification of the importance of non-lethal conditions on the public's health (Murray 1994).

4. *Describe the clinical picture of a disease*: epidemiological strategies can identify who is likely to get a disease such as capillariasis, the characteristic symptoms and signs, the extent of the epidemic, the risk factors, and the causative agent, and can help to determine the effectiveness of treatment and control efforts (Detels et al. 1969b).

5. *Identify factors that increase or decrease the risk of acquiring disease*: having specific characteristics increases the probability that individuals will or will not develop disease. These 'risk factors' may be social (smoking, drinking), genetic (ethnicity), dietary (saturated fats, vitamin deficiencies), and so on. Knowing these risk factors can often provide public health professionals with the necessary tools to design effective programmes to intervene before disease occurs. For example, descriptive, cross-sectional, case–control, cohort, and intervention studies have all shown that smoking is the biggest single risk factor for ill health, because

it is a major risk factor for cardiovascular disease, chronic respiratory disease, and many cancers (e.g. of the lung, nasopharynx, and bladder). Thus, smoking is the leading cause of disability and death in developed countries, if not the world. Health education campaigns and other strategies to stop or reduce smoking, based on these epidemiological studies, are now a major public health activity in most countries of the world.

6. *Identify precursors of disease and syndromes*: high blood pressure, a treatable condition, has been identified through case–control and cohort studies as a precursor to heart disease, stroke, and kidney disease (Joint National Committee on Prevention, Detection, Evaluation, and Treatment of High Blood Pressure 1997).

7. *Test the efficacy of intervention strategies*: a primary objective of public health is to prevent disease through intervention in the disease process. But a vaccine or other intervention programme must be proven effective and safe before it is used in the community. Double-blind placebo-controlled trials are a necessary step in developing an intervention programme, whether that programme is administration of a new vaccine, a behavioural intervention strategy to stop smoking, or a community intervention study to lower heart disease. Although it may be argued that injection of a saline placebo is no longer considered ethical, a proven vaccine, such as polio, can often be used as a placebo for a trial of a new vaccine for a different disease, as was used for trials of rubella vaccines in Taiwan (Detels et al. 1969a). Widespread use of an intervention not subjected to epidemiological studies of efficacy may result in implementation of an ineffective intervention programme at great public expense, and may actually result in greater morbidity and mortality because of an increased reliance on the favoured but unproven intervention and a reduced use of other strategies that are thought to be less effective but which are actually more effective.

Although an intervention such as a vaccine may have been demonstrated to have efficacy in double-blind trials, it may fail to provide protection when used in the community. Double-blind trials may demonstrate the 'biological efficacy' of the vaccine; but if the vaccine is not acceptable to the majority of the public, they will refuse to be vaccinated, and the 'public health effectiveness' of the vaccine will be very low. For example, the typhoid vaccine provided some protection against small infecting inocula, but the frequency of unpleasant side effects with the whole-cell vaccines and the need for multiple injections in the past influenced many people against being vaccinated (Chin 2000).

Another problem of inferring public health efficacy from small vaccine trials is that volunteers for these trials may not be representative of the general public, which needs to be protected against a specific disease. Thus, broad-based intervention trials also need to be carried out, to demonstrate the acceptability and public health effectiveness of a vaccine or other intervention to the entire population in need of protection.

As there are adverse effects associated with any vaccine, ongoing evaluations of the cost–benefit relationship of specific vaccines are important. By comparing the incidence of smallpox with the incidence of adverse effects from the smallpox vaccine, Lane et al. (1969) demonstrated that more disease resulted from routine use of the vaccine in the United States than by transmission from imported cases.

There are several epidemiological strategies that can be used for ongoing evaluation of intervention programmes. Serial cross-sectional studies can be used to determine if there has been a change in the prevalence of disease or of indicators of health status over time. The cohort design can be used to compare incidence of disease in comparable populations receiving and not receiving the prevention programme. The case–control design can be used to determine if there are differences in the proportion of cases and non-cases who received the intervention programme.

8. *Investigate epidemics of unknown aetiology*: epidemiological strategies were used to establish the extent, cause, modes of transmission, and risk factors for Ebola haemorrhagic fever, which first occurred in the Congo in 1976 (Feldmann et al. 1996; King 2013), and capillariasis in the Philippines in the mid 1960s (Detels et al. 1969b).

9. *Evaluate public health programmes*: departments of health are engaged in a variety of activities to promote the health of the community, ranging from surveillance and vaccination programmes to clinics for the treatment of specific diseases. Ongoing evaluation of such programmes is necessary to ensure that they continue to be cost-effective. Periodic review of routinely collected health statistics can provide information about the effectiveness of many programmes. For programmes for which relevant statistics are not routinely available, cohort studies and serial cross-sectional studies of the incidence and changing prevalence of the targeted disease in the populations which are the intended recipients of these programmes can measure whether the programmes have had an impact and are cost-effective. For example, most countries have established sexually transmitted infections (STI) clinics, but studies in Thailand (Prempree et al. 2007) and Beijing (Zhao et al. 2007) have demonstrated that the majority of the patients with STIs do not attend the government STI clinics.

10. *Elucidate mechanisms of disease transmission*: understanding the mechanisms of disease transmission can suggest ways in which public health professionals can protect the public by stopping transmission of the disease agent. Epidemiological studies of the various arboviral encephalitides have incriminated certain species of mosquitoes as the vectors of disease and specific animals as the reservoirs for the viruses. For example, public health efforts in California to prevent western equine encephalitis have concentrated on control of the mosquito vector and vaccination of horses, which are a reservoir of the virus. Although an effective vaccine for smallpox had been available for almost 200 years, eradication of the disease was not achieved until the recognition that the low infectivity of varicella virus and the relatively long incubation for development of smallpox could be used to develop a strategy of surveillance for cases, with identification and immediate vaccination of all susceptible contacts (containment). Using this containment strategy based on epidemiological principles, smallpox was eradicated through a worldwide effort in less than 10 years (Fenner et al. 1988).

11. *Elucidate the molecular and genetic determinants of disease progression*: epidemiological strategies helped to elucidate the changes in the human immune response by CD4 and CD8

cells that accompany infection and disease progression by disease agents (Detels et al. 1983; Fahey et al. 1984; Ho et al. 1995), and genetic factors (such as CCR5 absence or heterozygosity) that prevent HIV infection and slow progression of HIV disease (Liu et al. 2004).

12. *Implementation science*: recently the scientific community and policymakers have recognized the slow rate at which scientific advances are translated into public health policies and medical and public health practice. Thus, there is growing support for identifying and testing strategies that will speed up the process of translating science into action and practice. Epidemiological methods will play an important role in identifying and testing these strategies.

From the examples given in the preceding list, it should be clear that epidemiology functions as the backbone or core of evidence-based public health practices, as well as a key strategy for evaluating the effectiveness of both clinical and public health interventions. As such it is a particularly pertinent instrument for evidence-based policy formulation as well as a tool for building advocacy and resource justification for rational policies and programmes.

Applications of epidemiology

Specific epidemiological study designs are used to achieve specific public health goals. These goals range from identifying a suspected exposure–disease relationship to establishing that relationship, to designing an intervention to prevent it, and finally, to assessing the effectiveness of that intervention. The usual sequence of study designs in the identification and resolution of a disease problem is as follows:

- Ecological studies
- Cross-sectional (prevalence) surveys
- Case–control studies
- Cohort studies
- Experimental studies
- Adaptive trial design.

There are, however, many exceptions to the application of this sequence of study designs, depending on such factors as the prevalence and virulence of the agent and the nature of the human response to the agent.

The earliest suspicion that a relationship exists between a disease and a possible causative factor is frequently obtained by observing correlations between exposure and disease from existing data such as mortality statistics and surveys of personal or national characteristics. These can be correlations observed across geographical areas (ecological studies) or over time, or a combination of both. Many of the initial epidemiological investigations on chronic bronchitis used vital statistics data, particularly data on mortality. Case–control studies identified smoking as a possible causal factor for chronic bronchitis. Subsequent cohort studies confirmed the relationship. A decline in respiratory symptoms of chronic bronchitis and a concurrent but slower decline in lung function have been observed in individuals who cease smoking (Colley 1991). Using the information obtained from these studies,

public health has implemented vigorous antismoking campaigns and has used epidemiology to assess their effectiveness.

Although this is the usual sequence in which the various epidemiological study designs are applied, there are exceptions to this sequence. Furthermore, all study designs are not appropriate to answer all health questions. The usual applications of each of the epidemiological study designs and their limitations are, therefore, presented briefly in this subsection and in greater depth in subsequent chapters.

Ecological studies

The use of existing statistics to correlate the prevalence or incidence of disease in groups or populations to the frequency or trends over time of suspected causal factors in specific localities has often provided the first clues that a particular factor may cause a specific disease. These epidemiological strategies, however, document only the co-occurrence of disease and other factors in a population; the risk factors and the disease may not be occurring in the same people within the population. These types of descriptive studies are inexpensive and relatively easy to perform, but the co-occurrence observed may be merely due to chance. For example, the incidence of both heart disease and lung cancer has increased concurrently with the increased use of automatic washing machines in the United States. Few people, however, would attribute the increase in these two diseases to the use of automatic washing machines. Thus, ecological studies must be interpreted with caution. Nonetheless, they often reveal important relationships and can provide a strong rationale for undertaking more expensive analytic studies (see Chapter 5.2).

Cross-sectional/prevalence surveys

Cross-sectional/prevalence surveys establish the frequency of disease and other factors in a community. Because they require the collection of data, however, they can be expensive. They are useful to estimate the number of people in a population who have disease and can also identify the difference in frequency of disease in different subpopulations. This descriptive information is particularly useful to health administrators who are responsible for developing appropriate and effective public health programmes.

Cross-sectional studies can also be used to document the co-occurrence of disease and suspected risk factors not only in the population but also in specific individuals within the population. The cross-sectional study design is useful to study chronic diseases such as multiple sclerosis, which has a reasonably high prevalence, but an incidence that is too low to make a cohort study feasible (Detels et al. 1978). On the other hand, they are not useful for studying diseases that have a very low prevalence, such as SSPE or variant Creutzfeldt–Jakob disease. Cross-sectional studies are subject to problems of respondent bias, recall bias, and undocumented confounders. Further, unless historical information is obtained from all the individuals surveyed, the time-relationship between the factor and the disease is not known. Also, prevalence surveys identify people who have survived to that time point with disease, and thus, under-represent people with a short course of disease.

The cross-sectional study design is used in two special types of studies: field studies and surveillance. Field studies are usually investigations of acute outbreaks, which require immediate identification of the causative factors if effective public health interventions are to be implemented in a timely fashion. Surveillance is the monitoring of disease- or health-related factors over time and uses serial cross-sectional surveys to observe trends. Surveillance is important to identify diseases that are becoming an increasing public health problem, to assure that diseases already brought under control remain under control, and to evaluate the impact of public health intervention strategies (see Chapters 5.3, 5.4, and 5.17).

Case–control studies

The case–control study compares the prevalence of suspected causal factors between individuals with disease and controls who do not have the disease. If the prevalence of the factor is significantly different in cases than it is in controls, this factor may be associated with the disease. Although case–control studies can identify associations, they do not measure risk. An estimate of relative risk, however, can be derived by calculating the odds ratio. Case–control studies are often the analytic study design used initially to investigate a suspected association. Compared to cohort and experimental studies, they are usually relatively cheap and easy to perform. Cases can often be selected from hospital patients and controls either from hospitalized patients with other diseases or by using algorithms or formulas for selecting community (neighbourhood) or other types of controls. Selection bias, however, is often a problem, especially when using either hospitalized cases or controls. The participants are seen only once, and no follow-up is necessary. Although time sequences can often be established retrospectively for factors elicited by interview, they usually cannot be for laboratory test results. For example, an elevation in factor B may either be causally related, or it may be a result of the disease process and not a cause. Furthermore, factors elicited from interview are subject to recall bias; for example, patients are often better motivated to recall events than controls because they are concerned about their disease.

The case–control study is particularly useful for exploring relationships noted in observational studies. A hypothesis, however, is necessary for case–control studies. Relationships will be observed only for those factors studied. Case–control studies are not useful for determining the spectrum of health outcomes resulting from specific exposures, because a definition of a case is required in order to do a case–control study. On the other hand, these studies are the method of choice for studying rare diseases, and are often indicated when a specific health question needs to be answered quickly (see Chapter 5.5).

Cohort studies

Cohort studies follow defined groups of people without disease to identify risk factors associated with disease occurrence. They have the advantage of establishing the temporal relationship between an exposure and a health outcome, and thus measure risk directly. Because the population studied is often defined on the basis of its known likelihood of exposure to suspected factors, cohort studies are particularly suitable for investigating health hazards associated with environmental or occupational exposures. Further, these studies will measure more than one outcome of a given exposure, and therefore, are useful for defining the spectrum of disease resulting from exposure to a given factor. Occasionally, a cohort study is done to elucidate the natural history of a disease when a group that has a high incidence of disease, but in which specific

risk factors not previously known, can be identified. Although this cohort is not defined based on a known exposure, questions are asked and biological specimens are collected from which exposure variables can be identified concurrently or in the future.

Unfortunately, cohort studies are both expensive and time consuming. Unless the investigator can define a cohort in which risk factors were measured at some time in the past and has the assurance that the cohort has been completely followed up for disease outcomes in the interim (historical cohort), this design can take years to decades to yield information about the risks of disease resulting from exposure to specific factors. Ensuring that participants remain in a cohort study for such long periods of time is both difficult and expensive. Further, the impact of those who drop out of follow-up must be taken into account in the analysis and interpretation of these studies. Finally, exposures may vary over time, complicating the analysis of their impact.

Because of the cost and complexity of cohort studies, they are usually done only after descriptive, cross-sectional, and/or case–control studies have suggested a causal relationship. The size of the cohort to be studied is dependent, in part, on the anticipated incidence of the disease resulting from the exposure. For diseases with a very low incidence, population-based cohort studies are usually not feasible, either in terms of the logistics or of the expense of following very large numbers of people, or both. Cohort studies establish the risk of disease associated with exposure to a factor, but do not 'prove' that the factor is causal; the observed factor may merely be very closely correlated with the real causative factor or may even be related to the participants' choice to be exposed.

A variant of the cohort study that has become popular is the 'nested case–control study' (Gange et al. 1997). Cases arising from a cohort study are compared with individuals followed in the cohort who have not developed disease using the usual case–control analytic strategies. The advantage of this type of study is that the exposure variables are collected before knowledge of the outcome, and therefore, are unlikely to be tainted by recall bias (see Chapter 5.6).

Experimental studies

Experimental studies differ from cohort studies because it is the investigator who makes the decision about who will be exposed to the factor based on the specific design factors to be employed (e.g. randomization, matching, etc.). Therefore, confounding factors such as choice that may have led to the subjects being exposed in the cohort studies are usually not a problem in experimental studies. Because epidemiologists usually study human populations, there are few opportunities for an investigator to deliberately expose participants to a suspected factor. On the other hand, intervention studies of randomly assigned individuals (see Chapter 5.7) or communities (see Chapters 5.8–5.10) to receive or not receive an intervention programme that demonstrates a subsequent reduction in a specific health outcome in the intervention group do provide strong evidence, if not proof, of a causal relationship. Because of the serious implications of applying an intervention that may alter the biological status of an individual or the sociopolitical behaviour of a community, intervention studies should not be undertaken until the probability of a causal or risk relationship has been well established using the other types of study designs. A randomized clinical trial or vaccine trial is a typical example of an experimental study (see Chapters 5.7–5.10).

Meta-analysis

Because individual epidemiological studies rarely provide proof of causation and results of different studies can vary for a number of reasons, including small sample size, a recent trend has been to combine similar studies to increase the power of the analysis. This strategy for data synthesis is known as *meta-analysis*. It has been especially helpful in studying diseases with a low incidence or where similar studies have given conflicting results. But meta-analysis can yield opposite conclusions, especially if different sets of studies are used in the analysis. Meta-analysis investigates and identifies all available studies both quantitatively and qualitatively. The qualitative analysis excludes poor-quality studies that may be considered flawed by the investigators (Aschengrau and Seage 2008. As a result, meta-analysis is prone to heterogeneity problems as different case definitions and different sources of controls cannot be adjusted for in the analysis (Rothman et al. 2008) (see Chapter 5.15).

Adaptive trial designs

Adaptive trial designs provide a way to address uncertainty about choices made during the planning of a study and allow for planned modifications after initiation of the study at pre-specified time points or end points as data is accumulated within a study (Kairalla et al. 2012). This design provides flexibility and efficiency (smaller sample size) of study designs and increases the likelihood of a 'successful' trial that will yield the outcome of interest. However, improper adaptations can result in study bias. This type of study design can be applied in comparative effectiveness studies (Kairalla et al. 2012).

Methodological issues

Epidemiological studies, because they deal with humans, are subject to problems such as bias (deviation of results from truth), due to the strategies of recruiting participants or to differential recall among persons with and without disease, and confounding, due to factors which are associated with both the exposure variables and outcome variable under study. A cause may combine with another cause to produce an outcome (Susser et al. 2006). For example, a genetic abnormality can be modified by prenatal exposures, resulting in an adverse outcome (e.g. autism). This process is called interaction or effect modification and attempts are made to capture these with statistical measures (Susser et al. 2006). In the last several decades, many new techniques have been developed to reduce the effect of these factors, which can influence the outcome of a study and, in some instances, can cause apparent relationships to be observed which are in fact false (see Chapters 5.12 and 5.13).

Summary

Epidemiology is the core science of public health because it defines health and disease in human populations, describes disease aetiology, and evaluates public health control efforts. It achieves these goals through a variety of strategies and methods. Epidemiology is a dynamic science that is continually evolving new strategies and methods in support of public health goals.

References

Alter, M. (1976). Is multiple sclerosis an age-dependent host response to measles? *The Lancet*, 1(7957), 456–7.

Aschengrau, A. and Seage, G.R. (2008). *Essentials of Epidemiology in Public Health*. Sudbury, MA: Jones and Bartlett.

Chapman, S.W. and Henderson, H.M. (1994). New and emerging pathogens multiply resistant *Mycobacterium tuberculosis*. *Current Opinion in Infectious Diseases*, 7, 231–7.

Chin, J. (2000). *Control of Communicable Diseases Manual*. Washington, DC: American Public Health Association.

Colley, J.R.T. (1991). Major public health problems: respiratory system. In W.W. Holland, R. Detels, and G. Know (eds.) *Oxford Textbook of Public Health* (2nd ed.), pp. 227–48. Oxford: Oxford University Press.

Colley, J.R.T., Holland, W.W., Corkhill R.T., et al. (1974). Influence of passive smoking and parental phlegm on pneumonia and bronchitis in early childhood. *The Lancet*, 2(7888), 1031–4.

Communicable Disease Surveillance Centre (1994). Invasive group A streptococcal infections in Gloucestershire (England/Wales). *Communicable Disease Report*, 4, 97–100.

Detels, R., Fahey, J.L., Schwartz, K., et al. (1983). Relation between sexual practices and T-cell subsets in homosexually active men. *The Lancet*, 1(8325), 609–11.

Detels, R., Grayston, J.T., Kim, K.S., et al. (1969a). Prevention of clinical and subclinical rubella infection: efficacy of three HPV-77 derivative vaccines. *American Journal of Diseases of Children*, 118, 295–300.

Detels, R., Gutman, L., Jaramillo, J., et al. (1969b). An epidemic of intestinal capillariasis in man: a study in a barrio in northern Luzon. *American Journal of Tropical Medicine and Hygiene*, 18(5), 676–82.

Detels, R., McNew, J., Brody, J.A., et al. (1973). Further epidemiological studies of subacute sclerosing panencephalitis. *The Lancet*, 819, 11–14.

Detels, R., Muñoz, A., McFarlane, G., et al. (1998). Effectiveness of potent antiretroviral therapy on time to AIDS and death in men with known HIV infection duration. *Journal of the American Medical Association*, 280(17), 1497–503.

Detels, R., Visscher, B.R., Fahey, J.L., et al. (1987). Predictors of clinical AIDS in young homosexual men in a high-risk area. *International Journal of Epidemiology*, 16, 271–6.

Detels, R., Visscher, B.R., Haile, R.W., et al. (1978). Multiple sclerosis and age at migration. *American Journal of Epidemiology*, 108, 386–93.

Fahey, J., Prince, H., Weaver, M., et al. (1984). Quantitative changes in T-helper or T-suppressor/cytotoxic lymphocyte subsets that distinguish acquired immune deficiency syndrome from other immune subset disorders. *American Journal of Medicine*, 76, 95–100.

Feldmann, H., Slenczka, W., and Klenk, H.D. (1996). Emerging and reemerging of filoviruses. *Archives of Virology*, 11(Suppl.), 77–100.

Fenner, F., Henderson, D.A., Arita, I., et al. (1988). *Smallpox and its Eradication*. Geneva: World Health Organization.

Galea, S., Riddle, M., and Kaplan, G.A. (2010). Causal thinking and complex system approaches in epidemiology. *Internal Journal of Epidemiology*, 39, 97–106.

Gange, S., Munoz, A., Schrager, L.K., et al. (1997). Design of nested studies to identify factors related to late progression of HIV infection. *Journal of Acquired Immune Deficiency Syndromes and Human Retroviruses*, 15(Suppl.), S5–S9.

Hill, A.B. (1965). The environment and disease: association or causation? *Proceedings of the Royal Society of Medicine*, 58, 295–300.

Ho, D.D., Neumann, A.U., Perelson, A.S., et al. (1995). Rapid turnover of plasma virion and CD4 lymphocytes in HIV-1 infection. *Nature*, 373, 123–6.

Holland, W.W., Olsen, J., Florey, C.D.V., et al. (eds.) (2007). *The Development of Modern Epidemiology: Personal Reports from Those Who Were There*. Oxford: Oxford University Press.

Hypertension Detection and Follow-up Program Cooperative Group (1979). Five-year findings of the hypertension detection and follow-up program. I: reduction in mortality of persons with high blood pressure, including mild hypertension. *Journal of the American Medical Association*, 242, 2562–71.

Imagawa, D.T., Lee, M.H., Wolinsky, S.M., et al. (1989). Human immunodeficiency virus type 1 infection in homosexual men who remain seronegative for prolonged periods. *The New England Journal of Medicine*, 320, 1458–62.

Ji, G., Detels, R., Wu, Z., et al. (2006). Correlates of HIV infection among former blood/plasma donors in rural China. *AIDS*, 20(4), 585–91.

Joint National Committee on Prevention, Detection, Evaluation, and Treatment of High Blood Pressure. (1997). The sixth report of the Joint National Committee on Prevention, Detection, Evaluation, and Treatment of High Blood Pressure. *Archives of Internal Medicine*, 157, 2413–46.

Kairalla, J.A., Coffey, C.S., Thomann, M.A., and Muller, K.E. (2012). Adaptive trial designs: a review of barriers and opportunities. *Trials*, 13, 145.

King, J.W. (2013). *Ebola Virus Infection*. [Online] Emedicine.com, Inc. Available at: http://www.emedicine.com/MED/topic626.htm.

Lane, J.M., Ruben, F.L., Neff, J.M., et al. (1969). Complications of smallpox vaccination, 1968: national surveillance in the United States. *The New England Journal of Medicine*, 281, 1201–8.

Last, J. (ed.) (2001). *Dictionary of Epidemiology* (4th ed.). New York: Oxford University Press.

Lilienfeld, D.E. (1978). Definitions of epidemiology. *American Journal of Epidemiology*, 107, 87–90.

Liu, C., Carrington, M., Kaslow, R.A., et al. (2004). Lack of associations between HLA class II alleles and resistance to HIV-1 infection among white, non-Hispanic homosexual men. *Journal of Acquired Immune Deficiency Syndromes*, 37(2), 1313–17.

MacKenzie, W.R., Hoxie, N.J., Proctor, M.E., et al. (1994). A massive outbreak in Milwaukee of cryptosporidium infection transmitted through the public water supply. *The New England Journal of Medicine*, 331, 161–7.

Morris, J.N. (1957). *Uses of Epidemiology*. London: Churchill Livingstone.

Morris, J.N. (1975). *Uses of Epidemiology* (3rd ed.). London: Churchill Livingstone.

Murray, C.J. (1994). Quantifying the burden of disease: the technical basis for disability-adjusted life years. *Bulletin of the World Health Organization*, 72, 429–45.

Pearce, N. (2012). Classification of epidemiologic study designs. *International Journal of Epidemiology*, 41, 393–7.

Phair, J., Jacobson, L., Detels, R., et al. (1992). Acquired immune deficiency syndrome occurring within 5 years of infection with human immunodeficiency virus type-1: the Multicenter AIDS Cohort Study. *Journal of Acquired Immune Deficiency Syndromes*, 5, 490–6.

Polk, B.F., Fox, R., Brookmeyer, R., et al. (1987). Predictors of the acquired immunodeficiency syndrome developing in a cohort of seropositive homosexual men. *New England Journal of Medicine*, 316, 61–6.

Prempree, P., Detels, R., Ungkasrithongkul, M., et al. (2007). The sources of treatment of sexually transmissible infections in a rural community in central Thailand. *Sex Health*, 4(1), 17–19.

Rothman, K.J. (ed.) (1988). *Causal Inference*. Chestnut Hill, MA: Epidemiology Resources.

Rothman, K.J. and Greenland, S. (1998). *Modern Epidemiology* (2nd ed.). Philadelphia PA: Lippincott-Raven.

Rothman, K.J., Greenland, S., and Lash, T.L. (eds.) (2008). *Modern Epidemiology* (3rd ed.). Philadelphia, PA: Lippincott Williams & Wilkins.

Sackett, D.L., Haynes, R.B., Buyatt, G.H., et al. (1991). *Clinical Epidemiology: A Basic Science for Clinical Medicine*. London: Little, Brown.

Schwartz, J. and Zeger, S. (1990). Passive smoking, air pollution, and acute respiratory symptoms in a diary of student nurses. *American Review of Respiratory Disease*, 141, 62–7.

Susser, E., Schwartz, S., Morabia, A., and Bromet, E.J. (2006). *Psychiatric Epidemiology*. New York: Oxford University Press.

Tager, I.B., Weiss, S.T., Rosner, B., et al. (1979). Effect of parental cigarette smoking on the pulmonary function of children. *American Journal of Epidemiology*, 110, 15–26.

Tashkin, D.P., Clark, V.A., Simmons, M., et al. (1984). The UCLA Population Studies of Chronic Obstructive Respiratory Disease: VII. Relationship between parental smoking and children's lung function. *American Review of Respiratory Disease*, 129, 891–7.

Wu, Z. and Detels, R. (1995). HIV-1 infection in commercial plasma donors in China. *The Lancet*, 346, 61–2.

Wu, Z., Rou, K., Detels, R., et al. (2001). Prevalence of HIV infection among former commercial plasma donors in rural Eastern China. *Health Policy and Planning*, 16(2), 41–6.

Zhao, G., Detels, R., Gu, F., et al. (2007). The distribution of people seeking STD services in the various types of healthcare facilities in Chao Yang District, Beijing, China. *Sexually Transmitted Diseases*, 35, 65–7.

Ecological variables, ecological studies, and multilevel studies in public health research

Ana V. Diez Roux

Introduction to ecological variables and ecological studies

There has been much discussion in epidemiology about the utility of ecological variables and ecological studies. Most of these discussions centre on the limitations of ecological studies in drawing inferences regarding the relations between individual-level variables. These limitations are due to the presence of the ecological fallacy, that is, the well-established logical fallacy inherent in making inferences regarding individual-level associations based on group-level data (Piantadosi et al. 1988; Greenland 1992; Morgenstern 1995). Because of these limitations it is often argued that ecological studies should be limited to 'hypothesis generation', leaving the more esteemed process of 'hypothesis testing' to individual-level data.

A key notion that has received much attention in epidemiology over the last decade is that not all disease determinants can be conceptualized as individual-level attributes, hence the need to consider features of the groups to which individuals belong when studying the causes of ill health. This led epidemiologists and public health researchers to rethink the ideas on ecological studies and ecological variables traditionally espoused in epidemiology (Von Korff et al. 1992; Schwartz 1994; Susser 1994a, 1994b; Diez-Roux 1998; Blakely and Woodward 2000; Macintyre and Ellaway 2000; Diez Roux 2004; Subramanian et al. 2009). It has been recognized, and is now generally accepted, that constructs defined at the levels of groups or aggregates may be relevant to health. This has motivated researchers to consider the ways in which these group-level constructs can be examined in epidemiological studies. The characterization of group-level constructs often necessitates the use of group-level (or ecological) variables. In this chapter, the terms group-level or ecological will be used interchangeably to refer to variables that characterize groups. These variables can provide information that is not captured by individual-level variables. In addition, the desire to investigate the causal effects of group-level constructs on heath has implications for study design and analysis. The interest in the investigation of how group-level constructs

may affect health has been manifested, for example, in research and debate on the possible health effects of income inequality (Lynch et al. 2003; Subramanian and Kawachi 2003), social capital (Kawachi et al. 1999; Lynch et al. 2000), and neighbourhood characteristics (Pickett and Pearl 2001; Diez Roux 2004, 2007; Oakes 2004; Subramanian 2004). The renewed interest in the 'ecological', 'macro', or 'group-level' determinants of health occurred within a broader recognition of the need to consider multiple levels of organization (e.g. from molecules to society) in studying the determinants of health and disease.

The conceptual and analytical issues that arise when considering the uses of ecological studies and ecological variables derive from the presence of multiple levels of organization and nested data structures more generally. For example, many problems that arise when dealing with individuals nested within groups (e.g. persons nested within geographical areas), are also present when dealing with groups nested within larger groups (e.g. states nested within countries), persons nested within families, or multiple measurements on individuals over time (in this case the 'group' is the individual, and the 'individuals' are the measurement occasions). The need to deal with multiple levels of organization is the norm rather than the exception in epidemiology.

The presence of multiple levels has two important implications. First, the units of analysis (or observations for which independent and dependent variables are measured) can be defined at different levels. The unit of analysis determines the level at which variability is examined. For example, a study with individuals as the units of analysis (i.e. where each observation is an individual) can investigate the causes of interindividual variation in the outcome. A study with groups as the units of analysis (where observations are groups) can investigate the causes of intergroup variation in the outcome. A study involving repeated measures on individuals over time in which measures at different points in time are the units of analysis can investigate the causes of variability across measures. As we will see, the use of units of analysis at one level to make inferences about the causes of variability at a different level leads to a series of methodological problems.

The second implication of the presence of multiple levels is that constructs relevant to health can be conceptualized (and measured) at different levels. Constructs pertaining to a higher level may be important in understanding variability at a lower level, and, conversely, constructs defined at a lower level may be important in understanding variability at a higher level. For example, characteristics of the groups to which individuals belong may be important in explaining interindividual variability, and characteristics of the individuals composing the groups may be important in explaining intergroup variability. Analogously, when investigating multiple measures on individuals over time, individual characteristics may be important in understanding variability across measures, and factors specific to measurement occasions may be important in understanding variability across individuals.

This chapter discusses the use of ecological variables, ecological studies, individual-level and multilevel studies in epidemiology within the broader context of the implications of multiple levels of organization for understanding disease aetiology. Although the discussion will focus on the simple case of individuals nested within groups, it is generalizable to many other situations involving nested data structures, as noted earlier. The first section reviews the classic distinction between ecological and individual-level studies made in epidemiology and provides historical examples of the use of ecological studies in public health. The second section summarizes the sources of the 'ecological fallacy', placing this fallacy within the context of other fallacies that may arise when the presence of multiple levels is ignored. The third section discusses types of group-level or ecological variables and revisits the full range of possible study designs based on: (1) the units of analysis (and the level at which variability is examined) and (2) the levels at which relevant constructs are defined and measured. The final section highlights some challenges faced by epidemiology when it investigates the multilevel determinants of health.

Ecological studies and their use in public health

Epidemiology has traditionally distinguished two types of studies based on the units of analysis: ecological studies and studies of individuals. Ecological studies are studies in which groups are the units of analysis: both the dependent and the independent variables are measured for groups, and intergroup variability (and associations between independent and dependent variables across groups) is examined. For example, common ecological studies in public health involve measuring rates of disease for different geographic areas, and relating these rates to area social or physical characteristics (e.g. measures of area median income; levels of air pollution, water hardness, and radiation). Ecological studies are often cross-sectional with independent and dependent variables measured at the same point in time. However, ecological studies can also involve repeated measures on a group, or on several groups, over time, as in time-trend studies (Susser 1994a, 1994b; Morgenstern 1995). For example, an ecological study could examine yearly incidence rates of disease for different regions over a 10-year period and investigate the relation of these incidence rates to area characteristics that do and do not change over time. Ecological studies can also involve the analysis of groups randomized to receive or not receive an intervention. In many ecological studies the predominant analytic approach involves the estimation of correlation coefficients between the group-level exposure and the group-level outcome. However, many other analytic approaches are also possible, including the estimation of other measures of association (such as rate differences or rate ratios) using linear or log-linear models (Morgenstern 1995).

In contrast, in individual-level studies the units of analysis are individuals: both independent and dependent variables are measured for individuals and interindividual variation (and associations between independent and dependent variables across individuals) are investigated. Based on their design, individual-level studies can be cross-sectional (when both independent and dependent variables are measured at the same point in time), cohort (when individuals are followed over time to compare risk of the outcome in exposed and unexposed people), or case–control (when a sample of people with the outcome is compared with a sample of controls with regard to the presence of certain exposures).

Because the units of analysis differ in ecological and individual-level studies, the information they provide (and the information they lack) also differs. Ecological studies include information on group characteristics (which may sometimes be simply summaries of the characteristics of individuals in the group), but lack information on the cross-classification of individual-level characteristics within groups. For example, an ecological study may relate the percentage of smokers in different groups to mortality rates, but has no information on whether within groups, smokers were actually the ones more likely to die. On the other hand, individual-level studies focus on interindividual variation, and have information on individual-level characteristics but often lack information on characteristics of the groups to which individuals belong. Although the omission of relevant group-level characteristics in individual-level studies is rarely recognized as a problem, it also can lead to incorrect inferences, as will be discussed in more detail in the sections that follow.

Uses of ecological studies in public health

Descriptive ecological studies in which rates of disease or death are compared over time or across geographic areas have been a staple of epidemiology for centuries. Chadwick used an ecological approach in his famous *Report on an Inquiry into the Sanitary Condition of the Labouring Population of Great Britain* in 1842 (Chadwick 1965). Table 5.2.1 shows a portion of Chadwick's report,

Table 5.2.1 Death rates compared in three successive decades in a drained and an undrained town

The following has been the proportion of deaths to the population in the two towns:		
	Beccles	**Bungay**
Between the years 1811 and 1821	1 in 67	1 in 69
Between the years 1821 and 1831	1 in 72	1 in 67
Between the years 1831 and 1841	1 in 71	1 in 59

You will therefore see that the rate of mortality has gradually diminished in Beccles since it has been drained, whilst Bungay, notwithstanding its larger proportion of rural population, it has considerably increased.

Reproduced from John Snow, *On the Mode of Communication in Cholera*, Second Edition, John Churchill, New Burlington Street, London, UK, Copyright © 1854. Also published in Susser M., *Causal thinking in the health sciences*, Oxford University Press, New York, USA, © 1973.

in which mortality for a drained area is compared to mortality for an undrained area at three parallel points in time. By comparing mortality rates over time in both communities (one drained and the other undrained), he was able to draw inferences regarding the relationship between drainage and ill health. Drainage was the 'exposure', mortality the outcome, and communities the units of analysis. With these findings Chadwick had grounds to institute a system of sanitation nationwide. Although the miasmatic theory of disease causation which Chadwick espoused (and which he believed was supported by his data) was later shown to be mistaken, the method of sanitation that Chadwick introduced was probably as important as any other single measure in modern times (Susser 1973).

Early in his studies, John Snow also used an ecological approach in comparing cholera rates for London districts, and examining whether differences in these rates were related to differences in the sources of water (Susser 1973) (Table 5.2.2). The units of analysis were districts, and both the independent variable (source of water) and the dependent variable (cholera rates) were measured at the district level. At the beginning of the twentieth century, Goldberger and colleagues (Goldberger et al. 1920; Terris 1964) used an ecological approach to compare incidence rates of pellagra across villages. Their findings linking food availability at the village level to village pellagra rates contributed to the demonstration that pellagra was not an infectious disease, as was believed by many at the time.

More recently, ecological studies relating rates of cardiovascular disease across countries to risk factor prevalences (Ancel Keys's Seven Country Study) laid the foundation for future work on the epidemiology and causes of cardiovascular disease (Keys 1980). For example, data from the Seven Countries Study showed a relationship between the average proportion of calories derived from saturated fat and coronary heart disease mortality. Another recent example is provided by psychiatric epidemiology. Ecological studies have demonstrated that the incidence of acute transient psychoses varies dramatically across sociocultural

Table 5.2.2 Showing the mortality from cholera, and the water supply, in the districts of London in 1849. The districts are arranged in the order of their mortality from cholera

District	Population	Deaths from cholera	Deaths from cholera per 10,000 inhabitants	Annual value of house and shop room to each person (in #)	Water supply
Rotherhithe	17,208	352	205	4.238	Southwark and Vauxhall Water Works, Kent Water Works, and Tidal Ditches
St. Olave, Southwark	19,278	349	181	4.559	Southwark and Vauxhall
St. George, Southwark	50,900	836	164	3.518	Southwark and Vauxhall, Lambeth
Bermondsey	45,500	734	161	3.077	Southwark and Vauxhall
St. Saviour, Southwark	35,227	539	153	5.291	Southwark and Vauxhall
Newington	63,074	907	144	3.788	Southwark and Vauxhall, Lambeth
Lambeth	134,768	1618	120	4.389	Southwark and Vauxhall, Lambeth
Wandsworth	48,446	484	100	4.839	Pump-wells, Southwark and Vauxhall, river Wandle
Camberwell	51,714	504	97	4.508	Southwark and Vauxhall, Lambeth
West London	28,829	429	96	7.454	New River
Bethnal Green	87,263	789	90	1.480	East London
Shoreditch	104,122	789	76	3.103	New River, East London
Greenwich	95,954	718	75	3.379	Kent
Poplar	44,103	313	71	7.360	East London
Westminster	64,109	437	68	4.189	Chelsea
Whitechapel	78,590	506	64	3.388	East London
St. Giles	54,062	285	53	5.635	New River
Stepney	106,988	501	47	3.319	East London
Chelsea	53,379	247	46	4.210	Chelsea
East London	43,495	182	45	4.823	New River

(Continued)

Table 5.2.2 (Continued)

District	Population	Deaths from cholera	Deaths from cholera per 10,000 inhabitants	Annual value of house and shop room to each person (in #)	Water supply
St. George's, East	47,334	199	42	4.753	East London
London City	55,816	207	38	17.676	New River
St. Martin	24,557	91	37	11.844	New River
Strand	44,254	156	35	7.374	New River
Holborn	46,134	161	35	5.883	New River
St. Luke Kensington (expect Paddington)	110,491	260	33	5.070	West Middlesex, Chelsea, Grand Junction
Lewisham	32,299	96	30	4.824	Kent
Belgrave	37,918	105	28	8.875	Chelsea
Hackney	55,152	139	25	4.397	New River, East London
Islington	87,761	187	22	5.494	New River
St. Pancras	160,122	360	22	4.871	New River, Hampstead, West Middlesex
Clerkenwell	63,499	121	19	4.138	New River
Marylebone	153,960	261	17	7.586	West Middlesex
St. James, Westminster	36,426	57	16	12.669	Grand Junction, New River
Paddington	41,267	35	8	9.349	Grand Junction
Hampstead	11,572	9	8	5.804	Hampstead, West Middlesex
Hanover Square and May Fair	33,196	26	8	16.754	Grand Junction
London	2,280,282	14,137	62	–	

Reproduced from John Snow, *On the Mode of Communication in Cholera*, Second Edition, John Churchill, New Burlington Street, London, UK, Copyright © 1854. Also published in Susser M., *Causal thinking in the health sciences*, Oxford University Press, New York, USA, Copyright © 1973.

settings. In the World Health Organization's Ten-Country Study, for instance, the incidence of nonaffective acute remitting psychosis was tenfold higher in developing than in developed country settings (Susser and Wanderling 1994). These studies have led to testing of specific hypotheses about causation, including antecedent fever and culturally normative life events.

Much useful public health information has been obtained from ecological studies. However, as will be illustrated throughout this chapter, both studies of individuals and studies with groups as the units of analysis have their limitations. The degree to which a given study design is appropriate depends on the particular research problem. Snow's research provides an illustrative example. Four years after Snow's initial investigation (illustrated in Table 5.2.2), one of the companies, the Lambeth Company, had moved its waterworks to a point higher up on the Thames, thus obtaining a supply of water free from the sewage of London. This meant that within a single district, some houses were receiving water drawn from one place on the Thames and others were receiving water drawn from a different point. Thus, the district as the unit of analysis was no longer appropriate. In Snow's words, 'To turn this grand experiment into account, all that was required was to learn the supply of water to each individual house where a fatal attack of cholera might occur' (cited in Susser 1973, p. 59). Snow subsequently confirmed the conclusions drawn from his prior ecological analysis by examining the relation between source of

Table 5.2.3 Cholera death rates by company supplying household water

Company	Number of houses	Deaths from cholera	Deaths per 10,000 houses
Southwark and Vauxhall Company	40,046	1263	315
Lambeth Company	26,107	98	37
Rest of London	256,423	1422	59

Reproduced from John Snow, *On the Mode of Communication in Cholera*, Second Edition, John Churchill, New Burlington Street, London, UK, Copyright © 1854. Also published in Susser M., *Causal Thinking in the Health Sciences*, Oxford University Press, New York, USA, Copyright © 1973.

water and cholera risk with households, rather than districts, as the units of analysis (Table 5.2.3).

The next section, which focuses on 'fallacies' related to the existence of multiple levels of organization, discusses some of the limitations and potentialities of ecological studies and studies of individuals. The section begins with a discussion of the ecological fallacy because it is the fallacy most commonly mentioned in epidemiology. Other related fallacies that may occur even in studies with individuals as the units of analysis are also discussed.

The ecological fallacy and other fallacies related to the presence of multiple levels of organization

The ecological fallacy is the fallacy of drawing inferences at the individual level (i.e. regarding variability across individuals) based on group-level data. The most common example of the ecological fallacy involves situations in which group-level variables are used as proxies for unavailable individual level exposures. For example, in order to study the relation between exposure to substance X and cancer in the absence of individual level data, the prevalence of exposure to X in different areas is related to cancer rates in those areas. In this case, we do not have information on exactly who is exposed to X and who is not so the area prevalence of X is used as a rough approximation for the exposure of each area resident. Since we lack information on the joint distribution of exposure and outcome at the individual level (i.e. we do not know if persons who developed cancer were actually exposed to X) we cannot conclude that individuals exposed to X have a higher risk of lung cancer even if we find that areas with a higher percentage of people exposed to X have higher cancer rates. Another example is provided by attempts to draw inferences about the relation between income and obesity using countries as units of analysis and mean country income as a proxy for individual-level income data. Suppose a researcher finds that higher mean neighbourhood income is associated with higher mean body mass index (BMI). If he/she infers that at the individual level, higher income is associated with higher BMI, he/she may be committing the ecological fallacy, because there is no way of knowing whether within countries, individuals with higher income have higher BMI (in fact the opposite may be true, as we will discuss later in the chapter).

Sources of the ecological fallacy

The ecological fallacy arises when associations between two variables at the group level (or ecological level) differ from associations between analogous variables measured at the individual level. The typical ecological fallacy applies when aggregate measures for the group (e.g. the percentage of persons with a certain attribute or the mean attribute across persons) are used as proxies for individual-level data. These differences between individual-level and group-level associations for apparently analogous variables were first described for correlation coefficients (Robinson 1950) but may also be present for other measures of associations such as linear regression coefficients (Morgenstern 1982). Because the use of correlation coefficients raises additional complexities (and because of its limitations as a measure of association), the following discussion will focus on regression coefficients as the main measure of association estimated at both the group and the individual level.

The example on income and BMI used earlier is schematically illustrated in Fig. 5.2.1. At the group or country level, mean BMI increases with increasing mean income. At the same time, for individuals within countries, BMI decreases with increasing individual-level income. This situation arises because group-level mean income is related to BMI independently of individual-level income (or in other words because there is a group effect). Persons living in countries with higher mean income generally have higher BMIs than those living in countries with lower mean income, regardless of their individual level income.

Another situation is depicted in Fig. 5.2.2, where the relation between individual-level income and BMI differs by mean country income: in countries with higher mean income, individual-level income is strongly and inversely related to BMI, whereas this relation is nonexistent, or perhaps exists in the opposite direction, in countries with lower mean income. Here the group-level variable (average income of the country in which a person lives) modifies the effect of individual-level income on the outcome. In this case, group-level associations (the relation between mean country income and mean country BMI) will also differ from individual-level associations (the relationship between individual-level income and individual-level BMI). In addition, individual-level associations will differ from country to country, according to levels of mean country income. Thus, when a group-level variable is related to the outcome independently of the analogous variable measured at the individual level, or when the group-level variable modifies the effects of its individual-level analogue on the outcome, ecological associations (which express the

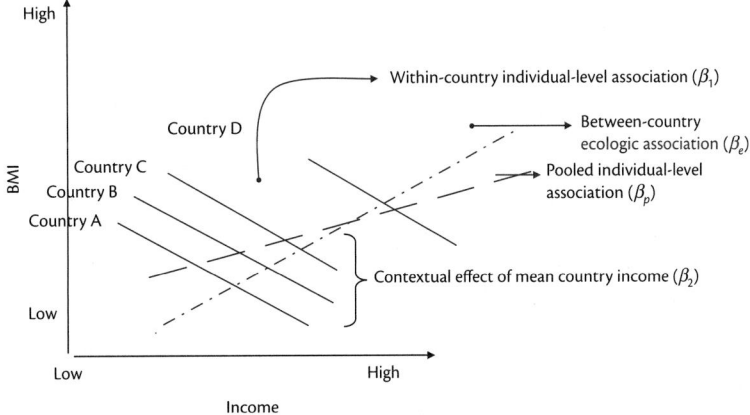

Figures are schematic and are not intended to accurately represent relative magnitudes of coefficients.

Fig. 5.2.1 Hypothetical associations of income with body mass index (BMI) within and between countries. Mean country income does not modify the effect of individual-level income.

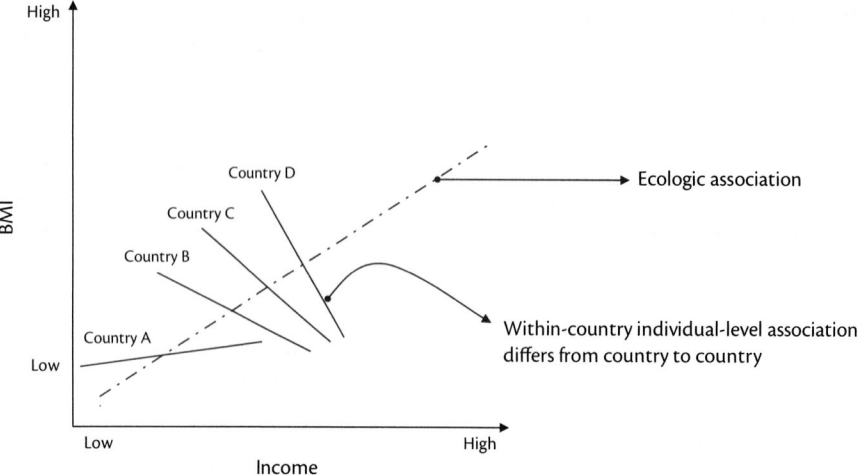

Fig. 5.2.2 Hypothetical associations of income with body mass index (BMI) within and between countries. Mean country income modifies the effect of individual-level income.

relationship between group-level variables and group-level outcomes) will differ from the corresponding individual-level associations (which express the relationship between individual-level variables and individual-level outcomes) (Hammond 1973; Firebaugh 1978; Greenland and Morgenstern 1989; Levin 1995).

The concepts just summarized can also be expressed mathematically. Suppose the 'true' relationship between country mean income, individual-level income, and individual-level BMI is reflected in Equation 5.2.1:

$$Y_{ij} = \beta_0 + \beta_1 X_{ij} + \beta_2 \overline{X}_j + U_j + e_{ij} \qquad (5.2.1)$$

where:

Y_{ij} = BMI for ith individual in jth country.

X_{ij} = income for ith individual in jth country.

$\overline{X}_j$ = mean X_{ij} in country j.

e_{ij} and U_j are individual-level and country-level errors, respectively.

β_1 = mean difference in individual-level BMI per unit difference in individual-level income.

β_2 = mean difference in individual-level BMI per unit difference in mean country income.

Thus, BMI for each individual is related not only to his or her own income, but also to the mean income for the country in which he or she lives. In Equation 5.2.1, β_1 reflects the individual-level relation between X_{ij} and Y_{ij}. Since it is 'adjusted' for the group effect (to the extent that between-group differences are entirely captured by β_2 and the group-level error U_j) it is equivalent to the within-group effect of individual-level income (or the average within-group effect if this varies across groups). β_1 is what we would like to estimate in order to quantify the individual-level effect of X_{ij} on Y_{ij}. β_2 reflects the relation between mean country income ($\overline{X}_j$) and Y_{ij}, after controlling for X_{ij} (i.e. the effect of mean country income on individual-level BMI after controlling for individual-level income). (Equation 5.2.1 can also be modified to allow interactions between X_{ij} and $\overline{X}_j$ as shown in Fig. 5.2.2. For

reasons of simplicity this situation will not be illustrated, but the discussion that follows applies as well.)

Suppose that instead of this full equation showing the relationship between BMI and individual-level income and mean country income, we fit the ecological equation shown as follows:

$$\overline{Y}_j = \beta_{e0} + \beta_{e1} \overline{X}_j + e_j \qquad (5.2.2)$$

where:

$\overline{Y}_j$ = mean BMI in country j.

$\overline{X}_j$ = mean income in country j.

β_{e1} = mean difference in mean country BMI per unit difference in mean country income. (The subscript e is used in this case because regression coefficients refer to ecological or group-level associations.)

In this case β_1 reflects the ecological relation between mean country income ($\overline{X}_j$) and mean country BMI ($\overline{Y}_j$). It is sometimes referred to as the between-group effect. Clearly, β_{e1} (the between-group effect) is not equivalent to β_1 (the within-group effect of X_{ij}) or β_2 (the effect of $\overline{X}_j$) in Equation 5.2.1. In fact both the individual-level within-group effect (β_1) and the effect of mean X_j (β_2) are confounded in the ecological regression coefficient (β_{e1}). In fact, β_e in Equation 5.22 is the sum of β_1 and β_2 in Equation 5.2.1 (Raudenbush and Bryk 2002)

Yet a third alternative is to fit a purely individual-level equation ignoring group membership:

$$Y_{ij} = \beta_{p0} + \beta_{p1} X_{ij} + e_{ij}. \qquad (5.2.3)$$

The subscript p is used in this case because regression coefficients refer to associations between individual-level variables pooled across groups. β_{p1} reflects the effect of X_{ij} on Y_{ij} pooling across groups and ignoring group membership (it is unadjusted for any potential group effects). When group effects are present, β_{p1} will differ from β_1 (the within-group effect) in Equation 5.21, and will also differ from β_{e1} (the ecological effect of $\overline{X}_j$) in Equation 5.2.2.

Both the within-group effects of X_{ij} and the effect of $\overline{X}_j$ on Y_{ij} are confounded in β_{p1}.

In the absence of group effects (e.g. when β_2 in Equation 5.2.1 equals 0) and when there is no interaction between $\overline{X}_j$ and X_{ij} (the group and individual-level variables), β_1 (within-group effect), β_{e1} (ecological effect), and β_{p1} (pooled individual effect) are all equivalent. However, in the presence of group effects, β_e does not equal β_1 or β_{p1} (source of the ecological fallacy). In addition, β_{p1} does not equal β_{e1} or β_2. When group effects are present, β_{p1} will be a weighted average of β_1 and β_{e1}, and will lie between them, although the order of magnitude of β_1 and β_{e1} cannot be predicted (Piantadosi et al. 1988). β_1 (the within-group effect), β_2 (the contextual effect), β_{e1}, and β_{p1} are schematically illustrated in Fig. 5.2.1. The typical explanation given for the ecological fallacy in many epidemiology textbooks (i.e. the absence of cross-classified information on exposure and outcome within groups) is precisely the reason why β_2 and β_1 are confounded in β_e, and hence the reason why β_e cannot reliably be used to make inferences about β_1 when β_2 is nonzero.

It is important to note that although results for correlation coefficients generally follow those for regression coefficients outlined above, individual-level (within-group) and ecological (between-group) correlation coefficients may differ even in the absence of group effects (i.e. even when $\beta_1 = \beta_{e1} = \beta_{p1}$) (Hammond 1973; Piantadosi et al. 1988). This is because correlations also depend on the relative dispersion of X and Y (Morgenstern 1982; Piantadosi et al. 1988).

As illustrated above, ecological associations will differ from individual-level associations in the presence of group effects, i.e. when β_2 in Equation 5.2.1 does not equal 0 (or when the interaction between X_{ij} and $\overline{X}_j$ in Equation 5.2.1 does not equal 0). The key to understanding the sources of the ecological fallacy therefore lies in specifying the conditions under which β_2 (the independent effect of $\overline{X}_j$) or the interaction between $\overline{X}_j$ and X_{ij} will differ from 0. Several different situations may result in nonzero values for β_2 or for the interaction term between X_{ij} and $\overline{X}_j$. These include: (1) situations where group mean X_{ij} ($\overline{X}j$) is a marker for omitted individual-level variables which individuals in a group tend to share, and (2) situations where mean X_{ij} at the group level measures a different construct than X at the individual level. Both situations will be discussed in more detail in the following subsections.

$\overline{X}_j$ is a marker for omitted individual-level variables that individuals in a group tend to share

It is possible that $\overline{X}_j$ is a marker for omitted individual-level variables that individuals in a group tend to share, that is, groups differ in the distribution of individual-level variables causally related to the outcome. In the earlier BMI example, unmeasured individual-level factors (e.g., diet, exercise, genetic factors) may vary from country to country, and their prevalence may be associated with mean country income. These individual-level factors may affect the risk of the outcome independently of individual-level income or may modify the association of individual-level income with the outcome. If these factors are unmeasured in the analyses, their effects will be reflected in the coefficient for mean income in Equation 5.2.1 (β_2) (or in the mean income by individual-level income interaction), and in the ecological regression coefficient relating mean income to mean BMI (β_{e1} in Equation 5.2.2). Thus, differences in

the distribution of these individual-level confounders or effect modifiers across groups may lead to discordances between the group-level and individual-level associations of income with BMI. Summary ecological measures of these individual-level factors for each group are sometimes available (e.g. percentage sedentary, or mean dietary fat). However, controlling for these summary measures in ecological analyses is often insufficient to account for the confounding effects of individual-level variables (although in some cases controlling for multiple summary measures of the same variable may reduce confounding to some extent) (Greenland and Morgenstern 1989; Greenland and Robins 1994; Morgenstern 1995). It is even possible for this ecological adjustment to actually increase bias (Greenland and Morgenstern 1989). The limitations of the use of summary measures are especially important when the relationship between individual-level factors and the outcome is nonlinear, when individual level factors interact or when there is measurement error (Greenland 1992; Greenland and Robins 1994; Piantadosi 1994).

An additional complexity arises from the fact that even an individual-level variable that is not a confounder at the individual level (because it is not associated with exposure within groups) may still operate as a confounder when ecological associations are used to draw individual-level inferences, if it is ecologically associated with the exposure prevalence across groups (Greenland and Morgenstern 1989; Greenland 1992). Similarly, even weak effect modifiers at the individual level may lead to important differences between ecological and individual-level associations, if their prevalence differs across groups (Greenland and Morgenstern 1989). On the other hand, a variable that is a confounder at the individual level (because it is associated with the exposure and the outcome within groups) may not confound the analogous ecological association if it is ecologically unassociated with the exposure across groups (Greenland and Robins 1994; Morgenstern 1995) (i.e. the grouping process itself may control for some confounding variables) (Morgenstern 1982). Brenner et al. (1992) have also shown that although nondifferential misclassification of a binary variable seriously hinders the ability to control for that variable in individual-level studies, it does not always reduce the ability to control for that variable in ecological studies. Thus in some cases, the ecological analysis may avoid the confounding present in individual-level analyses.

The absence of information on individual-level confounders (which may differ from group to group) and the limitations inherent in using ecological summaries (and interactions between ecological summaries) to control for individual-level confounders or account for nonlinearities in the individual-level effects, is the most common critique of ecological studies in epidemiology. A key assumption of this critique (which often goes unstated) is that the ecological measures (e.g. mean country income) and the individual-level measures (individual-level income) are indicators of the same construct. If it were somehow possible to control for the individual-level confounders and fully capture nonlinearities, it would be perfectly legitimate to draw inferences about associations between individual-level income and BMI based on the ecological association. But this assumption is not always true. Even if all possible individual-level confounders are controlled, ecological associations may differ from individual-level associations because the ecological measure of exposure and its individual-level namesake may be tapping into different constructs. This brings us to another important source of the ecological fallacy, discussed in the next subsection.

$\bar{X}_j$ and X_{ij} measure different constructs

An alternative interpretation of Fig. 5.2.1 (or Fig. 5.2.2) is that country mean income and individual-level income are measuring different constructs ($\bar{X}_j$ measures a group-level construct and X_{ij} measures a different individual-level construct), and the group-level construct is related to BMI independently of individual level income. Firebaugh (1978, p. 560) noted that 'The demystification of cross-level bias begins with the recognition that an aggregate variable often measures a different construct than its name-sake at the individual-level'. In this case, country mean income is a measure of a truly group-level attribute and not a proxy for individual-level income. Living in countries with high mean income places individuals at greater risk of having a high BMI regardless of their individual-level income (or modifies the relation between individual-level income and BMI, as in Fig. 5.2.2). Mean country income is said to exert a contextual effect on BMI. Both country-level and individual-level income provide distinct information, and both are needed to completely explain the distribution of BMI. In this case, the origin of the ecological fallacy lies in assuming that the group level measure is tapping into the same construct as the individual-level measure, when in fact it is not. Higher mean country income is associated with higher BMI, after controlling for individual-level income, but within countries, higher individual-level income is associated with lower BMI. In this situation the ecological fallacy can be thought of as a problem of construct validity: it arises because the aggregate measure is assumed to be measuring an individual-level construct when in fact it is measuring a group-level construct (Schwartz 1994).

The contextual effect of mean income may be due to a variety of different processes. For example, countries with higher mean income may rely to a greater extent on mass food production, and this may in turn be associated with higher calorie intake for all individuals. In addition, the higher mean income may be associated with differences in country occupational structures resulting in more sedentary occupations. Since disease is defined at the level of individuals, in order to affect health, contextual effects must ultimately be mediated through individual-level processes (i.e. through processes defined at a lower level of organization), just as the effects of individual-level behaviours, for example, are mediated through biological mechanisms. Mediators of a contextual effect do not necessarily involve the individual-level namesake of the group-level variable. In our BMI income example, for instance, the contextual effect of mean income may work through individual level variables other than income. It is also possible that the apparent contextual effect of the group-level variable is confounded by another group-level variable. For example, in our example higher mean income may not in itself be the cause of higher BMI. It may simply be associated with level of industrialization which is the truly causally relevant construct.

Grouping on the dependent variable

Hammond (1973) notes another (related) reason for differences between ecological and individual-level regression coefficients: grouping by the dependent variable. For example, if people are grouped into neighbourhoods based on their income (due to social processes driving economic residential segregation) and we are interested in estimating the relationship between race and income at the individual level, the ecological regression coefficient relating percentage of black and mean neighbourhood income would differ from the individual-level coefficient relating race to individual-level income because of the grouping process involved. Similarly, if people were grouped into neighbourhoods based on the presence of disease, and we are interested in the relationship between a certain risk factor and disease, the ecological relation between the percentage of people in the neighbourhood with the risk factor and the disease rate would be a biased estimate of the individual-level association between the risk factor and the probability of having the disease. Essentially, the grouping process generates a 'group effect' analogous to the contextual effects of mean group X described earlier.

Relationship between sources of the ecological fallacy

The three sources of the ecological fallacy described earlier all pertain to situations where there is some form of 'group-effect'. This includes situations where there is a failure to distinguish constructs at different levels (e.g. mean group X is assumed to measure the same thing as individual-level X), where something about the groups is associated with individual-level predictors of the outcome (mean group X is associated with other individual-level factors related to Y), or when some process results in grouping of persons by the dependent variable. It is important to emphasize that the simple presence of differences in the distribution of individual-level variables (e.g. diet and exercise in our example) across groups (countries in our example) may be an indication that group-level constructs play a causal role in the development of these individual-level factors. In common epidemiological discussions of the ecological fallacy, these group effects are viewed as a nuisance that makes it difficult for epidemiologists to draw inferences regarding individual-level associations based on group-level data. However, more recently, epidemiologists have become increasingly interested in investigating these group effects.

The previous discussion (like typical discussions of the ecological fallacy) focuses on the situation where the independent variable at the group level is an aggregate of characteristics of individuals in the group. Thus the group-level variable (mean income) has an individual-level namesake (individual-level income). However, other ecological variables do not involve aggregates of individual-level data (e.g. the existence of a certain law) and the problem of separating out contextual effects from individual-level effects of the variable (e.g. the effects of mean country income from that of individual-level income) is not an issue. In this situation it is obvious that the ecological variable is measuring a group-level construct. However, ecological studies relating these types of predictors to outcomes may still be limited in their ability to draw individual-level inferences because of the absence of information on individual-level confounders or effect modifiers which may differ from group to group.

Other reasons for differences between ecological and individual-level regression coefficients

In addition to the conceptual issues discussed previously, there are statistical considerations that may lead to a discrepancy between estimates from ecological and individual-level studies. The example used throughout this section (country mean income, individual-level income, and BMI) is based on a continuous individual-level dependent variable and highlights the limitations inherent in using a linear ecological model as a proxy for a linear individual-level model. Additional complexities arise when the individual-level outcome is binary. The use of a linear regression ecological model as a proxy for a nonlinear individual-level regression model (e.g. a log-linear or multiplicative model) may not always be appropriate. Fitting the aggregate or ecological regression model that directly corresponds to a nonlinear individual-level regression model is not always simple or possible with available ecological data (see Greenland 1992 for details). Failure to correctly specify the ecological model to be used as a proxy for the individual-level model (sometimes referred to as specification bias; Wakefield 2008) is another source of differences between individual-level and aggregate-level regression coefficients. However, all the sources of the ecological fallacy described in the preceding sections may still be present even if the form of the ecological model is appropriate for the individual-level model it is attempting to proxy.

It is important to emphasize that the degree to which ecological and individual-level coefficients differ may vary from situation to situation. The logical possibility of the ecological fallacy should not be taken as evidence that the fallacy necessarily occurs in all cases (Greenland and Robins 1994) or that when it occurs it has a critical impact. Some researchers have proposed strategies that may sometimes help reduce the ecological fallacy, particularly when the group-level aggregate exposure is simply a proxy for unavailable individual-level data. These strategies include selecting regions so as to minimize within-region variability and maximize between-region variability in individual-level exposure, comparing groups with similar covariate distributions, comparing results based on different specifications of the ecological model (Greenland 1992), two-phase designs that combine ecological data with samples of individual within groups (Wakefield and Haneuse 2008), and other statistical approaches (King 1997; Wakefield 2008). Many of these approaches assume that no other group-level effects are present or that the aggregate proxy is not serving as a proxy for group-level constructs. Despite these approaches, and for all the reasons outlined, the use of ecological studies to estimate individual-level relationships is often very challenging (Greenland 2001; Wakefield 2008).

Other fallacies related to the existence of multiple levels

The ecological fallacy is only one of a set of possible 'fallacies' that can result from the existence of multiple levels of organization (Diez-Roux 1998). Because, until relatively recently, epidemiologists have been mostly concerned with drawing inferences regarding the causes of interindividual variability, the ecological fallacy has received much more attention than its counterpart, the atomistic fallacy. The atomistic fallacy is the fallacy of drawing inferences regarding variability across groups based on individual-level data. The association of an individual-level predictor with an outcome in a study of individuals is not necessarily the same as the association of its group level namesake with the group-level outcome. Thus the use of individual-level associations to draw inferences regarding group-level associations may also lead to incorrect inferences. In the BMI example, β_{p1} (the relation between individual-level income and BMI pooling individuals across groups) does not equal β_{e1} (the ecological relation between country mean income and country mean BMI). In addition, β_1 (the within-group effect of individual-level income) does

not equal β_{e1} either. Moreover, the BMI example includes multiple groups (countries) and individuals within them, but many individual-level studies only include individuals from a single group. Factors that explain variability across individuals within groups are not necessarily the same as those that explain variability across groups. For example, if stress levels are relatively invariant within groups (e.g. communities or countries), stress may not be important in explaining variability in coronary heart disease within groups, but may be strongly associated with differences in coronary heart disease rates across groups. This is another reason why the use of individual-level associations to infer group-level associations may lead to incorrect inferences.

The ecological and atomistic fallacies can be thought of as methodological problems inherent in drawing inferences at one level when the data are collected at another level. These fallacies arise when the conceptual model being tested corresponds to one level, but the data are collected at another level, or in Riley's words when 'the methods fail to fit the model' (Riley 1963). We have seen that the sources of these problems lie in: (1) the lack of information on constructs pertaining to another level of organization, and (2) the failure to realize that a variable defined and measured at one level of organization may tap into a different construct than its namesake at another level, and that constructs at both levels may be relevant to the outcome studied.

More generally, careful consideration of the sources of the ecological and atomistic fallacies highlights the fact that even when making inferences about a given level, other levels of organization may need to be taken into account. The failure to consider group characteristics in drawing inferences regarding the causes of variability across individuals, and the failure to consider individuals in drawing inferences regarding the causes of variability across groups, gives rise to another set of fallacies, which are closely related to the ecological and atomistic fallacies described earlier. In these fallacies (which have been termed the psychologistic or individualistic and sociologistic fallacies), although the level at which data are collected may fit the conceptual model being investigated, important facts pertaining to other levels have been ignored, in Riley's words 'the methods may fail to fit the facts' (Riley 1963).

Ignoring relevant group-level variables in a study of individual-level associations may lead to what Riley has termed the psychologistic fallacy, that is, assuming that individual-level outcomes can be explained exclusively in terms of individual-level characteristics. For example, a study based on individuals might find that immigrants are more likely to develop depression than natives. But suppose this is only true for immigrants living in communities where they are a small minority. A researcher ignoring the contextual effect of community composition might attribute the higher overall rate in immigrants to the psychological effects of immigration per se or even to genetic factors, ignoring the importance of community-level factors and thus committing the psychologistic fallacy (Riley 1963; Valkonen 1969). (The term 'psychologistic fallacy' is not the most appropriate because the individual-level factors used to explain the outcome are not always exclusively psychological. Other authors have used the term 'individualistic fallacy' (Valkonen 1969), but because the term has also been used as a synonym of the 'atomistic fallacy' (Alker 1969; Scheuch 1969) it will be avoided here.)

Analogously, ignoring the role of individual-level factors in a study of groups may lead to what has been termed the sociologistic fallacy (Riley 1963). Suppose a researcher finds that communities with higher rates of transient population have higher rates of schizophrenia, and he/she concludes that higher rates of transient population lead to social disorganization, breakdown of social networks, and increased risk of schizophrenia among all community inhabitants. But suppose that schizophrenia rates are only elevated for transient residents (because transient residents tend to have fewer social ties, and individuals with few social ties are at greater risk of developing schizophrenia). That is, rates of schizophrenia are high for transient residents and low for nontransient residents, regardless of whether they live in communities with a high or a low proportion of transient residents. If this is the case, the researcher would be committing the sociologistic fallacy in attributing the higher schizophrenia rates to social disorganization affecting all community members rather than to differences across communities in the percentage of transient residents.

Both the psychologistic and the sociologistic fallacies arise because relevant variables pertaining to other levels have been excluded from the model leading to an inappropriate explanation for the association. Although it is didactically useful to distinguish both sets of fallacies (ecological and atomistic vs. psychologistic and sociologistic), they are closely interrrelated and are essentially different manifestations of the same phenomenon: the failure to recognize that constructs defined at different levels may be important in understanding the causes of variability within a given level, and the failure to adequately distinguish constructs defined at different levels.

The types of fallacies are summarized in Table 5.2.4.

The full range of epidemiological studies

In considering the most appropriate study design to answer a given research question, investigators need to consider two issues. The first issue is the level of organization about which inferences are to be made. For example, are we interested in drawing inferences regarding causes of variation in the outcome among groups or among individuals? The answer to this question will determine the most appropriate unit of analysis. The second issue is the level

Table 5.2.4 Types of fallacies

Unit of analysis	Level of inference	Type of fallacy
Group	Individuals	Ecological
Individual	Groups	Atomistic[a]
Individual (relevant group-level variables excluded)	Individuals	Psychologistic[a]
Group (relevant individual-level variables excluded)	Groups	Sociologistic

[a] Also called individualistic by some authors.

Reproduced with permission from Diez-Roux, A.V., Bringing context back into epidemiology: variables and fallacies in multilevel analysis, *American Journal of Public Health*, Volume 88, Number 2, pp. 216–22, Copyright © 1998 by the American Public Health Association*.

of organization at which the constructs of interest in explaining the outcome are conceptualized. The answer to this second question will determine the predictors to be investigated and the level at which they are conceptualized. Constructs relevant to health may be conceptualized, and measured, at different levels of organization (e.g. countries, states, neighbourhoods, peer groups, families, couples, persons, and measurement occasions). Factors defined at a higher level may be important in understanding variability at a lower level and, vice versa, factors defined at a lower level may be important in understanding variability at a higher level. Decoupling the unit of analysis from the level of organization of the constructs investigated may be helpful in discussing the full range of studies available to epidemiologists and the advantages and disadvantages of each for a particular research question.

Clearly specifying the constructs of interest is an important requirement of any study. Lack of clarity on exactly what constructs group-level or ecological variables are actually measuring underlies an important part of the confusion generated by the use of ecological studies and the interpretation of group-level or ecological associations. The next subsection reviews the use of group-level variables in epidemiology based on the constructs that they are intended to measure. The subsequent subsection considers study designs with different units of analysis in terms of the types of inferences that can be drawn from them and the types of constructs they are best suited to investigating.

Group-level variables in epidemiology

Group-level variables as proxies for individual-level variables

One of the most common uses of ecological variables in epidemiological studies is as proxies for individual-level variables, either because individual-level data are unavailable or because individual-level measurements are prone to measurement error. For example, in the absence of detailed information on smoking for individuals, the percentage of smokers in the area in which an individual lives may be used as a proxy. Of course, the use of these group-level proxies implies loss of information: we do not know whether a given person smokes or not; we use mean smoking levels in the area as an approximation. In this case the group-level measure is a second class alternative to the ideal individual-level measurement. The relevant construct (smoking) is defined at the individual level, but a group-level measurement is used as a proxy for it because direct individual-level measurements are unavailable. If a valid and reliable measure of individual-level exposure were available, it would be used instead.

Group-level variables are also used as proxies for individual-level data in cases in which individual-level measures are subject to a lot of measurement error, or when intraindividual variability makes a single measure a poor marker for the person's true exposure. For example, the mean yearly hours of sunlight in an area may be used as a proxy for individual-level exposure to sunlight and average per capita fat consumption in a group may be used as a proxy for the fat consumption of each member (due to limitations in characterizing an individual's fat intake based on a single, 1-day measurement). In these situations, the ecological measure is believed to be a better indicator of the 'true' individual level exposure than the individual level measure itself, because the ecological measure reduces the 'noise' associated with measurement error or intra-individual variation.

Group-level proxies for individual-level variables can be used in studies with individuals or groups as the units of analysis. Regardless of the study design in which they are used, the key assumption in the use of these variables is that the group-level measure is an adequate proxy for the individual-level construct, that is, even if there is measurement error, the construct that is being tapped into by the measure is an individual-level property rather than a group-level property. But this may not always be true: it is possible that the group-level measure is capturing information about a group-level attribute rather than about individual-level characteristics. For example, mean neighbourhood income could be used as a proxy for unavailable information on the income of residents. It is theoretically possible that areas with lower income have worse health not because people of low income have worse health but because there is something about areas with a lower income that places everyone in the area at higher risk regardless of their own income. Unless individual-level data are available, it will not be possible to differentiate the effects of individual-level income from the contextual effect of mean income (or other group-level properties associated with it). Thus, in considering the use of group-level variables as proxies of individual-level data, researchers should consider two issues: (1) the degree of measurement error in the individual-level construct inherent in using the group-level variable (e.g. misclassification of smokers as nonsmokers), and (2) the degree to which the group-level measure is tapping into a group-level construct rather than the individual-level construct it purports to proxy.

Group-level (higher-level) variables as measures of group-level (higher-level) constructs

Another application of ecological variables is to measure group-level constructs. Variables that reflect the characteristics of groups have been classified into two basic types (Valkonen 1969; Lazarsfeld and Menzel 1971; Blalock 1984; Von Korff et al. 1992; Morgenstern 1995): derived variables and integral variables. Derived variables (also termed analytical or aggregate variables) summarize the characteristics of individuals in the group (means, proportions, e.g. percentage of persons with incomplete high school, median household income). Although created through the aggregation of information from the individual members of a group, derived variables are often used as measures of group-level properties since they can provide information distinct from their individual-level analogue. For example, mean neighbourhood income, and individual-level income are indicators of two distinct constructs, each of which may be important to health. Mean neighbourhood income may be a marker for neighbourhood-level factors potentially related to health (such as recreational facilities, school quality, road conditions, environmental conditions, types of foods available, and their cost), and these factors may affect everyone in the community regardless of their individual-level income. Similarly, community unemployment level is a community-level property that may affect everyone in the community regardless of whether they are unemployed or not.

A special subset within derived variables is the average of the dependent variable within the group (Susser 1994a, 1994b). As noted by Ross in his theory of happenings (Ross 1916), for some types of events, the frequency of occurrence may depend on the number of individuals already affected. The prevalence of a given infection in the group to which a person belongs will affect his or her risk of infection, or may modify the relation between individual-level risk factors and the risk of disease (Halloran and Struchiner 1991; Koopman et al. 1991; Koopman and Longini 1994). The classic concept of herd immunity is a variant of this notion: the prevalence of immunity in a community will influence whether an epidemic of disease does or does not occur, and will therefore affect a nonimmune individual's risk of acquiring disease. The contextual effect of the dependent variable's prevalence within a group may also be important in understanding other health outcomes. For example, the prevalence of obesity in a community may influence the likelihood that an individual is obese. This effect may operate through several different mechanisms. The prevalence of obesity may itself generate societal norms regarding acceptability and desirability of obesity, which may influence an individual's risk of being obese. In addition, the probability of adopting behaviours conducive to obesity (e.g. certain types of diet or physical activity patterns) may be higher in situations where the behaviour is highly prevalent in the community. Although infrequently considered, these types of contextual effects may be important in understanding the distribution (and causes) of health-related behaviours.

Integral variables (also termed primary or global variables) describe group characteristics that are not derived from characteristics of its members (e.g. the existence of certain types of laws, availability of health care, political system, or population density). Integral variables do not have analogues at the individual level. They may be discrete and dichotomous (e.g. an intervention or a disaster, presence of a certain law), scaled and polychotomous (e.g. social disorganization, intensity of newborn care), or continuous (e.g. physicians per capita). A special type of integral variable refers to patterns and networks of contacts or interactions between individuals within groups. These patterns are derived from how individuals are connected to each other, and yet they are more than aggregates of individual characteristics. Lazarsfeld and Menzel (1971) have referred to these variables as structural variables although the term structural effects has also been used to refer to the effects of group-level properties more generally (Blau 1960). Patterns of interconnections among individuals may be important determinants of individual risk, particularly for infectious diseases, but possibly for many other health outcomes as well (Koopman et al. 1991; Koopman and Longini 1994; Koopman and Lynch 1999). In addition, these patterns of interconnections may modify the relation between certain individual-level attributes and risk of disease (Koopman et al. 1991). Patterns of interactions can be summarized in the form of group-level attributes such as network size or structure (Lazarsfeld and Menzel 1971; van den Eeden and Huttner 1982). Just as other 'group-level' variables can refer to groups of various sizes, these patterns of interactions may characterize a whole continuum of groups depending on the particular research problem: large groups, smaller groups within larger groups, or even pairs of individuals.

When group-level variables are used to characterize group-level properties there is no ambiguity in defining whether individuals are or are not exposed (as there is when group variables are used as proxies for individual level exposure data). The group level variable (whether derived or integral) applies equally to all individuals within the group: for example, all are 'exposed' to living in a neighbourhood with high unemployment regardless of whether they themselves are employed, all are 'exposed' to existing laws regarding seat belt use. Thus the measurement error problem that may be present when group measures are used as proxies for measures of individual-level constructs is not present (although there may of course be measurement error in the measure of the group-level construct itself, as there may be for any measure). When derived variables (such as area mean income or area unemployment) are used to capture group-level constructs, in the absence of individual-level data it will not be possible to distinguish a true group or contextual effect from an individual-level effect. But this problem does not arise with integral variables because no individual-level analogue exists. As we discuss later, group-level constructs can be investigated in studies with either individuals or groups as the units of analysis.

Study designs based on the units of analysis

Studies with groups as units of analysis

Studies with groups as the units of analysis (ecological studies) are most appropriate when investigators are interested in explaining variation between groups and the constructs of interest can be conceptualized as group-level properties. These group-level properties may be characterized using derived or integral variables. For example, numerous ecological studies have examined the relationship between area measures of deprivation (derived variables) and area disease or mortality rates (see, e.g. Townsend et al. 1988; Wing et al. 1992; Benach et al. 2001; Janghorbani et al. 2006). This analytical approach is most appropriate if the research question is formulated at the area (group)-level and the main construct investigated (deprivation) is conceptualized as an area or group-level attribute. In these cases, area deprivation is conceptualized as a group attribute that affects all individuals living within the community and the interest lies in drawing inferences regarding differences between areas.

An example involving integral group-level variables is provided by studies relating national legislation restricting tobacco advertising in different countries to country smoking rates: a country-level construct is examined and the interest lies in drawing country-level inferences. Ecological designs may also be appropriate for the evaluation of the effects of group-level interventions on group-level outcomes (Morgenstern 1982). For example, a study may want to investigate the relationship between the introduction of a mass media campaign to prevent teenage smoking (an integral variable) and the prevalence of teenage smoking in the area. Because the mass media campaign may affect all community inhabitants (regardless of whether they actually saw the ads or not) through mechanisms involving diffusion, peer pressure, etc., the intervention can be conceptualized as a group-level attribute.

As discussed earlier in the section on the ecological fallacy, these studies are limited in their examination of the role of individual-level constructs—as confounders, mediators, or effect modifiers of the group-level associations. In the earlier example, differences in the effects of the mass media campaign by individual-level characteristics (effect modification) could not be investigated. Neither could the impact of differences in individual exposures to the mass media campaign. In addition, in the case of ecological variables with individual-level analogues (e.g. area unemployment and individual-level unemployment), studies with groups as the units of analysis cannot differentiate the contextual effect of the variable from its individual-level effect. For example,

an ecological study showing that area unemployment is related to higher rates of adverse mental health outcomes could not differentiate whether the increased rate of mental illness is seen only in the unemployed or is present in all area inhabitants regardless of whether they are unemployed or not. However, from a public health perspective, the group-level association may itself be of great interest. If the association observed is causal, decreasing the unemployment rate would decrease the rate of mental illness regardless of whether the effect was due to the group or individual effect of unemployment. Similarly, the country-level relationship between income inequality and health may have important policy implications regardless of whether it is due to a contextual effect of income inequality itself, or to the fact that more unequal countries tend to have more people in the lower-income categories.

It is often argued that ecological studies may be particularly useful when investigating the health effects of individual-level attributes with little within-group variation but large between-group variation. For example, if dietary fat is homogeneous within countries but varies greatly from country to country, an individual-level study restricted to individuals from a single country may find no association between dietary fat and cardiovascular disease, but an ecological study comparing country rates to country average fat intake may find a strong relationship. From this perspective, the advantage of the ecological study results purely from the fact that it is able to include more variability in the exposure of interest. The same research question could be addressed in a study of individuals that included individuals from different countries and thus ensured sufficient variation in the exposure. But often this option is not feasible, whereas country-level measures may be available from standard sources. Of course, the presence of significant between-country differences in diet raises the important question of why countries differ in diet to begin with, and suggests that the diet of individuals has important country-level determinants. Despite the potential advantage of increasing variability in the exposure of interest, ecological studies of diet and health outcomes are subject to the limitations of ecological studies outlined earlier in terms of the inability to control for individual-level variables which may vary from group to group and the possibility of confounding by other group-level variables.

Although they will not be discussed here in detail, studies with groups as the units of analysis are subject to many of the same analytical issues as individual-level studies with respect to confounding, establishment of temporality, selection biases, etc. In addition, these types of analyses raise additional methodological issues, such as the need to have adequate numbers of groups as well as enough individuals per group, the need to account for differences in the variability of outcomes (i.e. estimated rates) for the different groups due to the fact that they may be based on different numbers of observations, and the possibility of multicollinearity between the predictors examined (which is often more of a problem in ecological studies than in individual-level studies) (Morgenstern 1982). In addition, studies in which the units of analysis are geographic areas may need to use statistical methods to account for the fact that areas geographically closer to each other may tend to be more similar (in outcomes) than those more distant from each other (due to unmeasured factors that cluster in space), which leads to violation of the assumption of independence of observations (e.g. Clayton et al. 1993; Zhu et al. 2006).

Time-trend studies also raise additional methodological issues related to time-series analyses generally (Morgenstern 1995).

Studies with individuals as units of analysis

Individual-level studies are most appropriate when investigators are interested in drawing inferences regarding variability across individuals, and all potential constructs of interest can be conceptualized as individual-level properties. The most common epidemiological studies are of this type. The assumption is that all constructs relevant to the outcome being studied are individual-level constructs.

Studies with individuals as the units of analysis and with information limited to individual-level constructs cannot examine the role of group-level constructs as antecedents of individual-level variables, as independent predictors of outcomes, or as confounders of individual-level associations. They cannot determine whether the effect of a given individual-level variable is only present in certain group contexts, or varies from group to group, as a function of group characteristics. In order to answer these questions, other types of studies are needed.

Studies limited to individuals from a single group are clearly unable to examine the role of group-level constructs in causing the outcome (or in interacting with individual-level variables), because group-level properties are invariant within groups (Schwartz and Carpenter 1999). If group-level factors are important in causing the outcome, studies focused on a single group may fail to detect important disease determinants. In the dietary fat example mentioned earlier, we noted that a study based on individuals from a single country would not detect dietary fat as a risk factor if it were invariant within countries. More fundamentally, the country-level factors that influence large variations in fat intake across countries is the salient variable that the individual-level study could not capture.

If the study involves individuals from many different groups, relevant group-level properties may be included in individual-level analyses. For example, group-level variables can be included in regression equations with individuals as the units of analysis. These types of analyses have been called contextual analyses (Blalock 1984; Iversen 1991). Susser (1994) has referred to studies that investigate the effects of group-level variables on individual-level outcomes as mixed studies. A simple example of the type of regression models fitted in contextual analysis is shown in Equation 5.2.4:

$$Y_{ij} = \beta_0 + \beta_1 C_j + \beta_2 X_{ij} + e_{ij} \qquad (5.2.4)$$

where:

Y_{ij} = outcome for ith individual in jth group.

C_j = group-level variable.

X_{ij} = individual-level variable.

e_{ij} = error for ith individual in jth group.

Contextual models can include multiple group-level and individual-level variables as well as their interactions. In the model shown in Equation 5.2.4, β_1 estimates the effect of the group-level characteristic on the individual-level outcome (after adjustment for X_{ij}) and β_2 estimates the effect of the individual-level variable on the outcome (after adjustment for C_j). Contextual models

can be used, for example, to investigate the effects of neighbourhood context on fertility outcomes by including characteristics of the neighbourhoods where individuals live (derived or integral variables) together with individual-level characteristics in individual-level regression models.

In these models, special methods may be necessary to account for residual within-group correlations in individual-level outcomes. Ignoring this correlation may lead to incorrect estimates of standard errors (Diggle et al. 2002). Efficiency of estimation may also be reduced (Diggle et al. 2002). One common approach to account for within-group correlations is to use marginal models (Zeger et al. 1988), also referred to as population-average models (Diggle et al. 2002) or covariance pattern models (Brown and Prescott 1999). Marginal or population-average models model the population-average response as a function of covariates without explicitly accounting for heterogeneity across groups (Zeger et al. 1988). In contrast to the multilevel models described in the next subsection, marginal models do not allow examination of group-to-group variability per se, or of the factors associated with it. Neither do they allow decomposition of total variability in the individual-level outcome into within- and between-group components. Although contextual analysis can be used to simultaneously investigate the effects of group-level and individual-level constructs in shaping individual-level outcomes it does not allow examination of group-to-group variability per se, or of the factors associated with it. The unit of analysis remains the individual and only interindividual variation is examined.

Studies with both groups and individuals as the units of analysis (multilevel studies)

Multilevel studies and multilevel analysis have gained increasing recognition and use in several fields including education, sociology, and public health (Mason et al. 1983; Hermalin 1986; Paterson and Goldstein 1991; DiPrete and Forristal 1994; Duncan et al. 1998; Kreft and deLeeuw 1998; Diez Roux 2000, 2002; Raudenbush and Bryk 2002; Subramanian 2003; Bingenheimer and Raudenbush 2004). Multilevel studies simultaneously examine groups (or samples of groups) and individuals within them (or samples of individuals within them). Variability at both the group level and the individual level can be simultaneously examined and the role of group-level and individual-level constructs in explaining variation between individuals and between groups can be investigated. For example, a study may have information on a series of country-level characteristics (e.g. gross national product, inequality in the distribution of income) and on the individual-level characteristics of a sample of individuals within each country (including health outcomes). Researchers may be interested in investigating how country-level and individual-level factors are related to health outcomes, as well as the extent to which between-country and between-individual variability in the outcomes are explained by variables defined at both levels. Thus, multilevel analysis allows researchers to deal with the micro-level of individuals and the macro-level of groups or contexts simultaneously (Duncan et al. 1998). Multilevel models can be used to draw inferences regarding the causes of interindividual variation and the extent to which it is explained by individual-level or group-level variables, but inferences can also be made regarding intergroup variation, whether it exists in the data, and to what extent it is accounted for by group and individual-level characteristics.

In the case of multilevel analysis involving two levels (e.g. individuals nested within groups), the model can be conceptualized as a two-stage system of equations. The case for a normally distributed dependent variable is illustrated in Equation 5.2.5. For reasons of simplicity, the illustration will focus on the case of only one independent variable at the individual and one independent variable at the group level (although models can of course be extended to include as many independent variables as needed).

In the first stage, a separate individual-level regression is defined for each group.

$$Y_{ij} = \beta_{0j} + \beta_{1j}I_{ij} + e_{ij} \qquad e_{ij} \sim N(0, \sigma^2) \qquad (5.2.5)$$

where:

Y_{ij} = outcome variable for ith individual in jth group (or context).

I_{ij} = individual-level variable for ith individual in jth group (or context).

β_{0j} is the group-specific intercept.

β_{1j} is the group-specific effect of the individual-level variable.

Individual-level errors (e_{ij}) within each group are assumed to be independent and identically distributed with a mean of 0 and a variance of σ^2. Regression coefficients (β_{0j} and β_{1j}) are allowed to vary from one group to another.

In a second stage, each of the group or context-specific regression coefficients defined in Equation 5.2.1 (β_{0j} and β_{1j} in this example) are modelled as a function of group-level variables:

$$\beta_{0j} = \gamma_{00} + \gamma_{01}C_j + U_{0j} \qquad U_{0j} \sim N(0, \tau_{00}) \qquad (5.2.6)$$

$$\beta_{1j} = \gamma_{10} + \gamma_{11}C_j + U_{1j} \qquad U_{1j} \sim N(0, \tau_{11}) \qquad (5.2.7)$$

$$\text{cov}\left(U_{0j}, U_{1j}\right) = \tau_{10}$$

where:

C_j = group-level or contextual variable.

γ_{00} is the common intercept across groups (where C_j is 0).

γ_{01} is the effect of the group-level predictor on the group-specific intercepts.

γ_{10} is the common slope associated with the individual-level variable across groups (where C_j is 0).

γ_{11} is the effect of the group-level predictor on the group-specific slopes.

The errors in the group-level equations (U_{0j} and U_{1j}), sometimes called 'macro errors', are assumed to be normally distributed with mean 0 and variances τ_{00} and τ_{11} respectively. τ_{01} represents the covariance between intercepts and slopes; for example, if τ_{01} is positive, as the intercept increases the slope increases. Thus, multilevel analysis summarizes the distribution of the group-specific coefficients in terms of two parts: a 'fixed' part which is unchanging

across groups (γ_{00} and γ_{01} for the intercept, and γ_{10} and γ_{11} for the slope) and a 'random' part (U_{0j} for the intercept and U_{1j} for the slope) which is allowed to vary from group to group.

By including an error term in the group-level equations (Equations 5.2.6 and 5.2.7), these models allow for sampling variability in the group-specific coefficients (β_{0j} and β_{1j}) and also for the fact that that the group-level equations are not deterministic (i.e. the possibility that not all relevant macro-level variables have been included in the model) (Wong and Mason 1985). The underlying assumption is that group-specific intercepts and slopes are random samples from a normally distributed population of group-specific intercepts and slopes (or equivalently, that the groups or macro errors are 'exchangeable') (DiPrete and Forristal 1994).

An alternative way to present the model fitted in multilevel analysis is to substitute Equations 5.2.6 and 5.2.7 in Equation 5.2.5 to obtain:

$$Y_{ij} = \gamma_{00} + \gamma_{01}C_j + \gamma_{10}I_{ij} + \gamma_{11}C_jI_{ij} + U_{0j} + U_{1j}I_{ij} + e_{ij} \qquad (5.2.8)$$

The model includes the effects of group level variables (γ_{01}), individual-level variables (γ_{10}) and their interaction (γ_{11}) on the individual-level outcome Y_{ij}. It also includes a random intercept component (U_{0j}), and a random slope component (U_{1j}), which together with the individual-level errors e_{ij} compose a complex error structure. Because of the presence of this complex error structure, special estimation methods must be used. Although multilevel or random effects models were first developed for continuous dependent variables, analogous methods have been developed for other types of outcomes (Wong and Mason 1985; Raudenbush and Bryk 2002; Hox 2010, Snijders and Bosker 2011; Goldstein 2011).

By simultaneously including information on both groups and individuals, multilevel models avoid the limitations of ecological studies and individual-level studies outlined in the earlier section on fallacies. Both individuals and groups are units of analysis and both intergroup and interindividual variability can be examined. Multilevel studies thus provide an opportunity to link traditional ecological and individual-level studies. Multilevel models allow investigation of a variety of interrelated research questions. They allow separation of the effects of context (i.e. group characteristics) and of composition (characteristics of the individuals in groups): do groups differ in average outcomes after controlling for the characteristics of individuals within them? Are group-level variables related to outcomes after controlling for individual-level variables? Multilevel models can also be used to examine the effects of individual-level variables: are individual-level variables related to the outcome after controlling for group-level variables? Do individual-level associations vary from group to group, and is this partly a function of group-level variables? Multilevel models also allow quantification of variation at different levels (e.g. within group and between group) (Merlo et al. 2006) and the degrees to which these sources of variation are 'statistically explained' by individual-level and group-level variables. For example, is there significant variation in group-specific intercepts or slopes (do τ_{00} and τ_{11} differ significantly from 0)? How does this variability change as individual-level or group-level variables are added? What percentage of the variability in individual-level outcomes is between and within groups?

Table 5.2.5 Types of study design used in public health based on unit of analysis, level at which variability is examined, and constructs most appropriately investigated

Type of study	Unit of analysis	Level at which variability is examined	Constructs investigated as potential 'causes' of variability	
			Group level	**Individual level**
Ecological	Groups	Groups (utility for interindividual variability limited)	Yes	Only group-level proxies
Individual level	Individuals	Individuals (utility for intergroup variability limited)	No (Yes in contextual)	Yes
Multilevel	Groups and Individuals	Groups and Individuals	Yes	Yes

The types of studies, the levels at which variability is examined, and the types of constructs which they are more suited to investigate are summarized in Table 5.2.5.

Challenges in multilevel studies

The investigation of the health effects of factors defined at multiple levels raises a number of conceptual and methodological challenges. A key requirement is to begin with a clearly articulated conceptual model of the levels and constructs most relevant to the health outcome being investigated. A multiplicity of different nested (or non-nested) groups or levels may be relevant for a particular research question. Specifying the relevant levels is part of the development of the theory that should precede the data collection and statistical analysis. An important methodological complexity is that the variance apportioned to a given level in multilevel models may be over- or underestimated if a relevant level is ignored in the analysis (Subramanian 2003). In addition, misspecification of the relevant level may result in incorrectly concluding that groups (or higher-level) effects are absent. For example, if the research question pertains to the impact of availability of healthy foods on diet, and neighbourhoods within a country are specified as the higher-level unit for which food availability is measured, the absence of an effect of neighbourhood food availability could be entirely consistent with a large effect of country-level food availability. The failure to include the country level in the analyses would lead the researcher to miss the country-level food availability effect (this situation is directly analogous to the inability of studies restricted to individuals from a single group to detect group effects (Schwartz and Carpenter 1999)).

The 'groups' relevant to a specific health outcome may be difficult to define (e.g. neighbourhoods) or have fuzzy and changing boundaries (e.g. friendship groups). Data is often unavailable for the theoretically relevant group of interest so a crude proxy is used (e.g. census tracts for neighbourhoods) (Diez Roux 2001, 2007; O'Campo 2003). This results in substantial misspecification

of the group and the group-level construct of interest. Whereas epidemiology has become very sophisticated at measuring individual-level attributes, the measurement of group level has only recently received comparable attention. In some cases the measurement of group-level constructs may be simple (e.g. the presence of a certain law), but in others (e.g. social capital, the structure of social networks, or features of neighbourhoods), it is not. In some cases relevant group-level constructs can be easily characterized using available data, for example, the presence of a certain type of tobacco legislation or the degree of income inequality. Other constructs (e.g. levels of social cohesion) may benefit from the use of surveys. Survey data can be aggregated to the group-level using empirical Bayes approaches to improve the measurement validity (Raudenbush and Sampson 1999; Mujahid et al. 2007). This approach also allows assessment of the measurement properties of the aggregated survey measure, including the agreement between respondents within a group and the reliability of the group-level measure for discriminating between groups (Raudenbush 2003; Mujahid et al. 2007). Other measures of group-level constructs may involve approaches that do not necessarily involve aggregation of individual measures (e.g. the structure of connections between individuals within a group or the use of 'geographic information systems' to develop measures of neighbourhood availability and accessibility of resources). The most appropriate measurement strategy will depend on the construct being assessed as well as practical issues regarding the availability of data.

Because group-level factors must ultimately affect individuals in order to influence health, their effects must necessarily be mediated through more proximate individual-level processes. At the same time, some individual-level factors may be confounders of group-level effects either because individuals are selected into groups based on their individual-level attributes (e.g. persons with low income are selected into disadvantaged neighbourhoods) or because individual-level factors and group-level factors are associated for other reasons (e.g. persons living in countries characterized by mass production of processed foods may also be less physically active). Indeed much of the effort in the estimation of group-level effects in multilevel studies goes into controlling appropriately for individual-level confounders of group effects (Duncan et al. 1998; Pickett and Pearl 2001). Residual confounding by mismeasured or unmeasured individual-level variables has long been a critique of studies of group effects (Hauser 1970; Diez Roux 2001; Oakes 2004). On the other hand, many of these individual-level factors may be mediators of group effects raising questions regarding whether or not group-level effects should be adjusted for these factors (Macintyre and Ellaway 2003). It has been noted that the use of multiple regression approaches to partition indirect and direct effects (e.g. the portion of a group effect that is mediated through a given variable and the portion that is not) may lead to incorrect conclusions regarding the presence and strength of direct effects (Robins and Greenland 1992; Cole and Hernan 2002). The extent to which the approach of estimating a direct effect by comparing a group-level effect before and after adjusting for a hypothesized mediator results in substantial bias is likely to vary from research problem to research problem depending on the extent to which adjustment for the mediator actually introduces substantial confounding by other unmeasured variables related to the mediator and the outcome (Blakely 2002;

Blakely et al. 2013). An additional analytical complexity arises in longitudinal analyses where a given individual-level variable can be both a mediator and a confounder of the neighbourhood effect (because it is affected by prior neighbourhood conditions and in turn influences subsequent exposure to certain neighbourhood conditions). Special methods such as marginal structural models have been developed to estimate the causal effects under these circumstances (Robins 1989; Robins et al. 2000). The extension of these emerging methods to multilevel data structures has grown in recent years (Cerdá et al. 2010; Nandi et al. 2010). Recent work has also extended multilevel analytical strategies to account for other dependencies in the data such as those generated by spatial autocorrelation (Verbitsky and Raudenbush 2009).

Observational multilevel studies face the same problems as other observational studies in estimating causal effects from observational data. The ability to draw causal inferences is based on the extent to which the methods used approximate the counterfactual comparison of interest. One important limitation of past work in this regard especially prevalent in research on neighbourhood health effects has been the reliance on group-level derived variables (e.g. neighbourhood mean income) as proxies for the relevant integral group-level variable of interest (Diez Roux 2001; Pickett and Pearl 2001; Macintyre et al. 2002). This has limited the extent to which the data available allow researchers to approximate the counterfactual contrast of interest, even within the limitations of observational studies. Better specification of the group-level factors of interest (e.g. moving from crude proxies to measures of the specific constructs of interest) and the testing of specific hypotheses improve the ability to draw causal inferences.

The extent to which group-level effects can be validly estimated through the use of multiple regression methods (including multilevel models) to control for individual-level confounders has been questioned (Oakes 2004). The adjusted comparison requires assumptions regarding the effects of the individual-level variable on the outcome across groups, and may involve extrapolations beyond the support in the data if there is little overlap in the distribution of the individual-level variable across groups (e.g. individual-level income across levels of neighbourhood disadvantage). The extent to which this is a problem is an empirical question and may vary from research problem to research problem (Diez Roux 2004). This is no different from similar situations involved in adjusted comparisons in individual-level studies. Propensity score matching (Rubin 1997), which has been increasingly used in multilevel contexts, is one way to ensure that inferences are well supported (Harding 2003; Subramanian et al. 2007) although it has its own set of limitations related to generalizability of the results and also assumes no unmeasured confounding.

Another complexity in observational studies of group effects is that certain group-level properties may be at least partly endogenous to the characteristics of the individuals that make up the group (Subramanian 2003; Oakes 2004). This makes the identification of these group-level effects from observational data problematic. The extent to which group-level properties are endogenous to individual-level properties is likely to vary for different group-level constructs and different research questions (Diez Roux 2004; Subramanian 2004). Endogeneity may appear more of a problem in the case of derived group-level variables (e.g. mean neighbourhood income) that are constructed by aggregating the characteristics of individuals within a group. However, as noted above, these variables are often used as proxies for a more clearly exogenous integral group-level property. Endogeneity is also a possibility for some integral group-level variables (e.g. dietary habits of residents may influence neighbourhood availability of healthy foods). However, it is unlikely that all group-level attributes are fully endogenous to the individual characteristics of persons of which the group is composed. Strategies to at least partly deal with the problem of endogeneity in the multilevel context have been proposed (Subramanian 2004) but in situations where endogeneity is a major concern other analytical strategies more appropriate for the analysis of dynamic systems may be more appropriate (Auchincloss and Diez Roux 2008).

Finally, sample size and power calculations in multilevel studies are complex and remain an area of active research (Raudenbush and Liu 2000; Raudenbush and Bryk 2002; Hox 2010; Snijders and Bosker 2011; Myers et al. 2012). In general, the power for estimating the individual-level regression coefficients depends on the total sample size (Hox 2010). The power for higher-level (group-level) effects and cross-level interactions (interactions between group and individual-level variables) depends more strongly on the number of groups than on the total sample size (Hox 2010). However, the power to estimate the ratio of between-group to total variability (the intraclass correlation coefficient) is affected by the number of groups and the number of persons per group in a different manner than the power to detect associations of group-level variables with individual-level outcomes (the fixed effects of group properties) (Snijders and Bosker 2011). Power and sample size calculations need to specify the key multilevel parameters of interest, and trade-offs may be involved.

Conclusion

In public health research, both predictors and outcomes may be conceptualized at different levels of organization, and understanding outcomes at a given level may require taking into account information pertaining to levels above or below it. Each system can be thought of as nested within another level, and dynamically interrelated with the levels above and below it. In addition, each level may acquire 'emergent' properties, unique characteristics confined to that level, which are different to the properties of its components. The selection of the appropriate study design should be based on the specific research question investigated, including the level of organization about which inferences are to be made, as well as the levels of organizations of the constructs of interest (including the main independent variables as well as potential confounders or effect modifiers of the association).

Problems related to the use of ecological studies and ecological variables in epidemiology often result from confusion regarding the level of organization to which the research question pertains, the level of organization at which the constructs of interest are defined and measured, and the sometimes inappropriate use of variables defined and measured at one level to proxy constructs defined at another level. Of course researchers must necessarily focus on certain aspects of the continuum of levels of organization and not all studies need (or can) span all levels. Rather than defending or critiquing one study design in favour of another, it is more useful to evaluate whether the level of analysis investigated and the constructs examined are appropriate for the specific question being asked. Because 'ideal' study designs are often not possible, the key lies in determining whether the particular design employed is 'good enough' for the question being asked. The issues reviewed in this chapter may be helpful in making this judgement.

References

Alker, H. (1969). A typology of ecological fallacies. In M. Dogan and S. Rokkam (eds.) *Socila Ecology*, pp. 69–86. Boston, MA: MIT Press.

Auchincloss, A.H. and Diez Roux, A.V. (2008). A new tool for epidemiology: the usefulness of dynamic-agent models in understanding place effects on health. *American Journal of Epidemiology*, 168(1), 1–8.

Benach, J., Yasui, Y., Borrell, C., Sáez, M., and Pasarin, M.I. (2001). Material deprivation and leading causes of death by gender: evidence from a nationwide small area study. *Journal of Epidemiology and Community Health*, 55(4), 239–45.

Bingenheimer, J.B. and Raudenbush, S.W. (2004). Statistical and substantive inferences in public health: issues in the application of multilevel models. *Annual Review of Public Health*, 25, 53–77.

Blakely, T. (2002). Commentary: estimating direct and indirect effects—fallible in theory, but in the real world? *International Journal of Epidemiology*, 31(1), 166–7.

Blakely, T., McKenzie, S., and Carter, K. (2013). Misclassification of the mediator matters when estimating indirect effects. *Journal of Epidemiology and Community Health*, 67(5), 458–66.

Blakely, T.A. and Woodward, A.J. (2000). Ecological effects in multi-level studies. *Journal of Epidemiology and Community Health*, 54(5), 367–74.

Blalock, H. (1984). Contextual-effects models: theoretical and methodological issues. *Annual Review of Sociology*, 10, 353–72.

Blau, P.M. (1960). Structural effects. *American Sociological Review*, 25, 178–93.

Brenner, H., Savitz, D.A., Jöckel, K.H., et al. (1992). The effects of nondifferential misclassification in ecologic studies. *Epidemiology*, 3, 85–95.

Brown, H. and Prescott, R. (1999). *Applied Mixed Models in Medicine*. New York: Wiley.

Cerdá, M., Diez-Roux, A.V., Tchetgen, E.T., Gordon-Larsen, P., and Kiefe, C. (2010). The relationship between neighborhood poverty and alcohol use: estimation by marginal structural models. *Epidemiology*, 21(4), 482–9.

Chadwick, E. (1965). *Report on the Sanitary Conditions of the Labouring Population of Great Britain*. Edinburgh: Edinburgh University Press.

Clayton, D.G., Bernardinelli, L., and Montomoli, C. (1993). Spatial correlation in ecological analysis. *International Journal of Epidemiology*, 22(6), 1193–202.

Cole, S.R. and Hernan, M.A. (2002). Fallibility in estimating direct effects. *International Journal of Epidemiology*, 31(1), 163–5.

Diez-Roux, A.V. (1998). Bringing context back into epidemiology: variables and fallacies in multilevel analysis. *American Journal of Public Health*, 88(2), 216–22.

Diez Roux, A.V. (2000). Multilevel analysis in public health research. *Annual Review of Public Health*, 21, 171–92.

Diez Roux, A.V. (2001). Investigating neighborhood and area effects on health. *American Journal of Public Health*, 91(11), 1783–9.

Diez Roux, A.V. (2002). A glossary for multilevel analysis. *Journal of Epidemiology and Community Health*, 56(8), 588–94.

Diez Roux, A.V. (2004a). Estimating neighborhood health effects: the challenges of causal inference in a complex world. *Social Science & Medicine*, 58(10), 1953–60.

Diez Roux, A.V. (2004b). The study of group-level factors in epidemiology: rethinking variables, study designs, and analytical approaches. *Epidemiologic Reviews*, 26, 104–11.

Diez Roux, A.V. (2007). Neighborhoods and health: where are we and where do we go from here? *Revue d'épidémiologie et de santé publique*, 55(1), 13–21.

Diggle, P.J., Heagerty, P.J., Liang, K.Y., and Zeger, S.L. (2002). *Analysis of Longitudinal Data*. New York: Oxford University Press.

DiPrete, T.A. and Forristal, J.D. (1994). Multilevel models: methods and substance. *Annual Review of Sociology*, 20, 331–57.

Duncan, C., Jones, K., and Moon, G. (1998). Context, composition and heterogeneity: using multilevel models in health research. *Social Science & Medicine*, 46(1), 97–117.

Firebaugh, G. (1978). A rule for inferring individual-level relationships from aggregate data. *American Sociological Review*, 43, 557–72.

Goldberger, J., Wheeler, G.A., and Sydenstricker, E. (1920). A study of the relation of factors of a sanitary character to pellagra incidence in seven cotton-mill villages of South Carolina in 1916. *Public Health Reports*, 35, 1701–24.

Goldstein, H. (2011). *Multilevel Statistical Models* (4th ed.). London: Wiley.

Greenland, S. (1992). Divergent biases in ecologic and individual-level studies. *Statistics in Medicine*, 11, 1209–23.

Greenland, S. (2001). Ecologic versus individual-level sources of bias in ecologic estimates of contextual health effects. *International Journal of Epidemiology*, 30, 1343–50.

Greenland, S. and Morgenstern, H. (1989). Ecological bias, confounding, and effect modification. *International Journal of Epidemiology*, 18(1), 269–74.

Greenland, S. and Robins, J. (1994). Ecologic studies – biases, misconceptions, and counter-examples. *American Journal of Epidemiology*, 139, 747–60.

Halloran, M.E. and Struchiner, C.J. (1991). Study designs for dependent happenings. *Epidemiology*, 2(5), 331–8.

Hammond, J. (1973). Two sources of error in ecological correlations. *American Sociological Review*, 38, 764–77.

Harding, D. (2003). Counterfactual models of neighborhood effects: the effect of neighborhood poverty on high school dropout and teenage pregnancy. *American Journal of Sociology*, 109, 676–719.

Hauser, R. (1970). Context and consex: a cautionary tale. *American Journal of Sociology*, 75, 645–64.

Hermalin, A. (1986). The multilevel approach: theory and concepts. *Population Studies Addendum Manual IX*, 66, 15–31.

Hox, J. J. (2010). *Multilevel Analysis: Techniques and Applications* (2nd ed.). New York: Hogrefe and Huber.

Iversen, G. (1991). *Contextual Analysis*. Newbury Park, CA: Sage Publications.

Janghorbani, M., Jones, R.B., and Nelder, R. (2006). Neighbourhood deprivation and excess coronary heart disease mortality and hospital admissions in Plymouth, UK: an ecological study. *Acta Cardiologica*, 61(3), 313–20.

Kawachi, I., Kennedy, B.P., and Glass, R. (1999). Social capital and self-rated health: a contextual analysis. *American Journal of Public Health*, 89(8), 1187–93.

Keys, A. (1980). *Seven Countries: A Multivariate Analysis of Death and Coronary Heart Disease*. Cambridge, MA: Harvard University Press.

King, G. (1997). *A Solution to the Ecological Inference Problem. Reconstructing Individual Behavior from Aggregate Data*. Princeton, NJ: Princeton University Press.

Koopman, J.S. and Longini, I.M. Jr. (1994). The ecological effects of individual exposures and nonlinear disease dynamics in populations. *American Journal of Public Health*, 84(5), 836–42.

Koopman, J.S., Longini, I.M. Jr., Jacquez, J., et al. (1991). Assessing risk factors for transmission of infection. *American Journal of Epidemiology*, 133(12), 1199–209.

Koopman, J.S. and Lynch, J.W. (1999). Individual causal models and population system models in epidemiology. *American Journal of Public Health*, 89(8), 1170–4.

Koopman, J.S., Prevots, D.R., Vaca Marin, M.A., et al. (1991). Determinants and predictors of dengue infection in Mexico. *American Journal of Epidemiology*, 133(11), 1168–78.

Kreft, I. and deLeeuw, J. (1998). *Introducing Multilevel Modeling*. London: Sage.

Lazarsfeld, P. and Menzel, H. (1971). On the relation between individual and collective properties. In A. Etzioni (ed.) *A Sociological Reader on*

Complex Organizations, pp. 499–516. New York: Holt, Rinehart, and Winston Inc.

Levin, B. (1995). Annotation: accounting for the effects of both group- and individual-level variables in community-level studies. *American Journal of Public Health*, 85, 163–4.

Lynch, J., Due, P., Muntaner, C., and Smith, G.D. (2000). Social capital—is it a good investment strategy for public health? *Journal of Epidemiology and Community Health*, 54(6), 404–8.

Lynch, J., Harper, S., and Davey Smith, G. (2003). Commentary: plugging leaks and repelling boarders—where to next for the SS income inequality? *International Journal of Epidemiology*, 32(6), 1029–36; discussion 1037–40.

Macintyre, S. and Ellaway, A. (2000). Ecological approaches: rediscovering the role of the physical and social environment. In L. Berkman and I. Kawachi (eds.) *Social Epidemiology*, pp. 332–48. New York: Oxford University Press.

Macintyre, S. and Ellaway, A. (2003). Neighborhoods and health: an overview. In I. Kawachi and L. Berkman (eds.) *Neighborhoods and Health*, pp. 20–44. New York: Oxford University Press.

Macintyre, S., Wong, G., and Entwisle, B. (2002). Place effects on health: how can we conceptualise, operationalise and measure them? *Social Science & Medicine*, 55(1), 125–39.

Mason, W., Wong, G., and Entwisle, B. (1983). Contextual analysis through the multilevel linear model. In S. Leinhardt (ed.) *Sociological Methodology*, pp. 72–103. San Francisco, CA: Jossey Bass.

Merlo, J., Chaix, B., Ohlsson, H., et al. (2006). A brief conceptual tutorial of multilevel analysis in social epidemiology: using measures of clustering in multilevel logistic regression to investigate contextual phenomena. *Journal of Epidemiology and Community Health*, 60(4), 290–7.

Morgenstern, H. (1982). Uses of ecologic analysis in epidemiologic research. *American Journal of Public Health*, 72(12), 1336–44.

Morgenstern, H. (1995). Ecologic studies in epidemiology: concepts, principles, and methods. *Annual Review of Public Health*, 16, 61–81.

Mujahid, M.S., Diez Roux, A.V., Morenoff, J.D., and Raghunathan, T. (2007). Assessing the measurement properties of neighborhood scales: from psychometrics to ecometrics. *American Journal of Epidemiology*, 165(8), 858–67.

Myers, N.D., Brincks, A.M., Ames, A.J., Prado, G.J., Penedo, F.J., and Benedict, C. (2012). Multilevel modeling in psychosomatic medicine research. *Psychosomatic Medicine*, 74(9), 925–36.

Nandi, A., Glass, T.A., Cole, S.R., et al. (2010). Neighborhood poverty and injection cessation in a sample of injection drug users. *American Journal of Epidemiology*, 171(4), 391–8.

Oakes, J.M. (2004). The (mis)estimation of neighborhood effects: causal inference for a practicable social epidemiology. *Social Science & Medicine*, 10, 1929–52.

O'Campo, P. (2003). Invited commentary: advancing theory and methods for multilevel models of residential neighborhoods and health. *American Journal of Epidemiology*, 157(1), 9–13.

Paterson, L. and Goldstein, H. (1991). New statistical methods for analysing social structures: an introduction to multilevel models. *British Educational Research Journal*, 17, 387–93.

Piantadosi, S. (1994). Invited commentary: ecologic biases. *American Journal of Epidemiology*, 139(8), 761–4; discussion 769–71.

Piantadosi, S., Byar, D.P., and Green, S.P. (1988). The ecological fallacy. *American Journal of Epidemiology*, 127(5), 893–904.

Pickett, K.E. and Pearl, M. (2001). Multilevel analyses of neighbourhood socioeconomic context and health outcomes: a critical review. *Journal of Epidemiology and Community Health*, 55(2), 111–22.

Raudenbush, S. (2003). The quantitative assessment of neighborhood social environments. In I. Kawachi and L. Berkman (eds.) *Neighborhoods and Health*, pp. 112–31. New York: Oxford University Press.

Raudenbush, S. and Bryk, A.S. (2002). Applications in organizational research. In *Hierarchical Linear Models: Applications and Data Analysis Methods*, pp. 99–159. Thousand Oaks, CA: Sage.

Raudenbush, S.W. and Liu, X. (2000). Statistical power and optimal design for multisite randomized trials. *Psychological Methods*, 5(2), 199–213.

Raudenbush, S.W. and Sampson, R.J. (1999). Ecometrics: toward a science of assessing ecological settings, with application to the systematic social observation of neighborhoods. *Sociological Methodology*, 29, 1–41.

Riley, M. (1963). Special problems of sociological analysis. In *Sociological Research I: A Case Approach*, pp. 700–25. New York: Harcourt, Brace, and World Inc.

Robins, J. (1989). The control of confounding by intermediate variables. *Statistics in Medicine*, 8(6), 679–701.

Robins, J.M. and Greenland, S. (1992). Identifiability and exchangeability for direct and indirect effects. *Epidemiology*, 3(2), 143–55.

Robins, J.M., Hernan, M.A., and Brumback, B. (2000). Marginal structural models and causal inference in epidemiology. *Epidemiology*, 11(5), 550–60.

Robinson, W. (1950). Ecological correlations and the behavior of individuals. *American Sociological Review*, 15, 351–7.

Ross, R. (1916). An application of the theory of probabilities to the study of a priori pathometry. Part I. *Proceedings of the Royal Society Series A*, 92, 204–30.

Rubin, D.B. (1997). Estimating causal effects from large data sets using propensity scores. *Annals of Internal Medicine*, 127(8 Pt 2), 757–63.

Scheuch, E. (1969). Social context and individual behavior. In M. Dogan and S. Rokkam (eds.) *Social Ecology*, pp. 133–55. Boston, MA: MIT Press.

Schwartz, S. (1994). The fallacy of the ecological fallacy: the potential misuse of a concept and its consequences. *American Journal of Public Health*, 84, 819–24.

Schwartz, S. and Carpenter, K.M. (1999). The right answer for the wrong question: consequences of type III error for public health research. *American Journal of Public Health*, 89(8), 1175–80.

Snijders, T.A.B. and Bosker, R.J. (2011). *Multilevel Analysis: An Introduction to Basic and Advanced Multilevel Modeling* (2nd ed.). London: Sage.

Subramanian, S. and Kawachi, I. (2003). Response: in defence of the income inequality hypothesis. *International Journal of Epidemiology*, 32(6), 1037–40.

Subramanian, S.V. (2004). The relevance of multilevel statistical methods for identifying causal neighborhood effects. *Social Science & Medicine*, 58(10), 1961–7.

Subramanian, S.V., Glymour, M.M., and Kawachi, I. (2007). Identifying causal ecologic effects on health: a methodological assessment. In S. Galea (ed.) *Macrosocial Determinants of Health*, pp. 301–32. New York: Springer Media.

Subramanian, S.V., Jones, K., and Duncan, C. (2003). Multilevel methods for public health research. In I. Kawachi and L. Berkman (eds.) *Neighborhoods and Health*, pp. 65–111. New York, Oxford University Press.

Subramanian, S.V., Jones, K., Kaffour, A., and Krieger, N. (2009) Revisiting Robinson: the perils of individualistic and ecologic fallacy. *International Journal of Epidemiology*, 38, 342–60.

Susser, E. and Wanderling, J. (1994). Epidemiology of nonaffective acute remitting psychosis versus schizophrenia: sex and sociocultural setting. *Archives of General Psychiatry*, 51, 294–301.

Susser, M. (1973). *Causal Thinking in the Health Sciences*. New York: Oxford University Press.

Susser, M. (1994a). The logic in ecological: I. The logic of analysis. *American Journal of Public Health*, 84(5), 825–9.

Susser, M. (1994b). The logic in ecological: II. The logic of design. *American Journal of Public Health*, 84(5), 830–5.

Terris, M. (1964). *Goldberger on Pellagra*. Baton Rouge, LA: Louisiana State University Press.

Townsend, P., Phillimore, P., and Beattie, A. (1988). *Health and Deprivation. Inequality and the North*. London: Routledge.

Valkonen, T. (1969). Individual and structural effects in ecological research. In M. Dogan and S. Rokkam (eds.) *Social Ecology*, pp. 53–68. Boston, MA: MIT Press.

Van den Eeden, P. and Huttner H.J. (1982). Multi-level research. *Current Sociology*, 30, 1–178.

Verbitsky Savitz, N. and Raudenbush, S.W. (2009). Exploiting spatial dependence to improve measurement of neighborhood social processes. *Sociological Methodology*, 39, 151–83.

Von Korff, M., Koepsell, T., Curry, S., and Diehr, P. (1992). Multi-level research in epidemiologic research on health behaviors and outcomes. *American Journal of Epidemiology*, 135, 1077–82.

Wakefield, J. (2008). Ecologic studies revisited. *Annual Review of Public Health*, 29, 75–90.

Wakefield, J. and Haneuse S. (2008). Overcoming ecologic bias using the two-phase study design. *American Journal of Epidemiology*, 167, 908–16.

Wing, S., Barnett, E., Casper, M., and Tyroler, H.A. (1992). Geographic and socioeconomic variation in the onset of decline of coronary heart disease mortality in white women. *American Journal of Public Health*, 82(2), 204–9.

Wong, G. and Mason, W. (1985). The hierarchical logistic regression model for multilevel analysis. *Journal of the American Statistical Association*, 80, 513–24.

Zeger, S.L., Liang, K.Y., and Albert, P.S. (1988). Models for longitudinal data: a generalized estimating equation approach. *Biometrics*, 44(4), 1049–60.

Zhu, L., Gorman, D.M., and Horel, S. (2006). Hierarchical Bayesian spatial models for alcohol availability, drug 'hot spots' and violent crime. *International Journal of Health Geographics*, 5, 54.

5.3

Cross-sectional studies

Manolis Kogevinas and Leda Chatzi

Introduction to cross-sectional studies

Cross-sectional studies examine the relationship between diseases (or other health-related characteristics) and other variables of interest as they exist in a defined population at a particular point in time (Last 2001). They could be defined as studies taking a snapshot of a society. Synonyms used for cross-sectional include prevalence studies and disease frequency studies.

The principal characteristic of cross-sectional studies is that they provide information on the *prevalence* of disease, that is, they include prevalent cases. In cross-sectional studies, exposure and disease are measured at the same point in time but this characteristic is shared by other epidemiological designs, for example, case–control studies. In many cross-sectional studies information on past exposures is not collected but this should not be regarded as a characteristic defining these studies. The outcome measured in cross-sectional studies can be a continuous variable such as blood pressure or forced expiratory volume in 1 second (FEV_1), as compared to a dichotomous outcome measured in case–control studies and, in most occasions, in cohort studies.

As is frequently the case in epidemiology, studies may use mixed designs. For example, a cross-sectional study may measure a biomarker referring to current exposure (e.g. vitamin E), may request information for the past (e.g. use of health services the last year), may identify older and recent cases (e.g. subjects having had asthma in childhood or those having their first attack of asthma in the last few months), and may convert into a cohort study if subjects included in the cross-sectional studies are followed up. The statistical analysis of cross-sectional studies depends on their hybrid design and is frequently similar to that of a case–control study using logistic regression and calculating (prevalence) odds ratios. Cross-sectional studies are extensively used to measure the prevalence of disease, exposures, or other health-related variables. On these occasions, the representativeness of the studied sample is a prerequisite.

In this chapter we will first describe the uses of cross-sectional studies in epidemiological and public health research and then discuss methodological issues concerning the design, the main biases of these studies including response rates, and how to improve participation in the studies. We will finally discuss issues related to the statistical analysis of cross-sectional studies. Many of these issues are also relevant to other epidemiological designs.

Uses of cross-sectional studies

Cross-sectional studies have been used to evaluate the prevalence of diseases and of health-related variables and also to evaluate the aetiology of diseases. Large, multipurpose, national cross-sectional studies are conducted in several countries for administrative reasons and to provide background documentation on the health status of a population.

National multipurpose surveys

National (or regional) multipurpose surveys are carried out routinely or ad hoc in several countries. The purpose and themes of these surveys are multiple and they may cover different health problems in successive years. The Health Survey in England collects data from a representative sample of approximately 8000 adults aged 16 and over and 2000 children in England (Department of Health 2012). Each year the survey consists of a series of core elements and also includes special topics. In 2012 the core survey covered general health, smoking, drinking, fruit and vegetable consumption, height, weight, blood pressure measurements, and collected blood and saliva samples. Special topics included were cardiovascular disease, hypertension, diabetes, social care, drinking, chronic pain, adult and child obesity, and information on well-being and dental health.

The National Health and Nutrition Examination Survey (NHANES) in the United States is the largest national multipurpose survey and is conducted on a routine basis (Centers for Disease Control and Prevention 2014). The NHANES is a programme of studies designed to assess the health and nutritional status of the civilian, non-institutionalized population of the United States. The survey examines a nationally representative sample of about 5000 persons each year and combines interviews and physical examinations.

Results of national health surveys can be used for several purposes, such as the evaluation of the prevalence of health-related behaviours or of symptoms, time trends in risk factors or health symptoms, the identification of causes of disease, and evaluation of health needs. Changes of health problems and risk factors in the population over time can be identified through repeated surveys. Repeated national multipurpose surveys may examine a sample of the same population, but not intentionally the same individuals. Thus, they are particularly useful for assessing changes in the same community, state, or nationally which may have undergone changes due to other factors, such as access to healthcare or population mixes. This type of information may allow health planning through the identification of needs and effectiveness of existing policies and interventions. Time trends in obesity and in levels of toxic substances such as lead in blood are examples of the use of these types of surveys. The prevalence of overweight and obesity has increased in recent years in both children and adults in many countries. Time trends and the effect of socioeconomic status on childhood obesity in the United States were examined using data from two large, nationally representative health surveys and data systems: the 1976–2008 National Health and Nutrition Examination Surveys (NHANES) and the 2003 and 2007 National Survey of Children's Health (NSCH) (Singh and Kogan 2010). The prevalence of overweight and obese children increased significantly in relation to decreased levels of household education and income in both 2003 and 2007 (Fig. 5.3.1). The prevalence of obesity for children with parents having fewer than 12 years of education was 30 per cent in 2007 compared to around 10 per cent for children whose parents had a college degree. The socioeconomic health disparities became wider in the period examined (Fig. 5.3.1).

The existence of a large national database has several advantages for the identification or confirmation of risk factors of a disease. Problems of cross-sectional studies that evaluate risk factors of diseases are discussed in the next section and particularly potential biases from the inclusion of prevalent cases and from frequent lack of information on past exposures. However, the evaluation of a national representative population sample, as is the case in several multipurpose surveys, has the advantage of capturing a global image of the society including population groups that may be omitted in other types of design. An example provided here is of a study on cleaners based on NHANES. The importance of this study lies, among others, in the fact that domestic cleaners are a population group that is very hard to identify through the usual designs applied, that in this case of occupational asthma would be industry-based cohorts.

Information on the population distribution of health problems and risk factors, provide important clues to researchers on the causes of disease and also may confirm previous hypotheses in large population samples. Arif and colleagues used data from the Third National Health and Nutrition Examination Survey (NHANES III) 1988–1994, to evaluate associations between occupation and work-related asthma and work-related wheezing among US workers (Arif et al. 2003). They identified several occupations that were at risk of developing work-related asthma with cleaners and equipment cleaners showing the highest risks. The population attributable risk for work-related asthma was 26 per cent. The study confirmed a previous hypothesis on asthma in cleaners (Kogevinas et al. 1999), provided an evaluation of asthma risk in other occupations in the US population, and also gave an estimate of the burden of occupational asthma.

By identifying the healthcare needs of the population, government agencies and private sector organizations can establish policies and plan research, education, and health promotion programmes that will help improve present health status and prevent future health problems.

Studies examining the prevalence of disease

Cross-sectional studies are, by definition, the appropriate design to evaluate the prevalence of diseases. An evaluation of the prevalence of a disease may be performed for administrative purposes or for reasons related to the evaluation of aetiological factors. The main issues regarding the conduct of these studies include the representativeness of the sample, the size of the sample, and the measurement of outcomes and exposures. The International Study of Asthma and Allergies in Childhood (ISAAC) is among the largest cross-sectional studies ever done.

The ISAAC study was designed to allow comparisons of the prevalence of allergic disorders in childhood between populations in different countries and their trends over time (Asher et al. 1995). In the early 1990s although it was generally perceived that asthma prevalence was increasing there existed very limited population-based estimates. The study included simple 'core' instruments for measuring the prevalence of allergic disorders, suitable for different geographical locations and languages: (1) written questionnaires on the prevalence and severity of asthma, rhinitis, and eczema for self-completion in 13–14-year-olds, or for completion by parents of 6–7-year-olds; and (2) video questionnaires on the prevalence and severity of asthma for self-completion by 13–14-year-old children. In phase I, children aged 13–14 years were studied in 155 centres in 56 countries (n = 463,801) and children aged 6–7 years were studied in 91 centres in 38 countries (n = 257,800) (Anonymous 1998). Up to 20-fold variations in the prevalence of 'current wheeze' (in the last 12 months) were observed between centres worldwide (range 1.8–36.7 per cent), with a sevenfold variation observed between the 10th and 90th percentiles (4.4 per cent; 30.9 per cent). The highest 12-month period prevalences were from centres in the United Kingdom, Australia, New Zealand, and the Republic of Ireland; the lowest prevalences were from centres in Eastern Europe, Albania, Greece, China, Taiwan, Uzbekistan, India, Indonesia, and Ethiopia.

Aetiological research

Cross-sectional studies are particularly valuable for the investigation of the aetiology of non-fatal diseases, degenerative diseases, diseases with no clear point of onset, for example, chronic

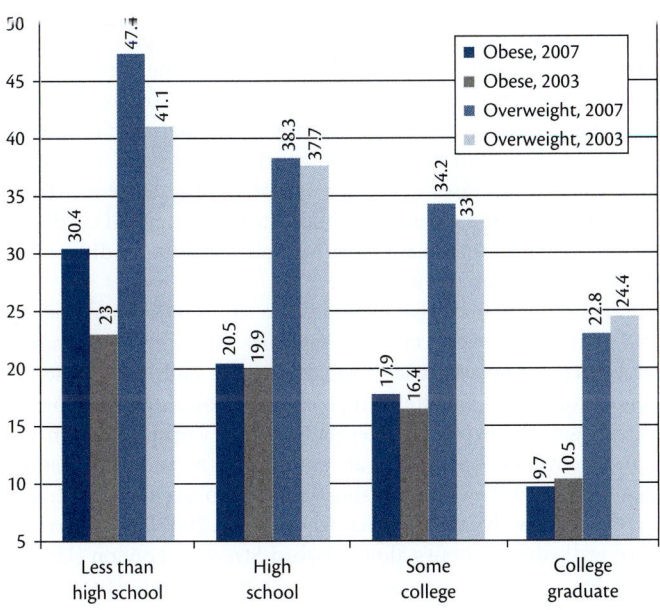

Fig. 5.3.1 Trends in the prevalence of overweight and obese children aged 10–17 years by parental education, United States, 2003–2007.
Reproduced from Singh, G.K. and Kogan, M.D., *Childhood Obesity in the United States, 1976–2008: Trends and Current Racial/Ethnic, Socioeconomic, and Geographic Disparities: A 75th Anniversary Publication*, Health Resources and Services Administration, Maternal and Child Health Bureau, Department of Health and Human Services, Rockville, Maryland, USA, 2010, available at: http://www.hrsa.gov/healthit/images/mchb_obesity_pub.pdf.

bronchitis, and effects on physiological variables, for example, forced vital capacity (FVC) or liver enzyme levels. In diseases with no clear point of onset it is difficult to identify incident cases and conduct cohort or incident case–control studies. The prevalence of a disease will be highest if it occurs relatively frequently and if the disease persists in time. A disease could be described as persistent if it is not rapidly fatal and if it does not usually manifest as a transitory condition. Diseases such as asthma and osteoarthritis that have a relatively high prevalence have frequently been examined in cross-sectional studies.

The European Community Respiratory Health Survey (ECRHS) is in many aspects similar in design to ISAAC and was initially conducted as an international cross-sectional study enrolling young adults mainly from European centres to evaluate the prevalence and aetiology of asthma and related diseases (Burney et al. 1994). In an initial screening short questionnaire, the ECRHS included information from around 140,000 individuals from 22 countries. A subsample of the study incorporated extensive questionnaires, measurement of atopic markers, spirometry, and methacholine challenge. The key findings of the study are the large geographical differences in the prevalence of asthma, atopy, and bronchial responsiveness in adults, with high prevalence rates in English-speaking countries and low prevalence rates in the Mediterranean region and Eastern Europe. Analyses of risk factors have highlighted the importance of occupational exposure for asthma in adulthood (Kogevinas et al. 1999). The association between sensitization to individual allergens and bronchial responsiveness was strongest for indoor allergens (mite and cat). Analysis of treatment practices has confirmed that the treatment of asthma varies widely between countries and that asthma is often undertreated (Janson et al. 2001). Subjects were subsequently followed up and the study was converted into a prospective study including subjects with and without asthma at the initial contact.

Design of cross-sectional studies

Main design issues in cross-sectional studies

The simplest form of a survey in a population is a one-time measurement of the prevalence of a disease (Checkoway et al. 2004). On some occasions, repeated surveys (panel studies) are conducted on the same or different individuals.

When evaluating the prevalence of a disease the sample studied should be representative of the base population from where subjects are recruited (internal validity). The random error of an estimate depends directly on the size of the study and standard techniques exist to calculate this error (see, e.g., free software such as Epi Info™ (Centers for Disease Control and Prevention (2013)). The measurement of outcomes may be particularly complicated since frequently prevalence studies are conducted for diseases that have a gradual onset and that are not fatal. In addition, problems may occur when comparisons of prevalence are done between countries that may have different systems for the identification of the disease or even different perceptions and oral descriptions of a disease. An example of this refers to the large prevalence studies conducted for the evaluation of the prevalence of children's asthma such as the ISAAC study (see earlier description). Wheezing is a key symptom defining asthma in childhood. However the perception of what is wheezing is not necessarily the same in different

countries and, further, some languages do not have a single word to describe what in English is called 'wheezing'.

Generalizability is another aspect of representativeness and refers to whether the findings in one population can be extrapolated to other populations (external validity). Generalizability is less of a problem when examining risk factors of disease since biological mechanisms through which an agent may provoke disease tend to be similar between populations. Generalizability may be, however, more difficult to ensure when examining prevalence since this may vary considerably within and between populations and extrapolations from one population to another can be problematic.

Panel studies apply a hybrid design that combines cross-sectional and cohort study methods. They are series of cross-sectional studies performed over time on the same group of individuals (measuring, however, prevalence rather than incidence), or in different groups of a population in subsequent time periods. The objective is to evaluate change in health status in relation to changes in exposure. Small groups, or panels, of individuals are followed over short time intervals, and health outcomes, exposure, and potential confounders are ascertained for each subject on one or more occasions. This design is especially useful for the study of physiological variables (i.e. pulmonary function, blood pressure), for which changes over several years may indicate early stages of disease processes. It is also useful to evaluate time trends in a disease.

The third phase of the ISAAC study (ISAAC, phase III) could be regarded as one form of a panel study. ISAAC-III was a repetition of the phase I survey after 5–10 years to examine time trends in the prevalence of allergic disorders in the same ages in centres and countries that participated in ISAAC phase I. The findings from ISAAC phase III indicate that international differences in asthma symptom prevalence have reduced with decreases in prevalence in English-speaking countries and Western Europe and increases in prevalence in regions where prevalence was previously low (Fig. 5.3.2). Although there was little change in the overall prevalence of current wheeze, the percentage of children reported to have had asthma increased significantly, possibly reflecting greater awareness of this condition and/or changes in diagnostic practice. The increases in asthma symptom prevalence in Africa, Latin America, and parts of Asia indicate that the global burden of asthma is continuing to rise, but the global prevalence differences are lessening (Pearce et al. 2007).

Panel studies may also evaluate the same individuals before and after an intervention or an exposure. These types of studies have been extensively used in occupational and environmental epidemiology to evaluate changes in symptoms or physiological parameters following an intervention in a workplace or in the general environment such as air pollution. An example is a study that examined the effects of short-term exposure to diesel traffic in 60 adults with asthma (McCreanor et al. 2007). Each participant walked for 2 hours along Oxford Street in London (United Kingdom) and, on a separate occasion, through Hyde Park, London. Physiological and immunological measurements were performed after each occasion. It was found that walking for 2 hours on Oxford Street induced consistent reductions of up to 6.1 per cent in FEV_1 and up to 5.4 per cent in FVC that were significantly larger than the reductions in FEV_1 and FVC after exposure in Hyde Park. Similar changes were also observed for markers of inflammation in the lungs.

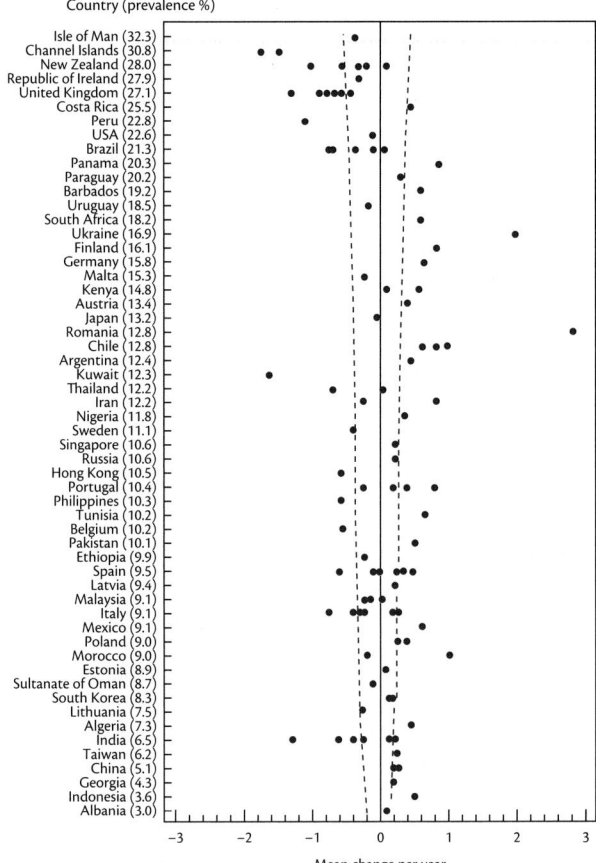

Country (prevalence %)

Fig. 5.3.2 Ranking plot showing the change per year in prevalence of current wheeze (wheeze in the past 12 months) in children aged 13–14 years for each centre by country, ISAAC-III study.

Reproduced from Pearce, N. et al., Worldwide trends in the prevalence of asthma symptoms: phase III of the International Study of Asthma and Allergies in Childhood (ISAAC), *Thorax*, Volume 62, Issue 9, pp. 758–66, ©2007, with permission from BMJ Publishing Group Ltd.

Panel studies, particularly when examining the same individuals, could be regarded as prospective studies and frequently this distinction between study designs is blurred. The study in Oxford Street is a cross-over study that includes aspects of a prospective experimental design and aspects of a cross-sectional study. The main difference between cross-sectional panel studies and prospective designs is that panel studies examine the prevalence of a disease or a physiological parameter rather than incidence.

Sampling and response rates

Cross-sectional studies aiming to identify the prevalence of a specific factor in a community should select a representative sample of that community. The same is, in principle, desirable in cohort and case–control studies but in these studies the main issue is internal validity rather than external validity (generalizability representativeness). In cohort studies the most important issue concerning subject selection and validity of results is completeness of follow-up. In case–control studies the crucial issue concerning selection of subjects is that cases and controls should be selected from the same study base; whether cases are representative of the general population is, by contrast, not crucial for the internal validity of a case–control study.

In a cross-sectional study, however, representative sampling is the only procedure that allows selection of subjects in a population that can be used as the basis of generalization. A sampling frame should be identified that allows the identification of any subject in a population that could be included in a sample. Different methods can then be applied to select the subjects. Sampling error estimation has been exhaustively addressed in statistics. This depends on the number of subjects included in a study and can be estimated. Non-sampling error refers to bias, and may be of considerably higher importance than sampling error. Enlarging the sample does not reduce non-sampling error. Non-response may be non-random and may, therefore, be related to factors of interest for a study such as education, ethnicity, or obesity.

Response rates and dealing with non-response

A response rate of 60 per cent has been frequently accepted as an adequate response in population surveys. However, the issue of non-response is complex and the acceptance of a fixed percentage as an adequate and probably unbiased response rate is an oversimplification. To some extent, this seems similar to the arbitrary acceptance of p <0.05 as the level for statistical significance (Timothy et al. 2012). There is a general perception, not only among epidemiologists, that it is becoming increasingly difficult in many industrialized countries to achieve high response rates in surveys (Hartge 2006). In an evaluation of 355 original epidemiological papers published in ten high-impact journals, it was found that average participation in epidemiological studies has fallen in the last 30 years and this has particularly affected controls in population-based studies (Morton et al. 2006). At least some information regarding participation was provided in 59 per cent of cross-sectional studies, 44 per cent of case–control studies, and 32 per cent of cohort studies. In 51 out of 86 cross-sectional studies that reported response rates, the mean participation was 74 per cent, ranging from 28 per cent to 100 per cent. In recent years, response rates among population controls of around 50 per cent are not uncommon. Participation in cross-sectional studies decreased by approximately 1 per cent per year from 1970 to 2003 (Morton et al. 2006).

The use of telephones as a means for defining a sampling frame has been rapidly decreasing. The main assumption for the use of random digit dialling (RDD) was that there was one working residential phone number per household. This assumption is no longer valid due to rapid changes in telecommunication, particularly the use of mobile phones. The rapid increase in the use of mobile phones throughout the world has made nearly impossible the identification of a roster of phones identified to a specific area through which a sample could be derived. In addition, in several countries the use of telephone contacts for commercial reasons has resulted in a decrease of response rates to any such type of contact. Computer-assisted telephone interviews are, however, an equally valid and efficient means of collecting information among subjects that have been contacted and agreed to participate.

Studies collecting biological samples

In recent years an increasing proportion of epidemiological studies collect biological samples, following the advances in molecular and genetic techniques and their application in large-scale studies. A recent review of 355 studies identified very high participation rates (above 90 per cent) in cohort and cross-sectional studies collecting biospecimens. However, only about a third of the studies reporting collection of biospecimens also reported response rates for the biological samples. A total of 134 of 355 (38 per cent) articles reported the collection of biological specimens to measure exposure or disease and the proportion of cohort and case–control studies that collected biological specimens increased over time while that of cross-sectional studies remained fairly constant (Morton et al. 2006). Large cross-sectional studies, such as the NHANES, are regularly collecting biological samples and the inclusion of the collection of biospecimens does not appear to influence the representativeness of the sample.

An increasing number of studies are collecting saliva or other biospecimens by mail. Several studies that have collected saliva samples by mail have obtained response rates that are not very different from those observed for paper-and-pencil questionnaires. In a study on 2994 subjects at Geneva University, Switzerland, the response rate for subjects requested to provide a mail questionnaire and saliva was 52 per cent while for those requested to complete only the mail questionnaire, it was 63 per cent; using financial incentives increased the response rates by 6–11 per cent (Etter et al. 2005). Sociodemographic factors may affect response rates in such a type of sampling. Self-collection of saliva was evaluated, concerning both response and quality of DNA retrieved in a random sample of 611 men (ages 53–87 years) in Sweden (Rylander-Rudqvist et al. 2006). The response rate was 80 per cent and varied from 89 per cent for those aged 67–71 years to 71 per cent in those aged 77–87 years. Similar to other studies, the DNA extracted was of high quality and could be used as an alternative to blood DNA in molecular epidemiological studies. There is little empirical evidence in several cultures to evaluate general tendencies concerning participation when biospecimens are collected. Whether non-response may differentially affect the analysis of biomarkers is unknown.

One study examined a series of genetic data (polymorphisms, haplotypes, and short tandem repeats) from 2955 individuals of three studies and found no evidence of differential results by participation (Bhatti et al. 2005). A note of caution, however, has been made against assuming that willingness to participate should not vary with a particular polymorphism or other forms of genetic variation (Hartge 2006).

Improving non-response

The difficulties in achieving high response rates and the potential biases resulting from self-selection makes indispensable the understanding of the reasons for non-response and the application of methods for limiting non-response. Numerous studies have evaluated factors affecting non-response in epidemiological and other types of studies. Most of the factors frequently identified such as age, sex, education, exposure status, method of recruitment, and type of questionnaire used may also be culture specific. This indicates that, in addition to some general guidelines, there is a need to verify main approaches to increase response in different sociocultural settings, and these may change in different time periods. Nevertheless, some general guidelines can be drawn up based on numerous observational and on randomized trials.

A comprehensive systematic review of available randomized trials from any relevant discipline (not restricted to medicine or epidemiology) evaluated factors that influence response to postal questionnaires (Edwards et al. 2002). Information from 292 randomized controlled trials that included 258,315 participants was reviewed. A total of 75 strategies that could influence response to postal questionnaires were reviewed. The review identified questionnaire length, use of monetary incentives particularly when not conditional on response, appearance of the package, layout of the questionnaire, type of follow-up, and registered delivery as the most influential factors in terms of participation rates. Fig. 5.3.3 shows effect estimates for the most influential factors. Contacting participants before sending questionnaires increased response as did follow-up contact. Questionnaires designed to be of more interest to participants were more likely to be returned but questionnaires containing questions of a sensitive nature were less likely to be returned. Questionnaires originating from universities were more likely to be returned than were questionnaires from other sources, such as commercial organizations. Overall, response to postal questionnaires can be improved by following strategies shown to be effective in other research.

Adjusting for non-response

The most important measure to deal with potential biases from non-response is to minimize, as much as possible, the number of non-responders. As already discussed, this is done through selecting adequate ways of contact and through repeated contacts with subjects. Several approaches have been described to evaluate and adjust estimates of prevalence taking into account non-response.

An evaluation of basic characteristics of non-responders is important and may give clues concerning the representativeness of the sample. Such characteristics may be derived from information known for the target population from other surveys, for example, percentage of smokers. They can also be derived from a subsample of non-responders followed up intensively. Estimates of prevalence can then be weighed using the data of respondents but

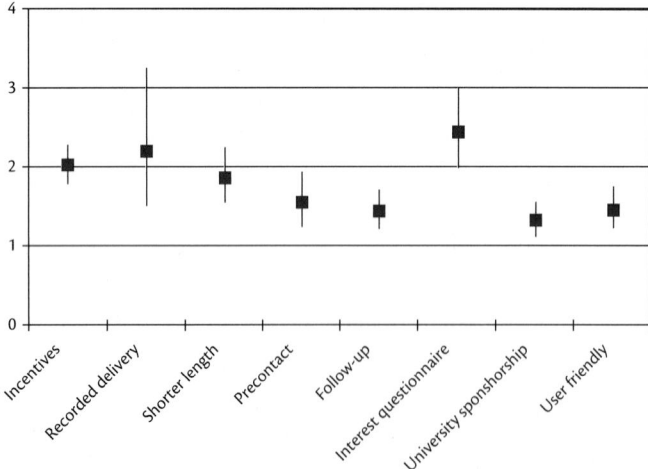

Fig. 5.3.3 Effects on questionnaire response (odds ratios and 95 per cent confidence intervals) of eight strategies where combined trials included over 1000 participants.

Source: data from Edwards, P. et al., Increasing response rates to postal questionnaires: systematic review, *British Medical Journal*, Volume 324, p. 1183, © 2002 BMJ Publishing Group Ltd.

taking into account information on variables known for responders and non-responders such as age, sex, residence, etc.

A usual procedure in prevalence surveys is to perform repeated contacts of subjects to increase response rates. The final estimates are derived from the total number of responders. In an alternative procedure it can be assumed that responders at different mailings or contacts are not representative of the population. Under this assumption, the overall prevalence estimates are modelled using the prevalence of each mailing. A cumulative response at the time of each mailing can be calculated taking into account different covariates (e.g. age, sex) of the samples responding in each mailing, and estimates of the prevalence of non-responders are derived through extrapolation.

Such modelling was conducted analysing responses of 13,007 subjects in the three English centres of the European Community Respiratory Health Survey (Chinn et al. 1995). Modelling responses to take into account centre, age, and sex had only small effects on estimated prevalence. For example, in Norwich, out of 440 eligible individuals aged 20–24 years, 141 responded to the first mailing (32 per cent), 58 to the second (cumulative response 45.2 per cent), and 45 to the third mailing (cumulative response 55.5 per cent). Prevalence of wheezing was modelled taking into account differences among responders and non-responders by age and sex and this gave an estimated prevalence of wheezing of 25.7 per cent. This estimate was further examined through modelling. In a model that included a parameter for a linear trend in prevalence with each mailing by age and sex group, an overall prevalence of 23.9 per cent was estimated. Overall in this study although several models gave statistically significant differences, in absolute terms the estimates of prevalence derived were rather similar. Such type of modelling is useful to explore the sensitivity of estimated prevalence to non-response bias. However, frequently changes due to such modelling are small and, in general, caution should be exerted when applying such models. In conclusion, the best way of adjusting for non-response is not having much of it.

Item non-response

Apart from the overall response rate the quality of the answers of participants deserves attention as well. The issue of item non-response has been little discussed and usually not reported. What is usually discussed and reported as 'non-response' refers to the non-contact with a selected person or the refusal of this person to participate (unit non-response). Failure of a responder to answer an individual question or provide a sample (item non-response) should also be considered and can equally affect the representativeness of specific analyses in a study. In a study on bladder cancer in Spain, the overall response rate to the main questionnaire was 85 per cent. However, the response to specific items was lower. For example, the questions on lifetime consumption of water and complete information on water quality in each of the residences of the subjects were available for 1479 out of a total of 2490 subjects (Villanueva et al. 2007). An evaluation of differences in sociodemographic characteristics of subjects included or excluded from the water analyses and also differences in the prevalence of known risk factors such as smoking indicated that on this occasion item non-response was not likely to bias results. Exclusion of subjects reduced, however, the statistical power of the study.

The inclusion of several variables in an analysis may result in a large amount of missing data due to item non-response. The pattern of missing data should be examined and, if possible, the causes of missing information determined. Multiple imputations methods are increasingly used to improve efficiency and minimize selection bias. It is frequently assumed that data are missing at random although this is not always easy to identify. Missing values are imputed and a set of complete data sets is generated that are further analysed individually to obtain a set of parameters and then combined into overall estimates (Rubin 1987). Several methods have been proposed to impute missing data and modern software has simplified the analysis of multiply imputed data (White et al. 2011; Cummings 2013).

Sampling methods

Different types of sampling may be applied in cross-sectional studies depending on the aims of the study, characteristics of the population studied, the available background information, and the means available in each study.

In a simple random sample, all subsets of the sampling frame are given an equal probability of being selected. What is used most frequently in large surveys is stratified sampling: this involves a first-stage selection of different categories of the population and subsequent selections at random within each stratum. The main reason for doing stratified sampling is efficiency, so as to secure adequate sampling of small population groups and avoid oversampling of larger groups. Several other probabilistic or non-probabilistic types of sampling have been applied such as 'cluster sampling' in which the unit selected is a group of persons (e.g. a city block) rather than individuals, and 'snowball sampling' and 'respondent-driven sampling' where a first set of study subjects ('seed participants') is used to recruit more subjects into the sample. These latter types are convenience sampling methods that are applied when a complete identification of the primary sampling population is not possible or hard to find (Magnani et al. 2005). Respondent-driven sampling is a variation of snowball sampling that allows a better control of the selection of the population examined, mainly by collecting information from recruiters on the size of their social network and on also on persons approached but who did not participate. The availability of such information, however, does not secure the selection of a random sample from members of a network (Heimer 2005). In addition, respondent-driven sampling is believed to have higher external validity than other convenience sampling methods because it may extend better to all potential members of a network (Magnani et al. 2005). The same approach has been used for the identification of samples for interventions in hard-to-reach populations. For example, respondent-driven sampling was used in a cluster-randomized trial in India to assess the effectiveness of HIV counselling and testing among men who have sex with men (Solomon et al. 2013).

Snowball sampling was applied in a study on the prevalence of depression among female sex workers of eastern Nepal (Sagtani et al. 2013). Snowball sampling is especially useful when the objective is to reach populations that are inaccessible or hard to find. The participants were 210 female restaurant-based and street-based sex workers in five cities of eastern Nepal. In countries like Nepal where commercial sex is illegal, the criminalized status of their work means that commercial sex workers are prone to harassment and violence. Under such conditions, identifying a base population and sampling from this population is impossible. Sex workers were contacted through snowball sampling. The first few respondents were traced with the help of a non-governmental organization working on HIV prevention in the study area. Face-to-face interviews were conducted and additional respondents were nominated. The prevalence of depression among respondents was 82 per cent. A major limitation of this type of sampling is that external validity of the study is questionable due to the unknown sampling frame.

Biased samples are samples where some members of the population are less likely to be included than others. (Note that some stratified samples are deliberately biased but the degree of bias can be estimated.) There are several classic examples of biased sampling. Among the most well known is a large opinion poll in the US presidential election in 1936 that erroneously predicted that the incumbent president, Franklin Roosevelt, would lose by a large margin. This poll of approximately 2 million persons was based on people who were readers of a magazine, supplemented by records of registered automobile owners and telephone users. The error was produced because the sample overrepresented more affluent people who were less likely to vote for the Democratic candidate.

Examples of different sampling procedures are listed in the following paragraphs, namely sampling in a large multipurpose survey (NHANES) in the United States, a large international prevalence survey (ISAAC), together with a local survey of a difficult-to-identify population of drug addicts in Spain.

The NHANES survey in the United States applies a multistage (four stages) probability sampling to select participants representative of the civilian, non-institutionalized US population (Centers for Disease Control and Prevention 2014). In stage 1, primary sampling units (mostly single counties) are selected. In the second stage, these units are divided up into segments (generally city blocks) and sample segments are selected taking size into account. In stage 3, households within each segment are listed and a sample is randomly drawn. In the final stage, individuals are randomly chosen from a list of all persons residing in the selected households within designated age–sex–race strata. NHANES is designed to sample larger numbers of certain subgroups of particular public health interest including African Americans, adolescents, and others.

In ISAAC, a combination of non-random and random methods was used. The areas participating within each country were not selected at random but instead qualitative criteria and convenience sampling were used. Stratified random sampling was then used within a given geographical area to select the school children. All schools in each geographical area centre were listed and a random sample was selected. The sampling unit was the school and non-participating schools were replaced. All children on a selected school within the two specified age groups (6–7 and 13–14 years of age) were included.

Web-based research and the use of wireless technologies

Web-based research has been expanding in recent years. The Internet has been used in research and clinical settings to enhance contact with participants. Prevalence surveys have traditionally been based on self-administered paper questionnaires, face-to-face or telephone interviews. Internet surveys have been proposed as having advantages compared to traditional approaches, for example, face-to-face or telephone interviews, regarding turnaround time and expenses. Internet-based surveys

similar to computer-assisted personal or telephone interviews have advantages concerning data management as compared to paper-and-pencil questionnaires.

The two main issues regarding the validity of use of Internet surveys are response rates and quality of the data collected. Several studies that focused on specific population groups with high indexes of Internet use have found comparable response rates between Internet-based questionnaires and more traditional approaches (Pealer et al. 2001). However, many of these studies report response rates for populations recruited through the Internet rather than for population-based samples. These results are therefore difficult to generalize, although they indicate that in specific populations, Internet-based surveys provide high-quality data.

Few studies exist that compare population-based data using both Internet and traditional type approaches. Results differ and depend crucially on the degree of education and computer literacy in different cultures, ages, and sociodemographic groups. Women referred for mammography at a Danish public hospital aged less than 67 years and without a history of breast cancer, were randomized to either receive a paper questionnaire, with a prepaid return envelope, or a guideline on how to fill in the Internet-based version online (Kongsved et al. 2007). The response rate was 18 per cent for the Internet group compared to 73 per cent for the paper questionnaire. An interesting aspect of this study was that after sending a reminder and offering the possibility of using the alternative questionnaire form (i.e. a paper questionnaire in the Internet group), the response rate for the Internet group became comparable to that of the group assigned the paper questionnaire. In the Millennium cohort (Smith et al. 2007) of military personnel in the United States, a similar proportion of the approximately 70,000 responders chose to respond using the Internet. Web responders were more likely to be male, to be younger, have a higher education, work in technical occupations, to be obese, and to smoke more cigarettes. They were less likely to be problem alcohol drinkers and to report occupational exposures. Several studies have evaluated quality of information from web-based studies and have found that it is similar to, if not better than, self-administered questionnaires. In the Danish mammography study mentioned earlier (Kongsved et al. 2007), the quality of the information was better in the Internet version with 98 per cent having no missing data compared to 63 per cent filling in a complete paper questionnaire. A study in Sweden (Bonn et al. 2013) compared web-based self-reports of bodyweight with weight measured at the study centre in a convenience sample of 149 individuals. As frequently happens with self-reported weight, overweight subjects (body mass index ≥ 25 kg/m^2) tended to underreport their weight and the overall mean difference between self-reported and measured weight was –1.2 kg. The Spearman correlation coefficient, however, between self-reported and measured weight was 0.98 (P <0.001) indicating that self-reported weight and perhaps other anthropometric measures via the web can be a valid method of data collection.

The use of wireless technologies and devices is rapidly increasing and it is expected that smartphone technology will become the most frequent way to access information in the World Wide Web. The ubiquity of mobile device ownership and the development applications allows new ways of contact and recording of health-related information in population studies. A study in

Barcelona used smartphone technology to improve environmental exposure assessment applying novel sensor technologies integrated with mobile phones (de Nazelle et al. 2013). Geographic location and physical activity patterns were tracked through a smartphone application in 36 subjects and were then linked to space–time air pollution mapping for improved air pollution exposure assessment. This information provides an accurate account of mobility of the subjects during the day and of physical activity. Mobile technologies also allow individuals to record and communicate behaviour in real time from any location. A study on 50 trained subjects evaluated the feasibility of using Twitter to capture dietary behaviour and reasons for eating over 3 consecutive days (Hingle et al. 2013). A list of hashtags representing food groups, for example, #fruit, and reasons for eating, for example, #mood, were provided to participants who were encouraged to annotate hashtags with photos, text, and links. A total of 773 tweets including 2862 hashtags were reported and eating behaviours were visualized through 'maps' of hashtag co-occurrences suggesting time-varying diet and behaviour patterns.

On the basis of existing evidence it appears that Internet-based surveys may provide high response rates in selected populations. In most general populations, however, Internet-based surveys do not yet seem to provide adequate response rates and this may lead to selected sampling. Several studies indicate that Internet surveys may be efficiently combined with traditional techniques to save resources and perhaps provide more complete answers. Clearly, more research is needed in the future in population-based surveys to evaluate changes in response in Internet-based research. While sensor-based applications in environmental epidemiology have been widely used and have been shown to improve exposure assessment, there is a lack of empirical evidence in public health research concerning the use of popular software applications such as Twitter.

Bias in cross-sectional studies

Cross-sectional studies may suffer from the same potential biases as other epidemiological designs: misclassification, selection bias, and confounding. Issues of particular concern in cross-sectional studies are the potential biases from the mixing of incident and prevalent cases, the frequent lack of information on past exposures and consequently on the time sequence of events, and the lack of representativeness in studies evaluating the prevalence of disease or of other health-related variables. Because of these difficulties, it has been recommended that cross-sectional studies examining the risk factors of disease are appropriate for diseases that produce little disability, and are also appropriate to the presymptomatic phases of more serious disorders (Coggon et al. 1997).

Incidence–prevalence bias (known as Neyman bias; also discussed as length-bias) is a type of selection bias due to the mix of incident and prevalent cases in cross-sectional studies. Incidence–prevalence bias refers specifically to the selection of a case group that is not representative of cases in the community. Fig. 5.3.4 (left graph) shows the hypothetical time of occurrence of disease and the duration of disease. A cross-sectional study would include a disproportionately high percentage of cases with long duration while those with more aggressive disease and hence short duration would have a lower probability of being sampled. The latter is exemplified in Fig. 5.3.4 (right graph). A bias would occur if survivors of a condition studied are atypical with respect to the exposure evaluated. If the exposure examined is not directly or indirectly related to survival, inclusion of prevalent cases would not bias any association. In addition, as noted by Hill et al. (2003), for diseases with extremely low case fatality (e.g. rheumatoid arthritis), studies based on prevalent cases are not subject to Neyman bias even if the risk factor under study produces increased mortality from other causes.

The association of smoking with Alzheimer's disease has been discussed as a potential effect of incidence–prevalence bias. Several cross-sectional studies have suggested that smoking exerts a protective effect on Alzheimer's disease. Evidence, however, from a few cohort studies is controversial. A cross-sectional study that included a prospective component suggested that part of the protective effect could be attributed to Neyman bias, specifically because smokers with dementia could have worse survival than

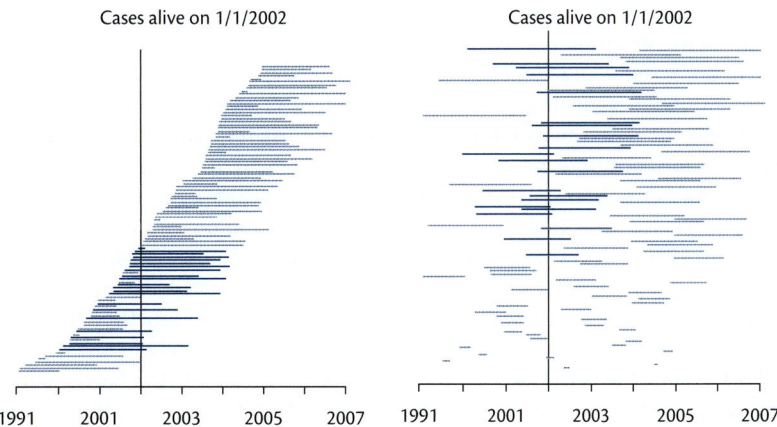

Fig. 5.3.4 Incidence–prevalence bias in cross-sectional studies. Note: the lines on this graph represent the duration of disease with the left end point representing the date that the disease was first diagnosed and the right end point representing the date that the patient died. In the left graph, subjects are ordered by time of initial diagnosis. A cross-sectional study in January 2002 selected those patients who were alive at that time (indicated with vertical line). Notice that patients diagnosed before 2002 with a short survival would have less probability of being selected compared to subjects diagnosed the same period but with a longer survival. In the graph on the right, patients with the shortest survival times appear at the bottom of the graph and the patients with the longest survival times appear at the top. Notice how rarely patients with short survival times appear among the prevalent cases.

Reproduced from *StATS: Neyman bias* (December 15, 2004), available from http://www.pmean.com/04/NeymanBias.html, with permission from Children's Mercy Hospital.

smokers without dementia. The study was a population-based cohort of 668 people aged 75–101 years in Sweden (Wang et al. 1999). Smoking was negatively associated with prevalent Alzheimer's disease (adjusted odds ratio = 0.6, 95% confidence interval (CI) 0.4–1.1). Over 3-year follow-up (1989–1992), the hazard ratio of incident Alzheimer's disease due to smoking was 1.1 (95% CI 0.5–2.4). In addition, mortality at follow-up was greater among smokers in demented (hazard ratio = 3.4) than non-demented subjects (hazard ratio = 0.8). The authors concluded that smoking does not protect against Alzheimer's disease and that the cross-sectional association might be due to differential mortality.

When examining prevalent cases an additional problem may occur if diseased persons modify their exposure or if disease affects measures of exposure, for example, the presence of disease distorting biomarker levels. Treatment with insulin of diabetes mellitus type 1 is an example. Before insulin was available, patients had a very poor survival of less than 1 year. At that time, a cross-sectional study would simply not identify many diabetics. With insulin treatment, survival has spectacularly increased to more than 20 years. A cross-sectional study evaluating diabetes and use of insulin would therefore find an association, simply because diabetics take insulin while non-diabetics do not. This bias has also been described as a type of Neyman bias (incidence–prevalence bias) but in reality it is rather a case of reverse causation provoked by misclassification due to an erroneous evaluation of timing of exposure.

In recent years there has been an increase in the number of studies using data from large surveys such as the NHANES. Experimental data suggest that phthalates, a widespread contaminant, could produce metabolic derangements that may lead to obesity. The association between urinary phthalate metabolites and body mass was examined in a cross-sectional analysis of 2884 children 6–19 years of age who participated in the 2003–2008 NHANES. Phthalates were measured at one time point and monoesters of phthalates typically have half-lives of around 24 hours. An association of phthalates with childhood obesity was identified among non-Hispanic black children while no significant associations were identified in any other ethnic groups. Making maximum use of a resource such as the NHANES is understandable and advisable given its cost and the population sampling and these findings should lead to additional research. However, making causal inferences from this type of cross-sectional data may be complex. Reverse causation may be a problem in cross-sectional analyses since both physiological aspects and behavioural pathways, for example, restricted mobility of subjects with disease, may influence measured exposures. The London bus drivers' study in the 1950s is a classic example of potential reverse causation.

The study by Jerry Morris on the incidence and prevalence of cardiovascular disease among London bus drivers and conductors (Morris and Dale 1955) is an example of selection bias in a cross-sectional study. Bus drivers in London were shown to have very different lipid profiles, blood pressure patterns, and eventually cardiovascular disease risk compared to bus conductors. Bus drivers were less physically active on the job than conductors, but could the difference in cardiovascular disease risk be ascribed to physical activity? One potential alternative explanation was that some characteristic of the persons such as obesity, could have led to self-selection in a job that was more (bus conductors) or less (bus drivers) active. The studies in London busmen were eventually the first to convincingly demonstrate the importance of physical activity for health.

The healthy worker effect may lead to an underestimation of an association in case–control studies that evaluate occupation and disease at a specific point in time (Checkoway et al. 2004). This happens because workers with health problems at work are more likely to change jobs than subjects without symptoms. In this case the selection is out of the job, contrary to what was a potential problem in busmen. Any cross-sectional evaluation will, therefore, not capture cases that have occurred in the past and will over-represent healthy individuals who have stayed in the job. An example of this was observed in a cross-sectional study on occupational asthma in Spain (Kogevinas et al. 1996). Subjects were asked about their current occupation and about current respiratory symptoms. The prevalence odds ratios (PORs) for asthma in subjects employed in high-risk occupations was 1.4 with 95% CI of 0.6–3.3. Subjects were also asked whether they had suffered respiratory symptoms in the past and, if yes, what type of job were they doing. The POR for employment in a high-risk occupation at the time of respiratory problems was 2.8 (95% CI 1.5–5.2) indicating that, indeed, the cross-sectional analysis failed to identify health risks due to the selective migration of subjects with respiratory symptoms out of high-risk jobs.

This type of bias is less of a problem if current exposure is a reliable surrogate for past exposure and is not a problem for non-changeable characteristics, for example, race, gender, and genetic variability. Case–control or cross-sectional studies are currently the most widely applied designs evaluating the effects of genetic susceptibility, such as the effects of SNPs (single nucleotide polymorphisms), on disease risk.

Social desirability bias has long been recognized and falls within the wider category of misclassification (Armstrong et al. 1994). Requesting information on behaviours that are regarded as sensitive by respondents may lead to refusal to participate or may lead to a tendency to over-report behaviours regarded as socially desirable (or, what is the same, under-report what is regarded as socially undesirable). This has become particularly evident in recent years in large surveys that inquire into health-related behaviours such as sexual activity and drug use.

There is extensive research showing that self-administered questionnaires lead to more valid information on socially sensitive issues compared to face-to-face interviews (Schuman and Presser 1981; Armstrong et al. 1994). In recent years the use of computers in soliciting information has considerably expanded. In addition to CAPIs (computer-assisted personal interviews) the technique of audio-computer-assisted self-interviewing (ACASI) has been proposed as an efficient method to enhance validity when evaluating behaviours that could be perceived as socially undesirable (Turner et al. 1998). In ACASI (also quoted as audio-CASI), respondents hear the questions through headphones and enter their responses directly into a computer. An experimental comparison of sexual behaviours in adolescent males using a paper-and-pencil self-administered questionnaire and ACASI identified an almost fourfold increase in the number of respondents reporting male–male sexual contact in the ACASI (5.5 per cent) as compared to 1.5 per cent in the paper-and-pencil questionnaire (Turner et al. 1998). Among the reported advantages of ACASI is that it reduces the literacy requirements of respondents compared to other forms of self-administered questionnaires (paper and pencil or computer assisted). ACASI has been tested in multiple settings and has generally been shown to provide higher estimates of prevalence of social undesirable behaviours compared to face-to-face interviews (Ghanem et al. 2005). Results are less consistent when comparing ACASI with self-administered questionnaires (Morrison-Beedy et al. 2006). Different computer-assisted methods (audio or text) may have little impact on reported socially undesirable behaviours and the choice of one method over another should be based on an evaluation of wider considerations on the study settings.

Analysis of cross-sectional studies

Prevalence is the ratio of the number of cases of a disease in a population at a particular time, to the size of the population at that time.

$$\text{Prevalence} = \frac{\text{number of existing cases of disease}}{\text{total population at a point in time}}$$

Point prevalence is estimated at one point in time, while period prevalence denotes the number of cases in a time interval (e.g. 1 year).

For example, in a given state in June 2007, there were 14,000 women with a diagnosis of breast cancer. The total female population in June 2007 was 1,558,000 women. The prevalence of breast cancer in this population on this specific date is 14,000/1,558,000, which equals 0.009 (or 0.9 per cent). This means that nearly 1 per cent of the women in June 2007 had breast cancer, a figure that corresponds to the actual prevalence of this disease in several industrialized countries. This estimate does not show how many new cases of breast cancer occur each year or when the 14,000 women had their disease diagnosed. In these types of estimates it is usually assumed that none of the persons diagnosed with a chronic disease is entirely cured, although such calculations could be incorporated into the estimation of prevalence.

Prevalence is, strictly speaking, a proportion although it is sometimes indicated, erroneously, as a rate. However, the term 'prevalence rate' should be regarded theoretically as an impossible concept (Elandt-Johnson 1975).

Prevalence reflects determinants of incidence as well as survival (duration of a disease). The prevalence of bladder cancer in the United States in January 2004 (377,523 persons alive with a history of bladder cancer) was higher than that of lung cancer (174,880 persons), even though the incidence of lung cancer (81.2 per 100.000) was clearly higher than that of bladder cancer (37.3/100.000). This is a reflection of the much better prognosis of bladder cancer (5-year relative survival rate of 79.5 per cent) compared to 15 per cent for lung cancer (National Cancer Institute n.d.).

In its most simple expression prevalence odds are equal to incidence rate times the duration of the disease:

$$\frac{P}{1-P} = I \times D$$

where P is prevalence, I is incidence, and D is duration (survival). This, however, is only true under stable conditions, that is, unchanging rates and population structure that are unlikely in most occasions in true populations. If two populations are compared, say 1 indicating the exposed and 0 the non-exposed, then the POR can be calculated as:

$$POR = \frac{P_1 / (1 - P_1) I_1 D_1}{P_0 / (1 - P_0) I_0 D_0}.$$

If the duration of the disease is expected to be equal in the exposed and unexposed, then the POR is equal to the incidence rate ratio (under steady conditions in the population). Under the same conditions, the ratio of prevalences (as compared to the ratio of prevalence odds) will only estimate the incidence rate ratio if the prevalence of the disease is low. In that occasion, $1 - P$ would be roughly equal to 1.

There has been some controversy whether cross-sectional studies should be calculating POR or prevalence ratios (Thompson et al. 1998; Pearce 2004). The choice of one or the other depends essentially on the purposes of the research, with the POR having advantages compared to the prevalence ratio if aetiological research is conducted. However, the prevalence ratio or probably the absolute difference in prevalences may be preferred if two populations are compared regarding the prevalence of disease.

Statistical analysis in cross-sectional studies is frequently limited to descriptive statistics through the use of standard statistical measures for proportions or a comparison of distributions (e.g. blood pressure) between an exposed and an unexposed group. Standard statistical tests comparing means of a distribution such as Student's t-test can be used. For the evaluation of multiple variables, standard techniques such as multiple linear regression can be used. For dichotomous outcomes, the POR is the most common effect measure estimated in cross-sectional studies comparing groups, with the application of logistic regression or equivalent techniques. A wide range of other analytical regression techniques is readily available for the modelling of prevalence ratios (Thompson et al. 1998; Barros and Hirakata 2003). The selection of the effect measure, that is, POR versus the prevalence ratio as the preferred effect measure, should, therefore, not depend on the availability of statistical tools (Pearce 2004), but rather on the objectives of the research.

Summary

Cross-sectional studies are among the most applied designs. The principal characteristic of cross-sectional studies is that they provide information on the prevalence of disease. In many cross-sectional studies information on past exposures is not collected but this should not be regarded as a characteristic defining these studies. On many occasions, cross-sectional studies tend to follow a hybrid design, an analysis incorporating aspects of cohort and of case–control studies. Repeated cross-sectional studies (panel studies) offer the possibility of assessing short-term and long-term physiological changes. Cross-sectional studies are extensively used to evaluate the prevalence of disease. Large cross-sectional studies are conducted in several countries to provide background information on health-related variables including health services use. In recent years these surveys have also incorporated the collection of biospecimens. In aetiological research, cross-sectional studies are suitable epidemiological means for studying non-fatal diseases and effects on physiological variables that do not have a clear time of onset. However, the design of cross-sectional studies makes them less appropriate than other study designs for investigating causal associations. Among the major limitations of cross-sectional studies are the inclusion of prevalent rather than incident cases and the frequent lack of information on past exposures and on the time sequence of events. The representativeness of the sample is crucial when evaluating prevalence of a disease and several policies have been developed to increase participation in studies, reduce non-response, and improve the quality of the recorded information.

References

Anonymous (1998). Worldwide variation in prevalence of symptoms of asthma, allergic rhinoconjunctivitis, and atopic eczema: ISAAC. The International Study of Asthma and Allergies in Childhood (ISAAC) Steering Committee. *The Lancet*, 351, 1225–32.

Arif, A.A., Delclos, G.L., Whitehead, L.W., Tortolero, S.R., and Lee, E.S. (2003). Occupational exposures associated with work-related asthma and work-related wheezing among U.S. workers. *American Journal of Industrial Medicine*, 44, 368–76.

Armstrong, B.K., White, E., and Saracci, R. (1994). *Principles of Exposure Measurement in Epidemiology*. New York: Oxford University Press.

Asher, M.I., Keil, U., Anderson, H.R., et al. (1995). International Study of Asthma and Allergies in Childhood (ISAAC): rationale and methods. *European Respiratory Journal*, 8, 483–91.

Barros, A.J. and Hirakata, V.N. (2003). Alternatives for logistic regression in cross-sectional studies: an empirical comparison of models that directly estimate the prevalence ratio. *BMC Medical Research Methodology*, 3, 21.

Bhatti, P., Sigurdson, A.J., Wang, S.S., et al. (2005). Genetic variation and willingness to participate in epidemiologic research: data from three studies. *Cancer Epidemiology, Biomarkers & Prevention*, 14, 2449–53.

Bonn, S.E., Trolle Lagerros, Y., and Bälter, K. (2013). How valid are web-based self-reports of weight? *Journal of Medical Internet Research*, 15(4), e52.

Burney, P.G., Luczynska, C., Chinn, S., and Jarvis, D. (1994). The European Community Respiratory Health Survey. *European Respiratory Journal*, 7, 954–60.

Centers for Disease Control and Prevention (2013). *Epi Info™*. [Online] Available at: http://wwwn.cdc.gov/epiinfo/.

Centers for Disease Control and Prevention (2014). National Health and Nutrition Examination Survey. Available at: http://www.cdc.gov/nchs/nhanes.htm.

Checkoway, H., Pearce, N., and Kriebel, D. (2004). *Research Methods in Occupational Epidemiology*. Oxford: Oxford University Press.

Chinn, S., Zanolin, E., Lai, E., Jarvis, D., Luczynska, C.M., and Burney, P.G. (1995). Adjustment of reported prevalence of respiratory symptoms for non-response in a multi-centre health survey. *International Journal of Epidemiology*, 24, 603–11.

Coggon, D., Rose, G., and Barker, D.J.P. (1997). *Epidemiology for the Uninitiated*. London: BMJ Publishing Group.

Cummings, P. (2013). Missing data and multiple imputation. *JAMA Pediatrics*, 13, 1–7.

De Nazelle, A., Seto, E., Donaire-Gonzalez, D., et al. (2013). Improving estimates of air pollution exposure through ubiquitous sensing technologies. *Environmental Pollution*, 176, 92–9.

Department of Health (2012). *Health Survey for England 2011*. Available at: https://www.gov.uk/government/publications/health-survey-for-england-2011.

Edwards, P., Roberts, I., Clarke, M., DiGuiseppi, C., Pratap, S., Wentz, R., and Kwan, I. (2002). Increasing response rates to postal questionnaires: systematic review. *BMJ*, 324, 1183.

Elandt-Johnson, R.C. (1975). Definition of rates: some remarks on their use and misuse. *American Journal of Epidemiology*, 102, 267–71.

Etter, J.F., Neidhart, E., Bertrand, S., Malafosse, A., and Bertrand, D. (2005). Collecting saliva by mail for genetic and cotinine analyses in participants recruited through the Internet. *European Journal of Epidemiology*, 20, 833–8.

Ghanem, K.G., Hutton, H.E., Zenilman, J.M., Zimba, R., and Erbelding, E.J. (2005). Audio computer assisted self-interview and face to face interview modes in assessing response bias among STD clinic patients. *Sexually Transmitted Infections*, 81, 421–5.

Hartge, P. (2006). Participation in population studies. *Epidemiology*, 17, 252–4.

Heimer, R. (2005). Critical issues and further questions about respondent-driven sampling: comment on Ramirez-Valles, et al. (2005). *AIDS and Behavior*, 9, 403–8.

Hill, G., Connelly, J., Hebert, R., Lindsay, J., and Millar, W. (2003). Neyman's bias re-visited. *Journal of Clinical Epidemiology*, 56, 293–6.

Hingle, M., Yoon, D., Fowler, J., et al. (2013). Collection and visualization of dietary behavior and reasons for eating using Twitter. *Journal of Medical Internet Research*, 15(6), e125.

Janson, C., Anto, J., Burney, P., et al. (2001). The European Community Respiratory Health Survey: what are the main results so far? European Community Respiratory Health Survey II. *European Respiratory Journal*, 18, 598–611.

Kogevinas, M., Anto, J.M., Soriano, J.B., Tobias, A., and Burney, P. (1996). The risk of asthma attributable to occupational exposures. A population-based study in Spain. Spanish Group of the European Asthma Study. *American Journal of Respiratory and Critical Care Medicine*, 154, 137–43.

Kogevinas, M., Anto, J.M., Sunyer, J., Tobias, A., Kromhout, H., and Burney, P. (1999). Occupational asthma in Europe and other industrialised areas: a population-based study. European Community Respiratory Health Survey Study Group. *The Lancet*, 353, 1750–4.

Kongsved, S.M., Basnov, M., Holm-Christensen, K., and Hjollund, N.H. (2007). Response rate and completeness of questionnaires: a randomized study of Internet versus paper-and-pencil versions. *Journal of Medical Internet Research*, 9, e25.

Magnani, R., Sabin, K., Saidel, T., Heckathorn, D. (2005). Review of sampling hard-to-reach and hidden populations for HIV surveillance. *AIDS*, 19(Suppl. 2), S67–72.

McCreanor, J., Cullinan, P., Nieuwenhuijsen, M.J., et al. (2007). Respiratory effects of exposure to diesel traffic in persons with asthma. *The New England Journal of Medicine*, 357, 2348–58.

Morris, J.N. and Dale, R.A. (1955). Epidemiology of coronary atherosclerosis. *Proceedings of the Royal Society of Medicine*, 48, 667–72.

Morrison-Beedy, D., Carey, M.P., and Tu, T. (2006) Accuracy of audio computer-assisted self-interviewing (ACASI) and self-administered questionnaires for the assessment of sexual behavior. *AIDS and Behavior*, 10, 541–52.

Morton, L.M., Cahill, J., and Hartge, P. (2006). Reporting participation in epidemiologic studies: a survey of practice. *American Journal of Epidemiology*, 163, 197–203.

National Cancer Institute (n.d.). *Cancer Stat Fact Sheets*. [Online] Available at: http://seer.cancer.gov/statfacts/.

Pealer, L.N., Weiler, R.M., Pigg, R.M., Jr., Miller, D., and Dorman, S.M. (2001). The feasibility of a web-based surveillance system to collect health risk behavior data from college students. *Health Education & Behavior*, 28, 547–59.

Pearce, N. (2004). Effect measures in prevalence studies. *Environmental Health Sciences*, 112, 1047–50.

Pearce, N., Ait-Khaled, N., Beasley, R., et al. (2007). Worldwide trends in the prevalence of asthma symptoms: phase III of the International Study of Asthma and Allergies in Childhood (ISAAC). *Thorax*, 62, 758–66.

Rubin, D.B. (1987). *Multiple Imputation for Nonresponse in Surveys*. New York: Wiley.

Rylander-Rudqvist, T., Hakansson, N., Tybring, G., and Wolk, A. (2006). Quality and quantity of saliva DNA obtained from the self-administered oragene method—a pilot study on the cohort of Swedish men. *Cancer Epidemiology, Biomarkers & Prevention*, 15, 1742–5.

Sagtani, R.A., Bhattarai, S., Adhikari, B.R., Baral, D., Yadav, D.K., and Pokharel, P.K. (2013). Violence, HIV risk behaviour and depression among female sex workers of eastern Nepal. *BMJ Open*, 3(6), e002763.

Schuman, H. and Presser, S. (1981). *Questions and Answers in Attitude Surveys: Experiments on Question Form, Wording, and Context*. San Diego, CA: Academic Press.

Singh, G.K. and Kogan, M.D. (2010). *Childhood Obesity in the United States, 1976–2008: Trends and Current Racial/Ethnic, Socioeconomic, and Geographic Disparities. A 75th Anniversary Publication*. Health Resources and Services Administration, Maternal and Child Health Bureau. Rockville, MD: U.S. Department of Health and Human Services.

Smith, B., Smith, T.C., Gray, G.C., and Ryan, M.A. (2007). When epidemiology meets the Internet: web-based surveys in the Millennium Cohort Study. *American Journal of Epidemiology*, 166, 1345–54.

Solomon, S.S., Lucas, G.M., Celentano, D.D., Sifakis, F., and Mehta, S.H. (2013). Beyond surveillance: a role for respondent-driven sampling in implementation science. *American Journal of Epidemiology*, 178(2), 260–7.

Thompson, M.L., Myers, J.E. and Kriebel, D. (1998). Prevalence odds ratio or prevalence ratio in the analysis of cross sectional data: what is to be done? *Occupational and Environmental Medicine*, 55, 272–7.

Timothy, P., Johnson, T.P., and Wislar, J.S. (2012). Response rates and non-response errors in surveys. *JAMA*, 307(17), 1805–6.

Turner, C.F., Ku, L., Rogers, S.M., Lindberg, L.D., Pleck, J.H., and Sonenstein, F.L. (1998). Adolescent sexual behavior, drug use and violence: increased reporting with computer survey technology, *Science*, 280, 867–73.

Villanueva, C.M., Cantor, K.P., Grimalt, J.O., et al. (2007). Bladder cancer and exposure to water disinfection by-products through ingestion, bathing, showering, and swimming in pools, *American Journal of Epidemiology*, 165, 148–56.

Wang, H.X., Fratiglioni, L., Frisoni, G.B., Viitanen, M., and Winblad, B. (1999). Smoking and the occurrence of Alzheimer's disease: cross-sectional and longitudinal data in a population-based study, *American Journal of Epidemiology*, 149, 640–4.

White, I.R., Royston, P., and Wood, A.M. (2011). Multiple imputation using chained equations: issues and guidance for practice. *Statistics in Medicine*, 30, 377–99.

5.4

Principles of outbreak investigation

Kumnuan Ungchusak and Sopon Iamsirithaworn

Introduction to principles of outbreak investigation

Knowledge of medicine and diseases has increased enormously over the last few decades. With the advance of knowledge, public health services in many countries can implement effective prevention programmes, and are able to protect people from many avoidable illnesses and death. However, people around the world still suffer and die from various known and unknown outbreaks of disease. Some outbreaks are old diseases that have re-emerged, some are newly identified or emerging, and some have been deliberately started. Outbreaks can occur anywhere, from a very remote area where no health facility exists to nosocomial outbreaks in a very sophisticated hospital where hundreds of health personnel are employed. Moreover, outbreaks may even spread across borders thereby threatening international health security. It is a challenge for governments and public health professionals of all countries to detect and control these outbreaks as early as possible. Outbreak investigations provide the opportunity to discover new aetiological agents, to understand factors that promote the spread of the diseases, and to identify the weaknesses of existing prevention and health programmes. For these reasons, all public health professionals should have the ability to detect, conduct, or play essential roles in supporting outbreak investigations.

This chapter provides a definition and describes the objectives of outbreak investigation, the methods for planning and conducting an investigation, and what needs to be done after the investigation has been completed. For simplicity, mainly examples of communicable disease investigations are discussed; however, the concepts and principles can also be applied to non-communicable diseases and injuries.

What is an outbreak?

The terms *outbreak* and *epidemic* can be used interchangeably. However, most people understand the term *outbreak*, which coveys a greater sense of urgency. Some epidemiologists prefer to use the term *epidemic* only in a situation that covers a very wide geographical area and involves large populations. For example, it is possible to use the term 'outbreak of HIV' to describe a sharply increasing HIV prevalence rate among commercial sex workers in a city where the normal rate was low in the previous year. However, the term *HIV epidemic* can be used when an abnormally high HIV prevalence is found among sex workers in many cities of the country.

In general, infectious diseases can be newly emerging and once the disease is able to sustain its transmission in the population of a geographical area we call it an endemic disease. Outbreak is used for a new emerging disease or situation when an endemic disease or health events occur at a greater frequency than normally expected within a specified period and place. There is often a misunderstanding that only communicable diseases can cause outbreaks. Non-communicable outbreaks such as mass sociogenic illnesses are sometimes reported as acute outbreaks of unexplained illness, especially in school settings (Centers for Disease Control and Prevention 1990, 1996). Another example of an event that can be called an outbreak and needs investigation is mass casualty. Following a fire in a pub on New Year's Eve 2009 in Thailand, an unprecedented number of 67 deaths and 153 hospitalizations resulted (Jongcherdchootrakul et al. 2010).

Because the criteria for judging an outbreak can be very subjective, it is useful to define the term in a more measurable manner. The criteria for judging that an outbreak has occurred can be one of the following:

1. The occurrence of a greater number of cases or events than normally occurs in the same place and during the same period as in past years. An example is detection of influenza outbreaks in the United States. The surveillance data from the 122 sentinel cities provides the seasonal baseline mortality attributed to influenza and pneumonia on a weekly basis, and an influenza outbreak is signalled by a rise of the mortality rates above the epidemic threshold. Another example is the epidemic of Kaposi's sarcoma, a manifestation of AIDS, confirmed in New York when almost 30 cases were reported in 1981, whereas only two or three cases had been reported in previous years (Biggar et al. 1988).

2. A cluster of cases of the same disease occurs that can be linked to the same exposure. The term *cluster* means aggregations of relatively uncommon events or diseases in space and/or time in amounts that are believed or perceived to be greater than could be expected by chance (Porta 2008). For example, in Denmark during August 2007, the Danish clinical notification system identified many cases of *Shigella sonnei* among employees of two companies. The patients had eaten in their workplace canteen, which were served by the same catering company (Lewis et al. 2009).

3. A single case of disease that has never occurred before or might have a significant implication for public health policy and practice can be judged as an outbreak that merits investigation. The first documented case of avian flu (H5N1) in the Hong Kong Special Administrative Region in a 3-year-old boy in May 1997 alerted the local authorities and scientists around the world to start a full-scale investigation (Lee et al. 1999).

How can an outbreak be detected?

Public health professionals need to maintain monitoring or surveillance of the disease situation in their local area or country, and also at the international level. It is possible to identify an outbreak by monitoring many sources of information, which will help to detect the abnormal occurrence of disease. Some useful sources are listed as follows.

Health personnel

Doctors and nurses in hospitals have a good opportunity to observe an abnormal increase in the number of patients with a particular disease or syndrome. A cluster of food poisoning in a northern province of Thailand was reported to an epidemiologist during a business telephone conversation with his colleague. The epidemiologist started an investigation and identified the first confirmed outbreak of *Clostridium botulinum* food poisoning associated with home-canned bamboo shoots in the country (Centers for Disease Control and Prevention 1999a). Without this personal contact, the outbreak would not have been investigated. Thus, public health authorities should maintain a cordial relationship with doctors and hospital staff, both in the governmental and private sectors. Conversely, doctors should report all suspected outbreaks to local public health authorities.

Laboratories

Every laboratory or network can serve as an excellent source of outbreak notification. The avian flu outbreak in the Hong Kong Special Administrative Region was first discovered by the Influenza Surveillance Network, which reported an abnormal influenza type A (H5N1) (Lee et al. 1999). Without the necessary laboratory capacity, avian flu might have been overlooked and not have triggered a field investigation. A public health professional should communicate regularly with laboratory technicians and vice versa. Laboratory scientists can prevent further spread if they report abnormal findings to public health authorities regularly and without delay.

Official disease notification systems

Most countries have official systems for notification of cases and deaths of epidemic-prone diseases in hospitals. The system was designed to detect outbreaks by comparing cases occurring in the current week or month with the average number of cases in the same area during the same period in past years.

For some diseases such as HIV/AIDS, a sentinel surveillance system was designed to monitor and detect abnormal trends in particular sentinel populations and sites. The first HIV sentinel serosurveillance in Thailand, which started in June 1989, detected HIV prevalence of 44 per cent among commercial sex workers in a popular northern tourist province. This finding was very alarming, and prompted a field investigation to confirm the high prevalence and to look for risk factors of HIV infection among sex workers (Siraprapasiri et al. 1991). The investigation confirmed the outbreak and revealed low levels of condom use, which led to a recommendation for promoting condom use in this high-risk population.

One of the most important functions that epidemiologists and public health professionals perform is regular analyses of reported disease data. Unfortunately, this task has been neglected, and the usefulness of disease reporting systems has been downgraded and often serves only as vital statistics reports. If this neglect of the reporting system can be overcome, the public health system will regain this powerful tool to detect and control outbreaks.

Newspapers and media

Public health professionals learn of outbreaks from the media more often than from the official surveillance system. Newspapers receive outbreak news directly from their journalists or people in the community, and are able to report them immediately. The Programme for Monitoring Emerging Diseases (ProMED) was the prototype for a communication system that monitors emerging infectious diseases globally, an initiative of the Federation of American Scientists co-sponsored by the World Health Organization (WHO), which obtains much of its outbreak news from the local or international media. Although timeliness is the strength of the media, the validity of the information is often of concern, so media reports require verification.

Village health volunteers

In rural areas where there are no health facilities and communication is limited, village leaders or village health volunteers can often help to recognize an abnormal increase in the numbers of some clinical diseases, such as diarrhoea, dysentery, measles, fever, deaths from unknown aetiology, etc. For example, between 2004 and 2005 there was a nationwide outbreak of avian influenza (H5N1) in poultry. The Thai Ministry of Public Health asked the village health volunteers to report any abnormal deaths of poultry to local health officers and the animal health authorities. With these notifications from villagers and a policy to provide compensation to households that lose chickens through culling of the suspected infected flock, Thailand was able to control the highly pathogenic avian influenza outbreak in chickens that then resulted in only 25 human cases.

Purposes of outbreak investigation

An outbreak investigation can have many purposes, but the critical ones are as follows.

Controlling the current outbreak

This should be the primary ultimate goal. If the investigation can start early, the findings can guide implementation of appropriate control measures to stop further spread. The avian influenza (H5N1) outbreak investigation found a link between infection and illness in chickens and humans. The same virus was found in both. There were a total of 18 cases and six deaths before the Hong Kong Special Administrative Region decided to kill all of the 1.5 million chickens in the islands within 3 days to end the outbreak (Lee et al. 1999). There have been no human cases in Hong Kong since then. However, the outbreaks of avian influenza (H5N1) in poultry

Sequence of events in outbreak detection and confirmation: scenario 1

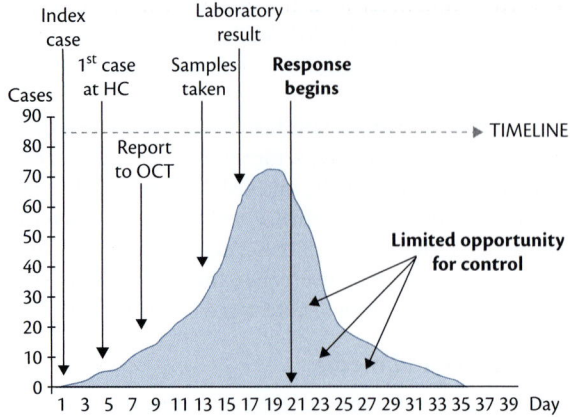

Sequence of events in outbreak detection and confirmation: scenario 2

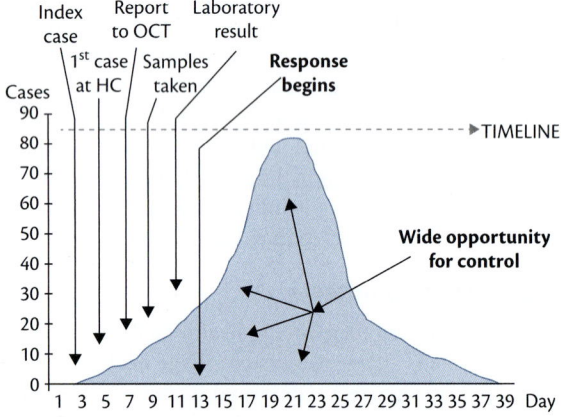

Fig. 5.4.1 The impact of early detection of and response to outbreak in reducing a disease burden.

Reproduced with permission from Connolly M.A (ed.), *Communicable Disease Control in Emergencies: A Field Manual*, World Health Organization, Geneva, Switzerland, Copyright © World Health Organization 2005, http://www.who.int/hac/techguidance/pht/communicable_diseases/field_manual/en/.

have re-emerged in several countries in Asia and other continents, with increasing numbers of human cases since late 2003. Up to 17 December 2012, there were 610 human cases of H5N1, including 360 deaths reported in 15 countries. To achieve the goal of controlling the current outbreak, it is necessary to eliminate the delay in detecting the outbreak, to start an investigation as soon as possible, and to immediately implement appropriate preventive and control measures indicated by the investigation results. With early cases detection and timely report to an outbreak response team, an opportunity of reducing a disease burden is potentially greater (Fig. 5.4.1).

Prevention of future outbreaks

Not all investigations start at the beginning or before the peak of the outbreak. The findings or lessons learned from the investigation may be too late to help fully control the current outbreak, but they can still contribute to prevention of future outbreaks. Through sound investigations, the weaknesses of the prevention programmes and/or necessary measures can be identified. If recommendations are taken seriously, the chance of recurrence of the

same outbreak or other diseases that share common risk factors can be reduced. There was a thorough investigation of a reported case of a neurological syndrome after eating a common local dish of fish-porridge in Bangkok during October 2002. The investigation revealed that the meat was from puffer fish, which is widely used as a substitute because it is less expensive and easy to obtain from large markets. The result of the investigation was presented to the authorities of the Thai Food and Drug Administration. A new regulation to prohibit selling of puffer fish was enacted to minimize a risk of tetrodotoxin poisoning from puffer fish consumption in the country (Samitsuwan et al. 2005).

Research to provide knowledge of the disease

Information about new diseases and their natural history, clinical spectrum, incubation periods, etc. can often be best learned during an outbreak investigation. Outbreak investigation can help ascertain new information, for example, modes of transmission, population at risk, and so on, and so provide essential information which can significantly contribute to the medical/public health literature. The outbreak of encephalitis in Malaysia, which continued until the end of April 1999 and resulted in 257 cases and 100 deaths, prompted an international outbreak investigation, resulting in the discovery of a new virus, Nipah (Centers for Disease Control and Prevention 1999b, 1999c). The mode of transmission was close contact with infected pigs through blood and secretions.

Evaluation of the effectiveness of prevention programmes

Investigation of an outbreak of disease, which is the target of a public health programme, may reveal weaknesses in that programme. Investigation of an outbreak of vaccine-preventable diseases often identifies populations that have not received the vaccine. For example, investigation of a measles outbreak that occurred in 1993 in Espindola, a rural community in the Peruvian Andes, revealed that more than a quarter of the 553 residents were affected, and that more than 3 per cent of those who contracted measles had died. One year before the outbreak, a national measles campaign targeting children younger than 15 years had been conducted. Although national data reported the coverage to be 78 per cent, the investigation revealed that only 4 per cent of the children in Espindola had actually been vaccinated (Sniadack et al. 1999).

Evaluation of the effectiveness of the existing surveillance system

Some aspects of the surveillance system can be evaluated during an outbreak, such as the timeliness, validity, sensitivity, appropriateness of case definitions, and utilization of the surveillance information.

Training of health professionals

The Epidemic Intelligence Service of the US Centers for Disease Control and Prevention (CDC) and over 50 field epidemiology training programmes around the world use real outbreaks as an opportunity for training health professionals, as well as to provide emergency services by investigating the causes and determinants of outbreaks. Recommendations and action taken by these applied epidemiology programmes resulted in a limited scale of outbreaks and improved the health of the public.

Responding to public, political, and legal concerns

In many situations, an investigation must be conducted because the media has publicized the complaints of people to politicians, or even rumours. The main objective for this kind of investigation is to verify the outbreak and diagnosis. If it is groundless, the investigator can supply the media with new information that can end the rumours. Conversely, if it is a true outbreak, investigators must decide on what steps need to be taken.

In general, for a real outbreak, many objectives can be achieved fully or at least partially. However, the ultimate goal is to control the current outbreak and to prevent future ones. It is unethical for investigators to compromise this ultimate goal with other goals such as training or non-essential research that does not directly contribute to control activities.

Components of an investigation team

In this chapter, the term *investigators* will represent people who are directly involved in planning and conducting outbreak investigations from start to finish. In principle, local health professionals at the district or provincial level should assume the role of investigators and start work as soon as possible. For complicated or difficult field investigations, additional disciplines or international experts can provide assistance. It is best to form an investigation team with a team leader in charge of the operation. A good investigation team should include the following:

1. A field epidemiologist who is technically competent to conduct field investigations systematically. The field epidemiologist usually serves as one of the primary investigators, and should be involved in all the investigative steps.

2. Disease control specialists who are experienced in implementing basic disease control measures such as food and environmental sanitation, vector control, and vaccination. If available, an educator who can provide essential knowledge to villagers in clear terms is also very useful for disease control implementation.

3. Laboratory technicians who are able to provide basic and advanced laboratory support to the investigation team. They might not need to travel to the field and collect the specimens themselves, except when a special collection procedure is required.

4. Specialists in particular areas (e.g. veterinary medicine) would be very helpful for an outbreak investigation of zoonotic diseases. An entomologist is a key team member for an outbreak investigation of vector-borne diseases. A social scientist with expertise in qualitative methods can help identify risk behaviours among affected populations and assess the acceptability of the recommended interventions.

5. Public health administrators who are good at providing logistic support, mobilizing resources, and providing administrative expertise for the team.

6. In certain situations, when the outbreak has caused panic or has gained the intense attention of the public, the investigation team should recruit or appoint a person to be in charge of public relations and press releases. This person should appropriately reassure and not unduly alarm the public.

In practice, all of these team members are not always available at the subdistrict or district level, due to limited human resources. Public health professionals and field epidemiologists need to have basic knowledge of all these relevant disciplines and be able to assume these tasks if needed. In the event of a technical problem or the need for consultation from the field, telecommunication equipment should be provided to field investigators.

Due to the sudden nature of a field investigation, it is best to establish in advance a list of people who will be on call and are ready to join an investigation team once an outbreak has occurred. The Thai Ministry of Public Health established 1030 Surveillance and Rapid Respond Teams to serve as investigation and control teams at all districts nationwide when the avian influenza outbreak occurred in early 2004. Public health officers received practical epidemiology training, and subsequently became frontline armies tracking outbreaks in their local area.

Issues to be considered before implementing an investigation

The team leader should consider all of the following issues before initiating a field investigation.

Assessing the existence of the outbreak

No matter how outbreak news is obtained, an investigator should confirm the validity of the information. The best way is to have direct communication with the responsible local health authority or field staff. It is not unusual for the information to be groundless. Sometimes, the outbreak has in fact occurred, but the media incorrectly quoted the name of the location. The investigator should carefully check with all other possible local health authorities so as not to overlook the outbreak.

Gathering available basic information

If the local health authority or field staff confirms the existence of the outbreak, the investigator should ask for additional information related to the situation and control measures being implemented. It is not necessary to gather all of the following listed information before leaving for the field, but having it will help investigators to plan an effective investigation.

Information related to the disease situation

1. What are the main symptoms and signs of the patients?

2. By whom and how was the diagnosis made; for example, using only clinical or also laboratory evidence?

3. How many patients were seen and how many died?

4. What was the average age of the patients and were there any differences in gender distribution?

5. Where did the patients come from? Are they clustered or scattered?

6. When was the increased number first observed and what is the trend at the moment?

Information related to control and response activities

1. What has already been done in terms of the field investigation and implementation of control activities?

2. Are there any serious constraints that compromise the field investigation and/or implementing control measures?

3. Who are the key people responsible for the investigation and control activities?

Ensuring that clinical specimens and suspected materials are collected in a timely and appropriate manner

It is absolutely critical to contact the doctors who saw the cases and made the diagnosis to obtain relevant clinical specimens such as serum and blood for future laboratory tests. The items to which the cases were exposed, such as food and water, should be collected immediately before anything is unintentionally destroyed. The investigator should contact the local and reference laboratories so that the necessary supplies and equipment can be obtained immediately.

Obtaining permission and adequate support from local and national authorities

The investigation team should ask the permission of the local health authorities, which will create a sense of shared responsibility and partnership. Usually local authorities are pleased to receive assistance. In a few situations, the local authority might be unhappy about having outsiders conduct the field investigation because of the sensitive nature of the problem. The investigator needs to convince local authorities that a thorough and sound investigation will incur more benefits than harm. The investigator should also request field support from the key authorities, such as field staff who will facilitate the fieldwork and provide transportation, medication, etc. In some situations, if the outbreak is possibly of international concern spelled out by the 2005 International Health Regulations, the principal investigator should inform national authorities so they are aware and can plan further necessary steps to report to WHO and deal with the media and international communities.

Planning the field operation

The investigator needs to have a short meeting with team members to summarize the situation, set up the objectives of the investigations, divide responsibility among team members, and check the readiness of laboratory and logistical support.

It is also important to plan the duration of the field investigation. The investigation team should stay in the field until all investigation processes such as data collection, analysis, interpretation, and the executive summary have been completed. Leaving the field without accomplishing all these objectives could delay the implementation of control measures. Most outbreak investigations should plan to obtain preliminary results and recommendations within a week of the start of the investigation to ensure that the findings will be timely enough for control of the current outbreak. Additional studies and subsequent investigations can be conducted later.

The investigation team should not spend too much time preparing a perfect plan, because of the urgency of the outbreak; rather, they should obtain what is most necessary and start the investigation as soon as possible.

Steps of outbreak investigation

An outbreak investigation is an observational study by nature, because the events have already occurred. Every outbreak investigation needs to start with a good descriptive study, followed by analytical studies whenever possible and necessary. Conclusions about the causes, sources, mechanisms, and determinants of the outbreak need to be drawn, based on sound epidemiological, clinical, laboratory, and environmental evidence.

A descriptive study can help to identify the risk population(s) and risk area(s) so that immediate interventions can be directed to those who need them the most. A good descriptive study can also generate hypotheses about how the outbreak has spread and what factors contributed to the abnormal occurrence of the disease. In theory, hypotheses derived from a descriptive study should be confirmed by further analytical study; in reality, this is not always possible, due to many constraints.

It is preferable to translate the methodology for outbreak investigation into steps of action. Gregg (1996) has divided the outbreak investigation process into ten steps; with a slight modification, this ten-step investigation process has been summarized in Box 5.4.1. Steps 1–4 use descriptive epidemiology to generate basic facts and hypotheses, steps 5–7 are processes to test the hypotheses and draw conclusions, and steps 8–10 emphasize the importance of communication of the results and follow-up of the recommendations.

This outline does not imply a strict course of action. In real outbreak investigations, many steps may be undertaken concurrently, depending on the situation.

Step 1: confirm the existence of an outbreak

The main question is: 'Is this a true outbreak?' Applying the definition of an outbreak outlined in this chapter, the investigator

---

Box 5.4.1 Ten steps to take in an outbreak investigation

1. Confirm the existence of the outbreak.

2. Verify the diagnosis and determine the aetiology of the disease.

3. Develop a case definition, start case finding, and collect information on cases.

4. Describe persons, places, and times, and generate hypotheses.

5. Test the hypotheses using an analytic study.

6. Carry out necessary environmental or other studies to supplement the epidemiological study.

7. Draw conclusions to explain the causes or the determinants of the outbreak, based on clinical, laboratory, epidemiological, and environmental studies.

8. Report and recommend appropriate control measures to concerned authorities at the local, national, and if appropriate, international levels.

9. Communicate the findings to educate other public health professionals and the general public.

10. Follow up the recommendations to ensure implementation of control measures.

Source: data from Gregg M.B. (ed.), Conducting a field investigation, p. 44–59, in *Field Epidemiology*, Oxford University Press, New York, USA, Copyright © Oxford University Press, Inc. 1996.

should be able to establish or refute the existence of the outbreak. Investigators should review the number of cases with the local health officers or hospital staff and compare it with the number found during the same period recorded in past years.

For example, the outbreak of trichinosis in North Rhine-Westphalia, Germany, was confirmed because there were 52 cases in a 3-month period between November 1998 and January 1999, compared with no more than ten cases annually during the same time period in the past 10 years (Centers for Disease Control and Prevention 1999d).

Step 2: verify the diagnosis and aetiology of the disease

If the number of cases fits the case criteria for the outbreak, the next related questions are:

1. What is the correct diagnosis and aetiology of the disease?

2. What can be done immediately to prevent new cases from occurring?

Knowing the exact diagnosis and aetiology of the disease will help to establish appropriate preventive measures immediately. This will protect susceptible people and allow the team to start educating villagers to avoid the risk factors. For example, many adults in a remote village were ill with fever, muscle and joint pain, rashes, etc. If the diagnosis and aetiology of the disease is unknown, the local public health officials will find it very difficult to educate the public or implement effective preventive programmes. Until the serology of some patients showed sharply rising immunoglobulin M (IgM) antibodies to dengue virus, control measures to destroy the larvae of the *Aedes* mosquito, the vector of dengue which breeds in water containers, could not be started.

In many situations, an unknown or unclear diagnosis can cause panic due to rumours. This was demonstrated by an outbreak of pneumonic plague in Surat, India in 1994, and of encephalitis in Malaysia in 1999, which resulted in severe panic among local people and foreign tourists. Thus, it is very important to obtain the exact diagnosis as rapidly as possible.

Investigators should have basic knowledge of the clinical diagnosis and how to confirm the aetiology of suspected disease by using well-established laboratory techniques. It is recommended that investigators visit and talk with some patients, review and visualize the signs and symptoms, and hold discussions with the attending doctors. The information from this step will help to develop a case definition to facilitate active case-finding. The information on aetiology will also help to interpret the findings from the later descriptive study and establish a causal association.

The investigators should also visit the laboratory facilities and ask for either positive or negative results of the testing of specimens. It is not necessary for all cases to be laboratory confirmed, but at least some of the apparent clinical cases or deaths should be confirmed. Once there are laboratory-confirmed cases, the investigator will find it more reasonable to assume that other cases with the same clinical manifestations in the same period and location are the same disease.

It is unfortunate that specimens from patients are often thrown away when the primary results (either positive or negative) are obtained. The investigators should plan with the doctors and laboratory scientists to perform further investigations on the specific strain, and to establish drug sensitivities, genetic markers, etc.

Many new laboratory technologies, such as serological testing, culture and isolation, and molecular techniques, are very powerful for diagnosing and tracking the connections between cases, even in different geographical areas. For example, outbreaks of *Shigella sonnei* infections in Denmark and Australia were detected during the same week in August 2007, and 215 laboratory-confirmed cases were reported in Denmark, with an additional 12 cases in Australia. Antibiotic resistance and pulsed field gel electrophoresis in isolates identified in those two outbreaks were indistinguishable. A hypothesis that the patients were exposed to the same implicated food item from the same original source was soon proved (Lewis et al. 2009).

Step 3: develop an appropriate case definition, start case finding, and collect information on cases

At this stage, the investigator needs to answer at least three questions:

1. Who should be counted as a case?

2. Are there more undetected cases in the hospitals and in the community?

3. What are the characteristics of cases?

To answer these three questions, the investigators must follow three steps.

Develop an appropriate case definition

It is important that the investigator develop a case definition, which will be applied consistently during the investigation. The definition should be sensitive or adequate at the beginning, in order to capture actual cases. A good case definition for investigative purposes should be specific to time and location. The case definition should not include any specific suspected exposure that the investigator plans to verify. This would create selection bias when the investigator generates the hypothesis or tests the hypothesis in the subsequent steps. Using the information obtained from the previous steps, the investigator can divide the case definition into different levels.

For example, in September 2012, when two patients with a novel coronavirus from Saudi Arabia and Qatar were found, WHO requested member states to start surveillance of the disease by using the interim case definitions as shown in Box 5.4.2.

Active case finding

In places where there is good surveillance, cases from all hospitals can be reported to the epidemiology unit at the district or provincial level. Investigators can apply the case definition and count the number of cases, and review data that are collected on the reporting form. If enough cases and basic information on cases have already been gathered, investigators can start descriptive epidemiology.

Conversely, if only a few cases have been seen at the health facility, the investigators should plan to search for more cases in the community. The investigator must start a process called *active case finding*. The objective of active case finding is to have enough cases to analyse. At the same time, this case finding will give a better picture of the magnitude of the outbreak. Investigators must frequently visit many hospitals in the outbreak area and review medical records themselves. Sometimes, they must search

Box 5.4.2 WHO interim case definitions for a novel coronavirus

1. Patients to be investigated (referred to as 'patient under investigation'):

- A person with an acute respiratory infection, which may include fever (≥38°C, 100.4°F) and cough; *and*

- Suspicion of pulmonary parenchymal disease (e.g. pneumonia or acute respiratory distress syndrome (ARDS)), based on clinical or radiological evidence of consolidation; *and*

- Travel to or residence in an area where infection with novel coronavirus has recently been reported or where transmission could have occurred (see updated area in WHO website) *and*

- Not already explained by any other infection or aetiology, including all clinically indicated tests for community-acquired pneumonia according to local management guidelines.

2. Probable case

- A person fitting the definition given in (1) of a 'patient under investigation' with clinical, radiological, or histo-pathological evidence of pulmonary parenchyma disease (e.g. pneumonia or ARDS) but no possibility of laboratory confirmation either because the patient or samples are not available or there is no testing available for other respiratory infections, *and*

- Close contact with a laboratory confirmed case, *and*

- Not already explained by any other infection or aetiology, including all clinically indicated tests for community-acquired pneumonia according to local management guidelines.

3. Confirmed case

A person with laboratory confirmation of infection with the novel coronavirus.

Reproduced with permission from World Health Organization, *Global Alert and Response (GAR): WHO Interim Case Definition—Novel Coronavirus*, as of 29 September 2012, Copyright © World Health Organization 2012, available from http://www.who.int/csr/disease/coronavirus_infections/case_definition_29092012/en/index.html.

for cases in each village by interviewing house to house, which is the true nature of outbreak field investigations and the way people learn epidemiology. This active case finding in the community also provides two more benefits:

1. Control measures can be implemented if the aetiology of the disease is known and treatable. During an investigation, using active case searching in a village that reported seven deaths from malaria in Kachin state in the Union of Myanmar, the investigator found 94 probable cases and 53 microscopically confirmed malaria infections. All of the probable and confirmed cases found by this active process were treated. Without this measure, there might have been more deaths later on (Dr Myint Win, personal communication, 1999).

2. Rapid environmental assessment can be started during the visit to the affected families or villages. From the direct interview with the cases, the investigators can develop hypotheses and implement necessary interventions immediately, such as sanitation improvement among food handlers and treatment of water to prevent a waterborne outbreak.

In situations in which the outbreak is not localized but widespread, the investigator might need to use the media to alert the public about the outbreak. People can then avoid suspected exposures and see a healthcare provider if they have developed symptoms compatible with the case definition.

Collecting information on cases

For each case, the investigator should collect at least four types of information:

1. Identifying information: name, hospital number, contact person, and address of contact. This additional information will help to avoid duplication of enumerated cases. The investigator can also maintain communication with these cases when more information is needed.

2. Demographic information: age, gender, occupation, religion, ethnicity, area of residence, place of employment, etc. This important information may help to determine the characteristics and distribution of cases.

3. Clinical information: symptoms and signs, date of onset, duration of illness, and results of diagnostic procedures. These data will help to confirm a true case, provide the pattern of clinical manifestations, and also the distribution of cases by time.

4. Suspected risk factors: investigators can ask for a history of exposure to factors before the disease developed. The timing of interest is usually one incubation period if the aetiology is known or suspected. Questions about contact with other patients who have similar clinical symptoms are also very helpful. If the diagnosis is not known, the investigator should collect this information in a qualitative manner.

The investigator should develop a questionnaire as a tool to collect the relevant information from the hospitals or during active case searching in the community. In practice, some of the information will not be available or not of good quality. The investigators should validate all data in doubt.

Step 4: describe the outbreak in person, place, and time, and hypotheses formation

In this step, investigators need to answer the following questions:

1. What are the main clinical features?

2. What population(s) is at risk?

3. What are the risk factors?

4. What are the most likely explanations of how the outbreak began?

A simple approach is to analyse clinical information from each case and see the distribution of cases in terms of person, place, and time. The analysis should be done using rates rather than absolute numbers; the investigator needs to obtain the denominators from an available source or to estimate them. Using rates, the investigator can compare and determine the populations and areas of highest risk. With the advent of computers, many software programs are available to analyse these data. A popular one is EpiInfo™, which is public domain software from the US CDC that is designed specifically for field investigations. In the absence of a computer, investigators can still analyse data manually. Individual questionnaires can be compiled into a line listing, which includes important variables of all cases. With this line listing, simple counts can be made. In this way, investigators will gain knowledge about populations and areas of risk. Resource and control measures can then be directed to the risk populations and risk areas. Enumeration will also produce information for hypothesis formation to explain how and why the outbreak occurred.

Clinical manifestations of cases

Signs and symptoms of cases can be analysed in percentages and presented in a summary table. In an outbreak of unknown aetiology, clinical information will help to establish the diagnosis. For an outbreak in which the aetiology is already known, the investigators still need to compare the clinical information found in the investigation with previous knowledge. Any discrepancy between the investigation and previous knowledge such as the attack rate, mortality rate, severity, and so on should be carefully examined, because this might indicate that a new strain or different specific host response is occurring. The high mortality rate of approximately 40 per cent in the Nipah encephalitis outbreak in Malaysia 1999 (Centers for Disease Control and Prevention 1999c) indicated that this outbreak might not be due to the usual endemic encephalitis.

Populations at risk

Investigators should analyse the characteristics of cases by gender, age, occupation, ethnicity, and so on. Initially this can be carried out by examining the proportion of all cases, but the specific attack rate by age and gender will be more useful for comparisons and hypothesis formation. The rates will provide useful indicators of the possible aetiology of the outbreak. In the Ebola haemorrhagic fever outbreak in Zaire in 1976, all ages and both genders were affected, but females slightly predominated. Age- and gender-specific attack rates indicated that adult females had the highest attack rate. This finding suggested that parenteral injection with unsterilized syringes and needles given during antenatal care in the local hospital was the means of transmission (World Health Organization 1978).

The outbreak of Nipah encephalitis in Malaysia in early 1999 was initially thought to be due to Japanese encephalitis alone. However, after careful analysis of the descriptive information, it was clear that the cases were mainly male, adult, involved in pig farming, and of Chinese ethnicity. This descriptive information did not fit the pattern for Japanese encephalitis, which mainly affects children of both genders, with no preference for a particular ethnicity. The investigator then began to suspect other organisms and to hypothesize that pig farming increased the risk of becoming ill.

Primary, index, and outlier cases

In infectious diseases, the first case on the epidemic curve is called the primary case. The primary case is important, because of the possibility that he/she brought the disease into the community either from the local area or from other locales. In investigations, sometimes the first case that draws the attention of the investigator is not the primary case. We call this the 'index case'. Index cases may be detected at the hospital or during the active case finding. The investigator may find the primary case among those who were sick in the community but did not seek medical care. Cases that appear at the very beginning or at the end of the epidemic who are markedly different from the rest of cases should also be given careful attention. These cases are called *outlier cases*, and can provide important information about the source and the way in which the disease is spread. A tourist who happened to be only a short time in the village during the outbreak and get sick is an example of an outlier.

Typically, the very first and very last cases in the epidemic curve should be critically appraised. The first case may not be the true index case because of misdiagnosis, a case unrelated to the epidemic, etc. The late cases may be due to misdiagnosis, a case unrelated to the epidemic, or a secondary case that had a different exposure than the majority of the cases in the epidemic.

During the outbreak of severe acute respiratory syndrome (SARS) in February 2003, the index case was identified as a 65-year-old medical doctor from Guangdong, mainland China, who stayed on the 9th floor of a hotel in Hong Kong (Fig. 5.4.2). He had treated patients with atypical pneumonia prior to his departure, and he was symptomatic upon arrival in Hong Kong. He infected over a dozen guests and international visitors. During the outbreak investigation, the investigators tried to identify contacts of this index case to prevent further transmission. A history and information of this index case obtained by the investigation team traced these cases back to previous atypical pneumonia outbreaks or undiagnosed SARS since late 2002 (World Health Organization Regional Office for the Western Pacific, 2006).

Location

Investigators can calculate attack rates of cases in different locations. These can be places of residence, places of employment, sites of exposure, etc. Locations with high attack rates often indicate the sources of infection or contamination. A spot map showing the locations of cases can give a very good idea of the source, as demonstrated by Snow in his classical investigation of a cholera outbreak in the Golden Square area of London between August and September 1854 (Frost 1936). In that investigation, Snow found most cases clustered around the Broad Street pump. From this information, Snow deduced that the Broad Street pump was probably the primary source of the outbreak.

If cases are scattered in many locations, investigators should explore the secular pattern of the cases over time, which will indicate whether the outbreak started in one area and spread to other areas, or whether people living in different places had a common exposure. The SARS outbreak is a good example of when cases are distributed worldwide originally from a single source of infection.

9th floor of the Metropole Hotel, 21 February 2003

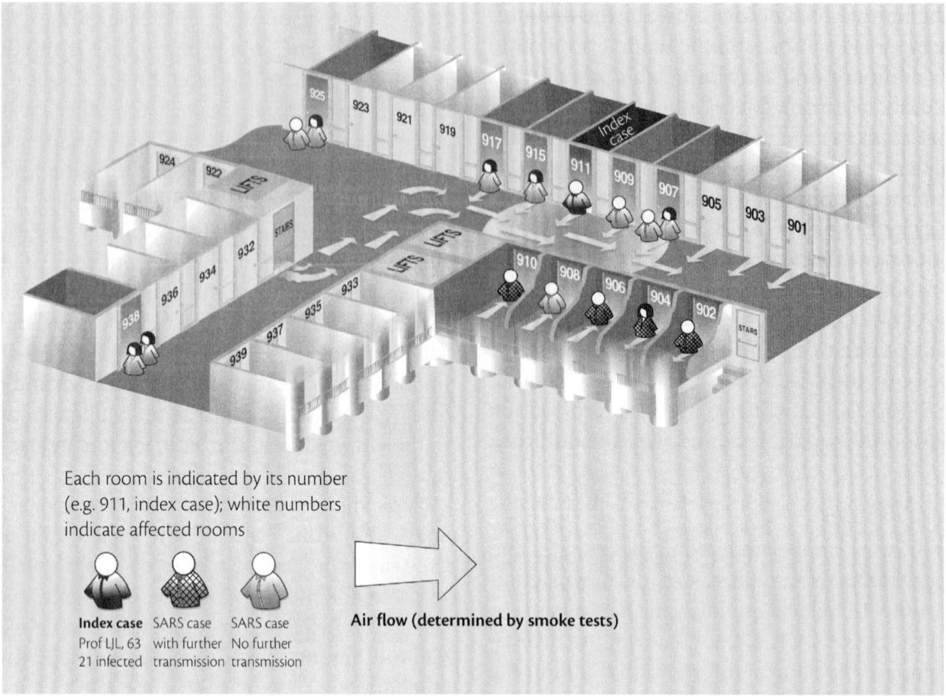

Fig. 5.4.2 Index case of SARS—Hong Kong, 2003.

Reproduced with permission from World Health Organization Regional Office for the Western Pacific, *SARS: How a Global Epidemic was Stopped*, World Health Organization, Western Pacific Region, Manila, Philippines, Copyright © 2006.

Time

The objective is to show the occurrence of cases over time and look for a pattern of occurrence. In general, there are two major types of outbreaks: a common source and a propagated source. The way to differentiate between these two patterns of outbreak is to draw an epidemic curve that shows the number of cases (on the *y*-axis) over time of onset (on the *x*-axis). The epidemic curve of each outbreak will suggest whether the mode of spread is by a common source or from person to person.

Common source outbreak

This kind of outbreak occurs when people are infected by exposure to the same source of infection. For example, a group of people contract viral hepatitis A because they ate the same contaminated food served during a wedding party. A common source outbreak can be divided into a point common source and a continuous common source:

1. A point common source outbreak occurs when there is a single source that exists for a very short time and all cases have common exposure to it at that particular time.

2. A continuous common source outbreak occurs when there is only one source that provides continuous or intermittent exposure over a longer period of time.

Epidemic curve of a point common source outbreak: the epidemic curve shows a sharp increase of many cases suddenly followed by a rapid decline, although not as rapid as at the beginning of the epidemic. Another criterion to judge a point common source is that the first and the last cases usually occur within one incubation period.

If the aetiology and the data of the incubation period of the disease are known, the investigators can then roughly estimate the probable time of the initial exposure. This can be done by identifying the peak of the epidemic from the curve and counting back on the *x*-axis the equivalent of the incubation period. The investigator can also use the first case and count back on the *x*-axis the duration of the minimum incubation period, which will also give a rough estimate of the time of exposure. In the opposite way, if the information on aetiologic agent and incubation period is unknown but the common exposure time is known, the mean incubation is the duration from exposure to the peak of the curve. The shortest incubation period is the duration from the time of exposure to the onset of the first case and the longest incubation period is the duration from the time of exposure to the onset of the last case.

If the aetiology of the disease is not known, but the epidemic curve fits well with a point common source outbreak, the investigator can estimate the average incubation period if he or she knows the times of common exposure.

Epidemic curve for a continuous common source outbreak: the epidemic curve shows an abrupt increase in the number of cases, but instead of having a peak and a decline within one incubation period, new cases persist for a longer time, with a plateau shape instead of a peak before decreasing. In the outbreak of food

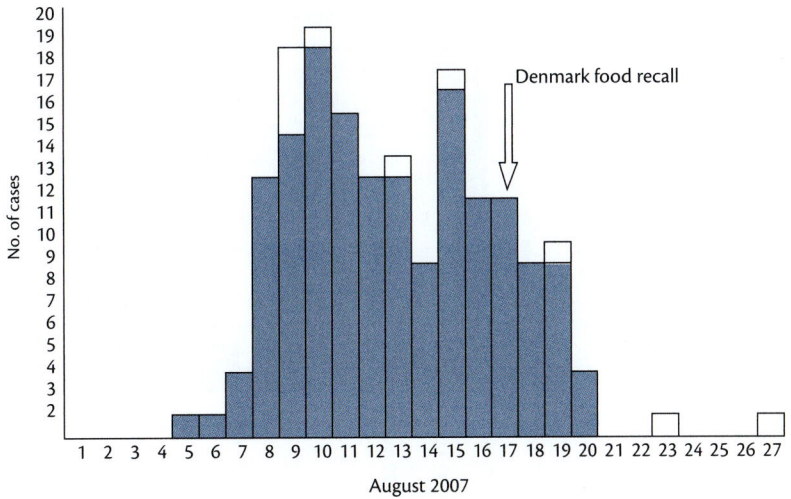

Fig. 5.4.3 Dates of illness onset for 163 cases in an outbreak of *Shigella sonnei* infections linked to consumption of imported raw baby corn in Denmark (■) and Australia (□) in August 2007.

From Lewis HC et al., Outbreaks of Shigella sonnei infections in Denmark and Australia linked to consumption of imported raw baby corn, *Epidemiology and Infection*, Volume 137, Special Issue 03, pp. 326–34, Copyright © 2009 Cambridge University Press, reproduced with permission, DOI: http://dx.doi.org/10.1017/S0950268808001829.

poisoning caused by *Shigella sonnei* infections linked to consumption of imported raw baby corn in Denmark and Australia in August 2007, the peak of the outbreak was observed 6 days after the onset date of the first case and gradually declined (Fig. 5.4.3). All of the cases developed symptoms within a 2-week period, and the outbreak subsided soon after a recall of the implicated batches of baby corn on 17 August 2007 (Lewis et al. 2009). However, if there are many peaks or irregular jagged curves, it suggests an intermittent common source.

Propagated outbreak

A propagated outbreak is caused by transmission from one person to another, and requires direct contact such as touching, biting, kissing, or sexual activity or via vector such as in vector-borne disease outbreak.

Epidemic curve of propagated source outbreak: the epidemic curve shows a slow increase in the number of cases, with progressive peaks approximately one incubation period apart. The investigators might observe an abrupt decrease in new cases, because everyone has already been infected. The span from the first to the last case will also last longer than several incubation periods.

The outbreaks of SARS in Singapore demonstrated the propagated source of transmission beginning from a young female who returned home from Hong Kong. This patient had stayed on the same hotel floor as the index case. She had initially infected many hospital staff before the disease spread for further generations (Kamps and Hoffmann 2003). The outbreak resulted in 238 cases and 33 deaths in a few months (Fig. 5.4.4).

Step 5: testing the hypotheses by an analytic study

In an outbreak of infectious disease, the investigator needs to answer the following questions:

1. What is the aetiology of the disease?

2. What is the source of infection?

3. What is the pattern of spread?

4. What are the risk factors for an individual to get the disease?

5. What are the determinants of the outbreak or the factors which, when combined together, result in the outbreak?

The aetiology of the disease should be derived from the laboratory study. The pattern of spread can be identified by a careful descriptive study. Sometimes it is not as simple as expected, and a descriptive study does not give enough clues. The investigator must carefully re-examine the descriptive information, carry out more active case-finding, and re-analyse the data. The investigator also needs to directly observe the location, lifestyle, and/or behaviour of the cases. These additional investigations usually help the investigator to generate some reasonable hypotheses.

A hypothesis needs to be tested by an analytical study design. The most common is a case–control study. The investigator needs to define the cases and measure the odds of suspected exposed factors found among cases in comparison to the odds of exposure found among appropriately selected controls. The case definition for the analytical study may be more specific than that used for a descriptive study in order to reduce misclassifying non-cases as cases. Conversely, the controls may also need to be tested to avoid classifying non-apparent cases as controls.

An example is the analytic study for identifying risk factors for haemolytic–uraemic syndrome in a large outbreak of Shiga toxin-producing *Escherichia coli* O104:H4 infections in Germany during May 2011 (Buchholz et al. 2011). A matched case–control study was carried out to obtain data from 26 case subjects with the haemolytic–uraemic syndrome and compared to data from

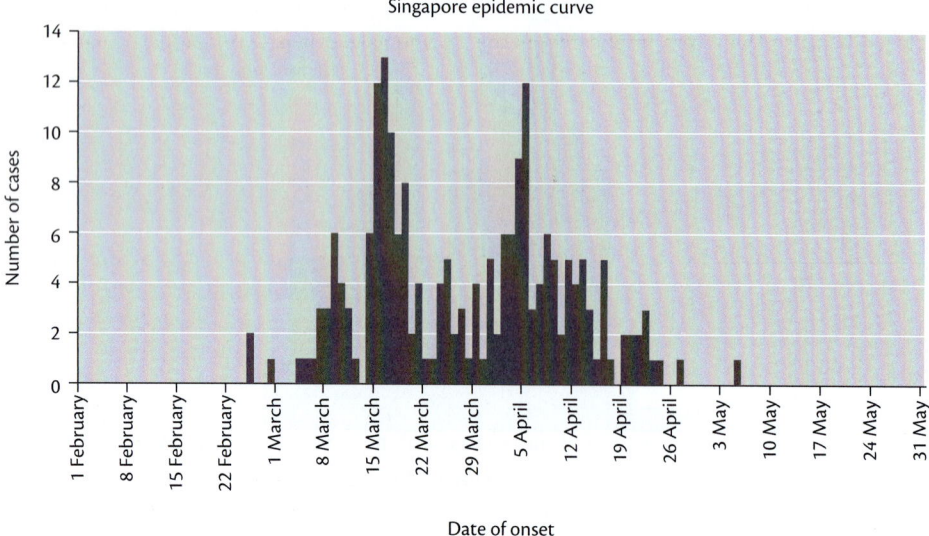

Fig. 5.4.4 SARS cases by date of onset—Singapore, 2003.

Reproduced with permission from World Health Organization Regional Office for the Western Pacific, *SARS: how a global epidemic was stopped*, World Health Organization, Western Pacific Region, Manila, Philippines, Copyright © 2006.

81 controls. The investigation revealed ingestion of raw sprouts as the vehicle of infection (matched odds ratio, 4.35; 95 per cent confidence interval, 1.05–18.0). A month after, a similar food poisoning outbreak of the same organism was detected in France (King et al. 2012). The investigators conducted a retrospective cohort study and they found an increased risk of developing the disease among adults who attended the buffet at the Children's Community Center Event on June 8, 2011 (relative risk, 5.1; 95 per cent confidence interval, 2.3–11.1) in multivariable analysis (Table 5.4.1).

Step 6: environmental or other studies to supplement epidemiological findings

Although an analytical study might be able to confirm a hypothesis, the investigator still needs to find environmental or other evidence to support and explain the epidemiological evidence. In an outbreak of unknown illness in a rural village of Egypt, in which the cases developed severe abdominal pain, persistent vomiting, and generalized weakness, the investigator was able to detect abnormally high blood lead levels among the cases. The analytical study revealed an association between high lead levels in the blood and eating flour from a particular mill factory. The mill implicated in the outbreak was visited, and upon arrival at the mill, the investigators noted a lead smelting pot in the corner of the mill. Lead was used by the miller to attach the crosspiece to the grinding stone. Occasionally the lead would break off and contaminate the flour. The miller reported using about 2 kg of lead per year. Analysis of grain from the mill showed no lead; however, lead was found in flour from the surface of the mill stone and in samples of flour after grinding was complete (Abdel-Nasser 1996).

Table 5.4.1 Multivariable Poisson regression with food-specific relative risks and 95 per cent confidence intervals among adults who attended the buffet at the Children's Community Center Event, France, June 2011 (n = 64)

Food item	RR	95% CI	P value[a]
Sprouts (any of the 3 kinds)	4.2	1.7–10.0	0.001
Gazpacho (tomato-based cold soup)	2.4	0.9–6.4	0.08
Carrots	2.3	0.8–7.1	0.14
Water (bottled)	2.0	0.8–5.2	0.14
Dip sauce (mayonnaise)	1.7	0.8–3.3	0.15
Lettuce	1.4	0.6–3.6	0.43
Green peppers	0.4	0.1–1.3	0.15

CI, confidence interval; RR, relative risk.

[a] All but 1 of the covariables in the presented final multivariable model have *P* values that are non-significant at the 0.05 level. These variables were left in the final model to ensure a sufficient numeric stability of the model.

Reproduced from King LA et al, Outbreak of Shiga toxin-producing Escherichia coli O104:H4 associated with organic fenugreek sprouts, France, June 2011, *Clinical Infectious Diseases*, Volume 54, Issue 11, pp. 1588–1594, Copyright © The Author 2012, published by Oxford University Press on behalf of the Infectious Diseases Society of America, by permission of Oxford University Press.

Step 7: establishing the causes of the outbreak

Once the hypothesis has been tested and other necessary studies have been carried out, the investigators can draw their conclusions about the causes of the outbreak. This conclusion is very important, because action should follow. Many restaurants or factories have been closed because they were implicated as the source of the outbreak. Outbreak investigations are naturally faced with constraints of time and other uncontrolled conditions that do not favour perfect design and methodology. The findings potentially include both random and systematic errors. Before drawing any conclusions, it is important that the investigator carefully examine the weaknesses or limitations of the investigation. In principle, the investigator must identify the cause of the outbreak based on the agreement of the following four pieces of evidence.

Laboratory evidence

The aetiology of the disease is identified in the patients and in the suspected source of infection. If the investigator cannot identify the aetiology from the suspected source, it is still possible to use certain markers to support their conclusions. For example, although a *Vibrio cholerae* type O1 could not be cultured from the drinking water supply of the affected community, the observation of human faecal coliform bacteria in the water helped to indicate that human faeces had contaminated the water.

Clinical evidence

It is necessary to verify that the incubation period and clinical manifestations of cases are compatible with the aetiological agents reported from the laboratory. In the SARS outbreak, most patients developed atypical pneumonia, with rapid progression to respiratory failure, and a fraction of them also had diarrhoea, which could be explained by the findings of SARS coronavirus both in the respiratory tract and stools of patients.

Environmental evidence

Careful investigation of the environment should reveal clues that the causative agent can pass from the source to the cases or the index case to subsequent cases. The investigation of early SARS cases revealed that the index case passed the virus to several people who stayed on the same floor and used the same elevator (Centers for Diseases Control and Prevention 2003).

For an outbreak of food poisoning, a cooking environment that is dirty or located close to the toilet is convincing evidence of food being contaminated by faeces. Crowding in bedrooms is very convincing evidence for a respiratory tract disease outbreak.

Epidemiological evidence

Epidemiological evidence found in the descriptive and analytical studies should clearly explain the following aspects:

• Pattern of spread, as described by an epidemic curve.

• Statistical strength of association between exposure and developing the disease.

• Dose–response relationship, which demonstrates a higher strength of association when the exposure is increasing.

• Exposure should precede an illness.

It is not uncommon to see some disagreement in the evidence from different sources. In this event, the investigator needs to verify the validity of each piece of evidence and discuss the data with people who have expertise in that particular area in order to obtain more information and draw a valid conclusion.

Step 8: on-site reporting to and recommendations for concerned authorities

The most important step leading to a timely response is to report the findings to the responsible individuals both at the local and national levels so that they can take appropriate action. Keeping this in mind, the investigators need to complete two tasks before leaving the outbreak area:

1. Complete analysis and data interpretation: leaving the field without completing these tasks will reduce the sense of urgency necessary to finish the work. Data are easier to retrieve when staying in the field rather than instructing field people to send them to the investigation team later.

2. Present the main findings with recommendations: some findings may be very sensitive because they reflect the weaknesses or mistakes of health personnel or other authorities. The investigator needs to select the appropriate approach, either formal or informal, with those responsible. Leaving the field without providing the information that the team obtains from the investigation will be detrimental to other people who could be prevented from becoming ill if the information were known. In many urgent situations, the findings and recommendations might be regularly given to the people responsible during the outbreak investigation process instead of waiting until the end. The investigators also need to present or communicate the findings and recommendations to the national authorities as soon as possible. The recommendations for action should be based on the findings of the investigation. These might include the following aspects.

What can be done to control the outbreak?

With timely investigation, some interventions can be implemented to stop further spread. In the outbreak of measles in a rural community in Peru, measles vaccines were given to children aged between 6 months and 15 years who were not measles cases, regardless of their previous immunization status. Using knowledge about the complication of measles in previous studies, the investigators estimated that the action prevented 87 cases of diarrhoea and 46 cases of pneumonia, and averted five deaths (Sniadack et al. 1999). Outbreaks can be controlled even if the disease aetiology is not known at the moment, but the mode of transmission is known from the investigation. One good example is the early story of the HIV/AIDS epidemic when sexual transmission was identified as a major mode of transmission among sexually active, young gay men.

How to prevent future outbreaks

In many instances, interventions cannot be implemented for the current outbreak, but the findings can be used to set up new practices or policies. These recommendations can help prevent future outbreaks. In Thailand, the recommendation was made to change practices of chicken farming and avoiding direct contact with sick poultry, which was recommended through the results of the investigation of human H5N1 cases. The Egyptian government, after reviewing the results of the investigation of lead contamination in flour mills, agreed to ban the use of lead in privately owned flour mills (Abdel-Nasser 1996).

How to improve the investigation

The investigator should review the performance of the investigation and identify the weaknesses of the methodology or the field operation so that improvements can be made. These might include a more appropriate case definition, a better investigative design, improved laboratory support, a different team composition, lower costs, a shorter time course, etc.

How to improve surveillance

The best time to evaluate the surveillance system is during an outbreak investigation. In most outbreaks, the investigator must review data from existing surveillance systems. With this direct involvement, the investigator will be able to evaluate the timeliness, completeness, validity of diagnosis, sensitivity of the system, and utilization of the surveillance information. The investigation of human cases of avian influenza (H5N1) in Thailand led to an improved definition of a human case in the areas experiencing an H5N1 virus outbreak in poultry.

Step 9: dissemination of information

In addition to on-site reporting, the investigator should disseminate information to educate the public health community and the general public. There may be many other communities that are also prone to a similar outbreak. The information will raise the awareness of health and government authorities to assess their own situation and implement measures to prevent possible outbreaks. Dissemination of information should occur in a timely manner through weekly or monthly reports. Release of important findings through the mass media is also very useful for educating the public. Before releasing the investigation results through the media, the investigator must ensure that all the facts are delivered in a constructive manner and do not result in blame of any organization. The investigator should also report the investigation results in an international journal or bulletin such as the *Weekly Epidemiological Record* of the WHO, the *Morbidity and Mortality Weekly Report* of the US CDC, the *Eurosurveillance* of the European Centre for Disease Prevention and Control, or the epidemiological bulletin of their own country. This practice is necessary to alert health professionals in other countries and keep them informed of the problem.

In recent years, sharing of information for outbreak detection and control through the Internet and email has been increasingly utilized for timely responses. Telecommunications played an important role in the outbreaks of SARS when the disease was spread rapidly by air transportation to countries on the other side of the world. An example is a teleconference on the clinical features and management of SARS that was held by the WHO, which united 80 clinicians from 13 countries worldwide (World Health Organization Regional Office for the Western Pacific 2006).

Step 10: follow-up to ensure implementation of control measures

Finally, the investigator should follow up the investigation by maintaining close communication with local health authorities. An absence of new cases for at least two incubation periods of the infectious disease under investigation could suggest that the outbreak is subsiding. A good investigator should follow up on the recommendations. An outbreak investigation is a waste of time if sound recommendations have not been implemented. The investigator should learn the reasons why the recommendations were or were not implemented. If the recommendations were implemented, the investigator can also learn the impact by observing the trend of the disease.

Cooperation for international outbreak investigation and preparedness

The world today is especially prone to outbreaks because of frequent cross-border movement, civil war and migration, rapid transportation, international trading, tourism, etc. An outbreak in one country can spread to other countries very easily. For example, in the multi-country SARS outbreak, international travellers were at risk of disease spreading from a single infectious case in a hotel (Centers for Disease Control and Prevention 2003). Ultimately, there were over 8000 cases reported in 26 countries worldwide. The world's experience with the SARS outbreak led to the commitment of countries around the world to improve surveillance and international joint investigation of emerging infectious diseases through new international health regulations that were adopted by the World Health Assembly in 2005.

A massive outbreak of botulism in northern Thailand in March 2006 tested the international capacity to respond to a public health emergency. Botulism poisoning due to contaminated home-canned bamboo shoots caused illness in 209 villagers, of whom 134 persons were hospitalized and 42 required mechanical ventilation. A global search for botulinum antitoxin began, involving international agencies, embassies, national laboratories, airlines, and commercial organizations in seven countries. Sufficient antitoxin was obtained from four sources for treatment of 90 patients, with a delay in treatment of 5–9 days from time of exposure. Rapid local outbreak detection and an effective international response likely prevented mortality and additional morbidity (World Health Organization 2007).

An outbreak anywhere in the world must therefore be treated as a threat to all countries. It is important for each country to build up its capacity for surveillance, outbreak preparedness, and investigation. In addition to the US CDC Epidemic Intelligence Services, over 50 countries have started training programmes and established a medical detective unit that is ready to investigate all kinds of outbreaks. These training programmes are known by different names, such as the Field Epidemiology Training Program (FETP) or the Field Epidemiology and Laboratory Training Program (FELTP), and The European Programme for Intervention Epidemiology Training (EPIET). Recently, ten countries under the Association of South East Asian Nations

(ASEAN) joined China, Japan and South Korea to establish the ASEAN+3 Field Epidemiology Training Network (ASEAN+3 FETN) to foster national and regional capacity-building in disease surveillance and outbreak responses. The WHO has supported the establishment of the Global Outbreak Alert and Response Network, a technical collaboration of existing institutions and networks to pool human and technical resources for the rapid identification, confirmation and response to outbreaks of international importance. It is a wise investment, and a commitment that is needed by the international community for information exchange and collaborative investigation of outbreaks in a timely manner.

Conclusion

Outbreak investigation is an essential function of public health professionals who care for the well-being of the community. It is an opportunity to gain new knowledge of diseases and to discover the weaknesses of current public health practices and systems. A good public health professional must always be alert to the possibility of outbreaks. Normal surveillance systems or unofficial sources, such as the mass media, can be a good source for detection of an outbreak. Before starting field investigations, investigators should organize the team, review previous knowledge, prepare the technical and management aspects, and start the investigation as soon as possible. The investigation can be conducted by following the ten steps outlined in this chapter. The investigation usually starts by confirming the existence of the outbreak, verifying the diagnosis, gathering case information, descriptive epidemiology, formulating and testing the hypothesis when necessary, conducting environmental surveys to supplement epidemiological evidence, and providing timely on-site reporting of the findings, with practical recommendations to local and national responsible authorities. Competent outbreak investigators combine sound scientific knowledge and good management skills. Direct participation in conducting the investigation is needed to gain the necessary skills. A good investigator should be a field-oriented person with strong levels of perseverance, scepticism, and common sense. The investigator should not end his or her work with the report, but should follow up on the recommendations and continue vigorous surveillance of the problem. In the future, increasing joint international investigations will be needed. Rich countries and resource-limited countries need to collaborate to detect and stop outbreaks before they get out of control. Through this cooperation, the world will be a safer place amidst the threat of old and emerging disease outbreaks.

Online materials

Additional online materials for this chapter are available online at ℘ www.oxfordmedicine.com

References

Abdel-Nasser, M.A. (1996). *Outbreak Investigation of an Unknown Illness in a Rural Village, Egypt, 1996.* Cairo: Field Epidemiology Training Programs.

Biggar, R.J., Nasca, P.C., and Burnett, W.S. (1988). AIDS-related Kaposi's sarcoma in New York City in 1977. *The New England Journal of Medicine*, 318, 252.

Buchholz, U., Bernard, H., Werber, D., et al. (2011). German outbreak of Escherichia coli O104:H4 associated with sprouts. *The New England Journal of Medicine*, 365(19), 1763–70.

Centers for Disease Control and Prevention (1990). Mass sociogenic illness in a day-care center, Florida. *Morbidity and Mortality Weekly Report*, 39, 301–4.

Centers for Disease Control and Prevention (1996). Outbreak of unexplained illness in a middle school—Washington, April 1994. *Morbidity and Mortality Weekly Report*, 45, 6–9.

Centers for Disease Control and Prevention. (1999a). Food-borne botulism associated with home-canned bamboo shoots—Thailand, 1998. *Morbidity and Mortality Weekly Report*, 48, 437–9.

Centers for Disease Control and Prevention (1999b). Outbreak of Hendra-like virus—Malaysia and Singapore, 1998–1999. *Morbidity and Mortality Weekly Report*, 48, 265–9.

Centers for Disease Control and Prevention (1999c). Outbreak of Nipah virus—Malaysia and Singapore, 1999. *Morbidity and Mortality Weekly Report*, 48, 335–7.

Centers for Disease Control and Prevention (1999d). Trichinellosis outbreaks—North Rhine-Westphalia, Germany, 1998–1999. *Morbidity and Mortality Weekly Report*, 48, 488–92.

Centers for Disease Control and Prevention (2003). Update: outbreak of severe acute respiratory syndrome—worldwide, 2003. *Morbidity and Mortality Weekly Report*, 52, 241–8.

Centers for Disease Control and Prevention (2010). Update: influenza activity—United States, 2009–10 Season. *Morbidity and Mortality Weekly Report*, 59, 901–8.

Connolly, M.A. (ed.) (2005). *Communicable Disease Control in Emergencies: A Field Manual.* Geneva: World Health Organization.

Frost, W.H. (1936). *Introduction to Snow on Cholera.* London: Oxford University Press and Commonwealth Fund.

Gregg M.B. (1996). Conducting a field investigation. In M.B. Gregg (ed.) *Field Epidemiology*, pp. 44–59. New York: Oxford University Press.

Jongcherdchootrakul, K., Henderson, A.K., and Jiraphongsa, C. (2011). Injuries and deaths at a pub fire in Bangkok, Thailand on New Year's Eve 2009. *Burns*, 37(3), 499–502.

Kamps, B.S. and Hoffmann, C. (2003). Epidemiology. In B.S. Kamps and C. Hoffmann (eds.) *SARS Reference* (3rd ed.), p. 71. Paris: Flying Publisher.

King, L.A., Nogareda, F., Weill, F.X., et al. (2012). Outbreak of Shiga toxin-producing Escherichia coli O104:H4 associated with organic fenugreek sprouts, France, June 2011. *Clinical Infectious Diseases*, 54(11), 1588–94.

Lee, S.Y., Mak, K.H., and Saw, T.A. (1999). The avian flu (H5N1): one year on. *Public Health and Epidemiology Bulletin*, 8, 1–8.

Lewis, H.C., Ethelberg, S., Olsen, K.E., et al. (2009). Outbreaks of *Shigella sonnei* infections in Denmark and Australia linked to consumption of imported raw baby corn. *Epidemiology and Infection*, 137(3), 326–34.

Porta M. (ed.) (2008). *A Dictionary of Epidemiology* (5th ed.). New York: Oxford University Press.

Samitsuwan, P., Sermkaew, T., and Laosiritaworn, Y. (2005). An outbreak of tetrodotoxin poisoning associated with puffer fishes, Bangkok, Thailand, 2002. *Journal of Health Science*, 14(1), 203–8.

Siraprapasiri, T., Thanprasertsuk, S., Rodklay, A., et al. (1991). Risk factors for HIV among prostitutes in Chiangmai, Thailand. *AIDS*, 5, 579–82.

Sniadack, D.H., Moscoso, B., Aguilar, R., et al. (1999). Measles epidemiology and outbreak response immunization in a rural community in Peru. *Bulletin of the World Health Organization*, 77, 545–52.

World Health Organization (1978). Report of the International Commission. Ebola hemorrhagic fever in Zaire, 1976. *Bulletin of the World Health Organization*, 56, 271–90.

World Health Organization (2007). The need for global planned mobilization of essential medicine: lessons from a massive Thai botulism outbreak. *Bulletin of the World Health Organization*, 85(3), 238–40.

World Health Organization (2012). *Global Alert and Response (GAR): WHO interim case definition—Novel Coronavirus, as of 29 September 2012.*

[Online] Available at: http://www.who.int/csr/disease/coronavirus_infections/case_definition_29092012/en/index.html.

World Health Organization Regional Office for the Western Pacific (2006). *SARS: How A Global Epidemic was Stopped*. Manila: World Health Organization, Western Pacific Region.

5.5

Case–control studies

Noel S. Weiss

Introduction to case–control studies

In 1971, Herbst and colleagues (Herbst et al. 1971) reported that mothers of seven of the eight teenage girls diagnosed with clear cell adenocarcinoma of the vagina in Boston, Massachusetts, during 1966–1969 claimed to have taken a synthetic hormone, diethylstilbestrol, while pregnant. None of the mothers of the 32 girls without vaginal adenocarcinoma, matched to the cases' mothers with regard to hospital and date of birth, had taken diethylstilbestrol during their pregnancy. Within a year, a New York study of five girls with and eight girls without vaginal cancer obtained similar results (Greenwald et al. 1971). The introduction of prenatal diethylstilbestrol use into obstetric practice in the United States during the 1940s and 1950s followed by the appearance of this hitherto unseen form of cancer some 20 years later supported a causal connection between *in utero* exposure to diethylstilbestrol and vaginal adenocarcinoma. The means by which *in utero* diethylstilbestrol exposure might predispose to the occurrence of clear cell vaginal adenocarcinoma was unknown in 1971. (It is now believed that diethylstilbestrol acts by interfering with normal development of the female genital tract, resulting in the persistence into puberty of vaginal adenosis in which adenocarcinoma can arise.) Nonetheless, a causal inference was made at that time by the Food and Drug Administration, which specified pregnancy as a contraindication for diethylstilbestrol use.

The investigation by Herbst et al. (1971) was a case–control study: a comparison of prior exposures or characteristics of ill people (cases) with those of people at risk for the illness in the population from which the cases arose. Generally, the prior experience of people at risk is estimated from observations of a sample of that population (controls). A difference in the frequency or levels of exposure between cases and control—that is, an association—may reflect a causal link.

A case–control, cohort, or any other form of non-randomized study has the potential to identify associations that are not causal, either because of chance or because of the influence of some other factor associated with both the exposure and outcome. Even so, the evidence that is provided by well-performed case–control studies can carry great weight when evaluating the validity of a causal hypothesis. Indeed, a number of causal inferences have been based largely on the result of case–control studies. These include, in addition to the diethylstilbestrol–vaginal adenocarcinoma relationship, the connection between aspirin use in children and the development of Reye's syndrome, and the use of absorbent tampons and the incidence of toxic shock syndrome.

One of the criteria used to assess the validity of a causal hypothesis is the strength of the association between exposure and disease, usually as measured by the ratio of the incidence rate in exposed and non-exposed people. In most case–control studies, it is not possible to measure incidence rates in either of these groups. Nonetheless, from the frequency of exposure observed in cases and controls, it is usually possible to estimate closely the ratio of the incidence rates.

To understand how this can be done, consider a cohort study in which exposed and non-exposed people are followed for a certain period of time. Table 5.5.1 summarizes their experience with regard to a particular disease.

The cumulative incidence of the disease in exposed and non-exposed people over a given period of follow-up is $a/(a + b)$ and $c/(c + d)$, respectively. The relative risk (RR) is the ratio of these:

$$RR = \frac{a/(a+b)}{c/(c+d)}.$$

If the incidence of the disease is relatively low during the follow-up period in both exposed and non-exposed people, then a will be small relative to b and c will be small relative to d. Therefore:

$$RR = \frac{a/(a+b)}{c/(c+d)} \approx \frac{a/b}{c/d} = \frac{a/c}{b/d}.$$

In this expression, the numerator (a/c) is the odds of exposure in people who develop the disease and the denominator (b/d) is the odds exposure in people who remain well. Therefore:

$$\text{Odds ratio (OR)} = \frac{a/c}{b/d}.$$

The numerator can be estimated from a sample of cases, and the denominator can be estimated from a sample of non-cases. Neither estimate is influenced by the proportion of cases among the subjects actually chosen for study.

In the hypothetical example shown in Table 5.5.2, assume that 100 of 10,000 people exposed to a particular substance or organism

Table 5.5.1 Data layout for a hypothetical cohort study involving a dichotomous exposure variable

Cases	Diseased	Non-diseased	Total
Exposed	a	b	a + b
Non-exposed	c	d	c + d

Table 5.5.2 Depiction of data from a hypothetical study of a possible association between exposure and disease in an entire population

Cases	Diseased	Non-diseased	Total
Exposed	100	9900	10,000
Non-exposed	300	89,700	90,000

Table 5.5.3 Depiction of the results of a case–control study conducted in the population from which Table 5.5.2 was derived

Cases	Diseased	Non-diseased
Exposed	$100 \times 0.5 = 50$	$9900 \times 0.01 = 99$
Non-exposed	$300 \times 0.5 = 150$	$89,700 \times 0.01 = 897$

developed a disease, compared with 300 of 90,000 non-exposed people:

Therefore:

$$RR = \frac{100 / 10000}{300 / 90000} = 3.00.$$

If a case–control study had been carried out in this population, in which 50 per cent of the cases were included but only 1 per cent of the non-cases, then the results shown in Table 5.5.3 would have been obtained.

In many studies, controls are chosen as they were in this example; that is, from people who have not developed the disease by the end of the same time period during which other people (the cases) have become ill. In such studies, the less common the disease in both the exposed and non-exposed people during the period, the better the odds ratio will estimate the ratio of cumulative incidence. In the example, only 0.1 per cent and 0.33 per cent of exposed and non-exposed people, respectively, developed the illness: so, the relative cumulative incidence and odds ratio are nearly identical (3 versus 3.02). However, it is also possible to choose controls from people free of disease only until the corresponding cases have been diagnosed; a person can appear in the study first as a control and later as a case. If this approach is used, the odds ratio will be a valid estimate of the ratio of incidence rates (i.e. cases divided by person-time at risk) irrespective of the disease frequency (Greenland and Thomas 1982; Pearce 1993).

Retrospective ascertainment of exposure status in cases and controls

Epidemiological studies seek to obtain information on exposures present during an aetiologically relevant period of time; that period varies across aetiological relationships. For example, although excess consumption of alcohol predisposes to both motor vehicle injuries and cirrhosis of the liver, it does so during considerably different time intervals before the occurrence of the injury or the onset of the illness, respectively.

Some case–control studies are nested within cohort studies in which specimens (e.g. blood or urine) have been obtained before diagnosis on all cohort members, but have not yet been analysed for the exposure(s) in question. When these analyses are carried out on cohort members who developed a particular illness and on controls selected from the cohort, the results obtained are not influenced by the events occurring after the diagnosis of the illness. (To avoid the possibility of occult illness in cases influencing levels of a suspected aetiological factor, many studies of this type exclude from the analyses specimens obtained in the period before diagnosis that might correspond to the preclinical stage of disease.) Also, among the large majority of case–control studies in which exposure status is not measured until the illness or injury has been diagnosed, some are concerned only with an exposure or characteristic that would have been the same at all times in a person's life. This is true for a genetically determined characteristic such as ABO blood type or the absence of glutathione transferase M_1 activity (an enzyme that metabolizes several potentially carcinogenic constituents of cigarette smoke). Clearly, these studies are no less valid for having had to measure exposure in retrospect.

However, most case–control studies are required to consider explicitly how best to assess in retrospect the subjects' exposure status during one or more possible aetiologically relevant time periods. Possible sources of exposure data include interviews or questionnaires, available records, and physical or laboratory measurements.

Interviews or questionnaires

For many exposures, a subject's memory is an excellent window to the past. A number of important aetiological relationships have been identified through interview-based case–control studies. Generally, study participants will report longer-term and more recent experiences with greater accuracy than shorter-term and more distant ones. Attention to the ways in which questions are asked (White et al. 2008), along with the use of visual aids when appropriate (e.g. pictures of medicines, or containers of household products, and calendars for important life events to enhance recall of the timing of other exposures), will maximize the accuracy of the information received. These efforts, along with the use of the same questions for cases and controls asked in the same way, will also minimize the potential for bias that could result from the subject's or interviewer's awareness of case or control status.

One advantage of exposure ascertainment via interview or questionnaire is that information can be sought for multiple points in the past. It is possible that a given exposure plays an aetiological role only if present at a certain age, for a certain duration, or at a certain time in the past. Because there is often little guidance before a study starts that suggests the most relevant age, length, or recency, key exposures are often elicited throughout much of the subject's lifetime. However, care must be taken not to include exposures that took place after the illness began. An instructive example is provided by Victora et al. (1989) in a case–control study of infant death from diarrhoea as related to the type of feeding. These investigators asked mothers whether their child was or was not being breastfed immediately before the onset of the fatal illness (mothers of controls were queried about type of feeding prior to a comparable point in time). Mothers were also asked if subsequent to the onset of the illness there had been any changes in the type of feeding; following the development of diarrhoea, many children were switched to formula and cow's milk. Relative to infants who were solely breastfed, those who were supplemented with powdered or cow's milk prior to their illness had about four times the risk of diarrhoeal death. However, the authors showed that if one inappropriately considered the feeding method that was present during the illness, about a 13-fold increase in risk associated with supplementation would have been estimated.

Records

Case–control studies have exploited the presence of vital, registry, employment, medical, and pharmacy records, to name a few, as a means of obtaining information on exposures. However, because the information contained in the records is usually assembled for purposes other than epidemiological research, they may not provide precisely the information desired by the epidemiologist. For example, a death certificate or an occupational record may state an individual's job, but often not his or her actual exposure to the substance(s) of interest to the study. A pharmacy record will indicate a prescription having been filled, but not necessarily whether the patient took the medication on a given day, or took it at all. This sort of imprecision will impair a study's ability to discern a true association between an exposure and a disease—the greater the imprecision, the greater the impairment.

Nonetheless, some very strong associations have been identified through record-based case–control studies. For example, Daling et al. (1982) conducted a tumour registry-based case–control study to test the hypothesis that homosexual men have a relatively high incidence of anal cancer. Although registry data do not specify a man's sexual preference, they do contain information regarding his marital status. The investigators found that three times more men with anal cancer than controls (men with colon or rectal cancer) had never been married. Being single is far from a perfect predictor of homosexuality, of course. Nonetheless, the presence of such a large case–control difference, given the very poor means of gauging the relevant exposure, was a stimulus to conduct interview-based studies that could elicit information regarding sexual history with greater precision. The latter studies showed an exceedingly strong association between anal cancer in men and a history of sexual intercourse with another man (Daling et al. 1987).

In case–control studies in which medical records are used to characterize exposure status, care must be taken to restrict the information obtained to that which precedes the case's diagnosis (and the presence of symptoms, if any, that led to the diagnosis). The records of controls must be truncated at similar points in time. Without this safeguard, it is possible that bias will arise because there are systematically more records available to review on cases than controls; the case's illness may have stimulated an enquiry by medical personnel into his or her past, whereas no corresponding enquiry would necessarily have occurred for control subjects.

Physical and laboratory measurements

The recognized limitations of interviews and records in characterizing a variety of potentially relevant exposures have stimulated the conduct of epidemiological studies that use laboratory and other methods of measurement. A woman cannot tell an investigator the level of her reproductive hormones, the concentration of various micronutrients in her blood, or whether her cervix is infected with human papillomavirus, but laboratory tests can. Unfortunately, such tests tell us what these things are only at the time that the specimens have been obtained. For some exposures, there will be a high correlation between the measured level following case and control identification, and that which was present during the aetiologically relevant time period. For example, lead enters and does not leave the dentine of teeth. Therefore, in young school-age children, lead dentine levels are an indicator of cumulative lead exposure, a good portion of which could be relevant to the development of intellectual impairment and other adverse neurological outcomes. In contrast, one would not rely on serum levels of reproductive hormones of postmenopausal cases of breast cancer and controls to indicate what their premenopausal levels were, much less their hormonal status during their very early reproductive years (at which time the hormones may be exerting their greatest impact on future risk of breast cancer).

Case definition

Ideally, the cases in a case–control study would comprise all (or a representative sample of) members of a defined population who develop a given health outcome during a given period of time. For studies of disease aetiology, that outcome is the disease incidence. For studies that seek to determine the efficacy of early disease detection or treatment, the outcome generally is the occurrence of complications of the disease or mortality; such studies have been described in detail elsewhere (Selby 1994; Weiss 1994), and will not be covered any further here.

The population from which cases are to be drawn may be defined geographically or on the basis of other characteristics such as membership in a prepaid healthcare plan or an occupational group. The identification of all newly ill people in a defined population can be facilitated by the presence of a reporting system such as a cancer or malformation registry that seeks to accomplish this identification for other purposes. Occasionally, care for the condition being studied may be centralized, so that it will be necessary to review the records of only one or a few institutions to identify all cases in the population in which those institutions are located. However, in many instances, it is not feasible to identify all cases that occur in a given population; therefore, case–control studies are often based on cases identified from hospital records, or from the records of selected providers from whom patients had sought healthcare. The study by Herbst et al. (1971) on vaginal adenocarcinoma was of this type. Whether or not the cases are derived from a defined population, it is necessary that they be drawn in an unselected manner with regard to exposure status; for example, by including in the study all otherwise eligible cases diagnosed or receiving care during a defined time period.

Although the goal of a case–control study of aetiology is to enrol incident cases, under some circumstances it may be necessary to enrol prevalent cases at a particular point in time, irrespective of when each one's illness had begun. For some conditions, the date of occurrence may simply not be known; for example, in the absence of very close sero-monitoring, one generally cannot determine when a person acquired an HIV infection. Furthermore, for uncommon diseases of long duration, an incidence series may yield too few cases for meaningful analysis. The disadvantages of using prevalent cases in a case–control study relate in part to the added problems of accurate exposure ascertainment. For prevalent conditions whose date of diagnosis is known, pre-illness exposure information on study subjects must be obtained for more distant points in the past, on average, than would be necessary for an incident series. For prevalent conditions whose date of occurrence is unknown (e.g. HIV infection), there will be uncertainty as to the best point in time before which one should elicit exposure information. Also, by studying people remaining alive with a given condition, one is simultaneously studying not only aetiological factors but also those that influence survival from the condition.

Ideally, the criteria used to identify and select individual cases for study should be objective with high sensitivity and specificity for the disease. Specificity is of particular concern, because the inadvertent inclusion of people without disease into the case group will generally obscure any true association with the exposure. With this in mind, in the case–control study of Reye's syndrome and antecedent analgesic use conducted by the Centers for Disease Control (Hurwitz et al. 1985), only cases with a substantial degree of neurological impairment (stage 2 or higher) were included. The use of this criterion minimized the chances that children with a disease other than Reye's syndrome, which generally would have a lesser degree of severity, would be included in the case group. It also was intended to serve as protection against selective misclassification of Reye's syndrome based on knowledge of exposure status, because the hypothesis of the association of aspirin with Reye's syndrome was well known by the time the study took place. Conceivably, the knowledge that the child had consumed aspirin could have led some doctors to diagnose Reye's syndrome in cases with an atypical illness.

Control definition

Occasionally, the proportion of ill people who have had a specific exposure is so high, unequivocally more than would be expected in the population from which they were derived, that the presence of an association (although not its magnitude) can be surmised from a case series alone (Cummings and Weiss 1998). For example, when it was learned that all cases of a form of pneumonia that was epidemic in Spain in 1981 had ingested adulterated rapeseed oil, a causal inference was drawn, leading to efforts to eliminate further use of this oil. This action was taken before any formal comparison of cases with controls was made (Tabuenca 1981).

However, in the vast majority of instances, an explicit control group is needed to estimate the frequency and degree of exposure that would have taken place among cases in the absence of an exposure–disease association. An ideal control group would be one that comprises individuals:

1. Selected from a population whose distribution of exposure is that of the population from which the cases arose.

2. Who are identical to the cases with respect to their distribution of all characteristics: (a) that influence the likelihood and/or degree of exposure, and (b) that, independent of their relation to the exposure, are also related to the occurrence of the illness under study or to its recognition.

3. In whom the presence of the exposure can be measured accurately and in a manner that is identical to that used for the cases.

If these criteria are not met in a particular study, then selection bias, confounding, or information bias, respectively, will be present.

Minimizing selection bias

If the cases identified in the study are all or a sample of those that occurred in a defined population, one can seek to achieve comparability by choosing as controls people sampled from that same population. For geographically defined populations, a number of different sampling methods have been used, including random digit dialling of telephone numbers, area sampling, neighbourhood sampling, voters' lists, population registers, motor vehicle licences, and birth certificates, among others. When cases are members of a prepaid healthcare plan who develop an illness or injury, a sample of people who were members of the health plan when the illness or injury occurred can serve as controls. When cases are ill or injured members of an employed population, controls can be selected from this same population.

Enumeration of the defined population from which the cases arose may require an innovative approach. For example, Smith et al. (2001) identified recreational boating fatalities in Maryland and North Carolina among persons 18 years and above during 1990–1998, seeking to determine the presence and magnitude of an association with alcohol consumption. Of 221 fatal cases on whom blood alcohol levels were measured, 55 per cent tested positive. To provide a basis for comparison, the investigators devised a plan to randomly sample recreational boats on the waterways of the two states, and then to obtain a breath sample for alcohol testing from the boat operator and a random sample of any passengers aboard (n = 3943). Only 17 per cent of these persons chosen as controls had a positive result, and the disparity between cases and controls grew with increasing alcohol levels.

If cases have not been selected from a definable population at risk for the disease, but from people treated for a particular illness at one or a few hospitals or clinics, then selection bias may be introduced if controls are not chosen from people who, had they developed the illness under study, would have received care at these hospitals or clinics, and if people who do and do not receive care from these sources differ with regard to the frequency or level of exposure. Therefore, when cases are chosen from a narrow range of healthcare providers, controls are often chosen from other ill people treated by these providers. Such ill controls may also be used if, irrespective of the source of the cases, there is no feasible way to sample from the population at large, or if sampling from the general population would result in a substantial level of non-response or information bias. For these reasons, in some studies of fatal illness, exposures in people with a given cause of death are compared with exposures in a sample of people who died from other causes.

However, the choice of ill or deceased controls can itself give rise to selection bias if the illnesses (causes of death) represented in the control group are in some way associated with the exposure of interest. For example, ill or recently deceased people tend to have been smokers of cigarettes more often than other people (McLaughlin et al. 1985), because smoking is associated with a variety of causes of illness and death. Because smoking histories of ill people overstate the use of cigarettes in the population from which the cases arose (even if that population cannot be defined), the odds ratio associated with smoking based on the choice of ill people as controls will be spuriously low.

To minimize selection bias related to having chosen ill or deceased controls, an attempt can be made to omit potential controls with conditions known to be related (positively or negatively) to the exposure. For example, in the analysis of a hospital-based case–control study of bladder cancer and earlier use of artificial sweeteners, the investigators excluded from their control group people who were admitted to hospital for obesity-related diseases (Silverman et al. 1983). They showed that without this restriction, the control group would have a spuriously high proportion of users of artificial sweeteners relative to the population from which their cases had actually come. This approach will succeed to the extent that one judges correctly which conditions are truly exposure related, and how accurately the presence of those conditions can be determined. For many exposures, this may pose little problem, and judicious exclusion will yield a control group capable of providing an unbiased result. For others, such as cigarette smoking or alcohol consumption, it has been shown that admitting diagnoses or statements of cause of death are incapable of identifying all people with illnesses related to these exposures (McLaughlin et al. 1985).

Some case–control studies simply compare exposure status among subgroups of patients with the same outcome. For example, Laumon et al. (2005) obtained blood samples of 10,748 drivers involved in fatal road accidents in France during 2001–2003, and had these analysed for a metabolite of cannabis. The investigators contrasted the proportion testing positive between drivers judged to have been at fault for the crash ('cases') and drivers judged not to have been at fault ('controls'). The results of such a study will be valid when it is possible to identify those drivers who were at fault. To the extent that this is not possible, the misclassification that ensues will tend to make the size of the observed association smaller than the true one.

Occasionally, controls are chosen from individuals who are tested for the presence of the disease under study and are found not to have it. For example, people demonstrated to have coronary artery occlusion on coronary angiography have been compared with angiography patients without occlusion with regard to potential risk factors (Thom et al. 1992). As another example, the prior use of oral contraceptives was compared between women diagnosed with venous thromboembolism and women seen at the same institution for suspected venous thromboembolism who were diagnosed as not having this condition (Bloemenkamp et al. 1999). It may be relatively inexpensive to select controls from people who receive the same diagnostic evaluation as do cases, and it is also possible to achieve case–control comparability with regard to the choice of a healthcare provider (and the correlates of that choice). This approach can have an impact on the study's validity if the frequency or degree of exposure differs between otherwise comparable members of a population who do and do not receive the test. It will increase the validity if the disease being investigated is generally asymptomatic, and so would not be detected in the absence of testing. Thus, the relation of the use of oral contraceptives with the incidence of *in situ* cancer of the cervix is best studied in women who have undergone cervical screening, by comparing oral contraceptive use between cases of *in situ* cancer and women with a negative screen. This is because:

◆ In most societies, women who use oral contraceptives are screened more commonly than women who do not.

◆ *In situ* cancers are asymptomatic and will not be identified in the absence of cervical screening.

Therefore, if controls are chosen from women in general, who may or may not have received cervical screening, an apparent excess of oral contraceptive users would be present among cases of *in situ* cancer even if no true association were present.

However, the choice of test-negative controls can detract from a study's validity if the large majority of the people who develop the disease would soon be diagnosed whether or not the test was administered. There was a controversy in the late 1970s regarding the suitability, in case–control studies of postmenopausal oestrogen use and endometrial cancer, of a control group restricted to women with no evidence of cancer on endometrial biopsy. Among women without endometrial cancer, oestrogen use differs greatly between those who have and have not undergone biopsy, because oestrogen use predisposes to uterine bleeding of non-malignant causes, which often leads to endometrial biopsy. Those investigators who believed that there was a great prevalence of occult endometrial cancer in the population suggested that the optimal control group ought to be women undergoing endometrial biopsy and found not to have cancer (Horwitz and Feinstein 1978). However, the majority of the investigators believed that no such large pool of prevalent, occult disease existed, and that choosing biopsy-negative controls would lead to a spuriously high estimate of oestrogen use in the population at risk, and thus, a spuriously low odds ratio (Shapiro et al. 1985).

No matter how controls are defined in a case–control study, selection bias may be introduced to the extent that exposure information is not obtained on all who have been selected to participate. The magnitude of this bias will increase in relation to the frequency of missing data and the degree to which exposure frequencies or levels differ between study subjects on whom exposure status is and is not known. The problem of incomplete ascertainment of exposure on study subjects is particularly common in interview- or questionnaire-based case–control studies. Strategies for minimizing the degree of non-response in case–control studies are discussed in detail elsewhere (White et al. 2008).

Minimizing confounding

Characteristics of confounding variables in case–control studies

Confounding occurs when the estimate of the relationship between an exposure and a disease is distorted by the influence of another factor. In any study design, confounding will occur to the extent that the other factor is associated with both the exposure (although not as a result of the exposure) and the disease or its recognition. In case–control studies alone, a factor may confound even if it is not associated with an altered risk of disease, if the proportions of cases and controls vary across levels or categories of the factor. For example, in a collaborative study of ovarian cancer and use of oral contraceptives (Weiss et al. 1981), an attempt was made to identify and interview all incident cases over several years in two American populations. In one of the populations (western Washington state), several controls per case were interviewed, whereas the control-to-case ratio in the other (Utah) was 1:1. Because oral contraceptive use was more common among women in Washington than in Utah, failure to take into account the state of residence in the analysis (e.g. by adjustment) would have led to a spuriously high estimate of the frequency of oral contraceptive use by controls relative to that by the cases.

Means of controlling for confounding

One straightforward way of preventing confounding is to restrict cases and controls to a single category or level of the potentially confounding variable. For example, in their study on physical activity and primary cardiac arrest, Siscovick et al. (1982) excluded people with conditions, such as clinically recognized heart disease, that could both predispose to cardiac arrest and might be expected to alter level of activity. A second way is to obtain information on exposures or characteristics that may differ between cases and controls, and then make statistical adjustments for those that are also found to be related to the exposure or characteristic under investigation (Rothman et al. 2008).

Finally, it is possible to match one or more controls to each case's category or level of a potentially confounding factor. It is appropriate to match if:

1. The variable is expected to be strongly related to both the exposure and disease. Thus, in a case–control study of breast cancer and use of hair dye, it would make sense to match on gender (if the study has not already been restricted to women) because use of dye is more common among women than men in most cultures. Although confounding by gender could be prevented even without matching by adjustment in the analysis, the statistical precision of the unmatched study would be substantially reduced relative to that of a case–control study having a more similar proportion of female cases and controls.

2. Information on possible matching variables can be obtained inexpensively. There are some means of control selection in which information regarding some confounders can be obtained at no cost. For example, from voters' lists or prepaid health-plan membership records, it would generally be possible to choose directly one or more controls who were identical to a given case's age. Conversely, if a population sampling scheme such as random digit dialling were being employed, the age of the respondent would not be known in advance of approaching him or her. Rather than omitting already contacted controls who did not match a particular case's age, the matching can be done much more broadly; additional control for finer categories of age can be accomplished in the data analysis.

3. Information on exposure status cannot be obtained inexpensively. The higher the cost of exposure ascertainment, the greater the incentive to limit the number of control subjects to the number of cases. Case–control differences regarding confounding factors particularly will reduce the statistical power of a study that does not have a surplus of controls. Enriching the group of controls selected with people more similar to the cases with regard to confounding factors (i.e. matching) can prevent this loss of statistical power.

In case–control studies of genetic characteristics as possible aetiological factors, some investigators have used a matched design in which a specific type of relative (e.g. parent, sibling, or cousin) is chosen as a control for each case (Yang and Khoury 1997; Witte et al. 1999). This approach has the advantage of minimizing potential confounding by other genetic characteristics with which the one of interest is associated. However, it has the disadvantage of excluding a possibly large fraction of cases for whom there is no relative available of the type needed to provide a sample for genetic analysis.

Table 5.5.4 Data layout in a hypothetical matched case–control study involving a dichotomous exposure variable

Cases	Controls	
	Exposed	Non-exposed
Exposed	a	b
Non-exposed	c	d

It should be remembered that matching alone is not sufficient to eliminate a variable's confounding influence: failure to consider a matching variable in the analysis of the study can lead to a biased result (Rothman et al. 2008). Analyses of studies that have matched controls to cases on a given characteristic can adjust for that characteristic as if no matching had taken place. Alternatively, these analyses can explicitly consider cases and controls as matched sets. In the instance of matched case–control pairs and a dichotomous exposure variable, Table 5.5.4 could be constructed.

Only the b pairs in which the case was exposed but not the matched control, and the c pairs in which the reverse was true, would enter the analysis. The odds ratio would be calculated as b/c. When there is more than one control per case, the matched odds ratio can be calculated as well (Breslow and Day 1980).

Minimizing information bias

For case–control studies in which information on exposure status is sought via an interview or questionnaire, the chief safeguards against information bias entail asking questions about events that are salient to the respondent, that are framed in an unambiguous way, and that are presented identically to both cases and controls. Employment of these safeguards, however, will not prevent differential accuracy of reporting between cases and controls in all circumstances. Some past exposures or events will simply be more salient to people with an illness, who might have dwelled on possible reasons for its occurrence, than to people without that illness. Other exposures may be viewed as socially undesirable, and there may be a difference between cases and healthy controls in their willingness to admit to them. If the anticipated difference in the quality of information between cases and otherwise appropriate controls is too great, a control group that is less than ideal in other respects may be selected instead so as to minimize the potential for information bias. For example, some studies of prenatal risk factors for a particular congenital malformation that utilize maternal interviews as the source of exposure data have selected as controls infants with other malformations (Rosenberg et al. 1983). This control group will provide a more valid result than a control group that consists of infants in general if mothers of malformed and mothers of normal infants report prenatal exposures to a different degree even in the absence of an association, and the exposure in question is not associated with the occurrence of the malformations present in control infants.

Similar reasoning led Daling et al. (1987), when conducting their case–control study on anal cancer and a history of anal intercourse, to eschew the geographic population from which their cases had arisen as a sampling frame for controls. They feared that interviews that sought information about prior anal intercourse might be more complete among men with cancer than men in the population at large. Thus, they chose as controls men with a cancer of a different site (colon), which they believed was unlikely to have been aetiologically related to prior anal intercourse.

When the exposure under consideration is sufficiently imprecise or is open to subjective interpretation, there may not be any control group that will provide information comparable to that provided by cases. An instructive example comes from a case–control study on Down's syndrome (Stott 1958), conducted shortly before the chromosomal basis for the aetiology of this condition had been learned. The study sought to determine whether emotional 'shocks' during pregnancy might be a risk factor. The author interviewed mothers of children with Down's syndrome with regard to the occurrence of a 'situation or event [that would be] stress- or shock-producing if this would have been its expected effect on an emotionally stable woman'. Identical interviews were administered to mothers of normal children, and also to mothers of children with mental retardation who did not have Down's syndrome. Even though it is not possible that an emotional shock in pregnancy could play any aetiological role in a condition already determined at conception, a far higher proportion of mothers of cases of Down's syndrome reported an emotional shock than did mothers of normal controls (RR estimated from the data, 17.0). The use of other children with mental retardation as controls only partially reduced the spuriously high relative risk, to a value of 4.3.

When conducting an interview-based study of a rapidly fatal disease, or a disease that impairs a person's ability to provide valid interview data, it is necessary to obtain information from at least some surrogate respondents; typically, these respondents are close relatives of the cases. In general, for purposes of comparability, similar information ought to be obtained from surrogates of controls, even though the control would be expected to provide more accurate data. Results of case–control studies based on exposure information provided by surrogate respondents need to be interpreted with particular caution. Although by no means present in every instance (Nelson et al. 1990; Campbell et al. 2007), there can be a large difference in the validity of the responses given by case and control surrogates. For example, Greenberg et al. (1985) investigated the basis for an apparent strong association between cancer mortality and 'nuclear' work among employees of a naval shipyard, which had been found during a comparison of work histories provided by surrogates of men who died from cancer and of those who died of other conditions. They observed that, regarding work in the nuclear part of the industry, surrogates of the cases generally provided information similar to that contained in employment records of the shipyard; in contrast, the surrogates of controls substantially misclassified the nature of their relatives' jobs as not involving radiation. Using the data provided by employment records, which included individual radiation dosimetry, little or no association was found between cancer mortality and radiation exposure received at the shipyard (Rinsky et al. 1981).

What was undoubtedly a spuriously negative association was found in a case–control study of lung cancer and passive cigarette smoking that used, for one analysis, information obtained from surrogate respondents (Janerich et al. 1985). In this analysis, the relative risk of lung cancer among non-smokers associated with a spouse's having smoked—0.33 (i.e. a 67 per cent reduction in risk)—would seem almost certainly due to a spurious minimization or the denial of smoking by spouses of cases, who may have feared their habit caused their spouse to develop lung cancer.

In most interview-based case–control studies, information is not sought from cases until days to months have elapsed following the diagnosis of their condition. These persons are queried regarding exposures that occurred during what is presumed to be the aetiologically relevant period prior to diagnosis. For controls, for whom there is no 'diagnosis' date, what is the appropriate time frame in which to focus the questions that are asked of them? If exposures that occurred some time in the past, or that occurred over an extended period, are most likely to be relevant, controls are generally asked about events during the same calendar time as the cases. However, when studying exposures that could act acutely to lead to illness, having the case recall events immediately prior to illness and the control do the same for the corresponding time in the past may lead to bias: only the cases will have the onset of their illness to help in recalling events that took place shortly prior to that time. This difference could lead to relatively more complete ascertainment of exposure among cases.

In response to this concern, some case–control studies investigating potentially rapidly acting exposures query controls about the time period prior to the date of interview instead of the date of their case's diagnosis (or, in an unmatched study, the date of a typical case's diagnosis). So, in a study of risk factors for meningococcal disease in adolescents (Tully et al. 2006), cases were asked about events during the 2 weeks prior to diagnosis (which occurred, on average, 53 days before the interview) and controls about events during the 2 weeks just prior to the interview itself. The investigators felt that the plausibility of case–control comparability on recall of exposures involved in transmission (e.g. 'intimate kissing with multiple partners') would be greater using this approach than one in which the controls were asked about a 2-week period ending 53 days prior to the interview. However, although a sound approach when trying to estimate the short-term influence of many exposures, this strategy can backfire if recall of an exposure diminishes over time to the same degree in cases and controls. For example, in the study of meningococcal disease, a far smaller proportion of cases than controls reported attending religious observances during their respective 2-week intervals (adjusted odds ratio = 0.1, 95 per cent confidence interval = 0.02–0.6). Almost certainly, this difference had more to do with relatively poorer recall of churchgoing among cases (who had to think back some 2 months) than to a genuine salutary effect of church attendance on the incidence of meningococcal disease.

Incomparable assessment of exposure status between cases and controls is not confined to interview- or questionnaire-based studies. Most laboratory-based studies seek to prevent this by testing samples blind to case and control status. If feasible, it is desirable to also carry out this blinding for studies in which exposure is to be determined from medical or other records. However, there are instances in which the nature of the information available in records has already been influenced by whether the subject is a case or a control. For example, it was found that among 100 infertile women who underwent laparoscopy (Stratby et al. 1982), 21 had endometriosis. Only 2 per cent of the 200 women who underwent laparoscopy for another indication, tubal ligation, were noted in the procedural records as having endometriosis. However, the interpretation of this association is unclear, because the identification and/or recording of endometriosis in cases and controls (women undergoing tubal ligation) may well have been incomparable—only in the infertile women was the laparoscopy expressly done as a diagnostic tool to investigate the possible presence of conditions such as endometriosis.

Estimating attributable risk from results of case–control studies

Occasionally, a case–control study identifies a large odds ratio relating an exposure to a disease, and for this and other reasons, a causal influence of the exposure may be suspected. The decision to seek to limit or eliminate that exposure requires weighing its negative and positive consequences. This weighing must be done in absolute, rather than in relative terms, because the same relative increase (or decrease) in risk is of far greater consequence for common than for rare outcomes. The absolute increase in the risk of disease believed to be due to a dichotomous exposure, sometimes referred to as the 'attributable risk' (AR), can be estimated directly from data gathered in cohort studies or randomized trials as the difference between the incidence among exposed (I_e) and non-exposed people (I_n). The formula $I_e - I_n$ can be rewritten as $RR(I_n) - I_n$, or as $I_n(RR - 1)$. Because the relative risk can be estimated from the results of a case–control study by means of the odds ratio, the only additional piece of information needed to estimate the attributable risk is an estimate of I_n. For the population in which the study has been conducted, I_n can be estimated if:

1. The overall incidence (I) of the disease in that population is known or can be approximated.

2. The frequency of exposure (P_e) in the controls selected for study reasonably reflects that of the population that gave rise to the cases.

Given (1) and (2):

$$I = I_e(P_e) + I_n(1 - P_e)$$
$$= I_n RR(P_e) + I_n(1 - P_e)$$
$$= I_n(P_e[RR - 1] + 1)$$

So:

$$I_n = \frac{I}{P_e(RR - 1) + 1}$$

Therefore:

$$AR = \frac{I(RR - 1)}{P_e + (RR - 1)} = \frac{I}{P_e + 1/(RR - 1)}.$$

For example, consider a disease with an incidence rate of 10 per 100,000 per year in a population in which 5 per cent of people have been exposed during a relevant period of time. Table 5.5.5 summarizes data from a case–control study conducted in that population.

The attributable risk that corresponds to the estimated 3.35-fold increase in risk is

$$\frac{10}{0.05 + 1/(3.35 - 1)} = 21.0 \text{ per } 100\,000 \text{ per year.}$$

Table 5.5.5 Depiction of results from a hypothetical case–control study involving a dichotomous exposure variable

Exposed	Cases (%)	Controls (%)	OR
Yes	15	5	3.35
No	85	95	1

From the results of case–control studies that suggest a causal relation, it is also possible to estimate the percentage of exposed people with the disease who developed it because of their exposure, rather than through one or more causal pathways not involving the exposure. This measure, often termed the 'attributable risk per cent' (AR per cent) among exposed people, is defined as

$$\frac{I_e - I_n}{I_e} \times 100.$$

It can be described in terms of the relative risk alone:

$$AR\% = \frac{I_e}{I_e} - \frac{I_n}{I_e} = 1 - \frac{1}{RR} = \frac{RR - 1}{RR} \times 100.$$

Therefore, the results of a case–control study that provide a valid estimate of the relative risk (via the odds ratio) can provide the attributable risk per cent as well, with no additional assumptions or sources of data. It is also possible to estimate the percentage of a disease's occurrence in the population as a whole that resulted from the actions of given exposure. This measure, the 'population attributable risk per cent' (PAR per cent) or 'aetiological fraction', is simply the attributable risk per cent multiplied by the proportion of cases in that population who were exposed (P_e):

$$PAR\% = AR\%P_e.$$

In the present example:

$$AR\% = \frac{3.35 - 1}{3.35} = 70.1\%$$

and

$$PAR\% = 70.1\% \left(0.15\right) = 10.5\%.$$

The role of case–control studies in understanding disease aetiology

Randomized trials will not be able to answer all questions regarding the reasons for disease occurrence. Many potential disease-causing or disease-preventing exposures cannot be manipulated, either at all—for example, most genetic characteristics—or in any practical way for purposes of a study. For many exposure–disease relationships, either the disease is too uncommon or the induction period is too long to conduct a randomized trial that is not unfeasibly large in size or long in duration. Finally, it generally will not be possible to conduct separate randomized trials to measure the impact of all potential types, amounts, and durations of a class of exposure.

Also, it is not possible to rely solely on cohort studies for answers. Just as with randomized trials, the disease outcome being studied may be too rare to allow a cohort approach to be useful. This explains why the aetiologies of vaginal adenocarcinoma and Reye's syndrome, for example, have been evaluated exclusively by case–control studies—these diseases are simply too uncommon for most cohort studies to generate any cases, even in 'exposed' individuals. Prospective cohort studies are also of limited use when the induction period for the exposure–disease relationship is either very short or very long. If the induction period is very short and the exposure status of an individual varies over time, a cohort study would need to assess exposure status repeatedly among cohort members. For this reason, studies of alcohol consumption and the occurrence of injuries typically are case–control in nature (Holcomb 1938). Similarly, unless information on exposure status can be ascertained retrospectively, it would not be feasible to initiate a cohort study of a suspected aetiological relation that requires a very long time (perhaps several decades) to manifest itself.

Although case–control studies may be of particular value in the evaluation of the aetiology of uncommon disease, they may have difficulty in obtaining statistically precise results if the frequency of the exposure in the population under study is either extremely common or extremely uncommon (Crombie 1981). Thus, only an association as strong as the one between cigarette smoking and lung cancer could have emerged reliably from case–control studies of several hundred British men conducted in the late 1940s (Doll and Hill 1950), given that well over 90 per cent of that population were cigarette smokers. For very uncommon exposures—for example, occupational exposure to a specific substance suspected of posing a risk to health, or an infrequently prescribed drug—barring a strong observed association based on a large number of subjects, even the best-designed case–control study will usually offer no more than a suggestion of the presence or absence of a relation with regard to the occurrence of a given illness.

Conclusion

♦ Case–control studies compare ill or injured persons (cases) with those at risk of the illness or injury (controls) in terms of prior exposures or characteristics.

♦ From most case–control studies of a given condition it is possible to obtain an estimate of the relative risk associated with an exposure by dividing the odds of exposure in cases by the odds of exposure in controls (odds ratio).

♦ The validity of the results of a case–control study can be compromised by differences between cases and controls with regard to exposures or characteristics that are also correlated with the likelihood or degree of the exposure in question.

♦ In most case–control studies, ascertainment of exposure status is undertaken after the cases have sustained their illness or injury. These studies will produce an unbiased estimate of an exposure–disease association to the extent that exposure status prior to disease onset can be ascertained with a high degree of sensitivity and specificity.

♦ In a setting in which (1) randomization of potential study participants is unethical or infeasible and (2) the outcome under study is an uncommon one, data from case–control studies may be the best available by which to judge a potential cause–effect relationship between the exposure and outcome.

Acknowledgements

The chapter has been adapted from Chapter 15, Case-Control Studies, pp. 374–402, in T.D. Koepsell and N.S. Weiss, *Epidemiologic Methods*, Oxford University Press, New York, USA, Copyright © 2003, by permission of Oxford University Press, Inc.

References

Bloemenkamp, K.W.M., Rosendaal, F.R., Buller, H.R., et al. (1999). Risk of venous thrombosis with use of current low-dose oral contraceptives is not explained by diagnostic suspicion and referral bias. *Archives of Internal Medicine*, 159, 65–70.

Breslow, N.E. and Day, N.E. (1980). *Statistical Methods in Cancer Research. Vol. 1: The Analysis of Case-Control Studies*. IARC Scientific Publication No. 32. Lyon: IARC Press.

Campbell, P.T., Sloan, M., and Kreiger, N. (2007). Utility of proxy versus index respondent information in a population-based case-control study of rapidly fatal cancers. *Annals of Epidemiology*, 17, 253–7.

Crombie, I.K. (1981). The limitations of case-control studies in the detection of environmental carcinogens. *Journal of Epidemiology and Community Health*, 35, 281–7.

Cummings, P. and Weiss, N.S. (1998). Case series and exposure series: the role of studies without controls in providing information about the etiology of injury or disease. *Injury Prevention*, 4, 34–57.

Daling, J.R., Weiss, N.S., Hislop, T.G. et al. (1987). Sexual practices, sexually transmitted disease, and the incidence of anal cancer. *The New England Journal of Medicine*, 317, 973–7.

Daling, J.R., Weiss, N.S., Klopfenstein, L.L., et al. (1982). Correlates of homosexual behavior and the incidence of anal cancer. *JAMA*, 247, 1988–90.

Doll, R. and Hill, A.B. (1950). Smoking and carcinoma of the lung. *British Medical Journal*, 2, 739–48.

Greenberg, E.R., Rosner, B., Hennekens, C., et al. (1985). An investigation of bias in a study of nuclear shipyard workers. *American Journal of Epidemiology*, 121, 301–8.

Greenland, S. and Thomas, D.C. (1982). On the need for the rare disease assumption in case-control studies. *American Journal of Epidemiology*, 116, 547–53.

Greenwald, P., Barlow, J.J., Nasca, P., et al. (1971). Vaginal cancer after maternal treatment with synthetic estrogens. *The New England Journal of Medicine*, 285, 390–3.

Herbst, A.L., Ulfelder, H., and Poskanzer, D.C. (1971). Adenocarcinoma of the vagina: association of maternal stilbestrol therapy with tumor appearance in young women. *The New England Journal of Medicine*, 284, 878–81.

Holcomb, R.L. (1938). Alcohol in relation to traffic accidents. *JAMA*, 111, 1076–85.

Horwitz, R.I. and Feinstein, A.R. (1978). Alternative analytic methods for case-control studies of estrogens and endometrial cancer. *The New England Journal of Medicine*, 299, 1089–94.

Hurwitz, E.S., Barren, M.J., Bregman, D., et al. (1985). Public Health Service Study on Reye's syndrome and medications. Report of the pilot phase. *The New England Journal of Medicine*, 313, 849–57.

Janerich, D.T., Thompson, W.D., Varela, L.R., et al. (1985). Lung cancer and exposure to tobacco smoke in the household. *The New England Journal of Medicine*, 323, 632–6.

Laumon, B., Godegbeku, B., Martin, J.L., et al. (2005). Cannabis intoxication and fatal road crashes in France: population-based case-control study. *British Medical Journal*, 331, 1371–4.

McLaughlin, J.K., Blot, W.J., Mehl, E.S., et al. (1985). Problems in the use of dead controls in case-control studies. II. Effect of excluding certain causes of death. *American Journal of Epidemiology*, 122, 485–94.

Nelson, L.M., Longstreth, W.T., Koepsell, T.D., et al. (1990). Proxy respondents in epidemiologic research. *Epidemiologic Reviews*, 12, 71–86.

Pearce, N. (1993). What does the odds ratio estimate in a case-control study? *International Journal of Epidemiology*, 22, 1189–92.

Rinsky, R.A., Zumwolde, R.D., Waxweiller, R.J., et al. (1981). Cancer mortality at a naval nuclear shipyard. *The Lancet* 1981(1), 231–5.

Rosenberg, L., Mitchell, A.A., Parsells, J.L., et al. (1983). Lack of relation of oral clefts to diazepam use during pregnancy. *The New England Journal of Medicine*, 309, 1282–5.

Rothman, K.J., Greenland, S., and Lash, T.L., (2008). *Modern Epidemiology* (3rd ed.). Philadelphia, PA: Lippincott Williams & Wilkins.

Selby, J.V. (1994). Case-control evaluations of treatment and program efficacy. *Epidemiologic Reviews*, 46, 91–101.

Shapiro, S., Kelly, J.P., Rosenberg, L., et al. (1985). Risk of localized and widespread endometrial cancer in relation to recent and discontinued use of conjugated estrogens. *The New England Journal of Medicine*, 313, 969–72.

Silverman, D.T., Hoover, R.N., and Swanson, G.M. (1983). Artificial sweeteners and lower urinary tract cancer: hospital vs. population controls. *American Journal of Epidemiology*, 117, 326–34.

Siscovick, D.S., Weiss, N.S., Hallstrom, A.P., et al. (1982). Physical activity and primary cardiac arrest. *JAMA*, 248, 3113–17.

Smith, G.S., Keyl, P.M., Hadley, J.A., et al. (2001). Drinking and recreational boating fatalities: a population-based case-control study. *JAMA*, 286, 2974–80.

Stott, D.H. (1958). Some psychosomatic aspects of casualty in reproduction. *Journal of Psychosomatic Research*, 3, 42–55.

Stratby, J.H., Molgaard, C.A., Coulam, C.B., et al. (1982). Endometriosis and infertility: a laparoscopic study of endometriosis among fertile and infertile women. *Fertility and Sterility*, 38, 667–72.

Tabuenca J.M. (1981). Toxic-allergic syndrome caused by ingestion of rapeseed oil denatured with aniline. *The Lancet*, 2, 567–8.

Thom, D.H., Grayston, J.T., Siscovick, D.S., et al. (1992). Association of prior infection with Chlamydia pneumoniae and angiographically demonstrated coronary artery disease. *JAMA*, 268, 68–72.

Tully, J., Viner, R.M., Coen, P.G. et al. (2006). Risks and protective factors for meningococcal disease in adolescents. *British Medical Journal*, 332, 445–50.

Victora, C.G., Smith, P.G., Vaughan, J.P., et al. (1989). Infant feeding and deaths due to diarrhea. *American Journal of Epidemiology*, 129, 1032–41.

Weiss, N.S. (1994). Application of the case-control method in the evaluation of screening. *Epidemiologic Reviews*, 16, 102–8.

Weiss, N.S., Lyon, J.L., Liff, J.M., et al. (1981). Incidence of ovarian cancer in relation to the use of oral contraceptives. *International Journal of Cancer*, 28, 669–71.

White, E., Armstrong, B.K., and Saracci, R. (2008). *Principles of Exposure Measurement in Epidemiology: Collecting, Evaluating and Improving Measures of Disease Risk Factors* (2nd ed.). Oxford: Oxford University Press.

Witte, J.S., Gauderman, W.J., and Thomas, D.C. (1999). Asymptotic bias and efficiency in case-control studies of candidate genes and gene–environment interactions: basic family designs. *American Journal of Epidemiology*, 149, 693–705.

Yang, Q. and Khoury, M.J. (1997). Evolving methods in genetic epidemiology. III. Gene–environment interaction in epidemiologic research. *Epidemiologic Reviews*, 19, 33–43.

Cohort studies

Alvaro Muñoz and F. Javier Nieto

Introduction to cohort studies

Cohort studies constitute one of the basic types of designs in epidemiological research. The key element of cohort studies is temporality (i.e. exposure preceding an outcome). Specifically, a cohort (i.e. group of individuals) is enrolled at the beginning of the study (baseline) to examine how characteristics (exposures) predict the occurrence of a discrete event (typically a disease onset) or changes in markers of health/disease status. In the former case, the cohort is typically formed by individuals who are free from the outcome of interest and have sufficiently heterogeneous profiles of putative risk factors (whose simplest form is as exposed or unexposed). In the latter case, the central aim is to characterize the heterogeneity of the change or trajectory of markers of disease progression according to constellations of putative risk factors.

The identification of exposures and risk factors for disease provides a basis for prevention. There are numerous examples of cohort-based exposure–disease associations that have resulted in beneficial prevention strategies: for instance, to prevent lung cancer, cigarette smoking should be avoided; to prevent infection with human immunodeficiency virus (HIV), high-risk sexual practices and injection with unsterile needles should be avoided; to prevent the development of acquired immune deficiency syndrome (AIDS) and death among individuals infected with HIV, antiretroviral therapy should be taken to suppress viral replication; to prevent heart disease, low levels of high-density and high levels of low-density lipids should be avoided (by diet, exercise, and/or lipid-lowering medications); to prevent cervical cancer, infection with human papilloma virus (HPV) should be avoided. Needless to say, there are instances in which the design of prevention strategies faces the complexity of multifactorial aetiology and of exposures that cluster so that exposures have to be taken into account jointly, and the lack of such recognition may lead to ascribing to a particular exposure an effect that is not appropriate. When an exposure is not a *sufficient* cause but a *component* of a more complex constellation of causal factors (Rothman et al. 2008; Szklo and Nieto 2012), acting only on that exposure may not result in successful prevention strategies; for example, based on data from cohort studies, high levels of beta-carotene markers (purportedly resulting from appropriate diets) have been associated with protection against cancer (Willett et al. 1984), but supplementation with beta carotene only has not resulted in a lower incidence of cancer in clinical trials (ATBC Cancer Prevention Study Group 1994; Virtamo et al. 2003).

Types of cohort studies

The observational cohort design shares with the experimental design or controlled clinical trial the temporal relationship between exposure and disease, of the putative cause with the supposed effect. The clinical trial design is a special type of cohort study in which the study subjects are randomly assigned to the different experimental (exposure) groups. Given the inherent limitation of observational designs to control for potential confounding variables unidentified by the investigator, the difference between these study designs lies on the validity of the conclusions regarding the potential causal relationships between exposure and disease. The role of randomization in clinical trials is to make the two groups comparable so that the effect of the therapy can be determined. But randomized controlled trials are not ethical or feasible when exploring the effects of potentially harmful exposures; moreover, the generalizability of results in highly selected trial participants is often limited. This is the reason why observational cohort studies, with all their limitations and caveats, will always be an important study design in epidemiological research.

In some studies, the investigator collects the data *concurrently* with the study being conducted, and in others, the data are available before the study is designed and the study is conducted to obtain that data (i.e. the data for the study precedes its conduct or the study is *non-concurrent*). This type of design is called 'retrospective study' by some authors (Kelsey et al. 1986; Vandenbroucke 1991), a term that can cause confusion because, as mentioned, it is also used for case–control studies. It is possible that studies collect data concurrently for some participants and non-concurrently (*historically*) for the remainder of the study population.

The simplest cohort design is to obtain exposure data at baseline and follow up individuals to only obtain data for when the event of interest occurs. A richer design includes regularly scheduled visits at which data on exposures are updated, and in many cases, biological samples are collected for testing to assess those exposures. Cohort studies with regularly scheduled visits for updating exposure information and/or determining outcomes are referred to as *panel studies* (Kelsey et al. 1986). When the outcome of interest is not an event but it is changes in the profile of a biomarker over time (e.g. change in kidney function measured by filtration rate), panel studies are often referred to as *longitudinal studies*.

Design issues in cohort studies

The nature of a cohort study provides the temporal structure necessary to associate a particular exposure with a subsequent event of interest. Documentation of the time sequences of exposures and events generates data upon which the course of event development can be modelled. Such data provide flexibility to define the study outcome based on the length of time elapsed between exposure and event. The time at which an exposure first occurs, placing individuals at risk for event development, is referred to as the *origin* (e.g. birth in population-level life-course epidemiology, infection with a virus or bacteria in infectious disease epidemiology). Ideally, a cohort study will have complete data of the time elapsed between the origin and the event of interest for as many participants as possible. However, in most studies, not all individuals are followed up from the origin: some will have been at risk for some time since the origin when enrolled into the cohort study. Those followed up from the origin are called the *incident* cohort and those entering the study after a certain duration from the origin are called the *prevalent* cohort. Implementation of the appropriate statistical methods to combine incident and prevalent cohorts may not only yield more efficient estimates but also provide the means for appropriately describing the timing of events beyond the study duration (Muñoz et al. 1997).

For some diseases, the origin is well defined and observable, such as employment into an occupation deemed to place workers at risk for health events. For others, the origin is well defined but difficult to observe, such as infection with a virus (e.g. sexual transmission of HPV, whose occurrence can be determined in a cohort study by following uninfected sexually active individuals with regularly scheduled visits at which the participants are tested for presence of antibodies to HPV). Still others do not have a well-defined origin, as in the case of coronary heart disease in which the origin may be the time of initiation of atherosclerotic plaques in the inner layer of the coronary arteries, the time when a certain level of coronary artery stenosis is reached, or the time when an atherosclerotic plaque ruptures and acutely occludes an arterial branch leading to clinical manifestations (angina or myocardial infarction). Cohort studies with data on individuals from origin to the event of interest as well as with baseline information and updated information on predictors at regular intervals between the origin and event provide the most complete data to describe the natural history of a disease (Muñoz et al. 1992; Muñoz and Xu 1996; Muñoz et al. 1997).

Study population

In a cohort design, the study population comprises individuals who are exposed or unexposed to the suspected risk factors and who are at risk for the disease of interest. Once the study population has been deemed to be free of the event whose occurrence is to be documented during the proposed follow-up, it should be ensured that the participants have enough variability in the presence and/or magnitude of exposure to the risk factor or factors of interest.

The cohort can be the totality (or almost the totality) of a geographically and temporally defined population. For example, Hoffmans et al. (1988) constructed a non-concurrent study of mortality among Dutch males born in 1932. This cohort included the totality of the 84,349 Dutch males who were 18 years old in 1950, when they were examined for eligibility to military service; the investigators used the data collected at baseline (when the individuals were 18 years old) to describe the relationship between obesity at 18 years and subsequent cause-specific mortality (Hoffmans et al. 1989).

Instead of the totality of a population, it is more common to include only a fraction or a sample of a population defined temporally and geographically. For instance, as outlined in Table 5.6.1, the Framingham study was initiated at the beginning of the 1950s in Framingham, Massachusetts, United States, with the goal of studying the incidence of and risk factors for cardiovascular diseases (Dawber 1980). From a list of residents aged 35–59 years (18,000 persons in total), 6507 adults were randomly selected, among whom 4469 agreed to participate in the initial examination. In order to compensate for the unexpectedly high rate of refusal, the investigators decided to include 734 individuals who, although not part of the random sample, had expressed interest in being part of the cohort. Of the resulting 5203 participants in the baseline examination, 76 persons were excluded for having clinical manifestations of cardiovascular disease, leaving a total of 5127 participants in the Framingham Heart Study cohort. The follow-up consisted of physical examinations every 2 years with comprehensive data collection particularly emphasizing diet, physical activity, and stress.

The generalization of results obtained from a cohort study whose participants are a sample from a sole population may have serious limitations, which are overcome by other studies that enrol participants from diverse populations. Indeed, the tradition initiated by the Framingham cohort study was complemented by three large cohort studies of cardiovascular disease conducted in the 1980s, which covered practically the whole spectrum of adults (≥18 years) as well as diverse ethnic and socioeconomic groups in the United States. Specifically, the CARDIA study (Friedman et al. 1988) recruited a total of 5115 persons between 18 and 30 years of age in four states; the ARIC study (ARIC Investigators 1989) cohort comprised 15,800 persons aged 45–64 years at the beginning of the study and residents of four states; and the CHS (Fried et al. 1991) followed up 2955 participants 65 years or older in another four communities of the United States.

In addition to strict temporal and geographic criteria, a cohort can also be defined by a group of individuals sharing common characteristics, which facilitates the follow-up and/or the accuracy and precision of the data to be collected. For example, the Multicenter AIDS Cohort Study (MACS) (Kaslow et al. 1987; Dudley et al. 1995) comprised homosexual men in four metropolitan areas of the United States with the overall aim of describing the natural history of HIV infection and AIDS (see Table 5.6.1), from the risk factors of infection with HIV to the hazard of death among those developing AIDS.

From April 1984 to March 1985, a cohort of 4954 men was recruited into the MACS in four metropolitan areas of the United States (Baltimore, Chicago, Los Angeles, and Pittsburgh). To increase minority enrolment, an additional 668 men, 69.3 per cent of whom were non-Caucasian, were recruited in 1987–1991. To address issues of long-term effectiveness of therapies and their putative adverse effects, 1350 men were additionally enrolled in 2001–2003. In 2010, an additional 47 men were recruited in Baltimore and Pittsburgh. Therefore, the entire MACS cohort as of September 2012 consisted of 7019 men with three primary inclusion criteria: men having sex with men, older than 18 years, and AIDS-free. Of them, 2905 (41 per cent) were seroprevalent for HIV at entry into the study. All men were followed up every 6 months

Table 5.6.1 Examples of cohort studies

	Framingham (Dawber 1980)	MACS (Kaslow et al. 1987; Dudley et al. 1995)	Norwegian electricians (Tynes et al. 1992)
Study aims	Incidence and risk factors for cardiovascular diseases and hypertension	Natural history of HIV infection and AIDS	Relationship between electromagnetic radiation and cancer incidence
Type of study	Concurrent	Concurrent	Non-concurrent
Date	1949–present	1984–present	1960–1991
Study population	Adults resident in Framingham, Massachusetts, USA	Homosexual men in four metropolitan areas of the USA	Electricians in 1960 census in Norway
Simple size	5127	7019	37,945
Sex	Male and female	Male	Male
Age at baseline (years)	30–62	18–70	20–70
Active follow-up	Study visits every 2 years including physical exam, electrocardiogram, and laboratory exams	Study visits every 6 months with extensive interviews including behaviour and medical care, physical exam, laboratory exams and collection of blood samples for national repository.	Not applicable
Passive follow-up	Clinical records (in case of hospitalization) Death certificates	Clinical records Death certificates National Death Index	Cancer registries Death certificates

Source: data from Dawber (1980), Kaslow et al. (1987), Dudley et al. (1995), and Tynes et al. (1992).

with repeat interviews, physical examinations, and collection of blood. Serological tests for HIV antibody were routinely carried out at each visit. Up to September 2012, the dates of last negative and first positive visits (i.e. seroconverters) were known for 704 men. Using blood samples collected at each semi-annual visit in order to characterize the level of HIV-induced immunosuppression, mononuclear cells were analysed by two-colour flow cytometry with antibodies specific for CD3, CD4, and CD8. Confirmation of AIDS diagnoses was made by obtaining physician and hospital summaries and by reviewing medical records; 1976 AIDS cases were observed up to September 2012. Deaths were monitored by follow-up and through an ongoing search of death records. A total of 2136 participants died before September 2012.

When a specific registry with baseline data is available, it provides the opportunity to conduct a non-concurrent cohort study. For example, Nieto et al. (1992) used a registry of physical examinations carried out on schoolchildren between 1933 and 1945 in Hagerstown (Maryland, United States) to assemble a non-concurrent cohort of about 13,000 children in order to study the relationship between childhood obesity and adult mortality; the baseline information obtained between 1933 and 1945 was linked to the mortality experience of the cohort up to 1985. In other historical cohorts, the study population is defined from the beginning as a function of the exposure factors to be investigated. Thus, participants are selected explicitly according to the presence or absence of the characteristics considered to be possible risk factors, such as a cohort of Norwegian electricians. As summarized in Table 5.6.1, this historical cohort of 37,945 workers was defined from the registry of occupations of the working population in Norway according to the 1960 census (Tynes et al. 1992).

With the increasing availability of electronic health records, new opportunities to use administrative healthcare databases as a basis for defining and conducting large-scale cohort studies are emerging (Phillips et al. 1999; Lau et al. 2007; Sterne et al. 2009; Manolio et al. 2012). These approaches offer the opportunity to carry out studies in large samples of tens or hundreds of thousands of individuals at relatively limited costs. They can be particularly powerful when combined with a comprehensive system of national registries, such as those offered by countries like Denmark (Frank 2000). These approaches may be limited, however, by the relative scarcity of 'negative' controls (i.e. healthy subjects) and by an under-representation of people who do not have access to (or choose not to take advantage of) healthcare services. In addition, the quality of the data collected for clinical purposes is variable, not usually subject to the rigours of standardization and quality typical in research settings, especially when studying phenomena that are not directly related to clinical care (e.g. upstream community determinants, psychosocial factors).

Finally, cohort studies can outlive themselves such as when the offspring of the cohort members are recruited into a so-called 'offspring' cohort, often with the purpose of conducting family and genetic studies. The Framingham Heart Study was again a pioneer in this methodology, when in the late 1970s the daughters and sons of the original cohort members (and their spouses) were recruited to constitute the Framingham Offspring Study (Kannel et al. 1979; Djoussé et al. 2002). Another example is the Beaver Dam Offspring Study, which recruited adult children (21 years or older) of the participants in the Epidemiology of Hearing Loss Study, a population sample based in the town of Beaver Dam, Wisconsin, United States (Cruickshanks et al. 2009).

Baseline visit

The objective of the baseline visit in a concurrent cohort study is generally the classification of the study participants according to the exposure factor or factors under investigation, as well as according to potentially relevant covariates (confounders) and/or effect modifiers. For example, Furth et al. (2006 and 2011) designed a cohort of children with chronic kidney disease to determine the risk factors for progression towards end-stage renal disease; for this, they recruited 586 children aged 1–16 years with an estimated glomerular filtration rate of between 30 and 90 mL/min/1.73 m^2, indicating a level of insufficiency in their kidney function that put them at risk of end-stage renal disease. Also important is the collection of information that facilitates the subsequent tracking of study participants during the follow-up including information on contacts.

In its simplest form, the baseline visit can take place over a single continuous time period until the desired sample size is reached. In many cases, however, more participants are recruited: (1) to replace those who have developed the event of interest or who have been lost to follow-up, (2) to include groups of individuals who were under-represented in the original recruitment, and/or (3) to respond to new scientific challenges due to the changing nature of the epidemiology of the disease of interest

Follow-up

The follow-up can be active, by repeated contacts via successive visits to a health centre, mailed questionnaires, or phone calls. Sometimes, the different forms of contacting participants are alternated. For example, in the follow-up of the ARIC study, participants were invited every 3 years to return to the clinic for a new physical examination and complementary assessments (ARIC Investigators 1989); in addition, each participant was called every year and asked about illnesses and hospitalizations occurring in the interim period since the last clinic visit. In the MACS, the visits are scheduled every 6 months and take place in dedicated settings instead of in a clinic. This is in contrast to clinic cohort studies in which visits take place according to the health needs of the participants.

For certain diseases and events (e.g. death, cancer), external sources (i.e. national death index, registries) can be used to record events occurring among the individuals enrolled in the study. The type and automation of the record linkage system is determined in each case by the availability of data and the characteristics of each particular registry (Oshima et al. 1979; Hole et al. 1981; Smith and Newcombe 1982; Newcombe 1984).

The quality of the information about the occurrence of events is fundamental for correct estimation of the incidence and its determinants. Therefore, in many cohort studies, a special effort is made to ensure that the information about disease occurrence or death is accurate. Generally, events recorded in interviews with study participants are verified by requesting documents such as the clinical records or death certificate of the subject, not only to verify the occurrence of the event but also to improve the information regarding diagnosis (e.g. to obtain the histological type in a study of lung cancer; to distinguish between thrombotic and haemorrhagic episodes in a study of cerebrovascular events). A major challenge in cohort studies with cause-specific mortality as the event of interest is the determination of the cause of death, which may require confirmation by inspecting clinical records or by interviewing the physician who attended to the participant before his or her death.

Types and measures of exposures

The classification of study participants according to exposure factors is one of the most complex challenges in a cohort study. *Exposure factor* means any attribute of the subject or any external agent that can influence his or her health (Armstrong et al. 1992).

Types of exposures

Exposure factors include host factors (such as age, sex, race, genetic factors, metabolic factors, and immune function) and environmental factors (such as viruses and bacteria, environmental pollutants, diet, alcohol, and/or tobacco consumption). Sometimes, an exposure factor represents a set of factors that are difficult to separate. For example, social class encompasses external environmental factors, related to individual behaviour, access to healthcare services, socioeconomic status, and others.

The exposures can be either fixed over time (e.g. sex) or variable. The latter could be exposures that change directly with time (e.g. age and calendar) or change at their own pace with time (e.g. cigarettes smoked per day, biological marker levels, diet). When exposures not only change over time but do so heterogeneously (i.e. change differently over time in different individuals), they are referred to as *internal* (i.e. at the individual level) time-dependent exposures. In contrast, exposures that change over time but affect groups or populations who are subject to the exposure in a similar way are referred to as *external* (i.e. at the population level) time-dependent exposures (i.e. they change equally over time for different individuals comprising a given population). The most common example of an external variable is calendar time, which is the same for the whole population. Other examples of external time-dependent exposures include the following: seasonal weather changes, levels of air pollution in a given region, supplements in the food and water supply, and medical therapies/procedures used in different calendar periods.

Follow-up visits in the setting of a cohort study provide the opportunity for collecting data to update internal time-dependent exposures. External time-dependent exposures may be obtained from external sources, but data obtained at the individual level can sometimes be used to define eras (i.e. calendar periods) when there are changes at the population level. For example, the MACS started in 1984 and has since been conducted concurrently with major advances in therapies effective against viral replication in HIV-infected individuals. In 1998, Detels et al. determined the effectiveness of the potent antiretroviral therapies introduced in 1995 by showing a doubling of the AIDS-free times under the conditions of the first two years (July 1995–July 1997) of the highly active antiretroviral therapy (HAART) era (Detels et al. 1998). In 2005, Schneider et al. determined the population effectiveness of prolonged use of HAART by showing that in the era when HAART was well established (i.e. July 2001–December 2005, 6–10 years after its introduction in July 1995), the median survival time after AIDS diagnosis increased tenfold from the 1.5 years in the era when no therapies were available (Schneider et al. 2005).

In cohort studies, two types of effects of interventions can be measured. The first can be termed 'individual effectiveness', which mimics clinical trials by using treatment data at the individual level. These analyses must overcome the lack of randomization and the confounding by indication, whereby those individuals at more advanced disease stages are the ones more likely to receive the therapies (Ahdieh et al. 2000). Measures of individual effect-iveness *supplement* (and typically support and extend) the results of clinical trials, but are usually subject to an unknown amount of residual confounding (Phillips et al. 1999). Data-analysis methods for individual effectiveness require the use of multivariate meth-ods of survival analysis, including the use of therapy as an internal time-dependent covariate; however, the complexity of the selec-tion of individuals receiving therapies may require the use of more elaborate methods for causal inferences (Robins et al. 2000; Cole et al. 2003). Randomized clinical trials are typically considered a standard study design for inference of the causal effect of an expo-sure on an outcome. However, when the exposure is predicted to be detrimental to health (e.g. abnormal birth history), an observa-tional study design is a suitable choice to investigate the effect of the exposure on an outcome. Established methods are available to attempt to mimic randomized experiments for the purpose of esti-mating causal effects in observational studies. These approaches include propensity score matching methods (Stuart 2010), inverse probability weights based on propensity scores (Robins et al. 2000), and marginal structural models (Hernán et al. 2001). The guiding principle of these approaches is to construct a sample in which two or more groups (e.g. exposed/unexposed) have identi-cal (or balanced) distributions of confounders (Stuart 2010).

There is growing interest in determining the effectiveness of the many therapies participants in cohort studies are observed to receive but there is strong confounding by indication as thera-pies tend to be given to individuals who fulfil guidelines for who and when to treat. Standard regression adjustments to compare outcomes of treated to those untreated seldom achieve control for the indication for receiving treatment. Alternative approaches include the use of inverse probability weights based on probabil-ity of receiving treatment. Inverse probability weights estimators provide an excellent means for estimating the causal effects of treatment among individuals with different covariate values at study baseline (Robins et al. 2000). However, covariates are often dynamic and changing values may alter the impact of therapy on the outcome. Further, marginal structural models are limited in their flexibility, becoming unstable if certain covariate values yield very large or very small probabilities of treatment. Inverse prob-ability weights methods offer powerful tools to deal with complex patterns of confounding, particularly in longitudinal data, where outcomes at one time point may influence both subsequent treat-ments and outcomes. More elaborate methods such as marginal structural models have been proposed to deal with these types of patterns, whereby the weights in these models are updated longi-tudinally using the complete past history. In addition, the weights are stabilized, resulting in improved performance. Many scientific initiatives present research questions involving strong confound-ers for which these approaches may overcome the limitations of classical multivariate regression methods. Although these meth-ods offer great potential (e.g. Kitahata et al. 2009), their imple-mentation could be problematic as it requires complex procedures and clear understanding of the required steps and algorithms to properly mimic a clinical trial in the setting of observational data (Hernán and Robins 2009). Furthermore, the attempts to analyse observational studies like randomized experiments (Hernán et al. 2008) can be controversial (Stampfer 2008; Willet et al. 2008) but may result in improvements of methods to compare groups and to characterize when a given exposure (e.g. years after menopause when hormone replacement therapy is initiated) may exert an effect on a health outcome (Hoover 2008; Prentice 2008).

The second type of effect that can be measured in a cohort study can be termed 'population effectiveness', which compares the occurrence of disease in the population when the most ill are treated to the occurrence of disease in the population when none or only few are treated with a given therapy. Because the introduc-tion and use of therapies are closely linked to calendar time, the primary comparison may be characterized by time periods. When periods are characterized by differential availability of therapies, they could then play the role of an *instrumental variable* (related to therapy but not to disease progression or markers indicative of therapy need) and thus provide an accurate effect of the ben-efits of therapy at the population level (Greenland 2000; Martens et al. 2006). To control for survival bias and overall disease pro-gression, this approach requires the comparison of groups reach-ing similar time at risk (e.g. duration of infection or time since disease diagnosis) in different eras of therapy defined by calendar periods (Hoover et al. 1994; Muñoz and Hoover 1995; Detels et al. 1998; Schneider et al. 2005). Measures of population effectiveness *complement* the efficacy measured in clinical trials and provide a key public health index: the amount of disease burden that is reduced when only some (typically the most ill) receive the ther-apy of interest (Muñoz et al. 2000). Comprehensive data collected by cohort studies are essential to eliminate possible ecological fal-laciousness (i.e. effectiveness due to changes over time other than changes in the therapies of interest). This includes not only pro-spectively collected data on therapy use, but also information on access, healthcare utilization and practices, and adherence at the population level.

Measures of exposures

The exposure can be defined as a quantitative (continuous) vari-able (e.g. blood pressure) or qualitative (categorical) variable (e.g. non-smoker, ex-smoker, current smoker).

When exposures are assessed repeatedly over time, the inves-tigators can take into account not only the amount (dose) but also the duration of the exposure (Armstrong et al. 1992). There are several ways of quantifying dose and duration: (1) cumula-tive exposure (e.g. number of pack-years of smoking, number of rad-years of exposure to a radioactive compound at work), (2) the average exposure during the latest years (e.g. average number of cigarettes per day, average number of rads in the work environ-ment), or (3) maximum exposure (e.g. maximum number of ciga-rettes per day, maximum level of radioactivity registered in the industry).

The most typical data-collection instruments in epidemio-logical practice are questionnaires, physical examination, and registries. Questionnaires allow not only the obtaining of infor-mation on demographic data, personal and family history, disease symptoms, behaviours, and attitudes, but also the recording of self-reported physical characteristics such as weight and height. They can be administered through personal or telephone inter-views, they can be completed by the participants themselves, or they can be administered by a computer-assisted method, which is particularly useful for the collection of sensitive data (e.g. sex-ual behaviour, drug abuse). Modern technologies are significantly expanding the range of possible modalities for data collection. Web-based instruments, smartphones, and other types of mobile devices are being used to collect information on dietary habits and other types of exposures (Illner et al. 2012). In addition, registries are external sources that can be used to complement the active follow-up and are particularly useful to obtain vital status events or diagnosis of a condition of interest (e.g. cancer registries).

Timescales and types of outcomes

The scientific aims of a cohort study should dictate the type of outcome or measure of disease occurrence that should be collected during follow-up. The most common measure of disease in cohort studies is the time individuals at risk take to develop an end point. To properly describe this time, the following need to be defined: (1) the origin, which marks the time at which individuals are placed at risk for the development of the particular event of interest; (2) the end point, which typically is the onset of a clinical condition or the occurrence of death; and (3) the scale of time.

Types of timescales

Traditionally, the timescale used in cohort studies is the time from the beginning of the study (when the cohort is identified and the baseline exam is conducted) until the event of interest (or censoring, as discussed in the next subsection) occurs. For example, in many of the analyses of the Framingham Study data, the origin (time 0) of the follow-up is defined as the date when the baseline interview/exam of each of the participants took place in or at around 1950. The fact that individuals start at different ages is dealt with in the analysis by statistically *controlling* for baseline age.

Whether or not an origin is well defined, the use of *age* as the timescale is an appealing alternative (Korn et al. 1997). The caveat of this approach when applied to a cohort of individuals entering at different ages (e.g. in adulthood) is that individuals are not under observation during the years from birth to the age at which they are recruited into the cohort. This needs to be handled in the analysis allowing for late entry (left truncation—see following subsection). This method was used, for example, in a study of the relation between sleep apnoea and cancer mortality in the Wisconsin Sleep Cohort (Nieto et al. 2012). Another application of age as the timescale was the characterization by Wada et al. (2013, 2014) of life expectancies of HIV-infected individuals in the era of HAART.

In most cases, even for groups of individuals with a persistent (e.g. fixed) exposure, the pattern of incidence of disease over the follow-up time is not the same at different durations at risk. An exposure whose deleterious effect monotonically accumulates over time will result in an incidence rate that increases with time (e.g. death after AIDS diagnosis in the absence of treatment). An exposure that first affects susceptible individuals so that those remaining free of the event over time represent resistance (i.e. some degree of immunity to the effects of exposure) will result in an increasing incidence followed by a decreasing incidence rate (e.g. a viral infection to which a subset of individuals are immune). An exposure that initially carries risk that ameliorates over time will result in a decreasing incidence rate (e.g. death after transplantation). A beneficial intervention that decreases the risk of death but whose effect is obliterated by other processes including old age will result in a bathtub hazard (Cox et al. 2013).

Incomplete observation from the origin and to the event

In some cohort studies, not all individuals are observed from the origin, but some enter the study after having been at risk for varying lengths of time. This type of incompleteness in the data is referred to as *late entries* or *staggered entries* and occurs when some individuals have experienced the origin that places them at risk for the event of interest at a date prior to their enrolment into a cohort study. Since these individuals have survived free of the event of interest from the origin to study enrolment, they have peers with similar origins who did not survive event-free and developed the event of interest prior to the cohort study enrolment, precluding their participation in the study. Such unseen individuals are *truncated*, and methods to adjust for these truncated observations need to be implemented by appropriately handling late entries. The presence of late entries in a study is a case of missing data, where missing data are the number and timing of the events of the truncated peers of those who entered late. Indeed, if an individual enters a cohort study w years after his/her time of origin, there are $[1 - S(w)] / S(w)$ truncated individuals who have not been included in the study. This is because the cohort would have needed to enrol a total of $1 / S(w)$ individuals for one of them to survive event-free for w years and be enrolled in the study.

With respect to the event, observations in a cohort study are incomplete because it is unfeasible for the investigator to observe the event in all participating individuals. This type of incompleteness in the data is called *censoring* and can be due to any of the following: individuals being observed as event-free on the date of analysis, sometimes called *administrative* censoring; individuals being lost to follow-up (prior to the date of analysis) before developing the event; or deaths due to unrelated causes, precluding the observation of the event of interest.

When the follow-up is ended by the investigators (e.g. because the source of funding for the study is exhausted), the participants still under follow-up without having experienced the event of interest are considered administrative losses. When participants emigrate during the course of the follow-up, change addresses or telephone numbers making them untraceable, or refuse to continue participating, they are considered censored observations due to follow-up losses. When death is the reason for censoring an event of interest, it is more appropriate to use methods of analysis based on competing risk models (Putter et al. 2007), which consider the deaths as exits or removals from the risk set as opposed to treating the deaths as observations that could have been observed had the participants not died before the event of interest occurred (Fine and Gray 1999; Checkley et al. 2010).

For the most part, subjects who are lost to follow-up are *right-censored*, which means that their exit from observation is the last possible time they contributed information to the study (i.e. on the timeline of their participation represented by a scale running from left to right, no data are available to the right of the time of censoring). Occasionally, information from sources external to the study (e.g. death certificates) are used to identify the interval of time during which individuals lost to follow-up and free of the event of interest are documented to have had the event because they died of the event of interest at some time point after the censoring. This interval is defined as the time between the date the individual was lost to follow-up and the date of death. Given that the individual died of the event of interest, the event must have occurred during this interval. These observations are called *interval-censored* observations. When using age as the timescale with mortality as the end point, censored observations are all interval censored as all individuals are expected to die by age 100 (Wada et al. 2013, 2014).

In the survival analysis section, we will discuss the issues regarding the relationships between the censoring mechanisms and the disease process, as well as the need for properly incorporating not only censoring (i.e. incomplete data on events) but also truncation resulting from late entries (i.e. incomplete data on origins) into the data analysis.

Time-to-event

The nature of a cohort study provides the temporal structure necessary to associate a particular exposure with a subsequent event of interest. Documentation of the time sequences of exposures and events generates data upon which the course of event development can be modelled. The use of time-to-event outcomes requires that the *time* variable be anchored at the origin, resulting in the characterization of the event incidence across the time since origin. In other words, the incidence of the event from 5 to 7 years past the origin will be handled differently in the analysis than the incidence from 9 to 11 years, even though both time periods equally span 2 person-years.

Examples of time-to-event outcomes used in epidemiological research include the following: (1) in clinical epidemiology, the classic time from diagnosis of a clinical condition to death or the time from initiating therapy to response; (2) in infectious disease epidemiology, the time from infection to overt disease (i.e. the incubation period); (3) in cancer epidemiology, the time from remission to relapse; (4) in behavioural epidemiology, the time from enrolment into a smoking cessation programme to the time the individual quits smoking; and (5) in occupational epidemiology, the time from employment to the occurrence of an occupationally related health outcome.

Change of biomarkers

In some cohort studies, the primary event is not an event but whether a marker of disease changes over time differently in individuals exposed to different risk factors. For example, in the cohort study of children with moderate kidney function insufficiency conducted by Furth et al. (2006), the primary objective was to identify the factors that predicted fast decline of kidney function (Pierce et al. 2011). Another example is the cohort study conducted

by Tager et al. (1983) in East Boston in the 1970s, showing the effect of maternal smoking on slowing the expected increase of pulmonary function in growing children. The study was seminal to the subsequent mounting evidence that second-hand (involuntary) smoking had detrimental health effects and guided the issuing of policies to ban smoking from work and public places as fundamental prevention measures for the health of the public. Furthermore, cohort studies have not only contributed substantially to the elucidation of disease aetiology but have also spurred the development of statistical methods to properly analyse data. For example, Rosner et al. (1985) developed methods for the analyses of data presented in their work in collaboration with Tager et al. (1983).

Analysis

A fundamental condition for valid epidemiological inferences is that for the disease to be (causally) linked to a given exposure, the exposed and unexposed groups should be comparable with respect to factors that are known to explain the heterogeneity of disease occurrence (i.e. no confounding). In cohort (observational) studies, comparability needs to be achieved by the use of appropriate analytical methods which often require approaches above and beyond classical stratification and/or regression methods. The goal of causal inference methods is to try to mimic randomization so as to assess the effect of a given exposure in groups of individuals who differ in the exposure of interest, but who are otherwise comparable with respect to all variables known to be associated with disease.

The type of outcome of interest determines the type of analytical technique most appropriate to yield a valid inference. Table 5.6.2 provides a succinct summary of the analytical methods reviewed here.

When the outcome data are collected as events in person-years, Poisson regression methods are apt for data analysis (outcome I in Table 5.6.2). These methods are particularly useful for the analysis of trends and changes in incidence of disease over calendar time; they are of great utility for data in which an origin is not well defined or not of interest, which will be the case if the rate of disease occurrence is assumed to be constant within a defined interval or period.

When the outcome data are times to event from a well-defined origin (outcome II in Table 5.6.2), the percentage of individuals remaining free of the event of interest at t units of time after the origin can be estimated by the Kaplan–Meier (Kaplan and

Table 5.6.2 Main methods for the analysis of cohort studies

Outcome		Summary measure	Comparison		Measure of association
			Exposed/unexposed (2-sample)	**Multiple (regression)**	
I	Events in person-years	Incidence rate	$(O-E)^2$/variance	Poisson	Relative incidence
II	Time to event	Kaplan–Meier/maximum likelihood estimates	Logrank or Mantel-Haenszel/ likelihood ratio test	Proportional hazards/parametric	Relative hazard/ relative time
III	Biomarker repeatedly measured at follow-up visits	Change	t-test for simple measures of change between baseline and last visit	Regression for correlated data; marginal, conditional, random effects	Differences in change over time

Meier, 1958) curve or by maximum-likelihood methods for the non-parametric and parametric (Cox et al. 2007) approaches, respectively. Two survival curves can be compared using the Mantel–Haenszel (Mantel and Haenszel, 1959) test or the likelihood ratio test (Cox et al. 2007). Regression analysis can be accomplished under the semi-parametric assumption of proportional hazards (Cox, 1972) or under richer parametric models (Cox et al. 2007) which lend themselves more directly to estimation of relative times quantifying not only how the hazard is modified by an exposure but also to what extent an exposure shortens (if deleterious) or extends (if beneficial) the event-free times. Software in several statistical packages to incorporate not only censoring but late entries is widely available (Cox et al. 2007).

When the outcome is a biomarker repeatedly measured at follow-up visits (outcome III in Table 5.6.2), regression methods for correlated data need to be used. This is so because the biomarkers measured in the same individual over the follow-up visits are correlated so that the standard methods of regression methods for statistically independent outcomes are inadequate.

Analysis based on person-time

Calculation of person-time and rates

The methods described in this subsection are useful for the analysis of the frequency of events in person-years in groups of individuals with different exposures and when anchoring at the origin is not important. The primary aim is to describe the heterogeneity of the incidence in subgroups of the population defined by exposures, often including age and calendar.

To illustrate the methods, we present data from the Precursors Cohort study. This cohort comprised 1337 medical students of the Johns Hopkins University, Baltimore, United States, who graduated between 1948 and 1964 (Klag et al. 1993). A total of 1271 students (95 per cent) completed a questionnaire and were examined during their stay at the school. In order to study the determining factors ('precursors') of general mortality and the occurrence of cardiovascular diseases, this cohort was followed up through mailed questionnaires. When the participants reported that they have had a myocardial infarction or another cardiovascular event, the hospital records were requested in order to validate the diagnosis. The vital status of the participants who did not respond was systematically investigated through calls to relatives and friends and through matching with the National Death Index. Table 5.6.3 shows data obtained in the follow-up for each of the groups (smokers and non-smokers), the column named 'person-years' showing the totality of time units lived by the members of the cohort between the indicated years of age. Thus, for example, the non-smokers in the cohort lived a total of 862.5 years while being 20–24 years old and 1929.5 years while being 25–29 years of age.

Univariate analysis

Internal comparison

The comparison of exposed and unexposed within a cohort can be done through the calculation of the standardized mortality ratio (SMR). Using data from the Precursors study, the last column of Table 5.6.3 shows the deaths 'expected' in the smokers if they had had the rates of the non-smokers. For example, the number of deaths expected in smokers aged 45–49 years old would be 0.00155 (deaths/year) $\times$ 2182.5 (person-years) = 3.4 deaths. The SMR is the ratio of total observed deaths to the total expected deaths in smokers (if the smokers had the same age-specific rates as the non-smokers), which in this case is 57/29.8 = 1.9.

Table 5.6.3 Internal comparison of the rates based on person-years in the Precursors Study. Occurrence of mortality (all-cause) until 1989, as a function of cigarette consumption at the baseline examination

| Age (years) | Non-smokers | | | Smokers | | | |
	Deaths	Person-years	Rate	Deaths	Person-years	Rate	Expected deaths[a]
20–24	1	862.5	0.00116	1	886.5	0.00113	1.0
25–29	2	1929.5	0.00104	2	2195.5	0.00091	2.3
30–34	0	2052	0	1	2360	0.00042	0
35–39	1	2064.5	0.00048	4	2354	0.00170	1.1
40–44	1	2029.5	0.00049	6	2280.5	0.00263	1.1
45–49	3	1940.5	0.00155	2	2182.5	0.00092	3.4
50–54	5	1501	0.00333	13	1819	0.00715	6.1
55–59	5	827	0.00605	11	1187	0.00927	7.2
60–64	4	370.5	0.01080	13	582	0.02234	6.3
65–69	0	103.5	0	4	106	0.03774	0
70–74	1	17.5	0.05714	0	23	0	1.3
75–79	0	1.5	0	0	0.5	0	0
Total	23			57			29.8

[a] Numbers of deaths that would occur in the group of smokers if they had the rate observed in the non-smokers.

Source: data from Klag MJ et al., Serum cholesterol in young men and subsequent cardiovascular disease, *New England Journal of Medicine*, Volume 328, pp. 313–18, Copyright © 1993 Massachusetts Medical Society. All rights reserved.

External comparison

In other situations, it can be of interest to compare the mortality in the study group with the mortality of the total population that is used as reference. In this case, it is necessary to obtain the expected number of deaths using population-level rates from demographic statistics. Thus, in the Precursors study, the observed mortality can be compared with the mortality of the population of white males in the United States, as shown in Table 5.6.4. The total number of observed deaths (23 + 57 = 80) divided by the total number of expected deaths based on the demographic statistics provides the SMR of the cohort in comparison with the general population, which in case of data from Table 5.6.4 is 80/148.1 = 0.54. This result implies that the mortality is almost half of what would be expected if the cohort had the same rates as that of the general population.

Multivariable analysis

The aim of multivariable analysis is to identify the constellation of exposures that explain the variability of incidence of disease, allowing for random variation under a probability distribution model. The Poisson distribution provides a useful and reasonable model to carry out the multivariable analysis of incidence rates observed in cohort studies. Ideally, the final regression model from a multivariable analysis should have an appropriate goodness of fit and be optimally parsimonious (i.e. with most regression coefficients being statistically significant).

Table 5.6.4 External comparison of the rates based on person-years in the Precursors Study. All-cause mortality until 1989, observed and expected according to national rates in 1980

Age (years)	National mortality rate[a]	Study cohort		
		Deaths	Person-years	Expected deaths[b]
20–24	0.001909	2	1749	3.3
25–29	0.001747	4	4125	7.2
30–34	0.001676	1	4412	7.4
35–39	0.002087	5	4418.5	9.2
40–44	0.003161	7	4310	13.6
45–49	0.005217	5	4123	21.5
50–54	0.008668	18	3320	28.8
55–59	0.013756	16	2014	27.7
60–64	0.021406	17	952.5	20.4
65–69	0.033121	4	209.5	6.9
70–74	0.050338	1	40.5	2.0
75–79	0.074685	0	2	0.1
Total		80	29,676	148.1

[a] Mortality rates in white males, U.S.A., 1980.

[b] According to national rates.

Source: data from Klag MJ et al., Serum cholesterol in young men and subsequent cardiovascular disease, *New England Journal of Medicine*, Volume 328, pp. 313–18, Copyright © 1993 Massachusetts Medical Society. All rights reserved.

Survival analysis

Time-to-event outcomes are used to accomplish the following epidemiological objectives: estimate the percentage of individuals that survive (i.e. remain event-free) for differing lengths of time from the origin, compare the survival of exposed and unexposed groups, and characterize the possibly multifactorial nature explaining observed heterogeneities in survival of different subgroups of individuals using multivariable analysis and regression methods.

Descriptors of the distribution of times-to-event

If T denotes the variable of time from origin to event, the simplest descriptor of the distribution of T is the *survival function* at time t (where t is a positive number), which is denoted by $S(t)$ and corresponds to the cumulative probability that an individual in the baseline cohort survives beyond time t. The survival function starts with a value of one and monotonically decreases towards zero. Its complement from $1 - S(t)$ is the cumulative incidence that an individual in the baseline cohort has the event before or at time t. The *pth percentile*, which is denoted by $t(p)$, is the time by which p per cent develop the event of interest; that is, when $1 - p = S(t(p))$. A widely used descriptor of survival times is the median, which is simply the 50th percentile, or the time since origin by which half of the individuals develop the event of interest.

The *hazard function* at t, which is denoted by $h(t)$, corresponds to the proportion of individuals who develop the event in the next unit of time among those who survive event-free until time t. That is, $h(t)$ equals the rate of decline of S at t divided by $S(t)$. The rate of decline of S is the *density function*, which is denoted by $f(t)$ and fulfils the equation $f(t) = h(t)S(t)$. It is important to note that $h(t)$ is a conditional probability and refers only to the subset of the cohort that survives event-free by time t.

Fig. 5.6.1 depicts the 25th percentile and hazard at $t = 12$ years of a survival function. The 25th percentile is 6 years (i.e. t (0.25) = 6 years), because it corresponds to the time by which 25 per cent of the individuals develop the event (i.e. 75 per cent survive). The hazard at $t = 12$ years is 10 per cent and corresponds to the ratio of 0.04/0.40, which is the value of the rate of decline of the survival function at $t = 12$ (i.e. the density $t = 12$) divided by the value of S at $t = 12$.

The accumulation of h from zero to t (i.e. the area under the curve described by h from zero to t) denoted by $H(t)$ is the 'summation' of all instantaneous hazards ($h(t)$) between zero and t. There is a close and useful relationship between the survival function and the cumulative hazard at t : $S(t) = \exp[-H(t)]$, or equivalently, $H(t) = -\log[S(t)]$. Therefore, the cumulative hazard does not equate to the cumulative incidence of events by time t because $-\log[S(t)]$ is not equal to $1 - S(t)$.

Estimation of the survival function

The presence of censored observations is a case of missing data, and the fundamental role of the assumption that censored observations are not a selected subgroup is that, at any time during the study, individuals who remain under observation *represent* those subjects who were censored beforehand. The observation of events beyond the time an individual is censored provides the data to estimate when the censored individual is expected to develop the event had she or he remained in the study. Furthermore, because the individuals who are observed to develop the event are

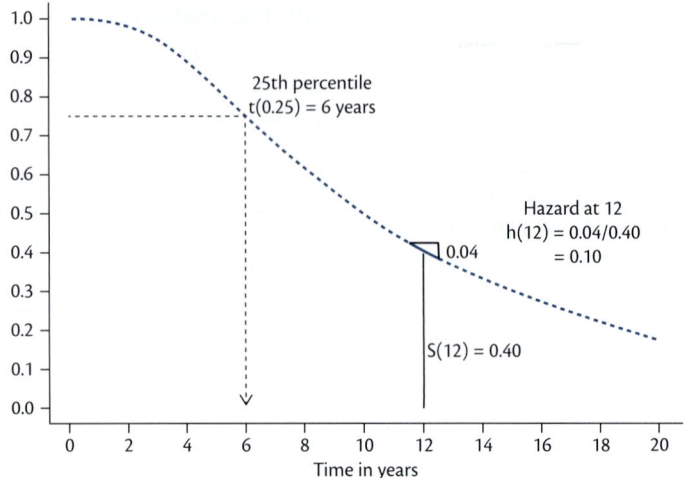

Fig. 5.6.1 Survival function, the 25th percentile (t(0.25)) and hazard at t = 12 years (h(12)).

representative of the observations censored before their time of event, estimates of the hazard functions based on the observed individuals are unbiased, and thus they represent the hazards that the censored individuals would have experienced had they remained under observation in the study. Indeed, this forms the basis of the Kaplan–Meier method (Kaplan and Meier 1958), based on the calculation of the survival probability through the product of one minus the instantaneous hazards. The standard error of the estimators of the Kaplan–Meier survival function can be obtained from methods proposed by Greenwood (1926).

Fig. 5.6.2 shows five Kaplan–Meier curves according to the number of copies of HIV detected in 500 mL of plasma measured by branched-DNA (bDNA) in HIV-infected individuals followed up in the MACS cohort (Mellors et al. 1997). It clearly shows the great predictive value that viral load has for the development of AIDS. Indeed, investigators in the MACS have developed methods to quantify the variability of time to AIDS explained by viral load and have shown that it alone explained approximately 50 per cent of the variability of time to AIDS (Mellors et al. 2007).

Univariate analysis

Graphical display of the survival curves is generally quite useful to obtain an overall comparison of the experiences of groups subjected to different exposures (Fig. 5.6.2). There are two different ways to measure the association between exposure and survival, which correspond to horizontal (i.e. relative time) and vertical comparisons (i.e. relative hazard) of survival curves. The first one is the relative times defined as $t_1(p)/t_0(p)$, where $t_i(p)$ corresponds to the time taken by p per cent of group i (for $i = 0,1$) to develop the event. The second one is the relative hazard, defined as $h_1(t)/h_0(t)$, where $h_i(t)$ is the hazard for the ith group (for $i = 0,1$) at time t. If exposure shortens survival, the relative time will be less than one and the relative hazard will be greater than one. If the relative times are independent of p and/or the relative hazards are independent of t, the times and/or the hazards are said to be proportional. In such cases, the relative times and/or hazards will be constant across all values of p and/or t, respectively. Since the percentiles are relative to the whole cohort but the hazard function is conditional on survivors, proportionality in one does not imply proportionality in the other. Methods based on parametric

models (e.g. lognormal regression) are more amenable to estimation and testing of relative times (e.g. to compare, for instance, the median survival time in exposed and unexposed) and they can also provide measures of relative hazards. Semi-parametric methods based on the proportionality of hazards focused attention to estimation and testing of relative hazards but caution must be exercised because proportionality of hazards is seldom attained.

There are hypothesis-testing procedures to assess whether the differences between two or more survival curves are statistically significant. The most commonly used is the logrank test (Peto et al. 1977), which assumes that the hazards are proportional and tests whether the relative hazard is equal to one. It is equivalent to the Mantel–Haenszel (Mantel and Haenszel, 1959) statistic for the combination of tables constructed at each time an event occurs whereby the table describes how many individuals were at risk at that time and how many of them developed the event from each group being compared.

Multivariable analysis

In the context of survival analysis, the most used method of multivariate analysis is the proportional hazards regression (Cox 1972). The semiparametric proportional hazards regression model corresponds to the hazard of the group with covariates representing exposures and confounders $x_1 = x_2 = \cdots = x_K = 0$ (i.e. the reference group) being completely arbitrary, and the hazard of the group characterized by any other values of x_1 to x_K being a fixed multiple of the hazard of the reference group according to a linear combination of the covariates. Specifically, the hazard of the group with covariates $x_1, x_2, \cdots, x_K$ denoted by $h_x(t)$ is $h_0(t) \exp(\beta_1 x_1 + \beta_2 x_2 + \cdots + \beta_K x_K)$. The interpretation of the parameters is directly linked to relative hazards. In particular, if we have two groups of individuals described by the constellation of covariates taking values x for one group and x^* for the other, the hazard at time t of the group described by x^* relative to the hazard at the same time of the group defined by x (i.e. the relative hazards) is given by $RH(t) \equiv \exp\left[\sum_{k=1}^{K} \beta_k (x_k^* - x_k)\right]$. Because such an expression does not depend on t, the relative hazard is constant (i.e. the hazards are proportional). In particular, if x and x^* only differ in one unit in the kth covariate

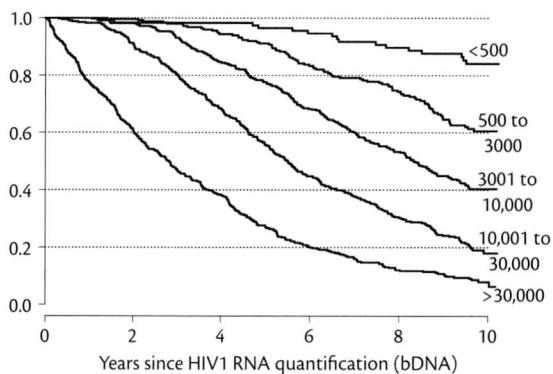

Fig. 5.6.2 Proportion AIDS-free by plasma HIV-RNA (copies/mL).
Source: data from Mellors JW et al., Prognostic Value of HIV-1 RNA, CD4 Cell Count, and CD4 Cell Count Slope for Progression to AIDS and Death in Untreated HIV-1 Infection, *Journal of the American Medical Association*, Volume 297, No. 21, pp. 2349–50, Copyright © 2007 American Medical Association. All Rights Reserved.

(i.e. $x^* = x_1, x_2, \cdots, x_k + 1, \cdots, x_K$), then the relative hazard of the x^* group to the x group is simply $RH(t) \equiv \exp(\beta_k)$.

When investigators from a cohort study are not only interested in relative hazards but also in describing the underlying hazard with the aim of characterizing mechanisms and the desire to quantify how exposures modify the magnitude of event-free times, parametric models are a more attractive option (Cox et al. 2007). To carry out parametric analyses of time-to-event data, the generalized gamma distribution offers a succinct yet flexible family of distributions. The generalized gamma distribution $GG(\beta, \sigma, \kappa)$ has three parameters whereby the location parameter β governs the value of the median for fixed values of σ and κ; the scale parameter σ determines the value of the interquartile ratio (i.e. IQR = 3rd quartile/1st quartile) for a fixed value of κ and independently of β; and the parameter κ determines the percentiles of the standard $\beta = 0$, $\sigma = 1$ generalized gamma. The generalized gamma contains commonly used parametric models in that the particular cases when κ is zero and one correspond to the lognormal and Weibull models, respectively. More importantly, the parameters κ and σ together determine the *type* of hazard function and yield a graphical taxonomy of the rich variety of hazards covered by the generalized gamma (Cox et al. 2007). Specifically, the taxonomy shows that the generalized gamma family includes all four of the common types of hazard functions: increasing, decreasing, U or bathtub shape, and inverted U or arch shape. More importantly, the pth percentile of the generalized gamma $t(p; \beta, \sigma, \kappa)$ can be expressed in terms of the three parameters by the simple equation $t(p; \beta, \sigma, \kappa) = e^\beta [t(p; 0, 1, \kappa)]^\sigma$ which dissects the role of each of the three parameters in determining the percentiles of the distribution (i.e. the pth percentile of the standard ($\beta = 0$ and $\sigma = 1$) generalized gamma with shape κ elevated to the power σ and multiplied by the antilog of β yields the pth percentile of $GG(\beta, \sigma, \kappa)$).

The conventional generalized gamma regression model corresponds to $GG(\beta'x, \sigma, \kappa)$, whereby the distribution of the times for the group of individuals with covariate vector x have different location parameters but same scale and shape. In this case, the relative times of the group with covariates x^* to the group with covariates x are constant (i.e. proportional times) and are equal to $\exp[\beta'(x^* - x)]$. Lack of proportionality of times can be easily incorporated by allowing σ to depend on covariates and full generalization of the model can be accomplished by further allowing κ to depend on covariates. Software is commonly available to implement generalized gamma regression in its full general form (e.g. streg command in STATA).

An example of the richness of parametric regression analyses for survival data is illustrated by Schneider et al. (2005), who used data from the MACS cohort of homosexual men and the WIHS cohort of women to characterize the changing pattern of survival after development of clinical AIDS from 1984 to 2004 when different antiretroviral therapies were introduced. Table 5.6.5 presents the relative hazards obtained from a multivariable Cox proportional hazards regression model and the relative times obtained from a multivariable Weibull regression model. Substantial differences in survival were seen between the last two HAART eras (July 1998–June 2001 and July 2001–December 2003) and the no/monotherapy era (prior to 1989); the time from AIDS to death (adjusted by age, sex, type of AIDS diagnosis, and CD4 cell count at diagnosis) expanded by eightfold and 11-fold in the two HAART eras, respectively. This analysis illustrates the role that cohort studies can play in providing measures of the effectiveness of interventions at the population level.

Longitudinal data analysis

The two analytical strategies explained in the preceding subsections (person-time and survival analysis) are the tools regularly utilized for the analysis of the results of a typical epidemiological cohort study when the dependent variable is the occurrence of an event such as disease or death. However, it is often the case that the dependent variable of interest in a cohort study is not the occurrence of an event but the trajectory of a determined biomarker such as blood pressure, weight, leucocyte count, viral load, glomerular filtration rate, pulmonary function, C-reactive protein, or CD4 cell count.

To illustrate the power of longitudinal data in cohort studies collecting data at regularly scheduled visits, we used data collected at semi-annual visits by the Multicenter AIDS Cohort Study from 1984 to 2006. The person-visits of interest were those happening after the first time individuals tested positive for antibodies to HIV and with data on therapy received, CD4 cell count (a marker of immunosuppression), and HIV-RNA (copies of HIV per mL of plasma). The objective was to describe the distribution of HIV-RNA in four categories of CD4 cell count using 200, 350, and 500 cells/mm³ as cut-off values and in four categories of therapy according to whether the participant at a given visit was not on any therapy, was just receiving antiretroviral therapy but not a triple combination, or was receiving triple combination therapy (HAART) and the visit occurred within 3 years or after 3 years from initiation. Two measures of HIV-RNA were used: (1) the median HIV-RNA and (2) the percentage of person-visits in a given category of CD4 cell count and therapy with undetectable HIV-RNA (i.e. <50 copies/mL). Fig. 5.6.3 uses a diamond-shaped equiponderant graphical display of the effects of CD4 cell count and therapy on HIV-RNA whereby the shaded area on each square is proportional to the HIV-RNA (Li et al. 2003). Both panels show the great effectiveness of HAART in suppressing viral replication in all categories of CD4 cell count.

Table 5.6.5 Descriptive statistics, adjusted relative hazards, and relative times for survival after an initial AIDS diagnosis in five calendar periods from July 1984 to December 2003

Variable	Calendar period				
	July 1984–Dec 1989	Jan 1990–Dec 1994	Jan 1995–June 1998	July 1998–June 2001	July 2001–Dec 2003
Therapy era	No/monotherapy	Monotherapy/combination therapy	HAART introduction	Short-term stable HAART	Moderate-term stable HAART
Number seen	633	660	472	496	464
% women	NA[a]	NA[a]	65%	72%	74%
Incident AIDS	633 (100%)	660 (100%)	472 (100%)	143 (29%)	57 (12%)
Median (IQR)[b] date of AIDS diagnosis	Oct 1987 (April 1986–Dec 1988)	April 1992 (Feb 1991–June 1993)	Jan 1996 (July 1995–Nov 1996)	Nov 1996 (Dec 1995–Sept 1998)	March 1997 (Jan 1996–Oct 1999)
Median (IQR)[b] age at AIDS diagnosis	36.5 (32.1–41.1)	39.7 (35.3–43.9)	39.7 (34.5–44.5)	39.8 (35.1–44.8)	40.1 (35.6–45.2)
Median (IQR)[b] CD4 cell count at AIDS diagnosis	141 (64–273)	90 (35–194)	196 (78–390)	241 (117–439)	268 (130–456)
Number of person-years	685	912	796	1156	992
Deaths number	388	445	109	71	44
% of person-years	57%	49%	14%	6%	4%
Relative hazard[c, e] (95% CI)	1	0.65 (0.55, 0.77)	0.21 (0.15, 0.28)	0.08 (0.06, 0.13)	0.06 (0.03, 0.10)
Relative time[d, e] (95% CI)	1	1.42 (1.24, 1.62)	3.57 (2.77, 4.61)	7.82 (5.86, 10.45)	10.65 (7.66, 14.80)

[a] NA, not applicable since WIHS began in October 1994.
[b] IQR, inter-quartile range.
[c] Results of Cox proportional hazards regression.
[d] Results of Weibull regression under the assumption of proportional survival times.
[e] Adjusted by age at AIDS diagnosis, type of AIDS diagnosis, gender, and CD4 within 1 year prior to AIDS diagnosis.

CI, confidence interval; NA, not applicable.

Reproduced with permission from Lippincott Williams and Wilkins/Wolters Kluwer Health from Schneider MF et al., Patterns of the hazard of death after AIDS through the evolution of antiretroviral therapy: 1984–2004, *AIDS*, Volume 19, Issue 17, pp. 2009–18, Copyright © 2005 Lippincott Williams & Wilkins, Inc.

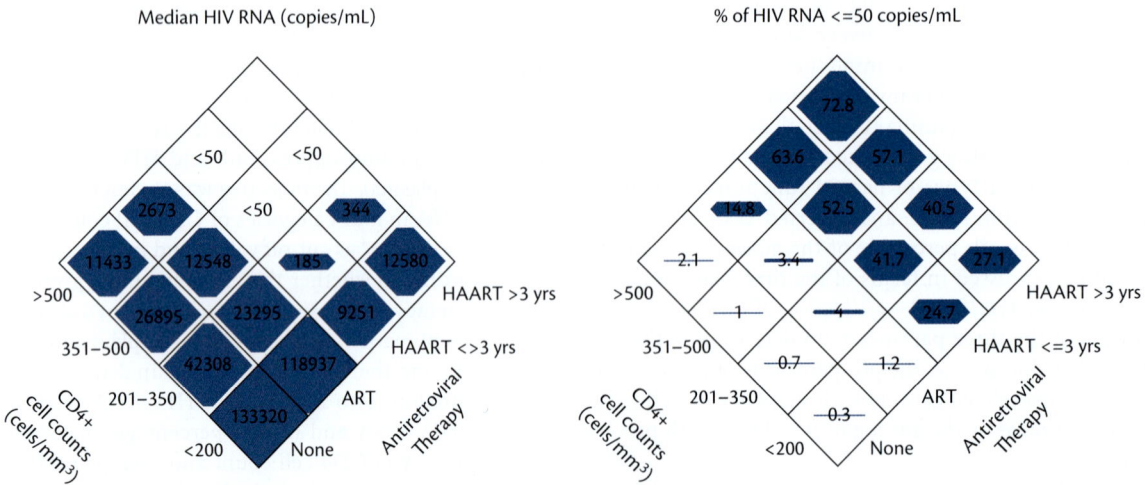

Fig. 5.6.3 Median HIV RNA (copies/mL) and per cent with HIV RNA ≤50 copies/mL in HIV infected individuals according to CD4 cell count and antiretroviral therapy. Multicenter AIDS Cohort Study, 1984–2006.

Methods for the analysis of longitudinal data can be broadly classified in three categories: marginal, conditional, and random effects models. The primary aim of the marginal approach is to combine the multiple cross-sections corresponding to visits so as to provide the most efficient summary of the cross-sectional relationships between exposure and disease. In this approach, the longitudinal component is typically incorporated by including age or time since baseline as a covariate for the regression component of the model. Approaches for the incorporation of the correlation between repeated measurements within individuals include parametric (Jennrich and Schluchter 1986) and non-parametric methods, the latter handling the correlation as a nuisance (Zeger and Liang 1992). The primary aim of conditional models is to regress current outcome on past values of the outcome, and current and previous exposures. Classical Markovian models for binary data were introduced in 1979 (Korn and Whittemore 1979) and applied in 1980 to a study of air pollution and asthma (Whittemore and Korn 1980). Extensions for continuous outcomes were used for the study of the effect of cigarette smoking on respiratory function (Rosner et al. 1985). The primary aim of the random effects models is to allow different individuals to have different intercepts and slopes according to components of variance and to provide direct averages of rates of change across individuals. Fig. 5.6.4 depicts the random effects model whereby the population average line has intercept α and slope β and the line for the ith individual has intercept $\alpha + a_i$ and slope $\beta + b_i$ with the departures being random effects. Methods for random-effects models have been provided for Gaussian outcomes (Laird and Ware 1982), binary outcomes (Kupper and Haseman 1978), and for event-in-person-years outcomes (Breslow 1984).

When data are longitudinal assessments of a biomarker (e.g. pulmonary function, blood pressure, viral load of an infectious agent), linear models for normally distributed biomarkers allowing for both fixed and random effects (i.e. mixed effects) are apt to describe the probabilistic structure of the data. In the simplest case of two groups (i.e. an exposure taking the value zero or one) with linear trends over time, the fixed effects describe the two average lines for each group. That is, for the unexposed group, the average biomarker trajectory is given by $\beta_0 + \beta_1 t$, and for the exposed group, the average biomarker trajectory is given by $(\beta_0 + \beta_0^*) + (\beta_1 + \beta_1^*)t$. In this case, β_0^* represents the fixed effect of exposure on the levels at baseline and β_1^* represents the fixed effects of exposure on the rates of change of the biomarker over time. The random effects allow individuals in each of the two groups to vary randomly around the average lines of the fixed effects (i.e. each individual has his or her own line that varies randomly from the average line as depicted in Fig. 5.6.4) (Laird and Ware 1982).

Joint analysis of survival and longitudinal data

Since the occurrence of an end point in a cohort study typically marks the end of follow-up in the study, the trajectories of participants who develop end points will typically be shorter than those who remain event-free. When subjects leave the study for reasons related to the effects of exposures and/or the progression of disease, the longitudinal data will be subjected to informative dropout. If the biomarkers of interest have greater changes among those who develop end points, a separate analysis of the longitudinal data may yield biased estimates of the rates of change of the biomarkers as they are unduly weighted towards longer and less changing trajectories. A joint model of the time-to-event data and the longitudinal biomarkers data aims to properly describe the relationships between exposures and the two distinct but related outcome processes. For longitudinal data, a joint model must take into account not only the dependence resulting from repeated measurement of the same outcome, but also the association between the different outcomes, all measured on the same individual. A solution to this problem has been provided by the development of shared-parameter models, in which the necessary

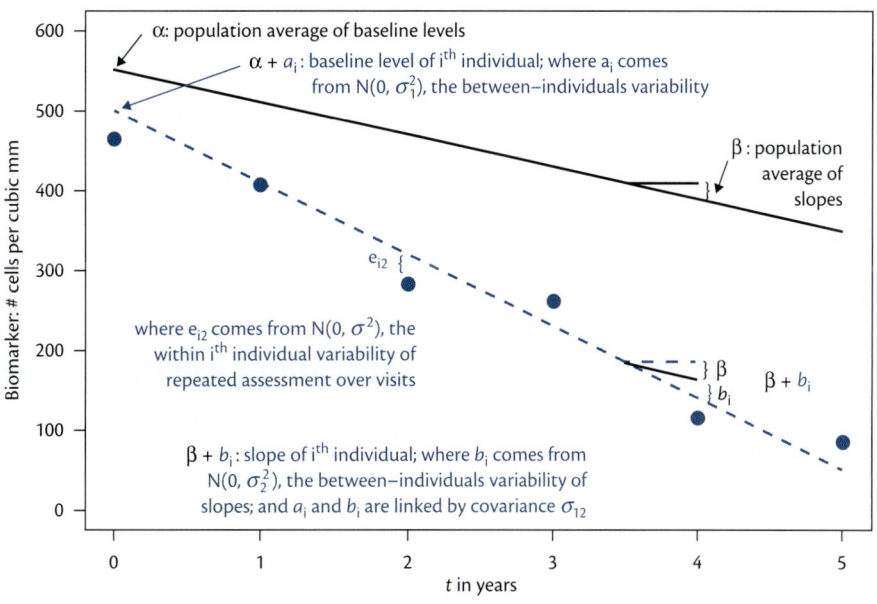

Fig. 5.6.4 Linear model with random intercepts and slopes for the analysis of longitudinal biomarkers data from cohort studies. Population averages in black and random departure of the line of the ith individual in grey.

dependence structure between the two types of data is provided by a vector of shared random effects that links all the measurements on the same individual. Typically the two outcomes (end point and markers) are assumed to be independent given the random effects, which results in a relatively simple factorization of the joint likelihood. Parametric models for the marginal distributions of each outcome, as well as the standard assumption of a multivariate normal distribution for the random effects, provide a complete description of the joint likelihood. Statistical software to fit these models is available in standard statistical software packages such as SAS and STATA.

Validity and biases

External validity

External validity refers to the extent to which the results of a cohort study can be extrapolated or generalized to the reference population. When the cohort is composed of volunteers, representativeness may be limited due to the fact that volunteers tend to be different from the general population.

The representativeness or the lack of representativeness of the cohort in relation to the general population is also determined by the inherent characteristics of the sampling framework. Thus, for instance, even in the case that the members of the Framingham cohort were a representative sample of the population of this small town in New England, it is more than dubious that this population was representative of the general population. A sample from Framingham might be representative of the population of New England, but perhaps not so of the population of the United States. To address this latter issue, the cohorts in studies of cardiovascular epidemiology undertaken in the latest decade in the United States (CARDIA, ARIC, CHS) included participants from several regions of the country, trying to include populations with diverse social and ethnic composition. Even in this case, the representativeness of these cohorts can be questioned if one intends to obtain inferences applicable to the overall population of the continent or the world.

Internal validity

Even when the representativeness of the cohort is dubious, it is possible that the internal comparison between cohort subgroups (e.g. exposed and unexposed) may be valid. In the Precursors Study, for example, it was observed that the standardized mortality ratio was 54 per cent (see Table 5.6.4), which indicates that the mortality in the cohort of the Precursors Study was almost half that of the general US population of the same sex, race, and age. Obviously, this is due to the fact that this cohort is formed by medical students belonging, in general, to higher socioeconomic strata than the average population, which limits the ability to generalize any estimates of the absolute values of incidence or mortality in this cohort. However, it is reasonable to assume that the *relative* comparison of the mortality in smokers and non-smokers in this population (see Table 5.6.3) is valid, or in other words, that the magnitude of the bias that affects the absolute value of mortality given the lack of representativeness of the cohort is proportionally similar in both groups; under these circumstances, even a non-representative cohort in the strict sense of the word, can yield unbiased estimates of the relative risk (or SMR in this case).

In cohort studies, the internal validity is based not only on the comparability of the selection process of exposed and unexposed when the cohort is established, but also on the comparability between the subjects who are lost to follow-up and those who continue under observation in the study. If the participants who are lost to follow-up have a different survival experience compared to those who remain under observation, the overall estimates of survival are biased (i.e. do not accurately represent the survival experience of the population in the original cohort) and special methods are required to avoid the biases due to informative censoring (Robins and Finkelstein 2000; Howe et al. 2011).

Biases

In the evaluation of the possibility of biases due to the losses to follow-up, it is important to consider which types of losses have occurred. The biases due to differential losses to follow-up in a cohort study are conceptually analogous to the *selection biases* that affect case–control or other types of epidemiological studies.

There are other biases than can affect the internal validity of a cohort study. Among the information biases, one type of bias that could affect these types of studies is *surveillance bias*. This bias is present when the persons exposed to a determined risk factor are more carefully monitored or watched over than the persons without that factor. If the disease has a long subclinical phase, this can make the magnitude of the association between that factor and the disease exaggerated. Thus, for example, diabetics are generally subject to periodical check-ups in which blood pressure is taken. Because in the natural history of hypertensive disease there exists a long asymptomatic phase and hypertension is much more likely to be diagnosed in diabetic persons given their periodical clinical assessment, it is possible that part of the strong association that exists between diabetes and hypertension is due in part to a surveillance bias. Even in cohort studies in which information is collected in a systematic form, if the observer knows the history of the participant, he/she can evaluate the presence of the disease in a biased form (*observer bias*). These biases are removed in large part in cohort studies in which a rigorous protocol for collection of information (preferably blinded) and well-trained observers exist.

As in all epidemiological studies, the presence of errors in classification of the participants regarding the presence of the exposure or the occurrence of the disease under study may generate *bias due to misclassification*. When the errors in the determination of disease occurrence are equal in exposed and non-exposed, or when the errors in measurement of the exposure are not differential between diseased and non-diseased, the bias is generally (but not always) conservative; that is, towards the underestimation of the true association (Flegal et al. 1991; Mertens 1993).

Applications and conclusions

Even with the potential limitations regarding internal and external validity discussed in the previous section, the cohort study constitutes the design of reference for all other designs in observational epidemiology. Cohort studies are free from certain types of biases that complicate the interpretation of cross-sectional and case–control studies (Schlesselman 1982), as, for example, recall bias (different recall of the exposure in cases and controls) and cross-sectional bias (when there is a different duration of disease in exposed and unexposed). The cohort design is more powerful for the establishment of the temporal relationship between cause and effect, one of the classical criteria for causality (Hill 1965).

Another advantage of cohort studies is the possibility of studying the occurrence of several events in addition to that initially planned. Thus, for instance, the Framingham cohort has been the basis for the investigation of several hypotheses in addition to those conceived in the initial aims of the study (Kannel 1990) as, for example, the relationship between several factors and cancer (Kreger et al. 1991), senile dementia (Bachman et al. 1993), cognitive function (Elias et al. 1993; Rhoda et al. 2006), osteoporosis (Hannan et al. 1992), hearing defects (Gates et al. 1990), kidney function (Culleton et al. 1999), pulmonary function (Wilk et al. 2009), healthcare preferences, and others. Furthermore, cohort studies are a platform to expand the initial scientific scope of the studies as new knowledge is acquired and new questions arise. For example, when the MACS was established in 1983, not even the causative infectious agent (HIV) had been identified. It was only in 1985, 2 years into the conduct of the study, that HIV was identified and only then baseline samples kept in a repository were tested to find out who at enrolment was infected with HIV. The whole investigation focused on the infectious aetiology as opposed to other potential causes including an environmental exposure or a nutritional aetiology. Another example is provided by the neurological complications of HIV, as at the beginning, there were no neurological manifestations of HIV but, in the course of the epidemic, cases of dementia were recognized among HIV-infected individuals. Thus, a completely new battery of tests and procedures were implemented in the MACS to respond to the challenge of in whom and when cognitive decline ensued in HIV-infected individuals.

Cohort studies have proven to be extremely valuable in many areas of medical research including cardiovascular disease (Dawber 1980), cancer (Doll and Hill 1952; Doll et al. 2005), and infectious diseases (Samet and Muñoz 1998). Cohort data may also be of great use for the development of public policy, such as treatment guidelines. Follow-up of cohorts before interventions are available provides the most appropriate data for the description of the natural history of disease. Furthermore, if these studies continue to collect data after interventions become available, three uses of these pre-intervention data are apparent: (1) as historical controls for assessing and/or confirming the effectiveness of interventions (Jacobson et al. 2002), (2) as a reference point to establish the effectiveness of interventions at the population level once the interventions have been widely implemented (Detels et al. 1998; Muñoz et al. 2000; Schneider et al. 2005), and (3) as a mechanism to identify the subgroups who should receive treatment once an intervention has been proven efficacious in clinical trials (Phair et al. 2002; Cole et al. 2004; Sterne et al. 2009). From the public health perspective, population effectiveness quantifies the reduction of disease achieved by treating the subset of the population that needs therapies the most. In doing so, cohort studies are at the cornerstone of public health and policy (Szklo and Nieto 2012).

References

Ahdieh, L., Gange, S., Greenblatt, R., et al. (2000). Selection by indication of potent antiretroviral therapy use in a large cohort of women infected with human immunodeficiency virus. *American Journal of Epidemiology*, 152, 923–33.

ARIC Investigators (1989). The Atherosclerosis Risk In Communities (ARIC) Study: design and objectives. *American Journal of Epidemiology*, 129, 687–702.

Armstrong, B.K., White, E., and Saracci, R. (1992). *Principles of Exposure Measurement in Epidemiology*. Oxford: Oxford University Press.

ATBC Cancer Prevention Study Group (1994). The effect of vitamin E and beta carotene on the incidence of lung cancer and other cancers in male smokers. *The New England Journal of Medicine*, 330, 1029–35.

Bachman, D.L., Wolf, P.A., Linn, R.T., et al. (1993). Incidence of dementia and probable Alzheimer's disease in a general population: the Framingham Study. *Neurology*, 43, 515–19.

Breslow, N. (1984). Extra-Poisson variation in log-linear models. *Applied Statistics*, 33, 38–44.

Checkley, W., Brower, R.G., and Muñoz, A. (2010). Inference for mutually exclusive competing events through a mixture of generalized gamma distributions. *Epidemiology*, 21, 557–65.

Cole, S.R., Hernán, M.A., Robins, J.M., et al. (2003). Effect of highly active antiretroviral therapy on time to acquired immunodeficiency syndrome or death using marginal structural models. *American Journal of Epidemiology*, 158, 687–94.

Cole, S.R., Li, R., Anastos, K., et al. (2004). Accounting for lead time in cohort studies: evaluating when to initiate HIV therapies. *Statistics in Medicine*, 23, 3351–63.

Cox, C., Chu, H., Schneider, M., et al. (2007). Parametric survival analysis and taxonomy of hazard functions for the generalized gamma distribution. *Statistics in Medicine*, 26, 4352–74.

Cox, C., Schneider, M., and Muñoz, A. (2013). Quantiles of residual survival. In M.L.T. Lee, M. Gail, R. Pfeiffer, G. Satten, T. Cai, and A. Gandy (eds.) *Risk Assessment and Evaluation of Predictions*, pp. 87–106. New York: Springer.

Cox, D. (1972). Regression models and life-tables. *Journal of the Royal Statistical Society*, B34, 187–202.

Cruickshanks, K.J., Schubert, C.R., Snyder, D.J., et al. (2009). Measuring taste impairment in epidemiologic studies: the Beaver Dam Offspring Study. *Annals of the New York Academy of Sciences*, 1170, 543–52.

Culleton, B.F., Larson, M.G., Evans, J.C., et al. (1999). Prevalence and correlates of serum creatinine levels: the Framingham Heart Study. *Archives of Internal Medicine*, 159, 1785–90.

Dawber, T.R. (1980). *The Framingham Study. The Epidemiology of Atherosclerotic Disease*. Cambridge, MA: Harvard University Press.

Detels, R., Muñoz, A., McFarlane, G., et al. (1998). Effectiveness of potent antiretroviral therapy on time to AIDS and death in men with known HIV infection duration. *Journal of the American Medical Association*, 280, 1497–503.

Djoussé, L., Rothman, K.J., Cupples, A., et al. (2002). Serum albumin and risk of myocardial infarction and all-cause mortality in the Framingham Offspring Study. *Circulation*, 106, 2919–24.

Doll, R. and Hill, A.B. (1952). A study of the aetiology of carcinoma of the lung. *British Medical Journal*, 2, 1271–86.

Doll, R., Peto, R., Boreham, J., et al. (2005). Mortality in relation to smoking: 50 years observations on male British doctors. *British Journal of Cancer*, 92(3), 426–9.

Dudley, J., Jin, S., Hoover, D., et al. (1995). The Multicenter AIDS Cohort Study: retention after 9-1/2 years. *American Journal of Epidemiology*, 142, 323–30.

Elias, M.F., Wolf, P.A., D'Agostino, R.B., et al. (1993). Untreated blood pressure level is inversely related to cognitive functioning: the Framingham Study. *American Journal of Epidemiology*, 138, 353–64.

Fine, J.P. and Gray, R.J. (1999). A proportional hazards model for the subdistribution of a competing risk. *Journal of the American Statistical Association*, 94, 496–509.

Flegal, K.M., Keyl, P.M., and Nieto, F.J. (1991). Differential misclassification arising from non-differential errors in exposure measurement. *American Journal of Epidemiology*, 134, 1233–44.

Frank, L. (2000). When an entire country is a cohort. *Science*, 287, 3298–9.

Fried, L.P., Borhani, N.O., Enright, P., et al. (1991). The Cardiovascular Health Study: design and rationale. *Annals of Epidemiology*, 1, 263–79.

Friedman, G.D., Cutter, G.R., Donahue, R.P., et al. (1988). CARDIA: study design, recruitment, and some characteristics of the examined subjects. *Journal of Clinical Epidemiology*, 41, 1105–16.

Furth, S.L., Abraham, A.G., Jerry-Fluker, J., et al. (2011). Metabolic abnormalities, cardiovascular disease risk factors, and GFR decline in children with chronic kidney disease. *Clinical Journal of the American Society of Nephrology*, 6, 2132–40.

Furth, S.L., Cole, S.R., Maxey-Mims, M., et al. (2006). Design and methods of the Chronic Kidney Disease in Children (CKID) prospective cohort study. *Clinical Journal of the American Society of Nephrology*, 1, 1006–15.

Gates, G.A., Cooper, J.C., Kannel, W.B., et al. (1990). Hearing in the elderly: the Framingham cohort, 1983–1985. Part I. Basic audiometric test results. *Ear and Hearing*, 11, 247–56.

Greenland, S. (2000). An introduction to instrumental variables for epidemiologists. *International Journal of Epidemiology*, 29, 722–9.

Greenwood, M. (1926). *The Natural Duration of Cancer*. Reports on Public Health and Medical Subjects, Number 33. London: Her Majesty's Stationery Office.

Hannan, M.T., Felson, D.T., and Anderson, J.J. (1992). Bone mineral density in elderly men and women: results from the Framingham Osteoporosis Study. *Journal of Bone and Mineral Research*, 7, 547–53.

Hernán, M.A., Alonso, A., Logan, R. et al. (2008). Observational studies analyzed like randomized experiments: an application to postmenopausal hormone therapy and coronary heart disease. *Epidemiology*, 19, 766–79, 789–92.

Hernán, M.A., Brumback, B.A., and Robins, J.M. (2001). Marginal structural models to estimate the joint causal effect of nonrandomized treatments. *Journal of the American Statistical Association*, 96, 440–8.

Hernán, M.A., and Robins, J.M. (2009). Letter to the Editor. RE: Early versus deferred antiretroviral therapy for HIV. *The New England Journal of Medicine*, 361, 822–3.

Hill, A.B. (1965). The environment and disease: association or causation? *Proceedings of the Royal Society of Medicine*, 58, 295–300.

Hoffmans, M.D.A.F., Kromhout, D., and Lezenne, C.C. (1988). The impact of body mass index of 78,612 18-year-old Dutch men on 32-year mortality from all causes. *Journal of Clinical Epidemiology*, 41, 749–56.

Hoffmans, M.D.A.F., Kromhout, D., and Lezenne, C.C. (1989). Body mass index at the age of 18 and its effects on 32-year-mortality from coronary heart disease and cancer. A nested case-control study among the entire 1932 Dutch male birth cohort. *Journal of Clinical Epidemiology*, 42, 513–20.

Hole, D.J., Clarke, J.A., Hawthorne, V.M., et al. (1981). Cohort follow-up using computer linkage with routinely collected data. *Journal of Chronic Diseases*, 34, 291–7.

Hoover, D.R., Muñoz, A., He, Y., et al. (1994). The effectiveness of interventions on incubation of AIDS as measured by secular increases within a population. *Statistics in Medicine*, 13, 2127–39.

Hoover, R.N. (2008). The sound and the fury: was it all worthy? *Epidemiology*, 19, 780–2.

Howe, C.J., Cole, S.R., Chmiel, J.S., et al. (2011). Limitation of inverse probability-of-censoring weights in estimating survival in the presence of strong selection bias. *American Journal of Epidemiology*, 173, 569–77.

Illner, A.K., Freisling, H., Boeing, H., et al. (2012). Review and evaluation of innovative technologies for measuring diet in nutritional epidemiology. *International Journal of Epidemiology*, 41, 1187–203.

Jacobson, L.P., Li, R., Phair, J.P., et al. (2002). Evaluation of the effectiveness of highly active antiretroviral therapy in persons with human immunodeficiency virus using biomarker-based equivalence of disease progression. *American Journal of Epidemiology*, 155, 760–70.

Jennrich, R.I. and Schluchter, M.D. (1986). Unbalanced repeated-measure models with structured covariance matrices. *Biometrics*, 42, 805–20.

Kannel, W.B. (1990). Contribution of the Framingham Study to preventive cardiology. *Journal of the American College of Cardiology*, 15, 206–11.

Kannel, W.B., Feinleib, M., McNamara, P.M., et al. (1979). An investigation of coronary heart disease in families: the Framingham offspring study. *American Journal of Epidemiology*, 110, 281–90.

Kaplan, E.L. and Meier, P. (1958). Non-parametric estimation from incomplete observations. *Journal of the American Statistical Association*, 53, 457–81.

Kaslow, R.A., Ostrow, D.G., Detels, R., et al. (1987). The Multicenter AIDS Cohort Study: rationale, organization, and selected characteristics of the participants. *American Journal of Epidemiology*, 126, 310–18.

Kelsey, J.L., Thompson, W.D., and Evans, A.S. (1986). *Methods in Observational Epidemiology*. New York: Oxford University Press.

Kitahata, M.M., Gange, S.J., Abraham, A.G., et al. (2009). Effect of early versus deferred antiretroviral therapy for HIV on survival. *The New England Journal of Medicine*, 360, 1815–26.

Klag, M.J., Ford, D.E., Mead, L.A., et al. (1993). Serum cholesterol in young men and subsequent cardiovascular disease. *The New England Journal of Medicine*, 328, 313–18.

Korn, E.L., Graubard, B.I., and Midthune, D. (1997). Time-to-event analysis of longitudinal follow-up of a survey: choice of the time-scale. *American Journal of Epidemiology*, 145, 72–80.

Korn, E.L. and Whittemore, A.S. (1979). Methods for analyzing panel studies of acute health effects of air pollution. *Biometrics*, 35, 795–802.

Kreger, B.E., Splansky, G.L., and Schatzkin, A. (1991). The cancer experience in the Framingham Heart Study cohort. *Cancer*, 67, 1–6.

Kupper, L.L. and Haseman, J.K. (1978). The use of a correlated binomial model for the analysis of certain toxicological experiments. *Biometrics*, 34, 69–76.

Laird, N.M. and Ware, J.H. (1982). Random-effects models for longitudinal data. *Biometrics*, 38, 963–74.

Lau, B., Gange, S.J., and Moore, R.D. (2007). Interval and clinical cohort studies: epidemiologic issues. *AIDS Human Research and Human Retroviruses*, 23, 769–76.

Li, X., Buechner, J.M., Tarwater, P.M., et al. (2003). A diamond-shaped equiponderant graphical display of the effects of two categorical predictors on continuous outcomes. *The American Statistician*, 57, 193–9.

Manolio, T.A., Weis, B.K., Cowie, C.C., et al. (2012). New models for large prospective studies: is there a better way? *American Journal of Epidemiology*, 175, 859–66.

Mantel, N. and Haenszel, W. (1959). Statistical aspects of the analysis of data from retrospective studies of disease. *Journal of the National Cancer Institute*, 22, 719–48.

Martens, E.P., Pestman, W.R., de Boer, A., et al. (2006). Instrumental variables, applications and limitations. *Epidemiology*, 17, 260–7.

Mellors, J.W., Margolick, J.B., Phair, J.P., et al. (2007). Prediction of CD4 cell decline and predictive value of HIV-1 RNA, CD4 cell count and CD4 cell slope for progression to AIDS and death in untreated HIV-1 infection. *Journal of the American Medical Association*, 297, 2349–50.

Mellors, J.W., Muñoz, A., Giorgi, J.V., et al. (1997). Plasma viral load and CD4+ lymphocytes as prognostic markers of HIV-1 infection. *Annals of Internal Medicine*, 126, 946–54.

Mertens, T.E. (1993). Estimating the effect of misclassification. *The Lancet*, 342, 418–21.

Muñoz, A., Carey, V., Taylor, J.M.G., et al. (1992). Estimation of time since exposure for a prevalent cohort. *Statistics in Medicine*, 11, 939–52.

Muñoz, A., Gange, S.J., and Jacobson, L.P. (2000). Distinguishing efficacy, individual effectiveness and population effectiveness of therapies. *AIDS*, 14, 754–6.

Muñoz, A. and Hoover, D. (1995). Use of cohort studies for evaluating AIDS therapies. In D. Finkelstein and D. Schoenfeld (eds.) *AIDS Clinical Trials*, pp. 423–66. New York: Wiley.

Muñoz, A., Sabin, C.A., and Phillips, A.N. (1997). The incubation period of AIDS. *AIDS*, 11, S69–S76.

Muñoz, A. and Xu, J. (1996). Models for the incubation of AIDS and variations according to age and period. *Statistics in Medicine*, 15, 2459–73.

Newcombe, H.B. (1984). Strategy and art in automated death searches [editorial]. *American Journal of Public Health*, 74, 1302–3.

Nieto, F.J., Peppard, P.E., Young, T., et al. (2012). Sleep-disordered breathing and cancer mortality. Results from the Wisconsin Sleep Cohort study. *American Journal of Respiratory and Critical Care Medicine*, 186, 190–4.

Nieto, F.J., Szklo, M., and Comstock, G.W. (1992). Childhood weight and growth as predictors of adult mortality. *American Journal of Epidemiology*, 136, 201–13.

Oshima, A., Sakagami, F., Hanai, A., et al. (1979). A method of record linkage. *Environmental Health Perspectives*, 32, 221–30.

Peto, R., Pike, M.C., Armitage, P., et al. (1977). Design and analysis of randomized clinical trials requiring prolonged observation of each patient. II: analysis and examples. *British Journal of Cancer*, 351, 1–39.

Phair, J.P., Mellors, J.W., Detels, R., et al. (2002). Virologic and immunologic values allowing safe deferral of antiretroviral therapy. *AIDS*, 16, 2455–9.

Phillips, A.N., Grabar, S., Tassie, J.M., et al. (1999). Use of observational databases to evaluate the effectiveness of antiretroviral therapy for HIV infection: comparison of cohort studies with randomized trials. EUROSIDA, the French Hospital Database on HIV and the Swiss HIV Cohort Study Groups. *AIDS*, 13, 2075–82.

Pierce, C.B., Cox, C., Saland, J.M., et al. (2011). Methods for characterizing differences in longitudinal GFR changes between children with glomerular and non-glomerular chronic kidney disease. *American Journal of Epidemiology*, 174, 604–12.

Prentice, R.L. (2008). Data analysis methods and reliability of analytical epidemiologic research. *Epidemiology*, 19, 785–7.

Putter, H., Fiocco, M., and Geskus, R.B. (2007). Tutorial in biostatistics: competing risks and multi-state models. *Statistics in Medicine*, 26, 2389–430.

Rhoda, A., Massaro, J.M., Wolf, P.A., et al. (2006). Association of white matter hyperintensity volume with decreased cognitive functioning: the Framingham Heart Study. *Archives of Neurology*, 63, 246–50.

Robins, J.M. and Finkelstein, D.M. (2000). Correcting for noncompliance and dependent censoring in an AIDS clinical trial with inverse probability of censoring weighted (IPCW) log-rank tests. *Biometrics*, 56, 779–88.

Robins, J.M., Hernán, M.A., and Brumback, B. (2000). Marginal structural models and causal inference in epidemiology. *Epidemiology*, 11(5), 550–60.

Rosner, B., Muñoz, A., Tager, I.B., et al. (1985). The use of an autoregressive model for the analysis of longitudinal data in epidemiologic studies. *Statistics in Medicine*, 4, 457–67.

Rothman, K.J., Greenland, S., and Lash, T.L. (2008). *Modern Epidemiology* (3rd ed.). Philadelphia, PA: Lippincott Williams & Wilkins.

Samet, J.M. and Muñoz, A. (1998). Evolution of the cohort study. *Epidemiological Reviews*, 20, 1–14.

Schlesselman, J.J. (1982). *Case-Control Studies*. New York: Oxford University Press.

Schneider, M.F., Gange, S.J., Williams, C.M., et al. (2005). Patterns of the hazard of death after AIDS through the evolution of antiretroviral therapy: 1984–2004. *AIDS*, 19, 2009–18.

Smith, M.E. and Newcombe, H.B. (1982). Use of the Canadian Mortality Database for epidemiological follow-up. *Canadian Journal of Public Health*, 73, 39–46.

Stampfer, M.J. (2008). ITT for observational data: worst of both worlds? *Epidemiology*, 19, 783–4.

Sterne, J., May, M., Costagliola, D., et al. (2009). Timing of initiation of antiretroviral therapy in AIDS-free HIV-infected patients: a collaborative analysis of 18 HIV cohort studies. *The Lancet*, 373, 1352–63.

Stuart, E.A. (2010). Matching methods for causal inference: a review and a look forward. *Statistical Science*, 25, 1–21.

Szklo, M. and Nieto, F.J. (2012). *Epidemiology, Beyond the Basics* (3rd ed.). Sudbury, MA: Jones & Bartlett Publishers.

Tager, I.B., Weiss, S.T., Muñoz, A., et al. (1983). Longitudinal study of the effects of maternal smoking on pulmonary function in children. *The New England Journal of Medicine*, 30, 699–703.

Tynes, T., Andersen, A., and Langmark, F. (1992). Incidence of cancer in Norwegian workers potentially exposed to electromagnetic fields. *American Journal of Epidemiology*, 136, 81–8.

Vandenbroucke, J.P. (1991). Prospective or retrospective: what's in a name? *British Medical Journal*, 302, 249–50.

Virtamo, J., Pietinen, P., Huttunen, J.K., et al. (2003). Incidence of cancer and mortality following alpha-tocopherol and beta-carotene supplementation: a post intervention follow-up. *Journal of the American Medical Association*, 290, 476–85.

Wada, N., Jacobson, L.P., Cohen, M., et al. (2013). Cause-specific life expectancies after age 35 for HIV-infected and HIV-negative individuals followed simultaneously in long-term cohort studies: 1984–2008. *American Journal of Epidemiology*, 177(2), 116–25. (Commentary by S. Coughlin on pp. 126–8; Response to invited commentary on pp. 129–30.)

Wada, N., Jacobson, L.P., Cohen, M., et al. (2014). Cause-specific mortality among HIV-infected individuals, by CD4+ cell count at HAART initiation, compared to HIV-uninfected individuals. *AIDS*, 28, 257–65. (Commentary by V. Miller and S. Hodder on pp. 273–4.)

Whittemore, A.S. and Korn, E.L. (1980). Asthma and air pollution in the Los Angeles area. *American Journal of Public Health*, 70, 687–96.

Wilk, J.B., Chen, T., Gottliebe, D.J., et al. (2009). A genome-wide association study of pulmonary function measures in the Framingham Heart Study. *PLoS Genetics*, 5, e1000429.

Willet, W.C., Manson, J.E., and Grodstein, F. (2008). Author's response, part II; re: observational studies analyzed like randomized experiments. *Epidemiology*, 19, 793.

Willett, W.C., Polk, B.F., Underwood, B.A., et al. (1984). Relation of serum vitamins A and E and arytenoids to the risk of cancer. *The New England Journal of Medicine*, 310, 430–4.

Zeger, S.L. and Liang, K.Y. (1992). An overview of methods for the analysis of longitudinal data. *Statistics in Medicine*, 11, 1825–39.

5.7

Methodology of intervention trials in individuals

Lawrence M. Friedman and Eleanor B. Schron

Introduction to methodology of intervention trials in individuals

An intervention trial, or a clinical trial, has been defined in various ways and may be of several kinds. The International Conference on Harmonisation (1996) defines a clinical trial as:

[A]ny investigation in human subjects intended to discover or verify the clinical, pharmacological, and/or other pharmacodynamic effects of an investigational product(s), and/or to identify any adverse reactions to an investigational product(s), and/or to study absorption, distribution, metabolism, and excretion of an investigational product(s) with the object of ascertaining its safety and/or efficacy. (p. 3)

This definition has the advantage of applying to all phases of a clinical trial (I–IV), as traditionally defined (Friedman et al. 2010). The International Conference on Harmonisation definition has the disadvantage of not including trials of non-pharmacological or non-device interventions (e.g. surgical procedures, diet, or exercise). To encompass trials of all kinds of interventions, and given that even many trials of drugs, devices, and biologics do not neatly fit into the usual phases, it makes sense to think about early and late phase trials. Early phase trials generally address questions such as proper dose or intervention approach, physiological response, tolerance, and toxicity in small numbers of participants. The participants are often healthy volunteers, but may also be people with disease who have not responded to other treatments. The early phase trials inform the design and conduct of subsequent late phase trials. This chapter will mainly address issues relating to late phase trials that use outcomes of clinical interest and are large enough to influence clinical practice. Such a clinical trial may be defined as 'a prospective study comparing the effect and value of intervention(s) against a control in human beings' (Friedman et al. 2010, p. 2).

Clinical trials are needed because only rarely is the precise pattern or outcome of a disease or condition known. It is not yet possible to identify all of the genetic and environmental factors that lead to disease progression, recovery, and relapse. Also rare is the treatment that is so overwhelmingly successful that even with a vague understanding of the course of the disease, it is possible to say, in the absence of a control group, that the treatment is obviously beneficial and has few major adverse effects. More often, the treatment, while useful, is less than perfect. Therefore, in order to determine the true balance of potential benefit and harm from a new treatment or intervention, it is necessary to compare people who have received the treatment with those who have not. Ideally, this comparison will be made in an unbiased manner so that, at the end, any difference seen between those treated and those not treated is most likely due to the treatment.

It has been said that except for systematic reviews, randomized clinical trials (RCTs) provide the highest level of evidence and an evidence pyramid has been developed (Pandis 2011). While true, it has also been acknowledged that RCTs do not have a monopoly on evidence and have limitations. Therefore, interpretation of clinical trial results must be viewed in the context of other kinds of clinical research.

This chapter can only cover some of the key issues in clinical trials. For more extensive discussions, the reader is referred to any of several textbooks (Pocock 1983; Meinert 1986; Piantadosi 2005; Hulley et al. 2006; Friedman et al. 2010) as well as journals such as *Clinical Trials* and *Statistics in Medicine*. The International Conference on Harmonisation documents (available at the official website: http://www.ich.org/) should also be consulted.

Ethical issues in intervention studies

The issue of the ethics of conducting clinical trials has generated considerable discussion and debate. Because interventions may be harmful, as well as helpful, and participants are asked to undergo potential hazards, discomforts, and expenditure of time, the question being addressed in any clinical trial must be important. Knowledge of the answer to the question must be worth these possible harms. This is particularly important since many clinical trials are conducted internationally, often with sites in developing countries. The question being addressed by the trial needs to be important in whatever site it is being performed, with the answer of relevance to that site. In addition, many accept that there must be what has been termed 'clinical equipoise' (Freedman 1987). That is, there must be uncertainty as to the usefulness of the intervention among those knowledgeable about the intervention. Individual investigators or doctors may have personal beliefs about the benefits of a new intervention. Those beliefs may prevent those investigators from participating in or entering participants into a clinical trial. The uncertainty in the medical community at large, however, and the importance of the question, are used to justify the conduct of the trial.

Informed consent of all study participants is essential. The nature of informed consent may differ in different countries and cultures, but the concept of individual choice to join or not join a trial must be universal (Nuremberg Code 1949; The National Commission for the Protection of Human Subjects of Biomedical and Behavioral Research 1979; Council for International Organization of Medical Sciences (CIOMS) 2002; World Medical Association 2013).

In addition to informed consent at the beginning of a trial, it is sometimes necessary either to modify the consent and/or to alert participants already in a trial to important new information. This can happen, for example, when an adverse effect that is important, but not so serious that a trial must be stopped, is noted. The Heart and Estrogen/Progestin Replacement Study (HERS), for example, observed an increase in thromboembolic events among the women taking the hormone therapy. This adverse outcome, which was not clearly stated in the consent form as a known risk, was uncommon, but serious. Rather than stop the trial, the investigators informed the participants of the findings and published the information in a 'Letter to the Editor' (Grady et al. 1997). It may also be necessary to re-inform participants when one clinical trial of a similar nature or question or intervention is reported while another is ongoing (US Department of Health and Human Services 2005).

The issue of conducting research in emergency settings or in other situations where informed consent is either not possible or must be delayed until after the intervention is started is a troublesome one. Such research can be extremely important, yet the imperative to only involve those who have understood the risks and volunteered to be subjects is considered by many to be unbreakable. The US Food and Drug Administration provides an exception from the informed consent requirement in limited settings, provided that certain policies are followed (US Food and Drug Administration 2006), as do other regulatory authorities (Interagency Advisory Panel on Research Ethics 2001; European Medicines Agency 2009).

Selection of the comparison group raises ethical issues. Clinical trials may compare a new or unproven intervention against standard or usual therapy, against no therapy, against a placebo, or in combination with standard therapy against placebo in combination with standard or usual therapy. Whenever the comparison is against no therapy or placebo, the ethics of not treating someone in the best possible way are raised. If indeed there is no good treatment, then it is not a problem. But if a treatment known to be beneficial exists, then a control consisting of no therapy or placebo must be carefully justified. This might be possible if there is no appreciable risk to health or discomfort for the time that effective therapy is withheld (Ellenberg and Temple 2000; Temple and Ellenberg 2000). Often, placebo-controlled trials or trials that have no treatment as the control use both the new intervention and the control (placebo or no treatment) in addition to the best-known treatment or standard care. In such trials, the intent of evaluating the new intervention is not to replace an existing one, but to add to it. The ethics of this situation are similar to those where there is no known effective therapy. A more difficult issue exists when a treatment is commonly used in practice, but it is either of unproven benefit or is not the best-known therapy. This latter situation may occur when practitioners do not accept the evidence for the best therapy or there are practical (including financial) barriers to implementing it (Dawson et al. 2009). Regardless of the reason for unproven or non-optimal treatment, some have advocated using usual therapy as a comparison, arguing that it provides the best test as to whether the new intervention is superior to what is being done (Eichacker et al. 2002). Investigators must consider the ethical issues of not using the best-known therapy as a control and the potential difficulties in interpretation of the results if the control group consists of a variety of interventions (some of which might be beneficial and others useless or even harmful).

Even when there is no known effective therapy, the ethics of using a placebo, and indeed of randomization, have been questioned (Hellman and Hellman 1991). The strictures of abiding by a study protocol reduce a clinician's freedom to do what he or she thinks is in the best interest of the patient. The interests of the individual study participant cannot be sacrificed for those of society. Conversely, it has been pointed out that a clinician's views as to the best treatment are often misguided, that hunches about treatment are not particularly helpful, and that trials can be designed to take into account participant needs (Passamani 1991).

This last point is crucial. Trial design needs to incorporate the highest ethical standards. Whenever there is a potential conflict between the needs of the participant and those of the study, the interests of the participant must take precedence.

Study question

Primary and secondary questions

The most important factor in selection of the study design, population, and outcome measures is the question that is posed. Each intervention study has a primary question that is specified in advance and is used to determine the sample size. As implied by its name, in the usual two-armed study there is typically just one primary question. It is a question that is important to answer and feasible to address. By feasibility is meant the ability to identify and enrol adequate numbers of participants, to employ the intervention in an effective and presumably safe manner, to ensure that there is adequate adherence to the protocol, and to measure the outcome accurately and completely. In addition to the primary question, there may be a variety of secondary questions. Secondary questions may be less important or less feasible to answer. There may be fewer outcomes or the outcomes may be harder to measure. They may help the investigator to understand the mechanism of action of the intervention by examining biochemical or physiological processes.

Study outcomes (also termed end points or response variables) may be of several sorts. One way of categorizing them is as either discrete or continuous. That is, they may consist of the occurrence of an event, such as a myocardial infarction or survival from cancer, or of a measurement, such as level of blood pressure or number of CD4 lymphocytes. For late phase trials, these outcomes are usually clinically important. That is, they may be fatal or serious non-fatal events, or other clinically meaningful conditions such as alleviation of pain, increased functional status, or change in an important risk factor such as cigarette smoking.

Often, primary outcomes are composites of two or more kinds of events. For example, in studies seeking to reduce the incidence of coronary heart disease (CHD), the outcome might be a combination of death from CHD and non-fatal myocardial infarction. Sometimes, occurrence of coronary revascularization procedures might be included. The reasons for using a composite outcome are that it adds events, and therefore will reduce the required sample size, and that the individual events all represent the same underlying disease. Interpretation of the results, however, can be challenging, particularly if the outcomes are of different clinical importance. It may be particularly challenging if the outcome perceived to be least important is most common, and dominates the analysis or if the comparisons between groups for the separate components trend in opposite directions (DeMets et al. 2006a).

Regardless of the primary outcome, several features pertain (Friedman et al. 2010). First, it must be specified in advance, written in a protocol. Second, it must be capable of being assessed in the same way in all participants. Third, it must be capable of unbiased assessment. Fourth, it must be assessed in all, or almost all, of the participants. As discussed later in this chapter, significant amounts of missing data can seriously affect the interpretation of the trial.

Biomarkers and surrogate outcomes

Clinical trials can require large numbers of participants, last for years, and be expensive. Trials with a continuous variable as the outcome require fewer participants than do trials with dichotomous outcomes. Also, if the outcome can be assessed before a clinical event has occurred, the study may be shorter in duration. Therefore, there is considerable interest in the use of outcomes that are continuous variables that may not, in of themselves, have clinical relevance, so-called biomarkers or surrogate outcomes. A surrogate outcome is one that substitutes for a clinical outcome; it may not, in itself, be important to the participant. An example is blood pressure. Elevated blood pressure is important primarily because it is a risk factor for stroke and heart disease, not because it is generally symptomatic. It has been shown in numerous clinical trials of both diastolic and isolated systolic hypertension that treatment reduces the occurrence of stroke and heart disease (SHEP Cooperative Research Group 1991; Psaty 1997; Staessen 1997). However, not all methods of reducing blood pressure are without risk or are equally effective in all people. Therefore, trials comparing different antihypertensive agents were conducted (ALLHAT Officers and Coordinators for the ALLHAT Collaborative Research Group 2002; Wing et al. 2003).

Similarly, we know that ventricular arrhythmias are associated with increased risk of sudden cardiac death (Bigger 1984). Therefore, for years it made sense to treat people with antiarrhythmic agents to reduce the occurrence of sudden death in those with heart disease and ventricular arrhythmias. Yet, when clinical trials of these agents were conducted, the results were sometimes unfavourable (The Cardiac Arrhythmia Suppression Trial (CAST) Investigators 1989; Waldo et al. 1995). Ventricular arrhythmia suppression is not a good surrogate for the clinical outcome of sudden cardiac death. Other examples of inadequate surrogate outcomes have been described (Fleming 1994; Fleming and DeMets 1996). Ideal characteristics of a surrogate outcome have been proposed (Prentice 1989) but these are unlikely to be fulfilled. Therefore, judgement as to the usefulness of a surrogate end point must be exercised. For early phase studies that do not attempt to address clinical questions, surrogate outcomes are entirely appropriate. For late phase trials, the kinds of issues that must be considered are the extent of correlation between the surrogate and the clinical event of interest, the ease or difficulty (and cost) of obtaining reliable surrogate outcome measurements on all of the participants, the feasibility of obtaining enough participants to conduct a clinical outcome study, the harm of a possibly wrong answer, and the

urgency of obtaining an answer. With regard to the possibility of an incorrect answer if a surrogate outcome is used, this may be justified in certain circumstances. For example, if the disease or condition is life-threatening, doctors and patients may require less evidence of clinical benefit and may be less concerned with possible harm from an intervention. The results of a trial with a surrogate outcome may be sufficiently persuasive to allow use of the new intervention. Similarly, in truly life-threatening situations, getting an early answer using a surrogate outcome may outweigh the interest in getting a better, but delayed, answer using a clinical outcome. Early trials in AIDS used surrogate outcomes. At that time, unlike the situation today, no proven treatments were available.

Many advocate the use of surrogate outcomes for rare genetic diseases. It may be important to obtain an answer regarding possible treatment efficacy quickly, given that the life expectancy of people with these conditions can be short. Also, it may be too difficult to find and enrol enough patients with the rare condition for a clinical event to serve as the primary outcome. This position is reasonable, but all (researchers, patients, families, regulatory agencies) should understand the limitations inherent in relying on surrogate outcomes.

Efficacy and effectiveness

Intervention studies are sometimes categorized as efficacy trials and effectiveness trials. An efficacy trial attempts to evaluate whether an intervention works under reasonably optimal circumstances. That is, if the active drug is taken as prescribed by essentially all in the intervention group, and if almost no one in the control group takes the active drug, will the drug alter some clinical outcome? An effectiveness trial allows for non-adherence to the assigned treatment; it resembles what is likely to happen in actual clinical practice. Many effectiveness trials may be termed 'practical', 'pragmatic', or 'practice-based' (Tunis et al. 2003). The intervention is typically one that can be easily administered and the outcome is easily measured. Some trials of this sort may have tens of thousands of participants and have therefore been called 'large, simple'. Because these trials are conducted in many sites, often by investigators with limited research experience, there may be less attention paid to quality control of data. It is assumed that randomization and large numbers will lead to balance and provide an unbiased assessment of the effect of the intervention. Unlike effectiveness trials, most efficacy trials will be relatively short, as longer trials would have trouble maintaining optimal adherence (Friedman et al. 2004). The distinction between efficacy and effectiveness trials may sometimes be unclear as it is a continuum.

Trial designs

Parallel design

In a parallel design study, participants are allocated to intervention or control groups and stay in that group until the end of the study. Although the typical study has two groups, one intervention and one control, many have more. Thus, there may be more than one intervention group and even more than one control group. When there are only two groups, the comparison is straightforward. When there are more than two groups, the comparisons can become complicated. For example, if there are three groups, two interventions and a control, there can be up to three main comparisons—each intervention against the control and one intervention against the other. This has implications for the overall type I error and therefore for the sample size. Conservatively, one would correct for the number of comparisons, in this case dividing the α level by 3. Instead of requiring a *p*-value of, for instance, 0.05 for significance, each comparison might require a *p*-value of 0.0167. To maintain adequate power to achieve this level of significance, the sample size will need to increase considerably. The possibly lower event rates in the two intervention groups (assuming benefit from the interventions) will also lead to the need for a larger sample size. If only the comparisons of the two interventions against the control are of interest, there is less penalty, and the three-arm design may be more efficient than initiating two individual studies, as the same control group can be used. Even here, as will be seen in the section on sample size, the control group may need to be larger than if there is only one intervention group.

Factorial design

If there is an interest in studying more than one intervention at a time, a factorial design study may be more efficient than a parallel design. The simplest factorial design is a two-by-two design. This design will have four groups: treatment A plus treatment B, treatment A plus the control for treatment B, control for treatment A plus treatment B, and control for treatment A plus control for treatment B. The last is the only group that has no exposure to either of the interventions being tested. When this design is analysed, there are two primary analyses: the two groups with treatment A versus the two groups without treatment A and the two groups with treatment B versus the two groups without treatment B. It is unlikely that there will be adequate power to look at a single group against another single group. This would usually only happen if both interventions show differences, and are additive. An example where this happened is the Second International Study of Infarct Survival (ISIS-2 (Second International Study of Infarct Survival) Collaborative Group 1988). Factorial designs need not be just two-by-two. There can be more than two groups for each factor, or even more than two factors. In addition to efficiency, an advantage to the factorial design is that one might derive suggestions of differential effect of treatment in the presence or absence of the other treatment. However, this is also a weakness. If these so-called interactions are present, they may make it difficult to discern an overall effect, particularly if they go in opposite directions (Brittain and Wittes 1989). Examples of successful factorial designs, in addition to the ISIS trials (ISIS-2 (Second International Study of Infarct Survival) Collaborative Group 1988; ISIS-3 (Third International Study of Infarct Survival) Collaborative Group 1992), are the Physicians' Health Study (Hennekens and Buring 1989) and the Women's Health Initiative (The Women's Health Initiative Study Group 1998). Interestingly, for a three-arm parallel design, it is generally thought appropriate to adjust the α level for the number of comparisons. For factorial design, however, the usual practice is not to make such an adjustment.

Cross-over design

In the cross-over design, each participant serves as his or her own control (Friedman et al. 2010). In the simplest case, half of the participants would receive intervention followed by control, and the other half the reverse. The major advantage of this design is the smaller sample size. Because each participant is on both intervention and control, half the number of participants are needed. The sample may be even smaller, because the variability is less than in the standard parallel design. There are disadvantages, however. The most obvious one is that the outcomes must be reversible. A cross-over design is not possible if the primary outcome is mortality or a clinical event. A second disadvantage is that there is an assumption of no carry-over effect from one period to the next. If the effect of the intervention persists into the period when the control is being administered, then the apparent effect may be less than the real one. Often, to minimize the likelihood of carry-over, a washout period is inserted between the actual cross-over periods. Unfortunately, it is difficult to prove that a carry-over effect is absent and a participant has truly returned to baseline.

Adaptive designs

Adaptive design can mean different things (Friedman et al. 2010). As indicated in the section on randomization procedures, it can refer to modifications in the randomization scheme in order to ensure balance among baseline characteristics or to efforts to maximize the number of participants in the study group that is trending better. Data monitoring can also lead to adaptive designs in the sense that trials may be ended earlier than scheduled because of greater than expected effects. A third use of the term refers to adjustment of sample size or study duration depending upon the overall event rate (study groups combined) or other factors used in the determination of sample size. Sometimes, a trial is designed to continue until a minimum number of outcome events has occurred (again, study groups combined), sometimes termed 'end point-driven' or 'event-driven' design

Studies of equivalency and non-inferiority

Studies of equivalency address whether the new intervention is similarly beneficial to an agent known to be worthwhile. Studies of non-inferiority look at whether the new intervention is at least as good as the standard therapy. Several factors need to be considered in the design and conduct of these kinds of trials. First, it is sometimes difficult to know that a comparison agent is worthwhile. Not all agents proven to be beneficial at some previous time will be so in all circumstances or to the same degree. Thus, what has been termed the 'constancy assumption' may not hold. This is the case with drugs such as antidepressants (Ellenberg and Temple 2000; Temple and Ellenberg 2000). Therefore, simply showing that a new intervention is no worse than the standard one may not truly prove that the new one is better than placebo. Second, 'equivalency' or 'non-inferiority' must be defined. It is not the same as failing to show a significant difference between the two agents. That could happen simply because the study has an insufficient number of participants, or because participants failed to adhere adequately to the treatments. Because the two agents cannot be shown to be identical (an infinite sample size would be needed), the new intervention must be shown to fall within some predefined boundary that is sufficiently close to the standard therapy. Many agents have been declared beneficial when they are shown superior to control by 20 or 25 per cent. Yet investigators often design non-inferiority trials with margins as large as 50 per cent. Defining how narrow the margin of non-inferiority should be will depend on the risks of inappropriately declaring the new agent to be as effective as the comparator and the feasibility of conducting a trial with a large enough sample size.

Analysis and interpretation of equivalency and non-inferiority trials is somewhat different from interpretation in superiority trials. Failing to show a difference in a superiority trial does not necessarily entitle one to claim non-inferiority to the control or superiority to no treatment. The breadth of the confidence intervals, and the pre-specified hypothesis must be considered. When conducting a non-inferiority trial, therefore, investigators must consider several factors (Friedman et al. 2010; DeMets and Friedman 2012; Piaggio et al. 2012). First, they should use the best available comparator. Using a control that might be less effective than another one, even if that one has been shown to be non-inferior to the best one, can yield misleading results. Second, investigators should select a margin of inferiority that is based on the best estimate of the effect of the comparator. Because the comparator may have been shown beneficial in trials conducted years before in somewhat different populations, conservative estimates are advised. It is essential to take into account what kind of difference between the comparator and the new agent is clinically important to exclude and how big a trial is practical. Third, one must conduct the best possible trial with high adherence and data completeness.

Interventions versus intervention strategies

Not all interventions need to consist of single treatments. Sometimes, intervention strategies may be tested. In some trials of hypertension treatment, a stepped care approach was used (Hypertension Detection and Follow-up Program Cooperative Group 1979; SHEP Cooperative Research Group 1991). The intent was to see if successful lowering of elevated blood pressure resulted in reduction of stroke or heart disease. If the first antihypertensive agent did not adequately lower the blood pressure, another drug was used or added. At the end of this kind of study, it may not be possible to say that a particular drug is responsible for the observed benefits, but rather a strategy. Sometimes, the strategy may incorporate non-pharmacological as well as pharmacological approaches (e.g. diet as well as drug in order to reduce blood pressure).

In trials that compared coronary artery bypass graft surgery against medical therapy (CASS (Coronary Artery Surgery Study) Principal Investigators and their Associates 1983), the comparison was not really coronary artery bypass graft versus medicine. Because, over the follow-up period, a large proportion of the participants in the medical arm received surgery, it was a strategy of early surgery versus surgery later if needed. Yusuf et al. (1994) reported 5-, 7-, and 10-year results from an overview of seven trials of coronary artery bypass graft surgery. At 5 years, 25 per cent of the participants assigned to the medical arms had received surgery; at 7 years 33 per cent had done so; at 10 years, 41 per cent had undergone surgery.

The Atrial Fibrillation Follow-up Investigation of Rhythm Management (AFFIRM) compared two strategies in patients with atrial fibrillation (AFFIRM Investigators 2002). One strategy attempted to correct the heart rhythm, using a variety of drugs; the other strategy was designed to control the heart rate. Despite the goal, only 62.6 per cent of the rhythm control group were actually in normal sinus rhythm at the end of 5 years, while 34.6 per cent of the rate control group were in sinus rhythm at the 5-year point. Nevertheless, the comparison of the two strategies addressed the appropriate and important clinical question of whether trying to convert those with atrial fibrillation to normal sinus rhythm was better than controlling the ventricular heart rate. At the end, the rate control group had mortality that was no worse than the rhythm control group, with fewer adverse effects.

These kinds of studies can be important and valid, but the objectives need to be clearly stated. Otherwise, the study may be criticized for not truly making the intended comparisons.

Quality of life, patient-reported outcomes, and cost-effectiveness

Not all study outcomes need be mortality or major morbidity. Increasingly, clinical trials have evaluated outcomes such as quality of life (QOL) (commonly referred to as health-related quality of life (HRQL), well-being, or patient satisfaction), a related concept called patient-reported outcomes (PROs), or the cost-effectiveness of administering a particular intervention as compared with another, either as primary or secondary outcomes.

There are many definitions of QOL. Essentially, QOL is a multidimensional concept that characterizes an individual's total well-being and includes psychological, social, and physical dimensions (Sartorius 1993). Numerous reliable and valid instruments have been developed for assessing QOL, both for a general population and for specific diseases and conditions (Ferrans and Powers 1985, 1992; Ware and Sherbourne 1992; Ware et al. 1995; McDowell 2006). Conceptual models have been developed that include factors that relate to QOL or HRQL (Wilson and Cleary 1995; Ferrans 1996; Guyatt et al. 2007). The key features may include biological and physiological variables, symptomatology, functional status, social and economic factors, and psychological and spiritual factors. Within each of these broad domains are various individual aspects, the nature of which will depend on the specific condition or disease being studied.

Over the past decade, there has been more attention paid to assessment of PROs. PROs are similar to QOL in that they refer to outcomes that the participant directly reports, without the investigator serving as an intermediary (US Food and Drug Administration 2009). Instruments that assess this seek to determine how the participant feels and what he or she is able to do (Cella et al. 2007; PROMIS® n.d.)

Assessment of QOL and PROs in clinical trials may be particularly valuable in cases when an intervention is not expected to alter survival but may affect a participant's perception of well-being. Cost-effectiveness evaluation may be important when interventions are expensive and where the difference between intervention and control on mortality or major morbidity is small. In a comparison of implantable cardiac defibrillators versus antiarrhythmic drugs, cost-effectiveness was a key secondary outcome. Patients with serious ventricular arrhythmias had a significant reduction in mortality from the defibrillator, but the costs were considerably greater (Larsen et al. 2002). Hlatky et al. (1997) compared quality of life, employment status, and medical care costs during 5 years of follow-up among patients treated with angioplasty or bypass graft surgery. Those in the surgical group had a better quality of life than those in the angioplasty group. Only in a subset of the participants was the cost lower in the angioplasty group.

There are ongoing improvements in methods of measuring and reporting these outcomes. The current status of HRQL (Guyatt et al. 2007), PROs (PROMIS® n.d.), and cost-effectiveness assessment, however, is sufficiently robust that they can be appropriately used as clinical trial end points.

Adverse effects

As noted at the beginning of this chapter, clinical trials are designed to assess the balance of benefits and harms from a new intervention, as compared with another intervention. Incidence of adverse effects comprises an important part of the harms. In the simplest case, adverse effects are simply the reverse of the hoped-for benefit in the primary outcome. But there are many other possible adverse effects, some of which are expected; others are either unexpected or, although expected, are more serious than anticipated. Assessment of adverse effects is complicated by several factors. First, because many are looked at, it may not be easy to say which ones are truly significantly increased and which ones are due to chance. This particularly the case with unexpected adverse effects. Although it is reasonable to demand clear statistical significance when deciding that a new intervention is beneficial, investigators will generally be less statistically rigorous when assessing safety of study participants. Second, serious but uncommon adverse effects may not occur often enough, even in large trials, to be properly evaluated. Furthermore, the trial may not last long enough for some kinds of adverse effects to appear. These might only be discovered after a drug has been marketed, when many people have been on it for a long enough time. Sometimes, only when a drug is being evaluated for another indication, requiring a larger sample size and a longer follow-up, will an adverse effect become clear. This occurred when COX-2 inhibitors, originally developed to treat inflammation due to arthritis, were studied for their effects on colon polyps (Bresalier et al. 2005; Solomon et al. 2006).

Often, adverse effects are uncovered not during a clinical trial, or even before approval of an intervention by a regulatory agency, but only after the intervention has been used for some time by many thousands or millions of people. Because of the time and size limitations of clinical trials in assessment of adverse effects, a combination of approaches is needed. In addition to careful monitoring of trials, post-trial follow-up may be important, as are meta-analyses of trial results, use of databases and observational studies, and the burgeoning field of pharmacogenetics.

Study population

A key part of defining the question to be answered is specifying the kinds of people who will be enrolled in the clinical trial. That is done by means of eligibility criteria, of which there are various sorts (Friedman et al. 2010). First, eligible participants must have the potential to benefit from the intervention. That is, they must have the condition that the intervention might affect. Implicit in this is having the degree of severity at a time in the disease process that is modifiable. Also, any change in the condition must be detectable. That is, it cannot be so mild or slowly progressing that to detect a change, the study must be too large or last too long to be feasible. Second, participants cannot have known

contraindications to the intervention. Third, they should not have other conditions which would make it difficult to detect changes in the condition of interest. An obvious example is someone who has both heart disease and cancer. If a 3-year study of an intervention for the heart disease is planned and the expected survival due to the cancer is less than that, it is unlikely that the person will contribute to answering the question about heart disease. Fourth, if the study requires participants to return for follow-up visits in order to assess the outcome, people who are unlikely to be able to do so should not be enrolled.

Fig. 5.7.1 shows how the study participants are derived from the general population. People are excluded at various stages, based on the entry criteria. The final stage indicates that there are identified eligible participants who are not enrolled. This is because participating is strictly voluntary as a result of informed consent. Many people decide that they would prefer not to enrol in the trial.

The issue of who is and who is not enrolled in a trial raises the concepts of validity, generalization, and representativeness (Friedman et al. 2010). A properly designed and analysed trial will yield a valid result. That is, it will be possible to say whether or not the intervention is different from or better than the control, in the setting of the kinds of participants who were enrolled.

Depending upon how narrow or broad the study sample is will determine how much the results can be generalized. If the eligibility criteria are highly selective, then the results might only apply to that sort of participant. If the eligibility criteria are broad, with many identifiable kinds of participants, then the results would be more broadly applicable. The reasons for performing one or the other type of study will depend partly on how much is known about the mechanism of action of the

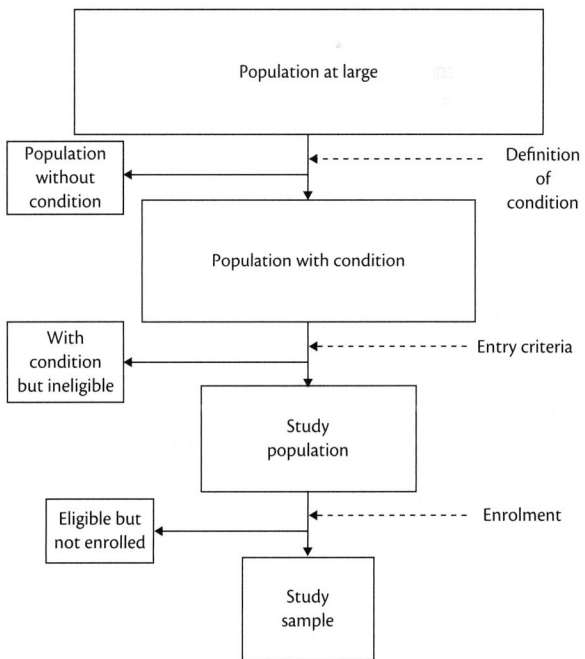

Fig. 5.7.1 Relationship of study sample to study population and population at large (those with and without the condition under study).
Reprinted from Friedman, L.M. et al. (Ed), *Fundamentals of Clinical Trials*, Fourth edition, p. 56, Springer, New York, USA, Copyright © 2010, with kind permission of Springer Science Business Media, http://www.springer.com/978-1-4419-1585-6.

intervention. Congestive heart failure may have several aetiologies. If it is known (or surmised) that the intervention only works in heart failure of a non-ischaemic origin, and therefore only such people are enrolled, then the results of the trial would only apply to people with non-ischaemic heart failure. Another reason for a narrowly defined study population might be concern over the risks versus benefits. For example, the first studies of blood pressure reduction were in people with quite elevated pressures (Veterans Administration Cooperative Study Group on Antihypertensive Agents 1967, 1970; Hypertension Detection and Follow-up Program Cooperative Group 1979). Any benefit from treatment would be easier to find because of the greater likelihood of clinical events in this high-risk group. Also, any adverse effects of the intervention would be more likely to be balanced by the benefits. Not until other trials were conducted in people with lower levels of blood pressure was it possible to say with certainty that such people should be treated. The first studies could not be extrapolated to the lower-risk population.

An example of a trial that successfully enrolled a broad population is the Heart Outcomes Prevention Evaluation Study (The Heart Outcomes Prevention Evaluation Study Investigators 2000). In that trial, an angiotensin-converting enzyme inhibitor was evaluated in over 9000 participants with either known vascular disease or diabetes plus a risk factor for cardiovascular disease, but without evidence of heart failure. Regardless of the type of patient, the intervention was found to be highly effective in reducing mortality and morbidity.

No clinical trial is truly representative of the population with the condition being studied. Investigators conduct trials in people to whom they have ready access, rather than a random sample of the population. Eligibility criteria exclude some people for study design reasons and not because it is thought that they would not respond to the intervention in the same way as those enrolled. Additionally, there are always differences between volunteers and non-volunteers. If one is rigid, the results would be applied only to people who are identical in all relevant ways to those in the trial. The key word is 'relevant'. Judgement must be used in deciding to whom the results reasonably apply. Are the characteristics of the patient whom one wishes to treat different in respects likely to alter the effect of the intervention as observed in the trial?

One also needs to ask if the setting or way in which the trial was conducted were so special as to preclude wide generalization of the results. Particularly for trials of surgical procedures or that require other specialized expertise, the trial investigators are likely to be more experienced than the average clinician who will implement the intervention if proven to be beneficial. Therefore, translation of the results of these trials into general practice must be done cautiously, and with due consideration of the skills of the investigators (Flather et al. 2006).

Randomization

The optimal way of allocating intervention or control to clinical trial participants is by means of randomization. Randomization does not guarantee balance in all factors between the groups, but the chances of balance are increased. Unknown as well as known and measured characteristics are likely to be comparable when there is randomization. A properly performed randomization procedure also reduces the opportunity for investigator bias in the allocation of intervention or control. Finally, randomization guarantees that statistical tests of significance will be valid.

Randomization does not require a one-to-one allocation to intervention or control, only that the allocation be unpredictable. Alternative assignment or assignment based on day of the month (e.g. odd or even) is predictable, and is not equivalent to randomization. Matching on the basis of important characteristics is also not considered randomization. Flipping an unbiased coin to determine whether a participant is assigned to group A or B can be a valid way of randomizing. In practice, however, tables of random numbers or computer-produced random numbers are more often used.

Randomized studies can, by definition, only have a concurrent control group. That is, a historical control study cannot have randomized allocation. This yields another advantage of randomization, namely that the participants are enrolled in the same time period in both the intervention and control groups. Therefore, temporal trends in care or in the nature of the condition being studied are equal in the two groups.

Randomization procedures

Several procedures for randomly assigning treatments to participants have been developed. The simplest are the fixed allocation procedures. If, for example, 20 participants are needed for a study, a coin may be tossed when each participant is entered. However, the likelihood that the number of participants in the two groups will be different (for instance, 12 to 8 or even more extreme) is about 50 per cent. As the sample size increases, the likelihood of such a large uneven split is reduced. If 100 participants are enrolled, the chance of a 60 to 40 split is only about 5 per cent (Friedman et al. 2010).

Blocked randomization is commonly used because of this problem. In blocked randomization, equal numbers of participants in the groups are guaranteed after every several are enrolled. For example, if the block size is 4, and the sample size is 12, then after 4, 8, and 12 participants are enrolled, there would be equal numbers in treatments A and B. This would be accomplished by specifying that each block of four would have two participants assigned to A and two to B. The order within the block of four would be randomized. Thus, it could be ABAB, AABB, ABBA, BABA, and so on. The hazard with this approach is that if the block size is known to the investigator and the treatments are not completely blinded, the last one of the block (and sometimes the last two) can be predicted. Therefore, often, the block size, as well as the order within the block, is random, and the investigator entering the participants is kept ignorant of the block size.

Another advantage of blocked randomization would be if participant entry criteria are modified partway through a trial. In the absence of blocking, even if at the end of entering all participants there are more or less equal numbers in the groups, there may be imbalance in numbers when only some of the participants have been entered. If, because of lagging participant entry, the eligibility criteria are loosened, different sorts of participants may enrol later during recruitment than enrolled earlier. As a result, the characteristics of the participants in group A may differ from those in group B. With blocked randomization, equal numbers are ensured throughout the enrolment period, and changes in entry criteria would not lead to imbalances between the groups in type of participant.

Stratified randomization is a special kind of blocked randomization. Here, the investigator wishes to ensure that there is balance between group A and B, not only in numbers of participants, but in kind of participant. If, despite the randomization process, there is concern that there will be imbalance between groups for one or two key highly prognostic variables, randomization can be stratified on those variables. Thus, within decades of age, for example, blocked randomization would occur. If sex is also a key variable, there would be blocked randomization within each age–sex category. The problem is that even with only two or three characteristics, each one having two or more factors, the number of strata can rapidly increase (Friedman et al. 2010). This can lead to unfilled cells unless many participants are being enrolled. If the sample size is large, randomization will generally lead to good balance, making stratification unnecessary. Therefore, stratified randomization should be done judiciously. If, after the trial is over, it is found that there is a major imbalance in a key factor, an adjusted analysis can be performed. In multicentre trials, randomization is usually done by centre, making the centre one of the important strata. This minimizes the chance that different sorts of participants or different medical practices among centres will confound the results.

In addition to the above fixed randomization procedures, there are various adaptive randomization procedures. In baseline adaptive procedures (also termed adaptive stratification or covariate adaptive randomization), the likelihood of randomization to A or B changes in order to reduce imbalances in selected characteristics. In response adaptive procedures, the likelihood of randomization to one or another group, changes based on the occurrence of study outcomes. Adaptive randomization procedures have not been used as frequently as fixed randomization. For more details of these procedures, see Friedman et al. (2010) and Rosenberger and Lachin (2002).

Blinding

Blinding, sometimes termed masking, is commonly used in clinical trials. In double-blind studies, neither the investigator nor the participant is aware of the intervention assignment. In single-blind trials, only the participant is not informed of the assignment. In unblinded, or open trials, all are aware of the assignment. Ideally, trials should be double-blind. This reduces the opportunity for bias in study management and outcome assessment. For most trials of procedures or lifestyle change, it is not feasible to have anything other than an unblinded design. Here, special efforts to ensure unbiased outcome assessment should be employed.

Sample size

Clinical trials should be designed with adequate power to answer the question being posed. That is, by the end of the trial, there should be enough events or, in the case of a continuous response variable, sufficient precision of the estimate to say with reasonable assurance that the intervention does or does not have the postulated effect. Several factors are considered in the calculation of sample size. For dichotomous outcome studies, these factors are event rate in the control group, expected benefit from the intervention, level of adherence to the intervention, level of adherence to the control regimen, α level, and power. For continuous outcome studies, the mean and variance of the control and intervention groups, plus the level of adherence, α level, and power, would be the relevant variables.

Various references provide formulas for calculating sample size (Lachin 1981; Lakatos 1986; Wu 1988), as does Chapter 8 in Friedman et al. (2010). In essence, the factors that lead to the need for larger sample sizes in the dichotomous outcome situation are lower control group event rate, smaller benefit from the intervention (or lesser difference that one wants to detect), smaller α, greater power to detect a real difference (smaller β), and poorer adherence (or greater cross-over). Alpha is commonly selected to be 0.05 (two-sided); power is typically 0.8–0.9.

As discussed later, the preferred method of analysis is by 'intention to treat'. This means that, in general, participants remain in the randomization group to which they have been assigned, regardless of their future actions or the degree to which they adhere to the assigned regimen. To the extent that those assigned to the intervention group fail to comply with the intervention, for example by not taking their medication (often called 'drop-out'), the expected benefit from the intervention is reduced. Similarly, to the extent that those assigned to the control group begin taking the intervention (often called 'drop-in'), the control group event rate is altered. The net effect of this non-adherence is a narrowing of the difference between the groups. This, in turn, leads to a larger sample size in order to maintain the same power to detect a real difference. Non-adherence can have an appreciable effect on sample size. A correction factor proposed by Lachin multiplies the needed sample size by $1/(1 - R_0 - R_1)^2$, where R_0 is the drop-out rate and R_1 is the drop-in rate. Because the factor is squared, the sample size increases rapidly as soon as the combined non-adherence rate goes over 20 per cent. Even a combined non-adherence rate of only 10 per cent means a sample size increase of almost a quarter. More complicated sample size formulas take into account the fact that most non-adherence is not linear, but is often greater earlier in a trial than later (Lakatos 1986; Wu 1988). Another factor sometimes considered in sample size calculations is the estimated time for an intervention to make the postulated biological changes. For example, if cholesterol-lowering drugs act at least partly by affecting arterial plaque, then the time for that process to occur (so-called lag time) implies a larger sample size (and a longer study).

As noted in the earlier section on study question, studies of equivalency and non-inferiority may require large sample sizes, depending on what is meant by 'equivalence'. Because the sample size formula contains the difference to be detected in the denominator, if zero difference is planned, the sample size would be infinite. Therefore, one typically specifies a difference δ. If the two treatments show differences less than this, they are considered equal, or at least they have differences that are unimportant. Sample size formulas for such studies are available (Blackwelder and Chang 1984). It should be emphasized that, unlike studies where a difference is being sought, an underpowered study of equivalence or non-inferiority will lead to the 'desired' outcome. That is, it will confirm the null hypothesis of no difference. Even more, poor adherence will enhance the likelihood of seeing no difference for either the primary outcome or for adverse effects.

The needed sample size is an estimate because factors such as event rate and adherence are rarely known for certain. It may be prudent, therefore, to be conservative in the assumptions that enter into calculating sample size. The disadvantage of being conservative is that increased size or duration leads to increased cost. Also, entering more people into a trial than is necessary to answer the question may put more people at risk than is appropriate. Just as randomization can be adjusted, based on observed outcomes, so can sample size. This chapter is not the place to discuss adaptive sample size methods in detail. Those interested should see Proschan et al. (2006).

Recruitment of participants

A rule of thumb for all late phase clinical trials is that participant recruitment is always more difficult than expected. With medical records and other ways of identifying study participants now being increasingly available electronically, screening can be conducted more efficiently than in the past. At the same time, however, there is increased attention in many countries to privacy concerns (National Institutes of Health 2003a; Peto et al. 2004; Trevena et al. 2006). Therefore, screening and contact of potential study participants must be conducted with proper consideration of privacy rights. This is particularly important in the age of social media. Investigators are beginning to use social media (e.g. Facebook, Twitter) in research to advertise studies, recruit and maintain contact with study participants, and disseminate findings but care must be taken to protect rights.

It is the uncommon clinical trial that finishes enrolment on schedule and the even rarer one that can do so without major recruitment strategy changes. Because recruitment is difficult, it is best to employ multiple strategies and to plan for back-up strategies in advance and to monitor progress closely throughout the enrolment period. Depending on the nature of the study population, back-up strategies would include adding sources of participants (e.g. clinics, hospital units) or disseminating information about the trial more widely, to both medical personnel and potential participants. If sufficient resources are available, the strategies might include adding staff whose primary responsibilities involve enhancing enrolment or increasing incentives. The latter raises ethical questions if the incentives are inappropriate in amount or kind. Paying so-called finder's fees, for example, would not be acceptable.

If participant enrolment remains slow, several options are available. One approach is to extend the time of enrolment. This has the advantage of not changing other study design factors, but the disadvantages of additional cost and delay in answering the question. A second approach is to accept the smaller sample size. Depending upon how large the shortfall is, the reduced power may not be too great. If the power goes from 90 to 85 per cent or even 80 per cent, that can be acceptable. However, if it falls much below 80 per cent, the study is likely to be underpowered. Some have argued that conducting even underpowered trials is useful, as cumulative meta-analyses of similar trials will yield the answers (Antman et al. 1992), but that approach is not recommended here. A third option is to change the entry criteria, so that more people are eligible. Depending on the original criteria, this might be feasible. However, care needs to be taken to make sure that other design assumptions, such as the expected effect of the intervention and the event rate, are not materially changed. In addition, as noted earlier, a blocked randomization scheme needs to be used to ensure that there is no gross imbalance between groups in participants enrolled before and after the criteria change.

A fourth option is to change the study outcome, so that fewer participants are needed to obtain the same number of events. A study may be originally designed with the outcome of death due to heart disease or non-fatal myocardial infarction. Because of limited resources, other remedies for slow participant accrual may not be feasible. It may be decided that the intervention is as likely to affect other important outcomes, such as need for coronary revascularization, as it is to affect myocardial infarction. Adding that event to the primary outcome would increase the event rate considerably, and allow for an answer with fewer participants. In another example, incidence of hypertension may be the outcome in a study looking at prevention of hypertension with weight loss. Instead of using incidence of hypertension as the primary event, mean blood pressure might be used. Going from a dichotomous outcome study to a study using a continuous variable as the outcome will reduce the needed sample size. These sorts of design changes should not be made lightly. They require considerable thought and review. A change in primary outcome should have no input from anyone or any group that is aware of the interim data by treatment assignment. If, because of these changes, the results are not persuasive to the outside community of practising clinicians, there is little point in undertaking them.

Adherence

As discussed in the earlier section on sample size, adherence (or compliance) on the part of participants is a key factor in clinical trials. It can reduce the power of a trial, and, if truly bad, can make the study results uninterpretable. Therefore, most investigators take steps when planning a study to minimize poor participant adherence. One is to design the study so that the regimen is as simple as possible. For medications, once-daily dosing is preferable to more frequent doses. For lifestyle interventions such as diet or exercise, simpler, more easily remembered programmes are better. Shorter trials have better chances of maintaining good adherence than longer ones. A second method is to select participants who are more likely to adhere. One way is by means of a run-in phase prior to randomization. Unless study participants must be enrolled immediately, for example, at the time of an acute event, a run-in period can be used to determine who adheres to the regimen. Potential participants might be given the active medication for several weeks. At the end of that time, only those who took at least 80 per cent (or some other reasonable amount) of the drug would be enrolled. The participants who could not adhere, even over the short term, would not be randomized. This approach has been successfully used in the Physicians' Health Study (Steering Committee of the Physicians' Health Study Research Group 1989; Glynn et al. 1994) and the Women's Health Study (Cook et al. 2005). Angiotensin-converting enzyme inhibitors may cause cough in some people. Therefore, to minimize the drop-out rate after randomization, studies of angiotensin-converting enzyme inhibitors have used a short run-in period to exclude those who might not tolerate the drug (Davis 1998). Excluding potential non-adherers on the basis of other demographic or psychosocial factors has been done, but the evidence that it successfully separates good from poor adherers is unclear (Dunbar-Jacob 1998). Educating potential participants about the trial is not only good practice from an informed consent standpoint, but is likely to lead to the enrolment of participants who are better adherers. Being unduly persuasive in enrolling participants may improve the recruitment figures, but it can lead to worse adherence statistics. Because the analysis is done on an intention-to-treat basis, the study is more harmed by someone who drops out after enrolment than by someone who does not enrol.

A variety of techniques to maintain good adherence have been tried. Those that appear to be useful are frequent contact and reminders, providing easy transportation and access to attractive facilities, providing continuity of care, providing special medication dispensers, such as calendar packs, and involving family members, particularly when the intervention is lifestyle change (Schron and Czajkowski 2001). Other techniques include attention to aspects of the trial regimen, such as single-dose formulation for medication, intervention schedules made similar to those in clinical practice, and the use of specially trained personnel.

Adherence monitoring has two purposes. One is to be able to advise participants who are not complying with their regimen on how they might improve. The second is to be able to interpret the results of the trial more accurately. The first requires knowledge of individual adherence; the latter only requires knowing how the groups are performing.

Monitoring individual adherence is important, but there is considerable debate about how accurately it can be done, except for interventions that take place entirely in clinics or hospitals (e.g. surgery, vaccine, periodic medication, food feeding studies). Self-reports are simple, but subject to considerable uncertainty. Participants may not remember accurately, and may have a desire to report better adherence than is truly the case. Assessment of activities such as nutritional intake and physical activity are particularly difficult. The use of diaries or other records may help, but still depend on accurate completion by the participant.

For studies involving medication, there are a variety of ways to assess adherence. Pill count is relatively simple, though there are studies that indicate that it over-reports adherence (Rand and Weeks 1998). Participants may forget to return the partially empty containers or may intentionally discard medication that was not taken. Laboratory measures of drug metabolites can be useful, but also may be misleading, as they do not reflect what was ingested long term or show the true pattern of medication usage. Use of special devices that register when a bottle cap is opened has been advocated (Rand and Weeks 1998). Electronic monitoring of this sort can provide a continuous record of dose taking. This probably provides a more accurate measure of adherence, but it is expensive. Even this technique does not prevent a participant from opening the bottle, removing a pill, and then discarding it.

Physiological or biochemical measures that reflect responses to the intervention can be used in some studies. For example, trials of cholesterol-lowering agents which have heart disease as the outcome would periodically measure lipid levels. These are not foolproof indicators of adherence, as individual responses vary, but they are particularly good at demonstrating that on average, after randomization, the intervention group has a different biochemical profile from the control group. One problem with using these sorts of measures as markers of individual adherence is that they may unmask the group to which a participant has been assigned.

Unless one is willing to go to considerable lengths and spend considerable resources, the simple measures of adherence are probably adequate for most purposes. They will certainly indicate gross problems overall, and allow the investigator to conclude, with reasonable assurance, that the intervention was or was not administered satisfactorily, and that there is or is not a difference between the groups in intermediate response variables or biomarkers. However, there is no single gold standard for measuring adherence. Furthermore in order to have a valid assessment of adherence, the use of more than one measure is recommended (DiMatteo 2004).

Data and safety monitoring

Data and safety monitoring is an essential part of any clinical trial. If the data become persuasive before the scheduled end of the trial, or if unexpected adverse events occur, the investigator is obligated either to stop the trial or to make necessary design changes. For many trials, the monitoring function is undertaken by a person or group external to the study investigator structure. For masked studies, this helps to keep the investigator blinded. But more importantly, for all trials, an outside group is less likely to have a bias and less likely to want the study to continue inappropriately because of financial or other reasons. The primary function of this group is to maximize participant safety. Secondarily, it helps ensure the integrity of the trial.

In the process of data and safety monitoring, several kinds of recommendations may be made. First, and most common, would be a recommendation to continue the trial without any change. Second would be a recommendation to modify the protocol in some way. Examples might be changing the participant entry criteria, changing the informed consent to take into consideration important new information, changing the frequency of certain tests to better ensure safety, or even dropping from the study certain types of participants for whom it may no longer be appropriate. Third, there might be reason to recommend extending the trial. This could occur if the participant accrual rate is slower than expected or if the overall event rate is much lower than expected. Fourth, there might be a recommendation to stop the trial early.

Data monitoring techniques

Regular data monitoring must be performed for ethical reasons. However, this carries a penalty:

> If the null hypothesis, H_0, of no difference between two groups is, in fact, true, and repeated tests of that hypothesis are made at the same level of significance using accumulating data, the probability that, at some time, the test will be called significant by chance alone will be larger than the significance level selected. That is, the rate of incorrectly rejecting the null hypothesis will be larger than what is normally considered to be acceptable. (Friedman et al. 2010, p. 299)

Therefore a variety of stopping boundaries or guidelines has been developed that maintain the overall prespecified α level. Biostatistics references can be consulted for the details of these methods. In essence, the methods fall into three categories: classical sequential, group sequential, and curtailed sampling. In the classical sequential approach (Whitehead 1997), there is no fixed sample size. Participant enrolment and the study end when boundaries for benefit or harm are exceeded. A theoretical advantage of the classical sequential approach is that fewer participants might need to be enrolled than in a fixed sample size design. This design requires study outcomes to occur relatively soon after enrolment, however, so that decisions about enrolment of new participants can be made. As a result, it may have limited usefulness.

The most commonly used monitoring techniques are the group sequential methods. Here, after a group of participants have been enrolled, or after a length of time, the data are examined. In order to conserve the overall α level, the study is not stopped early even if the nominal p-value (e.g. 0.05) is exceeded. More extreme p-values are required for early stopping. An example of such boundaries is that developed by O'Brien and Fleming (1979), which calls for very extreme results early in a study which gradually become less extreme towards the end. If the study goes to the expected end, the significance value is essentially what it would be without any interim monitoring. An approach proposed by Haybittle (1971) and Peto et al. (1976) uses a constant extreme value throughout the trial, with the usual p-value for significance at the end. Both of these techniques allow the final significance value to be what would be used without monitoring because of the low likelihood of stopping early, given the extreme nature of the boundaries. A modification of these techniques uses what is termed an α spending function (Lan and DeMets 1989). This technique allows for more flexible selection of the times when the data will be monitored.

Another modification of the group sequential methods employs asymmetric boundaries. For many trials, even those that are not one-sided tests of the hypothesis, it would be inappropriate to continue a trial until the intervention is proven harmful, using the usual p-value of 0.05. Therefore, instead of having the monitoring boundary for harm symmetric to the one for benefit, a less extreme monitoring boundary can be developed (DeMets and Ware 1982). Thus, if the one for benefit maintains the overall α at 0.05, the one for harm might maintain it at 0.1, or even less extreme. Even with one-sided tests of hypothesis, an advisory boundary for harm can be implemented, as was the case in the Cardiac Arrhythmia Suppression Trial (Pawitan and Hallstrom 1990).

Curtailed sampling addresses the probability of seeing a significant result if the trial were to continue to its end, given the data at the current time (that is, part way through the trial) (Lan and Wittes 1988). For example, if there is a strongly positive trend with three-quarters of the expected data in hand, one can examine the probabilities of having a statistically significant outcome under various assumptions regarding future data. A reasonable assumption might be that the control group event rate will continue, more or less, as it has been and that the null hypothesis is true. If, under those conditions, the outcome is still significant, there might be reason to stop the study. Conversely, if there is little or no benefit (or a trend towards harm) from the intervention, one might look at how large a benefit would be required from now on to see a significant benefit at the end. If there is little likelihood of that happening, the study might be stopped because continuation would be futile.

Descriptions of stopping decisions in clinical trials have been published (DeMets et al. 2006b). These include stopping early for overwhelming benefit, clear harm, or futility, or if evidence emerges that the study question has been answered elsewhere. A decision to stop a trial early is irrevocable; therefore, such a decision must be made carefully. Whenever a recommendation is made to stop a study early, factors other than whether or not the monitoring boundaries are crossed need to be considered (Friedman et al. 2010). Might the results be due to imbalance in baseline characteristics or to bias in ascertainment of the outcome? Might poor adherence or differential use of concomitant therapy be important? What might be the impact of outcomes other than the primary one on the interpretation of the conclusions? Are there major unexpected adverse effects that need to be considered? How might other ongoing research affect the results? Will the results be persuasive to others? The issues are not just statistical in nature. If they were, there would be little need for a monitoring committee. Instead, an algorithm could be created which would make the decision. But because the decisions depend on a complex interaction of statistics, understanding of the biological mechanism of action of the intervention, knowledge of other research findings, and judgement as to how the results will be received and interpreted, decisions to recommend continuation or stopping are rarely easy and often second-guessed.

Analysis issues

Whom to include

A purpose of assigning intervention or control by means of randomization is to ensure, as far as possible, that there is balance between the groups on both measured and unmeasured factors. Anything that alters that balance, such as removing from analysis some data from some participants, can induce bias. The reason is that it may be difficult to prove that the cause for the exclusion is unrelated to either a key baseline factor or to the intervention or control. Therefore, the general guideline for analysis is called 'intention to treat'. That is, once randomization has taken place, the data from all participants should be included and counted in the group to which they are assigned. This is in contrast to what has been termed 'per-protocol analysis'. Rather than 'per protocol', the phrase 'on treatment analysis' more accurately reflects what is done.

There are several reasons why one would want to withdraw participants or data from the analysis. First, it may be discovered, after enrolment, that a participant is not truly eligible for the trial. Therefore, that person would not contribute meaningfully to answering the question and, in fact, might confuse the issue by providing incorrect information. Also importantly, it might be hazardous for that person to be taking the intervention. Withdrawing such people from the study and the analysis might seem to be straightforward, but often it is not. If the decision that a person is ineligible is made after adverse effects or a clinical event has occurred, it might be viewed as an effort to manipulate the data. Eligibility criteria are commonly subjective and even in blinded trials there may be clues regarding the group to which the participant was assigned. Therefore, if participants are withdrawn from the trial because they are found to be ineligible, it must be done as soon as possible, before any events have occurred or follow-up measurements performed, and without knowledge of the treatment group. If that does not happen, then the best policy is to leave the participant in the study and analyse the data as if he or she is eligible. If it is possibly dangerous for the participant to be on the intervention, that can be discontinued without removing the person from the trial. If the percentage of ineligible people is small, that should not unduly affect the conclusions. If the percentage is large, such that the study integrity might be affected, then there is clearly a larger problem with the conduct of the trial.

A second reason for withdrawal of participants after randomization is poor adherence. As discussed in the sample size section, incomplete adherence to the protocol is best handled by increasing the number of people in the trial. Sometimes, however, it is decided to remove non-adherent participants from the analysis. The argument for doing this is that if they have not taken the intervention, there is no way that they can provide information as to its usefulness. The counter-argument is that lack of adherence may be a reflection of not being able to tolerate one or another of the treatments. Therefore, withdrawing poor adherers leads to an underestimate of the adverse effects. It also biases the analysis because those removed from one group are likely to be different from those removed from the other group. There have been attempts to adjust for non-adherence, but these approaches are questionable.

The classic example of how withdrawing poor adherers from analysis can lead to strange results is from the Coronary Drug Project, a trial of lipid lowering in heart disease patients. As expected, those assigned to the active medication group who did not take it fared worse than those who did. But those assigned to placebo who did not take the placebo also fared worse than those who did (Coronary Drug Project Research Group 1980). This outcome could not be accounted for by measured differences between the adherers and non-adherers. Therefore, unknown confounding factors must have been present, as the difference is not attributable to an inert substance. It is best to include the data from all participants, regardless of level of adherence, in the analysis. If, despite the best efforts of the investigator, adherence is so poor as to compromise the integrity of the trial, then that itself says something about the usefulness of the intervention.

Poor quality or, in the extreme case, missing data is a third reason for withdrawing participants from analysis. Every effort must be made to minimize these. If participants are lost to follow-up, or do not return for key outcome measurements, the data will be missing. To the extent that this constitutes more than a few per cent of the total data, the study is severely impaired. The reason, again, is that there is no assurance that the missing data are independent of the treatment. If participants do not return to the clinic because one of the treatments makes them feel unwell, the data in that group will only be from those who are healthier or better able to tolerate the treatment.

Various statistical methods have been proposed to take into account missing data, but none is perfect (Espeland et al. 1992; Proschan et al. 2001). In general, they make assumptions or a range of assumptions about the missing data (sensitivity analysis). They may use prior data from the individual or some average from the group to which that individual is assigned to impute the most likely values for the missing data. One assumption might be that all participants missing in one group had the most unfavourable results while all the other groups had the most favourable results, and vice versa. These techniques can be useful, but as with simply censoring missing data, are limited if the missing data are strongly related to treatment and there are large amounts of missing data. One hopes that regardless of the assumptions made, the overall conclusions are unchanged. If the amount of missing data is so great that, under reasonable assumptions, the conclusions vary, the investigator must question the validity of the study.

The same factors apply to poor-quality data or outliers. Ideally all analyses should be performed with and without including the outliers, as there may be important reasons for the apparently strange data that should not be ignored. One practice that is not encouraged is substituting data such as prior measurements from an individual for data that are thought to be incorrect or outlying.

Adjustment procedures

Despite best efforts, study groups may turn out to have imbalances in important factors at baseline. In such cases, it is tempting to adjust for these imbalances. Unless the imbalance is large and the factor is highly correlated with the outcome, however, adjustment is unlikely to make a major difference. Simply showing that there is a statistically significant difference in a baseline covariate is not sufficient reason to adjust on that factor. Conversely, large and potentially important differences may not be statistically significant because of small numbers. Furthermore, there may be several covariates that are imbalanced in a similar direction. Individually, they may not be important, but in the aggregate, they may lead to enough of an imbalance that adjustment is useful. In summary, adjustment for baseline imbalances is legitimate, and should be explored if there are apparent differences. Mostly, this is unnecessary. Certainly, if adjustment converts a non-significant result to a significant one, it needs to be interpreted cautiously.

Adjustment for post-randomization variables is strongly discouraged. Level of adherence is one example of such a variable. Others might be biomarkers or similar interim measures of the effect of the intervention, as well as concomitant therapy. Because such variables are, or may be, related to the intervention, unlike the baseline factors, adjustment for them can result in misleading interpretations. Response to an intervention can indicate better prognosis, even in the absence of the intervention (Coronary Drug Project Research Group 1980; Anderson et al. 1983). Adjustment on such a variable can make an intervention appear beneficial when it is not.

Subgroup analyses

In every clinical trial it is tempting to look at the effects of the intervention in subgroups of participants. This is particularly the case with trials that show no significant difference overall. Even without overall benefit, there might be some subsets that indeed benefit. The problem is that with enough creativity, one can almost always find a group that benefits (and a group that is harmed) from the intervention. Even in trials that have significant overall differences, there is a desire to find the types of participants who benefit the most.

It is generally the case that qualitative interactions are uncommon (Peto 1995). That is, an intervention is unlikely to be beneficial in one subgroup and harmful in another. Conversely, it is quite plausible that there are differential relative effects. Some kinds of people are indeed likely to be helped more than other kinds of people. The problem is that unless the subgroups of interest are specified in advance, it is likely that most of the observed differences are due to chance. The best way of confirming that subgroup differences are real is to examine an independent dataset, usually from another trial of the same question. Somewhat weaker is using independent data from the same trial. This can be done if, during data monitoring, a possible subgroup difference is identified. The data accrued during the remaining period of the trial on participants who have not yet had the event can be confirmatory. Other approaches, such as looking at trends in subgroups defined by continuous variables, especially where there is biological plausibility, can also be used.

As noted, with enough imagination, apparent subgroup differences can be uncovered. 'Fishing', or 'data-dredging' is a natural activity, as unexpected subgroup findings can be important sources of new information and new hypotheses. As opposed to raising new questions, however, conclusions should almost never be drawn from subgroups that are not prespecified. The examples of differences based on signs of the zodiac (ISIS-2 (Second International Study of Infarct Survival) Collaborative Group 1988) or similar characteristics are cautionary.

Meta-analyses

A separate chapter in this text is devoted to meta-analyses (Chapter 5.15). Therefore, only a brief summary is provided here. Meta-analyses can be important ways of synthesizing data. They enable researchers to incorporate multiple studies of the same question. Because of the added numbers of participants, they provide better estimates of intervention effects in subgroups. They allow one to put together several small studies to see if a larger study should be conducted to address a question more clearly. They do have potential limitations, however. Most important is the effort expended in collecting all of the relevant studies and the judgement that must go into selection of the studies to be combined. Studies that show benefit from an intervention are more likely to be published (Dickersin et al. 1987). Therefore, if meta-analyses are not done carefully with clear criteria, biases can be introduced. Another limitation is that only some outcomes can be used. Typically, mortality or major morbidity is the outcome of interest. When deciding on whether or not an intervention is useful, other outcomes, such as adverse effects and quality of life, may be important, but are rarely incorporated into published meta-analyses. The ability to perform meta-analyses easily may lead to several inadequately powered studies yielding an overall statistically significant p-value. Examples of probably misleading conclusions from these meta-analyses have been observed, once the single large trial was conducted (LeLorier et al. 1997). Any discouragement of the conduct of properly sized trials because of meta-analyses is unfortunate.

Reporting and interpretation

Several guidelines to the proper reporting of clinical trial results have been published and the Consolidated Standards of Reporting Trials (CONSORT) Statement should be consulted for updated guidelines (CONSORT Group 2010). In addition, many journals require that the trial be registered in any of a number of formal registries (De Angelis et al. 2004). In essence, the reporting guidelines call for objective recording of all pertinent aspects. It is recognized that space limitations restrict the amount of information that can be included in a publication. The advent of journal websites, however, allows for the dissemination of supplementary material.

Two related reporting issues concern authorship. Both 'guest authorship' (listing as authors those who did not contribute) and 'ghost authorship' (failure to credit those who actually wrote the paper) are unacceptable.

An ongoing issue is the development of open access online journals. This issue includes not just public access to the journal but access to the data. It should be noted that studies funded by the National Institutes of Health require data sharing plans (National Institutes of Health 2003).

Conclusion

It is not easy to conduct well-designed clinical trials, and there are ethical issues that must be considered. Nevertheless, there is no substitute for good clinical trials in providing important information for clinical use and public health about the possible benefits of interventions. As a result of the development of clinical trial technologies over the past several decades, more clinical decisions are evidence based. Improvements in trial design and analysis are continuing and will have further impacts, as will increasing knowledge about genetics, better understanding of disease aetiologies and processes, and pharmacology.

Acknowledgments

Text extracts from Friedman, L.M. et al. (Ed), *Fundamentals of Clinical Trials*, Fourth edition, Springer, New York, USA, Copyright © 2010, reproduced with kind permission of Springer Science Business Media, http://www.springer.com/978-1-4419-1585-6.

References

ALLHAT Officers and Coordinators for the ALLHAT Collaborative Research Group (2002). Major outcomes in high-risk hypertensive patients randomized to angiotensin-converting enzyme inhibitor or calcium channel blocker vs diuretic: The Antihypertensive and Lipid-Lowering Treatment to Prevent Heart Attack Trial (ALLHAT). *JAMA*, 288(23), 2981–97.

Anderson, J.R., Cain, K.C., and Gelber, R.D. (1983). Analysis of survival by tumor response. *Journal of Clinical Oncology*, 1(11), 710–19.

Antman, E.M., Lau, J., Kupelnick, B., et al. (1992). A comparison of results of meta-analyses of randomized control trials and recommendations of clinical experts. Treatments for myocardial infarction. *JAMA*, 268(2), 240–8.

Bigger, J.T. (1984). Identification of patients at high risk for sudden cardiac death. *The American Journal of Cardiology*, 54(9), 3–8D.

Blackwelder, W.C. and Chang, M.A. (1984). Sample size graphs for 'proving the null hypothesis'. *Controlled Clinical Trials*, 5(2), 97–105.

Bresalier, R.S., Sandler, R.S., Quan, H., et al., and the Adenomatous Polyp Prevention on Vioxx (APPROVe) Trial Investigators (2005). Cardiovascular events associated with rofecoxib in a colorectal adenoma chemoprevention trial. *The New England Journal of Medicine*, 352(11), 1092–102.

Brittain, E. and Wittes, J. (1989). Factorial designs in clinical trials: the effects of non-compliance and subadditivity. *Statistics in Medicine*, 8(2), 161–71.

CASS (Coronary Artery Surgery Study) Principal Investigators and their Associates (1983). Coronary artery surgery study (CASS): a randomized trial of coronary artery bypass surgery. Survival data. *Circulation*, 68, 939–50.

Cella, D. Yount, S., Rothrock, N., et al. on behalf of the PROMIS Cooperative Group (2007). The Patient-Reported Outcomes Measurement Information System (PROMIS): progress of an NIH Roadmap cooperative group during its first two years. *Medical Care*, 45, S3–S11.

CONSORT Group (2010). *The CONSORT Statement*. [Online] Available at: http://www.consort-statement.org.

Cook, N.R., Lee, I.M., Gaziano, J.M., et al. (2005). Low-dose aspirin in the primary prevention of cancer: the women's health study: a randomized controlled trial. *JAMA*, 294(1), 47–55.

Coronary Drug Project Research Group (1980). Influence of adherence to treatment and response of cholesterol on mortality in the coronary drug project. *The New England Journal of Medicine*, 303(18), 1038–41.

Council for International Organization of Medical Sciences (CIOMS) (2002). *International Ethical Guidelines for Biomedical Research Involving Human Subjects*. Geneva: World Health Organization.

Available at: http://www.cioms.ch/publications/layout_guide2002.pdf.

Davis, C.E. (1998). Prerandomization compliance screening: a statistician's views. In S.A. Shumaker, E.B. Schon, J.K. Ockene, and W.L. McBeem (eds.) *The Handbook of Health Behavior Change* (2nd ed.), pp. 485–90. New York: Springer.

Dawson, L., Zarin D.A., Emanuel E.J., et al. (2009). Considering usual medical care in clinical trial design. *PLoS Medicine*, 6(9), e1000111.

De Angelis, C.D., Drazen, J.M., Frizelle, F.A., et al. (2004). Clinical trial registration: a statement from the International Committee of Medical Journal Editors. *JAMA*, 292, 1363–4.

DeMets, D.L. and Friedman, L. (2012). Some thoughts on challenges for noninferiority study designs. *Drug Information Journal*, 46(4), 420–7.

DeMets, D.L., Furberg, C.D., and Friedman, L.M. (2006a). Lessons learned. In D.L. De Mets, C.D. Furberg, and L.M. Friedman (eds.) *Data Monitoring in Clinical Trials: A Case Studies Approach*, pp. 14–38. New York: Springer.

DeMets, D.L., Furberg, C.D., and Friedman, L.M. (2006b). *Data Monitoring in Clinical Trials: A Case Studies Approach*. New York: Springer.

DeMets, D.L. and Ware, J.H. (1982). Asymmetric group sequential boundaries for monitoring clinical trials. *Biometrika*, 69, 661–3.

Dickersin, K., Chan, S., Chalmers, T.C. et al. (1987). Publication bias and clinical trials. *Controlled Clinical Trials*, 8(4), 343–53.

DiMatteo, M.R. (2004). Variations in patients' adherence to medical recommendations: a quantitative review of 50 years of research. *Medical Care*, 42(3), 200–9.

Dunbar-Jacob, J. (1998). Predictors of patient adherence: patient characteristics. In S.A. Shumaker, E.B. Schon, J.K. Ockene, and W.L. McBeem (eds.) *The Handbook of Health Behavior Change* (2nd ed.), pp. 491–511. New York: Springer.

Eichacker, P.Q., Gersteinberger, E.P., Banks, S.M., et al. (2002). Meta-analysis of acute lung injury and acute respiratory distress syndrome trials testing low tidal volumes. *American Journal of Respiratory and Critical Care Medicine*, 166(11), 1510–14.

Ellenberg, S.S. and Temple, R. (2000). Placebo-controlled trials and active-control trials in the evaluation of new treatments. Part 2: practical issues and specific cases. *Annals of Internal Medicine*, 133(6), 464–70.

Espeland, M.A., Byington, R.P., Hire, D., et al. (1992). Analysis strategies for serial multivariate ultrasonographic data that are incomplete. *Statistics in Medicine*, 11(8), 1041–56.

European Medicines Agency (2009). *ICH Topic E6 (R1). Guidance for Good Clinical Practice*. [Online] Available at: http://www.ema.europa.eu/docs/en_GB/document_library/Scientific_guideline/2009/09/WC500002874.pdf.

Ferrans, C.E. (1996). Development of a conceptual model of quality of life. *Scholarly Inquiry for Nursing Practice*, 10(3), 293–304.

Ferrans, C.E. and Powers, M.J. (1985). Quality of life index: development and psychometric properties. *Advances in Nursing Science*, 8(1), 15–24.

Ferrans, C.E. and Powers, M.J. (1992). Psychometric assessment of the quality of life index. *Research in Nursing & Health*, 15(1), 29–38.

Flather, M., Deahunty, N., and Collinson, J. (2006). Generalizing results of randomized trials to clinical practice: reliability and cautions. *Clinical Trials*, 3(6), 508–12.

Fleming, T.R. (1994). Surrogate markers in AIDS and cancer trials. *Statistics in Medicine*, 13, 1423–35.

Fleming, T.R. and DeMets, D.L. (1996). Surrogate end points in clinical trials: are we being misled? *Annals of Internal Medicine*, 125(7), 605–13.

Freedman, B. (1987). Equipoise and the ethics of clinical research. *The New England Journal of Medicine*, 317, 141–5.

Friedman, L.M., Furberg, C.D., and DeMets, D.L. (2010). *Fundamentals of Clinical Trials* (4th ed.). New York: Springer.

Friedman, L.M., Simons-Morton, D.G., and Cutler, J.A. (2004). Comparative features of primordial, primary, and secondary prevention trials. In J.E. Manson, J.E. Buring, P.M. Ridker, and J.M. Gaziano (eds.) *Clinical Trials in Cardiovascular Disease* (2nd ed.), pp. 14–21. Philadelphia, PA: Elsevier Saunders.

Glynn, R.J., Buring, J.E., Manson, J.E., et al. (1994). Adherence to aspirin in the prevention of myocardial infarction. The physicians' health study. *Archives of Internal Medicine*, 154(23), 2649–57.

Grady, D., Hulley, S.B., and Furberg, C. (1997). Venous thromboembolic events associated with hormone replacement therapy. *JAMA*, 278(6), 477.

Guyatt, G.H., Ferrans, C.E., Halyard, M.Y., et al. (2007). Exploration of the value of health-related quality-of-life information from clinical research and into clinical practice. *Mayo Clinic Proceedings*, 82(10), 1229–39.

Haybittle, J.L. (1971). Repeated assessment of results in clinical trials of cancer treatment. *The British Journal of Radiology*, 44(526), 793–7.

Hellman, S. and Hellman, D.S. (1991). Of mice but not men. Problems of the randomized clinical trial. *The New England Journal of Medicine*, 324(22), 1585–9.

Hennekens, C.H. and Buring, J.E. (1989). Methodologic considerations in the design and conduct of randomized trials: The U.S. physicians' health study. *Controlled Clinical Trials*, 10(Suppl. 4), 142–50S.

Hlatky, M.A., Rogers, W.J., Johnstone, I., et al., and The Bypass Angioplasty Revascularization Investigation (BARI) Investigators (1997). Medical care costs and quality of life after randomization to coronary angioplasty or coronary bypass surgery. *The New England Journal of Medicine*, 336(2), 92–9.

Hulley, S.B., Cummings, S.R., Browner, W.S., and Grady D.G. (2006). *Designing Clinical Research: An Epidemiologic Approach* (3rd ed.). Philadelphia, PA: Lippincott Williams & Wilkins.

Hypertension Detection and Follow-up Program Cooperative Group (1979). Five-year findings of the hypertension detection and follow-up program. I. Reduction in mortality of persons with high blood pressure, including mild hypertension. *JAMA*, 242(23), 2562–71.

Interagency Advisory Panel on Research Ethics (2001). *Tri-Council Policy Statement (TCPS): Ethical Conduct for Research Involving Humans*. Government of Canada. (Amended 2010) [Online] Available at: http://www.pre.ethics.gc.ca/pdf/eng/tcps2/TCPS_2_FINAL_Web.pdf.

International Conference on Harmonisation of Technical Requirements For Registration Of Pharmaceuticals For Human Use (1996). *Guideline For Good Clinical Practice E6(R1)*. [Online] Available at: http://www.ich.org/fileadmin/Public_Web_Site/ICH_Products/Guidelines/Efficacy/E6_R1/Step4/E6_R1__Guideline.pdf

ISIS-2 (Second International Study of Infarct Survival) Collaborative Group (1988). Randomised trial of intravenous streptokinase, oral aspirin, both, or neither among 17 187 cases of suspected acute myocardial infarction: ISIS-2. *The Lancet*, 332(8607), 349–60.

ISIS-3 (Third International Study of Infarct Survival) Collaborative Group (1992). ISIS-3: a randomised comparison of streptokinase vs tissue plasminogen activator vs anistreplase and of aspirin plus heparin vs aspirin alone among 41 299 cases of suspected acute myocardial infarction. *The Lancet*, 339(8796), 753–70.

Lachin, J.M. (1981). Introduction to sample size determination and power analysis for clinical trials. *Controlled Clinical Trials*, 2(2), 93–113.

Lakatos, E. (1986). Sample size determination in clinical trials with time-dependent rates of losses and noncompliance. *Controlled Clinical Trials*, 7(3), 189–99.

Lan, K.K.G. and DeMets, D.L. (1989). Changing frequency of interim analysis in sequential monitoring. *Biometrics*, 45(3), 1017–20.

Lan, K.K.G. and Wittes, J. (1988). The B-value: a tool for monitoring data. *Biometrics*, 44(2), 579–85.

Larsen, G., Hallstrom, A., McAnulty, J., et al., and AVID Investigators (2002). Cost-effectiveness of the implantable cardioverter-defibrillator versus antiarrhythmic drugs in survivors of serious ventricular tachyarrhythmias: results of the Antiarrhythmics Versus Implantable Defibrillators (AVID) economic analysis substudy. *Circulation*, 105(17), 2049–57.

LeLorier, J., Gregoire, G., Benhaddad, A., et al. (1997). Discrepancies between meta-analyses and subsequent large randomized, controlled trials. *The New England Journal of Medicine*, 337(8), 536–42.

McDowell, I. (2006). *Measuring Health: A Guide to Rating Scales and Questionnaires* (3rd ed.). New York: Oxford University Press.

Meinert, C.L. (1986). *Clinical Trials Design, Conduct, and Analysis*. New York: Oxford University Press.

National Institutes of Health (2003a). *Clinical Research and the HIPAA Privacy Rule*. [Online] Available at: http://privacyruleandresearch. nih.gov/clin_research.rtf.

National Institutes of Health (2003b). *NIH Data Sharing Policy*. [Online] Available at: http://grants.nih.gov/grants/policy/data_sharing/.

Nuremberg Code (1949). *Trials of War Criminals Before the Nuremberg Military Tribunals Under Control Council Law No.10*. Washington, DC: US Government Printing Office. Available at: http://www.hhs. gov/ohrp/archive/nurcode.html.

O'Brien, P.C. and Fleming, T.R. (1979). A multiple testing procedure for clinical trials. *Biometrics*, 35(3), 549–56.

Pandis, N. (2011). The evidence pyramid and introduction to randomized controlled trials. *American Journal of Orthodontics and Dentofacial Orthopedics*, 140(3), 446–7.

Passamani, E. (1991). Clinical trials—are they ethical? *The New England Journal of Medicine*, 324(22), 1589–92.

Pawitan, Y. and Hallstrom, A. (1990). Statistical interim monitoring of the cardiac arrhythmia suppression trial. *Statistics in Medicine*, 9(9), 1081–90.

Peto, J., Fletcher, O., and Gilham, C. (2004). Data protection, informed consent, and research. *BMJ*, 328(7447), 1029–30.

Peto, R. (1995). Clinical trials. In P. Price and K. Sikora (eds.) *Treatment of Cancer* (3rd ed.), pp. 1039–43. London: Chapman and Hall.

Peto, R., Pike, M.C., Armitage, P., et al. (1976). Design and analysis of randomized clinical trials requiring prolonged observation of each patient. I. Introduction and design. *British Journal of Cancer*, 34(6), 585–612.

Piaggio, G., Elbourne, D.R., Pocock, S.J., et al. for the CONSORT Group (2012). Reporting of noninferiority and equivalence randomized trials: an extension of the CONSORT 2010 statement. *JAMA*, 308(24), 2594–604.

Piantadosi, S. (2005). *Clinical Trials. A Methodologic Perspective* (2nd ed.). New York: Wiley.

Pocock, S.J. (1983). *Clinical Trials. A Practical Approach*. New York: Wiley.

Prentice, R.L. (1989). Surrogate endpoints in clinical trials: definition and operational criteria. *Statistics in Medicine*, 8, 431–40.

PROMIS® (n.d.). *Dynamic Tools to Measure Health Outcomes from the Patient Perspective*. [Online] Available at: http://www.nihpromis.org.

Proschan M.A., Lan, K.K.G., and Wittes, J.T. (2006). Adaptive sample size methods. In M.P. Proschan et al. *Statistical Monitoring of Clinical Trials: A Unified Approach*, pp. 185–211. New York: Springer.

Proschan, M.A., McMahon, R.P., Shih, J.H., et al. (2001). Sensitivity analysis using an imputation method for missing binary data in clinical trials. *Journal of Statistical Planning and Inference*, 96, 155–65.

Psaty, B.M. (1997). Health outcomes associated with antihypertensive therapies used as first-line agents. A systematic review and meta-analysis. *JAMA*, 277(9), 739–45.

Rand, C.S. and Weeks, K. (1998). Measuring adherence with medication regimens in clinical care and research. In S.A. Shumaker, E.B. Schon, J.K. Ockene, and W.L. McBeem (eds.) *The Handbook of Health Behavior Change* (2nd ed.), pp. 114–32. New York: Springer.

Rosenberger, W.F. and Lachin, J.M. (2002). *Randomization in Clinical Trials: Theory and Practice*. New York: John Wiley and Sons.

Sartorius, N. (1993). A WHO method for the assessment of health-related quality of life (WHOQOL). In S. Walker and R. Rosser (eds.) *Quality of Life Assessment: Key Issues in the 1990s*, pp. 201–7. Boston, MA: Kluwer Academic Publishers.

Schron, E.B. and Czajkowski, S.M. (2001). Clinical trials. In L.E. Burke and I.S. Ockene (eds.) *Compliance in Health Care and Research*, pp. 219–33. New York: Future.

SHEP Cooperative Research Group (1991). Prevention of stroke by antihypertensive drug treatment in older persons with isolated systolic hypertension. Final results of the Systolic Hypertension in the Elderly Program (SHEP). *JAMA*, 265(24), 3255–64.

Solomon, S.D., Pfeffer, M.A., McMurray, J.J. et al., and APC and PreSAP Trial Investigators (2006). Effect of celecoxib on cardiovascular events and blood pressure in two trials for the prevention of colorectal adenomas. *Circulation*, 114(10), 1028–35.

Staessen, J.A. (1997). Randomised double-blind comparison of placebo and active treatment for older patients with isolated systolic hypertension. The Systolic Hypertension in Europe (Syst-Eur) Trial Investigators. *The Lancet*, 350(9080), 757–64.

Steering Committee of the Physicians' Health Study Research Group (1989). Final report on the aspirin component of the ongoing physicians' health study. *The New England Journal of Medicine*, 321(3), 129–35.

Temple, R. and Ellenberg, S.S. (2000). Placebo-controlled trials and active-control trials in the evaluation of new treatments. Part 1: ethical and scientific issues. *Annals of Internal Medicine*, 133(6), 455–63.

The Atrial Fibrillation Follow-up Investigation of Rhythm Management (AFFIRM) Investigators (2002). A comparison of rate control and rhythm control in patients with atrial fibrillation. *The New England Journal of Medicine*, 347(23), 1825–33.

The Cardiac Arrhythmia Suppression Trial (CAST) Investigators (1989). Preliminary report: effect of encainide and flecainide on mortality in a randomized trial of arrhythmia suppression after myocardial infarction. *The New England Journal of Medicine*, 321(6), 406–12.

The Heart Outcomes Prevention Evaluation Study Investigators (2000). Effects of an angiotensin-converting-enzyme inhibitor, Ramipril, on cardiovascular events in high-risk patients. *The New England Journal of Medicine*, 342(3), 145–53.

The National Commission for the Protection of Human Subjects of Biomedical and Behavioral Research (1979). *The Belmont Report: Ethical Principles and Guidelines for the Protection of Human Subjects of Research*. Washington, DC: Department of Health, Education, and Welfare. Available at: http://www.hhs.gov/ohrp/humansubjects/guidance/belmont.html.

The Women's Health Initiative Study Group (1998). Design of the women's health initiative clinical trial and observational study. *Controlled Clinical Trials*, 19(1), 61–109.

Trevena, L., Irwig, L., and Barratt, A. (2006). Impact of privacy legislation on the number and characteristics of people who are recruited for research: a randomised controlled trial. *Journal of Medical Ethics*, 32(8), 473–7.

Tunis S.R., Stryer D.B., and Clancy C.M. (2003). Practical clinical trials: increasing the value of clinical research for decision making in clinical and health policy. *Journal of the American Medical Association*, 290, 1624–32.

US Department of Health and Human Services (2005). *Protection of Human Subjects, Title 45 Code of Federal Regulations Part 46*. [Online] Available at: http://www.hhs.gov/ohrp/humansubjects/guidance/45cfr46.html.

US Food and Drug Administration (2006). *Exception from Informed Consent Requirements for Emergency Research; Title 21 CFR Part 50*. [Online] Available at: http://www.accessdata.fda.gov/scripts/cdrh/cfdocs/cfcfr/CFRSearch.cfm?fr=50.24.

US Food and Drug Administration (2009). *Guidance for Industry. Patient Reported Outcome Measures: Use in Medical Product Development to Support Labelling Claims*. Washington, DC: US Department of Health and Human Services, FDA. Available at: http://www.fda.gov/downloads/Drugs/GuidanceComplianceRegulatoryInformation/Guidances/UCM193282.pdf.2009.

Veterans Administration Cooperative Study Group on Antihypertensive Agents (1967). Effects of treatment on mortality in hypertension. Results in patients with diastolic blood pressures averaging 115 through 129 mm Hg. *JAMA*, 202, 1028–34.

Veterans Administration Cooperative Study Group on Antihypertensive Agents (1970). Effects of treatment on morbidity in hypertension. II. Results in patients with diastolic blood pressure averaging 90 through 114 mm Hg. *JAMA*, 213, 1143–52.

Waldo, A.L., Camm, A.J., deRuyter, H., et al. (1995). Survival with oral d-sotalol in patients with left ventricular dysfunction after myocardial infarction: rationale, design, and methods (the SWORD trial). *The American Journal of Cardiology*, 75(15), 1023–7.

Ware, J., Kosinski, M., Bayliss, M., et al. (1995). Comparison of methods for the scoring and statistical analysis of SF-36 health profile and summary measures: summary of results from the Medical Outcomes Study. *Medical Care*, 33(Suppl. 4), AS264–79.

Ware, J. and Sherbourne, C. (1992). The MOS 36-Item Short-Form Health Survey (SF-36). I. Conceptual framework and item selection. *Medical Care*, 30, 473–83.

Whitehead, J. (1997). *The Design and Analysis of Sequential Clinical Trials* (2nd ed.). Chichester: Wiley.

Wilson, I.B. and Cleary, P.D. (1995). Linking clinical variables with health-related quality of life: a conceptual model of patient outcomes. *Journal of the American Medical Association*, 273(1), 59–65.

Wing, L.M., Reid, C.M., Ryan, P., et al. for the Second Australian National Blood Pressure Study Group (2003). A comparison of outcomes with angiotensin-converting-enzyme inhibitors and diuretics for hypertension in the elderly. *The New England Journal of Medicine*, 348(7), 583–92.

World Medical Association (2013). *Declaration of Helsinki.* [Online] Available at: http://www.wma.net/en/20activities/10ethics/10helsinki/.

Wu, M.C. (1988). Sample size for comparison of changes in the presence of right censoring caused by death, withdrawal, and staggered entry. *Controlled Clinical Trials*, 9(1), 32–46.

Yusuf, S., Zucker, D., Passamani, E., et al. (1994). Effect of coronary artery bypass graft surgery on survival: overview of 10-year results from randomised trials by the Coronary Artery Bypass Graft Surgery Trialists Collaboration. *The Lancet*, 344(8922), 563–70.

Methodological issues in the design and analysis of community intervention trials

Allan Donner

Introduction to methodological issues in the design and analysis of community intervention trials

The purpose of this chapter is to address methodological issues that arise in community-based intervention trials. Although the word 'community' is often now used in the literature to encompass a wide variety of social groupings, including, for example, schools, workplaces, and religious organizations, the focus here will be largely, but not exclusively, on geographical groupings, such as villages, towns, or entire cities. An intrinsic feature of such trials is that both implementation and randomization at the community level is either the most natural choice or a virtual necessity. For example in mass education trials, it is difficult to provide advice concerning lifestyle modification to some people and not others in the same community without risking experimental contamination. Moreover the interventions administered in such trials often have the potential to affect all or most individuals in a community even though they are actually delivered to only a fraction of residents.

This notion has been recognized explicitly by researchers evaluating the effect of vaccines through the concept of 'herd immunity', where immunization is expected to reduce the attack rate among all residents of a community, even though only some individuals have been vaccinated. However, it also may be a factor in other community-based trials that rely on a variety of mechanisms governing human interaction to help modify health risk behaviour. For example, cities were the unit of randomization in the Community Intervention Trial for Smoking Cessation (COMMIT Research Group 1995), a randomized, controlled multicentre trial aimed at adult smokers, at least partly because it was expected that heavy smokers would find it easier to stop smoking in an environment where this practice was made less socially acceptable.

Methodological implications of community-based randomization

Trials that randomize communities or, more generally, 'clusters' of individuals to different intervention groups are almost always characterized by positive intracluster correlation, that is, the tendency for responses among individuals in the same cluster to resemble each other more than the responses of individuals in different clusters. This concept can be equivalently viewed as 'between-cluster variation', which reflects the natural variation among clusters that exists even in the absence of an intervention effect. That is, the higher the degree of intracluster correlation, the greater the degree of between-cluster variation.

The reasons for between-cluster variation are diverse, usually cannot be disentangled without an extensive quantity of empirical information, and may be induced either externally or internally. As an example of externally induced clustering effects, differences in smoking by-laws across communities may affect the relative success of smoking cessation programmes. As a second example, differences in socioeconomic status may be related to variation in the success of community-based education programmes. However, clustering effects may also be internally induced, as when individuals with respiratory problems migrate to dry climates or elderly individuals migrate to warm climates. Such effects may also arise simply through the interaction of individuals living in close proximity.

Whatever the source of the clustering, it is now well accepted that it must be accounted for at both the design and the analysis stages of the trial. Failure to account for the clustering in the estimation of trial power may lead to an elevated type II error (caused by a lower level of statistical power than planned for), while failure to account for it in the analysis stage may lead to an elevated type I error (higher rate of false significant differences than planned for). Thus there are two potential pitfalls operating on parallel tracks—if an important intervention effect is present, the probability of detecting it is reduced, while if the effect of intervention is non-existent, the probability of falsely detecting it is increased. As Cornfield (1978) stated, 'Randomization by cluster accompanied by an analysis by individual (without adjustment for clustering) is an exercise in self-deception, however, and should be discouraged' (p. 101). He might also have added a similar caution concerning the estimation of trial power.

A recent review of design and analysis strategies employed in cluster randomized trials was presented by Varnell et al. (2004), who surveyed 60 articles published in the *American Journal of Public Health* and *Preventive Medicine* from 1998 to 2002. Their review showed that only 15 per cent of these articles reported evidence of using appropriate methods of sample size estimation, while 54 per cent reported the use of appropriate analytic methods. These discouraging results are also fairly close to those found in a similar review published almost a decade earlier by Simpson et al. (1995).

Impact of the intracluster correlation

The intracluster correlation coefficient ρ may simply be defined as the standard Pearson product-moment correlation between any two observations in the same cluster. In community intervention trials, where negative values of ρ are usually regarded as implausible, ρ may be equivalently defined as the proportion of overall variance in the trial outcome that may be attributed to variation among clusters. More formally, we may define $\rho = \sigma_B^2 / \sigma_B^2 + \sigma_W^2$, where σ_B^2 represents the variance component among clusters and σ_W^2 represents the variance component within clusters. Letting $\sigma^2 = \sigma_B^2 + \sigma_W^2$ denote the overall variance of the outcome measure, we may then write $\sigma_W^2 = \sigma^2(1-\rho)$, showing how the degree of resemblance among responses within a cluster increases with ρ. Equivalently, higher values of ρ lead to increased variation among clusters for a fixed value of σ^2.

It is also possible to interpret clustering effects in community-based trials in terms of 'effective sample size'. Consider a trial randomizing k communities of size m to each of two intervention groups. If $N = km$ denotes the total number of individuals per group, then the effective sample size per group is given by $N/[1 + (m-1)\rho]$. Thus when ρ achieves its maximum value of 1.0, the total amount of information available from each cluster is no more than that provided by a single individual, while at $\rho = 0$ each individual in the trial provides an independent piece of information.

The factor VIF = $[1 + (m-1)\rho]$ is sometimes referred to as the 'variance inflation factor' or 'design effect', since it represents the factor by which the variance of a group mean or proportion must be multiplied to appropriately account for the randomization by cluster. It is thus clear that the impact of clustering in any one trial depends not only on the value of ρ, but also on the size of the randomized clusters. Unfortunately this has sometimes been a source of misunderstanding on the part of investigators who have ignored clustering effects simply because the estimated value of ρ was close to zero. Note, for example, that values of ρ less than 0.01 are not uncommon in cluster randomized trials. If such a trial were to randomize clusters containing 100 subjects each, the variance inflation factor is seen to be almost 2.0, implying that the effective sample size is only half that of an individually randomized trial enrolling the same number of subjects.

The effect on type I error of ignoring the VIF in testing the equality of two means using an unpaired t-test has been quantified by Scariano and Davenport (1987). For example, their results show that at $m = 100$ and $\rho = 0.01$, the true type I error rate at a nominal significance level of 0.05 is given by 0.1658, a more than threefold increase. Moreover the inflation in type I error rate for given values of m and ρ becomes even greater when an analysis of variance F-test is used to compare three or more means.

The actual value of ρ in practice will depend on both the outcome measure of interest as well as the size of the clusters randomized.

Although ρ is almost always small in size and positive, empirical evidence shows that it generally declines with cluster size, although relatively slowly. For example, in primary care settings ρ has been found to vary from about 0.01 to 0.05 (Campbell et al. 2000), while for very large communities values of ρ may be less than 0.001.

Some investigators may be tempted to perform a test of significance that attempts to rule out a positive value of ρ, interpreting a statistically non-significant result as an indication that clustering effects are absent. However this strategy is not only conceptually flawed ('absence of evidence does not imply evidence of absence') but is particularly weak in this context given the low power of such tests for detecting small but influential values of ρ.

A detailed discussion as to how to account for the impact of clustering in performing standard statistical tests is presented in the later section 'Analysis strategies in community-based intervention trials'.

Specifying the unit of inference

The previous discussion assumes that the unit of inference for the trial is at the individual level, while the unit of randomization is at the community (cluster) level. However, the literature shows that even for trials essentially evaluating the same intervention, there is considerable diversity in the choice of randomization unit. For example, West et al. (1991) report on a meta-analysis synthesizing the results of trials in which the allocation units included individuals, households, neighbourhoods, and entire communities. However, in each case the choice of randomization unit has been largely a matter of practicality or convenience—the aim of each of these trials has been to investigate the biological effect of vitamin A on child mortality. Therefore it is necessary in each of these trials to consider the impact of the variance inflation factor in both the design and the analysis.

However in other trials, particularly those developed from a policy perspective, the units of randomization and of inference may be the same. For example, Diwan et al. (1995) evaluated a policy of 'group detailing' on the prescribing of lipid-lowering drugs in a trial randomizing community health centres. A primary end point in this study was the number of appropriately administered prescriptions per month, with the health centre serving as the unit of analysis. Therefore standard methods of sample size and analysis were employed with no need to consider the role of the within-centre clustering effects. As a second example, the hospital-based rate of caesarean section was the primary end point in a trial designed to lower the rate of caesarean section at the hospital level in Latin America (Althabe et al. 2004). In trials such as these, where the observed results on any one subject are not of direct interest, the challenges that arise in design and analysis are essentially the same as those that which arise in individually randomized trials.

Failure of investigators to distinguish the primary unit of inference in the planning stages of a trial may lead to confusion in developing the trial protocol. Possibly related to this confusion is the terminology 'unit of analysis error', which implies that an analysis at the individual level is inevitably invalid when clusters are the unit of randomization. In fact, this is the case only if the clustering effects induced by the randomization are not appropriately accounted for.

The role of randomization

Randomized or non-randomized?

The discussion up to this point has assumed that communities will be assigned at random to different intervention groups. The advantages of randomization for community-based intervention trials are no different from those in any comparative trial, including the assurance that each eligible cluster has an equal chance of being assigned to a given intervention group, thus eliminating the risk of selection bias on the part of either the participants or the investigators. Randomization also tends to create groups that are comparable on factors (either known or unknown) that may influence response. Moreover this protection extends not only to community-level characteristics, such as size and geographic location, but also to individual-level baseline characteristics, such as age and gender, provided the entire community (or a random subset of residents) is randomized. However, the probability of substantive imbalance on such characteristics is higher than in individually randomized trials allocating the same number of subjects. Therefore it is important in any one trial to confirm the effectiveness of the randomization by comparing the distribution of both community-level and individual-level characteristics across groups.

In the absence of randomization it is almost impossible to rule out the possibility of selection bias in the allocation of communities to different intervention groups. As a result, the study findings run the risk of lacking credibility, particularly if they are unexpected. However non-randomized community-based trials are still frequently implemented, usually for a variety of practical or ethical reasons. For example, if an intervention has already been implemented on a major scale, or if resources for implementing a new intervention are only available in certain communities, randomization may not be viewed as feasible. In other cases, it may be perceived that non-randomized designs would be easier to explain to public officials and to gain public acceptance, given the resistance to assignment by chance that some individuals have. This points to the importance of being able to communicate the purposes and advantages of randomization to key stakeholders, and to possibly offer incentives for their participation.

There are also some arguments against randomization that are less cogent. For example it has sometimes been perceived that non-randomized designs may be preferable when the number of communities available for allocation is small. However, as pointed out by Koepsell et al. (1992), the availability of a limited number of clusters is not a strong reason to avoid randomization, since the increased probability of imbalance on important prognostic characteristics can be controlled by using stratification or pair-matching in the design. Moreover, the challenge of achieving balance when only a small number of communities in each group are available remains a problem whether randomization is employed or not.

In some studies, systematic allocation of geographically separated control and experimental communities has been seen as necessary to avoid experimental contamination, that is, the spread of an intervention effect to individuals in the control group or vice versa. However if the eligible communities are fairly large, this concern can be at least partially dealt with by subsampling participants within the centre of a randomized community while keeping track of any changes of residence (e.g. see Hayes 1998). Another approach sometimes used to deal with this problem is to combine groups of similar clusters into larger randomization units so as to reduce the extent to which individuals in different intervention groups are likely to mingle. For example, Moulton et al. (2001) describe the design of a vaccine trial conducted among American Indian populations in which two to four geopolitical units were combined into larger units 'so as to minimize social interaction between the units'. Thus the aim here was to sacrifice the potential gain in precision obtainable by choosing a smaller randomization unit in favour of reducing the possible bias due to cross-unit social interaction. Other practical methods of minimizing contamination while otherwise retaining strong internal validity in the context of randomization are discussed by Watson et al. (2004).

In spite of the lower quality of evidence usually obtained from non-randomized comparisons, it is clear that at the very least they may generate hypotheses that can be subsequently tested in a more rigorous experimental framework. Moreover in the initial stages of an evaluation there is undoubtedly greater scope for more widespread use of relatively advanced approaches such as time-series experiments (e.g. Biglan et al. 2000) when it is felt to be premature to launch a full-scale randomized trial.

Subsampling and the risk of selection bias

In some trials—for example, those randomizing worksites—all individuals in a cluster can be readily identified in advance and followed up. In this case, randomization by community will assure that both cluster-level and individual-level characteristics will be well-balanced between groups, that is, there will be no risk of selection bias at either of these levels. Such balance will also be preserved provided random subsamples of individuals are selected from communities after their initial randomization. However, for practical reasons or even out of necessity, subject recruitment is often done prospectively after randomization in an opportunistic manner, raising the possibility of intervention-related bias. For example, project staff who are responsible for recruiting participants to receive a new and promising intervention may be more enthusiastic or selective in their efforts than are individuals who are assigned to recruit participants into the control group. Torgerson (2001) has argued that such differential recruiting efforts could result in substantial imbalance between intervention groups with respect to both the number of the subjects recruited and their characteristics. Similar imbalances could result if willingness to participate differed by intervention group. In either case much of the benefit of the original randomization may be lost, since then it is only the community-level characteristics that will not be subject to selection bias. In the context of trials randomizing medical practices, where it is routine to identify eligible patients after their practice has been randomized, this phenomenon may be referred to as 'detect and treat bias'.

If eligible subjects in a community cannot be identified before randomization, it may be possible to reduce this bias by ensuring that subject recruitment is done by an individual, ideally one who is independent of the study, who does not have prior knowledge of the group allocation. However, if it is the investigator who has responsibility for identifying the trial participants, he/she should be blinded to group membership until a potential subject is judged as eligible. Jordhøy et al. (2002) describe how serious problems of selection bias arose in a cluster randomized trial of palliative care that did not involve blinded group allocation.

Pair-matching and stratification

The attraction of pair-matching as a design strategy

In some community-based trials it is desirable from both a methodological and logistical perspective not to impose any restrictions on the randomization scheme, that is, to adopt a 'completely randomized' design. For example, Sommer et al. (1986) investigated the impact of vitamin A supplementation on childhood mortality in a trial randomizing over 200 villages in Indonesia to each of two intervention groups. With these many clusters, unrestricted randomization can be expected to offer reasonable assurance that the intervention and control groups are well balanced with respect to important prognostic characteristics. Furthermore any remaining imbalance in either cluster-level or individual-level characteristics related to outcome can be controlled for in the analysis (see 'Adjusting for covariates' section).

However, in most community-based trials budgetary and other resource-based limitations simply do not allow a large number of communities to be randomized. Moreover, the smaller effective sample size characterizing such trials implies that the probability of imbalance on any one such characteristic will be greater than in an individually randomized trial that recruits the same total of subjects. Thus, pair-matching, although not a common design choice for individually randomized trials, has an obvious attraction. With this strategy, communities are first matched with respect to selected baseline characteristics, such as geographic area and size, which are expected to be related to outcome. One member of a pair is then randomly assigned to the new intervention, with the other member serving as a control, thus providing assurance that the groups compared are similar at the outset with respect to important prognostic characteristics.

An example of a matched-pair design is provided by the COMMIT smoking cessation trial first mentioned in the chapter introduction, in which the intervention program was randomly assigned to one of two cities in each of 11 matched pairs, ten in the United States and one in Canada. Matching was done with respect to several baseline characteristics, including community size, population density, demographic profile, and geographical proximity. It is also interesting to note that COMMIT enrolled more than three times the number of pairs that were recruited in the first generation of community-based trials, and, perhaps not coincidentally, was the first to use formal power considerations at the design stage.

Although the matching factors selected in any given trial will naturally vary according to the selected end points, two factors very frequently selected are community size (e.g. small, medium, large) and geographic area (e.g. urban vs. rural). Matching by size is particularly attractive since this factor may serve as a surrogate for other key prognostic factors that are more difficult to match on, such as socioeconomic status or access to healthcare resources (e.g. Lewsey 2004). For example, in trials conducted in developing countries larger communities may be advantaged with respect to certain outcomes simply because they are located closer to central health facilities than communities that are smaller in size. Matching by size is also an efficiency consideration since it provides assurance that the number of individuals assigned to each intervention group will be approximately the same.

Particularly large gains in efficiency may be achieved when it is possible to match on suitably categorized levels of the baseline version of the primary end point. For example, if this end point is an incidence rate, then the ability to match on the corresponding baseline incidence rate (or failing that, on a corresponding prevalence rate) can lead to considerable gains in precision. An interesting illustration of this effect is given by Todd et al. (2003) in the context of several HIV prevention studies conducted in East Africa.

A baseline survey that captures such information is also useful for other purposes, for example, in checking on some of the design assumptions that were used to estimate trial power, and in providing field experience to those staff who will be responsible for the final data collection. In making the decision as to whether it is worthwhile to conduct such a survey, Duffy et al. (1992) point out that pre-trial data may sometimes be obtained with a relatively minor increase in resources as compared to that required to secure the same amount of statistical power through increasing the study sample size. However, the decision as to how much baseline data should be collected should depend on how stable the outcome rates of interest have been in past years, as well as on the cost and ease of obtaining the required data retrospectively.

The efficiency of a matched-pair design is directly tied to the magnitude of the matching correlation ρ_m, which may be defined as the standard Pearson product-moment correlation coefficient between the members of a matched pair with respect to their observed end points. Since the actual gain in efficiency in reasonably large samples may be quantified by the factor $G = 1/(1 - \rho_m)$, it is clear that high values of ρ_m may bring large gains in precision. For example, the HIV prevention trial reported by Grosskurth et al. (1995) generated a matching correlation of 0.94 as a consequence of effective pair-matching of communities on prior rate of sexually transmitted disease, location (roadside, lakeshore, or island) and geographic proximity. However, this degree of success in pair-matching is unusual, and indeed in some trials efficiency may even be lost relative to that of a completely randomized design. This is because many community-based trials can afford to randomize only a small number of units per group, in which case the available degrees of freedom associated with the test statistic used to evaluate the effect of intervention plays an influential role. For example, a trial with k matched pairs is typically analysed using a paired t-statistic with $k - 1$ degrees of freedom, as compared to the $2(k - 1)$ degrees of freedom available for an unmatched analysis. While this difference may not be important if $k > 30$, Martin et al. (1993) have shown that it may have very tangible consequences in terms of power if $k < 10$. In this case they conclude that 'matching should be used only if the investigators are confident that the matching correlation is at least 0.20'.

Thus the question may arise as to the efficiency of performing an unmatched analysis of data arising from a matched-pair design. Diehr et al. (1995) have investigated this question, showing that for $k < 10$, breaking the matching and performing an unmatched analysis may in fact result in an increase in power for testing the effect of intervention. However, an important assumption here is that the decision to break the matches is made at the design stage of the trial. Thus it would be inappropriate to base the decision to break the matches on the basis of the observed matching correlation, as this would lead to an elevated type I error.

Another limitation of the matched-pair design that arises even in the presence of effective matching results from its inability to directly estimate the intracluster correlation coefficient. This limitation arises because estimation of ρ requires, by definition, an estimate of the natural variation in response among clusters that are treated the same. However, it is clear that the effect of an intervention within a matched pair is confounded with such variation. Hence in the presence of a positive intervention effect, the usual estimator of between-cluster variation, and hence of the intracluster correlation coefficient, will be biased upwards.

Although the inability to directly estimate ρ in a matched-pair design does not affect the ability of investigators to perform a test of the intervention effect, which is inevitably based on between-stratum information, the lack of a valid estimator of between-cluster variation may serve as a handicap in appropriately powering future trials randomizing the same or similar units. Moreover, as discussed by Klar and Donner (1997), constraints will be placed on the nature of several secondary analyses that can be performed, including the ability to make inferences concerning individual-level covariates.

Given the analytic complexities associated with the pair-matched design, a preferable option under many circumstances may be the 'stratified design', as discussed in the next section.

The stratified design

Stratified designs can be viewed as a more general form of the matched-pair design that allocates several communities in each stratum to either intervention or control. For example, the Pathways intervention trial for the prevention of obesity in American Indian schoolchildren (Caballero et al. 2003) used this design to allocate 41 schools to either a multicomponent intervention or to a control. The investigators created primary strata based on four distinct field centres in the study catchment area followed by the construction of two secondary strata within these centres based on a school's median body fat percentage. Half the schools within each stratum were then randomized to either the intervention group or the control group, resulting in 41 schools distributed among a total of eight strata. As stated by the authors, the choice of a stratified versus a paired design was made 'under the assumption that stratification would provide adequate control for the difference in percentage body fat'.

Unlike the matched-pair design, the stratified design allows some degree of cluster-level replication in each combination of treatment and stratum. As pointed out by Klar and Donner (1997), this provides greater flexibility in the statistical analysis, since stratum effects may simply be represented by indicator variables in a regression analysis that appropriately adjusts for clustering effects. As discussed in the 'Statistical approaches to estimating trial power' section, such modelling is not possible in a pair-matched design without making special assumptions.

Although in theory the stratified design offers less control over the influence of key baseline characteristics than a pair-matched design that enrols the same number of clusters, the difficulty in practice of securing adequate pair-matches for all eligible clusters may mitigate this advantage. Moreover, there is reason to believe that 'over-matching' is not uncommon, given that trials enrolling more than 50 matched pairs have been frequently reported in the literature. Since matching can only be effective to the extent that the baseline risk of an event varies across strata, the question may arise as to whether such a large number of distinct matches can actually be constructed in advance. This suggests, for example, that a stratified design enrolling four communities in each of 26 strata or eight communities in each of 13 strata, may be as efficient as a matched-pair design enrolling two communities in each of 52 strata, while at the same time offering increased flexibility in the analysis and more degrees of freedom for the estimation of error. Although a completely randomized design without any stratification would provide even more degrees of freedom, this may not lead to a gain in power if the strata are wisely chosen.

Other designs

The designs most frequently adopted in community-based research are the completely randomized, matched-pair, and stratified designs. However, increasing attention has been given recently to other designs that randomize communities. The first is the cluster-crossover design in which all participating clusters receive both treatment and control interventions in a sequence determined at random (Parienti and Kuss 2007). The principal advantage of this design is that it eliminates any confounding due to cluster level characteristics. Since each cluster is its own control, it also reduces the total number of clusters that need to be enrolled in the study, although with a considerable increase in study duration. As in standard crossover trials (essentially enrolling clusters of size one), its validity depends on the assumption that carryover effects are absent, that is, that the estimated effects of intervention are independent of the order in which they are assigned. From a practical perspective, it may also be difficult to assure a uniformly timed replacement of one intervention by the other over the course of the study. A review of methods for analysis of cluster-crossover designs is given by Turner et al. (2007).

The second design that is receiving increasing attention is the stepped wedge design which may be considered a variant of the cluster-crossover design (Hussey and Hughes 2007). For this design all clusters eventually cross over (to the alternate intervention), but at different time points. Moreover the clusters cross over in one direction only—typically from control to intervention. Instead what is randomized is the time at which a cluster begins the intervention. A principal advantage of this design is that clusters may be enrolled gradually over time which may be important from a logistical perspective.

The methodological development of both the cluster-crossover and stepped wedge designs is still evolving. For example, numerous approaches to the analysis have been proposed for both designs, with consensus on the optimal approach yet to be reached. We also need much more practical experience with both designs before they can be firmly recommended (Box 5.8.1).

Determining the required size of a trial

Statistical approaches to estimating trial power

The formal assessment of statistical power is now regarded as a fundamental step in the design of any comparative trial and is a staple of discussion in the clinical trial literature. Historically, however, many community-based intervention trials have been designed with little or no consideration of statistical power. This

---

Box 5.8.1 Common pitfalls in choice of a design

1. Failure to appropriately define the unit of inference.

2. Failure to define inclusion criteria at both the individual and cluster level.

3. Failure to consider matching or stratification, particularly in smaller trials.

4. Failure to appreciate the restrictiveness of a matched pair design on the subsequent statistical analysis.

5. Failure to consider the possibility of selection bias when subjects are recruited after randomization.

---

may be partly because any trial enrolling hundreds or even thousands of individuals may (erroneously) be perceived as obviously not lacking in power. However, even those investigators who recognized the issue of the smaller 'effective sample size' in cluster randomized trials did not have effective and easily accessible tools for dealing with this problem until the 1980s.

Appropriate sample size formulae are now easily available in both journals (e.g. Kerry and Bland 1998) and in textbooks (Murray 1998, pp. 305–320; Donner and Klar 2000). In their simplest form, they require that standard sample size formulae for comparing means or proportions be multiplied by an estimate of the likely variance inflation factor $VIF = 1 + (m - 1)\rho$. Thus for comparing either two means or two proportions, an investigator may use standard sample size formulas as would be applied in the design of individually randomized trials and multiply the result by an estimate of VIF.

As an example, let $Z_{\alpha/2}$ denote the two-sided critical value of the standard normal distribution corresponding to the desired type I error rate α, and Z_β denote the critical value corresponding to desired type II error rate β. Then, assuming the difference in sample means for the experimental and control groups can be regarded as approximately normally distributed, the number of subjects required per intervention group in a completely randomized design is given by

$$n = \frac{\left(Z_{\alpha/2} + Z_\beta\right)^2 \left(2\sigma^2\right)\left[1 + (m-1)\rho\right]}{\left(\mu_1 - \mu_2\right)^2},$$

where $\mu_1 - \mu_2$ denotes the magnitude of the difference to be detected and m denotes the average cluster size. Equivalently, the number of clusters required per group is given by $k = n/m$. For comparing two proportions P_1 and P_2, the required sample size may be obtained by replacing σ^2 in the formula by $P_1(1 - P_1) + P_2(1 - P_2)$.

For variable-sized clusters, Manatunga and Hudgens (2001) and Eldridge et al. (2006) have shown that this expression may be replaced by $VIF = 1 + ((cv^2(k - 1)/k + 1)\bar{m} - 1)\rho$, where the coefficient of variation $cv = S_m/\bar{m}$ and S_m is the standard deviation of the cluster sizes. Eldridge et al. (2006) also give some examples of the value of cv for sample sizes typically seen in cluster randomized trials.

In the presence of effective pair-matching or stratification, application of this formula may be expected to be conservative. However, if prior information concerning the matching correlation ρ_m is available, a more precise estimate of the required size

of sample for a matched-pair design may be obtained by multiplying n by $(1 - \rho_m)$. Donner and Klar (2000) provide examples of sample size estimation for each of the completely randomized, matched-pair, and stratified designs.

An alternative approach to estimate trial size is to formulate the problem directly in terms of the coefficient of variation between clusters rather than in terms of the intracluster correlation coefficient. A discussion of this approach is provided by Hayes and Bennett (1999), who also provide a sample size formula for trials in which outcomes are expressed as rates per person-year.

Ensuring the power is adequate

The requirement for an advance estimate of ρ in assessing the proper size of a cluster randomized trial is no different in principle than, for example, the need to have an advance estimate of the standard deviation of the primary outcome variable in an individually randomized trial. However until the 1990s, values of ρ obtained from previous trial data had not been readily available to investigators. Fortunately this problem is now less serious, with many investigators now routinely reporting the estimated value of ρ for a variety of randomization units and outcome variables. Indeed some investigators have now reported such estimates for a range of study results obtained in a particular research area (e.g. Agarwal et al. 2005; Parker et al. 2005; Gulliford et al. 2005).

The review by Gulliford et al. (2005) is particularly notable in that it reveals an approximate linear relationship which holds on the log scale between the prevalence of a trait and the corresponding value of ρ. This suggests that the anticipated prevalence of an outcome variable may be used in some research contexts to make an informed assumption about the magnitude of clustering effects.

It is important to recognize that any particular value of ρ must be interpreted in the context of the trial design and analysis. For example, estimates may be obtained either taking into account the trial stratification factors and/or the individual level covariates adjusted for in the analysis. It is also useful to note that unadjusted values of the intracluster correlation coefficient, which are those most frequently presented, will generally be larger than their adjusted counterparts, implying their future use in sample size estimation will be conservative.

Even with the availability of an appropriate estimate of required trial size, it is useful to conduct a sensitivity analysis exploring the effect on sample size by varying the values of the intracluster correlation, the number of clusters per intervention group, and the cluster (or cluster subsample) size.

The increased attention that has been paid more recently to the formal assessment of the required sample size in the design of community-based intervention trials is particularly welcome given that many of these studies have historically been underpowered and thus found to be inconclusive (e.g. Susser 1995). This is not only because many investigators have not had ready access to the statistical tools needed for this purpose, but also because community-based trials may be particularly susceptible to problems of low power given the nature of the interventions evaluated and the heterogeneity of the populations to which they are administered. For example, many interventions are applied over a wide area on a group basis with relatively little attention given to individual study participants. Thus the risk of both non-compliance and loss to follow-up is exacerbated, particularly since not only individuals but entire communities are subject to attrition. Moreover many community-based trials are also prevention trials whose aim is to reduce event rates that may already be quite low in a relatively healthy population. The lengthy follow-up time typically required in these trials places a further burden not only on the ability of study participants to show reasonable levels of compliance but also on the efforts of project staff who are administering the intervention over large geographic areas, often with only limited resources at their disposal. Thus it is perhaps not surprising, as stated by Susser (1995, p. 156), that 'generally the size of effects has been meager in relation to the effort expended'.

Some community intervention trials also have to contend with the immigration of new subjects after baseline, further complicating issues of ensuring that study power is adequate (Jooste et al. 1990). Further discussion of this issue in the context of cancer prevention trials is given by Byar (1988).

Since the power available in a given community-based trial is invariably limited by the degree of between-community heterogeneity, one strategy for increasing precision is to establish relatively narrow cluster-level eligibility criteria, for example, by randomizing communities of similar size and socioeconomic status. For example, LaPrelle et al. (1992) enrolled communities in a smoking cessation trial that were known to be similar with respect to racial and educational make-up, while acknowledging the corresponding risk of some loss in generalizability. Similarly, in the HIV intervention trial described in the section 'The attraction of pair-matching as a design strategy', clusters were deliberately selected to be homogeneous for the purpose of increasing statistical power.

For trials such as that described by LaPrelle et al. (1992), where there is some latitude in how the primary outcome variable can be defined, it is useful to recognize that continuous end points (e.g. number of cigarettes smoked per day) generally lead to much more statistical power than their dichotomous counterparts (e.g. quitting smoking or not), although issues of measurement error and ease of interpretability must also be considered here.

As mentioned in the section 'Specifying the unit of inference', some trials are also characterized by a degree of flexibility in the fundamental choice of the unit to be randomized. In this regard, Duan et al. (2000, p. 1470) have remarked that 'it is important to explore new conduits (such as churches) through which community-based interventions can be more effectively delivered to target subpopulations of heightened risk'. This argument recognizes that the choice of randomization unit may directly impact on statistical power through a variety of factors, both tangible and non-tangible.

A common rationale for avoiding individual randomization in the evaluation of a new intervention is to reduce the risk of experimental contamination. However, investigators have also recognized that power losses due to contamination may remain a problem even if intact social groups are randomized, particularly in the case of small adjacent clusters. Aside from its possible role in minimizing contamination, as discussed in the section 'Randomized or non-randomized?', selective subsampling can also be used more directly to increase power. For example, a decision could be made to enrol only neighbourhoods within a larger community that are known to have higher levels of risk factors than the community as a whole. From a statistical perspective, this strategy would be consistent with the well-known effect

on power of increasing the number of clusters in a trial versus increasing the sizes of these clusters. Thus in a trial allocating k clusters of size m to each of two intervention groups, the variance of an estimated event rate $\hat{p}$ is given by Var($\hat{p}$) = {$P(1 - P)$ $(1 + [m - 1])$}/k, where P is the value of the true event rate. It is therefore clear that increasing k for a fixed value of m steadily drives the value of this variance to zero, implying that the power of the trial can be increased indefinitely by increasing k. However it is also clear that as m increases for a fixed number of clusters k, Var($\hat{p}$) can only be reduced to a limiting threshold value given by $P(1 - P)/k$, thus constraining the maximum power that can be obtained. In fact even when clusters are (hypothetically) infinite in size, the power of a trial may be held below 80 per cent if k is not sufficiently large.

A useful rule of thumb in this regard is that very little increase in power will be obtained for a fixed number of clusters after m exceeds the value $1/\rho$ (Donner and Klar 2004). For example if $\rho = 0.01$, then the increased power obtained by enrolling more than 100 subjects per community will be small. Yet, as alluded to in the chapter introduction, investigators will often have practical reasons for enrolling very large numbers of subjects per community, even if not warranted from a strictly statistical perspective.

Torgerson (2001) and Farrin et al. (2005) have argued that the practice of randomizing intact social groups as a means of minimizing contamination effects may be overused. The argument made by these authors is that the loss of precision associated with cluster randomization often outweighs that which results from the contamination and subsequent dilution of intervention effect that can be expected under individual randomization. However, it must also be recognized that under individual randomization the presence of contamination will serve to bias the estimated intervention effect, a factor which must also be taken into account if the ultimate goal of the investigators is to estimate the magnitude of this effect when the intervention is applied in a non-experimental setting. Other factors to consider here include practical aspects involved in administering the intervention and the importance of reflecting 'real world' conditions while doing so.

If the correlation r between a baseline score and a follow-up score is fairly high, say 0.5 or larger, it would be more efficient to compare net changes in baseline between two intervention groups than it would be to compare the final scores alone. Moreover empirical findings reported by Murray et al. (2000) suggest that the value of ρ estimated from a net change from baseline may be considerably smaller than that corresponding to the final score, adding further to the gain in efficiency. An extension of this strategy would be to take repeated measurements over time in each community. This was done in the REACT trial (Luepker et al. 2000), where the slope of the linear trend over time was defined as the primary end point.

Similar gains in precision may accrue from the incorporation of relevant covariates in the context of regression modelling. The gain in precision obtained by covariate adjustment can be estimated using the correlation coefficient between the outcome variable and the covariate in question. Again denoting this correlation by r, the error variance in a standard model for continuous outcome variables will be reduced by the factor $1 - r^2$, a result also holding approximately for binary outcome variables. (For multiple covariates, r is replaced by the multiple correlation coefficient R.) It is thus seen that substantial gains in efficiency beyond that formally planned for can be secured if the appropriate covariates can be identified and measured in advance.

Trials allocating only one community to an intervention group and one to a control group are still occasionally reported in the literature. The flaw in these studies is not only one of low power but the questionable validity of the design itself. This is because any effect of intervention is totally confounded with intrinsic differences that are likely to exist between the two communities, even though on face value these communities may appear to be well matched. Thus it is impossible to develop a valid significance test for evaluating the effect of intervention, similar to the difficulty that would be faced in a clinical drug trial randomizing one patient to each of two treatments. Nonetheless this design might be helpful for pilot investigations whose main aim is to examine practical issues such as the acceptability of the intended intervention.

Once the appropriate sample size has been selected using statistical considerations, there remains the practical problem of ensuring that recruitment targets can actually be met. Shadish (2002) points out that this can be a particularly difficult challenge when researchers have had no previous experience with the communities to be enrolled, and cautions in this case that it is particularly important to conduct a pre-study survey that attempts to locate and count potential participants. This advice reflects continuing discussion in the literature that large-scale community-based intervention trials are sometimes launched without performing adequate feasibility studies of the complex intervention components and measurement instruments that tend to characterize these studies. An excellent example of how comprehensive feasibility studies can be used effectively in the planning stages of a large-scale community-based trial is given in a series of articles that describes the pilot phase of the Pathways obesity prevention study (Caballero et al. 2003) (Box 5.8.2).

Analysis strategies in community-based intervention trials

Basic methods of analysis

There are now many statistical procedures with an array of underlying assumptions that can be used to analyse data arising from cluster randomization trials. In this section we provide a limited discussion of some of these procedures. This will be done

---

Box 5.8.2 Common pitfalls in sample size estimation

1. Over-optimistic expectations regarding the anticipated effect size.

2. Failure to understand the relative roles of number of clusters enrolled versus average cluster size on trial power.

3. Interpreting values of the intraclass correlation (ICC) close to zero as ignorable for the purpose of sample size estimation.

4. Failure to do a sensitivity analysis with respect to the impact of the ICC on study power.

5. Failure to account for possible loss to follow-up and non-compliance at both the individual and cluster level.

---

separately for completely randomized, matched pair, and stratified designs.

Underlying this discussion are some fundamental principles that apply to most comparative trials. The first of these is that the 'intent-to-treat' approach will be used for the primary analyses, implying that all subjects will be counted in the group to which they have been assigned and that outcome data on all subjects will be included in the analyses. In the context of community-based trials, this implies that once a cluster has been randomized, it must be retained in the allocated intervention group. Thus, the intent-to-treat principle provides a 'real-world' assessment of the effectiveness of an intervention rather than an 'efficacy' assessment reflecting optimal conditions. However, secondary analyses in which certain clusters or cluster members are not counted can be particularly useful for either strengthening the trial conclusions or suggesting that caution be used in their interpretation.

To ensure that the final evaluation of intervention effect is not subject to bias, every effort should be made to obtain outcome data on subjects who, because of refusal or other factors, become characterized as 'dropouts'. Since in spite of an investigator's best efforts outcomes on some subjects will inevitably remain missing, satisfactory methods must be used to handle this problem, as reviewed, for example, by Shadish (2002). These include relatively simple methods of imputation, where a missing data point is replaced by the mean of the remaining observations to more sophisticated methods of multiple imputation (Little and Schenker 1995). A difficulty unique to community randomized trials is that entire clusters may be lost, in which case imputation at the analysis stage is generally not an alternative. Instead every effort must be made in the planning stages of the trial to motivate key decision-makers in each community to undertake all reasonable efforts to prevent a community from suspending their participation in the trial.

In some trials it has been the custom to perform a 'modified intent-to-treat analysis' in which certain subjects are removed on the grounds that treatment-related bias is highly unlikely, while statistical power will be improved. For example, in vaccine trials it is common to remove subjects who fail to receive even a single injection of the vaccine assigned. In this case it is always prudent to perform a secondary analysis that includes all subjects randomized.

The completely randomized and stratified designs

If a completely randomized design is adopted, k clusters (communities) are randomized to each of two groups, usually with a binary or continuous variable chosen as the primary outcome measure. In this case the simplest and perhaps most intuitive approach to the analysis would be to adjust standard procedures such as the chi-square test (for comparing proportions) or the t-test (for comparing means) to account for clustering effects.

We illustrate this approach by considering the comparison of proportions in a completely randomized design. A detailed description of methods for comparing both means and proportions in cluster randomized trials, including examples of all procedures discussed in this section, is given by Donner and Klar (2000, chapters 5–6).

Let m_{ij} denote the size of the jth community assigned to the ith group, $i = 1, 2; j = 1, 2 \ldots, k$, with $M_i = \sum_{j=1}^{k_i} m_{ij}$ denoting the total number of subjects in group i, and $\hat{P}_i$ denoting the corresponding value of the overall event rate in this group. Then the standard Pearson chi-square statistic with one degree of freedom may be written as $x_P^2 = \dfrac{\sum\limits_{i=1}^{2} M_i \left(\hat{P}_i - \hat{P}\right)^2}{\hat{P}\left(1 - \hat{P}\right)}$. However, application of this statistic to clustered data is invalid since the assumption of statistical independence required to ensure the validity of this test will be violated. In particular, the effect of applying x_P^2 to data arising from a cluster randomized trial will, in general, lead to an elevated type I error, implying that intervention effects declared as statistically significant may in fact not be significant if correctly evaluated.

Appropriate adjustment of x_P^2 for clustering effects requires an estimate of the underlying intracluster correlation coefficient ρ, which, under the null hypothesis of no intervention effect, may be assumed to be constant across intervention groups. The required estimate may be obtained by pooling the observations in both groups and then applying the 'analysis of variance approach' described by Donner and Klar (1994 and 2000, chapter 6). Let MSC and MSW denote the pooled mean square errors between and within groups, respectively. Then defining $\bar{m}_{Ai} = \sum\limits_{j=1}^{k_i} m_{ij}^2 / M_i$, we obtain:

$$\hat{\rho} = \left(MSC - MSW\right)/\left(MSC + \left[m_0 - 1\right]MSW\right),$$

where:

$$MSC = \sum_{i=1}^{2}\sum_{j=1}^{k} m_{ij}\left(\hat{P}_{ij} - \hat{P}_i\right)^2 \Big/ (k-2)$$

$$MSW = \sum_{i=1}^{2}\sum_{j=1}^{k_i} m_{ij}\hat{P}_{ij}\left(1 - \hat{P}_{ij}\right)\Big/ (M-k)$$

and $m_0 = \left[M - \sum\limits_{i=1}^{2}\bar{m}_{Ai}\right]\Big/(k-2)$.

The value of x_P^2 is then adjusted by applying a correction factor which depends on both $\hat{\rho}$ and the values of the m_{ij}. Letting $C_i = 1 + \left(\bar{m}_{Ai}\right)\hat{\rho}$, the adjusted chi-square statistic with one degree of freedom is given by $x_A^2 = \sum\limits_{i=1}^{2} \dfrac{M_i\left(\hat{P}_i - \hat{P}\right)^2}{C_i \hat{P}\left(1 - \hat{P}\right)}$.

At $\hat{\rho} = 0$ $(C_1 = C_2 = 1)$, it is clear that x_A^2 reduces to x_P^2, while if all clusters are of the same size m, it reduces to $x_P^2/[1+(m-1)\hat{\rho}]$.

As mentioned in the section 'Impact of the intracluster correlation', values of $\hat{\rho}$ computed as negative are usually truncated at zero, since negative clustering effects tend to be regarded as implausible in cluster randomization trials. It follows in this case that standard methods of statistical analysis may be applied to the trial data.

It is worth noting that the validity of this approach does not require the assumption that the correlation ρ between any two observations in the same cluster is constant (an assumption which in any case would be particularly dubious in the context of trials randomizing entire communities). Rather the only requirement

in this regard is that the average value of ρ is reasonably constant from cluster to cluster.

However, application of the statistic x_A^2 does require that the total number of clusters is sufficiently large to allow ρ to be estimated to a reasonable degree of accuracy. Thus for trials enrolling fewer than ten clusters per group, as is the case in many community-based studies, it may be preferable to restrict analyses to the cluster level, for example, by applying the standard two-sample t-test to comparing the mean event rates in the two groups. Although the required assumptions of normality and homogeneous variance for this procedure are clearly violated, particularly in the presence of variable cluster sizes, there is considerable evidence that the t-test is remarkably robust to such violations (e.g. Donner and Klar 1996).

An alternative is to apply nonparametric procedures such as the Wilcoxon rank sum test or Fisher's two-sample permutation procedure. While the Wilcoxon procedure is computationally simpler, the permutation test uses the actual values of the observed event rates rather than their ranks and therefore tends to be more powerful. Exact statistical inferences for these procedures can be conducted using programs such as Proc-StatXact® (Mehta and Patel 1997). However it is useful to note that both procedures require at least four clusters per group in order to achieve statistical significance at $p < 0.05$, reflecting their relatively weak power.

It is well known that the interpretation of results from any comparative trial is enhanced by their presentation in terms of confidence limits. Following the approach above, an approximate two-sided 95 per cent confidence interval about a difference in proportions may be readily obtained as:

$$\left(\hat{P}_1 - \hat{P}_2\right) \pm 1.96\sqrt{\frac{C_1 P_1\left(1 - P_1\right)}{M_1} + \frac{C_2 P_2\left(1 - P_2\right)}{M_2}}.$$

At $\hat{\rho} = 0$, $(C_1 = C_2 = 1)$, this expression reduces to the standard confidence interval about a difference between two proportions. However, the assumption of a common intracluster correlation coefficient, although guaranteed under the null hypothesis of no intervention effect, may not be appropriate for confidence interval construction. In this case separate estimates of ρ may be used in computing the variance inflation factors C_1 and C_2.

Since the stratified design may be viewed as a replication of the completely randomized design, straightforward extensions of the latter may be used to account for both stratification and clustering effects. For binary outcomes, Donner (1998) and Donner and Klar (2000, chapter 6) have shown how the well-known Mantel–Haenszel test for combining several two-by-two contingency tables may be applied to a stratified cluster randomized design (Mantel and Haenszel 1959). For continuous outcome measures, a weighted t-test procedure may be used, as described by Donner and Klar (2000, chapter 7).

As is the case for the completely randomized design, a stratified permutation test may be applied to this design when the number of clusters is small, as implemented using programs such as Proc-StatXact®. An example is given by Duan et al. (2000), who used this procedure to analyse data obtained from a church-based telephone-counselling trial, where the stratification factors were church characteristics thought to be strong predictors of the primary outcome variable.

In non-randomized community-based trials, the assumption of a common ρ may not be reasonable, although simulation studies performed by Jung et al. (2001) suggest that moderate differences in the value of ρ from group to group will only slightly disturb the properties of x_A^2. The ratio estimator approach, frequently used in the field of survey sampling (Rao and Scott 1992), requires no assumptions concerning the intracluster correlation coefficient and therefore may be preferred to x_A^2 in trials that have not employed random allocation. However, a practical disadvantage of this procedure is that it requires many more clusters per group (at least 20) to ensure its validity (Donner et al. 1994).

The matched-pair design

In a matched-pair design the intervention of interest is randomly assigned to one community within a pair (stratum), with the remaining community acting as a control. Since a measure of between-cluster variation is not directly available from the communities within a pair, the test of intervention effect is typically performed using cluster-level procedures such as the paired (one-sample) t-test, in which the error variance is estimated using between-stratum information.

This procedure is natural for testing the effect of intervention on a continuous outcome measure, where it is applied to the differences $d_j, j = 1, 2, \ldots k$, between the two means in the jth stratum, $j = 1, 2, \ldots k$. However it is also frequently used in the case of a binary outcome measure, since, as in the case of the two-sample t-test, research has shown (e.g. Gail et al. 1996) that the paired t-test is very robust to departures from the underlying assumption that the d_j are normally distributed with constant variance.

Let $d_j, j = 1, 2, \ldots k$, denote the difference in means or proportions in the jth stratum, with mean $\bar{d} = \sum_{j=1}^{k_i} d_j / k$ and variance $S_d^2 = \sum_{j=1}^{k_i} (d_j - \bar{d})^2 / (k-1)$. Then the paired t-statistic is given by $tp = (\bar{d}\sqrt{k}) / S_d$ with $(k-1)$ degrees of freedom.

This procedure was used to test for the effect of intervention in the community-based trial described in the section 'The attraction of pair-matching as a design strategy' that was designed to reduce the rate of HIV (Grosskurth et al. 1995). After transforming the observed HIV rates to the logarithmic scale to improve normality, the precision of the analysis was further improved by defining the primary end point as the difference between the baseline rate and the observed 2-year rate.

Some investigators avoid the need to make modelling assumptions in the analysis of data obtained from a matched-pair design by alternatively applying either the Wilcoxon signed rank test or Fisher's one-sample permutation test. Exact inferences for these procedures may again be obtained using Proc-StatXact®. However both procedures require at least six pairs in order to achieve statistical significance at $p < 0.05$.

Adjusting for covariates

The section 'Pair-matching and stratification' discusses how design-based strategies can be used to control for the influence of cluster-level covariates. An alternative is to adjust for both cluster-level and individual-level covariates in the statistical analysis using regression modelling. Although adjustment for aggregated versions of individual-level covariates can be achieved at the design stage (e.g. stratification by percentage of residents with high school education), statistical adjustment at the individual level for that covariate may bring greater efficiency as well as ease of interpretation due to the absence of the well-known

'ecological fallacy'. Moreover, since the likelihood of chance imbalance on any given covariate in a cluster randomized trial is greater than in an individually randomized trial enrolling the same number of individuals, regression modelling procedures may be essential for avoiding chance confounding. However, this is only possible if those covariates expected to have a strong relationship to outcome are measured at baseline. For example, Alexander et al. (1989) describe how failure to obtain baseline measures of socioeconomic status in a community-based breast cancer screening trial led to severe problems of interpretation.

Although standard modelling procedures such as multiple linear regression (for continuous outcomes) and multiple logistic regression (for binary outcomes) will yield valid estimates of regression coefficients in the presence of clustering effects, their associated standard errors will be underestimated, possibly leading to spurious statistical significance. We now discuss extensions of these procedures that may be used to account for these effects.

The completely randomized and stratified designs

An approach that has now become standard for the control of either cluster-level or individual-level covariates in a completely randomized cluster randomized trial having a continuous outcome measure is mixed effects regression modelling, as discussed by Donner and Klar (2000, chapter 7). The term 'mixed' in this expression arises because the model contains terms representing the fixed effect of intervention as well as random effects representing cluster effects and random error terms. Also referred to as either a two-stage nested or a repeated measures analysis of variance model, it may be written as

$$Y_{ijl} = \mu + G_i + V_{ij} + e_{ijl}, \ i = 1,2; j = 1,2\ldots,k_i; l = 1,2,\ldots,m_{ij} \quad (5.8.1)$$

The terms in this model include μ, the population mean response, and G_i, a constant representing the fixed effect of intervention group i ($i = 1,2$). Two random effects are also included in the model. Random cluster effects, denoted by V_{ij}, are assumed to be normally distributed with mean 0 and variance σ_A^2, that is, $V_{ij} \sim N(0, \sigma_A^2)$, while the remaining random error variation is modelled by assuming $e_{ijl} \sim N(0, \sigma_W^2)$.

The assumption that the cluster effects can be modelled as random variables implies that communities are theoretically obtained as a random sample from a well-defined population. This assumption is sometimes formally realized, as it was in the HIV prevention trial discussed in the section 'The attraction of pair-matching as a design strategy'. However, structured sampling schemes in which communities are selected at random are often not realistic. Indeed, as discussed in the section 'Ensuring the power is adequate', they may be selected instead with the express purpose of reducing between-cluster variability. In this case, the generalizabilty of the results on a wider scale must rest largely on non-statistical factors, including judgement and past experience.

Maximum likelihood estimates of the intervention effect, adjusted for the influence of covariates, may be obtained in practice using the SAS® procedure PROC MIXED. Stratification effects representing factors such as cluster size and geographic area can be easily added to the model given by Equation 5.8.1 by suitably incorporating indicator variables.

A more complicated model is required if multiple outcome measurements are obtained after baseline and it is of interest to test if the time course of changes in the intervention communities differs from that in the control communities. Such an analysis may be of particular interest for examining the mechanism of action over time induced by an intervention. This approach was adopted by Resnicow et al. (2001), who evaluated a multicomponent intervention designed to increase fruit and vegetable consumption among African Americans as delivered through black churches.

Further discussion of such models, which require treatment-by-interaction terms to be added to Equation 5.8.1, is given by Koepsell et al. (1991).

For binary outcome measures, two main approaches tend to be used. The first is that of generalized estimating equations (GEE), developed by Liang and Zeger (1986), which leads to an extension of standard logistic regression that adjusts for clustering effects. The most common strategy used for this purpose is 'robust variance estimation,' which implies that random sources of variability are estimated using between-cluster information, yielding what is often called the 'sandwich' estimator of variance. An attractive feature of this strategy is that although the within-cluster correlation structure must be specified in advance (the 'working correlation matrix'), subsequent statistical inferences will be valid even if this correlation structure is misspecified. The most common working correlation structure specified for cluster randomization trials is 'exchangeable,' implying that the correlation between any two responses in the same cluster is identical.

As a consequence of this property, the validity of robust variance GEE is assured only if the number of clusters is fairly large. However, the minimum number of clusters required depends on many factors, including the cluster sizes and the number of covariates in the model, although research suggests that this figure ranges between 20 and 40 (e.g. Feng et al. 1996; Pan and Wall 2002). Although several small-sample adjustments to robust variance GEE have been proposed in the statistical literature (e.g. Mancl and DeRoune 2001; Pan and Wall 2002), further research is required to assess their effectiveness under a wide range of practical settings. Therefore, as discussed by Murray et al. (2004), this greatly hampers the application of GEE to all but the largest community-based intervention trials.

The use of a 'model-based' estimator of variance rather than a robust variance estimator will allow inferences using GEE to be valid in samples of much smaller size. This desirable property arises since the resulting standard errors are now based on an assumed within-cluster correlation structure rather than on between-cluster variation. However, it is clear that in a trial randomizing moderately sized communities, it would be very difficult to specify any particular correlation structure in advance, with the consequent risk of bias in the estimation of standard errors. Thus robust variance estimators, sometimes referred to as 'sandwich estimators', are much more widely applied than model-based estimators, in spite of their reduced efficiency and unreliability in small samples.

The GEE approach may be characterized as 'population-averaged' in that it measures the expected ('marginal') change in a response over all clusters as the value of the covariate increases by one unit. Thus the regression coefficient estimating the effect of intervention estimates the difference in the expected response for subjects in the experimental communities as compared to subjects in the control communities, an interpretation similar to that for standard logistic regression. This is in contrast to an approach based on random effects or 'cluster-specific' models, which are characterized by the inclusion of parameters that are specific to each cluster, and which allows them to measure the expected change in response within a cluster as the value of a covariate increases by unit. Perhaps the most commonly used such model is the logistic-normal, which can be viewed as a standard logistic regression model with a normally distributed random effect. The interpretation of the resulting regression coefficients is then conditional on these effects. Unlike GEE, implementation of this procedure requires data that provides more than one observation per cluster.

Both population-averaged and random effects approaches can now be implemented using the SAS® procedures GENMOD and GLIMMIX, respectively, with analogous procedures available in Stata®. Although these approaches estimate the same population parameters when the outcome variable is normally distributed, this equivalence disappears in the case of a binary outcome variable, and thus their interpretation is different. As pointed out by Neuhaus (1992), interpretation of estimated covariate effects obtained from random effects models may be difficult when the covariate is defined at the cluster level, that is, takes on identical values within a cluster. This problem is most notable in cluster randomization trials, since the covariate of main interest tends to be the cluster-level intervention effect. Interpretation of such an effect using a cluster-specific model must formally rely on the notion of a subject within a given cluster changing his or her intervention status, clearly a non-observable event. This inability to provide internal validation has led Neuhaus (1992) to remark that random effects models are most suitable for testing the effect of covariates that vary within clusters (e.g. subject age or gender), while population-averaged models such as GEE are preferable for testing the effect of cluster-level covariates such as intervention status. However, it must also be noted that the differences between the two approaches disappear as the intracluster correlation coefficient approaches zero, and that more empirical work is needed to compare the advantages and disadvantages of the two approaches in practice. As pointed out by Omar and Thompson (2000), one advantage of the cluster-specific approach is that it provides direct estimates of variance components, and hence the intracluster correlation coefficient, quantities which are treated as nuisance parameters using the population-averaged approach. Moreover, it can also be extended to provide estimates of variance components at each of the multiple levels of clustering that arise in a natural hierarchy, such as villages selected from countries, or classrooms selected from schools that were in turn sampled from school districts. Some evidence also exists (e.g. Bellamy et al. 2000) that the logistic-modelling procedure performs better than GEE when the number of clusters is relatively small. However, the basic problem remains that clustering effects cannot be accurately estimated in this case, and thus the application of either approach to the adjustment of covariates in community-based intervention trials enrolling only a few communities is unfortunately limited in scope. An excellent non-technical discussion of the distinction between population-averaged and random effects models is given by Hanley et al. (2003).

The matched-pair design

A fairly simple but very general method that can be applied to incorporate the effect of covariates in a matched-pair design with a binary outcome variable has been described in the context of the COMMIT trial by Gail et al. (1992). The first step is to fit a multiple logistic regression model to the trial outcome data that contains the cluster-level and individual-level covariates of interest but which omits the variable representing intervention status. For each cluster the difference between the observed success rate and the expected success rate based on this 'null' model can be calculated by summing expectations over all individuals in the cluster. Then one can perform a paired *t*-test or one-sample permutation test on these residuals to test the null hypothesis of no intervention effect that takes into account the covariates at the first step. An analogous approach using multiple linear regression rather than multiple logistic regression may be used for the case of a continuous outcome variable.

While this approach may be used to control for the effect of both cluster-level and continuous-level covariates, it does not allow assessment of the independent effect of individual-level covariates on outcome. Such an assessment may be of interest when a secondary objective of the trial is to test the effect of covariates such as age or baseline blood pressure on outcome. Although aggregated versions of such covariates, such as mean baseline blood pressure, may be easily modelled at the cluster level using standard methods, modelling at the individual level may be of more direct interest. However, owing to the difficulty in estimating ρ this objective cannot be accomplished in a matched-pair design without making special assumptions.

One option available to investigators in this case is to break the matches and then perform a mixed model regression analysis as described in the section 'The completely randomized and stratified designs'. However, a theoretical objection to this strategy may be raised when both the outcome variable and the covariate(s) of interest vary with the remaining stratum effects, since the effect of such residual confounding may lead to an elevated type I error. Donner et al. (2007) have shown that this problem may indeed arise when a large number of small clusters are randomized. However, when a relatively small number of large clusters are randomized, as is the case in most community-based trials, the resulting test of significance for the independent effect of an individual-level covariate will in fact hold its significance level after the matches are broken. One caveat is that these results are restricted to the case of a continuous outcome variable and a single individual-level covariate, with the case of binary and multiple covariates requiring further research (Box 5.8.3).

Cohort versus cross-sectional designs

There has been considerable discussion in the literature as to the relative advantages of cohort versus cross-sectional designs for evaluating the effect of a community-based intervention. With the cohort approach, each individual is followed up over time, while for the cross-sectional design, different groups of individuals are independently sampled and assessed at each of several time periods. The former design is generally more powerful from a statistical perspective, since it permits an analysis that controls for individual baseline values, thus yielding a more precise estimate of the

---

Box 5.8.3 Common pitfalls in analysis

1. Indiscriminate use of relatively complicated multivariable methods without preliminary analysis of the data.
2. Application of generalized estimation equations or logistic-normal regression to trials enrolling fewer than 20 clusters.
3. Failure to recognize the relationship between mixed model regression and multilevel modelling.
4. Failure to appreciate the full efficiency of a cluster level analysis for a quantitative outcome variable when cluster sizes are equal.

---

intervention effect. This is not possible in cross-sectional designs, where covariate adjustment is restricted to cluster level summary measures. However, this theoretical advantage of a cohort design must be weighed against the risk of loss to follow-up that arises in any longitudinal study. If the loss to follow-up is different across intervention groups, the final estimate of intervention effect may be subject to substantial bias. Moreover, there may be substantial losses of efficiency relative to a cross-sectional design even when the subject attrition is unrelated to treatment assignment. Other disadvantages of the cohort design, as reviewed by Atienza and King (2002), include a loss of representativeness of the target population related to the ageing of the cohort, and 'learning effects' that may result from repeated assessments on the same individual.

From a conceptual perspective, the choice of design must also be considered in the light of how the primary question of scientific interest is posed. Thus if interest focuses mainly on change at the broader community level, cross-sectional designs may be the more natural choice while cohort designs may be more natural if change at the individual level is of most interest. Further discussion may be found in Feldman and McKinlay (1994).

Ethical issues in the design of community-based trials

Issues involving the need for informed consent

Guidelines for informed consent and other ethical issues are now well established for individually randomized clinical trials. Some of these guidelines apply to cluster randomized trials as well, such as the need for control group subjects to receive at least the current standard of local care and to be eligible to receive the new intervention on termination of the trial if it has been shown to be safe and effective. However, since the historical basis for such guidelines lies in the relationship between physician and patient, their direct application to cluster randomization trials, and community-based trials in particular, has proved to be controversial. As a result, ethical standards for such trials remain in the formative stage.

From this perspective, a distinctive feature of cluster randomized trials is that two levels of informed consent (and sometimes more) must be considered, one at the cluster level and one at the individual level. The first level of consent is generally provided by a key decision-maker such as a mayor or school principal on behalf of his/her constituents prior to randomization. In relatively small trials it also may be possible to obtain informed consent at the individual level prior to randomization. However, in many trials recruitment must instead be done prospectively after randomization due to an inability to identify all eligible subjects prior to randomization. In this case the development of appropriate consent procedures will be more complicated, since it involves consent to be followed up under a treatment regimen that has already been assigned. Post-randomization consent not only raises difficult ethical issues, but also the possibility of selection bias as discussed in the section 'Subsampling and the risk of selection bias'. Further complications arise when it is difficult or even impossible for a subject to withdraw from the study, as in the village-randomized trial described by Hutton (2001) that evaluated the efficacy of an insecticide spray.

Feasibility considerations alone will often present formidable obstacles to securing individual-level informed consent in community-based trials, as in trials that promote lifestyle changes through the media. In this case, where the intervention could be perceived as relatively benign, there may be little objection to the failure to secure informed consent at the individual level. Indeed the unawareness of the intervention programme on the part of community residents may in fact be perceived as a methodological strength of the study (Hutton 2001). However, more urgent challenges in securing informed consent may arise when relatively intrusive interventions are delivered, as in the case of trials delivering water fluoridation to all households in a community. In case of doubt, it seems reasonable to leave the decision to obtain informed consent to an independent committee, such as an Institutional Review Board (IRB). Unfortunately this solution may not always be straightforward, as most IRB guidelines do not distinguish clearly between consent at different levels.

A distinction made by Edwards et al. (1999) may be useful in clarifying these issues. These authors classify cluster randomization trials as either 'cluster-cluster' or as 'individual-cluster', depending on how the intervention is delivered. Thus in a cluster-cluster trial, the intervention is targeted at the entire community, as in the examples above, and it is difficult (although perhaps not impossible) for individuals to avoid. In this case, it may be argued that a 'guardian' or 'gatekeeper', such as a mayor or public health official, must not only provide permission for their cluster to be randomized, but should also sign a consent form clearly setting out the government's duties for safeguarding its constituents' interests. This approach can be seen to be consistent with guidelines for community-based research published by the World Health Organization and the Council for International Organizations of Medical Sciences (CIOMS 1993). However, other approaches have also been proposed, such as sampling the views of individual selected from the community (Eldridge et al. 2005). This approach might be particularly attractive when the decision-maker may not necessarily be a recipient of the intervention or may have special interest in the trial results (Hutton 2001). Further discussion of the role of gatekeepers in cluster randomization trials may be found in Gallo et al. (2012).

McRae et al. (2011) have set out a framework for addressing issues of informed consent in cluster randomized trials based on moral considerations and international regulatory provisions. They conclude that informed consent may not need to be secured if subjects cannot be approached at the time of randomization. However when potential subjects are approached after randomization, 'they must be provided with a detailed description of the interventions in the trial arm to which their clusters have been randomized; detailed information on interventions in other arms need not be provided'.

Cluster-cluster trials differ from individual-cluster trials in that for the latter it is possible to secure consent on an individual basis. As an example, a community-based prevention trial evaluating the effect of a new vaccine could allow any one individual the autonomy to accept or decline the intervention. Securing informed consent at the individual level should also be feasible in many health education trials and in trials administering supplementation by nutrients such as vitamin A, where the issues are very similar to those that arise in individually randomized trials. However for trials conducted in developing countries, it is recognized that procedures for securing such consent may vary somewhat depending on norms peculiar to the local setting (Hayes 1998).

The need for trial monitoring

It is largely ethical concerns that motivate the need for trial monitoring and interim analyses in individually randomized clinical trials. Thus data-dependent stopping plans, such as that proposed by O'Brien and Fleming (1979), have proved very helpful to researchers when termination of a study must be considered when one treatment shows unexpected early evidence of superior efficacy. The opportunity for early termination is particularly important for long-term trials having outcomes such as serious morbidity or mortality. However, it is interesting to note that cluster randomized trials in general, and community-based trials in particular, have not usually adopted formal procedures for trial monitoring. In some instances this may be due to the belief that unexpected early harm or benefit is unlikely given the nature of the interventions compared. Although this may be the case for some interventions, such as those designed to influence behavioural change, there are clearly many exceptions, as in long-term trials evaluating the effect of nutritional supplements such as vitamin A on child mortality.

A second reason for the failure to adopt formal stopping rules in cluster randomized trials is that the theory underlying the most frequently adopted plans has invariably assumed individual randomization. However, Zou et al. (2005) have recently shown that the most commonly adopted such plans may also be applied to cluster randomization trials with little difficulty. For trials that recruit communities prospectively, Lake et al. (2002) have also shown how an interim analysis of accumulating data can be used to re-estimate parameters such as the intracluster correlation coefficient, and hence ensure that the final trial power is of adequate size.

Reporting of results

Many of the reporting guidelines for community-based randomized trials are similar to those for cluster randomized trials in general, as discussed by Donner and Klar (2000, chapter 9) and by Campbell et al. (2004). A major contribution provided by the latter authors is an extension of the Consolidation of Standards for Reporting of Trials (CONSORT) Statement, developed over a decade ago as a template for reporting the results of individually randomized trials (Begg et al. 1996). A key element of CONSORT is a flow chart providing the number of subjects enrolled at each stage of randomization.

Some reporting guidelines have special relevance for community-based trials. For example, it was mentioned in the section 'The completely randomized and stratified designs' that the communities participating in a trial are rarely selected at random from a larger population of communities, with the risk of questions arising as to the likely generalizability of the conclusions (external validity). However, some understanding of this issue may be obtained by listing the number and characteristics of those communities that met the trial eligibility criteria but declined to participate. Similar reporting guidelines apply at the individual level if a subsampling strategy has been used to select residents within a community

The interventions evaluated in many community-based trials are frequently complex, with many components. This has led to a debate in the literature as to whether it should be the 'function and process' of the intervention that should be standardized rather than its specific components, thus allowing flexibility in its tailoring to the prevailing local conditions (Hawe et al. 2004). However, in either case, it is incumbent on investigators to adequately describe the content of the intervention as it is actually delivered, whether administered directly to individual subjects or implemented solely at the community level. This again allows the reader to more easily generalize the results as well as facilitating its application by policymakers.

With respect to the randomization procedure, both the timing and the method used should be described in the context of the selected design. For stratified designs, the number of communities in each combination of intervention group and stratum should be reported.

The first table in a publication reporting the results of an individually randomized trial is usually a description of baseline characteristics in the two intervention groups. In cluster randomization trials, two such descriptions are required, one at the cluster level, for characteristics such as size, geographic location, and so on, and the other at the individual level, with emphasis in both cases on those characteristics likely to be related to outcome.

The use of significance tests for comparing baseline characteristics in individually randomized trials is now widely discouraged, since under a properly executed randomization scheme the source of any observed baseline difference cannot be other than chance (e.g. Senn 1994). The problem will be compounded in community-based trials if these tests are performed without adjustment for clustering effects, since then the obtained p-values will be spuriously low. In any case, it should be the magnitude of such differences rather than their statistical significance that should be used to decide if covariate adjustment is required.

If experimental contamination can be regarded as a potential source of bias, a description of the steps taken to minimize this problem can allow a reader to judge its likely impact. For example, Grosskurth et al. (1995) describe how data on place of residence was used to track patterns of migration across communities in the HIV prevention trial described in the section 'The attraction of pair-matching as a design strategy'.

Differential loss to follow-up across intervention groups can be a threat to the internal validity of any trial. Therefore the reasons for such attrition, at both the cluster and individual level, should be provided. Reporting the overall individual loss to follow-up rate separately by cluster is also useful, since it allows the reader to

---

Box 5.8.4 Common pitfalls in reporting

1. Failure to describe the nature of the intervention in detail.
2. Failure to describe eligibility criteria at both the individual and cluster level.
3. Failure to present baseline characteristics by treatment group separately for individual level and cluster level characteristics.
4. Failure to report the observed value of the intracluster correlation coefficient or coefficient of variation.

---

understand if these losses are concentrated in communities having particular characteristics.

Since an assessment of between-cluster variation is crucial for sample size estimation, failure of investigators to report estimated values of the intracluster correlation coefficient handicaps the design of future trials in the same subject matter area. As mentioned in the section 'Ensuring the power is adequate', the magnitude of this problem has declined considerably over the last 15 years. However, a review of cluster randomization trials published from 1998 to 2002 indicates that there is still considerable room for improvement (Varnell et al. 2004).

Campbell et al. (2007) have reviewed the rapidly growing methodology available for handling clustering effects in both the sample size calculations and the analysis. Given the relative unfamiliarity of these methods, it is incumbent on authors to provide a clear statement of the procedures adopted, and, where appropriate, to provide accessible references (Box 5.8.4).

Conclusion

Despite the growing literature advising investigators on appropriate methodology, many community-based trials continue to be improperly designed and analysed. For example, failure to account for clustering effects at each of these stages can lead to serious problems of interpretation. Thus trials which fail to account for such effects in the assessment of sample size may fail to detect intervention effects having public health importance while those which fail to account for these effects in the analysis are prone to report spurious statistical significance.

We have also discussed issues related to the choice of design for studies randomizing intact communities, as well as the unique analytical and ethical issues that may emanate from this choice. More generally we have attempted to provide investigators with a better understanding of the many challenges involved in conducting a community-based trial and with guidelines for meeting these challenges.

Key points

- Clearly specify the unit of inference for the trial in terms of the stated objectives.
- Avoid the risk of selection bias if individuals are subsampled from communities.
- Be aware of the advantages and disadvantages of the completely randomized, pair-matched, and stratified designs.

◆ Ensure that the assessment of sample size and the approach to the statistical analysis adequately account for clustering effects.

◆ Use the CONSORT statement for cluster randomized trials as a guide to reporting trial results.

References

Alexander, F., Roberts, M.M., Lutz, W., and Hepburn, W. (1989). Randomization by cluster and the problem of social class bias. *Journal of Epidemiology and Community Health*, 43, 29–36.

Agarwal, G.G., Awasthi, S., and Walter, S.D. (2005). Intra-class correlation estimates for assessment of vitamin A intake in children. *Journal of Health, Population and Nutrition*, 23, 66–73.

Althabe, F., Belizan, J.M., Villar, J., et al. (2004). The Latin-American cluster randomized controlled trial of mandatory second opinion for the reduction of unnecessary caesarean sections. *The Lancet*, 363, 1934–40.

Atienza, A.A. and King, A.C. (2002). Community-based health intervention trials: an overview of methodological issues. *Epidemiologic Reviews*, 24, 72–79.

Begg, C., Cho, M., Eastwood, S., et al. (1996). Improving the quality of reporting of randomized controlled trials, the CONSORT statement. *Journal of the American Medical Association*, 276, 637–9.

Bellamy, S.L., Gibberd, R., Hancock, L., et al. (2000). Analysis of dichotomous outcome data for community intervention studies. *Statistical Methods in Medical Research*, 9, 135–59.

Biglan, A., Ary, D., and Wagenaar, A.C. (2000). The value of interrupted time-series experiments for community intervention research, *Prevention Science*, 1, 31–49.

Byar, D. (1988). The design of cancer prevention trials. *Recent Results in Cancer Research*, 111, 34–48.

Caballero, B., Clay, T., Davis, S.M., et al., for the Pathways Study Research Group (2003). Pathways: a school-based, randomized controlled trial for the prevention of obesity in American Indian schoolchildren. *American Journal of Clinical Nutrition*, 78, 1030–8.

Campbell, M.J., Donner, A., and Klar, N. (2007). Developments in cluster randomized trials and *Statistics in Medicine*. *Statistics in Medicine*, 26, 2–19.

Campbell, M.K., Elbourne, D.R., and Altman, D.G. for the CONSORT Group (2004). CONSORT statement: extension to cluster randomised trials. *British Medical Journal*, 328, 702–8.

Campbell, M.K., Mollison, J., Steen, N., et al. (2000). Analysis of cluster randomized trials in primary care: a practical approach. *Family Practice*, 17, 192–6.

COMMIT Research Group (1995). Community intervention trial for smoking cessation (COMMIT): I. Cohort results from a four-year community intervention. *American Journal of Public Health*, 85, 183–92.

Cornfield, J. (1978). Randomization by group: a formal analysis. *American Journal of Epidemiology*, 108, 100–2.

Council for International Organizations of Medical Sciences (CIOMS). (1993). *International Ethical Guidelines for Biomedical Research Involving Human Subjects*. Geneva: CIOMS.

Diehr, P., Martin, D.C., Koepsell, T., and Cheadle, A. (1995). Breaking the matches in a paired *t*-test for community interventions when the number of pairs is small. *Statistics in Medicine*, 14, 1491–504.

Diwan, V.K., Wahlström, R., Tomson, G., et al. (1995). Effects of 'Group Detailing' on the prescribing of lipid-lowering drugs: a randomized controlled trial in Swedish primary care. *Journal of Clinical Epidemiology*, 48, 705–11.

Donner, A. (1998). Some aspects of the design and analysis of cluster randomization trials. *Applied Statistics*, 47, 95–114.

Donner, A., Eliasziw, M., and Klar, N. (1994). A comparison of methods for testing homogeneity of proportions in teratologic studies. *Statistics in Medicine*, 13, 1253–64.

Donner, A. and Klar, N. (1994). Methods for comparing event rates in intervention studies when the unity of allocation is a cluster. *American Journal of Epidemiology*, 140, 279–89.

Donner, A. and Klar, N. (1996). Statistical considerations in the design and analysis of community intervention trials. *Journal of Clinical Epidemiology*, 49, 435–9.

Donner, A. and Klar, N. (2000). *Design and Analysis of Cluster Randomization Trials in Health Research*. New York: Oxford University Press.

Donner, A. and Klar, N. (2004). Pitfalls of and controversies in cluster randomization trials. *American Journal of Public Health*, 94, 416–21.

Donner, A., Taljaard, M., and Klar, N. (2007). The merits of breaking the matches: a cautionary tale. *Statistics in Medicine*, 26, 2036–51.

Duan, N., Fox, S.A., Derose, K.P., and Carson, S. (2000). Maintaining mammography adherence through telephone counseling in a church-based trial. *American Journal of Public Health*, 90, 1468–71.

Duffy, S.W., Rohan, T.E., and Day, N.E. (1992). Cluster randomization in large public health trials: the importance of antecedent data. *Statistics in Medicine*, 11, 307–16.

Edwards, S.J.L., Braunholtz, D.A., Lilford, R.J., and Stevens, A.J. (1999). Ethical issues in the design and conduct of cluster randomised controlled trials. *British Medical Journal*, 318, 1407–9.

Eldridge, S.H., Ashby, D., and Feder, G.S. (2005). Informed patient consent to participation in cluster randomized trials: an empirical exploration of trials in primary care. *Clinical Trials*, 2, 91–8.

Eldridge, S.H., Ashby, D., and Kerry, S. (2006). Sample size for cluster randomized trials: effect of coefficient of variation of cluster size and analysis method. *International Journal of Epidemiology*, 35, 1292–300.

Farrin, A., Russell, I., Torgerson, D., and Underwood, M. on behalf of the UK BEAM Trial Team (2005). Differential recruitment in a cluster randomized trial in primary care: the experience of the UK Back pain, Exercise, Active management and Manipulation (UK BEAM) feasibility study. *Clinical Trials*, 2, 119–24.

Feldman, H.A. and McKinlay, S.M. (1994). Cohort versus cross-sectional design in large field trials: precision, sample size, and a unifying model. *Statistics in Medicine*, 13, 61–78.

Feng, Z., McLerran, D., and Grizzle, J. (1996). A comparison of statistical methods for clustered data analysis with Gaussian error. *Statistics in Medicine*, 15, 1793–806.

Gail, M.H., Byar, D.P., Pechacek, T.F., and Corle, D.K. (1992). Aspects of statistical design for the community intervention trial for smoking cessation (COMMIT). *Controlled Clinical Trials*, 13, 6–21.

Gail, M.H., Mark, S.D., Carroll, R.J., et al. (1996). On design considerations and randomization-based inference for community intervention trials. *Statistics in Medicine*, 15, 1069–92.

Gallo, A., Weijer, C., White, A., et al. (2012). What is the role and authority of gatekeepers in cluster randomization trials in health research? *Trials*, 13, 116–30.

Grosskurth, H., Mosha, F., Todd, J., et al. (1995). Impact of improved treatment of sexually transmitted diseases on HIV infection in rural Tanzania: randomized controlled trial. *The Lancet*, 346, 530–6.

Gulliford, M.C., Adams, G., Ukoumunne, O.C., et al. (2005). Intraclass correlation coefficient and outcome prevalence are associated in clustered binary data. *Journal of Clinical Epidemiology*, 58, 246–51.

Hanley, J.A., Negassa, A., Edwardes, M.D., and Forrester, J.E. (2003). Statistical analysis of correlated data using generalized estimating equations: an orientation. *American Journal of Epidemiology*, 157, 364–75.

Hawe, P., Shiell, A., and Riley, T. (2004). Complex interventions: how 'out of control' can a randomised controlled trial be? *British Journal of Medicine*, 328, 1561–3.

Hayes, R. (1998). Design of human immunodeficiency virus intervention trials in developing countries. *Journal of the Royal Statistical Society, Series A*, 161, 251–63.

Hayes, R.J. and Bennett, S. (1999). Simple sample size calculation for cluster-randomized trials. *International Journal of Epidemiology*, 28, 319–26.

Hussey, M.A. and Hughes, J.P. (2007). Design and analysis of stepped wedge cluster randomized trials. *Contemporary Clinical Trials*, 28, 182–91.

Hutton, J.L. (2001). Are distinctive ethical principles required for cluster randomized controlled trials? *Statistics in Medicine*, 20, 473–88.

Jooste, P.L., Yach, D., Steenkamp, H.J., et al. (1990). Drop-out and newcomer bias in a community cardiovascular follow-up study. *International Journal of Epidemiology*, 19, 284–9.

Jordhøy, M.S., Fayers, P.M., Ahlner-Elmqvist, M., and Kaasa, S. (2002). Lack of concealment may lead to selection bias in cluster randomized trials of palliative care. *Palliative Medicine*, 16, 43–9.

Jung, S., Ahn, C., and Donner, A. (2001). Evaluation of an adjusted chi-square statistic as applied to observational studies involving clustered binary data. *Statistics in Medicine*, 20, 2149–62.

Kerry, S. and Bland, J.M. (1998). Analysis of a trial randomized in clusters. *British Medical Journal*, 316, 549.

Klar, N. and Donner, A. (1997). The merits of matching in community intervention trials. *Statistics in Medicine*, 16, 1753–64.

Koepsell, T.D., Martin, D.C., Diehr, P.H., et al. (1991). Data analysis and sample size issues in evaluations of community-based health promotion and disease prevention programs; a mixed-model analysis of variance approach. *Journal of Clinical Epidemiology*, 44, 701–13.

Koepsell, T.D., Wagner, E.H., Cheadle, A.C., et al. (1992). Selected methodological issues in evaluating community-based health promotion and disease prevention programs. *Annual Review of Public Health*, 13, 31–57.

Lake, S., Kammann, E., Klar, N., and Betensky, R. (2002). Sample size re-estimation in cluster randomized trials. *Statistics in Medicine*, 21, 1337–50.

LaPrelle, J., Bauman, K.E., and Koch, G.C. (1992). High intercommunity variation in adolescent cigarette smoking in a 10-community field experiment. *Evaluation Review*, 16, 115–30.

Lewsey, J.D. (2004). Comparing completely and stratified randomized designs in cluster randomized trials when the stratifying factor is cluster size: a simulation study. *Statistics in Medicine*, 23, 897–905.

Liang, K.-Y. and Zeger, S.L. (1986). Longitudinal data analysis using generalized linear models. *Biometrika*, 73, 13–22.

Little, R.J. and Schenker, N. (1995). Missing data. In G. Arminger, C.C. Clogg, and M.E. Sobel (eds.) *Handbook of Statistical Modeling for the Social and Behavioral Sciences*, pp. 39–75. New York: Plenum Press.

Luepker, R.V., Raczynski, J.M., Osganian, S., et al. (2000). Effect of a community intervention on patient delay and emergency medical service use in acute coronary heart disease: The Rapid Early Action for Coronary Treatment (REACT) Trial. *JAMA*, 284, 60–7.

Manatunga, A.K. and Hudgens, M.G. (2001). Sample size estimation in cluster randomized studies with varying cluster size. *Biometrical Journal*, 43, 75–86.

Mancl, L. and De Rouen, T.A. (2001). A covariance estimator for GEE with improved small sample properties. *Statistics in Medicine*, 57, 126–34.

Mantel, N. and Haenszel, W. (1959). Statistical aspects of the analysis of data from retrospective studies of disease. *Journal of the National Cancer Institute*, 22, 719–48.

Martin, D.C., Diehr, P., Perrin, E.B., and Koepsell, T.D. (1993). The effect of matching on the power of randomized community intervention studies. *Statistics in Medicine*, 12, 329–38.

McRae, A.D., Weijer, C., Bink, A., et al. (2011). When is informed consent required in cluster randomized trials in health research? *Trials*, 12, 202.

Mehta, C. and Patel, N. (1997). *Proc-StatXact for SAS Users, Statistical Software for Exact Nonparametric Inference User Manual*. Cambridge, MA: CYTEL Software Corporation.

Moulton, L.H., O'Brien, K.L., Kohberger, R., et al. (2001). Design of a group-randomized Streptococcus pneumoniae vaccine trial. *Controlled Clinical Trials*, 22, 438–52.

Murray, D.M. (1998). *Design and Analysis of Group-Randomized Trials*. New York: Oxford University Press.

Murray, D.M., Clark, M.H., and Wagenaar, A.C. (2000). Intraclass correlations from a community-based alcohol prevention study: the effect of repeat observations on the same communities. *Journal of Studies on Alcohol*, 61, 881–90.

Murray, D.M., Varnell, S.P., and Blitstein, J.L. (2004). Design and analysis of group-randomized trials: a review of recent methodological developments. *American Journal of Public Health*, 94, 423–32.

Neuhaus, J.M. (1992). Statistical methods for longitudinal and clustered designs with binary responses. *Statistical Methods in Medical Research*, 1, 249–73.

O'Brien, P.C. and Fleming, T.R. (1979). A multiple testing procedure for clinical trials. *Biometrics*, 34, 549–56.

Omar, R.Z. and Thompson, S.G. (2000). Analysis of a cluster randomized trial with binary outcome data using a multi-level model. *Statistics in Medicine*, 19, 2675–88.

Pan, W. and Wall, M.M. (2002). Small sample adjustments in using the sandwich variance estimator in generalizing estimating equations. *Statistics in Medicine*, 21, 1429–41.

Parienti, J.-J. and Kuss, O. (2007) Cluster-crossover design: a method for limiting cluster level effects in community-intervention studies. *Contemporary Clinical Trials*, 28, 316–23.

Parker, D.R., Evangelou, E., and Eaton, C.B. (2005). Intraclass correlation coefficients for cluster randomized trials in primary care: the cholesterol education and research trial (CEART). *Contemporary Clinical Trials*, 26, 260–7.

Rao, J.N.K. and Scott, A.J. (1992). A simple method for the analysis of clustered binary data. *Biometrics*, 48, 577–85.

Resnicow, K., Jackson, A., Wang, T., et al. (2001). A motivational interviewing intervention to increase fruit and vegetable intake through black churches: results of the Eat for Life trial. *American Journal of Public Health*, 91, 1686–93.

Scariano, S.M. and Davenport, J.M. (1987). The effects of violations of independence assumptions in the one-way ANOVA. *The American Statistician*, 41, 123–9.

Senn, S. (1994). Testing for baseline balance in clinical trials. *Statistics in Medicine*, 13(17), 1715–26.

Shadish, W.R. (2002). Revisiting field experimentation: field notes for the future. *Psychological Methods*, 1, 3–18.

Simpson, J.M., Klar, N., and Donner, A. (1995). Accounting for cluster randomization: a review of primary prevention trials, 1990 through 1993. *American Journal of Public Health*, 85, 1378–82.

Sommer, A., Tarwotjo, I., Djunaedi, E., et al. (1986). Impact of vitamin A supplementation on childhood mortality. *Lancet*, 1, 1169–73.

Susser, M. (1995). Editorial: The tribulations of trials—intervention in communities. *American Journal of Public Health*, 85, 156–8.

Todd, J., Carpenter, L., Li, X., et al. (2003). The effects of alternative study designs on the power of community randomized trials: evidence from three studies of human immunodeficiency virus prevention in East Africa. *International Journal of Epidemiology*, 32, 755–62.

Torgerson, D.J. (2001). Contamination in trials: is cluster randomisation the answer? *British Medical Journal*, 322, 355–7.

Turner, R.M., White, I.R., and Croudace, T. (2007). Analysis of cluster randomised cross-over trial data: a comparison of methods. *Statistics in Medicine*, 26, 274–89.

Varnell, S.P., Murray, D.M., Janega, J.B., and Blitstein, J.L. (2004). Design and analysis of group-randomized trials: a review of recent practices. *American Journal of Public Health*, 94, 393–9.

Watson, L., Small, R., Brown, S., et al. (2004). Mounting a community-randomized trial: sample size, matching, selection, and randomization issues in PRISM. *Controlled Clinical Trials*, 25, 235–50.

West, K.P., Pokhrel, R.P., Katz, J., et al. (1991). Efficacy of vitamin A in reducing preschool child mortality in Nepal. *The Lancet*, 338, 67–71.

Zou, G., Donner, A., and Klar, N. (2005). Group sequential methods for cluster randomization trials with binary outcomes. *Clinical Trials*, 2, 479–85.

5.9

Community intervention trials in high-income countries

John W. Farquhar and Lawrence W. Green

Introduction to community intervention trials in high-income countries

As background on theories and methods underlying successful multilevel, multimethod, *community-based, health promotion intervention trials*, this chapter first reviews community organizational and mass media intervention developments in the first half of the twentieth century and the origin of randomized trials outside laboratory settings early in that century. It then reviews specific health examples from tuberculosis mobile X-ray and immunization campaigns in the 1950s and 1960s, family planning programmes in the 1960s and 1970s, and HIV/AIDS in the 1980s. We then turn to the most prominent and influential community health intervention trials for the remainder of the twentieth century as touchstones for development of twenty-first-century public health challenges, such as obesity and diabetes control, substance abuse prevention, and cancer control. These touchstones were the cardiovascular disease prevention and risk reduction trials (including most notably hypertension, tobacco, dyslipidaemia, and physical inactivity) mounted in California with the Stanford Three-Community Study and in North Karelia, Finland in 1972. Parallel national and statewide successes in hypertension control in the 1970s, and tobacco control in the 1980s and beyond, have drawn significantly on these and subsequent exemplary trials from North America, Europe, Australia, and elsewhere.

These later trials exemplify the scope and innovation of *experimental* epidemiology in advancing disease prevention and health promotion science, involving total populations of communities, initiated often following insights from *observational* epidemiology, or from *randomized clinical trials* in smaller populations. Some were derived from 'natural experiments' that studied the impact of policies and programmes not initiated by academic investigators.

The earliest of mid-century trials were often in developing countries, designed to reduce social development problems associated with communicable diseases and high birth rates. The communicable disease studies in Western countries gave opportunities to test new polio vaccines and their adoption, and later by emergence of new infectious diseases, particularly HIV/AIDS. Other studies increasingly addressed risk factors for cardiovascular disease (CVD), cancer, and other chronic diseases as the rising mortality curve of chronic diseases crossed the declining curve of communicable diseases in the mid-twentieth century. All relied on locally available mass communication channels, community organizing, and other policy advocacy and educational methods, using relatively low-cost approaches with potentials to change lifestyles or specific behaviours.

One study examined alcohol-involved trauma using only community organizing to promote adherence to existing laws, rather than public education for policy-change advocacy (Holder et al. 1997). Another study, designed to reduce consumption of dietary trans fats, used primarily new laws and regulations (Angell et al. 2009). By community organizing we mean collaborating and seeking support from community leaders and other channels of communication. The World Health Organization characterized this as community participation or participatory planning (Green 1983), and as 'maximum feasible participation' (Moynihan 1969) for community projects under President Kennedy's 'New Frontier', and Lyndon Johnson's 'New Society' legislation. But this spin on community organization assumed lay communities set the goals (Green 1989). This orientation was recently termed 'community-based participatory research' when organizing was undertaken collaboratively at the initiative of the community or by academic or external health agencies (George et al. 1996; Minkler and Wallerstein 2008). Following further definition of community and community organizing for health, we review this history to identify some prominent precedents in the public health and community health promotion literature.

Definitions of community and community organizing for health

A community-based programme was defined historically as one organized locally, and promoted through the community's institutions and communication channels.

'*Community-based*' has become more broadly labelled, including both community-initiated and community-administered following initiation from external agencies. Programmes were termed '*community-placed*' when conceived, sponsored by, or driven from organizations outside the community and applied with or without community participation.

The traditional definition of a 'community' is a residential area with legally defined geographic boundaries, where a *local* governmental system regulates many aspects of schools, businesses, law enforcement, transportation, and recreational activities. A community is usually the last designated jurisdiction in a nation's official or governmental regulatory chain, where education and implementation must ultimately occur. In rural areas the county or district becomes the agent for education and other official governance. For programmes funded by non-governmental organizations, local agencies or branch organizations are the implementing agents within communities.

The following summarizes changing precedents in effectiveness trials of community health promotion, reviewed by twentieth-century decades. It illustrates that technologies for solving emerging public health problems led to research in high-income countries, developing theories, and evidence needed for community interventions for large segments of the population at risk.

Some converging developments for community health trials

Table 5.9.1 summarizes a chronology of community trials that dominated eras of action research across seven decades of the twentieth century, and a few citations of works illustrating trial types and theoretical and epidemiological problems they tested, either as proof-of-concept trials, or as health promotion model evaluations.

The origin of randomized controlled trials (RCTs) is usually attributed to Sir Ronald Fisher (1925) for its application to field trials comparing effectiveness of alternative cultivation methods (Fisher 1926). Some rural sociologists began in the 1930s to study the spread among farmers of new hybrid seeds, providing technical assistance to farmers by agricultural extension agents. This led to the first publication of the diffusion model describing the normal-curve pattern of adoption of new ideas, behaviour, or innovations in populations (Ryan and Gross 1943). The diffusion model and its theoretical framing of social and behavioural change in populations has been chronicled by the rural sociologist Everett Rogers (2003), through five editions of his book, *Diffusion of Innovations*, and specifically for public health applications (Green et al. 2009). Rogers converged at Stanford with others who brought their various sociobehavioural and health disciplines to bear on development of the first large-scale, interdisciplinary US trial in community-based cardiovascular risk factor reduction. Table 5.9.1 recapitulates this history of community trials leading to and including the cardiovascular trials and beyond to tobacco control and now obesity control.

Tobacco control successes, from the 1960s through to the 1990s

Of all chronic disease prevention and health promotion efforts, tobacco control is the most cited as a great success of health

Table 5.9.1 Decades in which community trials of particular types dominated in development of a body of evidence, methods, and theories

Decade	Influential community trials	Examples and reviews
1930s	Agricultural extension trials and diffusion studies	Fisher 1926; Ryan and Gross 1943; Rogers 2003; Green et al. 2009
1940s	Mass media and war-years' propaganda studies; advertising, radio and film studies	Hovland 1948; Maccoby 1951; Michael and Maccoby 1953
1950s	Community mobile X-ray and various immunization studies	Hochbaum 1958; Rosenstock et al. 1959; World Health Organization 1954; Green 1970
1960s	Community family planning and polio immunization campaign trials	Stycos 1962, pp. 481–482; Berelson 1966; Bogue 1962; Northcutt et al. 1964; D'Onofrio 1966; Gray et al. 1966; Green et al. 1972
1970s	The first cardiovascular community risk-factor prevention trials	Farquhar et al. 1977; Puska et al. 1981
1980s	The HIV/AIDS and substance abuse prevention trials	Miller et al. 1990; Ruiz et al. 2000; Cain et al. 2001; Darrow et al. 2009; Kagan et al. 2012
1990s	Culmination of four decades of tobacco control	Centers for Disease Control and Prevention 1999; Rogers 2010; Levy et al. 2012
2000s	Obesity control	Institute of Medicine 2010a, 2010b, 2012a, 2012b

behaviour change on a population scale. Ironically, at least in North America, Europe, Australia, and New Zealand, this success, initially, was not the direct application of controlled trials, either clinical or community. It followed many planned media and educational events, popular media, policy initiatives and the environmental changes associated with them, and their evaluation through yearly measures of tobacco consumption. The mass media 'softened' public opinion, denormalizing smoking in public places, and assisting smoking cessation policy changes (Fig. 5.9.1).

These associations offer 'lessons' from tobacco control for chronic disease control at the population level, demonstrating that changing risk *conditions* in the social and physical environment is needed for behaviour change.

In addition to denormalization, research shows other policies and programmes have additive or multiplicative effects on reducing tobacco consumption and its premature mortality. The greatest impacts include tobacco price increases, high-intensity media campaigns, comprehensive cessation treatments, strong health warnings, stricter smoke-free air regulations, advertising bans, and youth access laws (e.g. Levy et al. 2012). Price increases have an independent effect; but the last three depend on both laws and their enforcement. These, in turn, have depended on building an informed and activated electorate through community-level organizing and communications, because community policies

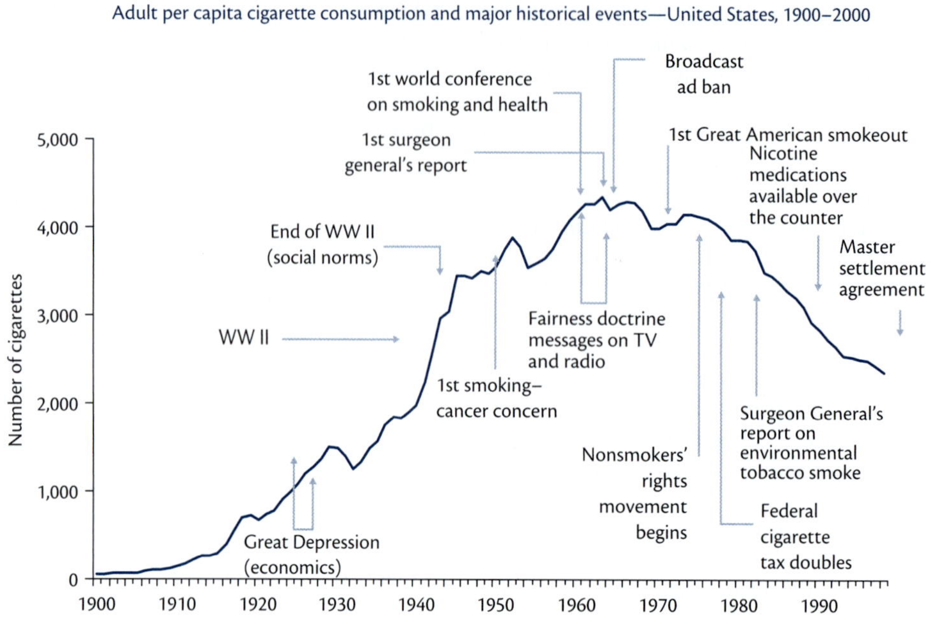

Adult per capita cigarette consumption and major historical events—United States, 1900–2000

Fig. 5.9.1 Linkage in tobacco consumption trends with historical events in the social, economic, and policy environments.
Adapted from US Department of Health and Human Services, *Reducing Tobacco Use: A Report of the Surgeon General*, US Department of Health and Human Services, Centers for Disease Control and Prevention, National Center for Chronic Disease Prevention and Health Promotion, Office on Smoking and Health, Atlanta, Georgia, USA, 2000, available from http://www.cdc.gov/tobacco/data_statistics/sgr/2000/complete_report/pdfs/fullreport.pdf

controlling tobacco promotions and smoking in public places could be passed locally when they could not overcome industry lobbying at state and national levels.

Lessons drawn from the last seven decades of the twentieth century

We draw 'lessons' or generalizations for community prevention and health promotion interventions from seven decades of trials and natural experiments just reviewed, drawing especially on CVD trials and adoption and cessation trends of tobacco seen during the twentieth century (Fig. 5.9.1). Many 'lessons', derived from the tobacco consumption trends, were more readily adoptable within the CVD community trials, which began in the 1970s, and included smoking prevention and cessation. The tobacco experiences were also then seen as applicable to other risk behaviours at the community level. Finally lessons from these CVD trials lead to a description of the mix and sequence of the intervention steps needed.

The economic imperative

Cigarettes became increasingly popular and inexpensive in the century's first three decades after manufacturing 'advances' reduced mass production costs, accounting for a steep rise in consumption. Consumption plummeted in the late 1920s during the Great Depression. This strong association in usage was early evidence for the wisdom of suppressing consumption through tobacco excise taxation. It demonstrated that even an addictive product is sensitive to price relative to disposable income. The argument for excise taxes gained momentum as evidence accumulated. A 10 per cent increase in cigarette price, on average, reduces consumption by about 4 per cent (Chaloupka et al. 2002),

and more for young, lower-income and pregnant smokers (Hyland et al. 2006).

Two other advantages spurred more cigarette tax initiatives. One is that revenues can finance statewide *and* community tobacco control programmes, making cigarette taxes even more palatable to the public, thus launching and sustaining some very successful programmes. The other is growing evidence that tobacco consumption increases healthcare expenditures, and since taxes decrease tobacco use, healthcare costs may eventually fall by billions of dollars in a state the size of California (Max et al. 2013).

The economic imperative also relates to obesity control and diabetes prevention, partly due to decades of increasing agricultural efficiency, causing progressive food price decreases. Food manufacturers and vendors have increased portion sizes, thus many have become accustomed to consuming larger portions and more frequent indulgences of cheaper, unhealthful food; much of it processed rather than home-cooked, and often with empty calories. These trends have led a contemporary movement advocating taxation of sugar-sweetened beverages (e.g. Novak and Brownell 2011).

The social normative or denormalization imperative

Two early notable changes in the trajectory of tobacco consumption were acceleration during the Second World War, and a less dramatic but significant rise during the First World War (Fig. 5.9.1). These are partly attributable to official condoning, facilitating, and even encouraging of smoking among soldiers to reduce boredom, and cope with stress, and smoking became integrated with their camaraderie. A modest drop in smoking occurs following the Second World War as soldiers' social networks fragment. Later recognition of these social norm changes led to using mass media to portray smoking as less glamorous, less fashionable, less smart, and portrayed the tobacco industry as deceiving and exploiting the public. Experiments within the community CVD trials began to highlight use of social influence strategies and media use to provide role models for changing behaviours, such as smoking (Ramirez et al. 1995).

The public health education and informed electorate imperative

Before mass media were used to create denormalization, most public health education was limited to smoking's health hazards, which had effects as noted. In 1954 a single mass media message created a precipitous drop in tobacco use. That year, *The Reader's Digest*, a popular and credible magazine with the American public, featured an article showing that tar of tobacco residues induced cancerous tumours when painted on mice. Although dramatic in its drop, consumption soon bounced back and continued upwards with continued tobacco industry advertising (Fig. 5.9.1).

As the public became more aware and cautious about tobacco, America was ready for the first Surgeon General's Report on Tobacco and Health in 1965, the peak of tobacco consumption growth. This and subsequent events led to legislation restraining the tobacco industry (e.g. the Fairness Doctrine requiring equal broadcast media time for anti-tobacco and pro-tobacco advertising). This indicated that public health education's most powerful method, certainly in relation to tobacco, was creation of an informed electorate—more supportive of regulations restraining industry advertising, promotion, and sales of a harmful product, and raising tobacco products' taxes.

The surveillance imperative

The tracking of tobacco consumption illustrates how helpful a consistently measured outcome or risk-factor metric related to particular chronic diseases can be. Ideally, such measures should be collected on whole populations and also on smaller subpopulations requiring particular attention. Regrettably, such surveillance—nearly universal for communicable diseases—remains sparse for most chronic disease risk factors. They are usually absent at the community level, so special surveys are needed for community intervention effects on behavioural and environmental issues. This expense alone makes trials prohibitively costly and dependent on a national government's funding.

The comprehensiveness imperative

The major tobacco consumption declines, following the first Surgeon General's Report on Smoking and Health in 1965, reflect the historical creation of national policies and programmes supportive of state and local efforts to create comprehensive programmes (Centers for Disease Control and Prevention 1999, 2007). Two states in particular (California and Massachusetts) in the late 1980s and early 1990s increased tobacco taxes, with a portion of the revenue earmarked for statewide and community tobacco control, including use of the social normative approach through schools, worksites, and mass media. These programmes achieved tobacco consumption reductions that doubled and then tripled decline rates of the other 48 states within a few years. Given results of these and later statewide and community trials, and success in measuring and tracking their effects, the Centers for Disease Control and Prevention's Office on Smoking and Health published in 1999 and updated in 2007 the 'Best Practices' document cited earlier, guiding other states' comprehensive statewide programme development.

The formative evaluation and tailoring imperative

Formative evaluation must begin before and be continued throughout implementation of any planned community intervention campaign. Success requires programmes well designed in mix and sequence, delivered through varied channels, adjusted for audience responses. This integration, with goals set in advance and adjustments from early results, is analogous to a commercial marketing campaign, hence the term 'social marketing'. (Ironically, *commercial* marketing has adopted many novel methods from academic research on *social* marketing.) It includes recognition of audience segmentation, or tailoring of messages and appeals to the varied motives, needs, and preferences of subpopulations (Slater and Flora 1991). Needs analysis, message design, and pre-testing are formative evaluation phases. Message sequences should first increase awareness, then knowledge, then motivation, and last provide training in the skills and resources to enable adoption and maintenance of new behaviours (Bandura 1986). Electronic media can furnish the first two parts of this sequence and stimulate use of more information-dense print media of newspapers, booklets, CDs, and websites, which are inherently more effective in *skills training* than are electronic media (Flora et al. 1997).

The ecological imperative

Health behaviours and health status are influenced by economic, political, cultural, and socioeconomic factors, all non-biological (Schooler et al. 1997; Best et al. 2003; Trickett et al. 2011). Healthcare's reliance on clinical services can neither prevent most chronic disease nor reach large population segments. Therefore, changing behaviour and improving health need to include family, cultural, and social contexts of these populations. A primary tenet of community prevention programmes is the opportunity to intervene in multiple settings and domains (Poland et al. 2000), and at multiple levels from individuals to families, organizations, and whole populations. This ecological approach honours the 'Comprehensiveness Imperative', but also urges communities to encompass interdependencies among environmental, social, and individual factors and the potential for public health strategies to interact with individually tailored therapeutic and medical strategies (Shea and Basch 1990; Schooler et al. 1997; Green et al. 2012; Farquhar in press). This principle is known as the ecological approach to community or population programmes (Green et al. 1996; Kok et al. 2008; Golden and Earp 2012), and has been a central tenet of the Ottawa Charter for Health Promotion (World Health Organization et al. 1986).

Community-based programmes offer opportunities to approximate the ideal multicomponent and multilevel approach by coordinating population-based policy and mass health communication and education strategies with individual-based clinical intervention. Social norms and community attributes greatly impact health. Community governmental and private institutions influence health behaviours by controlling, for example, health, recreational (e.g. Kokko et al. 2008), and transportation services (Mosquera et al. 2012) and youth access to tobacco. The health and safety policies and worksite health promotion practices of businesses can also affect health. Stores and restaurants also shape health according to the food they sell (Schooler et al. 1997) and whether menus provide information on calories and ingredients.

The ideal programme design, then, would include programmes developed within or channelled through multiple and coordinated worksites, schools, recreation sites, libraries, churches, local business organizations, and other sites to supplement and expand the effects of policy and health education approaches and appropriate delivery of healthcare (Farquhar et al. 1985; Kokko et al. 2006; Dooris 2009). This broad reach into the community is critically appropriate to chronic disease prevention and injury control because most people are at some level of risk for these and will benefit from interventions to predispose, enable, and reinforce healthful behaviour, leading to creating a *population* impact on prevalent risk factors. Indeed, most CVD does not occur among the relatively few adults at highest risk, but among many at moderate risk (Blackburn 1979; Puska et al. 1985; Schooler et al. 1997). Therefore, population health promotion must reach a community's entire population, including those who are neither engaged with the health system nor motivated to reduce a possible distant development of chronic disease.

While some behaviour change reflects individuals recognizing and reducing a risk, a population-wide impact always requires diffusion of behaviour change from a social process—individuals learning about new behaviours from neighbours, or individuals being encouraged to adopt new behaviours by those in their social networks. Such social diffusion results best from increasing opportunities to learn about and implement new behaviours, plus increased social expectations for doing so. The tobacco control literature calls this the social norms approach, 'denormalizing', by making both tobacco smoking and the tobacco industry's practices socially unacceptable, an approach central to California's successful Tobacco Control Program (Rogers et al. 2010).

This social normative and total community approach requires building an environment that coherently and consistently favours behaviour change. In addition to policy changes and mass communications campaigns, this total environmental change may be aided by entrepreneurs recognizing a need and developing products to accelerate behaviour change, through workplaces providing incentives for adherence to wellness programmes (Volpp et al. 2009), through schools that modify food available to children and require physical activity (Lynagh et al. 1997; Michaud 2003; Louriero 2004), through sports clubs (Kokko et al. 2006), and through programmes in other community settings. The goal is to create a behaviour change cascade, arising from synergistic interactive effects when many components are embedded in total community-based programmes that encourage institutional change, leaves space for entrepreneurs, and includes mass media and environmental change (Schooler et al. 1997).

Several synergies arise from combining multicomponent, multilevel (ecological) community intervention approaches with clinical services of physicians and other health professionals (Green et al. 2012). Adherence to dietary and exercise advice is more readily followed when family members, friends, and colleagues are modelling, enabling, and reinforcing these behaviours. Medication adherence improves when others in the patient's social network have learned, for example, about the need to control blood pressure and blood lipids. Health professionals, and their practice sites, potentially contribute to the 'total push' for better health, for example, by supplying print materials on health and alerting their patients to forthcoming community health events.

Comprehensive community-based efforts may modify the environment to support healthful or inhibit unhealthful individual actions, create organizational and institutional support for programmes, and influence the knowledge, attitudes, and behaviours of individuals (Schooler et al. 1997). However, a pragmatic view on implementing community-based programmes includes healthy scepticism about depending on institutions if reducing the CVD burden is not central to their primary missions. For workplaces, schools, and other community organizations the advantages may be made more evident when improved health increases performance or reduces absenteeism, for example, of students or employees.

Committing limited resources from community-level organizations to programmes may be unsustainable if incentives are weak or if interventions are too complex to implement and maintain, leading to dissipation despite early enthusiasm (Thompson et al. 2000). For example, businesses that have insurance incentives to reduce smoking and obesity might invest in CVD prevention programmes, but few precedents exist for long-term sustainability and effectiveness even in high-income countries—and the potential incentives for businesses in low- and middle-income countries are less certain. However, recent findings suggest that financial incentives increase effectiveness of many worksite programmes, with evidence limited so far to their use in large worksites (Volpp et al. 2009). Similarly, physical activity is greatly needed in schools, but may not be implementable, given competition for limited educational resources and their primary academic mission. The infrastructure and capacity may be even more fragile in less formalized community organizations. More knowledge is needed on methods to create programmes and disseminate or scale them up in low- and middle-income countries.

'Best processes' to complement 'best practices'

Community intervention trials are typically funded to determine *efficacy*; multi-community trials test *effectiveness*, that is, what might result when applied to different populations with different community structures. The generalizability from these to many varieties of communities and populations involves external validity (Green et al. 2009). Adaptation is an assessment and planning *process* which considers the history, culture, demographic and political structure, attitudes, community needs, and diversity of a particular community.

Features of this planning, implementation, and evaluation process approach are shown procedurally in models such as PRECEDE-PROCEED (Green and Kreuter, 2004), which was informed by community trials following on Stanford and North Karelia, and the PATCH programme model of CDC (Green and Kreuter 1992).

Message characteristics

Messages must arouse interest in health improvement and disease prevention and appeal to individuals with varied backgrounds and knowledge. They must surmount indifference caused by the public's exposure to an *extreme* advertising overload. Since the 1990s, the average adult's annual exposure in the United States was 35,000 television advertisements, equalling 292 hours of personal exposure (Fortmann et al. 1995). They must arouse interest and awareness and have production qualities able to capture the public's attention. Formative evaluation must continue to match message content to the population's readiness. Early campaign messages must raise awareness and increase knowledge; later messages should increase motivation, provide direction to access resources, and develop needed skills—with resultant behaviour change (Schooler et al. 1997).

For adolescents, for example, the following enhanced success: parents and teachers whose personal habits were role models; and amount and quality of school-based education on tobacco, fitness, and nutrition. Also, certain personal characteristics were influential—for example, the person's baseline *self-efficacy* toward one's behaviour-change abilities (Fortmann et al. 1995). Finally, as Perry, of the Minnesota Heart Health Project (Perry 2000) explained, if a peer-led smoking prevention curriculum reduced smoking onset among youth, effect preservation required other support: 'The careful links of behavioural curricula, parental involvement, community support and peer participation and leadership, with messages that are consistent and coordinated, have demonstrated efficacy beyond the implementation of a single strategy' (p. 122). This lesson is very germane for developing countries, given their proportionately high adolescent population.

The multiplicity and multilevel dimensions of community supports are shown in Table 5.9.2 as channels and mediators, referring to the individuals through whom the interventions can be personally or organizationally adopted and converted into reasons to act themselves, and then to influence others to change behaviour. They connect in the third column to the receiver's social cognitive change processes (Bandura 1986).

Prominent theories applied in community-based interventions

Community-based health education carried out by SPRC and some analogous projects has been guided by two major theories (community organizing and health communication–behaviour change), with success depending on their judicious blend (Flora et al. 1989; Farquhar et al. 1991).

Community organizing theory

This describes how to identify the community's health problem (and resources needed or available), and how to mobilize the community's opinion leaders and organizations. It describes the need to form coalitions, begin and maintain educational programmes, achieve regulatory changes, and *empower communities* to reach and maintain their goals. See 'Functions (for the sender)' in Table 5.9.2. Community organizing has elements central to concepts of 'community self-development' (Green and Kreuter 2005; Minkler 2005) and includes elements of diffusion theory (Rogers 2003)—which has shown how innovations are adopted through natural social networks, aided by a community's opinion leaders. Rogers strongly advised to ensure that these leaders play an important role, given their perceived trustworthiness (Rogers 2003).

Health communication–behaviour change theory

Health communication–behaviour change theory describe the basis for educating the population and its subgroups considering their health needs, cultural attributes, social networks, media habits, attitudes, motivation, knowledge, and self-management skills (see Table 5.9.1). It describes principles underlying education's success, including social cognitive theory (Bandura 1986), which emphasizes an individual's capacity for self-directed change. Bandura's research builds on the long-standing educational principle that 'learning by doing' is more effective than 'learning from observing' (modelling a behaviour), and both are more effective than an 'information-only' approach. Bandura described these principles as *social cognitive theory*: proposing that guided practice in a new behaviour can increase self-efficacy and behaviour change beyond the usual (Bandura 1986). The health communication–behaviour change theory includes efficient ways to reach total populations using methods described earlier in this chapter as 'social marketing' (Kotler 1975; Lefebvre and Flora 1988). The goal of a comprehensive, multi-component, community-based intervention is to achieve 'community efficacy', just as 'self-efficacy' occurs for an individual after a successful behaviour change programme (Bandura 1986).

Specific methods for CVD community-based interventions

Problem identification

The first task is to identify the problem, initiated from within or outside the community. Local (community) interventions ideally interact with national programmes and link to scientific support

Table 5.9.2 The components of health communication–behaviour change

Communication inputs	Functions (for the sender)	Behaviour objectives (for the receiver)
Face-to-face messages	Determine receiver's needs	Become aware
Mediated messages	Gain attention (set the agenda)	Increase knowledge
Community events	Provide information	Increase motivation and interest
Environmental cues	Provide incentives	Take action, assess outcomes
Training for community sources of influence (parents, employers, etc.)	Provide training to enable and reinforce others	Maintain action, practise self-management skills
Diffusion and influence beyond the primary receivers	Provide cues to action, including environmental change	Become an opinion leader (exert peer-group influence)

Adapted from Farquhar, J.W. et al., Methods of communication to influence behavior, in Holland WW, Detels R, and Knox G (eds) *Oxford Textbook of Public Health*, Second Edition, Volume 2, Oxford University Press, Oxford, UK, Copyright © 1991, by permission of Oxford University Press.

from national or international levels, as noted with the family planning and HIV/AIDS histories. CVD prevention (World Health Organization 1986) and alcohol sales control (Holder and Wallack 1986) are problems requiring local action, and any chronic disease requiring widespread education for changing 'lifestyle' behaviours (such as exercise, diet, and cigarette use) will require analogous methods.

Formation of partnerships

Key opinion leaders as well as relevant organizations usually need to form a coalition or at least a network of strategic partnerships (Green et al. 2001) to assure coordinated agreement on needs assessments, planning and implementation, development of a community resource inventory, and mobilization of populace support for policy changes and enforcement. Relevant organizations, particularly in developed countries, include the following: the County Medical Society, or its equivalent, the local public health department, municipal hospital community affairs departments, city parks and recreation departments and voluntary health agencies (e.g. the local branches of national heart, lung, cancer and diabetes organizations). Any organization that will act as a conduit for the public's education should also be represented (e.g. television and radio stations, local newspapers, schools, churches, libraries, pharmacies, clinics, and physicians' and dentists' offices). As the coalition-partner numbers proliferate, a 'steering committee', preferably limited to six members, is needed for more detailed planning, including formation of expert groups ('task forces') in education and evaluation and other topics (Flora et al. 1989; Farquhar et al. 1991).

Matching for comparison

Assuming the high likelihood of a non-randomized or cluster-randomized small number of communities, and therefore a 'quasi-experimental' design (Flora et al. 1989; Mercer et al. 2007), successful implementation requires close matching of intervention communities (treatment) with comparison (control) communities on relevant demographic and socioenvironmental factors, while also minimizing shared media channels (Farquhar et al. 1985). Many community trials have not followed these important principles.

Intervention components

The goals include providing behaviour-change skills training, supplementing goals of increasing knowledge. They should enlist multiple sectors beyond health organizations in health improvement campaigns, including changes in social and built environments, and regulations that promote access to facilities and resources needed for healthful physical activity. Multiple communication channels can facilitate reaching subgroups with differing needs. Comprehensive interventions should involve schools, worksites, senior citizens' centres, churches, and facilities for sport, recreation, and health. Voluntary health agencies (such as the local branches of any national organization that deal with cardiovascular disease, diabetes, and cancer) should be involved. These can serve as education conduits, with the community's electronic and print mass media organizations assisting in message design, content, and delivery. The Internet's community education role (digital health) is now a major force (Baker et al. 2003) and can reach and benefit more than traditional channels—an emerging variant of mass media. Interactive computer learning, including

hand-held computers (King et al. 2008) ('mobile health') now provides new points of entry.

The intervention 'dose'

For future community intervention planning, an important question is how much amount and duration of intervention (the 'dose') is needed? Although outcome evaluations measure change achieved in health or disease risk, this 'dose' is rarely measured, thus cost-effectiveness remains a mystery. Dose measurement is difficult, the usual report gives only the intervention's duration and a cursory description of the educational inputs (Farquhar 2014), with little attention to reach or intensity (exposures). One can, at least, measure print and electronic media distributed, all converted to time, as was done uniquely in the Stanford Five City Project (Farquhar et al. 1990). Public health policy would be served if this were done more commonly.

The community transformative phase

This begins early in the community-organizing period, preceding the intervention, but accelerates throughout, particularly in the terminal period when external support diminishes or ceases (Farquhar et al. 1985). Enhancing a community's programme adoption for intervention sustenance is a major goal. This begins earlier, but becomes more definitive toward cessation of educational forces extrinsic to the community. A concurrent goal is to facilitate policy and regulatory changes that foster long-term goals and provide supportive physical infrastructures. The preferred outcome sees a continuing role for the original external academic advisors for community assistance, including the county's health agencies, to create new disease prevention programmes, as new technologies emerge. The ideal long-term outcome is that the 'transformed' community will advocate for local, regional, and national governmental regulations and laws increasing local intervention effects, such as smoke-free places, and extend them beyond the community.

The case of comprehensive community health promotion for CVD

The history of seven decades of twentieth-century community trials described has encompassed a mid-twentieth-century shift from public health and medical strategies appropriate to communicable diseases that accounted for the majority of deaths to those appropriate to a growing chronic disease burden. It outlined a series of formal research projects designed to affect health of communities, and illustrative CVD risk factors. The CVD trials have involved entire populations of at least one *education* community, compared to at least one *control* community. Three projects are described in greater detail here as case studies to provide examples of their methods and results. Dissemination worldwide into practical applications of community organizing and mass communication technologies, derived in part from these projects, occurred throughout these decades, with a relatively small number using research methods analogous to those described here.

Two examples: the first decade of CVD community-based projects

The first example is the Stanford Three-Community Study (3CS) in three small agricultural marketing towns in California (total population 45,000). The second is the North Karelia Study (NKS) in two adjoining predominantly rural Finnish counties (North Karelia population about 180,000). Both projects began in 1972.

The first of two Stanford projects, 3CS, was carried out from 1972 to 1975 in both English and Spanish, comparing effects of 2 years of mass media plus ten-session risk reduction classes for 1 year for some high-risk adults in one community with the effects in a comparison community having 2 years of mass media alone, and a third as a control having neither (Farquhar et al. 1977; Schooler et al. 1997). Groups exposed to varied education amounts showed a dose–response change in levels of smoking, blood pressure, and blood cholesterol. Spanish-speaking residents had a proportionately larger effect than did the Anglo majority. A composite measure of CVD risk reduction at 2 years of about 23 per cent and 30 per cent occurred in the mass media-only and mass media-plus classroom conditions, respectively. The risk score (a probability) was derived from each adult's 'before–after' risk levels. These risk parameters predicted the 12-year future probability of a coronary heart disease event, using the scoring system derived from the long-term Framingham Heart Study (Truett et al. 1967). Thus, a relatively modest amount of mass media alone over 2 years (about 30 television and radio 'spots', weekly newspaper columns on heart health, and four separate mass mailings of booklets) was sufficient to change the population's coronary disease risk by 23 per cent. The education followed the principles outlined in the earlier section 'Prominent theories applied in community-based interventions' for prominent theories of community organizing and health communication-behaviour change.

In Finland, NKS evaluated two unmatched rural counties that contained many villages with farming and lumbering as their main occupations. North Karelia (which has a population of about 180,000, with the highest CVD rates in Finland) received an education campaign that began in 1972, continuing to the present and expanded to the entire country. After 10 years, CVD risk factor changes comparable to the 3CS occurred, and significant net reductions in CVD events occurred (Puska et al. 1985; Schooler et al. 1997). Extensive community organizing, resulting in strong partnerships with residents and their organizations marked this study. The NKS influence on Finland's national policies was unequalled among the CVD projects, giving its most important lesson—that a well-executed project led by respected scientists can change an entire country. Examples included Finland's food and agricultural industries making large changes: fertilizers were supplemented with selenium (a substance needed for health, but low in Finland's soil), milk pricing previously based on fat content converted to protein-based pricing, programmes were created to replace dairy farms with berry farms, a new canola industry replaced jobs lost in dairying, and increased production of low-saturated fat foods occurred (Puska et al. 1985, 1995). In 1972, population-wide nutrition change and smoking cessation interventions were an innovation internationally, which may partly explain the success of both 3CS and NKS (Green and Richard 1993).

Early international diffusion, 1977–1983

Building on the 3CS and NKS were studies carried out in various countries:

◆ Italy (The Martignacco Project, 1977–1983, one treatment, mass media and screening, one control—CHD risk fell in men only).

◆ Australia (The North Coast Project, 1978–1980, similar to 3CS, one mass media, one mass media plus classes—effects on smoking, greater in the mass media 'plus' community).

◆ Switzerland (two treatment, two control pairs, German and French speaking, with mass media, classes and environmental changes—small effects on smoking, blood pressure, and obesity).

◆ South Africa (similar to 3CS, one mass media, one mass media plus classes plus community events—decreased CHD risk, blood pressure, smoking; both treatments were equivalent).

All of these studies, reviewed in Schooler et al. (1997), reported significant risk factor changes, adding evidence both for the effectiveness of the 3CS model, and for the external validity of the evidence. In all, a predominately community-wide mass media campaign was effective, but a supplemental face-to-face instruction usually adds effects (Farquhar et al. 1991). A noteworthy qualification is that all these studies were done in rather small communities (population sizes of about 12,000 to 15,000 residents), thus achieving these effects may be more difficult in larger and more complex cities.

The second and third decades—projects begun in the 1980s and 1990s

The third case study, the Stanford Five-City Project (5CP) (California, United States), had an intervention phase of slightly more than 5 years, 1980–1986, and extended 3CS methods to larger populations (total population of about 360,000) with multifactor CVD prevention directed at two northern California cities, no intervention in three control cities (Farquhar et al. 1990). It differed from 3CS in larger community sizes, in greater use of community organizing, in greater collaboration with the communities' health, media and educational organizations in planning and implementing programmes, and in offering extensive continuing collaboration with Stanford. It was similar in its generous use of mass media, both print and electronic. The *proportion* of message sources received by the average adult over 5 years of education included: television and radio 67 per cent, newspaper 28 per cent, other print (such as booklets and 'tip' sheets) 4 per cent, and face-to-face 1 per cent. This dose measurement method, more fully described elsewhere (Farquhar 2014), was unique among all reported CVD community intervention programmes in measuring total education dose. In the intervention communities this amounted to about 5 hours/year and about 100 exposure episodes/year to all forms of media and classroom education (Flora et al. 1989; Farquhar et al. 1990). This method's use increased evaluation costs, almost two-thirds of total expenses. This expense may explain why others have not used it to similar degrees. Public health education would be served were more campaigns analysed in this way (Brown et al. 2012).

The first year of 5CP's television messages (characterized as 'high reach/low involvement') led to the public's later use of print media, which contained more specific instructions than from television in skills needed for changing smoking, diet, exercise, or weight control (Flora et al. 1997). Television, however, was also quite effective in skills training. For example, the 5CP presented an 8-week 'live' smoking cessation TV programme, demonstrating smoking cessation skills (Altman et al. 1987). The results of an antismoking campaign of a 'quit smoking' contest, the television and face-to-face classes, and a widely distributed print 'Quit Kit' were analysed separately. The highest cost-effectiveness was achieved by the low-cost print component (Altman et al. 1987). Results were comparable to the 3CS (about a 15 per cent fall in

Framingham composite risk of CVD) (Truett et al. 1967), with a major impact on blood pressure (4–5 per cent) and smoking (13 per cent) (Farquhar et al. 1990). The usually timid health policy experts might gain courage from the 5CP's evidence that only 3 hours/year of high-quality television health education can counteract the public's relatively intimidating exposure to about 100 hours/year of television advertising devoted to unhealthful nutrition. The US population's exposure is estimated as 292 hours of TV advertisement as measured by the Nielsen monitoring system (Farquhar 2014). Michael Jacobson, from the Center for Science in the Public Interest, identified that one-third of these promoted unhealthful nutrition (personal communication).

Compared to similar projects, 5CP's greater effects at relatively low cost, support that communication–behaviour change theory's predicted effects may be explained by mass media presentation components, including adaptation of skills training aspects of Bandura's social cognitive theory. An important lesson for policymakers is that adult quitters saved over three times more money from their cessation of cigarette purchases (2860 quitters @ $274/quitter/year) than the cost of the entire population-wide campaign ($4/adult/year), which would justify cigarette taxes as the campaign's payment. Savings are retained life-long by the community's smoker-quitters, not counting long-term health costs' savings, and absenteeism from the individual's employment decreases, all accruing to the whole community. The intervention's relatively low cost is again emphasized, since the total yearly cost of cigarettes to the 22,000 smokers (over $6 million) was 23 times greater than the yearly campaign costs (about $260,000/year). Additionally, the county's Health Department adopted 5CP's technologies, applying them to seatbelt promotion, changing restaurants' saturated fat use, violence prevention, and adolescent pregnancy prevention.

More variably sized CVD projects occurred in the 1980s and 1990s in the United States, Sweden, Denmark, Canada, Germany, the Czech Republic, and China, including World Health Organization-sponsored projects (Schooler et al. 1997). The Minnesota Heart Health Project (MHHP) (Luepker et al. 1994) emerged as an important innovation source, pioneering introduction of antismoking contests (Lando et al. 1990), and demonstrating synergism in school health intervention effects when multiple schools in a community are involved within a comprehensive community intervention (Perry 2000). Many projects borrowed heavily from and often received training from either the Stanford or the North Karelia groups, although changes seen were often less than in those two projects. Reasons for lower success may defy explanations (e.g. the magnitude of the interventions was incompletely described). For many, the cause was likely due to inadequate use of inherently cost-effective mass media.

To summarize lessons learned, a five-step approach emerges from community trials, much derived from the Stanford 5CP, and some from various worldwide trials. Generalizability, of course, has limitations inherent in the nature of such trials, including designs, locales and methods:

1. Define the problem. Choose behaviour and environment change goals following community consultation.

2. Implement a 2-year campaign. Provide 3–5 hours of multichannel education/year. Year 1: 70 per cent electronic media, 15 per cent print, 15 per cent community classes, contests, health fairs. Year 2: change to 40 per cent, 35 per cent, and 25 per cent.

3. Evaluate. Use formative, process, and summative evaluations, tracking exposure, and effects of each intervention type. Use repeated cohort surveys to best measure effects, avoiding greater variance and in-migration's dilution effect. Repeated independent sample designs are feasible if in-migration dilution is less than 5 per cent/year.

4. Institutionalize. Continue intervention. Create a community demonstration project as a regional resource centre.

5. Leverage. Advocate for local, regional, and national governmental regulations to magnify intervention effects.

Conclusions

Six decades of applying the 'total community' health promotion approach in developed countries show unequivocally that considerable change is achievable at reasonable cost. Well-designed projects have transferred educational technologies and social-behavioural intervention skills to a community's infrastructure (public health, media, schools, etc.), resulting in significant improvements in health risk factors and conditions of populations (Schooler et al. 1997). Although many studies were done in small communities, recent successes in New York City (Angell et al. 2009), suggest that success occurs in large urban populations. Adherence to theory is key: gains in self-efficacy of many individuals through education results in *community efficacy*, enhancing changed institutional policy and practice, thus maintaining and extending community change. Changing communities through organizing and education requires *advocacy, activism, partnership building*, and *leadership*; success is enhanced by *regulatory change*. When needed laws and regulations come from state, provincial or national governments, local changes are enhanced. Both local and broad governmental approaches are needed to succeed in preventing chronic disease, which is particularly important for developing countries (Institute of Medicine 2010a). Adding well-planned, well-integrated digital health programmes, as yet untried, can likely increase effectiveness at decreased cost.

References

Altman, D.G., Flora, J.A., Fortmann, S.P., and Farquhar, J.W. (1987). The cost-effectiveness of three smoking cessation programs. *American Journal of Public Health*, 77, 162–5.

Angell, S.Y., Silver, L.D., Goldstein, G.P., et al. (2009). Cholesterol control beyond the clinic: New York City's trans fat restriction. *Annals of Internal Medicine*, 151, 129–34.

Baker, L., Wagner, T.H, Singer, S., and Bundorf, M.K. (2003). Use of the internet and e-mail for health care information: results from a national survey. *Journal of the American Medical Association*, 289, 2400–6.

Bandura, A. (1986). *Social Foundations of Thought and Action: A Social Cognitive Theory*. Englewood Cliffs, NJ: Prentice-Hall.

Berelson, B. (ed.) (1966). *Family Planning and Population Policies: A Review of World Developments*. Chicago, IL: University of Chicago Press.

Best, A., Stokols, D., Green, L., et al. (2003). An integrative framework for community partnering to translate theory into effective health promotion strategy. *American Journal of Health Promotion*, 18, 168–76.

Blackburn, H. (1979). Diet and mass hyperlipidemia: public health considerations – a point of view. In R.R.B. Levy, B. Dennis, and N. Ernst (eds.) *Nutrition, Lipids, and Coronary Heart Disease*, pp. 309–47. New York: Raven Press.

Brown, D.R., Soares, J., Epping, J.M., et al., (2012) Community Preventive Services Task Force. Stand-alone mass media campaigns to increase physical activity. A community guide updated review. *American Journal of Preventive Medicine*, 43, 551–61.

Cain, R.E., Schyulze, R.W., and Preston, D.B. (2001). Developing a partnership for HIV primary prevention for men at high risk for HIV infection in rural communities. *Promotion and Education: International Journal of Health Promotion and Education*, 8(2), 75–8.

Centers for Disease Control and Prevention (1999). *Best Practices for Comprehensive Tobacco Control Programs* (1st ed.). Atlanta, GA: US Department of Health and Human Services, Centers for Disease Control and Prevention, National Center for Chronic Disease Prevention and Health Promotion, Office on Smoking and Health.

Centers for Disease Control and Prevention (2007). *Best Practices for Comprehensive Tobacco Control Programs* (2nd ed.). Atlanta, GA: US Department of Health and Human Services, Centers for Disease Control and Prevention, National Center for Chronic Disease Prevention and Health Promotion, Office on Smoking and Health.

Chaloupka, F.J., Cummings, K.M., Morley, C., and Horan, J. (2002). Tax, price and cigarette smoking: evidence from the tobacco documents and implications for tobacco company marketing strategies. *Tobacco Control*, 11, i62–72.

Darrow, W.W., Montanea, J.E., and Sánchez-Braña, E. (2009). Coalition contract management as a systems change strategy for HIV prevention. *Health Promotion Practice*, 11, 867–75.

D'Onofrio, C.N. (1966). *Reaching our Hard to Reach—The Unvaccinated*. Berkeley, CA: California State Department of Public Health.

Dooris, M. (2009). Holistic and sustainable health improvement: the contribution of the settings-based approach to health promotion. *Perspectives in Public Health*, 129, 29–36.

Farquhar, J.W. (2014). Community-based health promotion. In. W. Ahrens and I. Peugot (eds.) *Handbook of Epidemiology* (2nd ed.), 419–38. Berlin: Springer.

Farquhar, J.W., Fortmann, S.P., Flora, J.A., et al. (1990). The Stanford Five-City Project: effects of community-wide education on cardiovascular disease risk factors. *Journal of the American Medical Association*, 264, 359–65.

Farquhar, J.W., Fortmann, S.P., Flora, J.H., et al. (1991). Methods of communication to influence behaviour. In W.W. Holland, R. Detels, and G. Knox (eds.) *Oxford Textbook of Public Health* (1st ed.), pp. 331–44. Oxford: Oxford University Press.

Farquhar, J.W., Maccoby, N., Wood, P., et al. (1977). Community education for cardiovascular health. *Lancet*, 1, 1192–5.

Farquhar, J.W., Maccoby, N., and Wood, P.D. (1985). Education and communication studies. In W.W. Holland, R. Detels, and G. Knox (eds.) *Oxford Textbook of Public Health* (1st ed.), pp. 207–21. Oxford: Oxford University Press.

Fisher, R.A. (1925). *Statistical Methods for Research Workers*. Edinburgh: Oliver & Boyd.

Fisher, R.A. (1926). The arrangement of field experiments. *Journal of the Ministry of Agriculture of Great Britain*, 33, 505–13.

Flora, J.A., Maccoby, N., and Farquhar, J.W. (1989). Communication campaigns to prevent cardiovascular disease: the Stanford studies. In R. Rice and C. Atkin (eds.) *Public Communication Campaigns*, pp. 233–52. Beverly Hills, CA: Sage.

Flora, J.A., Saphir, M.N., Schooler, C., and Rimal, R.N. (1997). Toward a framework for intervention channels: reach, involvement and impact. *Annals of Epidemiology*, S7, S104–12.

Fortmann, S.P., Flora, J.S., Winkleby, M., et al. (1995). Community intervention trials: reflections on the Stanford Five-City Project. *American Journal of Epidemiology*, 142, 576–86.

George, M.A., Daniel, M. and Green, L.W. (1998–99). Appraising and funding participatory research in health promotion. *International Quarterly of Community Health Education,* 18(2), 181–97.

Golden, S.D. and Earp, J.A. (2012). Social ecological approaches to individuals and their contexts: twenty years of *Health Education & Behavior* health promotion interventions. *Health Education & Behavior*, 39, 364–72.

Gray, R.M., Kesler, J.P., and Moody, P.M. (1966). The effects of social class and friends' expectations on oral polio vaccination participation. *American Journal of Public Health*, 56, 2028–32.

Green, L.W. (1970). *Status Identity and Preventive Health Behavior*. Pacific Health Education Reports No. 1. Berkeley, CA: University of California School of Public Health.

Green, L.W. (1983). New policies in education for health. *World Health* April–May, 13–17.

Green, L.W. (1989). The theory of participation: a qualitative analysis of its expression in national and international health policies. In R.D. Patton and W.B. Cissell (eds.) *Community Organization: Traditional Principles and Modern Applications*, pp. 48–62. Johnson City, TN: Latchpins Press.

Green, L.W., Brancati, F.L., Albright, A., Primary Prevention of Diabetes Working Group (2012). Primary prevention of diabetes: integrative public health and primary care opportunities, challenges and strategies. *Family Practice*, 29(Suppl. 1), i13–23.

Green, L.W., Daniel, M., and Novick, L. (2001). Partnerships and coalitions for community based research. *Public Health Reports*, 116, 15–26.

Green, L.W., Gustafson, H.C., Griffiths, W., and Yaukey, D. (1972). *The Dacca Family Planning Experiment*. Berkeley, CA: School of Public Health, University of California.

Green, L.W. and Kreuter, M.W. (1992). CDC's planned approach to community health as an application of PRECEDE and an inspiration for PROCEED. *Journal of Health Education* 23(3), 140–7.

Green, L.W. and Kreuter, M.W. (2005). *Health Program Planning: An Educational and Ecological Approach* (4th ed.). St. Louis: McGraw-Hill Publishing Co.

Green, L.W., Ottoson, J.M., Garcia, C., and Hiatt, R. (2009). Diffusion theory and knowledge dissemination, utilization and integration. *Annual Review of Public Health*, 30, 151–74.

Green, L.W., Potvin, L., and Richard, L. (1996). Ecological foundations of health promotion. American *Journal of Health Promotion*, 10(4): 270–81.

Green, L.W. and Richard L. (1993). The need to combine health education and health promotion: the case of cardiovascular disease prevention. *Promotion and Education: International Journal of Health Promotion and Education*, 1, 11–17.

Hochbaum, G. (1958). *Public Participation in Medical Screening Programs*. Public Health Service Publication No. 572. Washington, DC: US Government Printing Office.

Holder, H.D., Salz, R.F., Grube, J.W., et al., (1997). Summing up: lessons from a comprehensive community prevention trial. *Addiction*, 92(S2), S293–S301.

Holder, H.D. and Wallack, L. (1986). Contemporary perspectives for prevention of alcohol problems: an empirically-derived model. *Journal of Public Health Policy* 7, 324–30.

Hovland, C.I. (1948). Social communication. *Proceedings of the American Philosophical Society*, 92, 371–5.

Hyland, A., Laux, F., Higbee, C., et al. (2006). Cigarette purchase patterns in four countries and the relationship with cessation: findings from the International Tobacco Control (ITC) Four Country Survey. *Tobacco Control*, 15(Suppl. 3), iii59–64.

Institute of Medicine (2010a). *Promoting Cardiovascular Health in the Developing World: A Critical Challenge to Achieve Global Health*. Washington, DC: National Academies Press.

Institute of Medicine (2010b). *Bridging the Evidence Gap in Obesity Prevention: A Framework to Inform Decision Making*. Washington, DC: National Academies Press.

Institute of Medicine (2012a). *An Integrated Framework for Assessing the Value of Community-Based Prevention*. Washington, DC: National Academies Press.

Institute of Medicine (2012b). *Measuring Progress in National and Community Efforts in Obesity Control*. Washington, DC: National Academies Press.

Kagan, J.M., Rosas, S.R., Siskind, R.L., et al. (2012). Community–researcher partnerships at NIAID HIV/AIDS clinical trials sites: insights for evaluation and enhancement. *Progress in Community Health Partnerships*, 6, 311–29.

King, A.C., Ahn, D.K., Oliveira, B.M., et al. (2008). Promoting physical activity through hand-held computer technology. *American Journal of Preventive Medicine*, 34, 138–42.

Kok G., Gottlieb, N.H., Commers, M., and Smerecnik, C. (2008). The ecological approach in health promotion programs: a decade later. *American Journal of Health Promotion*, 22, 437–42.

Kokko, S., Kannas, L., and Villberg J. (2006). The health promoting sports club in Finland—a challenge for the settings approach. *Health Promotion International*, 21, 219–29.

Kotler, P. (1975). *Marketing for Nonprofit Organizations*. Englewood Cliffs, NJ: Prentice Hall.

Lando, H.A., Loken, B., Howard Pitney, B., et al. (1990). Community impact of a localized smoking cessation contest. *American Journal of Public Health*, 80, 601–3.

Lefebvre, R.C. and Flora, J.A. (1988). Social marketing and public health interventions. *Health Education Quarterly*, 15, 299–315.

Levy, D., Gallus, S., Blackman, K., et al. (2012). Italy SimSmoke: the effect of tobacco control policies on smoking prevalence and smoking attributable deaths in Italy. *BMC Public Health*, 12, 709.

Louriero, I. (2004). A study about effectiveness of health promoting schools network in Portugal. *Promotion and Education* 11(2), 85–92.

Luepker, R.V., Murray, D.M., Jacobs, D.R., et al. (1994). Community education for cardiovascular disease prevention: risk factor changes in the Minnesota Heart Health Program. *American Journal of Public Health*, 84, 1383–93.

Lynagh, M., Schofield, M.J., and Sanson-Fisher, R.W. (1997). School health promotion programs over the past decade: a review of the smoking, alcohol and solar protection literature. *Health Promotion International*, 12, 43–59.

Maccoby, E.E. (1951). Television: its impact on school children. *Public Opinion Quarterly*, 15, 425.

Max, W., Sung, H.-Y., and Lightwood, J. (2013). The impact of changes in tobacco control funding on healthcare expenditures in California, 2012–2016. *Tobacco Control*, 22(e1), e10–15.

Mercer, S.M, DeVinney, B.J., Fine, L.J., et al. (2007). Study designs for effectiveness and translation research: identifying trade-offs. *American Journal of Preventive Medicine*, 33(2), 139–54.

Michael, D.N. and Maccoby, N. (1953). Factors influencing verbal learning from films under varying conditions of audience participation. *Journal of Experimental Psychology*, 46, 411–18.

Michaud, P.-A. (2003). Prevention and health promotion in school and community settings: a commentary on the international perspective. *Journal of Adolescent Health*, 33, 219–25.

Miller, H.G., Turner, C.F., and Moses, L.E. (eds.) (1990). *AIDS: The Second Decade*. Washington, DC: National Academies Press.

Minkler, M. (ed.) (2005). *Community Organizing and Community Building for Health* (2nd ed). New Brunswick, NJ: Rutgers University Press.

Minkler, M. and Wallerstein, N. (2008). *Community-Based Participatory Research for Health* (2nd ed.). San Francisco, CA: Jossey-Bass.

Mosquera, J., Para, D.C., Gomez, L.F., et al. (2012). An inside look at active transportation in Bogotá: a qualitative study. *Journal of Physical Activity and Health*, 9, 776–85.

Moynihan, D.P. (1969). *Maximum Feasible Misunderstanding: Community Action in the War on Poverty*. New York: Free Press.

Northcutt, T.J., Jenkins, C.D., and Johnson, A.L. (1964). Factors influencing vaccine acceptance. In J.S. Neill and J.O. Bond (eds.) *Hillsborough County Oral Polio Vaccine Program*. Monograph No. 6. Jacksonville, FL: Florida State Board of Health.

Novak, N.L. and Brownell, K.D. (2011). Taxation as prevention and as a treatment for obesity: the case of sugar-sweetened beverages. *Current Pharmaceutical Design*, 17(12), 1218–22.

Perry, C. (2000). Commentary: the school as a setting for health promotion. In B.D. Poland, L.W. Green, and I. Rootman (eds.) *Settings for Health Promotion: Linking Theory to Practice*, pp. 120–6. Thousand Oaks, CA: Sage.

Poland, B.D., Green, L.W., and Rootman, I. (2000). Reflections on settings for health promotion. In B. Poland, L.W. Green, and I. Rootman (eds.) *Settings for Health Promotion: Linking Theory and Practice*, pp. 341–51. Newbury Park, CA: Sage.

Puska, P. (1995). Experience with major subprogrammes and examples of innovative interventions. In P. Puska, A. Nissinen, and E. Vartianinen (eds.) *The North Karelia Project*, pp. 159–67. Helsinki: Helsinki University Printing House.

Puska, P., Nissinen, A., Tuomilehto, J., et al. (1985). The community-based strategy to prevent coronary heart disease: conclusions from the ten years of the North Karelia Project. *Annual Review of Public Health*, 6, 147–93.

Puska, P., Tuomilehto, J., Salonen, J., et al. (1981). *The North Karelia Project: Evaluation of a Comprehensive Community Programme for Control of Cardiovascular Diseases in 1972–1977 in North Karelia, Finland*. Copenhagen: World Health Organization.

Ramirez, A.G., McAlister, A., Gallion, K.J., and Villarreal, R. (1995). Targeting Hispanic populations: future research and prevention strategies. *Environmental Health Perspectives*, 103(Suppl. 8), 287–90.

Rogers, E. (2003). *Diffusion of Innovations* (5th ed.). New York: Free Press.

Rogers, T. (2010). The California Tobacco Control Program: introduction to the 20-year retrospective. *The Quarter that Changed the World: Celebrating 20 Years of California Tobacco Control Program, special issue of Tobacco Control*, 19 (Suppl. 1), i1–i2.

Rosenstock, I.M., Derryberry, M., and Carriger, B.A. (1959). Why people fail to seek poliomyelitis vaccination. *Public Health Reports*, 74, 98–103.

Ruiz, M.S., Gable, A.R., Kaplan, E.H., et al. (2000). *No Time to Lose: Getting More from HIV Prevention*. Washington, DC: National Academies Press.

Ryan, B. and Gross, N.C. (1943). The diffusion of hybrid seed corn in two Iowa communities. *Rural Sociology*, 8, 15–24.

Schooler, C., Farquhar, J.W., Fortmann, S.P., and Flora, J.A. (1997). Synthesis of findings and issues from community prevention trials. *Annals of Epidemiology*, S7, S54–68.

Shea, S. and Basch, C.E. (1990). A review of five major community-based cardiovascular disease prevention programs. Part I. Rationale, design, and theoretical framework. *American Journal of Health Promotion*, 4, 203–13.

Slater, M.D. and Flora, J.A., (1991). Health lifestyles: audience segmentation analysis for public health interventions. *Health Education Quarterly*, 18, 221–33.

Stycos, J.M. (1962). A critique of the traditional planned parenthood approach in underdeveloped areas. In C.V. Kiser (ed.) *Research in Family Planning*, pp. 477–501. Princeton, NJ: Princeton University Press.

Thompson, B., Lichtenstein, E., Corbett, K., et al. (2000). Durability of tobacco control efforts in the 22 Community Intervention Trial for Smoking Cessation (COMMIT) communities 2 years after the end of intervention. *Health Education Research*, 154, 15(3), 353–66.

Trickett, E.J., Beehler, S., Deutsch, C., et al. (2011). Advancing the science of community-level interventions. *American Journal of Public Health*, 101, 1410–19.

Truett, J., Cornfield, J., and Kannel, E. (1967). Multivariate analysis of the risk of coronary heart disease in Framingham. *Journal of Chronic Disease*, 20, 511–24.

US Department of Health and Human Services (2000). *Reducing Tobacco Use: A Report of the Surgeon General*. Atlanta, GA: US Department of Health and Human Services, Centers for Disease Control and Prevention, National Center for Chronic Disease Prevention and Health Promotion, Office on Smoking and Health. Available at: http://

www.cdc.gov/tobacco/data_statistics/sgr/2000/complete_report/index.htm.

Volpp, K.G., Troxel, A.B., Pauly, M.V., et al. (2009). A randomized, controlled trial of financial incentives for smoking cessation. *The New England Journal of Medicine*, 360, 699–709.

World Health Organization (1954). *Expert Committee on Health Education of the Public*. WHO Technical Report Series No. 89. Geneva: World Health Organization.

World Health Organization (1986). *Report of a WHO Expert Committee. Community Prevention and Control of Cardiovascular Disease*. Technical Report Series No. 732. Geneva: World Health Organization.

World Health Organization, Health and Welfare Canada, and Canadian Public Health Association (1986). *Ottawa Charter for Health Promotion: An International Conference on Health Promotion—The Move Towards a New Public Health, Nov. 17–21, Ottawa*. Geneva: World Health Organization.

5.10

Community-based intervention trials in low- and middle-income countries

Sheena G. Sullivan and Zunyou Wu

Introduction to community-based intervention trials

In recent years, community-based intervention trials have been increasingly used to evaluate public health interventions to control disease and promote health. They can provide reliable data on the efficacy and cost-effectiveness of disease control strategies to inform policymakers in developing health policy and allocating resources. Typically, community-based interventions use lifestyle interventions that reflect community norms and are thus more readily integrated into current practices.

Community-based interventions were first used in high-income countries for reducing risk factors for cardiovascular and other chronic diseases. They began to be used in low- and middle-income countries in the late 1980s, initially to test programmes addressing maternal and child health. Early interventions targeted increasing immunization coverage (Desgrees du Lou et al. 1995; Brugha and Kevany 1996), decreasing general childhood mortality (Bang et al. 1990; Pandey et al. 1991; West et al. 1991), and maternal mortality (Fauveau et al. 1991), with a strong focus on reducing the impact of communicable diseases. More recently, the use of community-based intervention trials has increased considerably and the focus expanded to include non-communicable conditions, including cardiovascular disease (Dowse et al. 1995; Fang et al. 1999; Jafar et al. 2009), obesity (Kain et al. 2004; Li et al. 2008), mental health (Jacob et al. 2007; Pronyk et al. 2006), and cancer (Ramadas et al. 2003). These types of studies are now used to such an extent there are systematic reviews on specific types of community-based interventions in low- and middle-income countries (Lassi et al. 2010; Sguassero et al. 2012).

The results of these trials have been used in many cases to influence clinical and public health practice not only in the countries in which they are conducted, but also in other countries, including developed nations. For example, community-based sexually transmitted disease (STD) treatment trials in Uganda and Tanzania demonstrated that syndromic treatment of STDs could reduce the incidence of HIV infection at the early stage of an HIV/AIDS epidemic (Grosskurth et al. 1995; Wawer et al. 1998; Kamali et al. 2003), a strategy that was later recommended by the Joint United Nations Programme on HIV/AIDS (UNAIDS) and

adopted widely; a strategy to increase face-washing to reduce trachoma that was tested in Tanzania (West et al. 1995) and another to control fly populations in Gambia (Emerson et al. 1999) have since been incorporated into the World Health Organization's (WHO) SAFE strategy for trachoma control (surgery, antibiotics, facial cleanliness and environmental improvement), widely implemented in Africa (Ngondi et al. 2008).

In contrast, in some cases quality may be compromised to such an extent that the results cannot be used to influence health policy (Li et al. 2008). These trials are often complicated and expensive. Due to the scarcity of resources available in middle-income and particularly in low-income countries, community-based intervention trials have design and methodological features that may be different from similar studies in high-income countries. This chapter reviews community-based intervention trials in low- and middle-income countries. The chapter discusses study design, study population, intervention activities and quality of intervention, ethical issues, measurement issues, and interpretation and translation of results of community-based intervention trials conducted in low- and middle-income countries.

Design

Confusingly, community-based intervention trials can include a range of different study designs. Although the community, however defined, is the unit of intervention, evaluation may be done at either the community or individual level. Moreover, evaluation may be through cross-sectional survey or a cohort may be established, the choice of which has important implications for analysis.

Defining communities

Communities are generally classified along geographical or administrative lines, which in low- and middle-income countries is often a village, urban district, neighbourhood, census tract, or some other locally relevant administrative area. For example, in a study to examine the effect of vitamin A and β-carotene supplementation on postpartum illness in Nepal, randomization was by ward, a subunit of the study district consisting of several small subdistricts (Christian et al. 2000). Entire regions are also sometimes randomized, as was done in four regions of southern Guatemala for a study evaluating the effectiveness of information, education, and communication strategies to increase maternal awareness about pregnancy (Perreira et al. 2002). Hospitals or hospital departments may also serve as the unit of intervention, as was done in a large, multicountry trial to evaluate a multidimensional approach for prevention of ventilator-associated pneumonia in intensive care unit patients of adult (Rosenthal et al. 2012b) and paediatric hospitals (Rosenthal et al. 2012a). For interventions among children, schools often provide a suitable environment in which to conduct intervention activities. In China, for example, there have been a number of attempts to conduct intervention trials to reduce overweight and obesity among schoolchildren, with the unit of intervention being either class groups within schools or entire schools (Li et al. 2008). The reality, of course, is that in many low- and middle-income settings, interventions targeting only schools or hospitals will miss a sizeable portion of the target population, most notably the very poor. However, targeting a comprehensive range of subcommunities is a strategy that has been used to overcome this problem, such as in a Vietnamese trial to control dengue vectors, where local leaders, health volunteer teachers, and schoolchildren were all targeted (Kay et al. 2002).

Regardless of what unit of 'community' is chosen, the unit should be well defined and variations within and between communities should be low. However, in reality this is often not the case. The size of the communities selected and factors that can potentially interfere with the outcomes often vary between selected study venues. It is important to understand the maximum tolerance of heterogeneity among selected study venues. The tolerance of venue variation should be based on appropriate statistical consideration.

Selection of study sites

The first stage of any study is to select an appropriate site for launching a trial. Several issues need to be considered. First, study sites must have a reasonably high prevalence of the events of interest, particularly sufficient high incidence. A high event rate is important to increase the cost-efficiency of the study and to reduce the duration of the trial. In low- and middle-income countries disease incidences are frequently high, particularly infectious diseases. Early community trials of STD treatment for HIV prevention in Africa were in part able to be conducted because of the very high rates of key STDs and HIV compared with other countries: in Mwanza, the average prevalence of syphilis was 15.6 per cent and the average prevalence of HIV was 4.1 per cent (Grosskurth et al. 1995); in Rakai, these figures were 10 per cent for syphilis and 15.9 per cent for HIV (Wawer et al. 1998); and in Mataka, they were 13.1 per cent and 9.8 per cent (Kamali et al. 2003).

Second, existing resources, when available, should be used as much as possible; otherwise the intervention will be expensive and will not be sustainable when the trial is completed. Traditional birth attendants have long been used in interventions to reduce neonatal mortality (Bang et al. 1990). In a community drug prevention study in China, schools, families, communities, and health service infrastructures were all used (Wu et al. 2002). A re-evaluation in 2007 indicated that intervention village residents continued to have higher HIV/AIDS knowledge than control village residents, and the villages were still using educational

programmes and cultural activity rooms established during the trial (Lee 2010).

Third, study sites should be representative of most communities affected by the diseases of interest. This is important because the intervention strategies and measures being tested in the trial should be expanded to other communities or even to the whole country or other countries if they are successful.

Fourth, study sites should be separated from each other in defined minimum distances in order to avoid contamination between intervention and control sites. However, given rapid economic and social development in low- and middle- income countries, people move from one place to another frequently. It is also true that the Internet has created a way for people to communicate almost with no boundaries. These factors should be considered in the study design stage.

Understanding the setting

Prior to attempting any kind of study, it is important to understand the community's dynamics, administrative structures, cultural characteristics, and existing infrastructure. In some settings, census information or public records may be available, although they may be out of date (Eder et al. 2012). Usually little background information about study communities is available in low- and middle-income countries.

Qualitative methods are effective tools for collecting the necessary background information to develop a suitable intervention. It is important to interview key informants in the community. Key informants include community administrative leaders, community religious leaders, opinion leaders, and, importantly, members of the target community. Information can also be sought from these people through focus group discussion. Wacira et al. (2007), in designing an intervention to increase the use of insecticide-treated bednets in Kenya, conducted interviews and focus group discussions with representatives from government ministries, companies, and non-governmental organizations as well as employers and community members. Bhandari et al. (2003), in designing an intervention to improve perinatal and neonatal health outcomes, used qualitative methods to collect information about community characteristics, children's nutritional status, feeding practices, and reasons children may not be breastfed.

On-site observation can also be used to understand community dynamics. This method was used in the National Institute of Mental Health (NIMH) Collaborative HIV/STD Prevention Trial study in five countries (NIMH Collaborative HIV/STD Prevention Trial Group 2007a). Anthropologists observed daily activity in food markets from 6 a.m. when the markets opened until 6 p.m. when they closed. Their major objectives were to identify the most influential individuals within the markets who could be selected and trained for delivery of the intervention and to identify existing social networks among food market vendors that could be used for diffusion of the intervention.

For interventions which target specific groups or venues, researchers may also use mapping tools to identify where and when target groups congregate. An intervention to promote condom use among Lao *Kathoy*, for example, first mapped all the venues where they congregated and the peak periods of activity to develop their sampling framework for administering evaluation questionnaires (Longfield et al. 2011).

The amount of effort that should be put into a qualitative study prior to a trial varies from study to study and depends on how complex the proposed intervention is, how complex the communities involved in the trial are, how much background information already exists, the prior experience of the investigators, and how much money is available for the study.

Community consultation

Complementing the qualitative study should be a comprehensive consultation with the community. Different communities include different subgroups of people, each with its own characteristics, interests, and needs. Comprehensive consultation with different subgroups is an important part of project planning and design that can influence whether or not a project is in fact successful. In a review of 12 community-based intervention studies, 11 reported that community involvement had enhanced the quality of the intervention; two thought that it had improved the outcomes; eight believed it had improved enrolment; four noted better research methods and dissemination; and three described better descriptive measures (Agency for Healthcare Research and Quality 2003). Those members of the community who are consulted may include any person or organization relevant to the trial. For example, a drug prevention study in China consulted a wide range of people, including government leaders in education, health, public security, culture and entertainment, agriculture technology, ethnics group management, and poverty alleviation, as well as community leaders, youth leaders, women leaders, student leaders, teachers, village health workers, and drug users (Wu et al. 2002). Multisite interventions may choose to consult different community members in the different sites.

Ethical concerns with the conduct of research in low- and middle-income countries have led to calls that studies organize a formal community advisory board (CAB), which is consulted to ensure communities are not exploited (Emanuel et al. 2004). Their role extends to include: providing community support for a trial; identifying priority health concerns; assessing the value of research; planning, conducting, and overseeing the research; integrating the results into the healthcare system; respecting the community's values, culture, and social practices; and ensuring that communities benefit from the research (Emanuel et al. 2004). There is no clear consensus on the composition of a CAB, but specific funding bodies or trial groups may have their own requirements. The AIDS Clinical Trials Groups, for example, requires CABs to include people infected with HIV and trial participants and suggests inclusion of patient advocates, parents, community-based healthcare providers, religious leaders, and representatives of underserved communities (AIDS Clinical Trials Group 2012). Even with guidelines, the CAB elected may be ineffective. For example, in Tanzania, initial efforts to establish a CAB for a site for malaria drug and vaccine trials as well as tuberculosis and HIV research met with many problems: village leaders who were asked to recommend individuals to represent their village elected themselves, leading to an overly-male CAB—entirely inappropriate for studies largely targeting women and children—whose attendance was very low, thus compromising training requirements and the establishment of easily-recognized CAB representatives, and who hindered study coordination because of their own political interests (Shubis et al. 2009). While CABs in high-income countries were often developed by activists and researchers who demanded their involvement in research, in low- and middle-income countries CABs are manned by community representatives who are asked to become involved and who therefore may have different expectations, including monetary expectations (Shubis et al. 2009). Efforts to instil a sense of empowerment can help CAB members to perceive that they are respected by the investigators, that they share the ownership of the project, and, therefore, that they share the responsibility for the success of the project. It is important to promote the perception that the project is the community's project, that it will benefit the community, and that everyone has a responsibility to participate.

The comparison group

Community-based intervention trials typically follow one of two formats: (1) an intervention/control or intervention/intervention comparison or (2) a pre-/post-intervention comparison. The simplest approach is the latter; that is, to compare baseline prevalence of a disease or behaviour with the prevalence post intervention. In some situations, this may be the best option available. For example, in 1987, the Senegal government introduced immunization programmes into Bandafassi, an isolated area that previously had had no regular immunization programmes. Since regular immunizations were the only change introduced into the area during this period, it was possible to assess the impact of immunization on childhood mortality by comparing mortality rates before and after the immunization programme was introduced (Desgrees du Lou et al. 1995). In a study promoting consistent condom use among female sex workers in China, high mobility among the sex workers precluded the researchers' ability to identify a suitable control group (Wu et al. 2007). Sex workers would frequently work in several establishments at the same time or quickly move between establishments. Those sex workers coming from an intervention establishment to a control establishment who shared their new knowledge with co-workers would dilute the intervention effect and could incorrectly lead to the conclusion that condom promotion had had no effect, a process known as contamination. Studies that use the mass media are particularly affected by contamination and necessitate a pre-/post-intervention comparison. In Burkina Faso, an intervention to distribute drugs against schistosomiasis was preceded by a nationwide information campaign utilizing television and radio to ensure high compliance with the treatment, eliminating any possibility of using a control group (Gabrielli et al. 2006).

A more robust design is to have a control group; a group which was comparable with the intervention group at baseline and who, for the duration of the intervention, experienced none of the intervention activities, but did experience other phenomena which may have led to an improvement in the desired outcome anyway. This last point is impossible to control in pre-/post-intervention comparisons. Intervention and control communities may be assigned, as in a quasi-experimental design, or may be randomly allocated, as in a cluster-randomized controlled design (discussed further in the next section).

Studies do not have to be limited to testing one intervention against a control. Multiple interventions can be tested and compared with controls to determine which combination of activities leads to the greatest impact. In Honduras, a programme to increase the use of healthcare services compared four groups: (1) money given directly to households, (2) resources to local health teams combined with a community-based nutrition intervention, (3) both packages, and (4) neither package (Morris et al. 2004). In some cases it may be deemed unethical or impractical to have a control group, in which case it may be possible to compare two different interventions. In the study of trachoma in Tanzania, intervention villages received free treatment and health education while 'control' villages received the treatment only (West et al. 1995). The addition of health education carried an additional cost but the study showed it would be worth implementing on a wider scale since children in intervention communities were 60 per cent less likely to develop trachoma. Alternatively, the design may include a wait-listed control, where the control communities receive the intervention once it has been shown to be effective. This was done in a programme that combined microfinance and gender/HIV training in South Africa (Pronyk et al. 2006). Communities were pair-matched, then randomized to receive the intervention at study onset or 3 years later.

Randomization, matching, and stratification

Well-designed randomized controlled trials are recognized as the gold standard for the evaluation of public health interventions. With randomization, unmeasured confounding factors are expected to be equally distributed in the intervention and comparison groups. Unbiased effect-estimates and valid confidence intervals can therefore, in theory, be obtained. The extension of this in community-based trials is to randomize at the community level, following the cluster- or group-randomized trial design, where the unit of randomization is the community rather than the individual. The number of units of randomization in community-randomized trials is usually smaller than in individually randomized trials, although the number of individuals may be large. In Nepal, studies to improve postpartum outcomes randomized 270 wards in 30 villages to one of two intervention groups or a control but the total number of individuals enrolled in the study was more than 15,000 (Christian et al. 2000). Often, community trials have fewer communities available for randomization. When the number of units is very small, randomization is less likely to achieve comparability between intervention and control groups at baseline.

To overcome dissimilarity between intervention and control communities, researchers may consider matching, which involves matching communities on factors highly associated with the outcome variable, and then randomizing within the matched pair. For example, in the study of the effect of face-washing on trachoma, three paired villages were matched on the level of maternal education, baseline prevalence of clean faces in young children, and trachoma status. Within each pair, one village was randomized to the intervention and the other to the control group (West et al. 1995). The rationale for matching is to improve power in randomized studies. However, if matching variables are not strongly associated with the outcome, matching actually reduces study power through loss of degrees of freedom with a small number of experimental units (Martin et al. 1993).

An alternative to matching is stratification, where communities may be grouped rather than paired by variables associated with the outcome and later randomized within strata. In both matching and stratification, the degrees of freedom are reduced, but this can be offset by the decrease in the variance between communities, which in turn can reduce the design effect and improve power. The results of

the three landmark STD/HIV community-randomized trials conducted in Africa (Grosskurth et al. 1995; Wawer et al. 1998; Kamali et al. 2003) were compared to examine the differential effects of stratification or matching (Todd et al. 2003). In Mwanza (Grosskurth et al. 1995) and Masaka (Kamali et al. 2003), matching and stratification reduced between-community variance and improved the power of the study compared with an unmatched or unstratified design. In the Rakai trial (Wawer et al. 1998), where communities had been selected to be relatively homogeneous, matching reduced the variance between communities but did not increase power.

In certain circumstances, randomization of intervention units may not be possible. This may occur, for example, when study villages are adjacent to one another and the risk of contamination is high. In a community-based intervention trial to reduce childhood mortality from pneumonia, random allocation was not performed (Bang et al. 1990). The intervention included mass education about childhood pneumonia and case management of pneumonia by village health workers and traditional birth attendants. A total of 102 villages in one contiguous area were studied, of which 58 villages were assigned to the intervention group and 44 villages were in the control group. The two groups were separated by a small 'buffer' zone of a few villages. In this example, given the geographic proximity of the intervention and control communities and the use of mass education, the other choices available to the researchers were randomization without using mass education, or using the mass media without a control area.

Where randomization is chosen, investigators should follow the guidelines found in the CONSORT (Consolidated Standards of Reporting Trials) statement (Campbell et al. 2004). This statement was initially designed to guide the reporting of randomized clinical trials and has since been updated to provide guidance on the reporting of cluster-randomized trials. It includes a flow diagram and a 22-point checklist to remind researchers to include important information necessary for objective interpretation of the results, such as the intracluster correlation, design effect, and power and sample size calculations. Many medical journals now require adherence to the statement as a condition for publication.

Cohort versus repeated cross-sectional samples

Whether a study design uses a pre/post or intervention/control design, measuring the effect of the intervention is usually done at the individual level. Ideally, all individuals in the target population are sampled. Two early studies to reduce childhood mortality in India (Bang et al. 1990) and Nepal (Pandey et al. 1991) were able to carry out a census of all children under 5 years at the beginning of the study and enumerate all births and deaths during the study. However, conducting a census is expensive and often not logistically possible. Thus, researchers in low- and middle-income countries have generally needed to make a choice between one of two study designs: (1) a cohort study design, where a selected group of individuals is followed up for changes over the course of the study; or (2) a repeated (serial) cross-sectional survey design where different groups, usually randomly selected, are assessed at each time period. This decision depends on the characteristics of the outcome variable, the information-collecting system available at the study sites, the ability to follow the sample population, and the amount of funds available for the study.

Cohort studies are statistically more powerful than cross-sectional surveys, since individual baseline characteristics can be controlled, which reduces sampling error. Moreover, the change in disease frequency or knowledge, attitudes, and beliefs can be compared both between intervention and control and pre/post intervention. For example, the Chilean intervention to prevent childhood obesity enrolled children at intervention and control schools, measured various adiposity indices at baseline and again at 6-month follow-up, and was able to measure the *relative* changes between intervention and control schools over the 6-month study period (Kain et al. 2004). Sometimes results based solely on a cohort may not be representative of the target population due to selection bias. The cohort sample is often a self-selected subset of that group who are willing to be followed up. Attrition throughout the study may also decrease the external validity of the sample, particularly if the participants who leave the study are disproportionately reached by the intervention. Moreover, repeated measurement may act as a kind of intervention in itself, increasing participants' knowledge and confounding the results.

Cross-sectional studies also have their own strengths and weaknesses. Given that the target population for community-based interventions is often the wider community, it could be argued that cross-sectional surveys are more appropriate to see changes in the communities targeted. They may include people who have had extensive or limited exposure to the intervention, thus giving a more representative picture of the intervention's reach. On the other hand, this may also be seen as a weakness, especially when limited exposure is associated with in-migration and a related short duration of exposure, rather than limited reach (Feldman and McKinlay 1994). Cross-sectional surveys are often used to assess mass-media campaigns, since it may be impossible to find an unexposed control group. In a systematic review of 24 media campaigns to change HIV/AIDS-related behaviours in developing countries, 15 used cross-sectional surveys to measure the impact of the campaign (Bertrand et al. 2006). There are other circumstances where cohorts are almost impossible to establish, such as in areas of high migration. In the trial to promote condom use among sex workers in China, repeated cross-sectional surveys were the only feasible choice given the high turnover of sex workers in the study site (Wu et al. 2007).

Sometimes a retrospective cohort can be reconstructed in repeated cross-sectional surveys. In the study of prevention of drug use in China (Wu et al. 2002), the incidence of drug use among adolescents and young adults was estimated based on a reconstructed retrospective cohort derived from repeated cross-sectional surveys. This was possible because there was very little migration in or out of the villages and the village leader was responsible for recording all in- and out-migrations.

In some cases, both a cohort and a cross-sectional survey have been used simultaneously. In China, an intervention to improve the quality of life of people living with HIV that comprised both an intervention for patients and a popular-opinion model targeting the community enrolled a cohort of people with HIV among whom changes in perceived and felt stigma could be measured, and conducted serial cross-sectional surveys of the community to assess the impact of the community campaign to reduce stigma towards people living with HIV (Xu et al. 2008).

Sample size and statistical power

The estimation of sample size in any study depends on the availability of background information on the prevalence of the disease or behaviour of interest, the size of the source population, and the likely refusal rate. This can be achieved through reviewing data available from similar studies in the target group. For example, a study to prevent childhood obesity in Chile used average body mass index values from an earlier survey of nutrition and obesity in Chilean schoolchildren (Kain et al. 2004). Alternatively, census data may be available, although this can sometimes be out of date. A group re-evaluating an intervention in Bolivia, for example, discovered too late that the census data they had used to develop their sampling frame did not reflect the real number of households in each village, resulting in recruitment of 73 per cent of the intended number of households (Eder et al. 2012). National estimates may also be used, such as those for neonatal mortality and birth rates, which were used to determine sample size in a Nepali study of a participatory intervention to reduce neonatal mortality (Manandhar et al. 2004).

The method used to estimate sample size is of course dependent on the study design. In the community intervention trials discussed in this chapter, the designs varied: the number of communities involved ranged from one (self-controls) to a comparison of two communities to a comparison of many communities either assigned or randomized to receive the intervention(s) or control condition. For example, in the Mauritius non-communicable disease prevention study, it was not feasible to use a control area in the small island, therefore only one unit was used, assessed by pre- and post-intervention cross-sectional surveys including 5080 and 5162 participants, respectively (Dowse et al. 1995). Emerson et al. (1999) used two pairs of villages (1124 children enrolled at baseline) to study control of trachoma and diarrhoea in Gambia. In such non-randomized studies, the sample calculation is straightforward and estimates the number of community members to be recruited. However, when multiple communities are used there are other parameters to consider, and methods for cluster-randomization should be employed. Individuals within a community are more similar to each other than to individuals from another community and are therefore more likely to have the same outcome. This violates the assumption of independence between observations, which is essential in most statistical analyses. Thus, the correlation between individuals within communities can greatly affect the sample size (Kerry and Bland 1998a). For example, a study which has enrolled 2000 people in 50 clusters may note that individuals within those clusters are all very similar in terms of key covariates, so the effective sample size is actually closer to 50 than it is to 2000. The sum of the variance between subjects in a cluster and the variance between clusters, is used to calculate the intracluster correlation and is used to calculate the design effect (Kerry and Bland 1998b). This is the ratio of the total number of subjects required using cluster randomization to the number that would be required if individual randomization were used. It is used to estimate how much larger the sample size (of individuals) needs to be to achieve statistical power. For example, if the design effect is 1.17, then the number of participants needs to be increased by 17 per cent (Todd et al. 2003). In estimating the required sample size these parameters need to be known a priori and can be estimated from previous studies or existing data on the study communities. However, such information is often unavailable or incompletely described (Kerry and Bland 1998a).

To a certain extent, increasing the number of individual observations in a cluster can reduce the variability within communities and increase statistical power, but at a certain point this effect plateaus and the number of clusters needs to be increased. In general, if communities are particularly homogeneous, a larger number of small communities should be considered. However, the advantages of increasing the number of communities needs to be balanced with the feasibility and costs associated with targeting more communities. In the South African study to reduce intimate-partner violence, the number of clusters was limited to four in each study arm because of operational constraints, including the time required for recruitment and follow-up, the need to enrol all households in a village before expansion, and ethical concerns about withholding the intervention from control villages (Pronyk et al. 2006). Conversely, a smaller number of communities can be used if communities are relatively heterogeneous. In either case, the number of individuals required in cluster-randomization is larger than would be needed for individual randomization and failure to do so comes at the expense of power to detect a difference between groups. For example, in a study to promote exclusive breastfeeding in Mexico City, 39 clusters with two to four city blocks each were randomized to one of two intervention conditions or a control. A total of 125 children were enrolled in each arm, which met the minimum required sample size of 120, based on $\alpha = 0.05$ (one-sided), and giving 86 per cent power to detect a 20 per cent absolute difference in exclusive breastfeeding between intervention and control groups (24 per cent versus 4 per cent) if there was no design effect; accounting for a design effect of 1.2, power was reduced to 76 per cent (Morrow et al. 1999).

An alternative to increasing the sample size in an individual study or site is to pool data from different trials or run multisite trials. Pooling data from trials that were not planned together requires they have comparable outcome measures and can be difficult to achieve. Even multisite trials may find it difficult to preserve the study design. The NIMH Collaborative HIV/STD Prevention Trial is a community-level study conducted in five countries—China, India, Peru, Russia, and Zimbabwe—to assess the efficacy of an intervention involving popular-opinion leaders to reduce the incidence of HIV/STDs (NIMH Collaborative HIV/STD Prevention Trial Group 2007b, 2010). The trial used comparable intervention strategies and data collection instruments to allow the pooling of data to increase power, although individual sites were also powered to observe an effect. Site-specific sources of variance need to be taken into account when determining sample size and power and in analysing the results.

Further discussion on sample size calculations for cluster randomized trials can be found in Chapter 5.8.

Ethical issues

There are several ethical issues unique to community-based interventions, some of which can affect the study design. Foremost is the issue of informed consent. Obtaining informed consent from every individual in a target community to be exposed to an intervention is often impractical and can compromise the validity of the trial by artificially raising awareness of the problem being addressed. Moreover, individuals may not be able to realistically avoid exposure to an intervention, such as when the mass media is used to deliver the intervention (Sim and Dawson 2012). Community consultation with different stakeholders and approval from a CAB may be seen by some as seeking the consent of the community to conduct a trial (Edwards et al. 1999), while others believe that an internal review board's review should be sufficient (Sim and Dawson 2012).

Where individuals in a community are enrolled in a cohort to receive specific intervention components, consent can be sought from those individuals. However, unlike a drug trial, which can be double-blinded and where participants are aware that they may receive treatment or placebo, community trials often involve educational or other programmes and participants know whether they are receiving the intervention or not. By fully informing participants in the control group about the intervention during the informed consent process, contamination may be introduced by prompting the controls to seek out the information that their counterparts in the intervention group are receiving. Contamination can be reduced by using geographically distant communities, but this may lead to incomparability between comparison groups. If controls are receiving routine care, then it may be considered acceptable to withhold information regarding the intervention from them. In this way, individual consent to participate in intervention activities is sought only from those in the intervention communities, and consent for data collection and to be contacted for follow-up is taken from all parties (Edwards et al. 1999). There is a balance between ensuring study validity and protecting participants; contamination could reduce the efficacy of a trial, and conducting a methodologically-poor study may be perceived as being unethical (Sim and Dawson 2012).

The problem of whether to fully inform controls about the intervention is further complicated when monetary incentives are introduced. In many low- and middle-income countries, financial or other incentives, such as free food, washing powder, or other household consumables, are provided for participation in a trial. Any financial or other incentive may be viewed as coercion given the poor financial situation of most eligible participants in low- and middle-income countries, but in many of these settings incentives are expected. The nature and amount of such incentives should be described in the study protocols submitted to ethics review committees, which will ultimately decide if the incentive implicates voluntary participation. Where controls are concerned, fairness and justice may be compromised. Both intervention and control participants would normally receive reimbursement for data collection activities, but controls would not normally participate in any intervention activities, such as skills training, so would not be eligible for any associated reimbursements. In addition, there is some risk that incentives increase the intervention effect by creating a motivation to participate that artificially increases exposure.

In some instances it may be unethical to even have a control group at all, such as when an intervention is already known to be effective. Instead, two interventions may be compared, a waitlisted control used, or researchers may need to consider a pre-/post-intervention comparison within intervention communities only. In some low- and middle-income countries, communities do not understand the need for controls, or believe them not to be cost-effective because of the expenses involved in maintaining such communities. Similarly, they may not accept the process of randomization. In these situations it is important to educate the government or communities about the need for controls and randomization in yielding scientifically valid findings, and alternative study designs may need to be considered.

As researchers from high-income countries intensify their research activity in low- and middle-income countries, and as researchers from low- and middle-income countries increasingly bid for foreign funding, adherence to international ethical guidelines has become increasingly important. This includes the establishment of institutional structures, such as institutional review boards (IRBs) or ethics committees that can monitor the progress of the research and protect the people enrolled in the trials. International Guidelines for Epidemiological Studies (CIOMS 2009) have been developed to help guide these institutional bodies. But questions may remain (Weijer et al. 2011). For example, would an IRB in a developing country really understand the ethical issues posed by a study for a community in a low-income setting and be able to assess the appropriateness of informed consent procedures? Conversely, would an IRB in a developed country have sufficient, well-trained epidemiologists to assess the methodological quality of a trial? Where interventions have been successful in developed countries, their translation to low-income settings may compromise their efficacy. And where they prove effective, who will fund the continued implementation of the intervention? Greater debate is needed among high-, middle-, and low-income countries to understand the ethical issues peculiar to each setting and to develop ethical guidelines for the conduct of community-based interventions.

Intervention activities

Types of interventions

The content of community interventions can include changes in public policy, the environment, community norms, or personal behaviours at both the individual and community levels. In broad terms, intervention programmes can be grouped into four types: (1) individual-level programmes, such as self-study manuals, one-to-one communication or counselling, and peer education programmes; (2) group interventions such as educational programmes in schools or with informal groups such as support organizations of drug users or sex workers; (3) mass media campaigns such as radio and television advertisements or newspaper stories; (4) public policy changes, such as mandated non-smoking areas in public places and the use of seat belts; and (5) structural interventions, such as the building water and sanitation infrastructure and public exercise equipment. Often community-wide interventions include programmes of each type. Choosing which types of interventions to use should be determined by the characteristics of the communities, the diseases of interest, cost, feasibility, and other factors.

Individually targeted, intensive interventions may be of limited use in community trials because participation in these kinds of programmes is low, and thus the population-level impact will be small. Group intervention may also have limited reach, though have additional benefits such as development of support groups. On the other hand, mass media campaigns can have a wide reach at low cost, but necessarily have a broad message which may be unable to correct misconceptions and may be lost among the plethora of media options now available (Wakefield et al. 2010). Policy changes, if enforced, can have tremendous impact, but may need to be accompanied by media messaging or information dissemination to make people aware of the change (Wongkhomthong et al. 1995).

Generally, a combined approach is more likely to be effective than one which uses only one approach because the combined approach will reach a wider audience. For example, the Indian intervention to promote exclusive breastfeeding employed a combination of interventions, namely: (1) individual counselling by traditional birth attendants, immunization clinic nurses, and healthcare workers; (2) meetings between the healthcare workers and community representatives who in turn held neighbourhood meetings to promote breastfeeding among women in the community; and (3) printed educational materials including pamphlets, posters in clinics, flip books for health workers, and counselling guides to solve common breastfeeding problems (Bhandari et al. 2003). In Guatemala, an intervention to increase awareness of danger signs during pregnancy, delivery, and the postpartum period used: (1) a clinic-based programme which trained health providers on prenatal counselling and provided educational media to patients, (2) a community-based programme consisting of radio messages about obstetric complications, and (3) education sessions conducted through women's groups (Perreira et al. 2002). The components of a health, water, and sanitation intervention in Bolivia that targeted improving health and nutritional status of vulnerable women and children used: (1) community health promoters who provided one-on-one and group-based health and nutrition education, (2) school breakfasts, (3) engagement of parents in school feeding activities, (4) establishment of school gardens, (5) culturally-sensitive maternal and child health activities to address harmful traditional health practices, and (6) used food as compensation for the time spent participating in intervention activities (Eder et al. 2012).

Appropriateness of intervention messages

Community interventions, particularly those that try to change people's behaviour, need to be carefully tailored to the target audience. Even those interventions that test treatments requiring only a minor change in behaviour encounter difficulties in ensuring compliance among patients. Thus the sensitivities of the target population should be integrated into intervention messages. For example, sex workers may be more receptive to HIV/sexually transmitted infection prevention messages when they are put in the context of fertility (Liao et al. 2003). However, in many cases knowledge and information is not enough to create change and structural or policy interventions may be needed. An example is antismoking education among health professionals, which has largely failed on its own, while strategies that have included policy interventions, such as regulations prohibiting smoking in hospital settings, have been more effective in stopping health professionals from smoking around clinical settings (Smith et al. 2005).

Difficulties in message framing are often exacerbated in low- and middle-income countries by limited education. For example, people may not understand how chronic behaviour, such as long-term smoking, can lead to adverse health consequences many years later. Thus the literacy levels of the population should also be taken into account.

Religion can pose a barrier, an obvious example being proscription by the Catholic Church of condom use to prevent HIV/STD infection. However, there are some examples where religion has successfully been incorporated into intervention activities. For example, harm reduction for drug users in Muslim communities has been advocated on the basis that it is the lesser of two harms (Kamarulzaman and Saifuddeen 2010).

Intensity of the interventions

How much intervention is less than enough, how much is just enough, and how much is more than enough depends on such variables as the nature of the intervention, the characteristics of the target population, and the cultural characteristics of the society or community. Thus no guidelines can be formulated to cover all circumstances. Answering this question can be incorporated into the study design. For example, in the study to promote exclusive breastfeeding in Mexico City, two intervention groups with different counselling frequencies, six visits and three visits, were compared with a control group that had no intervention (Morrow et al. 1999). Infants were followed up until 3 months of age to assess the effect of the peer education programme on promoting exclusive breastfeeding and on the incidence of diarrhoea among children. Exclusive breastfeeding was achieved in 67 per cent in the six-visit group, 50 per cent in the three-visit group, and 12 per cent in the control group.

Often a community health intervention trial can be designed, funded, and implemented in a place where other health-related programmes may already be under way with public and/or private sponsorship in both experimental and control communities. Many community intervention trials may be testing only an incremental increase in the general level of health promotion in intervention communities, not the effectiveness of the intervention alone. Any community intervention programme must be sufficiently potent to be 'heard' beyond the background noise of ongoing health promotion activities. Thus an intervention programme should direct resources toward interventions that are relatively unique and not available in control communities.

Sustainability of interventions

The sustainability of an intervention is one of the most important issues in conducting community-based interventions in low- and middle-income countries. Several factors likely affect sustainability. First, the cost-effectiveness of the intervention. The cheaper the intervention is, the more sustainable the programme is likely to be. In the Mwanza STD study, during the 2 years of follow-up, 11,632 cases of STDs were treated in the intervention health units; 252 HIV infections were averted each year in the intervention group compared with control group. The average per capita cost was US$0.39. It was estimated that the average cost per disability-adjusted life year (DALY) saved was US$10 (range: US$2.51–47.86). The estimated cost-effectiveness of the intervention, that is, improved treatment services for STDs, compared favourably with the cost of childhood immunization programmes, US$12–17 per DALY (Gilson et al. 1997). If the intervention can generate profits, community may be more likely to sustain it after study completion.

Second, the simpler the intervention is, the more sustainable the programme will be. In a study on reducing childhood mortality in Nepal (Pandey et al. 1991), the intervention programme focused on active case detection. Every day each health worker visited 10–15 households with children under 5 years of age, most within a half-hour walk from the worker's home. The worker completed a round of the target households (about 160) under his/her responsibility every 2 weeks. The intervention occupied about half his/ her time and allowed him/her to continue his/her regular farming activities.

Third, the higher the proportion of people in the community covered by the intervention, the more likely the programme will be sustained. In the Rakai STD study, all consenting adults were given treatment (Wawer et al. 1998); that is, the STD rate in the community was reduced for the period of the trial and this would have at least a medium-term impact on keeping levels of infection low. However, without continued availability of free treatment to address new infections, the long-term sustainability is limited.

Fourth, the higher the intensity of the intervention, the less likely the programme will be sustained because maintaining high intensity is usually expensive, difficult, and often results in 'burn-out'. However, if the intensity is not high enough, the programme may not be able to produce changes.

A careful review of what really makes interventions sustainable appears to be unavailable, probably because few research groups return to their study site years later to examine the sustained effect of the intervention. Researchers may be unable to source the necessary funding to conduct a re-evaluation many years later and may have moved on to other fields. Many interventions are conducted with donor support and do not follow a rigorous scientific method. Donors may require some limited evaluation, but do not require very long-term evaluation. One group in Bolivia returned to villages 6 years after a comprehensive donor-funded health, nutrition, water and sanitation intervention had ended to evaluate whether the intervention practices had been sustained (Kain et al. 2004). Compared with control communities, intervention communities continued to have more functional water systems, that were better maintained, but maintenance of latrines in households was less impressive. In addition, more intervention households continued to practise positive maternal and child health behaviours. Communities which had received both development and health investments were better off than those which received only health or development assistance. This type of long-term follow-up should be done more often to assess the true, long-term impact of an intervention.

Measurement

While the unit of intervention in community-based trials is the community, the unit of measurement is often the individual. Since the overall aim of a community-based intervention programme is generally to reduce mortality and/or morbidity, these two measures are commonly used indicators of the impact of the intervention. In the childhood mortality studies in Nepal (Pandey et al. 1991; Manandhar et al. 2004) and India (Bang et al. 1990) neonatal, infant, and child mortality was used as the outcome variable. Maternal mortality was an outcome in an antenatal care intervention in Bangladesh (Bang et al. 1990) and Nepal (Manandhar et al. 2004). In three STD studies conducted in Africa, the incidence rates of STDs and HIV infection were used to evaluate intervention effects (Grosskurth et al. 1995; Wawer et al. 1998; Kamali et al. 2003). Morbidity may also be measured not only as disease incidence measured through biological methods, but also by using psychosocial measures. A number of these now exist to measure quality of life, addiction, depression, and other psychological symptoms, many of which have been translated and tested in the context of low- and middle-income countries. In India, the effectiveness of a day-care programme for the elderly was measured using standardized scales for assessing psychiatric morbidity and quality of life (Jacob et al. 2007).

Direct measures of outcome variables, such as disease incidence or mortality, provide valid data to assess the effectiveness of an intervention programme. However, determining them is often expensive. The high cost of individual-level measurements may limit the number of surveys that can be done and thus the statistical power of the evaluation. The high cost of measuring incidence often precludes long-term monitoring for latent effects, which can be important since the time lag between programme implementation and individual-level effects is often uncertain and may be long. Costs can be reduced to a certain extent by taking advantage of local health services records and using passive case detection, rather than surveying participants at specific times. In Ghana, an intervention to prevent malaria in children was measured by the incidence of malaria and anaemia as detected when children were hospitalized at any one of 11 health clinics in the study site (Chandramohan et al. 2005). In many low- and middle-income countries, however, health services may not be established well enough to make this feasible. Serial cross-sectional surveys may also reduce costs as they are usually less expensive than incidence studies.

Because of these problems, other measures are often used as surrogate markers for morbidity. Examples of surrogate or intermediate outcomes that are measured in a variety of behavioural intervention studies include knowledge, attitudes, beliefs, intentions, behavioural skills, and behaviours. In such studies, the assumption is that increasing knowledge and changing attitudes will lead to reduced risk behaviours and by reducing risk behaviours the likelihood of developing the disease is also reduced. In community-based HIV/AIDS education interventions, knowledge, sexual behaviours, and condom use behaviours may be used as outcome variables to assess the impact of the interventions. Self-reported data are cheaper because they avoid costly clinical tests. Moreover, changes in behaviour may be expected to be seen to a larger extent than changes in the frequency of disease, making sample size calculations smaller and reducing overall study expenditure.

However, data collected through self-report are less robust than objective measures such as biological testing because they may be affected by recall bias and social-desirability bias. Ideally, where funding is sufficient, self-reported behaviours are verified by more objective data, such as biological data, to verify that the changes in behaviour lead to the desired outcome, at least in the short term. Studies of condom use to prevent HIV infection will often ask participants about their risk behaviours but may verify this through biological assessments, such as testing for STDs (which generally have a higher incidence and infectivity than HIV, and hence are more likely to yield an observable change in prevalence), or observing whether participants can demonstrate correct condom use.

Other general measures can include distribution of intervention materials or demand for services. In the nationwide schistosomiasis campaign launched in Burkina Faso, the number of immunizations was one outcome used to measure coverage (Gabrielli et al. 2006). Environmental factors can also act as objective measures of the success of an intervention. In a study to increase knowledge and modify behaviours related to dengue vectors in Vietnam, the main outcome was the prevalence of the *Aedes aegypti* mosquito larvae in water storage containers (Vu et al. 2005).

Interpretation

Interpretation of results is sometimes difficult. Cautious interpretation must be made especially when no control group is used. The Matlab study of maternal mortality in Bangladesh concluded that maternal mortality was significantly lower in areas with maternal and child healthcare programmes and family planning programmes (MCH-FP) than in the control area (Fauveau et al. 1991). However, continued observation indicated that there was no sustained difference between the MCH-FP and comparison areas (Ronsmans et al. 1997). The authors thus concluded that the introduction of the maternity-care programme coincided with declining trends in direct obstetric mortality in the areas covered by the programme, although it is also possible that the effectiveness of the intervention declined.

Even with a control group, sometimes the relative benefits of an intervention are not observable. This may be because the investigators have failed to accommodate secular trends in the community under study. Conducting a pre-baseline survey before randomization can provide data to help interpret the influence of secular trends. Qualitative data can also help to interpret secular trends. In the South Africa study, qualitative data and analytic methods that could control for secular trends were used to detect reductions in intimate-partner violence (Pronyk et al. 2006).

Appropriate statistical analysis

A key issue in interpreting results from a community-based trial is using the correct data analysis, particularly when cluster-randomization has been used. Because the analysis is complicated—requiring that both individual-level and group-level characteristics be accommodated—few researchers use the correct statistical analyses, even in high-income countries. A review of 56 papers in seven peer-reviewed journals identified few that had appropriate study designs or used the appropriate methods of analysis (Ukoumunne et al. 1999). Often, researchers fail to take into account the group or design effect and data are analysed at the individual level. By ignoring the group effect, the relative benefits of the intervention are exaggerated and the intervention may seem more effective than it really is (Donner and Klar 2000). Accounting for group and individual-level covariates can be achieved using a multilevel or hierarchical model which includes a parameter for the correlation of observations within a cluster. A number of texts now exist describing how to perform these types of analysis using commonly-used statistical programs, making these methods more accessible to researchers. (See also Chapter 5.8.)

Translating scientific studies to programme settings

Often, the scientific environment in which a study is conducted is quite different from programme settings. Investigators will often choose a study environment that will allow methodological robustness. For example, communities with low emigration are often used in scientific studies to maximize the likelihood of good follow-up of participants for the duration of the study. Scientific studies are also generally able to expend more resources (financial, human, and time) than would be feasible if the project were later institutionalized in the routine healthcare system in low- and middle-income countries. The capacity of health workers is a key issue in scaling up evidence-based interventions. In many low- and middle-income countries, health workers, particularly those in rural areas, have only had some high-school education, with additional training in first aid and preventive medicine. Intervention activities need to be within the capabilities of the health human resources that are reasonably available or that require a level of training that is realistic given local health budgets.

In low- and middle-income countries, trials are often done to determine their effectiveness, rather than their efficacy. The differences between these two objectives are important when considering whether or not to scale up an intervention. Efficacy measures the benefits of an intervention among those who take advantage of it or the benefits of an intervention given under fairly ideal conditions; effectiveness measures the benefits of an intervention among those offered or under programmatic or 'real-life' conditions. When scaling up a community intervention programme, the overall effectiveness of a programme is more important than knowing how good it could be if people were to use it, especially when trying to determine how best to use limited resources. However, a programme is unlikely to prove effective if it has not been demonstrated to be efficacious. This extends to structural barriers that prevent people from using an intervention. In the study from Honduras that compared giving monetary incentives to women to use primary healthcare services with direct transfer of resources to local health teams, it was found that the household-level intervention had a large impact, but the transfer of resources could not be implemented properly because of legal complications (Morris et al. 2004). While the researchers acknowledged this limited interest in their findings, they stressed that their objective was to test effectiveness, rather than efficacy; the inability of the government to successfully transfer resources was therefore an important observation because of its implications for scale-up. Sometimes in community trials, particularly those conducted in low- and middle-income countries, *feasibility* is the most important study outcome.

Feasibility is greatly aided by community consultation. As mentioned earlier, consultation with key community members in the design phase of a project can aid translation of research into policy by ensuring that the study asks questions which the community regard as important. Continued communication with these parties is essential for creating the sense of ownership required for politicians and government officials to support scale-up of an intervention. Strategies that facilitate the development of relationships among members in different, responsible sectors can facilitate this process of persuasion. They are especially important when recommending the scale-up of interventions that benefit marginalized or stigmatized members of the population.

Conclusion

Community intervention trials are now used in low- and middle-income countries more than ever before and cover an increasing range of public health issues, including infectious diseases, neonatal mortality, malnutrition, and unhealthy behaviours, as well as chronic diseases. Their use is likely to continue to increase in coming years as concern grows over the evaluation of the delivery of health services, public education, and social policy. One advantage of conducting community intervention trials in low- and middle-income countries is that they often address urgent preventable health problems in these countries. However, it is often more challenging to implement community intervention trials in these countries because of the lack of background information, lack of infrastructure, and lack of trained and experienced resource personnel. Several criteria need to be considered before beginning community intervention trials in low- and middle-income countries:

◆ Study sites should have a reasonably high incidence of the health events of interest.

◆ A qualitative study of the social and cultural characteristics of the community may need to be conducted.

◆ Community consultation should be carried out before finalizing the intervention plan.

◆ Local resources should be used for the intervention to ensure sustainability.

◆ The type, intensity, and quality of the intervention must be considered acceptable and culturally sensitive to the communities.

◆ Simplicity, affordability, and sustainability of intervention strategies should always be emphasized.

Community interventions have been demonstrated to be effective in low- and middle-income countries but more trials are needed for the many public health problems still affecting these countries.

Acknowledgements

The authors are especially grateful to Professors Roger Detels and Mary Ann Lansang for their comments, suggestions, and helpful editing. The authors would also like to thank Ms Linc Handlos-Neerup for her assistance with the literature review.

References

Agency for Healthcare Research and Quality (2003). *Community-Based Participatory Research: Assessing the Evidence*. Washington, DC: Agency for Healthcare Research and Quality, US Department of Health and Human Services.

AIDS Clinical Trials Group. *Joint Recommendation of the ACTG Executive Committee, the ACTG Network Community Advisory Board (NCAB), and ACTG Community Advisory Board (CAB) Members for the Effective Operation of Community Advisory Boards* [Online]. Available at: https://actgnetwork.org/community/general-information/gcab/guidelines.

Bang, A.T., Bang, R.A., Tale, O., et al. (1990). Reduction in pneumonia mortality and total childhood mortality by means of community-based intervention trial in Gadchiroli, India. *The Lancet*, 336, 201–6.

Bertrand, J.T., O'Reilly, K., Denison, J., Anhang, R., and Sweat, M. (2006). Systematic review of the effectiveness of mass communication programs to change HIV/AIDS-related behaviors in developing countries. *Health Education Research*, 21, 567–97.

Bhandari, N., Bahl, R., Mazumdar, S., Martines, J., Black, R.E., and Bhan, M.K. (2003). Effect of community-based promotion of exclusive breastfeeding on diarrhoeal illness and growth: a cluster randomised controlled trial. *The Lancet*, 361, 1418–23.

Brugha, R.F. and Kevany, J.P. (1996). Maximizing immunization coverage through home visits: a controlled trial in an urban area of Ghana. *Bulletin of the World Health Organization*, 74, 517–24.

Campbell, M.K., Elbourne, D.R., and Altman, D.G. (2004). CONSORT statement: extension to cluster randomised trials. *British Medical Journal*, 328, 702–8.

Chandramohan, D., Owusu-Agyei, S., Carneiro, I., et al. (2005). Cluster randomised trial of intermittent preventive treatment for malaria in infants in area of high, seasonal transmission in Ghana. *British Medical Journal*, 331, 727–33.

Christian, P., West, K.P., Jr., Khatry, S.K., et al. (2000). Vitamin A or beta-carotene supplementation reduces symptoms of illness in pregnant and lactating Nepali women. *Journal of Nutrition*, 130, 2675–82.

CIOMS (2009). *International Ethical Guidelines for Epidemiological Studies*. Geneva: CIOMS.

Desgrees du Lou, A., Pison, G., and Aaby, P. (1995). Role of immunizations in the recent decline in childhood mortality and the changes in the female/male mortality ratio in rural Senegal. *American Journal of Epidemiology*, 142, 643–52.

Donner, A. and Klar, N. (2000). *Design and Analysis of Cluster Randomization Trials in Health Research*. London: Arnold Publishing Company.

Dowse, G.K., Gareeboo, H., Alberti, K.G., et al. (1995). Changes in population cholesterol concentrations and other cardiovascular risk factor levels after five years of the non-communicable disease intervention programme in Mauritius. Mauritius Non-communicable Disease Study Group. *British Medical Journal*, 311, 1255–9.

Eder, C., Schooley, J., Fullerton, J., and Murguia, J. (2012). Assessing impact and sustainability of health, water, and sanitation interventions in Bolivia six years post-project. *Revista Panamericana de Salud Pública*, 32, 43–8.

Edwards, S.J., Braunholtz, D.A., Lilford, R.J., and Stevens, A.J. (1999). Ethical issues in the design and conduct of cluster randomised controlled trials. *British Medical Journal*, 318, 1407–9.

Emanuel, E.J., Wendler, D., Killen, J., and Grady, C. (2004). What makes clinical research in developing countries ethical? The benchmarks of ethical research. *Journal of Infectious Diseases*, 189, 930–7.

Emerson, P.M., Lindsay, S.W., Walraven, G.E., et al. (1999). Effect of fly control on trachoma and diarrhoea. *The Lancet*, 353, 1401–3.

Fang, X.H., Kronmal, R.A., Li, S.C., et al. (1999). Prevention of stroke in urban China: a community-based intervention trial. *Stroke*, 30, 495–501.

Fauveau, V., Stewart, K., Khan, S.A., and Chakraborty, J. (1991). Effect on mortality of community-based maternity-care programme in rural Bangladesh. *The Lancet*, 338, 1183–6.

Feldman, H.A. and McKinlay, S.M. (1994). Cohort versus cross-sectional design in large field trials: precision, sample size, and a unifying model. *Statistics in Medicine*, 13, 61–78.

Gabrielli, A.F., Toure, S., Sellin, B., et al. (2006). A combined school- and community-based campaign targeting all school-age children of Burkina Faso against schistosomiasis and soil-transmitted helminthiasis: performance, financial costs and implications for sustainability. *Acta Tropica*, 99, 234–42.

Gilson, L., Mkanje, R., Grosskurth, H., et al. (1997). Cost-effectiveness of improved treatment services for sexually transmitted diseases in preventing HIV-1 infection in Mwanza Region, Tanzania. *The Lancet*, 350, 1805–9.

Grosskurth, H., Mosha, F., Todd, J., et al. (1995). A community trial of the impact of improved sexually transmitted disease treatment on the HIV epidemic in rural Tanzania: 2. Baseline survey results. *AIDS*, 9, 927–34.

Jacob, M.E., Abraham, V.J., Abraham, S., and Jacob, K.S. (2007). The effect of community based daycare on mental health and quality of life of elderly in rural south India: a community intervention study. *International Journal of Geriatric Psychiatry*, 22, 445–7.

Jafar, T.H., Hatcher, J., Poulter, N., et al. (2009). Community-based interventions to promote blood pressure control in a developing country: a cluster randomized trial. *Annals of Internal Medicine*, 151, 593–601.

Kain, J., Uauy, R., Albala, Vio, F., Cerda, R., and Leyton, B. (2004). School-based obesity prevention in Chilean primary school children: methodology and evaluation of a controlled study. *International Journal of Obesity and Related Metabolic Disorders*, 28, 483–93.

Kamali, A., Quigley, M., Nakiyingi, J., et al. (2003). Syndromic management of sexually-transmitted infections and behaviour change interventions on transmission of HIV-1 in rural Uganda: a community randomised trial. *The Lancet*, 361, 645–52.

Kamarulzaman, A. and Saifuddeen, S.M. (2010). Islam and harm reduction. *International Journal of Drug Policy*, 21, 115–18.

Kay, B.H., Nam, V.S., Tien, T.V., et al. (2002). Control of aedes vectors of dengue in three provinces of Vietnam by use of Mesocyclops (Copepoda) and community-based methods validated by entomologic, clinical, and serological surveillance. *American Journal of Tropical Medicine and Hygiene*, 66, 40–8.

Kerry, S.M. and Bland, J.M. (1998a). The intracluster correlation coefficient in cluster randomisation. *British Medical Journal*, 316, 1455.

Kerry, S.M. and Bland, J.M. (1998b). Sample size in cluster randomisation. *British Medical Journal*, 316, 549.

Lassi, Z.S., Haider, B.A., and Bhutta, Z.A. (2010). Community-based intervention packages for reducing maternal and neonatal morbidity and mortality and improving neonatal outcomes. *Cochrane Database of Systematic Reviews*, 11, CD007754.

Lee, D. (2010). *Long-term follow-up of community-based drug and HIV prevention intervention in Yunnan, China*. PhD, University of California.

Li, M., Li, S., Baur, L., and Huxley, R. (2008). A systematic review of school-based intervention studies for the prevention or reduction of excess weight among Chinese children and adolescents. *Obesity Reviews*, 9, 548–59.

Liao, S.S., Schensul, J., and Wolffers, I. (2003). Sex-related health risks and implications for interventions with hospitality women in Hainan, China. *AIDS Education and Prevention*, 15, 109–21.

Longfield, K., Panyanouvong, X., Chen, J., and Kays, M.B. (2011). Increasing safer sexual behavior among Lao kathoy through an integrated social marketing approach. *BMC Public Health*, 11, 872.

Manandhar, D.S., Osrin, D., Shrestha, B.P., et al. (2004). Effect of a participatory intervention with women's groups on birth outcomes in Nepal: cluster-randomised controlled trial. *The Lancet*, 364, 970–9.

Martin, D.C., Diehr, P., Perrin, E.B., and Koepsell, T.D. (1993). The effect of matching on the power of randomized community intervention studies. *Statistics in Medicine*, 12, 329–38.

Morris, S.S., Flores, R., Olinto, P., and Medina, J.M. (2004). Monetary incentives in primary health care and effects on use and coverage of preventive health care interventions in rural Honduras: cluster randomised trial. *The Lancet*, 364, 2030–7.

Morrow, A.L., Guerrero, M.L., Shults, J., et al. (1999). Efficacy of home-based peer counselling to promote exclusive breastfeeding: a randomised controlled trial. *The Lancet*, 353, 1226–31.

Ngondi, J., Matthews, F., Reacher, M., Baba, S., Brayne, C., and Emerson, P. (2008). Associations between active trachoma and community intervention with Antibiotics, Facial cleanliness, and Environmental improvement (A,F,E). *PLOS Neglected Tropical Diseases*, 2, e229.

NIMH Collaborative HIV/STD Prevention Trial Group (2007a). Design and integration of ethnography within an international behavior change HIV/sexually transmitted disease prevention trial. *AIDS*, 21(Suppl. 2), S37–48.

NIMH Collaborative HIV/STD Prevention Trial Group (2007b). Methodological overview of a five-country community-level HIV/sexually transmitted disease prevention trial. *AIDS*, 21(Suppl. 2), S3–18.

NIMH Collaborative HIV/STD Prevention Trial Group (2010). Results of the NIMH collaborative HIV/sexually transmitted disease prevention trial of a community popular opinion leader intervention. *Journal of Acquired Immune Deficiency Syndromes*, 54, 204–14.

Pandey, M.R., Daulaire, N.M., Starbuck, E.S., Houston, R.M., and McPherson, K. (1991). Reduction in total under-five mortality in western Nepal through community-based antimicrobial treatment of pneumonia. *The Lancet*, 338, 993–7.

Perreira, K.M., Bailey, P.E., De Bocaletti, E., et al. (2002). Increasing awareness of danger signs in pregnancy through community- and clinic-based education in Guatemala. *Maternal and Child Health Journal*, 6, 19–28.

Pronyk, P.M., Hargreaves, J.R., Kim, J.C., et al. (2006). Effect of a structural intervention for the prevention of intimate-partner violence and HIV in rural South Africa: a cluster randomised trial. *The Lancet*, 368, 1973–83.

Ramadas, K., Sankaranarayanan, R., Jacob, B.J., et al. (2003). Interim results from a cluster randomized controlled oral cancer screening trial in Kerala, India. *Oral Oncology*, 39, 580–8.

Ronsmans, C., Vanneste, A.M., Chakraborty, J., and Van Ginneken, J. (1997). Decline in maternal mortality in Matlab, Bangladesh: a cautionary tale. *The Lancet*, 350, 1810–14.

Rosenthal, V.D., Alvarez-Moreno, C., Villamil-Gomez, W., et al. (2012a). Effectiveness of a multidimensional approach to reduce ventilator-associated pneumonia in pediatric intensive care units of 5 developing countries: International Nosocomial Infection Control Consortium findings. *American Journal of Infection Control*, 40, 497–501.

Rosenthal, V.D., Rodrigues, C., Alvarez-Moreno, C., et al. (2012b). Effectiveness of a multidimensional approach for prevention of ventilator-associated pneumonia in adult intensive care units from 14 developing countries of four continents: findings of the International Nosocomial Infection Control Consortium. *Critical Care Medicine*, 40(6), 497–501.

Sguassero, Y., De Onis, M., Bonotti, A.M., and Carroli, G. (2012). Community-based supplementary feeding for promoting the growth of children under five years of age in low and middle income countries. *Cochrane Database of Systematic Reviews*, 6, CD005039.

Shubis, K., Juma, O., Sharifu, R., Burgess, B., and Abdulla, S. (2009). Challenges of establishing a Community Advisory Board (CAB) in a low-income, low-resource setting: experiences from Bagamoyo, Tanzania. *Health Research Policy and Systems*, 7, 16.

Sim, J. and Dawson, A. (2012). Informed consent and cluster-randomized trials. *American Journal of Public Health*, 102, 480–5.

Smith, D.R., Zhang, X., Zheng, Y., and Wang, R.S. (2005). Tobacco use among public health professionals in Beijing: the relationship between smoking and education level. *Australian and New Zealand Journal of Public Health*, 29, 488–9.

Todd, J., Carpenter, L., Li, X., Nakiyingi, J., Gray, R., and Hayes, R. (2003). The effects of alternative study designs on the power of community randomized trials: evidence from three studies of human immunodeficiency virus prevention in East Africa. *International Journal of Epidemiology*, 32, 755–62.

Ukoumunne, O.C., Gulliford, M.C., Chinn, S., Sterne, J.A., and Burney, P.G. (1999). Methods for evaluating area-wide and organisation-based interventions in health and health care: a systematic review. *Health Technology Assessment*, 3, iii-92.

Vu, S.N., Nguyen, T.Y., Tran, V.P., et al. (2005). Elimination of dengue by community programs using Mesocyclops (Copepoda) against Aedes aegypti in central Vietnam. *American Journal of Tropical Medicine and Hygiene*, 72, 67–73.

Wacira, D.G., Hill, J., McCall, P.J., and Kroeger, A. (2007). Delivery of insecticide-treated net services through employer and community-based approaches in Kenya. *Tropical Medicine & International Health*, 12, 140–9.

Wakefield, M.A., Loken, B., and Hornik, R.C. (2010). Use of mass media campaigns to change health behaviour. *The Lancet*, 376, 1261–71.

Wawer, M.J., Gray, R.H., Sewankambo, N.K., et al. (1998). A randomized, community trial of intensive sexually transmitted disease control for AIDS prevention, Rakai, Uganda. *AIDS*, 12, 1211–25.

Weijer, C., Grimshaw, J.M., Taljaard, M., et al. (2011). Ethical issues posed by cluster randomized trials in health research. *Trials*, 12, 100.

West, K.P., Jr., Pokhrel, R.P., Katz, J., et al. (1991). Efficacy of vitamin A in reducing preschool child mortality in Nepal. *The Lancet*, 338, 67–71.

West, S., Munoz, B., Lynch, M., et al. (1995). Impact of face-washing on trachoma in Kongwa, Tanzania. *The Lancet*, 345, 155–8.

Wongkhomthong, S., Kaime-Atterhog, W., and Ono, K. (1995). *AIDS in the Developing World: a Case Study of Thailand*. Bangkok: ASEAN Institute for Health Development, Mahidol University.

Wu, Z., Detels, R., Zhang, J., Li, V., and Li, J. (2002). Community-based trial to prevent drug use among youths in Yunnan, China. *American Journal of Public Health*, 92, 1952–7.

Wu, Z., Rou, K., Jia, M., Duan, S., and Sullivan, S.G. (2007). The first community-based sexually transmitted disease/HIV intervention trial for female sex workers in China. *AIDS*, 21(Suppl. 8), S89–94.

Xu, J., Sullivan, S.G., Xu, C., et al. (2008). *A Community-Randomised Intervention Trial to Reduce HIV Stigma in Rural China*. AIDS 2008. Mexico: International AIDS Society.

5.11

Clinical epidemiology

Vivian A. Welch, Kevin Pottie, Tomás Pantoja, Andrea C. Tricco, and Peter Tugwell

Introduction to clinical epidemiology

In many university settings there is often a differentiation between social or public health epidemiology and clinical epidemiology. Clinical epidemiology emerged as the application of epidemiology principles for the study of individuals in clinical settings.

Clinical epidemiology was defined by Alvan Feinstein in 1968 as: 'the clinicostatistical study of diseased populations. The intellectual activities of this territory include the following: the occurrence rates and geographic distribution of disease; the patterns of natural and post-therapeutic events that constitute varying clinical courses in the diverse spectrum of disease; and the clinical appraisal of therapy' (Feinstein 1968).

The *Journal of Clinical Epidemiology*, a leading journal in its field, believes its role is to promote the quality of clinical epidemiological and patient-oriented health services research through advancement and application of innovative methods of conducting and presenting primary research; synthesizing research results; disseminating results; and translating results into optimal clinical practice. While clinical epidemiology originally intended to focus on studies that would inform clinical practice, recently clinical epidemiology methods have informed pragmatic trials that are an important part of public health intervention research. Pragmatic trials are designed to evaluate the effectiveness of interventions in real-life conditions, whereas efficacy trials aim to test whether an intervention works under optimal conditions. Pragmatic trials are attractive for public health in that they produce results that can be generalized and applied in various communities. A shift in recent years to pragmatic trials reflects a desire for more generalizable research. However, there are limitations to pragmatic trials such as high cost for large trials.

While epidemiology is focused on the study of distribution of disease and determinants (Last 1996), clinical epidemiology involves extrapolating results from best available evidence (including experimental studies such as randomized trials as well as non-randomized studies) to individual patients in a clinical setting. Clinical epidemiology evolved to also extrapolate results to populations. For example, the Framingham study on cardiovascular risk factors was designed to inform decisions about both individuals and populations. Clinical epidemiology was disseminated widely throughout low- and middle-income countries by the International Clinical Epidemiology Network (INCLEN), an initiative funded by the Rockefeller Foundation in 1980 (Box 5.11.1).

In the 1990s, the term 'evidence-based medicine' was coined by Gordon Guyatt, and subsequently defined by Dave Sackett in 1996 as: 'Evidence based medicine is the conscientious, judicious and explicit use of current best evidence in making decisions about the care of individual patients. The practice of evidence-based medicine means integrating individual clinical expertise with the best available external clinical evidence from systematic research' (Sackett et al. 1996). In 1993, the Cochrane Collaboration was formally launched with the mission to assemble the best available evidence about effects of healthcare interventions. Although this work was initially primarily focused on synthesizing evidence from randomized trials, the Cochrane Collaboration has formally recognized the importance of non-randomized studies for particular questions, such as studying upstream public health interventions.

Indeed, there is a growing emphasis within the Collaboration on evidence-informed decision-making for public health. The Cochrane Public Health Group was registered in 2008, with a mandate to assess effects of social and structural interventions on population health such as the effects of obesity prevention messages, social housing improvements, social policies, and transport interventions. The World Health Organization (WHO) Commission on Social Determinants of Health included a Measurement and Evidence Network which promoted the role of systematic reviews in providing the evidence base for action on health equity and social determinants of health. In the United States, the Community Guide, associated with the Centers for Disease Control and Prevention, has developed explicit methods to develop evidence-based preventive guidelines on topics such as obesity prevention, traffic injuries, and improving population mental health. The National Institute for Health Research in the United Kingdom asks all grant submissions to refer to existing systematic reviews on the topic to establish the need for further research in light of these reviews, including the Public Health Research Programme.

Evidence-informed public health has been defined as: 'The process of distilling and disseminating the best available evidence from research, practice and experience and using that evidence to inform and improve public health policy and practice' (Ciliska et al. 2010). There is an increasing application of clinical epidemiology methods to appraise evidence about public health interventions such as handwashing, obesity prevention, and vaccination. For example, one of us (AT) is involved in a review of the efficacy of influenza vaccines in healthy adults when the antigens in the vaccine do not match those of circulating strains (Tricco et al. 2012). Mismatched strains

Box 5.11.1 The International Clinical Epidemiology Network (INCLEN)

INCLEN (http://www.inclentrust.org) began as a strategy funded by the Rockefeller Foundation in 1980 to improve healthcare by providing health professionals, mostly physicians, with the necessary tools to plan, measure, and evaluate clinical care. Healthcare professionals, empowered in such a fashion, would provide an essential link to help develop functional health and health research systems in low- and middle-income countries. Currently with over 1500 members, the network has trained physicians and other health specialists at a Master's degree level in clinical epidemiology, social sciences, biostatistics, or clinical economics. This strategy has built a global resource network to support fundamental changes in the way physicians, medical educators, and policymakers think about health and disease. INCLEN has semi-autonomous regional networks in Africa, India, China, South East Asia, Latin America, Europe–Mediterranean, and Canada–United States.

INCLEN's long-range goals are to strengthen national health systems and to improve healthcare practice globally by providing health professionals with the tools to analyse the efficacy, effectiveness, efficiency, and equity of health interventions and preventive measures.

A recent series of articles in the *Journal of Clinical Epidemiology* highlights the continued contributions of INDIAclen to public health in the areas of measurement tools for developmental delay in children, pneumococcal infections, and tuberculosis (Thomas 2013).

occur frequently—there was a mismatched influenza B strain in the influenza vaccine for six of the 11 previous flu seasons in the United States (Centers for Disease Control and Prevention 2012). This review is of relevance to public health, because mismatched strains can lead to reduced vaccine effectiveness, which may result in reduced uptake of influenza vaccination and subsequently, more severe influenza epidemics.

The application of clinical epidemiology to both public health and clinical questions requires structured methods to consider effects on health equity. For example, a theory-based approach is suggested to consider plausible mechanisms of action of public health interventions on health inequity (Anderson et al. 2011). The use of visual logic models or analytic frameworks may help to describe the causal pathways and assumed mechanisms of action for complex public health interventions.

For public health, as in clinical medicine and healthcare, evidence must be assessed according to whether it is 'fit for purpose', rather than using an evidence hierarchy (Tugwell 2010). However, the different non-randomized studies need to be assessed for risk of bias, particularly due to confounding (Higgins and Green 2011). Higgins and Green define non-randomized study designs as 'any quantitative study estimating the effects of an intervention (harm or benefit) that does not use randomization to allocate units to comparison groups' (Higgins and Green 2011). Recent reporting guidelines for equity-focused systematic reviews, many of which are focused on public health questions such as obesity prevention, recommends reporting the justification for including different types of study designs (Welch et al. 2012).

In some areas of public health, there is conflict between non-randomized and randomized studies. For example, meta-analysis of prospective cohort studies found that people with higher dietary salt intake have a greater risk of stroke compared to people with lower salt intake. In contrast, a recent Cochrane review of seven randomized evaluations of advice to reduce salt intake found insufficient evidence of effects on all-cause mortality, cardiovascular mortality, or blood pressure due to sparse data (Taylor et al. 2011). Similarly, the Institute of Medicine in the United States convened an expert panel to assess the evidence from a comprehensive review of both observational and randomized studies and concluded that reduced dietary salt intake may increase adverse effects in some subgroups and there is little evidence to support salt reduction for preventing mortality or cardiovascular disease (Strom et al. 2013). The two recent reviews both concluded further research with sufficient power and appropriate design is needed to assess the effects of salt reduction on mortality. Thus, in public health, there is a need to consider different types of evidence and to critically appraise the risk of bias for the outcomes of interest.

For some public health questions, non-randomized studies which are designed to control for confounding may be better suited to providing evidence about effectiveness. For example, in a review of interventions to improve water quality, 39 out of 44 studies of effectiveness of environment and sanitation measures were non-randomized studies (Snilstveit and Waddington 2009). However, it is important to assess the risk of bias in these studies. Another example of including non-randomized studies is a recent Cochrane systematic review of obesity prevention for children which found that educational and behavioural interventions are effective at reducing body mass index in children from lower socioeconomic status settings, and there was no evidence of increases in health inequalities (Waters et al. 2011). A third example is a review of policies to reduce child consumption of sugar-sweetened beverages, such as reduced accessibility of vending machines in schools and price regulation through taxes (Levy et al. 2011). This review also included non-randomized studies, and found that price increases through taxation reduce consumption and may be more effective for children at greatest risk of overweight and from lower income families.

Systematic reviews on public health interventions and policies are increasingly available. For example, the Health Evidence database (http://www.healthevidence.org/) now contains over 3000 quality-appraised systematic reviews related to public health identified from searches of the Cochrane Database of Systematic Reviews, MEDLINE, Sociological abstracts, PsychINFO, and handsearching of 46 public health and health promotion journals.

In the next section, we will use the equity–effectiveness framework to illustrate six steps of evidence-informed public health that highlight the interface between public health and clinical epidemiology of assessing the burden of illness (need), the effects on population health and health inequity, economic evaluation, implementation, monitoring, and reassessment.

Interfaces between clinical epidemiology and public health

Other functions of clinical epidemiology that contribute or interface with public health include screening programmes, health technology assessment, and standards setting (through practice guidelines and quality improvement).

Screening is an important part of primary care, typically done by family physicians and nurse practitioners. Good examples of an evidence-based approach to this include the Canadian Task Force on the Periodic Health Exam, Canadian Task Force on Preventive Healthcare (http://canadiantaskforce.ca/), the US Preventive Services Task Force (http://www.ahrq.gov/clinic/uspstfix.htm), and guidelines for disease promotion in immigrants and refugees in Canada (Pottie et al. 2011). Many of these screening clinical actions need to be integrated with public health services.

Health Technology Assessment, defined by Battista as the bridge between science and policy, also bridges clinical epidemiology and public health. Indeed one of us (PT) has used the same stepwise iterative loop approach to systematizing the methods (Tugwell et al. 1995). Health equity impact assessment is gaining interest as a method to explicitly consider effects of policies and programmes on health equity (Povall et al. 2013).

Standards setting through practice guidelines and quality assurance in clinical epidemiology also has many parallels with public health, especially public health units. Clinical guidelines are only as good as the evidence and judgements they are based on. For example, the international GRADE initiative has been developed for users of clinical practice guidelines and other recommendations to provide them with the information needed to know how much confidence they can place in the recommendations. Systematic and explicit methods of making judgements can reduce errors and improve communication. The GRADE system grades the quality of evidence and the strength of recommendations that can be applied across a wide range of interventions and contexts. Judgements about the strength of a recommendation require consideration of the balance between benefits and harms, the quality of the evidence, translation of the evidence into specific circumstances, and the certainty of the baseline risk. It is also important to consider costs (resource utilization) before making a recommendation. Inconsistencies among systems for grading the quality of evidence and the strength of recommendations reduce their potential to facilitate critical appraisal and improve communication of these judgements. This system for guiding these complex judgements balances the need for simplicity with the need for full and transparent consideration of all important issues. These are being used not only for clinical guidelines but also to assess quality of evidence for each outcome in a systematic review and at the policy level. For example, the WHO used GRADE to assess the evidence for antivirals for avian influenza (Schunemann et al. 2007) and cryotherapy for cervical cancer prevention (Santesso et al. 2012).

An example of a public health guideline is the *Treating Tobacco Use and Dependence: 2008 Update* clinical practice guideline (Fiore et al. 2008). This initiative was sponsored by the Public Health Service and conducted by collaborative efforts among eight US federal government and not-for-profit organizations, including the Agency for Healthcare Research and Quality (AHRQ). The guideline was based upon a comprehensive systematic review, for which over 8700 titles and abstracts were screened. Three strength of evidence ratings were applied to each of the recommendations, with well-conducted randomized clinical trials being the highest level of evidence and consensus being the lowest level of evidence. Meta-analyses were conducted on 11 pre-defined topics and ten key guideline recommendations were formulated. These included encouraging all smokers to try effective counselling interventions, such as telephone and group counselling, as well as medications, such as nicotine gum and varenicline. In order to increase the uptake of the clinical practice guideline, executive summaries were tailored for health policymakers, clinicians, and patients. Furthermore, smokers are provided with access to a website to help them quit smoking, as well as a phone number for a quitline service. Such knowledge translation strategies increase the likelihood that key recommendations will reach the target audience.

The equity–effectiveness framework to assess the interface between clinical epidemiology and public health

Clinical epidemiology and its derivative—the evidence-based medicine movement—have many parallels with public health. Indeed many clinicians with clinical epidemiology training develop research projects and subsequently research programmes that move beyond clinical decision-making to include a population focus. This stimulated one of us (PT) and his colleagues to address this process systematically through an iterative measurement loop framework (Tugwell et al. 1985). The focus was on evidence-based, action-oriented epidemiology based upon the health needs of the relevant individuals and their community.

This has been updated with an 'equity lens' to ensure that disadvantaged populations are explicitly considered (Tugwell et al. 2006a) (see Fig. 5.11.1). What was the stimulus to incorporate explicit attention by clinical epidemiologists to the disadvantaged? This was due to the realization that average improvement can hide important inequitably worse health effects amongst the disadvantaged. For example, impressive gains in health during the twentieth century, showing dramatic increases in average life expectancy in rich and poor countries (WHO 1999), would meet the criteria we initially recommended in the 1985 paper, but there is a critical component missing. These averages obscure the fact that health in both high- and low-income countries is unevenly distributed according to socioeconomic position; health and longevity are highest for the richest, and decrease steadily with decreasing socioeconomic status (Wilkins and Adams 1983; Wilkinson 1996). Where these inequalities in health are avoidable by action or policies and they are considered unfair, they meet the criteria for being considered health inequities (Whitehead 1990). The judgement of fairness is normative and depends on context. For example, in countries where health is viewed as a commodity not a right, the judgement about the fairness of health inequalities or disparities may differ.

These social gradients in health, or socioeconomic inequalities in health, are pervasive in all countries of the world (Diderichsen et al. 2001) and hold true for most diseases, injuries, and health behaviours. For example, globally, childhood obesity has increased dramatically since 1990 from 4 per cent to 7 per cent. The association of childhood obesity with socioeconomic status varies depending on gender, age, and country. Those with low socioeconomic status in higher-income countries and those with higher socioeconomic status in lower-income countries have higher exposure to energy-dense diets and higher risk of obesity (Wang and Lim 2012). In the United States, the prevalence of childhood obesity in boys is 21 per cent in those living below 130 per cent of the poverty level compared to 12 per cent in boys from families at 350 per cent above the poverty level (Ogden et al. 2010). Modern health policy must increasingly be oriented not only to

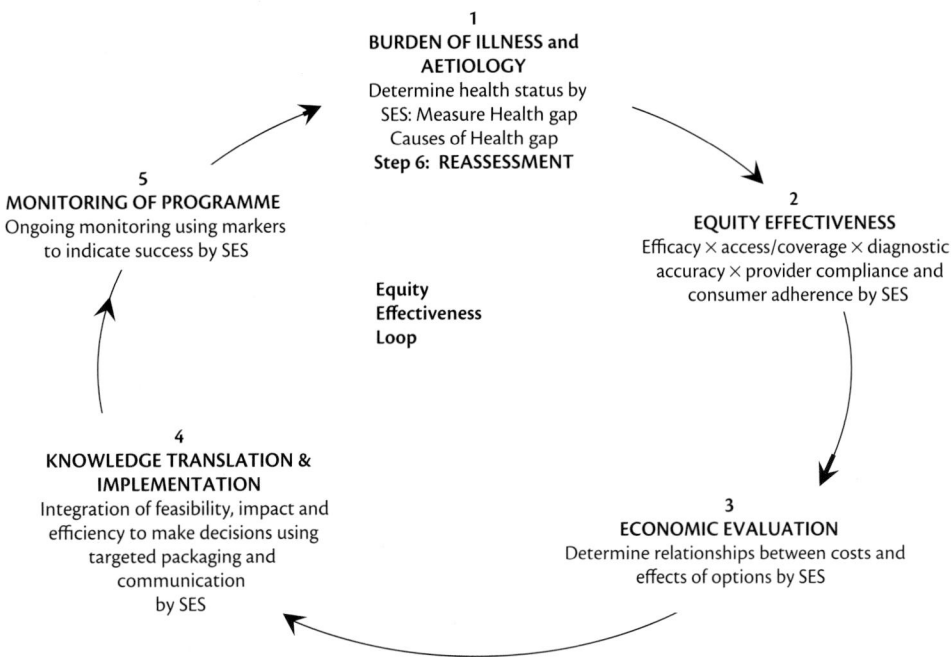

Fig. 5.11.1 Equity–effectiveness framework. SES: socioeconomic status.

the production of health, but also to the distribution of health and health equity (Gwatkin 2003). The WHO Commission on Social Determinants of Health and the recent Rio Commission meeting drew attention to the need for an improved evidence base to tackle avoidable and unfair inequalities in health.

The 'equity–effectiveness iterative framework', was developed to address this need for evidence about both improving population health and reducing health inequities. This framework has been expanded to provide a logical way to apply an 'equity lens' as one moves from assessing needs and burden of disease through to assessing effectiveness, and cost-effectiveness, of interventions, leading to the development and evaluation of evidence-based health policy, as well as scaling up from proof of concept to a population level. This framework integrates the concepts of individual risk and socioeconomic status with intervention effectiveness from a population health perspective.

Step 1: burden of illness

This step measures the burden of illness and its gradient by socioeconomic status. This includes downstream (individual) and upstream (societal) determinants of health (biological, cultural, political, psychosocial, and environmental). Health information systems and routinely collected data are important for assessing not only the overall burden of illness but also differences across socioeconomic status and other factors associated with inequities in health such as sex/gender and urban versus rural settings.

Step 2: differential equity–effectiveness

Controlled studies provide estimates of efficacy and effectiveness; efficacy measures how well an intervention can work in ideal circumstances (Sackett et al. 1985). Effectiveness measures how well an intervention works in real settings and systems at the community level. Community effectiveness is often substantially lower than efficacy because of a staircase effect with four 'steps': (1) the result of lower awareness, access, or coverage; (2) screening, diagnosis, or targeting; (3) compliance of providers; and (4) adherence of consumers. Poor people may have circumstances that reduce efficacy at all four steps and therefore a greater staircase effect may be observed compared to the least poor people. There is a need to assess equity issues across each step to identify barriers to implementation related to gradients in wealth.

Step 3: economic evaluation

This step assesses the efficiency (health benefits such as number of disability-adjusted life years avoided for a specific cost that includes direct, indirect, and where possible intangible costs) of the intervention. Assessing the efficiency requires adequate evidence of efficacy and valid estimates of cost. Assessing the equity issues related to cost-effectiveness implies a trade-off between cost efficiency and population health equity. Priority funding of interventions with the best cost-effectiveness ratios might increase differences between the richest (or least poor) and poorest because the cost of reaching poor people may be higher and health benefits may be lower. Four approaches to this have been proposed (Drummond et al. 2006). One promising method to assess equity issues related to cost-effectiveness is the development of an equity and quality-adjusted life year (EQ-QALY), as a complement to established measures of the difference between rich and poor, such as the concentration index (Wagstaff 2002).

Step 4: knowledge translation and implementation

Translation of knowledge is defined as the process that transfers research results from producers of knowledge to its users, for the benefit of the population. Moving beyond the traditional domain of academic publication, it comprises three interlinked components of uptake and translation: exchange, synthesis, and ethically sound application of knowledge (Birdsell et al. 2002). This step entails uptake and translation of knowledge into action (Grimshaw et al. 2001; Birdsell et al. 2002; Davis et al. 2003).

There is therefore a need to develop new, effective means of packaging and communicating evidence on effectiveness across wealth gradients to the different policy, community, and practitioner groups or individuals responsible for each of the components of community effectiveness—access, diagnostic accuracy, compliance of providers, and adherence of consumers (Giuffrida et al. 2000; Zwarenstein and Bryant 2000; Briggs et al. 2001; Mowatt et al. 2001). Evidence that interventions using knowledge translation are efficacious is currently lacking in most sectors. One exception is the work of INCLEN (see Box 5.11.1), which is developing methods explicitly to consider equity issues in developing and applying clinical guidelines (INCLEN 2004). By targeting the wealth gradient in knowledge translation strategies, we support the operational research agenda for optimizing the benefits to the poor of key interventions.

Steps 5 and 6: monitoring and reassessment

Monitoring identifies the importance of process assessments and intermediate outcomes to assess success in affecting mortality and morbidity by socioeconomic group and deciding whether further remediable need exists; if so, an additional iteration of the equity–effectiveness loop is needed. The Whitehall cohort study, for example, showed that, even with equitable access to cardiac care, the social deprivation gradient still produces disparities in outcomes (Britton et al. 2004), indicating a need to tackle other causes, or 'steps', of disparities.

Applying the equity–effectiveness framework step by step

We elaborate on the application of the equity–effectiveness loop using the example of school lunch and breakfast programmes for disadvantaged children. School feeding programmes are described by the World Food Programme as tools to combat hunger, nutritional deficits, educational attendance, and gender inequalities (www.wfp.org/school-meals/in-depth). They are considered a transfer to impoverished families (Alderman and Bundy 2012). However, there is some controversy about school feeding programmes because of the epidemiological transition leading to increased obesity in disadvantaged children in both high-income countries and lower-income countries. We will examine the effects of school feeding in detail using the equity–effectiveness framework.

Step 1: burden of illness

Undernutrition is the largest cause of global burden of disease and predominantly affects children. Childhood undernutrition is responsible for a third of mortality and disease burden in children under 5 years old. It also has long-term effects on physical and cognitive development. Childhood malnutrition is inversely associated with income in all developing countries, and meets the criteria of being inequitable since child malnutrition is both avoidable and unfair (Van de Poel et al. 2008). Burden of illness

can be measured by household surveys or by routinely collected health data. There is increasing attention to also collecting indicators of socioeconomic status alongside health data to allow an assessment of differences in health status between different populations and settings.

Step 2: efficacy, community effectiveness, and differential equity–effectiveness

When asking questions about effectiveness and efficacy, clinical epidemiology provides critical appraisal tools to identify studies at the lowest risk of bias for the question of interest. For example, non-randomized studies of school feeding have shown larger effects on weight gain and cognition, partly because they are unable to control for bias in the measurement of outcomes.

For a public health decision to be evidence-informed, policymakers should follow clear steps in: (1) formulating a question, (2) seeking the best available evidence, (3) determining the quality of that evidence, and (4) determining the applicability of the evidence to their settings.

1. *Formulating a question*: any well-designed question should be composed of the following four criteria: PICO—Population, Intervention, Control, and Outcome. Some questions, particularly those related to public health, may need to specify context, study design or time of follow-up.

   a. For school feeding, in disadvantaged children (population), does school feeding (intervention) improve health, cognition, and attendance (outcome) in comparison to control (control)? This structured question addresses all of the important components of an answerable question.

2. Seeking *the best available evidence*: for the purpose of this chapter, we searched the Health Evidence database which is a collection of systematic reviews that address public health questions (Tirilis et al. 2011). We used the terms: 'school AND (feeding OR lunch OR breakfast OR meal OR snack)'. We identified 25 reviews with these terms.

3. *Determining the quality of the evidence*: we then assessed the relevance of each systematic review in answering our question. Only one review was relevant to our question (Kristjansson et al. 2007). This review is rated as strong quality using the Health Evidence quality appraisal tool (score of 10 on a scale where the maximum possible is 10). If no systematic review exists, then you may need to search for primary studies and apply the same steps, or consider conducting a systematic review. Guidance for conducting a systematic review, including how to develop a search strategy, can be found from the Cochrane Collaboration handbook (Higgins and Green 2011).

4. *Applying the findings to the target populations*: this Cochrane systematic review found that children who received school feeding had a 13.5 per cent increase in growth rate relative to a control group, measured as an absolute difference of 0.39 kg (95 per cent confidence interval of 0.11–0.67 kg). Implementation of school feeding requires consideration of a number of factors (Greenhalgh et al. 2007) such as local context and preferences, possible leakage to family members, and substitution or displacement of a child's regular meals at home.

Differential effectiveness

Controlled studies provide estimates of efficacy, that is, how well an intervention can work in ideal circumstances. The equity–effectiveness framework takes efficacy as the anchor point representing the maximum benefit that can be achieved. Community effectiveness is the measure of how well an intervention does work when delivered in real-life settings and systems at the community level. This 'community effectiveness' is often substantially lower than the expected efficacy because of four systemic factors: awareness/access/coverage, screening/diagnosis/targeting, provider compliance, and consumer adherence.

School feeding is a good example of differential effectiveness across socioeconomic status

The relative improvement in growth of 13 per cent is expected to be the same for both poorest and least poor children. However, there are differences in access (estimated by school participation rate) and consumer adherence (increased rates of leakage and substitution in the poorest families). These two factors lead to a reduction in community effectiveness from 10 per cent in the least poor (most advantaged) to 4 per cent in the poorest (Table 5.11.1).

Step 3: economic evaluation

This step assesses the efficiency (health benefits (number of lives saved, number of quality/disability-adjusted life years avoided)) obtained for a specific cost (direct, indirect, and where possible the intangible costs expressed in monetary units such as dollars, euros, or pounds) of the intervention. That is, whether the intervention is being delivered to those who would benefit from it with an optimal use of resources. Assessment of efficiency should not be done in the absence of adequate evidence of efficacy and valid estimates of cost. Application of an equity lens to this step implies a trade-off between cost-efficiency and population health equity. Priority funding of interventions with the best cost-effectiveness ratios might increase rich–poor differences because the cost of reaching the poor may be higher (e.g. distance to care) and health benefits may be lower. The concept of using equity-adjusted traditional utility metrics such as an EQ-QALY needs to be developed, as described earlier.

For the case of school feeding, cost studies were conducted to assess the cost per child and cost per outcome, based on a Cochrane systematic review (Galloway et al. 2009). The results show the cost per extra day of attendance of $4.7 to $15.8 and the cost per extra kilogram of weight ranged from $112 to $252. Comparability of these results to other health and education interventions will be enhanced when the cost analyses for different interventions are performed using the same methods and the same outcomes.

Step 4: implementation

The implementation of school feeding is critical to the success of the programme. For example, school feeding programmes designed with community involvement and palatability testing were more successful. Furthermore, there is a need to minimize substitution by using snacks which are less likely to lead to meal substitution.

The science of implementation overlaps substantially with the recently burgeoning 'knowledge translation' initiatives—see the following 'Knowledge translation and innovation' section.

Steps 5 and 6: monitoring and reassessment

Monitoring identifies the importance of process assessments and intermediate outcomes (putting the human and physical resources in place, monitoring the identification, and treatment of those at risk/in need). The main purpose of these steps in the equity–effectiveness framework is to assess success in affecting mortality and morbidity by socioeconomic group and deciding whether further remediable need exists; if so, there needs to be an additional iteration of the framework.

Monitoring of any scaled-up programme for school feeding is essential; just applying the evidence alone will be insufficient. For example, monitoring is needed to assess acceptability of food, unintended consequences, and substitution of meals at home by meals at school.

An example of an equity-focused approach to monitor health programmes is the Equity Gauge of the Global Equity Gauge Alliance, funded by Rockefeller Foundation. This group developed 'equity gauges' as a means of tracking gaps in health at the national or sub-national levels (McCoy et al. 2003). This approach to equity includes three pillars: (1) measuring key indicators, (2) public participation, and (3) advocacy. Inclusion of all three pillars aims at bringing about evidence-based action. Equity Gauges have been or are being developed in Bangladesh, Chile, China, Ecuador, Kenya, South Africa, Thailand, Uganda, Zambia, and Zimbabwe (McCoy et al. 2003).

The WHO has developed a Health Metrics Network to enable performance-based monitoring of interventions and health systems. The Network aims to build transparency and accountability, and ensure that policy decisions are based upon evidence. Equity is central to the proposed data indicators (AbouZahr and

Table 5.11.1 Equity–effectiveness framework applied to school feeding

	Efficacy	Efficacy modifiers				Community effectiveness	Least poor: poor equity–effectiveness ratio
		Access	Diagnostic accuracy	Provider compliance	Consumer adherence		
• Least poor	13%	97%	95%	90%	91%	10%	2.5
• Poorest	13%	73%	95%	80%	49%	4%	

Boerma 2005). The Institute for Health Metrics and Evaluation led by Dr Chris Murray has recently published updated global burdens of disease and their association with 67 risk factors. These country-wide data can be used to monitor changes over time in burden of disease in populations. For example, the recent analyses show an increase in non-communicable diseases in adults, relative to a decreasing burden of communicable diseases in children (Lim et al. 2012).

Our stepwise illustration of the equity–effectiveness framework concludes here, showing the interface between clinical epidemiology and public health.

Knowledge translation and innovation

This is an aspect of clinical epidemiology that has developed in the last 10 years, stimulated in part by being singled out for funding by agencies such as the Canadian Institutes of Health Research (CIHR). This is highly relevant to public health and warrants discussion here.

The CIHR defines knowledge translation as a 'dynamic and iterative process that includes synthesis, dissemination, exchange and ethically-sound application of knowledge to improve the health of Canadians, provide more effective health services and products and strengthen the health care system' (Straus et al. 2009). This involves uptake and translation of knowledge into ethically sound action. To do this, tailored interventions are needed to reach a range of target groups, including researchers, local and national policymakers, professionals, affected communities, industry, media, and the general public. However, one of the primary challenges facing these initiatives is to determine the most effective strategies to promote the use and application of research.

In public health, there is an important role of legislation and regulation in knowledge translation. For example, smoking bans have been showcased as an intervention that has been effective in many different settings for reducing smoking prevalence. However, there is a need to balance the evidence of effectiveness with any infringement on moral values such as individual autonomy or injustice in the distribution of effects of the interventions. For example, workplace smoking bans have been shown to increase inequalities in smoking across socioeconomic status (Lorenc et al. 2012). The widely publicized initiative by the city of New York to ban the sale of soft drinks in sizes larger than 16 ounces was overruled on the basis that the mayor exceeded his legislative authority (Saul 2013). There is an increasing need for policy innovations in law and regulation to tackle global problems such as the increasing burden of non-communicable disease, and these need to include multiple stakeholders such as government, private sector, and civil society (Gostin et al. 2013).

There are numerous models and frameworks for developing knowledge translation strategies, depending on the target audience as well as other characteristics. We next describe two case studies of knowledge translation: (1) Canadian Collaboration for Immigrant and Refugee Health Knowledge Exchange Network (CCIRH KEN), and (2) Evidence into Policy Network (EVIPNet).

Case Study: Canadian Collaboration for Immigrant and Refugee Health Knowledge Exchange Network

The CCIRH KEN (http://www.ccirhken.ca) began in 2007, funded by the Public Health Agency of Canada. Its strategy was to improve the healthcare of a vulnerable population by providing primary healthcare practitioners with the necessary evidence-based guidelines to effectively manage newly arriving immigrant and refugee patients. Newly arriving immigrants and refugees depend on community-based primary healthcare practitioners for decision support and healthcare system navigation. In addition, immigrant communities often connect to national and international diaspora networks for decision supports and resources. Thus, a long-range objective of the evidence-based initiative was to create guidelines and decision support tools to assist vulnerable migrants that could be used in Canada and in other migrant-receiving counties.

Currently with over 400 members, the CCIRH KEN has provided clinical guidelines, methods, narrative podcasts, and e-learning programmes for physicians and other health practitioners as well as medical and graduate students. The network has also begun to work with leaders in Australia, Europe, and the United States as it builds trust and momentum for international evidence-based migrant health.

Vision

CCIHR KEN aims to strengthen primary health systems and improve the quality and delivery of primary healthcare for vulnerable migrant populations. To meet this goal, it will use evidence- and equity-based methods, migrant community engagement, and partnerships with international organizations such as the International Organization of Migration and the Cochrane Collaboration.

Mission

The CCIRH KEN including specialists, primary care practitioners, researchers, policymakers, and immigrant community leaders each dedicated to improving the health of immigrants and refugees. CCIRH KEN is a knowledge translation initiative aimed at improving the health of immigrants and refugees. It is designed to provide practical evidence-based recommendations and high-quality education and community resources to primary care practitioners and medical students, immigrant community champions and health advocates, and health and immigration policymakers.

Examples of CCIRH outputs with public health implications

The Evidence Based Guidelines initiative (Pottie et al. 2011) of the CCIRH was a 6-year interdisciplinary collaboration involving primary care practitioners, specialists, researchers, immigrant community champions, and policymakers that brought an evidence-based lens to the emerging discipline of migrant health. CCIRH produced 20 systematic reviews and formulated 26 evidence-based guidelines for primary care practitioners that covered a broad range of infectious diseases (tuberculosis, HIV, hepatitis B, hepatitis C, varicella, malaria, intestinal parasites, MMR (measles, mumps and rubella), DTP (diphtheria, tetanus, pertussis)), mental health and physical and emotional maltreatment (depression, post-traumatic stress disorder, child maltreatment, intimate partner violence), chronic non-communicable diseases (diabetes, dental disease, vision disorders, iron deficiency anaemia), and women's health (cervical cancer, unmet contraceptive needs and pregnancy), conditions identified by practitioners across Canada working with immigrants and endorsed by immigrant community champions.

These internationally unique guidelines were made possible thanks to the development of new methods developed by methodologists from the GRADE Working Group, Cochrane Collaboration, and the Canadian Task Force on Preventive Health Care. These methods used an equity–effectiveness approach whereby literature was first synthesized focusing on the PICO question to determine effectiveness (benefits and harms) and then a literature review provided equity consideration to inform the formulation of GRADE recommendations. The equity lens included: Baseline Risk for Population; Culture, Diet, Genetic Differences; Practitioner adherence; Patient adherence (Tugwell et al. 2011).

In an effort to support implementation of the evidence and guideline, CCIRH KEN launched a Knowledge Exchange Website (http://www.ccirhken.ca). To introduce student and resident doctors to global health competencies and the CCIRH guidelines, we launched an Open Access Refugees and Global Health e-Learning Program (http://ccirhken.ca/eLearning). Currently this programme and its certification quiz are being used in eight universities across Canada and one in the United States to help prepare students to work with vulnerable populations. Most recently, CCIRH KEN has launched its Evidence Based Checklist E-Learning (http://ccirhken.ca/eLearning) with Narrative Podcasts and Decision Tables. This open-access evidence-based tool allows practitioners to access the CCIRH-Cochrane Immigrant Health Narrative Podcasts as well as providing a practical checklist for seven world regions. The site also provides an RSS feed targeting evidence-based migrant health news and publication, and a Twitter feed to push out new publications and emerging concerns related to vulnerable migrant populations.

The CCIRH KEN is now initiating Health Impact Assessments (HIAs) to support equity-based improvements in policy, programme, and service design relevant for low-income migrants. This decision support tool will build on previous HIA work, but will be unique in its focus on migrant populations, its implementation of new equity methods, and its link to migrant health methods and data from a new repository emerging from the International Organization for Migration (IOM). This initiative will be initiated in collaboration with decision-maker partners and will aim to promote World Health Assembly priorities on health of migrants: monitoring of migrant health, promote conducive policy and legal frameworks on the health of migrants, promote migrant-inclusive health systems, promote partnerships, networks and multicountry frameworks.

Knowledge translation and global health

Knowledge translation is particularly important for low- and middle-income countries where the burden of disease is much higher and there are less resources for research. For example, INCLEN developed Knowledge Plus Packages in 2003, to focus on getting evidence intro practice and policy. These packages were developed with consideration for equity and effectiveness.

Knowledge translation at the policymaking level: the case of EVIPNet

Low- and middle-income countries have scarce resources to address their health system challenges and need high-quality scientific evidence to use those resources efficiently. If health sector managers and policymakers ignore evidence on the root causes of problems or what works best to address them, they risk wasting precious resources on inadequately designed programmes and policies. The direct consequence of ignoring this evidence is poor population health.

In the last decade, there have been recurrent calls from a number of international organizations for using evidence to strengthen policy and practice. For instance, the WHO in 2004, in its *World Report on Knowledge for Better Health*, mentioned that 'stronger emphasis should be placed on translating knowledge into action to improve public health by bridging the gap between what is known and what is actually being done' (WHO 2004). However a number of challenges in this 'translation' process have been identified: (1) research evidence competes with many other factors in policymaking, (2) research evidence is not valued enough by policymakers as an information input, (3) research evidence is not relevant to the policy issues that policymakers face, and (4) research evidence is not easy to use (Lavis et al. 2006). Therefore, any initiative aimed to bridge this gap should consider ways to address those challenges in a meaningful and efficient way.

The EVIPNet is an initiative—sponsored by WHO—that promotes the systematic use of health research evidence in policymaking (http://global.evipnet.org/). Focusing on low- and middle-income countries, EVIPNet promotes partnerships at the country level between policymakers, researchers, and civil society in order to facilitate both policy development and policy implementation through the use of the best scientific evidence available. EVIPNet comprises networks that bring together country-level teams, which are coordinated at both regional and global levels. The initiative was launched in 2005 and currently includes 38 countries in four WHO Regions (Africa, Americas, Asia, and Eastern Mediterranean) (Hamid et al. 2005; EVIPNet 2008).

EVIPNet activities at the country level are jointly led by local policymakers and researchers and are designed to meet the specific needs of each country. Country activities currently supported under the EVIPNet umbrella include:

◆ Production of policy briefs and other user-friendly formats for research synthesis and discussions of policy options.

◆ Establishment of priority-setting mechanisms for policy-relevant research syntheses and primary research.

◆ Production of research syntheses.

◆ Organization of 'safe haven' deliberative forums involving policymakers, researchers, and citizens' groups to stimulate context-specific, evidence-informed local action.

◆ Investigation of the potential of clearinghouses, observatories, and rapid response mechanisms that might provide timely, high-quality research syntheses and research relevant to policy.

In addition, at the regional and global levels EVIPNet supports:

- Capacity strengthening and empowerment of policymakers, researchers, and representatives of civil society to enable them to make better use of evidence in policy-making and advocacy.

- Interactive learning processes building on experiences to improve evidence-to-policy methods.

- Monitoring and evaluation processes that document the lessons learned from the use of an array of evidence-to-policy processes in different contexts.

- Information exchange—disseminating successful methods and tools, experiences, and best practices among partners and other countries, mostly through the EVIPNet Portal—an Internet-based platform, and WHO country offices.

Although it was launched 7 years ago, most of the country teams have only begun implementing different 'translation' activities in the last 3 years. Therefore, we cannot yet draw definitive conclusions about what works, in which context and for whom. However, an evaluation team has been collecting data from some of the country initiatives (mostly in Africa) identifying some initial 'lessons learned' from the process. (Lavis and Panisset 2010). Strategic alliances and continuous dialogue between policymakers and researchers were considered crucial. Likewise, training and the availability of local technical support in evidence-informed policy-making tools were deemed important facilitators. On the other hand, limited funding and concerns about the sustainability of the initiative at the country level were the most frequently mentioned barriers.

Summing up, the 'EVIPNet model' has allowed the development of formal strategies to address some of the challenges in linking evidence to policymaking in low- and middle-income countries, as well as building capacity of both scientists and decision-makers to engage in evidence-informed decision-making. Although it is still too early to assess the impact of this 'living laboratory', promising lessons have been identified and will eventually be incorporated in the implementation plans of the different country teams around the world.

Conclusion

In summary:

- Clinical epidemiology has adopted many public health methods; conversely, it has contributed to methods for tackling public health problems.

- Clinical epidemiology training has led to many clinicians and other healthcare providers developing research programmes addressing public health problems.

- Health equity, with a special focus on effectiveness, has recently become a focus of clinical epidemiology, and complements the longstanding concern for this in public health.

- The equity–effectiveness framework is just one approach for systematically organizing the clinical epidemiological approach to public health problems.

- Clinical epidemiology has a contribution to make to public health.

Acknowledgements

We would like to acknowledge the leadership and contributions from Dr Ed Mills and Dr Jason Busse to the previous edition of this chapter.

References

AbouZahr, C. and Boerma, T. (2005). Health information systems: the foundations of public health. *Bulletin of the World Health Organization*, 83, 578–83.

Alderman, H. and Bundy, D. (2012). School feeding programs and development: are we framing the question correctly? *World Bank Research Observer*, 27(2), 204–21.

Anderson, L.M., Petticrew, M., Rehfuess, E., et al. (2011). Using logic models to capture complexity in systematic reviews. *Research Synthesis Methods*, 2, 33–42.

Birdsell, J.M., Atkinson-Grosjean, J., and Landry, R. (2002). *Knowledge Translation in Two New Programs: Achieving 'The Pasteur Effect'*. Ottawa: Canadian Institutes of Health Research.

Briggs, C.J., Capdegelle P., and Garner, P. (2001). Strategies for integrating primary health services in middle- and low-income countries: effects on performance, costs and patient outcomes. *Cochrane Database of Systematic Reviews*, 4, CD003318.

Britton, A., Shipley, M., Marmot, M., et al. (2004). Does access to cardiac investigation and treatment contribute to social and ethnic differences in coronary heart disease? Whitehall II prospective cohort study. *British Medical Journal*, 329, 318–20.

Centers for Disease Control and Prevention (2012). *Seasonal Influenza (Flu)- Past Weekly Surveillance Reports*. Atlanta, GA: Centers for Disease Control and Prevention.

Ciliska, D., Thomas, H., and Buffett, C. (2010). *An Introduction to Evidence-Informed Public Health and A Compendium of Critical Appraisal Tools for Public Health Practice*. Prepared for the National Collaborating Centre for Methods and Tools. McMaster University. 2008 (updated November 2010). Available at: http://www.nccmt.ca/pubs/2008_07_IntroEIPH_compendiumENG.pdf.

Davis, D., Evans, M., Jadad, A., et al. (2003). The case for knowledge translation: shortening the journey from evidence to effect. *British Medical Journal*, 327, 33–5.

Diderichsen, F., Evans, T., and Whitehead, M. (2001). The social basis of disparities in health. In T. Evans, M. Whitehead, F. Diderichsen, et al. (eds.) *Challenging Inequities in Health. From Ethics to Action*, pp. 13–23. New York: Oxford University Press.

Drummond, M., Weatherly, H., Claxton, K., et al., (2006). *Assessing the Challenges of Applying Standard Methods of Economic Evaluation to Public Health Interventions*. Report prepared for the Department of Health by the Public Health Research Consortium, University of York. Available at: http://www.york.ac.uk/phrc/D1-05_FR.pdf.

EVIPNet Americas Secretariat (2008). EVIPNet Americas: informing policies with evidence. *Lancet*, 372, 1130–1.

Feinstein, A.R. (1968). Clinical epidemiology. I. The populational experiments of nature and of man in human illness. *Annals of Internal Medicine*, 69, 807–20.

Fiore, M.C., Jaén, C.R., Baker, T.B., et al. (2008). *Treating Tobacco Use and Dependence: 2008 Update*. Clinical Practice Guideline. Rockville, MD: U.S. Department of Health and Human Services.

Galloway, R., Kristjansson, E., Gelli, A., Meir, U., Espejo, F., and Bundy, D. (2009). School feeding: outcomes and costs. *Food and Nutrition Bulletin*, 30(2), 171–82.

Giuffrida, A., Gosden, T., Forland, F., et al. (2000). Target payments in primary care: effects on professional practice and health care outcomes. *Cochrane Database of Systematic Reviews*, 3, CD000531.

Gostin, L.O., Friedman, E.A., Buse, K., et al. (2013). Towards a framework convention on global health. *Bull World Health Organ*, 91(10), 790–3. doi: 10.2471/BLT.12.114447.

Greenhalgh, T., Kristjansson, E., and Welch, V. (2007). Realist review to understand the efficacy of school feeding programmes. *British Medical Journal*, 335, 858–61.

Grimshaw, J.M., Shirran, L., Thomas, R., et al. (2001). Changing provider behavior: an overview of systematic reviews of interventions. *Medical Care*, 39(Suppl. 2), I12–I45.

Gwatkin, D. (2003). How well do health programmes reach the poor? *Lancet*, 361, 540–1.

Hamid, M., Bustamante-Manaog, T., Viet-Dung, T., et al. (2005). EVIPNet: translating the spirit of Mexico. *Lancet*, 366, 1758–9.

Higgins, J.P.T. and Green, S. (eds.) (2011). *Cochrane Handbook for Systematic Reviews of Interventions Version 5.1.0* [updated March 2011]. The Cochrane Collaboration. Available at: http://www.cochrane-handbook.org.

INCLEN (2004). *Knowledge Translation to Policy and Practice: INCLEN's Knowledge 'Plus' Program.* Available at: http://www.inclentrust.org/page.php?id=185.

Kristjansson, B., Petticrew, M., MacDonald, B., et al. (2007). School feeding for improving the physical and psychosocial health of disadvantaged students. *Cochrane Database of Systematic Reviews*, 1, CD004676.

Lavis, J.N., Lomas, J., Hamid, M., and Sewankambo, N. (2006). Assessing country-level efforts to link research to action. *Bulletin of the World Health Organization*, 84, 620–8.

Lavis, J.N. and Panisset, U. (2010). EVIPNet Africa's first series of policy briefs to support evidence-informed policymaking. *Int J Technol Assess Health Care*, 26(2), 229–32. doi: 10.1017/S0266462310000206.

Levy, D.T., Friend, K.B., and Wang, Y.C. (2011). A review of the literature on policies directed at the youth consumption of sugar sweetened beverages. *Adv Nutr*, 2(2), 182S–200S. doi: 10.3945/an.111.000356.

Lim, S.S., Vos, T., Flaxman, A.D., et al. (2012). A comparative risk assessment of burden of disease and injury attributable to 67 risk factors and risk factor clusters in 21 regions, 1990–2010: a systematic analysis for the Global Burden of Disease Study 2010. *Lancet*, 380(9859), 2224–60.

Lorenc, T., Petticrew, M., Welch, V., and Tugwell, P. (2013). What types of interventions generate inequalities? Evidence from systematic reviews. *Journal of Epidemiology and Community Health*, 67(2), 190–3.

McCoy, D., Bambas, L., Acurio, D., et al. (2003). Global equity gauge alliance: reflections on early experiences. *Journal of Health and Population Nutrition*, 21, 273–87.

Mowatt, G., Grimshaw, J.M., Davis, D.A., et al. (2001). Getting evidence into practice: the work of the Cochrane effective practice and organization of care group (EPOC). *The Journal of Continuing Education in the Health Professions*, 21, 55–60.

Ogden, C.L., Lamb, M.M., Carroll, M.D., and Flegal, K.M. (2010). *Obesity and Socioeconomic Status in Children: United States 1988–1994 and 2005–2008*. NCHS data brief no. 51. Hyattsville, MD: National Center for Health Statistics.

Pottie, K., Greenaway, C., Feightner, J., et al. (2011). Evidence-based clinical guidelines for immigrants and refugees. *Canadian Medical Association Journal*, 183(12), E824–925.

Povall, S.L., Haigh, F.A., Abrahams, D., and Scott-Samuel, A. (2013). *Health Promot Int*, Feb 28. [Epub ahead of print]. Health equity impact assessment.

Sackett, D.L., Haynes, R.B., Guyatt, G.H., and Tugwell, P. (1991). *Clinical Epidemiology: A Basic Science for Clinical Medicine*. Boston: Little, Brown.

Sackett, D.L., Rosenberg, W.M., Gray, J.A., et al. (1996). Evidence based medicine: what it is and what it isn't. *British Medical Journal*, 312, 71–2.

Santesso, N., Schünemann, H., Blumenthal, P., et al. (2012). World Health Organization guidelines: use of cryotherapy for cervical intraepithelial neoplasia. *International Journal of Gynecology & Obstetrics*, 118(2), 97–102.

Saul, M. (2013). Judge cans soda ban. *The Wall Street Journal*, 11 March.

Schunemann, H.J., Hill, S.R., Kakad, M., et al. for the WHO Rapid Advice Guideline Panel on Avian Influenza (2007). Rapid Advice Guidelines for pharmacological management of sporadic human infection with avian influenza A (H5N1) virus. *Lancet Infectious Diseases*, 7, 21–31.

Snilstveit, B. and Waddington, H. (2009). Effectiveness and sustainability of water, sanitation, and hygiene interventions in combating diarrhoea. *Journal of Development Effectiveness* 1, 295–335.

Straus, S.E., Tetroe, J., and Graham, I. (2009). Defining knowledge translation. *Canadian Medical Association Journal*, 181(3–4), 165–8.

Strom, B., Yaktine, A.L., and Oria, M. (eds.) (2013). *Sodium Intake in Populations: Assessment of Evidence*. Washington, DC: National Academies Press.

Taylor, R.S., Ashton, K.E., Moxham, T., Hooper, L., and Ebrahim, S. (2011). Reduced dietary salt for the prevention of cardiovascular disease. *Cochrane Database of Systematic Reviews*, 7, CD009217.

Thomas, K. (2013). Introduction: challenges to clinical epidemiology in India. *Journal of Clinical Epidemiology*, 66(1), 4–5.

Tirilis, D., Husson, H., DeCorby, K., and Dobbins, M. (2011). Missing and accounted for: gaps and areas of wealth in the public health review literature. *BMC Public Health*, 11, 757.

Tricco, A.C., Chit, A., Soobiah, C., et al. (2013). Comparing influenza vaccine efficacy against mismatched and matched strains: a systematic review and meta-analysis. *BMC Medicine*, 25(11), 153.

Tugwell, P., Bennett, K., Sackett, D.L., et al. (1985). The measurement iterative loop: a framework for the critical appraisal of need, benefits and costs of health interventions. *Journal of Chronic Diseases*, 38, 339–51.

Tugwell, P., de Savigny, D., Hawker, G., et al. (2006). Applying clinical epidemiological methods to health equity: the equity effectiveness loop. *British Medical Journal*, 332, 358–61.

Tugwell, P., Petticrew, M., Kristjansson, E., et al. (2010). Assessing equity in systematic reviews: realising the recommendations of the Commission on Social Determinants of Health. *BMJ*, 341, c4739. doi: 10.1136/bmj.c4739.

Tugwell, P., Pottie, K., Welch, V., et al. (2011). Evaluation of evidence based literature and formulation of recommendations for clinical preventative guidelines for immigrant and refugees in Canada. *Canadian Medical Association Journal*, 183(12), E933–8.

Tugwell, P., Sitthi-Amorn, C., O'Connor, A., et al. (1995). Technology assessment. Old, new, and needs-based. *International Journal of Technology Assessment in Health Care*, 11, 650–62.

Van de Poel, E., Hosseinpoor, A.R., Speybroeck, N., Van Ourti, T., and Vega, J. (2008). 1. Socioeconomic inequality in malnutrition in developing countries. *Bulletin of the World Health Organization*, 86(4), 282–91.

Wagstaff, A. (2002). Inequality aversion, health inequalities and health achievement. *Journal of Health Economics*, 21, 627–41.

Wang, Y. and Lim, H. (2012). The global childhood obesity epidemic and the association between socio-economic status and childhood obesity. *Int Rev Psychiatry*, 24(3), 176–88. doi: 10.3109/09540261.2012.688195.

Waters, E., de Silva-Sanigorski, A., Hall, B.J., et al. (2011). Interventions for preventing obesity in children. *Cochrane Database Syst Rev*, (12):CD001871. doi: 10.1002/14651858.CD001871.pub3.

Welch, V., Petticrew, M., Tugwell, P., et al. (2012). PRISMA-Equity 2012 extension: reporting guidelines for systematic reviews with a focus on health equity. *PLoS Medicine*, 9(10), e1001333.

Welch, V., Tugwell, P., and Morris, E.B. (2008). The equity-effectiveness loop as a tool for evaluating population health interventions. *Revista de Salud Pública*, 10, 83–96. Available at: http://www.scielosp.org/scielo.php?script=sci_arttext&pid=S0124-00642008000600008&lng=en&nrm=iso.

Whitehead, M. (1992). The concepts and principles of equity and health. *Int J Health Serv*, 22(3), 429–45.

Wilkins, R. and Adams, O. (1983). *Healthfulness of Life*. Montreal: Institute for Research on Public Policy.

Wilkinson, R.G. (1996). *Unhealthy Societies. The Afflictions of Inequality*. London: Routledge.

World Health Organization (1999). *The World Health Report 1999: Making a Difference*. Geneva: WHO.

World Health Organization (2004). *World Report on Knowledge for Better Health*. Geneva: WHO.

Zwarenstein, M. and Bryant, W. (2000). Interventions to promote collaboration between nurses and doctors. *Cochrane Database of Systematic Reviews*, 2, CD000072.

5.12

Genetic epidemiology

Elizabeth H. Young and Manjinder S. Sandhu

Introduction to genetic epidemiology

What is genetic epidemiology?

Classical epidemiology asks whether, across a study population, a measured exposure is consistently associated with an observed disease or trait. Similarly, *genetic* epidemiology in its simplest paradigm asks whether a *genetic* exposure is associated with a disease or health outcome in a given population. To expand on this, genetic epidemiology can be defined as population-based research that focuses on the aetiological role of genes in the occurrence of disease, in order to provide insights into disease biology and mechanism by unpicking the causal pathway from genes to disease.

Over the last decade there has been an extraordinary pace of change in genetic epidemiology driven by rapid advances in technology. These changes have revolutionized the scope and scale of what can be done, ranging from studies of single gene variants measured in small samples through to the emergence of high-throughput genotyping, genome-wide association studies (GWAS), and next-generation whole-genome sequencing technologies which produce information on millions of genetic variants in thousands of individuals. In parallel, as these genomic technologies provide new opportunities to better understand disease and develop targeted therapeutics for patients, it is becoming increasingly apparent that a knowledge of genomic medicine will be essential for public health practitioners in meeting the public's future healthcare needs.

Genetic epidemiology and public health practice

Ultimately, the goal of genetic epidemiology lies in the application of research findings to clinical care and improved health for the population. The discovery and confirmation of genetic variants associated with diseases and traits may have translational implications—such as advances in treatment and genetic risk prediction. First, the identification of genetic determinants of traits, together with a better understanding of the underlying physiology and regulation, should help inform drug development and improve therapeutic effectiveness. Secondly, in relation to risk prediction, as more disease loci are identified it may be useful to assess whether genetic testing could improve risk prediction of disease beyond traditional risk factors. Additionally, use of genetic data makes risk stratification possible at a young age, when signs and symptoms of disease are not yet present—the clinical and ethical implications of this must be carefully considered. Thus, in this twenty-first-century era of genetic epidemiology and genomic science, public health practitioners cannot overlook the impact of genetic epidemiology on our understanding of models of disease, individualized medicine, and the relationship between individuals and populations, treatment, and prevention strategies.

Heredity, genetics, and disease

DNA, RNA, and proteins: the structure and function of genes

The human genome carries the chemical information that allows the exact transmission of genetic information from one cell to its daughter cells and from one generation to the next. Our genome is made up of deoxyribonucleic acid (DNA), which consists of a long sequence of nucleotide bases of four types: adenosine (A), cytosine (C), guanine (G), and thymine (T). Strong covalent bonds bind the bases together along a single strand, and weaker hydrogen bonds pair A with T, and C with G, between the two strands in their double-helix form. The double-stranded DNA acts as a template for its own replication: separation of the two strands, and construction of a new complementary strand for each, results in two identical copies of the original.

DNA also acts as a template for its transcription and translation into proteins. The precise order (the 'sequence') in which nucleotide bases are arranged along the DNA strand determines the amino acid sequences of the proteins. First, a single strand of DNA can act as a template for a complementary strand of ribonucleic acid (RNA), through the process of *transcription*. Importantly, in certain regions of DNA, which can be called genes, the transcribed RNA encodes instructions that tell the cell how to assemble amino acids to make proteins through a process known as *translation*. Thus, just as DNA directs the sequence of RNA, so RNA directs the sequence of amino acids and proteins. Only 1–2 per cent of these RNA transcripts encode for protein; the vast majority are transcribed as non-coding RNA which has important biological functions that influence gene expression through a variety of mechanisms (Amaral and Mattick 2008; Kaikkonen et al. 2011).

At its simplest, a *gene* can be thought of as a length of DNA containing the code for the amino acid sequence of a protein. However, few genes exist as continuous coding sequences; rather, most genes contain one or more non-coding regions, called introns, that interrupt the coding regions, or exons. It was previously assumed that non-coding regions of DNA had no biological function. However, we now know that many types of non-coding DNA sequences may have active roles in the regulation of protein-coding sequences and gene modulation (The ENCODE Project Consortium 2011).

The complete human DNA sequence is the human genome, and contains around 3 billion DNA base pairs. The human genome is distributed among 46 chromosomes, composed of 23 pairs: 22 homologous pairs of autosomes, and one pair of sex chromosomes (X and Y). In each pair of autosomes, one chromosome is inherited from the mother and the other from the father. Chromosomal DNA will contain many genes, with DNA segments of varying length between them. A given gene may exist in alternative forms, differing in DNA sequence, known as *alleles*. The *genotype* of an individual refers to the combination of two alleles inherited (one inherited maternally, the other paternally) at a specific locus—for example, AA, AG, TC, GG, etc. If the alleles are the same, the genotype is homozygous; if different, heterozygous.

Generating genetic diversity

The DNA of the human genome is subject to a variety of different types of genetic variation, defined as any change in the nucleotide sequence or arrangement of DNA. Some genetic variants may have no phenotypic effect and, therefore, no clinical consequences. Other variants will profoundly alter disease susceptibility or, in extreme instances, be incompatible with life.

Genetic variants can be inherited from a parent, or acquired during a person's lifetime (somatic). They may be caused by radiation, viruses, and mutagenic chemicals, as well as errors that occur during meiosis (cell division) or DNA replication, or induced by cellular processes within an organism. Globally, human populations show structured genetic diversity as a result of geographical dispersion, selection and drift (Campbell and Tishkoff 2008; McCarthy et al. 2008; Novembre and Ramachandran 2011). Understanding this genomic variation can provide insights into our human origins and the evolutionary processes that shape variation in phenotypic traits and disease risk.

In the context of genetic epidemiology, we are concerned with understanding how disease susceptibility may be conferred by different kinds of genetic variation. Within an individual, genetic variation can occur at three levels:

♦ *Genome variation*: changes that affect the number of intact chromosomes in the cell.

♦ *Chromosome variation*: changes that alter the structure of individual chromosomes.

♦ *Genetic variation*: changes that alter the sequence of nucleotide bases in a length of DNA.

Genetic variants

Gene variants are alterations in DNA sequence. Different versions of a particular DNA sequence at one specific chromosomal location (locus) are called alleles. When a particular allele is rare—conventionally, with a frequency of less than 1 per cent in the general population—it is known as a *rare variant* or *mutation*. By contrast, where an allele is found in more than 1 per cent of the population it is called a *genetic polymorphism* (literally, 'many forms') or *common variant*. There are many different types of DNA sequence variants, that can range from a change in a single nucleotide base to a change in many thousands of base pairs (Bochud 2012).

The most studied class of variant is the *single nucleotide polymorphism* (SNP, pronounced 'snip'; also known as a point mutation), where the DNA sequence varies in a single base—for example, A is present instead of T, C is present instead of G. SNPs are the most common type of variant; as of June 2012, there are around 38 million known SNPs in the human genome (dbSNP database; National Center for Biotechnology Information n.d.). SNPs lying in protein-coding regions of the gene can alter the code for an amino acid sequence and may (or may not) in turn affect the function or availability of a protein and cause disease. Non-coding SNPs, occurring in intronic (non-coding sequence of a gene) or intergenic (sequence of DNA between genes) regions of the genome can also cause disease, by affecting gene transcription and function. In addition to SNPs, there are also other types of structural variations in the human genome such as variable number tandem repeats (VNTRs), insertions and deletions of DNA bases, and copy number variants (CNVs), which have been used successfully to identify disease genes (Bochud 2012).

Patterns of inheritance, genotypes, and phenotypes

An individual's *genotype* can be understood as the combination of alleles present at a specific position (known as a locus) occupied by a gene on a chromosome. A *phenotype* is an observable, measurable characteristic or trait (biochemical, physiological, morphological, or behavioural) of an individual, other than its genotype. A phenotype could be a quantitative characteristic (such as systolic blood pressure) or a binary disease state (presence or absence of hypertension).

Many variations at the genotype level result in little or no observable variation in phenotype. If, however, a phenotype is present in individuals with just one copy of an abnormal allele, the allele is dominant. By contrast, if the phenotype is only expressed in the presence of two abnormal alleles, the allele is said to be recessive.

Reduced penetrance and variable expressivity are additional factors that influence the phenotypic expression of a particular genetic change. The *penetrance*, or positive predictive value, of a given genotype is the percentage of people with a disease-associated genotype who develop the disease. In cases where all individuals with a particular genotype develop the disease, the gene shows 100 per cent penetrance. In contrast to this, some phenotypes are not expressed in all genotypically predisposed individuals; here, the gene is said to show *reduced penetrance*.

The concept of penetrance is often confused with *variable expressivity*, which is the variation in the severity of expression of a phenotype. Although some genetic disorders exhibit little variation, most have signs and symptoms that differ among affected individuals, in some instances ranging from mild symptoms through to life-threatening complications. Variable expressivity refers to the range of severity of clinical features that occur in different people who have the same genotype.

Single-gene disorders

Single-gene, or monogenic, disorders run in families and are caused by a single mutated gene. Single-gene disorders are often called 'Mendelian' because they display obvious and characteristic patterns of inheritance as described by the nineteenth-century scientist Gregor Mendel, in his study of how traits were passed from one generation of garden peas to the next. Mendelian disorders are usually characterized by extreme phenotypes in rare patient subgroups that are linked to causal genes with rare mutations. These disorders, whilst individually rare and not contributing substantially to the global burden of disease, might collectively cause significant disease and death in a population. They can also provide invaluable insights into the underlying biology of disease and help to inform the search for susceptibility genes for more common diseases and traits.

Complex multifactorial diseases

Familial aggregation

In contrast to monogenic disorders, genetic disorders may also be complex (also known as multifactorial, or polygenic or non-Mendelian), meaning they are likely to be associated with the effects of multiple genes in combination with lifestyle and environmental factors, with no clear mode of inheritance. Multifactorial disorders include many common diseases such as cancers, heart disease, and diabetes, and quantitative traits such as height, weight, blood pressure and blood chemistries. Patterns of inheritance for complex disorders do not fit simple patterns as with Mendelian diseases. This makes it difficult to determine a person's risk of inheriting or passing on these disorders. Complex disorders are also difficult to study and treat because the specific factors that cause most of these disorders have not yet been identified.

However, this does not mean that the genes cannot eventually be located and studied. Because relatives share a greater proportion of their genes with one another than with unrelated individuals in the population, a primary feature of diseases or traits with a genetic basis is that affected individuals tend to cluster in families. Of course, familial aggregation does not necessarily mean there must be a genetic contribution; family members may develop a disease or trait simply by chance alone, particularly if it is common in the general population, or as a result of a shared environmental exposure. Given this, a helpful measure of familial aggregation is the *recurrence risk ratio* (λ_r), which takes into account the population prevalence of a disease. λ_r estimates the ratio of the risk of developing disease when a relative already has the disease compared to the risk in the general population (i.e. background prevalence).

The correlation of a trait or disease among relatives provides another useful estimate of genetic influence, on the assumption that the degree of similarity in the values of trait (e.g. body mass index (BMI)) measured among relatives is proportional to the number of alleles they share at the loci for that trait. Based on this premise, the more closely related the individuals are in a family the more likely they are to share alleles at loci and—in this instance—the more strongly correlated will be their BMI values. Thus a tendency for BMI to be more similar among relatives than among the general population is further evidence for a genetic aetiology. Familial correlations can also be used to calculate the *heritability* (h^2) of a trait, a measure that quantifies the percentage of phenotypic variation in a trait that is attributable specifically to genotypic differences. The higher the heritability, the greater the contribution of genetic variation among people in causing the variability of a trait for a given population.

Twin studies

To help disentangle the relative contributions of genes and environment in the aetiology of disease, twin and adoption studies are used (Boomsma et al. 2002). Comparison of disease concordance rates in identical (monozygotic (MZ)) and non-identical (dizygotic (DZ)) twins helps to assess the genetic influences on a disease. MZ twins are genetically identical, sharing the same alleles at every locus. DZ twins, on the other hand, share on average half the alleles at all loci, like all siblings. MZ twins provide an opportunity to study disease occurrence when genetic factors are held constant, by measuring concordance in relatives with identical genotypes who may or may not be reared together in the same environment. Concordance in MZ twins in early life can be the result of genes or a shared environment. However, in later life most twins live apart and concordance at that stage may suggest a genetic component to the disease. Concordance less than 100 per cent in MZ twins is strong evidence that non-genetic factors are involved in disease aetiology.

DZ twins reared together provide an opportunity to study disease occurrence when genetic differences are present but environmental factors are shared. Greater concordance in MZ versus DZ twins is strong evidence of a genetic component to the disease. Comparison of concordance rates in MZ versus DZ twins can be used to estimate the heritability of a disease.

As with family studies, twin studies are not without their limitations. First, despite being referred to as 'identical', MZ twins do not have identical gene expression of their identical genotypes; for example, somatic rearrangements will differ between MZ twins, which may give rise to phenotypic discordance and differences in disease susceptibility. Secondly, environmental exposures may not be the same for twins; even the intrauterine environment may differ within a twin pair (e.g. differential placental blood supply in MZ twins). Furthermore, studies comparing MZ to DZ twins are based on the assumption that they differ only by the number of genes they share and that within each pair the exposure to environment factors is identical; yet it is likely that MZ twins share more of their environment than DZ twins (particularly compared to opposite-sex DZ twins). Ascertainment bias poses an additional limitation, where twins who are very alike will tend to participate in studies more than twins who are very discordant for a phenotype. Studies of twins reared apart are easier to conduct than adoption studies, and similarly are an effective way of investigating the influence of shared genes and different environments. However, even with MZ twins separated at birth, intrauterine environmental influences cannot be distinguished from genetic influences.

Adoption studies

Adoption studies provide another valuable source of information about the genetic component of a disease. In this study design, a disease or trait is identified in adoptees and then studied in both their adoptive family (shared environmental factors only) and biological family (shared genetic factors only). Whilst undoubtedly providing the best way of separating out genetic and environmental influences, adoption studies carry obvious difficulties: information may be lacking about the biological family, compounded by their wish not to be identified and approached for details. In addition, relatively small sample sizes for which both adoptive and biological parents are available have limited the use of these studies.

The results of family studies must be interpreted with care. Importantly, familial aggregation of a continuous trait or discrete disease—however measured—does not indicate that genes are wholly responsible. Families share many factors besides their genes, such as common environmental exposures, cultural attitudes, and behaviours. This means that family studies are likely to overestimate the genetic component of a disease, and the strong environmental component to many complex, multifactorial diseases, must not be overlooked.

Role of the environment and gene–environment interactions

Nearly all human diseases originate in large part from a complex interplay between genetic susceptibility factors and modifiable environmental exposures (including chemical, physical, infectious, nutritional, and behavioural factors). Therefore, in understanding the aetiology of disease and assessing the role of susceptibility alleles in disease risk, it is important to examine genetic factors *and* environmental factors and—importantly—the relation between the two: so-called gene–environment interactions.

Studies of gene–environment interactions present a number of methodological challenges (Hunter 2005). The assessment of the relation between genes and environment requires information on both components. Gene–environment interaction may be measured by the different effects of an environmental exposure on disease risk among individuals with different genotypes, or by the different effects of a genotype on disease risk among individuals with different environmental exposures (Yang and Khoury 1997). However, the power of studies to detect statistically relevant interactions is highly dependent on the precision with which genetic and non-genetic exposures are measured. As discussed elsewhere in this chapter, with the advent of next-generation genotyping and sequencing technologies, it is now possible and affordable to generate massive genomic datasets. By contrast, a challenge still remains to achieve accurate and objective measures of environmental exposures such as dietary intake or physical activity that are feasible to collect in a large-scale epidemiological context.

In addition, the need for suitably large sample sizes is a major obstacle to overcome in the design of interaction studies (Hunter 2005). The sample size required to detect the joint effect of two variables is much larger than the size required to evaluate the main effect of each variable; given that many epidemiological studies are underpowered to detect main effects, these studies will be substantially underpowered to detect interactions. Careful consideration of study design, and the accurate and detailed assessment of genetic factors, environmental exposures, and disease phenotypes, is therefore crucial for planning interaction studies that will yield meaningful results.

Determining the details of gene–environment interactions will help us to understand the aetiology of disease and might lead to opportunities for targeted prevention strategies for some high-risk individuals (Hunter 2005; Khoury et al. 2005). Indeed, there may be significant public health benefits in using genetic information to improve existing approaches to identify and modify environmental risk factors, including stratifying the allocation of environmental interventions that prevent disease (Khoury et al. 2005). It may be, for example, that individuals with a certain genotype are particularly susceptible to the negative consequences of specific lifestyle behaviours, and that they would have most to gain from a targeted preventive intervention programme. Understanding how to detect these individuals and which environmental factors a programme should attempt to manipulate is a major goal of studies that attempt to unravel gene–environment interactions.

Finding disease genes: methods in genetic epidemiology

From monogenic to multifactorial disease

A number of strategies have been used to try and uncover genes involved in the aetiology of common, multifactorial disease (Table 5.12.1). Non-Mendelian disorders may depend on the interplay of common variants—polymorphisms—in several susceptibility genes together with a variable contribution from the environment. These genetic variants are presumed to have only modest effects accounting for a small percentage of variation in a trait, at least when examined individually; however, they may play a more important role through interaction with other gene variants and be responsible for significant population attributable risk for disease.

Linkage studies, fine mapping through mutation screening, and case–control and cohort-based association studies of patients—combined with data from animal models—have uncovered the genes causing many Mendelian, or monogenic, disorders. In turn, a knowledge of the genetic basis of these Mendelian disorders has helped further our understanding of human physiology and played a vital part in establishing the causal role for disease risk factors and in the development of drug targets. In recent years there has been considerable progress in mapping—that is, identifying and localizing—loci that influence susceptibility to common human diseases.

Genetic linkage scans

Linkage analysis is often the first stage in the genetic investigation of a trait, since it can be used to identify broad chromosomal regions of the genome (as opposed to specific alleles) that might contain a disease gene (Teare and Barrett 2005; Altshuler et al. 2008). Genetic linkage is the tendency of genes that are located close to each other on a chromosome to be transmitted together to offspring. Genes that are positioned nearer to each other are less likely to be separated onto different parts of the chromosome during *genetic recombination* (the breakage and rejoining of DNA strands to produce new combinations of alleles, encoding a novel set of genetic information) and are therefore said to be genetically linked. On this basis, susceptibility or causal genes can be localized by searching for genetic markers that co-segregate with the disease trait; if an allele of gene A causes disease, but is otherwise undetectable, whereas the allele of gene B can be easily detected and distinguished, gene B can be used as a marker of the inherited disease. Linkage studies use DNA from family members to identify areas of the genome that show evidence of containing the unknown disease-related genetic variant on the basis of correlation with DNA variation. Polymorphic markers positioned across the genome are genotyped in families, followed by calculating the degree of linkage of the marker to a disease trait. An advantage of linkage analysis is that this approach attempts to map genes purely by position and does not presume any a priori hypotheses about their location, biological function, or number.

Table 5.12.1 Common strategies for finding disease genes

Study design	Participants	Strengths	Limitations
Linkage studies	Relatives: large pedigrees, affected sib-pairs, or discordant sib-pairs	Can study multiple genetic markers simultaneously Good for rare traits	Only defines a locus or region, not specific genes
Family-based association studies	Parent–child trios, siblings	Less prone to population stratification Provides a rich context for evaluating shared genetic and environmental influences	Difficult to separate genetic from environmental influences Challenging for outcomes of older age: finding families with more than one affected generation will be difficult Findings may not be applicable to general population
Candidate gene association studies	Unrelated individuals	Powerful study design for common traits	Led by the state of current knowledge: success depends on selecting the right candidate gene
Genome-wide association studies	Unrelated individuals	Genotyping platforms developed to simultaneously examine hundreds of thousands of genetic variants	Lots of false positives; association does not equate to causation Replication of initial results is a challenge
Sequencing studies	Unrelated individuals	Good for identifying rare variants	Limited by costs and existing technological capabilities

Linkage analyses have proved highly successful for finding genes causing Mendelian disorders. However, linkage studies only work well if the phenotype of interest is caused by variation in the same gene region, and have generally been unsuccessful at identifying genes for common disorders where multiple genes are implicated (Hirschhorn and Gajdos 2011). Linkage analyses can only identify large regions and, whilst a very strong candidate gene might exist within the linkage region, such regions may contain hundreds of genes, many of which are biologically plausible candidates. To refine any association may require extensive genotyping—both time-consuming and expensive—and potentially produce many false positive results.

Association studies

Genetic association studies provide an alternative approach to finding disease genes, which overcome some of the limitations of linkage studies. Genetic association studies aim to detect an association between an allele and trait (unlike linkage studies, which focus on a genetic locus as the unit of analysis regardless of the alleles present at that locus). Association differs from linkage in that the same allele (or alleles) is associated with the trait in a similar manner across the whole population, while linkage allows different alleles to be associated with the trait in different families. Whereas linkage studies can only be conducted using family data, association analyses can be done using unrelated and/or related people. Association studies can be conducted at the level of a candidate gene (candidate gene association study), or at the level of the entire genome (GWAS).

Candidate gene association studies

The candidate gene approach has many parallels with identifying and ranking risk factors in an epidemiological study (Tabor et al. 2002): from a large number of potential factors, researchers must pick those factors that are most likely to be associated with the outcome of interest. The selection of candidate genes focuses the search onto specific susceptibility genes that are identified a priori on the basis of their presumed biological relevance to the disease or trait of interest. Once a candidate has been selected, common variants—usually SNPs—in the gene are then identified

(either *de novo* from sequencing/mutation screening, or based on previously published work). The SNPs are then genotyped and tested for association with the outcome of interest. In the case of a binary outcome, SNPs will be genotyped in cases and controls to assess whether the variants are associated with the phenotype of interest; where the outcome of interest is a quantitative trait, SNPs are typed in population cohorts. A strength of this gene-centric method is that it is a highly efficient way of identifying susceptibility genes if biological plausibility is high. Conversely, a drawback of the method is that it is, by definition, limited by the state of current knowledge. Thus countless genes may be overlooked because biological candidacy has not yet been established. Issues of multiple testing and false positives remain limitations of the candidate gene approach.

Genome-wide association studies

GWAS have recently emerged as a powerful new tool for identifying the genetic variants related to common, complex diseases by effectively combining the association and linkage approaches to gene identification (McCarthy et al. 2008; Hirschhorn and Gajdos 2011). The basic paradigm of GWAS is to catalogue thousands of very common SNP markers located throughout the human genome, and then to genotype them in large numbers of unrelated humans who have already been carefully characterized for a wide variety of common diseases and traits. The GWAS approach affords the possibility of exploring the whole genome without any a priori knowledge of underlying disease biology. This allows for hypothesis-free testing of a substantial fraction of common genetic variation for a role in determining disease risk, and potentially enables the discovery of unexpected genetic factors or pathways for common diseases.

A central factor in the development of GWAS is having a comprehensive map of carefully selected SNPs (Box 5.12.1). Over the last two decades, a number of international efforts have successfully done this, creating denser and denser genetic maps. As these have emerged, it has become apparent that many SNPs are strongly correlated (Palmer and Cardon 2005). Consequently, if the pattern of allelic association can be described, direct assay of all existing polymorphisms is unnecessary, because genotypes of

---

Box 5.12.1 International scientific efforts to describe common human genetic diversity

The Human Genome Project, the SNP Consortium, the International HapMap Project, and the 1000 Genomes Project have collectively identified around 10 million common genetic variants in humans. Knowledge of these SNPs and their patterns of correlation have enabled GWAS which have successfully identified hundreds of novel disease genes (Donnelly 2008; International HapMap 3 Consortium 2010).

Completed in 2003, the *Human Genome Project* was an international collaborative research programme whose goal was to discover all the estimated 20,000–25,000 human genes and map the complete sequence of the 3 billion DNA bases (International Human Genome Mapping Consortium 2001; International Human Genome Sequencing Consortium 2001; International SNP Map Working Group 2001; Roberts et al. 2001; Collins et al. 2003). The official Human Genome Project was meant to have been a 15-year project spanning 1990–2005, but progress was faster than expected. Conducted on an industrial scale at a few large genome centres across the world, genetic maps were developed ahead of the original schedule, and the final stage of large-scale DNA sequencing was facilitated by developments in automated high-throughput sequencing techniques. The need to manage and store the huge amounts of sequencing data that were being produced led to the development of large electronic databases. Importantly, a key aim of this endeavour was to make these genomic data publicly available and accessible to the scientific community at large.

The *SNP Consortium* was established in 1999 as public–private partnership of several companies and institutions to produce a public resource of SNPs in the human genome (Kruglyak 2008). The initial goal was to discover 300,000 SNPs in 2 years, but the final results exceeded this, as 1.4 million SNPs had been released into the public domain at the end of 2001.

The SNP Consortium subsequently joined forces with the *International HapMap Project*. Launched in 2002, the HapMap Project is a global consortium of scientists and researchers with the aim of providing a public resource to inform and accelerate genetic medical research. Specifically, the project set out to describe the common patterns of human DNA sequence variation across the human genome in order to find genes affecting health, disease, and responses to drugs and environmental factors. Whereas the SNP Consortium was concerned with individual SNPs, the HapMap Project focused on examining combinations of SNPs that are inherited together, known as haplotypes. By 2007, the project had genotyped more than 3 million SNPs which captured the majority of all common variants with frequencies above 5 per cent (International HapMap Consortium 2007). In its current phase, 'HapMap 3', the project is expanding its scope to identify rarer genetic variants that may be implicated in human disease and achieve a higher resolution map of human genetic variation (International HapMap 3 Consortium 2010).

The *1000 Genomes Project* (1000 G) was launched in 2008 as an extension of the HapMap project. Its aim is to create a public reference database containing an even more detailed characterization of the human genome by extending the catalogue of human genetic variants to include 95 per cent of rarer variants, occurring at frequency of 1–5 per cent (The 1000 Genomes Project Consortium 2010). As of November 2012, using a combination of whole-genome sequencing and exome sequencing, the architecture and functional spectrum of human genetic variation has now been characterized in the genomes of 1092 individuals from 14 populations (The 1000 Genomes Project Consortium 2012).

---

common SNPs may be inferred from knowledge of only a few representative SNPs. This is the principle underlying the tagging-SNP method: that it is possible to select the maximally informative set of polymorphisms (tagSNPs) to genotype in an association study such that all known SNPs are either directly genotyped or exceed a threshold level of association with a tagSNP. Given the practical limitations on genotyping, selection of tagging SNPs can usefully decrease the amount of genotyping required and thus improve the cost-effectiveness of studies. Inevitably, there is a trade-off between this improved efficiency and the loss of power that occurs when SNPs are discarded. However, by specifying various parameters (e.g. the level of allelic correlation, and the likelihood of genetic linkage) it is possible to try and maximize efficiency whilst maintaining statistical power.

In 2007, the Wellcome Trust Case Control Consortium (WTCCC) set the benchmark for GWAS of common disease on an unparalled scope and scale. Representing a UK-wide collaboration of more than 50 research groups and 200 scientists in the field of human genetics, the WTCCC genotyped over 500,000 SNPs in DNA samples from 17,000 people across the United Kingdom. Over 2 years, they analysed almost 10 billion pieces of genetic information, and substantially increased the number of genes known to play a role in the development of some of our most common diseases such as heart disease, hypertension, Crohn's disease, and diabetes. Many of these genes that have been found are in areas of the genome not previously thought to have been related to the diseases (Wellcome Trust Case Control Consortium 2007). More recently, advances from commercial companies such as Affymetrix and Illumina in the availability of dense genotyping chips with approximately 5 million SNPs are making even larger GWAS both cost-effective and feasible, and there has been considerable progress in the search for disease-related loci and genetic variants using the GWAS approach.

Searching for rare variants

GWAS have now been completed for many common human diseases and related traits, identifying a wealth of common gene variants. However, GWAS have a number of limitations: first, their scope is defined by the current knowledge of existing genetic variants that are included on a specific genotype chip. Second, most of the disease-associated SNPs found in GWAS have very small effect sizes, and explain only a modest fraction of the genetic component of human disease. This is to be expected if much of the missing heritability is due to gene variants that are less common or too rare to be detected by GWAS and have relatively modest effect sizes (Cirulli and Goldstein 2010). On this basis, gene discovery efforts have in recent years expanded to search for rare genetic variants.

To capture such rare variants, it will be necessary to use large samples sizes (thousands of individuals) and sequence entire genomes, rather than genotype a catalogue of variants. Until recently, this was technically unfeasible. However, the technological advances of the last couple of years (so-called next-generation sequencing technology) have made this possible (Metzker 2010; Zhang et al. 2011): now, billions of DNA bases can be sequenced in a matter of days. The most complete study of rare disease variants will require *whole-genome sequencing* in large sample sizes of human participants. At present, despite the rapid pace of technological development and the precipitant fall in the costs, it is likely that the shift to whole-genome sequencing association studies on a massive scale may still not be feasible.

In the meantime, *targeted sequencing* and *exome sequencing* offer more affordable strategies for finding rare genetic variants. Targeted sequencing is focused on genomic regions of specific interest—rather than the whole genome—and enables a systematic assessment of the full spectrum of genetic variation, including common and rare variants, for high-throughput sequencing at a lower cost per sample. Similarly, selectively sequencing only the exome constitutes a powerful and efficient alternative to whole-genome sequencing (Bamshad et al. 2011). Approximately 85 per cent of all disease-causing variants in humans can typically be found in the subset of the human genome that is protein coding—known as the exome. With the availability of next-generation sequencing technology, exome sequencing has become a cost-effective method for the identification of rare sequence variants (Choi et al. 2009; Ng et al. 2009; Pussegoda 2010). This strategy (also known as targeted exome capture) has been used successfully to identify disease-causing variants for a number of rare Mendelian disorders (Choi et al. 2009; Ng et al. 2010; Bamshad et al. 2011) and is an effective technique to detect causal variants associated with disease even when few individuals with disease are sequenced (Cirulli and Goldstein 2010). Although this method has only been used in the study of Mendelian disorders, these studies have provided the framework for the application of this method to the study of complex diseases (Cirulli and Goldstein 2010).

Generating genomic data: analytical issues

At present GWAS typically generate information on several million genetic variants, on many thousands of individuals. Many computational and analytical steps are required to translate massive raw genomic data into usable, high-quality data, and may include techniques for genotype imputation. Imputation is the term used to describe the substitution of some value for missing data. In the context of GWAS data, genotype imputation is the process of predicting or imputing genotypes that are not directly assayed in a study sample of individuals, based on reference panels of SNPs (Li et al. 2009). These *in silico* genotypes can then be used to increase the total number of SNPs that can be analysed for association, thus improving the statistical power of the study. Handling such vast datasets, and identifying the few true association signals amongst the masses of false positive signals, requires extensive computing and storage infrastructure, and advances in computational resources and statistical techniques for processing, analysis, and interpretation (Hunter and Kraft 2007).

A key determinant of the quality in any association study—genetic or non-genetic—is its sample size (Ioannidis et al. 2003).

This is particularly pertinent in genetic studies, which must be powered to detect variants that have only modest associations with the outcome of interest. Small initial studies rarely find the correct result and, even when they do, are likely to overestimate the true effect size (Ioannidis et al. 2003; Lohmueller et al. 2003; Wacholder et al. 2004). An implication of looking at modest effect sizes of genetic variants is the need for sufficiently large sample sizes to avoid underpowered studies with false negative results (Lohmueller et al. 2003; Ioannidis et al. 2006). In addition to ensuring adequate samples sizes, care must be taken to ensure optimal ascertainment of cases and controls, to improve study power—for example, by selecting cases with minimal phenotypic heterogeneity, or focusing on extreme phenotypes such as early-onset severe disease in order to enrich for disease-causing alleles (Hattersley and McCarthy 2005).

Multiple testing is also an issue for these large datasets: when testing so many SNP–disease associations simultaneously, the probability of a nominally significant result from within the entire experiment occurring by chance is higher than the individual *p*-value associated with that result, because of random variation in the data and the large number of tests that are performed (Thomas and Clayton 2004). In other words, there is an increased chance of false positives, and one cannot be certain at the outset whether there are any true associations to be found at all. Consequently, the individual *p*-values of the tests may not be an appropriate guide to actual statistical significance.

There are several statistical techniques which may be used to correct for multiple testing, including a reduction in the number of tests, or the setting of a more stringent *p*-value, or permutation testing (Hirschhorn and Daly 2005). When adjusting for multiple testing, larger samples will be required so that if an initial association is statistically significant, it will remain significant after correction (Benjamini and Hochberg, 1995; Hirschhorn and Daly 2005). Where GWAS findings indicate an association between a genetic variant and a trait or disease, validation and replication studies are essential to determine whether the result of the initial study represents a true reproducible association with genome-wide statistical significance (McCarthy et al. 2008; Ioannidis et al. 2009).

Causal inference

In observational epidemiological studies, causal inferences are potentially susceptible to problems of bias and confounding that, in addition to chance, provide alternative explanations for an observed association between an exposure and a disease. Likewise, the assessment of causality in gene–disease associations is vulnerable to possible other explanations (Geneletti et al. 2011). The role of *bias* must be considered in any observed gene–disease association. In contrast to studies of non-genetic exposures, which are potentially prone to recall bias, an individual's genotype is an exposure that is fixed at conception—thus the association between genetic variants and disease outcomes will not usually be biased in this way. However, a key potential bias in genetic association studies is the differential genotyping of cases and controls. Wherever possible this can be minimized by randomly allocating cases and controls in the genotyping process, so that systematic genotyping errors affecting solely cases or controls are unlikely to occur. Selection bias due to non-comparable cases and controls may also explain the observed associations. Bias, though, need not necessarily be a problem: it can also be used positively to enhance a study. For instance, one might deliberately select cases enriched for genetic variants (e.g. based on their family history of a disease or trait), in order to improve the power of a study to detect a statistically significant association.

In the context of genetic association studies, classical *confounding* variables such as age and sex are not usually relevant. This is because in order to confound the association between genotype and phenotype, these characteristics would need to be associated with both the genotype and the specific outcome. In the case of genetic association studies this is not applicable, based on the assumption of random assortment—that is, during gamete formation alleles are allocated arbitrarily from parent to offspring independently of other traits. This results in population distributions of genetic variants that are generally independent of behavioural and environmental factors that typically confound epidemiological associations between risk factors and disease.

Nevertheless, we cannot ignore confounding as a result of *undetected population stratification* due to ethnic admixture, which can mimic the signal of association and give rise to false positives and produce associations of disease with genotype at loci that are not linked to any locus that affects disease susceptibility (Hoggart et al. 2003; Freedman et al. 2004; Marchini et al. 2004). Ethnic admixture refers to the presence of multiple subgroups within a larger population, caused by non-random mating, which have differing allele frequencies. This can have implications for studies of gene–disease association if the subgroups have different genotypic distributions (Fig. 5.12.1). If cases and controls are drawn differentially from two or more subpopulations in which marker allele frequencies *and* disease prevalence differ across subpopulations, this will result in an over-representation of one or more genetic subgroups among individuals chosen as disease cases in an association study. In this instance, any SNP with allele proportions that differ between the subgroup and the general population will be associated with disease status. Although the association is real from a statistical point of view, it is regarded as spurious since it does not yield any information about the biology of the phenotype or about the genomic location of the disease-modifying locus; rather, the association between the allele and the disease is confounded by the existence of genetic heterogeneous subpopulations (Wacholder et al. 2000; Ziv and Burchard 2003).

There are a number of different ways of addressing population stratification, such as matching cases and controls according to ethnicity and geographical origin. This matching can be difficult to achieve, and several different control populations might have to be used in any given study. To address this problem, a variety of statistical methods that infer genetic ancestry may be used to control for confounding by population stratification (Cordell and Clayton 2005; Balding 2006; Price et al. 2010). A commonly used statistical method for controlling population stratification is *genomic control*, in which the test statistic is corrected using an inflation factor (lambda, λ). To do this, associations between marker loci across the genome and traits or diseases are used to assess population structure and determine an average effect of population structure across the whole genome. The residual effects of stratification for all investigated markers are then adjusted by a uniform λ. Thus the further λ deviates from the value 1, the greater the correction, and the more evidence for presence of population stratification or

other biases; conversely, the closer λ is to 1, the more unlikely it is that stratification is present.

An alternative method is to use *principal components analysis* (PCA) to correct for stratification, which can be carried out using software such as EIGENSTRAT. PCA explicitly models ancestry differences between cases and controls. The resulting genomic correction factor, λ, is specific to a candidate marker's variation in frequency across ancestral populations, minimizing spurious associations while maintaining power to detect true associations. Other approaches include family-based tests such as the transmission disequilibrium test, and mixed models—the latter having the additional advantage of simultaneously addressing population stratification along with other systematic differences, such as family structure or relatedness, that may be present in the data (Price et al. 2010).

Even after many convincing replications of a SNP–disease association, causality may not be inferred; the causal variant may still need to be identified. In this instance, the parallels with classic epidemiology are clear: an association between a SNP and trait might exist if: (1) the SNP with the observed association has a causal role; (2) the SNP has no causal role but is highly correlated (associated) with the true causal variant. It is also possible that the currently identified SNPs might not fully describe genetic diversity, as a result of *incomplete capture of genetic variation*. One therefore cannot exclude the possibility that the unidentified and untyped variants might have shown statistically significant associations with disease and might include among them the true causal variant. Ultimately, to refine the association signal at a locus of interest requires knowledge of the SNP correlations in that region which, in turn, depends on the genetic variation in the region being fully characterized (Ioannidis et al. 2009).

The need for functional validation

For conclusive evidence of causality, the epidemiological approaches just described need to be complemented by efforts to establish which regions of the human genome sequence truly have a biological function and thus may be relevant to disease mechanism and human health. The recent discoveries from genome-wide studies represent a significant advance in our unravelling of the genetic basis of common human disease (Kruglyak 2008). Despite the large number of loci and the robustness of their associations with diseases or disease traits, these loci tend to have small individual effects on phenotype, and even collectively tend to explain only a small fraction of the heritable component. Moreover, it is not yet clear what most of the causal variants or even the causal genes are at these loci. Thus, whether the GWAS approach can yield biologically relevant insights into human physiology remains to be established.

A next step is to identify and validate functional variants through studies of gene expression, in order to clarify the biological role of proteins or other gene products encoded by specific genomic regions and to understand how they influence biological processes and confer disease risk; an example of this is the ENCODE project (Box 5.12.2).

Problematically, some genes may only be expressed locally—for example, in specific brain nuclei—and so attaining samples for physiological studies may prove unfeasible. *In vitro* studies of gene activity, as well as *in vivo* overexpression and knockout studies in experimental animal models, will continue to play an

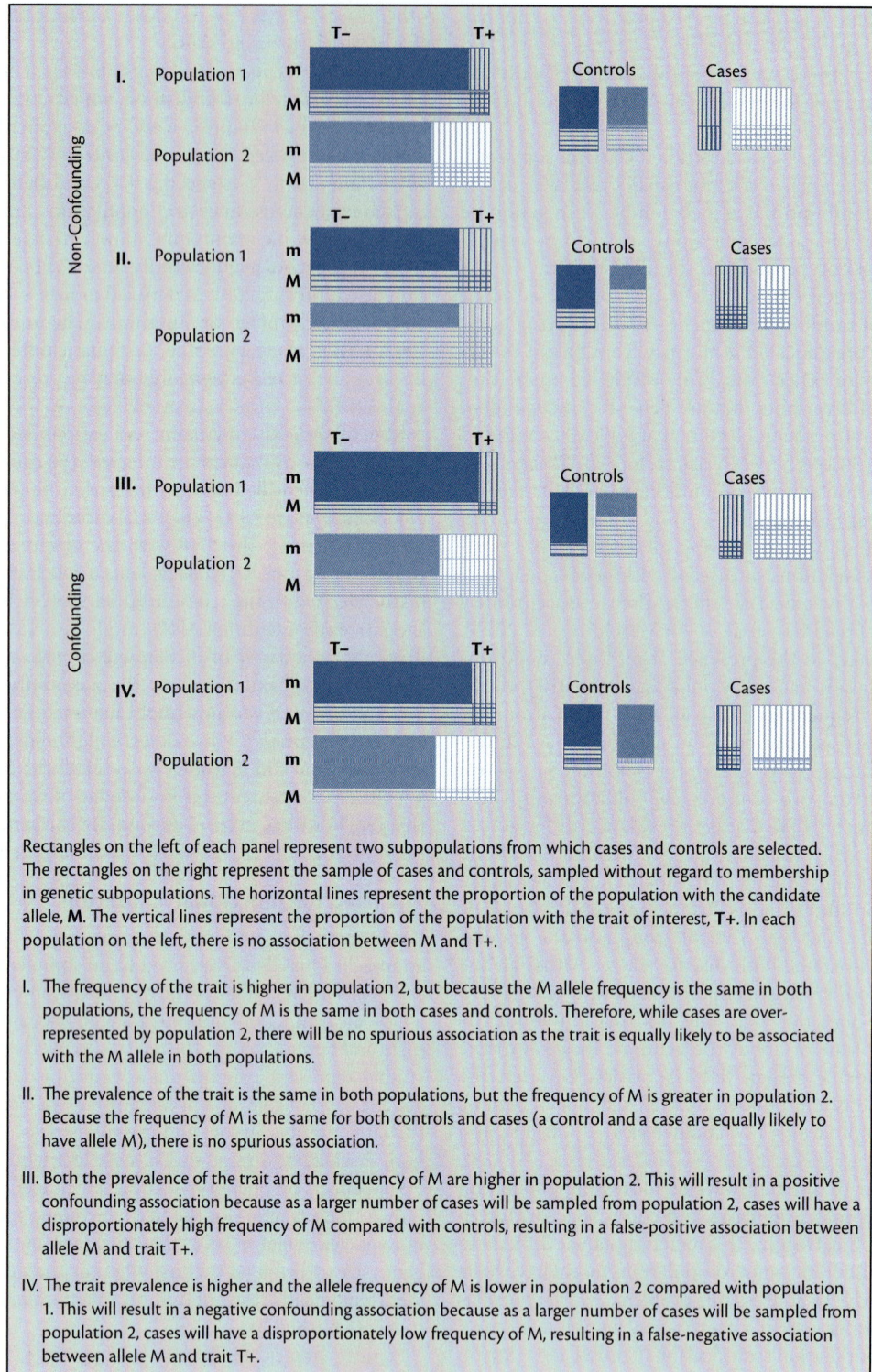

Rectangles on the left of each panel represent two subpopulations from which cases and controls are selected. The rectangles on the right represent the sample of cases and controls, sampled without regard to membership in genetic subpopulations. The horizontal lines represent the proportion of the population with the candidate allele, **M**. The vertical lines represent the proportion of the population with the trait of interest, **T+**. In each population on the left, there is no association between M and T+.

I. The frequency of the trait is higher in population 2, but because the M allele frequency is the same in both populations, the frequency of M is the same in both cases and controls. Therefore, while cases are over-represented by population 2, there will be no spurious association as the trait is equally likely to be associated with the M allele in both populations.

II. The prevalence of the trait is the same in both populations, but the frequency of M is greater in population 2. Because the frequency of M is the same for both controls and cases (a control and a case are equally likely to have allele M), there is no spurious association.

III. Both the prevalence of the trait and the frequency of M are higher in population 2. This will result in a positive confounding association because as a larger number of cases will be sampled from population 2, cases will have a disproportionately high frequency of M compared with controls, resulting in a false-positive association between allele M and trait T+.

IV. The trait prevalence is higher and the allele frequency of M is lower in population 2 compared with population 1. This will result in a negative confounding association because as a larger number of cases will be sampled from population 2, cases will have a disproportionately low frequency of M, resulting in a false-negative association between allele M and trait T+.

Fig. 5.12.1 Spurious associations as a result of population stratification.

Adapted from Ziv E, and Burchard EG. Human population structure and genetic association studies, *Pharmacogenomics*, Volume 4, pp. 431–41, Copyright 2003, with permission from Future Medicine Ltd.

important role in elucidating the specific molecular pathways that are relevant to human physiology and validating GWAS results. If functional studies can confirm a causal role for genetic variants, these results may help identify potential new drug targets.

Using genetic epidemiology to identify new environmental exposures

A key challenge of classical epidemiology is establishing whether an association between an exposure and a disease outcome is

Box 5.12.2 The ENCODE project: identifying functional properties of the human genome sequence

ENCODE, the Encyclopedia of DNA Elements, is an international collective effort to interpret the human genome sequence and make this information available for medical and scientific communities to apply it to understand disease biology and improve human health (The ENCODE Project Consortium 2011). The project aims to define and annotate the functional elements encoded in the human genome sequence, such as those regions that regulate transcription from DNA into RNA, or regulate the expression of genes. In its initial pilot phase in 2003–2007, the ENCODE investigators set out to annotate functional elements in a defined 1 per cent of the human genome. In 2007, the ENCODE project was expanded to study the entire human genome, to locate and describe discrete regions of the genome with a specific biological function. All data and derived results are readily available through a freely accessible public database. In September 2012, the project released an extensive set of results, in 30 papers published simultaneously in several journals, including *Nature, Genome Biology*, and *Genome Research*. As part of ENCODE's expansion, a subproject named GENCODE was launched, run by an international team led by the Wellcome Trust Sanger Institute, specifically to annotate the genes within the human genome with even higher accuracy (Harrow et al. 2012).

causal or not. Given the observational nature of epidemiological research, an association may also be completely explained by confounding. In this scenario, the relationship is explained by a third factor that is associated with both the exposure and disease risk; the exposure is not independently or causally linked to disease risk. Epidemiological approaches generally use multivariable statistical analysis to reduce confounding. However, because of residual confounding (as a result of measurement error) and unknown confounders, standard observational epidemiology cannot resolve whether an observed association has a causal basis. The conceptual ambiguity of any disease mechanism (specifically, defining mediators and confounders) also limits statistical modelling to reduce confounding. Furthermore, the observed association may be due to reverse association/causation—that is, the relationship between biomarker and disease could be the result of undiagnosed or early disease rather than the risk factor, and thus a consequence of disease rather than a cause.

Establishing the causal inference of environmental risk factors can be strengthened by the *Mendelian randomization* approach, in which the biology underpinning genetic epidemiology can be exploited to make causal inferences and establish aetiological associations (Davey Smith and Ebrahim 2003; Lawlor et al. 2008; Sandhu et al. 2008). The assignment of alleles from parents to offspring that occurs during gamete formation and conception tends to be random, and not correlated either with environmental exposures or with alleles at other loci. This means that the inheritance of one trait is independent of (that is, randomized with respect to) the inheritance of other traits, and characteristics that may confound any association between an exposure and disease are equally distributed among the relevant genetic variants. Thus the association between a disease and a genetic variant is generally

much less susceptible to reverse causation or confounding by classical or environmental risk factors.

Given this, a comparison of groups of individuals defined by a genetic variant, based on a Mendelian randomization design, is equivalent to a randomized comparison, with only the relevant exposure differing across the relevant genetic variant. Examining the relationship between variants in the genome that show unequivocal associations with the relevant exposure and disease risk is therefore a potential method of assessing whether an exposure might be causally linked to disease (Fig. 5.12.2).

One example of the success of the Mendelian randomization approach is its role in providing evidence of a causal association between lipoprotein(a) and coronary heart disease. Lipoprotein(a) is a composite particle comprising low-density lipoprotein (LDL) cholesterol linked to apolipoprotein(a) and has long been studied as a possible cardiovascular risk factor. Despite large-scale meta-analyses previously demonstrating an association between lipoprotein(a) and disease risk (Emerging Risk Factors Collaboration et al. 2009), it remained unclear whether the observed association reflected a causal relationship or simply an unexplained correlation. However, more recently, a Mendelian randomization study of around 40,000 participants demonstrated that the magnitude of heart attack risk associated with genetically raised concentrations of lipoprotein(a) was consistent with that associated with an equivalent difference in measured lipoprotein(a) levels (Danesh and Erqou 2009; Kamstrup et al. 2009). These findings are consistent with a causal association between lipoprotein(a) and increased risk of heart disease, and highlight lipoprotein(a) as a potential therapeutic target for the management of cardiovascular disease risk. Mendelian randomization analyses have since been used to investigate a number of biomarkers of coronary heart disease—for example, to provide evidence that genetic variants

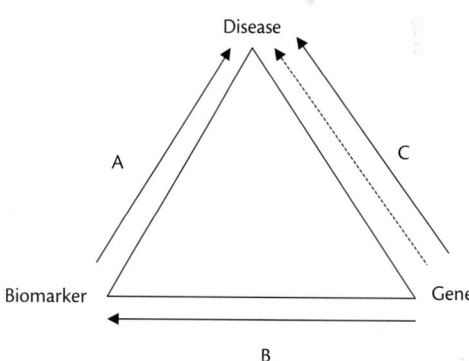

Fig. 5.12.2 Mendelian randomization. The Mendelian randomization design provides a strategy to help clarify whether there is a causal relation between an exposure and disease. Information on the magnitude of the association between the exposure and disease, A, combined with information on the magnitude of the association between the genetic variant and the exposure, B, is used to estimate the expected magnitude of the association between the genetic variant and disease risk (dashed line in C). Based on several assumptions, including a linear association between the exposure and disease, the direct assessment of C (indicated by the solid line) provides an unconfounded assessment of the association between the exposure and disease risk, A.
Adapted from Springer, *Diabetologia*, Volume 51, Issue 2, 2008, pp. 211–13, Mendelian randomisation studies of type 2 diabetes: future prospects, Sandhu MS et al, Figure 1, Copyright © Springer-Verlag 2007, with kind permission of Springer Science and Business Media.

underlying triglycerides are likely to be causal and, conversely, to refute a causal role for high-density lipoprotein (HDL) cholesterol in coronary heart disease (Triglyceride Coronary Disease Genetics Consortium and Emerging Risk Factors Collaboration et al. 2010; Voight et al. 2012).

As with all genetic epidemiology studies, there are problems associated with the need for large sample sizes (Ebrahim and Davey Smith 2008). Mendelian randomization studies, like other genetic epidemiological studies, require reliable identification of statistical associations between genetic variants and biomarkers and disease risk. Importantly, the principal requirement is the ability of Mendelian randomization studies to detect an association of equivalent magnitude to that predicted by a proportional change in the relevant trait or risk factor. Given that individual genetic variants are likely to explain only a very small proportion of the variation in a biomarker trait or risk factor, these assessments will require very large sample sizes. Mendelian randomization findings may also be limited by the effects of biological compensation (also known as canalization) and pleiotropy (Davey Smith and Ebrahim 2003; Lawlor et al. 2008). Canalization refers to the process by which potentially disruptive influences on normal development from genetic variations are buffered by compensatory developmental and physiological adaptations. This developmental compensation can lead to inconsistencies in the magnitude of the triangulated associations. Furthermore, the pleiotropic nature (multiple biological and phenotypic effects) of some genetic variants may produce confounded associations between genetic variants and phenotypes. Despite these limitations, Mendelian randomization provides a potential research framework using genetic variants to make causal inferences about modifiable (non-genetic) risk factors for disease and health-related outcomes. These studies, when correctly performed, will provide insights into aetiological mechanisms and causality, informing potential therapeutic and preventative strategies.

Why is genetic epidemiology important for public health?

Genetics has increasingly become an essential part of the epidemiology paradigm. As we have seen, the integration of epidemiological methods with genome-wide technologies has provided unprecedented insights into the aetiology of complex traits and diseases in human populations and has made substantial and independent contributions to the identification of genetic loci associated with a broad range of complex traits and diseases, including diabetes, heart disease and cancer (Visscher et al. 2012). In parallel, there has been increasing speculation and expectation over how these findings may translate into practical applications for improving human health and lead to public health benefit.

The integration of human genomics discoveries into clinical and public health practice raises a number of questions. Public health is, by its very definition, concerned with improving health from a population perspective (Khoury et al. 2011a, 2011b). How does genomic discovery translate into population health benefit and provide new tools for achieving public health goals? After all, public health prevention and health promotion initiatives have, conventionally, focused on risk factors that are modifiable whereas genetic risk factors are unmodifiable. As we make the case in this section, the discovery and confirmation of genetic variants associated with diseases and traits may have translational implications and major impacts on both individual and population health: first, through elucidation of underlying disease biology and advances in therapeutics and, second, through risk prediction and personalized medicine. In addition, *genetic testing*—undertaken in order to diagnose an inherited disease that is caused by a specific genetic mutation—represents another application of genomic medicine, and is briefly mentioned here for completeness; for a full discussion of the topic, see Chapter 2.5.

Drug discovery and development

The aetiological mechanisms underpinning complex disorders almost certainly involve a combination of many factors: multiple susceptibility genes of modest effect, gene–gene interactions, gene–environment interactions, and heterogeneity of genetic and environmental exposures. The most beneficial application of genetic association studies is likely to be in unravelling the complex biological mechanisms of disease and providing novel insights into disease pathways. In turn, a better understanding of human biology may offer new possibilities for treatment and prevention at the population level (Kingsmore et al. 2008; McCarthy et al. 2008).

Clinical advances in novel therapeutic targets

First, the identification of susceptibility genes for common diseases and traits, together with a better understanding of their underlying functional properties and advances in knowledge of human physiology, should help inform drug development and help determine whether changes in gene activity have pharmacological potential. This is likely to have broad application at the population level (Table 5.12.2). For example, if overexpression of

Table 5.12.2 Examples of matches between GWAS traits and drugs licensed for clinical use

Drug name or class	Gene	Drug indication	GWAS trait
Immunosuppressants and immunomodulators	IL2RA	Relapsing-remitting multiple sclerosis	Multiple sclerosis
Antidiabetic drugs	KCNJ11	Type 2 diabetes	Type 2 diabetes
Statins	HMGCR	Hypercholesterolaemia	LDL cholesterol
Lipid-regulating drugs	LPL	Hyperlipidaemia	HDL cholesterol
Gonadotrophins	FSHR	Female infertility	Polycystic ovary syndrome

a variant gene product was protective against hypercholesterol-aemia, then—even if the effect size was small among carriers—a drug which mimicked and inflated the biological effect of the causal variant might be an effective therapy for treatment of raised blood cholesterol. Such a drug could confer clinical benefit across the cholesterol range, and could be used in the general population irrespective of a person's genotype. Such translational opportunities present very real benefits for public health, although expectation must be tempered with realism: the time from gene discovery to an approved and marketable drug takes, on average, at least 10 years. Thus whilst the greatest impact of genomic medicine is likely to result from its application to novel biological pathways and new therapies, the full success of this will only be appreciable in decades to come (Hirschhorn and Gajdos 2011).

Improved responses to existing drug treatments

A second, and more immediate, application of genomic data may be for drug repositioning—that is, the identification or refining of clinical indications for existing drugs (Sanseau et al. 2012). To do this, a first step would be to identify genes that are already being pursued as drug targets and the diseases that these drugs are currently being used to treat. Next, by utilizing data from GWAS, one can see whether those genes may be associated with additional traits or disease, which in turn could be explored as new potential drug indications. As an illustration, denosumab is a drug currently licensed for the treatment of osteoporosis, bone metastases, and rheumatoid arthritis. It acts by targeting the gene *TNFSF11*. In GWAS, the *TNFSF11* gene has been associated with Crohn's disease and thus it is reasonable to speculate that denosumab may have a therapeutic role in the management of Crohn's disease (Sanseau et al. 2012). Taking this approach thus affords translational opportunities for repositioning existing drugs for many common diseases with widespread benefit to public health.

Pharmacogenomics

Patients can vary in their response to prescribed drugs; some patients do not respond at all to certain drug treatments, and for other drugs the dose required to achieve a therapeutic effect can vary (Daly 2010). Personalized treatment for diseases according to genotype might be feasible where risk alleles predict an individual's response to treatment or susceptibility to adverse drug reactions—for example, those genes that influence the effect of coumarin anticoagulant drugs such as warfarin. Warfarin is widely prescribed to reduce blood clotting and is used to protect high-risk patients from stroke, pulmonary embolism, and thrombosis. However, there is a large variation in the dose required to achieve safe yet effective anticoagulation; thus, reducing the uncertainty in establishing the therapeutic dose for individual patients would improve the safety and efficacy of anticoagulation therapy and potentially avoid the clinical complications associated with under- or over-coagulation. Warfarin is metabolized by the hepatic cytochrome P450 enzyme expressed by the *CYP2C9* gene. Its anticoagulant effect is mediated by the enzyme VKORC1, which is the target enzyme inhibited by warfarin. Among Caucasians, warfarin dosing is more strongly correlated with genetic variation in the *VKORC1* and *CYP2C9* genes than other patient-related factors (Cooper et al. 2008; Takeuchi et al. 2009; Teichert et al. 2009; Jorgensen et al. 2012). Common variants in *CYP2C9* are associated with slower metabolism of warfarin, higher warfarin concentrations, decreased dose requirements, and susceptibility

to bleeding. Polymorphisms in *VKORC1* lead to hypocoagulable states, and necessitate lower dosage.

The translational applications of these observations are not yet fully established. In principle, an individual's genotype could, potentially, be used as a predictor of warfarin dosage. Indeed, several studies have suggested that combining genetic information on variants in *VKORC1* and *CYP2C9* together with clinical data of a patient may help better predict the warfarin dosage—both for initiation of therapy and for maintenance—required to achieve satisfactory anticoagulation (Hatch et al. 2008; International Warfarin Pharmacogenetics Consortium et al. 2009; Horne et al. 2012; Tatarunas et al. 2012). To date, though, genotype-guided dosing algorithms are not widely used, as they have not yet been shown to be cost-effective in preventing adverse events. However, a number of large clinical trials are now underway, designed specifically to assess whether using genetic data to inform warfarin dosing will improve outcomes for patients being treated with warfarin.

Another example of how genomic information has been successfully applied to understanding drug responses is in the treatment of chronic hepatitis C infection. Standard therapy for the last decade has been a combination of pegylated interferon and ribavirin. It has been well documented that treatment response has only limited efficacy, even for more responsive viral genotypes. However, there is increasing evidence that marked variation in prognosis and response to hepatitis C treatment may be due to differences in human genome diversity; in particular, polymorphisms at the *IL28B* gene locus, encoding interferon-λ-3 (IFN-λ-3), predict response to interferon with genome-wide significance (Ge et al. 2009; Thomas et al. 2009).

A number of other GWAS on pharmacogenomics have identified several novel genetic variants that may affect drug responses or reactions, although many of these associations have failed to reach statistical significance probably due to insufficient sample sizes (Daly 2010). Nevertheless, these findings potentially could be used to develop genetic tests to determine the most appropriate drug for treatment or the optimum dose to prescribe. Whilst it is too early to say if this is of clinical relevance in terms of predicting the trajectory of disease, the prospect of individually tailored treatment in the future raises exciting possibilities—see later for further discussion. Genotype-based randomized controlled clinical trials will be needed to formally evaluate the potential utility of genotype-specific treatment (Manolio et al. 2009; Marteau et al. 2010b).

Risk prediction, stratified medicine, and the emergence of personalized medicine

The emergence of genomic medicine represents a shift from traditional medical genetics—with its focus on rare genetic diseases—towards improved risk prediction and, potentially, greater personalization in the practice of medicine and prevention of common diseases.

Complex diseases and traits—including coronary heart disease, diabetes, hypertension, and most cancers—are caused by multiple genetic and environmental factors. For such conditions, individual risk assessment is an important component of clinical decision-making, potentially identifying people who might benefit from earlier or more intensive interventions. However, individual risk assessment is multifaceted, involving an evaluation of risks and benefits to the individual and to society (British Medical Association Board of Science

2005; Grosse and Khoury 2006). It is also complicated by the debate over statistical methods to assess the utility of risk factors (including genetic variants) for disease risk prediction (Fig. 5.12.3) (Wood and Greenland 2009; Romanens et al. 2010; Talmud et al. 2010). Ultimately—and crucially—the utility of predictive models depends on their ability to alter clinical management which in turn relies on the availability of clinical interventions that are universally indicated but might be beneficial or cost-effective for higher-risk patient subgroups (Hirschhorn and Gajdos 2011).

The identification of several genetic variants, each independently impacting on disease risk, has led to a reassessment of whether these variants improve risk prediction. To date, genetic variants identified for complex diseases explain only a small proportion of the total variation in disease risk. Accordingly, currently identified genetic susceptibility loci do not have the discriminatory power to substantially improve disease risk prediction (Kraft et al. 2009). However, with large-scale studies and new genomic sequencing technologies, there is the potential to identify new susceptibility loci. Could these variants improve clinical risk prediction? Data indicate that the variation in disease risk explained by many of these unidentified genetic variants may be very small; their detection may always be beyond the resolution of genomic research strategies and

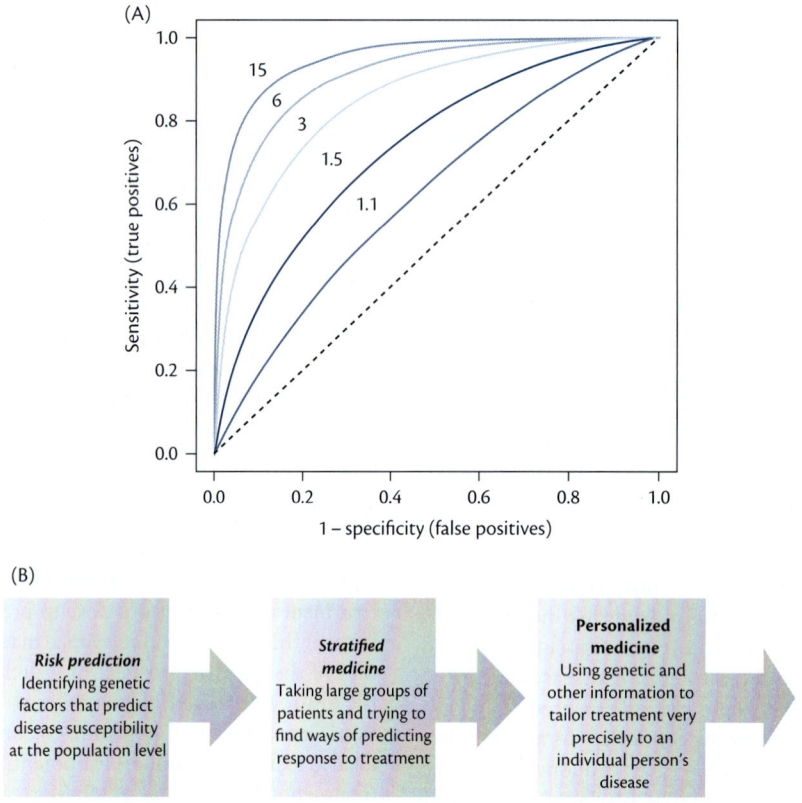

Fig. 5.12.3 Genomic risk prediction and personalized medicine. (A) *Individual disease risk prediction from theoretical ROC curves for familial relative risk.* Measures of risk discrimination include the sensitivity (the proportion of people who develop disease who were correctly categorized as having a high risk of disease) and specificity (the proportion of people who do not go on to develop disease who were correctly categorized as having a low risk of disease) of the test.

These metrics are usually presented in a receiver operator characteristic (ROC) curve, and an overall assessment is given by the area under the ROC curve. This area is equal to the probability that a random person with disease has a higher value of predicted risk than a random person without disease; thus the larger the area, the better the test.

These metrics can be used to determine the positive predictive value—the proportion of people categorized as high risk that go on to develop disease.

The figure shows ROC curves for various values of FRR. For a given disease prevalence, when the FRR is high (for example, FRR=15), the curve rises steeply, indicating the test has a relatively high sensitivity and specificity; the corresponding area under the ROC curve increases. As the FRR drops, sentitivity and specificity fall and the area under the curve decreases. For lower FRRs (for example, FRR=1.1), the curve approaches the diagonal dotted line, indicating a test with only 50% probability of correctly predicting risk of disease.

(B) *The spectrum of genomic medicine.* In practice the three elements of risk prediction, stratified medicine, and personalized medicine, are not distinct but form a continuum of patient management. *Genomic risk prediction* involves identifying genetic variants that predict disease risk within a population. Futher along the spectrum lies *stratified medicine*, which potentially allows targeting of treatments to specific disease pathways, identification of treatments effective for particular groups of patients, and development of diagnostics to ensure the right patient gets the right treatment at the right time. In the context of genomic medicine, individuals with disease are tested for a genetic marker which indicates whether a patient is likely to show a response to therapy. A further refinement of this approach takes us to *personalized (individualized) medicine*, where patients receive custom-made treatment.

Adapted from *The Lancet*, Volume 376, Issue 9750, Sandhu M. et al., Genomic risk prediction, pp. 1366–67, Copyright © 2010, with permission from Elsevier, http://www.sciencedirect.com/science/journal/01406736.

available sample sizes. Hence, a small proportion of the heritability of a disease may not be identified (Clayton 2009; Wray et al. 2010).

At the population level, the familial relative risk (FRR) represents the risk prediction achievable if all relevant loci were identified—assuming that the magnitude of the FRR is accurate and that it primarily reflects shared genetic variants rather than environments (Xu et al. 2009; Wray et al. 2010). With these caveats, for rare or common diseases with greater heritability the discovery of all disease susceptibility variants might provide opportunities to more reliably identify people at greater risk of disease (Fig. 5.12.3). However, for common diseases, such as type 2 diabetes, heart disease, and some cancers, with relatively small FRRs, it is unlikely that the discovery of all susceptibility loci will achieve the necessary predictive accuracy to provide clinically useful information (Wald et al. 1999; Ware 2006; Park et al. 2010).

The ultimate utility of genomic risk prediction in the context of complete genome sequencing will depend on the underlying genetic architecture, the proportion of the variation in disease attributable to genetic factors, and the disease prevalence. Population-wide, it seems unlikely that genomic risk prediction alone will attain the discriminatory resolution to predict individual disease-risk for many common diseases with only modest heritability. However, the use of genomic factors for individual disease risk prediction in conjunction with conventional risk factors, or for identifying subgroups for screening, remains unclear (Pharoah et al. 2008; Xu et al. 2009). Whilst at present we lack the ability to provide clinically useful risk prediction, as more disease loci are identified it may be beneficial to re-assess whether genetic testing could improve risk prediction of common disease beyond traditional risk factors.

In addition to risk prediction and a better understanding of disease aetiology, genetic data may be increasingly used in the field of stratified medicine (Fig. 5.12.3). Patient response to drug treatments and therapeutic interventions varies markedly across the population as a result of differing underlying mechanisms of disease and patient responses to both disease and treatment. Stratified medicine can be described as identifying the different strata within a disease using a biomarker or genotype, in order to identify a patient subpopulation which is more likely to benefit or experience an adverse reaction in response to a given therapy. This approach—with patients better matched to therapies—is anticipated to have a major effect on both clinical practice and the development of new drugs and diagnostics (Trusheim et al. 2007). At the extreme of this patient matching are 'personalized' medicines, which by definition vary for each individual's unique genetic make-up, such as customized stem-cell based therapies. However, the logistical, clinical and ethical implications of this must be carefully considered.

Limitations and challenges of genetic epidemiology

Human genetics has advanced at an extraordinary pace during the last 20 years. The number of, and the ease with which, genetic markers of disease are being discovered has gone from dozens to millions. As we enter the era of next-generation high-throughput genotyping and sequencing, it is important to remember the limitations of this knowledge in order to have realistic expectations of what it can, and cannot, deliver and to apply it appropriately and responsibly.

Ethical, legal, and social implications

The generation of genetic information has contributed greatly to our understanding of the molecular basis of disease and, increasingly, to the development of effective treatments. In parallel, there are concerns about the ethical, legal, and social implications of this knowledge on the well-being of individuals and populations (Box 5.12.3).

Accounting for unexplained variation

Despite the success of GWAS in identifying disease genes, a substantial proportion of the heritability of disease traits remains unexplained (Manolio et al. 2009). So far, loci shown to be associated with disease only account for a small fraction of the total genetic contribution; the great majority of susceptibility loci remain to be identified. How do we account for this remaining variation? Unexplained heritability may be due to unknown common variants of small effect, or rare variants with larger effects, or influences by environmental factors. To better understand the missing heritability of disease traits, larger-scale studies are required, using denser SNP arrays. In addition, exome sequencing, whole genome sequencing, or whole genome association studies in large populations will be needed to identify all potential variants within a gene or locus. Sequencing candidate genes in individuals at the extremes of a quantitative trait (e.g. the extremes of lipid levels) may identify new variants, common or rare, and help further our understanding of disease biology and prevention.

Genetic epidemiology in low- and middle-income countries

To date, most human genomics research has been done in populations of European ancestry, and has successfully provided new insights into the biology of chronic diseases and their risk factors in these populations. However, the relevance of many recent genomic findings to populations in low- and middle-income countries (LMICs) is not known. It may be difficult to meaningfully apply the findings from Western populations to LMIC populations, where both genetic and non-genetic susceptibility may be different.

To fully appreciate the impact of a genetic variant on disease risk it will be important to establish whether the findings from one population apply to other populations of different ancestry. Globally, human populations show structured genetic diversity as a result of geographical dispersion, selection and drift (Campbell and Tishkoff 2008; Novembre and Ramachandran 2011). Accordingly, among many populations in LMICs there is marked genomic diversity—in particular, among populations of African descent, where there is more human genetic diversity than anywhere else (Tishkoff et al. 2009). Given this, understanding the genomic basis of common diseases and their risk factors in LMICs is likely to provide additional insights into disease aetiology and potential therapeutic strategies (Hill 2006; Campbell and Tishkoff 2008; Novembre and Ramachandran 2011).

Thus the value of GWAS will be enhanced further by including populations with greater genetic diversity and less correlation between variants, and will benefit from more precise

---

Box 5.12.3 Examples of some of the ethical, legal, and social implications of genetic epidemiology

Genetic discrimination

A primary concern is that genetic information could be harmful and could lead to discrimination such as: (1) denial of health insurance or employment, based on genetic susceptibility; and (2) stigmatization of a specific ethnic group.

Genetic determinism

This stems from a misconception about the causal relationship between genetics and behaviour, and the erroneous belief that genetic information is somehow more predictive and certain than other types of health information because 'you cannot change your genes'. This can lead to an unhelpful and inaccurate sense of inevitability and the use of genetic determinism to explain health disparities.

Data protection

The generation of vast amounts of genetic data, and its potential identifiability of individuals, raises significant issues around the storage of genetic data, data processing, data access, and confidentiality. Additional concerns exist around sharing sensitive data with other family members, such as in the context of reproductive choice.

Return of individual research findings (including incidental findings)

Disclosing study results and presenting clinical risk information can have important effects on health outcomes and health behaviours among study participants. Understanding probability information about disease risk and the benefits of intervention is a vital component of an individual's decision-making capacity. The obligation of the health professional to return genetic findings—particularly when the clinical validity and utility is unclear—needs to be considered. Additionally, disclosing results for which treatments may be unavailable or prohibitively expensive raises particular ethical issues.

Informed consent

National and international research guidelines agree that valid consent to participate in research must be consent that is informed in a manner that is linguistically and culturally appropriate and is understood by the study participant. This can be particularly challenging in the context of genomics research which is complex and often difficult to understand, and where the implications of research findings are largely unknown (including incidental findings which are not relevant to the original research question but may have clinical significance). An additional challenge is to resolve issues around individual consent versus family consent, including the right 'not to know' the findings of genetic studies.

Fair distribution of benefits from research

As with all fields of research, particular individuals, groups, or communities should neither bear an unfair share of the direct burdens of participating in research, nor should they be unfairly excluded from the potential benefits of research participation. This is particularly pertinent when genetic research is conducted in countries where genetic services are not available or may not be readily accessed. Inclusiveness in genetic research and fair distribution of benefits and burdens should be important considerations for researchers, research ethics boards, and sponsors. Issues of fair and equitable treatment arise in deciding whether and how to include individuals, groups or communities in research, and the basis for the exclusion of some.

---

characterization of phenotypes and environmental exposures (Manolio et al. 2009). Ultimately, large-scale international collaborations will facilitate studies in different global populations and help to determine whether loci identified in initial GWAS (usually done in populations of European ancestry) are relevant in non-European individuals. As a result of such studies, our ability to treat disease and reduce risk will be much more complete.

In addition to studies of the human genome, techniques from genetic epidemiology can also be used to examine pathogen genomes, yielding important applications for human health—for example, in helping to understand the causes of resistance to malaria treatment. First-line treatment for uncomplicated falciparum malaria is artemisinin-based combination therapy (ACT), which has been highly effective in treating this disease. However, in recent years, resistance to artemisinin has become increasingly prevalent in Cambodia and Thailand, characterized by slow parasite clearance from the blood (Uhlemann and

Fidock 2012). Antimalarial drug resistance hinders malaria control and is a major public health threat to global initiatives to control and eliminate the disease. Using a variety of techniques, including targeted association studies of candidate genes for ACT and genotyping of variants across the malaria genome, a number of studies have identified that resistance to artemisinins is, in part, genetically determined by variants in the malaria-parasite genome and conclude that parasite genetics have a central role in determining parasite clearance rates (Cheeseman et al. 2012; Phyo et al. 2012). Furthermore, these studies report that the heritability (h^2)—that is, the contribution of parasite genetics that explains the variation in parasite clearance—has increased from 30 per cent in 2001–2004 to 66 per cent in 2007–2010 (Phyo et al. 2012). The mechanisms underlying the reported associations are not yet known, but understanding these biological processes could potentially inform new approaches for effective malaria treatment in the future.

The application of genetic epidemiology and genomic research to public health practice merits specific discussion in the context of LMICs—where the global burden of infectious and chronic, complex diseases is greatest. Additionally, in LMICs healthcare is often severely constrained by limited financial and human resources and a lack of appropriate infrastructure (Burke et al. 2010). It would be simplistic to suggest that because of the great health needs of LMICs—overwhelmingly determined by economic and social factors—genomics is an irrelevance and has no role to play in improving health. Rather, to omit genomic discoveries from the healthcare agenda of LMICs would serve only to promote existing inequities between rich and poor, between economically advantaged and disadvantaged. Public health professionals have an essential role to play in leading the response to genomic medicine in LMICs, ensuring that healthcare providers and policymakers are informed by a strong evidence base for the effectiveness of genomic approaches in improving population health.

Improving phenotypic characterization and classification of disease

Associations between genetic variants and phenotypes are limited by the accuracy with which each is measured. The ability to measure genotypes now far exceeds our ability to measure phenotypes (Altshuler et al. 2008). We need to match this with more detailed, and more accurate, assessments of clinical phenotypes. Indeed, carefully designed GWAS with thorough phenotypic characterization have the potential to redefine disease classification (Kingsmore et al. 2008). In some cases, it will become increasingly possible to unpick the phenotypic complexity of diseases that involve several pathological processes and allow us to establish whether genetic factors distinctly contribute to different phenotypes of the condition. A recent example of this is in the area of coronary artery disease (CAD), where GWAS have successfully discriminated genetic variants for distinct CAD phenotypes—suggestive of distinct underlying pathological mechanisms (Reilly et al. 2011). This opens up avenues for patient stratification and personalized treatments.

Conversely, for other complex diseases that have previously been regarded as distinct clinical entities, GWAS findings may point to common underlying disease processes and a shared pathogenesis. To illustrate, a recent GWAS of Crohn's disease and ulcerative colitis found a sizeable overlap in susceptibility loci for the two diseases. With such a degree of sharing of genetic risk, it seems likely that many of the biological mechanisms involved in one disease have some other role in the other (Jostins et al. 2012). These studies provide a rich source of clues to the biological mechanism underlying complex disease. However, the translation of such GWAS discoveries into prognostic and therapeutic benefit will need greater insights into the relation between each loci and the different phenotypes.

Risk communication

The extent to which genetic information will play a role in 'personalized medicine' will depend not only on whether predictive accuracy beyond conventional measure can be attained, but also on whether there are interventions whose effectiveness is improved by knowledge of a genetic result. A key challenge will therefore be to find effective ways to communicate information on small incremental risk increases conferred by genetic markers for disease risk, in order to prompt changes in lifestyle that will ultimately confer health gain to individuals. At present, it is not clear if personal genomic information is likely to beneficially impact public health through motivation of lifestyle behavioural change. Risk perception and risk communication are complex processes, and are shaped by social and cultural values, assumptions, and beliefs held at the individual and societal level.

An individual's ability to make sense of genetic information will involve an understanding of the concepts of genes, genetics, ancestry and heritability, in a manner that is culturally relevant and acceptable. Most of the information we have on genetic susceptibility to disease is, at best, incomplete as discussed earlier in this chapter; health professionals' advice to people will have to change as more robust evidence on risk factors comes to light, sometimes seeming to conflict with, or even to contradict, previous knowledge. Conveying this uncertainty is a difficult and challenging task.

The creation of personal genomic risk profiles, that predict an individual's lifetime risk of various common diseases, raises the possibility that public health promotion could potentially be directed at susceptible individuals/groups of people in the population based on their genomic risk profile. This marks a departure from conventional public health practice which has tended to focus on social and environmental determinants of disease and health, and allows a focus on preventing disease, disability and mortality among people with specific genotypes that increase their disease risk. It is tempting to think that knowledge of individual risk of a given disease, as predicted by genome-wide profiling, will motivate individuals to change their behaviour and promote greater adherence to a healthy lifestyle or treatment regimen in order to reduce their risk; however, human behaviour is complex and risk estimates are difficult to communicate meaningfully to patients (Loos 2011). Recent studies, including a Cochrane review, seem to indicate that genetic testing may not result in individuals changing their behaviour in any significant or sustained way (Marteau et al. 2010a; Bloss et al. 2011).

Conclusions

It is clear that public health practice cannot ignore the impact of genetic epidemiology and the knowledge derived from genomics research. The results from genetic epidemiological research have two broad translational applications which have the potential to contribute to population health and well-being. First, as our understanding of disease aetiology and its underlying biological mechanisms increases, there is the potential for new drug development and improved therapeutic strategies to manage disease. Second, in parallel, there is growing interest in the use of these genetic variants to predict individual disease risk over and above classical risk factors, and to develop stratified and personalized approaches to diagnosis and disease management. The public health community has a central leadership role to play in critically and systematically evaluating these discoveries for their potential use in disease prediction, prevention, and treatment response. Furthermore, public health practice must ensure that the benefits of genomics are applied with equity across the population.

As our understanding of the molecular basis of disease increases, there is a need for public health practitioners to have a degree of knowledge about genetic susceptibility and to understand the scientific basis of genetic epidemiology and the benefits it can afford, as well as to be aware of the limitations of this knowledge. The ultimate goal of public health is to promote and improve the health and well-being of the population. A public health approach to genetic epidemiology should assess the contribution of genomics to health in the context of wider determinants of disease and health, and provide a robust evidence-base to inform healthcare policymakers, health service commissioners, and providers.

References

Altshuler, D., Daly, M.J., and Lander, E.S. (2008). Genetic mapping in human disease. *Science*, 322, 881–8.

Amaral, P.P. and Mattick, J.S. (2008). Noncoding RNA in development. *Mammalian Genome*, 19, 7–8.

Balding, D.J. (2006). A tutorial on statistical methods for population association studies. *Nature Reviews Genetics*, 7, 781–91.

Bamshad, M.J., Ng, S.B., Bigham, A.W., et al. (2011). Exome sequencing as a tool for Mendelian disease gene discovery. *Nature Reviews Genetics*, 12, 745–55.

Benjamini, Y. and Hochberg, Y. (1995). Controlling the false discovery rate: a practical and powerful approach to multiple testing. *Journal of the Royal Statistical Society: Series B*, 57, 289–300.

Bloss, C.S., Schork, N.J., and Topol, E.J. (2011). Effect of direct-to-consumer genomewide profiling to assess disease risk. *The New England Journal of Medicine*, 364, 524–34.

Bochud, M. (2012). Genetics for clinicians: from candidate genes to whole genome scans (technological advances). *Best Practice & Research Clinical Endocrinology & Metabolism*, 26, 119–32.

Boomsma, D., Busjahn, A., and Peltonen, L. (2002). Classical twin studies and beyond. *Nature Reviews Genetics*, 3, 872–82.

British Medical Association Board of Science (2005). *Population Screening and Genetic Testing. A Briefing on Current Programmes and Technologies*. London: British Medical Association.

Burke, W., Burton, H., Hall, A.E., et al. (2010). Extending the reach of public health genomics: what should be the agenda for public health in an era of genome-based and 'personalized' medicine? *Genetics in Medicine*, 12, 785–91.

Campbell, M.C. and Tishkoff, S.A. (2008). African genetic diversity: implications for human demographic history, modern human origins, and complex disease mapping. *Annual Review of Genomics and Human Genetics*, 9, 403–33.

Cheeseman, I.H., Miller, B.A., Nair, S., et al. (2012). A major genome region underlying artemisinin resistance in malaria. *Science*, 336, 79–82.

Choi, M., Scholl, U.I., Ji, W., et al. (2009). Genetic diagnosis by whole exome capture and massively parallel DNA sequencing. *Proceedings of the National Academy of Sciences of the United States of America*, 106, 19096–101.

Cirulli, E.T. and Goldstein, D.B. (2010). Uncovering the roles of rare variants in common disease through whole-genome sequencing. *Nature Reviews Genetics*, 11, 415–25.

Clayton, D.G. (2009). Prediction and interaction in complex disease genetics: experience in type 1 diabetes. *PLoS Genetics*, 5, e1000540.

Collins, F.S., Morgan, M., and Patrinos, A. (2003). The Human Genome Project: lessons from large-scale biology. *Science*, 300, 286–90.

Cooper, G.M., Johnson, J.A., Langaee, T.Y., et al. (2008). A genome-wide scan for common genetic variants with a large influence on warfarin maintenance dose. *Blood*, 112, 1022–7.

Cordell, H.J. and Clayton, D.G. (2005). Genetic association studies. *The Lancet*, 366, 1121–31.

Daly, A.K. (2010). Genome-wide association studies in pharmacogenomics. *Nature Reviews Genetics*, 11, 241–6.

Danesh, J. and Erqou, S. (2009). Risk factors: lipoprotein(a) and coronary disease—moving closer to causality. *Nature Reviews Cardiology*, 6, 565–7.

Davey Smith, G. and Ebrahim, S. (2003). 'Mendelian randomization': can genetic epidemiology contribute to understanding environmental determinants of disease? *International Journal of Epidemiology*, 32, 1–22.

Donnelly, P. (2008). Progress and challenges in genome-wide association studies in humans. *Nature*, 456, 728–31.

Ebrahim, S. and Davey Smith, G. (2008). Mendelian randomization: can genetic epidemiology help redress the failures of observational epidemiology? *Human Genetics*, 123, 15–33.

Emerging Risk Factors Collaboration, Erqou, S., Kaptoge, S., et al. (2009). Lipoprotein(a) concentration and the risk of coronary heart disease, stroke, and nonvascular mortality. *Journal of the American Medical Association*, 302, 412–23.

Freedman, M.L., Reich, D., Penney, K.L., et al. (2004). Assessing the impact of population stratification on genetic association studies. *Nature Genetics*, 36, 388–93.

Ge, D., Fellay, J., Thompson, A.J., et al. (2009). Genetic variation in IL28B predicts hepatitis C treatment-induced viral clearance. *Nature*, 461, 399–401.

Geneletti, S., Gallo, V., Porta, M., Khoury, M.J., and Vineis, P. (2011). Assessing causal relationships in genomics: from Bradford-Hill criteria to complex gene-environment interactions and directed acyclic graphs. *Emerging Themes in Epidemiology*, 8, 5.

Grosse, S.D. and Khoury, M.J. (2006). What is the clinical utility of genetic testing? *Genetics in Medicine*, 8, 448–50.

Harrow, J., Frankish, A., Gonzalez, J.M., et al. (2012). GENCODE: the reference human genome annotation for The ENCODE Project. *Genome Research*, 22, 1760–74.

Hatch, E., Wynne, H., Avery, P., Wadelius, M., and Kamali, F. (2008). Application of a pharmacogenetic-based warfarin dosing algorithm derived from British patients to predict dose in Swedish patients. *Journal of Thrombosis and Haemostasis*, 6, 1038–40.

Hattersley, A.T. and McCarthy, M.I. (2005). What makes a good genetic association study? *The Lancet*, 366, 1315–23.

Hill, A.V. (2006). Aspects of genetic susceptibility to human infectious diseases. *Annual Review of Genetics*, 40, 469–86.

Hirschhorn, J.N. and Daly, M.J. (2005). Genome-wide association studies for common diseases and complex traits. *Nature Reviews Genetics*, 6, 95–105.

Hirschhorn, J.N. and Gajdos, Z.K.Z. (2011). Genome-wide association studies: results from the first few years and potential implications for clinical medicine. *Annual Review of Medicine*, 62, 11–24.

Hoggart, C.J., Parra, E.J., Shriver, M.D., et al. (2003). Control of confounding of genetic associations in stratified populations. *American Journal of Human Genetics*, 72, 1492–504.

Horne, B.D., Lenzini, P.A., Wadelius, M., et al. (2012). Pharmacogenetic warfarin dose refinements remain significantly influenced by genetic factors after one week of therapy. *Thrombosis and Haemostasis*, 107, 232–40.

Hunter, D.J. (2005). Gene–environment interactions in human diseases. *Nature Reviews Genetics*, 6, 287–98.

Hunter, D.J. and Kraft, P. (2007). Drinking from the fire hose—statistical issues in genomewide association studies. *The New England Journal of Medicine*, 357, 436–9.

International Hapmap Consortium (2007). A second generation human haplotype map of over 3.1 million SNPs. *Nature*, 449, 851–62.

International HapMap 3 Consortium (2010). Integrating common and rare genetic variation in diverse human populations. *Nature*, 467, 52–58.

International Human Genome Mapping Consortium (2001). A physical map of the human genome. *Nature*, 409, 934–41.

International Human Genome Sequencing Consortium (2001). Initial sequencing and analysis of the human genome. *Nature*, 409, 860–921.

International SNP Map Working Group (2001). A map of human genome sequence variation containing 1.42 million single nucleotide polymorphisms. *Nature*, 409, 928–33.

International Warfarin Pharmacogenetics Consortium, Klein, T.E., Altman, R.B., et al. (2009). Estimation of the warfarin dose with clinical and pharmacogenetic data. *New England Journal of Medicine*, 360, 753–64.

Ioannidis, J.P.A., Thomas, G., and Daly, M.J. (2009). Validating, augmenting and refining genome-wide association signals. *Nature Reviews Genetics*, 10, 318–29.

Ioannidis, J.P.A., Trikalinos, T.A., and Khoury, M.J. (2006). Implications of small effect sizes of individual genetic variants on the design and interpretation of genetic association studies of complex diseases. *American Journal of Epidemiology*, 164, 609–14.

Ioannidis, J.P.A., Trikalinos, T.A., Ntzani, E.E., and Contopoulos-Ioannidis, D.G. (2003). Genetic associations in large versus small studies: an empirical assessment. *The Lancet* 361, 567–71.

Jorgensen, A.L., Fitzgerald, R.J., Oyee, J., Pirmohamed, M., and Williamson, P.R. (2012). Influence of CYP2C9 and VKORC1 on patient response to warfarin: a systematic review and meta-analysis. *PLoS ONE*, 7, e44064.

Jostins, L., Ripke, S., Weersma, R.K., et al. (2012). Host–microbe interactions have shaped the genetic architecture of inflammatory bowel disease. *Nature*, 491, 119–24.

Kaikkonen, M.U., Lam, M.T.Y., and Glass, C.K. (2011). Non-coding RNAs as regulators of gene expression and epigenetics. *Cardiovascular Research*, 90, 430–40.

Kamstrup, P.R., Tybjaerg-Hansen, A., Steffensen, R., and Nordestgaard, B.G. (2009). Genetically elevated lipoprotein(a) and increased risk of myocardial infarction. *Journal of the American Medical Association*, 301, 2331–9.

Khoury, M.J., Bowen, M.S., Burke, W., et al. (2011a). Current priorities for public health practice in addressing the role of human genomics in improving population health. *American Journal of Preventive Medicine*, 40, 486–93.

Khoury, M.J., Davis, R., Gwinn, M., Lindegren, M.L., and Yoon, P. (2005). Do we need genomic research for the prevention of common diseases with environmental causes? *American Journal of Epidemiology*, 161, 799–805.

Khoury, M.J., Gwinn, M., Clyne, M., and Yu, W. (2011b). Genetic epidemiology with a Capital E, ten years after. *Genetic Epidemiology*, 35, 845–52.

Kingsmore, S.F., Lindquist, I.E., Mudge, J., Gessler, D.D., and Beavis, W.D. (2008). Genome-wide association studies: progress and potential for drug discovery and development. *Nature Reviews Drug Discovery*, 7, 221–30.

Kraft, P., Wacholder, S., Cornelis, M.C., et al. (2009). Beyond odds ratios—communicating disease risk based on genetic profiles. *Nature Reviews Genetics*, 10, 264–9.

Kruglyak, L. (2008). The road to genome-wide association studies. *Nature Reviews Genetics*, 9, 314–18.

Lawlor, D.A., Harbord, R.M., Sterne, J.A.C., Timpson, N., and Davey Smith, G. (2008). Mendelian randomization: using genes as instruments for making causal inferences in epidemiology. *Statistics in Medicine*, 27, 1133–63.

Li, Y., Willer, C., Sanna, S., and Abecasis, G. (2009). Genotype imputation. *Annual Review of Genomics and Human Genetics*, 10, 387–406.

Lohmueller, K.E., Pearce, C.L., Pike, M., Lander, E.S., and Hirschhorn, J.N. (2003). Meta-analysis of genetic association studies supports a contribution of common variants to susceptibility to common disease. *Nature Genetics*, 33, 177–82.

Loos, R.J.F. (2011). Genome-wide risk profiles—will they change your life(style)? *Nature Reviews Endocrinology*, 7, 252–4.

Manolio, T.A., Collins, F.S., Cox, N.J., et al. (2009). Finding the missing heritability of complex diseases. *Nature*, 461, 747–53.

Marchini, J., Cardon, L.R., Phillips, M.S., and Donnelly, P. (2004). The effects of human population structure on large genetic association studies. *Nature Genetics*, 36, 512–17.

Marteau, T.M., French, D.P., Griffin, S.J., et al. (2010a). Effects of communicating DNA-based disease risk estimates on risk-reducing behaviours. *Cochrane Database of Systematic Reviews*, 6, CD007275.

Marteau, T.M., Munafo, M.R., Aveyard, P., et al. (2010b). Trial protocol: using genotype to tailor prescribing of nicotine replacement therapy: a randomised controlled trial assessing impact of communication upon adherence. *BMC Public Health*, 10, 680.

McCarthy, M.I., Abecasis, G.R., Cardon, L.R., et al. (2008). Genome-wide association studies for complex traits: consensus, uncertainty and challenges. *Nature Reviews Genetics*, 9, 356–69.

Metzker, M.L. (2010). Sequencing technologies—the next generation. *Nature Reviews Genetics*, 11, 31–46.

National Center for Biotechnology Information (n.d.). *DbSNP Database*. Available at: http://www.ncbi.nlm.nih.gov/projects/SNP/snp_summary.cgi.

Ng, S.B., Buckingham, K.J., Lee, C., et al. (2010). Exome sequencing identifies the cause of a mendelian disorder. *Nature Genetics*, 42, 30–5.

Ng, S.B., Turner, E.H., Robertson, P.D., et al. (2009). Targeted capture and massively parallel sequencing of 12 human exomes. *Nature*, 461, 272–6.

Novembre, J. and Ramachandran, S. (2011). Perspectives on human population structure at the cusp of the sequencing era. *Annual Review of Genomics and Human Genetics*, 12, 245–74.

Palmer, L.J. and Cardon, L.R. (2005). Shaking the tree: mapping complex disease genes with linkage disequilibrium. *The Lancet*, 366, 1223–34.

Park, J.H., Wacholder, S., Gail, M.H., et al. (2010). Estimation of effect size distribution from genome-wide association studies and implications for future discoveries. *Nature Genetics*, 42, 570–5.

Pharoah, P.D.P., Antoniou, A.C., Easton, D.F., and Ponder, B.A.J. (2008). Polygenes, risk prediction, and targeted prevention of breast cancer. *The New England Journal of Medicine*, 358, 2796–803.

Phyo, A.P., Nkhoma, S., Stepniewska, K., et al. (2012). Emergence of artemisinin-resistant malaria on the western border of Thailand: a longitudinal study. *The Lancet*, 379, 1960–6.

Price, A.L., Zaitlen, N.A., Reich, D., and Patterson, N. (2010). New approaches to population stratification in genome-wide association studies. *Nature Reviews Genetics*, 11, 459–63.

Pussegoda, K. (2010). Exome sequencing: locating causative genes in rare disorders. *Clinical Genetics*, 78, 32–3.

Reilly, M.P., Li, M., He, J., et al. (2011). Identification of ADAMTS7 as a novel locus for coronary atherosclerosis and association of ABO with myocardial infarction in the presence of coronary atherosclerosis: two genome-wide association studies. *The Lancet*, 377, 383–92.

Roberts, L., Davenport, R.J., Pennisi, E., and Marshall, E. (2001). A history of the Human Genome Project. *Science*, 291, 1195.

Romanens, M., Ackermann, F., Spence, J.D., et al. (2010). Improvement of cardiovascular risk prediction: time to review current knowledge, debates, and fundamentals on how to assess test characteristics. *European Journal of Cardiovascular Prevention and Rehabilitation*, 17, 18–23.

Sandhu, M., Wood, A., and Young, E. (2010). Genomic risk prediction. *The Lancet*, 376, 1366–7.

Sandhu, M.S., Debenham, S.L., Barroso, I., and Loos, R.J. (2008). Mendelian randomisation studies of type 2 diabetes: future prospects. *Diabetologia*, 51, 211–13.

Sanseau, P., Agarwal, P., Barnes, M.R., et al. (2012). Use of genome-wide association studies for drug repositioning. *Nature Biotechnology*, 30, 317–20.

Tabor, H.K., Risch, N.J., and Myers, R.M. (2002). Candidate-gene approaches for studying genetic traits: practical consideration. *Nature Reviews Genetics*, 3, 1–7.

Takeuchi, F., McGinnis, R., Bourgeois, S., et al. (2009). A genome-wide association study confirms *VKORC1*, *CYP2C9*, and *CYP4F2* as principal genetic determinants of warfarin dose. *PLoS Genetics*, 5, e1000433.

Talmud, P.J., Hingorani, A.D., Cooper, J.A., et al. (2010). Utility of genetic and non-genetic risk factors in prediction of type 2 diabetes: Whitehall II prospective cohort study. *British Medical Journal*, 340, b4838.

Tatarunas, V., Lesauskaite, V., Veikutiene, A., Grybauskas, P., Jakuska, P., and Benetis, R. (2012). The combined effects of clinical factors and CYP2C9 and VKORC1 gene polymorphisms on initiating warfarin treatment in patients after cardiac valve surgery. *Journal of Heart Valve Disease*, 21, 628–35.

Teare, M.D. and Barrett, J.H. (2005). Genetic linkage studies. *The Lancet*, 366, 1036–44.

Teichert, M., Eijgelsheim, M., Rivadeneira, F., et al. (2009). A genome-wide association study of acenocoumarol maintenance dosage. *Human Molecular Genetics*, 18, 3758–68.

The 1000 Genomes Project Consortium (2010). A map of human genome variation from population-scale sequencing. *Nature*, 467, 1061–73.

The 1000 Genomes Project Consortium (2012). An integrated map of genetic variation from 1,092 human genomes. *Nature*, 491, 56–65.

The ENCODE Project Consortium (2011). A user's guide to the Encylopedia of DNA Elements (ENCODE). *PLos Biology*, 9, e1001046.

Thomas, D.C. and Clayton, D.G. (2004). Betting odds and genetic associations. *Journal of the National Cancer Institute*, 96, 421–3.

Thomas, D.L., Thio, C.L., Martin, M.P., et al. (2009). Genetic variation in IL28B and spontaneous clearance of hepatitis C virus. *Nature*, 461, 798–801.

Tishkoff, S.A., Reed, F.A., Friedlaender, F.R., et al. (2009). The genetic structure and history of Africans and African Americans. *Science*, 324, 1035–44.

Triglyceride Coronary Disease Genetics Consortium and Emerging Risk Factors Collaboration, Sarwar, N., Sandhu, M.S., et al. (2010). Triglyceride-mediated pathways and coronary disease: collaborative analysis of 101 studies. *The Lancet*, 375, 1634–9.

Trusheim, M.R., Berndt, E.R., and Douglas, F.L. (2007). Stratified medicine: strategic and economic implications of combining drugs and clinical biomarkers. *Nature Reviews Drug Discovery*, 6, 287–93.

Uhlemann, A.C. and Fidock, D.A. (2012). Loss of malarial susceptibility to artemisinin in Thailand. *The Lancet*, 379, 1928–30.

Visscher, P.M., Brown, M.A., Mccarthy, M.I., and Yang, J. (2012). Five years of GWAS discovery. *American Journal of Human Genetics*, 90, 7–24.

Voight, B. F., Peloso, G. M., Orho-Melander, M., et al. (2012). Plasma HDL cholesterol and risk of myocardial infarction: a mendelian randomisation study. *The Lancet*, 380, 572–80.

Wacholder, S., Chanock, S., Garcia-Closas, M., El Ghormli, L., and Rothman, N. (2004). Assessing the probability that a positive report is false: an approach for molecular epidemiology studies. *Journal of the National Cancer Institute*, 96, 434–42.

Wacholder, S., Rothman, N., and Caporaso, N. (2000). Population stratification in epidemiologic studies of common genetic variants and cancer: quantification of bias. *Journal of the National Cancer Institute*, 92, 1151–8.

Wald, N.J., Hackshaw, A.K., and Frost, C.D. (1999). When can a risk factor be used as a worthwhile screening test? *British Medical Journal*, 319, 1562–5.

Ware, J.H. (2006). The limitations of risk factors as prognostic tools. *The New England Journal of Medicine*, 355, 2615–17.

Wellcome Trust Case Control Consortium (2007). Genome-wide association study of 14,000 cases of seven common diseases and 3,000 shared controls. *Nature*, 447, 661–78.

Wood, A.M. and Greenland, P. (2009). Evaluating the prognostic value of new cardiovascular biomarkers. *Disease Markers*, 26, 199–207.

Wray, N.R., Yang, J., Goddard, M.E., and Visscher, P.M. (2010). The genetic interpretation of area under the ROC curve in genomic profiling. *PLoS Genetics*, 6, e1000864.

Xu, J., Sun, J., Kader, A.K., et al. (2009). Estimation of absolute risk for prostate cancer using genetic markers and family history. *Prostate*, 69, 1565–72.

Yang, Q. and Khoury, M.J. (1997). Evolving methods in genetic epidemiology. III. Gene–environment interaction in epidemiologic research. *Epidemiologic Reviews*, 19, 33–43.

Zhang, J., Chiodini, R., Badr, A., and Zhang, G. (2011). The impact of next-generation sequencing on genomics. *Journal of Genetics and Genomics*, 38, 95–109.

Ziv, E. and Burchard, E.G. (2003). Human population structure and genetic association studies. *Pharmacogenomics*, 4, 431–41.

Validity and bias in epidemiological research

Sander Greenland and Tyler J. VanderWeele

Introduction to validity and bias in epidemiological research

Some of the major concepts of validity and bias in epidemiological research are outlined in this chapter. The contents are organized in four main sections: validity in statistical interpretation, validity in prediction problems, validity in causal inference, and special validity problems in case–control and retrospective cohort studies. Familiarity with the basics of epidemiological study design and a number of terms of epidemiological theory, among them risk, competing risks, average risk, population at risk, and rate, is assumed. A number of textbooks provide more background and depth than can be given here; see, for example, Kelsey et al. (1996), Koepsell and Weiss (2003), Checkoway et al. (2004), and Rothman et al. (2008).

Despite similarities, there is considerable diversity and conflict among the classification schemes and terminologies employed in various textbooks. This diversity reflects that there is no unique way of classifying validity conditions, biases, and errors. It follows that the classification schemes employed here and elsewhere should not be regarded as anything more than convenient frameworks for organizing discussions of validity and bias in epidemiological inference. Many types of bias can be qualitatively illustrated with causal diagrams, which reveal the relationships among confounding and selection bias; for example, see Greenland et al. (1999), Cole and Hernán (2002), Hernán et al. (2004), Glymour and Greenland (2008), and Pearl (2009).

Several important study designs, including randomized trials, prevalence (cross-sectional) studies, and ecological studies, are not discussed in this chapter. Such studies require consideration of the validity conditions mentioned earlier and also require special considerations of their own. Further details of these and other designs can be found in the general textbooks cited in the preceding paragraphs. For discussions of the problems of ecological studies, see Greenland (2001, 2002a, 2004a) and Morgenstern (2008). Meta-analytic methods are discussed by Eddy et al. (1992), Greenland and O'Rourke (2008), and Borenstein et al. (2009). A number of central problems of epidemiological inference are also not covered, including choice of effect measures, problems of induction, and causal modelling. For critical discussions of effect measures by the present authors, see Greenland et al. (1986, 1991, 1999), Greenland (1987, 1999, 2002b), Greenland and Robins (1988), Rothman et al. (2008, chapter 4), and VanderWeele (2012).

Greenland (1998a, 1998b) and Rothman et al. (2008, chapter 2) discuss problems of inductive and probabilistic inference, Greenland and Brumback (2002) review causal modelling in epidemiology, and Rothman et al. (2008, chapter 2) discuss broader issues in causal inference and philosophy.

Among the deeper problems not discussed here are the failure of conventional statistical methods to account for non-random sources of uncertainty, and the tendency of people (including scientists) to make overconfident and biased inferences in the face of uncertainty (Gilovich et al. 2002). Analytical approaches to these problems are discussed by Eddy et al. (1992), Greenland (2005), Greenland and Lash (2008), and Lash et al. (2009, 2014).

Inference and validity

Epidemiological inference is the process of drawing inferences from epidemiological data, such as prediction of disease patterns or identification of causes of diseases or epidemics. These inferences must often be made without the benefits of direct experimental evidence or established theory about disease aetiology. Consider the problem of predicting the risk and incubation (induction) time for acquired immunedeficiency syndrome (AIDS) among persons infected with type 1 human immunodeficiency virus (HIV-1). Unlike an experiment, in which the exposure is administered by the investigator, the date of HIV-1 infection cannot be accurately estimated in most cases; furthermore, the mechanism by which 'silent' HIV-1 infection progresses to AIDS is not known with certainty. Nevertheless, some prediction must be made from the available data if one is to prepare effectively for future healthcare needs.

As another example, consider the problem of estimating how much excess risk of coronary heart disease (if any) is produced by coffee drinking. Unlike an experimental exposure, coffee drinking is self-selected; it appears that persons who drink coffee are more likely to smoke than non-drinkers and probably tend to differ in many other behaviours as well (Greenland 1993). As a result, even if coffee use is harmless, we should not expect to observe the same pattern of heart disease in users and non-users. Thus, small effects of coffee drinking are very difficult to disentangle from the effects of other behaviours. Nevertheless, because of the high prevalence of coffee use and the high incidence of heart disease, any effect of coffee on heart disease risk may be of considerable public health importance.

In both these examples, and in general, inferences will depend on evaluating the validity of the available studies; that is, the degree to which the studies meet basic logical criteria for absence of bias. When (as is usually the case) aspects of validity cannot be guaranteed by successful design strategies, such as blinded random assignment (which ensures that baseline non-comparability is random), we must evaluate the magnitude of bias that would arise from plausible violations of validity conditions.

Because biases due to misinterpretation of statistics are often neglected in textbooks yet pervade the health-sciences literature, the next subsection will describe common misinterpretations to be alert for when examining reports or analysing data. The remaining subsections will outline and illustrate major concepts of validity and bias in epidemiological research as applied in three settings: prediction from one population to another, causal inference from cohort studies, and causal inference from case–control and retrospective cohort studies. Parallel aspects of each application will be emphasized. In particular, each problem requires the consideration of comparison bias (better known as confounding), follow-up bias (i.e. loss-to-follow-up or censoring bias), bias due to mismeasurement, bias due to erroneous statistical models, and bias due to erroneous statistical interpretation. (The term 'bias' is, here, used in the informal epidemiological sense, and corresponds to the formal statistical concept of inconsistency.) Case–control studies require the additional consideration of case-selection bias and control-selection bias, and are often subject to additional sources of measurement error beyond those occurring in prospective cohort studies. Similar problems arise in retrospective cohort studies.

Misinterpretations of statistics

Severe consequences can arise from failure to properly interpret statistical outputs, and failure to recognize when the output is the result of a statistical method breaking down. Unfortunately, few textbooks discuss these problems in detail, even though they can result in inferential errors as severe as those from the more familiar biases discussed in the following subsections.

Two problems very common in the health-sciences literature are briefly described here. Both problems as well as many others can be avoided with certain Bayesian statistical approaches. Detailed arguments for Bayesian approaches can be found in Berger and Berry (1988), Greenland (1998b, 2006), and Thomas et al. (2007). For an introduction to Bayesian methods that can be carried out with ordinary software, see Greenland (2007) and Sullivan and Greenland (2013). The remainder of this subsection concerns only conventional 'frequentist' methods of significance tests, confidence intervals (CIs), *p*-values, and model fitting.

Misinterpretations of statistical significance

Many authors have noted that significance testing is very difficult to interpret correctly, so difficult that otherwise expert epidemiologists and even statisticians routinely make dramatic mistakes (Altman et al. 2000; Greenland 2004b, 2011, 2012a; Greenland and Poole 2011). Perhaps the largest source of misreporting and misjudgement in the scientific literature, however, is the simple confusion of presence or absence of an association with presence or absence of statistical significance (Altman and Bland 1995; Rothman et al. 2008, chapter 10; Greenland 2011). A common

consequence of this confusion is the mistaken reporting of non-significant results as 'confirming' the null, when in reality the results are completely ambiguous. For example, a study that results in 95 per cent confidence limits for a relative risk (RR) of 0.80 and 2.0 is non-significant. Even if perfectly valid, however, it would not support the null hypothesis any more than it would support the hypothesis that the true relative risk is 1.5 (a 50 per cent increase in risk). Misinterpreting non-significant results as null is easily avoided by paying attention to the confidence limits (Rothman 1978; Altman et al. 2000; Poole, 2001; Rothman et al. 2008, chapter 10). The limits of 0.80 and 2.0 show that the results are not 'significantly' different at the 0.05 level from any relative risk between 0.80 and 2.0. Unfortunately, mistaken claims that non-significant results support the null hypothesis of no association still pervade the field, especially in important policy and legal applications of statistics to epidemiology (Greenland 2004b, 2011, 2012a; Greenland and Poole 2011).

A converse misinterpretation is to say that two groups showed different results because they had different statistical significance. As an example, one article abstract (Park et al. 2007) reported that an inverse association with colorectal cancer was 'seen for total vitamin D intake in men (RR = 0.72, 95 per cent CI: 0.51, 1.00; *p* for trend = 0.03) but not in women' (the estimate compares the highest quintile of vitamin D intake to the lowest). Examination of table 3 of the paper reveals, however, that the corresponding relative risk for women was 0.89 with 95 per cent confidence limits of 0.63 and 1.27, which means that the association for women was in fact inverse, just as in men (0.89 = 11 per cent lower risk in the highest quintile than in the lowest). Although it was not significantly different at the 0.05 level from 1 (the null), it was also not significantly different from the relative risk of 0.72 seen for men; nor was it significantly different from any relative risk from 0.63 to 1.27. One way to summarize these results would have been to state that an inverse association was observed in both men and women, but that it was weaker and non-significant for women. An even better interpretation is that the study had too few subjects to detect whether men and women actually differ with respect to the relation of vitamin D to colorectal cancer. Such honest reports of study weaknesses are not common, however. This issue is especially problematic in the interpretation of subgroup analyses in randomized trials (Rothwell 2005; Wang et al. 2007).

An opposite misinterpretation of the one just illustrated is to claim that two results are not significantly different because their confidence intervals overlap. It is true that they will not be significantly different if the interval from either group contains the point estimate from the other group (as in the preceding example, in which the men's point estimate of 0.72 falls within the women's limits of 0.63 and 1.27), and that the two groups will be significantly different if their confidence intervals do not overlap. Nonetheless, if the intervals overlap but neither interval contains both point estimates, one cannot determine significance without conducting a direct test of the difference in results.

Misinterpretations such as just described arise in part from the conventional use of a cut-off value such as 0.05 to declare presence or absence of significance, and the corresponding use of 95 per cent to determine the width of a confidence interval (which is just the collection of all values that are not significant at the 0.05 level). In reality, there is a continuum of degrees of significance, as measured by the *p*-value ('significance level'), and any cut-off value is both arbitrary and distortive (Rothman et al. 2008, chapter 10). Thus, some authors have encouraged a movement away from classifying associations 'significant' or 'non-significant', towards presenting instead the actual *p*-value for the tested hypothesis and for other values of interest (see Poole 1987a, 1987b; Goodman 1993; Greenland and Poole 2013a, 2013b).

Even if one presents *p*-values, however, the complexities and subtleties of determining and interpreting significance become even worse when multiple tests are involved (the 'multiple comparisons' problem). Here, adjustments for the multiplicity of tests can worsen certain problems even as they address others, for example, by worsening power even as it protects the validity (alpha level) of the tests. They may also shift the null hypothesis being tested to one that, if understood, might be seen as irrelevant to the scientific question at hand. For a discussion of these issues and further references, see Rothman et al. (2008, chapter 10) and Greenland and Poole (2011). Many of these problems can be avoided by shifting to a multilevel (hierarchical) approach for the analysis (Greenland 2000a, 2000b).

Sparse-data bias

Most epidemiological studies collect data on so many variables that any thorough stratification (tabulation) of the data on those variables will result in 'sparse data', in which many if not most cell counts may be very small. Classical epidemiological methods such as standardization break down in the face of this sparsity. Although modelling was developed to address problems of sparse data, it is not a sure fix. Conventional methods for fitting risk and rate models such as maximum likelihood (ML), weighted least squares, and generalized estimating equations are 'large-sample' (asymptotic) techniques, meaning that they have sample-size requirements for valid performance. In the context of say logistic regression (the most common method in epidemiology), this means that among other things there are sufficient numbers of cases and non-cases observed at all levels of categorical variables in the model.

A serious problem is that when there are too few cases or non-cases in a given category a coefficient estimate based on that category may 'blow up', taking on a value that is much too large in absolute magnitude. This problem can arise in both unconditional and conditional logistic regression (Greenland et al. 2000). In a similar fashion, certain estimates may become inflated when there are too many variables in the model relative to the number of cases and non-cases. This hazard is especially severe when the data are divided into subgroups for separate analysis, for example, separating men and women instead of modelling effects with a variable for gender, or when 'interaction' (product) terms are used in the model. In almost all reports, the inflated estimates if 'statistically significant' are misinterpreted as representing strong effects rather than being recognized as statistical artefacts.

To spot these problems, investigators should check tables of the variables in the model against the outcome, and beware of estimates obtained when the observed numbers in each category fall below 4 or 5, or when the ratios of the number of cases and non-cases to the number of variables in the model fall below 4 or 5. Various methods for shrinkage estimation (including random-coefficient, hierarchical, multilevel, ridge, penalized, and Bayesian regression) can be used as an alternative to collapsing categories or deleting variables from the model to avoid

sparse-data bias (Greenland 2000b, 2007; Sullivan and Greenland 2013).

Validity and bias in prediction problems

Turning now to more traditional topics, the following prediction problem will be used to illustrate several basic concepts of validity. A health clinic for homosexual men is about to begin enrolling HIV-1-negative men in an unrestricted programme that will involve retesting each participant for HIV-1 antibodies at 6-month intervals. We can expect that, in the course of the programme, many participants will seroconvert to positive HIV-1 status. Such participants will invariably ask difficult questions, such as: What are my chances of developing AIDS over the next 5 years? How many years do I have before I develop AIDS? In attempting to answer these questions, it will be convenient to refer to such participants (i.e. those who seroconvert) as the target cohort. Even though membership of this cohort is not determined in advance, it will be the target of our predictions. It will also be convenient to refer to the time from HIV-1 infection until the onset of clinical AIDS as the AIDS incubation time. We could provide reasonable answers to a participant's questions if we could accurately predict AIDS incubation times, although we would also have to estimate the time elapsed between infection and the first positive test.

There might be someone who responds to the questions posed here with the following anecdote: 'I've known several men just like the ones in this cohort, and they all developed AIDS within 5 years after a positive HIV-1 test.' No trained scientist would conclude from this anecdote that all or most of the target cohort will develop AIDS within 5 years of seroconversion. Of course, one reason is that the men in the anecdote cannot be 'just like' men in our cohort in every respect: they may have been older or younger when they were infected; they may have experienced a greater degree of stress following their infection; they may have been heavier smokers, drinkers, or drug users; and so on. In other words, we know that the anecdotal men and their post-infection life events could not have been exactly the same as the men in our target cohort with respect to all factors that affect AIDS incubation time, including measured, unmeasured, and unknown factors. Furthermore, it may be that some or all of the men referred to in the anecdote had been infected long before they were first tested, so that (unlike men in our target cohort) the time from their first positive test to AIDS onset was much shorter than the time from seroconversion to AIDS onset.

Any reasonable predictions must be based on observing the distribution of AIDS incubation times in another cohort. Suppose that we obtain data from a study of homosexual men who underwent regular HIV-1 testing, and we then assemble from these data a study cohort of men who were observed to seroconvert. Suppose also that most of these men were followed for at least 5 years after seroconversion. We cannot expect any member of this study to be 'just like' any member of our target cohort in every respect. Nevertheless, if we could identify no differences between the two cohorts with respect to factors that affect incubation time, we might argue that the study cohort could serve as a point of reference for predicting incubation times in the target cohort. Thus, we shall henceforth refer to the study cohort as our reference cohort.

Note that our reference and target cohorts may have originated from different populations; for example, the clinic generating the target cohort could be in New York, but the study that generated the reference cohort may have been in San Francisco. Of course, for both the target and reference cohorts, the actual times of HIV-1 infection will have to be imputed, based on the dates of the last negative and the first positive tests.

Suppose that our statistical analysis of data from the reference cohort produces estimates of 0.05, 0.25, and 0.45 for the average risk of contracting AIDS within 2, 5, and 8 years of HIV-1 infection. What conditions would be sufficient to guarantee the validity of these figures as estimates or predictions of the proportion of the target cohort that would develop AIDS within 2, 5, and 8 years of infection? If by 'valid' we mean that any discrepancy between our predictions and the true target proportions is unbiased or purely random (unpredictable in principle), the following conditions would be sufficient:

(C) *Comparison validity*—the distribution of incubation times in the target cohort will be approximately the same as the distribution in the reference cohort.

(F) *Follow-up validity*—within the reference cohort, the risk of censoring (i.e. follow-up ended by an event other than AIDS) is not associated with risk of AIDS.

(M) *Measurement validity*—all measurements of variables used in the analysis closely approximate the true values of the variables. In particular, each imputed time of HIV-1 infection closely approximates the true infection time, and each reported time of AIDS onset closely approximates a clinical event defined as AIDS onset.

(Sp) *Specification validity*—the distribution of incubation times in the reference cohort can be closely approximated by the statistical model used to compute the estimates. For example, if one employs a lognormal distribution to model the distribution of incubation times in the reference cohort, this model should be approximately correct.

The first condition concerns the external validity of making predictions about the target cohort based on the reference cohort. The remaining conditions concern the internal validity of the predictions as estimates of average risk in the reference cohort. The following subsections will explore the meaning of these conditions in prediction problems.

Comparison validity

Comparison validity is probably the easiest condition to describe, although it is difficult to evaluate. Intuitively, it simply means that the distribution of incubation times in the target cohort could be almost perfectly predicted from the distribution of incubation times in the reference cohort, if the incubation times were observed without error and there was no loss to follow-up. Other ways of stating this condition are that the two cohorts are comparable or exchangeable with respect to incubation times, or that the AIDS experience of the target cohort can be predicted from the experience of the reference cohort.

Confounding

If the two cohorts are not comparable, some or all of our risk estimates for the target cohort based on the reference cohort will be biased as a result. This bias is sometimes called *confounding*. There has been much research on methods for identifying and adjusting for such bias; see the textbooks cited earlier.

To evaluate comparison validity, we must investigate whether the two cohorts differ on any factors that influence incubation time. If so, we cannot reasonably expect the incubation time distributions of the two cohorts to be comparable. A factor responsible for some or all of the confounding in an estimate is called a confounder or confounding variable, the estimate is said to be confounded by the factor, and the factor is said to confound the estimate.

To illustrate these concepts, suppose that men infected at younger ages tend to have longer incubation times and that the members of the reference cohort are on average younger than members of the target cohort. If there were no other differences to counterbalance this age difference, we should then expect that members of the reference cohort will on average have longer incubation times than members of the target cohort. Consequently, unadjusted predictions of risk for the target cohort derived from the reference cohort would be biased (confounded) by age in a downward direction. In other words, age would be a confounder for estimating risk in the target cohort, and confounding by age would result in underestimation of the proportion of men in the target cohort who will develop AIDS within 5 years.

Now suppose that we can compute the age at infection of men in the reference cohort, and that within 1-year strata of age, for instance, the target and reference cohorts had virtually identical distributions of incubation times. The age-specific estimates of risk derived from the reference cohort would then be free of age confounding and so could be used as unconfounded estimates of age-specific risk for men in the target cohort. Also, if we wished to construct unconfounded estimates of average risk in the entire target cohort, we could do so via the technique of age standardization.

To illustrate, let P_x denote our estimate of the average risk of AIDS within 5 years of infection among members of the reference cohort who become infected at age x. Let W_x denote the proportion of men in the target cohort who are infected at age x. Then the estimated average risk of AIDS within 5 years of infection, standardized to the target cohort's age distribution, is simply the average of the age-specific reference estimates P_x weighted by the age distribution (at infection) of the target cohort; algebraically, this average is the sum of the products $W_x P_x$ over all ages and is denoted by $\sum_x W_x P_x$. Considered as an estimate of the overall proportion of the target cohort that will contract AIDS within 5 years of HIV-1 infection, the standardized proportion $\sum_x W_x P_x$ will be free of age confounding.

The preceding illustration brings forth an important and often overlooked point: when one employs standardization to adjust for potential biases, the choice of standard distribution should never be considered arbitrary. In fact, the standard distribution should always be taken from the target cohort or the population about which inferences will be made. If inferences are to be made about several different groups, it may be necessary to compute several different standardized estimates.

Methods for removing bias in estimates by taking account of variables responsible for some or all of the bias are known as adjustment or covariate control methods. Standardization is perhaps the oldest and simplest example of such a method; methods based on multivariate models are more complex. See also Cole and Stuart (2010) for an alternative approach to such adjustment using weighting.

Unmeasured confounders

If all confounders were measured accurately, comparison validity could be achieved simply by adjusting for these confounders (although various technical problems might arise when attempting to do so). Nevertheless, in any non-randomized study, we would ordinarily be able to think of a number of possible confounders that had not been measured or had been measured only in a very poor fashion. In such cases, it may still be possible to predict the direction of uncontrolled confounding by examining the manner in which persons were selected into the target and reference cohorts from the population at large. If the cohorts are derived from populations with different distributions of predictors of the outcome, or the predictors themselves are associated with admission differentially across the cohorts, these predictors will become confounders in the analysis.

To illustrate this approach, suppose that HIV-1 infection via an intravenous route (e.g. through needle sharing) leads to shorter incubation times than HIV-1 infection through sexual activity. Suppose also that the reference cohort had excluded all or most intravenous drug users, whereas the target cohort was non-selective in this regard. Then incubation times in the target cohort will on average be shorter than times in the reference cohort owing to the presence of intravenously infected persons in the target cohort. Thus we should expect the results from the reference cohort to underestimate average risks of AIDS onset in the target cohort.

Random sampling and confounding

Suppose, for the moment, that our reference cohort had been formed by taking a random sample of the target cohort. Can predictions about the target made from such a random sample still be confounded? With the definition of confounding given here, the answer is yes. To see this, note for example that by chance alone men in our sample reference cohort could be younger on average than the total target; this age difference would in turn downwardly bias the unadjusted risk predictions if men had longer incubation times at younger ages.

Nevertheless, random sampling can help to ensure that the distribution of the reference cohort is not too far from the distribution of the target cohort. In essence, the probability of severe confounding can be made as small as necessary by increasing the sample size. Furthermore, if random sampling is used, any confounding left after adjustment will be accounted for by the standard errors of the estimates, provided that the correct statistical model is used to compute the estimates and standard errors. We shall examine the latter condition under the subsection on specification validity.

Follow-up validity

In any cohort study covering an extended period of risk, subjects will be followed for different lengths of time. Some subjects will be lost to follow-up before the study ends. Others will be removed from the study by an event that precludes AIDS onset, which in this setting is death before AIDS onset from fatal accidents, fatal myocardial infarctions, and so on. Because subjects come under study at different times, those who are not lost to follow-up or who die before developing AIDS will still have had different lengths of follow-up when the study ends; traditionally, a subject still under follow-up at the end of study is said to have been 'withdrawn from study' at this time.

Suppose that we wish to estimate the average risk of AIDS onset within 5 years of infection. The data from a member of the reference cohort who is not observed to develop AIDS but is also not followed for the full 5 years from infection are said to be censored for the outcome of interest (AIDS within 5 years of infection). Consider, for example, a subject killed in a car crash 2 years after infection but before contracting AIDS: the incubation time of this subject was censored at 2 years of follow-up.

Follow-up validity means that over any span of follow-up time, risk of censoring is unassociated with risk of the outcome of interest. In our example, follow-up validity means that over any span of time following infection, risk of censoring (loss, withdrawal, or death before AIDS) is unassociated with risk of AIDS. All common methods for estimating risk from situations in which censoring occurs (e.g. person-years, life table, and Kaplan–Meier methods) are based on the assumption of follow-up validity. Given follow-up validity, we can expect that, at any time t after infection, the distribution of incubation times will be the same for subjects lost or withdrawn at t and for subjects whose follow-up continues beyond t.

Violations of follow-up validity can result in biased estimates of risk; such violations are referred to as follow-up bias or biased censoring. To illustrate, suppose that younger reference subjects tend to have longer incubation times (i.e. lower risks) and are lost to follow-up at a higher rate than older reference subjects. In other words, lower-risk subjects are lost at a higher rate than higher-risk subjects. Then, after enough time, the average risk of AIDS in the observed portion of the reference cohort will tend to be overestimated; that is, higher than the average risk occurring in the full reference cohort (as the latter includes both censored and uncensored subject experience).

The follow-up bias in the last illustration would not affect the age-specific estimates of risk (where age refers to age at infection). Consequently, the age bias in follow-up would not produce bias in age-standardized estimates of risk. More generally, if follow-up bias can be traced to a particular variable that is a predictor of both the outcome of interest and censoring, bias in the estimates can be removed by adjusting for that variable. Thus, some forms of follow-up bias can be dealt with in the same manner as confounding.

Measurement validity

An estimate from a study can be said to have measurement validity if it suffers from no bias due to errors in measuring the study variables. Unfortunately, there are sources of measurement error in nearly all epidemiological studies, and nearly all sources of measurement error will contribute to bias in estimates. Thus, evaluation of measurement validity primarily focuses on identifying sources of measurement error and attempting to deduce the direction and magnitude of bias produced by these sources.

To aid in the task of identifying sources of measurement error, it can be useful to classify such errors according to their source. Errors from specific sources can then be further classified according to characteristics that are predictive of the direction of the bias they produce. One classification scheme divides errors into three major categories, according to their source:

1. *Procedural error*: arising from mistakes or defects in measurement procedures
2. *Proxy-variable error*: arising from using a 'proxy' variable as a substitute for an actual variable of interest
3. *Construct error*: arising from ambiguities in the definition of the variables.

Regardless of their source, errors can be divided into two basic types, differential and non-differential, according to whether the direction or magnitude of error depends on the true values of the study variables. Two different sources of error may be classified as dependent or independent, according to whether or not the direction or magnitude of the error from one source depends on the direction or magnitude of the error from the other source. Finally, errors in continuous measurements can be factored into systematic and random components. As described in the following subsections, these classifications have important implications for bias.

Procedural error

Procedural error is the most straightforward to imagine. It includes errors in recall when variables are measured through retrospective interview (e.g. mistakes in remembering all medications taken during pregnancy). It also includes coding errors, errors in calibration of instruments, and all other errors in which the target of measurement is well defined and the attempts at measurement are direct but the method of measurement is faulty. In our example, one target of measurement is HIV-1 antibody presence in blood. All available tests for antibody presence are subject to error (false negatives and false positives), and these errors can be considered to be procedural errors of measurement.

Proxy-variable error

Proxy-variable error is distinguished from procedural error in that use of proxies necessitates imputation and hence virtually guarantees that there will be measurement error. In our example, we must impute the time of HIV-1 infection. For instance, we might take as a proxy the infection time computed as 6 weeks before the midpoint between the last negative test and the first positive test for HIV-1 antibodies. Even if our HIV-1 tests are perfect, this measurement incorporates error if (as is certainly the case) time of infection does not always occur 6 weeks before the midpoint between the last negative and first positive tests.

Construct error

Construct error is often overlooked, although it may be a major source of error. Consider our example in which the ultimate target of measurement is the time between HIV-1 infection and onset of AIDS. Before attempting to measure this time span, we must unambiguously define the events that mark the beginning and end of the span. While it may be reasonable to think of HIV-1 infection as a point event, the same cannot be said of AIDS onset. Symptoms and signs may gradually accumulate, and then it is only by convention that some point in time is declared the start of the disease. If this convention cannot be translated into reasonably precise clinical criteria for diagnosing the onset of AIDS, the construct of incubation time (the time span between infection and AIDS onset) will not be well defined let alone accurately measurable. In such situations, it may be left to various clinicians to improvise answers to the question of time of AIDS onset, and this will introduce another source of extraneous variation into the final 'measurement' of incubation time.

Differential and non-differential error

Errors in measuring a variable are said to be differential when the direction or magnitude of the errors tend to vary across the true values of other variables. Suppose, for example, that recall of drug use during pregnancy is enhanced among mothers of children with birth defects. Then, a retrospective interview about drug use during pregnancy will yield results with differential error, as false-negative error will occur more frequently among mothers whose children have no birth defects.

Another type of differential error occurs in the measurement of continuous variables when the distribution of errors varies with the true value of the variable. Suppose, for example, that women more accurately recall the date of a recent cervical-smear (Papanicolaou) test than the date of a more distant test. Then, a retrospective interview to determine length of time since a woman's last cervical smear test would tend to suffer from larger errors when measuring longer times.

Errors in measuring a variable are said to be non-differential with respect to another variable if the magnitudes of errors do not tend to vary with the true values of the other variable. Measurements are usually assumed to be non-differential if neither the subject nor the person taking the measurement knows the values of other variables. For example, if drug use during pregnancy is measured by examining pre-partum prescription records for the mother, it would ordinarily be assumed that the error will be non-differential with respect to birth defects discovered postnatally. Nevertheless, such 'blind' assessments will not guarantee non-differential error if the measurement scale is not as fine as the scale of the original variable (Flegal et al. 19991; Wacholder et al. 1991) or if there is a third uncontrolled variable that affects both the measurement and the other study variables.

Dependent and independent error

Errors in measuring two variables are said to be dependent if the direction or magnitude of the errors made in measuring one of the variables is associated with the direction or magnitude of the errors made in measuring the other variable, conditional on the true variables. If there is no such association of errors, the errors are said to be independent.

In our example, errors in measuring age at HIV-1 infection and AIDS incubation time are dependent. Our measure of incubation time is equal to our measure of age at AIDS onset minus our measure of age at infection; hence, overestimation of age at infection will contribute to underestimation of incubation time, and underestimation of age at infection will contribute to overestimation of incubation time. In contrast, in the same example, it is plausible that the errors in measuring age at infection and age at onset are independent.

Systematic and random components of error

For well-defined measurement procedures on continuous variables, measurement errors can be subdivided into systematic and random components. The systematic component (sometimes called the bias of the measurement) measures the degree to which the procedure tends to underestimate or overestimate the true value on repeated application. The random component is the residual error left after subtracting the systematic component from the total error.

To illustrate, suppose that in our study HIV-1 infection time was unrelated to time of antibody testing and that the average time of HIV-1 seroconversion was 8 weeks after infection. Then, even if one used a perfect HIV-1 test, a procedure that estimated infection time as 6 weeks before the midpoint between the last negative and first positive test would on average yield an estimated infection time that was 2 weeks later than the true time. Thus, the systematic component of the error of this procedure would be +2 weeks. Because AIDS incubation time is AIDS onset time minus HIV-1 infection time, use of this procedure would add –2 weeks (i.e. a 2-week underestimation) to the systematic component of error in estimating incubation time.

Each of the components of an error, systematic and random, may be differential (i.e. may vary with other variable values) or non-differential, and may or may not be independent of the error components in other variables. We shall not explore the consequences of the numerous possibilities. However, one important (but semantically confusing) fact is that, for certain quantities, independent and non-differential systematic components of error will not harm measurement validity in that they will produce no bias in estimation (Poole 1985).

To illustrate, suppose that in our example we wish to estimate the degree to which AIDS incubation time depends on age at HIV-1 infection. Suppose also that the systematic components of the measurements of incubation time and age of infection are –2 weeks and +2 weeks (as mentioned), and do not vary with true incubation time or age at measurement (i.e. the systematic components are non-differential). Then, the systematic components, being equal, will cancel out when we compute differences in incubation time and differences in age at infection. Because only these differences are used to estimate the association, the observed dependence of incubation time on age at infection will not be affected by the systematic components of error (although it may be biased by the random components of error).

Specification validity

All statistical techniques, including so-called 'distribution-free' or 'non-parametric' methods as well as basic contingency table methods, are derived by assuming the validity of a sampling model or error distribution. A common example is the binomial model, which is discussed in all the textbooks cited in the introduction. For parametric methods, the sampling model is a mathematical formula that expresses the probability of observing the various possible data patterns as a function of certain unknown constants (parameters). Although the parameters of this model may be unknown, the mathematical form of this model incorporates only known or purely random aspects of the data-generation process; unknown systematic aspects of this process (such as most follow-up and selection biases) will not be accounted for by the model.

All parametric statistical techniques also assume a structural model, which is a mathematical formula that expresses the parameters of the sampling model as a function of study variables. A common example is the logistic model (Kelsey et al. 1996; Hosmer and Lemeshow 2000; Checkoway et al. 2004; Jewell 2004; Greenland 2008a, 2008b). The structural model is most often incorporated into the sampling model, and the combination is referred to as the statistical model. An estimate can be said to have specification validity if it is derived using a statistical model that is correct or nearly so.

If either the sampling model or the structural model used for analysis is incorrect, the resulting estimates may be biased. Such bias is sometimes called specification bias, and the use of an incorrect model is known as model misspecification or specification error. Even when misspecification does not lead to bias, it can lead to invalidity of statistical tests and confidence intervals.

The true structural relation among the study variables is almost never known in studies of human disease. Furthermore, in the absence of random sampling and randomization, the true sampling process (i.e. the exact process leading people to enter and stay in the study groups) will also be unknown. It follows that we should ordinarily expect some degree of specification error in an epidemiological analysis. Minimizing such error largely consists of contrasting the statistical model against the data and against any available information about the processes that generated the data, such as prior information on demographic patterns of incidence.

Many statistical techniques in epidemiology are based on assuming some type of logistic model. Examples include all the popular adjusted odds ratios, such as the Woolf, ML, and Mantel–Haenszel estimates, as well as tests for odds ratio heterogeneity. Classical 'indirect' adjustment of rates and other comparisons of standardized morbidity ratios depend on similar multiplicative models for their validity (Breslow and Day 1987).

The degree of bias in traditional epidemiological analysis methods when the model assumptions fail has not been extensively studied. A few traditional methods, such as directly standardized comparisons and the Mantel–Haenszel test, remain valid under a wide variety of structural models. In addition, risk regression has been extended to situations involving more general models than assumed in classical theory (Breslow and Day 1987; Hastie and Tibshirani 1990). Leamer (1978) and White (1993) give more details on the effects of specification error in multiple regression problems, and Maldonado and Greenland (1994) and Greenland and Maldonado (1994) examine the implications of specification error in epidemiology.

Summary of prediction example

The example in this subsection provides an illustration of the most common threats to the validity of predictions. The unadjusted estimates of AIDS risk may be confounded if the target and reference cohorts differ in composition, and may also be biased by losses to follow-up or use of an incorrect statistical model. Finally, our predictions are likely to be compromised by errors in measurements. These sources of error should be borne in mind in any attempt to predict AIDS incidence.

Validity and bias in causal inference

All the bias problems in prediction arise in studies of causation; confounding, follow-up bias, measurement errors, and specification errors must be considered. In fact, as we shall see, problems of causal inference can be viewed as a special type of prediction problem, namely prediction of what would happen (or what would have happened) to a population if certain characteristics of the population were (or had been) altered (Greenland, 2012b).

To illustrate the validity issues in causal inference, we shall consider the hypothesis that coffee drinking causes acute myocardial infarction. This hypothesis can be operationally interpreted in a number of ways, such as

> 1. There are people for whom the consumption of coffee results in their experiencing a myocardial infarction sooner than they might have, had they avoided coffee.

Although this hypothesis is appealingly precise, it offers little practical guidance to an epidemiological researcher. The problem lies in our inability to recognize an individual whose myocardial infarction was caused by coffee drinking. It is quite possible that myocardial infarctions precipitated by coffee use are clinically and pathologically indistinguishable from myocardial infarctions due to other causes. If so, the prospect of testing this hypothesis with purely physiological evidence is not good.

We could overcome this impasse by examining a related epidemiological hypothesis; that is, a hypothesis that refers to the distribution of disease in populations. One of many such hypotheses is

> 2. Among five-cup-a-day coffee drinkers, cessation of coffee use will lower the frequency of myocardial infarction.

This form not only involves a population (five-cup-a-day coffee drinkers) but also asserts that a mass action (coffee cessation) will reduce the frequency of the study disease. Thus, the form of the hypothesis immediately suggests a strong test of the hypothesis: conduct a randomized intervention trial to examine the impact of coffee cessation on myocardial infarction frequency. This solution has some profound practical limitations, not least of which would be persuading anyone to give up or take up coffee drinking to test a speculative hypothesis.

Having ruled out intervention, we might consider an observational cohort study. In this case, our epidemiological hypothesis must refer to natural conditions, rather than intervention. One such hypothesis is

> 3. Among five-cup-a-day coffee drinkers, coffee use has elevated the frequency of myocardial infarction.

There have been many conflicting cohort and case–control studies of coffee and myocardial infarction. The present discussion will be confined to the issues arising in the analysis of a single study. For a review of issues arising in the analysis of multiple studies (meta-analysis) see Greenland (1994) and Greenland and O'Rourke (2008).

Consider a cohort study of coffee and first myocardial infarction. At baseline, a cohort of people with no history of myocardial infarction is assembled and classified into subcohorts according to coffee use (e.g. never-drinkers, ex-drinkers, occasional drinkers, one-cup-a-day drinkers, two-cup-a-day drinkers, etc.). Other variables are measured as well: age, gender, smoking habits, blood pressure, and serum cholesterol. Suppose that at the end of 10 years of monitoring this cohort for myocardial infarction

events, we compare the five-cup-a-day and never-drinker subcohorts, and obtain an unadjusted estimate of 1.22 for the ratio of the person-time incidence rates of first myocardial infarction among five-cup-a-day drinkers and never-drinkers (with 95 per cent CIs of 1.00 and 1.49). In other words, it appears that the rate of first myocardial infarction among five-cup-a-day drinkers was 1.22 times higher than the rate among never-drinkers. (Hereafter, myocardial infarction means first myocardial infarction, risk means average risk, and rate means person-time incidence rate.)

The estimated rate ratio of 1.22 may not seem large. Nevertheless, if it accurately reflects the impact of coffee use on the five-cup-a-day subcohort, this estimate implies that persons drinking five cups a day at baseline suffered a 22 per cent increase in their myocardial infarction rate as a result of their coffee use. Given the high frequency of both coffee use and myocardial infarction in many populations, this could represent a substantial health impact. Therefore, we would want to perform a careful evaluation of possible bias in the estimate.

As in the AIDS example, we can proceed by examining a series of conditions sufficient for validity of the estimate as a measure of the effect of coffee:

(C) *Comparison validity (no confounding)*—if the members of the five-cup-a-day subcohort had instead never drunk coffee, their distribution of myocardial infarction events over time would have been approximately the same as the distribution among the never-drinkers.

(F) *Follow-up validity*—within each subcohort, the risk of censoring (i.e. follow-up ended by an event other than myocardial infarction) is not associated with the risk of myocardial infarction.

(M) *Measurement validity*—all measurements of variables used in the analysis closely approximate the true values of the variables.

(Sp) *Specification validity*—the distribution of myocardial infarction events over time in the subcohorts can be closely approximated by the statistical model on which the estimates are based.

These four conditions are sometimes called *internal validity conditions* because they pertain only to estimating effects within the study cohort rather than to generalizing results to other cohorts. They are sufficient but not necessary for validity, in that certain violations of the conditions will not produce bias in the effect estimate (although most violations will produce some bias).

The meaning of these conditions for an observational cohort study of a causal hypothesis is explored in the following subsections. An important phenomenon known as *effect modification*, which is relevant to both internal validity and generalizability, will also be discussed following comparison validity.

Comparison validity

In our example, comparison validity means that the distribution of myocardial infarctions among never-drinkers accurately predicts what would have happened in the coffee-drinking groups had the members of these groups never drunk coffee. Another way of stating condition C is that the five-cup-a-day and never-drinker subcohorts would be comparable or exchangeable with respect to myocardial infarction times if no one had ever drunk coffee, or that there is no confounding (Greenland et al. 1991; Rothman et al. 2008, chapter 4).

Despite its simplicity, comparison validity depends on the hypothesis of interest in a very precise way. In particular, the research hypothesis (hypothesis 3 in the preceding subsection) is a statement about the impact of coffee among five-cup-a-day drinkers. Thus, this subcohort is the target cohort, and never-drinkers serve as the reference cohort for making predictions about this target.

To illustrate further the correspondence between comparison validity and the hypothesis at issue, suppose for the moment that our research hypothesis was:

4. Among never-drinkers, five-cup-a-day coffee use would elevate the frequency of myocardial infarction.

In examining this hypothesis, the never-drinkers would be the target cohort and the coffee drinkers would be the reference cohort. Thus, the comparison validity condition would have to be replaced by a condition such as

(C') If the never-drinkers had drunk five cups of coffee per day, their distribution of myocardial infarctions would have been approximately the same as the distribution among five-cup-a-day drinkers.

Other ways of stating condition C' are that the five-cup-a-day and never-drinker subcohorts would be comparable or exchangeable with respect to time to myocardial infarction if everyone had been five-cup-a-day drinkers, and that the myocardial infarction experience of five-cup-a-day drinkers accurately predicts what would have happened to the never-drinkers if the latter had drunk five cups a day.

Confounding

Failure to meet condition C results in a biased estimate of the effect of five-cup-a-day coffee drinking on five-cup-a-day drinkers, a condition sometimes referred to as confounding of the estimate. Similarly, failure to meet condition C' results in a biased estimate of the effect that five-cup-a-day drinking would have had on never-drinkers.

To evaluate potential confounding, we must check whether the subcohorts differed at baseline on any factors that influence time to myocardial infarction. If so, we could not reasonably expect the myocardial infarction distributions of the subcohorts to be comparable, even if the subcohorts had the same level of coffee use. In other words, we could not expect condition C (or C') to hold, and so we should expect our estimates to suffer from confounding. This is so, regardless of whether adjustment appears to change the association of coffee use and myocardial infarction (Greenland et al. 1999).

Some studies have found a positive association between cigarette smoking (an established risk factor for myocardial infarction) and coffee use (Greenland 1993). It also seems a priori sensible that a person habituated to a stimulant such as nicotine would be attracted to coffee use as well. Thus, we should expect to see a higher prevalence of smoking among coffee users in our study.

Suppose then that, in our cohort, smoking is more prevalent among five-cup-a-day subjects than never-drinkers. This elevated smoking prevalence should have led to elevated myocardial infarction rates among five-cup-a-day drinkers, even if coffee had

no effect. More generally, we should expect the myocardial infarction rate among never-drinkers to underestimate the myocardial infarction rate that five-cup-a-day drinkers would have had if they had never drunk coffee. The result would be an inflated estimate of the impact of coffee on the myocardial infarction rate of five-cup-a-day drinkers. Similarly, we should expect the myocardial infarction rate among five-cup-a-day drinkers to overestimate the myocardial infarction rate that never-drinkers would have had if they had drunk five cups a day.

Adjustment for measured confounders

As in the prediction problem, we can stratify the data on potential confounders with the objective of creating strata within which confounding is minimal or absent. We can also employ standardization to remove confounding from estimates of overall effect. Again, some care in the selection of the standard is required.

To illustrate, let R_{xz} denote the estimated rate of myocardial infarction among cohort members who drank x cups of coffee per day and smoked z cigarettes per day at baseline, with R_{0z} denoting the estimated rate among never-drinkers. Let W_{xz} denote the proportion of person-time among x-cup-per-day drinkers that was contributed by z-cigarette-per-day smokers. Finally, let R_{xc} be the unadjusted rate observed among cohort members who drank x cups per day at baseline, with R_{0c} denoting the estimated unadjusted rate among never-drinkers.

Suppose for the moment that any change in coffee-use patterns would have negligible impact on the person-time distribution of smoking in the cohort. The predicted (i.e. expected) rate among five-cup-a-day drinkers had they never drunk coffee, adjusted for confounding by smoking, is the average of the smoking-specific estimates from the never-drinker (reference) subcohort weighted by the smoking distribution of the five-cup-per-day (target) cohort. Algebraically, this average is the following sum (over z):

$$\Sigma_z W_{5z} R_{0z}.$$

This sum is commonly termed the rate in the never-drinkers standardized to the distribution of smoking among five-cup-a-day drinkers. Such terminology obscures the fact that the sum is a prediction about the five-cup-a-day drinkers, not the never-drinkers.

Given the last computation, a smoking-standardized estimate of the increase in myocardial infarction rate produced by coffee drinking among five-cup-per-day drinkers is the rate ratio standardized to the five-cup-per-day smoking distribution:

$$\Sigma_z W_{5Z} R_{5Z} / \Sigma_z W_{5Z} R_{0z}.$$

This formula reveals a property common to a simple standardized rate ratio: The same weights W_{xz} must be used in the numerator and denominator sums. Some insight into this formula can be obtained by noting that the unadjusted rate R_{5c}, among the five-cup-a-day drinkers, is equal to

$$\Sigma_z W_{5z} R_{5z},$$

so that the standardized rate ratio can be rewritten as:

$$R_5 / \Sigma_z W_{5z} R_{0z}.$$

This version shows that the ratio is a classical observed unadjusted rate over the rate expected without exposure, or standardized morbidity ratio (SMR). Another standardized rate ratio is:

$$\Sigma_z W_{0z} R_{5z} / \Sigma_z W_{0z} R_{0Z}.$$

This differs from the previous standardized ratio in that the weights are taken from the never-drinkers (W_{0z}) instead of five-cup-a-day drinkers (W_{5z}). Insight into this formula can be obtained by noting that the numerator sum is simply a prediction (expectation) of what would have happened to the never-drinkers if they had been five-cup-a-day drinkers, and the denominator sum is equal to the unadjusted rate R_{0c}, among never-drinkers. Thus, the last standardized ratio is a smoking-standardized estimate of the increase in the myocardial infarction rate that five-cup-a-day drinking would have produced among the never-drinkers.

Standardization is appealingly simple in both justification and computation. Unfortunately, if the number of cases occurring within the confounder categories tends to be small (under five or so), the technique will be subject to various technical problems including possible bias. These problems can be avoided by broadening confounder categories or by not adjusting for some of the measured confounders. Unfortunately, both these strategies are likely to result in incomplete control of confounding. To avoid having to adopt these strategies, many researchers attempt to control confounding by using a multivariate model. This remedy has problems of its own, some of which we shall address in the subsection on specification validity.

Another problem is that standardized procedures (as well as typical modelling procedures) take no account of potential exposure effects on the adjustment variables or their distribution. Thus, in the preceding example, to justify use of the fixed weights W_{xz} we had to invoke the dubious assumption that changes in coffee use would only negligibly affect the smoking distribution. We shall briefly discuss this issue in the subsection on intermediate variables.

Unmeasured confounders

Among the possible confounders not measured in our hypothetical study are diet and exercise. Suppose that 'health conscious' subjects who exercise regularly and eat low-fat diets also avoid coffee. The result will be a concentration of these lower-risk subjects among coffee non-users and a consequent overestimation of coffee's effect on risk.

Confounding by unmeasured confounders can sometimes be minimized by controlling variables along the pathways of their effect. For example, if exercise and a low-fat diet lowered myocardial infarction risk only by lowering serum cholesterol and blood pressure, control of serum cholesterol and blood pressure would remove confounding by exercise and dietary fat. Unfortunately, such control may also generate bias if the controlled variables are intermediates between our study variable and our outcome variable.

If external information is available to indicate the relationship in our study between an unmeasured confounder and the study variables, we can attempt to use an indirect method to adjust for the confounder; even if external information is unreliable or unavailable, we can examine the sensitivity of our results to unmeasured confounders (Greenland and Lash 2008;

VanderWeele and Arah 2011). Sometimes we can also predict the direction of the bias resulting from confounding (VanderWeele 2008; VanderWeele et al. 2008). Finally, we can evaluate the impact that uncertainty about unmeasured confounders should have on our final inferences about the effect (Greenland and Lash 2008; Lash et al. 2009).

Randomization and confounding

Suppose, for the moment, that the level of coffee use in our cohort had been assigned by randomization and that the participants diligently consumed only their assigned amount of coffee. Could our estimates of coffee effects from such a randomized trial still be confounded? By our earlier definition of confounding, the answer is yes. To see this, note for example that by chance alone the five-cup-a-day drinkers could be older on average than the never-drinkers; this difference would in turn result in an upward bias in the unadjusted estimate of the effect of five cups a day, because age is an important risk factor for myocardial infarction.

Nevertheless, randomization can help to ensure that the distributions of confounders in the different exposure groups are not too far apart. In essence, the probability of severe confounding can be made as small as necessary by increasing the size of the randomized groups. Furthermore, if randomization is used and subjects comply with their assigned treatments, any confounding left after adjustment will be accounted for by the standard errors of the estimates, provided that the correct statistical model is used to compute the effect estimates and their standard errors (Robins 1988; Greenland 1990).

Intermediate variables

In effect estimation, we must take care to distinguish intermediate variables from confounding variables. Intermediate variables represent steps in the causal pathway from the study exposure to the outcome event. The distinction is essential, for control of intermediate variables can increase the bias of estimates.

To illustrate, suppose that coffee use affects serum cholesterol levels (as suggested by the results of Curb et al. (1986)). Then, given that serum cholesterol affects myocardial infarction risk, serum cholesterol is an intermediate variable for the study of the effects of coffee on this risk. Now suppose that we stratify our cohort data on serum cholesterol levels. Some coffee drinkers will be in elevated cholesterol categories because of coffee use and so will have an elevated risk of myocardial infarction, yet these subjects will be compared with never-drinkers in the same stratum who are also at elevated risk due to their elevated cholesterol. Therefore, the effect of coffee on the risk of myocardial infarction via the cholesterol pathway will not be apparent within the cholesterol strata, and so cholesterol adjustment will contribute to underestimation of the effect of coffee on risk of myocardial infarction. Analogously, if coffee affected the risk of myocardial infarction by elevating blood pressure, blood pressure adjustment will contribute to underestimation of the effect of coffee. Such underestimation can be termed overadjustment bias.

Intermediate variables may also be confounders and thus present the investigator with a severe dilemma. Consider that most of the variation in serum cholesterol levels is not due to coffee use and that much (perhaps most) of the association between coffee use and cholesterol is not due to the effects of coffee, but rather to factors associated with both coffee and cholesterol (such as exercise and dietary fat). This means that serum cholesterol may also be viewed as a confounder for the coffee–myocardial infarction study and that estimates unadjusted for serum cholesterol will be biased unless they are also adjusted for the factors contributing to the coffee–cholesterol association.

Suppose that a variable is both an intermediate and a confounder. It will usually be impossible to determine how much of the change in the effect estimate produced by adjusting for the variable is due to introduction of overadjustment bias and how much is due to removal of confounding. Nevertheless, a qualitative assessment may be possible in some situations. For example, if we know that the effects of coffee on serum cholesterol are weak and that most of the association between coffee and serum cholesterol is due to confounding of this association by uncontrolled factors (such as exercise and diet), we can conclude that the cholesterol-adjusted estimate is probably the less biased of the two. Alternatively, if we have accurately measured all the factors that confound the coffee–cholesterol association, we can control these factors instead of cholesterol to obtain an estimate free of both overadjustment bias and confounding by cholesterol. Finally, if we have multiple measurements of coffee use and cholesterol over time, techniques are available that adjust for the confounding effects of cholesterol but do not introduce overadjustment (Hernán et al. 2000; Robins et al. 2000).

Direct and indirect effects

Often, one may wish to estimate how much of the effect under study is indirect relative to an intermediate variable (in the sense of being transmitted through the intermediate), or how much of the effect is direct relative to the intermediate (i.e. not mediated by the intermediate). For example, we might wish to estimate how much of the effect of coffee on myocardial infarction risk is due to its effect on serum cholesterol, or how much is due to the effects of coffee on cardiovascular variables other than cholesterol.

One common approach to this problem is to adjust the coffee–myocardial infarction association for serum cholesterol level via ordinary stratification or regression methods and then use the resulting estimate as the estimate of the direct effect of coffee. This procedure is potentially biased as it may introduce new confounding by determinants of serum cholesterol, even if these determinants did not confound the total (unadjusted) association (Robins and Greenland 1992, 1994; Cole and Hernán 2002; Glymour and Greenland 2008). Nonetheless, given sufficient data, it is possible to obtain separate estimates for direct and indirect effects using special stratification or modelling techniques (Robins and Greenland 1994; Kaufman et al. 2005; Vansteelandt 2010, 2012; Valeri and VanderWeele et al. 2013), but again these techniques make much stronger assumptions than those for total effects. These assumptions can be assessed to a certain extent using sensitivity analysis (VanderWeele 2010).

Effect modification (heterogeneity of effect)

Estimation of effects usually requires consideration of effect-measure modification, which is also known as effect modification, effect variation, or heterogeneity of effect. As an example, suppose that drinking five cups of coffee a day elevated the myocardial infarction rate of men in our cohort by a factor of 1.40 (i.e. a 40 per cent increase), but elevated the myocardial infarction rate

of women by a factor of only 1.10 (i.e. a 10 per cent increase). This situation would be termed modification (or variation or heterogeneity) of the rate ratio by gender, and gender would be called a modifier of the coffee–myocardial infarction rate ratio.

As another example, suppose that drinking five cups of coffee a day elevated the myocardial infarction rate in men in our cohort by a factor of 400 cases per 100,000 person-years but elevated the rate in women by a factor of only 40 cases per 100,000 person-years. This situation would be termed modification of the rate difference by gender, and gender would be called a modifier of the coffee–myocardial infarction rate difference.

As a final example, suppose that drinking five cups of coffee per day elevated the myocardial infarction rate in our cohort by a factor of 1.22 in both men and women. This situation would be termed homogeneity of the rate ratios across gender.

Effect modification and homogeneity are not absolute properties of an effect, but instead are properties of the way that the effect is measured. For example, suppose that drinking five cups of coffee per day elevated the myocardial infarction rate in men from 1000 cases per 100,000 person-years to 1220 cases per 100,000 person-years, but elevated the rate in women from 400 cases per 100,000 person-years to 488 cases per 100,000 person-years. Then the gender-specific rate ratios would both be 1.22, homogeneous across gender. In contrast, the gender-specific rate differences would be 220 cases per 100,000 person-years for males and 88 cases per 100,000 person-years for females, and so are heterogeneous or 'modified' by gender. Examples such as this one show that one should not equate effect modification with biological concepts of interaction such as synergy or antagonism (Greenland and O'Rourke 2008; VanderWeele 2009).

Effect modification can be analysed by stratifying the data on the potential effect modifier under study, estimating the effect within each stratum, and comparing the estimates across strata. There are several potential problems with this approach. The number of subjects in each stratum may be too small to produce stable estimates of stratum-specific effects, particularly after adjustment for confounder effects. Estimates may fluctuate wildly from stratum to stratum owing to random error. A related problem is that statistical tests for heterogeneity in stratified data have extremely low power in many situations, and therefore are likely to miss much if not most of the heterogeneity when used with conventional significance levels (such as 0.05). Finally, the amount of bias from confounding, loss to follow-up, measurement error, and other sources may vary from stratum to stratum, in which case the observed pattern of modification will be biased.

Effect modification and generalizability

Suppose that we succeed in obtaining approximately unbiased (internally valid) estimates from our study. We can then confront the issues of generalizability (external validity) of our results. For example, we can ask whether they accurately reflect the effect of coffee on myocardial infarction rates in a new target cohort. We can view such a question as a prediction problem in which the objective is to predict the strength of the effects of coffee in the new target cohort. From this perspective, generalizability of an effect estimate involves just one additional validity issue, namely confounding of the predicted effect by effect modifiers.

Suppose that the rate increase (in cases per 100,000 person-years) produced by coffee use is 400 for males and 40 for females among five-cup-a-day drinkers in both our study cohort and the new target. If our study cohort is 70 per cent male, while the new target is only 30 per cent male, the average increase among five-cup-a-day drinkers in our study cohort would be $0.7 \times 400 + 0.3 \times 40 = 292$, whereas the average increase in the new target would be only $0.3 \times 400 + 0.7 \times 40 = 148$. Thus, any valid estimate of the average increase in our study cohort will tend to overestimate greatly the average increase in the new target. In other words, modification of the effect of coffee by gender confounds the prediction of its effect in the new target. This bias can be avoided by making only gender-specific predictions of effect or by standardizing the study results to the gender distribution of the new target population.

Follow-up validity

In our example, follow-up validity means that follow-up is valid within every subcohort being compared. In other words, over any span of time during follow-up, risk of myocardial infarction within a subcohort is unassociated with censoring risk in the subcohort. Given follow-up validity, we can expect that, at any follow-up time t, the myocardial infarction rates in a subcohort will be the same for subjects lost or withdrawn at t and subjects whose follow-up continues beyond t.

In fact, we should expect follow-up to be biased by cigarette smoking: smoking is associated with mortality from myocardial infarction and from many other causes; the association of smoking with socioeconomic status might also produce an association between smoking and loss to follow-up. The result would be elevated censoring among high-risk (smoking) subjects. As a consequence, unadjusted estimates of the risks of myocardial infarction will underestimate those risks in the complete subcohorts (as the latter includes both censored and uncensored subject experience). If the degree of underestimation varies across subcohorts, bias in the relative-risk estimates will result.

In fact, the degree of underestimation should vary in this example because of the variation in the prevalence of smoking across subcohorts. Nevertheless, this variation is not necessary for smoking-related censoring to produce biased estimates of absolute effect. For example, if smoking-related censoring produced a uniform 15 per cent underestimation of the myocardial infarction rate in each subcohort, all rate differences would also be underestimated by 15 per cent.

Analogous to control of confounding, any bias produced by the association of smoking with myocardial infarction and censoring can be removed by smoking adjustment. As before, if adjustment is by standardization, the standard distribution should be chosen from the target subcohort.

Because the same correction methods can sometimes be applied, some authors classify follow-up bias as a form of confounding. Nevertheless, the two phenomena are reversed with respect to the causal ordering of the third variable responsible for the bias: confounding arises from an association of the study exposure (coffee use) with other exposures (such as smoking) that affect outcome risk; in contrast, follow-up bias arises from an association between the risk of the study outcome (myocardial infarction) and risks of other end points (such as other-cause mortality or loss to follow-up) that are affected by exposure, and thus is classified as a form of selection bias by many authors (Kelsey et al. 1996; Hernán et al. 2004). In this regard, note that certain forms of follow-up bias cannot be removed by adjustment, and

thus do not resemble confounding (Hernán et al. 2004; Glymour and Greenland 2008). These problems are discussed in the statistics literature under the topic of dependent competing risks (Slud and Byar 1988) and resemble the selection-bias problems of case–control studies, which are discussed later.

Measurement validity

Unlike gender, the continuous variables of coffee use, cigarette use, blood pressure, cholesterol, and age are time-dependent covariates. With the exception of age (whose value at any time can be computed from birth date), this fact adds considerable complexity to measuring these variables and estimating their effects.

Consider that we cannot reasonably expect a single baseline measurement, no matter how accurate, to summarize adequately a subject's entire history of coffee drinking, smoking, blood pressure, or cholesterol. Even if the effect of a subject's history could be largely captured by using a single summary number (e.g. total number of cigarettes smoked), the baseline measurement may well be a poor proxy for this ideal and unknown summary. For these reasons, we should expect proxy-variable errors to be very large in our example.

Proxy-variable error in the study variables

The degree of proxy-variable error in measuring the study variables depends on the exact definitions of the variables that we wish to study. In turn, this definition should reflect the hypothesized effect that we wish to study. To illustrate, consider the following acute-effect hypothesis:

> Drinking a cup of coffee produces an immediate rise in short-term myocardial infarction risk. In other words, coffee consumption is an acute risk factor.

This hypothesis does not exclude the possibility that coffee use also elevates long-term risk of myocardial infarction, perhaps through some other mechanism; it simply does not address the issue of chronic effects.

One way to examine the hypothesis would be to compare the myocardial infarction rates among person-days in which one, two, three, or more cups were drunk with the rate among person-days in which no coffee was drunk (adjusting for confounding and follow-up bias). If we had only baseline data, baseline daily consumption would have to serve as the proxy for consumption on every day of follow-up. This would probably be a poor proxy for daily consumption at later follow-up times where more outcome events occur. A 'standard' analysis, which only examines the association of baseline coffee use with myocardial infarction rates, is equivalent to an analysis that uses baseline consumption as a proxy for consumption on all later days. Thus, estimates from a standard analysis would suffer large bias if considered as estimates of the acute effects of coffee.

The proxy-variable error in this example could easily be differential with respect to the outcome: person-days accumulate more rapidly in early follow-up, where the error from using baseline consumption as the proxy is relatively low; in contrast, myocardial infarction events accumulate more rapidly in later follow-up, where the error is probably higher. This difference in accumulation illustrates an important general point: errors in variables can be differential, even if the variables are measured before the outcome event. Such phenomena occur when errors are associated with risk factors for the outcome; in our example, the error is associated with follow-up time and hence age. In turn, such associations are likely to occur when measurements are based on proxy variables.

Suppose now that we examine the following chronic-effect hypothesis:

> Each cup of coffee drunk eventually results in a long-term elevation of myocardial infarction risk.

This hypothesis was suggested by reports that coffee drinking produces a rise in serum lipid levels (Curb et al. 1986); it does not address the issue of acute effects. One way to examine the hypothesis would be to compare the myocardial infarction rates among person-months with different cumulative doses of coffee (perhaps using a lag period in calculating dose; e.g. one might ignore the most recent month of consumption). If we had only baseline data, however, baseline daily consumption would have to be used to construct a proxy for cumulative consumption at every month of follow-up. This construction could be done in several different ways. For example, we could estimate the subjects' cumulative doses up to a particular date by multiplying their baseline daily consumption by the number of days that they had lived between age 18 and the date in question. This estimate assumes that coffee drinking began at age 18 and the baseline daily consumption is the average daily consumption since that age. We should expect considerable error in such a crude measure of cumulative consumption.

The degree of bias in estimating chronic effects could be quite different from the degree of bias in estimating acute effects. Furthermore, as discussed in the following, the errors in each proxy will make it virtually impossible to discriminate between acute and chronic effects.

Misclassification and bias towards the null

Although measurement errors can bias effect estimates, in some cases one may be able to predict the direction of the bias. Measurement of a binary (dichotomous) variable is called better than random if, regardless of the true value, the probability that the measurement yields the true value is higher than the probability that it does not. In other words, the measurement is better than random if it is more likely to be correct than incorrect, no matter what the true value is. Given two binary variables, better-than-random measurements with independent non-differential errors cannot inflate or reverse the association observed between the variables. In other words, any bias produced by independent non-differential error in better-than-random measurements can only be towards the null value of the association (which is one for a relative-risk measure) and not beyond.

If either variable has more than two levels, then (contrary to assertions in most pre-1990 literature) the preceding conditions are not sufficient to guarantee that the resulting bias will only be towards the null and not beyond (Dosemeci et al. 1990). Despite this insufficiency, knowing that errors are independent and non-differential can increase the plausibility that any resulting bias is towards the null, although it should not increase the plausibility that the observed association is in the correct direction (Weinberg et al. 1994). For further discussions of measurement error and bias towards the null, see Flegal et al. (1991), Wacholder et al. (1991), Weinberg et al. (1994), Rothman et al.

(2008, chapter 9), VanderWeele and Hernán (2012), and Gustafson and Greenland (in press).

There is one important situation in which the assumption of independent non-differential measurement error and hence bias towards the null have particularly high plausibility: in a double-blind clinical trial with a dichotomous treatment and outcome, successful blinding of treatment status during outcome evaluation should lead to independence and non-differentiality of treatment and outcome measurement errors. Successful blinding thus helps to ensure (although it does not guarantee) that any bias produced by measurement error contributes to underestimation of treatment differences (conservative bias).

Measurement error and confounding

If a variable is measured with error, estimates adjusted for the variable as measured will still be somewhat confounded by the variable. This residual confounding arises because measurement error prevents construction of strata that are internally homogeneous with respect to the true confounding variable (Greenland 1980).

To illustrate, consider baseline daily cigarette consumption. This variable can be considered a proxy for consumption on each day of follow-up or can be used to construct an estimate of cumulative consumption (analogous to the cumulative coffee variable discussed in the preceding). Suppose that we stratify the data on a cumulative smoking index constructed from the baseline smoking measurement. Within any stratum of the index, there would remain a broad range of cumulative cigarette consumption. For example, two subjects who were age 40 and smoked one pack a day at baseline would receive the same value for the smoking index and so end up in the same stratum. However, if one of them stopped smoking immediately after baseline, while the other continued to smoke a pack a day, after 10 years of follow-up the former subject would have ten fewer pack-years of cigarette consumption than the continuing smoker.

Suppose now that cumulative cigarette consumption is positively associated with cumulative coffee consumption. Then, even within strata of the smoking index, we should expect subjects with high coffee consumption to exhibit elevated myocardial infarction rates simply by virtue of having higher levels of cigarette consumption. As a consequence, the estimate of the effect of coffee adjusted for the smoking index would still be confounded by cumulative cigarette consumption.

In some cases, a study variable may appear to have an effect (or no effect) only because of poor measurement of an apparently unimportant confounder. This can occur, for example, when an important confounding variable is measured with a large amount of non-differential error. Such an error would ordinarily reduce the apparent association of the variable with the exposure, and would also make the variable appear to be a weak risk factor, perhaps weaker than the study exposure. This in turn would make the variable appear to be only weakly confounding, in that adjustment for the variable as measured would produce little change in the result. However, this appearance would be deceptive because adjustment for the variable as measured would eliminate little of the actual confounding by the variable.

As an example, suppose that coronary proneness of personality was measured only by the baseline yes or no question: Do you consider yourself a hard-driving person? Such a crude measure of the original construct would be unlikely to show more than a weak association with either coffee use or myocardial infarction, and adjusting for it would produce little change in our estimate of the effect of coffee. Suppose, however, that coronary-prone personalities have an elevated preference for coffee. Such a phenomenon would lead to a concentration of coronary-prone persons (and hence, a spuriously elevated myocardial infarction rate) among coffee drinkers, even after stratification on the response to the question.

One would ordinarily expect adjustment for a non-differentially misclassified confounder to produce an estimate lying somewhere between the unadjusted estimate and the estimate adjusted for the true values of the confounder (Greenland 1980). Unfortunately, if the true confounder has more than two levels, it is possible for adjustment by the misclassified confounder to be more biased than the unadjusted estimate (Brenner 1993); this can even happen with confounders with two levels if the confounder affects the exposed and unexposed subjects in opposite directions (Ogburn and VanderWeele 2012). It is also possible for adjustment by factors that affect misclassification to worsen bias (Greenland and Robins 1985). If however the effect of the confounder is in the same direction regardless of exposure, and its misclassification is independent and non-differential with respect to the exposure and outcome, adjustment for the misclassified confounder will on average produce an estimate between the unadjusted estimate and the estimate adjusted for the true confounder values (Ogburn and VanderWeele 2012, 2013).

Measurement error and separation of effects

Because of their impact on the effectiveness of adjustment procedures, measurement errors can severely reduce our ability to separate different effects of the study variable. Suppose in our example that we wished to estimate the relative strength of acute and chronic effects of coffee. To do so, we must take account of the fact that acute and chronic effects will be confounded. When examining acute effects, person-days with high coffee consumption will occur most frequently among persons with high cumulative coffee consumption. As a consequence, if cumulative coffee consumption is a risk factor, it will be a confounder for estimating the acute effects of coffee consumption. By similar arguments, if coffee consumption has acute effects, these will confound estimates of the chronic effects of cumulative consumption.

Unfortunately, both cumulative and daily consumption are measured with considerable error. As a result, any effect observed for one may be wholly or partially due to the other, even if the other has little or no apparent effect.

Repeated measures

One costly but effective method for reducing the degree of proxy-variable error in measuring time-dependent variables is to take repeated (serial) measurements over the follow-up period and ask subjects to report their pre-baseline history of such variables at the baseline interview. In our example, subjects could be asked about their age at first use and level of consumption at different ages for coffee and cigarettes; they could then be recontacted every year or two to assess their current consumption. Of course, not all subjects may be willing to cooperate with such active follow-up, but the penalties of some extra loss may be far outweighed by the benefit of improved measurement accuracy.

Errors in assessing incidence

An important form of measurement error in assessing incidence is misdiagnosis of the outcome event. In the AIDS example, a false-positive diagnosis of AIDS would result in underestimation of incubation time, whereas a false-negative diagnosis would result in overestimation. In the present example, false-positive errors would result in overestimation of myocardial infarction rates, whereas false-negative errors would result in underestimation. These errors will be of particular concern when the study depends on existing surveillance systems or records for detection of outcome events.

There are special cases in which the errors will induce little or no bias in estimates, provided the errors have little effect on the person-time observed. If the only form of misdiagnosis is false-negative error, the proportion of outcome events missed in this fashion is the same across cohorts, and if there is no follow-up bias, then the relative-risk estimates will not be distorted by the underdiagnosis. Suppose in our example that all recorded myocardial infarction events are true myocardial infarctions, but that in each subcohort 10 per cent of myocardial infarctions are missed. The myocardial infarction rates in each subcohort will then be underestimated by 10 per cent; nevertheless, if we consider any two of these rates, say R_0 and R_5, the observed rate ratio will be:

$$\frac{0.9R_5}{0.9R_0} = \frac{R_5}{R_0}$$

which is undistorted by the underdiagnosis of myocardial infarction. Nonetheless, if coffee primarily induced 'silent' myocardial infarctions and these were the most frequently undiagnosed events, the effect of coffee would be underestimated.

Analogously, if the only form of misdiagnosis is false-positive error, the rate of false positives is the same across cohorts, and if there is no follow-up bias, then rate differences will not be distorted by the overdiagnosis. Suppose that the rate of false positives in our example is R_f in all subcohorts; then, if we consider any two true rates, say R_0 and R_5, the observed rate difference will be:

$$\left(R_s + R_f\right) - \left(R_0 + R_f\right) = R_s + R_0$$

which is undistorted by the overdiagnosis of myocardial infarction. However, if there is non-differential underdiagnosis of myocardial infarction, as is probably the case in our example, the rate difference will be underestimated.

Specification validity

As noted earlier, the use of a statistical method based on an incorrect model (specification error) can lead to bias in estimates and improper performance of statistical tests and interval estimates. All statistical techniques, including non-parametric methods, must assume some sort of model for the process generating the data; however, in the absence of randomization or random sampling, it will rarely be possible to identify a 'correct' sampling model. In addition, structural assumptions are rarely (if ever) exactly satisfied. Thus, some specification error should be expected. As before, minimization of specification error must rely on checking the model against the data and against background information about the processes generating the data.

Recall that the unadjusted rate ratio estimates for five-cup-a-day versus never-drinkers is 1.22 in the present example, with 95 per cent confidence limits of 1.00 and 1.49, and a *p*-value of 0.05. Suppose that these figures were obtained by conventional person-time methods (Rothman et al. 2008, chapter 14). These methods are based on a binomial sampling model for the number of cases who drank five cups a day at baseline, given the combined total number of cases among five-cup-a-day and never-drinkers. In our example, the validity of this model depends on the assumption that the myocardial infarction rate remains constant within subcohorts over the follow-up period. It follows that the model (and hence the statistics given earlier) cannot be valid in our example; the subcohort members grow older over the follow-up period, and hence the myocardial infarction rates must increase with follow-up time.

The invalidity just noted can be rectified by stratifying either on follow-up time or the variable responsible for the change in rates over follow-up time (here, age). The stratification need only be fine enough to ensure that the myocardial infarction rate change within strata is negligible over follow-up. As noted earlier, however, we must also adjust for smoking and perhaps other factors responsible for confounding or follow-up bias. If we stratify finely enough to remove all the bias from these sources, the resulting estimates would be undefined or so unstable that they would tell us nothing about the association of coffee and myocardial infarction.

The standard solution to such problems is to compute adjusted estimates using regression models. These are structural models representing a set of assumptions (usually rather strong ones) about the joint effects of the study variables. Such models allow estimates and tests to be extracted from what would otherwise be hopelessly sparse data, at a cost of a greater risk of bias arising from violations of the assumptions underlying the models (Robins and Greenland 1986). For further details of cohort modelling, see Breslow and Day (1987), Hosmer and Lemeshow (2000), Kelsey et al. (1996), Checkoway et al. (2004), Jewell (2004), and Greenland (2008a, 2008b).

Summary of cohort example

The example used in this subsection provides an illustration of the most common threats to the validity of effect estimates from cohort studies. The unadjusted estimates of the effect of coffee on myocardial infarction will be confounded by many variables (such as smoking), and there will be follow-up bias. As a result, the number of variables that must be controlled is too large to allow adequate control using only stratification. The true functional dependence of myocardial infarction rates on coffee and the confounder is unknown, so that estimates based on multivariate models are likely to be biased. Even if this bias is unimportant, our estimates will remain confounded because of our inability to measure the key confounders accurately. Finally, our inability to summarize coffee consumption accurately would further bias our estimates, making it impossible to separate acute and chronic effects of coffee use reliably.

Given that there are several sources of bias of unknown magnitude and different directions, it would appear that no conclusions about the effect of coffee could be drawn from a study such as the one described in the preceding, other than that coffee does not appear to have a large effect. This type of result—inconclusive,

other than to rule out very large effects—is common in thorough epidemiological analyses of observational data. In particular, inconclusive results are common when the data being analysed were collected for purposes other than to address the hypothesis at issue, for such data often lack accurate measurements of key variables.

Special issues in case–control studies

The practical difficulties of cohort studies have led to extensive development of case–control study designs. The distinguishing feature of such designs is that sampling is intentionally based on the outcome of individuals. In a population-based or population-initiated case–control study, one first identifies a population at risk of the outcome of interest, which is to be studied over a specified period of time or risk period. As in a cohort study, one attempts to ascertain outcome events in the population at risk. Nevertheless, unlike a cohort study, one selects persons experiencing the outcome event (cases) and a 'control' sample of the entire population at risk for ascertainment of exposure and covariate status.

In a case-initiated case–control study, one starts by identifying a source of study cases (e.g. a hospital emergency room is a source of myocardial infarction cases). One then attempts to identify a population at risk such that the source of cases provides a random or complete sample of all cases occurring in this population. Study cases recruited from the source occur over a risk period; controls are selected in order to ascertain the distribution of exposure in the population at risk over that period. Case–control studies may also begin with an existing series of controls (Greenland, 1985). Regardless of how a case–control study is initiated, evaluation of validity must ultimately refer to a population at risk that represents the target of inference for the study.

Relative-risk estimation in case–control studies

The control sample may or may not be selected in a manner that excludes cases. If persons who become cases over the risk period are ineligible for inclusion in the control group (as in traditional case–control designs), a 'rare disease' assumption may be needed to estimate relative risks from the case–control data. In contrast, if persons who become cases over the risk period are also eligible for inclusion in the control group (as in newer case–control designs), the rare disease assumption can be discarded. These points are discussed in the textbooks cited at the beginning of this chapter.

The basics of case–control estimation will be illustrated using the following example. We wish to study the effect of coffee drinking on rates of first myocardial infarction and we have selected a population for study (e.g. all residents aged 40–64 in a particular town) over a 1-year risk period. At any point during the risk period, the population at risk comprises persons in this selected population who have not yet had a myocardial infarction.

Suppose that the average number of never-drinkers in the population at risk was 20,000 over the risk period, the average number of five-cup-a-day drinkers was 10,000, there were 120 first myocardial infarctions among never-drinkers, and there were 90 first myocardial infarctions among five-cup-a-day drinkers. Then, if one observed the entire population without error, the estimated rates among never-drinkers and five-cup-a-day drinkers would be:

$$\frac{120}{20,000 \text{ person-years}} = \frac{90}{10,000 \text{ person-years}}.$$

Thus, if we observed the entire population, the estimated rate ratio would be:

$$\frac{90/10,000 \text{ person-years}}{20,000 \text{ person-years}} = \frac{90/120}{10,000/20,000 \text{ person-years}} = 1.50.$$

This estimate depends on only two figures: the relative prevalence of five-cup-a-day versus never-drinkers among cases (90/120), and the same relative prevalence in the person-years at risk (10,000/20,000). These two relative prevalences are often called the case exposure odds and the population exposure odds.

The first relative prevalence (numerator) could be estimated by interviewing an unbiased sample of all the new myocardial infarction cases that occur over the risk period, and the second relative prevalence (denominator) could be estimated by interviewing an unbiased sample of the population at risk over the risk period. The ratio of relative prevalences from the case- and control-sample interviews would then be an unbiased estimate of the population rate ratio of 1.50. This estimate is called the sample odds ratio.

Three points about the preceding argument should be carefully noted. First, no rare disease assumption was made. Second, the control sample of the population at risk was accumulated over the entire risk period (rather than at the end of the risk period); such sampling is called density sampling (Rothman et al. 2008, chapter 8) or risk-set sampling (Breslow and Day 1987). Third, because of the density sampling, someone may be selected for the control sample, and yet have a myocardial infarction later in the risk period and become part of the case sample as well. Methods for carrying out density sampling can be found in the textbooks cited at the beginning of this chapter.

Validity conditions in case–control studies

The primary advantages of case–control studies are their short time frame and the large reduction in the number of subjects needed to achieve the same statistical power as a cohort study. The primary disadvantage is that more conditions must be met to ensure their validity (in addition to the four listed in the cohort study example), and hence, there are more opportunities for bias to arise.

Suppose that our case–control study data yield an unadjusted rate-ratio estimate (odds ratio) of 1.50, with 95 per cent confidence limits of 1.00 and 2.25. The following series of conditions would be sufficient for the validity of this figure as an estimate of the effect of drinking five cups of coffee a day (versus none) on the myocardial infarction rate:

(C) *Comparison validity*—if five-cup-a-day drinkers in the population at risk had instead drunk no coffee, their distribution of myocardial infarction events over time would have been approximately the same as the distribution among never-drinkers.

(F) *Follow-up validity*—within each subpopulation defined by coffee use, censoring risk (i.e. population membership ended by an event other than myocardial infarction, such as emigration or death from another cause) is not associated with myocardial infarction risk.

(Se) *Selection validity*—this has two components:

1. *Case-selection validity*—if one studies only a subset of the myocardial infarction cases occurring in the population over the risk period (e.g. because of failure to detect all cases), this subset provides unbiased estimates of the prevalence of different levels of coffee use among all cases occurring in the population over the risk period.
2. *Control-selection validity*—the control sample provides unbiased estimates of the prevalences of different levels of coffee use in the population at risk over the risk period.

(Sp) *Specification validity*—the distribution of myocardial infarction events over time in the subpopulations can be closely approximated by the statistical model on which the estimates are based.

(M) *Measurement validity*—all measurements of variables used in the analysis closely approximate the true values of the variables.

Issues of comparison validity, follow-up validity, specification validity, effect modification, and generalizability in case–control studies parallel those in follow-up studies, and so will not be discussed here. Case–control studies are vulnerable to certain problems of measurement error that are less severe or do not exist in prospective cohort studies. We shall discuss these problems first, and then examine selection validity and modelling. Finally, we shall briefly discuss analogous issues in retrospective cohort studies.

Retrospective ascertainment

A special class of measurement errors arises from the retrospective ascertainment of time-dependent variables; that is, attempting to measure past values of the variables. Retrospective ascertainment must be based on individual memories, existing records of past values, or some combination of the two. Therefore, such ascertainment usually suffers from faulty recall, missing or mistaken records, or lack of direct measurements in existing records.

Retrospective ascertainment may be an important component of a cohort study. For example, the cohort study of coffee and myocardial infarction discussed earlier could have been improved by asking subjects about their coffee use and smoking prior to the start of follow-up. This information would allow one to construct better cumulative indices than could be constructed from baseline consumption alone, although the resulting indices would still incorporate error due to faulty recall.

Unless records of past measurements are available for all subjects, measurements on cases and controls must be made after the time period under study as subjects are not selected for study until after that period. Thus, unlike cohort studies, most case–control studies of time-dependent variables depend on retrospective ascertainment. Considering our example, there may be much more error in determining daily coffee consumption ten years before interview than one month before interview; one might then expect case–control studies to be more accurate for studying acute effects than for studying chronic effects. Nonetheless, if acute and chronic effects are heavily confounded, the elevated inaccuracies of long-term recall will make it impossible to disentangle short-term from long-term effects. As illustrated earlier, this confounding can arise in a cohort study. Nevertheless, in a cohort study, such confounding can be minimized by taking repeated measurements. In contrast, such confounding would be unavoidable in a case–control study based on recall, even if detailed longitudinal histories were requested from the subjects.

The preceding observations should be tempered by noting that some case–control studies have access to exposure measurements of the same quality as found in cohort studies and that the exposure measurements in some cohort studies may be no better than those used in some case–control studies. For example, a cohort study in which measurements are derived by abstracting routine medical records would suffer from no less measurement error than a case–control study in which measurements are derived by abstracting the same records.

Outcome-affected measurements

One common potential problem in case–control studies is outcome-affected recall, often termed *recall bias*. This term refers to the differential measurement error that originates when the outcome event affects recall of past events. Examples arise in case–control studies of birth defects, for instance. If the trauma of having an affected child either enhances recall of prenatal exposures among case mothers or increases the frequency of false-positive reports among them, estimates of relative risk will be upwardly biased by effects of the outcome on case recall. This bias may be counterbalanced by other biases, such as recall bias among controls, making the final direction and magnitude of bias due to faulty measurements hard to predict (Drews and Greenland 1990).

One method commonly proposed for preventing bias due to outcome-affected recall is to restrict controls to a group believed to have recall similar to the cases. Unfortunately, one usually cannot tell to what degree this restricted selection corrects the bias from outcome-affected recall. Even more unfortunately, one usually cannot tell if the selection bias produced by such restriction is worse than the recall bias one is attempting to correct (Swan et al. 1992; Drews et al. 1993).

A problem similar to outcome-affected recall can occur when the outcome event affects a psychological or physiological measurement. This is of particular concern in case–control studies of nutrient levels and chronic disease. For example, if colon cancer leads to a drop in serum retinol levels, the relative risk for the effect of serum retinol will be underestimated if serum retinol is measured after the cancer develops. Errors of this type can be viewed as proxy-variable errors in which the post-outcome value is a poor proxy for the pre-outcome value of interest.

Selection validity

Selection validity is straightforward to understand but can be extraordinarily difficult to verify. A violation of the selection validity conditions is known as selection bias. Many case–control designs and field methods are devoted to avoiding such bias (Kelsey et al. 1996; Koepsell and Weiss 2003; Rothman et al. 2008, chapter 8).

In some instances, it may be possible to identify a factor or factors that affect the chance of selection into the study. If in such instances we have accurate measurements of one of these factors,

we can stratify on (or otherwise adjust for) the factor and thereby remove the selection bias due to the factor. Because of this possibility, some authors classify selection bias as a form of confounding. Nevertheless, there are some forms of selection bias that cannot be removed by adjustment. These points will be illustrated in the following subsections.

Case-selection validity

Case-selection bias can be minimized (although may still be large due to non-participation) if one can identify every case that occurs in the population at risk over the risk period. This requires a surveillance system for the outcome of interest, such as a population-based disease registry. In our coffee–myocardial infarction example, we would probably have to construct a myocardial infarction surveillance system from existing resources, such as emergency room admission records, ambulance service records, and paramedic records.

Even if all cases of interest can be identified, selection bias may arise from failure to obtain information on all the cases. In our example, many cases would be dead before interview was possible. For such cases, there are only two alternatives: attempt to obtain information from some other source, such as next of kin or co-workers, or exclude such cases from the study. The first alternative increases measurement error in the study. The second alternative will introduce bias if coffee affects risk of fatal and non-fatal myocardial infarction differently, or if coffee affects risk of myocardial infarction survivorship. To illustrate, suppose that coffee drinking reduced one's chance of reaching the hospital alive when a myocardial infarction occurred. Then, the prevalence of coffee use among myocardial infarction survivors would under-represent the prevalence among all myocardial infarction cases. Underestimation of the rate ratio would result if fatal myocardial infarction cases were excluded from the study.

It might seem possible to remove the case-selection bias in this example by redefining the study outcome as non-fatal myocardial infarction. This does not remove the bias, however; it only leads to its reclassification as a bias due to differential censoring (here classified as a form of follow-up bias). In a study of non-fatal myocardial infarction, fatal myocardial infarction is a censoring event associated with risk of non-fatal myocardial infarction; if fatal myocardial infarction is also associated with coffee use, the result will be underestimation of the rate ratio for non-fatal myocardial infarction. More generally, it is usually not possible to remove bias by placing restrictions on admissible outcomes.

Unfortunately, exclusion is the only alternative for cases that refuse to participate or cannot be located. In our example, if such cases tend to be heavier coffee users than others, underestimation of the rate ratio would result. However, suppose that, within levels of cigarette use, such cases were no different from other cases with respect to coffee use. Then, adjustment for smoking would remove the selection bias induced by refusals and failures to locate cases. (Of course, such adjustment would require accurate smoking measurement, which is a problem in itself.)

Bias that arises from failure to detect certain cases is sometimes called detection bias. If our surveillance system used only hospital admissions, many out-of-hospital myocardial infarction deaths would be excluded, and a detection bias of the sort described here could result.

Control-selection validity

Control-selection bias can be minimized (although may still be large due to non-participation) if one can potentially identify every member of the population at risk at every time during the risk period. In such a situation, one could select controls with one of many available probability sampling techniques, using the entire population at risk as the sampling frame. Unfortunately, such situations are exceptional.

Many studies attempt to approximate the ideal sampling situation through use of existing population lists. An example is control selection by random digit dialling; here, the list (of residential telephone numbers) is not used directly but nevertheless serves as a partial enumeration of the population at risk. This list excludes people without telephone numbers. In our example, if people without telephones drink less coffee than people with telephones, a control group selected by random digit dialling would over-represent coffee use in the population at risk. The result would be underestimation of the rate ratio.

One could redefine the population at risk in the previous example so that the telephone-related selection bias did not exist by restricting the study to persons with telephones. This would require excluding persons without telephones from the case series. The resulting relative-risk estimate would suffer no selection bias. The only important penalty from this restriction is that the resulting estimate might apply only to the population of persons with telephones, which is a problem of generalizability rather than a problem of selection validity. In a similar fashion, it is often possible to prevent confounding or selection bias by placing restrictions on the population at risk (and hence, the control group). In such instances, however, one must take care to apply the same restrictions to the case series and avoid using restrictions based on events that occur after exposure (Poole 1999; Rothman et al. 2008, chapter 8).

Even if all members of the population at risk can be identified, selection bias may arise from failure to obtain information on all people selected as controls. The implications are the reverse of those for case-selection bias. In our example, if controls who refuse to participate or cannot be located tend to be heavier coffee users than other controls, overestimation of the rate ratio would result. This should be contrasted with the underestimation that results from the same tendency among cases.

More generally, one might expect an association of selection probabilities with the study variable to be in the same direction for both cases and controls. If so, the resulting case- and control-selection biases would be in opposite directions and so, to some extent, they would cancel one another out, although not completely. To illustrate, suppose that among cases the proportions who refuse to participate are 0.05 for five-cup-a-day drinkers and 0.02 for never-drinkers, and among controls the analogous proportions are 0.20 and 0.10. These refusals will result in the odds of five-cup-a-day versus never-drinkers among cases being underestimated by a factor of $0.95/0.98 = 0.97$; this in turn results in a 3 per cent underestimation of the rate ratio. Among controls, the odds will be underestimated by a factor of $0.80/0.90 = 0.89$; this results in a $1/0.89 = 1.12$, or a 12 per cent overestimation of the rate ratio. The net selection bias in the rate ratio estimate will then be $0.97/0.89 = 1.09$, or 9 per cent overestimation.

For further discussions of control-selection validity, see the textbooks cited in the beginning of this chapter, and also Savitz

and Pearce (1988), Schlesselman (1992), Swan et al. (1992), and Wacholder et al. (1992).

Matching

In cohort studies, matching refers to selection of exposure sub-cohorts in a manner that forces the matched factors to have similar distributions across the subcohorts. If the matched factors are accurately measured and the proportion lost to follow-up does not depend on the matched factors, cohort matching can prevent confounding by the matched factors, although there are statistical reasons to control the matched factors in the analysis (Weinberg 1985).

In case–control studies, however, matching refers to selection of subjects in a manner that forces the distribution of certain factors to be similar in cases and controls. Because the population at risk is not changed by case–control matching, such matching does not by itself prevent confounding by the matched factors. In fact, it is now widely recognized that case–control matching is a form of selection bias (Glymour and Greenland 2008; Rothman et al. 2008, chapter 11). This bias can be removed by adjusting for the matching factor; to the extent the factor has been closely matched and accurately measured, this adjustment also controls for confounding by the factor.

As an example, suppose that our population at risk is half male, that the men tend to drink less coffee than the women, and that about 75 per cent of our cases are men. Unbiased control selection should yield about 50 per cent men in the control group. However, if we matched controls to cases on gender, about 75 per cent of our controls would be men. Because men drink less coffee than women and men would be over-represented in the matched control group, the matched control group would under-represent coffee use in the population at risk. Note, however, that matching does not affect the gender-specific prevalence of coffee use among controls, and so the gender-specific and gender-adjusted estimates would be unaffected by matching. In other words, the selection bias produced by matching could be removed by adjustment for the matching factor.

The conclusion to be drawn is that matching can necessitate control of the matching factors. Thus, in order to avoid increasing the number of factors requiring control unnecessarily, one should limit matching to factors for which control would probably be necessary anyway. In particular, matching is usually best limited to known strong confounders, such as age and gender in the preceding example (Rothman et al. 2008, chapter 11).

More generally, the primary theoretical value of matching is that it can sometimes reduce the variance of adjusted estimators. However, there are circumstances in which matching can facilitate control selection and so is justified on practical grounds. For example, neighbourhood controls may be far easier to obtain than unmatched general population controls. In addition, although neighbourhood matching would necessitate use of a matched analysis method, the neighbourhood-matched results would incorporate some control of confounding by factors associated with the neighbourhood (such as socioeconomic status and air pollution).

Special control groups

It is not unusual for investigators to select a special control group that is clearly not representative of the population at risk if they can argue that: (1) the group will adequately reflect the distribution of the study factor in the population at risk; or (2) that the selection bias in the control group is of the same magnitude of (and so will cancel with) the selection bias in the case group. The first rationale is common in case–control studies of mortality in which persons dying of other selected causes of death are used as controls; in such studies, selection validity can be assured only if the causes of death of controls are unrelated to the study factor. The second rationale is common in studies using hospital cases and controls; in particular, selection validity can be assured in such studies if the control conditions are unrelated to the study factor, and the study disease and the control conditions have proportional exposure-specific rates of hospital admission (Schlesselman 1992).

Selection into a special control group usually requires membership in a small and highly select subset of the population at risk. Thus, use of a special control group requires careful scrutiny for mechanisms by which the study factor may influence entry into the subset. See Schlesselman (1992) and Kelsey et al. (1996) for discussions of practical issues in evaluating special control groups, and Rothman et al. (Rothman et al. 2008, chapter 8) for validity principles in mortality case–control studies (so-called proportionate mortality studies).

Case–control modelling

The most popular model for case–control analysis is the logistic model. Details of logistic modelling for case–control analysis are covered in many textbooks, including Breslow and Day (1980), Schlesselman (1992), Kelsey et al. (1996), Hosmer and Lemeshow (2000), and Jewell (2004), and Greenland (2008b).

One important aspect of case–control modelling is that matched factors require special treatment. For example, suppose that matching is done on age in 5-year categories and age is associated with the study exposure. To control for the selection bias produced by matching, one must either employ conditional logistic regression with age as a stratifying factor, or else enter indicator variables for each age-matching category into an ordinary logistic regression (the latter strategy has the drawback of requiring about ten or more subjects per age stratum to produce valid estimates). Simply entering age into the model as a continuous variable may not adequately control for the matching-induced bias.

Summary of case–control example

The example in this subsection provides an illustration of the most common threats to validity in case–control studies (beyond those already discussed for cohort studies). After adjustments for possible confounding and follow-up bias (along the lines described for the cohort study), there may still be irremediable selection bias, especially if we use only select case groups (e.g. myocardial infarction survivors) or control groups (e.g. hospital controls). In addition, retrospective ascertainment will lead to greater measurement error than prospective ascertainment, and some of this additional error may be differential.

Given the even greater number of potential biases of unknown magnitude and different directions, it would appear that (as in the cohort example) no conclusions about the effect of coffee could be drawn from a study such as the one described, other than that coffee does not have a large effect. Again, this is a common result in thorough epidemiological analyses of observational data.

Special issues in retrospective cohort studies

Two major types of cohort studies can be distinguished depending on whether members of the study cohort are identified before or after the follow-up period under study. Studies in which all members are identified before their follow-up period are called *concurrent* or *prospective* cohort studies, and studies in which all members are identified after their follow-up period are called *historical* or *retrospective* cohort studies.

Similar to case–control studies, retrospective cohort studies often require special consideration of retrospective ascertainment and selection validity. In particular, retrospective cohort studies that obtain exposure or covariate histories from post-event reconstructions are vulnerable to bias from outcome-affected measurements. Suppose, for example, that a study of cancer incidence at an industrial facility had to rely on company personnel to determine the location and nature of various exposures in the plant during the relevant exposure periods. If these personnel were aware of the locations at which cases worked (as when a publicized 'cluster' of cases has occurred), biased exposure assessment could result. Such problems can also occur in a prospective cohort study if exposure or covariate histories are based on post-event reconstructions.

Retrospective cohort studies can also suffer from selection biases analogous to those found in case–control studies. Suppose, for example, that a retrospective cohort study relied on company records to identify members of the cohort of plant employees. If retention of an employee's records (and hence identification of the employee as a cohort member) were associated with both the exposure and outcome status of the employee, the exposure–outcome association observed in the incomplete study cohort could poorly represent the exposure–outcome association in the complete cohort of plant employees.

Conclusion

Uncertainty about validity conditions is responsible for most of the inconclusiveness inherent in epidemiological studies. This inconclusiveness can be partially overcome when multiple complementary studies are conducted; that is, when new studies are conducted under conditions that effectively limit bias from one or more of the sources present in earlier studies. Ideally, after enough complementary studies have been conducted, each known or suspected source of bias might have been rendered unimportant in at least one study. If at this point all the study results appear consistent with one another (which is not the case for coffee and myocardial infarction, although the studies of smoking and lung cancer provide a good example), the epidemiological community may reach some consensus about the existence and strength of an effect.

Even in such ideal situations, however, one should bear in mind that consistency is not validity. For example, there may be some unsuspected source of bias present in all the studies, so that they are all consistently biased in the same direction. Alternatively, all the known sources of bias may be in the same direction, so that all the studies remain biased in the same direction if no one study eliminates all known sources of bias. Such problems can be addressed tentatively via sensitivity analysis or the more elaborate methods of risk analysis and bias analysis (Eddy et al. 1992;

Greenland and Lash 2008; Lash et al. 2009; VanderWeele and Arah 2011; Greenland 2014). For these and other reasons, many authors have warned that all causal inferences should be considered tentative, at least if drawn from observational epidemiological data alone, although such tentativeness does not in any way rule out interventions when it is clear that the probable cost of failing to act far outweighs the probable cost of intervention (Rothman 1988; Rothman et al. 2008, chapter 2).

Acknowledgements

The authors wish to thank I. Hertz-Picciotto, K. Hoggatt, P. Kass, J. Kelsey, G. Maldonado, S. Norrell, J. Schlesselman, and A. Walker for their helpful comments on earlier versions of this chapter.

References

Altman, D.G. and Bland, J.M. (1995). Absence of evidence is not evidence of absence. *British Medical Journal*, 311, 485.

Altman, D.G., Machin, D., Bryant, T.N., et al. (eds.) (2000). *Statistics with Confidence*. London: BMJ Books.

Berger, J.O. and Berry, D.A. (1988). Statistical analysis and the illusion of objectivity. *American Scientist*, 76, 159–65.

Borenstein, M., Hedges, L.V., Higgins, J.P.T., and Rothstein, H.R. (2009). *Introduction to Meta-analysis*. New York: Wiley.

Brenner, H. (1993). Bias due to nondifferential misclassification of a polytomous confounder. *Journal of Clinical Epidemiology*, 46, 57–63.

Breslow, N.E. and Day, N.E. (1980). *Statistical Methods in Cancer Research. I: The Analysis of Case Control Studies*. Lyon: IARC.

Breslow, N.E. and Day, N.E. (1987). *Statistical Methods in Cancer Research. II: The Analysis of Cohort Data*. Lyon: IARC.

Checkoway, H., Pearce, N., and Kreibel, D. (2004). *Research Methods in Occupational Epidemiology* (2nd ed.). New York: Oxford University Press.

Cole, S.R. and Hernán, M.A. (2002). Fallibility in estimating direct effects. *International Journal of Epidemiology*, 31, 163–5.

Cole, S.R. and Stuart, E.A. (2010). Generalizing evidence from randomized clinical trials to target populations: the ACTG-320 trial. *American Journal of Epidemiology*, 172, 107–15.

Curb, J.D., Reed, D.M., Kautz, J.A., et al. (1986). Coffee, caffeine, and serum cholesterol in Japanese men in Hawaii. *American Journal of Epidemiology*, 123, 648–55.

Dosemeci, M., Wacholder, S., and Lubin, J.H. (1990). Does nondifferential misclassification of exposure always bias a true effect towards the null value? *American Journal of Epidemiology*, 132, 746–8.

Drews, C.D. and Greenland, S. (1990). The impact of differential recall on the results of case-control studies. *International Journal of Epidemiology*, 19, 1107–12.

Drews, C.D., Greenland, S., and Flanders, W.D. (1993). The use of restricted controls to prevent recall bias in case-control studies of reproductive outcomes. *Annals of Epidemiology*, 3, 86–92.

Eddy, D.M., Hasselblad, V., and Schacher, R. (1992). *Meta-analysis by the Confidence Profile Method*. New York: Academic Press.

Flegal, K.M., Keyl, P.M., and Nieto, E.J. (1991). Differential misclassification arising from nondifferential errors in exposure measurement. *American Journal of Epidemiology*, 134, 1233–44.

Gilovich, T., Griffin, D., and Kahneman, D. (2002). *Heuristics and Biases: The Psychology of Intuitive Judgment*. New York: Cambridge University Press.

Glymour, M.M. and Greenland, S. (2008). Causal diagrams. In K.J. Rothman, S. Greenland, and T.L. Lash (eds.) *Modern Epidemiology* (3rd ed.), pp. 183–211. Philadelphia, PA: Lippincott Williams & Wilkins.

Goodman, S.N. (1993). P-values, hypothesis tests, and likelihood: implications for epidemiology of a neglected historical debate. *American Journal of Epidemiology*, 137, 485–96.

Greenland, S. (1980). The effect of misclassification in the presence of covariates. *American Journal of Epidemiology*, 112, 564–9.

Greenland, S. (1985). Control initiated case-control studies. *International Journal of Epidemiology*, 14, 130–4.

Greenland, S. (1987). Interpretation and choice of effect measures in epidemiologic analyses. *American of Journal of Epidemiology*, 125, 761–8.

Greenland, S. (1990). Randomization, statistics, and causal inference. *Epidemiology*, 1, 421–9.

Greenland, S. (1993). A meta-analysis of coffee, myocardial infarction, and coronary death. *Epidemiology*, 4, 366–74.

Greenland, S. (1994). A critical look at some popular meta-analytic methods. *American Journal of Epidemiology*, 140, 290–6.

Greenland, S. (1998a). Induction versus popper: substance versus semantics. *International Journal of Epidemiology*, 27, 543–8.

Greenland, S. (1998b). Probability logic and probabilistic induction. *Epidemiology*, 9, 322–32.

Greenland, S. (1999). The relation of the probability of causation to the relative risk and the doubling dose: a methodologic error that has become a social problem. *American Journal of Public Health*, 89, 1166–9.

Greenland, S. (2000a). Principles of multilevel modelling. *International Journal of Epidemiology*, 29, 158–67.

Greenland, S. (2000b). When should epidemiologic regressions use random coefficients? *Biometrics*, 56, 915–21.

Greenland, S. (2001). Ecologic versus individual-level sources of confounding in ecologic estimates of contextual health effects. *International Journal of Epidemiology*, 30, 1343–50.

Greenland, S. (2002a). A review of multilevel theory for ecologic analyses. *Statistics in Medicine*, 21, 389–95.

Greenland, S. (2002b). Causality theory for policy uses of epidemiologic measures. In C.J.L. Murray, J.A. Salomon, C.D. Mathers, et al. (eds.) *Summary Measures of Population Health*, pp. 291–302. Cambridge, MA: Harvard University Press/WHO. (Reprinted as Greenland, S. (2005). Epidemiologic measures and policy formulation: lessons from potential outcomes (with discussion). *Emerging Themes in Epidemiology*, 2, 1–4.)

Greenland, S. (2004a). Ecologic inference problems in studies based on surveillance data. In D.F. Stroup and R. Brookmeyer (eds.) *Monitoring the Health of Populations: Statistical Principles and Methods for Public Health Surveillance*, pp. 315–40. New York: Oxford University Press.

Greenland, S. (2004b). The need for critical appraisal of expert witnesses in epidemiology and statistics. *Wake Forest Law Review*, 39, 291–310.

Greenland, S. (2005). Multiple-bias modeling for analysis of observational data (with discussion). *Journal of the Royal Statistical Society, Series A*, 168, 267–308.

Greenland, S. (2006). Bayesian perspectives for epidemiologic research. I: foundations and basic methods. *International Journal of Epidemiology*, 35, 765–8.

Greenland, S. (2007). Bayesian methods for epidemiologic research. II: regression analysis. *International Journal of Epidemiology*, 36, 195–202.

Greenland, S. (2008a). Introduction to regression models. In K.J. Rothman, S. Greenland, and T.L. Lash (eds.) *Modern Epidemiology* (3rd ed.), pp. 381–417. Philadelphia, PA: Lippincott Williams & Wilkins.

Greenland, S. (2008b). Introduction to regression modeling. In K.J. Rothman, S. Greenland, and T.L. Lash (eds.) *Modern Epidemiology* (3rd ed.), pp. 418–57. Philadelphia, PA: Lippincott Williams & Wilkins.

Greenland, S. (2011). Null misinterpretation in statistical testing and its impact on health risk assessment. *Preventive Medicine*, 53, 225–8.

Greenland, S. (2012a). Nonsignificance plus high power does not imply support for the null over the alternative. *Annals of Epidemiology*, 22, 364–8.

Greenland, S. (2012b). Causal inference as a prediction problem: assumptions, identification, and evidence synthesis. Ch. 5 in: C. Berzuini, A.P. Dawid and L. Bernardinelli (eds.) *Causal Inference: Statistical Perspectives and Applications*, pp. 43–58. John Wiley and Sons, Chichester, UK.

Greenland, S. (2014). Sensitivity analysis and bias analysis. Ch. 19 in W. Ahrens and I. Pigeot (eds.) *Handbook of Epidemiology* (2nd ed.), pp. 1087–159. New York: Springer.

Greenland, S. and Brumback, B.A. (2002). An overview of relations among causal modelling methods. *International Journal of Epidemiology*, 31, 1030–7.

Greenland, S. and Lash, T.L. (2008). Bias analysis. Ch. 19 in K.J. Rothman, S. Greenland, and T.L. Lash (eds.) *Modern Epidemiology* (3rd ed.), pp. 345–80. Philadelphia, PA: Lippincott Williams & Wilkins.

Greenland, S., Maclure, M., Schlesselman, J.J., et al. (1991). Standardized coefficients: a further critique and a review of alternatives. *Epidemiology*, 2, 387–92.

Greenland, S. and Maldonado, G. (1994). The interpretation of multiplicative model parameters as standardized parameters. *Statistics in Medicine*, 13, 989–999.

Greenland, S. and O'Rourke, K. (2008). Meta-analysis. In K.J. Rothman, S. Greenland, and T.L. Lash (eds.) *Modern Epidemiology* (3rd ed.), pp. 652–82. Philadelphia, PA: Lippincott Williams & Wilkins.

Greenland, S., Pearl, J., and Robins, J.M. (1999). Causal diagrams for epidemiologic research. *Epidemiology*, 10, 37–48.

Greenland, S. and Poole, C. (2011). Problems in common interpretations of statistics in scientific articles, expert reports, and testimony. *Jurimetrics*, 51, 113–29.

Greenland, S. and Poole, C. (2013a). Living with P-values: resurrecting a Bayesian perspective. *Epidemiology*, 24, 62–8.

Greenland, S. and Poole, C. (2013b). Living with statistics in observational research. *Epidemiology*, 24, 73–8.

Greenland, S. and Robins, J.M. (1985). Confounding and misclassification. *American Journal of Epidemiology*, 122, 495–506.

Greenland, S., and Robins, J.M. (1988). Conceptual problems in the definition and interpretation of attributable fractions. *American Journal of Epidemiology*, 128, 1185–97.

Greenland, S., Robins, J.M., and Pearl, J. (1999). Confounding and collapsibility in causal inference. *Statistical Science*, 14, 29–46.

Greenland, S., Schlesselman, J.J., and Criqui, M.H. (1986). The fallacy of employing standardized regression coefficients and correlations as measures of effect. *American Journal of Epidemiology*, 123, 203–8.

Greenland, S., Schwartzbaum, J.A., and Finkle, W.D. (2000). Problems from small samples and sparse data in conditional logistic regression analysis. *American Journal of Epidemiology*, 151, 531–9.

Gustafson, P. and Greenland, S. (in press). Misclassification. In W. Ahrens and I Pigeot (eds.) *Handbook of Epidemiology* (2nd ed.). New York: Springer.

Hastie, T. and Tibshirani, R. (1990). *Generalized Additive Models.* New York: Chapman and Hall.

Hernán, M.A., Brumback, B., and Robins, J.M. (2000). Marginal structural models to estimate the causal effect of zidovudine on the survival of HIV-positive men. *Epidemiology*, 11, 561–70.

Hernán, M.A., Hernandez-Diaz, S., and Robins, J.M. (2004). A structural approach to selection bias. *Epidemiology*, 15, 615–25.

Hosmer, D.W. and Lemeshow, S. (2000). *Applied Logistic Regression* (2nd ed.). New York: Wiley.

Jewell, N. (2004). *Statistics for Epidemiology.* Boca, FL: Chapman and Hall/CRC.

Kaufman, S., Kaufman, J.S., MacLehose, R.F., et al. (2005). Improved estimation of controlled direct effects in the presence of unmeasured confounding by intermediate variables. *Statistics in Medicine*, 24, 1683–702.

Kelsey, J.L., Whittemore, A.S., Evans, A.S., et al. (1996). *Methods in Observational Epidemiology* (2nd ed.). New York: Oxford University Press.

Koepsell, T.D. and Weiss, N.S. (2003). *Epidemiologic Methods.* New York: Oxford University Press.

Lash, T.L., Fox, M.P., and Fink, A.K. (2009). *Applying Quantitative Bias Analysis to Epidemiologic Data.* Boston, MA: Springer Publishing Company.

Lash, T.L., Fox, M.P., MacLehose, R.F., et al. (2014). Good practices for quantitative bias analysis. *International Journal of Epidemiology*, 43, 1–17.

Leamer, E.E. (1978). *Specification Searches.* New York: Wiley.

Maldonado, G. and Greenland, S. (1994). A comparison of the performance of model-based confidence intervals when the correct model form is unknown. *Epidemiology*, 5, 171–82.

Morgenstern, H. (2008). Ecologic studies. In K.J. Rothman, S. Greenland, and T. L. Lash (eds.) *Modern Epidemiology* (3rd ed.), pp. 511–31. Philadelphia, PA: Lippincott Williams & Wilkins.

Ogburn, E.L. and VanderWeele, T.J. (2012). On the nondifferential misclassification of a binary confounder. *Epidemiology*, 23, 433–9.

Ogburn, E.L. and VanderWeele, T.J. (2013). Bias attenuation results for nondifferentially mismeasured ordinal and coarsened confounders. *Biometrika*, 100(1), 241–8.

Park, S.Y., Murphy, S.P., Wilkens, L.R., et al. (2007). Calcium and vitamin D intake and risk of colorectal cancer: the Multiethnic Cohort Study. *American Journal of Epidemiology*, 165, 784–93.

Pearl, J. (2009). *Causality: Models, Reasoning and Inference* (2nd ed.). Cambridge: Cambridge University Press.

Poole, C. (1985). Exceptions to the rule about nondifferential misclassification (abstract). *American Journal of Epidemiology*, 122, 508.

Poole, C. (1987a). Beyond the confidence interval. *American Journal of Public Health*, 77, 197–9.

Poole, C. (1987b). Confidence intervals exclude nothing. *American Journal of Public Health*, 77, 492–3.

Poole, C. (1999). Controls who experienced hypothetical causal intermediates should not be excluded from case-control studies. *American Journal of Epidemiology*, 150, 547–51.

Poole, C. (2001). Low P-values or narrow confidence intervals: which are more durable? *Epidemiology*, 12, 291.

Robins, J.M. (1988). Confidence intervals for causal parameters. *Statistics in Medicine*, 7, 773–85.

Robins, J.M. and Greenland, S. (1986). The role of model selection in causal inference from nonexperimental data. *American Journal of Epidemiology*, 123, 392–402.

Robins, J.M. and Greenland, S. (1992). Identifiability and exchangeability for direct and indirect effects. *Epidemiology*, 3, 143–5.

Robins, J.M. and Greenland, S. (1994). Adjusting for differential rates of prophylaxis therapy for PCP in high- versus low-dose AZT treatment arms in an AIDS randomized trial. *Journal of the American Statistical Association*, 90, 737–49.

Robins, J.M., Hernán, M.A., and Brumback, B. (2000). Marginal structural models and causal inference in epidemiology. *Epidemiology*, 11(5), 550–60.

Rothman, K.J. (1978). A show of confidence. *The New England Journal of Medicine*, 299, 1362–3.

Rothman, K.J. (ed.) (1988). *Causal Inference.* Chestnut Hill, MA: Epidemiology Resources.

Rothman, K.J., Greenland, S., and Lash, T.L. (eds.) (2008). *Modern Epidemiology* (3rd ed.). Philadelphia, PA: Lippincott Williams & Wilkins.

Rothwell, P.M. (2005). Subgroup analysis in randomised controlled trials: importance, indications, and interpretation. *The Lancet*, 365, 176–86.

Savitz, D.A. and Pearce, N. (1988). Control selection with incomplete case ascertainment. *American Journal of Epidemiology*, 127, 1109–17.

Schlesselman, J.J. (1992). *Case-Control Studies: Design, Conduct, Analysis.* New York: Oxford University Press.

Slud, E. and Byar, D. (1988). How dependent causes of death can make risk factors appear protective. *Biometrics*, 44, 265–70.

Sullivan, S. and Greenland, S. (2013). Bayesian regression in SAS software. *International Journal of Epidemiology*, 42, 8–17.

Swan, S.H., Shaw, G.R., and Schulman, J. (1992). Reporting and selection bias in case-control studies of congenital malformations. *Epidemiology*, 3, 356–63.

Thomas, D.C., Witte, J.S., and Greenland, S. (2007). Dissecting complex mixtures: who's afraid of informative priors? *Epidemiology*, 18, 186–90.

Valeri, L. and VanderWeele, T.J. (2013). Mediation analysis allowing for exposure-mediator interactions and causal interpretation: theoretical assumptions and implementation with SAS and SPSS macros. *Psychological Methods*, 18(2), 137–50.

VanderWeele, T.J. (2008). The sign of the bias of unmeasured confounding. *Biometrics*, 64, 702–6.

VanderWeele, T.J. (2009). Sufficient cause interactions and statistical interactions. *Epidemiology*, 20, 6–13.

VanderWeele, T.J. (2010). Bias formulas for sensitivity analysis for direct and indirect effects. *Epidemiology*, 21, 540–51.

VanderWeele, T.J. (2012). Confounding and effect modification: distribution and measure. *Epidemiologic Methods*, 1, 55–82.

VanderWeele, T.J. and Arah, O.A. (2011). Bias formulas for sensitivity analysis of unmeasured confounding for general outcomes, treatments and confounders. *Epidemiology*, 22, 42–52.

VanderWeele, T.J. and Hernán, M.A. (2012). Results on differential and dependent measurement error of the exposure and the outcome using signed DAGs. *American Journal of Epidemiology*, 175, 1303–10.

VanderWeele, T.J., Hernán, M.A., and Robins, J.M. (2008). Causal directed acyclic graphs and the direction of unmeasured confounding bias. *Epidemiology*, 19, 720–8.

VanderWeele, T.J. and Vansteelandt, S. (2010). Odds ratios for mediation analysis with a dichotomous outcome. *American Journal of Epidemiology*, 172, 1339–48.

Vansteelandt, S. (2012). Estimation of direct and indirect effects. In C. Berzuini, A.P. Dawid, and L. Bernardinelli (eds.) *Causal Inference: Statistical Perspectives and Applications*, pp. 126–50. Chichester: John Wiley and Sons.

Wacholder, S., Dosemeci, M., and Lubin, J.H. (1991). Blind assignment of exposure does not always prevent differential misclassification. *American Journal of Epidemiology*, 134, 433–7.

Wacholder, S., McLaughlin, J.K., Silverman, D.T., et al. (1992). Selection of controls in case-control studies. *American Journal of Epidemiology*, 135, 1019–50.

Wang, R., Lagakos, S.W., Ware, J.H., Hunter, D.J., and Drazen, J.M. (2007). Statistics in medicine—reporting of subgroup analyses in clinical trials. *The New England Journal of Medicine*, 357, 2189–94.

Weinberg, C.R. (1985). On pooling across strata when frequency matching has been followed in a cohort study. *Biometrics*, 41, 103–16.

Weinberg, C.R., Umbach, D., and Greenland, S. (1994). When will non-differential misclassification preserve the direction of the trend? *American Journal of Epidemiology*, 140, 565–71.

White, H. (1993). *Estimation, Inference, and Specification Analysis*. New York: Cambridge University Press.

5.14

Causation and causal inference

Katherine J. Hoggatt, Sander Greenland, and Tyler J. VanderWeele

Introduction to causation and causal inference

This chapter offers an introduction to causal inference theory as relevant to public health research. Causal inference can be viewed as a prediction problem, addressing the question of what the likely outcome under one action versus an alternative action is. Although asking these types of questions is very natural, answering them requires careful thought in both the statement of the causal hypothesis and the techniques used to attempt an answer. This chapter discusses these complexities, with further discussion in Chapter 5.13. More thorough coverage of these issues can be found in chapters 2, 4, and 9 of Rothman et al. (2008).

The chapter reviews considerations that have been invoked in discussions of causality based on epidemiological evidence. It then describes the potential-outcome (counterfactual) framework for cause and effect, showing how measures of effect and association are distinguished in that framework. The framework illustrates problems inherent in attempts to quantify the changes in health expected under different actions or interventions. The chapter concludes with a discussion of how research findings may be translated into policy.

The study of cause and effect

Starting in childhood, people acquire a notion of cause and effect that is based on the observation of one event always or often following another. Children observe that flipping a switch consistently results in the light going on and readily assign a cause and effect interpretation to these relations. Nonetheless, such naïve equation of 'variation in tandem' with causation will too often conflate causation with mere association.

The emergence of modern science has led to increasingly sophisticated observational and experimental methods to distinguish causal from non-causal association, aided by formal theories of causation. A formal theory of causation facilitates application of deductive reasoning to the process of causal inference. Of great importance, it allows us to define precisely the difference between causation and association and gives guidance on how to pose causal questions and test causal hypotheses; it does not, however, provide a basis for 'proving' causality, nor can it model the entire process of causal inference.

As Hume (1739) realized and discussed at length, there is no deductive way to prove causality. Thus, causal inference can only be a speculative, inductive process whose output is a theory of cause and effect. Indeed, the history of science shows that all theories, including causal ones, are necessarily provisional and that future evidence may lead to rejecting previously 'established' causal relations (Kuhn 1970). A key feature of several formal theories of causation is that they provide comparative predictions about the consequences of alternative interventions (e.g. dietary supplementation versus none) rather than singular predictions of events assuming no intervention (e.g. forecasts of flu epidemics) (Greenland 2012).

Those working in public health or policy must often make decisions on how to proceed in the face of equivocal evidence. The question then arises of how to weigh the evidence in favour of cause and effect to determine, say, whether smoking should be banned in bars to prevent lung cancer in bar workers, whether pregnant women should be told to take folic acid to prevent neural tube defects in their offspring, or whether postmenopausal women should be prescribed hormone replacement therapy (HRT) to prevent heart disease. In each of these cases, the final decision by health or policy professionals was made in the absence of definitive proof of causality, relying instead on the imperfect evidence gleaned from scientific studies.

Because of its central importance, causal inference is often confused with the more complex process of rational decision-making. While causal inference is a crucial input to decision-making, decision-making also depends on the costs and benefits of the outcomes. For example, it is believed that banning smoking in bars is likely to have health benefits that will more than outweigh any negative economic impacts. This perceived imbalance favouring benefits over costs is a major basis for a proposed ban. In contrast, recommendations that doctors prescribe HRT for the prevention of heart disease must acknowledge that HRT could have serious side effects on women's health. The recommendations are easily challenged if the costs are shifted according to individual preferences and values.

Such examples show that multiple effects should be considered when policymakers evaluate the evidence of cause and effect based on epidemiological studies. Nonetheless, most attempts to formalize the process of causal inference focus on single end points. This single-end point view must be understood thoroughly before considering multiple end points.

Hill's considerations

Many authors have attempted to list considerations that should be weighed when advancing causal arguments. Among these, the best known in epidemiology are by Sir Austin Bradford Hill (Hill 1965), which are closely related to the considerations found in the first US Surgeon General's report on smoking and health (1964). Hill's article has been widely misinterpreted as providing necessary conditions ('criteria') for causation to be inferred; see Phillips and Goodman (2004) for a discussion of this and other misinterpretations. In Hill's own words, the considerations were not meant to be a checklist or set of criteria, but rather simply 'points to consider', namely: (1) strength, (2) consistency, (3) specificity, (4) temporality, (5) biological gradient, (6) plausibility, (7) coherence, (8) experimental evidence, and (9) analogy; we shall discuss each of these in turn. In fact, the only one of these considerations that is necessary is temporality (time order).

Strength

The strength of an association may be considered important because it is harder to explain away strong effects as complete artefacts of biases such as confounding. There is no general rule for how large an association needs to be to provide compelling evidence for an effect, but, for example, it has been reported that many epidemiologists would be sceptical of a identifying a new risk factor for cancer if its risk ratio were less than 3 (Taubes 1995). Nonetheless, there are many smaller associations that are generally agreed to reflect causal effects. This is in part because they have been replicated in a variety of populations using different designs and in part because of considerations other than strength. Examples include the association between smoking and heart disease and between environmental tobacco smoke and lung cancer. Similarly, there are several well-known examples of relatively strong non-causal associations. One example is the association between birth order and Down's syndrome: maternal ageing, which is strongly associated with infant birth order, has since been accepted as the actual cause of the syndrome responsible for the association. Sensitivity and bias analysis can be used along with external information to estimate or quantitatively speculate on the extent to which possible bias sources have affected the strength of an observed association (Greenland and Lash 2008; Lash et al. 2009; VanderWeele and Arah 2011; Greenland 2014).

Consistency

A consistent finding is an association reported across multiple populations, over time, and using different study designs. Although the presence of a consistent result is often taken as a compelling argument for causality, the argument can be specious; for example, an inverse association of beta-carotene with cancer was seen across epidemiological studies but failed to be replicated in subsequent randomized trials. Conversely, the absence of consistency does not imply the absence of a causal effect. Acute effects may be submerged in studies that examine only chronic exposure, and some agents may operate only in highly susceptible subpopulations. Nonetheless, consistency across studies of a similar design helps rule out chance as an explanation for an observed association. Consistency across studies of different designs can provide evidence against specific biases but cannot rule out bias entirely unless all reasonably possible biases have been addressed.

Specificity

In Hill's formulation, specificity can refer either to a cause having a single effect or an effect having a single cause. The limitations of this criterion are apparent even in the case of smoking and lung cancer. Although the smoking and lung cancer association is stronger (on the ratio scale) than the association between smoking and, say, heart disease, there is general agreement today that smoking can increase the risk of many diseases, including heart disease and other cancers.

Specificity can strengthen a causal inference if a competing non-causal hypothesis would predict a non-specific association. For example, some have argued that screening for certain cancers is ineffective in and of itself for reducing cancer mortality, and the apparent protective effect after adjustment for lead-time reflects the fact that those people who choose to undergo regular screenings are generally more health conscious and therefore at a lower risk for cancer due to their 'healthy lifestyle'. If a specific screening instrument, say a mammogram, were shown to be associated with lower mortality from breast cancer but not lower mortality due to cancers in other sites, it could strengthen the inference that mammography is indeed useful in preventing deaths from breast cancer; this approach is sometimes referred to as one of using 'negative controls' (Lipsitch et al. 2010). Although such issues can in theory also be addressed via randomized trials, the controversy surrounding trials of mammography (Freedman et al. 2004) shows that in practice similar considerations will arise even with randomized treatment assignment.

Temporality

Temporality means that a cause must necessarily precede its effect. This positive assertion is inarguable, but it is also possible that in some instances a putative cause (X) is followed by the hypothesized effect (Y), whereas in other instances the putative cause (X) precedes and does cause the effect (Y). Thus an observation that Y preceded X in a specific case is not an argument against causality in cases where Y followed X. Temporality is a definitive criterion for non-causality only if we know that X *cannot* come before Y. Temporality is, however, a necessary condition for assertion of causality in any given case. If X and Y vary over time, it is also possible that there is feedback between such that both affect each other. If data are available on multiple measurements of these variables, contemporary methods from causal inference can help evaluate such feedback (Robins et al. 1999).

Biological gradient

A biological gradient is a dose–response relation between an exposure and an outcome. Though most epidemiologists think of a 'linear' or monotonic dose–response association as strengthening a causal inference, this need not be the case. There may be a sharp increase in risk for specific outcomes at low to moderate doses of a given exposure that tapers off at higher doses, or there may be no adverse effect until saturation of detoxification mechanisms is reached, resulting in increased risk only at higher doses.

Many substances show non-monotonic trends with outcomes in a manner consistent with their hypothesized biological effects; for example, very low and very high doses of certain vitamins may increase the risk of death, a fact consistent with what we know about the biological properties of these vitamins. In addition, an apparent monotonic dose–response relation (risk always increasing with exposure or risk always decreasing with exposure) does not prove the observed associations are genuine rather than artefacts of confounding. If an uncontrolled confounder is monotonically associated with the exposure and monotonically associated with the disease, an apparent dose–response relation between exposure and outcome could simply reflect the dose–response relation between the confounder and outcome (Weiss 1981). Sensitivity analysis can clarify the extent to which a dose–response relationship contributes to evidence of causality (Rosenbaum 2003).

Plausibility

A plausible association is one that conforms to the current scientific understanding of the relation between a putative cause and its effect. This understanding can be informed by other epidemiological studies, animal studies, biology, toxicology, etc. The limitation of plausibility as a criterion for assessing causality is that current scientific understanding can be incomplete or wrong. The observation that cholera occurs in outbreaks does not demonstrate that cholera is caused by miasmas, despite miasma theory being the dominant idea in the early nineteenth century for how infectious agents were transmitted.

Coherence

Hill used the term 'coherence' to mean that the hypothesized causal relation of exposure to disease is not in conflict with the current scientific understanding of the disease process. Hill emphasized that an absence of coherent information was not a strong argument against causality. If an observed association apparently conflicts with current scientific understanding of a disease process, it may be that the understanding is mistaken rather than that the association is non-causal. For example, at the time it was made, the observation that shallow inhalers of cigarette smoke had increased rates of lung cancer relative to deep inhalers seemed to contradict the understanding of lung cancer aetiology. Subsequent research on lung cancer, however, found that the cells affected by cigarette smoke tended to be in the upper respiratory tract, which was in fact consistent with the observed association for shallow inhalers.

Conversely, coherence is a very fallible argument in support of causality. The theory that the inverse association of beta-carotene with cancers observed in epidemiological studies represented a preventive effect was quite coherent with contemporary theories of antioxidants and cancer, but this theory was nonetheless refuted by subsequent randomized trials.

Experimental evidence

In modern discussions, 'experimental evidence' often refers to either human or animal experiments, which themselves are very different categories of evidence. This type of evidence may be limited or absent. For many exposures, human experimentation is impractical or unethical, and, for many disease processes, no suitable animal model exists.

Hill seemed to have a different notion of experiment in mind, however, one more akin to classical writers such as Mill (1862). Hill discussed the evidence for causality that can be obtained by examining the association between exposure and disease when the potentially harmful exposure has been reduced or removed. These types of before-and-after comparisons may provide compelling evidence, although they can mislead if there are uncontrolled time-varying confounders that drive the observed associations.

Analogy

Analogy refers to drawing inferences about the association between a given exposure and disease based on what is known about other exposure–disease relations. Based on what is known about the health effects of cigarette smoking, we might expect that inhalation of other combustibles (e.g. marijuana) would have similar effects, even in the absence of studies on the subject. Analogy can be a useful scientific tool for generating new hypotheses about disease processes; however, its utility for assessing causality is limited by the understanding and imagination of the scientist.

Summary

For reasons such as those just discussed, Hill and other critical thinkers have discouraged taking his 'viewpoints' as a checklist for causality. Hill's considerations may be useful in generating testable hypotheses that can bear on a discussion of causality, but none of them is sufficient to justify a causal inference, and only one, temporality, is a necessary condition for claiming that an observed association is causal.

Despite the ongoing popularity of Hill's considerations—sometimes in modified form—there is no general agreement on which considerations should be used or how they should be used in making causal inferences (Weed and Gorelic 1996; Kaufman and Poole 2000; Holman et al. 2001). Some have argued that such aids to inference amount to refined common sense, which if taken as rigid criteria may harm the inferential process (Lanes and Poole 1984; Phillips and Goodman 2004, 2006; Rothman et al. 2008, chapter 2). Others have used the considerations to develop general deductive formats for evaluating causal hypotheses (Maclure 1985; Weed 1986; Susser 1991). Finally, researchers may use different considerations or deploy them differently based on the specifics of the inferences being made, suggesting that, in practice, most of the considerations are more like values than objective inferential tools (Poole 2001).

Formal approaches to causal inference

Implicit in the discussion of causal considerations is the idea that there is a well-defined notion of what constitutes cause and effect. Perhaps the oldest non-circular set of definitions arises from the potential-outcome or counterfactual framework. The potential-outcome or counterfactual model (Rosenbaum 2002; Morgan and Winship 2007; Rothman et al. 2008 chapter 4; Pearl 2009) specifies what happens to individuals or populations under alternative actions or interventions and also makes explicit the problems in operationally defining causes (Greenland 2002, 2005; Hernán 2005). This model of causation is also useful in defining methodological concepts such as confounding; this is discussed further in Chapter 5.13 and also in chapter 4 of Rothman et al. (2008).

Potential outcomes and counterfactual causality

Causal inference can be viewed as a prediction problem. For example, a public health researcher may wish to predict how the rates of lung cancer among bar workers would change if an indoor smoking ban was enacted. The potential-outcome model allows us to formalize questions such as 'Will a smoking ban decrease the rates of lung cancer in 10 years beyond what can be expected in the absence of a ban?'.

In discussions of potential outcomes, three components must be defined:

- A target of interest, either an individual or group, that will be the subject of the study of causation.

- A list of possible interventions or actions (x_0, x_1, etc.) that could have been applied to the target over some time span of interest.

- An outcome measure (Y) taken after implementation of the intervention or action.

If x_a is the action taken from among possible actions $x_0, x_1, ..., x_n$, a potential-outcome model posits that there is a well-defined outcome, $Y(x_a)$, that would have followed from that specific action x_a. This outcome is often termed a 'potential outcome'.

As an example, suppose the treatment of interest is sending to members of an insurance plan, on their fiftieth birthday, a mail-in home sampling kit to screen for stool blood, a possible indicator of colon cancer. Suppose $X = 1$ if the kit is supplied to a person, and $X = 0$ if not. Ordinary analyses might examine one outcome variable, such as $Y = 1$ if the person dies of colon cancer by age 60 and $Y = 0$ if the person does not die by this age. But a potential-outcome analysis considers one outcome variable for every treatment being compared: for $X = 1$, we consider the outcome $Y(1) = 1$ if the person dies of colon cancer by age 60 *when sent the kit* and $Y(1) = 0$ if the person does not die *when sent the kit*. Similarly, for $X = 0$ we consider the outcome $Y(0) = 1$ if the person dies of colon cancer by age 60 *when not sent the kit* and $Y(0) = 0$ if the person does not die *when not sent the kit*. Offering the kit is then beneficial for the person with respect to these outcomes if $Y(1) = 0$ but $Y(0) = 1$, which is to say if the person would not die of colon cancer by age 60 if sent the kit but *would so die* if the kit *was not sent*. Presumably, such a benefit would arise because the kit, if sent, would be received, used, and would lead to detection of and intervention for an otherwise fatal tumour.

The potential-outcome model is widely used in statistical discussions of causality, and it has become increasingly popular in epidemiology and other fields. Yet, it is not without controversy, largely because at most only one potential-outcome variable can be observed for each person. That observable potential outcome is the one corresponding to the treatment actually received; all the other potential outcomes are unobserved, and hence are 'missing data'. Understandably, the incompleteness of the data under the model is upsetting to practitioners, and the inevitable missingness requires reconsideration of many conventional statistical methods. Such reconsiderations have, however, led to innovative methods for previously intractable problems, such as the estimation of effects of time-varying treatment regimens (Robins et al. 1999).

There are also a number of aspects of the model that are often misrepresented as limitations but are not. For example, the model does *not* require that outcomes be well defined for any possible intervention; it simply requires that the outcomes be well defined for those interventions of interest. If, in a study of motorcycle crash fatalities, we wish to estimate the effect of a helmet law mandating fines for non-use versus no law, we do not need to specify any other actions (such as a law mandating jail time for non-use). Also, and contrary to some misunderstandings, the potential-outcome model is not inherently deterministic: although the model is quite often introduced and taught using deterministic language, a potential outcome could instead be the parameter of a probability distribution, for example the probability of disease.

Causes and effects

The term 'effect' is sometimes used to specify the outcome of a causal process. A researcher may describe lung cancer or heart disease as two possible effects of cigarette smoking. A quantitative definition of an effect is a numerical contrast in outcome measures corresponding to different actions or interventions, for example, $Y(x_1)$ and $Y(x_0)$. The numerical contrast is called a *measure of effect*. In the earlier example, if x_1 is the absence of a helmet law and x_0 is the presence of a helmet law, then $Y(x_1) - Y(x_0)$ could be the fatality-rate difference for motorcycle crashes and $Y(x_1)/Y(x_0)$ could be the fatality-rate ratio.

Thus, under a potential-outcome model, an effect is a contrast in outcomes corresponding to *two* different actions in *one* single target. Effects must be defined with respect to a clearly specified alternative or reference condition. To say that smoking one pack of cigarettes a day increases the risk for lung cancer and heart disease would be incorrect without specifying the alternative: smoking one pack a day may be harmful relative to not smoking, the implicit reference condition, but may be protective relative to smoking two packs a day. Statements about the effects of causes can be ambiguous or meaningless unless both the index and reference actions are stated explicitly.

It follows that an action cannot be considered inherently causal, and it can only be deemed causal when the outcome associated with it is compared to the outcome associated with an alternative action. Consider a person with depression who is prescribed an antidepressant medication. The weeks following initiation of treatment are thought to be periods of increased risk for suicide. If this person commits suicide in the period following treatment initiation, some would say the antidepressant caused the suicide. Given that the person was depressed to begin with, it is possible that he would have committed suicide even if he had not been prescribed the medication, in which case the antidepressant did not cause the suicide in reference to the alternative of no prescription. If instead of being prescribed an antidepressant, however, the individual had been hospitalized, he may not have committed suicide, in which case the antidepressant treatment may be considered a cause of his suicide, but only in reference to the alternative action of hospitalization.

A second important point is that because an effect is a contrast in outcomes for one target, we can observe at most one of the actions and its corresponding outcome. The other treatments, which are not observed, are *counterfactual* (contrary to fact), and as a consequence their corresponding potential outcomes are not observed; for example, $Y(x_0)$ is unobserved (missing data) for all persons receiving treatment x_1. These alternative potential outcomes can only be estimated.

If the index and reference actions lead to identical outcomes, then the index action is said to have no effect on the target. When an action has an effect, describing it as causal or preventive depends on which outcome we are referring to. If smoking a pack a day for 20 years (versus none) causes an individual to die at age 70, then this smoking also prevents survival past age 70. In parallel, if not smoking prevents death at age 70 relative to smoking a pack a day for 20 years, it causes that individual to survive past age 70.

Confounding and measures of association

Our inability to observe the potential outcome of more than one action fundamentally limits our ability to make causal inferences. In any attempt to estimate a causal effect, at least one potential outcome, corresponding to a counterfactual action, must be estimated or predicted rather than measured. In practice, this is accomplished by measuring outcomes in other individuals who actually experience the reference action. In experiments and in cohort studies, these individuals are often called the control subjects.

As an example, on 1 July 2000, Florida weakened its existing motorcycle helmet use law to exempt individuals over the age of 21 who had at least US$10,000 in insurance in case of an accident. To estimate the effect of weakening the helmet law in Florida, we could compare (contrast) the rates of motorcycle crash fatalities before and after the change. Instead of the fatality rate in 2001, had the law not been changed, we use the fatality rate in 1999 before the law changed. This is no longer a measure of effect, because it is not a contrast of the outcomes of two different actions in a single group. Instead, it is a *measure of association*, which is a contrast of outcomes in two or more different groups. We use this measure of association as a substitute for the corresponding measure of effect. The amount of *confounding* is the difference between the measure of association and the measure of effect that it is intended to represent.

Confounding is a serious threat to our ability to make causal inferences. Nonetheless, we can often determine factors that contribute to the difference between the measure of association and the measure of effect. In our example, these would be reasons why the motorcycle fatality rates in 1999 would differ from those in 2001, had the helmet law never changed. These factors are commonly known as *confounders*. When confounders are measured, analytic methods can be used to minimize the amount of confounding from those factors and thus strengthen our inferences. The most basic methods are based on stratifying the observations on values of these confounders. *Standardization* then averages across outcomes in the index and reference groups using a shared (standard) weighting scheme (Rothman et al. 2008). Other methods make special assumptions to combine measures of association across strata. In all these approaches, the resulting summary comparison across the strata is said to be *adjusted* for the confounders used to create the stratification.

An adjusted measure of association will be a good estimate for the desired measure of effect only insofar as we have controlled for (e.g. stratified on) the important confounding factors. If there are other factors that contribute to important differences between the

counterfactual (alternative) outcome and the observed outcome used as a substitute, then the measure of association will remain a biased estimate for the measure of effect. In the case of the helmet law and the motorcycle crash fatalities, one would have to ask if all the important factors contributing to changes in the rate of crash fatalities *other than the change to the helmet law* had been measured and properly controlled. To the extent we are uncertain or doubtful about our measurement and control of important confounders, we would have to doubt the validity of the adjusted association as an estimate of the measure of effect (see Chapter 5.13).

Practical uses of causal inference

Academic discussions of cause and effect often focus on the 'effects' of changes that have no realistic interpretation as actions (e.g. elimination of lung cancer) or actions that are not realistic options (e.g. achieving a 'smoke-free society'). Even when discussions focus on the impact of feasible interventions, they are often based on unrealistic assumptions about their consequences, for example, assuming 100 per cent compliance with a given treatment or behaviour-modification programme.

As an extreme example, some discussions centre on the expected health impact if a given disease or outcome could be removed. Such discussions are irrelevant and often misleading for policy formulation. For example, in a discussion of the 'burden of disease due to lung cancer', a rough ranking of actions and questions from irrelevant and unrealistic to most relevant would be:

◆ Directly eliminating lung cancer (e.g. 'How many deaths could be prevented if we could eliminate lung cancer?').

◆ Removing risk factors for lung cancer (e.g. 'How many deaths could be prevented if we could eliminate cigarette smoking?').

◆ Applying an intervention to an entire population (e.g. 'If we could implement a given smoking-cessation programme to the entire smoking population of a nation, how many deaths could be prevented?').

◆ Applying an intervention that will produce a small change in risk behaviours in part of a population (e.g. 'If we could implement a given smoking-cessation programme in a targeted group of motivated individuals, how many deaths could be prevented?').

We will discuss each of these actions in turn.

Removing outcomes

Discussions of the burden of disease often focus on the expected change in population health that might be expected if certain diseases or outcomes could be removed from a population, for example, in discussions of survival if one could 'eliminate' a certain type of cause-specific mortality. For example, suppose Y represents cause of death, with $Y = y_1$ for death from myocardial infarction (MI) and $Y = y_0$ for death from other causes ('competing risks'). An individual will eventually experience one but not both of these outcomes, so at least one must be counterfactual.

Now suppose Z represents years of survival past age 50. Z is a measure of the burden of MI among those who reach age 50. The value Z will take depends not only on the value of Y but also on how that value (y_1 or y_0) is brought about. Suppose a man with a sedentary lifestyle and poor diet died from an MI at age 54, so that we observe $Z(y_1) = 4$ (the number of years lived past the age of 50). The value of $Z(y_0)$ would then be the number of years lived past age 50 *if the MI death had been prevented*. This value would depend critically on how the MI death was prevented. If the man had taken up a regimen of physical activity and a healthy diet in his twenties, $Z(y_0)$ could be considerably larger than $Z(y_1)$ because the regimen would lower his risk of many causes of death besides MI. If instead the MI death was prevented by medical care at the time the MI occurred, $Z(y_0)$ and $Z(y_1)$ may not differ by much because the man would remain at an increased risk for future MI, cancer, and other potentially fatal diseases.

When the outcomes are not directly manipulable, any prediction based on the hypothesized removal of the outcomes needs to consider not just the fact of the outcome removal but also the method used to remove it (Greenland 2002, 2005; Kalbfleisch and Prentice 2002; Hernán 2005; Hernán and VanderWeele 2011). Even if we can define a realistic intervention for removal of the outcome with few side effects, there is little basis to assume that removal of a particular outcome in a given group yields a risk profile similar to that for other individuals who did not have the intervention yet do not experience the removed outcome. Unfortunately, standard statistical procedures for analysing these types of data make the assumption that the risk profiles are similar (an assumption of 'independent competing risks'). Thus, it is reasonable to expect that even if we can conceive of an intervention that will prevent a specific outcome, estimates of effect in light of this outcome removal will likely be biased if estimation is based on the experience of those who do not experience the outcome in the absence of the intervention. In sum, to estimate the effects of outcome removal, one must study successfully treated individuals.

Removing risk factors

Consider the debate on obesity and mortality. Numerous studies have reported increases in mortality associated with having a body mass index (BMI) over 30 (the cutpoint for obesity) relative to a 'normal' BMI of 20–24.9. Some authors have used these findings to ascribe a causal role for obesity in mortality and have gone on to assert that getting people to lose weight will save lives. But suppose not all individuals who go from a BMI of over 30 to a BMI of (say) 24 lose weight in the same way. Some might start exercising and eating more healthfully, in which case lower mortality may in fact result. Others might undergo gastric bypass surgery or become chronic users of amphetamines, each of which are known to confer some mortality risk.

Unfortunately, studies that examine only the association of BMI with mortality tell us nothing about the impact of different interventions to change BMI. To obtain a relevant causal inference, one must specify an intervention aimed at reducing BMI and then compare the mortality outcomes under that intervention to outcomes under a reference intervention (such as no intervention). The resulting measure of association, as an estimate of a measure of effect, would *not* be a contrast in outcomes of persons at different levels of BMI; it would be a contrast in outcomes under *specific interventions* among persons who started with the same BMI.

The very idea of the 'health effects of BMI' suffers from confusion of the effects of interventions (e.g. a diet and exercise regimen) with the downstream results of intermediate outcomes (e.g. changes in BMI). At best, mortality rates across BMI groups are averages taken across a range of *unknown* interventions that brought about the observed BMI levels. As a consequence, comparisons of these rates correspond to comparing average outcomes under differing distributions of unknown interventions (VanderWeele and Hernán 2013), and even this limited interpretation holds only under very strong assumptions. A change in BMI is not an intervention, thus one cannot unambiguously define the causal effect of a change in BMI. A similar problem arises if one considers the effect on lung cancer incidence if more people were non-smokers. As with BMI, a researcher would need to specify an intervention (e.g. nicotine patches, hypnotherapy, medication, etc.) before discussing the possible result of getting smokers to quit.

When conceptualizing exposures in observational studies as interventions, as opposed to protocols in clinical trials, there are limitations to how detailed the description can be, making vagueness about the hypothetical intervention unavoidable (Robins and Greenland 2000). Nevertheless, moving away from thinking of outcomes such as BMI as potential causes—as opposed to intermediates—is necessary for making policy-relevant causal inferences from observational data.

A related problem arises in discussing the causal effects of personal characteristics. For example, considerable debate has surrounded the question of whether it is meaningful to speak about factors such as race or sex as being possible causes of effects (Holland 1986; Greenland 2005; Kaufman 2008; VanderWeele and Hernán 2012). Although it might seem natural to ask whether the risk of a disease like hypertension is affected by a person's race, studies that contrast rates of hypertension in different racial groups do not adequately address this question. To ameliorate the racial disparities in hypertension, we would first need to identify feasible interventions. For this goal, discussing race as a cause is of no help, because changing the race of individuals is not a clearly defined action let alone a feasible intervention. Such associations can identify disparities but will usually not pinpoint their causes (Kaufman 2008).

Identifying and evaluating feasible interventions

Even when an exposure is an intervention, the discussion of its effects can be complicated if there is treatment non-compliance. In practice, apart from occasional mandates, treatments are only prescribed or recommended, therefore prescription or recommendation is all that can be studied and implemented. What a subject actually chooses to do in response to the assigned treatment is a function not only of the assignment but also of other factors, many if not most of which are infeasible to modify (such as the subject's age).

If the researcher wishes to understand the effects of received treatment rather than treatment assignment, it is important to realize that received treatment is an outcome, not an intervention, and is thus subject to the problems described earlier for intermediate outcomes such as BMI. Special techniques are available for studying the effects of received treatment (e.g. instrumental variables, g-estimation; see Greenland 2000 and Greenland et al. 2008 for elementary discussions of these topics). Nonetheless, effects estimated by these techniques are those expected under ideal conditions and will likely overestimate the effects that will be seen in field implementation. The most relevant causal hypotheses for policymakers and health practitioners concern the changes in outcome to be expected under the implementation of feasible interventions, subject to all their compliance problems.

Estimating field effects of feasible interventions is difficult but doing so at least avoids the unrealism and biases that arise from pretending that subject characteristics or behaviour are under direct or perfect control of health practitioners or society. In studying these types of interventions, the effect measure of interest will be a contrast in outcomes corresponding to different levels of the intervention (e.g. whether or not to fund a given programme), rather than the 'received treatment' discussed earlier. Thus the question is not what would happen if people were to comply with the intervention they were assigned, but rather what would result if people were offered a given treatment at a given cost.

Studies that address causal hypotheses about feasible interventions face profound methodological difficulties. If the intervention is not assigned at random (e.g. if individuals who participate in a given intervention are volunteers, and their outcomes are compared to those who chose not to participate), the resulting measure of association is likely to be confounded and will therefore be a poor estimate of the desired measure of effect. The measure of association can also be distorted due to refusals, loss to follow-up, and measurement error, among other things. These threats to validity are discussed in Chapter 5.13 and in epidemiological methods texts such as Rothman et al. (2008).

Problems in generalizing the results from a particular study to the target population of interest are not given detailed attention in many textbooks, yet they are of great concern for policymaking. The target populations for policy are always different from study populations, for at the very least the target population is defined in terms of future experience, whereas study results are always based on the past. Even if there are no time trends, however, factors such as the compliance rate and response to the intervention may depend on the characteristics of the individuals involved in a given study. The results from a study may therefore not be applicable to other populations, each of which may be composed of a different mix of individuals.

This problem of population heterogeneity of effect is sometimes framed as an issue of 'effect measure modification', meaning that the measure of the intervention effect depends on characteristics of the individual or the population (see Rothman et al. 2008, chapter 4). In theory, the solution is to identify factors responsible for the heterogeneity, stratify on these factors, estimate effect measures within the stratified groups, and predict the likely impact of an intervention in a target population by standardizing the stratified estimates based on the distribution of the factors in the target population. This approach is not wholly satisfactory, however, because it can be difficult to identify all the important sources of heterogeneity, and there are always severe data limitations on the number of factors that can be studied in this fashion.

From research to policy and beyond

This chapter has reviewed some of the considerations necessary in making causal inferences relevant to public health. These considerations are not crucial in all or even most studies, especially if the explicit goal of the study is to report associations and thus provide data for subsequent evaluations, rather than to estimate causal effects (Greenland et al. 2004). In fact, results from epidemiological studies are rarely the sole basis for policy decisions, although they

are important inputs for policy and judicial decisions. To name just a few examples, studies on the link between smoking and lung cancer have led to labelling of cigarette packs and bans on indoor smoking; results linking air pollutants to disease and mortality have informed emissions standards; and findings on the connection between vitamin deficiencies and adverse health outcomes have led to fortification of milk, cereals, and flour. In all these examples, decisions were based not only on multiple epidemiological studies but also on evidence from laboratory and clinical studies and considerations of mechanistic theories.

It is thus important for public health researchers as well as policymakers to understand the fundamentals of causal inference, especially the often neglected issues of defining meaningful and feasible interventions. It is equally important for researchers to understand that scientific research is done to inform policymaking, not to set policy, and that causal inference represents a synthesis of multiple evidence streams. Apart from perhaps outbreak investigations or large, well-executed randomized trials, no single study is capable of establishing a causal relation; furthermore, randomized trial populations must be reasonably representative of target populations in order to fully inform clinical or policy decisions. Those decisions should be based on a careful consideration of the entire relevant scientific and policy literature and must address cost–benefit considerations as well as purely scientific issues.

References

Freedman, D.A., Petitti, D.B., and Robins, J.M. (2004). Point-counterpoint. On the efficacy of screening for breast cancer. *International Journal of Epidemiology*, 33, 43–55.

Greenland, S. (2000). An introduction to instrumental variables for epidemiologists. *International Journal of Epidemiology*, 29, 722–9. (Erratum: 2000, 29, 1102).

Greenland, S. (2002). Causality theory for policy uses of epidemiologic measures. In C.J. Murray, J.A. Salomon, C.D. Mathers, et al. (eds.) *Summary Measures of Population Health*, pp. 291–301. Cambridge, MA: Harvard University Press/World Health Organization.

Greenland, S. (2005). Epidemiologic measures and policy formulation: lessons from potential outcomes (with discussion). *Emerging Themes in Epidemiology*, 2, 1–4.

Greenland, S. (2012). Causal inference as a prediction problem: assumptions, identification, and evidence synthesis. In C. Berzuini, A.P. Dawid, and L. Bernardinelli (eds.) *Causal Inference: Statistical Perspectives and Applications*, pp. 43–58. Chichester: John Wiley and Sons.

Greenland S. (2014). Sensitivity analysis and bias analysis. In W. Ahrens and I. Pigeot (eds.) *Handbook of Epidemiology* (2nd ed.), pp. 685–706. New York: Springer.

Greenland, S., Gago-Domiguez, M., and Castellao, J.E. (2004). The value of risk-factor ('black-box') epidemiology (with discussion). *Epidemiology*, 15, 519–35.

Greenland, S., Lanes, S.F., and Jara, M. (2008). Estimating efficacy from randomized trials with discontinuations: the need for intent-to-treat design and g-estimation. *Clinical Trials*, 5, 5–13.

Greenland S. and Lash T.L. (2008). Bias analysis. In K.J. Rothman, S. Greenland, and T.L. Lash (eds.) *Modern Epidemiology* (3rd ed.), pp. 345–80. Philadelphia, PA: Lippincott.

Hernán, M.A. (2005). Hypothetical interventions to define causal effects—afterthought or prerequisite? *American Journal of Epidemiology*, 162, 618–20.

Hernán M.A. and VanderWeele T.J. (2011). Compound treatments and transportability of causal inference. *Epidemiology*, 22, 368–77.

Hill, A.B. (1965). The environment and disease: association or causation? *Proceedings of the Royal Society of Medicine*, 58, 295–300.

Holland, P.W. (1986). Statistics and causal inference. *Journal of the American Statistical Association*, 81, 945–60.

Holman, C.D.J., Arnold-Reed, D.E., de Klerk, N., McComb, C., and English, D.R. (2001). A psychometric experiment in causal inference to estimate evidential weights used by epidemiologists. *Epidemiology*, 12, 246–50.

Hume, D. (1739). *A Treatise of Human Nature*. L. A. Selby-Bigge (ed.) (1888). Oxford: Oxford University Press.

Kalbfleisch, J.D. and Prentice, R.L. (2002). *The Statistical Analysis of Failure-Time Data* (2nd ed.). New York: Wiley.

Kaufman, J.S. (2008). Epidemiologic analysis of racial/ethnic disparities: some fundamental issues and a cautionary example (with discussion). *Social Science & Medicine*, 66, 1659–80.

Kaufman, J.S. and Poole, C. (2000). Looking back on causal thinking in the health sciences. *Annual Review of Public Health*, 21, 101–19.

Kuhn, T.S. (1970). *The Structure of Scientific Revolutions* (2nd ed.). Chicago, IL: University of Chicago Press.

Lanes, S.F. and Poole, C. (1984). 'Truth in packaging?' The unwrapping of epidemiologic research. *Journal of Occupational Medicine*, 26, 571–4.

Lash, T.L., Fox, M.P., and Fink, A.K. (2009). *Applying Quantitative Bias Analysis to Epidemiologic Data*. Boston, MA: Springer Publishing Company.

Lipsitch, M., Tchetgen Tchetgen, E.J., and Cohen, T. (2010). Negative controls: a tool for detecting confounding and bias in observational studies. *Epidemiology*, 21, 383–8.

Maclure, M. (1985). Popperian refutation in epidemiology. *American Journal of Epidemiology*, 121, 343–50.

Mill, J.S.A. (1862). *System of logic, ratiocinative and inductive* (5th ed.). London: Parker, Son and Bowin. (Cited in: Clark, D.W., and MacMahon, B. (eds.) (1981). *Preventive and Community Medicine* (2nd ed.). Boston, MA: Little, Brown.

Morgan, S.L. and Winship, C. (2007). *Counterfactuals and Causal Inference: Methods and Principles for Social Research*. New York: Cambridge University Press.

Pearl, J. (2009). *Causality: Models, Reasoning and Inference* (2nd ed.). Cambridge: Cambridge University Press.

Phillips, C.V. and Goodman, K.J. (2004). The missed lessons of Sir Austin Bradford Hill. *Epidemiologic Perspectives and Innovation*, 1, 3.

Phillips, C.V. and Goodman, K.J. (2006). Causal criteria and counterfactuals; nothing more (or less) than scientific common sense. *Emerging Themes in Epidemiology*, 3, 5.

Poole, C. (2001). Causal values. *Epidemiology*, 12, 139–41.

Robins, J.M. and Greenland, S. (2000). Comment on 'Causal inference without counterfactuals' by A.P. Dawid. *Journal of the American Statistical Association*, 95, 477–82.

Robins, J.M., Greenland, S., and Hu, F. (1999). Estimation of the causal effect of time-varying exposure on the marginal means of a repeated binary outcome (with discussion). *Journal of the American Statistical Association*, 94, 687–712.

Rosenbaum, P.R. (2002) *Observational Studies* (2nd ed.). New York: Springer.

Rosenbaum, P.R. (2003). Does a dose–response relationship reduce sensitivity to hidden bias? *Biostatistics*, 4, 1–10.

Rothman, K.J., Greenland, S., and Lash, T.L. (2008). *Modern Epidemiology* (3rd ed.). Philadelphia, PA: Lippincott Williams & Wilkins.

Susser, M. (1991). What is a cause and how do we know one? A grammar for pragmatic epidemiology. *American Journal of Epidemiology*, 133, 635–48.

Taubes, G. (1995). Epidemiology faces its limits. *Science*, 269, 164–9.

United States Department of Health, Education and Welfare. (1964). *Smoking and Health: Report of the Advisory Committee to the Surgeon General of the Public Health Service*. PHS Publ No. 1103. Washington, DC: Government Printing Office.

VanderWeele, T.J. and Arah, O.A. (2011). Bias formulas for sensitivity analysis of unmeasured confounding for general outcomes, treatments and confounders. *Epidemiology*, 22, 42–52.

VanderWeele, T.J. and Hernán, M.A. (2012). Causal effects and natural laws: towards a conceptualization of causal counterfactuals for non-manipulable exposures with application to the effects of race and sex. In C. Berzuini, A.P. Dawid, and L. Bernardinelli (eds.) *Causal Inference: Statistical Perspectives and Applications*, pp. 101–13. Chichester: John Wiley and Sons.

VanderWeele T.J. and Hernán M.A. (2013). Causal inference under multiple versions of treatment. *Journal of Causal Inference*, 1(1), 1–20.

Weed, D.L. (1986). On the logic of causal inference. *American Journal of Epidemiology*, 123, 965–79.

Weed, D.L. and Gorelic, L.S. (1996). The practice of causal inference in cancer epidemiology. *Cancer Epidemiology, Biomarkers & Prevention*, 5, 303–11.

Weiss, N. (1981). Inferring causal relationships: elaboration of the criterion of 'dose–response'. *American Journal of Epidemiology*, 113, 487–90.

5.15

Systematic reviews and meta-analysis

Jimmy Volmink and Mike Clarke

Introduction to systematic reviews and meta-analysis

Reviewing and summarizing existing knowledge from studies that have addressed a particular topic (sometimes referred to as research, or evidence, synthesis) has long been recognized as an important scientific activity. At a meeting in 1884, Lord Rayleigh, a Professor of Physics at Cambridge University, noted, 'If, as is sometimes supposed, science consisted in nothing but the laborious accumulation of facts, it would soon come to a standstill, crushed, as it were, under its own weight. . . Two processes are thus at work side by side, the reception of new material and the digestion and assimilation of the old; and as both are essential we may spare ourselves the discussion of their relative importance' (Rayleigh 1885).

These remarks underscore the importance of understanding the cumulative nature of science, implying that new research should be guided by what is already known and that new research findings should be interpreted in the context of the totality of available evidence (Chalmers et al. 2002). In practice this means that new research should begin and end with an adequate review of other relevant research (Clark and Horton 2020; Clarke et al. 2010).

Reviews also play a critical role in guiding practitioners, policymakers, and consumers to make well-informed decisions and choices. The massive expansion in the volume of biomedical literature, beginning in the middle of the twentieth century, has made it increasingly difficult for healthcare decision-makers to keep up with the findings of individual studies. Reviews of the literature are thus important for taking stock of existing knowledge and making informed choices about healthcare and resource allocation (Mulrow 1995; Sackett et al. 1997; Chalmers and Glasziou 2009).

To the extent that they provide reliable summaries of research evidence, reviews can be extremely valuable. However, poorly conducted reviews drawing incorrect conclusions from the literature have the potential to cause serious harm to patients and populations, and waste much-needed resources (Chalmers 2003).

Rationale for systematic reviews

A number of obstacles to carrying out scientifically sound reviews have been identified. First, research reports are very widely dispersed and relevant papers may be hard to find. In the mid 1990s, it was estimated that some two million articles were published annually in more than 20,000 biomedical journals (Mulrow 1995) and there have been further increases since then. Furthermore, other useful scientific information is distributed in the 'grey literature' (e.g. books, theses, conference abstracts government and company reports) and on the Internet. Added to this, access to research is often biased (Hopewell et al. 2007b, 2009; Dwan et al. 2008). For instance, studies with 'negative' or 'disappointing' findings are less likely to be published. If they are, they are less likely than 'positive' studies to be published in full, in journals that are widely read, or in English. This means that limiting one's efforts to easily accessible studies may result in an over-optimistic view of reality. Another problem is that studies addressing the same question frequently produce conflicting findings which will require explanation, and careful efforts to compare and contrast different studies. Such inconsistencies in findings can be due to factors such as differences in study characteristics (participants, interventions, and outcomes), flaws in study conduct, or reporting (bias) or random error (the play of chance). To address these challenges, sound methods to identify, assess, and synthesize study findings are needed.

Unfortunately, scientific rigour has not always received sufficient attention in the conduct of literature reviews. A seminal study published in the 1980s demonstrated that reviews published in leading medical journals failed to use scientific methods for synthesizing research evidence (Mulrow 1987). Subsequent research showed that these shortcomings were widespread, often leading to recommendations that were not based on the best available evidence, and to inadequate healthcare being offered with deleterious effects on health outcomes. For example, in the field of cardiovascular medicine it was found that poorly conducted research syntheses had contributed to substantial delays in adopting effective interventions, while allowing other interventions to remain in use long after research had demonstrated that they were ineffective or harmful (Antman et al. 1992). Similar findings have been documented across a range of healthcare fields (Egger et al. 2001; Chalmers 2003; Oxman et al. 2007).

In recent years, the 'systematic review' has emerged as a response to these deficiencies (Chalmers and Altman 1995; Glasziou et al. 2001; Higgins and Green 2011; Khan et al. 2011). Systematic reviews use systematic, explicit, and reproducible methods to identify relevant studies, assess the risk of bias in primary studies, extract information, and synthesize findings. Systematic reviews often employ statistical methods to combine data from similar

Table 5.15.1 Comparison of systematic and traditional reviews

Systematic review	Traditional review
States the methods of the review	Often does not state the methods of the review
Answers a focused question or tests a hypothesis; usually narrow in scope	May have a clear question but it often involves general discussion with no stated hypothesis; often very broad in scope
Attempts to locate all relevant studies to minimize publication and other biases	Usually does not attempt to locate all relevant studies
Uses explicit eligibility criteria to determine which studies will be included in the review to prevent selection bias on behalf of the reviewer	Usually does not specify why some studies are included and others excluded
Systematically appraises the methods of the included studies to determine possibility of bias in these studies and sources of heterogeneity between the study results	Often does not assess the risk of bias in the studies or acknowledge differences in their methods
Bases results on studies that are most methodologically sound	Often does not distinguish between methodologically sound and unsound studies
May combine study results statistically in a meta-analysis	Often does not pool results in a meta-analysis
Results illustrate true level of heterogeneity of data, allowing quantification of uncertainty	Results often presented in black and white terms without indicating uncertainty or variability

Source: data from Needleman IG, A guide to systematic reviews, *Journal of Clinical Periodontology*, Volume 29, Issue Supplement 3, pp. 6–9, Copyright © 2002 and Petticrew M., Systematic reviews from astronomy to zoology: myths and misconceptions, *British Medical Journal*, Volume 322, pp. 98–101, Copyright © 2001.

studies (known as meta-analysis) in order to obtain more precise estimates than those derived from the individual studies included in reviews. Table 5.15.1 provides a comparison of the typical characteristics of systematic versus more traditional reviews.

In recent years, systematic reviews have gained wide recognition as an essential tool for evidence-based decision-making in healthcare (Petticrew 2001; McMichael et al. 2005; Lavis 2009; Dickersin 2010). For instance, when evaluating the effects of interventions they are considered as the 'gold standard', occupying the top of the 'hierarchy of evidence'. This hierarchy is typically depicted in the form of a pyramid with expert opinion at its base, followed by various types of observational studies, then randomized trials and finally systematic reviews. Because the risk of bias decreases when moving from the bottom to the top of the pyramid, the position of systematic reviews in the hierarchy reflects the fact that they are regarded as the most reliable form of evidence. A further indication of their general acceptance into the mainstream comes from two other developments: funding agencies are beginning to require that investigators provide evidence from up-to-date systematic reviews that a new trial is justified, and some journals now require authors of new trials to report the findings from a systematic review which puts their trial into context (Clark and Horton 2010).

In this chapter, we describe the steps involved in conducting a systematic review: formulation of a review question, identification of relevant studies, extraction of data, assessment of bias in included studies, synthesis of the data, interpreting the evidence, and writing up and updating the review. Further details on each of these steps can be found in published handbooks and guidelines (Liberati et al. 2009; Higgins and Green 2011), as well as in various texts on systematic reviews (Glasziou et al. 2001; Borenstein et al. 2009; Higgins and Green 2011; Khan et al. 2011).

The review protocol

As should be the case for any new piece of scientific research, a systematic review begins with the preparation of a protocol in which the objectives and proposed methods are documented. In a systematic review this is important for reducing bias that may result from reviewers making judgements during the review process that are influenced by their knowledge of individual study findings.

Publication of the review protocol in a publicly accessible register is encouraged (Liberati et al. 2009; *PLoS Medicine* Editors 2011; Stewart et al. 2012). This not only improves transparency and allows detection of any changes to the protocol that may have occurred during the process of the review, but also reduces the likelihood of unnecessary duplication of effort and facilitates peer review of the intended methods (Silagy et al. 2002; Straus and Moher 2010; Booth et al. 2011). PROSPERO, developed by the Centre for Reviews and Dissemination at the University of York, England (Booth et al. 2011) and the *Cochrane Database of Systematic Reviews* (http://www.thecochranelibrary.com) are examples of registers of systematic reviews. Certain funders, such as the National Institutes of Health Research in the United Kingdom and the Canadian Institutes of Health Research, now require that all systematic reviews they support are registered (Stewart et al. 2012).

Formulating the review question

The most critical step in preparing a systematic review is the formulation of a clearly defined question, since this influences all subsequent steps of the review. Review questions may address a wide variety of issues, such as the incidence or prevalence of disease (Pendlebury and Rothwell 2009), accuracy of a diagnostic test (Doust et al. 2004), disease aetiology (Renehan et al. 2008), effects of curative or preventive interventions (Siegfried et al. 2009), economic evaluations (Pérez Velasco et al. 2012), or disease prognosis (Damman et al. 2007). These questions typically lead to the search for, and synthesis of, quantitative studies.

Systematic reviews of qualitative studies, despite presenting some unique methodological challenges, are also possible and are growing in popularity (Britten et al. 2002; Munro et al. 2007; Atkins et al. 2008). Such reviews tend to focus on the framing of a health problem (Mays 2005; Lavis et al. 2009) or explore barriers to, and facilitators of, policy or programme implementation (Innvaer 2002; Child 2012). These may be helpful for explaining why certain interventions do or do not work.

The review question may have a broad or narrow scope. For example, when evaluating the effects of interventions to promote adherence to therapy, a review could assess all interventions in any patient using chronic medication. Alternatively, the review question may be limited to a particular kind of intervention (e.g. economic support) in a particular group (e.g. adults) with a specific disease (e.g. tuberculosis) and explore a specific outcome (e.g. cure or treatment completion).

Decisions about a review's scope will be influenced by considerations such as the purpose, intended relevance and envisaged impact of the review, the theoretical, biological, and epidemiological rationale, and the potential for obtaining valid answers to the review question or for generalizing the findings of the review (O'Connor et al. 2011). Often, the scope will depend on the resources available for conducting the review. Although reviews with a broad scope tend to be more useful than those with a limited scope for generalizing findings across different participants, interventions, and settings, they may present a higher risk of heterogeneity ('mixing apples and oranges'), which can make it difficult to interpret their findings (O'Connor et al. 2011).

Regardless of how wide the intended scope of a review may be, it is always important to formulate the question as precisely as possible. The reason for this is that the question has a direct impact on all subsequent aspects of the review process, in particular the eligibility criteria for including or excluding studies and the efficiency of the search for relevant studies. A review question that is imprecise or unfocused may result in the reviewer finding a large amount of potentially relevant literature, which will take a long time to screen in order to find the truly relevant articles for answering the question.

A well-structured question for a review of the effects of an intervention will typically specify the following key components: participants (*p*opulation or problem), *i*ntervention (or indicator), comparator (*c*ontrol), and *o*utcome(s) of interest. The acronym 'PICO' is therefore often used as a reminder of these specific aspects of the question and its use can be illustrated as follows: 'In patients receiving treatment for clinical tuberculosis (P) does a policy of direct observation of treatment (I) versus a policy of self-treatment (C) lead to different treatment success rates (O)?'

The PICO approach can also be used for formulating review questions that are not related to the benefits or harms of interventions. Regarding aetiology or risk, one might, for example, ask: 'Are women (P) who smoke during pregnancy (I) compared to women who do not smoke (C) more likely to give birth to children who develop asthma during the first 5 years of life (O)?'

Once a review question has been constructed, it can be converted into one or more specific review objectives. Thus, with reference to the first example of a review question given earlier, the objective could be: 'To compare directly observed therapy with self-administration of treatment on treatment success rates in patients receiving treatment for clinically active tuberculosis.'

Identifying relevant literature and setting eligibility criteria

The most time-consuming step of a systematic review is usually the identification of studies which should be included in the review. This requires the development of an efficient search strategy, a process which begins with the choice of study eligibility criteria.

Building on the defined review question and associated objectives, eligibility criteria for inclusion or exclusion of studies in the review can be specified. These eligibility criteria are usually defined in terms of the type of participants, interventions, and comparisons (and less frequently the outcomes). In addition to these 'PICO' components, the types of study to be included in the review are usually also specified at this stage. Describing each of these components in some detail will assist the development of the search strategy, as well as the selection of relevant studies. An example of this is provided in Box 5.15.1.

Defining the participants or problem (P)

Participants could be described in terms of sociodemographic characteristics, such as age, sex, ethnicity, and educational status,

---

Box 5.15.1 Study eligibility criteria specified in a review of adenoidectomy versus non-surgical management or tympanostomy tubes in children with otitis media

- (P) The participants included children up to 18 years of age diagnosed with otitis media.
- (I/C) Studies that compared adenoidectomy versus non-surgical management only (defined as watchful observation and medical treatment): adenoidectomy and unilateral tympanostomy tube versus unilateral tympanostomy tube only; and adenoidectomy with bilateral tympanostomy tubes versus bilateral tympanostomy tubes only.
- (O) The primary outcome was the proportion of time children had effusion, diagnosed with or without tympanometry. Secondary outcomes were occurrence of acute otitis media, occurrence of otitis media with effusion, and the mean hearing level. Occurrence of the condition was defined as the number of episodes per year, number of days per episode per year, and the proportion of children with recurrent episodes.
- (S) Only randomized trials were considered for inclusion and only those that had follow-up of participants of at least 6 months.

Source: data from Van den Aardweg MTA et al., Adenoidectomy for otitis media in children, *Cochrane Database of Systematic Reviews* 2010, Issue 1, Art. No.:CD0077810, Copyright © 2010 The Cochrane Collaboration. Published by John Wiley & Sons, Ltd.

as well as the setting in which the study occurred (e.g. hospital or community based). It may also be important to provide a specific definition of the target health condition under consideration. Where restrictions based on population characteristics (e.g. people living in low- and middle-income countries) are used, these need to be explained clearly. It is often better to include studies covering a wide spectrum of participants, because differences across different groups can always be explored in the review at a later stage. If a narrow range of patients is specified at the outset of the review, there will be no such variability to explore at later stages of the review.

Defining the types of interventions (I) and comparisons (C)

For reviews of the effects of interventions, it is important to clearly define the intervention being evaluated: what is being delivered, at what intensity, how often, who delivers it, for how long, when it is delivered and what training was given to people involved in the delivery?

Reviewers also need to specify whether the intervention will be compared with an inactive or 'neutral' control intervention (e.g. placebo, standard care, no treatment) or an active control intervention (e.g. different regimen of the same drug or a different kind of therapy).

Defining the types of outcomes (O)

All outcomes that are relevant to end-users of the review, such as patients, healthcare practitioners, and policymakers, should ideally be included. For this reason, outcomes usually do not form part of the eligibility criteria for deciding whether or not an individual study should be included in the review. Reviewers are encouraged to include important outcomes even if they have not been addressed in the original studies, because this could help identify gaps in the evidence base that need to be addressed in future research.

Further, it may be necessary to consider whether the outcomes of interest are measured objectively (e.g. death or number of strokes) or subjectively as rated by clinician, patient, or carer (e.g. disability scales), and whether measuring instruments would have required validation. The timing of outcome measurement may also be important to define, for example, short-term compared to long-term outcomes.

It is advisable to separate outcomes into primary outcomes that are critical for informing decision-making (or that can be measured objectively) and secondary (additional) outcomes that may be of interest for other reasons (or that are less objectively assessed). Reviews should evaluate at least one desirable (beneficial) and one undesirable (adverse) outcome as both are important for making informed healthcare decisions. Various frameworks to evaluate adverse effects in systematic reviews have been proposed (Loke et al. 2007; Guyatt et al. 2011). Reviewers should also consider using pre-defined core outcome sets to help them to decide which outcomes to use in their review (Williamson et al. 2012; Kirkham et al. 2013).

Defining the study design (S)

Based on the review question, a determination needs to be made about the types of study design that are likely to provide the most reliable answers. For instance, it may be appropriate to limit the review to randomized trials in the case of questions about the effects of an intervention, to cross-sectional studies for reviews of diagnostic accuracy, or to cohort studies if the intention is to answer a question about disease prognosis. Reasons for including and excluding specific study designs need to be made explicit in the review.

In the real world, researchers sometimes conduct reviews using study designs that are not ideally suited to a particular question, perhaps because more reliable studies do not exist. This can pose challenges to the interpretation of the evidence, because of inconsistency of the findings, which limits decision-making. The case of male circumcision as a public health intervention for the prevention of HIV acquisition in heterosexual men provides an instructive example of such a scenario. In 1995, a Cochrane Review commissioned by the World Health Organization assessed all 37 observational studies that had studied this relationship (Siegfried et al. 2005). Although many studies showed an association between male circumcision and HIV prevention, the review documented substantial between-study variation in the findings. This was particularly marked in studies conducted in the general population, as opposed to those conducted among high-risk groups. The authors, because of their concerns about residual confounding in these studies, concluded that the evidence available was insufficient to guide policy and that the findings of randomized trials should be awaited. A few years later, a Cochrane Review update (Siegfried et al. 2009) evaluated the results of the three trials which had been completed subsequent to the publication of the original review. It found strong evidence that medical male circumcision reduces the acquisition of HIV by heterosexual men by between 38 per cent and 66 per cent over 24 months, with a low incidence of adverse events. Fig. 5.15.1 presents the findings of the observational studies and trials conducted in the general population, showing the marked differences in consistency in their results, as well as the results of the subsequent randomized trials.

Search strategy

Once the study eligibility has been determined, the reviewer can proceed to the development of the search strategy. The aim should be to develop a search strategy which has high sensitivity (defined as the number of relevant reports identified divided by the total number of all relevant reports in existence) and high precision (i.e. the number of relevant reports identified divided by the total number of reports identified) (Lefebvre et al. 2011). In order to reduce the impact of reporting biases, it is important to search for articles published in any language, as well as those that are unpublished or available only in the grey literature (Hopewell et al. 2007c).

In the biomedical sciences, there are three key electronic sources of published reports of clinical trials: MEDLINE (http://www.ncbi.nlm.nih.gov/pubmed), EMBASE (http://www.elsevier.com/online-tools/embase), and CENTRAL (Cochrane Central Register of Controlled Trials) (http://www.thecochranelibrary.com). A comprehensive search strategy requires each of these databases to be searched (Lefebvre et al. 2011) and others as appropriate to the review. As these three databases tend to have a North American and European bias, it might also be worth searching other databases such as LILACS (Latin American Caribbean

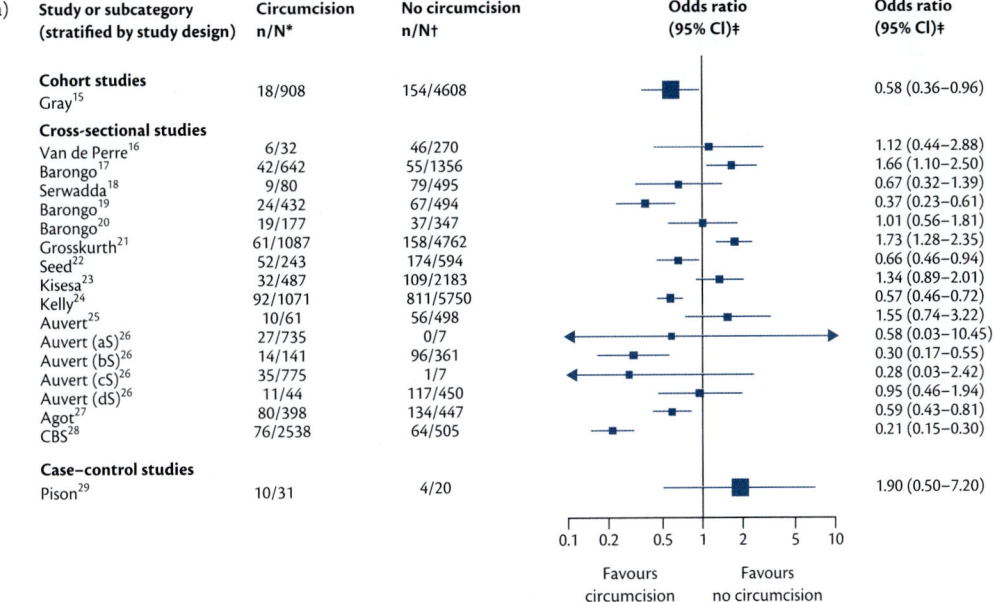

Fig. 5.15.1 The relationship between male circumcision and heterosexual acquisition of HIV in men in studies conducted in the general population. (a) Observational studies. Reprinted from *The Lancet Infectious Diseases*, Volume 5, Issue 3, Siegfried N et al., HIV and male circumcision–a systematic review with assessment of the quality of studies, pp.165–73, Copyright © 2005, with permission from Elsevier, http://www.sciencedirect.com/science/journal/14733099/5/3 (b) Randomized trials. Reproduced with permission from Siegfried N, Muller M, Deeks JJ, Volmink J, *Male circumcision for prevention of heterosexual acquisition of HIV in men. Cochrane Database of Systematic Reviews* 2009, Issue 2. Art. No.: CD003362. Copyright © 2009 The Cochrane Collaboration. Published by John Wiley & Sons, Ltd.

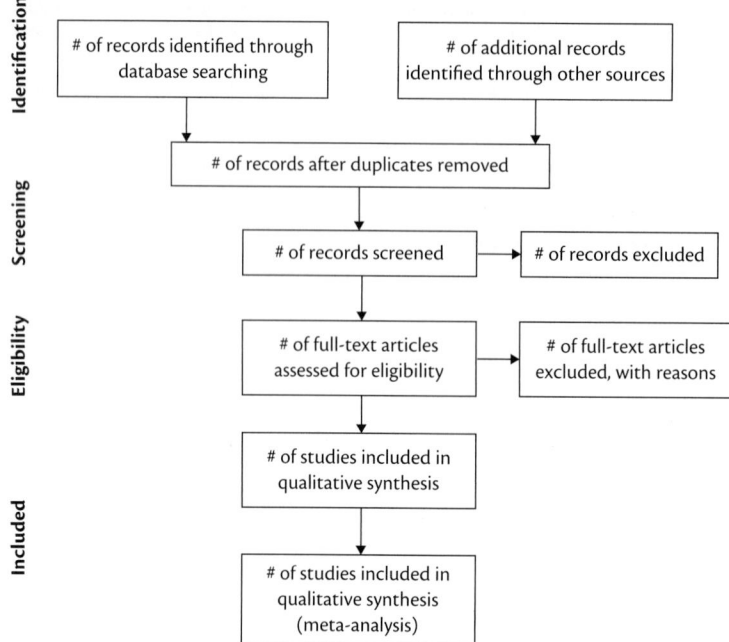

Fig. 5.15.2 Flow diagram of study selection process (from PRISMA guidelines).

Health Sciences Literature) (http://lilacs.bvsalud.org/en/) and African HealthLine (http://www.nisc.co.za/databases?id=62). It may also be important to include subject-specific databases, such as PsycINFO (www.apa.org/pubs/databases/psycinfo/index.aspx) (for psychology and related behavioural and social sciences), as well as Internet search engines, such as Google Scholar (http://scholar.google.co.uk/).

Strategies can be used to identify both free-text words in the database, and controlled terms (called MeSH, or Medical Subject Headings, in MEDLINE and EMTREE in EMBASE) which are used as keywords. Search strategies need to include the key terms in the review question, and use the Boolean operators ('AND', 'OR') to produce a search that is most likely to find relevant studies. Because of the complexities inherent in designing search strategies, it is advisable to seek assistance from librarians or information specialists before embarking on a literature search (Lefebvre et al. 2011).

The next step in searching for relevant articles involves screening of reference lists of all studies identified from the electronic search, including previously published reviews, to identify any missed studies (Horsley et al. 2011). It is also legitimate to conduct handsearching of specific journals that are not indexed in electronic databases to make sure that no studies that meet the review inclusion criteria have been missed (Hopewell et al. 2007a). Finally, unpublished studies and 'grey literature' such as conference abstracts, research reports, policy documents, dissertations, book chapters, and personal correspondence, should be sought by contacting authors of identified papers and relevant organizations, including pharmaceutical companies and by searching websites (Hopewell et al. 2007c). It is also important to identify ongoing studies, for example, by searching prospective trials registers, as these may be needed for future updates of the review (Ghersi et al. 2009).

Application of the search strategy typically identifies many (sometimes thousands of) potentially relevant papers. At this stage, two reviewers should read the title and abstract of each report to determine whether the study should be included or excluded based on whether or not it meets the pre-specified eligibility criteria (Edwards et al. 2002). Where there is uncertainty, a copy of the full paper needs to be obtained for further scrutiny. The two reviewers should compare their results, and resolve any differences through consensus or by using a third person to arbitrate when required (Higgins and Deeks 2011). The search strategy should be carefully conducted to ensure reproducibility and its outcome clearly presented, ideally by means of a flowchart as recommended by PRISMA (Fig. 5.15.2) (Liberati et al. 2009).

Data collection and extraction

Deciding on what data to collect

The specific items of data to be collected from included studies will be influenced by the goals of the systematic review. However, the following items should generally be considered (Higgins and Deeks 2011):

◆ Eligibility of the study for inclusion or reason for exclusion.

◆ Study methods, such as study design and duration, as well as items that will be used to assess the risk of bias, such as sequence generation, allocation concealment, and blinding.

◆ Data regarding participants (e.g. sex, age, ethnicity, and education level) and setting (e.g. institution and geographic location) which may influence the size of the effect estimate or assist in assessing the applicability of results.

◆ The number of intervention groups and the details of the specific interventions involved. Any information relating to the fidelity with which the intervention was administered (i.e. the extent to which it was implemented as planned) should be obtained.

This is particularly important in preventive or complex interventions, which are usually implemented under 'real-world' conditions.

◆ Information regarding the outcomes such as their definitions, time points at which they were measured, and units of measurement should be collected. Usually, this is done only for those outcomes pre-specified in the review protocol. However, listing all other outcomes reported in the included study may enable analysis of risk of bias due to selective outcome reporting.

◆ Results should be collected only for those outcomes pre-specified in the protocol. For a meta-analysis it is also necessary to collect the data for analysis (see next section on data extraction).

◆ Other information to be collected could include funding source, details of ethics approval, name of contact of authors, citations, etc.

Once the data to be collected have been identified, it is necessary to design appropriate data collection forms. These may be electronic or paper-based, depending on the preference of reviewers. Paper-based forms allow extraction of data anywhere, and they are easier to create and use, whereas electronic forms offer the advantages of data extraction and entry in one step, programming of forms, and better storage, sorting, and retrieval of data in reviews with large number of studies (Higgins and Deeks 2011). Usually several forms, serving different purposes, are used.

Data extraction

Data extraction refers to the process of recording all the relevant data from the included studies onto data collection forms. Piloting data collection forms using a representative sample of studies is recommended. This will help to identify data that may not initially have been considered for collection, and to detect coding that might be unclear (Higgins and Deeks 2011).

To reduce the risk of errors during data extraction, it is advisable that at least two reviewers, working independently, are involved in extracting the data. Any disagreements between the reviewers should be resolved through consensus or arbitration by a third person. Blinding data extractors to study details, such as names of authors and results, may decrease the risk of bias (Jadad et al.

1996). However, as the evidence for this practice is not conclusive (Berlin 1997), routine blinding of data extractors is not currently recommended.

It is important to keep in mind that a single study may have been reported in more than one paper. Reviewers should be vigilant to the existence of the often covert practice of reporting the same data in different journals or even in the same journal at different times (Von Elm et al. 2004). The inclusion of duplicate publications with repeated observations in a systematic review will introduce bias on account of undue weight given to the findings concerned (Tramer et al. 1997). Where multiple papers arising from the same study report different data, it is, however, necessary to include all relevant articles in order to ensure that data extraction is complete.

The type of summary data needed for subsequent meta-analysis will vary according to the type of outcome involved. For dichotomous outcomes, the numbers of participants who did and did not experience the outcome in each intervention group should be extracted. In the case of continuous outcomes, the mean and standard deviation, as well as the number of participants in each group, will be needed.

Where the desired summary measures are not reported, they may be derived from other statistics. For example, numbers of participants may be derived from percentages or effect estimates, such as odds ratios. Sometimes study authors will have to be contacted for clarification.

Assessing risk of bias

Once the data extraction is completed, each study should be carefully assessed for the risk of bias in the design, conduct, analysis, or reporting of a study. The main aim of this exercise is to guide interpretation of the findings of the review. In extreme cases, one may choose to exclude a study which is so fundamentally flawed that its results are not valid.

There are several methods for assessing the risk of bias. The Cochrane Collaboration recommend a 'domain-based evaluation' for clinical trials in which judgements are made about the risk of bias in each of the following domains: selection bias, performance bias, detection bias, attrition bias, reporting bias, and other bias (Table 5.15.2).

Table 5.15.2 Domain-based scheme for classification of bias in included studies

Type of bias	Description	Relevant domains
Selection bias	Systematic differences in the baseline characteristics of the groups that are compared	• Sequence generation • Allocation concealment
Performance bias	Systematic differences between groups in the care that is provided, or in exposure to factors other than the interventions of interest	• Blinding of participants, personnel and outcome assessors • Other potential threats to validity
Attrition bias	Systematic differences between groups in withdrawals from study	• Incomplete outcome data • Blinding of participants, personnel and outcome assessors
Detection bias	Systematic difference between groups in how outcomes are determined	• Blinding of participants, personnel and outcome assessors • Other potential threats to validity
Reporting bias	Systematic differences between reported and unreported findings	• Selective outcome reporting

Adapted with permission from Higgins JPT, Altman DG, and Sterne JAC on behalf of the Cochrane Statistical Methods Group and the Cochrane Bias Methods Group, Chapter 8 'Assessing risk of bias in included studies' in Higgins JPT and Green S (eds), *Cochrane Handbook for Systematic Reviews of Interventions*, Version 5.1.0 updated March 2011, The Cochrane Collaboration, Copyright © 2011, available from http://www.cochrane-handbook.org.

A judgement relating to the risk of bias for each item is assigned, which is supported by a description of what was done in the study. The judgement is indicated by answering a pre-specified question (e.g. 'Was the allocation sequence adequately generated?') which requires a 'yes' representing a low risk of bias, 'no', a high risk of bias, and 'unclear' an unclear or unknown risk of bias. Criteria for judging the risk of bias are provided in The Cochrane Collaboration's 'risk of bias tool'. The final step involves the risk of bias assessments being summarized across all domains for each study, and across all studies by indicating the proportion of domains studies with low, unclear, or high risk of bias.

Risk of bias is assessed based on the information in the reports of trials. Sometimes, the reported information may be insufficient to make critical judgements about the methods of a study. In these cases, it is important to contact the study authors to clarify any issues regarding study design or missing data that are not described clearly in the report (Mullan et al. 2009; Higgins et al. 2011).

Summarizing the evidence

One of the reasons for conducting a systematic review is that the individual studies are too small to provide a reliable and robust answer on their own. The review seeks to bring together the studies of relevance to the question in order to avoid undue emphasis on the findings of any single study, to minimize bias and to maximize statistical power by combining all the relevant data if this would be appropriate. This will help to overcome the biases of focusing on the findings of individual studies, and the effects of chance that may lead to an over- or underestimate of the true effect. Even when a randomized trial is well conducted and has minimized the possibility of biases that might overwhelm any true difference between the interventions being compared in that study, it is still susceptible to the effects of chance and the mathematical testing that is done to assess this cannot provide certainty on whether or not the result was distorted by chance, or on the size or direction of any distortion. However, combining the data from multiple studies in a meta-analysis will serve to minimize the effects of chance, such that any over- or underestimate is likely to be smaller than that in a single study. Even when the mathematical combination of the results of studies is not done, presenting them all in the same place and in the same way helps the reader to compare and contrast the studies in the review.

This provision of a summary of the evidence helps the systematic review fulfil the purpose of placing existing research in context, ensuring that new research is designed and implemented in the most appropriate way. And, when systematic reviews are used as part of the presentation of the findings of a new study, it ensures that those findings are seen in proper context (Clarke et al. 2010).

In deciding on how to summarize the evidence identified for the review, the reviewer might use a quantitative approach seeking to combine the results in a meta-analysis, a qualitative approach in which each study's findings are kept separate, or both. The choice about these techniques depends to some extent on the heterogeneity in the outcomes measured across the studies, since if there is too much variation in the outcomes that were measured, the measurement tools that were used, how or when they were used, or in how the results are made available, it might be impossible to combine the data. Efforts are underway in many areas of healthcare to help overcome this by reaching consensus on standardized core outcome sets, and the COMET Initiative is bringing such examples together and facilitating the development of further core outcome sets (Williamson et al. 2012), but the challenges in the existing literature can be substantial. These challenges, which might prevent the combining of data in the review, can also make it much more difficult to compare and contrast the included studies.

Regardless of whether they will do a meta-analysis, reviewers need to decide how much or how little information to extract and report for each study, and the sources to be used, especially if published reports are inadequate (Clarke and Stewart 1994). In compiling as complete a dataset as feasible and sensible, the principles of minimizing systematic biases and chances effects must be applied. If a meta-analysis is to be done, compatible data should be sought for all relevant trials and, if these data are not available, the proportion of missing data needs to be small enough to allow the reviewer and the reader to feel confident that the review's findings are robust. In particular, the reviewers need to consider whether the unavailability of the data is due to results-related bias. If it is, the meta-analysis of available data will itself be biased, leading to potentially misleading overall findings and conclusions.

There are several benefits of doing a meta-analysis if it is appropriate so to do. It provides a more precise estimate of the treatment effect, helping one to be more confident about the size of any effect. There is more statistical power to detect small effects, which may be clinically significant; and it helps in the evaluation of the applicability of the results to other settings. However, one of the important decisions that a reviewer has to take is whether the trials are similar enough that averaging their results is meaningful. This is done by considering whether there is excessive heterogeneity in the design of the studies (including the interventions and participants studied). Statistical tests are also available to assess whether the results of a series of trials might differ from each other by more than chance (Higgins et al. 2003).

In seeking data and other information from the original researchers to prepare their summary, the reviewers might try to gather aggregate data, for example, by asking the original researchers to complete a table; or they might seek data at a finer level, such as that for individual participants. This gathering of data from the original researchers might make the dataset available for the review more complete, up to date, and accurate than anything that was previously available. It also helps the review to perform standardized analyses across the studies (Stewart et al. 1995).

A variety of techniques for combining results from separate studies in a meta-analysis is available to the reviewer (Cooper and Rosenthal 1980; Deeks 2002). The overriding principle of most of these is that each study is analysed separately and the overall result for the review comes from combining these results from the individual statistics. In this two-step approach, participants in one study are only directly compared with others in the same study and it is now fairly standard for the results of these analyses to be shown as a forest plot (e.g. Fig. 5.15.1). This allows the reader to see the contribution of each study (Lewis and Clarke 2001; Glasziou and Sanders 2002; Higgins et al. 2003).

In planning and conducting the statistical analyses for any review, careful consideration needs to be given to the types of analyses, the options available for these analyses, and the reliability of the overall average. Once again, the effects of chance and bias should be considered carefully. This is for the overall results and for any subgroup analyses that are conducted; especially if decisions about the analyses to conduct and present are due to fore-knowledge of the likely findings (Counsell et al. 1994). This can be a particular problem for systematic reviews, since they are retrospective research and some or all of the findings of the included studies might already be known to the reviewers before they reach the stage of planning or conducting the analyses.

Subgroup analyses present the reviewer with the dilemma that having brought together the data from multiple studies, they might now wish to break it apart again into subgroups to explore the effects in different patients or settings, or when different interventions were used. This needs to be done with caution because of the possibility that spurious, chance results will be obtained; which will be misinterpreted as being of importance in making decisions about healthcare (Counsell et al. 1994; Clarke and Halsey 2001; Bender et al. 2008). Even if there is an a priori reason to expect a subgroup analysis to show something different to the overall result, this is no guarantee that a statistically significant difference is reliable clinically. This is because the more analyses are done, the more likely it is that statistically significant results will be found, even when there is truly no difference between the subgroups. Subgroup analyses in a systematic review should be regarded as a way of showing that the direction of effect is the same across different types of patient or as a generator of a hypothesis for testing in future research. Regardless of whether subgroup analyses are done, it is often more reliable to assume that the overall result is as good, and if not a better, estimate of the relative effects of treatments in the particular type of patient than that obtained by looking at the results for just these types of patient in the review. This is because the effect of chance will be smaller for the overall result than it would be on the result in any subgroup.

Systematic reviews might also include sensitivity analyses, which ideally should also be planned in advance. A sensitivity analysis is used to determine how sensitive the results of the systematic review are to the decisions that the reviewer took about how the review was done. They are particularly useful where there is uncertainty about the choices that a reviewer needs to make. For example, sensitivity analyses could be used to determine the effect of including studies published in languages other than English, of using data from studies assessed to be of poor quality, or of choosing one statistical technique over another.

The multiplicity which might arise in a systematic review because of the variety of outcomes, and measures of these outcomes, available is compounded further by the variety of ways to analyse these in order to obtain an estimate of the difference between the intervention and the comparator. If a meta-analysis is done, this multiplicity will arise at the level of the overall estimate of effect. If the results of each study are kept separate, with no combination of these in a meta-analysis, it arises at the study level. Typical effect measures in systematic reviews that use dichotomous, or binary, data are estimates of risk (either a ratio or absolute difference) and odds (almost always a ratio).

The decision on which effect measure to use should, ideally, be taken when the systematic review is being planned. It should be based on the mathematical appropriateness of the effect measure for the type of data to be analysed. As with any of the decisions when conducting a systematic review, changes to this a priori plan should be kept to a minimum, and should be documented and reported. Any changes that are made because of the reviewers' preference for one result over another need to be treated with particular caution, because of the risk of bias. In meta-analyses of dichotomous data, it is most common for the odds ratio, risk ratio, or both to be used (Deeks and Altman 2001).

In some cases, the original intention for the effect measure will turn out to be mathematically inappropriate or suboptimal because of the nature of the data identified for inclusion in the review. This should be dealt with and described in a transparent way by the reviewers. They should avoid conducting multiple exploratory analyses using different effect measures and then focusing on the analysis that generates their preferred result. In circumstances where a variety of effects measures are appropriate, the different analyses may be conducted, and all that are conducted should be reported. The greatest confidence in the findings of the review would then arise if there is consistency among the results from the different effect measures. If the results differ in important ways, the reviewers and the users of the review need to be cautious.

If the meta-analysis uses continuous data, the typical effect measure will be the mean difference. If the data from the included studies relate to the same outcome but they were measured in different ways, for example, by using a variety of scales to measure satisfaction with the provision of care, this needs to be standardized. The reviewers might also have the option of dividing the continuous data into 'high' and 'low' in order to dichotomize the outcome and, thereby, use effect measures such as the risk ratio or odds ratio. Particular caution is needed in such circumstances, especially if there is no natural or well-accepted threshold for this splitting of the data.

Writing up the review

In recent years, there has been increasing recognition of the value of guidelines on the reporting of a wide variety of types of research study, including randomized trials (Schulz et al. 2010), observational research (von Elm et al. 2007), and studies of diagnostic test accuracy (Bossuyt et al. 2003). The principal guide for the reporting of systematic reviews is PRISMA (Moher et al. 2009), which updated the QUOROM statement (Moher et al. 1999).

This section of this chapter outlines some of the key elements in the reporting of a review, which should help both with the preparation of the report and with its use. When preparing a report of a systematic review, though, it is important to bear in mind what the reader will be looking for. The traditional format of scientific papers of Introduction, Methods, Results, and Discussion is used in the following, but the reports of some reviews might change this order, or move some content to appendices or supplementary papers, depending on the interests and needs of their readers.

Title for the review

The title might flow naturally from the question for the review, containing elements relating to the population being studied, interventions or actions, the outcome of most interest, the study designs incorporated into the review, and the fact that the research being reported is a systematic review. The title should help the reader to decide whether the review is potentially relevant to them and might be particularly important in ensuring that the review is retrieved by people searching for research in the particular area. Some titles might be declarative, very briefly summarizing the main finding of their review, but this might not be possible in reviews covering more than one intervention, population, or outcome, where there are multiple important findings.

Question and purpose for the review

One of the distinguishing features of systematic reviews over more traditional reviews is the use of a clear research question at the design stage of the review. Formulating and clarifying the question at the outset of the review and at the start of its report is important for the reviewer, and then for the reader. The question will also help to reveal the purpose of the review, which might have been to provide evidence to guide future practice, or to map out existing research to help design a new, definitive study. For example, the question might be 'What are the effects of an incentive scheme to encourage exercise in the adult population?', or 'What types of incentive scheme to encourage exercise in the adult population have been tested in trials?', or 'How have trials of incentive schemes to encourage exercise in the adult population been assessed?'.

A systematic review might contain more than one question and comparison, and this should also be made clear early in the report. For example, the review might cover the comparison of an intervention with usual care, comparisons of different forms of the intervention, or comparisons (direct or indirect) between the intervention and alternative strategies.

Background

Setting the scene for the review will help orientate the reader to the topic and is also an opportunity to explain the importance and relevance of the review. The Background section might provide details on how common the circumstances or condition under investigation are; how the intervention was developed, how it might work and how common it is in practice; and any relevant studies that are already likely to be well known. Information on the consequences and severity of the outcomes being assessed might be helpful. It might also be important to set out the reasons for conducting the review in a particular way, especially if there are alternatives that might be in the minds of the reader. If the review had a pre-prepared protocol or was prospectively registered, this could also be stated in the background section.

Inclusion and exclusion criteria

In providing the eligibility criteria for a review, it may be important to be clear that these are what the reviewers sought, which will not necessarily be matched completely by what they found and were able to include in the review. For example, the review might have looked for a variety of interventions to protect factory workers from noise but found that only a few of the commonly used strategies had been tested in research (Verbeek et al. 2012). For most reviews, the eligibility criteria can be set out under domains, as discussed earlier in the chapter in relation to the use of PICO. This would identify the types of participants, interventions, actions or strategies, outcome measures, and types of study design.

The types of participants should include information on the types of people that would be eligible. This might contain information about personal characteristics such as sex, age, socioeconomic group, and diagnosis, as well as information about their

setting. The types of interventions, actions, and strategies covers what was to happen to the participants, and needs to contain information on any interventions, actions, and strategies that were used for comparative purposes. Types of outcome measures might be divided into primary and secondary outcome measures. It may also be helpful to distinguish 'outcomes' (e.g. depression) from 'outcome measures' (e.g. the instrument used to measure depression and the timing and application of the instrument). If there is a core outcome set relevant to the circumstance of the review, this might be referred to in this section (Williamson et al. 2012). Finally, the types of studies sets out which research designs were eligible for review.

Within the eligibility criteria, providing both inclusion and exclusion criteria can help clarify what would definitely be eligible for the review, and what would not be. This should not simply include 'mirror images' of the inclusion criteria in the exclusion criteria. For example, if the inclusion criteria require that people were living in residential care homes, it is superfluous to mention the exclusion of people who live in other settings. Rather, the exclusion criteria might be used to note that a subpopulation of people who would otherwise be eligible are not eligible, such as people in the care homes who are under the age of 60 years.

Methods

The authors of the review should describe what they had intended to do, and what they were able to do given the material that they found for their review. If they had a protocol for the review, this could be referred to here. As a minimum, the Methods section should provide details of the search strategy, how eligibility was determined, methods for data extraction or collection, and the techniques used to summarize the findings, which—as discussed earlier—might be quantitative, qualitative or both. Strategies used within the review to minimize bias, such as blinding during data extraction, checking of reference lists and obtaining unpublished data, and to minimize error, such as independent assessment for eligibility should be described. Changes to the methods between the original plans or the protocol for the review, and the final review should be noted and explained.

Results

The Results section might begin with details of what was found for the review, separating studies that had been judged to be eligible, ineligible, and eligible but ongoing (with results not available). This might include the PRISMA flow diagram to show the attrition at each stage in the process from original search to final inclusion in the review's analyses. Details should be provided on each included study, which might vary in depth from a thorough description of several features of each study, to a brief summary and details of sources of more information, such as the citation for a published report, link to a study website or to the entry for the study in a research register.

Studies that were judged eligible but were excluded, and studies which readers might expect to have been included but weren't, should be reported along with a reason for their exclusion. This reassures the reader that these studies were identified by the reviewers. Failure to mention them might raise concerns in the reader's mind about, for example, the robustness of the searches for the review or the potential for reporting bias.

Whether or not the review includes quantitative or qualitative synthesis of the included studies, if the reviewer presents sufficient detail for each study and its findings, this would allow the reader to repeat such syntheses for themselves, perhaps changing how the studies are grouped or leaving out some studies. The use of forest plots for each meta-analysis is a fairly straightforward way to both show the proportional contribution of each study and present its numerical results (Lewis and Clarke 2001).

Conclusions

The next section in this chapter goes into more detail on the interpretation of the findings of a systematic review but some of the things for the reviewers to consider in their Discussion section are outlined here. They need to be cautious about introducing new evidence at this point to answer the question if, for example, there was insufficient information available in the studies included in the review. Having been so careful in planning the systematic review itself, it may be undermined by non-systematic approaches to introducing alternative sources of evidence for the review's primary question in the Conclusion section. Where relevant, the reviewers' conclusions might be separated into their opinions on the implications of their review for practice and for further research. The latter might include specific suggestions on the types of study that are needed now, given the existing research that has been summarized in the review (Brown et al. 2006; Clarke et al. 2007).

In a complex or large review of the effects of interventions, the reviewers might choose to summarize their conclusions by highlighting where they have found convincing evidence of which interventions are beneficial, harmful, are lacking in evidence and need more research, or are lacking in evidence from the studies in their review but which probably do not warrant more research. If the review is not about interventions but concerns, for example, the relationship between characteristics of people and their behaviour, a similar categorization of the conclusions on the basis of confidence about a positive or negative relationship, one that is unproven and worthy of more research, and one that is unproven but does not justify more research, might be helpful. This categorization of the interventions might help policymakers to focus in on those that might be introduced or reinforced, abandoned (Garner et al. 2013), or restricted to use in research.

Interpreting the findings

When interpreting the findings of a review, either as the person preparing the review or someone reading it, it is important to remember some of the key principles underpinning evidence-based healthcare (Sackett et al. 1997). The systematic review is a source for one part of the evidence needed for well-informed decision-making. In the context of systematic reviews of the effects of interventions, this will be an estimate of the difference between the alternative interventions. In the context of, for example, associations between the presence of a characteristic, such as social deprivation, and an outcome, such as diabetes, it will be the estimate of the strength of this association. Other types of evidence are also needed to make a well-informed decision, including information on diagnosis, expertise, feasibility, values, and preferences. Some of this evidence might be provided

by additional systematic reviews of other types of research, which could be incorporated into the main review, but some will come from the target population to whom the review will be applied. This makes it important for the review to provide the information needed to use its findings in practice and to interpret the findings and recommendations cautiously.

One way to decide on the potential relevance of the review to settings other than those in the included studies, is to consider whether there are any strong reasons why the participants in the studies included in the review, the interventions assessed in these studies, and the outcome measures reported are not sufficiently similar to the people, interventions, and outcome measures of relevance in other circumstances and the values and preferences of the population for whom the results will be applied.

Some examples of the decisions that might need to be made about the possible applicability of the findings of the review are if the evidence in the review is from research done in academic research hospitals in large cities but it will be used in decisions for clinics in rural settings; the trials were done in North America and the burden of the problem is greatest in Africa; or the patients in the trials were from a particular, high socioeconomic group but the findings will need to be applied to other groups.

Earlier in this chapter, the challenges of subgroup analyses were noted and one possibility for applying the results of a heterogeneous review to a target population is to consider the results within the target population subgroup. As noted, this needs to be done with caution because of the problems of lessening statistical power, multiplicity, and bias. In fact, the more reliable guide to the effects for a patient in the subgroup of interest might be the overall average from the meta-analysis, rather than the specific result from the subgroup analysis. One way to assess this and to decide between the overall result and the result of a specific subgroup is to consider whether the rationale for the subgroup analysis is to identify different effects among the subgroups or to identify similarities. For instance, do the subgroup analyses provide reassurance that the difference between the treatments is similar regardless of specific patient characteristics (such as age, setting, or socioeconomic group)? Or, do they show that one intervention will be beneficial in one type of patient but harmful in another? This might happen if a treatment has a beneficial effect for one outcome but increases the risk for another. The treatment might be regarded as beneficial, on average, for people with few risk factors for the latter; but harmful in those at high risk of it.

As well as considering whether or not there are substantial differences between the participants in the studies in the review and people for whom it will be applied, it is also important to consider whether the interventions in the review are similar enough to the ones that would be used in practice. This might be straightforward if the interventions were drugs that can be administered in a standard way but it might be more difficult for interventions that are more skill based, such as surgery or psychotherapy; or for complex interventions, such as a community intervention strategy to reduce criminal behaviour or a training programme for nurses. An additional challenge here is that information on how the drug should be administered might be well described in the included studies and the review, while the details on a complex intervention might be inadequate for implementation.

Assessing the quality of a systematic review

There are a number of guides to help readers assess the quality of systematic reviews (Katrak et al. 2004). Three of the commonest ways to assess the quality of systematic reviews are tools based on the Overview Quality Assessment Questionnaire (OQAQ) developed by Andy Oxman and Gordon Guyatt (1991), the PRISMA checklist (Liberati et al. 2009; Moher et al. 2009), and the AMSTAR tool (Shea et al. 2007, 2009). As part of the appraisal of the systematic review and when deciding upon its relevance to a health or social care decision, the user should also consider whether the review is sufficiently up to date. To be truly up to date, a systematic review would need to have been completed just before its findings were to be used and would need to include all the relevant research available at that time. This is not practical. It would require reviews to be revised as soon as new evidence became available. Although this might be possible if updating the findings of a systematic review simply involved the insertion of data from the latest evidence into a meta-analysis, the separate chapter on systematic reviews shows that the review process is more complex than the statistical combination of the results of the included studies. Reviewers need to apply their eligibility criteria, appraise the quality of the studies, make decisions about the suitability of the outcome data, and draw conclusions about their findings. This will take time. It also needs to be preceded by searching for studies and the assessment of the retrieved records for potential relevance. In considering how up to date a review is, it is also important to consider whether the review is so early in the evaluation of an intervention that the availability of studies for it was influenced by time-lag bias (Hopewell et al. 2007b), meaning that the conclusions are likely to change as this bias is corrected by increased availability of studies with less favourable findings.

Updating systematic reviews

Unless reviews are regarded as historical documents summarizing the evidence up to the time point of the review, reviewers and commissioners of reviews need to consider how the review might be kept up to date, so that it remains a valid source of knowledge for decision-makers in the future. For example, the intention for Cochrane Reviews is that these will be updated periodically and, at least, every 2 years or annotated to explain why this has not been done. The ideal, of course, might be that a review includes all relevant research available at the time that it is being used to inform a decision but this is not practical without a process for new evidence to be continually incorporated into existing reviews. The updating process takes time and can also serve to maintain the contemporary relevance of the review. This may be especially important if the review uses information that changes over time, such as economic costs, the organizational structures for delivering healthcare or the processes in which decisions are made about healthcare.

Acknowledgement

We thank Solange Durao of the South African Cochrane Centre for her help in preparing this chapter.

References

Address by the Rt. Hon. Lord Rayleigh (1885). In *Report of the Fifty-Fourth Meeting of the British Association for the Advancement of Science*, held at Montreal in August and September 1884. London: John Murray. Available at: http://www.jameslindlibrary.org.

Antman, E.M., Lau, J., Kupelnick, B., Mosteller, F., and Chalmers, T.C. (1992). A comparison of results of meta-analyses of randomized control trials and recommendations of clinical experts. *Journal of the American Medical Association*, 268, 240–8.

Atkins, S., Lewin, S., Smith, H., Engel, M., Fretheim, A., and Volmink, J. (2008). Conducting a meta-ethnography of qualitative literature: lessons learnt. *BMC Medical Research Methodology*, 8(21), 1471–2288.

Bender, R, Bunce, C., Clarke, M., et al. (2008). Attention should be given to multiplicity issues in systematic reviews. *Journal of Clinical Epidemiology*, 61, 857–65.

Berlin, J.A. (1997). Does blinding of readers affect the results of meta-analyses? University of Pennsylvania Meta-analysis Blinding Study Group. *Lancet*, 350, 185–6.

Booth, A., Clarke, M., Ghersi, D., Moher, D., Petticrew, M., and Stewart, L. (2011). An international registry of systematic-review protocols. *Lancet*, 377, 108–9.

Borenstein, M., Hedges, L.V., Higgins, J.P.T., and Rothstein, H.R. (eds.) (2009). *Introduction to Meta-Analysis*. Hoboken, NJ: Wiley and Sons.

Bossuyt, P.M., Reitsma, J.B., Bruns, D.E., et al. (2003). The STARD statement for reporting studies of diagnostic accuracy: explanation and elaboration. *Annals of Internal Medicine*, 138(1), W1–12.

Britten, N., Campbell, R., Pope, C., Donovan, J., Morgan, M., and Pill, R. (2002). Using meta ethnography to synthesise qualitative research: a worked example. *Journal of Health Services & Research Policy*, 7(4), 209–15.

Brown, P., Brunnhuber, K., Chalkidou, K., et al. (2006). How to formulate research recommendations. *British Medical Journal*, 333, 804–6.

Chalmers, I. (2003). Trying to do more good than harm in policy and practice: the role of rigorous, transparent, up-to-date evaluations. *Annals of the American Academy of Political and Social Science*, 589, 22–40.

Chalmers, I. and Altman, D.G. (eds.) (1995). *Systematic Reviews*. London: BMJ Publishing Group.

Chalmers, I. and Glasziou, P. (2009). Avoidable waste in the production and reporting of research evidence. *Lancet*, 374(9683), 86–9.

Chalmers, I., Hedges, L.V., and Cooper, H. (2002). A brief history of research synthesis. *Evaluation & the Health Professions*, 25, 12–37.

Child, S., Goodwin, V., Garside, R., Jones-Hughes, T., Boddy, K., and Stein, K. (2012). Factors influencing the implementation of fall-prevention programmes: a systematic review and synthesis of qualitative studies. *Implementation Science*, 7, 91.

Clark, S. and Horton, R. (2010). Putting research into context—revisited. *Lancet*, 376(9734), 10–11.

Clarke, L., Clarke, M., and Clarke, T. (2007). How useful are Cochrane reviews in identifying research needs? *Journal of Health Services Research and Policy*, 12, 101–3.

Clarke, M. and Halsey, J. (2001). DICE 2: a further investigation of the effects of chance in life, death and subgroup analyses. *International Journal of Clinical Practice*, 55, 240–2.

Clarke, M., Hopewell, S., and Chalmers, I. (2010). Clinical trials should begin and end with systematic reviews of relevant evidence: 12 years and waiting. *Lancet*, 376, 20–1.

Clarke, M.J. and Stewart, L.A. (1994). Systematic reviews: obtaining data from randomised controlled trials: how much do we need for reliable and informative meta-analyses? *British Medical Journal*, 309, 1007–10.

Cooper, H.M. and Rosenthal, R. (1980). Statistical versus traditional procedures for summarizing research findings. *Psychological Bulletin*, 87, 442–9.

Counsell, C.E., Clarke, M.J., Slattery, J., and Sandercock, P.A.G. (1994). The miracle of DICE therapy for acute stroke: fact or fictional product of subgroup analysis? *British Medical Journal*, 309, 1677–81.

Damman, K., Navis, G., Voors, A.A., et al. (2007). Worsening renal function and prognosis in heart failure: systematic review and meta-analysis. *Journal of Cardiac Failure*, 13(8), 599–608.

Deeks, J.J. (2002). Issues in the selection of a summary statistic for meta-analysis of clinical trials with binary outcomes. *Statistics in Medicine*, 21, 1575–600.

Deeks, J.J. and Altman, D.G. (2001). Effect measures for meta-analysis of trials with binary outcomes. In M. Egger, G. Davey Smith, and D.G. Altman (eds.) *Systematic Reviews in Health Care: Meta-Analysis in Context*, pp. 313–35. London: BMJ Books.

Dickersin, K. (2010). To reform US health care, start with systematic reviews. *Science*, 329, 516–17.

Doust, J.A., Glasziou, P.P., Pietrzak, E., and Dobson, A.J. (2004). A systematic review of the diagnostic accuracy of natriuretic peptides for heart failure. *Archives of Internal Medicine*, 164(18), 1978–84.

Dwan, K., Altman, D.G., Arnaiz, J.A., et al. (2008). Systematic review of the empirical evidence of study publication bias and outcome reporting bias. *PLoS One*, 3(8), e3081.

Edwards, P., Clarke, M., DiGuiseppi, C., Pratap, S., Roberts, I., and Wentz, R. (2002). Identification of randomized controlled trials in systematic reviews: accuracy and reliability of screening records. *Statistics in Medicine*, 21, 1635–40.

Egger, M., Davey Smith, G., and Altman, D.G. (eds.) (2001). *Systematic Reviews in Health Care: Meta-Analysis in Context* (2nd ed.). London: BMJ Publishing Group.

Garner, S., Docherty, M., Somner, J., et al. (2013). Reducing ineffective practice: challenges in identifying low-value health care using Cochrane systematic reviews. *Journal of Health Services Research and Policy*, 18, 6–12.

Ghersi, D. and Pang, T. (2009). From Mexico to Mali: four years in the history of clinical trial registration. *Journal of Evidence Based Medicine*, 2(1), 1–7.

Glasziou, P., Irwig, L., Bain, C., and Colditz, G. (2001). *Systematic Reviews in Healthcare: A Practical Guide*. Cambridge: Cambridge University Press.

Glasziou, P.P. and Sanders, S.L. (2002). Investigating causes of heterogeneity in systematic reviews. *Statistics in Medicine*, 21, 1503–11.

Guyatt, G.H., Oxman, A.D., Kunz, R., et al. (2011). GRADE guidelines: 2. Framing the question and deciding on important outcomes. *Journal of Clinical Epidemiology*, 64, 395–400.

Higgins, J.P.T., Altman, D.G., Sterne, J.A.C., on behalf of the Cochrane Statistical Methods Group and the Cochrane Bias Methods Group. (2011). Assessing risk of bias in included studies. In J.P.T. Higgins and S. Green (eds.) *Cochrane Handbook for Systematic Reviews of Interventions Version 5.1.0* [updated March 2011]. The Cochrane Collaboration. Available at: http://www.cochrane-handbook.org.

Higgins, J.P.T. and Deeks, J.J. (2011). Selecting studies and collecting data. In J.P.T. Higgins and S. Green (eds.) *Cochrane Handbook for Systematic Reviews of Interventions Version 5.1.0* [updated March 2011]. The Cochrane Collaboration. Available at: http://www.cochrane-handbook.org.

Higgins, J.P.T. and Green, S. (eds.) (2011). *Cochrane Handbook for Systematic Reviews of Interventions Version 5.1.0* [updated March 2011]. The Cochrane Collaboration. Available at: http://www.cochrane-handbook.org.

Higgins, J.P.T., Thompson, S.G., Deeks, J.J., and Altman, D.G. (2003). Measuring inconsistency in meta-analyses. *British Medical Journal*, 327, 557–60.

Hopewell, S., Clarke, M.J., Lefebvre, C., and Scherer, R.W. (2007a). Handsearching versus electronic searching to identify reports of randomized trials. *Cochrane Database of Systematic Reviews*, 2, MR000001.

Hopewell, S., Clarke, M.J., Stewart, L., and Tierney, J. (2007b). Time to publication for results of clinical trials. *Cochrane Database of Systematic Reviews*, 2, MR000011.

Hopewell, S., Loudon, K., Clarke, M.J., Oxman, A.D., and Dickersin, K. (2009). Publication bias in clinical trials due to statistical significance or direction of trial results. *Cochrane Database of Systematic Reviews*, 1, MR000006.

Hopewell, S., McDonald, S., Clarke, M.J., and Egger, M. (2007c). Grey literature in meta-analyses of randomized trials of health care interventions. *Cochrane Database of Systematic Reviews*, 2, MR000010.

Horsley, T., Dingwall, O., and Sampson, M. (2011). Checking reference lists to find additional studies for systematic reviews. *Cochrane Database of Systematic Reviews*, 8, MR000026.

Innvaer, S., Vist, G., Trommald, M., and Oxman, A. (2002). Health policy-makers' perceptions of their use of evidence: a systematic review. *Journal of Health Services Research & Policy*, 7(4), 239–44.

Jadad, A.R., Moore, R.A., Carroll, D., et al. (1996). Assessing the quality of reports of randomized clinical trials: is blinding necessary? *Controlled Clinical Trials*, 17, 1–12.

Katrak, P., Bialocerkowski, A., Massy-Westropp, N., Kumar, V.S., and Grimmer, K. (2004). A systematic review of the content of critical appraisal tools. *BMC Medical Research Methodology*, 4, 22.

Khan, K., Kunz, R., Kleijnen, J., and Antes, G. (2011). *Systematic Reviews to Support Evidence-based Medicine* (2nd ed.). New York: CRC Press, Taylor & Francis Group.

Kirkham, J.J., Gargon, E., Clarke, M., and Williamson, P.R. (2013). Can a core outcome set improve the quality of systematic reviews? A survey of the Co-ordinating Editors of Cochrane review groups. *Trials*, 14, 21.

Lavis, J.N. (2009). How can we support the use of systematic reviews in policy making? *PLoS Medicine*, 6(11), e1000141.

Lefebvre, C., Manheimer, E., Glanville, J., on behalf of the Cochrane Information Retrieval Methods Group (2011). Searching for studies. In J.P.T. Higgins and S. Green (eds.) *Cochrane Handbook for Systematic Reviews of Interventions Version 5.1.0* [updated March 2011]. The Cochrane Collaboration. Available at: http://www.cochrane-handbook.org.

Lewis, S. and Clarke, M. (2001). Forest plots: trying to see the wood and the trees. *British Medical Journal*, 322, 1479–80.

Liberati, A., Altman, D.G., Tetzlaff, J., Mulrow, C., and Gøtzsche, P.C. (2009). The PRISMA statement for reporting systematic reviews and meta-analyses of studies that evaluate health care interventions: explanation and elaboration. *PLoS Medicine*, 6(7), e1000100.

Loke, Y.K., Price, D., Herxheimer, A., for the Cochrane Adverse Effects Methods Group (2007). Systematic reviews of adverse effects: framework for a structured approach. *BMC Medical Research Methodology*, 7, 32.

Mays, N., Pope, C., and Popay, J. (2005). Systematically reviewing qualitative and quantitative evidence to inform management and policy-making in the health field. *Journal of Health Services Research & Policy*, 10(Suppl. 1), 6–20.

McMichael, C., Waters, E., and Volmink, J. (2005). Evidence-based public health: what does it offer developing countries? *Journal of Public Health*, 27(2), 215–21.

Moher, D., Cook, D.J., Eastwood, S., Olkin, I., Rennie, D., and Stroup, D.F. (1999). Improving the quality of reports of meta-analyses of randomised controlled trials: the QUOROM statement. Quality of Reporting of Meta-analyses. *Lancet*, 354(9193), 1896–900.

Moher, D., Liberati, A., Tetzlaff, J., Altman, D.G., and The PRISMA Group (2009). Preferred Reporting Items for Systematic Reviews and Meta-Analyses: The PRISMA Statement. *PLoS Medicine*, 6(7), e1000097.

Mullan, R.J., Flynn, D.N., Carlberg, B., et al. (2009). Systematic reviewers commonly contact study authors but do so with limited rigor. *Journal of Clinical Epidemiology*, 62, 138–42.

Mulrow, C.D. (1987). The medical review article: state of the science. *Annals of Internal Medicine*, 106, 485–8.

Mulrow, C.D. (1995). Rationale for systematic reviews. In I. Chalmers and D.G. Altman (eds.) *Systematic Reviews*, pp. 1–8. London: BMJ Publishing Group.

Munro, S.A., Lewin, S.A., Smith, H.J., Engel, M.E., Fretheim, A., and Volmink, J. (2007). Patient adherence to tuberculosis treatment: a systematic review of qualitative research. *PLoS Medicine*, 4(7), e238.

Needleman, I.G. (2002). A guide to systematic reviews. *Journal of Clinical Periodontology*, 29(Suppl. 3), 6–9.

O'Connor, D., Green, S., and Higgins, J.P.T. (2011). Defining the review question and developing criteria for including studies. In J.P.T. Higgins and S. Green (eds.) *Cochrane Handbook for Systematic Reviews of Interventions Version 5.1.0* [updated March 2011]. The Cochrane Collaboration. Available at: http://www.cochrane-handbook.org.

Oxman, A.D. and Guyatt, G.H. (1991). Validation of an index of the quality of review articles. *Journal of Clinical Epidemiology*, 44, 1271–8.

Oxman, A.D., Lavis, J.N., and Fretheim, A. (2007). Use of evidence in WHO recommendations. *The Lancet* 369, 1883–9.

Pendlebury, S.T. and Rothwell, P.M. (2009). Prevalence, incidence, and factors associated with pre-stroke and post-stroke dementia: a systematic review and meta-analysis. *The Lancet Neurology*, 8(11), 1006–18.

Pérez Velasco, R., Praditsitthikorn, N., Wichmann, K., et al. (2012). Systematic review of economic evaluations of preparedness strategies and interventions against influenza pandemics. *PLoS ONE*, 7(2), e30333.

Petticrew, M. (2001). Systematic reviews from astronomy to zoology: myths and misconceptions. *British Medical Journal*, 322, 98–101.

PLoS Medicine Editors (2011). Best practice in systematic reviews. The importance of protocols and registration. *PLoS Medicine*, 8(2), e1001009.

Renehan, A.G., Tyson, M., Egger, M., Heller, R.F., and Zwahlen, M. (2008). Body-mass index and incidence of cancer: a systematic review and meta-analysis of prospective observational studies. *The Lancet*, 371(9612), 569–78.

Sackett, D.L., Richardson, W.S., Rosenberg, W., and Haynes, B.R. (1997). *Evidence-Based Medicine: How to Practice & Teach EBM*. New York: Churchill Livingstone.

Schulz, K.F., Altman, D.G., and Moher, D. (2010). CONSORT 2010 Statement: updated guidelines for reporting parallel group randomised trials. *PLoS Medicine*, 7(3), e1000251.

Shea, B.J., Grimshaw, J.M., Wells, G.A., et al. (2007). Development of AMSTAR: a measurement tool to assess the methodological quality of systematic reviews. *BMC Medical Research Methodology*, 7, 10.

Shea, B.J., Hamel, C., Wells, G.A., et al. (2009). AMSTAR is a reliable and valid measurement tool to assess the methodological quality of systematic reviews. *Journal of Clinical Epidemiology*, 62, 1013–20.

Siegfried, N., Muller, M., Deeks, J., et al. (2005). HIV and male circumcision—a systematic review with assessment of the quality of studies. *Lancet Infectious Diseases*, 5(3), 165–73.

Siegfried, N., Muller, M., Deeks, J.J., and Volmink, J. (2009). Male circumcision for prevention of heterosexual acquisition of HIV in men. *Cochrane Database of Systematic Reviews*, 2, CD003362.

Silagy, C.A., Middleton, P., and Hopewell, S. (2002). Publishing protocols of systematic reviews: comparing what was done to what was planned. *Journal of the American Medical Association*, 287, 2831–4.

Stewart, L., Clarke, M., for the Cochrane Collaboration Working Group on meta-analyses using individual patient data (1995). Practical methodology of meta-analyses (overviews) using updated individual patient data. *Statistics in Medicine*, 14, 2057–79.

Stewart, L., Moher, D., and Shekelle, P. (2012). Why prospective registration of systematic reviews makes sense. *Systematic Reviews*, 1, 7.

Straus, S. and Moher, D. (2010). Registering systematic reviews. *Canadian Medical Association Journal*, 182, 13–14.

Tramer, M.R., Reynolds, D.J., Moore, R.A., and McQuay, H.J. (1997). Impact of covert duplicate publication on meta-analysis: a case study. *British Medical Journal*, 315, 635.

Van den Aardweg, M.T.A., Schildre, A.G.M., Herket, E., Boonacher, C.W.B., and Rovers, M.M. (2010). Adenoidectomy for otitis media in children. *Cochrane Database of Systematic Reviews*, 1, CD0077810.

Verbeek, J.H., Kateman, E., Morata, T.C., Dreschler, W.A., and Mischke, C. (2012). Interventions to prevent occupational noise-induced hearing loss. *Cochrane Database of Systematic Reviews* 10, CD006396.

Von Elm, E., Altman, D.G., Egger, M., Pocock, S.J., Gotzsche, P.C., and Vandenbroucke, J.P. (2007). The Strengthening the Reporting of Observational Studies in Epidemiology (STROBE) statement: guidelines for reporting observational studies. *Annals of Internal Medicine*, 147(8), 573–7.

Von Elm, E., Poglia, G., Walder, B., and Tramer, M.R. (2004). Different patterns of duplicate publication: an analysis of articles used in systematic reviews. *Journal of the American Medical Association*, 291, 974–80.

Williamson, P., Altman, D., Blazeby, J., Clarke, M., and Gargon E. (2012). Driving up the quality and relevance of research through the use of agreed core outcomes. *Journal of Health Services Research and Policy*, 17(1), 1–2.

5.16

Statistical methods

Gail Williams

Introduction to statistical methods

Statistics is the study of mathematically based techniques used to collect, analyse, and interpret quantitative data. In public health, this occurs in a complex of biological, clinical, epidemiological, social, ecological, and administrative systems. Sometimes we want to describe, explore, or summarize data without extending our findings beyond the coverage of the data we have—that is, the sample. More usually, however, we want to extend, or generalize, our findings from the sample to a larger group, sometimes called the 'target' population. In this situation, we need to consider carefully two aspects of our data collection. Firstly, what was the actual source of our data, and how did we select the sample from the population? If we deliberately excluded some people in our sampling, or made it more difficult for some rather than others to be included in our sample, then the sample may not represent the population equitably—we may have a *biased* sample. Secondly, we expect that if we repeat the data collection, even under identical conditions, we will get somewhat different results. This variability, called *sampling variability*, needs to be taken into account in deciding how precisely findings from our sample reflect what is happening in the population.

We now have access to a wider range of statistical techniques than ever before. It is important that analytical methods used are appropriate to the sampling strategy, the type of data collected, and the research questions to be answered. We usually want to generalize our results to a population. The process of using samples to draw conclusions about populations is called *statistical inference*.

In this chapter, I discuss basic concepts underpinning data analysis and statistical inference. The ideas of probability theory are heavily involved in random sampling, which takes place under the assumption that a probability model governs the selection of the sample. Probability models are also involved in helping quantify uncertainty in sample estimates. I will also discuss a range of statistical techniques in common usage, outlining the underlying assumptions, and focusing on interpretation.

Basic concepts

Populations, samples, and sampling

For the purpose of discussing statistical methods, a *population* is the complete set of entities we want to consider in our enquiry. The entities may, for example, be free-living humans, hospital patients, disease vectors, communities, or health services. A *sample* is defined generally as a subset of a population. The sample may not

be of interest in itself; its use is to provide information about the population, such as to estimate the incidence of malaria or to compare the risk of lung cancer among smokers and non-smokers. By taking a sample from the population instead of enumerating the entire population, we save resources and time. We may choose to spend some of these savings on achieving greater quality of measurement, or better follow-up of those we select. The price paid, however, is that we cannot make an absolute statement about the population; we have only an estimate—the sample incidence, or the excess of lung cancer in our sample of smokers.

Probability and random sampling

The solution to the concerns of obtaining an unbiased estimate and being able to quantify uncertainty entails the notion of 'fairness' in the sample selection process. A 'fair' method of sampling does not favour or discriminate against any member of the population. However, if we can quantify any 'unfairness', we can correct for this in the analysis, and so still obtain an unbiased estimate. For example, if males are twice as likely as females to be selected from a population that contains equal numbers of each sex, we can compile the data so that females have twice the weight. Thus, what actually matters is that we know how likely it is that each individual in a population is selected for the sample—i.e. the *probability of selection* of each person.

We measure probability with a single number, which has particular properties, some of which are as follows:

- Probabilities lie between 0 and 1 (or 0 and 100 per cent).

- If the probability of the event is 0, there is no chance of the event occurring.

- If the probability of the event is 1, the event is certain to occur.

- The combined probability of a complete collection of events is 1.

A process whose outcome is unpredictable and governed by rules of probability is termed *random*. If we are drawing random lots to select one person from 100 people, we can say (before sampling) that the probability of inclusion of an individual is 1 in 100, but we cannot predict exactly which individuals will be included. Other classic random processes are outcomes of coin tosses or rolls of a die. We know that in the long run, the chance or probability of a head is 0.5 or 50 per cent on any one toss of an unbiased coin, but the outcome of any particular toss is unpredictable.

The word 'random' as used in statistics has a specialized meaning. It is used to describe a process whose outcome (in this case, getting selected for the sample or not) is governed by the play of chance. Random does not mean 'haphazard' or 'arbitrary'.

A sample in which each person in the population has the same chance of selection is called a *simple random sample*. This can be achieved by listing all the members of the population (this list is called a *sampling frame*), applying an unbiased random process of selection, such as drawing lots or using computer-generated random numbers, and obtaining a sample of the required size. In practice, compiling a sampling frame can be difficult. More generally, a sample for which we know the probability of selection (whether the same or not) for each person in the population is called a *probability* or *random sample*.

Recommended sampling techniques usually require identifying a population as the source of our sample. Thus, to obtain a sample of 7-year-old children to estimate the prevalence of childhood asthma, we might begin by obtaining school class lists. It is important to be clear about the population for which we want to draw conclusions. Is it the population of 7-year-old school children or is it all 7-year-olds? It may only be feasible to sample formally a restricted population (school children), but we really want to make conclusions about a wider population (all school-aged children). This wider population is sometimes referred to as the *target population*. Whether conclusions can be extrapolated to a wider population than actually sampled is then a matter of judgement.

If someone has no chance of being selected in the sample, and they are different with respect to the characteristics we are measuring, or if individuals vary in both their chances of selection and the characteristics of interest, we expect to have a biased sample. We often have no way of predicting how individuals vary in the characteristics being measured, but if we can control, and therefore know, the probability of selection, we can control the potential for bias. Sampling which does not follow these rules is termed *non-probability sampling*. Here we do not know the probability of inclusion of population units. Sometimes we cannot define the population sampled. These methods include convenience samples (people waiting in outpatient departments) or haphazard samples ('people in the street').

Critically, a sample is termed a random sample because of its method of selection. We cannot determine whether a sample is random by examining it, we must know the process by which it was obtained. Examining a sample for observations which are deviant in some respect or comparing its characteristics with those of a target population cannot ascertain randomness.

Thus, 'random' does not equal 'representative' (although using a random method of selection, in some sense, decreases our chances of non-representativeness). In summary, the reasons for using random sampling are to:

◆ Enable quantification of the sampling variation using probability theory.

◆ Ensure that a statistically unbiased estimator of the quantity of interest is obtained.

Complex sampling

Complex sampling is the term used to describe probability sampling which is not simple. A variety of methods, or their combination, may be used. *Stratified sampling* is used when the population consists of a number of subpopulations or strata which vary in the quantity of interest. We sample randomly within each strata separately, in order to control the stratum-specific numbers, or to take into account large variability across strata. For example, typically (but not universally) urban areas have larger populations than rural areas. For sampling such a population we might first wish to stratify by rural/urban status, to achieve predetermined numbers or sampling fractions in each region. If sampling fractions differ for each stratum, the overall sample will not be a simple random sample, because the probability of selection will vary across strata; it will, however, be a probability or random sample because we can, knowing the sampling fractions within strata, calculate the probability of selection of any unit. If we control the stratum sizes to exactly reflect those in the population we can achieve greater precision than a method which ignores strata. In designing a stratified sampling scheme, we need to be clear about our priorities—do we want to disproportionately increase the numbers in a particular stratum, or do we want to control optimally for interstrata variability?

If we select a simple random sample from a large city, individuals selected would be widely scattered and costly to reach if we have to conduct face-to-face interviews, for example. *Cluster sampling* involves selecting groups of individuals, rather than individuals themselves, to increase logistical efficiency. A random sample of people in a city could be achieved by first selecting a simple random sample of census collection districts, and including all people living within the selected districts. The disadvantage is that the sample may be artificially 'homogeneous'; the selected people may be more alike than if we had used a simple random sample. This statistical inefficiency is measured by what is known as the *design effect*, which must be estimated in the analysis phase.

Two-stage sampling is similar to cluster sampling except that a sample of the cluster is taken instead of the whole cluster. This helps overcome the problem of 'homogeneity' to some extent, but creates a more complex process, as there are two sampling stages.

In some cases, the sampling fractions for selecting clusters and selecting from them are carefully manipulated so that the overall probability of each population unit being selected is the same. One such method is called *sampling proportional to size*—clusters are selected with a probability proportional to their size (larger clusters have larger chance of selection) and then a fixed number of individuals is selected randomly from each selected cluster. Another method is *proportional sampling* in which clusters are selected with equal probability, and a fixed sampling fraction is used to select individuals from each selected cluster. Cluster sampling and two-stage sampling do not require an explicit sampling frame for the whole population. In two-stage sampling we need a list of first-stage units (e.g. census districts) and then a list within only each first-stage unit actually selected. This is an advantage, particularly if sampling poorly documented populations. Two-stage sampling can be extended to three or more stages, for example, districts, towns, households, and individuals.

Stratified, cluster, or multistage sampling strategies provide opportunities to measure entities at all levels. Thus, factors may be relevant at the village level (presence of a health centre, degree of remoteness), the household level (family income, access to piped water), or the individual level (age, sex).

Complex sampling allows individuals to have different probabilities of inclusion in a sample. It is imperative that we can calculate each person's probability of inclusion, otherwise we cannot make the necessary analytical adjustments. All information relevant to probability of inclusion must be documented in the course of the sample selection.

Complex sampling schemes require expertise and care to design and analyse. It is usually necessary to seek advice from a professional statistician. Most statistical software has appropriate analytical procedures, and these may have particular requirements in the construction of the data set.

I next consider the issue of characterizing information collected on our sample. This involves categorizations of variable types, crucial in deciding how to present or analyse data.

Describing variables

A primary distinction is made between *quantitative* and *categorical* variables, because these are analysed using different techniques. The distinction is based on the kinds of *values* a variable may take. For the purpose of statistical analysis, what matters is the type of measurement of the variables, specifically whether they are measured on a numerical scale (such as age) or in categories (male or female). Sometimes a numerical variable (e.g. blood pressure in mmHg), is subsequently categorized (hypertensive or not hypertensive), but it is important to realize that it is the final form (numerical or categorical) of the variable that matters for analysis.

Categorical variables

A categorical variable is one whose values are expressed in mutually exclusive categories (e.g. survival status, social class, sex, religion, extent of disability). These are further subdivided into *nominal* and *ordinal*. A nominal variable has values that are categories, with no implicit ordering of the categories (e.g. sex, religion). A variable with two levels only (e.g. sex) is referred to as a

binary, or *dichotomous* variable. Categories of an *ordinal variable* have an underlying order (e.g. social class, extent of disability). Categorical variables are usually described by *frequencies* and *percentages* in each value category, and presented in tabular or graphical form, such as bar charts or pie charts. For example, a study of child mortality examined the types of birth attendant at delivery of children in the study. This can be presented in a table (Table 5.16.1), or graphically in various ways (Fig. 5.16.1).

Table 5.16.1 Community-based sample of children under 5 years of age in Bohol Province, the Philippines, 1984–1986, by birth attendant at delivery

Birth attendant	Number of deliveries (n = 511)	Percentage of deliveries (%)
Untrained TBA	8	1.6
Trained TBA	224	43.8
Midwife	186	36.4
Nurse	3	0.6
Physician	34	6.7
Unknown	56	11.0
Total	511	100.0

TBA, traditional birth attendant.

Source: data from *Acute Respiratory Infection Research Project*, funded by the Australian International Development Assistance Bureau, Bohol, Philippines, Copyright © 1986–1992.

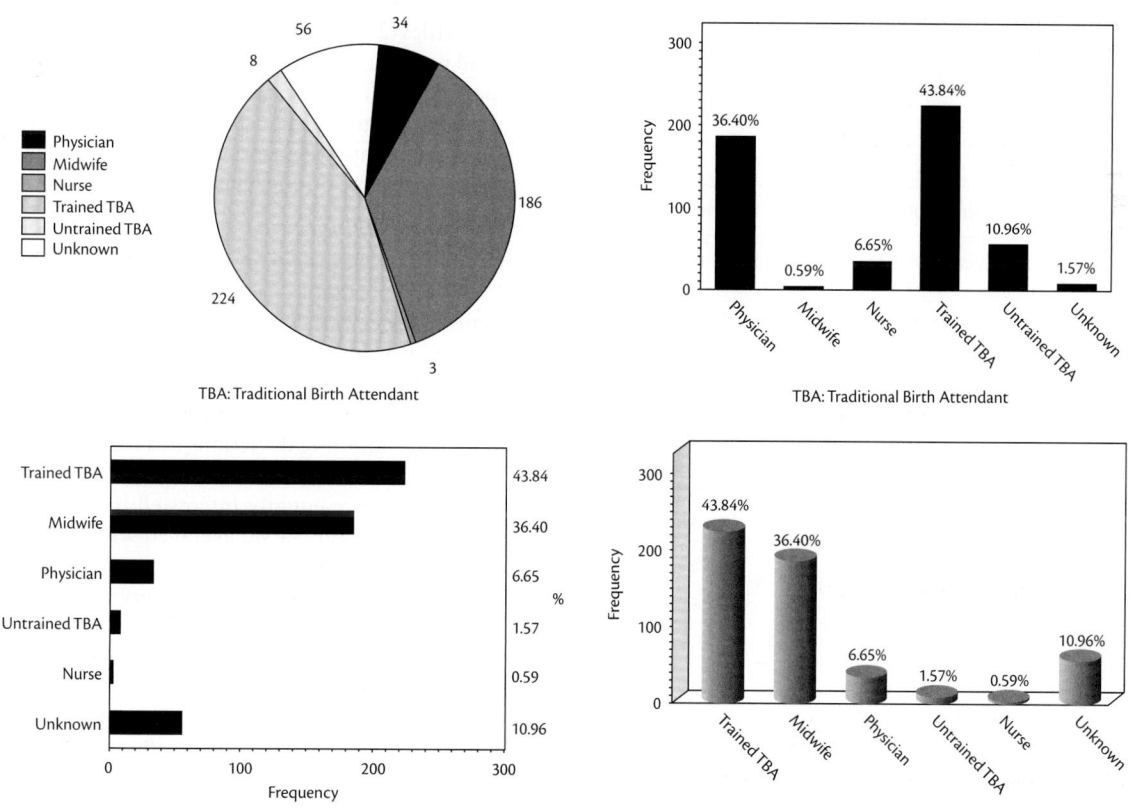

Fig. 5.16.1 Community-based sample of children under 5 years of age in Bohol Province, the Philippines, in 1984–86, by birth attendant at delivery. Alternative graphical methods of presentation.

Although the choice of graphical presentation is partly a matter of taste, bar charts tend to be used for ordinal variables (as the bars can be ordered appropriately) and pie charts used for nominal variables (to de-emphasize order).

Quantitative variables

Quantitative variables express values in numerical measurement (e.g. height, age, number of births), and are further subdivided into *discrete* and *continuous* variables. A discrete variable takes only certain distinct values, usually whole numbers (e.g. number of births). A continuous variable take all values within the observable range (e.g. age, birthweight, serum cholesterol). It is essential to specify units of measurement.

Frequency distributions

Quantitative variables are usually described, at least initially, in a frequency distribution, which tabulates, in mutually exclusive and contiguous groups, the number or percentage in each group. For example, a study documents birthweights (kg) of children born at a major obstetric hospital in Brisbane, Australia, using a sample of 500 full-term babies (gestation of at least 39 weeks). A frequency distribution portrays this (Table 5.16.2), after cut-off points for groups of birthweight are chosen.

Choice of cut-off points for groups is to some extent arbitrary. We usually want at least eight groups, and prefer them to be evenly spaced, although this is not strictly necessary. Some recommend using $\sqrt{N}$ (square root of N) groups, where N is the sample size. We may use cut-offs defined for other purposes (e.g. using 2.5 kg as a cut-off identifies 'low' birthweight babies, as commonly defined). If we want to compare with a frequency distribution from another study, we use the same cut-off points. A frequency distribution is often graphed in a histogram (Fig. 5.16.2A). This usually requires a large number of values to provide a picture of the shape of the distribution, which may be important when we are choosing a method of analysis. Not all distributions are symmetric. A variable may have a negatively (Fig. 5.16.2B) or positively (Fig. 5.16.2C) skewed distribution, when the peak is pushed to the right or left, respectively.

Measures of location

The measure most commonly used to summarize the magnitude of a quantitative variable is the *mean* (the usual arithmetic mean, or average). When some values need to be given more or less weight, a *weighted* mean may be used. When distributions are positively skewed, *geometric means* are typically used. The *median* of a variable is the middle value of its distribution; that is, half the distribution is below, and half is above, the median. The mean for the distribution of 500 birthweights given in Fig. 5.16.2A is 3.49 kg, and the median is 3.47 kg; these are very similar because of the symmetry of the distribution.

When data are 'skewed', as shown in Fig. 5.16.2B,C, the median is usually considered preferable to the mean (i.e. a better representative of the data), because the 'extreme' values may unduly influence the mean, whereas the median is little affected. In positively skewed data, the mean is greater than the median; in negatively skewed data, the reverse is true. The *mode* is the most frequently occurring value; a variable will have two modes if the distribution has two peaks (this can be checked using histogram plots as in Fig. 5.16.2). The mode has few useful applications in health statistics, as well as being difficult to handle mathematically. A *quantile* is a value cutting off a specified proportion of values of a random variable. Common particular cases are tertiles (two cut-off points, dividing the distribution into three equal areas of 33.3 per cent each), quartiles (25 per cent), quintiles (20 per cent), deciles (10 per cent), and percentiles (1 per cent). Note that the median is also the 2nd quartile, the 5th decile, and the 50th percentile. An extremely useful method of graphical display of a continuous variable is the *box plot*. These compactly incorporate information about location, variability, and shape of a distribution, as well as about outliers.

Measures of variability

From a statistical viewpoint, describing the variability of a quantity is just as important as describing its average value. The most useful measures of variability depend on the difference between individual values and the mean value (deviations). If all values equal the mean (no variability at all), all deviations are zero; large deviations indicate greater variability.

One way of combining deviations in a single measure is to first square the deviations and then average the squares. Squaring is done because we are equally interested in negative deviations and positive deviations; if we averaged without squaring, negative and positive deviations would 'cancel out'. This measure is called the *variance* of the set of observations. It is 'the average squared deviation from the mean'. Because the variance is in 'square' units, a second measure is derived by taking the square root of the variance. This is the *standard deviation* (SD), and is the most commonly used measure of variability in practice. The SD for the distribution of 500 birthweights given in Fig. 5.16.2A is 0.45 kg. The *range* of a variable is defined as the difference between the largest and the smallest values. For the birthweight data in Fig. 5.16.2A, the range is (from the raw data) 4.71 − 2.34 = 2.37 kg. The range is susceptible to extreme values and depends on the number of observations; in general, the

Table 5.16.2 Sample of births in Brisbane, Australia, 1981, by birthweight

Birthweight (kg)	Number of babies (n = 500)	Percentage of babies (%)
2.3–2.49	6	1.2
2.5–2.69	10	2.0
2.7–2.89	19	3.8
2.9–3.09	63	12.6
3.1–3.29	71	14.2
3.3–3.49	94	18.8
3.5–3.69	78	15.6
3.7–3.89	65	13.0
3.9–4.09	41	8.2
4.1–4.29	26	5.2
4.3–4.49	20	4.0
4.5–4.69	6	1.2
4.7–4.89	1	0.2
Total	500	100.0

Source: data from Najman, J.M. et al., Cohort profile: the Mater-University of Queensland Study of Pregnancy (MUSP), *International Journal of Epidemiology*, Volume 34, Issue 5, pp. 992–7, Copyright © 2005.

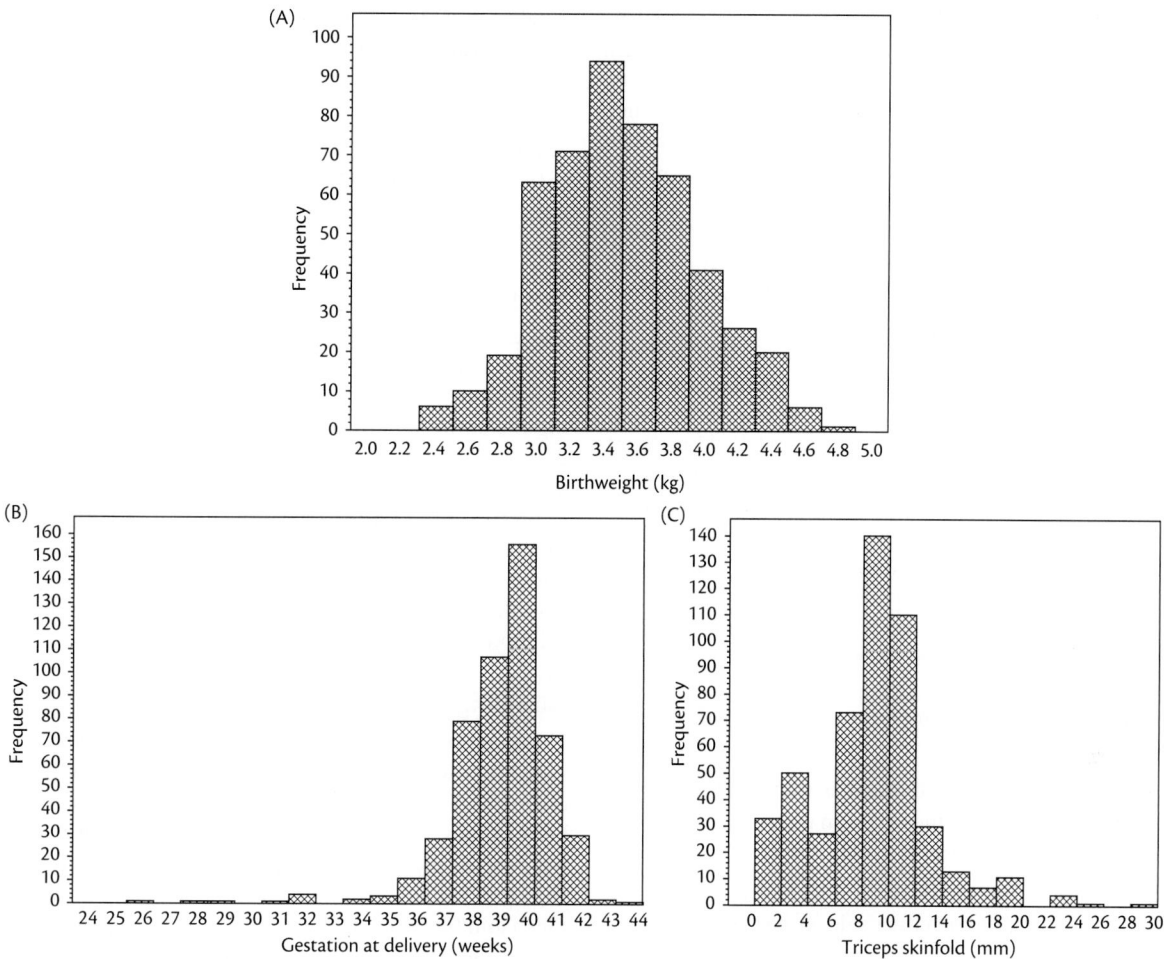

Fig. 5.16.2 Frequency distributions of characteristics of 500 babies born in Brisbane, Australia, 1981. (A) birthweight (kg), (B) gestation at delivery (weeks) for 500 babies, and (C) triceps skinfold thickness for 500 5-year-olds.

more observations, the greater the range. In practice, reporting the smallest to the largest values (2.34 to 4.71 kg) is more useful than the range itself.

The *coefficient of variation* is the ratio of the SD to the mean, usually written as a percentage. It thus expresses variation in relation to location or size. For the birthweight data, the coefficient of variation is 0.45 kg/3.49 kg = 0.129 or 12.9 per cent: the SD is 12.9 per cent of the mean birthweight.

Probability distributions

Just as a sample mean or SD (if the sample is randomly drawn) reflect the population mean or SD, so the observed distribution in the sample reflects the distribution of values in the population. In practice, it is found that certain distribution shapes re-occur. It turns out to be extremely useful to give a particular mathematical form to these characteristic shapes, which can then serve as 'models' to enable further conclusions from samples.

The normal distribution

The distribution of birthweight for a sample of 500 full-term babies born in Brisbane, Australia, followed a roughly symmetric and bell-shaped curve. The empirical observation that distributions of continuous variables often follow this shape prompted

mathematicians to work on finding a mathematical or idealized representation to describe this.

The smooth curve so discovered has the mathematical formula:

$$f(X) = \frac{1}{\sqrt{2\pi} \times (SD)} \exp\left(-\frac{1}{2 \times (SD)^2}(X - Mean)^2\right)$$

where 'exp' is the exponential (or antilog) function, and π ('pi') = 3.14159. X is the symbol given to the value of the variable in question (e.g. birthweight). Note the dependence on the mean of the population and its SD. This formula is known as the normal distribution and is a specific instance of a probability distribution; a mathematical description of the behaviour of a random variable (a variable whose values cannot be predicted with certainty). It can be thought of as an 'idealized' description of data, and can serve as a model upon which we base an analytical approach. The purpose of having an idealized model may be to 'smooth' the data or acquire some insight into the processes that underlie the generation of observations, by allowing us to test data against a given model. Once we have sample estimates for the mean and SD, we can fit this distribution to the sample. The mean controls the location of the central peak and the SD controls the extent of variability.

Many statistical procedures depend upon assuming an underlying probability model. Checking actual observations against these predictions can provide us with insight: if the probability model 'fits', then we can use features of the model to make further inferences or predictions about the population. If the model does not 'fit', then we need to find a more appropriate one. We would not regard the normal distribution a 'good' model for all distributions, such as those shown in Fig.5.16.2B,C. Other probability distributions may be used in such instances; they may be more complex, because they incorporate additional information about the extent and type of skewness.

The usefulness of the normal model lies in the fact that its properties have been well studied. Specifically, for example, we know that approximately two-thirds of the distribution is enclosed by 1 SD either side of the mean, and approximately 95 per cent of the distribution is enclosed by 2 SDs either side of the mean. Fig. 5.16.3 shows the normal model fitted to the mean and SD of the sample of birthweight.

Within this normal model, 2 SDs either side of the mean takes us from 3.49 – (2 × 0.45) kg = 2.59 kg to 3.49 + (2 × 0.45) kg = 4.39 kg. The area (or the area under the curve) between 2.59 and 4.39 kg in Fig. 5.16.3 (the outer set of vertical lines) is approximately 95 per cent of the total area.

In summary, the descriptive properties of the normal distribution are as follows:

- It describes a continuous variable across the entire numerical scale, although in practice values from an assumed normal distribution will be confined to a particular range.

- It is bell-shaped, and symmetrical about its mean value; that is, half of the distribution lies on either side of the mean.

- It is determined completely by its mean and SD.

- Limits sets by the number of SDs either side of the mean predict the proportion of the distribution enclosed by these limits—for 1 SD, the area is 68 per cent of the distribution; for 1.96 SDs (≈2 SDs), it is 95 per cent; and for 2.56 SDs, it is 99 per cent. The number of SDs corresponding to different proportions is calculated from the standard normal distribution, which has zero mean and a SD of 1.

The purpose of fitting a distribution in this way may simply be to obtain a 'smoothed' picture of a distribution. But we can use this 'smoothed' representation as a model for further calculations, such as estimating: (1) the proportion of babies whose birthweights are within a particular range or (2) the value of birthweight that cuts off a certain proportion of birthweights.

Sampling variability

The concept of sampling variability lies at the heart of what is known as *statistical inference*. Using a sample to estimate a mean or a proportion relating to a population, as opposed to examining the entire population, results in a considerable reduction in cost. This, however, results in some uncertainty about our estimate. Mathematical rules have been established which enable us to predict, within limits of probability, the sampling variability inherent in an estimation process based on random sampling. These rules contribute to the well-known practice of estimating confidence intervals (CIs), testing hypotheses, and fitting statistical models.

Sampling distributions

The *sampling distribution* of an estimate describes the chance variability we would expect to see in the distribution of sample estimates if we were to repeat our sampling process a large number of times. In practice we only have one sample and one estimate (of the mean, for example) and so must rely on mathematical theory to tell us the properties of the sampling distribution of the mean and therefore its precision.

Consider the example of taking a random sample of births, in order to estimate mean birthweight. As random sampling favours neither high nor low birthweights (i.e. it is unbiased), we expect that any particular sample mean will be as likely to be above the mean as below it. So, the first property governing the behaviour of random sampling is:

1. Irrespective of sample size, the sampling distribution of a mean has the same mean as the population mean.

Next, consider the size of the sample. Given an estimate is unbiased, how close is it likely to be to the true population value (i.e. the value we would obtain if we measured everyone in the population)? Intuitively, we would expect a random sample of 1000 members of a population to provide a 'better' or more precise estimate than a sample of 100. This results in the second property governing the behaviour of random sampling: governing the behaviour of random sampling:

2. The sampling distribution of a mean has variability (i.e. standard deviation) which decreases with the size of the sample.

The practical implication of (1) and (2) is that as the sample size N becomes larger, our sample estimate is more likely to be closer to the population mean.

Both properties of the sampling distribution of the mean have been mathematically demonstrated and further quantified. An important mathematical discovery related the expected SD of a sample mean to the sample size and the SD of the variable within

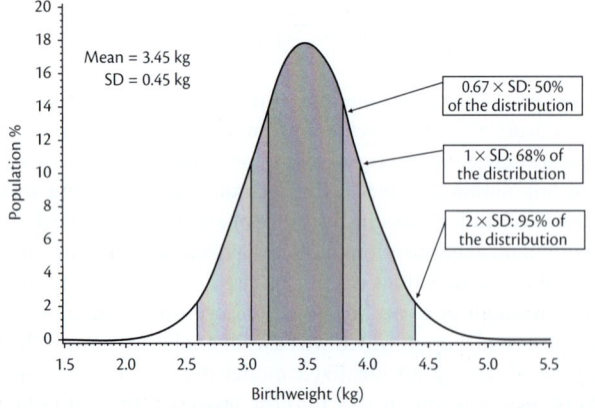

Fig. 5.16.3 A normal distribution fitted using the sample of 500 birthweights (mean = 3.49 kg, SD = 0.448 kg) showing areas enclosed by 0.67, 1, and 2 standard deviations (SDs) either side of the mean.

the population. The SD of a mean is more usually referred to as the *standard error of the mean* (SE).

The variability in the sample mean is defined by

$$
\text{SD of the means} = \text{Standard error of the mean} = \frac{\text{SD of the population}}{\sqrt{N}}
$$

where N is the size of the sample.

This shows that the larger the sample size, the less variable are the means, and that the greater the variability in the original measurements in the population, the more variable are the means.

In a remarkable mathematical result (the Central Limit Theorem), Pierre-Simon Laplace showed, in 1810, that the sampling distribution of the mean follows a normal distribution, once N becomes large enough, even when the original distribution itself does not follow a normal distribution! This puts us in a powerful position to predict the behaviour of sampling variability.

Confidence intervals
Confidence interval for a mean

The sample mean provides us with an estimate of the unknown population mean. Using the previous theory, we now know what to expect of its sampling variability.

Using our example of birthweights, and $N = 64$, we have an expected SE of 0.07 kg. Using the assumption of a normal distribution for sample means (the Central Limit Theorem), there is a 95 per cent chance that the error of our estimate is less than 0.14 kg (1.96×0.07). Another way of putting this is to say that there is a 95 per cent chance that:

- Sample mean – population mean < 0.14 kg, if the sample mean is greater than the population mean; and

- Population mean – sample mean < 0.14 kg, if the population mean is greater than the sample mean.

Reorganizing these, with 95 per cent probability, equivalent statements are:

1. Sample mean – 0.14 kg < population mean, if the sample mean is greater than population mean; and

2. Sample mean + 0.14 kg > population mean, if the population mean is greater than the sample mean.

Combining (1) and (2), we can say, with 95 per cent probability, that the limits (sample mean – 0.14 kg, sample mean + 0.14 kg) enclose the true (unknown) population mean. This is known as the *95 per cent CI for the mean*. We use other values (from the standard normal distribution) to obtain the CIs corresponding to different percentages. Generally:

$$
\text{CI for a mean} = \left(\text{sample mean} - k \times \text{SE}, \text{sample mean} + k \times \text{SE} \right)
$$
$$
\text{where SE} = \text{standard error of mean} = \frac{\text{SD}}{\sqrt{N}}
$$

where $k = 1.28$, 1.645, 1.96, and 2.56 for a 80 per cent, 90 per cent, 95 per cent, and 99 per cent CI, respectively.

In expressing this results we say 'there is a 95 per cent probability that the interval (3284 g, 3516 g) contains the true mean birthweight', *not* that 'there is a 95 per cent probability that the population mean lies within (3284 g, 3516 g)'.

In practice, we do not know the SD of the population and usually replace it with the sample SD. This introduces very little error if the sample size is 50 or more. If the sample is small, we use a different multiplier for the standard error (i.e. a different k); this multiplier is obtained from the *t*-distribution (i.e. not the standard normal distribution), available in statistical software. We need to specify another parameter called *degrees of freedom* (df), which depends on the sample size: for sample size N, df = $N - 1$. Therefore, for $N = 30$, df = 29; for a 95 per cent CI, we use $k = 2.045$, instead of $k = 1.96$.

Note that a CI combines information regarding the size (location) of the parameter, the variability of values within a population, and the sample size used to estimate the parameter. It is thus a very useful quantity to summarize sample results.

Confidence interval for a proportion

We can also obtain a CI for proportions. The concept of a CI for a mean extends to a proportion, or indeed other epidemiological measures. Let us return to the birth attendant data from the Philippines (Table 5.16.1). We estimate that 224 of the 511 babies (43.8 per cent) were delivered by trained traditional birth attendants (TBAs). The principles underlying consideration of sampling errors for proportions are the same as for the mean. The Central Limit Theorem again assures us that, provided samples are large enough, sample proportions will have, approximately, a normal distribution.

The only different feature of the process of obtaining a CI for a proportion is the formula for the standard error of the estimate. The standard error of a proportion is

$$
\text{Standard error of a proportion (SEP)} = \sqrt{\frac{p \times (1-p)}{N}}
$$

where p is the sample proportion, and N is the sample size.

In our example, we have $N = 511$, $p = 0.438$:

$$
\text{Standard error of a proportion (SEP)} = \sqrt{\frac{0.438 \times (1 - 0.438)}{511}} = 0.022.
$$

The formula for a CI for a proportion is then completely analogous to that for a mean. The 95 per cent CI for the proportion of babies delivered by TBAs is then $0.438 - (1.96 \times 0.022)$, $0.438 + (1.96 \times 0.022)$, or (0.395, 0.481). Expressing the result in percentages, an estimated 43.8 per cent of babies are delivered by TBAs, with a 95 per cent CI of (39.5 per cent, 48.1 per cent).

Basic principles and methods of comparative analysis

This section deals with some of the basic methods of analysis. Firstly, we consider situations in which we want to compare a set of mutually exclusive groups. This comparison may be on a number of different variable types, such as categorical or continuous health outcome, or the prevalence or mean of a risk factor. Secondly, we introduce models, aimed at examining associations of variables, or patterns of risk factors.

Group comparisons

Many research questions in public health involve comparing groups. This may be in the context of an experimental or intervention study, a designed analytical study such as a cohort, case–control, or cross-sectional studies. Such analyses proceed in two phases: first we describe the pattern of the data *within* each group, using methods such as those described above, and then we evaluate the comparisons *between* groups.

The comparison between groups may initially be descriptive, but then we usually want an evaluation of the 'significance' of the differences we see; that is, are the differences compatible with sampling variability alone, or are there 'real' differences between the groups, which might be due to biological or other effects? If the differences are not attributed to chance, are they important from a clinical or public health perspective? We also often want to determine whether differences are due to 'causal' factors, and whether these causal factors are modifiable and so provide a basis for prevention or management. The judgement of causality involves additional evidence other than statistical analysis, such as biological plausibility, magnitudes of effects, and considerations of confounding. Although statistical analysis, particularly multivariable analysis (see later), can help provide some information, the final judgement of causality is a complex one.

Some examples of research questions, how they might be framed, and the nature of the variables involved are shown in Table 5.16.3.

If a relationship is being examined, it is usually important to consider whether variables have a role (or potential role) as 'outcome', 'explanatory', or 'predictor' variables. In Table 5.16.3, birthweight, length of labour, and stage of disease are outcome variables; mother's height, number of previous births, and distance from the health centre are potentially explanatory variables ('potentially' because if it turns out there is no relationship, then one variable can hardly 'explain' the other). A variable may take on different roles in different questions; for example, number of years of schooling is an outcome variable in question 6 and an explanatory variable in question 7. So, for the purpose of classifying variables as outcome or explanatory, what matters is the orientation of the question (which event comes first?).

Analyses of relationships depend on the types of variables involved, and there may be several valid methods from which to choose.

Comparing proportions or percentages

The first step in examining the relationship between two categorical variables is usually to cross-classify them; that is, break down one variable by the values of another. This is usually displayed in a contingency table, which shows all combinations of values. Consider an example (Table 5.16.4) taken from a study of skin cancer in Queensland, Australia (Green et al. 1999).

Table 5.16.3 Some research questions that involve relationships between two variables

Question	Variable combination
1. Does **height** influence the **birthweight** of her child?	Continuous–Continuous
2. Is there an association between **length of labour** and the **number of previous births** a woman has had?	Continuous–Discrete
3. Do people present at a later **stage of disease** if they live a greater **distance from the health centre**?	Ordinal–Continuous
4. Do different **ethnic groups** have different **calcium intake**?	Nominal–Continuous
5. Does the **number of sunburns** a person has experienced predict the **number of skin cancers** they have?	Discrete–Discrete
6. Does the **number of years of schooling** a child acquires depend on his or her **birth order** in the family?	Discrete–Ordinal
7. Does the **number of years of schooling** a girl acquires influence her **paid employment status** in later life?	Discrete–Nominal
8. Do different **socioeconomic groups** present with different degrees of **disease severity**?	Ordinal–Ordinal
9. Does **diagnosis at presentation** depend on **socioeconomic group**?	Nominal–Ordinal
10. Does susceptibility to **skin cancer** depend on **skin colour**?	Nominal–Nominal

Table 5.16.4 Numbers of people with a non-melanoma skin cancer (NMSC) diagnosed on a sun-exposed site in the period 1993–2006, by skin type, as reported in 1992

	No NMSC	One NMSC lesion only	Multiple NMSC lesions	Total
Always burn	236 (69.4)	50 (14.7)	54 (15.9)	340
Burn, then tan	866 (78.8)	112 (10.2)	121 (11.1)	1099
Tan only	148 (82.7)	16 (8.9)	15 (8.4)	179
Total	1250 (77.3)	178 (11.0)	190 (11.7)	1618

Figures in parentheses are percentages within each skin type.

Source: data from *The Lancet*, Volume 354, Issue 9180, Green, A. et al., Daily sunscreen application and betacarotene supplementation in prevention of basal-cell and squamous-cell carcinoma of the skin; a randomised controlled trial, pp. 72–5, Copyright © 1999 Elsevier Ltd. All rights reserved.

A contingency table should include *all* combinations of *all* categories of each variable. The overall incidence of skin cancer in the follow-up period is 22.7 per cent (combining single and multiple lesions), but incidence is higher in those reporting a skin type that sunburns, with or without tanning (21.2 per cent and 30.6 per cent, respectively), than in those whose skin tans without burning (17.3 per cent).

If we repeat the skin cancer study with another sample of 1600 or so participants, we will obtain slightly different results, even if we follow exactly the same procedures. This is due to sampling variability: within our study population, individual people with the same characteristics will have different skin cancer outcomes. How do we take this into account in our interpretation of findings? To simplify the example, consider the comparison of the three skin types, combining single and multiple lesions. The first step is to calculate what we would expect to see if people with different skin types produced on average, the *same distribution of responses*. In other words, what would we expect to see if sampling variability was the *only* factor operating to produce variability in responses? The answer is: the same distribution of skin cancer within each skin type. The results of calculating these 'expected' results are shown in Table 5.16.5.

The figures in parentheses in the table are called *expected frequencies*; that is, the numbers expected if skin type is unrelated to skin cancer. Note that the marginal totals of observed and expected frequencies are the same. We have observed more skin cancer in the 'Always burn' group (about 27 more cases) than expected on the basis of no difference between skin types and less in the 'Tan only' group (10 fewer cases). These differences relate either to:

1. Sampling variability alone (i.e. no additional risk of skin cancer associated with skin type).

2. Sampling variability *plus* an additional risk of skin cancer associated with skin type.

The statement that, in the study population, skin type is unrelated to skin cancer is called the *null hypothesis*, and is the first step in any formal evaluation of the role of chance.

The Pearson chi-squared test

The statistic called the *chi-squared test statistic*, developed by Karl Pearson, enables us to summarize the differences between observed and expected frequencies, so we can make a decision as to the significance of these. Calculations are shown in Table 5.16.6.

Table 5.16.5 Numbers of people with a non-melanoma skin cancer (NMSC) diagnosed on a sun-exposed site in the period 1993–2004, by skin type, as reported in 1992, and numbers expected (in parentheses) if the distributions of skin types are the same in each group

	No NMSC lesions	One or more NMSC lesions	Total
Always burn	236 (262.7)	104 (77.3)	340
Burn, then tan	866 (849.0)	233 (250.0)	1099
Tan only	148 (138.3)	31 (40.7)	179
Total	1250	368	1618

Table 5.16.6 Calculation of the chi-square statistic for data in Table 5.16.5

	No lesions	One or more lesions
Always burn	$\frac{(236-262.7)^2}{262.7} = 2.71$	$\frac{(104-77.3)^2}{77.3} = 9.22$
Burn, then tan	$\frac{(866-849.0)^2}{849.0} = 0.34$	$\frac{(233-250.0)^2}{250.0} = 1.16$
Tan only	$\frac{(148-138.3)^2}{138.3} = 0.68$	$\frac{(31-40.7)^2}{40.7} = 2.31$

Sum of all $\dfrac{(\text{Observed Frequency} - \text{Expected Frequency})^2}{\text{Expected Frequency}}$

$= 2.71 + 9.22 + 0.34 + 1.16 + 0.68 + 2.31$

$= 16.42$

The formula for the chi-squared statistic is:

$$X^2 = \sum_{i=1}^{i=k} \frac{(O_i - E_i)^2}{E_i}$$

where k is the number of cells in the table.

The following is observed:

♦ The smallest value of X^2 that can occur is 0, when all individual terms have their smallest value as 0 and corresponding expected and observed frequencies are exactly equal.

♦ The value of X^2 increases as differences between observed and expected frequencies increase.

♦ The larger the sample, the larger the value of X^2, for a given strength of association: if we double the sample size, for example, we double the calculated value of X^2.

So, the measure (X^2) increases as the observed frequencies increasingly depart from the expected frequencies. Thus small values of X^2 are consistent with (1) above, but increases in X^2 suggest that (2) is the underlying explanation.

The calculated value of X^2 is 16.42 (Table 5.16.6). But how large does X^2 need to be before we can decide in favour of (2) over (1)? Is there a cut-off point? The mathematics of this question have been solved: for any given value of X^2 we can find the probability that this value, or one larger than it, will occur if the observed differences are due to chance alone; that is, if (1) is true. The relationship between values of X^2 and the probability of such values occurring is expressed in the *chi-squared distribution*. Tables for the chi-squared distribution are available in standard textbooks, or values can be obtained from statistical software. The probabilities depend on another parameter, the df, which depends on the number of row and column categories in the contingency table. If the table has r rows and c columns, df $= (r-1) \times (c-1)$. For Table 5.16.6, there are three rows and two columns: df $= (3-1) \times (2-1) = 2$.

The probability, referred to as the *p*-value, of getting $X^2 = 16.42$, or larger, is 0.0003. So if (1)—sampling variability—is the sole explanation for the observed treatment difference, the probability of seeing such a large value of X^2 is 0.0003, or 0.03 per cent or 1 chance in 3333. Because this is very small, we would feel inclined to reject (1) in favour of (2). In practice, the most common cut-off point to use in order to make this decision is $p = 0.05$ or 5 per cent.

We then say that there is a *statistically significant difference* between skin types in risk of skin cancer ($p = 0.0003$). From Table 5.16.6, we see that the 'Always burn' skin type contributes by far the most to the value of X^2, so we could conclude that this category is responsible for most of the statistically significant finding.

Limitations of the Pearson chi-squared test

The use of the *Pearson chi-squared test* involves an important underlying assumption—that the observed frequencies are independent. If, for example, instead of skin type we were comparing pre- and post-intervention incidence of skin cancer within the same sample of people, the observations would not be independent, because outcomes for the same person would be expected to be related and the Pearson chi-squared test should not be used.

The chi-squared test also depends on samples being 'large enough' to be valid. For contingency tables, 'large enough' has been found to depend on the size of the expected frequencies. The rule of thumb has emerged that if around 1 in 5 (or 20 per cent), or more, of expected frequencies are less than 5, then the test is not valid. Statistical software provides simulation or permutation tests which give an estimated *p*-value directly, which is then interpreted in the usual way.

We had decided to reject the null hypothesis based on a probability cut-off point in order to distinguish between (1) and (2). This decision might have been incorrect. It is unlikely (about 1 chance in 3333), not impossible, that a value of $X^2 = 16.42$, or larger, could occur if (1) were true. Rejecting the null hypothesis, concluding there is a significant difference when there is not, is a *type 1 error*. The reverse error, failing to reject the null hypothesis when it is false or concluding there is no difference when there really is, is called a *type 2 error*. This error typically arises when we have a small sample size, and our data are insufficient to detect a difference.

Table 5.16.7 summarizes the four possible outcomes from a statistical test of a hypothesis, according to whether there is a real effect (e.g. a real difference) and whether the test statistic is significant (i.e. the *p*-value is small). A type 1 error is a false-positive finding and a type 2 error is a false-negative finding.

Asserting that a difference, or an association, is 'significant' does not mean that the association is 'strong' or that it is causal.

Table 5.16.7 Type 1 and type 2 errors

		True effect	
		Null hypothesis true	**Null hypothesis not true**
Statistically significant effect (reject null hypothesis)	No	✓	Type 1 error (false-positive)
	Yes	Type 2 error (false-negative)	✓

A statistically significant finding means that the size of the difference or association is larger than would be likely to occur by chance alone (i.e. sampling variability alone) in the absence of any real association. These techniques can be applied to larger contingency tables, although sometimes further examination of the data may be needed to identify the nature of the differences.

The chi-squared test explores all variability in proportions in a contingency table. However, sometimes we want to examine a more specific type of association, and the chi-squared test may not be the best one to use. An example of such a situation occurs when we want to examine trends in proportions.

Suppose we regarded the skin type groups (in order) in Table 5.16.5 as indicative of an increasing inflammatory reaction to sun exposure and wanted to test a hypothesis about increasing risk of skin cancer with increasing inflammatory response (rather than just variability in risk with skin type, whatever the pattern). That is, we want to treat the variable as ordinal rather than nominal—we need a statistical test that specifically looks for a trend pattern. Various options are available, which usually involve assigning an increasing score to the categories of the ordinal variable. Tests for these will be discussed in the subsection for regression modelling of binary variables.

Comparing means

Suppose we want to examine whether a child's birthweight depends upon his or her mother's marital status. We know that the distribution of birthweight, a continuous variable, can be summarized by its mean and standard deviation. So we examine these summary measures within values of the categorical variable (marital status, a nominal variable) to see how the continuous variable varies with the categorical variable. Table 5.16.8 shows the results.

If the frequency distribution of a continuous variable is approximately normal (as it is for birthweight), then it is described fully by its mean and SD, which is why we use these measures in the example. In other cases, such as skewed distributions, we might use the median or the geometric mean as a measure of location and the interquartile range as a measure of variability, and present these instead of, or along with, the mean and standard deviation.

These results show that, compared to 'Married' women, women who have 'Never married' have slightly heavier babies (by 0.07 kg), whereas women 'Living together' and 'Other' have slightly lighter babies (by 0.19 kg and 0.17 kg, respectively). These differences seem comparatively small, but would be regarded as important differences (by comparison with other risk factors that decrease birthweight, e.g. smoking). The mean for married women is very close to the overall mean, because they make up most (363/500 = 72.6 per cent) of the sample. We now need to make an assessment of the role of chance in producing the observed differences. We know that some variability in observed means is due to sampling error, but could sampling error be the complete explanation? The crucial question is whether the means differ more than would be expected by chance alone.

The sampling variability of a mean is assessed by its standard error of the mean (SE) which has earlier been used to derive a CI for the true mean. We can apply these techniques to the data in Table 5.16.8, examining mothers' marital status and birthweight (Table 5.16.9).

Table 5.16.8 Mean, standard deviation (SD), and range of birthweight, by marital status of mother, for a group of Brisbane babies born in 1984–1988

Marital status	N	Mean (kg)	SD (kg)	Minimum (kg)	Maximum (kg)
Married	363	3.57	0.42	2.33	4.85
Never married	70	3.64	0.44	2.34	5.06
Living together	53	3.38	0.42	2.27	4.18
Other	14	3.40	0.40	2.86	4.28
Total	500	3.56	0.43	2.27	5.06

Source: data from Najman, J.M. et al., Cohort profile: the Mater-University of Queensland Study of Pregnancy (MUSP), *International Journal of Epidemiology*, Volume 34, Issue 5, pp. 992–7, Copyright © 2005.

Table 5.16.9 Mean birthweight (kg), standard errors (SE), and 95 per cent confidence intervals (CI), by marital status of mother, for a sample of Brisbane babies born in 1984–1988

Marital status	N	Mean (kg)	SE (kg)	95% CI
Married	363	3.57	0.022	(3.53, 3.62)
Never married	70	3.64	0.052	(3.53, 3.74)
Living together	53	3.38	0.058	(3.27, 3.50)
Other	14	3.40	0.108	(3.16, 3.63)
Total	500	3.56	0.019	(3.52, 3.59)

Source: data from Najman, J.M. et al., Cohort profile: the Mater-University of Queensland Study of Pregnancy (MUSP), *International Journal of Epidemiology*, Volume 34, Issue 5, pp. 992–7, Copyright © 2005.

Note the variability in the standard errors due to the variability in the sample size: the largest group ('Married' women) has the smallest standard error and the smallest group ('Other') has the largest standard error. Correspondingly, the CIs vary greatly in their widths. For 'Married' and 'Never married' mothers the CIs overlap considerably, but the 'Married' group has a very narrow CI, which does not overlap the 'Living together' category. We might feel that the difference among 'Married' and the 'Never married' could be explained by sampling variability, but that the difference between 'Married' and 'Living together' categories could not. Sometimes overlap or non-overlap of CIs is used in this way, but if we wish to make a formal statement about the difference between means then we must make a formal statistical test.

The two-sample *t*-test

The first step of a formal statistical test is to formulate a null hypothesis. In this case, the null hypothesis is that (true) mean birthweights do not vary among marital status groups. First consider the difference between birthweights of children of 'Married' (3.57 kg) and 'Never married' (3.64 kg) mothers—a difference of 0.07 kg. The next step involves assessing the role of chance in producing this observed difference if there is no difference in the population means. As before, we need to obtain the probability of getting a difference of 0.07 kg, by chance, if the null hypothesis is true. We evaluate this by first calculating a *t*-statistic. Perhaps not surprisingly, the test statistic depends on:

♦ The size of the difference between the means.

♦ The standard errors of the means.

Therefore:

$$t = \frac{\text{Difference between the means}}{\sqrt{\text{Sum of (SE)}^2}}$$

with degrees of freedom (df) = sum of sample sizes – 2.

This is called the *two-sample t-test*. The larger the difference between the two sample means, and the smaller the standard errors (or the larger the samples), the larger the value of *t*. As for the chi-squared test, once we have a calculated value and a value for the degrees of freedom, we obtain a *p*-value using statistical software.

For the comparison of birthweights of children whose mothers are 'Married' or 'Never married', we have:

$$t = \frac{3.57 - 3.64}{\sqrt{0.002^2 + 0.052^2}} = -1.24$$

with degrees of freedom (df) = 363 + 70 – 2 = 431.

From statistical tables, we see that the *p*-value is > 0.10 (using df = infinity (∞)). The probability that such a difference could occur by chance is quite high. We then attribute the observed difference to sampling variability and conclude the difference is not significant.

Analysis of variance

For the example of mothers' marital status and birthweight, we could carry out more *t*-tests, looking at the difference between other pairs of groups. However, it is considered bad practice to 'search' for significance in this way. A more acceptable practice is to carry out a 'global' test on the set of four means, to see if there is any significant variability among the means as a set, without specifying any particular pair of means. Pairwise differences may then be examined post hoc, once overall variability has been established. The technique used for this global test on a set of means is called *analysis of variance* (ANOVA). The null hypothesis is that there is no variation in the population means for all groups. Effectively, we assume all mothers, irrespective of marital status, belong to the same population, as far as their babies' birthweights are concerned. No new conceptual issues arise in this analysis.

Again we work out a test statistic, now called an *F*-statistic. This test statistic depends on:

♦ The variability among the means.

♦ The standard errors of the means.

Now we have 2 df to work out: the so-called 'numerator' df is the number of groups minus 1 and the 'denominator' df is the total sample size minus the number of groups being compared.

We would usually use statistical software for ANOVA, which will also give us a p-value. In this case, the F-statistic is 14.01, with df = (3,497), and p = 0.0029. This is smaller than our usual cut-off point of 0.05, and we conclude that there are significant differences in birthweight among the marital status groups. These differences obviously arise from the 'Living together' and 'Other' groups.

If we had decided not to reject the null hypothesis, the matter would have ended there. When we do reject the null hypothesis, we might want to examine the pairwise differences using t-tests. Although opinions vary, sometimes modified versions of the t-test are used to take into account the multiple comparisons that might be involved in such examination. Multiple comparisons increase the overall risk of a type 1 error (i.e. finding at least statistically significant result just by chance).

Assumptions of the two-sample t-test and ANOVA

The two-sample t-test and ANOVA have important underlying assumptions. These are as follows:

- If the sample is small, the mean is based on a variable with a normal distribution; if the variable does not have a normal distribution, the sample is large enough for the Central Limit Theorem to apply to the distribution of the mean.

- The SDs within each group are approximately equal.

- The samples are independent observations; that is, separate groups of individuals.

We have already established that the distribution of birthweight is quite close to a normal distribution, so the first assumption has been met. What about the second? Inspection of the 'SD' column in Table 5.16.8 confirms this—the SDs vary only slightly.

A statistical test, called Bartlett's test, can be used to determine whether SDs are significantly different. Some statistical software automatically carries out this test when an ANOVA is requested. Alternative tests are available in such a situation.

There are two main options for dealing with non-normal distributions: transformations and non-parametric tests.

Transformations: it is sometimes possible to transform the variable to make a normal distribution, and then carry out the t-test or ANOVA on the transformed variable. If a variable has a positively skewed distribution, the log transformation is sometimes used to give a more symmetric distribution, closer to the normal distribution. Many transformations are available, but there is no guarantee that any will work in any particular case. The distribution of the transformed variable needs to be examined to confirm this.

Non-parametric tests: if a transformation cannot be found, it is possible to use a non-parametric test. These do not require the first two assumptions, but still require independence between observations (the third assumption). Instead of a t-test, we use the Wilcoxon–Mann–Whitney test to get a p-value for comparing two means; instead of ANOVA, we use the Kruskal–Wallis analysis of variance to obtain a p-value for comparing two means.

If the assumptions are met and non-parametric tests are used, these tests will have less ability to detect differences between means; that is, they will result in larger p-values than the t-test or ANOVA and be less likely to reject the null hypothesis. Usually researchers want to make the maximal use of their data, and carry out the most sensitive tests possible, so they prefer to use tests based on the normal distribution if possible.

Repeated measurements of a quantitative variable

The questions in Table 5.16.3 are about relationships between two variables, each of which is essentially different from the other. Sometimes our question relates to whether a single variable changes over time. Suppose we are investigating the effectiveness of an intervention to improve the nutritional status of children. In this case, we might measure the nutritional status of each child within the sample of children before and after the intervention. At first sight, this looks similar to the previous case: there are two variables, nutritional status before intervention and nutritional status after intervention. But this is different because we are really observing one variable at two different times. We expect measurements taken on the same individual at two different times to be related. This relationship needs to be taken into account when the effect of a second variable (intervention) is being evaluated.

In a trial to examine the effectiveness of a dietary intervention, 17 participants had vitamin A intake (in micrograms) assessed at baseline and 6 months later, to see whether the dietary intervention helped increase vitamin A intake over the 6-month period (Table 5.16.10). At first sight, we might see this as a situation for a two-sample t-test, comparing mean vitamin A intake at baseline

Table 5.16.10 Vitamin A intake levels (micrograms) at baseline and 6 months post-intervention

Person	Baseline	6 months	Change (6 months − baseline)
1	120	124	4
2	122	135	13
3	126	140	14
4	131	130	−1
5	135	169	34
6	157	189	32
7	160	176	16
8	181	196	15
9	195	223	28
10	200	254	54
11	205	267	62
12	211	289	78
13	215	301	86
14	220	227	7
15	246	305	59
16	255	278	23
17	278	299	21
Mean (SD)	185.7 (49.6)	217.8 (65.4)	32.1 (26.3)

and at 6 months. This is not appropriate because the third assumption for the two-sample *t*-test—independence of the groups being compared—has not been met.

Almost all 6-month values are higher than baseline values, although some individual differences are quite small. The appropriate summary statistic to compare paired repeated measurements of a continuous variable is the *mean change* within individuals. For each participant, we subtract baseline vitamin A levels from 6-month values. The mean and SD of these individual changes are then calculated. Hence, for matched data, we finally deal with one variable (i.e. change after intervention) and not two variables. In this example, the mean change in vitamin A levels was 32.1 micrograms, with a range of changes from –1 to +86 micrograms and a SD of 26.3 micrograms. Where the distribution of the observed changes is not normal, a more valid summary would be the median.

To get a 95 per cent CI for the mean change, we first calculate the standard error of the mean change in vitamin A intake, which is

$$\text{SE(change)} = \frac{\text{SD(change)}}{\sqrt{N}} = \frac{26.3}{\sqrt{17}} = 6.4 \text{ micrograms}.$$

The 95 per cent CI = (mean change – 1.96 × SE(mean change), mean change + 1.96 × SE(mean change)) = (19.5, 44.6).

Notice that the lower limit of this 95 per cent CI is well above zero, so we have considerable confidence that the change is positive, at least.

We can formally test the null hypothesis that the true increase is zero by calculating a *t*-statistic, as follows:

$$t = \frac{\text{mean change}}{\text{SE(change)}}.$$

This is referred to as the *paired or one-sample t-test*, because it assumes paired measures, and we want to evaluate the significance of the change (or more generally, the difference) within the paired values. The larger the mean change, and the smaller the standard error (or the larger the sample), the larger the value of *t*.

Once *t* and its df are calculated, we obtain a *p*-value from *t*-tables or statistical software. For the paired *t*-statistic on *N* pairs, the df is *N* – 1. We calculate *t* = 5.02, with 16 df, for which *p* = 0.0001. It is extremely unlikely that such a difference could occur by chance, or sampling variability, alone, with no effect attributable to the intervention. So we reject the null hypothesis and conclude that the intervention has increased dietary intake by an estimated 32.1 micrograms per day, with a 95 per cent CI of (19.5 micrograms, 44.6 micrograms).

Again, this *t*-test is based on the assumption that the change in vitamin A level is normally distributed. If this assumption cannot be made, a non-parametric counterpart test can be used—the Wilcoxon signed-rank test.

Correlation and regression

We now examine similar questions, when both variables being considered are continuous. This leads to some different measures of data presentation, and different techniques for assessing the significance and size of associations.

Scatter plots

Suppose we are interested in the relationship between birthweight and maternal weight prior to pregnancy, both continuous variables. An efficient method of displaying such a relationship visually is to use a scatter plot in which each point represents a particular mother (weight)–child (birthweight) pair. Fig. 5.16.4 shows that heavier mothers tend to have heavier babies. Although such a pictorial representation of the relationship is useful, we usually summarize the relationship more concisely, with a 'coefficient of association'.

Coefficients of association

Various coefficients of association have been developed for quantitative measures, with some common properties. These include the following:

◆ A value of zero for the coefficient means no association.

◆ A negative value for the coefficient means that one variable increases as the other decreases.

◆ A positive value for the coefficient means that the variables increase or decrease together.

◆ The range of the coefficient is from –1 to +1. Attainment of –1 or +1 is said to be 'perfect association'.

For the relationship shown in Fig. 5.16.4, we would expect a measure of association to be a positive value, somewhat less than 1.

Pearson correlation coefficient

The most commonly used measure of association is the Pearson correlation coefficient (*r*), used to describe the linear relationship between two continuous variables. If values of both variables increase together, *r* will be positive. If values of one variable increase as those of the other decrease, *r* will be negative. In the earlier example, '*Y*' is birthweight and '*X*' is maternal weight, corresponding to our scatter plot in Fig. 5.16.4. The correlation coefficient is estimated as +0.50. Is this a 'high' or 'strong' correlation? As a rough guide, in biostatistics, 0–0.15 is usually regarded as

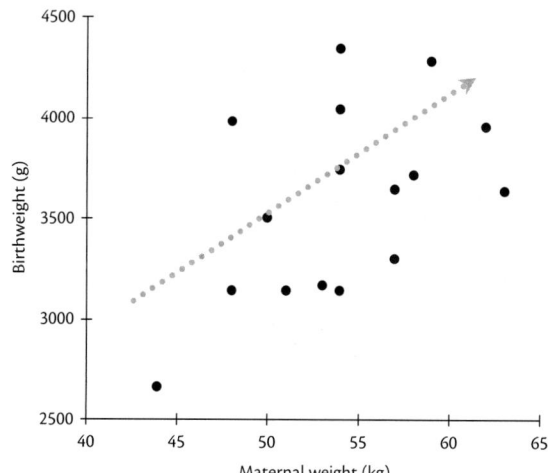

Fig. 5.16.4 Scatter plot and regression line of birthweight (g) and maternal pre-pregnancy weight (kg) fitted by least squares for a group of 16 term Brisbane babies, born in 1984–1988.

Source: data from *The Lancet*, Volume 354, Issue 9180, Green, A. et al., Daily sunscreen application and betacarotene supplementation in prevention of basal-cell and squamous-cell carcinoma of the skin; a randomised controlled trial, pp. 72–5, Copyright © 1999 Elsevier Ltd. All rights reserved.

a 'low' correlation, 0.16–0.4 as a 'modest' correlation, 0.41–0.7 a 'moderate' correlation, and above 0.7 a 'high' correlation, although context usually matters.

Significance of the correlation coefficient

The value of 0.5 obtained may be considered moderate in magnitude. A separate issue is that of significance. This examines the role of chance or sampling variability in observing a coefficient of this size. We need to obtain the probability that a coefficient as large as 0.5 would be observed by chance in a sample of this size if maternal weight and birthweight had no true relationship (a true correlation coefficient of 0).

In the case of the Pearson correlation coefficient, the p-value is obtained directly from tables or statistical software. As before, we need to calculate the df parameter which depends on the sample size N. In this case, df $= N - 2$, or $16 - 2 = 14$. This gives $p = 0.048$, just less than the conventional cut-off. So the correlation coefficient could be described as 'significant' or, more completely, as 'significantly different from zero'.

Types of association and correlation

Fig. 5.16.5 shows various types of association and how they would be described. It is important to note that the correlation coefficient measures only linear relationships; alternatively, we might say the correlation coefficient only measures that part of the relationship which is linear. A linear relationship is one in which a straight line approximates the relationship.

Note that the lower right graph in Fig. 5.16.5 would give a correlation close to zero correlation for the Pearson coefficient. The reason for this is that the data are non-linear, even though there

appears to be a relationship between the two variables. Thus, the Pearson coefficient only measures strength of a linear relationship. If we wanted to estimate strength of association for a non-linear relationship, we would have to specify a particular non-linear form.

Regression

To illustrate the regression approach to analysis, we use the data in Fig. 5.16.4. We wish to 'model' the association between the two variables by fitting a straight line to the data, as follows. A linear model involving one dependent and one independent variable is expressed as:

$$Y = \alpha + \beta X + e.$$

In setting up a regression model, one variable, usually denoted Y, called the *dependent variable* (or *outcome*), is the variable to be predicted or modelled. The other variable, usually denoted X, is sometimes called the *independent variable* (or better, the *predictor* or *explanatory variable*) and is the variable used to predict or explain Y. The formula of the model assumes Y has a straight-line relationship with X. The symbols α and β represent the intercept and the slope, respectively, of the line on a scatter plot of Y versus X. The parameter β is called the *regression coefficient*, and is a measure of how much Y changes for a unit (e.g. 1 kg of maternal weight) change in X; α is usually not of interest. The quantity e measures the 'error'—given that it is very unlikely such a simple model will describe data such as that in Fig. 5.16.4, we allow for the 'error' to have a distribution. In this case, for each value of X, the errors are assumed to have a normal distribution about the predicted value $\alpha + \beta X$.

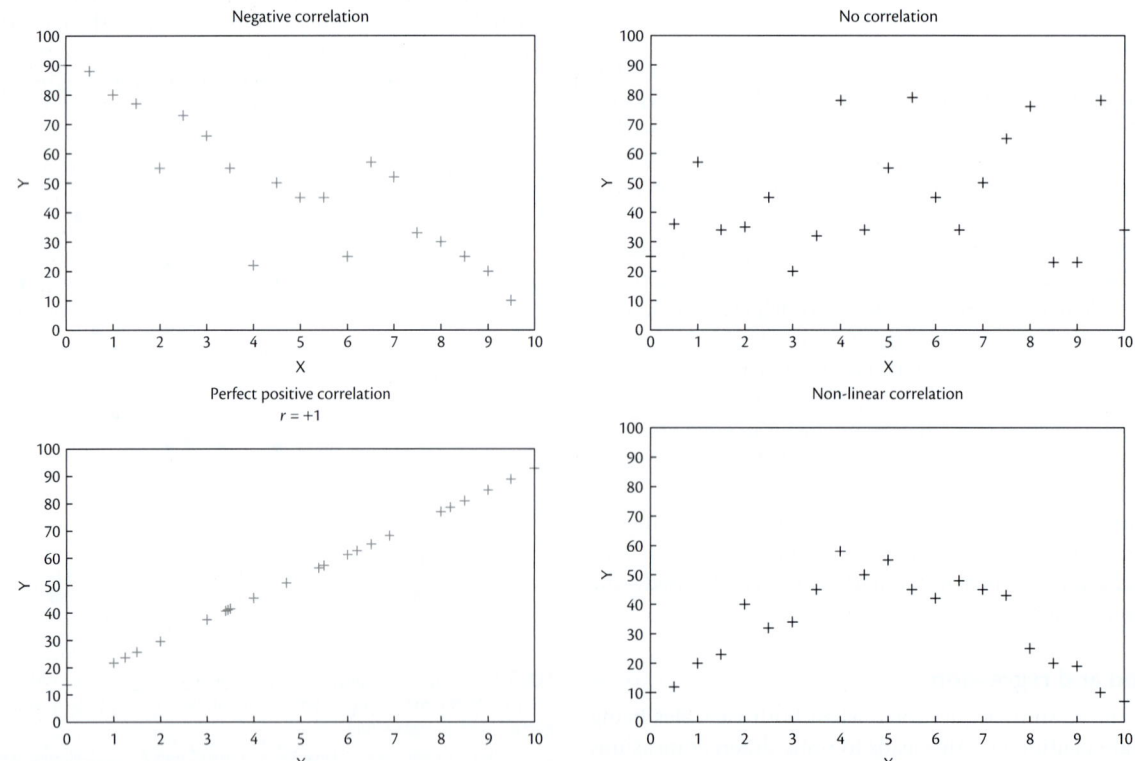

Fig. 5.16.5 Types of association.

A mathematical algorithm is need to estimate α and β—the simplest of these is the *method of least squares* which minimizes the squared differences between observed values and those predicted by the model.

For the birthweight data in Fig. 5.16.4, we obtain the following model:

$$Y = 1,124 + 45.5X.$$

That is, birthweight increases by 45.5 g for every 1 kg of mother's weight. So mothers who differ by, say, 10 kg in their pre-pregnancy weight would expect to have babies, on average, who differ by 455 g in birthweight. Standard errors and CIs can be calculated for a regression coefficient. In this case, the 95 per cent CI for the regression coefficient is (4.5, 86.5). Although this CI is quite wide, it excludes the value 0, which would correspond to no relationship between mother's weight and child's birthweight (a horizontal line on Fig. 5.16.4).

We can also formally test for the statistical significance of the regression coefficient, using statistical software. For this example $p = 0.03$, which is small enough to conclude the relationship is significant.

The model can be used for prediction. If a pregnant woman has a pre-pregnancy weight of 50 kg, we can predict that her infant will have a birthweight of $Y = 1124 + (45.5 \times 50) = 3399$ g.

Assumptions of correlation and regression analyses

Correlation and regression coefficients are estimated on an assumption of a linear association. To make inferences (test hypotheses or calculate CIs), however, you need to make additional assumptions. These are as follows:

- For correlation analyses, the two variables involved have joint normal distributions.

- For regression analyses, the outcome (dependent variable) has a normal distribution.

- For correlation and regression analyses, the samples are independent observations; that is, all pairs of observations are independent.

We have already established that the distribution of birthweight is quite close to a normal distribution, so the second assumption needed for regression analysis is met. What about the others? What do we do if the assumptions are not met? Again there are two main options: transformations and non-parametric correlation coefficients.

- *Transformations*: transformations can be used, as described in the subsection on *t*-tests and ANOVA.

- *Non-parametric correlation coefficients*: if a transformation cannot be found, it is possible to use a non-parametric test instead. These do not require either of the two distribution assumptions mentioned here. Instead of a Pearson correlation, we use the Kendall (τ or tau) or Spearman correlation coefficient (r_s).

The successful fitting of a straight line to the data does not establish causality. Although we predict that babies whose mothers' weights differ by 1 kg will have birthweights differing on average by 45.5 g, we cannot predict that increasing a mother's weight by 1 kg will cause an increase of 45.5 g in her child's birthweight. Observing an association between an outcome and a potential risk factor is, however, the first step in examining causality; we then have to consider possible explanations, which include chance, bias, and confounding. The results of a significance test enable us to assess the role of chance, but bias and confounding are crucial to consider. Multivariable statistical modelling is one approach to examining confounding; and is dealt with later in this chapter.

Survival data

In a cohort study, if an event or disease of interest is likely to occur in most participants, then interest centres on the actual time till the event, rather than the occurrence of the event itself. Examples include time to death following a diagnosis of breast cancer, time to remission of disease following treatment, or time to cessation of breastfeeding, in a cohort of infants. Such data are referred to as *survival data* or *failure time data*. A person's 'survival time' is his or her time from entry in the study until the occurrence of the event. The distribution of survival times is often very skewed and may be bimodal (e.g. if significant postoperative mortality is followed by increased then gradually decreasing prospects of survival).

Survival data may be *censored* if there are participants who do not experience an event because the study ends before this occurs, are 'lost to follow-up' (because of, e.g. migration or death), experience another type of event which precludes the event of interest (e.g. death from another cause), or cease to be eligible for the study (e.g. in a study of under-5s, children are ineligible after their fifth birthday). In such instances, the person's survival time cannot be known precisely, only that it is *at least* a certain amount. *Survival analysis* enables use of all of a person's 'at-risk' time, irrespective of whether an event is experienced. An additional feature is that it allows the incidence rate to vary for the entire period of observation.

The Worcester Heart Attack Study (WHAS) examined factors associated with survival rates following acute myocardial infarction (MI) (Tonne et al. 2005). Data were collected from 1975 to 2001, on 500 MI patients' hospital admissions in the Worcester, Massachusetts Standard Metropolitan Statistical Area. Data analysis focuses on time from admission to death, or time from admission to the last-follow-up, if the patients were still alive. Of the 500 patients, 215 (43 per cent) died within their follow-up period.

The analytical approach is to divide the follow-up time into short periods, called *risk sets*, and count events that occur within each risk set, as a fraction of all people who were in the study for that period. The latter is particularly important: people will drop out of the analysis because they have experienced the event (died) or had finished their follow-up period. These fractions are then manipulated in a process attributed to Kaplan and Meier (1958) to form a curve that shows the estimated probability of survival to that time. Results for fitting this curve to the WHAS data overall and to two subgroups (with and without complications at admission) are shown in Fig. 5.16.6, with 95 per cent CIs.

'Notice that mortality is highest immediately after the initial MI, with only about 70 per cent surviving the first year, but flattens a little at about 2 years. This analysis yields more information than simply examining mortality rates. The survival curve can also be used to estimate the median survival, the length of time corresponding to 50 per cent survival: project from a horizontal line at survival = 0.5 to the horizontal axis to give an estimated 50 per cent of people survive to 5 years or more (i.e. the 5-year survival is 50 per cent).

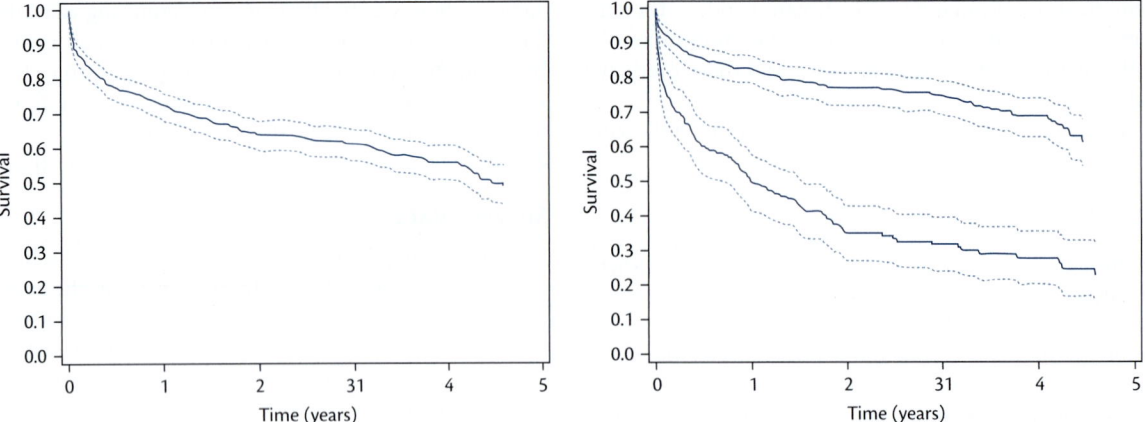

Fig. 5.16.6 Survival curves for patients with MI, overall and according to presence or absence of complications at time of admission (Worcester Heart Attack Study). Those without complications is the upper graph on the right.

Source: data from Tonne C, et al., Long-term survival after acute myocardial infarction is lower in more deprived neighborhoods, *Circulation*, Volume 111, pp. 3063–70, Copyright © 2005 American Heart Association, Inc. All rights reserved.

Other quantiles can similarly be estimated. Kaplan–Meier survival curves can be formally compared using the Wilcoxon or logrank tests (Martinez et al. 2010)' (Doi and Williams 2013).

Additional comments on censoring

'Whenever a participant experiences an event which precludes them from experiencing the event of interest, they are censored at that point. For example, if, in the WHAS, the event of interest is death from cardiovascular disease, then a patient who experiences death from cancer is considered censored at the time of death. We also assume that censoring is independent—that is, that people with censored observations have the same future risk as those that are not censored. This is quite a strong assumption. For example, suppose we are examining survival of patients admitted to an intensive care unit. If follow-up ceases at discharge then, given that those discharged are more likely to have a better prognosis than those not discharged, censored observations would be likely to have a lower risk. If drop-outs differ from non-drop-outs this is also likely to lead to dependent censoring.

A specific example of this occurs in 'competing risk' models. In the example given earlier for death from cardiovascular disease, and censoring by death from cancer, we need to consider whether a person who dies from cancer would have the same future risk (had she/he not died from cancer) of death from cardiovascular disease. This may seem plausible. However if, in a series of patients with obesity, the event of interest is death from cardiovascular disease, death from diabetes would be a competing event, since it is likely that risks of these outcomes would be associated. In such instances it is argued that the methods described earlier would result in biased estimates of survival. The appropriate analyses are complex, essentially involving the joint analysis of the cumulative incidence of both the event of interest and any competing event(s)' (Doi and Williams 2013).

Multivariable analysis

This section deals with the situation where we have more than one variable predicting an outcome variable. The term 'multivariable' is used in preference to 'multivariate' which is commonly also used to describe this situation. Classical statistical usage for the term 'multivariate' is in describing analyses which are required to predict more than one outcome variable simultaneously, such as when one has a set of items purporting to measure a common dimension, for example, depression or anxiety, or when measurement of outcomes is repeated over time. We consider various models which arise, as a consequence of different outcome variables or study designs. As we shall see, these models share a common framework, the generalized linear model, which is a generalization of the simple regression model discussed earlier; models differ only where necessary to incorporate their different assumptions. We begin with models based on the normal distribution.

Normal theory regression

Having established that birthweight and maternal weight are associated, and having estimated the regression coefficient, we might be interested in further exploring the prediction of birthweight. We could perform the same analyses on a range of other variables, such as family income, tobacco, or alcohol consumption. In each case, a regression model provides us with a measure of the size of the effect (the regression coefficient, at a 95 per cent CI) and its statistical significance (*p*-value). In this way, we might identify a collection of predictors or 'risk factors'. It is likely that these relationships will themselves be related: consider the following example, now based on a sample of 500 births.

Regression of birthweight upon maternal pre-pregnancy weight yields:

Birthweight (g) = 2832 + 11.3 × maternal weight (kg).

Birthweight increases by 11.3 g per kg of maternal weight.

Regression of birthweight upon number of previous pregnancies yields:

Birth weight (g) = 3453 + 29.5 × number of previous pregnancies.

Birth weight increases by 29.5 g per previous pregnancy.

But if a woman's weight increases with increasing number of pregnancies, then these two findings might be related; for example, does birthweight increase with increasing number of pregnancies because of the increasing weight of the mother, or is the effect separate?

To examine this, we set up a multivariable linear model such as:

$$Y = \alpha + \beta_1 X_1 + \beta_2 X_2 + e$$

where β_1 and β_2 are regression coefficients indicating the dependence of Y upon variables X_1 and X_2, X_1 being maternal weight and X_2 being the number of previous pregnancies. This model is fitted in the same way as before, to obtain:

Birth weight (g) = 2830 + 11.0 × maternal weight (kg) + 16.9 × number of previous pregnancies.

We see that the maternal weight effect remains virtually the same, but the effect of number of previous pregnancies has about halved, and is no longer significant. To see why this has happened, we use our multivariate model to assess the effect of a difference in maternal weight of 1 kg on birthweight. Suppose a woman A has a pre-pregnancy weight of 50 kg and one previous pregnancy. Her baby's predicted birthweight (g) is 2830 + 11.0 × 50 (kg) + 16.9 × 1.

Suppose a second women B has a pre-pregnancy weight of 49 kg and no previous pregnancies. The latter has an effect on birthweight, so B is not comparable to A. The prediction model can make A and B comparable in terms of pregnancy history, by setting B to have one previous pregnancy. The predicted birthweight for B's baby (if she had one previous pregnancy) is 2830 + 11.0 × 49 (kg) + 16.9 × 1.

Subtracting these two equations to obtain the difference in predicted birthweight for these two women, gives a predicted difference of 11.0 g, the regression coefficient for maternal weight in the multivariable model. Thus, the regression coefficient of 11.0 g represents the effect of an additional 1 kg of maternal weight, after controlling (or adjusting) for number of previous pregnancies.

Reciprocally, the regression coefficient for number of previous pregnancies reflects the association between birthweight and number of previous pregnancies, after adjusting for the effect of maternal weight in the multivariate model. As this effect has been much decreased to the point of non-significance, we would conclude that the significant effect we saw in the first, separate analysis was due to confounding by maternal weight.

A *confounding variable* is one that is associated with both the outcome variable and a predictor variable. In summary, a multivariable regression model yields estimates of the separate or 'adjusted' relationships between the outcome variable and the predictor variables.

Essentially, no new principles emerge when this process is extended to more predictors or risk factors. We obtain a series of estimated regression coefficients, and confidence limits for the parameters, and p-values, each reflecting the association between the outcome and the predictor, after adjusting for all other predictors included in the fitted model.

If an outcome variable is continuous, but the normal distribution for errors does not apply, the outcome variable can sometimes be transformed, so that the normal assumption is satisfied. Typical transformations include the log or square root transform, which can correct skewness. While these are useful statistical devices, they can sometimes make results more difficult to interpret.

Logistic regression

Logistic regression is used in similar situations to normal theory regression, but where the outcome variable is binary (e.g. dead/alive, having a specific disease or not) and we want to model the risk of this outcome (death, diseased) according to certain predictors or risk factors. The difference is that we use a transformation, called the *logit* transformation, to account for the binary nature of the variable. This is seen on the left hand side of the following formula:

$$\log(p) = \log\big(p / (1 - p)\big) = \alpha + \beta_1 X_1 + \beta_2 X_2 + e$$

where log is the logarithm function to base e, p is the predicted proportion of people with the outcome of interest, given particular values of the predictor variables X_1 and X_2. Note that the left hand side is now modelling the log(odds of outcome), where odds of outcome may be estimated by the number with the outcome, divided by the number without the outcome. The error distribution on the right hand side (e) is assumed to follow a binomial distribution, which is a probability distribution describing the number of times an outcome occurs, in a set number of individuals at risk. The regression coefficients β_1 and β_2 now need to be re-interpreted in the light of the transformation. When the model is fitted to data, and the regression coefficients back-transformed by exponentiating (taking anti-logs), we obtain odds ratios for the association between the outcome and the risk factor. The odds ratio is the odds of the outcome (defined earlier) within those who have the risk factor, divided by the odds of the outcome within those who do not have the risk factor. It is a widely used measure of association between a risk factor and an outcome. An odds ratio of one indicates no association between risk factor and outcome; odds ratios of greater than one or less than one indicate an increased or decreased risk of the outcome associated with the risk factor, respectively.

As an example, suppose we are interested in examining the predictors of overweight in adolescent girls, using data on 1823 14-year-old girls born into a cohort study (Najman et al. 2005). Of these we note that 466, or 26 per cent, are overweight at age 14, and also that being overweight at age 14 is associated with parental weight at the child's birth. A girl was more likely to be overweight at 14 if her mother was overweight at the start of the pregnancy (51 per cent of daughters of overweight mothers were overweight, compared to 21 per cent of non-overweight mothers). Calculating from first principles, the odds ratio for the association between mothers and daughters being overweight is (0.51/(1 − 0.51))/(0.21/(1 − 0.21)) = 3.9. A similar, but not quite so marked, result was noted for fathers'- weight: 39 per cent of daughters of overweight fathers were overweight, compared to 21 per cent of daughters of non-overweight fathers. These data are displayed in Table 5.16.11.

In addition, girls who were overweight at age 14 had a mean birthweight of 3.4 kg, compared to 3.3 kg for those who were not. We could surmise (and can conform by additional analyses) that the mother's pre-pregnant weight, the father's weight at the time of pregnancy, and the daughter's birthweight are likely to be positively associated, resulting in some confounding of their effects. In order to sort out the separate contributions of these three predictors we use a logistic regression model as follows. We would

Table 5.16.11 Association between maternal pre-pregnant overweight status and daughters' overweight status at age 14

Risk factor		N	Daughters overweight	Odds ratio (OR) for daughter overweight and risk factor (1 = reference category)
Mother overweight	No	1545	324 (21%)	Reference
	Yes	278	142 (51%)	3.9
Father overweight	No	1381	293 (21%)	Reference
	Yes	442	173 (39%)	2.4

Source: data from Mamun, A.A., Lawlor, D.A., O'Callaghan, M.J. et al. Family and early life factors associated with changes in overweight status between ages 5 and 14 years: findings from the Mater University Study of Pregnancy and its outcomes. *International Journal of Obesity (London)*, 29(5):475–82.

Table 5.16.12 Logistic regression: predicting overweight in adolescent girls from maternal and paternal overweight status prior to pregnancy, and birthweight

Risk factor		Odds ratio (OR) for daughter overweight and risk factor (95% confidence intervals)		
		Unadjusted	Adjusted for other parental overweight	Adjusted for other parental weight and birthweight
Mother overweight	No	Reference	Reference	Reference
	Yes	3.9 (3.0–5.1)	3.5 (2.7–4.6)	3.4 (2.6–4.5)
Father overweight	No	Reference	Reference	Reference
	Yes	2.4 (1.9–3.0)	2.1 (1.6–2.6)	2.1 (1.6–2.6)
Birth weight	(kg)	1.4 (1.1–1.7)		1.2 (1.0–1.5)

Source: data from Mamun, A.A., Lawlor, D.A., O'Callaghan, M.J. et al. Family and early life factors associated with changes in overweight status between ages 5 and 14 years: findings from the Mater University Study of Pregnancy and its outcomes. *International Journal of Obesity (London)*, 29(5):475–82.

typically begin with a model which uses one risk factor at a time, then a multivariable model, or series of them which examines the effects of adjusting for other risk factors. As before, effects obtained from multivariable models are adjusted for all other variables (risk factors) in the model. When this is done for this example, we find the various effect estimates and 95 per cent CIs as shown in Table 5.16.12.

Our multivariable analyses (last two columns) show some reduction in effect estimates after adjustment, indicating that the effects of maternal and paternal overweight are largely separate effects. Adjusting for birthweight makes very little difference to the magnitude of parental effects. Notice that the effect of birthweight, as a continuous variable, is expressed differently to the categorical variables of parental overweight. The odds ratio for birthweight gives the increase in odds of the daughter being overweight at age 14, for a unit (1 kg) increase in birthweight, that is, a child who was 4 kg at birth is predicted to have 40 per cent increase in odds of being overweight at 14, compared to a child who was 3 kg at birth. This same relative increase applies when comparing a 3.5 kg child with a 2.5 kg child. When we include continuous variables in a logistic model we assume that the relative effect, per unit change in the variable, is constant. This is an assumption that should be checked.

Poisson regression

Poisson regression (named after the French mathematician who first described a probability distribution for count data) is used when the outcome variable is a count variable (e.g. number of deaths over a period, or number of incident cases of disease). There two differences, compared to normal theory regression. The first is that we apply a log transformation to our count data, and the second is that we (usually) have to incorporate an 'offset' variable' which measures the period of time at risk, over which the events are accumulated. This model is expressed according to the following formula:

$$\log(\text{number of events})$$
$$= \alpha + \beta_1 X_1 + \beta_2 X_2 + \log(\text{person} - \text{time at risk}) + e$$
$$\text{or, equivalently,}$$
$$\log(\text{event rate}) = \alpha + \beta_1 X_1 + \beta_2 X_2 + e.$$

The error distribution on the right hand side (e) is assumed to follow a Poisson distribution, which is a probability distribution describing a 'count' of a number of independent events. As for logistic regression, the regression coefficients β_1 and β_2 need to be re-interpreted in the light of the log transformation. When the model is fitted to data, and the regression coefficients back-transformed by exponentiating (taking anti-logs), we obtain rate ratios for the association between the outcome and the risk factor. The rate ratio in this context is the rate of the outcome (as a person-time rate) within those who have the risk factor, divided by the rate of the outcome within those who do not have the risk factor. Again a rate ratio of one indicates no association between risk factor and outcome; rate ratios of greater than one or less than one indicate an increased or decreased risk of the outcome associated with the risk factor, respectively.

As an example, consider the results of a Poisson regression applied to examining risk factors for the occurrence of a particular form of skin cancer (squamous cell carcinoma (SCC)) in a cohort study. Because participants dropped out of the study at different stages throughout the 12-year period of follow-up, it was necessary to take account of each individual's person-time of follow-up. This leads to the offset variable described earlier. The outcome of this analysis was whether or not a participant had a new SCC lesion detected in the follow-up period. Note that an individual only appears once in the analysis. Subsequent new SCC lesions did not contribute. This is an important assumption of Poisson regression, that is, that the outcomes are independent of each other—it is likely that SCCs will tend to cluster within individuals, and therefore subsequent events within the same individual will not be independent. An alternative model (e.g. negative binomial regression) must be used if one wants to consider multiple events within an individual. Variables to be considered in a multivariable analysis for predicting SCC included sex, age, skin colour, history of skin cancer, and skin response to exposure to the sun. The results of this analysis are shown in Table 5.16.13.

The first column of rate ratios indicates the increase in risks associated with each risk factor (and their 95 per cent CIs), taken one at a time. The second column of rate ratios shows the increases in risks when each risk factor is adjusted for the effects of the others, and any associations among risk factors. We see that the general tendency is for rate ratios to reduce, after adjustment for confounding. Most notably, the RR associated with a previous history of skin cancer drops from 5.08 (3.55–7.20) to 2.50 (1.69–3.71) when adjusted for other risk factors; this is because factors (such as age, skin response to the sun) will be associated both with a past history and future risk of skin cancer. When these factors are taken into account, some of the effect of history

of skin cancer, as a single factor is reduced. Note also that the age effect appears modest—RR = 1.06 (1.05–1.08)—but one needs to take into account that this is the increase in risk, per year of age. Over a decade of age this translates to a cumulative rate ratio of 1.84 (1.64–2.23).

Cox proportional hazards regression

'The Cox proportional hazards model (Cox 1972) is a widely used method for multivariable analysis of survival data. It can be thought of as a combination of the Kaplan–Meier method which involves dividing the follow-up time into small intervals, and the Poisson regression model approach which formulates a model within each of these time periods.

Consider the WHAS data referred to in Fig. 5.16.6. Suppose our follow-up time is divided into intervals determined by the time points t1, t2, t3, etc. We imagine a regression model within each of these intervals (t1, t2) etc., which relates the probability of death within the interval to a risk factor, such as complications of a myocardial infarct. From such a model we can obtain an effect estimate (a relative risk of death in this case, associated with having complications) for that time interval. This relative risk would vary over time. However, we begin by making a simplifying assumption that the risk ratio (usually termed hazard ratio in this context) is constant over time—this is called the proportional hazards assumption.

We now consider a Poisson model', to cover the time period from t to t+1, as follows (Doi and Williams 2013).

$$\log(\text{event rate at time t}) = \alpha + \beta_1 X_1 + \beta_2 X_2 + e$$

Conceptually, this model is then fitted for each time period (with the constraint that the estimates β_1 and β_2 are, the same for each period). This occurs by a process called partial likelihood. The resultant parameter estimates then the log of the hazard ratio.

Table 5.16.13 Comparison of unadjusted and multivariable Poisson regression for risk factors for SCC: rate ratios

Risk factor		Rate ratios (RR) for incidence of SCC (95% confidence intervals)	
		Unadjusted	Multivariable analysis
Sex	Female	Reference	Reference
	Male	1.53 (2.17–5.72)	1.39 (0.98–1.99)
Age	Years	1.08 (1.06–1.10)	1.06 (1.05–1.08)
Skin colour	Olive	Reference	Reference
	Medium	1.33 (0.52–3.40)	1.22 (0.47–3.14)
	Fair	2.11 (0.86–5.21)	1.60 (0.63–4.07)
History of skin cancer	No	Reference	Reference
	Yes	5.08 (3.55–7.20)	2.50 (1.69–3.71)
Skin response to sun	Tans	Reference	Reference
	Burns, then tans	1.13 (0.59–2.20)	1.45 (0.74–2.86)
	Burns, never tans	2.33 (1.17–4.62)	2.12 (1.02–4.39)

The usual form of the model expresses the 'intercept' as a log of a 'baseline hazard', this being the predicted death rate for the reference category of the predictor variable:

$$
\begin{aligned}
\log\big(\text{event rate at time t}\big) \\
= \log \, (\text{event rate at time t for} \\
\text{reference categories for } X_1 \text{ and } X_2) \\
+ \beta_1 X_1 + \beta_2 X_2 + e.
\end{aligned}
$$

Thus the hazard ratios β_1 and β_2 give the multipliers of the baseline hazard associated with being in particular risk groups. You can see that the hazard ratios 'multiply', since the above model, after exponentiating both sides becomes:

$$
\begin{aligned}
\text{Event rate at time t} = \text{ event rate at time t for reference} \\
\text{categories for } X_1 \text{ and } X_2 \times \beta_1 X_1 \times \beta_2 X_2.
\end{aligned}
$$

When we fit a Cox model to the WHAS data, using the predictors of patient's sex, age (years), and presence of complications, we find the following, as shown in Table 5.16.14.

The 'unadjusted' hazard ratios represent separate models, one at a time. The multivariable analysis gives hazard ratios which are mutually adjusted for other variables in the model. Thus we see the sex effect reduces when age and complications are taken into account. The magnitude of the complications effect reduces but remains quite strong.

The proportional hazards assumption and time-dependent variables

As noted earlier, the formulation of the above model assumes a constant hazard ratio. We can formally test this assumption and alter the model to accommodate some variation in the hazard ratio. We can also include time-dependent risk factors. For example if we want to include alcohol intake as a risk factor, we could include alcohol intake measured at baseline (time constant) or at any point in time, when it might change (time-dependent). While the process for doing this is a little complicated, no new concepts emerge in terms of interpreting results.

Variations and extensions to other probability models

Logistic regression has been extended to the situation where one has a categorical outcome with more than two outcomes. This

Table 5.16.14 Cox regression for mortality after a myocardial infarct by patient age at MI, sex and presence/absence of CHF complications

Risk factor		Hazard ratios (RR) for death (95% confidence intervals)	
		Unadjusted	**Multivariable analysis**
Sex	Female	Reference	Reference
	Male	1.46 (1.12–1.92)	0.86 (0.65–1.13)
Age	Years	1.07 (1.06–1.08)	1.06 (1.05–1.08)
Complications	No	Reference	Reference
	Yes	3.31 (2.53–4.34)	2.41 (1.82–3.19)

Source: data from Tonne, C., Schwartz, J., Mittleman, M., Melly, S., Suh, H., and Goldberg, R. (2005). Long-term survival after acute myocardial infarction is lower in more deprived neighborhoods. *Circulation*, 111, 3063–70.

is known as a multinomial (as opposed to a binomial) model and leads to *multinomial regression*. A standard multinomial model will require more than just a single odds ratio parameter associated with each risk factor level, since now there are more outcome levels to deal with. For example, suppose an outcome variable has three levels (no disease, moderate level severity disease, severe disease), and we are evaluating a binary risk factor (history of tobacco use, no history). A multinomial model will involve an odds ratio quantifying the increased risk associated with smoking for moderate-level severity disease, and another quantifying the increased risk for severe disease. If the outcome variable is an ordinal variable (such as in the current example), then the multinomial model can be simplified by assuming that the odds ratios associated with moving from no disease to moderate-level severity disease, and from moderate disease to severe disease are the same. This is referred to as *cumulative logit regression*. The assumption of a common odds ratio is called a proportional odds assumption and should be checked for validity as it is quite a strong assumption. It is sometimes considered that a disadvantage of logistic regression is that it results in odds ratios, which are often not good measures of relative risks, particularly in dealing with outcomes which occur commonly. *Log-binomial regression* has been proposed to deal with this situation, since it assumes a binomial distribution of errors (as does logistic regression) but the use of a log rather than logit distribution results in estimated effects which are interpreted as risk ratios. However, fitting these models can sometimes be technically problematic.

As mentioned earlier, Poisson regression assumes that the outcomes of interest are independent. There are many instances when this is not the case. In the SCC example given earlier, individuals will probably have a propensity to develop SCC which is not fully explained by the risk factors we include in a model, leading to a failure of the assumption of independence. In modelling the occurrence of episodes of an infectious disease, this will also be a problem—while we can 'explain' some of the aggregation of episodes within individuals by our predictor variables (nutritional status, environmental exposure, etc.), we are unlikely to explain this completely, as unmeasured and unknown factors will affect the risk of an episode. One of the most common alternatives to use is *negative-binomial regression* which posits a somewhat more complex mechanism for development of an episode, that is that each individual has a particular propensity for the outcome (e.g. a skin cancer), and that given this propensity, an individual's number of episodes will have a Poisson distribution. Once this more complex process is taken into account, the results of a negative-binomial distribution are very similar to those of a Poisson distribution, that is, one obtains rate ratios for episodes of the outcome of interest. Other alternatives are also used, which include *zero-inflated regression* models. These are based on models such as the Poisson or negative-binomial but particularly assume that there are more values of zero counts (numbers of episodes) than would be predicted by those models. This would be particularly appropriate in the case of a vector-borne disease, for example, where the population may include a large subpopulation who have no exposure to the relevant vector, and a smaller subpopulation who have varying, but non-zero, exposure.

Study designs which have a hierarchical nature often use *random effect regression* models. These may involve different types of probability models, but have the defining feature that they include factors (covariables) which are considered themselves to have distributions. For example, one may design a study to examine the relationship between air pollution and child health. A number of sites are chosen which are close to air pollution monitoring stations, and a sample of schools is selected within a defined radius of the monitoring sites. Children are chosen from each school and their lung function measured. In this case a regression model with lung function as the outcome would be appropriate, and the primary risk factor would be the air pollution level, with perhaps other covariables (socioeconomic status, age, sex, etc.) also used in a multivariable model. However, variation among schools needs also to be taken into account. Given that we had taken a sample of schools, we would regard this effect as random, in the sense that we want to regard the study schools as representative of all schools. This contrasts with the more usual 'fixed' effects, such as for smoking status where we have levels of non-smoking or smoking and there is no sense in which we have a sample of levels of smoking. A consequence of a random effects regression model is that we can allow for effects (such as the mean lung function or the regression coefficient linking lung function and air pollution) to vary by school. Our model than examines the variability of these effects and estimates a mean across schools. Thus one has within-school effects and between-school effects.

The multivariable models so far considered have the common property that they either consider individual records to be independent, or, as in the negative-binomial or the random effects model, incorporate non-independence into the probability model itself. Non-independences occur in many study designs. These include repeated measures designs, hierarchical designs, or spatial designs. Regression models applied to such designs incorporate a non-independence correlation structure which allows the correlations between measures within the same individuals over time, or within the same subpopulation, or the same spatial unit, to be estimated and taken into account. Depending on the software used, a variety of options is available for this structure, such as a constant correlation, an exponentially decaying correlation over time or space, and others. Complex designs are often fitted using the method of *generalized estimating equations* (GEEs), which is an extremely flexible approach to fitting models, and has an added advantage of coping somewhat better with missing data than classical fitting approaches.

Generalized additive regression models (GAMs) have been used particularly to explore non-linearity in effects. A simple regression model assumes, for example, that the relationship between a continuous outcome variable (birthweight) and a predictor (maternal weight) is linear—the increase in birthweight per unit of maternal weight is constant over the range of maternal weight. This is a strong assumption and will often need to be explored. A GAM is constructed in a very similar fashion to a generalized linear model except that one may specify a predictor as a collection of curvilinear functions fitted over various subranges of the predictor variable. The complexity of the non-linearity may be specified. This is a very sensitive and flexible approach to exploring curvilinearity of effects, or in the case of a confounding variable which has non-linear effects, ensuring minimal residual confounding.

Summary

Modern statistics and software offer a wide array of approaches to statistical analyses. The key to appropriate and efficient analysis lies in clarity around the study design and the questions to be answered, thorough preliminary analyses of the data available and selection of the appropriate techniques to be used, and a critical approach to presentation and interpretation of results. Common errors include applying techniques that are not appropriate to variable types or their distributions, ignoring design features (such as repeated or hierarchical sampling), and misinterpretation of computer output. Unfortunately, the availability of statistical software that can perform sophisticated analyses is likely to make these errors more frequent, rather than the opposite. There is little substitute for consulting a qualified statistician, particularly with complex study designs.

Acknowledgments

Text extracts reproduced from Springer, *Methods of Clinical Epidemiology*, Chapter 10 Modelling Binary Outcomes and Chapter 11 Modelling Time-to-Event Data, pp. 173–77, Gail M. Williams and Robert Ware, Copyright © Springer-Verlag Berlin Heidelberg 2013. With kind permission of Springer Science+Business Media.

References

Cox, D.R. (1972). Regression models and life tables. *Journal of the Royal Statistical Society*, 34, 187–220.

Doi, Suhail A.R. and Williams, Gail M. (Eds.) (2013). *Methods of Clinical Epidemiology*. Springer Series on Epidemiology and Public Health, Springer, Verlag, Germany.

Green, A., Williams, G.M., Neale, R., et al. (1999). Daily sunscreen application and betacarotene supplementation in prevention of basal-cell and squamous-cell carcinoma of the skin; a randomised controlled trial. *The Lancet*, 354 (9180), 72–5.

Kaplan, E.L. and Meier, P. (1958). Nonparametric estimation from incomplete observations. *American Statistical Association*, 53, 457–81.

Martinez, R.L.M.C. and Naranjo, J.D. (2010). A pretest for choosing between logrank and Wilcoxon tests in the two-sample problem. *METRON—International Journal of Statistics*, LXVIII(2), 111–25.

Najman, J.M., Bor, W., O'Callaghan, M., Williams, G.M., Aird, R., and Shuttlewood, G. (2005). Cohort profile: the Mater-University of Queensland Study of Pregnancy (MUSP). *International Journal of Epidemiology*, 34, 992–7.

Tonne, C., Schwartz, J., Mittleman, M., Melly, S., Suh, H., and Goldberg, R. (2005). Long-term survival after acute myocardial infarction is lower in more deprived neighborhoods. *Circulation*, 111, 3063–70.

5.17

Measuring the health of populations: the Global Burden of Disease study methods

Theo Vos and Christopher J. L. Murray

Introduction to measuring the health of populations

Over the last two decades, the global health landscape has undergone rapid transformation. People around the world are living longer than ever before, and populations are getting older. Many countries have made remarkable progress in preventing child deaths. As a result, disease burden is increasingly defined by disability as opposed to being dominated by premature mortality. The leading causes of death and disability are shifting from communicable diseases in children to non-communicable diseases in adults. These global trends differ across regions. Notably, in sub-Saharan Africa, communicable, maternal, and newborn diseases and nutritional deficiencies continue to dominate. While low- and middle-income countries are tackling this 'unfinished agenda' of largely poverty-related diseases, increasingly, they also need to prepare their health services for a growing burden of non-communicable diseases and injuries, which some have called the 'double burden' or 'triple burden' (Bradshaw et al. 2003; Marshall 2004; Boutayeb 2006). In high-income countries, health budgets are steadily increasing relative to gross domestic product due to ageing of the population, an ever-expanding array of medical technologies, and greater demands of consumers for healthcare services (Smith et al. 2009). For governments and other healthcare providers to be able to respond to these challenges, high-quality comparable data on the size and trends in mortality and morbidity are essential. The word 'comparable' is of paramount importance. Commercial and professional interests often lead to implausible claims of the number of deaths or cases affected by a particular disease. The only way to deal with these exaggerated claims is to make a comprehensive assessment of the health of each population by ensuring that all deaths by cause add up to the total number of deaths and a similar rigor applied to classifying cases of disease. The two more prominent examples of independent assessments of population health statistics are the Child Epidemiology Reference Group of the World Health Organization (WHO) which has made global estimates of childhood deaths (Black et al. 2010) and the successive iterations of the Global Burden of Disease study (GBD—a full list of abbreviations is given in Table 5.17.1) (Murray and Lopez 1996; Mathers et al. 2008; Lozano et al. 2012; Murray et al. 2012a). The latter endeavour is the only one to estimate health loss across the age spectrum and for all diseases and injuries. After the initial GBD assessment for 1990, updates until 2008 have largely continued to use the same methods with piecemeal improvements. In 2007, the Bill & Melinda Gates Foundation funded the Global Burden of Diseases, Injuries, and Risk Factors Study 2010 (GBD 2010) which endeavoured to re-think methods and assumptions underlying population health measurement while making use of the vastly improved health data and computational resources. This chapter describes the methods underlying the GBD 2010 study.

About GBD 2010

The GBD approach is a systematic, scientific effort to quantify the comparative magnitude of health loss due to diseases, injuries, and risk factors by age, sex, and geography for specific points in time. GBD 2010 was published in a series of papers in *The Lancet* in December 2012. The information is made available as a global public good that will be useful for informing the design of health systems and the creation of public health policy. GBD 2010 estimated premature death and disability from 291 diseases and injuries, 1160 sequelae (direct consequences of disease and injury), and 67 risk factors for 20 age groups and both sexes in 1990, 2005, and 2010. The study produced estimates for 187 countries and 21 regions and generated nearly 1 billion estimates of health outcomes.

GBD 2010 was a collaborative effort among 488 researchers from 50 countries and 303 institutions. The Institute for Health Metrics and Evaluation (IHME) acted as the coordinating centre for the study. The collaboration strengthened both the data-gathering effort and the quantitative analysis by bringing together some of the foremost minds from a wide range of disciplines. The intention is to build on this collaboration by enlarging the network in

Table 5.17.1 Abbreviations

CODEm	Cause of death ensemble model
DALY	Disability-adjusted life year
DFLE	Disability-free life expectancy
DW	Disability weight
GBD	Global Burden of Disease
HALE	Health-adjusted life expectancy or health life expectancy
ICD	International Classification of Diseases and Related Health Problems
IHME	Institute for Health Metrics and Evaluation
$_5q_0$	Probability of dying before 5th birthday
$_{45}q_{15}$	Probability of dying between 15th and 60th birthday
QALY	Quality-adjusted life year
UNAIDS	Joint United Nations Programme on HIV/AIDS
VA	Verbal autopsy
WHO	World Health Organization
YLD	Years lived with disability
YLL	Years of life lost

years to come. IHME and its collaborators will expand the list of diseases, injuries, and risk factors included in GBD and routinely update the GBD estimates. Continual updates will ensure that the international community can have access to high-quality estimates in the timeliest fashion. Through sound measurement, it will provide the foundational evidence that will lead to improved population health.

Value choices and population health metrics

Several metrics that combine mortality and morbidity are in use. They all have in common that health loss or health gain is measured in units of time. There are two classes of population health measures: health expectancies and health gap measures. Health expectancies extend the concept of life expectancy, a composite measure of age-specific mortality rates in a given year in a population, and adjust years in a life table for loss of health from non-fatal conditions. Demographers calculate life expectancy in a life table by applying the currently prevailing mortality rates in a population to a hypothetical birth cohort. In each row of the life table deaths and survivors of the birth cohort are tracked at successive age groups until a top age category (e.g. 80+ or 100+) in which everyone is assumed to die. In each age group the average number of years lived is calculated and the sum of years lived over all ages divided by the initial size of the assumed birth cohort is the average life expectancy. A common interpretation of life expectancy is 'the average number of years a child born today can expect to live'. Of course, this interpretation only holds if the currently prevailing mortality rates at each age would continue to apply for the total life span of the birth cohort. In reality, mortality rates are changing considerably over time. As mortality rates are declining at almost all ages in most countries, the true life expectancy in a

population is higher than the figures that are frequently used in health statistics. However, it is a popular and frequently used statistic because it is an easy way to summarize in one number a lot of detailed information on mortality rates by age and because users have an intuitive understanding how to interpret a life expectancy measure (even if that interpretation is not quite right).

Health expectancies are an adaptation of life expectancy taking into account that not all years of remaining life expectancy are lived in good health. The coarsest version of health expectancy is the disability-free life expectancy (DFLE) which classifies disability in a dichotomous way: those above the threshold contribute no time to DFLE and those below contribute a full year to the measure (Murray 2002). Health-adjusted life expectancy (HALE), also sometimes referred to as healthy life expectancy, grades the severity of disability across several categories or the full spectrum and adjusts time lived at each age in a life table by the severity-weighted prevalence of disability. The attractions of health expectancies are that they capture health of a population in a single number and that the concept is relatively easy to explain to policymakers. Its main uses are ranking lists by country or subpopulations within a country, and tracking of change over time for the same population. The downside of health expectancies is that it is not easy to attribute a population's health to underlying diseases, injuries, or risks.

The disability-adjusted life year (DALY) is a health gap measure that was created to allow measurement of a population's health with the ability to express the contribution of diseases, injuries, and risks as a proportion of the total burden of disease. It is called a health gap measure as it quantifies loss of health from mortality and morbidity in a population against a stated ideal that 'everyone should live until a ripe old age, free of disease'. A number of social value choices are incorporated into the DALY, all of which have been reconsidered by a panel of ethicists and philosophers for GBD 2010 (Murray et al. 2012b).

The first inevitable choice in constructing a health gap measure concerns the choice of the standard for length of life. In earlier versions of GBD, a standard life table was chosen that mirrored life expectancy of Japanese women in the early 1990s. This was Coale and Demeny's West level 26 female model life table with a life expectancy at birth of 82.5 years (Coale and Demeny 1966). A choice was made to set a slightly lower standard for men, postulating a biological difference in life expectancy between men and women. As there was no male model life table in the Coale and Demeny series that came close to the chosen female life table, the West level 25 female model life table with life expectancy at birth of 80 years was chosen for men. Use of a standard life table essentially is a weighting for age at death: infant deaths are considered equivalent to a loss of the number of years of life expectancy at birth; a death at age 20 is equivalent to the loss of the remaining life expectancy at that age. It also follows that even deaths at the oldest age groups still account for some years of life lost. The panel of ethicists and philosophers advised that there was no clear rationale for a difference between males and females and that it would be fitting to update the standard to achievable levels of life expectancy in 2010. A choice was made to create a new standard life table consisting of the lowest observed mortality rates in any age group in any population greater than 5 million. This is a standard life table with life expectancy at birth of 86.0 years. The full list of life expectancy at each age from the standard life table can be found in the web appendix to one of the GBD 2010 papers published in *The Lancet* (Murray et al. 2012a).

A second choice is whether to apply the same standard life table to all populations and over time. From a principle of wishing to compare 'like with like' and for the sake of making meaningful comparisons of changes in health status of populations over time, GBD uses a single model life table to measure years of life lost, regardless of whether the death occurred in a population currently experiencing high or low mortality rates.

A third choice that has to be made in a summary measure like the DALY is how to value health loss from non-fatal conditions relative to the loss of health from deaths. The previous two choices determined how counts of death are translated into a number of years of life lost. To translate non-fatal health loss in a population into a comparable time measure of 'lost healthy years' a severity weighting for each disease or consequence of disease and injury is needed. The original GBD study in the 1990s derived these 'disability weights' (DWs) from a panel of international health experts who valued 22 tracer conditions with person trade-off methods. Subsequently, they were asked to interpolate all remaining health states by indicating a distribution across seven classes of severity after binning the valuations for the 22 tracer conditions (Murray and Lopez 1996). DWs ranged from a low of 0.005 for mild anaemia and a high of 0.85 for a number of severe congenital anomalies. Since then, national burden of disease studies (Melse et al. 2000; Begg et al. 2008) have continued to use these DWs but supplemented them with a new set of DWs developed for the Dutch burden of disease study (Stouthard et al. 2000), as well as a number of ad hoc derivations of DWs for new conditions. As this had led to a lack of consistency between DWs and because there had been criticism of depending on the values of a small panel of health experts, for GBD 2010 population surveys were conducted in Peru, Indonesia, Bangladesh, Tanzania, and the United States, as well as an open-access Internet survey. More than 30,000 respondents took part from 167 countries. To minimize the cognitive burden a simplified method of pair-wise comparisons was adopted. Each time, a respondent was asked to decide between two health states 'who is the healthier?'. The health states were described in short lay descriptions capturing the essential domains of loss of function in fewer than 35 words, as pilot testing indicated this was the maximum of information respondents were able to absorb. Valuations were obtained for a parsimonious set of 220 health states covering all 1160 sequelae. In addition, respondents to the Internet survey were asked to answer a small number of population health equivalence questions to anchor the values from the pair-wise comparison on a 0–1 scale, where 0 represents no health loss and 1 represents health loss equivalent to being dead. All DWs were estimated with an uncertainty interval. The least severe DW of 0.005 was for mild hearing loss and a mild infectious disease episode while the worst DW of 0.756 was given to the acute, psychotic phase of schizophrenia. Further methods and details of all lay descriptions and DWs can be found in Salomon et al. (2012a).

Two other choices that had been used in previous GBD studies, discounting and age-weighting, were rejected by the panel of ethicists and philosophers. Both these choices had been subject to criticism in the academic literature (Anand and Hanson 1997; Tsuchiya 2001; Arnesen and Kapiriri 2004) but also were difficult to explain to policymakers. With discounting a future stream of lost health, greatest value is given to loss of health in the year of interest while years into the future gets valued less and less. Previous GBD studies used an instantaneous discount rate of 3 per cent which meant that a female infant death with a standard life expectancy of 82.5 years would translate into 30.5 years of life lost. Age-weighting was a further complication incorporated into the DALY of previous GBD studies. The age-weighting function gives less value to health loss at young and older ages and greater value to health loss in young adults arguing that the latter have a social duty to look after the young and the old.

A further general choice is whether to generate estimates of non-fatal health loss from incident or prevalent cases. Previous GBD studies have used an incidence approach arguing that it fits better with the measurement of lost years from deaths and that it would suit policymaking about prevention, as the future stream of health lost in an incident case of disease reflects the potential health gain from prevention (Murray and Lopez 1996). However, it was difficult to explain to policymakers that the burden of disease in a particular year was not reflecting the health loss from current cases of disease. The most important consideration to adopt a prevalence approach to non-fatal health loss measurement in GBD 2010 was that it would have been computationally nigh impossible to correct for co-morbidity with an incidence approach, as it would have to deal with a large combination of lost health streams of different durations. A corollary of choosing a prevalence approach is also that by definition you cannot apply discounting, but that was a decision already made.

This was a long introduction about the metrics used in burden of disease and how key assumptions have changed over time. It is important to point out that any change in these value choices means using a different metric that is no longer comparable to another. For that reason, in GBD 2010 estimates were explicitly re-estimated for 1990 to avoid anyone making comparisons with the original GBD 1990 estimates. While not necessarily pertinent to this chapter, it seems wise to explain the difference between DALYs used in burden of disease and DALYs that are used in economic evaluations. In economic evaluations DALYs are no longer defined as a health gap measure quantified against the standard life expectancy. Instead, the mortality rates are used that apply to the population of interest for which the cost-effectiveness of one or more health interventions is being evaluated. Similar to the use of quality-adjusted life years (QALYs), economic evaluation models using DALYs compare the future health consequences between a population getting a particular health intervention and a population receiving an alternative (e.g. 'current practice' or no intervention). In both arms of such models the amount of time lived is recorded and time lived with non-fatal health outcomes is multiplied by one minus a DW in DALYs and by a utility weight in QALYs. The difference between disability-adjusted or quality-adjusted time lived between the two arms of the model determines the health gain (or loss) attributed to the health intervention of interest. A list of key terms is found in Box 5.17.1.

Estimation principles

The GBD cause list is a set of mutually exclusive and collectively exhaustive categories. The 291 causes included in GBD 2010 were chosen based on considerations of their relevance to global health policymaking and/or the size of their expected contribution to mortality and/or morbidity burden.

Box 5.17.1 Key terms

Years of life lost (YLLs): years of life lost due to premature mortality.

Years lived with disability (YLDs): years of life lived with any short-term or long-term health loss.

Disability-adjusted life years (DALYs): the sum of YLLs and YLDs. DALYs are also defined as years of healthy life lost.

Healthy life expectancy, or health-adjusted life expectancy (HALE): the number of years that a person at a given age can expect to live in good health if current rates of mortality and disability would remain constant.

Sequelae: consequences of diseases and injuries.

Health states: groupings of sequelae that reflect key differences in symptoms and functioning.

Disability weights: number on a scale from 0 to 1 that represents the severity of health loss associated with a health state.

Uncertainty interval: a range of values that is likely to include the correct estimate of health loss for a given cause.

All quantities of interest are estimated arguing that an uncertain estimate even when data are sparse or not available is preferable to no estimate. No estimate is often taken to mean no burden from that condition.

To convey to users the strength of the evidence for each quantity, uncertainty distributions for each quantity are reported in various metrics of uncertainty such as 95 per cent uncertainty intervals.

An important component of the analytical work on GBD is to ensure that the set of results are internally consistent. The sum of cause-specific mortality must equal all-cause mortality: 'you only die once'. Deaths are assigned following International Classification of Diseases and Related Health Problems (ICD) rules on underlying cause. The sum of cause-specific estimates of impairments such as blindness and anaemia must equal estimates of all-cause blindness and anaemia. Where conditions are in equilibrium, incidence, prevalence, remission, and duration must be internally consistent.

Burden of disease estimation should be seen as an iterative process. New data and methodological innovation will lead to revision of estimates. Revisions should re-estimate the entire time series so that results are always available over time using consistent data and methods.

Data synthesis

The emphasis in the GBD 2010 is on systematically identifying all published and unpublished data sources. Published literature is a good source for some conditions such as epilepsy. For many others, national data systems such as vital registration, hospital discharges, national surveys, and surveillance data are equally important sources. By starting with the universe of all measurements, we can avoid publication or selection bias where different groups pick and choose between data sources.

Making use of all available data requires careful consideration of non-sampling error due to variation in case definition, diagnostic technology, study design, training of data collectors, recall periods (1 month, 12 months, lifetime), etc. For example, review

of diabetes prevalence studies found 18 different case definitions in use and review of myocardial infarction data showed marked differences in rates using heart-related serum creatine kinase fraction or troponin tests. Across studies or measurements, sampling error is a much smaller contributor to observed variance than these sources of non-sampling error. The GBD approach is to identify and correct for bias.

Key areas in cause of death data concern mapping across variants of the ICD, redistribution of ill-defined or 'garbage' codes, and validity of verbal autopsy (VA) diagnoses (attribution of cause of death based on interviews with relatives of a deceased). For epidemiological data, statistical methods are used to quantify the relationship between different types of measurement such as variations in case definitions, diagnostic technologies, or recall periods. Setting a 'desired' reference measurement definition allows adjustments of all available data ('crosswalks') into comparable units, definitions, or categories. Where possible, uncertainty in these mappings is propagated into the uncertainty interval for the measurement. Some measurements may have to be excluded because they cannot be made comparable to the rest of the measurements or have fundamental problems of validity. For instance, measures of lifetime prevalence were rejected as invalid measures of disease occurrence due to recall bias. A few exceptions to this rule were made for conditions where exclusion of such estimates would leave little other information for making estimates.

After adjusting the data into comparable units, appropriate statistical methods are used that are designed to handle both sampling and non-sampling error. Covariates are added to the models to improve predictions where data are sparse by borrowing strength across time or geography. All estimates in GBD are generated with 1000 draws reflecting uncertainty from sampling error, non-sampling error, methods of correcting data, and where possible, model specification. Ideally, the validity of the data synthesis approach is determined using out-of-sample predictive validity. This has been fully implemented for mortality and causes of death but not for the synthesis of data on disease sequelae. Computational limitations and sparse data have so far limited the extent to which formal out-of-sample predictive validity can be evaluated for disease sequelae.

The analytical steps of GBD

The GBD approach contains 22 distinct components, as outlined in Fig. 5.17.1. The components of GBD are interconnected. For example, when new data are incorporated into the age-specific mortality rates analysis (components 2 and 3), other dependent components must also be updated, such as rescaling deaths for each cause (component 9), healthy life expectancy, or HALE (component 17), YLLs (component 18a), and estimation of YLLs attributable to each risk factor (component 22a). A brief description of these key components follows. More detailed descriptions of each component are included in published articles (Black et al. 2010; Lim et al. 2012; Lozano et al. 2012; Murray et al. 2012a, 2012b; Salomon et al. 2012a, 2012b; Vos et al. 2012).

1. Covariates

Where data are sparse, extensive use is made of a database of covariates that guide statistical methods on borrowing strength across time or geography. The more than 200 covariates cover

GBD Data and Model Flow Chart

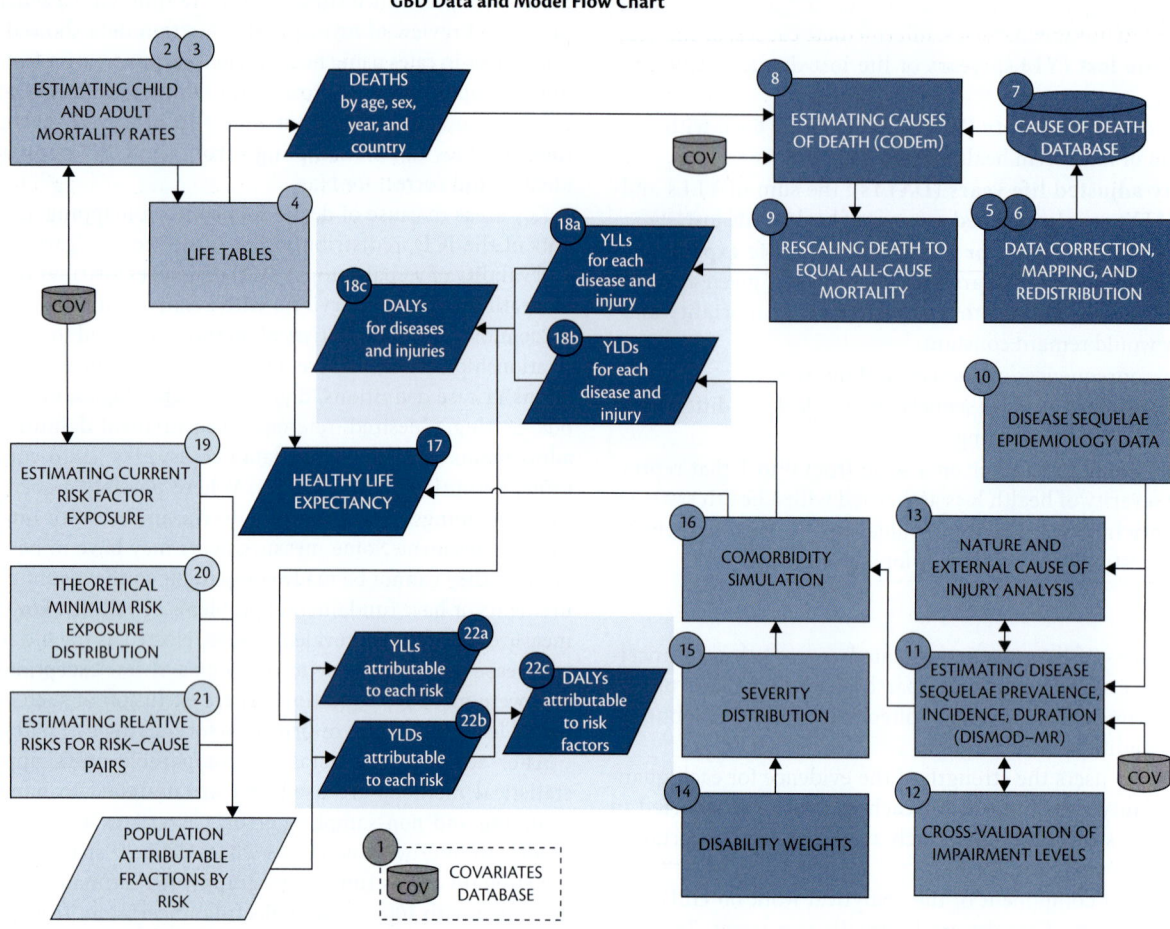

Fig. 5.17.1 The 22 components of the Global Burden of Disease study.

socioeconomic factors (e.g. gross domestic product), demography (e.g. population density, total fertility rate), behaviours (e.g. mean consumption of alcohol, tobacco, and a range of foods), and health system characteristics (vaccination coverage or a composite measure of health systems access). Essential is that values are available for all populations and years of analysis. The information largely comes from international databases, national censuses, and surveys. Where information is missing for a time period or particular population, imputation techniques are used to fill in the gaps.

2. Estimating mortality in children under 5

Sources of under-5 mortality data include vital and sample registration systems as well as surveys and censuses that ask mothers about live births and deaths of their children. All available data are processed to address biases and estimate the probability of death between ages 0 and 5 ($_5q_0$) using Gaussian process regression.

3. Estimating adult mortality

Sources of adult mortality include vital and sample registration systems as well as surveys and censuses that ask about deaths among siblings. Similar methods to those for childhood deaths are used to estimate the probability of dying between ages 15 and 60 ($_{45}q_{15}$).

4. Life tables

The estimates of $_5q_0$ and $_{45}q_{15}$ are entered into a model life table system to determine age-specific mortality rates by sex for each country between 1970 and 2010 with life expectancy at birth estimates and counts of death by age, sex, country, and year as outputs.

5. Cause of death data sources

Information on causes of death comes primarily from vital registration systems and VA studies. VA is a means of ascertaining the cause of death in populations with incomplete vital registration systems. With a structured questionnaire, interviewers ask relatives about the signs and symptoms of a recently deceased individual. Validation studies suggest that VA performs reasonably well for many causes of death (Lozano et al. 2011). For selected causes, additional sources such as police records for homicides and road traffic accidents, surveillance systems for maternal mortality and cancer registries provide further information.

6. Data correction, mapping, and redistributions

A first task to make cause of death data comparable is the mapping across various revisions and national variants of the ICD. Algorithms have also been developed to deal with the problem of ill-defined coding in vital registration and VA data where deaths are assigned to unknown causes, intermediate causes, or immediate causes of death rather than the underlying cause of death. For comparisons between countries and over time it is undesirable to have varying numbers of death in such 'garbage' code categories. The GBD approach is to reassign such deaths to more specific causes. The allocation of these garbage codes across target causes is done on the basis of published scientific literature, expert judgement, or statistical analysis. In some cases, deaths in garbage codes are reassigned proportionately across all causes. Full details can be found in the web appendix to the GBD paper on causes of death by Lozano et al. (2012).

7. Cause of death database

The GBD 2010 cause of death database contains 2798 site-years of vital registration data from 130 countries and 486 site-years of VA data across 66 countries, of which 10 per cent were nationally representative. For the estimation of mortality from cancer, 2715 site-years of cancer registry incidence data across 93 countries were included. From registries that also track cancer mortality, mortality-to-incidence ratios were derived. The log of the mortality-to-incidence ratios for each type of cancer was modelled as a function of national income per capita with random effects for country, year, and age. The ratios were then applied to the incidence figures and the resulting cancer death estimates added to the cause of death database. For injuries, information on the proportions of deaths due to injuries was added from 32 site-years of burial and mortuary data in 11 African countries and from 21 site-years of data on deaths in health facilities. Multiple demographic and health surveys, other surveys, and censuses provided data on the fraction of deaths in the reproductive age groups that are pregnancy-related. Sibling history data from 1609 survey years covering 61 countries were identified. Another eight countries had nationally representative maternal mortality surveillance systems.

8. Estimating causes of death

GBD 2010 used a new statistical approach, named CODEm (Cause of Death Ensemble model), to determine the number of deaths from each cause by age, sex, country, and year. Ensemble modelling was made famous by the recipients of the Netflix Prize, BellKor's Pragmatic Chaos, in 2009, who engineered the best algorithm to predict how much a person would like a film, taking into account their past movie preferences.

The basis of CODEm is that the analyst takes no firm position on what the best statistical method and choice of predictive covariates are but rather tests a large range of plausible statistical models and determines which single model or combination of models performs best. Four families of statistical models are used: mixed effects linear and spatial-temporal Gaussian process regression models of either the log of the death rate or the logit of the cause fraction. These four families of statistical models are run with multiple combinations of covariates. Based on published studies, plausible relationships between covariates and each cause are identified and tested. All models where the sign on the coefficient for a covariate is in the direction expected based on the literature and the coefficient is statistically significant are retained.

Next, the performance of single models and blends of various models, so-called ensembles, is evaluated using out-of-sample predictive validity tests. This is done by running the models on 70 per cent of the data and comparing predictions for the remaining data withheld from the model-building exercise with the actual observed data. Tests of out-of-sample performance include the root-mean-squared error of the log of the cause-specific death rate, the direction of the trend in the prediction compared to the data, and the validity of the 95 per cent uncertainty interval. The best performing model or ensemble is selected on the basis of out-of-sample predictive validity.

Typically for each cause of death, several hundred single models were run and ensembles created of five to 20 best-performing individual models, but for some causes almost 100 models contributed to the final ensemble.

CODEm was not used for a number of conditions, including infectious diseases such as HIV/AIDS, measles, whooping cough, and congenital syphilis, which are known to be subject to considerable misclassification bias. Instead, natural history models were created based on incidence, prevalence, and case-fatality rates. Estimates of HIV/AIDS deaths were taken directly from UNAIDS. For another 27 causes with very low numbers of death for which stable ensemble models could not be created, negative binomial models were run with a choice of plausible covariates. Information on deaths due to conflict and natural disasters from international databases was used to incorporate sudden peaks in mortality from these two causes.

9. Rescaling deaths to equal all-cause mortality

The number of deaths from all causes in a sex, age, country, and year category are scaled to ensure their sum equals the total number of deaths estimated in the GBD demographic analysis of steps 2 to 4.

10. Systematic review of the epidemiology of disease sequelae

A large effort by 44 expert groups and the core research team went into the systematic review of published and unpublished data on the prevalence, incidence, remission, mortality risk, and duration of 289 diseases and injuries and their 1160 sequelae. The systematic reviews were supplemented with analyses of household survey data, antenatal clinic surveillance, reportable disease notifications, disease registries, hospital admissions data, outpatient visit data, population-based cancer registries, active screening data, and other administrative data. As with data on causes of death, a considerable effort has gone into documenting factors that influence the quality and comparability of all data points, such as different case definitions, diagnostic technologies, and sampling strategies (Vos et al. 2012).

11. Estimating disease sequelae prevalence by Bayesian meta-regression

For the task of developing estimates for disease prevalence by age, sex, year, and country, a Bayesian meta-regression tool was specifically developed for GBD: DisMod-MR. This tool was designed to process data presented with a wide variety of age intervals; to predict values for countries and regions with sparse data; to correct data from studies with different case definitions, diagnostic technology, or sampling strategies; and to ensure internal consistency between related epidemiological parameters such as incidence, prevalence, excess mortality, and duration. DisMod-MR estimates a generalized negative binomial model for all epidemiological data. The model includes the following: covariates that predict variation in true rates; covariates that predict variation across studies because of measurement bias; super-region, region, and country random intercepts; and age-specific fixed effects. When appropriate, the rates were assumed to have been constant over time, which allowed data for incidence, prevalence, excess mortality, and cause-specific mortality to inform prevalence estimates. The differential equations governing the relation between the parameters of incidence, remission, mortality, prevalence, and duration are well characterized (Barendregt et al. 2003). More detail is provided elsewhere on the development and application of DisMod-MR (Vos et al. 2012).

An additional part of the analysis has been to try and deal with selection bias intrinsic to some data sources, such as hospital discharges where access to care influences the number of discharges in a population or antenatal clinic data on HIV prevalence. More elaborate natural history models were used for some causes, such as HIV and hepatitis, which require multiple stages of disease progression to be accounted for.

12. Cross-validation of impairment levels

There are no data sources we can use to set all-cause disability in a population similar to the all-cause mortality rates from demographic data sources that determine the 'envelope' of deaths. However, there are a number of impairments for which there are data collections of the overall prevalence in a population. In GBD 2010 this was the case for vision loss, hearing loss, anaemia, infertility, heart failure, intellectual disability, and epileptic seizures. In these cases, the quality and extent of data on the overall impairment level was considered stronger than the disease-specific estimates of the same impairments.

13. External cause and nature of injury analysis

Injuries are classified in the cause list according to the external cause such as a road injury, animal bite, or drowning, whereas the disability from injury is determined by the nature of injury such as brain trauma, hip fracture, or spinal cord lesion. The injury analysis was carried out in six steps. First, household survey and hospital discharge data were analysed using DisMod-MR to generate estimates of incidence for each external cause by age, sex, country, and year. Survey data included recall of injuries that led to hospital admission and other levels of medical attention. The meta-regression included a covariate for whether an individual was admitted to hospital or not, which was used to generate predictions both for injury warranting hospital admission and injury warranting outpatient care. Second, negative binomial models were used to analyse hospital data from 28 countries that had dual coding of discharges by external cause and nature of injury after ICD-9 and ICD-10. This led to matrices of external codes and nature of injury categories by age and sex, for high-income and low/middle-income countries and separately for injuries that were treated in emergency departments and those that led to admission. Third, for each nature of injury the prevalence of short-term disability was estimated from incidence and expert estimates of duration. Fourth, the probability of individuals developing long-term disability was estimated in a re-analysis of follow-up data from four rare studies in two high-income countries that documented outcomes of injuries after 1 year. Fifth, DisMod-MR was used again to estimate the prevalence of individuals in the population who have disability from a previous injury. Prevalence was estimated from incidence assuming zero remission and a relative risk of death compared with the general population based on available studies. In the last step, the YLDs due to prevalent cases of long-term injury were attributed back to external causes in proportion with the contributions of these causes to every type of injury.

14. Disability weights

DWs used in GBD 2010 have already been discussed in the earlier section on value choices.

15. Severity distributions

For 41 diseases, the sequelae of the disease have been linked to more than one health state (often classified as mild, moderate, and severe) including stroke, anxiety, major depressive disorder, dementia, and asthma. DWs across these severity levels were measured in population surveys for individuals without co-morbidity. Therefore, estimates of the distribution of severity need to be controlled for co-morbidity, otherwise the severity distribution would be systematically biased towards more severe symptoms. For example, if individuals with stroke are also likely to have diabetes and kidney disease, the reported distribution of functional health status would be shifted towards the more severe end.

For some diseases for which data are available for the distribution of severity by age, sex, and region, we pooled proportions in each health state using DisMod-MR or simple meta-analysis methods. Data for severity distributions are often scarcer and of poorer quality than data for prevalence of disorders. Because of the heterogeneity of the available evidence for disease severity, disease-specific reviews had to be supplemented with an analysis of three high-income country data sources which combined a range of diagnostic information and health status data. These sources allowed the assessment of the severity distributions, taking into account co-morbidity.

16. Co-morbidity simulation

In past GBD studies, YLDs were estimated for each disease and sequela and then simply added, implicitly assuming that disability from different conditions is additive. At the level of an individual this can lead to a person with several severe impairments having a combined level of DWs exceeding one, that is, being worse than dead. The 2003 Australian Burden of Disease study (Begg et al. 2008) introduced a method to simulate hypothetical populations with a correction for co-morbidity using a multiplicative rather than additive function to combine DWs. A similar approach was adopted for GBD 2010.

For each age, sex, country, and year, we used a Monte Carlo simulation of 20,000 individuals to estimate the co-occurrence of sequelae using the prevalence data with uncertainty intervals as probabilities. In simulated individuals with two or more sequelae a combined DW was calculated with a multiplicative function and then parsed back proportionately to each co-morbid sequela. The mean reduction across all individuals with a particular sequela was taken as the co-morbidity correction.

Tests on real data from the US Medical Expenditure Panel Surveys (Agency for Healthcare Research and Quality 2000) suggested that this multiplicative model was the most appropriate and that after correcting for independent co-morbidity (i.e. just based on prevalence), taking further into account that some conditions are dependent (i.e. more likely to co-occur in the same individual) made little additional difference to the co-morbidity corrections.

17. Healthy life expectancy

The life tables developed in component 4 for each country and the output of the co-morbidity simulations were combined to estimate healthy life expectancy for 187 countries. Healthy life expectancy is a single summary metric of population health that is not affected by population age structure. It can be thought of as equivalent to the expectation of life at birth in full health given the currently observed age-specific death rates and prevalence of disease and injury sequelae.

18. Calculation of YLDs, YLLs, and DALYs

YLLs are simply the multiplication of the deaths by cause, age, sex, country, and year with the relevant value from the standard life table for the age at death. YLDs are the product of prevalence of a sequel and the co-morbidity-corrected DW. DALYs are the simple addition of YLLs and YLDs. Each quantity in GBD 2010 is estimated with uncertainty by generating 1000 draws. A thousand values of each summary measure are computed by taking the first draw for each quantity, then the second draw and so on until 1000 estimates are calculated. Thus, the correlation across age and over time for causes of death sequelae prevalence is retained.

19. Estimating risk factor exposure

In GBD 2010, risk factors were chosen based on their likely importance to disease burden or policy; availability of sufficient data and methods to enable estimation of exposure distributions by country; sufficient evidence for causal effect and to estimate outcome-specific effect sizes; and evidence to support generalizability of effect sizes to populations other than those included in epidemiological studies.

Analogous to the same principles used for work on disease sequelae, a database of published and unpublished sources on the prevalence of exposure was created. For some risks, innovative sources such as satellite imagery have been used. For a number of risk factors, primary survey data have been collated and re-analysed along with published studies.

20. Theoretical minimum risk factor distribution

The tradition in risk factor epidemiology is to assess attributable burden by estimating a counterfactual scenario where exposure to a risk factor in the past is set to a counterfactual distribution. Attributable deaths, YLLs, YLDs, or DALYs are then the difference between observed burden of disease and the counterfactual scenario. Following the framework for comparative risk assessment (Murray and Lopez 1999), counterfactuals are set to the lowest risk distribution that has been observed or is theoretically possible—the theoretical minimum risk exposure distribution.

21. Estimating relative risks for risk factor–disease pairs

For each risk–disease pair, relative risks for specific disease outcomes have been taken from published meta-analyses or updated meta-analyses that have been undertaken as part of GBD 2010. Special analyses have been undertaken for water and sanitation, all sources of particulates less than 2.5 microns, and the components of diet. Standardized approaches to the attenuation of relative risks with age for cardiovascular disease outcomes have been included. Uncertainty in the relative risks for each risk–disease pair by age and sex have been propagated into the final estimates. Full details on the risk factor estimation are provided in Lim et al. (2012).

22. Estimating deaths, YLDs, YLLs, and DALYs attributable to risk factors

Risk factor burden is assessed using the distributions of burden for each disease associated with a risk factor. Uncertainty from the prevalence of exposure, relative risks, and where appropriate the theoretical minimum risk exposure distribution, are all propagated into the final risk factor uncertainty. Final uncertainty reflects both the uncertainty for an age–sex group from the process of disease and injury estimation and the uncertainty in the population attributable fractions. We assume that uncertainty in the population attributable fractions is uncorrelated with uncertainty in disease and injury burden. For the computation of clusters of risk factors (e.g. diet), we have assumed that the combined effects of risk factors are multiplicative and independent.

Exploring GBD results

The GBD is considered a 'public good'. To guide policymakers, researchers, students, and interested individuals through the large amount of results, IHME has created innovative visualization tools to explore health trends for different countries and regions. The visualization tools allow people to view GBD estimates through hundreds of different dimensions. To explore the IHME website to use the GBD data visualization tools, visit http://www.healthmetricsandevaluation.org/gbd/visualizations/country.

The *Mortality* and *Causes of Death* visualizations show the results, data inputs, and data transformations of all mortality estimates. *GBD Compare* shows results of deaths, YLLs, YLDs, and DALYs by diseases and risk factors. The main view is a 'tree map' which is basically a square pie chart showing the proportional distribution of the overall burden by underlying causes. Additional views can be added showing a map of the world, time plots, or age plots. Each can interactively be explored by country, age, sex, year, cause, or risk factor. Data are available as counts, rates, and proportions of total. Rates can be shown by age for all ages combined and age standardized to the 2001 WHO world standard population (Ahmad et al. 2001). The former is most useful to explore the amount of disease burden health systems need to address. The latter helps to understand the underlying epidemiological trends, that is, after taking out population growth and ageing as drivers of differences in burden estimates. *GBD Arrow Diagram* allows the user to compare ranking lists for countries and world regions between 1990 and 2010. As with *GBD Compare*, changes in ranking and rates can be viewed with and without age standardization.

GBD Cause Patterns is the tool of choice to compare country results with any grouping of other countries. It can also be used to explore age patterns. *GBD Heatmap* is a different method of showing rankings of diseases or risk factors between countries and regions of choice. Top ranking causes are coloured in deep red and successively shaded in lighter hues that change to yellow, green, and blue further down the ranking. This tool quickly shows areas of progress or concern in a particular country in comparison to others. The *GBD Uncertainty Visualization* tool graphically shows the width of the uncertainty intervals for quantities of interest and allows a quick scan of the importance of differences in ranks. The *Healthy Life Years vs Life Expectancy* tool graphs these two summary measures of population health and how they have changed over time for each country. Lastly, there is the *GBD Insight* tool which shows summary country profiles.

Key GBD results

A comparison of the top 20 causes of DALYs in the world between 1990 and 2010 shows a shift from communicable, maternal, neonatal, and nutritional disorders (dark blue) to non-communicable diseases (blue) and injuries (light blue) (Fig. 5.17.2). Ischaemic heart disease and stroke have become the leading and third-leading causes, displacing lower respiratory infections, diarrhoeal diseases, and pre-term birth complications. Among the major infectious diseases, only malaria and HIV/AIDS increased in rank and size. The growing importance of disability contributing to the burden of disease globally is illustrated by the prominent and rising positions of low back pain and major depressive disorder, both responsible for large amounts of YLDs but no mortality (Fig. 5.17.2).

The column on the right of Fig. 5.17.2 shows the median proportion change in DALYs (with a 95 per cent uncertainty interval) between 1990 and 2010. Some of the change is due to population increase, some due to ageing of the world's populations, and some due to a change in the epidemiological trends. Fig. 5.17.3 shows the same top-20 ranking of DALYs but based on age-standardized rates. In this figure the column on the right reflects the change in epidemiological rates over time having removed the demographic drivers of changes in the numbers of DALYs. Apart from a shift in the ranks of some conditions the greater difference is in the median proportion change column. For instance, the increase in stroke DALYs was entirely due to demographic changes, while the epidemiological rates actually dropped by 23 per cent, as seen in Fig. 5.17.3. Similarly, the DALYs for low back pain increased by 43 per cent, while the rate showed just a trivial change. Both measures have their own use. Changes in the volume of disease (as in Fig. 5.17.2) inform policymakers about health service planning. The epidemiological changes tell us something about the impact of prevention and cure on the occurrence of disease.

The shift from communicable diseases largely affecting children to non-communicable disease in adults is further illustrated by the change over time in the ranking order of the main risk factors (Fig. 5.17.4). Childhood underweight has been replaced by dietary risks (a combination of 14 component dietary factors such as low fruit or vegetable intake or high sodium intake). High blood pressure and high body mass (overweight and obesity) have increased in rank and amount of disease burden. The small overall

1990

Mean rank (95% UI)	
1.0 (1 to 2)	1 Lower respiratory infections
2.0 (1 to 2)	2 Diarrhoeal diseases
3.4 (3 to 5)	3 Pre-term birth complications
3.8 (3 to 5)	4 Ischaemic heart disease
5.2 (4 to 6)	5 Stroke
6.3 (5 to 18)	6 COPD
8.0 (6 to13)	7 Malaria
9.8 (7 to 13)	8 Tuberculosis
10.1 (7 to14)	9 Protein-energy malnutrition
10.2 (7 to 15)	10 Neonatal encephalopathy
11.7 (8 to 15)	11 Road injury
11.9 (7 to 17)	12 Low back pain
12.8 (8 to 16)	13 Congenital anomalies
15.0 (8 to 18)	14 Iron-deficiency anaemia
15.2 (11 to 18)	15 Major depressive disorder
15.2 (3 to 37)	16 Measles
15.3 (8 to 24)	17 Neonatal sepsis
17.3 (15 to 19)	18 Meningitis
20.0 (17 to 25)	19 Self-harm
20.6 (18 to 26)	20 Drowning
21.1 (18 to 25)	21 Diabetes
23.0 (19 to 28)	23 Falls
32.7 (26 to 38)	32 HIV/AIDS

2010

	Mean rank (95% UI)	Median % change
1 Ischaemic heart disease	1.0 (1 to 2)	30 (21 to 34)
2 Lower respiratory infections	2.0 (1 to 3)	−44 (−48 to −39)
3 Stroke	3.2 (2 to 5)	21 (5 to 26)
4 Diarrhoeal diseases	4.8 (4 to 8)	−51 (−57 to −45)
5 HIV/AIDS	6.5 (4 to 9)	353 (293 to 413)
6 Malaria	6.7 (3 to 11)	18 (−9 to 63)
7 Low back pain	7.1 (3 to 11)	43 (38 to 48)
8 Pre-term birth complications	7.9 (5 to 11)	−27 (−37 to −16)
9 COPD	8.1 (5 to 11)	−2 (−9 to 5)
10 Road injury	8.4 (4 to 11)	33 (11 to 63)
11 Major depressive disorder	10.8 (7 to 14)	37 (25 to 49)
12 Neonatal encephalopathy	13.3 (11 to 17)	−17 (−30 to −1)
13 Tuberculosis	13.4 (11 to 17)	−18 (−34 to −5)
14 Diabetes	14.2 (12 to 16)	70 (59 to 77)
15 Iron-deficiency anaemia	15.2 (11 to 22)	−3 (−6 to −1)
16 Neonatal sepsis	15.9 (10 to 26)	−4 (−25 to 27)
17 Congenital anomalies	17.3 (14 to 21)	−28 (−43 to −9)
18 Self-harm	18.7 (15 to 26)	24 (−1 to 42)
19 Falls	19.7 (16 to 25)	37 (20 to 55)
20 Protein-energy malnutrition	19.9 (16 to 26)	−42 (−51 to −33)
25 Meningitis	24.4 (20 to 27)	−22 (−32 to −12)
32 Drowning	32.9 (27 to 38)	−33 (−40 to −5)
56 Measles	56.3 (28 to 94)	−80 (−85 to 74)

Communicable, maternal, neonatal, and nutritional
Non-communicable
Injuries

—— Ascending order in rank
----- Descending order in rank

Fig. 5.17.2 Global top-20 ranking of diseases and injuries in DALYs, 1990 and 2010.

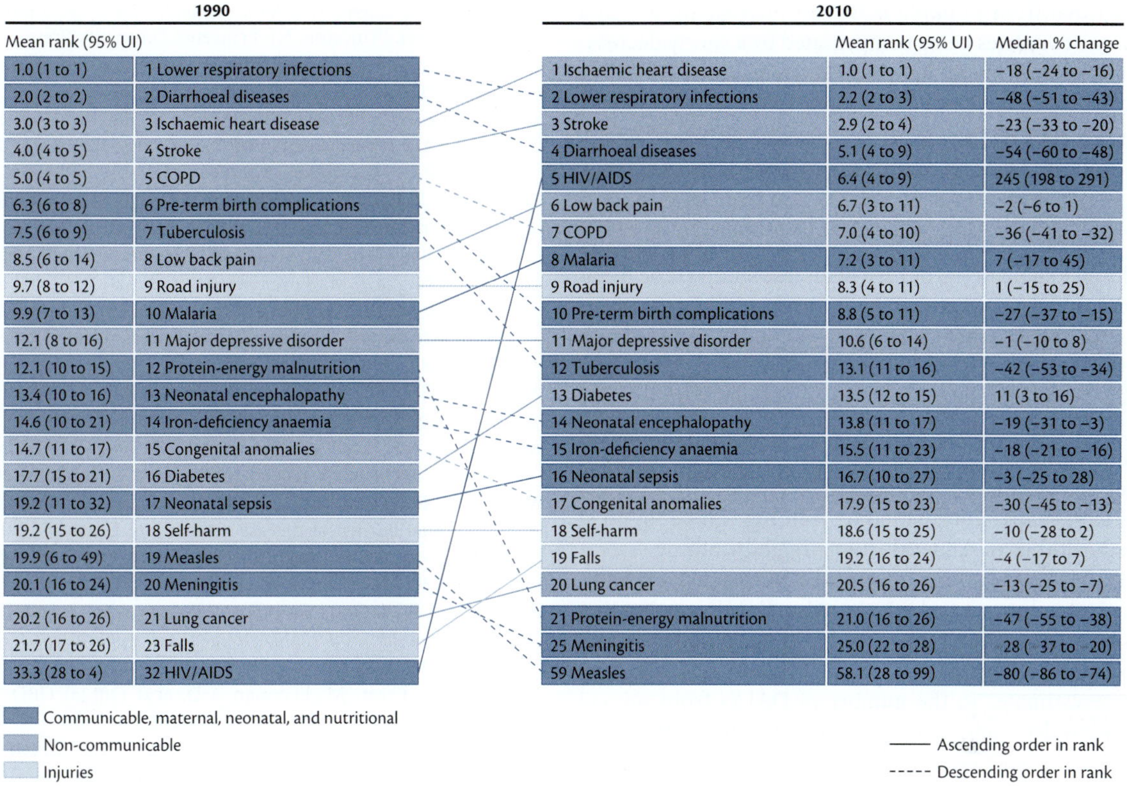

1990

Mean rank (95% UI)

Mean rank (95% UI)	Disease/Injury
1.0 (1 to 1)	1 Lower respiratory infections
2.0 (2 to 2)	2 Diarrhoeal diseases
3.0 (3 to 3)	3 Ischaemic heart disease
4.0 (4 to 5)	4 Stroke
5.0 (4 to 5)	5 COPD
6.3 (6 to 8)	6 Pre-term birth complications
7.5 (6 to 9)	7 Tuberculosis
8.5 (6 to 14)	8 Low back pain
9.7 (8 to 12)	9 Road injury
9.9 (7 to 13)	10 Malaria
12.1 (8 to 16)	11 Major depressive disorder
12.1 (10 to 15)	12 Protein-energy malnutrition
13.4 (10 to 16)	13 Neonatal encephalopathy
14.6 (10 to 21)	14 Iron-deficiency anaemia
14.7 (11 to 17)	15 Congenital anomalies
17.7 (15 to 21)	16 Diabetes
19.2 (11 to 32)	17 Neonatal sepsis
19.2 (15 to 26)	18 Self-harm
19.9 (6 to 49)	19 Measles
20.1 (16 to 24)	20 Meningitis
20.2 (16 to 26)	21 Lung cancer
21.7 (17 to 26)	23 Falls
33.3 (28 to 4)	32 HIV/AIDS

2010

Disease/Injury	Mean rank (95% UI)	Median % change
1 Ischaemic heart disease	1.0 (1 to 1)	−18 (−24 to −16)
2 Lower respiratory infections	2.2 (2 to 3)	−48 (−51 to −43)
3 Stroke	2.9 (2 to 4)	−23 (−33 to −20)
4 Diarrhoeal diseases	5.1 (4 to 9)	−54 (−60 to −48)
5 HIV/AIDS	6.4 (4 to 9)	245 (198 to 291)
6 Low back pain	6.7 (3 to 11)	−2 (−6 to 1)
7 COPD	7.0 (4 to 10)	−36 (−41 to −32)
8 Malaria	7.2 (3 to 11)	7 (−17 to 45)
9 Road injury	8.3 (4 to 11)	1 (−15 to 25)
10 Pre-term birth complications	8.8 (5 to 11)	−27 (−37 to −15)
11 Major depressive disorder	10.6 (6 to 14)	−1 (−10 to 8)
12 Tuberculosis	13.1 (11 to 16)	−42 (−53 to −34)
13 Diabetes	13.5 (12 to 15)	11 (3 to 16)
14 Neonatal encephalopathy	13.8 (11 to 17)	−19 (−31 to −3)
15 Iron-deficiency anaemia	15.5 (11 to 23)	−18 (−21 to −16)
16 Neonatal sepsis	16.7 (10 to 27)	−3 (−25 to 28)
17 Congenital anomalies	17.9 (15 to 23)	−30 (−45 to −13)
18 Self-harm	18.6 (15 to 25)	−10 (−28 to 2)
19 Falls	19.2 (16 to 24)	−4 (−17 to 7)
20 Lung cancer	20.5 (16 to 26)	−13 (−25 to −7)
21 Protein-energy malnutrition	21.0 (16 to 26)	−47 (−55 to −38)
25 Meningitis	25.0 (22 to 28)	28 (37 to 20)
59 Measles	58.1 (28 to 99)	−80 (−86 to −74)

▮ Communicable, maternal, neonatal, and nutritional
▮ Non-communicable
▮ Injuries

—— Ascending order in rank
---- Descending order in rank

Fig. 5.17.3 Global top-20 ranking of diseases and injuries in age-standardized DALY rates, 1990 and 2010.

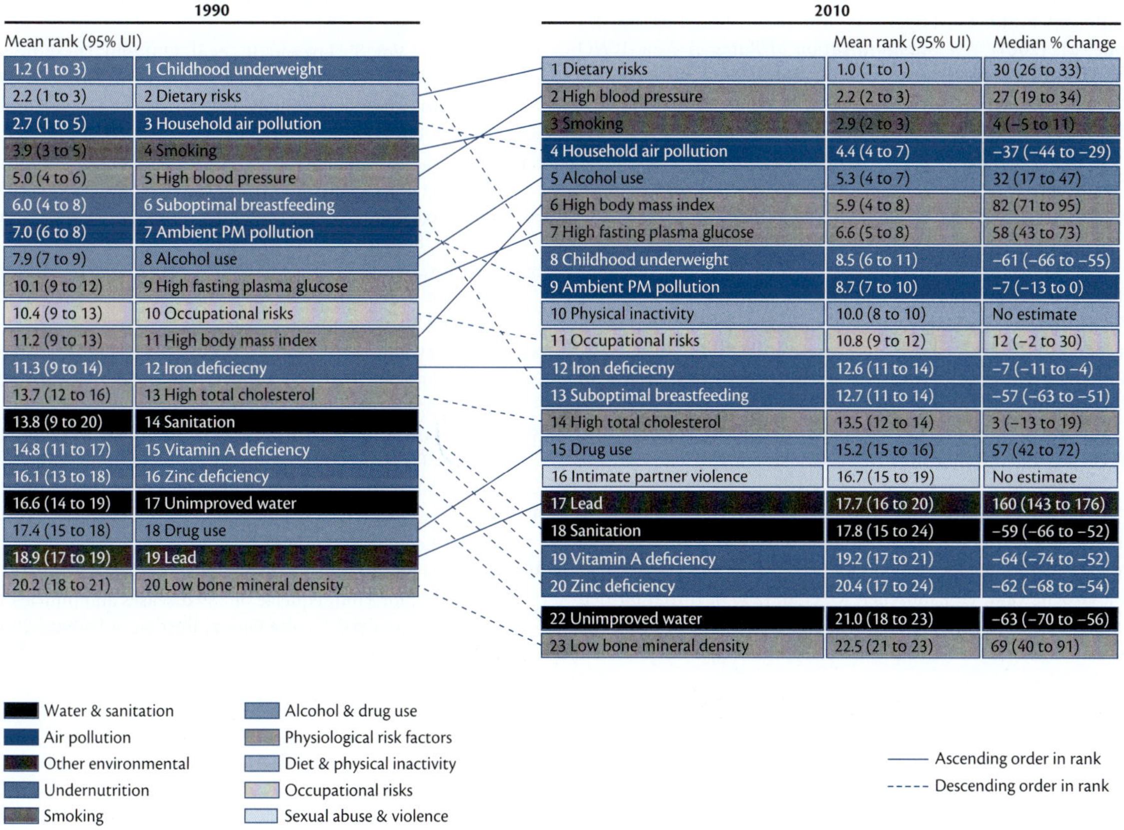

1990

Mean rank (95% UI)

Mean rank (95% UI)	Risk factor
1.2 (1 to 3)	1 Childhood underweight
2.2 (1 to 3)	2 Dietary risks
2.7 (1 to 5)	3 Household air pollution
3.9 (3 to 5)	4 Smoking
5.0 (4 to 6)	5 High blood pressure
6.0 (4 to 8)	6 Suboptimal breastfeeding
7.0 (6 to 8)	7 Ambient PM pollution
7.9 (7 to 9)	8 Alcohol use
10.1 (9 to 12)	9 High fasting plasma glucose
10.4 (9 to 13)	10 Occupational risks
11.2 (9 to 13)	11 High body mass index
11.3 (9 to 14)	12 Iron deficiency
13.7 (12 to 16)	13 High total cholesterol
13.8 (9 to 20)	14 Sanitation
14.8 (11 to 17)	15 Vitamin A deficiency
16.1 (13 to 18)	16 Zinc deficiency
16.6 (14 to 19)	17 Unimproved water
17.4 (15 to 18)	18 Drug use
18.9 (17 to 19)	19 Lead
20.2 (18 to 21)	20 Low bone mineral density

2010

Risk factor	Mean rank (95% UI)	Median % change
1 Dietary risks	1.0 (1 to 1)	30 (26 to 33)
2 High blood pressure	2.2 (2 to 3)	27 (19 to 34)
3 Smoking	2.9 (2 to 3)	4 (−5 to 11)
4 Household air pollution	4.4 (4 to 7)	−37 (−44 to −29)
5 Alcohol use	5.3 (4 to 7)	32 (17 to 47)
6 High body mass index	5.9 (4 to 8)	82 (71 to 95)
7 High fasting plasma glucose	6.6 (5 to 8)	58 (43 to 73)
8 Childhood underweight	8.5 (6 to 11)	−61 (−66 to −55)
9 Ambient PM pollution	8.7 (7 to 10)	−7 (−13 to 0)
10 Physical inactivity	10.0 (8 to 10)	No estimate
11 Occupational risks	10.8 (9 to 12)	12 (−2 to 30)
12 Iron deficiency	12.6 (11 to 14)	−7 (−11 to −4)
13 Suboptimal breastfeeding	12.7 (11 to 14)	−57 (−63 to −51)
14 High total cholesterol	13.5 (12 to 14)	3 (−13 to 19)
15 Drug use	15.2 (15 to 16)	57 (42 to 72)
16 Intimate partner violence	16.7 (15 to 19)	No estimate
17 Lead	17.7 (16 to 20)	160 (143 to 176)
18 Sanitation	17.8 (15 to 24)	−59 (−66 to −52)
19 Vitamin A deficiency	19.2 (17 to 21)	−64 (−74 to −52)
20 Zinc deficiency	20.4 (17 to 24)	−62 (−68 to −54)
22 Unimproved water	21.0 (18 to 23)	−63 (−70 to −56)
23 Low bone mineral density	22.5 (21 to 23)	69 (40 to 91)

▮ Water & sanitation
▮ Air pollution
▮ Other environmental
▮ Undernutrition
▮ Smoking
▮ Alcohol & drug use
▮ Physiological risk factors
▮ Diet & physical inactivity
▮ Occupational risks
▮ Sexual abuse & violence

—— Ascending order in rank
---- Descending order in rank

Fig. 5.17.4 Global top-20 ranking of risk factors in DALYs, 1990 and 2010.

change in burden from smoking masks an increase in low- and middle-income countries being compensated by a slowly decreasing burden from smoking in high-income countries.

The future of GBD

GBD will be updated annually. The intention is to expand the network of collaborators to include country researchers, staff of ministries of health, and IHME to strengthen national estimates and to undertake subnational burden of disease studies. Local epidemiological assessment is crucial for informing local priorities.

IHME is seeking partners interested in conducting in-depth studies of the burden of disease in countries. Through such partnerships, IHME is helping governments and donors gain insights into localized health trends to inform planning and policymaking. IHME is committed to building capacity for GBD analysis in countries around the world, and will be conducting a variety of training workshops. Information on training can be found at http://www.healthmetricsandevaluation.org/gbd/training.

Currently, IHME is working to expand GBD to track expenditure for particular diseases and injuries. Also, IHME is estimating utilization of outpatient and inpatient facilities and other health services for specific diseases and injuries. Side-to-side comparisons of these estimates to the number of DALYs from myriad causes will allow decision-makers to better evaluate health system performance and priorities.

References

Agency for Healthcare Research and Quality (2000). *United States Medical Expenditure Panel Survey*. Rockville, MD: Agency for Healthcare Research and Quality.

Ahmad, O., Boschi-Pinto, C., Lopez, A., Murray, C.J.L., Lozano, R., and Inoue, M. (2001). *Age Standardization of Rates: A New WHO Standard*. GPE Discussion Paper Series: No. 31. Geneva: World Health Organization.

Anand, S. and Hanson, K. (1997). Disability-adjusted life years: a critical review. *Journal of Health Economics*, 16, 685–702.

Arnesen, T. and Kapiriri, L. (2004). Can the value choices in DALYs influence global priority-setting? *Health Policy*, 70, 137–49.

Barendregt, J.J., van Oortmarssen, G.J., Vos, T., and Murray, C.J.L. (2003). A generic model for the assessment of disease epidemiology: the computational basis of DisMod II. *Population Health Metrics*, 1, 4.

Begg, S.J., Vos, T., Barker, B., Stanley, L., and Lopez, A.D. (2008). Burden of disease and injury in Australia in the new millennium: measuring health loss from diseases, injuries and risk factors. *Medical Journal of Australia*, 188, 36–40.

Black, R.E., Cousens, S., Johnson, H.L., et al. (2010). Global, regional, and national causes of child mortality in 2008: a systematic analysis. *The Lancet*, 375, 1969–87.

Boutayeb, A. (2006). The double burden of communicable and non-communicable diseases in developing countries. *Transactions of the Royal Society of Tropical Medicine and Hygiene*, 100, 191–9.

Bradshaw, D., Groenewald, P., Laubscher, R., et al. (2003). Initial burden of disease estimates for South Africa (2000). *South African Medical Journal*, 93, 682–8.

Coale, A. and Demeny, P. (1966). *Regional Model Life Tables and Stable Populations*. Princeton, NJ: Princeton University Press.

Lim, S.S., Vos, T., Flaxman, A.D., et al. (2012). A comparative risk assessment of burden of disease and injury attributable to 67 risk factors and risk factor clusters in 21 regions, 1990–2010: a systematic analysis for the Global Burden of Disease Study 2010. *The Lancet*, 380, 2224–60.

Lozano, R., Lopez, A.D., Atkinson, C., et al. (2011). Performance of physician-certified verbal autopsies: multisite validation study using clinical diagnostic gold standards. *Population Health Metrics*, 9, 32.

Lozano, R., Naghavi, M., Foreman, K., et al. (2012). Global and regional mortality from 235 causes of death for 20 age groups in 1990 and 2010: a systematic analysis for the Global Burden of Disease Study 2010. *The Lancet*, 380, 2095–128.

Marshall, S.J. (2004). Developing countries face double burden of disease. *Bulletin of the World Health Organization*, 82, 556.

Mathers, C., Fat, D.M., and Boerma, J.T. (2008). *The Global Burden of Disease: 2004 Update*. Geneva: World Health Organization.

Melse, J.M., Essink-Bot, M.L., Kramers, P.G., and Hoeymans, N. (2000). A national burden of disease calculation: Dutch disability-adjusted life-years. Dutch Burden of Disease Group. *American Journal of Public Health*, 90, 1241–7.

Murray, C.J.L. (2002). *Summary Measures of Population Health, 2002: Concepts, Ethics, Measurement and Applications*. Geneva: World Health Organization.

Murray, C.J.L., Ezzati, M., Flaxman, A.D., et al. (2012a). GBD 2010: design, definitions, and metrics. *The Lancet*, 380, 2063–6.

Murray, C.J.L. and Lopez, A.D. (1996). *The Global Burden of Disease: A Comprehensive Assessment of Mortality and Disability from Diseases, Injuries, and Risk Factors in 1990 and Projected to 2020*. Boston, MA: Harvard School of Public Health on behalf of the World Health Organization and the World Bank.

Murray, C.J.L. and Lopez, A. (1999). On the comparable quantification of health risks: lessons from the Global Burden of Disease Study. *Epidemiology*, 10, 594–605.

Murray, C.J.L., Vos, T., Lozano, R., et al. (20120b). Disability-adjusted life years (DALYs) for 291 diseases and injuries in 21 regions, 1990–2010: a systematic analysis for the Global Burden of Disease Study 2010. *The Lancet*, 380, 2197–223.

Salomon, J.A., Vos, T., Hogan, D.R., et al. (2012a). Common values in assessing health outcomes from disease and injury: disability weights measurement study for the Global Burden of Disease Study 2010. *The Lancet*, 380, 2129–43.

Salomon, J.A., Wang, H., Freeman, M.K., et al. (2012b). Healthy life expectancy for 187 countries, 1990–2010: a systematic analysis for the Global Burden Disease Study 2010. *The Lancet*, 380, 2144–62.

Smith, S., Newhouse, J.P., and Freeland, M.S. (2009). Income, insurance, and technology: why does health spending outpace economic growth? *Health Affairs (Millwood)*, 28, 1276–84.

Stouthard, M.E.A., Essink-Bot, M.-L., and Bonsel, G.J. (2000). Disability weights for diseases: a modified protocol and results for a Western European region. *European Journal of Public Health*, 10, 24–30.

Tsuchiya, A. (2001). *The Value of Health at Different Ages*. York: Centre for Health Economics, University of York.

Vos, T., Flaxman, A.D., Naghavi, M., et al. (2012). Years lived with disability (YLDs) for 1160 sequelae of 289 diseases and injuries 1990–2010: a systematic analysis for the Global Burden of Disease Study 2010. *The Lancet*, 380, 2163–96.

Mathematical models of transmission and control of infectious agents

Alex Welte, Brian Williams, and Gavin Hitchcock

Introduction to mathematical models of transmission and control of infectious agents

Mathematical modelling plays a key role in the design, implementation, and evaluation of public health interventions. Here we clarify what mathematical modelling is, show how it has been used successfully in the past, and discuss ways in which it can be used to interpret epidemiological trends and project trends into the future.

It is important at the outset to distinguish between static models, which often rely on sophisticated statistical analyses, and dynamical models, which more often depend on computer-based simulations. The recurrent theme in dynamical modelling, which is the focus of this chapter, is the interplay between what can be known about the nature and course of an infection in an individual, and what can be known about disease trends in a community. It is remarkable that it is possible to move between these scales at all; but the beauty of mathematics is that it allows us to capture fundamental patterns and relations between rates and numbers. These may be the rates at which people are born, die, become infected, are cured, or recover; and the numbers of people in different classes, age groups, or stages of infection. Einstein observed that 'the supreme goal of all theory is to make the irreducible basic elements as simple and as few as possible without having to surrender the adequate representation of a single datum of experience' (Einstein 1934); that is, for modellers: always start with the simplest possible assumptions and the smallest number of parameters, adding complexity only where provoked and justified by specific data or key hypotheses about cause and effect, seeking always to bring to light the essential underlying patterns and the dominant processes and mechanisms.

While epidemiological data can be collected among individuals, and clinical trials can measure the response of individuals to different treatments or interventions, public health is usually concerned with the dynamics of disease over time, in specified population groups, under varied conditions, and under different interventions. In public health, many factors—biological, psychological, sociological, and economic—are involved in understanding what is likely to work, how people will respond, whether an intervention will be acceptable, how much it will cost, and what the impact is likely to be. Models are now being used not only to understand the natural history of disease but also to advise and guide public health policy and resource allocation. Mathematical modelling has become an indispensable part of public health.

The uses of models in public health are many and varied, both as concerns the nature of the models and the range of the problems to which they are applied. Good recent introductions to modelling infectious diseases are by Bacaër (2010), Vynnycky and White (2010), Brauer et al. (2008), and Keeling and Rohani (2008). Models have become important, especially in contexts where good empirical data are not readily available, for predicting changes over time in disease burden and treatment requirements, hence warranting projections of counterfactuals in quasi-experimental impact evaluation designs, and power calculations for experimental study designs (Delva et al. 2012). Recent applications include determining optimal responses to emerging pathogens (Riley et al. 2003), clarifying the requirements for eradication of polio (Grassly et al. 2006), exploring the impact of control measures and quantifying uncertainty in predictions for influenza pandemics (Fraser et al. 2009; Keeling and Danon 2009), evaluating intervention strategies for malaria (Griffin et al. 2010), and re-evaluating investment strategies in HIV programmes (Salomon et al. 2005; Granich et al. 2009; Schwartländer et al. 2011). The unprecedented attention and funding which the HIV/AIDS epidemic has attracted has brought infectious disease modelling to prominence in this field. Increasing reliance on mathematical modelling has been shown by agencies which fund, coordinate, and evaluate HIV prevention efforts: the World Bank, the Global Fund, the World Health Organization (WHO), the United Nations Joint Programme on HIV and AIDS (UNAIDS), and the President's Emergency Plan for AIDS Relief (PEPFAR). Lately, while spending on HIV has levelled off and might even be declining (Kaiser Family Foundation 2011), some important discoveries have been made, notably that antiretroviral therapy (ART) can dramatically reduce infectiousness in HIV-positive individuals (Cohen et al. 2011). The many questions that this provokes, and in particular the extent to which early treatment can stop the epidemic of HIV, can be approached most effectively by mathematical modelling

(Montaner et al. 2006; Granich et al. 2009; Delva et al. 2012). Examples include: (1) how funding should be reallocated in the light of new data (Granich et al. 2009), (2) deciding the importance or otherwise of the acute phase of HIV infection in the dynamics of the epidemic (Cohen et al. 2012), (3) how to evaluate the threat of drug resistance to the effectiveness of treatment (Wagner et al. 2010), and (4) how best to measure the impact of existing programmes (Hallett et al. 2007).

Brief historical overview

Perhaps the first application of dynamical mathematical modelling in public health was carried out in 1760 by Daniel Bernoulli to understand the efficacy of inoculating people with smallpox to prevent their developing the disease later. Bernoulli used what we would now call an 'SR model' (of susceptible and removed elements) to elucidate the variations in the size of susceptible and removed subpopulations over time (Bernoulli 1760/2004; Dietz and Heesterbeek 2002; Bacaër 2010). Bernoulli concluded that, while inoculation carried some risk, it could substantially increase life expectancy, not only by trading the risks and benefits for individuals but (crucially) also by reducing overall transmission in the population.

More than one hundred years after Bernoulli's seminal work, Ronald Ross showed in 1895 and 1899 that malaria infects people through the bites of mosquitoes, and for this discovery he was awarded the Nobel Prize for Physiology or Medicine in 1902. In fact, Ross may have been a better mathematician than he was an entomologist. He developed one of the first mathematical models of disease transmission based on differential equations to support his claim, in the face of considerable scepticism, that malaria could be eradicated by reducing the mosquito population to below a critical level. The notion that there are critical thresholds on dynamical parameters, below which disease transmission cannot persist, could be called 'the central dogma of epidemiology'. This is most famously embodied in the concept of R_0, the basic reproduction number, about which there is more later in this chapter. A crucial example of such a 'tipping point', which can only be understood through the collective dynamics of a population, is the attainment of 'herd immunity' at partial coverage of an imperfect vaccine—that is, the effect that, while there are still infected and susceptible individuals in a population, the prevalence is doomed to decline if transmission is not efficient enough to replace cases as quickly as they are naturally removed (@* see online appendix for more details).

Ross's model, published in the second edition of his book *The Prevention of Malaria* (Ross 1910, 1923), became the basis for subsequent modelling of vector-borne infections and is a good illustration of how such a mathematical model is formulated. It consists of two differential equations expressing the rates of change of I (the number of infected humans) and i (the number of infected mosquitoes), in terms of I, i, N (the total human population in the area of concern), and a few other parameters. Ross's work and later developments have been discussed in detail by Smith et al. (2012). Ross made a number of explicit assumptions, encapsulated in the constancy of the parameters: the total number of mosquitoes n; the biting frequency of mosquitoes b; the transmission probabilities p, and p', per bite, of malaria, from mosquito to human, and vice versa; the rate a at which humans recover from malaria; and

the mortality rate m of mosquitoes. This model implies a relationship between malaria prevalence, I/N, and the ratio of numbers of mosquitoes to humans, n/N. There is a critical threshold value for this ratio, below which prevalence tends to zero in the long run, and above which the endemic prevalence of infection in people would increase rapidly, before beginning to level off at about 50 per cent. Importantly, this levelling off helps to explain how it was that no correlation had been previously observed between mosquito numbers and malaria prevalence. While the threshold itself is very sensitive to changes in the biting rate b, Ross observed that the basic overall shape of the curve does not change. He concluded, as cited in Bacaër (2010):

> As a matter of fact all epidemiology, concerned as it is with the variation of disease from time to time or from place to place, must be considered mathematically, however many variables are implicated, if it is to be considered scientifically at all. To say that a disease depends upon certain factors is not to say much, until we can also form an estimate as to how largely each factor influences the whole result. And the mathematical method of treatment is really nothing but the application of careful reasoning to the problems at issue.

In the late 1920s and 1930s, William Kermack and Anderson McKendrick introduced continuous-time epidemic models that incorporated stochastic (random) elements of infection and recovery (McKendrick 1926; Kermack and McKendrick 1927; Harvey 1943; Bacaër 2010). They showed how to include age or time since infection as continuous variables, and how to generalize models to deal with time-dependent infectiousness and recovery rates. Together with Hamer, Soper, and Ross, they laid the early foundations for modern mathematical modelling in epidemiology. Crucially, they realized that epidemics are driven by the rate of contact between susceptible and infectious individuals. Because the simplest models do not distinguish between individuals, all uninfected people are equally likely to be infected and the probability that a susceptible person is infected is simply proportional to the number of people who are already infected. The so-called principle of mass-action, first formulated to model the rates of chemical reactions, now found applications in infectious disease epidemiology. It simply captures the idea of two populations being so perfectly mixed that the 'contact rate' is proportional to each population size individually.

A major theme in twentieth-century modelling was analysing the existence and implications of critical thresholds, already introduced above. When considering the control of transmissible diseases, the single most import concept is the basic reproduction number, conventionally written as R_0 and most commonly thought of as the number of secondary cases produced by a single primary case introduced into an otherwise entirely uninfected population. The roots of this concept can be traced through the work of Alfred Lotka, Ronald Ross, and others, but its first modern application in epidemiology was by George Macdonald (1957), in constructing population models of the spread of malaria. The concept was extended and developed by Dietz (1980) and by Anderson and May (1991) and their various colleagues and coworkers. The collaboration of Anderson and May culminated in their definitive book *Infectious Diseases of Humans: Dynamics and Control* (1991).

The last decade has seen dramatic developments in the role of modelling in informing public health policy and funding decisions. This may be illustrated by two reviews of modelling in the context of HIV, the first, by Stover in 2000, exhorting, and the other, by Johnson and White in 2011, almost exulting, while still urging better modelling practice and clarity in communication:

> Better mechanisms to translate modelling results into information that is usable by policy makers are needed to enhance the impact of modelling research on HIV and AIDS policies and programs. (Stover 2000)
>
> Mathematical models can assist policy makers in comparing the relative impact and cost-effectiveness of different interventions, generalising the results of randomised controlled trials to the local setting, identifying threats to programme success, identifying opportunities for maximizing intervention impact/efficiency and evaluating the extent to which observed trends in HIV prevalence are attributable to HIV/AIDS programme success. (Johnson and White 2011)

A number of other reviews of modelling in epidemiology have recently been published (Grassly and Fraser 2008; Temime et al. 2008; Keeling and Danon 2009; Garnett et al. 2011; Wilson and Garnett 2011; Eaton et al. 2012). While the proportion of published papers on epidemiological modelling, recorded in the Web of Science database, roughly quadrupled from 2000 to 2010, the growth in citations of this work has not been commensurate, notwithstanding the third bullet point below, which relates to a particular subfield. This highlights the need to make epidemiological modelling more accessible to a wider audience (see Box 5.18.1). In an interesting review, 'The rising impact of mathematical modelling in epidemiology: antibiotic resistance research as a case study' (Temime et al. 2008), the authors found:

- 'A general interest in applied mathematical epidemiological models outside the fields of mathematics or epidemiology.'

Box 5.18.1 Basic concepts crucial to the modelling of infectious agents (@+ see online appendix for more detailed discussion)

- *(Disease) mortality:* rate of death (usually probability per year).
- *Basic reproduction number:* number of new cases directly produced by one case in a purely susceptible population.
- *Case detection rate:* proportion of cases detected (within a time frame), or probability per unit time of detection.
- *Disease duration:* length of time individuals spend in an infected state.
- *Epidemic growth rate:* (usually relative) growth rate of prevalence.
- *Equilibrium:* a scenario in which the state of the model world is unchanged by time.
- *Herd immunity:* collective ability of a population to resist or extinguish an outbreak, despite containing susceptible individuals.
- *Incidence:* rate of occurrence of infections.
- *Initial doubling time:* time taken for an early prevalence to double.
- *Model scenario:* 'model world' history with fully specified initial conditions and rules.
- *Parameter:* a variable which expresses a rule—a model input.
- *Prevalence:* proportion of a population affected by a condition at a point in time.
- *State variable:* a variable capturing a model output.

- 'Heightened attention and acceptance accorded to these methods (modelling) by the scientific community.'

- A 'high citation impact...for most modelling articles, compared to other articles published in the same journals' (Temime et al. 2008).

What is a mathematical model?

A model can be any, necessarily simplified, representation of reality, such as a two-dimensional picture, a three-dimensional model, a sketch, a plan, a schema, a mind map, a flow diagram, a graphical diagram, a computer code, or a set of equations. The idea of mathematical modelling was first fully developed in physics and could be said to have its roots in Galileo's breathtakingly simple yet ground-breaking combination of observation, algebra, and geometry, applied to a basic human experience—a stone falling under gravity. For Galileo in 1623, philosophy is written in the book of nature, but to understand it we have to master the language in which it is written—mathematics; without mathematics we will be lost and grasp nothing (Galileo 1623/1957). His fundamental insight was to transform the question about the falling stone from the qualitative, philosophical 'Why?' to the quantitative, observation-oriented, and empirical 'How?' and to see the value of carefully selected measurable parameters under dramatically simplifying assumptions. Galileo started by assuming constant acceleration, on grounds of simplicity. In order to handle the matter in a scientific way, it was necessary to 'cut loose' from such irksome difficulties as friction or air resistance. Once we have discovered our theorems about the stone, assuming there is no resistance, 'we can correct them or apply them with limitations as experience will teach'. 'It seems we shall not be far wrong if we put the increment of speed as proportional to the increment of time' (Galileo 1638/1914). Galileo's basic principles of observation, quantitative questioning, simplifying assumptions, graphical representation, and hypothesis-making and testing lie at the heart of all modern science, and the mathematical modelling that he pioneered is now used in almost every field of intellectual pursuit.

In the context of public health, a mathematical model serves as a conceptual tool for thinking about the behaviour of complex systems and learning how to describe, observe, predict, and control the behaviour of such systems. Such a model is expected to mirror, in useful ways, some of the reality that it represents, and is constructed to imitate selected aspects of this reality. For modelling infections in human populations, models based on algebra and calculus have been widely deployed over a long time. But as the applications become more complex and detailed, analytical solutions become less tractable and computer simulation is increasingly important.

A mathematical model is a set of explicit assumptions about features to be modelled and hence abstracted, together with selected mathematical modes of expression and analysis including variables, functional dependencies, flow diagrams, recurrence relations, differential equations, programming code, and so on. This reductionist approach can give rise to fears that the models are too simplistic and therefore unrealistic. But, as illustrated earlier by Galileo's primal act of modelling, it is this reductionism that is the key to the success of much science. Far from aspiring to capture reality in all its complexity, the modeller addresses each specific question by careful selection and abstraction of those elements of reality requisite for the task. A powerful though simple conceptual device in maintaining a clear boundary between real and modelled scenarios, and exploring a 'model world' in its own right, is to think separately about three realms, or objects of our attention: (1) the real world, (2) the abstracted 'model world' per se, where things are simple and fully specified, and (3) the mathematical tool box for manipulating and analysing events in the model world. The point here is to discuss the mathematical and analytical activities by reflecting on their interpretation within the model world.

The value of a mathematical model lies in the extent to which it suggests new insights into the nature and mechanisms of the processes being modelled, or in its ability to make predictions which can be tested and which stand up well to such testing. The model is 'calibrated' by estimating its parameters using known data; the model is 'validated' either by comparing its predictions with appropriately collected data resulting from experiments or trials different from those used in the initial model calibration, or by comparisons with other models' predictions. The fruitful interaction between abstract theory and real-world data is intrinsic to the process of good modelling practice, which we will focus on in the final two sections.

What kinds of questions are we trying to understand?

A primary purpose of modelling is to help us understand the natural history of the infection or disease that we are studying. Fig. 5.18.1 gives the trends in the number of cases of various diseases reported in England and Wales between 1930 and 1985 as presented by Anderson and May (1991).

It is clear from Fig. 5.18.1 that the dynamics of the various diseases are quite different. Diphtheria cases remain high but variable from 1930 to 1940, then decline rapidly, and by 1950 diphtheria is essentially eliminated from England and Wales. The number of measles cases fluctuates with up to fourfold increases, and declines from one year to the next. But what is most striking is the very regular 2-year cycle from 1950 to 1960. Acute polio (paralytic poliomyelitis and polioencephalitis) trickles along steadily until 1941, increases tenfold in 1942, fluctuates for the next 10 years and then declines rapidly to eradication by about 1965. Scarlet fever falls steadily, with some fluctuations, from 1930 to 1985 but is never quite eliminated. Typhoid and paratyphoid seem to come down very rapidly from a high point in 1940, but, since this appears to be an outlier, one might wish

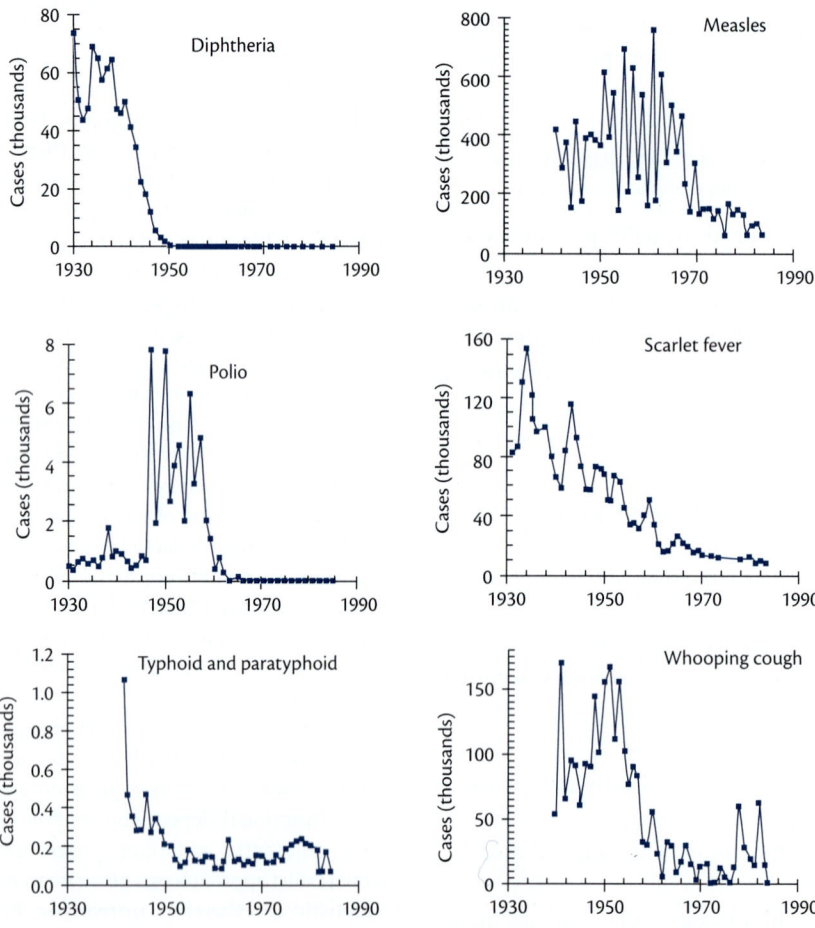

Fig. 5.18.1 Disease trends in England and Wales. The data give the number of cases per thousand people of various diseases from 1930 to 1985.

Adapted from Anderson, R.M. and May, R.M., *Infectious diseases of humans: dynamics and control*, pp. 42–43, Oxford University Press, Oxford, UK, Copyright © Roy M. Anderson and Robert M. May, 1991, by permission of Oxford University Press Inc. Contains data from Topics A-Z, Health Protection Agency, available online at http://www.hpa.org.uk/Topics/InfectiousDiseases/InfectionsAZ.

to exclude it. The number then reaches a low but steady level in 1950 with no significant change after that. Whooping cough is particularly interesting. Numbers are very high in the 1950s, fall dramatically in the 1960s and 1970s but then show two 'outbreaks' in 1978 and 1982.

Before we can begin to make models to explain these different trends, we need a better understanding of the individual diseases. Diphtheria is a bacterial infection of the upper respiratory tract, transmitted through contact with saliva, with case fatality rates of 5–10 per cent with higher rates in young children and old people. Vaccination with diphtheria toxin was developed over the course of the twentieth century. The United Kingdom proposed the introduction of mass childhood diphtheria immunization in 1940 (Mortimer 2011) and this led to the elimination of diphtheria by 1950. Only about ten cases are now reported each year in England and Wales.

Measles is a viral disease of the respiratory tract, transmitted by aerosols from infected people. It is highly contagious and almost all those without immunity through previous exposure or vaccination will be infected. There is an asymptomatic incubation period lasting for about ten days after infection and people are infectious for approximately one week. In developed countries about 0.3 per cent of measles cases will die (Orenstein et al. 2004), but in countries with high rates of malnutrition and poor healthcare or in people with HIV (Sension et al. 1988) the case-fatality rates can be up to 30 per cent. The measles vaccine, which confers lifetime immunity, was licensed in 1968, after which the number of cases started to decline. There was a further decline after 1988 when the combined MMR (measles, mumps, and rubella) vaccine was introduced.

Polio is a viral disease and may soon be the second disease, after smallpox, to be eradicated worldwide; in 2011 there were only 650 cases in the world. Polio is highly contagious, transmitted mainly via the faecal–oral route when people consume contaminated water or food. In endemic areas, it once infected virtually the entire population. Virus particles are excreted in the faeces for several weeks following infection. Three doses of the live attenuated oral polio vaccine produce protective antibodies to all three poliovirus types in more than 95 per cent of recipients and this was licensed for use in 1962.

Scarlet fever is caused by a toxin produced by a bacterium, most commonly in 4- to 8-year-old children. It is spread mainly by inhalation, and 15–20 per cent of school-age children may be asymptomatic carriers. A vaccine is not available but scarlet fever can be treated with antibiotics.

Typhoid is a bacterial disease, transmitted by the ingestion of food or water contaminated with the faeces of an infected person. Partially protective vaccines are available, but the disease is best prevented through good sanitation and hygiene. Oral rehydration therapy provides a simple way to prevent many of the deaths of diarrhoeal diseases in general and this applies to both typhoid and cholera.

Pertussis, or whooping cough, is a highly contagious bacterial disease and treatment is of little benefit. Vaccination gives protection for 5–10 years, covering childhood—the time of greatest exposure and greatest risk of death. In the 1970s there were suggestions that the vaccine might cause permanent brain damage in very rare cases. Further studies found no connection of any kind between the vaccine and permanent brain injury. However a few well-publicized anecdotal reports of permanent disability were blamed on the vaccine. Consequently, the immunization rate fell in Great Britain from 80 per cent in 1972 to 30 per cent in 1978. Coverage rates then increased slowly again and reached 90 per cent by 1992.

We can now think about ways in which modelling might help us to understand the patterns of disease shown in Fig. 5.18.1. Diphtheria is fairly straightforward, but we may want to ask why the prevalence in the early twentieth century seemed to be stable at about 60,000 cases per year. We note that, although vaccines were developed prior to 1940, it was only with the introduction of mass vaccination of children that diphtheria was effectively eliminated. We could collect data on coverage over time and see if this helps to explain the rate of decline between 1940 and 1950. We could also model the effect of vaccinating children at different ages.

Measles is particularly interesting. Since the infectious period is very short and infection confers lifelong immunity, measles can only persist because it is highly infectious. This means that it can spread very rapidly, but, since infected people either die or are immune for life, it is also unstable and can burn itself out, leading to the oscillations seen in Fig. 5.18.1. The modelling question is then: why is there this tendency to oscillate with a period of 1 year? The broad answer is that in a small, closed population the introduction of measles will lead to an epidemic that burns out and never recurs. For the epidemic to recur requires new susceptibles and these arise from new births. In England and Wales the birth rate in the 1950s was such that it took about a year to acquire enough susceptibles to sustain another epidemic. So the modelling prediction is that the inter-epidemic period should be shorter where the birth rate is higher and vice versa. We could further take into account that for the first year of life children are protected from measles by maternal antibodies, and that contact rates and spatial heterogeneity also affect the details of the epidemic pattern (Earn 2004). However, we see that after the introduction of vaccination in 1968, measles began to decline, but the *coup de grâce* was only delivered in 1988 with the introduction of the MMR vaccine in that year. The modelling question here would be to compare coverage in the period 1968–1988 and see if this explains the decline.

Polio is still not fully understood even as we approach final eradication of the virus. The tenfold increase after 1940 still demands an explanation. A common explanation is as follows: we know that polio is transmitted through water or food contaminated by the faeces of people with polio and we know that adolescents are much more likely than infants to develop paralytic or acute polio. The suggestion, then, is that improved sanitation and hygiene reduced transmission rates and delayed the age at which people acquired polio, leading to the dramatic increase in 1940. At first glance, this seems unlikely, since improvements in sanitation and hygiene would have happened slowly and 1941 was not a critical year in this regard. An equally sudden upsurge was recorded in the United States, but there the upsurge occurred in 1907, not 1941 (Nathanson and Martin 1979).

Furthermore, there seemed to be no shift in the age distribution of people developing acute polio before and after the sudden change. The explanation for the rise remains open. The very rapid decline after the introduction of the oral polio vaccine in 1962 makes sense. In 2012 there were 222 cases of polio in Pakistan, Afghanistan, and Nigeria combined, five in Chad, and one in

Niger, so that the more interesting modelling question now involves ways to achieve final eradication and to be certain that it has happened (World Health Organization 2013).

Scarlet fever cannot be prevented but it can be treated with antibiotics, and the steady decline, albeit with some residual variability, raises interesting questions for modellers. Early treatment with antibiotics might have reduced the effective infectious period of the disease, but antibiotics only became widely available after the Second World War, and the decline seems to have predated the war. It has been suggested (Londish and Murray 2008) that improved living conditions (particularly with regard to nutrition and housing), implementation of control strategies, and possibly reduced virulence of circulating strains (perhaps the result of a natural evolutionary process favouring diminished pathogenicity to maximize onward transmission) may have had a bigger impact on scarlet fever than the availability of effective treatments.

Typhoid is also transmitted through food or water contaminated by the faeces of infected people, and the decline up to 1950 may well have been the result of improved sanitation and hygiene. One would like to have data on the extent to which sanitation and hygiene improved over this period and perhaps compare it with similar time-series data in other countries.

Pertussis was very common in the United Kingdom, but the introduction of the DPT (diphtheria, pertussis, and tetanus) vaccine in the 1950s, with about 80 per cent of children being vaccinated before their second birthday by 1972, led to dramatic falls in the number of cases. However, with the ultimately unfounded scare that the pertussis vaccine was associated with brain damage in children, coverage rates fell to about 30 per cent and there were substantial outbreaks in 1972, 1984, and 1986. As coverage rates rose again, pertussis came close to elimination (Ramsay 2012). An interesting question for modellers is to explore the relationship between vaccine coverage and cases of pertussis.

When is mathematical modelling appropriate?

It is important to clarify the relationship between modelling and other types of study design. In particular, we will attempt to indicate where dynamical modelling is or is not useful, and what it is uniquely capable of doing. There are some kinds of questions that are more naturally answered by conducting an appropriate epidemiological, clinical, or laboratory study. For example: is malaria prevalence likely to be higher in areas where the prevalence of HIV is higher? Are individuals who share cigarettes at increased risk of chronic bronchitis? Does passive smoking increase one's risk of lung cancer? Does taking aspirin reduce one's risk of heart attack? Do high doses of vitamin C reduce one's risk of cancer? Does washing one's hands regularly reduce one's risk of influenza? Given the incidence time series, what was the food item responsible for a food-borne disease outbreak? In short, in many situations modelling is not the right tool for answering simple factual questions which are at heart biological, or about specific incidents. But there are many important questions, such as questions about the interaction of observations, rules, or assumptions, which cannot be given a satisfactory answer without appealing to dynamical modelling. It is increasingly important in the multidisciplinary world of epidemiology for researchers to sense when they have reached the limits of alternative methods and it is time to call in

the modellers. On the other hand, mathematical modelling can perform a truly useful function in infectious disease study and control only if good epidemiological and statistical methods are applied at all relevant stages of data collection, cleaning, management, and analysis, and in all theory testing.

Identifying which questions are better answered by using dynamical modelling rather than any other method of investigation—systematic reviews, meta-analysis, quasi-experimental design, randomized controlled trials (RCTs), observational studies, ecological analyses, and so forth—is not always easy. To help us think about this we might ask the following: could data feasibly be collected to answer the question directly and without modelling? Is there an underlying process that would produce changing patterns that we might be able to analyse mathematically? Are we trying to move from one scale to another—from individuals to populations, or from populations to individuals? Sometimes the issue is determined by what data are available for attempting an answer. For example, estimating just how protective a vaccine is from clinical trials alone is an epidemiological problem, but estimating protectiveness from population-level data is a modelling problem. Knowing that HIV causes AIDS is a clinical problem, but working out by how much we would need to reduce transmission to eliminate HIV altogether is a modelling problem.

The following points highlight some important general categories of applications of mathematical modelling in the framework of public health to illustrate its power and versatility. Modelling is useful for:

◆ Encapsulating the quantifiable essence of a complex situation in a simple framework which can then be used to make estimates. Dual infection or co-infection is a good example; the HIV epidemic has transformed the dynamics of malaria (Abu-Raddad et al. 2006) and of tuberculosis (TB) (Cohen et al. 2006). In particular, we know that people with HIV are at about ten times greater risk of TB, on average, than people who are not infected with HIV. The HIV epidemic has consequently driven up the incidence of TB, in some countries by five or more times (but with a delay of about 5 years between the rise in HIV and the rise in TB). This can in turn be explained by the notion that once an individual is infected with HIV, the risk of developing TB increases with time, only reaching very high values after about 5 years.

◆ Translating descriptions of behaviour at one scale (e.g. individual-level epidemiology of a disease) into descriptions at another scale (e.g. population dynamics). For instance, Ross's question about malaria was this: given a certain level of risk (measured as effective biting rate) at the individual level, what outcome might we expect to see at the population level? Using a mathematical model, he found conditions for equilibrium that fitted the data well, and saw how this could be reversed: if one could characterize this equilibrium, then something about individual-level parameters could be inferred, setting useful targets for mosquito control.

◆ Enabling extrapolation, with quantified uncertainty, from data measured over a relatively short term to a projection of what is likely to happen in the long-term evolution over time, or from the results of randomized control trials to a particular local setting. The HPTN-052 study (Cohen et al. 2011) showed that ART reduces a person's infectiousness to others by about

96 per cent, but we need models to tell us what the consequences of this would be for controlling the epidemic of HIV in populations.

◆ Synthesizing data from different fields into a single framework, thus enabling checks on consistency. In modelling the impact of HIV on TB, we need clinical information concerning the rate of progression of AIDS; we need cellular information concerning the way in which CD4[+] cell counts decline with time since infection; we need epidemiological data concerning time trends in the epidemic of HIV; we need data on the way in which the incidence of TB varies with CD4[+] cell counts; we need trial data concerning the extent to which ART reduces the risk of developing TB; and we need economic data if we are to assess the cost-effectiveness of possible interventions against either TB or HIV.

◆ Providing clear guidelines for new data collection strategies when trying to answer specific questions where critical features are missing from the data. This may include identifying what type of data, how much data, and at what temporal and spatial resolution it should be collected, within limited funding constraints.

◆ Identifying the factors that sustain an infection within a population and estimating the relative importance of parameters, thus informing control and prevention programmes. In the case of HIV, factors include sexual behaviour, the use of condoms, the use of contaminated needles among drug users, the extent of intergenerational sex, and the age at sexual debut. Modellers might seek, for example, to compare the effects on HIV transmission of sexual heterogeneity, concurrency, and different mixing patterns.

◆ Making predictions over time of the probable dynamics of prevalence, incidence, and infection-related mortality, under different interventions.

◆ Comparing the impacts and synergies of different combinations of interventions.

◆ Identifying threats to the success of an existing intervention.

◆ Maximizing cost-effectiveness of interventions, hence enabling optimization of use of resources to combat an infection, whether within a hospital, an isolated community, a country, or globally.

◆ Evaluating the economics of different control strategies, and deciding whether programmes should re-allocate funding in response to the new data or scientific breakthroughs (such as the recent finding that ART can substantially reduce the infectiousness of HIV-infected individuals (Cohen et al. 2011)).

Modelling policy choices

In this section we give specific examples of important modelling work in HIV and TB, drawing heavily on the review by Johnson and White (2011). The aim is to showcase the scope and power of modelling in one field at least, to encourage readers to identify where such modelling might be applicable in their own fields of interest, and to indicate where more details may be found.

◆ Who should be tested for HIV? Who should be prioritized for ART? Should we offer ART to everyone or only to those with low CD4[+] cell counts? How shall we spend the available funds (Dodd et al. 2010; Kahn et al. 2011; Delva et al. 2012; Eaton et al. 2012)?

◆ Can observed trends in HIV prevalence be attributed to intervention success or failure? More specifically, how much of the observed reductions in HIV prevalence can be attributed to behaviour change programmes or other interventions? Can HIV prevalence be expected to decline in the absence of interventions? In early epidemics, can HIV prevalence rise even in the presence of partially effective prevention programmes? Can we estimate what would have happened in the absence of interventions (a 'counterfactual' scenario) (White et al. 2004; Korenromp et al. 2005; Hallett et al. 2006, 2009; Boily et al. 2008)?

◆ Have HIV prevention programmes had an impact on HIV prevalence in South African youth (Actuarial Society of South Africa 2011)?

◆ In which risk groups is most HIV transmission occurring (Brown and Peerapatanapokin 2004; Johnson et al. 2009)?

◆ Can we translate individual-level efficacy of a hypothetical vaccine in the United States, modelling transmission in heterosexuals, men who have sex with men (MSM), and injecting drug users (IDUs), to population-level impact (Long et al. 2009)?

◆ Can vaccines be beneficial (in terms of reducing mortality) even if they do not reduce susceptibility to HIV (Anderson and Hanson 2009)?

◆ When will the number of AIDS orphans peak in South Africa (Actuarial Society of South Africa 2011)?

◆ Can we project for another few decades the number of person years of ART provision in South Africa (Granich et al. 2009)?

◆ Which would be most cost-effective in increasing life expectancy in an African country with limited ART provision: (1) changing ART initiation CD4[+] count from current WHO level to 200 or 350, (2) introducing second-line ART, or (3) replacing stavudine with tenofovir in first-line ART (Walensky et al. 2010)?

◆ Which of three different feeding recommendations for HIV-positive mothers should be recommended: (1) exclusive breastfeeding for 6 months, (2) replacement feeding, (3) mixed breastfeeding for 24 months (Piwoz and Ross 2005)?

◆ What is the risk, in a 'real-world' setting where HIV testing is less frequent (as opposed to an RCT setting), that women receiving an ART drug-based microbicide could rapidly develop drug-resistant HIV if they become infected while on the microbicide (Wilson et al. 2008)?

◆ Can male circumcision programmes significantly benefit women (indirectly) by reducing the chance that their partners are infected (Auvert et al. 2005; Nagelkerke et al. 2007; Anderson et al. 2009; Londish and Murray 2008; Hankins et al. 2009; UNAIDS/WHO/SACEMA Expert Group et al. 2009)?

◆ Can vaginal microbicides significantly benefit men (indirectly), because of their partners having a lower HIV risk (Wilson et al. 2008)?

◆ How would the cumulative number of HIV infections averted in non-IDUs compare with the number averted in IDUs, under a programme of provision of syringes and condoms to IDUs (Foss et al. 2006)?

- Would the impact on HIV incidence of treating sexually transmitted infections be the same if the intervention had been introduced at different stages in the epidemic (White et al. 2008)?

- What would have happened if the rate at which secondary sexual behaviour patterns (concurrency) are acquired were reduced to zero, at different stages in the HIV epidemic (Johnson and White 2011)?

- What will be the effect of risk compensation behaviour following the introduction of highly active ART for an MSM group (Bezemer et al. 2008)?

- What is the effect of pre-exposure prophylaxis on HIV incidence (Abbas et al. 2007)?

- Is there a significant risk of a self-sustaining epidemic of drug-resistant HIV (Smith et al. 2010)?

- Could the widespread use of isoniazid preventive therapy for HIV-infected adults lead to the accumulation of drug-resistant TB and have only short-term benefit (Cohen et al. 2006)?

- Is regular viral load testing the best strategy for initiating, monitoring, and discontinuing ART (Baggaley et al. 2006)?

- What would be the effect of different strategies (reducing patient length of stay, and forcing staff and patients to use masks, or both) for controlling extensively drug-resistant TB (Basu et al. 2007)?

Types of mathematical models

In this section we give conceptual definitions of, and brief remarks on, some of the most important model types encountered in disease modelling. The list is far from a systematic review, and skirts controversy about type demarcation. Note that quite a few of these categories cut across each other—for example, compartmental models may be deterministic or stochastic, and they may be discrete or continuous, in any combination.

Individual-based models (also sometimes referred to as 'agent-based' models and 'microsimulation' models): in these, individual players (mainly people) exist as distinct entities able to experience changes in state (such as infection, relationships, fertility, and death). These models make it possible to implement complex rules, and to ask nuanced questions about important sequences of events, such as the ordering of condom use cessation, pregnancy, HIV exposure, declining health, and so on.

Compartmental models: these, the workhorses of applied mathematics, express a system in terms of 'amounts' (volumes, masses, or numbers and counts) of items or material in a number of categories, or 'compartments'. They can range from models of water in a system of tanks, to money in portions of a portfolio, or people in regions, or population groups—such as infected, immune, risk groups, and so on.

In vivo *models*: models of biological processes within an individual, from cell and antigen life cycles to pharmakinetic and pharmadynamic models, are often referred to as '*in vivo*' models. This categorization refers only to the real-world regime of which it is an analogue, namely biological processes, and does not determine what kind of mathematical form the model takes (e.g. continuous versus discrete).

Population-level models: in contrast to biological-level (*in vivo*) models (earlier in this list), population-level models focus on a higher-level view. Usually this point is not explicitly noted, as most epidemiological models disregard complex biological details.

Discrete models (or discrete aspects of models): models with features which jump in discrete steps, such as time or other quantities expressing the state of the model world.

Continuous models (or aspects of models): models with features which vary continuously, being able, in principle, to take any value in some sensible range. This can readily apply to quantities, like population sizes, which are in reality discrete, without necessarily implying any inconsistencies. Note that it is not at all unusual for individual models simultaneously to conceive of some aspects continuously and others discretely—for example, discrete jumps in population states occurring against a continuous timeline and continuously varying risk factors.

Deterministic models: here the outcome is entirely determined by an 'initial condition' and the choice of dynamical rules and parameters. Mathematically, the model 'output' will be some sort of specification of the 'model state' over a range of times.

Stochastic models: here there is intrinsic randomness in the unfolding of continuous processes, or occurrence of events. Some such models are implicit in conventional data analysis, but these usually focus on modelling an experimental process which captures the random effects of sample selection and measurement error. We wish to draw attention to models where epidemiological processes are understood to involve chance, especially around transmission-related events. A fully fledged 'stochastic model output' will contain some sort of summary of possible ranges of outcomes, rather than merely example outputs which are 'consistent with', or 'representative of', the underlying rules. This can rapidly lead to great complexity and deep technical challenges, not to mention difficulties in presentation and interpretation. However, with the growth of computational power and the development of suitable programmes, stochastic models have increasing relevance and importance.

Static models: occasionally this term is applied to model worlds in which nothing at all happens, so that the model is just a static picture of a situation which may be useful in showing the instantaneous, or long enduring state of a system—such as a map of the world showing HIV prevalence estimates at a point in time. More typically, the term refers to a stable 'context' in which rules affecting individuals are static, and where we can still model individual life trajectories involving costs and benefits of health system interactions; here 'static' indicates the lack of accounting for impact (feedback) of factors like health system interventions on the overall context in which individuals will find themselves. Such a model can help focus on how individuals are expected to experience one or other health programme, implemented in a particular way and context which is readily specified, without entertaining complex dynamical questions about the inevitable evolution of the context itself.

Dynamical models: this can broadly refer to models in which parameters may change with time. However, a model may be called 'dynamical' when you wish to emphasize, for example, that an intervention which directly affects the well-being of people who receive it, can then potentially reduce infectious pressure; and that this is taken into account in computing the changing risk of infection over time. This may be crucial when long-term costs and benefits are estimated.

Some simple examples

This section is a demonstration of elementary models which capture the essence of dynamical modelling, with some conceptual digressions. The motivation for including it in this chapter is the subtextual message that modelling is really not something sinister or mystical, accessible only to a closed circle of initiates or specialists. Even though the illustrations are simple—and useful epidemiological models can be complex (though often need not be)—they form a valid basis for approaching most population dynamic models and, hence, disease transmission models. Readers with no prior modelling experience, but who are familiar with advanced high school mathematics, and have a willingness to suspend disbelief in their abilities, should be able to follow most, if not all, of the details of these examples. Those with some prior knowledge of elementary calculus but no experience of disease modelling should find here a foundation for a deeper reading of the modelling literature.

Modelling 'exponential' growth or decline

The notion of 'exponential growth' is one of the most important recurring themes of dynamical modelling—from pure sciences like physics to highly applied social science like population dynamics. It has little to do with the popular notion that something has 'grown exponentially', which often simply means that something has 'grown enormously'. Technically, what is meant is that some quantity grows at a rate proportional to how large it currently is, with size and growth ever adjusting to maintain this relationship.

> *Question 1.* Given a population of 1 million individuals, with individual mortality risk (m) of 0.001 per year, how many will be alive after 10 years?

Following our noses, we first build a discrete-time model, letting time, t, take discrete values $1, 2, 3, \ldots$ (years in our population-based example, but it could be days, seconds, and so forth). We let N_t denote the population after t years, and we assume that

◆ no births or immigration take place, and

◆ the same proportion, m, of the population N_t dies in each time step $[t, t+1]$.

The second point is really a foundational and widely recurring assumption—namely that the individual-level risk or probability of death can be directly taken, within each time step, to be the actual population proportion which dies. In truth, risks are expressions of averages (formally 'expected values') and for large populations, the actually realized proportions are usually very close to the appropriately defined average individual-level risk.

Throughout this section we will ignore models which consider how the 'realized' population dynamic 'fluctuates' around the

'expected' dynamic, and we will simply calculate the expected dynamic. This is a widely followed practice, which, firstly, is necessary in order to move ahead without drowning in technical complexity, and, secondly, is remarkably robust in many areas of science and engineering, including disease modelling. That is not to imply that random effects in population processes are irrelevant, merely that a large body of knowledge about dynamical processes can be developed by analysing the averages of these random effects. The study of variation around expected effects lies at the heart of statistics and formal data analysis.

The flipside, then, of the assumption about the proportion of deaths, m, per time step, is that a proportion $(1-m)$ of the population survives each year. Hence we have the following equations expressing the population in each year in terms of the population at the start:

$$N_1 = (1-m)N_0,$$

$$N_2 = (1-m)(1-m)N_0,$$

and so forth. These equations follow from the general expression governing the population dynamic, which gives the population 1 year later in terms of the population at time t:

$$N_{t+1} = (1-m)N_t.$$

It readily follows that, for any positive integer t, the population after t years is given by

$$N_t = (1-m)^t N_0. \tag{1}$$

Fig. 5.18.2 shows the decline of a population over successive years with the annual mortality increased substantially relative to our example, in order to show the effect more starkly in a small number of steps.

Even without mathematical analysis we might expect that, as the number of years grows indefinitely large (tends to infinity), the population becomes indefinitely small (tends to zero). This is

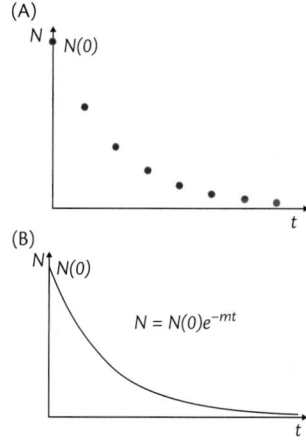

Fig. 5.18.2 (A) Exponential decline of a population, observed in regular time steps with a (percentage) attrition in each step. (B) Continuously observed exponential decline of a population or general quantity. A key property of exponential functions is that a simple rescaling, or inversion, of the axes, without any further shape adjustment, generates all possible exponential functions.

reflected in the formulae, in that the population size after t steps (years) is the original population size, multiplied by t copies (or t th power) of the factor $(1 - m)$, and that $(1 - m)$ is positive but less than one. A key concept in algebra and analysis is that powers of any number less than one can be made as close to zero as we want, by taking a high enough power. This property that, in each time step, the population sheds a number of members in proportion to how large the population was at the beginning of that time step, is the exponential decline of the population. According to the discrete model, then, the concrete answer to Question 1 is given, to the nearest whole number, by:

$$N_{10} = (1 - 0.001)^{10} 10^6 = (0.999)^{10} 10^6 = 990,044.9 = 990,045. \quad (2)$$

Now let time t vary continuously from zero to infinity. Assume again that no births or immigration take place but that there is a constant per capita mortality rate m. We will use the standard notation of calculus, but develop the argument intuitively rather than formally.

The fundamental concept in continuous-time modelling is to consider what happens as the time t advances by a very small increment dt. The nearly vacuous Fig. 5.18.3 is a sufficiently useful crutch for us to recommend it be drawn whenever continuous models are being developed. In reality, it becomes more and more likely that no notable events occur, as we consider ever smaller time windows, and the very idea of a time increment or window of size dt is of one that is small beyond all measurement and practical meaning. However, the crucial conceptual leap here is to recall that we are modelling not the actual number of events in some system realization, but rather the average number of events which are expected to occur in this time increment. As dt is intended to be tiny, the expected number of events is some tiny fraction, although the underlying real-world concept has no fractional population members or events. In continuously varying model worlds, populations vary smoothly in size and take on any numerical values which are needed to follow the locally applicable smooth dynamical rules.

Extending the argument of the large (or macroscopic) time step argument considered earlier in the discrete model, we declare that, between time t and time $t + dt$, there will be $mN(t)dt$ deaths. (Previously, we just used a time step of one unit, instead of giving it a named size, dt.) Thus we have a (negative) increment in the population, which we call dN. These two alternative expressions for the small difference in population, known as its 'differential', can be equated, yielding what is called a 'differential equation':

$$dN = -mN(t)dt,$$

which is usually written as:

$$\frac{dN}{dt} = -mN. \quad (3)$$

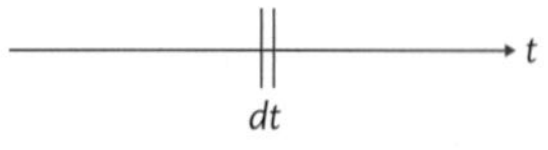

Fig. 5.18.3 The fundamental diagram of dynamical modelling in continuous time. By focusing on what happens during a small interval of time, between t and $t + dt$, we are enabled to derive differential equations whose solution will describe how the system evolves over time.

The meaning of dN/dt, known as a 'derivative', is, by analogy with the concept of gradient or slope, an expression for the rate of change of N with the passage of time. This equation can be solved (technically, 'integrated') by standard methods developed in any calculus course, to yield an expression for the population $N(t)$ after time t:

$$\begin{aligned} N(t) &= N(0)(e^{-m})^t \\ &= N(0)e^{-mt} \\ &= N(0)\left(\frac{1}{e^m}\right)^t. \end{aligned} \quad (4)$$

The symbol e denotes the 'base of the natural logarithm', a number (approximately 2.718) which, for analytical convenience, is the preferred base through which to define powers. Setting $N(0) = 10^6$, $m = 0.001$, $t = 10$, we can calculate the answer to Question 1 given by the continuous model, as follows, rounded to the nearest whole number:

$$N(10) = 10^6 e^{-0.001 \times 10} = 10^6 e^{-0.01} = 990,050. \quad (5)$$

This differs slightly from the answer given by the discrete model in Equation 2, and the respective solutions will diverge more as the number of years increases. This somewhat fine but important point is not an error per se in either method, or a sign of some fundamental incompatibility of approaches, and certainly not a reason for concern about the formal manipulations we have performed. In fact, it simply reflects our imprecise use of the fundamental notion of annual risk of death, a concept which is explored separately in the online appendix to this chapter, along with other fundamental modelling concepts. For now, we should note that the definition of a hazard rate like m needs to be carefully stated as applying to a particular period, such as a year. The value of m in Equation 3 in the continuous-time model is the intrinsic risk per unit time, and it is a theorem of calculus that this translates into the risk, $R(T)$ over a particular period, T, according to the expression:

$$R(T) = 1 - e^{-mT}. \quad (6)$$

Using the corresponding value for $1 - R(t)$, the probability of surviving for t years, in place of $(1 - m)^t$ in Equation 1, we can make the discrete-time model solution correspond exactly to the continuous-time model solution in Equation 4. (We note too, that $1 - m$ is an increasingly accurate approximation of the exponential function e^{-m} as m approaches zero.) In this simple case, the only difference is whether we intended to evaluate the discrete-time model for non-whole-numbered values of t.

The models we have just constructed also apply to a susceptible population being infected at a constant rate, which might then be called 'force of infection', 'incidence', or 'hazard rate'. Similar problems may be framed in many other contexts, modelled by essentially the same equations: an infected population with constant rate of recovery, the mass of water remaining in a towel drying on a clothes line, the temperature (relative to room-temperature) of a cooling cup of coffee, the decaying mass of a radioactive substance.

Discrete versus continuous models

It is not necessary here to explore in detail how continuous and discrete-time models differ or correspond in less simple cases, but the following remarks may be helpful. Continuous-time models, though they may be daunting to people who are not comfortable with calculus, are in fact usually mathematically much simpler than discrete-time models. The rules which apply over an 'infinitesimally' small period of time, dt, do not need to be updated over this period of time, because the system itself accrues irrelevantly small (infinitesimal) changes in this interval. Hence, without much technical effort, we can usually solve for the state of the system at the end of an infinitesimal time step, relative to a specified initial state, by simply translating the rules of our model world from words into algebra. Thus we derive 'differential equations'. Then, if we want to know how the system changes over a substantial period of time, we invoke the tools of calculus to 'solve' the differential equations. These 'solutions' are not values of populations at particular times, in the sense that 'values' are 'solutions' to the more familiar 'algebraic' equations. Solutions to differential equations are 'functions', that is, fully specified formal relations between population states and time.

Discrete models may require either extra sophistication or additional assumptions of convenience, in order for the fundamental time-step relations to be written down. These are called 'difference equations', and their solutions too are mathematical functions (of time) which are intended to be evaluated at discrete times. Sometimes these discrete time steps need to be taken seriously, and it will not be possible or sensible to simply read off the system state at non-whole-number times. For instance, it may be possible to build a year-on-year model of an insect population, which accounts for the net result of a brief breeding season with many births and deaths but does not attempt nor claim to describe the intermediate states when many eggs, larvae, and pupae are formed and eliminated. Similarly, seasonal models of human disease may not be intended to model the details of brief outbreaks, but merely account for net impact of typical outbreaks in terms of mortality, morbidity, vaccines used, accumulated immunity, and so forth.

Often, indeed usually, neither differential nor difference equations can be neatly solved with explicit formulae. Then it becomes necessary to use computational means to provide numerical approximations, graphical representations, and the like. These numerical methods form a mature and robust field of knowledge in their own right, and can deal routinely with most epidemiologically interesting models. On the other hand, sizeable challenges may arise with computational power and run-times required for in-depth investigations. Exploring many alternative scenarios in an attempt to 'fit' models to data, and exploring the sensitivity of outcomes to inputs and assumptions, may demand quite sophisticated use of data management technology and computer clusters.

To avoid proliferation of analysis, the remaining examples in this section will be demonstrated with the continuous formulation, chosen for its conceptual clarity and pedagogic value. The development of intuition about the applicability of calculus is a powerful problem solving capacity.

Question 2. What will happen to the population of Question 1, with death rate of 0.1 per cent per year, if there is immigration of individuals at an average rate of 200 per year?

Assume a constant per capita mortality rate m (a probability per unit time of death) as before, and a constant immigration rate b (a number of people coming in per unit time). In a small time increment dt, the change in population is given by:

$$dN = b\,dt - mN\,dt.$$

Hence the derivative (rate of change) is given by:

$$\frac{dN}{dt} = b - mN. \tag{7}$$

This 'differential equation' can be solved, by relatively elementary methods of calculus, to yield:

$$N(t) = \frac{b}{m} + \left(N(0) - \frac{b}{m} \right) e^{-mt}. \tag{8}$$

Note that the second term of the solution has the previously noted 'exponential decline' structure. Whatever value is taken for the initial population $N(0)$, this second term fades after a large period of time, so that, as time t tends to infinity, the population size tends to a constant equilibrium value, namely $N_E = b/m$, which in our case is 200,000. The key point is that this is the eventual state of the system no matter what the (positive) initial value was (see Fig. 5.18.4). A corollary to this is that, for our particular original population size to be maintained, an average influx of 1000 individuals per year would be required, since then $N_E = b/m = 1000/0.001 = 1,000,000$. Indeed, Equation 7 shows directly, without passing through the formalities of obtaining a solution, that the rate of change of the population will be zero when $N = b/m$. This idea of exploring the behaviour of dynamical (difference, or differential) equations in their own right, without working with potentially complicated solutions, is a normal, and very informative part of the investigation of the properties of model worlds.

The volume of water in a vertical-sided tank can be used as a helpful concrete mental image for this model, also making for a cheap and informative physical demonstration. Consider the water filling the tank to a level above a small outlet from which the rate of flow is proportional to the pressure at the outlet, and so to the height of the water level above the outlet, and hence also proportional to the volume $N(t)$ of water above the outlet (see Fig. 5.18.5). If the tap is shut, the water level will exponentially decay down to the level of the hole. If the tap produces a steady stream of water, the level in the tank will approach an equilibrium value at which the outflow matches the (fixed) inflow. In principle, the

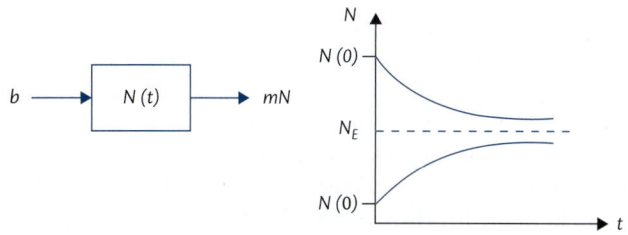

Fig. 5.18.4 Question 2. Stable equilibrium.

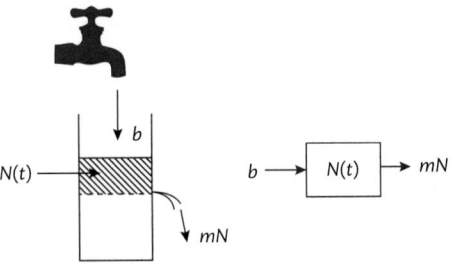

Fig. 5.18.5 Flow diagram and water-tank model for population $N(t)$ at time t, with constant inflow rate b and variable outflow rate $mN(t)$. Question 1: No inflow, set $b = 0$. Question 2: Inflow or immigration rate b per year

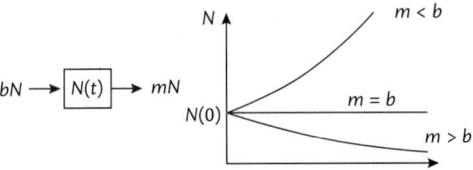

Fig. 5.18.6 Question 3. Exponential growth/decline, and equilibrium.

tank may overflow if the hypothetical equilibrium water level is higher than the top of the tank.

This inflow–outflow model can be applied to the population of red blood cells in a human body. Bone marrow normally produces about 2×10^6 cells per second, or 1728×10^8 per day, while a nearly constant proportion of cells die daily. If we assume the body maintains an equilibrium population of about 2×10^{13} (20 trillion) red blood cells at any moment, that mortality rate can easily be calculated from our model.

> *Question 3.* What will happen to the population of Question 1, with a per capita death rate of 0.001 per year, if there is no immigration, but a constant per capita birth rate of 0.004?

Once more we assume a constant per capita mortality rate m (again a probability per unit time of death) and constant per capita birth rate b, that is, a probability per unit time that an existing population member produces a new population member. This is a rather crude model of fertility, but the fertility rate b can be chosen to produce some reasonable dynamics. Certainly, a nuanced discussion of fertility, and other demographic processes like changing age structure of a country over time, cannot be aided by models lacking explicit age structure, but these kinds of complications are mainly about proliferation of detail, not mainly about new concepts. As ever, we have to understand what happens during a small time increment or time step of size dt. The change in population is given by:

$$dN = bNdt - mNdt, \tag{9}$$

hence the derivative (rate of change) is given by:

$$\frac{dN}{dt} = (b - m)N. \tag{10}$$

This can be solved to give:

$$N(t) = N(0)e^{(b-m)t}. \tag{11}$$

In Question 3 we proposed values of $m = 0.001$, $b = 0.004$, so that $N(t) = N(0)e^{0.003t}$, which describes exponential growth. The model predicts exponential increase when $m < b$, a constant population when $m = b$, and exponential decline when $m > b$ (see Fig. 5.18.6). Exponential growth or decline is also called 'geometric' increase or decline. When there is exponential growth, it is easy to show that there is a fixed population 'doubling time', and in the case of exponential decline there is a fixed population 'halving-time', sometimes called the 'half-life'.

That populations, even under much less simplistic assumptions, tend to increase geometrically was first observed and studied by Euler in the mid-eighteenth century, before being more famously explored by Thomas Malthus in 1798. Although exact exponential relations such as those presented here arise only under idealized conditions, their conceptual importance and wide applicability can hardly be overstated. With a technically small but far-reaching mathematical twist, they also form the basis of much modelling in pure science and engineering, including the study of oscillations and waves.

Susceptible–infectious compartmental models

The introduction of multiple health or disease states into our model worlds is naturally crucial to modelling disease transmission and progression. We will also need to expand our options for thinking about rates. Thus far, the populations in our example models have been allowed to:

◆ grow by fixed in- or out-flows (the immigration and mortality previously considered) or

◆ experience growth or decline processes scaled in proportion to the instantaneous population size (our fertility and mortality models).

Next, we consider the basic model of transmission, previously noted as the principle of mass action. Thus, the number of new infections occurring in a time window of duration dt is proportional to the number of infection-susceptible individuals, and also proportional to the number of infectious individuals, and hence proportional to the product of the two. The constant of proportionality can be understood to capture the probability per unit time of any one member of one group coming into contact with any one member of the other, and the ordinary probability (not per unit time) of such a contact leading to transmission of infection.

> *Question 4.* How can we describe the prevalence of gonorrhoea in a closed sexually active population?

Let $S(t)$ and $I(t)$ denote the numbers of susceptible and infectious people at time t. Assume that individuals mix randomly, people are infectious as soon as they are infected, and they recover at a constant per capita rate r per day, after which they again become susceptible.

In a small increment of time, dt, the increments in numbers of susceptible and infectious individuals are:

$$dS = -\beta I(t)S(t)dt + rI(t)dt, \qquad dI = \beta I(t)S(t)dt - rI(t)dt, \tag{12}$$

where β is the just noted mass action proportionality constant. Seen from the point of view of an individual, this indicates that the risk $\lambda(t)$ of infection at time t is given by $\beta I(t)$ (see also Fig. 5.18.7).

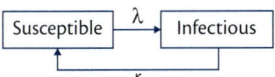

Fig. 5.18.7 Basic model of gonorrhoea transmission and recovery. Individuals move from the susceptible class to the infected or infectious class with incidence λ, arising dynamically from contacts with individuals in the infectious class according to the principle of mass action (perfectly random mixing), while they move in the opposite way through natural recovery. The dynamics are captured in Equation 12.

The system of differential equations describing the dynamics of $I(t)$ and $S(t)$ is:

$$\frac{dS}{dt} = -\beta I(t)S(t) + rI(t),$$
$$\frac{dI}{dt} = \beta I(t)S(t) - rI(t).$$

These equations can be subjected to some instructive detailed analysis beyond our immediate scope. Hethcote and Yorke (1984) noted that the model has prevalence declining to zero for plausible estimates of the average partner change rate, the transmission probability per partnership, and the duration of infection. Indeed, certain types of models, such as those involving infections for which survival or cure confers immunity, or for which infection is incurable, generically predict that epidemics die out (potentially after temporarily rising to a peak) unless there is a sufficient source of new susceptible individuals. In this model, the cured individuals recover to be susceptible again, so, in principle, an endemic equilibrium might have been produced. As it was, the model led to a conundrum in the context of data on gonorrhoea as it could not reasonably explain the low, stable equilibrium prevalence in the United States in the 1980s.

Question 5. How can we model an observed low endemic prevalence of gonorrhoea in a closed sexually active population?

Hethcote and Yorke (1984) went on to build a further model (Fig. 5.18.8) in which they divided the sexually active population into two groups: low activity (the majority) and high activity—2 per cent of the population with higher partner change rate. They showed that with plausible estimates of the relevant parameters they could convincingly model the low gonorrhoea prevalence shown by the data. It is very common that simple first models of systems sensibly capture initial insights and data, but fail to reproduce crucial

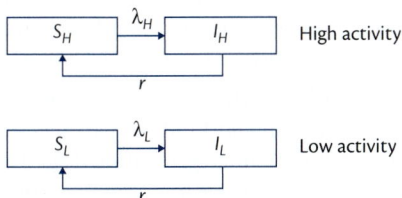

Fig. 5.18.8 Model of gonorrhoea transmission with contact heterogeneity. The population is divided into a high- and low-activity class. Within each, individuals move from the susceptible class to the infected or infectious class with incidence λ, arising dynamically from contacts with individuals in the infectious class according to the principle of mass action. Meanwhile, individuals move in the opposite direction through natural recovery.

features which are known to arise in the real system. It is also very typical that one seeks to address this by identifying some important further refinement of population classes. This will require thinking about estimates of sub-population sizes, and details of contact and mixing rules. The work of Cooke, Hethcote, Nold and Yorke (Cooke and Yorke 1973; Yorke et al. 1978; Hethcote et al. 1982; Hethcote and Yorke 1984) highlighted the importance of incorporating in modelling both risk-heterogeneity and the class of asymptomatic individuals. The implications of their work helped to inform US control policy for sexually transmitted infections in the 1980s.

Other important classes of models

Our somewhat technical examples have only considered:

♦ Single populations experiencing in- and out-flows.

♦ Simple structured populations with susceptible and infected classes, and high or low contact tendencies.

Other key population structures which may be important to consider are:

♦ Gender.

♦ Age.

♦ Location.

♦ Relationship status.

♦ Finely resolved disease states such as exposed but clinically healthy and uninfectious, or detailed viral and immunological markers.

♦ Treatment access and utilization.

Putting to one side the list of potential complications, we want to return to our opening remarks for this section. Model building and interpretation, while deserving care and attention, and benefiting from technical skill and experience, should not be seen as obscure activities left to the strange practices of a secret society.

The role of models is to formalize our understanding of, or hypotheses about, data and processes, so that we can tap into powerful tools developed by mathematicians over many years. This allows us to restate our thoughts about systems in an orderly fashion, demonstrating details of their internal workings, in the context of tough political and technical questions about investment in, and management of, public health systems.

Modelling as a process

In all good science there is an inescapable cycle of observation, hypothesis, and testing; of interactive theory-making and experimentation, reformulation of theory, and retesting. Ideally, mathematical modellers in the public health arena apply well-educated intuition to painstaking observations and interrogations of nature and human society. The aim is to frame the most interesting possible answers to important questions as quantitative hypotheses that can in principle be tested. This process entails choices about what kind of model to build, and the identification of parameters that can be varied, and perhaps later estimated, to determine specific model behaviour. Then there is the actual construction, logical analysis, and deduction within the model world; the interpretation, leading to reflections on, or predictions about, the real world; the testing of predictions against data, recalibration, and retesting; and the possible revisiting of model design, statistical analysis, or the data itself. The modeller aims for validation (albeit provisional) and optimization of the model before reporting to peers and appropriate scientific and policy forums.

Basic principles of model selection

Following the quote from Einstein in the introduction, the first rule of modelling is: a model should be as simple as possible, provided it fits the data within the limits of accuracy. The nature and complexity of the model depends on the answers to some basic preliminary questions: what questions are we trying to answer? What scale are we working at? What data are available, and within what limits of accuracy? What degree of generality or precision is required? How soon are results needed?

Another rule of thumb for modellers is: even a simple model can be useful. Here 'useful' might mean yielding some qualitative insight, such as the basic shape of the prevalence graph (as in Ross's malaria model), or the indispensability of heterogeneity of sexual activity in plausibly modelling sexually transmitted infections, as illustrated in the previous section. All models are imperfect by definition. Baran and Sweezy (1968) coming from the world of economics, capture well the philosophical essence of all good modelling, insisting that science progresses by building very partial models of reality. By selecting the decisive elements to gain a clear focus on, and abstracting from non-essentials, good models—while apparently unrealistic in a sense—offer us keys to understanding reality.

Comparing the utility of different models hinges on questions such as these: what is the purpose of this model? What can we get out of this model? Why should anybody believe its conclusions or predictions? What difference would it make if they did? On the need to balance simplicity and complexity in ecological models, Koella (1991) wrote:

> On the one hand, the more variables…in a model the closer the predictions…agree with observations, simply because more degrees of freedom are involved. However, a close agreement between prediction and observation does not necessarily imply an agreement between the structure of the model and the biological processes. …(Q)ualitative predictions of simple models may be more biologically meaningful than the precise quantitative predictions of complex models…(M)ore detailed models do not necessarily result in greater predictive power…(and)…more complex models may be less reliable than…simple (models). As one includes more detail…the number of assumptions about interactions increases exponentially,…the probability of making a wrong and critical assumption increases rapidly, and…the predictive power…declines after some level of detail has been exceeded.

Choosing a model is often a delicate compromise. It is good modelling practice to allow the nature, quantity, and quality of the available data to inform the choice of model. The following examples serve to illustrate this principle. The archetypal wrong way to model a situation is to shoehorn the problem into a favoured model in which much prior effort has been invested. It is far better, as pioneered in the physical sciences, and applied successfully in epidemiology, to start with what is observed—the data—and ask specific pertinent questions that probe the data for patterns. The next step is to formulate hypotheses, or plausible narratives, that might help to make sense of the data and provide answers to the questions. For asking the right questions, for arriving at fruitful hypotheses, as well as for any serious testing of the hypotheses, a prerequisite is relevant and reliable data—collected, scrutinized, and analysed with substantial biological, epidemiological, and statistical understanding. Only then can a relevant model be constructed. The mathematical modeller cannot contribute meaningfully in isolation, but the modeller's work can be of great value in improving the subsequent design of trials and collection of relevant data, and in generating more refined questions; and so the cycle continues. Although the interactions are not strictly sequential or cyclical, we will formulate this modelling process very roughly below as consisting of four steps, illustrated by some typical fundamental questions, about measles, influenza, and HIV, thus developing further the discussion in the section 'What kinds of questions are we trying to understand?'.

Step 1: asking questions

Question 1. Why do measles epidemics oscillate?

Question 2. Why do flu epidemics burn out but come back at rather irregular intervals?

Question 3. Why is the prevalence of HIV declining rapidly in Zimbabwe, but not in Malawi, Zambia, or Botswana?

Question 4. Why is HIV so much worse in southern Africa than anywhere else?

Question 5. It seems that Cambodia now has only about 10,000 HIV-positive people with about 1000 new cases per year. How can we drive it to extinction?

Step 2: making hypotheses, learning to guess

Whether we are analysing a data set or building a model this cannot be done in a conceptual vacuum, so we need to decide what might be going on before we even start. Here are some ideas:

1. A measles epidemic seems to burn out rather rapidly but then re-establish itself at regular intervals. This could be because it is being driven by something external like climate. Or it could be something to do with the natural history of measles. Perhaps it has something to do with high-contact subgroups, associated with periodic school terms.

2. Once infected, a person is immune for the rest of that flu season, but there seems to be renewed susceptibility at the next flu season. Perhaps the host loses immunity, or perhaps the virus mutates.

3. Perhaps behavioural change, allied to educational levels and targeted educational programmes, is a significant factor in the different HIV dynamics observed in Zimbabwe, as also in Uganda.

4. Are people in southern Africa engaging in more sex, having more partners, and different kinds of partners, more concurrent partners, and more inter-generational sex than people in other countries? Is oscillating migration centred on the gold mines—an enduring legacy of apartheid—a significant driver of the epidemic?

5. In Cambodia there is the prospect of eliminating HIV completely. How can we best locate the few remaining cases? Are there useful parallels with smallpox or polio eradication?

The point about these 'hypotheses' is not that they should be right but only that they should be testable. If we can show that one particular explanation does not fit, we have made great progress by narrowing the possibilities.

Step 3: engaging with the biology, epidemiology, and statistics

Apart from high-level considerations, we need to learn as much as we can about the natural history of the disease and associated quantitative parameters: disease duration, case fatality, symptom duration, infectiousness, latent period, immunity (partial or complete), rates of increase (time), rates of spread (geography), susceptibility (by age, gender), periodicity, and geography. We then need to do some statistics to see if we can identify (or exclude) interesting relationships between variables.

1. Do measles epidemics occur annually in equatorial places where there is much less seasonality? What calendar correlations can be observed in countries with reliable data on measles outbreaks?

2. What trustworthy data can we access on the duration of flu epidemics and their frequency of occurrence? What's known about phylogenetics and viral evolution? Is flu a zoonosis? That is to say, are there hosts for the virus other than man?

3. Have any studies explored correlations between HIV prevalence or incidence and significant differences in the backgrounds of various African population groups relating to history, geography, genetics, politics, religion, sociology, culture, migration, education, and health intervention? How can we explore the possible effects of behavioural change, whether as a consequence of educational programmes or perceived mortality?

4. What is the evidence that HIV is so much worse in southern Africa, and are there other places where it is equally severe? Can we identify factors that are peculiar to southern Africa? Oscillating migration? Sexual norms of behaviour?

5. We need to find very rare events. Should we do the equivalent of ring vaccination—when we find a person with HIV, test everyone in that person's area, school, or social network? Should we do contact tracing—ask individuals to identify their sexual partners?

Step 4: choosing and building a mathematical model

It is usually the case that we do not have enough information to build a very detailed model, but starting from a very simple model may help us to focus our thoughts and identify those things that we need to understand if we are to model the transmission dynamics more accurately.

1. For measles, and for other viral and bacterial infections that commonly afflict children, such as rubella, mumps, pertussis, and diphtheria, a great deal is known. These infections have much in common from a modelling point of view: a direct route of transmission, lifelong immunity, and readily available techniques for detecting past or current infection. Measles periodicity might demand a model with positive feedback or a delay process to model the oscillations.

2. Since immunity is for life and we find that there are animal hosts (pigs and ducks), perhaps we should consider what is happening in the pigs and ducks. Does the virus mutate? Should we think about some kind of multispecies model?

3. We can build a model incorporating parameters describing delayed changes in sexual behaviour resulting from perceived HIV mortality. Can we, by varying parameters, achieve some kind of fit to known data on HIV prevalence, incidence, and mortality in Zimbabwe?

4. Data on sexual behaviour may reveal that this behaviour does not differ greatly among populations but that the network structure does. We might consider a network model.

5. For polio and smallpox the disease duration is rather short and this suggests that ring vaccination is a good idea; for HIV the disease duration is rather long so this suggests that contact tracing might be better. Think about network models and also about stochastic extinction.

Some important lessons may be drawn by would-be mathematical modellers, from these examples. First, to contribute significantly to infectious disease modelling, one must start with a specific, clearly defined question, and attain familiarity with the natural history of the disease. Second, if sufficient time and trouble is taken to understand the problem, the mathematical approach will often more or less suggest itself.

Principles of good practice in modelling

In order to promote good practice in epidemiological modelling in support of public health decision-making, of which a flip side is to facilitate interpretation of such models by non-modellers, a set of nine principles was recently distilled (Delva et al. 2012) out of a process involving the World Bank and the HIV Modelling Consortium (The HIV Modelling Consortium 2012). Though the immediate questions of that process were contextualized by the HIV epidemic, the principles themselves are completely general. We briefly outline them here, although a deeper engagement with these issues will benefit from a close reading of the full article and, even more, from a practice of habitual interaction with modellers.

Principle 1: clear rationale, scope, and objectives

A modelling study report should clarify, and appropriately refer to, the following three points, intrinsic to the interpretation of the study: (1) the precise questions the study aims to address; (2) justification for why epidemiological modelling is appropriate for the problem, rather than, or in addition to, some other study design (e.g. systematic review, meta-analysis, quasi-experimental design, randomized controlled trial); and (3) a profile of the intended readership. These three serve to ensure alignment of aims, model, results, and interpretation, and act as criteria for judging all modelling decisions.

Principle 2: explicit model structure and key features

A complete description of the model used in the analysis should be given (perhaps as an online technical appendix, including computer code) to permit replication of findings and projections. This description should cover the basic structure (a flow diagram is helpful) and main features, cross-referenced to the scope and objectives, and a clear justification for choice of model type. The selection of model structure involves explicit choices about which factors (demographic, behavioural, biological, clinical, or epidemiological) to include and which to exclude, based on assumptions (which must be stated) or on research results (which must be quoted).

Principle 3: well-defined and justified model parameters

Among the assumptions to be explicitly listed in any modelling study are the nature and values of each parameter, for example, the annual population growth rate, or the probability of HIV transmission per sex act for an individual on ART. This listing should include, for each parameter: its name, the mathematical symbol (where relevant), its meaning in plain language, the value(s) assigned to it (a point estimate and range or confidence interval as appropriate), and a contextual justification for these values, whether the parameter is fitted in the model or is derived from another (referenced) source.

Principle 4: alignment of model output with data

The relative caution or confidence with which results of a model should be received depends on demonstrating the model's capacity to reproduce observed patterns. But of such 'validation', it has to be asked: were input parameters chosen to maximize the correspondence of outputs to data, or did these correspondences emerge naturally from choosing externally justified inputs? It is impressive when a model that has been fitted to a 'training' data set is shown to be capable of producing output in close correspondence with additional 'testing' data, especially when the second data set has independent origin or is markedly different. On the other hand, it may be quite unrealistic to expect a model to extend its predictive power to data emerging from a fundamentally different scenario, and the uncritical use of models that have not been calibrated to local data can mislead policymakers.

Sometimes a model's failure to fit data (without resorting to implausible assumptions about parameters) can lead to new scientific insights, through diagnosis of fundamental model limitations. And even when there are insufficient data to construct scenarios allowing credible predictions of future outcomes, modelling can still help to explore important questions such as what performance characteristics of a public health programme would be required for certain goals to be achieved.

Principle 5: clear presentation of results, including uncertainty

The presentation of model outputs, through judicious use of tables and graphs, warrants substantial investment of thought and effort, because the quantity of information in modern models (potentially run many times under carefully chosen conditions) easily becomes too vast for readers to absorb. It is the responsibility of modellers to highlight some particularly informative views of the results, in addition to providing all information for full replication (see Principle 2).

All assumptions, whether involving the structure of the model, the parameter estimates, or the data, will have uncertainties, and it is important to show how these propagate through to key model outputs (Blower and Dowlatabadi 1994). Uncertainty in a particular parameter may be benign—all credible assumptions give the same result—therefore meriting increased confidence in the model's use of this parameter. In other cases, different, superficially credible values for a parameter (or choices of model structure or interpretations of data) will lead to different results, perhaps not all plausible. For example, the simulated impact of an HIV intervention can be quite sensitive both to the assumed degree of heterogeneity in sexual behaviour and to the assumed patterns of sexual mixing, and the associated parameters are not easy to estimate even from good data.

Principle 6: exploration of model limitations

Model consumers may misunderstand the reductionist and minimalist approach of mathematical modelling, which (as explained earlier) proceeds by careful selection and abstraction of elements of reality requisite for answering specific questions. Effective dialogue can take place only if the modeller gives a full catalogue of model limitations alongside the results, so that model consumers are assisted to recognize both the weaknesses and the strengths of the model. On the other hand, consumers of models, looking for guidance in decision-making, should be alert to the possibility that the limitations are critical to their specific needs, and aware that open discussion by modellers of the limitations of their work is by no means a confession of ineptitude, or a sign of a model's irrelevance.

Principle 7: contextualization with other modelling studies

When different modelling groups appear to be addressing the same research question, but apply different model structures, with different assumptions, apparent conflicting results in the modelling literature may lead consumers of models to distrust their use in decision-making. To support an understanding of their differences, modelling results should always be set in the context of earlier relevant work, clarifying exactly where there is agreement and disagreement (Hankins et al. 2009; Kretzschmar et al. 2009; UNAIDS/WHO/SACEMA Expert Group et al. 2009; Hankins et al. 2011; Eaton et al. 2012).

Principle 8: application of epidemiological modelling to health economic analyses

In considering interventions, public health decision-makers generally seek to maximize cost-efficiency in some way. When cost-effectiveness, affordability, and returns on investments are of crucial interest, the most understandable and relevant modelling studies will be those that have integrated into cost-effectiveness analyses, providing outputs such as the number of incident infections or deaths averted, quality-adjusted life years gained, or disability-adjusted life years averted. Good examples appear in Vickerman et al. (2006), Anderson et al. (2009), Long et al. (2010), and Alistar et al. (2011), and guidelines have been developed for the production, submission, and review of health economic analyses by the *British Medical Journal* (Drummond et al. 1996). Conversely, it is important for those seeking guidance in health economic analyses to critique the scenarios in which indicators have been calculated, and in particular to probe whether a suitable level of self-consistency has been applied to modelling the overall epidemiological dynamic, incorporating possible population-level feedback that is likely to be triggered through the proposed intervention itself, rather than a static view in which individual-level costs and effects are modelled in terms of an initial status quo.

Principle 9: clear language

For results to be considered by policymakers, it is important that modellers use language that supports effective communication. Such clarity is desirable at two distinct levels: the internal technical description of the model, and the intended real-world interpretation and application. Precision about model assumptions will help consumers assess the model on its own terms. Clarifying correspondence to real-world features and scenarios will help evaluate the impact of potential policy implications and interventions. Speaking as modellers, we particularly caution against overconfident statements like: 'This modelling exercise shows that a consequence of the intervention will be...'

Conclusion

Modelling the transmission and control of infectious agents spans a very broad range of activities, from microscopic models of biological processes, to population-level projections of the consequences of large public health interventions. Stripping away layers of technical complexity, modelling is ultimately, when practised with discipline, little more than consistently clarifying relationships between data and assumptions. Often, modelling has been seen as a niche activity, but, encouragingly, there is increasing engagement and discourse with a range of disciplines, from clinical, laboratory, and social science to funding and policymaking. Modelling is becoming an important unifying discipline which enables disparate areas of knowledge and expertise to be brought to bear on key decisions in public health.

Acknowledgements

Text extract from Bacaër, Nicolas, *A Short History of Mathematical Population Dynamics*, Springer-Verlag, London, UK, Copyright © 2011, reproduced with kind permission of Springer Science and Business Media, http://www.springer.com/978-0-85729-114-1.

Text extract from *Acta Tropica*, Volume 49, Issue 1, Jacob C. Koella, On the use of mathematical models of malaria transmission, pp. 1–25, Copyright © 1991, reprinted with permission from Elsevier, http://www.sciencedirect.com/science/journal/0001706X.

Further reading

Among the references, the following books provide more detail on the topics of this chapter: Bacaër (2010); Vynnycky and White (2010); Keeling and Rohani (2008); Brauer et al. (2008); Anderson and May (1991). There are four excellent introductory articles on mathematical modelling of infectious diseases, by Mark Lewis, Marjorie Wonham, Fred Brauer and David Earn, in *Pi in the Sky*, Issue 8 (December 2004). It can be downloaded from: http://www.pims.math.ca/pi. The following survey and review articles among the references may also be found helpful: Johnson and White (2011), Garnett et al. (2011), Wilson and Garnett (2011), Keeling and Danon (2009), Grassly and Fraser (2008).

Online materials

The online appendix to this chapter, containing definitions and discussion of key modelling concepts, may be found at ✆ www.oxfordmedicine.com

References

Abbas, U., Anderson, R., and Mellors, J. (2007). Potential impact of antiretroviral chemoprophylaxis on HIV-1 transmission in resource-limited settings. *PLoS One*, 19(9), e875.

Abu-Raddad, L., Patnaik, P., and Kublin, J. (2006). Dual infection with HIV and malaria fuels the spread of both diseases in sub-Saharan Africa. *Science*, 314(5805), 1603–6.

Actuarial Society of South Africa (2011). *ASSA 2008 AIDS and Demographic Model*. [Online] Available at: http://aids.actuarialsociety.org.za.

Alistar, S., Owens, D., and Brandeau, M. (2011). Effectiveness and cost effectiveness of expanding harm reduction and antiretroviral therapy in a mixed HIV epidemic: a modeling analysis for Ukraine. *PLoS Medicine*, 8(3), e1000423.

Anderson, J., Wilson, R., Templeton, D., Grulich, A., Carter, R., and Kaldor, J. (2009). Cost-effectiveness of adult circumcision in a resource-rich setting for HIV prevention among men who have sex with men. *Journal of Infectious Diseases*, 15(12), 1803–12.

Anderson, R. and Hanson, M. (2005). Potential public health impact of imperfect HIV type 1 vaccines. *Journal of Infectious Diseases*, 191(Suppl. 1), S85–96.

Anderson, R.M. and May, R.M. (1991). *Infectious Diseases of Humans: Dynamics and Control*. Oxford: Oxford University Press.

Auvert, B., Taljaard, D., Lagarde, E., Sobngwi-Tambekou, J., Sitta, R., and Puren, A. (2005). Randomized, controlled intervention trial of male circumcision for reduction of HIV infection risk: the ANRS 1265 trial. *PLoS Medicine*, 2(11), e298.

Bacaër, N. (2010). *A Short History of Mathematical Population Dynamics*. London: Springer-Verlag.

Baggaley, R., Garnett, G., and Ferguson, N. (2006). Modelling the impact of antiretroviral use in resource-poor settings. *PLoS Medicine*, 3(4), e124.

Baran, P. and Sweezy, P. (1968). *Monopoly Capital: An Essay on the American Economic and Social Order*. New York: Monthly Review Press.

Basu, S., Andrews, J., Poolman, E., et al. (2007). Prevention of nosocomial transmission of extensively drug-resistant tuberculosis in rural South African district hospitals: an epidemiological modelling study. *The Lancet*, 370(9597), 1500–7.

Bernoulli, D. (1760). Essai d'une nouvelle analyse de la mortalité causée par la petite vérole et des avantages de l'inoculation pour la prévenir. In *Histoire de l'Académie Royale des Sciences (Paris) avec Mém des Math et Phys and Mém*, pp. 1–45. (English translation by Blower, S. (2004). An attempt at a new analysis of the mortality caused by smallpox and of the advantages of inoculation to prevent it. *Reviews in Medical Virology*, 14, 275–88.)

Bezemer, D., de Wolf, F., Boerlijst, M., et al. (2008). A resurgent HIV-1 epidemic among men who have sex with men in the era of potent antiretroviral therapy. *AIDS*, 22(9), 1071–7.

Blower, S. and Dowlatabadi, H. (1994). Sensitivity and uncertainty analysis of complex models of disease transmission: an HIV model, as an example. *International Statistical Review/Revue Internationale de Statistique*, 62(2), 229–43.

Boily, M., Pickles, M., Vickerman, P., et al. (2008). Using mathematical modelling to investigate the plausibility of attributing observed antenatal clinic declines to a female sex worker intervention in Karnataka state, India. *AIDS*, 22(Suppl. 5), S149–64.

Brauer, F., Allen, L., van den Driessche, P., and Wu, J. (2008). *Lecture Note in Mathematics: Mathematical Epidemiology*. Mathematical Biosciences Subseries no. 1945. Berlin: Springer-Verlag.

Brown, T. and Peerapatanapokin, W. (2004). The Asian Epidemic Model: a process model for exploring HIV policy and programme alternatives in Asia. *Sexually Transmitted Infections*, 80(Suppl. 1), i19–24.

Cohen, M., Chen, Y., McCauley, M., et al. (2011). Prevention of HIV-1 infection with early antiretroviral therapy. *The New England Journal of Medicine*, 365(6), 493–505.

Cohen, M., Dye, C., Fraser, C., Miller, W.C., Powers, K., and Williams, B. (2012). HIV treatment as prevention: debate and commentary—will early infection compromise treatment-as-prevention strategies? *PLoS Medicine*, 9(7), e1001232.

Cohen, T., Lipsitch, M., Walensky, R., and Murray, M. (2006). Beneficial and perverse effects of isoniazid preventive therapy for latent tuberculosis infection in HIV-tuberculosis coinfected populations. *Proceedings of the National Academy of Sciences of the United States of America*, 103(18), 7042–7.

Cooke, K. and Yorke, J. (1973). Some equations modelling growth processes and gonorrhea epidemics. *Mathematical Biosciences*, 16, 75–101.

Delva, W., Eaton, J., Meng, F., et al. (2012). HIV treatment as prevention: optimising the impact of expanded HIV treatment programmes. *PLoS Medicine*, 9(7), e1001258.

Delva, W., Wilson, D., Abu-Raddad, L., et al. (2012). HIV treatment as prevention: principles of good HIV epidemiology modelling for public health decision-making in all modes of prevention and evaluation. *PLoS Medicine*, 9(7), e1001239.

Dietz, K. (1980). Models for vector-borne parasitic diseases. In C. Barigozzi (ed.) *Vito Volterra Symposium on Mathematical Models in Biology* (Vol. 2), pp. 264–77. Berlin: Springer.

Dietz, K. and Heesterbeek, J. (2002). Daniel Bernoulli's epidemiological model revisited. *Mathematical Biosciences*, 180, 1–21.

Dodd, P., Garnett, G., and Hallett, T. (2010). Examining the promise of HIV elimination by 'test and treat' in hyperendemic settings. *AIDS*, 24(5), 729–35.

Drummond, M., Jefferson, T. on behalf of the The Economic Evaluation Working Party (1996). Guidelines for authors and peer reviewers of economic submissions to the BMJ. *British Medical Journal*, 313(7052), 275–83.

Earn, D. (2004). Mathematical modelling of recurrent epidemics. *Pi in the Sky*, 8, 14–17.

Eaton, J., Johnson, L., Salomon, J., et al. (2012). HIV treatment as prevention: systematic comparison of mathematical models of the potential impact of antiretroviral therapy on HIV incidence in South Africa. *PLoS Medicine*, 9(7), e1001245.

Einstein, A. (1934). On the method of theoretical physics. *Philosophy of Science*, 1(2), 163–9. (First published as *On the method of theoretical physics: The Herbert Spencer Lecture*, delivered at Oxford, 10 June 1933.)

Foss, A., Watts, C., Vickerman, P., et al. (2006). Could the CARE–SHAKTI intervention for injecting drug users be maintaining the low HIV prevalence in Dhaka, Bangladesh? *Addiction*, 102(1), 114–25.

Fraser, C., Donnelly, C., Cauchemez, S., et al. (2009). Pandemic potential of a strain of influenza A (H1N1): early findings. *Science*, 324(5934), 1557–61.

Galileo Galilei (1623). *Il Saggiatore*. Rome. (Translated by Drake, S. (1957). *Discoveries and Opinions of Galileo*, pp. 237–8. New York: Anchor Books.)

Galileo Galilei (1638). *Discorsi e dimostrazioni matematiche, intorno a due nuove scienze attentanti alla meccanica ed a muovementi localli*. Leiden. (The work was completed by Galileo in 1636; relevant passages are in Crew, H. and de Salvio, A. (trans.) *Dialogues Concerning Two New Sciences*. New York: Macmillan (1914), pp. 161–76, reprinted New York: Dover (1952), pp. 251–7.)

Garnett, G., Cousens, S., Hallett, T., Steketee, R., and Walker, N. (2011). Mathematical models in the evaluation of health programmes. *The Lancet*, 378(9790), 515–25.

Granich, R., Gilks, C., Dye, C., de Cock, K., and Williams, B. (2009). Universal voluntary HIV testing with immediate antiretroviral therapy as a strategy for elimination of HIV transmission: a mathematical model. *The Lancet*, 373(9657), 48–57.

Grassly, N. and Fraser, C. (2008). Mathematical models of infectious disease transmission. *Nature Reviews Microbiology*, 6(6), 477–87.

Grassly, N., Fraser, C., Wenger, J., et al. (2006). New strategies for the elimination of polio from India. *Science*, 314(5802), 1150–3.

Griffin, J., Hollingsworth, T., Okell, L., et al. (2010). Reducing plasmodium falciparum malaria transmission in Africa: a model-based evaluation of intervention strategies. *PLoS Medicine*, 7(8), e1000324.

Hallett, T., Aberle-Grasse, J., Bello, G., et al. (2006). Declines in HIV prevalence can be associated with changing sexual behaviour in Uganda, urban Kenya, Zimbabwe, and urban Haiti. *Sexually Transmitted Infections*, 82(Suppl. 1), i1–8.

Hallett, T., Gregson, S., Mugurungi, O., Gonese, E., and Garnett, G. (2009). Assessing evidence for behaviour change affecting the course of HIV epidemics: a new mathematical modelling approach and application to data from Zimbabwe. *Epidemics*, 1(2), 108–17.

Hallett, T., White, P., and Garnett, G. (2007). Appropriate evaluation of HIV prevention interventions: from experiment to full-scale implementation. *Sexually Transmitted Infections*, 83(Suppl. 1), i55–60.

Hankins, C., Glasser, J., and Chen, R. (2011). Modeling the impact of RV144-like vaccines on HIV transmission. *Vaccine*, 29(36), 6069–71.

Hankins, C., Hargrove, J., Williams, B., et al. (2009). Male circumcision for HIV prevention in high HIV prevalence settings: what can mathematical modelling contribute to informed decision making? *PLoS Medicine*, 6(9), e1000109.

Harvey, W. (1943). A.G. McKendrick 1876–1943. *Edinburgh Medical Journal*, 50, 500–6.

Hethcote, H. and Yorke, J. (1984). *Lecture Notes in Biomathematics: Gonorrhea Transmission Dynamics and Control* (Vol. 56). Berlin: Springer-Verlag.

Hethcote, H., Yorke, J., and Nold, A. (1982). Gonorrhea modeling: a comparison of control methods. *Mathematical Biosciences*, 58(1), 93–109.

Johnson, L., Dorrington, R., Bradshaw, D., Pillay-van Wyk, V., and Rehle, T. (2009). Sexual behaviour patterns in South Africa and their association with the spread of HIV: insights from a mathematical model. *Demographic Research*, 21(11), 289–340.

Johnson, L. and White, P. (2011). A review of mathematical models of HIV/AIDS interventions and their implications for policy. *Sexually Transmitted Infections*, 87(7), 629–34.

Kahn, J., Marseille, E., Williams, B., Granich, R., et al. (2011). Cost-effectiveness of antiretroviral therapy for prevention. *Current HIV Research*, 9(6), 405–15.

Kaiser Family Foundation (2011). *International AIDS assistance from donor governments: commitments and disbursements, 2002–2010*. [Online] Available at: http://facts.kff.org/chart.aspx?ch=946.

Keeling, M. and Rohani, P. (2008). *Modeling Infectious Diseases in Humans and Animals*. Princeton, NJ: Princeton University Press.

Keeling, Y. and Danon, L. (2009). Mathematical modelling of infectious diseases. *British Medical Bulletin*, 92(2), 33–42.

Kermack, W. and McKendrick, A. (1927). Contributions to the mathematical theory of epidemics I. *Proceedings of the Royal Society of London. Series A*, 700–21. (Reprinted in *Bulletin of Mathematical Biology* (1991), 141(843), 94–122.)

Koella, J. (1991). On the use of mathematical models of malaria transmission. *Acta Tropica*, 49(1), 2.

Korenromp, E., White, R., Orroth, K., et al. (2005). Determinants of the impact of sexually transmitted infection treatment on prevention of HIV infection: a synthesis of evidence from the Mwanza, Rakai, and Masaka intervention trials. *Journal of Infectious Diseases*, 191(Suppl 1), S168–78.

Kretzschmar, M., Turner, K., Barton, P., Edmunds, W., and Low, N. (2009). Predicting the population impact of chlamydia screening programmes: comparative mathematical modelling study. *Sexually Transmitted Infections*, 85(5), 359–66.

Lamagni, T., Dennis, J., George, R., and Efstratiou, A. (2008). Analysis of epidemiological patterns during a century of scarlet fever. In *Proceedings of the European Scientific Conference on Applied Infectious*

Disease Epidemiology. Berlin. Available at: http://www.hpa.org.uk/webc/HPAwebFile/HPAwebC/1229594253740.

Londish, G. and Murray, J. (2008). Significant reduction in HIV prevalence according to male circumcision intervention in sub-Saharan Africa. *International Journal of Epidemiology*, 37(6), 1246–53.

Long, E., Brandeau, M., and Owens, D. (2009). Potential population health outcomes and expenditures of HIV vaccination strategies in the United States. *Vaccine*, 27(39), 5402–10.

Long, E., Brandeau, M., and Owens, D. (2010). The cost-effectiveness and population outcomes of expanded HIV screening and antiretroviral treatment in the United States. *Annals of Internal Medicine*, 153(12), 778–89.

Macdonald, G. (1957) *The Epidemiology and Control of Malaria*. Oxford: Oxford University Press.

McKendrick, A.G. (1926). Applications of mathematics to medical problems. *Proceedings of the Edinburgh Mathematical Society*, 44(1), 98–130.

Montaner, J., Hogg, R., Wood, E., et al. (2006). The case for expanding access to highly active antiretroviral therapy to curb the growth of the HIV epidemic. *The Lancet*, 368(9534), 531–6.

Mortimer, P. (2011). The diphtheria vaccine debacle of 1940 that ushered in comprehensive childhood immunization in the United Kingdom. *Epidemiology and Infection*, 139(4), 487–93.

Nagelkerke, N., Moses, S., de Vlas, S., and Bailey, R. (2007). Modelling the public health impact of male circumcision for HIV prevention in high prevalence areas in Africa. *BMC Infectious Diseases*, 7, 16.

Nathanson, N. and Martin, J. (1979). The epidemiology of poliomyelitis: enigmas surrounding its appearance, epidemicity, and disappearance. *American Journal of Epidemiology*, 110(6), 672–92.

Orenstein, W., Perry, R., and Halsey, N. (2004). The clinical significance of measles: a review. *Journal of Infectious Diseases*, 189(Suppl. 1), S4–16.

Piwoz, E. and Ross, J. (2005). Use of population-specific infant mortality rates to inform policy decisions regarding HIV and infant feeding. *The Journal of Nutrition*, 135(5), 1113–19.

Ramsay, M. (2012). *Epidemiology of Whooping Cough (Pertussis)*. Health Protection Agency. Available at: http://www.hpa.org.uk/webc/HPAwebFile/HPAweb_C/1317136329151.

Riley, S., Fraser, C., Donnelly, C., et al. (2003). Transmission dynamics of the etiological agent of SARS in Hong Kong: impact of public health interventions. *Science*, 300(5627), 1961–6.

Ross, R. (1910). *The Prevention of Malaria* (2nd ed.). London: John Murray.

Ross, R. (1923). *Memoirs: With a Full Account of the Great Malaria Problem and its Solution*. London: John Murray.

Salomon, J., Hogan, D., Stover, J., et al. (2005). Integrating HIV prevention and treatment: from slogans to impact. *PLoS Medicine*, 2(1), e16.

Schwartländer, B., Stover, J., Hallett, T., et al. (2011). Towards an improved investment approach for an effective response to HIV/AIDS. *The Lancet*, 377(9782), 2031–41.

Sension, M., Quinn, T., Markowitz, L., et al. (1988). Measles in hospitalized African children with human immunodeficiency virus. *American Journal of Diseases of Children*, 142(12), 1271–2.

Smith, D., Battle, K., Hay, S., Barker, C., Scott, T., and McKenzie, F. (2012). Ross, Macdonald, and a theory for the dynamics and control of mosquito-transmitted pathogens. *PLoS Pathogens*, 8(4), e1002588.

Smith, R., Okano, J., Kahn, J., Bodine, E., and Blower, S. (2010). Evolutionary dynamics of complex networks of HIV drug-resistant strains: the case of San Francisco. *Science*, 327(5966), 697–701.

Stover, J. (2000). Influence of mathematical modeling of HIV and AIDS on policies and programs in the developing world. *Sexually Transmitted Diseases*, 27(10), 572–8.

Temime, L., Hejblum, G., Setbon, M., and Valleron, A. (2008). The rising impact of mathematical modelling in epidemiology: antibiotic resistance research as a case study. *Epidemiology and Infection*, 136(3), 289–98.

The HIV Modelling Consortium Treatment as Prevention Editorial Writing Group (2012). HIV treatment as prevention: models, data, and questions—towards evidence-based decision-making. *PLoS Medicine*, 9(7), e1001259.

UNAIDS/WHO/SACEMA Expert Group on Modelling the Impact and Cost of Male Circumcision for HIV Prevention (2009). Male circumcision for HIV prevention in high HIV prevalence settings: what can mathematical modelling contribute to informed decision making? *PLoS Medicine*, 6(9), e1000109.

Vickerman, P., Kumaranayake, L., Balakireva, O., et al. (2006). The cost-effectiveness of expanding harm reduction activities for injecting drug users in Odessa, Ukraine. *Sexually Transmitted Diseases*, 33(10), S89–102.

Vynnycky, E. and White, R. (2010). *An Introduction to Infectious Disease Modelling*. Oxford: Oxford University Press.

Wagner, B., Kahn, J., and Blower, S. (2010). Should we try to eliminate HIV epidemics by using a 'test and treat' strategy? *AIDS*, 24(245), 775–6.

Walensky, R., Wood, R., Ciaranello, A., et al. (2010). Scaling up the 2010 World Health Organization HIV Treatment Guidelines in resource-limited settings: a model-based analysis, *PLoS Medicine*, 7(12), e1000382.

White, R., Orroth, K., Glynn, J., et al. (2008). Treating curable sexually transmitted infections to prevent HIV in Africa: still an effective control strategy? *Journal of Acquired Immune Deficiency Syndromes*, 47(3), 346.

White, R., Orroth, K., Korenromp, E., et al. (2004). Can population differences explain the contrasting results of the Mwanza, Rakai, and Masaka HIV/sexually transmitted disease intervention trials? A modeling study. *Journal of Acquired Immune Deficiency Syndromes*, 37(4), 1500–13.

Wilson, D., Coplan, P., Wainberg, M., and Blower, S. (2008). The paradoxical effects of using antiretroviral-based microbicides to control HIV epidemics. *Proceedings of the National Academy of Sciences of the United States of America*, 105(28), 9835–40.

Wilson, D. and Garnett, G. (2011). Introduction to recent developments in HIV epidemic modeling. *Current Opinion in HIV and AIDS*, 6(2), 91–3.

World Health Organization (2013). *Polio Eradication*. [Online] Available at: http://www.polioeradication.org/Dataandmonitoring/Poliothisweek.aspx.

Yorke, J., Hethcote, H., Nold, A., et al. (1978). Dynamics and control of the transmission of gonorrhoea. *Sexually Transmitted Diseases*, 5(2), 51–6.

Public health surveillance

James W. Buehler and Ann Marie Kimball

Introduction to public health surveillance

Public health surveillance provides the epidemiological foundation for modern public health practice. The ongoing monitoring of disease or health trends within populations informs what public health actions are taken and reflects whether those actions are effective. Surveillance may involve monitoring of diseases and other health-related conditions as well as their antecedents, characteristics, and consequences. Surveillance can guide the local response to individual cases of disease or more broadly inform public health programmes and policies. A key function of surveillance is to identify circumstances that merit further public health scrutiny, such as groups or locations that are disproportionately affected or changes in disease occurrence or severity. Person, place, and time are the key epidemiological attributes of disease distribution in populations, and knowledge of these attributes afforded by surveillance allows targeting of public health programmes. General principles that underlie the practice of surveillance are essentially the same for all countries, regardless of economic development. Defining surveillance objectives depends on programme goals and on what information is needed, who needs it, and how it will be used. Desirable but potentially competing attributes of surveillance include completeness, timeliness, representativeness, high predictive value, acceptability, flexibility, simplicity, and low cost. Public health surveillance is conducted in many ways, depending on the nature of the health event under surveillance, the nature of healthcare and information infrastructures, the population involved, resources available, and information needs. The widespread and expanding use of the Internet, electronic media, communication technologies, and mobile computing have enabled innovations in public health surveillance that reach far beyond traditional methods. Surveillance systems should be periodically assessed to determine whether information needs are being fulfilled and whether the resources are being used effectively. Although surveillance methods were originally developed as part of efforts to control infectious diseases, basic concepts of surveillance have been applied to all areas of public health.

In many resource-poor countries, challenges to meeting needs for population health information are heightened and include potential tensions between the perspectives of external funders and in-country officials, between the interests of those responsible for disease-specific 'categorical' programmes and those interested in strengthening general surveillance infrastructures, and between advocates for using limited resources to strengthen information capacities versus those who would focus spending to address urgent service needs. At the same time, recent innovations hold promise for improving surveillance in resource-poor settings, where precedents in developed countries that can impede innovation are absent or less established.

Definition

People who are responsible for protecting and promoting the health of populations need ongoing, timely, and reliable information about the health of the populations they serve. The term 'surveillance' encompasses the multiple processes that public health agencies employ to meet this need for information. Surveillance can include information about specific diseases or health risks or more general indicators of overall population health. As an integral part of public health practice, surveillance is an ongoing, systematic process of information collection, analysis, interpretation, visualization, dissemination, and connection to public health programmes (Thacker and Berkelman 1988). Surveillance systems are organized networks of people and activities dedicated to managing and maintaining surveillance for specific conditions. Surveillance systems can operate at various levels within countries, from local to national, or on a global scale.

In 1963, Langmuir established the modern concept of surveillance as 'the continued watchfulness over the distribution and trends of incidence through the systematic collection, consolidation, and evaluation of morbidity and mortality reports and other relevant data' together with timely and regular dissemination to those who 'need to know' (Langmuir 1963, pp. 182–183). In 1968, the twenty-first World Health Assembly described surveillance as the systematic collection and use of epidemiological information for the planning, implementation, and assessment of disease control; in short, surveillance implied 'information for action' (World Health Organization 1968). Over time, the scope and methods of surveillance have been adapted to meet the information needs of public health programmes that address a broad spectrum of infectious and non-infectious diseases and acute and chronic conditions. For brevity, the term 'diseases' or 'conditions' will be used as shorthand throughout this chapter for diseases, injuries, risk factors, and other health-related events that are the focus of public health programmes and surveillance systems.

Surveillance can include monitoring of the incidence, prevalence, antecedents (such as behavioural risks or hazardous exposures), characteristics, and outcomes of disease and other health conditions of public health importance. According to the US Centers for Disease Control and Prevention (CDC), a 'public health surveillance system is useful if it contributes to the prevention and control of adverse health-related events…and can be useful in contributing to [public health program] performance measures, including health indicators that are used in needs assessments and accountability systems' (CDC 2001). Surveillance should begin when there exists, or is likely to exist, a public health problem that merits attention, and it should be discontinued or revamped when the information it yields is no longer needed or useful.

Objectives of surveillance

The purpose of surveillance is to meet the needs of public health programmes for information about the health of the populations they serve (Box 5.19.1). These needs usually include a description of the temporal and geographical trends in the occurrence of a disease in a particular population. Questions addressed by surveillance can be summarized using epidemiological measures of time (when), place (where), person (who), and disease characteristics (what):

◆ *Time*: are disease trends upwards, downwards, or stable? Do downward trends coincide with interventions, such as the introduction of a vaccine, treatment, or prevention programme? Do upturns coincide with aggravating situations? Changes in trends might reflect the underlying health of populations or they might reflect changes in how surveillance is conducted or changes in medical or public concern about particular conditions. A key purpose of surveillance is to recognize changes in trends that might herald the onset of an outbreak or epidemic, prompting investigations to confirm the observed upturn in disease and, if so, identify the likely cause and guide interventions.

◆ *Place*: where is disease occurring or not occurring? Understanding geographic variations in incidence or prevalence can inform where investigations and interventions should be directed and can provide important clues to environmental, occupational, water- or food-borne, behavioural, or other risk factors. Alternatively, geographic variations might reflect differences in detection of disease resulting from variations in the availability, quality, or use of public health or healthcare services.

◆ *Person*: who is affected? Understanding the characteristics and commonalities of affected people, such as their age,

gender, occupation, race, ethnicity, habits, customs, or social or economic status, provides further insights into potential exposures or behaviours that can affect the risk of disease. Combined with information about the characteristics of the population at large, as from census data or population surveys, surveillance can provide critical insights into variations in the rates of disease among different groups. For example, in 1981, shortly after the disease later named acquired immunedeficiency syndrome (AIDS) was recognized and before the aetiological agent (human immunodeficiency virus (HIV)) was identified, by describing the sexual, blood-related, or perinatal exposures of affected people, surveillance combined with early epidemiological investigations helped to determine the infectious nature of the disease, identify probable modes of transmission, inform early prevention recommendations, and calm fears about the potential for widespread transmission through casual contact with affected people (Jaffe et al. 1983).

◆ *Disease characteristics*: what are the characteristics of disease, such as the clinical or laboratory manifestations, severity, and outcomes? For example, understanding the prevalence of the sensitivity or resistance of infectious agents to antimicrobial drugs is critical to informing healthcare and public health responses, and monitoring the prevalence of different microbe strains can be important for understanding the spread of different infectious or for vaccine development. Global influenza surveillance is used to anticipate which strains of influenza virus will be most prevalent during upcoming influenza seasons and to develop annual influenza vaccines (Cox et al. 1994). Differences in the spectrum or severity of disease among affected people might pinpoint differences among groups in genetic susceptibility, the co-occurrence of other illnesses, or access to healthcare.

Taken together, population-level measures of time, place, person, and disease characteristics can lead to an understanding of the impact of various diseases and insights into individual and social determinants of their occurrence. Surveillance might lead to hypotheses that can be tested in more definitive investigations and can identify individuals who could be enrolled in further epidemiological studies. In some instances, surveillance alone can provide compelling evidence of the impact of prevention programmes, such as the sharp decline in the incidence of a vaccine-preventable disease coincident with the widespread use of a new vaccine (Seward et al. 2002). In other situations, surveillance can contribute to evaluating the impact of interventions, but more detailed investigations are necessary to explain trends that are shaped by multiple factors. Low incidence or prevalence does not necessarily mean that certain diseases do not deserve public health attention, including continuation of surveillance, since this might reflect the impact of successful prevention efforts that must be sustained in order to prevent re-emergence.

Information on disease trends gained through surveillance, when combined with other information, can also be used to predict future disease trends. For example, with the ageing of the 'baby boom' population in countries such as the United States, projections of disease prevalence in the elderly, such as the anticipated prevalence and cost of dementia (Hurd et al. 2013), are garnering increased attention.

Box 5.19.1 Purposes of public health surveillance

To define public health priorities.

   To characterize disease patterns by time, place, person, and disease characteristics.

   To detect epidemics.

   To suggest hypotheses for further investigation.

   To identify cases for epidemiological research.

   To guide and evaluate prevention and control programmes, including assessment of effectiveness and/or adverse consequences.

   To facilitate planning, including projection of future trends and healthcare needs.

Setting priorities

An important use of surveillance is to help set public health priorities. In addition to recent measures of incidence or prevalence, other factors that can shape priority setting include likely future trends, the potential for public health or other interventions to have an impact, severity, disparities and attendant social justice concerns, and public interest. To the extent that surveillance data are used in priority setting, deliberations may give rise to concerns about surveillance methods, how surveillance data are queried and analysed, and the accuracy of estimates of disease impact. For example, even though mortality monitoring is the oldest form of surveillance and remains important in assessing the impact of different diseases (Thacker 2010), different agencies using mortality data may arrive at different conclusions, depending on the use of overall mortality measures, age-specific measures, or approaches that seek to integrate measures of mortality and wellness. Table 5.19.1 provides two estimates of the number of deaths (in millions) for leading causes of death globally in 2010, one from the Institute for Health Metrics and Evaluation (IHME) and another from the World Health Organization (WHO) (Liu 2000). Such estimates from different organizations rarely line up, and disparities in estimates can cause consternation among donors and national governments seeking to prioritize interventions.

In addition to using age-specific mortality measures, the impact of deaths among younger age groups can be further illuminated using a measure of years of potential life lost (cumulative years of life lost before a particular age such as 65 or 75 years). These measures can be further adjusted to account for the impact of diseases on the quality of life or disabilities. For example, in 1993, the World Bank Development Report, *Investing in Health*, adopted the approach of using disability-adjusted life years (DALYs) lost to consider not only the impact of premature death but also the impact on ill health or disability for specific diseases, in effect combining the mortality and morbidity into a single measure (World Bank 1993).

More recently, the IHME (Murray et al. 2012), experts convened by the WHO (2008), and groups focused on specific diseases have published estimates of DALYs to assess the impact of different conditions. As with overall mortality estimates, DALYs estimates from different organizations rarely align.

Formal burden of disease estimates rely on diverse datasets and sophisticated modelling. Cross-sectional surveys such as the Demographic and Health Surveys (DHS) financed by the United States Agency for International Development (USAID) (USAID 2013), the Multiple Indicator Cluster Survey (MICS) sponsored by the United Nations International Children's Emergency Fund (UNICEF) (UNICEF 2013), and the Malaria Indicator Survey sponsored by USAID (Malaria Surveys 2013) along with special academic research studies provide country-specific data. Information on causes of death is enhanced by the inclusion of 'verbal autopsy' modules within some of the larger cross-sectional surveys. Data from these sources are then modelled to account for missing data points and to create locality- or country- and disease-specific estimates of DALYs.

Such efforts to estimate the impact of different diseases can be done periodically as data and the resources to analyse them become available, but this approach does not lend itself to frequent and ongoing monitoring where disease patterns are shifting because: (1) data quality is highly variable from different surveys or settings and often repurposed from its original collection goal; (2) cross-sectional survey information typically becomes available 1–2 years after surveys are completed; (3) estimates for very remote and information-poor geographic locations are often based on imputed data from neighbouring localities, and little 'ground truthing' is done to verify imputed data; and (4) assignment of causes of death, especially when based on verbal autopsies, is plagued with potential misclassification.

Establishing a surveillance system

Establishing a surveillance system requires a statement of objectives, definition of the disease or condition under surveillance, and implementation of procedures for collecting information (or obtaining information from existing sources), managing, analysing, visualizing, interpreting, and disseminating the information. In addition, as the number of surveillance systems increases, attention should be given to whether there are multiple systems

Table 5.19.1 Estimates of the global number of deaths, by cause, 2010, Institute of Health Metrics and Evaluation (IHME) and World Health Organization (WHO)

Cause of death	IHME Deaths (millions) (95% CI)	WHO Deaths (millions) (95% CI)
Pneumonia/lower respiratory infections	0.847 (0.736–0.981)	1.396 (1.189–1.642)
Diarrhoeal diseases	0.666 (0.544–0.763)	0.801 (0.555–1.182)
Malaria	0.676 (0.445–1.002)	0.564 (0.432–0.709)
HIV/AIDS	0.126 (0.105–0.150)	0.159 (0.131–0.185)
Neonatal sepsis or meningitis	0.514 (0.318–0.841)	0.573 (0.388–0.789)
Total deaths in children <5 years of age	6.841 (6.439–7.302)	7.622 (no CI is given)

CI, confidence interval.

Source data from Institute of Health Metrics and Evaluation, University of Washington, Seattle, WA, USA (unpublished report) and WHO via Child Health Epidemiology Reference Group, Department of International Health, Johns Hopkins Bloomberg School of Public Health, Baltimore, MD, USA; *The Lancet*, Volume 379, Issue 9832, Liu L. et al., Global, regional, and national causes of child mortality: an updated systematic analysis for 2010 with time trends since 2000, pp. 2151–61, Copyright © 2000.

collecting information within a population and, if so, whether these systems collect common data elements and adhere to shared information standards. This is important to allow for information sharing across systems, to minimize duplication of effort, and to simplify the work of those who are asked to report to these systems. As surveillance becomes more automated and draws upon health information that is stored and transmitted electronically, adherence to information standards will become increasingly important. Attention should also be given to whether surveillance for a particular condition can be done similarly in different locations, increasing the likelihood that comparison of disease incidence or prevalence across multiple localities or countries is meaningful.

Surveillance systems are information loops, or cycles, that involve healthcare providers, public health agencies, and the public in a process of information collection, analysis and interpretation, and feedback. The cycle begins when events of public health concern occur and is completed when information about these events is made available and applied in public health programmes. This may involve multiple levels that should be specified in developing a surveillance system, ranging from the anticipated local response to individuals with cases of disease to the use of information aggregated from multiple localities to inform national policies. The delivery of information to constituents and policymakers (Langmuir 1963) is essential to the completion of the surveillance cycle. To the extent that surveillance data can be released without compromising privacy or confidentiality, they should be placed in the public domain to allow full use and benefits, with appropriate documentation.

Weaknesses in any part of the information chain can affect the entire surveillance process, and potential constraints should be anticipated. For example, when surveillance draws upon information arising from the use healthcare services, surveillance will be affected by the availability and quality of those services, including laboratory and other diagnostic services (Berkelman et al. 1994) and by the accuracy with which diagnoses are recorded or coded.

No information resource is perfect, and establishing surveillance requires consideration of options, each with strengths and limitations, for how surveillance should be conducted at each step in the surveillance cycle. Having data that are complete and without error is desirable, but the effort required to obtain such data in a timely manner may not be feasible or sustainable. To assist in the design and evaluation of surveillance systems, the US CDC has identified a series of desirable but potentially conflicting attributes of surveillance. Deciding which of these attributes to prioritize will shape how surveillance is conducted:

◆ *Completeness*: ideally, surveillance data are complete, or stated in epidemiological terms, they have high *sensitivity*. Completeness will be a priority when it is essential to identify all people with a particular condition, such as a highly transmissible and severe infectious disease for which treatment is effective and can interrupt further transmission, or when it is important to have an accurate assessment of the impact of a particular condition.

◆ *Representativeness*: if surveillance is not complete, then ideally, it is representative of affected people within a population. Representativeness will be a priority when it is important to know where or among which groups to target interventions.

Representativeness can be affected by variations in reporting or by variable access to healthcare services. When surveillance depends on sampling of individuals or facilities, statistically defined sampling is ideal. But, rigorous sampling might not be feasible to implement, or response rates may be so low as to obviate the value of rigorous sampling. An alternative is convenience sampling, using informed judgement and best efforts to maximize representativeness in selecting sites to conduct surveillance.

◆ *Predictive value*: ideally, cases or reports represented in surveillance, indeed people with the disease or condition of interest, i.e. the data have a high positive predictive value. Predictive value is likely to be affected by the criteria used to define reporting requirements, resources available to make accurate diagnoses, the level of expertise and training of surveillance staff, or the nature of surveillance information resources. When diagnostic capacities are limited, surveillance often depends on syndromic criteria defined on the basis of symptoms or disease manifestations. Having the ability to conduct validations of syndromic diagnoses, at least in a sample of instances, can help to refine syndromic criteria or understand their limitations. The term 'predictive value' can also be used to characterize statistical alerts that disease trends have exceeded a predefined threshold indicating a possible disease outbreak. In this context, a high predictive value would mean that a high proportion of such alerts actually indicate the occurrence of outbreaks (CDC 2004).

◆ *Timeliness*: surveillance data need to be 'in time' to be useful, and timeliness depends on the intended use of the information. For example, a surveillance system that is aimed at detecting disease outbreaks as quickly as possible may need to monitor events within hours or a day of their occurrence. For disease where the use of prophylactic medications can prevent illness among contacts of affected people, surveillance must be sufficiently prompt to allow follow-up within the window of time that prophylaxis is likely to be effective. In contrast, for chronic diseases, such as cancer or cardiovascular disease trends, important trends unfold over a period of years, and annual data may be sufficient. Efforts to hasten the surveillance process are likely to come at the expense of other desirable attributes, such as completeness or predictive value. The metric of timeliness can be used to characterize the entire sequence of steps in the 'cycle of surveillance' as well as the promptness with which surveillance can identify aberrant disease trends.

◆ *Acceptability*: surveillance systems typically depend on the goodwill of many to sustain them over the long term. If reporting procedures are cumbersome, if the data are perceived as going into a 'black hole' without demonstrable use or value, if surveys take too long to administer, if information technologies that support surveillance are difficult to use, etc., then the *acceptability* and eventually the quality of surveillance will suffer. Public and political goodwill is also critical to sustaining funding and the necessary legal authorities to conduct surveillance. This requires that surveillance is conducted ethically, that confidentiality is protected, and that intrusions into the privacy of individuals are justified by the larger public good that arises from surveillance. Allowing public access to surveillance data (constrained as needed to protect confidentiality) can broaden the use of surveillance by researchers, students, journalists, community advocates, and others and can enhance public support for surveillance.

◆ *Simplicity*: simplicity is desirable and can affect acceptability at each stage in the surveillance cycle. Like other measures, simplicity is a relative standard. For example, some users will prefer simple and quickly digestible reports that they can read quickly. Others will need to delve into the full complexity of surveillance in order to use it effectively, but simplifying access to the data and essential documentation would be desirable.

◆ *Flexibility*: information needs and the context in which surveillance occurs often changes over time, requiring flexibility to adapt to new circumstances. The epidemiology, diagnosis, or treatment of disease may evolve in ways that require changes in how surveillance is conducted. For example, in the decades following the initiation of AIDS surveillance in 1981 in the United States, the causative agent was identified, the treatment of HIV infection shifted from hospital to outpatient settings, immunological monitoring became part of routine patient care, an increasing proportion of infections among women and injection drug users was associated with changes in the spectrum of common disease manifestations, and the introduction of increasingly effective antiretroviral drugs altered the course of HIV infection. Taken together, these changes required multiple updates to the surveillance definition for AIDS (CDC 2008). In addition, disease coding schemes, such as the International Classification of Diseases, are periodically updated, and surveillance systems must adapt to these changes. Infrastructures established for the surveillance of one disease can be adapted to benefit surveillance of others, as illustrated by efforts to use capacities established for polio and measles surveillance to improve surveillance for meningitis and encephalitis in China, Bangladesh, and India (CDC 2012a).

◆ *Stability*: because most surveillance systems operate over long periods of time, stability in how surveillance is conducted is desirable to increase the likelihood that observed trends reflect the health of the monitored population and not fluctuations in how surveillance is conducted. This attribute can be at odds with flexibility. For example, while the 1993 revision to the surveillance definition for AIDS was necessary to accommodate changes in HIV/AIDS care and epidemiology, implementation of the new definition was associated with an abrupt increase in reported AIDS cases, requiring the use of complex mathematical approaches to discern underlying trends in the epidemic (Neal et al. 1997).

◆ *Interoperablity*: although not one of the attributes considered in the CDC guidelines, interoperability of surveillance systems is becoming increasingly important as the number and automation of surveillance systems increases. If a system differs from others in how comparable information is categorized or coded or if it uses electronic information exchange standards that differ from others, then participants are likely to be frustrated by the extra effort required to accommodate multiple systems and/or to combine information from multiple systems. The term 'interoperability' describes the ability to combine or share information across multiple surveillance systems. As the use of electronic health records and electronic laboratory information systems expands, then consideration of interoperability extends

to the ability of public health surveillance systems to exchange information electronically with these clinical information systems. Similarly, if surveillance systems involve the use of mobile electronic devices to collect, store, or transmit surveillance information, those devices must be sufficiently compatible to allow for the desired exchange of information.

◆ The last attribute is *cost*, which can be measured in fiscal terms or in terms of the effort that is needed to sustain surveillance. Because public health and healthcare resources are limited, cost is often an important determinant of how surveillance is conducted and the need to minimize costs can constrain the ability to maximize other desirable attributes of surveillance.

Public health surveillance in under-resourced countries: special considerations

General principles that underlie the practice of surveillance are essentially the same for all countries. These include the steps of system design and the principle of collecting and using information for action. Of interest, the revised international health regulations, which were adopted by the WHO in May 2005 and came into force in June 2007, provide a powerful mandate to strengthen surveillance systems globally (Baker and Fidler 2006). However, information and other surveillance resources vary widely among countries.

Tracking disease trends, particularly infectious diseases, has been the main reason surveillance systems have been initiated in under-resourced countries. Surveillance data are also needed to establish rational public health priorities and to evaluate the impact of large-scale prevention and treatment programmes, such as those established for malaria, tuberculosis, and HIV/AIDS. Many infectious diseases and other conditions of public health import occur in settings with only rudimentary healthcare and few laboratory resources. With large-scale treatment programmes underway, the need for an adequate laboratory infrastructure has become even more critical, in large part to assure that the treatment is appropriate, that diagnoses are accurate, that microbes are not becoming resistant to therapies, or that viral or bacterial strains represented in vaccines are not being replaced by other strains. Lack of definitive diagnoses may hinder surveillance and response efforts as well as resulting in inappropriate therapy and adverse consequences, such as increases in drug resistance.

The success of surveillance depends on having sufficient resources, the simplicity of reporting procedures, personal rapport among people in the network, regular feedback, and the visibility of actions taken in response to case reports or analyses of surveillance data. For example, programmes to eradicate polio make extensive use of surveillance to monitor progress and focus efforts towards reaching their goals. A major accomplishment of the polio eradication programme has been to develop an integrated global virological surveillance network to track the genetic profile and transmission patterns of circulating polio viruses (Pallansch and Sandhu 2006). Eradication programmes must rely on such highly targeted surveillance, which becomes more important (and expensive) as eradication of the target disease approaches.

In many under-resourced countries, the absence of an effective vital event registration systems for births and deaths shapes how surveillance is conducted. Use of the verbal autopsy, based on interviews to determine the cause of death, may assist in following mortality patterns in places without routine death registration (Kumar et al. 2006). The sensitivity of this approach in classifying causes of death may be lower for acute febrile conditions such as malaria, than for maternal deaths, injuries, tuberculosis, and AIDS. In addition, different techniques in conducting verbal autopsies may result in different sensitivities of classifications for specific conditions (Setel et al. 2006). A potentially simple and rapid alternative to such mortality surveillance is to monitor severe morbidity through periodic surveys of hospitals for the number of admissions attributed to particular conditions. Again, the success of such surveys is largely dependent on the accuracy of diagnoses.

Other sources of health information may include UNICEF, WHO, international conferences, non-governmental organizations, and population laboratories (e.g. the International Centre for Diarrhoeal Disease Research, Bangladesh). Although some health problems are similar in many under-resourced settings, relying on data from other countries or districts can often create major problems when there are large geographical differences in the incidence of specific conditions.

The design of surveillance systems must consider the security and safety of surveillance staff, geography and accessibility, population dispersion and mobility, type of health system, and literacy. Problems (more common but not unique to under-resourced countries) may include limited personnel available for public health, coincident operation of multiple surveillance systems within a target population, lack of laboratory capacity, and infrastructure and communications constraints (e.g. lack of equipment, supplies, or electrical power).

Solutions to address the lack of personnel for public health and prevention have included voluntary systems (using community health workers, traditional birth attendants, or village volunteers). More familiar solutions are public health training programmes designed to meet human resource gaps. Concerns about the cost-effectiveness of short-term training have resulted in establishing long-term programmes to build capacity within countries. Applied field epidemiology training programmes have been applauded for boosting the number of trained personnel (Cardenas et al. 2002).

Concurrently, the increase in availability of computers to analyse and transmit surveillance data and the decrease in the cost of such technology offer increased opportunities for surveillance. Epi Info™ is a freely available computer program designed to assist public health data management and analysis (CDC 2013a); this tool has been used successfully in both well-resourced and under-resourced countries, and is available in multiple languages. Epi Info™ and other information systems should be seen as tools to be used to provide data to policymakers and others to inform decisions that will improve health. The use of mobile phones and hand-held devices is proving useful in many areas. By leveraging the availability of mobile telephone networks and international telecommunication systems, few additional resources are needed to provide for collection of information and for two-way exchange of information needed for response.

Target population

The population under surveillance may be defined on the basis of where people live, work, attend school, consume water or food, or use healthcare services. Alternatively, the population may be defined on the basis of where health events occur. For example, surveillance of traffic injuries aimed at identifying roadway hazards could include all injuries that occur in a target community, regardless of whether affected people live in that community.

In some cases, target populations for public health surveillance may be animals. For example, animal surveillance systems for West Nile virus and avian influenza have been developed, recognizing that these pathogens of concern to human health also infect animals and may alert public health authorities of potential transmission to humans.

Constituents of surveillance systems

Surveillance systems are likely to have many constituents, including healthcare providers, public health professionals, researchers at academic health centres, politicians, the media, the public, and others with diverse perspectives and uses for surveillance data. Because these diverse needs cannot always be satisfied, the primary or most important constituents should be identified as the system is established.

Nature of public health programmes

The objectives of surveillance systems will be shaped by the public health programmes they serve. For example, a programme to eradicate an infectious disease requires intensive surveillance in the later stages of the campaign that emphasizes identification of all people with the disease (Hinman and Hopkins 1998). In contrast, an educational programme to influence health-related behaviours may depend on a surveillance system that describes the practices of a sample of people in a community.

Health problems under surveillance

It is necessary to decide exactly what disease or health problem will be under surveillance. Surveillance may frequently be conducted for any of several points along a spectrum, ranging from exposure to an adverse outcome. It is important to consider which manifestations or stages of a disease should be under surveillance. For example, manifestations of ischaemic heart disease include angina pectoris, acute myocardial infarction, and (sudden) death, and precursors may include hypertension or behavioural risk factors such as tobacco use, unhealthy dietary habits, or lack of exercise.

Case definition

The case definition is fundamental to any surveillance system because it is the formal declaration of what is to be monitored. The case definition is primarily a criterion for determining who or what is to be counted but can also serve other objectives, such as providing a guide to clinicians for diagnoses. Where feasible, consistent use of case definitions across geographical areas permits comparison of disease rates. The case definition should be sufficiently inclusive (sensitive) to identify people who require public health attention or to monitor trends reliably but sufficiently exclusive (specific) for surveillance to have adequate predictive value.

Case definitions must be crafted so that they can be applied in a given surveillance context, reflecting the level of expertise of those who report and collect surveillance data and the extent of information that is likely to be available. Surveillance case definitions may also be layered to include those with possible, suspected, presumptive, or confirmed diagnoses, depending on the urgency of need to respond to certain diseases before diagnoses are definitively established. For infectious diseases, confirmation of the diagnosis typically requires a positive laboratory test. But, if laboratory testing is not routinely available, syndromic criteria might be sufficient to guide treatments and to monitor disease trends. For example, in the United States, surveillance criteria for sexually transmitted diseases such as gonorrhoea or syphilis, incorporate both clinical and laboratory criteria (CDC 2011a), reflecting the routine availability of diagnostic testing. However, in many countries, routine access to such tests is not available, and syndrome-based criteria have been developed to treat and monitor conditions such as urethritis or cervical infection, based on prior assessments that included laboratory testing and informed presumptions regarding likely diagnoses and effective treatments (WHO 2003).

A similar range of possible case definitions also exists for surveillance systems that focus on adverse health exposures or risk behaviours. Body mass index (BMI), calculated using a person's weight and height, is commonly used in surveillance systems that track trends in the proportion of people who are obese or overweight. The use of self-reported height and weight, as in telephone surveys, or measured height and weight, which requires staff and equipment to perform the measurements, will affect the cost, coverage, and other attributes of surveillance in varying ways. BMI itself is a proxy measure for more direct measures of body fat that require weighing people underwater or sophisticated whole-body x-ray scans—measures that are unlikely to be feasible for surveillance purposes (CDC 2011b).

The flow of information

Surveillance may rely on data acquired explicitly for surveillance purposes or on secondary uses of data obtained from existing information sources. Regardless, there is a flow of information throughout the surveillance process, which should be planned.

Reporters

For surveillance systems that depend on reporting individual cases of disease or tabulations of disease counts, people responsible for reporting may be all or selected healthcare providers in a defined area, including laboratories. Reporters may also be asked to collect specimens needed by public health agencies for laboratory confirmation or characterization of specific diseases or exposures.

Data collection instruments

The desire to collect detailed information must be tempered by the need to limit data collection to information that can be reliably and consistently collected and used over the long term. Forms, questionnaires, or other data collection instruments that are too extensive will not be welcomed by those on whom the surveillance system must depend. While computerized systems may permit more detailed data collection, collecting large volumes of data may exceed the capacity of public health agencies to make effective use of those data. Standards for exchanging electronic health information are critical as healthcare information systems and public health surveillance systems become increasingly automated. In the United States, the Health Information Technology for Economic and Clinical Health (HITECH) Act in 2009 provides incentives for healthcare providers to adopt electronic health records and requires that doctors and hospitals use their electronic health record systems to report quality-of-care measures to government-sponsored healthcare insurance programmes for the elderly and poor and immunization service and certain disease data to state and local public health programmes, using national information standards (HealthIT.gov 2013).

Timing

Surveillance systems collect and provide data on a regular basis, ranging from daily to annually or, in some instances, every few years when surveillance depends on information from surveys that are conducted intermittently. This periodicity should be specified. For surveillance of a given disease or condition, acceptable intervals between the occurrence of events of interest and the eventual availability of reports from surveillance systems will depend on the nature of the targeted condition and how data are needed and used to inform public health actions.

Aggregation of data

Surveillance data may be in the form of individual patient records or aggregate counts and tabulations. In some instances, there may be a need at the local level to maintain records on individual people to direct follow-up services but for regional or national reports to be in the form of aggregate counts. Individual-level data permit more flexibility of analysis than aggregate data. This can be useful when routine analyses raise questions that require more detailed analyses.

Data transmission

The mode of data transmission will depend on both the need for timeliness and availability of resources. While reliance on postage of paper forms or facsimile transmission continues, there is growing use of telecommunications and the Internet to transmit surveillance information. In places where Internet access remains limited, the use of handheld mobile devices and mobile telephones for data collection and transmission is growing. In 2012, the World Bank estimated that three-quarters of the world's population have access to a mobile telephone, providing a relatively inexpensive and widely available technology to improve access to health information and public health surveillance (World Bank 2012).

Data management

Critical to the ongoing nature of surveillance is the management of surveillance data, including the maintenance of historical data and procedures for incorporating new information into surveillance databases. In particular, the following should be considered as part of data management procedures.

Updating records

Surveillance data often need to be updated. Information that was initially missing may become available; follow-up investigations may yield supplemental information; people initially classified as meeting or not meeting a case definition may be reclassified; errors may be identified and corrected; and duplicate case reports may be recognized and culled. One approach to handling these and other changes is to maintain both provisional and final records.

Selecting measures for time and place

A case report may include dates, such as those of the onset of disease, diagnosis, report to local health authorities, or report to regional or national health authorities. Analyses of surveillance data may be based on the date of any of these events. However, if there are long delays between dates of diagnosis and report, analyses of trends based on date of diagnosis will be unreliable for the most recent periods. Similarly, surveillance data may be tabulated on the basis of the site of occurrence of the health event (e.g. the place of exposure, disease onset, or injury), the place of diagnosis, or place of residence. Classification of case events by place of residence of affected people allows for calculation of disease rates using census data.

Confidentiality/privacy

Because public health surveillance involves the collection and maintenance of information about the health of individuals, it represents a certain degree of government intrusion into personal health matters. This intrusion is minimized when data are collected anonymously or as aggregate counts and increased when data collection includes the names or other identifying information or when follow-up investigations are conducted that involve contacting affected people or reviewing medical records. In surveillance practice, the term 'privacy' describes expectations that others are not looking into our health status, and 'confidentiality' refers to the use and protection of health information held by public health agencies. The laws that authorize public health agencies to intrude on individual privacy for the benefit of both individuals and the larger community generally determine what information they are allowed to collect as well as requirements for protecting the confidentiality of public health records.

Preventing inappropriate disclosure of surveillance data is essential both to protect the privacy of people with reported cases of disease and to the trust of participants in the surveillance system. The protection of confidentiality begins with limiting collection of identifying information and transmission to a necessary minimum and includes ensuring the physical security of surveillance records, the discretion of surveillance staff, and legal safeguards. Uses of surveillance data should arise from a broad consensus of stakeholders in clinical medicine, public health, and the community (Fairchild et al. 2007).

Physical protection of records is accomplished by rules of conduct for people involved in the design, development, operation, or maintenance of any surveillance system. For automated surveillance systems, technical requirements for protecting data security should be part of information standards.

Users of data containing identifiers of individuals or establishments should be held to the minimum number deemed essential to perform public health functions. Those entrusted to use these data must be trained and accept responsibility to protect against inappropriate release. When surveillance data are reported, categories, such as those for age or place of residence, should be sufficiently broad to avoid inadvertent identification of an individual person or institution. The principle of making data as widely available as possible needs to be balanced with the protection of confidentiality. This can involve the development of public-access databases in which steps are taken to de-identify individual records. Even when efforts are made to de-identify records, data-use agreements may be necessary to prohibit efforts to re-identify data, which is increasingly possible using sophisticated analytic tools (Brownstein et al. 2006)

Initiating and maintaining participation

Whether required by law, voluntary, or (rarely) financially rewarded, reporting to or sharing information with public health takes time and effort. Even with automated electronic reporting, efforts are needed to install, validate, maintain, and periodically update the requisite information technologies. Minimizing the time and simplifying procedures for reporting is likely to increase adherence to reporting procedures. Dissemination of reports that demonstrate the usefulness of surveillance is likely to be a key to initiating and maintaining participation.

Public health laws provide the authority to conduct surveillance, and legal mandates that require that certain diseases or conditions be reported are an important approach to initiate and maintain reporting. In general, public health agencies have been reluctant to enforce these laws through penalties or fines because of concerns that such an approach would alienate healthcare providers—whose collaboration and partnership is essential not just for surveillance but for many public health interventions as well.

Organizational structure

Surveillance systems require an organizational structure that defines the roles and responsibilities of participants in all stages of the surveillance cycle, including participants at different levels of government (local, state, regional, national, or international). This includes articulation of procedures for alerting those responsible for prevention and control activities when surveillance data identify situations that merit further attention, such as an upturn in observed disease incidence that might herald the onset of an outbreak.

Types of surveillance systems and data

Historically, information sources for surveillance have fallen into two broad categories: information that arises from the use of healthcare service and population surveys. A third source is largely developmental: unstructured data that is culled from the Internet or other large electronic data repositories or from direct public participation in Internet-based social networks.

Surveillance might involve a mix of complementary sources that provide information on different facets of a disease. For example, influenza surveillance is often multifaceted and includes measures of morbidity (e.g. office or hospital emergency department visits for 'influenza-like illness' or hospitalizations among people with laboratory-confirmed influenza), mortality (e.g. deaths attributed to 'pneumonia and influenza'), and laboratory-based indicators (e.g. viral isolates from participating laboratories where virus type, alignment with vaccine strains, or sensitivity to antiviral medications can be tested) (CDC 2012b).

Healthcare-based surveillance

Notification systems

Notifiable disease reporting is the approach traditionally used by public health programmes, based on laws or regulations that require reporting of selected diseases or conditions to public health departments. People or institutions responsible for reporting often include doctors, other healthcare providers, coroners and medical examiners, laboratories, clinics, and hospitals. With the emergence of large, often commercial, laboratories that serve multiple providers across relatively large geographic areas, public health agencies are increasingly emphasizing laboratory-based reporting. This approach increases the timeliness and completeness of case reporting for diseases that require a laboratory test to diagnose. Because clinical information that accompanies specimens submitted to laboratories is often limited, however, follow-up with the providers who order laboratory tests or with patients themselves is often needed to complete case reporting (Ackers et al. 2000).

The overall completeness of notifiable disease surveillance depends on a succession of events: affected people must be sufficiently ill to seek healthcare, diagnostic tests are performed (which might not occur if patients are treated empirically), and positive results are reported. This approach may be relatively passive, meaning that public health staff do not reach out to healthcare providers to encourage reporting, or more active, meaning that public health staff may contact or visit providers to prompt reporting or assist in the reporting process. In general, more active approaches to surveillance will result in more complete and timely reporting. For example, in the late 1970s, a relatively large shigellosis outbreak in Washington, District of Columbia, United States, was not recognized by the health department's surveillance system because fewer than a third of outbreak-associated cases had been reported as required. A review of the surveillance system found that surveillance was not only incomplete but also not representative because reporting varied considerably among different facilities. In hindsight, adherence to reporting requirements lagged because the health department had taken a very passive approach and had done little to inform and remind local healthcare providers of their reporting requirements (Kimball et al. 1980).

Completeness of reporting may be affected for multiple other reasons: if patients and doctors seek to conceal the occurrence of diseases that carry a social stigma, if healthcare providers are unaware of regulations, or if interest in particular diseases is limited. Even if reporting is incomplete, temporal trends and geographic patterns can be determined as long as the proportion of cases detected remains consistent over time and across geographical areas. Conversely, lack of representativeness and heterogeneity of reporting further limit the usefulness of incomplete data (Lowndes et al. 2004).

Example: notifiable disease surveillance in China

The China Infectious Disease Automated-alert and Response System (CIDARS) is an extension of the nationwide electronic system for notifiable disease reporting that was initiated in 2004 following the severe acute respiratory system (SARS) outbreak. The system focuses on 39 infectious diseases or syndromes that clinicians are required to report to the Ministry of Health. CIDARS added a formal process for analysis and follow-up that specified statistical thresholds for prompting alerts, based on the number of cases relative to historical precedents or temporal–spatial clustering; procedures for notifying responsible local officials via mobile telephone when those thresholds were exceeded within a locality; responsibility for preliminary assessments and, if indicated, more definitive field investigations; and responsibility for documenting and reporting the results of those assessments and investigations.

In an initial evaluation of CIDARS conducted in a sample of ten provinces, for nine relatively rare but potentially severe infections, 308 alerts were identified during a 2-year period in 2008–2010, of which 69 (22 per cent) merited a field investigation, leading to detection of nine cholera outbreaks. For other more common but less severe diseases, there were more than 100,000 statistical alerts, of which 1.4 per cent were deemed to merit further attention, leading to detection of 167 disease outbreaks (Yan et al. 2012).

Healthcare provider networks

Networks of healthcare providers have been organized for several decades, primarily to gather information on selected health events. Most have been organized by practising doctors on a voluntary basis; in many European countries, these networks have formed firm relationships with both public health authorities and academic centres. The strengths of sentinel provider systems include the commitment of the participants, the possibility of collecting longitudinal data, the flexibility to address a changing set of conditions, and the potential to conduct focused studies of the incidence, prevalence, care, or outcomes of various conditions, typically in primary care settings (Fleming et al. 2003). The main limitation of this type of system is that the population served by participating doctors may not be representative of the population.

Laboratory surveillance

Laboratory surveillance may be conducted as part of a notifiable diseases system, sentinel surveillance system, or other system. In addition to supporting routine case reporting, laboratory-based surveillance can allow for the use of molecular epidemiological tools, more detailed evaluation of microbe strains or types, and monitoring of drug sensitivity. The use of molecular tools to enhance surveillance of pathogens is growing in many countries to facilitate outbreak detection, especially in situations where disease is associated with widely distributed food products, where the number of cases of illness due to a particular infection is insufficient to prompt attention, but where epidemiological linkage of geographically disparate cases allows detection of distinctive outbreak-associated pathogen strains. In the United States, PulseNet is a network of public health laboratories that performs DNA 'fingerprinting' on bacteria that may be foodborne (Swaminathan et al. 2001). The network permits rapid comparison of these 'fingerprint' patterns through an electronic database and has detected multiple outbreaks that likely would have been otherwise unrecognized. For example, in 2008–2009, PulseNet detected and enabled tracking of an outbreak of salmonellosis associated with contaminated peanut butter with over 500 cases of illness detected in 43 states (CDC 2009). Molecular methods are also increasingly applied in surveillance of the HIV epidemic. For example, surveillance systems in Canada (Jayaraman et al. 2006) routinely characterize newly diagnosed HIV infections with respect to the HIV subtype.

Disease registries

Registries are comprehensive longitudinal listings of people with particular conditions. They often include detailed information about diagnostic classification, treatment, and outcome. Registries were initially established primarily for epidemiological research on individual diseases or conditions to develop aetiological hypotheses and to identify cases for further research (Weddell 1973). Registries have also been used to ensure the provision of appropriate care and to evaluate changing patterns of medical care; unlike other disease information systems, they cut across the different levels of severity of illness and may provide information over time about individual people. Registries can also be valuable for monitoring disease incidence and distribution.

To focus on selected diseases or conditions, registries often develop a constituency that promotes participation and reporting. Most registries rely on numerous sources of data for case detection including, but not limited to, hospitals, laboratories, and death records; few registries rely primarily on doctor notification.

Example: birth defects

Surveillance for birth defects was first initiated in response to the thalidomide tragedy in the late 1950s and early 1960s; registries were established to provide reliable baseline rates for specific birth defects and to detect increases in the prevalence of birth defects as a means to identifying human teratogens. The CDC has conducted birth defects surveillance in metropolitan Atlanta, Georgia, United States, since 1967 by using multiple sources of ascertainment of all serious birth defects observed in stillborn and liveborn infants and recognized by signs and symptoms apparent in the first year of life (Correa-Villasenor et al. 2003).

The International Clearinghouse for Birth Defects Surveillance and Research consists of 40 registries globally (Botto et al. 2006). The International Clearinghouse conducts a spectrum of surveillance activities that includes monitoring of selected conditions, and the exchange of information about birth defects clusters under investigation, findings of unpublished studies, and rumours about the occurrence of birth defects. Clearinghouse participants work at the intersection of surveillance and research in their assessment of the potential teratogenicity of first-trimester use of medications.

Healthcare information systems

Surveillance systems often depend on existing health data collection systems; these systems may be either integral to surveillance or serve as an adjunct to surveillance for specific diseases or conditions. Examples include use of hospital discharge databases and insurance claims data. Because these databases are often established for monitoring the use of healthcare services or to support billing or payment for healthcare, they allow not only for the assessment of the prevalence of multiple diseases but also for assessment of their impact on healthcare use and costs. For example, as part of a multifaceted approach to diabetes surveillance, the CDC uses data from a national hospital discharge database to track lower extremity amputations among people with diabetes—a severe complication arising from long-term inadequate management of diabetes (CDC 2012c).

The advantage of this approach is that it involves use of information systems that have been previously established for other purposes and can be tapped for surveillance applications for relatively little additional expense. In addition, these information systems often represent very large numbers of people. The main limitation is that diagnoses may be inaccurately or variably recorded or coded. For example, workers' compensation claims have been useful for surveillance of occupational injuries and illnesses in specific geographical locales. However, because regulations governing reporting of such events differ among jurisdictions, data

derived from these systems in different locations cannot easily be compared and the incidence or prevalence of various conditions is likely to be underestimated (Fan et al. 2006).

In areas where a growing number of healthcare providers are using electronic health records, local or regional organizations are being developed to foster automated exchange of information from patients' medical records. The primary aim of these efforts is to facilitate providers' access to information about their patients, including information stored in other providers' record systems. Ideally, this can lead to improved efficiency of health care by reducing the time needed for retrieving patients' information from other providers, reduce medical errors, and reduce redundant use of diagnostic tests. From the public health perspective, these 'health information exchanges' provide a focal point for obtaining surveillance information within communities and for providing feedback to clinicians (Public Health Informatics Institute 2005).

A variation on the use of health information systems is the creation of 'distributed' networks of healthcare providers or insurers who maintain electronic healthcare or billing records. In these systems, participating institutions or organizations agree to extract and maintain selected data on an ongoing basis. Rather than share these data in a centralized repository, participating institutions agree to analyse their data and share the results using standardized queries. Examples include the Vaccine Safety DataLink system coordinated by the CDC to monitor and assess potential adverse reactions to vaccines and the Sentinel network supported by the US Food and Drug Administration to characterize adverse reactions to medications. Because these systems comprise very large numbers of patients, they can be used to track relatively rare events (DeStefano 2001; Behrman et al. 2011).

Vital statistics

In countries with well-established vital event registration systems, monitoring trends for various causes of death is a long-standing part of surveillance for life-threatening conditions. Despite the well-recognized limitations in how causes of death are classified on death certificates, monitoring cause-specific mortality trends overall and by age, gender, and geographic location provides a useful, broad-brush picture of the impact and trends for multiple conditions.

There is frequently a lengthy interval between death and collection and analysis of death certificates, which may make such vital statistics less useful for surveillance purposes when more current data are needed. However, summary vital data can be rapidly collected. For example, weekly reporting of deaths from 122 cities to the CDC has been integral to the surveillance of influenza epidemics in the United States (Fig. 5.19.1), providing an indication of the timing and severity of annual seasonal influenza relative to historical norms (Choi and Thacker 1981; CDC 2009).

Medical examiner and coroner reports

For more detailed descriptions of the circumstances surrounding deaths (including autopsy reports, toxicology studies, and police reports), medical examiner and coroner records may be useful. These reports are typically representative of unexpected or medically unattended deaths or deaths caused by intentional and unintentional injuries and have been used for surveillance of such conditions as heatwave-related mortality and alcohol-related

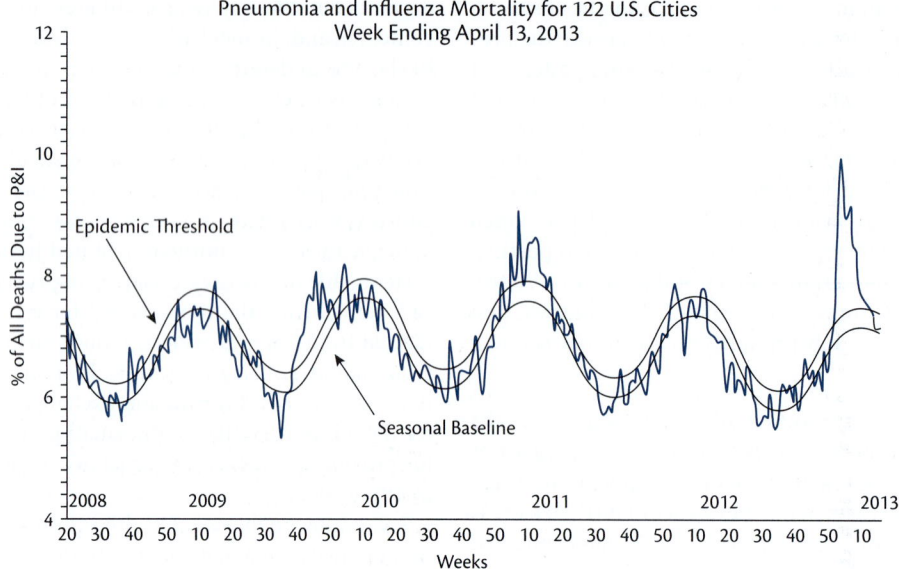

Fig. 5.19.1 Percentage of deaths attributed to pneumonia and influenza (P&I) reported by the 122 Cities Mortality Reporting System, by week and year—United States, 2008–2013.

Reproduced from *FluView, 2013–2014 Influenza Season Week 3 ending January 18, 2014*, Pneumonia and Influenza (P&I) Mortality Surveillance, available from http://www.cdc.gov/flu/weekly/#S2.

injuries. Systematic necropsy examinations have also been useful in ascertaining the contribution of tuberculosis to mortality of HIV-infected individuals in West Africa. Antibody determinations performed on postmortem medical examiner samples may be useful for estimating population prevalence of infectious diseases (e.g. dengue) (Rigau-Perez et al. 2006).

Syndromic surveillance

A growing number of public health agencies have been prompted by concerns about the threat of bioterrorism to invest in automated 'syndromic surveillance' to detect epidemics more quickly than possible using traditional approaches (CDC 2004; Mandl et al. 2004). This involves monitoring trends in healthcare use for relatively non-specific syndromes (e.g. febrile respiratory illness or gastrointestinal symptoms) or other manifestations of illness (e.g. medication purchases, work or school absenteeism) that may be apparent and can be monitored before diagnoses are established. Because these systems emphasize timeliness of the entire surveillance process, often enabling tracking of events within a day or less of their occurrence, they generally rely on data from electronic health information systems. These systems use automated methods to harvest electronically stored data, apply statistical tools to detect aberrant trends, and develop visual displays of geospatial disease trends. Despite this emphasis on automation, these systems still require human judgement to interpret reports and determine what level of further assessment or response is warranted when statistical alerts are generated.

Population health surveys

Behavioural data can be collected from samples of the population at large, from populations at particular risk for the health condition of interest, and from populations affected by the health condition of interest (Davy 2006). When conducted in person, objective

measures of health can also be obtained, such as measurements of height, weight, blood pressure, or collection of specimens for laboratory testing. Population-wide household surveys, such as the National Health Interview Survey in the United States (CDC 2013b) or the General Household Survey in England and Wales (Twigg 1999), have provided information on personal health practices such as alcohol use and smoking, disabilities, and doctor encounters.

In countries where most residents have telephones, telephone interviews have the advantage of lower cost per interview, allowing for wider geographic coverage and more local estimation of the prevalence of various health indicators. For example, in the United States, all states conduct the Behavioral Risk Factor Surveillance System (BRFSS) to monitor a spectrum of health-related behaviours at the state, and in many instances local level. The BRFSS, like all telephone-based surveys, has had to adapt to the declining use of landline telephones and the increasing use of mobile telephones, trends that have varied among demographic groups within the population (CDC 2013c).

Inclusion of behavioural measures has been advocated by the WHO for HIV and sexually transmitted infection surveillance programmes. Increasingly, demographic and health surveys are conducted to include both behavioural and biological measures, and to use sampling methods that provide representative data on a population level (Kenya Central Bureau of Statistics et al. 2004).

Surveys of populations at special risk may also play an important role in guiding public health response. Such systems may be relatively simple, in the form of episodic surveys of convenience samples (e.g. episodic convenience samples of men who have sex with men attending gay bars in Scotland) (Williamson et al. 2006) or may be formalized as ongoing surveillance systems. Such surveys can provide data on levels of risk behaviours, on adoption of desired preventive behaviours, and on exposure to public health prevention messages.

Unstructured data

Internet-based approaches to surveillance

The widespread use of the Internet and electronic media has led to innovations in population health monitoring that reach far beyond traditional surveillance methods. In 1994, the International Society for Infectious Diseases launched the Program for Monitoring Emerging Diseases (ProMed), which allowed individuals to post reports and updates on disease events on a public-access Internet site, with a moderator assuring the professionalism of the website. Information posted on ProMed includes alerts, reports of epidemics, and local observer reports, with over 30,000 subscribers worldwide (Madoff and Woodall 2005). For example, the earliest public notice of the outbreak later known as SARS was in the form of a query posted on ProMed in early 2003 by a physician who learned from an acquaintance of widespread severe respiratory illness in Guangzhou, China. This report and other updates to ProMed alerted the global public health community to this epidemic and played a key role in charting its course of spread to multiple countries (Yu and Madoff 2004).

The Global Public Health Intelligence Network (GPHIN) is managed by the Public Health Agency of Canada and is geared to providing early warning for potential threats to public health worldwide. GPHIN uses an ongoing, automated process to monitor online media reports in six languages worldwide for early indicators of events such as disease outbreaks, natural disasters, food or water contamination, potential biological or chemical terrorism, and other threats. GHIN operates 24 hours a day, 7 days a week in 'near real time.' Access to GPHIN is limited to agencies determined to have a legitimate public health mandate, as determined by the WHO and Health Canada (Public Health Agency of Canada, 2013). The Google.org Flu Trends monitors trends in Internet searches using terms that have been observed to correlate with influenza activity. While this approach yields trends that parallel other indicators of influenza-like illness, its public health application is yet to be determined (Valdivia et al. 2010).

The growing use of the Internet, including use of mobile phones that provide mobile Internet access, is enabling a form of public 'participatory epidemiology' or 'crowd sourcing' where interested members of the public or members of online communities interested in specific health problems are encouraged to post reports of illness or disease outbreaks. The application of such utilities and services is an area of ongoing development and evaluation (Freifeld et al. 2010).

Analysis of surveillance data

Uses of surveillance data begin with descriptive analyses according to the basic epidemiological parameters of time, place, and person, including the use of standard tests for statistical significance. Typically, public health surveillance data are completed, summarized, and reported over specified time intervals (days, weeks, months, or years) and for specific geopolitical jurisdictions (cities, counties, states, provinces, nations, etc.). Incidence or prevalence rates can be calculated using various population denominators, typically census data, and comparisons of rates over time or across geographic areas should be adjusted using standard methods to account for differences in population characteristics, such as differences in the age distribution of populations. The use of maps or graphics is common to illuminate differences in disease incidence or prevalence by time, place, or personal characteristics such as age or gender.

Analyses of trends are generally designed to determine whether current or recent levels of disease differ from levels that would be expected based on historical precedent, which may be defined over a period of years to days, depending on the availability of historical data and the epidemiology of different diseases or conditions. Detection of epidemics or evaluation of suspected epidemics is a key function of surveillance. Nonetheless, many epidemics are first recognized by astute healthcare providers who observe an increase in disease occurrence, instead of being detected by surveillance systems, because the cycle of surveillance has not had time to detect an upturn. Even in such instances, however, surveillance can be useful to help assess whether recently observed cases of disease exceed expected levels. Surveillance is most likely to provide the initial recognition of potential epidemics in situations where cases are occurring over a sufficiently large geographic area or time period so that the increase would not be apparent to individual practitioners.

The key to discerning whether observed trends are in excess of expected trends is excluding the possibility of random variations or 'noise' in observed disease levels. One approach to resolving this dilemma is to employ various techniques to 'smooth' the data, especially for graphic displays of temporal trends (Devine and Parrish 1998), including the use of moving averages or the aggregation of data points into longer but still relevant time intervals (e.g. by week instead of by day or by month instead of by week). A spectrum of advanced analytic techniques for evaluating trends in surveillance data has evolved to model various types of historical trends, such as seasonal variations or long-term secular trends, to estimate predicted or expected levels of disease based on those trends, and to determine whether observed levels are statistically different from expected levels (Brookmeyer and Stroup 2003). The use of geographic information systems extends the traditional use of maps to display surveillance data by allowing for analyses that allow geospatial assessment of disease and locations of risk exposures or preventive or therapeutic services (Waller and Gotway 2004). Recognition of clusters of disease is common but often difficult to distinguish from random variation, giving rise to various statistical techniques to detect and characterize clusters (Kulldorff 1997). The increasing automation of the surveillance process, especially for systems of syndromic surveillance that track daily trends in disease and seek to detect changes in disease trends quickly, has spawned the development of statistical methods and computer software algorithms for automatic trend aberration detection, including techniques that are derived from cluster detection and industrial quality control methods (Burkom 2007).

Regardless of whether analyses involve straightforward descriptive statistics or advance modelling techniques, any analyses of surveillance data must take into account potential limitations of the data, including variations in their completeness, representativeness, timeliness, or data quality over time or among different locations.

Linkage of surveillance data to other information sources

Given the complexity of establishing new data and information systems, there is increasing interest in the combination of existing databases for surveillance purposes. This allows the combination of information about individual case-patients from multiple sources. For example, linkage of birth certificates (which include the birth weight and information on other infant or maternal characteristics) and death certificates (which include information on the age and cause of death) allows determination of neonatal or postneonatal deaths rates for infants in different birth-weight or gestational age groups (Buehler et al. 2000). Linkage of HIV and tuberculosis records enables surveillance for the co-occurrence of these two infections (Ahmed et al. 2007).

Techniques involved in data linkage are based on comparing records from different information systems, assessing the likelihood that records from two different sources represent the same individual, and combining the data for those individuals whose records match (Clark 2004). In using linked record systems, assessments should be done to determine what proportion of linked records do not actually represent the same individual and, conversely, what proportion of records should have been but were not correctly linked.

Dissemination of surveillance information

Communication of surveillance data is an essential step in the surveillance chain. Appropriate feedback must be given to those providing the data, such as analyses that allow them to compare their experience to that of the community at large and other reports that enable them to see the value of the information resource to which they contributed. When appropriate, people or institutions providing the data should be credited for their contributions and acknowledged. Public health professionals, policymakers, or others who may be responsible for taking action or setting the direction of public health programmes in response to surveillance data must receive the information that they need from the surveillance system on a timely basis and in an appropriate format for their use. In addition, these data should be available as widely as possible to all who may be interested in analysis and interpretation of these data. Websites are increasingly used to disseminate surveillance data as with the US CDC's *Morbidity and Mortality Weekly Report* (http://www.cdc.gov/MMWR), the WHO's *Weekly Epidemiological Record* (http://www.who.int/wer), and the European *Eurosurveillance* (http://www.eurosurveillance. org/).

The data must be provided on a regular basis, with the frequency of surveillance reports commensurate with the nature of the surveillance system, the characteristics of the disease under surveillance, and information needs. To improve the timeliness of surveillance data, provisional or preliminary data may be released, with appropriate caveats, in advance of completion of more definitive reports.

The format for dissemination varies with the target audience; a creative design will help to make the information stand apart from other documents and receive greater attention. Most policymakers and clinicians would prefer to see the data interpreted using graphics that provide a quick visual image that highlights key observations, accompanied by an abbreviated summary text. The important role that graphs and maps can play in visually decoding large quantities of data has been clearly demonstrated, with graphic displays giving the reader an understanding of large and complex datasets not conveyed easily in other ways (Tukey

1977; Tufte 1983). In contrast, many epidemiologists and other scientists will find access to more detailed data to be most useful.

Evaluation of surveillance systems

Surveillance systems should be periodically evaluated to ensure that important public health problems are under surveillance, that the information provided is useful, and that resources dedicated to surveillance are being used wisely. Such evaluations may include a mix of quantitative and qualitative assessments (CDC 2001, 2004; Silk and Berkelman 2005; Buehler et al. 2009). Evaluation may also be considered in a broader strategy of continuous quality assurance (Krause 2006). Reflecting the steps that are taken in establishing a surveillance system, an evaluation of a surveillance system should include a review of its objectives, a detailed description of its operation, an assessment of its performance using the surveillance attributes as a guide, and recommendations.

Conclusion

Public health surveillance has historically galvanized and guided prevention and control programmes for infectious diseases, ranging from smallpox eradication, immunization campaigns to prevent childhood diseases, programmes to prevent HIV infection and AIDS, and responses to emergent diseases such as SARS or pandemic influenza. Surveillance has also taken on increased visibility and importance in evaluating and guiding prevention and control efforts for a broad spectrum of non-infectious diseases and conditions. Surveillance provides a stimulus to keep prevention and control activities moving in the right direction, guiding the response to individual cases as well as public policy.

Effective public health interventions depend upon a continuing and reliable source of information; resources should be allocated for the maintenance of the surveillance systems and for their regular evaluation. The data must be timely and representative of the population; they must be analysed and interpreted with feedback to the reporters and disseminated as widely as possible, including to those formulating and implementing public health policy. Allocation of resources devoted to surveillance for the purpose of informing prevention and control activities must be balanced with resources needed to implement those activities.

Acknowledgements

The authors thank Drs Ruth L. Berkelman, Donna Stroup, and Patrick L. Sullivan for their contributions as authors of previous editions of this chapter.

References

Ackers, M.-L., Puhr, N.D., Tauxe, R.V., and Mintz, E.D. (2000). Laboratory-based surveillance of salmonella serotype typhi infections in the United States: antimicrobial resistance on the rise. *Journal of the American Medical Association*, 283(20), 2668–73.

Ahmed, A.B., Abubakar, I., Delpech, V., et al. (2007). The growing impact of HIV infection on the epidemiology of tuberculosis in England and Wales. *Thorax*, 62, 672–6.

Baker, M.G. and Fidler, D.P. (2006). Global public health surveillance under new international health regulations. *Emerging Infectious Diseases*, 7, 1058–65.

Behrman, R.E., Benner, J.S., Brown, J.S., McClellan, M., Woodcock, J., and Platt, R. (2011). Developing the sentinel system—a national resource for evidence development. *The New England Journal of Medicine*, 364(6), 498–9.

Berkelman, R.L., Bryan, R.T., Osterholm, M.T., et al. (1994). Infectious disease surveillance: a crumbling foundation. *Science*, 264, 368–70.

Botto, L.D., Robert-Gnansia, E., Siffel, C., et al. (2006). Fostering international collaboration in birth defects research and prevention: a perspective from the International Clearinghouse for Birth Defects Surveillance and Research. *American Journal of Public Health*, 96, 774–80.

Brookmeyer, R. and Stroup, D.F. (2003). *Monitoring the Health of Populations: Statistical Principles and Methods for Public Health Surveillance*. Oxford: Oxford University Press.

Brownstein, J.S., Cassa, C.A., and Mandl, K.D. (2006). No place to hide—reverse identification of patients from published maps. *The New England Journal of Medicine*, 355(16), 1741–2.

Buehler, J.W., Prager, K., and Hogue, C.J. (2000). The role of linked birth and infant death certificates in maternal and child health epidemiology in the United States. *American Journal of Preventive Medicine*, 19(Suppl. 1), 3–11.

Buehler, J.W., Whitney, E.A., Smith, D., Prietula, M.J., Stanton, S.H., and Isakov, A.P. (2009). Situational uses of syndromic surveillance. *Biosecurity and Bioterrorism: Biodefense Strategy, Practice, and Science*, 7(2), 165–77.

Burkom, H. (2007). Alerting algorithms for biosurveillance. In J.S. Lombardo and D.L. Buckeridge (eds.) *Disease Surveillance: A Public Health Informatics Approach*, pp. 143–92. Hoboken, NJ: John Wiley & Sons.

Cardenas, V.M., Roces, M.C., Wattanasri, S., et al. (2002). Improving global public health leadership through training in epidemiology and public health: the experience of TEPHINET. Training Programs in Epidemiology and Public Health Interventions Network. *American Journal of Public Health*, 92, 196–7.

Centers for Disease Control and Prevention (2001). Updated guidelines for evaluating public health surveillance systems. *Morbidity and Mortality Weekly Report*, 50, 1–35.

Centers for Disease Control and Prevention (2004). Framework for evaluating public health surveillance systems for early detection of outbreaks. Recommendations from the CDC Working Group. *Morbidity Mortality Weekly Report*, 53(RR05), 1–11.

Centers for Disease Control and Prevention (2008). Revised surveillance case definitions for HIV infection, incorporating the HIV classification system and the AIDS case definition for adults and adolescents, HIV infection among children aged <18 months, and HIV infection and AIDS among children >18 months but <13 years, United States, 2008. *Morbidity and Mortality Weekly Report*, 57(RR10), 1–8.

Centers for Disease Control and Prevention (2009). Multistate outbreak of Salmonella infections associated with peanut butter and peanut butter-containing products—United States, 2008–2009. *Morbidity and Mortality Weekly Report*, 58(4), 85–90.

Centers for Disease Control and Prevention (2011a). *STD Surveillance Case Definition*. Available at: http://www.cdc.gov/std/stats10/app-casedef.htm.

Centers for Disease Control and Prevention (2011b). *About BMI for Adults*. Available at: http://www.cdc.gov/healthyweight/assessing/bmi/adult_bmi/index.html.

Centers for Disease Control and Prevention (2012a). Expanding poliomyelitis and measles surveillance networks to establish surveillance for acute meningitis and encephalitis syndromes—Bangladesh, China, and India, 2006–2008. *Morbidity and Mortality Weekly Report*, 61(49), 1008–11.

Centers for Disease Control and Prevention (2012b). *Overview of Influenza Surveillance in the United States*. Available at: http://www.cdc.gov/flu/weekly/overview.htm.

Centers for Disease Control and Prevention (2012c). *Diabetes Complications*. Available at: http://www.cdc.gov/diabetes/statistics/complications_national.htm.

Centers for Disease Control and Prevention (2013a). *Epi Info™*. Available at: http://wwwn.cdc.gov/epiinfo/.

Centers for Disease Control and Prevention (2013b). *National Health Interview Survey*. Available at: http://www.cdc.gov/NCHS/NHIS.htm.

Centers for Disease Control and Prevention (2013c). *Behavioral Risk Factor Surveillance System*. Available at: http://www.cdc.gov/brfss.

Choi, K. and Thacker, S.B. (1981). An evaluation of influenza mortality surveillance, 1962–1979. I. Time series forecasts of expected pneumonia and influenza deaths. *American Journal of Epidemiology*, 113, 215–26.

Clark, D.E. (2004). Practical introduction to record linkage for injury research. *Injury Prevention*, 10, 186–91.

Correa-Villasenor, A., Cragan, J., Kucik, J., et al. (2003). The Metropolitan Atlanta Congenital Defects Program: 35 years of birth defects surveillance at the Centers for Disease Control and Prevention. *Birth Defects Research. Part A, Clinical and Molecular Teratology*, 67, 617–24.

Cox, N., Brammer, T.L., and Regnery, H. (1994). Influenza: global surveillance for epidemic and pandemic variants. *European Journal of Epidemiology*, 10(4), 467–70.

Davy, M. (2006). Time and generational trends in smoking among men and women in Great Britain, 1972–2004/05. *Health Statistics Quarterly*, 32, 35–43.

DeStefano, F. (2001). The Vaccine Safety Datalink project. *Pharmacoepidemiology and Drug Safety*, 10(5), 403–6.

Devine, O. and Parrish, R.G. (1998). Monitoring the health of a population. In D.S. Stroup and S.M. Teutsch (eds.) *Statistics in Public Health*, pp. 59–91. New York: Oxford University Press.

Fairchild, A.L., Gable, L., Gostin, L.O., et al. (2007). Public goods, private data: HIV and the history, ethics, and uses of identifiable public health information. *Public Health Reports*, 122(Suppl. 1), 7–15.

Fan, Z.Y., Bonauto, D.K., Foley, M.P., et al. (2006). Underreporting of work-related injury or illness to workers' compensation: individual and industry factors. *Journal of Occupational and Environmental Medicine*, 48, 914–22.

Fleming, D.M., Schellevis, F.G., and Paget, W.J. (2003). Health monitoring in sentinel practice networks: the contribution of primary care. *The European Journal of Public Health*, 13(Suppl. 1), 80–4.

Freifeld, C.C., Chunara, R., Mekaru, S.R., et al. (2010). Participatory epidemiology: use of mobile phones for community-based health reporting. *PLoS Medicine*, 7(12), e1000376.

HealthIT.gov (2013). *HITECH Act*. Available at: http://www.healthit.gov/policy-researchers-implementers/hitech-act-0.

Hinman, A.R. and Hopkins, D.R. (1998). Lessons from previous eradication programs. In W.R. Dowdle and D.R. Hopkins (eds.) *The Eradication of Infectious Diseases*, pp. 19–32. New York: Wiley.

Hurd, M.D., Martorell, P., Delavande, A., Mullen, K.J., and Langa, K.M. (2013). Monetary costs of dementia in the United States. *The New England Journal of Medicine*, 368(14), 1326–34.

Jaffe, H.W., Choi, K., Thomas, P.A., et al. (1983). National case control study of Kaposi's sarcoma and *Pneumocystis carinii* pneumonia in homosexual men: epidemiologic results. *Annals of Internal Medicine*, 99, 293–8.

Jayaraman, G.C., Archibald, C.P., Kim, J., et al. (2006). A population-based approach to determine the prevalence of transmitted drug-resistance HIV among recent versus established HIV infections: results from the Canadian HIV strain and drug resistance surveillance program. Journal of *Acquired Immune Deficiency Syndromes*, 42, 86–90.

Kenya Central Bureau of Statistics, Ministry of Health (MOH) and ORC Macro (2004). *Kenya 2003 Demographic and Health Survey: Key Findings*. Calverton MD, USA, MOH and ORC Macro. Available at: http://www.measuredhs.com/pubs/pdf/SR104/SR104KE03.pdf.

Kimball, A.M., Thacker, S.B., and Levy, M.E. (1980). Shigella surveillance in a large metropolitan area: assessment of a passive reporting system. *American Journal of Public Health*, 70(2), 164–6.

Krause, G. (2006). From evaluation to continuous quality assurance of surveillance systems. *Eurosurveillance*, 11(11), 204–5.

Kulldorff, M. (1997). A spatial scan statistic. *Communications in Statistics—Theory and Methods*, 26(6), 1481–96.

Kumar, R., Thakur, J.S., Rao, B.T., et al. (2006). Validity of verbal autopsy in determining causes of adult deaths. *Indian Journal of Public Health*, 50, 90–4.

Langmuir, A.D. (1963). The surveillance of communicable diseases of national importance. *The New England Journal of Medicine*, 268, 182–92.

Liu, L., Johnson, H.L., Cousens, S., et al. (2000). Global, regional, and national causes of child mortality: an updated systematic analysis for 2010 with time trends since 2000. *The Lancet*, 379(9832), 2151–61.

Lowndes, C.M. and Fenton, K.A. (2004). Surveillance systems for STIs in the European Union: facing a changing epidemiology. *Sexually Transmitted Infections*, 80, 264–71.

Madoff, L.C. and Woodall, J.P. (2005). The Internet and the global monitoring of emerging diseases: lessons from the first 10 years of ProMED-mail. *Archives of Medical Research*, 36, 724–30.

Malaria Surveys (2013). *Malaria Indicator Surveys 2013*. Available at: http://malariasurveys.org/index.cfm.

Mandl, K.D., Overhage, J.M., Wagner, M.M., et al. (2004). Implementing syndromic surveillance: a practical guide informed by the early experience. *Journal of the American Medical Informatics Association*, 11, 141–50. Available at: http://www.pubmedcentral.nih.gov/picrender.fcgi?artid=353021&blobtype=pdf.

Murray, C.J.L., Vos, T., Lozano, R., et al. (2012). Disability-adjusted life years (DALYs) for 291 diseases and injuries in 21 regions, 1990–2010: a systematic analysis for the Global Burden of Disease Study. *The Lancet*, 380(9859), 2197–223.

Neal, J.J., Fleming, P.L., Green, T.A., and Ward, J.W (1997). Trends in heterosexually acquired AIDS in the United States, 1988 through 1995. *Journal of Acquired Immune Deficiency Syndromes*, 14(5), 465–74.

Pallansch, M.A. and Sandhu, H.S. (2006). The eradication of polio—progress and challenges. *The New England Journal of Medicine*, 355, 2508–11.

Public Health Agency of Canada (2013). *The Global Public Health Intelligence Network (GPHIN)*. Available at: http://www.phac-aspc.gc.ca/gphin/.

Public Health Informatics Institute (2005). *Public Health Opportunities in Health Information Exchange. Topics in Public Health Informatics (2005)*. Available at: http://www.phii.org/sites/default/files/resource/pdfs/Opportunities_0605.pdf.

Rigau-Perez, J.G., Torres, J.V., Hayes, J.M., et al. (2006). Medical examiner samples: a source for dengue surveillance. *Puerto Rico Health Sciences Journal*, 25, 67–9.

Setel, P.W., Rao, C., Hemed, Y., et al. (2006). Core verbal autopsy procedure with comparative validation results from two countries. *PLoS Medicine*, 3, e268.

Seward, J.F., Watson, B.M., Peterson, C.L., et al. (2002). Varicella disease after introduction of varicella vaccine in the United States, 1995–2000. *Journal of the American Medical Association*, 287(5), 606–11.

Silk, B. and Berkelman, R.L. (2005). A review of strategies to enhance completeness of reporting. *Journal of Public Health Management and Practice*, 11, 191–200.

Swaminathan, B., Barrett, T.J., Hunter, S.B., et al. and the CDC PulseNet Task Force (2001). PulseNet: The Molecular Subtyping Network for Foodborne Bacterial Disease Surveillance, United States. *Emerging Infectious Diseases*, 7, 382–9.

Thacker, S.B. (2010). Historical development. In L.M. Lee, S.M. Teutsch, S.B. Thacker, and M.S. Louis (eds.) *Principles and Practice of Public Health Surveillane*, pp. 1–17. Oxford: Oxford University Press.

Thacker, S.B. and Berkelman, R.L. (1988). Public health surveillance in the United States. *Epidemiologic Reviews*, 10, 164–90.

Tufte, E.R. (1983). *The Visual Display of Quantitative Information*. Cheshire, CT: Graphics Press.

Tukey, J.W. (1977). *Exploratory Data Analysis*. Reading, MA: Addison-Wesley.

Twigg, L. (1999). Choosing a national survey to investigate smoking behavior: making comparisons between the General Household Survey, the British Household Panel Survey and the Health Survey for England. *Journal of Public Health Medicine*, 21, 14–21.

UNICEF (2013). *Multiple Indicator Cluster Survey 2013*. Available at: http://www.unicef.org/statistics/index_24302.html.

United States Agency for International Development (2013). *Demographic and Health Surveys 2013*. Available at: http://www.measuredhs.com.

Valdivia, A., López-Alcalde, J., Vicente, M., Pichiule, M., Ruiz, M., and Ordobas, M. (2010). Monitoring influenza activity in Europe with Google Flu Trends: comparison with the findings of sentinel physician networks—results for 2009–10. *Eurosurveillance*, 15(29), 2–7.

Waller, L.A. and Gotway, C.A. (2004). *Applied Spatial Statistics for Public Health Data*. Hoboken, NJ: John Wiley & Sons.

Weddell, J.M. (1973). Registers and registries: a review. *International Journal of Epidemiology*, 2, 221–8.

Williamson, L.M., Dodds, J.P., Mercey, D.E., et al. (2006). Increases in HIV-related sexual risk behaviour among community samples of gay men in London and Glasgow: how do they compare? *Journal of Acquired Immune Deficiency Syndromes*, 42, 238–41.

World Bank (1993). *World Development Report 1993: Investing in Health*. Oxford: World Bank and Oxford University Press.

World Bank (2012). *2012 Information and Communications for Development: Maximizing Mobile*. Washington, DC: World Bank.

World Health Organization (1968). *Report of the Technical Discussions at the 21st World Health Assembly on 'National and Global Surveillance of Communicable Diseases'*. Geneva: World Health Organization.

World Health Organization (2003). *Guidelines for the Management of Sexually Transmitted Infections*. Geneva: World Health Organization. Available at: http://www.who.int/hiv/pub/sti/pub6/en/.

World Health Organization (2008). *Global Burden of Disease: 2004 Update*. Geneva: World Health Organization.

Yan, W., Nie, S., Xu, B., Dong, H., Palm, L., and Diwan, V. (2012). Establishing a web-based integrated surveillance system for early detection of infectious disease epidemic in rural China: a field experimental study. *BMC Medical Informatics and Decision Making*, 12(1), 4.

Yu, V.L. and Madoff, L.C. (2004). ProMED-mail: an early warning system for emerging diseases. *Clinical Infectious Diseases*, 39(2), 227–32.

5.20

Life course epidemiology and analysis

Diana Kuh, Yoav Ben-Shlomo, Kate Tilling, and Rebecca Hardy

Introduction: what is life course epidemiology?

A life course approach in epidemiology investigates the biological, behavioural, and social pathways that link physical and social exposures and experiences during gestation, childhood, adolescence, and adult life, and across generations, to later life health and disease risk (Kuh and Ben-Shlomo 1997, 2004). Initially, the focus was on chronic diseases, particularly cardiometabolic and respiratory disease, where the life course perspective was used to integrate and extend three broad and apparently conflicting theories of disease aetiology: (1) fetal or developmental origins of adult disease (Barker 1998; Gluckman and Hanson 2006), (2) adult lifestyle (Krieger 2013), and (3) social causation theories (Marmot et al. 1984; Krieger 2013). Life course epidemiology then widened its gaze to a broader set of later life health outcomes that emphasized changes in function at the individual and physiological systems levels, through their period of development, maturation, and age-related decline. What had previously been seen as risk factors for subsequent later disease, were themselves seen as outcomes that required a fuller understanding of their natural history as well as life course determinants. The emphasis has been in exploiting the scientific value of the maturing birth cohort studies (Power et al. 2013) and other life course studies that have collected information on more than one phase of the life course. This has enabled researchers to test to what extent pre-adult factors influence later health, function, and disease risk, and whether the risk factor burden on these outcomes may be modified by early life risk and vice versa. In building its conceptual frameworks and models, life course epidemiology has built on relevant theories and concepts from scientists in other disciplines where a life course or developmental perspective was initiated earlier than it was for chronic disease epidemiology (Ben-Shlomo and Kuh 2002; Kuh et al. 2003). It has also discovered its roots in epidemiology and public health before the adult lifestyle model came to dominate chronic disease epidemiology in the second half of the twentieth century (Kuh and Davey Smith 1997). Now in the twenty-first century, a new interdisciplinary consensus is building, based on a life course approach to health and the changes in health with age in response to environmental challenges (Alwin 2012; Hertzman 2013; Kuh et al. 2014). By health, we mean how

people feel and function (at the individual, body systems, or cellular levels) and the disease risks they develop across life. In this chapter we describe these developments, update and elaborate our life course conceptual frameworks and models in response, and present examples that illustrate the application of life course methods that are a strength of life course epidemiology. We end by bringing up to date our reflections on the policy implications of taking a life course approach.

Background to life course epidemiology

A catalyst for the development of life course epidemiology was David Barker's imaginative studies that linked growth *in utero* or infancy to cardiometabolic and respiratory disease in later life (Barker 1998) which were interpreted as evidence for a critical developmental period with long-term consequences for chronic disease. Here, the life course approach encouraged three developments. The first was the replication and then systematic review of the growing epidemiological evidence that birthweight (a marker of fetal growth) or infant size was associated with adult blood pressure (Huxley et al. 2002), cardiovascular disease (Huxley et al. 2007), and diabetes (Whincup et al. 2008). This included investigating whether the associations between early life growth and adult disease were confounded by socioeconomic circumstances—generally they were not (Vagero and Leon 1994; Rich-Edwards et al. 1997; Hardy et al. 2003)—and what factors in adult life mediated or modified this early life risk; few adult cardiovascular risk factors were found to be mediators of the birthweight association with cardiovascular disease or mortality (Koupilova et al. 1999; Lawlor et al. 2004).

Second, life course epidemiologists also drew attention to potentially sensitive periods in childhood and adolescence, or during biological or social transitions in adult life, when the effects of physical and social exposures on long-term disease risk may be more marked than at other times. Here they drew on growing evidence from maturing birth cohort studies, as did Barker, so that the original fetal origins hypothesis widened to become more inclusive and was adapted to the developmental origins of adult disease (Gluckman and Hanson 2006). The emphasis was on fetal, childhood, and adolescent physical growth in relation to chronic diseases and their adult risk factors (e.g. Cooper et al. 2001; Hardy et al. 2004; Barker et al. 2005).

Third, in respect of the adult lifestyle or social causation theories of chronic disease, life course epidemiology drew attention to the early acquisition of lifestyle and its cumulative effects (Schooling and Kuh 2002; Clennell et al. 2008; Cooper et al. 2011b), and to the impact of the socioeconomic environment in childhood as well as in adult life on later health and health inequalities (Davey Smith and Lynch 2004; Kuh et al. 2004). Here, there was extensive documentation of the impact of early socioeconomic position (SEP) on cardiovascular and respiratory disease, operating independently and/or cumulatively with the effects of adult SEP (Galobardes et al. 2004; Power and Kuh 2004; Singh-Manoux et al. 2004; Power et al. 2013). The extent to which social gradients in health and disease are explained by adult behavioural factors has long been a subject of investigation and debate; for example, a recent study has shown that better longitudinal characterization of health behaviours increased the power to explain the social gradients in mortality (Stringhini et al. 2010). But early life SEP acts as a cause of causes, through effects on the development and maintenance of health behaviours or through influencing adult social destinations (Phelan et al. 2004).

Other ways that early SEP was hypothesized to 'get under the skin' and affect adult health and health inequalities, was through socially patterned exposures and experiences leaving imprints (or being 'biologically embedded' (Hertzman and Boyce 2010)) in the structure and function of body systems during sensitive periods of development or biological transitions. Evidence for early life developmental risk explaining social gradients in health and disease was sought for—and in many cases found (Boyce et al. 2012). It may be that pathways associated with neurodevelopment are particularly pertinent in relation to early social adversity. In the related field of cognitive epidemiology (Deary 2012), there is growing evidence that childhood and adolescent cognitive ability is associated with adult mortality, morbidity, and better health. Whether these associations are explained by lifetime SEP, and whether both SEP and cognitive associations are driven by neurodevelopmental processes is of research interest.

From chronic disease to functional trajectories

The gaze of life course epidemiology has widened since the term was first coined in 1997, to include a whole range of other health outcomes—for example, studies have investigated the role of early life risk factors on the development of cancers (Potischman et al. 2004) and neuropsychiatric disorders (Factor-Litvak and Susser 2004) (where there was already a strong research tradition on childhood origins), and aspects of body function, such as musculoskeletal (Kuh et al. 2006a, 2006b), cognitive (Richards and Sacker 2003; Richards et al. 2004), and reproductive function (Kuh and Hardy 2002; Mishra et al. 2007; Rich-Edwards et al. 2010).

Studying biological function is a way of looking at health across the life before diseases are manifest, and estimating the impact of social and physical hazards that leave imprints on the function of body systems. These imprints reflect the ability of the organism to respond adaptively to ever changing environmental challenges,

and provide clues to aetiology. Functional trajectories provide a more dynamic concept than a simple dichotomous mortality or disease end-point categorization, incorporating the natural history and physiological trajectory of biological systems. Many functional measures are outcomes in their own right (e.g. lung, muscle, and cognitive function) as well as risk factors for later disease. Groups or classes of individuals who display different life course functional patterns can be considered and their lifetime determinants investigated (Silverwood et al. 2011; Mishra and Kuh 2012; Wills et al. 2012). Most functions display rapid growth and development in the early stages of life until a peak or plateau is reached at maturity, followed by a gradual decline with age (Fig. 5.20.1). These trajectories may reflect: (1) normal development and decline (trajectory A), (2) the influence of exposures or genetic factors that result in suboptimal development resulting in a reduced functional reserve at maturity (trajectory B), (3) the influence of exposures or genetic factors acting post maturity that result in accelerated age-related decline (trajectory C), and (4) a combination of trajectories B and C (trajectory D). There are also body functions that display different life course trajectories; for example, systolic blood pressure shows a rapid increase in adolescence, a gentle increase through early adulthood, a midlife acceleration beginning around the mid-30s, and a slowing and reversal of these increases into old age (Wills et al. 2011). However it is possible to reconceptualize the increase in midlife systolic blood pressure as reflecting age-related loss in arterial wall elasticity due to wear and tear from repeated pulsatile expansion and contraction (McEniery et al. 2010). The terminal decline in the oldest subjects remains more controversial and may reflect the composite effects of a healthy survivor effect, medication, heart failure, and failure of central neural control.

Life course epidemiology also has developed an interest in modelling physical and cognitive developmental trajectories that may provide clues to the imprinting of nutritional influences, infections, and other early life exposures either acting during critical or sensitive periods or accumulating over time. A natural extension of understanding functional trajectories is to try and explain biological ageing, the progressive generalized impairment of function

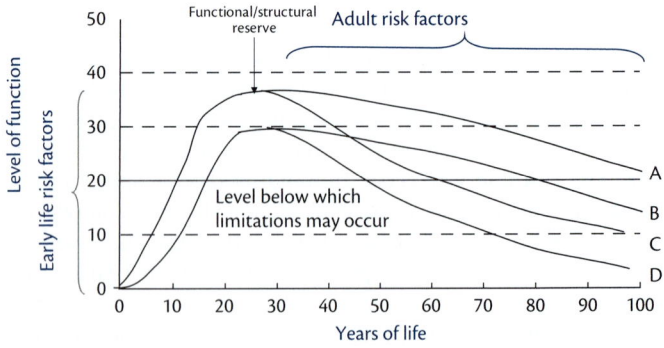

Fig. 5.20.1 Life course trajectories. A = normal development and decline; B = exposure during development reducing functional reserve at maturity; C = exposure acting post maturity accelerating age-related decline; D = combination of B and C.

Adapted from Kuh D, and Ben-Shlomo Y, *A Life Course Approach to Chronic Disease Epidemiology: Tracing the Origins of Ill-Health from Early to Adult Life*, Second Edition. Oxford: Oxford University Press, Oxford, UK, Copyright © 2004, by permission of Oxford University Press.

('senescence') that occurs post maturity, and healthy biological ageing (Kuh et al. 2014), that is, the maintenance of optimal functioning for the longest period of time. The rate of functional decline reflects growing impaired physiological responses to environmental and behavioural challenges.

Environmental, behavioural, and physiological risk factors acting earlier in life may leave imprints on the development of peak function or the rate of decline, whereas these factors acting later in life can only affect the rate of decline or the ability to recover after an initial loss of function, for example, degree of heart failure after a myocardial infarction. A life course conceptual framework hypothesizes the relationships between biological, psychological, and social risk factors and health outcomes over time, taking into account their potential confounding, mediating, or interactive effects. A set of life course models hypothesizes how risk factors influence disease and functional outcomes (Kuh et al. 2003; Ben-Shlomo et al. 2013); Mishra and colleagues (Mishra et al. 2009) have developed a novel structured approach to distinguish critical, sensitive and accumulation models (see section on 'Analytical challenges of life course epidemiology'). Now these life course frameworks and methods are being extended to investigate age at onset, duration and trajectories of these risk factors, and how they inter-relate in dynamic ways with functional trajectories of interest. They utilize a range of methodological approaches (see section on 'Analytical challenges of life course epidemiology') for modelling repeat continuous and binary outcome measures and link these to later outcomes or trajectories.

Historical and interdisciplinary perspectives

We have written extensively elsewhere to show that the idea that early life factors have long-term effects that stretch into adult life was the conventional wisdom in public health in the first half of the twentieth century (Kuh and Davey Smith 1993) and lay behind social welfare policies for mothers, babies, and young children that developed at this time (Dwork 1987). These early ideas in public health were influenced by biological and behavioural research into critical periods of animal and human development; and which influenced a new field of developmental science and the setting up of several US cohort studies of growth and development in the 1920s and 1930s (Kuh and Davey Smith 2004).

Epidemiological and public health interest in early life factors for adult health waned in the post-Second World War era as population cohort studies monitoring the development of coronary heart disease and cancers among middle-aged individuals became fashionable. However, pockets of interest remained: for example, in relation to the childhood origins of chronic bronchitis (Reid 1969; Colley et al. 1973), hypertensive and cardiovascular diseases (Abraham et al. 1971; Forsdahl 1977), and neuropsychiatric disorders (Stein et al. 1975). But it was the link that Barker postulated between nutritional experience *in utero* and adult chronic disease (Barker 1990, 1995), that really caught the scientific imagination and acted as a catalyst for further research, at a time of growing disenchantment with the adult lifestyle model of chronic disease. While initially built on evidence from ecological and historical cohort studies, investigations into the developmental origins of adult disease increasingly focus on potential

biological mechanisms; for example, studies of placental shape and function (Burton and Barker 2010) and epigenetics (Godfrey et al. 2011). In parallel, Boyce, Hertzman, and others are generating interest in a revitalized and interdisciplinary developmental science, 'the developmental biology of social adversity', which combines insights from disciplines such as neuroscience, genetics, and epigenetics, together with data from birth cohort and life course studies, to elucidate the biological pathways that link early experience to later health and health inequalities (Boyce et al. 2012; Hertzman 2013).

Scientists in life course epidemiology, and this new developmental science, acknowledge the relevant and influential research undertaken by Sir Michael Rutter and colleagues in the field of developmental psychopathology to understand continuities and discontinuities between childhood adversity and early disorders, and adult psychopathology (Rutter 1989, 2012b; Rutter et al. 2006). His work has revealed the great heterogeneity in how children respond to environmental adversity—when it may be good, tolerable, or harmful—and the need to understand resilience as a dynamic concept (Rutter 2012a).

More broadly, many disciplines champion a life course or a lifespan conceptual framework for organizing research on human development, maturation, and ageing and are increasingly identifying what they have in common, rather than their distinctive features. Life course sociology and lifespan psychology are examples (Mayer 2003; Alwin 2012). Life course sociology and life course epidemiology share an interest with demographers in understanding group differences through cohort effects that may reveal the impact of earlier life experiences on adult health and social outcomes (Myrskyla 2010).

Modern evolutionary approaches to science and medicine are highly relevant to all these disciplines. For example, Gluckman and colleagues have placed the developmental origins of adult disease within an evolutionary framework (Gluckman et al. 2009). They postulate how responses to environmental challenges can operate over different time scales: the role of homeostasis to restore equilibrium in the short term, the role of developmental plasticity in the early years to adapt to the environment and maximize the chance of reproductive success, and the force of natural selection over generations and millennia (Gluckman et al. 2009). Kirkwood and Austad (2000), Austad (2008), and others have provided evolutionary explanations for why we age, due to the decline in the force of natural selection in the post-reproductive phase of life which leaves the organism increasingly less able to repair the accumulating molecular and cellular damage. Here again heterogeneity and resilience, this time in older people, is of particular interest.

Life course conceptual models and their relationship to ageing

Our original life course models (Ben-Shlomo and Kuh 2002; Kuh et al. 2003; Kuh and Ben-Shlomo 2004) were developed to test the importance of timing and duration of exposures on later disease risk. They included: (1) a 'critical or sensitive period model' (mentioned earlier) when an exposure in earlier life has lifelong effects on structure or function that are either not modified or are modified by later experience and (2) the 'accumulation of risk models' (Fig. 5.20.2, models a and b) shown here where there is

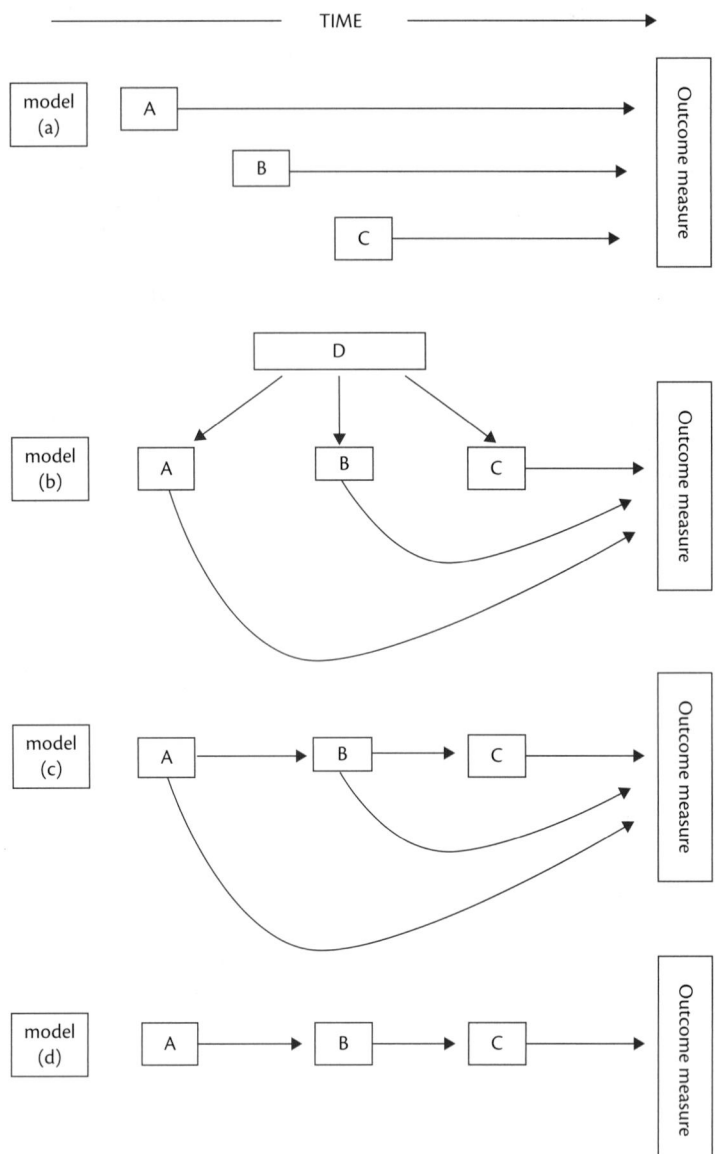

Fig. 5.20.2 Life course conceptual models.
Reproduced from Kuh D et al., *Journal of Epidemiology Community Health*, Life course epidemiology, Volume 57, Issue 10, pp. 778–83, Copyright © 2003, with permission from BMJ Publishing Group Ltd.

cumulative damage to biological systems over the life course or a 'chain of risk model' (Fig. 5.20.2, models c and d) where there is a sequence of linked exposures that lead to impaired function either through an accumulation of adverse effects across exposures or by the sequence leading to a 'trigger' exposure whilst the antecedent exposures are themselves of no direct consequence.

We have previously presented these as different classes of models though it is more sensible to view critical or sensitive period models as special subsets of an accumulation model (Ben-Shlomo et al. 2013)—hence the effects of exposures over different time periods do not add up in a simple additive fashion but differ in the strength of effect in a quantitative sense (sensitive period) or in a qualitative sense so that they can only be observed in one time period (critical period). For example, duration of obesity may increase risk of breast cancer in women in a simple linear dose–response relationship (accumulation). If, however, being

obese during puberty further increased cancer risk independent of duration, this would suggest that puberty is a sensitive period of exposure for future carcinogenic risk. Finally, if one only observed an increased risk with obesity in puberty and being obese outside this period was not related to cancer risk then there would be evidence for a critical period effect. In this case women who were obese in puberty but remained obese outside this time window would have the same risk as those who were only obese during puberty—hence there would be no evidence in support of accumulation of effect.

These life course models do not accurately represent the complexities of life course epidemiology as practised today when researchers are interested in the dynamic interplay of developmental, risk factor (behavioural or environmental), and ageing-related trajectories. The challenge is to model the characteristics of risk factors over time (age at onset, duration, and change with age) with changes in the functional outcomes of interest. While there is now considerable experience in modelling risk factor trajectories, such as physical growth, there is much more limited experience in investigating how functional outcomes change with age, and the lifetime determinants that drive this change, in addition to those that establish the initial level (Wills et al. 2012; Lawlor and Hardy 2014).

Furthermore, given that there is great heterogeneity in biological ageing, our models need to be able to take into account this variation in resilience to environmental challenges with age. We identify two sources of resilience to ageing post maturity. The first is intrinsic 'compensatory reserve'; this may reflect structural factors, for example, size of heart muscle, functional capacity, that is, the efficiency of the heart to generate cardiac output or recuperative function, in other words, the ability of body systems to compensate physiologically or repair damage with varying degrees of success when faced with acute or chronic low-level challenges. We envisage compensatory reserve as an intrinsic biological phenomenon which preserves function but deteriorates with age, probably in a non-linear fashion and possibly in parallel across multiple domains (e.g. vascular, neurological, immune, homeostatic systems) in those who will become frail. For example, the degree of heart failure subsequent to a heart attack will not only depend on the location of the infarction but also on the premorbid structure and function and the ability to open up collateral circulation in

the immediate postinfarction period thereby salvaging cardiac muscle and function.

The second aspect of resilience in ageing is the individual's extrinsic responses or adaptations when faced with age-related declines, by altering behaviour or the environment to modify the effect on, or slow the rate of, functional decline. So, for example, the 'use it or lose it' hypothesis argues that continued cognitive stimulation will maintain synaptic connectivity despite neurodegenerative changes and hence slow down decline or maintain cognitive function due to enhanced cognitive reserve (Stern 2002).

Ferrucci and Studentski (2012) identified four key ageing phenotypes where growing disequilibrium or dysfunction in response to environmental challenges can lead to frailty, and where conversely, maintenance would represent healthy biological ageing: (1) central nervous system (CNS) integrity or neurodegeneration, (2) homeostatic regulation or age-related dysregulation in signalling pathways that maintain homeostasis (encompassing both the endocrine and immunological systems), and the extent of age-related changes in (3) body composition (muscle, fat, and bone), and (4) in energy capacity and consumption.

An integrated life course model of ageing is illustrated in Fig. 5.20.3. From a life course perspective we are particularly interested in how growth and development (box 1 in Fig. 5.20.3) impact these four phenotypes (box 2), related physiological systems such

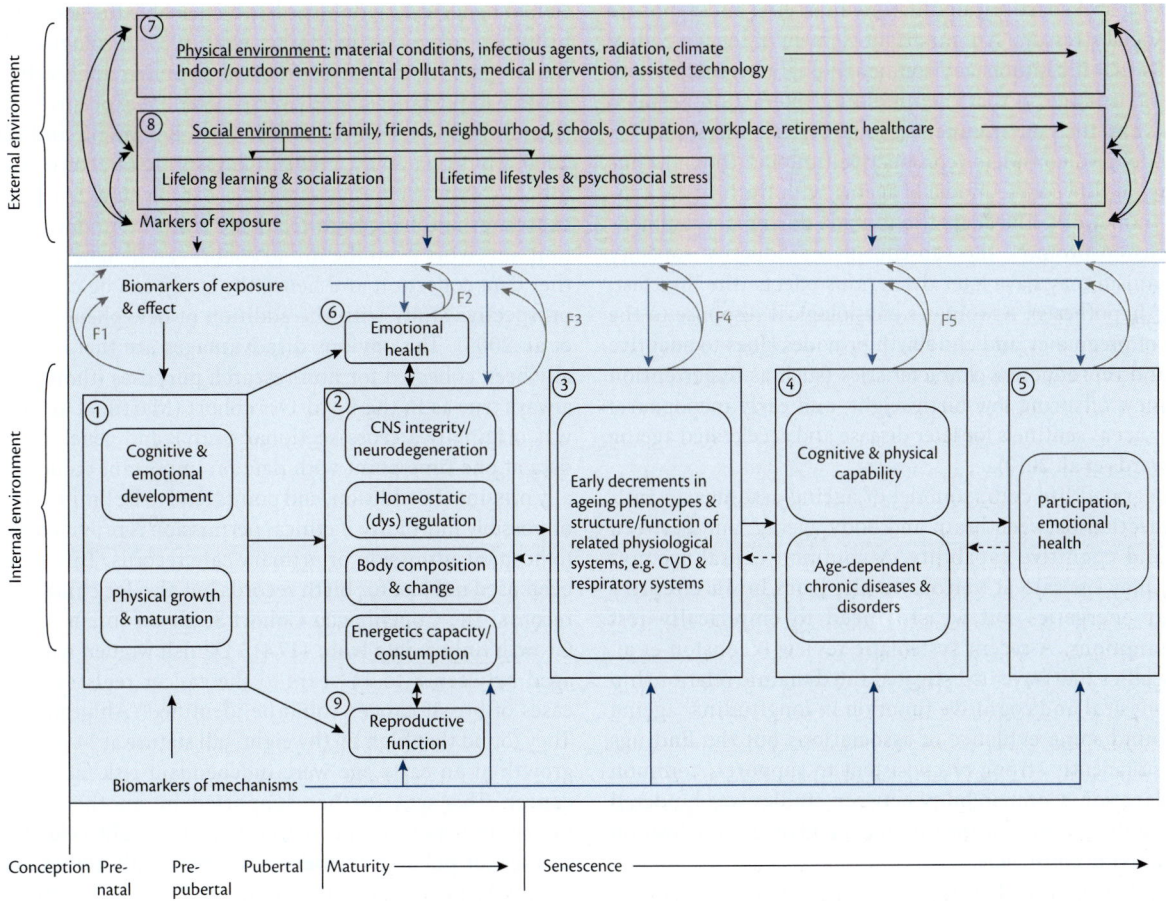

Fig. 5.20.3 Integrated life course model of ageing.
Adapted from Kuh D et al. (eds), *A Life Course Approach to Healthy Ageing*, Oxford University Press, Oxford, Copyright ©2014, by permission of Oxford University Press.

as the cardiovascular and respiratory systems (box 3), and the phenotypic emergence of their consequences for physical and cognitive capability (the capacity to undertake the physical and mental tasks of daily living) (box 4). Being able to detect early markers of an accelerated trajectory of decline, and before it is manifest in adverse changes to physical and cognitive capability, is one of the cornerstones of the life course perspective on ageing because it offers an opportunity to delay the onset of decline or its rate of change through preventive strategies.

Our life course model of ageing also encompasses the emotional health of older people and their continued participation in society as a health phenotype in its own right (box 5) which may be threatened by functional decline. But emotional health is intertwined with physiological ageing, as both a determinant and a consequence (box 6). Early emotional development predicts adult emotional health and life chances, and lifetime emotional health influences physiological ageing as well as determines individual capacity for psychological and social adaptation. The feedback loops in the diagram (labelled F1–5) illustrate the possibility of physiological compensation, or psychological and social adaptation through modifying behaviour or the surrounding environment.

In our model, we have separated out lifetime physical and social environments (boxes 7 and 8) but show strong links between the two. The social environment is shown to influence the ageing trajectory not only through exposures to material conditions and other aspects of the physical environment, but also through lifelong learning and socialization, lifetime lifestyles, and exposure to psychosocial stressors. An important element of the life course approach is that it captures environmental characteristics before impairments emerge so that the unfolding interaction between individuals and their environments can be better understood.

This model also considers reproductive function (box 9), thus integrating our life course model of ageing with the broader evolutionary framework. The adaptations made during developmental plasticity to promote the subsequent reproductive capacity of the organism may have later deleterious effects (the 'live fast, die young' hypothesis). A woman's physiological response to the challenge of pregnancy and childbirth provides clues to adaptive capacity and reproductive characteristics (such as hypertension in pregnancy, offspring low birthweight, and early menopause) which may act as sentinels for later disease and accelerated ageing (Rich-Edwards et al. 2010).

This integrated life course model of ageing assumes an intimate connection between brain and body ageing, and between physical and cognitive capability. A common causal account of ageing may operate at various levels, from brain circuitry to cellular energetics but we still need to empirically test these assumptions. A recent systematic review (Clouston et al. 2013) of studies that have investigated the dynamic relationship between physical and cognitive function in longitudinal ageing cohorts found some evidence of associations but the findings were not sufficiently strong or consistent to support a common cause explanation. Comparability between studies was hindered because of differences in the measurement and operationalization of the underlying constructs.

The stochastic nature of ageing—the nature of chance—means that this integrated life course model is unlikely to predict individual outcomes, but it may explain group differences in ageing. It provides insight into the lifetime characteristics of individuals and their environments that drive ageing, and that could be targeted to extend healthy active lives. The development of more refined markers or biomarkers of exposure and effect, and biomarkers of underlying mechanisms would facilitate such investigations. For example, we simplify repeated measures by aggregating them into a mean summary measure. But the variability of measures may also add information. So, Rothwell et al. (2010) have demonstrated that not just mean blood pressure but blood pressure variability for a given mean level independently increases risk of cardiovascular disease. It is unclear whether greater variability reflects additional structural changes (e.g. arterial stiffness) which are harmful or is a marker of failing homeostatic mechanisms that maintain blood pressure within a limited range. Similar observations have been seen for gait speed in the elderly whereby a larger standard deviation of gait speed rather than mean level predicts future falls risk and probably reflects underlying neurological dysfunction as this is also seen with disorders such as Parkinson's disease (Frenkel-Toledo et al. 2005).

Study designs for life course epidemiology

Any epidemiological design can in theory be used for life course studies as long as exposures in an earlier period can be related to future outcomes. The rise in life course epidemiology followed on directly from both ecological studies and the ingenious identification of historical birth records which enable the construction of a historical cohort study (Barker et al. 1989). Ecological designs as well as time trend analyses remain a popular approach to test the relative importance of early versus later life exposures such as SEP (Ben-Shlomo and Davey Smith 1991; Bengtsson and Lindstrom 2000; Myrskyla 2010). Epidemiologists are often attracted to historical cohort studies as outcomes can be quickly related to past exposures and hence are relatively cheap to undertake. In addition, survivors from the initial cohort can then be invited for further data collection and hence the study can be converted into a prospective study with the addition of new phenotypes (Syddall et al. 2005). The obvious disadvantages are that data have usually been collected for non-research purposes (though this is not always true as in the Boyd-Orr cohort (Martin et al. 2005) which was originally a cross-sectional study), and generally only have data at one time point with data on important confounders usually missing. In addition, end points tend to be limited to mortality or possibly morbidity if ethical permission is provided to link data to hospital admission or primary care records. This approach has been used not just for birth records but also for childhood growth records. The Copenhagen Cohort Study on Infant Nutrition and Growth linked data from 117,415 Danish women when they were aged between 8 to 14 years to the cancer registry so that 3340 cases of breast cancer could be identified (Ahlgren et al. 2004). They found that high birthweight, tall stature at 14 years, and peak growth at an early age were independent risk factors for breast cancer. This was further supported by another school-based follow-up which found that early peak height velocity, a proxy marker for puberty, was also associated with higher insulin-like growth factor 1 (IGF-1) (Sandhu et al. 2006a). The latter is known to be anti-apoptotic and has been associated with increased risk of premenopausal breast cancer (Renehan et al. 2004).

The conventional prospective cohort study is usually more suited for life course epidemiology, but traditionally studies of chronic disease would only recruit adults in midlife hence the availability and maturation of the UK birth cohorts have provided ideal datasets to test may life course hypotheses. Birth cohorts are costly but they provide a very rich dataset that can test a wide range of hypotheses and the integration of genetic and epigenetic data makes them extremely valuable resources.

Another approach has been the use of natural experiments and the long-term follow-up, usually unplanned at the time of design, of past randomized trials. The best known example of the former has been the series of studies on the survivors of the Dutch famine. The timing of the famine imposed by the German troops on the inhabitants of Amsterdam enabled researchers to test whether the timing (early, mid, late gestation) of severe nutritional deprivation during pregnancy had an effect on early childhood development (Stein et al. 1975), and more recently cardiovascular, metabolic disease (Ravelli et al. 1998), and a range of traits including epigenetic methylation patterns (Heijmans et al. 2008). Follow-up of conventional randomized controlled trials has also been undertaken but here only a single hypothesis related to the specific intervention can be tested, though the problem of confounding may be overcome assuming no systematic loss to follow-up by randomization status. For example, Singhal and colleagues followed-up premature babies who were randomized to either breast versus formula feeding or high- versus low-nutrient feeds (Singhal et al. 2001). In these studies the response rate at follow-up was low (around 20 per cent) though there do not appear to be major differences at baseline between those who re-attended compared to those who did not at baseline. From these data they suggested more rapid growth in the immediate postnatal period may be deleterious in terms of adolescent risk factors ('growth acceleration hypothesis') (Singhal et al. 2004). In contrast, a village-based stepped wedge cluster trial in Hyderabad, India, found that children who received nutritional supplementation were taller at follow-up, indicating some effect on development and had better insulin function as well as less stiff arteries, though the differences were modest (Kinra et al. 2008).

Family-based designs have traditionally been used by psychologists in their efforts to explain how much of a trait such as intelligence, can be explained by genetic or the shared and non-shared environment (Plomin and Daniels 2011). Within the context of life course epidemiology, they have regained interest as a method to disentangle causal from confounded associations. Comparing relationships within and between family members—between generations or siblings or twins, for example—can help to clarify the mechanisms underlying associations in life course studies and help to determine causality (Lawlor and Mishra 2009). Prenatal influences can be studied by comparing the relationship between the exposure experienced by the mother during pregnancy and outcome in the offspring with that between the experience of the father to the same exposure and offspring outcome (Davey Smith et al. 2009a). In the Avon Longitudinal Study of Parents and Children (ALSPAC), the effect of maternal smoking on childhood obesity was of a similar magnitude to the effect of paternal smoking (Leary et al. 2006) suggesting that maternal smoking does not have a direct intrauterine effect on childhood obesity, but rather that any association may be due to the confounding effects of lifestyle in parents who smoke unlike birthweight which was much more strongly associated with maternal smoking. The use of maternal versus paternal comparisons with offspring outcomes has been further extended with the use of genetic information as instrumental variables. Lawlor and colleagues (Lawlor et al. 2008) tested the developmental overnutrition hypothesis which argues that the increase in childhood adiposity reflects the cumulative inter-generational effect of obese mothers having more obese children who in turn become obese mothers. This study not only used maternal and paternal body mass index but also the maternal FTO genotype which is associated with body mass index but not associated with the usual socioeconomic confounders (see discussion of Mendelian randomization in 'Analytical challenges of life course epidemiology'). They found stronger maternal than paternal associations, even after accounting for a 10 per cent non-paternity rate, but there was no FTO offspring obesity association conditional on offspring FTO status. The use of genetic and environmental interactions or epigenetic effects on fetal development is likely to further expand opportunities for hypothesis testing. Many past studies have failed to find an association between maternal alcohol drinking during pregnancy and offspring IQ but mothers who drink more tend to have higher SEP which would mask any association. Lewis and colleagues in the ALSPAC cohort were able to show that a risk allele score using four alcohol metabolizing genes was associated with worse cognition but only if the mother reported moderate drinking (1–6 units per week) whilst there was no effect of the genetic score amongst abstainers (Lewis et al. 2012).

Life course epidemiologists have formed research collaborations that involve a number of cohort studies, such as HALCyon (Healthy Ageing across the Life Course, http://www.halcyon. ac.uk) (Kuh et al. 2012), and FALCon (Function Across the Life Course) to increase the sample size and power to investigate lifetime risk factors on longitudinal phenotypes, and to test whether findings are replicated across cohorts in a systematic way. The collaborations have developed experience in data harmonization to derive comparable phenotypes across the cohorts, and in cross cohort methods (Cooper et al. 2011a; Wills et al. 2011; Hardy et al. 2013).

Cross-cohort comparisons also enable one to examine for generalizability or unique birth cohort effects and can help disentangle causal from confounded associations as confounding structures may vary in different populations. A two-cohort comparison was undertaken between the UK-based ALSPAC cohort and the Brazilian Pelotas cohort as in the former higher SEP was associated with greater breastfeeding whilst in Pelotas there was no socioeconomic association (Brion et al. 2011). Not surprisingly, the ALSPAC study demonstrated an association between breastfeeding and lower blood pressure, lower body mass index (BMI) and higher cognition even after adjustment for a wide range of confounders. In contrast there was no association between breastfeeding and blood pressure or BMI in Pelotas but the association with cognition remained and is supported by findings from the PROBIT randomized trial of breastfeeding (Kramer et al. 2008). Thus it can be concluded that associations of breastfeeding with child blood pressure and BMI are likely to reflect residual confounding, while breastfeeding may have causal effects on cognitive function. In this example both cohorts had subjects of a similar age but it is more common to have cohorts with subjects of very different ages. In this scenario, one can still use the comparisons to triangulate across clinical and subclinical end points. For example, we could test whether breastfeeding is protective for cardiovascular disease by seeing if in the oldest cohorts (ages greater than 60 years) breastfeeding is associated with cardiovascular mortality and morbidity whilst younger cohorts (ages less than 60) could examine for preclinical surrogates such as carotid intimal medial thickness or echocardiographic changes to the heart. The consistency of findings across the life course both supports a causal explanation (as the confounding structure may differ by secular period) as well as providing insights into the onset of the pathophysiological process.

Analytical challenges of life course epidemiology

The statistical analysis of life course data is complex and challenging as it aims to study how risk factors from across the whole of life jointly influence later health and increasingly how life course risk factors influence patterns of functional change across the life course (see section entitled 'From chronic disease to functional trajectories'). Whatever statistical model is used, analyses attempting to disentangle the life course effects still require understanding of the underlying biology, and careful consideration of confounding, intermediate variables, and potential biases.

Exposures which are measured repeatedly over time (e.g. when relating infant weight gain to later outcomes) present three related analytical problems: (1) repeated measures on the same individual are likely to be correlated, (2) the potential high dimensionality of the resulting exposure (e.g. six repeated measures of weight over the first year of life (Tilling et al. 2011a)), (3) specifying the hypothesis to be tested (e.g. is average weight gain related to the later outcome? Maximum weight gain? Total weight gained?). One way of dealing with the first two problems is to derive simple summary measures such as an area under a growth curve (Li et al. 2004), the length of time an individual has been overweight (Wills et al. 2010; Silverwood et al. 2013), or the number of time points an individual has been in a disadvantaged SEP (Davey Smith et al. 1997; Wamala et al. 2001). However, this approach assumes an underlying model, does not test alternatives and does not address the impact of timing of an exposure. For example, age at onset of obesity was associated with blood pressure at 53 years, but whether duration of obesity or BMI at 53 years was the main driver of this association could not be teased out (Wills et al. 2010).

In order to distinguish a critical period, or more likely a sensitive period, model from an accumulation model, Mishra et al. (2009) operationalized these models algebraically. First, a saturated model is fitted, in which each of the possible life course trajectories is allowed to influence the outcome in a different way. Each alternative life course model is then tested against this saturated model, using a *p*-value-based approach to choose the best-fitting model. This approach was developed in the context of repeated measures of a binary classification of occupational social class (e.g. high versus low SEP). The ability to distinguish between the various models is limited by the variability in trajectories within any dataset, and the timing and spacing of the measurement points. In the original paper, measures that spanned three relatively equal-spaced time periods were used, whereas in an application with only childhood and adult SEP, the adult SEP exposure

covered a much longer time period than the childhood measure (Birnie et al. 2011).

When considering a continuous repeated exposure (such as body size), several methods for relating change to later outcomes have been proposed. Simple methods, including z-score plots showing standardized growth measures over time in different outcome groups, and methods based on multivariable regression have been widely used to address early growth and health. Life course plots were developed to visualize both size and growth, and consist of plotting the regression coefficients from a model relating the outcome to all body size measures simultaneously against their respective measurement ages and joining the points (Cole 2007). To address the issue of uninformative ages and collinearity between measures, ages where the measure appears unrelated to the outcome may be removed and the model refitted and a new plot produced. Cole provides an example where weight at ages 4 and 6 are uninformative in relation to subsequent age at menarche (Cole 2007), and the final life course plot includes positive coefficients for weight at birth and 2 years and a negative coefficient for weight at 7 years. The interpretation is thus suggestive of two separate processes: one acting early in life where above-average weight delays puberty and the second in later childhood where a slow rate of weight gain relative to peers is related to later puberty. This practice of adjusting for a later measure of body size when interpreting the association between an earlier measure of body size and outcome has been the subject of much debate. If birthweight has a positive association with later body size, which is itself positively related to the outcome, then the association between birthweight and outcome can change from positive to negative on conditioning on the later body size variable (termed the 'reversal paradox' (Tu et al. 2005)). To avoid this problem, conditional change measures have been proposed, whereby residuals from models of each body size measure regressed on previous body size measures are derived (Adair et al. 2009). By definition, these residuals are all independent of each other and can be included in the same regression model. It is then possible to test whether change in one period has a stronger association with the outcome than change in other periods (Wills et al. 2010). Alternatively, path analysis can be used to model simultaneously the direct and indirect effects of an early body size measure on an outcome (Gamborg et al. 2009). The saturated path model is a combination of the conditional change model parameterization and the size model parameterization (Wills and Tilling 2014). As well as the need for careful interpretation, a major disadvantage of all these methods is that measurements must be taken on all study members at the same age and that individuals are dropped from analysis if they have missing measurements (unless multiple imputation (e.g. De Stavola et al. 2004) or other procedures are carried out).

To overcome the need for balanced data, and to shed light on the relative importance of exposure at different times, estimates of change from growth curves (using multilevel or mixed-effects models) have been used to summarize repeated exposures. Growth curves may be smooth (e.g. using natural or cubic splines (Silverwood et al. 2009), fractional polynomials (Wen et al. 2012), or extended splines (Pan and Goldstein 1998)) or connected periods of approximately linear growth (e.g. using linear splines (Tilling et al. 2011a)). Linear spline random effects models have been fitted to repeated measurements of weight between birth and 5 years of age in the Barry Caerphilly Growth Study (Ben-Shlomo et al. 2008). A model was fitted with two knots (selected in this case to be at 5 months, and 1 year and 9 months) allowing different gradients in the three time periods. The between-subject random effects (i.e. birthweight and each of the three slopes defined as immediate postnatal, infant, and child weight velocities) were then related to blood pressure in young adulthood and suggested that low birthweight and rapid postnatal growth were associated with higher systolic blood pressure, but that only immediate postnatal weight gain was associated with higher diastolic blood pressure. The periods into which time is partitioned may be driven by model fit (e.g. by choosing the combinations of knots), from a specified set, which provide the best fit as assessed by measures such as the AIC (Akaike information criterion) or BIC (Bayesian information criterion) or, a priori, based on biological changes in growth patterns. Aspects of the growth curve other than estimates of change can be derived, such as the location of the BMI peak between 5 and 13 years (Silverwood et al. 2009). A study examining growth between 9 and 18 years and with up to 65 repeat measurements derived maximal velocity and age at peak height velocity, which was used as a surrogate for the timing of puberty (Sandhu et al. 2006b) showing that younger age at peak height velocity was associated with higher adult IGF-1 levels. A more recent analysis of the same anthropometric data using the SuperImposition by Translation And Rotation (SITAR) model (Cole et al. 2010) identified three random effects for each individual which summarized their growth patterns; these represent size, growth tempo, and growth velocity. This model was able to explain 99 per cent of the variance in growth patterns and then each parameter was related to adult levels of IFG-1. Many of these models can also be fitted as joint models using structural equation models (De Stavola et al. 2006) or multivariate multilevel models (Goldstein and Kounali 2009; Macdonald-Wallis et al. 2012).

As an alternative to relating derived aspects of a growth trajectory to an outcome, individuals can be classified into groups of people with similar trajectories (using latent class analysis (Nagin and Tremblay 2001; Nagin and Odgers 2010) or growth mixture modelling), and class membership related to the outcome. Latent class analysis was used to summarize childhood overweight patterns in relation to kidney function (Silverwood et al. 2013) and wheezing phenotypes in the first 6 years of life in relation to atopy and lung function in later childhood (Henderson et al. 2008). One study, however, suggested that the latent trajectory classes (extracted using growth mixture models) of midlife change in blood pressure contained the same information as the intercept and slope from a random effects models, when predicting angina (Wills et al. 2012). The latent classes derived may not always coincide with hypotheses of interest, and there must be a priori reasons for thinking that distinct subpopulations (or classes) exist (Tilling et al. 2011b).

In situations when we are interested in two body size measurements, there is a third variable of interest (the difference or growth) that is a linear function of the other two and this has been termed the *duality of size and growth* (Cole 2007; Wills and Tilling 2014). This duality means it is impossible to estimate mutually distinct effects for all three parameters and is analogous to the problem of disentangling age, period and cohort effects. Partial least squares (PLS) regression has been used to attempt to overcome this problem by extracting functions of the exposures which explain the highest percentage of variance in the outcome (Tu et al. 2010;

Heys et al. 2013). This method was used to relate blood pressure at 11 years to height and weight during childhood, and showed that systolic blood pressure was related to size at birth, 3 months and 11 years, as well as change in BMI between 3 months and 11 years (Heys et al. 2013).

To be of policy relevance the causal nature of observed associations needs to be established. Directed acyclic graphs (Greenland et al. 1999; Greenland and Brumback 2002) can be used to articulate assumptions made about potential confounding and mediating variables, and to help identify variables to be controlled for in analyses (Hernan et al. 2002). Path analysis or structural equation models can be used to parameterize the causal graph (Greenland and Brumback 2002). Given the time frame over which associations operate in life course epidemiology, the potential for confounding by multiple variables across the life course is great. Methods available to adjust for the bias due to confounding in observational studies include: adjustment for confounders in regression models, stratification by confounders, use of propensity score (Rosenbaum and Rubin 1983) (or other matching) methods to mimic randomized trials by creating subgroups of individuals with similar likelihood of having the exposure, and instrumental variable methods (Greenland 2000). Because an instrumental variable is related to the outcome only through the exposure, and is unrelated to any confounders of exposure and outcome, the relationships between instrument and outcome and between instrument and exposure can be used to derive an unconfounded estimate of the causal effect of exposure on outcome. Examples of instrumental variables in epidemiology include offspring BMI as an indicator of own BMI in analysis relating BMI and mortality to avoid reverse causation (Davey Smith et al. 2009b) and age-specific retirement incentives as an instrument to relate retirement to later health (Behncke 2012). A more common use is of genetic instrumental variables in Mendelian randomization (Davey Smith and Ebrahim 2004; Didelez and Sheehan 2007). For example, although greater adiposity was associated with increased odds of psychological distress, Mendelian randomization analysis using genetic variants robustly associated with adiposity suggested an inverse association (Lawlor et al. 2011). In contrast, Mendelian randomization analysis suggested a causal link between childhood BMI and age at menarche (Mumby et al. 2011). A two-step epigenetic Mendelian randomization method has now been proposed as an extension which may help establish the causal role of epigenetic processes in pathways to disease (Relton and Davey Smith 2012).

An added complication, called time-dependent confounding, occurs in life course analyses when confounders are themselves measured repeatedly over time, and early exposures influence these later confounders (Daniel et al. 2012). Standard statistical models may be biased when there is time-dependent confounding, and this bias may not be removed by adjusting for either the baseline value of the covariate, or the time-updated covariate (Daniel et al. 2012). Methods such as marginal structural models, g-estimation, or the g-computation formula may be used to estimate the effect of an exposure on an outcome in the presence of time-dependent confounding (Robins 1986; Robins et al. 1992, 2000; Daniel et al. 2012).

In all the methods described, long-running population-based studies inevitably result in missing data and measurement error which may bias findings. Methods for dealing with missing data are well developed, although implementation can be complex in a life course setting. Multilevel models (estimated using maximum likelihood) allow for missing data, provided that the data are missing at random (Steele 2008), and thus have an advantage over regression-based methods (Peters et al. 2012). In ageing research, because of the high mortality rates and the increased likelihood of missing data being non-ignorable, the potential bias induced must be considered (Enders 2011).

Public health implications

There is a growing interest in the policy implications of the accumulating evidence from life approaches in epidemiology and other disciplines that factors across life shape adult health and health differentials (Butland 2007; Barondess 2008a, 2008b; Foresight Mental Capital and Wellbeing Project 2008; Shonkoff et al. 2009; Marmot 2010; Scientific Advisory Committee 2011; Halfon 2012; Shonkoff et al. 2012). Currently, there seems to be more emphasis in the United States on calling for early life interventions, and somewhat more emphasis in the United Kingdom on interventions across life.

In looking for some broad principles on which to base a life course approach, we would suggest that a risk-based model of medicine that starts in midlife is too late. Clearly from a life course perspective we should aim to maximize the level of peak function achieved by maturity as well as modifying the age at onset and rate of functional decline. The primary prevention of risk factors is a priority, coupled with 'earlier, more vigorous and longitudinally maintained management of risk factors' linked to greater integrated care, both vertically and horizontally (Barondess 2008b). This means that in offering individuals help to manage their health, service providers need to take account of prior life and health experiences as well as complex preventive or care needs that cut across clinical specialities, or across health and social domains. Life course interventions to promote adult health and reduce health inequalities need to enable the best early nurturing environments as well as recognizing opportunities to take advantage of later life modifiability, plasticity, and resilience, especially during later biological and social transitions (e.g. during adolescence, pregnancy, becoming a parent, and during the menopausal and retirement transitions).

At the population level, many of the policy implications would appeal to a broad constituency: removing unnecessary physical and social environmental hazards (such as contaminated food) and creating health-promoting neighbourhoods in which individuals live and work must remain priorities. The message from a life course perspective is that these types of improvements to the environment are likely to have long-term as well as short-term health benefits; this can be a difficult message where political interests are often focused on short-term gains. The evidence for these long-term effects will continue to come from observational studies, increasingly using study designs that are more able to confer causal inference, as setting up randomized control trials to study such long-term effects is not practical nor, in many cases, ethical.

Reports that take a life course perspective in recommendations to reduce health inequalities are clearly relevant to this debate. For example, the Marmot Review has six policy objectives for reducing health inequalities: giving every child the best start in life; enabling all children, young people, and adults to maximize their capabilities and have control over their lives; create fair employment and good work for all; ensure a healthy standard of living for all; create and develop healthy and sustainable places and communities; and strengthen the role and impact of ill-health prevention (Marmot 2010). Other UK reports, for example, on mental capital and well-being (Foresight Mental Capital and Wellbeing Project 2008), obesity (Butland 2007; Department of Health 2011), and reproductive health (Scientific Advisory Committee 2011), also champion a life course perspective.

In adulthood, there are risk factors that are common to many later life health outcomes, which have themselves been shaped by exposures and experiences from early life onward. For example, a recent assessment of the risk factors for dementia and cognitive decline (Anonymous 2010) showed the best evidence for midlife obesity, high blood pressure and elevated cholesterol, and smoking. The strongest evidence for modifiable factors that protected against dementia or cognitive decline was for physical activity and moderate alcohol intake; there was also some evidence that following a Mediterranean diet and being socially active were protective. These risk and protective factors are clearly relevant for many other ageing outcomes (Kuh et al. 2014).

The principles and objectives of a life course approach to improve lifelong health and reduce health inequalities may be fairly straightforward to postulate. But designing, implementing, and evaluating effective interventions that operate at one or more key life stages is clearly challenging, as is creating the political will to fund interventions and to implement those that are successful across the wider society, especially during economic recessions (McKee et al. 2012). There is a danger of interventions generating further inequalities; this is more likely in individual-based rather than structural-based interventions (White et al. 2009). Effective interventions require input from those with skills in translation or implementation in population sciences and public health (Ogilvie et al. 2009; Lobb and Colditz 2013), working with researchers and policy and practice stakeholders, and using all types of evidence, from basic science and epidemiology to evaluation, to build a strong evidence base.

Public health in the twenty-first century needs a dynamic and life course concept of health that reflects the 'ability to adapt and self-manage' (Huber et al. 2011) based on resilience to cope and maintain and restore one's integrity, equilibrium, and sense of well-being. The next phase of the life course epidemiology research agenda will be to measure and characterize compensation and adaptation effectively, and investigate how they change over time, their consequences, and life course determinants. Life course epidemiologists need to respond to this challenge, and to the challenge of translating these findings into effective interventions and public health policy.

References

Abraham, S., Collins, G., and Nordsieck, M. (1971). Relationship of childhood weight status to morbidity in adults. *HSMHA Health Reports*, 86, 273–84.

Adair, L.S., Martorell, R., Stein, A.D., et al. (2009). Size at birth, weight gain in infancy and childhood, and adult blood pressure in 5 low- and middle-income-country cohorts: when does weight gain matter? *American Journal of Clinical Nutrition*, 89(5), 1383–92.

Ahlgren, M., Melbye, M., Wohlfahrt, J., et al. (2004). Growth patterns and the risk of breast cancer in women. *The New England Journal of Medicine*, 351(16), 1619–26.

Alwin, D.F. (2012). Integrating varieties of life course concepts. *The Journals of Gerontology Series B Psychological Sciences and Social Sciences*, 67(2), 206–20.

Anonymous (2010). *Your Guide to Reducing the Risk of Dementia*. [Online] Available at: http://news.bbc.co.uk/1/hi/health/8484868.stm.

Austad, S. (2008). Making sense of biological theories of aging. In V.L. Bengston, M. Silverstein, N.M. Putney, and D. Gans (eds.) *Handbook of Theories of Aging* (2nd ed.), pp. 163–78. New York: Springer.

Barker, D.J., Osmond, C., Forsen, T.J., et al. (2005). Trajectories of growth among children who have coronary events as adults. *The New England Journal of Medicine*, 353(17), 1802–9.

Barker, D.J.P. (1990). The fetal and infant origins of adult disease. *British Medical Journal*, 301, 1111.

Barker, D.J.P. (1995). Fetal origins of coronary heart disease. *British Medical Journal*, 311, 171–4.

Barker, D.J.P. (1998). *Mothers, Babies and Health in Later Life* (2nd ed.). Edinburgh: Churchill Livingstone.

Barker, D.J.P., Winter, P.D., Osmond, C., et al. (1989). Weight in infancy and death from ischaemic heart disease. *The Lancet*, ii, 577–80.

Barondess, J.A. (2008a). Toward healthy aging: the preservation of health. *Journal of the American Geriatrics Society*, 56(1), 145–8.

Barondess, J.A. (2008b). Toward reducing the prevalence of chronic disease: a life course perspective on health preservation. *Perspectives in Biology and Medicine*, 51(4), 616–28.

Behncke, S. (2012). Does retirement trigger ill health? *Health Economics*, 21(3), 282–300.

Bengtsson, T. and Lindstrom, M. (2000). Childhood misery and disease in later life: the effects of mortality in old age of hazards experienced in early life, southern Sweden, 1760–1894. *Population Studies*, 54, 263–77.

Ben-Shlomo, Y., Mishra, G., and Kuh, D. (2013). Life course epidemiology. In W. Ahrens and I. Pigeot (eds.) *Handbook of Epidemiology* (2nd ed.), pp. 1521–50. Berlin: Springer.

Ben-Shlomo, Y. and Davey Smith, G. (1991). Deprivation in infancy or adult life: which is more important for mortality risk? *The Lancet*, 337, 530–4.

Ben-Shlomo, Y. and Kuh, D. (2002). A life course approach to chronic disease epidemiology: conceptual models, empirical challenges and interdisciplinary perspectives. *International Journal of Epidemiology*, 31(2), 285–93.

Ben-Shlomo, Y., McCarthy, A., Hughes, R., et al. (2008). Immediate postnatal growth is associated with blood pressure in young adulthood: the Barry Caerphilly Growth Study. *Hypertension*, 52(4), 638–44.

Birnie, K., Cooper, R., Martin, R.M., et al. (2011). Childhood socioeconomic position and objectively measured physical capability levels in adulthood: a systematic review and meta-analysis. *PLoS ONE*, 6(1), e15564.

Boyce, W.T., Sokolowski, M.B., and Robinson, G.E. (2012). Toward a new biology of social adversity. *Proceedings of the National Academy of Sciences of the United States of America*, 109(Suppl. 2), 17143–8.

Brion, M.J., Lawlor, D.A., Matijasevich, A., et al. (2011). What are the causal effects of breastfeeding on IQ, obesity and blood pressure? Evidence from comparing high-income with middle-income cohorts. *International Journal of Epidemiology*, 40(3), 670–80.

Burton, G.J. and Barker, D.J.P. (eds.) (2010). *The Placenta and Human Developmental Programming*. Cambridge: Cambridge University Press.

Butland, B. (2007). *UK Government's Foresight Programme—Tackling Obesities: Future Choices—Project Report*. London: The Government Office for Science.

Clennell, S., Kuh, D., Guralnik, J.M., et al. (2008). Characterisation of smoking behaviour across the life course and its impact on decline in lung function and all-cause mortality: evidence from a British birth cohort. *Journal of Epidemiology and Community Health*, 62(12), 1051–6.

Clouston, S.A.P., Brewster, P., Kuh, D., et al. (2013). The dynamic relationship between physical function and cognition in longitudinal aging cohorts. *Epidemiologic Reviews*, 35(1), 33–50.

Cole, T. (2007). The life course plot in life course analysis. In A. Pickles, B. Maughan, and M. Wadsworth (eds.) *Epidemiological Methods in Life Course Research*, pp. 137–55. Oxford: Oxford University Press.

Cole, T.J., Donaldson, M.D., and Ben-Shlomo, Y. (2010). SITAR—a useful instrument for growth curve analysis. *International Journal of Epidemiology*, 39(6), 1558–66.

Colley, J.R.T., Douglas, J.W.B., and Reid, D.D. (1973). Respiratory disease in young adults: influence of early childhood lower respiratory tract illness, social class, air pollution, and smoking. *British Medical Journal*, 2, 195–8.

Cooper, C., Eriksson, J.G., Forsen, T., et al. (2001). Maternal height, childhood growth and risk of hip fracture in later life: a longitudinal study. *Osteoporosis International*, 12, 623.

Cooper, R., Hardy, R., Aihie, S.A., et al. (2011a). Age and gender differences in physical capability levels from mid-life onwards: the harmonisation and meta-analysis of data from eight UK cohort studies. *PLoS ONE*, 6(11), e27899.

Cooper, R., Mishra, G.D., and Kuh, D. (2011b). Physical activity across adulthood and physical performance in midlife: findings from a British birth cohort. *American Journal of Preventative Medicine*, 41(4), 376–84.

Daniel, R.M., Cousens, S.N., De Stavola, B.L., et al. (2012). Methods for dealing with time-dependent confounding. *Statistics in Medicine*, 32(9), 1584–618.

Davey Smith, G. and Ebrahim, S. (2004). Mendelian randomization: prospects, potentials, and limitations. *International Journal of Epidemiology*, 33(1), 30–42.

Davey Smith, G., Hart, C., Blane, D., et al. (1997). Lifetime socioeconomic position and mortality: prospective observational study. *British Medical Journal*, 314, 547–52.

Davey Smith, G., Leary, S., Ness, A., et al. (2009a). Challenges and novel approaches in the epidemiological study of early life influences on later disease. *Advances in Experimental Medicine and Biology*, 646, 1–14.

Davey Smith, G. and Lynch, J. (2004). Life course approaches to socioeconomic differentials in health. In D. Kuh and Y. Ben-Shlomo (eds.) *A Life Course Approach to Chronic Disease Epidemiology* (2nd ed.), pp. 77–116. Oxford: Oxford University Press.

Davey Smith, G., Sterne, J.A., Fraser, A., et al. (2009b). The association between BMI and mortality using offspring BMI as an indicator of own BMI: large intergenerational mortality study. *British Medical Journal*, 339, b5043.

Deary, I.J. (2012). Looking for 'system integrity' in cognitive epidemiology. *Gerontology*, 58(6), 545–53.

De Stavola, B.L., dos Santos Silva, I., McCormack, V., et al. (2004). Childhood growth and breast cancer. *American Journal of Epidemiology*, 159, 671–82.

De Stavola, B.L., Nitsch, D., dos Santos Silva, I., et al. (2006). Statistical issues in life course epidemiology. *American Journal of Epidemiology*, 163(1), 84–96.

Department of Health (2011). *Healthy Lives, Healthy People: A Call to Action on Obesity in England*. [Online] Available at: https://www.gov.uk/government/publications/healthy-lives-healthy-people-a-call-to-action-on-obesity-in-england.

Didelez, V. and Sheehan, N. (2007). Mendelian randomization as an instrumental variable approach to causal inference. *Statistical Methods in Medical Research*, 16(4), 309–30.

Dwork, D. (1987). *War is Good for Babies and Other Young Children. A History of the Infant and Child Welfare Movement in England 1989–1918*. London: Tavistock.

Enders, C.K. (2011). Analyzing longitudinal data with missing values. *Rehabilitation Psychology*, 56(4), 267–88.

Factor-Litvak, P. and Susser, E. (2004). A life course approach to neuropsychiatric outcomes. In D. Kuh and Y. Ben-Shlomo (eds.) *A Life Course Approach to Chronic Disease Epidemiology* (2nd ed.), pp. 324–45. Oxford: Oxford University Press.

Ferrucci, L. and Studenski, S. (2012). Clinical problems in aging. In D. Longo, A. Fauci, D. Kasper, S. Hauser, J. Jameson, and J. Loscalzo (eds.) *Harrison's Principles of Internal Medicine* (18th ed.), pp. 570–85. New York: McGraw-Hill.

Foresight Mental Capital and Wellbeing Project (2008). *Final Project Report*. London: The Government Office for Science.

Forsdahl, A. (1977). Living conditions in childhood and adolescence and important risk factor for arteriosclerotic heart disease? *British Journal of Preventive and Social Medicine*, 31, 91–5.

Frenkel-Toledo, S., Giladi, N., Peretz, C., et al. (2005). Effect of gait speed on gait rhythmicity in Parkinson's disease: variability of stride time and swing time respond differently. *Journal of Neuroengineering and Rehabilitation*, 2, 23.

Galobardes, B., Lynch, J.W., and Davey Smith, G. (2004). Childhood socioeconomic circumstances and cause-specific mortality in adulthood: systematic review and interpretation. *Epidemiologic Reviews*, 6, 7–21.

Gamborg, M., Andersen, P.K., Baker, J.L., et al. (2009). Life course path analysis of birth weight, childhood growth, and adult systolic blood pressure. *American Journal of Epidemiology*, 169(10), 1167–78.

Gluckman, P., Beedle, A., and Hanson, M. (2009). *Principles of Evolutionary Medicine*. New York: Oxford University Press.

Gluckman, P.D. and Hanson, M.A. (2006). *Developmental Origins of Health and Disease*. Cambridge: Cambridge University Press.

Gluckman, P.D., Hanson, M.A., Bateson, P., et al. (2009). Towards a new developmental synthesis: adaptive developmental plasticity and human disease. *The Lancet*, 373(9675), 1654–7.

Godfrey, K.M., Sheppard, A., Gluckman, P.D., et al. (2011). Epigenetic gene promoter methylation at birth is associated with child's later adiposity. *Diabetes*, 60(5), 1528–34.

Goldstein, H. and Kounali, D. (2009). Multilevel multivariate modelling of childhood growth, numbers of growth measurements and adult characteristics. *Journal of the Royal Statistical Society: Series A (Statistics in Society)*, 172(3), 599–613.

Greenland, S. (2000). An introduction to instrumental variables for epidemiologists. *International Journal of Epidemiology*, 29(4), 722–9.

Greenland, S. and Brumback, B. (2002). An overview of relations among causal modelling methods. *International Journal of Epidemiology*, 31(5), 1030–7.

Greenland, S., Pearl, J., and Robins, J.M. (1999). Causal diagrams for epidemiologic research. *Epidemiology*, 10(1), 37–48.

Halfon, N. (2012). Addressing health inequalities in the US: a life course health development approach. *Social Science & Medicine*, 74(5), 671–3.

Hardy, R., Cooper, R., Sayer, A., et al. (2013). Body mass index, muscle strength and physical performance in older adults from eight cohort studies: the HALCyon programme. *PLoS ONE*, 8(2), e56483.

Hardy, R., Kuh, D., Langenberg, C., et al. (2003). Birth weight, childhood social class and change in adult blood pressure in the 1946 British birth cohort. *The Lancet*, 362, 1178–83.

Hardy, R., Kuh, D., Langenberg, C., et al. (2004). Birth weight, childhood growth and blood pressure at 43 years in a British birth cohort. *International Journal of Epidemiology*, 33, 121–9.

Heijmans, B.T., Tobi, E.W., Stein, A.D., et al. (2008). Persistent epigenetic differences associated with prenatal exposure to famine in humans. *Proceedings of the National Academy of Sciences of the United States of America*, 105(44), 17046–9.

Henderson, J., Granell, R., Heron, J., et al. (2008). Associations of wheezing phenotypes in the first 6 years of life with atopy, lung function and airway responsiveness in mid-childhood. *Thorax*, 63(11), 974–80.

Hernan, M.A., Hernandez-Diaz, S., Werler, M.M., et al. (2002). Causal knowledge as a prerequisite for confounding evaluation: an application to birth defects epidemiology. *American Journal of Epidemiology*, 155(2), 176–84.

Hertzman, C. (2013). Commentary on the symposium: biological embedding, life course development, and the emergence of a new science. *Annual Review of Public Health*, 34, 1–5.

Hertzman, C. and Boyce, T. (2010). How experience gets under the skin to create gradients in developmental health. *Annual Review of Public Health*, 31, 329–47.

Heys, M., Lin, S.L., Lam, T.H., et al. (2013). Lifetime growth and blood pressure in adolescence: Hong Kong's 'children of 1997' birth cohort. *Pediatrics*, 131(1), e62–72.

Huber, M., Knottnerus, J.A., Green, L., et al. (2011). How should we define health? *British Medical Journal*, 343, d4163.

Huxley, R., Neil, A., and Collins, R. (2002). Unravelling the fetal origins hypothesis: is there really an inverse association between birthweight and subsequent blood pressure? *The Lancet*, 360(9334), 659–65.

Huxley, R., Owen, C.G., Whincup, P.H., et al. (2007). Is birth weight a risk factor for ischemic heart disease in later life? *The American Journal of Clinical Nutrition*, 85(5), 1244–50.

Kinra, S., Rameshwar Sarma, K.V., Ghafoorunissa, et al. (2008). Effect of integration of supplemental nutrition with public health programmes in pregnancy and early childhood on cardiovascular risk in rural Indian adolescents: long term follow-up of Hyderabad nutrition trial. *British Medical Journal*, 337, a605.

Kirkwood, T.B. and Austad, S.N. (2000). Why do we age? *Nature*, 408(6809), 233–8.

Koupilova, I., Leon, D.A., McKeigue, P.M., et al. (1999). Is the effect of low birth weight on cardiovascular mortality mediated through high blood pressure? *Journal of Hypertension*, 17(1), 19–25.

Kramer, M.S., Aboud, F., Mironova, E., et al. (2008). Breastfeeding and child cognitive development: new evidence from a large randomized trial. *Archives of General Psychiatry*, 65(5), 578–84.

Krieger, N. (2013). *Epidemiology and the People's Health: Theory and Context*. New York: Oxford University Press.

Kuh, D. and Ben-Shlomo, Y. (1997). *A Life Course Approach to Chronic Disease Epidemiology: Tracing the Origins of Ill-Health from Early to Adult Life*. Oxford: Oxford University Press.

Kuh, D. and Ben-Shlomo, Y. (2004). *A Life Course Approach to Chronic Disease Epidemiology: Tracing the Origins of Ill-Health from Early to Adult Life* (2nd ed.). Oxford: Oxford University Press.

Kuh, D., Ben-Shlomo, Y., Lynch, J., Hallqvist, J., and Power, C. (2003). Life course epidemiology. *Journal of Epidemiology and Community Health*, 57(10), 778–83.

Kuh, D., Cooper, R., Hardy, R., Richards, M., and Ben-Shlomo, Y. (eds.) (2014). *A Life Course Approach to Healthy Ageing*. Oxford: Oxford University Press.

Kuh, D., Cooper, R., Richards, M., Gale, C., von Zglinicki, T., and Guralnik, J. (2012). A life course approach to healthy ageing: the HALCyon programme. *Public Health*, 126(3), 193–5.

Kuh, D. and Davey Smith, G. (1993). When is mortality risk determined? Historical insights into a current debate. *Social History of Medicine*, 6, 101–23.

Kuh, D. and Davey Smith, G. (1997). The life course and adult chronic disease: an historical perspective with particular reference to coronary heart disease. In D. Kuh and Y. Ben-Shlomo (eds.) *A Life Course Approach to Chronic Disease Epidemiology: Tracing the Origins of Ill-Health from Early to Adult Life*, pp. 15–44. Oxford: Oxford University Press.

Kuh, D. and Davey Smith, G. (2004). The life course and adult chronic disease: an historical perspective with particular reference to coronary heart disease. In D. Kuh and Y. Ben-Shlomo (eds.) *A Life Course Approach to Chronic Disease Epidemiology* (2nd ed.), pp. 15–41. Oxford: Oxford University Press.

Kuh, D. and Hardy, R. (2002). *A Life Course Approach to Women's Health*. Oxford: Oxford University Press.

Kuh, D., Hardy, R., Butterworth, S., et al. (2006a). Developmental origins of midlife grip strength: findings from a British cohort study. *Journal of Gerontology: Medical Sciences*, 61A, 702–6.

Kuh, D., Hardy, R., Butterworth, S., et al. (2006b). Developmental origins of midlife physical performance: evidence from a British birth cohort. *American Journal of Epidemiology*, 164, 110–21.

Kuh, D., Power, C., Blane, D., et al. (2004). Socioeconomic pathways between childhood and adult health. In D. Kuh and Y. Ben-Shlomo (eds.) *A Life Course Approach to Chronic Disease Epidemiology* (2nd ed.), pp. 371–95. Oxford: Oxford University Press.

Lawlor, D.A., Ben-Shlomo, Y., and Leon, D.A. (2004). Pre-adult influences on cardiovascular disease. In D. Kuh and Y. Ben-Shlomo (eds.) *A Life Course Approach to Chronic Disease Epidemiology* (2nd ed.), pp. 41–77. Oxford: Oxford University Press.

Lawlor, D.A., Harbord, R.M., Tybjaerg-Hansen, A., et al. (2011). Using genetic loci to understand the relationship between adiposity and psychological distress: a Mendelian randomization study in the Copenhagen General Population Study of 53,221 adults. *Journal of Internal Medicine*, 269(5), 525–37.

Lawlor, D.A. and Hardy, R. (2014). A life course approach to metabolic and vascular function. In D. Kuh, R. Cooper, R. Hardy, M. Richards, and Y. Ben-Shlomo (eds.) *A Life Course Approach to Healthy Ageing*, pp. 146–61. Oxford: Oxford University Press.

Lawlor, D. and Mishra, G. (2009). *Family Matters: Designing, Analysing and Understanding Family Based Studies in Life Course Epidemiology*. Oxford: Oxford University Press.

Lawlor, D.A., Timpson, N.J., Harbord, R.M., et al. (2008). Exploring the developmental overnutrition hypothesis using parental–offspring associations and FTO as an instrumental variable. *PLoS Medicine*, 5(3), e33.

Leary, S.D., Davey Smith, G., Rogers, I.S., et al. (2006). Smoking during pregnancy and offspring fat and lean mass in childhood. *Obesity (Silver Spring)*, 14(12), 2284–93.

Lewis, S.J., Zuccolo, L., Davey Smith, G., et al. (2012). Fetal alcohol exposure and IQ at age 8: evidence from a population-based birth-cohort study. *PLoS One*, 7(11), e49407.

Li, X., Li, S., Ulusoy, E., et al. (2004). Childhood adiposity as a predictor of cardiac mass in adulthood: the Bogalusa Heart Study. *Circulation*, 110(22), 3488–92.

Lobb, R. and Colditz, G.A. (2013). Implementation science and its application to population health. *Annual Review of Public Health*, 34, 235–51.

Macdonald-Wallis, C., Lawlor, D.A., Palmer, T., et al. (2012). Multivariate multilevel spline models for parallel growth processes: application to weight and mean arterial pressure in pregnancy. *Statistics in Medicine*, 31(26), 3147–64.

Marmot, M. (2010). *Fair Society, Healthy Lives: The Marmot Review*. London: UCL Institute of Health Equity.

Marmot, M.G., Shipley, M.J., and Rose, G. (1984). Inequalities in death—specific explanations of a general pattern? *The Lancet*, 5, 1003–6.

Martin, R.M., Gunnell, D., Pemberton, J., et al. (2005). Cohort profile: the Boyd Orr cohort—an historical cohort study based on the 65 year follow-up of the Carnegie Survey of Diet and Health (1937–39). *International Journey of Epidemiology*, 34(4), 742–9.

Mayer, K. (2003). The sociology of the life course and life span psychology: diverging or converging pathways? In U. Staudinger and U. Lindenberger (eds.) *Understanding Human Development: Dialogues with Lifespan Psychology*, pp. 463–81. New York: Kluwer Academic.

McEniery, C.M., Spratt, M., and Munnery, M. (2010). An analysis of prospective risk factors for aortic stiffness in men: 20-year follow-up from the Caerphilly prospective study. *Hypertension*, 56(1), 36–43.

McKee, M., Basu, S., and Stuckler, D. (2012). Health systems, health and wealth: the argument for investment applies now more than ever. *Social Science & Medicine*, 74(5), 684–7.

Mishra, G., Hardy, R., and Kuh, D. (2007). Are the effects of risk factors for timing of menopause modified by age? Results from a British birth cohort study. *Menopause*, 14(4), 717–24.

Mishra, G.D. and Kuh, D. (2012). Health symptoms during midlife in relation to menopausal transition: British prospective cohort study. *British Medical Journal*, 344, e402.

Mishra, G., Nitsch, D., Black, S., et al. (2009). A structured approach to modelling the effects of binary exposure variables over the life course. *International Journal of Epidemiology*, 38(2), 528–37.

Mumby, H.S., Elks, C.E., Li, S., et al. (2011). Mendelian randomisation study of childhood BMI and early menarche. *Journal of Obesity*, 2011, 180729.

Myrskyla, M. (2010). The relative effects of shocks in early- and later-life conditions on mortality. *Population and Development Review*, 36(4), 803–29.

Nagin, D.S. and Odgers, C.L. (2010). Group-based trajectory modeling in clinical research. *Annual Review of Clinical Psychology*, 6, 109–38.

Nagin, D.S. and Tremblay, R.E. (2001). Analyzing developmental trajectories of distinct but related behaviors: a group-based method. *Psychological Methods*, 6(1), 18–34.

Ogilvie, D., Craig, P., Griffin, S., et al. (2009). A translational framework for public health research. *BMC Public Health*, 9, 116.

Pan, H. and Goldstein, H. (1998). Multi-level repeated measures growth modelling using extended spline functions. *Statistics in Medicine*, 17(23), 2755–70.

Peters, S.A., Bots, M.L., den Ruijter, H.M., et al. (2012). Multiple imputation of missing repeated outcome measurements did not add to linear mixed-effects models. *Journal of Clinical Epidemiology*, 65(6), 686–95.

Phelan, J.C., Link, B.G., Diez-Roux, A., et al. (2004). 'Fundamental causes' of social inequalities in mortality: a test of the theory. *Journal of Health and Social Behaviour*, 45(3), 265–85.

Plomin, R. and Daniels, D. (2011). Why are children in the same family so different from one another? *International Journal of Epidemiology*, 40(3), 563–82.

Potischman, N., Troisi, R., and Vatten, L. (2004). A life course approach to cancer epidemiology. In D. Kuh and Y. Ben-Shlomo (eds.) *A Life Course Approach to Chronic Disease Epidemiology* (2nd ed.), pp. 260–81. Oxford: Oxford University Press.

Power, C. and Kuh, D. (2004). Life course development of unequal health. In J. Siegrist and M. Marmot (eds.) *Socioeconomic Position and Health: New Explanations and Their Policy Implications*, pp. 27–54. Oxford: Oxford University Press.

Power, C., Kuh, D., and Morton, S. (2012). Developmental origins of adult disease to life course research on adult disease and aging: insights from birth cohort studies. *Annual Review of Public Health*, 34, 7–28.

Ravelli, A.C.J., van der Meulen, J.H.P., Michels, R.P.J., et al. (1998). Glucose tolerance in adults after prenatal exposure to famine. *The Lancet*, 351, 173–7.

Reid, D.D. (1969). The beginnings of bronchitis. *Proceedings of the Royal Society of Medicine*, 62, 311–16.

Relton, C.L. and Davey Smith, G. (2012). Two-step epigenetic Mendelian randomization: a strategy for establishing the causal role of epigenetic processes in pathways to disease. *International Journal of Epidemiology*, 41(1), 161–76.

Renehan, A.G., Zwahlen, M., Minder, C., et al. (2004). Insulin-like growth factor (IGF)-1, IGF binding protein-3, and cancer risk: systematic review and meta-regression analysis. *The Lancet*, 363, 1346–53.

Richards, M. and Sacker, A. (2003). Lifetime antecedents of cognitive reserve. *Journal of Clinical and Experimental Neuropsychology*, 25(5), 614–24.

Richards, M., Shipley, B., Fuhrer, R., et al. (2004). Cognitive ability in childhood and cognitive decline in mid-life: longitudinal birth cohort study. *British Medical Journal*, 328, 552–4.

Rich-Edwards, J.W., McElrath, T.F., Karumanchi, S.A., et al. (2010). Breathing life into the lifecourse approach: pregnancy history and cardiovascular disease in women. *Hypertension*, 56(3), 331–4.

Rich-Edwards, J.W., Stampfer, M.J., Manson, J.E., et al. (1997). Birth weight and risk of cardiovascular disease in a cohort of women followed up since 1976. *British Medical Journal*, 315(7105), 396–400.

Robins, J.M. (1986). A new approach to causal inference in mortality studies with a sustained exposure period-application to control of the healthy worker survivor effect. *Mathematical Modelling*, 7, 1393–512.

Robins, J.M., Blevins, D., Ritter, G., et al. (1992). G-estimation of the effect of prophylaxis therapy for *Pneumocystis carinii* pneumonia on the survival of AIDS patients. *Epidemiology*, 3(4), 319–36.

Robins, J.M., Hernan, M.A., and Brumback, B. (2000). Marginal structural models and causal inference in epidemiology. *Epidemiology*, 11(5), 550–60.

Rosenbaum, P. and Rubin, D. (1983). The central role of the propensity score in observational studies for causal effects. *Biometrika*, 70(1), 41–55.

Rothwell, P.M., Howard, S.C., Dolan, E., et al. (2010). Prognostic significance of visit-to-visit variability, maximum systolic blood pressure, and episodic hypertension. *The Lancet*, 375(9718), 895–905.

Rutter, M. (1989). Pathways from childhood to adult life. *Journal of Child Psychology and Psychiatry*, 30, 25–51.

Rutter, M. (2012a). Achievements and challenges in the biology of environmental effects. *Proceedings of the National Academy of Sciences of the United States of America*, 109(Suppl. 2), 17149–53.

Rutter, M. (2012b). Resilience as a dynamic concept. *Development and Psychopathology*, 24(2), 335–44.

Rutter, M., Kim-Cohen, J., and Maughan, B. (2006). Continuities and discontinuities in psychopathology between childhood and adult life. *Journal of Child Psychology and Psychiatry*, 47(3–4), 276–95.

Sandhu, J., Davey Smith, G., Holly, J., et al. (2006a). Timing of puberty determines serum insulin-like growth factor-I in late adulthood. *Journal of Clinical Endocrinology and Metabolism*, 91(8), 3150–7.

Sandhu, J., Davey Smith, G., Holly, J., et al. (2006b). Timing of puberty determines serum insulin-like growth factor-I in late adulthood. *Journal of Clinical Endocrinology and Metabolism*, 91(8), 3150–7.

Schooling, M. and Kuh, D. (2002), A life course perspective on women's health behaviours. In D. Kuh and R. Hardy (eds.) *A Life Course Approach to Women's Health*, pp. 279–303. Oxford: Oxford University Press.

Scientific Advisory Committee (2011). *Opinion Paper 27: Why Should We Consider a Life Course Approach to Women's Health Care?* London: Royal College of Obstetricians and Gynaecologists.

Shonkoff, J.P., Boyce, W.T., and McEwen, B.S. (2009). Neuroscience, molecular biology, and the childhood roots of health disparities: building a new framework for health promotion and disease prevention. *The Journal of the American Medical Association*, 301(21), 2252–9.

Shonkoff, J.P., Garner, A.S., The Committee on Psychosocial Aspects of Child and Family Health, et al. (2012). The lifelong effects of early childhood adversity and toxic stress. *Pediatrics*, 129(1), e232–e246.

Silverwood, R., Pierce, M., Thomas, C., et al. (2013). Association between younger age when first overweight and increased risk for CKD. *Journal of the American Society of Nephrology*, 24(5), 813–21.

Silverwood, R.J., De Stavola, B.L., Cole, T.J., et al. (2009). BMI peak in infancy as a predictor for later BMI in the Uppsala Family Study. *International Journal of Obesity*, 33(8), 929–37.

Silverwood, R.J., Nitsch, D., Pierce, M., et al. (2011). Characterizing longitudinal patterns of physical activity in mid-adulthood using latent class analysis: results from a prospective cohort study. *American Journal of Epidemiology*, 174(12), 1406–15.

Singhal, A., Cole, T.J., Fewtrell, M., et al. (2004). Is slower early growth beneficial for long-term cardiovascular health? *Circulation*, 109(9), 1108–13.

Singhal, A., Cole, T.J., and Lucas, A. (2001). Early nutrition in preterm infants and later blood pressure: two cohorts after randomised trials. *The Lancet*, 357, 413–19.

Singh-Manoux, A., Ferrie, J.E., Chandola, T., et al. (2004). Socioeconomic trajectories across the life course and health outcomes in midlife: evidence for the accumulation hypothesis? *International Journal of Epidemiology*, 33(5), 1072–9.

Steele, F. (2008). Multilevel models for longitudinal data. *Journal of the Royal Statistical Society: Series A (Statistics in Society)*, 171(1), 5–19.

Stein, Z., Susser, M., Saenger, G., et al. (1975). *Famine and Human Development. The Dutch Hunger Winter of 1944–45*. New York: Oxford University Press.

Stern, Y. (2002). What is cognitive reserve? Theory and research application of the reserve concept. *Journal of the International Neuropsychological Society*, 8(3), 448–60.

Stringhini, S., Sabia, S., Shipley, M., et al. (2010). Association of socioeconomic position with health behaviors and mortality. *Journal of the American Medical Association*, 303(12), 1159–66.

Syddall, H.E., Sayer, A.A., Dennison, E.M., et al. (2005). Cohort profile: the Hertfordshire Cohort Study. *International Journal of Epidemiology*, 34, 1234–42.

Tilling, K., Davies, N.M., Nicoli, E., et al. (2011a). Associations of growth trajectories in infancy and early childhood with later childhood outcomes. *American Journal of Clinical Nutrition*, 94(Suppl. 6), 1808S–13S.

Tilling, K., Howe, L.D., and Ben-Shlomo, Y. (2011b). Commentary: methods for analysing life course influences on health—untangling complex exposures. *International Journal of Epidemiology*, 40(1), 250–2.

Tu, Y.K., West, R., Ellison, G.T., et al. (2005). Why evidence for the fetal origins of adult disease might be a statistical artifact: the 'reversal paradox' for the relation between birth weight and blood pressure in later life. *American Journal of Epidemiology*, 161(1), 27–32.

Tu, Y.K., Woolston, A., Baxter, P.D., et al. (2010). Assessing the impact of body size in childhood and adolescence on blood pressure: an application of partial least squares regression. *Epidemiology*, 21(4), 440–8.

Vagero, D. and Leon, D. (1994). Ischaemic heart disease and low birth weight: a test of the fetal origins hypothesis from the Swedish town registry. *The Lancet*, 343, 260–2.

Wamala, S.P., Lynch, J., and Kaplan, G.A. (2001). Women's exposure to early and later life socioeconomic disadvantage and coronary heart disease risk: the Stockholm Female Coronary Risk Study. *International Journal of Epidemiology*, 30, 275–84.

Wen, X., Kleinman, K., Gillman, M.W., et al. (2012). Childhood body mass index trajectories: modeling, characterizing, pairwise correlations and socio-demographic predictors of trajectory characteristics. *BMC Medical Research Methodology*, 12, 38.

Whincup, P.H., Kaye, S.J., Owen, C.G., et al. (2008). Birth weight and risk of type 2 diabetes: a systematic review. *Journal of the American Medical Association*, 300(24), 2886–97.

White, M., Adams, J., and Heywood, P. (2009). How and why do interventions that increase health overall widen inequalities within populations? In S. Babones (ed.) *Social Inequality and Public Health*, pp. 65–82. Bristol: The Policy Press.

Wills, A.K., Hardy, R.J., Black, S., et al. (2010). Trajectories of overweight and body mass index in adulthood and blood pressure at age 53: the 1946 British birth cohort study. *Journal of Hypertension*, 28(4), 679–86.

Wills, A.K., Lawlor, D.A., Matthews, F.E., et al. (2011). Life course trajectories of systolic blood pressure using longitudinal data from eight UK cohorts. *PLoS Medicine*, 8(6), e1000440.

Wills, A.K., Lawlor, D.A., Muniz-Terrera, G., et al. (2012). Population heterogeneity in trajectories of midlife blood pressure. *Epidemiology*, 23(2), 203–11.

Wills, A. K. and Tilling, K. (2013). Modelling repeat exposures: some examples from life course epidemiology. In D. Kuh, R. Cooper, R. Hardy, M. Richards, and Y. Ben-Schlomo (eds.) *A Life Course Approach to Healthy Ageing*, pp. 91–108. New York: Oxford University Press.

SECTION 6

Social science techniques

6.1

Sociology and psychology in public health

Stella R. Quah

Introduction to sociology and psychology in public health

The disciplines of sociology and psychology have common links both conceptually and methodologically but they also differ in interesting ways. They differ in overall scope: psychology typically focuses on the individual while sociology examines the individual's social action (agency) and the community's social and physical context (structure) within which they live, interact, work, and play. One important similarity between sociology and psychology is that both disciplines have a dedicated subfield for the study of health and illness. These subfields are, respectively, medical sociology and health psychology. Thus, in line with the objective of this volume, the focus of this chapter is on the contributions to public health by medical sociology and health psychology, the two subfields most relevant to public health.

One plain but important notion about illness runs across the three fields of knowledge, medical sociology, health psychology, and public health. That notion is that infectious disease may begin with one individual but, if left unchecked, it can affect entire continents. This principle was highlighted by a British physician, Southwood Smith, in the nineteenth century. Smith (1866) was alerting the health authorities on the need to investigate and control infectious diseases. By the twenty-first century, sociology and psychology have accumulated a wealth of research on the impact of individual and collective social behaviour on health to show that Southwood Smith's notion applies also to people's behaviour and social conditions associated with non-infectious diseases and, indeed, to health-related phenomena as a whole.

The discussion that follows is presented in four sections: sociology and public health, psychology and public health, the contribution of both disciplines to public health training, and conclusion. The sections on sociology and psychology cover the same three themes: the highlights of their respective theoretical contributions, the main methodological approaches that are relevant to public health, and a succinct summary of areas of research that illustrate the contributions of medical sociology and health psychology to the field of public health. The list of references documents the arguments made in the text and serves as further reading on the historical as well as most current information on what medical sociology and health psychology offer to public health researchers and practitioners.

Sociology in public health

The sociological analysis of health and illness can be traced back to the beginnings of sociology as an area of systematic knowledge in the late 1800s. Sociology's pioneers in Europe investigated the influence of cultural, socioeconomic, and political conditions in the community on individuals' social action. Two of the pioneers were Emile Durkheim (1858–1917) in France and Max Weber (1864–1920) in Germany. In the midst of the development of sociological theorizing, while sociology pioneers were examining the nature and dynamics of society and social action, the spread of infectious diseases was exerting a heavy toll in Europe. The damage caused by epidemics alerted some British and European medical authorities to the possible connection of three phenomena hitherto seen as unrelated by medical experts: social conditions in the community, social behaviour, and public health. Among the first physicians to presume that connection existed were Virchow and Billings. A notable German pathologist, Rudolf Virchow (1812–1902), seen as 'a dominant figure in German medicine' (Shryock 1974, p. 202) was perhaps the first medical scientist who considered medicine as a social science (Elling and Sokołoska 1978, p. 14). John Shaw Billings, an American surgeon and the first publisher of the *Index Medicus*, wrote on the link between 'hygiene and sociology' around 1879 (Shryock 1974, pp. 182–183; Cockerham, 2010b, p. 2). In a 1894 article on the social factors of illness another physician, Charles McIntyre, used for the first time the term 'medical sociology' (Cockerham 2010b, p. 2).

The initial phase of medical sociology was rooted in research by sociologists working in medical academic settings and in public health or biomedical clinical settings (Elling and Sokołoska 1978). Medical sociology research and publications paved the way to the inclusion of medical sociology courses in the medical curriculum at American and British universities after the Second World War (Elling and Sokołoska 1978; Cockerham 2010, pp. 2–3), as I explain later. Some of the signposts of the formalization of medical sociology as a subdiscipline of sociology are the establishment of the Medical Sociology Section of the American Sociological Association in 1959, the Research Committee on Medical Sociology of the International Sociological Association in 1963,[1] and the Medical Sociology Research Network in the British Sociological Association in 1969 (Reid 1976).

Research publications in medical sociology include journal articles and books. Among the most important domain-specific international refereed journals are the *Journal of Health and Social Behaviour* (*JHSB*), the dedicated medical sociology journal of the American Sociological Association; *Social Science & Medicine* (*SSM*); *Sociology of Health and Illness*; and *Health Sociology Review*, the journal of the Health Sociology Section of the Australian Sociological Association. There are several textbooks in medical sociology; one of the most established is Cockerham's (2010b), already in its 11th edition. Among serial books is the *New Blackwell Companion to Medical Sociology* (with editions published in 2001, 2005, and 2010) and the *Handbook of Medical Sociology* (HMS). The first edition of the HMS was published in 1963 (Freeman et al. 1963) and it discussed 'the *potential* of the sociological enterprise for understanding the etiology, diagnosis, and treatment of diseases; the ways health care is provided and funded; the societal and communal commitment to the support of health activities; and, indeed, the very definitions of health and illness'. Looking back at the first three editions of 1963, 1972, and 1979, the editors of the fourth edition wrote that, 'the promise of medical sociology [is now] replaced by hard evidence as to its utility' (Freeman and Levine 1989, p. 1). These authors correctly pointed out that medical sociology uses the full range of sociological theories and methodologies (1989, p. 7).

In concert with the increase in research and publications by the 1980s, medical sociologists were also 'actively involved in public health programs, and. . . accredited schools of public health in the United States were required to provide formal training in the social and behavioral sciences' (Coreil 2008, p. 102) and there were calls to increase medical sociology input in the training of public health practitioners not only in the United States (Gordon and McFarlane 1996) but also in Canada (Massé and Moloughney 2011) and elsewhere. I return to this issue later.

Sociological theories and public health

Historically, the twin theoretical roots of sociology are philosophy and science as they developed in the seventeenth and eighteenth centuries in Europe with the writings of thinkers such as Charles Montesquieu (1689–1755) and Jean Jacques Rousseau (1712–1778) on social forces, power, and social facts; Immanuel Kant (1724–1804) on the systematic analysis of cause and effect; and Henri de Saint-Simon (1760–1825) about industry, the need for social reforms, and the scientific study of society and social life. Philosophers such as René Descartes (1596–1650), Thomas Hobbes (1588–1679), and John Locke (1632–1704) aimed at 'grand, general, and very abstract systems of ideas that made rational sense', but other thinkers were more concerned with testing those ideas against their 'real world' experiences or more specifically, 'to combine empirical research with reason' following the path of science (Ritzer 1992, pp. 6–11). The latter trend 'led to the application of the scientific method to social issues' seeking to identify possible laws governing social behaviour just as Newtonian physics demonstrated that physical laws rule the physical world (Ritzer 1992, pp. 10–11). This embryonic tension and subsequent symbiosis between the two approaches—a purely theoretical outlook vis-à-vis the imperative to test assumptions empirically—remain at the core of sociology as a field of knowledge today.

Sociology grew from those early ideas into a distinct discipline in the context of wide-ranging social change. Two founding fathers of the discipline were born at the time of the Industrial Revolution and the rise of capitalism in the nineteenth century.

The first was the French thinker August Comte (1798–1857) who contributed his treatise on a new discipline that he labelled 'sociology' and envisaged it as the systematic analysis of society following the model of physics. The second pioneer thinker was Comte's compatriot Emile Durkheim (1858–1917), who promoted the symbiosis of theory and empirical research. Durkheim paid particular attention to, on the one hand, the study of disorder, conflict and its consequences in society; and on the other hand, to the importance of social facts for the study and planning of social reform to reduce social disorder. Durkheim 'legitimized sociology in France' (Ritzer 1992, p. 17). Durkheim's treatise on the systematic analysis of social facts and his study of social factors associated with suicide are seminal works in sociology. Two of Durkheim's most influential books are *Suicide* (1897/1951), demonstrating the link between individual behaviour and society's socioeconomic conditions, and *The Rules of Sociological Method* (1895/1964). Durkheim's emphasis on both sociological theory and empirical research paved the way for today's evidence-based research. His conceptual contribution on the notions of 'the socially *normal* and *abnormal*' set the path for 'twentieth century medical sociology' along 'the enlightenment inspired *normal/pathological* bifurcation in medicine' (Thomas 2012, p. 216).

Two other pioneers in sociology were German: Georg Simmel (1858–1918) and Max Weber (1864–1920). Simmel and Weber were cofounders of the German Sociological Society. Simmel's key contribution is his notion of reciprocity and uncertainty in social interaction (Gerhardt 1989, p. 17). Max Weber's theory of social action, authority systems, and bureaucratization, are among many other seminal contributions in his large body of work, and form part of the foundation of contemporary sociology (Ritzer 1992, pp. 25–29). Among Weber's contributions is his ground-breaking theory of social action and social systems (1921/1968), a classical theory in sociology. In medical sociology, Weber's conceptual contributions are applied to a wide range of studies including, for example, the analysis of the bureaucratization of healthcare systems and organisations (Fox 1989; Germov 2005), the analysis of power and authority of the medical profession (Starr 1982; Freidson 1988); and the impact of life chances and lifestyle on health-related behaviour (Cockerham 2010b).

The body of theory in sociology has grown exponentially over the past century. Sociological theories may be classified into two types: general theories that address all human behaviour and have 'universal' applicability; and 'middle-range' theories that have limited applicability. The most relevant general theories for the sociological analysis of health and illness are: structural-functional theory, symbolic interactionism, conflict theory, and phenomenology/ethnomethodology. Given the space constraints of this chapter, only the general theories are discussed.

The structural-functional theory (now neo-functionalism) is the contribution of American sociologist Talcott Parsons (1937). This theory addresses societies as social systems and proposes that all components of society whether they are individuals, groups, communities, nations, or global organizations, have functions—both manifest and latent—for their maintenance and growth. The dominant trend in social organizations, groups, and social interactions is the maintenance of balance or equilibrium. Consequently, conflict is considered dysfunctional to the development of organizations and social relationships, and dysfunctions need to be rectified or balanced through normative values and the correction of unanticipated consequences of action (Ritzer 1992). Parsons (1937) approached the analysis of health-related phenomena from the perspective of structural-functionalist systems theory, offering two 'models of illness': the 'deviance' model and the 'sick-role' or 'capacity' model, both of which incorporate the micro- and macro-levels of the social structure. The 'deviance' model presents illness as a state of dependency for the person affected whereby therapy is expected but seen as a social control system and the physician as an agent of social control. The 'capacity' model proposes that illness is a breakdown of normality leading to the individual's total or partial incapacity to perform normal social roles, and brings the person into the 'sick-role'. The sick-role is a social position with different rights and obligations within the social structure that includes the doctor–patient interaction and the doctor's role with specific rights and obligations (Parsons 1937; Gerhardt 1989, pp. 1–67).

The second influential general theory is symbolic interactionism. It proposes that the individual's subjective perception of the situation through meanings and symbols has a significant impact on his/her behaviour. In contrast to structural-functionalism that is predominantly associated with one theorist—Talcott Parsons—symbolic interactionism represents the conceptual contributions of several theorists and offers two models of illness: the 'labelling' model and the 'negotiation' or 'crisis' model. The labelling model proposes that illness may be socially defined or labelled through a process of normative evaluation. Correspondingly, the negotiation model proposes that patients have control over their illness through negotiation: diagnoses and treatments by the medical profession may be negotiated and treatment involves the patient's active participation (Gerhardt 1989, pp. 73–173). Some analysts consider symbolic interactionism as playing an important part in current medical sociology through qualitative methodological designs such as participant observation (Cockerham and Scambler 2010, p. 8).

Conflict theory is the third general sociological theory of relevance for public health. It proposes that the potential for conflict is a normal component of social relationships, thus, negotiation and bargaining are key elements of social interaction. When applied to health phenomena, conflict theory offers two models, the 'loss' or 'stress' model and the 'domination–deprivation' model. The 'loss' or 'stress' model proposes that there is a strong connection between stress and illness; the loss of required social support increases the likelihood of illness; and vulnerability to illness is unequally distributed in society. The body of sociological research on the stress–illness connection was initiated in the 1950s and continues growing today (Pearlin 1989; Thois 2010). The 'domination–deprivation' model argues that the medical profession occupies a dominant position in society by virtue of its expertise vis-à-vis the patient's position of dependence given the patient's lack of specialized knowledge. The domination–deprivation model is also applied to the analysis of social inequality and socioeconomic deprivation in society (Gerhardt 1989, pp. 249–348). Conflict theory as a school of thought has been particularly influential in the analysis of health policy: 'one of conflict theory's most important assets for medical sociology [is] the capacity to explain the politics associated with health reform' (Cockerham and Scambler 2010, p. 10).

A fourth theoretical position is that of phenomenology/ethnomethodology which proposes, as Ritzer (1992, p. 388) summarizes it, that 'people are the product of the very society they create'. This phenomenology model regards illness as belonging to 'a broad category of disturbing occurrences. . . which breach the taken-for-granted peace of everyday routines' (Gerhardt, 1989, p. 190). Compared to the other theories, and particularly, to the abundance of empirical research generated by the other three conceptual orientations—structural-functionalism, symbolic interactionism, and conflict theory—the phenomenology/ethnomethodology school of thought has contributed relatively less to empirical research in medical sociology (Cockerham and Scambler 2010).

Sociological research relevant to public health

At the most abstract level, there are two distinctive contributions of medical sociology to the study of health and illness in general and public health in particular. The first contribution is the systematic examination of the link between individual and community and 'the social organizational factors that shape the behaviour of groups' (Thorlindsson 2011, p. 21). The second main contribution is 'that health care systems are organizations . . . embedded within larger institutions, which have been shaped by historical precedents and operate within a specific cultural context' (Quadagno 2010). Medical sociology research relevant to public health can be found within the framework of these two key contributions. The most significant social aspects that exemplify the link between individuals and groups in the context of public health are cultural and social class influences on health-related behaviour of individuals and communities; lifestyles; and the creation and transformation of healthcare systems. Cultural values rooted in ethnic and religious ethos together with social class differences shape people's beliefs and attitudes on health and illness and their lifestyles. Healthcare systems originate, develop and change as part of the interplay of socioeconomic, cultural, and political factors. Let us discuss each of these aspects—culture, lifestyle, social class, and health systems—in more detail.

Culture and public health

Culture is a key term that refers to values and beliefs emanating from one's ethnic and/or religious ethos, typically transmitted across generations as part of the community's identity or 'design for living'. In addition to the influence of the physical and socioeconomic environment on the risk of infectious diseases (Armelagos and Harper 2010) and chronic illness (Charmaz and Rosenfeld 2010), the impact of culture on public health is manifold and it is manifested in at least three main ways: health behaviour, that is, what people do regarding health risks; health attitudes and beliefs, that is, how people feel and think about health and illness; and people's perceptions of and responses to health authorities' public health guidelines and recommendations (Fox 1989; Quah 2007a, 2007b, 2010). Perhaps the best example of this threefold impact is the influence of cultural and/or religious norms and traditions on people's food preparation and diet. Irrespective of what public health authorities advise on food consumption (Harvey 2008, p. 62), ethnic and/or religious groups differ in this regard as they tend to follow their traditionally sanctioned diet, such as vegetarian cuisine, avoidance of pork, the use of animal fat or refined vegetable oils in food preparation, or the avoidance of fried food at all; preferred beverages; and level of sugar consumption, among other aspects (Seow 2008, p. 193; Cockerham 2010b, pp. 29–32; Idler 2010).

Cultural norms and traditions also guide people's preference for some types of health services over others. For example, cultural healing traditions such as traditional Chinese medicine and Ayurveda represent, respectively, essential aspects of Chinese and Indian cultures and thus the population's preference for and use of these therapeutic practices must be taken into consideration in public health policy (Quah 2003, 2008; Etkin et al. 2008).

Yet another contribution of medical sociology research on the impact of culture on public health and the wider healthcare system is the analysis of the provision of healthcare from two perspectives: the micro-cosmos of clinician–patient interaction, and its permutation into the macro-cosmos of the interaction of health authorities with communities and groups. Two examples suffice. It has been found that social stereotypes held by practitioners (whether clinicians or public health practitioners) distort clinical decisions and interactions with their subjects of care and lead to linking 'certain diagnoses to certain patients' (Smith et al. 2012, p. 162). The second example is a related version of the latter phenomenon: the impact of 'medical constructs', that is, when a physical or mental condition is defined by the health authorities 'as a "disease"' while the same condition is considered normal by the community or at least not a condition that requires medical attention. When this clash of the expert versus lay interpretations occur, the official classification 'has consequences for the social legitimacy of the symptoms, access to treatment, and costs to the health care system' (Conrad and Barker 2010; Rosich and Hankin 2010, p. S4). One illustration of this problem from the field of epidemic prevention is the opposition to mandatory culling of poultry or livestock by some farming communities who fail to appreciate the connection between disease and the destruction of what for them are healthy farm animals and their families' source of livelihood (Quah 2007a).

Lifestyle and health

Medical sociology research provides evidence of another significant influence—related to but distinct from culture—on what people do about health risks: their lifestyle. Cockerham, (2010a, p. 159) defines health lifestyles as 'collective patterns of health-related behaviour based on choices from options available to people according to their life chances'. Life chances is a concept proposed by Max Weber (1968) to represent choices, that is, opportunities and constraints imposed on individuals by their relative position in society. People's lifestyle shapes their patterns of leisure and physical activity: some people have no time for leisure; others are sedentary or engaged in extreme sports; some frequent gyms as networking and thus do regular exercise; others are regularly involved in alcohol drinking, cigarette smoking, and/or hard drugs consumption. Likewise, a person's lifestyle is associated with the risk of serious injuries and the likelihood of contracting infectious diseases. Consequently, it is not surprising to find persistent differences in morbidity and mortality across ethnic groups that are basically of social rather than biological or genetic origin (Krieger 1987; Link and Phelan 1995; Anderson and Whyte 2008; Williams and Sternthal 2010). Considering that lifestyles vary for men and women particularly in Asia, gender differences are clearly discernible in morbidity and mortality figures

(Quah 2011). The importance of culture for public health policy and practice is becoming better recognized and has led some analysts to recommend that public health practitioners be equipped with 'cultural competence' (Perez and Luquis 2008; Waters et al. 2008).

A person's lifestyle is shared and reinforced by his/her social network. Medical sociology research demonstrates the active link between social relationships—also known as social ties—on the one hand, and health behaviours and outcomes on the other hand (Umberson and Montez 2010). Social ties and social networks significantly influence health-related behaviour leading to obesity, cigarette smoking, 'recreational' drug use, and alcohol consumption, among other risk behaviours (Cockerham 2010a; Jones et al. 2011). However, while the most visible influence of social networks on health is negative, social networks can be mobilized in public health policy for the promotion of healthy habits and health risk-avoidance in the community (Mechanic and Tanner 2007; Umberson and Montez 2010; Brown et al. 2011).

Social class, social stratification, and public health

Social class, a fundamental sociological construct, depicts the relative position of an individual in the social hierarchical system of prestige in his/her society (Weber 1968). In sociological research, a person's social class—socioeconomic status or SES—is ascertained by means of a composite index of three or more indicators, the most common of which are personal income level, years of formal education completed, and occupational prestige.[2] The resultant SES scores may be used as a continuous scale (usually standardized scores ranging from 0 to 100) or as a set of discrete categories based on the arithmetic mean and standard deviation. The simplest presentation of SES scores is a three-level description of lower class, middle class, and upper class. However, quantitative and continuous SES scores are preferred in sociological studies of class differences and patterns of stratification in society (Bendix and Lipset 1966; Nam and Powers 1983; Phelan et al. 2010).

The nearly universal phenomenon of social class differences influencing the person's access to and utilization of healthcare services is supported by sociological research findings: the higher a person's social class, the greater his/her access to healthcare services (Heggenhougen and Quah 2008; Lahelma 2010; Rosich and Hanki 2010; Brown et al. 2011). A country's socioeconomic conditions lead to 'persistent health inequalities among social groups' (Rosich and Hankin 2010), inequalities which normally are 'deeply rooted in society' (Phelan et al. 2010). Research findings indicate that social class reinforces the influence of lifestyle on health behaviour. However, under certain conditions, social class—mostly due to the influence of education and occupation—may have a stronger impact than cultural beliefs and norms on health behaviour, on access to health services, and on a person's exposure to occupational hazards. Indeed, workers have differential exposure to dangerous repetitive tasks, risk of industrial accidents, and environmental pollution, among other health risks embedded in the nature of the job. Consequently, sociologists examine the health impact of each SES component separately: occupational prestige, income level and educational level as well as the strength of SES as a predictor of health behaviour.

The influence of social class on health status, health behaviour, access to and use of health services, is one of the earliest and most examined social influences on health. Summarizing the advances of medical sociology in the study of social class and health in the last fifty years, Phelan et al. (2010, p. S29) report that their data support 'the theory of fundamental causes'. This theory states that social class 'influences multiple disease outcomes. . . through multiple risk factors'; impacts 'access to resources that can be used to avoid risks or minimize the consequences of disease once it occurs'; and that those influences tend to persist over time. Their research findings support the theory and have implications for public health policy that are different from results in studies applying 'an individually oriented risk-factor approach'. Thus, these authors recommend that social class-induced health inequalities 'can be reduced by instituting health interventions that automatically benefit individuals irrespective of their own resources or behaviors' (Phelan et al. 2010, p. S37).

Two additional contributions of the sociological study of occupations and professions that increase our understanding of health and illness in society are the analysis of occupational hazards and the role of the medical profession. On the one hand, the comparative analysis of health outcomes, disease prevalence and disease incidence across the wide spectrum of occupations in society consistently reveals clear variations derived mainly from the nature of work performed and occupational hazards (see, e.g. Christ et al. 2012). On the other hand, sociologists also examine the biomedical profession and traditional healing occupations in terms of their relative prestige, their training, internal composition and dynamics, and their impact on the health of populations (e.g. Starr 1982; Freidson 1988; Quah 2003, 2008). Research findings indicate that the ideal trust-based and confidential doctor–patient relationship is corporatized today as the medical profession is overwhelmed by 'the healthcare industry' dominated by employers' 'guidelines, pre-authorization, centralization and financial awards for increased output' (Starr 1982; Freidson 1988; Timmermans and Oh 2010; Vanderminden and Potter 2010, pp. 356–7).

Healthcare systems and public health

In addition to the analysis of the impact of culture and social class on public health, another illustration of the contributions of medical sociology is the study of the nature, dynamics, and evolution of healthcare systems at the national and transnational level. When sociologists study healthcare systems they include the approaches taken by nation-states towards the creation, organization, distribution, and management of their healthcare resources. Thus, health policy and healthcare reform are integral parts of this type of studies. Some cross-national and comparative research findings on healthcare systems suggest that in many countries today 'too much priority has been given to hospital care at the expense of the development of primary care, community care and public health' (Stevens 2010, p. 435).

One of several aspects of healthcare systems that have received increased attention by medical sociologists in the past decade is the analysis of flaws in health systems that distort the link between cost and utilization of health services, thus the urgency of healthcare reform (Mechanic and McAlpine 2010). One sector of the healthcare system that has a significant input in healthcare costs is the role of stakeholders such as the pharmaceutical industry in the promotion of medicalization, particularly through the use of market opportunities and marketing methods to sell their products (Rosich and Hankin 2010, pp. S4–S5).

Another illustration of medical sociology analyses of health systems is the area of health services research. There is a vast literature of studies documenting the influence of social class and ethnic differences on unequal access to and utilization of health services. Three types of studies illustrate this research area. The first type of study shows that unequal access to healthcare services is preserved by institutions and policies that constrain and enable 'the actions of health services organizations, health care providers, and consumers' (Wright and Perry 2010, p. S109). Those studies of multiple dysfunctions of health systems challenge international policymakers and are the subject of social policy interventions based on social science research such as the Disease Control Priorities Project jointly conducted by the World Health Organization, the US National Institutes of Health, and the World Bank (Laxminarayan et al. 2006). The second type of health systems research study is the comparative analysis of health financing approaches and systems in terms of their suitability to the socioeconomic needs and demographic characteristics of the population. One example of this type of research is the study of insurance plans by Zaslavsky and Epstein (2005). The third type of study represents the direct input of medical sociologists on public policy; one recent example is the analysis of changes in state regulations on the collection and access to health relevant population data for research purposes (Hynes 2011).

In addition to the relevance of the analysis of culture, lifestyle, social class, and social systems for public health, medical sociology also examines the interaction of these and other factors in the analysis of disease incidence and prevalence in the community. For example, Anderson et al. (2011, p. 390) found that 'social, cultural, and biological issues should all be considered in the assessment of differences in breast cancer survival'. Brown et al. (2011, p. 941) discuss the relevance of social factors in the diagnosis and management of obesity, diabetes, and asthma. A wealth of studies on the social factors of disease is found in medical sociology journals mentioned earlier such as *JHSB*, *SSM*, and *Sociology of Health and Illness* and numerous other international refereed journals on health research.

Sociological research methods and public health

Medical sociology applies the full range of sociological approaches and methodological tools to the study of socioeconomic, cultural, and demographic characteristics of populations and individuals that impact their health (Rosich and Hankin 2010; Smith et al. 2012). Indeed, referring to the analysis of epidemics and health behaviour in general, Hedges et al. (2002) argue that 'social science knowledge in theory and methodology has guided public health research for several decades'. One illustration of this influence is the application of sociological approaches to the analysis of income inequality and health in most of the articles compiled in the book on that topic by Kawachi et al. (1999).

The fundamental position of sociology in general, and medical sociology in particular, regarding scientific research is well articulated by Vogt (2007, p. 5) when he highlights the critical tasks of collecting and analysing evidence for the purpose of creating knowledge. In this regard, there is clear compatibility between the goals of research in both fields of knowledge, medical sociology, and public health. Still, there are three important characteristics of sociological research methodology that must be taken into consideration: (1) the kinds of data used in sociology, (2) the levels of measurement applied, and (3) the types of research design followed. Let us consider each characteristic in turn.

What kinds of data are used in sociology? Two kinds of evidence or data are used: *primary* and *secondary* data. Primary data are data collected first-hand by the investigator, for example, data on people's attitudes and behaviour obtained through personal interviews, observation, experiments, or surveys; or data extracted by means of first-hand analyses of documents, letters, records, or other types of 'raw' data. In contrast, secondary data are data previously collected by others, for example, official statistics, population censuses, or databases with processed or coded data sets from surveys or completed studies. Many research institutions keep databases of secondary data, usually codified data from survey research studies that can be purchased by other researchers together with the respective codebook for secondary and longitudinal analyses (Miller and Salkind 2002, pp. 346–53). Many data archives are now accessible online.

What levels of measurement are used in sociology? Sociological research uses four levels of measurement: nominal, ordinal, interval, and ratio levels. The most rudimentary is the *nominal* level which uses names or labels to depict different categories of the phenomenon under study (e.g. the labels 'male' and 'female' to record a subject's gender; the labels 'Muslim', 'Hindu', 'Christian', 'other religion' and 'no religion', to record the subject's religious affiliation). Each name or category may be assigned a numerical code but the numbers have no quantitative meaning, they are only labels. *Ordinal* measurement assigns ranks to categories of the observed phenomenon (example: 'slender', 'plump', 'obese' to record body appearance) but 'the distances between ranks in an ordinal scale are not necessarily equal'. *Interval* measurement uses ranks with a standard and measurable distance between categories but 'have no meaningful zero point'. The typical illustration of an interval level of measurement is the Fahrenheit temperature scale. A common sociological example is the range of a person's attitudes towards a problem or situation. Here are two sociological interview questions that illustrate the *interval* scale: 'Would you say you are very confident, only slightly confident, slightly anxious, or very anxious about what needs to be done to handle the patient?'; 'How would you rate your quality of life? "Very poor", "Poor", "Neither poor nor good", "Good", or "Very good"?' Yet another illustration of interval scales is the questionnaire used for the analysis of people's 'quality of life' comprising the Quality of Life scale by the World Health Organization (2004). The interval scale is more accurate than the nominal or ordinal levels of measurement, but less precise than the *ratio* scale that has both 'equal intervals between categories and a true zero point' (Vogt 2007, pp. 9–10). Examples of ratio scales in sociology are: the measurement of the subject's age in years, income in dollars earned per month, formal education in number of years of completed schooling, number of children, and years of marriage.

What types of research designs are used in sociology? Depending on the nature of the phenomena under investigation and on the investigator's preferred level of measurement, sociologists may use qualitative or quantitative designs or a combination of both. Researchers who have a preference for qualitative research tend to steer clear of measurement altogether or use only nominal levels of measurement. Some of the most common qualitative research designs are participant and non-participant observation of social phenomena, and conversations with research subjects individually or in small groups (Schwartz and Jacobs 1979). One modality of the small-group method is the focus group approach whereby the researcher, acting as moderator, gathers together a small group of people—preferably not acquainted with each other—to discuss a particular topic. The focus group method is probably the weakest approach and it should be used with extreme caution and perhaps only in exploratory research, due to its three most serious limitations: (1) considering that the conversation is public, that is, in front of strangers, the researcher cannot guarantee confidentiality to the focus group participants, but confidentiality is an important component of informed consent required when conducting research with human subjects (Citro et al. 2003); (2) the validity and reliability of data collected in focus group discussions are low or non-existent; and (3) focus group participants are typically influenced by social pressure given the dynamics of small-group interactions.

In contrast to qualitative designs, a quantitative research design may involve all four levels of measurement but mostly interval and ratio levels of measurement of social phenomena. Similarly, a quantitative research design may include one or more methods of data collection: document analysis, observation, personal interviews with structured or unstructured questionnaires, surveys, experiments or quasi-experiments (Boudon 1993, pp. 158–71; Vogt 2007, pp. 8–10). Naturally, as it happens in all fields of knowledge, research methods have their limitations and researchers need to consider the suitability of the methods selected and take steps to reduce as much as possible the probability of error. With the objective of error reduction in mind, medical sociologists may use in the same study a combination of methods from the array available: participant and non-participant observation; in-depth unstructured interviews; and structured interviews using questionnaires with a variety of question formats, from open-ended questions to attitudinal scales. Structured questionnaires are usually the main instrument of data collection in survey research. Survey research is a methodological design in sociology created by Paul Lazarsfeld (Boudon 1993). A prominent sociologist, Paul Lazarsfeld (1901–1976) identified three phases in the history of surveys. The earliest phase was before 1930, when surveys were used for 'the collection of factual information which could help to improve social conditions'. The second phase covered the period 1930 to 1948 when surveys were used to collect data on public opinion and consumer preferences. The third phase, from 1949 onwards, started with the publication of the seminal sociological study *The American Soldier* when the survey method became an important sociological tool for the collection of 'a large body of data' that could be 'made coherent and meaningful by careful statistical analysis' (Lazarsfeld 1968, pp. vii–x; Boudon 1993).

Sociologists using quantitative research methods aim to ascertain and reduce the level of error in the calculation of correlations among phenomena and in inferences drawn from representative samples to the total population (inferential type I and type II errors). This objective is facilitated by the application of statistical analysis models ranging in complexity and sophistication from simple measures of association such as chi-square, Pearson's coefficient, analysis of variance (ANOVA) and path analysis, to multilevel models such as ordinal logistic regression, structural equation modelling, and hierarchical linear modelling, among others. Examples of some of the most recent medical sociology studies applying multilevel models are: the impact of alcohol drinking on academic performance of secondary school students (Crosnoe et al. 2012), perceived discrimination and health among adolescents and young adults (Grollman 2012), the influence of social networks in the management of hypertension (Cornwell and Waite 2012), and factors leading to sleep disturbance among US adults (Ailshire and Burgard 2012).

Another important aspect of sociological research that must be mentioned is the commitment that mainstream sociology shares with all other fields of scientific research: to pay serious attention to data validity and reliability. Reliability means consistency in the measurement: getting the same results every time the phenomenon is measured with the same instrument. The relation between validity and reliability is important: a reliable instrument may have low validity (Vogt 2007, p. 118). Validity has two general dimensions: internal and external. Internal validity focuses on the research question. The most elementary form of internal validity is content validity and it addresses the question: is the instrument measuring what it intends to measure or something else? There are two additional types of internal validity: criterion-related validity and construct validity. The second dimension is external validity; that is, 'the potential for a study's findings to be generalized from one setting to others' (Burchett et al. 2011, p. 238).

This brings us to the matter of sampling. From the perspective of public health, perhaps one of the most relevant methodological features of sociology, and in particular, medical sociology, is the study of population trends through the analysis of representative samples, also known as probability samples. A representative sample is a sample drawn from the target population following a procedure that gives each individual in the target population the same probability of being selected. Probability samples allow the researcher to make inferences to the total population while non-probability samples do not. The application of inferential statistical tests such as chi-square, t-test, and ANOVA indicate the probability that what was found in the sample does not reflect the situation in the population but it is due to chance or sampling error (Neuman 2000, p. 217; Vogt 2007, p. 12).

On the matter of sampling, two caveats are in order. The first caveat is that there are research topics and research situations for which random sampling is impossible to obtain or is unsuitable. This is the case of health conditions socially seen as stigmatizing, or deviant, so that the affected subjects and/or their families refuse participation in the study; or there is no comprehensive and reliable record of all members of the target population that could be used as the sampling frame to draw a random sample. In situations like these, the researcher may opt for a non-probability sample.

The 'purposive sample' is one form of non-probability sample whereby subjects are selected based on specific criteria, rather than randomly (Vogt 2007, p. 81). Naturally, non-probability samples preclude any inferences to the total population as only a probability sample has external validity (Vogt 2007, p. 82).

The second caveat is on the size of the sample. Besides the options of representative or purposive sampling of large populations, there is also the case study approach whereby the researcher studies only one or a few 'cases' of the social phenomenon under investigation. This approach is useful in at least two ways. First, in emergency situations, a case study may be conducted when rapid information about a condition is required, for example, the case study of a person or a family affected by a rare or 'new' illness that may be potentially contagious; or a unique event that could seriously affect large numbers of people. Second, in non-emergency situations, a case study approach is commonly used in exploratory research: that is in situations where the social phenomenon is new or never studied before and the researchers wish to familiarize themselves with the nature of the phenomenon in order to plan a more comprehensive and systematic study (Ragin and Becker 1992).

Psychology in public health

It is generally agreed that the discipline of psychology was born in the late nineteenth century (Norcross and Karpiak 2012) as a continuation of the discovery of 'the neurophysiological location of psychological faculties' among other advances in the study of the human body (Greenwood 2009). The period 1890–1910 was particularly fruitful for the discipline: it produced the seminal book *Principles of Psychology* by American William James in 1890, and Sigmund Freud's *Die Traumdeutung* published in 1900, often deemed as the framework of psychoanalysis and of Freud's subsequent studies of the thread linking personality, mind, and illness (Friedman 2002).

Just as the subfield of medical sociology plays an important role within the discipline of sociology, the most relevant area of specialization in psychology for public health is health psychology (Luecken and Gallo 2008). Health psychology is also referred to by some analysts as clinical psychology or clinical health psychology (Boyer and Paharia 2008), and as a distinct and growing subfield (Romanow and Marchildon 2003). Health psychology has a relatively recent history (Albery and Munafò 2008). Introducing his *Health Psychology* textbook, Howard S. Friedman wrote that although health psychology has 'its roots in the fields of medical sociology. . . public health' and other fields, 'until the late 1970s, there were no programs of study in health psychology' (Friedman 2002, p. 23). The formal introduction of health psychology as a subdiscipline of psychology is highlighted by three chronological signposts: 1974 when health psychology was first proposed as a new subject in the curriculum at the University of California–San Francisco School of Medicine; 1977 when Health Psychology was approved as a new division of the American Psychological Association; and 1984 when the 'First International Symposium of Health Psychology' was held (Stone 1991, p. 3). As Friedman reports, the number of health psychologists has been growing rapidly not only in the United States but in many other countries (2002, p. 23).

However, until about one decade ago health psychology had traditionally 'maintained. . . a pronounced unidimensional focus on mental health' (Arnett 2001, p. 38). Arnett argued that the field of health psychology 'would be significantly enhanced by a more comprehensive understanding of the epidemiology, pathophysiology, and natural history of the wide range of health disorders amenable to psychological interventions' (Arnett 2001, 43). Among the health areas that Arnett suggested could be studied by health psychology—in addition to mental health—are weight control, and addictions to alcohol, nicotine, and hard drugs (Arnett 2001, p. 41). Health psychology has developed significantly since the 1970s although at different paces in different countries. Sweden is seen as a pioneer based on the development of 'psychophysiology of stress at the Karolinska Institute in Stockholm' in the early 1970s (Stone 1991, p. 9).

Psychological theories and public health

One of the best known names in the history of psychology is Sigmund Freud (1859–1939). Freud was trained as a physician. He launched a new 'school' of psychoanalysis in psychology with his colleague Joseph Breuer promoting the idea that neuroses had a psychological, not a physiological basis (Ritzer 1992, p. 32). Freud based his theories on his observation of patients, making general inferences from individual cases.

In its early development, psychology had a similar concern found in sociology: a positivist trend following the goals of science, to identify universal laws 'expressed in theories that allowed prediction and explanation' (Looren de Jong 2010, p. 746). Over the years this quest promoted a range of theories including psychoanalysis, neuropsychology and various personality theories some of them spanning the disciplines of sociology and psychology, usually clustered into four groups. These clusters are: (1) social cognition models addressed to the explanation of individuals' health-related behaviour and comprising the theory of planned behaviour, the health belief model, the trans-theoretical model, and the health action process model; (2) self-regulation models focus on risk behaviours and include cognitive adaptation theory, the self-regulation model, and the model of self-efficacy; (3) the psycho-physiological models cluster that 'describes how psychological processes, particularly in response to stressors, can influence physiological functioning', and includes the gate control theory of pain, the cognitive perceptual model, and the general adaptation syndrome, among others; (4) the fourth and final cluster is the environmental models cluster that includes the operant learning theory, conservation of resources theory, and the demand-control model of work stress (Weinman et al. 2007a, xxx–xxxv). Given the space constraints of this chapter, this is only a summary of the main theories but it conveys the idea of the large and growing array of conceptual perspectives underpinning research in psychology today. Marshall H. Becker and his colleagues (Becker et al. 1977/2007) provide an excellent discussion of the conceptual collaboration between sociology and psychology in the analysis of health behaviour and the fruits of that collaboration in the form of conceptual models and abundant research.

Seen from a different and more abstract perspective, psychology—and all its subfields including health psychology—is engaged in a debate between two contrasting positions: a contemporary version of the positivistic approach termed 'rational reconstruction and theory building' and 'critical deconstructivism'. The latter approach 'focuses on theory as dialogue and critique' and on 'the collective construction of meaning, not the discovery of objective facts about the mind' (Looren de Jong 2010, 747–8). The two positions are seen as the bases for 'two research traditions within academic psychology, that is, social constructionism and cognitive neuroscience' (Praetorius 2003).

The debate over theoretical paths that can strengthen psychology's contribution to science and psychologists' professional identity continues unabated (Romanow and Marchildon 2003), but it has produced some intermediate schools of thought that

coexist with 'mainstream psychological research' (Looren de Jong 2010). At the same time, some psychologists like C.R. Cooper and J. Denner have recommended the inclusion of culture in the discipline's research repertoire acknowledging that culture affects behaviour. Their recommendation springs from the engagement of psychologists in interdisciplinary research and the fact that culture is a long-standing subject of investigation in sociology and other social sciences but has not received sufficient attention in psychology (Cooper and Denner 1998). Another reason is their concern with the problem of external validity in psychology. They wrote, 'Psychologists continue to generalize beyond their samples; while studying only their own countries. . . they assume that psychological phenomena are universal enough to make such studies representative' (Cooper and Denner 1998, p. 579).

Psychological research and services relevant to public health

The general scope of health psychology research was well delineated by Canadian psychologist John L. Arnett (2001, p. 45) thus: 'the diagnosis and prevention of illness, the promotion of health, and the amelioration of suffering related to the whole range of health conditions. . . across the whole spectrum of health'.

Clinical/health psychologists provide direct healthcare but their actual clinical practice is determined by government regulations and, more broadly, by the political system and ideology guiding the healthcare system. American psychologists succeeded in obtaining official licensing and getting federal statutes modified 'to gain autonomous inclusion in most federal programs' providing paid healthcare and to practise in managed healthcare organizations. However, for most of the twentieth century, the training and practice of psychology and health psychology did not attend to the profession's participation in the public policy process or in 'programs that. . . address society's public health priorities and perceived needs' (DeLeon et al. 1995, p. 493). This situation is common in other countries but it has been changing. For example, in most OECD (Organization for Economic Cooperation and Development) countries, people have access to paid psychotherapy services only if provided by physicians specialized in psychiatry. However, while both psychologists and psychiatrists can provide psychotherapy, 'PhD-level clinical psychologists receive far more extensive training and education in psychotherapy than physician-trained psychiatrists' (Romanow and Marchildon 2003, p. 286). In the realm of ideology, in countries with 'centralized planning for healthcare' or in community-based healthcare programmes such as Cuba, Costa Rica, and India, 'the concept of health psychology appeared early and its approach tended to be community-oriented', in contrast to the individual orientation of the field in the European tradition (Stone 1991, pp. 12–13).

The practice areas among health psychologists also vary across countries. In the first two decades of the field, while clinical work was the most common area of activity in the United States and the United Kingdom, the main work of health psychologists in Germany, Austria, France, and Argentina was teaching at medical schools (Stone 1991, p. 10). An overview of current health psychology work relevant to public health is suggested in the 2010 study of American health psychologists by Norcross and Karpiak (2012). These researchers found that the most common area of professional work among American health psychologists is psychotherapy practised either on individuals or as group therapy. Indeed, 76 per cent of the professional health psychologists spent about 35 per cent of their professional activity in psychotherapy in 2010, and it has been the most common area of work since 1986 when comparative data collection started. The four other main professional activities are: diagnosis/assessment (58 per cent), teaching (49 per cent), clinical supervision (47 per cent), and research/writing (47 per cent) (Norcross and Karpiak 2012, pp. 5–6).

Psychologists propose that some of the services they offer do increase the productivity of health services by lowering public health expenditure. One illustration of this type of services is the provision of individual or group psychotherapies for breast cancer patients, and the treatment of depression and addiction-related conditions through cognitive behaviour therapies (Romanow and Marchildon 2003). Another example is 'evidence-based parenting interventions' to assist parents with the effective management of children and adolescents affected by 'behavioural and emotional problems' (Sanders, 2010). In his Presidential address to the Canadian Psychological Association, M.R. Sanders suggested that psychologists could offer evidence-based parenting interventions as a 'public health approach' because the aim of his proposal was 'to reduce the prevalence rates of inadequate parenting at. . . [the]. . . population level', a drastic departure from the traditional focus of psychology on 'individual clinical interventions' (Sanders 2010, p. 17). Similar intervention programmes have been tried in the United States, England, and several European countries.

One of the relevant areas of health psychology for public health is stress management. An interesting input was borne out of the collaboration between a public health practitioner and a psychologist: preventive stress management programmes for corporations based on the 'theory of preventive stress management (TPSM)' devised by J.C. Quick and J.D. Quick in 1979 and focused on both physiological stress and organizational stress (Hargrove et al. 2011). According to the TPSM, individuals and organizations react to stressors either positively or negatively. The response to a stressor, or distress, 'is the psychophysiological response of the individual as well as. . . of a group or organization to fight or to flee'; the outcomes of that response may be 'either positive, such as a heightened alertness and enhanced performance, or negative, such as medical, psychological and behavioural distress' (Hargrove et al. 2011, pp. 182–3). As mentioned earlier, research on stress management was one of the earliest contributions in the field of health psychology by Sweden's Karolinska Institute. Swedish researchers analysed the impact of stressors produced by the individual's social and physical environment including the work setting, home environment, transportation, and retirement among other factors (Stone 1991, p. 9).

Family psychotherapy is yet another area of psychology that is relevant to public health. It involves various modalities two of which are perhaps the best well known. They are family therapy involving children and adolescents, and family therapy with older adults. Family psychotherapy involving children and youth is typically offered in collaboration with the school system in the community and deals with children's mental illness as well as with behavioural problems including drug abuse, truancy, and academic performance issues among other aspects. Family psychotherapy involving older adults is gaining ground in countries with a growing elderly population. Psychologists involved in family psychotherapy with older adults deal with a wide range of issues

from dementia and other mental illness to intergenerational conflict, the significance of home setting, pain management, mobility, and physical impairment, among other problems (Curtis and Dixon 2005). In their review of recent developments in family psychotherapy with older adults in the United Kingdom, Curtis and Dixon found 'a lack of empirical research into family therapy with late life families' that needs to be addressed and an insufficient number of family psychotherapists doing this type of work compared to the larger number involved in family therapy with children and younger adults (2005, pp. 56–7).

Change in health-related behaviour is another area of work of health psychologists that is relevant to public health. Psychologists apply one or more social cognition theories (used in sociology as well) in individual and group therapy interventions with youth and adults to modify risk-taking behaviours such as alcohol drinking and cigarette smoking, and to reinforce preventive health behaviours such as condom use and healthy diet (Thirlaway and Upton 2009).

Psychological research methods relevant to public health

A distinguishing feature of psychology is its permanent state of critical introspection. This situation applies to its research methodology. Discussing the methodological landscape in psychology, Lambdin (2012, p. 68) argues that a dominant feature is the rift between two camps: experimental psychologists who claim their work 'is science because it is experimental' and the work of their non-experimental colleagues. Both psychology camps are searching for ways to advance the discipline and correct research gaps and bias. But, as Lambdin rightly points out, common sources of bias are found in all scientific research—irrespective of the knowledge area, whether it is psychology, sociology, biomedicine, or any other: 'the results of any study can be preordained by the selection of stimuli, how variables are operationally defined, the construction of the experimental protocol, the level at which the data are aggregated, or the particular analysis the researcher chooses to utilize' (2012, p. 69). Lambdin suggests that researchers should explain their findings 'without reference to inferential statistics'; and advises applying instead 'a lot of hard thinking and critical reasoning' and focusing on 'effect sizes and confidence intervals which. . . are together far more informative and meaningful' (2012, pp. 70–1).

The use of statistical inference is only one of several aspects under discussion within the field of psychology. Four main fundamental issues that impact research are actively discussed today: the 'scientific versus humanistic' cultures in psychology; two ontological issues, the 'subjective–objective' and the 'individual–collective tensions'; 'the problem of evaluative criteria'; and 'the problem of competing worldviews or value systems' (Goertzen 2008). The beneficial ongoing debate ranges from critiques of conceptual schools of thought in psychology to practice-oriented assessment of diagnostic material, including approaches to improve the *Diagnostic and Statistical Manual of Mental Disorders,* the internationally recognized prime classification of psychopathology published periodically by the American Psychiatric Association (Acton and Zodda 2005).

Most if not all health psychologists are inclined to see conclusions obtained from an experimental design, also known as a randomized clinical trial, as significantly better than findings from case studies, but unfortunately it is not possible to use random allocation and true experiments in health psychology (Friedman 2002, p. 21). Thus, in addition to other forms of systematic observation, psychologists have traditionally used attitudinal scales and questionnaires to collect systematic responses from subjects in laboratory situations or one-to-one interviews or small-group contexts. In addition to this long-established psychological methodology, some psychologists may occasionally borrow methods from other fields to study psychological phenomena. For example, in their investigation of people's beliefs about medicine, Kienhues and Bromme (2012) used a survey technique by sending a questionnaire online to 284 higher school students.

The distinction made between quantitative and qualitative methods of research—discussed above—is the same as in sociology. Thus, in general, psychologists have a preference for quantitative methods and for the application of advanced statistical models in data analysis. However, Weinman and colleagues (2007b) suggest that qualitative methods are used now more often than before and discuss several methods that are undergoing improvement. Three examples suffice. The first illustration is studies of health-related behaviour where investigators may use 'self-report, observation by video or audio recording'. Subjects' self-reports are the most common method of data collection in psychology 'but it is open to problems of error and bias'; thus this method is under close scrutiny and efforts are underway to improve it with a view to make it more 'psychometrically sound'. The second illustration is the assessment of stress as the occurrence of negative life events and emotional changes using attitudinal scales such as the 'Impact of Event Scale' and the 'Hospital Anxiety and Depression Scale' or HADS. The third illustration is the measurement of 'health and illness cognitions' such as the perception of health risks through the use of questionnaire scales such as the Multi-dimensional Health Locus of Control scale and the Illness Perception Questionnaire (Weinman et al. 2007b). As is the pattern in sociology, psychologists dedicate considerable effort at examining and improving the validity and reliability of their research instruments (Sutton 2007).

Formalizing the contributions of sociology and psychology to public health training

The relevance of sociology and psychology to public health is amply recognized today not only in public health research and practice but also in public health education, particularly graduate training in public health.

Some researchers maintain that the United Kingdom was the first country to formalize the field of public health (Paccaud et al. 2011, p. 68). It is not surprising then, that the first training programme in public health was launched in 1871 in the United Kingdom. That programme was the Diploma in Public Health comprising only three subjects, 'epidemiology, population statistics and communicable diseases', and given 'a growing interest in how social determinants of health and illness interacted with disease since the 1930's', sociology and psychology were 'incorporated into public health education' in the United Kingdom in the 1960s (Cole et al. 2011, pp. 89–90).

The incorporation of sociology and psychology in public health curricula has been sluggish in European countries but in the United States, two private universities included both fields as the forerunners of graduate training in public health: Johns Hopkins and Harvard (Paccaud et al. 2011, p. 69). The American framework for public health training at the university level—the origins of which can be traced back to the Welch-Rose Report published in 1915—implemented in schools of public health include social and behavioural sciences as one of five core areas of the curriculum. The five areas are required by the Council on Education for Public Health (CEPH) that regulates Masters and Doctoral Public Health programmes in the United States (Gebbie et al. 2007; Calhoun et al. 2011, pp. 152–3; CEPH 2011, pp. 14, 17; Imperato et al. 2011; Rosenstock et al. 2011, pp. 43–6).

The past two decades have seen serious efforts to improve the quality of medical education curricula worldwide (WHO 2005). Other international organizations such as the World Federation for Medical Education are leading the improvement of medical education standards by incorporating in the graduate public health curriculum 'basic biomedical, behavioral and social sciences, general clinical skills, clinical decision skills, communication abilities and medical ethics' (World Federation for Medical Education 2003, pp. 5–10). As part of that effort to improve public health training, the experience of the University of North Carolina–Charlotte (UNC) is illustrative of the trend towards inclusion of health behaviour in the curricula of public health graduate and undergraduate programmes accredited by the CEPH. At UNC the expansion of the public health curricula was motivated by the aim to establish 'a thriving research base that emphasized population health and health behavior research' and 'responsive and progressive health and human service training programmes' within an interdisciplinary model (Thompson et al. 2009, p. 3). The UNC's current 45-credit curriculum for the Master of Science in Public Health consists of professional practice and research in epidemiology, biostatistics, research methods, 'behavioral and environmental determinants of health' as well as programme planning and evaluation; and the core curriculum includes 'Social and Behavioral Foundations of Public Health' (Thompson et al. 2009, p. 6). A case was made as well for the inclusion of health sociology modules in the Columbia University Medical Center's curricula for internal medicine residents to expose them to 'important societal health issues such as health disparities, social determinants of health and health literacy' (Fiebach et al. 2011, p. S268).

Public health programmes in Europe have followed the same trend of incorporating social and behavioural sciences as core subjects in graduate schools of public health following accreditation requirements set by the European Agency for Accreditation in Public Health Education (Otok et al. 2011; Tulchinsky and McKee 2011). Outside the Western sphere, however, the incorporation of social and behavioural sciences into the public health curriculum started only recently. Today, medical sociology and health psychology are standard components of many graduate public health programmes in some non-Western countries (Bangdiwala et al. 2011; Pino and Solimano 2011).

A final word is in order. The development of multidisciplinary research on human subjects involving biomedicine, sociology, and psychology in various combinations, has led regulatory agencies to support collaboration by creating and expanding ethical guidelines. This effort also reinforces the fact that research ethics is as important in medical sociology and health psychology research as it is in biomedical research. Two of the most relevant dedicated guidebooks have been published by the National Academies Press: *Protecting Participants and Facilitating Social and Behavioral Sciences Research* (Citro et al. 2003) and *Conducting Biosocial Surveys* (Hauser et al. 2010).

Conclusions

The preceding pages present a succinct description of what two social sciences, sociology and psychology, and their respective subfields, medical sociology and health psychology, offer to the discipline of public health. Perhaps the strongest tie binding medical sociology and health psychology is their interest in the systematic analysis of health-related behaviour and their attention to applicability of research findings to the solution of health-related problems in the community.

The essential focus of sociology is on the individual's social behaviour, that is, the person's actions and motives addressed to the actions and motives of others in primary and formal relations, as well as in collective entities ranging from small groups to institutions, social systems, nations, and global organizations. Therefore, medical sociology analyses actions, beliefs, attitudes, and knowledge of individuals on matters of health and illness; health-related activities of groups, organizations, and institutions at all levels of society; and the impact of the socioeconomic, cultural, political, and physical environment upon the actions, attitudes, and beliefs of individuals and collective entities of any size. Consequently, medical sociology involves the study of both the micro-level and the macro-level spheres of social action: from the trilogy of individual action (preventive health behaviour, illness behaviour, sick-role behaviour), to dyads and primary groups (e.g. doctor–patient relations, family's health, impact of small social networks on health risks), to large and complex organizations and social systems (e.g. the analysis of healthcare organizations, insurance and pharmaceutical corporations, the medical profession, government health policies, and impact of ideologies on the distribution of health resources in the population).

Health psychology's original focus was on the analysis of the individual's mental health. However, over the past two decades health psychology has re-oriented its attention to the analysis of all other aspects of health behaviour in addition to and beyond mental illness. This re-alignment of research interests is a positive development for public health because public health practitioners may now benefit not only from the growing body of knowledge produced by medical sociology and health psychology, but they also benefit from the conceptual and methodological expertise of both disciplines.

Knowledge production in the twenty-first century is increasingly leaning towards multidisciplinary collaboration across knowledge domains. This modality presents a unique challenge: multidisciplinary collaboration works well as long as each participating discipline has something distinct to offer to the collaborative enterprise. Each discipline must continue to push the boundaries of knowledge to increase its own expertise. Medical sociology and health psychology continue creating knowledge in their respective areas of interest through research and constant critical examination of their own theories and methodological approaches. At the same time, both disciplines collaborate actively with each other, with public health, and with other biomedical fields for the improvement of people's health. The collaboration involves both applied and theoretical knowledge. The increasing pace of collaboration among medical sociology, health psychology, and public health is already evident not only in the joint authorship of scientific publications in books and refereed journals, but also in the multidisciplinary composition of the faculty in schools of public health around the world. Indeed, high-ranking public health schools tend to have a greater proportion of faculty from different disciplines.

Notes

1. The name of the ISA Research Committee was changed from 'Medical Sociology' to 'Sociology of Health' in 1986 but the work and objectives of the ISA Research Committee remained the same.
2. Sociological research over the past six decades around the world has demonstrated with systematic empirical evidence a universal phenomenon first hinted at by French sociology pioneer Henri de Saint-Simon in 1819: different occupations are allocated different levels of prestige or deference and rewarded accordingly financially (from low-paid, unskilled occupations such as street cleaners or bricklayers, to high-salary, highly skilled occupations such as neuroscientists). Occupational prestige is measured by means of population surveys whereby each person from a representative sample of the total population is asked to rate in a five-point scale (5 'excellent standing', 4 'good standing', 3 'average standing', 2 'below average standing', and 1 'poor standing') a comprehensive list of occupations in their society.

References

Acton, G.S. and Zodda, J.J. (2005). Classification of psychopathology. Goals and methods in an empirical approach. *Theory & Psychology*, 15(3), 373–99.

Ailshire, J.A. and Burgard, S.A. (2012). Family relationships and troubled sleep among US adults: examining the influences of contact frequency and relationship quality. *Journal of Health and Social Behavior*, 53(2), 248–62.

Albery, I.P. and Munafò, M. (2008). *Key Concepts in Health Psychology*. London: Sage Publications.

Anderson, B.O., Cazap, E., Saghir, N.S.E., et al. (2011). Optimization of breast cancer management in low-resource and middle-resource countries: executive summary of the Breast Health Global Initiative consensus, 2010. *Lancet Oncology*, 12, 378–98.

Anderson, I.P.S. and Whyte, J.D. (2008). Populations at special health risk: indigenous populations. In H.K. Heggenhougen and S.R. Quah (eds.) *International Encyclopedia of Public Health* (Vol. 5), pp. 215–24. Oxford: Elsevier.

Armelagos, G.J. and Harper, K.N. (2010). Emerging infectious diseases, urbanization, and globalization in the time of global warming. In W.C. Cockerham (ed.) *The New Blackwell Companion to Medical Sociology*, pp. 291–311. New York: Wiley-Blackwell.

Arnett, J.L. (2001). Clinical and health psychology: future directions. *Canadian Psychology/Psychologie Canadienne*, 42(1), 38–48.

Bangdiwala, S.I., Tucker, J.D., Zodpey, S., et al. (2011). Public health education in Indian and China: history, opportunities, and challenges. *Public Health Reviews*, 33(1), 204–24.

Becker, M.H., Haefner, D.P., Kasl, S.V., Kirsh, J.P., Maiman, L.A., and Rosenstock, I.M. (2007). Selected psychosocial models and correlates of individual health-related behaviors. In J. Weinman, M. Johnston, and Molloy, G. (eds.) *Health Psychology. Vol. 1. Theoretical Models and Frameworks*, pp. 3–26. London: Sage Publications. [Originally published in 1977 in *Medical Care*, XV(5), 27–46.]

Bendix, R. and Lipset, S.M. (eds.) (1966). *Class, Status, and Power. Social Stratification in Comparative Perspective* (2nd ed.). London: Routledge & Kegan Paul.

Boudon, R. (ed.) (1993). *Paul F. Lazarsfeld—On Social Research and Its Language*. Chicago, IL: The University of Chicago Press.

Boyer, B.A. and Paharia, M.I. (eds.) (2008). *Comprehensive Handbook of Clinical Health Psychology*. New York: John Wiley & Sons.

Brown, P., Lyson, M., and Jenkins, T. (2011). From diagnosis to social diagnosis. *Social Science & Medicine*, 73, 939–43.

Burchett, H., Umoquit, M., and Dobrow, M. (2011). How do we know when research from one setting can be useful in another? A review of external validity, applicability and transferability frameworks. *Journal of Health Services Research & Policy*, 16, 238–44.

Calhoun, J.G., Wrobel, C.A., and Finnegan, J.R. (2011). Current state in the U.S. Public Health competence-based graduate education. *Public Health Reviews*, 33(1), 148–67.

Charmaz, K. and Rosenfeld, D. (2010). Chronic illness. In W.C. Cockerham (ed.) *The New Blackwell Companion to Medical Sociology*, pp. 312–33. New York: Wiley-Blackwell.

Christ, S.L., Fleming, L.E., Lee, D.J., Muntaner, C., Muenning, P.A., and Caban-Martinez, A.J. (2012). The effects of a psychosocial dimension of socioeconomic position on survival: occupational prestige and mortality among US working adults. *Sociology of Health & Illness*, 34(7), 1103–17.

Citro, C.F., Ilgen, D.R., and Marrett, C.B. (eds.) (2003). *Protecting Participants and Facilitating Social and Behavioral Sciences Research*. Washington, DC: National Academies Press.

Cockerham, W.C. (2010a). Health lifestyles—bringing structure back. In W.C. Cockerham (ed.) *The New Blackwell Companion to Medical Sociology*, pp. 159–83. Oxford: Wiley-Blackwell.

Cockerham, W.C. (2010b) *Medical Sociology* (11th ed.). London: Pearson.

Cockerham, W.C. and Scambler, G. (2010). Medical sociology and sociological theory. In W.C. Cockerham (ed.) *The New Blackwell Companion to Medical Sociology*, pp. 3–26. Oxford: Wiley-Blackwell.

Cole, K., Sim, F., and Hogan, H. (2011). The evolution of public health education and training in the United Kingdom. *Public Health Reviews*, 33(1), 87–104.

Conrad, P. and Barker, K.K. (2010). The social construction of Illness: key insights and policy implications. *Journal of Health and Social Behavior*, 51(S), S67–79.

Cooper, C.R. and Denner, J. (1998). Theories linking culture and psychology: universal and community-specific processes. *Annual Review of Psychology*, 49, 559–84.

Coreil, J. (2008). Social science contributions to public health: overview. In H.K. Heggenhougen and S.R. Quah (eds.) *International Encyclopedia of Public Health* (Vol. 6), pp. 101–14. Oxford: Elsevier.

Cornwell, E.Y. and Waite, L.J. (2012). Social network resources and management of hypertension. *Journal of Health and Social Behavior*, 53(2), 215–31.

Council on Education for Public Health (2011). *Accreditation Criteria—Schools of Public Health. Amended June 2011*. Washington, DC: CEPH.

Crosnoe, R., Benner, A.D., and Schneider, B. (2012). Drinking, socioemotional functioning, and academic progress in secondary school. *Journal of Health and Social Behavior*, 53(2), 150–4.

Curtis, E.A. and Dixon, M.S. (2005). Family therapy and systematic practice with older people: where are we now? *Journal of Family Therapy*, 27, 43–64.

DeLeon, P.H., Frank, R.G., and Wedding, D. (1995). Health psychology and public policy: the political process. *Health Psychology*, 14(6), 493–9.

Durkheim, E. (1951). *Suicide*. New York: Free Press. (Work originally published in 1897.)

Durkheim, E. (1964). *The Rules of Sociological Method*. New York: Free Press. (Work originally published in 1895.)

Elling, R.H. and Sokołoska, M. (eds.) (1978). *Medical Sociologists at Work*. New Brunswick, NJ: Transaction Books.

Etkin, N.L., Baker, J.D., and Busch, J.N. (2008). Cultural factors influencing therapeutic practice. In H.K. Heggenhougen and S.R. Quah (eds.) *International Encyclopedia of Public Health* (Vol. 2), pp. 56–9. Oxford: Elsevier.

Fiebach, N.H., Rao, D., and Hamm, M.E. (2011). A curriculum in health systems and public health for internal medicine residents. *American Journal of Preventive Medicine*, 41, (4S3), S264–9.

Fox, R.C. (1989). *The Sociology of Medicine. A Participant Observer's View*. Englewood Cliffs, NJ.: Prentice Hall.

Freeman, H.E. and Levine, S. (1989). *Handbook of Medical Sociology*. (4th ed.) Englewood-Cliffs, NJ: Prentice-Hall.

Freeman, H.E., Levine, S., and Reeder, L.G. (eds.) (1963). *Handbook of Medical Sociology*. Englewood Cliffs, NJ: Prentice-Hall.

Freidson, E. (1988). *Profession of Medicine. A Study of the Sociology of Applied Knowledge*. Chicago, IL: University of Chicago Press.

Friedman, H.S. (2002). *Health Psychology* (2nd ed.). Upper Saddle River, NJ: Prentice Hall.

Gebbie, K., Goldstein, B.D., Gregorio, D.I., et al. (2007). The National Board of Public Health Examiners: credentialing public health graduates. *Public Health Reports*, 122(4), 435–40.

Gerhardt, U. (1989). *Ideas about Illness. An Intellectual and Political History of Medical Sociology*. New York: New York University Press.

Germov, J. (2005). Managerialism in the Australian public health sector: towards the hyper-rationalisation of professional bureaucracies. *Sociology of Health & Illness*, 27(6), 738–58.

Goertzen, J.R. (2008). On the possibility of unification: the reality and nature of the crisis in psychology. *Theory & Psychology*, 18(6), 829–52.

Gordon, L.J. and McFarlane, D.R. (1996). Public health practitioner incubation plight: following the money trail. *Journal of Public Health Policy*, 17(1), 59–70.

Greenwood, J.D. (2009). Materialism, strong psychological continuity, and American scientific psychology. *Theory & Psychology*, 19(4), 545–64.

Grollman, E.A. (2012). Multiple forms of perceived discrimination and health among adolescents and young adults. *Journal of Health and Social Behavior*, 53(2), 199–214.

Hargrove, M.B., Quick, J.C., Nelson, D.L., and Quick, J.D. (2011). The theory of preventive stress management: a 33-year review and evaluation. *Stress and Health*, 27, 182–93.

Harvey, T.S. (2008). Cultural issues in health communication. In H.K. Heggenhougen and S.R. Quah (eds.) *International Encyclopedia of Public Health* (Vol. 2), pp. 60–5. Oxford: Elsevier.

Hauser, R.M., Weinstein, M., Pool, R., and Cohen, B. (eds.) (2010). *Conducting Biosocial Surveys: Collecting, Storing, Accessing, and Protecting Biospecimens and Biodata*. Washington, DC: National Academies Press.

Hedges, L.V., Johnson, W.D., Semaan, S., and Sagolow, E. (2002). Theoretical issues in the synthesis of HIV prevention research. *Journal of Acquired Immune Deficiency Syndrome*, 30(Suppl. 1), S8–14.

Heggenhougen, H.K. and Quah, S.R. (eds.) (2008). *International Encyclopedia of Public Health*. Oxford: Elsevier.

Hynes, M.M. (2011). Sociology, health data, and health equity: one state agency as a site of social change. *Current Sociology*, 60(2), 161–77.

Idler, E.L. (2010). Health and religion. In W.C. Cockerham (ed.) *The New Blackwell Companion to Medical Sociology*, pp. 133–58. New York: Wiley-Blackwell.

Imperato, P.J., LaRosa, J.H., Kavaler, F., Benker, K., and Schechter, L. (2011). The establishment of the School of Public Health at the State University of New York, Downstate Medical Center: the first nationally accredited School of Public Health in a public university in New York City. *Journal of Community Health*, 36, 1–13.

Jones, I.R., Papacosta, O., Whincup, P.H., Wannamethee, S.G., and Morris, R.W. (2011). Class and lifestyle 'lock-in' among middle-aged and older men: a multiple correspondence analysis of the British Regional Heart Study. *Sociology of Health & Illness*, 33(3), 399–419.

Kawachi, I., Kennedy, B.P., and Wilkinson, R.G. (eds.) (1999) *Income Inequality and Health. The Society and Population Health Reader*. New York: The New Press.

Kienhues, D. and Bromme, R. (2012). Exploring laypeople's epistemic beliefs about medicine—a factor-analytic survey study. *BMC Public Health*, 12, 759–74.

Krieger, N. (1987). Shades of difference: theoretical underpinnings of the medical controversy on black/white differences in the United States, 1830–1870. *International Journal of Health Services*, 17, 259–78.

Lahelma, E. (2010). Health and social stratification. In W.C. Cockerham (ed.) *The New Blackwell Companion to Medical Sociology*, pp. 71–96. New York: Wiley-Blackwell.

Lambdin, C. (2012). Significance tests as sorcery: science is empirical—significance tests are not. *Theory & Psychology*, 22, 67–90.

Laxminarayan, R., Mills, A.J., Breman, J.G., et al. (2006). Advancement of global health: key messages from the Disease Control Priorities Project. *The Lancet*, 367, 1193–208.

Lazarsfeld, P.F. (1968). Foreword. In M. Rosenberg (ed.) *The Logic of Survey Analysis*, pp. vii–x. New York: Basic Books.

Link, B.G. and Phelan, J. (1995). Social conditions as fundamental causes of disease. *Journal of Health and Social Behavior*, 35, 80–94.

Looren de Jong, H. (2010). From theory construction to deconstruction: the many modalities of theorizing in psychology. *Theory & Psychology*, 20(6), 745–63.

Luecken, L.J. and Gallo, L.C. (eds.) (2008). *Handbook of Physiological Research Methods in Health Psychology*. Los Angeles, CA: Sage Publications.

Massé, R. and Moloughney, B. (2011). New era for schools and programs of public health in Canada. *Public Health Reviews*, 33(1), 277–88.

Mechanic, D. and McAlpine, D.D. (2010). Sociology of health care reform: building on research and analysis to improve health care. *Journal of Health and Social Behavior*, 51(S), S147–59.

Mechanic, D. and Tanner, J. (2007). Vulnerable people, groups, and populations: societal view. *Health Affairs*, 26, 1220–30.

Miller, D.C. and Salkind, N.J. (2002). *Handbook of Research Design & Social Measurement* (6th ed.). London: Sage Publications.

Nam, C.B. and Powers, M.G. (1983). *The Socioeconomic Approach to Status Measurement (With a Guide to Occupational and Socioeconomic Scales)*. Houston, TX: Cap and Gown Press.

Neuman, W.L. (2000). *Social Research Methods. Qualitative and Quantitative Approaches*. Boston, MA: Allyn and Bacon.

Norcross, J.C. and Karpiak, C.P. (2012). Clinical psychologists in the 2010s: 50 years of the APA Division of Clinical Psychology. *Clinical Psychology: Science and Practice*, 19(1), 1–12.

Otok, R., Levin, I., Sitko, S., and Flahault, A. (2011). European accreditation of Public Health education. *Public Health Reviews*, 33(1), 30–8.

Paccaud, F., Weihofen, A., and Nocera, S. (2011). Public health education in Europe: old and new challenges. *Public Health Reviews*, 33(1), 66–86.

Parsons, T. (1937). *The Structure of Social Action*. New York: McGraw-Hill.

Pearlin, L.I. (1989). The sociological study of stress. *Journal of Health and Social Behavior*, 30, 241–56.

Perez, M.A. and Luquis, R.R. (2008). *Cultural Competence in Health Education and Health Promotion*. San Francisco, CA: Jossey-Bass.

Phelan, J.C., Link, B.C., and Tehranifar, P. (2010). Social conditions as fundamental causes of health inequalities: theory, evidence, and policy implications. *Journal of Health and Social Behavior*, 51(Extra Issue), S28–40.

Pino, P. and Solimano, G. (2011). The School of Public Health at the University of Chile: origins, evolution, and perspectives. *Public Health Reviews*, 33(1), 315–22.

Praetorius, N. (2003). Inconsistencies in the assumptions of constructivism and naturalism: an alternative view. *Theory & Psychology*, 13(4), 511–39.

Quadagno, J. (2010). Institutions, interest groups, and ideology: an agenda for the sociology of health care reform. *Journal of Health and Social Behavior*, 51, 125–36.

Quah, S.R. (2003). Traditional healing systems and the ethos of science. *Social Science and Medicine*, 57(10), 1997–2012.

Quah, S.R. (ed.) (2007a). *Crisis Preparedness: Asia and the Global Governance of Epidemics*. Stanford, CA: Shorenstein Asia-Pacific Research Centre, Stanford University.

Quah, S.R. (2007b). Public image and governance of epidemics: comparing HIV/AIDS and SARS. *Health Policy*, 80, 253–72.

Quah, S.R. (2008). In pursuit of health: pragmatic acculturation in everyday life. *Health Sociology Review*, 17(4), 419–21.

Quah, S.R. (2010). Health and Culture'. In W.C. Cockerham (ed.) *The New Blackwell Companion to Medical Sociology*, pp. 27–46. New York: Wiley-Blackwell.

Quah, S.R. (2011). Gender and the burden of disease in ten Asian countries: an exploratory analysis. *Asia Europe Journal*, 8, 499–512.

Ragin, C.C. and Becker, H.S. (eds.) (1992). *What is a Case? Exploring the Foundations of Social Inquiry*. Cambridge: Cambridge University Press.

Reid, M. (1976). *The Development of Medical Sociology in Britain*. Discussion Papers in Social Research No. 13. Glasgow: University of Glasgow.

Ritzer, G. (1992). *Sociological Theory* (3rd ed.). New York: McGraw-Hill.

Romanow, R.J. and Marchildon, G.P. (2003). Psychological services and the future of health care in Canada. *Canadian Psychology/Psychologie Canadienne*, 44(4), 283–95.

Rosenstock, L., Heksing, K., and Rimer, B.K. (2011). Public health education in the United States: then and now. *Public Health Reviews*, 33(1), 39–65.

Rosich, K.J. and Hankin, J.R. (2010). What do we know? Key findings from 50 years of Medical Sociology – Executive Summary. *Journal of Health and Social Behavior*, 51, S1–9.

Sanders, M.R. (2010). Adopting a public health approach to the delivery of evidence-based parenting interventions. *Canadian Psychology*, 51 (1), 17–23.

Schwartz, H. and Jacobs, J. (1979). *Qualitative Sociology. A Method to the Madness*. New York: The Free Press.

Seow, A. (2008). Dietary guidelines, international. In H.K. Heggenhougen and S.R. Quah (eds.) *International Encyclopedia of Public Health* (Vol. 2), pp. 190–4. Oxford: Elsevier.

Shryock, E.H. (1974). *The Development of Modern Medicine. An Interpretation of the Social and Scientific Factors Involved*. Madison, WI: University of Wisconsin Press.

Smith, M., Saunders, R., Stuckhardt, L., and McGinnis, J.M. (2012). *Best Care at Lower Cost: The Path to Continuously Learning Health Care in America*. Washington, DC: National Academies Press.

Smith, S. (1866). *The Common Nature of Epidemics, and their Relation to Climate and Civilization*. Philadelphia, PA: J.B. Lippincott.

Starr, P. (1982). *The Social Transformation of American Medicine. The Rise of a Sovereign Profession and the Making of a Vast Industry*. New York: Basic Books.

Stevens, F. (2010). The convergence and divergence of modern health care systems. In W.C. Cockerham (ed.) *The New Blackwell Companion to Medical Sociology*, pp. 434–54. New York: Wiley-Blackwell.

Stone, G.C. (1991). An international review of the emergence and development of health psychology. In M.A. Jansen and J. Weinman (eds.) *The International Development of Health Psychology*, pp. 3–17. Philadelphia, PA: Hardwood Academic Publishers.

Sutton, S. (2007). Predicting and explaining intentions and behavior: how well are we doing? In J. Weinman, M. Johnston, and G. Molloy (eds.) *Health Psychology. Vol. 3. Methods and Measurement*, pp. 3–21. London: Sage Publications.

Thirlaway, K. and Upton, D. (2009). *The Psychology of Lifestyle: Promoting Healthy Behaviour*. London: Routledge.

Thois, P.A. (2010). Stress and health: major findings and policy implications. *Journal of Health and Social Behavior*, 51(5), 541–53.

Thomas, C. (2012). Theorising disability and chronic illness: where next for perspectives in medical sociology? *Social Theory & Health*, 10(3), 209–28.

Thompson, M.E., Harver, A., and Eure, M. (2009). A model for integrating strategic planning and competence-based curriculum design in establishing a public health programme: the UNC Charlotte experience. *Human Resources for Health*, 71(7), 1–10.

Thorlindsson, T. (2011). Bring in the social context: towards an integrated approach to health promotion and prevention. *Scandinavian Journal of Public Health*, 39(Suppl. 6), 19–25.

Timmermans, S. and Oh, H. (2010). The continued social transformation of the medical profession. *Journal of Health and Social Behavior*, 51(S), S94–106.

Tulchinsky, T.H. and Mc Kee, M. (2011). Education for a public health workforce in Europe and globally. *Public Health Reviews*, 33(1), 7–15.

Umberson, D. and Montez, J.K. (2010). Social relationships and health: a flashpoint for health policy. *Journal of Health and Social Behavior*, 51(S), S54–66.

Vanderminden, J. and Potter, S.J. (2010). Challenges to the doctor–patient relationship in the twenty-first century. In W.C. Cockerham (ed.) *The New Blackwell Companion to Medical Sociology*, pp. 355–72. New York: Wiley-Blackwell.

Vogt, W.P. (2007). *Quantitative Research Methods for Professionals*. Boston, MA: Pearson.

Waters, E., Gibbs, L., Riggs, E., Priest, N., Renzaho, A., and Kulkens, M. (2008). Cultural competence in public health. In H.K. Heggenhougen and S.R. Quah (eds.) *International Encyclopedia of Public Health* (Vol. 2), pp. 38–43. Oxford: Elsevier.

Weber, M. (1968). *Economy and Society*. Totowa, NJ: Bedminster Press. (Work originally published in 1921.)

Weinman, J., Johnston, M., and Molloy, G. (eds.) (2007a). *Health Psychology. Volume 1. Theoretical Models and Frameworks*. London: Sage Publications.

Weinman, J., Johnston, M., and Molloy, G. (eds.) (2007b). *Health Psychology. Volume 3. Methods and Measurement*. London: Sage Publications.

Williams, D.R. and Sternthal, M. (2010). Understanding racial-ethnic disparities in health: sociological contributions. *Journal of Health and Social Behavior*, 51(S), S15–27.

World Federation for Medical Education (2003). *Basic Medical Education. WFME Global Standards for Quality Improvement*. Copenhagen: World Federation for Medical Education.

World Health Organization (2004). *WHOQOL-BREF*. Geneva: WHO.

World Health Organization (2005). *Accreditation of Medical Education Institutions. Report of a Technical Meeting*. Schæffergården, Copenhagen: World Health Organization-World Federation for Medical Education Task Force on Accreditation.

Wright, E.R. and Perry, B.L. (2010). Medical sociology and health services research: past accomplishments and future policy challenges. *Journal of Health and Social Behavior*, 51(S), S107–19.

Zaslavsky, A.M. and Epstein, A.M. (2005). How patients' sociodemographic characteristics affect comparisons of competing health plans in California on HEDIS® quality measures. *International Journal of Quality in Health Care*, 17(1), 67–74.

Sexuality and public health

Richard Parker, Jonathan Garcia, Miguel Muñoz-Laboy, Marni Sommer, and Patrick Wilson

Introduction to sexuality and public health

Over the course of the past 25–30 years, there has been an explosion of public health research and programmes focusing on sexuality. Never before in the history of public health have sex and sexual issues been seen as more worthy of attention. In countries and communities around the world, researchers, practitioners, and policymakers have sought to develop new knowledge, to design new programmes, and to articulate and implement new policies focusing on sexuality and sexual health.

This recent interest in sexuality and public health contrasts significantly with the ways in which sexuality was addressed in earlier times. In the late nineteenth and early twentieth centuries, sexuality was considered at best to be a marginal concern, with attention focused primarily on seeking to control what at the time were called venereal diseases (Brandt 1987). Approaches to such diseases in both medicine and public health were characterized by prevailing moral values of the time, and the primary concern seemed to be with protecting mainstream society from the threat posed by such sexually transmitted diseases.

Over the course of the mid-twentieth century, this situation gradually changed, as growing interest began to focus not so much on sexually transmitted diseases, but on the wider range of what might be thought of as 'normal' sexual behaviours of both men and women—less with the goal of protecting them from disease than to seek to promote their health and well-being. This focus reached its zenith in the late 1940s, and the early 1950s with the publication of the Kinsey studies in the United States (Kinsey et al. 1948, 1953). Yet the significant controversy that surrounded the publication of the Kinsey reports, especially in the cold war political climate of the 1950s, quickly led to an almost total curtailment of work on (and financial support for) the topic of sexuality during the ensuing decades (Corrêa et al. 2008).

It was only in the wake of the emerging human immunodeficiency virus (HIV) epidemic in the early 1980s that the consequences of this long-term neglect of public health work focusing on sexuality became apparent. As the devastating proportions of acquired immune deficiency syndrome (AIDS)—a global epidemic transmitted primarily through sexual contact—began to be perceived, the urgent need for greater understanding of sexual behaviour and for innovative new approaches to sexual health promotion quickly became evident. Public health researchers and practitioners quickly began to seek to address such issues, with a sense of urgency that perhaps could only be generated by such a widespread global crisis, and a new wave of public health research, intervention, and sexual health promotion began and continued to gain strength over the course of the 1990s and the 2000s.

A major aspect of sexuality research has not only focused on a two-dimensional examination of how identities lead to behaviours, but also on the role of desire in grasping the public health implications of sexuality. The collective need to categorize others, as well as the individual need for self-understanding and belonging to a particular community, have created a range of sexual identities throughout the world that are associated with a variety of behaviours and desires. These range from the very Western-centred political identity of being 'gay' and 'out of the closet', to 'queer' identities that proliferated with the development of multicultural societies, to socioeconomically and even caste-related alternative sexualities (e.g. *Hijras* in India), to individual-centred identities defining subcultures within the lesbian, gay, bisexual, transgender, and queer (LGBTQ) framework (e.g. dykes, bois, drama queens). Strategic identities such as that of 'sex worker' have in fact empowered some subcultures by reframing categories to diminish the stigma associated to 'prostitution'. Throughout this chapter we explore some of the implications of this three-dimensional perspective on sexuality (i.e. identity, behaviour, and desire) for heterosexuals as well as non-heterosexuals and among both youth and adults.

This chapter seeks to provide an overview of this rapidly growing body of work in public health. It describes the initial public health response to sexuality in the context of HIV and AIDS, as well as the ways in which the response has been gradually broadened over time in order to provide a more comprehensive approach to sexual health and well-being. It also focuses on both the local and the global dimensions of this work, in both developed and developing countries, and as much in the work of local communities struggling to respond to the needs of their own populations, as well as on the part of a range of international agencies that are increasingly seeking to address a range of challenges to sexual health.

The impact of AIDS

The emergence of the HIV and AIDS epidemic in the early 1980s led to a major transformation in the ways in which public health has addressed issues of sexuality. During the early years of the HIV epidemic, one of the most frequently repeated laments of public health officials was the lack of data on sexual behaviour and the need to rely on findings from studies, such as the work of Kinsey and his colleagues in the United States, that were nearly 50 years out of date. The urgent need to respond to the epidemic with more contemporary knowledge on sexual behaviour provided the justification for a massive increase in research funding for work on sexuality among diverse population groups, and made the development of public health interventions to reduce the risk of sexual transmission of HIV an urgent priority (Turner et al. 1989).

Driven by epidemiological concerns, research on sexuality in relation to HIV and AIDS was initially developed in medical institutions, and was shaped by Western biomedical assumptions. Much of the early research carried out in response to the epidemic focused on surveys of risk-related sexual behaviours and on the knowledge, attitudes, and practices linked to risk of HIV infection. Most studies collected quantitative data on numbers of sexual partners, specific sexual practices, sexually transmitted infections (STIs), and similar topics related to transmission of HIV. Behavioural research sought to build a scientific foundation for public health policies and intervention programmes that would more effectively prevent HIV infection (Parker et al. 1991).

Very early in the epidemic, however, critical public health and social science research also highlighted the extent to which HIV and AIDS needed to be understood as what Paula Treichler described as 'an epidemic of signification' (1988). Such work emphasized the ways in which complex cultural meanings shaped social understandings of the epidemic and surrounded it in deeply rooted forms of stigma, discrimination, and denial (Parker and Aggleton 2003). It highlighted the importance of critically examining epidemiological and biomedical categories as well as popular understandings related to the epidemic, and emphasized the need to investigate local sexual cultures and the social organization of sexual practices in different social and cultural contexts (Parker 2001).

In early work on HIV among gay and bisexual men, for example, it became clear that many men who have sex with other men may not identify themselves as homosexual on the basis of this behaviour, and that Western biomedical categories such as 'homosexuality', 'bisexuality', or 'heterosexuality' might not adequately describe the lived sexual experience of many individuals. Increasingly, descriptive categories such as 'men who have sex with men' (or 'MSM') were adopted both in research and in public health practice in order to avoid imposing culturally inaccurate or inappropriate labels and classifications. This led, in turn, to important work rethinking the relationship between sexual orientation, sexual identity, and sexual behaviour. Based on this work, it became evident that assumptions about the relationship between sexual desire, sexual behaviour, and sexual identity—in particular, the assumption that feeling desire necessarily led to enacting behaviour, and that enacted behaviour necessarily led to forming a distinct sexual identity based on that behaviour—needed to be re-examined and investigated empirically (Dowsett 2003).

Work on homosexuality and MSM opened the way for a broader critique of other key categories that had been used in seeking to understand the epidemiology of HIV infection. Research on 'prostitution', for example, highlighted extensive cross-cultural diversity in the ways in which sex is exchanged for money, gifts, or favours, and emphasized the importance of sex work and sex workers, on the one hand, and other forms of transaction that might characterize many sexual relationships without constituting sex work or identifying those involved as sex workers or clients (de Zalduondo 1991). Similarly, while the female sexual partners of male injecting drug users (or the male sexual partners of female injecting drug users) might constitute meaningful epidemiological categories, they have little or no sociological significance, and members of groups identified through such categories have little or no sense of self-identity or group identification based on these circumstances, making them largely useless for purposes of health promotion and HIV prevention (Kane and Mason 1992). As a result of HIV and AIDS, then, the ways in which public health has approached issues of sexuality have changed significantly, and a new understanding of sexual health promotion has been developed that has important consequences for other areas of sexual health, independent of HIV and AIDS.

Public health research on marginalized populations such as female sex workers and male and female injecting drug users and their sexual partners also focused growing attention on the broader synergy that exists in many societies between poverty, racial or ethnic discrimination, gender power inequality, and vulnerability to HIV infection (Farmer et al. 1996). It became increasingly clear that sexual behaviour is not somehow isolated or free-floating, separate from other forms of social experience and social structure. On the contrary, sexuality exists embedded in social hierarchies, and sexual behaviour can only be understood within the context of social processes. One of the lasting lessons of the HIV/AIDS epidemic for understanding sexuality in relation to public health more broadly was therefore that sexual risk behaviour must be understood not just as 'behavioural risk' but as 'social risk'—and, indeed, that the concept of 'risk' should perhaps be abandoned altogether in favour of a greater emphasis on 'social vulnerability' that would be more useful in seeking to understand the social drivers of the epidemic (Parker et al. 2000).

The various insights derived from work on sexuality in the context of HIV and AIDS have continued to shape public health approaches to sexuality over the course of the last two decades. They have been especially important in seeking to develop both research and programmes aimed at promoting sexual health among young people, heterosexual women and men, as well as sexual communities and populations outside the mainstream of society that often face special forms of vulnerability due to emerging forms of social marginalization and exclusion. Work on sexuality in relation to population health has also heightened awareness of the complex ways in which sexual experience is socially regulated, with consequences that can be highly diverse. A broader focus not just on the absence of disease, but on a fuller realization of true health and well-being, in relation to sexuality as in relation to other aspects of health, requires a broader focus on the relationship between sexual health and sexual rights (Parker 2007). Notably, the work of public health has been shaped, through setting a political agenda, cultural framings, and outright displays of indignation with the status quo stemming from AIDS social movements throughout the world (Altman and Buse 2012). The AIDS social movement has been significant in addressing cultural, structural, and social determinants of health not only to increase access to essential medications, but also to give a sense of hope and commitment (a type of sociocultural resiliency) to the study of sexuality in the realm of public health (Parker 2011).

In the following sections of this chapter, we will seek to address the development of work on these various dimensions of sexuality and public health, explore ways in which sexuality intersects with public health issues such as mental health and violence, and to highlight the ways in which this rapidly growing field of work is developing in the early twenty-first century.

Youth, sexuality, and gendered experience

The definition of 'youth' and the timing of a young person's first experience of sexuality are two important considerations for public health researchers and practitioners designing sexual health interventions. The biologically defined developmental stages of youth tend to place an important emphasis on puberty as the beginning stage of human sexuality (Patton and Viner 2007). The onset of puberty brings with it numerous physiological changes and new social pressures for young people transitioning into young adulthood within any given society. Along with adjusting to the new biological changes that are experienced, including the development of secondary sexual characteristics, young people must adjust to the social responses of peers, family, and communities to their obvious physical and emotional sexual maturation. As societies shift from rural to urban, as the advent of formal schooling incorporates greater populations of young people, as influences from globalization and new technologies shape the experience of childhood and young adulthood, and as gender norms continue to evolve, the sexual socialization of young people is being altered and transformed (Blum 2007).

Girls and boys experience puberty differently biologically and socioculturally. Puberty is not only experienced at different ages according to gender, but may be marked by differing rites of passage (broadly defined) that depend on contextual and structural factors. Sexual differentiation moulded by social norms can shape the transformation of gendered expectations and sexual opportunities for girls and boys. The socializing norms influencing young people's development, perceived societal roles, and ultimately their restraint or engagement in sexual risk-taking behaviours are closely linked to the femininity and masculinity norms shaping or constraining their choices and experiences, which we will also address in relation to adult heterosexual relations. In some cultures, girls are de-sexualized at a young age through procedures such as female genital excision, or what has been widely framed by the feminist human rights movement as female genital mutilation (Boyle 2005). Emphasis is generally placed on fertility as the representation of femininity. Boys also undergo sexual rites of passage, but these are often more 'empowering', signifying the acquisition of manhood and emphasizing the importance of virility. Whereas women are sometimes denied sexual pleasure through these procedures, boys that experience male circumcision are ascribed a role in their communities that associates their sexuality with power and responsibility (World Health Organization 2000).

In recent decades, attention has shifted to the social construction of sexuality for understanding the ways in which young people's sexuality and gendered experience are influenced by the societal pressures and traditions around them (Freud 1994). This differentiation based on the social construction of sexuality has concrete implications for gendered disparities in human development related to both education and health. A gendered division of labour presents significant barriers to closing the gap in illiteracy and access to essential health services in resource-poor settings (Blum and Mmari 2006). In addition, girls are often married-off to older men, and boys are sometimes forced to migrate from rural to urban settings to find work. Both intergenerational sex and migration are factors that contribute to sexual risk.

As young people transition into young adulthood, sexual and reproductive health becomes a priority health issue. This is particularly true for young women in low-income countries, for whom adolescent pregnancy presents particular risks of maternal mortality and morbidity (such as obstetric fistula), infection with HIV and AIDS, and other STIs (Hindin and Fatusi 2009). Adolescent pregnancy makes girls vulnerable to dropping out of school and to mental health problems. Campaigns to prevent STIs and HIV are only beginning to target youth facing structural barriers. The risk of sexual violence is an additional challenge, particularly in societies where gendered power dynamics place young women in positions of little negotiation around sexual relations, and where masculinity norms promote aspects of virility and strength for young men.

Moreover, it is important to question the assumption that sexuality actually begins at puberty. Some studies have shown that sexual experimentation and initiation might begin before this biological landmark (Bankole et al. 2007). Masturbation is a major part of sexual experimentation, and access to pornography on the Internet is widespread. The international community has paid increasing attention to the effects of globalization on trafficking in children and sex work as major public health problems in the contemporary world. This protection of the rights of children is the responsibility of families, communities, and nation-states.

Much of sex education for youth is regulated through kinship networks and schools (Barker 2007). The family and 'traditional values' play an important role in sex education for boys and girls. The age of sexual debut continues to change around the world with influences of modernization and delays in the age of marriage secondary to the advent of formal schooling. The quality of communication between parents and youth influences the ways in which youth are sexually socialized. Religious values that condemn condom use are particularly influential in shaping the types of messages youth receive from their families and in schools. International debates about what constitutes sex education are shaped by progressive advocates for comprehensive approaches (which might include the distribution of condoms to youth for STI and HIV prevention), and by conservatives who believe that sex education should be limited to teaching sexual abstinence until marriage.

More recently, debates over sex education have begun to discuss sexual orientation because at a very young age children begin to experience bullying, especially in schools and on the Internet. School and cyberbullying can lead to increased sexual risk, mental health problems, and substance use among youth. Structural interventions that target school policies are crucial for the formulation and implementation of comprehensive sex education to prevent bullying based on sexuality (Jones et al. 2009).

Heterosexual relations

Public health research on heterosexuality has been relatively limited when compared to the focus on non-heterosexuality. Kinsey's studies began to uncover the gradients of sexuality, as opposed to a dichotomous divide between heterosexuality and homosexuality—yet, the curiosity for deconstructing the accepted norms was in some ways even aimed at showing the non-existence of an authentic heterosexuality. Historically, the field of sexuality research is laden with bias towards studying 'deviations' from the sexual norm rather than at seeking to more fully understand the ways in which dominant normative patterns of experience are produced and organized (Wilkinson and Kitzinger 1994). Paradoxically, daily experience—ranging from the ways sexuality is produced in the media to our interpersonal relations at work, schools, religious institutions, etc.—shows that a notion of heterosexuality exists almost pervasively and that this cultural norm has meaningfully strategic uses in regulating power dynamics in most societies. The concept of 'heteronormativity' has been used in critical public health frameworks to describe the ways in which men and women form both casual and steady partnerships, which are moulded by social and cultural norms (Kitzinger 2005). This concept has theoretical traction for understanding patterns of sexual behaviour with important implications for public health outcomes.

The fact that heterosexuality is employed as a form of normative domination at the same time that it has largely escaped the gaze of scientific inquiry calls our attention to how public health can benefit from highlighting recent explorations of heterosexuality. Reproduction, gendered relations of power, masculine/feminine ideologies, marriage, and parenting have more recently begun to be explored at the intersection between sexuality and public health. In large part as a result of the HIV and AIDS epidemic, there has also been growing attention to what can be described as the political economy of heterosexual relationships: the ways in which economic exchange relations shape heterosexual interactions far beyond the context of what is traditionally understood as prostitution or sex work (Hunter 2002). The examination of the transactional nature of heterosexual relations has received special attention in sub-Saharan Africa as a result of research seeking to respond to the need for fuller understanding of vulnerability in relation to the heterosexual transmission of HIV (Leclerc-Madlala 2003; Swidler and Watkins 2007), but is clearly an important, albeit highly variable, part of the organization of partner relations between women and men across widely varying social and cultural contexts that requires increased attention in seeking to develop the field of sexuality in public health more broadly.

Another key area of research that focuses on heterosexual relations has been related to human procreation. According to the World Health Organization, reproductive health relates to having a 'responsible, satisfying and safe sex life and. . . the capability to reproduce and the freedom to decide if, when and how often to do so', safely, effectively, and affordably, and through access to health services (World Health Organization 2011a). This discourse comes after decades of public health policies in countries throughout the world, such as those that supported the mass sterilization of women, with a focus on population control as a means to reduce poverty and increase economic growth. These 'structural' determinants of health severely limited women's sexual agency and sexual decision-making.

Moreover, in heterosexual partnerships these asymmetric gendered power dynamics occur not only at a structural level, but they also have effects on individual health outcomes for both

women and men. Ideologies of masculinity have vast implications for public health outcomes globally. Preserving a sense of heterosexual manhood and invincibility has been a barrier to seeking health services (Gough 2013). This has been particularly challenging for public health movements advocating for prostate cancer screening, and heterosexual men are often more averse to anally invasive prostate exams (Gray et al. 2002). The concept of 'machismo' or male chauvinism has often been used to analyse the effects of Latin American heterosexual masculinity and its implications for health. Although studies on machismo have associated this ideology with sexual risk behaviours and intimate partner violence, the concept of machismo has been criticized for stereotyping Latino men (Torres 2002). A more complex understanding of Latin American and Latino male sexuality shows that sexual behaviours are dependent on social and interpersonal context. Same-sex socialization among heterosexual men (Kandel and Davies 1991; Ramirez et al. 2012) has been linked to higher levels of sexual risk-taking with women, drug use, and sexual violence.

At the same time, femininity has also been shown to have effects on the health of women. Forms of the ideal 'sexy' woman certainly vary across the globe, among cultures, and often depend on social factors such as race and ethnicity. However, there is an overwhelming prevalence of this context-dependent sexualized ideal, which even in its multiform instantiations has impacts on how women perceive themselves. The epidemics of eating disorders are one of the clearest examples of how heteronormative femininity affects women's health. Public health research has shown that heterosexual women are affected by eating disorders such as anorexia nervosa and bulimia more so than non-heterosexual women (Meyer et al. 2001). Heteronormative femininity is a 'social determinant' of women's sexual health according to the Healthy People 2020's definition, which lists the factors that limit the 'availability of resources to meet daily needs, such as educational and job opportunities, living wages, or healthful foods' (Healthy People 2020 2011), such as violence and discrimination.

Furthermore, heterosexual relations, procreation, and partnerships often result in men and women taking on the responsibility of parenthood. Although parenting is not solely a heteronomative phenomenon in the current world order, public health studies have focused on the negative effects of single motherhood and absent fathers on the sexual and mental well-being of younger generations (East et al. 2007; Ishida 2010). For many, maintaining the institution of *heteronomative* marriage as both religiously and socially stable is a solution to potential health problems associated with heterosexual relations (Mahoney et al. 2008). However, the more critical public health research has associated ideologies with heteronormative marriage with infidelity, intimate partner violence, and sexual risk (Hirsch et al. 2007).

The purpose of this section was to highlight the absence of a necessary critique of heterosexual relations by considering political, economic, cultural, social, and interpersonal determinants of health. Both methodologically and analytically, heterosexuality has mostly been treated as the 'referent' category in public health work on sexuality. Our critique is not of heterosexuality in itself, but of the multiple forms of inequalities that result from male dominant power relations that are overall unfavourable for women and men.

Sexual diversity and alternative sexualities

Framing sexual diversity in public health is methodologically and epistemologically complicated, particularly because of how sexual desires, behaviours, and identities converge and diverge. Addressing sexual *identities* might be easier in social and behavioural research because there is more reliability in measures when the respondent identifies either to themselves or openly to society about being a LGBTQ individual. Alternative sexualities go beyond identity, however, and a person who practises same-sex sexual behaviours or sex work might not identify with a particular group culture. It becomes even more complicated when speaking of desire that does not necessarily translate into behaviour or identity formation, as we mentioned earlier. Research questions vary depending on these dimensions of sexual diversity and alternative sexualities, and public health has often collaborated closely with social movements to set research agendas.

The broader framework of sexual health has been employed to study health problems related to populations characterized by sexual diversity (Parker et al. 2004). Much of public health research has focused on behaviour change towards the practice of safer sex (e.g. through condom use and reduction in sexual partners), especially considering the disproportionately high impact of HIV and AIDS on gay and bisexual communities (Cow et al. 2011; Millett et al. 2012). Scholars have also focused on the intersections of mental and sexual health. Using theories such as 'minority stress' scholars have focused on distal and proximal factors that affect depression, anxiety, and healthcare utilization (Meyer 2003). Fear of disclosure of having same-sex desires or of practising alternative sexualities, for instance, can have important implications on the ways people interact with their healthcare providers (Klitzman and Greenberg 2002). Sexual diversity interacts with other social factors, such as race and poverty, which lead to differential access to healthcare and exposure to disease (Díaz et al. 2001).

In the sexual health literature, there have been disputes over how to create epidemiological categories that capture sexual diversity. The categories men who have sex with men (MSM), men who have sex with men and women (MSMW), and women who have sex with women (WSW), behaviourally bisexual, bisexual, gay, and non-heterosexual are all used in the field of public health depending on the research question involved. Some of these categories, such as MSM, attempt to capture self-identified gays and bisexuals as well as those who practise same-sex sexualities but that do not self-identify as gay or bisexual. The category MSM might strip away the social and political implications of public health work on alternative sexualities, which has been a prominent claim among public health activists. Categorizing populations such as MSM and WSW might be understood as an attempt to objectively perform science. Those advocating for LGBTQ health are part of a public health social movement that contends that understanding non-heterosexuality as having vast variation in sexual performance is central to a notion of well-being that hinges on social rights. The epidemiological use of categories such as MSM and WSW, among others, does not fully take into consideration that 'community, networks, and relationships in which same-gender pairings mean more than merely sexual behavior', and these categories have been criticized by the public social movement as heterosexist (Young and Meyer 2005). Another trend in public health

that has been disputed is having sex on the 'down low' (Millett et al. 2005). Sex on the down low describes patterns of secrecy and discretion that facilitate extra-marital sex, keeping a heterosexual identity while having same-sex sexual relations, and sexual concurrency.

There has been less attention to the particular health disparities that affect lesbians and women who have sex with women in the public health literature (Bauer and Jairam 2008). This gap is probably due to the lesser impact that HIV and AIDS has had on these populations, when compared to other 'risk' groups. This has led to gaps in research for women who are vulnerable to HIV, although other STIs such as HPV (which causes cervical cancer in women) have been addressed in non-heterosexual women populations (Charlton et al. 2011). Bisexual women and women who have sex with women and men (WSWM) have had some attention particularly regarding their sexual health. There are important concerns about the unmet needs of lesbians, bisexual women, and WSWM in healthcare due to stigma and discrimination when seeking health (Stevens et al. 1988). This is especially the case when they fear disclosing their sexualities. Lesbians and bisexuals have been identified as having a higher rate of cigarette smoking than heterosexuals in national studies (Ryan et al. 2001). The health concerns of lesbians are more proximal to those of heterosexual women (relative to comparing gay men with heterosexual men). However, non-heterosexual women encounter barriers in sexual and reproductive health, as well as in making important life decisions, such as child-bearing that make them particularly vulnerable to stigma and discrimination (Dahl et al. 2013).

The mental and physical health of transgender men and women has drawn special attention in public health, especially in discussions about gender modification procedures, the formal classification of transgender individuals in the *Diagnostic and Statistical Manual of Mental Disorders*, and their access to health more generally (Lombardi 2001; De Cuypere et al. 2010). Illegal hormone and silicone injection has been of particular concern due to the high cost of gender transformation (Wiessing et al. 1999). Moreover, stigma and discrimination are probably most prevalent for transgender individuals, limiting their employment and education opportunities. These are social aspects of their gender identities that directly affect their risk for HIV and AIDS and mental health problems, especially because many transgender women resort to commercial sex work because of their limited opportunities (Abdullah et al. 2012). In some countries, such as Brazil and Cuba, public health policy debates about government funding for gender modification are being couched in human rights frameworks and public health safety (Gorry 2010).

Moreover, male and female sex workers are among the most vulnerable populations for HIV infection, sexual violence, and drug use (Mayhew et al. 2009). The public health implications of sex work (and the shift to applying a human rights framework) have been explored through a variety of methods, including qualitative and ethnographic techniques. Innovative public health research and interventions have studied sexual risk and mental health risks throughout the world (Kempadoo 2003). Sex work, intergenerational sex, and gift-exchange for sex have been documented throughout the world, and it has been linked to factors such as food insecurity (Weiser et al. 2007). Progressive public health has shown that sex workers can no longer be thought to be merely victims, but have come to take on the role of the human rights advocates throughout the world pointing to the elements of structural stigma and discrimination that led to their condition.

It is a challenge to study sexual desire and behaviour in populations where assuming an identity puts the person at sociocultural, political economic, and even legal disadvantages. Because of the stigma and discrimination associated with non-heterosexual sexualities, non-politicized alternative sexual communities and/or individuals are often 'hidden' or hard to reach. Such populations have a number of distinctive characteristics, including the fact that no sampling frame exists for them because their boundaries and their size are unclear or unknown. Perhaps even more importantly, members of these populations may often be unwilling to cooperate with research activities or public health programmes because of their understandable fear of experiencing stigma and discrimination as a result of their participation. Widely used research methods, such as household or neighbourhood surveys, are therefore ineffective (as well as inefficient because of the fact that the number of persons in such hidden populations is typically relatively small) (Ramirez-Valles et al. 2005).

Public health studies and interventions on hidden populations are among the most methodologically innovative. Snowball sampling or chain-referral sampling are common techniques in achieving a theoretically defined number of participants in qualitative research in fields such as anthropology and sociology. Respondent-driven sampling is a type of chain-referral sampling in which study participants refer others to the study, beginning with key informants or seeds that can be randomly selected. This form of chain-referral provides a dual incentive for the participant and weights the sample. Respondent-driven sampling lends itself to social network analysis if referral systems and patterns are tracked. In fact, this can be particularly useful in public health to study sexual networks, networks of drug users, or sex workers (Ramirez-Valles et al. 2005). More researchers are beginning to bridge the gap between qualitative and quantitative approaches, as well as forging interdisciplinary perspectives, precisely because they acknowledge the complexities of studying sexual diversity in public health. It is now more common for studies with large probability samples to explore multilevel research questions that require a complementary approach of ethnography and survey methods.

Social regulation of sexuality

The social regulation of sexuality impacts how public health studies are conceptualized, designed, and executed. A range of formal and informal institutions and community structures define socially accepted expressions of sexuality, delineating cultural and social psychological norms. Social regulation might occur to enforce moral 'tradition', especially when relating sexuality with heteronormative reproductive practices.

Legal frameworks are regulations with implications on sexual practices as well as on gender roles. Throughout the world, laws determine the ways in which sexuality affects economic and political issues, such as through the institution of marriage, which marginalizes non-heterosexuals. Laws that ban sodomy or that deny adoption privileges based on sexual orientation target non-heterosexuals and punish the unmarried. Legal systems also dictate who has control over the female body, what women are allowed to wear, how women are inherited through generations

of men in some countries, the kinds of sexual pleasure women should be granted, and in some cases laws sanction gender-based violence.

Social networks might regulate sexuality through 'soft' mechanisms such as gossip or 'harder' mechanisms such as ostracism from communities if non-conforming sexualities or gender roles are expressed. Families and schools are among the most important institutions in directly providing sex education for children and adults throughout the world. While families are often thought of as spaces for social support, conservative family values that condemn homosexuality, for example, might create structural vulnerabilities to mental health problems, including depression, substance use, and thoughts of suicide among LGBTQ youth. Schools and their political agendas on sexuality vary, having a major impact on the sexual formation of the individual and her/his interaction with peers. Policy interventions, such as those that ban bullying in schools, might have vast implications for public health outcomes.

Community-based groups and civil society organization such as faith-based organization have varied on their position on sexuality and public health. Some religious traditions, such as Pentecostal evangelicals—which have been proliferating in numbers throughout the world in the twentieth and twenty-first centuries, have been the most adamant proponents of public health campaigns that promote the reduction of sex partners, faithful relationships, and waiting until marriage, among other more conservative approaches to regulating sexuality at the expense of excluding non-heterosexuals and gender non-conforming individuals from their messages and flocks. In research on Afro-descendent religions in countries such as Brazil, some faith-based organizations have been shown to embrace alternative sexualities and sexual diversity, as well as have a strong platform for women's equality and rights (Garcia and Parker 2011).

Also noteworthy, the Internet is among the most influential social/virtual institutions in contemporary life that shape and regulate sexuality and sexual norms. The pornography industry is ever growing and few public health studies have systematically analysed the association between exposure to pornography and sexual behaviour, some finding that increased exposure to pornography is associated with higher sexual risk-taking (Eaton et al. 2012). Social networks and smartphone applications (apps) such as Grindr (which uses advanced GPS systems to locate proximal partners in the vicinity of the individual essentially to meet up and have sex) are often used to meet new sexual partners and fulfil sexual fantasies that were once only imagined. Even though the Internet has been more liberating than limiting in its forms of social regulation, conservative civil society groups are ever present on the worldwide web with moralizing, normalizing, and moderating tendencies that often make people afraid of having excessive sexual pleasure.

The public health implications of the social regulation of sexuality are extensive. Regulatory groups and mechanisms include not only legal frameworks, but also the family, schools, religious groups/institutions, formal community leadership structures, informal structures that generate social (and virtual) capital, just to name a few, which have been considered important in public health studies and interventions related to sexuality. When considering the possibility of targeting sexual behaviours through community and ecological interventions and studies, we call for new methodologies that analyse both heterosexual and non-heterosexual practices and pleasures. For example, cellular phone technologies and innovative forms of ethnographic mapping that examine trends on how virtual social networks on the Internet could contribute to a greater understanding of how sexual desires are enacted. These technologies can also be used to target vulnerable populations that might be excluded from participation in civil society organizations through self-selection or through social sanctioning.

Sexual health and sexual rights

The notion of sexual rights is the counterpart to social regulation. The emphasis on sexual rights has helped to constitute a fairly new field of public health and this framework draws on interdisciplinary and intersectoral approaches to improving collective health outcomes in what can be considered a public health social movement. Even though international mobilization has dominated the use of the term 'sexual rights' as a rallying framework in global activism, sexual rights are often only regulated effectively as they are interpreted and understood on the local level in families, at schoolyards, by community-based groups and non-governmental organizations (Garcia and Parker 2006).

The language of sexual rights in public health stems greatly from the application of a human rights framework to addressing not only individual, but also social and structural vulnerabilities. Human rights are generally understood as universal and fundamental rights deserved equally by all people. The International Conference on Population and Development (ICPD) held in Cairo in 1994 was a watershed moment for the transnational dissemination of discourses of sexual rights, although the official document of the ICPD did not include in it a clear mention of the term 'sexual rights' after much heated debate among conservatives and progressives (Petchesky 2000).

Although public health leaders have partnered with activists throughout the world to push for sexual equality to be considered part of our fundamental rights, it has been difficult to include sexual rights as part of framing documents at the level of the United Nations because of their contentious nature. International discourses about reproductive and sexual rights have been rooted primarily in Western individualism, even though notions of bodily integrity and personhood have a long history in non-Western contexts, in which they are more intertwined with social and cultural norms and collective rights (Corrêa and Petchesky 1994). To address vulnerabilities that are contingent on context, culture, and structures, it is paramount to include access to resources and the community-level conditions that might enable or restrict sexuality and health.

Moreover, sexual rights emerged under the umbrella of reproductive rights (which focused primarily on gender inequality, violence against women, and population control, among other heterocentric issues), but health rights activists and LGBTQ groups have pushed the envelope to develop a concept that goes beyond human reproduction and addresses non-heterosexual health and rights-based issues (Miller 2000). Although sexual health is often confounded with reproductive health, there has been an attempt to differentiate the two by the World Health Organization. These include the right of all persons, free of coercion, discrimination and violence, to: 'a state of physical, mental and social well-being in relation to sexuality. It requires a positive and respectful approach to sexuality and sexual relationships, as well as the possibility of having pleasurable and safe sexual experiences' (World Health Organization 2011b).

While sexuality can include all of these dimensions, not all of them are always experienced or expressed. The 'responsible' exercise of human rights requires that all persons respect the rights of others. Within the framework elaborated by WHO, sexual and reproductive health are central aspects of life at all ages and encompass sex, gender identities and roles, sexual orientation, pleasure, and reproduction. Sexuality is experienced and expressed in thoughts, fantasies, desires, beliefs, attitudes, values, behaviours, practices, roles, and relationships. Sexuality-related vulnerabilities highlight why these issues ought to be framed as inextricably tied to other human rights, political and civil liberties, and economic rights.

The protection from harm, be it for heterosexual or non-heterosexual populations, has been the main focus of the sexual rights movement. Nonetheless, sexual pleasure has also been conceptualized as an integral part of sexual rights by activists and also by progressive public health campaigns. One example of harnessing the power of the sensual in social marketing is the eroticization of the condom. Rather than showing the condom in isolation as a prophylactic barrier to natural sex, campaigns throughout the world have used sex symbols to entice safer sex—almost as a form of harm reduction in which people are assumed to be having sex in any case, so these campaigns make 'safer', sexy. Sexual rights frameworks that are emerging throughout the world are giving birth to new debates about gender and sexual equality that goes beyond reproduction (not to downplay the utmost importance of debates about new reproductive technologies that are more inclusive of non-heterosexuals).

Conclusion

Especially during the closing decades of the twentieth century and the beginning of the twenty-first, the field of sexuality and public health has taken shape as one of the fastest growing areas of research and intervention in relation to population health. It is a field that has been characterized historically as highly polemical, often marked by controversy and disagreement based on conflicts in relation to fundamental values and ethical positions. But at least since the emergence of the HIV/AIDS epidemic in the early 1980s, we have also realized that ignoring issues of sexuality, sweeping them under the carpet or leaving them hidden away in the closet, does nothing to promote the realization of true sexual health and well-being. This is especially worrisome when sexual norms, as we have pointed out, lead to grave disparities in health. On the contrary, it is only by bringing sexuality out into the open, by freeing it of stigma, prejudice, and discrimination, and by building a culture of sexual rights, freedoms, and protections, that we can truly advance the cause of sexual health and well-being. In this sense, it is clear that public health work on sexuality in the early twenty-first century both grows out of and is aligned with the long tradition of public health as a social movement—a movement based on principles of social justice and human rights, capable of promoting health for all based on a foundational set of ethical and political principles. Far from a peripheral concern related to a taboo topic, few areas of work are so central to a public health project for the present.

References

Abdullah, M.A., Basharat, Z., Kamal, B., et al. (2012). Is social exclusion pushing the Pakistani Hijras (Transgenders) towards commercial sex work? A qualitative study. *BMC International Health and Human Rights,* 12(1), 32.

Altman, D. and Buse, K. (2012). Thinking politically about HIV: political analysis and action in response to AIDS. *Contemporary Politics,* 18(2), 127–40.

Bankole, A., Biddlecom, A., Guiella, G., Singh, S., and Zulu, E. (2007). Sexual behavior, knowledge and information sources of very young adolescents in four sub-Saharan African countries. *African Journal of Reproductive Health,* 11(3), 28–43.

Barker, G. (2007). *Adolescents, Social Support and Help-Seeking Behavior: An International Literature Review and Programme Consultation with Recommendations for Action.* Geneva: World Health Organization.

Bauer, G.R. and Jairam, J.A. (2008). Are lesbians really women who have sex with women (WSW)? Methodological concerns in measuring sexual orientation in health research. *Women & Health,* 48(4), 383–408.

Blum, R. and Mmari, K. (2006). *Risk Protective Factors Affecting Adolescent Reproductive Health in Developing Countries: An Analysis of Adolescent Sexual and Reproductive Health Literature from Around the World.* Geneva: World Health Organization.

Blum, R.W. (2007). Youth in sub-Saharan Africa. *Journal of Adolescent Health,* 41(3), 230–8.

Boyle, E.H. (2005). *Female Genital Cutting: Cultural Conflict in the Global Community.* Baltimore, MD: Johns Hopkins University Press.

Brandt, A. (1987). *No Magic Bullet: A Social History of Venereal Disease in the United States since 1880.* New York: Oxford University Press.

Charlton, B.M., Corliss, H.L., Missmer, S.A., et al. (2011). Reproductive health screening disparities and sexual orientation in a cohort study of U.S. adolescent and young adult females. *Journal of Adolescent Health,* 49(5), 505–10.

Chow, E.P., Wilson, D.P., and Zhang, L. (2011). What is the potential for bisexual men in China to act as a bridge of HIV transmission to the female population? Behavioural evidence from a systematic review and meta-analysis. *BMC Infectious Disease,* 11(242), 1–17.

Corrêa, S. and Petchesky, R. (1994). Reproductive and sexual rights: a feminist perspective. In G. Sen, A. Germaine, and L. Chen (eds.) *Population Policies Reconsidered: Health, Empowerment, and Rights,* pp. 107–22. Boston, MA: Harvard University Press.

Corrêa, S., Petchesky, R., and Parker, R. (2008). *Sexuality, Health and Human Rights.* London: Routledge.

Dahl, B., Margrethe Fylkesnes, A., Sørlie, V., and Malterud, K. (2013). Lesbian women's experiences with healthcare providers in the birthing context: a meta-ethnography. *Midwifery,* 29(6), 674–81.

De Cuypere, G., Knudson, G., and Bockting, W. (2010). Response of the World Professional Association for Transgender Health to the proposed DSM 5 criteria for gender incongruence. *International Journal of Transgenderism,* 12(2), 119–23.

de Zalduondo, B.O. (1991). Prostitution viewed cross-culturally: toward recontextualizing sex work in AIDS intervention research. *Journal of Sex Research,* 22(2), 223–48.

Díaz, R.M., Ayala, G., Bein, E., Henne, J., and Marin, B.V. (2001). The impact of homophobia, poverty, and racism on the mental health of gay and bisexual Latino men: findings from 3 US cities. *American Journal of Public Health,* 91(6), 927–32.

Dowsett, G.W. (2003). Some considerations on sexuality and gender in the context of AIDS. *Reproductive Health Matters,* 11(22), 21–9.

East, L., Jackson, D., and O'Brien, L. (2007). 'I don't want to hate him forever': understanding daughter's experiences of father absence. *Australian Journal of Advanced Nursing,* 24(4), 14–18.

Eaton, L.A., Cain, D.N., Pope, H., Garcia, J., and Cherry, C. (2012). The relationship between pornography use and sexual behaviours among at-risk HIV-negative men who have sex with men. *Sexual Health,* 9(2), 166–70.

Farmer, P., Connors, M., and Simmons, J. (eds.) (1996). *Women, Poverty and AIDS: Sex, Drugs and Structural Violence.* Monroe, ME: Common Courage Press.

Freud, S. (1994). The social construction of gender. *Journal of Adult Development,* 1(1), 37–45.

Garcia, J. and Parker, R. (2006). From global discourse to local action: the makings of a sexual rights movement? *Horizontes Antropológicos,* 12(26), 13–41.

Garcia, J. and Parker, R.G. (2011). Resource mobilization for health advocacy: Afro-Brazilian religious organizations and HIV prevention and control. *Social Science & Medicine,* 72(12), 1930–8.

Gorry, C. (2010). Transgender health in Cuba: evolving policy to impact practice. *MEDICC Review,* 12(4), 5–9.

Gough, B. (2013). The psychology of men's health: maximizing masculine capital. *Health Psychology,* 32(1), 1–4.

Gray, R.E., Fitch, M.I., Fergus, K.D., Mykhalovskiy, E., and Church, K. (2002). Hegemonic masculinity and the experience of prostate cancer: a narrative approach. *Journal of Aging and Identity,* 7(1), 43–62.

Healthy People 2020 (2011). *Determinants of Health.* [Online] Available at: http://www.healthypeople.gov/2020/about/DOHAbout.aspx.

Hindin, A. and Fatusi, A. (2009). Adolescent sexual and reproductive health in developing countries: an overview of trends and interventions. *International Perspectives on Sexual and Reproductive Health,* 35(2), 58–62.

Hirsch, J.S., Meneses, S., Thompson, B., Negroni, M., Pelcastre, B., and Del Rio, C. (1007). The inevitability of infidelity: sexual reputation, social geographies, and marital HIV risk in rural Mexico. *American Journal of Public Health,* 97(6), 986–96.

Hunter, M. (2002). The materiality of everyday sex: thinking beyond 'prostitution'. *African Studies,* 61, 99–120.

Ishida, K. (2010). The role of ethnicity in father absence and children's school enrollment in Guatemala. *Population Research and Policy Review,* 29(4), 569–91.

Jones, N., Moore, K., Villar-Marquez, E., and Broadbent, E. (2009). *Painful Lessons: The Politics of Preventing Sexual Violence and Bullying at School.* London: Overseas Development Institute.

Kandel, D. and Davies, M. (1991). Friendship networks, intimacy, and illicit drug use in young adulthood: a comparison of two competing theories. *Criminology,* 29(3), 441–69.

Kane, S. and Mason, T. (1992). 'IV drug users' and 'sex partners': the limits of epidemiological categories and the ethnography of risk. In G. Herdt and S. Lindenbaum (eds.) *In the Time of AIDS: Social Analysis, Theory and Method,* pp. 199–222. Newbury Park, CA: Sage.

Kempadoo, K. (2003). Globalizing sex workers' rights. *Canadian Woman Studies,* 22(3), 143–50.

Kinsey, A., Martin, C.E., Gebhard, R.H., and Pomeroy, W. (1953). *Sexual Behavior in the Human Female.* Philadelphia, PA: Saunders.

Kinsey, A., Martin, C.E., and Pomeroy, W. (1948). *Sexual Behavior in the Human Male.* Philadelphia, PA: Saunders.

Kitzinger, C. (2005). Heteronormativity in action: reproducing the heterosexual nuclear family in after-hours medical calls. *Social Problems,* 52(4), 477–98.

Klitzman, R.L. and Greenberg, J.D. (2002). Patterns of communication between gay and lesbian patients and their health care providers. *Journal of Homosexuality,* 42(4), 65–75.

Leclerc-Madlala, S. (2003). Transactional sex and the pursuit of modernity. *Social Dynamics – A Journal of the Centre for African Studies University of Cape Town,* 29, 213–33.

Lombardi, E. (2001). Enhancing transgender health care. *American Journal of Public Health,* 91(6), 869–72.

Mahoney, A., Pargament, K.I., Tarakeshwar, N., and Swank, A.B. (2008). Religion in the home in the 1980s and 1990s: a meta-analytic review and conceptual analysis of links between religion, marriage, and parenting. *Psychology of Religion and Spirituality,* S(1), 63–101.

Mayhew, S., Collumbien, M., Qureshi, A., et al. (2009). Protecting the unprotected: mixed-method research on drug use, sex work and rights in Pakistan's fight against HIV/AIDS. *Sexually Transmitted Infections*, 85(Suppl. 2), ii31–6.

Meyer, C., Blissett, J., and Oldfield, C. (2001). Sexual orientation and eating psychopathology: the role of masculinity and femininity. *International Journal of Eating Disorders*, 29(3), 314–18.

Meyer, I.H. (2003). Prejudice, social stress, and mental health in lesbian, gay, and bisexual populations: conceptual issues and research evidence. *Psychological Bulletin*, 129(5), 674–97.

Miller, A.M. (2000). Sexual but not reproductive: exploring the junction and disjunction of sexual and reproductive rights. *Health and Human Rights*, 4(2), 68–109.

Millett, G., Malebranche, D., Mason, B., and Spikes, P. (2005). Focusing 'down low': bisexual black men, HIV risk and heterosexual transmission. *Journal of the National Medical Association*, 97(Suppl. 7), 52S–59S.

Millett, G.A., Peterson, J.L., Flores, S.A., et al. (2012). Comparisons of disparities and risks of HIV infection in black and other men who have sex with men in Canada, UK, and USA: a meta-analysis. *The Lancet*, 380(9839), 341–8.

Parker, R. (2001). Sexuality, culture and power in HIV/AIDS research. *Annual Review of Anthropology*, 30, 163–79.

Parker, R. (2007). Sexuality, health, and human rights. *American Journal of Public Health*, 97(6), 972–3.

Parker, R. (2011). Grassroots activism, civil society mobilization and the politics of the global HIV/AIDS epidemic. *Brown Journal of World Affairs*, 17(2), 21–37.

Parker, R. and Aggleton, P. (2003). HIV and AIDS-related stigma and discrimination: a conceptual framework and implications for action. *Social Science & Medicine*, 7(1), 13–24.

Parker, R., Di Mauro, D., Filiano, B., Garcia, J., Muñoz-Laboy, M., and Sember, R. (2004). Global transformations and intimate relations in the 21st century: social science research on sexuality and the emergence of sexual health and sexual rights frameworks. *Annual Review of Sex Research*, 15, 362–98.

Parker, R., Easton, D., and Klein, C. (2000). Structural barriers and facilitators in HIV prevention: a review of international research. *AIDS*, 14(Suppl. 1), S22–32.

Parker, R.G., Herdt, G., and Carballo, M. (1991). Sexual culture, HIV transmission, and AIDS research. *The Journal of Sex Research*, 28, 77–98.

Patton, G. and Viner, R. (2007). Pubertal transitions in health. *The Lancet*, 369, 1130–9.

Petchesky, R.P. (2000). Sexual rights: inventing a concept, mapping an international practice. In R.G. Parker, R.M. Barbosa, and P. Aggleton (eds.) *Framing the Sexual Subject*, pp. 81–103. Berkeley, CA: University of California Press.

Ramirez, M., Paik, A., Sanchagrin, K., and Heimer, K. (2012). Violent peers, network centrality, and intimate partner violence perpetration by young men. *Journal of Adolescent Health*, 51(5), 503–9.

Ramirez-Valles, J., Heckathorn, D.D., Vázquez, R., Diaz, R.M., and Campbell, R.T. (2005). From networks to populations: the development and application of respondent-driven sampling among IDUs and Latino gay men. *AIDS and Behavior*, 9(4), 387–402.

Ryan, H., Wortley, P.M., Easton, A., Pederson, L., and Greenwood, G. (2001). Smoking among lesbians, gays, and bisexuals: a review of the literature. *American Journal of Preventive Medicine*, 21(2), 142–9.

Stevens, P.E. and Hall, J.M. (1988). Stigma, health beliefs and experiences with health care in lesbian women. *Image Journal of Nursing Scholarship*, 20(2), 69–73.

Swidler, A. and Watkins, S. (2007). Ties of dependence: AIDS and transactional sex in rural Malawi. *Studies in Family Planning*, 38, 147–62.

Torres, J.B., Solberg, V.S.H., and Carlstrom, A.H. (2002). The myth of sameness among Latino men and their machismo. *American Journal of Orthopsychiatry*, 72(2), 163–81.

Treichler, P.A. (1988). AIDS, homophobia and biomedical discourse: an epidemic of signification. In D. Crimp (ed.) *AIDS: Cultural Analysis and Cultural Activism*, pp. 31–70. Cambridge MA: The MIT Press.

Turner, C.F., Miller, H.G., and Moses, L.E. (eds.) (1989). *AIDS: Sexual Behavior and Intravenous Drug Use*. Washington, DC: National Academy Press.

Weiser, S.D., Leiter, K., Bangsberg, D.R., et al. (2007). Food insufficiency is associated with high-risk sexual behavior among women in Botswana and Swaziland. *PLoS Medicine*, 4(10), 1589–98.

Wiessing, L.G., Van Roosmalen, M.S., Koedijk, P., Bieleman, B., and Houweling, H. (1999). Silicones, hormones and HIV in transgender street prostitutes. *AIDS*, 13(16), 2315–16.

Wilkinson, W. and Kitzinger, C. (1994). The social construction of heterosexuality. *Journal of Gender Studies*, 3(3), 307–17.

World Health Organization (2000). *What About Boys? A Literature Review on the Health and Development of Adolescent Boys*. Geneva: World Health Organization.

World Health Organization (2011a). *Reproductive Health*. [Online] Available at: http://www.who.int/topics/reproductive_health/en/.

World Health Organization (2011b). *Sexual Health*. [Online] Available at: http://www.who.int/topics/sexual_health/en/.

Young, R.M. and Meyer, I.H. (2005). The trouble with 'MSM' and 'WSW': erasure of the sexual-minority person in public health discourse. *American Journal of Public Health*, 95(7), 1144–9.

Demography and public health

Emily Grundy and Michael Murphy

Introduction to demography and public health

The health and healthcare needs of a population cannot be measured or met without knowledge of its size and characteristics. Demography is concerned with this and with understanding population dynamics—how populations change in response to the interplay between fertility, mortality, and migration. This understanding is a prerequisite for making the forecasts about future population size and structure which should underpin healthcare planning. Such analyses necessitate a review of the past. The number of very old people in a population, for example, depends on the number of births eight or nine decades earlier and risks of death at successive ages throughout the intervening period. The *proportion* of very old people depends partly on this numerator but more importantly on the denominator, the size of the population as a whole. The number of births in a population depends on current patterns of family building, and also on the number of women 'at risk' of reproduction—itself a function of past trends in fertility and mortality. Similarly, the number and causes of deaths are strongly influenced by age structure.

Demography is largely concerned with answering questions about *how* populations change and their measurement. The broader field of population studies embraces questions of *why* these changes occur, and with what consequences.

This chapter presents information on demographic methods and data sources and their application to health and population issues, together with information on demographic trends and their implications and the major theories about demographic change, in order to elucidate the complex interrelationship between population change and human health.

Global issues

Fig. 6.3.1 shows that the world's population has recently been growing at an unprecedented rate and was estimated to be 7.05 billion at mid 2012 (UN 2011). While it took an estimated 123 years (from 1804 to 1927) for the world to increase its population from 1 to 2 billion, the increase from 6 to 7 billion was achieved in a tenth of the time (1999–2011). The United Nation's (UN's) medium projection suggests a further increase of some 2.3 billion by 2050 (UN 2011). Beyond this, there is a good chance that global population growth will cease by the end of the twenty-first century (Lutz and Samir 2010).

This prospect of global population stability masks huge differences between regions and between richer and poorer countries. Between 1950 and 2000, 77 per cent of world population growth occurred in countries currently designated by the UN as less developed (excluding the least developed, see Box 6.3.1 for definitions); 13 per cent in least developed countries and 11 per cent in more developed regions. Between 2000 and 2050, medium-term projections suggest that population growth in more developed regions will account for only 4 per cent of the total with 63 per cent occurring in less developed countries and 33 per cent in the least developed countries. These projections imply that by 2050 the share of the world's population living in currently more developed regions will account for only 14 per cent of the total world population—compared with 32 per cent a century earlier—while the representation of those in the poorest countries will have increased from 8 per cent of the total in 1950 to 19 per cent in 2050.

These hugely differing rates of growth arise from differences in vital rates, and associated large variations in age structures, which are illustrated for regions and selected countries within them in Table 6.3.1. In a number of European countries and some Asian

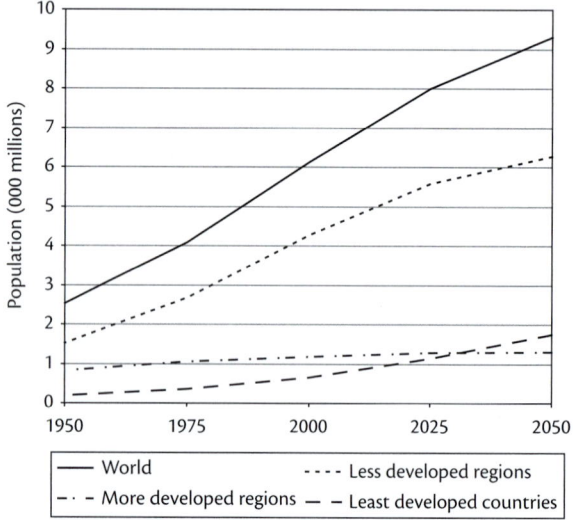

Fig. 6.3.1 Population and projected population of the world and more, less, and least developed regions, 1950–2050.

Source: data from United Nations, *World Population Prospects: The 2010 Revision*, United Nations, New York, USA, Copyright © 2011, available from http://esa.un.org/unpd/wpp/Excel-Data/population.htm.

Box 6.3.1 Country and regional classifications by level of development

The UN classifies countries into 'more' and 'less' developed and also identifies a group of 50 'least developed' countries. The more developed category includes all of Europe, North America, Australia, New Zealand, and Japan. The least developed countries are mostly in sub-Saharan Africa but also include Afghanistan, Bangladesh, Cambodia, and Myanmar. The classification has some anomalies in that some wealthy Asian and Near Eastern countries are counted as less developed (e.g. South Korea, Singapore, Cyprus, Israel) whereas some poorer former Eastern bloc countries are treated as more developed (e.g. Albania, Belarus, Bulgaria).

The World Bank employs a classification based on gross national income per capita which divides countries into high-, middle-, and low-income groups, with a subdivision of the middle into upper and lower. Some of the countries (principally from Eastern Europe) classified by the UN as developed fall into middle-income categories, while some of the UN less developed group are classified by the World Bank as middle income (principally Latin American) or high income (some South East Asian).

Membership of the Organisation for Economic Cooperation and Development (OECD) is also sometimes used as an indicator of developed country status; members include Russia and Mexico, both of which are classified by the World Bank as middle- rather than high-income countries.

The Human Development Index compiled by the UN Development Programme takes into account factors other than income, such as school enrolment, literacy, and levels of mortality.

Regional groupings employed by different international agencies also vary slightly. Further details of all these classifications are available on the relevant organizations' websites.

While some regions grapple with the needs of rapidly growing populations, such as large increases in requirements for child health services and schools, others face challenges of population ageing and, in some cases, population decline. By 2025, nearly a quarter of the Western European population is expected to be aged 65 or more and in some countries, such as Japan, South Korea, Spain, and Italy, projections suggest that a third or more of the population will be aged 65 and over by 2050 (UN 2011).

Table 6.3.1 Indicators of age structure, fertility, and mortality: world regions and selected countries, 2011

Region/country		Proportion (%) of population aged:		Total fertility rate	Life expectancy at birth (years)
		<15	65 and over		
Africa		41	3	4.6	58
	Sub-Saharan	43	3	5.0	56
	Northern	33	5	3.1	70
Asia		25	7	2.2	70
	India	30	5	2.6	67
	China	18	9	1.5	75
	Japan	14	23	1.4	84
	Indonesia	27	6	2.3	71
	South Korea	16	11	1.2	79
Australia		18	14	1.8	82
Europe		15	16	1.6	76
	Italy	14	20	1.4	82
	Poland	15	14	1.3	76
	Germany	13	21	1.4	80
	Sweden	15	20	1.7	81
	Ukraine	14	15	1.3	69
	UK	17	16	1.9	80
Latin America and Caribbean		27	7	2.2	74
	Brazil	25	7	1.8	73
	Chile	22	9	1.9	78
	Guatemala	38	4	3.3	71
North America		19	14	2.0	79
	United States	20	13	2.1	78
World		26	8	2.4	68

Source: data from United States Census Bureau, Population Division, International Programs Center, International Data Base, available from http://www.census.gov/population/international/data/idb/informationGateway.php.

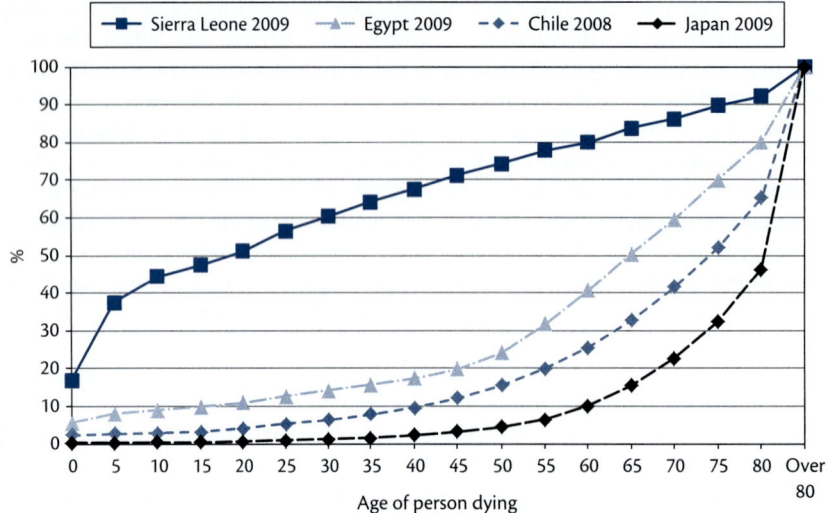

Fig. 6.3.2 Cumulative distribution of deaths by age; Sierra Leone 2009, Egypt 2009, Chile 2008, Japan 2009.

Source: data from United Nations Department of Economic and Social Affairs, Demographic Yearbook 2011, ST/ESA/STAT/SER.R/41, United Nations, New York, USA, Copyright © United Nations 2012, available from http://unstats.un.org/unsd/demographic/products/dyb/dybsets/2011.pdf

countries, such as Japan, women on average have only 1.4 children or fewer (see Box 6.3.2 for derivation of total fertility rate), and people aged 65 and over outnumber children under 15. In sub-Saharan Africa, women on average have five children each, 40 per cent or more of the population is aged 15 or under, and only 3 per cent aged 65 or more.

Levels of mortality, and associated differences in age and cause distribution of death, also vary markedly. In some high-income countries, average life expectancy at birth is above 80, while in some sub-Saharan countries it is below 50, substantially because of HIV/AIDS. As shown in Fig. 6.3.2, in Sierra Leone, 40 per cent of all deaths in a year are of infants and children aged under 5, compared with 0.3 per cent in Japan. Conversely, of all deaths, 70 per cent in Japan and 50 per cent in Chile, a middle-income country, are of people aged 75 and over; equivalent proportions for Egypt and Sierra Leone are

20 per cent and 8 per cent respectively. These variations have enormous implications for health and healthcare priorities in, and beyond, the populations concerned. Divergence in population growth between regions of the world is also fuelling mass migration, which itself has implications for global population health (Fernandes et al. 2007).

Closely related to variations in the distribution of deaths by age are differences in the cause structure of death. As shown in Table 6.3.2, communicable diseases, maternal and perinatal conditions, and nutritional deficiencies account for 67 per cent of all deaths in sub-Saharan Africa but only 5 per cent in Europe. Conversely, non-communicable diseases are responsible for 25 per cent of deaths in sub-Saharan Africa, 66 per cent in Asia, but 88 per cent in Europe. While in parts of the world, communicable diseases and reproductive and child health present the most pressing public health problems, concerns about the prevalence

Table 6.3.2 Distribution of deaths (%) by cause group and world region, 2010

	Communicable	Non-communicable	Injuries
Global	24.9	65.5	9.6
Europe	5.1	88.3	6.6
North America	5.3	88.0	6.8
High-income Asia and Pacific	11.4	81.1	7.5
Oceania	15.1	78.1	6.9
Latin America and Caribbean	14.2	69.0	16.8
North Africa and Middle East	16.2	75.2	8.6
Asia (excl. high-income and Middle East)	23.3	66.2	10.4
sub-Saharan Africa	66.5	24.9	8.6

Source: data from Global Burden of Disease Study 2010, Mortality Results 1970–2010, Institute for Health Metrics and Evaluation (IHME), Seattle, Washington, USA, Copyright © 2012, available from http://ghdx.healthdata.org/record/global-burden-disease-study-2010-gbd-2010-mortality-results-1970-2010.

of age-related chronic degenerative diseases predominate in others. In sub-Saharan Africa, 1.2 million deaths are due to HIV/AIDS. Although the numbers of such deaths are estimated to have peaked globally around 2005 (UNAIDS 2012), they still represent a substantial and long-term burden (UN 2011).

The process that separates populations with high fertility, relatively high mortality, young age structures, and rapid growth from those with low vital rates, older age structures, and slow or no growth, is conceptualized as the demographic transition. Identifying, and explaining, this and associated profound changes in health has been a central preoccupation of modern demography (Lee 2003). Before turning to these issues, the basic methods and materials of demographic analysis must be considered and the issue of population dynamics—*how* populations change—addressed.

Demographic data and methods of analysis

In the seventeenth century, John Graunt, a London merchant, used data from the London Bills of Mortality to devise an early life table, leading to him being dubbed the 'father of modern demography'. However, while Graunt had information on *numbers* of deaths, he lacked data on the population at risk and could not compute death *rates*. Essentially all demographic analysis requires data both on the population 'stock' and on 'flows' in and out—births, deaths, and migration. The traditional sources of information on the former are population censuses and, for the latter, vital registration systems.

Population censuses

The first 'modern' censuses were undertaken in Scandinavia in the eighteenth century. Censuses spread throughout Europe during the nineteenth century and most of the rest of the world in the twentieth. As well as basic questions about age, sex, marital status, and place of residence, data on other characteristics such as employment, education and housing are often collected. The UN recommends that censuses be conducted at least decennially in years ending in 0 or 1.

Censuses have many strengths and are often the only source of data for small areas or population subgroups. Although primarily a tool for collecting data on population 'stock', censuses have also been used to find out about vital events. Many countries use censuses to provide data on recent internal migration (through questions on place of residence 1 or more years earlier) and immigration (through questions on country of birth and/or date of entry for those born elsewhere). Indirect estimation techniques developed by Brass and others mean that questions on number of children born and number who have died, on widowhood, and orphanhood are widely used to assess mortality levels and trends using both censuses and surveys in countries with deficient vital registration systems (Preston et al. 2001).

However, censuses involve huge costs and the challenge of ensuring acceptable data quality. Approaches to reducing cost (and improving quality) include use of sample censuses, either for the census as a whole, as in China, or for more detailed questions, as in the United States. Census taking requires not only a reasonable administrative infrastructure, but also the cooperation of the population to be enumerated. Some countries have given up taking censuses because the latter is lacking and now rely on large-scale surveys or 'virtual censuses' based on population registration data. The twenty-first century is seeing more countries adopting alternatives as the information required by governments becomes more complex and the difficulties of mass data collection escalate. In 2010, only 11 of the 27 current European Union members conducted traditional censuses (Valente 2010).

When censuses are taken, difficulties arising from errors and omissions are common, even in countries with a long history of census taking. Young, geographically mobile adults, recent (especially unauthorized) immigrants, members of minority ethnic groups, infants, and the very old are those most likely to be under-enumerated—some of the very groups that policymakers and health professionals may be most keen to know about.

Groups such as seasonal migrants, military personnel, people temporarily away from home, and those with more than one residence also present problems. Not only are they more likely to be missed, but a decision has to be made about whether they should be assigned to their place of usual or legal residence (assuming it can be determined), or counted as belonging to the place of enumeration. The former system is termed *de jure*, the latter *de facto*. The issue of assigning people to some place of usual residence is important as often resources are allocated based on population size and characteristics. Moreover, it is essential to try and ensure that demographic events recorded in one system (vital registration) are attributed to the population actually 'at risk' of experiencing them. In richer countries, for example, most deaths occur in hospitals which may draw patients from a wide area. If these decedents are not assigned to the locality where they lived prior to hospital admission, areas including large hospitals will appear to have very high mortality rates while in others, recorded mortality will be artificially low.

Under-enumeration is usually assessed through census validation surveys (surveys of a sample of census addresses in which intensive efforts are made to contact non-respondents and check information supplied by respondents) and comparisons with population estimates from other sources. Beyond ensuring near-complete enumeration, the quality of the data collected is also a major concern.

In many populations, people may not always know their exact age and some approximation is reported or made by an enumerator. 'Heaping' on ages ending in 0 or 5 is a common result. Heaping can be detected by looking at the age distribution and applying various tests of consistency and such data are normally adjusted before publication. More serious problems arise when reported age is based on other characteristics, such as marital status, number of children or grandparent status, as clearly any analysis of, for example, age at first marriage, will be biased if people's report of their age is influenced by their marital status.

Vital registration

Data on demographic events, as well as on population characteristics, are needed. In richer countries these are drawn from vital registration. Compulsory registration of births and deaths was established in most European countries during the nineteenth century. In England and Wales, for example, civil registration was introduced in 1837. Subsequent improvements to the system included those following the 1874 *Births and Deaths Registration Act* which made parents legally responsible for registering births and required attending physicians to supply information on cause of death. Other revisions have since been made, for example, the inclusion of first mother's and later father's age and in 2012, recording of all children previously born, rather than just legitimate ones, on the confidential section of birth certificates. Most high-income countries have well-established registration systems with complete, or very near complete, coverage. In poorer parts of the world, however, vital registration systems are frequently seriously incomplete or non-existent, although there are exceptions and some countries, including India and China, have sample registration systems for selected areas. Currently only about a third of deaths estimated to occur globally are registered and reported to the World Health Organization, although if the sample registration systems in India and China are considered as sufficiently representative of their national populations, this proportion rises to 72 per cent (Mathers et al. 2005).

The quality of the information supplied and coded is of course very important. No one registers their own death and the information obtained from proxy informants may be inaccurate. Differential reporting of age, occupation, marital status, or other characteristics in the census and in other sources, such as death certificates, presents a further difficulty. Numerator–denominator discrepancies may introduce serious bias into the analysis of mortality at advanced ages, or by characteristics such as occupationally defined social class, marital status, or ethnicity (Williams et al. 2006). The Nordic and some other European countries avoid these problems by maintaining well-developed register-based systems that link vital registration data to population, occupational, and educational registers. One study of marital status differences in mortality at older ages found marked differences in results for countries using traditional and register-based systems (Murphy et al. 2007).

Cause of death

Death certificates are the major source of information on cause of death. In richer countries, cause of death is generally certified by a physician and coded according to the International Classification of Diseases (ICD) which originated from work undertaken by the nineteenth-century British medical statistician, William Farr. The tenth revision of the ICD came into use from 1994 and included nearly twice as many codes as ICD-9. ICD-11 is in preparation and is expected to come into use in 2015. National preferences, as well as ICD revisions, may influence assignment of cause of death, as illustrated in a number of classic papers in which case studies of deaths were distributed to physicians in different countries. Growing awareness of particular conditions may also influence coding practices. In the United States, Australia, and elsewhere, for example, there have been large increases in mentions of Alzheimer's disease and other dementias on death certificates since 2000. These partly reflect some changes associated with the introduction of ICD-10 but also effects of increased awareness and some specific campaigns to increase recognition of these conditions (Moschetti et al. 2012).

Older people, now the vast majority of decedents in low-mortality populations, are more likely to suffer multiple pathologies and the number of conditions recorded on death certificates has been increasing. Choice of one over another as the 'true' underlying cause of death is bound to be partially arbitrary. In the United Kingdom, for example, between 1984 and 1992 some 25 per cent fewer deaths were allocated to respiratory diseases purely as a result of changes in the rules used to select underlying cause of death (Griffiths and Brock 2003). Multiple coding of death certificates and analyses by all mentions of a condition may be more informative but such data are available in only a few countries (Anderson 2011). Variations in death certificate coding reflecting differences in medical knowledge and diagnosis, in the extent to which autopsies are used, in classification systems, and the quality of registration systems are a major factor complicating analyses of trends over time or between countries.

Deaths assigned to symptoms, signs and ill-defined conditions such as 'old age' or 'senility' or other causes lacking diagnostic meaning, sometimes referred to as 'garbage codes', present a particular problem. Mathers et al. (2005) in an investigation of coverage and quality of cause of death coding in 2003, found that in some countries over 40 per cent of deaths were assigned to these 'causes'. Only 23 countries met their definition of high quality of data with coverage of at least 90 per cent and fewer than 10 per cent of deaths assigned to ill-defined codes.

Variations in coding practices and use of ill-defined codes complicate comparisons over time, as well as between countries. Preston (1976) argued that there was an inverse association between the proportions of deaths assigned to circulatory diseases and to ill-defined causes, and that part of the apparent twentieth-century epidemic in heart disease mortality in richer countries may have been an artefactual consequence of improvements in death certification. A review of the proportion of all deaths in England and Wales assigned to circulatory diseases and to ill-defined causes in age groups over 65 from 1911–1915 to 2001–2010 is instructive. Early in the twentieth century, large proportions of deaths among the very old were assigned to ill-defined categories and declines in this proportion were associated with increases in the proportion attributed to circulatory diseases. The proportion of ill-defined deaths in the oldest group aged 80 and over was, however, slightly higher in 2001–2010 than in the preceding period, reflecting increased assignment to 'old age' as a cause. Reasons for this are unclear, although the cessation in 1993 of further enquiry into vague causes of death may have been a small contributory factor. Use of this 'cause of death' is likely to be reversed again in response to the 2000–2005 public enquiry into the case of Harold Shipman, a British family doctor whose serial murder of over 250 elderly patients was not detected for many years; an illustration of the importance of surveillance of deaths for reasons other than epidemiological or demographic investigation.

In countries which lack adequate certification and registration systems, data on deaths by cause are seriously limited. Attempts have been made to develop verbal autopsies, protocols for collecting information from lay informants which can be reviewed by physicians and used to assign cause of death (Wang et al. 2007). This approach has been useful in a number of small investigations and is being employed on a larger scale, for example, in India (Gajalakshmi and Peto 2011). However, a recent study tested physician-certified verbal autopsies in six sites in four poorer countries against gold standard assessment and found a concordance of less than 50 per cent, with substantial variability by cause and physician (Lozano et al. 2011). In the absence of routinely recorded data, estimates may be obtained by modelling. This has been used for the important issue of establishing the number of deaths from HIV/AIDS. The most ambitious exercise is the Global Burden of Disease programme which has used a large array of sources and methods, including expert knowledge, vital registration, field surveys, surveillance, and police and mortuary data to derive estimates of cause-specific mortality by age and sex for 235 separate causes for every country in the World (Wang et al. 2012).

Other data sources

Many countries have a range of surveys which provide more detailed information on, for example, health-related behaviour, family building strategies, reasons for migration, or information on biomarkers that would be impossible to collect in a census. In poorer countries, where other data sources are scarcer, surveys often present the best source of data on basic demographic parameters. Data quality is potentially better in a survey than a census, as it is more likely that well-trained interviewers can be used. The World Fertility Survey (WFS), an international population research programme launched in 1972 to determine fertility levels throughout the world, and its successor, the Demographic and Health Survey Programme (DHS), have been particularly valuable in providing demographic and health data for a range of poorer countries. Other approaches include multi-round surveys, in which respondents are asked about events since last contact, and dual-record systems which involve two independent data collection systems (one often a multi-round survey), the results of which are then combined. This method allows some estimation of missed events, but is expensive. These approaches are described in more detail in most demographic textbooks (Preston et al. 2001; Rowland 2003; Siegel and Swanson 2004).

The raw materials of demography relate to individuals' most personal experiences—sexual activity, family formation, birth control, reproduction, marital breakdown, illness, and death. All of these occur in a social framework which attaches value to some of these behaviours and stigmatizes others. Not surprisingly, respondents in censuses and surveys may be reluctant to disclose non-marital pregnancies, illegal abortions, undocumented migration, or deaths of relatives from AIDS. Concealment has also been the policy of some national governments which have treated demographic data as official secrets. Additionally, the enormous potential complications arising from people's uncertainties about age or other 'basic' characteristics including children ever-born; uncertain recollections of prior events and the vast scope for administrative errors have to be considered. The demographer's traditional obsession with data quality is hence understandable. Differences in perceptions and reporting of health status are also problematic and have bedevilled attempts to make international comparisons of health status as, even if questions are harmonized, the ways people respond to them are not (Ritu et al. 2002).

The statistics produced in series like the *United Nations Demographic Yearbooks* have their origins in what is or has been *done* by millions of people, mediated by what is *said* about these events and experiences, further filtered by how this is *recorded*, processed and analysed. Some assessment of data quality is given in the *United Nations Demographic Yearbooks*, but sometimes users may pay insufficient attention to this. A number of other organizations also produce international reference works and databases including the World Health Organization (WHO), the World Bank, the Organisation for Economic Cooperation and Development (OECD), Eurostat, The United States Census Bureau International Data Base (United States Census Bureau n.d.), and the Human Mortality Database. In most cases, these are available free of charge online.

The analysis of demographic data

A standard array of techniques and measures forms the basis of much demographic analysis; the most common of these are described briefly here. Further detail is supplied in a number of textbooks (Preston et al. 2001; Rowland 2003; Siegel and Swanson 2004). Analysis involves not just the application of a particular technique, but also decisions about what units of analysis to use and how to group them. A major distinction is between *period* and *cohort* analysis. Period analysis deals with events of a particular time period (e.g. mortality rates from 2005 to 2010) while cohort analyses follow the experience of individuals through time. Cohorts in this sense are defined as groups of people who have experienced the same significant event at the same time. Thus birth cohorts comprise people born in a particular year or group of years and marriage cohorts those marrying at a particular time. Cohort and life-course approaches to analysing mortality and other indicators of population health have an intuitive appeal and are increasingly used, both fuelling and fuelled by a growing number of longitudinal studies. Cohort analysis of time series data may be used in the absence of specially collected longitudinal data.

Cohort and period are two of the dimensions which 'place' persons in time; the third is age. Duration effects (such as duration of marriage, proximity to death, or length of exposure to a particular pathogen) may also be important. Cohort effects may be substantial and, unless allowed for, may mask relationships between age and various risks. Differences in the smoking behaviour of cohorts, for example, have a major effect on the relationships between age and smoking-related disease observed at different periods (Grundy 1997).

Decisions about whether to use individuals, families, households, or geographic areas as units of analysis are often constrained by data availability. Until relatively recently, most census data were only available as aggregate tabulations, but individual-level information is increasingly available. Other innovations include the development of samples including linked census, vital registration, and in some cases health service data such as the Longitudinal Studies available for countries of the United Kingdom and a number of others (Young et al. 2010). In these data sets, individuals' census records are linked with their vital registration records so numerator–denominator biases in, for example, the analysis of mortality are avoided. In Nordic countries, the whole population has been assigned personal identification numbers facilitating linkage of information from a range of registers. Linkage to use of health and care services is also available in some countries, such as Finland.

These advances have greatly extended the material available for analyses of variations in demographic behaviour, and their consequences. They have also raised complex security and confidentiality issues fuelling debate over appropriate restrictions on access to data.

The measurement of fertility

Fertility means the childbearing performance of a woman, couple, or population. Generally only live births are included. The term fecundity, by contrast, is used to refer to the physiological capability of producing a live-born child. A rough idea of fertility may be gained from using census or survey data to calculate child–woman ratios: the ratio of 0–4-year-olds to women aged 15–49. However, the survival of infants (and their mothers) and the age structure of the female population affects these ratios, so they are generally only used if no other data are available.

The simplest measure of fertility commonly used is the crude birth rate—the number of births in a particular year per 1000 population. As the denominator of this includes those not 'at risk' of giving birth (women outside reproductive age groups and men), it is really a ratio rather than a rate. Crude birth rates are influenced by the age structure of the population, but less seriously so than crude death rates. In 2005–2010 crude birth rates ranged from less than 10 per 1000 in parts of Europe to nearly 50 per 1000 in the highest fertility countries of sub-Saharan Africa.

Slightly more sophisticated is the general fertility ratio—births per 1000 women of reproductive age (generally defined as aged 15–49 or 15–44). Where data allow, age-specific fertility rates (births per 1000 women of a particular age or age group) are preferred. These are frequently summarized using the total fertility rate (TFR). Where, as is usually the case, period data are used to calculate this, it indicates how many children women in a hypothetical cohort would have if they experienced current age-specific fertility rates throughout their reproductive life. This measure is sometimes explicitly denoted TPFR (total period fertility rate). In low-mortality populations, a TFR of 2.1 is taken to indicate *replacement level* fertility as, under this regime, a cohort of women would be succeeded by a cohort of daughters of the same size (after some allowance for mortality and the fact that 105–106 boys are born for every 100 girls).

One difficulty with the TFR is that it is affected by changes in the 'tempo' as well as the 'quantum' of childbearing. If women start delaying their fertility but 'catch up' later, there will be a divergence between cohort and period measures, as the latter will be based partly on the behaviour of earlier cohorts whose timing of births was different. Similarly, if women have children earlier, TFRs will rise, even if eventual family sizes remain unchanged. This means that period measures are much more volatile than cohort ones. For example, the US TFR, having risen in the early parts of this century, fell by more than 10 per cent, from 2.12 to 1.89, between 2007 and 2011 (Hamilton et al. 2012). For these reasons, many statistical offices use cohort, rather than period, measures of fertility as the basis for projections.

More sophisticated measures of fertility include parity progression ratios. These indicate the probability of proceeding from one birth to another (e.g. what proportion of mothers with two children progress to having a third). Parity progression ratios are normally calculated for cohorts who have completed, or nearly completed, their childbearing but it is also possible to use data on births by birth order to derive period progression ratios (Bongaarts and Feeney 1998).

In the past, demographers often preferred to calculate age-specific *marital* fertility rates (and TFRs and other measures) on the grounds that the unmarried population is not 'at risk' (or at reduced risk) of childbearing. Changes in marital fertility indicative of deliberate attempts to limit family size are regarded as one of the defining features of the fertility 'transition' (see later) and so distinguishing these from changes due to variations in the 'at risk' (married population) has been particularly emphasized. However, rises in non-marital childbearing, which now account for over 40 per cent of births in countries such as France, the United States, and United Kingdom, mean that restricting analyses to marital fertility is generally no longer appropriate.

Reproduction rates

In the absence of migration and with fixed mortality, populations will grow if mothers replace themselves with more than one (surviving) daughter and decline if they have fewer than one. Theoretically, it would also be possible to measure the replacement of fathers by sons, but in practice the difficulties involved in obtaining paternity data make this infeasible. Reproduction rates thus relate only to female fertility—births of daughters. The gross reproduction rate (GRR) is derived in the same way as the TFR except that age-specific birth rates based only on births of daughters are used in the calculation. The net reproduction rate (NRR) makes an allowance for mortality; specifically the chance that a daughter will herself survive to childbearing age. The NRR cannot be calculated unless both age-specific fertility and mortality data are available (although it can be approximated using the GRR and appropriate life table survival data). Changes in either fertility or mortality (or both) will mean a divergence between period measures (based on the experience of a hypothetical cohort) and the experiences of real cohorts.

Summary information on measures of fertility and reproduction is shown in Boxes 6.3.2 and 6.3.3.

The measurement of mortality

As for fertility, the simplest measure of mortality is the crude mortality rate, deaths per 1000 population. This is strongly influenced by age structure. Although life expectancy at birth in the more developed regions of the world in 2005–2010 was some 10 years longer than in less developed regions (76 years and 66 years respectively), crude death rates—deaths per 1000 population of all ages—were higher in the more developed regions (10.0 compared with 8.0 in less developed regions) (UN 2011). Age (and sex) specific rates, or measures based on them, are therefore much to be preferred if data are available to calculate them. Both direct and indirect standardization are sometimes used to make comparisons between populations with different age and sex structures. Standardized mortality ratios (SMRs) are calculated using indirect standardization. This involves selecting a set of 'standard' age-specific mortality rates, for example, those for a national population, and applying these to the numbers of people in the relevant age groups in the subpopulation of interest—for example, the population of a particular region. This yields an 'expected' number of deaths—the number of deaths there would be in the subpopulation if age-specific death rates were the same as those in the standard population. The ratio of observed to expected deaths gives the SMR. Thus an SMR of 1.24 indicates that mortality in the sub population is 24 per cent higher than in the standard population, after allowing for age differences. SMRs are useful summary measures of differences in mortality, but give no indication of the *level* of mortality. In direct standardization, widely used by WHO and national statistical offices, age and sex specific rates are applied to an external 'standard' population, such as the European Standard Population, to produce an overall standardized (weighted) death rate.

Box 6.3.2 Fertility measures

Definitions

Fertility: the childbearing performance of individuals, couples, or populations.

Fecundity: the physiological capability of producing a live birth.

Parity: the number of children previously born alive (or sometimes number of previous confinements) to a woman or couple. Nulliparous women are those who have borne no children.

Measure

Crude birth rate: the ratio of births in a year (other specified period) to the average population in the same year/period (mid-year population), expressed per 1000:

$$CBR = \frac{\text{number of births}}{\text{mid-year population}} \times 1000.$$

General fertility rate: births to women aged 15–44/49 in a year/period per 1000 women aged 15–44/49 in the same period:

$$GFR = \frac{\text{number of births to women aged } 15-44/49}{\text{mid-year population of women aged } 15-44/49} \times 1000.$$

Age-specific fertility rate (ASFR): number of births to women aged x (or x to x + n) per 1000 women aged x (or x to x + n). 'n' refers to the length of an age interval.

ASFRs are frequently calculated for 5-year age groups from 15–19 to 40–44 or 45–49.

$$ASFR = \frac{\text{births to women aged x}}{\text{mid-year population of women aged x}} \times 1000.$$

Total (period) fertility rate (TFR/TPFR): the sum of the age-specific fertility rates for all reproductive age groups for a particular period (usually a year), conventionally expressed per woman. The TFR indicates how many children a woman would have if throughout her reproductive life, she had children at the age-specific rates prevalent in the specified year or period.
x = 49:

$$TFR = \sum_{x=15}^{x=49} f_x$$

where 'f_x' is the age-specific fertility rate at age x. If rates for age groups, rather than single years, are used then the sum of the age-specific rates must be multiplied by the number of single ages included in the group (usually five).
x = 45–49:

$$TFR = 5 * \sum_{x=15-19}^{x=45-49} f_x.$$

Parity progression ratio: the probability of a women of parity x progressing to parity x + 1.

Box 6.3.3 Reproduction rates

Measures

Gross reproduction rate (GRR): the sum of the age-specific female fertility rates (births of daughters), for all reproductive age groups for a particular period (usually a year) conventionally expressed per woman. The GRR indicates how many *daughters* a woman would have if, throughout her reproductive life, she had children at the age-specific rates prevalent in the specified year of period. The GRR can be calculated either by summing female age-specific fertility rates (relating to births of daughters rather than all births) or using the formula:

$$GRR = TFR \times \text{proportion of female births}.$$

The proportion of female births can be taken as 0.488 (100/205) in the absence of more detailed information.

Net reproduction rate (NRR): the average number of daughters that would be borne, according to specified rates of mortality and of bearing daughters, by a female subject through life to these rates. The NRR employs the same fertility data as the GRR, but also takes into account the effects of mortality. An NRR of 1.0 indicates that a population's fertility and mortality levels would result in exact replacement of mothers by daughters.

Age-specific death rates are calculated using the numbers of deaths at age x (or between ages x and x + n) in a particular year as the numerator and the mid-year population of the same age as the denominator. The rate is conventionally expressed per 1000 or per 100,000 population. The mid-year population is used as a measure of the average population at risk on the assumption that deaths are evenly distributed throughout the year. For some age groups, notably infants, this assumption is invalid. In low-mortality populations, deaths in the first 3 days of life may account for half or more of all deaths in the first year of life. Moreover, information on the size of population aged less than 1 normally comes from birth data (as in 9 out of 10 years relevant census data will not be available). For these reasons live births in a particular year are conventionally used as the denominator of the infant mortality rate while deaths to infants aged less than 1 constitute the numerator. Some infants dying in a given year will have been born in the previous year and some born in the year in question will die the following year. This can cause distortions if there are large annual fluctuations in numbers of births (or infant deaths) and often 3-year averages are preferred. Deaths at very old ages are also not evenly distributed throughout the year and an adjustment is often made to allow for this.

Infant mortality rates (IMRs) were very high in some parts of historical Europe—with 300 or even 400 deaths per 1000 live births in regions of Russia and Germany at the end of the nineteenth century (van de Walle 1986). In England and Wales at the start of the twentieth century, there were some 140 infant deaths per 1000 live births. Infant mortality in high-income countries is now extremely low—fewer than five infant deaths per 1000 live births in many European countries, Australia, Japan, South Korea, Hong Kong, and Singapore. There have also been huge falls

---

Box 6.3.4 Mortality measures

Measures

Crude death rate: the ratio of deaths in a year (other specified period) to average population in the same year/period (mid-year population), expressed per 1000:

$$CBR = \frac{\text{number of deaths}}{\text{mid-year population}} \times 1000.$$

Age-specific mortality rate (ASMR): number of deaths to persons aged x (or x to x + n) per 1000 persons aged x (or to x + n):

$$ASMR = \frac{\text{deaths to persons aged x}}{\text{mid-year population of persons aged x}} \times 1000.$$

Standardized mortality ratio (SMR): the ratio of observed to expected deaths in a study population. Expected deaths are calculated by applying a set of standard age-specific mortality rates to the age distribution of the study population. Standardized ratios are only useful for comparisons. They have no intrinsic meaning.

Infant mortality rate (IMR):

$$\frac{\text{number of deaths to infants ages} < 1 \text{ year}}{\text{number of live births}} \times 1000.$$

Sometimes decomposed into *neonatal mortality rates* (deaths of live born infants during the first 4 weeks) and *post-neonatal* mortality (from 4 to 52 weeks).

The *perinatal mortality rate* measures late fetal deaths (stillbirths) and early neonatal deaths relative to live births.

Perinatal mortality rate

$$= \frac{\text{stillbirths + deaths under 1 week}}{\text{still + live births}} \times 1000.$$

Stillbirths used to refer to deaths of fetuses of 28 or more weeks' gestation; however, an earlier threshold of 24 weeks is now more generally used.

Box 6.3.5 Life table measures and notation

x = age attained last birthday.

l_0 = the radix of the life table (hypothetical number of babies), usually 100,000.

l_x = number of survivors at age x, so l_{65} is the number of persons alive at age 65 in the hypothetical life table population.

$_nq_x$ = probability of dying between age x and x + n, so $_4q_1$ is the probability of dying between age 1 and 5 for a person aged 1.

$_np_x$ = probability of surviving between ages x and x + n, so $_{20}p_{65}$ is the probability of surviving from age 65 to age 85 for a person aged 65.

$_nd_x$ = number of deaths between age x and x + n.

$_nL_x$ = number of person years lived between x and x + n.

T_x = total number of person years lived after age x.

e_x = expectation of life at age x, so e_0 is expectation of life at birth.

---

and other demographic processes. Life tables show the probability of dying (and surviving) between specified ages. They also allow the calculation of various other indicators, including expectation of life. If complete data on the mortality of a birth cohort are available, then a cohort life table may be constructed. However, the use of cohort life tables is obviously only possible retrospectively. More commonly, period life tables, based on mortality rates at a particular time, are calculated. These life tables show death (and survival) probabilities for a hypothetical cohort with an arbitrary radix (number of babies at the beginning) usually set to 10,000, 100,000 or some other multiple of 100.

Specific notation, summarized in Box 6.3.5, is used in life table analysis. The basis of the table is a set of probabilities of dying—$_nq_x$—which are calculated from age-specific death rates; x here refers to age at the start of an interval whose length is specified by n. Thus $_5q_{50}$ refers to the probability of someone alive at 50 dying between age 50 and age 55. The complement of $_nq_x$—the probability of surviving—is denoted $_np_x$. The (hypothetical) number of survivors at each age is given by l_x; thus l_0 equals the radix (of 100,000) and l_{75} the number of survivors at age 75. The number of person years lived in an interval ($_nL_x$) and the total number of person years lived after a particular age (T_x) are often not shown in published tables but are steps on the way to the calculation of e_x—life expectancy at age x.

This measure provides an indicator of mortality which is very largely independent of the age structure of the population since it depends only on age-specific mortality rates. This makes it more useful than either a standardized mortality ratio (which gives no indication of level) or a crude death rate (which is strongly influenced by age structure). Life expectancy either at birth (e_0) or further life expectancy at a particular age, say 65 (e_{65}), is calculated by dividing the total person years lived after age 0 or 65 (T_0 or T_{65}) by the number of survivors aged 0 (l_0) or 65 (l_{65}).

Values of life expectancy at birth are sometimes (mis)interpreted as indicators of usual age at death in a particular population. In very low-mortality populations where most deaths occur within a relatively small range of ages (see the example of Japan in Fig. 6.3.2); there will be a close correspondence between median and modal ages of death and life expectancy at birth (which is a mean value). However, in populations such as Sierra Leone where

---

in infant mortality in many poorer countries; in 2011 China and India had reported IMRs of 13 and 47 respectively (WHO 2013). Rates remain high in some of the very poorest countries—over 100 deaths per 1000 live births.

Variations on this scale have substantial demographic impacts. Infant mortality has also attracted particular interest because of links with fertility behaviour and as an indicator of public health conditions. Particularly in this latter context, perinatal, early and late neonatal and post neonatal mortality rates are often distinguished where data allow (see Box 6.3.4).

Life tables

Life table analysis is a core demographic technique and life tables provide one of the most powerful tools for analysing mortality

so many deaths occur in infancy, there will be a wide divergence. There is also sometimes confusion about the interpretation of values of further life expectancy at a particular age. This is derived from information about the probabilities of death and survival at *subsequent* ages, and so is not influenced by deaths at earlier ages and it is erroneous to think that, for example, the further life expectancy of someone aged 65 will equal life expectancy at birth minus 65. The higher the mortality rates at young ages the greater will be this divergence. In 2008, for life example, female life expectancy at birth in the United States was 80.6 years but the further life expectancy of women aged 65 was 20.0 years. The equivalent figures in 1900–1901 were 49 years and 12.0 years.

Model life tables
Patterns of age-specific death rates show similarities whatever the level of mortality. Death rates tend to be higher in infancy than later childhood and rise with age from around the age of puberty, although in the oldest age groups rates of increase tend to flatten out. Because of the tendency for death rates at one age to be associated with death rates at other ages in a given population, it is possible to derive hypothetical schedules, called *model life tables*, describing variations in mortality by age and sex, normally in terms of a limited number of parameters which allow for particular features of the mortality pattern of the population considered. Model life tables are derived from empirical data from countries where these are available. They are extremely useful aids for the estimation of mortality by age in populations with defective data. They are also used (in conjunction with fertility data) to show the outcomes of particular fertility and mortality regimes on, for example, population age structure and for making population projections. All demographic texts give further details of their derivation and application.

Other applications of life table analysis
Life tables are widely used to analyse probabilities associated with events other than death, such as risks of divorce or contraceptive use failure and discontinuation rates, and in estimates of disability-free or healthy life expectancy. Many chronic conditions associated with ageing, such as musculoskeletal and sensory impairments, may have serious implications for health status but are not directly life-threatening. Life table methods are used to decompose total life expectancy into 'healthy' and 'unhealthy' or 'disabled' components. This can be done using cross-sectional data on morbidity prevalence in conjunction with mortality data, although this has some limitations. More sophisticated (and data demanding) multistate approaches which allow transitions both to and from disabled states have also been developed (Manton et al. 2006). Despite these technical advances, there is still controversy about *trends* in indicators of the health status of populations, including disability. To a large extent this debate arises from measurement problems and the difficulties involved in making comparisons between health indicators derived in different ways, a further reminder of the importance of data quality and measurement.

Multiple decrement life tables allow 'decrements' from more than one event—for example, different causes of death. Cause elimination life tables are also used to identify the 'pure' severity of a particular cause of death. Multistate models allow analysis of a range of transitions, particularly those where re-entries into a particular state, such as being married or living in a certain region, are possible. These more sophisticated applications of course require more detailed data.

The measurement of migration
In many countries migration is the predominant influence on the spatial distribution of the population. In Asia and Latin America recent rural-to-urban migration has resulted in the phenomenal growth of cities, often lacking the infrastructure to meet the needs of the expanding population for basic services such as sanitation and power. In 2010, 52 per cent of the world's population lived in urban areas compared with 29 per cent in 1950 (UN 2012).

Measuring migration represents particular difficulties. The classical definition of internal migration is a permanent or semi-permanent move across an administrative boundary, which means that the extent of migration recorded depends partly on the size of administrative areas. For example, in a country divided into many small areas, a move over 5 kilometres will count as migration, which would not be the case for countries divided into larger ones. Hence, international comparison of internal migration rates is potentially misleading. Even the distinction between international and internal migration may be problematic if boundaries are contested or changing. The temporal dimension to migration presents further difficulties; what constitutes permanent or semi-permanent and how should groups such as seasonal migrants be treated?

The reason for defining migration as a move over a boundary is largely pragmatic. Often only moves of this kind are recorded; moreover this is the information required by local administrations. For research purposes, analyses of *all* moves (preferably with an indication of distance moved) may often be preferred. Some countries have registration systems in which changes of address are recorded. More commonly, censuses are used to find out about migration. Questions on usual address 1 or 5 years ago allow the proportion of *movers* in the population to be measured (except for those aged less than 1 or 5). These data also allow inflows *and* outflows between pairs of areas to be measured. *Moves*, as opposed to *movers*, are not directly measured as someone moving several times in the reference period cannot be distinguished from someone moving only once. Those leaving an address and later returning to it cannot be identified either. This means that the length of the reference period used is important; the proportion of movers in the 5 years preceding a census will *not* equal five times the proportion moving in 1 year before the same census.

In the absence of direct census data, estimates of migration can be made indirectly using the 'balancing equation' referred to in the following subsection. Differences in the size of a population at two points in time not accounted for by natural change (i.e. births minus deaths) must be due to migration (or data errors). If vital registration data are available, then both births and deaths can be taken into account. If they are lacking, then the survival of groups enumerated in the first of a pair of censuses must be estimated from a life table and the number of expected survivors compared with the number enumerated in the second census (obviously ageing must be allowed for, so the number of 20–29-year-olds in the first census will be compared with 30–39-year-olds 10 years later). These methods only allow estimation of *net* migration (balance between in-migration and out-migration). Their major weakness lies in the fact that the residual population balance assumed to be due to migration may in fact reflect differences in the quality of the two censuses considered or errors in the estimates of survival used.

Survey data are also used to measure migration and potentially provide illuminating information on the reasons for, and consequences of, migration. However, as migration over long distances is a relatively rare event, even large general population samples may yield relatively few migrants. A similar problem besets samples of international travellers, such as the UK International Passenger Survey, designed to estimate flows of international migrants through port or border surveys. Tourists and business travellers comprise the vast bulk of people entering or leaving so surveys are an inefficient way of identifying immigrants and emigrants. Unfortunately, other data are often lacking as legal and administrative record systems are frequently concerned with citizenship and right of abode rather than international migration per se (and virtually never with emigration). Estimates of the size of immigrant populations depend on whether the measure used is based on place of birth or on nationality—the size of the latter is influenced by policies on acquisition of citizenship.

Population dynamics

Any population comprises those who have made an entry and not yet exited. When whole populations of defined geographic areas are considered, the only means of entry are birth or immigration and the only means of exit death or emigration.

The most basic method of demographic analysis is the decomposition of overall population change ($P_t - P_0$) into its components (B, D, I, E):

$$P_t - P_0 = B - D + I - E$$

where P_t = population at an end of period; P_0 = population at the beginning of a period; and B, D, I, E represent respectively births, deaths, immigrations, and emigrations during the same period (B – D is referred to as natural increase and I – E as net migration). Population subgroups may be similarly defined in terms of entries and exits. In the absence of migration, entry to the population aged 75–84 is through ageing (passage from 74 to 75) exit is through further ageing (84 to 85) or death. This simple accounting equation is an important one, both methodologically and as a formal reminder of the need to consider *past* as well as current events.

Of the three demographic determinants of population size, structure, and growth, fertility has historically been of much greater importance than either mortality or migration. Every birth represents not just an addition to the current generation of children, but also potentially an exponentially increasing augmentation in the size of future generations. Death carries no such promise of future return. Births increase the population only at age zero, so making it younger, whereas deaths are spread across the whole age range and so have much less impact on age structure. The third determinant—migration—is generally not of significant magnitude to have a major impact on most national populations, although there are exceptions especially when natural increase is close to zero. Increased levels of immigration to many European countries since the 1990s have had quite an effect on population size and age structure; the population of Spain for example,

increased by 10.2 per cent between 1999 and 2006 and over 90 per cent of this increase was due to migration (Sobotka 2008).

For social and biological reasons fertility, mortality, and migration have interactive effects. Decreases in mortality among those with reproductive potential, for example, influence not just the size of the age group affected at the time, but also the size of succeeding generations. Declines in male mortality, particularly in populations where large age differences between spouses are common and remarriage of widows is rare, will similarly tend to increase fertility by effectively increasing the proportion of women of reproductive age who are still married. Conversely, reductions in fertility clearly reduce the risk of maternal mortality and may have further positive effects on the survival of mothers, infants or both. Age at motherhood also influences rates of population growth. The average age of mothers at the birth of their daughters is termed the mean length of a generation and is generally around 29 years. A shorter interval will mean more rapid generational succession (and faster population growth).

Migration affects other demographic parameters because migrants differ from the general population. International migrants are generally young and in good health and often move from relatively high- to low-fertility populations. Consequently, immigrants may serve to (temporarily) 'rejuvenate' the host population and, at least initially, have higher fertility and lower mortality. In England and Wales, for example, 24 per cent of births in 2011 were to mothers themselves born outside the United Kingdom. Despite the disadvantages they often face, mortality of immigrant groups is often lower than that of host populations because of the differential selection of immigrants. The degree of selection tends to vary according to difficulties and distance to be overcome in making an international move. For all these reasons, the demographic characteristics of population subgroups largely comprising immigrants and their immediate descendants may vary substantially from those of the population as a whole.

Population projections

Population projections represent one of the most widely used outputs of demographic analysis. Strictly speaking, a projection simply represents the outcome of applying various assumptions about future fertility, mortality, and migration and so differs from a *forecast*, which implies prediction. However, projections are often treated as forecasts and the degree of uncertainty inherent in them is not always sufficiently recognized, although the production of probabilistic forecasts, as in the latest UN projections, makes this more explicit. The most common method of projection is the component method, based on the balancing equation ($P_t = P_0 + B - D + I - E$). Assumptions are made about the three components of change—births, deaths, and migration—and applied to age and sex groups within the initial population to give a projection of future size and structure. To a large extent assumptions are based on recent trends together with other information, for example, survey data on fertility intentions or (sometimes) models of change in particular causes of death. Forecasting fertility has generally been regarded as the most problematic area of projection but recently greater attention has been paid to the errors that have been made in forecasting mortality in developed countries. This has little effect on age groups in which survival is high, but can have quite substantial impacts on forecasts of the number of older people. Migration may be an important element and may be underestimated, if projections do not take into account feedback loops whereby migrant populations tend to generate further migration (Bongaarts and Bulatao 2000). International migration is also difficult to forecast as it is affected by events outside the country, is often a sensitive political issue and may be volatile. Partly for these reasons, immigration levels have been consistently under-projected in forecasts in many European countries (Alders et al. 2007).

Population growth

Changes in the size of a population produced by the surplus (or deficit) of births over deaths are termed natural increase (or decrease). A common indicator of growth is the crude rate of natural increase—the difference between the crude birth rate (annual births per 1000 population) and the crude death rate (annual deaths per 1000 population). If net migration is zero, this will be the same as the growth rate of the population—the overall annual change in the population divided by the population size—(conventionally expressed as a percentage). In several European countries deaths outnumbered births in the period 2005–2010, with the largest deficits in Ukraine, Bulgaria, Latvia, Belarus, Hungary, Lithuania, and the Russian Federation. In some others births still outnumber deaths even though fertility rates have been below the level required for *long-term* replacement for 40 years or so. This apparent paradox largely reflects the fact that the number of births is a function of the number of potential mothers, to which immigration may also contribute, as well as of their fertility patterns. If the former is increasing so too may the numbers of births, even if women have fewer children each.

The young age structures of many populations in the developing world mean that these populations have a huge built-in potential for growth. Population *momentum* is the measure which gives the ratio of the ultimate size a given population would achieve to current population size if fertility were to immediately fall to replacement level. Even allowing for the effect of HIV/AIDS-related mortality, the population of sub-Saharan Africa is expected to increase from 0.86 billion to 1.96 billion between 2010 and 2050 (UN 2011), a consequence of both population momentum and high levels of fertility. In some low-fertility countries there are now concerns about 'negative momentum'—the prospect of decline in population even if fertility rates increase somewhat because of successively smaller cohorts of women in childbearing age groups.

Intrinsic rate of natural increase: stable population theory

Early in the twentieth century, Lotka (1907) demonstrated mathematically that a population closed to migration and subject to unchanging age-specific fertility and mortality rates for a long period would eventually have a fixed age structure (in which the proportion in each age group remained unchanged) and would grow at a constant rate. This type of population is called a *stable* population. The fixed age structure of a stable population is independent of the initial age structure—two very different populations subject to the same unchanging rates for a long period would eventually assume the same structure. A particular case of a stable population is a *stationary* population—one in which birth and death rates are constant and in balance and so population growth is zero. The L_x column of the life table is an example of a stationary

population. The number of births is fixed (the radix) and the age distribution is also fixed. In non-stationary stable populations, the age structure is also fixed but the size of every age group is growing at the same constant rate as the overall population and the number of births. This is called the *intrinsic rate of natural increase* and is a function of the net reproduction rate and the mean length of a generation (approximated by the mean age of childbearing). Non-stationary stable populations can be calculated by adjusting the L_x values of a particular life table to allow for the intrinsic rate of growth. These are often published in conjunction with model life tables to show the effects of particular (unchanging) fertility and mortality regimes.

Although stable and stationary populations are theoretical constructs, real populations at various times have met the model requirements closely enough to allow stable population theory to be used to develop methods for indirectly estimating fertility and mortality in populations lacking adequate directly derived data. Stable population models are also widely used for insurance, pension, and personnel planning. One of the important results of the work of Lotka and his successors was to show theoretically the important influence of fertility on age structure.

Age structure

Population pyramids graphically illustrate the current structure of populations and in so doing, also provide insights into both the future and the past of the population. High fertility populations have a pyramid shape with each successive cohort being larger than its predecessor. The population pyramid for Bangladesh (Fig. 6.3.3A) shows a typical pattern for a population with a history of high fertility but a recent downturn. Each successive cohort is larger than the preceding one, with the exception of the youngest. 'Old' populations, such as that of England and Wales (Fig. 6.3.3B), are more rectangular with a gradual tapering at the top. Bulges in population pyramids due to high numbers of births have 'echo' effects when members of large cohorts themselves have children. Thus the baby boom experienced in many populations in the post-Second World War period (precise timing varied between countries) had an echo effect in the 1980s.

Historically, and apparently paradoxically, improvements in mortality in those European populations which now have high proportions of old people in fact served to *offset* the trend towards population ageing, as they chiefly benefited the young—and led to increases in the proportions surviving to have children themselves. However, although fertility has the greatest *potential* impact on age structure and population growth, in some circumstances mortality (or migration) may become a more important influence. Many populations in richer countries now have fertility at or below replacement level, life expectancies at birth close to 80 and near universal survival to the end of the (female) reproductive span. In these conditions, further improvements in mortality have the greatest impact at old ages and further population ageing occurs from the apex, rather than, or in addition to, the base of the population pyramid. Mortality changes are now the main motor of the further ageing of a number of populations with already old age structures (Preston and Stokes 2012). Population age structures and associated rates of growth or decline, changes in age structures such as population ageing, and the speed and stage of age structural change all have important economic and

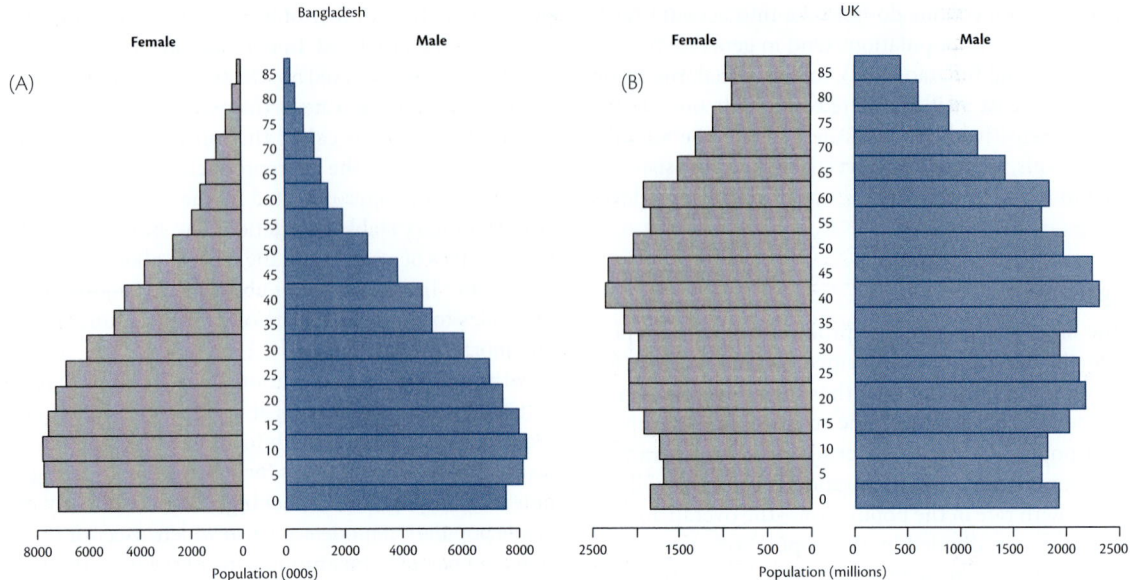

Fig. 6.3.3 Distribution of the population of (A) Bangladesh and (B) the UK by age and sex, 2010.
Source: data from United Nations, *World Population Prospects: The 2010 Revision*, United Nations, New York, USA, Copyright © 2012, available from http://esa.un.org/wpp/documentation/pdf/WPP2010_Volume-I_Comprehensive-Tables.pdf

health implications which have attracted considerable debate and controversy.

Many economists have pointed out that population growth has often provided a spur to human ingenuity and economic growth. Less positively, the countries which now have the youngest age structures and most rapid rates of population growth are already suffering from land degradation and in many cases, constrained agricultural potential (Alexandratos 2005). Large and growing child populations also hamper efforts at improving human capital through education or improved health (Casterline 2010).

Reduced fertility initially produces a 'demographic dividend' or 'window' when the ratio of children to adults falls and those in prime productive ages, the survivors of larger birth cohorts, account for a higher proportion of the population. It has been argued that this dividend of lower child dependency and higher representation of adults in the prime working age groups played an important part in the rapid economic development of the 'East Asian Tigers', like South Korea and also China (Bloom et al. 2000). The next phase, involving high and increasing representation of older people may, it has been suggested, also bring some economic benefit in the form of increased savings (by the large number of older people) and so greater capital available for investment (Mason and Lee 2006). However, population ageing is more often perceived as a challenge with potentially negative implications for both the economy and for population health (OECD 1999).

The major concerns arising from increases in the proportions of older people relate to effects on productivity and need for support systems of various kinds, including pensions, healthcare and long-term care. In OECD countries, healthcare expenditure is typically three to five times as high for those aged 65 and over as for those aged under 65. However there is considerable international variation in the proportion of GDP devoted to healthcare spending for older people which bears little obvious relationship to the proportion of older people in the population concerned.

In populations which have more recently moved to low fertility and low mortality regimes, the pace of demographic change has been much faster than occurred historically in Europe. The proportion of the Japanese population aged 65 and over doubled, from 7 per cent to over 14 per cent, between 1970 and 1996. In France a similar increase took 130 years to achieve and in Sweden 85 years (Kinsella and Phillips 2005). More recently ageing populations have thus had a much shorter period in which to adapt to new public health priorities. The origins of these age structure changes lie in the demographic transition.

The demographic transition

Towards the end of the nineteenth century (earlier in France) birth and death rates started falling in a number of European countries. Between 1871–1875 and 1911–1915 the TFR for England and Wales, for example, dropped from 4.8 to 2.8; by the early 1930s it was below replacement level, a development which was viewed with alarm and led to the first Royal Commission on Population. Although modern methods of contraception were lacking, it was clear that this huge drop in fertility was the result of the deliberate limitation of family size. Half of couples married in the 1870s had six or more children compared with 12 per cent of couples married in 1911–1915 (Coleman and Salt 1992). Expectation of life at birth, meanwhile, increased by some 15 years between the end of the nineteenth century and the early 1930s.

Researchers attempting to relate such shifts in demographic regimes to economic and social changes, originated the theory of the demographic transition. The 'classical' view propounded by Notestein (1945) and others was that in 'traditional' societies fertility and mortality are both high and roughly in balance. Change is driven by economic advance which results in lower mortality. Fertility initially remains high, resulting in a rapid period of population growth. After this lag, however, fertility also falls in response to falling mortality and the erosion of 'traditional' pro-natalist values.

This classical view has since been considerably modified (Lee 2003). Coale and his collaborators in an ambitious project to track the transition in historical Europe suggested that no economic 'threshold' for fertility decline could be identified and that the pattern of decline seemed to follow regional groupings, suggesting a cultural rather than a socioeconomic dimension (Coale and Watkins 1986). Falls in infant mortality, assumed to be a particularly important stimulus to fertility decline, sometimes followed rather than preceded changes in fertility. For example, Woods et al. (1989) argued that declines in fertility led to reductions in infant mortality, rather than vice versa in England and Wales. In short, the role of mortality decline as a trigger and the dominance of economic change have both been questioned. Caldwell (1982) additionally argued that in non-European countries, it was not so much socioeconomic modernization but 'Westernization' involving increased emphasis on the nuclear family and a change in intergenerational wealth flows (resulting in the costs of children outweighing their potential benefits) that was the important trigger of fertility transition.

Research on the historical demographic transition in Europe may seem of limited relevance to contemporary problems. However, this research was fuelled by post-war fears about population growth. By 1950, significant mortality declines had been achieved or initiated throughout the world. In China, for example, expectation of life at birth increased from 43 in 1960 to over 75 by 2010. Even in sub-Saharan Africa, a gain of nearly 10 years—from 43 to 52—was achieved between 1950 and 1990, sadly since reversed although now starting to increase again (World Bank 1993; UN 2011). In this context it seemed imperative to discover the causes of fertility decline and use this knowledge to accelerate fertility 'adjustment' to falling mortality. Was 'development the best contraceptive' as concluded at the stormy 1974 World Population Conference; could change be achieved through intensive family planning programmes, as the experience in Taiwan and South Korea seemed to suggest; or was some combination of these and other factors the key to fertility transition? Studies of societies in which the fertility transition had occurred seemed to offer the best prospect of an answer to these questions. While simple answers to complex questions are rarely forthcoming, Coale (1973) identified three factors which he considered prerequisites for fertility decline in contemporary populations. These were: that potential parents must think it acceptable to balance the advantages and disadvantages of another child, that some advantage must be gained from reduced fertility, and that effective techniques of fertility control must be available.

Trends in fertility in the second half of the last century and early part of this century have shown considerable divergence and shed some light on these debates. TFRs are highest in sub-Saharan Africa, with Uganda, Somalia, Mali, Timor-Leste, and Niger having TFRs above 6.3 in 2005–2010. In all other world regions there was clear evidence of onset of a transition to lower fertility by the 1970s or 1980s; Japan was the first non-Western country to experience a fertility transition starting after the Second World War. Globally, the estimated TFR in 2005–2010 was 2.52, with 48 per cent of the world population living in countries with below-replacement fertility levels (UN 2011). Substantial fertility declines have occurred in a number of countries which at that time had only a limited amount of development, such as Sri Lanka, Thailand, China, and more recently Bangladesh. One of the largest and fastest fertility declines took place in the Islamic Republic of Iran where fertility fell from 7.0 in 1980 to 1.9 in 2006 (Abbasi-Shavazi et al. 2009) defying assumptions that socially and religiously conservative Muslim societies with low rates of female employment would be resistant to fertility change.

Recent interpretations of fertility change have reverted to considering development—in its broadest sense rather than restricted to consideration of average incomes—a stronger influence in contemporary populations than ideational changes, although the relevance and role of cultural and policy related factors is recognized (Bryant 2007). Common factors identified in poor rural populations where fertility has fallen significantly are well-established education systems, improvements in healthcare and in child survival, some form of extra-familial welfare, well-organized local government, and an organized family planning programme. Potential benefits of investing more resources in fewer children, as a consequence of increasing opportunities in urban or industrial livelihoods, also seem to be important (McNicoll 2006; Bryant 2007). The education of women has been identified as a particularly significant influence on both falling fertility and improved infant survival (Cleland 1990; Hobcraft 1993) and female education and empowerment were recognized as key policy objectives at the 1994 International Conference on Population and Development (UNFPA 1995).

As noted earlier, fertility rates remain high in much of sub-Saharan Africa. Continuing expressed preferences for large families and other family and social characteristics of African populations have led some to conclude that the model of change seen in Asia and Latin America may not be applicable to Africa, or at least not to all regions of Africa (Caldwell et al. 1992). There is nevertheless evidence of unmet demand for family planning and a strong case can be made, on the grounds of improving maternal and child health, for renewed investment in family programmes which in some places faltered as the policy focus and funding shifted to the HIV/AIDs crisis (Cleland et al. 2006).

Recent trends have also made it clear that the end point of fertility transition is not necessarily a fertility level around the 'replacement rate'. In some countries, such as Guatemala, Peru, Egypt, Turkey and Ghana, fertility declines 'stalled' (sometimes temporarily) at a level higher than two children per woman (Bongaarts 2005). In others they have continued downward spiralling, giving rise to a new set of concerns about 'lowest low' fertility.

Lowest low fertility and the second demographic transition

In contrast to the scenario of high fertility and rapid population growth in some of the poorest countries, a growing number of high-income countries now have concerns about the implications of low fertility. Many of these countries experienced a post-Second World War 'baby boom' during the 1950s and early 1960s followed by a 1970s 'baby bust' when fertility declined to very low levels. In Scandinavia, France, the United Kingdom, the United States, and other English-speaking countries fertility rates have since fluctuated at levels between 1.6 and replacement level with something of an increase in the first decade of this century—a pattern also seen in many other industrialized countries—however, this may turn out to be a temporary phenomenon particularly given current economic conditions. These populations have also experienced a range of family-related behavioural changes, included marked increases in cohabitation, non-marital childbearing, divorce, postponed childbearing, and increased levels of childlessness, described by some as a 'Second Demographic Transition' (Lesthaeghe and Neidert 2006). Such behaviours, which have become more usual among Northern European cohorts born from around the 1950s onwards, are much less prominent in Southern and Eastern Europe and the richer countries of South and East Asia. However, it is mainly in these latter countries that 'lowest low' fertility—rates below 1.3—has been prevalent with 21 countries from these regions having TFRs below 1.3 in 2003 (Goldstein et al. 2009). The recent increase in fertility in developed societies meant that only three of these countries, South Korea, Slovakia, and Singapore, had average values below 1.3 in the period 2005–2010 (UN 2011). However, the TFR remained below 1.5 in a large number of other countries including Poland, Japan, Germany, Italy, Ukraine, Spain, and the Russian Federation in 2005–2010. An important determinant of very low fertility in many of these societies has been a precipitous fall in marriage rates (Billari and Kohler 2004). Japan, for example, has been transformed from a society with near universal marriage in the early and mid twentieth century to one in which a fifth of the population will remain never-married at age 45 (Retherford et al. 2001). In this case the erosion of arranged marriages after the Second World War has played a part; changing gender roles may also be important. In some countries with very low fertility, explicit pro-natalist polices are under discussion or have been introduced, however these remain controversial and of unclear effectiveness.

The proximate determinants of fertility

One of the contributions of research into the fertility transition has been improved understanding of biosocial influences on reproduction. A huge range of social, economic, cultural, and psychological factors may influence decisions about family building strategies and family size. However, these can only have effect if they are translated into patterns of behaviour or physiological characteristics that influence the risks of conception or delivery.

Conversely, other patterns of behaviour with potentially important influences on fertility may be adopted with little or no thought to these consequences. Davis and Blake (1956) distinguished a series of 'intermediate fertility variables': factors influencing exposure to risk of pregnancy (marriage and coital frequency), risk of pregnancy (such as contraception), and pregnancy outcome (spontaneous and induced abortion). The most influential refinement of this work is the Bongaarts decomposition model (Bongaarts 1978), which identified four elements chiefly responsible for observed fertility variations:

◆ The proportion of women married (exposed to risk).

◆ Contraceptive use.

◆ Induced abortion.

◆ Post-partum non-susceptibility to conception (largely determined by breastfeeding practice).

The TFR is dependent on the interactive effect of these variables and hypothetical maximum fertility. In modern 'post-transition' populations, fertility decisions are normally couple- (or woman-) based and are implemented through contraception and abortion. In non-contracepting populations, biosocial factors, notably marriage patterns, breastfeeding practices, sexual frequency and, in some populations, the prevalence of infertility, are of major importance.

The social reproductive span, from entry to end of marriage or any sexual union, nearly always starts later, often much later, than menarche. Fecundity—the potential for bearing children—decreases after the third decade, more sharply after the age of 35 and in most non-contracepting populations the average age at last birth is around 40. Social factors, as well as biological ones, are important influences. Sexual activity may cease before menopause because of widowhood or separation. In some African populations, childbearing after becoming a grandmother is disapproved of.

For those within the effective reproductive span—biologically capable of childbearing and in a sexual union—overall fertility is largely a function of length of intervals between births, itself largely determined by breastfeeding patterns. Among non-breastfeeding women, average duration of post-partum amenorrhea is only 1.5–2 months, compared with 18 months or more with protracted breastfeeding, particularly in some populations where sexual activity is proscribed for breastfeeding mothers.

Longer birth intervals and increased breastfeeding also have positive effects on infant and child health. Overall deaths before the age of 5 might be reduced by as much as 30 per cent in some countries if closely spaced births were delayed (World Bank 1993; Cleland et al. 2006).

The epidemiological transition

Transitions from relatively high- to low-mortality regimes have in all populations been associated with transformations in the age, cause, and sex structure of death. Omran (1971) coined the phrase 'epidemiological transition' to describe this process. Changes in the response of societies to health and disease processes also need consideration. The term 'health transition' has been proposed as one which embraces both these phenomena.

Substantial falls in death rates from infectious and parasitic diseases and maternal mortality are hallmarks of the epidemiological transition. In England and Wales, over half the gain in life expectancy at birth between 1871 and 1911 was due to reduced infectious disease mortality. Some 20 per cent of the total gain was due to reduced death rates from tuberculosis (Caselli 1991). Declines in these causes of death were greater among the young, hence deaths at older ages accounted for a larger share of all deaths; the epidemiological transition has also been consistently associated with larger falls in mortality among women than men. Changes in the intra-household allocation of resources, declines in causes of death primarily affecting women (such as maternal mortality and respiratory tuberculosis), gender differences in health-related behaviour and in exposure to occupational hazards, and the possibly greater susceptibility of men to stresses associated with socioeconomic changes, may all be underlying factors.

The relative contribution of various eighteenth- and nineteenth-century developments in promoting the historical epidemiological transition in the West remains a matter of debate. Improved nutrition, better housing and living conditions, public sanitation schemes, and specific public health initiatives, such as smallpox inoculation, all have their adherents. In the early twentieth century, improved personal hygiene practices and better infant care were also important. A common thread linking most of these factors is their relationship to overall social and economic development and improvements in standards of living. During the twentieth century, however, developments in medical technology and vector control offered the potential for 'exogenous' mortality decline less dependent on a particular country's level of income and development. One consequence was that the relationship between per capita income and life expectancy has shifted to the right (Preston 1975, 2007). In 1901, for example, life expectancy in the United States was 49 and income per capita was about US$7300 (2005 purchasing power parity). In 2009, income per capita in China was almost identical ($7400) but life expectancy was 73 years (http://www.gapminder.org/).

Many poor countries have been able to achieve remarkable falls in mortality, especially child mortality, through behavioural change, improved education of women, and introduction of relatively cheap treatments and interventions, such as vaccination and antibiotics (Cutler et al. 2006). Between 1975–1980 and 2005–2010 life expectancy at birth increased from 53 to 68 in Bangladesh and from 56 to 68 in Indonesia (UN 2011) and there are now a number of poor or middle-income countries with life expectancies at birth as high as in the United States.

The process of the epidemiological transition (or at least the initial phases) is now complete or under way in much of the world and non-communicable causes of death predominate in all regions except sub-Saharan Africa (see Table 6.3.2). However, some recent changes have been less benign and new challenges or reversals have emerged, notably the HIV/AIDS epidemic and the health consequences of the collapse of the former Soviet Union (Olshansky et al. 1997; Murphy 2011). Partly because of these challenges, there are signs that after a period in which risks of mortality in different parts of the world showed a tendency to converge (i.e. poorer countries caught up with richer ones), more recently there has been a trend towards divergence. Another factor in this may be that recent successes in richer countries in, for example, lowering mortality from heart disease, have partly been achieved through treatments which are harder to 'transfer' to poor countries because of infrastructure and cost limitations (Vallin and Mesle 2004; Ford et al. 2007).

Recent demographic trends and public health

Population size, growth, and age structure are all outcomes of variations in demographic behaviours and all have implications for population health and well-being. Population ageing will almost certainly be the predominant demographic issue of the twenty-first century in nearly all richer and a growing number of poorer countries. The strong association between age and risks of health impairment and disability imply growing needs for support services, even if levels of disability fall. In those countries which are growing old before they grow rich, changes in family support systems for older people may pose additional challenges. A range of strategies for responding to these challenges has been proposed, including encouraging longer working lives through review of retirement and pensions policies, better organization of acute and long-term care services, and initiatives to promote healthy ageing (Rechel et al. 2013).

Changes in marriage and family patterns also have other public health implications. In North America and North West Europe (and also Latin America and the Caribbean) high rates of divorce and non-marital childbearing mean that increasing proportions of children are spending at least part of their childhood in lone-parent families. Although causal pathways are difficult to elucidate because of various selection effects, there is evidence indicating poorer health among lone mothers and their children, and among unmarried (especially divorced) people more generally, so these trends have some negative implications.

Continuing improvement in child and adult mortality is projected for the poorer world, based on optimistic assumptions about the course of the HIV/AIDS epidemic. In the poorest countries the interaction of rapid population growth, environmental degradation and conflict pose continuing health problems and the 'unfinished agenda' in terms of health includes providing access to contraception for women who wish to space or limit their children (Cleland et al. 2006). In other middle- and low-income countries, patterns of tobacco use are likely to have a substantial effect on health trends in coming decades (West 2006).

Issues such as international migration, economic and cultural 'globalization', and climate change all have substantial health implications for the rest of the twenty-first century; all interact with demographic patterns and processes. Measuring these trends and assessing their effect on health and demand for healthcare requires an understanding of population dynamics and population-based measures, and suitable demographic data. Demography is thus an essential component of public health.

References

Abbasi-Shavazi, M., McDonald, P., and Hosseini-Chavoshi, M. (2009). *The Fertility Transition in Iran: Revolution and Reproduction.* Dordrecht: Springer.

Alders, M., Keilman, N., and Cruijsen, H. (2007). Assumptions for long-term stochastic population forecasts in 18 European countries. *European Journal of Population*, 23(1), 33–69.

Alexandratos, N. (2005). Countries with rapid population growth and resource constraints: issues of food, agriculture and development. *Population and Development Review*, 31, 237–58.

Anderson, R.N. (2011). Coding and classifying causes of death. In R.G. Rogers and E.M. Crimmins (eds.) *International Handbook of Adult Mortality*, pp. 47–490. Dordrecht: Springer.

Billari, F. and Kohler, H.P. (2004). Patterns of low and lowest-low fertility in Europe. *Population Studies*, 58, 161–76.

Bloom, E., Canning, D., and Malaney, P. (2000). Demographic change and economic growth in Asia. *Population and Development Review*, 26(Suppl.), 257–90.

Bongaarts, J. (1978). A framework for analysing the proximate determinants of fertility. *Population and Development Review*, 4, 105–32.

Bongaarts, J. (2005). *The Causes of Stalling Fertility Transitions.* Working Paper 204. New York: The Population Council.

Bongaarts, J. and Bulatao, R.A. (eds.) (2000) *Beyond Six Billion: Forecasting the World's Population.* Washington, DC: National Academies Press.

Bongaarts, J. and Feeney, G. (1998). On the quantum and tempo of fertility. *Population and Development Review*, 24, 271–91.

Bryant, J. (2007). Theories of fertility decline and the evidence from development indicators. *Population and Development Review*, 33, 101–27.

Caldwell, J. (1982). *Theory of Fertility Decline*. New York: Academic Press.

Caldwell, J.C., Orubuloye, I.O., and Caldwell, P. (1992). Fertility decline in Africa: a new type of transition? *Population and Development Review*, 18, 211–42.

Caselli, G. (1991). Health transition and cause specific mortality. In R. Schofield, D. Reher, and A. Bideau (eds.) *The Decline of Mortality in Europe*, pp. 68–96. Oxford: Clarendon Press.

Casterline, J.B. (2010). *Determinants and Consequences of High Fertility: A Synopsis of the Evidence*. Washington, DC: World Bank.

Cleland, J. (1990). Maternal education and child survival: further evidence and explanations. In J. Caldwell, S. Findley, P. Caldwell, et al. (eds.) *What Do We Know About Health Transition? The Cultural, Social and Behavioural Determinants of Health*, pp. 400–19. Canberra: Health Transition Centre, Australian National University.

Cleland, J., Bernstein, S., Ezeh, A., Faundes, A., Glasier, A., and Innis, J. (2006). Family planning: the unfinished agenda. *The Lancet*, 368, 1810–27.

Coale, A. (1973). The demographic transition reconsidered. In *International Union for the Scientific Study of Population, International Population Conference 1973*, pp. 53–72. Liège: Ordina.

Coale, A. and Watkins, S.C. (eds.) (1986). *The Decline of Fertility in Europe*. Princeton, NJ: Princeton University Press.

Coleman, D. and Salt, J. (1992). *The British Population: Patterns, Trends and Processes*. Oxford: Oxford University Press.

Cutler, D., Deaton, A., and Lleras-Muney, A. (2006). The determinants of mortality. *Journal of Economic Perspectives*, 20(4), 97–120.

Davis, K. and Blake, J. (1956). Social structure and fertility: an analytic framework. *Economic Development and Cultural Change*, 4, 211–35.

Fernandes, A., Carballo, M., Malheiros, J., and Pereira Miguel, J. (eds.) (2007). *Challenges for Health in the Age of Migration*. Conference on Health and Migration in the EU, Lisbon, Portugal, 27–28 September 2007.

Ford, E.S., Ajani, U.A., Croft, J.B., et al. (2007). Explaining the decrease in U.S. deaths from coronary heart disease, 1980–2000. *The New England Journal of Medicine*, 356, 2388–98.

Gajalakshmi, V. and Peto, R. (2011) Verbal autopsy of 80,000 adult deaths in Tamilnadu, South India. *BMC Public Health*, 4, 47.

Goldstein, J.R., Sobotka, T., and Jasilioniene, A. (2009). The end of 'lowest-low' fertility? *Population and Development Review*, 35(4), 663–99.

Griffiths, C. and Brock, A. (2003). Twentieth century mortality trends in England and Wales. *Health Statistics Quarterly*, 18, 5–16.

Grundy, E. (1997). The health of older adults 1841–1994. In J. Charlton and M. Murphy (eds.) *The Health of Adult Britain 1841–1994* (Vol. II), pp. pp. 183–204. London: The Stationery Office.

Hamilton, B.E., Martin, J.A., and Ventura, S.J. (2012). Births: preliminary data for 2011. *National Vital Statistics Reports*, 61(5), 1–20.

Hobcraft, J. (1993). Women's education, child welfare and child survival: a review of the evidence. *Health Transition Review*, 3, 159–73.

Institute for Health Metrics and Evaluation (IHME) (2012). *Global Burden of Disease Study 2010 (GBD 2010) Mortality Results 1970–2010*. Seattle, WA: IHME. Available at: http://www.healthmetricsandevaluation.org/ghdx.

Kinsella, K. and Phillips, D. (2005). The challenge of global aging. *Population Bulletin*, 60(1), 5–41.

Lee, R. (2003). The demographic transition: three centuries of fundamental change. *Journal of Economic Perspectives*, 17, 167–90.

Lesthaeghe, R.J. and Neidert, L. (2006). The second demographic transition in the United States: exception or textbook example? *Population and Development Review*, 32, 669–98.

Lotka, A. (1907). Relation between birth and death rates. *Science*, 26, 21–2.

Lozano, R., Lopez, A.D., Atkinson, C., et al. (2011). Performance of physician-certified verbal autopsies: multisite validation study using clinical diagnostic gold standards. *Population Health Metrics*, 9, 32.

Lozano, R., Mohsen Naghavi, M., Foreman, K., et al. (2012). Global and regional mortality from 235 causes of death for 20 age groups in 1990 and 2010: a systematic analysis for the Global Burden of Disease Study 2010. *The Lancet*, 380, 2095–128.

Lutz, W. and Samir, K.C. (2010). Dimensions of global population projections: what do we know about future population trends and structures? *Philosophical Transactions of the Royal Society B*, 365, 2779–91.

Manton, K.G., Gu, X., and Lamb, V.L. (2006). Long-term trends in life expectancy and active life expectancy in the United States. *Population and Development Review*, 32, 81–105.

Mason, A. and Lee, R. (2006). Reform and support systems for the elderly in developing countries: capturing the second demographic dividend. *Genus*, LXII, 11–36.

Mathers, C.D., Ma Fat, D., Inoue, M., Rao, C., and Lopez, A.D. (2005). Counting the dead and what they died from: an assessment of the global status of cause of death data. *Bulletin of the World Health Organization*, 83, 171–7.

McNicoll, G. (2006). Policy lessons of the East Asian demographic transition. *Population and Development Review*, 32, 1–25.

Moschetti, K., Cummings, P.L., Sorvillo, F., and Kuo, T. (2012). Burden of Alzheimer's disease-related mortality in the United States, 1999–2008. *Journal of the American Geriatrics Society*, 60(8), 1509–14.

Murphy, M. (2011). Adult mortality in the former Soviet Union. In R.G. Rogers and E.M. Crimmins (eds.) *International Handbook of Adult Mortality*, pp. 83–100. Dordrecht: Springer.

Murphy, M., Grundy, E., and Kalogirou, S. (2007). The increase in marital status differences in mortality up to the oldest age in seven European countries, 1990–99. *Population Studies*, 61(3), 287–98.

Notestein, F.W. (1945). Population: the long view. In T.W. Schulz (ed.) *Food for the World*, pp. 36–57. Chicago, IL: University of Chicago Press.

Olshansky, S.J., Carnes, B., Rogers, R.G., and Smith, L. (1997). *Infectious Diseases—New and Ancient Threats to World Health*. Population Bulletin 52. Washington, DC: Population Reference Bureau.

Omran, A.R. (1971). The epidemiologic transition: a theory of the epidemiology of population change. *Millbank Memorial Fund Quarterly*, 49, 509–38.

Organisation for Economic Co-operation and Development (1999). *Maintaining Prosperity in an Ageing Society*. Paris: OECD.

Preston, S.H. (1975). The changing relation between mortality and level of economic development. *Population Studies*, 29, 231–48.

Preston, S.H. (1976). *Mortality Patterns in National Populations*. New York: Academic Press.

Preston, S.H. (2007). Response: on 'The changing relation between mortality and level of economic development'. *International Journal of Epidemiology*, 36(3), 502–3.

Preston, S.H., Heuveline, P., and Guillot, M. (2001). *Demography: Measuring and Modelling Population Processes*. Oxford: Blackwell Publishers.

Preston, S.H. and Stokes, A. (2012). Sources of population aging in more and less developed countries. *Population and Development Review*, 38(2), 221–36.

Rechel, B., Grundy, E., Robine, J.M., et al. (2013). Ageing in Europe. *The Lancet*, 381(9874), 1312–22.

Retherford, R.D., Ogawa, N., and Matsukura, R. (2001). Late marriage and less marriage in Japan. *Population and Development Review*, 27, 65–102.

Ritu, S.R., Mathers, C.D., Lopez, A.D., Murray, C.L.J., and Iburg, K.M. (2002). Comparative analyses of more than 50 household surveys on health status. In C.J.L. Murray, J.A. Salomon, C.D. Mathers, and A.D. Lopez (eds.) *Summary Measures of Population Health Concepts, Ethics, Measurement and Applications*, pp. 369–86. Geneva: WHO.

Rowland, D.T. (2003). *Demographic Methods and Concepts*. Oxford: Oxford University Press.

Siegel, J.S. and Swanson, D.A (eds.) (2004). *The Methods and Materials of Demography* (2nd ed.). San Diego, CA: Academic Press.

Sobotka, T. (2008). The rising importance of migrants for fertility in Europe. *Demographic Research*, 19, 225–48.

UNAIDS (2012). *Global Report: UNAIDS Report on the Global AIDS Epidemic 2012*. New York: Joint United Nations Programme on HIV/AIDS.

UNFPA (1995). *International Conference on Population and Development—ICPD—Programme of Action. Report of the International Conference on Population and Development*. A/CONF.171/13/Rev.1. New York: UN.

United Nations (2011). *World Population Prospects: The 2010 Revision*. New York: UN. Available at: http://esa.un.org/unpd/wpp/Excel-Data/population.htm.

United Nations (2012). *World Urbanization Prospects, the 2011 Revision: Highlights*. New York: United Nations.

United States Census Bureau, Population Division, International Programs Center (n.d.). *International Data Base*. [Online] Available at: http://www.census.gov/population/international/data/idb/information Gateway.php.

United Nations Department of Economic and Social Affairs (2012). *Demographic Yearbook 2011, ST/ESA/STAT/SER.R/41*. New York: UN. Available at: http://unstats.un.org/unsd/demographic/products/dyb/dyb2009-2010.htm.

Valente, P. (2010). Census taking in Europe: how are populations counted in 2010? *Population and Societies*, 467, 1–4.

Vallin, J. and Mesle, F. (2004). Convergences and divergences in mortality: a new approach to health transition. *Demographic Research*, Special collection 2, 12–43. Available at: http://www.demographic-research.org/special/2/2.

van de Walle, F. (1986). Infant mortality and the European demographic transition. In A.J. Coale and S.C. Watkins (eds.) *The Decline of Fertility in Europe*, pp. 201–33. Princeton, NJ: Princeton University Press.

Wang, L., Yang, G., Jiemin, M., et al. (2007). Evaluation of the quality of cause of death statistics in rural China using verbal autopsies. *Journal of Epidemiology and Community Health*, 61, 519–26.

West, R. (2006). Tobacco control: present and future. *British Medical Bulletin*, 77–8, 123–36.

Williams, G.M., Najman, J.M., and Clavarino, A. (2006). Correcting for numerator/denominator bias when assessing changing inequalities in occupational class mortality, Australia 1981–2002. *Bulletin of the World Health Organisation*, 84(3), 198–203.

Woods, R.I., Watterson, P.A., and Woodward, J.H. (1989). The causes of rapid infant mortality decline in England and Wales, 1861–1921 (Part II). *Population Studies*, 43, 113–32.

World Bank (1993). *World Development Report 1993: Investing in Health, World Development Indicators*. Oxford: Oxford University Press.

World Health Organization (2013). *Global Health Observatory Data Repository Mortality and Burden of Disease: Child Mortality*. Available at: http://apps.who.int/gho/data/#.

Young, H., Grundy, E., O'Reilly, D., and Boyle, P. (2010). Self-rated health and mortality in the UK: results from the first comparative analysis of the England and Wales, Scotland, and Northern Ireland Longitudinal Studies. *Population Trends*, 139, 11–36.

6.4

Health promotion, health education, and the public's health

Simon Carroll and Marcia Hills

Health promotion, health equity, and action on the determinants of health: an introduction

Previous attempts (Green and Raeburn 1988; Tones and Tilford 1994; Tones 2002) to situate health promotion within the broad field of public health have often used 'health education' as the starting point. This is an entirely sensible approach which we will discuss but it tends to underemphasize the *radical* departure health promotion aims to make from traditional public health approaches in general. Without claiming health promotion means everything all at once, thereby leaving its lofty rhetoric in the realm of the aspirational yet ineffectual, we aim to place health promotion more centrally in the ongoing saga of an increasingly globally aware public health. As one of the acknowledged founders and innovators of the modern health promotion movement has unceasingly argued, health promotion, at its most persistent and radical, heralds a 'new public health', not merely a more fine-tuned and effective tool-box for a less paternalistic health education (Kickbusch 1989, 2007).

We will begin with a clear definition of health promotion. Then, by unpacking the dense and sometimes opaque wording that define the elements of health promotion as a concept, we intend to open up some of its central, yet often hidden, connections to much broader themes in contemporary social and political movements and ideas.

Next, we situate health education and its internal critique as an important part of the history of health promotion, while providing more context concerning the specific historical/national trajectories that made the genesis of the modern health promotion movement a mixture of different influences, of which health education is only one.

We will consider how health promotion manages its ambiguous relationship with the history and ideological background of public health, and how it sees itself in relation to the past, present, and future of public health.

We suggest there is a new opportunity for health promotion to reconnect with the avant-garde in public health, which can be examined along two broad dimensions, namely how to achieve health equity, and the question of health in a global political-economic context. Particular attention will be paid to the recent work following up the World Health Organization (WHO) Commission on the Social Determinants of Health, led by Sir Michael Marmot, and the renewal of the *Ottawa Charter* action area of 'healthy public policy' in the *Health in All Policies* global movement, spearheaded by the WHO.

In a previous version of this chapter (Hills and Carroll 2009), we argued that there was an under-analysed political economy of health promotion; in this revision, we argue that this is partly to do with the relative lack of engagement with social theory within the health promotion field. We offer some suggestions and map out potential pathways towards more serious reflection on this missing social-theoretical base. Finally, we consider the emerging role of complexity theory and systems thinking in health promotion research.

In general, this chapter on health promotion is *critical* in the positive sense of the word. Previous surveys of the concept and practice of health promotion that provide excellent guidance to the field are referenced. However, we consider that practitioners and researchers in public health can benefit from a reflexive inquiry into the rich ambiguities and tensions that are embedded in the discourse and practice of health promotion. This is particularly the case if, as we argue, the development of health promotion *is* the development of a 'new public health'.

'Health promotion': a definition and conceptual critique

In this chapter, we will follow the *Ottawa Charter for Health Promotion* (WHO 1986) definition of health promotion as 'the process of enabling people to increase control over, and to improve their health'. However, we will also draw upon the expanded definition in the updated *Health Promotion Glossary*:

> Health promotion represents a comprehensive social and political process, it not only embraces actions directed at strengthening the skills and capabilities of individuals, but also action directed towards changing social, environmental and economic conditions so as to alleviate their impact on public and individual health. Health promotion is the process of enabling people to increase control over *the determinants of health* and thereby improve their health. (WHO 1998, our emphasis)

Here, the 'how' and 'why' *ideology* is linked to the 'what' of the *determinants of health* (WHO 1998). This is crucial, because if health promotion is about anything, it is about *action* taken across the broad spectrum of health determinants, particularly directed towards the social, environmental, and economic conditions that support health (WHO 1984).

The *Glossary* also emphasizes that 'participation is essential to sustain health promotion action', and identifies the three *Ottawa Charter* strategies for health promotion: '*Advocacy* for health to create the essential conditions for health indicated above; *enabling* all people to achieve their full health potential; and *mediating* between the different interests in society in the pursuit of health.'

These strategies are supported by five priority action areas as outlined in the *Ottawa Charter*:

1. Build healthy public policy.

2. Create supportive environments for health.

3. Strengthen community action for health.

4. Develop personal skills, and

5. Re-orient health services. (WHO 1986)

As one can see from these definitions, we already have started the 'unpacking'. A more nuanced analysis of some of the key elements in this definition is described in the following subsections: the 'process' of health promotion; 'enabling' and 'empowering'; and for what, the outcome, 'improved health'. This will be followed by an analysis of the *Ottawa Charter strategies* and its *priority action areas* (often called 'action strategies').

As soon as we begin, we find ourselves in murky waters, though not without some guidance. Ironically, although health promotion is, as Tones (2004) noted, an 'essentially contested concept', there has been a remarkable degree of effort, and consensus, concerning its ostensive definition. Few, if any, health promoters dispute the *Ottawa Charter*'s now canonical phrasing (WHO 2005).

The real ambiguity that surrounds the concept of health promotion is embedded in the elision of the concrete meaning of the elements that make up its agreed upon definition.

Health promotion as a process

The emphasis on *process* is important, if only because it warns against reducing health promotion to merely a technical function of public health. It connotes the wider meaning of the concept by signalling that the radical departure and critique of traditional public health lies in its advocacy for changing the *way* we do public health, just as much as *what* we change and *why* we change.

Health promotion, whether it be generated from an internal critique of health education or from other dissatisfactions with the way public health was being practised, is fundamentally concerned with change and, specifically, with the failure of traditional, paternalistic, and professionally dominated public health processes to bring about positive changes in health, particularly for those groups that suffer disproportionately negative health outcomes and the consequent disadvantages. What is substituted is a call for health promoters to create a dynamic, participatory engagement with individuals and communities, to help or 'enable' them to take control over the determinants of their own health.

The first ambiguity we meet when trying to analyse this 'process' turns on whether one interprets the health promotion process as, primarily: a revamped tool-box of health education techniques and social marketing devices, with a rhetorically efficient participatory gloss; or, as a values-based process of communicative interaction that has as its central premise the ethical foundation of respect for human dignity and autonomy. These are certainly polar extremes and there is no doubt that there is room for both aspects in a broad, ecumenical attitude to a diverse field of practical action. Yet, because health promotion is a process often dominated by professionals, in a context where its supposed beneficiaries are often those in a position of relative powerlessness, the tendency for professionals to retreat to an insulated cocoon of technical expertise is strong. The essence of the health promotion process is a focused shift of power from professionals to the community and to individuals within their communities who historically have had less power. To do this, it is crucial that the 'process' we focus on is the one that involves negotiating values, principles, ethics, and power, not the less complicated one of transferring a packet of new skills and technical tools to a community that is presumed to lack capacity. In order to achieve this shift in power, health promoters need to begin by examining their own values and assumptions that inform their actions.

Beliefs and assumptions underlying health promotion

Health promotion practice is influenced by the beliefs and assumptions we hold. While a detailed discussion of this topic is beyond the scope of this chapter, we outline how certain beliefs and assumptions influence how we act in health promoting ways in given situations.

Beliefs are learned through life experiences; they are what we hold as 'true'. They are convictions that influence the way we think, feel, and act. Health promotion practice relies on a set of underlying assumptions that guide those who work in the field. Hartrick et al. (1994) contend health promotion is a 'way of being' that requires certain convictions in order to act in health promoting ways. These include:

1. All people have strengths and are capable of determining their own needs, finding their own answers, and solving their own problems.

2. Every person and family lives within a social-historical context that helps shape their identity and social relationships.

3. Diversity is positively valued.

4. People without power have as much capacity as the powerful to assess their own needs (people are their own experts).

5. Relationships between people and groups need to be organized to provide an equal balance of power (this includes professional/client relationships).

6. The power of defining health problems and needs belongs to those experiencing the problem.

7. The people disadvantaged by the way that society is currently structured must play the primary role in developing the strategies by which they gain increased control over valued resources.

8. Empowerment is not something that occurs purely from within (only I can empower myself), nor is it something that can be done to others (we need to empower the group). Rather, empowerment describes our intentional efforts to create more equitable

relationships where there is greater equality in resources, status, and authority.

9. Shared power relations do not deny health professionals their specialized expertise and skills. Rather, professional expertise and skills are used in new ways that result in greater power equity in interpersonal and social relations. (Hartrick et al. 1994, p. 87)

So, for example, if we consider the first assumption in the list, believing that people are able to find their own answers and solve their own problems leads one to act in empowering ways because of the belief that people have this capacity to figure things out. On the other hand, if one believes that people need to be told what to do, or that they are not able to figure out issues on their own, it is more difficult to create conditions that are enabling. For some, it might even feel irresponsible to put people in these circumstances or to allow them to have control over these types of decisions.

Enabling and empowerment

At the time of the *Ottawa Charter*, the word 'enabling' was favoured, although later this tended to be replaced with the more direct and comprehensive concept of 'empowerment'. Essentially, this meant that a prerequisite for the new approach was that individuals and communities were to directly participate in the planning and implementation of health promotion activities. The assumption was based on the notion that only by genuinely participating in the health promotion process would people be 'enabled' or 'empowered' to take control of what determined their health. However, the concept of 'enabling' also referred to the more general process of changing the social, economic, and environmental conditions that made it difficult for people to become empowered. There is a deep ambiguity here: it is not clear, for some commentators, whether more macro-scale action, at a policy level, also requires active participation of local communities. There is some room for an interpretation that tends to retain a traditional paternalism when it comes to healthy public policy, leaving the 'participatory' aspect of health promotion to the realm of 'community action'. As will be argued throughout this chapter, health promotion is constantly at risk of sliding back into this paternalistic approach, leaving the more 'complex' and high-level 'technical' decisions to the experts. Yet, if there is a direct link between human dignity, autonomy, and equity, then *all* aspects of health promotion must integrate the fundamental perspective of participation. In fact, it is argued that the rhetoric of 'empowerment' often masks a continuing bureaucratic and professional dominance of the process of improving public health (Baum 2007).

A key aspect of this ambiguity can be seen when we consider the link to health inequity. Without a genuinely participatory, empowering process, it is those worst off who are left further behind as they suffer, not only a failure to affect those conditions most important to their health, but also a direct assault on their human dignity (Sennett 2003). Those who tend to manage any gains from processes that lack true participation are usually segments of the population that already have access to positions of status and the resources and capacities to take advantage of the interventions on offer. The distinction here is between a situation where already disadvantaged people are assumed to be too ignorant or incapable of participating and thus have solutions imposed on them, and a situation where people of a privileged status delegate, as equals, to professional experts. This is not to say that a participatory process is not better for everyone, regardless of class position or status; rather, it is to emphasize that non-participatory processes have a disproportionate adverse effect on disadvantaged groups.

On the positive side, an empowering health promotion process leaves the ownership and control of a health promotion activity or programme in the hands of the community itself. This is particularly important in communities that have suffered historical social injustices and have thus been actively 'disempowered' (an ugly but accurate term). Allowing people to participate in a genuine way in determining not only *what* they want but *how* they want to get it is demonstrably the most effective strategy for change. It is also the *only* strategy for sustaining progress in improving health and shifting control back to the community and away from a negative dependence on bureaucratic and professional power. In this model, professionals are not demons; they are just transformed from arrogant experts into supportive servants of the will of the community.

There is in these simple terms ('enable' or 'empower') the entire, complex, and ambiguous story of health promotion. All the themes that will be touched upon in this chapter can be traced back to just what is at stake in the ostensive goal of 'empowering' people to take control over what determines their health.

What is the 'health' in health promotion?

Understanding how we conceptualize health is a key reflective step in health promotion. How we think about health largely determines the types of action we take to promote health. We see below how different historical conceptions of health still shape the contemporary health landscape and continue to sustain ambiguities in how people approach health promotion itself. In the twentieth century, due to the relative success of the sanitation approach to public health and the emergent hegemony of the germ theory of disease, an implicit biomedical definition of health as *the absence of disease* dominated, and along with it, a narrow, individual treatment focus, centred on the healthcare system, was the preferred solution. The WHO had, in 1946, introduced the *positive* definition of health as 'a state of complete physical, mental, and social well-being and not merely the absence of disease or infirmity' (WHO 1946). Nevertheless, this definition had little concrete impact on actual health systems, leaving the absence of disease approach to health as the default option when governments turned their attention to the public's health.

The Lalonde Report, an official document produced by the Canadian Department of Health and Welfare (Lalonde 1974), marked a significant change in thinking about health. Although the report is recognized internationally as the first government document to suggest that health promotion could be a key strategy for improving health, its other, more significant contribution, was to redefine how we view health. Lalonde's report argued that the healthcare system plays only a small part in determining health, and suggested that health was determined by the interplay between human biology, healthcare organization, environment, and lifestyle. This view of health became known as the 'lifestyle or behavioural approach to health', partly because the 'environmental' dimension was either ignored or treated narrowly.

With the publication of the discussion paper on concepts and principles of health promotion (WHO 1984) and the endorsement of the *Ottawa Charter for Health Promotion* (1986), a third

Table 6.4.1 From concept to action: different approaches to health

	Medical approach	**Behavioural approach**	**Socioecological approach**
Health concept	Biomedical; absence of disease or disability	Individualized; physical-functional ability, physical well-being	Positive state connectedness; ability to do things that are important or have meaning; psychological well-being
Health determinant	Disease categories, physiological risk factors (e.g. hypertension)	Behavioural risk factors (e.g. unsafe sex)	Psychological risk factors (e.g. isolation) and socioenvironmental risk conditions (e.g. poverty)
Principal strategy	Surgery, drugs, therapy, illness care, medically managed behavioural change	Advocacy for healthy lifestyle choices	Personal empowerment, small group development, community organization, coalition advocacy, political action
Programme development	Professionally managed	Negotiated with communities and professionals	Managed by community in critical dialogue with supporting professionals and agencies

view of health arose: the socioecological approach. This approach defined health as 'a resource for everyday life, not the objective of living'. 'Health is a positive concept emphasizing social and personal resources as well as physical capacities' (1986, p. 1). In order to reach this state of physical, mental, and social well-being, people must be able to identify and realize their aspirations, to satisfy their needs and to change, or cope, with their environment. This inextricable link between people and their environment provides the conceptual basis for this socioecological perspective on health and it forms the conceptual base for health promotion practice.

At first glance, these different views of health may appear to be developmental or historical. However, Labonté and others (Labonté 1993; Rootman and Raeburn 1994; Raeburn and Rootman 2007) argue that, in fact, all three views of health (along with many other definitions) continue to be endorsed by different people in the field of health promotion and, furthermore, that the view of health one holds influences one's health promotion practice. Table 6.4.1 illustrates this connection between how we think about health, our view of health, and our actions (health promotion practice). For example, if we hold a view that health is the absence of disease, we are likely to talk about disease processes and risk factors and to manage the problem professionally by prescribing a treatment. If we hold a socioecological view of health, we are more likely to focus on the conditions in which the person is living, the factors that are influencing their ability to meet their needs, and to use enabling strategies to assist the person to have more control over their health.

The *Ottawa Charter* strategies

The three strategies mentioned in the *Ottawa Charter* are: *to advocate*, *to enable*, and *to mediate*. We have already reflected upon the second strategy, as it is part of the definition of health promotion. However, a few words need to be said about the other two strategies.

The concept of *advocacy* receives very little elaboration in the *Ottawa Charter*. In the *Health Promotion Glossary*, it is stated that advocacy 'can take many forms including the use of the mass media and multi-media, direct political lobbying, and community mobilization through, for example, coalitions of interest around defined issues. Health professionals have a major responsibility to act as advocates for health at all levels in society' (WHO 1998, p. 6). This raises one of the many thorny issues that come

up when professionals are caught between highly mobilized and often highly critical communities and a state bureaucracy that is extremely reticent about providing funding that sanctions and supports the capacity for critical attention to its policies and programmes. Even at the level of independent professional organizations, the participation and funding provided by government bodies creates a tension around the organization taking strong critical perspectives. Another aspect of this strategy, as defined in the glossary and glossed over, is the potential contradiction between activities such as 'political lobbying' and 'community mobilization'. Often, the same organization or individual will be less effective as a political lobbyist to the extent they are perceived to be directly associated with community mobilization efforts that the powerful are either indifferent to, or actively disfavour.

Mediation is an even more delicate strategy for health professionals. Its original *Glossary* definition in relation to health promotion was: 'A process through which the different interests (personal, social, economic) of individuals and communities and different sectors (public and private) are reconciled in ways that promote and protect health' (WHO 1986). In the expanded definition of 1998, more explicit emphasis is given to the potential conflicts that often arise between the competing interests mentioned in the original definition. However, the goal of mediation as 'reconciliation' is left unchanged. While there is nothing inherently wrong with the idea of reconciliation, professionals should be extremely self-critical and reflexive when operating with this strategy. Two dangers are apparent with the strategy. First, in striving for 'reconciliation', one may simply paper over a conflict for the purposes of short-term peace, while leaving the principal reasons behind the conflict intact, thereby creating the potential for longer-term embitterment and strategic action by all parties, which ultimately undermines the appearance of agreement. Second, a very real threat to equity can arise when professionals reconcile a conflict between the powerful and the powerless and end up re-enforcing the powerful at the expense of the powerless. This tendency is very strong given the fact that professionals have little to gain personally from any radical re-structuring of power relations. Despite these important caveats, mediation has become even more critical for the success of health promotion in the future, especially in relation to the new global, multilayered context of health governance that the *Bangkok Charter* (WHO 2005) has set out to address and which will be discussed later.

The *Ottawa Charter* action areas

The priority action areas of the *Ottawa Charter* were identified as those areas that were seen at the time of the charter (and still to this day) as critical arenas for health promotion's strategic activities. We will not try and survey the myriad accomplishments of health promotion activity; rather, consistent with our general approach, we will offer a few critical comments on each action area:

Building healthy public policy

There are three elements of healthy public policy emphasized in the *Ottawa Charter*:

1. If, as the Lalonde Report (1974) argued, the determinants of health lay mainly outside healthcare itself, then policy action must come from policy sectors other than health. The health sector would still play an important, but not exclusive, role in public policy action to support health.

2. Healthy public policy requires the coordinated use of all policy levers available, including 'legislation, fiscal measures, taxation, and organizational change' (WHO 1986).

3. Healthy public policy requires the identification and removal of obstacles to the adoption of such policies in non-health sectors.

Without going into a long list of efforts and results in this area, the progress made can be summed up as substantial and encouraging in regard to changes in the rhetoric and discourse around health, in both developed nations and in many of the global institutions responsible for improving health and development worldwide. Conversely, one can equally characterize progress as ephemeral and demoralizing when it comes to the concrete goal of 'coordinated action that leads to health, income and social policies that foster greater equity' (WHO 1986). For a variety of reasons discussed in the later subsection on the political economy of health promotion, given the increasingly urgent crisis of widening inequities in health both between and within societies, the collective policy response of the most powerful countries on earth has been miserly and despicable. To call it 'inadequate' is a gross understatement and an unconscionable euphemism.

When *action* finally starts to catch up with some of the lofty rhetoric behind the calls for 'health in all policies' (Ståhl et al. 2006), health promotion can begin to find some satisfaction in the area of building healthy public policy. Since the last version of this chapter we have seen this contradiction intensify, as the global economic crisis brought on by the 2008 financial crash has led to some very regressive shifts in fiscal policy and thus social supports for a healthy public policy; meanwhile, at the level of rhetoric, global institutions, such as the WHO, have been increasingly supportive of the conceptual logic of healthy public policy. We will discuss some of the latter recent developments in relation to the *Health in All Policies* movement in a later section.

Creating supportive environments

This area forms the basis for what is called the *socioecological* approach to health. Here it is asserted that both the natural and built environments are inextricably linked with people's health. It is crucial to understand that the conceptualization of supportive environments given here is consistent with the expanded, positive understanding of health as a 'resource for everyday life'. It is not merely about threats to physical health, but involves creating conditions that allow people to have 'living and working conditions that are safe, stimulating, satisfying, and enjoyable'. This entails the complex relationships between rapidly changing technologies, working conditions, resource use, climate change, urbanization, and health (amongst others).

In considering progress, past endeavours, and future prospects in this area, one must take into account the lofty ambition (and some would say naïvety) of this programme of action. As a project of knowledge development, its referral to the 'complex interrelatedness' of contemporary societies is but a cipher for the entire corpus of theoretical and empirical dispute and debate within the social sciences over how to characterize what are now acknowledged to be multiple, interrelated, global, national, regional, and local processes of socioeconomic and cultural change (Held et al. 1999). Later we consider some recent moves toward adopting complexity science and systems thinking to more adequately address this complex interrelatedness.

In the real world, we are not able to coordinate all the best knowledge sources available and neatly calculate what is best for health. Instead, we are left with tools like 'health impact assessment' (HIA) (Kemm 2006). The action area of creating supportive environments can be seen as a great boon to academic productivity, both theoretical and empirical; yet, before the final judgements of the academy can be handed down, actions must be taken and decisions must be made.

Communities and developers, politicians, and bureaucrats must decide whether to build this or that highway, license this or that mining operation, enact this or that employment regulation, and build this or that oil pipeline. We are thus forced, by the necessity to decide and act, into an inevitable reduction of complexity. The question is not whether this is a good or bad thing; it is *how*, by what *process*, is complexity reduced? Whither participation and empowerment in a field dominated by professional expertise and the cloistered secrecy of executive and administrative decision-making in both the public and private sectors?

We argue *against* the implication that instruments like HIA inevitably vitiate participatory processes (Kemm 2006). The natural tendency is always to define ahead of time, objectively, what elements of the built or natural environment are most important for enhancing people's health. From a utilitarian perspective, locally defined needs and wishes may even legitimately be ignored in the name of some greater good for a larger population. However, health promotion should always err primarily on the side of the fundamental value of the autonomy and the dignity of people and their communities. In this mode, participation is foundational, even in what are prima facie obvious areas for the guidance of refined professional expertise. In enquiring into the best way to protect and enhance the built and natural environment for health, the first step is to find out what people actually identify as the things that would make life 'safe, stimulating, satisfying, and enjoyable'. From the professional perspective this route has one incontestable drawback: people are inevitably confused, ignorant, inconsistent, contradictory, and even just 'wrong'. 'People' will disagree with each other; will get annoyed or, even worse, angry; will disrespect experts, politicians, lawyers, and any number of people who 'actually know' about the issue. What is feared here is what is fondly called deliberative politics; in other words, the foundation of democratic civil society.

We are, as is universally acknowledged in the health promotion community, a long way from creating supportive environments for health, especially for those suffering gross inequities in social conditions and in consequent health outcomes. What is less often acknowledged is that part of the reason this is so difficult is that we consistently exclude the very people we are meant to be helping from determining the goals, and strategies necessary to move from here to there. Once again, we are led to believe that the ends can justify the means; we can have non-participatory processes as long as we intend to make changes to enhance the lives of the less fortunate. That we end up in a place we did not intend, is inextricably linked to the fact that, at crucial junctures, when inevitable changes of directions and compromises are made (local development processes are a prime example), the people who have an inherent interest in speaking up for the powerless (the powerless themselves) are nowhere to be seen, or are barely heard.

Strengthening community action

This action area is at the very heart of health promotion; in fact, it can be argued that this action area is the one where the basic principles of health promotion lie. You can imagine (wrongly) participation, equity, and empowerment to be contingent add-ons to the other action areas; with strengthening community action the essential unity of all the values of health promotion are embedded as necessary features of its realization. Indeed, what we see in this area is the place where the true spirit of health promotion is anchored in community development as a process. In fact, in the *Ottawa Charter* itself, there is a strange ellipsis where the term community development is introduced in the section on strengthening community action. It is as if one missed something: there is no linking phraseology relating community development to strengthening community action. This, we surmise, is no error: strengthening community action quite simply *is* community development.

Consider the definition of community development as agreed upon at the International Association for Community Development at a meeting in Budapest in 2004. Community development is a:

> way of strengthening civil society by prioritising the actions of communities, and their perspectives in the development of social, economic and environmental policy. It seeks the empowerment of local communities, taken to mean both geographical communities, communities of interest or identity and communities organizing around specific themes or policy initiatives. (Craig 2005, p. 3)

For a more sustained treatment of the need to recognize the central place processes of community development and empowerment should play in health promotion, Raeburn and Rootman's *People-Centred Health Promotion* is an essential reference (Raeburn and Rootman 1998). Raeburn and Rootman draw heavily, in their chapter on community development, on Meridith Minkler's important piece, 'Improving health through community organization' (1990). In this seminal piece, Minkler outlines the five principles she sees as foundational to community organization or development:

- Empowerment
- Community competence
- Participation
- Issue selection
- Creating 'critical consciousness'.

As is now obvious, we have run into some of these principles already, the key to which is that the community itself has collective control over the process of identifying issues and planning how to address them. In addition, the important notion of 'critical consciousness' is raised. This refers to the need for critical dialogue in the Freirian sense (Freire 1972); this is particularly important when working with historically oppressed or disadvantaged communities.

Developing personal skills

The new wave of health promotion has often downgraded attention to this critical aspect of its mandate. The *Ottawa Charter* tells us that health promotion 'supports personal and social development through providing information, education for health, and enhancing life skills'. However, since the *Ottawa Charter*, health promoters, with some exceptions, have tended to either ignore or aim strong criticism at the developing personal skills area. This has come about for three reasons. First, as part of the critique of health education, it was argued that individually focused education approaches were generally ineffective in bringing about health promoting behavioural change; instead, a switch to an emphasis on the *social* factors that influence health was necessary to overcome the limitations of traditional counselling and other interventions circumscribed by the discipline of psychology. Second, the emphasis on developing personal skills was associated with the 'victim-blaming' element that many health promoters saw as the consequence of an interpretation of the Lalonde report and other government documents (particularly, the approach taken in the United Kingdom under the Thatcher governments) in the context of the neo-liberal rolling back of the state's commitment to a strong social safety net. Finally, although developing personal skills is a central mechanism for empowering individuals to take control over their own health, many worried that, in this narrow approach, the *collective* strengthening of communities was adversely effected by too much emphasis on individual empowerment.

All of these concerns are legitimate, though in each of them there is a high risk that we will miss important opportunities by mistaking what are contingent tendencies for essential features.

As has recently been argued, the ignorance of, or even hostility to, work in this area may seriously damage health promotion's potential impact (Godin 2007). First, while many health education and behaviour change approaches are limited in their effectiveness, there are some demonstrably effective interventions that should not be ignored (Kok et al. 1997). Furthermore, we can learn and are learning about why some approaches in this area have not been effective. Second, the fact that this area of health promotion can be enlisted as part of a more general 'victim-blaming' culture of health promotion, does not mean it must be enlisted; in fact, to the extent that genuinely empowering health education is taken seriously, the resulting improvements in self-esteem should work against victim blaming. Third, individual and community empowerment should not be a zero sum trade-off. It is only when an exclusive focus on individuals is emphasized that we will have the phenomenon of rescuing survivors from a sinking ship.

In summary, while we must be vigilant against the temptation and limitations of an individually focused, skills development approach, we must also re-engage with the most advanced and progressive elements in this area of work. If we fail to do this, we will jeopardize a key aspect of health promotion.

Reorienting health services

While we have made some important gains in the previous four areas, reorienting health services has proved more difficult. In general, throughout the world, health services remain medically dominated, cure and treatment focused, and individualistic. The *Ottawa Charter* states 'the role of the health sector must move increasingly in a health promotion direction, beyond its responsibility for providing clinical and curative services'. However, 'across the world, there appears to have been a stubborn resistance to systematic change in healthcare services and only limited examples of effective and sustainable health services reorientation' (Wise and Nutbeam 2007). Health services need to embrace an expanded mandate which is sensitive and respects cultural needs. This mandate should support the needs of individuals and communities for a healthier life, and open channels between the health sector and broader social, political, and physical environmental components.

Health services are broad and far-reaching, with the most complex service for health promotion being the acute care hospital setting. There has been some advancement in this area with the creation of the healthy hospital settings movement, with some research evidence that it is possible to practice from a health promotion perspective even within this particularly medically dominated environment, for nurses at least (Hills 1998). However, we want to focus in this chapter on the area where health promotion should flourish but has not as yet—primary healthcare. Many who work in health promotion would argue that the *Alma Ata Declaration* (WHO 1978) was the precursor for the *Ottawa Charter*. These two documents share the same values, principles, and basic tenets; the *Alma Ata Declaration* addresses health systems more particularly while the *Ottawa Charter* has a broader mandate. But it is their relationship that provides the key to reorienting health services. That is, primary healthcare is a place for health promotion to focus its energy in terms of reorienting health services. In fact, the more that health promotion disassociates itself from primary healthcare, the more we give the impression that it is in the domain of medicine, not health. 'The more health promotion becomes distinct from the world of curative care, the more the latter is allowed to continue to be seen as the real work of medicine' (MacDonald 1992).

We want to be clear that when we are talking about primary healthcare, we are not talking about primary care. These terms are often confused or used interchangeably. Primary healthcare refers to the philosophy and principles articulated in the *Alma Ata Declaration* (WHO 1978). It calls for universal access to health services (universality) and the removal of geographic, social, economic, or cultural barriers to access (accessibility); it demands community participation in planning, operation, and evaluation of health services (participation); it requires integration across health and other sectors such as housing, education, and employment; it recognizes the power of multidisciplinary teams working as equal partners for the health of the community; it focuses on a range of services, determined by the community, that include health promotion, primary prevention, rehabilitative, and curative (essentiality); and, it demands a commitment to equity concerning issues of power and resources (equity and access). Therefore, primary healthcare resists the conceptual and operational separation of treatment and prevention which fits the engineering model of healthcare, with prestige and often scarce resources going to clinical medicine to the neglect of prevention, promotion, and rehabilitation (MacDonald 1992).

People who work in health promotion and understand its philosophy and principles must be involved in the development and implementation of primary healthcare. Many people working in health promotion are of the opinion that health promotion and healthcare are distinct and separate entities. They are critical of health promoters who talk about healthcare or health service delivery at the same time that they are talking about health promotion. We have a different opinion: it is necessary, not only to talk but to act as health promoters to facilitate primary healthcare reform.

Besides the *Ottawa Charter* outlining our responsibility to take up this challenge, there are two other reasons why it must be people who work in health promotion who participate in the reorientation of health systems to primary healthcare.

First, the health system is controlled by the powerful. There is a hegemony that supports a predominant treatment/cure paradigm. Power resides in these structures and with the health professionals who work in those systems. So, as advocates for equity and social justice, health promoters have a responsibility to take up this challenge. If we continue to work only in the community where we are comfortable, we will avoid confronting one of the greatest challenges of our times: creating a health system that is based on the principles of health promotion. We are not neutral in this process. As Paulo Freire (1972) said, 'washing one's hands of the conflict between the powerful and the powerless, means to side with the powerful, not to be neutral'. Kickbusch (1989) confirms this concern. She states, 'herein lies the great historical opportunity and challenge. Maybe health promotion can break the deadlock of the health policy debate that is basically about medical care and provider dominance' (p. 14). As she suggests, we are well beyond the burden of proof needed to claim that health promotion is successful—we have demonstrated this through our change in attitudes towards smoking, drinking, and nutrition—even if these are mainly concerns of the middle class and of high-income countries. 'Accountability and the burden of proof should now lie with the medical system' (Kickbusch 1989, p. 14).

The second reason that health promoters must take up this challenge can be summarized in one question: if health promoters do not advocate for primary healthcare based on the principles of the *Alma Ata Declaration* and the *Ottawa Charter*, what model of primary healthcare will dominate our countries?

Health promotion: history and influences

Health education

Health education plays a profound role in the history of health promotion. While it is true that health promotion is an 'essentially contested concept' claimed by a variety of different interests and actors (Green and Raeburn 1988), many of its most prolific commentators, particularly in the area of health promotion research and knowledge development, have been from the field of health education (Green and Kreuter 2005).

These writers have often been concerned with the failure of traditional health education approaches to help motivate individuals to act on health information. Following Tones, we adopt his definition of health education as: 'Any intentional activity which is designed to achieve health or illness-related learning, that is, some permanent change in an individual's capability or disposition' (Tones 2004, p. 7). This refers to what knowledge, attitudes, or skills can be acquired by individuals through a variety of health education processes. In relation to health promotion, key health educators have radically restructured the traditional approaches to influencing health behaviour. Most of this work has revolved around challenging what are now seen to be simplistic and mechanical models of health belief and health decision-making. At the centre of this change has been an adoption of the concept of empowerment and an advocacy for using participatory learning processes that break down the power imbalances between health professionals and lay members of society. Crucially, the relationship between devolving control, developing self-esteem, and bridging the gap between knowledge, attitude, and behaviour is highlighted.

In relation to the overall theme of health equity, the move away from traditional health education models has been critical. Without the concept of empowerment, and the development of capacities and self-esteem, the traditional 'health action model' of raising awareness and changing attitudes to health behaviours tended to exacerbate health inequalities, as the 'prepared' middle classes quickly adopted the new healthy practices of more exercise, less smoking, and a healthy diet. The efforts to help population groups that had both the worst health outcomes and the most intransigent health-related social conditions have not been nearly as successful.

A detailed account of these changes can be found in Tones (2004). One very important aspect of his account is how health promoters can learn, as professionals, to overcome the social gap in both power and understanding between them and the groups and individuals they aim to enable and empower. As Tones notes, the 'holy trinity' of counselling (respect, empathy and genuineness) is pertinent here. Often the more socioecological accounts of the health promotion process gloss over this crucial interactive aspect of health promotion. Whether it is with individuals or with groups, health promoters cannot act effectively without using highly developed skills of empathic understanding and facilitation. Particularly with group interactions, where often highly charged community issues are discussed, the professionals striving for neutrality and objectivity will find themselves unable to cope with the anger and resentment felt by people who perceive a history of grave social injustice behind their 'health' problems. It is important that these basic counselling skills are imparted to health promoters-in-training before they go out into communities and work with them on issues relevant to their health.

This shift in health education from an information-giving, pamphlet distribution approach to an empowerment liberatory approach has brought renewed interest in Freire's emancipatory education paradigm (1972). Health promoters in several countries, most notably those in Brazil, have reclaimed and embraced his basic premises and have employed his dialogical problem-posing teaching strategies that help make health education more consistent with the principles and values of health promotion and the 'new' public health. Freire's (1972) model of empowerment education describes a three-stage methodology consisting of listening, participatory dialogue, and action. Freire proposes that the main strategy of empowerment education, critical dialogue, requires us to engage in a process of problem-posing rather problem-solving.

Problem-posing is different from problem-solving because it does not seek immediate solutions to problems. Rather, generative themes arising from the listening phase are 'codified' and posed as problematics to raise group consciousness about specific issues. Wallerstein and Hammes (1991) contend that this process recognizes the complexity and the time needed to create effective solutions to societal issues. 'An effective code shows a problematic situation that is many sided, familiar to participants and open-ended without solutions' (Wallerstein and Bernstein 1988, p. 383). Freire describes these as 'generative' themes because they generate energy and motivate people to act. Freire contends that, through a process of dialogue that reflects on the generative themes raised through listening, people become masters of their own thinking in interaction with others (1972, p. 95). As Wallerstein and Bernstein explain: 'The goal of group dialogue is critical thinking by posing problems in such a way as to have participants uncover root causes of their place in society—the socioeconomic, political, cultural, and historical contexts of personal lives' (1988, p. 382).

Freire cautions that 'the liberating educator has to be very aware that transformation is not just a question of methods and techniques' (1972, p. 35). If that were the case, we could simply substitute one set of methods for another. 'The question is in a different relationship to knowledge and to society' (1972, p. 35).

Public health

Many health promotion researchers preface their scholarly remarks on the birth and development of health promotion with a discussion of its relationship to its older, more developed discipline, public health (Kickbusch 1986; Terris 1992). How this history is understood is perhaps the most telling aspect of how health promotion and its progress are viewed as a contemporary phenomenon. The argument developed below is that there has been a tendency within health promotion to tell a story of public health as a 'fall from grace'—a fall from its original reforming, perhaps even zealous, focus on the social and environmental causes of ill health, to a more restrictive, preventive biomedical era, and finally, to a broader scale but narrower scope in the 'lifestyles' approach focused on individual risk factors and behavioural change (Kickbusch 1986). Health promotion steps into the story to herald the era of a 'new public health', as a sort of re-emergence of the spirit of the nineteenth-century socioenvironmental model, with a modern gloss on the more subtle socioeconomic determinants of health. The purpose of this critical analysis is to challenge this tendency to nostalgia, and to explicate some of its continuing consequences for health promotion's rather schizophrenic relationship to public health. The 'golden age' of public health was influenced by a particular philosophical and political outlook that still finds its expression today in its most modern and rigorous proponents.

The history of health promotion conventionally begins with the publication of the Lalonde Report, entitled *A New Perspective on the Health of Canadians* (Lalonde 1974). The report was the first high-level national government document in the world to advocate for health promotion as a basic strategy for improving population health. It was influential internationally and set the stage for future debate with its concept of the *health field* as the articulation of the argument that the medically dominated healthcare system was only one and perhaps the least significant determinant of health, alongside biology, the physical and social environment, and individual lifestyles. The Lalonde Report relied explicitly for its argumentation on such critiques of the healthcare system found in 'social medicine' as those comprehensively outlined by (McKeown 1976), but which had their roots in the classic public health tradition of William Petty, Johann Frank, Rudolf Virchow, and William Farr (White 1991). The report contains not only the notable tension between an emphasis on individual lifestyles and the subsequently neglected socioenvironmental factors, but also an equal tension, given its own chapter heading, of 'Science versus Health Promotion'. Here it is made very clear that the 'science base' of the health field concept is epidemiology and, in this context, health promotion is seen as that type of action that must be taken even though the pertinent scientific questions have yet to be definitively answered. In some ways, this attitude allowed some initial breathing space for health promotion to prosper; however, by setting up this dichotomy, it ensured that, eventually, when 'science' made its accounting, health promotion would have its day of reckoning with epidemiology.

Meanwhile, many in the health promotion community, especially in Europe and Canada, were starting to develop an independent conceptual basis for their work, based on a rigorous reflection on the type of actions necessary to most effectively promote the health of individuals and communities. Much of this work evolved out of a complex internal critique of the failure of traditional health education approaches and a more sophisticated understanding of behavioural change (Kickbusch 1986; Tones 1993). Yet, in some countries, such as Canada, the absence of a strong health education tradition contributed strongly to a more socioecological approach to promoting health (with some of its most influential leaders being sociologists and nurses, rather than psychologists and health educators). Furthermore, for a variety of complex reasons (including, again, individual leadership), much of the discourse of contemporary social movements (new leftist, feminist, gay/lesbian, environmentalist) found its way onto the official agenda of major institutions such as the WHO and Health and Welfare Canada (Labonté 1994). As has been recognized by one of the leaders in health promotion internationally, Canada provided a hybrid and fertile mixture of traditional welfare state values and innovative community activism that seemed to provide the perfect ground for a push for the new socioenvironmental approach to health promotion (Kickbusch 1994). Out of this productive interaction between European 'health promotion tourists' (Kickbusch 1986, 1994) and many able Canadian activist/public health practitioners, grew the idea and finally the accomplishment of the *Ottawa Charter for Health Promotion* (1986).

To fully understand the impact that the *Ottawa Charter* had and continues to have, it is important to see that there was a crucial transformation from the epidemiological and bureaucratic dominance of the Lalonde Report to the emerging 'more pluralistic (and messier) social-science paradigm of human and social relations' embedded in the *Ottawa Charter* (Labonté 1994, p. 86). This shift is key to understanding the constant tension between a 'scientific' approach to health promotion and the 'values' underlying the *Ottawa Charter* that is renewed whenever health promoters are asked to more rigorously account for their activities. It raises the uncomfortable question for those who, correctly, see the importance of reconnecting health promotion to the new public

health, of just how 'new' the new public health is willing to be, when it comes to its underlying philosophical commitments.

This same tension underlies some of the confusion within the health promotion research community about how to relate to the more recent (Evans and Stoddard 1990) emphasis on 'population health' (Labonté 1997; Poland et al. 1998; Raphael and Bryant 2002). On the one hand, there is a justified admiration for the advocates of population health for their influential arguments about socioeconomic determinants of health, even so far as to single out progressive population health researchers such as John Frank (Raphael and Bryant 2002). On the other hand, there is the well-articulated angst about the lack of health promotion principles within the population health perspective. The critiques of the population health perspective for its lack of emphasis on values, its weak or non-existent orientation to action, and its somewhat imperious attitude to what is to count as proper 'knowledge', are all cogent and well-aimed. The question is: why should this be a surprise? It is not enough to point out the baleful influence of a replacement ideology for health promotion. Where did it come from, and why is it so influential? Furthermore, is this newly emergent approach (Evans and Stoddard 1990) really so new? How far is it simply a modern, sophisticated renaissance of that very same 'golden era' of public health that health promoters so often return to as their intellectual and moral heritage?

Although health promoters themselves (especially Canadians, who were the ones facing this challenge directly) reacted strongly and were able to defend the rationale for keeping a health promotion focus, the more incisive critiques were often too 'reactionary' and came off rhetorically as overly defensive. A more accommodating response came from within Health Canada itself with Hamilton and Bhatti (1996) introducing the concept of *population health promotion*. This was clearly an attempt to marry these two potentially adversarial positions and to cement the term health promotion as an integral component of population health that could not be ignored.

Why is it that health promotion often seems 'behind the game' in the science debate? Partly, this is due to the fact that, as Labonté says and a *Companion to Social Theory* attests (Turner 2000), the social science world is 'messy'. However, it may also be partially true that, for too long, health promotion has neglected its need to develop an independent 'science base' having unconsciously bought into that original Lalonde dichotomy. This is becoming increasingly clearer as many of the leading proponents in the field are pushing for more intensive theoretical development, a pressure that has become especially acute as the need for demonstrating effectiveness has increased (McQueen 2001; McQueen and Jones 2007; McQueen and Kickbusch 2007). To understand why health promotion has such a complex and ambiguous relationship to public health, it is necessary to dig more deeply into the foundations of modern public health and to unpack its driving philosophy and world view.

Politics and philosophy in public health and epidemiology

It is crucial to understand that the roots of the modern public health epidemiologists' focus on individual risk factors and randomized controlled trials (RCTs) is not in contradiction with or a deviation from the Edwin Chadwicks, the John Simons, and the John Snows of the classical public health. Rather, the full flowering of a utilitarian calculus, an uncompromising economism, and an obdurate scepticism of anything but positivistic scientific knowledge, can be seen as the late fruit of more than three centuries of development in public health and epidemiology.

There is a dilemma and prima facie paradox that health promotion faces when confronting its genealogy in the history of public health. In terms of lives saved and healthy years lived, the early public health interventions to combat the spread of deadly and debilitating communicable diseases cannot be underestimated. However, it is no accident that once the environmental risk factors of the major communicable diseases were effectively neutralized, a shift in focus took place to providing preventive, immunization measures. As Kerr White (1991) so convincingly puts it, the history of public health and epidemiology can be read as successive and iterative 'redefinings of the unacceptable'. Public health has always been concerned with an economistic and utilitarian approach to the health of the population; when things start to 'cost too much', the unacceptable becomes miraculously 'visible'. To understand this history, one has to ignore the facile disciplinary chasm between public health and economics, which has only recently and tentatively been bridged (Evans et al. 1994). While economics became progressively theoretical and mathematical, public health continued the original classical liberal tradition of reformist, practical utilitarianism, most powerfully apparent in the Benthamite tradition's attempt to rationalize government and public services. There is a great irony that the humanitarian idealism (an idealism at the core of health promotion's values base) of the British 'public health doctors', such as Haygarth, Heysham, Thackrah, Baker, and Millar, was never the driving force behind concentrated public health action (Fraser 1973).

As we will discuss in the subsection on health promotion and social justice, public health shares with economics a default, often merely implicit, utilitarian ethics. This shared history is seldom acknowledged, but it is a history that health promotion must confront explicitly. Fortunately, and ironically, recent developments in public health have brought into question the utilitarian approach, finding it inadequate, particularly in relation to the question of health inequity (Anand et al. 2004). The argument fleshed out below is that health promotion must forcefully engage in helping public health move in the direction advocated for by Amartya Sen and others (Anand et al. 2004).

Social movements

In this section, we briefly review one of the constitutive ambiguities at the heart of health promotion—many public health practitioners in the 1970s and early 1980s were increasingly cognizant of the lack of participatory involvement of the 'public' in public health programming.

A strong feature of the so-called 'new social movements' in the post-1968 period was a trenchant critique of bureaucratic structures and an increasingly administered society alongside the traditional leftist critique of capitalism. Some public health institutions, particularly urban public health units, decided to transform local public health practice by integrating a participatory model of programming that was heavily influenced by this anti-bureaucratic critique (Labonté 1994). However, as Dupéré et al. (2007) argue, despite its ambitions, health promotion is still not accurately described as a 'social movement', but rather a 'professional movement that had successfully advanced a

discourse about health and the production of health'. Yet, despite this acknowledged status, health promoters have recognized that much of their effectiveness depends on very high levels of social engagement. The more recent emphasis on health in the context of globalization (Labonté 2007) makes the necessity for health promotion to engage with larger social movements, particularly on the global development agenda, even more apparent.

Nevertheless, we find health promotion once again suspended between its constitutive desire to become one with the 'community' and its real position as a mediating professional fraction, often acting on behalf of formal public institutions. In the future, health promotion will have to sacrifice some of its cherished professional neutrality to choose sides, especially in its responsibility to advocate for health. While this new form of activist engagement must be balanced with the legitimacy attained from professional status, the balance must shift quite radically, given the growing threats to health represented by the inequity of contemporary societies in a globalized world.

Health promotion, health inequities, and social justice

We have, throughout this chapter, alluded to the commitment health promotion has to the principle of health equity. This is a fundamental and central value for health promoters and is often the touchstone for deciding why, where, and how to enact health promoting practice and policy. Yet, despite this nearly constant refrain, there is still confusion within health promotion about the theoretical and conceptual basis for its concern with health equity. While most, if not all health promoters, would see health equity as a basic goal of health promotion, seldom is the specific normative dimension that underlies this commitment fleshed out. The basic understanding is that health inequities are undesirable and should be eliminated because they are a set of systematic inequalities in health outcomes that are based on *unjust* inequalities of access to resources that provide for health. The *Health Promotion Glossary* describes what equity in health entails: 'That all people have an equal opportunity to develop and maintain their health, through fair and just access to resources for health.'

However, this definition begs many key questions, such as: what is 'fair' and 'just' access? And, what are 'resources for health'? While health promoters have often reflected deeply on health inequity, much of the appeal has been to an intuitive basis for supporting the elimination of inequity. We argue that this stance is no longer good enough. Health promotion must fully engage with recent work in political philosophy, particularly in the arguments surrounding the concept of social justice that have been developing since the publication of John Rawls' *A Theory of Justice* (1971). Since Rawls' groundbreaking work, an ongoing debate has taken place concerning what is the proper approach to justice for whole societies (Kymlicka 1990; Aveneri and de-Shalit 1992). More recently this debate has been expanded to consider how we are to think of justice in the global context (Nussbaum 2006). Health promoters should pay close attention to what is at stake in these debates for two reasons.

First, without an awareness of these important arguments, health promotion is liable to accept a default utilitarianism that it inherits from public health, which in turn the latter shares with orthodox economics. It is argued here that this unacknowledged utilitarianism is in direct contradiction to two profound moral intuitions that form the core of health promotion values: that it is wrong to increase overall health at the expense of the least well off; and, that human dignity and personal autonomy are overriding values.

Second, important developments in these debates are directly relevant to concerns with acting on the social determinants of health. Recent arguments have been refined concerning why and how we should address the issue of health inequity, both within and between societies (Anand et al. 2004; Nussbaum 2000). As health promoters, charged with the responsibility to advocate, enable, and mediate for equity in health, we should be armed with the very best arguments supporting our position.

We argue here that the one of the most promising theoretical developments in political philosophy that have implications for health promotion are in the evolving 'capabilities' approach to social justice and equity (Nussbaum and Sen 1993; Nussbaum 2000, 2006). This approach most nearly matches the health promotion approach to health as a 'resource for everyday living'; according to this doctrine, the 'social bases for health' would count as a primary good, or capability that should, by right, be provided to all citizens (and by extension, all human beings) at a minimum standard (Nussbaum 2006). It cannot be assumed that arguments for equity in health are unassailable and intuitively obvious for two reasons. First, without some substance behind what is meant by equity and what kinds of resources are to be distributed equitably, the demand for equity in health can be dismissed as either empty or naïvely utopian. Second, differing conceptions of what is just will lead to different outcomes in terms of actions to promote health. For example, unless we are very clear, 'equal opportunity' can be understood in an absolute minimalist sense and can allow powerful institutions to continue to support vast inequities in resources for everyday living. As we will see below, how we conceive of social justice has a profound impact on the types of actions we can imagine as solutions to the gross inequities in health we find across the world. Specifically, it has become apparent that the goals of health promotion are intimately related to the goals of a socially just global development agenda. Next we focus on an important element that tends to be lost in much of the discourse on health equity: what are the political, economic and social mechanisms by which the social determinants of health are reproduced as unequal resources for health? This is followed by considering one emerging global initiative aimed at policy solutions in this area: the *Health in All Policies* agenda.

The political economy of health promotion

Much good work has been done on the 'political economy of health' (the analysis of how different politico-economic social structures affect health outcomes), yet an enormous amount is still required (Navarro and Shi 2001; Navarro 2002; Langille 2003; Raphael 2003). Furthermore, there have been some excellent analyses of the 'political economy of healthcare' (the analysis of the effect of different political and economic arrangements on the quality and differential access to health services). In this subsection, we outline a different question: what is it about our contemporary political and economic structures that vitiates against the implementation of health promotion strategies and actions as they are conceived in the *Ottawa Charter*?

To begin to answer this question, we need to consider the three fundamental dimensions to health promotion: empowering communities and individuals, building health public policy, and creating supportive environments.

As has already been argued, empowerment is a key dimension of health promotion. By its very nature, empowerment aims to rebalance existing power arrangements by enabling those currently without power to gain access to the resources necessary to live fulfilled and happy lives. In order to do this with any success, health promoters must do two things: they must have a clear-headed view of existing power structures and relations; and, they must recognize, as professionals, how they themselves fit into those power relations and how they help, often unconsciously, to reproduce them. One way of seriously addressing this issue is to pay more attention to the concepts of class and status mentioned on the section on social justice and health promotion.

Health promotion, to be successful, must rely on concerted action by governments around the world, both within their own territories and in cooperation to address needs that require global action, such as on climate change. However, while these wishes are often articulated (WHO 2005), seldom are we offered an analysis of the structure and dynamics of the contemporary state system in a global context. A more reflective perspective is important here, as theorists of the state argue that certain issues and certain groups, using specific strategies, are more or less likely to be successful changing the nature of hegemonic projects and reversing the direction of state policies (Jessop 2002). Health promotion must become more strategic in how it operates vis-à-vis the state; it must recognize in an explicit way the limitations and opportunities available and integrate theoretical perspectives and practical actions in regard to one of its key areas: building health public policy.

Finally, creating a supportive environment is even more wrapped up in the dynamics of global capitalism than all the other areas combined. The fundamental prerequisites for health as outlined in the *Ottawa Charter* are: peace, shelter, education, food, income, a stable ecosystem, sustainable resources, social justice, and equity. These are the elements that, when in adequate supply, make up many of the properties of a supportive environment for health. Yet, each of these elements is in large part determined by the particular structure and dynamics of our global socioeconomic system.

It is necessary to develop an awareness of the fundamental political and economic drivers behind the dynamics of contemporary societies in both the developed and developing worlds. If equity in health relies on the fundamental fairness of social, political, and economic institutions, then ignoring these basic realities is no longer an option for a serious approach to health promotion. These important insights should no longer be gained in an ad hoc way but should be seen as part of what should constitute core knowledge for competent health promoters.

Social theory and health promotion

Recently, particularly following the report of the WHO Commission on Social Determinants of Health (2008), there has been a raft of activity by both academia and governments aimed at developing knowledge about the social determinants of health. There has also been a marked (and needed) shift of emphasis to what types of *action* societies need to take to address the consequences of the iniquitous distribution of resources that support health. Less prominent are attempts to confront theoretically the main causal mechanisms that produce and reproduce the social inequalities that lead to health inequities. While there have been recent attempts by some health promotion researchers to re-engage with fundamental debates in social theory (McQueen et al. 2007), for the most part the public health community as a whole, and health promotion by proxy, is still dominated by the narrowly focused methodological lens of epidemiological science. This failure to confront the ghost of social theory's past is most apparent in the way that the categories of *class* and *status* are dealt with in health promotion and public health discourse. Where they are mentioned at all, they tend to be conceptualized as epidemiological variables that measure an individual or group's socioeconomic attributes or properties (e.g. income, education level, wealth, job status), not as social processes that reproduce structural disadvantages for most and accumulate power and privilege for a few (see Scambler (2012) for an excellent review of this problem). The key elements of social theory that should be at the forefront of debate in health promotion circles are considered more extensively in two recent sources (McQueen et al. 2007; Carroll 2012).

The *Health in All Policies* Movement

Launched as Finland's main theme of its 2006 European Presidency, *Health in All Policies* (HiAP) is a strategy to help link health and other policy sectors in an over-arching intersectoral approach to improving health and well-being and reducing health inequity (Stähl et al. 2006). It is an attempt to reinvigorate the original emphasis in the *Ottawa Charter* on healthy public policy, and to follow up on the work done at the WHO conference in Adelaide, Australia in 1988 (WHO, 1988). Since that meeting, there has been much reflection on both the details of how to implement healthy public policy and the particular challenges posed by integrated, coherent, intersectoral action for health. More recently, the WHO reconvened in Adelaide to produce an international statement on HiAP called the 'Adelaide statement on health in all policies: moving toward a shared governance for health and well-being' (WHO, 2010). It is no coincidence that it lays heavy emphasis on 'governance'. This was followed by two important publications in 2012, also focusing on governance (Kickbusch and Gleicher 2012; McQueen et al. 2012). The central challenge of implementing HiAP has been the difficulty of managing the governance and accountability structures necessary to sustain both vertical (levels of government, non-governmental and private sector) and horizontal (cross-ministry, inter-departmental) intersectoral collaboration. We are only now beginning in public health and health promotion circles to appreciate the different type of knowledge base required to assess the effectiveness of policy implementation. We are still largely stuck in an outmoded attempt to squeeze what are really matters for political science, economic sociology and the sociology of the state into the narrow methodological confines of standard epidemiological research designs. Some emerging work (Lawless et al. 2012; Carroll et al. 2013) examines case studies of HiAP in order to better understand the key mechanisms underlying success and failure, but this is in its infancy. Clearly, HiAP is required to move forward on the intersectoral action agenda outlined in the *Ottawa Charter*; however, there is a large knowledge gap concerning implementation and sustainability that needs to be addressed in the future.

Since the last version of this chapter, little has changed in the field that might signify a shift in this direction. Training in health promotion still lacks any real engagement with scholarly debates in the social science disciplines that have insight into these key problems.

Complexity, context, and causality in health promotion research

Over the past 15 years, a series of publications have charted the specific methodological challenges for evaluating the effectiveness of health promotion interventions (IUHPE 1999; Rootman et al. 2001; Zaza et al. 2005; McQueen and Jones 2007). There has been some scepticism about applying the methodological protocols of evidence-based medicine (EBM) and RCTs as the gold standard because of the problems of complexity and context (McQueen 2007). One emerging alternative has been to use different methods for synthesizing evidence, such as the realist (Pawson et al. 2005) or meta-narrative (Greenhalgh et al. 2005) review approaches. A more detailed treatment of these latter approaches is beyond the scope of this chapter; however, one further potential for advancing beyond traditional EBM-type methods, is in the use of so-called 'systems thinking' or 'complexity science' to understand the rich complexity and contextual subtlety of the settings within which health promotion interventions take place, and of the interventions themselves.

Key to understanding the critique of EBM and some of the proposed alternative strategies is the different nature of how causality is conceptualized. The realist alternative has a direct, philosophical critique of the underlying empiricist-positivism of EBM's approach to causality (Bhaskar 2008). Conversely, systems thinking and complexity science approaches are more concerned with EBM's inability to take account of the interactive, emergent, and non-linear dynamics of causation that are crucial to understanding health promotion interventions as complex adaptive systems that intervene in the context of settings that are themselves complex adaptive systems.

Some health promotion researchers have started to take seriously the potential for a complexity or systems approach to health promotion interventions (Rickles et al. 2007; Shiell et al. 2008; Hawe et al. 2009; Trickett et al. 2011). These emergent attempts to apply complexity science have yet to show fruit (though systems thinking in public health has a longer pedigree), yet they hold much potential to transcend the current impasses in health promotion effectiveness research.

The role of social media

Finally, an important emerging issue, and one that has attracted much attention, is the potential role of social media in public health. The pervasive use and influence of the Internet and social media in nearly all parts of the world, presents new opportunities and challenges for health promotion and health education (see Chapter 4.3). A key feature that differentiates social media from more traditional communication processes is its interactive nature, where communications are not a one-way process, and where users also play an active role. This allows the formation of new online communities, which can enable virtual participation and collaboration among its members.

In this way, social media can provide resources as well as social support for patients with specific diseases or individuals with specific needs. In view of this, social media is emerging as a key platform for the dissemination of preventive health information. This can provide additional scientific information for individuals and communities, which can facilitate and enable greater public participation in the discussion about how the evidence base could be best used for the community. However, there are risks too that social media platforms could be used as avenues of persuasion by industry and other players who have vested interests in promulgating specific points of view.

Nevertheless, social media can also be used as a tool to listen to a much wider range of individuals and groups within the community and internationally. This can provide very useful inputs that could balance the traditional, more top-down, nature of public health programming. As a corollary, social media provides a major platform for health advocacy and activism that could lead to the strengthening of community action, the transformation of personal skills, and draw attention to health issues arising from social inequalities.

Conclusion

We have chosen not to give a technical survey of the health promotion field for which there are many excellent sources available (Tones and Green 2004; Green and Kreuter 2005). Two global perspectives on health promotion have been published, covering substantive areas and technical research problems concerning health promotion effectiveness (McQueen and Jones 2007).

Instead, we have attempted to offer the reader a chance to reflect on a set of core conceptual issues that underlie the health promotion problematic. The five key messages we want to impart about health promotion are listed here:

- Health promotion is a complex, often ambiguous concept and set of practices. Health promotion finds its core values and principles in the Ottawa Charter which bears careful examination to comprehend the essence of health promotion.

- Health promotion has an intimate connection to health education, with many of its most important and prolific thinkers having a health education background. The revolution in health education practice is directly connected to the birth of health promotion but beyond this, health promotion has its roots in the deep history of public health and has been invigorated by contemporary social movements.

- Health promotion is fundamentally about ethics, values, and social justice. Only secondarily is it about technical strategies for behaviour change. The foundational principles of health promotion are *equity*, *participation*, and *empowerment*.

- Health promotion is a professionally dominated movement. This requires health promotion professionals to be critical and reflexive in their practice; they must acknowledge power imbalances that favour professional dominance and work to restore power to individuals and communities.

- Health promotion must take its duty to enable people to control the determinants of their health seriously. To do this it must engage more directly with contemporary arguments in political philosophy and it must be aware of the dynamics of the global political economy and its effect on the potential for health promotion.

Some of these issues are well known, such as the problem of professional dominance; while others, such as the political economy of health promotion, or the engagement with political philosophy, are not addressed or require much deeper reflection.

We have argued that, at its heart, health promotion is about a radical shift in values for public health. It is not that public health was never concerned with equality or alleviating the misery of the poor; arguably, the so-called 'golden age' was driven by exactly these moral questions. However, these intuitive commitments were not sufficiently followed through when it came to not just *what* outcomes to change but *how* to change them. Too much of public health, for too long, was driven by a benevolent paternalism that, particularly when it came to dealing with chronic diseases and with vulnerable populations, ended up being counterproductive. Indeed, not only was this paternalism ineffective in many areas, it was unethical. It assumed the authority of experts and professionals, not only to determine technical solutions, but to determine needs. If we are to take the concepts of equity and empowerment seriously, they have profound implications for how we do public health interventions. We have learned that by addressing needs without first establishing a participatory framework that enables individuals and communities to determine those needs for themselves, we fatally undermine one of the most crucial capacities for health: human dignity and self-respect. This is particularly so in communities that have suffered historical social injustices. As Richard Sennett says, people subjected to this disempowering process, experience 'that peculiar lack of respect which consists of not being seen, not being accounted as full human beings' (Sennett 2003, pp. 12–13).

We hope to have demonstrated that there are many barriers to realizing this change in power relations; yet, there are also very important opportunities, such as with the Millennium Development Goals and the Commission on the Social Determinants of Health, where there is an increasing clamour for action to redress health inequities through empowering processes. It is notable that even the World Bank, often the subject of brutal criticism for exacerbating inequalities (Stiglitz 2003), has made significant moves toward recognizing the importance of reducing inequity in human development and has integrated an empowerment approach (World Bank 2006). It remains to be seen whether these gains can be translated into major policy changes and effective implementation; nevertheless, it is at this level where health promoters and all public health practitioners and researchers must have a strong advocacy position.

We hope that it is apparent that, in our interpretation, health promotion is much more than a set of technical public health interventions aimed at revamping traditional health education for the twenty-first century. We cannot let go of the core competencies built up by health education and other contributing fields, but we cannot be limited in our vision either. Health promotion has to face up to the fact that, while it may only be a junior partner in the global struggle to develop a more just and equitable world, when it comes to a key human capability and resource, *health*, it must take a lead role in making the argument for equity, develop and present the evidence for what *action* is necessary to achieve equity in health, and finally, to hold the powerful accountable where they fail to live up to the demands of justice for health. Embedded in health promotion is an imperative to act ethically and justly. In this case, unlike most, there is no choice.

Acknowledgements

Text extracts from Hartrick, G. et al. Family nursing assessment: meeting the challenge of health promotion, *Journal of Advanced Nursing*, Volume 20, Issue 1, pp. 85–91, Copyright © 1994, reproduced with permission from John Wiley & Sons, Inc.

Text extracts from World Health Organization, *Health Promotion Glossary* (WHO/HPR/HEP/98.1), WHO, Geneva, Switzerland, Copyright © 1998, reproduced with permission from the World Health Organization, http://www.who.int/healthpromotion/about/HPR%20Glossary%201998.pdf?ua=1.

References

Anand, S., Peter, F., and Sen, A. (eds.) (2004). *Public Health, Ethics, and Equity*. Oxford: Oxford University Press.

Aveneri, S. and de-Shalit, A. (eds.) (1992). *Communitarianism and Individualism*. Oxford: Oxford University Press.

Baum, F. (2007). Cracking the nut of health equity: top down and bottom up pressure for action on the social determinants of health. *Promotion & Education*, 14, 90–5.

Bhaskar, R. (2008). *A Realist Theory of Science*. New York: Routledge.

Carroll, S. (2012). Social theory and health promotion. In I. Rootman, S. Dupéré, A. Pederson, and M. O'Neill (eds.) *Health Promotion in Canada* (3rd ed.), pp. 33–52. Toronto: Canadian Scholar's Press.

Carroll, S., Hills, M., Miller, G., Geneau, R., Mitic, W., and Foster, L. (2013). *Intersectoral Action for Health: The Case of BC*. Presentation at the 21st IUHPE World Conference on Health Promotion, Pattaya, Thailand, 28 August.

Commission on the Social Determinants of Health (2008). *Closing the Gap in a Generation: Health Equity Through Action on the Social Determinants of Health*. Geneva: WHO. Available at: http://www.who.int/social_determinants/final_report/en.

Craig, G. (2005). *Community Capacity-Building: Definitions, Scope, Measurements and Critiques*. OECD Paper, Prague, Czech Republic, 8 December 2005.

Dupéré, S., Ridde, V., Carroll, S., et al. (2007). Conclusion: the rhizome and the tree. In M. O'Neill, A. Pederson, S. Dupéré, and I. Rootman (eds.) *Health Promotion in Canada*, pp. 371–88. Toronto: Canadian Scholar's Press.

Evans, R., Barer, M., and Marmor, T. (eds.) (1994). *Why are Some People Healthy and Others not?* New York: Aldine de Gruyter.

Evans, R. and Stoddart, G. (1990). Producing health, consuming health care. *Social Science & Medicine*, 31, 1347–63.

Fraser, D. (1973). *The Evolution of the British Welfare State*. London: Macmillan Press Ltd.

Freire, P. (1972). *Pedagogy of the Oppressed*. Harmondsworth: Penguin.

Godin, G. (2007). Has the individual vanished from Canadian health promotion? In M. O'Neill, A. Pederson, S. Dupéré, and I. Rootman (eds.) *Health Promotion in Canada*, pp. 367–70. Toronto: Canadian Scholar's Press.

Green, L. and Kreuter, M. (2005). *Health Promotion Planning: An Educational and Ecological Approach*. Toronto: McGraw-Hill Higher Education.

Green, L. and Raeburn, J. (1988). Health promotion. What is it? What will it become? *Health Promotion International*, 3, 151–9.

Greenhalgh, T., Robert, G., Macfarlane, F., Bate, P., Kyriakidou, O., and Peacock, P. (2005). Storylines of research in diffusion of innovation: a meta-narrative approach to systematic review. *Social Science & Medicine*, 61, 417–30.

Hamilton, N. and Bhatti, T. (1996). *Population Health Promotion: An Integrated Model of Population Health and Health Promotion*. Ottawa: Health Promotion Development Division, Public Health Agency of Canada. Available at: http://www.phac-aspc.gc.ca/ph-sp/phdd/php/php.htm.

Hartrick, G., Lindsey, A., and Hills, M. (1994). Family nursing assessment: meeting the challenge of health promotion. *Journal of Advanced Nursing*, 20, 85–91.

Hawe, P., Shiell, A., and Riley, T. (2009). Theorising interventions as events in systems. *American Journal of Community Psychology*, 43(3–4), 267–76.

Held, D., McGrew, A., Goldblatt, D., et al. (1999). *Global Transformations*. Cambridge: Polity Press.

Hills, M. (1998). Student experiences of nursing health promotion practice in hospital settings. *Nursing Inquiry*, 5, 164–73.

Hills, M. and Carroll, S. (2009). Health promotion, health education, and the public's health. In R. Detels, J. McEwen, R. Beaglehole, and H. Tanaka (eds.) *The Oxford Textbook of Public Health* (4th ed.), pp. 752–66. Oxford: Oxford University Press.

IUHPE (1999). *The Evidence of Health Promotion Effectiveness: Shaping Public Health in a New Europe*. Brussels: European Commission.

Jessop, R. (2002). *The Future of the Capitalist State*. Cambridge: Polity Press.

Kemm, J. (2006). Health impact assessment and Health in All Policies. In T. Ståhl, M. Wismar, E. Ollila, E. Lahtinen, and K. Leppo (eds.) *Health in all Policies: Prospects and Potentials*, pp. 189–208. Helsinki: Ministry of Social Affairs and Health.

Kickbusch, I. (1986). Health promotion: a global perspective. *Canadian Journal of Public Health*, 77, 321–6.

Kickbusch, I. (1989). Back to the future: moving public health into the 90's. In *Proceedings from National Symposium on Health Promotion*, pp. 1–5. Victoria: BC Ministry of Health.

Kickbusch, I. (1994). Introduction: tell me a story. In A. Pederson, M. O'Neill, and I. Rootman (eds.) *Health Promotion in Canada: Provincial, National & International Perspectives*, pp. 8–17. Toronto: W.B. Saunders Canada.

Kickbusch, I. (2007). Health promotion: not a tree but a rhizome. In M. O'Neill, A. Pederson, S. Dupéré, and I. Rootman (eds.) *Health Promotion in Canada*, pp. 363–6. Toronto: Canadian Scholar's Press.

Kickbusch, I. and Gleicher, D. (2012). *Governance for Health in the 21st Century*. Copenhagen: WHO.

Kok, G., Van Den Borne, B., and Dolan Mullen, P. (1997). Effectiveness of health education and health promotion: meta-analyses of effect studies and determinants of effectiveness. *Patient Education and Counseling*, 30, 19–27.

Kymlicka, W. (1990). *Contemporary Political Philosophy: An Introduction*. Oxford: Oxford University Press.

Labonté, R. (1993). Community development and partnerships. *Canadian Journal of Public Health*, 84, 237–40.

Labonté, R. (1994). Death of program, birth of metaphor: the development of health promotion in Canada. In A. Pederson, M. O'Neill, and I. Rootman (eds.) *Health Promotion in Canada: Provincial, National & International Perspectives*, pp. 72–90. Toronto: W.B. Saunders Canada.

Labonté, R. (1997). The population health/health promotion debate in Canada: the politics of explanation, economics and action. *Critical Public Health*, 7(1 and 2), 7–27.

Labonté, R. (2007). Promoting health in a globalized world: the biggest challenge of all? In M. O'Neill, A. Pederson, S. Dupéré, and I. Rootman (eds.) *Health Promotion in Canada*, pp. 207–22. Toronto: Canadian Scholar's Press.

Lalonde, M. (1974). *A New Perspective on the Health of Canadians*. Ottawa: Health and Welfare Canada.

Langille, D. (2003). The political determinants of health. In D. Raphael (ed.) *Social Determinants of Health: Canadian Perspectives*, pp. 283–96. Toronto: Canadian Scholar's Press.

Lawless, A., Williams, C., Hurley, C., Wildgoose, D., Sawford, A., and Kickbusch, I. (2012). Health in All Policies: evaluating the South Australian approach to intersectoral action for health. *Canadian Journal of Public Health*, 103(Suppl.1), S15–19.

MacDonald, J. (1992). *Primary Health Care: Medicine in its Place*. London: Earthscan Publications Ltd.

McKeown, T. (1976). *The Role of Medicine: Dream, Mirage or Nemesis.* London: Nuffield Provincial Hospitals Trust.

McQueen, D. (2001). Strengthening the evidence base for health promotion. *Health Promotion International*, 16, 261–8.

McQueen, D. (2007). Evidence and theory. In McQueen, D. and Jones, C. (eds.) (2007). *Global Perspectives on Health Promotion Effectiveness*, pp. 281–303. New York: Springer Publications.

McQueen, D. and Jones, C. (eds.) (2007). *Global Perspectives on Health Promotion Effectiveness.* New York: Springer Publications.

McQueen, D., Kickbusch, I., Potvin, L., et al. (2007). *Health and Modernity: The Role of Theory in Health Promotion.* New York: Springer Publications.

McQueen, D., Wismar, M., Lin, V., Jones, C., and Davies, M. (2012). *Intersectoral Governance for Health in All Policies: Structures, Actions and Experiences.* Copenhagen: WHO, European Observatory on Health Systems and Policies.

Minkler, M. (1990). Improving health through community organization. In K. Glanz, F. Lewis, and B. Rimer (eds.) *Health Behavior and Health Education*, pp. 257–85. San Francisco, CA: Jossey-Bass.

Navarro, V. (ed.) (2002). *The Political Economy of Social Inequalities: Consequences for Health and Quality of Life.* Amityville, NY: Baywood Press.

Navarro, V. and Shi, L. (2001). The political context of social inequalities and health. *Social Science & Medicine*, 52, 481–91.

Nussbaum, M. (2000). *Women and Human Development.* Cambridge: Cambridge University Press.

Nussbaum, M. (2006). *Frontiers of Justice: Disability, Nationality, Species Membership.* Cambridge, MA: Harvard University Press.

Nussbaum, M. and Sen, A. (eds.) (1993). *The Quality of Life.* Oxford: Clarendon Press.

Pawson, R., Greenhalgh, T., Harvey, G., and Walshe, K. (2005). Realist review—a new method of systematic review for complex policy interventions. *Journal of Health Services and Policy Research*, 10(Suppl 1), 21–34.

Poland, B., Coburn, D., Robertson, A., et al. (1998). Wealth, equity, and health care: a critique of a population health perspective on the determinants of health. *Social Science & Medicine*, 46, 785–98.

Raeburn, J. and Rootman, I. (1998). *People-Centred Health Promotion.* Chichester: John Wiley.

Raeburn, J. and Rootman, I. (2007). A new appraisal of the concept of health. In M. O'Neill, A. Pederson, S. Dupéré, and I. Rootman (eds.) *Health Promotion in Canada*, pp. 19–32. Toronto: Canadian Scholar's Press.

Raphael, D. (ed.) (2003). *Social Determinants of Health: Canadian Perspectives.* Toronto: Canadian Scholar's Press.

Raphael, D. and Bryant, T. (2002). Putting the population into population health. *Canadian Journal of Public Health*, 91, 9–12.

Rawls, J. (1971). *A Theory of Justice.* Cambridge, MA: Harvard University Press.

Rickles, D., Hawe, P., and Shiell, A. (2007). A simple guide to chaos and complexity. *Journal of Epidemiology and Community Health*, 61(11), 933–7.

Rootman, I., Goodstadt, M., Hyndman, B., McQueen, D., Potvin, L., and Springett, J. (2001). *Evaluation in Health Promotion: Principles and Perspectives.* Copenhagen: WHO.

Rootman, I. and Raeburn, J. (1994). The concept of health. In A. Pederson, M. O'Neill, and I. Rootman (eds.) *Health Promotion in Canada: Provincial, National & International Perspectives*, pp. 72–90. Toronto: W.B. Saunders Canada.

Scambler, G. (2012). Review article: health inequalities. *Sociology of Health & Illness*, 34(1), 130–46.

Sennett, R. (2003). *Respect: The Formation of Character in an Age of Inequality.* London: Penguin.

Shiell, A., Hawe, P., and Gold, L. (2008). Complex interventions or complex systems? Implications for health economic evaluation. *British Medical Journal*, 336(7656), 1281–3.

Ståhl, T., Wismar, M., and Ollila, E. (eds.) (2006). *Health in All Policies: Prospects and Potentials.* Helsinki: Ministry of Social Affairs and Health.

Stiglitz, J. (2003). *Globalization and its Discontents.* New York: W.W. Norton & Company.

Terris, M. (1992). Concepts of health promotion: dualities in public health theory. *Journal of Public Health Policy*, 13, 267–76.

Tones, K. (1993). Changing theory and practice: trends in methods, strategies and settings in health education. *Health Education*, 52, 125–39.

Tones, K. (2002). Health promotion, health education, and the public health. In R. Detels, J. McEwen, R. Beaglehole, and H. Tanaka (eds.) *The Oxford Textbook of Public Health* (4th ed.), pp. 865–76. Oxford: Oxford University Press.

Tones, K. and Green, L. (2004). *Health Promotion: Planning and Strategies.* London: Sage.

Tones, K. and Tilford, S. (1994). *Health Promotion: Effectiveness, Efficiency and Equity.* London: Chapman and Hall.

Trickett, E., Beehler, S., Deutsch, C., et al. (2011). Advancing the science of community level interventions. *American Journal of Public Health*, 101(8), 1411–19.

Turner, B. (ed.) (2000). *The Blackwell Companion to Social Theory.* Malden, MA: Blackwell Publishers.

Wallerstein, N. and Bernstein, E. (1988). Empowerment education: Freire's ideas adapted to health education. *Health Education Quarterly*, 15, 379–84.

Wallerstein, N. and Hammes, M. (1991). Problem posing: a teaching strategy for improving the decision-making process. *Health Education*, 22, 250–3.

White, K.L. (1991). *Healing the Schism: Epidemiology, Medicine, and the Public's Health.* New York: Springer-Verlag.

Wise, M. and Nutbeam, D. (2007). Enabling health systems transformation: what progress has been made in re-orienting health services? *Promotion & Education*, Suppl. 2, 23–7.

World Bank (2006). *World Bank Development Report 2006: Equity and Development.* Washington, DC: World Bank.

World Health Organization (1946). *Constitution.* Geneva: WHO.

World Health Organization (1978). *Declaration of Alma-Ata.* International Conference on Primary Health Care, Alma-Ata, USSR, 6–12 September 1978. Geneva: WHO.

World Health Organization (1984). *Health Promotion: A Discussion Document on the Concept and Principles.* Copenhagen: WHO, European Regional Office for Europe.

World Health Organization (1986). *Ottawa Charter for Health Promotion.* Ottawa: WHO.

World Health Organization (1988). *The Adelaide Recommendations on Healthy Public Policy.* Geneva: WHO.

World Health Organization (1998). *Health Promotion Glossary.* Geneva: WHO.

World Health Organization (2005). *The Bangkok Charter for Health Promotion in a Globalized World.* Geneva: WHO.

World Health Organization (2010). *The Adelaide Statement on Health in All Policies*, Geneva: WHO.

Zaza, S., Briss, P., and Harris, K. (2005). *Guide to Community Preventive Services: What Works to Promote Health?* New York: Oxford University Press.

Development and evaluation of complex multicomponent interventions in public health

Rona Campbell and Chris Bonell

Introduction to development and evaluation of complex multicomponent interventions

The need for a better evidence base in public health to support decision-making in policy and practice has been acknowledged by government, policy bodies, and researchers (UK Clinical Research Collaboration 2008; House of Commons Health Committee 2009; House of Lords Science and Technology Sub-Committee 2011; Katikireddi et al. 2011) and recent funding initiatives in the United Kingdom have been specifically designed to enhance the quality and quantity of research in public health and to support research capacity development (UK Clinical Research Collaboration 2013; National Institute for Health Research School for Public Health Research (n.d.). A number of consistent themes have emerged. First is a concern that when new public health initiatives are introduced little thought is given to evaluation. The result is that opportunities for baseline data collection, the identification of suitable control conditions, and the possibility of randomizing to intervention and control conditions are missed. A second is that new initiatives and policy interventions are introduced in too rushed a way with little time for development, piloting, fine tuning, and bedding in before they are replaced by something else. A third theme is the need for researchers and practitioners to work together more closely in order to integrate evaluations from the outset so that the evidence base of what works in public health is built and can inform decisions about policy, practice, and resource allocation at local, national, and international levels. In this chapter, we consider how these concerns can be addressed as we describe methods for developing and evaluating complex public health interventions. We begin by examining what complexity means in the context of public health.

Definition and scope of the concept of a 'complex intervention'

A complex intervention is generally held to comprise a number of synergistic interrelated components where effects cannot be attributed to a single 'active ingredient' (Medical Research Council 2000). Updated guidance provided by the UK's Medical Research Council (MRC) further suggests that complexity derives from: the number and difficulty of behaviours required by those delivering or receiving the intervention, the number of groups or organizational levels targeted by the intervention, the number and variability of outcomes, and the degree of flexibility or tailoring of the intervention permitted (Craig et al. 2008). By contrast, a simple intervention tends to be characterized as involving a straightforward pathway from the single component intervention, such as a drug treatment, to the intended outcome (Petticrew 2011). According to this distinction between simple and complex, many public health interventions and programmes are complex, although arguably vaccination programmes and some screening programmes (e.g. for phenylketonuria in the newborn) could be considered simple interventions. Recently, however, it has been suggested that the issue of complexity is not necessarily to do with the intervention but is about both the complexity of the settings (e.g. family, school, community, country) in which interventions are implemented and whether the research question being examined by evaluators of the intervention requires a simple (e.g. 'does this work?') or a complex answer (e.g. 'for whom does this work and under what circumstances?') (Petticrew 2011).

Complex interventions or complex settings, contexts, or systems

Interventions with a number of interrelated parts, it has been suggested, may be more helpfully thought of as complicated rather than complex. Complexity, so the argument runs, is a property of the system that an intervention is trying to change, not an inherent feature of the intervention itself (Shiell et al. 2008). Complex systems are said to be 'built up from very large numbers of mutually interacting subunits (that are often composites themselves) whose repeated interactions result in rich, collective behaviour that feeds back into the behaviour of the individual parts' (Rickles et al. 2007, p. 933). For example, Project Northland in the United States used schools as a setting for a health promotion intervention to discourage alcohol use by young people. It involved making changes to elements of the school curriculum, changing the school environment, and engagement with parents and the wider community to restrict both access to and demand for alcohol (Perry et al. 2002). The intervention is clearly a complicated one, but is also complex. Schools were not simply the context for the delivery of this intervention but comprised a complex system, involving a whole series of different types of subunits (e.g. students, teaching staff, classes, buildings), which the intervention aimed to transform. The schools were also part of a wider community, another complex system, on which the intervention was also intended to have an impact. The intention was that the action in both systems would be mutually reinforcing and produce a reduction in alcohol use.

When developing a public health intervention, it can be instructive to understand something of the nature of complex systems, and to think of an intervention as something that is intended to disrupt the system. Doing so can help ensure that the likely mechanisms for achieving change, the potential consequences of disrupting the system (both intentional and unintentional), and the interaction between the intervention and the context in which it is being implemented, are all carefully considered from the outset.

Standardized or flexible interventions?

When the UK MRC first published a framework for the development and evaluation of complex interventions (MRC 2000) it adapted the phases undertaken in drug development and testing and proposed a five-stage schema comprising: (1) 'pre-clinical' theoretical phase; (2) phase I—modelling: defining the components of the intervention; (3) phase II—exploratory trial: defining the trial and intervention design; (4) phase III—definitive randomized controlled trial (RCT); (5) phase IV—long-term implementation (Campbell et al. 2000). Phase II was specified as the stage at which the intervention could be adapted and changed but it was made clear that 'once the RCT has begun, the intervention must not evolve, as the RCT results will be unusable if later participants experience a different intervention than earlier ones. Fidelity to treatment protocols or quality standards may be essential to effectiveness. Monitoring will be essential to ensuring that individual styles and evolution in treatment do not render results from different groups of participants incomparable or excessively reduce the effectiveness of the intervention' (MRC 2000, p. 11). This emphasis on testing a standardized intervention, implemented with a high degree of fidelity, caused some concern because, it was thought, some public health interventions might be maximally effective if they actively encouraged appropriate tailoring to local circumstances. Such a view led some to conclude that randomized trials were therefore not a suitable method for evaluating public health and health promotion interventions (McNulty et al. 2014). As Hawe and colleagues (Hawe et al. 2004) pointed out, however, this concern was based on a misconception of what is standardized. She argued that what should be standardized is the function of the intervention and the steps in the process by which change is to be achieved, not that all the components of an intervention have to be delivered in exactly the same way to each person, or in each setting. Hawe and colleagues did not reject the randomized trial as a method of evaluation but argued that 'instead of mimicking trial phases which assume that the "best" or the "ideal" comes from the laboratory and gets progressively compromised in real world applications, community trial design would start by trying to understand communities themselves as complex systems and how the health problem or phenomena of interest is recurrently produced by that system' (Hawe et al. 2004, p. 1562). However, it is an empirical question rather than a matter of principle whether standardized or adapted interventions are more effective, and one which will depend on the intervention. This matter is discussed in further detail in the later subsection on fidelity.

Simple or complex research questions

As already mentioned, evaluations can address simple or complex questions (Petticrew 2011). For example, you might wish to evaluate the effectiveness of a multicomponent programme to reduce childhood obesity in a local authority area which includes: a health promotion intervention for pregnant women to encourage breastfeeding and healthy weaning; work with nursery schools, child minders, and day care providers to ensure provision of healthy food and sufficient opportunity for physical activity; a classroom-based intervention for primary schools aimed at teaching children about good nutrition and being physically active which also involves parents; and a health promotion intervention via large, local spectator sports clubs to encourage fathers to be physically active with their children and to eat healthily. As the commissioner of the programme, you may simply wish to know whether or not it has been effective in reducing the percentage of children who are obese or overweight and that the investment was worthwhile. Or you may wish to know: for which subpopulations of children and in what settings it was effective or ineffective; whether there were important secondary outcomes such as a reduction in obesity in adults or an improvement in educational attainment in the children; whether there were intervention synergies or feedback loops which made it more effective than it might otherwise have been; or whether there were externalities (changes outside the system but of interest) such as a reduction in the number of fast food outlets in the locality due to a drop in demand, or tipping points where, for example, increased pressure from parents and local community groups to provide better outdoor play facilities for children resulted in the local authority upgrading play parks resulting in them being more heavily used by families.

Intervening at different levels to improve the health of populations

The importance of multilevel and multifaceted interventions was set out in both the 1986 *Ottawa Charter for Health Promotion* (Rickles et al. 2007) and the later *Bangkok Charter* (Anonymous 2006) so that interventions aim both to address individual, 'downstream' determinants of health such as knowledge and attitudes, as well as community and societal 'upstream' determinants, such as access to health benefiting and health harming goods and services and social inequalities in wealth and power. When designing complex public health interventions, the socioecological approach to public health described by McLeroy and colleagues (Kenneth et al. 1988) but with its origins in the work of Bronfenbrenner (1974) on ecological systems theory, can provide a useful framework for thinking about the different levels of intervention. This socioecological framework was designed to focus attention on both social and environmental factors as targets for health promotion. It identifies five complementary levels of change, targets and approaches which are set out in Table 6.5.1.

Historical evidence suggests that the greatest improvements in public health have been achieved through non-medical interventions, such as improved sanitation, welfare benefits,

Table 6.5.1 Socioecological framework

Level of change	Target	Approach
Intrapersonal	Individuals	Changing individuals by changing their knowledge, attitudes, values, motives, skills and behaviour
Interpersonal	Small groups such as the family, work colleagues, friendship groups	Achieving change through formal and informal social networks and peer groups by changing group norms or the group culture
Institutional	Organizational settings such as schools, colleges, and workplaces	Achieving change via organizational policies and rules, and by creating healthier organizational cultures and environments
Communities as mediating structures, relationships amongst organizations and as geographical entities with political power	Neighbourhoods, community organizations	Achieving change through collective action by working with community organizations that are sources of social capital, coordination and coalition building between organizations, and increasing the representation of disadvantaged population groups on community decision-making bodies
Public policy	Whole populations at local, regional, national, and international level	Achieving structural change through the development and implementation of health promoting local-, regional-, country-, and international-level policy and legislation

Adapted with permission from McLeroy, K.R. et al., An Ecological Perspective on Health Promotion Programs, *Health Education Quarterly*, Volume 15, Issue, pp. 351–77, Copyright © 1988 by Society for Public Health Education, DOI: 10.1177/109019818801500401.

and improved workplace safety (McKeown 1976). Current evidence also indicates that multifaceted and multilevel interventions are more effective than those operating at a single level (Greaves et al. 2011), and that environmental level interventions are more likely to be cost-effective than individually targeted clinical or non-clinical prevention interventions (Chokshi and Farley 2012). Recent reviews of the use of socioecological models in health promotion since the late 1980s have, however, suggested that published evaluations still tend to focus on one or two levels of intervention (Richard et al. 2011; Golden and Earp 2012), although there has been a notable increase, particularly in the last few years, in interventions with multiple and more 'upstream' targets, such as the community or political environment (Richard et al. 2011).

Health inequalities

Public health has the dual goals of improving population health and reducing health inequalities. One approach is to target interventions at disadvantaged groups or those at high risk of morbidity or mortality. This can be problematic, both because it can sometimes be stigmatizing and even harmful, but also because even if effective in reducing these groups' risk it may be insufficient in bring about substantial population-level reductions in risk because, as Geoffrey Rose pointed out (Rose 1981), where disease risks follow a bell-shaped curve (as is the case with almost all non-communicable disease), the majority of cases of a disease will arise from those at low or medium risk (because there are simply more of them). However, universalist approaches which do not address the 'upstream' determinants of disease and only address individual behaviour may have the potential for widening inequalities because of the 'inverse prevention law' (Gordon et al. 1999) whereby socioeconomically advantaged groups are able to benefit disproportionately from universal interventions. Progressive universalism has been advocated, for example, by the *Marmot Review*, as a way of avoiding these difficulties by ensuring that action on health inequalities both addresses 'the causes of the causes' but also by ensuring that the scale and intensity of

more downstream interventions are proportionate to the level of disadvantage (Marmot 2010).

These matters must be examined empirically within evaluations. A recent evaluation of the free swimming initiative for children, introduced in England as part of an intended legacy of the 2012 Olympic Games, is a good example of an evaluation examining whether the inverse prevention law was operating. The findings indicated that uptake was not socioeconomically stratified but was higher among girls and older children. The authors concluded that by ending the initiative after two years, an opportunity had been lost to promote physical activity across the social gradient (Audrey et al. 2012).

When developing public health interventions, it is therefore important to consider their potential for narrowing or widening health inequalities, and to ensure that evaluations formally test whether factors such as socioeconomic status, gender, or ethnicity moderate (statistically interact with) intervention effects. The PROGRESS acronym (Evans and Brown 2003) indicates disadvantage may be related to place of residence, race/ethnicity, occupation, gender, religion, education, socioeconomic status, and social capital and is a helpful prompt to thinking about which factors are relevant to the population for which the intervention is being designed.

Stages in the development of complex interventions

Review of existing quantitative and qualitative evidence

The first practical step in developing a complex intervention, whether designing something new or modifying an existing approach, is to review the available evidence. If there are already relevant systematic reviews, then it may only be necessary to read these or update them. But if not, you may need to conduct your own review (see Chapter 5.15 for further information about systematic reviews). While quantitative systematic reviews will tell you what is known about the effectiveness of a particular intervention, it is also useful to review relevant qualitative research which may provide important knowledge about the likely acceptability of your proposed intervention and identify potential barriers and facilitators to implementation. It will also be useful to learn about risk and protective factors, both 'downstream' and 'upstream' for the outcome of interest, again preferably drawing on systematic reviews, to consider if existing interventions are comprehensive in addressing these.

Involving policy and practice partners from the outset

Consulting or collaborating with key stakeholders at this early stage will also provide useful insights into exactly what is seen to be required from the policy and practice perspective. Involving stakeholders from the outset is also more likely to result in its successful translation from research into routine practice if the subsequent evaluation of the intervention shows it to be effective and cost-effective (see Chapter 6.1 for details of social science research methods including interviews and focus groups).

Public involvement from the outset

Similarly, working directly with those whose health it is hoped will be improved by the planned intervention is also vital in ensuring that it is relevant and acceptable. In the health and social care sectors, pre-existing groups represent particular patient and client groups, which can be engaged as partners in research. In public health, identifying representative groups, particularly for universalist interventions, may be more challenging. There is, however, guidance available on how to approach this and examples of good practice. INVOLVE is part of the National Institute for Health Research in the United Kingdom and its role is to encourage and support increased public involvement in health research (INVOLVE 2012) and its website provides ample guidance for researchers (http://www.invo.org.uk) and the public. Involvement in public health research can and should include specific population groups such as children and young people (Bird et al. 2013) and there are specialist groups being set up who can provide such input. The ALPHA group (Advice Leading to Public Health Advancement) is one such example. This specially trained group of young people meets monthly to provide input into research undertaken by the DECIPHer public health research centre and other research organizations (DECIPHer n.d.).

Importance of theory

Pawson and Tilley (1997) suggest that all interventions are in essence 'theories incarnate' because they assume that a certain intervention will involve a particular causal process leading to particular outcomes. In the absence of proper theory, the assumptions made by intervention planners, providers, or evaluators remain implicit. Recent guidance on developing complex interventions advocates using explicit theories of change to inform their design (Campbell et al. 2007; Craig et al. 2008; Glanz and Bishop 2010). While interventions formulated without recourse to theory can and do work, there is increasing evidence that they are more likely to be effective when informed by theory (Noar et al. 2008; Glanz and Bishop 2010). The ASSIST peer-led smoking prevention intervention is an example of a successful theory-based smoking prevention intervention (Campbell et al. 2008). Students aged 12–13, identified by class mates at secondary school as being influential, are trained to have conversations with their peers about the benefits of not smoking (Audrey et al. 2004). The intervention was informed by diffusion of innovations theory (Rogers 1983) with the peer supporter's role being to diffuse new attitudes and new norms of behaviour relating to smoking throughout the year group. A cluster RCT conducted in south Wales and south-west England showed a 22 per cent overall reduction in the odds of being a smoker in intervention compared with control schools. The research also included an evaluation of the process of delivering ASSIST to facilitate understanding what factors make the programme successful. This process evaluation found that ASSIST was implemented with a high degree of fidelity and was acceptable to schools and school teachers (Audrey et al. 2008; Holliday et al. 2009), and to the young people who received it. More detailed follow-on research on the peer supporters found that those who are asked to work informally, rather than under the supervision of teaching staff, engaged more effectively with the task they have been asked to undertake and more effectively diffused the health-promotions messages, in this case smoking prevention (Noar et al. 2008).

Reviews of which theories have been utilized most frequently in relation to public health interventions show that the field is dominated by psychological theories (Glanz and Bishop 2010; Davis et al. 2014). However, as we have already indicated, effective public health intervention is likely to require action at more than just the level of the individual and the National Institute for Health and Care Excellence's 2007 guidance on behaviour change concluded interventions would be more effective if they did so (National Institute for Health and Care Excellence 2007). Public health intervention research may therefore need to draw on theories from a variety of disciplines. There are useful resources available which provide compendia of theories but the range of theories included in each reflects the disciplines involved or the contexts examined (Glanz and Rimmer 1997; Conner and Sparks 2005; Nutbeam et al. 2010).

Development of intervention logic models

An understanding of intervention theory, that is, how an intervention is intended to produce its effect, is critical to planning a process evaluation. Logic models are diagrammatic representations of the logical relationships, for example, between an intervention's inputs, activities, outputs, and outcomes, although there is scope for flexibility regarding the precise categories used (Cooksy et al. 2001; Kellogg Foundation 2004). Intervention theory and logic models are useful tools in clarifying how an intervention is to be delivered and to what ends, and thereby provide a focus for evaluating process (and outcomes). Fig. 6.5.1 provides an example of a recent logic model. It is for the INCLUSIVE intervention which was designed to reduce bullying and aggression in secondary schools (Bonell et al. 2013). The intervention's theory of change is informed by Markham and Aveyard's theory of human functioning and school organization (Markham and Aveyard 2003). Its tenets inform a diagrammatic logic model consisting of inputs, processes, institutional changes, intermediate impacts, and health outcomes. Inputs include training staff in 'restorative practice' (RP) as an approach to preventing and managing student aggression and misbehaviour, as well as an external facilitator who

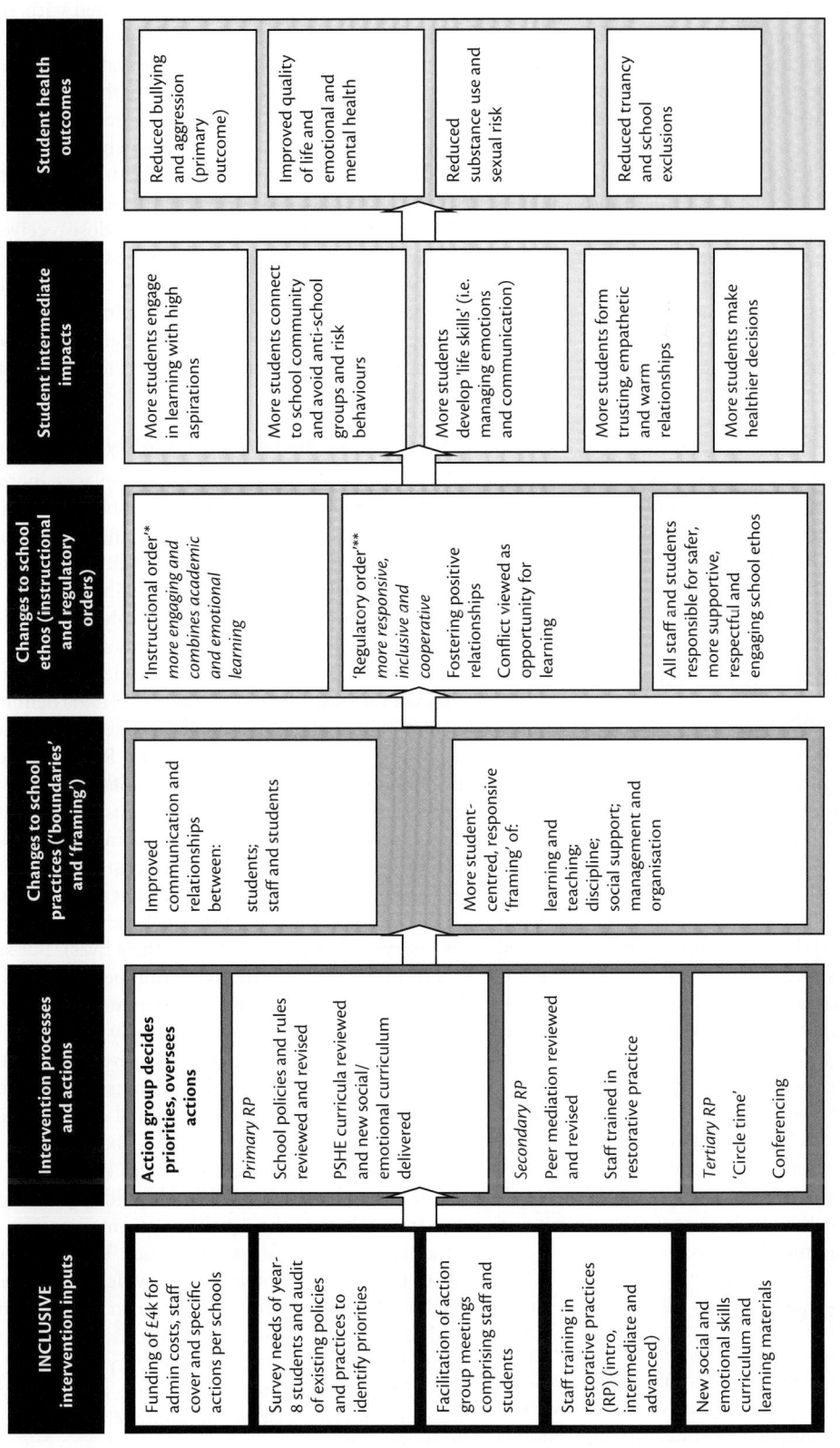

Fig. 6.5.1 Logic model for the INCLUSIVE intervention to reduce bullying and aggression in secondary schools.

* i.e. learning and teaching in school ** i.e. discipline, social support and sense of community in school

Reproduced with permission from Bonell, C. et al., A pilot randomized controlled trial of the INCLUSIVE intervention for initiating change locally in bullying and aggression through the school environment: final report, *BMC Public Health*, Copyright © 2013 BioMed Central.

would convene meetings of students and staff to review data on student needs in order to plan and deliver school-specific actions. These inputs are intended to enable processes, such as improved personal, social, and health education (PSHE) and the use of RP in schools, as well as the review and revision of school policies and rules by staff and students working collaboratively. In turn these processes are intended to modify various 'boundaries' within the school, such as the quality of staff–student relationships, and how schooling is framed, for example, to render decision-making more student-centred. These processes are ultimately theorized as transforming the ethos of the school so that more students are committed to the school's instructional order (teaching) and the regulatory order (discipline and school sense of community) and are thus less likely to become committed to anti-school peer groups and behaviours such as bullying and substance use.

Using theory effectively in the design of interventions although highly recommended is an area where good guidance is still somewhat lacking. How to identify relevant theories from the many disciplines that relate to public health, how to use them to develop a logic model specifying the mechanisms by which change is to be achieved, and then how to translate this model into a practical public health intervention is a challenge and one for which few exemplars of good practice exist. We hope though that this is a challenge that researchers and practitioners will rise to and that there is a consequent increase in the development of effective complex public health interventions.

Evaluation of complex interventions

Piloting and feasibility studies

Before embarking on a definitive RCT or some other evaluation of the effects of an intervention, it is wise to undertake a pilot or feasibility study. These terms have tended to be used interchangeably (Arain et al. 2010) but the National Institute for Health Research Evaluation, Trials and Studies Coordinating Centre (NETSCC) has proposed a helpful distinction (NETSCC 2014). A pilot study is in effect a miniature version of the main trial and is designed to test that both the intervention and the evaluation can be implemented as intended. If the pilot is successful and no changes are made then data from it can be incorporated into the main trial (this is termed an internal pilot as opposed to an external one where data cannot be incorporated into the main trial). In contrast, feasibility studies are intended to indicate whether or not a definitive trial is feasible and to examine important areas of uncertainty such as the willingness of participants to be randomized, response rates to questionnaires collecting outcome data, or the standard deviation of the primary outcome measure required for the sample size calculation. Such studies can have a much more flexible format and need not necessarily be randomized.

Process evaluation methods

Process evaluation is as important as outcome evaluation. Process evaluation can provide valuable insight not only within feasibility and pilot studies, but also within definitive RCTs as well as in studies examining implementation of scaled-up interventions after effectiveness trials have been completed. Process evaluations can examine how interventions are planned, delivered, and received (Bonell et al. 2006; Oakley et al. 2006).

There is no single, agreed definition of process evaluation. The UK MRC states that process evaluations 'can be used to assess fidelity and quality of implementation, clarify causal mechanisms and identify contextual factors associated with variation in outcomes' (Craig et al. 2008); more specific guidance is currently being drafted. Other priority areas have been identified. One of the most widely cited frameworks is that of Steckler and Linnan (2002) which identified priority areas for process evaluation, including: fidelity (the extent to which the intervention is delivered as intended), reach (whether an intervention is received by all those it targeted), dose delivered (the amount or number of units of intervention offered to participants, dose received (the extent of participants' active engagement in the scheme), and context (local factors which impact implementation). Thus, process evaluation can explore whether those whom an intervention targets actively engage with it, an important consideration for social interventions. The following subsections consider some of these priority areas in more depth.

Intervention delivery and fidelity

The importance of process evaluation was increasingly recognized during the 1980s, spurred by publication of a paper on 'type 3 error', defined as concluding that an intervention is ineffective when a lack of effect actually reflects it is not being implemented as intended (Basch et al. 1985). Initially, the main aim of process evaluations was therefore to assess intervention fidelity, in order to determine whether outcomes evaluation could represent valid assessment of an intervention's underlying theory. Fidelity is defined variously. Moncher and Prinz (1991) define fidelity as confirmation that manipulation of the independent variable occurred as planned. Within the context of a RCT or other comparative evaluation, this requires assessment of the integrity of both delivery within the intervention arm and its differentiation from what occurred in the control arm. Later definitions of fidelity, for example, by Lichstein and colleagues (Lichstein et al. 1994), saw this as also encompassing receipt (participant uptake of the intervention) and enactment (the extent to which participants apply the lessons of interventions into practice in their lives). But such definitions begin to blur the useful distinction between fidelity and factors such as dose, acceptability and even outcomes, so most researchers continue to define fidelity narrowly in terms of delivery.

Assessments of fidelity generally involve quantitative measurement, for example, using observations, video-recording, or provider self-assessments to audit actual delivery against what was intended to occur. However, fidelity should not be viewed only in terms of ticking boxes on simple checklists. Steckler and Linnan (2002) argue that when evaluating fidelity, it is also important to assess whether the 'spirit' of an intervention is delivered in practice, and not just its mechanics. For example, when evaluating motivational interviewing, which is counselling aimed at enabling clients to recognize their own motivations for behaviour and to modify behaviour where this is not in line with their own goals, it is important to evaluate fidelity not merely as a cook-book list of techniques, but also whether the underlying empathic, patient-centred spirit of the approach is achieved (Miller and Rollnick 2009).

Another important consideration when evaluating fidelity is the degree to which interventions should be standardized. Advocates of strict fidelity (Mihalic 2004) argue that this is essential if effective interventions are to be replicated, especially when an intervention's 'active ingredient' may not be known. They present evidence which suggests that high fidelity is associated with greater impact for some interventions (Mihalic 2004). Advocates of local adaptation (Dane and Schneider 1998) argue that interventions need to be tailored to local circumstances. Durlak and DuPre (2008) propose a compromise whereby an intervention's 'core components' should be delivered in standard form but less central intervention components or features can be modified to fit local needs. They present research which suggests that a balance between fidelity and adaptation is likely to be most effective, with the precise balance dependent on the specific intervention. As noted earlier in this chapter, Hawe and colleagues go further to argue that with complex interventions characterized by synergistic interactions between multiple components, too much attention has been paid to standardizing the *form* of intervention components (what precise actions are delivered) and more attention should be given to standardizing the *function* of intervention components (what the aim of each component is and how it contributes to the overall aim of the intervention) (Hawe et al. 2004). Consider the case of the INCLUSIVE intervention described earlier. Fidelity of form might be measured by determining whether the training in RP was delivered as planned and whether the facilitator convened a sufficient number of staff–student meetings. In contrast, fidelity of function might be measured by determining whether teachers were equipped to deliver RP and whether staff and students felt involved in the process of reviewing school policies.

Intervention reach, dose, and acceptability

Steckler and Linnan conceive of evaluating intervention reach and dose, and participants' responses to an intervention largely in quantitative terms (Steckler and Linnan 2002). Reach and dose are commonly examined quantitatively using methods such as questionnaire surveys exploring participants' exposure to and satisfaction with an intervention. However, receipt can also be seen in qualitative terms as exploring participants' reports of an intervention in their own terms. Qualitative research can be useful in examining how participants perceive an intervention in unexpected ways which may not be fully captured by researcher-developed quantitative constructs. Qualitative research can also explore how providers or participants exert 'agency' (willed action) in engaging with the intervention rather than merely receiving it passively (Oakley et al. 2006). For example, process evaluation of a youth work intervention to reduce teenage pregnancy in England reported how some youth workers and teachers responded to onerous recruitment and retention targets by transforming the intervention from one delivered out of school hours to one delivered as a partial alternative to normal school time, which may have explained its ineffectiveness (Wiggins et al. 2006).

Context

Context is a critical aspect of process evaluation. Although there is no consistent definition, context can be taken to mean anything that was in place before the intervention itself was implemented. This could include factors such as the needs of participants, the infrastructure within which interventions will be delivered, the skills and attitudes of providers, and the attitudes and cultural norms of potential participants. In Steckler and Linnan's (2002) framework, context is largely considered in terms of factors which

may help or hinder implementation. For example, an intervention may be delivered poorly in some areas, but well in others, because of better provider capacity or more receptive community norms in some areas. Others consider context also in terms of how it influences outcomes. For example, 'realist' evaluators place great emphasis on whether interventions work more effectively in some contexts than others and how this might be explained by interactions between contextual factors and the mechanism of action of the intervention. Context can be measured quantitatively in order to inform 'moderator' analyses but this occurs rarely and inconsistently between studies (Bonell et al. 2012). Qualitative research allows for a different understanding of the importance of context, for example, examining how intervention providers or recipients describe the interaction between their context and their own agency in explaining their actions (Oakley et al. 2006).

Intervention mechanism of action

Assessing an intervention's mechanisms of effects involves assessing whether the validity of the theory of change does indeed explain its operation. Such analysis can explain why an intervention is found to be effective or ineffective within an outcome evaluation. This might be critically important in refining an intervention found to be ineffective or in understanding the potential generalizability of interventions found to be effective. Quantitative data can be used to undertake mediator analyses to assess whether intervention outputs or intermediate outcomes appear to explain intervention effects on health outcomes (Gardner et al. 2006). Qualitative data can be used to examine such pathways and this is particularly useful when the pathways in question have not been comprehensively examined using quantitative data, as well as when pathways are too complex (e.g. using multiple steps or feedback loops) to be assessed adequately using quantitative analyses. This was, for example, the case with an assessment of possible causal pathways underlying an intervention to modify school environments in order to reduce student substance use, which appeared to involve feedback loops whereby student participation within certain intervention activities increased student commitment to the intervention which in turn increased student participation within other components (Bonell et al. 2010).

However, such analyses can be challenging. First, as suggested earlier, quantitative analyses require evaluators to have correctly anticipated what data is needed to examine causal pathways and to have collected these. For example, the evaluation of the youth work intervention aiming to prevent teenage pregnancy reported a higher rate of pregnancies among those receiving the intervention. It was hypothesized that this apparent adverse outcome resulted from the intervention bringing together young people engaged in risk behaviours so that pro-risk social norms were amplified. However, data on these were not collected so that this hypothesis could not be tested (Wiggins et al. 2008). A second challenge involves using qualitative alongside quantitative data to understand causal pathways. If qualitative data are analysed in order to explain quantitative findings, this may bias interpretation (Wight 2002). Furthermore, quantitative and qualitative methods originate from different research paradigms. Qualitative research is inductive and generalizations are made from particular circumstances making the external validity of the findings somewhat uncertain. As Munro and Bloor (2010) put it: 'process evaluations do indeed enrich our understanding of the social processes involved in the delivery and receipt of complex interventions', they provide 'interpretations to which a degree of indeterminacy is always attached that cannot be expressed in probabilistic terms. . . The continuing tension between positivist and interpretive paradigms within that research design pose problems of understanding and reporting. Not so much "paradigm peace" as "paradigm truce"'.

While we advocate process evaluation as an important evaluative tool it should not be seen as a panacea for answering all the questions an outcome evaluation cannot, nor is its use unproblematic. The range of possible domains it can focus on (delivery, fidelity, reach, dose, acceptability, context, sustainability) is wide, and resources may not be available to collect the data required to examine them all. Some may be a greater priority than others depending on the nature of the intervention and its stage of development. For example, the acceptability of an intervention is something that should predominantly be explored in a pilot or feasibility study rather than leaving it till the definitive trial, where understanding mechanism of effects may be a more pressing matter for a process evaluation to examine.

Implementation issues

Sustainability

The implementability and sustainability of new public health interventions beyond the scale required for a robust evaluation of effectiveness, to a scale capable of population impact is an important consideration. For example, it may be that a group of health promotion specialists, substance misuse experts and youth workers have been specially assembled to deliver a new intervention in secondary schools to reduce substance and alcohol misuse. This intervention is shown in a cluster RCT to be effective. The issue then becomes how can that delivery model be replicated and sustained outside of the trial so that effectiveness is maintained. The 'RE-AIM' framework (reach, effectiveness, adoption, implementation, maintenance) is useful in conceptualizing this (Glasgow et al. 1999). Its originators argue that those commissioning public health services need to know not only that an intervention is effective but that it is capable of being adopted by provider agencies and implemented by them as planned, and will reach sufficient people to achieve a population health impact that can be maintained over time (Glasgow et al. 2001).

From research into practice

The impact of research on policy and practice is increasingly recognized to occur through a gradual and indirect process of enlightenment rather than via direct effects of single studies or even reviews on single decisions (Weiss 1986; Graham et al. 2006). However, while empirically accurate this is normatively disappointing for those advocating a more direct role for evidence in informing policy (Davies et al. 2000). Now there is recognition that to be influential, research needs to engage reciprocally with policy and practice. Earlier in this chapter we highlighted the need to consult key policy and practice stakeholders and the public early in the development and evaluation of complex public health interventions. This approach is now being extended by some into a process whereby evidence is co-produced through a knowledge exchange partnership between researchers, policymakers, and practitioners using transdisciplinary action research

(Daker-White et al. 2013). This method involves academics from a variety of relevant disciplines working with policymakers and practitioners to identify what research is required, develop research questions, conduct evaluations, synthesize evidence, and implement and maintain evidence-based public health practice. The advantage of this approach is that if evaluations indicate that changes to practice are producing the desired outcomes then the capacity building necessary to sustain that whole system change is built into the approach. There are a number of examples of promising interventions (de Silva-Sanigorski et al. 2010; Chittleborough et al. 2013), including the INCLUSIVE intervention in England (Bonell et al. 2013) and the Gatehouse project in Australia, where this approach has been taken (Bond et al. 2001, 2004).

Discussion and future direction

Public health interventions can comprise policy-level initiatives implemented at a national or international level, for example the World Health Organization's Healthy Cities programme (World Health Organizations n.d.), through to brief individual behaviour change interventions to encourage reduced alcohol consumption delivered in primary care populations (Kaner et al. 2007). Interventions may be programmatic in nature with many different components such as the Northland project in secondary schools to reduce alcohol consumption, or it may be very simple, as in the example of human papilloma virus vaccination which involves three injections over a 12-month period to reduce substantially the chances of a woman having cervical cancer. Given this huge variability there is no 'one-size-fits-all' approach to their development and evaluation. What we have identified in this chapter are the key issues to be considered and the range of methods available to tackle them.

We conceive of the development and evaluation of complex public health interventions as distinct elements but ideally part of an overall symbiotic and cyclical process rather than sequential phases. Knowledge exchange partnerships between researchers and public health practitioners and policymakers are a potential way of achieving this ideal, but their effectiveness has yet to be the subject of systematic evaluation.

References

Anonymous (2006). The Bangkok Charter for Health Promotion in a Globalized World. *Health Promotion International*, 1, 10–14.

Arain, M., Campbell, M.J., Cooper, C.L., and Lancaster, G.A. (2010). What is a pilot or feasibility study? A review of current practice and editorial policy. *BMC Medical Research Methodology*, 10, 67.

Audrey, S., Cordall, K., Moore, L., Cohen, D., and Campbell, R. (2004). The development and implementation of a peer-led intervention to prevent smoking among secondary school students using their established social networks. *Health Education Journal*, 63, 266–84.

Audrey, S., Holliday, J., and Campbell, R. (2008). Commitment and compatibility: teachers' perspectives on the implementation of an effective school-based, peer-led smoking intervention. *Health Education Journal*, 67, 74–90.

Audrey, S., Wheeler, B.W., Mills, J., and Ben-Shlomo, Y. (2012). Health promotion and the social gradient: the free swimming initiative for children and young people in Bristol. *Public Health*, 126, 976–81.

Basch, C.E., Sliepcevich, E.M., Gold, R.S., Duncan, D.F., and Kolbe, L.J. (1985). Avoiding type III errors in health education program evaluations: a case study. *Health Education & Behavior*, 12, 315–31.

Bird, D., Culley, L., and Lakhanpaul, M. (2013). Why collaborate with children in health research: an analysis of the risks and benefits of collaboration with children. *Archives of Disease in Childhood – Education and Practice*, 98, 42–8.

Bond, L., Glover, S., Godfrey, C., Butler, H., and Patton, G.C. (2001). Building capacity for system-level change in schools: lessons from the Gatehouse Project. *Health Education & Behavior*, 28, 368–83.

Bond, L., Patton, G., Glover, S., et al. (2004). The Gatehouse Project: can a multilevel school intervention affect emotional wellbeing and health risk behaviours? *Journal of Epidemiology and Community Health*, 58, 997–1003.

Bonell, C., Fletcher, A., Fitzgerald-Yau, N., et al. (in press). A pilot randomized controlled trial of the INCLUSIVE intervention for initiating change locally in bullying and aggression through the school environment: final report.

Bonell, C., Fletcher, A., Morton, M., and Lorenc T. (2012). 'Realist Randomised Controlled Trials': a new approach to evaluating complex public health interventions. *Social Science and Medicine*, 75(12), 2299–306.

Bonell, C.P., Sorhaindo, A.M., Allen, E.E., et al. (2010). Pilot multimethod trial of a school-ethos intervention to reduce substance use: building hypotheses about upstream pathways to prevention. *Journal of Adolescent Health*, 47, 555–63.

Bronfenbrenner, U. (1974). Development research, public policy and the ecology of childhood. *Child Development*, 45, 1–5.

Campbell, M., Fitzpatrick, R., Haines, A., et al. (2000). Framework for design and evaluation of complex interventions to improve health. *British Medical Journal*, 321, 694–6.

Campbell, N.C., Murray, E., Darbyshire, J., et al. (2007). Designing and evaluating complex interventions to improve health care. *British Medical Journal*, 334, 455–9.

Campbell, R., Starkey, F., Holliday, J., et al. (2008). An informal school-based peer-led intervention for smoking prevention in adolescence (ASSIST): a cluster randomised trial. *The Lancet*, 371, 1595–602.

Chittleborough, C.R., Nicholson, A.L., Young, E., Bell, S., and Campbell, R. (2013). Implementation of an educational intervention to improve hand washing in primary schools: process evaluation within a randomised controlled trial. *BMC Public Health*, 13, 757.

Chokshi, D.A. and Farley, T.A. (2012). The cost-effectiveness of environmental approaches to disease prevention. *The New England Journal of Medicine*, 367, 295–7.

Conner, M. and Sparks, P. (eds.) (2005). *Predicting Health Behaviour: Research and Practice with Social Cognition Models*. Buckingham: Open University Press.

Cooksy, L.J., Gill, P., and Kelly, A. (2001). The program logic model as an integrative framework for a multimethod evaluation. *Evaluation and Program Planning*, 24, 119–28.

Craig, P., Dieppe, P., MacIntyre, S., Michie, S., Nazareth, I., and Petticrew, M. (2008). Developing and evaluating complex interventions: the new Medical Research Council guidance. *British Medical Journal*, 337, a1655.

Daker-White, G., Donovan, J., and Campbell, R. (2013). Redefined by illness: meta-ethnography of qualitative studies on the experience of rheumatoid arthritis. *Disability and Rehabilitation*, September 3. [Epub ahead of print.]

Dane, A.V. and Schneider, B.H. (1998). Program integrity in primary and early secondary prevention: are implementation effects out of control? *Clinical Psychology Review*, 18, 23–45.

Davies, H.T.O., Nutley, S.M., and Smith, P.C. (2000). Learning from the past, prospects for the future. In H.T.O. Davies, S.M. Nutley, and P.C. Smith (eds.) *What Works? Evidence-based Policy and Practice in Public Services*, pp. 351–66. Bristol: Policy Press.

Davis, R., Campbell, R., Hildon, Z., Hobbs, L., and Michie, S. (2014). Theories of behaviour and behaviour change across the social and behavioural sciences: a scoping review. *Health Psychology Review*, DOI :10.1080/17437199.2014.941722.

DECIPHer (n.d.). *ALPHA – Advice Leading to Public Health Advancement* [Online]. Available at: http://decipher.uk.net/en/content/cms/about-decipher/public-involvement/alpha%20researchers/.

de Silva-Sanigorski, A., Prosser, L., Carpenter, L., et al. (2010). Evaluation of the childhood obesity prevention program Kids—'Go for your life'. *BMC Public Health*, 10, 288.

Durlak, J.A. and Dupre, E.P. (2008). Implementation matters: a review of research on the influence of implementation on program outcomes and the factors affecting implementation. *American Journal of Community Psychology*, 41, 327–50.

Evans, T. and Brown, H. (2003). Road traffic crashes: operationalizing equity in the context of health sector reform. *International Journal of Injury Control and Safety Promotion*, 10, 11–12.

Gardner, F., Burton, J., and Klimes, I. (2006). Randomised controlled trial of a parenting intervention in the voluntary sector for reducing child conduct problems: outcomes and mechanisms of change. *Journal of Child Psychology and Psychiatry*, 47, 1123–32.

Glanz, K. and Bishop, D.B. (2010). The role of behavioral science theory in development and implementation of public health interventions. *Annual Review of Public Health*, 31, 399–418.

Glanz, K. and Rimmer, B.K. (1997). *Theory at a Glance: A Guide for Health Promotion Practice*. Bethesda, MD: National Cancer Institute.

Glasgow, R.E., McKay, H.G., Piette, J.D., and Reynolds, K.D. (2001). The RE-AIM framework for evaluating interventions: what can it tell us about approaches to chronic illness management? *Patient Education and Counseling*, 44, 119–27.

Glasgow R.E., Vogt, T.M., and Boles, S.M. (1999). Evaluating the public health impact of health promotion interventions: the RE-AIM. *American Journal of Public Health*, 89, 1322–7.

Golden, S.D. and Earp, J.A.L. (2012). Social ecological approaches to individuals and their contexts: twenty years of Health Education & Behavior health promotion interventions. *Health Education & Behavior*, 39, 364–72.

Gordon, D., Shaw, M., Dorling, D., Davey-Smith, G., and Townsend, P. (1999). *Inequalities in Health: The Evidence Presented to the Independent Inquiry into Inequalities in Health, Chaired by Sir Donald Acheson*. Bristol: Policy Press.

Graham, I.D., Logan, J., Harrison, M.B., et al. (2006). Lost in knowledge translation: time for a map? *Journal of Continuing Education in the Health Professions*, 26, 13–24.

Greaves, C., Sheppard, K., Abraham, C., et al. (2011). Systematic review of reviews of intervention components associated with increased effectiveness in dietary and physical activity interventions. *BMC Public Health*, 11, 119.

Hawe, P., Shiell, A., and Riley, T. (2004). Complex interventions: how 'out of control' can a randomised controlled trial be? *British Medical Journal*, 328, 1561–3.

Holliday, J., Audrey, S., Moore, L., Parry-Langdon, N., and Campbell, R. (2009). High fidelity? How should we consider variations in the delivery of school-based health promotion interventions? *Health Education Journal*, 68, 44–62.

House of Commons Health Committee (2009). *Health Inequalities HC286-1. Third Report of Session 2008–09*. London: The Stationery Office.

House of Lords Science and Technology Sub-Committee (2011). *Health Behaviour Change*. London: Stationery Office.

INVOLVE (2012). *Briefing Notes for Researchers: Involving the Public in NHS, Public Health and Social Care Research*. Eastleigh: INVOLVE.

Kaner, E.F., Beyer, F., Dickinson, H.O., et al. (2007). Effectiveness of brief alcohol interventions in primary care populations. *Cochrane Database of Systematic Reviews*, 18, CD004148.

Katikireddi, S.V., Higgins, M., Bond, L., Bonell, C., and MacIntyre, S. (2011). How evidence based is English public health policy? *British Medical Journal*, 343, d7310.

Kellogg Foundation, W.K. (2004). *Logic Model Development Guide*. Battle Creek, MI: W.K. Kellogg Foundation.

Lichstein, K.L., Riedel, B.W., and Grieve, R. (1994). Fair tests of clinical trials: a treatment implementation model. *Advances in Behaviour Research and Therapy*, 16, 1–29.

Markham, W.A. and Aveyard, P. (2003). A new theory of health promoting schools based on human functioning, school organisation and pedagogic practice. *Social Science & Medicine*, 56, 1209–20.

Marmot, M. (2010). *Fair Society, Healthy Lives: The Marmot Review: Strategic Review of Health Inequalities in England Post-2010*. London: University College London.

McKeown, T. (1976). *The Role of Medicine: Dream, Mirage, or Nemesis?* London: Nuffield Provincial Hospitals Trust.

McLeroy, K.R., Bibeau, D., Steckler, A., and Glanz, K. (1988). An ecological perspective on health promotion programs. *Health Education Quarterly*, 15, 351–77.

McNulty, C.A.M., Hogan, A.H., Ricketts, E.J., et al. (2014). Increasing chlamydia screening tests in general practice: a modified Zelen prospective cluster randomised controlled trial evaluating a complex intervention based on the theory of planned behaviour. *Sexually Transmitted Infections*, 90(3), 188–94.

Medical Research Council (2000). *A Framework for Development and Evaluation of RCTs for Complex Interventions to Improve Health*. London: MRC.

Mihalic, S. (2004). The importance of implementation fidelity. *Emotional & Behavioral Disorders in Youth*, 4, 83–105.

Miller, W.R. and Rollnick, S. (2009). Ten things that motivational interviewing is not. *Behavioural and Cognitive Psychotherapy*, 37, 129–40.

Moncher, F.J. and Prinz, R.J. (1991). Treatment fidelity in outcome studies. *Clinical Psychology Review*, 11, 247–66.

Munro, A. and Bloor, M. (2010). Process evaluation: the new miracle ingredient in public health research? *Qualitative Research*, 10, 699–713.

National Institute for Health and Care Excellence (2007). *Behaviour Change: The Principles for Effective Interventions (PH6)*. London: NICE. Available at: http://www.nice.org.uk/PH6.

National Institute for Health Research Evaluation, Trials and Studies Coordinating Centre (2014). *Glossary*. [Online]. Available at: http://www.netscc.ac.uk/glossary/.

National Institute for Health Research School for Public Health Research (n.d.). *Research Themes*. [Online]. Available at: http://sphr.nihr.ac.uk/research.

Noar, S.M., Chabot, M., and Zimmerman, R.S. (2008). Applying health behavior theory to multiple behavior change: considerations and approaches. *Preventive Medicine*, 46, 275–80.

Nutbeam, D., Harris, E., and Wise, M. (2010). *Theory in a Nutshell: A Guide to Health Promotion Theory*. Sydney: McGraw Hill.

Oakley, A., Strange, V., Bonell, C., Allen, E., and Stephenson, J. (2006). Process evaluation in randomised controlled trials of complex interventions. *British Medical Journal*, 332, 413–16.

Pawson, R. and Tilley, N. (1997). *Realistic Evaluation*. London: Sage.

Perry, C.L., Williams, C.L., Komro, K.A., et al. (2002). Project Northland: long-term outcomes of community action to reduce adolescent alcohol use. *Health Education Research*, 17, 117–32.

Petticrew, M. (2011). When are complex interventions 'complex'? When are simple interventions 'simple'? *The European Journal of Public Health*, 21, 397–8.

Richard, L., Gauvin, L., and Raine, K. (2011). Ecological models revisited: their uses and evolution in health promotion over two decades. *Annual Review of Public Health*, 32, 307–26.

Rickles, D., Hawe, P., and Shiell, A. (2007). A simple guide to chaos and complexity. *Journal of Epidemiology and Community Health*, 61, 933–7.

Rogers, E. (1983). *Diffusion of Innovations*. New York: The Free Press.

Rose, G. (1981). Strategy of prevention: lessons from cardiovascular disease. *British Medical Journal*, 282, 1847–51.

Shiell, A., Hawe, P., and Gold, L. (2008). Complex interventions or complex systems? Implications for health economic evaluation. *British Medical Journal*, 336, 1281–3.

Steckler, A. and Linnan, L. (2002). *Process Evaluation for Public Health Interventions and Research*, San Francisco, CA: Jossey-Bass.

UK Clinical Research Collaboration (2008). *Strengthening Public Health Research in the UK. Report of the UK Clinical Research Collaboration Public Health Research Strategic Planning Group*. London: UK Clinical Research Collaboration.

UK Clinical Research Collaboration (2013). *Public Health Research* [Online]. Available at: http://www.ukcrc.org/research-coordination/joint-funding-initiatives/public-health-research/.

Weiss, C.H. (1986). The circuitary of enlightenment: diffusion of social science research to policy-makers. *Knowledge: Creation, Diffusion, Utilization*, 8, 274–81.

Wiggins, M., Bonell, C., Burchett, H., et al. (2008). *Young People's Development Programme Final Report*. London: Institute of Education.

Wiggins, M., Sawtell, M., Austerberry, H., Burchett, H., Strange, V., and Bonell, C. (2006). *Evaluation of the Young People's Development Programme Second Interim Report*. London: Social Institute of Education.

Wight, D. and Obasi, A. (2002). Unpacking the black box: the importance of process data to explain outcomes. In J. Stephenson, J. Imrie, and C. Bonell (eds.) *Effective Sexual Health Interventions: Issues in Experimental Evaluation*, pp. 151–66. Oxford: Oxford University Press.

World Health Organization (n.d.). *Types of Healthy Settings: Healthy Cities* [Online]. Available at: http://www.who.int/healthy_settings/types/cities/en/index.html.

Economic appraisal in public healthcare: assessing efficiency and equity

David Parkin, Stephen Morris, and Nancy Devlin

What is economic appraisal?

Planning healthcare services to meet the health needs of a population always has to recognize a constraint on its aims, which is the finite availability of resources with which to meet them. There are many choices that must be made, for example, which public health and healthcare services are to be provided, in what ways, and to whom. Economic appraisal (EA) is a systematic way of analysing the consequences of such choices. It is one element of Health Technology Assessment (HTA), the uses of which include pharmaceutical and other healthcare pricing and reimbursement decisions, planning of the location of healthcare facilities, and priority setting. EA is not the only element of HTA, but it is an important one.

Similarly, the discipline of economics is not the only contributor to EA. It also requires other public health relevant disciplines such as epidemiology, statistics, and operational research. Economics contributes the rationale for EA, an overall framework for analysis, and some measurement principles and methods.

The term 'economic appraisal' describes a set of techniques that weigh up the costs of an action, such as providing a particular type of healthcare to a segment of a population such as a group of patients, against the benefits that it may provide. The term 'economic evaluation' is also used. The distinction between the two terms is that appraisal is undertaken before the action is taken, to help in deciding whether or not and how the action is to be done, and evaluation is undertaken after the action, to judge its effects. This distinction is often forgotten and these terms are used interchangeably in much of health economics. The expression 'evaluation' is now most commonly used in the health economics literature, but appraisal is used here because that more accurately describes the main purpose for which economic analysis in healthcare is applied in practice. The usual label given to this activity in economics is cost–benefit analysis (CBA). However, that term is often reserved in health EA for a particular technique, which is explained later in this chapter.

The principles of EA can be applied to all kinds of health interventions, from intervention at the level of the individual patient to population-based programmes, all of which may be of interest to public health practitioners. This chapter therefore does not restrict itself to activities conventionally labelled as public health,

and it also includes interventions that are not usually thought of as healthcare, such as health promotion. It does highlight the special issues that EA generally faces in evaluating public health activities, and finishes with a specific examination of those issues.

The economics of economic appraisal

EA should not be confused with financial appraisal. A financial appraisal is concerned with the monetary implications of a proposed action, such as investment in a healthcare facility or the provision to a population of one or more interventions. It examines cash expenditures and available funding to ensure that the actions taken are viable and provide a reasonable return. These cash flows are measured using accounting principles. EA shares some of the methods and principles of financial appraisal, but its aim is a more general assessment of costs and benefits and has some measurement principles derived from economic concepts. The most important of these are *opportunity cost, social cost, marginal cost, efficiency,* and *equity.*

In practice, these theoretical principles are hard and occasionally impossible to adhere to, but they provide a guide as to what are the best sources of cost and benefit data and to the reliability of the numbers actually used.

Opportunity cost

As with any good or service, production of healthcare requires resources such as personnel (often referred to as labour), equipment and buildings (often referred to as capital), land, and raw materials. There is a finite amount of such resources available to be converted into goods and services at any particular time, so it is not possible to produce everything that everyone in a population might want. In this sense, resources are scarce relative to the demands for them. In the economy as a whole, there are not enough scarce resources to meet all of the wants that people have, so we have to choose which wants are met and which are not met. Similarly, in the healthcare system there are not enough healthcare resources to meet all of the health needs that people have, so we have to choose which needs are met and which are not met. Of course, it might be argued that if we cannot meet all health needs, resources should be diverted from other parts of the economy, and it is legitimate for public health practitioners to advocate that. But it would not be possible to do that indefinitely and at some point the opportunity cost would be in terms of health, not just education, welfare, and other goods and services in the public and private sectors of the economy.

Economics suggests that scarcity and the resulting necessity to choose are ubiquitous and unavoidable. This observation leads directly to an important and fundamental economics concept, which is *opportunity cost*. If scarce resources are used to produce a good or service, those resources cannot be used to produce other goods or services. Opportunity cost derives from the benefits that are forgone by not producing those other goods. Because there are many possible uses for resources, the opportunity cost of using resources in a particular way is defined as the benefits that would have resulted from their best alternative use.

When economists refer to costs, they usually mean opportunity costs. This is quite different to the more familiar concept of financial costs, the costs of goods and services and of scarce resources in terms of money. Very often, financial costs are used to measure opportunity costs, but this is not always the case. Opportunity cost and financial costs are different ways of thinking about costs, rather than separate elements of overall costs; it would make no sense to calculate them separately and add them together, for example.

Measuring opportunity costs is often difficult in practice. It is preserved in good EA practice by the separation of costing services into measuring the quantity of resources required to provide that service and calculating the value of those resources, by, for example, examining the prices of each type of resource. This is also good practice for ensuring that research can be generalized to other settings where quantities and prices may differ. For example, different countries may have very different ways of providing services, with different combinations of different kinds of personnel, facilities, and locations, as well as differing relative costs of those resources.

Social costs and benefits

A financial appraisal of a proposed action takes into account only costs that are incurred by the person or organization taking the action and benefits to the person or those who are the organizations' clients. These are referred to as *private* costs and benefits. However, in some kinds of EA it is in principle essential to take account of all costs and benefits to society, whatever they are and whoever incurs them. In particular, it is essential to take account of *social* costs and benefits in a CBA that examines the impact on the economy as a whole. For example, the total costs of a medical intervention would include not only costs incurred within the health sector, but also those incurred in subsequent personal care and support, whether by organizations or private carers. However, it is arguable that such wider costs should not be included in a cost-effectiveness analysis (CEA), in which the aim is to maximize healthcare outcomes within a limited budget.

A special example of the difficulties involved in this is *transfer payments*, for example, social security payments and other state benefits paid out of taxation. Except for the costs involved in administering them, these are not costs to society as a whole. Rather, they are transfers between different members of society, since the recipients derive benefits from them that match the costs

to taxpayers. However, from the state's point of view such expenditure may be regarded as a use of tax revenues which has an opportunity cost in terms of other government expenditure.

Again, this principle is almost impossible to follow perfectly because of information limitations. However, it is preserved in good practice in health EA by examining costs and benefits according to who bears them, in three categories: the health service, patients and their families, and the rest of society. It is also embodied in the recommendation that any analysis should make clear the perspective from which the analysis is conducted, for example, society, the government, or the health sector.

Marginal costs and benefits

The total cost of any activity is likely to depend on how much of it is carried out, for example, the total cost of a vaccination scheme will depend on the number of people to be vaccinated. In estimating these total costs, an obvious solution is to multiply *average* costs per unit of activity, which are the accounting data most usually made available, by the number of units. However, in some circumstances that may mislead, and what are required are *marginal* costs. Again, the same is true for benefits.

The definition of a marginal change is that it is a change in an economic variable, such as the measure of benefit or cost that is caused by the smallest possible change in another variable. For example, the marginal cost of a good is most widely defined as the extra cost incurred in producing one more unit of it. Note that marginal does not mean small or unimportant; instead it means at the margins of an existing state of affairs, for example, the cost or benefit that will be incurred or gained by changing the allocation of resources slightly. That cost could actually be rather large, even though the change in the amount of the good is small. As an extreme example, suppose that the good is a particular screening programme and the screening centre processing the test material has reached full capacity. Screening an extra person could only be carried out if a new screening centre was built, so its marginal cost would be very high. By contrast, the marginal cost of the last test performed within the existing capacity may have been quite small, simply the cost of performing the test. This demonstrates another important point. Marginal cost may vary considerably with respect to the same size of change in the other variable, depending on the level of that other variable, in this case the number of people screened.

An example of the importance of looking at marginal costs is the impact of schemes designed to lower hospital inpatient surgical costs by reducing length of stay through earlier discharge. Hospitals may have information on the average cost of an inpatient stay, which can be used to calculate an average cost per day. However, the costs of an inpatient day are not constant. In particular, they may be much smaller than the average towards the end of the stay, because the average includes a share of the costs of treatment and perhaps of high dependency care that took place towards the beginning of an inpatient stay. So, reducing the number of low dependency days at the end of the stay will save far fewer resources than would be expected by examining the average. Marginal costs calculated with respect to an increase or decrease in the number of days would give a correct estimate of the likely savings.

Similarly, it will be important to examine marginal benefit, for example, as the extra benefit gained by the consumption of one more unit of a good. An example of the importance of looking at marginal rather than average benefits is a screening programme that can be carried out with different numbers of sequential tests. The more tests, the more cases are detected. A programme that used two tests might yield 11 cases per 1000 people tested, which could look reasonable. But suppose that a one-test programme would discover ten cases. If instead of analysing these as a one-test screen and a two-test screen, the two-test programme is analysed as one test followed by another, the marginal benefit is only one case, which does not look so good.

To give a real example, Torgerson and Spencer (1996) illustrated the importance of marginal analysis by analysing data on the cost-effectiveness of biochemical screening for Down's syndrome as a replacement for screening by maternal age. An estimate had been published that introducing biochemical screening in a population of 20,000 pregnant women would cost £413,501 and might prevent 11 affected births, giving a cost-effectiveness ratio of £37,591 per affected fetus identified. Torgerson and Spencer pointed out that for the same number of women, existing antenatal screening procedures based on maternal age and additional tests already cost £79,500 with four births potentially prevented. So, the true cost-effectiveness of biochemical screening was (£413 500 − £79 000)/(11 − 4) = £334,500/7 = £47,786, a much higher cost per affected fetus identified than for the estimate based on average cost.

Efficiency and equity

Economic analysis is usually employed to judge the way in which scarce resources are employed according to two main criteria: efficiency and equity. These two concepts have technical definitions, which will be described in the following subsections, but in very broad terms efficiency refers to obtaining the greatest output for a given set of resources and equity refers to a fair distribution of that output amongst the population. The term 'output' is very general and in our context we usually mean the additional amount of healthcare or health produced.

Efficiency

It is necessary to give a warning about definitions of efficiency. Economists, as specialists in the analysis of efficiency, largely agree about what it means and how different types of efficiency may be defined, but the labels they give to those types vary. The same concept may be given different names and the same name given to different concepts. Here we use the labels and definitions given in Morris et al. (2012).

Knapp (1984) gave a very broad definition of efficiency as 'the allocation of scarce resources that maximizes the achievement of aims'. This is a useful start, because it suggests the very benign nature of the desire to achieve efficiency. If we have scarce resources and competing uses for them, our aim will be to obtain the best set of uses, with 'best' defined in whatever way we want. If we decide that the aim of the health system is to improve the health of the population and we have a fixed healthcare budget, we will obtain the biggest health gain if the allocation of scarce healthcare resources is efficient.

For practical purposes, we require more precise and technical definitions of efficiency. However, it is useful first to understand a slightly abstract idea, called Pareto efficiency (named after the nineteenth-century economist Vilfredo Pareto who introduced the concept), which is also (though not consistently) called allocative efficiency. This arises from an attempt to create a widely acceptable criterion for judging different allocations of resources to different ends. The suggestion is that we would be able to say that one allocation is better than another if at least one person is better off under the first allocation and no one is worse off. This is called the Pareto criterion. If we change from one allocation of resources to another, for example, if it were possible to make changes to the healthcare system in terms of the kind of care that is made available, and this means that some people benefit and no one is made worse off, then this is described as a Pareto improvement. If it is not possible to make any such changes, then we have achieved a Pareto optimum. Another way to view the Pareto optimum is that it is a position where it is not possible to make anyone better off without making someone else worse off.

If our aim is to make people as well off as possible and we are not concerned about whether some people are better off than others, then a Pareto optimum is efficient. We cannot further improve the achievement of our aim because even if we can make someone, or even many people, better off, we do not know if this is outweighed by those who are made worse off. Of course, there are many allocations of resources that would be Pareto optimal, some of which would imply great inequalities between different people. If our aims also took account of the undesirability of inequalities, then we might not view all Pareto optimums as efficient. Nevertheless, ideas of efficiency in economics do derive from this concept of Pareto efficiency. Here, we define three types: technical, economic, and social.

Technical efficiency is a concept that is used in considering how health and healthcare, which we may call 'output', are produced from scarce resources, or 'inputs'. Technically efficient production is achieved if we are producing most output from a set of inputs, or producing a set amount of output using the fewest inputs. For example, the number of people that can be vaccinated against influenza in a general practice clinic depends on the number of nursing staff that are available and other inputs. If the most that can be provided by three practice nurses is 100 vaccinations each day, then it is technically inefficient to provide 99 vaccinations with that number of nurses or to provide 100 vaccinations with more nurses.

Another way of viewing technical efficiency, which is consistent with Pareto efficiency, is that the practice cannot vaccinate more people without employing at least one more nurse. More generally, production is technically efficient for a given set of inputs if it is only possible to produce more by employing more of at least one input.

In practice, EA does not directly address technical efficiency, though as will be explained it is an essential underlying assumption in most cases.

Economic efficiency has a number of different labels, including cost-effectiveness, though that term should be used carefully, as will be explained below. Technical efficiency is defined with respect to the physical numbers of inputs, but economic efficiency is interested in the cost of those inputs. Economic efficiency is achieved if we are producing most output for a given cost, or producing a set amount of output at the lowest possible cost. Using the earlier example, suppose that people could be vaccinated by different grades of nurses, but at least one senior nurse must be part of the team. It might be equally technically efficient for 100 people to be vaccinated each day by employing one senior and two junior nurses, one junior and two senior nurses, or three senior nurses. But senior nurses are more expensive to employ than junior nurses, so it will be economically efficient to use the first of these staff mixes. This demonstrates that although achieving technical efficiency is necessary to achieve economic efficiency, not all technically efficient ways of producing are economically efficient.

Another way of viewing economic efficiency, which is consistent with Pareto efficiency, is that given the costs of employing nursing staff, the practice cannot undertake more treatments without them costing more to provide. More generally, production is economically efficient for a given set of input prices if it is only possible to produce more by incurring greater costs.

In practice, economic efficiency is the dominant type of efficiency analysed in EA. However, there are different ways in which this is done, as will be explained below.

Social efficiency is a much broader concept than technical and economic efficiency. If there is economic efficiency in production in every part of the economy, there is *allocative efficiency in production* for the economy as a whole. There is an equivalent concept relating to the consumption of goods and services called *allocative efficiency in consumption* where, given prices of goods and services, consumers maximize the benefit that they derive from those goods and services. If *both* of these are achieved, then there is allocative efficiency in the economy as a whole, which is also known as social efficiency. This is the same as the Pareto efficiency described earlier.

Obviously, social efficiency according to this strict definition is not a concept likely to be of practical use in health economics. However, it is important because it underlies CBA, whose aim in theory is to move the economy closer to social efficiency.

Equity

Equity is an important criterion for allocation of resources, and it is particularly important in health systems because it is observable that people attach more importance to fairness in health and healthcare than to the distribution of many other goods and services. Almost every healthcare system in the world has equity as an important policy objective. However, economic analysis of equity is less clear than that of efficiency, except for how equity might be measured, and there is less agreement amongst economists about it.

Equity means fairness, and in the context of healthcare this means fairness in the distribution of health and healthcare between people and in the burden of financing healthcare. It is not a synonym for equality, which means an equal distribution. It may not always be fair to be equal, for example, it might be thought to be unfair if both healthy and sick people are given the same amount of healthcare. But equality is often used to define equity, as, for example, in the principles of *horizontal equity*—the equal treatment of equals—and *vertical equity*—the unequal treatment of unequals. An example often used in healthcare is the proposal that there should be equal access to healthcare for people with the same level of healthcare needs.

However, that is not the only possible definition of healthcare equity, and more generally there is no single definition of what equity is. Moreover, ideas about equity are not mainly founded on economics principles, rather on philosophy, ethics, law, and other forms of enquiry. An example is the equity principle of procedural justice, which in this context might mean that the process used to decide on the allocation of healthcare resources between people should be fair. This is an important principle in deciding how HTA is applied, but it is not especially based in economics. Culyer and Bombard (2012) have suggested that one way to incorporate the plurality of approaches to equity in HTA is to use a 'checklist' to ensure that decision-makers take all aspects into account.

It is necessary to consider what it is that we wish to be equitable about. Three areas in which equity may be considered are the finance of healthcare, the distribution of healthcare, and the distribution of health.

Analysis of equity in the finance of healthcare mainly concentrates on vertical equity, with a particular emphasis on whether or not healthcare is financed according to people's ability to pay. Horizontal equity in financing considers whether or not people, who have the same income, and therefore the same ability to pay for healthcare, make the same payments.

Horizontal equity in the distribution of healthcare mainly examines whether or not people with the same need for healthcare make the same use of healthcare services. Vertical equity in the distribution of healthcare is usually interpreted to mean whether individuals with different levels of ill health have different levels of use that are appropriate to that difference.

Equity in the distribution of health is almost always expressed in terms of inequalities in health. Health inequalities, particularly those that demonstrate that health levels vary systematically and inversely with socioeconomic status, are always of some importance in health policy debates and a major concern of some governments, depending on their political preferences. It may be argued that this is in fact the only real equity concern, since a concern for equity in healthcare derives solely from a concern about the distribution of health.

Formulating an economic appraisal

One way to look at how an appraisal is carried out is to consider it as a process with stages, as follows:

1. Defining the problem to be analysed. The problem is always the starting point of an appraisal. This may seem obvious, but in fact it is often solutions that are, wrongly, regarded as the starting point. From an appraisal point of view, the problem is not whether a fluoridation programme is cost-effective, but what is the most cost-effective way to deal with the problem of dental caries.

2. Specifying the alternatives, which include different ways of dealing with the problem defined in the first stage. It is important to select the most relevant alternative whatever it is, for example, promotion of tooth-friendly nutrition amongst children, or doing nothing.

3. Assessing costs and benefits which has three elements:

   ◆ *Enumeration* of costs and benefits, which means the drawing up of a descriptive list of the costs and benefits that are to be included in the appraisal.

   ◆ *Measurement*, which means obtaining data to describe the levels of costs and benefits for the different alternatives.

   ◆ *Valuation*, which is required to convert the data into values. For example, data on resource use should be converted into costs by applying to those data the value of the resources.

4. Calculating results means combining the data on costs and benefits into the results that will be presented. The exact nature of this will depend on the type of appraisal that is carried out and how uncertainty over the results is dealt with.

5. Making a decision. The endpoint is when a decision is taken on the basis of the appraisal. This will not be taken by an appraiser, but by someone who has the responsibility to make a decision. However, appraisers often do recommend a decision which is based on their own appraisal, or imply such a recommendation. This is legitimate if the relevant decision rules are known. For example, there might be an accepted decision rule that states that if the benefits of a health intervention exceed its cost then it should be provided to the population. A finding, for a particular intervention, that its benefits did exceed its costs may then lead to a recommendation that it should be provided.

One important factor in this is that an appraisal should be formulated and carried out with full awareness of which viewpoint is being taken. This arises because different actors in the health system—patients, health professionals, and government, for example—may have different interests and concerns, so that what is efficient from one point of view may not be from another. This is important because it determines which type of appraisal is to be used, what constitutes a benefit and a cost and how these are to be valued. Most appraisals will take the viewpoint of the health service, since that embodies most of those who have the legitimacy to decide which healthcare is to be provided. However, they may also take the viewpoint of society as a whole, since that defines the recipients of healthcare as well as the ultimate funders of it. Whatever viewpoint is adopted, researchers should be explicit about which it is. In EAs of public health interventions, a broader perspective is frequently taken, to account for costs and benefits that occur outside the health system.

Types of economic appraisal

Although there are several different types of EA, we will concentrate here on those most likely to be encountered in healthcare and other public health activities. Unfortunately, there are different ways in which these types can be classified. This leads to occasional disputes about how results of a particular type of appraisal should be interpreted or used. One way is to classify them according to what kind of efficiency they analyse. A second way is to classify them according to which costs and benefits are measured and how this is done. A third way is to classify them according to the type of decision that they apply to. Although we will discuss all three types here, the most widespread and popular classification in health economics is given by Drummond et al. (2005), which uses both the measurement and decision type principles.

In what follows, we refer to what is being appraised as alternatives, reflecting the use of EA in healthcare in decision-making about alternative ways of using healthcare resources. This includes many kinds of decisions, including different ways of delivering healthcare, different types of healthcare and different treatment options.

Cost–benefit analysis

In economics more generally, CBA starts with an inventory of all of the costs and benefits of each of the alternatives, whatever they are and whoever incurs them. This can be regarded as a balance sheet in which costs and benefits are weighed up against each other.

However, in healthcare appraisals CBA is usually defined, following Drummond et al. (2005), as a technique in which all costs and benefits are measured in terms of money. The rationale for this is that it is only possible to weigh up all of the costs and benefits if they are measured in the same unit. Although in principle any common unit could be used, in practice money is the obvious and natural choice, as it is the measure of value most used in modern economies. The result of such a CBA would be to establish which of the alternatives has the greatest net benefit, the difference between benefits and costs, which could of course be negative.

The main decision rule for CBA is that an activity should be undertaken if the sum of the benefits is greater than the sum of the costs or, identically, if the net benefit is positive. If only one activity with a positive net benefit can be undertaken (because, for example, there are limited funds), then the rule is to choose the activity with the highest net benefit.

CBA is based on economics theory, because if all of the costs and benefits are measured in the correct way—for example, all costs measure their true opportunity costs—and an alternative has a net benefit, it will lead to a Pareto improvement. The way that this has been interpreted by Drummond et al. (2005) is that CBA is therefore appropriate for answering questions about whether or not a healthcare programme should be implemented or a treatment should be used, rather than which of a number of alternative programmes or interventions is the most efficient.

Because CBA requires benefits to be measured in financial or monetary terms and to cover a very wide range of costs and benefits, it is rarely used. An example in public health is Wang et al. (2005), who estimated a limited range of costs and benefits of using bike and pedestrian trails to reduce healthcare costs arising from inactivity. They calculated that the annual cost per person of using the trails was US$209.28 and the resulting reduction in medical costs was $564.41. This gives a net benefit of $355.13 per person.

Investment appraisal

Investment appraisal in the context of healthcare can be explained using the example of a specific technique called by the United Kingdom's finance ministry (the Treasury) *option appraisal*. This is described in the guidance that it gives to public bodies about how they should appraise and evaluate projects that are to be paid for from public funds; the distinction between appraisal and evaluation is carefully kept to in this case. It is a process in which different options for meeting an objective, defined by the aim of meeting some public need, are generated; CBA is applied to these options; and the best solution for meeting the aims is chosen on the basis of the results. For example, an appraisal of a project for setting up a new national programme for measuring obesity among schoolchildren would not start as a comparison of the new programme with the existing circumstances. It would start with the need to understand the extent of obesity among schoolchildren, generate different options for dealing with that need, which might include a new measurement programme, examine the costs and benefits of each alternative, and from this derive the economic case for the new programme, if it was found to be the best alternative. The economic case for the project would simply be part of a more general project appraisal including affordability and achievability and various types of impact assessment including on health, the environmental and health and safety.

Cost–consequences analysis

Cost–consequences analysis (CCA) is a form of CBA which does not try to put all of the costs and benefits into the same units. In particular, it accepts that there are different types of benefits that cannot be measured in the same units. This distinguishes it from CEA, which is discussed in the following subsection. The assumption is that in making decisions based on a CCA, different decision-makers will place their own weights on the different benefits and on costs, implicitly if not explicitly. CCA is of particular interest in public health because it is argued that it is more suitable for population health issues involving a wide range of agencies and of differing and incommensurable outcome indictors. For example, the National Institute for Health and Care Excellence (NICE) in England permits CCA to be used for public health interventions, unlike other healthcare. CCA is often referred to as a disaggregated approach, because the benefits and costs are not combined into a single indicator such as net benefit or a cost-effectiveness ratio, which are defined below.

Cost-effectiveness analysis

Cost-effectiveness derives from the analysis of economic efficiency, where one alternative is preferred to another if it provides greater benefit at the same or lower cost, or lower cost for the same or greater benefit. This definition leaves open the question of which of two alternatives is more efficient if one provides greater benefit than the other, but at a lower cost. However, under certain conditions, for example, that the alternatives can be reduced or increased in size to produce any level of total cost or benefit, such comparisons can be made. A cost-effectiveness ratio (CER), defined as costs divided by benefits, can be calculated in order to do this. The CER most often used in health economics is called an incremental CER, or ICER, where the costs and benefits of each alternative are calculated compared with their next best alternative, rather than with a common alternative.

The measurement principle for CEA is that costs are measured in terms of money, but that benefits are measured in units other than money. However, unlike CCA, all of the benefits are measured in the same units, usually because only one type of benefit is considered. The obvious consequence of this is that costs and benefits are not weighed against each other. The ICER simply shows the cost of obtaining a unit of benefit. Whether that cost is worth incurring is a different question. So, unlike CBA, which tells us whether or not health programmes or treatment are an efficient use of resources, CEA tells us which of the possible ways of providing those is the most efficient.

Drummond et al. (2005) restrict the use of the term CEA in two ways. First, they regard CEA as being applicable only when both the costs and benefits differ between alternatives. The case where benefits are the same but costs differ is called *cost-minimization analysis* (CMA). In practice, this term is rarely used to describe analyses that have been carried out, although such analyses may well be quite widespread. Secondly, they restrict the measurement of benefits to be in what they call *natural units*, such as numbers of cases detected, changes in clinical measures like blood pressure or changes in undesirable biological markers. This contrasts with

the measurement of benefits in terms of changes in health-related quality of life, which is often given the label *cost–utility analysis* (CUA), discussed in the following subsection.

The first decision rule for this kind of CEA is that we should reject any alternatives that are *dominated* by another alternative or combination of alternatives. This is economic efficiency in the strict sense described earlier, where the dominated alternative has a greater cost with no greater benefits or lower benefits with the same or greater costs. The choice between non-dominated alternatives is more complex. Where only one alternative can be chosen, that with the lowest ICER should be chosen, but only if it is below a *ceiling ratio*, which is a level of the ICER which any alternative must meet if it is to be regarded as cost-effective. Where combinations of more than one alternative can be used, it is in principle necessary to calculate the ICERs for every possible combination to decide which is most efficient and if any meet the ceiling ratio requirement.

These issues are often illustrated using a *cost-effectiveness plane* diagram (Black 1990), as in Fig. 6.6.1. ICERs are presented graphically as a combination of the costs and the effects of a health intervention, described in Fig. 6.6.1 as a treatment, compared to some alternative. Costs are conventionally placed on the north–south axis and effects on the east–west axis. In both cases, these effects can be negative, zero or positive.

The ceiling ratio can be also be demonstrated using a cost-effectiveness plane diagram, where it is often referred to as demonstrating *cost-effectiveness acceptability*, as in Fig. 6.6.2.

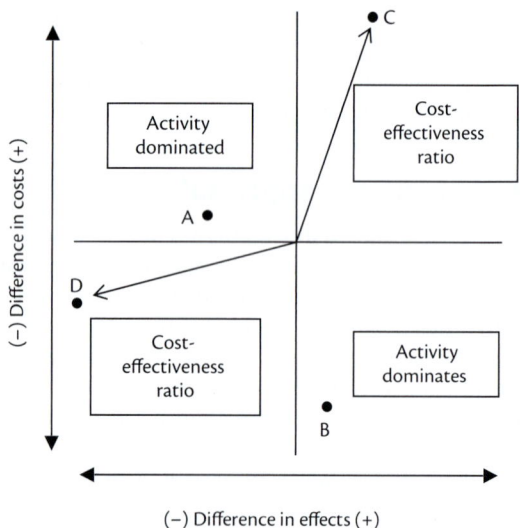

Fig. 6.6.1 The cost-effectiveness plane. An intervention can be placed anywhere on this diagram according to its incremental costs and benefits. If it lies in the north-west quadrant, such as point A, the costs of the intervention are higher than the alternative, and its benefits are lower. It is therefore unambiguously worse, and is said to be dominated by the alternative. Similarly, in the south-east quadrant, at a point such as B, costs are lower and benefits are higher, so the treatment dominates its alternative. In the north-east quadrant, at a point such as C, higher benefits are gained at a net cost over the alternative. So, we can calculate an ICER, the cost per unit of effect gained, measured as the slope of the line from the origin to the point. In the south-west quadrant, at a point such as D, lower costs are possible, but at the expense of lower benefits. Again, we can calculate an ICER, although this now refers to a cost saving per unit of effect lost, which is again measured as the slope of the line from the origin to the point.

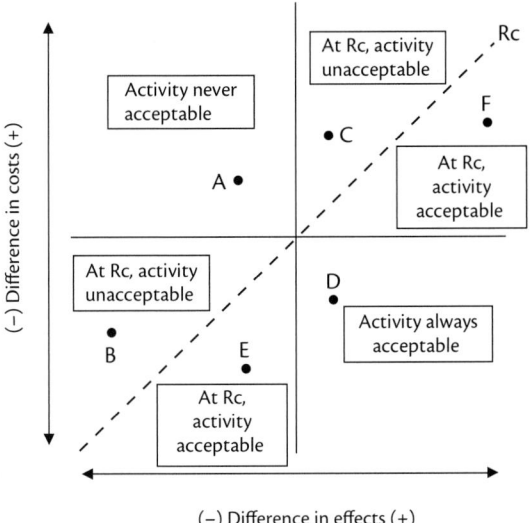

Fig. 6.6.2 Cost-effectiveness acceptability. In this diagram, the dotted diagonal line marked Rc represents the ceiling ratio. If an intervention lies above the line, it will not be acceptable on cost-effectiveness grounds. This is either because it is dominated by the alternative, whatever the ceiling ratio is, as in point A, or its ICER does not satisfy the actual ceiling ratio, as in points B and C. It should be noted that in the south-west quadrant, this means that the ICER is below the ceiling ratio, as in point B, while in the north-east quadrant it is above, as in point C. Below the line it will be acceptable. This is either because it dominates the alternative, as in point D, or its ICER satisfies the ceiling ratio, as in points E and F. In this case, the ICER is above the ceiling ratio in the south-west quadrant, as in point E, or below it in the north-east quadrant, as in point F.

Cost-effectiveness acceptability is also important because it is one way in which uncertainty in EA is dealt with, which is explained later in this chapter.

Cost–utility analysis

CUA is a term often used in the United Kingdom and elsewhere, though rarely in the United States, to refer to a special form of CEA in which health benefits are measured in terms of quality-adjusted life years (QALYs). QALYs are a composite measure of gains in life expectancy and health-related quality of life, described in more detail in the 'Measuring benefit in terms of health gain' subsection, along with disability-adjusted life years (DALYs). The distinctive outcome of a CUA is the calculation of an ICER in terms of the extra cost per QALY gained (CQG), which may also be thought of as the price of obtaining one extra QALY using a particular healthcare intervention or programme. An example is described in Box 6.6.1.

The rationale for CUA is more complex than that of CEA more generally. QALYs in themselves are regarded by many as a better outcome indicator than the 'natural' units of CEA when appraising therapeutic alternatives for the same condition. This is because they deal with efficiency in the production of health itself rather than simply of healthcare. But CUA also offers something that CEA more generally cannot, which is the possibility of comparing across treatments for different conditions. In principle, it is possible to compare interventions for, say, eating more healthily to reduce weight with, say, reducing alcohol consumption, to determine which is the most efficient at producing health gain in the form of QALYs. Of course, this is controversial. For a CEA

Box 6.6.1 A cost–utility analysis of vaccinating schoolgirls against HPV infection

Anonychuk et al. (2009) investigated the cost-effectiveness of vaccinating 12-year-old girls against human papillomavirus (HPV) types 16 and 18 to prevent cervical cancer. The vaccine also cross-protects against other HPV types, and its overall effectiveness is determined by herd immunity effects, the consequent reduction in the risk of infection to non-vaccinated people. For each 100,000 girls vaccinated, between 390 and 633 cases of cervical cancer and 168 and 175 deaths would be prevented, depending on whether or not herd immunity and cross-protection effects are included. This would generate QALY gains of 0.0083 to 0.0095 per person over the group's lifetime. There would be an increase in cost of Can$256 to Can$263 per person. For the base case of no herd immunity or cross-protection effects, Table 6.6.1 shows the costs and effects with and without vaccination.

This gives an extra cost per QALY gained (CQG) of Can$263/0.0083 = Can$31 687. With cross-protection, the CQG was Can$26,947; with herd immunity Can$27,849; and with both Can$18,672. The authors concluded that the vaccine reduced cancer cases and mortality and was cost-effective, though that conclusion does depend on an assumption about the size of the ceiling ratio.

Table 6.6.1 Incremental costs and QALY gains from vaccination

	Non-vaccinated	Vaccinated	Difference
Total cost (Can$)	476	739	263
Total QALYs	30.5015	30.5098	0.0083

Source: data from Anonychuk et al., A cost-utility analysis of cervical cancer vaccination in preadolescent Canadian females, *BMC Public Health*, Volume 9, Issue 1, pp. 401, Copyright © 2009 Anonychuk et al. licensee BioMed Central Ltd. Reproduced under the Creative Commons Attribution License 2.0.

restricted to different treatments for a particular condition, it can be assumed that the patients receiving the treatments are the same people, but this will not be true of comparisons across conditions.

CUA has, in principle, the ability to compare across all health interventions. A contentious implication of this is that it can be used to allocate healthcare resources between different health programmes, and therefore be used to determine healthcare priorities. That would overcome the principal problem that CEA has compared with CBA, because it would indicate whether or not the healthcare benefits from a particular type of healthcare should be realized, rather than simply which is the best way of achieving those benefits. Some people therefore regard CUA as a limited form of CBA rather than a special form of CEA. Viewed in this way, CUA is better than CBA, because it avoids having to measure benefits in terms of money.

To explain this further, recall that a decision rule for CEA is that the ICER of the best alternative is compared to a ceiling ratio. In the case of CUA the ICER is the CQG, so the ceiling ratio is the amount that we think it is reasonable to pay to gain a QALY. This is sometimes referred to as a CQG *threshold*, because it is the dividing line between healthcare that is regarded as cost-effective and that which is not. NICE has a threshold, which it regards as deriving from the limited budget that the National Health Service has, which determines what can be afforded. This is known as the shadow price of a QALY. Alternatively, it could be set according to what the population is willing to pay for health gain. This is known as the social value of a QALY. But either way, if this is known, it can in principle be used as a means of converting costs to QALYs or vice versa. This puts costs and benefits into the same units, enabling the calculation of net benefits in the same way as for CBA.

Net benefits can be calculated in terms of either money or QALYs. Suppose that an intervention has incremental costs of £30,000 and incremental benefits of 2 QALYs. The ceiling ratio can be regarded as the price that it is acceptable to pay for a QALY, and therefore represents the money value of a QALY. Suppose that the ceiling ratio is £20,000 per QALY gained. If we decide to analyse cost-effectiveness in monetary terms, we first multiply the QALY gain by the ceiling ratio to give the money value of the QALY gain, in this case 2 × £20,000 = £40,000. The net cost is then subtracted from this to give a net monetary benefit of £40,000 – £30,000 = £10,000. Alternatively, we could convert the costs to their QALY gain equivalent by dividing the ceiling ratio by them. This would give a net cost equivalent of £30,000/£20,000 = 1.5 QALYs, and an overall net health benefit of 2 – 1.5 = 0.5 QALYs. Because these are positive—and they must always have the same sign—the intervention is deemed cost-effective.

Of course, this is exactly the same result as if we had calculated the ICER to be £30,000/2 = £15,000 and observed that it is below the ceiling ratio of £20,000. However, this net-benefit approach does have an advantage if we do not know the ceiling ratio, since we can calculate net benefits for any value of the ceiling ratio.

Measuring costs

As suggested earlier in the chapter (see 'Formulating an economic appraisal'), the process of costing involves three steps: identifying and describing resource use changes; quantifying them in physical units; and valuing them.

In general, there are two types of costing: macro or top–down costing and micro- or bottom–up costing. These are distinguished by the level of disaggregation at which individual resources are measured and valued. In its pure form, macro-costing starts with the total costs incurred by, for example, a hospital and calculates the costs of, for example a specialty, by allocating a proportion of the total costs to it using some indicator of the costliness of that specialty compared with others. For example, if a specialty had 20 per cent of the hospital's cases, 20 per cent of the costs would be allocated to it. At the extreme, micro-costing would examine every item of service and every consumable used by every patient. Each item of service would be costed by examining all of the time spent on it by every member of staff as well as the time spent using every piece of equipment. In practice, these extremes are not found. Moreover, it is common for mixed methods to be used for different elements of cost.

The time at which resources are utilized is an important consideration, as not all costs are incurred at the same time. There are two important elements to this. First, if costs occur in different years, then they should be adjusted for any inflation or deflation that has occurred. This is to make the figures comparable over different years and to ensure that it is the value of resources that is considered, which may be unaffected by the rate of inflation. The best practice is to select 1 year's unit costs and apply them to different years' resource use. But that is rarely possible for many items of cost, so the procedure is to deflate yearly costs by a cost index. This also means that if there are any cost projections, these should not take account of projected inflation.

Secondly, although inflation-adjusting means that each year's costs are measured in the same units of value for each year, this does not mean that every year's costs are of the same value when viewed from a particular year. In particular, people in general prefer to postpone costs if they can, and therefore a cost now has a higher weight than exactly the same money cost incurred in the future. Looked at another way, costs in the future have a lower value now. This is dealt with by *discounting*, which is a time weight applied to costs, which diminishes the further in the future the cost is. In practice, what is done is to apply a discount rate, which can be viewed as the inverse of an interest rate. Applying an interest rate to an investment means that the value grows over time even if it is fixed. Applying a discount rate means that the value falls over time. In an EA, if costs are summed over time, then discounting all future costs back to the present gives a present value.

The issue of timing may be very important in healthcare, because of the long-lasting effects of many interventions. (Benefits in the future may also have a lower value now, requiring the same approach; this is discussed later in the chapter, see 'Measuring benefit in terms of health gain'). Of particular public health interest is the problem that prevention incurs costs now, and even if it reduces costs in the future by a greater amount, there may not be a net cost saving if the future costs are discounted. Even if there is a net cost saving, it will have a lower value than if discounting was not used. In the extreme, measures to deal with maternal nutrition to reduce illness in the later adult life of their babies, as suggested by the Barker hypothesis (Barker 1992), might see cost reductions so many years in the future that discounting would reduce them to a negligible value.

There is some dispute about exactly what the discount rate to be used should be, and how it should be obtained. There are two competing theories to guide this. One is the social opportunity cost approach, which assumes that public and private investments compete for resources, so the public sector should use market rates of borrowing. The other is the social rate of time preference, which measures what people are willing to receive in compensation for delaying consumption from one year to the next.

Measuring benefits

Measurement of benefits in terms of 'natural' units in a CEA does not require any special economic analysis, and the measurement of diverse benefits within a CCA is too diverse to be dealt with here. This section therefore concentrates on the measurement of *health gain* for use in a CUA, and the measurement of *monetary gain* for use in a CBA.

However, a third technique, which does not fit neatly into these two categories, is becoming increasingly important, the *discrete choice experiment* (DCE). In this, respondents are offered a choice between different interventions, which are described according to attributes that may include health outcomes and price. The choices made reveal the relative values of different attributes. This might be used to ascribe a value to different interventions, or to calculate values in terms of money or to obtain values for different health states. The last of these is described in the following subsection.

Measuring benefit in terms of health gain

There are many different ways in which health and improvements in health can be measured. Different concepts and measurement techniques are appropriate for different uses. The approaches that are adopted for use in EA are largely determined by the requirements that their use for appraisal purposes dictates.

First, appraisal is attempting to obtain an unambiguous measure of benefit. This implies that the measure of health should be a single number representing all relevant aspects. Secondly, because appraisal looks at the use of scarce resources that could be devoted to all sorts of healthcare, the measure of health should be capable of comparing those different uses of resources. This implies that a generic measure of health should be used. Thirdly, appraisal compares costs, which represent the value of resources used with benefits, which implies that the measure of health should also be capable of being interpreted as a value.

One measure that meets these requirements is the QALY. This combines length of life and quality of life into a single indicator. Depending on the type of health gain, QALYs can be thought of as a quality adjustment to years of life gained or the length of time for which quality of life is improved or both. It is important to remember that the benefit of a health intervention is the gain in QALYs that it produces. A similar measure is the DALY. This chapter does not describe DALYs fully; such details can be found in Chapter 5.17, which compares the two measures. Essentially, however, the DALY is a population-based measure that combines life expectancy in a population with the prevalence of disability to generate an estimate of a 'health gap'.

Fig. 6.6.3 illustrates how in principle QALYs are calculated, for a highly stylized description of prognoses for a disease with and without treatment. For example, suppose that with a particular disease, the prognosis is that a person will live for a further 10 years. During the first two of those, their health-related quality of life (HRQOL) will deteriorate at a constant rate from 80 per cent of full health to 60 per cent and during the last eight will deteriorate more slowly to 30 per cent by the time of their death. This is represented in the diagram by the solid line, with HRQOL

values of 0.8 at time t, 0.6 at $(t + 2)$ and 0.3 at $(t + 10)$. With treatment, life expectancy will rise to 12 years, in each of which the patient will enjoy full health. This is shown by the dashed line with HRQOL = 1.0 from time t to $(t + 12)$.

The QALY gain can be calculated by subtracting the total QALYs for an untreated patient from the total that they would have if treated. Without the treatment, the patient has 2 years at an average HRQOL of 0.6 = 1.4 QALYs, plus 8 years at an average of 0.45 = 3.6 QALYs, making a total of 5 QALYs. With the treatment, the patient has 12 years at full health, which is 12 QALYs. The gain is therefore 7 QALYs. Equivalently, we can calculate the total gain by summing the gains within each time period. The first 2 years have a HRQOL improvement from an average of 0.7 to 1 = 0.3, giving a QALY gain of 0.6. The next 8 years have an improvement from an average of 0.45 to 1 = 0.55, giving a QALY gain of 4.4. The final 2 years are additional years at full health, which is a gain of 2 QALYs. The total gain is as before 7 QALYs.

One of the big advantages of the QALY is that it can, in principle, be applied to any kind of intervention, whether it raises life expectancy without improving quality of life, improves quality of life without affecting longevity, improves both or improves one at the expense of lowering the other. However, to some people this is a weakness of QALYs, as they argue that length and quality of life cannot or should not be compared in the same metric.

Before looking at how QALYs are calculated in practice, it should be noted that if QALYs are gained, or indeed lost, at different times, then in principle they should be discounted if they are to be added together, in exactly the same way as costs, if they are to be used in an economic evaluation. There has been a considerable debate about this and there are arguments in favour of discounting both costs and QALYs at the same rate, discounting costs but not QALYs, and discounting them both, but at different rates.

In what follows, the concern is only with the quality of life element of the QALY, since the measurement of life expectancy has no special economic aspects attached to it except for discounting.

In carrying out an appraisal, QALYs can be calculated in a number of different ways. One is to measure the value that patients attach to their quality of life directly. Another is to apply a conversion factor to other indicators of health that will estimate from the indicator a quality of life value. However, an approach which has become most popular, and indeed is recommended by NICE, is to obtain from patients a measure of their health state using a generic health status measure, such as the EQ-5D (Brooks 1996; Herdman et al. 2011), and to apply to the resulting health profile data a value for each state that has been measured for a standard population. The intention is that those values should represent the values of society as a whole.

These sets of values are derived from population surveys. There are different techniques that are used to obtain values, of which the main four are rating or visual analogue scales (VAS), time trade-off (TTO), standard gamble (SG), and the DCE. A VAS usually consists of a single line drawn with verbal and numerical descriptors at each end, describing the meaning of the two ends, such as 'Best possible health' and 'Worst possible health'. Scale markers are often added to the line to denote distance along the line, and these are sometimes also numbered. Respondents are presented with a set of health states and are asked to rate the desirability of each by placing it at some point on the line on or between the two end points.

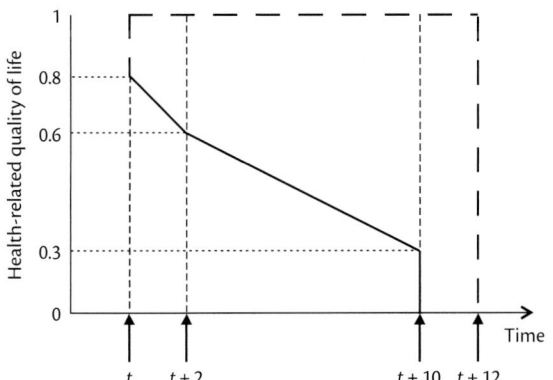

Fig. 6.6.3 Calculating gains in quality-adjusted life years.

In the TTO method, respondents are offered a choice between a number of years in full health and a number of years in a particular health state and asked to choose between them. Slightly different versions of this are used depending on whether the states are chronic or acute state and whether the respondent believes them to be better or worse than being dead. For a chronic health state preferred to death, different numbers of years in full health are offered for a fixed number of years in a health state, until the respondent cannot choose between the alternatives. The value for the health state is then determined by the ratio of the number of years in full health to the number of years in the health state. This calculation is based on the assumed equivalence of the number of QALYs generated by the two alternatives.

In the SG method, respondents are offered a choice between the certainty of being in a particular health state and a gamble whose outcomes are full health with a certain probability and death, and asked to choose between them. Again, slightly different versions of this are used depending on whether the states are chronic or acute and whether the respondent believes them to be better or worse than being dead. For a chronic health state preferred to death, different probabilities of being in full health are offered, until the respondent cannot choose between the alternatives. The value for the health state is equal to the probability at that point of indifference. This calculation is based on the *expected values* of the two alternatives, which is discussed later in the chapter (see 'Economic appraisal models and uncertainty').

DCEs applied to health state valuation are undertaken by offering respondents a choice between two, or sometimes more, health states and recording their choice. This technique does not measure any individual respondent's valuations of health states, but infers from the responses of a group their collective valuation.

Generic health state measures are usually accompanied by sets of values for each health state that they define. Because they have so many health states, the values are usually generated by a model, which may be called a *multiattribute utility model*, though that label is not explicitly used in some cases and its use in some cases may be disputed. Essentially, health states are decomposed into attributes. Generic health measures usually describe health states using different dimensions, in which people can be at different levels, which form the attributes.

The attributes are combined using a mathematical function. For example, the widely used EQ-5D has attached to it a number of value sets that have been calculated and published (Szende et al. 2007). The mathematical form used is additive, which means that the attributes are weighted and added together.

Measuring benefit in monetary terms

Monetary measures of benefits can be based on *revealed preference* or *stated preference*. Revealed preference techniques use observations from people's behaviour to infer monetary values. As an example, it is possible to examine the value that people place on the avoidance of death or injury by looking at the wages that are paid to people to undertake jobs that differ in the risk of these occurring but are otherwise identical. Stated preference techniques rely on surveys and experiments in which people are essentially asked what monetary value they place on healthcare, or health states or on other aspects of health benefits. They are not usually asked that question directly, but are given choices between different alternatives, from which money values are inferred.

Such stated preference studies are sometimes called *willingness-to-pay* studies, although that description is not entirely accurate for all of them. The economic theory underlying these kinds of studies is the measurement of what are called compensating variation and equivalent variation. In the context of measuring the money value of health benefits, these mean monetary payments made by or to a person to compensate for a change in their health, either an improvement or a deterioration, and *not* having a change in their health, respectively. Willingness to pay refers to compensation paid *by* the person, either for obtaining an improvement in their health or not having their health deteriorate. Willingness to accept refers to compensation paid *to* the person, either for having their health deteriorate or not obtaining an improvement in their health.

Although stated preference methods used vary, best practice in economics more generally is to use the *contingent valuation* method. Contingent valuation requires the survey or experiment to describe a plausible market in which the choices made by respondents about goods reveal the values that are required. The values are said to be contingent on that description. One way to do this is to use a DCE in which price is one of the attributes that the goods have.

Economic appraisal models and uncertainty

In theory, it is possible that an EA could be carried out using one source of data, for example, a clinical trial in which resource use, costs, and quality of life are all measured for individual patients. This would have all of the advantages of a clinical trial in terms of the reliability of results. In practice, EAs are usually based on different sources of data, which have to be linked together. There are many calculations behind the estimates of costs and benefits, which are embodied in what is called an EA *model*, and in practice all healthcare EAs involve some modelling. In fact, economic modelling is regarded by many as superior to a trial-based EA as it may overcome the problems that trials have in terms of generalizability and speed of producing usable results. Of course, models may use data from trials, but only as one input.

A simple model might be regarded simply as a balance sheet in which the data used to calculate costs and benefits are combined to give figures for total costs and total benefits. However, many EAs cannot use such simple models, and these are no longer regarded as acceptable in the context of technology appraisals examined by bodies such as NICE. The reasons are, first, that treatment options are not always straightforward and clinical decision-making may involve strategies for management, rather than a simple choice between using and not using a single therapy; and secondly, that there is usually some uncertainty about both the model and the data.

As a result, modelling usually uses *decision analysis* (see, e.g. Briggs et al. 2006). This deals both with the complexity issue, by imposing a structure on the implied clinical decision-making, and some aspects of uncertainty. However, there is one aspect of uncertainty that is not dealt with directly by decision analysis, which is uncertainty about the values that data take. A number of techniques have been developed in recent years to deal with this, which are briefly described.

The problem that is dealt with can be encapsulated by the observation that summaries of effectiveness data, such as changes in blood pressure resulting from some intervention, are usually presented as both a point estimate and an interval estimate, or confidence interval, reflecting variability in the data; we should have a similar summary for cost-effectiveness data. When this is done as part of a trial-based analysis it is called *stochastic CEA*. Unfortunately, there are two problems with this. First, many of the data used in an EA model are not based on sampling, and therefore do not have a variance that can be used to create an interval estimate. Secondly, the summary index of cost-effectiveness is the ICER, which as a ratio has special problems, such that in general it is not possible to estimate a confidence interval even if all of the data that are used to calculate it do have variability. This second problem applies equally to trial-based and model based EAs.

Sensitivity analysis

The usual way in which uncertainty is dealt with when using a model is *sensitivity analysis*. This is a set of techniques that analyse how sensitive the results are to changes in the model, for example, in the data that are contained within it or the way that the data are combined. Some sensitivity analysis techniques are described below. In these, the model that has the best assumed structure and data is called the *base case*, and the assumptions and data that we wish to test are referred to as the *parameters* of the model.

One-way sensitivity analysis means looking at how sensitive results are to changes in one parameter. If, for example, a new screening programme is appraised using a model, one of the parameters of the model may be the unit cost of the test used. The base case will use the best estimate that the analyst has of the unit cost as an input to the calculated ICER. One-way sensitivity analysis will calculate the ICER for different values of the unit costs, showing whether the cost makes a lot of or a little difference to the result.

Of course, what is meant by a lot or a little should really be defined. One way to do this is to use the ceiling ratio. If at every possible value of the parameter the ICER remains above or alternatively remains below the ceiling ratio, then the result remains the same, and the decision is not sensitive to the value of the uncertain parameter. In other cases, it may be that at some levels of the parameter for example when the unit cost is low—the ICER will be below the ceiling ratio, but at others—for example, when the unit cost is high the ICER will be above. At some point the ICER will be equal to the ceiling ratio, and at that point called a threshold—a change in the preferred option occurs. This is known as threshold analysis. If the base case and the threshold are very different, then the results are not sensitive to the values of the parameter.

But again, what does very different mean? One way to deal with this is to define upper and lower plausible values for the parameter; for example, with a base case cost of £100 per unit, it may be thought unlikely that the cost could be as high as £200 or as low as £10. This will give a plausible range to the calculated ICER, and if the threshold is within that range, then the results are sensitive to the assumption made.

This can be extended to vary more than one parameter at the same time and to observe the combined impact on the ICER. The ceiling ratio can again be used to define a threshold, and plausible ranges for the ICER can be calculated from the plausible values of the variables, taken in combination. Such multiway analysis is essential, because it is possible that separate one-way analyses of the parameters might suggest that the results are not sensitive to their value, but in combination they might be.

Statistical sensitivity analysis

Plausible range methods are not very satisfactory because their basis is often unclear and not testable. Using statistical methods is better because, as suggested, the base case cost-effectiveness results can be seen as a point estimate and sensitivity analysis as an interval estimate. When this is done as part of a decision analysis model, it is called *probabilistic sensitivity analysis*.

In this, Monte Carlo simulations are used to generate an ICER distribution. A distribution for each of the model's parameters is assumed, if it is not known. Samples are taken from each distribution, and the ICER is calculated from those simulated data using the model. This is repeated many times to generate an ICER distribution, from which, in principle, a variance might be calculated, and therefore a confidence interval.

Unfortunately, in practice that might still not be possible, because of another problem with ICERs. It is quite possible that the distribution of the ICERs generated by simulation might include both positive and negative values. These mean such different things—a negative value means dominance rather than a true ICER—that a confidence interval calculated from them is meaningless.

There are two possible solutions to this. One is essentially to get rid of the ICER by using the net benefit approach described earlier. Because net benefit is a single number, not a ratio, there is no problem with using simulation to generate a distribution of it and to calculate a variance and therefore an interval estimate.

Another solution is to generate a *cost-effectiveness acceptability curve* (CEAC), which retains the CER, but uses a method of describing uncertainty which is different to the confidence interval (van Hout et al. 1994). The simulated ICER values are each compared with a ceiling ratio, and a count is obtained of the proportion of simulated values that are acceptable at that ratio. This is repeated for each possible value of the ceiling ratio, and the proportion that is acceptable will be different for each of those values. A CEAC plots these together, as in Fig. 6.6.4. In this illustrative example, the proportion 25 per cent of the simulations of cost and outcomes for a particular therapy are acceptable if the ceiling ratio is £4500 per QALY gained; 50 per cent if £11,500 and

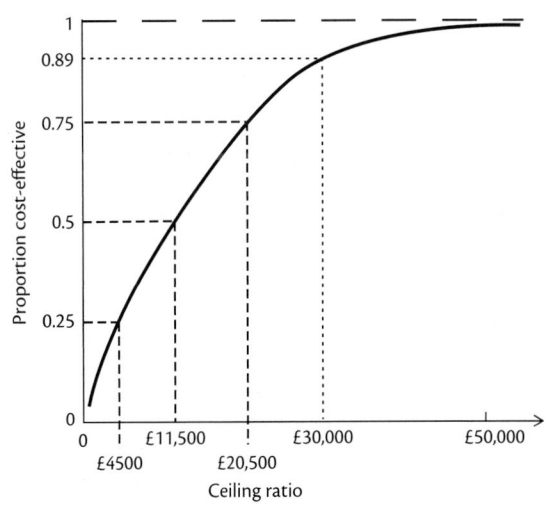

Fig. 6.6.4 Cost-effectiveness acceptability curve.

75 per cent if £20,500. At the ceiling ratio £30,000, 89 per cent are acceptable. Under certain conditions, which are beyond the scope of this chapter to describe, the proportions may be interpreted using a Bayesian approach as probabilities, such that at a ceiling ratio of £30,000, there is a 0.89 probability that the therapy is cost-effective.

Decision analysis

Decision analysis is used when the outcomes of decisions are not certain, but the probabilities of different outcomes are known. For example, the treatment of cases detected by a screening programme may not be effective in every case, but is known to work in 80 per cent of cases. It is of particular value when decisions involve strategies with different actions. For example, if some members of the population do not respond to a whole population screening initiative, then they may be targeted to increase uptake. Decision analysis is a way of structuring the different options in order to calculate which of the strategies is best.

Decision analysis relies on the concept of *expected values*. We can think of the expected value of something as its average value when it is repeated a large number of times. For example, if a treatment produces a gain of 2 QALYs per person in 80 per cent of cases and a gain of 1 QALY per person in the remaining 20 per cent, then out of 100 patients the total gain will be $(2 \times 80) + (1 \times 20) = 180$, giving an average of 1.8 QALYs gained per patient. This is the expected value. Of course, in reality the nature of uncertainty is such that it is unlikely that the probabilities of 0.8 and 0.2 would produce exactly 80 and 20 in a population of 100, which is why an assumption of large numbers is made. More generally, the expected value is calculated as the sum over all possible outcomes of the probability of the outcome multiplied by the value of the outcome.

Decision analysis calculates the expected values of both costs and benefits and also, though this is a more complicated issue, ICERs. It usually takes the following form, which may be compared with the more general formulation of an EA given earlier:

1. Structure the problem by constructing a mathematical model of decision-making, usually a decision tree. Identify the decision alternatives; list the possible outcomes of each alternative; and specify the sequence of events.

2. Assign probabilities to chance events.

3. Assign values to all possible outcomes of chance events.

4. Calculate the expected value of each strategy.

5. Perform sensitivity analyses by systematically changing the assumptions in (1)—(3) to see the impact on the result of (4).

An extension of decision analysis, which is however not yet well-established in practical decision-making, is *value of information analysis*. Decision analysis is based on choosing the alternative that has the highest expected value given current information. The value of information approach analyses the consequences of making the wrong choice with the aim of assessing how much it is worth spending to improve information so that we do not make the wrong choice. If an incorrect choice is made, the loss incurred is the outcome from the option chosen minus the expected value of the best alternative option. Multiplying this loss by the probability that the incorrect option is chosen gives its expected value.

This gives the *value of perfect information*; it is worth paying up to this value to avoid making the incorrect choice and therefore investing in research into probabilities of events, quality of life, and costs. Using statistical information on levels of significance and power, it is also possible to estimate the *value of sample information*, which gives the amount that it is worth paying for a sample of given size to improve information.

Economic appraisal and equity

In discussing equity, we noted that Culyer and Bombard (2012) have suggested using a checklist to ensure that decision-makers take all aspects of equity into account. Here we describe only a narrow range of equity analyses, related to EAs and concerning the distribution of healthcare resources and outcomes between people.

The impact of healthcare interventions is ultimately on individual people, and it is always relevant to examine equity at that level. However, in practice inequities are mostly observed between population groups defined by particular characteristics, for example, people who have serious ill health or are poor, aged, or children. This is particularly important for public health interventions, which are usually conducted at the population level.

Similarly, although it is always relevant to look at the distributional consequences of decisions about every kind of healthcare, it may be of particular importance for public health interventions, since they may be designed specifically to reduce inequalities in population health. It may be that some interventions that target individuals or groups who are disadvantaged would not be regarded as cost-effective relative to many other interventions. It may also be that some public health interventions, such as those designed to enhance health-promoting lifestyles, may be less effective for those who are disadvantaged, thereby increasing health inequalities. In each case an analysis of the implied trade-off between efficiency and equity is essential.

Despite the near-universal acceptance that assessment of equity is as important as efficiency in EA, this has not been matched by practice. In a systematic review, Sassi et al. (2001) were unable to find any satisfactory equity analyses as part of EAs of healthcare in general; Weatherly et al. (2009) found the same for public health interventions.

Cookson et al. (2009) proposed four possible approaches to analysing equity:

1. Reviewing existing inequalities related to the topic being appraised. This is not in itself evaluative, but it provides background information and therefore some context to decision-making that is based on an efficiency-oriented EA.

2. Measuring the redistributive impact of a decision about healthcare, that is a quantitative description of who gains and who loses, and the size of gains and losses. Baeten et al. (2010) proposed that for interventions targeted on a particular group, appraisal might assess outcomes in absolute terms for the targeted group but also relative to groups who are not targeted. Sassi et al. (2001) made similar suggestions for assessing the distributional effects for subgroups: the effect of competing interventions; the effect of selectivity; and the effect of prioritizing over other interventions.

3. If an intervention generates greater equity, but at the expense of a larger health gain overall, measuring its opportunity cost. This cost is not measured in terms of money, but of health, for example, the number of QALYs that would be lost for the population overall by targeting a particular group.

4. Cost-effectiveness with equity weights applied to the outcomes for different groups. An example which is in practice applied is the 'end-of-life premium' used by NICE in England, which weights more highly QALYs generated by interventions where survival without the intervention is short, even if the length of the gain from the intervention is itself short. Baeten et al. (2010) also proposed a variant of this in the form of multi-criteria decision analysis (MCDA). In MCDA, decision-makers consider many relevant characteristics of an intervention and explicitly incorporate trade-offs within and between them in the form of relative weights. The proposal is that both efficiency and equity consequences are included in characteristics of intervention, thereby taking both into account. Unlike the other three proposed approaches, explicit weighting requires an extra source of data to generate the weights, rather than using data available from an efficiency-based appraisal.

Baeten et al. (2010) illustrated their proposal with an assessment of equity for breast cancer screening. They applied the redistributive impact assessment and both variants of the equity weighting approach; these gave very similar conclusions in favour of selectivity on both efficiency and equity grounds.

Economic appraisal of public health interventions

This chapter has highlighted some issues that arise in applying EA to specifically public health interventions. The state of the art in addressing these is currently less advanced than for other healthcare programmes. But there are many examples that demonstrate both the value of EA in public health and the value of public health interventions themselves.

In reviewing the state of the art in EA of public health interventions, Weatherly et al. (2009) outlined four key methodological challenges, one of which, the specific concern that public health has for equity, we have already discussed. Of the others, one is the kind of evidence that public health interventions are based on. Guidelines for HTA of interventions with individual patients emphasize that the best source of scientific data is the randomized controlled trial (RCT). However, not only are there fewer RCTs for public health interventions, they are inherently more difficult to conduct. We discussed one of the reasons for this in relation to discounting (see 'Measuring costs'); the impact of public health interventions may be on a longer time scale than an RCT could plausibly encompass. Other problems include that it may be infeasible to establish controls for population-based interventions such as screening and that pathways of causation between intervention and outcome are often less direct than individual treatments, for example, health education programmes. It is therefore necessary to use other ways of establishing evidence, and to rely on extensive use of modelling.

A second concerns the way in which outcomes are specified and measured. Cost-effectiveness analyses use QALYs or other health measures as their outcome measure and it is arguable that is the correct measure where health gain to individual patients are the main aim. However, in public health interventions not only is health gain difficult to measure, because of the difficulties of establishing evidence that we have discussed, but also because the intervention may have additional goals, or important side effects. These include improving public knowledge and awareness, and the benefit of reassurance, as well as possible unintended adverse consequences such as false reassurance and raised anxiety over possible health problems.

The third concerns the boundaries given to the costs and benefits that are included in an EA. Previously we stated that a social perspective would include all of these (see 'Social costs and benefits'), whatever they are and whoever bears them, but it may be essential to restrict their scope depending on the perspective that is taken. For example, as our discussion of the NICE threshold implies (see 'Cost–utility analysis'), an HTA for interventions that are paid for by a health agency that has a fixed budget is justified in restricting the scope of costs to those incurred by that agency. However, public health interventions typically have much wider effects on the public sector than the health sector, and indeed on the economy as a whole. In turn, those could impact on health; Weatherly et al. (2009) suggest as an example that 'improvements in housing could reduce illness and injuries, with consequent reductions in health care utilization'.

Despite these problems, there are reasons to be optimistic both about the possibilities of undertaking EA in public health and also about the results from such analyses. Owen et al. (2011) examined the economic analyses that formed the evidence base for public health guidance by NICE issued from 2006 and 2010, an example of which is described in Box 6.6.2. Of 200 cost-effectiveness analyses, 30 of the interventions both improved outcomes and lowered costs, in other words dominated the alternative and were in the south-east quadrant of the cost-effectiveness plane. One hundred and forty-one had cost-effectiveness ratios below NICE's official stated 'lower threshold' of £20,000 per QALY gained, with a median of £1,020; a further seven were below the 'upper threshold' of £30,000, with a median of £25,150; and 11 were above that, with a median of £90,786. Eleven were dominated, that is in the north-west quadrant where costs are higher and benefits lower.

Of course, this sample is only from England, and the coverage may not be representative of the broad range of public health interventions; 127 of them were related to smoking and other interventions may not have been selected for evaluation if they were considered unlikely to be cost-effective. Nevertheless, they did cover very different types of interventions to very different sections of the population. One finding was that interventions aimed at the population as a whole produced the lowest costs per QALY gained.

Efficiency and equity in the economics sense are not the only considerations for decisions in public health or healthcare in general, and EA is only one of the types of evidence that are relevant to them. However, EA is a powerful way of assessing evidence about important consequences of such decisions, and in particular helps in considering how to manage scarce healthcare resources. In advocating that public health should receive a fair share of those resources, it is essential to base arguments that are as strong as those for other types of healthcare and to use equally powerful techniques for analysing them.

Box 6.6.2 Economic analysis of interventions to prevent smoking among schoolchildren

An example is the evidence review underlying NICE guidance on public health interventions to prevent the uptake of smoking among schoolchildren (Jit et al. 2009). A literature review was undertaken and no published economic evaluations of school-based smoking prevention programmes in the United Kingdom were identified. It was argued that studies based in other countries were of limited relevance to the United Kingdom because of differences in the populations being studied and the methodological framework used. In addition, most studies assumed that school-based smoking prevention programmes achieved a lasting reduction in smoking prevalence beyond school age, and this finding was not supported by evidence used to produce the guidance. As a consequence, the authors undertook new research to evaluate whether or not the implementation of a school-based smoking prevention initiative would be cost-effective.

Survey data were used to quantify the association between the age at which smoking was initiated and the probability of quitting smoking quit in later life (older age at initiation was significantly associated with an increased likelihood of quitting in later life). A systematic review was undertaken to quantify the impact of smoking prevention programmes on decreasing smoking uptake in the long term and delaying the onset of smoking, and whether these effects varied by the age of the participants.

These data were combined with cost and other data in an economic model and used to calculate the cost-effectiveness of school-based smoking prevention programmes. Results were presented for a generic programme delivered to 11-year-old students. Assuming an intervention cost of £38.50 per participant the CQG was estimated to be £2030–12,700, depending on assumptions made about the persistence of effect of the programme over time. The results were fairly robust to changes in key model parameters concerning the association between age of smoking initiation and probability of smoking in later life, mortality in smokers and non-smokers, health-related quality of life in smokers, lifetime medical costs of smokers, and the quality of the studies used to inform the models. In few cases was the extra CQG greater than the ceiling ratio, which was assumed to be £20,000 per QALY gained.

References

Anonychuk, A.M., Bauch, C.T., Merid, M.F., Van Kriekinge, G., and Demarteau, N. (2009). A cost-utility analysis of cervical cancer vaccination in preadolescent Canadian females. *BMC Public Health*, 9(1), 401.

Baeten, S., Baltussen, R., Uyl-de Groot, C., Bridges, J., and Niessen, L. (2010). Incorporating equity-efficiency interactions in cost-effectiveness analysis—three approaches applied to breast cancer control. *Value in Health*, 13(5), 573–9.

Barker, D.J.P. (ed.) (1992). *Fetal and Infant Origins of Adult Disease*. London: BMJ Books.

Black, W.C. (1990). The cost-effectiveness plane: a graphic representation of cost-effectiveness. *Medical Decision Making*, 10, 212–15.

Briggs, A., Sculpher, M., and Claxton, K. (2006). *Decision Modelling for Health Economic Evaluation*. Oxford: Oxford University Press.

Brooks, R. (1996). EuroQoL: the current state of play. *Health Policy*, 37, 53–72.

Cookson, R., Drummond, M., and Weatherly, H. (2009). Explicit incorporation of equity considerations into economic evaluation of public health interventions. *Health Economics, Policy and Law*, 4(2), 231–45.

Culyer, A. and Bombard, Y. (2012). An equity framework for health technology assessments. *Medical Decision Making*, 32(3), 428–41.

Drummond, M.F., Sculpher, M.J., Torrance, G.W., O'Brien, B., and Stoddart, G.L. (2005). *Methods for the Economic Evaluation of Health Care Programmes* (3rd ed.). Oxford: Oxford University Press.

Herdman, M., Gudex, C., Lloyd, A., et al. (2011). Development and preliminary testing of the new five-level version of EQ-5D (EQ-5D-5L). *Quality of Life Research*, 20, 1727–36.

Jit, M., Barton, P., Chen, Y.-F., Olalekan, U., Aveyard, P., and Meads, C. (2009). *School-Based Interventions to Prevent the Uptake of Smoking Among Children and Young People: Cost-Effectiveness Model*. Birmingham: West Midlands Health Technology Assessment Collaboration.

Knapp, M. (1984). *The Economics of Social Care*. London: Macmillan.

Morris, S., Devlin, N., Parkin, D., and Spencer, A. (2012). *Economic Analysis in Health Care* (2nd ed.). London: Wiley & Sons.

Owen, L., Morgan, A., Fischer, A., Ellis, S., Hoy, A., and Kelly, M.P. (2011). The cost-effectiveness of public health interventions. *Journal of Public Health*, 34(1), 37–45.

Sassi, F., Archard, L., and Le Grand, J. (2001). Equity and the economic evaluation of healthcare. *Health Technology Assessment*, 5(3), 1–138.

Szende, A., Oppe, M., and Devlin, N. (2007). *EQ-5D Value Sets: Inventory, Comparative Review and User Guide*. Dordrecht, Netherlands: Springer.

Torgerson, D. and Spencer, A. (1996). Marginal costs and benefits. *British Medical Journal*, 312, 35–6.

Van Hout, B.A., Al, M.J., Gordon, G.S., and Rutten, F.F.H. (1994). Costs, effects and C/E ratios alongside a clinical trial. *Health Economics*, 3, 309–19.

Wang, G., Macera, C., Scudder-Soucie, B., Schmid, T., Pratt, M., and Buchner, D. (2005). A cost-benefit analysis of physical activity using bike/pedestrian trails. *Health Promotion Practice*, 6, 174–9.

Weatherly, H., Drummond, M., Claxton, K., et al. (2009). Methods for assessing the cost-effectiveness of public health interventions: key challenges and recommendations. *Health Policy*, 93(2–3), 85–92.

6.7

Behavioural economics and health

Judd B. Kessler and C. Yiwei Zhang

Introduction to behavioural economics and health

Behavioural economics is a field at the intersection of economics and psychology. Standard economic theory is built on the assumption that individuals are fully rational, completely selfish, forward-thinking decision-makers. This set of assumptions has allowed economists to predict behaviour using simple and tractable analytical models. But research from both economics and psychology has demonstrated that individuals regularly deviate from the predictions of standard economic theory and do so in systematic ways. Behavioural economics aims to: (1) explain why individuals deviate from the assumptions of standard economic theory and (2) use these insights to advance our models of individual behaviour.

By improving our models, behavioural economics allows policymakers to design interventions—like the health interventions that are described in this chapter—to more effectively achieve policy goals. In this way, behavioural economics is both descriptive, giving us a better picture of what behaviour looks like (and why it looks that way), and prescriptive, suggesting how policy can most effectively impact individual decision-making.

In this chapter, we discuss four major topic areas within economics and behavioural economics: (1) reward incentives, (2) information and salience, (3) context and framing, and (4) social forces. We will address each topic area with a section of the chapter. Within each section, we will highlight some of the topic area's most influential papers—including some from outside the health domain, which we believe provide relevant background.

Throughout the chapter, we describe research on a number of important health behaviours, including: medication adherence, obesity and weight control, and medical donation. While we touch on a number of other health behaviours in the chapter, we describe these three (and the reasons we find them of particular interest) in the following section.

It is worth noting that this chapter is by no means exhaustive in its coverage of the behavioural economics insights that might influence health behaviours or of the health behaviours that might be subject to the insights we discuss. Instead, we have picked a few illustrative settings where we have seen fruitful application of behavioural economics research and expect to see more in the coming years.

Externalities

Since many papers described in this chapter analyse interventions that affect health behaviours, it is worth outlining in broad strokes what standard economic theory says about when policymakers should be intervening in the health domain. This exercise provides a baseline for thinking through the additional policy interventions that might be justified by results from behavioural economics.

As already noted, standard economic theory models individuals as fully rational, selfish, and forward thinking. Individuals who satisfy these assumptions (who we simply call 'rational' throughout) are usually better off when left to their own devices. If a rational individual fails to take his doctor-prescribed medication, his decision is likely best for him, since by assumption he has thought through all the costs and benefits and decided that the costs (e.g. the cost of purchasing his medication and the pain of the side effects) outweigh the potential benefits (e.g. his lower risk of a heart attack).

Under the assumption that individuals are rational, there are generally only two reasons for intervention. First, if the rational individual suffers from a constraint that prevents him from implementing his preferred choice (e.g. he cannot afford to purchase his medication even though he would like to take it) then a policymaker may want to help the individual by loosening those constraints (e.g. providing him with a loan to help pay for his medication). Second, a policymaker may want to intervene if a decision creates *externalities*. Externalities are indirect effects on other agents that an individual does not fully consider when making his decisions. For example, if the patient in the earlier example cannot afford his cost of care for his heart attack, then when he fails to take his medication he forces society (i.e. the government and thus all tax payers) to cover some of his higher costs. Consequently, his decision about whether or not to take his medication affects people beside himself. That individuals fail to consider the costs imposed on other agents (or the benefits incurred by other agents) generally leads to socially inefficient outcomes.

Externalities are the key rationale for policy interventions across a number of domains both inside and outside of health. The government taxes pollution created by companies and individuals since pollution imposes negative externalities on those exposed to it. Regulation that forbids individuals from blasting music at 3 a.m. is designed to discourage the negative externality a rowdy party might have on neighbours who want to go to sleep.

As hinted above, a number of activities in the health domain create externalities. Some of the externalities are obvious while others are not. On the obvious end of the spectrum, medical donations (e.g. donations of blood, bone marrow, tissues, and organs) create positive externalities since they clearly benefit other people. Individuals who receive donor kidneys can expect better health outcomes than if they remained on dialysis. Some forms of preventative care are both beneficial to the recipient and create positive externalities for the health of other people. Receiving a flu shot or a vaccine helps keep the recipient from getting sick but also plays an important role in preventing the spread of disease since inoculated individuals are less likely to spread a virus. At the less obvious end of the spectrum, many activities that make a person healthier (e.g. healthy eating, exercise, medication adherence, and smoking cessation) can generate positive externalities for society since most individuals do not pay the full cost of their medical care and are instead covered in part by health insurance, the government, or a combination of the two. Consequently, requiring less care or staying healthy for longer (and requiring care later in life) makes the individual better off and lessens the cost paid by others in insurance premiums and taxes.

Given that many health activities have positive externalities, it may be socially beneficial to encourage individuals to engage in them. Economics and behavioural economics can provide strategies to most effectively encourage people to eat healthy, take their medication, donate their organs, get flu shots, and so on.

Behavioural biases

When rational individuals do not face constraints that restrict their choice and do not impose externalities with their actions, then there is little scope for intervention, even if we disagree with individuals' choices. An individual who can afford his medication and pays for all his health costs out of pocket may choose not to take his medication because he simply prefers not to. If he is fully informed about the costs and benefits and he is rational, we can do no better than to trust his judgement.

Behavioural economics has demonstrated, however, that individuals are not fully rational in the way standard economic theory predicts. Individuals who are not fully rational (who we will call 'behavioural') might suffer from biases that make it difficult for them to achieve the behaviour they actually prefer. This introduces another rationale for intervention: helping individuals achieve their own desired behaviour.

For example, one way in which behavioural individuals may make suboptimal choices is by displaying *present bias*. In particular, individuals often overweight costs and benefits incurred today (i.e. the present) relative to the costs and benefits incurred tomorrow (i.e. the future). This type of bias can lead individuals to forgo healthy behaviours and do so in a way that is inconsistent across time. Imagine an individual deciding whether to go to the gym, which has a cost today in terms of time and fatigue but has health benefits in the future. When considering his choice today, he may overweight the time and fatigue costs—since they are incurred in the present—and so decide to skip the gym. When considering his choice for tomorrow, however, he would not overweight those costs. When considering tomorrow, he may prefer to go to the gym and even believe that he will do so. When tomorrow arrives, however, it has become the present, and he again overweights the time and fatigue costs and again skips the workout.

This inconsistent behaviour is not unique to going to the gym. It can explain why individuals procrastinate about eating healthily, quitting smoking, or getting a flu shot. Each of these activities features a present cost (e.g. sacrificing something you enjoy, giving

up time, incurring physical discomfort) and a delayed benefit (e.g. better health) and so individuals might perpetually wait to incur those costs until a never-arriving tomorrow. If our patient from the medication example described earlier was present biased, he might skip taking his pill because he overweights the small costs he faces today like paying for the prescription and experiencing side effects. We consider these examples mistakes because if the behavioural agent could commit today to force himself to go to the gym (or eat the apple, or quit smoking, or get the flu shot, or take his pill) tomorrow, he would choose to do so. Behavioural individuals may want help making choices and following through with them.

Present bias is just one of many behavioural phenomena that might make individuals deviate from their own desired behaviour. For example, a behavioural individual might forget to take his medication, which a rational agent would not do. A behavioural individual might not attend to all the relevant data needed to make an informed decision about whether to take the pill or might fail to aggregate the data he does consider.

Behavioural economics can help identify cases where individuals might have trouble (e.g. due to present bias or forgetfulness) and suggest strategies to help individuals achieve their ideal behaviours (e.g. commitment contracts or reminders, discussed later in the chapter). As we go through each topic area, we will describe the way individual behaviour differs from the predictions of standard economic theory. We will then describe interventions—suggested by economics and behavioural economics—that can encourage individuals to improve their own decision-making and generate better health outcomes for the decision-maker and better outcomes for society at large.

Health behaviours

Here we highlight three health behaviours that we reference repeatedly throughout the chapter. We think these behaviours are of particular interest for interventions motivated by behavioural economics.

Medication adherence

The failure of individuals to properly adhere to medication regimens prescribed by their doctors is a major issue in healthcare. Non-adherence can often lead to serious health consequences as well as increased healthcare costs down the road. Estimates from Osterberg and Blaschke (2005) suggest that around half of all medication-related hospital admissions in the United States are a result of failure to adhere properly to medication. These hospital admissions are estimated to cost approximately $100 billion a year. While medication expense may be part of the explanation, non-adherence is a problem even among patients who face zero co-pays and so can get their medication for free (see Doshi et al. 2009). Cutler and Everett (2010) suggest various reasons why people fail to adhere to medication including: lifestyle, psychological issues, health literacy, support systems, and side effects. Behavioural economics interventions that help individuals overcome some of the common barriers to adherence can generate better health outcomes and lower cost of care.

Obesity and weight control

Obesity is a major problem in healthcare and is blamed for over 110,000 deaths a year in the United States alone (Flegal et al.

2007). Flegal et al. (2010) calculate that 68 per cent of Americans are overweight or obese. Schroeder (2007) suggests that decreasing obesity—along with decreasing smoking—can lead to substantial improvements in the state of health in the United States. Individuals often have trouble controlling their weight. DellaVigna and Malmendier (2006) find that individuals buy expensive monthly gym memberships but go so infrequently that paying per visit would cost less. This result suggests that individuals have trouble making it to the gym even though they want to and intend to go. Behavioural economics can help explain the difficulty individuals have in sticking to a weight-loss regimen and can provide strategies or interventions to help people succeed.

Medical donation

There are a number of forms of medical donation, including blood and plasma donation, bone marrow donation, and organ and tissue donation. Medical donation is an important area of health research since these donations can have a substantial impact on health outcomes (Schnitzler et al. 2005a, 2005b) and cost of care (Dew et al. 1997) and there is often significant need. As of July 2014 over 123,000 individuals in the United States were on the waiting list for an organ transplant (United Network for Organ Sharing n.d.). Registered organ donors make their organs available for transplant upon their death, and one deceased donor can provide up to eight life-saving organs. However, fewer than 50 per cent of Americans over the age of 18 are registered as organ donors (Donate Life America 2014). Behavioural economics interventions may be particularly relevant in motivating medical donation since monetary incentives are often not allowed in medical donation (Roth 2007).

Reward incentives

Reward incentives are a natural place to start an investigation of how economic and behavioural economic forces impact health behaviours. Reward incentives show how traditional economic interventions work and how these interventions can be improved by insights from behavioural economics.

In standard economic theory, individuals value money and other tangible rewards and engage in effort to get them. People go to work to earn money and we expect them to work harder when there is more money at stake. Consequently, standard economic theory suggests that reward incentives—particularly monetary incentives—can motivate individuals to engage in behaviours that they otherwise would avoid. We begin this section by describing interventions that utilize standard reward incentives in the health domain.

Behavioural economics has made two important advances with regard to reward incentives and how they affect behaviour. First, it has suggested that not all incentives are created equal. Individuals overweight small probability events and feel losses more severely than equivalent gains. A reward incentive that leverages these biases might be more effective for the same expected value. Second, and much more troubling for standard economic theory, behavioural economics has shown that in certain domains individuals respond in perverse ways to reward incentives. In some settings, monetary incentives lead individuals to respond with *less* effort rather than more.

After describing settings where standard reward incentives motivate health behaviours, we catalogue examples of interventions that leverage behavioural biases in designing reward incentives. Finally, we describe settings where reward incentives backfire.

Standard reward incentives

There are a number of health domains where standard reward incentives have been shown to successfully influence health behaviours. Here we highlight their use in three domains: obesity and weight control, smoking cessation, and medical donation.

In the context of obesity and weight control, researchers have used monetary and non-monetary incentives to encourage more frequent gym attendance. Charness and Gneezy (2009) report the results of two such studies on incentives and gym attendance. In the first study, they compare the gym attendance of three groups of college students participating in a randomized experiment. One group was provided only with information regarding the value of exercise. A second group was provided with the same information and received an additional $25 if they visited the gym once in the following week. A third group was treated like the second group but received an additional $100 if they visited the gym eight more times in the following 4 weeks. The authors find that individuals respond to monetary incentives. Those who were paid to go to the gym were much more likely to do so, and those who were paid for more visits went more often. The second study took a similar form but included biometric measures to better gauge health improvements. The study found that individuals paid to go to the gym more often had lower body fat, lower body mass index, and improved on a number of other health measures. The authors provide evidence that the effects from both studies persist; those who were paid to go to the gym continued to do so at higher rates for a few months after the incentives were removed. This result suggests that these individuals may have formed a habit of gym attendance. As will be seen throughout this section, this potential habit formation is quite rare in the context of reward incentives.

A similar study by Acland and Levy (2013) also finds that individuals were more likely to go to the gym when paid to do so. They also observe that the effect persists in the weeks after the incentive was removed. After a semester break, however, the group that had seemed to form a habit for gym attendance was no longer more likely to attend, suggesting that the habit was short-lived.

In the context of smoking cessation, Volpp et al. (2009) report the results from an experiment at a multinational company. Half of the employees in their sample were given information about smoking cessation programmes while the other half received the same information plus incentives worth a total of $750 for enrolling in a programme, quitting smoking within 6 months, and staying quit for an additional 6 months. Individuals with the incentives were significantly more likely to complete the programme, quit, and stay quit.

In the context of medical donation, the use of monetary incentives is often restricted. For example, the National Organ Transplant Act of 1984 prohibits the use of 'valuable consideration' to induce organ donation. Fortunately, standard economic theory does not require that reward incentives be monetary for them to be effective. In the context of medical donation, a variety of non-monetary reward incentives have been shown to generate increased willingness to donate.

Individuals are more likely to donate blood when provided with coupons for merchandise (Ferrari et al. 1985), lottery tickets

(Goette and Stutzer 2008), and other incentives (for a summary of blood donation incentives, see Goette et al. (2010)). Lacetera et al. (2012) do an extensive empirical analysis of participation in American Red Cross blood drives and find that drives with non-monetary incentives for blood donation (including blankets, T-shirts, mugs, and coupons to retailers) generate more donors. In addition, the larger the economic value of the incentive, the bigger the increase in donors. They caution, however, that some of the increase in donation may be the result of substitution away from nearby drives that do not have incentives. A review of a variety of blood donation research supports the claim that incentives increase blood donation without affecting quality (Lacetera et al. 2013). Related work has demonstrated that individuals are more likely to become bone marrow donors when legislation that provides donors with paid leave and tax incentives is in place (Lacetera et al. 2014).

A particular non-monetary incentive that might motivate individuals to register as organ donors is priority on organ donation waiting lists for those who register but end up needing organs rather than being in a position to provide them. This non-monetary incentive—a higher likelihood of receiving a transplantable organ or receiving a transplantable organ more quickly—can be given to registered donors simply by changing the way organs are allocated. Both Israel and Singapore currently provide priority on organ donor waiting lists to registered donors. Kessler and Roth (2012) investigate the effect of a priority rule on a laboratory game designed to look like organ donor registration and show that it substantially increases the likelihood of donation.

Early data from Israel, which implemented the policy fully in 2012, suggests that the policy may have increased the number of deceased organ donors and the organ donation rate (Lavee et al. 2013). One quirk of the Israeli policy, however, is that it has the potential for a loophole that allows individuals to receive priority without ever being in a position to donate their organs. A follow-up study (Kessler and Roth 2014a) investigates the effect of a loophole and finds that in a laboratory setting, such a loophole can eliminate the beneficial effect of the priority rule. Allowing individuals to receive the priority without paying the costs of donation completely eliminates the effectiveness of the priority rule. In addition, when subjects receive feedback about the use of the loophole they become less likely to register as donors than when no priority system is available, suggesting that how these priority systems are implemented can be crucial to their success.

Designing incentives using behavioural economics

As noted earlier, behavioural economics has shown that individuals overweight small probability events, feel losses more severely than equivalent gains (called *loss aversion*, see Kahneman and Tversky (1979)), and do not like to feel regret (called *regret aversion*).

Lotteries can take advantage of the fact that individuals overweight small probability events. For example, providing a 1 per cent chance of winning $100 might motivate people more substantially than offering them $1 directly, even though the two have the same expected value.

Combining probability weighting with loss aversion and regret aversion, some studies have motivated individuals to take health actions using *regret lotteries*. In a regret lottery, all individuals are entered into the lottery and informed about whether their name is picked. If an individual fails to take a required action, however, she fails to earn the lottery prize when picked. Even if a 1 per cent chance of winning $100 is not enough to motivate an individual to take an action (e.g. going to the gym today), she might go to the gym to avoid the potential distress of knowing she would have won $100 but lost it by skipping her workout. The regret lottery leverages overweighting of small probabilities through the lottery, loss aversion by framing the earnings as money that is lost, and regret aversion since it threatens individuals who fail to take the rewarded action with feelings of regret.

Regret lotteries have successfully influenced behaviour in a variety of health domains. In the context of medication adherence, Volpp et al. (2008) find that providing a regret lottery worth either $3 or $5 in expected value significantly increases the likelihood that individuals correctly take their prescribed medications. In the context of weight loss, Volpp et al. (2008) find that subjects lose significantly more weight when provided with a regret lottery that pays out an expected $3 per day (in the form of a 20 per cent chance of winning $10 plus a 1 per cent chance of winning $100) if the subject is on track to his or her weight loss goal.

Another way to leverage loss aversion with monetary incentives is to provide individuals the opportunity to make *commitment contracts* (also called *deposit contracts*) in which they put up their own money. This money is then forfeited if they fail to achieve a certain goal, such as reaching a weight loss target or attending the gym a specified number of times in a week or month. This strategy allows individuals to create monetary incentives for themselves and leverage loss aversion simultaneously. Volpp et al. (2008) also find that a commitment contract (in which committed funds were matched one to one by researchers to increase take up) was effective at achieving weight lost by study participants.

One concern with monetary incentives of any form is that they may generate short-term effects. Once the monetary incentives are removed, individuals may backslide into their unhealthy behaviours. In Volpp et al. (2008) once the regret lottery or commitment contract was removed, both groups regained a significant amount of the weight they had lost during the study. John et al. (2011) run a longer study in which some subjects have a commitment contract to lose weight (also with a one-to-one match) for a period of 24 weeks. They find that subjects with the commitment contract lose significantly more weight but much of the weight is regained in the 8 weeks after the incentive is removed. At the end of those 8 weeks, the weight of the group that previously had the contract was no different from the control group that never had the contract.

On the other hand, Giné et al. (2010) find that the effects of a 6-month commitment contract on smoking cessation can persist over the long run. In particular, they find that smokers who were randomly offered the contract were significantly more likely to pass a urine test for nicotine and cotinine (by-products of tobacco use), and they remained significantly more likely to pass another (surprise) urine test administered 6 months after the removal of the incentive. Examples of behavioural economics in action are given in Box 6.7.1.

There are other ways in which incentives can be altered to take advantage of forces uncovered by behavioural economics. One example is to bundle something desirable (or addictive) with a behaviour you want to encourage. The old adage 'a spoonful of

Box 6.7.1 Behavioural economics in action

Behavioural Insights Team (BIT)

Established in 2010 by UK Prime Minister David Cameron, the BIT (nicknamed the 'Nudge Unit') uses insights from behavioural economics and psychology in developing and testing different public policy measures. For example, inspired in part by Giné et al. (2010), the BIT is considering using loss-aversion and commitment contracts in their countrywide efforts to reduce smoking (BIT 2010).

StickK.com

The brainchild of several economists, StickK.com is a website that allows individuals to create and enter into their own commitment contracts to help them achieve personal goals. Common personal goals include losing weight, exercising regularly, and quitting smoking. Individuals determine how much money, if any, to put at stake and designate another individual to verify the goal outcome. Should an individual fail to reach his or her goal, the forfeited money goes to a charity of their choice or to an 'anti-charity' that the individual does not want to support, making failure to meet the commitment feel even more costly.

sugar helps the medicine go down' can help explain why some vitamins are candy-coated. In this spirit, Milkman et al. (2014) developed an incentive for gym attendance using an activity that they deemed to be desirable and possibly addictive. In their study, researchers provided each subject in their treatment groups with a loaner-iPod loaded with popular books-on-tape that were considered relatively addictive (e.g. *The Hunger Games* and *The Da Vinci Code*). For one treatment group, the iPods were stored in lockers at the gym and could only be accessed if the subject was at the gym. The authors found a significant increase in gym attendance in this group over the control group, but also found that the effect deteriorated over time.

Crowding out

Researchers in a number of disciplines across the social sciences have uncovered some perverse effects of incentives. In particular, financial incentives have been shown at times to decrease effort rather than increase it. This phenomenon has been called *crowding out of intrinsic motivation* as the monetary incentive is thought to replace the intrinsic motivation to engage in an action (see Gneezy et al. (2011) for a summary).

For example, Gneezy and Rustichini (2000a, 2000b) find a number of crowding out results in domains outside of health. They find that paying people a small amount for each correct IQ problem solved can lead to fewer solved problems than if no monetary incentive is in place. They also find that paying money to volunteers (e.g. 1 per cent or 10 per cent of the amount of money collected while door-to-door fundraising) can decrease the amount of money volunteers collect. Finally, imposing a monetary fine for being late to pick up children from day care led parents to be late more often rather than less. Similarly, it has been shown that paying people for a short while to take a certain action and then removing

the incentive can lead individuals to provide less effort than before the incentive was introduced (Deci 1971).

In the context of medical donation, Titmuss (1971) argued that providing a monetary incentive for blood donation might decrease the amount of blood received. Mellstrom and Johannesson (2008) find some weak evidence of this crowding out in blood donation in response to an incentive worth about $7. In their experiment, they offer the incentive to subjects to complete a health examination that was required to become a blood donor. In one treatment the incentive could only be taken in cash while in another treatment the subjects had the option to have the money donated to charity. They do not see crowding out in response to the incentive on average, but they do see it among women. Interestingly, crowding out is only present when the incentive must be taken in cash and donation rates return to the control treatment levels when the money can be donated to charity.

Reward incentives: discussion

One disadvantage of financial interventions is that pay-for-performance schemes like providing monetary incentives to engage in health behaviour are viewed by many as unfair or unethical (see, e.g. Long et al. 2008). There may be a way to mitigate this concern by making the incentives non-monetary. In the context of blood donation, individuals report a larger willingness to donate for a 10-euro voucher (to purchase books or food) rather than for 10 euros in cash (Lacetera and Macis 2010a).

As seen throughout this section, another potential disadvantage of reward incentives is that they may fail to build enduring habits. While very effective when in place, monetary incentives regularly fail to motivate continued behaviour change after they are removed. Only a few studies we've discussed—Charness and Gneezy (2009), Volpp et al. (2009), Giné et al. (2010), and Acland and Levy (2013)—have found evidence that paying subjects to engage in a health behaviour had a lasting impact. In addition, Acland and Levy (2013) suggest that an exogenous break in attendance (a semester break for students) eliminated this effect. One solution to this problem is to keep monetary incentives in place indefinitely, a possibility using variation in premiums allowed under the Patient Protection and Affordable Care Act (Volpp et al. 2011).

The inability for monetary incentives to lead to sustained behaviour change may be in part a function of the potential crowding out effects of such incentives, although there is still much work to be done to better understand crowding out effects and habit formation in health behaviours.

Salience and information

An assumption made by standard economic theory is that individuals have no limitation in their ability to make decisions, either in terms of the cognitive capacity to solve complex problems or the amount of time needed to do so.

To illustrate, imagine an individual who enters a shop to purchase groceries. According to standard economic theory, this individual considers all the goods he expects to be available for purchase in the shop (including all their prices or, if the prices are too costly to discover, what he expects their prices to be) and calculates which basket of goods would be best for him to buy. In doing so, the individual also considers items in others stores that he could potentially buy instead, factoring in the time and cost it would take to drive to those shops to continue his shopping.

In reality, we have finite mental resources available to make our decisions so we are prone to ignore much of the information available and to take shortcuts in aggregating what information we do attend to. An actual individual walking into the grocery shop might forget to pick up his vitamins, be distracted by a prominent display of sweets, or simply not realize that a healthier snack alternative is available on a bottom shelf.

Another way to put this is that individuals are *boundedly rational*. Simon (1957) suggested that because individuals are limited by their cognitive capacity, as well as by information and time constraints, they lack the resources to make a truly optimal decision. Any decisions made by a boundedly rational individual are at best optimal within his or her constraints.

Bounded rationality can influence individual behaviour in several ways. For instance, individuals may exhibit forgetfulness (i.e. limited memory), may fail to pay attention (i.e. inattention), and may make decisions without collecting all the relevant information available (i.e. imperfect information). We address these three phenomena and their applications to health behaviours in turn in the following subsections.

Limited memory

No one likes to forget things. During the course of a day, however, many different pieces of information are presented to us, and we must exert mental energy to remember the important ones.

In the health realm, this limited ability to perfectly store and process information can help explain the difficulty many individuals have in adhering to a prescribed course of treatment. One potential explanation for poor medication adherence is that individuals are forgetful. Several studies have investigated interventions designed to remind people to take their medication. In theory, the ideal intervention requires no additional cognitive resources.

To this end, electronic reminders are increasingly being used to address poor medication adherence rates. These reminders alert individuals by either providing an audio or visual reminder or by sending an automatic electronic message such as a text message. Electronic reminders present two distinct advantages over other types of reminders. First, these electronic reminders *actively* remind individuals to take their medication. In contrast, passive reminders such as day-of-the-week pillboxes or blister packaging provide information that medication should be taken but are not helpful reminders if they are not seen. Active reminders are better suited for individuals whose main reason for poor adherence is forgetfulness whereas passive reminders assist individuals who need help remembering the correct dosage and combination of medication to take. Second, these reminders can be automated to arrive at a specific time. For example, if an individual is liable to forget to take his medication, a reminder provided when he is not with his pills might also be forgotten and fail to improve adherence. Third, these reminders are relatively inexpensive because they can be automated. Alternative reminders such as personal phone calls can increase adherence but often require costly time investment and commitment by healthcare providers.

Vervloet et al. (2012) review 13 randomized control trials that test the effectiveness of different electronic reminders on adherence to various types of chronic medication. They find evidence suggesting that electronic reminders encourage medication adherence in the short run (less than 6 months) but are less effective over the long run. Furthermore, effectiveness can vary across medications for a given type of electronic reminder. While text messages are an effective tool for increasing adherence among adult patients with HIV (Hardy et al. 2011; Pop-Eleches et al. 2011) or children requiring influenza vaccinations (Stockwell et al. 2012), they have mixed effects on adherence for women taking oral contraceptives (Hou et al. 2010; Castano et al. 2012).

Forgetfulness can influence other health decisions as well. A large number of preventative care measures require individuals to remember not only to set up an appointment but also to follow through with it. The Centers for Disease Control and Prevention recommend numerous preventative screening measures such as checks for high blood pressure and diabetes screenings. Many individuals fail to take the recommended preventative care measures, even when the monetary costs of doing so are effectively zero. Forgetfulness may help to explain why individuals fail to take these recommended preventative care measures.

The difficulty in remembering to engage in recommended health behaviours has prompted both individuals and employers to seek out ways to outsource the task of remembering. The company Evive Health, LLC keeps track of when the employees of their clients are due for preventative screenings and sends personalized reminders at the appropriate times, encouraging employees to make appointments and providing information on how to do so. That employers are willing to pay companies such as Evive highlights the importance of these behavioural consequences on health outcomes.

Inattention

The salience of a given piece of information, or the degree to which that piece of information stands out relative to other information, can affect whether an individual considers it in her decision-making process. If a piece of information is not particularly salient, it might be overlooked or more easily forgotten. Consider two individuals who must remember to take their medication. The first individual has a toothache and experiences acute pain when he forgets his medication. The second individual suffers from high cholesterol and does not discern any noticeable difference in discomfort if he forgets. Because the pain of forgetting is more salient for the individual with a toothache, he may be more likely to remember his medication than the individual with high cholesterol. In this case, the salience of individual health symptoms can influence whether or not an individual remembers to take his medication.

Salience may also play a role by affecting the actual act of remembering. A person who programmes a reminder into their calendar for their next doctor's appointment is effectively making that appointment more salient. Milkman et al. (2011) report the results of a field experiment to test whether suggesting individuals write down when they intend to get an influenza vaccine (i.e. making it more salient) increases rates of vaccination. The authors study the behaviour of employees who receive a reminder mailing that provides information on the times and locations of free on-site vaccination clinics. Treated subjects were randomly assigned to receive a prompt to write down either: (1) the date the employee plans to get vaccinated or (2) both the date and the time the employee plans to get vaccinated. The authors find that the vaccination rate for employees with the date and time prompt was significantly higher than for the control group that was not prompted to write down anything. The rate for employees with the date only prompt was directionally, but not significantly, higher than the control group. These results suggest that encouraging individuals to make a more concrete plan—making the plan more salient—can increase the likelihood of compliance.

Imperfect information

Regardless of whether a person is rational or is subject to behavioural biases, information is necessary for making optimal decisions. Consequently, decisions often change as more information becomes available. Bounded rationality can influence this process if it prevents individuals from optimally gathering or aggregating information.

In the past two decades, a growing literature has emerged looking at the effects of providing nutritional or caloric information on nutrient intake, the consumption of food, and other health outcomes. Such information could affect behaviour if individuals do not otherwise have all the information they need to make their food consumption decisions.

Several papers have studied the impact of the Nutrition Labeling and Education Act (NLEA), which mandated the nutrition labelling of all pre-packaged foods in the United States beginning in 1994. Prior to the NLEA, nutritional labelling was voluntary with the exception of products that contained added nutrients or made nutritional claims. These studies find that the enactment of the NLEA was associated with decreased body weight (for some groups) and lower probability of obesity (Variyam and Cawley 2006), increased fibre and iron intake (Variyam 2008), and lower calorie intake (Kim et al. 2000; Abaluck 2011).

Other papers in the literature have instead focused on the provision of information on the calorie content of foods. Several cities in the United States, such as New York and Philadelphia, currently require chain restaurants to post the caloric content of their menu items. These laws are in part a reaction to the concern that individuals may have imperfect information as to the true nutritional value of the items they purchase, which may in turn lead to suboptimal food consumption. Wisdom et al. (2010) conducted a field experiment at a fast-food sandwich chain to study the effects of providing calorie information. They find that total calorie consumption significantly decreases by 60 calories on average when information on calorie content is provided. Wisdom et al. (2012) find that making healthier sandwiches a more convenient choice relative to less healthy sandwiches has significant decreases on total calorie consumption but only when the intervention is relatively heavy-handed. While these findings suggest that consumers do in fact change their consumption decisions when given more information, evidence from other studies is more mixed (Elbel et al. 2009; Bollinger et al. 2011; Finkelstein et al. 2011). In addition, many of these studies are limited by the fact that individuals who are induced to consume less due to an experimental treatment may consume more at a later meal when the experimenter can no longer observe them.

Salience and information: discussion

The extent to which we care that individuals are boundedly rational depends on whether (and by how much) individuals are made worse off because of their cognitive limitations. In the realm of healthcare, the cognitive limitations faced by boundedly rational individuals might have important ramifications for health and their overall well-being.

Despite the research in this field, a great deal remains unknown about bounded rationality in the health domain and how to best address cognitive resource limitations. We do not yet understand in which settings the behaviours will be most affected by bounded rationality. For example, the likelihood of forgetting (and thus the effectiveness of reminders) may depend on the size of the costs to non-adherence. On one hand, the likelihood of forgetting to take a medication may be higher when a disease is serious and an individual does not want to think about it—suggesting reminders may be most valuable when the consequences of non-adherence are relatively large. Alternatively, the likelihood of forgetting might be higher when the stakes are lower—suggesting reminders will help most when the consequences of non-adherence are small.

Additionally, it is hard to trace back from a given behaviour to a particular behavioural bias or cognitive limitation, which makes it hard to identify what intervention will be most effective. For example, an individual may fail to make a mammogram appointment not because she is forgetful but instead because the costs associated with figuring out where to make an appointment are too great, or because she lacks full information on the risks of breast cancer, or because she perpetually plans to do it tomorrow. Knowing how to most successfully impact behaviour requires a better understanding of its underlying cause.

Context and framing

According to standard economic theory, rational individuals make the optimal choice given the set of options available and the constraints they face. The way in which options are presented does not influence the decision made by a rational agent. For example, a rational individual choosing between two different types of over-the-counter pain relievers is not influenced by the order in which he sees the pain relievers when walking down the pharmacy aisle. Likewise, a rational individual deciding whether to enrol in one of three healthcare plans is not influenced by the fact that his employer defaulted him into one of them.

If an individual behaves as standard economic theory predicts, her choices reflect her true preferences. But behavioural economics suggests that context and framing can play an important role in subtly influencing how we make decisions. Evidence of this influence exists across a wide range of domains, including many high-stakes environments where one might think individuals would be properly motivated to implement their optimal choices. In this section, we discuss three examples of how individuals are influenced by context and framing. First, individuals demonstrate a strong tendency to exhibit inertia around default options. Second, individuals are easily influenced by visual cues. Third, individual decisions depend on the manner in which the choice set is presented or *framed*. Understanding the contextual influences to which individuals are susceptible is critical for understanding individual behaviour and for effectively designing behavioural interventions.

Default effects

One example of the effect of context on behaviour is the strong tendency of individuals to exhibit inertia around default options.

Specifically, individuals tend to remain with their default choice even in cases where the default is randomly assigned. This *default effect* is well documented in empirical work across many different choice settings, from retirement savings decisions (Samuelson and Zeckhauser 1988; Madrian and Shea 2001; Choi et al. 2004; Carroll et al. 2009) to prescription drug home delivery enrolment (Beshears et al. 2013), to Internet privacy agreements (Bellman et al. 2001, 2004).

In a classic study on default effects outside of the health domain, Johnson et al. (1993) investigate whether individuals remain in the auto insurance plan into which they were defaulted. The authors were motivated by evidence from choices in the 1990s when the states of New Jersey and Pennsylvania introduced auto insurance plans with lower rates but limited rights to sue. Drivers in Pennsylvania were defaulted into the more expensive 'full right' plan whereas drivers in the neighbouring state of New Jersey were defaulted into the less expensive 'limited right' plan. Because the underlying choices—the full right plan on one hand and the limited right plan on the other—were the same across states, whether drivers were defaulted into one plan or the other was not expected to impact behaviour. However, a reported 75 per cent of Pennsylvania drivers stayed with their 'full right' plan whereas only 20 per cent of New Jersey drivers switched to the 'full right' plan.

Defaults play an important role in many health domains, including insurance plan choice. For example, people who remain eligible for Medicare Part D are defaulted into their prescriptive drug coverage plan from the previous year. Ericson (forthcoming) shows that few enrolees switch from their plan from the previous year, even when relative prices of plans change. Likewise, Handel (2013) looks at the behaviour of enrolees in a Preferred Provider Organization (PPO) health insurance plan after relative prices of plans changed significantly. As a result of the price changes, the current plan of some enrolees became strictly dominated by an alternative PPO health insurance plan (that is, for any possible level and type of medical expenditure, their current plan would require higher combined premium and out-of-pocket costs than the alternative PPO plan). Despite these enrolees' plans being strictly dominated, Handel finds that 89 per cent of the enrolees choose the default: to remain in their current plan. Default effects can similarly be found in employee contributions to health-care flexible spending accounts (Schweitzer et al. 1996).

Default rules often affect whether individuals participate in certain programmes. Default rules generally either require explicit consent (e.g. an opt-in rule) or presume consent (e.g. an opt-out rule). In the United States, deceased organ donation follows an opt-in rule, requiring explicit consent from the deceased (e.g. having previously joined a state registry) or consent from the deceased's next-of-kin. But not all countries follow an opt-in rule. A number of European countries follow an opt-out rule where individuals are automatically assumed to be a donor unless they previously chose to remove themselves from the registry. So long as the costs to opting in or opting out are small, the default rule should have little influence on donor registration rates. Johnson and Goldstein (2003, 2004) show, however, that there is considerable variation in organ donor registration rates by the default rule. They report that at the time of their research the effective consent rate was around 17 per cent in the United Kingdom, which followed an opt-in rule, and was 98 per cent in Belgium, which followed an opt-out rule. Of the countries surveyed by the authors, the difference in participation rate between the highest opt-in and lowest opt-out countries was nearly 60 percentage points.

In a corresponding hypothetical choice experiment about organ donation, Johnson and Goldstein randomly assigned individuals to one of three default conditions: (1) opt-in, (2) opt-out, and (3) neutral. Under the third condition, individuals were not defaulted into or out of the donor pool but were instead asked to make an 'active choice' between either donating or not donating. They find that the average participation rate by individuals under the opt-out condition is significantly higher than that of individuals under the opt-in condition. Johnson and Goldstein also find that the neutral condition is not significantly different from the opt-out condition, suggesting that asking individuals to make an active choice might be more effective at generating organ donor registrations than the opt-in policy. Similar arguments about organ donation are made in the popular press (Thaler 2009). The United Kingdom and a number of US states (including, notably: Illinois, California, and New York) have changed the request for organ donor registration from opt-in to active choice.

However, it is too soon to tell whether these changes will increase organ donor registration rates. Experimental evidence on real organ donor registrations finds that the active choice frame does not improve registration rates over an opt-in frame, and may lead to lower consent rates from next-of-kin (Kessler and Roth 2014b).

There are a number of explanations for why individuals tend to exhibit inertia around default options. Traditional economic theory suggests that the default effect could be accounted for by the presence of switching or transaction costs. These costs do not have to be monetary in nature but can also include time and effort that individuals have to expend to switch away from the default. If the costs to switching are large enough, individuals will actually prefer not to switch from their default option. Inertia around default options could also be rational behaviour if individuals believe the default option is an implicit recommendation by the person who chose the default. For example, an individual may view a default health plan choice as an implicit recommendation from her employer.

Default effects are often present even when the apparent costs to switching are negligible and the likelihood of the default being viewed as an implicit recommendation is small. An alternative behavioural explanation for such an effect is the bounded rationality of individuals. For example, an individual may be enrolled in the same prescription drug plan as the previous year (the default option) because after the initial enrolment period, he paid little attention to any changes in circumstances that might induce him to switch. Because of this inattention, the individual fails to make a conscious choice and so is automatically enrolled into his plan from the previous year.

Alternatively, people may simply exhibit *status quo bias*, a preference for the current status quo independent of whatever the best option is, or *omission bias*, a preference for inaction over action. Any combination of these explanations could lead to inaction and thus the observed default effect. Regardless of what the true underlying mechanism is, however, it remains that defaults can have a significant influence on individual choices.

Visual cues

Visual cues and other environmental factors can also play a role in individual decision-making. Benartzi and Thaler (2007) find that the number of lines displayed on an investment elections form influenced the number of funds into which individuals invested their retirement savings. Individuals were randomly given either a form with eight lines or a form with only four lines (but a nearly costless way to increase the number of lines). Of the individuals given the four-line form, only 10 per cent invested in more than four funds. By comparison, approximately 40 per cent of individuals given the eight-line form invested in more than four funds.

Within the realm of health, there is an extensive literature looking at how visual cues can affect food consumption and food choices. Everything from the visibility or salience of food to the size and shape of food packaging can influence individual consumption. For example, people consume more food when they are given larger serving bowls (Wansink and Cheney 2005) or there is greater perceived variety (Rolls et al. 1981; Kahn and Wansink 2004). They pour 30 per cent more alcohol when using short, wide glasses rather than tall, narrow glasses (Wansink and van Ittersum 2007).

The environment in which we eat can also affect food consumption choices. An individual purchasing groceries may be more likely to buy tempting goods, such as chocolate bars, if they are located near the register where the effort cost of adding them to the purchase is low than if they are located at the opposite end of the shop. In this example, the convenience of the chocolate bars may influence the likelihood of purchase. Hanks et al. (2012) studied whether the conversion of a cafeteria lunch line into a 'convenience line' that only offered healthy food options influenced the consumption of healthy (versus unhealthy) foods. The authors find that following the introduction of a convenience line, the consumption (measured in grams) of healthy foods chosen did not change but the consumption of unhealthy foods decreased significantly by 27.9 per cent. The share of total consumption from healthy foods increased on average while the share from unhealthy foods decreased.

Framing

Another assumption about rational economic actors is that their preferences are consistent. This consistency implies that the way a set of choices is framed or presented does not influence the individual's decision so long as no additional information is conveyed by the frame.

In a famous example, Tversky and Kahneman (1981) demonstrated that framing affects choices using a hypothetical life-or-death scenario. Their study asked participants to consider a scenario where the United States is preparing for the outbreak of a disease, which is expected to kill 600 people. There are two proposed programmes to combat the disease. The first set of respondents to the survey were told:

- If Programme A is adopted, 200 people will be saved.

- If Programme B is adopted, there is 1/3 probability that 600 people will be saved, and 2/3 probability that no people will be saved.

The second set of respondents were instead told:

- If Programme C is adopted, 400 people will die.

- If Programme D is adopted, there is 1/3 probability that nobody will die, and 2/3 probability that 600 people will die.

Both groups were then asked which of the two programmes they would favour. The first programme for each group involves no risk (the outcome is presented with certainty) whereas the second programme involves some risk-taking. Of the respondents in the first group, 72 per cent chose Programme A over Programme B. Of the respondents in the second group, 78 per cent chose Programme D over Programme C. The authors point out, however, that Programme A and Programme C are equivalent, as are Programme B and Programme D.

When the estimates of the consequences of each of the programmes were framed in terms of lives saved, respondents preferred the programme that offered the certain outcome. Yet when the consequences were instead framed in terms of lives lost, respondents preferred the programme that involved risk-taking. As it turns out, in situations involving risk, individuals often exhibit such preference reversals depending on whether the outcome is framed in terms of gains or losses. Individuals are generally risk averse when facing gains and risk seeking when facing losses (Kahneman and Tversky 1979).

While the proposed scenario of a disease outbreak was hypothetical, such framing effects have been shown to have consequences for individuals making real decisions regarding their health. McNeil et al. (1982) find that individuals are more likely to prefer surgery to radiation therapy (which has no risk of death during treatment) when told that surgeries face a 90 per cent survival rate as opposed to a 10 per cent mortality rate. In another study, women's attitudes towards potential side effects of tamoxifen, a medication taken by high-risk women to help prevent the first-time development of breast cancer, varied depending on whether they were informed that 2.8 out of 100 women experience cardiovascular problems as a side effect versus 28 out of 1000 women (Zikmund-Fisher et al. 2008). While the information presented is the same in either case, participants were more concerned about the potential side effects when randomly informed of the risk statistic using the larger denominator. The way in which this information is framed can significantly affect the decision-making process.

Context and framing: discussion

Recognizing the influence that context and framing can have on individual behaviour is important, especially when the choices lead to significantly different outcomes—some of which might make individuals better off. It is often difficult to separately identify the effects of context and framing from other factors that may come into play, and so any estimates of the effects of these cues on behaviour and welfare must be considered carefully. Even with this caveat, however, it is clear that context and framing can significantly influence individual choices and outcomes. For example, Handel (2013) finds that, on average, individuals who are defaulted into their health plan choice from the previous year (but are given an option to switch) forgo roughly $2000 in implied savings by staying in their default plan rather than choosing an alternative option. If individuals choose to stay in the same plan because they were defaulted into it, rather than due to switching costs, the decision can represent a substantial loss to individuals. Furthermore, if defaults lead to low levels of switching, the factors that influence individuals in their initial decision can end up having long-term effects.

One way to reduce the influence of default effects, visual cues, and framing is to help individuals overcome these biases while making their decisions. For example, providing information that lessens the complexity of a decision can decrease default effects. Enrolees in prescription drug plans who are provided with information regarding the relative costs of each of the available plans are much more likely to switch from their current plan (the default) than those who do not receive such information (Kling et al. 2012).

Similarly, rather than requiring individuals to either opt in or opt out of participation or enrolment in a programme, an alternative solution is to require that these individuals actively consider the decision being made. This can be achieved either by designing the choice environment so that individuals are forced to consider whether they really want to opt in (or out) or by requiring that they make an active choice.

It is sometimes difficult or impossible, however, to design an environment that does not influence behaviours in some way. And in many scenarios involving public health, it may actually be preferable to use behavioural economics to design choice environments so as to encourage certain behaviours. For example, it is extremely difficult to design a cafeteria environment that does not influence food consumption decisions. Food items must be placed in some order and in some location, and so influencing food consumption is unavoidable. Often the current design of an environment is simply one potential design option (just the one into which the policymaker has been defaulted).

Box 6.7.2 discusses approaches to regulatory policy based on the insights of behavioural economics.

Although contextual influence has long been recognized, Thaler and Sunstein (2008) popularized the topic with their discussion of *choice architecture*—the design of the environments in which individuals make choices. As they note, behavioural economics can be a useful tool in nudging individuals towards behaviours that are beneficial while still allowing individuals complete autonomy

---

Box 6.7.2 Behavioural economics and lessons for regulatory policy

Cass R. Sunstein, co-author of *Nudge* (2008) and Administrator of the White House Office of Information Regulatory Affairs (2009–2012), suggests four promising approaches to regulatory policy based on the insights of behavioural economics:

1. 'Using disclosure as a regulatory tool, especially if disclosure policies are designed with an appreciation of how people process information.
2. Simplifying and easing choices through appropriate default rules, reduction of complexity and paperwork requirements and related strategies.
3. Increasing the salience of certain factors or variables.
4. Promoting social norms through private–public partnerships and other approaches that operate in the service of agreed-upon public goals.'

These approaches address some of the commonly cited behavioural biases studied in behavioural economics and mentioned in this chapter.

---

in making their choice. A choice architect may choose to use an opt-out rule when there is underutilization of something seen as beneficial. For example, influenza vaccinations are often encouraged in part because individuals who do not receive the vaccination impose a negative externality on other individuals. In such instances, designing a behavioural intervention where individuals must opt-out of receiving a vaccination can increase overall vaccination rates (Chapman et al. 2010; Keller et al. 2011). Similarly, a school may design the food display in their cafeteria so that salad options are placed before dessert options, and an employer may encourage savings by requiring individuals to opt out of contributing to a savings plan.

Social forces

Humans are social animals who mirror the actions of others, behave differently when they know that others will learn about their actions, and respond to requests. These features of human behaviour suggest three predictions. First, individuals informed about the actions of others will tend to conform to others' behaviour. Second, individuals who become aware that they are being observed will take actions that make them appear more favourably in the eyes of others (e.g. they will take actions that make them look more generous or more responsible). Third, individuals will be more likely to take an action when asked to do so by someone else. These social forces—which can be partially justified by the rational model and which we think of partially as behavioural—influence a wide variety of behaviours, including a number in the health domain. For each of the following three subsections, we provide evidence from health and non-health settings. As will be discussed at the end of this section, we believe social forces to be an area of behavioural health economics that has the opportunity to grow in the coming years.

Responding to the actions of others

It has been well documented that individuals informed about the actions of others tend to conform to others' behaviour. One way in which researchers have established this fact is to provide experimental subjects with *social information*: specific information about the actions of other people. Individuals who are provided with such information respond by taking actions that are more similar to the behaviour of others.

Outside of the health domain, this effect of social information has been observed in settings including charitable giving, environmental protection, and job choice. Individuals are more likely to donate to charity when they are told that others also donate. Frey and Meier (2004) find that students are more likely to make charitable donations to student funds at the University of Zurich when they are told that 64 per cent of students donate to the funds (64 per cent was a recent semester's average) rather than being told that 46 per cent of students donate to the funds (where 46 per cent was a 10-year average). Individuals also donate more money to a charity when they are told that others donated larger amounts. Shang and Croson (2009) find that the amount of money donated to a public radio campaign increases when donors who have called in to make a gift are told of a large recent donation of $300 rather than being told of a smaller donation of $75 or being told no information about a previous donation. This effect on donation amount works even more strongly in the negative direction;

people donated significantly less when the donation amount cited is below what they gave in the previous year (Croson and Shang 2008). Individuals are also more likely to engage in environmental protection when they are told that others engage in environmental protection. In a study on towel reuse, Goldstein et al. (2008) find that hotel guests are significantly more likely to reuse their towel—saving the water and electricity required to wash it—when they are told that 75 per cent of hotel guests reuse their towels rather than being given a generic environmental appeal. As with the charity examples, information can also impact the extent to which an individual engages in environmental protection. In a related setting, Allcott (2011) finds that sending households report cards comparing their electricity use to the electricity use of similarly sized households can decrease electricity usage by as much as an 11–20 per cent short-run price increase. On job choice, Coffman et al. (2014) find that individuals are more likely to accept a job as a school teacher when they are told that 84 per cent of accepted applicants took the job in the previous year.

That individuals respond to the actions of others has been shown to be important in the health domain as well. Here we focus on binge drinking and smoking, contexts in which individuals have been shown to conform to the behaviours of those around them.

Most students across the country have beliefs about the drinking habits of other students that are 'too high'—they think their peers drink more heavily than their peers actually do. Researchers have shown that beliefs about peer alcohol consumption correlate with own alcohol consumption. Perkins et al. (2005) perform a multivariate analysis of survey data from 130 schools and find overestimates of alcohol consumption among peers and a strong statistical relationship between those beliefs and own alcohol consumption, controlling for all available demographic variables. A similar approach has found a correlation between the smoking behaviour of adolescents and their perceptions of other teens smoking (Eisenberg and Forster 2003).

This correlational evidence is suggestive of a causal link in which individuals respond directly to their beliefs about others' drinking or smoking habits when making their own decision of whether to drink or smoke. This correlational evidence, however, is far from conclusive. It is quite possible that the causal link goes in the opposite direction. For example, teens may drink or smoke in groups; those who smoke may be more likely to observe others drinking and smoking and thus generate estimates about the prevalence of those behaviours among the rest of their peers that are too high. Similarly reported beliefs about others' drinking may be influenced by own drinking and the assumption that others are similar to oneself, leading those who drink or smoke more to believe that others drink or smoke more as well.

A true experiment that manipulates the information provided to individuals could more successfully show a causal link. For the case of alcohol consumption, DeJong et al. (2006) provide this experimental demonstration in a study involving 18 institutions of higher learning across which they randomized whether the schools ran a 3-year social norms marketing campaign (SNMC). These SNMCs educated college students about the actual alcohol consumption of students at the school. Many colleges and universities had previously implemented these types of SNMCs to inform students of the actual drinking behaviours of their students and so one aim of the research was to experimentally test their effectiveness.

The authors gathered self-reported beliefs about the alcohol consumption of other students and the self-reported own consumption from the Survey of College Alcohol Norms and Behaviour conducted before and after the 3-year SNMCs. Students surveyed at schools that were randomly selected to have a campaign reported larger decreases in drinking from pre survey to post survey on a number of dimensions (including a composite drinking scale, recent maximum consumption, and drinks consumed when partying). This decrease was associated with a decrease in reported beliefs about the drinking of others at the school. The authors also note that the decrease in drinking was more pronounced at schools with more intensive SNMCs.

When others are watching

Both inside and outside the health domain, individuals take actions that make them look more generous and more responsible when they believe that they are being observed. These effects are stronger when individuals care more about the person or persons observing them.

Outside of the health domain, being observed affects voting, charitable giving, and providing other public goods (i.e. taking costly actions that benefit others). On voting, Gerber et al. (2008) show that informing individuals that whether or not they vote is public record (and that their voting is being watched by researchers) increases the likelihood of voting over a standard message. Voting rates are even higher when individuals are told that their voting records will be sent to their neighbours after the upcoming election. In charitable giving, individuals care about what others learn about their donations. Harbaugh (1998) demonstrates that when a prestigious law school switches reporting all donations to reporting donations by category, donations become significantly more clustered at the lowest amount that achieves a certain level of recognition (e.g. many more donations at $500 when the reported category is $500–999). Similarly, Kessler et al. (2014) show that alumni of a large university are more likely to donate in consecutive years when they know they will receive public recognition for doing so.

In the health domain, image concerns affect individuals' willingness to engage in charitable health donation behaviours, including donating blood. Lacetera and Macis (2010b) looked at donation records from an Italian town; they found an increase in likelihood of blood donation as individuals approach the threshold for a symbolic prize (a medal) for their donations, but only if the winners of the medals are announced in the local newspaper and awarded publicly.

Combining social forces with monetary incentives can potentially strength the effect of an intervention. Haisley et al. (2012) increase the percentage of employees who complete a health risk assessment by combining a regret lottery (described earlier in 'Designing incentives using behavioural economics') with a social component where individuals could earn more if other employees—whose identities they knew—also completed the assessment. This treatment worked better than a standard reward incentive of a similar expected value.

Requests from others

Individuals are more likely to take an action when asked by someone else to do so. Encouragement or discouragement from others (also known as *peer pressure*) is a powerful social force that can influence individual behaviour inside and outside of health contexts.

Outside of the health domain, Meer and Rosen (2011) show that being more likely to be called on the phone in a university fundraising campaign makes donors much more likely to make a donation. Similarly, DellaVigna et al. (2012) show that individuals are less likely to answer to the door and less likely to make a donation in a door-to-door fundraising campaign when they are warned that an individual is coming to make a request. They interpret this result as individuals being worried about facing peer pressure and choosing to opt out when they know they will be asked to donate. Freeman (1997) reports that people are much more likely to volunteer when asked by a friend.

A number of health interventions attempt to leverage individuals' favourable responses to requests from others. Campbell et al. (2008) report on the results of a randomized controlled trial on teen smoking using 59 schools and 10,730 students aged 12–13 in Wales. Control schools received the standard smoking education. Treated schools had a special programme that included peer mentors: students who were trained to have informal conversations with their peers in which they discouraged smoking. Treated schools showed a decrease in the likelihood that students smoked 1 year later. By the second year after the intervention, the effect is attenuated (and no longer statistically significant), although students at the treated schools are still directionally less likely to smoke.

Kelly et al. (1991) report that training individuals identified as opinion leaders in their communities to endorse safe sex among gay men at risk of HIV drastically decreased the extent to which gay men engaged in unprotected anal intercourse (as measured by surveys before and after the intervention). Control cities that did not have individuals trained to endorse behaviour change did not show a decrease in unsafe sex during the same time period.

Long et al. (2012) investigate a peer mentoring treatment on glucose control for individuals with diabetes. In one treatment, subjects with poor diabetes control are paired with mentors who previously had poor control but have since improved. On average the mentor–mentee pairs talk once a week at the start of the study and once every 2 weeks at the end of the study 6 months later. The peer mentor group shows a large and significant improvement in glucose control. The authors found that this group also outperformed a financial incentive treatment where individuals were paid $100 or $200 for decreasing their glucose level. Similarly, the Geisinger Health System has been able to achieve better patient outcomes by having nurses follow-up with patients to monitor medication use and address possible questions and concerns (Cutler and Everett 2010).

Social forces: discussion

Social forces have been shown to have a powerful effect on behaviour in a number of domains outside of health, including charitable giving, environmental protection, voting, and job choice. The growing evidence on how social forces impact behaviour in health domains suggests that these forces may be particularly effective in affecting health behaviours as well.

If shown to be effective, social forces have a number of particular benefits in the health domain. First, leveraging social forces can be significantly less expensive than monetary incentives and thus may provide a very cost-effective way to affect behaviour (Hollingworth et al. 2012). Second, while we have yet to see many studies with long follow-up periods to test for the effectiveness of social treatments in the long term, there is reason to believe that social forces might build sustaining habits for healthy behaviour. Unlike a monetary incentive, which is either on or off, social incentives might have lingering effects. Once someone has been told that fewer people drink than he suspected, he may hold on to that information and it may still affect him months or years later. A peer mentor might continue to provide mentorship even after a study intervention period is over. In this way, social forces have the potential to provide longer-lasting effects. Additional research is needed to investigate the sustainability of these forces—research that we hope to see conducted in the coming years.

Conclusion

This chapter outlines findings from behavioural economics, highlighting four topic areas: reward incentives, salience and information, context and framing, and social forces. Results from each of these topic areas suggest interventions that can affect health behaviours.

As emphasized in the introduction, policymakers must be responsible with when and how they use available interventions to affect health behaviours. Policymakers must look for constraints, externalities, or behavioural biases to justify intervention. Fortunately, some individuals with behavioural biases may explicitly ask for interventions. They may recognize that they need help to engage in certain desirable behaviours like going to the gym, eating healthily, or taking their medications. In these cases, individuals will happily sign up for studies designed to test ways to impact behaviour, allowing us to conduct more research. In addition, they will happily opt in to programmes policymakers design to effectively encourage behaviour change.

Previous research has provided us with some insights into how to motivate behaviour, but exciting work remains to be done. One open question of particular importance—the proverbial Holy Grail of behavioural economics research in health behaviour—is how to create habit formation among individuals who want to engage in healthy behaviours and have trouble doing so. In this chapter, we saw examples in which a treatment that was in place for a while and then removed might have created a habit for visiting the gym, at least for a short while (Charness and Gneezy 2009; Acland and Levy 2013). In addition, we saw success in breaking the hold of an addictive behaviour like smoking (Volpp et al. 2009, Giné et al. 2010). But there are many more examples of interventions failing to help subjects form healthy habits that persist after the intervention is removed. By better understanding habit formation we can develop interventions that can be cost effective and have significant policy appeal.

References

Abaluck, J. (2013). *Naïveté, Projection Bias, and Habit Formation in Gym Attendance*. Unpublished manuscript.

Acland, D. and Levy, M. (2011). *Habit Formation, Naivete, and Projection Bias in Gym Attendance*. Unpublished manuscript.

Allcott, H. (2011). Social norms and energy conservation. *Journal of Public Economics*, 95(9–10), 1082–95.

Behavioural Insights Team (2010). *Applying Behavioural Insight to Health*. [Online] London: Crown. Available at: https://www.gov.uk/government/uploads/system/uploads/attachment_data/file/60524/403936_BehaviouralInsight_acc.pdf.

Bellman, S., Johnson, E.J, Kobrin, S.J., et al. (2004). International differences in information privacy concerns: a global survey of consumers. *Information Society*, 20(5), 313–24.

Bellman, S., Johnson, E.J., and Lohse, G.L. (2001). To opt-in or opt-out? It depends on the question. *Communications of the ACM*, 44(2), 25–7.

Benartzi, S. and Thaler, R.H. (2007). Heuristics and biases in retirement savings behavior. *Journal of Economic Perspectives*, 21(3), 81–104.

Beshears, J., Choi, J.J., Laibson, D., et al. (2013). *Active Choice and Health Care Costs: Evidence from Prescription Drug Home Delivery.* Unpublished manuscript.

Bollinger, B., Leslie, P., and Sorensen, A. (2011). Calorie posting in chain restaurants. *American Economic Journal: Applied Economics*, 3(1), 91–128.

Campbell, R., Starkey, F., Holliday, J., et al. (2008). An informal school-based peer-led intervention for smoking prevention in adolescence (ASSIST): a cluster randomised trial. *The Lancet*, 371(9624), 1595–602.

Carroll, G.D., Choi, J.J., Laibson, D., et al. (2009). Optimal defaults and active decisions. *Quarterly Journal of Economics*, 124(4), 1639–74.

Castano, P.M., Bynum, J.Y., Andres, R., et al. (2012). Effect of daily text messages on oral contraceptive continuation: a randomized controlled trial. *Obstetrics & Gynecology*, 119(1), 14–20.

Chapman, G.B., Li, M., Colby, H., et al. (2010). Opting in vs opting out of influenza vaccination. *Journal of the American Medical Association*, 304(1), 43–4.

Charness, G. and Gneezy, U. (2009). Incentives to exercise. *Econometrica*, 77(3), 909–31.

Choi, J.J., Laibson, D., Madrian, B.C., et al. (2004). For better or worse: default effects and 401(k) savings behavior. In D.A. Wise (ed.) *Perspectives on the Economics of Aging*, pp. 81–121. Chicago, IL: University of Chicago Press.

Coffman, L., Featherstone, C.R., and Kessler, J.B. (2014). *Can Social Information Affect What Job You Choose and Keep?.* Unpublished manuscript.

Croson, R. and Shang, J. (2008). The impact of downward social information on contribution decisions. *Experimental Economics*, 11, 221–33.

Cutler, D.M. and Everett, W. (2010). Thinking outside the pillbox—medication adherence as a priority for health care reform. *The New England Journal of Medicine*, 362(17), 1553–5.

Deci, E.L. (1971). Effects of externally mediated rewards on intrinsic motivation. *Journal of Personality and Social Psychology*, 18(1), 105–15.

DeJong, W., Schneider, S.K., Towvim, L.G., et al. (2006). A multisite randomized trial of social norms marketing campaigns to reduce college student drinking. *Journal of Studies on Alcohol*, 67(6), 868–79.

DellaVigna, S., List, J.A., and Malmendier, U. (2012). Testing for altruism and social pressure in charitable giving. *Quarterly Journal of Economics*, 127(1), 1–56.

DellaVigna, S. and Malmendier, U. (2006). Paying not to go to the gym. *American Economic Review*, 96(3), 694–719.

Dew, M.A., Switzer, G.E., Goycoolea, J.M., et al. (1997). Does transplantation produce quality of life benefits? A quantitative analysis of the literature. *Transplantation*, 64(9), 1261–73.

Donate Life America (2014). *Annual Update.* [Online] Richmond: Donate Life America. Available at: http://donatelife.net/.

Doshi, J.A., Zhu, J., Lee, B.Y., et al. (2009). Impact of a prescription copayment increase on lipid-lowering medication adherence in veterans. *Circulation*, 119(3), 390–7.

Eisenberg, M.E. and Forster, J.L. (2003). Adolescent smoking behavior: measures of social norms. *American Journal of Preventive Medicine*, 25(2), 122–8.

Elbel, B., Kersh, R., Brescoll, V.L., et al. (2009). Calorie labeling and food choices: a first look at the effects on low-income people in New York City. *Health Affairs (Millwood)*, 28(6), 1110–21.

Ericson, K.M.M. (forthcoming). Consumer inertia and firm pricing in the Medicare Part D prescription drug insurance exchange. *American Economic Journal: Economic Policy.*

Ferrari, J.R., Barone, R.C., Jason, L.A., et al. (1985). The use of incentives to increase blood donations. *Journal of Social Psychology*, 125(6), 791–3.

Finkelstein, E.A., Strombotne, K.L., Chan, N.L., et al. (2011). Mandatory menu labeling in one fast-food chain in King County, Washington. *American Journal of Preventive Medicine*, 40(2), 122–7.

Flegal, K.M., Caroll, M.D., Ogden, C.L., et al. (2010). Prevalence and trends in obesity among US adults, 1999–2008. *Journal of the American Medical Association*, 303(3), 235–41.

Flegal, K.M., Graubard, B.I., Williamson, D.F., et al. (2007). Cause-specific excess deaths associated with underweight, overweight, and obesity. *Journal of the American Medical Association*, 298(17), 2028–37.

Freeman, R.B. (1997). Working for nothing: the supply of volunteer labor. *Journal of Labor Economics*, 15(1), S140–66.

Frey, B.S. and Meier, S. (2004). Social comparisons and pro-social behavior: testing 'conditional cooperation' in a field experiment. *American Economic Review*, 94(5), 1717–22.

Gerber, A.S., Green, D.P., and Larimer, C.W. (2008). Social pressure and voter turnout: evidence from a large-scale field experiment. *American Political Science Review*, 102(1), 22–48.

Giné, X., Karlan, D., and Zinman, J. (2010). Put your money where your butt is: a commitment contract for smoking cessation. *American Economic Journal: Applied Economics*, 2(4), 213–35.

Gneezy, U., Meier, S., and Rey-Beil, P. (2011). When and why incentives (don't) work to modify behavior. *Journal of Economic Perspectives*, 25(4), 191–210.

Gneezy, U. and Rustichini, A. (2000a). Pay enough or don't pay at all. *Quarterly Journal of Economics*, 115(3), 791–810.

Gneezy, U. and Rustichini, A. (2000b). A fine is a price. *Journal of Legal Studies*, 29(1), 1–17.

Goette, L. and Stutzer, A. (2008). *Blood Donations and Incentives: Evidence From a Field Experiment.* IZA Discussion Paper, No. 3580. Institute for the Study of Labor.

Goette, L., Stutzer, A., and Frey, B.M. (2010). Prosocial motivation and blood donations: a survey of the empirical literature. *Transfusion Medicine and Hemotherapy*, 37(3), 149–54.

Goldstein, N.J., Cialdini, R.B., and Griskevicius, V. (2008). A room with a viewpoint: using social norms to motivate environmental conservation in hotels. *Journal of Consumer Research*, 35, 472–82.

Haisley, E., Volpp, K.G., Pellathy, T., and Loewenstein, G. (2012). The impact of alternative incentive schemes on completion of health risk assessments. *American Journal of Health Promotion*, 26(3), 184–8.

Handel, B. (2013). Adverse selection and inertia in health insurance markets: when nudging hurts. *American Economic Review*, 103(7), 2643–82.

Hanks, A.S., Just, D.R., Smith, L.E., et al. (2012). Healthy convenience: nudging students toward healthier choices in the lunchroom. *Journal of Public Health*, 34(3), 370–6.

Harbaugh, W.T. (1998). What do donations buy? A model of philanthropy based on prestige and warm glow. *Journal of Public Economics*, 67(2), 269–84.

Hardy, H., Kumar, V., Doros, G., et al. (2011). Randomized controlled trial of a personalized cellular phone reminder system to enhance adherence to antiretroviral therapy. *AIDS Patient Care and STDS*, 25(3), 153–61.

Hollingworth, W., Cohen, D., Hawkins, J., et al. (2012). Reducing smoking in adolescents: cost-effectiveness results from the cluster randomized ASSIST (A Stop Smoking In Schools Trial). *Nicotine & Tobacco Research*, 14(2), 161–8.

Hou, M.Y., Hurwitz, S., Kavanagh, E., et al. (2010). Using daily text-message reminders to improve adherence with oral contraceptives: a randomized controlled trial. *Obstetrics & Gynecology*, 116(3), 633–40.

John, L.K., Loewenstein, G., Troxel, A.B., et al. (2011). Financial incentives for extended weight loss: a randomized, controlled trial. *Journal of General Internal Medicine*, 26(6), 621–6.

Johnson, E.J. and Goldstein, D.G. (2003). Do defaults save lives? *Science*, 302(5649), 1338–9.

Johnson, E.J. and Goldstein, D.G. (2004). Defaults and donation decisions. *Transplantation*, 78, 1713–16.

Johnson, E.J., Hershey, J., Meszaros, J., et al. (1993). Framing, probability distortions, and insurance decisions. *Journal of Risk and Uncertainty*, 7, 35–51.

Kahn, B.E. and Wansink, B. (2004). The influence of assortment structure on perceived variety and consumption quantities. *Journal of Consumer Research*, 30(4), 519–33.

Kahneman, D. and Tversky, A. (1979). Prospect theory: an analysis of decision under risk. *Econometrica*, 47(2), 263–92.

Keller, P.A., Harlam, B., Loewenstein, G., et al. (2011). Enhanced active choice: a new method to motivate behavior change. *Journal of Consumer Psychology*, 21(4), 376–83.

Kelly, J.A., St. Lawrence, J.S., Diaz, Y.E., et al. (1991). HIV risk behavior reduction following intervention with key opinion leaders of population: an experimental analysis. *American Journal of Public Health*, 81(2), 168–71.

Kessler, J.B., Milkman, K.L., and Zhang, C.Y. (2014) *Social Recognition in Charitable Giving: In Pursuit of Perfection*. Unpublished manuscript.

Kessler, J.B. and Roth, A.E. (2012). Organ allocation policy and the decision to donate. *American Economic Review*, 102(5), 2018–47.

Kessler, J.B. and Roth, A.E. (2014a). Loopholes undermine donation: an experiment motivated by an organ donation priority loophole in Israel. *Journal of Public Economics*, 114, 19–28.

Kessler, J.B. and Roth, A.E. (2014b). *Don't Take 'No' for an Answer: An Experiment with Actual Organ Donor Registrations*. Unpublished manuscript.

Kim, S., Nayga, Jr. R.M., Capps, Jr. O. (2000). The effect of food label use on nutrient intakes: an endogenous switching regression analysis. *Journal of Agricultural and Resource Economics*, 25(1), 215–31.

Kling, J.R., Mullainathan, S., Shafir, E., et al. (2012). Comparison friction: experimental evidence from Medicare drug plans. *Quarterly Journal of Economics*, 127(1), 199–235.

Lacetera, N. and Macis, M. (2010a). Do all material incentives for pro-social activities backfire? The response to cash and non-cash incentives for blood donations. *Journal of Economic Psychology*, 31(4), 738–48.

Lacetera, N. and Macis, M. (2010b). Social image concerns and prosocial behavior: field evidence from a nonlinear incentive scheme. *Journal of Economic Behavior and Organization*, 76(2), 225–37.

Lacetera, N., Macis, M., and Slonim, R. (2012). Will there be blood? Incentives and displacement effects in pro-social behavior. *American Economic Journal: Applied Economics*, 4(1), 186–223.

Lacetera, N., Macis, M., and Slonim, R. (2013). Economic rewards to motivate blood donations. *Science*, 340(6135), 927–8.

Lacetera, N., Macis, M., and Stith, S.S. (2014). Removing financing barriers to organ and bone marrow donation: the effect of leave and tax Legislation in the U.S. *Journal of Health Economics*, 33, 43–56.

Lavee, J., Ashkenazi, T., Stoler, A., et al. (2013). Preliminary marked increase in the national organ donation rate in Israel following implementation of a new organ transplantation law. *American Journal of Transplantation*, 13(3), 780–5.

Long, J.A., Helweg-Larsen, M., Volpp, K.G. (2008). Patient opinions regarding 'pay for performance for patients.' *Journal of General Internal Medicine*, 23(10), 1647–52.

Long, J.A., Jahnie, E.C., Richardson, D.M., et al. (2012). Peer mentoring and financial incentives to improve glucose control in African American veterans: a randomized trial. *Annals of Internal Medicine*, 156(6), 416–24.

Madrian, B. and Shea, D.F. (2001). The power of suggestion: inertia in 401(k) participation and savings behavior. *Quarterly Journal of Economics*, 116(4), 1149–525.

McNeil, B.J., Pauker, S.G., Sox, H.C., et al. (1982). On the elicitation of preferences for alternative therapies. *The New England Journal of Medicine*, 306(21), 1259–62.

Meer, J. and Rosen, H.S. (2011). The ABCs of charitable solicitation. *Journal of Public Economics*, 95(5–6), 363–71.

Mellstrom, C. and Johannesson, M. (2008). Crowding out in blood donation: was Titmuss right? *Journal of the European Economic Association*, 6(4), 845–63.

Milkman, K.L., Beshears, J., Choi, J.J., et al. (2011). Using implementation intentions prompts to enhance influenza vaccination rates. *Proceedings of the National Academy of Sciences of the United States of America*, 108(26), 10415–20.

Milkman, K.L., Minson, J.A., and Volpp, K.G. (2014). Holding the Hunger Games hostage at the gym: an evaluation of temptation bundling. *Management Science*, 60(2), 283–99.

Osterberg, L. and Blaschke, T. (2005). Adherence to medication. *The New England Journal of Medicine*, 353(5), 487–97.

Perkins, H.W., Haines, M.P., and Rice, R. (2005). Misperceiving the college drinking norm and related problems: a nationwide study of exposure to prevention information, perceived norms and student alcohol misuse. *Journal of Studies on Alcohol*, 66(4), 470–8.

Pop-Eleches, C., Thirumurthy, H., Habyarimana, J.P., et al. (2011). Mobile phone technologies improve adherence to antiretroviral treatment in a resource-limited setting: a randomized controlled trial of text message reminders. *AIDS*, 25(6), 825–34.

Rolls, B.J., Rowe, E.A., Rolls, E.T., et al. (1981). Variety in a meal enhances food intake in man. *Physiology & Behavior*, 26(2), 215–21.

Roth, A.E. (2007). Repugnance as a constraint on markets. *Journal of Economic Perspectives*, 21(3), 37–58.

Samuelson, W. and Zeckhauser, R.J. (1988). Status quo bias in decision making. *Journal of Risk and Uncertainty*, 1, 7–59.

Schnitzler, M.A., Lentine, K.L., and Burroughs, T.E. (2005a). The cost effectiveness of deceased organ donation. *Transplantation*, 80(11), 1636–7.

Schnitzler, M.A., Whiting, J.F., Brennan, D.C., et al. (2005b). The life-years saved by a deceased organ donor. *American Journal of Transplantation*, 5(9), 2289–96.

Schroeder, S.A. (2007). We can do better—improving the health of the American people. *The New England Journal of Medicine*, 357(12), 1221–8.

Schweitzer, M., Hershey, J.C., and Asch, D.A. (1996). Individual choice in spending accounts: can we rely on employees to choose well? *Medical Care*, 34(6), 583–93.

Shang, J. and Croson, R. (2009). A field experiment in charitable contribution: the impact of social information on the voluntary provision of public goods. *Economic Journal*, 119, 1422–39.

Simon, H.A. (1957). *Models of Man: Social and Rational—Mathematical Essays on Rational Human Behavior in a Social Setting*. New York: Wiley.

Stockwell, M.S., Kharbanda, E.O., Martinez, R.A., et al. (2012). Effect of a text messaging intervention on influenza vaccination in an urban, low-income pediatric and adolescent population: a randomized controlled trial. *Journal of the American Medical Association*, 307(16), 1702–8.

Sunstein, C.R. (forthcoming). Nudges.gov: behavioral economics and regulation. In E. Zamir and D. Teichman (eds.) *Oxford Handbook of Behavioral Economics and the Law*. New York: Oxford University Press.

Thaler, R.H. (2009). Opting in versus opting out. *New York Times*, 26 September. [Online] Available at: http://www.nytimes.com/2009/09/27/business/economy/27view.html.

Thaler, R.H. and Sunstein, C.R. (2008). *Nudge: Improving Decisions about Health, Wealth, and Happiness*. New Haven, CT: Yale University Press.

Titmuss, R.M. (1971). *Gift Relationship: From Human Blood to Social Policy*. New York: Pantheon.

Tversky, A. and Kahneman, D. (1981). The framing of decisions and the psychology of choice. *Science*, 211(4481), 453–58.

United Network for Organ Sharing (n.d.). *Data Resources*. [Online] Richmond: United Network for Organ Sharing. Available at: http://www.unos.org/donation/index.php?topic=data_resources.

Variyam, J.N. (2008). Do nutrition labels improve dietary outcomes? *Health Economics*, 17(6), 695–708.

Variyam, J.N. and Cawley, J. (2006). *Nutrition Labels and Obesity*. NBER Working Paper, No. 11956. National Bureau of Economic Research.

Vervloet, M., Linn, A.J., van Weert, J.C.M., et al. (2012). The effectiveness of interventions using electronic reminders to improve adherence to chronic medication: a systematic review of the literature. *Journal of the American Medical Informatics Association*, 19(5), 696–704.

Volpp, K.G., Asch, D.A., Galvin, R., et al. (2011). Redesigning employee health incentives—lessons from behavioral economics. *The New England Journal of Medicine*, 365(5), 388–90.

Volpp, K.G., John, L., Troxel, A.B., et al. (2008). Financial incentive-based approaches for weight loss: a randomized trial. *Journal of the American Medical Association*, 300(22), 2631–7.

Volpp, K.G., Loewenstein, G., Troxel, A.B., et al. (2008). A test of financial incentives to improve warfarin adherence. *BMC Health Services Research*, 8, 272.

Volpp, K.G., Troxel, A.B., Pauly, M.V., et al. (2009). A randomized, controlled trial of financial incentives for smoking cessation. *The New England Journal of Medicine*, 360(7), 699–709.

Wansink, B. and Cheney, M.M. (2005). Super bowls: serving bowl size and food consumption. *Journal of the American Medical Association*, 293(14), 1727–8.

Wansink, B. and van Ittersum, K. (2007). Portion size me: downsizing our consumption norms. *Journal of the American Dietetic Association*, 107(7), 1103–6.

Wisdom, J., Downs, J.S., and Lowenstein, G. (2010). Promoting healthy choices: information versus convenience. *American Economic Journal: Applied Economics*, 2(2), 164–78.

Zikmund-Fisher, B., Fagerlin, A., Roberts, T., et al. (2008). Alternate methods of framing information about medication side effects: incremental risk versus total risk occurrence. *Journal of Health Communication*, 13(2), 107–24.

6.8

Governance and management of public health programmes

Eng-kiong Yeoh

Introduction to governance and management of public health programmes

In the 2007 publication of the World Health Organization (WHO), *Everybody's Business: Strengthening Health Systems to Improve Health Outcomes*, a critical question asked is 'Why aren't health systems working better?' (WHO 2007). The publication begins with the observation: 'The world has never possessed such a sophisticated arsenal of interventions and technologies for curing disease and prolonging life. Yet the gaps in health outcomes continue to widen. The power of existing interventions is not matched by the power of health systems to deliver them to those in greatest need in a comprehensive way, and on an adequate scale' (p. iii). The WHO proposes a framework for action to strengthen health systems. In the health systems framework, governance and leadership, also referred to as stewardship, is the critical function. Governance refers to 'the wide range of functions carried out by governments as they seek to achieve national health policy objectives', and involves overseeing and guiding the whole health system (WHO 2007). It is pivotal in ensuring that the different components of the system function effectively together to achieve objectives and goals. Good governance and effective management is critical to the performance of health systems (Lauer 2001; WHO 2002, 2007; Mills et al. 2006; Institute on Governance 2011). *Governance Matters*, a global study on governance by the World Bank, found empirical evidence of a strong causal relationship between better governance and better developmental outcomes (Kaufmann et al. 1999). The study was based on a new database of over 300 governance indicators compiled from different sources in over 150 countries. The elements of governance examined were: how governments were selected, ability to formulate and implement sound policies, and the institutions which govern interactions with the state. There was a strong causal relationship of good governance and higher per capita incomes, lower infant mortality, and higher literacy. In a subsequent study of health system efficiency, the WHO also found a positive correlation between both the health and overall efficiency measures and 'index of government effectiveness' (Lauer 2001; Mills et al. 2006). There have been an increasing number of studies that have found that effective or good governance is a critical factor for achieving the goals and objectives of an organization (Institute on Governance 2011).

In the current world order, governance of public health programmes can no longer be considered in isolation from the wider system of public health governance, impervious to influences in the wider context (WHO 2007). Public health programmes vary enormously in size, scope, and coverage, and may originate locally from community groups and organizations or be commissioned by provincial or national governments and non-government organizations (NGOs) and foundations. The programmes may also be part of a growing number of huge global health initiatives (GHIs) that is changing the whole global health governance landscape. Globally, development assistance for health grew from US$5.6 billion in 1990 to US$21.8 billion in 2007 (Ravishankar et al. 2009). In 2012, 10 years after it was set up, The Global Fund to Fight AIDS, Tuberculosis and Malaria (GFATM) channelled US$3 billion annually (GFATM 2013). These global public health programmes are multinational and disbursements of funds are channelled increasingly through NGOs and in direct bilateral assistance to governments rather than the traditional intergovernmental agencies such as the agencies of the United Nations (UN), the UN Population Fund (UNFPA), the UN Children's Fund (UNICEF), and the WHO (Ravishankar et al. 2009). Issues have arisen and concerns been expressed that national health priorities may be distorted by global health priorities. National health systems with limited capacity in their infrastructure find it difficult to cope with the competing priorities of different donors with varying requirements for governance structures and mechanisms and reporting. Governance and management of public health programmes must be understood and studied in the wider context of public health management and governance.

Evolution of the concept of governance

The concept of governance and its applications have evolved, since the origins of the word derived from the fourteenth-century Latin *gubernantia* which meant 'to steer'. In subsequent usage it became equated with the exercise of authority and a system of government. The *Oxford English Dictionary* describes governance as 'the act or manner of governing, of extending control or authority over the actions of subjects; a system of regulations'. In recent usage, the concept of governance is no longer understood to be synonymous with government (Rosenau 1995; UNDP 1997). Government-the-state is conceived as one form of governance, which is highly formalized (Dodgson et al. 2002). Governance transcends the state, and incorporates the private sector and civil society (Rosenau 1995; UNDP 1997). This is a reflection of the changes in the relationship between the 'governing' and the 'governed' in current society where the 'governing' need to seek the consent of the 'governed' to secure its legitimacy. It also reflects the prominent roles and the increasing influence of two other institutions of society—the for-profit private sector and civil society—in all aspects of social pursuits. The Institute on Governance observed that the concept of 'governance' had evolved in its application to be used as a fundamental consideration in most disciplines in the last two decades (Institute on Governance 2011). Governance has been conceptualized from different perspectives in a broad range of disciplines—political, social, policy and health sciences, law, and international relations and has been applied to diverse aspects of social endeavour and scholarly inquiry. This has led to a proliferation of definitions consistent with their respective conceptualization and application. Two definitions of governance are of particular relevance to, and reflect the essence of, public health. The first, the United Nations Development Programme (UNDP), defines governance as 'the exercise of political, economic administrative authority of a country's affairs at all levels'. Governance comprises the complex mechanisms, processes, and institutions through which citizens and groups articulate their interests, mediate their differences, and exercise their legal rights (UNDP 1997). The UNDP definition recognizes the political and economic nature of social life, and the roles and interdependencies of the pillars of organized society such as the state, private sector, and civil society. The UNDP conception of governance incorporates the basic premise of democratic societies of the relationship between state and citizens. A common theme of the different conceptions of democracy is the exercise of collective self-determination of communities based on the consent of the governed (Scholte 2005). Governance in democratic societies emphasizes the source legitimacy, limits of authority, the purpose for which authority given should be applied for, and accountability in its exercise. A second, even broader, definition of governance in a conceptual review of global health governance is 'the action and means adopted by a society to promote collective action and deliver collective solutions in the pursuit of common goals' (Dodgson et al. 2002). This recognizes the whole range of cooperative endeavours undertaken in society, from informal arrangements and agreements by groups of individuals in the community to the highly formalized form of established rules, conduct, and procedures institutionalized in government. There are virtually infinite mechanisms, many of which fall outside the realms of government, all contributing in important ways to the collective actions of society in the pursuit of common goals. These two conceptions of governance are of particular relevance to public health, which as defined by Acheson, and adopted in this publication is 'the science and art of preventing disease, prolonging life, and promoting health through the organized efforts of society' (Acheson 1988, p. 1). A mono focus on the role of the state in health governance neglects the equally important roles and influence of civil society and the private sector in contributing to efforts to promote and improve health. It has been argued that an exclusive focus on the state in governance, undermines our ability to govern effectively (Ollila 2005; Kempa et al. n.d.; Renukumar n.d.).

Public health governance: conception

The broader conceptions of governance will underpin the approach used in this paper as they enable a holistic perspective and better understanding of the mechanisms in government, the private sector, and civil society, their interactions and interdependencies, their complex and dynamic nature, and how they influence and enable the goal of improving the health of people. This is reflected in the two following definitions: 'Health governance concerns the actions and means adopted by a society to organize itself in the promotion and protection of the health of its population' (Dodgson et al. 2002, p. 6); 'Public health governance is the means by which society collectively seeks to assure the conditions under which the population can live with the highest possible level of health and well being' (Bennett et al. 2009, p. 207). Public health concerns health of populations in societies; public health governance is health governance and the two terms will be used interchangeably in this chapter. Health governance is multilayered with mechanisms at: (1) supranational, that is, global, regional, and international; and (2) national, that is, federal, provincial, and local levels, with close and complex interactions between the different levels. Public health programmes may be initiated at every one of these levels and are not only closely interrelated but also integrated in many facets. Supranational global initiatives inter-digitate with local programmes, and regional with provincial. The proliferation of GHIs initiated by private donors, foundations, and donor countries for different diseases and health problems influence priority setting of national health programmes. In addition, the multiplicity of competing demands of the different donors can create pressures for local health systems with limited planning and delivery capacity. A discussion of governance of public health has to examine the structures and mechanisms at each of the levels, their interactions, and interdependencies.

Public health governance: a systems framework

Governance has been applied to specific and a relatively narrow scope of collective actions such as in clinical and corporate governance, and to the broader concept of global health governance (Dodgson et al. 2002). A systems framework and typology is useful in understanding this complex and developing field of inquiry. Systems theory has enabled the development of a new conceptual underpinning for studying and understanding social systems which are inherently complex. Systems theory has been applied in the WHO's framework to strengthen health systems which comprises six components, referred to as 'building blocks' (Fig. 6.8.1). The six system building blocks which are core functions of every health system are: (1) service delivery; (2) health workforce; (3) information; (4) medical products, vaccines, and technologies; (5) financing; and (6) leadership and governance (WHO 2007). These six building blocks are interdependent and interrelated components of the health system, and need to be coordinated to

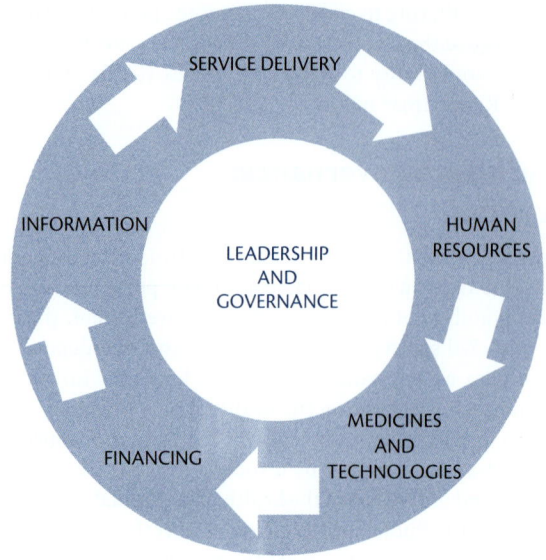

Fig. 6.8.1 The WHO health system framework.

Reproduced with the permission from *Everybody's Business: Strengthening Health Systems to Improve Health Outcomes: WHO's Framework for Action*, World Health Organization, Geneva, Switzerland, Copyright © 2007, available from http://www.who.int/healthsystems/strategy/everybodys_business.pdf.

function together as a whole. Strengthening health systems, that is, making them more effective, involves improving these components and managing their interactions. Systems theory provides the conceptual basis for studying, understanding, and researching how these six building blocks interrelate, and how their interdependencies can be better managed to strengthen health systems to improve health outcomes. The systems approach will also enable the definition of the desirable attributes of health systems needed for effectiveness.

Systems theory has also been applied in understanding global health governance as a complex adaptive system (Hill 2011). Complexity theory provides a frame for understanding of, and providing insights into, the complex and constantly evolving polyvalent relationships of the diverse actors, and the reconfigurations of influence in the multitude of networks, in global health governance. The key concepts of general systems theory can be applied to health governance as a system, and comprise the following (Kast and Rosenzweig 1972):

1. A system is composed of interrelated parts which are interconnected.

2. A system is not the sum of the components, and can only be explained in totality.

3. Systems may be open or closed, social systems are inherently open.

4. Systems have boundaries which distinguish them from their environments; however, boundaries are very difficult to define in social systems.

5. There is a hierarchical relationship between the components of a system, with subsystems, and both are part of a suprasystem.

6. Open systems are in a dynamic relationship with their environment, receiving inputs which are transformed into outputs which are exported.

7. Systems are subject to the forces of entropy; in open systems, however, the process can be arrested or may be reverted to a state of negative entropy by virtue of its ability to import resources from its environment and transform them into outputs.

8. Information relating to the outputs of a system, feedback into the system, and facilitating changes in the transformation process.

9. Open systems tend to become more differentiated, organized, and elaborated.

10. Social systems comprise individuals and subunits, with different values and objectives and seek multiple goals.

11. Equifinality is a characteristic of open systems, which achieve their respective objectives with diverse inputs and different processes.

A public health governance system is part of the wider governance system of human societies (the suprasystem), wherein lie the mechanisms and actions which define the social determinants of health. The components (the subsystems) of health governance are the entities of the state or government, the private for-profit sector, and civil society, and their respective institutions, structures, and mechanisms (subunits). The health governance functions of these three entities interact and are interrelated and are in a dynamic relationship with the environment of the wider governance system in society. A framework for public health governance provides a theoretical basis for studying and understanding the complex mechanisms and processes of health governance within the three component entities, and the interactions and interrelations between them. It also provides a conceptual basis for appreciating and studying the evolutionary changes in health governance which are observed over time resulting from the interactions and feedback to the system. The prominence of civil society, the powerful influence of the private sector, and the redefined role of the state in governance can be better appreciated with this frame. Table 6.8.1 shows the framework and typology which will be used in this chapter.

Public health governance can be conceived as a complex system of the interactions and interdependencies of the institutions of current society—the entities of the state, private sector, and civil society—in collectively seeking to assure the conditions under which populations can live with the highest possible level of health and well-being. These three entities can be conceived as horizontal

Table 6.8.1 Public health governance—a systems framework

Levels	Entities/components	Structure
Supranational:	Government/state	Institutions
Global	Private [for-profit] sector	Organization
Regional	Civil society	Instruments/tools
International	Hybrids of government:	Mechanisms/processes
National:	Private	
Federal	Civil society	
Provincial		
Local		

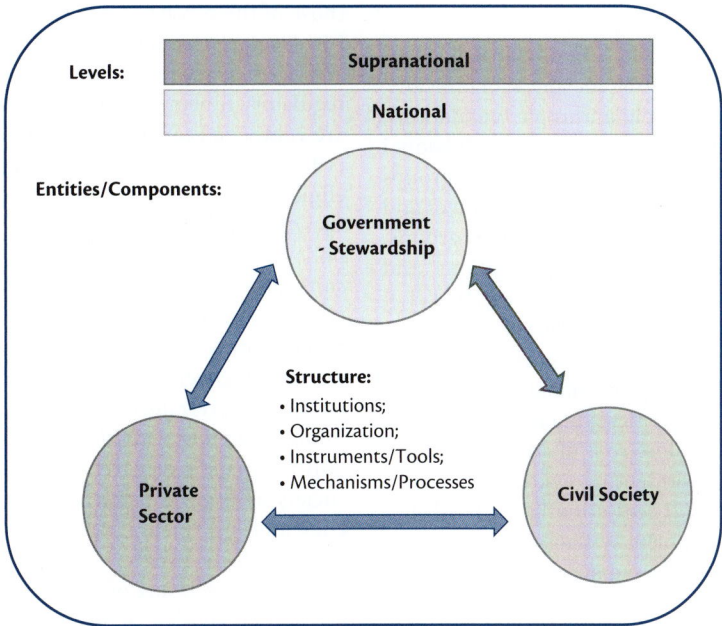

Fig. 6.8.2 Public health governance system—the entities of government, private sector, and civil society.

components or subsystems each with distinct structures, institutions, organization, instruments and tools of influences, mechanisms, and processes for interactions within and between the component entities. The interactions and interdependencies of these three horizontal entities, inter-digitate in a second, hierarchical dimension at either the national or supranational levels. The organizational context of governance within the three component entities and at the two hierarchical levels is a third dimension of the system. These distinctions provide the basis of defining the distinct characteristics of each of these component subsystems (Fig. 6.8.2).

The private sector

The private sector refers to all the private business organizations and enterprises, including the informal market sector, with a profit objective. The private sector creates jobs and generates income, and influences socioeconomic policies and politics, to create an environment which is conducive for markets and enterprise (UNDP 1997). The organization of the sector varies considerably, comprising a diversity of arrangements from the family-based informal sector to highly organized, vertically integrated and horizontally diversified corporations, at national, multinational, and transnational levels. Different organization forms have also emerged, reflecting the dynamic environment of the complex nature of social systems, and include: strategic alliances, partnerships, and collaborative networks, both within the private sector and with civil society and government.

The governance instruments available to the private sector are wide-ranging, and include a number of those available to government: exhortation, expenditure, direct provision and regulations. The significant difference is, in traditional application of these instruments by the private sector, it is without the authority of the state, and in particular the coercive power of the state to impose penalties, withhold benefits, and restrict individual decisions.

However, even this has changed, with the evolving role of government and hybrid forms of public–private governance, the private sector may be given authority normally bestowed to the state, either through the contracts to the private sector in ensuring compliance with state regulatory functions or outright delegation which may be explicit and embodied in the law (Freeman 2000; Kempa et al. n.d.). One example is the passage of legislation in the US Congress requiring hospitals to be accredited by the Joint Commission on Health Care and Accreditation of Health Organizations (JCAHO) as a condition for participation in the federal social insurance programme, Medicare. Another prevalent practice is the delegation of health professional regulations to health professions. These hybrid roles have been referred to as 'the privatization of governance' (Scholte 2005). Corporations have been described as the most influential and powerful organizations in contemporary governance. They have available substantial controlling resources, ability to frame and influence discourses, flexibility in pursuing their objectives and enterprise in finding niches (Freeman 2000; Kempa et al. n.d.). 'Private government' has been used to describe the powerful influence of the private sector in 'governing states' through the threat of flight of capital as a means of getting governments to enact socioeconomic policies which are conducive to corporate profit maximizing, and in governance of security in non-state spaces, which are privately owned but open to public access, to varying degrees, such as shopping complexes, parks, and golf courses, where the police of the state are mobilized to do the 'bidding' of private security (Kempa et al. n.d.). The private sector's role in health governance is pervasive, as providers, financiers, marketers, commissioners, and employers.

The proliferation of GHIs initiated by private donors, foundations, and donor countries have a strong influence on priorities of national health programmes and can create significant pressures for local health systems.

Civil society

Civil society comprises individuals, and formally organized or informal groups of individuals, interacting socially, economically, and politically. Civil society includes philanthropic foundations, labour unions, business forums and associations, professional associations, academic institutions, think tanks, religious groups and organizations, social and recreational clubs, cooperatives and community groups, environmental movements, lobby groups, women's networks, youth associations, relief organizations, and media outlets. Political parties are excluded if it is viewed that civil society organizations should not seek public office (UNDP 1997; Emmerij et al. 2001; Scholte 2005). In health governance, academic institutions, professionals, and professional organizations in public health have a unique and critical function. The public health community has been at the forefront of advocacy and in empowering civil society, by: (1) presenting evidence of health issues, and effective interventions; (2) demystifying technical subjects and the complexities of government systems and policy processes, by providing information to the public; and (3) facilitating engagement of members of the community. Civil society is the intermediary institution between the individual and the state and has a critical role in providing the checks and balance on government power and demands for greater accountability and transparency of public office. Civil society networks facilitate social and political interaction and communication. Civil society groups and organizations are effective channels of communications between individuals and business and the state, and are powerful groups for influencing public policies, and allocation of public resources that better reflect community needs. The origins of governance can be traced to civil society. Individuals in society group to take collective action, and deliver collective solutions in pursuit of common goals. Collective behaviour may be based on expectations and understanding of members of the group and rules and procedures may be informal. They may also be more organized with structures and agreed mechanisms for decision and criteria and procedures for membership. The range of arrangements from the informal to the formal depends on the purpose for which the group was created, the dynamics between members, and the context of the wider community environment. Many of the groups will cease after they have accomplished the goals for which they were created, or have been unable to make much progress, or members have lost their initial interest. A number will continue to develop and agreements and rules become institutionalized, and may even become legal entities—NGOs. NGOs may establish alliances among themselves or with other members of civil society, private and public sector agencies, to strengthen their influence and further their goals. These alliances may be temporary or may evolve into policy networks and other more formal arrangements. Linkages may also be established with international NGOs, particularly those with similar missions. The historical roots of present government emerged through these societal arrangements and developed over the millennia. Governance systems, like all complex systems, comprise components, or subsystems which are interrelated. The interactions and interrelationships of the principal components of governance systems are dynamic, with feedback which enables emergent forms to evolve. This is evident in the emergence of the powerful influence of the private sector and civil society in contemporary governance, particularly in global space. The instruments of influence of civil society are similar to those of the private sector: exhortation, resource, and provision. In addition, it has a long-standing tradition of hybrid governance arrangements with government, particularly in implementing regulatory functions of the state. In many states, welfare benefits are contracted to NGOs, which are given the leeway to interpret criteria to determine the eligibility of applicants, such as in the eligibility for admission and transfers to nursing homes. Civil society actions in advocacy campaigns, public demonstrations, policy briefs, investigative journalism, and public interest lawsuits have become established tools for exhortation. In extreme circumstances civil unrest and disobedience may result in government backing down on unpopular policies, or may even lead to changes in government. In a World Bank paper entitled *Demand for Good Governance in the World Bank: Conceptual Evolution, Frameworks and Activities* (Demand for Good Governance Team 2010), demand-side governance tools which seek to empower civil society in its governance role are categorized under: (1) transparency and information, (2) accountability, and (3) participation. Tools in the transparency and information category include provisions for disclosure of relevant documents, right to information legislation, and mechanisms to demystify technical papers, and dissemination of information. Accountability tools include grievance redress mechanisms which can be formal, such as complaints office, appeals committee, ombudsman system, and local courts, and informal arrangements such as citizen grievance committees. Accountability tools can also be in the form of third-party monitoring of public sector activities and independent verification of outcomes of public policy, such as public service surveys and consumer satisfaction and client feedback surveys. In the third category of demand-side governance tools, mechanisms to enable participation include user committees and training and capacity building for stakeholder participation. Mechanisms to engage members of the community are necessary complements in the application of these tools, to recruit, mobilize, and motivate individuals and groups to actively participate.

Government

The structure for public health governance at the national level is determined by basic dimensions in government structures. In federal forms of government, such as in Canada, Australia, Germany, India, and the United States, the provinces or states share power with the federal government. The provisions in the Constitution delineate the authority and responsibilities of the federal and provincial government. The responsibility for financing may be a federal function and provision of services and regulation of providers a provincial or local function. Interpretation of the constitutional provisions may be contentious and may be challenged and subjected to adjudication by the courts, as in the recent example of the ruling by the Supreme Court on the healthcare reforms proposed by President Obama which mandated healthcare insurance for all individuals in the United States. In Canada, by Constitution, the majority of healthcare responsibilities were given to the Provinces, but the provisions for public health were not clearly allocated. Public health was considered to be under provincial jurisdiction under a section of the Constitution which gives the provinces property and civil rights, and subsequent legal interpretations have recognized this. This has created a dilemma for the federal government, which has resorted to other provisions in the Constitution to pass legislation to protect the public's health, such as in the control of transmission of health risks (Wilson 2004). The ambiguity creates challenges in the coordination of public health responses, as each province has the authority to enact policies and pass legislation as it deems appropriate. Gaps and duplications in carrying out public health functions are potential problems (Office of the Auditor General of Canada 1999). Similar issues of jurisdictional clarity between different levels of government in responding to public health emergencies were also reported in an analysis of federalism, rights, and public health laws in Australia (Bennett 2009). Variability in standards of public health practice in these jurisdictions where public health responsibilities are primarily located in the provinces may also raise concerns. In nations with federal systems of government, public health institutions may be under the jurisdiction of different levels of government and accountable to elected officials of different political affiliations, with the potential for conflict. In unitary forms of government, all the powers reside at the national level and are delegated to the provinces and local levels as the government in power sees fit. In systems of unitary government, coordination of public health responses and conflicts between central and provincial and local governments does not have the constitutional and political challenges of federal forms, although there may still be problems from the organizational and managerial contexts. Another basic dimension of government structure which is a critical determinant of governance structure is the separation of executive, legislative and judicial powers. In Presidential systems, the chief executive and legislature are elected separately, and legislation and budgets proposed by the executive have to be passed by the legislature which also has the function of oversight of executive actions. Governance responsibilities and structures are constructed to reflect this. Designated committees in the legislature to debate, discuss, scrutinize, amend, endorse, or reject proposed public health policies are a usual structure. In parliamentary forms of government, such as in England, Singapore, and Malaysia, where the chief executive is chosen by the legislature, although budget, legislative, and policy proposals are also debated and have to be passed by the legislature, in practice the passage is usually achieved as the chief executive is normally chosen from the ruling majority and has its confidence and support. An independent judiciary is important, to ensure that the government of the day acts within the law and does not exceed the powers provided by law, and to ensure that laws are justly and fairly applied. The judiciary also adjudicates on constitutional issues between the different levels of government and between the people and the state, protecting the rights of the individual as enshrined in the constitution and other laws of the land. It has also an important function of interpreting laws. Many important public health policies are enacted in law, and the courts have been called upon to adjudicate when parties affected by public health policies believe they have been aggrieved by the enactment. The legal challenges by the tobacco industry to delay, subvert, and undermine public health legislation intended to reduce smoking have been well documented (Brandt 2007; Weishaar et al. 2012). The basis generally used to justify public health regulation is the 'harm principle' which was originally framed for medical treatment and services, which is that 'the law should only intervene in an individual's choice and behaviours only where those choices or behaviours pose a risk or harm to other persons' (Gostin and Gostin 2009). Legislation providing for the detention and quarantine of individuals, in the control of communicable diseases,

was premised on this principle. However, more recent legislation which aimed to control injuries and non-communicable diseases overrides individual choice for the protection of the individual and that of the population. The argument put forward is that governments have an ethical mandate to intervene to protect individuals and populations at risk of harm; the consequence for not doing so would be greater illness, and health inequalities which would divide communities (Gostin and Gostin 2009).

A feature of both federal and unitary forms of government is the structure of the executive branch, comprising a political and an administrative arm. The political structure is under the leadership of the elected chief executive, the President, or the Prime Minister and is supported by a cabinet of ministers who have responsibilities for different portfolios. Individuals, experts in their fields and external to the cabinet, may also be appointed to serve as 'national advisers' in providing input in specific areas considered necessary. Advisory boards and councils composed of experts and/or representatives of different professional and community groups may also feature as part of the mechanisms of the governance system that seek to interact with civil society. In federal systems, the structures are replicated at the provincial level. The Minister for Health is the cabinet minister who assumes responsibility for public health. The civil service normally houses the administrative arm. The cabinet ministers are supported by the civil service department heads of the respective portfolios, and different designations are given to these officials. In the public health portfolio, the lead official could carry a title such as Chief Medical Officer or Permanent Secretary for Health. The corresponding department would be the Department of Health, which provides support to the minister in: formulating health policies; developing strategies; assessing health needs and determining priorities; defining regulatory frameworks; commissioning, monitoring, and evaluating public health programmes; and collecting and seeking health data, information and intelligence. At all levels of government, horizontal structures are required for coordinating functions and interacting with and engaging the principal partners in governance, the private sector, and civil society. Many of the socioeconomic determinants of health are not under the policy responsibility of the health minister. Efforts to address health inequalities require cabinet action under the leadership of the chief executive. The health minister needs to work across cabinet colleagues and secure the support of the chief executive to give priority to public health strategies and programmes. At the administrative level, cross-departmental structures and processes need to be in place to coordinate the work required. In the political context of a government with a policy for democratic participation, and a recognition of the need for public health governance to incorporate political and public accountability, the Public Health and Health Professions Department of the Welsh Assembly Government is developing an integrated system of governance to improve public health (Jewell and Wilkinson 2008). The structures designed for cross-departmental collaboration comprise a permanent secretary's business group for all the heads of departments in government to meet on a weekly basis, and a strategy delivery and performance board for corporate decisions. The model of integrated governance for public health incorporates mechanisms and structures of interaction with: (1) the Welsh Ministers and local government, (2) regulators, (3) media, (4) voluntary sector, (5) public, (6) individuals, (7) professions, and (8) United

Kingdom and global policy. The interactions with regulatory bodies focus on strengthening the collaboration and coordination between the bodies inspecting, regulating, and auditing health and social care. At the local level, community governance is evolving as the roles and functioning of local government are changing as with the other levels of government. There is recognition of the need to engage citizens and communities in decision-making on the design and delivery of local social services in order to benefit from local knowledge and networks (Pillora and McKinlay 2011). A development in community governance initiated by the UK government was the introduction of a Localism Bill in the year 2000, which provided for 'community budgets', which would enable communities to have more control of their funding streams, enabling them to combine different sources of public funding to tackle cross-cutting issues in a particular locality. This revolutionary initiative of enabling local control over local spending would be pioneered in different areas in the country, with the aim of making it available throughout the country in 2013 (Pillora and McKinlay 2011). Strong civic leadership has been identified as a key component of community governance, required to mobilize communities and external stakeholders. New methods of community engagement involving active collaboration between groups with different knowledge bases are more likely to be successful and could facilitate the development of long-term alliances among members of the community from different backgrounds and affiliations. The policies and innovations in empowering and enabling civil society of local communities and service users to participate in policy options for services and resources has also been referred to as citizen-centred governance (Barnes et al. 2008). The fundamental change in community governance requires innovations in the mechanisms of enabling local communities to prioritize their needs, and how these needs will be met and public sector services improve the quality of their lives. The new mechanisms to involve individual members of the community and service users, and NGOs and community organizations are both in consultation and decision-making processes. The participation could be through formal appointments to community boards, management committees and as governors to National Health Service Foundation Trusts, serving alongside other private and public sector members. To strengthen local accountability, the National Health Service has innovated a new form of public organization, a 'public benefit corporation'. The foundation trust is structured to include three constituencies—the public, patients, and staff. Each constituency elects governors to represent their interests. Twenty-four of the 33 governors are elected by the three constituencies. Nine of the remaining governors are nominated by key stakeholders of the trust, the local authority, primary care trusts, and the university. The specific responsibilities of the governors include participating in the appointment of the trust's chair, non-executive directors, chief executive, and auditors. The governors meet in a consultative council and comment on the plans of the board of directors, the accounts, and annual report of the trust. A separate board of directors of executive and non-executive members is responsible for the strategic management and operations of the trust. There are also other forms of innovative governance which do not have a formal legal status, such as partnerships of public, private, voluntary, and community sectors in an 'unincorporated association' whose finances and contracts are managed on its behalf by a legally incorporated authority, trust, or agency (Barnes et al. 2008).

These innovations in governance which benefit from local knowledge are of particular relevance for disadvantaged communities and for implementing programmes to address poverty, social exclusion, and inequality, all key issues for public health.

The instruments used by government to influence society have been classified in a range of approaches, using different criteria. A classification by Hood (1986) groups these by government resource, namely nodality, authority, treasure, and organization. Another classification by Deber of policy instruments of government, is based on the degree of coercion in the means utilized. In this classification, the means of government influence from the least coercive to the most coercive are: exhortation, taxation, expenditure, regulations, and public ownership (Deber et al. 2004). Exhortation is often the first instrument used by government in governance, seeking initially to persuade with information and rationale (and may also include inferences of more coercive action if this does not have the effect intended). Health messages and information on health risks, interventions, and services are examples. This is frequently accompanied or followed by more coercive instruments, such as expenditure for a comprehensive programme of health education. Taxation is viewed as only slightly coercive. Providing tax incentives or disincentives, encourages or discourages targeted behaviours respectively. Provision of tax exemptions for not-for-profit organizations has encouraged the growth of NGOs in civil society, many of whom are engaged in social and health endeavours and services. Charities and charitable foundations are exempted from tax and in most countries make a substantial contribution to health initiatives. Tax disincentives, such as tax on tobacco and tobacco products, have been effective in reducing smoking rates. Expenditure is considered moderately coercive. This financial instrument can be cash or in-kind support such as providing meeting rooms for patient groups, and organizations to conduct patient support programmes. Contracts and direct payments to NGOs to operate health services and programmes for the care, treatment, and support of patients with HIV/AIDS, would be an example of the use of this vehicle. Indirect means can also be used, such as subsidies for vaccines to encourage uptake of an immunization programme to prevent an outbreak of seasonal influenza. The use of vouchers has also been used to improve access and encourage utilization of health services. The fourth category of instruments, regulations, is more coercive. The definitions of regulations used are 'all mechanisms of intentional and unintentional control' (Saltman and Russe 2002), 'setting rules of behaviour backed up directly by sanctions and penalties of the state' (Doern and Phidd 1992). Powers of regulations accrue to the three branches of government, the executive, legislative, and judicial, and can be in the forms of administrative decree, legislation, and judicial orders. Regulations on drugs and biological products seek to protect the public, ensuring the safety and quality of these products. The regulatory function may be administered by the government directly or by a public agency, such as a National Drug Administration or Agency. Regulation of health professions has been assigned by the state to the professions, in state-endorsed self-regulation, which is usually backed up by sanctions normally available only to governments. This hybrid form of governance arrangement, in which the private sector is able to use instruments of the state, is one instance of the evolving environment of health governance. The potential benefit of this arrangement is that the professional knowledge of a group of peers will enable effective ways of regulating conduct and behaviour and should reduce the cost of compliance, as compared to having government regulating. The disadvantage is the potential for 'regulatory capture' when professions use the process to protect their own interests over the public's. The fifth and last category of policy instruments in Deber's classification is public ownership. This is seen as the most coercive as government has 'full' control of the organization, product, or service it owns or provides. A National Health Service, providing health services to all the citizens of the country, enables governments to determine the types, scope, quality, and quantity of health services available, and where they will be available and how they will be accessed.

The policy instruments of government are one of the principal categories of the instruments of public sector governance; two other categories relate to structure and processes that foster coherence, collaboration, and partnership, within government and with civil society and the private sector (St-Pierre 2008). The cabinet of ministers of executive government is a key structure for coherence and consistency of national policies and intersectoral collaboration in policy development. Standing and ad hoc interdepartmental committees and task forces are structures within the administration which coordinate the work of different government departments. Structures for interactions and engagement with the private sector and civil society include advisory boards and consultative committees. New structures have been introduced to facilitate community- or citizen-centred governance, to engage the community in local governance. Examples of these include deliberative forums, citizens' juries, and community conferences (Pillora and McKinlay 2011). Networks of public officials with individuals, groups, and organizations in the private sector and civil society are a flexible structural mechanism for interaction. Participation in networks is voluntary; the interactions are informal and facilitate mutual understanding and development of common goals (St-Pierre 2008). The more recent innovative hybrid structures of 'unincorporated associations' of partnerships of the public, private, voluntary, and community sectors, is an organizational form. Appointment of community members and organizations are also structural forms of governance instruments. The third category of governance instruments of the government is processes (St-Pierre 2008). Different approaches to engage the community are needed to mobilize participation. In the United Kingdom, public and patient members for the constituency for governors in the National Health Service are advertised.

Supranational health governance

Health governance at the supranational level comprises three configurations: (1) an international configuration formed by a voluntary agreement of national governments and governed by formal rules of engagement, decision-making procedures and conduct, typified by organizations such as: the UN and the agencies within its ambit such as UNDP, and WHO, and a host of other international organizations such as World Bank, International Monetary Fund, World Trade Organization, G8 and G20; (2) regional groupings of sovereign states governed under different mechanisms and arrangements, ranging from the most formal, the European Union, with a formal constitution within which member states are obliged to act, to geo-political groupings of nations for economic and security discourse and agreements, such as Asia Pacific

Economic Cooperation, North Atlantic Treaty Organization and the Association of South East Asian Nations; and (3) a transnational global formation, comprising not only international and regional organizations and nation states, but also transnational and multinational business corporations and social movements and organizations of civil society. The challenges and issues in global health and the global health governance have generated considerable discourse and research, not only in public health, but also in international relations, political and social sciences, and international law. Global health and how it is governed affects every nation on the globe and the health of all of humanity.

Globalization, an intensification of the connections between populations enabled by the growth in the flows of people, goods, services, and ideas across countries, has been associated with a concomitant globalization of health determinants (Dodgson et al. 2002: Magnusson 2009; Kruk 2012). The health of populations has improved indirectly due to the benefits of globalization on the broader social determinants, although the benefits have not been spread equally within populations and between nations. In parallel, with globalization the transnational nature of the risk of infectious diseases associated with the increased flows of people and goods has been well documented, exemplified by the spread of HIV/AIDS in the last quarter of the twentieth century and of SARS in 2003. Although not receiving the same attention, there has also been globalization of risk factors for chronic diseases (Magnusson 2009). Non-communicable diseases accounted for 59 per cent of global mortality, with 54 per cent of all deaths in low- and middle-income countries, and 87 per cent in high-income countries. Economic growth is increasing incomes, urbanization, and a trend to more sedentary lifestyles. Intense global marketing of processed foods with transnational investments in supermarkets has also been associated with a change from traditional to diets richer in salt, sugar, and fats. The marketing of tobacco globally is hampering the efforts of national governments to control its use to reduce the harmful health effects. Climate change, an ecological impact of environmental change, is global. The global nature of health determinants restricts the capacity of national governments to address them on their own and international and global strategies are required. Global health, and its priorities, policies, and governance, are defined by the metaphors of how global health is framed. At least five metaphors have been identified. Global health framed as foreign policy is based on politicians using global health policies to foster trade, alliances, economic growth, stability, and democracy. The priority diseases targeted would be infectious diseases and HIV/AIDS. The second metaphor frames global health as security, the goals would be to combat bioterrorism and infectious diseases. Priority diseases targeted would include avian influenza, AIDS, and multidrug-resistant tuberculosis. The third frame is as charity, with the goal of fighting absolute poverty. Priority diseases to be addressed would be malnutrition, HIV/AIDS, malaria, and tuberculosis. The next frame is as investment, and how to maximize its value. Priority diseases would be HIV/AIDS and malaria. The fifth metaphor frames global health as public health, the goal would be to maximize health effect. The priority would be reducing the worldwide burden of disease (Stuckler and Mckee 2008). In a discussion of the concept and definition of global health, a consortium of universities advocated that global health should also address tobacco control, micronutrient deficiencies, obesity, injury prevention, migrant-worker health, and migration of health workers (Koplan et al. 2009). They also drew a distinction between global health, international health and public health. As discussed, how global health is framed will define policies, priorities and governance. On this premise alone, global health must be public health. The challenge of how this could and should be addressed has stimulated debate on global health governance. The policies and programmes to address transglobal risk factors for chronic diseases effectively are beyond the capacities and mandates of national governments on their own. Strategies and policies to address changing dietary habits require engagement with the food system, from primary production, manufacture, through to retail, catering, and advertising, agriculture, and trade, at national and international levels.

In the last one and a half decades, there has been a substantial increase of stakeholders in health with considerable influence on the global stage, and a consequential change in the configuration of the relationships, roles, and influence of the civil society, the private sector, and the state in health governance. Development Assistance for Health (DAH), defined as all disbursements for health from private and public institutions whose primary purpose is to provide development assistance to low- and middle-income countries, grew from US$5.1 billion in 1990 to US$21.8 billion in 2007 (GFATM 2013). DAH rose sharply after 2002, both from public and private funding. The US government was the largest public source of donations, followed by the United Kingdom, Japan, Germany, France, Netherlands, Canada, Sweden, Norway and Italy. The financial flows from low- and middle-income countries including China, and non-OECD high-income countries were not included in the assessment. The increases from private sources, from both philanthropic foundations and donors, and in-kind contributions from the private corporate sector which included donations of equipment and drugs from the pharmaceutical industry, amounted to approximately 50 per cent of the total disbursements for most years. The sources of funding from private donors and foundations increased, accounting for a growing share of DAH, from 19 per cent in 1998 to 26.7 per cent in 2006. In 2007, the Bill and Melinda Gates Foundation (BMGF) alone, was estimated to have spent US$2 billion on global health, comparable to the US$3.3 billion budget of the WHO (Kruk 2012). Equally significant, the proportion of funds channelled through UN agencies and development banks decreased, while NGOs and the GFATM, and the Global Alliance for Vaccines and Immunization (GAVI) accounted for an increasing share of DAH (GFATM 2013).

The significance of the changes in the flow of funds is not only in the relative role of UN agencies such as the WHO and UNICEF, but the fact that these agencies have to compete with NGOs for a share of the voluntary contributions which make up a growing proportion of their total expenditure. The powerful influence of the private sector in the changing global landscape is also evident in the strategies and tactics employed by the private corporate sector. There is well-documented research about how corporate strategies and actions at local, national, and global levels hindered the development of comprehensive approaches to tobacco control (Weishaar et al. 2012; GFATM 2013). Global tactics were employed by transnational tobacco corporations to undermine the development of the WHO Framework Convention on Tobacco Control (FCTC) (Weishaar et al. 2012). The research was based primarily on internal industry documents made public through litigation in the United States and a comprehensive literature review of the tobacco industry's strategies to influence the FCTC. The research demonstrated how the industry was able to develop and employ a comprehensive, multipronged strategy across multiple jurisdictions at a global level (for further detail, see Chapter 9.1). They highlight the flexible and varied approaches used by the industry, often ahead of the efforts of a weak system of international health governance, which is dependent on the voluntary participation of national governments and on their capacity to implement approaches they have committed to, in their respective states.

In the discussions of chronic disease and the challenge of global health governance, Magnusson also examined the nature of international health law and draws a similar conclusion: 'International health law, where it exists, takes the form of international agreements whose substantive obligations nation states have signed on to voluntarily, following a process of negotiation in a multilateral forum'. An important exception is the International Health Regulations (IHRs), which binds members on an 'opt-out' rather than an 'opt-in' basis (Magnusson 2009). The pace and extent to which individual states execute national policies to meet their substantive obligations is determined largely by the capacity and political commitment of the state, the only external influence is the normative pressure brought to bear by the international and global communities, notably, civil society. Understanding the prominent roles of the multinational corporations, and of civil society in global health requires an examination of the global governance environment. Many scholars from different fields have engaged in this pursuit.

Jan Aart Scholte puts forward the notion of globalization as 'deterritorialization' or 'supraterritoriality', and 'globality' as a unique social space, that transcends territorial place, distance, and borders, where there is no single source of authority (Scholte 2005). Geographical territoriality is determined by sovereign statehood which has jurisdiction over a designated territorial space. He goes further, arguing that territorialist governance is no longer practicable as national governments are no longer able by themselves to regulate effectively in the face of global mass media, ecological challenges, and finance. In this global governance space, unfettered by the absence of a 'world government', the roles and influence of the non-state institutions of society, namely the private sector and civil society, are transformed from those in sovereign states. In the absence of a single source of authority, the powers and influence of the corporate sector and civil society are considerable and arise from: (1) the resources at their command, (2) the capacity to frame and influence global health issues, (3) the flexibility in regularly incorporating new organization forms for governance in response and in anticipation of the rapidly changing environment, and (4) the ability to capitalize on new hybrid structures of partnerships of private–public governance which make available traditional public sector instruments for governance (Rosenau 1995; Kickbusch 2002; Loughlin and Berridge 2002; Kohlmorgen 2005; Scholte 2005; Kruk 2012). In contrast, the powers and influence of the state are muted. The traditional structures for governance of the state are lacking, the instruments of the state are also blunted, acting primarily through international bodies, the effectiveness of which has been limited. Fidler refers to the phenomenon of 'old-school anarchy' to describe the environment of international governance in which collective action taken by states is characterized by protracted negotiations, as states generally prefer to limit their obligations and restrictions to their sovereignty, and retain greater flexibility to pursue their own national priorities and interests (Fidler 2007). Fidler concluded that there was not a single global governance structure or distinct architecture and coined the term 'open-source anarchy' for the governance space which is equally accessible to state and non-state actors. The overlapping roles of international agencies in health governance have been significant and compound the phenomenon of the fragmentation of the influence of nation states in international and global health governance. The World Bank, WHO, and UNAIDS are three different forms of intergovernmental organizations with overlapping roles in global health governance. This governance space of open source anarchy, which is not under the jurisdiction of sovereign states, presents unprecedented opportunities for stakeholders in the global stage to define the new world order. The private corporate sector is the most powerful entity in the current environment of global health governance (Kempa et al. n.d.), with its flexibility to adapt to the changing terrain, entrepreneurial capabilities to innovate new mechanisms for influence, and market expertise to capitalize on the untapped potential in this new governance space. Even international organizations and states are capitalizing on the global 'open space anarchy' to further their own interests. In addition to its international role in global health governance, the United States has also taken bilateral, multilateral and unilateral roles. The United States provides one-third of the total bilateral global aid to health (Ollila 2005). One recent prominent example of its many roles is the President's Emergency Plan For AIDS, launched in 2004 providing US$15 billion over 5 years to fight HIV/AIDS; US$9 billion for new bilateral programmes, US$5 billion for existing programmes in 75 countries and US$1 billion for the GFATM (Kohlmorgen 2005). The unilateral role in global health and the links with its own domestic policies and interests and repositioning, has been the subject of some discussion (Kickbusch 2002). The United States is not unique in its multiprong approaches in global health. Many wealthy nation states are active in bilateral aid, including the more recent additions of India and China. Many multilateral initiatives of the powerful states either on their own or in partnership with private foundations and corporations have proliferated (Kickbusch 2002; Kohlmorgen 2005). Global health governance has been characterized as unstructured, pluralistic, and multicentric (Kickbusch 2002; Ollila 2005; Kruk 2012). The role and influence of private foundations and multistakeholder initiatives in defining and funding global health priorities has gained prominence in the last two decades. Kruk reported that there are now 100 GHIs, multistakeholder initiatives generally focused on a specific disease, product, or population, such as the GFATM, GAVI, and US President's Emergency Plan for AIDS Relief (PEPFAR). This has been paralleled by the emergence of major, extremely well-resourced GHIs by private foundations, such as the BMGF, the Clinton Foundation, and the Rockefeller Foundation (Ollila 2005; Kruk 2012). The plethora of GHIs has generated discussions about how these should be governed, and about global health governance in general. The issues of concern pertain to: (1) the composition and governance of the different GHIs and partnerships, their representative legitimacy, accountability, competence, and transparency in the decision-making process; (2) GHIs may differ from national health priorities; (3) the limited capacity of the health system infrastructure in many developing countries requires augmentation to enable delivery of the global health

programme; and (4) the transaction costs of applying for funding from the different funds, the burden of planning for the dissimilar programmes, and the need to meet the requirements of multiple donors in reporting progress, and financial and management information and evaluation methodologies (Brugha and Walt 2001; Ollila 2005). In recognition of these issues, efforts have been made to coordinate the global programmes. Health 8 (connotations of G8) comprising a grouping of GHIs and international agencies: WHO, World Bank, UNICEF, UNFPA, UNAIDS, GAVI, GFATM, and BMGF and International Health Partnerships, a grouping of seven donor countries, were formed as informal partnerships to facilitate coordination (2012). Global health governance is multicentric, with multiplicity of stakeholders' interests defining multiple frameworks (Hill 2011) and characterized as unstructured plurality (Fidler 2007). New governance forms of public–private partnerships of international bodies and agencies, national governments, civil society, and transnational corporations have emerged (Magnusson 2009; Hill 2011). Hill discusses global health governance as a complex adaptive system, with rich dynamic interactions, non-linearity of the relationships, and the relative interdependence of other elements within the system (Hill 2011). Studying global health governance as a chronic adaptive system provides a model for deeper understanding of the relationships and interactions of the components and the capacity to track, study, and research the changes that will emerge and evolve, reminiscent of the phenomenon 'back to the future', how governance evolved through the millennia to its form today of government, civil society and the private corporate sector.

Good health governance

Governance is a neutral concept. The UNDP defines it as the exercise of political, economic, and administrative authority in the management of a country's affairs at all levels (1997). It is how the authority is exercised which is the basis of good or bad governance. The UNDP has identified eight attributes of good governance, namely: participation, rule of law, transparency, responsiveness, consensus oriented, equity and inclusiveness, effectiveness and efficiency, and accountability.

The World Bank's approach to identify good governance is based on measurement of subjective perceptions of a set of over 300 governance indicators, in polls of experts and cross-country survey of residents. The World Bank's definition of governance is 'the traditions and institutions by which authority in a country is exercised' (Kaufmann et al. 1999). This includes '(1) the process by which governments are selected, monitored and replaced, (2) the capacity of the government to effectively formulate and implement sound policies, and (3) the respect of citizens and the state for the institutions that govern economic and social interactions among them' (Kaufmann et al. 1999). These were used to organize a subset of governance indicators into six clusters. Two clusters under the titles 'Voice and Accountability' and 'Political Instability and Violence' are key aspects of 'the process by which governments are selected, monitored and replaced'. The next two clusters titled 'Government Effectiveness' and 'Regulatory Burden' are aspects of 'the capacity of the state to formulate and implement sound policies'. The final two clusters under 'Rule of Law' and 'Graft', are derived from 'the respect of citizens and the state for the rules which govern their interaction'. The data was collected from over 150 countries. The quality of governance was correlated with developmental outcomes in cross-country comparisons. The study concluded that there was 'empirical evidence of a strong causal relationship from better governance to better development outcome' (Kaufmann et al. 1999).

In health governance, a recent attempt to identify the attributes and indicators of 'good health governance' was made by the Eastern Mediterranean Regional Office of WHO, in conjunction with Johns Hopkins University, Pakistan Health Policy Forum, Heartfile, and the Country Office of WHO in Pakistan. The goal was to develop a framework for assessing health governance as a gateway for good governance of health systems (Siddiqi et al. 2009). The group studied four frameworks developed for analysis of national governance, namely the UNDP's principles of good governance, the World Bank's six basic aspects of governance, the Pan American Health Organization's (PAHO) essential public health functions, and the WHO domains of stewardship. The group examined the PAHO's 11 essential public health functions in developing the framework because they were based on the principles of public health, and included the collective intervention of the state and civil society to protect and improve the health of the population, and the responsibilities of the steering role of government. The WHO in the *World Health Report 2000*, recognized stewardship of health systems as a key responsibility of the government (WHO 2000). The group concurred that the concept of stewardship is very similar to governance and that the terms were used interchangeably, but the group preferred the term 'governance' as the performance of health systems depends on overall governance of a country, and the many international development institutions and agencies had delineated attributes of governance that were understood and had been applied in assessment of governance, and governance is more familiar and better understood. The three stewardship tasks—defining the vision and direction, exerting influence, and collecting and using intelligence—were also governance functions and were included in the analysis. The group concluded that the UNDP governance principles provided a useful basis for developing the analytical framework for assessing health systems governance as it enabled a direct approach for the purpose and tools could be developed for more in-depth assessment. However there was a need to adapt the approach to include aspects unique to health. This was achieved by incorporating health-specific components of governance embodied in the stewardship functions proposed by WHO and PAHO's essential public health functions. Some aspects of the World Bank's principles of governance were also incorporated. The group proposed ten governance principles for assessing health governance: strategic vision, participation and consensus orientation, rule of law, transparency, responsiveness, equity and inclusiveness, effectiveness and efficiency, accountability, intelligence and information, and ethics. The ten principles were subsequently disaggregated into domains, from which were derived broad questions, leading to specific questions. The approach permitted an expression of the full meaning of the principle and how it could be operationalized. A total of 63 broad questions were developed and were related to context, description, process, and outcomes. The assessment framework has been applied to low- and middle-income countries

Stewardship, governance, and good governance

As discussed earlier, the concept of stewardship and governance in the WHO documents are similar and used interchangeably. In the conceptualization of health governance by the WHO, 'Governance in the health sector refers to a wide range of steering and rule making related functions carried out by governments/decision makers as they seek to achieve national health policy objectives that are conducive to universal coverage' (WHO 2013). The WHO's approach to health governance has evolved from the concept of stewardship in the *World Health Report 2000*, which was defined as a 'function of a government responsible for the welfare of the population, and concerned about the trust and legitimacy with which its activities are viewed by the citizenry' (WHO 2000). In a subsequent publication in 2007, *Everybody's Business: Strengthening Health Systems to Improve Health Outcomes*, 'leadership and governance of health systems' are 'also called stewardship' (WHO 2007). It is about the role of government in health and its relation to other actors whose activities impact on health. Health governance and public health governance as defined (Bennett et al. 2009), is the collective means adopted by society in attaining the conditions for health, and recognizes the partnerships of civil society, private sector, and the state in governance. In this conceptualization, stewardship described by WHO is in fact the Health Ministry's role and function in the context of government's responsibilities in the tripartite governance model. The stewardship role of government in health governance is to oversee and guide the whole health system in improving the health of the population. In fulfilling its responsibility as stewards in health governance, WHO has identified six key functions for stewardship as follows (WHO 2007):

1. Policy guidance: defining goals, directions and priorities, developing strategies, and establishing the roles of the public, and private sectors and civil society.

2. Intelligence and oversight: on responsiveness, financial protection and health outcomes of the health system, policy options, effects of policies and reforms, and on trends and differentials in inputs, access, coverage and safety of health services.

3. Collaboration and coalition building: across government, and with civil society and the private sector, to facilitate action which improves health and to generate support for health policies.

4. Regulations and incentives: should be designed, and fairly enforced to support strategies, goals and priorities.

5. Systems design: to ensure a fit between strategy and structure, minimizing duplication and fragmentation.

6. Accountability mechanisms: to be applied to all the components of the health system, transparency being a prerequisite.

WHO's description of the attributes of how the role and function should be performed effectively spells out the 'Good Stewardship role of Government in Public Health Governance'. In a similar way, in the context of global health governance, the WHO would be an appropriate body to have the stewardship role from its mandate in international health.

Governance and management in public health organizations

Good effective management in public health organizations is critical for success in developing and implementing strategies and programmes to improve the health of populations. Two key characteristics of public health programmes that create the context in which the governance and management in public health organizations should be considered are: (1) the majority of public health programmes involve the public sector, and not-for-profit organizations, and community organizations and groups with a wide range of formal and informal governance arrangements and capabilities, and (2) public health programmes range in scale from transnational and international programmes and initiatives, such as the global programme for HIV/AIDS, to discrete local programmes to improve health knowledge in local communities.

This organizational context of public health organizations creates the need for: (1) different governance and management systems appropriate for the legal incorporation status, size, complexity, and organizational formality of the NGOs and community organizations and groups; and (2) different management roles for public health officers depending on how the programme was initiated (De la Peza and Perry 2010). The civil society organizations and groups could be: (1) established NGOs, legally incorporated with formal board structures and policies and procedures for how they function; (2) recently incorporated NGOs originating from a small group of volunteers committed to a social cause, and supported by a handful of staff; and (3) largely informal community groups and networks of community groups and organizations, the majority without legal incorporation, working collectively for a common objective

Governance in legally incorporated public health organizations

The Institute on Governance in its work with the public sector and not-for-profit organizations defines governance as processes and a set of practices which enable an organization to achieve its goals. This is a system that defines how authority, decision-making, and accountability are exercised, and within which the organization determines its directions, monitors performance, and allocates power and resources (Institute on Governance 2011). Management is the process of planning, organizing, leading, and controlling the efforts of organization members and of using organizational resources to achieve stated organizational goals (Longest and Darr 2008). Management and governance are integral aspects of an organization, and enable it to accomplish the objectives and goals for the purpose for which it was set up. Although the roles can be segregated and functions differentiated, they need to be understood as interdependent and interrelated components in the continuum of systems and processes of the organization. The ultimate powers, authority, and accountability reside in the governance function of boards of incorporated organizations, and in the exercise of its powers in defining how authority, decision-making, and accountability will be exercised, it must do so in a manner which enables management to function effectively and efficiently, to accomplish the goals and objectives set. Conversely, management also has a responsibility to support governance to fulfil its duties and obligations setting directions and in the design of

systems with the categories of information required for monitoring of performance.

The process of developing the governance system should commence with examination of the legislative framework under which it was incorporated. Depending on the jurisdiction, they may be required to register as voluntary organizations or societies or be legally incorporated under the company's ordinance, with corresponding regulations under which they are required to operate. The organizations whose mission is not-for-profit, which would be the majority of public health community organizations, would be eligible to apply for tax exemption status. This would impose additional legal regulations with which the NGO would have to comply. The articles of incorporation specify the powers, responsibilities, and roles of the general membership and of the directors. The structure, composition, and procedures for the formation of the board, and rules and procedures for conducting meetings of the general membership or assembly and appointments of officers such as auditors and legal advisors may be specified either in the articles of incorporation or in the bylaws under which the organization should operate. The articles of incorporation serve as the 'constitution' under which the organization functions, sections of which are legally mandated under the relevant governing legislation and cannot be altered. The sections that are optional are within the discretion of the members of the organization, but any amendments require the approval of the general membership. The bylaws supplement the articles of incorporation, defining the rules, processes, and conduct under which it operates. Compliance to both the articles of association and bylaws is required.

Function of the board of directors

The first function of the board of directors is to determine the structures and procedures under which it will operate, within the requirements of the law, to define the policies and conduct under which it will function, and the values which will guide decision-making.

The second function of the board is to clarify its roles and define how this will relate to the roles of the chief executive and management team, and determine the decision-making process.

The third function of the board is to define how it will fulfil its responsibilities by examining four aspects of governance (De la Peza and Perry 2010):

1. Setting direction—the organization defines the mission, the purpose for its creation, and serves to align the board, management, and staff, providing meaning for its work. The mission is supported by defining a shared vision, representing where the organization aspires to be and provides the focus for the development of a strategic plan.

2. Overseeing organizational effectiveness and providing support—involves appointing a chief executive officer with the attributes to lead the organization, competencies to implement policies and execute plans, capacities to work collaboratively with the board to enable the board to fulfil its responsibilities, and conduct and values compatible with the organization's mission. The board needs to ensure that: the decision-making processes in the organization are transparent, the organization's resources are used rationally, efficiently and effectively, financial oversight is effective, the organization is financially sustainable, and quality of services are continuously improved.

3. Maintaining good external relationships—strategies, structures and mechanisms need to be established to engage and communicate with the community, donors, partners, and the government. Stakeholders need to be informed, their expectations need to be met, and their support needs to be solicited.

4. Maintaining the effectiveness of the board—this is enabled by having a composition of members with the skills, experience, diversity, commitment, and integrity, supported by an education and development programme, effective board structures and processes, and a system for evaluating and improving board performance.

A fourth function of the board is to consider 'intelligence systems' that will enable understanding, encoding, and tracking of the 'informal governance' mechanisms which are present in all organizations. Informal governance refers to traditions, organizational values, founding principles, and culture that are typically unwritten but that nonetheless prevail in the organization (Institute on Governance 2011). These traditions and values have a significant impact on how decisions are made, and how the decisions are affected.

The governance system in smaller NGOs with limited human resources, scale, and scope of work, has to be designed to suit their requirements. In these organizations, transitioning from voluntary initiatives and shared commitment to a common objective and functioning with informal rules, to the formal organization environment of a legal incorporation requires substantial support. In the process of transition, the founders who have been intimately involved with every aspect of the endeavour may have difficulty in separating governance and management roles. Resultant gaps in fulfilling governance functions required by law may be even more problematic. Complex, elaborate mechanisms are inappropriate. Simplified models based on principles of good corporate governance, and appropriate external support from organizations in civil society with a mission to promote governance, such as the Institute on Governance, academic and training institutions, and foundations.

Governance in public health organizations lacking legal incorporation

The governance mechanisms of largely informal community groups and networks of community groups and organizations, the majority not legally incorporated, are structurally distinct. These collaborations and partnerships are based on voluntary participation and authority is derived from the consent of the members. A study of governance in public–private community health partnerships reported a wide range of governing characteristics in the 25 partnerships involved in the community care network (Alexander et al. 1998). The study concluded that: (1) there is no single best way of governing community partnerships, and (2) governance structures and progress towards governance goals could be related to organization, composition, location, and type of collaborative activity of the partnership. Effective governance in these networks have as their foundations a commitment to a shared vision of community health and leadership in the governing bodies, and building of trust in incremental steps which would be the basis of changing governance practices. The range of governance arrangements and practices reflects a developmental continuum of different pathways.

Some will evolve to more formal organizations with better alignment of the objectives of the remaining partners, a number will continue to operate under network governance based on commitment to a common purpose and trust, and a few may be disengaged either because the purpose of the collaborative partnership has been dealt with as far as it was possible under the arrangements or progress was not made with loss of interest among the members.

Governance–management collaboration

The management roles of executives and public officials in public health organizations in supporting and facilitating good governance of groups and organizations in civil society is one facet of the governance–management interdependence which is critical for effectiveness of public health organizations and programmes.

The interdependence of governance and management functions is evident in the need for collaboration between management and governance, to enable the board to fulfil its responsibilities and management to understand the organization's mission and to be guided in its decisions by its values and vision. There are corresponding responsibilities of the board and management in developing the four key components of governance function of the organization in setting direction, overseeing organizational effectiveness and providing support, maintaining good external relationships, and maintaining the effectiveness of the board

Management of public health organizations

Management is the process of planning, organizing, leading, and controlling the efforts of organization members and of using all other resources to achieve stated organizational goals. Management has also been described as the science of getting things done through people. Management science is applied: (1) in the management of the organizations; (2) in the management of a function, for example, governance function in public health, 'Public health management'; and (3) in the management of a task, project, or programme, for example, 'Programme management in public health'.

General management principles apply to all organizations, but the application of the principles in the practice of public health also needs to be understood to enable effective management. Public health management functions in diverse contexts.

Public health management

Public health management, defined as 'the optimal use of the resources in society and its health services towards the improvement of the health experience' (Alderslade and Hunter 1994), has epidemiology at its core, and requires management capabilities and capacity. The conceptualization of the WHO has been driven by the knowledge that although significant health gains can be attained through systems and innovative approaches in health promotion and disease prevention, and by more effective management of clinical care, health systems are grossly underperforming in terms of improving the health of populations relative to what is feasible.

Another observation that has driven the approach is that the public health agenda has not been given the priority it should have, and this has been attributed to insufficient political commitment, marginalization of public health in health systems, and the limited capacity of public health to influence policymakers to make the changes necessary (WHO 2002). Public health management is based on the premise of a public health infrastructure, embedded in the health system, effecting interventions to improve the health of the population through the different components of the system in a holistic approach. This should enable health systems to be transformed from 'disease systems' to truly 'health systems'.

The principles of a public health management approach include (WHO 2002):

◆ 'Public health can find a legitimate place within an integrated set of provider services and hence be strongly supported within a provider framework.

◆ Critical to the success of this integration is strong central government commitment to public health outcomes for all provider services thus reinforcing the contributions public health can make to an integrated provider system.

◆ Contracting for outputs/outcomes, with ring fencing of public health funding, is one means of achieving this.

◆ Organized primary care is a key service division of an integrated district health system, with symbiotic relationships with public health.'

WHO has characterized the distinguishing features and roles of public health management (Table 6.8.2).

Public health management is a tool of governance that can bring about fundamental changes in the system at the national policy and local management level. At the national policy level the key considerations are: (1) developing a vision for coordinated 'joined up' policies in government which complement the policies to improve the health of populations, and for the vision to be effectively communicated and institutionalized in the decision-making structure; (2) ministerial leadership role in influencing other relevant government ministries and departments; (3) systems, mechanisms, and processes for integrated policymaking and implementation; and (4) cross-service and cross-agency collaboration for horizontal integration at local, provincial, national, and supranational levels and integration of these levels.

At the local operational level, the key considerations are: (1) developing and implementing a national policy framework which adopts a health outcome focus, (2) organizational options for coordination of providers and networks, (3) funding models to enable public health focus in integration, and (4) strategic purchasing and management. New Zealand is an example of a country which has an integrated system which is based on a broader conception of public health. Public health remains a central component of an integrated provider system, linked to primary care. All services—primary, secondary, and traditional public health—are population based (WHO 2002).

Programme management in public health

Programmes in public health range in scale and complexity, from global and multinational programmes and initiatives such as the multibillion GFATM covering specific country-level programmes in different nations across the globe, to discrete modest initiatives of local NGOs to improve health knowledge. Different governance structures and mechanisms are required for these two extremes of programmes, and the management approach would have to be tailored accordingly. However, principles of programme management apply to both.

The objective of programme management in public health is to organize and direct public health workers in the implementation of scientifically sound interventions, and appropriate strategies towards specific health problems (Bernard and Turnock 2013). The approach seeks to integrate the knowledge in public health with the scientific approaches in management in planning, organizing, leading, and controlling interventions to improve health. Success of a programme is not judged only by the programme's goals to improve health but also by criteria of efficiency and effectiveness. The programme management cycle comprises planning, implementation (organizing and leading), and evaluation (controlling). The three management processes should not be viewed as discrete phases, since feedback at all stages of the cycle should be used to make appropriate changes to the plans. There are continuous changes in both the internal and external environment,

Table 6.8.2 Distinguishing features and roles of public health management

Distinguishing features of public health management	Roles of public health management
Is multisectoral and professional	Advocacy and management roles
Combines knowledge and action	Knowledge and action
Has epidemiology at its core	Managerial capacity and infrastructure
Is influential across all health determinants	Networking to create partnerships across organizations and disciplines
Involves public health reporting, leading to health strategy development	Broad involvement of people and skills
Communicates with politicians, professionals, and the public	Infrastructure and curricula for education
Is influential organizationally and financially	Evidence-based policy and practice
Lies at the heart of the civic society	An outcome-based focus
	A national agenda for health and health services research

which have an impact on the planned intervention and require a modification of implementation strategies. The strategy for evaluation should be considered at the planning phase, based on identifying measures which would enable assurance of attaining critical milestones throughout the programme management cycle.

The approach to programme management can be framed in terms of asking five key questions: (1) Where are we? This involves examining the state of the current problem, identifying the effective interventions available, and the resources available; (2) Where do we want to be? This is the desired outcome to be accomplished; (3) Should we do something? This requires a decision on the extent of a health problem that warrants intervention; (4) What should we do? This is the process of establishing a work plan that incorporates the tasks and activities that are required, the resources that need to be committed and measures to track progress. This would also lead to development of a programme budget and the process of organizing the intervention. Programme structure, systems, and processes need to be designed, responsibilities and accountabilities assigned, and coordination and control mechanisms built in; and (5) How do we know that we are getting there? The key is to establish measurable milestones in time and direction that assure that the tasks are on track, the process objectives are achieved, and the intended health outcomes are attained.

Management in public health organizations

The four management processes of planning, organizing, leading, and controlling can be applied to every organization and facilitate the achievement of organizational goals (Longest and Darr 2008). Planning refers to deciding what to do, what is to be achieved, strategies for the task, and committing the resources required. Organizing is the design of an organization to execute the plans by establishing work units/clusters, allocating resources (including human) and responsibilities, delegating authority, establishing accountability, coordination of work processes, procedures, communications, as well as integration of work produced, systems, and structures.

Leading means leading, directing, and motivating people in the organization to achieve its plans and objectives. The last management process on controlling is to ensure the organization, work plans, and objectives are achieved through establishing and measuring performance standards, detecting deviations, and correcting performance. Not-for-profit (NGO) public health organizations vary considerably in their mission, scope of operations, and complexity of organization. Smaller NGOs have limited management and governance capacities. Board members may be volunteers who have a strong sense of purpose, and a hands-on approach to the operations. Conversely, boards may have evolved with time from the original founders and may not be able to commit the time to fulfil good governance requirements. The role of management to support the board to enable it to perform its function and fulfil its responsibilities is crucial. Good management will understand that an effective board in fact facilitates its work. The commissioners of public health programmes also have a key role in the management of NGOs contracted, in facilitating the development of management–governance relationships and capacities. This is being increasingly recognized by GHIs, which are now providing support to local NGOs, to enhance their management and governance capacities (Ravishankar et al. 2009).

Conclusions

Good governance and effective management are critical to the performance of health systems and of public health programmes. Public health programmes vary greatly in size, scope, and coverage, and operate in an environment of changing global landscape and national priorities and systems. Public health governance and management have to be understood as a whole in order to appreciate the rich, dynamic interactions and complexities that characterize it. Systems theory provides a conceptual basis for understanding, studying, and researching health governance as a system and the interactions and relationships within the wider environment of governance in society. Government, the private for-profit sector, and civil society are the institutions of society which make up the three components (subsystems) of the system with distinct structures, institutions, organizations, instruments and tools of influence, and mechanisms and processes for governance. The interactions and interdependencies of the three entities of public health governance are dynamic and evolving. This is evident in global health governance, where roles and influence of the private sector and civil society have gained prominence in the last decade and a half, and new governance forms have emerged such as public–private partnerships and the 'privatization' of governance. The principles of public health management and programme management are tools to enhance governance and management of public health organizations. The structure and mechanisms for the governance and management of public health organizations have to be appropriate for their context including considerations such as legal incorporation status, size, complexity, and organizational formality. Governance–management collaboration is critical for organizational effectiveness and complementary roles can be structured to facilitate this. Good governance and effective management ensure that the right things are done right, in the right way.

Acknowledgements

Text extracts from World Health Organization, *Everybody's Business: Strengthening Health Systems to Improve Health Outcomes: WHO's Framework for Action*, World Health Organization, Geneva, Switzerland, Copyright © 2007, reproduced with permission from the World Health Organization, available from http://www.who.int/healthsystems/strategy/everybodys_business.pdf.

Text extracts from Kaufmann, D. et al., *Governance Matters*, Policy Research Working Paper 2196, The World Bank Development Research Group, Macroeconomics and Growth and World Bank Institute Governance, Regulation and Finance, Copyright © 1999, reproduced with permission of the World Bank, available from http://info.worldbank.org/governance/wgi/pdf/govmatters1.pdf.

Text extracts from World Health Organization, *Public Health Management: World Health Organization—University of Durham meeting report*, World Health Organization, Geneva, Switzerland, Copyright © 2002, reproduced with permission from the World Health Organization, available from http://www.who.int/chp/knowledge/publications/PH_management7.pdf.

References

Acheson, D. (1988). *Public Health in England: The Report of the Committee of Inquiry into the Future Development of the Public Health Function.* London: HMSO.

Alderslade, R. and Hunter, D.J. (1994). Commissioning and public health. *Journal of Management and Medicine*, 8(6), 20–31.

Alexander, J.A., Comfort, M.E., and Weiner, B.J. (1998). Governance in public–private community health partnerships: a survey of the community care network demonstration sites. *Nonprofit Management & Leadership*, 8(4), 311–22.

Barnes, M., Skelcher, C., Beirens, H., Dalziel, R., Jeffares, S., and Wilson, L. (2008). *Designing Citizen-Centred Governance.* Birmingham: Joseph Rowntree Foundation.

Bennett, B. (2009). Legal rights during pandemics: federalism, rights and public health laws—a view from Australia. *Public Health*, 123(3), 232–6.

Bennett, B., Gostin, L., Magnusson, R., and Martin, R. (2009). Health governance: law, regulation and policy. *Public Health*, 123(3), 207–12.

Bernard, J. and Turnock, M. (2013). *Program Management in Public Health.* [Online] Available at: http://www.uic.edu/sph/prepare/courses/ph440/mods/ph441text.

Brandt, A.M. (2007). *The Cigarette Century.* New York: Basic Books.

Brugha, R. and Walt, G. (2001). A global health fund: a leap of faith. *British Medical Journal*, 323, 152–4.

Deber, R., Topp, A., and Zakus, D. (2004). *Private Delivery and Public Goals: Mechanisms for Ensuring that Hospitals Meet Public Objectives.* Toronto: University of Toronto.

De la Peza, L. and Perry, C.P. (2010). Promoting good governance in public and private health organizations. In *Health Systems in Action: An eHandbook for Leaders and Managers*, pp. 3.1–3.44. Medford, MA: Management Sciences for Health, Inc.

Demand for Good Governance Team (2010). *Demand for Good Governance in the World Bank: Conceptual Evolution, Frameworks and Activities.* Washington, DC: World Bank Social Development Department.

Dodgson, R., Lee, K., and Drager, N. (2002). *Global Health Governance: A Conceptual Review.* Geneva: World Health Organization and London School of Hygiene and Tropical Medicine.

Doern, G. and Phidd, R. (1992). *Canadian Public Policy: Ideas, Structure, Process* (2nd ed.). Toronto: Nelson Canada.

Emmerij, L., Jolly, R., and Weiss, T.G. (2001). Governance, good governance, and global governance. In *Ahead of the Curve? UN Ideas and Global Challenges*, pp. 183–204. Bloomington, IN: Indiana University Press.

Fidler, D.P. (2007). Architecture amidst anarchy: global health's quest for governance. *Global Health Governance*, 1(1), 1–17.

Freeman, J. (2000). The private role in public governance. *New York University Law Review*, 75(101), 543–675.

Gostin, L.O. and Gostin, K.G. (2009). A broader liberty: J.S. Mill, paternalism and the public's health. *Public Health*, 123, 214–21.

Hill, P.S. (2011). Understanding global health governance as a complex adaptive system. *Global Public Health*, 6(6), 593–605.

Hood, C. (1986). *The Tools of Government.* Chatham, NJ: Chatham House Publishers.

Institute on Governance (2011). *Governance.* [Online] Available at: http://iog.openconcept.ca/en/about-us/governance.

Jewell, T. andWilkinson, J. (2008). Health and social care regulation in Wales: an integrated system of political, corporate and professional governance for *improving* public health. *The Journal of the Royal Society for the Promotion of Health*, 128(6), 306–12.

Kast, F.E. and Rosenzweig, J.E. (1972). General systems theory: applications for organization and management. *Academy of Management Journal*, 15(4), 447–65.

Kaufmann, D., Kraay, A., and Zoido-Lobaton, P. (1999). *Governance Matters.* Policy research working paper. The World Bank.

Kempa, M., Shearing, C., and Burris, S. (n.d.). *Changes in Governance: A Background Review.* [Online] Available at: http://www.temple.edu/lawschool/phrhcs/salzburg/Global_Health_Governance_Review.pdf.

Kickbusch, I. (2002). Influence and opportunity: reflections on the U.S. role in global public health. *Health Affairs*, 21(6), 131–41.

Kohlmorgen, L. (2005). *International Organisations and Global Health Governance. The Role of the World Health Organization, World Bank and UNAIDS. The Salzburg Seminar on the Governance of Health.* Salzburg: German Overseas Institute.

Koplan, J.P., Bond, T.C., Merson, M.H., et al. (2009). Towards a common definition of global health. *The Lancet*, 373, 1993–5.

Kruk, M.E. (2012). Globalisation and global health governance: implications for public health. *Global Public Health*, 7(S1), S54–62.

Lauer, J.A. (2001). Determinants of performance. In C. Murray and J. Frenk (eds.) *Health System Performance: Concepts, Measurement and Determinants*, pp. 1–16. Geneva: World Health Organization.

Longest, B.B. and Darr, K., Jr. (2008). *Managing Health Services Organizations and Systems* (5th ed.). Baltimore, MD: Health Professions Press.

Loughlin, K. and Berridge, V. (2002). *Global Health Governance: Historical Dimensions of Global Governance.* Geneva: World Health Organization and London School of Hygiene and Tropical Medicine.

Magnusson, R.S. (2009). Rethinking global health challenges: towards a 'global compact' for reducing the burden of chronic disease. *Public Health*, 123(3), 265–74.

Mills, A., Rasheed, F., and Tollman, S. (2006). Strengthening health systems. In D.T. Jamison, J.G. Breman, A.R. Measham, et al. (eds.) *Disease Control Priorities in Developing Countries*, pp. 87–102. Washington, DC: The World Bank.

Office of the Auditor General of Canada (1999). *1999 September Report of the Auditor General of Canada. Chapter 14: National Health Surveillance—Diseases and Injuries.* Ottawa: Office of the Auditor General of Canada and the Commissioner of the Environment and Sustainable Development.

Ollila, E. (2005). Global health priorities—priorities of the wealthy? *Global Health*, (1)6.

Pillora, S. and McKinlay, P. (2011). *Evolution in Communitity Governance: Building on What Works: Literature Review.* Sydney: Australian Centre of Excellence for Local Government, Sydney UoT.

Ravishankar, N., Gubbins, P., Cooley, R.J., et al. (2009). Financing of global health: tracking development assistance for health from 1990 to 2007. *The Lancet*, 373(9681), 2113–24.

Renukumar, N. (n.d.). *Good Governance: Concepts and Components.* [Online] Centre for Good Governance. Available at: http://www.scribd.com/doc/45724301/Good-Governance.

Rosenau JN. (1995). Governance in the twenty-first century. *Global Governance*, 1(1), 13–43.

Saltman, R. and Russe, R. (2002). Balancing regulation and entrepreurialism in Europe's health sector theory and practice. In R. Saltman, R. Russe, and E. Mossialos (eds.) *Regulating Entrepreneurial Behaviour in European Health Care Systems*, pp. 1–52. Buckingham: Open University Press.

Scholte, J.A. (2005). Civil society and democracy in global governance. In R. Wilkinson (ed.) *The Global Governance Reader*, pp. 322–40. New York: Routledge.

Siddiqi, S., Masud, T.I., Nishtar, S., et al. (2009). Framework for assessing governance of the health system in developing countries: gateway to good governance. *Health Policy*, 90(1), 13–25.

St-Pierre, L. (2008). *Governance Tools and Framework for Health in All Policies.* Montréal: National Collaborating Centre for Healthy Public Policy.

Stuckler, D. and Mckee, M. (2008). Five metaphors about global-health policy. *The Lancet*, 372, 95–7.

The Global Fund to Fight AIDS, Tuberculosis and Malaria (2013). Website. [Online] Available at: http://www.theglobalfund.org/en/.

United Nations Development Programme (1997). *Governance for Sustainable Human Development:A UNDP Policy Document.* [Online] United Nations Development Programme. Available at: http://mirror.undp.org/magnet/policy/.

Weishaar, H., Collin, J., Smith, K., Grüning, T., Mandal, S., and Gilmore, A. (2012). Global health governance and the commercial sector: a documentary analysis of tobacco company strategies to influence the WHO Framework Convention on Tobacco Control. *PLoS Medicine*, 9(6), e1001249.

Wilson, K. (2004). The complexities of multi-level governance in public health. *Canadian Journal of Public Health*, 95(6), 409–12.

World Health Organization (2000). *World Health Report 2000. Health Systems: Improving Performance.* Geneva: WHO.

World Health Organization (2002). *Public Health Management. University of Durham Meeting Report.* Geneva: WHO.

World Health Organization (2007). *Everybody's Business: Strengthening Health Systems to Improve Health Outcomes: WHO's Framework for Action.* Geneva: WHO.

World Health Organization (2013). *Health Systems: Governance.* World Health Organization. [Online] Available at: http://www.who.int/healthsystems/topics/stewardship/en/.

Implementation science and translational public health

Kedar S. Mate, Theodore Svoronos, and Dan W. Fitzgerald

Introduction to implementation science and translational public health

As the armamentarium of available technologies and services to improve health and healthcare in low- and middle-income countries grows, there has been a well-recognized gap between the health gains that could be achieved and those that are being realized around the world (World Health Organization 2007). This is not a problem unique to resource-poor countries—some investigators have estimated delays in implementing evidence-based care of up to 17 years in rich countries (Balas-Eltes 2000). Well-known, evidence-based health technologies are not reliably implemented in any context. As the editors of the journal *Implementation Science* wrote in their inaugural issue, 'Uneven uptake of research findings—and thus inappropriate care—occurs across settings, specialties and countries' (Eccles and Mittman 2006, p. 1).

In 2001, the Institute of Medicine (IOM) in the United States noted that, 'between the healthcare we have and the care we could have lies not just a gap, but a chasm' (Committee on Quality of Health Care in America 2001, p. 1). Scientists and researchers, policymakers, and advocates had concluded that inadequate or incomplete implementation of evidence-based practices in US hospitals had resulted in more than 99,000 avoidable deaths annually. These delays are likely longer and cause more avoidable death and injury in resource-poor settings. Tuberculosis (TB) is an illustrative example: despite knowing the cure for TB for more than 60 years, 1.4 million people died of TB in 2011 (World Health Organization 2012). While the clinical evidence has clearly demonstrated that antiretroviral (ARV) treatment for patients living with TB/HIV co-infection is effective, only 48 per cent of these patients received these life-saving medications in 2011 (World Health Organization 2012).

Implementation science is the study of strategies undertaken to implement evidence-based technologies, services, diagnostics, or therapeutics (referred to henceforth as 'healthcare interventions') in 'real-life' populations and contexts. The subject of study, as described by the National Institutes of Health (NIH), is the implementation method itself or the 'strategies to adopt and integrate evidence-based health interventions and change practice patterns within specific settings' (NIH 2011). The editors of *Implementation*

Science go further in their initial description by suggesting the purpose of this new field of investigation: 'Implementation research is the scientific study of methods to promote the systematic uptake of research findings and other evidence-based practices into routine practice, and, hence, to improve the quality and effectiveness of health services and care' (Eccles and Mittman 2006, p. 1). Thus there is an important link between the study of implementation and healthcare quality and effectiveness—a link made by the Institute of Medicine in its *Chasm* report (Committee on Quality of Health Care in America 2001).

The primary aim of implementation science is an optimistic one—focused on finding the opportunities to improve health and healthcare for all populations where gaps in care currently persist. In 2009, the African Academies of Science described one such opportunity when they wrote, 'If coverage of essential MNCH [maternal, newborn, and child health] interventions reached all families in sub-Saharan Africa and everyone received high quality care, nearly 4 million mothers, newborns, and children could be saved each year' (African Academies of Sciences 2009, p. 3). The goal of implementation science is not only to inform policymakers that create guidelines and new regulations, but also to examine how and why these guidelines, policies, and regulations too often fail at the front lines of service delivery (Schackman 2010; Padian et al. 2011).

Two examples from the HIV clinical world illustrate the need for implementation science clearly. High rates of preventable HIV infection illustrate gaps in translating research into bedside and community-level results. Preventive health technologies, including ARV medications, can now reduce the risk of perinatally acquired HIV from approximately 25 per cent to less than 2 per cent, and global calls for eliminating perinatal HIV transmission have been issued by the World Health Organization (WHO) and the United Nations (Lindegren et al. 1999; Centers For Disease Control and Prevention 2007; McKenna and Hu 2007; UNAIDS 2011). Yet, despite the promise of these interventions, only 50 per cent of pregnant women are tested for HIV in the highest-burden countries in east and southern Africa, and only 68 per cent of pregnant women living with HIV receive therapy containing ARV medications in these countries (WHO 2010). Failure to deliver well-established prevention of mother-to-child HIV transmission (PMTCT) interventions contributes to the nearly 370,000 babies

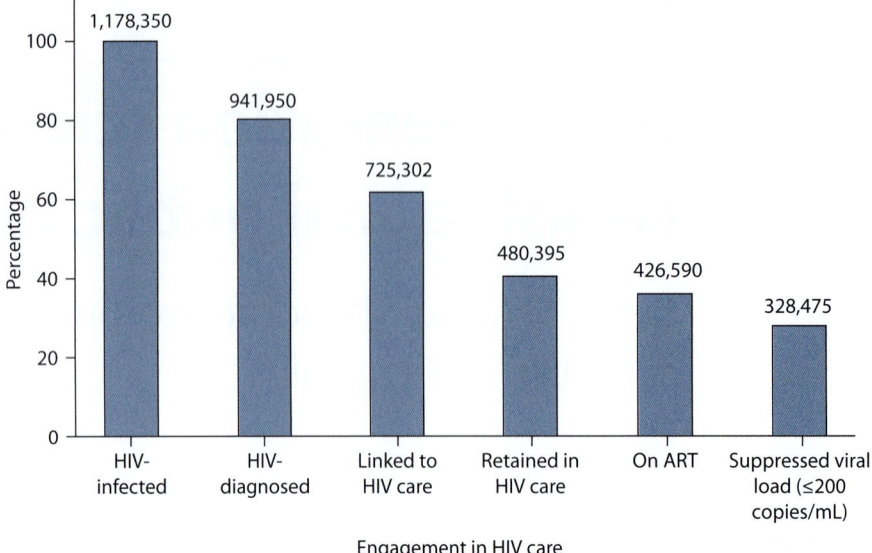

Fig. 6.9.1 Number and percentage of HIV-infected people engaged in selected stages of the continuum of HIV care—United States. ART, antiretroviral therapy; HIV, human immunodeficiency virus.

Reproduced from Centers for Disease Control and Prevention (CDC), Vital signs: HIV prevention through care and treatment: United States, *Morbidity and Mortality Weekly Report* (MMWR), Volume 260, Issue 47, pp. 1618–1623, 2011, available from http://www.cdc.gov/mmwr/preview/mmwrhtml/mm6047a4.htm.

infected with HIV each year (United Nations 2000; WHO 2010). Such findings highlight the differences between results obtained in controlled research settings and those recorded in 'real-life' health systems with constrained resources and inadequate systems.

Similarly for the clinical management of HIV infection, investigators have described a cascade of interventions from diagnosis to effective treatment that are needed for an HIV-infected individual to improve his or her chances of long-term survival (Fig. 6.9.1) (Centers for Disease Control and Prevention 2011). The points along this cascade represent opportunities for patients to become 'lost to follow-up'. As the graph clearly shows there are major losses at each step, which represent opportunities for further investigation for implementation scientists.

The purpose of implementation science is to study the myriad approaches to implementation that are taken with any given healthcare technology or service with the goal of understanding how to close gaps between 'what we know' (evidence-based interventions) and 'what we actually do' at the front lines of healthcare. In the case of each country, the conditions of the context are different—budgets will vary, healthcare personnel will be limited, distribution channels may be fraught, but community assets might be stronger, families more engaged, policies more favourable. Each country and each community will be different, and these differences will in turn affect the implementation approach taken and the consequent evaluation approach. For the purposes of this chapter, we discuss low- and middle-income countries as one block and high-income countries as another block, but we recognize that these groups of dozens of countries and many thousands of communities represent a great deal of heterogeneity that will affect the implementation of any healthcare intervention at the front lines.

Finally, implementation science investigators seek to ensure that the approaches taken to close the gaps described above are based as much on evidence and careful study as the healthcare technologies and services they seek to implement. The audiences

for this evidence on implementation strategies are policymakers, programme managers, health system designers, and global health practitioners. But, most importantly, the audience is the front-line healthcare workers who seek to more rapidly and reliably deliver the fruits of modern medical science to their patients every day.

Locating implementation science

Therapeutic discovery occurs in phases which the NIH has classified as translational steps (Fig. 6.9.2). With each advancing phase the number of clinical subjects that are part of the research study gets larger as confidence in the investigational therapeutic grows. Phase IV trials, included under the 'translation to practice' step, are meant to be large-scale studies across multiple heterogeneous practice environments, translating phase III therapeutic efficacy into effective public health programming at scale.

While this image locates implementation science in the third translation, we would argue that the study of implementation is also salient to the fourth translation, 'to population health'. The order of magnitude is different, but the study of methods and approaches to implementing a healthcare technology or service 'at scale' is an important part of the study of implementation. Thus we believe that implementation science ought to span both the third and fourth translations in the conventional research sequence shown in Fig. 6.9.2.

The NIH defines implementation research as a context-sensitive science, explaining that:

> Implementation research studies should distance from prior assumptions that empirically-supported interventions can be transferred into any service setting without attention to local context and that a unidirectional flow of information (e.g. publishing a guideline) is sufficient to achieve practice change. Relevant studies should develop a knowledge base about 'how' interventions are transported to real-world practice settings, which will likely require more than the dissemination of information about the interventions. (NIH 2012)

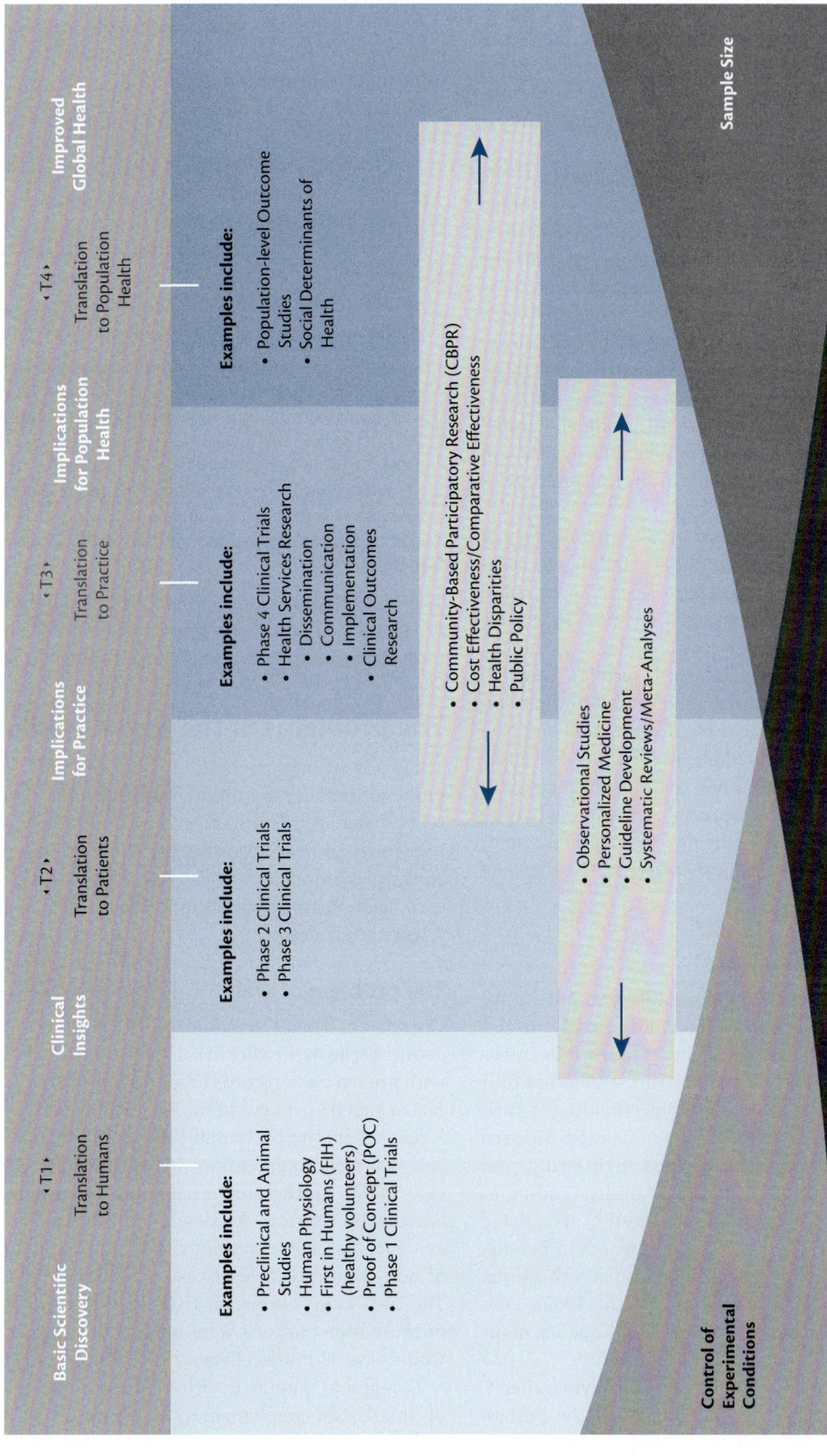

Fig. 6.9.2 Clinical and translational research spectrum.

Reproduced with permission from Harvard Catalyst, *Clinical and Translational Research Spectrum*, Copyright © 2014 by the President and Fellows of Harvard College, available from http://catalyst.harvard.edu/pathfinder/.

Implementation science as a science

Scientific methods and approaches are as vital to the study of implementation successes and failures as they are to the discovery of new diagnostics and therapeutics. Failure to subject the implementation approaches taken to the discipline of scientific testing and analysis will ensure that the current inadequate delivery systems will prevail, leaving the medicines and technologies of modern scientific discovery to reach patients heterogeneously and by chance.

When new evidence-based technologies are introduced, the healthcare delivery system must be adjusted to take advantage of what the new technology can now offer. This adjustment does not happen automatically without deliberate attention to how the health system must change. In fact, as new therapeutic, diagnostic, and preventative technologies are introduced the gap between what is possible and the actual performance of health systems may grow wider (Victora et al. 2000). This 'technology-to-systems gap' means that clinically important discoveries are often held hostage to the inability of our health systems to deliver them. Parallel investment in the study of implementation in health systems will ensure that all patients can reap the benefits of clinically meaningful new technologies.

The tools of today's research community—controlled study designs, randomization, methods to limit bias, and match comparison groups—are perfectly designed to science conducted under the microscope or in clinical research settings. Such tools may not be well suited to study the services provided in hospitals, clinics, or the complex adaptive public health systems in which these organizations operate. However, in resource-limited settings, if we are to create a future that is different from the past with its persistent implementation failures, we will need to apply the rigours of scientific process to a new set of implementation problems. The study of implementation remains foremost a science and requires the discipline of developing new ideas, predicting or hypothesizing their impact, and rigorously assessing the effects of these new ideas in context.

Origins of implementation science

Implementation science shares both quantitative and qualitative analytic traditions as part of its history. W. Edwards Deming's system of profound knowledge lies at the heart of the implementation intellectual tradition (Deming 1993). This system has four central aspects: understanding of systems, understanding of variation, theory of knowledge, and psychology of change. Modern operations research science, industrial process engineering, and the management sciences inform our current understanding of systems. The health systems research agenda, recently articulated at the Global Symposium on Health Systems Research in Beijing, is the best representation of this pursuit of systems thinking. Quantitative studies of practice variation from the 1980s, economic decision analysis, and aspects of industrial quality management form the backbone of understanding variation.

Ethnography, cognitive behavioural sciences, behavioural economics, sociology, and psychology have informed the human factors considerations that are critical to understanding why patients and providers act on certain ideas and reject others. The NIH notes that implementation science fundamentally, 'seeks to understand the behaviour of healthcare professionals and support staff, healthcare organizations, healthcare consumers and family members, and policymakers in context as key variables in the sustainable adoption, implementation and uptake of evidence-based interventions' (NIH 2012).

Finally, emerging evaluative techniques, including realist and adaptive trial designs, have been slowly reshaping the design of implementation research evaluation. This transformation in how we know what we know forms Deming's final building block on theory of knowledge or epistemology. Implementation science combines quantitative and qualitative analytic traditions into methods that allow learning from the context in which the process of care delivery is actually occurring.

Importantly, implementation science differs from the routine monitoring and evaluation that is common in donor-financed programmes in resource-limited countries. This difference has been most clearly described by Hirschorn et al. who wrote:

> In general, the objectives of monitoring and evaluation programs and implementation are similar: to understand what is working well, what is not working, and why. However, most monitoring and evaluation activities necessarily focus on measuring the services provided rather than on the barriers to implementation. The scientific rigor of implementation research broadens the scope of monitoring and evaluation activities to understand the etiology of gaps between expected results and observed outcomes. (Hirschhorn et al. 2007, p. S528)

Thus despite similarities in objectives and data sources to routine programme monitoring, implementation science remains foremost a rigorous hypothesis-driven investigational activity.

The problems of the new discipline

The study of implementation is complicated by four important problems that are not unique to implementation science, but present particular dilemmas that must be overcome in the design of implementation science studies. These are the problems of scale, context, methods, and overconfidence which are addressed in turn before turning our attention to the details of implementation science study design.

The problem of scale

Current challenges in public health, particularly in resource-poor countries, lie in the effective delivery and scale-up of interventions with proven track records (Victora et al. 2011). A recent study estimated that 63 per cent of the 7.6 million deaths in children under 5 years of age are preventable if just 23 evidence-based preventive and treatment interventions were implemented universally (Jones et al. 2003). Much of maternal and newborn premature mortality is avoidable (African Academies of Sciences 2009). Cost-effective, evidence-based interventions exist to prevent and limit the impact of non-communicable diseases (NCDs) (Beaglehole et al. 2008). The 2007 *Lancet* series on NCDs estimated that if a small subset of these interventions were universally applied in 23 nations, it would save 32 million lives by 2015 (Beaglehole et al. 2007).

The global public health literature is replete with studies of small-scale implementation where a particular problem is addressed using a well-resourced, robust implementation strategy that produces a successful 'pilot' result under study circumstances. This now 'evidence-based' intervention is then appropriately selected by practitioners and policymakers to be replicated elsewhere. Yet, as the intervention is spread and implemented in multiple different contexts, facing different constraints, and without the carefully controlled study circumstances of the pilot study, the intervention's results are often not replicated.

Take, for example, rapid response systems—clinical interventions designed to provide an earlier bedside response in the hospital setting to a patient's changing haemodynamics and to nursing, patient, or family concerns about changes in the patient's condition (Devita et al. 2006). Several studies in pilot sites found significant impacts of this clinical intervention on inpatient mortality, cardiopulmonary arrest rates, and deaths not in intensive care units (Bristow et al. 2000; Buist et al. 2002). Seizing on these results, numerous organizations sought to actively promote and scale-up the use of rapid response systems, but the pilot testing results could not be replicated reliably elsewhere (Steel and Reynolds 2008).

In a heated exchange in the literature, rapid response teams were criticized severely and the validity of the earlier studies was called into question (Winters et al. 2006). What was overlooked, however, was the fact that the implementation itself—the design of the rapid response teams themselves, the systems in which they were deployed, the culture of the implementing hospitals, and the leadership support (or lack thereof)—was rarely systematically documented, analysed, and interpreted. Without this careful study of the implementation of this complex intervention, a conclusion about the effectiveness of rapid response teams cannot be easily reached.

The problem of context

Scaling up requires a nuanced understanding of how the implementation of efficacious interventions varies across social, economic, and political contexts. It requires an accounting of how these contextual details might exert as much influence on uptake of an intervention as the specific details of the healthcare technology itself (Arifeen et al. 2004).

The problem of context has been well documented by leading epidemiologist John Ioannidis, who studied 45 'evidence-based' medical practices and found that fully a third could not be duplicated in new contexts (Ioannidis 2005). This was illustrated further by Parry et al., 'Simply copying models, without taking account of local context, does not guarantee successful widespread improvement' (Parry et al. 2013). Healthcare technologies found to be effective in a carefully designed trial may not be as effective in contexts that are dissimilar to the one in which they were initially studied. Indeed, as the implementation context varies further from the context of the original efficacy study, the chances of implementation success may diminish further. Efforts to study, measure, and understand the role of context and its influence on implementation are underway (Kaplan et al. 2010; Svoronos and Mate 2011).

In addition to the social, economic, and political contexts in which healthcare interventions are deployed, one must also consider that healthcare organizations are themselves constantly changing which may influence the uptake of an intervention. In order to better inform service delivery, ongoing evaluations of implementation effectiveness will need to provide implementers with real-time continuous feedback on how they are changing to affect outcomes (Rowe 2009; Victora et al. 2011). Summative evaluations that spend years collecting baseline data and reporting on results after the conclusion of the intervention are no longer adequate. Going back

to the example provide earlier, one commentator noted, 'An RRS (rapid response system) is not a drug treatment, a hospital is not a body. Both are continually changing, complex social interventions' (Øvretveit and Suffoletto 2007).

The problem of method

Despite some understanding of these needs, the techniques and methods for studying implementation across contexts and at scale remain underdeveloped and underreported in the literature (Victora et al. 2004, 2011). Instead, study designs built to evaluate the efficacy of a clinical intervention in a controlled setting or to study a biomedical compound in the laboratory are often mistakenly applied to study and interpret the effectiveness of both the intervention and the implementation approach (Oxman et al. 1995; Øvretveit and Gustafson 2003). These designs, including the fixed-protocol randomized controlled trial, are primarily capable of assessing an intervention in controlled situations that rarely imitate 'real life'.

Methods for studying the variety of approaches that may be taken to implement a new diagnostic technique or therapeutic across heterogeneous contexts remains scarcely documented. The journal *Implementation Science* was introduced only in 2006 and it remains the only journal dedicated to advancing the methodology of studying implementation. The journal, 'aims to publish research relevant to the scientific study of methods to promote the uptake of research findings into routine healthcare in clinical, organizational or policy contexts' (*Implementation Science* 2014). Such approaches are welcome, but need to be expanded and further developed. Additionally, although *Implementation Science* encourages contributions from developing countries, only a small fraction of the studies appearing in the journal describe implementation studies from resource-limited contexts.

The problem of overconfidence and unintended variation

Finally, despite multiple documented failures of implementation of evidence-based technologies in high- and low-income settings, we continue to place undue faith in our clinical practitioners—insisting that when confronted with the evidence and mounting guidelines, they will make the right decisions and will deliver all necessary care to everyone in a timely and reliable manner. The principles of authority, autonomy, and independent responsibility for services to the individual patient are deeply embedded in the psychology of the practitioner and in the psychology of many patients who seek the expert counsel of their doctors (Berwick 2009).

This compact between patient and doctor is in many ways the foundations of the profession, but variations in clinical practice for even common conditions like pneumonia, heart failure, and myocardial infarction are now a well-documented phenomenon (Wennberg 1998; Fisher et al. 2009). Physician decisions are influenced by their peers, by their patients, and by their professional societies. Reliable implementation is destabilized by these external forces which must be measured in order to be successfully brought under control. The sobering data describing enormous practice variation for even the most basic of evidence-based practices serves as a persistent reminder not of the failure of intention on the part of physicians, but failures of systems design to support practitioners to make the right thing to do, the default thing to do.

Implementation science study design

We review the core elements of study design including: understanding the subject of study, identifying the primary research question, planning measures, and selecting the format for the study including considerations of control groups and strategies for eliminating bias. These are not unique to implementation science studies, but in the context of studying implementation they do have unique features.

Understanding the subject of implementation science: the approach to implementation

Before proceeding further it is worth describing the subject of study further. Implementation science focuses upon the approaches used to implement a healthcare technology, service, diagnostic, or therapeutic. The units of study may be individual patients, but more often the units of study are health facilities, hospital wards, health districts, or geographic populations where different approaches are used to provide a healthcare technology. As a clinical researcher studies new interventions and tries to characterize and control for the variability between individual patients, the implementation scientist studies new approaches to provide an existing technology and tries to characterize and control for variability between units of study (health facilities, hospital wards, health districts, etc.).

The implementation scientist may or may not be involved in the implementation effort itself. While it may be cleaner to have the implementation effort be conducted by one group and the study of the implementation approach done separately by an unbiased individual or organization, there are often many situations in which this separation is unrealistic and impossible, especially in resource-constrained settings.

There are many approaches to implementation of a healthcare technology, service, diagnostic, or therapeutic. The healthcare intervention itself is not under study (e.g. antibiotic, diagnostic test, procedure)—these are studied elsewhere using conventional biomedical and clinical research tools described in great detail in textbooks of clinical research methods. Implementation science is the study of the approaches taken to reliably providing these technologies across heterogeneous contexts. A non-exhaustive list of examples of implementation approaches might include:

1. Executive mandate—the quintessential top-down approach where a chief executive requires, or mandates, a group of individuals, an organization, or a geopolitical entity to implement a healthcare intervention.

2. Guidelines—also known as 'clinical practice guidelines', these are practice recommendations developed by a discipline's governing academic society or group of expert practitioners. Guidelines are often amalgamated from the clinical trials results and are thus referred to as being 'evidence based'.

3. Clinical protocols or pathways—based on clinical practice guidelines and standards, but locally adapted, these protocols or pathways are the literal step-by-step translation of the guidelines to help local practitioners provide guideline-based care to their patients. Protocols or pathways often are represented as flow charts, algorithms, or other similar diagrams.

4. Training—an important implementation approach that focuses primarily in providing knowledge to clinicians, healthcare workers, patients, and families. There are many more specific approaches to training including train-the-trainer approaches, on-the-job training (hands-on), variations based on who the trainer and trainee are, and many variations of how the training is delivered (e.g. didactic, workshop, online, in-person, team-based, etc.).

5. Task shifting—often the approach to improvement may involve changing the types of personnel or locale where a health technology is provided. For example, vaccines may be more efficiently distributed to a population in pharmacies than in physicians' offices.

6. Checklists—a tool which provides a simplified visual reminder of aspects of a clinical protocol or pathway. Checklists are designed to improve consistency and reliability of implementation (Haynes et al. 2011).

7. Campaigns—similar to political campaigns, public health campaigns have been used to spread evidence-based clinical practices to a large region. Historically used in low-resource settings to improve delivery of vaccines, ARV medications for HIV (the WHO's '3 by 5' Initiative), and simple surgical procedures (male medical circumcision, cataract surgery). More recently campaigns have been used in the United States and Europe to improve patient safety and reduce hospital-acquired infections (Berwick et al. 2006; McCannon et al. 2007b; Motsoaledi 2010).

8. Laws and regulation—similar to executive mandate, legal and regulatory mechanisms work to enforce implementation of healthcare practices. National governments can legislate the right to basic primary healthcare services for their citizens as a primary method for implementation.

9. Pay-for-performance and use of incentives and penalties—incentives or disincentives for implementing a procedure or conducting a service is a hotly debated approach to improving implementation consistency and reliability. 'Payment' can come in many forms including financial, public recognition, or other forms of penalty or reward (less frequent licensure visits, faster reimbursement, etc.).

10. Process improvement—derived from management sciences, this approach views dynamic healthcare systems as complex processes which can be systematically improved using a combination of tools to diagnose system failures (e.g. process maps), an incremental problem-solving approach (e.g. Plan–Do–Study–Act cycles), and time-series measurement and evaluation techniques. (See Box 6.9.1 for more detail.)

This is far from an exhaustive list, but it gives the reader an impression of the heterogeneity of approaches that are taken to improve implementation. These approaches, alone or in combination, along with myriad variations, are the focus of study in implementation science. Further, the reader can begin to understand the complexity of characterizing and controlling for the variability between units of study which are often large organizations or populations.

Box 6.9.1 The quality improvement approach

The quality improvement (QI) approach is an implementation method that is grounded in operations research and management science, two well-established fields that have combined the disciplines of statistics, psychology, systems engineering, and iterative learning, to have major impacts on systems performance across countries and industries. QI seeks to design systems for maximum effectiveness, efficiency, and adaptability and to actively disseminate the best models for health service delivery at a rapid rate. Specialized, evidence-based tools aimed at rapid-cycle iterative testing of changes, networked collaborative learning, development of institutional capability for continuous improvement, and frameworks to guide large-scale change have been developed to facilitate this process. The QI approach supports a shift in provider attitudes and practice from a prescriptive mode to one that supports critical thinking and problem-solving skills with continuous review and improvement of service provision.

Healthcare quality improvement principles and the model for improvement (Fig. 6.9.3) provide an effective approach to help close implementation gaps. The approach places a premium on data-driven front-line decision-making, peer-to-peer knowledge exchange, local adaptation of clinical protocols, and highly participative management. Originally developed in the United States and widely adopted in the United Kingdom and other high-income nations, these efforts have increasingly found their way into global health applications in low- and middle-income countries.

Application of the QI approach to health systems of low- and middle-income countries shows considerable promise. Efforts in the Russian Federation have reduced neonatal mortality by 60 per cent (Quality Assurance Project 2001); in Niger, malnutrition-related fatality was halved in a single year (Catsambas et al. 2008); in

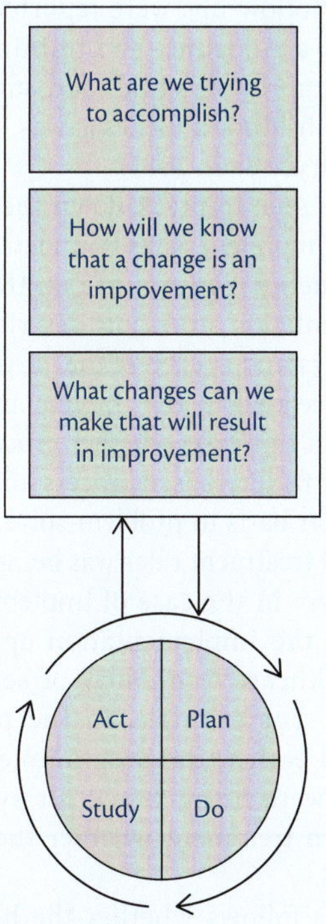

Fig. 6.9.3 Model for improvement.
From Langley, G.L. et al., *The Improvement Guide: A Practical Approach to Enhancing Organizational Performance*, Second edition, Jossey-Bass Publishers, San Francisco, USA, Copyright © 2009. Reproduced with permission from John Wiley & Sons Ltd.

Ecuador, an essential obstetric care collaborative substantially reduced the incidence of postpartum haemorrhage (Hermida et al. 2005); in projects in South Africa, rapid scale-up of access to HIV care and treatment services and falling rates of mother-to-child transmission of HIV at a district level have been demonstrated (Barker et al. 2007; Doherty et al. 2009).

Traditionally this approach is used following policy formulation and where some programme implementation experience has already been established. This often means that healthcare providers have to unlearn what they have been doing for years and replace with new enabling and empowering approaches that involve critical thinking and problem-solving skills, which have the added advantage of application to other health challenges facing the facility or service.

Identifying the primary research question

As already described, the focus of an implementation science study is on *whether* a particular approach to implementing a healthcare technology or service is successful or *why* it has succeeded or failed. Researchers may investigate *what* combinations of approaches work best or what sequence is optimal, *who* should provide a service, or *where* a service is best delivered. Alternatively, researchers may explore why the same approach succeeds in one context but fails in another.

An analysis, both qualitative and quantitative, of the barriers and challenges to implementation may make up the formative research that is needed to decide on what particular approach would be most successful to implement a healthcare technology or service in a specific context. In addition, a local contextual analysis may help guide implementers to the likely adaptations to a healthcare intervention that will be needed to improve its local implementation.

Implementation scientists can also guide the implementers to sequence their effort in a way that allows for more effective study of the implementation approach. As an example, in Andhra Pradesh, India, a newly legislated health insurance system for high-cost surgical procedures for the poor was rolled out in stages throughout the 23 districts in the state which allowed investigators to exploit differences in rollout times to study the impacts of the system on the intended beneficiaries (Fan et al. 2012).

Planning measures

The measurement framework for an implementation science study will be a composite of input, process, outcome, and impact measures.

Input measures will measure whether the specific components of the implementation approach are delivered to the organization or population as needed. For example, in a study of a process improvement implementation approach for delivering syphilis testing and treatment to pregnant women in Haiti, the number of basic trainings on process improvement for the participating sites and monthly follow-ups were reported (Severe et al. 2013). Similarly, inputs to a guideline- and training-based implementation approach to improving childhood survival, the Integrated Management of Childhood Illness, was described in Ghana, Benin, and Mali (Bryce et al. 2010).

Process measures seek to break down the implementation process itself into its component parts to understand whether they are carried out with fidelity. For example, in the syphilis testing and treatment implementation study just described, process measures would seek to understand at each of the participating sites whether specific processes related to the implementation approach were being carried out: in this case, whether process mapping had been conducted, whether facility-based process improvement teams were meeting on a regular basis to problem-solve, and whether data on syphilis testing and treatment rates was being tracked over time.

Outcome measures in the case of implementation science will focus on whether the implementation approach succeeded in delivering the healthcare technology or service to the intended target population. For example, in the process improvement example described earlier, the programme focused on whether pregnant women were being tested for syphilis and for those requiring penicillin treatment whether they were receiving the needed medication.

Impact measures follows whether the healthcare technology or service produces the patient-level results that it is designed to produce. The gold standard for impact assessment are the results produced by healthcare technologies and services under tightly controlled randomized controlled trial circumstances. In the example of syphilis testing and treatment, impact measures would include an assessment of the overall rates of congenital syphilis in the clinic's catchment areas and a comparison to the rates that might have been achieved in the original controlled efficacy studies of penicillin for prevention of congenital syphilis.

Selecting a study format

The gold standard of study design is the randomized controlled trial. In implementation science, 'cluster' randomization is often used as the units of study are villages or health facilities where different approaches to provide a service are tested. A fixed-protocol randomized-controlled trial design reduces bias, limits contamination and confounders, and tests a single hypothesis. Unfortunately, while it is the gold standard, randomized trials are often not feasible or practical in the conduct of implementation science. They are large, costly, and conducted over long periods of time with significant delay between initial study conceptualization and realization of results (Berwick 2007). Therefore, a number of other study approaches have been developed. These are briefly described as follows.

Several authors have proposed alternative methodologies to evaluate large-scale interventions and implementation approaches. Pawson and Tilley's 'realistic evaluation' method proposes a framework that is best summarized by the equation 'context + mechanism = outcome' (Pawson and Tilley 1997). Briefly, this framework suggests that the impact ('outcome') of an intervention is the product of the pathway through which an intervention produces change (its 'mechanism') and how that pathway interacts with the target organization's existing reality ('context').

Realist evaluations embrace the notion that all studies are driven by an implicit theory about the implementation approach that is needed to drive improvements in healthcare outcomes in a population. It uses techniques to make these 'implementation theories' explicit by identifying them and subjecting them to hypothesis testing. In order to do this, the evaluation must capture not only data about the impact of the healthcare intervention on the population, but also data on the fidelity of the specific implementation approach to prove or disprove the implementation theory. By analogy to clinical studies, researchers must show the 'adherence' to the implementation approach under study.

Alternative evaluation frameworks have been proposed as a way of shortening delays between study concept and result with the idea of capturing data in real time to aid and nuance the implementation approach that is being tested. The integrated continuous survey methodology proposed by Rowe et al. suggests a regular data review of key systems performance and implementation indicators that are closely tied to decision-making at the local level. Focused audit studies generally involve periodically assessing the progress of the implementation of an intervention by monitoring key variables over time. Multiple case studies take the opposite approach, randomly choosing several successful recipients of an intervention and studying the implementation approaches used in each case in detail (Harvey and Wensing 2003). Process evaluations involve studying the implementation approaches for the primary purpose of understanding if each stage of implementation was successful (Oakley et al. 2006). Examples of process evaluations include programme impact pathways and results chain evaluations (Victora et al. 2004).

Alongside these methodologies, 'theory-based evaluation' has been proposed to further understand the details of the actual process of change that an intervention seeks to produce, rather than relying exclusively on quantitative data before and after the intervention. For example, evaluating a behaviour change programme must involve specifying how particular components (mass media advertisements, information sessions, etc.) will lead to the desired changes in population behaviour. Such evaluations typically rely on qualitative study designs and require that any quantitative data that is captured be interpreted through the lens that this qualitative data is used to produce.

Finally, in order to capture the subtleties of why a particular implementation approach succeeds or fails in a given healthcare context, implementation scientists often used qualitative techniques. These techniques allow for the development and refinement of explanatory theories for implementation success or failure. Ethnographic and system documentation tools, like the driver diagram, can be used to facilitate this process (Svoronos and Mate 2011).

Control groups

As with clinical research, the study of implementation approaches faces questions about how to limit or reduce bias and how to establish adequate counterfactuals and control groups that would provide appropriate comparisons. With clinical research studies, randomization is often regarded as the predominant tool to reduce or eliminate bias—in this case by spreading confounders evenly throughout the intervention and control arms of the study.

With implementation science, often randomization is neither possible nor practical and may have a diminished impact on reducing bias. In a detailed examination of this issue, English et al. describe several problems with randomization in implementation studies. In sum these include:

◆ Number: with increasing size, fewer and fewer health units are available for randomization.

◆ Balancing confounders: with fewer and more complex health units, the ability to balance confounders between control and intervention arm may not be possible.

◆ Complexity: with increasingly complicated multistep implementation interventions, the opportunities for bias and confounding at each step become legion and it may not be possible to account for this complexity in the randomization. In particular, it may be difficult to account for this complexity a priori before the implementation study is underway and the contextual complexity becomes apparent.

◆ Contamination: in complex, real-life scenarios, health units randomized to the control arm may be shifted towards the intervention by geopolitical forces beyond the control of the investigators.

The point here is not to dismiss or devalue randomization—it is an important and effective tool for trying to reduce bias. However, one should not overestimate the effects of randomization, particularly in the study of implementation approaches where the power of randomization alone to reduce bias may be limited.

A number of other strategies have been developed to establish control groups. We outline these in Table 6.9.1. In lieu of starting out with a priori controls, quasi-experimental designs add and subtract factors considered to affect outcomes sequentially over time (Rogers 2000; Victora et al. 2004; Walshe 2007). Stepped wedge designs where the intervention is rolled out in stages to increasing numbers of health units are particularly useful approaches (Hussey and Hughes 2007). In these stepped wedge designs, a number of health units are divided into groups or 'steps' ahead of time and the intervention is sequentially introduced to each step at predetermined points in time. The health units that have received the intervention are in the intervention arm and those in the 'steps' that await intervention form a natural concurrent control group. Over time with each 'step', the intervention group expands to include additional health units and the control arm decreases in size.

Where concurrent controls are not possible (e.g. in a large-scale nationwide campaign to provide vaccines to children), historical comparisons will be needed to detect whether implementation approaches are demonstrating improved health system performance and outcomes. Continuous or interrupted time series studies, and segmented regression analysis can be used in these circumstances to provide the statistical support needed (Finison and Finison 1996; Wagner et al. 2002; Thor et al. 2007).

Table 6.9.1 Study design and control groups in implementation science

Study design	Description of control group	Strengths and weaknesses
Randomized controlled trial	This is the gold standard method to limit bias and confounders. Health units are randomized to receive the experimental implementation approach(es) or not. The groups are then compared after time	There may not be sufficient numbers of health units to randomize or the large number required makes the trial impractical. There may be contamination across randomization group. The size of these trials makes them expensive and lengthy
Stepped wedge	A number of health units are divided into groups or 'steps' and the intervention under study is sequentially introduced to each step at predetermined points in time. Units that have not yet received the intervention serve as controls	There may be contamination across groups as 'step' groups learn about the new approach and implement it before the predetermined time. Concurrent changes in context over time, unrelated to the study, may impact study outcome and confound results
Time series (continuous, sequential, interrupted)	Health units serve as their own controls as interventions are introduced continuously, sequentially, or in discrete interrupted pattern. Feedback may permit further adjustment and improvement of approach	While improvement can be measured and established, asserting causality between the individual interventions and the improvement is difficult
Case–control	Health units (facilities, wards, villages) that have successfully implemented change are compared to health units that have not. Researchers compare implementation approach or context characteristics of successful versus unsuccessful health units. Simple and fast study design	This design can be used to generate associations and hypothesis but given the complexity of implementation approaches and characteristics of health units, there are numerous potential confounders
Historical control	A comparison of outcomes in a group of health units before and after an intervention has been introduced	Subject to implementation 'placebo' effect. Health units tend to do better when someone is watching regardless of the intervention under study. Concurrent changes in context over time, unrelated to the study, may impact study outcome and confound results

In addition, such designs and analytic techniques can provide the type of constant feedback needed for implementation activities to be further adjusted and improved within prevailing contextual circumstances (Nelson et al. 2004; Speroff and O'Connor 2004).

The optimal evaluation of an implementation approach will be a mixed methods approach drawing on the quantitative techniques described above to examine whether the implementation approach under study is succeeding or not, along with qualitative techniques that will provide the context-specific detail to explain how and why the implementation approach produced the result that it did.

Review of implementation science in low- and middle-income countries

Implementation science studies from low- and middle-income countries have been reported in the literature since the late 1990s, initially focused on strengthening health promotion and changing healthcare provider behaviours. The literature on implementation research was dramatically accelerated by the launch of the journal *Implementation Science* in 2006. However, reports from low- and middle-income countries became more prevalent after 2008 when the US government's President's Emergency Plan For AIDS Relief (PEPFAR) made implementation research a core part of its strategy (Padian et al. 2011). In addition, the literature expanded as countries worked to implement evidence-based practices to achieve the Millennium Development Goals. Implementation science studies from low- and middle-income countries are thus particularly strong in three dimensions: HIV, maternal and child health, and health systems strengthening.

HIV

Implementation research has been used to study HIV prevention including methods to prevent mother-to-child HIV transmission (De Cock et al. 2000), improve uptake of male medical circumcision (Kebaabetswe et al. 2003), and reduce HIV risk from drug use through needle exchange syringe distribution, ARV treatment programmes for active drug users, and opioid substitution therapy (Wood et al. 2008).

ARV treatment programmes for HIV have also been the subject of implementation science studies. Once run through central urban tertiary care centres, HIV programmes throughout the world are now being decentralized to ensure wider and more equitable access to ARVs. However, shortages of trained healthcare workers and challenges of integrating HIV/AIDS care into routine primary healthcare remain barriers to reliable provision of ARVs. Implementation studies have evaluated clinical guideline adaptation and training, such as the PALSA PLUS programme in South Africa and the PALM PLUS programme in Malawi (Schull et al. 2011). These studies suggest that despite variations in health systems, the principal obstacles to decentralization can be overcome by a combination of improving healthcare worker retention and satisfaction while improving the quality of care.

In addition, HIV treatment expansion efforts require new personnel to prescribe and deliver life-saving ARVs. Implementation science studies have helped to demonstrate that nurse-initiated and -managed antiretroviral treatment (NIMART) is both feasible and acceptable in the South African health service (Cameron et al. 2012). Formative implementation research into NIMART described workload and capacity constraints, the logistical and infrastructural challenges faced, the training and support needed, and the new working and referral relationships between health staff that would be needed. These formative results optimized the intervention design and allowed a more nuanced selection of implementation approaches including a combination of clinical guidelines tailored to nurses, and significant health services reorganization (Georgeu et al. 2012).

PEPFAR has welcomed implementation science and the US Agency for International Development has twice released programme statements seeking implementation science proposals to improve HIV service delivery in low- and middle-income country settings. The HIV research community has welcomed the advent of this field, signified by the launch of a new section on 'Implementation and Operational Research' in 2010 in the *Journal of Acquired Immunodeficiency Syndrome*. However, in order for implementation science to gain further ground, there will need to be better coordination and integration of the findings from this research and the programme delivery efforts themselves (Norton et al. 2009; Schackman 2010).

Maternal and child health

A second area of focus for implementation scientists in low- and middle-income countries is efforts to improve the delivery of care for mothers and children. Several implementation approaches have been tested in varying contexts. First, promotion of clinical practice guidelines has met with varied results in Burkina Faso, Ghana, and Tanzania (Baker et al. 2012). WHO's Integrated Management of Childhood Illness, which combines evidence-based care protocols with a train-the-trainer programme, has been studied carefully by implementation scientists seeking to understand what contextual and programmatic factors have led to implementation success and failure (Bryce et al. 2010). Efforts by Spector and Gawande to develop a safe childbirth checklist build on successful applications of checklist reminder systems in other contexts (operating room care, critical care, etc.) (Spector et al. 2012).

Kangaroo mother care (KMC) is a safe, cost-effective method of caring for low-birth weight infants and improving newborn survival rates. *KMC Ghana*, an initiative to scale up KMC in four regions in Ghana, utilized two implementation approaches: (1) train healthcare facilities that conduct deliveries with the necessary skills for KMC practice and (2) use validated KMC-specific data collection tools to monitor progress and provide facility-level feedback (Bergh et al. 2012). In Ecuador, the Quality Assurance Project (QAP) and the USAID Health Care Improvement Project (HCI) assisted in the adoption, scaling up, and institutionalization of active management of the third stage of labour (AMTSL) for prevention of postpartum haemorrhage via a continuous quality improvement implementation approach. This approach used techniques adopted from industrial process engineering to improve patient flow, streamline care delivery processes, and remove operational barriers (Hermida et al. 2012).

Various implementation approaches have been taken to improve the delivery and uptake of evidence-based vaccinations. Mass-immunization campaigns have been used in a number of settings, particularly with the recent efforts to eradicate polio infection (Institute for International Programs, 2008a, 2008b, 2008c). A number of strategies have been used to improve communication to parents and children about the benefits of vaccination. To organize these efforts and to study their effects on childhood immunization rates, the Communicate to Vaccinate (COMMVAC) project has been established. This project studies communication strategies aimed at improving communication with parents about vaccines (Lewin et al. 2011). Child health programmes have used campaigns in a variety of other contexts as well as to deliver key health interventions on a broad range of topics such as breastfeeding promotion (Bosnjak et al. 2004), insecticide-treated nets (Institute for International Programs 2008a, 2008b, 2008c), and interventions to prevent congenital syphilis (Saraceni and Leal 2003).

Financial incentives have been well studied by implementation scientists for their potential impacts on the implementation of evidence-based care for mothers and children. Several studies examined the impact of financial or other material incentives provided to mothers and families upon achievement of certain caregiving behaviour such as vaccination (Institute for International Programs 2008c), in-facility delivery (Chiwuzie et al. 1997; Bhat et al. 2007; Lim et al. 2010), antenatal and/or postnatal visits (Mushi et al. 2003; Morris et al. 2004; Bhat et al. 2007; Moloney, 2010), and education attainment (Morris et al. 2004; Fernald et al. 2008). In India, a government-sponsored conditional cash transfer was associated with fewer perinatal deaths (Lim et al. 2010). But not all financial incentives seem to work. In the Accelerated Child Survival and Development programme in Mali, incentives to improve childhood vaccination did not improve child survival in intervention versus control areas (Institute for International Programs 2008c).

Health systems strengthening

Interest in strengthening health systems has led to renewed interest in studying implementation efforts that would also lead to stronger health systems (WHO 2007). While the majority of this literature is also related to HIV and maternal and child health implementation studies, two types of studies deserve specific mention. The first are efforts to study the translation of evidence-based research into policy. While the focus of implementation science is on the study of the uptake of research findings into clinical practice, a growing body of evidence is beginning to describe the challenges in translating evidence-based findings into policy (El-Jardali et al. 2012; Lavis et al. 2012; Lewin et al. 2012). Solutions are emerging as well, including dynamic new social networks such as the EVIPNet, sponsored by the WHO, to improve collaboration between researchers and policymakers (Lavis and Panisset 2010).

Finally, implementation scientists have been determined to approach implementation at scale. Strategies for taking a healthcare intervention to scale—whether through the mass media, social networks or the use of technology, or more conventional approaches to community organizing, facility-level investment, health camps, or campaigns—are now under scientific scrutiny thanks to the efforts of implementation scientists (McCannon et al. 2007a). Importantly, implementation scientists seek to understand both whether the scale-up approach was successful and why it succeeded. This tacit knowledge, often poorly documented, includes a practical understanding of the settings and the contexts in which the intervention was scaled up and may lead to improved implementation and scale-up in the future (Massoud et al. 2012).

A review of implementation science in high-income countries

Implementation science has found an increasingly prominent role in health services research in high-income countries. Given the wide variation in both the cost and quality of health services in the United States, there is considerable interest in understanding how evidence-based guidelines can be translated into effective care. Support for such initiatives has come from governmental agencies (Agency for Health Care Research and Quality), health providers (Kaiser Permanente), academic journals (*British Medical Journal Quality and Safety*), and insurers (Blue Cross) among others (Rubenstein and Pugh 2006). Though still a nascent discipline, implementation research has facilitated several successful health interventions on a large scale. For example, Lorig et al. (2001) found significant gains from a chronic disease self-management training programme, primarily focusing on the diffusion of best practices for self-care among arthritis patients. The success of this intervention, studied both as a randomized trial and using quasi-experimental methods, has led to its widespread implementation across the United Kingdom. A comparable programme focused on diabetes prevention through community health workers also achieved significant improvement in both glucose levels and weight (Katula et al. 2011). Again, the initial success of this programme was supplemented with multiple study replications in various settings. These replications were largely able to mimic the findings of the initial efficacy trial. Perhaps more importantly, they provided insights as to how this intervention could best be adapted to various community settings and with varying levels of resources (Glasgow et al. 2012).

The US Veterans Affairs Quality Enhancement Research Initiative (QUERI) is particularly useful in revealing the various strengths of implementation research. This programme was created to address the gap between evidence and clinical practice in health service provision within the Veterans Health Administration, with an emphasis on quality improvement (Stetler et al. 2008b). QUERI was the focus of a series of articles published in *Implementation Science*, ranging from theoretical frameworks to empirical studies. For example, Stetler et al. (2008a) presented the organizational framework underlying QUERI, which focused on cultural norms, resource capacity, and supportive infrastructures as the three contextual determinants of implementation success. These principles were used in the rollout of programmes aimed at reducing HIV risk (Goetz et al. 2008), treating schizophrenia (Brown et al. 2008), and improving eye care for diabetic patients (Krein et al. 2008).

Despite these notable examples of implementation science in practice in high-income settings, disagreements persist in the terminology and theoretical frameworks underlying implementation science. For example, a 2009 article identified over 30 distinct definitions of dissemination and implementation, and questioned whether the discipline could progress before reconciling them (Proctor et al. 2009). Many have emphasized the need for unifying theoretical models as a way to unify these definitions (Rubenstein and Pugh 2006), while others have emphasized the distinctive methodological needs of the discipline (Wallace and Legro 2008; Mdege et al. 2011). The Cochrane Effective Practice and Organization of Care (EPOC) Group, a review group of the Cochrane Collaboration, has the potential to resolve these differences. By taking a meta-analytic approach to interventions focused on improving the delivery of healthcare services, EPOC is well placed to find unifying trends in the implementation science literature.

Conclusion

The study of approaches to implementing care at the bedside and in the community is a field in rapid evolution. The discipline is new and the approaches and methods used are under active development. At the moment, despite the availability of useful alternatives, conventional approaches to study design and analysis, designed for clinical research trials, are often applied to the study of implementation approaches.

Implementation science requires a deep understanding of health systems, of variation in behaviours and outcomes over time, of psychology of patients and practitioners, and of the way knowledge is developed and spread. It seeks to understand the complexities of how and why healthcare delivery succeeds and fails at the bedside and in our communities.

Acknowledgements

Text extract from Lisa R. Hirschhorn et al., Research for Change: Using Implementation Research to Strengthen HIV Care and Treatment Scale-Up in Resource-Limited Settings, *Journal of Infectious Diseases*, Volume 1956, Supplement 3, pp. S516–S522, Copyright © 2007 Infectious Diseases Society of America, by permission of Oxford University Press.

References

African Academies of Sciences (2009). *Science In Action: Saving the Lives of Africa's Mothers, Newborns, and Children*. Cape Town: African Academies of Sciences.

Arifeen, S., Blum, L., Hoque, D., and Chowdhury, E. (2004). Integrated Management of Childhood Illness (IMCI) in Bangladesh: early findings from a cluster-randomised study. *The Lancet*, 364, 1595–602.

Baker, U., Tomson, G., Some, M., et al. (2012). 'How to know what you need to do': a cross-country comparison of maternal health guidelines in Burkina Faso, Ghana and Tanzania. *Implementation Science*, 7, 31.

Balas-Eltes, A. (2000). Managing clinical knowledge for health care improvement. *Yearbook of Medical Informatics*, 65–9.

Barker, P.M., McCannon, C.J., Mehta, N., et al. (2007). Strategies for the scale-up of antiretroviral therapy in South Africa through health system optimization. *Journal of Infectious Diseases*, 196(Suppl. 3), S457–63.

Beaglehole, R., Ebrahim, S., Reddy, S., Voute, J., and Leeder, S. (2007). Prevention of chronic diseases: a call to action. *The Lancet*, 370, 2152–7.

Beaglehole, R., Epping-Jordan, J., Patel, V., et al. (2008). Improving the prevention and management of chronic disease in low-income and middle-income countries: a priority for primary health care. *The Lancet*, 372, 940–9.

Bergh, A.M., Manu, R., Davy, K., et al. (2012). Translating research findings into practice—the implementation of kangaroo mother care in Ghana. *Implementation Science*, 7, 75.

Berwick, D. (2007). *Eating Soup With a Fork*. Keynote address. IHI National Forum, Orlando, Florida, 11 December.

Berwick, D.M. (2009). What 'patient-centered' should mean: confessions of an extremist. *Health Affairs (Millwood)*, 28, 555–65.

Berwick, D.M., Calkins, D.R., Mccannon, C.J., and Hackbarth, A.D. (2006). The 100,000 lives campaign: setting a goal and a deadline for improving health care quality. *Journal of the American Medical Association*, 295, 324–7.

Bhat, R., Singh, A., Maheshwari, S., and Somen, S. (2007). *Maternal Health Financing: Issues and Options: A Study of Chiranjeevi Yojana in Gujarat*. Ahmedabad: Indian Institute of Management Ahmedabad.

Bosnjak, A., Batinica, M., Hegedus-Jungvirth, M., Grgurić, J., and Bozikov, J. (2004). The effect of baby friendly hospital initiative and postnatal support on breastfeeding rates—Croatian experience. *Collegium Antropologicum*, 28, 235–43.

Bristow, P.J., Hillman, K.M., Chey, T., et al. (2000). Rates of in-hospital arrests, deaths and intensive care admissions: the effect of a medical emergency team. *Medical Journal of Australia*, 173, 236–40.

Brown, A.H., Cohen, A.N., Chinman, M.J., Kessler, C., and Young, A.S. (2008). EQUIP: implementing chronic care principles and applying formative evaluation methods to improve care for schizophrenia: QUERI Series. *Implementation Science*, 3, 9.

Bryce, J., Gilroy, K., Jones, G., Hazel, E., Black, R.E., and Victora, C.G. (2010). The Accelerated Child Survival and Development programme in west Africa: a retrospective evaluation. *The Lancet*, 375, 572–82.

Buist, M.D., Moore, G.E., Bernard, S.A., Waxman, B.P., Anderson, J.N., and Nguyen, T.V. (2002). Effects of a medical emergency team on reduction of incidence of and mortality from unexpected cardiac arrests in hospital: preliminary study. *British Medical Journal*, 324, 387–90.

Cameron, D., Gerber, A., Mbatha, M., Mutyabule, J., and Swart, H. (2012). Nurse-initiation and maintenance of patients on antiretroviral therapy: are nurses in primary care clinics initiating ART after attending NIMART training? *South African Medical Journal*, 102, 98–100.

Catsambas, T.T., Franco, L.M., Gutmann, M., Knebel, E., Hill, P., and Lin, Y.-S. (2008). *Evaluating Health Care Collaboratives: The Experiences of the Quality Assurance Project*. Bethesda, MD, University Research Corporation.

Centers For Disease Control and Prevention (2007). *HIV/AIDS Surveillance Report, 2005*. Atlanta, GA: US Department of Health and Human Services.

Centers For Disease Control and Prevention (2011). Vital signs: HIV prevention through care and treatment—United States. *MMWR: Morbidity and Mortality Weekly Report*, 60(47), 1618–23.

Chiwuzie, J., Okojie, O., Okolocha, C., et al. (1997). Emergency loan funds to improve access to obstetric care in Ekpoma, Nigeria. The Benin PMM Team. *International Journal of Gynecology & Obstetrics*, 59(Suppl. 2), S231–6.

Committee on Quality of Health Care in America (2001). *Crossing the Quality Chasm: A New Health System for the 21st Century*. Washington, DC: Institute of Medicine.

De Cock, K.M., Fowler, M.G., Mercier, E., et al. (2000). Prevention of mother-to-child HIV transmission in resource-poor countries: translating research into policy and practice. *Journal of the American Medical Association*, 283, 1175–82.

Deming, W.E. (1993). *The New Economics for Industry, Government, Education*. Cambridge, MA: Massachusetts Institute of Technology, Center for Advanced Engineering Study.

Devita, M.A., Bellomo, R., Hillman, K., et al. (2006). Findings of the first consensus conference on medical emergency teams. *Critical Care Medicine*, 34, 2463–78.

Doherty, T., Chopra, M., Nsibande, D., and Mngoma, D. (2009). Improving the coverage of the PMTCT programme through a participatory quality improvement intervention in South Africa. *BMC Public Health*, 9, 406.

Eccles, M.P. and Mittman, B.S. (2006). Welcome to Implementation Science. *Implementation Science*, 1, 1.

El-Jardali, F., Lavis, J.N., Ataya, N., Jamal, D., Ammar, W., and Raouf, S. (2012). Use of health systems evidence by policymakers in eastern Mediterranean countries: views, practices, and contextual influences. *BMC Health Services Research*, 12, 200.

Fan, V.Y., Karan, A., and Mahal, A. (2012). State health insurance and out-of-pocket health expenditures in Andhra Pradesh, India. *International Journal of Health Care Finance and Economics*, 12, 189–215.

Fernald, L.C., Gertler, P.J., and Neufeld, L.M. (2008). Role of cash in conditional cash transfer programmes for child health, growth, and development: an analysis of Mexico's Oportunidades. *The Lancet*, 371, 828–37.

Finison, L. and Finison, K. (1996). Applying control charts to quality improvement. *Journal for Healthcare Quality*, 18, 32–41.

Fisher, E.S., Bynum, J.P., and Skinner, J.S. (2009). Slowing the growth of health care costs—lessons from regional variation. *The New England Journal of Medicine*, 360, 849–52.

Georgeu, D., Colvin, C.J., Lewin, S., et al. (2012). Implementing nurse-initiated and managed antiretroviral treatment (NIMART) in South Africa: a qualitative process evaluation of the STRETCH trial. *Implementation Science*, 7, 66.

Glasgow, R.E., Vinson, C., Chambers, D., Khoury, M.J., Kaplan, R.M., and Hunter, C. (2012). National Institutes of Health approaches to dissemination and implementation science: current and future directions. *American Journal of Public Health*, 102, 1274–81.

Goetz, M.B., Bowman, C., Hoang, T., et al. (2008). Implementing and evaluating a regional strategy to improve testing rates in VA patients at risk for HIV, utilizing the QUERI process as a guiding framework: QUERI Series. *Implementation Science*, 3, 16.

Harvey, G. and Wensing, M. (2003). Methods for evaluation of small scale quality improvement projects. *Quality and Safety in Health Care*, 12, 210–14.

Haynes, A.B., Regenbogen, S.E., Weiser, T.G., et al. (2011). Surgical outcome measurement for a global patient population: validation of the Surgical Apgar Score in 8 countries. *Surgery*, 149(4), 519–24.

Hermida, J., Salas, B., and Sloan, N.L. (2012). Sustainable scale-up of active management of the third stage of labor for prevention of postpartum hemorrhage in Ecuador. *International Journal of Gynaecology & Obstetrics*, 117, 278–82.

Hermida, J.R.M., Vaca, L., Ayabaca, P., Romero, P., and Vieira, L. (2005). *Scaling Up and Institutionalizing Continuous Quality Improvement in the Free Maternity and Child Care Program in Ecuador: Latin America and Caribbean Regional Health Sector Reform Initiative Report*. Bethesda, MD: University Research Co LLC.

Hirschhorn, L.R., Ojikutu, B., and Rodriguez, W. (2007). Research for change: using implementation research to strengthen HIV care and treatment scale-up in resource-limited settings. *Journal of Infectious Diseases*, 196(Suppl. 3), S516–22.

Hussey, M.A. and Hughes, J.P. (2007). Design and analysis of stepped wedge cluster randomized trials. *Contemporary Clinical Trials*, 28, 182–91.

Implementation Science (2014). About *Implementation Science*. [Online] Available at: http://www.implementationscience.com/about.

Institute For International Programs (2008a). *Final Report: The Retrospective Evaluation of ACSD: Benin*. Baltimore, MD: Johns Hopkins University Bloomberg School of Public Health.

Institute For International Programs (2008b). *Final Report: The Retrospective Evaluation of ACSD: Ghana*. Baltimore, MD: Johns Hopkins Bloomberg School of Public Health.

Institute For International Programs (2008c). *Final Report: The Retrospective Evaluation of ACSD: Mali*. Baltimore, MD: Johns Hopkins Bloomberg School of Public Health.

Ioannidis, J.P. (2005). Contradicted and initially stronger effects in highly cited clinical research. *Journal of the American Medical Association*, 294, 218–28.

Jones, G., Steketee, R.W., Black, R.E., Bhutta, Z.A., and Morris, S.S. (2003). How many child deaths can we prevent this year? *The Lancet*, 362, 65–71.

Kaplan, H.C., Brady, P.W., Dritz, M.C., et al. (2010). The influence of context on quality improvement success in health care: a systematic review of the literature. *Milbank Quarterly*, 88, 500–9.

Katula, J.A., Vitolins, M.Z., Rosenberger, E.L., et al. (2011). One-year results of a community-based translation of the Diabetes Prevention Program: Healthy-Living Partnerships to Prevent Diabetes (HELP PD) Project. *Diabetes Care*, 34, 1451–7.

Kebaabetswe, P., Lockman, S., Mogwe, S., et al. (2003). Male circumcision: an acceptable strategy for HIV prevention in Botswana. *Sexually Transmitted Infections*, 79, 214–19.

Krein, S.L., Bernstein, S.J., Fletcher, C.E., et al. (2008). Improving eye care for veterans with diabetes: an example of using the QUERI steps to move from evidence to implementation: QUERI Series. *Implementation Science*, 3, 18.

Lavis, J.N. and Panisset, U. (2010). EVIPNet Africa's first series of policy briefs to support evidence-informed policymaking. *International Journal of Technology Assessment in Health Care*, 26, 229–32.

Lavis, J.N., Rottingen, J.A., Bosch-Capblanch, X., et al. (2012). Guidance for evidence-informed policies about health systems: linking guidance development to policy development. *PLoS Medicine*, 9, e1001186.

Lewin, S., Bosch-Capblanch, X., Oliver, S., et al. (2012). Guidance for evidence-informed policies about health systems: assessing how much confidence to place in the research evidence. *PLoS Medicine*, 9, e1001187.

Lewin, S., Hill, S., Abdullahi, L.H., et al. (2011). 'Communicate to vaccinate' (COMMVAC). Building evidence for improving communication about childhood vaccinations in low- and middle-income countries: protocol for a programme of research. *Implementation Science*, 6, 125.

Lim, S., Dandona, L., Hoisington, J., James, S., Hogan, M., and Gakidou, E. (2010). India's Janani Suraksha Yojana, a conditional cash transfer programme to increase births in health facilities: an impact evaluation. *The Lancet*, 375, 2009–23.

Lindegren, M.L., Byers, R.H., Jr., Thomas, P., et al. (1999). Trends in perinatal transmission of HIV/AIDS in the United States. *Journal of the American Medical Association*, 282, 531–8.

Lorig, K.R., Ritter, P., Stewart, A.L., et al. (2001). Chronic disease self-management program: 2-year health status and health care utilization outcomes. *Medical Care*, 39, 1217–23.

Massoud, M.R., Mensah-Abrampah, N., Sax, S., et al. (2012). Charting the way forward to better quality health care: how do we get there and what are the next steps? Recommendations from the Salzburg Global Seminar on making health care better in low- and middle-income economies. *International Journal for Quality in Health Care*, 24, 558–63.

McCannon, C.J., Berwick, D.M., and Massoud, M.R. (2007a). The science of large-scale change in global health. *Journal of the American Medical Association*, 298, 1937–9.

McCannon, C.J., Hackbarth, A.D., and Griffin, F.A. (2007b). Miles to go: an introduction to the 5 Million Lives Campaign. *Joint Commission Journal on Quality and Patient Safety*, 33, 477–84.

McKenna, M.T. and Hu, X. (2007). Recent trends in the incidence and morbidity that are associated with perinatal human immunodeficiency virus infection in the United States. *American Journal of Obstetrics & Gynecology*, 197, S10–16.

Mdege, N.D., Man, M.S., Taylor Nee Brown, C.A., and Torgerson, D.J. (2011). Systematic review of stepped wedge cluster randomized trials shows that design is particularly used to evaluate interventions during routine implementation. *Journal of Clinical Epidemiology*, 64, 936–48.

Moloney, A. (2010). Difficulties hit Bolivia's programme for pregnant women. *The Lancet*, 375, 1955.

Morris, S.S., Flores, R., Olinto, P., and Medina, J.M. (2004). Monetary incentives in primary health care and effects on use and coverage of preventive health care interventions in rural Honduras: cluster randomised trial. *The Lancet*, 364, 2030–7.

Motsoaledi, A. (2010). *Outline of the National HIV Counselling and Testing (HCT) Campaign*. [Press release]. Pretoria: Department of Health.

Mushi, A.K., Schellenberg, J.R., Mponda, H., and Lengeler, C. (2003). Targeted subsidy for malaria control with treated nets using a discount voucher system in Tanzania. *Health Policy and Planning*, 18, 163–71.

National Institutes of Health (2011). *Dissemination and Implementation Research in Health*. Bethesda, MD: National Institutes of Health.

National Institutes of Health (2012). *Dissemination and Implementation Research in Health*. PAR-10-038. Bethesda, MD: National Institutes of Health. Available at: http://grants.nih.gov/grants/guide/pa-files/PAR-10-038.html.

Nelson, E., Splaine, M., Plume, S., and Batalden, P. (2004). Good measurement for good improvement work. *Quality Management in Healthcare*, 13, 1.

Norton, W.E., Amico, K.R., Cornman, D.H., Fisher, W.A., and Fisher, J.D. (2009). An agenda for advancing the science of implementation of evidence-based HIV prevention interventions. *AIDS and Behavior*, 13, 424–9.

Oakley, A., Strange, V., Bonell, C., Allen, E., and Stephenson, J. (2006). Process evaluation in randomised controlled trials of complex interventions. *British Medical Journal*, 332, 413–16.

Øvretveit, J. and Gustafson, D. (2003). Using research to inform quality programmes. *British Medical Journal*, 326, 759–61.

Øvretveit, J. and Suffoletto, J.A. (2007). Improving rapid response systems: progress, issues, and future directions. *Joint Commission Journal on Quality and Patient Safety*, 33, 512–19.

Oxman, A.D., Thomson, M.A., Davis, D.A., and Haynes, R.B. (1995). No magic bullets: a systematic review of 102 trials of interventions to improve professional practice. *Canadian Medical Association Journal*, 153, 1423–31.

Padian, N.S., Holmes, C.B., Mccoy, S.I., Lyerla, R., Bouey, P.D., and Goosby, E.P. (2011). Implementation science for the US President's Emergency Plan for AIDS Relief (PEPFAR). *Journal of Acquired Immune Deficiency Syndromes*, 56, 199–203.

Parry, G., Carson-Stevens, A., Luff, D.F., McPherson, M., and Goldmann, D. (2013). Recommendations for evaluation of health care improvement initiatives. *Academic Pediatrics*, 13(6), S23–S30

Pawson, R. and Tilley, N. (1997). *Realistic Evaluation*. London: Sage Publications.

Proctor, E.K., Landsverk, J., Aarons, G., et al. (2009). Implementation research in mental health services: an emerging science with conceptual, methodological, and training challenges. *Administration and Policy in Mental Health*, 36, 24–34.

Quality Assurance Project (2001). *Improving the System of Care for Neonates Suffering from Respiratory Distress Syndrome in Tver Oblast*. Bethesda, MD: University Research Corporation.

Rogers, P. (2000). Causal models in program theory evaluation. *New Directions for Evaluation*, 2000, 47–55.

Rowe, A. (2009). Potential of integrated continuous surveys and quality management to support monitoring, evaluation, and the scale-up of health interventions in developing countries. *The American Journal of Tropical Medicine and Hygiene*, 80, 971–9.

Rubenstein, L.V. and Pugh, J. (2006). Strategies for promoting organizational and practice change by advancing implementation research. *Journal of General Internal Medicine*, 21(Suppl. 2), S58–64.

Saraceni, V. and Leal, M.C. (2003). [Evaluation of the effectiveness of the congenital syphilis elimination campaigns on reducing the perinatal morbidity and mortality: Rio de Janeiro, 1999–2000]. *Cad Saude Publica*, 19, 1341–9.

Schackman, B.R. (2010). Implementation science for the prevention and treatment of HIV/AIDS. *Journal of Acquired Immune Deficiency Syndromes*, 55(Suppl. 1), S27–31.

Schull, M.J., Cornick, R., Thompson, S., et al. (2011). From PALSA PLUS to PALM PLUS: adapting and developing a South African guideline and training intervention to better integrate HIV/AIDS care with primary care in rural health centers in Malawi. *Implementation Science*, 6, 82.

Severe, L., Benoit, D., Chou, X.K., Pape, J.W., Fitzgerald, D., and Mate, K.S. (2013). Rapid-testing technology and systems improvement for the elimination of congenital syphilis in Haiti: overcoming the 'technology to systems gap'. *Journal of Sexually Transmitted Diseases*, 2013, 247901.

Spector, J.M., Agrawal, P., Kodkany, B., et al. (2012). Improving quality of care for maternal and newborn health: prospective pilot study of the WHO safe childbirth checklist program. *PLoS One*, 7, e35151.

Speroff, T. and O'Connor, G. (2004). Study designs for PDSA quality improvement research. *Quality Management in Healthcare*, 13, 17.

Steel, A.C. and Reynolds, S.F. (2008). The growth of rapid response systems. *Joint Commission Journal on Quality and Patient Safety*, 34, 489–95.

Stetler, C.B., Mcqueen, L., Demakis, J., and Mittman, B.S. (2008a). An organizational framework and strategic implementation for system-level change to enhance research-based practice: QUERI Series. *Implementation Science*, 3, 30.

Stetler, C.B., Mittman, B.S., and Francis, J. (2008b). Overview of the VA Quality Enhancement Research Initiative (QUERI) and QUERI theme articles: QUERI Series. *Implementation Science*, 3, 8.

Svoronos, T. and Mate, K.S. (2011). Evaluating large-scale health programmes at a district level in resource-limited countries. *Bulletin of the World Health Organization*, 89, 831–7.

Thor, J., Lundberg, J., Ask, J., Olsson, J., Carli, C., Härenstam, K., and Brommels, M. (2007). Application of statistical process control in healthcare improvement: systematic review. *Quality & Safety in Health Care*, 16, 387–99.

UNAIDS (2011). *Global Plan Towards the Elimination of New HIV Infections among Children by 2015 and Keeping Their Mothers Alive*. Geneva: UNAIDS.

United Nations (2000). *UN Millennium Declaration. A/RES/55/2, Section II*. New York: UN.

Victora, C., Black, R., Boerma, J., and Bryce, J. (2011). Measuring impact in the Millennium Development Goal era and beyond: a new approach to large-scale effectiveness evaluations. *The Lancet*, 377, 85–95.

Victora, C., Habicht, J., and Bryce, J. (2004). Evidence-based public health: moving beyond randomized trials. *American Journal of Public Health*, 94, 400–5.

Victora, C.G., Vaughan, J.P., Barros, F.C., Silva, A.C., and Tomasi, E. (2000). Explaining trends in inequities: evidence from Brazilian child health studies. *The Lancet*, 356, 1093–8.

Wagner, A.K., Soumerai, S.B., Zhang, F., and Ross-Degnan, D. (2002). Segmented regression analysis of interrupted time series studies in medication use research. *Journal of Clinical Pharmacy and Therapeutics*, 27, 299–309.

Wallace, C.M. and Legro, M. W. (2008). Using formative evaluation in an implementation project to increase vaccination rates in high-risk veterans: QUERI Series. *Implementation Science*, 3, 22.

Walshe, K. (2007). Understanding what works—and why—in quality improvement: the need for theory-driven evaluation. *International Journal for Quality in Health Care*, 19(2), 57–9.

Wennberg, D.E. (1998). Variation in the delivery of health care: the stakes are high. *Annals of Internal Medicine*, 128, 866–8.

Winters, B.D., Pham, J., and Pronovost, P.J. (2006). Rapid response teams—walk, don't run. *Journal of the American Medical Association*, 296, 1645–7.

Wood, E., Kerr, T., Tyndall, M.W., and Montaner, J.S. (2008). A review of barriers and facilitators of HIV treatment among injection drug users. *AIDS*, 22, 1247–56.

World Health Organization (2007). *Everybody's Business: Strengthening Health Systems to Improve Health Outcomes: WHO's Framework for Action* [Online]. Geneva: WHO. Available at: http://www.who.int/healthsystems/strategy/everybodys_business.pdf.

World Health Organization (2012). *Global Tuberculosis Report 2012*. Geneva: WHO.

World Health Organization and UNICEF (2010). *Towards Universal Access: Scaling up Priority HIV/AIDS interventions in the Health Sector 2010 Progress Report*. Geneva: WHO.

SECTION 7

Environmental and occupational health sciences

Environmental health issues in public health

Chien-Jen Chen

Environment and health: historical perspective

Human beings live in a complex environment. The importance of environmental factors in human health has been recognized since antiquity. Hippocrates, in his classical writing *On Airs, Waters and Places*, emphasized the relevance of the environment to human health (Hippocrates 1950). He pointed out the influence of seasons and weather, location of residence, and nature of water on human health, and the occurrence of *epidemics*. Since ancient times, the seasonality of infectious diseases and the geographical clustering of endemic diseases have been documented worldwide. Several hypotheses had been advanced to explain the unique distribution of various diseases in time and place. The contagion theory proposed that both direct and indirect contact with sick people or animals might transmit diseases and hence both isolation and quarantine had been suggested to prevent the spread of diseases. Although they might have reduced the risk of spread of infectious diseases by ships, the strategies evolved from the contagion theory had not stopped the outbreak of many infectious diseases.

The miasma theory proposed that dirty living environments, unclean drinking water, and poor ventilation due to overcrowding might cause various diseases (Hamlin 1998). This led to environmental sanitary reforms aimed at removing miasma by contributing to a cleaner environment in Europe. The hygienic movement emphasized the importance of implementing a safe drinking water supply and sewage disposal system. The Public Health Act enacted in Britain in 1848 was considered the first example of governmental involvement in public health affairs. However, a large outbreak of cholera still occurred in London despite its well-constructed sewage disposal system and much improved environmental sanitation in the 1850s. Through a carefully designed survey, John Snow published his famous epidemiological study on cholera in 1855 (Snow 1936) while the germ theory was still in its infancy. He identified the consumption of contaminated drinking water as the cause of the cholera outbreak. The removal of the handle which pumped contaminated water 'magically' prevented the spread of the disease. The relocation of sources of drinking water successfully controlled the cholera outbreak. This was a pioneering epidemiological study in the identification of environmental factors in a disease outbreak.

In late nineteenth century, the development of germ theory led to the discovery of many specific infectious agents for human diseases. It also led to the development of several drugs for treatment of diseases, and improvements in sanitation and disinfection to control outbreaks of diseases. Koch's postulates (Koch 1891), which emphasized a one-to-one relationship between cause and disease, were well accepted as criteria for the identification of causal agents of infectious diseases. Effective control of several infectious diseases through identification of specific agents, discovery of chemical and biological drugs, and invention of preventive and therapeutic vaccines had improved life quality and longevity of human beings. The discovery of animal reservoirs and vectors of infectious agents led to the control of vectors through environmental sanitation and disinfection. More and more biological and mechanical vectors have been identified for various viral, bacterial, and parasitic diseases since then. Control of vectors in the environment using pesticides became an important task for the prevention of infectious diseases. For example, malaria was eradicated in Taiwan through the detection and treatment of infected cases and use of the insecticide DDT. However, the widely used pesticides polluted the environment and became hazardous to wild animals and humans.

Life expectancy in most countries increased significantly after the 1950s, when conventional infectious diseases had been controlled through the widespread use of various vaccines and antibiotics. The major diseases that threaten human life have since gradually shifted from infectious to chronic non-communicable diseases. Environmental factors with exposures through lifestyle habits, dietary intakes, and environmental pollution play important roles in the development of chronic diseases such as cancers, cardiovascular diseases, and neurological disorders. There are multiple risk factors in the complex pathogenesis of chronic diseases. For examples, risk factors for ischaemic heart disease included hypertension, diabetes, hyperlipidaemia, cigarette smoking, obesity, lack of exercise, and environmental pollutants. Some environmental pollutants may cause several chronic diseases in multiple organ systems. For example, arsenic in drinking water has been documented to induce cancers of the skin, bladder, kidney, and lung, blackfoot disease, ischaemic heart disease, stroke, hypertension, diabetes, erectile dysfunction, mental retardation, neurological disorder, cataract, and pterygium. The classical Koch's postulates for judging the cause of disease are less applicable to chronic diseases. Hill's criteria including the strength, dose–response relation, temporality, specificity, and biological plausibility of the association between risk factor and disease have been widely adopted for the identification of causes of various diseases (Hill 1953).

Endemic diseases are often characterized by their unique geographical clustering. This clustering may be associated with biological or chemical agents prevailing in local environments. Some parasitic diseases such as schistosomiasis remain endemic in areas where the ecological system maintains the life cycle of the parasites. The interruption of the life cycle through the identification and treatment of affected patients, eradication of vectors, and improvement of environmental sanitation may decrease the prevalence of these endemic parasitic diseases. Some endemic diseases such as goitre and blackfoot disease are caused by the deficient or excessive intake of certain chemicals in the environment. High concentration of fluoride and arsenic in well water has been identified as the cause of fluorosis and blackfoot disease, respectively. The replacement of well water with surface water with low concentration of these chemicals had decreased the occurrence of the associated diseases. In the case of endemic goitre caused by low dietary intake of iodine, salt iodization has been implemented to effectively prevent it.

There has been a long-standing recognition that the workplace environment can induce occupational diseases. Ramazzini published his seminal treatise on diseases of workers (Raffle et al. 1987). Scrotum cancer had long been considered a disease of chimney sweeps. The poor working environment in the nineteenth century sparked reform attempts in Europe, but specific regulations to protect workers against occupational diseases were mostly implemented in the twentieth century. Occupational hazards may spread from the workplace to its adjacent environments. For example, a major gas and chemical leak incident in a pesticide plant in Bhopal, India in 1984, and the 1986 accident at the Chernobyl nuclear power plant in Ukraine resulted in environmental disasters. In addition to the immediate casualties, both events also increased the risk of a number of chronic diseases in residents living in the vicinity. The health hazards induced by long-term exposure to industrial wastes are usually more insidious than those resulting from acute environmental disasters. Environmental pollution by industrial waste has been well documented to cause Itai-itai disease and Minamata disease in Japan. Chronic poisoning by heavy metals in industrial waste has become an important issue in environmental health. Soil and water contamination by widely used agricultural chemicals have brought significant threats to human health, wild animal life, and ecological sustainability. Air pollution has increased the risk of pulmonary diseases including asthma and chronic bronchitis, as well as ischaemic heart disease.

Natural disasters including snow-storms, hurricanes, floods, sand-storms, and forest fires have had serious consequences for public health. Other environmental disasters including earthquakes, tsunamis, and landslides are also detrimental to human health. The explosions that occurred at the Fukushima nuclear power plants in the aftermath of the major earthquake and tsunami in Fukuoka, Japan in 2011, resulted in a multiple environmental disaster. In addition to the heavy immediate casualties, natural environmental disasters threaten the function and efficiency of food, water and electricity supply systems, ambulance and health care systems, sewage and waste disposal, and the control of infectious diseases. Protecting public health through proper environmental management is becoming a lasting challenge.

Causes of human diseases: host–agent interaction in the environment

Both host and environmental factors are involved in the development of human diseases, and the relative importance of environmental to host factors varies as a continuous spectrum for different diseases. Environmental factors seem to play a small role in the development of genetic diseases compared with infectious diseases or accidents. However, exposure to environmental factors may trigger the clinical manifestation of genetic diseases such as phenylketonuria and glucose-6-phosphate dehydrogenase deficiency. Environmental influences on human health are exerted through exposures to physical, chemical, and biological risk factors, and through related changes in human behavioural responses to those factors. The World Health Organization has released a country-by-country analysis of the impact of environmental factors on health (Pruss-Ustun and Corvalan 2006). These data show huge inequalities but also demonstrate that in every country, people's health could be improved by reducing environmental risks including pollution, hazards in the work environment, ultraviolet radiation, noise, agricultural risks, climate, and ecosystem change. It is estimated that 13 million deaths worldwide could be prevented every year by making environments healthier. Reducing environmental risks could save as many as 4 million lives a year in children alone, mostly in developing countries. In some countries, more than one-third of the disease burden could be prevented through environmental improvements. In 23 countries worldwide, more than 10 per cent of deaths were due to two environmental risk factors: unsafe water, including poor sanitation and hygiene; and indoor air pollution due to solid fuel used for cooking. Around the world, children under 5 years were the main victims and made up 74 per cent of deaths due to diarrhoea and lower respiratory infections. Proper environmental management is the key to prevent the quarter of all illnesses which are directly caused by environmental factors.

Human beings live in environments with many causes of diseases as shown in Table 7.1.1. Environmental causes for human diseases include physical, chemical, and biological agents. The physical component includes non-ionizing and ionizing radiation, noise, vibration, pressure, humidity, temperature, earthquake, landslides, typhoons and hurricanes, snow-storms, and sand-storms. Ionizing radiation includes alpha and beta particles, gamma rays and X-rays. Ionizing radiation may induce spontaneous abortion, congenital malformation, cancers, and haematopoietic disorders through its effects on DNA damage and chromosomal aberrations. Non-ionizing radiation includes ultraviolet rays, visible light, infrared rays, microwaves, and electromagnetic fields. Ultraviolet rays may induce skin cancer and cataract; while electromagnetic fields may induce some cancers. The chemical component includes heavy metals, organic solvents, agricultural chemicals, polycyclic hydrocarbons, and chlorinated organic compounds. Their health effects may be classified as acute toxigenicity, subacute toxigenicity, chronic toxigenicity, carcinogenicity, mutagenicity, and teratogenicity. Some chemicals may persist in the environment and result in bioaccumulation. The biological component includes viruses, bacteria, fungi, parasites, allergens, arthropods, as well as plant and animal toxins. A number of infectious diseases of various organ systems are caused by biological agents. In addition to the acute and subacute symptoms and signs, these infectious agents may also induce chronic diseases such as cancers of the nasopharynx, stomach, liver, bladder, cervix, uteri, and lymphoid and soft tissue, pulmonary diseases, cardiovascular diseases, as well as neurological disorders.

Host components in response to environmental components are also important in the determination of a number of human diseases

Table 7.1.1 Environmental components of causes for human diseases

Component	Category
Physical	Ionizing radiation (α-particles, β-particles, γ-rays, X-rays)
	Non-ionizing radiation (ultraviolet rays, visible light, infrared rays, microwaves, electromagnetic fields)
	Noise
	Vibration
	Pressure
	Humidity and temperature
	Earthquakes and landslides
	Typhoons and hurricanes
	Snow-storms and sand-storms
Chemical	Heavy metals
	Organic solvents
	Agricultural chemicals
	Polycyclic hydrocarbons
	Chlorinated organic compounds
Biological	Viruses
	Bacteria
	Fungi
	Parasites
	Allergens
	Arthropods
	Animal and plant toxins

Table 7.1.2 Host components of causes for human diseases

Component	Category
Behavioural	Substance abuse (alcohol, tobacco, betel, drugs)
	Dietary intake (malnutrition, over-nutrition)
	Personal hygiene
	Occupational protection practice
	Stressful life events
	Sports and exercise
	Personal communication and networking
Social	Housing and home safety
	Water supply system
	Sewage and waste disposal
	Transportation system
	Agricultural and irrigational methods
	Working environment
	Industrial hygiene and safety
	Anthropogenic pollution and climate changes
	Ecosystem degradation
	Schooling system
	Healthcare system
	Social welfare and criminal prevention

as shown in Table 7.1.2. Social components of human diseases include built environments, occupational settings, agricultural methods and irrigation schemes, transportation systems, water supply systems, sewage and waste disposal, schooling systems, healthcare systems, social welfare and criminal prevention systems, anthropogenic climate changes, and ecosystem degradation. Behavioural components include substance use, dietary intake, personal hygiene including hand-washing, occupational safety, safe sex, sports and exercise, personal communication and networking, and response to stressful life events. All these host components play very important roles in the development of environmental health hazards. For example, using cleaner fuel such as gas or electricity, using better cooking devices, improving ventilation, or keeping children away from smoke could have a major impact on respiratory infections and diseases among women and children. As estimated by the World Health Organization, reducing levels of air pollution (measured by PM10) as set out in the Air Quality Guidelines would save an estimated 865,000 lives per year. The household interventions could dramatically reduce the death rate. Interventions at the community or national level would involve promoting household water treatment and safe storage, and introducing energy policies, which favour development and health.

Several causal models have been proposed to describe the host–environment interaction in human diseases as shown in Table 7.1.3. The traditional epidemiological triangle emphasizes the equal importance of host, agent, and environment, which are located in three angles of the epidemiological model. Host factors may include the biological characteristics, sociodemographic characteristics and behavioural characteristics listed in Table 7.1.3. The agent factor includes the physical, chemical, biological, and social characteristics of causal agent of disease. Environmental factors include living and working environments such as family, school, workplace, and recreation place. The epidemiological triangle model is widely used to develop various strategies to prevent the occurrence of diseases. Host factors may be strengthened through the improvement in nutritional status, optimal rest and exercise, personal hygiene, active and passive immunization, immunomodulation, chemoprevention, and so forth. Agent factors may be controlled through disinfection and sterilization, antibiotic use, prevention of drug resistance, and antiviral therapy. Environmental factors may be improved through clean housing and workplaces, safe water and food supply, hygienic sewage and waste disposal, and others.

The epidemiological triangle model emphasizes the unique causal agent of a specific disease. This model is most appropriate for infectious diseases because the infectious agent is the necessary (unique) cause of a given infectious disease, even though the infectious agent may not be sufficient to cause the given disease. For many infectious agents, not all infected individuals will develop the disease. The one-to-one causal relation between agent (cause) and disease (outcome) may not be observed under this circumstance. The triangle model is not appropriate for most chronic non-communicable diseases. Most chronic diseases have multiple causes. A single agent is neither necessary nor sufficient to cause the disease. The ecological wheel model shown in Table 7.1.3 was proposed to describe the host–environment interaction for human diseases. The wheel model includes an axle (host factors) surrounded by a tyre (environmental factors). No unique single agent is specified for a disease in this model. Environmental factors are further classified into those from the physicochemical environment including energy and chemical substances, living and working infrastructure, and public facilities; biological environmental factors including infectious agents,

Table 7.1.3 Causal models describing host–environment interaction in human diseases

Model	Illustration	Components	Characteristics
Epidemiological triangle	Host / Agent / Environment	Host	Biological: age, gender, race, genetic composition, nutritional status, immune status, anthropometric characteristics
			Sociodemographic: marital status, education, occupation, profession, socioeconomic status
			Behavioural: dietary habits, lifestyles, personality, social activities
		Agent	Physical
			Chemical
			Biological
			Social
		Environment	Family
			School
			Working place
			Recreation place
Ecological wheel	PE / H / BE / SE	Host	Genes
			Behaviours
		Physicochemical environment	Energy and chemical substances
			Living and working infrastructure
			Public facilities
		Biological environment	Infectious agents
			Animal reservoir
			Vectors
			Infected carriers
		Social environment	Culture
			Customs
			Social networks
Evolutionary spiral	Host / Environments	Chronology/stage	Initiation→ Promotion→ Progression
		Health effects/lesions	Molecules→ Cells→ Tissues→ Organs → Systemic illness
		Host	Genes
			Behaviours
		Environments	Physicochemical environment
			Biological environment
			Social environment

animal reservoirs, vectors, and infectious carriers; and social environmental factors including culture, customs, and social networks. Genetic factors are located in the core of the host with the rest of the host factors including lifestyle, personality, dietary intake, and immunity. This causal model emphasizes the importance of ecological balance in the maintenance of the health status of a host. The relative importance of host and various environment factors varies by diseases. For example, genetic factors are most important for the highly inheritable diseases; the biological environment for various infectious diseases; and the social environment for accidents. This wheel model also describes the interactions among host and various environment components.

The ecological wheel does not take the time dimension of disease development into consideration. The development of both acute and chronic diseases follows a specific temporal sequence. This usually starts from contact of causal agent with target cells, through the structural and functional changes as well as proliferation of causal agent and transformed cells, the development of lesions in

affected tissues or organs, the onset of clinical symptoms and signs, to the development of systemic illness. There are various agents and environment factors involved at different stages of the pathological progression. For example, the multistage process of carcinogenesis may be classified into initiation, promotion, progression, invasion, and metastasis. An evolutional spiral model has been proposed to describe host–environment interactions over the entire natural history of disease as shown in Table 7.1.3 (Chen 1999). At the initial stage, both cause and molecular or cellular change are simple and small, and causal relationship tends to be one-to-one. With disease progression, however, both causes and affected lesions become more and more complicated and involve complex host–environment interactions at different stages.

The evolutional spiral model is most appropriate for the description of multistage pathogenesis of a disease with a multifactorial aetiology. As shown in Fig. 7.1.1, the development of hepatocellular carcinoma is a multistage process with the involvement of multiple risk factors. A healthy individual may be infected by

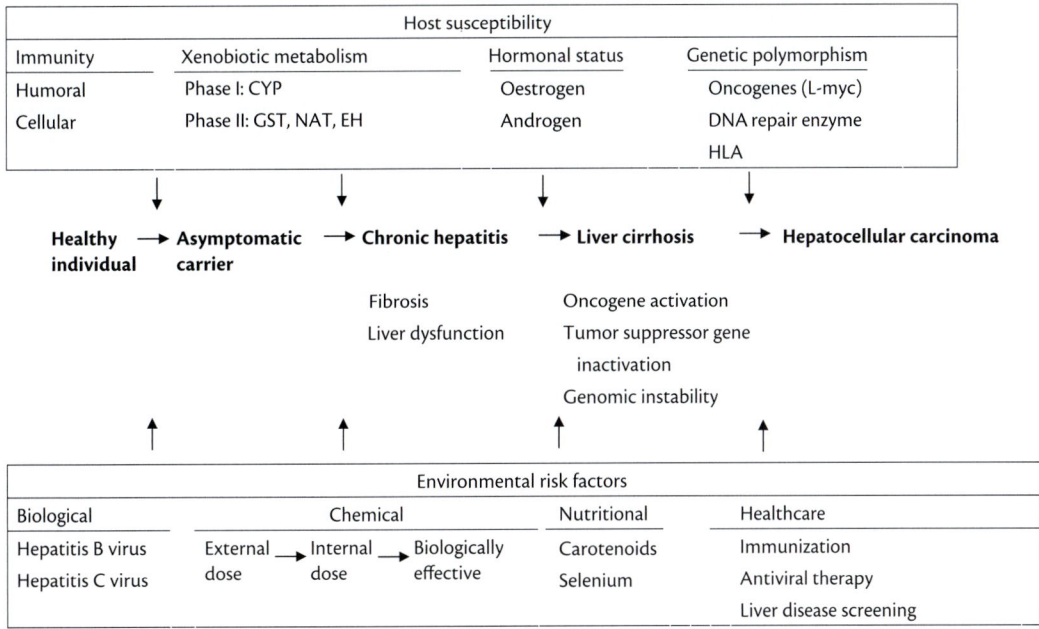

Fig. 7.1.1 Multistage hepatocarcinogenesis with a multifactorial aetiology.

infectious agents such as hepatitis B virus (HBV) and hepatitis C virus and become an asymptomatic carrier. With the long-term progression of the viral hepatitis, the carrier may start to develop chronic hepatitis, liver fibrosis, cirrhosis, and even hepatocellular carcinoma. During the disease development period, there are host and environmental factors that may influence the disease progression at various stages. Chemical carcinogens including aflatoxins, benzo(a)pyrene, and 4-aminobipheyl as well as micronutrients such as carotenoids and selenium are involved in hepatocarcinogenesis. Host factors including humoral and cellular immunity, xenobiotic metabolism, hormones, and susceptibility genes can modify the progression of chronic hepatitis B. Healthcare factors including immunization, antiviral therapy and abdominal ultrasonographic screening may be used to stop or slow the pathogenic process. This example illustrates how physicochemical, biological, and social environments are important in the entire hepatocarcinogenesis process.

Ecological studies: identification of environmental health hazards at aggregate level

Geographical clustering of endemic diseases in a small area is the most important characteristic of environmental health hazards. An extremely high prevalence of an endemic disease in a confined area always leads to the search for unique environmental risk factors. Ecological studies are often used to compare the morbidity or mortality of environmental disease between endemic and non-endemic areas. In ecological studies, aggregate attributes such as the morbidity of residents in exposed and unexposed areas, rather than individual attributes such as the health status of exposed and unexposed subjects, are analysed and compared. Ecological studies tend to compare health indices in areas with and without the environmental exposure, or to examine quantitatively the correlation between health indices and environmental

exposure in many areas. Some environmental characteristics or co-morbidity rates may be used as surrogate indicators of the causal agents to elucidate the relation between the disease risk and the causal agent. The interpretation of ecological studies may be limited by the potential existence of ecological fallacy, when the agent–disease correlation observed at the aggregate level may not consistently be found at the individual level. However, ecological studies are frequently used to explore environmental component of causes for human diseases.

As an illustrative example, blackfoot disease is an endemic peripheral vascular disorder confined to a limited area on the southwest coast of Taiwan. Clinically the disease starts with numbness or coldness of one or more extremities and intermittent claudication, which progresses to black discoloration, ulcer and gangrene. In end stages of the disease, spontaneous amputation of the distal parts of the affected extremities is common. The disease was hyperendemic in four neighbouring townships in southwestern Taiwan. As the water from shallow wells (6–8 metres in depth) in this area had high salinity, residents in some villages had started to use water from artesian wells (100–200 metres deep) since 1920s. The use of artesian well water was found to be associated with the occurrence of the blackfoot disease, and water samples from artesian wells of the endemic area were found to have high arsenic concentrations which ranged from 0.35 to 1.14 mg/L. Based on the analysis of mortality data, residents in the endemic area of blackfoot disease had significantly elevated mortality from cancers of the bladder, kidney, skin, lung, and liver as shown in Table 7.1.4. Compared with the general population in Taiwan, the standardized mortality ratios for cancer of the bladder, kidney, skin, and lung were threefold greater among residents in the endemic area (Chen et al. 1985).

As the four townships in this endemic area had different prevalence of blackfoot disease, cancer mortality was further compared among townships. It was found that the higher the blackfoot disease prevalence of a township, the greater the age-standardized

Table 7.1.4 Age-standardized mortality ratios[1] of skin and internal cancers in villages of arseniasis-endemic area in southwestern Taiwan by blackfoot disease prevalence and drinking water source

Cancer	Gender	Blackfoot disease endemic area	Township by blackfoot disease endemicity[2]				Village by blackfoot disease endemicity[3]			Village by types of wells as major drinking water source[4]		
			Very high	High	Medium	Low	High	Medium	Low	Artesian only	Both	Shallow only
Skin	Male	5.3	8.4	8.3	5.3	1.3	11.2	6.5	2.2	10.9	6.5	2.2
	Female	6.5	6.8	15.7	3.6	1.9						
Bladder	Male	11.0	13.8	15.6	10.7	6.1	40.3	17.2	3.8	26.3	11.2	4.5
	Female	20.1	38.0	34.6	16.1	5.6						
Kidney	Male	7.7	14.0	12.44	8.2	4.8	14.9	7.7	3.2	9.2	7.5	3.3
	Female	11.2	14.7	22.5	8.5	3.2						
Lung	Male	3.2	3.8	5.3	2.6	1.7	6.2	3.1	1.8	4.6	2.8	1.8
	Female	4.1	6.3	6.8	3.3	1.9						
Liver	Male	1.7	1.6	1.9	1.7	1.6	3.0	1.5	1.3	2.0	1.8	1.4
	Female	2.3	1.8	2.3	2.5	2.4						

[1] Mortality rates of general population in Taiwan were used as the standard rates to calculate standardized mortality ratio (Taiwan = 1.0).

[2] Four townships including Peimen, Husehchia, Putai and Ichu with blackfoot disease prevalence of 5.67, 3.87, 2.02 and 0.64 per 1,000, respectively. Age-standardized mortality ratios were calculated for males and females, respectively.

[3] A total of 84 villages were classified into three groups by blackfoot disease prevalence: 0, 0.1–5.0 and >5.0 per 1000, respectively. Age–gender-standardized mortality ratios were calculated.

[4] A total of 84 villages were classified into three groups by type of wells used as major drinking water source: artesian wells only, both artesian and shallow wells, and shallow wells only. Age–gender-standardized mortality ratios were calculated.

Reproduced with permission from Chen CJ et al., Malignant neoplasms among residents of a blackfoot disease-endemic area in Taiwan: High-arsenic artesian well water and cancers, *Cancer Research*, Volume 45, pp. 5895–5899, Copyright © 1985 American Association for Cancer Research.

mortality ratios for cancers of the skin, bladder, lung, and liver. As 84 villages in these four townships also had different prevalence of blackfoot disease and used different types of well water, more refined analyses of cancer mortality at village level were carried out. A significant dose–response relationship between the prevalence of blackfoot disease and the age–sex-standardized mortality ratios for cancers of the skin, bladder, kidney, lung and liver was observed at the village level as shown in Table 7.1.4. Furthermore, biological gradients of cancer mortality were also found by the type of wells used as drinking water source with the highest cancer mortality in villages where only artesian wells were used and the lowest in villages which used only shallow wells. As both blackfoot disease and artesian well use were significantly associated with the arsenic in drinking water, they were used as the surrogate environmental variable for arsenic exposure. It was thus implied that arsenic in drinking water might increase the risk of both skin and internal cancers. However, the best way to assess the cancer risk associated with arsenic in drinking water is to obtain the arsenic levels in drinking water from wells.

The arsenic levels in water of shallow and artesian wells in 42 villages of the blackfoot disease endemic area were available for further analysis of the association between arsenic in drinking water and cancer mortality. As shown in Table 7.15, there was a significant dose–response relation between arsenic in drinking water and age-adjusted mortality for cancers of the bladder, kidney, lung, skin, liver, and prostate at the village level (Chen et al. 1988a). A significant dose–response relationship was also observed between arsenic in drinking water and age-adjusted mortality for cardiovascular diseases and peripheral vascular diseases at the village level (Wu et al. 1989). In another ecological correlation study on age-adjusted

cancer mortality of 314 precincts and townships in Taiwan (Chen and Wang 1990), the arsenic level in water of 83,656 wells was tested to derive the average arsenic level in well water in each precinct or township. Both cancer deaths and mid-year population in all study precincts and townships were obtained from the national death certification and household registration system. Based on the weighted multiple regression analysis, there were significant correlations between the average arsenic level in well water and the age-adjusted mortality rates of cancers of the liver, nasal cavity, lung, skin, bladder, kidney, and prostate at the precinct/township level, after adjustment for indices of industrialization and urbanization. In these ecological correlation studies, both disease risk and environmental exposure were measured at a group (village or precinct/township) level. The findings have to be further validated by studies at the individual level, in which potential ecological fallacy and confounding effects of extraneous factors such as cigarette smoking habit are limited.

Ecological studies have also been used to explore possible associations between infectious agents and cancer. Chronic hepatitis B is a worldwide public health challenge. Despite the availability of an effective vaccine, an estimated 350–400 million people are chronically infected with the HBV. Chronic hepatitis B is particularly prevalent in the Asia-Pacific and sub-Saharan Africa regions, where infection is predominantly acquired either during the perinatal period or in the early childhood years. The countries with high incidence of liver cancer are also clustered in the Asia-Pacific and sub-Saharan Africa regions. The significant ecological correlation between the mortality from liver cancer and the prevalence of chronic hepatitis B was also observed among townships in Taiwan. These ecological study findings suggest the importance of chronic

Table 7.1.5 Age-standardized mortality (per 100,000) from skin and internal cancers in villages of arseniasis-endemic area in southwestern Taiwan by arsenic level in well water

Cancer	Gender	Arsenic level in drinking water in arseniasis-endemic villages			General population in Taiwan
		0.60+	0.30–0.59	<0.30	
Skin	Male	28.0	10.7	1.6	**0.8**
	Female	15.1	10.0	1.6	0.8
Bladder	Male	89.1	37.8	15.7	3.1
	Female	91.5	35.1	16.7	1.4
Kidney	Male	21.6	13.1	5.4	1.1
	Female	33.3	12.5	3.6	0.9
Lung	Male	87.9	64.7	35.1	19.4
	Female	83.8	40.9	26.5	9.5
Liver	Male	68.8	42.7	32.6	28.0
	Female	31.8	18.8	14.2	8.9

Reproduced from *The Lancet*, Volume 1, Number 8582, Chen CJ et al., Arsenic and cancers (letter), pp. 414–415, Copyright © 1988, with permission from Elsevier, http://www.sciencedirect.com/science/journal/01406736.

hepatitis B in the development of liver cancer, specifically hepatocellular carcinoma. The seroprevalence of antibodies against *Helicobacter pylori* was found to be associated with the mortality from gastric cancer in Taiwan, suggesting *Helicobacter pylori* infection may be a causal agent of gastric cancer. However, the ecological correlation observed at the aggregate level needs further validation by studies at the individual level.

Cross-sectional surveys and longitudinal studies: assessment of environmental health hazards at individual level

Several different study designs have been used to assess the environmental health hazards at the individual level as shown in Table 7.1.6. Based on the time of the collection of disease risk (outcome) and environmental exposure (cause) data, they may be classified into cross-sectional and longitudinal studies. Cross-sectional studies collect the data on disease and exposure at the same time. The most common type of cross-sectional studies is the environmental health survey, in which participants are enrolled from exposed and unexposed areas to collect the

information on health status, exposure to environmental factors, and potential confounding factors. Morbidity estimates from cross-sectional surveys represent disease prevalence rather than incidence. As the disease and exposure data are collected simultaneously, the causal temporality of disease and exposure needs further evaluation. If the environmental exposure is quite consistent over a long period of time before the onset of the disease, the causal temporality may be considered correct. Longitudinal studies may be further classified into case–control and cohort studies according to the enrolment of study participants. Conventional case–control studies recruit incident cases and matched controls from healthcare institutions or the community, and collect the history of exposure to environmental factors through questionnaire interviews. While the causal temporality is accounted for, the information on environmental exposure history may be subject to recall and other biases. If there were detailed records of long-term exposure history, the bias may be reduced significantly. Conventional cohort studies recruit exposed and unexposed healthy participants from community or workplace, and follow the cohort until an adequate proportion of participants develop the disease under study. While there is no recall bias of the exposure information, it may be limited by participants being lost to follow-up. If data from disease registration systems or health insurance databases were available, the loss to follow-up may be solved through computerized data linkage.

Returning to blackfoot disease as an illustrative example, in a community-based cross-sectional survey of 40,421 residents in 37 villages in the endemic area in southwestern Taiwan, the relationship between status of skin cancer and blackfoot disease in participants, and arsenic in well water was examined (Tseng 1977). As shown in Fig. 7.1.2 there was a significant dose–response relationship between skin cancer and blackfoot disease, and arsenic concentrations in the drinking water for most age and sex groups. There was a significant coexistence of both skin cancer and blackfoot disease. In a community-based case–control study, a total of 353 pairs of blackfoot disease cases and matched controls were interviewed (Chi and Blackwell 1968). The length of residing in the endemic villages was significantly associated with the risk of developing blackfoot disease in a dose–response relation. While all 353 (100 per cent) blackfoot disease cases had ever used artesian well water as the principal source of drinking water during the 15 years before onset, only 233 (66 per cent) matched controls had consumed artesian well water ($p < 0.001$). Blackfoot disease cases had lower educational level and socioeconomic status than matched controls. In another case–control study on 241 blackfoot disease patients and 759 matched healthy controls, questionnaire

Table 7.1.6 Major study designs of investigation on environmental health hazards at individual level

Temporality between disease and exposure	Collection of disease and exposure data	Study subjects selection	Limitations	Association estimates
Cross-sectional	Simultaneous	Random sample of population	Temporal correctness	Odds ratio
Longitudinal	Retrospective (retrieval of previous exposure)	Affected cases and unaffected controls	Recall bias	Odds ratio
Longitudinal	Prospective (follow-up of future disease)	Exposed and unexposed cohorts	Loss of follow-up	Hazard ratio

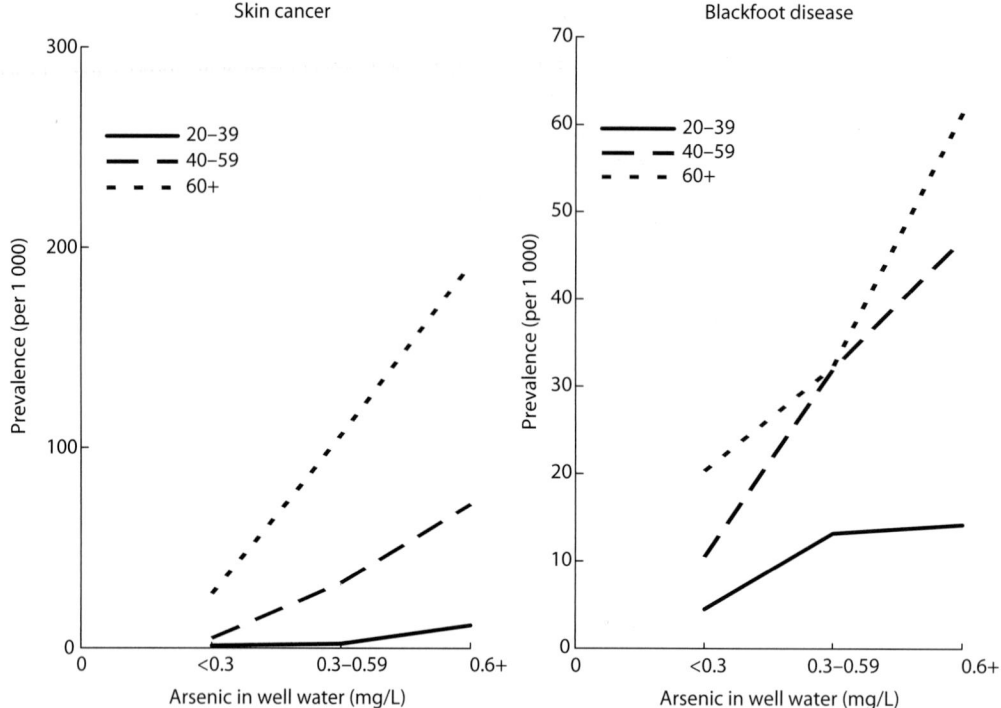

Fig. 7.1.2 Dose–response relationship between arsenic in well water and prevalence of skin cancer and blackfoot disease.
Reproduced from Tseng, W.P., Effects and dose-response relationships of skin cancer and blackfoot disease with arsenic, *Environmental Health Perspectives*, Volume 19, pp. 109–19, Copyright © 1977.

interviews were carried out to obtain information on the history of consuming artesian well water, diet, alcohol intake and cigarette smoking, as well as the presence of arsenic-induced skin keratosis and cancer, and blackfoot disease in first-degree relatives (Chen et al. 1988b). There was a significant dose–response relationship between the risk of developing blackfoot disease and the duration of consumption of artesian well water. In addition, arsenic-induced skin lesions, family history of blackfoot disease, and undernourishment were also associated with the development of blackfoot disease independent of the duration of consuming artesian well water.

In a cohort study of cause-specific mortality of 789 blackfoot disease patients followed for 15 years (Chen et al. 1988b), age–sex-standardized mortality ratios were derived for blackfoot disease patients using the mortality rates of the general population in Taiwan and the blackfoot disease endemic area as the standard rates, respectively. As shown in Table 7.1.7, patients of blackfoot disease had significantly increased mortality from cardiovascular disease and cancers of the bladder, skin, lung, and liver compared to two reference populations. In another case–control study on cancers of bladder, lung, and liver in the endemic area of blackfoot disease (Chen et al. 1986), the duration of consuming artesian well water was significantly associated with three cancers in a dose–response relationship after adjustment for age and sex.

A community-based health survey study was carried out in three blackfoot disease-hyperendemic villages to examine the associations between arsenic in drinking water and various chronic diseases. A total of 1571 residents aged over 30 years were interviewed by public health nurses, and 1071 of them had health examinations. Residents in these villages started using artesian wells as the

Table 7.1.7 Age-standardized mortality ratios for cancers and vascular diseases for blackfoot disease patients in comparison with two populations

Disease	Standardized mortality ratio in blackfoot disease patients	
	Taiwan population as reference[1]	Endemic area population as reference[2]
Skin cancer	28.5**	4.5*
Bladder cancer	38.8***	2.6**
Kidney cancer	19.5	1.6
Lung cancer	10.5***	2.8**
Liver cancer	4.7***	2.5**
Prostate cancer	17.3	2.7
Peripheral vascular disease	12.4***	3.5***
Cardiovascular disease	2.1***	1.6**
Cerebrovasular disease	1.2	1.1

[1] Mortality rates of general population in Taiwan were used as the standard rates (Taiwan = 1.0)

[2] Mortality rates of population in blackfoot disease-endemic area were used as the standard rates (endemic area = 1.0)

* P < 0.5, ** P < 0.01, *** P < 0.001

Reproduced with permission from Chen CJ et al., Atherogenicity and carcinogenicity of high-arsenic artesian well water: Multiple risk factors and related malignant neoplasms of blackfoot disease, *Arteriosclerosis, Thrombosis, and Vascular Biology*, Volume 8, pp. 452–460, Copyright © 1988 American Heart Association, Inc. All rights reserved. DOI: 10.1161/01. ATV.8.5.452.

principal drinking source in early 1910s, and shifted to the public water supply system using surface water from a distant reservoir in early 1970s. The arsenic level in water of artesian wells of the blackfoot disease-hyperendemic villages was surveyed in the early 1960s. As residents in a given village shared a few wells together, the median arsenic level of the water from the shared wells was used as the level of arsenic in drinking water for residents of the village. As a participant might migrate from one village to another, a detailed life history of residence and consumption of artesian well water was obtained through a structured questionnaire interview. The cumulative arsenic exposure was derived by the formula $\Sigma(C_i \times D_i)$; where C_i was the median arsenic level in water of shared wells of a village in which the participant lived, and D_i was the duration of drinking artesian well water in the village during the consecutive period i. The average arsenic exposure level in drinking water of a participant was derived by $\Sigma(C_i \times D_i)/\Sigma(D_i)$. Residents in hyperendemic villages of blackfoot disease had a significantly higher age-specific prevalence of diabetes mellitus (Lai et al. 1994) and hypertension (Chen et al. 1995) than residents in non-endemic areas. Furthermore, there was a significant dose–response relationship between the cumulative arsenic exposure and prevalence of diabetes mellitus (Lai et al. 1994), hypertension (Chen et al. 1995), peripheral vascular disease based on Doppler ultrasonography

(Tseng et al. 1996), carotid atherosclerosis based on duplex ultrasonography (Wang et al. 2002), electrocardiogram-based ischaemic heart disease (Tseng et al. 2003), cataract (See et al. 2007), and pterygium (Lin et al. 2008) as shown in Table 7.1.8. Follow-up studies also found a significant biological gradient of incidence of skin cancer (Hsueh et al. 1997) and lethal ischaemic heart disease (Chen et al. 1996a) with increasing cumulative arsenic exposure as also shown in Table 7.1.8.

Table 7.1.8 also shows summary data from another survey of well-water arsenic and health status in northeastern Taiwan that involved a total of 8102 residents in four townships. Residents in these townships had their own tube wells in their backyards. The arsenic levels in well water of these households were tested in early 1990s. The public water supply system using surface water was introduced in this area in early 1990s, and its coverage was as high as 95 per cent in the year 2000. Cerebrovascular disease, especially cerebral infarction, was identified from home-visit personal interviews and ascertained through the review of hospital medical records (Chiou et al. 1997). These revealed a dose-related increase in the risk of cerebral infarction with higher cumulative arsenic exposure.

In several cohort studies of participants enrolled from the endemic areas of arseniasis in southwestern and northeastern

Table 7.1.8 Dose–response relationship between cumulative arsenic exposure and risk of various diseases. Figures are relative risks (95 per cent confidence intervals)

Disease/cause of death	Cumulative arsenic exposure			
	Low	Medium	Medium high	High
Skin cancer[1]	1.0 (referent)	2.8 (0.3–31.9)	2.6 (0.3–22.9)	7.6 (1.0–60.3)
Hypertension[2]	1.0 (referent)	0.9 (0.2–3.3)	2.4 (0.8–6.9)	3.6 (1.4–9.6)
Ischaemic heart disease death[3]	1.0 (referent)	2.5 (0.5–11.4)	4.0 (1.0–15.6)	6.5 (1.9–22.2)
Cataract (posterior subcapsular opacity)[4]	1.0 (referent)	2.2 (0.4–12.1)	4.8 (1.0–22.2)	5.7 (1.2–26.3)
	Low	Medium	High	
Diabetes mellitus[5]	1.0 (referent)	6.6 (0.9–51.0)	10.1 (1.3–77.9)	
Electrocardiogram-based ischaemic heart disease[6]	1.0 (referent)	1.6 (0.5–5.3)	3.6 (1.1–11.7)	
Doppler ultrasonography-based peripheral vascular disease[7]	1.0 (referent)	2.8 (0.9–9.1)	4.3 (1.3–14.5)	
Duplex ultrasonography-based carotid atherosclerosis[7]	1.0 (referent)	1.8 (0.8–3.8)	3.1 (1.3–7.4)	
Cerebral infarction[8]	1.0 (referent)	2.7 (1.2–5.8)	3.4 (1.4–8.1)	
Pterygium[9]	1.0 (referent)	3.1 (1.8–5.6)	4.1 (2.2–7.4)	

[1] Follow-up study in southwestern Taiwan, arsenic level stratified as 0, 0.1–10.6, 10.7–17.7, >17.7 mg/L-years

[2] Survey in southwestern Taiwan, arsenic level stratified as 0, 0.1–6.3, 6.4–10.8, 10.9–14.7 mg/L-years (two groups >14.7 mg/L-years are not shown here)

[3] Follow-up study in southwestern Taiwan, arsenic level stratified as 0, 0.1–9.9, 10.0–19.9, >19.9 mg/L-years

[4] Survey in southwestern Taiwan, arsenic level stratified as 0, 0.1–12.0, 12.1–20.0, >20.0 mg/L-years

[5] Survey in southwestern Taiwan, arsenic level stratified as 0, 0.1–15.0, >15.0 mg/L-years

[6] Survey in southwestern Taiwan, arsenic level stratified as 0, 0.1–14.9, >14.9 mg/L-years

[7] Survey in southwestern Taiwan, arsenic level stratified as 0, 0.1–19.9, >19.9 mg/L-years

[8] Survey in northwestern Taiwan, arsenic level stratified as <0.1, 0.1–4.9, >4.9 mg/L-years

[9] Survey in southwestern Taiwan, arsenic level stratified as 0, 0.1–15.0, >15.0 mg/L-years

Source data from: skin cancer (Hsueh et al. 1997), hypertension (Chen et al. 1995), ischaemic heart disease death (Chen et al. 1996a), cataract (See et al. 2007), diabetes mellitus (Lai et al. 1994), electrocardiogram-based ischaemic heart disease (Tseng et al. 2003), Doppler ultrasonography-based peripheral vascular disease (Tseng et al. 1996), duplex ultrasonography-based carotid atherosclerosis (Wang et al. 2002), cerebral infarction (Chiou et al. 1997), and pterygium (Lin et al. 2008).

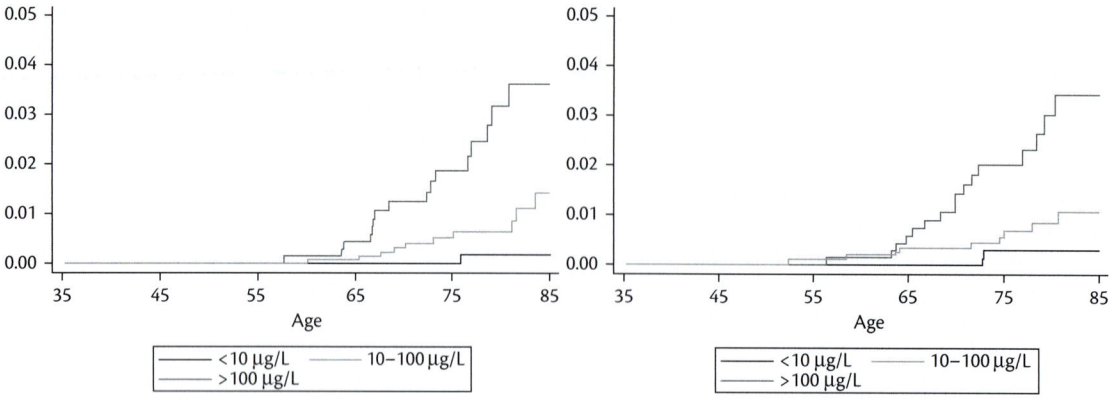

Fig. 7.1.3 Life time risk of lung cancer (left) and urothelial carcinoma (right) in arseniasis-endemic area in northeastern Taiwan by arsenic level in well water.
Reproduced from *Journal of Asian Earth Sciences*, Volume 77, Yang TY et al., Lifetime risk of urothelial carcinoma and lung cancer in the arseniasis-endemic area of northeastern Taiwan, pp. 332–337, Copyright © 2013, with permission from Elsevier, http://www.sciencedirect.com/science/journal/13679120.

Taiwan, the occurrence of cancers was identified and ascertained through computerized data linkage with national cancer registry and death certification profiles. A dose–response relation was observed between long-term arsenic exposure from drinking well water and incidence of urothelial carcinoma (Chiou et al. 2001) and lung cancer (Chen et al. 2004). Based on follow-up data from northeastern Taiwan, the cumulative lifetime risk of lung cancer and urothelial carcinoma was found to increase with the arsenic concentration in well water (Fig. 7.1.3) (Yang et al. 2013). It is important to be aware of the possibility of temporal variations in concentration of the causal agent in various environmental media, individual variations in frequency and quantity of contact with the contaminated environmental media, and variations in detection limit of various exposure assessment methods. It is essential to ensure accuracy in the assessment of exposure to environmental factors in all cross-sectional surveys, case–control studies, and cohort studies in order to identify and characterize the environmental health hazards efficiently and effectively.

Several case–control studies have assessed the association between risk of hepatocellular carcinoma, chronic hepatitis B infection, and seropositivity of hepatitis B surface antigen (HBsAg) (Chen et al. 1997; You et al. 2004). A statistically significant association between hepatocellular carcinoma and HBsAg serostatus was found in all cross-sectional case–control studies. It should be noted that the HBsAg serostatus determined at the time of the diagnosis of hepatocellular carcinoma, might not reflect the serostatus long before the onset of the cancer. However, since most HBsAg-seropositive participants become chronic carriers in early childhood, this would support a longer-standing temporal association between HBsAg seropositivity and hepatocellular carcinoma in such cases. Another case–control study further evaluated the importance of hepatitis B e antigen (HBeAg) in the development of hepatocellular carcinoma (Chen et al. 1991). The relative risk of hepatocellular carcinoma was 58-fold higher for those who were seropositive for both HBsAg and HBeAg, 17-fold higher for seropositives for HBsAg only, as compared with those who were seronegative on both markers as reference. As both HBsAg and HBeAg disappear gradually with increasing age, their seroprevalence estimated at the onset of hepatocellular carcinoma is much lower than those in childhood or young adulthood. An insurance-based cohort study of 3,454 chronic HBsAg carriers

and 19,253 non-carriers in northern Taiwan had confirmed the high risk of hepatocellular carcinoma for chronic HBsAg carriers compared with the non-carriers, with a relative risk greater than 100-fold (Beasley et al. 1981). Another community-based cohort study on 2361 carriers and 9532 non-carriers of HBsAg in seven townships in Taiwan showed the importance of HBeAg serostatus in the development of hepatocellular carcinoma in addition to HBsAg serostatus (Yang et al. 2002). These observational studies suggest the most effective and efficient ways to reduce the risk of hepatocellular carcinoma in Taiwan are vaccination to prevent hepatitis B infection and appropriate antiviral treatment of patients with chronic hepatitis B infection.

Intervention trials: validation of environmental health hazards through preventive intervention

It is unethical to carry out experimental studies on human beings to validate the suspected effects of environmental health hazards identified from observational studies discussed earlier. However, intervention trials may be used to evaluate possible effects of environmental agents on disease risk by removing the agents from the environment. Intervention trials may be classified as individual or cluster trials depending on whether individual subjects or clusters such as households, schools, or communities are allocated to the intervention. Intervention trials may also be classified as controlled and uncontrolled trials depending on the inclusion of a comparable control group or not. In controlled trials, the effect of intervention on environmental health hazards is evaluated by the comparison of disease occurrence between experimental and control groups. In uncontrolled trials, the effect of intervention is assessed by the comparison of disease occurrence of the experimental group before and after the intervention.

The implementation of a public water supply system, which used uncontaminated surface water from distant reservoirs, in the blackfoot disease-endemic area of southwestern Taiwan was started in the early 1960s and completed in the 1970s. The arsenic-induced health hazards identified from observational studies could thus be validated through the comparison of the secular changes in morbidity and mortality of arsenic-induced diseases in the endemic and non-endemic areas. In a series of studies, cause-specific standardized mortality ratios of residents in the blackfoot disease endemic from 1971 to 2003 were calculated using the general population in Taiwan as the standard population. Cumulative sum techniques were used to detect the occurrence of changes in the standardized mortality ratios. A significant decline in mortality from ischaemic heart disease (Chang et al. 2004), renal disease (Chiu and Yang 2005), peripheral vascular disease (Yang 2006), and cancers of the lung (Chiu et al. 2004b), kidney (Yang et al. 2004), and bladder (Yang et al. 2005) was observed for both males and females in the southwestern endemic area of blackfoot disease. A significant decline in mortality from liver cancer (Chiu et al. 2004a) and diabetes mellitus (Chiu et al. 2006) was observed for females but not males. Based on the reversibility criterion, it was concluded that associations between arsenic exposure and various health effects was very likely to be causal. Although the findings are quite consistent with observational studies mentioned earlier, there are several issues which need further clarification: (1) classification of underlying causes of death may vary by area and time. It is necessary to examine whether the variations in the classification of underlying causes in death certificates are comparable in different areas over the study period. (2) Competing causes of death may be quite different between the endemic area and Taiwan as a whole. Arsenic has a pleiotropic health effect that induces various cancers, circulatory diseases, diabetes mellitus, hypertension, renal disease, and so forth. A person may die with several arsenic-induced diseases. It is thus difficult to select an underlying cause of death for an arsenic-exposed person. (3) Mortality associated with a disease is a function of the incidence and fatality of the disease. High mortality may imply an increased incidence and/or an elevated fatality rate. It is better to analyse incidence rather than mortality to clarify the causal association between agent and disease. (4) Risk factors other than arsenic may be important confounding factors, such as habits of cigarette smoking and alcohol drinking, chronic infection with hepatitis viruses, and obesity. They are not taken into consideration in the mortality analysis. It is thus more convincing to compare the secular changes in the incidence of arsenic-induced diseases after the implementation of public water supply system. Furthermore, age-cohort-period analysis may also help the identification of susceptible ages at exposure to arsenic and the assessment of reversibility effect of intervention.

A nationwide vaccination programme aimed at eradicating HBV infection was launched on 1 July 1984 in Taiwan (Chien et al. 2006). It was the first universal hepatitis B vaccination programme for newborns in the world. During the first 2 years (July 1984 to June 1986) of the programme, only newborns born to high-risk (HBsAg-positive) mothers were vaccinated. Since July 1986, however, all newborns were vaccinated. The programme was further extended to the preschool children who had not received vaccination as neonates since 1987. There has been a dramatic decrease in the HBsAg carrier rate and HBV infection rate among children and adolescents born after 1984 demonstrating the programme not only successfully prevented the perinatal transmission of HBV but also reduced the risk of horizontal transmission of HBV among children (Hsu et al. 1999). Recent studies in Taiwan also demonstrated a significant decline in the mortality from fulminant hepatitis in infants (Kao et al. 2001) and the incidence of hepatocellular carcinoma (Chang et al. 1997) in children since the nationwide hepatitis B vaccination programme was launched. Even more striking has been the effectiveness of the national hepatitis B vaccination programme in reducing long-term risk of infant fulminant hepatitis, chronic liver disease, and hepatocellular carcinoma, as shown by the data from a recent report, which are summarized in Table 7.1.9 (Chiang et al. 2013). These important findings demonstrated that hepatitis B vaccination not only protected children from becoming chronic HBV carriers but also protected them from developing fulminant hepatitis, chronic liver diseases, and hepatocellular carcinoma. These are among the first studies to demonstrate the prevention of human cancer through vaccination. Through the strong evidence of a striking decline in childhood incidence of hepatocellular carcinoma after the introduction of the national vaccination programme, the causal relation of chronic hepatitis B infection with hepatocellular carcinoma is well confirmed. However, the elucidation of the failure of hepatitis B vaccination to eliminate all childhood hepatocellular carcinoma requires further study at the individual rather than national level.

Before the Second World War, endemic goitre was highly prevalent in mountainous areas in Taiwan. A national survey showed a prevalence as high as 70 per cent in some aboriginal townships in mountainous areas. The prevalence of goitre in pigs was found to be significantly higher in the goitre-endemic area than non-endemic area. It was debated whether dietary deficiency in iodine or goitrogenic foodstuff intake was the major cause of the endemic goitre. The use of iodine tablets to supplement dietary iodine intake was found to be effective in lowering the prevalence of endemic goitre in school children, but it was considered costly and inconvenient. In order to identify an effective and efficient prevention strategy at the community level, a controlled community intervention trial on iodized salt was carried out in two townships in northern Taiwan (Chen et al. 1976). All the dietary salt used in experimental and control townships was strictly provided by the research team. Before the implementation of the community trial, the endemic goitre prevalence among schoolchildren was similarly high. One year after the trial, the prevalence of endemic goitre in the experimental township was significantly lower than in the control township. While the study did not rule out the possible effects of the intake of goitrogenic foodstuff, iodine deficiency was confirmed to be the most important risk factor for endemic goitre in Taiwan. A nationwide salt iodization programme supported by UNICEF was implemented, and the goitre prevalence has been drastically reduced since then. As there may be changes in dietary intake of iodine other than iodized salt, it is essential to monitor and adjust the level of iodine in the salt to prevent thyroid toxicity due to excessively high intakes of iodine.

Gene–environment interaction in environmental health hazards: identification and application of molecular and genomic biomarkers

The risk of developing an environmental disease may vary in different persons exposed to the same environment. In other

Table 7.1.9 Decline in mortality rates of infant fulminant hepatitis, chronic liver diseases, and hepatocellular carcinoma and incidence rates of hepatocellular carcinoma of birth cohorts born before and after the launch of the hepatitis B immunization program in 1984 in Taiwan

Birth years	Infant fulminant hepatitis		Chronic liver diseases		Hepatocellular carcinoma			
	Mortality rate per 100,000 person-years	Sex-adjusted rate ratio (95% CI)	Mortality rate per 100,000 person-years	Age–sex-adjusted rate ratio (95% CI)	Mortality rate per 100,000 person-years	Age–sex-adjusted rate ratio (95% CI)	Incidence rate per 100,000 person-years	Age–sex-adjusted rate ratio (95% CI)
1977–1980	5.76	1.00 (reference)	0.65	1.00 (reference)	0.81	1.00 (reference)	1.14	1.00 (reference)
1981–1984	5.09	0.88 (0.65–1.21)	0.39	0.65 (0.53–0.79)***	0.56	0.70 (0.59–0.83)***	0.77	0.73 (0.63–0.85)***
1985–1988	2.64	0.46 (0.31–0.69)***	0.13	0.40 (0.28–0.57)***	0.30	0.43 (0.33–0.55)***	0.37	0.48 (0.38–0.60)***
1989–1992	2.67	0.46 (0.31–0.69)***	0.02	0.12 (0.05–0.28)***	0.17	0.27 (0.19–0.39)***	0.23	0.37 (0.27–0.51)***
1993–1996	0.66	0.11 (0.06–0.24)***	0.07	0.39 (0.02–0.73)**	0.12	0.21 (0.13–0.34)***	0.22	0.43 (0.30–0.62)***
1997–2000	0.36	0.06 (0.02–0.17)***	0.03	0.16 (0.05–0.50)**	0.12	0.21 (0.12–0.38)***	0.17	0.37 (0.21–0.62)***
2001–2004	0.22	0.04 (0.01–0.16)***	0.02	0.11 (0.02–0.80)*	0.05	0.08 (0.02–0.34)***	0.09	0.20 (0.06–0.65)*
2005–2008	0.39	0.07 (0.02–0.21)***	–	–	–	–	–	–
2009–2011	0.19	0.03 (0.01–0.24)**	–	–	–	–	–	–

CI, confidence interval. *P < 0.5, **P < 0.01, ***P < 0.001.

Reproduced with permission from Chiang CJ et al, Effectiveness of national programs on hepatitis B immunization and viral hepatitis therapy in Taiwan, *Journal of American Medical Association*, in press, Copyright © 2014 American Heart Association, Inc.

words, there exists a host variation in the susceptibility to diseases caused by environmental factors. The individual susceptibility may come from genetic or behavioural components. For example, poor nutritional status and arsenic methylation capability may modify the risk associated with arsenic-induced health hazards including cancers and cardiovascular diseases. Multiple risk factors including cigarette smoking, aflatoxin exposure, antioxidant deficiency, and serum androgen levels are all important risk factors to hepatitis B-induced hepatocellular carcinoma. Some environmental co-factors are difficult to detect and quantify unless biomarkers are used. Many studies have been carried out in recent decades on changes in the structures and functions of macromolecules, cells, tissues, and organ systems in response to exposures to environmental risk factors, to ascertain if the preclinical lesions of environmental diseases could be detected at an early stage which would allow more timely intervention. More recently, the dramatic advances in genomic research technologies have enabled more extensive investigations into the polymorphisms and mutations of genes of host and biological agents and the effects of gene–gene and gene–environment interactions.

Various biomarkers of exposure, effect, and susceptibility of human diseases have been identified and applied in studies on environmental health hazards. The biomarkers for the exposure to environmental risk factors include molecular dosimetry of internal dose and biologically effective dose. The biomarkers for the effect include early biological changes, altered structures and functions of target organs, and preclinical lesions. The susceptibility biomarkers include both genetic and acquired susceptibility. As an illustration, since the development of chronic arsenic poisoning is a multistage pathogenesis, a series of biomarkers of arsenic-induced health hazards have been developed and applied as shown in Table 7.1.10 (Chen et al. 2005). There are several biomarkers of short-term internal dose for ingested arsenic including levels of arsenic in blood, urine, hair, and finger or toe nails. Arsenic in urine, hair, and nails are better biomarkers for short-term exposure than arsenic in blood. The cumulative arsenic exposure to arsenic from drinking water was found to be significantly associated with relative proportion of monomethylarsonic acid and dimethylarsinic acid in urine; but not with urinary levels of arsenite, arsenate, and organic arsenic. Skin hyperpigmentation and palmoplantar hyperkeratosis, characteristic dermatological lesions induced by long-term exposure to arsenic, are excellent clinical biomarkers for long-term exposure to ingested arsenic. The proportion of monomethylarsonic acid in total urinary arsenic level is an important marker for the biologically effective dose of ingested arsenic. The biomarkers of molecular changes induced by ingested arsenic include plasma levels of reactive oxidants and inflammatory molecules such as chemokine C-C motif ligand 2/monocyte chemotactic protein-1 (CCL2/MCP1). The arsenic-induced cellular changes include sister chromatid exchanges, micronuclei and chromosomal aberrations in peripheral lymphocytes and urothelial cells; as well as chromosomal loss and gain detected by comparative genomic hybridization and loss of heterozygosity in urothelial cells. Biomarkers of subclinical changes include carotid atherosclerosis, QT prolongation, and increased dispersion detected by electrocardiogram, retarded peripheral neural conduction, and retarded neurobehavioral function. The biomarkers

Table 7.1.10 Molecular and genomic biomarkers of exposure, effect, and susceptibility of arsenic-induced health hazards

Category	Group	Biomarkers
Exposure	Internal dose	
	Short term	Arsenic in urine, hair, and nail
	Long term	Relative proportion of monomethylarsonic acid and dimethylarsinic acid in urine
		Skin hyperpigmentation and hyperkeratosis
	Biologically effective dose	Monomethylarsonic acid in urine
Effect	Molecular changes	Reactive oxidants in blood
		Inflammatory molecules in blood
	Cellular changes	Sister chromatid exchanges, micronuclei,
		chromosomal aberrations in target cells
		Chromosomal loss/gain and loss of heterozygosity in target cells
	Subclinical changes	QT abnormality in electrocardiogram
		Carotid atherosclerosis
		Retarded peripheral neural conduction
		Retarded neurobehavioural function
Susceptibility	Genetic susceptibility	Xenobiotic metabolism enzymes
		Arsenic methylation enzymes
		DNA repair enzymes
		Oxidative stress-related enzymes
		Serum carotene level
	Acquired susceptibility	

of susceptibility to arsenic-induced health hazards include low serum level of carotenes and genetic polymorphisms of enzymes involved in xenobiotic metabolism, arsenic methylation, oxidative stress, and DNA repair.

In the multistage hepatocarcinogenesis of chronic hepatitis B, there are many other risk factors that modify the risk of developing hepatocellular carcinoma (Chen and Chen 2002). Biomarkers associated with hepatitis B-induced hepatocellular carcinoma are shown in Table 7.1.11. HBV infection markers include HBsAg, HBeAg, antibodies against hepatitis B core antigen (anti-HBc), antibodies against HBsAg (anti-HBs), antibodies against e antigen (anti-HBe), as well as serum levels of HBV DNA (viral load) and HBsAg. Different HBV infection markers have different associations with the development of hepatocellular carcinoma. In addition to the seropositivity of HBsAg and HBeAg, serum HBV DNA level is associated with an increasing risk of cirrhosis and hepatocellular carcinoma in a dose–response relation (Chen et al. 2006; Iloeje et al. 2006). Different genetic characteristics of HBV are also associated with different risk of liver cirrhosis and hepatocellular carcinoma. The genotype C, basal core promoter A1762T/G1764A mutant, and pre-S mutant of HBV are significantly associated with an increased risk of liver diseases; while the precore stop codon

Table 7.1.11 Molecular and genomic biomarkers associated with hepatitis B virus-caused hepatocellular carcinoma

Category	Group	Biomarkers
Exposure	Hepatitis B virus	HBsAg/HBeAg seropositivity
		Serum HBV DNA level (viral load)
		Genotype
		Mutants
		Serum HBsAg level
	Aflatoxins	Urinary levels of metabolites and guanine adducts
		Serum level of albumin adducts
	Tobacco smoke	DNA adducts of 4-aminobiphenyl and polyaromatic hydrocarbons
		HBsAg-seropositivity and normal ALT
Effect	Asymptomatic carriers	Elevated ALT, liver fibrosis
	Chronic hepatitis	Liver fibrosis, cirrhosis, failure
	Cirrhosis	Anti-HBs-seropositivity
		Serum levels of androgen and oestrogen
		HLA
Susceptibility	Immunity	Xenobiotic metabolism enzymes
	Hormonal status	DNA repair enzymes
	Genetic polymorphisms	Hormone metabolism enzymes and receptors
		Serum levels of carotenoids and selenium
	Nutritional intake	

G1896A mutant is associated with a decreased risk. Both quantitative and qualitative characteristics of HBV are important in the development of hepatocellular carcinoma.

Dietary exposure to aflatoxins and habits of cigarette smoking, alcohol drinking, and betel quid chewing have been found to increase the risk of hepatitis B-related hepatocellular carcinoma. Due to the difficulties in measuring dietary exposure to trace amount of aflatoxins and environmental exposures to tobacco smoke, several biomarkers are used for the molecular dosimetry of aflatoxin and tobacco smoke exposures. These include metabolites in urine as biomarkers for internal dose, and macromolecular adducts as biomarkers for biologically effective dose. The hepatic DNA adducts of 4-amino-biphenyls and polyaromatic hydrocarbons are used to measure the biologically effective dose of exposures to tobacco smoke, while DNA and albumin adducts of aflatoxin B_1 were used as biomarkers of biologically effective dose. There is a dose–response relation between exposure to hepatotoxins and risk of hepatocellular carcinoma. There are significant synergistic effects on hepatocellular carcinoma between chronic hepatitis B and environmental hepatotoxins. The hepatocarcinogenesis process progresses from asymptomatic carrier status, chronic hepatitis, cirrhosis, to hepatocellular carcinoma. There are several biomarkers which may be used for the detection of various precancerous lesions.

The effect of environmental hepatotoxins on the hepatitis B-induced hepatocellular carcinoma is modified by genetic polymorphisms of enzymes related to xenobiotic metabolism. Genetic polymorphisms of cytochrome P450 (CYP) enzymes 1A1 and 2E1, glutathione S-transferase (GST) M1 and T1, N-acetyltransferase 2 were found to modify the associations with hepatocellular carcinoma for chemical carcinogen exposure and low micronutrient intake among those with chronic HBV infection. As shown in Fig. 7.1.4 a significant dose–response relation between risk of hepatocellular carcinoma and serum level of aflatoxin B_1 albumin adducts is observed in chronic HBV carriers with null genotype of glutathione S-transferase (GST) M1 or T1, but no dose–response relation is observed for carriers with wild genotypes (Chen et al. 1996b). Elevated serum testosterone level is associated with an increase in the risk of HCC. This association

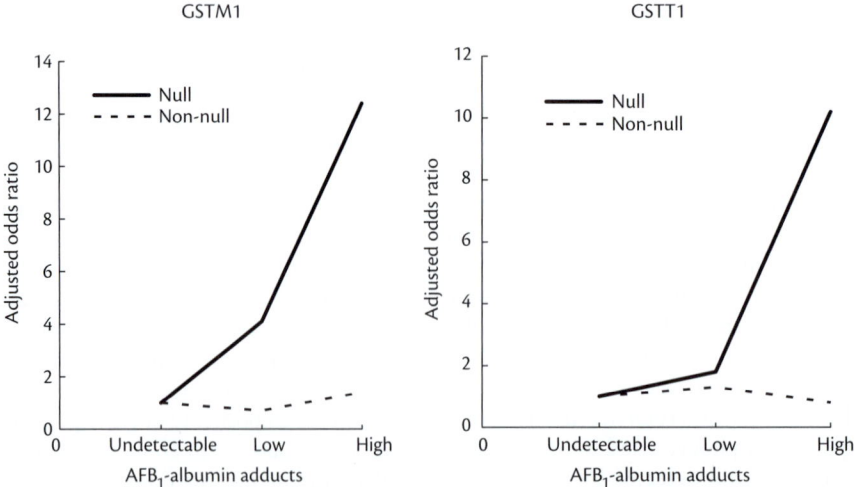

Fig. 7.1.4 Modifying effect of genotypes of glutathione S-transferase (GST) M1 and T1 on the dose–response relationship between serum level of aflatoxin B1(AFB1)-albumin adducts and risk of hepatocellular carcinoma.

Reproduced from *The American Journal of Human Genetics*, Volume 59, Issue 1, Chen CJ et al., Chronic hepatitis B carriers with null genotypes of glutathione S-transferase M1 and T1 polymorphisms who are exposed to aflatoxins are at increased risk of hepatocellular carcinoma, pp. 128–134, Copyright © 1996 by The American Society of Human Genetics, with permission from Elsevier, http://www.sciencedirect.com/science/journal/00029297.

is modified by genetic polymorphisms of androgen receptor (Yu et al. 2000). The highest risk of hepatitis B-related hepatocellular carcinoma was observed among those who have elevated serum level of testosterone and high-risk genotype of androgen receptor. Furthermore, the combination of putative high-risk genotypes of androgen receptor, CYP17, and steroid 5α-reductase is associated with highly elevated risk of hepatocellular carcinoma suggesting a significant additive effect of gene–gene interaction in the human host (Yu et al. 2001). Low serum levels of micronutrients including carotenoids and selenium are associated with an increased risk of HBV-caused hepatocellular carcinoma. The interactive effects on human health between biological and chemical agents in the environment are complicated and deserve further scrutiny.

Risk calculators of human diseases: combination of multiple biomarkers for prediction of long-term risk of disease

The prediction of disease risk is important for the planning and evaluation of public health programmes aimed at controlling the disease. Risk calculators of many diseases, especially cardiovascular diseases, have been developed and widely applied. As there are many risk predictors for most diseases, it is necessary to integrate several predictors into one measure of absolute risk using a regression model. Uncertainty about clinical interpretation of a single abnormal biomarker may be improved by the development of risk calculators based on the combination of multiple biomarkers. The risk calculator also allows for appropriate recognition of clinically important risk in persons with several but seemingly marginal risk factors that individually may otherwise not raise clinical concerns.

As described earlier, there are several risk predictors of hepatocellular carcinoma in patients affected with chronic hepatitis B. Based on the long-term follow-up findings of a community-based prospective cohort study to elucidate the natural history of chronic hepatitis B (REVEAL-HBV study), several risk calculators for predicting long-term risk of hepatocellular carcinoma have been developed and validated (Yang et al. 2010, 2011). In the most updated risk calculator derived from the REVEAL-HBV Study (Lee et al. 2013), age, sex, family history of hepatocellular carcinoma, serum alanine transaminase (ALT) level, HBeAg serostatus, serum HBV DNA, serum HBsAg level, and HBV genotype are included in the regression model. Integer risk scores are assigned to different categories of various risk predictors as shown in Table 7.1.12. The nomogram showing 5-, 10-, and 15-year cumulative risk of hepatocellular carcinoma by sum of risk score is illustrated in Fig. 7.1.5 For example, a 64-year-old man with a serum ALT level > 45 IU/L, a family history of hepatocellular carcinoma, and a HBeAg-seropositive status with genotype C infection has a sum of risk score of 6 + 2 + 2 + 2 + 7 = 19. His cumulative risk of developing hepatocellular carcinoma after 5, 10, and 15 years is estimated at around 40 per cent, 80 per cent, and 90 per cent, respectively. This risk calculator was found to have a high sensitivity, specificity, and discriminating capability. The risk calculators for many other diseases may also be developed if there were good large-scale long-term cohort studies on the diseases.

Table 7.1.12 Risk scores assigned to predictors of long-term risk of hepatocellular carcinoma caused by chronic hepatitis B

Baseline hepatocellular carcinoma predictor	Risk score
Age	
30–34	0
35–39	1
40–44	2
45–49	3
50–54	4
55–59	5
60–64	6
Sex	
Female	0
Male	2
Levels of alanine transaminase (IU/L)	
<15	0
15–44	1
45+	2
Family history of hepatocellular carcinoma	
No	0
Yes	2
HBeAg/HBV DNA/HBsAg/genotype	
Negative/<10^4/< 100/any type	0
Negative/<10^4/100–999/any type	2
Negative/<10^4/1000+/any type	2
Negative/10^4–< 10^6/<100/any type	3
Negative/10^4–< 10^6/100–999/any type	3
Negative/10^4–< 10^6/1000+/any type	4
Negative/10^6+/any level/B or B+C	5
Negative/10^6+/any level/C	7
Positive/any level/any level /B or B+C	6
Positive/any level/any level /C	7

Adapted from Lee MH et al., Models predicting long-term risk of liver cirrhosis and hepatocellular carcinoma in chronic hepatitis B patients: risk scores integrating characteristics of host and hepatitis B virus, *Hepatology*, Volume 58, Issue 2, pp. 546–554, Copyright © 2013 by the American Association for the Study of Liver Diseases. Reproduced with permission from John Wiley & Sons Ltd.

Promotion of public health through environmental health intervention

With increasing globalization, environmental pollution or infectious disease outbreaks in one country may result in environmental disasters and health hazards in both adjacent and remote countries. Public health can be promoted through environmental health interventions including the prevention of air, water, and soil pollution with chemicals or biological agents; the reduction in exposures to ultraviolet, ionizing radiation, noise,

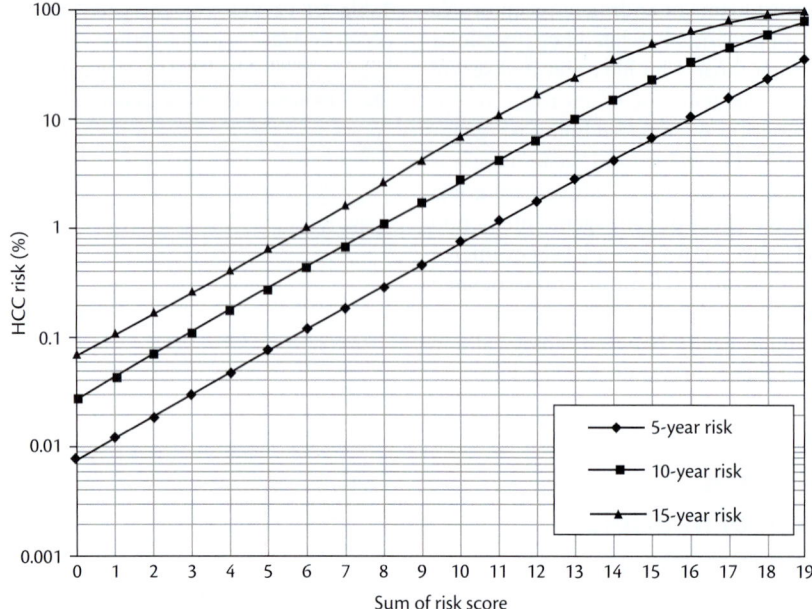

Fig. 7.1.5 Nomogram for the predicted risk of hepatocellular carcinoma caused by chronic hepatitis B.

From Lee MH et al., Models predicting long-term risk of liver cirrhosis and hepatocellular carcinoma in chronic hepatitis B patients: risk scores integrating characteristics of host and hepatitis B virus, *Hepatology*, Volume 58, Issue 2, pp. 546–554, Copyright © 2013 by the American Association for the Study of Liver Diseases. Reproduced with permission from John Wiley & Sons Ltd.

and electromagnetic fields; improvement of built environments including housing, land use patterns, and roads; minimization of carbon dioxide emission, global warming, severe climate change, and ecosystem deterioration; optimization of agricultural methods and irrigation schemes; and promotion of occupational safety and security, and so forth. Many environmental health interventions are more cost-effective compared with other kinds of health-sector efforts. These interventions often yield long-term benefits in addition to immediate health improvements. Reduction in the burden of environmental diseases may help the eradication of extreme poverty and hunger, the achievement of universal primary education, the promotion of gender equality and women's empowerment, the reduction in child mortality, the improvement in maternal health, the maintenance of environmental sustainability, and the control of epidemics including AIDS/HIV, malaria, tuberculosis, and other infectious diseases. Global partnerships need to be strengthened to achieve interrelated goals of health, environmental sustainability, and development.

References

Beasley, R.P., Hwang, L.Y., Lin, C.C., et al. (1981). Hepatocellular carcinoma and hepatitis B virus: a prospective study of 22,707 men in Taiwan. *The Lancet*, 2, 1129–33.

Chang, C.C., Ho, S.C., Tsai, S.S., and Yang, C.Y. (2004). Ischemic heart disease mortality reduction in an arseniasis-endemic area in southwestern Taiwan after a switch in the tap-water supply system. *Journal of Toxicology and Environmental Health, Part A*, 67, 1353–61.

Chang, M.H., Chen, C.J., Lai, M.S., et al. (1997). Nationwide hepatitis B vaccination and the incidence of hepatocellular carcinoma in children in Taiwan. *The New England Journal of Medicine*, 336, 1855–9.

Chen, C.J. (1999). *Epidemiology: Principles and Methods*. Taipei: Lian-Chin.

Chen, C.J. and Chen, D.S. (2002). Interaction of hepatitis B virus, chemical carcinogen and genetic susceptibility: multistage hepatocarcinogenesis with multifactorial etiology (Editorial). *Hepatology*, 36, 1046–9.

Chen, C.J., Chiou, H.Y., and Chiang, M.H. (1996a). Dose–response relationship between ischemic heart disease mortality and long-term arsenic exposure. *Arteriosclerosis, Thrombosis, and Vascular Biology*, 16, 504–10.

Chen, C.J., Chuang, Y.C., Lin, T.M., and Wu, H.Y. (1985). Malignant neoplasms among residents of a blackfoot disease-endemic area in Taiwan: high-arsenic artesian well water and cancers. *Cancer Research*, 45, 5895–9.

Chen, C.J., Chuang, Y.C., You, S.L., Lin, T.M., and Wu, H.Y. (1986). A retrospective study on malignant neoplasms of bladder, lung and liver in blackfoot disease endemic area in Taiwan. *British Journal of Cancer*, 53, 399–405.

Chen, C.J., Hsu, L.I., Shih, W.L., et al. (2005). Biomarkers of exposure, effect and susceptibility of arsenic-induced health hazards in Taiwan. *Toxicology and Applied Pharmacology*, 206, 198–206.

Chen, C.J., Hsueh, Y.M., Lai, M.S., Hsu, M.P., Wu, M.M., and Tai, T.Y. (1995). Increased prevalence of hypertension and long-term arsenic exposure. *Hypertension*, 25, 53–60.

Chen, C.J., Kuo, T.L., and Wu, M.M. (1988a). Arsenic and cancers (letter). *The Lancet*, 1, 414–15

Chen, C.J., Liang, K.Y., Chang, A.S., et al. (1991). Effects of hepatitis B virus, alcohol drinking, cigarette smoking and familial tendency on hepatocellular carcinoma. *Hepatology*, 13, 398–406.

Chen, C.J. and Wang, C.J. (1990). Ecological correlation between arsenic level in well water and age-adjusted mortality from malignant neoplasms. *Cancer Research*, 50, 5470–4.

Chen, C.J., Wu, M.M., Lee, S.S., Wang, J.D., Cheng, S.H., and Wu, H.Y. (1988b). Atherogenicity and carcinogenicity of high-arsenic artesian well water: multiple risk factors and related malignant neoplasms of blackfoot disease. *Arteriosclerosis, Thrombosis, and Vascular Biology*, 8, 452–60.

Chen, C.J., Yang, H.I., Su, J., et al. (2006). Risk of hepatocellular carcinoma across a biological gradient of serum hepatitis B virus DNA level. *Journal of the American Medical Association*, 295, 65–73.

Chen, C.J., Yu, M.W., and Liaw, Y.F. (1997). Epidemiology and multifactorial etiology of hepatocellular carcinoma. *Journal of Gastroenterology and Hepatology*, 12, S294–308.

Chen, C.J., Yu, M.W., Liaw, Y.F., et al. (1996b). Chronic hepatitis B carriers with null genotypes of glutathione S-transferase M1 and T1 polymorphisms who are exposed to aflatoxins are at increased risk of hepatocellular carcinoma. *American Journal of Human Genetics*, 59, 128–34.

Chen, C.L., Hsu, L.I., Chiou, H.Y., et al. (2004). Ingested arsenic, cigarette smoking and lung cancer risk: a follow-up study in arseniasis-endemic areas in Taiwan. *Journal of the American Medical Association*, 292, 2984–90.

Chen, K.P., Lee, T.Y., Hsu, P.Y., et al. (1976). Studies on the effect of salt iodization on endemic goiter, Taiwan. I. Mass survey on goiter of school children. *Journal of the Formosan Medical Association*, 75, 471–82.

Chi, I.C. and Blackwell, R.Q. (1968). A controlled retrospective study of blackfoot disease, an endemic peripheral gangrene disease in Taiwan. *American Journal of Epidemiology*, 88, 7–24.

Chiang, C.J., Yang, Y.W., You, S.L., et al. (2013). Thirty-year outcomes of the national hepatitis B immunization program in Taiwan. *Journal of the American Medical Association*, 310, 974–6.

Chien, Y.C., Jan, C.F., Kuo, H.S., and Chen, C.J. (2006). Nationwide hepatitis B vaccination program in Taiwan: effectiveness in 20 years after it was launched. *Epidemiologic Reviews*, 28, 126–35.

Chiou, H.Y., Chiou, S.T., Hsu, Y.H., et al. (2001). Incidence of transitional cell carcinoma and arsenic in drinking water: a follow-up study of 8,102 residents in an arseniasis-endemic area in northeastern Taiwan. *American Journal of Epidemiology*, 153, 411–18.

Chiou, H.Y., Huang, W.I., Su, C.L., Chang, S.F., Hsu, Y.H., and Chen, C.J. (1997). Dose–response relationship between prevalence of cerebrovascular disease and ingested inorganic arsenic. *Stroke*, 28, 1717–23.

Chiu, H.F., Chang, C.C., Tsai, S.S., and Yang, C.Y. (2006). Does arsenic exposure increase the risk for diabetes mellitus? *Journal of Occupational and Environmental Medicine*, 48, 63–7.

Chiu, H.F., Ho, S.C., Wang, L.Y., Wu, T.N., and Yang, C.Y. (2004a). Does arsenic exposure increase the risk for liver cancer? *Journal of Toxicology and Environmental Health, Part A*, 67, 1491–500.

Chiu, H.F., Ho, S.C., and Yang, C.Y. (2004b). Lung cancer mortality reduction after installation of tap-water supply system in an arsenic-endemic area in Southwestern Taiwan. *Lung Cancer*, 46, 265–70.

Chiu, H.F. and Yang, C.Y. (2005). Decreasing trend in renal disease mortality after cessation from arsenic exposure in a previous arseniasis-endemic area in southwestern Taiwan. *Journal of Toxicology and Environmental Health, Part A*, 68, 319–27.

Hamlin, C. (1998). *Public Health and Social Justice in the Age of Chadwick: Britain, 1800–1854*. Cambridge: Cambridge University Press.

Hill, A.B. (1953). Observation and experiment. *The New England Journal of Medicine*, 248, 995–1001.

Hippocrates (1950). *Airs, Waters, Places*. In J. Chadwick and W.N. Mann (trans.) *The Medical Works of Hippocrates*, pp. 90–111. Springfield, IL: C.C. Thomas.

Hsu, H.M., Lu, C.F., Lee, S.C., et al. (1999). Seroepidemiologic survey for hepatitis B virus infection in Taiwan: the effect of hepatitis B mass immunization. *Journal of Infectious Diseases*, 179, 367–70.

Hsueh, Y.M., Chiou, H.Y., Huang, Y.L., et al. (1997). Serum beta-carotene level, arsenic methylation capability and incidence of arsenic-induced skin cancer. *Cancer Epidemiology, Biomarkers & Prevention*, 6, 589–96.

Iloeje, U.H., Yang, H.I., Su, J., Jen, C.L., You, S.L., and Chen, C.J. (2006). Predicting cirrhosis risk based on the level of circulating hepatitis B viral load. *Gastroenterology*, 130, 678–86.

Kao, J.H., Hsu, H.M., Shau, W.Y., et al. (2001). Universal hepatitis B vaccination and the decreased mortality from fulminant hepatitis in infants in Taiwan. *Journal of Pediatrics*, 139, 349–52.

Koch R. (1891). Ueber bakteriologische Forschung. *Verhandlungen des X. Internationalen Medicinischen Congresses Berlin, 4–9 August 1890*, pp. 35–47. Berlin: Hirschwald.

Lai, M.S., Hsueh, Y.M., Chen, C.J., et al. (1994). Ingested inorganic arsenic and prevalence of diabetes mellitus. *American Journal of Epidemiology*, 139, 484–92.

Lee, M.H., Yang, H.I., Liu, J., et al. (2013). Models predicting long-term risk of liver cirrhosis and hepatocellular carcinoma in chronic hepatitis B

patients: risk scores integrating characteristics of host and hepatitis B virus. *Hepatology*, 58, 546–54.

Lin, W., Wang, S.L., Wu, H.J., et al. (2008). Associations between arsenic in drinking water and pterygium in southwestern Taiwan. *Environmental Health Perspectives*, 116, 952–5.

Pruss-Ustun, A. and Corvalan, C. (2006). *Preventing Disease through Healthy Environments: Towards an Estimate of the Environmental Burden of Disease*. Geneva: World Health Organization.

Raffle, P.A.B., Lee, W.R., McCallum, R.I., and Murray, R. (1987). *Hunter's Diseases of Occupations*. Boston, MA: Little Brown.

See, L.C., Chiou, H.Y., Lee, J.S., et al. (2007). Dose–response relationship between ingested arsenic and cataract among residents in southwestern Taiwan. *Journal of Environmental Science and Health, Part A*, 42, 1843–51.

Snow, J. (1936). *Snow on Cholera*. New York: Commonwealth Fund.

Tseng, C.H., Chong, C.K., Chen, C.J., and Tai, T.Y. (1996). Dose–response relationship between peripheral vascular disease and ingested inorganic arsenic among residents in blackfoot disease endemic villages in Taiwan. *Atherosclerosis*, 120, 125–33.

Tseng, C.H., Chong, C.K., Tseng, C.P., et al. (2003). Long-term arsenic exposure and ischemic heart disease in arseniasis-hyperendemic villages in Taiwan. *Toxicology Letters*, 137, 15–21.

Tseng, W.P. (1977). Effects and dose–response relationships of skin cancer and blackfoot disease with arsenic. *Environmental Health Perspectives*, 19, 109–19.

Wang, C.H., Jeng, J.S., Yip, P.K., et al. (2002). Biological gradient between long-term arsenic exposure and carotid atherosclerosis. *Circulation*, 105, 1804–9.

Wu, M.M., Kuo, T.L., Hwang, Y.H., and Chen, C.J. (1989). Dose–response relation between arsenic concentration in well water and mortality from cancers and vascular diseases. *American Journal of Epidemiology*, 130, 1123–32.

Yang, C.Y. (2006). Does arsenic exposure increase the risk of development of peripheral vascular diseases in humans? *Journal of Toxicology and Environmental Health, Part A*, 69, 1797–804.

Yang, C.Y., Chiu, H.F., Chang, C.C., Ho, S.C., and Wu, T.N. (2005). Bladder cancer mortality reduction after installation of a tap-water supply system in an arsenious-endemic area in southwestern Taiwan. *Environmental Research*, 98, 127–32.

Yang, C.Y., Chiu, H.F., Wu, T.N., Chuang, H.Y., and Ho, S.C. (2004). Reduction in kidney cancer mortality following installation of a tap water supply system in an arsenic-endemic area of Taiwan. *Archives of Environmental Health*, 59, 484–8.

Yang, H.I., Lu, S.N., You, S.L., et al. (2002). Hepatitis B e antigens and the risk of hepatocellular carcinoma. *The New England Journal of Medicine*, 347, 168–74.

Yang, H.I., Sherman, M., Su, J., et al. (2010). Nomograms for risk of hepatocellular carcinoma in patients with chronic hepatitis B virus infection. *Journal of Clinical Oncology*, 28, 2437–44.

Yang, H.I., Yuen, M.F., Chan, H.L., et al. (2011). Risk estimation for hepatocellular carcinoma in chronic hepatitis B (REACH-B): development and validation of a predictive score. *Lancet Oncology*, 12, 568–74.

Yang, T.Y., Hsu, L.I., Chen, H.C., et al. (2013). Lifetime risk of urothelial carcinoma and lung cancer in the arseniasis-endemic area of northeastern Taiwan. *Journal of Asian Earth Sciences*, 77, 332–7.

You, S.L., Yang, H.I., and Chen, C.J. (2004). Seropositivity of hepatitis B e antigen and hepatocellular carcinoma. *Annals of Medicine*, 36, 215–24.

Yu, M.W., Cheng, S.W., Lin, M.W., et al. (2000). Androgen-receptor CAG repeat, plasma testosterone levels, and risk of hepatitis B-related hepatocellular carcinoma. *Journal of the National Cancer Institute*, 92, 2023–8.

Yu, M.W., Yang, Y.C., Yang, S.Y., et al. (2001). Hormonal markers and hepatitis B virus-related hepatocellular carcinoma risk: a nested case-control study among men. *Journal of the National Cancer Institute*, 93, 1644–51.

Radiation and public health

Leeka Kheifets, Adele Green,
and Richard Wakeford

Introduction to radiation and public health

The electromagnetic spectrum encompasses frequencies that range from above approximately 10^{20} hertz (Hz) for ionizing radiation at the high end of the spectrum to static fields and power frequencies of 50–60 Hz at the low end. Between the two ends of the spectrum, in order of decreasing frequency, are ultraviolet radiation, visible light, infrared radiation (IR), microwaves, and radio waves (Fig. 7.2.1). This chapter reviews sources and health effects of human exposure to ionizing and non-ionizing radiation and reviews policies for limiting human exposure where appropriate.

The focus of research and our knowledge of the health effects of these forms of energy have been driven, at least partly, by the prevalence of exposure to the general public, although valuable additional information has been derived from occupational studies of high exposure. Our understanding varies: for ionizing radiation, ultraviolet radiation, and extremely low-frequency (ELF) fields numerous state-of-the art epidemiological and toxicological investigations, encompassing a variety of end points, have been undertaken; a lot of the recent research has been on radiofrequency (RF) fields, but focused on the cell phone use and tumours of the head and neck, with less attention to other sources and outcomes; although numerous studies of static fields have been completed, here too, much of the key research is yet to be done; for IR and intermediate frequencies only scant information is available.

Technological developments involving exposure to electromagnetic fields (EMFs) bring social and economic benefits to large sections of society but the health consequences of these developments can be difficult to predict and manage. As countries increase their capacity to generate and distribute electricity and take advantage of the many new technologies—such as telecommunications—to improve lifestyle and work efficiency, exposures to electric and magnetic fields from 0 to 300 GHz (non-ionizing radiation) have been increasing rapidly. In this chapter, our main emphasis is on exposures common in everyday life rather than occupational exposures. When relevant, we also consider separately exposures from medical applications, as these exposures are commonly higher, but carry a different risk/benefit ratio for the exposed individuals.

Static fields

Sources and environmental levels

For a steady current in a circuit corresponding to zero-frequency (static fields), the charge density at any point of the circuit is constant, and therefore, the electric fields are constant in time. Since magnetic fields are created by moving electric charges, magnetic fields are also constant for static fields. The unit of measurement for magnetic fields is tesla (T). Another commonly used unit in engineering sciences is gauss (G); one T is equivalent to 10,000 G. Environmental exposure levels are described in microtesla (μT), or 10^{-6} T.

There is a natural static magnetic field that originates from the electric current flowing in the upper layer of the Earth's core, as well as solar activity and atmospheric processes. There are significant local differences in the strength of this field: the vertical component of the field reaches a maximum of about 70 μT at the magnetic poles, and approaches zero at the magnetic equator; conversely the horizontal component is close to zero at the poles and is a maximum of just over 30 μT at the magnetic equator.

In addition to the earth's magnetic field are man-made magnetic fields of significantly higher strength. Major sources of exposure to the general public are transportation and magnetic resonance imaging (MRI). In general, electrified railway systems produce some of the largest static field levels encountered by the general public. Static fields up to several tens of microtesla have been reported inside trams operating on direct current (European Commission 1996). Modern magnetic levitation (maglev) systems use very high fields (around 1 T) directly on the rails; inside the trains fields vary between 50 μT and 10 mT depending on the cabin design. MRI systems have proliferated in recent years and there are currently many thousands worldwide. The static magnetic fields are in the range of 0.2–3 T for systems for routine clinical use. MRI also utilizes much smaller time-varying gradient magnetic fields and radiofrequency radiation. Medical applications with the potential of using fields up to 10 T have been developed and are beginning to be used (Gowland 2005).

Sources of exposure that are either relatively uncommon or small include steel construction materials, high-voltage direct current (DC) transmission lines, headphones and telephone speakers, and steel-belted radial tyres. Use of magnetic plasters, blankets, and mattresses for therapeutic properties have surface magnetic flux densities of about 50 mT but decay quickly within a few millimetres and are not used widely (European Commission 1996). High occupational exposures to static fields are encountered in several industrial processes including aluminium and chlorine production, gas welding, and in accelerator research.

Health effects

The three established biophysical mechanisms are magnetic induction, and magneto-mechanical and electronic interactions.

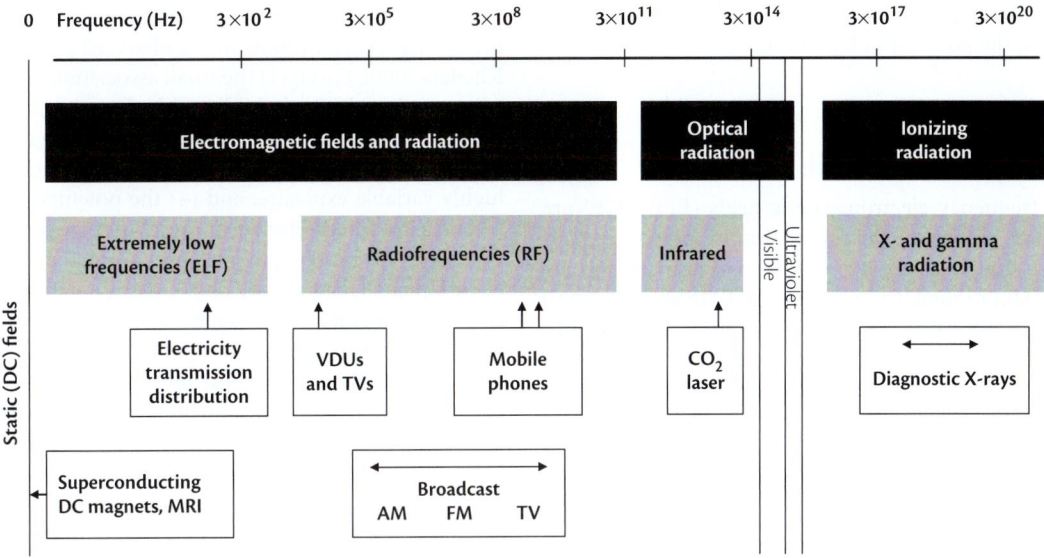

Fig. 7.2.1 Major sources of radiation and electromagnetic spectrum.

Laboratory studies of animals show aversive responses and field avoidance at 4 T or higher, probably vestibular in nature. Thresholds for motion-induced vertigo are estimated to be 1 T per second for greater than 1 second.

Cancer

The few epidemiological studies published to date leave a number of issues unresolved concerning the possibility of increased cancer risk from exposure to static magnetic fields. These studies have been carried out almost exclusively on workers exposed to static magnetic fields generated by equipment using large DC fields. Assessment of exposure has been poor, and the number of participants in the studies has been very small. Most of the studies were conducted in aluminium or other smelter plants. The limitations of these studies in providing useful information are supported by their lack of clear evidence for increased risk due to other, more established, carcinogenic factors present in some of these work environments: aluminium reduction creates coal tar, pitch volatiles, fluoride fumes, sulphur oxides, and carbon dioxide. Although some welders are exposed to relatively high static fields in some processes, they are also exposed to fumes and ELF and RF magnetic fields. Furthermore, most of the studies on welders do not provide enough information to determine the type of welding used, limiting the usefulness of these data in a review of potential health effects of static magnetic field exposure. Other work environments with a potential for high fields, for example, MRI technicians, have not been adequately evaluated, but have been identified as a high research priority by the World Health Organization (WHO 2006). In short: there is insufficient information for proper risk assessment of the impacts of static magnetic fields on cancer. Evidence from animal carcinogenesis studies is inconclusive, in the few studies that have been carried out (van Rongen et al. 2007).

Other outcomes

Even less information is available on other outcomes such as reproductive outcomes. One study examined fertility and pregnancy outcomes in female MRI operators, where the potential for exposure to relatively large static fields of up to approximately 1 T may have existed. The risk of miscarriage for pregnancies during MRI work was slightly increased compared to work in other jobs and was considerably higher than the risk of homemakers (Evans et al. 1993), but the study was methodologically weak. Several indicators of reproductive health were studied in aluminium and metal workers with inconsistent results in a study with numerous methodological limitations. No adverse effects have been demonstrated in animal studies, but there are few good studies, especially with exposures in excess of 1 T (WHO 2006).

Policy and prevention (static fields)

Exposure to equipment generating large static electric fields is uncommon. Exposures to large static magnetic fields (up to several tens of mT) occur as a result of the industrial use of DC electric currents, for example, in welding and electrolytic processes, and less commonly in high-energy physics laboratories and experimental fusion reactors. Few countries have developed exposure guidance.

However, exposure may be becoming more common. With the advent of superconductor technology in the latter part of the twentieth century, it has been possible to develop large electromagnets capable of generating fields in excess of 1 T. Patient exposure to fields of 1–3 T during clinical MRI diagnostic procedures is now routine, and will increase in the future as technology develops. Most MRI use involves relatively short scans of less than 1 hour, and there are usually clear benefits to the person being scanned, hence the approach to guidance on exposure is different from that adopted for occupational and public exposure, because of the different risk/benefit ratio to those concerned.

The International Commission on Non-Ionizing Radiation Protection (ICNIRP) recommended a spatial peak magnetic field of 2 T for head and trunk, which can be raised to 8 T for limbs or in a controlled environment (ICNIRP 2009). For the general public, a recommendation that exposure should not exceed 400 mT is given. Special consideration should be given to patients, whose whole-body exposure should be limited to 4 T in normal mode, and go up to 8 T in a controlled mode. More caution is recommended above 8 T, which is considered experimental and should be accompanied by clinical monitoring. Further, to avoid vertigo and nausea, patients should move or be moved slowly during the MRI procedures and in the presence of high fields.

Extremely low frequency

Sources and environmental levels

Extremely low-frequency electromagnetic fields (ELF EMF) are associated with all aspects of the production, transmission, and use of electricity. The fields are imperceptible to humans and are ubiquitously present in modern societies. ELF EMF are composed of two separate components, electric fields and magnetic fields. Electric fields are created by electric charges and are measured in volts/metre (V/m). Typical residential exposure levels are under 10 V/m. In the immediate vicinity of electric appliances, exposure levels can reach as high as several hundred V/m, whereas exposure levels immediately under high-tension power lines can reach several thousand V/m.

Average magnetic field exposures in the workplace have been found to be higher in electrical occupations which include power and telephone line workers, electricians, and electrical engineers, among others, than in other occupations such as office workers. Exposures range from 0.4 to 0.6 μT for electricians and electrical engineers to approximately 1 μT for power line workers and above 3 μT for welders, railway engine drivers, and textile workers. By contrast, typical residential exposure levels are around 0.1 μT. In the immediate vicinity of electric appliances that are in use, magnetic fields could be as high as several hundred μT but are usually only of short duration.

Health effects

Since the late 1970s, numerous epidemiological studies of varying quality have investigated possible health risks from residential and occupational exposure to both electric and magnetic fields.

Cancer

An association between higher-than-average magnetic field exposure levels and leukaemia risk is reported in most of the approximately 30 epidemiological studies investigating childhood leukaemia and ELF EMF. However, most of them are based on a small number of highly exposed cases and, thus, lack precision. A robust biological hypothesis to explain this association is lacking. In 2000, two independently conducted pooled analyses of previously published studies showed a statistically significant, approximately twofold increase in childhood leukaemia risk for average residential exposure levels above 0.3 or 0.4 μT, compared to the lowest exposure category of 0.1 μT or lower (Ahlbom et al. 2000; Greenland et al. 2000). More recently, Kheifets et al. (2010a) identified 14 studies published since the two previous 2000 pooled analyses, of which seven met their inclusion criteria. The odds ratios for exposure above 0.3 μT compared to lower than 0.1 μT was 1.44 (95 per cent confidence interval (CI): 0.88–2.36). Without the most influential study, from Brazil, which is suspected to be particularly prone to bias, the odds ratios increased and became similar to previous pooled analyses. Risk increases this small are notoriously hard to evaluate in epidemiology because it is usually difficult to achieve enough precision to distinguish a small risk from no risk. Such small effect estimates, compared to larger ones, are also more likely to result from inadvertent error, or bias, that can occur in epidemiological studies (Greenland and Kheifets 2006). Selection bias,

which can arise in the process used to select or enrol study participants, might explain some of the observed association (Mezei and Kheifets 2006). Given (1) the small associations observed in studies of magnetic fields and childhood leukaemia, (2) a limited understanding of causal risk factors for childhood leukaemia, (3) methodological difficulties in an assessment of a non-memorable and highly variable exposure, and (4) the potential for selection bias, a conclusive interpretation of these findings remains a challenge. The lack of a robust biophysical mechanism that would explain how environmental magnetic fields could cause cancer and a lack of support from laboratory investigations also indicates that the findings might be a result of study design and measurement issues rather than being truly causal. However, the remarkable consistency of epidemiological studies is difficult to dismiss, or explain away.

Kheifets et al. performed a similar pooled analysis for childhood brain tumours (2010b). In contrast to childhood leukaemia, there was little indication of an elevation in risk in the highest exposure category, and much less of a monotonic exposure–response relationship (with risk ratios below one in intermediate exposure categories). Results for other cancers, such as adult leukaemia and brain cancer (occupational exposures mostly) are less consistent than those for childhood leukaemia (Kheifets et al. 2008). For breast cancer a biological mechanism has been proposed but has not been confirmed in recent epidemiologic studies which strongly argue against an association (WHO 2007).

Other health outcomes

A number of additional health outcomes, particularly neurodegenerative disease, reproductive outcomes, and cardiovascular disease, have also been investigated in epidemiological studies. Motor neuron diseases and reproductive outcomes have not been sufficiently investigated, and studies that have been conducted are characterized by methodological difficulties. In a recent meta-analysis of occupational studies of exposure to ELF EMF and neurodegenerative disease, investigators found weak associations for proxies of occupational magnetic field exposures with Alzheimer's disease (AD) and motor neuron diseases (MND) (Vergara et al. 2013). MND risk was associated with electric occupations but not with magnetic fields, while AD risk was associated with estimated magnetic field levels. Disease misclassification, particularly for AD, and imprecise exposure assessment affected most studies. The epidemiological results are thus inconsistent and lack supportive laboratory evidence.

Epidemiological investigation of cardiovascular diseases has been motivated by biologically based hypotheses which stemmed from two independent lines of evidence: (1) magnetic fields were reported to reduce the normal heart rate variability in human experiments, and (2) several prospective cohort studies have suggested that reductions in some components of heart rate variability are associated with increased risk for heart disease, overall mortality rate in survivors of myocardial infarction, and sudden cardiovascular death. Thus, it was hypothesized that occupational exposure to magnetic fields increases the risk for cardiac arrhythmia-related conditions and acute myocardial infarction, but not chronic cardiovascular disease. Although an initial study appeared to support this hypothesis, recent larger and more rigorous studies have found no effects and have failed to confirm earlier findings, which suggest that ELF magnetic fields do not play a role in the development of cardiovascular diseases (Kheifets et al. 2007).

Policy and prevention

During the past decade, a number of national and international expert panels, including ones assembled by the United States National Institute of Environmental Health Sciences, the International Agency for Research on Cancer (IARC) and the WHO have reviewed the evidence on the potential relationship between exposure to ELF EMF and various adverse health outcomes (National Institute of Environmental Health Sciences 1999; IARC 2002; WHO 2007). Evaluations by these expert panels generally agree that short-term, adverse effects do not occur at exposures to magnetic fields below 100 µT. Current guidelines (recently revised) are based on induced internal electric fields and use a threshold for an induction of magnetic phosphines. For general public exposure, the reference levels for power frequency (50 Hz) electric and magnetic fields are of the order of 5 kV/m and 200 µT, respectively. These values are well above levels encountered in most environments.

Based on these intensive reviews IARC and WHO classified ELF magnetic (but not electric) fields as a 'possible human carcinogen', or a Group 2B carcinogen. This classification was based both on epidemiological evidence showing a consistent association between exposure to ELF magnetic fields and childhood leukaemia even though laboratory studies in animals and cells do not support an association between exposure to ELF magnetic fields and cancer.

Several risk characterization attempts have indicated that the public health impact of residential magnetic fields on childhood leukaemia is likely to be limited (Kheifets et al. 2006). Positing sensitivity and bias models for methodological problems in the epidemiologic studies and accounting for uncertainties regarding field levels that may have effects, suggest that, in light of the available data, both no public health impact and a large impact remain possibilities (Greenland and Kheifets 2006).

The combination of widespread exposures, established biological effects from acute, high-level exposures, and the possibility of leukaemia in children from low-level, chronic exposures have made it necessary but difficult to develop consistent public health policies. In view of these uncertainties, it might be advisable to adopt general no- and low-cost measures to reduce exposure (WHO 2007).

Intermediate frequency

Intermediate frequency (IF) exposures occur in the range 300 Hz to 10 MHz, partially encompassing frequencies also assigned to very low-frequency (VLF; 0.3–30 kHz) and high (3–30 MHz) ranges.

Because few biological studies of exposures to intermediate frequencies have been conducted, exposure guidelines have largely been extrapolated from the encompassing ELF (at the low end) and RF (at the high end) limits.

Sources and environmental levels

Intermediate frequency exposures are common from occupational appliances such as induction heaters (used in the heating of metals prior to manipulation) and plasma heaters. Smaller exposures occur from induction heating elements in residential cooking appliances. Television, radio, and other communications transmitters can emit IF, but they are discussed in the section on RF, which constitutes the much more common wavelengths of exposure from such sources. Indirect exposures from medical equipment (e.g. MRI machines and magnetic bone stimulators where pulses may drop to IF levels) may occur rarely. Direct exposures to IF may also occur from surgical equipment used for tissue cutting and cauterizing. Common exposures to IF occur in proximity to devices that read magnetic cards or buttons for identification purposes (Polichetti and Vacchia 1996), and similarly, from antitheft devices that read magnetic identification tags. Very small exposures are obtained from television screens (and CRT computer monitors). Use of antitheft technologies, device tagging and identification is increasing rapidly, exposures immediately beside RFID reader antennas can be locally higher, and simultaneous exposures can come from a variety of IF sources, locations of which may be unknown (ICNIRP 2008).

Health effects

Since exposure level and proximity to the source together determine the IF levels in tissue, knowledge of both is important in determining the biological effects of IF exposure levels in humans.

Biological effects in humans can be either thermal, when frequency is sufficient to induce a heating response, or non-thermal (i.e. cell membrane excitation or electroporation), when frequency does not induce a heating response.

Studies of the impact of IF on human health, particularly with exposure from new technologies, are currently lacking.

Policy and prevention

Because of the lack of data, currently there are no specific recommendations for limiting exposure to IF, other than those extrapolated from EMF at extremes of the IF range (ELF and RF). As use of IF fields and subsequent exposure to the population is increasing, there is an increased interest in characterizing exposure and health effects in the IF range. GERoNiMO is: http://www.crealradiation.com/index.php/en/geronimo-home.

Radiofrequency radiation

Sources and environmental levels

With rapid advances in EMF technologies and communications, people are increasingly exposed to frequencies in the RF range. RF fields are produced by radio and TV broadcasts, mobile phone base stations, and other communication infrastructure. The most prevalent exposure is to handheld mobile telephones. This technology typically uses frequencies from 450 to 2500 MHz, although new technology has broadened this band. Other sources of exposure to the general population are radio and television transmitters which operate at between 200 kHz and 900 MHz. Radio and TV signals are broadcast to a large area from comparatively few sites (Neubauer et al. 2007). Compared to radio and TV transmitters, mobile phone base stations cover a smaller area, and produce much lower emissions, but are vastly more common in many countries. Residential exposures also come from wireless monitors used in children's cribs, cordless phones, and wi-fi (wireless Internet connections) commonly used at home and in schools. Occupational exposures include RF PVC welding machines, plasma etchers, and military and civil radar systems. All operate at different frequencies.

Handheld mobile phones available since the late 1980s became widely used by the general population only in the late 1990s. Currently there are more than 5 billion mobile phone users worldwide, with a penetration in some countries reaching 120 per cent (i.e. many people have more than one phone). Use of mobile phones has changed markedly over recent years, concomitant with the development of new technologies (e.g. 2G to 3G, power control, handover management, and novel uses of smartphones). Phones operating under 2G and 3G can have significantly different output power; 3G is thought to be around 1 per cent of the power emitted by a phone operating under 2G. In addition, modes of mobile phone use are constantly changing as texting, web-surfing, playing games, and listening to music on mobile phones are becoming more and more common. Exposure from mobile phones is concentrated closest to the handset and the antenna. Absorption of RF from mobiles is localized and depends on the position of the phone during use. This represents a very important determinant of exposure: only calls made with the mobile phone close to the head result in absorption of RF energy inside the head.

Exposures from mobile phone base stations are several orders of magnitude lower than from the phones. For whole-body exposure, mobile phone base stations can be the largest individual source of RF, but other sources such as radio or TV transmitters can result in comparable exposures depending on where the measurements are taken. For RF sources other than mobile phones, typical power densities outdoors would be 0.01–1 mW/m^2, but could be orders of magnitude higher (i.e. 100 mW/m^2 and above). Indoor levels are often lower than outdoor exposures by orders of magnitude; for example, in Europe, a median indoor power density of 0.005 mW m^{-2} has been reported. Note that the exposure from base stations differs from that of mobile phones; base stations expose the whole body, but the exposure duration is considerably longer. Perhaps more importantly, base station exposure has been a subject of much concern to the public because it is not under the control of the public and its presence is not perceived to be of direct individual benefit.

Population exposure to RF fields has been less completely characterized than exposures to ELF fields. This is due to: (1) technical challenges, (2) the rapid evolution of RF-related technology (frequency, coding schemes), and (3) changing patterns of use (duration of calls, text messaging, web surfing, etc.).

Health effects

Since RF radiation induces heating in body tissues and imposes a heat load on the whole body, prevention of excessive heating serves as a basis for most international guidelines for human exposure. Studies of the interaction of RF with tissue in the range used for mobile phones have led to the proposal of many different non-thermal mechanisms for RF interaction. Generally, it is thought that non-thermal interactions are unlikely to be biologically significant at the RF levels below guidance values, but much of the ongoing research is directed towards non-thermal mechanisms.

Cancer

Epidemiological studies of health effects related to RF exposure from mobile phones have primarily focused on cancer, especially brain tumours. While over the past 10 years there have been a large number of studies focusing on mobile phones, studies with long-term exposure with sufficient latency are still limited. Currently it is only possible to evaluate short- to medium-term effects of mobile phone exposure; the majority of studies have found no effects on either brain or parotid gland tumour risk (Swerdlow et al. 2011). Exposure assessment remains problematic: substantial random error has been shown for even short-term recall of mobile phone use; and information bias appears to affect at least the reporting of the side of the head where the phone is commonly used. Also,

some studies may be compromised by a non-representative control group, caused by an increased participation of mobile phone users. Results for acoustic neuroma are more suggestive albeit inconsistent (Swerdlow et al. 2011). Recently, a few studies have examined other cancers, such as leukaemia, non-Hodgkin's lymphoma, and uveal and testicular cancers. Results are unremarkable, but subject to the same limitations as brain tumour studies. So far only one study has examined the possible association between brain tumours and use of mobile phones in children (Aydin et al. 2012). Small and imprecise risks were reported in the high exposure categories, which became more pronounced in a subgroup of about one-third of the subjects for whom objective operator data was available. However, due to methodological limitations, some internal inconsistencies, and most importantly, lack of increases in the brain tumour rates for children in the registry, the authors consider their data to argue against causality. Clearly, more studies of children are needed.

A few studies have assessed cancer risk in relation to radio and TV transmitters (Ahlbom et al. 2004). Often driven by a previously identified cancer cluster, these analyses are based simply on distance from the source and often include an extremely small number of cases. It is therefore not surprising that such studies have been uninformative. Four recent case–control studies of cancer risk related to mobile phone base stations (Ha et al. 2007; Merzenich et al. 2008; Elliott et al. 2010; Li et al. 2012) have employed improved methods both in terms of design and exposure assessment. While reporting some positive associations for disease and exposure subgroups, overall these studies provide no consistent evidence of association between exposure from base stations and other transmitters and risk of childhood cancer. However, numerous methodological limitations remain, including the inability to detect small increases in risk.

Although occupational studies have been performed over a longer time period, we are only beginning to measure and learn about RF exposures in various occupations, and the exposure may not always be relevant for an assessment of effects of mobile phone frequencies. Although some increased risks have been found in certain studies, there is no consistent evidence of risk increases for any cancer sites. The studies have several methodological weaknesses: (1) none of the studies have made measurements of the actual RF exposure for the subjects included, (2) exposure classification has often been based on the job title alone, and (3) no or only limited control of confounding has been made (Ahlbom et al. 2004).

All of the studies have reported null results for carcinogenicity in normal animals at exposure levels compatible with mobile phones; however, co-carcinogenicity studies have been suggestive (IARC 2012). As a result, the IARC classified RF as possibly carcinogenic to humans based on limited evidence in humans (from studies of glioma and acoustic neuroma in relation to mobile phones) and limited evidence in animals (based on co-carcinogenicity studies).

Other outcomes

It is well established in animal studies that hyperthermia during pregnancy can cause embryonic death, abortion, growth retardation, and developmental defects; development of the central nervous system is especially susceptible. Serious health effects of hyperthermia in humans are associated only with greatly elevated body temperatures (> 40°C), and such temperature rises are well above those generated by the maximum allowable level for public RF exposure.

Numerous studies have evaluated developmental effects of RF fields on mammals, birds, and other non-mammalian species (Heynick and Merritt 2003; Independent Advisory Group on Non-Ionizing Radiation 2003). These studies have shown that RF fields are teratogenic at exposure levels that are high enough to cause significant increases in temperature. There is no consistent evidence of effects at non-thermal exposure levels, although a few studies have evaluated possible effects on postnatal development using sensitive end points, such as behavioural effects.

Several studies of occupational RF exposure, primarily to physiotherapists, have reported an increased risk of congenital malformations, but no specific type of malformation has been consistently reported, and there is a potential for recall bias in these studies (Larsen 1991). Exposure to RF during sensitive periods of development in early life may lead to lasting effects on health (Kheifets et al. 2005). No association was found between mobile phone use during pregnancy and early neurodevelopment in very young children in two studies (Vrijheid et al. 2010; Divan et al. 2011). A Danish study has raised the hypothesis that pregnancy and childhood exposure to mobile phones may result in common childhood behavioural problems (Divan et al. 2008). Behavioural problems related to cell phone use in children stand out as the only association independently confirmed in several studies (Abramson et al. 2009; Thomas et al. 2010; Divan et al. 2012). Prospective evaluations of this association in large cohorts are needed.

Possible health effects based in part on anecdotal reports of numerous symptoms such as headaches and sleep disturbance from continuous whole-body RF exposure from base stations is an area of major public concern. Because of numerous methodological shortcomings, data regarding effects of such RF exposure on symptoms are inadequate for assessment at present.

Policy and prevention

Guidance on exposure for the general public is intended to restrict local tissue temperature rises to acceptable levels and currently is set to 0.08 Wkg^{-1}, for the whole body, and 2 Wkg^{-1}, for the head. Mobile telephones have only been in widespread use for a relatively short time and therefore, the possibility remains that long-term RF exposures from mobile telephony can have adverse health effects. More importantly, many of the health outcomes are yet to be studied and research on potential detrimental effects on children is particularly sparse.

The need for public health policy coupled with the paucity of data, particularly for children regarding the long-term health effects of mobile phone use, suggests that low-cost precautionary measures are appropriate. Mobile phone use is increasingly common among school children, and teenagers may be among the heaviest mobile phone users today with some exposures close to guideline limits (Kheifets et al. 2010c). Exposure can be reduced by users restricting the length of their calls, or by using 'hands-free' devices to keep mobile phones away from the head and body.

Infrared radiation

Sources and environmental levels

Wavelengths between 780 nm and 1 mm are classified as IR. The IR spectrum is conventionally broken down into three separate categories: IR 'A' (780nm –1.4 μm); IR 'B' (1.4–3 μm); and far-IR 'C' (3 μm–1mm). Besides solar radiation and fire as common natural sources, artificial sources of IR include a variety of therapeutic and domestic applications such as heating devices, lights, 'infrared saunas', and industrial sources related to heat production such as in steel/iron industries. Lasers comprise a special group that emit IR radiation over one or more extremely narrow wavelength bands, not covered in detail here.

Health effects

IR penetrates human skin and ocular tissues, namely the cornea, lens, and retina, to varying depths depending on wavelength, ranging from several millimetres (IR-A) to only superficial absorption (IR-C). Humans have protective aversion responses to thermal pain and to the bright light/visible radiation that is often also present, so that potentially hazardous exposure can be avoided. When harmful effects of IR in humans do occur, most studies suggest that the main mechanism of action is thermal injury, with little evidence of photochemical or other biological interactions.

Harmful effects

Harmful effects of any episode of hyperthermia of the skin depend on the intensity and the duration of the IR exposure (Moritz et al. 1947). When the temperature of the skin is held at 44°C, around 6 hours is required before irreversible skin damage is sustained, while at surface temperatures of 70°C or higher, less than 1 second is required to cause epidermal necrosis (Moritz et al. 1947). In industrial settings, whole-body heat stress tends to limit the duration of exposure to IR radiation, keeping it under the threshold for thermal damage to the skin, and so only very brief exposures to very high irradiances pose a thermal hazard. Chronic IR exposure of the skin without burning (such as repeatedly sitting with exposed skin close to open fires—common in the past) can cause a distinctive red-brown mottling of the skin known as erythema ab igne. IR is not considered relevant in the initiation of skin cancer although it has been hypothesized that IR might accelerate UV-induced skin carcinogenesis (Edwards et al. 1999), possibly by reducing DNA repair ability (Dewhirst et al. 2003), or by triggering damage by reactive oxygen species, but supportive evidence is scant.

The main detrimental effect of high IR exposure is to the eye due to the sensitivity of the cornea, iris, lens, and retina to thermal damage, though damage thresholds for these tissues vary greatly depending on the precise wavelength and exposure duration. For example, with laser irradiation at 1.315 μm, the cornea is the most sensitive of the tissues to continuous wave exposure. The retina, lens, and iris are sensitive to short exposure durations of approximately 0.1–1.0 seconds, and the retina is the eye tissue most sensitive to damage by sub-millisecond laser pulses (Zuclich et al. 2007). When incident IR radiation is absorbed by the cornea it is converted into heat which is conducted to the lens with marked decreases in lens proteins whose aggregation is thought to lead to the lens opacity of cataract (Aly and Mohamed 2011). There is considerable evidence of IR-induced cataract in industries with extremely high exposures (e.g. glass workers (Lydahl and Philipson 1984) and iron and steel workers (Wallace et al. 1971)). Most non-industrial exposures to IR appear insufficient to cause cataract or other eye damage however.

Workers exposed to high levels of IR contend with whole-body hyperthermic effects (rise in body temperature causing heat-stress) which are similar to those in any industry involving physical activity in warm environments. The same is likely true of risks of excessive exposure to far-IR saunas or warming cabins. Thus, the exposure limits in these situations will rely mainly on ensuring that safe body temperatures are maintained.

In summary, there have been relatively few studies of the health effects of IR, but current evidence suggests that harmful effects are few and due to acute high-intensity exposure or to chronic exposure, causing ocular damage and heat-related illness in certain situations.

Beneficial effects

A single review of the health benefits of far-IR saunas has been carried out, restricted to evidence from randomized controlled trials, non-randomized trials, and cohort studies (Beever 2009). Far-IR (around 10 μm wavelength) saunas are popular because they operate at lower temperatures than traditional saunas and promote greater sweating since skin penetration by IR is greater than by hot air. The review found moderate, limited evidence to support far-IR saunas in normalizing blood pressure and treating congestive heart failure, very limited evidence supporting decrease in chronic pain, and only weak evidence for benefit in chronic fatigue syndrome and obesity (Beever 2009).

Policy and prevention

There are various international standards for limiting exposure to IR that are provided separately for IR-A, B, and sometimes C (ICNIRP 2006). These limits, based on combinations of wavelength and time of exposure, are most appropriate for industrial applications where exposures are extreme and measurable. The heat-generating effects of IR tend to be avoided when humans react to minimise exposure before thermal injury to the skin occurs. This is not true for exposures causing cataract, so specific recommendations exist for wearing protective eye coverings and limiting exposure to IR. Again this applies largely to occupational settings with extreme exposures and assumes that any exposure of the eye to IR is potentially harmful.

There are currently no recommendations for limiting or avoiding exposures to IR in saunas and other recreational settings other than to limit exposure to avoid heat-related illness.

Ultraviolet radiation

Sources and environmental levels

Ultraviolet (UV) radiation is categorized as UVA (400–320 nm), UVB (320–280 nm), and UVC (280–250 nm), and the sun is the natural source. All UVC and much of the UVB emitted by the sun are absorbed by the earth's atmosphere such that the midday sun comprises about 95 per cent UVA and 5 per cent UVB, although in recent decades depletion of ozone in the stratosphere by man-made chlorofluorocarbons has resulted in greater levels of UVB on the earth's surface in some temperate and arctic regions. Solar UVB levels increase with decreasing latitude and increasing altitude and are highest in the summer and in the middle hours of the day; levels of ambient UVA mostly parallel UVB levels. Light cloud cover prevents about 50 per cent of solar UV energy from reaching the earth's surface (Diffey 1991), while very heavy cloud cover can virtually eliminate UV radiation. Reflectance from light-coloured surfaces such as concrete, snow, and to a lesser degree, water, increases terrestrial UVB.

There are a variety of sources of artificial UV found in occupational and medical settings and these include mercury vapour lamps, arc-welding, commercial germicidal UV lamps, and dental

polymerizing equipment. In addition, over the last two decades the sunbed industry has emerged as a prevalent source of community UV exposure, sought after by fair-skinned people, particularly adolescents and young adults, seeking to acquire a tan by artificial means (Olsen and Green 2012).

Health effects

The penetration of human tissues by UV radiation and the ensuing health effects are not only wavelength-dependent with longer UVA wavelengths penetrating human tissues more deeply than UVB, but also age dependent. The structure of juvenile skin may result in increased UV dosage and more damage to target cells than in adult skin, with increased childhood susceptibility to long-term carcinogenic effects (Green et al. 2011); for example, in the juvenile eye, the crystalline lens allows UV transmission to the retina and choroid, whereas after around 25 years of age the adult lens and cornea filter almost all UV (Lerman 1984).

Harmful effects

Acute exposure to UVB causes inflammation of the skin (sunburn) and eye (photokeratitis of the cornea) and immunosuppression (Young 2006). Chronic UV exposure of the skin causes photoaging, benign keratinocytic skin tumours (actinic keratoses), and skin cancer (basal cell and squamous cell carcinomas (BCC and SCC) and melanoma) (IARC 2012). Skin colour determines sensitivity to the acute and chronic effects of UV radiation on the skin, with white Caucasians bearing most of the burden of harmful effects compared with those with black or olive skin. Chronic UV exposure of the eye causes a range of degenerative effects, for example, pterygium, cataract, macular degeneration, as well as cancer (SCC and ocular melanoma) regardless of skin and eye colour.

The carcinogenic effects of solar UV radiation derive from the combined action of UVB and UVA: direct damage by UVB and to a less extent by UVA to DNA through cyclobutane pyrimidine dimer formation as well as the indirect oxidative damage induced by UVA, modulated by the efficiency of DNA repair pathways such as nucleotide excision repair (Ikehata and Ono 2007). UV radiation also suppresses the immune system by inducing immunosuppressive mediators and by interfering with immune responses of antigen-presenting cells (Halliday and Rana 2008).

A multitude of epidemiological studies support the causation of cancers of the skin by solar UV radiation in white populations (IARC 2012), ranging from descriptive studies showing positive associations with birth and/or residence at low latitudes and rare occurrence at non-sun exposed body sites, to analytic studies indicating that biological indicators of excessive sun exposure, namely multiple sunburns (throughout life, but especially in childhood) and actinic keratoses, are significant risk factors (Whiteman et al. 2001; Fears et al. 2002; Chang et al. 2009). Further, there is now evidence from randomized controlled trials that regular application of a broad-spectrum sunscreen to the skin to filter at least 95 per cent of UVB and a proportion of UVA, protects against actinic keratoses, SCC, and melanoma (Thompson et al. 1993; Green et al. 1999, 2011). Convincing evidence is now also available from cohort studies and meta-analyses that the use of tanning beds increases the risks of all three major skin cancers—BCC, SCC, and melanoma—particularly if exposure occurs during the first three decades of life (IARC 2007; Boniol et al. 2012; Olsen and Green 2012; Wehner et al. 2012; Zhang et al. 2012).

Beneficial effects

Besides the modest photoprotection of pale skin against further UV-induced skin damage that is provided by a suntan, UV exposure enhances vitamin D synthesis which is essential to bone health. Conclusive evidence of benefit of UV radiation beyond bone health, mediated through vitamin D or otherwise, is not presently available, however (National Research Council of the National Academies 2011; Thacher et al. 2011; Allinson et al. 2012). When a systematic review of vitamin D and cancer was performed by the IARC in 2008, benefits were inconclusive and did not outweigh the harms (IARC 2008), and later systematic reviews have been consistent with this (Gandini et al. 2011).

Policy and prevention

Limiting exposure to solar UV

The Global Solar UV Index (UVI) is a unitless quantity estimated on a daily basis that describes the maximum intensity of solar UV radiation received on the earth's surface (Allinson et al. 2012). Originally introduced by the WHO, the United Nations Environment Programme, the World Meteorological Organization, and the International Commission for Non-Ionizing Radiation Protection (ICNIRP) as a measure to monitor changes in terrestrial UV irradiation (caused, for example, by ozone depletion), the UVI has had its utility since expanded to serve as a public awareness tool about the amount of harmful UV radiation present at a specified location (WHO 2002). Guidance about appropriate sun protection measures is also provided in line with standard recommendations of cancer control agencies worldwide on how best to avoid solar UV exposure in order to facilitate the primary prevention of skin cancer. These are: limit exposure during midday hours; seek shade; wear protective clothing including a broad-brimmed hat to protect the eyes, face, and neck; protect the eyes further with wrap-around sunglasses with side panels; use and reapply broad-spectrum sunscreen of sun protection factor (SPF) 15+ liberally; and protect babies and young children (WHO 2002). The specific use of at least sunscreen is advocated as an adjunct to physical protection measures (shade, clothing cover) and sunscreen should be reapplied after sweating, swimming, and long periods in the sun. Despite much evidence from ecological and observational studies about sun exposure, vitamin D, and human health outcomes, currently there is an absence of evidence from randomized controlled trials about their quantitative relationships, and thus, there is as yet no established basis on which to include vitamin D considerations in sun protection recommendations (Allinson et al. 2012).

Limiting exposure to sunbeds

Many countries have enacted legislation to more tightly regulate the sunbed industry and limit people's exposure to this source of UV radiation. Sunbeds are banned in Brazil, and legislation prohibiting use by those under 18 is in place in France, Spain, Portugal, Germany, Austria, Belgium, England, Wales, Northern Ireland, and Scotland, and parts of Australia, Canada, and the United States (Pawlak et al. 2012). These regulations need to be reinforced by warnings from health professionals and educators about the risks of indoor tanning, so that young people in particular are aware that their use of sunbeds for short-term cosmetic tanning materially raises their skin cancer risk (Olsen and Green 2012).

Limiting occupational exposures

The ICNIRP recommends upper limits of exposure to UV in occupational settings, outdoor and indoor, to protect both the skin and the eyes of workers (ICNIRP 2004). It is recognized that the risks of UV exposure of the skin differ greatly depending on skin colour: skin protection must be emphasized for white-skinned people, while higher average threshold exposure is allowed for Asian and black skin types. Eye protection against UV is emphasized for all skin types.

For the outdoor worker, exposure of the skin depends upon the work tasks and posture, exposure duration, the particular environment, time of day, and season, and all of these factors need to be taken into account in establishing appropriate control measures. Under most situations, ocular UV exposure does not exceed the limits for even long exposure duration unless in environmental conditions where ground reflectance is unusually high (ICNIRP 2010). Standard protective clothing and headwear can be complemented by application of broad-spectrum sunscreen, while UV protective goggles can effectively reduce ocular UV exposure from high-reflectance surfaces like snow. For indoor workers' exposure to artificial sources such as UVC-emitting lamps for sterilizing work areas in hospitals, the food industry, and laboratories, or UV lasers, safety precautions include engineering (structural) and administrative controls and personal protective equipment and training. Educating individual workers about the risks of excessive UV exposure is also of paramount importance (ICNIRP 2010).

Ionizing radiation

Ionizing radiation consists of high-frequency electromagnetic radiation—X-rays and gamma-rays—or of subatomic particles such as alpha-particles (^{4}He nuclei), beta-particles (electrons), neutrons, protons, pions, and muons. For radiation to be ionizing it must have high enough energy to eject electrons from atoms or molecules, thus creating electrically charged ions. Electrically charged particles (e.g. alpha- and beta-particles) are directly ionizing, whereas electrically neutral particles (e.g. gamma-rays and neutrons) are ionizing because they produce charged particles on interacting with matter. The energy deposited in matter by ionizing radiation is measured in gray (Gy), 1 Gy being 1 J/kg, which is the absorbed dose of radiation (National Research Council of the National Academies 2006; International Commission on Radiological Protection (ICRP) 2007; United Nations Scientific Committee on the Effects of Atomic Radiation 2008, 2010).

The amount of energy transferred by particles per unit track length when passing through matter is called the linear energy transfer (LET) of the radiation. For example gamma- and X-rays, electrons and muons are sparsely ionizing—low-LET—radiations because relatively few ionization events occur along their paths. On the other hand, alpha-particles, neutrons, and accelerated heavy charged nuclei (e.g. ^{12}C) generated by synchrotrons are termed high-LET radiations because they transfer a relatively large amount of energy per unit track length, producing a high density of ionizations. Measurement units commonly used are defined and listed in Table 7.2.1 (ICRP 2007).

For the purposes of radiological protection, in the context of low doses (< 100 mGy of low-LET radiation) or low dose-rates (< 0.1 mGy/min, as an hourly average, of low-LET radiation), the absorbed dose is weighted by the different ionization capabilities of

Table 7.2.1 Quantities and dose units of ionizing radiation

Quantity dose	Unit	Definition
Absorbed dose	gray (Gy)	Energy deposited in matter (= 1 J/kg)
	Rad (obsolete unit)	1 rad = 100 erg/g = 0.01 Gy = 1 cGy
Equivalent dose	sievert (Sv)	Absorbed dose multiplied by the radiation weighting factor, w_R, for the particular type of radiation
	Rem (obsolete unit)	1 rem = 0.01 Sv = 1 cSv
Effective dose	sievert (Sv)	Sum of equivalent doses, each multiplied by the tissue weighting factor, w_T, for the particular tissue irradiated
Collective effective dose	Person-Sv	Sum of the individual effective doses for a population
Committed effective dose	sievert (Sv)	Cumulative effective dose to be received over a given period from a given intake of radioactive material
Radioactivity	becquerel (Bq)	One radioactive disintegration per second
	Curie (Ci) (obsolete unit)	37 billion disintegrations per second (= 37 GBq)

Source: data from International Commission on Radiological Protection (ICRP), *The 2007 Recommendations of the International Commission on Radiological Protection*, ICRP Publication 103, Copyright © 2007.

the various types of radiation and by the different radiosensitivities of the various human tissues, reflecting the overall health detriment posed by such exposures. The equivalent dose is given by the sum of the absorbed doses (averaged over a tissue) each multiplied by the radiation weighting factor for the particular types of radiation involved, and the effective dose is the sum of the equivalent doses received by different tissues with each equivalent dose weighted by

the tissue weighting factor—both equivalent and effective doses are measured in sievert (Sv). For low-level exposure, the effective dose gives the same overall risk of an adverse health effect as a whole-body dose of gamma radiation. It is used in radiological protection when different organs/tissues receive different doses, possibly from radiations with different radiation weighting factors (ICRP 2007).

Sources and environmental levels

Exposure to natural background radiation is ubiquitous. Additional exposure occurs from anthropogenic sources, mainly for the purposes of medical diagnosis. Overall, the world-averaged individual effective dose from naturally occurring sources is about 2.4 mSv/year, with a typical range of 1.0 to 13 mSv/year (United Nations Scientific Committee on the Effects of Atomic Radiation 2010). This represents about 80 per cent of the global average individual effective dose, the approximately 0.6 mSv/year received from artificial sources being dominated by medical exposures (United Nations Scientific Committee on the Effects of Atomic Radiation 2010). The different sources contribute the fractional amounts as summarized in Fig. 7.2.2. The rapid advance in radiodiagnostic technology (such as computed tomography (CT) scanning) has led to a comparatively large increase in doses from medical sources in developed countries (United Nations Scientific Committee on the Effects of Atomic Radiation 2010).

Naturally occurring sources

In addition to external sources of radiation, such as cosmic-rays originating from outside the Earth and terrestrial gamma-rays from naturally occurring radioactive materials in the environment, radionuclides are inhaled or ingested, irradiating the body from within, and the inhalation of the radioisotopes of radon and their radioactive decay products contributes on average more than 50 per cent of the effective dose from natural sources. Radon-222 is the main source of radon exposure and is produced by the decay of radium-226, which is a component of the radioactive decay chain of naturally occurring uranium-238; rarer radon-220 is part of the decay chain of naturally occurring thorium-232. When radon is inhaled the dose is largely from alpha-particles to the bronchial

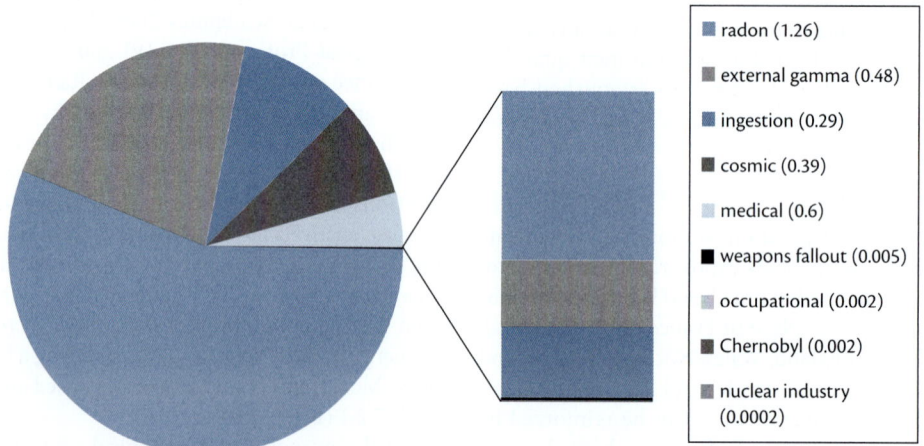

radon (1.26)

external gamma (0.48)

ingestion (0.29)

cosmic (0.39)

medical (0.6)

weapons fallout (0.005)

occupational (0.002)

Chernobyl (0.002)

nuclear industry (0.0002)

Fig. 7.2.2 Worldwide average annual individual effective dose (mSv).
Source: data from United Nations Scientific Committee on the Effects of Atomic Radiation, *UNSCEAR 2008 Report to the General Assembly, with Scientific Annexes*, United Nations, New York, USA, Copyright © 2010.

epithelium, with a consequent risk of lung cancer. The ingestion of naturally occurring radionuclides is mainly through the presence of the decay products of uranium-238 and thorium-232, and of long-lived radionuclides such as potassium-40, in food and drink. When cosmic-rays strike the upper atmosphere, radionuclides are formed, mainly tritium (hydrogen-3) and carbon-14, and these enter the body largely through the consumption of food and drink.

There are important variations in the natural background dose depending on factors such as the nature of rock and soils, building materials, and altitude. There exist on Earth high natural background radiation areas where annual effective doses can exceed 10 mSv and even 100 mSv (77). These elevated levels may be due to gamma radiation, such as from the monazite sands of the coast of Kerala in India, but mainly they are due to gaseous radon entering buildings and producing high concentrations in air. Radon concentrations in some houses in the most affected areas of the world are sufficiently raised that remediation measures are necessary to reduce the consequent risk of lung cancer to acceptable levels. Cosmic radiation levels are increased at high altitudes due to decreased shielding by the atmosphere—air travel therefore raises the dose received from cosmic-rays, but with the exception of frequent travellers, this forms a relatively small increase in the overall dose from natural sources of radiation (Table 7.2.2).

Man-made radiation sources

The main man-made global contribution to environmental exposure has come from radioactive fallout from the testing of nuclear weapons in the atmosphere, mainly during the late 1950s and early 1960s. The world average annual effective dose reached a peak of 0.11 mSv in 1963, and since then it has decreased to about 0.005 mSv in 2000, most of this dose now coming from carbon-14 (United Nations Scientific Committee on the Effects of Atomic Radiation 2010). Other contributions are from the generation of electricity from nuclear energy and the production of nuclear weapons, and also from naturally occurring radionuclides in the discharges from fossil-fuelled power stations and other industrial plants, such as phosphate processing factories. Doses to members of the public from these exposures are now generally low at around 1 μSv. Doses to workers in the nuclear industry and in other occupations (e.g. industrial radiographers) have fallen over the years with improved radiological protection measures. The world-wide average annual dose in the nuclear industry is now about 1 mSv (Table 7.2.2). Modern technological advances have led to other sources of exposure, such as smoke detectors and security scanners, although the doses received from these are almost always minute.

Some potential sources of exposure have raised public concern, such as lost medical or industrial radiation sources, deliberate contamination of items such as foodstuffs with radioactive materials, or 'dirty bombs'. 'Dirty bombs' (a type of 'radiological dispersion device') spread radioactive materials by using conventional explosives (Amaldi and Kraft 2006), but it is difficult to assess just how dangerous these terrorist weapons would be in terms of radiological effects, and it is likely that the greatest impact would be psychological as a result of fear and panic.

Exposure from medical procedures

Modern diagnostic radiography assures earlier, more precise diagnosis and monitoring the progression of a large number of diseases. Screening procedures (such as mammography) are beneficial for specific populations who are at a higher risk from certain diseases. Diagnostic radiography using conventional X-ray examination, CT scanning, and positron emission tomography (PET) have significantly improved the staging and accuracy of diagnosis. In addition, a number of interventional radiologically driven procedures (such as angioplasty) introduced in the last 10–20 years, contribute significantly to the effectiveness of treatment of serious diseases of the cardiovascular and central nervous systems and other organs. Such technological improvements can be critically important in effecting cures, but involve relatively high exposure, and therefore should be used with care.

In recent years the use of nuclear medicine and in particular CT scanning has increased to a marked extent in economically developed countries. This increase is illustrated by the average annual effective dose to members of the population of the United States from medical procedures (mainly from diagnostic exposures), which was 0.53 mSv in the early 1980s, but had risen to 3.0 mSv in 2006, a level that is comparable to the average annual effective dose received from natural sources. The doses received from medical procedures are dependent on economic development: world-averaged individual dose from medical exposures during 1997–2007 was 0.62 mSv/year, but in countries with advanced healthcare systems it was 1.92 mSv/year (United Nations Scientific Committee on the Effects of Atomic Radiation 2010). The number of procedures carried out in the United States during 2006 in each category of diagnostic and interventional procedures, together with the average effective dose received per procedure, is given in Table 7.2.3 (National Council on Radiation Protection and Measurements 2009).

Table 7.2.2 Global occupational radiation exposures

Source of exposure	Average annual effective dose (mSv)	Number of monitored workers worldwide (thousands)
Man-made sources[a]		
Nuclear fuel cycle (including uranium mining)	1.0	660
Industrial uses of radiation	0.3	869
Military activities	0.1	331
Medical uses of radiation	0.5	7440
Miscellaneous	0.1	565
Total from man-made sources	0.4	9865
Enhanced natural sources[b]		
Aircrew	3.0	300
Mining (other than coal)	3.0	4600
Coal mining	2.4	6900
Other workplaces	4.8	1250
Total from natural sources	2.9	13,050

[a] 2000–2002.
[b] 1995–2002.

Source: data from United Nations Scientific Committee on the Effects of Atomic Radiation, *UNSCEAR 2008 Report to the General Assembly, with Scientific Annexs*, United Nations, New York, USA, Copyright © 2010.

Table 7.2.3 Estimated number of procedures, and the average effective dose received, in each category of diagnostic and interventional procedures carried out in the United States during 2006

Category	Number of procedures (million)	Average effective dose per procedure (mSv)	Collective dose (person-Sv)
Computed tomography	67	6.6	440,000
Conventional radiography and fluoroscopy	293	0.3	100,000
Interventional fluoroscopy	17	7.5	128,000
Nuclear medicine	18	12.8	231,000
Total	395	2.3	899,000

Source: data from National Council on Radiation Protection and Measurements, *Ionizing Radiation Exposure of the Population of the United States. NCRP Report No. 160*, National Council on Radiation Protection and Measurements, Bethesda, Maryland, USA, Copyright © 2009.

Radiation therapy is based on the ability of ionizing radiation to kill cells, and radiation can be targeted at a particular group of cells, such as cancerous cells. Radiotherapy saves many lives every year, and in the case of palliative treatment, substantially reduces suffering. There are also some non-malignant diseases whose treatment by radiation is also a method of choice. Most of the side effects of conventional radiotherapy are predictable and expected, arising from the unintentional irradiation of cells outside the target tissues, and one of the aims of modern intensity-modulated radiation therapy is to reduce the side effects to a minimum by sparing normal tissues (Hall 2006). However, radiotherapy inevitably leads to some degree of irradiation of healthy tissues and to some consequent risk of adverse health effects arising from this exposure. This is particularly relevant for deeply seated tumours, tumours closely located to critical organs, and paediatric tumours. One newly emerging method is the use of charged particles (e.g. protons and ^{12}C ions), with their positive physical and radiobiological properties, which allows highly conformal treatment of various kinds of tumours while delivering minimal doses to large volumes of surrounding healthy tissues. This means that they can cause severe damage to the DNA in cancer cells while sparing both traversed and deeper healthy tissue. This characteristic also enables them to be used for a more accurate irradiation of the tumour (Rosen 2001).

Recommendations for medical exposure

Medical exposures are intended to provide a direct benefit to the exposed individual. If the practice is justified and the protection optimized, the dose in the patient will be as low as is compatible with the medical purposes. Therefore dose limits are generally not applied to medical exposures. However, there is considerable opportunity for dose reductions in diagnostic radiology using the techniques of optimization of protection, and this is important since the second largest exposure to individuals is from medical exposures, and this is increasing particularly in the developed countries.

The risk from diagnostic radiography is a particularly important consideration for children—they are still developing and are more sensitive to radiation-induced cancer than adults; in addition, they have a longer prospective life span, and hence, the period over which potential long-term side-effects may arise is greater (Brenner et al. 2001; WHO 2005). Therefore, care should be taken to minimize the number of unnecessary X-ray examinations, including dental X-ray examinations, and in optimizing the CT exposure settings when this procedure is indicated.

Health effects

Ionizing radiation causes two categories of adverse health effects: tissue reactions (also known as deterministic effects) and stochastic effects (ICRP 2007). Tissue reactions are caused by the ability of radiation to kill cells—if sufficient cells are killed then the tissue reaction occurs—and tissue reactions are characterized by a threshold dose below which the effect does not occur and above which the tissue reaction increases in severity. Stochastic effects are caused by non-lethal cell modification, which may develop into a cancer if the affected cell is somatic or into a hereditary abnormality if the affected cell is germ. Stochastic effects are understood to have no threshold dose, and at low doses or low dose-rates the risk is assumed to be directly proportional to the received dose, although this is not universally accepted. The overall risk of stochastic effects is dominated by the risk of cancer in the exposed individual (ICRP 2007).

Ionizing radiation causes damage to DNA either through direct physical interaction with DNA or through the nearby creation of free radicals that then chemically react with DNA. These interactions cause strand breaks in the DNA, and ionizing radiation is particularly efficient at producing clustered (i.e. localized) damage and consequently double-strand breaks. DNA repair mechanisms attempt to deal with the strand breaks caused by ionizing radiation, but double-strand breaks are especially difficult to repair accurately. Heavy damage to DNA from high acute doses of radiation often leads to a loss of DNA integrity that is sufficiently serious to lead to cell death, and when a particular proportion of cells in a tissue is killed then a tissue reaction occurs; the greater this proportion the more severe the tissue reaction. A cell may survive the DNA damage caused by radiation because the DNA is repaired correctly, but a cell may also survive with the DNA damage unrepaired or misrepaired, and this is understood to be the origin of the risk of cancer (in somatic cells) and hereditary effects (in germ cells).

The dose–response for stochastic effects is conventionally thought to be produced by a combination of the single traversal of the cell nucleus by a track of radiation and multiple traversals by independent tracks. The former occurs at low doses or low dose-rates of sparsely ionizing radiation and produces a linear term in the dose–response, while the latter occurs at moderate and high doses delivered at a high dose-rate and leads to an upward curving quadratic term; this is the mechanistic origin of the dose and dose-rate effectiveness factor (DDREF) of greater than 1 (conventionally, a value of 2). At high doses, cell killing becomes more likely, and the slope of the dose–response reduces as a consequence (since dead cells cannot contribute to the risk of stochastic effects). The linear no-threshold dose–response assumes that at low doses or low dose-rates the risk of non-lethal DNA damage of relevance to stochastic effects is directly proportional to the dose, and therefore, to the overall number of tracks crossing cell nuclei.

For high-LET radiations, the density of ionizations is such that the passage of a single particle through a cell nucleus does sufficient damage to the DNA that only a linear term in the dose–response is apparent. Indeed, at the cellular level, the passage of a single alpha-particle track is a high-dose event, with a reasonable probability of inducing cell death, so the passage of two alpha particles is most likely to kill the cell. Thus, the dose–response for high-LET radiations is characterized by linearity, with a slope greater than that for the same absorbed dose produced by low-LET radiations, followed by a reduction in slope at high doses due to cell killing.

However, this picture is a greatly simplified version of reality, the biological mechanisms involved being very complex. For example, it assumes that DNA repair following acute low doses, producing just a few electron traversals of a cell nucleus, is not much more efficient (conventionally, twice as efficient—a DDREF of 2) than that following acute moderate doses, producing many electron traversals, and this assumption may not be correct. Further, there is evidence that epigenetic mechanisms may play a role in radiation-induced risk, in a way that is as yet unclear, and that these mechanisms may differ between high doses and low doses.

Some argue that since low doses produce a degree of DNA damage that is comparable to the level of damage that is constantly occurring through background biochemical processes, it is unlikely that low doses are harmful because the radiation-induced damage is 'swept up' by routine repair. Going even further, some argue that low doses of radiation stimulate the immune system, and so are beneficial (so-called 'radiation hormesis'). On the other hand, some mechanisms of damage may be more effective at low doses than at moderate doses, leading to a supra-linear dose–response, and the bystander effect (whereby a cell hit by radiation adversely influences neighbouring cells that were not directly hit) is one example of such a mechanism because it affects more bystander cells at low doses than at moderate doses, where the effect is saturated because nearly all cells are hit. This serves to illustrate the complexity of radiobiology, and why risk estimates are still dominated by empirical epidemiological findings (ICRP 2007).

Cancer

It has been known for many decades that brief exposure to a dose of several gray leads to death through the killing of sufficient numbers of cells in vital tissues such as the red bone marrow, that is, death is caused by tissue reactions in radiosensitive tissues. An example from recent decades is the 28 emergency workers attending the Chernobyl accident in 1986 who died within a few months as a result of the high doses they received over a short period. Other tissue reactions include permanent and temporary sterility, depression of haematopoiesis, and eye lens opacities and cataracts.

Radiation has always been a natural part of our environment, and the types of radiation emitted from anthropogenic sources are fundamentally the same as those emitted from natural sources. At present it is not possible to distinguish between cancers resulting from radiation exposure (whether from man-made or naturally occurring sources) and those arising from other causes (National Research Council of the National Academies 2006; ICRP 2007; United Nations Scientific Committee on the Effects of Atomic Radiation 2008, 2010; IARC 2012). Consequently, in the absence of being able to determine the risk to human health from exposure to ionizing radiation from fundamental radiobiological principles, risk estimates must be derived empirically from epidemiological studies of suitably exposed groups of humans, augmented by an incomplete knowledge of radiobiological mechanisms. The evidence

that has been constructed from radio-epidemiological studies is substantial, and with the possible exception of tobacco, no other exposure has been studied so extensively. These epidemiological studies fall into four broad categories: studies of the Japanese survivors of the atomic bombings, those exposed for medical purposes either therapeutically or diagnostically, occupational exposure, and those exposed environmentally (National Research Council of the National Academies 2006; ICRP 2007; United Nations Scientific Committee on the Effects of Atomic Radiation 2008, 2010; IARC 2012).

The experience of the survivors of the atomic bombings of Hiroshima and Nagasaki in 1945 provides the principal (but certainly not the only) epidemiological evidence on which radiation risk estimates are based. A large cohort study, the Life Span Study (LSS), was established from information gathered during the Japanese national census in October 1950, and analyses of data generated by the LSS continue today (Preston et al. 2007; Ozasa et al. 2012; Hsu et al. 2013). The LSS consists of about 93,500 survivors, around 86,500 of whom have individually estimated tissue-specific doses—considerable effort has been expended on the reconstruction of tissue-specific doses received during the bombings (mainly from gamma-rays, but a component from neutrons), the latest database being the Dosimetry System 2002 (DS02). Of the LSS subjects, approximately 48,000 received non-trivial doses (>5 mSv), and of these approximately 18,000 received doses greater than 100 mSv, and approximately 2400 doses greater than 1 Sv; almost two-thirds of the non-trivially exposed survivors received doses less than 100 mSv (i.e. low doses). At the end of the last mortality follow-up (2003), 58 per cent of the LSS subjects had died, and 24 per cent of the deaths were due to cancer (Ozasa et al. 2012); 527 solid cancer deaths (8 per cent of such deaths among non-trivially exposed survivors) are estimated to be attributable to radiation exposure during the atomic bombings. As well as mortality, cancer incidence is ascertained in the LSS through two specialist registries, the most recent analysis of solid cancer incidence covering the period 1958–1998 (Preston et al. 2007), while the latest findings of the incidence of leukaemia, lymphoma, and multiple myeloma are from an analysis of covering the period 1950–2001 (Hsu et al. 2013). In a subset of the LSS, the Adult Health Study (AHS), survivors participate in regular medical examinations to record clinical parameters such as blood pressure. Other relevant cohorts are those who were exposed *in utero* and the offspring of survivors who were conceived after the bombings, the latter group providing information on the risks of the heritable effects of exposure.

Early support for the initial findings of the studies of the Japanese atomic-bomb survivors came from investigations of long-term health effects among patients treated with radiotherapy, in particular British patients irradiated for ankylosing spondylitis and US women treated with radiation for cancer of the uterine cervix (United Nations Scientific Committee on the Effects of Atomic Radiation 2008). Now there is evidence deriving from a wide range of radiotherapeutic treatments such as various groups of cancer survivors, children irradiated for ringworm of the scalp or haemangioma of the skin or for an enlarged thymus, and patients injected with radium-224. Patients exposed to radiation for diagnostic purposes are providing increasingly useful information as the use of CT scans increases, but those X-rayed to monitor treatment for tuberculosis or for scoliosis, and fetuses exposed during an abdominal X-ray examination of the pregnant mother, have already provided valuable evidence on the risks of low-level exposures. A recent large cohort study of British children who received at least one CT scan found evidence of an increased risk of brain tumours and leukaemia that was related to the dose of radiation estimated to have been received from the scans (Pearce et al. 2012). An interesting group of patients is those injected with the radiographic contrast medium Thorotrast, which unfortunately was thorium-based and therefore radioactive and gave large doses to certain tissues, such as the liver and red bone marrow.

Radiologists and radiographers have been subjects of study since the early uses of radiation in medicine, and US radiologists provided the first indication that radiation could cause leukaemia (March 1944). Of particular interest are groups of underground hard-rock miners (e.g. uranium and tin miners) who inhale the radioactive gas radon and its decay products, which irradiate the lungs (mainly with alpha-particles); and in the past, exposures have been high. Workers (mainly young women) who applied radium-based luminous paint to watch and instrument dials inadvertently ingested radium (an alpha-emitter) through the habit of licking the tips of paintbrushes ('tipping'), and some workers ingested large quantities of radium, which deposits in bones. Of increasing importance is the evidence obtained from the study of groups of nuclear industry workers, especially those who worked during the early years of the industry when doses were comparatively high relative to those received today. Large worker studies are providing valuable information on the effects of protracted low-level exposure, and international collaborations have the potential to produce statistically powerful results. Special cases are those workers involved in dealing with emergencies, such as the 'liquidators' who were brought in to deal with the aftermath of the Chernobyl accident in 1986, and those from the early years of operations at the Mayak nuclear complex in Russia who were particularly highly exposed to both external sources of radiation and plutonium, an alpha-emitter that was inhaled in relatively large amounts during early weapons production.

Radon in homes has been a subject of substantial scientific attention because globally this is the source of the largest exposure to radiation for the great majority of people. Large case–control studies that take into account the important contribution of risk posed by cigarette smoking, have examined the risk of lung cancer arising from residential exposure to radon, and appropriately combined findings from these studies have produced radon-related risk estimates that are compatible with those obtained from underground hard-rock miners (IRCP 2010). Exposure to other sources of natural background radiation, in particular terrestrial gamma radiation, has also been studied, notably in those parts of the world where such exposures are materially greater than the global average. A well-designed study of cancer incidence in Kerala (India) has not found an excess cancer risk related to radiation exposure (Nair et al. 2009), although findings are, as yet, compatible with those of the LSS. A large British case–control study concentrating on childhood leukaemia has found evidence of an excess risk from background gamma radiation that is consistent with risk models derived from the Japanese atomic-bomb survivors (Kendall et al. 2013).

Radioactive contamination from accidental and routine discharges from nuclear installations has been another area of study, radioactive iodine releases from the accident at Chernobyl and substantial pollution of the Techa River by liquid effluent from the Mayak complex being notable examples. The releases during

the Fukushima accident in 2011 provide another opportunity for study, although it would appear that doses are not sufficiently large for any effects to be detectable (WHO 2012a, 2012b). Fallout from atmospheric nuclear weapons testing, especially at its peak in the late 1950s and early 1960s, has provided another source of exposure for study, and those resident in the vicinity of weapons testing sites (such as the Semipalatinsk Testing Site in present-day Kazakhstan) are of particular interest. Finally, a group of Taiwanese residents was irradiated by gamma radiation from ^{60}Co-contaminated steel accidentally used in building construction, and this group is being followed.

Epidemiological studies have clearly established that acute exposure to moderate and high doses of ionizing radiation (> 100 mGy of sparsely ionizing radiation) increases the risk of cancer (National Research Council of the National Academies 2006; ICRP 2007; United Nations Scientific Committee on the Effects of Atomic Radiation 2008, 2010; IARC 2012). However, all types of cancer do not have equal sensitivity to radiation induction—acute leukaemia, thyroid, and female breast cancer have a high sensitivity, whereas chronic lymphocytic leukaemia, Hodgkin's lymphoma, and malignant melanoma of the skin have a low sensitivity, with other cancers falling somewhere in between from higher (e.g. lung and colon cancers) to lower (e.g. pancreatic and prostate cancers) sensitivity. Leukaemia was the first cancer to be definitively linked to radiation exposure when a clear excess risk of the malignant disease was detected in the Japanese atomic-bomb survivors in the early 1950s (although unusually high numbers of cases were reported by alert clinicians in the late 1940s), and there had been earlier reports of elevated levels of leukaemia among radiologists (March 1944), which had been difficult to interpret at the time. As the follow-up of the atomic-bomb survivors progressed, raised mortality and incidence of other cancer sites were found to be related to exposure, and this evidence was supplemented by other exposed groups, such as an increased risk of a number of solid cancers among patients treated with radiotherapy for a variety of diseases, a marked excess of bone cancer among those groups with high intakes of radium, an excess risk of lung cancer among underground hard-rock miners exposed to radon, and an excess risk of liver cancer among the Thorotrast patients with high body burdens of thorium. Recently, the Chernobyl accident has produced a notable excess risk of thyroid cancer among those who as children inhaled and ingested high levels of radioactive iodine released during the accident, an excess that is compatible with that found among those exposed as children to external sources of radiation.

The most recent analysis of leukaemia mortality among the LSS cohort found that a linear-quadratic dose–response best described the data, and that the excess relative risk was 3.1 (95 per cent CI: 1.8–4.3) at 1 Gy red bone marrow dose and 0.15 (95 per cent CI: −0.01–0.31) at 0.1 Gy, based on 318 deaths (Ozasa et al. 2012). About half of the leukaemia deaths among the non-trivially exposed (> 5 mGy) survivors are attributed to irradiation during the bombings. However, modelling demonstrates a marked variation of risk with age-at-exposure and time-since-exposure: for young children, the excess relative risk (ERR, the proportional increase in risk) rises to a peak of approximately 50 some 7 years after exposure and then falls away to approximately 5 some 30 years after exposure—a temporal wave of excess risk—while for exposed adults this wave is hardly apparent, with the ERR remaining below 5 at all times after exposure. From the latest datasets for the mortality and incidence of all solid cancers (malignant diseases other than leukaemia, lymphoma, and multiple myeloma) among the survivors, a linear dose–response fits the data best, with a slope of the ERR for solid cancer mortality for a survivor exposed at age 30 years and at an attained age of 70 years of 0.47 (95 per cent CI: 0.38–0.56) Gy^{-1}, based upon almost 11,000 deaths. The ERR coefficients for leukaemia and solid cancer incidence are similar to those for mortality (Preston et al. 2007; Ozasa et al. 2012; Hsu et al. 2013). However, as already mentioned, there is notable variation in the ERR/Gy for individual sites of cancer, the ERR for the incidence of breast, thyroid, and non-melanoma skin cancers being high while that for cancers of the rectum and uterus are low.

Risk models have been developed from the cancer data for the Japanese atomic-bomb survivors, supplemented by other data sources where these are found to make a useful contribution to evidence, such as for leukaemia and for thyroid and breast cancers following exposure for medical therapy. Lung cancer among radon-exposed underground hard-rock miners has provided a valuable source of information on the risk of radon-induced lung cancer, which is compatible with the risk of lung cancer among those exposed residentially to, in general, much lower levels of radon. The influence of tobacco smoke upon the risk of lung cancer is especially important to take into account in such studies, and it would appear that radiation and cigarette smoke interact to produce a combined risk of lung cancer that is more than additive, so that smokers are at a greater risk of radon-induced lung cancer than non-smokers.

In general, the findings of the studies of the Japanese atomic-bomb survivors are compatible with those from other exposed groups, although comparisons are often not straightforward. For example, doses from radiotherapy are usually localized and high, with the objective of killing the target cells, but the unintentional irradiation of healthy cells can also lead to their being killed and thereby to a reduction in the risk per unit dose of cancer. Doses away from the target are received from scattered radiation and are difficult to compute accurately, although modern dose reconstruction methods are improving dose estimates. Of growing importance are studies of acute low doses or protracted low dose-rates, because these exposure circumstances directly test the assumptions required for everyday radiological protection. Preliminary findings of such studies, for example, of patients receiving CT scans, those living in areas affected by radioactive contamination, or nuclear industry workers, indicate that there is an increased risk from low doses/dose-rates (at least, for some types of cancer, notably leukaemia), but that this risk is not greatly different from the predictions of conventional risk models.

Other outcomes

Epidemiological studies have failed to produce definitive evidence that exposure to ionizing radiation increases the risk of heritable genetic effects in the descendants of those exposed (ICRP 2007). Even the follow-up of more than 30,000 offspring of the Japanese atomic-bomb survivors who were conceived after the bombings has not provided clear evidence of an inherited effect from parental exposure. Nonetheless, large experiments involving laboratory animals, mainly mice, have produced unambiguous evidence that irradiation of parents does raise the risk of hereditary effects in offspring. The risk of radiation-induced hereditary effects in humans derived from this evidence suggests that this risk is much lower than the risk of cancer in the exposed individual.

The lens of the eye is sensitive to radiation-induced cataracts, and recent evidence indicates that the threshold for the production of cataracts, at around 500 mGy of low-LET radiation, is much lower than the 5 Gy previously considered as a threshold dose (ICRP 2012). This evidence comes from the Japanese atomic-bomb survivors, the Chernobyl 'liquidators', and medical staff.

The embryo and fetus are sensitive to radiation-induced developmental effects, such as, early in pregnancy, congenital malformations (although death may occur before birth defects become likely) (ICRP 2007). Severe mental retardation was found among Japanese atomic-bomb survivors exposed *in utero* to high doses during 8–15 weeks of gestation, and less so at 16–25 weeks.

An issue requiring resolution is whether low doses/dose-rates are capable of raising the risk of non-cancer somatic diseases, in particular diseases of the blood circulatory system, such as heart attack and stroke (ICRP 2012). It has been known for some time that high doses can lead to an excess risk of these diseases, and this was attributed to tissue damage produced during such exposure, but epidemiological evidence is mounting for an effect at lower doses. However, a mechanism has yet to be identified, and the confounding effects of major (non-radiation) risk factors cannot yet be reliably eliminated as responsible for the association. Nonetheless, the potential risk of circulatory disease following low-level exposure to radiation is considered sufficiently important that significant research effort is being devoted to its investigation.

Policy and prevention

The ICRP, in its latest assessment of evidence, provides detriment-adjusted nominal risk coefficients for all cancers combined: 5.49 per cent Sv^{-1} for the whole population and 4.07 per cent Sv^{-1} for the working population (ICRP 2007). The detriment-adjusted nominal risk coefficients for hereditary effects are: 0.2 per cent Sv^{-1} for the general population and 0.12 per cent Sv^{-1} for a working population. Consequently, the aggregated detriment-adjusted nominal risk coefficients for stochastic effects following low-level exposure to radiation are 5.7 per cent Sv^{-1} for a general population and 4.2 per cent Sv^{-1} for a working population. These risk coefficients form the technical basis of the current framework of radiological protection recommended by the ICRP, and give rise to dose limits: for workers, the limit is an effective dose of 20 mSv per year averaged over a defined period of 5 years (with a maximum of 50 mSv in any one year), and for the general public the limit is an effective dose of 1 mSv in a year (although in special circumstances a higher dose could be received in any one year provided the annual average is 1 mSv over a 5-year period). These limits do not apply to medical or naturally occurring sources of exposure, although residential exposure to radon and its radioactive decay products in some areas of the world are assessed to produce a sufficiently high risk of lung cancer that remediation measures are required to reduce the exposure.

The three key principles of radiological protection remain: (1) the justification of activities that could cause or affect radiation exposures, (2) the optimization of protection in order to keep doses as low as reasonably achievable, and (3) the application of dose limits (ICRP 2007). The recommendations state:

1. No practice involving exposures to radiation should be adopted unless it produces sufficient benefit—to the exposed individuals or to society—to offset the detriment it causes.

Table 7.2.4 Recommended dose limits

Type of limit	Occupational	Public
Effective dose	20 mSv per year, averaged over defined periods of 5 years, with a maximum of 50 mSv in any one year[a]	1 mSv in a year
Annual equivalent dose in: Lens of the eye	20 mSv per year, averaged over defined periods of 5 years, with a maximum of 50 mSv in any one year	15 mSv
Skin	500 mSv	50 mSv
Hands and feet	500 mSv	–

[a] The basis for the control of the occupational exposure of women who are not pregnant is the same as that for men. However, once pregnancy has been declared, the embryo/fetus is protected—the effective dose limit for the embryo/fetus is 1 mSv.

Source: data from International Commission on Radiological Protection (ICRP), *The 2007 Recommendations of the International Commission on Radiological Protection*, ICRP Publication 103, Copyright © 2007.

2. In relation to any particular source within a practice, the magnitude of individual doses, the number of people exposed, and the likelihood of incurring exposures (where these are not certain to be received) should all be kept as low as reasonably achievable, economic and societal factors being taken into account.

3. The exposure of individuals resulting from the combination of all the relevant practices should be subject to dose limits, or to some control of risk in the case of potential exposures; hence, ensuring that no individual is exposed to radiation risks that are judged to be unacceptable from these practices in any normal circumstances. Dose (or risk) constraints are used to restrict to upper bounds the dose received (or potentially received) from a specific source.

Restrictions on effective dose sufficient to ensure the avoidance of deterministic effects in all body organs and tissues, and that limit the risk of stochastic effects to acceptable levels, are shown in Table 7.2.4.

Conclusions

The nature, frequency, and severity of adverse effects on human health caused by exposure to ionizing and non-ionizing radiation vary depending on the intensity and other exposure parameters, and are highly frequency dependent. Potential effects range from rapidly fatal injuries to birth and hereditary defects, cancer, and other chronic diseases. Many effects occur only at high levels and are controlled or reduced by applicable exposure standards. In this chapter, our main emphasis is on exposures common in everyday life and on long-term effects, which are typically of most concern to the public.

The IARC classified ionizing radiation and UV radiation as a 'known' or Group 1 carcinogen, while ELF magnetic fields and RF fields have been classified as a 'possible human carcinogen', or a Group 2B, and static fields as well as ELF electric fields have been assigned Group 3 (not classifiable as to carcinogenicity to humans). Intermediate frequencies and infrared radiation have not yet been classified as to their carcinogenic potential.

As it is not possible to eliminate exposure to ionizing radiation, these exposures are kept to a practical minimum. Most recommend

avoiding solar UV exposure in order to facilitate the prevention of skin cancers. Because recent literature suggests beneficial effects of solar UV exposure it is critical to develop and adopt a well-balanced set of recommendations regarding this exposure. For ELF magnetic fields, given exposure prevalence, considerable scientific uncertainty, and limited public health impact, no- and very low-cost precautionary measures are justified. For RF, potential risk could affect a large number of people because of the ubiquitous nature of the exposure. Thus, given the important gaps in knowledge and availability of no- to low-cost measures, such as use of hands-free devices to reduce exposures from mobile phones, such measures can and should be adopted.

Rigorous studies capable of addressing knowledge gaps are urgently needed, particularly for rapidly growing technologies such as mobile phones, MRI exposures, IF anti-theft and device tagging, and modern magnetic levitation (maglev) systems.

Acknowledgements

We are grateful to Dr Madhuri Sudan for help in manuscript preparation and to Drs Myles Cockburn and Manjit Dosanjh who co-authored this chapter in the previous edition.

References

Abramson, M.J., Benke, G.P., Dimitriadis, C., et al. (2009). Mobile telephone use is associated with changes in cognitive function in young adolescents. *Bioelectromagnetics*, 30(8), 678–86.

Ahlbom, A., Day, N., Feychting, M., et al. (2000). A pooled analysis of magnetic fields and childhood leukaemia. *British Journal of Cancer*, 83(5), 692–8.

Ahlbom, A., Green, A., Kheifets, L., Savitz, D., Swerdlow, A.; ICNIRP (International Commission for Non-Ionizing Radiation Protection) Standing Committee on Epidemiology (2004). Epidemiology of health effects of radiofrequency exposure. *Environmental Health Perspectives*, 112(17), 1741–54.

Allinson, S., Asmuss, M., Baldermann, C., et al. (2012). Validity and use of the UV Index: report from the UVI Working Group, Schloss Hohenkammer, Germany, 5–7 December 2011. *Health Physics*, 103(3), 301–6.

Aly, E.M. and Mohamed, E.S. (2011). Effect of infrared radiation on the lens. *Indian Journal of Ophthalmology*, 59(2), 97–101.

Amaldi, U. and Kraft, G. (2006). Particle accelerators take up the fight against cancer. *CERN Courier*, 6 December [Online] Available at: http://cerncourier.com/cws/article/cern/29777.

Aydin, D., Feychting, M., Schuz, J., Roosli, M., and CEFALO study team (2012). Childhood brain tumours and use of mobile phones: comparison of a case-control study with incidence data. *Environmental Health*, 11, 35.

Beever, R. (2009). Far-infrared saunas for treatment of cardiovascular risk factors. *Canadian Family Physician*, 55(7), 691–6.

Boniol, M., Autier, P., Boyle, P., and Gandini, S. (2012). Cutaneous melanoma attributable to sunbed use: systematic review and meta-analysis. *British Medical Journal*, 345, e4757.

Brenner, D., Elliston, C., Hall, E., and Berdon, W. (2001). Estimated risks of radiation-induced fatal cancer from pediatric CT. *AJR American Journal of Roentgenology*, 176(2), 289–96.

Chang, Y.M., Barrett, J.H., Bishop, D.T., et al. (2009). Sun exposure and melanoma risk at different latitudes: a pooled analysis of 5700 cases and 7216 controls. *International Journal of Epidemiology*, 38(3), 814–30.

Dewhirst, M.W., Viglianti, B.L., Lora-Michiels, M., Hanson, M., and Hoopes, P.J. (2003). Basic principles of thermal dosimetry and thermal thresholds for tissue damage from hyperthermia. *International Journal of Hyperthermia*, 19(3), 267–94.

Diffey, B.L. (1991). Solar ultraviolet radiation effects on biological systems. *Physics in Medicine and Biology*, 36(3), 299–328.

Divan, H.A., Kheifets, L., Obel, C., and Olsen, J. (2008). Prenatal and post-natal exposure to cell phone use and behavioral problems in children. *Epidemiology*, 19(4), 523–9.

Divan, H.A., Kheifets, L., Obel, C., and Olsen, J. (2012). Cell phone use and behavioural problems in young children. *Journal of Epidemiology and Community Health*, 66(6), 524–9.

Divan, H.A., Kheifets, L., and Olsen, J. (2011). Prenatal cell phone use and developmental milestone delays among infants. *Scandinavian Journal of Work, Environment & Health*, 37(4), 341–8.

Edwards, C., Gaskell, S.A., Hill, S.A., Heggie, R., Pearse, A.D., and Marks, R. (1999). Effects on human epidermis of chronic suberythemal exposure to pure infrared radiation. *Archives of Dermatology*, 135(5), 608–9.

Elliott, P., Toledano, M.B., Bennett, J., et al. (2010). Mobile phone base stations and early childhood cancers: case-control study. *British Medical Journal*, 340, c3077.

European Commission (1996). *Non-Ionizing Radiation; Sources, Exposure and Health Effects*. B-1049. Brussels: European Commission.

Evans, J.A., Savitz, D.A., Kanal, E., and Gillen, J. (1993). Infertility and pregnancy outcome among magnetic resonance imaging workers. *Journal of Occupational Medicine*, 35(12), 1191–5.

Fears, T.R., Bird, C.C., Guerry, D.T., et al. (2002). Average midrange ultraviolet radiation flux and time outdoors predict melanoma risk. *Cancer Research*, 62(14), 3992–6.

Gandini, S., Boniol, M., Haukka, J., et al. (2011). Meta-analysis of observational studies of serum 25-hydroxyvitamin D levels and colorectal, breast and prostate cancer and colorectal adenoma. *International Journal of Cancer*, 128(6), 1414–24.

Gowland, P.A. (2005). Present and future magnetic resonance sources of exposure to static fields. *Progress in Biophysics and Molecular Biology*, 87(2–3), 175–83.

Green, A., Williams, G., Neale, R., et al. (1999). Daily sunscreen application and betacarotene supplementation in prevention of basal-cell and squamous-cell carcinomas of the skin: a randomised controlled trial. *The Lancet*, 354(9180), 723–9.

Green, A.C., Wallingford, S.C., and McBride, P. (2011). Childhood exposure to ultraviolet radiation and harmful skin effects: epidemiological evidence. *Progress in Biophysics and Molecular Biology*, 107(3), 349–55.

Green, A.C., Williams, G.M., Logan, V., and Strutton, G.M. (2011). Reduced melanoma after regular sunscreen use: randomized trial follow-up. *Journal of Clinical Oncology*, 29(3), 257–63.

Greenland, S. and Kheifets, L. (2006). Leukemia attributable to residential magnetic fields: results from analyses allowing for study biases. *Risk Analysis*, 26(2), 471–82.

Greenland, S., Sheppard, A.R., Kaune, W.T., Poole, C., and Kelsh, M.A. (2000). A pooled analysis of magnetic fields, wire codes, and childhood leukemia. Childhood Leukemia-EMF Study Group. *Epidemiology*, 11(6), 624–34.

Ha, M., Im, H., Lee, M., et al. (2007). Radio-frequency radiation exposure from AM radio transmitters and childhood leukemia and brain cancer. *American Journal of Epidemiology*, 166(3), 270–9.

Hall, E.J. (2006). Intensity-modulated radiation therapy, protons, and the risk of second cancers. *International Journal of Radiation Oncology, Biology, Physics*, 65(1), 1–7.

Halliday, G.M. and Rana, S. (2008). Waveband and dose dependency of sunlight-induced immunomodulation and cellular changes. *Photochemistry and Photobiology*, 84(1), 35–46.

Heynick, L.N. and Merritt, J.H. (2003). Radiofrequency fields and teratogenesis. *Bioelectromagnetics*, Suppl. 6, S174–86.

Hsu, W.L., Preston, D.L., Soda, M., et al. (2013). The incidence of leukemia, lymphoma and multiple myeloma among atomic bomb survivors: 1950–2001. *Radiation Research*, 179(3), 361–82.

Ikehata, H. and Ono, T. (2007). Significance of CpG methylation for solar UV-induced mutagenesis and carcinogenesis in skin. *Photochemistry and Photobiology*, 83(1), 196–204.

Independent Advisory Group on Non-Ionizing Radiation (2003). *Health Effects from Radiofrequency Electromagnetic Fields*. Chilton: National Radiological Protection Board.

International Agency for Research on Cancer (2002). *IARC Monographs on the Evaluation of Carcinogenic Risks to Humans. Non-Ionizing Radiation, Part 1: Static and Extremely Low-Frequency (ELF) Electric and Magnetic Fields*. Lyon: IARC.

International Agency for Research on Cancer (Working Group on Artificial Ultraviolet Light and Skin Cancer) (2007). The association of use of sunbeds with cutaneous malignant melanoma and other skin cancers: a systematic review. *International Journal of Cancer*, 120(5), 1116–22.

International Agency for Research on Cancer (2008). *Vitamin D and Cancer*. Lyon: IARC.

International Agency for Research on Cancer (2012). *IARC Monographs on the Evaluation of Carcinogenic Risks to Humans. Radiation. Volume 100 D. A Review of Human Carcinogens*. Lyon: International Agency for Research on Cancer.

International Commission on Non-Ionizing Radiation Protection (2004). Guidelines on limits of exposure to ultraviolet radiation of wavelengths between 180 nm and 400 nm (incoherent optical radiation). *Health Physics*, 87(2), 171–86.

International Commission on Non-Ionizing Radiation Protection (2006). ICNIRP statement on far infrared radiation exposure. *Health Physics*, 91(6), 630–45.

International Commission on Non-Ionizing Radiation Protection (2008). ICNIRP statement on EMF-emitting new technologies. *Health Physics*, 94(4), 376–92.

International Commission on Non-Ionizing Radiation Protection (2009). Amendment to the ICNIRP 'Statement on Medical Magnetic Resonance (Mr) Procedures: Protection of Patients'. *Health Physics*, 97(3), 259–61.

International Commission on Non-Ionizing Radiation Protection (2010). ICNIRP statement – protection of workers against ultraviolet radiation. *Health Physics*, 99(1), 66–87.

International Commission on Radiological Protection (2007). *The 2007 Recommendations of the International Commission on Radiological Protection*. ICRP Publication 103. Oxford: Elsevier.

International Commission on Radiological Protection (2010). *Lung Cancer Risk from Radon and Progeny and Statement on Radon*. ICRP Publication 115. Oxford: Elsevier.

International Commission on Radiological Protection (2012). *2012 ICRP Statement on Tissue Reactions / Early and Late Effects of Radiation in Normal Tissues and Organs—Threshold Doses for Tissue Reactions in a Radiation Protection Context*. ICRP Publication 118. Oxford: Elsevier.

Kendall, G.M., Little, M.P., Wakeford, R., et al. (2013). A record-based case-control study of natural background radiation and the incidence of childhood leukaemia and other cancers in Great Britain during 1980–2006. *Leukemia*, 27(1), 3–9.

Kheifets, L., Afifi, A.A., and Shimkhada, R. (2006). Public health impact of extremely low-frequency electromagnetic fields. *Environmental Health Perspectives*, 114(10), 1532–7.

Kheifets, L., Ahlbom, A., Crespi, C.M., et al. (2010a). Pooled analysis of recent studies on magnetic fields and childhood leukaemia. *British Journal of Cancer*, 103(7), 1128–35.

Kheifets, L., Ahlbom, A., Crespi, C.M., et al. (2010b). A pooled analysis of extremely low-frequency magnetic fields and childhood brain tumors. *American Journal of Epidemiology*, 172(7), 752–61.

Kheifets, L., Ahlbom, A., Johansen, C., Feychting, M., Sahl, J., and Savitz, D. (2007). Extremely low-frequency magnetic fields and heart disease. *Scandinavian Journal of Work, Environment & Health*, 33(1), 5–12.

Kheifets, L., Monroe, J., Vergara, X., Mezei, G., and Afifi, A.A. (2008). Occupational electromagnetic fields and leukemia and brain cancer: an update to two meta-analyses. *Journal of Occupational and Environmental Medicine*, 50(6), 677–88.

Kheifets, L., Repacholi, M., Saunders, R., and van Deventer, E. (2005). The sensitivity of children to electromagnetic fields. *Pediatrics*, 116(2), e303–13.

Kheifets, L., Swanson, J., Kandel, S., and Malloy, T.F. (2010c). Risk govern-ance for mobile phones, power lines, and other EMF technologies. *Risk Analysis*, 30(10), 1481–94.

Larsen, A.I. (1991). Congenital malformations and exposure to high-frequency electromagnetic radiation among Danish physiothera-pists. *Scandinavian Journal of Work, Environment & Health*, 17(5), 318–23.

Lerman, S. (1984). Biophysical aspects of corneal and lenticular transpar-ency. *Current Eye Research*, 3(1), 3–14.

Li, C.Y., Liu, C.C., Chang, Y.H., Chou, L.P., and Ko, M.C. (2012). A population-based case-control study of radiofrequency exposure in relation to childhood neoplasm. *The Science of the Total Environment*, 435–6, 472–8.

Lydahl, E. and Philipson, B. (1984). Infrared radiation and cataract II. Epidemiologic investigation of glass workers. *Acta Ophthalmologica*, 62(6), 976–92.

March, H.C. (1944). Leukemia in radiologists. *Radiology*, 43(3), 275–8.

Merzenich, H., Schmiedel, S., Bennack, S., et al. (2008). Childhood leukemia in relation to radio frequency electromagnetic fields in the vicinity of TV and radio broadcast transmitters. *American Journal of Epidemiology*, 168(10), 1169–78.

Mezei, G. and Kheifets, L. (2006). Selection bias and its implications for case-control studies: a case study of magnetic field exposure and child-hood leukaemia. *International Journal of Epidemiology*, 35(2), 397–406.

Moritz, A.R. and Henriques, F.C. (1947). Studies of thermal injury: II. The relative importance of time and surface temperature in the causation of cutaneous burns. *The American Journal of Pathology*, 23(5), 695–720.

Nair, R.R., Rajan, B., Akiba, S., et al. (2009). Background radiation and cancer incidence in Kerala, India-Karanagappally cohort study. *Health Physics*, 96(1), 55–66.

National Council on Radiation Protection and Measurements (2009). *Ionizing Radiation Exposure of the Population of the United States*. NCRP Report No. 160. Bethesda, MD: National Council on Radiation Protection and Measurements.

National Institute of Environmental Health Sciences (1999). *NIEHS Report on Health Effects from Exposure to Power-Line Frequency Electric and Magnetic Fields*. Research Triangle Park, NC: National Institutes of Health.

National Research Council of the National Academies (2006). *Health Risks from Exposure to Low Levels of Ionizing Radiation: BEIR VII Phase 2*. Washington, DC: The National Academies Press.

National Research Council of the National Academies (2011). *Dietary Reference Intakes for Calcium and Vitamin D*. Washington, DC: The National Academies Press.

Neubauer, G., Feychting, M., Hamnerius, Y., et al. (2007). Feasibility of future epidemiological studies on possible health effects of mobile phone base stations. *Bioelectromagnetics*, 28(3), 224–30.

Olsen, C.M. and Green, A.C. (2012). More evidence of harms of sunbed use, particularly for young people. *British Medical Journal*, 345, e6101.

Ozasa, K., Shimizu, Y., Suyama, A., et al. (2012). Studies of the mortality of atomic bomb survivors. Report 14, 1950–2003: an overview of cancer and noncancer diseases. *Radiation Research*, 177(3), 229–43.

Pawlak, M.T., Bui, M., Amir, M., Burkhardt, D.L., Chen, A.K., and Dellavalle, R.P. (2012). Legislation restricting access to indoor tanning throughout the world. *Archives of Dermatology*, 148(9), 1006–12.

Pearce, M.S., Salotti, J.A., Little, M.P., et al. (2012). Radiation exposure from CT scans in childhood and subsequent risk of leukaemia and brain tumours: a retrospective cohort study. *The Lancet*, 380(9840), 499–505.

Polichetti, A. and Vacchia, P. (eds.) (1998). *Exposure of the General Public to Low- and Medium-Frequency Electromagnetic Fields. Proceedings of the 3rd COST 244bis Workshop on 'Intermediate Frequency Range'*; 25–26 April 1996, Paris. Florida: CRC Press.

Preston, D.L., Ron, E., Tokuoka, S., et al. (2007). Solid cancer incidence in atomic bomb survivors: 1958–1998. *Radiation Research*, 168(1), 1–64.

Rosen, N.S. (2001). Taking care of children. *AJR American Journal of Roentgenology*, 177(3), 715–17.

Swerdlow, A.J., Feychting, M., Green, A.C., et al. (2011). Mobile phones, brain tumors, and the interphone study: where are we now? *Environmental Health Perspectives*, 119(11), 1534–8.

Thacher, T.D. and Clarke, B.L. (2011). Vitamin D insufficiency. *Mayo Clinic Proceedings Mayo Clinic*, 86(1), 50–60.

Thomas, S., Heinrich, S., von Kries, R., and Radon, K. (2010). Exposure to radio-frequency electromagnetic fields and behavioural problems in Bavarian children and adolescents. *European Journal of Epidemiology*, 25(2), 135–41.

Thompson, S.C., Jolley, D., and Marks, R. (1993). Reduction of solar kera-toses by regular sunscreen use. *The New England Journal of Medicine*, 329(16), 1147–51.

United Nations Scientific Committee on the Effects of Atomic Radiation (2008). *UNSCEAR 2006 Report to the General Assembly, with Scientific Annexes*. New York: United Nations.

United Nations Scientific Committee on the Effects of Atomic Radiation (2010). *UNSCEAR 2008 Report to the General Assembly, with Scientific Annexes*. New York: United Nations.

Van Rongen, E., Saunders, R.D., van Deventer, E.T., and Repacholi, M.H. (2007). Static fields: biological effects and mechanisms relevant to expo-sure limits. *Health Physics*, 92(6), 584–90.

Vergara, X., Kheifets, L., Greenland, S., Oksuzyan, S., Cho, Y.S., and Mezei, G. (2013). Occupational exposure to extremely low-frequency mag-netic fields and neurodegenerative disease: a meta-analysis. *Journal of Occupational and Environmental Medicine*, 55(2), 135–46.

Vrijheid, M., Martinez, D., Forns, J., et al. (2010). Prenatal exposure to cell phone use and neurodevelopment at 14 months. *Epidemiology*, 21(2), 259–62.

Wallace, J., Sweetnam, P.M., Warner, C.G., Graham, P.A., and Cochrane, A.L. (1971). An epidemiological study of lens opacities among steel workers. *British Journal of Industrial Medicine*, 28(3), 265–71.

Wehner, M.R., Shive, M.L., Chren, M.M., Han, J., Qureshi, A.A., and Linos, E. (2012). Indoor tanning and non-melanoma skin cancer: systematic review and meta-analysis. *British Medical Journal*, 345, e5909.

Whiteman, D.C., Whiteman, C.A., and Green, A.C. (2001). Childhood sun exposure as a risk factor for melanoma: a systematic review of epidemio-logic studies. *Cancer Causes & Control*, 12(1), 69–82.

World Health Organization (2002). *Global Solar UV Index: A Practical Guide. A joint recommendation of World Health Organization, World Meteorological Organization, United Nations Environment Programme and the International Commission on Non-Ionizing Radiation Protection*. Geneva: WHO.

World Health Organization (2003). *Radiological Dispersion Device (Dirty Bomb)*. Geneva: WHO. Available at: http://www.who.int/ionizing_radi ation/en/WHORAD_InfoSheet_Dirty_Bombs21Feb.pdf.

World Health Organization (2005). *The International Radon Project*. Geneva: WHO. Available at: http://www.who.int/ionizing_radiation/ env/radon/en.

World Health Organization (2006). *Static Fields. Environmental Health Criteria*, 232. Geneva: WHO.

World Health Organization (2007). *Extremely Low Frequency (ELF) Fields. Environmental Health Criteria*, 238. Geneva: WHO.

World Health Organization (2012a). *Health Risk Assessment from the Nuclear Accident after the 2011 Great East Japan Earthquake and Tsunami, Based on a Preliminary Dose Estimation*. Geneva: WHO.

World Health Organization (2012b). *Preliminary Dose Estimation from the Nuclear Accident after the 2011 Great East Japan Earthquake and Tsunami*. Geneva: WHO.

Young, A.R. (2006). Acute effects of UVR on human eyes and skin. *Progress in Biophysics and Molecular Biology*, 92(1), 80–5.

Zhang, M., Qureshi, A.A., Geller, A.C., Frazier, L., Hunter, D.J., and Han, J. (2012). Use of tanning beds and incidence of skin cancer. *Journal of Clinical Oncology*, 30(14), 1588–93.

Zuclich, J.A., Lund, D.J., and Stuck, B.E. (2007). Wavelength dependence of ocular damage thresholds in the near-ir to far-ir transition region: pro-posed revisions to MPES. *Health Physics*. 92(1), 15–23.

7.3

Environmental exposure assessment: modelling air pollution concentrations

John Gulliver and Kees de Hoogh

Introduction to environmental exposure assessment

Epidemiological studies ideally would have access to information on continuous lifetime air pollution exposures at the individual level that are suitably resolved in space and time for studying specific diseases. Air pollution exposures are a function of the indoor and outdoor locations (i.e. micro-environments) that people visit during their daily routines, are variable over hours, days, and weeks due to routine work and leisure patterns, and change over months and years due to activities associated with different stages of childhood and adulthood. Over different periods of life the sources of air pollution can be many and variable; they occur at home (cooking, heating), outdoors and during journeys (traffic, industry, shipping, aircraft), and work (i.e. various 'occupational' exposures). Capturing representative information on exposures, particularly for active population subgroups, for even relatively short periods of life, is thus challenging.

Air pollution monitoring has been ongoing in developed countries for decades. The United Kingdom, for example, has a network of air pollution monitors for black smoke (BS) and sulphur dioxide (SO_2) in operation since 1955. In the last 20 years technology has been developed to allow automatic monitoring of a range of air pollutants (e.g. nitrogen dioxide, particulates, ozone) at high temporal resolution (i.e. < 1 hour) using different measurement techniques depending on the type of pollutant. Many medium-to-large cities typically have continuous measurement of air pollutants at one or more dedicated (i.e. fixed-site) locations. Some mega-cities have detailed networks of air pollution monitors; London, for example, has over 100 measurement site locations as part of the national 'Automatic Urban and Rural Network' (AURN) and is supplemented by local government sites. These sites provide the basis both for monitoring changes in air quality to provide information to the public on the air that they breathe and as a policy tool for assessing emissions interventions and controls (e.g. low emissions zones, congestion charging). To what extent these sites provide information representative of air pollution exposures in an epidemiological context is questionable. Using the nearest air pollution monitor, for example, has been shown to be a poor marker for exposure (Gulliver et al. 2011), especially in urban areas that are characterized by complex air pollution surfaces due to dense transport networks, buildings, industrial sources, and terrain.

Portable air pollution sensors if sufficiently small and lightweight offer an opportunity to measure more 'personalized' exposures (e.g. the VE³SPA study; Montagne et al. 2013). These sensors are becoming more portable and cost-effective and can be used on a relatively small number of individuals (e.g. cohort or panel studies). For large numbers of individuals air pollution monitoring is not practical.

For large cohorts or population-wide studies the alternatives are models or proxies of exposures. Most exposure assessments have, however, been simple and crude, providing proximity measures (e.g. distance from road) or relying on extrapolation from measurements of air pollution concentrations. Methods such as spatial interpolation (e.g. inverse-distance weighting, splines, trend surface analysis) and geo-statistical techniques (e.g. Kriging) can provide large geographical scale surfaces from monitored concentrations (Jerrett et al. 2005), but have been shown to perform poorly where monitoring networks are sparse or over complex urban surfaces (Gulliver et al. 2011). Combining background air pollution measurements with information on proximity to locally varying sources (e.g. roads) can improve spatial resolution of exposure estimates (Hoek et al. 2001), but this does not allow for consideration of the variations in source emissions over time.

Two techniques have been developed which are now widely used to undertake air pollution exposure assessment: dispersion modelling and land use regression (LUR) modelling (also known as regression mapping). Whilst dispersion modelling would likely be the preferred method as it simulates the physical characteristics of the dispersion environment (Carruthers et al. 2000), it is often impractical for exposure assessment for the following reasons: (1) most areas do not have detailed emissions inventories for different air pollutants, (2) it is computationally intensive for large geographical areas, and (3) most dispersion models are run without considering the spatially varying influence of land cover (types of land use, buildings etc.).

Epidemiological studies thus increasingly turn to LUR modelling as an alternative to dispersion modelling. LUR modelling, developed by Briggs et al. (1997, 2000) in the United Kingdom, uses proximity measures such as distance and circular buffers of varying sizes to summarize around point locations (i.e. monitoring sites, addresses) geographical features (e.g. land use, road networks, traffic, terrain, etc.) which explain variability in monitored concentrations. The intersection of buffers with geographical features and measures of distance to sources are undertaken in a geographical information system (GIS). A typical model might have 50–100 variables being considered for inclusion. The variables are assessed one by one, or grouped by variables type (e.g. roads), in regression analysis in terms of their correlation with monitored concentrations of air pollution and then in combination to find the best set of variables (i.e. variables that collectively explain the highest proportion of variation in monitored concentrations). Models are typically developed against a set of 'training' monitoring sites and evaluated on a set of 'test' (i.e. held-out) monitoring sites from the same monitoring network.

Many different LUR models have been developed over the last 15 years. Two substantive reviews of the structure and application of LUR models have been done in recent years (Ryan and LeMasters 2007; Hoek et al. 2008). In many locations it is not possible, however, to develop LUR models due to a lack of information on monitored concentrations of pollutants and/or information on source emissions. One option is to consider using a model developed elsewhere or from a different time period. These reviews raise questions about the transferability of LUR models in space (between different cities, from small areas to larger areas etc.) and time (i.e. back extrapolation), but so far these issues have not received much attention. Important considerations in the transfer of LUR models are threefold: (1) are the types and resolution of source data comparable between the area where the model was developed and the area where it will be applied, (2) have the sources of air pollution changed over space and/or time, (3) is there air pollution monitoring data in the area where the LUR model will be applied to either evaluate the transfer of an existing model or calibrate the model for the target area/time period?

This chapter describes how to undertake the various steps in LUR modelling from initial data collection through to model evaluation (see 'Developing land use regression models' section); the goal is to provide practical guidelines (i.e. dos and don'ts) for undertaking LUR modelling. The 'Transferability of LUR models in space and time' section addresses the issue of transferring land use regression models in space and time between different areas (i.e. city-wide or regional models) of the United Kingdom, and extrapolating models to different time periods both within areas where models have been developed and to other areas without locally developed models.

Developing land use regression models

Requirements for LUR modelling

It is firstly important to understand the data and software requirements for LUR:

1. Monitoring site coordinates (X, Y) with monitored concentrations of air pollutants for the period of study (i.e. months, years) (these data are used to develop and evaluate the performance (i.e. validation) of the resulting LUR model).

2. GIS data that represent the emissions sources (e.g. road geography, traffic flows, area of industrial land, housing, and population) and characteristics of the dispersion environment (altitude, terrain, meteorology, buildings).

3. GIS software for developing and extracting information on potential explanatory variables and multivariate statistical software for regression analysis.

Monitored concentrations of air pollutants

Many cities have either their own municipal monitoring networks (e.g. http://www.londonair.org) or contain monitoring sites which are part of a national network (e.g. http://www.airquality.co.uk) usually administered by government agencies. For some pollutants (e.g. fine particulates) there often will only be a handful of monitoring sites within even larger cities and many small-to-medium urban areas will not have air pollution monitoring. It is therefore often necessary to undertake bespoke air pollution monitoring campaigns, particularly in relation to epidemiological studies (Cyrys et al. 2012; Eeftens et al. 2012b), to obtain a sufficiently dense network of monitoring sites to get a representative sample of air pollution variability across the population being studied. There is no rule on the minimum numbers of sites that are needed to develop an LUR model, but typically a minimum of 30–40 sites will be used; it may be possible to develop models with as few as 20 sites where the study area is relatively small or the emissions sources and geographical characteristics of the dispersion environment are fairly homogeneous. Indeed, in the Netherlands, LUR models were shown to be valid when 20–30 air pollution measurement sites were used to develop models (Wang et al. 2012).

Ideally, monitoring sites will represent a range of site types (e.g. roadside, industrial land, urban background, remote/rural, coastal/inland) with a focus on residential areas if the purpose of the LUR model is for population exposure assessment. Roadside sites should furthermore be representative of the range of traffic flows in the area and characteristics such as street canyons, arterial roads in open suburbia, etc.

Predictor variables

GIS data needs to be of sufficient spatial resolution to accurately depict emission sources and the dispersion environment with respect to the geographical units being used for exposure assessment (e.g. address, postcode, census tract). Ryan and LeMasters (2007) provide a review of the different types of variables used in different studies over the first 10 years after LUR was introduced.

Road traffic is the major source of air pollution in many urban areas and is often ubiquitous because of dense road networks. Ready-made data on road geography is commonplace and some areas will also have access to information on traffic volumes on main roads. Data on land cover is also usually available or can be derived using remote sensing techniques or digitized from aerial photographs. Although there may be highly resolved land cover data at the local level, where harmonized LUR approaches (i.e. consistent exposure assessment) are needed at national or international level (e.g. multicity cohort studies) more coarse land cover data might be used; for example, in the ESCAPE project (Eeftens et al. 2012a; Beelen et al. 2013; de Hoogh et al. 2013) the CORINE pan-European land cover data set was used to provide a harmonized data input for all areas even though better data was available in some study areas.

Many LUR models include data on population as a surrogate for emissions related to domestic heating, domestic wood burning, or perhaps emissions from minor road sources not included in traffic data sets. Some LUR models include information on both population and land cover categories for housing from the same zones, but this raises questions about 'double-counting' of emissions sources as population and housing density overlap.

Traffic and land cover classes for the built environment (housing, industry, etc.) are expected to have a positive direction of effect (i.e. increase) on air pollution concentrations. Sometimes 'natural' rural land cover classes are included in LUR models to have a negative effect on pollutant concentrations (i.e. decrease). Open areas of water or woodland, for example, may be useful in LUR to represent locations with no source emissions. Some rural land cover classes might on the other hand represent areas associated with pollution emissions (e.g. farming, bio-composting etc.).

Many countries have digital models of terrain (DTM) and elevation (DEM) through national mapping agencies, typically of spatial resolution between 10 and 100 m from which altitude can be derived for point (e.g. monitoring site) locations. Where not available locally there are international models at coarser resolution (e.g. SRTM 90 m Digital Elevation Data (http://srtm.csi.cgiar.org/)).

GIS software

Preparing data and extracting variables from GIS for LUR modelling is relatively straightforward due to the major improvements in computing power and menu-driven GIS software. There are a wide range of commercially available GIS software with a growing number of freely available open-source GIS. Moreover, open-source statistical software (e.g. R) means that LUR modelling is open to everyone who can obtain both data representative of emissions sources and the dispersion environment and modest computing power.

Developing land use regression models

The typical set of steps involved in developing and applying an LUR model are: (1) extract predictor variables for different monitoring site locations, (2) use regression analysis to determine the 'best' set of predictor variables and associated coefficients (i.e. 'weights'), and (3) apply the model at locations for exposure assessment. Fig. 7.3.1 summarizes the steps taken to develop an LUR model with variables on traffic and housing.

Variables for LUR are normally extracted from digital data in a GIS. Each variable type (e.g. roads, land cover) is usually summarized using circular 'buffers' of increasing radii (i.e. using GIS tool/functions) to represent the distances up to which (i.e. sphere of influence) source emissions should affect concentrations at each location (i.e. air pollution monitoring sites). Variables for road length, for example, might be summarized in circular buffers (i.e. sum of road length) at 50 m intervals up to 1000 m, but it is unlikely in most situations that roads beyond this distance would directly influence air pollution concentrations. In addition to circles, measures of distance (e.g. distance to road, distance to coast etc.) can be calculated in GIS for LUR using standard functions (i.e. 'NEAR').

Regression analysis

The next stage is to undertake the regression analysis to select variables for inclusion in the model. Variables extracted for each monitoring site location in a GIS are usually exported to statistical software for the regression analysis. The goal of regression analysis is to select the variable(s) that explain the highest proportion of variability in pollutant concentrations at monitoring site locations. The

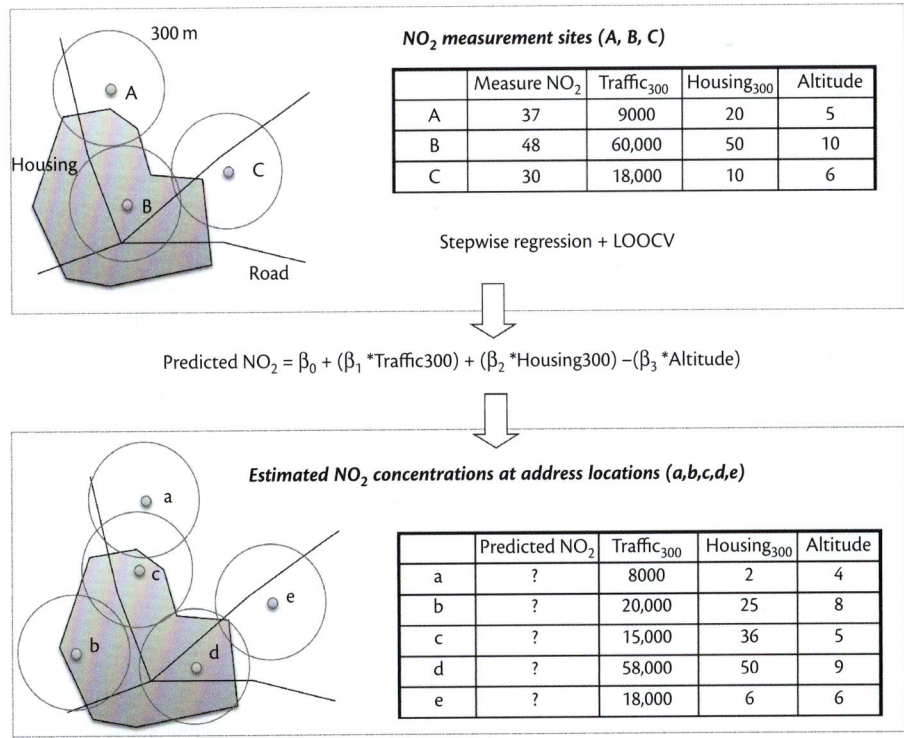

Fig. 7.3.1 Steps undertaken in a GIS to extract and summarize predictor variables.

focus of this procedure is thus to maximize the correlation between the predictions and observations whilst minimizing model errors.

There is no singly recognized process for regression analysis, but a general set of 'rules' has evolved for the development of LUR models as shown in Box 7.3.1 (see also Hoek et al. 2008).

Su et al. (2009) suggested a formalized procedure for the development of LUR called ADDRESS: 'A Distance Decay REgression Selection Strategy'. This method is essentially the same as the one described in Box 7.3.1 but ADDRESS used a graphic representation of the changes in the correlation (R^2) between each variables and measured concentrations with different buffer distances.

The most common statistical measure used to assess the process of model building is the coefficient of determination, and commonly referred to as R^2 (pronounced as 'R-squared'). In essence, this is a measure of error between observations (e.g. pollutant concentrations) and predictions expressed as a proportion of the overall variability in observations:

$$R^2 = \frac{SSE}{SSy} = 1 - \frac{\sum\limits_{i=1}^{n}(O_C - P_C)^2}{\sum\limits_{i=1}^{n}(O_C - \bar{O}_C)^2} \quad (7.3.1)$$

Where:

SSE is the sum of the square of errors between observations and model predictions.

SSy is the sum of the squares of the observations (e.g. measured concentrations)—in other words, the sum of the squared differences between each observation and the mean of all observations (i.e. similar to variance).

O_C is each observation (e.g. measured concentration).

P_C is each model prediction (i.e. prediction at each monitoring site from a given set of LUR variables).

$\bar{O}_C$ is the mean of observations.

Values of R^2 range from 0 to 1. Thus, R^2 will tend towards a value of 1 if errors are small relative to the variance in measured concentrations of pollutants; conversely, if errors are large relative to the variance in measured concentrations then R^2 will tend towards zero. Values of r^2 (i.e. 'r' for a single variable) are the same as the square of Pearson's correlation coefficient (r) when an intercept is included in the model and the outcome (i.e. measured concentration) is predicted from only one explanatory variable. If an intercept is included and there are multiple variables then the coefficient of determination (R^2) is used.

A variant of R^2 is the adjusted R^2 (i.e. adj.R^2). A model with ten variables is likely to be less robust (i.e. it is unlikely that, e.g. variables 6 to 10 are very strong predictors) than a model with three to four strong variables. Thus the adj.R^2 penalizes the R^2 for the number of parameters in the model:

$$adj.R^2 = 1 - \left[\frac{(1 - R^2)(n-1)}{n-k-1}\right] \quad (7.3.2)$$

where:

n is the number of observations (outcomes) in the regression.

k is the number of parameters in the regression not counting the constant.

Box 7.3.1 Guidelines for creating regression models

1. Before the LUR model development perform descriptive analyses:
   a. Plot distributions of concentrations and predictor variables (e.g. boxplots to assess variation and outliers).
   b. Check for normality of measured concentrations (consider log-transformation of data for skewed distributions).
   c. Correlation between predictor variables to check for collinearity.
2. Try to enter explanatory variables in a supervised stepwise manner, so that you include your most important predictors first.
3. The sign for each coefficient in the model must conform to the expected direction of effect (i.e. positive values for emissions sources and negative values for variables which represent areas without emissions sources, e.g. semi-natural land).
4. Variable with highest increase in adjusted R^2 should be included if:
   a. increase in adjusted R^2 > 1 per cent (a typical threshold)
   b. β coefficient has pre-specified direction
   c. direction for other variables does not change.
5. Each variable in the model should be significant (e.g. $p < 0.05$).
6. Following point 2, variables entered later in the process should not be maintained if they cause variables already in the model to invalidate guidelines 3, 4, or 5.
7. Avoid double counting by excluding overlapping buffers. For example, including roads in 0–20 m and 20–40 m is valid, but including roads in 0–20 m and 0–40 m is not.
8. Gaps in the buffers should also be avoided. For example, roads in 20–40 m should not be included unless roads in 0–20 m is already in your model.
9. Final model checked for:
   a. influential observations: Cook's D
   b. heteroscedasticity of the residuals
   c. normality of the residuals
   d. spatial autocorrelation of the residuals (kriging or Moran's I).

As Equation 7.3.2 implies, the larger the number of parameters (k) in the model then the lower the adj.R^2. Adjusted R^2 is not normally used in model evaluation (see later) as the comparison then is univariate (i.e. the predicted concentrations compared to the measured concentrations).

In seeking as high as possible correlation between the predictor variables and the observations, the goal is also to reduce the model prediction errors; errors are commonly assessed in model development by the standard error of the estimate (SEE). SEE is defined in Equation 7.3.3:

$$SEE = \frac{\sqrt{\sum(Y - Y')^2}}{N} \quad (7.3.3)$$

where:

Y is the observed value (measurement concentration at a monitoring site).

Y' is the prediction for a given set of variables.

N is the number of pairs of observations and predictions.

One concern in multiple-regression is collinearity between model variables (i.e. 'double-counting'). The variance inflation factor (VIF) is a useful indicator of collinearity between variables at each stage of model development. As a general rule, values of VIFs less than 5 are acceptable but LUR models often use a more stringent threshold (e.g. maximum VIF of 3); that is, as applied in the ESCAPE study (e.g. Eeftens et al. 2012a; Beelen et al. 2013). In LUR, collinearity might occur when overlapping buffers are used (e.g. road length in buffers 0–100 m and 0–200 m) or variable types are included more than once (e.g. urban land within 1000 m and housing within 1000 m), hence the guidelines for handling variables in LUR shown in Box 7.3.1.

Cook's distance is a method of identifying outliers in model development. For example, one or two sites might supress the predictive capacity of a particular variable because their site characteristics are unusual; Cook's distance is particularly useful to filter out problematic sites when the number of sites used for model development is relatively small.

Model errors should be checked for heteroscedasticity (i.e. model errors should be proportionally the same over the range of pollutant concentrations) and normally distributed—prerequisites of regression modelling. Finally it is useful to map model residuals (standardized by concentration) to see whether models perform poorly in a particular part of the study area (i.e. clustering of residuals). Moran's I (Getis and Ord 1992) is commonly used, and available in some GIS software, as a quick, 'one-shot' assessment of whether model residuals are spatially dependent; in other words, Moran's I (denoted by 'Z') is used to detect whether there are clusters of relatively large residuals from the LUR model. A value of −1 represents complete dispersion, a value of zero represents a completely random distribution of residuals, and a value of 1 represents complete clustering of residuals. A value of Moran's I tending towards 1 and statistically significant ($p < 0.05$), indicates that the model is not working well in a particular part of the study area, which may relate to one or more weak variables in the model.

Evaluating model performance

In convincing the rest of the world that your model is valid for use in exposure assessment, it is commonplace to compare predicted concentrations from models with measured concentrations from fixed-site air pollution monitors. The most useful assessment of model performance is to make predictions for locations that were not used to develop the parameters in the model (i.e. an independent test).

One possibility is to select some of the 'pool' of sites for model development and reserve some sites for model evaluation. The evaluation sites are often referred to as 'out-of-sample' or 'held-out' based on methods development in statistics. In the development of national scale models for historic exposure assessment of BS and SO_2 Gulliver et al. (2011), for example, made a stratified random sample of 75 per cent of sites to be used for model development and used the remaining 25 per cent of sites for model evaluation. The stratification was to ensure a representative numbers of each monitoring location by site type (i.e. residential, industrial, rural, etc.) and by geographic location (i.e. region) both in the training and evaluation sets. Out-of-sample evaluations are often constrained, however, by the number of available monitoring sites so other approaches are

needed for model evaluation. In situations where the number of sites available for LUR modelling is relatively low (e.g. 20–40) then cross-validation is often applied. Leave-one-out-cross-validation (LOOCV) has been used in several LUR studies with limited monitoring sites (Basagaña et al. 2012; Wang et al. 2012). LOOCV operates, as the name suggests, by re-running the regression analysis with one monitoring site removed from the training data each time ($n − 1$ sites) to derive new coefficients for model variables and then predict the pollutant concentration for the removed site. This is repeated for all sites in turn and then model performance is assessed on the LOOCV predictions.

A range of performance statistics have been used to evaluate LUR models. Commonly used measures are summarized in Table 7.3.1 including a description of their purpose.

Case study on model development and evaluation

This next section applies the procedures just described to develop and evaluate an LUR model for a real-world example. As part of the multicentre ESCAPE (European Study of Cohorts and Air Pollution Effects) project, a bespoke measurement campaign for particulate matter (PM_{10}, $PM_{2.5}$, PM_{coarse}, $PM_{2.5}$ absorbance) and oxides of nitrogen (NO_X, NO_2) was undertaken in the Thames Valley region (i.e. London and the surrounding area towards Oxford) during 2010 as the basis for developing LUR models (Cyrys et al. 2012; Eeftens et al. 2012b). Routine monitoring sites were not used in the ESCAPE study because they are not comparable across Europe (i.e. different measurement techniques) and the location of routine monitoring sites do not capture the full extent of intra-urban variation of air pollution. The Thames Valley study area lies in the South East of England and has a total population of approximately 15.5 million with around 8 million people living in the area known as Greater London (Fig. 7.3.2). The area is characterized by road traffic—especially in the cities of London, Oxford, and Reading—housing, commercial buildings, light industry, and mainly covers gently undulating, lowland terrain.

Monitoring sites were chosen to reflect areas with different geographical characteristics and the distribution of population, hence the highest concentration of sites in the Thames Valley study is in London (see Fig. 7.3.2).

The measurement data collected for NO_2 in the Thames Valley area are used here to demonstrate the main processes involved in developing an LUR model. During ESCAPE, air pollution monitoring was also undertaken in Bradford. The Bradford study area (Fig. 7.3.2) encompasses the metropolitan borough of Bradford, which includes surrounding centres like Keighley and Bingley. Bradford is the fourth largest metropolitan district in England with a population of 2.4 million and is located on the eastern foothills of the Pennine hills in West Yorkshire. Data from the Bradford monitoring sites are used in the 'Transferability of land use regression models in space and time' section to illustrate the transferability of LUR models. Forty sites in Thames Valley were identified in different locations (i.e. roadside, urban background, suburban, remote/rural) for deploying passive samplers (Ogawa, http://www.ogawausa.com) (Roosbroeck van et al. 2006) to measure concentrations of NO_2 over 2 weeks at three times (warm, cold, and one other period) during 2010. Values of NO_2 were averaged over all periods to create long-term (i.e. annual) concentrations of NO_2 for each

Table 7.3.1 Performance statistics used to evaluate LUR models.

Performance statistic	Description	Equation	Comments
R	Correlation coefficient	$$\dfrac{\sum_{i=1}^{n}(O_C-\overline{O}_C)(P_C-\overline{P}_C)}{\sqrt{\sum_{i=1}^{n}(O_C-\overline{O}_C)^2\sum_{i=1}^{n}(P_C-\overline{P}_C)^2}}$$	This is the formula for the commonly used Pearson's correlation coefficient. Alternatively, Spearman's correlation is used where ranking is important or where the observed data are not normally distributed
R^2	Coefficient of determination	$$1-\dfrac{\sum_{i=1}^{n}(O_C-P_C)^2}{\sum_{i=1}^{n}(O_C-\overline{O}_C)^2}$$	The proportion of variation in measured (observed) concentrations explained by the model. In other words, one minus the sum of squares of the residuals divided by the total sum of squares (proportional to the variance of the measured concentrations). This is not the same as $(R)^2$ returned by some statistical software, which is simply the square of the correlation coefficient
MSE	Mean squared error	$$\dfrac{1}{n}\sum_{i=1}^{n}(O_C-P_C)^2$$	The mean of the squares of residuals. Also used as the numerator in MSE-based R^2
MSE-based R^2	MSE rescaled to be comparable to R^2	$$1-\dfrac{MSE}{\dfrac{1}{n}\sum_{i=1}^{n}(O_C-\overline{O}_C)^2}$$	Equivalent to the coefficient of determination but differently written to be applied in model evaluation for comparison around the 1:1 line
RMSE	Root mean squared error	$$\sqrt{\dfrac{1}{n}\sum_{i=1}^{n}(O_C-P_C)^2}$$	The average error and is comparable to absolute concentrations
FAC2	Factor of 2	$$\dfrac{1}{2}O_C\le P_C\le 2O_C$$	The percentage of predictions in the range of one half and double the observed concentrations
FB	Fractional bias	$$2\left(\dfrac{\overline{O}_C-\overline{P}_C}{\overline{O}_C+\overline{P}_C}\right)$$	A measure of overall bias by comparing the mean of the observations with the mean of the predictions
IOA	Index of agreement	$$1-\dfrac{\sum_{i=1}^{n}(O_C-P_C)^2}{\sum_{i=1}^{n}[(O_C-\overline{O}_C)+(P_C-\overline{O}_C)]^2}$$	The index is based on squared differences between predicted and observed values and it varies between 0 (complete disagreement) and 1

O_C, observed concentration; P_C predicted concentration; $\overline{O}_C$, mean of observed concentrations; $\overline{P}_C$, mean of predicted concentrations.

measurement location. LUR models were developed in 36 ESCAPE areas for NO_2 using harmonized digital data to develop predictor variables. Further details of the measurements and models can be found in Cyrys et al. (2012), Eeftens et al. (2012a, 2012b), Beelen et al. (2013), and de Hoogh et al. (2013).

For the Thames Valley area, 80 different variables were created including information on distance to the nearest road, traffic flow on the nearest road, and circular buffers for road length, traffic intensity (the sum of road length multiplied by traffic flow on each road), low- and high-density housing, industry, population counts, and urban green space. For land cover variables, the pan-European CORINE data set was used (http://www.eea.europa.eu). Variables relating to roads were developed from a central data set (Eurostreets version 3.1 digital road network (1:10,000 resolution) derived from the TeleAtlas MultiNet) for the year 2008. Traffic composition was obtained in the United Kingdom from the Department of Transport. Road and traffic intensity variables were extracted in circular buffers of 25, 50, 100, 300, 500, and 1000 m reflecting the local influence of these sources on air pollution levels. Land cover variables were extracted in buffer distances of 100, 300, 500, 1000, and 5000 m. Buffer distances of 1000 m and more were included to reflect regional influences, not picked up by the smaller buffers.

An LUR model was developed for Thames Valley according to the procedure described in the 'Developing land use regression models' section (also see Box 7.3.1). Table 7.3.2 shows model development from the first stage (i.e. the initial strongest variable) to the final model, which includes three variables. Values of β represent the coefficients (i.e. 'weights') applied to each variable and values for the statistical significance are denoted by 'Sig. (*p*)'. Each model includes a constant (i.e. intercept) to represent 'background' concentrations; in other words, the constant is the value of NO_2 concentration at locations where there are assumed to be no detectable source emissions.

As shown in Table 7.3.2, the strongest predictor variable at stage 1 is 'HEAVYTRAFLOAD50' (i.e. the sum of the number of heavy goods vehicles multiplied by road length within 50 m) which explains approximately 67 per cent of the variability in measured concentrations of NO_2. At stage 2 a variable for road length within 500 m is added to the model which increases the adjusted R^2 to approximately 83 per cent. At stage 3 a variable for housing (HLDRES5000) is added to represent the diffuse emission from housing and minor roads otherwise not included in the model. At stage 4, the previously strongest variable (HEAVYTRAFLOAD50) is removed from the model (p > 0.1) and replaced by a similar

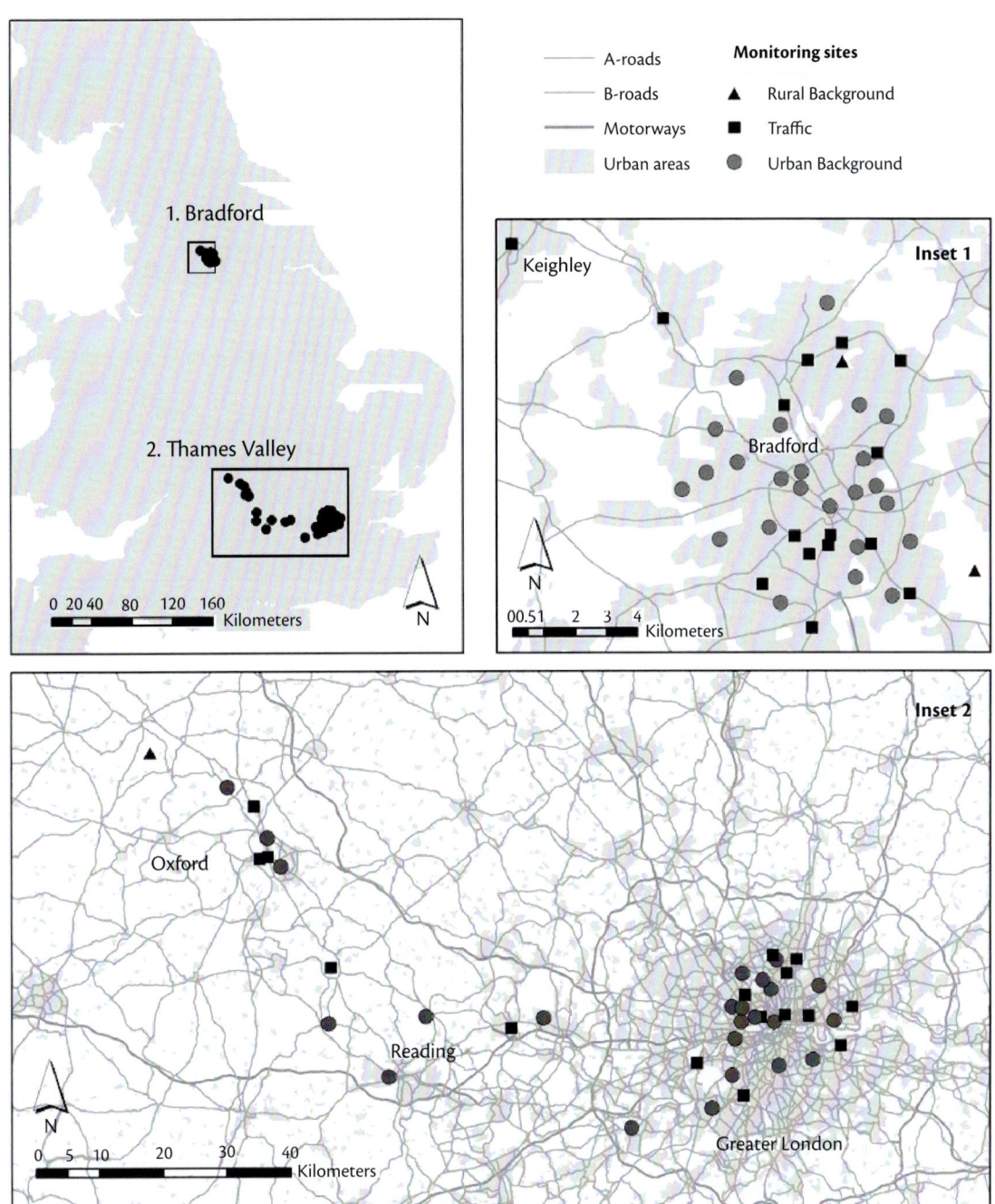

Fig. 7.3.2 Monitoring site locations for the Thames Valley and Bradford study areas.
Source: data from *Atmospheric Environment*, Volume 62, Cyrys, J. et al., Variation of NO_2 and NO_x concentrations between and within 36 European study areas: results of the ESCAPE project Atmos, pp. 374–390, Copyright © 2012 Elsevier Ltd and *Atmospheric Environment*, Volume 62, Eeftens, M. et al., Spatial variation of PM2.5, PM10, PM2.5 absorbance and PMcoarse concentrations between and within 20 European study areas and the relationship with NO2—Results of the ESCAPE project, pp. 303–317, Copyright © 2012 Elsevier Ltd.

variable for all traffic (TRAFMAJORLOAD50) rather than heavy vehicles alone (NB: there was very little difference in the explained variability of these two variables at stage 1: approximately 67 per cent); variables for heavy traffic and all traffic on major roads within 50 m buffers are highly correlated as indicated by high values of VIFs (> 10). As with most LUR models, the variables added at later stages tend to increase the adjusted R^2 by decreasing amounts, until no variable can add more than 1 per cent to the adjusted R^2.

The final model (stage 4) includes three variables: traffic load within 50 m, road length within 50 m, and residential housing within 5000 m. Logically, road length within 50 m is an indicator of emissions from the nearest road(s), traffic load within 500 m is an indicator of the magnitude of traffic emissions in the wider area (i.e. beyond the nearest road), and housing within 5000 m represents emissions from domestic sources but may also represent traffic emissions from minor roads which are otherwise not included in the model. The model explains approximately 89 per cent of the

Table 7.3.2 Stages of model development for the Thames Valley LUR model (n = 40)

Stage	Variable	B	R^2	Adj.R^2	Sig. (p)	VIF	SEE
1	(Constant)	30.19	0.671	0.662	0.000	–	10.40
	HEAVYTRAFLOAD50	0.0001500			0.000	1.000	
2	(Constant)	10.8515519	0.837	0.828	0.003	–	7.42
	ROADLENGTH500	0.0016410			0.000	1.120	
	HEAVYTRAFLOAD50	0.0001242			0.000	1.120	
3	(Constant)	9.90	0.864	0.852	0.004	–	6.89
	HLDRES5000	0.0000002			0.011	1.768	
	HEAVYTRAFLOAD50	0.0001204			0.000	1.136	
	ROADLENGTH500	0.0011237			0.001	1.805	
4	(Constant)	8.51	0.892	0.883	0.005	–	6.59
	TRAFMAJORLOAD50	0.0000073			0.000	1.082	
	ROADLENGTH500	0.0010971			0.000	1.806	
	HLDRES5000	0.0000002			0.000	1.747	

Source: data from *Atmospheric Environment*, Volume 72, Beelen, R., et al., Development of NO_2 and NO_x land use regression models for estimating air pollution exposure in 36 study areas in Europe—the ESCAPE project, pp. 10–23, Copyright © 2013 Elsevier Ltd.

Table 7.3.3 Performance statistics from LOOCV for the Thames Valley LUR model

β_0 (constant)	β_1	95% CI	R^2	MSE-R^2	RMSE	FB	p	Moran's I
1.12	0.97	0.84, 1.09	0.89	0.89	5.81	0.000	0.000	Z = 0.37 (p = 0.71)

Source: data from *Atmospheric Environment*, Volume 72, Beelen, R., et al., Development of NO_2 and NO_x land use regression models for estimating air pollution exposure in 36 study areas in Europe—the ESCAPE project, pp. 10–23, Copyright © 2013 Elsevier Ltd.

variability in monitored concentrations. The variables are associated with low values of VIF (i.e. < 2), values of statistical significance are all substantially less than 0.05.

Due to the relatively low number of sites available in the Thames Valley area, the ESCAPE NO_2 LUR model was evaluated using LOOCV. The LOOCV R^2 (as shown in Table 7.3.3) is the same ($R^2 = 0.89$) as for model development ($R^2 = 0.89$). Table 7.3.3 also shows some of the more informative of the summary statistics that are described in Table 7.3.1. Also included is the slope of the regression line (β) and 95 per cent confidence intervals associated with the regression fit. A good model performance will result in the lower and upper bounds of the confidence intervals intersecting with a value of 1.

Table 7.3.3 also shows performance statistics for Moran's I (Getis and Ord 1992) which is a measure of spatial autocorrelation in the model residuals. In the case of the Thames Valley model evaluation, Moran's I of 0.37 was returned indicating slight clustering of residuals, but this was not statistically significant (p = 0.71).

Figure 7.3.3 shows a comparison of predictions (x-axis) and measured values (y-axis). In the perfect model, all points would lie on the 1:1 line shown on the graph. The regression line represents the best-fit line for the model predictions. In essence, the closer the

best fit line lies to the 1:1 line then the better the fit of the model; the aim is for beta to have a value close to 1 and the constant to be small (i.e. $y = \beta_0 + X\beta_1$). As Table 7.3.3 shows, the slope of the regression line (measured $NO_2 = 1.119 + (0.968 \times LOOCV\ NO_2)$) means the model evaluation is close to 1:1. As shown in Fig. 7.3.3 and via the summary statistics in Table 7.3.3 the LUR model appears valid for exposure assessment in Thames Valley.

Transferability of land use regression models in space and time

In order to develop LUR models it is necessary to collect/obtain both measured concentrations for the pollutant of interest and GIS predictor variables covering the entire study area. It may be possible to convert an LUR model developed for one pollutant to another (e.g. $PM_{2.5}$ to NO_X) for the same area if the pollutants are known to be highly correlated, or there is an established method to convert between them (e.g. receptor modelling; Stedman et al. 2001). It may also be possible to transfer LUR models developed in one area to another in both space and time. This does, however, raise concerns about the 'transferability' of models due to differences in source emissions and geographical characteristics of the distribution of sources (i.e. urban form).

The transferability of LUR models in space and time is illustrated here with an example from the recent ESCAPE study. Some cohorts within this study were intended for a larger area than the study area (i.e. the area where measurements took place). In the United Kingdom, for example, the LUR models based on measurement in Thames Valley (see Fig. 7.3.2) were intended to provide exposure estimates for three cohorts, a proportion of which live or have moved outside the study area.

An analysis was undertaken to see if the Thames Valley LUR model for NO_2 could be applied to measurement sites outside the study area—transferability in space. Moreover, the timeline

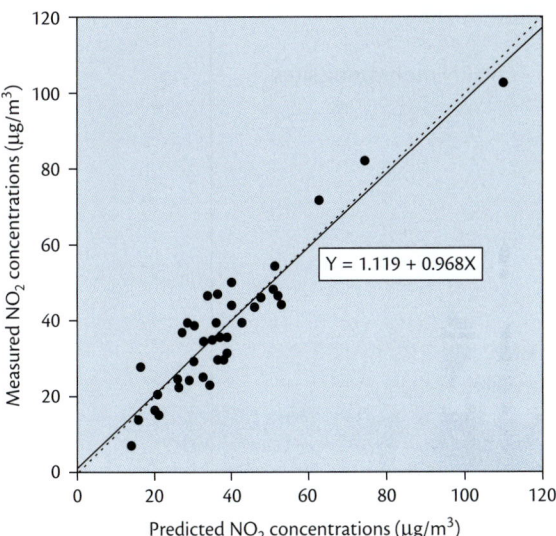

Fig. 7.3.3 Predicted versus measured NO_2 concentrations from LOOCV.
Source: data from *Atmospheric Environment*, Volume 72, Beelen, R., et al., Development of NO_2 and NO_x land use regression models for estimating air pollution exposure in 36 study areas in Europe—the ESCAPE project, pp. 10–23, Copyright © 2013 Elsevier Ltd.

Table 7.3.4 Summary statistics from transfer of the Thames Valley model to Bradford measurement sites.

R^2	MSE-R^2	RMSE	Regression line
0.42	0.00	15.01	Y = 13.10 + X*1.01

Table 7.3.5 Performance of the Thames Valley LUR model both within and outside the study area and over time (2010 to 1999) at AURN monitoring sites

Year	≤10 km		>10–≤100 km		>100–≤200 km		> 200 km	
	R^2	n	R^2	n	R^2	n	R^2	n
2010	0.856	12	0.591	31	0.716	28	0.555	29
2009	0.908	12	0.526	31	0.785	27	0.517	25
2008	0.891	14	0.533	33	0.745	22	0.531	27
2007	0.856	12	0.587	29	0.817	20	0.531	24
2006	0.582	19	0.498	30	0.790	23	0.450	23
2005	0.581	22	0.494	28	0.792	21	0.423	20
2004	0.601	21	0.503	29	0.757	27	0.327	21
2003	0.659	16	0.389	26	0.748	24	0.213	18
2002	0.608	20	0.433	27	0.748	23	0.247	18
2001	0.545	22	0.430	24	0.709	22	0.225	18
2000	0.557	22	0.518	21	0.741	21	0.117	12
1999	0.616	23	0.584	16	0.442	20	0.149	12

of cohorts (start-up, first follow-up, second follow-up, etc.) rarely coincides with the time period of the measurement data used to develop the LUR model. For example, the ESCAPE LUR model represents annual mean NO_2 concentrations for 2010, whereas EPIC Oxford, one of the cohorts in the ESCAPE study, started in 1993 and had follow-ups in 2001/2002 and 2007/2008. We therefore also had to assess how well the LUR model for 2010 predicts air pollution exposures going back in time—transferability in time. In order to investigate both these issues (space and time) we used monitoring sites from the Automatic Urban Rural Network (AURN; http://www.airquality.co.uk) covering the whole of the United Kingdom, measured over a long period (1994 to present), and independent from the model development.

Table 7.3.4 shows the performance statistics resulting from applying the Thames Valley model to the Bradford monitoring sites. The R^2 (0.42) is substantially reduced compared to the R^2 (0.89) from the within-area model evaluation (see Table 7.3.3). The other performance statistics further suggest that there are problems in transferring the Thames Valley model to Bradford. A mean squared error (MSE)-R^2 of zero and the equations of the regression line show that, when transferred, the model provides a poor fit around unity (i.e. 1:1). Because the correlations are moderate to good rather than poor it would still be possible to calibrate the model transfer if there were some monitoring sites (i.e. AURN) within the target area. Otherwise the Thames Valley model under-predicts concentrations of NO_2 in Bradford by approximately 13 micrograms/m^3.

The analysis was extended to a national assessment of the transferability of the Thames Valley model in space and time. Table 7.3.5 shows the performance (R^2, n) of the Thames Valley model applied to AURN sites located inside the Thames Valley area (i.e. the area within 10 km of the area encompassing the ESCAPE measurement sites) and by distance bands radiating from the edge of the study area, from 2010 (i.e. ESCAPE NO_2 measurement year) back to 1999. Fig. 7.3.4 shows the location of AURN sites and the distance bands radiating from the edge of the Thames Valley study

area. The performance of the Thames Valley model at AURN sites within the study area is similar to that obtained in model evaluation (i.e. LOOCV shown in Table 7.3.3) for 2007–2010. For earlier years, model performance weakens (R^2: ~0.55–0.62) but is still in the range of what modellers would deem to be 'good' performance. The Thames Valley model performance is weaker at sites outside the study area for more recent years (i.e. 2007–2010). Model performance is broadly similar back in time in the middle distance bands (i.e. > 10–≤100km and > 100–≤ 200 km) but is much weaker for earlier years for sites further away from the Thames Valley area. It must be borne in mind, however, that performance measures for earlier years were calculated on relatively few sites, which might raise concern about robustness of the assessment. Furthermore, direct comparisons between years should be treated with caution as the site list changes over time (e.g. some sites present in 1999 were no longer in existence in later years; new sites have been deployed in later years).

Discussion

The transferability of LUR models in space and time (back-extrapolation) is a relatively recent pursuit motivated by the needs of epidemiological studies.

Some studies have transferred models in space either from one city to another (i.e. as shown here for the transfer of the Thames Valley model to Bradford) or have evaluated national-scale models in specific locations. A National LUR model for Switzerland (Liu

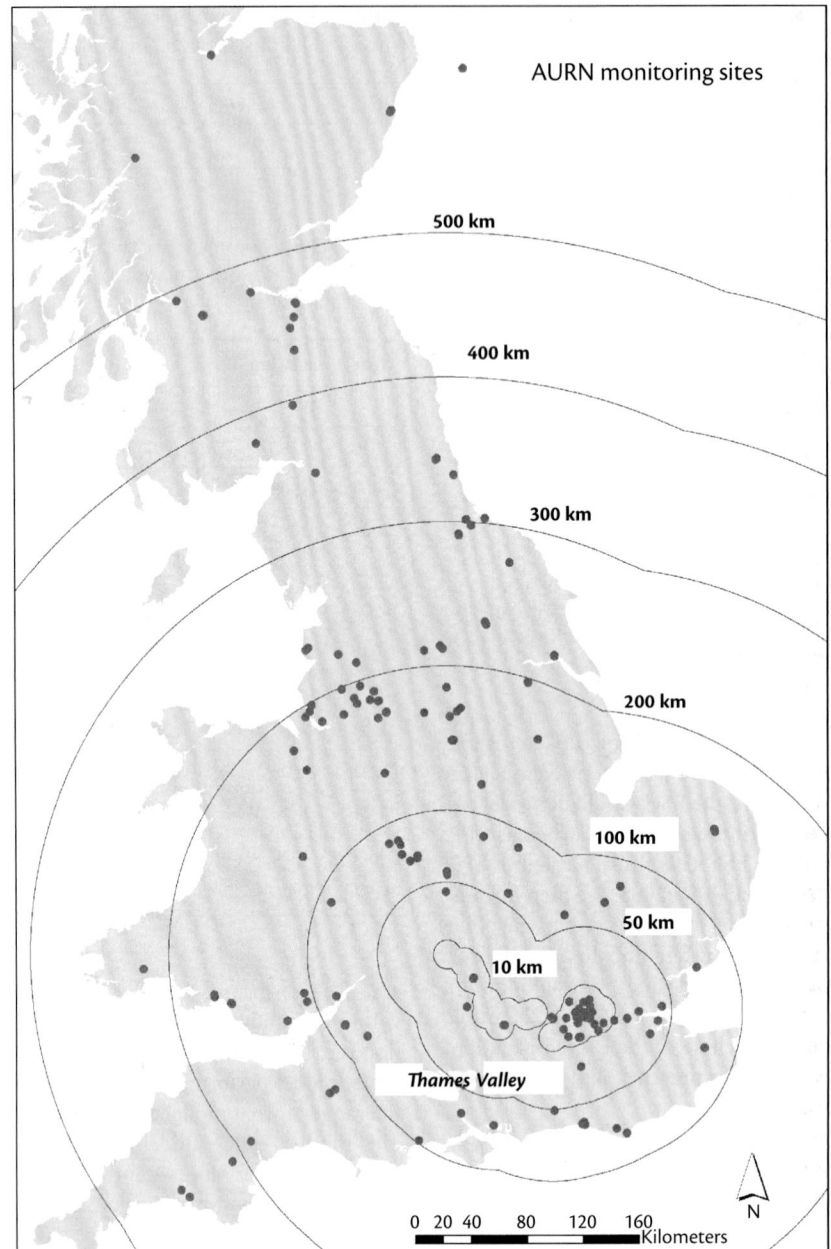

Fig. 7.3.4 Distance bands and location of UK routine monitoring sites

Source: data from Department for Environment, Food and Rural Affairs (DEFRA), *Interactive monitoring networks map*, © Crown Copyright 2014, and Defra via http://uk-air.defra.gov.uk/ licensed under the Open Government Licence, available from http://uk-air.defra.gov.uk/interactive-map?network=aurn.

et al. 2012) performed well in back-extrapolation to the early 1990s (R^2: ~0.80–0.84) but did not fit individual areas well (R^2: ~0.02–0.61). A national LUR model ($R^2 = 0.73$) in Canada (Hystad et al. 2011) was shown to be much weaker in some areas when evaluated against independent city-specific monitoring sites (R^2: ~0.18–0.60). It was suggested that differences in topography and meteorology led to weak model performance in some areas. Conversely, it was shown that one LUR model in the Netherlands (Eeftens et al. 2011) was sufficient to capture spatial variation in 1999/2000 and 2007, yielding model R^2 of 0.85 and 0.86, respectively, which may relate to fewer differences in topography and homogeneity of sources. Vienneau et al. (2010) showed that national models for

Great Britain and the Netherlands weakened when transferred but still provided satisfactory performance ($r^2 > 0.5$). Results of these assessments are mixed so care should be taken in transferring LUR models in space.

A few studies have transferred LUR models in time. An LUR model developed for 2007 NO_2 concentrations in Rome (Cesaroni et al. 2012) had strong linear correlation ($r = 0.83$) with measured NO_2 concentrations at the same monitoring locations ($n = 67$) 12 years earlier. In the Netherlands, LUR NO_2 models were transferred for 1999/2000 forward to 2007, and 2007 models back to 1999/2000; models slightly weakened when applied to other years but still explained 81 per cent and 77 per cent of the variation in monitored concentrations of NO_2, respectively (Eeftens et al. 2011). In the United Kingdom, back extrapolation of four different 2009 NO_2 models to 1991 monitoring sites (i.e. independent sites not used in model development) yielded values of MSE-R^2 of ~0.52–0.55 (Gulliver et al. 2013).

It is clear that models tend to perform less well when transferred in space and time than their performance in the study area where they were developed, but performance may still be acceptable. It is important in all cases, however, to consider a range of performance statistics. Taking the correlation (e.g. R, R^2) alone might be misleading as model transfer may result in a large degree of under- or overprediction, as seen here in the example of applying the Thames Valley model to the Bradford measurement sites. It is advisable to produce a range of performance statistics and plot the predictions against observations. Where possible also look at performance by different site types and if applying models over large geographical areas look at the performance stratified by space (e.g. regions or distance bands). LUR is a powerful and relatively easy to apply tool for exposure assessment, but it must be applied so that models reflect the sources contributing to air pollution concentrations and should be evaluated with a rigorous set of performance criteria. Even an LUR model that performs well will only provide information about outdoor air pollution at the address. 'Dynamic' models that both account for time-weighted exposures in different microenvironments and are applicable to cohorts or population wide studies are not yet available.

References

Basagaña, X., Rivera, M., Aguilera, I., et al. (2012). Effect of the number of measurement sites on land use regression models in estimating local air pollution. *Atmospheric Environment*, 54, 634–42.

Beelen, R., Hoek, G., Vienneau, D., et al. (2013). Development of NO_2 and NO_x land use regression models for estimating air pollution exposure in 36 study areas in Europe—the ESCAPE project. *Atmospheric Environment*, 72, 10–23.

Briggs D.J., Collins S., Elliott P., et al. (1997). Mapping urban air pollution using GIS: a regression-based approach. *International Journal of Geographical Information Science*, 11, 699–718.

Briggs, D.J., de Hoogh, C., Gulliver, J., et al. (2000). A regression-based method for mapping traffic-related air pollution: application and testing in four contrasting urban environments. *Science of the Total Environment*, 253(1–3), 151–67.

Carruthers D.J., Edmunds H.A., Lester A.E., McHugh C.A., and Singles R.A. (2000). Use and validation of ADMS-Urban in contrasting urban and industrial environments. *International Journal of Environmental Pollution*, 14, 1–6.

Cesaroni, G., Porta, D., Badaloni, C., et al. (2012). Nitrogen dioxide levels estimated from land use regression models several years apart and association with mortality in a large cohort study. *Environmental Health*, 11, 48.

Cyrys, J., Eeftens, M., Heinrich, J., et al. (2012). Variation of NO_2 and NO_x concentrations between and within 36 European study areas: results of the ESCAPE project. *Atmospheric Environment*, 62, 374–90.

de Hoogh, K., Wang, M., Adam, M., et al. (2013). Development of land use regression models for particle composition in 20 study areas in Europe. *Environmental Science & Technology*, 47(11), 5778–86.

Eeftens, M., Beelen, R., de Hoogh, K., et al. (2012a). Development of land use regression models for PM(2.5), PM(2.5) Absorbance, PM(10) and PM(coarse) in 20 European Study Areas; results of the ESCAPE Project. *Environmental Science & Technology*, 46(20), 11195–205.

Eeftens, M., Beelen, R., Fischer, P., Brunekreef, B., Meliefste, K., and Hoek, G. (2011). Stability of measured and modelled spatial contrasts in NO_2 over time. *Occupational and Environmental Medicine*, 68(10), 765–70.

Eeftens, M., Tsai, M., Ampe, C., Anwander, B., Brunekreef, B., and Hoek, G. (2012b). Spatial variation of PM2.5, PM10, PM2.5 absorbance and PM coarse concentrations between and within 20 European study areas and the relationship with NO_2—results of the ESCAPE project. *Atmospheric Environment*, 62, 303–17.

Getis, A. and Ord, J. K. (1992). The analysis of spatial association by use of distance statistics. *Geographical Analysis*, 24(3), 189–206.

Gulliver, J., de Hoogh, K., Hansell, A., and Vienneau, D. (2013). Development and back-extrapolation of NO_2 land use regression models for historic exposure assessment in Great Britain. *Environmental Science & Technology*, 47(14), 7804–11.

Gulliver, J., Vienneau, D., Fecht, D., de Hoogh, K., and Briggs, D. (2011). Comparative assessment of GIS-based methods and metrics for estimating long-term exposure to air pollution. *Atmospheric Environment*, 45(39), 7072–80.

Hoek, G., Beelen, R., de Hoogh, K., et al. (2008). A review of land-use regression models to assess spatial variation of outdoor air pollution. *Atmospheric Environment*, 42, 7561–78.

Hoek, G., Brunekreef, B., Goldbohm, S., Fischer, P., and van den Brandt, P.A. (2001). Association between mortality and indicators of traffic-related air pollution in the Netherlands: a cohort study. *The Lancet*, 360(9341), 1203–9.

Hystad, P., Setton, E., Cervantes, A., et al. (2011). Creating national air pollution models for population exposure assessment in Canada. *Environmental Health Perspectives*, 119(8), 1123–9.

Jerrett, M., Arain A., Kanaroglou, P., et al. (2005). A review and evaluation of intraurban air pollution exposure models. *Journal of Exposure Science & Environmental Epidemiology*, 15, 185–204.

Liu, L.J.S., Tsai, M., Keidel, D., et al. (2012). Long-term exposure models for traffic related NO_2 across geographically diverse areas over separate years. *Atmospheric Environment*, 46, 460–71.

Montagne, D., Hoek, G., Nieuwenhuijsen, M., et al. (2013). Agreement of land use regression models with personal exposure measurements of particulate matter and nitrogen oxides air pollution. *Environmental Science & Technology*, 47(15), 8523–31.

Roosbroeck, S., van Wichmann, J., Janssen, N.A.H., et al. (2006). Long-term personal exposure to traffic-related air pollution among school children, a validation study. *Science of the Total Environment*, 368, 565–73.

Ryan, P.H. and LeMasters, G.K. (2007). A review of land-use regression models for characterizing intraurban air pollution exposure. *Inhalation Toxicology*, 19(Suppl. 1), 127–33.

Stedman, J.R., Linehan, E., Conlan, B. (2001). Receptor modelling of PM10 concentrations at a United Kingdom national network monitoring site in central London, *Atmospheric Environment*, 2001, 35(2), 297–304.

Su, J.G., Jerrett, M., Beckerman, B., Wilhelm, M., Ghosh, J.K., Ritz, B. (2009). Predicting traffic-related air pollution in Los Angeles using a distance decay regression selection strategy, *Environmental Research*, 109(6), 657–70.

Vienneau, D., de Hoogh, K., Beelen, R., Fischer, P., Hoek, G., and Briggs, D. (2010). Comparison of land-use regression models between Great Britain and the Netherlands. *Atmospheric Environment*, 44, 688–96.

Wang, M., Beelen, R., Eeftens, M., Meliefste, K., Hoek, G., and Brunekreef, B. (2012). Systematic evaluation of land use regression models for NO_2. *Environmental Science & Technology*, 46(8), 4481–9.

Occupational health

David Koh and Tar-Ching Aw

Introduction to occupational health

The World Health Organization (WHO) estimated in 2007 that the global labour force (about 3300 million) was half of the world's population (WHO 2007a). The officially registered working population includes 60–70 per cent of the world's adult males and 30–60 per cent of adult females. Most people between the ages of 22 and 65 spend approximately 40 per cent of their waking hours at work (Leigh et al. 1997).

Occupational health, as defined by a joint committee of the WHO and the International Labour Organization (ILO), involves the 'promotion and maintenance of the highest degree of physical, mental and social wellbeing of workers in all occupations' (Forsmann 1983). This definition emphasizes the term health rather than disease, and further implies a multidisciplinary responsibility as well as a mechanism for the provision of health services for the working population. As practised today, the main components of occupational health practice are reduction of risks from exposure to workplace hazards, placement of workers with existing ill health or impaired function in jobs that will not pose an added risk to the individual or to others, and health protection and health promotion for those at work. In many countries, such activities extend beyond the worker to include provision of treatment and prevention for family members. For a summary of key points on occupational health see Box 7.4.1.

History and development

The Italian physician Bernardino Ramazzini (1633–1714) is often described as the 'Father of Occupational Medicine'. His publication in 1700, *De Morbis Artificum Diatriba*, was the seminal text in occupational medicine. Ramazzini stated that according to Hippocratic teaching, 'When you come to a patient's house, you should ask him what sort of pain he has, what caused them, how many days he has been ill, whether the bowels are working and what sort of food he eats' (Ramazzini 1713/1964). Following this citation, Ramazzini wrote: 'I may venture to add one more question: *What occupation does he follow?*' Ramazzini described many occupational illnesses that are still seen today, and the principles for their control.

The Industrial Revolution and occupational health

The major event that profoundly influenced the development of occupational health was the Industrial Revolution in the eighteenth century. Engineering and scientific innovations in the Western world, related to newly introduced industrial processes and the setting up of factories, led to dramatic social changes. Previously, work was done mainly by craftsmen in rural cottage industries. The Industrial Revolution resulted in work being carried out in factories in urban centres.

Effects were seen both within the community, as well as in the individual worker. Family life was disrupted, with men leaving their families and moving to work in new industrial areas. In these new areas, health and social problems emerged, for example, poor housing and sanitation, alcoholism, prostitution, and poverty. Inside factories, individuals were exposed to long hours of work and uncontrolled occupational hazards, and the risk of accidents. Child labour and apprenticeship of young children were commonplace, and there was an absence of labour legislation.

As problems of industrialization grew, people of influence and political power campaigned to improve working conditions. Occupational health legislation appeared towards the end of the eighteenth century, and progressively developed to protect the health and rights of workers.

Today, the phenomena seen during the Industrial Revolution are being replicated in some rapidly developing nations. Even in industrialized nations, similar problems are still encountered by migrant workers and other deprived sectors of society.

Occupational health legislation

Many countries today have comprehensive occupational health legislation. For example, in the United States, the Occupational Safety and Health Act was passed by Congress in 1970. Its goal was to assure safe and healthy working conditions for working men and women. The UK Health and Safety at Work Act 1974, provided a broad legislative framework for the protection of workers. The European Union (EU) adopted a policy in 1989 on the 'Fundamental Social Rights of Workers', emphasizing the need for safety and health protection in the workplace, improvements in living and working conditions, and provision of social protection for workers. Over 180 countries belong to the ILO. This is a United Nations (UN) agency that produces and promulgates international labour standards, and promotes social justice and human and labour rights.

A historical development was the passing of legislation to ensure that employers do not discriminate against job applicants and employees with disabilities. One example of such legislation is the Disability Discrimination Act 1995 in the United Kingdom. The equivalent legislation in the United States is the Americans with Disabilities Act, 1990 (ADA). In 2006, the UN adopted a Convention on the Rights of People with Disabilities (ILO 2006a).

Occupational diseases, injury, and work-related ill health

The ILO reported that in 2008, 2.34 million people died from work-related accidents or diseases (ILO 2011). The majority (2.02 million) were caused by various types of disease, while 321,000 deaths resulted from work-related accidents. On average, more than 6300 work-related deaths occur every day. An analysis of the causes of work-related mortality revealed that 29 per cent were due to malignant neoplasms, 25 per cent were due to communicable diseases, 21 per cent were due to circulatory diseases, 14 per cent were due to occupational injuries, and 7 per cent were due to respiratory disease (ILO 2011).

Workplace hazards are responsible for a significant proportion of global morbidity. It has been estimated that 37 per cent of back pain, 16 per cent of hearing loss, 13 per cent of chronic obstructive pulmonary diseases, 11 per cent of asthma, 10 per cent of injuries, 10 per cent of lung cancers, and 2 per cent of leukaemias are related to work (Concha-Barrientos et al. 2004).

In total, work-related accidents and diseases have been estimated to result in a 4 per cent loss of the global gross domestic product. However, these statistics offer only a partial picture and most likely underestimate the true extent of the problem. This is because limited or no data for non-fatal occupational illness and injury are available from most countries.

Over 100 occupational diseases have been classified according to the tenth revision of the International Classification of Diseases and Related Health Problems (ICD-10), and the list is expected to grow with the current efforts in developing ICD-11. Occupational diseases are usually classified by the target organs affected, for example, respiratory, musculoskeletal, cardiovascular, reproductive, neurotoxic, skin and psychological disorders, or by effects, for example, hearing loss, occupational infections, and cancer.

Major types of occupational disease and injury

Occupational illness can affect virtually every organ system. Occupational diseases of the lung and skin are common since these organs have substantial surface areas in direct contact with toxic substances. Noise-induced hearing loss and musculoskeletal disorders are among the most common disorders arising from physical factors in the workplace. Occupational cancer is a major concern because of the high mortality associated with many forms of cancer. Increasing attention has been paid in recent years to stress and work-related mental ill health, and diseases affecting the neurological, reproductive, and immunological systems.

Occupational lung diseases

The respiratory system is an easily accessible target organ for airborne toxic agents. Major categories of occupational lung disease include the pneumoconioses ('dust diseases' of the lungs), lung cancer, occupational asthma, chronic bronchitis and other effects of respiratory irritants, and occupational pulmonary infections. Silicosis is the most common form of pneumoconiosis worldwide. Exposure to silica occurs in a wide variety of occupations such as sandblaster, miner, miller, pottery worker, foundry worker, and workers using abrasives. In the United States, over 1 million workers are at risk of developing silicosis each year. From 1968 to 2005, silicosis was recorded as the underlying cause of death in over 7000 death certificates (Centers for Disease Control and Prevention 2008). Exposure to silica dust in the construction of the Hawk's Nest tunnel in West Virginia (1930–1931) was responsible for the highest recorded number of silicosis deaths from a single construction activity in the United States (Cherniak 1986). The International Agency for Research on Cancer (IARC) has classified crystalline silica as a known human carcinogen (IARC 1997).

Asbestos is another important cause of lung diseases that include mesothelioma, lung cancer, and asbestosis (a form of progressive pulmonary fibrosis). Historical asbestos consumption per head of population is related to an increase in asbestos-related diseases (Lin et al. 2007), and asbestos is responsible for over 100,000 deaths per year worldwide (Takala 2003). It has been estimated that there will be more than half a million disability-adjusted life years globally due to asbestos-induced malignant mesothelioma (Driscoll et al. 2005). Given the long latency, the future burden of mortality resulting from asbestos will be substantial even if all future exposure were to be eliminated completely.

Bronchial asthma affects about 300 million people worldwide, with an increasing prevalence every decade. More than 10 per cent of the population in developed countries are affected (Braman 2006). Population-based estimates suggest that 10–25 per cent of new-onset asthma cases in adults are work related (Kogevinas et al. 2007). In some jurisdictions, occupational asthma has become the most prevalent occupational lung disease, exceeding silicosis and asbestosis. Even so, prevalence studies of occupational asthma usually underestimate the number of affected workers because these workers tend to quit jobs where they suffer such symptoms, although their asthma symptoms and signs may continue even after leaving work.

Many gases, fumes, and aerosols are directly toxic to the respiratory tract, causing acute inflammation. Examples include soluble irritants, for example, hydrogen chloride, ammonia, and sulphur dioxide, which produce effects in the eyes, nasopharynx, and large airways. Less soluble irritants (e.g. nitrogen dioxide, ozone, phosgene) produce few upper-respiratory symptoms, but following high exposure can cause delayed pulmonary oedema.

Occupational cancer

Occupational carcinogens include chemical substances, for example, benzene and asbestos; physical hazards, for example, ionizing radiation; and biological hazards, for example, viruses. It is estimated that approximately 16 million workers in the EU are exposed to carcinogens at work. The most common cancers due to these workplace exposures are cancers of the lung, bladder, skin, and liver.

Occupational cancer accounts for about 4–20 per cent of all cancers in developed countries. Variability in the estimates arises from differences in data sets used and assumptions applied. The most commonly accepted estimate is 4 per cent with a plausible range, based on the best quality studies, being 2–8 per cent. However, if one considers only the adult population in which exposure to occupational carcinogens occurs almost exclusively, the proportion of cancer attributed to occupation would increase to about 20 per cent among those exposed (Pearce et al. 1998).

Occupational skin disorders

Skin disorders are among the most commonly reported occupational diseases. The annual incidence rate for work-related skin disease in the United Kingdom is 136/100,000 (Health and Safety Executive (HSE) 2011a). The most common occupational skin disorder is irritant contact dermatitis. Although skin disorders are relatively easily diagnosed, occupational skin diseases are believed to be under-reported, so that the actual rate is many times higher than officially reported (European Agency for Safety and Health at Work 2008). Occupational skin disorders are unevenly distributed between industries. Florists, hairdressers and barbers, metal workers, and maintenance fitters are occupations at risk. In general, a worker in agriculture, forestry, fishing, or manufacturing has a much greater risk of developing a work-related skin disease compared to a worker in other industries. This is likely to be due to their exposure to a wider range of substances known to be irritants or allergens.

Occupational infections

Much attention about infectious diseases has focused on healthcare settings, although infections can be transmitted in other work places, such as research laboratories and animal processing facilities. In healthcare settings, awareness has grown about the risk of infection from hepatitis B, the human immunodeficiency virus (HIV), and tuberculosis (*Mycobacterium tuberculosis*). Needlestick injuries accounted for about 40 per cent of hepatitis B and hepatitis C infections and 4.4 per cent of HIV infections in healthcare workers (Pruss-Ustun et al. 2005). An increased risk of HIV infection has been shown to exist in settings in which workers may be exposed to blood or body fluids (National Institute for Occupational Safety and Health (NIOSH) 1996).

Transmission of *M. tuberculosis* is a recognized risk in healthcare facilities. After years of declining incidence rates, multidrug-resistant tuberculosis has re-emerged as a major occupational and public health problem globally (Morens et al. 2004; Shah et al. 2007; WHO 2007b).

Emerging infectious diseases also pose a risk to healthcare workers. One example is severe acute respiratory syndrome (SARS), caused by a novel coronavirus. In the 2003 worldwide outbreak of SARS, 20 per cent of patients were healthcare workers (Koh et al. 2003). Concerns about the risk of infection among healthcare workers also apply to a range of other infections such as respiratory syncytial virus and influenza A (H1N1).

Infectious diseases can be especially prevalent in developing countries, resulting in higher risks for workers in these countries.

Some of the infections result directly from the work, while others are indirectly related to work. Examples include vector-borne diseases, for example, malaria, dengue haemorrhagic fever, Lyme disease, and anthrax; water and food-borne diseases resulting from poor sanitation and inadequate potable water, for example, cholera and typhoid; and zoonoses among veterinarians, farmers, agricultural and forestry workers, for example, leptospirosis and rabies.

Occupational reproductive disorders

The overall contribution of occupational exposures to reproductive disorders is not known because there has been scant research in this area. Few studies are available especially on physical and biological agents that may affect fertility and pregnancy outcomes in humans.

Occupational exposure to chemical agents such as lead (Pb) and the pesticide dibromochloropropane (DBCP) have been documented to cause testicular effects with resultant reduction in sperm count. Pb can also cross the placenta in a pregnant woman to cause adverse effects in the developing fetus. Other substances associated with documented adverse reproductive outcomes include metal compounds (e.g. methyl mercury), solvents (e.g. carbon disulphide), oestrogenic agents, anaesthetic gases, antineoplastic drugs, carbon monoxide, ethylene oxide, ethylene glycol ethers, polychlorinated biphenyls, and physical agents (e.g. ionizing radiation).

Occupational exposures can cause a wide range of reproductive disorders in both males and females (Kumar 2004; Jensen et al. 2006). Effects of exposures in males include reduced sperm count, aberrant sperm shape, altered sperm function; and lowered hormone levels or libido. Exposures in females may cause menstrual cycle irregularities, infertility, chromosomal aberrations, reduced breast milk production, early onset of menopause, and suppressed libido.

Reproductive disorders also include adverse effects on the offspring of the exposed worker. Potential fetal and developmental effects from maternal exposures include preterm delivery, fetal loss, prenatal death, low birth weight, altered sex ratio of live births, congenital malformations, childhood malignancies, and neurobehavioural disorders in the offspring.

Occupational noise-induced hearing loss

High levels of occupational noise are a persistent problem all over the world. In the United States, up to 30 million workers are exposed to hazardous noise levels at work (NIOSH 2011). In Germany, 12–15 per cent of the workforce are exposed to hazardous noise levels (Concha-Barrientos et al. 2004). In most developing countries, noise-induced hearing loss (NIHL) is one of the most commonly reported occupational disorders. Twenty per cent of workers in the EU indicate exposure to high levels of noise for at least half of their working hours. Noise exposure is especially high in the manufacturing and construction industries.

Industries such as manufacturing, mining, construction, transportation, agriculture, and the military are at the highest risk for NIHL. In developed countries, increasing awareness has led to greater implementation of protective measures, whereas in developing countries, industrialization may herald an increase in exposure to noise (Loney and Aw 2012).

Occupational traumatic injuries

These injuries include such events as amputations, fractures, severe lacerations, eye losses, acute poisonings, and burns. In 2008, approximately 317 million workers were injured in accidents at work that resulted in an absence of 4 days or more from work. This translates to an annual accident incidence of 10,600 per 100,000 workers, or 850,000 injuries per day. For every fatal accident there are another 500–2000 injuries, depending on the occupation (ILO 2002). In Great Britain, the rate of non-fatal major injuries reported in 2005 to 2006 was 100.3 per 100,000 workers. European Statistics at Work reported about 4.7 million accidents at work in the EU which resulted in 3 or more days away from work in 2001, and about 4900 fatal accidents at work (Eurostat 2010).

Work-related diseases

Work-related diseases are diseases in which occurrence may be associated with workplace factors, but these need not be the only risk factor in each case. They occur more commonly than pure 'occupational diseases', and the term is also used to refer to aggravation of a pre-existing medical condition by workplace factors. While prevention of occupational diseases is possible by the elimination of the workplace hazard, work-related diseases cannot be entirely prevented by only addressing occupational hazards. Common work-related diseases include hypertension, ischaemic heart disease, psychosomatic illnesses, musculoskeletal disorders, and non-specific respiratory disease. Two examples are given in the following subsections.

Work-related musculoskeletal disorders

In developed countries, acute and chronic work-related musculoskeletal disorders are a major cause of morbidity affecting workers. The term 'work-related musculoskeletal disorders' encompasses a range of conditions from back pain, upper and lower limb disorders, neck and shoulder symptoms, hand–arm vibration syndrome (HAVS), carpal tunnel syndrome, repetitive strain injury, and other effects on the musculoskeletal system. Musculoskeletal disorders, in particular low back pain, rank alongside mental and behavioural disorders as major causes of long-term sickness absence in the United Kingdom. For 2010/2011, around three-quarters of new cases of work-related conditions in the United Kingdom were due to either musculoskeletal disorders or stress, depression or anxiety (HSE 2012). In the EU, musculoskeletal problems were the most commonly reported work-related health problem accounting for 60 per cent of reports (European Commission 2010). In the United States, musculoskeletal disorders account for 34 per cent of all non-fatal occupational injuries and illnesses involving days away from work (NIOSH 2007). This is also true in many other developed countries. More than half of the working population experience low-back injury at some time in their working career.

Stress-related ill health

Job stress has been defined as the 'harmful physical and emotional responses that occur when the requirements of the job do not match the capabilities, resources or needs of the worker' (NIOSH 1999). NIOSH reports that in the United States:

◆ 25 per cent of employees view their jobs as the main stressor in their lives.

◆ 75 per cent of employees believe the worker has more on-the-job stress than a generation ago.

◆ Problems at work are more strongly associated with health complaints than any other life stressor—more than even financial or family problems.

◆ Workers who take time off work because of stress, anxiety, or a related disorder will be off the job for about 20 days.

Individual and situational factors, such as balance between work and family life, social support, individual outlook, and personality can affect the likelihood of developing stress. However, working conditions often play a significant and sometimes major role in the causation of stress.

Workplace stress-related hazards consist of factors in both work content as well as context (Leka et al. 2003). Work content encompasses job content (e.g. meaningless, unpleasant tasks), workload (under- as well as overload) and working under time pressure, work schedules (e.g. long, unsociable, inflexible working schedules), degree of participation in decision-making, and lack of control of work. Work context includes concerns about career development, status and salary, the individual's role in the organization, issues relating to interpersonal relationships, the organizational culture/climate, and conflict or lack of support in the home–work interface.

The clinical manifestations of occupational stress are indistinguishable from stress caused by non-work factors. Stress can present as emotional lability, anxiety, depression, insomnia and even attempts at suicide. Adverse health outcomes of job stress are wide ranging, from increased risk of cardiovascular disease, musculoskeletal symptoms, impaired immune function, and gastrointestinal disorders, for example, peptic ulcers and irritable bowel syndrome (Barbara et al. 2004). The impact of workplace stress on an organization may include a decrease in work commitment, reduced productivity, lowered staff morale and increase in absenteeism, increasing staff and customer complaints, and a poor public image for the company.

General diseases affecting the working population

General diseases prevalent in every community include infections such as HIV/AIDS, tuberculosis and malaria, or non-communicable diseases and lifestyle-related diseases, for example, diabetes mellitus, cardiovascular disease, cancer, and malnutrition. These diseases may not be directly caused by occupational exposures, but can invariably affect work productivity. Workplace factors can also influence the progress and prognosis of these diseases.

Estimates of costs and economic loss

Total economic losses due to occupational injuries and illnesses are large. The ILO estimated that overall economic losses from work-related injuries and illnesses in 1997 were approximately 4 per cent of the world's gross national product (GNP). According to recent estimates, the cost of work-related health loss and associated productivity loss may amount to several per cent of total GNP of a country. For example, the HSE has estimated the cost of occupational illness and injury to the British economy to be £14 billion in 2009–2010 (HSE 2011b). The main contributors to these estimated costs are provision of medical care, rehabilitation and compensation, loss of working days (over 25 million days a year) and therefore productivity for the organization and loss of income for the affected individual, and associated costs of concurrent damage to property and equipment. There are also non-financial 'costs' from pain, grief, and suffering.

In the United States, the direct cost of the most disabling workplace injuries and illnesses in 2008 was estimated to be US$53 billion, with substantial additional indirect costs ranging up to 4.5 times the direct costs, and the indirect costs ranging from US$137.4 to US$229 billion (Occupational Health and Safety Administration 2012).

Under-recognition of occupational ill health

Although recording of workplace injuries is reasonably accurate in most developed countries, this is not so for occupational illnesses where there are substantial under-estimates of actual cases. One explanation for this is the inherent difficulty in diagnosing occupational diseases and in establishing cause-and-effect relationships. The link between occupation and disease may sometimes be unclear, because most occupational diseases are not distinct clinically and pathologically from diseases associated with non-occupational aetiologies. For example, skin cancer caused by polycyclic aromatic hydrocarbons is similar in appearance to that caused by excessive exposure to sunlight. Similarly, solvent-induced encephalopathy may easily be confused with effects of advancing age. Only for a very limited number of diseases, for example, mesothelioma (caused by asbestos), and angiosarcoma of the liver (caused by vinyl chloride monomer) is the causal association between occupational exposure and disease readily established initially primarily on clinical grounds, and mainly based on a good occupational history documenting exposure.

Another cause of the under-recognition of occupational disease is that the majority of chemicals in commerce have never been fully evaluated in regards to their potential toxicity. Only a small percentage of the approximately 80,000 chemicals currently used in industry have been screened for toxicity. Such toxicity testing often concentrates primarily on high-dose, acute effects and on the long-term cancer risk. Toxicity testing for reproductive, neurological, immunological, and other adverse effects remains quite limited.

The long latency which typically elapses between occupational exposure and onset of illness is a third factor which may obscure the occupational aetiology of chronic disease. For example, occupational cancers rarely appear within 10 or even 20 years of first exposure to a carcinogen. Similarly, chronic neurotoxic effects of solvents may become evident only after decades of exposure. In such instances, it is unlikely that the worker will be diagnosed as having a disease of occupational origin.

Lack of awareness among health practitioners about the hazards found at work is a fourth cause of underestimation of occupational disease, reflecting the fact that most physicians are not adequately trained to suspect work as a cause of disease. With competing demands for time in the medical curriculum from an increasing number of disciplines and subject areas, most medical schools now only allocate limited time to teaching medical students to take a proper occupational history, to recognize symptoms of common industrial toxins, or to recall known associations between occupational exposures and disease. In the United Kingdom, there has been a progressive decline in the total number of hours allocated for occupational medicine in medical schools (Wynn et al. 2002).

Compounding a lack of medical awareness is the limited ability of many workers to provide an accurate report of their exposures. Workers may have had multiple toxic exposures in a variety of jobs over a working lifetime. In most countries, there are no requirements to inform workers of the hazard of the materials with which they work. In the United States, employers' reporting requirements remain limited under the Hazard Communication Standard and state right-to-know laws. In many instances, a patient may not know or may not be able to remember all his or her past occupational exposures.

Finally, given the potential financial liability associated with the finding that a disease is of occupational origin, employers may be reluctant to recognize the work-relatedness of a disorder, especially in cases where personal habits or non-occupational pursuits are possible contributory factors. Since employers are often in the best position to recognize causal associations between workplace exposures and disease, this conflict of interest represents an obstacle to obtaining accurate estimates of the burden of occupational illness.

The changing work and health landscape

The global economy has expanded rapidly in the past few decades, but many of the estimated 3.5 billion workers in the world (China alone has a labour force of over a billion workers) continue to be employed in conditions which do not meet international health and safety standards and guidelines. These workers are exposed to high levels of dust, dirt, noise, toxic chemicals, and biological substances. Their health and livelihood, and sometimes their lives are at risk. In developed countries where there has been some success in the control of exposure to chemical and physical hazards, work stress and work-related musculoskeletal disorders have become major causes of ill health and sickness absence.

Globalization has reshaped the world with the introduction of new materials and procedures, advances in technology, improved communication tools, and greater flexibility in responding to production demands. However, the rapidly changing working conditions, new employment patterns and evolving labour relations can also pose challenges to the protection of workers' health. New global health threats have also emerged, such as the risk of epidemic and pandemic diseases (e.g. SARS and influenza A (H1N1) infection). These infections have affected occupational groups from healthcare workers to farmers. Global spread of infection has been facilitated by ease of international travel and increasingly porous health borders.

Other pressing concerns which impact the health of workers are international and internal migration of workers, a growing informal sector (where defined terms of employment and workers' benefits may be weak or non-existent), and discrimination at the workplace. These are often associated with unhealthy, unsafe, and unfair working conditions.

Despite the existence of protective legislation in many countries, the burden of injury and illness on workers remains significant. There is a need for international coordination of occupational health protection for workers, given the increasing globalization of the world economy. Several initiatives have been proposed to address this issue. This includes the harmonization of health, safety, and environmental standards in a way that does not unfairly impose a competitive disadvantage on the newly industrialized nations. Governments and multinational corporations must be prepared to share advances in control technology, expertise, and resources. Instead of allowing industries to manufacture products in other countries when these are banned for use in their own country, governments in developed nations could provide incentives for their industries to develop and export safer products and technologies. At a minimum, international systems should be established to ensure complete notification of potential hazards, including labelling the contents of raw materials and products.

Special populations of workers

Workplace hazards affect some worker populations disproportionately, for example, those in developing nations, child labourers, women employees, and impaired workers. These populations are especially vulnerable because of the interaction between their work roles and broader roles in society, as well as by their particular exposures in the workplace.

Workers in developing nations

More than 80 per cent of workers in the global workforce are from the developing world (Rosenstock et al. 2005). Workers' health should be viewed in the context of national development. Occupational health policymakers in many nations must consider a balance between adverse impacts on workers' health and the economic advantages of rapid development by allowing foreign investigators access to low-cost labour and weak labour protection provisions.

The relationship between workers' health and development is complex. For example, workers in many developing countries may be affected by poor nutrition or endemic diseases, such as malaria, in which work may aggravate the condition, or which make the worker more susceptible to the effects of workplace exposures. Workers in these countries also generally have lower educational backgrounds and are often inadequately trained to handle the new technologies and potential hazards. There may be high turnover with little management investment in worker training.

Working conditions in tropical developing countries (as in South East Asia), and countries with desert environments (as in the Middle East and North Africa) may present special hazards because of climatic conditions, building ventilation design, and equipment and production facilities. The importation of production equipment from developed countries can pose some difficulty with the availability of replacement parts and service. The machinery could be pre-owned or dated and possibly considered obsolete for use in the developed countries, while new and safer equipment may be unavailable or too expensive for developing countries.

The social organization of work in developing countries also affects workers' health. In addition to the large number of workplaces with a small number of workers, large proportions of the workforce work in the 'informal' sector. This sector consists of small, often home-based businesses that have no government registration and oversight. For example, recent estimates of the proportion of informal non-agricultural employment were about 58 per cent for Latin America and 75 per cent in sub-Saharan Africa. The informal economy accounts for 90 per cent of women working in non-agricultural sectors in India and Indonesia, and 95 per cent in Benin, Chad, and Mali (Rosenstock et al. 2005).

Finally, countries of the developing world may have access to advanced industrial technologies from the developed world, but they have little in the way of legal or administrative infrastructure to control the adverse impacts from these new technologies on the workforce. Even if developing countries adopt standards and legislation from more developed nations, there is often a shortage of trained personnel to recognize and manage workplace hazards.

Child labour

The ILO estimates that the global number of child workers is 215 million, with a large number involved in hazardous work (IPEC 2012). Child labour has become an important issue because the children are vulnerable to exploitation in the workplace and may be denied basic human rights, such as decent wages or access to education. Poverty is the primary reason why children work. Poor households need the money, and children in employment can contribute to family income. Unfortunately, if the family has a tradition of engaging in a hazardous occupation, it is likely that the children will continue in the trade.

Children in hazardous occupations are at greater risk of suffering ill effects than adult workers. They may have greater exposure to hazards than adult workers in the same occupation because children tend to be given the most menial jobs, which can involve higher exposures to toxic substances. Children are more susceptible to the same hazards faced by adult workers because they differ from adults in their physical, physiological, and psychological characteristics. Children using hand tools designed for adults run a higher risk of fatigue and injury. Personal protective equipment (PPE) designed for adults do not fit children, and therefore do not provide adequate protection. Furthermore, children may not be as aware as adults of workplace dangers, or as knowledgeable of precautions to be taken at work. Children are also more vulnerable to psychological and physical abuse than are adults, and suffer deeper psychological damage when they are denigrated or bullied.

The International Programme on the Elimination of Child labour (IPEC 2011) launched in 1992 was aimed at the elimination of child labour, giving priority to its worst forms. The 'worst forms' comprise all forms of slavery or practices similar to slavery; the use, procurement, or offering of a child for prostitution or production of pornography; the use, procurement, or offering of a child for illicit activities; and work which is inherently likely to harm the health, safety, or morals of children. Withdrawing children from the worst forms of child labour requires improved legislation and enforcement, improved methodologies for identifying the children, rehabilitation of the children, provision of viable alternatives to the children, and raising awareness at all societal levels.

The efforts of IPEC in the elimination of child labour are beginning to pay off, with a decline in the proportion of child labourers. Unfortunately, the rate of child labour continues to be disparately high in sub-Saharan Africa (ILO 2006b).

Women workers

Women in many countries of the world are often at a disadvantage compared to men in various spheres of society. As a result, gender issues have traditionally lacked visibility, and this includes women at work (WHO 2011).

About 42 per cent of the global workforce is female (Messing 2006). There is significant interplay between women's roles in society, socioeconomic condition, and occupation. Women's roles in traditional societies are defined in relation to child bearing and upbringing of children and responsibility for the care and comfort of the family. Paid employment of women has increased in most countries, but this has led to a conflict between the necessity to be at work and women's traditional home and family responsibilities. In many societies, early marriage, repeated pregnancies, large families, low educational status, and poverty all disproportionately impact on women workers (Loewenson 1999). The dual roles of women as workers and unpaid caregivers is especially challenging for sole-support mothers, who comprise 20–30 per cent of households worldwide.

Employment of women in most societies is characterized by occupational segregation, under-employment (often involved in doing seasonal and part-time work below their level of education), and barriers to advancement. Occupational segregation means that women tend to be clustered into a small number of occupations while being under-represented in most others (Stellman 1999). For example, professional women tend to be in teaching, nursing, and other healthcare specialities. In manufacturing, women tend to have jobs in assembly and small machine operations. Women in developing countries tend to be employed in sectors such as agriculture, textiles and clothing, food processing, and social services (Loewenson 1999). Compared with men, women work for smaller industries or organizations, have less opportunity for work control, and face the psychological demands of people-oriented or machine-paced work (Paltiel 1998). Women are more likely to work in the informal sector, in specific types of informal work such as domestic work, street vending, and sex work, with their accompanying low social status and lack of legislative protection. While many countries have enacted laws prohibiting gender discrimination, some countries still have formal restrictions on women's employment. Gender differences are also observed in the rates of occupational injuries and illnesses, but these differences are primarily because of differences in the conditions of work or exposures, rather than due to genetic differences (Stellman 1999).

Impaired workers

A large proportion of individuals with disabilities are in the working age group, and they are able to make constructive contributions in the workplace despite physical impairment. Legislation in some countries prohibits employers from discriminating against individuals with disabilities, and encourages employers to make reasonable accommodation for those with a known impairment.

France and Germany impose quotas on enterprises to employ a certain percentage of disabled people. India and Japan use employment promotion measures to ensure workplace accessibility and provide employment services in the form of job placement agencies. Singapore provides tax reductions as a financial incentive to compensate employers for any financial burden resulting from the employment of disabled people.

Reasonable accommodations are changes made to the work environment, job responsibilities, or conditions of work that provide opportunities for workers with special needs to perform essential job functions. These measures may include technical assistance devices; customization, including PPE and clothing; and changes to processes, location, or timing for essential job functions.

The chemical company DuPont showed that employees with disabilities perform as well as or better than comparable employees with no disabilities. Additional adjustments in the workplace were required by only 4 per cent of disabled people of employable age (ILO 2007a).

Migrant workers

There are an estimated 150–190 million migrants in the world—2 per cent of the world's population—including migrant workers, refugees, asylum seekers, and permanent immigrants. The number has increased dramatically with globalization. The vast majority of this migration is from developing to developed countries. Three-quarters of all migrants lived in 28 countries in 2005, with one in five migrants living in the United States. Many migrants move to seek work.

According to the UN, 'migrant workers' are people who are to be engaged, are engaged, or have been engaged in remunerated activities in a State of which they are not nationals (UN 1990). Some migrant workers stay permanently in their new countries, while many return to their original homes after working for a period of time. The latter are strictly not true migrants, as they may have intentions of returning to their home countries after a period of gainful employment in a foreign land. Hence a more appropriate term for this group of workers is 'expatriate workers'.

Expatriate workers are a particularly vulnerable population for many of the same reasons that were described for workers in developing countries, for example, they may be affected by poor nutrition and endemic diseases, they often have lower educational backgrounds, and they are inadequately trained to deal with potential work hazards. This is especially true for expatriate manual workers. Many face additional obstacles because they do not speak the language of the host country adequately. They are often not familiar with local health and safety practices and regulations. The accommodation available for them can be temporary and often crowded with limited shared facilities and restricted access to medical care and other social services. Expatriate workers may encounter racism, xenophobia, and exploitation because they do not have full legal status or awareness of their rights in the host country (Holmes 2006; McKay et al. 2006).

Shift workers

Shift work and irregular work hours have increased significantly among those who are employed. The ILO found that 20 per cent of workers worldwide put in more than 48 hours of work a week, often earning only a bare minimum wage (ILO 2007b). A similar proportion of workers in the EU countries engage in shift work or night work (Eurostat 2010). The recent evaluation by the IARC regarding shift work and breast cancer indicating shift work that involves circadian disruption as probably carcinogenic to humans (Group 2A carcinogen) poses a challenge for occupational health and public health advice and intervention (IARC 2010). This finding has implications for occupational groups as varied as air crew, journalists, physicians, laboratory technicians, and telephone operators (Weiderpass et al. 2011).

Assessing the risk of work

Health protection begins with an assessment of risk. Risk assessment is a structured and systematic procedure that is dependent upon the correct identification of hazards and an appropriate estimation of the risks arising from them (HSE 1995). The purpose of risk assessment is to ensure that a valid decision can be made for measures necessary to control exposure to substances hazardous to health arising in the workplace. Risk assessments are legal requirements in many countries. It can be a qualitative or quantitative process.

Expertise, effort, and detail required for risk assessment depends on the nature and degree of risk, and the complexity of the work process. Adequate controls are determined based on several factors: the toxicity of substances, numbers exposed, acceptability of risk, legal requirements, costs, and availability of control measures.

Hazard and risk

In occupational health practice, an understanding of the difference between the terms 'hazard' and 'risk' is essential.

Hazard refers to a substance, agent, or physical situation with a potential for harm in terms of injury or ill health, damage to property, damage to the environment, or a combination of these. Hazards can be physical, chemical, biological, ergonomic, or psychosocial in nature.

Physical hazards include exposure to extremes of temperature, light, noise, vibration, electricity, and radiation. Chemical hazards cover a range of organic (aliphatic or aromatic) and inorganic chemicals. Biological hazards are those due primarily to infectious organisms (e.g. viruses, bacteria, rickettsia), and also prions and proteins. Ergonomic and mechanical hazards result from poor design of work stations and disorganized systems of work, and psycho-social hazards are those that contribute to and cause workplace stress. Hazard identification is the process of recognizing that a hazard exists and defining its characteristics.

Risk relates to the likelihood of the harm or undesired event occurring, and the consequences of its occurrence. It is the probability that the substance or agent will cause adverse effects under the conditions of use and/or exposure, and the possible extent of harm. It is thus a function of both exposure to the hazard and the likelihood of effects on health from the hazard. Extent of risk covers the population that might be affected by the risk, the numbers exposed, and the consequences.

Risk assessment

Risk assessment is the process of estimating the magnitude of risk, and deciding if the risk is tolerable or acceptable. A tolerable risk may not always be acceptable. It merely refers to a willingness to live with a risk to secure certain benefits, and in the confidence that the risk is being properly controlled (Sadhra and Rampal 1999). The levels of tolerability of risk are different for different countries, and in different working populations and the general public. The views on tolerability depend to a large extent on the populations that might be affected by the risk.

Risk assessment and risk management must take into account both routine and non-routine activities and conditions, including foreseeable emergency situations. Hazards that are intrinsic to these situations, or generated by such activities should be recognized. Exposed people should be identified, including non-employees and those who are susceptible and therefore at higher risk because of illness or other medical conditions. Existing control measures, if any, need to be evaluated.

The health risks from the hazards should be determined and assessed, and a decision made on whether the risk is acceptable or tolerable. Unacceptable risks have to be eliminated or reduced with new or improved control measures, and their effectiveness monitored. Such a process requires a team effort, involving the workers themselves as well as personnel with the relevant expertise. It is important to inform workers of the hazards, risks, and appropriate measures that have been and can be taken to protect them.

The steps for risk assessment for chemical, biological, ergonomic, and psychosocial hazards may differ, as illustrated by the following examples. The assessments for chemical or physical exposures are generally more objective and precise than the assessment for psychological stressors. As an example, an initial assessment for a chemical exposure might include the following steps:

1. List substances in the area to be assessed.

2. Determine which substances are actually used, and in what quantities, and the frequency and duration of use.

3. Evaluate workers' concerns.

4. Assess the tasks of workers, their exposure, and methods of handling.

5. Obtain suppliers' data sheets.

6. Evaluate data sheets.

7. Inspect places where the substances are handled.

8. Evaluate method of control.

9. Perform environmental monitoring for the chemical if needed.

10. Decide on acceptability or tolerability of risk, and if further control measures are needed.

The assessment of psychosocial factors at work is more complex. It may include the evaluation of organizational dysfunction, work conditions, as well as a study of indicators such as sickness absence, staff turnover, and measurement of stress-related illness among employees. Possible work stressors are poor design of tasks, aggressive management style, inadequate interpersonal relationships, unclear work roles, limited career prospects, and adverse environmental conditions at the workplace. The extent of work stress can be assessed by use of validated questionnaires administered to staff; for example, the General Health Questionnaire (Jackson 2007), the Finnish Occupational Stress Questionnaire (Elo et al. 1992), or the NIOSH Generic Work Stress Questionnaire (NIOSH 2008).

Assessing exposure

Environmental monitoring

Environmental or ambient monitoring in the workplace is undertaken to measure external exposure to harmful agents. The monitoring is to ensure that exposure is kept within 'permissible levels' so as to prevent the occurrence of disease. The concept of permissible levels assumes that for each substance there is a level of exposure at or below which the exposed worker does not suffer any health impairment.

Permissible levels or occupational exposure limits

These are standards that have been set for commonly encountered physical, chemical, and biological hazards in workplaces. There are variations in exposure limits from different countries and different agencies. Much depends on factors such as the philosophy and rationale for the standards, the process of standard setting, nomenclature and applicability, and whether economic considerations and technical feasibility are taken into account.

In the United States, threshold limit values (TLVs) for chemical substances and physical agents are set and reviewed annually by the American Conference of Governmental Industrial Hygienists (ACGIH). These TLVs are one of the best known and widely used of the occupational exposure limits (OELs). They are derived using information from industrial experience, as well as studies in both animal and human populations. These standards are adopted by many countries, especially those without their own occupational exposure standard setting mechanism.

The US also has recommended exposure limits (RELs) produced by NIOSH, and permissible exposure limits (PELs) from the Occupational Health and Safety Administration (OSHA). The United Kingdom has Workplace Exposure Limits (WELs), and in Germany there are two groups of OELs: (1) technical guidance concentrations (TRKs), and (2) maximum concentration for a chemical substance in the workplace (MAK).

Permissible levels have their limitations. For example, a 'safe' level of exposure can be difficult to determine for agents such as allergens and carcinogens. As such every effort must be made to keep exposure levels as low as reasonably practicable and the permissible level is then a level above which exposure must not occur. This level may be mandated by legislation. Concerns regarding health risks have arisen from substances assumed previously to be safe, for example, glycol ethers in the electronic industry associated with the risk of spontaneous abortions have led to further investigations into whether retention or lowering of the current occupational exposure levels is warranted. Standards that are set for an 8-hour working day would not be applicable for a 12-hour work shift. Furthermore, exposure to several hazards simultaneously does occur. In such situations, there can be possible synergistic or additive effects. This would then require more stringent control of each individual hazard.

The methods for environmental monitoring require choice of the correct collecting devices, sampling strategy, and analysis of the collected samples in accredited laboratories. Variations in age, gender, pre-existing disease, genetic makeup, and social habits, for example, smoking, influence individual susceptibility and have to be considered in applying the findings from exposure assessment to the exposed population. Despite these limitations, sensible use of environmental standards can often result in practical control of many common workplace hazards so that the majority of workers are protected.

Biological monitoring

Biological monitoring refers to the measurement and assessment of workplace agents or their metabolites either in tissues, secreta, excreta, expired air, or any combinations of these to evaluate exposure and health risk compared to an appropriate measure. The specific chemical or its breakdown product can be measured to detect the total body burden of the substance. The method of measurement of these substances must be validated and there should be a means to interpret the results obtained in terms of the extent of exposure, and risk to health.

Biological monitoring and environmental monitoring complement each other in the assessment of health risk in the exposed worker. One major feature of biological, as compared to environmental, monitoring is that for a particular individual, it takes into account exposure from all routes of absorption. For example, for workplace exposure to organic solvents, skin absorption may be a significant route of entry of the solvent into the body, and ambient environmental air monitoring might be less useful as an indicator of exposure than biological monitoring. Furthermore, environmental monitoring at the workplace would not account for non-occupational or extra-occupational exposures. A person exposed to organic solvents at work may have additional exposure at home as a result of hobbies or other non-occupational activity.

While the term 'biological monitoring' has previously been used to also include clinical procedures (e.g. periodic X-rays, blood tests, symptom enquiry, etc.) for monitoring the health status of exposed workers, it is preferable to make a clear distinction between the terms 'biological monitoring' (used for assessing exposure), and 'biological effects monitoring' and 'health surveillance' (used for detecting effects).

Biological monitoring standards

A set of values has been developed by the ACGIH, for interpreting results of biological monitoring (as well as biological effects monitoring). The Biological Exposure Index (BEI) is described as representing the 'levels of determinants that are most likely to be observed in specimens collected from healthy workers who has been exposed to chemicals to the same extent as workers with inhalation exposure at the TLV' (ACGIH 2012). Exceptions would be made for chemicals for which TLVs are based on non-systemic effects, for example, irritation; and for chemicals with significant routes of entry via additional routes of entry (usually percutaneous absorption).

The ACGIH cautions that BEIs are not able to clearly distinguish hazardous from non-hazardous exposures. Biological variation in individuals may sometimes result in measurements in individuals to exceed recommended BEI levels without an increased health risk (ACGIH 2012). It further states that BEIs are not intended for use as a measure of adverse effect or diagnosis of occupational disease. However, if measurements of the individual or group of workers persistently exceed the BEIs, the cause of the excessive values should be investigated, and measures should be taken to reduce the exposure.

The UK HSE has similar values for a smaller number of compounds. These are termed biological monitoring guidance values (BMGV).

Assessing health effects

Biological effect monitoring

This refers to the measurement and assessment of early biological effects, of which the relationship to health impairment has not yet been established, in exposed workers to evaluate exposure and/or other health risk compared to an appropriate reference. Some examples include detection of alterations in enzyme levels (e.g. cholinesterase for workers exposed to organophosphorus or carbamate pesticides), or other biochemical changes such as delta-aminolaevulinic acid in urine of workers exposed to inorganic lead, or beta-2 microglobulin in the urine of cadmium exposed workers. These changes do not necessarily lead to any direct overt pathological damage in an individual, but may reflect effects that are often reversible on removal of the worker from further exposure.

Recent technological advances in molecular biology have resulted in the development of newer molecular biomarkers of exposure, response, and genetic susceptibility. These include measurements for structural gene damage, gene variation, and gene products in cells and body fluids, for example, oncogenes and tumour suppressor genes, DNA adducts, gene products and genetic polymorphisms, and metabolic phenotypes in environmentally exposed populations (Koh et al. 1999). The availability of genetic tests to identify susceptible workers raises issues of ethics, individual privacy, right to work, and the relevance of such tests. Given the limitations of individual molecular biomarkers in assessing health risk, and the multifactorial nature of environmental disease, it is likely that a combined approach which examines several of these biomarkers simultaneously will increase our understanding of the complex issue of disease mechanisms and further refine the process of occupational risk assessment.

Health surveillance

This refers to the detection of health effects through the periodic physiological or clinical examination of exposed workers with the objective of protecting and preventing occupationally related diseases. Examples are audiometry for noise exposed workers, and clinical examination for skin lesions in workers exposed to polycyclic aromatic hydrocarbon compounds in tar, pitch, and bitumen. The use and limitations of periodic medical examinations are discussed further in the section on secondary prevention.

Managing the risk of work and promoting health at work

Prevention of occupational disease can take place at various levels, such as at the national level, at the level of the workplace itself, or measures directed at the individual worker.

Primary prevention aims at reducing the occurrence of disease by eliminating the causal factors contributing to disease or reducing workplace exposure to safe levels. Examples are banning the use of asbestos to prevent asbestosis, mesothelioma, and lung cancer, and reduction of noise at its source to levels that do not cause noise-induced deafness. Primary prevention with regard to chemicals requires either: (1) elimination of toxic materials and their replacement by less hazardous substitutes or (2) use of safe systems of work, and controls such as complete enclosure or local exhaust ventilation at the source of aerosol generation.

Secondary prevention aims to detect over-exposure, or early reversible effects of disease in order to take corrective action. For example, regular monitoring of blood lead levels among exposed workers could indicate a potential for lead poisoning, or regular audiograms among noise-exposed workers may show temporary threshold shift (TTS). Removal of workers with TTS from further noise exposure, and subsequent containment of the source of the noise can allow recovery of hearing, and a return to regular work duties. Successful secondary prevention depends on the ability to identify work-related illness early and effectively through screening workers at high risk for occupational disease.

Tertiary prevention aims to minimize the consequences in people who already have established disease. This activity is primarily a curative and rehabilitative function and depends on availability of appropriate treatment. However, even for acute poisonings, there are very few specific effective antidotes available. Hence, the focus should be on primary or secondary prevention.

Prevention at all three levels requires information on the nature and extent of exposure, and knowledge of the potential effects of these exposures.

Primary prevention

Control of new hazards

Laboratory toxicology studies using animal models and/or cell lines are used to predict potential effects of hazardous materials on humans. The findings from such studies determine whether substances or groups of substances are marketed for use in industry and/or in the community. The European Union's REACH (Registration, Evaluation, Authorisation, and Restriction of Chemicals) regulations which came into force in June 2007 placed an obligation on manufacturers, importers, and users of chemicals in Europe to register and provide information on hazardous chemicals and risk reduction measures (European Chemicals Agency 2012). The regulations also promote the use of methods of risk assessment that reduce the need for animal testing

Control of known hazards

Several countries have legislation to ban the use of substances known to be harmful to human health. The UN has compiled a consolidated list of products whose consumption and sale have been banned, withdrawn, severely restricted, or not approved by governments. This publication constitutes a tool that helps governments keep up to date with regulatory decisions taken by other governments and assists them in considering the scope for eventual regulatory action. The United Nations Environment Programme (UNEP) in 1989 has evolved a procedural mechanism of prior informed consent (PIC) to inform government of banned agents such that these governments could take appropriate action for their control. By such means, the UN system attempts to prevent importing countries from unknowingly using substances banned in other countries for health reasons. At the national level, there may be rules that regulate the import, storage, sale, and transport of legislated substances through a licensing system, for example, for pesticides. Some substances may be subjected to import controls.

Control measures within the workplace

Within the workplace, a hierarchy of control measures is often invoked for reducing occupational hazards. This consists of considering the following steps listed according to order of priority:

1. Hazard elimination or substitution.

2. Engineering controls.

3. Redesign of the workstation or work process.

4. Administrative controls and worker education.

5. Use of personal protective equipment.

Elimination of the hazard or substitution with a safer alternative

This option eliminates the health risk completely, and has been used for substances that are carcinogenic—such as asbestos and benzene, or those that can cause serious health effects such as heavy metals. For example, it is possible to produce new soldering materials that contain little or no cadmium at all, and the HSE in the United Kingdom has produced legislation for this elimination (Mason et al. 1999).

Substitution of the hazard with a less toxic alternative is another option. In the case of processes which use solvents, such as degreasing operations, a less toxic solvent such as 1,1,1 trichloroethane can be used, instead of the comparatively more toxic trichloroethylene or tetrachloroethylene.

Selection of a less hazardous process or equipment also represents a meaningful control strategy. For example, substitution of a continuous process by an intermittent process almost invariably results in a decrease in exposure. Instead of replacing an entire work process to reduce hazards, equipment substitution may achieve the desired reduction in exposure. An example is use of a degreaser with a hoist instead of dipping components into solvents by hand.

Engineering controls

Automation, enclosure, or segregation of a work process, and the use of dampeners or mufflers to reduce vibration or noise have been successful engineering control measures used.

Improved ventilation is also an effective and widely used control measure. Control of hazards by ventilation can be through local exhaust ventilation or general ventilation. The approach for implementing ventilation controls is firstly to conduct an engineering study to evaluate sources of exposure; secondly, to develop an engineering design; thirdly, to install a system based on the design; and lastly, to evaluate the completed system to ensure that the air contaminant has been effectively controlled.

Isolation is defined as the interposing of a barrier between a hazard and workers who might be injured or made ill by the hazard. Isolation may refer to storage of materials, such as flammable liquids, enclosure or removal of equipment to another area (such as noisy generators), or isolation of processes or of the workers themselves (e.g. by enclosing a sawmill worker in a soundproof ventilated booth to protect them from noise and wood dust). The petroleum industry, for example, uses automated remote processing in plants based on centralized computer control of process equipment. Workers are thus largely isolated from hazards except in maintenance operations and during process upsets.

Suppressing the substance by 'wetting' of dusty operations is another example of effective engineering control. Alteration of work practices can help to reduce exposure to hazards. An example is vacuuming cotton lint off spinning machines rather than blowing it off with compressed air, a practice which creates airborne dust particles.

Redesign of the workstation or work process

Workstation redesign to reduce unnecessary and repetitive bending, or poor postures can minimize ergonomic hazards. Among computer operators, use of adjustable equipment, positioning of the workstation to reduce glare, and provision of appropriate work rest periods can prevent the occurrence of visual and musculoskeletal complaints.

Administrative controls and worker education

Administrative controls may be a viable alternative or an additional measure to reduce worker exposure to occupational hazards. This could take the form of job enlargement or job rotation, restriction of hours of work at a hazardous operation, or temporary job reassignment.

With administrative controls, the level of exposure to the hazard is not diminished; instead, the duration of exposure is reduced. For example, mandatory rest periods and shorter work hours for outdoor workers during extremely hot weather (as in desert environments) have helped to reduce the likelihood of heat stress. Another example is the reduction of overall noise exposure through rotation of tasks. Given the typical demands of production and the potential for misuse, administrative methods of controls should never be a first-line choice for control of hazards.

Training of workers to recognize work hazards, to work safely, and to know what to do in the event of an emergency is another important aspect of prevention. There may be considerable variability in exposure even amongst a group of workers supposedly performing the same work tasks (Symanski et al. 2001). This variation

can be explained by differences in hazard awareness, attitude, and practice of safe working techniques in different workers.

Programmes for encouraging personal hygiene constitute another approach to reducing exposure. The provision and use of showers and a change to clean clothes at the end of the working day is a practical personal hygiene measure. Indeed, US OSHA standards, such as the occupational lead standard, require management to provide such facilities. A subtle but potentially important route of exposure is ingestion of toxic agents through eating or smoking, at the workplace. To prevent such exposure, separate facilities for consumption of food away from production lines should be provided.

Use of personal protective equipment

It is axiomatic that use of personal protective devices to prevent occupational ill health should be considered as a last resort after all other methods for minimizing exposure to workplace hazards have been tried. PPE can never be as efficient a means of protection as engineering or process controls. Nevertheless, the use of PPE is often widely practised, perhaps because it is seen as a relatively low-cost measure that puts much of the onus on the worker for compliance with use. PPE can be useful for short-term (as for emergency rescue work) or infrequent exposure to occupational hazards. Respirators, gloves, protective clothing, ear plugs, and muffs are all common forms of PPE in use throughout industry. They can play an important role, provided that carefully designed PPE programmes are in place and that the devices are frequently and regularly checked.

Protective devices should be properly selected to be effective against specific hazards, for example, the choice of an appropriate glove for use with a particular solvent. Workers have to be trained to use the equipment correctly and to ensure that it is working effectively, such as respirator fit testing in the use of respirators. Worker compliance in the use of these devices has to be high, or its protective effects may be less than desired. Compliance can be an issue, because of discomfort, especially for workers in hot and humid climates. Protective devices also have to be properly maintained and replaced when necessary.

Secondary prevention

Secondary prevention aims to detect situations of early effects of disease before they manifest as clinical symptoms and signs. Upon early detection, corrective action can be taken, such as removal of the worker from further exposure. In most instances, early effects of disease can be reversed if corrective action is promptly taken.

Pre-employment examinations

The often stated aim of these assessments is to detect any mismatch between the job applicant's health and the intended job. A decision can then be made by management as to whether or not the person should be hired. Cost considerations and concerns about inability to carry out the full range of work tasks and possible harm to third parties are often given as reasons for rejection of an applicant. In practice, the detection rate for relevant clinical abnormalities is low (2 per cent in prospective healthcare workers in the United Kingdom) (Whitaker and Aw 1995), such that the cost-effectiveness of the process is questionable. There is an element of selection bias since individuals who are in poor health with existing clinical abnormalities are unlikely to be seeking employment. Pre-employment examinations probably constitute one of the most frequent procedures performed by occupational health departments especially in developing countries. In many developed countries there are laws prohibiting discrimination on the basis of health status. Individuals are hired primarily on the basis of their credentials and ability, and subsequent adjustments to the job tasks or work environment can then be made if indicated for health reasons.

Where they are performed, the pre-employment examination or the pre-placement assessment can be used as an occasion to obtain baseline data on health status or fitness, to inform and educate the new worker about potential hazards in their work and the preventive measures that can be taken to safeguard their health. Immunization against diseases that may possibly be contracted on the job, and for which an effective vaccine is available, should also be given. An example is the immunization of healthcare personnel exposed to the hepatitis B virus. Some genetic disorders which can be identified at the pre-employment stage may enable suitable advice to be given in regards to special care in handling chemicals at work, for example, people with glucose-6-phosphate dehydrogenase deficiency are at risk of haemolytic anaemia on exposure to naphthalene and fava beans. People with serum total alpha-1-antitrypsin deficiency may be susceptible to smoke, fumes, and other respiratory irritants (Koh and Jeyaratnam 1998).

Periodic medical examinations

The aim of statutory medical examinations is to prevent special groups of 'at-risk' workers from developing serious occupational diseases. Regular health examinations, which are specific for the type of hazard the worker is exposed to, are conducted. Workers found to have signs of overexposure to the hazard or with early signs of disease can be removed from further exposure. They can be given alternative work until they are fit to return to their former jobs. Furthermore, if signs of overexposure are detected, additional control measures can be taken to reduce the exposure at source, and prevent other workers from being similarly affected.

Special groups of workers are required to undergo periodic medical examinations for protecting the health of the public, for example, professional drivers and food handlers.

In many countries, employment laws require specified categories of employees to undergo statutory periodic medical examinations, for example, for workers exposed to known hazards such as noise, radiation, asbestos, silica, and heavy metals. In principle, this approach to prevention sounds reasonable, that is, to detect health effects from occupational exposure early in order to take preventive action. In practice the usefulness of such regular procedures is questionable. For example, examining radiation workers for the early effects of radiation exposure or performing annual chest X-rays on workers exposed to fibrogenic or carcinogenic dusts (asbestos, silica) has little beneficial effect on prevention. This is because radiological changes in the chest as a result of exposure to these dusts occur after a long latent period, and by the time the changes are detected, irreversible damage has already occurred. The prospects for effective treatment are often limited. The prevention of disease in other exposed workers would need to involve control measures instituted at a much earlier stage before X-ray changes appear.

For the countries that require statutory periodic medical examinations, these are often only to be carried out by qualified health personnel, with additional postgraduate training in occupational health. There is usually stipulation for the results of the examinations to be kept for a specified period of time, and copies of examination or investigation findings need to be sent to the relevant government agency.

Post-illness or -injury evaluation

An evaluation of the health status of the employee returning to work after a prolonged absence from work due to illness or injury can help ensure that the worker has sufficiently recovered, and is fit to return to work duties. Several issues to consider are:

1. Can the worker perform his/her duty without compromising his/ her health and safety or that of fellow workers and others?

2. Is the worker capable of performing the work efficiently despite any residual impairment of function that has resulted from the illness?

3. Could the worker benefit from some adjustment to the work process, provision of additional or modified equipment, or alteration to the system of work?

4. Should he/she return to previous full-time unrestricted duty, or should alternative work be considered?

Notification of occupational diseases

Most countries require the statutory notification of occupational diseases to the government. This allows investigation, confirmation, and follow-up of cases by the authorities, and an analysis of trends over time. A single notified case may indicate poor control of work hazards that can pose a risk to other workers in the same work environment. Thus, it fits in with the concept of secondary prevention in that the sentinel 'notified' case may enable exposure to be further controlled before overt disease occurs in other exposed workers. The responsibility for notification has involved doctors, employers, or employee representatives, and varies between countries. Many countries produce a list of notifiable occupational diseases. This can be different from a list of prescribed diseases for which individuals may obtain financial compensation.

Notification serves as an additional means of control of occupational diseases. It should initiate a chain of events, starting from investigation and confirmation of the index case, and active case finding of other affected people. Recommendations for specific preventive measures at the workplace are then prescribed. The authorities would follow up by ensuring that the recommendations have been implemented. If necessary, further evaluation of the effectiveness of the preventive measures can be made.

Tertiary prevention

Tertiary prevention involves mainly early treatment and rehabilitation. For occupational ill health, affected workers should be removed from further exposure, and the appropriate medical treatment given as necessary. Examples of appropriate treatment include the rendering of first aid promptly after an injury, chelation for severe cases of heavy metal poisoning, atropine and aldoximes for organophosphate poisoning, antidotes for cyanide poisoning, use of calcium gluconate for hydrofluoric acid burns, and hyperbaric treatment for cases of compressed air illness. Treatment would also include prompt provision of clinical supportive measures.

Planning for emergency response

Occupational health personnel can assist in developing plans to cope with disasters in the workplace that may also affect the surrounding community. In addition to first aid and acute healthcare provisions, other aspects such as fire and emergency response services are essential. Planning and practice drills should be done jointly with the relevant local community agencies.

Rehabilitation

Rehabilitation of workers is another important aspect of occupational health practice. Management, co-workers, occupational health professionals, and the injured worker have to work together to ensure that suitable alternative duties are provided, and that any work restrictions or physical limitations are understood. There should be clear short- and long-term goals in rehabilitation, and alternative duties should be meaningful and contribute to production (Australasian College of Occupational Medicine and Australian College of Rehabilitation Medicine 1987). Sometimes, the use of external rehabilitation resources may be needed.

Workers' compensation

In many countries, workers who are injured at work or fall ill from hazardous work exposures are eligible for compensation. Workers' compensation is designed to provide income support, medical payments, and rehabilitation payments to workers injured on the job, as well as to provide benefits to the family and dependants of fatally injured workers. Most industrialized countries have workers' compensation programmes. In some countries, certain categories of workers, for example, domestic helpers are excluded. In many countries, employers have social insurance to give protection to employment injury victims. The principle of social insurance is that of sharing of risks and pooling financial resources. A social insurance scheme establishes a public channel through a government department or government supervised body, which oversees procedures of screening, determination of award and payment of benefits.

Benefits are payable for temporary incapacity or permanent incapacity, and include survivors' benefits for those killed at work. Guidelines for assessment of disability are available in most countries. The final assessments for disability are made when the worker's medical condition has stabilized, and not likely to improve or deteriorate further. Besides workers' compensation and social insurance schemes, injured workers can sue their employer for negligence through common law. This can be a lengthy process in some countries (although not in the United Kingdom), acceptance of benefits from a state or federal workers' compensation scheme requires waiver of the right to sue the employer.

Health promotion at the workplace

The WHO defines health promotion in its broadest sense as 'the process of enabling people to increase control over, and to improve their health'. Health promotion is an integral part of a comprehensive occupational healthcare system (WHO 1988).

It is a process of activating communities, policymakers, professionals, and the public for health supportive policies, systems, and ways of living. It is manifested by promoting healthy lifestyles and community action for health, and by creating conditions that make it possible to live a healthy life. The workplace is a suitable venue to develop and provide health promotion for individuals and for groups of workers. These activities include cessation of smoking, providing dietary advice, encouraging exercise and physical activity, promoting healthy lifestyles, reducing cardiovascular and other risks, and emphasizing compliance with health and safety measures at the workplace.

Table 7.4.1 Comparison of occupational health and environmental health

Occupational health	Environmental health
Hazards in workplace environment	Hazards in community environment
Hazards largely in air	Hazards in air, soil, water, and food
Hazards are physical, chemical, biological, and psychosocial	Hazards are physical, chemical, biological, and psychosocial
Route of exposure: inhalation and dermal	Route of exposure: ingestion, inhalation, and dermal
Exposure period: 8 hours/day for working life	Exposure period: 24 hours a day, lifelong
Exposed population: adults, usually healthy	Exposed population: children, adults, elderly (includes the sick and infirm)

Source: data from American Conference of Governmental Industrial Hygienists (ACGIH), *TLVs and BEIs, Threshold Limit Values for Chemical Substances and Physical Agents: Biological Exposure Indices*, American Conference of Governmental Industrial Hygienists, Inc. Cincinnati, USA, Copyright © 2012.

From occupational health to environmental health

Occupational health practice today has evolved to include consideration of environmental health issues. There are several reasons for the increasing convergence of the two disciplines. Firstly, many sources of pollution originate from the workplace. Secondly, especially in regards to work and health, there can be an overlap between the work environment, the home environment, and the general environment, for example, in agriculture and in cottage and small-scale industries. In these examples, there is often no clear demarcation between the workplace and the home. Thirdly, there are several areas of common ground between occupational and environmental health. Table 7.4.1 compares the factors in the work environment that influence the health of the working population (occupational health) with that of the general environment affecting the health of the community (environmental health).

Occupational health practitioners have the necessary skills in clinical medicine, toxicology, hygiene, epidemiology, and preventive health to contribute to the management of environmental health concerns, especially those resulting from workplace activity. The success of both occupational health and environmental health in regards to investigations, interventions, and implementation of prevention relies heavily on good communication between the professionals and the stakeholders.

Conclusion

Workers suffer a broad range of injuries and illnesses caused by hazards encountered in the workplace. In the practice of occupational health, prevention of work-related and occupational disease is a key objective. It also includes efforts for preventing occupational injury. Prevention can be at the primary, secondary, or tertiary level. Reducing exposure to occupational hazards in the workplace is the mainstay for reducing the burden of occupational ill health. The workplace is also an ideal setting for health promotion activities, although the benefits from health promotion will only be realized if occupational hazards are first controlled.

The importance of occupational health lies in its emphasis on prevention, and in this respect it shares common objectives and strategies with public health. Occupational health focuses mainly on a specific group in the community—those in employment. Public health covers the health interests of the whole community. There is much merit and scope for closer links between occupational health, environmental health, and public health.

References

American Conference of Governmental Industrial Hygienists (2012). *TLVs and BEIs. Threshold Limit Values for Chemical Substances and Physical Agents. Biological Exposure Indices*. Cincinnati, OH: ACGIH.

Australasian College of Occupational Medicine and Australian College of Rehabilitation Medicine (1987). *Occupational Rehabilitation. Guidelines on Principles and Practice*. Melbourne: ACOM and ACRM.

Barbara, G., De Giorgio, R., Stanghellini, V., Cremon, C., Salvioli, B., and Corinaldesi, R. (2004). New pathophysiological mechanisms in irritable bowel syndrome. *Alimentary Pharmacology & Therapeutics*, 20(Suppl. 2), 1–9.

Braman, S.S. (2006). The global burden of asthma. *Chest*, 130(1), 45–125.

Centers for Disease Control and Prevention (2008). Silicosis-related years of potential life lost before age 65 years. United States, 1968–2005. *Morbidity and Mortality Weekly Report*, 57(28), 771–5.

Cherniak, M. (1986). *The Hawk's Nest Incident: America's Worst Industrial Disaster*. New Haven, CT: Yale University Press.

Concha-Barrientos, M., Campbell-Lendrum, D., and Steenland, K. (2004). *Occupational Noise: Assessing the Burden of Disease from Work-Related Hearing Impairment at National and Local Levels*. WHO Environmental Burden of Disease Series, No. 9. Geneva: WHO.

Concha-Barrientos, M., Nelson, D.I., Driscoll, T., et al. (2004). Selected occupational risks. In M. Ezzati, A. Lopez, A. Rodgers, and C.J.L. Murray (eds.) *Comparative Quantification of Health Risks: Global and Regional Burden of Disease Attributable to Selected Major Risk Factors*, pp. 1652–801. Geneva: WHO.

Driscoll, T., Nelson, D.I., Steenland, K., et al. (2005). The global burden of disease due to occupational carcinogens. *American Journal of Industrial Medicine*, 48, 419–31.

Elo, A.-L., Leppanen, A., Lindstrom, K., and Ropponen, T. (1992). *OSQ-Occupational Stress Questionnaire: User's Instructions*. Helsinki: Finnish Institute of Occupational Health.

European Agency for Safety and Health at Work (2008). *Occupational Skin Diseases and Dermal Exposure in the European Union (EU-25): Policy and Practice Overview*. Luxembourg: Office for Official Publications of the European Communities.

European Chemicals Agency (2012). *Understanding REACH*. [Online] Available at: http://echa.europa.eu/web/guest/regulations/reach/understanding-reach.

European Commission (2010). *Health and Safety at Work in Europe (1997–2007)*. Luxembourg: Publications Office of the European Union.

Eurostat (2010). *Health and Safety at Work in Europe (1999–2007)*. Luxembourg: Publications Office of the European Union. Available at: http://epp.eurostat.ec.europa.eu/cache/ITY_OFFPUB/KS-31-09-290/EN/KS-31-09-290-EN.PDF.

Forsmann, S. (1983). Occupational health. In L. Parmeggiani (ed.) *Encyclopaedia of Occupational Health and Safety* (3rd ed.), pp. 1491–3. Geneva: ILO.

Health and Safety Executive (1995). *Generic Terms and Concepts in the Assessment and Regulation of Industrial Risks*. London: HMSO.

Health and Safety Executive (2011a). *Costs to Britain of Workplace Injuries and Work-Related Ill-Health*. London: HSE. Available from http://www.hse.gov.uk/statistics/.

Health and Safety Executive (2011b). *Work-Related Skin Disease*. London: HSE. Available at: http://www.hse.gov.uk/statistics/.

Health and Safety Executive (2012). *Annual Statistics Report 2010/11*. London: HSE.

Holmes, S.M. (2006). An ethnographic study of the social context of migrant health in the United States. *PLoS Medicine*, 3(10), e448.

International Agency for Research on Cancer (1997). *IARC Monographs on the Evaluation of Carcinogenic Risks to Humans: Silica, Some Silicates, Coal Dust and Para-Aramid Fibrils*. Lyon: IARC.

International Agency for Research on Cancer (2010). *IARC Monographs on the Evaluation of Carcinogenic Risks to Humans: Painting, Firefighting, and Shiftwork*. Lyon: IARC.

International Labour Organization (2002). *Press Release: Work Related Fatalities Reach 2 million Annually*. ILO Reference No. ILO/02/23. Geneva: ILO.

International Labour Organization (2006a). *Press Release: ILO Welcomes New UN Convention on Rights of People with Disabilities*. ILO Reference No. ILO/06/58. Geneva: ILO.

International Labour Organization (2006b). *The End of Child Labour: Within Reach. Global Report Under the Follow-Up to the ILO Declaration on Fundamental Principles and Rights at Work*. Geneva: ILO.

International Labour Organization (2007a). *Equality at Work: Tackling the Challenges. Global report under the follow-up to the ILO Declaration on Fundamental Principles and Rights at Work*. Geneva: ILO.

International Labour Organization (2007b). *Press Release: Working Time Around The World*. ILO Reference No. ILO/07/29. Geneva: ILO.

International Labour Organization (2011). Introductory report: global trends and challenges on occupational safety and health. In *XIX World Congress on Safety and Health at Work*, Istanbul, Turkey, 11–15 September, 2011.

International Programme on the Elimination of Child Labour (2011). *Children in Hazardous Work. What We Know. What We Need To Do*. Geneva: International Labour Organization.

International Programme on the Elimination of Child Labour (2012). *IPEC Action Against Child Labour 2011–2012: Progress and Future Priorities*. Geneva: International Labour Office.

Jackson, C. (2007). The General Health Questionnaire. *Occupational Medicine*, 57, 79.

Jensen, T.K., Bonde, J.P., and Joffe, M. (2006). The influence of occupational exposure on male reproductive function. *Occupational Medicine*, 56(8), 544–53.

Kogevinas, M., Zock, J.P., Jarvis, D., et al. (2007). Exposure to substances in the workplace and new-onset asthma: an international prospective population-based study (ECRHS-II). *The Lancet*, 370, 336–41.

Koh, D. and Jeyaratnam, J. (1998). Biomarkers, screening and ethics. *Occupational Medicine*, 48, 27–30.

Koh, D., Lim, M.K., Chia, S.E. (2003). SARS: health care work can be hazardous to health. *Occupational Medicine*, 53(4), 241–3.

Koh, D., Seow, A., and Ong, C.N. (1999). New techniques in molecular epidemiology and their relevance to occupational medicine. *Occupational and Environmental Medicine*, 56, 725–9.

Kumar, S. (2004). Occupational exposure associated with reproductive dysfunction. *J Occupational Health*, 46, 1–19.

Leigh, J.P., Markowitz, S.B., Fahs, M., Shin, C., and Landrigan, P.J. (1997). Occupational injury and illness in the United States. *Archives of Internal Medicine*, 157, 1557–68.

Leka, S., Griffiths, A., and Cox, T. (2003). *Work Organization and Stress*. Protecting Workers' Health Series No. 3. Geneva: WHO.

Lin, R.T., Takahashi, K., Karjalainen, A., et al. (2007). Ecological association between asbestos-related diseases and historical asbestos consumption: an international analysis. *The Lancet*, 369(9564), 844–9.

Loewenson, R.H. (1999). Women's occupational health in globalization and development. *American Journal of Industrial Medicine*, 36, 34–42.

Loney, T. and Aw, T.C. (2012). Occupational noise and health. *Health and Safety Middle East*, 10, 39–45.

Mason, H.J., Williams, N., Armitage, S., et al. (1999). Follow up of workers previously exposed to silver solder containing cadmium. *Occupational and Environmental Medicine*, 56, 553–8.

McKay, S., Craw, M., and Chopra, D. (2006). *Migrant Workers in England and Wales: An Assessment of Migrant Worker Health and Safety Risks*. Suffolk: HSE Books.

Messing, K. (2006). *Gender Equality, Work and Health: A Review of the Evidence*. Geneva: WHO.

Morens, D.M., Folkers, G.K., and Fauci, A.S. (2004). The challenge of emerging and re-emerging infectious diseases. *Nature*, 430, 242–9.

National Institute for Occupational Safety and Health (1996). *National Occupational Research Agenda Update*. DHHS (NIOSH) Publication No. 96-115. Cincinnati, OH: NIOSH.

National Institute for Occupational Safety and Health (1999). *Stress at Work*. DHSS (NIOSH) Publication No. 99-101. Cincinnati, OH: NIOSH.

National Institute for Occupational Safety and Health (2007). *NORA (National Occupational Research Agenda): Disease and Injury. NORA Priority Research Areas*. Cincinnati, OH: NIOSH. Available at: http://www.cdc.gov/niosh/docs/96-115/diseas.html.

National Institute for Occupational Safety and Health (2011). *Hearing Loss Prevention (NIOSH Program Portfolio)*. Cincinnati, OH: NIOSH. Available at: http://www.bls.gov/iif/oshwc/osh/os/ostb1481.pdf.

National Institute for Occupational Safety and Health (2008). *NIOSH Generic Job Stress Questionnaire (Organization of Work: Measurement Tools for Research and Practice)*. Cincinnati, OH: NIOSH. Available at: http://www.cdc.gov/niosh/.

Occupational Health and Safety Administration (2012). *Injury and Illness Prevention Programs*. White Paper. [Online] OHSA. Available at: http://www.osha.gov.

Paltiel, F. (1998). Shifting paradigms and policies. In J. Stellman (ed.) *Encyclopaedia of Occupational Health and Safety* (4th ed.), pp. 24.1–24.21. Geneva: ILO.

Pearce, N., Boffetta, P., and Kogevinas, M. (1998). Cancer—introduction. In J. Stellman (ed.) *Encyclopaedia of Occupational Health and Safety* (4th ed.), pp. 2.1–2.18. Geneva: ILO.

Pruss-Ustun, A., Rapiti, E., and Hutin, Y. (2005). Estimation of the global burden of disease attributable to contaminated sharps injuries among health-care workers. *American Journal of Industrial Medicine*, 38, 482–90.

Ramazzini, B. (1964). *De Moribs Artificum Diatriba* (W. Cave Wright, trans.). New York: Hafner Publishing Co. (Work originally published in 1713.)

Rosenstock, L., Cullen, M.R., and Fingerhut, M. (2005). Advancing worker health and safety in the developing world. *Journal of Occupational and Environmental Medicine*, 47, 132–6.

Sadhra, S. and Rampal, K.G. (eds.) (1999). *Occupational Health. Risk Assessment and Management*. Oxford: Blackwell Science Ltd.

Shah, N.S., Wright, A., Bai, G.-H., et al. (2007). Worldwide emergence of extensively drug-resistant tuberculosis. *Emerging Infectious Diseases*, 13(3), 380–7.

Stellman, J. (1999). Women workers: the social construction of a special population. *Occupational Medicine*, 14, 559–80.

Symanski, E., Sallsten, G., Chan, W., and Barregard, L. (2001). Heterogeneity in sources of exposure variability among groups of workers exposed to inorganic mercury. *Annals of Occupational Hygiene*, 45(8), 677–87.

Takala, J. (2003). ILO and asbestos. In *Asbestos Conference*, Dresden, 3 September. Available at: http://www.ilo.org/safework.

United Nations (1990). *Convention on the Protection of the Rights of All Migrant Workers and Members of Their Families*. Ratified 1 July 2003. Available at: http://www.ohchr.org/english/law/cmw.htm.

Weiderpass, E., Meo, M., and Vainio, H. (2011). Risk factors for breast cancer, including occupational exposures. *Safety and Health at Work*, 2, 1–8.

Whitaker, S. and Aw, T.C. Audit of pre-employment assessments by occupational health departments in the National Health Service. *Occupational Medicine*, 45(2), 75–80.

World Health Organization (1988). *Health Promotion for Working Populations*. Technical Report Series 765. Geneva: WHO.

World Health Organization (2007a). *Workers' Health: Draft Global Action Plan. Sixtieth World Health Assembly, Provisional Agenda item 12.13*. Geneva: WHO.

World Health Organization (2007b). *The Global MDR-TB and XDR-TB Response Plan*. Geneva: WHO.

World Health Organization (2011). *Gender, Work and Health*. Geneva: WHO.

Wynn, P.A., Aw, T.C., Williams, N.R., and Harrington, M. (2002). Teaching of occupational medicine to undergraduates in UK schools of medicine. *Medical Education*, 36, 1–5.

7.5

Toxicology and risk assessment in the analysis and management of environmental risk

David Koh, Tar-Ching Aw, and
Bernard D. Goldstein

Introduction to toxicology and risk assessment in the analysis and management of environmental risk

Toxicology is the study of the science of poisons. In theory, any substance can cause harm to health. To paraphrase the immortal words of the physician alchemist Paracelsus, 'It is only the dose that distinguishes a poison from a remedy'. To that we can also add that the route of entry into the body can also determine the extent of injury or ill health. In practice, most poisons are either chemicals or biological materials that cause severe effects in relatively small doses. Poisonous substances that contaminate the environment can lead to an increased risk of ill health in exposed populations. The level of risk is a function of the extent of exposure and the susceptibility of those exposed. An understanding of toxicology is essential in determining and managing environmental risk.

The goal of this chapter is to synthesize toxicology and risk assessment as a basis for evaluating human health risks posed by chemical, biological, and physical agents in the environment. Disciplines other than toxicology, such as epidemiology and exposure assessment, are also required to better understand risk, and for many specific agents will provide the major basis for the information underlying risk assessment and risk management.

Environmental risk analysis is a broad field, encompassing risks to ecosystems and materials as well as to human health. Only human health risks will be considered in this chapter. However, the link between human and environment health is obvious. Risk to ecosystems can often serve as a warning about human health risk. As an example, the concern about the impact of acid deposition on trees and lakes preceded by about two decades the recognition that relatively low atmospheric concentrations of fine particulates as part of acid deposition are a human health risk. Another related example is the impact of global climate change on human health (see Box 7.5.1).

Toxicology has two important roles in environmental risk management:

1. The ascertainment of cause and effect relationships linking chemical and physical agents to adverse effects in humans or the general environment.

2. The development of techniques capable of preventing these problems.

Toxicologists usually approach questions of disease causation by starting with the chemical or physical agent and studying its effects in laboratory animals or in test-tube systems. An exciting aspect of modern toxicology is the development of tools, primarily through molecular biology and advanced computational techniques, capable of probing the extent to which a given disease in an individual is caused by a chemical or other environmental factor. This reversal of approach, in which we start with disease and move towards determining the cause, is enabled by the increasing ability of epidemiology to link subtle biological markers indicative of early effects to biological markers indicative of exposure.

Toxicology is also an important discipline in the primary and secondary prevention of human health effects. Understanding the mechanisms by which chemical agents cause biological effects can result in toxicological tests useful to prevent the development of harmful chemicals, or the early detection of potential adverse effects.

General concepts of toxicology relevant to risk assessment

Knowledge about poisons extends back to the beginning of history as humans became aware of the toxicity of natural food components. The bible contains injunctions concerning poisons, including how to avoid them. Greek and Roman history gives evidence of the use of poisons as an instrument of statecraft, an approach that was extended in the Middle Ages with such notable practitioners

Box 7.5.1 Case study: global climate change and human health

Unprecedented social and demographic changes and evolving patterns of economic activity have resulted in large-scale and systemic environmental impacts. One such impact is the rapid increase of greenhouse gas emissions and the resulting global climate change (McMichael 2013).

Human health can be impacted by direct biological consequences of extreme weather events, for example heatwaves, through temperature-enhanced levels of urban air pollutants; and via increased health risks from changes in biophysically and ecologically based processes and systems, for example, food yields, water flows, infectious-disease vectors, and intermediate-host ecology for zoonotic diseases. There are also more diffuse and indirect effects, such as mental health problems in failing farm communities, displaced groups, disadvantaged indigenous and minority ethnic groups, and consequences of tension and conflict owing to climate change-related declines in basic resources (water, food, timber, living space).

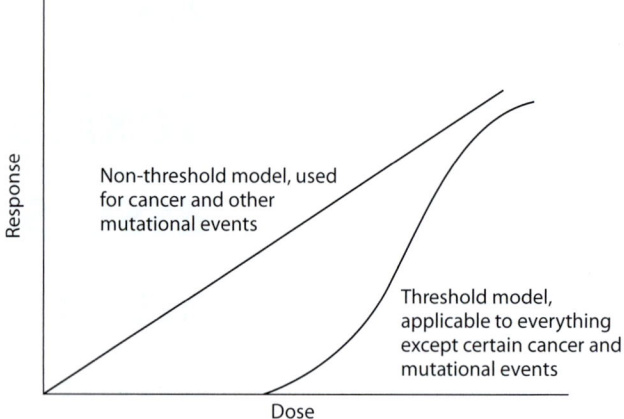

Fig. 7.5.1 Dose–response curve.

as the Borgias. Toxicologists credited Paracelsus with the first law of toxicology, that the dose makes the poison. There are two other major maxims that underlie modern toxicology: that chemicals have specific biological effects, a maxim that has been credited to Ambrose Pare (Goldstein and Gallo 2001); and that humans are members of the animal kingdom.

The 'laws' of toxicology

The following subsections discuss 'laws' and general concepts of toxicology pertinent to understanding how a chemical or physical agent acts in a biological system. The focus will be on the biological response, rather than on the intrinsic properties of the agent. The three 'laws' of toxicology are:

1. The dose makes the poison.

2. Chemicals have specific effects.

3. Humans are animals.

The first law: the dose makes the poison

Central to toxicology is the exploration the relation between dose and response. As a generalization, there are two main types of dose–response curves (Fig. 7.5.1). One is an S-shaped curve that is characterized by having at lowest doses no observed effect and, as the dose increases, the gradual development of an increasing response. This is followed by a linear phase of increase in response in relation to dose and, eventually, a dose level at which no further increase in response is observed. Of particular pertinence to environmental toxicology is that this curve presumes that there is a threshold level—below which no harm whatsoever is to be expected. There is ample scientific basis for the existence of thresholds for specific effects. For example, if one drop of undiluted sulphuric acid is splashed onto the skin it is capable of producing a severe burn. Yet one drop of pure sulphuric acid in a bathtub of water is sufficiently dilute to be without effect. Thresholds for an adverse effect will differ among individuals based upon a variety of circumstances, some of which are genetically determined and others may represent

stages of life or specific circumstances. In the example of sulphuric acid on the skin, there are genetically determined differences in susceptibility related to the protective presence of skin hair; babies will be more susceptible than adults; and skin that is already damaged will be at particular risk. This S-shaped dose–response curve is assumed to fit all toxic effects except those that are produced by direct reaction with genetic material.

The second general type of dose–response curve covers end points caused by persistent changes in the genes. This occurs in cancer, in which a somatic mutation occurring in a single cell results in a clone of cancer cell progeny. Another example is inherited mutations of the genetic components of cells involved in reproduction. It is believed that a single change in DNA can alter the genetic code in such a way to lead to a mutated cell. It therefore follows that any single molecule of a carcinogenic chemical or packet of physical energy such as ionizing radiation, that can alter DNA is theoretically capable of causing a persistent mutation. The presumption that every single molecule or ionizing ray has the possibility of changing a normal cell to a cancerous cell implies that there is no absolutely safe dose. The resultant dose–response curve starts at a single molecule, that is, it has no threshold below which the risk is zero. As a further simplification, the shape of the curve can be linearly related to dose in that the risk of two molecules of a DNA-altering chemical causing a mutation is conceivably twice that of one molecule, and so on, until a dose level results in dead cells.

Features of both the S-shaped and linear dose–response curves occur in the body's response to allergens. It is likely that a relatively large dose of an allergen is required to sensitize an individual (i.e. with a threshold dose for sensitization that may vary with the agent and the individual). However, once sensitized, the affected person may react to molecules of the causative agent with no apparent threshold for elicitation of a reaction.

There are also a few chemicals that have a U-shaped dose–response curve. This is where high levels of exposure cause harm and insufficient amounts lead to deficiency which results in ill health. Examples are fat-soluble vitamins and essential trace minerals. Excess vitamin D intake causes hypervitaminosis D, and vitamin D deficiency leads to rickets and osteomalacia. There is therefore an ideal range for vitamin D levels which results neither in deficiency nor poisoning.

The second law: specificity of effects

That chemical and physical agents have specific effects is in essence no different than recognizing that possession of a gun does not make one a murder suspect if the victim has been stabbed to death. The law of specificity is well understood by the general public in terms of drugs: aspirin will help with your headache but is useless for constipation, while laxatives have the opposite effect. However, various surveys suggest that the selectivity of effects of environmental chemicals is not well understood by the lay public; many believing that a chemical that can cause cancer in a particular organ can cause cancer and other diseases anywhere in the body. Some chemicals may cause malignancy in more than one body site (e.g. asbestos as a cause of lung cancer, peritoneal mesothelioma, and laryngeal cancer), but in general, chemical and physical agents are highly specific in their effects.

The specificity of effects is due both to chemistry and to biology. Understanding the relationship between chemical structure and biological effect has been central to both pharmacology and toxicology. Structure–activity relationships (SARs) are often used as a means to design a chemical with a specific effect that might be useful as a therapeutic agent. SARs are also used to predict whether a new chemical being readied for manufacture might be of potential harm. While SARs are a useful tool which is being improved through modern computational approaches, their predictive values remain too limited to be used without recourse to additional testing of a potentially toxic agent. For example, only one simple methyl group separates toluene from benzene, with only the latter known to cause bone marrow damage and leukaemia; ethanol from methanol, the latter causing metabolic acidosis, renal failure, and blindness; and n-hexane from either n-heptane or n-pentane, with only n-hexane being responsible for peripheral nerve damage. These examples of specificity reflect both the formation of toxic metabolites, such as active species derived from the metabolism of benzene, and the interaction of a chemical or its metabolite within specific biological niches, such as the diketone metabolite (2,5-hexanedione) of n-hexane within neuronal axons.

Specificity of effects is also conferred by cellular processes that lead certain cells to be more susceptible to environmental agents. For example, red blood cells have the iron-containing protein haemoglobin that is responsible for the transport of oxygen. Toxicity through alteration of efficient oxygen delivery occurs through certain specific mechanisms. One is through the oxidation of the reduced ferrous form to the ferric form of iron, known as methaemoglobin, which can no longer carry oxygen. This occurs with a limited number of agents (e.g. nitrates and phenols) that once within the red blood cell are capable of oxidizing intracellular iron. Another specific mechanism of interference is exemplified by carbon monoxide. This otherwise relatively inert gas has a physical chemistry that sufficiently resembles oxygen so that it is able to tightly combine with the oxygen combining site of haemoglobin, thereby displacing oxygen. There are many other examples in which in essence a normal body process is disrupted by an exogenous chemical through a specific chemical alteration, such as oxidation or covalent addition, or by fitting into a niche designed through evolution to accommodate a necessary internal chemical which it superficially resembles.

The third law: humans are animals

The conceptual foundation for extrapolating from animals to humans is a central facet of modern toxicology. The basic principles of cell function are common to all of biology. All cells must obtain energy, build structure, and release waste. Cell function in complex organisms such as humans is highly specialized, but there is still a great deal of similarity in cellular and organ function among mammals facilitating extrapolation of effects from one species to another. In general, the specificity of toxic effects is relatively similar across mammals, for example, a kidney poison in one species is likely to be a kidney poison in another, although there are certainly exceptions. Arsenic is an example of a human carcinogen where the animal evidence for carcinogenicity is lacking. However, dose–response considerations often vary substantially, reflecting differences in absorption, distribution, metabolism, excretion, function, and target organ susceptibility between species. Understanding the factors responsible for inter-species differences greatly facilitates extrapolation from animals to humans. Once elucidated, the role of different absorption rates, metabolism, or other factors can be taken into account, often through a mathematical approximation that has come to be called physiologically based pharmacokinetics (or toxicokinetics). One of the greatest threats to the public health value of toxicological sciences comes from animal rights activists who in their arguments against animal research intentionally ignore the major positive impact of animal toxicology on the well-being and lifespan of animals, including pet dogs and cats.

Pathways of exogenous chemicals within the body

The four major processes governing the impact of an exogenous chemical within the human body are absorption, distribution, metabolism, and excretion. All can vary greatly among different individuals, and within the same individual depending upon, for example, stage of life and state of health. These variations are among the major reasons for differences among humans in susceptibility to risks from exposure to chemical and physical agents. The increased understanding of how the human genotype and phenotype affects absorption, distribution, metabolism, and excretion of external agents, including foods, is providing insight into answers to the oldest human question about disease: 'Why is this happening to me?' (Omenn 2000).

Absorption

Absorption of a chemical into the body occurs through ingestion, inhalation, and across the skin. Depending upon the specific chemical, the route of exposure can have major implications on the extent of absorption and the resultant toxicity. For example, almost 100 per cent of inhaled lead-containing fine particles are absorbed into the body as compared to a much smaller percentage of ingested lead. Internal factors also can affect absorption, particularly from the gastrointestinal tract. In the case of lead absorption, iron and calcium deficiencies both produce an increase in absorption of ingested lead. The matrix of the exposure agent also may have an effect. For example, the rate at which benzene in gasoline is absorbed through the skin will likely be increased by oxygenated components of the gasoline mixture; and the absorption of dioxins from contaminated soil can vary enormously (Umbreit et al. 1986). The American Conference of Governmental Industrial Hygienists (2013) provides a 'skin' notation for chemicals that can be absorbed through the skin to cause systemic effects following exposure.

Often, a single route of absorption is dominant. But, in many instances, more than one route is important. For example, exposure to chlorinated disinfection products in drinking water systems, or gasoline contamination of well water through a leaky underground storage tank, is usually thought of solely in terms of the ingestion of water. However, during showering there is likely to be both inhalation and transdermal absorption, and if groundwater is contaminated there can be off-gassing from soil into the home. Epidemiological studies of the potential adverse consequences of water contamination need to take all of these exposure routes into account (Arbuckle et al. 2002).

Other less common routes of absorption can be through the intravenous, intramuscular, intraperitoneal, or sublingual route, or via suppositories. These occur mainly in animal experiments or in human drug delivery. A novel route of absorption is the translocation of nanoparticles deposited in the nasal area via the olfactory nerves directly into the brain (Oberdörster et al. 2004).

Distribution

Once inside the body, distribution of the chemical occurs through different pathways. In part, this depends upon the route of absorption. Most compounds absorbed in the gastrointestinal tract go directly to the liver and may go no further. The liver has a strong capacity to detoxify many absorbed chemicals. This first-pass effect occurs when a toxin or drug is absorbed by the digestive system and enters the hepatic portal system into the liver before it reaches the rest of the body. Enzymes of the gastrointestinal bacteria, lumen, gut wall, and liver contribute to the first-pass effect, which may greatly reduce the bioavailability of the toxin or drug in the systemic circulation. On the other hand, inhaled agents first go to the lung or other parts of the respiratory tract and then to the general circulation without being impacted by the first-pass effect.

Distribution also depends upon the chemical and physical properties of the agents. Small inhaled particles tend to be distributed deep within the respiratory tract while larger particles get filtered out in the nose or are trapped and cleared by the bronchiolar mucociliary escalator. Particles sized less than 2.5 microns are most likely to penetrate to the lower respiratory tract and alveoli. Chemicals that are poorly soluble in water, for example, oils, usually distribute within fatty tissues. Only certain types of compounds, for example, alcohols are able to cross the blood–brain barrier. Organ-specific factors are also important, for example, a specific pump located in the thyroid gland facilitates uptake of iodine and makes the thyroid particularly vulnerable to the adverse impact of radioactive iodine.

Metabolism

Metabolism in the narrowest sense of the term refers to alteration of chemicals by the body. The major metabolic function of the body is to alter food into energy or structural materials. Metabolism of xenobiotics (chemical compounds that are foreign to a living organism) is often protective, converting unwanted absorbed materials into chemical forms that are readily excretable. Thus, a fat-soluble agent can often be converted into water-soluble agents capable of being excreted in the urine. However, for certain classes of chemicals, metabolism results in conversion of relatively inactive compounds into harmful agents. For example, some carcinogens, including polycyclic organic hydrocarbon components of soot and benzene, require metabolic activation from a 'pro-carcinogen' to the 'ultimate carcinogen'.

All organs appear to have metabolic capability, often related both to organ function and to susceptibility to toxic agents. Understanding the specifics of the enzyme and enzyme families responsible for metabolism within cell types is important to the question of why chemicals have specific effects in specific organs.

In the case of benzene, about 50 per cent of the body burden is exhaled unchanged as the parent compound and the rest is metabolized to potentially toxic metabolites. Slowing down benzene metabolism leads to an increase in the relative amount that is exhaled rather than metabolized, and thus a decrease in bone marrow toxicity An apparent genetically determined increase in benzene metabolism to toxic metabolites, or a decrease in the detoxification of these metabolites, increases haematological risk in humans—with both polymorphisms together appearing to be at least additive and perhaps multiplicative in increasing risk (Rothman et al. 1997; Kim et al. 2007). The application of genomics and proteomics to metabolism is often known as 'metabolomics'.

Excretion

Excretion from the body can occur through a variety of different routes, primarily the gastrointestinal tract for unabsorbed compounds and for compounds dissolved in bile; and via the renal tract in urine for water-soluble agents of appropriate molecular weight and charge. Significant loss of volatile compounds can occur through the respiratory tract. Other routes of excretion include sweating and lactation, the latter unfortunately putting the breastfed infant at risk.

Interactions in multiple and combined exposures

Many toxicological studies of absorption, distribution, metabolism, and excretion are performed for single chemicals. Yet in real-life exposures, multiple and combined exposures are the norm rather than the exception. For such situations, the possibility of additive or synergistic effects, or potentiation or antagonism of effects has to be considered.

For example, in terms of interaction, exposure to two organophosphate insecticides may cause a simple additive adverse effect. In the case of exposure to carbon tetrachloride and ethanol, or asbestos exposure and cigarette smoking the combined effects are synergistic. The hepatotoxic effect of carbon tetrachloride can be potentiated by concurrent exposure to isopropanol (which by itself does not cause hepatotoxicity).

Antagonism could take various forms. Functional antagonism is exemplified by the opposing functional effects of a combination of barbiturate and norepinephrine. An example of chemical antagonism is the addition of BAL (British anti-Lewisite) to inactivate metal ions through chelation. The principle of dispositional antagonism is utilized in the treatment of poisoning with charcoal, or by use of an emetic or a diuretic. Receptor antagonism is seen in the case of the treatment of morphine overdose with naloxone.

Risk assessment

Risk assessment has evolved from two separate streams of toxicological reasoning: (1) for toxic agents implicitly or explicitly assumed to have a threshold, and (2) for carcinogens. The safety assessment of chemicals developed from simplified approaches such as studies on laboratory animals in which the dose (expressed usually as mg/kg body weight) capable of killing 50 per cent of the test animals (the LD_{50}); or the concentration (expressed as parts per million of the substance in air or water or other medium, i.e. the LC_{50}) were determined. This observed dose was used as a basis for extrapolating to permissible levels in humans, often using several tenfold 'safety factors'. These protective factors were based on the concern that humans could be more sensitive as a species than were laboratory animals; that there was a greater variability in sensitivity among humans than among genetically inbred laboratory animals all raised in a similar environment; and that there could be adverse non-lethal effects that should be avoided. A presumptive tenfold safety factor has been added specifically to protect children in recognition of their greater risk to certain chemicals compared to adults (National Research Council 1993).

The inherent assumption in the 'safety factor' approach is that there is a threshold dose level below which there are no adverse effects. However, for carcinogenesis a single mutation could be the basis for the entire cancer process. As each molecule of a carcinogen at least theoretically could cause this mutation, a threshold could not be assumed, and, as a simplification, there is no level of exposure that is without risk.

Almost all DNA damage is repaired by efficient cellular processes. Some unrepaired mutations are lethal to the cell. As dead cells do not reproduce this cannot be the basis for cancer or for inherited abnormalities. The majority of mutations are silent in that they have no discernible effects. Accordingly, the risk of any one molecule actually causing cancer is infinitesimally small—literally trillions of molecules of carcinogens are inhaled with every cigarette, yet not all cigarette smokers develop cancer. The assumption that the risk is not zero has a major impact on communicating to the public about cancer risk due to chemical and physical carcinogens.

There are circumstances in which cancer causation does depend upon exceeding a threshold level of a chemical (e.g. the mechanism by which saccharin causes bladder cancer in laboratory animals appears to proceed through the precipitation of saccharin in the bladder which requires a dose sufficient to exceed the physicochemical processes determining saccharin solubility). However, the prudent management of cancer risk usually assumes that the carcinogen is 'guilty until proven innocent' of having no risk-free level. In essence, the burden of proof is on industry to demonstrate scientifically that their cancer-causing chemical does have a threshold.

The four major components of risk assessment and their definitions are shown in Box 7.5.2.

Box 7.5.2 Components of risk assessment

Hazard identification: the determination of whether a specific chemical or physical agent is causally linked to a specific end point of concern; that is, specificity, or the second law of toxicology.

Dose–response evaluation: the determination of the relation between the magnitude of exposure and the probability of occurrence of the specific end point of concern; that is, the dose makes the poison, or the first law of toxicology.

Exposure evaluation: the determination of who and how many people will be exposed; through which routes; and the magnitude, duration, and timing of the exposure.

Risk characterization: the description of the nature and often the magnitude of the human risk, including attendant uncertainty.

Hazard identification

Hazard is the potential to cause harm. It is an intrinsic property of a substance or situation. Risk is the likelihood of harm occurring (and the severity of the resulting effect). It is a function of both hazard and exposure; for example, asbestos fibres sealed in a ceiling of an office have the potential to cause health effects, but the likelihood of that occurring is low if the ceiling is left intact. However, if the ceiling is demolished and dust containing the asbestos fibres is released, the risk to health can be considerable. The risk has changed because of the circumstances of exposure. The identification of the presence of a hazard is just one step in risk assessment; the subsequent steps such as exposure evaluation are key to determining what preventive action needs to be taken to reduce the risk.

A weight of evidence approach is often used by regulatory and quasi-scientific bodies to identify a hazard. In essence, a panel of scientists is asked to judge whether sufficient evidence exists to identify an agent or condition as having a risk of a specific effect in humans, or in some other target such as an ecosystem. The US approach to permitting the marketing of a new chemical is to have an internal Environmental Protection Agency scientific group review the chemical structure and other data submitted by industry. Similarly, the US Food and Drug Administration relies heavily on an advisory committee process to review evidence of efficacy and toxicity before approving a new pharmaceutical agent or medical device.

Formal weight-of-evidence approaches have been particularly useful in evaluating potential human carcinogens. The International Agency for Research on Cancer (IARC) of the World Health Organization categorizes carcinogens using this approach. IARC convenes expert panels to evaluate the evidence for carcinogenicity of specific chemical compounds or defined mixtures (e.g. diesel fuel, wood dust). The effort is focused on the weight of the evidence for carcinogenicity based upon carefully framed criteria considering animal toxicology, epidemiology, mechanistic information, and exposure data—but not on the potency of the compound as a cancer-causing agent. IARC has increased the weight it places on understanding toxicological mechanisms in assigning its score (Cogliano 2004). The information produced by IARC is used by many countries to decide governmental regulatory approaches at the workplace or general environment. In the United States, the IARC listing of carcinogens has no official status but carries much weight with US regulators as does a similar process used by the National Toxicology Program for its semi-annual Report on Carcinogens (National Toxicology Program 2011).

Relatively few chemicals have been reported as capable of causing cancer in humans. Of the perhaps 70,000–100,000 chemicals in commerce, about 100 are known to be human carcinogens. To an extent this represents the success of environmental health science in providing tools that guide chemical manufacturers away from new chemicals that are potentially carcinogenic. Early application in the chemical development process of simple test batteries evaluating the potential for mutagenesis or other predictors of cancer causation provides a responsible chemical industry with the means to avoid producing carcinogens or other potentially harmful products—and the means to avoid the regulatory and toxic tort consequences of harming the public. The value of this primary preventive approach depends upon the availability of effective toxicological test batteries. Such tests are based upon a basic understanding of the chemical and biological processes underlying toxic effects. Unfortunately, the investment in using standardized test batteries for high production volume chemicals, and the major increase in such investments due to the new requirements such as the EU REACH legislation (see later) has not been accompanied by recognition of the need to develop better and more effective tests to protect the public. Advances in molecular toxicology provide many opportunities to improve these test batteries (National Research Council 2007).

Dose–response evaluation

The key issues in dose–response evaluation involve how to extrapolate from the high doses at which an effect is observed in an animal or epidemiological study, to the usually much lower levels of risk which are of public or policy concern. Crucial to extrapolation are assumptions about the shape of the dose–response curve, that is, threshold, linear non-threshold, sublinear, or supralinear. It must be emphasized that the levels of risk desired by our society, for example, in the range of less than 1 in 10,000 to less than 1 in 1 million lifetime, are usually too low to be scientifically verifiable. This is particularly true as the end points of concern cannot be solely attributed to the environmental hazard under consideration, as illustrated in Box 7.5.3.

Box 7.5.3 Case study: benzene and leukaemia in the United States

Based upon extrapolation from both epidemiological and animal studies, the potency of benzene is estimated to result in a range of 2.2–7.8 in 1 million increase in the lifetime risk of leukaemia of an individual who is exposed for a lifetime to 1 microgram/m^3 benzene in air (US Environmental Protection Agency 2007).

In the case of the United States, a reasonable average benzene outdoor level is approximately 3 micrograms/m^3, which would predict a risk of 6.6–23.4 in 1 million lifetime caused by this benzene exposure. Regulatory approaches that decrease that outdoor background level by two-thirds to 1.0 micrograms/m^3 benzene nationwide would be estimated to decrease the risk of benzene-induced leukaemia by two-thirds. This would mean that nationwide there would be 4.4–15.6 less cases of leukaemia lifetime for every 1 million Americans, or approximately 10 in 1 million lifetime. Assuming a 70-year lifetime, and 350 million Americans, one can estimate that there would be 50 fewer cases of leukaemia a year nationwide as a result of a two-thirds decrease in outdoor benzene levels. This is a very small percentage of the 48,610 new cases of leukaemia in 2013 (http://www.cancer.gov/cancertopics/types/leukemia) estimated by the National Cancer Institute. While preventing that number of leukaemia cases is socially desirable, there are no current epidemiological or animal toxicology methods that could scientifically validate these assumptions.

A further complication is that for most of the US population, unregulated and highly variable indoor exposure to benzene, as well as to many other volatile organic compounds, far exceeds outdoor exposure. In fact, the major reason for a decrease in personal benzene exposure in the United States has been the decline in cigarette smoking for smokers, and its restriction from public places for non-smokers (Goldstein et al. 2011).

Exposure evaluation

Exposure evaluation is central to the management of environmental risks. Prevention of human exposure to a harmful chemical is synonymous with reduction of human risk. New advances in the field of exposure science are particularly crucial to understanding aggregate and cumulative risk (International Life Sciences Institute 1999; US Environmental Protection Agency 2003). Aggregate risk takes into account the different pathways of exposure for the same chemical. Cumulative risk describes the multiple effects of different agents through different routes, in essence an assessment of the impact of the mix of external synthetic and natural chemicals in which we all live. Cumulative risk assessment is particularly pertinent to environmental justice considerations.

The importance of exposure assessment in understanding risk is exemplified by investigations of potential adverse health consequences resulting from man-made events such as the attack on the World Trade Center in New York in September 2001, or natural disasters such as the earthquake and tsunami that destroyed the Fukushima nuclear plant in March 2011. Careful evaluation of disease end points in relation to exposure will help unravel the highly political and litigious issue of whether responders or the general public have an increased incidence of disease from such exposures generated by the explosion or in the process of cleaning up. New protocols and tools to assess exposures resulting from man-made or natural disasters may help in better evaluation of the exposure–effect relationship (Lioy et al. 2006).

Risk characterization

Many challenges are presented through the seemingly straightforward process of characterizing the risk estimated through the hazard identification, dose–response evaluation, and exposure evaluation steps. First, those doing the characterization are given an opportunity to put their 'spin' on the findings, for example, the public is likely to respond differently to the characterization that something is '99 per cent free of risk' than to the numerically equivalent characterization that there is a '1 per cent likelihood of a serious consequence including death'.

There is also the challenge of characterizing who is at risk (the denominator). Reporting the risk in terms of the entire exposed general public can trivialize the risk to a highly sensitive subpopulation, such as asthmatics.

Risk can also be displaced from one country to another, as was observed when the dumping of hazardous waste, illegally sent from Europe to the Côte d'Ivoire, was reported to have caused 9000 acute illnesses and six deaths in Abidjan (Greenpeace 2006, 2012). Compounding the issue is that the Côte d'Ivoire, not having its own expertise, had to use its scanty funds to hire a European company to retrieve, ship, and process the toxic waste (United Nations Environmental Programme 2006). The European company involved in the incident made a series of payments to the Ivorian government and individual claimants in relation to the case without admitting liability. In July 2010, the company was found guilty of illegally exporting toxic waste from Amsterdam and concealing the nature of the cargo by a Dutch court. The company was fined 1 million euros (BBC 2012)

There is also a long-standing debate on the extent to which numerical uncertainty, rather than a simple qualitative statement of the major sources of uncertainty, should be a routine part of risk characterization. Those in favour of routinely providing numerical boundaries that quantify the extent of uncertainty point out that the many estimates and default assumptions in a risk assessment provide wide ranges of uncertainty that should be presented to the risk manager and the general public.

Those in favour of a more restricted use of quantitative uncertainty analysis point out that most risk assessments are scoping activities aimed at considering alternatives or developing priorities. Further, major societal decisions are made on numerical estimates for which no uncertainty factors are given (e.g. the gross domestic product, unemployment estimates). The qualitative issues underlying uncertainty in a risk analysis should always be transparent to the risk manager and to the affected stakeholders.

The future of risk assessment

Risk assessment as a formal process to evaluate environmental agents has been evolving, particularly during the last few decades where more sophisticated approaches to cancer risk assessment and to cumulative and aggregate risk have developed. Using molecular toxicology to replace standard default assumptions is particularly promising (National Research Council 2007). Just as in other natural sciences, newer advances in data handling and informatics provide the opportunity to assess larger and more complex databases. Advances in epidemiologic methodology using biological indicators of exposure and effect based upon ecogenetics and other molecular biological techniques should be particularly fruitful (Omenn 2000). Conceptually, our genetic make-up is what loads the gun—but it is the environment that pulls the trigger. Identification of subpopulations sensitive to environmental factors will challenge regulatory and legal interpretation of the many environmental health laws that are aimed at protecting susceptible populations. Global harmonization of risk assessment has been under way for decades and will particularly be needed to avoid the use of environmental health principles as a façade for trade barriers. The application of evidence-based approaches to toxicology as is now increasingly used in medicine is a welcome development. It will be a challenge to use such processes for risk assessments that depend heavily on extrapolation to levels of risk below those that are readily observable, that is, the evidence will be indirect.

The regulatory approach to protecting worker health from toxic chemicals is often based upon both a measurable workplace standard and a subtle measure of effect. Thus for benzene, there is a 1 part per million, 8-hour time-weighted average workplace air standard as well as a requirement for routine blood counts. The latter informs the former both in terms of whether unmeasured exposures may be occurring, and whether a reconsideration of the allowable external standard is needed. As red cell, white cell, and platelet counts can be affected by a variety of common conditions, for example, infections and iron-deficiency anaemia, surveillance findings must be carefully evaluated before ascribing any observations to benzene exposure. In contrast, environmental standards are almost always measures of external pollutant emissions or ambient levels. Such standards are surrogates for the desired goal of avoiding adverse consequences to human health and the environment. Achieving a level of scientific knowledge that would permit the direct evaluation of subtle biological precursors of adverse effects would be a desired route to develop emission standards that

are truly protective. There is much work in progress in this field of environmental health indicators.

Human history of protecting against the consequences of environmental agents in essence is the history of catching up on the adverse effects of otherwise beneficial new technology—starting with the human use of fire. One of the more challenging new technologies with potential for beneficial and adverse consequences is that of nanotechnology. Decreasing the size of particles can result in unexpected new physico-chemical properties, in part due to a very high surface-to-volume ratio (Helland et al. 2007). Concern has been expressed as to what nano particles may do at the cellular level. The debate is unresolved about whether current toxicological testing schemes and regulatory processes are adequate to protect against the potential harm of nanotechnology products. However, toxicological principles are still relevant and central to the risk assessment process, as shown in Box 7.5.4.

The precautionary principle and/or/ versus risk assessment

A key issue facing risk management is how to proceed in the presence of hazard data with limited or no evidence of human toxicity. Application of the precautionary principle could be one approach for such an issue while additional scientific information is being gathered.

Box 7.5.4 Case study: potential environmental health effects of nanosilver

An area of concern identified by scientists has been the release of nanomaterials in consumer products to the environment. Nanosilver is one such product which has been used for treating socks that are marketed as non-odour producing as it confers antimicrobial properties. Benn and Westerhoff (2008) reported that six types of nanosilver treated socks leached silver nanoparticles when soaked in distilled water. This study raised concerns that nanosilver released from consumer products may enter wastewater systems and disrupt aquatic ecosystems. While ionic silver is known to be toxic to aquatic life, it is known that the speciation of silver affects its toxicity. Silver that is bound to sulphur or organic ligands is very much less toxic than free Ag ions. The alpha phase of silver sulphide, $\alpha\text{-}Ag_2S$ (found in nature as the mineral acanthite) is one of most insoluble Ag minerals known, in contrast to metallic Ag nanoparticles which are an efficient source of Ag ions in water.

In the environment, sources of silver can be from industry (e.g. mining, photographic, electronic) or from consumer products containing silver and nanosilver. In water, there could be dissolved Ag ions, bound Ag, Ag nanoparticles, coarser particles, and compounds, for example, $AgCl_2$. During the process of waste water treatment, the silver is converted mainly to the insoluble alpha phase of silver sulphide ($\alpha\text{-}Ag_2S$). However, what happens to the silver when it is discharged into the natural waterways is still unknown. It is uncertain whether surface modifications and coatings of Ag engineered nanoparticles make it more mobile and resistant to transformation reaction and produce less $\alpha\text{-}Ag_2S$ formation (Nowack 2010).

The precautionary principle was given impetus by the 1992 Rio Declaration on the Environment and Development which provided the following statement (United Nations Environmental Programme 1992): 'In order to protect the environment, the precautionary approach shall be widely applied by States according to their capabilities. Where there are threats of serious or irreversible damage, lack of full scientific certainty shall not be used as a reason for postponing cost-effective measures to prevent environmental degradation.' The Rio Declaration statement includes qualifying language such as 'according to their capabilities' and 'postponing cost-effective measures'. Furthermore, the triple negative notion—that the *absence* of rigorous proof of danger does *not* justify *inaction* is viewed by some as rather weak (World Commission on the Ethics of Scientific Knowledge and Technology 2005). The statement forces the consideration of precautionary intervention but does not necessarily require such intervention.

There are many variants of this definition and an extensive literature devoted to developing a more rigorous definition of the precautionary principle. To some, the precautionary principle is merely a means to build more public health protection into quantitative risk analysis, with additional prudent defaults and safety factors to protect at risk populations, and a further focus on uncertainty. To others, the precautionary principle is a new way of addressing environmental risk and for dealing with complexity and uncertainty. Its use is more likely to provide timely and preventive interventions (Tickner and Ketelson 2001; Martuzzi 2007). Some of the important approaches advocated by the precautionary principle, such as transparency and involvement of stakeholders, have also been advocated by many under the rubric of risk assessment and management.

A working definition of the precautionary principle has been proposed by UNESCO (World Commission on the Ethics of Scientific Knowledge and Technology 2005; italics in the original) (Box 7.5.5). This includes the firm statement that actions based upon the precautionary principle should be subject to continuous analysis and review

In addition to definitional issues, a number of major concerns have been raised about the precautionary principle. These are summarized in Box 7.5.6. First, what does the precautionary principle add to standard public health concepts? The precautionary principle is very welcome as an enthusiastic restatement of these concepts which provides an impetus and rallying point for actions that protect public health and the environment, even if nothing new is added to our understanding of the forces responsible for public health action and inaction.

The precautionary principle is said to be pertinent in situations where the scientific evidence is uncertain (Box 7.5.7). An often-cited example of this is the management of the health and environmental risks of endocrine disruptors, a particularly challenging problem in view of the need to consider the interactive effects of multiple chemicals with a wide range of additive, synergistic, and antagonistic interactions (Kortenkamp 2007). Yet it should be noted however, that the United States banned the production of polychlorinated biphenyls (PCBs) in 1976 despite the opposition, then and now, of industry on the grounds of uncertain science. The continual decline in body burdens of PCBs and dioxins have been accomplished based on regulatory decisions that were made without recourse to the precautionary principle. Advancing the science needed for decision-making must remain a major goal

---

Box 7.5.5 Working definition of the precautionary principle

'When human activities may lead to morally unacceptable harm that is scientifically plausible but uncertain, actions shall be taken to avoid or diminish that harm. *Morally unacceptable harm* refers to harm to humans or the environment that is

- threatening to human life or health, or
- serious and effectively irreversible, or
- inequitable to present or future generations, or
- imposed without adequate consideration of the human rights of those affected.

The judgment of *plausibility* should be grounded in scientific analysis. Analysis should be ongoing so that chosen actions are subject to review.

Uncertainty may apply to, but need not be limited to, causality or the bounds of the possible harm.

Actions are interventions that are undertaken before harm occurs that seek to avoid or diminish the harm. Actions should be chosen that are proportional to the seriousness of the potential harm, with consideration of their positive and negative consequences, and with an assessment of the moral implications of both action and inaction. The choice of action should be the result of a participatory process.'

Reproduced with permission from COMEST (World Commission on the Ethics of Scientific Knowledge and Technology), *The Precautionary Principle*, Copyright © 2005 United Nations Educational, Scientific and Cultural Organization, available from http://unesdoc.unesco.org/images/0013/001395/139578e.pdf.

Box 7.5.6 Questions about the precautionary principle

What does it add to standard public health concepts?

Is it true that complex scientific questions are unsolvable and, if so, is the precautionary principle needed to act in the face of scientific uncertainty?

In view of its alleged use to justify trade barriers, is it still possible to advocate the precautionary principle as an antidote to biased decision-making?

---

for environmental public health, including actions taken under the precautionary principle (Foster et al. 2000; Goldstein and Carruth 2003a, 2003b; Grandjean et al. 2004).

An example that may provide practical insight into the often confusing debate about the precautionary principle versus risk assessment is how the European Union (EU) and other countries evaluate the safety of chemicals. The EU promulgated the Registration, Evaluation, Authorisation and Restriction of Chemical Substances (REACH) regulations, after much debate, with its proponents focusing on the precautionary principle as a rationale for the new legislation. REACH requires industry to develop data, assess risk, and provide information about virtually all chemicals in use, including constituents of product mixtures. No distinction is made between newly developed chemicals or those long available in commerce—a contrast with the US Toxic Substances Control Act whose weakness in this regard has led to the inadequate testing of compounds such as the gasoline additive—methyl tert-butyl ether (MTBE) before its

Box 7.5.7 Case study: the precautionary principle and bisphenol A

Worldwide, over 3 million tons of bisphenol A (BPA) are produced annually. BPA can be found in many consumer products. These include reusable water bottles, baby bottles, implantable medical devices, and dental sealants. BPA is also a component of epoxy resins, which are used to overlay the inside of food and beverage cans, in cardboard and papers used for food wrapping, in some plastic water pipes, and in paints and cigarette filters. Of concern is the fact that BPA leaches out from these consumer products, even under normal use conditions. The leaching is increased under high temperatures, and with exposure to acidic or basic solutions.

Animal studies have shown that BPA may alter male and female reproductive tract development, the brain, and the mammary glands. In large-scale human population studies in various parts of the world, BPA has been detected in urine, blood, saliva, breast milk, and tissues and fluids associated with pregnancy at levels similar to those that have been shown to cause damage in animals.

In Canada, a study of over 5000 people showed that over 90 per cent had detectable levels of BPA in urine, with a geometric mean concentration of 1.16 ng/mL (Bushnik et al. 2010). Health Canada has stated that precaution is warranted, since it is not possible to dismiss the potential harmful effects of bisphenol A (Health Canada 2010). With this statement, Canada is the first country to declare BPA a health hazard, but additional regulatory action has yet to be taken (Vandenberg 2011).

inappropriate release into the environment (Goldstein and Erdal 2000).

The cost of implementing REACH is estimated at about US\$3–6 billion over the first 11 years for obtaining data and registering compounds. Risk assessment, based on both toxicity and exposure, is used extensively throughout the process, including setting priorities for data needs and making decisions on regulatory approaches. Unfortunately, there appears to be no uniform coordinated effort to develop the research where toxicological data is scant.

Unfortunately, the precautionary principle has been tainted through disagreements on its application. The United States, Canada, and other countries have disagreed with the EU on the extent of risk to health from consumption of hormone-treated beef or genetically modified foods. The EU's use of the precautionary principle to establish a stringent aflatoxin standard to the detriment of exports of sub-Saharan countries has been criticized as the misuse of public health principles for trade protectionism (Goldstein 2007). The risk of exposure to electromagnetic fields from use of mobile phones is another contentious and confused issue resulting in advice based on a mix of the precautionary principle and on the scientific evidence.

The primary missing ingredient in the approach to ever more complex environmental challenges, including such broader issues as global warming, is a systems-based approach incorporating the best science focusing on the most important questions. Unfortunately, the fragmented national and international approaches to environmental issues are producing piecemeal efforts that are falling further behind in protecting public health and the environment. Perhaps the need to respond to the

challenges of global climate change will lead to a more systematic and coordinated international effort.

Conclusion

Understanding the web of environmental cause and effect relations is an increasing challenge in a shrinking globe. Advances in toxicology, filtered through an appropriate appreciation of the optimal approaches to analyse and present risks to an involved public, are crucial to protecting public health and the environment.

References

American Conference of Governmental Industrial Hygienists (2013). *Threshold Limit Values for Chemical and Physical Agents and Biological Exposure Indices*. Cincinnati, OH: ACGIH.

Arbuckle, T.E., Hrudey, S.E., Krasner, S.W., et al. (2002). Assessing exposure in epidemiologic studies to disinfection by-products in drinking water: report of an international workshop. *Environmental Health Perspectives*, 110(Suppl 1), 53–60.

BBC News (2012). Amnesty and Greenpeace in Trafigura investigation call. *NEWS Africa*, 25 September. [Online] Available at: http://www.bbc.co.uk/news/world-africa-19706163.

Benn, T.M. and Westerhoff, P. (2008). Nanoparticle silver released into water from commercially available sock fabrics. *Environmental Science & Technology*, 42, 4133–9.

Bushnik, T., Haines, D., Levallois, P., et al. (2010). Lead and bisphenol A concentrations in the Canadian population. *Health Reports*, 21, 7–18.

Cogliano, V.J. (2004). Current criteria to establish human carcinogens. *Seminars in Cancer Biology*, 14, 407–12.

Foster, K.R., Vecchia, P., and Repacholi, M.H. (2000). Science and the precautionary principle. *Science*, 288, 979–81.

Goldstein, B.D. (2007). Problems in applying the precautionary principle to public health. *Occupational and Environmental Medicine*, 64, 571–4.

Goldstein, B.D. and Carruth, R.S. (2003a). Implications of the precautionary principle to environmental regulation in the United States: examples from the control of hazardous air pollutants in the 1990 Clean Air Act Amendments. *Law and Contemporary Problems*, 66, 247–61.

Goldstein, B.D. and Carruth, R.S. (2003b). Implications of the precautionary principle: is it a threat to science? *European Journal of Oncology*, 2, 193–202.

Goldstein, B.D. and Erdal, S. (2000). MTBE as a gasoline oxygenate: lessons for environmental public policy. *Annual Review of Energy and the Environment*, 25, 765–802.

Goldstein, B.D. and Gallo, M.A. (2001). Paré's law: the second law of toxicology. *Toxicological Sciences*, 60, 194–5.

Goldstein, B.D., Liu, Y., Wu, F., and Lioy, P.J. (2011) Comparison of the effects of the US Clean Air Act and of smoking prevention and cessation efforts on the risk of acute myelogenous leukemia. *American Journal of Public Health*, 101, 2357–61.

Grandjean, P., Bailar, J.C., Gee, D., et al. (2004) Implications of the precautionary principle in research and policy-making. *American Journal of Industrial Medicine*, 45, 382–5.

Greenpeace (2006). *Toxic Waste in Abidjan*. [Online] Available at: http://www.greenpeace.org/international/news/ivory-coast-toxic-dumping/toxic-waste-in-abidjan-green.

Greenpeace (2012). *The Toxic Truth*. [Online] Available at: http://www.greenpeace.org/international/en/publications/Campaign-reports/Toxics-reports/The-Toxic-Truth/Publication.

Health Canada (2010). Order adding a toxic substance to Schedule 1 to the Canadian Environmental Protection Act, 1999. *Canada Gazette*, 2010, 144.

Helland, A., Wick, P., Koehler, A., et al. (2007) Reviewing the environmental and human health knowledge base of carbon nanotubes. *Environmental Health Perspectives*, 115, 1125–31.

International Life Science Institute (1999). *A Framework for Cumulative Risk Assessment; Workshop Report*. Washington, DC: ILSI Risk Science Institute.

Kim, S., Lan, Q., Waidyanatha, S., et al. (2007) Genetic polymorphisms and benzene metabolism in humans exposed to a wide range of air concentrations. *Pharmacogenetics and Genomics*, 17, 789–801.

Kortenkamp, A. (2007). Ten years of mixing cocktails: a review of combination effects of endocrine-disrupting chemicals. *Environmental Health Perspectives*, 115(Suppl. 1), 98–105.

Lioy, P., Pellizzari, E., and Prezant, D. (2006). The World Trade Center aftermath and its effects on health: understanding and learning through human exposure science. *Environmental Science and Technology*, 40, 6876–85.

Martuzzi, M. (2007). The precautionary principle: in action for public health. *Occupational and Environmental Medicine*, 64, 569–70.

McMichael, A.J. (2013) Globalization, climate change and human health. *The New England Journal of Medicine*, 368, 1335–43.

National Research Council (1993) *Pesticides in the Diets of Infants and Children*. Washington, DC: National Academies Press.

National Research Council (2007). *Toxicity Testing in the 21st Century*. Washington, DC: National Academies Press.

National Toxicology Program (2011). *Report on Carcinogens*. [Online] Available at: http://ntp.niehs.nih.gov/?objectid=03C9AF75-E1BF-FF40-DBA9EC0928DF8B15.

Nowack, B. (2010). Nanosilver revisited downstream. *Science*, 330, 1054–5.

Oberdörster, G., Sharp, Z., Atudorei, V., et al. (2004). Translocation of inhaled ultrafine particles to the brain. *Inhalation Toxicology*, 16(6–7), 437–45.

Omenn, G.S. (2000). Public health genetics: an emerging interdisciplinary field for the post-genomic era. *Annual Review of Public Health*, 21, 1–13.

Rothman, N., Smith, M.T., Hayes, R.B., et al. (1997). Benzene poisoning, a risk factor for hematological malignancy, is associated with the NQO1 609C –>T mutation and rapid fractional excretion of chlorzoxazone. *Cancer Research*, 57, 2839–42.

Tickner, J. and Ketelson, L. (2001). Democracy and the precautionary principle. *Science and Environmental Health Network*, 6, 1–6.

Umbreit, T.H., Hesse, E.J., and Gallo, M.A. (1986). Bioavailability of dioxin in soil from a 2,4,5-T manufacturing site. *Science*, 232, 497–9.

United Nations Environmental Programme (1992). *Rio Declaration on Environment and Development, Principle 15*. [Online] Available at: http://www.unep.org/Documents.Multilingual/Default.asp?DocumentID=78&ArticleID=1163.

United Nations Environmental Programme (2006). *Liability for Cote d'Ivoire Hazardous Waste Clean-Up*. [Press release] Available at: http://www.unep.org/Documents.Multilingual/Default.asp?DocumentID=485&ArticleID=5430&l=en.

US Environmental Protection Agency (2003). *Framework for Cumulative Risk Assessment*. EPA/630/P-02/001F. Washington, DC: Risk Assessment Forum. Available at: http://www.epa.gov/raf/publications/pdfs/frmwrk_cum_risk_assmnt.pdf.

US Environmental Protection Agency (2007). *Integrated Risk Information System: Benzene CASRN 71-43-2*. Available at: http://www.epa.gov/iris/subst/0276.htm#carc.

Vandenberg, L.N. (2011). Exposure to bisphenol A in Canada: invoking the precautionary principle. *Canadian Medical Association Journal*, 183(11), 1265–70.

World Commission on the Ethics of Scientific Knowledge and Technology (2005). *The Precautionary Principle*. [Online] Available at: http://unesdoc.unesco.org/images/0013/001395/139578e.pdf.

7.6

Risk perception and communication

Baruch Fischhoff

Introduction to risk perception and communication

Sound health risk decisions require understanding the risks and benefits of possible actions. Some of those choices are personal. They include whether to wear bicycle helmets and seat belts, whether to read and follow safety warnings, whether to buy and use condoms, and how to select and cook food. Other choices are made as citizens. They include whether to protest the siting of hazardous waste incinerators and halfway houses, whether to support fluoridation and 'green' candidates, and what to include in sex education.

Sometimes, single choices have large effects (e.g. buying a safe car, taking a dangerous job, getting pregnant). Sometimes, small effects accumulate over multiple choices (e.g. exercising, avoiding trans-fats, wearing seatbelts, using escort services). Sometimes, health-related choices focus on health; sometimes, they do not (e.g. purchasing homes that require long commutes, choosing friends who exercise regularly, joining religious groups opposed to vaccination).

This chapter reviews the research base for assessing and improving individuals' understanding of the risks and possible benefits of health-related choices. Following convention, these pursuits are called *risk perception* and *risk communication*, respectively, even though the same basic behavioural principles apply to the benefits that all risk decisions entail, if only the benefits of reducing risks (Fischhoff et al. 2011). Psychologists sometimes reserve the term 'perception' for direct physiological responses to stimuli, using 'judgement' for the translation of those responses into observable estimates. A perennial research topic is identifying the conditions under which judgement surrenders to perception, and when emotions play little role because people know what they want to do (Slovic et al. 2005). This chapter emphasizes judgement, hoping to expand the envelope of deliberative processes in personal and public health decisions.

Inaccurate judgements about risks can harm people. So can inaccurate beliefs about those judgements. If their understanding is overestimated, then people may face impossibly hard choices (e.g. among unfamiliar medical alternatives, without adequate counselling). If their understanding is underestimated, then people may be needlessly denied the right to choose. As a result, the chapter assumes: (1) that descriptive statements about people's beliefs must be underpinned by empirical evidence and (2) that evaluative statements about the adequacy of people's understanding must be

founded on rigorous analysis of what they need to know, in order to make a sound decision. To these ends, the chapter emphasizes methodological safeguards against misguided assessments.

The next section, 'Quantitative assessment', considers beliefs about how large risks are. The following section, 'Qualitative assessment', treats beliefs about the processes that create and control risks, on the basis of which people produce and evaluate quantitative estimates. Both sections address both measurement issues and barriers to understanding. The next section, 'Creating communications,' provides a structured approach for developing communications about health-related decisions, focused on individuals' information needs. The 'Conclusion' section considers the strategic importance of risk communication in public health. Access to research on complementary social and emotional processes might begin with Breakwell (2007), Krimsky and Golding (1992), and Peters and McCaul (2005).

Quantitative assessment
Estimating risk magnitude

A common complaint among experts is that 'the public doesn't realize how small (or large) Risk X is'. There is empirical evidence demonstrating such biases (Slovic 2001). However, that evidence has often been collected in settings designed to reveal biases. Looking for problems is a standard strategy in experimental sciences, designed to reveal the processes creating those problems, but not their prevalence or magnitude in specific domains of everyday life. Generalizing from research decisions to real-world ones requires matching the conditions in each. Looking at the details of one widely cited study shows how that matching process might proceed, while introducing some general principles and results.

Participants

Lichtenstein et al. (1978) asked members of a civic group in Eugene, Oregon, to estimate the annual number of deaths in the United States from 30 causes (e.g. botulism, tornadoes, motor vehicle accidents). They were older than the college students often studied by psychologists. Age could affect *what* people think, as a result of differences in their education and life experience. It is less likely to affect *how* they think. Many cognitive processes are widely shared, once people pass middle adolescence, unless they suffer some impairment (Fischhoff 2008; Reyna and Farley 2006; Finucane and Gullion 2010).

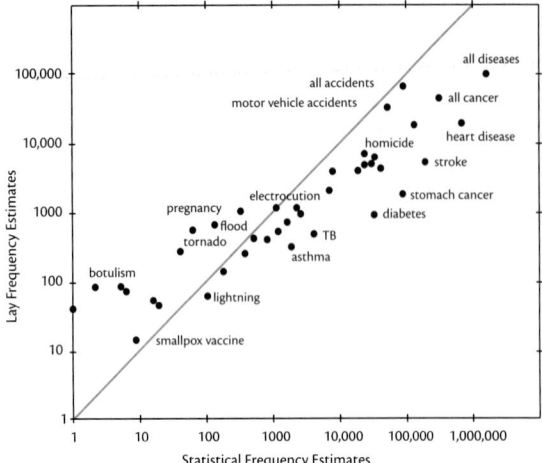

Fig. 7.6.1 Best quadratic fit line to geometric mean judgements of the annual toll from 40 causes of death in the United States, compared to best available statistical estimates.

Reproduced from Fischhoff, B. and Kadvany, J., *Risk: A Very Short Introduction*, Figure 12, p. 92, Oxford University Press, Oxford, UK, Copyright © Baruch Fischhoff and John Kadvany 2011, by permission of Oxford University Press.

One widely shared class of cognitive processes relies on judgemental *heuristics* to infer unknown quantities (Kahneman et al. 1982; Gilovich et al. 2003). One well-known heuristic is *availability*, whereby people assess an event's probability by how easily instances come to mind. Although more available events are often more likely, media coverage (among other things) makes some events disproportionately available, thereby inducing biased judgements—unless people take into account how appearances can be deceiving. *How* people generate instances of events, using their memory and imagination, should reflect widely shared general cognitive processes. *What* those memories and images contain, as well as what faith people place in information sources, should vary with their experiences.

Lichtenstein et al. (1978) elicited judgements with two *response modes*. One asked people to pick the more frequent of two paired causes of death (e.g. asthma, botulism) and then to estimate the ratio of their frequencies. The second asked for the number of deaths, after providing the value for one cause (either electrocution or motor vehicle accidents) in order to give respondents a feeling for annual death rates—after pretests found that many people had little idea about what range of numbers to give. Fig. 7.6.1 shows results with the second method, which are typical of such studies.

Results

1. Judgements of the *relative* risk from different causes were similar however the question was asked. Risks assigned higher frequency estimates were typically judged more likely when paired with risks with lower frequency estimates. Ratios of the direct estimates were similar to directly estimated ratios. Thus, these people seemed to have an internal 'scale' of relative risk, which they expressed consistently even with these unfamiliar tasks.

2. Judgements of *absolute* risk, however, were affected by the procedure. People told that 50,000 people die annually from auto accidents gave estimates two to five times higher than did people told that 1000 die annually from electrocution. Thus, people seemed

to have less feeling for absolute frequency, rendering them sensitive to implicit cues given by how questions are posed (Poulton 1989; Schwarz 1999; Fagerlin and Peters, 2011).

3. Absolute risk judgements were less dispersed than were the corresponding statistical estimates. Although the latter varied over six orders of magnitude, individuals' estimates typically ranged over three to four. That 'compression' could reflect another judgemental bias, called *anchoring*, whereby judgements are drawn toward an initial value that draws their attention. With these anchors (electrocution, motor vehicle accidents), people overestimated small frequencies and underestimated large ones. That pattern might change with other anchors. For example, a lower anchor (e.g. botulism) should reduce (or perhaps eliminate) the overestimation of small frequencies, while increasing the underestimation of large ones.

4. Relative and absolute risk judgements seemed to reflect availability bias. Some causes of death (e.g. flood, homicide, tornadoes) received higher estimates than did others with similar statistical frequency. Typically, there were causes that were disproportionately reported in the news media. When told about the possibility of availability bias, participants could not improve their judgements, consistent with the finding that tracking frequency is such an automatic process that people do not realize how observations shape their perceptions (e.g. Koriat 1993).

Thus, Lichtenstein et al. (1978) found some response patterns that were affected by the procedure that was used (e.g. absolute estimates) and some that were not (e.g. relative risk judgements). A century of psychophysics research (Poulton 1989) has identified many other procedural details that can affect quantitative judgements. Determining how much those details affect any specific judgement requires studies examining their relative impact in that context. How important that effect (or any bias) is depends on the decision. Shifting fatality estimates by a factor of two to five might tip some decisions, but not others.

Fischhoff and MacGregor (1983) provide another example of response mode effects. They asked about the chances of dying (in the United States) among people afflicted with various maladies (e.g. influenza), in four ways: (1) how many people die out of each 100,000 who get influenza; (2) how many people died out of the 80 million who caught influenza last year; (3) for each person who dies of influenza, how many have it and survive; (4) 800 people died of influenza last year, how many survived? As in Lichtenstein et al. (1978), relative risk judgements were consistent across response modes, while absolute estimates varied greatly (over one to two orders of magnitude). They also found that people liked format (3) much less than the others—and were much less able to remember statistics reported that way. That format also produced the most discrepant estimates, identifying it as a poor way to elicit or communicate risks.

Evaluative standards

Risk judgements can be evaluated in terms of their *consistency* or their *accuracy*. Evaluating consistency requires asking logically related questions and comparing the answers (e.g. do risk estimates increase with increasing exposure?). Evaluating accuracy requires asking questions that are sufficiently precise to be compared to sound risk estimates (e.g. Chapter 7.5). Without sound scientific estimates, individuals' judgements may be compared to a standard that they would reject. For example, after the 9/11 attacks in New York by terrorist-commandeered aeroplanes, some observers claimed that some Americans had increased their risk level by driving, rather than flying. These claims were based on historical risk statistics. However, it was difficult to ascertain the safety of aviation at that time as the US aircraft fleet was grounded, whereas the historical statistics used for driving encompassed all drivers, including the young, elderly, and drinkers, and were not specific to those drivers who had changed their transportation modes. Even if these historical statistics were valid, other factors must have affected the drivers' decisions such as the cost and hassle of flying during that period. As a general rule, one cannot infer risk judgements from risk decisions without knowing the other factors involved.

Probability judgements

The sensitivity of quantitative judgements to methodological details might suggest avoiding them in favour of verbal quantifiers (e.g. likely, rare). Indeed, some researchers hesitate to elicit probabilities at all, fearing that the questions will exceed laypeople's cognitive capabilities. That hesitation is strengthened by evidence of lay innumeracy (Fagerlin and Peters 2011). However, even imperfect measures can have value, if their strengths and weaknesses are understood. The research literature on eliciting probability judgements is vast (O'Hagan et al. 2006). Findings relevant to public health researchers and practitioners include:

1. People often prefer to provide verbal judgements and receive numeric ones, given that numeric responses require more effort and incur greater accountability (Erev and Cohen 1990).

2. Verbal quantifiers are often interpreted differently across people and situations (e.g. rare disease vs. rare sunny day), making it hard to know what those terms mean, in situations without established usage norms (Budescu and Wallsten 1995; Schwarz 1999).

3. People can use well-designed numeric scales as well as verbal ones. For example, Woloshin et al. (1998) found similar performance and satisfaction with linear and log-linear probability scales as with verbal ones.

4. Numeric probability judgements often have good *construct validity*, in the sense of correlating sensibly with other variables. For example, Fischhoff et al. (2000) found that teens who gave higher probabilities of becoming pregnant also reported more sexual activity; teens giving higher probabilities of getting arrested also reported more violent neighbourhoods.

5. Misinformation and mistaken inferences can bias probability judgements, as when one's own care in driving is more available that that of other drivers, making one feel safer than average.

6. Probability judgements can be deliberately biased, when people respond strategically. For example, Christensen-Szalanski and Bushyhead (1993) found that physicians overestimated the probability of pneumonia, fearing that unlikely cases might be neglected. Weather forecasters may overstate the probability of precipitation, in order to keep people from being caught unprotected (Lichtenstein et al. 1982).

7. Transient emotions can affect judgements. For example, anger increases optimism, fear the opposite (Lerner and Keltner 2001), with effects large enough to tip close decisions.

8. Judgements of the probability of being correct are moderately correlated with how much people actually know. For example, Fischhoff et al. (1977) had people choose the larger of two causes of death (from Lichtenstein et al. 1978), and then give the probability of having chosen correctly. In relative terms, people were correct more often when they were more confident. In absolute terms, *overconfidence* (e.g. being 90 per cent confident with 75 per cent correct choices) is typical with hard tasks, underconfidence with easy ones.

9. Probability judgements can vary by response mode (e.g. odds vs probabilities, probabilities vs relative frequencies, judgements of individual or grouped items) (Griffin et al. 2003).

10. Some numeric values are treated specially. For example, people seldom use fractional values; when uncertain what to say, people sometimes say 50 in the sense of 50–50, rather than a numeric probability (Bruine de Bruin et al. 2000).

11. Probability judgement processes mature by middle adolescence. For example, teens are no more likely than adults to believe in their own adolescent invulnerability (Quadrel et al. 1993); indeed, unlike adults, many teens greatly exaggerate their probability of premature death (Fischhoff et al. 2000).

12. People differ in their ability to use probabilities, with lower ability correlated with poorer performance on other tasks and with life outcomes that require decision-making competence (Bruine de Bruin et al. 2007b).

13. The use of probabilities can sometimes be improved with even a single round of prompt, intense feedback (Lichtenstein and Fischhoff 1980).

14. Experts' judgements are often imperfect, when forced to go beyond established knowledge and calculations (O'Hagan et al. 2006).

A test of any measure is its predictive validity. Even though risk decisions often involve choices among options with non-risk outcomes (which might outweigh risk concerns), Brewer et al. (2007) found that risk judgements alone have predictive value. Similarly, teens' probability judgements predict major events in their lives (e.g. pregnancy, incarceration), one to 5 years hence (Fischhoff 2008). Pointing to probability judgements that are higher than actual risks, some researchers have argued that public health communications have worked too well, producing exaggerated fears of smoking (Viscusi 1992) and breast cancer (Black et al. 1995).

Defining risk

Studies like Lichtenstein et al. (1978) measure 'risk' perceptions, if 'risk' means 'chance of death'. However, even among experts, 'risk' has multiple meanings (Fischhoff et al. 1984; National Research Council 1996). 'Risk' might mean just death or it might also include other outcomes, such as morbidity and trauma. Even if 'risk' only considers fatalities, it might be measured in terms of probability of death, expected life years lost, or deaths per person exposed (or per hour of exposure). Each definition entails an ethical position. For example, *probability of death* treats all deaths (and lives) equally, whereas *life-years lost* places extra weight on deaths of young people and from injury (e.g. drowning, driving, workplace hazards), as each incurs many lost years, compared to deaths from chronic illnesses. Adding morbidity and trauma would heighten concern for alcohol and illegal drugs, which can ruin lives without ending them.

Without clear, shared definitions, people can unwittingly speak at cross purposes, when addressing 'risks'. Clarifying definitions has long been central to risk research. Before considering that research, it is worth noting that 'risky' (or 'safe') is sometimes used as a discrete variable, treating activities as risky (or safe) or not. Such shorthand says little, without defining the threshold of concern. Calls for 'safe' products can be unfairly ridiculed, if the demand for reasonable risk is equated with zero risk. Such demands are seen in the various *precautionary principles*, identifying risks seen as too great to countenance (DeKay et al. 2002). However, even those calls may be more about uncertainty than risk, reflecting aversion to hazards that science does not understand (Löfstedt et al. 2002).

Catastrophic potential

One early risk perception study asked experts and laypeople to estimate the 'risk of death' from 30 activities and technologies (Slovic et al. 1979). These judgements correlated more strongly with statistical estimates of average-year fatalities for experts than they did for laypeople. However, when asked to estimate 'fatalities in an average year', experts and laypeople responded similarly. Comparing the two sets of judgements suggested that lay respondents interpreted 'risk of death' as including catastrophic potential, reflecting the expected deaths in non-average years. If so, then experts and laypeople agreed about the risk of routine (average year) deaths (for which the science is often good), but disagreed about possible anomalies (for which the science is naturally much weaker). Thus, when experts and laypeople disagree about risks, they might be seeing the facts differently or they might be looking at different facts, ones relevant to their definition of 'risk' (National Research Council 1989). People might consider catastrophic potential because they care more about lives lost at once than lost individually or because catastrophic potential suggests hazards that might spin out of control (Slovic et al. 1984).

Dimensions of risk

Beginning with Starr (1969), many features, like uncertainty and catastrophic potential, have been suggested as affecting definitions of risk (Lowrance 1976). In order to reduce that set to a manageable size, Fischhoff et al. (1978) asked members of a liberal civic organization to rate 30 hazards on nine such features. Factor analysis on mean ratings identified two *dimensions*, which accounted for 78 per cent of the variance. Fig. 7.6.2 plots factor scores in this 'risk space'. Similar patterns emerged with students, members of a conservative civic organization, and risk experts, suggesting that

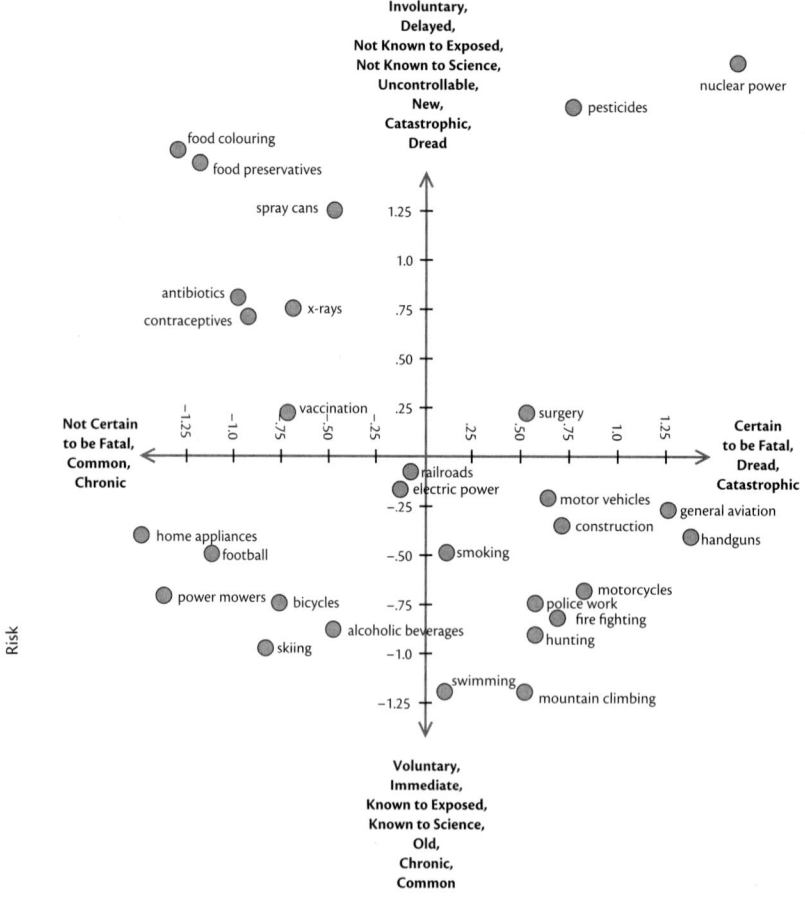

Fig. 7.6.2 Location of 30 hazards within the two-factor space obtained from members of a civic group who rated each activity or technology on each of nine features. Ratings were subjected to principal components factor analysis, with a varimax rotation.

people think similarly about such factors, even when they disagree about how specific hazards stack up.

Hazards high on the vertical factor (e.g. food colouring, pesticides) were rated as new, unknown, and involuntary, with delayed effects. Hazards high on the horizontal factor (e.g. nuclear power, commercial aviation) were rated as fatal to many people, if things go wrong. The factors were labelled *unknown* and *dread*, respectively, and might be seen as capturing cognitive and emotional aspects of people's concern.

Many studies following this 'psychometric paradigm' have found roughly similar dimensions, using differing elicitation modes, scaling techniques, items, and participants (Slovic 2001). When a third dimension emerges, it typically reflects the scope of the threat, labelled *catastrophic potential*. The position of hazards in the space correlates with attitudes towards them, such as how stringently they should be regulated. Analyses of mean responses, as in the figure, are best suited to predicting aggregate (societal) responses. Individual differences have also been studied (e.g. Vlek and Stallen 1981; Arabie and Maschmeyer 1988).

Risk comparisons

The multidimensionality of risk means that hazards similar on some dimensions can still evoke quite different responses. This fact is neglected in appeals to accept one risk because one has accepted another risk with some similarities (Fischhoff et al. 1984). A common kind of such 'risk comparison' presents the statistical risks from many hazards in common terms (e.g. arguing that people who eat peanut butter should accept nuclear power because both a tablespoonful of peanut butter and 50 years living by a nuclear power plant create a one-in-a-million risk of premature death). (For a summary of the problems with such risk comparisons, see National Research Council (2006).)

One way to improve the legitimacy of risk comparisons is to involve users in setting them. The US Environmental Protection Agency (1993) followed this strategy in facilitating dozens of regional, state, and national 'risk-ranking exercises', in which participants identified the dimensions important to them, then deliberated priorities, supported by technical staff providing relevant evidence. Letting participants choose the dimensions made their exercise more relevant, but reduced comparability across exercises. Florig et al. (2001) developed a method for standardizing such comparisons, based on the risk dimensions research (Table 7.6.1). The UK government has endorsed a variant (HM Treasury 2005).

Qualitative assessment
Event definitions

Once adequately defined, 'risk' can be estimated. For risk assessors, that means specifying such details as the frequency and timing of intercourse, contraceptives used, and partners' physical state—when estimating the risk of pregnancy. Two experts with different definitions may see the same data and produce different estimates. So may laypeople asked for their perceptions of risk, but forced to guess at what exactly is meant. Consider this question from a prominent national survey: 'How likely do you think it is that a person will get the AIDS virus from sharing plates, forks, or glasses with someone who has AIDS?' After answering this question, US college students were asked what they had inferred about the kind and amount of sharing. Most agreed about the kind, with 82 per cent selecting 'sharing during a meal' from a set of options. However, they disagreed about the frequency, with 39 per cent selecting 'a single occasion', 20 per cent 'several occasions', 28 per cent 'routinely', and 12 per cent uncertain (Fischhoff 1996). Respondents making different assumptions were, in effect, answering different questions, whose meaning researchers must guess, if they are to offer any conclusions about lay risk perceptions.

Laypeople are, similarly, left guessing when experts communicate about risks ambiguously (Fischhoff 1994). For example, McIntyre and West (1992) found that teens knew that 'safe sex' was important, but disagreed about what it entailed. Downs et al. (2004b) found that teens interpret 'it can only take once' as meaning that they will get pregnant after having sex once. If they do not, some infer that they are infertile, encouraging unsafe sex. Murphy et al. (1980) found people divided over whether '70 per cent chance of rain' referred to: (1) the area receiving rain, (2) the time it would rain, (3) the chance of some rain anywhere, or (4) the chance of some rain at the weather station (the correct answer). Fischhoff (2005a) describes procedures for making sure that experts and laypeople are talking about the same thing, when they communicate about risks.

Supplying details

The details that people infer, when given ambiguous and incomplete risk questions or messages, reveal their intuitive theories. For example, teens who thought aloud while judging the probabilities of ambiguous events (like that about sharing plates, etc., with someone with AIDS), noticed many unstated details, including ones that would affect scientific risk estimates (Fischhoff 1994). For example,

Table 7.6.1 A standard multidimensional representation of risks

Number of people affected	Degree of environmental impact	Knowledge	Dread
Annual expected number of fatalities: 0–**450**–600 (10% chance of zero)	Area affected by ecosystem stress or change **50** km²	Degree to which impacts are delayed **1–10** years	Catastrophic potential **1000** times expected annual fatalities
Annual expected number of person-years lost: 0–**9000**–18,000 (10% chance of zero)	Magnitude of environmental impact **Modest** (15% chance of large)	Quality of scientific understanding **Medium**	Outcome equity **Medium** (ratio = 6)

Source: data from Willis, H.H. et al., Aggregate and disaggregate analyses of ecological risk perceptions, *Risk Analysis*, Volume 25, Issue 2, pp. 405–428, Copyright © 2005.

they wondered about the 'dose' of most risks (e.g. the amount of drinking and driving, when judging the probability of an accident), when it was missing from a question. An exception was not thinking about the amount of sex involved, when judging the risks of pregnancy and HIV transmission. Teens seemed to believe that an individual is either vulnerable or not, making the number of exposures immaterial. Sometimes they considered variables unrelated to risk, such as how well partners know one another. In order to dispel such misunderstanding, Downs et al. (2004a) explicitly addressed how partners could fail to self-diagnose sexually transmitted infections (STIs)—in an interactive DVD that successfully reduced adolescent sexual risks.

Cumulative risk—a case in point

There is no full substitute for directly studying the beliefs that people bring to and take away from risk messages, especially when recipients come from cultures and social circumstances different than those of the communicators. However, the research literature provides a basis for anticipating those beliefs (Fischhoff et al. 2011). For example, optimism bias is so widespread that one can assume that people see themselves as facing less risk than other people, whenever some personal control seems feasible. Similarly, teens' insensitivity to the amount of sex, when judging STI risks, reflects a well-known insensitivity to how risks accumulate over repeated exposures. Thus, people cannot be expected to infer the cumulative accident risk from repeatedly driving without a seat belt (Slovic et al. 1978) or the pregnancy risk from having sex without effective contraceptives (Shaklee and Fischhoff 1990). One corollary of this insensitivity is not realizing the cumulative impact of small differences in single-exposure risks (e.g. slightly better contraceptives, wearing a seat belt). People similarly underestimate exponential growth (e.g. Wagenaar and Sagaria 1975; Frederick 2005).

For example, Linville et al. (1993) had college students judge the probability of transmission from an HIV-positive man to a woman from 1, 10, or 100 cases of protected sex. For one case, the students' median estimate was 0.10, much higher than then-current public health estimates—despite using a log-linear response mode that facilitated expressing very low probabilities (Woloshin et al. 1998). The median estimate for 100 contacts was 0.25, a more accurate estimate, but much too small given their one-case estimates. Given the inconsistency in these beliefs, researchers studying risk perceptions must ask about both, in order to get a full picture, and educators seeking to inform risk beliefs need to communicate them both, in order to create a full picture.

Mental models of risk processes

The role of mental models

As mentioned, when people lack explicit information about the magnitude of a risk (or benefit), they must infer it. Judgemental heuristics, like availability, provide one class of inferential rules for deriving specific estimates from general knowledge. A second class of inferential rules draws on individuals' *mental models* of the general processes that create and control risks in order to estimates those risks, follow discussions about them, and generate choice options. The term 'mental model' refers to the intuitive theories supporting such inferences. Mental models have a long history in psychology, having been studied for topics as diverse as how people understand physical processes, international tensions, complex equipment, energy conservation, climate change, interpersonal

relations, and drug effects (Meyer et al. 1985; Ericsson and Simon 1993; Sterman and Sweeney 2002).

However sound these inferences, they can produce erroneous conclusions when mental models contain flawed assumptions (or 'bugs'). For example, not realizing how quickly the risks of pregnancy and STIs accumulate over sex acts could make other knowledge seem irrelevant. Bostrom et al. (1992) found that many people knew that radon was a colourless, odourless, radioactive gas, but overestimated its risks because they also thought that radioactivity meant permanent contamination. However, radon's by-products (or 'progeny') have short half-lives, meaning that once intrusion of the gas stops, the problem disappears. However, while it persists, rapid decay means rapid energy release. Homeowners unaware of these facts might reasonably decide not to test for radon—the problem doesn't seem urgent and there is nothing to do anyway if they find a problem.

Morgan et al. (2001) offer a general approach appropriate to studying mental models for complex, uncertain processes, like those of many public health risks. The approach begins by creating a formal (or 'expert') model, summarizing relevant scientific knowledge, with enough conceptual precision to allow computing quantitative predictions, were its data needs met (Fischhoff et al. 2006). A common formalism is the influence diagram (Howard 1989). Fig. 7.6.3 shows such a diagram for radon. An arrow means that the value of the variable at its head depends on the value of the variable at its tail. Thus, the lungs' particle clearance rate depends on individuals' smoking history. Other examples include STIs (Fischhoff et al. 1998), breast implants (Byram et al. 2001), sexual assault (Fischhoff 1992), Lyme disease, falls, sexual assault, breast cancer, vaccination, infectious disease, and nuclear energy sources in space (Morgan et al. 2001; Fischhoff 2005b; Downs et al. 2008).

The research continues with open-ended one-on-one interviews, structured around the model, eliciting lay beliefs in their intuitive formulation. Those 'mental model' interviews begin with general questions, asking respondents what they believe about the topic, then to elaborate on each issue raised. The interviews are non-judgemental, seeking to understand, not evaluate respondents' perspectives. After exhausting responses to general questions, interviewers ask increasingly pointed ones, starting with general processes (e.g. exposure, effects, mitigation), and proceeding to specific issues (e.g. 'How does the amount of sex (or number of partners) affect HIV risk?'; 'What does 'safe sex' mean?'). A variant has people think aloud while sorting photographs by their relevance, hoping for insights into topics that were otherwise missed. For example, seeing a supermarket produce section prompted some respondents to say that radon might contaminate plants (Bostrom et al. 1992).

Once transcribed, interviews are coded into the formal model, adding new elements raised by respondents, marked as either misunderstandings or expertise (e.g. knowledge about how equipment really works). The precision of the formal model typically allows reliable coding. Once mapped, lay beliefs can be analysed in terms of their accuracy, relevance, specificity, and focus. Coding for accuracy can reveal beliefs that are correct and relevant, wrong, vague, peripheral, or general (e.g. radon is a gas). For example, Bostrom et al. (1992) found that most respondents, drawn from civic groups, knew that radon is a gas (88 per cent), which concentrates indoors (92 per cent), is detectable with a test kit (96 per cent), comes from underground (83 per cent), and can cause cancer

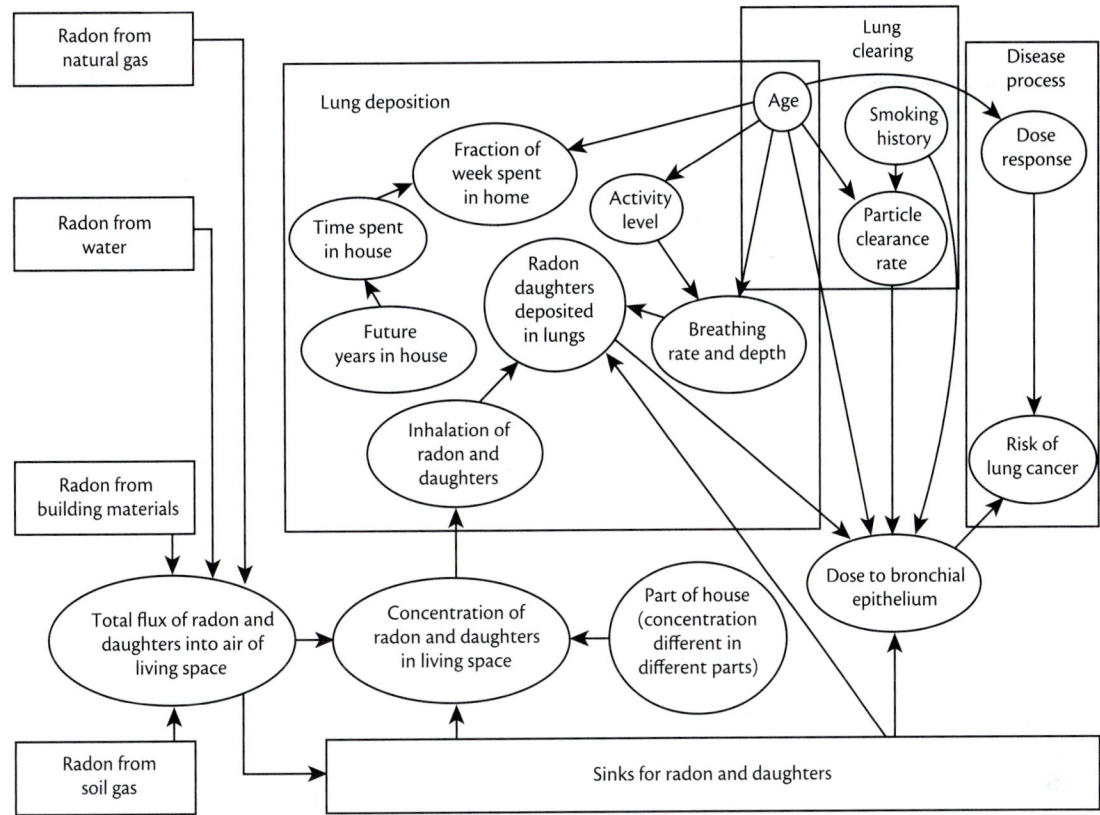

Fig. 7.6.3 Expert influence diagram for health effects of radon (in a home with a crawl space). This diagram was used as a standard and as an organizing device to characterize the content of lay mental models.

Reprinted with permission from Morgan, M.G. et al., Communicating Risk to the Public: First, Learn what people know and believe, *Environmental Science and Technology*, Volume 26, pp. 2048–56, Copyright © 1992, American Chemical Society.

(63 per cent). However, many also believed erroneously that radon affects plants (58 per cent), contaminates blood (38 per cent), and causes breast cancer (29 per cent). Few (8 per cent) mentioned that radon decays. The interviews led to a structured survey suited to assessing the prevalence of beliefs in larger samples, with questions having ecological validity, in the sense of sampling the key topics in the formal model (Bruine de Bruin et al. 2007a).

From risk beliefs to risk decisions

The adequacy of risk perceptions depends on the decisions that depend on them. Some decisions require precise estimates, others just a rough idea. For example, von Winterfeldt and Edwards (1986) showed that many decisions with continuous options (e.g. invest US$X) are insensitive to the precise values assigned to the probabilities and utilities of possible outcomes. Dawes et al. (1989) showed that choices with discrete options (e.g. choosing graduate candidates) are often insensitive to exactly how predictors or outcomes are weighted, meaning that simple linear (weighted-sum) models may do as well as more complicated ones. Thus, any model that considers the probability and magnitude of consequences should have some success in predicting behaviour, if researchers have some idea about the topics on decision-makers' minds. On the other hand, because many such models will do reasonably well, they provide little insight regarding the underlying processes.

Feather (1992) provides a general account of such *expectancy-value* (probability-consequence) models, which predict decisions by multiplying ratings of the likelihood and desirability of potentially relevant consequences. The health-belief model and the theory of reasoned action fall into this general category. For example, Bauman (1980) had seventh graders rate the importance, likelihood, and valence (positive or negative) of 54 possible consequences of using marijuana. A 'utility structure index', computed from these three judgements, predicted about 20 per cent of the variance in respondents' reported marijuana usage.

The template for studying these perceptions is a *decision tree* with the options, relevant outcomes, and uncertain events linking the two. Fig. 7.6.4 shows a simple decision tree, for men considering the dietary supplement, saw palmetto, for symptomatic relief of benign prostatic hyperplasia. The choice (the square node on the left) leads to a sequence of events (the circular *uncertain event* nodes), resulting in the outcomes (or consequences) on the right. The success of a structured model (e.g. Bauman 1980) depends on how well it captures the issues that occupy decision-makers. In identifying those elements, researchers can draw on previous research, convention, or intuitions—or by eliciting them from decision-makers. The greater the social distance between the experts and the decision-makers, the more important such elicitation becomes—lest experts miss options, uncertainties, or outcomes that occupy decision-makers, but would never occur to them, or vice versa.

Effective elicitation typically requires prompting different ways of looking at a decision, so that respondents do not get locked into a narrower perspective than would occur in life (Schwarz 1999).

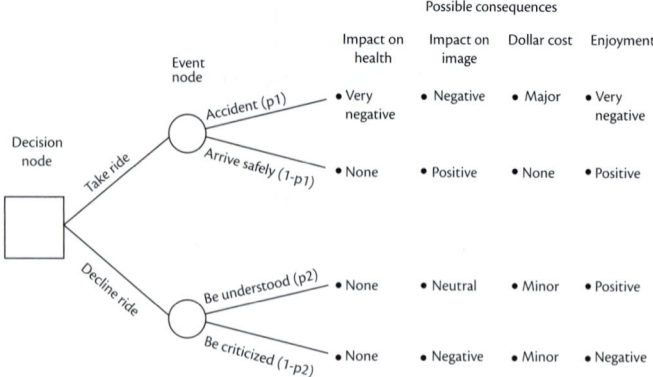

Fig. 7.6.4 A simple decision tree for whether to take saw palmetto for benign prostatic hyperplasia.
Reproduced From Fischhoff, B. and Quadrel, M.J. Adolescent alcohol decisions, *Alcohol Health and Research World*, Volume 15, pp. 43–51, 1991.

For example, Beyth-Marom et al. (1993) had teens work out possible consequences of either accepting a risky option (e.g. drinking and driving, smoking marijuana) or rejecting it. Although accepting and rejecting are formally complementary actions, they can stimulate different thought processes. In this study, participants who thought about accepting risky options produced more consequences (suggesting that action is more evocative than inaction), a higher ratio of bad to good consequences (suggesting that risks are more available from that perspective), and fewer references to social consequences (suggesting that social pressure is more salient when resisting temptation than when yielding to it). When participants thought about making choices repeatedly, rather than just once, they often produced different consequences (e.g. repeatedly 'accepting an offer to smoke marijuana at a party' evoked more mentions of social reactions than did thinking about doing it once). Parents of these teens cited similar possible outcomes, except for being more likely to mention long-term consequences (e.g. ruining career prospects). From this perspective, if parents and teens see the choices differently, it is not because they see different outcomes as possible, but because they disagree about how likely and important those outcomes are. These different perspectives would be hidden with structured surveys that elicit ratings of fixed, predetermined consequences.

Fischhoff (1996) reports a study imposing even less structure, with 105 teens asked to describe three difficult personal decisions in their own words. These descriptions were coded in terms of their content (which choices trouble teens) and structure (how they were formulated). For example, none of the teens mentioned a choice about drinking-and-driving, while many described drinking decisions. Few of their decisions had option structures as complicated as Fig. 7.6.4. Rather, most had but one option (e.g. whether to attend a party with drinking). Judging by Beyth-Marom et al.'s (1993) results, teens looking at that option saw different decisions than did teens focusing on other possible options (e.g. going somewhere else) or multiple options. Experimental research has found that the opportunity costs (foregone benefits) of neglected options are less visible than are their direct consequences (Thaler 1991). For example, the direct risks of vaccinating children can loom

disproportionately larger than the indirect risks of not vaccinating them (Ritov and Baron 1990).

Different methods for eliciting decision-makers' perspective have different, often complementary strengths and weaknesses (Ericsson and Simon 1993). Structured methods (e.g. surveys) can omit important aspects of decisions or express them in unfamiliar terms. Open-ended methods (e.g. mental models interviews) allow people to say whatever is on their minds in their own terms, but require tight control lest researchers influence what is said. Combining methods can provide a rounded picture, especially when a formal analysis ensures their comprehensiveness. Unlike commercial research, scientific studies rarely use focus groups, except for the initial generation of ideas. Indeed, the inventor of focus groups, Robert Merton (1987) rejected them as sources of evidence, given the unnatural discourse of even the best-moderated group, the difficulty of hearing individuals out, and the impressionistic coding of contributions. He preferred *focused interviews*, akin to mental models interviews without the normative analysis. Whichever methods researchers use, they are likely to miss the mark unless they listen to decision-makers' perspectives, before imposing structured methods or designing communications.

Creating communications

Selecting information

Communication design begins by selecting content. The gold standard is a normative analysis, identifying the information most relevant to the choices that the communication is meant to inform. In practice, though, the content-selection process often is ad hoc, with experts intuiting 'what people ought to know' (Nickerson 1999). Poorly selected information can waste recipients' time, take the place of relevant content, or bury facts that people need to know among others that might only be nice to know. Poorly selected information can erode recipients' faith in the experts responsible for communications (and in the institutions employing them), by showing insensitivity to their informational needs ('Why are you telling me X, when I need to know Y?'). It can also undermine experts' faith in their audience, if they fail to realize that their messages have missed the mark. For example, Florig and Fischhoff (2007) found that it was impractical for many individuals to secure and store items on official lists of emergency provisions. Recipients of such advice might ask why they were being asked to do the impossible (Fischhoff, 2011).

The logic of setting information priorities is straightforward: begin with the facts that will have the greatest impact, if they are properly understood. In economics terms, that means creating a 'supply curve' for facts, ordered by their importance. That task can be formalized in 'value of information analysis' (vonWinterfeldt and Edwards 1986; Sox et al. 2007), as used by Merz et al. (1993) in setting priorities when securing informed consent for medical procedures, with carotid endarterectomy as a case study. Scraping out the main artery to the brain can reduce stroke risk, but also cause many problems, including strokes. Attempting to communicate all these risks could easily overwhelm patients. The research identified the risks that mattered most by creating a population of hypothetical patients, varying in their physical condition and health preferences, all of whom would want the procedure were there no side effects (and were money no object). The analysis then asked what percentage of these patients should decide against the surgery, upon learning about each possible side effect. It found that only three of the many side effects (death, stroke, facial paralysis) were sufficiently likely and severe to change many decisions. Although nothing should be hidden, communications should be sure to get the few key facts across.

At times, people are not required to make a specific choice, but are just trying to understand a situation that could pose many decisions (e.g. a newly diagnosed disease, food-borne illness). The same logic of prioritization applies here as well. Communications should focus on the information that is most useful for predicting the outcomes that matter most (e.g. the critical signs of health problems, the key determinants of food safety). That information completes the *mental model* that people need to monitor their environment, generate action options, and follow discussions on the topic (Morgan et al. 2001). Here, too, building on individuals' existing knowledge allows focusing communications on critical gaps (while also demonstrating that the experts know what their audience already knows). For example, Downs et al. (2004a) found that most teens knew so much about HIV/AIDS that communications could focus on a few critical gaps, such as how risks mount through repeated exposure and how hard it is for sexual partners to self-diagnose their own disease status.

An essential part of the content of any communication is the strength of the evidence supporting it (O'Hagan et al. 2006; Politi et al. 2007). The most dangerous beliefs are those held with too great or too little confidence, leading to overly risky or overly cautious actions. Campbell (2011) shows ways to represent uncertainty graphically. Schwartz and Woloshin (2011) showed how much can be conveyed with text describing the quality of the data (e.g. the length, size, and quality of clinical trials). Funtowicz and Ravetz (1990) showed how to characterize the quality of the underlying science, including its *pedigree* (e.g. the extent to which empirical patterns are supported by theory). As an example of how an assessment of uncertainty can inform choices, a meta-analysis (Fortney 1988) concluded, with great confidence, that oral contraceptives may increase a non-smoking woman's life expectancy by up to 4 days and decrease it by up to 80 days. Moreover, the research base was so large that no conceivable study could materially change those bounds.

Formatting information

Once selected, information must be presented. Reimer and Van Nevel (1999) and Wogalter (2006) provide important pointers on research on alternative displays. They note, for example, that comprehension improves when: (1) text has a clear structure, corresponding to recipients' intuitive representation; (2) there is a clear hierarchy of information; and (3) readers receive *adjunct aids*, such as highlighting, advanced organizers (showing what to expect), and summaries.

Scientifically established design principles provide a point of departure for arranging information. These are better 'best guesses' than those informed merely by intuition. Their success in any specific application is an empirical question, though, which can be studied with standard usability testing procedures, such as seeing how long it takes users to find designated pieces of information, how often they reach the wrong information, and how likely they are to realize that (Wogalter 2006). Riley et al. (2001) developed a general method for evaluating the adequacy of communications, drawing on basic research into search patterns. Taking methylene

chloride-based paint stripper as a case study, the method begins by identifying critical information (in this case the steps that most effectively reduce exposures to the chemical and its by-products). It then evaluates product labels by seeing what risk-related information would be found by users who search in different ways. For example, a label might reveal critical information to someone who reads the first five items, but not someone who only reads the instructions or just highlighted material. Actual experience will depend on the prevalence of these search patterns (e.g. what percentage of users look at black box warnings or have instructions read to them). Unless the communication format fits users' natural search patterns, its information might be hidden in plain sight. Riley et al. found that some paint stripper products made critical, useful precautionary information accessible to any reader, while some helped only some readers (e.g. those who read warnings first), and some omit critical information altogether.

Evaluating communications

However sound their theoretical foundations, communications must be empirically evaluated (National Research Council 1989; Slovic 2001). One should no more release an untested health communication than an untested drug. Indeed, communications are part of any medical product or procedure, shaping when it is chosen, how it is used, and whether problems are noticed in time to be remedied and reported. Arguably, evidence about the effectiveness of such communications should be part of the evidence submitted when requesting approval of a product, or when conducting post-licensing surveillance of its benefits and risks in actual use.

A communication is *adequate* if it:

- Includes the information that recipients need, in order to make decisions about risks.
- Affords them access to that information, given their normal search patterns.
- Allows them to comprehend that information, with a reasonable effort.

Applying each of these three tests requires evidence. Knowing what information people need requires learning their goals, which may differ from those of the experts providing the information. Knowing whether people can find the information that is there requires observing how they search. Knowing how much they comprehend requires seeing how well they have mastered the content.

As seen in the references to this chapter, applying these tests to a publication standard is a serious undertaking, requiring professional training. However, simple versions of each test are within the reach of any communicator. The US Food and Drug Administration's *Communicating Risks and Benefits: An Evidence-Based User's Guide* (Fischhoff et al. 2011) ends each chapter with a section on how to conduct evaluations at no cost, a small cost, and a cost commensurate with the stakes riding on effective communication. Central to all forms of evaluation is listening, without presuming to know recipients' goals, beliefs, uncertainties, emotions, or modes of expression. In order to identify individuals' information needs, ask how they see the risks in the context of their lives. In order to see how easily people can access information, watch as they search for it in existing sources (e.g. online) and drafts of proposed communications (Downs et al. 2008). In order to assess a communication's comprehensibility, ask people to recall it, paraphrase it, make inferences from it, or create scenarios using it (Bruine de Bruin et al. 2009).

These are all structured ways of conducting conversations about technical topics of mutual interest, designed to bridge some of the social distance between experts and lay people. For these methods to succeed, they also need to bridge any perceived status difference. Thus, they must be framed as testing the communications, not the recipients, in order to help experts to help the public. Almost any open-minded data collection is better than none. Thus, even a few open-ended, one-on-one interviews might catch incomprehensible or offensive material. The core presumption of risk communication should be that, if lay people have not learned facts that matter to them, the expert community must have failed to get that information across to them. Only if scientific resources have been exhausted should it be assumed that laypeople are incapable of learning the required information. The stakes riding on facilitating lay decision-making should justify that investment and humility. Amateurish, unscientific communications can be worse than nothing, by holding audience members responsible for failing to understand risks when the information was missing, inaccessible, or incomprehensible.

The science of communication can guide both *persuasive communications*, designed to influence individuals to act in ways determined by the communicator, and *non-persuasive communications*, designed to help individuals identify actions in their own best interest. The two kinds of communication converge when persuasive communicators establish that they are influencing people in ways that they would accept as being 'for their own good' (Thaler and Sunstein 2009). Without studying people's goals, however, one risks imposing experts' views on them. For example, in a study mentioned earlier, Bostrom et al. (1992) found people who rejected persuasive communications that advocated testing for radon because they wanted to avoid creating evidence that could complicate selling their homes. Fischhoff (1992) reports on the conflicting advice given to women about reducing the risk of sexual assault, reflecting differences in the goals that experts attribute to the women (and in beliefs regarding the effectiveness of self-defence strategies) (Farris and Fischhoff, 2012). Slovic and Fischhoff (1983) describe how reasonable individuals may 'defeat' safety measures by gaining more benefit from a product (e.g. driving faster with a car that handles better), frustrating policymakers concerned solely with safety.

Managing communication processes

In order to communicate effectively, organizations require four kinds of expertise:

1. *Subject matter specialists*, who can identify the processes that create and control risks (and benefits).

2. *Risk and decision analysts*, who can estimate the risks (and benefits) most pertinent to decision-makers (based on subject matter specialists' knowledge).

3. *Behavioural scientists*, who can assess decision-makers' beliefs and goals, guide the formulation of communications, and evaluate their success.

4. *Communication practitioners*, who can create communication products and manage communication channels, getting messages to audiences and obtaining feedback from them.

The work of these experts must be coordinated, so that they play appropriate roles. For example, behavioural scientists should not revise text (trying to improve its comprehensibility) without having subject matter specialists check that the content is still accurate; subject matter specialists should not slant the facts according to their pet theories of how the public needs to be alarmed or calmed. Without qualified experts, these roles will be filled by amateurs, imperilling the organization and its public.

Conclusion

Effective risk communication is essential to managing risks in socially acceptable ways. Without it, individuals are denied the best possible chances of making sound choices—before, during, and after problems arise. As a result, they may suffer avoidable injury, along with the insult of feeling that the authorities have let them down, by not creating and disseminating the information that they needed, in a timely, comprehensible way. One should no more expose individuals to an untested risk communication than to an untested medical product or procedure.

Effective risk communication focuses on the decisions that people face. Without that focus, one cannot know what information they need. Sound risk management requires not only communicating that information, but also creating it, both through risk analyses, summarizing existing research (see Chapter 7.5), and new research creating the basis for risk analyses (most other chapters in this textbook). As a result, effective risk communication cannot be just an afterthought, letting the public know what the authorities have decided. Rather, it must be central to risk management, as part of disciplined, continuing, two-way communication between decision-makers and the authorities.

This chapter has focused on measurement, rather than on general theories about how people perceive and respond to risks. That is because critical details vary across risk decisions and decision-makers. Sweeping generalizations about what 'people do' or 'people think' or 'people want' undermine the attention to detail that responsive risk communications require. Separate research programmes could be dedicated to communicating the science presented in many chapters in the textbook, ensuring that the public gets full value from that science. However, the methods for studying judgement and decision-making are sufficiently general and well understood that they could be applied in any domain, and for any form of information dissemination. Given a well-characterized decision or risk, it is relatively straightforward, if technically demanding, to assess lay (or expert) perceptions. If decision-makers' risk (and benefit) perceptions have been measured well, their choices can often be roughly predicted with simple linear models (Dawes et al. 1989). More precise prediction requires more detailed understanding of the cognitive processes shaping these beliefs, as well as an understanding of the emotional, social, economic, and other factors impinging on specific decisions. Prediction may not be that important, when the public health goal is helping people to make the best choices or empowering them to change their circumstances.

Meeting the challenge of effective risk communication requires coordinating the activities of four kinds of experts: subject matter specialists, risk and decision analysts, behavioural scientists, and communication practitioners. Assembling those teams requires leadership, seeing communication as being essential to the public health mission. The research itself is inexpensive, relative to the stakes riding on sound risk decision-making, both for individuals and for the public health organizations expected to serve them. There is no good reason for the measurement of risk perceptions and the evaluation of risk communications to use less than the readily available methods described here. There is no good reason to ignore well-established results, such as the multidimensional character of 'risk', the problems with verbal quantifiers, and the need to help people to understand how risks mount up through repeated exposure. Ad hoc communications might reflect sound intuition, but they deserve less trust than scientifically developed ones.

By definition, better risk communication should help its recipients to make better choices. It need not make the communicators' lives easier—recipients may discover bona fide disagreements with the communicators and their institutions. What it should do is avoid conflicts due to misunderstanding, increasing the light-to-heat ratio in risk management, leading to fewer but better conflicts (Fischhoff 1995).

Acknowledgement

The preparation of this chapter was supported by the Center for Climate and Energy Decision Making (SES-0949710) through a cooperative agreement between the National Science Foundation and Carnegie Mellon University. The views expressed are the author's.

References

Arabie, P. and Maschmeyer, C. (1988). Some current models for the perception and judgment of risk. *Organizational Behavior and Human Decision Processes*, 41, 300–29.

Bauman, K.E. (1980). *Predicting Adolescent Drug Use: Utility Structure and Marijuana*. New York: Praeger.

Beyth-Marom, R., Austin, L., Fischhoff, B., et al. (1993). Perceived consequences of risky behaviors. *Developmental Psychology*, 29, 549–63.

Black, W.C., Nease, R.F., and Tosteson, A.N.A. (1995). Perceptions of breast cancer risk and screening effectiveness in women younger than 50 years of age. *Journal of the National Cancer Institute*, 8, 720–31.

Bostrom, A., Fischhoff, B., and Morgan, M.G. (1992). Characterizing mental models of hazardous processes: a methodology and an application to radon. *Journal of Social Issues*, 48(4), 85–100.

Breakwell, G.M. (2007). *The Psychology of Risk*. Cambridge: Cambridge University Press.

Brewer, N.T., Chapman, G.B., Gibbons, F.X., et al. (2007). Meta-analysis of the relationship between risk perception and health behavior: the example of vaccination. *Health Psychology*, 26, 136–45.

Bruine de Bruin, W., Downs, J.S., Fischhoff, B., and Palmgren, C. (2007a). Development and evaluation of an HIV/AIDS knowledge measure for adolescents focusing on misconceptions. *Journal of HIV/AIDS Prevention in Children and Youth*, 8(1), 35–57.

Bruine de Bruin, W., Fischhoff, B., Halpern-Felsher, B., et al. (2000). Expressing epistemic uncertainty: it's a fifty-fifty chance. *Organizational Behavior and Human Decision Processes*, 81, 115–31.

Bruine de Bruin, W., Güvenç, Ü., Fischhoff, B., Armstrong, C.M., and Caruso, D. (2009). Communicating about xenotransplanation: models and scenarios. *Risk Analysis*, 29, 1105–15.

Bruine de Bruin, W., Parker, A., and Fischhoff, B. (2007b). Individual differences in adult decision-making competence (A-DMC). *Journal of Personality and Social Psychology*, 92, 938–56.

Budescu, D.F. and Wallsten, T.S. (1995). Processing linguistic probabilities: general principles and empirical evidence. In J.R. Busemeyer, R. Hastie, and D.L. Medin (eds.) *Decision Making from the Perspective of Cognitive Psychology*, pp. 275–316. New York: Academic Press.

Byram, S., Fischhoff, B., Embrey, M., et al. (2001). Mental models of women with breast implants regarding local complications. *Behavioral Medicine*, 27, 4–14.

Campbell, P. (2011). Understanding the receivers and the receptions of science's uncertain messages. *Philosophical Transactions of the Royal Society*, 369, 4891–912.

Christensen-Szalanski, J. and Bushyhead, J. (1993). Physicians' misunderstanding of medical findings. *Medical Decision Making*, 3, 169–75.

Dawes, R.M., Faust, D., and Meehl, P. (1989). Clinical versus actuarial judgment. *Science*, 243, 1668–74.

DeKay, M.L., Small, M.J., Fischbeck, P.S., et al. (2002). Risk-based decision analysis in support of precautionary policies. *Journal of Risk Research*, 5, 391–417.

Downs, J.S., Bruine de Bruin, W., and Fischhoff, B. (2008). Patients' vaccination comprehension and decisions, *Vaccine*, 26, 1595–607.

Downs, J.S., Bruine de Bruin, W., Murray, P.J., et al. (2004b). When 'it only takes once' fails: perceived infertility predicts condom use and STI acquisition. *Journal of Pediatric and Adolescent Gynecology*, 17, 224.

Downs, J.S., Murray, P.J., Bruine de Bruin, W., et al. (2004a). An interactive video program to reduce adolescent females' STD risk: a randomized controlled trial. *Social Science and Medicine*, 59, 1561–72.

Eggers, S.L. and Fischhoff, B. (2004). Setting policies for consumer communications: a behavioral decision research approach. *Journal of Public Policy and Marketing*, 23, 14–27.

Erev, I. and Cohen, B.L. (1990). Verbal versus numerical probabilities: efficiency, biases and the preference paradox. *Organizational Behavior and Human Decision Processes*, 45, 1–18.

Ericsson, K.A. and Simon, H.A. (1993). *Verbal Reports as Data*. Cambridge, MA: MIT Press.

Fagerlin, A. and Peters, E. (2011). Quantitative information. In B. Fischhoff, N.T. Brewer, and J.S. Downs (eds.) *Communicating Risks and Benefits: An Evidence-Based User's Guide*, pp. 53–64. Washington, DC: US Food and Drug Administration.

Farris, C. and Fischhoff, B. (2012). A decision science informed approach to sexual risk and non-consent. *Clinical and Translational Science*, 5, 482–5.

Feather, N. (1982). *Expectancy, Incentive and Action*. Hillsdale, NJ: Erlbaum.

Finucane, M.L. and Gullion, C.M. (2010). Developing a tool for assessing the decision-making competence of older adults. *Psychology & Aging*, 25, 271–88.

Fischhoff, B. (1992). Giving advice: decision theory perspectives on sexual assault. *American Psychologist*, 47, 577–88.

Fischhoff, B. (1994). What forecasts (seem to) mean. *International Journal of Forecasting*, 10, 387–403.

Fischhoff, B. (1995). Risk perception and communication unplugged: twenty years of process. *Risk Analysis*, 15, 137–45.

Fischhoff, B. (1996). The real world: what good is it? *Organizational Behavior and Human Decision Processes*, 65, 232–48.

Fischhoff, B. (2005a). Cognitive processes in stated preference methods. In K.G. Mäler and J. Vincent (eds.) *Handbook of Environmental Economics*, pp. 937–68. Amsterdam: Elsevier.

Fischhoff, B. (2005b). Decision research strategies. *Health Psychology*, 21, S9–16.

Fischhoff, B. (2008). Assessing adolescent decision-making competence. *Developmental Review*, 28, 12–28.

Fischhoff, B. (2011). Communicating the risks of terrorism (and anything else). *American Psychologist*, 66, 520–31.

Fischhoff, B., Brewer, N.T., and Downs, J.S. (eds.) (2011). *Communicating Risks and Benefits: An Evidence-Based User's Guide*. Washington, DC: US Food and Drug Administration.

Fischhoff, B., Bruine de Bruin, W., Guvenc, U., et al. (2006). Analyzing disaster risks and plans: an avian flu example. *Journal of Risk and Uncertainty*, 33, 133–51.

Fischhoff, B., Downs, J., and Bruine de Bruin, W. (1998). Adolescent vulnerability: a framework for behavioral interventions. *Applied and Preventive Psychology*, 7, 77–94.

Fischhoff, B. and Kadvany, J. (2001). *Risk: A Very Short Introduction.* Oxford: Oxford University Press.

Fischhoff, B. and MacGregor, D. (1983). Judged lethality: how much people seem to know depends upon how they are asked. *Risk Analysis*, 3, 229–36.

Fischhoff, B., Parker, A., Bruine de Bruin, W., et al. (2000). Teen expectations for significant life events. *Public Opinion Quarterly*, 64, 189–205.

Fischhoff, B., Slovic, P., and Lichtenstein, S., (1977). Knowing with certainty: the appropriateness of extreme confidence. *Journal of Experimental Psychology: Human Perception and Performance*, 3, 552–64.

Fischhoff, B., Slovic, P., Lichtenstein, S., et al. (1978). How safe is safe enough? A psychometric study of attitudes towards technological risks and benefits. *Policy Sciences*, 8, 127–52.

Fischhoff, B., Watson, S., and Hope, C. (1984). Defining risk. *Policy Sciences*, 17, 123–39.

Florig, K. and Fischhoff, B. (2007). Individuals' decisions affecting radiation exposure after a nuclear event. *Health Physics*, 92, 475–83.

Florig, H.K., Morgan, M.G., Morgan, K.M., et al. (2001). A deliberative method for ranking risks. *Risk Analysis*, 21, 913–22.

Fortney, J. (1988). Contraception: a life long perspective. In *Dying for Love*, pp. 33–8. Washington, DC: National Council for International Health.

Frederick, S. (2005). Cognitive reflection and decision making. *Journal of Economic Perspectives*, 19(4), 25–42.

Funtowicz, S.O., and Ravetz, J. (1990). *Uncertainty and Quality in Science for Policy.* London: Kluwer.

Gilovich, T., Griffin, D., and Kahneman, D. (eds.) (2003). *Judgment Under Uncertainty II: Extensions and Applications.* New York: Cambridge University Press.

Griffin, D., Gonzalez, R., and Varey, C. (2003). The heuristics and biases approach to judgment under uncertainty. In A. Tesser and N. Schwarz (eds.) *Blackwell Handbook of Social Psychology*, pp. 207–35. Boston, MA: Blackwell.

HM Treasury (2005). *Managing Risks to the Public.* London: HM Treasury.

Howard, R.A. (1989). Knowledge maps. *Management Science*, 35, 903–22.

Kahneman, D., Slovic, P., and Tversky, A. (eds.) (1982). *Judgment Under Uncertainty: Heuristics and Biases.* New York: Cambridge University Press.

Koriat, A. (1993). How do we know that we know? *Psychological Review*, 100, 609–39.

Krimsky, S. and Golding, D. (1992). *Theories of Risk.* New York: Praeger.

Lerner, J.S. and Keltner, D. (2001). Fear, anger, and risk. *Journal of Personality and Social Psychology*, 81, 146–59.

Lichtenstein, S. and Fischhoff, B. (1980). Training for calibration. *Organizational Behavior and Human Performance*, 26, 149–71.

Lichtenstein, S., Fischhoff, B., and Phillips, L.D. (1982). Calibration of probabilities. In D. Kahneman, P. Slovic, and A. Tversky (eds.) *Judgment Under Uncertainty: Heuristics and Biases*, pp. 306–39. New York: Cambridge University Press.

Lichtenstein, S., Slovic, P., Fischhoff, B., et al. (1978). Judged frequency of lethal events. *Journal of Experimental Psychology: Human Learning and Memory*, 4, 551–78.

Linville, P.W., Fischer, G.W., and Fischhoff, B. (1993). AIDS risk perceptions and decision biases. In J.B. Pryor and G.D. Reeder (eds.) *The Social Psychology of HIV Infection*, pp. 5–38. Hillsdale, NJ: Erlbaum.

Löfstedt, R., Fischhoff, B., and Fischhoff, I. (2002). Precautionary principles: general definitions and specific applications to genetically modified organisms (GMOs). *Journal of Policy Analysis and Management*, 21, 381–407.

Lowrance, W.W. (1976). *Of Acceptable Risk: Science and the Determination of Safety.* Los Altos, CA: William Kaufman.

McIntyre, S. and West, P. (1992). What does the phrase 'safer sex' mean to you? Understanding among Glaswegian 18 year olds in 1990. *AIDS*, 7, 121–6.

Merton, R.F. (1987). The focussed interview and focus groups. *Public Opinion Quarterly*, 51, 550–66.

Merz, J., Fischhoff, B., Mazur, D.J., et al. (1993). Decision-analytic approach to developing standards of disclosure for medical informed consent. *Journal of Toxics and Liability*, 15, 191–215.

Meyer, D., Leventhal, H., and Gutmann, M. (1985). Common-sense models of illness: the example of hypertension. *Health Psychology*, 4, 115–35.

Morgan, M.G., Fischhoff, B., Bostrom, A., et al. (1992). Communicating risk to the public. *Environmental Science and Technology*, 26, 2048–56.

Morgan, M.G., Fischhoff, B., Bostrom, A., et al. (2001). *Risk Communication: The Mental Models Approach.* New York: Cambridge University Press.

Murphy, A.H., Lichtenstein, S., Fischhoff, B., et al. (1980). Misinterpretations of precipitation probability forecasts. *Bulletin of the American Meteorological Society*, 61, 695–701.

National Research Council (1989) *Improving Risk Communication.* Washington, DC: National Academy Press.

National Research Council (1996). *Understanding Risk: Informing Decisions in a Democratic Society.* Washington, DC: National Academy Press.

National Research Council (2006). *Scientific Review of the Proposed Risk Assessment Bulletin from the Office of Management and Budget.* Washington, DC: National Academy Press.

Nickerson, R.A. (1999). How we know—and sometimes misjudge—what others know: imputing our own knowledge to others. *Psychological Bulletin*, 125, 737–59.

O'Hagan, A., Buck, C.E. Daneshkhah, A., et al. (2006). *Uncertain Judgements: Eliciting Expert Probabilities.* Chichester: Wiley.

Peters, E. and McCaul, K.D. (eds.) (2005). Basic and applied decision making in cancer. *Health Psychology*, 24(4), S3.

Politi, M.C., Han, P.K.J., and Col. N. (2007). Communicating the uncertainty of harms and benefits of medical procedures. *Medical Decision Making*, 27, 681–95.

Poulton, E.C. (1989). *Bias in Quantifying Judgment.* Hillsdale, NJ: Lawrence Erlbaum.

Quadrel, M.J., Fischhoff, B., and Davis, W. (1993). Adolescent (in)vulnerability. *American Psychologist*, 48, 102–16.

Reimer, B., and Van Nevel, J.P. (eds.) (1999). Cancer risk communication. *Journal of the National Cancer Institute Monographs*, 19, 1–185.

Reyna, V. and Farley, F. (2006). Risk and rationality in adolescent decision making: implications for theory, practice, and public policy. *Psychology in the Public Interest*, 7(1), 1–44.

Riley, D.M., Fischhoff, B., Small, M., et al. (2001). Evaluating the effectiveness of risk-reduction strategies for consumer chemical products. *Risk Analysis*, 21, 357–69.

Ritov, I. and Baron, J. (1990). Status quo and omission bias. Reluctance to vaccinate. *Journal of Behavioral Decision Making*, 3, 263–77.

Schwartz, L.M. and Woloshin, S. (2011). Communicating uncertainties about prescription drugs to the public: a national randomized trial. *Archives of Internal Medicine*, 171, 1463–8.

Schwarz, N. (1999). Self reports. *American Psychologist*, 54, 93–105.

Shaklee, H. and Fischhoff, B. (1990). The psychology of contraceptive surprises: judging the cumulative risk of contraceptive failure. *Journal of Applied Psychology*, 20, 385–403.

Slovic, P. (2001). *Perception of Risk.* London: Earthspan.

Slovic, P. and Fischhoff, B. (1983). Targeting risk. *Risk Analysis*, 2, 231–8.

Slovic, P., Fischhoff, B., and Lichtenstein, S. (1978). Accident probabilities and seat-belt usage: a psychological perspective. *Accident Analysis and Prevention*, 10, 281–5.

Slovic, P., Fischhoff, B., and Lichtenstein, S. (1979). Rating the risks. *Environment*, 21(4), 14–20, 36–9.

Slovic, P., Lichtenstein, S., and Fischhoff, B. (1984). Modeling the societal impact of fatal accidents. *Management Science*, 30, 464–74.

Slovic, P., Peters, E., Finucane, M.L., et al. (2005). Affect, risk and decision making. *Health Psychology*, 24, S35–40.

Sox, H.C., Blatt, M.A., Higgins, M.C., et al. (2007). *Medical Decision Making.* Philadelphia, PA: American College of Physicians.

Starr, C. (1969). Societal benefit versus technological risk. *Science*, 165, 1232–8.

Sterman, J. and Sweeney, J. (2002). Cloudy skies: assessing public understanding of climate change. *System Dynamics Review*, 18, 207–40.

Thaler, R. (1991). *Quasi-Rational Economics*. New York: Russell Sage Foundation.

Thaler, R. and Sunstein, C. (2009). *Nudge: Improving Decisions about Health, Wealth and Happiness*. New Haven, CT: Yale University Press.

USEPA (1993). *A Guidebook to Comparing Risks and Setting Environmental Priorities*. Washington, DC: USEPA.

Viscusi, K. (1992). *Smoking: Making the Risky Decision*. New York: Oxford University Press.

Vlek, C. and Stallen, P.J. (1981). Judging risks and benefits in the small and in the large. *Organizational Behavior and Human Performance*, 28, 235–71.

Von Winterfeldt, D. and Edwards, W. (1986). *Decision Analysis and Behavioral Research*. New York: Cambridge University Press.

Wagenaar, W. and Sagaria, S.D. (1975). Misperception of exponential growth. *Perception & Psychophysics*, 18, 416–22.

Willis, H.H., DeKay, M.L., Fischhoff, B., et al. (2005). Aggregate and disaggregate analyses of ecological risk perceptions. *Risk Analysis*, 25, 405–28.

Wogalter, M. (2006). *The Handbook of Warnings*. Hillsdale, NJ: Lawrence Erlbaum Associates.

Woloshin, S., Schwartz, L.M., Byram, S., et al. (1998). Scales for assessing perceptions of event probability: a validation study. *Medical Decision Making*, 14, 490–503.

SECTION 8

Major health problems

Epidemiology and prevention of cardiovascular disease

Nathan D. Wong

Introduction to epidemiology and prevention of cardiovascular disease

Cardiovascular disease (CVD) is the leading cause of morbidity and mortality, accounting for 17.3 million deaths globally each year and this figure is expected to grow to 23.6 million by the year 2030; 80 per cent of these deaths occur in lower- and middle-income countries (Mendis et al. 2011). It is the largest contributor to non-communicable diseases (NCDs) that are now responsible for the largest share of morbidity and mortality worldwide. The incidence of CVD, including coronary heart disease, heart failure, and stroke, as well as the prevalence of key risk factors, varies greatly according to geographical region, gender, and ethnic background. Multiple longitudinal epidemiological studies have provided valuable insights into the natural history and risk factors associated with the development and prognosis of CVD. Randomized clinical trials have demonstrated the value of management of several key risk factors for both the primary and secondary prevention of CVD. This chapter discusses the epidemiology of CVD, its associated risk factors and evidence for their control, assessment of CVD risk, and the evidence behind the control of CVD risk factors for the prevention of CVD.

Definitions, incidence, and distribution

CVD comprises many conditions, including coronary heart disease, heart failure, rheumatic fever/rheumatic heart disease, stroke, and congenital heart disease. Ischaemic heart disease, consisting principally of coronary heart disease (CHD), is the predominant manifestation of CVD and is responsible for 46 per cent of deaths due to CVD in men and 38 per cent in women, followed closely by cerebrovascular disease at 34 per cent and 37 per cent, respectively (Fig. 8.1.1). While the burden of CVD was highest in Western countries during much of the twentieth century, the highest rates of CVD now occur among certain Asian and Middle Eastern regions (Fig. 8.1.2). By country, total death rates (per 100,000) from CVD, CHD, and stroke are highest in the Russian Federation for both men (1185, 659, and 308, respectively) and women (463, 221, and 158, respectively) and among the lowest in Israel for men (133, 72, and 24, respectively) and in France for women (51, 12, and 14, respectively), with intermediate rates in the United States (250, 143, and 30, respectively, in men and 124, 56, and 22, respectively, in women) (Go et al. 2013).

In the United States, the overall prevalence of CVD (including hypertension) increases dramatically from 12.8 per cent in men between the ages of 20 to 39 years to 83.0 per cent for men above 80 years old; the corresponding figures for women are 10.1 per cent and 87.1 per cent (Go et al. 2013).

Of note, however, is the substantial reduction in CVD mortality rates in the United States over the past three decades, both in men and in women, although absolute mortality from CVD in women since 1985 has exceeded that observed in men. These declines have been attributed both to improved treatments for CVD and its associated risk factors, as well as to improvements in lifestyle factors such as substantial declines in cigarette smoking, although the increasing obesity epidemic is expected to negate some of these reductions in CVD.

Myocardial infarction, angina pectoris, and sudden coronary death are the major clinical manifestations of CHD. CHD initially presents as sudden coronary death in approximately one-third of cases. Other forms of documented CHD include procedures performed as a result of documented significant atherosclerosis, such as coronary artery bypass grafting (CABG) or percutaneous coronary interventions (PCI), including angioplasty and stenting. People with documented significant disease from a coronary angiogram, echocardiogram, nuclear myocardial perfusion, magnetic resonance imaging, or computed tomography (CT) angiographic or coronary calcium scan can also designate the presence of CHD; however, because the definitions used to define significant CHD vary and these findings often do not result in hospitalization or hard CHD events, such people are not normally counted as incident or prevalent CHD, particularly for the purposes of end points in epidemiological studies or clinical trials. Non-fatal or fatal myocardial infarction or sudden coronary death are most typically included as 'hard' CHD end points, while 'total' CHD may additionally include angina requiring hospitalization as well as PCI or CABG.

CHD prevalence rates vary dramatically by age and gender in the United States. The most recent statistics from 2007 to 2010 showed that 15.4 million US adults aged 20 years and greater have CHD; this varies widely by race and gender within the United States. For example, for males, while the overall prevalence was 7.9 per cent, the prevalence in non-Hispanic white males was 8.2 per cent, in black males 6.8 per cent, and in Mexican-American males 6.7 per cent. The corresponding figures for females were 5.1 per cent overall, 4.6 per cent in non-Hispanic white females, 7.1 per cent in

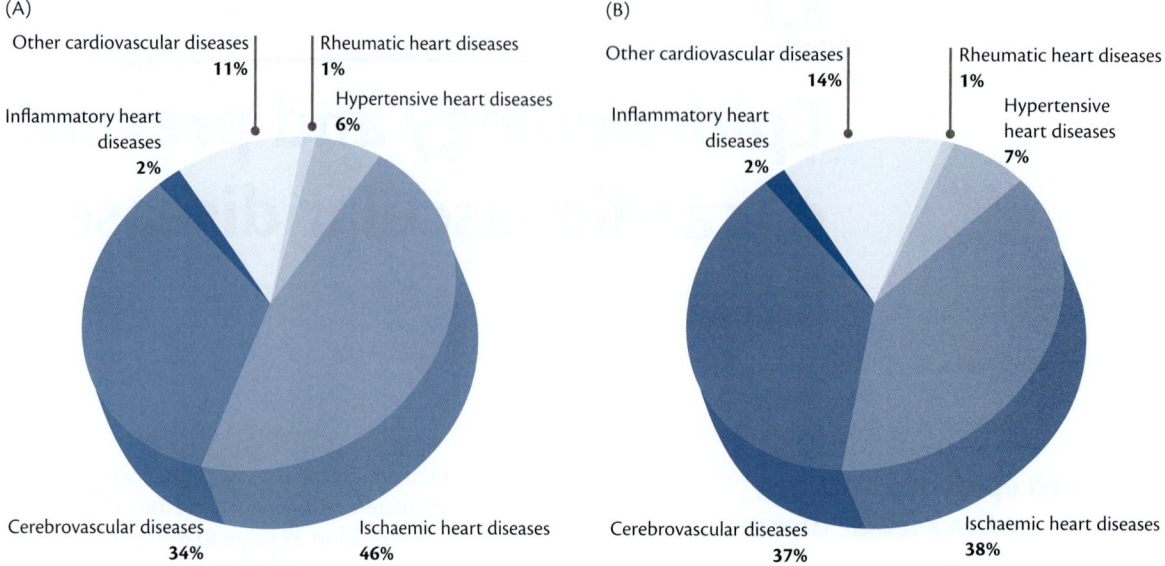

Fig. 8.1.1 Proportion of deaths from cardiovascular disease (CVD) due to ischaemic heart disease, cerebrovascular disease, and other CVD causes in males (A) and females (B).

Reproduced with permission from Mendis S, Puska P, and Norrving B (eds), *Global Atlas on Cardiovascular Disease Prevention and Control*, World Health Organization, Geneva, Switzerland, Copyright © 2011, available from http://www.who.int/cardiovascular_diseases/publications/atlas_cvd/en/.

black females, and 5.3 per cent in Mexican-American females. In the United States, there is a heart attack every 44 seconds. CHD makes up more than half of all CVD deaths in men and women under 75 years of age, with a lifetime risk of developing CHD after age 40 years, of 49 per cent for men and 32 per cent for women (Go et al. 2013).

Other important manifestations of CVD include cerebrovascular disease (including stroke and transient ischaemic attacks), heart failure, atrial fibrillation, and peripheral arterial disease, in particular. Somewhat less common but still of significance are valvular heart disease, rheumatic heart disease, and bacterial and valvular endocarditis.

Cerebrovascular disease includes stroke and transient ischaemic attacks (TIAs). Stroke prevalence in the United States ranges from less than 1 per cent in those under 40 years of age to 14 per cent in both genders in those aged 80 years and over. An estimated 6.8 million Americans aged 20 years and over have had a stroke; each year an estimated 795,000 people experience a new or recurrent stroke, with approximately 610,000 of these cases being first attacks. Of all strokes, about 87 per cent are ischaemic and 10 per cent are intracerebral haemorrhagic strokes, and 3 per cent subarachnoid haemorrhage strokes (Go et al. 2013). The self-reported prevalence of physician-diagnosed TIAs is about 2.3 per cent, translating to approximately 5 million people, but the true prevalence is likely to be greater as many with neurological symptoms consistent with TIA fail to report them to their healthcare provider. About 15 per cent of all strokes are preceded by a TIA.

While mortality rates due to total CVD, and especially CHD and stroke, have declined substantially over the past 30 years, hospitalizations due to total CVD have increased, much of this fuelled by the more than doubling in the number of hospitalizations due to heart failure between 1980 and 2010 (1,023,000 in 2010 in the United States). It is projected that this will increase by another 25 per cent by the year 2030. The prevalence of heart failure ranges

from less than 1 per cent in those under age 40 to 9 per cent of men and 12 per cent of women aged 80 years and over.

Peripheral arterial disease is highly prevalent affecting approximately 8.5 million Americans aged 40 years and over and is associated with significant morbidity and mortality; it is most common in older people over age 55 and is asymptomatic in most cases, being diagnosed by a Doppler tool measuring the ankle–brachial index (ABI), where a value of less than 0.9 is diagnostic of peripheral arterial disease. The estimated prevalence in the US population is 4.6 per cent; only about 10 per cent of those with peripheral arterial disease actually have the classic symptoms of intermittent claudication (or leg pain) (Go et al. 2013).

Estimates of the prevalence of valvular heart disease, which includes aortic, mitral, and tricuspid valve disorders, range from less than 1 per cent in those under the age of 45 years to 12–13 per cent in those aged 75 years and over. Rheumatic heart disease while uncommon in developed countries, affects more than 15 million individuals in Africa, Asia, and the Pacific, causing over 200,000 deaths annually. Infective endocarditis is relatively rare and results from formation of nonbacterial thrombotic endocarditis on the surface of a cardiac valve, bacteraemia, and adherence of the bacteria in the bloodstream; the estimated risk in the general population is as low as one case per 14 million dental procedures (Go et al. 2013).

Risk factors for cardiovascular disease

The Framingham Heart Study, the seminal epidemiological study of CVD, is a large longitudinal investigation that started in 1948 in the small town of Framingham, Massachusetts, United States. The original cohort of 5209 participants aged 30–62 years of age received biennial physical examinations, risk factor assessments, and surveillance for CVD events (Wong and Levy 2013). The

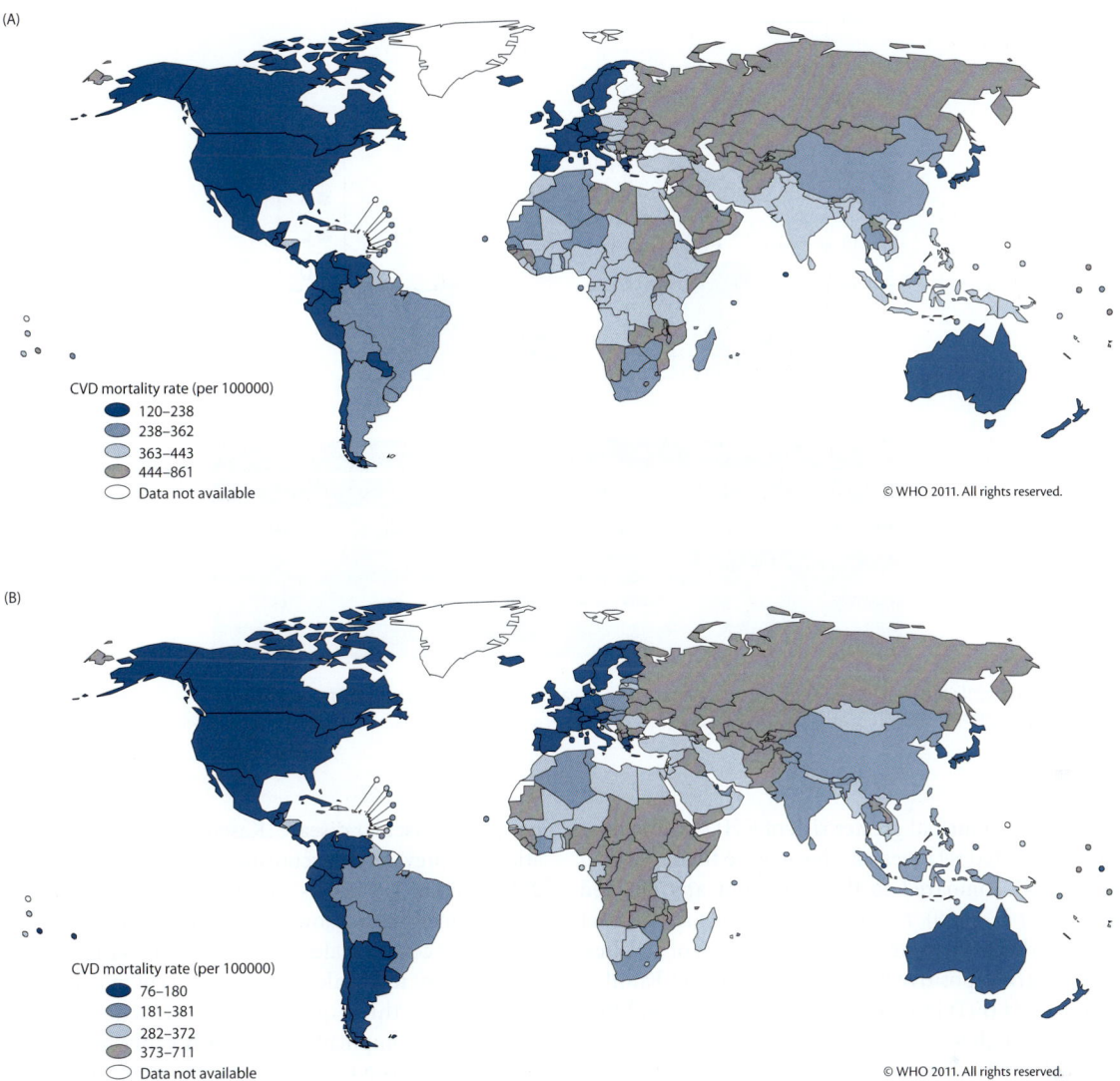

Fig. 8.1.2 Global distribution of CVD mortality rates in males (A) and females (B), age-standardized per 100,000.

Reproduced with permission from Mendis S, Puska P, and Norrving B (eds), *Global Atlas on Cardiovascular Disease Prevention and Control*, World Health Organization, Geneva, Switzerland, Copyright © 2011, available from http://www.who.int/cardiovascular_diseases/publications/atlas_cvd/en/.

Framingham study was instrumental in the original identification of many of the factors that are associated with an increased risk of CVD and, in 1961, coined for the first time the term 'risk factors' that is widely utilized in many different fields of medicine today (Kannel et al. 1961). The increased awareness of major risk factors for CVD initially identified by the Framingham Heart Study and by other researchers provided the impetus for important public health initiatives against smoking in the 1960s, hypertension in the 1970s, and hypercholesterolaemia in the 1980s. More recently, obesity and physical inactivity have also been recognized as key risk factors for CVD. Diabetes is also now widely regarded as a CHD risk equivalent and the importance of a clustering of major cardiometabolic risk factors, commonly referred to as the metabolic syndrome, has received significant attention from the research and clinical community (Grundy et al. 2005). Risk factors often cluster together, and the number of risk factors present and their co-occurrence are directly related to the incidence of CHD (Fig. 8.1.3). Importantly, it was the Framingham Heart Study that

first introduced the concept of multivariable or global risk assessment for coronary heart disease (see also 'Global risk scores for cardiovascular disease risk assessment') (Wilson et al. 1998).

Family history and genomics

A family history of premature CHD is a well-established, but unmodifiable risk factor for future CHD, and can sometimes be the crucial and single most important risk factor in predisposing an individual to early CHD (Hopkins et al. 2000; Williams et al. 2001). A large proportion of heart attacks or strokes occurring at a young age are felt to be attributable to inherited or familial predisposition. Hence, knowledge of an individual's family history can help guide preventive efforts. A family history of premature CHD is generally defined as having a male first-degree relative experiencing a first manifestation of CHD under the age of 45, or a female first-degree relative experiencing CHD under the age of 55. The number of affected relatives with premature CHD is also felt to be an important factor, since those with one affected relative

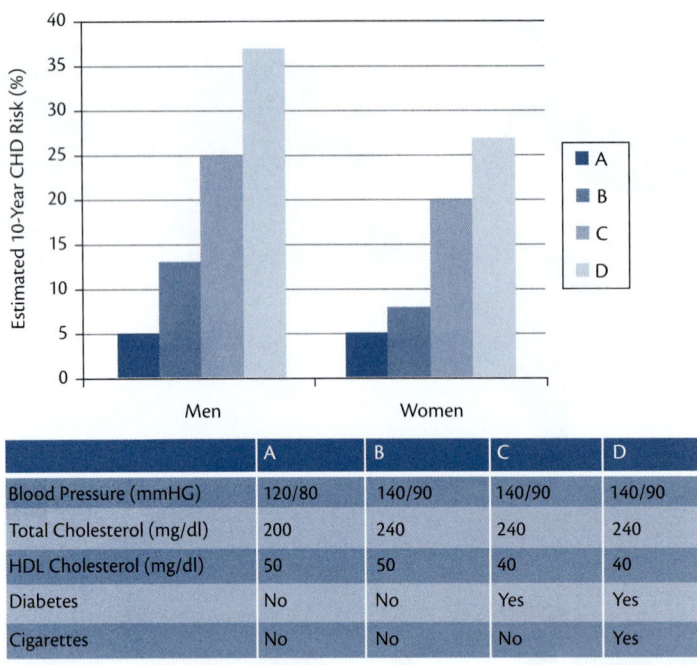

Fig. 8.1.3 Estimated 10-year CHD risk in 55-year-old adults according to levels of various risk factors: Framingham Heart Study.
Source: data from Wilson PWF et al., Prediction of Coronary Heart Disease Using Risk Factor Categories, *Circulation*, Volume 97, pp. 1837–1847, Copyright © 2008 American Heart Association, Inc. All rights reserved.

	A	B	C	D
Blood Pressure (mmHG)	120/80	140/90	140/90	140/90
Total Cholesterol (mg/dl)	200	240	240	240
HDL Cholesterol (mg/dl)	50	50	40	40
Diabetes	No	No	Yes	Yes
Cigarettes	No	No	No	Yes

can be shown to have a fourfold greater risk of CHD, while those with two or more affected relatives may have more than a 12-fold greater risk of CHD compared to those without any affected relatives (Hopkins et al. 2000). Moreover, it has been shown that 35 per cent of all early CHD occurs in just 3.2 per cent of families, all of whom have a strong positive family history of CHD. Familial hypercholesterolaemia (FH) is an autosomal dominant condition associated with very high levels of total and low-density lipoprotein cholesterol (LDL-C) (total cholesterol levels exceeding 500 are commonly reported) where individuals inherit from one or both parents (homozygous) a defective LDL-C receptor gene. Affected individuals have been known to have heart attacks and die by the age of 20 and FH is among the most widely studied genetic conditions responsible for CHD. Other genetic defects responsible for hypertension, obesity, diabetes, and other major cardiovascular risk factors have also been identified and are the subject of major investigations (Williams et al. 2001).

In recent years, with the ability to sequence the entire human genome, key single-nucleotide polymorphisms (SNPs) have been identified and linked to the likelihood of CHD, although with a much higher threshold required to confirm a statistically significant relationship ($p = 10^{-8}$) (Schunkert et al. 2011). One region that has received significant attention is 9p21 because of its strong association with CHD (Palomaki et al. 2010). However, the utility of such SNPs in improving the ability to predict CHD over traditional risk factors is only modest and current guidelines have not recommended genomic screening due to the thus far limited demonstrated clinical utility.

Diabetes and metabolic syndrome

Diabetes mellitus is a major risk factor for CVD, and is associated with a greater risk for CHD, stroke, chronic kidney disease, and peripheral vascular disease (Kaseta et al. 2005). There are wide variations in prevalence according to gender and ethnicity. In 2009–2010, among US adults, the prevalence of physician-diagnosed diabetes mellitus was lowest in white people (6.2 per cent in females and 7.7 per cent in males) and highest in non-Hispanic black people (15.4 per cent in females and 13.5 per cent in males).

More than three-quarters of those with diabetes die of cardiovascular complications, most notably myocardial infarction and stroke. Given this point, the National Cholesterol Education Program designated diabetes as a CHD risk equivalent (Expert Panel on Detection, Evaluation, and Treatment of High Blood Cholesterol in Adults 2001) because the risk of CHD in those with diabetes without known heart disease had been shown to be similar to recurrent CHD events in those with CHD (but without known diabetes), although more recent studies are showing that this is not always the case. Most population-based studies have shown about a twofold greater risk of CHD in men with diabetes as compared to men without diabetes, but in women, the corresponding figure is a three- to seven-fold greater risk of CHD.

Diabetes is typically diagnosed by a glycated haemoglobin (HbA1c) level of 6.5 per cent or greater, fasting glucose of 126 mg/dL (7 mmol/L) or above, or glucose level of at least 200 mg/dL (11.1 mmol/L) from the non-fasting state or after a 2-hour post-load glucose challenge test (American Diabetes Association 2013). Pre-diabetes is diagnosed by a fasting glucose of 100–125 mg/dL or casual glucose of 140–199 mg/dL.

Clinical trial evidence to show whether intensive glycaemic control in people with diabetes lowers CVD event rates has shown mixed results. The United Kingdom Prospective Diabetes Study (UKPDS) originally showed a borderline, non-significant ($p = 0.052$) 16 per cent reduction in risk of myocardial infarction among those with newly diagnosed type 2 diabetes who were treated with intensive glucose lowering therapy, but the 10-year post-interventional follow-up of this study, which was recently published, showed that these benefits continued with a 15 per cent significant ($p = 0.01$) reduction in risk of myocardial infarction (Holman et al. 2008). A similar, extended post-interventional follow-up of the Diabetes Control and Complications Trial of Type 1 diabetes, which did not initially show a significant reduction in CVD events at the end of the randomized trial, showed years later a continued effect of the original intensive glucose-lowering treatment, with a 42 per cent reduction in the risk of any cardiovascular event (Nathan et al. 2005). Such a continued post-trial effect of the randomized glycaemic therapy has been termed a 'glycaemic legacy' effect. More recently, however, three important randomized clinical trials (the Action to Control Cardiovascular Risk in Diabetes (ACCORD), ADVANCE, and the Veterans Affairs Diabetes Trial (VADT)) failed to show that intensive glucose lowering to a HbA1c range of 6–6.5 per cent significantly reduced CVD event rates, as compared to more standard maintenance of the HBA1c in the 7–9 per cent range. In fact, those randomized to the intensive therapy group in ACCORD actually had a higher rate of CVD mortality (Action to Control Cardiovascular Risk in Diabetes Study Group et al. 2008), although this increased risk was restricted to those with prior macrovascular disease and where there was unsuccessful lowering of the glucose as a result of the intensive therapy. Those with less complicated diabetes (e.g. patients who were more recently diagnosed and without prior macrovascular disease) actually showed a benefit in the primary end point. Moreover, an important lipid substudy of ACCORD tested the efficacy of adding the fibric acid derivative fenofibrate or placebo to ongoing statin therapy and found no benefit in terms of reducing CVD event rates (although there was a benefit seen in the subgroup with high triglycerides and low high-density lipoprotein cholesterol (HDL-C)) (ACCORD Study Group 2010a). In addition, in the blood pressure substudy of ACCORD, intensive blood pressure therapy to achieve a systolic blood pressure less than 120 mmHg, as compared with less than 140 mmHg, was also found to provide no significant benefit in terms of CVD risk reduction, although there was a significant benefit in stroke reduction (ACCORD Study Group 2010b).

Of particular interest in the past decade has been the designation of metabolic syndrome, referring to a constellation of cardiometabolic risk factors that are associated with a greater risk of developing future diabetes and CVD. This clinical condition has been useful for the purposes of defining those with multiple risk factors which place them at greater CVD risk, and who may benefit from a more intensified, unified approach at risk factor modification. Studies have documented that 30–40 per cent of adults have metabolic syndrome in the United States, with even higher prevalence rates in some countries such as in the Middle East. Certain definitions of the metabolic syndrome place insulin resistance or abdominal obesity as the necessary condition, with additional conditions including elevated blood pressure, low HDL-C, elevated triglycerides, and impaired fasting glucose making up the definition. The American Heart Association (AHA)/National Heart Lung and Blood Institute definition (Grundy et al. 2005) requires the presence of at least three of the following five criteria: abdominal obesity defined by a waist circumference greater than 35 inches (89 cm) in women or greater than 45 inches (115 cm) in men; HDL-C less than 40 mg/dL in men or less than 50 mg/dL in women, fasting triglycerides of 150 mg/dL or above; elevated blood pressure of 130 mmHg systolic or above, or 85 mmHg diastolic or above, or on hypertensive therapy; or impaired fasting glucose defined as at least 100 mg/dL (5.6 mmol/L) or on hypoglycaemic therapy. It is important to recognize that other definitions exist, such as that from the International Diabetes Federation which requires the presence of abdominal obesity as measured by lower waist circumference cut-off points in European Caucasians (> 94 cm in men and > 80 cm in women), and among most Asian groups and those of Central and South American ancestry (where > 80 cm in women and > 90cm in men define increased waist circumference) (Alberti et al. 2005).

Numerous studies have shown an increased risk of future CVD events in people with the metabolic syndrome. Among adults in the United States (Malik et al. 2004), a stepwise increase in risk for CHD, CVD, and total mortality has been shown relating to the presence of metabolic syndrome alone, metabolic syndrome with diabetes or pre-existing CVD, and metabolic syndrome with both CVD and diabetes (Fig. 8.1.4).

Hypertension

Elevated blood pressure, and particularly systolic blood pressure, is strongly and positively related to the risk of future CHD and stroke. Hypertension is currently defined as a systolic blood pressure of 140 mmHg or higher, diastolic blood pressure of 90 mmHg or higher (or on pharmacological treatment to lower blood pressure). Elevated blood pressure at levels of 140–159 mmHg systolic or 90–99 mmHg diastolic is defined as stage 1 hypertension, and levels of 160 mmHg or higher systolic or 100 mmHg or higher diastolic is defined as stage 2 hypertension. In 2010, the prevalence of hypertension in US adults aged 20 years and over was 33.6 per cent in men and 32.2 per cent in women, ranging from 18.7 per cent among Asians to 47 per cent in Non-Hispanic black females (Go et al. 2013). Prevalence ranges from under 10 per cent in those younger than 35 years of age and progressively increases with age to more than 70 per cent in those aged 75 years and over with higher prevalences in men before age 55, but higher prevalences in women after age 65 (reaching 80 per cent among those aged 75 years and over). Of note, isolated diastolic hypertension (systolic blood pressure of < 140 mmHg but diastolic blood pressure of 90 mmHg or higher) is the most common form of hypertension under age 50, while isolated systolic hypertension (systolic blood pressure of 140 mmHg or higher, but diastolic blood pressure < 90 mmHg) predominates over the age of 60 years (Franklin et al. 2001). The Seventh Joint National Committee on Prevention, Detection, Evaluation and Treatment of High Blood Pressure (Chobanian et al. 2003) also defines those with a level of blood pressure of 120–139 mmHg systolic or 80–89 mmHg diastolic as 'pre-hypertensive' because of the greater future risk for these people to develop hypertension (one-sixth to one-third of such people will become clinically hypertensive in the next 4 years). Approximately one-third of US adults are pre-hypertensive. Blood pressure is not considered normal unless it is less than 120 mmHg systolic *and* <80 mmHg diastolic. For every blood pressure increase of 20/10 mmHg (systolic/diastolic) above 115/75 mmHg, the risk of death from CHD, stroke or CVD doubles (Lewington et al. 2002). While there have been major improvements in the treatment of hypertension, only about one-third of adult patients with hypertension are adequately controlled. This varies substantially

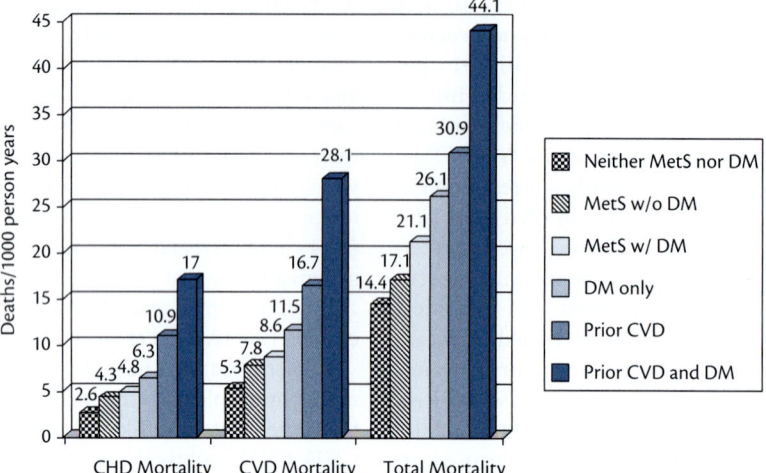

Fig. 8.1.4 Relative risks for mortality from coronary heart disease, cardiovascular disease, and all causes in United States adults associated with the presence of metabolic syndrome with and without diabetes: NHANES II: 1976–1980 follow-up study (mean 13 years follow-up).
Reproduced from Malik S. et al., Impact of the metabolic syndrome on mortality from coronary heart disease, cardiovascular disease, and all causes in United States Adults, *Circulation*, Volume 110, Issue 10, pp. 1239–1244, Copyright © 2004 American Heart Association, Inc. All rights reserved., with permission from Lippincott Williams and Wilkins.

by ethnicity and gender, ranging from a low of 38 per cent in Mexican-American males to as high as 56.8 per cent among white females (Go et al. 2013).

Numerous clinical trials have shown that lowering blood pressure substantially decreases the risk of future cardiovascular events, stroke, and end-stage renal disease. A large meta-analysis of active treatment (with initial low dose diuretic, beta blocker, angiotensin-converting enzyme (ACE) inhibitor or calcium antagonist) compared to placebo showed significant reductions in the risk for heart failure (36 per cent), stroke (33 per cent), CHD (16 per cent), CVD death (15 per cent), overall CVD (25 per cent), and total mortality (12 per cent) (Elliott 2005).

Dyslipidaemia

Increased levels of total and LDL-C have long been recognized as major risk factors for CHD. A direct curvilinear relation exists between total and LDL-C and the risk of CHD. For example, compared to those with total cholesterol levels of 200 mg/dL, those with levels of 240 mg/dL are at approximately twofold greater risk, while those with levels of 300 mg/dL have a fourfold increased risk. A population optimal LDL-C level has been designated as less than 100 mg/dL with levels of 130 mg/dL, 160 mg/dL, or 190 mg/dL often considered the thresholds for beginning lipid-lowering therapy in those at high, intermediate, or low CHD risk, respectively (Expert Panel on Detection, Evaluation, and Treatment of High Blood Cholesterol 2001). However, there is significant overlap in total or LDL-C levels between those who experience CHD events versus those who do not and approximately one-third of heart attacks occur in people with 'normal' levels of total cholesterol below 200 mg/dL. Importantly, a low level of HDL-C (typically defined as < 40 mg/dL in men and < 50 mg/dL in women), regardless of level of total cholesterol, is strongly associated with an increased risk of CHD (Castelli et al. 1986). For example, across levels of total cholesterol from less than 200 mg/dL to 260 mg/dL or above, the 14-year incidence of CHD varies only from 11.2 to 12.5 per cent, whereas when HDL-C is less than 60 mg/dL, these rates are 3.7 to 3.8 per cent respectively.

Other lipid abnormalities include elevated serum triglyceride levels (the normal level is considered to be < 150 mg/dL), small particle size LDL-C (known as small dense LDL-C) and elevated lipoprotein (a) levels. There has also been recent interest in non-HDL-C since it captures all the atherogenic apolipoprotein B-containing lipoproteins and does not require, unlike LDL-C, measurements to be made after fasting. Several epidemiological studies have demonstrated a stronger relationship of non-HDL-C compared to LDL-C with incidence of CHD.

Table 8.1.1 shows the prevalence of elevated total and LDL-C and low HDL-C levels among US adults aged 20 years and over in 2010 (Go et al. 2013).

Numerous primary and secondary prevention clinical trials have documented the efficacy of lowering LDL-C, particularly with HMG-CoA reductase inhibitor drugs ('statins'), which can lead to approximately 25–35 per cent reductions in CHD and CVD incidence, where the lower the LDL-C achieved, the lower were the event rates (Rosensen 2004). These trials also showed no threshold level of LDL-C reductions where the CVD event rates begin to flatten. A large meta-analysis of 14 statin trials comprising 90,056 subjects showed that over a 5-year treatment period, every mmol/L reduction (approximately 40 mg/dL) in LDL-C achieved, was associated with reductions in all-cause mortality of 12 per cent, coronary mortality of 18 per cent, myocardial infarction and CHD death of 23 per cent, stroke incidence of 17 per cent, all major vascular events of 21 per cent, and with no difference (relative risk 1.00) in cancer incidence (Baigent et al. 2005). Importantly, several trials have shown the additional benefit of reducing the LDL-C, with high-dose statin therapy, to levels below 100 mg/dL. The largest of these, the Treat to New Targets (TNT) study showed that the achieved LDL-C of 77 mg/dL with high dosage atorvastatin therapy, when compared to achieved LDL-C of 101 mg/dL with low-dose atorvastatin therapy, resulted in an additional 22 per cent reduction in major cardiovascular events (LaRosa 2005).

Given that most randomized clinical trials of LDL-C lowering have demonstrated no more than 40 per cent reductions in CVD incidence, addressing the remaining 'residual' risk has been of

Table 8.1.1 Prevalence of elevated total and LDL-C and low HDL-C by gender and ethnicity, US adults aged 20 years and over: National Health and Nutrition Examination Survey 2010

Population	Total cholesterol ≥ 200 mg/dL	Total cholesterol ≥ 240 mg/dL	LDL-C ≥ 130 mg/dL	HDL-C < 40 mg/dL
All	43.4%	13.8%	31.1%	21.8%
Males	41.3%	12.7%	31.9%	31.8%
Females	44.9%	14.7%	30.0%	12.3%
White males	40.5%	12.3%	30.1%	33.1%
White females	45.8%	15.6%	29.3%	12.4%
Black males	38.6%	10.8%	33.1%	20.3%
Black females	40.7%	11.7%	31.2%`	10.2%
Mexican-American males	48.1%	15.2%	39.9%	34.2%
Mexican-American females	44.7%	13.5%	30.4%	15.1%

great interest. One factor that has been specifically investigated has been whether the raising of HDL-C levels will provide further benefit in reducing CVD events beyond that afforded by LDL-C lowering, given the strong protective effect of increased HDL-C levels suggested by observational studies. The AIM-HIGH Trial (AIM-HIGH Investigators et al. 2011) was designed to be a rigorous test of the HDL hypothesis, randomizing 3414 men and women with a prior CVD event and low HDL-C, and who had well-controlled LDL-C levels averaging 74 mg/dL on a statin, to extended-release niacin or placebo. LDL-C levels were kept similar between the groups, and the on-treatment HDL-C level averaged 5 mg/dL higher in those on niacin. However, the trial was discontinued early due to futility, with no significant reduction in CVD events observed (hazard ratio = 1.02, $p = 0.79$). The failure of this trial, as well as that of a second much larger niacin trial, HPS2-Thrive and one involving a novel cholesterol ester transferase protein (CETP) inhibitor, dalcetrapib, have raised significant questions as to the benefit of raising HDL-C levels, particularly in patients who are already well-controlled on statins. Additionally, the use of fibrate therapy to address the residual risk associated with low HDL-C and elevated triglycerides, while initially showing benefit in the HDL Intervention Trial (HIT) among veterans with known CHD, has not been shown to provide added benefit over the background of statin therapy in the recent ACCORD Lipid Trial among people with diabetes (ACCORD Study Group 2010a).

Cigarette smoking

Tobacco smoking is among the leading preventable causes of death globally (see also Chapter 9.1). Numerous studies have linked tobacco use to the incidence of, and mortality from, CVD, with approximately half a million deaths annually in the United States being attributed to tobacco use. Further, environmental tobacco smoke ('second-hand smoke') is responsible for approximately 40,000 deaths from heart disease annually in the United States. Cigarette smokers are 2 to 4 times more likely to develop CHD than non-smokers. Also, their risk of stroke is doubled and risk for peripheral vascular disease is more than ten times higher

than that of non-smokers (Luepker and Lando 2005). The most recent data among US adults in 2010 show an overall prevalence of smoking of 19.0 per cent, with a wide variation by ethnic/gender groups, ranging from 5.5 per cent in Asian females to 24.6 per cent in American Indian/Alaska Native men (Go et al. 2013).

Obesity and physical inactivity

Recent estimates showed that two-thirds of US adults are overweight or obese (body mass index of 25 kg/m² or higher), with 30 per cent being obese (body mass index of 30 kg/m² or higher). Since the 1960s, there has been a dramatic nearly three-fold increase in obesity prevalence among men from 10.7 per cent to 34.4 per cent and more than a twofold increase in women from 15.7 per cent to 36.1 per cent. Moreover 18.8 per cent of children aged 6–11 and 18.2 per cent aged 12–17 are defined to be obese based on latest survey data from 2007 to 2010. Further recent estimates from 2007–2010 showed that barely a third of the US adult population (44.2 per cent of men and 36.2 per cent of women; and only one-third of African American women) met nationally recommended amounts of physical activity (150 minutes of moderate, or 90 minutes of vigorous activity or an equivalent combination per week) (Go et al. 2013).

Obesity has been shown by numerous studies to be associated with an approximate 1.5- to twofold increase in risk of death from CHD, with the increase in risk beginning below the 25 kg/m² cut-off point for overweight. Numerous studies also show approximately 20–40 per cent lower risks of mortality and cardiovascular events associated with increased levels of physical activity or measured fitness. Several cardiovascular risk factors are linked to obesity, including hypertension, dyslipidaemia (including low HDL-C levels), type 2 diabetes, obstructive sleep apnoea, and hyperinsulinaemia. Increases in physical fitness have also been shown to be linked to increases in HDL-C levels and reductions in systolic and diastolic blood pressure, insulin resistance, and glucose intolerance. Abdominal obesity, most commonly indicated by a waist circumference of greater than 40 inches (102 cm) in men or greater than 35 inches (89 cm) in women, is a major component of the metabolic syndrome. Studies demonstrate that weight loss can substantially improve many cardiometabolic risk factors (McCowen and Blackburn 2005).

The National Institutes of Health's Obesity Educational Initiative provides guidelines on the identification, evaluation, and treatment of overweight and obese adults. Assessment includes measurement of body mass index, waist circumference, as well as other accompanying risk factors. Moderate hypocaloric diets of 1000–1200 kcal per day are generally recommended to provide moderate, sustained weight loss. Incorporating diet and exercise together has been shown to result in longer-term success in weight control (National Institutes of Health 1998). More recent guidelines for obesity management from the ACC/AHA have also been published, recommending regular assessment of body mass index, and in those who are overweight, waist circumference. It is emphasized that even moderate weight loss of 3–5 per cent of body weight can result in important reductions in cardiometabolic risk factors (Jensen et al. 2014). Reduced caloric intake, involving 1200–1500 kcal/d for women and 1500–1800 kcal/d for men is recommended for those who would benefit from weight loss. They also point out the importance of high intensity weight loss interventions (ideally at least 14 sessions over a 6 month period) with a lifestyle interventionalist to maximize potential for weight loss.

Measures of cardiovascular health and CVD risk

In recent years, the AHA (Go et al. 2013) has promoted a goal to improve the cardiovascular health of all Americans by 20 per cent while reducing mortality from heart disease and stroke by 20 per cent by the year 2020. These goals introduce the concept of promoting cardiovascular health which is more positive and motivating than the concept of preventing *cardiovascular disease*, and have focused on examining the proportion of individuals (and the relation to CVD risk) who achieve one or more 'ideal levels' based on the following seven metrics (also known as AHA's Life's Simple Seven™): (1) cigarette smoking (non-smoking is ideal); (2) physical activity (150 minutes or more moderate intensity or equivalent exercise per week is ideal); (3) body mass index (< 25 kg/m² is ideal); (4) healthy diet (achieving at least four of five key dietary components focusing on fruit/vegetable, fish, fibre, and sodium intake and sweetened beverage intake); (5) cholesterol (< 200 mg/dL ideal in adults, < 170 mg/dL in children); (6) blood pressure (< 120/80 mmHg is ideal); and (7) fasting plasma glucose (< 100 mg/dL is ideal). Fewer than 20 per cent of adults and only about 40 per cent of children meet five or more of these criteria for ideal cardiovascular health and fewer than 1 per cent of adults are at ideal levels of all seven metrics of cardiovascular health. Moreover, CVD incidence varies more than tenfold according to the number of cardiovascular health behaviours and factors that are present (Folsom et al. 2011) (Fig. 8.1.5).

Risk factors for stroke

Important risk factors for stroke include elevated blood pressure, diabetes mellitus, disorders of heart rhythm, low HDL-C, cigarette smoking, family history, and chronic kidney disease (Go et al. 2013). Elevated blood pressure is the most important risk factor for both ischaemic stroke and intracranial haemorrhage, with about 77 per cent of those with a first stroke having a blood pressure of 140/90 mmHg or higher. The Framingham Heart Study demonstrated the importance of mid-life antecedent hypertension as well as systolic hypertension as important predictors of stroke (Romero and Wolf 2013). Even pre-hypertension is associated with incident stroke. Randomized clinical trials consistently show the efficacy of blood pressure control for prevention of stroke. Diabetes is also a strong predictor of stroke, although mainly before 55 years of age in black people and before 65 years of age in white people. Atrial fibrillation is another powerful risk factor for stroke, independently increasing risk approximately fivefold at all ages, with nearly one-quarter of strokes attributable to atrial fibrillation in the ninth decade of life. While elevated total cholesterol levels are not strongly predictive of stroke, some studies have found low HDL-C levels to predict risk, but clinical trials of statin therapy consistently show

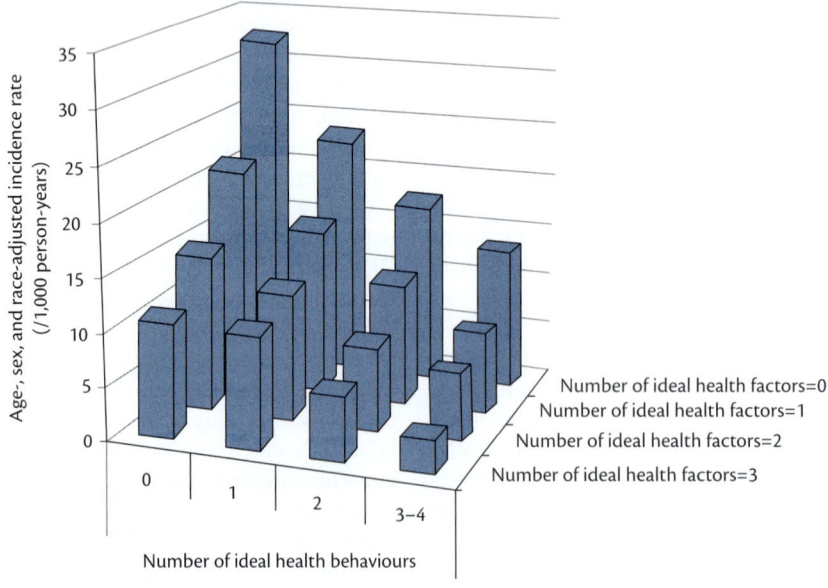

Fig. 8.1.5 Incidence of CVD according to the number of ideal health behaviours and health factors.

Reprinted from *Journal of the American College of Cardiology*, Volume 57, Issue 16, Folsom AR, et al., Community prevalence of ideal cardiovascular health by the American Heart Association definition and relation with cardiovascular disease incidence, pp. 1690–1696, Copyright © 2011, with permission from Elsevier, available from http://www.sciencedirect.com/science/journal/07351097.

benefits of such therapy for preventing stroke. Prospective studies have also shown moderate to vigorous physical activity to be associated with an overall 35 per cent reduction in risk of ischaemic stroke compared with no physical activity. A family history of parental ischaemic stroke before the age of 65 has also been shown to be associated with a three-fold increase in ischaemic stroke in offspring, even after adjustment for other risk factors. Finally, increased levels of creatinine and reduced glomerular filtration rate have been shown to predict future stroke and symptoms (Go et al. 2013).

Risk factors for heart failure

Hypertension is among the most prominent of risk factors for heart failure, followed by a preceding myocardial infarction, elevated B-type natriuretic peptide levels, and urinary albumin-to-creatinine ratio (Go et al. 2013). In the Physicians Health Study, the lifestyle risk of heart failure was greater in those with hypertension and less in those with healthy lifestyle factors, including normal weight, not smoking, regular exercise, moderate alcohol intake, consumption of breakfast cereals, fruits, and vegetables (Djousse et al. 2009). The Framingham Heart Study was key in demonstrating the poor prognosis associated with heart failure in the community, with one of two individuals dying within 5 years of diagnosis and the strong association of hypertension conferring nearly an eightfold risk in men and fourfold risk in women for developing heart failure. They also documented other predictors of new onset heart failure, including elevated plasma natriuretic peptide levels, asymptomatic left ventricular systolic dysfunction, and increased left ventricular diastolic dimension (Mahmood and Wang 2013).

Risk factors for peripheral arterial disease

Peripheral arterial disease shares many of the same risk factors that coronary heart disease does, although diabetes and cigarette smoking are stronger risk factors for peripheral arterial disease than for coronary heart disease with odds ratios in the range of 3–4. Another study showed hypertension, diabetes, chronic kidney disease, and smoking were associated with incident peripheral arterial disease. Pooled data from 11 studies showed that peripheral arterial disease, defined by an ABI of less than 0.9, is an independent risk factor for all-cause mortality (relative risk 1.6, 95 per cent confidence interval (CI) = 1.3–2.0) as well as cardiovascular mortality (relative risk 2.0, 95 per cent CI = 1.5–2.6) (Go et al. 2013).

Cardiovascular disease risk assessment

Global risk scores for cardiovascular disease risk assessment

In order to understand an individual's risk of CVD or CHD, it is important to understand an individual's 'global risk' of developing the condition. Most typically, this involves determination of the future risk of developing CHD in the next 10 years. This can be done by various 'risk assessment' algorithms. Most commonly used for this purpose are the Framingham Risk Algorithms that are recommended to assess an individual's 10-year risk of CHD (Kaseta and Sowers 2005) for the purposes of appropriate stratification for

risk factor management, especially for the initiation or intensification of lipid management. From knowing an individual's age, gender, systolic blood pressure (and treatment status), current smoking status, total cholesterol, and HDL-C, for which each factor is assigned a certain number of points according to its presence (and degree) or absence, a total score is obtained which corresponds to a probability of suffering a hard CHD event in the next 10 years based on Framingham follow-up data. If the projected 10-year risk of CHD is less than 10 per cent, the individual is generally considered to be at low risk of CHD, 10–20 per cent intermediate risk, and if greater than 20 per cent is judged to be at high risk, and in fact, a CHD risk-equivalent (a condition or combination of risk factors conferring a future risk or prognosis similar to that of diagnosed CHD). Use of these algorithms have been recommended for those with at least two major risk factors out of the following: family history of premature CHD (< 45 years in male or < 55 years in female first-degree relative), low HDL-C, hypertension, cigarette smoking, and advanced age (male 55 years or older or female 65 years or older). Those with fewer than two risk factors are felt to be generally at lower risk where treatment would not typically be warranted. Those with diabetes, CHD, or other atherosclerotic disease would also be designated at high risk for aggressive treatment, so such a calculation has not been recommended for such individuals (Expert Panel on Detection, Evaluation and Treatment of High Blood Cholesterol 2001).

There is, however, great heterogeneity in the end point predicted by various risk scores. For example, the 10-year CHD risk score recommended by the Third Adult Treatment Panel of the National Cholesterol Education Program (Expert Panel on Detection, Evaluation and Treatment of High Blood Cholesterol 2001) includes only hard CHD (myocardial infarction and CHD death) as its end point, thus does not include other forms of CHD (such as angina or revascularization) as well as other forms of CVD such as stroke, heart failure, and peripheral arterial disease, which are also important CVD manifestations of concern which should be included in such risk scores. Other algorithms such as the European SCORE or German PROCAMM risk scores are utilized mainly outside the United States. More recently, algorithms for total CVD risk from Framingham have been developed, which are more global as they incorporate the combined risk for CHD, stroke, heart failure, and peripheral arterial disease (D'Agostino et al. 2008). Most recently, the American College of Cardiology (ACC) and American Heart Association (AHA) released new guidelines for cardiovascular risk assessment which call for the use of a pooled cohort risk score (Goff et al. 2013). These new risk scores are based on 4 major US population-based cohort studies comprising over 25,000 black and white adults with at least 10 years of follow-up for atherosclerotic cardiovascular disease (ASCVD) events. The risk calculator provides both 10-year and lifetime risk estimates for ASCVD consisting of nonfatal myocardial infarction, CHD death, and stroke (http://tools.cardiosource.org/ASCVD-Risk-Estimator/).

In those where a global risk estimate is obtained, depending on the risk status, the appropriate intensity of treatment for given risk factors is considered. For instance, if an individual is found to be at high risk or to have a CHD risk equivalent, treatment for dyslipidaemia would be recommended to reduce the LDL-C level to less than 100 mg/dL. If at intermediate risk or low risk, however, these goals would be less than 130 mg/dL and less than 160 mg/dL, respectively.

While estimation of global risk as described earlier is recommended, it may be best considered a starting point in risk assessment. The presence of other risk factors not included in the risk algorithms, such as abdominal obesity, elevated triglycerides (if severe enough), impaired fasting glucose, or a strong positive premature family history, if present, however, could be used by the clinician to stratify an individual's risk or required intensity of treatment upward. Others have also recommended novel risk factors, such as C-reactive protein, a measure of systemic inflammation, or the presence of subclinical atherosclerosis, such as coronary artery calcium or carotid intimal media thicknesses, to aid in risk stratification. If these are present to a significant degree, they are being suggested as indicators for stratifying an individual's required intensity of treatment upward. The most recent American College of Cardiology/American Heart Association risk assessment guideline notes that when the treatment decision is uncertain, evaluation of premature family history of CHD, hs-C-reactive protein, ankle brachial index, or coronary calcium scoring may be considered for further risk stratification (Goff et al. 2013).

Inflammatory measures for cardiovascular disease risk

High levels of inflammatory markers, including high-sensitivity C-reactive protein (hs-CRP), a marker of systemic inflammation, as well as lipoprotein phospholipase associated A2 (LpPla2), a measure of vascular inflammation, have been shown in numerous studies to be independently related to the risk of future cardiovascular events. Interleukin-6, other interleukins, myeloperoxidase, and tumour necrosis factor-alpha (TNF-alpha) also have inflammatory activity and have been shown to be associated with cardiovascular events in some studies, as have other biomarkers such as brain natriuretic peptide (BNP) and troponin levels. Levels of C-reactive protein exceeding 3 mg/L have been designated to be associated with increased CVD risk, levels in the range of 1–3 mg/L with intermediate risk, and low risk levels have been designated as less than 1 mg/L (Pearson et al. 2003). Modest recommendations have been provided for the measurement of hs-CRP in older adults (men ≥ 50 years or women ≥ 60 years) with LDL-C less than 130 mg/dL (class IIa) or in those below these ages who are at intermediate risk (class IIb), for the purposes of guiding the initiation or intensification of therapy. A similar class IIb recommendation is given for the measurement of LpPla2 in asymptomatic intermediate risk adults. There are no recommendations for the measurement of other inflammatory markers or biomarkers for the assessment of CVD risk in asymptomatic adults, however (Greenland et al. 2010).

Subclinical cardiovascular disease assessment

The ability to image or directly measure the atherosclerotic burden has been of great interest but whether these measures provide added value over less expensive and easier traditional office-based risk factor measures (including global risk assessment scores) has been an important question in cardiovascular epidemiology and prevention over the past 15 years (Greenland et al. 2010). Such measures must have a high level of sensitivity and specificity for detection of the disease, must be reproducible and cost-effective, and should provide added clinical utility over current office-based risk assessment.

Increased carotid intima medial thickness (CIMT) as measured from carotid B-mode ultrasound, has been shown to be related to the risk of future CVD events from numerous prospective epidemiological studies over the past 25 years, including the Atherosclerosis Risk in Communities (ARIC), Cardiovascular Health Study (CHS), and the Multiethnic Study of Atherosclerosis (MESA). CIMT has also been used as a surrogate end point in numerous clinical trials involving lipid-lowering and other interventions. Moreover, the presence of carotid plaques provides additional information and together with CIMT measurements have modest clinical utility for reclassification of risk in asymptomatic intermediate risk adults. Individuals with CIMT levels of 1 mm or higher or in the highest quartile for age-specific values are generally considered to be at increased risk. While persons at intermediate risk were previously given a class IIa recommendation for the measurement of CIMT (Greenland et al. 2010), more recent guidelines no longer recommend CIMT measurement for risk assessment (Goff et al. 2013).

ABI measured from ankle and arm blood pressures utilizing a Doppler, provides for an assessment of peripheral arterial disease, which is diagnosed to be present when the ABI is less than 0.9. A low ABI has also been shown to be related to increased total and CVD mortality in numerous observational studies. However, as the prevalence of a low ABI tends to be very low until after the age of 60 years, it is therefore most useful as a screening tool for peripheral arterial disease in older people. It is also a class IIa recommendation for assessment in intermediate risk individuals (Greenland et al. 2010).

Measures of coronary artery calcium (CAC) as assessed by CT, have been shown in numerous prospective studies, to be associated with the future risk of CHD and CVD events, independent of standard risk factors (Detrano et al. 2008). CAC measures also provide incremental predictive value and added reclassification of risk over global risk assessment for the prediction of cardiovascular events. In the MESA study, it has been shown to provide greater incremental risk prediction among intermediate risk individuals (from C-statistic improvement) than any other major biomarker or subclinical disease screening test (Yeboah et al. 2012). CAC testing also receives a class IIa recommendation for assessment of risk in asymptomatic subjects at intermediate risk (Greenland et al. 2010).

There are also numerous other tests which have varying levels of evidence relating them to CVD event risk. These include assessments of endothelial function, pulse wave velocity, brachial artery reactivity, and imaging of soft plaque such as by CT coronary angiography. Most of these other tests, however, do not have the quantity, strength, or consistency of evidence that CIMT, ABI, or CAC assessment do, and hence there is not the same level of consensus for recommending their use for the screening of asymptomatic adults (Greenland et al. 2010).

Preventive strategies for cardiovascular disease risk reduction

Cardiovascular epidemiology and disease prevention encompasses an extensive field investigating the distribution and variation of CVD conditions, most notably coronary heart disease and stroke, their risk factor determinants, and strategies at the population and individual level aimed at preventing the development or recurrence of CVD. Epidemiological approaches to studying CVD provide us with the tools for preventive efforts at the individual and population level. *Primordial prevention* is aimed at prevention of the risk factors for CVD, such as efforts aimed to prevent hypertension, obesity, or dyslipidaemia. *Primary prevention,* which focuses on the modification of these and other known risk factors, is aimed at preventing the clinical manifestations of CVD, such as myocardial infarction and stroke. *Secondary prevention* focuses on those who already have manifestations of disease, but where aggressive control of risk factors can have a major impact in preventing recurrences of disease. Concerted efforts between governmental agencies, the community, and the private sector are required to best address the continuing epidemic of CVD.

Preventive strategies can be considered using the 'ABCDE' approach addressing aspirin/antiplatelet therapy (A), blood pressure and hypertension (B), cholesterol and dyslipidaemia (C), diet and nutrition (D), and exercise and physical activity (E). For secondary prevention among people with pre-existing CVD, guidelines have been published by the AHA/American College of Cardiology (Smith et al. 2011).

Aspirin and antiplatelet therapy

Aspirin prophylaxis (81–162 mg/day) has been recommended for people at intermediate risk, for the prevention of CHD in men and prevention of stroke in women, including those with diabetes or metabolic syndrome (Expert Panel on Detection, Evaluation, and Treatment of High Blood Cholesterol in Adults 2001; Grundy et al. 2005). Additionally, among those with pre-existing CVD, aspirin is recommended in combination with clopidogrel due to the added benefit in prevention of secondary events. The use of alternative antiplatelet therapies is also discussed (Smith et al. 2011).

Blood pressure control

The JNC-7 guidelines (Chobanian et al. 2003) have recommended the standard blood pressure goal of treatment of those with hypertension to be less than 140/90 mmHg, usually starting with a diuretic or beta blocker and considering additional therapy as needed to reach the goal, in most uncomplicated subjects. Recently, however, the American Diabetes Association modified the target blood pressure to less than 140/80 mmHg for most patients with diabetes (given the results of recent clinical trials such as the blood pressure substudy in ACCORD that did not demonstrate benefits from lower blood pressure goals in such patients) and continued the recommendation for using an ACE inhibitor or angiotensin receptor blocker as the preferred therapy due to their renal protective effects (Expert Panel on Detection, Evaluation, and Treatment of High Blood Cholesterol in Adults 2001). The JNC-7 guidelines additionally recommend beginning with combination therapy (including fixed dosage combinations) for people who are 20 mmHg or more systolic or 10 mmHg or more diastolic blood pressure away from the treatment goal. This takes into account the fact that, based on prior trials, for most patients, two or three medications will be needed to achieve adequate blood pressure control. Additionally, both the JNC-7 and AHA note a normal blood pressure optimal for the population to be less than 120/80 mmHg. A more recent report from members appointed to the JNC-8, however, has raised the threshold for treatment and goal to below 150/90 mmHg in adults aged 60 years and over (James et al. 2013), although this has not been endorsed by other recent guidelines.

Cholesterol and lipid control

Previous National Cholesterol Education Program (NCEP) goals for treatment of elevated LDL-cholesterol include achieving levels of < 100 mg/dL in those with the highest risk (pre-existing CHD or other CHD risk equivalents such as those with diabetes or other atherosclerotic disease or a calculated global risk of greater than 20 per cent for CHD in 10 years); less than 130 mg/dL in those with two or more risk factors; and <160 mg/dL in those with less than two risk factors (see section on risk assessment) (Expert Panel for Detection, Evaluation and Treatment of Blood Cholesterol 2001). Optional goals for lowering LDL-C to less than 70 mg/dL have been recommended for those at the very highest risk (e.g. pre-existing CVD plus diabetes or other uncontrolled risk factors, or with acute coronary syndromes) (Smith et al. 2011). The NCEP has also recommended non-HDL-C targets that are 30 mg/dL higher than the respective LDL-C targets for those with triglyceride levels of 200 mg/dL or greater as such people may have other atherogenic lipoproteins present and/or where the calculation of LDL-C is less accurate. While triglycerides less than 150 mg/dL and HDL-C levels of 40 mg/dL or greater in men and 50 mg/dL or greater in women are considered to be desirable, these are not specific therapeutic targets due to the lack of demonstrated benefit from clinical trials on CVD end points. Statins (HMG-CoA reductase inhibitors) are the preferred first-line therapeutic approach after lifestyle modification (see 'Exercise and physical activity' and 'Food and nutrition'), given the strength of the evidence from numerous clinical trials. There are currently no recommendations for the addition of fibrate therapy or niacin given the lack of incremental benefit over statins as shown by recent clinical trials. Most recent American College of Cardiology/American Heart Association Guidelines for the Management of Blood Cholesterol (Stone et al. 2013) have revised the approach for management of dyslipidaemia to include four statin eligible groups: 1) those with known atherosclerotic cardiovascular disease, 2) those with LDL-cholesterol of 190 mg/dl or higher, 3) those with diabetes, and 4) those with a 10-year pooled cohort risk of atherosclerotic cardiovascular disease of 7.5 per cent or greater (Stone et al. 2013) with LDL-C monitoring recommended only for evaluation of therapeutic response and adherence to statin therapy.

Cigarette smoking prevention and intervention

Smoking cessation has long been documented to reduce the risk of CVD. The risk of CHD is reduced by 50 per cent within 1 year of smoking cessation and to that of a never-smoker within 15 years. It is recommended that at each consultation with a healthcare provider the visit should be used as an opportunity to address the 5As of smoking cessation counselling which include 'Ask' (assess tobacco use at every visit), 'Advise' (strongly urge quitting), 'Attempt' (try to identify smokers ready to quit), 'Assist' (aid the patient in quitting), and 'Arrange' (for follow-up contacts). Interventions for smoking are varied. For youth, school, and community-based prevention programmes, state and federal initiatives, as well as cessation assistance are available. For adults, behavioural treatment, self-help approaches, and pharmacological therapy are used, with varying levels of success. For example quit rates vary from 6 per cent with physician advice only to 40 per cent in those who participate in group programmes (Luepker and Lando 2005).

Diabetes control

Recommendations for the treatment of diabetes to optimize cardiovascular risk reduction are available from a variety of sources. For example, the latest recommendations from the American Diabetes Association (Expert Panel on Detection, Evaluation, and Treatment of High Blood Cholesterol in Adults 2001) address antiplatelet therapy, glycaemic control, blood pressure control, lipid control (discussed earlier), weight control, and lifestyle management. Moreover, similar guidelines have been published by the European Association for the Study of Diabetes. Multifactorial intervention focusing on lipid, blood pressure, and glycaemic control has been shown to decrease the risk of future CVD events by more than 50 per cent (Gaede et al. 2008). This is a very important message given that in recent reports, only one tenth of those with diabetes have achieved target treatment levels for HbA1c, blood pressure, and LDL-C (Wong et al. 2012). While the goal of glycaemic control is a HbA1c level of less than 7 per cent in most uncomplicated diabetics, and even 6–6.5 per cent if achievable without side effects, given the results of recent trials, HbA1c levels of less than 8 per cent are accepted as an appropriate goal for those with pre-existing micro or macro-vascular disease or difficult-to-control diabetes (American Diabetes Association 2013). For optimal control, the recommended lipid targets from the American Diabetes Association are for the LDL-C to be less than 100 mg/dL (< 70 mg/dL if known macrovascular disease is present) and blood pressure of less than 140/80 mmHg for most people. More recent recommendations from the ACC/AHA have called for statin use in those with diabetes whose LDL-C is at least 70 mg/dL and a high-intensity statin in those who additionally have a 10-year ASCVD risk of 7.5 per cent or greater (Stone et al. 2014). Moreover, members appointed to the JNC-8 have recommended a threshold for treatment and goal for blood pressure to be set at 140/90 mmHg (James et al. 2014).

Exercise and physical activity

The ACC/AHA currently recommends 3 to 4 sessions a week, lasting on average 40 minutes per session, and involving moderate- to vigorous-intensity physical activity (Eckel et al. 2014). Regular physical activity can help maintain healthy blood pressure, weight, lipid levels, low levels of inflammation (C-reactive protein) and insulin sensitivity. A pedometer can be an effective tool for intervention with one guideline, for example, recommending walking at least 10,000 steps a day. For secondary prevention, a prescribed exercise programme is recommended, and participation initially in a supervised cardiac rehabilitation programme is advised for those recovering from a recent CHD event.

Food and nutrition

The National Cholesterol Education Program recommended the Therapeutic Lifestyle Change (TLC) diet which focuses on fresh vegetables and fruits and wholegrain products and consumption of monounsaturated fatty acids. A goal is to keep total fat intake to 25–35 per cent of total calories, monounsaturated fat intake to up to 20 per cent of total calories, fibre intake at 20–30 g per day, and balancing energy intake and expenditure. Use of stanol ester margarine supplements and fish oil supplementation can provide additional benefits on lipid levels and other cardiovascular risk factors. Most recent ACC/AHA guidelines focus on recommending a dietary pattern that emphasizes intake of vegetables, fruits, and wholegrains; includes low-fat dairy products, poultry, fish, legumes, nontropical vegetable oils and nuts; and limits intake of sweets, sugar-sweetened beverages, and red meats (Eckel et al. 2014). Additional recommendations include consumption of no more than 2400 mg of sodium per day, or at least a 1000 mg reduction in daily sodium intake.

Specific additional recommendations for secondary prevention of CVD

Besides lipid control, blood pressure, antiplatelet, diabetes control, and lifestyle recommendations discussed in previous subsections, guidelines for secondary prevention also include therapy with a beta blocker, renin angiotensin and aldosterone system blockers, as well as annual influenza vaccination (Smith et al. 2011). Specific systems implemented in the hospital setting, such as pre-printed discharge instructions, reminders on charts (which can be automated in the case of electronic medical records systems) are key to ensure maximal adherence to recommended therapies for secondary prevention of CHD.

Conclusions

CVD accounts for the greatest burden of morbidity and mortality worldwide, both in developed and in developing countries. Key cardiovascular risk factors, including hypertension, cigarette smoking, high blood glucose, physical inactivity, obesity, and elevated cholesterol are (in that order) the top leading causes of death worldwide. It has been estimated that elimination of obesity, unhealthy diets, and physical inactivity could reduce up to 80 per cent of heart disease, stroke, and diabetes (Mendis et al. 2011).

In a recent Presidential Advisory (Smith et al. 2012) issued by the presidents of the World Heart Federation, European Society of Cardiology, AHA, and other leading cardiac societies, the call to reduce NCD deaths by 25 per cent by the year 2025 was noted (of which nearly half are due to CVD) and key global targets recommended for adoption were: (1) a 10 per cent reduction in the prevalence of insufficient physical activity, (2) a 25 per cent reduction in the prevalence of raised blood pressure, (3) a 30 per cent reduction in salt/sodium intake with a recommended goal of achieving lower than 5 g salt intake (2000 mg sodium) per day, and (4) a 30 per cent relative reduction in the prevalence of current tobacco smoking. Also receiving support was a reduction of saturated fat intake by 15 per cent, halving the prevalence of obesity, reducing alcohol intake by 10 per cent, reducing elevated cholesterol by 20 per cent, increasing by 50 per cent the number of people eligible to receive drug therapy to prevent heart attacks and strokes, and increasing availability of basic technologies and generic essential medicines for prevention of CVD.

Concerted global efforts aimed at coordinating care for those with pre-existing CVD (secondary prevention), primary prevention, identifying people with cardiovascular risk factors and getting them the necessary treatments, as well as primordial prevention aimed at prevention of obesity and other major risk factors in the first place, are critical for reducing the morbidity and mortality associated with CVD.

References

ACCORD Study Group (2010a). Effects of combination lipid therapy in type 2 diabetes mellitus. *The New England Journal of Medicine*, 362, 1563–74.

ACCORD Study Group (2010b). Effects of intensive blood-pressure control in type 2 diabetes mellitus. *The New England Journal of Medicine*, 362, 1575–85.

Action to Control Cardiovascular Risk in Diabetes Study Group, Gerstein, H.C., Miller, M.E., et al. (2008). Effects of intensive glucose lowering in type 2 diabetes. *The New England Journal of Medicine*, 358, 2545–59.

AIM-HIGH Investigators, Boden, W.E., Probstfield, J.L., et al. (2011). Niacin in patients with low HDL cholesterol levels receiving intensive statin therapy. *The New England Journal of Medicine*, 365, 2255–67.

Alberti, K.G., Zimmet, P., and Shaw, J. (2005). IDF Epidemiology Task Force Consensus Group: the metabolic syndrome – a new worldwide definition. *The Lancet*, 366, 1059–62.

American Diabetes Association (2013). Executive Summary: Standards of Medical Care in Diabetes 2013. *Diabetes Care*, 36(Suppl. 1), S4–S10.

Baigent, C., Keech, A., Kearney, P.M., et al. (2005). Cholesterol Treatment Trialists' (CTT) Collaborators. Efficacy and safety of cholesterol-lowering treatment: prospective meta-analysis of data from 90,056 participants in 14 randomised trials of statins. *The Lancet*, 366, 1267–78.

Castelli, W.P., Garrison, R.J., Wilson, P.W., Abbott, R.D., Kalousdian, S., and Kannel, W.B. (1986). Incidence of coronary heart disease and lipoprotein cholesterol levels. The Framingham Study. *Journal of the American Medical Association*, 256(20), 2835–8.

Chobanian, A.V., Bakris, G.L., Black, H.R., et al. (2003). The seventh report of the Joint National Committee on Prevention, Detection, Evaluation, and Treatment of High Blood Pressure: the JNC7 Report. *Journal of the American Medical Association*, 289, 2560–72.

D'Agostino, R.B., Ramachandran, S.V., Pencina, M.J., et al. (2008). General cardiovascular risk profile for use in primary care: the Framingham Heart Study. *Circulation*, 117, 743–53.

Detrano, R., Guerci, A.D., Carr, J.J., et al. (2008). Coronary calcium as a predictor of coronary events in four racial or ethnic groups. *The New England Journal of Medicine*, 358, 1336–45.

Djousse, L., Driver, J.A., and Gaxiano, J.M. (2009). Relation between modifiable lifestyle factors and lifetime risk of heart failure. *Journal of the American Medical Association*, 302, 394–400.

Eckel, R.H., Jakicic, J.M., Ard, J.D., et al. (2014). American College of Cardiology/American Heart Association Task Force on Practice Guidelines. 2013 AHA/ACC guideline on lifestyle management to reduce cardiovascular risk: a report of the American College of Cardiology/American Heart Association Task Force on Practice Guidelines. *J Am Coll Cardiol*, 63(25 Pt B), 2960–84.

Elliott, W.J. (2005). Cardiovascular events in clinical trials of antihypertensive drugs vs. placebo/no treatment: a meta-analysis. *Journal of Hypertension*, 23(Suppl. 2), S273.

Expert Panel on Detection, Evaluation, and Treatment of High Blood Cholesterol in Adults (2001). Executive Summary of the Third Report of the National Cholesterol Education Program (NCEP) Expert Panel on Detection, Evaluation, and Treatment of High Blood Cholesterol in Adults (Adult Treatment Panel III). *Journal of the American Medical Association*, 285, 2486–97.

Folsom, A.R., Yatsuya, H., Nettleton, J.A., et al. (2011). Community prevalence of ideal cardiovascular health by the American Heart Association definition and relation with cardiovascular disease incidence. *Journal of the American College of Cardiology*, 57, 1690–6.

Franklin, S.S., Jacobs, M.J., Wong, N.D., L'Italien, G.L., and Lapuerta, P. (2001). Predominance of isolated systolic hypertension among middle-aged and elderly US hypertensives—analysis based on NHANES III. *Hypertension*, 37, 869–74.

Gaede, P., Lund-Andersen, H., Parving, H.H., and Pedersen, O. (2008). Effect of multifactorial intervention on mortality in type 2 diabetes. *The New England Journal of Medicine*, 358, 580–91.

Go, A.S., Mozaffarian, D., Roger, V.L., et al. (2013). American Heart Association Statistics Committee and Stroke Statistics Subcommittee. Heart disease and stroke statistics—2013 update: a report from the American Heart Association. *Circulation*, 127, e6–e245.

Goff, D.C. Jr., Lloyd-Jones, D.M., Bennett, G., et al. (2014). American College of Cardiology/American Heart Association Task Force on Practice Guidelines. 2013 ACC/AHA guideline on the assessment of cardiovascular risk: a report of the American College of Cardiology/American Heart Association Task Force on Practice Guidelines. *J Am Coll Cardiol*, 63(25 Pt B), 2935–59.

Greenland, P., Alpert, J.S., Beller, G.A., et al. (2010). 2010 ACCF/AHA Guideline for Assessment of Cardiovascular Risk in Asymptomatic Adults: A Report of the American College of Cardiology Foundation/American Heart Association Task Force on Practice Guidelines. *Journal of the American College of Cardiology*, 56, 50–103.

Grundy, S.M., Cleeman, J.I., Daniels, S.R., et al. (2005). Diagnosis and management of the metabolic syndrome. An American Heart Association/National Heart, Lung, and Blood Institute Scientific Statement. *Circulation*, 112, 2735–52.

Holman, R.R., Paul, S.K., Bethel, M.A., et al. (2008). 10-year follow-up of intensive glucose control in type 2 diabetes. *The New England Journal of Medicine*, 359, 1577–89.

Hopkins, P.N., Hut, S.C., and Wu, L.L. (2000). Family history and genetic factors. In N.D. Wong, H.R. Black, and J.M. Gardin (eds.) *Preventive Cardiology: A Practical Approach*, pp. 94–128. New York: McGraw Hill.

James, P.A., Oparil, S., Carter, B.L., et al. (2014). 2014 evidence-based guideline for the management of high blood pressure in adults: report from the panel members appointed to the Eighth Joint National Committee (JNC 8). *JAMA*, 311(5):507–20.

Jensen, M.D., Ryan, D.H., Apovian, C.M., et al. (2014). American College of Cardiology/American Heart Association Task Force on Practice Guidelines; Obesity Society. 2013 AHA/ACC/TOS guideline for the management of overweight and obesity in adults: a report of the American College of Cardiology/American Heart Association Task Force on Practice Guidelines and The Obesity Society. *J Am Coll Cardiol*, 63(25 Pt B), 2985–3023.

Kannel, W.B., Dawber, T.R., Kagan, A., et al. (1961). Factors of risk in development of coronary heart disease—six year follow-up experience: the Framingham Study. *Annals of Internal Medicine*, 55, 33–50.

Kannel, W.B., Doyle, J.T., Ostfeld, A.M., et al. (1984). Optimal resources for primary prevention of artherosclerotic diseases. Atherosclerosis Study Group. *Circulation*, 70(Suppl. A), 155A–205A.

Kaseta, J. and Sowers, J.R. (2005). Diabetes and the metabolic syndrome. In N.D. Wong, H.R. Black, and J.M. Gardin (eds.) *Preventive Cardiology: A Practical Approach* (2nd ed.), pp. 212–32. New York: McGraw Hill.

LaRosa, J.C., Grundy, S.M., Waters, D.D., et al. (2005). Treating to New Targets (TNT) Investigators. Intensive lipid lowering with atorvastatin in patients with stable coronary disease. *The New England Journal of Medicine*, 352, 1425–35.

Lewington, S., Clarke, R., Qizilbash, N., Peto, R., Collins, R.; Prospective Studies Collaborative (2002). Age-specific relevant of usual blood pressure to vascular mortality: a meta-analysis of individual data for one million adults in 61 prospective studies. *The Lancet*, 360, 1903–13.

Luepker, R.V. and Lando, H.A. (2005). Tobacco use, passive smoking, and smoking cessation interventions. In N.D. Wong, H.R. Black, and J.M. Gardin (eds.) *Preventive Cardiology: A Practical Approach* (2nd ed.), pp. 217–50. New York: McGraw Hill.

Mahmood, S.S. and Wang, T.J. (2013). The epidemiology of congestive heart failure: contributions from the Framingham Heart Study. *Global Heart*, 8, 77–82.

Malik, S., Wong, N.D., Franklin, S.S., et al. (2004). Impact of the metabolic syndrome on mortality from coronary heart disease, cardiovascular disease, and all causes in United States Adults. *Circulation*, 110, 1239–44.

McCowen, K.C. and Blackburn, G.L. (2005). Obesity and weight control. In N.D. Wong, H.R. Black, and J.M. Gardin (eds.) *Preventive Cardiology: A Practical Approach* (2nd ed.), pp. 233–55. New York: McGraw Hill.

Mendis, S., Puska, P., and Norrving, B. (eds.) (2011). *Global Atlas on Cardiovascular Disease Prevention and Control*. Geneva: World Health Organization.

Nathan, D.M., Cleary, P.A., Backlund, J.Y., et al. (2005). Intensive diabetes treatment and cardiovascular disease in patients with type 1 diabetes. *The New England Journal of Medicine*, 353, 2643–53.

National Institutes of Health (1998). *Obesity Education Initiative. Clinical Guidelines on the Identification, Evaluation, and Treatment of Overweight and Obese Adults. Executive Summary*. Bethesda, MD: NIH.

Palomaki, G.E., Melillo, S., and Bradley, L.A. (2010). Association between 9p21 genomic markers and heart disease. A meta-analysis. *Journal of the American Medical Association*, 303, 648–56.

Pearson, T.A., Mensah, G.A., Alexander, R.W., et al. (2003). Markers of inflammation and cardiovascular disease: Application to clinical and public health practice. A statement for healthcare professionals from the Centers for Disease Control and Prevention and the American Heart Association. *Circulation*, 107(3), 499–511.

Romero, J.R. and Wolf, P.A. (2013). Epidemiology of stroke. Legacy of the Framingham Heart Study. *Global Heart*, 8, 67–75.

Rosensen, R.S. (2004). Statins: can the new generation make an impression? *Expert Opinion on Emerging Drugs*, 9(2), 269–79.

Schunkert, H., Konig, I.R., and Kathiresan, S. (2011). CARDIoGRAM Consortium. Large scale association analysis identifies 13 new susceptibility loci for coronary artery disease. *Nature Genetics*, 43, 333–8.

Smith, S.C. Jr., Benjamin, E.J., Bonow, R.O., et al. (2011). AHA/ACCF secondary prevention and risk reduction therapy for patients with coronary and other atherosclerotic vascular disease: 2011 update: a guideline from the American Heart Association and American College of Cardiology Foundation endorsed by the World Heart Federation and the Preventive Cardiovascular Nurses Association. *Journal of the American College of Cardiology*, 58, 2432–46.

Smith, S.C. Jr., Collins, A., Ferrari, R., et al. (2012). Our time: a call to save preventable death from cardiovascular disease (heart disease and stroke). *Journal of the American College of Cardiology*, 60, 2343–8.

Stone, N.J., Robinson, J.G., Lichtenstein, A.H., et al. (2014). American College of Cardiology/American Heart Association Task Force on Practice Guidelines. 2013 ACC/AHA guideline on the treatment of blood cholesterol to reduce atherosclerotic cardiovascular risk in adults: a report of the American College of Cardiology/American Heart Association Task Force on Practice Guidelines. *J Am Coll Cardiol*, 63(25 Pt B), 2889–934.

Williams, R.R., Hunt, S.C., Heiss, G., et al. (2001). Usefulness of cardiovascular family history data for population-based preventive medicine and medical research (The Health Family Tree Study and the NHLBI Family Heart Study). *American Journal of Cardiology*, 87, 129–35.

Wilson, P.W.F., D'Agostino, R.B., Levy, D., Belanger, A.M., Silbershatz, H., and Kannel, W.B. (1998). Prediction of coronary heart disease using risk factor categories. *Circulation*, 97, 1837–47.

Wong, K., Glovaci, D., Malik, S., et al. (2012). Comparison of demographic factors and cardiovascular risk factor control among US adults with type 2 diabetes by insulin treatment classification. *Journal of Diabetes and its Complications*, 26, 169–74.

Wong, N.D. and Levy, D. (2013). Legacy of the Framingham Heart Study: rationale, design, initial findings and implications. *Global Heart*, 8(1), 3–9.

Yeboah, J., McClelland, R.L., Polonsky, T.S., et al. (2012). Comparison of novel risk markers for improvement in cardiovascular risk assessment in intermediate-risk individuals. *JAMA*, 308(8), 788–95.

8.2

Cancer epidemiology and public health

Zuo-Feng Zhang, Paolo Boffetta, Alfred I. Neugut, and Carlo La Vecchia

Introduction to cancer epidemiology and public health

Classification of neoplasms is based on the International Classification of Diseases—Oncology (World Health Organization (WHO) 1976; Fritz et al. 2000) into topographical categories (according to the organ where the neoplasm arises) and morphological categories (according to the characteristics of the cells).

Further, they can be characterized by abnormal growth that can be distinguished in humans by localization, morphology, molecular characteristics, clinical behaviour, and response to therapy.

Benign and malignant tumours

Benign neoplasms represent localized growths of tissue with predominantly normal characteristics: in many cases they cause minor symptoms and are amenable to surgical therapy. They can be fatal because of their clinical importance when they occur in organs in which compression is possible and surgery cannot be easily performed (e.g. benign brain tumour), and when they produce hormones or other substances with a worsening systemic effect (e.g. adrenaline (epinephrine) produced by benign phaeochromocytoma). Because relatively little is known about the distributions and causes of most benign neoplasms, they will not be further discussed in this chapter.

Malignant neoplasms are characterized by progressive growth of abnormal cells with structural and functional alterations with respect to the normal tissue. In some cases, the alterations can be so serious that it becomes difficult to identify the tissue of origin. A peculiarity of most malignant tumours is the ability to invade the nearby tissue, and to migrate and colonize other organs via blood and lymph vessel penetration and transport. The presence, extension, and control of metastases are often the critical factors to determine the success of therapy and the survival of cancer patients.

Carcinogenesis

Increasingly, neoplasms are characterized at the molecular level according to phenotypic aspects (e.g. presence of receptors, expression of genes) and genetic alterations (e.g. mutation in a given gene).

The understanding of the molecular and cellular mechanisms of carcinogenesis has greatly advanced in recent years. According to a widely accepted model, cells have to acquire six characteristics to become fully malignant (Hanahan and Weinberg 2011). These include the ability to produce growth signals (several known oncogenes mimic growth signalling), the lack of sensitivity to antigrowth signals (the retinoblastoma (RB) protein and its homologues play a key role in the ability of the cell to decide whether to proliferate, to be quiescent, or to enter into a post-mitotic state, based on external signalling), resistance towards programmed cell death or apoptosis (in many cases via inactivation of the p53 protein), immortalization (normal cells have a limited replication potential that is related to the length of the telomeres: in malignant cells, overexpression of telomerase circumvents it), stimulation of blood vessel production (by changing the balance of angiogenesis inducers and countervailing inhibitors), and ability to invade and metastasize. The acquisition of these neoplastic characteristics typically occurs by alterations of relevant genes, but an inability to maintain genomic integrity (so-called genomic instability, which includes reduced ability to repair DNA damage) is an additional feature of malignant cells, as accumulation of random mutations in genes involved in all the functions just mentioned would be a too rare event for the development of cancer during the normal lifespan. Inflammation also fosters multiple hallmark functions, and consequently promotes carcinogenesis. A final point to consider is the heterogeneity of neoplastic genetic alterations: the acquisition of the different biological capabilities of the neoplastic cell can appear at different times, and the particular sequence in which capabilities are acquired can vary widely, even among the same type of tumours. In addition, tumours contain a repertoire of normal cells, which contribute to create the tumour microenvironment.

Several inherited conditions carry a very high risk of one or several cancers. High-penetrance genes (or high-risk genes) are identified through family-based and other linkage studies. These conditions, however, are rare and explain only a small proportion of human cancers. Genetic factors, however, are likely to play an important role in interacting with non-genetic factors to determine individual cancer risk.

The long process of carcinogenesis justifies the efforts to develop and apply screening approaches for early detection of selected subclinical neoplasms in healthy individuals.

Cancer epidemiology and distribution

The development of cancer epidemiology has formed the basis for knowledge about the causes and the possible preventive strategies which has greatly advanced during the last several decades. The identification of the determinants of cancer relies on two complementary approaches, the epidemiological and the experimental.

Table 8.2.1 reports the ratio of the 80th to the 20th percentile as well as the highest to the lowest of the ranking of country-specific incidence rates of selected cancers, as estimated in the Globocan 2012 project (Ferlay et al. 2013). For overall cancer (excluding skin), the ratios of 80 per cent versus 20 per cent are 3.16 for men and 1.97 for women. For men, the lowest ratio of 80 per cent versus 20 per cent is 2.68 for non-Hodgkin's lymphoma. For women, the lowest ratio is 2.21 for ovary cancer. For gall bladder, lung, kidney, and testis cancers in men, multiple myeloma in women, malignant melanoma and Kaposi sarcoma for both genders, the ratios are over 10. This comparison is based on stable figures, but masks larger variations among very-high-risk and very-low-risk areas. The highest to

Table 8.2.1 Ratio of the 20th/80th percentile and highest/lowest in the ranking of country-specific estimated age standardized incidence rates of selected cancers (Globocan 2012)

Cancer	Men		Women	
	20th/80th	Highest/lowest	20th/80th	Highest/lowest
All cancer, excluding skin	3.16	6.80	1.97	4.72
Oral cavity	3.27	75.75	2.46	105.50
Thyroid	5.75	173.00	6.17	886.00
Nasopharynx[a]	9.50	106.00	8.00	39.00
Other pharynx	7.50	149.00	5.00	33.00
Larynx	3.75	47.33	8.00	30.00
Oesophagus	4.69	94.00	8.50	208.00
Stomach	3.95	47.92	3.04	49.40
Colorectum	5.98	41.07	4.84	35.80
Liver	3.20	81.50	3.37	87.29
Pancreas	5.13	39.67	5.78	79.00
Gall bladder	19.00	78.00	7.67	128.00
Lung	10.19	191.50	8.56	188.00
Melanoma	13.25	405.00	11.00	331.00
Breast			2.73	24.33
Cervix			3.82	37.95
Corpus uteri			4.63	341.00
Ovary			2.21	18.63
Prostate	6.26	189.33		
Testis	14.33	122.00		
Bladder	6.24	103.33	3.89	24.67
Kidney	12.00	241.00	7.83	105.00
Brain, nervous system	7.00	127.00	9.20	107.00
Kaposi sarcoma[b]	26.00	464.00	11.00	236.00
Non-Hodgkin's lymphoma	2.68	36.20	3.26	36.50
Hodgkin's lymphoma	5.50	42.00	9.00	36.00
Leukaemia	3.16	125.00	3.35	57.50
Multiple myeloma	7.50	76.00	10.50	54.00

[a] Female: 20% vs 78%.

[b] Male: 10% vs 72%; female, 10% vs 47%.

Source: data from Ferlay J, et al. GLOBOCAN 2012 v1.0, *Cancer Incidence and Mortality Worldwide: IARC CancerBase No. 11*, International Agency for Research on Cancer, Lyon, France, Copyright © IARC 2013, available from http://globocan.iarc.fr.

the lowest ratios in Table 8.2.1 represent extreme geographic differences that deserve epidemiological investigation into environmental and genetic factors in the development of cancer.

Analytical studies (case–control and cohort) have shown the causal role of specific exposures in the aetiology of several malignant neoplasms. One limitation of the epidemiological approach, which may prove of critical importance in trying to detect comparatively small increases in risk, as in the case of environmental pollutants, is that even in the best conditions it is impossible to confidently identify by epidemiological means an increase in risk smaller than about 10 per cent to 20 per cent and serious problems arise in the interpretation of increases below 50 per cent, as the biases inherent in any observational study are of at least this order of magnitude (Lagiou et al. 2008).

The identification of carcinogens via the laboratory relies on three types of tests: (1) long-term (often lifetime) carcinogenicity tests in experimental animals, most commonly rodents (mice, rats, and hamsters); (2) short-term tests assessing the effects of chemical agents on a variety of end points belonging to three general classes: DNA damage, mutagenicity, and chromosome damage; and (3) mechanistic tests, aimed at identifying the intermediate steps in the compound-specific carcinogenic process.

These tests are valuable to the extent that such effects may reflect underlying events in the carcinogenic process. Indeed, consistent positivity in tests measuring DNA damage, mutagenicity and chromosomal damage is usually regarded as indicating potential carcinogenicity of the tested agent. In addition, a number of factors, including hormones and overweight/obesity, show carcinogenic effects through non-genotoxic pathways, for which mechanisms of carcinogenesis are less well defined and their biomarkers are sparse (Boffetta and Islami 2013).

Results of laboratory tests constitute useful supporting evidence when adequate epidemiological data for the carcinogenicity of an environmental agent exists, but they become all the more essential when the epidemiological evidence is non-existent or inadequate in quality or in quantity. In the latter case, although no universally accepted criteria exist to automatically translate data from long-term animal tests or short-term tests to cancer risk in humans, an evaluation of the risk can be made on a judgemental basis using all available scientific evidence. This policy has been applied by the International Agency for Research on Cancer (IARC) in a systematic programme of evaluation of the carcinogenic risk of chemicals to man. Agents are commonly classified in group 1 when the evidence of their carcinogenicity in humans, derived from epidemiological studies, is considered sufficient, and are classified in group 2A when the evidence in humans is limited and the agent is an experimental carcinogen. Agents in group 2B include mainly experimental carcinogens for which the human evidence is inadequate or non-existent (IARC 2006). Since 1972, IARC has published 100 volumes presenting evaluations and re-evaluations for 968 chemical, physical, and biological agents and groups of agents, as well as exposure circumstances, such as occupations. A total of 111 agents have been classified in group 1, 66 in group 2A, and 285 in group 2B, 505 in group 3 (not classifiable as to its carcinogenicity to humans), and one in group 4 (probably not carcinogenic to humans). The complete list of agents, with their evaluations can be found on the Monographs website (IARC 2014).

Temporal changes in incidence rates, particularly when they take place over a few decades, are incompatible with a genetic explanation.

However, the possibility of environmental exposure changes as well as their possible interaction with genetic factors might contribute partially to temporal changes in incidence rates. Recorded incidence rates are affected by diagnostic changes and mortality rates are, in addition, affected by changes in treatment effectiveness; however, marked trends like the one for lung cancer mortality (Malvezzi et al. 2013) are most likely to reflect real changes in cancer rates, pointing to the importance of environmental factors.

Aetiological risk factors of cancer

A number of factors are associated with an increased risk of malignant neoplasms, but their importance varies in different settings and for neoplasms at different sites.

Tobacco smoking

This is the single major cause of human cancer worldwide (IARC 2004a). Tobacco-related cancers include cancers of the lung, nasal cavity, larynx, oral cavity, pharynx, oesophagus, stomach, liver, pancreas, colorectum, ovary, uterine cervix, kidney, and bladder, as well as of myeloid leukaemia. In high-income countries, tobacco smoking has been estimated to cause approximately 30 per cent of all human cancers (Doll and Peto 2005). In many medium- and low-income countries, the burden of tobacco-related cancer is still lower, given the relatively later start of the tobacco epidemics, which will result in a greater number of cancers in the near future. The IARC has classified tobacco smoking as a group 1 carcinogen and determined that 81 carcinogens in mainstream cigarette smoke have sufficient evidence for carcinogenicity in humans or laboratory animals, including 11 carcinogens in group 1, 14 in group 2A, and 56 in group 2B (IARC 2004a; Smith et al. 2003).

Diet and obesity

Despite considerable research efforts in recent years, the exact role of dietary factors in causing or protecting against human cancer remains largely unquantified. There is sufficient evidence of an increased risk of liver cancer with exposure to aflatoxin, a carcinogen in diet produced by some fungi in certain tropical areas. According to a recent comprehensive review on nutrition and cancer, high intake of red meat as well as processed meat were considered to have convincing evidence for an increased risk of colorectal cancer. There is convincing evidence that weight gain is associated with increased risk of cancers of the oesophagus (adenocarcinoma), pancreas, colorectum, post-menopausal breast cancer, endometrium, and kidney (World Cancer Research Fund and American Institute for Cancer Research (WCRF and AICR) 2007).

Alcohol drinking

As a group 1 carcinogen by IARC, alcohol drinking was considered to have sufficient evidence of carcinogenesis. Alcohol drinking at high levels increases the risk of cancers of the oral cavity, pharynx, larynx, oesophagus, liver, pancreas, colorectum, and female breast (Baan et al. 2007).

Infectious agents

These are considered the second most important factors for cancer risk in the world. Nine infectious agents have been classified as group 1 carcinogens (8.1 per cent), including six viruses associated with the origin of certain types of human cancers (Table 8.2.2): Epstein–Barr virus (EBV) with an attributable fraction (AF) of 97.9 per cent for nasopharyngeal cancer, 45.9 per cent for

Table 8.2.2 Assessment of associations between infections and human cancer, from IARC Monographs

	Evidence[a]	Target organs[b]	IARC Monographs Vol.
Viruses			
Hepatitis B virus	S	Liver, bile duct (leukaemia/lymphoma)	59, 100B
Hepatitis C virus	S	Liver, bile duct, leukaemia/lymphoma	59, 100B
Hepatitis D virus	I	Liver	59
Human papilloma virus type 16	S	Cervix, vulva, vagina, penis, anus, oral cavity, tonsil, pharynx, (larynx)	64, 90, 100B
Human papilloma virus type 18	S	Cervix, (oral cavity), (penis), (anus), (vulva)	64, 90, 100B
Human papilloma virus types 31, 35, 39, 45, 51, 52, 56, 58, 59	S	Cervix	64, 90, 100B
Human papilloma virus type 33	S	Cervix, (anus), (vulva)	64, 90, 100B
Human papilloma virus types 6, 11	I	(Larynx)	90, 100B
Human papilloma virus types 26, 53, 66, 67, 68, 70, 73, 82	L	(Cervix)	100B
Human papilloma virus types 30, 34, 69, 85, 97	I		100B
Human papilloma virus, genus-beta types (except 5 and 8) and gamma types	I	(Skin)	90, 100B
Human papillomavirus types 5, 8 (in patients with epidermodysplasia verruciformis)	L	(Skin)	100B
Human immunodeficiency virus 1	S	Anus, Kaposi sarcoma, cervix, eye, leukaemia/lymphoma, (liver/bile duct), (skin), (vulva), (vagina), (penis)	67, 100B
Human immunodeficiency virus 2	L	Kaposi sarcoma, non-Hodgkin's lymphoma	67
Human T-cell lymphotrophic virus I	S	Adult T-cell leukaemia/lymphoma	67, 100B
Human T-cell lymphotrophic virus II	I		67
Epstein–Barr virus	S	Nasopharynx, leukaemia/lymphoma, (stomach)	70, 100B
Human herpes virus 8	S	(Kaposi's sarcoma), leukaemia/lymphoma	70, 100B
Merkel cell polyomavirus	L	(Skin)	104
Bacterium			
Helicobacter pylori	S	Stomach, leukaemia/lymphoma	61, 100B
Parasites			
Schistosoma haematobium	S	Bladder	61, 100B
Schistosoma japonicum	L	(Colorectum, liver/bile duct)	61
Schistosoma mansoni	I		61
Opistorchis viverrini	S	Liver/bile duct	61, 100B
Opistorchis felineus	I		61
Clonorchis sinensis	L	Liver/bile duct	61, 100B
Malaria (*Plasmodium falciparum*)	L	(Leukaemia/lymphoma)	104
Plants			
Plants containing aristolochic acid	S	Renal pelvis and ureter	82, 100A

[a] I, inadequate; L, limited; S, sufficient.

[b] Established target organs without brackets; suspected target organs in brackets.

Source: data from International Agency for Research on Cancer (IARC), *IARC Monographs on the Evaluation of the Carcinogenic Risks to Humans*, International Agency for Research on Cancer, Lyon, France, Copyright © IARC 2014 International Agency for Research on Cancer, available from http://monographs.iarc.fr/. Specific volumes: Volume 59, *Hepatitis Viruses* (IARC, 1994a); Volume 61, *Schistosomes, Liver Flukes and Helicobacter Pylori* (IARC, 1994b); Volume 64, *Human Papillomaviruses* (IARC 1995); Volume 67, *Human Immunodeficiency Viruses and Human T-Cell Lymphotropic Viruses* (IARC 1996); Volume 70, *Epstein–Barr Virus and Kaposi's Sarcoma Herpes Virus/Human Herpesvirus 8* (IARC 1997); Volume 82, *Some Traditional Herbal Medicines, Some Mycotoxins, Naphthalene, and Styrene* (IARC 2002); Volume 90, *Human Papillomaviruses* (IARC 2007), Volume 100 (A), *Pharmaceuticals* (IARC 2012a); Volume 100 (B), *Biological Agents* (IARC 2012b); and Volume 104, *Malaria and Some Polyomaviruses* (IARC 2013).

Hodgkin's lymphoma, and 2.2 per cent for non-Hodgkin's lymphoma (NHL); human papillomavirus (HPV) with AFs of 100 per cent for cervical cancer, 55.7 per cent for anogenital cancer, 4.4 per cent for mouth and oral-pharyngeal cancers; hepatitis B virus (HBV) and hepatitis C virus (HCV) with an AF of 83.9 per cent for liver cancer; human immunodeficiency virus type 1 (HIV-1) with an AF of 12 per cent for NHL, and human T-lymphotropic virus type 1 (HTLV-1) with an AF of 1.1 per cent for NHL; as well as the bacterium *Helicobacter pylori* (AF of 63.6 per cent for stomach cancer), and parasites *Schistosoma haematobium* (AF of 3 per cent for bladder cancer) and *Opisthorchis viverrini* (liver flukes, AF of 0.4 per cent for liver cancer) (Parkin, 2006).

Occupation and pollution

While some carcinogens (e.g. *bis*-chloro methylethers) represent today a historic curiosity, exposure is still widespread for carcinogens such as asbestos, arsenic, and silica. Estimates of the global burden of cancer attributable to occupation in high-income countries result in figures on the order of 2–3 per cent (Steenland et al. 2003; Doll and Peto 2005).

Ionizing and non-ionizing radiation

The estimates of the contribution of ionizing radiation to human cancer in high-income countries are on the order of 3–5 per cent (Colditz et al. 2000; Doll and Peto 2005). Several neoplasms, in particular acute lymphocytic leukaemia, acute and chronic myeloid leukaemia, and cancers of the breast, lung, bone, brain, and thyroid are produced as a result of this radiation (IARC 2000).

Genetic factors

A number of inherited mutations of a high-penetrance cancer gene increase dramatically the risk of some, yet, in some populations, the number of cases attributable to them is small.

The global burden of neoplasms

The number of new cases of cancer which occurred worldwide in 2012 has been estimated at about 14,090,000 of which it was projected that 4,653,000 deaths occurred in men and 3,547,000 in women in the same year. In more developed and less-developed regions of the world, approximately 2,878,000 and 5,323,000 cancer deaths have resulted, respectively. Among men, lung, liver, stomach, colorectal, and oesophageal cancers are the most common causes of cancer deaths, while breast, lung, colorectal, cervix uteri, and stomach cancers are the most common causes of cancer deaths among women (GLOBOCAN 2012: Ferlay et al. 2013).

One complementary approach in assessing the global burden of neoplasms is to weigh the years of life with disability and add them to the years lost because of premature death (disability-adjusted life-years (DALYs)). According to the Global Burden of Disease Study 2010, lung cancer was responsible for 32.4 million DALYs, liver cancer for 19.1 million, breast cancer for 12.0 million, stomach cancer for 16.4 million, and colorectal cancer for 14.4 million (Murray et al. 2012).

Distribution, aetiology, and prevention of selected cancers

We report estimates for 2012 since more recent data are available only for selected regions and countries. The cancer site is ordered based on numbers of specific cancer deaths based on Globocan 2012 (Ferlay et al. 2013).

Lung cancer

In 2012 lung cancer was the most frequent cancer in the world as there were 1,824,701 new lung cancer cases, accounting for approximately 13.0 per cent of the global cancer burden (GLOBOCAN 2012: Ferlay et al. 2013). Lung cancer was also the most common cause of cancer death, causing 1,589,800 deaths in 2012.

Incidence and mortality rates for lung cancer are approximately twice as high among men as among women. Lung cancer is the most common cancer in men worldwide (1.2 million new cases, 16.7 per cent of the total), with the highest age-standardized incidence rates observed in Central and Eastern Europe (53.5 per 100,000) as well as Eastern Asia (50.4 per 100,000) (GLOBOCAN 2012). The geographic pattern of incidence rates among women is slightly different, and generally lower, reflecting historic tobacco consumption patterns. The highest age-standardized incidence rates for women are observed in North America (33.8 per 100,000) and Northern Europe (23.7 per 100,000) (GLOBOCAN 2012). The geographical patterns in mortality closely follow those in incidence due to the high fatality and relative lack of variability in survival in different regions of the world.

The geographical and temporal patterns of lung cancer incidence are to a large extent determined by consumption of tobacco.

Principal histological types of lung cancer include squamous cell carcinoma, small cell carcinoma, adenocarcinoma, and large cell carcinoma; the last decades have witnessed a decrease in the predominant squamous cell carcinoma type and an increase in adenocarcinomas.

A carcinogenic effect of tobacco smoke on the lung was demonstrated in the 1950s and has been recognized by public health and regulatory authorities since the mid 1960s (IARC 2004a). The risk of lung cancer among smokers relative to the risk among never-smokers is on the order of over 20- to 40-fold. As compared to continuous smokers, the excess risk levels off in ex-smokers after quitting, but a small excess risk is likely to persist in long-term quitters throughout life. An association has been shown in many studies between exposure to involuntary smoking and lung cancer risk in non-smokers. The magnitude of the excess risk among non-smokers exposed to involuntary smoking is on the order of 20 per cent (IARC 2004a).

The UK Million Women Study demonstrated that the relative risks (RRs) of lung cancer were 10.5 for current smokers of ten cigarettes per day, 22.0 for 15, and 36.0 for 20 or more cigarettes per day (Pirie et al. 2013). Thus, even moderate smokers have substantial excess lung cancer mortality. This overall risk reflects the contribution of the different aspects of tobacco smoking: average consumption, duration of smoking, time since quitting, age at start, type of tobacco product, and inhalation pattern, with duration being the dominant factor.

The cumulative risk of lung cancer of a continuous smoker is 16 per cent and it is reduced to 10 per cent, 6 per cent, 3 per cent, and 2 per cent among those who stopped at ages 60, 50, 40, and 30, respectively (Peto et al. 2000). Among women in the United Kingdom, quitting smoking before age 40 years could avoid more than 90 per cent of the excess mortality caused by continuing smoking (Pirie et al. 2013). In the United States, stopping smoking before the age of 40 years would reduce the risk of death associated with continued smoking by about 90 per cent (Jha et al. 2013).

An increase in tobacco consumption is paralleled some decades later by an increase in the incidence of lung cancer; similarly, a decrease in consumption is followed by a decrease in incidence, as observed in the United States. The highest incidence rates in men (> 80/100,000) are recorded among black people from the United States (American Cancer Society (ACS) 2013). Incidence rates are also high (> 40/100,000) in the North American and European countries where a significant decline is shown among US white men and among men in the United Kingdom and Northern Europe with the lowest revealed in Africa. Comparably, rates in women are high in these regions (> 30/100,000) apart from Africa and Central Asia where the prevalence of smoking only increased recently. A notable exception is China, with high rates being recorded despite a low prevalence of smoking (20.4/100,000) (GLOBOCAN 2012: Ferlay et al. 2013).

The risk of lung cancer is increased among workers employed in several industries and occupations.

For several of these high-risk workplaces, the agent (or agents) responsible for the increased risk have been identified. Of these, asbestos and combustion fumes are the most important. Occupational agents were responsible in the past for an estimated 5–10 per cent of lung cancers in industrialized countries, though this proportion is likely to be smaller in recent years.

Pulmonary tuberculosis has demonstrated an increased risk to lung cancer, although it is not coherent whether it is due to the chronic inflammatory status of the lung parenchyma or the specific action of the *Mycobacterium*. High levels of fibres and dusts might result in lung fibrosis (e.g. silicosis and asbestosis), along with chronic bronchitis and emphysema, conditions that also entail an increase in the risk of lung cancer.

Other concerns relate to the presence of urban air posing as a susceptible risk factor; however, the excess is unlikely to be larger than 20 per cent in most urban areas (Speizer and Samet 1994).

A protective effect noted against lung cancer is the intake of cruciferous vegetables, possibly due to their high content of isothiocyanates (IARC 2004b). However, despite the many studies of intake of other foods, such as cereals, eggs, and dairy products, for example, it is inadequate to formulate a judgement pertaining to evidence describing a carcinogenic or protective effect.

Currently, genome-wide association studies (GWAS) with large sample size have identified polymorphisms of genes located within 15q25 (*CHRNA3* and *CHRNA5*), 5p15.33 (*TERT-CLPTM1L*), and 6p21.33 (*BAT3*) to be associated with the risk of lung cancer. However, significant future studies are still needed to identify heritable risk factors and molecular pathways and signature of lung carcinogenesis (Marshall and Christiani 2013).

There is conclusive evidence that exposure to ionizing radiation increases the risk of lung cancer (IARC 2000). Atomic bomb survivors and patients treated with radiotherapy for ankylosing spondylitis or breast cancer are at moderately increased risk of lung cancer, while studies of nuclear industry workers exposed to relatively low levels, however, provided no evidence of an increased risk of lung cancer. Underground miners exposed to radioactive radon and its decay products, which emit α-particles, have been consistently found to be at increased risk of lung cancer (IARC 2001). The risk increased with estimated cumulative exposure and decreased with attained age and time since cessation of exposure

(Lubin et al. 1994). It was estimated that annual low-dose computed tomography (CT) scan was associated with a 5.5 per cent increased risk of lung cancer among smokers (Brenner, 2004).

Prevention of lung cancer

Control of tobacco smoking (including involuntary smoking) remains the key strategy for the prevention of lung cancer. Reduction in exposure to occupational and environmental carcinogens (in particular indoor pollution and radon), as well as increase in consumption of fruits and vegetables are additional preventive opportunities. The recent US National Lung Cancer Screening Trial reported a 20 per cent reduction of lung cancer mortality using low-dose CT scan; however, longer follow-up of this and other cohorts is needed to evaluate other possible side effects of the low-dose CT scan (Sarma et al. 2012; Field et al. 2013).

Cancer of the liver

The estimated worldwide number of new cases of liver cancer in 2012 is 782,000, of which 83 per cent are from developing countries (50 per cent from China alone) (GLOBOCAN 2012: Ferlay et al. 2013). Most low-income regions of the world, with the exception of South-Central and Western Asia, reflect a high incidence of liver cancer. The highest rates (above 30/100,000 in men and above 10/100,000 in women) are recorded in Eastern and South-Eastern Asia, Northern and Western Africa, and Melanesia. The lowest rates are in Northern Europe and South-Central Asia, where age-standardized rates are below 5/100,000 in men and 2.5/100,000 in women. Intermediate rates (5–10/100,000 in men) are observed in areas of Southern Europe and North America. Rates are two- to threefold higher in men than women, and the difference is stronger in high-incidence than in low-incidence areas.

Chronic infections with hepatitis B virus (HBV) and hepatitis C virus (HCV) are the main causes of HCC. The risk increases with early age at infection (in high-risk countries, most HBV infections occur perinatally or in early childhood), and the presence of liver cirrhosis is a pathogenic step. The estimated relative risk of developing HCC among infected subjects, compared to uninfected, ranged between 10 and 50 in different studies. On a global scale, the fraction of liver cancer cases attributable to HBV is 54 per cent, the one attributable to HCV is 31 per cent (Parkin 2006). Overall, over 75 per cent of liver cancer cases are related to infection (de Martel et al. 2012).

Ecological studies have shown that the incidence of HCC correlates not only with HBV and HCV infection, but also with contamination of foodstuffs with aflatoxins, a group of mycotoxins produced by the fungi *Aspergillus flavus* and *Aspergillus parasiticus*, which cause liver cancer in many species of experimental animals (Turner et al. 2012). Contamination originates mainly from improper storage of cereals, peanuts, and other vegetables and is prevalent in particular in Africa, South-East Asia, and China. The investigation of the carcinogenic role of aflatoxins in humans has been complicated by the inadequacy of traditional methods of exposure assessment (e.g. questionnaires). During the last decades, however, prospective studies have shown a strong association between biological markers of aflatoxin exposure in serum or urine and risk of subsequent liver cancer. A carcinogenic role for aflatoxins, in particular of aflatoxin B_1, has therefore been confirmed and shown to be independent from—and to interact with—that exerted by HBV infection (London and McGlynn 2006).

(Alcoholic) cirrhosis is probably the most important risk factor for HCC in populations with low prevalence of HBV and HCV infection and low exposure to aflatoxins, such as North America and Northern Europe (La Vecchia 2007). The association between tobacco smoking and HCC is now established, with a RR of the order of 1.5 to 2 for tobacco smoking on liver carcinogenesis (IARC 2004a).

Use of oral contraceptives (OC) increases the risk of liver adenomas, and is associated with the risk of HCC, although the absolute risk is likely to be small. Case reports have associated use of anabolic steroids with development of liver cancer, but the evidence is not conclusive (Cibula et al. 2010).

Diabetes is also related to an excess risk of HCC, and the increased prevalence of overweight and obesity, and consequently of diabetes, in several populations may have had some role in recent unfavourable trends of HCC in North America and other areas of the world. Combined exposure to overweight at diabetes led to a RR of HCC of 4.75, after allowance for hepatitis, alcohol, and other recognized possible confounding factors (Turati et al. 2013a).

The excess risk of liver cancer associated with overweight/obesity and diabetes has been related to the development of non-alcoholic fatty liver disease (NAFLD) (Sanyal et al. 2010). NAFLD is characterized by excess fat accumulation in the liver, and ranges from isolated hepatic steatosis to non-alcoholic steatohepatitis (NASH), the more aggressive form of fatty liver disease, which can progress to cirrhosis and HCC. However, NAFLD/NASH increases HCC risk even in the absence of cirrhosis (Turati et al. 2013a).

Prevention of liver cancer

In high-prevalence areas, HBV vaccination has to be introduced in the perinatal period. In the last few decades, many countries from Asia, Southern Europe, and, to a lesser extent, Africa have expanded their national childhood vaccination programme to include HBV. Reduction of the incidence of liver cancer in young adults was observed in Qidong, a high risk area of liver cancer in China, because of both HBV vaccination and aflatoxin B_1 reduction in foods (Sun et al. 2013). A similar primary preventive approach is not available for HCV. Control of transmission is, however, feasible and medical treatment of carriers with interferon or newer antiviral drugs might represent an alternative approach, which is also available for HBV carriers.

Control of aflatoxin contamination of foodstuffs represents another important preventive measure. While this is easily achieved in high-income countries, its implementation is limited by economic and logistic factors in many high-prevalence regions. Control of alcohol drinking and tobacco smoking represent additional primary preventive measures.

Since about half of HCC, but not normal adult liver, secrete the fetal antigen α-fetoprotein, the detection of this marker has been proposed as a screening method. However, no population-based studies are currently available showing a decreased mortality from liver cancer in screened populations.

Cancer of the stomach

Accounting for approximately 951,000 new cases or 6.8 per cent of the global cancer burden, stomach cancer is the fifth most frequent cancer in the world (GLOBOCAN 2012: Ferlay et al. 2013) and the third most common cause of cancer death worldwide (723,000 deaths in 2012, 8.9 per cent) in 2012. This marks a substantive decrease in incidence since 1975 when stomach cancer was the most common neoplasm worldwide. Incidence rates are about twice as high in men as in women, with age-standardized rates highest (above 35/100,000 in men and 10/100,000 in women) in Eastern Asia, Eastern and Central Europe, and South America. Low-incidence areas include Africa, North America, and Northern Europe. The majority of cases occur in developing countries (677,000), with over 40 per cent of all new cases coming from China alone (404,996).

An increased risk of gastric cancer is associated with *Helicobacter pylori* infection. The biological plausibility of a causal association is also supported by a strong association between *H. pylori* and precancerous lesions, including chronic and atrophic gastritis and dysplasia. Given that the prevalence of infection is very high, especially in developing countries and among older cohorts, *H. pylori* can explain a large proportion of all new cases of gastric cancer that occur, or over 5 per cent of all cancer cases globally (Parkin 2006). However, only a small fraction of infected individuals were diagnosed as having stomach cancer. Persistent *H. pylori* infection due to a combination of virulence factors and immune subversion and manipulation mechanisms is associated with gastric carcinogenesis (Salama et al. 2013).

Another important cause of stomach cancer is tobacco smoking. Smokers have a 50–60 per cent increased risk of stomach cancer, as compared to non-smokers. This relationship would indicate that smoking is responsible for approximately 10 per cent of all cases (IARC 2004a).

Throughout the world there is a consistent correlation between consumption of salt and salted foods and stomach cancer incidence. A large number of studies that have examined this relationship have generally found an increased risk of approximately twofold for frequent consumption of salt and salted foods. The relationship is biologically plausible, given that salt may lead to damage to the protective mucosal layer of the stomach.

A notably striking feature of gastric cancer is the dramatic decline in its incidence and mortality which has been observed in most high-income countries over the past century. The decline is apparent for both sexes, and has occurred earlier in countries which currently have a low risk. This continuous dramatic decline, as well as the results from migrant studies, suggests a strong environmental influence on the disease.

Reasons for the generalized decline in gastric cancer rates are complex and not completely understood. Almost certainly, these include a more varied and affluent diet and better food conservation, including refrigeration, as well as the control of *H. pylori* infection. Whether improved diagnosis and treatment have also played some role on the favourable trends in gastric cancer, particularly over most recent calendar periods, however, remains open to question.

GWAS on stomach cancer was mainly conducted in Asian populations. In Japanese populations, polymorphisms in the *PSCA* gene, which may possibly be involved in regulating gastric epithelial cell proliferation, were found to be associated with diffuse-type gastric cancer (Sakamoto et al. 2008). In Chinese populations, multiple variants at the 10q23 region (*PLCE1*) have been identified to be associated with cardia gastric cancer (Abnet et al. 2010), and two novel susceptibility loci at 5p13.1 (*PTGER4* and *PRKAA1*) and 3q13.31 (*ZBTB20*) were found to be associated with non-cardia gastric cancer (Shi et al. 2011). These genes might regulate cell growth, differentiation, apoptosis and angiogenesis and be associated with the development of stomach cancer.

Other intervention trials conducted in a Chinese population known to be micronutrient deficient observed that a combination supplement of beta-carotene, vitamin E and selenium did result in a small reduction in the risk of stomach cancer (Blot 1997), but recent findings on the issue on other, better nourished populations, are largely negative (Plummer et al. 2007). More chemoprevention trials are needed for stomach cancer (Ford 2011).

Primary prevention of stomach cancer by dietary means is feasible by encouraging high-risk populations to decrease consumption of cured meats and salt preserved foods. Prevention may also be feasible through eradication of *H. pylori* infection, particularly in childhood and adolescence, and by avoiding mother to child transmission. Screening and early detection of stomach cancer have been developed in Japan with the use of X-ray photofluorography to identify early lesions, followed by gastroscopy.

Colorectal cancers

Cancers of the colon and rectum accounted in 2012 for an estimated 1,361,000 new cases and 694,000 deaths worldwide (GLOBOCAN 2012: Ferlay et al. 2013). They represent the third most frequent malignant disease in terms of incidence and the fourth for mortality. Colorectal cancer is the third most common cancer in men (746,000 new cases, 10 per cent total) and the second most common cancer in women (614,000 new cases, 9.2 per cent of the total).

The majority (55 per cent) of cases of colorectal cancer occur in high-income regions of the world, and geographical patterns are very similar in men and women. Generally, rates are slightly higher among men than women. The highest age-standardized rates are observed in Australia and New Zealand (44.8/100,000 for men and 32.2/100,000 for women), followed by western, southern, and northern Europe. There is considerable geographical variation in incidence of colorectal cancer, and the lowest rates in the world are observed in western Africa (4.5/100,000 for men and 3.8/100,000 for women) (GLOBOCAN 2012: Ferlay et al. 2013). A small increase in the incidence of colon cancer has been observed during the last few decades in most populations, but Western Europe over the last two decades (Fernandez et al. 2005; Siegel et al. 2014). Studies of migrant populations have shown that the risk of colon cancer approaches that of the country of adoption within one generation; the incidence is higher in urban than in rural populations.

The predominant histological type of malignant neoplasms of the colon is adenocarcinoma. This neoplasm is usually preceded by an adenomatous polyp, or adenoma, less frequently by a small area of flat mucosa exhibiting various grades of dysplasia. The malignant potential of an adenoma is increased by a surface diameter greater than 1 cm, by villous (rather than tubular) organization and by severe cellular dysplasia. Carriers of one adenoma larger than 1 cm have a two to four times increased risk of developing colon cancer; this risk is further doubled in carriers of multiple adenomas. On a topographical basis, the prevalence of adenomas detected during colonoscopy closely parallels the incidence of colon cancer.

Several studies have associated tobacco smoking with an increased risk of colonic adenoma. For colon cancer, a modest increased risk following prolonged heavy smoking has been shown in some of the largest prospective studies (IARC 2004a). Excessive alcohol consumption (50 g alcohol/day) has been associated with moderately increased risk of colon cancer (Baan et al. 2007).

Patients with ulcerative colitis and Crohn's disease are at increased risk of colon cancer. The overall RR has been estimated in the range of 5–20, and it is higher for young age at diagnosis, severity of the disease, and presence of dysplasia. The contribution of shared genetic and environmental factors in the genesis of the two inflammatory conditions and of colon cancer is not known. Diabetes and cholecystectomy have been associated with a moderate (1.5–2-fold) increased risk of (right-sided) colon cancer, possibly due to continuous secretion of bile. Patients with one cancer of the colon have a twofold risk to develop a second primary tumour in the colon or rectum, and the relative (though not the absolute) risk is greater for early age at first diagnosis. In women, an association has been shown also with cancers of the endometrium, ovary, and breast, possibly due to shared hormonal or dietary factors.

Several pathways which incorporate genetic instability (chromosomal instability (CIN) and microsatellite instability (MSI)), and inherited mutations of the adenomatous polyposis coli (*APC*) gene and mismatch repair genes pose as risk factors for colon cancer (Arends, 2013). More than 20 variants have been identified from regions at the 8q24 locus and genes within the TGF-β and Wnt signalling pathways. *CRAC1* on 15q13 and *SMAD7* on 18q21.1 were highlighted in multiple GWAS (Fernandez-Rozadilla et al. 2013; Peters et al. 2013). The majority of colorectal cancer GWAS were conducted in European descendants, with only two studies focused on East Asian populations (Cui et al. 2011; Jia et al. 2013).

Several rare hereditary conditions are characterized by a very high incidence of colon cancer. Familial adenomatous polyposis, due to inherited or *de novo* mutation in the *APC* gene on chromosome 5, is characterized by a very high number of colonic adenomas and a cumulative incidence of colon or rectal cancer close to 100 per cent by age 55. Gardner's syndrome, Turcot syndrome, and juvenile polyposis feature among the rarer diseases having this association. All these hereditary conditions, although very serious for the affected patients, account for no more than 1 per cent of colon cancers in the general population.

Lynch syndrome I is characterized by an increased risk of cancer of the proximal (right) colon, and is due to inherited mutation in one of two genes involved in DNA repair. Contrastingly, Lynch syndrome II has also an increased risk of extra-colonic neoplasms, mainly of the endometrium and the ovary. Overall, hereditary non-polyposis colon cancer may account for a sizeable proportion of cases of colon cancer in Western populations. In addition to these hereditary conditions, first-degree relatives of colon cancer patients have a two- to threefold increased risk of developing a cancer of the colon or the rectum.

Recent evidence from prospective studies provides only limited evidence in favour of a role of specific foods and nutrients (Marques-Vidal et al. 2006). The strongest evidence concerning dietary factors responsible for a substantial proportion of colorectal cancers demonstrate an increased risk for high intake of meat and of smoked, salted, or processed foods (Huxley et al. 2009).

Vitamin D, and in particular its most active form, 25(OH) D, has been inversely related to colorectal cancer risk (Giovannucci 2005). The preventive effect is only possible when the vitamin D receptor (VDR) is present so that the mechanisms to increase VDR expression would enhance the preventive ability of vitamin D (Stubbins et al. 2012). Reduction of the incidence of colorectal cancer is also associated with the increased use of aspirin and other nonsteroidal anti-inflammatory drugs (Bosetti et al. 2012; Ferrández, et al. 2012). Additionally, hormone therapy in menopause and other female hormones, including OC, have been inversely related to colon cancer risks, and hence may also play some protective role (ACS 2011a).

Prevention of colorectal cancer

Increased physical activity, avoidance of overweight and obesity, reduced alcohol drinking, and quitting smoking are the main tools for the primary prevention of colorectal cancer. While aspirin use could prevent colorectal cancer as well, its use is not routinely recommended because of its spectrum of side effects.

Surveillance via flexible colonoscopy, involving removal of adenomas, is a secondary preventive measure. An additional approach consists in the detection of faecal occult blood. The method suffers from low specificity and, to a lesser extent, low sensitivity, in particular in the ability to detect adenomas. However, randomized trials have shown a reduced mortality from colorectal cancer after an annual test, although this is achieved at a high cost due to an elevated number of false positive cases. Current recommendations for individuals aged 50 and over include either annual faecal occult blood testing or one colonoscopic examination which does not need to be repeated in 10 years if results are normal (Boyle et al. 2003; ACS 2011a). Randomized trials have also demonstrated

the efficacy of sigmoidoscopy in reducing colorectal cancer mortality, primarily for the distal colon.

Cancer of the breast

Breast cancer is the most important cause of cancer death among women, and accounted for an estimated 521,000 deaths worldwide in 2012 (GLOBOCAN 2012: Ferlay et al. 2013). The incidence of breast cancer is relatively low (less than 25/100,000) in most countries of Middle Africa, in China, and a few other countries of East and South-Central Asia. The highest rates (70–90/100,000) are recorded in North America, Australia and New Zealand, Northern and Western Europe, as well as in the Bahamas, Argentina, Uruguay, Lebanon, and Armenia. The incidence of breast cancer has grown rapidly during the last few decades in many low-resource countries and slowly in high-income countries. In high-income countries, age-specific incidence rates increase sharply after age 45 and the rate in women aged 65+ is over 250/100,000. However, incidence rates in medium- and low-income countries are between 50 to 100/100,000 after age 45 (Fig. 8.2.1). Mortality rates remained fairly stable between 1960 and 1990 in most of Europe and the Americas; appreciable declines have occurred since the early 1990s. Incidence appears to increase linearly with age up to menopause, after which a further increase is less distinct (in high-income countries) or almost absent (in low-income countries). Women from high social class have consistently higher rates (about 30–50 per cent) than women from low social class.

The combined evidence from reproductive factors points towards an important role for endogenous hormones in breast carcinogenesis. A direct assessment of the role of oestrogens and testosterone is also available from recent prospective studies collecting data from biological samples. Oestradiol concentrations in the blood have been directly associated with breast cancer risk in post-menopausal women, whereas data are fewer and results are less consistent in pre-menopausal women. The association might be stronger with oestrogen and progesterone receptor positive

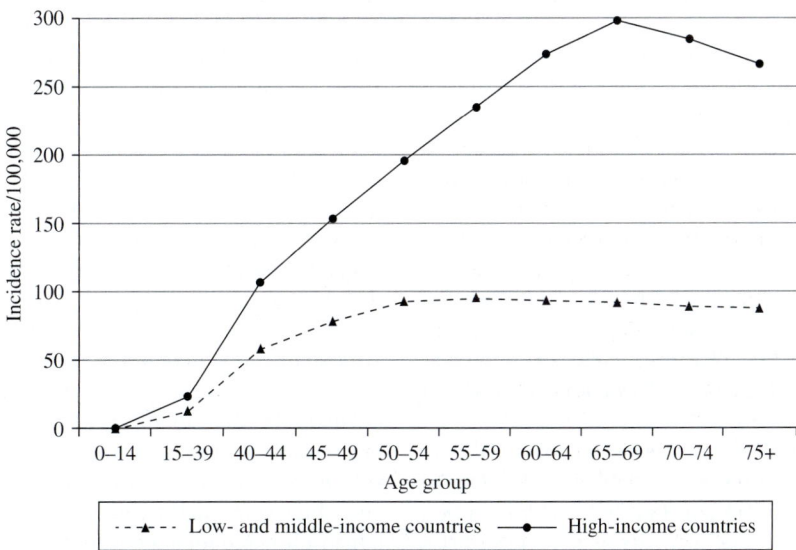

Fig. 8.2.1 Age-specific incidence of breast cancer by region of the world, 2012.

Source: data from Ferlay, J., et al. GLOBOCAN 2012 v1.0, *Cancer Incidence and Mortality Worldwide: IARC CancerBase No. 11*, International Agency for Research on Cancer, Lyon, France, Copyright © IARC 2013, available from http://globocan.iarc.fr.

tumours. Comparable findings have been reported for measures of testosterone and other androgens, but the data are inconsistent for all endogenous hormones across major cohort studies.

Less than 1 per cent of all cases of breast cancer occur in men. The incidence provides limited evidence of geographical and interracial variations, with no clear correlation with incidence in women. Conditions involving high oestrogen levels, such as gonadal dysfunction, alcohol abuse, and obesity, are likely risk factors for breast cancer in men. BRCA2 mutations are more frequent than BRCA1 in male familial breast cancers.

Women suffering from the two most common benign breast diseases, fibrocystic disease and fibroadenoma, carry a two- to three-fold increased risk of breast cancer. While these lesions are not likely to represent pre-neoplastic conditions, they share with breast cancer epithelial proliferation, linked to hormonal alterations.

A history of breast cancer in first-degree relatives is associated with a two- to threefold increased risk of the disease. Most of the role of familial history is likely to result from low-penetrance genes associated with hormonal metabolism and regulation, and DNA damage and repair. In the family linkage studies, breast cancer risk is greatly increased in carriers of mutations of several high-penetrance and low-frequency genes, including BRCA1, BRCA2, PTEN, and TP53. The mutations of these genes are associated with high risk of breast cancer, defined as inherited breast cancer syndrome. Although the cumulative lifetime risk in carriers of these genes is over 50 per cent, they are rare in most populations and explain only a small fraction (2–5 per cent) of total cases. There are exceptions, however, such as Ashkenazi Jews, among whom high-risk BRCA1 or BRCA2 mutations are responsible for an estimated 12 per cent of breast cancers. In addition, a group of low penetrance and low frequency DNA repair genes are related to moderate risk of breast cancer, including CHEK2, ATM, BRIP, and PALB2. Both high- and moderate-risk genes account for approximately 25 per cent of cases with family history of breast cancer. Recent GWAS of breast cancer identified single nucleotide polymorphisms (SNPs) in several novel genes, including TNRC9, FGFR2, MAP3K1, H19, and LSP1, and these genes are related to metabolism, apoptosis, cell cycle regulation, and mitochondrial functions (Fanale et al. 2012).

There are similarities and differences in risk profiles between triple negative (TNBC) and ER+ breast cancer based on results of the Women's Health Initiative study. Similar risk factors included BMI, lack of physical activity, and breast density (Phipps et al. 2011a, 2012). Nulliparity was associated with decreased risk of TNBC but increased risk of ER+ breast cancer. Among parous women, the number of births was positively associated with TNBC and inversely associated with ER+ disease. Ages at menarche and menopause were modestly associated with risk of ER+ but not TNBC (Phipps et al. 2011b). Tobacco smoking was not associated TNBC, but a risk factor for ER+ disease. Alcohol drinking was protective for TNBC, but a risk factor of ER+ breast cancer (Kabat et al. 2011).

Many lifestyle factors have been investigated as possible causes of breast cancer. Alcohol drinking is an established aetiological factor for breast cancer by IARC (Baan et al. 2007). Consumption of three or more alcoholic drinks per day carries an increased risk on the order of 30–50 per cent, with each daily drink accounting for about a 10 per cent higher risk. It is likely that both overweight and heavy alcohol drinking act on breast cancer through mechanisms involving hormonal level or metabolism. Tobacco smoking does not carry an increased risk of breast cancer. A high level of physical activity, on the other hand, is likely to moderately decrease the risk in post-menopausal women (Kruk and Czerniak 2013). Studies of occupational factors and of exposure to organochlorine pesticides have failed to provide evidence of an aetiological role (Salehi et al. 2008).

Survival from breast cancer has slowly increased in high-income countries, such as the United States, Canada, Sweden, Cuba, and Japan, where improvements in screening practices and treatments have achieved 5-year survival rates of 80 per cent. In contrast, 5-year survival rates are between 60 per cent and 79 per cent in middle-income countries and below 60 per cent in low-income countries (Coleman et al. 2008). In the United States, breast cancer survival in the black population is consistently poorer than the white population (Allemani et al. 2013).

Prevention of breast cancer

Primary prevention of breast cancer has been attempted via nutritional intervention, involving reduction of energy intake, reduction of the proportion of calories from fat, and increase in fruit and vegetable consumption. No evidence of efficacy has been produced so far. However, control of weight gain, particularly of post-menopausal women, would have favourable implications in breast cancer risk.

The most suitable approach for breast cancer control is secondary prevention through mammography. The effectiveness of screening by mammography in women older than 50 years has been demonstrated, and programmes have been established in various countries (Boyle et al. 2003). The effectiveness in women younger than 50 is not yet demonstrated. Other screening techniques, including breast self -examination, have not been proven to reduce breast cancer mortality (US Preventive Services Task Force 2009).

Cancer of the oesophagus

Approximately 456,000 new cases and 400,000 deaths of oesophageal cancer occurred worldwide in 2012 (GLOBOCAN 2012: Ferlay et al. 2013). The geographical distribution of oesophageal cancer is characterized by very wide variations within relatively small areas. Very high rates (over 50/100,000) are recorded for both men and women in northern Iran, various provinces of eastern China, and certain areas of Kazakhstan (Wei et al. 2011; Igissinov et al. 2012). Intermediate rates in men (10–50/100,000) occur in South Africa, Eastern Africa, Eastern Asia, some provinces in China, and regions of Central Asia.

In all these high-risk areas, squamous cell carcinoma (SqCC) is the predominant histological type. Ethnic factors are suggested by the fact that populations at higher risk in Central Asia are of Turkish or Mongolian origin. Generally, rates in men are two- to fourfold higher than in women, although men and women have comparable rates in the very high-risk populations. In many high-risk areas, a decrease in the incidence of SqCC of the oesophagus has occurred during recent decades. In northern Europeans and white people in the United States, an increase in incidence was largely observed for adenocarcinoma of the lower oesophagus.

Tobacco smoking and alcohol drinking account for 90 per cent or more of the cases of oesophageal SqCC in Western Europe and North America. However, this proportion is lower in developing countries, particularly in selected high-risk areas of Asia and South America. In a large case–control study in China, both tobacco smoking and alcohol drinking accounted for only 40 per cent of SqCC cases (Wu et al. 2011a).

The risk in heavy smokers relative to non-smokers is on the order of 5–10 in the Western populations. However, the RR estimate is much lower in the Asian populations. A recent large case–control study in Jiangsu, China reported that for individuals smoking more than 30 pack-years, the adjusted OR was 1.85 (1.49–2.29) (Wu et al. 2011b). A strong relationship has been shown for the duration of smoking and average consumption. Quitting smoking substantially reduces the risk: the RR declines within 5 years after quitting, remains substantially elevated at least 10 years after cessation, and declines by 40 per cent thereafter (Bosetti et al. 2006; Wu et al. 2011b). Thus, cessation of smoking could have an appreciable impact in reducing SqCC oesophageal cancer, and represents an obvious priority for prevention and public health purposes. Smoking black tobacco, high-tar, and hand-rolled cigarettes, as well as pipes, might exert a stronger effect than smoking other products. Chewing tobacco represents an important risk factor in India and southern Africa, but its role has not been confirmed in central Asia. In the latter region, smoking and eating opium may be (or may have been in the past) a reason for the high incidence rates (Shakeri et al. 2012). Snuff use has also been related to an excess risk of oesophageal cancer, with RR of 3.5 for SqCC in a Swedish cohort study based on ten non-smoking cases (Zendehdel et al. 2008; Lee 2011).

Areca nut chewing has been reported as an independent risk factor for SqCC in Asia and it may have additive interactions with tobacco smoking on the risk of the disease. Carcinogenic nitrosamines derived from areca nut are formed in the saliva of chewers and have been suggested as a risk factor for oral cancer and oesophageal cancer (Akhtar 2013).

In a meta-analysis of 40 case–control and 13 cohort studies, the pooled RRs for oesophageal SqCC were 1.38 for light drinking (< 12.5 g/day), 2.62 for 12.5–50 g/day, and 5.54 for greater than 50 g/day. Among never smokers, there was no association for light drinkers, but the RR rose to 3.1 for heavy drinkers. The association with alcohol might be modified by genetic factors such as aldehyde dehydrogenase 2 (ALDH2) polymorphisms in Asian populations (Islami et al. 2011; Wu et al. 2013). It is unclear whether there are differences in the carcinogenic potency of different alcoholic beverages, but the most common beverage in each population is the most strongly related one. A reduction in the excess risk of oesophageal SqCC is suggested 15–20 years after quitting. Furthermore, the effect of alcohol is independent from the effect of tobacco, and the interaction between the two exposures fits a multiplicative or additive model (Wu et al. 2011b).

Familial aggregation of oesophageal cancer has been occasionally shown, with joint segregation of a gene responsible for keratosis palmaris et plantaris (tylosis). Studies of families without the tylosis gene have not provided evidence of an important role of other high-penetrance genetic susceptibility factors in oesophageal cancer. However, recent GWAS studies in Chinese and Japanese populations implicate certain low-penetrance genes in oesophageal cancer development. Reported genes encoded enzymes involved in the metabolism of alcohol or tobacco, DNA damage repair, and other carcinogenesis pathways (Cui et al. 2009; Wang et al. 2010; Wu et al. 2011).

Other active carcinogens might be mycotoxins or N-nitroso compounds. Mycotoxins, including fumonosin B1, have also been detected in mouldy corn from high-risk areas in China and southern Africa. In addition, in Japan, eating bracken fern has been associated with an elevated oesophageal cancer risk. The elucidation of dietary factors implicated in oesophageal carcinogenesis, in particular the possible role of mycotoxins and N-nitroso compounds (including endogenously formed nitrosamines), would represent an important step in the understanding and prevention of this disease. Oesophageal cancer is related to ionizing radiation, in particular in women irradiated for breast cancer.

Reduced intake of fresh fruits and vegetables also appears to represent a risk factor for oesophageal cancer. A similar effect has been suggested for low intake of fish, and high intake of red and processed meat. In general, a dietary pattern rich in foods from animal origin and poor in vitamins and fibre appears to increase oesophageal cancer risk (Bravi et al. 2012). The available data do not, however, allow us to establish the potentially preventive role of specific micronutrients from fruits and vegetables, and the results of most chemo-preventive trials with retinol, riboflavin, vitamin E, zinc and selenium have failed to show a benefit.

Patients suffering from Plummer–Vinson syndrome, a sideropenic dysphagia due to deficit of iron, riboflavin, and other vitamins, had an increased incidence of hypopharyngeal and oesophageal cancers. Oesophageal cancer risk is also increased among coeliac disease patients, possibly because of nutritional deficiencies. Subjects with a family history of oesophageal cancer have about threefold excess risk after adjustment for tobacco and alcohol, and the RR rose to over 100-fold in heavy drinkers and smokers with positive family history in first-degree relatives (Garavello et al. 2005).

Adenocarcinoma occurs in the lower third of the oesophagus. Its incidence has sharply increased in the last four decades in most Western countries and has largely affected white people and high social class individuals. Barrett's oesophagus, a columnar metaplasia of the epithelium, is strongly associated with the subsequent development of adenocarcinoma. The main risk factor for Barrett's oesophagus and oesophageal adenocarcinoma is persistent reflux oesophagitis. It is predominantly seen in countries such as the United States or Scotland.

Overweight, obesity, lack of physical activity, and gastro-oesophageal reflux are featured risk factors in adenocarcinoma. In a meta-analysis of 22 studies (Turati et al. 2013b) compared with normal weight individuals, the pooled RR was 1.7 for overweight (body mass index (BMI) 25–30) and 2.3 for obese ones (BMI > 30). The increased prevalence of overweight and inactivity in North America and northern Europe may partly or largely, explain the increased frequency of adenocarcinoma (La Vecchia et al. 2002; Buas and Vaughan 2013).

Tobacco smoking has also shown a consistent association with oesophageal adenocarcinoma. The pooled RR from a meta-analysis of 33 studies was 1.8 for ever smokers and 2.36 for current smokers (Tramacere et al. 2011; Buas and Vaughan 2013). In contrast, there is no material association between alcohol drinking and oesophageal adenocarcinoma (Tramacere et al. 2012). Epidemiological evidence suggests a protective role for high intake of fruits and vegetables and an unfavourable role for intake of salty food.

Prevention of oesophageal cancer

Avoidance of tobacco smoking and elevated alcohol drinking remains the main preventive approach in reducing the burden of oesophageal SqCC in Western populations. Improved diet, in particular increased consumption of fresh fruits and vegetables, might also contribute to prevention. Avoidance of tobacco, control of obesity, increased physical activity, and treatment of reflux are considered the main issues for the prevention of oesophageal adenocarcinoma. Incomplete understanding of the role of other factors complicates the elaboration of preventive strategies in many high-risk regions, although decreasing intake of extremely hot drinks and slowing down eating speed might be important (Wu et al. 2011a).

Cancer of the pancreas

The great majority of malignant neoplasms of the pancreas are adenocarcinomas which originate from the exocrine portion secreting digestive enzymes. Rare pancreatic neoplasms include tumours (of uncertain clinical behaviour) of the endocrine portion, which secrete insulin and glucagon, as well as lymphomas and sarcomas.

Geographical and temporal variations exist in the sensitivity and specificity of clinical diagnosis and in the proportion of histological verification of pancreatic cancer cases. Even when comparing populations living in the same place at the same time (e.g. different social classes or age groups), differential access to healthcare might affect incidence and mortality data.

The median of 5-year survival was 5.2 per cent with a range of 2.2–9.6 per cent in countries with different economic status (ACS 2011b). Given its very poor survival, mortality rates closely parallel incidence rates. Rates are about 50 per cent higher in men than in women. An increase in incidence and mortality has taken place since the 1970s, particularly in Europe, that can be attributed in part to diagnostic improvements. However, incidence and mortality have levelled off and declined over recent years in men in the United States, Canada and United Kingdom (Levi et al. 2003; Ferlay et al. 2010; Malvezzi et al. 2013).

The disease accounts for an estimated 337,000 new cases in 2012, 55 per cent of which (187,000) occurred in more developed regions (GLOBOCAN 2012: Ferlay et al. 2013) where the highest rates are recorded among black people in the United States (about 16.9/100,000 in men and 13.9/100,000 in women) and European countries. The lowest rates, which may suffer from under-diagnosis, are recorded in South-Central Asia and Middle and Eastern Africa (below 2/100,000 in men and 1/100,000 in women). In the United States, the ratios of incidence of black versus white people were 1.26 and 1.36 for men and women, respectively (ACS 2013).

Urban populations have higher rates than rural ones, but this may again reflect differences in quality of diagnosis. Migrant population studies suggest that first-generation migrants from low- to high-risk areas experience, after 15 or 20 years, rates that are even higher than those of the country of migration, suggesting an important role of environmental exposures occurring late in life (Anderson 2006).

The best known risk factor for pancreatic cancer is tobacco smoking. The risk in smokers is two- to threefold higher than that in non-smokers, and a dose–response relationship and a favourable effect of quitting smoking have been shown in many populations. It has been estimated that 20–30 per cent and 10 per cent of cases relating to pancreatic cancer in men and women are attributable to tobacco smoking (IARC 2004a; Iodice et al. 2008).

Some of the features of the descriptive epidemiology of pancreatic cancer (that is, a high incidence among black people in the United States as compared to a low incidence in Africa, and a higher risk among men and urban residents) can be explained by differences in smoking habits.

Several medical conditions have been studied with respect to their associations with subsequent risk of pancreatic cancer. A history of pancreatitis increases the risk more than tenfold, with little difference between the alcoholic and non-alcoholic forms of the disease. An increased risk has also been shown in several studies of diabetic patients; the RR is likely to fall in the range of 1.5–2 and is higher in the short term after diagnosis of diabetes. Gastrectomy patients are at a two- to threefold increased risk of pancreatic cancer; the association does not appear to be confounded by tobacco smoking.

A familial history of cancer of the pancreas is present in 8–10 per cent of patients, suggesting a possible role for genetic factors. Specific hereditary conditions carrying an increased risk of pancreatic cancer include the Li–Fraumeni syndrome, hereditary non-polyposis colon cancer, and a group of rare hereditary pancreatitis that involve deficiency in enzyme metabolism: these conditions, however, explain only a small proportion of cases in the general population.

Although there were six GWAS conducted on pancreatic cancer (four on Caucasians, one on Japanese, and one on Chinese), results were rather inconsistent and may need further confirmation (Amundadottir et al. 2009; Diergaarde et al. 2010; Low et al. 2010; Petersen et al. 2010; Willis et al. 2012; Wu et al. 2012a). Interestingly, one recent GWAS has identified genetic variation at the 11p15.4 region (*SBF2*) to be associated with overall survival in patients with pancreatic adenocarcinoma in both European and Asian populations (Wu et al. 2012b).

Studies have reported on the significant association between alcohol and pancreatic cancer; however, not all have addressed it. The current evidence suggests a possible weak effect of heavy alcohol drinking, but the evidence is not sufficient (Lucenteforte et al. 2012).

Nutritional and dietary factors have been suggested to be related to pancreatic cancer, including obesity and low physical activity, low intake of foods containing folate, red meat and a low intake of vegetables and fruit (WCRF and AICR 2007). The issue of nutrition, diet, and pancreatic cancer remains, however, largely undefined. Early reports of an association between coffee consumption and pancreatic cancer risk have not been confirmed by larger, more recent investigations (WCRF and AICR 2007). There is no effective cure for pancreatic cancer, with the exception of surgery for a small number of patients. Screening methods are not available. Primary prevention is the only available tool for this disease: avoidance of smoking is the major practicable way for reducing the number of cases. Control of obesity may be another potential preventive measure.

Head and neck cancer (cancers of oral cavity, pharynx, and larynx)

Tumours of the oral cavity, pharynx, and larynx are defined as a group named head and neck cancer because of shared histology (the majority are squamous cell carcinoma) and aetiological factors (tobacco smoking and alcohol drinking). However, tumours of the lip, naso-pharynx, and salivary glands have distinct aetiological factors. We will focus our discussion on head and neck cancer in this section.

There were an estimated 600,000 new cases of cancers of the head and neck worldwide in 2012. The estimated number of deaths was 325,000 (GLOBOCAN 2012: Ferlay et al. 2013).

Cancer of the oral cavity, oropharynx, and hypo-pharynx

The incidence of cancers of the oral cavity varies over 20-fold between high-risk areas (e.g. Papua New Guinea, Maldives, Sri Lanka, Pakistan, Bangladesh, and India) and low-risk areas (e.g. China, Vietnam, Korea, and Haiti) (GLOBOCAN 2012: Ferlay et al. 2013). In all populations, rates in the oral cavity and pharynx in men exceed those in women by a factor of 2–8. Incidence rates of both sites increased in Europe and the Americas until the late 1980s and have levelled off or declined in most countries over the last decade. When looking at subsites within the oral cavity and the pharynx, cancer of the oropharynx and hypo-pharynx account for as many or more cases than cancer of the oral cavity in high-risk European populations. Cancers of the tongue, floor of the mouth, and other parts of the oral cavity represent the majority of cases in India and the United States.

Tobacco and alcohol are the most important risk factors for cancer of the oral cavity and pharynx. In Western populations, smoking represents the main use of tobacco, and the RRs of oral cancer among smokers compared to non-smokers are on the order of 3–10. The risk is higher for heavy smokers, long-term smokers, and smokers of black tobacco or high-tar cigarettes. Cigar and pipe smoking also poses a risk, while stopping smoking is followed by a decrease in risk. In India, chewing tobacco is the main risk factor for oral cancer, although *bidi* and cigarette smoking also contribute to the risk. In the United States and Europe, use of smokeless tobacco has also been implicated in the development of oral cancer (Boffetta et al. 2008).

Consumption of alcoholic beverages increases the risk of oral and pharyngeal cancer (Baan et al. 2007; Goldstein et al. 2010). Relative to abstainers and light drinkers, the RR in heavy drinkers is on the order of 10. The effects of tobacco smoking and alcohol drinking are multiplicative or larger; that is, the effect of exposure to both is close to or greater than the product of their individual effects. The combined effect of tobacco smoking and alcohol drinking accounts for almost 80 per cent of cancers of the oral cavity and pharynx in the West. Similarly, tobacco chewing and smoking and their combination are responsible for a large proportion of these cancers in India.

With reference to alcohol drinking, additional issues are worth discussing. First, oral cancer risks show a clear decline after stopping smoking. The pattern of risk after stopping drinking remains unclear, though it appears that an appreciable excess risk persists for several years. Second, although ethanol is the main carcinogenic ingredient in alcoholic beverages, it remains unclear whether different types of alcohol beverages have different influences on oral carcinogenesis. For example, spirits may be associated with higher risks than beer or wine (Boffetta and Hashibe 2006; Baan et al. 2007). This could explain some of the exceedingly high rates in countries like Hungary or Slovakia, where fruit-derived hard spirits are commonly consumed.

Human papilloma virus (HPV) DNA, detected in pre-neoplastic and neoplastic lesions of the oropharynx, is associated with over a 100-fold excess risk of oropharyngeal cancer (IARC 2007). The association is less strong for cancer of the oral cavity and is suspected as an aetiological factor for cancer of the hypo-pharynx. The role of HPV in head and neck cancer has become increasingly important since the 1990s in Europe and North America, mainly because of changes in sexual practices, while it remains less important in other regions of the world. The role of other oral cancer risk factors, as well as diagnosis and disease management, is smaller than that of tobacco or alcohol, and remains largely undefined. For example, dietary and nutritional factors, such as fruit and vegetable consumption, have shown a protective effect on oral cancer risk. Moreover, earlier diagnosis and improved treatment on oral cancer survival may have favourably influenced oral cancer death rates over time.

Poor oral hygiene and ill-fitting dentures are likely additional risk factors for oral cancer. Several occupations have been sporadically reported to confer an increased risk of oral and pharyngeal cancer. The evidence is consistent only for employment as a waiter and/or bartender, probably reflecting an increased consumption of alcohol and exposure to environmental tobacco smoke (ETS).

The role of genetic susceptibility in oral carcinogenesis is probably modest. High-risk families have been reported only occasionally. However, a role is likely for low-penetrance factors, such as increased sensitivity to mutagens and genetic polymorphisms of enzymes implicated in the metabolism of alcohol (alcohol dehydrogenase and aldehyde dehydrogenase) (Lewis and Smith 2005). GWAS in Caucasian populations have identified five variants, including three variants located within the alcohol dehydrogenase genes (*ADH7*, *ADH1B*, and *ADH1C*), one 4q21 variant located near DNA repair genes *HEL308* and *FAM175A*, and one 12q24 variant located near the *ALDH2* gene to be associated with head and neck cancer (Mckay et al. 2011). One GWAS with limited sample size conducted in an Indian population on chewing tobacco-related oral cancers did not identify any variant which reached genome-wide significance level (Bhatnagar et al. 2012). GWAS on head and neck cancer are relatively limited and replication studies in populations other than Caucasians are needed.

Prevention of oral and pharyngeal cancers

Avoidance of tobacco (smoking, chewing and snuffing) and avoidance of excessive alcohol drinking represent the main preventive measures for cancers of the oral cavity and pharynx. Primary prevention through prophylactic HPV vaccination is promising and would involve both girls and boys (Kreimer 2014). It is unclear whether additional benefits might be obtained from an increase in fruit and vegetable intake and improvement of oral hygiene. Avoidance of excessive exposure to solar radiation would represent the main preventive approach for lip cancer. In populations at high risk of nasopharyngeal cancer from China and possibly other countries, avoidance of salted fish and other preserved food, in particular as weaning food, should be recommended.

Oral inspection aimed to identify pre-neoplastic lesions might be an effective approach for secondary prevention of oral cancer. The inspection can be performed by medically certified professionals, but also, in particular in high-risk areas from developing countries, such as India, by specifically trained health workers. A large-scale preventive trial demonstrated a reduction in oral cancer mortality during its 15-year follow-up, with larger reductions in those adhering to repeated rounds of screening (Sankaranarayanan et al. 2013).

Cancer of the larynx

More than 90 per cent of cancers of the larynx are squamous cell carcinomas; the majority originate from the supraglottic and glottic regions of the organs. The incidence in men is high (10/100,000 or more) in Cuba, Armenia, Hungary, Kazakhstan, Romania, Bulgaria and Moldova, while the lowest rates (< 1/100,000) are recorded in Benin, Burkina Faso, Cote d'Ivoire, Ethiopia, Guinea-Bisseau, and Haiti. The incidence in women is ≤ 1/100,000 in most populations. In most high-income countries, rates have declined in men over the last two decades. An estimated 157,000 new cases occurred worldwide in 2012, of which 88 per cent occurred among men (GLOBOCAN 2012: Ferlay et al. 2013). In addition, laryngeal cancer accounted for about 83,000 deaths.

Up to 80 per cent of cases of laryngeal cancer in high-income countries are attributable to tobacco smoking, alcohol drinking, and the interaction between the two factors (Olshan, 2006). The effect of tobacco, with risks in smokers on the order of 10 relative to non-smokers, seems to be stronger for glottic than supraglottic neoplasms. Studies in several populations have shown a dose–response relationship and a beneficial effect of quitting smoking (Pelucchi et al. 2008). Smoking black-tobacco cigarettes confers a stronger risk than smoking blond-tobacco cigarettes. Studies from India have also reported an effect of chewing tobacco-containing products. The effect of alcohol is stronger for supraglottic tumours than for tumours at other sites. It is not clear, however, whether different alcoholic beverages exert a different carcinogenic effect.

There are suggestions of a protective effect exerted by a high intake of fruits and vegetables, although the evidence is not conclusive and the data regarding specific micronutrients, such as carotenoids and vitamin C, are inadequate. Data concerning a possible effect of other foods are not consistent.

Occupational exposure to mists of strong inorganic acids, in particular of sulphuric acid, is an established risk factor for laryngeal cancer. An increased risk following inhalation of asbestos fibres is plausible. A possible effect has been suggested for other occupational exposures, including nickel and ionizing radiation, but the evidence is not conclusive.

An aetiological role of HPV infection in laryngeal cancer has been suggested. First, laryngeal papillomatosis, a condition characterized by multiple benign papillomas caused by infection with HPV types 6 and 11, confers an increased risk of laryngeal cancer. Second, a meta-analysis of studies assessing the presence of HPV DNA reported strong associations between HPV infection and laryngeal squamous cell carcinoma, with a summary odds ratio (OR) of 5.39 (95 per cent confidence interval (CI) 3.25–8.94). A similar association was observed for HPV-16 (OR 6.07; 95 per cent CI 3.44–10.70) (Li et al. 2013).

There is no evidence of strong genetic factors in laryngeal carcinogenesis. However, polymorphisms for enzymes implicated in the metabolism of alcohol and tobacco and DNA repair might represent susceptibility factors (Lewis and Smith 2005; McKay et al. 2011).

Survival from laryngeal cancer is fair. Five-year survival rates are on the order of 65 per cent in high-income countries and 40 per cent in developing countries (Ellis et al. 2012). These patients are at very high risk of developing a second primary tumour in the oral cavity, pharynx, and lung. While shared risk factors are likely to play an important role, it is plausible that host factors are also partially responsible. For example, an increased sensitivity to mutagens has been shown in lymphocytes of laryngeal cancer patients, in particular those with multiple tumours, as compared to controls. A report indicated that p53-related genes are related to susceptibility of second primary cancer in patients with primary head and neck cancer (Jin et al. 2013)

Control of tobacco smoking and excessive alcohol drinking, possibly together with an increased intake of fruits and vegetables, would prevent the majority of cases of laryngeal cancer in most populations. Control of exposure to known and suspected occupational carcinogens is an additional measure for exposed workers. Prophylactic HPV vaccination is promising (Kreimer 2014). No screening methods are currently available for laryngeal cancer.

Prostate cancer

Prostate cancer is the second most common cancer and the fifth leading cause of death from cancer in men worldwide with an estimated 1,111,000 newly diagnosed cases and 307,000 deaths in 2012 (GLOBOCAN 2012: Ferlay et al. 2013). Almost 70 per cent of the cases (759,000) occurred in more developed regions. It is the most common malignant neoplasm in men from Australia/New Zealand (111.6/100,000), North America (97.2/100,000), and Western Europe (94.9/100,000). The incidence is 69.5/100,000 in high-income regions and 14.5/100,000 in low- and middle-income regions. The rates remain the lowest in South-Central Asia (4.5) and Eastern Asia (10.5) (GLOBOCAN 2012: Ferlay et al. 2013). Mortality rates of prostate cancer show less variability among regions, suggesting that the number of non-fatal cases diagnosed in different countries varies depending on screening and other diagnostic procedures.

The incidence of prostate cancer is highly dependent on the adoption of prostate-specific antigen (PSA) testing. Prostate cancer incidence has shown substantial changes following the introduction of PSA testing, with major increases due to the detection of large number of prevalent cases, followed by substantial declines. The changes in trends have been much smaller for mortality, but both in the United States and in Western Europe, peak rates were observed in the early 1990s, with a levelling off and a decline thereafter, approaching 20 per cent in the EU (Bosetti et al. 2011).

The recent trends in prostate cancer mortality in Europe are consistent with a favourable impact of improved diagnosis, as well as of advances in therapy, on prostate cancer mortality in Western Europe and North America (Bosetti et al. 2011).

Prospective studies failed to provide convincing evidence of an increased risk linked to increased level of testosterone or other sexual hormones. Similarly, an increased risk of prostate cancer was reported in retrospective studies following a history of benign prostatic hypertrophy, but no excess risk was found in prospective studies. If an association exists between prostatic hypertrophy and cancer, it can be due to shared aetiological factors or to a common pathological process.

Carriers of *BRCA1* and *BRCA2* mutations have a four- to fivefold increased risk of prostate cancer with especially a two- to threefold increased risk of developing the same neoplasm in first-degree relatives. It is also similarly identified in small magnitudes in breast and colon cancers. Genetic variants entailing an increased risk of prostate cancer have been identified within the 8q24 and possibly the 17q12 region (Amundadottir et al. 2006; Gudmundsson et al. 2007; Haiman et al. 2007; Yeager et al. 2007). This was also confirmed recently, in over 20 GWAS studies, including chromosome 3, 7, 17, 22, and X, and explains 13 per cent of the total genetic variance of prostate cancer risk (Kim et al. 2010; Chen et al. 2013). Although the majority of the studies were conducted in European descendants, the 8q24 region continues to be the most implicated region in prostate cancer risk in other race/ethnic groups, including Japanese, Latinos, Chinese, and African American (Takata et al. 2010; Ishak and Giri 2011; Cheng et al. 2012; Xu et al. 2012).

It has been suggested that the risk of the disease increases with number of sexual partners and number of encounters with prostitutes, and with a previous history of syphilis and gonorrhoea. Serological studies of HPV 16 and HPV 18 have shown an increased risk among positive subjects, but the findings are inconsistent. It is not clear at present, however, whether syphilis and HPV are causal factors or markers of infection with sexually transmitted agents, and hence general markers of inflammation.

A possible protective role of high intake of vegetables has been suggested in a few studies; high intake of meat, dairy products, total fat, and saturated fat might represent a risk factor. The evidence concerning other dietary factors, including fruit intake and intake of specific micronutrients, is, however, largely inconclusive at present. These include lycopene, a retinoid present in particular in tomatoes which has been found to be associated with a reduced risk in a few (but not other) studies, and calcium which has been associated with an elevated risk, possibly on account of its influence on vitamin D balance. There is, in fact, biological evidence that the most active form of vitamin D, 25(OH) D, has a favourable role on prostate cancer, but epidemiological data are inconsistent (Giovannucci 2005; Gilbert et al. 2011). Vitamin D may prevent prostate cancer progression, and hence the most aggressive forms of the disease (Li et al. 2007), and there is also an observation by a meta-analysis that an increased risk exists among individuals with elevated serum level of insulin-like growth factor 1 (Chen et al. 2009). An increased risk of the advanced prostate cancer has been reported among subjects with a high BMI (Platz and Giovannucci 2006; Discacciati et al. 2012). Data on nutrition, diet, and prostate cancer are, however, largely inconsistent.

The wide geographical variability of prostate cancer suggests that environmental factors likely related to diet and other lifestyle factors, such as physical activity, are important determinants of the disease. Primary prevention, however, is hampered by the fragmentary knowledge of its precise causes. Secondary prevention has been proposed, based on measurement of PSA and digital rectal examination. There is little evidence from controlled trials that either procedure decreases the mortality from prostate cancer (Boyle and Brawley 2009; Welch and Albertsen 2009). Despite this lack of evidence, these procedures, in particular the PSA testing, have gained popularity in many countries, and are the cause of the steep increase in number of diagnosed cases since the mid 1980s in North America and other high-income countries. It is unclear how much of the decrease in mortality reported since the mid 1990s in the United States and in Western Europe can be attributed to a beneficial effect of (unplanned) use of PSA testing, but it is likely due mainly to improved management and treatment of the disease, including better surgery, radiotherapy

and medical therapy. The United States Preventative Services Task Force (USPSTF) made a final recommendation against PSA based screening for healthy men because there is 'moderate or high certainty that the service has no benefit or that the harms outweigh the benefits'. The USPSTF issued a Grade D to discourage the use of the test by men of all ages for screening purpose.

Cancer of the uterine cervix

The estimated worldwide burden of cervical cancer in 2012 was approximately 528,000 new cases and 266,000 deaths (GLOBOCAN 2012: Ferlay et al. 2013). Cervical cancer is a major public health problem in less developed regions, where about 84 per cent of cases (445,000) and 86 per cent of deaths (230,000) occurred in 2012. The number of estimated cervical cancer deaths in these regions is third to breast cancer (324,000) and lung cancer (281,000) among women (Ferlay et al. 2013). Incidence rates are high (over 30/100,000) in Eastern, Southern, and Middle Africa and Melanesia. Rates are lowest in Australia/New Zealand (5.5), Western Asia (4.4), Middle-East (6.4), Northern American (6.6), and Northern Africa (6.6). Incidence and mortality rates have decreased steadily in high-income countries, but an upturn in incidence had been observed among young women in a few of these. Few data on temporal trends are available from middle- and low-income countries, but incidence has likely decreased during recent decades in those areas of the world, too. In high-income countries, rates increase up to age 60, while in middle and low-income countries there is little increase above age 50. Cervical cancer hits preferentially women of lower education and social class.

Most cervical cancers originate from the area of squamous metaplasia called the transformation zone, which is adjacent to the junction between the columnar epithelium of endometrial origin and the characterizing epithelium of vaginal origin. Most invasive cancers are SqCC or mixed adeno-squamous tumours. Invasive carcinoma is preceded by inflammatory and condylomatous atypia, mild dysplasia (also called cervical intraepithelial neoplasia of grade 1, or CIN 1), moderate dysplasia (CIN 2), severe dysplasia and carcinoma *in situ* (CIN 3) (Schiffman and Hildesheim 2006).

Chronic infection with HPV is a necessary cause of cervical cancer. Using sensitive molecular techniques, virtually all tumours are positive for the HPV (Clifford et al. 2005). Different types of HPV exist, and those associated with cervical cancer are mainly types 16, 18, 31, 45, and 58 where HPV 16 is the main cervical carcinogen in most populations, while the distribution of other types varies by geographical region (Fig. 8.2.2). The host response to HPV infection is important in determining its carcinogenic effect; immunosuppression, as present in transplanted patients and HIV infected women, increases the risk of dysplasia, carcinoma *in situ*, and invasive neoplasms.

Sexual histories of women (early age at first intercourse and increased number of sexual partners) and of their male partners (high number of sexual partners, presence of genital diseases, and contact with prostitutes) are risk factors for cervical cancer in many populations. They reflect an increased likelihood of HPV infection, as well as the duration of HPV infection. As for most carcinogens, in fact, duration of exposure is the major determinant of subsequent cancer risk (Plummer et al. 2012).

Tobacco smoking has also an independent effect on cervical carcinogenesis with a RR of 1.5–1.6 for current smokers, also

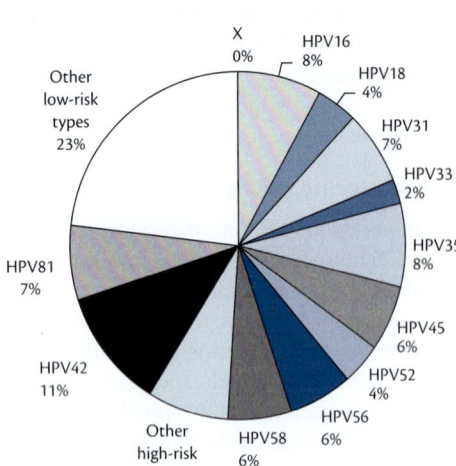

Sub-Saharan Africa (319 infections)

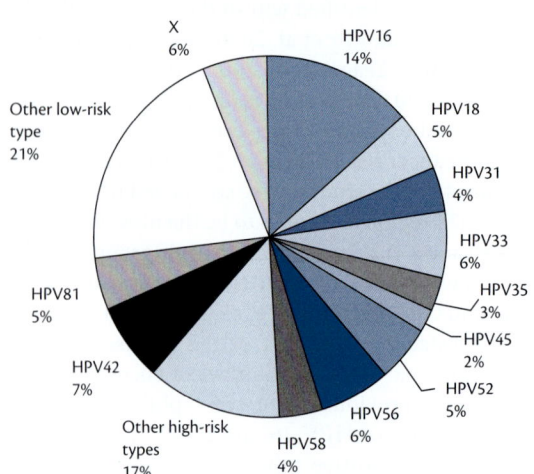

Asia (669 infections)

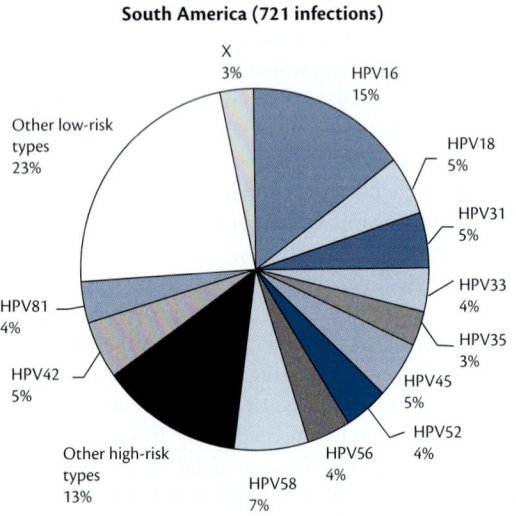

South America (721 infections)

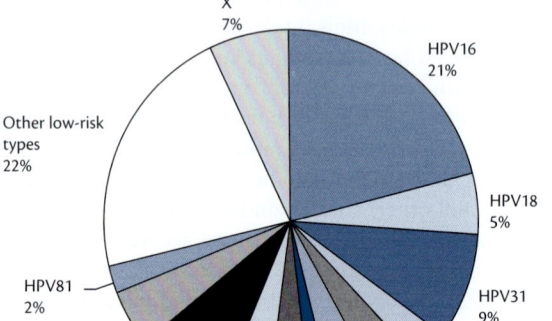

Europe (294 infections)

Fig. 8.2.2 Most common HPV types in 14,097 cases of invasive cervical cancer by region.

Reprinted from *The Lancet*, Volume 366, Issue 9490, Clifford, G.M. et al. Worldwide distribution of human papillomavirus types in cytologically normal women in the International Agency for Research on Cancer HPV prevalence surveys: a pooled analysis, pp. 991–998, Copyright © 2005, with permission from Elsevier, http://www.sciencedirect.com/science/journal/01406736.

once HPV infection is taken into account (IARC 2004a; Moralejo 2009). A possible protective effect of a diet rich in fruits and vegetables has been suggested in a few studies, but the role of diet on cervical cancer risk is probably modest and largely undefined.

Cytological examination of exfoliated cervical cells (the Papanicolaou smear, Pap test) is effective in identifying precursor lesions, resulting in a substantial decrease in incidence of and mortality from invasive cancer. Cytological smears are not largely applicable, however, in countries with limited availability of cytologists and pathologists, including many countries with a high prevalence of HPV infection and high incidence of invasive cancer. Alternative approaches for secondary prevention have therefore been proposed, including visual inspection of the cervix with possible enhancement of precursor lesions by acetic acid (VIA). VIA performs as well as the Pap test in terms of sensitivity and specificity and can be used in low-income areas (Bradford and

Goodman 2013). Use of HPV-DNA testing appears now, however, to be more specific and sensitive than the Pap test, and is, therefore, likely to replace the Pap smear as the first screening method in the near future. The primary method for prevention of cervical cancer for future generations, however, is likely to become HPV vaccination. One vaccine against HPV 16, 18 (as well as 6 and 11, linked to genital warts) is now available, and another against HPV 16 and 18 only (FUTURE II Study Group 2007). Vaccines including larger numbers of HPV strains (i.e. eight strains) are in the late stage of testing. The final impact of the effect of such vaccination is complicated by the geographical variations in the distribution of HPV types. In addition, smoking cessation may play a role since tobacco smoking is an independent aetiological factor of cervical cancer.

Studies of infection with other agents, in particular *Chlamydia* and herpes simplex 2, have failed to provide consistent evidence of an effect independent from HPV. An increased risk, on the order of twofold, has been detected among long-term current or recent users of OC, which is not completely explained by sexual behaviour or HPV infection. However, there is no residual association 5–10 years after stopping OC use. Consequently, the public health implications of OC use on cervical cancer risk are limited in time (La Vecchia and Bosetti 2003; Cibula et al. 2010). Condom and (perhaps) diaphragm use, on the other hand, exert a protective effect, possibly via prevention of HPV infection.

GWAS identified multiple loci within the MHC region at 6p21.3 to be associated with cervical cancer, indicating the importance of impaired immune response in cervical cancer development (Chen et al. 2013; Shi et al. 2013).

Principles of primary and secondary cancer prevention

Primary prevention

Many determinants of malignant neoplasms, including UV radiation, ionizing radiation, tobacco smoking, alcohol drinking, overweight, a number of viruses and parasites, and a number of chemicals, industrial processes and occupational exposures, are sufficiently well established to constitute logical priorities for preventive action. Two more reasons add weight to this priority: some of the agents are responsible for sizeable proportions of the cancers occurring today, and for many agents it is, in principle, feasible to reduce or even to completely eliminate exposure. If this is taken as the objective of preventive action, some practical points are helpful in guiding such action.

First, although epidemiological data in most cases do not allow a direct estimate of the risk of cancer at low doses, it is reasonable (at least from a preventive point of view) to assume that the dose (exposure)–risk relationships for agents acting through damage to DNA are linear with no threshold (Peto et al. 1991). Second, the carcinogenic effect is not equally dependent on the dose rate (dose per unit of time) and on duration of exposure. For example, in regular smokers, the incidence rate of lung cancer depends more strongly on duration of exposure, increasing with the fourth power of it, than on dose rate, increasing only with the first or second power of it.

Furthermore, as illustrated earlier, the carcinogenic process may be represented as a succession of stages, taking place in the time span from first exposure to a carcinogenic agent to the appearance of clinical cancer. In its simplest form, as first brought out in mouse skin carcinogenesis experiments, the multistage process reduces to two stages: an irreversible 'initiation' stage inducing malignant cells, and a 'promotion' stage which propagates these cells into a malignant growth. A third stage of 'progression', characterized by an increased rate of growth and metastases, as well as an increase in chromosomal changes in the cell, has also been observed. Formal statistical multistage models of carcinogenesis have provided a useful framework to interpret on a common basis of (postulated) mechanisms both experimental and epidemiological observations. As the stages are assumed to occur in a specific sequence, some may be described as 'early' and some as 'late'. Epidemiological observations indicate that, for example, smoking has both an early stage effect, as indicated by the existence of a minimum interval of several years before an increase in risk of lung cancer becomes manifest, and a late stage effect, as indicated by the decrease in risk (with respect to continuous smokers) soon after stopping smoking.

Cancer prevention strategies have evolved from a predominant environmental and lifestyle approach to a model that matches individual-oriented actions with public health interventions. Advances in identifying, developing, and testing agents with the potential either to prevent cancer initiation, or to inhibit or reverse the progression of initiated lesions support this approach. Encouraging laboratory and epidemiological studies, along with studies of secondary end points in prevention trials, have provided a scientific rationale for the hypothesis. Promising results have been reported for various types of cancer, in particular among high-risk individuals (Greenwald 2005; Dunn and Greenwald 2010).

Secondary and chemoprevention

Given the limitations still constraining the primary prevention of many cancers, early detection needs to be considered as a secondary and alternative option, based on the reasonable expectation that the earlier the diagnosis and the stage at which a malignancy is discovered, the better the prognosis. This implies that an effective treatment for the disease exists and that the less advanced the cancer at the pre-clinical stage, the better the scope for treatment, and the better the prognosis. This latter aspect cannot be taken for granted.

Before a screening programme can be adopted on a large scale, a number of other requirements need to be fulfilled. First of all, a screening test (that is, a relatively simple and rapid test aimed at the presumptive identification of pre-clinical disease) must be available that is capable of correctly identifying cases and non-cases. In other words, both sensitivity and specificity should be high, approaching 100 per cent. While high sensitivity is obviously important, given that the very purpose of screening is to pick up, if possible, all cases of a cancer in its detectable pre-clinical phase, it is specificity that plays a dominant role in the practical utilization of the test within a defined population. As the prevalence of a pre-clinical cancer to be screened in well-defined populations is often in the range of 1 to 10 per 1000, if a test is used with a specificity of 95 per cent, then 5 per cent of results will be false positives. In other words, for every case which will turn out at the diagnostic work-up to be a true cancer (assuming 100 per cent sensitivity), there will be 5–50 cases falsely identified as such and ultimately found not to be cancers. This situation is likely to prove unacceptable due to too high psychological and economic costs. One solution is an increase in specificity, for example, by developing better tests or combinations of tests, or by changing the criterion of positivity of a given test to make it more stringent (this necessarily decreases sensitivity). In addition, one might select populations with relatively high prevalence of the cancer ('high-risk' groups), so as to increase the number of the true positives. Whatever the group on which the programme operates, additional requirements are that the test is safe, easily and rapidly applicable, and acceptable in a broad sense to the population to be examined. It has also to be cheap, but what is or is not cheap is better evaluated within a cost-effectiveness analysis of different ways of preventing a cancer case or death, an issue not further discussed here.

If these requirements are met, still nothing is known about the possible net benefit in outcome deriving from the screening programme (in fact, screening test plus diagnostic work-up plus treatment, as applied in a given population). To evaluate benefit, several measures of outcome can be assessed. An early one, useful but not sufficient, is the distribution by stage of the detected cancer cases which, if the programme is ultimately to be beneficial, should be shifted to earlier, less invasive stages of the disease in comparison with the distribution of the cases discovered through ordinary medical care. A second measure of outcome is the survival of cases detected at screening compared with the survival of cases detected through ordinary medical care. This is a superficially attractive but usually equivocal criterion, to the extent that screening may only advance the time of diagnosis (and therefore the apparent survival time), without postponing the time of death ('lead time bias'). A final outcome (and the main test of the programme) is the site-specific cancer mortality in the screened population compared with the mortality in the unscreened population.

Correct, unbiased comparison of this outcome, and thus unbiased measure of the effect of the screening programme, should in principle be made within the framework of a randomized controlled trial, in which two groups of subjects are randomly allocated to the screening programme and to no screening (that is, receiving only the existing medical care system) or to two alternative screening programmes, for instance, entailing different tests or different intervals between periodical examinations. Unfortunately, largely due to pressures to adopt on a large scale screening programmes hoped to be effective, a situation has often arisen where withholding screening to a group has been regarded as unethical or socially unacceptable, thus preventing the conduct of a proper experiment. Very few randomized trials evaluating the effectiveness of screening programmes are available. Comparisons are made through non-randomized experiments or through observational studies.

In addition to lead-time bias, three types of bias are peculiar to the assessment of screening programmes. Because of self-selection, persons who elect to receive early detection may be different from those who do not: for instance, they may belong to better educated classes, be generally healthier and health conscious, and this could produce a longer survival independent of any effect of early detection. In addition, cancers with longer pre-clinical phases, which may mean less biological aggressiveness and better prognosis, are, in any case, more likely to be intercepted by a programme of periodic screening than cancers with a short pre-clinical phase, and a rapid, aggressive clinical course (length bias). Finally, because of criteria of positivity adopted to maximize yield of early cases, a number of lesions which in fact would never become malignant growths are included as 'cases', thus falsely improving the survival statistics (over-diagnosis bias) (Croswell et al. 2010).

Chemoprevention can also be considered for primary and secondary prevention of cancer, but data are negative or inconsistent for most micronutrients or other substances considered.

Conclusions

Neoplasms are a group of diverse diseases with complex distributions in human populations and with different aetiological factors. Current knowledge of the causes of human neoplasms and the development of control strategies have led to the elaboration of lists of recommendations for their prevention (Box 8.2.1).

Box 8.2.1 European Code Against Cancer (Boyle et al. 2003)

Many aspects of general health can be improved, and many cancer deaths prevented, if we adopt healthier lifestyles:

1. Do not smoke; if you smoke, stop doing so. If you fail to stop, do not smoke in the presence of non-smokers.

2. Avoid obesity.

3. Undertake some brisk, physical activity every day.

4. Increase your daily intake and variety of vegetables and fruits: eat at least five servings daily. Limit your intake of foods containing fats from animal sources.

5. If you drink alcohol, whether beer, wine, or spirits, moderate your consumption to two drinks per day if you are a man or one drink per day if you are a woman.

6. Care must be taken to avoid excessive sun exposure. It is specifically important to protect children and adolescents. For individuals who have a tendency to burn in the sun, active protective measures must be taken throughout life.

7. Apply strictly regulations aimed at preventing any exposure to known cancer-causing substances. Follow all health and safety instructions on substances which may cause cancer. Follow advice of National Radiation Protection Offices.

8. There are public health programmes that could prevent cancers developing or increase the probability that a cancer may be cured. Women from 25 years of age should participate in cervical screening. This should be within programmes with quality control procedures in compliance with *European Guidelines for Quality Assurance in Cervical Screening*.

9. Women from 50 years of age should participate in breast screening. This should be within programmes with quality control procedures in compliance with *European Guidelines for Quality Assurance in Mammography Screening*.

10. Men and women from 50 years of age should participate in colorectal screening. This should be within programmes with built-in quality assurance procedures.

11. Participate in vaccination programmes against hepatitis B virus infection.

A comprehensive strategy for cancer control might lead to the avoidance of a sizeable proportion of human cancers, and the greatest benefit can be achieved via tobacco control. However, such a strategy would imply major cultural, societal, and economic changes. More modest objectives for cancer prevention should focus on the neoplasms and the exposures that are prevalent in any given population. For example, vaccination of children against HBV is likely to be the most cost-effective cancer prevention action in many countries of Africa and Asia.

Neoplasms will continue to be a major source of human disease and death. Considerable efforts are made in the public and private domains to develop effective therapeutic approaches. Even if major discoveries in the clinical management of cancer patients will be accomplished in the near future, the changes will mainly affect the affluent part of the world population. Prevention of the known causes of cancer remains the most promising approach to reducing the consequences of cancer, in particular in countries with limited resources. Control of tobacco smoking and of smokeless tobacco products, moderation in alcohol intake, reduced overweight and obesity, increased physical activity, avoidance of exposure to solar radiation, control of known occupational carcinogens, and vaccination against known carcinogenic infectious agents are the main approaches.

References

Abnet, C.C., Freedman, N.D., Hu, N., et al. (2010). A shared susceptibility locus in PLCE1 at 10q23 for gastric adenocarcinoma and esophageal squamous cell carcinoma. *Nature Genetics*, 42, 764–7.

Akhtar, S. (2013). Areca nut chewing and esophageal squamous-cell carcinoma risk in Asians: a meta-analysis of case-control studies. *Cancer Causes and Control*, 24, 257–65.

Allemani, C., Sant, M., Weir, H.K., et al. (2013). Breast cancer survival in the US and Europe: a CONCORD high-resolution study. *International Journal of Cancer*, 132, 1170–81.

American Cancer Society (2011a). *Colorectal Cancer Facts & Figures 2011–2013*. Atlanta, GA: American Cancer Society.

American Cancer Society (2011b). *Global Cancer Facts & Figures* (2nd ed.). Atlanta, GA: American Cancer Society.

American Cancer Society (2013). *Cancer Facts & Figures for African Americans 2013–2014*. Atlanta, GA: American Cancer Society.

Amundadottir, L., Kraft, P., Stolzenberg-Solomon, R.Z., et al. (2009). Genome-wide association study identifies variants in the ABO locus associated with susceptibility to pancreatic cancer. *Nature Genetics*, 41, 986–90.

Amundadottir, L.T., Sulem, P., Gudmundsson, J., et al. (2006). A common variant associated with prostate cancer in European and African populations. *Nature Genetics*, 38, 652–8.

Anderson, K.E. (2006). Cancer of the pancreas. In D. Schottenfeld and J.F. Fraumeni (eds.) *Cancer Epidemiology and Prevention*, pp. 721–62. New York: Oxford University Press.

Arends, M.J. (2013). Pathways of colorectal carcinogenesis. *Applied Immunohistochemistry & Molecular Morphology*, 21, 97–102.

Baan, R., Straif, K., Grosse, Y., et al. (2007). Carcinogenicity of alcoholic beverages. *The Lancet Oncology*, 8, 292–3.

Bhatnagar, R., Dabholkar, J., and Saranath, D. (2012). Genome-wide disease association study in chewing tobacco associated oral cancers. *Oral Oncology*, 48, 831–5.

Blot, W.J. (1997). Vitamin/mineral supplementation and cancer risk: international chemoprevention trials. *Proceedings of the Society for Experimental Biology and Medicine*, 216, 291–6.

Boffetta, P. and Hashibe, M. (2006). Alcohol and cancer. *The Lancet Oncology*, 7, 149–56.

Boffetta, P., Hecht, S., Gray, N., Gupta, P., and Straif, K. (2008). Smokeless tobacco and cancer. *The Lancet Oncology*, 9, 667–75.

Boffetta, P. and Islami, F. (2013). The contribution of molecular epidemiology to the identification of human carcinogens: current status and future perspectives. *Annals of Oncology*, 24, 901–8.

Bosetti, C., Bertuccio, P., Chatenoud, L., Negri, E., La Vecchia, C., and Levi, F. (2011). Trends in mortality from urologic cancers in Europe, 1970–2008. *European Urology*, 60, 1–15.

Bosetti, C., Gallus, S., Garavello, W., and La Vecchia, C. (2006). Smoking cessation and the risk of oesophageal cancer: an overview of published studies. *Oral Oncology*, 42, 957–64.

Bosetti, C., Rosato, V., Gallus, S., Cuzick, J., and La Vecchia, C. (2012). Aspirin and cancer risk: a quantitative review to 2011. *Annals of Oncology*, 23, 1403–15.

Boyle, P., Autier, P., Bartelink, H., et al. (2003). European Code Against Cancer and scientific justification: third version. *Annals of Oncology*, 14, 973–1005.

Boyle, P. and Brawley, O.W. (2009). Prostate cancer: current evidence weighs against population screening. *CA: A Cancer Journal for Clinicians*, 59, 220–4.

Bradford, L. and Goodman, A. (2013). Cervical cancer screening and prevention in low-resource settings. *Clinical Obstetrics and Gynecology*, 56, 76–87.

Bravi, F., Edefonti, V., Randi, G., et al. (2012). Dietary patterns and the risk of esophageal cancer. *Annals of Oncology*, 23, 765–70.

Brenner, D.J. (2004). Radiation risks potentially associated with low-dose CT screening of adult smokers for lung cancer. *Radiology*, 231, 440–5.

Buas, M.F. and Vaughan, T.L. (2013). Epidemiology and risk factors for gastroesophageal junction tumors: understanding the rising incidence of this disease. *Seminars in Radiation Oncology*, 23, 3–9.

Chen, D., Juko-Pecirep, I., Hammer, J., et al. (2013). Genome-wide association study of susceptibility loci for cervical cancer. *Journal of the National Cancer Institute*, 105, 624–33.

Chen, R., Ren, S., and Sun, Y. (2013). Genome-wide association studies on prostate cancer: the end or the beginning? *Protein & Cell*, 4(9), 677–86.

Chen, W., Wang, S., Tian, T., et al. (2009). Phenotypes and genotypes of insulin-like growth factor 1, IGF-binding protein-3 and cancer risk: evidence from 96 studies. *European Journal of Human Genetics*, 17, 1668–75.

Cheng, I., Chen, G.K., Nakagawa, H., et al. (2012). Evaluating genetic risk for prostate cancer among Japanese and Latinos. *Cancer Epidemiology, Biomarkers & Prevention*, 21, 2048–58.

Cibula, D., Gompel, A., Mueck, A.O., et al. (2010). Hormonal contraception and risk of cancer. *Human Reproduction Update*, 16, 631–50.

Clifford, G.M., Gallus, S., Herrero, R., et al. (2005). Worldwide distribution of human papillomavirus types in cytologically normal women in the International Agency for Research on Cancer HPV prevalence surveys: a pooled analysis. *The Lancet*, 366, 991–8.

Colditz, G.A., Atwood, K.A., Emmons, K., et al. (2000). Harvard report on cancer prevention volume 4: Harvard Cancer Risk Index. Risk Index Working Group, Harvard Center for Cancer Prevention. *Cancer Causes and Control*, 11, 477–88.

Coleman, M.P., Quaresma, M., Berrino, F., et al. (2008). Cancer survival in five continents: a worldwide population-based study (CONCORD). *The Lancet Oncology*, 9, 730–56.

Croswell, J.M., Ransohoff, D.F., and Kramer, B.S. (2010). Principles of cancer screening: lessons from history and study design issues. *Seminars in Oncology*, 37, 202–15.

Cui, R., Kamatani, Y., Takahashi, A., et al. (2009). Functional variants in ADH1B and ALDH2 coupled with alcohol and smoking synergistically enhance esophageal cancer risk. *Gastroenterology*, 137, 1768–75.

Cui, R., Okada, Y., Jang, S.G., et al. (2011). Common variant in 6q26-q27 is associated with distal colon cancer in an Asian population. *Gut*, 60, 799–805.

De Martel, C., Ferlay, J., Franceschi, S., et al. (2012). Global burden of cancers attributable to infections in 2008: a review and synthetic analysis. *The Lancet Oncology*, 13, 607–15.

Diergaarde, B., Brand, R., Lamb, J., et al. (2010). Pooling-based genome-wide association study implicates Delgamma-glutamyltransferase 1 (GGT1) gene in pancreatic carcinogenesis. *Pancreatology*, 10, 194–200.

Discacciati, A., Orsini, N., and Wolk, A. (2012). Body mass index and incidence of localized and advanced prostate cancer—a dose-response meta-analysis of prospective studies. *Annals of Oncology*, 23, 1665–71.

Doll, R. and Peto, R. (2005). Epidemiology of cancer. In D.A. Warell, T.M. Cox, and J.D. Firth (eds.) *Oxford Textbook of Medicine* (4th ed.), pp. 193–218. Oxford: Oxford University Press.

Dunn, B.K. and Greenwald, P. (2010). Cancer prevention I: introduction. *Seminars in Oncology*, 37, 190–201.

Ellis, L., Rachet, B., Birchall, M., and Coleman, M.P. (2012). Trends and inequalities in laryngeal cancer survival in men and women: England and Wales 1991–2006. *Oral Oncology*, 48, 284–9.

Fanale, D., Amodeo, V., Corsini, L.R., Rizzo, S., Bazan, V., and Russo, A. (2012). Breast cancer genome-wide association studies: there is strength in numbers. *Oncogene*, 31, 2121–8.

Ferlay, J., Parkin, D.M., Curado, M.P., et al. (2010). *Cancer Incidence in Five Continents, Volumes I to IX: IARC CancerBase No. 9*. [Online] Available at: http://ci5.iarc.fr.

Ferlay, J., Soerjomataram, I., Ervik, M., et al. (2013). *GLOBOCAN 2012 v1.0, Cancer Incidence and Mortality Worldwide: IARC CancerBase No. 11*. [Online] Available at: http://globocan.iarc.fr.

Fernandez, E., La Vecchia, C., Gonsalez, J.R., Lucchini, F., Negri, E., and Levi, F. (2005). Converging patterns of colorectal cancer mortality in Europe. *European Journal of Cancer*, 41, 430–7.

Fernandez-Rozadilla, C., Cazier, J.B., Tomlinson, I.P., et al. (2013). A colorectal cancer genome-wide association study in a Spanish cohort identifies two variants associated with colorectal cancer risk at 1p33 and 8p12. *BMC Genomics*, 14, 55.

Ferrández, A., Piazuelo, E., and Castells, A. (2012). Aspirin and the prevention of colorectal cancer. *Best Practice & Research Clinical Gastroenterology*, 26, 185–95.

Field, J.K., Oudkerk, M., Pedersen, J.H., and Duffy, S.W. (2013). Prospects for population screening and diagnosis of lung cancer. *The Lancet*, 382, 732–41.

Ford, A.C. (2011). Chemoprevention for gastric cancer. *Best Practice & Research Clinical Gastroenterology*, 25, 581–92.

Fritz, A., Percy, C., Jack, A., et al. (eds.) (2000). *International Classification of Diseases for Oncology (ICD-O)* (3rd ed.). Geneva: WHO.

FUTURE II Study Group (2007). Quadrivalent vaccine against human papillomavirus to prevent high-grade cervical lesions. *The New England Journal of Medicine*, 356, 1915–27.

Garavello, W., Negri, E., Talamini, R., et al. (2005). Family history of cancer, its combination with smoking and drinking, and risk of squamous cell carcinoma of the esophagus. *Cancer Epidemiology, Biomarkers & Prevention*, 14, 1390–3.

Gilbert, R., Martin, R.M., Beynon, R., et al. (2011). Associations of circulating and dietary vitamin D with prostate cancer risk: a systematic review and dose-response meta-analysis. *Cancer Causes and Control*, 22, 319–40.

Giovannucci, E. (2005). The epidemiology of vitamin D and cancer incidence and mortality: a review (United States). *Cancer Causes and Control*, 16, 83–95.

Goldstein, B.Y., Chang, S.C., Hashibe, M., La Vecchia, C., and Zhang, Z.F. (2010). Alcohol consumption and cancers of the oral cavity and pharynx from 1988 to 2009: an update. *European Journal of Cancer Prevention*, 19, 431–65.

Greenwald, P. (2005). The future of cancer prevention. *Seminars in Oncology Nursing*, 21, 296–8.

Gudmundsson, J., Sulem, P., Steinthorsdottir, V., et al. (2007). Two variants on chromosome 17 confer prostate cancer risk, and the one in TCF2 protects against type 2 diabetes. *Nature Genetics*, 39, 977–83.

Haiman, C.A., Patterson, N., Freedman, M.L., et al. (2007). Multiple regions within 8q24 independently affect risk for prostate cancer. *Nature Genetics*, 39, 638–44.

Hanahan, D. and Weinberg, R.A. (2011). Hallmarks of cancer: the next generation. *Cell*, 144, 646–74.

Huxley, R.R., Ansary-Moghaddam, A., Clifton, P., Czernichow, S., Parr, C.L., and Woodward, M. (2009). The impact of dietary and lifestyle risk factors on risk of colorectal cancer: a quantitative overview of the epidemiological evidence. *International Journal of Cancer*, 125, 171–80.

Igissinov, S., Igissinov, N., Moore, M.A., Kalieva, Z., and Kozhakhmetov, S. (2012). Epidemiology of esophageal cancer in Kazakhstan. *Asian Pacific Journal of Cancer Prevention*, 13, 833–6.

International Agency for Research on Cancer (1994a). *IARC Monographs on the Evaluation of the Carcinogenic Risks to Humans. Volume 59. Hepatitis Viruses*. Lyon: International Agency for Research on Cancer.

International Agency for Research on Cancer (1994b). *IARC Monographs on the Evaluation of the Carcinogenic Risks to Humans. Volume 61. Schistosomes, Liver Flukes and Helicobacter Pylori*. Lyon: International Agency for Research on Cancer.

International Agency for Research on Cancer (1995). *IARC Monographs on the Evaluation of the Carcinogenic Risks to Humans. Volume 64. Human Papillomaviruses*. Lyon: International Agency for Research on Cancer.

International Agency for Research on Cancer (1996). *IARC Monographs on the Evaluation of the Carcinogenic Risks to Humans. Volume 67. Human Immunodeficiency Viruses and Human T-Cell Lymphotropic Viruses*. Lyon: International Agency for Research on Cancer.

International Agency for Research on Cancer (1997). *IARC Monographs on the Evaluation of the Carcinogenic Risks to Humans. Volume 70. Epstein-Barr Virus and Kaposi's Sarcoma Herpes Virus/Human Herpesvirus 8*. Lyon: International Agency for Research on Cancer.

International Agency for Research on Cancer (2000). *IARC Monographs on the Evaluation of Carcinogenic Risks to Humans. Volume 75. Ionizing Radiation, Part 1: X-radiation and Gamma-radiation, and Neutrons*. Lyon: International Agency for Research on Cancer.

International Agency for Research on Cancer (2001). *IARC Monographs on the Evaluation of Carcinogenic Risks to Humans. Volume 78. Ionizing Radiation, Part 2: Some Internally Deposited Radionuclides*. Lyon: International Agency for Research on Cancer.

International Agency for Research on Cancer (2002). *IARC Monographs on the Evaluation of the Carcinogenic Risks to Humans. Volume 82. Some Traditional Herbal Medicines, Some Mycotoxins, Naphthalene, and Styrene*. Lyon: International Agency for Research on Cancer.

International Agency for Research on Cancer (2004a). *IARC Monographs on the Evaluation of the Carcinogenic Risks to Humans. Volume 83. Tobacco Smoke and Involuntary Smoking*. Lyon: International Agency for Research on Cancer.

International Agency for Research on Cancer (2004b). *IARC Handbooks of Cancer Prevention. Volume 9. Cruciferous Vegetables, Isothiocyanates and Indoles*. Lyon: International Agency for Research on Cancer.

International Agency for Research on Cancer (2006). *IARC Monographs on the Evaluation of Carcinogenic Risks to Humans: Preamble to the IARC Monographs* [Online] Available from: http://monographs.iarc.fr/ENG/Preamble/index.php.

International Agency for Research on Cancer (2007). *IARC Monographs on the Evaluation of the Carcinogenic Risks to Humans. Volume 90. Human Papillomaviruses*. Lyon: International Agency for Research on Cancer.

International Agency for Research on Cancer (2012a). *IARC Monographs on the Evaluation of the Carcinogenic Risks to Humans. Volume 100 (A). Pharmaceuticals*. Lyon: International Agency for Research on Cancer.

International Agency for Research on Cancer (2012b). *IARC Monographs on the Evaluation of the Carcinogenic Risks to Humans. Volume 100 (B). Biological Agents.* Lyon: International Agency for Research on Cancer.

International Agency for Research on Cancer (2013). *IARC Monographs on the Evaluation of the Carcinogenic Risks to Humans. Volume 104. Malaria and Some Polyomaviruses (SV40, BK, JC, and Merkel Cell Viruses).* Lyon: International Agency for Research on Cancer.

International Agency for Research on Cancer (2014). *IARC Monographs on the Evaluation of Carcinogenic Risks to Humans: Carcinogen Classifications* [Online]. Available at: http://monographs.iarc.fr/ENG/Classification/.

Iodice, S., Gandini, S., Maisonneuve, P., and Lowenfels, A.B. (2008). Tobacco and the risk of pancreatic cancer: a review and meta-analysis. *Langenbeck's Archives of Surgery*, 393, 535–45.

Ishak, M.B. and Giri, V.N. (2011). A systematic review of replication studies of prostate cancer susceptibility genetic variants in high-risk men originally identified from genome-wide association studies. *Cancer Epidemiology, Biomarkers & Prevention*, 20, 1599–610.

Islami, F., Fedirko, V., Tramacere, I., et al. (2011). Alcohol drinking and esophageal squamous cell carcinoma with focus on light-drinkers and never-smokers: a systematic review and meta-analysis. *International Journal of Cancer*, 129, 2473–84.

Jha, P., Ramasundarahettige, C., Landsman, V., et al. (2013). 21st-century hazards of smoking and benefits of cessation in the United States. *The New England Journal of Medicine*, 368, 341–50.

Jia, W.H., Zhang, B., Matsuo, K., et al. (2013). Genome-wide association analyses in East Asians identify new susceptibility loci for colorectal cancer. *Nature Genetics*, 45, 191–6.

Jin, L., Sturgis, E.M., Zhang, Y., et al. (2013). Genetic variants in p53-related genes confer susceptibility to second primary malignancy in patients with index squamous cell carcinoma of head and neck. *Carcinogenesis*, 34, 1551–7.

Kabat, G.C., Kim, M., Phipps, A.I., et al. (2011). Smoking and alcohol consumption in relation to risk of triple-negative breast cancer in a cohort of postmenopausal women. *Cancer Causes and Control*, 22, 775–83.

Kim, S.T., Cheng, Y., Hsu, F.C., et al. (2010). Prostate cancer risk-associated variants reported from genome-wide association studies: meta-analysis and their contribution to genetic variation. *Prostate*, 70, 1729–38.

Kreimer, A.R. (2013). Prospects for prevention of HPV-driven oropharynx cancer. *Oral Oncology*, 50(6), 555–9.

Kruk, J. and Czerniak, U. (2013). Physical activity and its relation to cancer risk: updating the evidence. *Asian Pacific Journal of Cancer Prevention*, 14, 3993–4003.

Lagiou, P., Trichopoulos, D., and Adami, H.O. (2008). Concepts in cancer epidemiology and etiology. In H.O. Adami, D. Hunter, and D. Trichopoulos (eds.) *Textbook of Cancer Epidemiology*, pp. 127–54. New York: Oxford University Press.

La Vecchia, C. (2007). Alcohol and liver cancer. *European Journal of Cancer Prevention*, 16, 495–7.

La Vecchia, C. and Bosetti, C. (2003). Oral contraceptives and cervical cancer: public health implications. *European Journal of Cancer Prevention*, 12, 1–2.

La Vecchia, C., Negri, E., Lagiou, P., and Trichopoulos, D. (2002). Oesophageal adenocarcinoma: a paradigm of mechanical carcinogenesis? *International Journal of Cancer*, 102, 269–70.

Lee, P.N (2011). Summary of the epidemiological evidence relating snus to health. *Regulatory Toxicology and Pharmacology*, 59, 197–214.

Levi, F., Lucchini, F., Negri, E., and La Vecchia, C. (2003). Pancreatic cancer mortality in Europe: the leveling of an epidemic. *Pancreas*, 27, 139–42.

Lewis, S.J. and Smith, G.D. (2005). Alcohol, ALDH2, and esophageal cancer: a meta-analysis which illustrates the potentials and limitations of a Mendelian randomization approach. *Cancer Epidemiology, Biomarkers & Prevention*, 14, 1967–71.

Li, H., Stampfer, M.J., Hollis, J.B., et al. (2007). A prospective study of plasma vitamin D metabolites, vitamin D receptor polymorphisms, and prostate cancer. *PLoS Medicine*, 4, e103.

Li, X., Gao, L., Li, H., et al. (2013). Human papillomavirus infection and laryngeal cancer risk: a systematic review and meta-analysis. *Journal of Infectious Diseases*, 207, 479–88.

London, W.T. and McGlynn, K.A. (2006). Liver cancer. In D. Schottenfeld and J.F. Fraumeni (eds.) *Cancer Epidemiology and Prevention*, pp. 763–86. New York: Oxford University Press.

Low, S.K., Kuchiba, A., Zembutsu, H., et al. (2010). Genome-wide association study of pancreatic cancer in Japanese population. *PLoS One*, 5, e11824.

Lubin, J.H., Liang, Z., Hrubec, Z., et al. (1994). Radon exposure in residences and lung cancer among women: combined analysis of three studies. *Cancer Causes and Control*, 5, 114–28.

Lucenteforte, E., La Vecchia, C., Silverman, D., et al. (2012). Alcohol consumption and pancreatic cancer: a pooled analysis in the International Pancreatic Cancer Case-Control Consortium (PanC4). *Annals of Oncology*, 23, 374–82.

Malvezzi, M., Bertuccio, P., Levi, F., La Vecchia, C., and Negri, E. (2013). European cancer mortality predictions for the year 2013. *Annals of Oncology*, 24, 792–800.

Marques-Vidal, P., Ravasco, P., and Ermelinda Camilo, M. (2006). Foodstuffs and colorectal cancer risk: a review. *Clinical Nutrition*, 25, 14–36.

Marshall, A.L. and Christiani, D.C. (2013). Genetic susceptibility to lung cancer—light at the end of the tunnel? *Carcinogenesis*, 34, 487–502.

McKay, J.D., Truong, T., Gaborieau, V., et al. (2011). A genome-wide association study of upper aerodigestive tract cancers conducted within the INHANCE consortium. *PLoS Genetics*, 7, e1001333.

Moralejo, D. (2009). Smoking increased risk of cervical cancer, independent of infection with high-risk HPV types. *Evidence-Based Nursing*, 12, 122.

Murray, C.J., Vos, T., Lozano, R., et al. (2012). Disability-adjusted life years (DALYs) for 291 diseases and injuries in 21 regions, 1990–2010: a systematic analysis for the Global Burden of Disease Study 2010. *The Lancet*, 380, 2197–223.

Olshan, A.F. (2006). Cancer of the larynx. In D. Schottenfeld and J.F. Fraumeni (eds.) *Cancer Epidemiology and Prevention*, pp. 627–37. New York: Oxford University Press.

Parkin, D.M. (2006). The global health burden of infection-associated cancers in the year 2002. *International Journal of Cancer*, 118, 3030–44.

Pelucchi, C., Gallus, S., Garavello, W., Bosetti, C., and La Vecchia, C. (2008). Alcohol and tobacco use, and cancer risk for upper aerodigestive tract and liver. *European Journal of Cancer Prevention*, 17, 340–4.

Peters, U., Jiao, S., Schumacher, F.R., et al. (2013). Identification of genetic susceptibility loci for colorectal tumors in a genome-wide meta-analysis. *Gastroenterology*, 144, 799–807.e724.

Petersen, G.M., Amundadottir, L., Fuchs, C.S., et al. (2010). A genome-wide association study identifies pancreatic cancer susceptibility loci on chromosomes 13q22.1, 1q32.1 and 5p15.33. *Nature Genetics*, 42, 224–8.

Peto, R., Darby, S., Deo, H., Silcocks, P., Whitley, E., and Doll, R. (2000). Smoking, smoking cessation, and lung cancer in the UK since 1950: combination of national statistics with two case–control studies. *BMJ*, 321, 323–9.

Peto, R., Gray, R., Brantom, P., and Grasso, P. (1991). Effects on 4080 rats of chronic ingestion of N-nitrosodiethylamine or N-nitrosodimethylamine: a detailed dose–response study. *Cancer Research*, 51, 6415–51.

Phipps, A.I., Buist, D.S., Malone, K.E., et al. (2012). Breast density, body mass index, and risk of tumor marker-defined subtypes of breast cancer. *Annals of Epidemiology*, 22, 340–8.

Phipps, A.I., Chlebowski, R.T., Prentice, R., et al. (2011a). Body size, physical activity, and risk of triple-negative and estrogen receptor-positive breast cancer. *Cancer Epidemiology, Biomarkers & Prevention*, 20, 454–63.

Phipps, A.I., Chlebowski, R.T., Prentice, R., et al. (2011b). Reproductive history and oral contraceptive use in relation to risk of triple-negative breast cancer. *Journal of the National Cancer Institute*, 103, 470–7.

Pirie, K., Peto, R., Reeves, G.K., Green, J., Beral, V.; Million Women Study Collaborators (2013). The 21st century hazards of smoking and benefits of stopping: a prospective study of one million women in the UK. *The Lancet*, 381, 133–41.

Platz, E.A. and Giovannucci, E. (2006). Prostate cancer. In D. Schottenfeld and J.F. Fraumeni (eds.) *Cancer Epidemiology and Prevention*, pp. 1128–50. New York: Oxford University Press.

Plummer, M., Peto, J., Franceschi, S.; International Collaboration of Epidemiological Studies of Cervical Cancer (2012). Time since first sexual intercourse and the risk of cervical cancer. *International Journal of Cancer*, 130, 2638–44.

Plummer, M., Vivas, J., Lopez, G., et al. (2007). Chemoprevention of pre-cancerous gastric lesions with antioxidant vitamin supplementation: a randomized trial in a high-risk population. *Journal of the National Cancer Institute*, 99, 137–46.

Sakamoto, H., Yoshimura, K., Saeki, N., et al. (2008). Genetic variation in PSCA is associated with susceptibility to diffuse-type gastric cancer. *Nature Genetics*, 40, 730–40.

Salama, N.R., Hartung, M.L., and Müller, A. (2013). Life in the human stomach: persistence strategies of the bacterial pathogen Helicobacter pylori. *Nature Reviews Microbiology*, 11, 385–99.

Salehi, F., Turner, M.C., Phillips, K.P., Wigle, D.T., Krewski, D., and Aronson, K.J. (2008). Review of the etiology of breast cancer with special attention to organochlorines as potential endocrine disruptors. *Journal of Toxicology and Environmental Health Part B: Critical Reviews*, 11, 276–300.

Sankaranarayanan, R., Ramadas, K., Thara, S., et al. (2013). Long term effect of visual screening on oral cancer incidence and mortality in a randomized trial in Kerala, India. *Oral Oncology*, 49, 314–21.

Sanyal, A., Poklepovic, A., Moyneur, E., and Barghout, V. (2010). Population-based risk factors and resource utilization for HCC: US perspective. *Current Medical Research and Opinion*, 26, 2183–91.

Sarma, A., Heilbrun, M.E., Conner, K.E., Stevens, S.M., Woller, S.C., and Elliott, C.G. (2012). Radiation and chest CT scan examinations: what do we know? *Chest*, 142, 750–60.

Schiffman, M.H. and Hildesheim, A. (2006). Cervical cancer. In D. Schottenfeld and J.F. Fraumeni (eds.) *Cancer Epidemiology and Prevention*, pp. 1044–67. New York: Oxford University Press.

Shakeri, R., Kamangar, F., Nasrollahzadeh, D., et al. (2012). Is opium a real risk factor for esophageal cancer or just a methodological artifact? Hospital and neighborhood controls in case-control studies. *PLoS One*, 7, e32711.

Shi, Y., Hu, Z., Wu, C., et al. (2011). A genome-wide association study identifies new susceptibility loci for non-cardia gastric cancer at 3q13.31 and 5p13.1. *Nature Genetics*, 43, 1215–18.

Shi, Y, Li, L., Hu, Z., et al. (2013). A genome-wide association study identifies two new cervical cancer susceptibility loci at 4q12 and 17q12. *Nature Genetics*, 45, 918–22.

Siegel, R., Ma, J., Zou, Z., and Jemal, A. (2014). Cancer statistics, 2014. *CA: A Cancer Journal for Clinicians*, 64, 9–29.

Smith, C.J., Perfetti, T.A., Garg, R., and Hansch, C. (2003). IARC carcinogens reported in cigarette mainstream smoke and their calculated log P values. *Food and Chemical Toxicology*, 41, 807–17.

Speizer, F.E. and Samet, J.M. (1994). Air pollution and lung cancer. In J.M. Samet (ed.) *Epidemiology of Lung Cancer*, pp. 131–50. Volume 74, Lung Biology in Health Disease. New York: Marcel Dekker.

Steenland, K., Burnett, C., Lalich, N., Ward, E., and Hurrell, J. (2003). Dying for work: the magnitude of US mortality from selected causes of death associated with occupation. *American Journal of Industrial Medicine*, 43, 461–82.

Stubbins, R.E., Hakeem, A., and Núñez, N.P. (2012). Using components of the vitamin D pathway to prevent and treat colon cancer. *Nutrition Reviews*, 70, 721–9.

Sun, Z., Chen, T., Thorgeirsson, S.S., et al. (2013). Dramatic reduction of liver cancer incidence in young adults: 28 year follow-up of etiological interventions in an endemic area of China. *Carcinogenesis*, 34, 1800–5.

Takata, R., Akamatsu, S., Kubo, M., et al. (2010). Genome-wide association study identifies five new susceptibility loci for prostate cancer in the Japanese population. *Nature Genetics*, 42, 751–4.

Tramacere, I., La Vecchia, C., and Negri, E. (2011). Tobacco smoking and esophageal and gastric cardia adenocarcinoma: a meta-analysis. *Epidemiology*, 22, 344–9.

Tramacere, I., Pelucchi, C., Bagnardi, V., et al. (2012). A meta-analysis on alcohol drinking and esophageal and gastric cardia adenocarcinoma risk. *Annals of Oncology*, 23, 287–97.

Turati, F., Talamini, R., Pelucchi, C., et al. (2013a). Metabolic syndrome and hepatocellular carcinoma risk. *British Journal of Cancer*, 108, 222–8.

Turati, F., Tramacere, I., La Vecchia, C., and Negri, E. (2013b). A meta-analysis of body mass index and esophageal and gastric cardia adenocarcinoma. *Annals of Oncology*, 24, 609–17.

Turner, P.C., Flannery, B., Isitt, C., Ali, M., and Pestka, J. (2012). The role of biomarkers in evaluating human health concerns from fungal contaminants in food. *Nutrition Research Reviews*, 25, 162–79.

US Preventive Services Task Force (2009). Screening for breast cancer: U.S. Preventive Services Task Force Recommendation Statement. *Annals of Internal Medicine*, 151, 716–26.

Wang, L.D., Zhou, F.Y., Li, X.M., et al. (2010). Genome-wide association study of esophageal squamous cell carcinoma in Chinese subjects identifies susceptibility loci at PLCE1 and C20orf54. *Nature Genetics*, 42, 759–63.

Wei, W.Q., Yang, J., Zhang, S.W., Chen, W.Q., and Qiao, Y.L. (2011). Esophageal cancer mortality trends during the last 30 years in high risk areas in China: comparison of results from national death surveys conducted in the 1970's, 1990's and 2004–2005. *Asian Pacific Journal of Cancer Prevention*, 12, 1821–6.

Welch, H.G. and Albertsen, P.C. (2009). Prostate cancer diagnosis and treatment after the introduction of prostate-specific antigen screening: 1986–2005. *Journal of the National Cancer Institute*, 101, 1325–9.

Willis, J.A., Olson, S.H., Orlow, I., et al. (2012). A replication study and genome-wide scan of single-nucleotide polymorphisms associated with pancreatic cancer risk and overall survival. *Clinical Cancer Research*, 18, 3942–51.

World Cancer Research Fund and American Institute for Cancer Research (2007). *Food, Nutrition, Physical Activity and the Prevention of Cancer: A Global Perspective*. Washington, DC: AICR.

World Health Organization (1976). *International Classification of Diseases for Oncology*. Geneva: WHO.

Wu, C., Hu, Z., He, Z., *et al.* (2011). Genome-wide association study identifies three new susceptibility loci for esophageal squamous-cell carcinoma in Chinese populations. *Nature Genetics*, 43, 679–84.

Wu, C., Kraft, P., Stolzenberg-Solomon, R., et al. (2012b). Genome-wide association study of survival in patients with pancreatic adenocarcinoma. *Gut*, 63, 152–60.

Wu, C., Miao, X., Huang, L., et al. (2012a). Genome-wide association study identifies five loci associated with susceptibility to pancreatic cancer in Chinese populations. *Nature Genetics*, 44, 62–6.

Wu, M., Chang, S.C., Kampman, E., et al. (2013). Single nucleotide polymorphisms of ADH1B, ADH1C and ALDH2 genes and esophageal cancer: a population-based case-control study in China. *International Journal of Cancer*, 132, 1868–77.

Wu, M., Van't Veer, P., Zhang, Z.F., et al. (2011a). A large proportion of esophageal cancer cases and the incidence difference between regions are attributable to lifestyle risk factors in China. *Cancer Letters*, 308, 189–96.

Wu, M., Zhao, J.K., Zhang, Z.F., et al. (2011b). Smoking and alcohol drinking increased the risk of esophageal cancer among Chinese men but not women in a high-risk population. *Cancer Causes and Control*, 22, 649–57.

Xu, J., Mo, Z., Ye, D., et al. (2012). Genome-wide association study in Chinese men identifies two new prostate cancer risk loci at 9q31.2 and 19q13.4. *Nature Genetics*, 44, 1231–5.

Yeager, M., Orr, N., Hayes, R.B., et al. (2007). Genome-wide association study of prostate cancer identifies a second risk locus at 8q24. *Nature Genetics*, 39, 645–9.

Zendehdel, K., Nyrén, O., Luo, J., et al. (2008). Risk of gastroesophageal cancer among smokers and users of Scandinavian moist snuff. *International Journal of Cancer*, 122, 1095–9.

Chronic obstructive pulmonary disease and asthma

Jeroen Douwes, Marike Boezen, Collin Brooks, and Neil Pearce

Introduction to chronic obstructive pulmonary disease and asthma

The most common non-malignant respiratory conditions characterized by airway dysfunction are referred to collectively as obstructive airway diseases, and include chronic obstructive pulmonary disease (COPD) and asthma. Both conditions are highly prevalent and have increased dramatically in the past few decades, in Western and non-Western societies. They have a profound impact on quality of life for patients and their families, and COPD accounts for several million premature deaths per year worldwide (Lopez et al. 2006a).

COPD is usually defined as airflow obstruction due to inflammation of the peripheral airways and lung parenchyma, in which the airflow limitation is not fully reversible and progresses over time. Asthma is a heterogeneous chronic inflammatory disorder of the airways involving airflow limitation which is variable and reversible. Thus, the critical difference between both conditions is whether airflow obstruction is reversible. However, there is increasing evidence that reversibility of airflow obstruction may be observed in COPD, and that some asthmatics have irreversible obstruction. This has been described as 'overlap syndrome' (Gibson and Simpson 2009).

In this chapter we will describe both COPD and asthma in parallel. We first consider definitions, possible mechanisms, time trends, and population patterns of prevalence. Then we consider the evidence regarding risk factors for exacerbations as well as the initial development of both diseases.

Definitions

COPD

Traditionally COPD has been defined as irreversible airflow obstruction due to chronic bronchitis and emphysema which progresses over time (Petty 2006). Emphysema was already described in the seventeenth and eighteenth centuries (Petty 2006), and one of the first reports of chronic bronchitis as a serious and disabling disorder appeared in 1814 (Badham 1814). It was only a few years later that Laënnec made the observation that chronic bronchitis and emphysema often occurred in the same subject at the same time (Laennec 1821; Petty 2002, 2006). However, it was not until about 150 years later that Burrows et al. (1966) suggested labelling the spectrum of chronic bronchitis and emphysema as 'chronic obstructive lung disease', or COPD. A few years previously, the Ciba Guest Symposium (Ciba Foundation Guest Symposium 1959) and the American Thoracic Society symposium (Committee on Diagnostic Standards for Nontuberculous Respiratory Diseases 1962) proposed the first definitions of chronic bronchitis and emphysema respectively. Current definitions are still largely based on these initial definitions, that is, chronic bronchitis is defined clinically as the presence of chronic productive cough for at least 3 consecutive months in 2 consecutive years; emphysema, on the other hand, is defined in pathological terms as an increase in the size of the distal airspaces and destruction of their walls without obvious fibrosis (American Thoracic Society Committee on Diagnostic Standards 1962).

The most recent definitions of COPD as reported in the American Thoracic Society (ATS), European Respiratory Society (ERS), and the Global Initiative for Chronic Obstructive Lung Disease (GOLD) guidelines (Rabe et al. 2007) emphasize the inflammatory response to noxious particles and gases as the predominant pathological feature of the disease, and have parted from the definition of COPD as being a syndrome of chronic bronchitis and emphysema. The widely accepted GOLD definition (Rabe et al. 2007) states that COPD is:

> a preventable and treatable disease with some significant extrapulmonary effects that may contribute to the severity in individual patients. Its pulmonary component is characterised by airflow limitation that is not fully reversible. The airflow limitation is usually progressive and associated with an abnormal inflammatory response of the lung to noxious particles or gases. (Rabe et al. 2007)

Although no longer specifically included in the definition, it is still recognized that chronic bronchitis and emphysema are important causes of the chronic airflow limitation characteristic of COPD. The three main components (inflammation, airflow limitation that is not fully reversible, and a gradual loss of lung function over time) represent the major pathophysiological events leading to the symptoms typically expressed by those with COPD: chronic and progressive cough, sputum production, and dyspnoea. Cough and sputum production may precede the development of airflow limitation, but fixed airflow obstruction may also develop without these symptoms (Petty 2006).

Clinical COPD

Spirometry is an essential tool in the clinical diagnosis of COPD and there are well accepted standardized guidelines (Miller et al. 2005). In COPD the maximum volume of air that can be forcibly expired (forced vital capacity (FVC)) is generally unaffected, or only marginally affected; however, the volume of air exhaled in the first second of expiration (forced expiratory volume in 1 second (FEV_1)) is significantly reduced. COPD is therefore defined based on the post-bronchodilator FEV_1/FVC ratio. A cut-point of 0.7 (i.e. 70 per cent) is widely used (Rabe et al. 2007), but this has not been clinically validated. Also, it is well recognized that using a fixed FEV_1/FVC ratio to define COPD independent of age has the potential for significant misclassification, with under-diagnosis in younger adults and over-diagnosis in the elderly (Medbo and Melbye 2007). Bronchodilator treatment prior to spirometry is important since it establishes whether obstruction is irreversible and distinguishes it from asthma in which obstruction is mostly reversible.

The degree of severity of COPD (defined as a $FEV_1/FVC < 70$ per cent) is usually based on the patient's FEV_1. The 2006 GOLD criteria classify COPD severity into four stages (Rabe et al. 2007) (see Box 8.3.1).

Recently these GOLD guidelines were revised, recognizing that although spirometry is still important for making a clinical diagnosis of COPD, it should be included as part of a combined assessment taking symptoms, spirometry, and history of exacerbations into account (Vestbo et al. 2012).

Despite the well-accepted guidelines for diagnosis, and the availability of inexpensive and convenient hand-held spirometers, COPD remains a significantly under-diagnosed disease particularly in younger people and women (Chapman et al. 2001; Watson et al. 2003; Halbert et al. 2006). This is largely because those with mild COPD often have no symptoms, or they have symptoms that are not perceived by patients and healthcare providers as abnormal, therefore not warranting a spirometric assessment. Similarly, subjects may be less likely to be diagnosed with COPD if there is no history of smoking, one of the best-known risk factors for COPD.

Defining COPD in epidemiological surveys

In population-based surveys, COPD is often defined on the basis of: (1) self-report of a doctor diagnosis of COPD, bronchitis or emphysema; (2) self-report of respiratory symptoms; and (3) spirometry with or without prior bronchodilator treatment. It has repeatedly been shown that self-reports of a clinical diagnosis significantly underestimate the true disease prevalence (Chapman et al. 2006; Halbert et al. 2006). This is probably largely due to underdiagnosis of COPD by most general practitioners (see 'Clinical COPD').

Spirometric assessment to define COPD is therefore superior to a clinical assessment without spirometry, or a self-report of doctor-diagnosed COPD. However, the use of bronchodilators significantly complicates large population-based spirometry surveys, and many studies therefore do not collect post-bronchodilator measurements. The implications of failing to check for reversibility of airflow obstruction (using pre- and post-bronchodilator spirometry) may, however, result in an overestimation of the prevalence. For example, in a study in a random population sample of 2235 adults, the prevalence of COPD based on post-bronchodilator measurements was 7.0 per cent compared to 9.6 per cent for pre-bronchodilator measurements (Johannessen et al. 2005). Thus, the use of post-bronchodilator spirometry to determine the diagnosis of COPD in population-based studies is strongly recommended.

Asthma

The word 'asthma' comes from a Greek word meaning 'panting' (Keeney 1964), but reference to asthma-like symptoms can also be found in ancient Egyptian, Hebrew, and Indian medical writings (Ellul-Micallef 1976). There were clear observations of patients experiencing attacks of asthma in the second century, and evidence of disordered lung anatomy as far back as the seventeenth century (Willis 1678).

The definition of asthma initially proposed at the Ciba Foundation conference in 1959 (Ciba Foundation Guest Symposium 1959) and endorsed by the American Thoracic Society in 1962 (American Thoracic Society Committee on Diagnostic Standards 1962) is that 'asthma is a disease characterized by wide variation over short periods of time in resistance to flow in the airways of the lung'. Although these features receive lesser prominence in some current definitions, as the importance of airways inflammation is recognized, they are still integral to the current Global Initiative for Asthma (GINA) description of asthma as:

a chronic inflammatory disorder of the airways in which many cells and cellular elements play a role. The chronic inflammation is associated with airway hyperresponsiveness that leads to recurrent episodes of wheezing, breathlessness, chest tightness, and coughing, particularly at night or in the early morning. These episodes are usually associated with widespread, but variable, airflow obstruction within the lung that is often reversible either spontaneously or with treatment. (GINA 2006)

Box 8.3.1 GOLD criteria of COPD severity

- Stage I, mild: $FEV_1 \geq 80\%$ predicted.

- Stage II, moderate: $50\% \leq FEV_1 \geq 80\%$ predicted.

- Stage III, severe: $30\% \leq FEV_1 \geq 50\%$ predicted.

- Stage IV, very severe: $FEV_1 < 30\%$ predicted *or* $FEV_1 < 50\%$ predicted *plus* chronic respiratory failure (i.e. arterial pressure of oxygen (PaO_2) < 8.0 kPa (60 mm Hg) with or without arterial pressure of CO_2 ($PaCO_2 > 6.7$ kPa (50 mm Hg)) while breathing air at sea level).

Reproduced with permission from Rabe, K.F. et al., Global strategy for the diagnosis, management, and prevention of chronic obstructive pulmonary disease: GOLD executive summary, *American Journal of Respiratory and Critical Care Medicine*, Volume 176, Number 6, pp. 532–55, Copyright © 2007 The American Thoracic Society, DOI: 10.1164/rccm.200703-456SO.

These three components—chronic airways inflammation, reversible airflow obstruction, and enhanced bronchial reactivity—therefore form the basis of current definitions of asthma. They also represent the major pathophysiological events leading to the symptoms of wheezing, breathlessness, chest tightness, cough, and sputum by which physicians clinically diagnose this disorder.

Clinical asthma

There is no single test or pathognomonic feature which defines the presence or absence of asthma. Furthermore, the variability of the condition means that evidence of it may or may not be present at assessment. Thus, a diagnosis of asthma is made on the basis of the clinical history, combined with physical examination and respiratory function tests over a period of time. Several studies have found the prevalence of physician-diagnosed asthma to be substantially lower than the prevalence of asthma symptoms in the community (e.g. Asher et al. 1998). This is not surprising since a clinical diagnosis of asthma can only be made if a person presents him- or herself to a doctor. This requires an initial self-assessment of the symptoms, as well as access to a doctor once a self-assessment has been made. Several further medical consultations may be required. Thus, diagnosed asthma is dependent not only on morbidity, but also on a patient's symptom perception, physician practice, and healthcare availability. Furthermore, there are several disorders which have signs and symptoms (such as wheeze) which can be confused with or mimic aspects of asthma, including COPD, dysfunctional breathing, eosinophilic bronchitis, vocal cord dysfunction, and bronchiectasis (King and Moores 2008).

There are, however, a number of tests that may facilitate the diagnosis and monitoring of asthma. Measurements of lung function are the most frequently used and provide important information on airflow variability, reversibility, and severity. Airflow limitation is generally measured using spirometry or a peak expiratory flow (PEF) meter. PEF meters are inexpensive and easy to use, but they are less precise than spirometry, and may underestimate the degree of airflow limitation (Aggarwal et al. 2006), therefore spirometry is preferred. Recent guidelines have emphasized the importance of conducting spirometry both before and after bronchodilator treatment when assessing lung function in asthma (Bateman et al. 2008). This is important since it establishes if obstruction is irreversible, and allows distinction from COPD. Reversibility of FEV_1 of $\geq$ 12 per cent and $\geq$ 200mL from the pre-bronchodilator value is generally accepted as a valid indication of asthma (GINA 2006). However, due to the highly variable nature of the condition, repeated lung function tests are required, as some patients may not display reversibility when their asthma is well controlled (McCormack and Enright 2008). Moreover, although asthma is generally associated with reversible airflow obstruction, it has been estimated that between 35 and 50 per cent of asthmatics have at least some degree of irreversible obstruction (Bel 2004). Additionally, reversibility may be present in non-asthmatics (van Vugt et al. 2012).

In subjects with asthma symptoms but normal lung function, bronchial hyperresponsiveness (BHR) testing may be used as a diagnostic aid. BHR constitutes airway narrowing to non-specific stimuli, such as exercise, cold air, and chemical irritants, and can be measured as airway responsiveness to histamine, methacholine, adenosine-5'-monophosphate (AMP), hypertonic saline, exercise challenge (de Meer et al. 2004a), and mannitol powder (Parkerson and Ledford 2011). However, although BHR is related to asthma, it may occur independently of asthma, and vice versa (Pearce et al. 2000a), which makes the BHR test of limited use for individual asthma diagnostics.

More recently an increasing number of tests are available to measure non-invasive markers of airway inflammation including sputum induction tests (Simpson et al. 2006), exhaled nitric oxide tests (Taylor et al. 2006) and measurements of inflammatory markers in exhaled breath condensate (Kharitonov and Barnes 2006). Whilst these tests may be useful in establishing asthma phenotypes (Douwes et al. 2002b; Simpson et al. 2006) and identifying patients who are more likely to respond to optimal treatment (Donohue and Jain 2013), they have as yet to be convincingly demonstrated to aid in asthma diagnosis, although it has been suggested that fractional exhaled nitric oxide measurements had a stronger asthma diagnostic capability (88 per cent sensitivity) than either peak flow or spirometric assessment (between 0 and 47 per cent sensitivity) (Smith et al. 2004).

There have been several approaches used to categorize asthma (Wenzel 2012). However, until recently, asthma has most commonly been clinically classified on the basis of severity using GINA criteria (GINA 2006), which subdivided asthma into four categories (intermittent, mild persistent, moderate persistent, and severe persistent). More recent guidelines (GINA 2013) have suggested that clinical categorization should be based on the current level of asthma control (controlled, partly controlled, and uncontrolled), which may more adequately address the individual clinical needs of the patient.

Overlap syndrome

Although reversibility of airway obstruction (or the lack thereof) is the primary clinical characteristic used to define either asthma or COPD, it is increasingly recognized that irreversible or only partially reversible airway obstruction may be observed in some asthmatics (Vonk et al. 2003), and conversely, some COPD patients may show a measurable degree of reversibility (Calverley et al. 2003). It is therefore difficult to clearly distinguish and diagnose the two conditions, particularly in older patients. This has led to the description of 'overlap syndrome', in which obstructive respiratory disease shows features of both asthma and COPD (Gibson and Simpson 2009). In fact, it has been previously suggested that COPD and asthma should not be considered as separate diseases, but rather as different expressions of the same disease entity. This theory, proposed in 1961 and known as the *Dutch hypothesis*, has since been heavily debated (Kraft 2006; Barnes 2006).

To date, there have been few epidemiological studies examining the incidence and prevalence of the overlap of COPD and asthma. However, it has been suggested that between 15 and 20 per cent of patients with obstructive airway diseases have evidence of overlap (Soriano et al. 2003), and this is most commonly seen in those with a history of smoking (Gibson and Simpson 2009).

Defining asthma in epidemiological surveys

Defining and diagnosing asthma in population-based epidemiological surveys poses even greater difficulties than defining asthma in individuals. Because of this, asthma prevalence surveys usually focus on self or parental-reported 'asthma symptoms' rather than diagnosed asthma (Burney et al. 1994; Asher et al.

1995). This approach allows a large number of participants to be rapidly surveyed without great cost. Of the symptoms clinically associated with asthma, epidemiological studies have shown that wheezing is the most important symptom for the identification of asthma, and thus the majority of questionnaires used to assess asthma prevalence are based on this symptom (Pearce et al. 1998).

An alternative approach to symptom questionnaires has been to use more 'objective' measures such as BHR testing, either alone or in combination with questionnaires. In particular, it has been suggested that asthma should be defined in epidemiological studies as symptomatic BHR (Toelle et al. 1992). However, some have criticized the use of BHR, and have questioned whether it is more valid than symptoms questionnaires (Pearce et al. 2000a). Furthermore, due to the variability of asthma, BHR may not be present at the time of assessment (Shaw et al. 2012).

Mechanisms, prevalence, and risk factors of COPD

Mechanisms of COPD

COPD encompasses emphysema, chronic bronchitis, or a combination of both conditions. Emphysema is characterized by loss of lung tissue elasticity and destruction of alveolar architecture. As a result of this the small airways collapse during exhalation, leading to air trapping and impaired ability to exhale. Chronic bronchitis involves inflammation of the airways, resulting in thick mucus which makes it difficult to efficiently inhale air into the lungs. In COPD, this airway inflammation is characterized by (non-allergic) T-helper 1 (TH_1)-associated CD8+ T cell and neutrophilic involvement (Chrysofakis et al. 2004; Simpson et al. 2013).

COPD is largely (but not exclusively) attributable to smoking. An exception is the genetically mediated alpha-1-antitrypsin (AAT) deficiency, where carriers need no environmental smoke exposure to develop COPD. However, AAT -deficiency accounts for a minimal number of COPD cases worldwide (<1 per cent). Thus, the majority of COPD cases are due to smoking. Despite this, genetics also likely plays a role, as only a small proportion of smokers develop COPD. These 'susceptible smokers' show premature onset of lung function decline and, to a lesser extent, more rapid rates of decline later in life (Tager et al. 1988). In non-smokers, FEV_1 declines at a mean rate of approximately 30 mL/year during adult life, whereas in smokers, this is increased to 30–45 mL/year. Within a subset of susceptible cigarette smokers the rate of decline is 80–100 mL/year, and only 10–20 per cent of Caucasian chronic heavy cigarette smokers develop symptomatic COPD.

The deleterious effect of smoking is due to the fact that cigarette smoke contains a large amount of free radicals which disturbs the reduction/oxidation balance in the lungs, leading to elevated oxidative stress. Such an oxidant overdose can injure lung tissue directly by oxidation of cellular components, or indirectly by promoting neutrophilic inflammation and tissue degradation, subsequently affecting lung function (MacNee 2005; Kirkham and Rahman 2006).

Prevalence of COPD

COPD is a major global cause of mortality and morbidity, with exacerbations leading to frequent hospitalization. Despite the large personal, societal, and economic burden (Rennard et al. 2002) only about 30 prevalence surveys of COPD had been reported until 2001 (Chapman et al. 2006). The establishment of the Burden Of Obstructive Lung Disease (BOLD) Initiative (see later), and other recent international initiatives to assess the global burden of COPD, allow more valid comparisons of the prevalence of COPD over time and across nations in the near future. Below, the most important studies currently available are summarized.

European epidemiological studies of COPD show prevalence estimates for COPD of 4–11 per cent (Vestbo 2004). These differences in prevalence estimates are presumed to be attributable to differences in risk exposures or population characteristics, but methods and definitions used to measure COPD may also play a role. Definitions of COPD used in these studies vary from a doctor's diagnosis of COPD, to more rigid definitions based on pathology and/or pulmonary lung function testing.

Halbert and co-workers (Halbert et al. 2006) assessed the reasons for conflicting prevalence estimates described in the literature. They selected studies that had: (1) estimated population-based COPD prevalences and (2) clearly described the methods used to obtain these estimates. In total, 32 studies presenting prevalence data for COPD were identified and reviewed, representing 17 countries and eight WHO regions. Prevalence estimates were based on spirometry (11 studies), respiratory symptoms (14 studies), patient-reported disease (10 studies), or expert opinion. The reported prevalence of COPD ranged from 0.23 to 18.3 per cent, with the lowest prevalences (0.2 to 2.5 per cent) being those based on expert opinion. Sixteen studies had measured rates that could confidently be extrapolated to an entire region or country. All of these 16 studies were conducted in Europe or North America, and in most the prevalence was between 4 per cent and 10 per cent. However, in some studies, COPD prevalence may be higher than this. For example, preliminary data from 13,301 participants in the LifeLines cohort study performed in the Netherlands showed that 1920 out of 13,301 subjects had GOLD stage I or higher (14 per cent) (i.e. 1402 had GOLD stage I, 494 GOLD stage II, and 24 GOLD stage III/IV).

Although the most accurate prevalence data are from Western countries, estimates suggest that about half of the approximately 2.7 million deaths in 2000 were in the Western Pacific Region, with the majority occurring in China. About 400,000 deaths occur each year from COPD in Western countries (Lopez et al. 2006b). Lopez and co-workers recently noted that the reported increase in global COPD deaths between 1990 and 2000 (0.5 million) is partially real, and partially due to better diagnostic methods and more extensive data availability in 2000. The regional COPD prevalence in adults in 2000 was estimated to vary from 0.5 per cent in parts of Africa to 3–4 per cent in North America (Soriano et al. 2000).

Halbert and co-workers (Halbert et al. 2006) quantified the global prevalence of COPD by performing a systematic review and random effects meta-analysis. For the 1990–2004 period they identified 101 prevalence estimates from 28 countries. The pooled prevalence of COPD was 7.6 per cent; the prevalence of chronic bronchitis alone was 6.4 per cent, and the prevalence of emphysema alone was 1.8 per cent. The pooled prevalence of COPD based on spirometry was 8.9 per cent.

The BOLD initiative developed standardized methods for estimating COPD prevalence and is currently one of only a few studies with truly comparable international prevalence estimates (Buist et al. 2007). This study included 9425 participants from 12 centres in 12 countries including China, Turkey, Austria, South Africa, Iceland, Germany, Poland, Norway, Canada, the United States, Philippines, and Australia. Using identical methods, the study showed considerable variation in COPD prevalences, with GOLD stage II or higher COPD in women ranging from 5.1 per cent in Guangzhou, China, to 16.7 per cent in Cape Town, South Africa. In men it ranged from 8.5 per cent in Reykjavik, Iceland, to 22.2 per cent in Cape Town, South Africa. Using a similar study design, the Latin American Project for the Investigation of Obstructive Lung Diseases (PLATINO) studied the prevalence of COPD in 5315 study participants in five Latin American centres (Mexico, Venezuela, Brazil, Chile, and Uruguay) (Menezes et al. 2005). Crude prevalence rates of COPD ranged from 7.8 per cent in Mexico City, Mexico, to 19.7 per cent in Montevideo, Uruguay. Age and smoking did not fully explain the international variation in disease prevalence, suggesting a role for additional risk factors.

Although COPD is mainly observed in the elderly, it is not a disease of the elderly alone. In the Confronting COPD Study, the presence of COPD in younger age groups has also been described (Rennard et al. 2002); a phenomenon confirmed in the European Community Respiratory Health Survey, which verified COPD diagnosis using spirometric testing in random population samples of younger age (<45 years) (Vestbo 2004).

Future prevalence and burden of COPD

Assessing the future prevalence and burden of COPD requires the consideration of changing population distributions and smoking habits. For example, Feenstra and co-workers (Feenstra et al. 2001) in 2003 used a dynamic multistage life table model to compute projections for the Netherlands. Changes in population size and composition were predicted to cause COPD prevalence to increase from 21/1000 in 1994 to 33/1000 in 2015 for men, and from 10/1000 to 23/1000 for women. Changes in smoking behaviour would reduce the projected prevalence to 29/1000 for men, but would increase it to 25/1000 for women. The overall increases in COPD were estimated to be 43 per cent in men and 142 per cent in women.

Vestbo et al. examined survival after admission due to COPD in 267 men and 220 women who had participated in the Copenhagen City Health Study, and who were hospitalized with a discharge-diagnosis of COPD. The crude 5-year survival rate after a COPD admission was higher in women (52 per cent) than in men (37 per cent). However, estimations of the overall mortality due to COPD in the next decade showed that COPD mortality within women was expected to exceed that of men, with a similar trend observed in the United States. Thus, with the expected global increase in female mortality from COPD, mortality rates for females will soon equal or exceed those for males (Crockett et al. 1994; Mannino et al. 1997; Vestbo et al. 1998; Vestbo 2002; Watson et al. 2003).

Risk factors for COPD

In the past few decades, the environmental risk factors for COPD, that is, smoking, air pollution, occupational exposure, childhood respiratory illness, diet, and exposure to respiratory allergens, have been studied in detail. Also, the presence of respiratory symptoms, increased numbers of blood eosinophils, a family history of asthma, and increased airway responsiveness were all found to be significant predictors of reduced level of FEV_1 (Wang et al. 2004; de Marco et al. 2013).

Cigarette smoking

The WHO has estimated that 73 per cent of all COPD mortality in high-income countries is caused by smoking; the estimate for low- and middle-income countries was 40 per cent (Lopez et al. 2006a). Tobacco smoke therefore is the most important cause of COPD. In fact, there is a well-established association between current and cumulative smoking and COPD, and several cohort studies have shown that adult smokers experience a faster FEV_1 decline than non-smokers. This excess decline in lung function may return to normal levels of ageing-related decline after smoking cessation (Camilli et al. 1987). Women and children are considered to be particularly sensitive to the effects of inhaled tobacco smoke (Xu et al. 1994) and significant reductions in FEV_1 due to environmental tobacco smoke among children with smoking parents have been shown (Tager et al. 1983).

What is most striking about the epidemiology of COPD has been the change in prevalence in women in the past decade (Lopez and Murray 1998). Due to increased smoking rates in women and women taking up smoking at younger ages in recent decades (Kemm 2001; Watson et al. 2003), the prevalence of COPD in women in the United Kingdom reached the same level as that of men in the previous decade (Lopez et al. 2006b). A similar pattern is seen in the United States, and this is expected to be reflected in other European countries in the near future (Halbert et al. 2003). Nonetheless, as noted earlier, women with COPD remain less likely to be diagnosed and treated (Miravitlles et al. 2005). General practitioners, in particular, consider the diagnosis of COPD less frequently in women than in men presenting with the same risk factors and clinical symptoms (Miravitlles et al. 2006).

Few data are available on the incidence of COPD according to smoking habits. Analysis of the Copenhagen City Heart Study confirmed a higher incidence of COPD in smokers than non-smokers, with 27 per cent of participants who continued to smoke over a 25-year period developing COPD as defined by GOLD stage II–IV COPD, compared with 5.7 per cent of non-smokers (Lokke et al. 2006). The longitudinal Vlagtwedde/Vlaardingen Cohort Study (with a follow-up of 25 years) also showed that persistent cigarette smokers (odds ratio (OR) = 1.99, 95 per cent confidence interval (CI) = 1.68–2.35), recidivist smokers (OR = 1.96, 95 per cent CI = 1.34–2.86), variable pipe/cigar smokers (OR = 2.11, 95 per cent CI = 1.52–2.91), and subjects who stopped smoking (OR = 1.39, 95 per cent CI = 1.08–1.80) had an increased risk of developing COPD compared to never smokers. The risks of developing COPD in sustained ex-smokers (OR = 0.98, 95 per cent CI = 0.79–1.22), starters (OR = 1.62, 95 per cent CI = 0.87–2.99), brief smokers (OR = 1.22, 95 per cent CI = 0.76–1.94) and persistent pipe/cigar smokers (OR = 1.41, 95 per cent CI = 0.98–2.04) were not significantly different. Therefore, it was concluded that, taking longitudinal smoking habits into account, subjects who quit smoking between two successive surveys still had an increased risk of developing COPD compared with never smokers, whereas sustained ex-smokers were no longer at risk of developing COPD.

Other environmental risk factors

Although cigarette smoking is considered to be the main risk factor for COPD development, recent estimations are that 25–45 per cent of COPD patients have never smoked (Salvi and Barnes 2009). Some of these never-smoking COPD patients may have previously been diagnosed with asthma, as a history of asthma has been shown to be a risk factor for COPD in some studies (Silva et al. 2004). However, other environmental exposures (e.g. occupational exposures and air pollution) are also important risk factors, specifically in non-Westernized countries.

Occupational exposure to dusts, gases, and fumes have been shown to be associated with the rate of decline in FEV_1 and the development of COPD. In fact, an ad hoc committee of the American Thoracic Society that reviewed occupational studies on COPD estimated that 15–20 per cent of COPD was caused by occupational factors (Balmes 2005), and other studies suggest that these estimates could even be higher. For example, analyses of data collected in the Third National Health and Nutrition Examination Survey in the United States suggest that approximately 20 per cent of COPD cases in the United States are attributable to work-related exposures (Hnizdo et al. 2002). The proportion was even higher (approximately 30 per cent) in never smokers. Combined exposures to smoking and occupational factors have been shown to have greater than additive effects (Trupin et al. 2003). Some examples of occupational risk factors for COPD are coal dust, silica dust, oil mists, welding fumes, and organic dusts including cotton, grain, and wood (Balmes 2005).

Indoor air pollutants are another important risk factor for COPD, particularly in low-income countries where biomass fuels (wood and crop residues) and coal fuels are often used for heating and cooking without appropriate ventilation (Liu et al. 2007). WHO estimates suggest that indoor smoke from biomass fuels may cause 35 per cent of all COPD cases in low- and middle-income countries (Lopez et al. 2006a). COPD is also related to outdoor pollution levels, but the attributable risk is expected to be relatively small (Tashkin et al. 1994).

Genetic risk factors

Since COPD is predominantly expressed in later years, genetic factors are difficult to study, as the parents of individuals with COPD have often already died, and the children of subjects with COPD are likely to be too young to have significant fixed airway obstruction (van Diemen and Boezen 2007). Initial genetic studies on COPD included small numbers of subjects and applied different definitions of disease, hampering a valid comparison between studies and increasing the likelihood of spurious results. Many positive results from genetic studies of COPD have therefore not been replicated (Boezen and Postma 2007). Furthermore, lack of replication might also be due to the apparent difficulties of extrapolating results from one population to another, such as Asians and Caucasians, as a result of lower prevalences of particular polymorphisms in Caucasians (Boezen and Postma 2007).

More recently, several large population-based cohort studies have been conducted in which excess decline in lung function leading to development of COPD was studied prospectively. Such studies may allow assessment of different mechanisms that can lead to poor lung function. For example, subjects may have experienced an unusually high rate of decline in lung function, may not have attained the normal maximal level of lung function, or the age of onset of decline may have been unusually early. Genetic factors may affect any one, or a combination, of these different patterns of lung function loss. Therefore, it is of importance to study

the genetic contribution to lung function loss using a longitudinal study design, covering the time span during which these different patterns and their underlying causes evolve (van Diemen and Boezen 2007).

Candidate gene studies on COPD

Most studies on genetics of COPD have focused on genes that are involved in the processing of various tobacco smoke products, oxidative stress, or in the protease/antiprotease balance. In particular, variations in the genes encoding enzymes that detoxify cigarette smoke products (and are thus protective against oxidative stress) may explain why only a proportion of smokers develop COPD.

Candidate genes identified in this way include *EPHX1*, *ADAM33*, *MMP1*, *GSTP1*, *GSTT1*, *GSTM1*, *HMOX1*, and *SERPINA1* (Postma et al. 2011). However, two recent meta-analyses showed that there are only a few genes with statistically significant associations with COPD, namely: *GSTM1*, *TGFB1*, *TNF*, *SOD3*, *IL1RN*, *VNTR*, *TNFA*, *GSTP1*, and *EPHX1* (Smolonska et al. 2009; Castaldi et al. 2010). Of interest, these genes are positioned in biologically plausible pathways of oxidative stress response and defence against oxidative stress, like *GSTM1*, *TGFB1*, *TNF*, *SOD3*, *TNFA*, *GSTP1*, and *EPHX1* (Postma et al. 2011).

Genome-wide association studies on COPD

Genome-wide association (GWA) studies are applied to identify genetic loci that are associated with disease using markers throughout the genome, rather than selected on the basis of their assumed biological function (Boezen 2009). Using GWA study approaches, several novel loci have now been identified for COPD.

The first COPD GWA study identified variants in the nicotinic acetylcholine receptor (nAChR) subunit genes, *CHRNA3/5* (Pillai et al. 2009) and this was confirmed in later studies (Wilk et al. 2012). SNPs in this nicotinic cluster have previously been related to smoking habits and addiction. Another recent GWA study identified a new locus on chromosome 19q13 which was associated with COPD and severe COPD. This region includes *RAB4B*, *EGLN2*, *MIA*, and *CYP2A6*, and has previously also been identified in association with cigarette smoking behavior (Cho et al. 2012). The identification of loci involved in smoking habits and smoking addiction have triggered some discussion whether these genes are directly involved in lung function loss leading to COPD per se, or indirectly through the effects of nicotine addiction (Budulac et al. 2012).

Other recent GWA studies showed associations between several loci and reduced FEV_1 and FEV_1/FVC ratio, some of which indicated developmental genes like *HHIP* (Hancock et al. 2010).

Mechanisms, prevalence, and risk factors of asthma

Until recently, asthma was widely regarded as an allergic disease involving IL-5-mediated eosinophilic airways inflammation (Douwes et al. 2002b). As a consequence, asthma is often grouped together with other 'allergic diseases' such as rhinitis and eczema. This assumption has, however, been challenged (Pearce et al. 1999; Ronchetti et al. 2007; Weinmayr et al. 2007), and it is now increasingly accepted that asthma is a heterogenous syndrome that may be associated with different types of inflammation (Wenzel 2012). In particular, there has been growing interest in other non-allergic/ non-eosinophilic mechanisms underlying asthma (Douwes et al. 2002b; Simpson et al. 2007).

Allergic asthma

Allergic asthma is caused by IgE-mediated (or atopic) inflammatory mechanisms in which a large number of cells play a role including mast cells, eosinophils, T-lymphocytes, dendritic cells, and macrophages. Briefly, the sensitization process involves the interaction of allergens with dendritic cells in the airway mucosa, which subsequently migrate to the regional lymph nodes, where allergen epitopes are presented to B and T cells. This results (through T-helper-2 (Th$_2$) responses) in the production of allergen-specific IgE. Once allergic, a subject can develop symptoms minutes after being exposed, which is known as the early-phase allergic reaction. In the early phase, symptoms are a result of allergen-IgE antibody cross-linking at the surface of the mast cells, leading to degranulation and release of vasoactive and inflammatory mediators, causing contraction of bronchial smooth muscle and oedema in the airways. Clinically this results in a decreased lung function and symptoms of wheeze, shortness of breath, chest tightness, and coughing.

During the late phase of the allergic reaction (4–8 hours after exposure), eosinophil-related inflammatory reactions are particularly important. A critical step in this late phase reaction is the activation of Th$_2$ cells, which release several pro-inflammatory cytokines including IL-5, resulting in the influx and activation of eosinophils. This reaction is characterized by the development of a non-specific BHR that can continue for several days. Repeated exposures may result in more permanent BHR.

Non-allergic asthma

A systematic review of population-based studies (Pearce et al. 1999) found that the proportion of asthma cases that are attributable to atopy is usually less than half (Table 8.3.1). Standardized comparisons across populations or time periods also show only weak and inconsistent associations between the prevalence of asthma and the prevalence of atopy (Priftanji et al. 2001). For example, the International Study on Allergies and Asthma in Children (ISAAC; see later) showed that the association between atopy and asthma symptoms differed strongly among populations, but increased with economic development (Weinmayr et al. 2007). In this study, the fraction of current wheeze attributable

Table 8.3.1 Summary of nine population-based studies in children and seven population-based studies in adults: proportions of asthmatics and non-asthmatics who are atopic and % of asthma cases attributable to atopy

Age-group	% Non-atopic	% atopic	Pooled relative risk	% cases attributable to atopy
Children	29	58	3.4	38
Adults	24	54	3.7	37

Source: data from Pearce, N., et al., How much asthma is really attributable to atopy?, *Thorax*, Volume 54, Issue 3, pp. 268–72, Copyright © 1999 BMJ Publishing Group Ltd & British Thoracic Society. All rights reserved.

to atopy ranged from 0 per cent in Ankara (Turkey) to 93.8 per cent in Guangzhou (China) (Fig. 8.3.1); the overall proportion of asthma cases that were attributable to atopy was only 40.7 per cent in affluent countries and 20.3 per cent in non-affluent countries. The European Community Respiratory Health Survey (see later) showed that asthma attributable to atopy in adults ranged from 4 to 61 per cent between individual study centres with an overall estimate of only 30 per cent for all centres combined (Sunyer et al. 2004).

Several studies have also shown that patients may have severe and persistent asthma in the absence of eosinophilic inflammation, and may experience an exacerbation of asthma without an increase in eosinophilic inflammation (Turner et al. 1995). Furthermore, recent studies have demonstrated that less than 50 per cent of asthma cases are attributable to eosinophilic airway inflammation, the hallmark of allergic asthma (Douwes et al. 2002a; Simpson et al. 2006).

Thus, evidence from studies of eosinophilia and asthma is consistent with that from studies of atopy and asthma: in both instances, at most about one-half of asthma cases appear to be due to 'allergic' mechanisms.

The underlying mechanisms of non-eosinophilic/non-allergic asthma have yet to be fully elucidated. Some studies suggest that it may involve innate-like pathology, with increased airway neutrophil influx and expression of innate receptors such as Toll-like receptors (Simpson et al. 2007). There is also some evidence for combined activation of both innate (neutrophils) and allergic (eosinophils) inflammatory mechanisms in asthma. This has led to suggestions that asthma can be characterized into four inflammatory subtypes on the basis of sputum eosinophil and neutrophil proportions: eosinophilic asthma, neutrophilic asthma, mixed granulocytic asthma, and paucigranulocytic asthma (Simpson et al. 2006) (Fig. 8.3.2).

The pathophysiological mechanisms involved in paucigranulocytic asthma are not clear, but it is possible that they may involve remodelling rather than active inflammation (Holgate 2012).

There have been contradictory findings reported regarding the clinical characteristics of eosinophilic asthma (EA) and non-eosinophilic asthma (NEA) in adults. Some studies have shown eosinophilic airway inflammation in adult asthma in association with increased symptom severity and frequency (Gibson et al. 2000; Jatakanon et al. 2000). Despite this, NEA has been observed across the spectrum of clinical severity (Pavord et al. 1999; Wenzel et al. 1999), and several studies have shown very few clinical differences between EA and NEA (Simpson et al. 2006; Berry et al. 2007). However, there are also distinct differences: in particular, non-eosinophilic asthmatics appear less atopic, have normal subepithelial layer thickness, and perhaps most importantly, they have a poor short-term response to treatment with inhaled corticosteroids (Berry et al. 2007). NEA is also more likely to be associated with smoking history (Chalmers et al. 2001) and obesity (Sutherland et al. 2009). Thus, despite some clinical similarities, eosinophilic and non-eosinophilic asthma appear to represent distinct pathological phenotypes.

Asthma time trends

It has long been suspected that the prevalence of asthma has been increasing not only in industrialized countries, but also in developing countries (Pearce et al. 2000b). However, this has been a

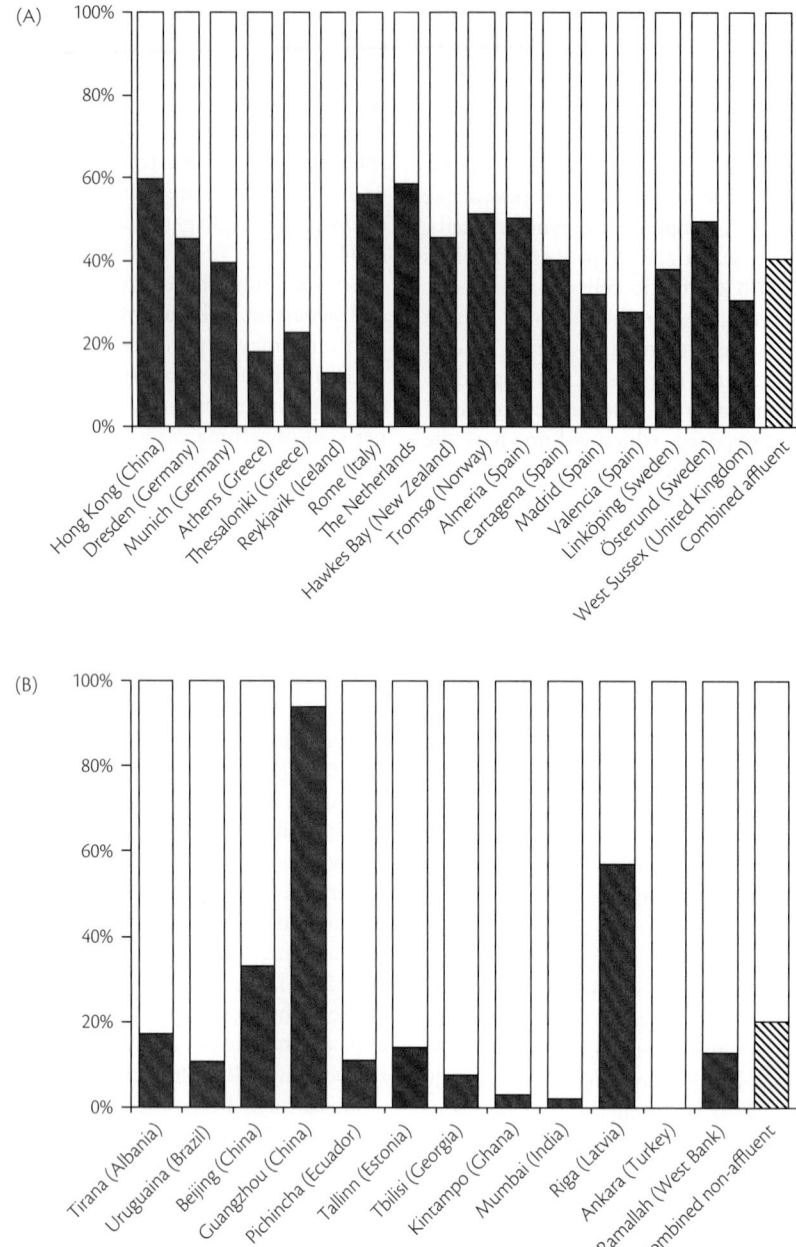

Fig. 8.3.1 The ISAAC phase II estimated attributable fractions (%) of current wheeze due to atopy for all affluent countries (A), and non-affluent countries (B).

Source: data from Weinmayr, G. et al., Atopic sensitization and the international variation of asthma symptom prevalence in children, *American Journal of Respiratory and Critical Care Medicine*, Volume 176, Issue 6, pp. 565–74, Copyright © 2007 The American Thoracic Society.

particularly difficult issue to resolve because of the lack of systematic standardized studies measuring changes in asthma prevalence over time, with some reviewers arguing that the increases in reported prevalence are largely due to increased awareness and diagnosis of asthma symptoms (Magnus and Jaakkola 1997). Nevertheless, most studies which have determined the prevalence of asthma symptoms using the same methodology in the same community at different times, have reported that asthma prevalence has increased in recent decades, and that the magnitude of the increase has in some cases been substantial (Table 8.3.2).

One of the most informative studies to date is that of Haahtela et al. (1990) who analysed the medical examination reports of

approximately 900,000 conscripts to the Finnish defence forces during 1966–1989, and a proportion of those examined in 1926–1961. During 1926–1961 the prevalence of asthma recorded at call-up examinations was in the range of 0.02 per cent to 0.08 per cent. However, asthma prevalence increased from 0.29 per cent in 1966 to 1.79 per cent in 1989. The authors concluded that the increase was unlikely to be simply due to improved diagnostic methods. This conclusion was strengthened by a concomitant rise (from 0.12 per cent in 1966 to 0.75 per cent in 1989) in exemptions and discharges due to asthma. This study is consistent with other evidence showing that the increases in asthma prevalence in industrialized countries appear to have

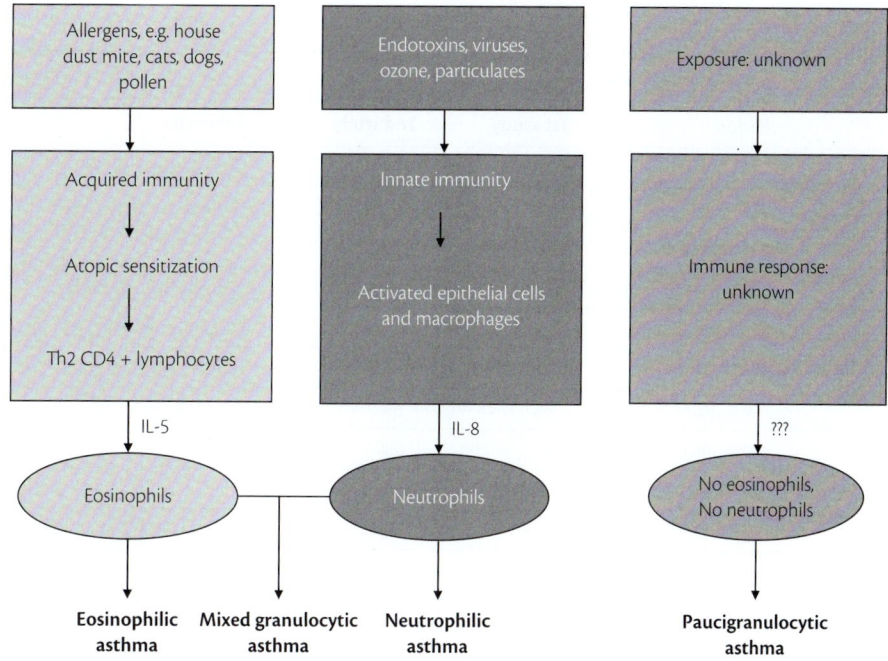

Fig. 8.3.2 The inflammatory pathways of various asthma phenotypes.

commenced after the Second World War, particularly in the 1960s and 1970s (Table 8.3.2).

However, several recent studies in affluent countries have reported either no increase, or even a decrease, in asthma prevalence over the last decade. For instance, Bollag et al. (2005) found that overall consultations for asthma in primary care in Switzerland increased from 1989 to 1994, then stabilized, and have declined since 2000. The observation that asthma incidence might be falling is in agreement with several other studies showing similar time trends for asthma and hay fever (Pearce and Douwes 2005).

International prevalence comparisons

The causes of the international time trends in the prevalence of asthma are unclear, and are currently under intensive investigation. An important component of this research process involves the use of standardized international prevalence comparisons (Pearce et al. 1998), which involve the compilation of information from large numbers of people in random samples collected in a comparable manner across social groups, regions, and countries. This approach has been used in the international survey of asthma prevalence in adults (Burney et al. 1994), and in the International Study of Asthma and Allergies in Childhood (Pearce et al. 1993; Asher et al. 1995; Ellwood et al. 2005).

The European Community Respiratory Health Survey

In each centre of the European Community Respiratory Health Survey (ECRHS), a representative sample of 3000 adults, aged 20–44 years, completed a Phase I screening questionnaire assessing asthma symptoms and medication use (Burney et al. 1994). Individuals answering 'yes' to waking with an attack of shortness of breath, an attack of asthma or current asthma medications were defined as 'asthmatic'. A random subsample of 600 subjects and an additional sample of up to 150 'asthmatic' individuals were then studied in more detail in Phase II, with measurements of skin prick tests to common allergens, serum total and specific IgE, bronchial responsiveness to inhaled methacholine, as well as an additional questionnaire on asthma symptoms and medical history, occupation and social status, smoking, the home environment and the use of medications and medical services. The Phase I results (Burney et al. 1996) included data from 48 centres, predominantly in Western Europe, with only nine centres from six countries (Algeria, Iceland, India, New Zealand, Australia, and the United States) outside of Europe. Phase II was conducted in 37 centres in 16 countries (Burney et al. 1996).

The International Study of Asthma and Allergies in Childhood

The International Study of Asthma and Allergies in Childhood (ISAAC) (Asher et al. 1995; Ellwood et al. 2005) had a similar study design, with a simple Phase I survey and a more in-depth Phase II survey. However, in order to obtain the maximum possible participation across the world, Phase I (which was conducted in 155 centres in 56 countries) was separated from Phase II (which was conducted in a smaller number of centres), and the Phase I questionnaire modules were designed to be simple and inexpensive to administer. In addition, a video presentation of clinical signs and symptoms of asthma was developed (Shaw et al. 1995) in order to minimize translation problems. The population of interest was schoolchildren aged 6–7 years and 13–14 years. ISAAC Phase II was conducted by 30 centres in 22 countries and involved parental questionnaires (n = 54,439), skin prick tests (n = 31,759) and serum IgE measurements (n = 8951). House dust samples to measure indoor allergens were also collected (Weinmayr et al. 2007). Phase III involved a repeat of the phase I survey after an interval of 5–10 years in 106 centres in 56 countries in children aged 13–14 years (n = 304,679) and in 66 centres in 37 countries in children aged 6–7 years (n = 193,404) (Asher et al. 2006; Pearce et al. 2007).

Table 8.3.2 Changes in asthma prevalence in children and young adults

Country	Asthma prevalence			
	Period	1st study	2nd study	Reference
Australia	1964–1990	19.1%	46.0%	(Robertson et al. 1991)
	1982–1992	10.4%	28.6%	(Robertson et al. 2004)
	1992–2002	28.6%	23.7%	
	1987–1992	5.6%	9.3%	(Campbell et al. 1992)
	1992–1995	9.3%	11.4%	(Adams et al. 1997)
	1993–2002	27.2%	20.2%	(Robertson et al. 2004)
	1966–1975	6%	6%	(James et al. 2010)
	1975–1981	6%	8%	
	1981–2005	8%	19%	
Canada	1980–1983	3.8%	6.5%	(Infante-Rivard et al. 1987)
	1980–1990[c]	140/10,000	256/10,000[a]	(Manfreda et al. 1993)
		125/10,000	254/10,000[b]	
England	1956–1975	1.8%	6.3%	(Smith 1976)
	1966–1990	18.3%	21.8%	(Whincup et al. 1993)
	1973–1986	2.4%	3.6%	(Burney et al. 1990)
	1978–1991	11.1%	12.8%	(Anderson et al. 1994)
England & Wales	1970–1981	11.6%	20.5%[a]	(Fleming and Crombie 1987)
		8.8%	15.9%[b]	
Finland	1961–1986	0.1%	1.8%	(Haahtela et al. 1990)
France	1968–1982	3.3%	5.4%	(Perdrizet et al. 1987)
Germany	1991/2–1995/6	3.7%	4.1%	(von Mutius et al. 1998)
Israel	1986–1990	7.9%	9.6%	(Auerbach et al. 1993)
Italy	1974–1992	5.5%	12.2%	(Ronchetti et al. 2001)
	1992–1998	12.2%	12.0%	
	1983–1993/5	2.9%	4.4%	(Ciprandi et al. 1996)
Japan	1982–1992	3.3%	4.6%	(Nishima 1993)
	1992–2002	4.6%	6.5%	(Nishima et al. 2009)
Netherlands	1989–1993	13.4%	13.3%	(Mommers et al. 2005)
	1993–1997	13.3%	11.9%	
	1997–2001	11.9%	9.1%	
New Zealand	1969–1982	7.1%	13.5%	(Mitchell 1983)
	1975–1989	26.2%	34.0%	(Shaw et al. 1990)
Norway	1985–1995	9.3%	13.2%	(Selnes et al. 2005)
	1995–2000	13.2%	13.8%	
Papua New Guinea	1973–1984	0.0%	0.6%	(Dowse et al. 1985)
Scotland	1964–1989	10.4%	19.8%	(Ninan and Russell 1992)
	1989–1994	19.8%	25.4%	(Omran and Russell 1996)
Spain	1994–2003	9.3%	9.3%	(Garcia-Marcos et al. 2004)
Sweden	1971–1981	1.9%	2.8%	(Aberg 1989)
	1979–1999	2.5%	5.7%	

(continued)

Table 8.3.2 Continued

Country	Asthma prevalence			
	Period	**1st study**	**2nd study**	**Reference**
	1985–1995	10%	14.5%	(Kalvesten and Braback 2008)
	1995–2005	14.5%	14.2%	
	1996–2006	11.7%	13.0%	(Bjerg et al. 2010)
	1990–2008	20%	16%	(Bjerg et al. 2011)
Switzerland	1992–1995	8.8%	7.8%	(Grize et al. 2006)
	1995–1998	7.8%	6.4%	
	1998–2001	6.4%	7.4%	
Tahiti	1979–1984	11.5%	14.3%	(Liard et al. 1988)
Taiwan	1974–1985	1.3%	5.1%	(Hsieh and Shen 1988)
United Kingdom	1991–1998	33.9%	27.5%	(Anderson et al. 2004)
	1991–1993	17.7%	22.0%	(Rizwan et al. 2004)
	1993–1998	22.0%	29.8%	
United States	1964–1983[d]	183/100,000	284/100,000	(Yunginger et al. 1992)
	1971–1976	4.8%	7.6%	(Gergen et al. 1988)
	1981–1988	3.1%	4.3%	(Weitzman et al. 1992)
	1983–1992	9.2%	15.9%	(Farber et al. 1997)
Wales	1973–1988	4.0%	9.0%	(Burr et al. 2006)
	1988–2003	15.2%	19.7%	

[a] Men, [b] women, [c] prevalence rates per 10,000 subjects, [d] incidence rates per 100,000 subjects.

What do the ECRHS and ISAAC studies show?

Firstly, both studies show striking international differences in asthma symptom prevalence with a particularly high prevalence of reported asthma symptoms in English-speaking countries (Fig. 8.3.3), that is, the British Isles, New Zealand, Australia, the United States, and Canada (Burney et al. 1996; Asher et al. 1998; Beasley et al. 1998). This appears to be unlikely to be entirely due to translation problems, since the same pattern was observed with the ISAAC video questionnaire (Asher et al. 1998).

Secondly, the ISAAC survey showed that centres in Latin America also had particularly high symptom prevalence (Fig. 8.3.3). This finding is of particular interest in that the Spanish-speaking centres of Latin America showed higher prevalences than Spain itself, in contrast to the general tendency for more affluent countries to have higher prevalence rates.

Thirdly, amongst the non-English-speaking European countries, both studies show high asthma prevalence in Western Europe, with lower prevalences in Eastern and Southern Europe. For example, in the ISAAC survey, there is a clear Northwest–Southeast gradient within Europe, with the highest prevalence being in the United Kingdom, and some of the lowest prevalences in Albania and Greece (Asher et al. 1998). The West–East gradient was particularly strong; in particular there was a significantly lower prevalence in the former East Germany than in the former West Germany.

Fourthly, Africa and Asia generally showed relatively low asthma prevalence (Fig. 8.3.3). In particular, prevalence was low in developing countries such as China and Indonesia whereas more affluent Asian countries such as Singapore and Japan showed relatively high asthma prevalence rates. Perhaps the most striking contrast is between Hong Kong and Guangzhou which are close geographically, and involve the same language and predominant ethnic group; Hong Kong (the more affluent city) had a 12-month period prevalence of wheeze of 12.4 per cent, compared with 3.4 per cent in Guangzhou (the less affluent city).

Fifthly, in contrast to the asthma findings, the highest prevalences of rhinitis symptoms were reported from centres scattered throughout most regions of the world, including Western Europe, Africa, North America, and South East Asia. Thus, although the prevalences of these conditions were correlated, the association was not particularly strong, suggesting that the major risk factors are different for these related disorders, or that they involve different latency periods and time trends.

Sixthly, the ISAAC Phase II study showed that the link between atopic sensitization and asthma symptoms differed strongly between populations and increased with economic development (Weinmayr et al. 2007); the association between atopy and flexural eczema was also weak and positively linked to gross national income (Flohr et al. 2008).

Finally, the asthma prevalence in many affluent countries has peaked or even begun to decline, whereas asthma symptom

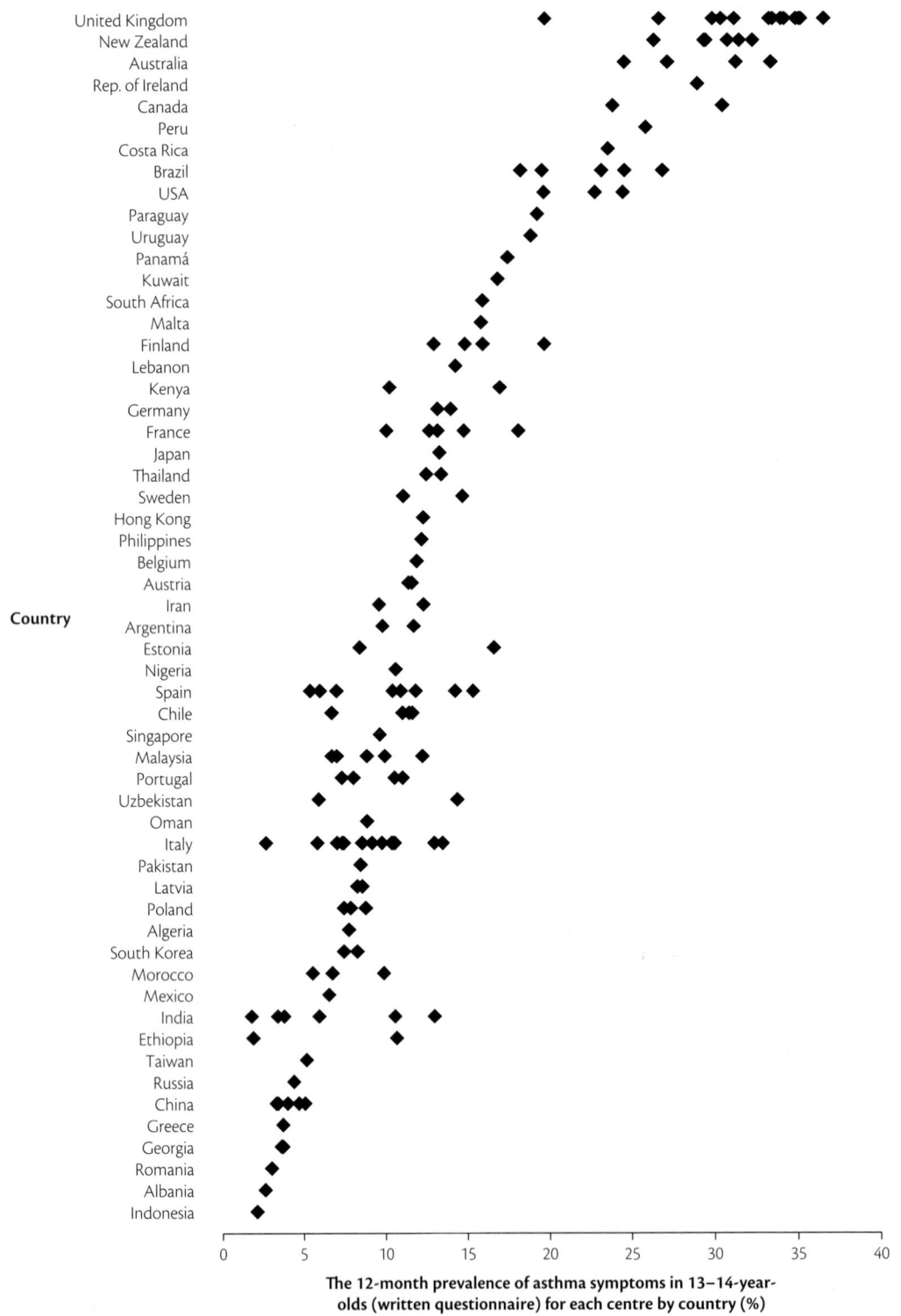

Fig. 8.3.3 Wheeze in the previous 12 months for each centre by country ordered according to the mean prevalence for all centres in the country.

Source: data from ISAAC Steering Committee, Worldwide variations in the prevalence of asthma symptoms: the International Study of Asthma and Allergies in Childhood (ISAAC), *The European Respiratory Journal*, Volume 12, Issue 2, pp. 315–35, Copyright © ERS Journals Ltd 1998.

prevalence continues to rise in less affluent countries. In particular, ISAAC Phase III showed that international differences in asthma symptom prevalence have reduced, particularly in 13–14-year-olds, with decreases in prevalence in English speaking countries and Western Europe and increases in prevalence in regions where prevalence was previously low including Africa, Latin America, and parts of Asia (Fig. 8.3.4) (Asher et al. 2006; Pearce et al. 2007). Similarly, Phase II of the ECRHS found no further increase in current or severe asthma symptoms (Chinn et al. 2004). Nonetheless, a significant increase in diagnosed asthma was observed which most

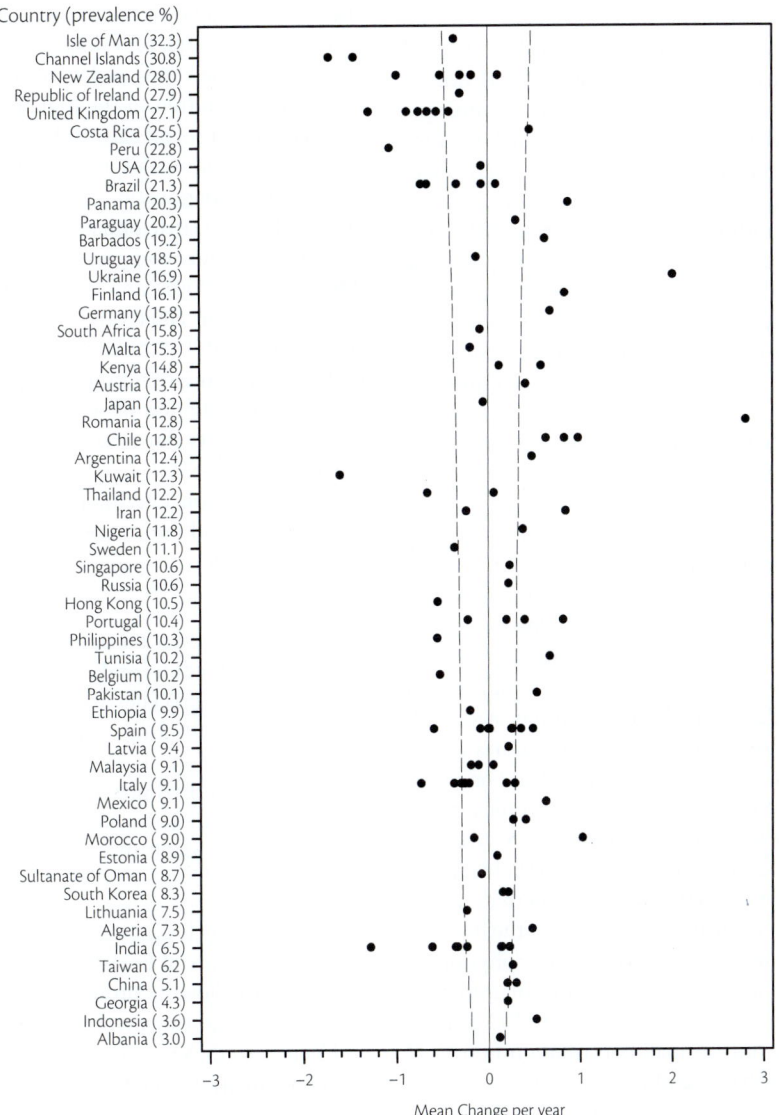

Fig. 8.3.4 Ranking plot showing the change per year in prevalence of current wheeze (wheeze in the last 12 months) in 13–14-year-old children for each centre by country, with countries ordered by their average prevalence (for all centres combined) across Phase I and Phase III (the plot also shows the confidence interval about zero change for a given level of prevalence (i.e. the average prevalence across Phase I and Phase III) given a sample size of 3000 and no cluster sampling effect).

Reproduced from Thorax, Pearce N. et al., Worldwide trends in the prevalence of asthma symptoms: phase III of the International Study of Asthma and Allergies in Childhood (ISAAC), Volume 62, Issue 9, pp. 758–66, Copyright © 2007 BMJ Publishing Group Ltd and the British Thoracic Society, with permission from BMJ Publishing Group Ltd.

likely reflects changes in diagnostic labelling and/or medical treatment for mild and/or moderate asthma (Weiland and Pearce 2004).

Risk factors for asthma

These striking findings from the ISAAC and ECRHS surveys, together with recent studies within Western countries, are challenging established theories of the development of asthma, and facilitating the search for new theoretical paradigms. In this section we review evidence on traditional risk factors as well as some more recently suggested risk factors for asthma.

Atopy

As noted earlier, atopy is strongly associated with asthma within populations. However, the proportion of asthma cases that are

attributable to atopy is usually less than one-half (Pearce et al. 1999) and an even lower population attributable risk (~20 per cent) was found in less affluent populations (Weinmayr et al. 2007). Also, comparisons across populations suggest that the association between atopy and asthma is relatively weak and highly variable between populations (Sunyer et al. 2004; Weinmayr et al. 2007). Furthermore, although atopy may be a risk factor for asthma, it is not a classic environmental 'exposure' (e.g. indoor allergen exposure, smoking, air pollution) which could by itself explain increases in asthma prevalence. Rather it represents a biological response to various exposures (e.g. allergen exposure) which is modified by susceptibility factors (genetic and/or environmental).

Genetic factors

The heritable component of asthma has been variously estimated to be between 35 and 95 per cent (Ober and Yao 2011). However, asthma is multifactorial in origin and influenced by multiple genes and environmental factors. Thus, it is not inherited in a simple Mendelian fashion, and particular genetic factors may affect one or more aspects of the complex aetiological processes potentially involved in asthma including atopic sensitization, BHR, airway inflammation, and innate immunity. Investigating possible genes for these individual aetiological factors is also fraught with difficulties, as control of these factors is also multifactorial (Zamel et al. 1996). Another issue is that asthma development, exacerbations and progression may all involve different environmental triggers and genetic factors.

Despite the considerable heterogeneity observed, a number of genome linkage and GWA studies have identified several chromosomal regions significantly associated with asthma susceptibility. Regions with the strongest evidence include chromosome 2q, 5q, 6q, 11q, 12q, and 13q (Bierbaum and Heinzmann 2007). A more recent GWA study of 10,365 physician-diagnosed asthmatics supported some of these associations, and also provided evidence of asthma susceptibility linkage with chromosomes 8, 15, and 22 (Moffatt et al. 2010). From these studies, a large number of asthma-susceptibility candidate genes have been implicated, with only some confirmed in subsequent independent studies (Todd et al. 2011). These include IL4, IL13, CD14, and ADRB2 on chromosome 5; HLA-DRB1, HLA-DBQ1, and TNF on chromosome 6; IL33 on chromosome 9; FCER1B on chromosome 11; SMAD3 on chromosome 15; IL4RA on chromosome 16; ORMDL3/GSDMB on 17q21; and ADAM33 on chromosome 20 (Bierbaum and Heinzmann 2007; Moffatt et al. 2010). In many cases, the involvement of the products of these genes in asthma pathophysiology is feasible, as they are associated with a variety of inflammatory or epithelial/cell-contact pathways. However, in the GWA studies described, these genes make only a small contribution to overall disease risk on an individual basis, and there may be issues due to the use of different asthma classifications in different studies (Todd et al. 2011). Furthermore, some gene variants may only be associated with certain asthma subtypes, such as that observed between ORMDL3/GSDMB and childhood-onset asthma (Moffatt et al. 2010).

Demographic factors

There are a variety of demographic factors which are associated with asthma including age, gender (Anderson et al. 1992), and ethnicity (Pattemore et al. 2004).

Asthma incidence and prevalence are consistently lower in females than in males before age 12 years, whereas during adolescence and adulthood there is evidence of higher incidence and prevalence in females (Kimbell-Dunn et al. 1999). The reasons for this are unclear, but could be related to later age of asthma onset in childhood and adolescence in females and differences between boys and girls in exposures, airway size, and frequency and severity of lower respiratory tract illnesses. On the other hand, these differences could be due to hormonal influences on allergic predisposition, airway size, inflammation, and smooth muscle vascular functions (Redline and Gold 1994). Premenstrual asthma may be especially relevant to the hormonal involvement of asthma since it may not only cause asthma exacerbations but may thereby affect the frequency and duration of asthma symptoms, resulting in an increase in the prevalence of 'current asthma'.

Studies in the 1960s and 1970s suggested that asthma is more common in children in the higher social classes. There has been less evidence of social class differences as the diagnosis of asthma has become more widespread (Littlejohns and Macdonald 1993), even though diagnostic labelling of wheezing in adults differs by social class (Littlejohns et al. 1989). However, severe asthma appears to be more common in children in the lower social classes (Stewart et al. 2001) and in some disadvantaged ethnic groups (Pattemore et al. 2004), and low socioeconomic status is associated with hospital admissions for asthma (Watson et al. 1996) and with reduced lung function in adults. This could represent either a greater prevalence of asthma in disadvantaged groups, or increased severity due to environmental factors (e.g. second hand tobacco smoke (SHS), nutrition, occupational exposures) (Eagan et al. 2002; Ellison-Loschmann et al. 2007) or inadequate disease management and poor access to healthcare (Ellison-Loschmann and Pearce 2006).

Obesity

Studies have shown an association between body weight and asthma in both adults and children, and prospective studies suggest that obesity precedes asthma (Ronmark et al. 2005; Noal et al. 2011). However, findings supporting this have not been entirely consistent (Noal et al. 2011). The evidence linking obesity and atopy is also conflicting with some studies suggesting that obesity is associated with asthma independent of atopy (Loerbroks et al. 2008; Visness et al. 2010).

Diet

Many studies including several infant cohort studies have investigated the effects of breastfeeding on allergies and asthma with some studies showing protective effects, some showing no effect, and others suggesting that breastfeeding is a risk factor (Friedman and Zeiger 2005; Kramer et al. 2007; Matheson et al. 2007).

Other nutritional factors may also play a role in the aetiology of asthma. In particular, it has been speculated that the increase in asthma prevalence may be due to a change in dietary patterns in the past few decades, that is, as cultures have become more 'Westernized' they have shifted from growing and consuming locally grown foods to consuming more processed foods, as well as a reduction in the intake of fresh produce. This is supported by results from the ISAAC Phase II and other studies (Chatzi and Kogevinas 2009; Nagel et al. 2010), which found that fruit, vegetable, and fish consumption was associated with a lower prevalence of current wheeze and asthma. Trans-fatty acids and burger consumption, on the other hand may be associated with an increased risk (Asher et al. 2010). Some studies have found that development of some atopic disorders was associated with exposures to n-6 versus n-3 fatty acids, but this finding was not consistent for all atopy/allergies (Almqvist et al. 2007; Notenboom et al. 2011). Maternal folate supplementation during pregnancy has also been suggested as a risk factor for asthma in childhood.

Vitamin D

There is an increasing number of studies suggesting an association between vitamin D and asthma with several studies based on dietary questionnaire findings showing a protective effect of higher levels of maternal vitamin D on the development of asthma in children (Muehleisen and Gallo 2013). In a recent study in which vitamin D levels were measured in cord blood, a similar protective effect of vitamin D was found with an inverse association with wheezing at the age of 15 months, 3 years and 5 years, but not for incident asthma by the age of 5 years (Camargo et al. 2011). Low serum vitamin D levels in asthmatic children and adults have also been associated with asthma severity and poor asthma control (Majak et al. 2011; Korn et al. 2013). However, the evidence has been mixed with some studies showing that infant vitamin D supplementation may be associated with an increased risk of atopy and allergic rhinitis in adulthood (Hypponen et al. 2004) and high maternal vitamin D levels with an increased risk of atopic eczema and asthma in children (Gale et al. 2008).

Outdoor air pollution

The role of outdoor air pollutants (particulate matter, ozone, nitrogen dioxide, and sulphur dioxide) in asthma has been extensively studied. An association between measures of distance to major roads or traffic density and asthma symptoms has been demonstrated in a number of European countries (World Health Organization 2005). Also, a large number of studies have reported associations between direct measurements of air pollution levels and exacerbation of pre-existing asthma, both in children and adults (Boezen et al. 1999; World Health Organization 2005). Some studies, including a birth cohort study (Brauer et al. 2007), have also suggested that air pollution may cause *new onset* of asthma and allergic disease. In particular, several large prospective studies have suggested a role for ozone (McDonnell et al. 1999; McConnell et al. 2002), although significant associations with some asthma outcomes were also shown for PM2.5, soot, and NO2 (Brauer et al. 2007).

Tobacco

The evidence for a role of tobacco smoke in asthma is strongest for increases in severity in children who already have asthma. However, an increasing number of studies also show positive associations between SHS and the initial occurrence of asthma (incidence) (Accordini et al. 2012). Earlier reviews and meta-analyses differed in their conclusions about the role of SHS (US EPA 1992; Office of Environmental Health Hazard Assessment 1997; US DHHS 2006; Strachan and Cook 1998), but a more recent meta-analysis including studies published between 1970 and 2005 concluded that household SHS exposure was positively and consistently associated with the incidence of new onset asthma (Vork et al. 2007) not only in younger, but also older children. A subsequent review and meta-analysis confirmed this conclusion, and suggested that SHS may increase the incidence of wheeze and asthma in children and young people by at least 20 per cent (Burke et al. 2012). Thus, despite some conflicting data (Eagan et al. 2002; Accordini et al. 2012), it generally appears that SHS causes new-onset asthma in children, and active smoking is causing asthma exacerbations, but may also be involved in the development of asthma itself in adolescents and adults.

Indoor air pollution

Little is currently known about the contribution of indoor air pollutants (other than SHS) to the incidence and prevalence of asthma. Nitrogen dioxide from burning fossil fuels has received the most attention while sulphur dioxide from burning sulphur-containing coal or gas, mosquito coil smoke, and formaldehyde from wood

preparation have also been considered. Particulates from open or closed wood and coal burning fires have received less attention in developed countries, but have been studied in developing countries where very high indoor levels have been encountered. Damp indoor environments and indoor fungal exposure may also play a role as demonstrated in a large number of studies conducted across many geographical regions (Douwes and Pearce 2003), with a 2011 report concluding that there is sufficient evidence for an association between indoor dampness and asthma development (Mendell et al. 2011).

Occupational exposures

Occupational asthma is the most common occupational respiratory disease in developed countries. For example, asthma accounted for 28 per cent of cases reported to the United Kingdom Surveillance of Work-related and Occupational Respiratory Diseases (SWORD) project (Meredith et al. 1991). Estimates of the total proportion of adult asthma which is thought to be occupational in origin range from 2 to 15 per cent in the United States, 15 per cent in Japan (Chan-Yeung and Malo 1994), 5 per cent in Spain (Kogevinas et al. 1996), 2–3 per cent in New Zealand (Fishwick et al. 1997), and 2–6 per cent in the United Kingdom (Meredith and Nordman 1996). A recent study in the United States estimated that new-onset asthma may be caused by occupational exposures in as many as one of six adult patients (Mazurek et al. 2013). More than 250 agents have been identified as causes of occupational asthma (State of New Jersey Department of Health (n.d.). Some of the most common occupational asthmagens include flour/grain dusts, wood dusts, latex allergens, and isocyanates.

Respiratory viral infections

Viral infections are common causes of exacerbations of asthma, and associated with hospital admissions in both children and adults (Johnston et al. 1995). In fact, respiratory viral infections are detected in the majority of asthma exacerbations; of these, about 60 per cent are rhinoviruses (Johnston 2007). Viral infections may also be involved in the development of asthma, but the evidence is less clear. Several long-term longitudinal studies have shown that respiratory syncytial virus (RSV) infections increase the risk of subsequent recurrent wheezing and asthma in early childhood (Sigurs et al. 2005). However, this risk may progressively decrease with increasing age (Stein et al. 1999). Other viruses have also been associated with asthma development including human rhinovirus (HRV) which may in fact be a more important risk factor than RSV (Lemanske et al. 2005). The mechanisms of viral-induced asthma are poorly understood, but it is possible that impaired innate immune responses may play a crucial role (Johnston 2007).

Paracetamol

It has been reported that prenatal paracetamol (or acetaminophen) use during pregnancy was a risk factor for asthma and wheezing in the offspring at 6–7 years of age (Shaheen et al. 2002, 2005). Similarly, several cross-sectional and longitudinal studies have reported that paracetamol use was associated in a dose-dependent manner with an increase in asthma in children and new-onset asthma in adults (Shaheen et al. 2000; Barr et al. 2004). Furthermore, national per capita consumption of acetaminophen was ecologically associated with the prevalence of wheeze, diagnosed asthma, and BHR in Western Europe (Newson et al.

2000). Some of these associations may have been due to confounding (e.g. confounding by indication), but this is unlikely to fully explain the positive associations in birth cohort studies (Shaheen et al. 2002, 2005), and longitudinal studies in adults that focused on new-onset asthma (Barr et al. 2004). The underlying mechanisms are unclear, but it has been suggested that paracetamol decreases glutathione levels in the lung, which may predispose to oxidative injury, bronchospasm, and an increased Th$_2$ response (Shaheen et al. 2002).

Allergens

Indoor allergens, particularly house dust mite allergens, are perhaps the group of possible asthma risk factors that have received the greatest attention. It is well established that in sensitized asthmatics, allergen exposure can trigger asthma attacks, and that prolonged exposure can lead to the prolongation and exacerbation of symptoms. However, most studies in children show only weak associations between allergen exposure and current asthma, even when the analyses are restricted to atopic patients and allergen avoidance has been accounted for (Pearce et al. 2000c). Also, secondary intervention trials have had mixed results (Gotzsche et al. 1998).

Furthermore, the evidence linking allergen exposure with new-onset asthma is weak (Pearce et al. 2000c). The key study linking allergen exposure in infancy to the subsequent development of asthma is that of Sporik et al. (1990) who followed 67 children with a family history of atopy. However, more recent longitudinal birth cohort studies found little or no association between early dust mite allergen exposure and asthma later in childhood (Burr et al. 1993; Corver et al. 2006; Tepas et al. 2006). For example, Burr et al. (1993) conducted a longitudinal study among 453 infants in South Wales with a family history of allergic diseases. Doctor diagnosed asthma and wheezing at age 7 was neither associated with mite allergen exposure as determined in the first 12 months nor at 7 years of age (ORs were not given). Similarly, in the German Multicentre Allergy Study, levels of mite and cat allergens in early life remained strongly related to specific sensitization at age 3–7 years (Lau et al. 2000, 2002), but no dose–response relationship between allergen exposure and any measure of asthma/wheeze at 7 years of age was found (Lau et al. 2000, 2002). Dust mite allergens are therefore unlikely to play a major role in the initial development of asthma. The evidence for a causal role of other allergens including cat, dog, cockroach and *Alternaria* allergens is even weaker (Pearce et al. 2000c).

Can the traditional risk factors explain the international patterns and time trends?

There is little evidence that the traditional risk factors can account for the global prevalence increases, or the international prevalence patterns observed. Furthermore, genetic factors alone are unlikely to account for a substantial proportion of asthma cases (Douwes and Pearce 2002) as the asthma prevalence increases have occurred too rapidly, although genetic susceptibility to changing environmental exposures may play an important role.

The global patterns of asthma prevalence are also inconsistent with the hypothesis that air pollution is a major risk factor for the development of asthma (Asher et al. 1998, 2006; Beasley et al. 1998). Regions such as China and Eastern Europe where there are some of the highest air pollution levels generally have lower asthma prevalence than the countries of Western Europe, North America, and Oceania, which have lower levels of pollution. It also appears unlikely that the international prevalence patterns can be explained by differences in smoking (Mitchell et al. 2002), or occupational exposures.

Allergen exposure is the risk factor that has perhaps received the most attention. In particular, it has been suggested that increases in indoor allergen exposures, through changes in lifestyle associated with Westernization, could account for the global increases in asthma prevalence (Sporik et al. 1990). However, the only study of English homes at two time points (1979 and 1989) did not demonstrate any change in house dust mite allergen levels (Butland et al. 1997), although marked increases have been observed in Australian studies (Peat et al. 1996).

The ISAAC (Asher et al. 1998) and ECRHS studies (Burney et al. 1996) have consistently found uniformly high levels of asthma prevalence in English-speaking countries, despite wide variation in house dust mite levels across these countries (Martinez 1997). In geographical areas in which dust mite exposure is very low or absent, including desert regions and mountainous regions the prevalence of asthma is as high as or even higher than that in other areas where house dust mite exposure is high (Martinez 1997).

Other available evidence on the association between allergen exposure and the subsequent risk of asthma at the population level is also less than persuasive. For example, Fig. 8.3.5 shows data from seven Australian surveys in centres with widely differing levels of mite allergen exposure; the overall prevalences of sensitization and asthma were both unrelated to the levels of house dust mite allergen (Der p 1) exposure in the six centres. The dominant

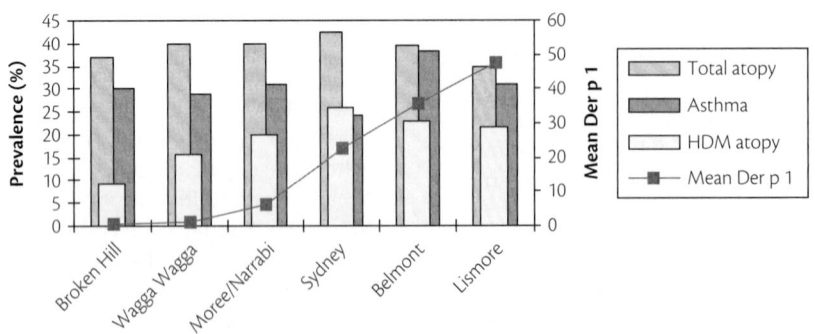

Fig. 8.3.5 Mean Der p 1 levels and prevalence (%) of house dust mite atopy, total atopy, and asthma in six areas of Australia.

Source: data from Peat JK et al. House dust mite allergens: A major risk factor for childhood asthma in Australia, *American Journal of Respiratory and Critical Care Medicine*, Volume 153, Issue 1, pp. 141–6, Copyright © 1996 American Thoracic Society. All Rights Reserved.

allergen varied between regions, but there was little overall difference in the prevalence of sensitization or of asthma despite the major differences in mite allergen levels.

The other asthma risk factors (e.g. diet, obesity, and/or paracetamol) may significantly contribute to the observed time trends and international patterns of asthma prevalence, but current evidence for this is scant.

Towards a new paradigm

Thus, although many of the traditional risk factors may exacerbate pre-existing asthma, the evidence that they may be involved in the initial development of asthma is limited. Also, there is little evidence that these factors account for the global prevalence increases.

Recent research has therefore shifted attention to factors that may 'programme' the initial susceptibility to asthma. This also involves a shift of attention from risk factors for asthma to protective factors, and the possible role of the loss of protective factors in the global increases in asthma prevalence (Pearce et al. 2000b). In particular, the increase in allergy and asthma contrasts strongly with a reduced prevalence of infectious diseases and corresponding decreased exposure to non-infectious microorganisms. This has been hypothesized as a possible explanation for the allergy and asthma epidemic (Eder et al. 2006), and is commonly referred to as the 'hygiene hypothesis'. The hygiene hypothesis has been prompted by evidence that overcrowding and unhygienic conditions were associated with a lower prevalence of atopy, eczema, hay fever, and asthma (Strachan 1989). Having a large number of siblings (especially older siblings) and attendance at daycare centres were determined to be particularly protective (Ball et al. 2000).

Several studies have shown associations between viral, bacterial or parasitic infections (e.g. hepatitis A, measles, *Schistosoma mansonii*) or Bacille Calmette–Guérin (BCG) immunization and a lower prevalence of atopy and allergies (Shaheen et al. 1996; Matricardi et al. 1997; Flohr et al. 2006), although findings have been inconsistent (Alm et al. 1998; Matricardi et al. 2000). It is possible that protection is specific to certain infections, at particular times of life. For example, one study found that croup (OR = 0.3; 95 per cent CI 0.12–0.72) and repeated ear infections (OR = 0.58; 95 per cent CI 0.35–0.98) in the first 12 months of life were inversely associated with atopy, whilst bronchiolitis was positively associated with asthma (OR = 2.77; 95 per cent CI 1.23–6.22) (Ramsey et al. 2007). Furthermore, it remains unclear as to what is the most important factor in protection from allergies and asthma; dose, route (oral–faecal versus airborne), type of infection (viral versus bacterial versus parasitic) or location (upper versus lower airways or digestive tract).

Environmental exposures to pro-inflammatory microbial agents (such as bacterial endotoxin) have also been suggested to be protective (Douwes et al. 2004). Studies have reported a significant inverse association between indoor endotoxin levels and atopic sensitization, hay fever, and atopic asthma (Braun-Fahrlander et al. 2002; Bottcher et al. 2003; Douwes et al. 2006). Recent work from ISAAC Phase II supports this, that is, combined across countries, household endotoxin levels were inversely related with asthma ever (OR = 0.53; 95 per cent CI 0.29–0.96) and current wheeze (0.77; 95 per cent CI 0.64–0.93) although the association with atopy was weaker (Gehring et al. 2008). However, the

available data regarding endotoxin are inconsistent with some studies showing an increased risk (Bolte et al. 2003; Perzanowski et al. 2006).

Exposures to different types of non-pathogenic bacteria may have differential effects on atopy and asthma. One birth cohort study showed that exposure to both Gram-positive and Gram-negative bacteria was inversely associated with asthma, whereas only Gram-negative bacteria were associated with allergic sensitization (Sordillo et al. 2010). More recently, studies in farming and non-farming environments have suggested that diversity of microbial species, rather than exposure to one particular microbial component, may be particularly protective (Heederik and von Mutius 2012). Consistent with these findings are recent observations that daycare centres—known to be associated with a lower prevalence of allergies and asthma in attending children—have been shown to be associated with considerable bacterial diversity (Lee et al. 2007) as have households with daycare attendees, or with cats and dogs (Maier et al. 2010).

In addition to specific agents with potential protective effects, subpopulations have been identified with low atopy and asthma rates compared to the general population. In particular, several studies have found consistently low prevalences of allergies and asthma in farmers' children, in both high- and low-income countries (Douwes et al. 2009; Genuneit 2012). These protective effects have also been observed in adult farmers (Douwes et al. 2007), despite increased risks of other respiratory conditions such as COPD (Schenker et al. 1998). The observed protective effects of farming on allergies and asthma have been particularly strong for animal contact (Douwes et al. 2008) or unpasteurized farm milk consumption (Loss et al. 2011), although the evidence for farm animals is mixed (Brunekreef et al. 2012). It remains unclear which specific factors are most important, but microbial exposures may play a role either through ingestion (lactobacilli, particularly through raw milk) or inhalation (endotoxin and other microbial components; see earlier). Whey proteins in raw milk may also be important (Loss et al. 2011). Protection conferred by farm residence may be dependent upon the type of farming conducted. For example, Ege et al. (2007) found that atopic asthma was inversely associated with animal exposures and raw milk consumption, but an effect for non-atopic asthma was only observed with silage exposure and agricultural farming. Recent data also suggest that farming may protect against asthma independent of atopy (Fuchs et al. 2012).

Furthermore, exposure to domestic animals may also confer protection. For example, pet ownership has been shown to be inversely associated with atopy and asthma in children and adults (de Meer et al. 2004b). This effect may be particularly strong with multiple pet exposures (Mandhane et al. 2009). In other parts of the world (Guinea-Bissau and Nepal) it has been shown that pigs and cattle in the home are associated with less atopy (Shaheen et al. 1996; Melsom et al. 2001). This is consistent with observations that animal contact in farmers' children may confer protection, and as hypothesized for the farmers' children, increased microbial exposures may play a role (Douwes et al. 2002b).

Although the specific immune mechanisms are not clear, it is believed that microbial exposures activate pattern recognition receptors (PRRs), such as Toll-like receptors (TLRs). This process is hypothesized to lead to downstream suppression of TH_2 cell expansion and therefore TH_2-mediated diseases, including allergic asthma, hay fever, and eczema (Douwes et al. 2002a). Originally this was believed to function simply through altering the TH_1/TH_2 balance, that is, growing up in a more hygienic environment with less microbial exposure would enhance atopic (TH_2) immune responses, whereas microbial pressure would drive the response of the immune system—which is known to be skewed in an atopic TH_2 direction during foetal and perinatal life—into a TH_1 direction and away from its tendency to develop atopic immune responses (Martinez and Holt 1999). This model now appears to be oversimplistic, as demonstrated by parasitic infections which are associated with powerful TH_2 responses, but protect against atopy (described earlier). An alternative model has been proposed involving altered immunoregulatory mechanisms whereby microbial modulation (either directly or indirectly) of regulatory T cells may result in reduced expression of both TH_1 and TH_2 immunity. Some evidence for this was provided by a study in newborns (Schaub et al. 2009) and animal studies (Schabussova et al. 2012). However, at this stage the immunological mechanisms underlying the observed epidemiological associations remain largely unclear

Can the 'hygiene hypothesis' explain the international patterns and time trends?

With the large proportion of asthma that is not attributable to atopy/allergy it is questionable whether the 'hygiene hypothesis' on its own can explain the large increases observed over the last decades or the global prevalence patterns, particularly since there is some evidence that non-atopic asthma may have increased more than atopic asthma (Thomsen et al. 2004). Also, although housing conditions are unlikely to have become more hygienic in inner city populations in the United States, asthma prevalence has increased significantly in those populations, particularly among African Americans living in poverty (Crater et al. 2001). Finally, the hygiene hypothesis is unlikely to explain why asthma prevalence is now apparently falling in some affluent countries (Chinn et al. 2004; Asher et al. 2006; Pearce et al. 2007), as exposures to factors that have previously been identified as being 'protective' (family size, endotoxin exposure, infectious diseases, pets, etc.) are likely to have decreased in more recent times rather than increased.

Thus, the hygiene hypothesis may not fully explain the current time and geographical trends in asthma prevalence. Nevertheless, whatever mechanism is involved, it is becoming increasingly clear that the 'package' of changes associated with Westernization may be contributing to the global increases in asthma susceptibility and prevalence.

Conclusions

What do these epidemiological findings tell us about the major causes of asthma and COPD?

The prevalence of COPD is still increasing particularly in women, and future projections indicate that the global burden of COPD will increase even further. The major causal risk factor is tobacco smoke, but a substantial proportion of COPD is also caused by occupational and indoor exposures, particularly in middle- and low-income countries. Only a minority of persistent smokers develop COPD, that is, those that are likely to be genetically susceptible for cigarette smoking. Similar to asthma, large international differences are observed in COPD prevalence even

when identical assessment methods are used, and these are not explained by age or cigarette smoking alone. Further understanding is required why some smokers develop COPD, and others don't, and what causes the striking differences in the global prevalence of COPD. However, we do know how to prevent COPD in the majority of cases, that is, smoking cessation is the most effective way to prevent the development of COPD and reduce disease progression.

In contrast, there remain major gaps in our current understanding of asthma aetiology. Although atopic sensitization is strongly associated with asthma, it appears to account for less than one-half of all cases, and there is little evidence that the traditional environmental asthma risk factors account for international prevalence increases. Recent decades have seen decreasing family size, increased hygiene, shift in dietary patterns, as well as increasing use of medical interventions such as immunization, antibiotics, and paracetamol. It seems that as a result of this 'package' of changes in the intrauterine and infant environment, we are seeing an increased susceptibility to the development of asthma and/or allergy. However, more recently the increase in asthma prevalence appears to have levelled off in many high-income countries, with some even showing a decrease. The reasons for this are unclear. Understanding why these changes are occurring, and ascertaining which elements of the 'package' of twentieth-century economic development and lifestyle changes are responsible, is essential in order to develop effective intervention programmes to halt the current global asthma epidemic.

Acknowledgements

The Centre for Public Health Research is supported by a Programme Grant from the Health Research Council of New Zealand.

References

Aberg, N. (1989). Asthma and allergic rhinitis in Swedish conscripts. *Clinical & Experimental Allergy*, 19, 59–63.

Accordini, S., Janson, C., Svanes, C., et al. (2012). The role of smoking in allergy and asthma: lessons from the ECRHS. *Current Allergy and Asthma Reports*, 12, 185–91.

Adams, R., Ruffin, R., Wakefield, M., et al. (1997). Asthma prevalence, morbidity and management practices in South Australia, 1992–1995. *Australian & New Zealand Journal of Medicine*, 27, 672–9.

Aggarwal, A.N., Gupta, D., and Jindal, S.K. (2006). The relationship between FEV_1 and peak expiratory flow in patients with airways obstruction is poor. *Chest*, 130, 1454–61.

Alm, J.S., Lilja, G., Pershagen, G., et al. (1998). BCG vaccination does not seem to prevent atopy in children with atopic heredity. *Allergy*, 53, 537.

Almqvist, C., Garden, F., Xuan, W., et al. (2007). Omega-3 and omega-6 fatty acid exposure from early life does not affect atopy and asthma at age 5 years. *Journal of Allergy and Clinical Immunology*, 119, 1438–44.

American Thoracic Society Committee on Diagnostic Standards (1962). Definitions and classification of chronic bronchitis, asthma and pulmonary emphysema. *American Review of Respiratory Disease*, 85, 762–8.

Anderson, H.R., Butland, B.K., and Strachan, D.P. (1994). Trends in prevalence and severity of childhood asthma. *BMJ*, 308, 1600–4.

Anderson, H.R., Pottier, A.C., and Strachan, D.P. (1992). Asthma from birth to age 23—incidence and relation to prior and concurrent atopic disease. *Thorax*, 47, 537–42.

Anderson, H.R., Ruggles, R., Strachan, D.P., et al. (2004). Trends in prevalence of symptoms of asthma, hay fever, and eczema in 12–14 year olds in the British Isles, 1995–2002: questionnaire survey. *BMJ*, 328, 1052–3.

Asher, M.I., Anderson, H.R., Stewart, A.W., et al. (1998). Worldwide variations in the prevalence of asthma symptoms: International Study of Asthma and Allergies in Childhood (ISAAC). *European Respiratory Journal*, 12, 315–35.

Asher, M.I., Keil, U., Anderson, H.R., et al. (1995). International Study of Asthma and Allergies in Childhood (ISAAC): rationale and methods. *European Respiratory Journal*, 8, 483–91.

Asher, M.I., Montefort, S., Bjorksten, B., et al. (2006). Worldwide time trends in the prevalence of symptoms of asthma, allergic rhinoconjunctivitis, and eczema in childhood: ISAAC Phases One and Three repeat multicountry cross-sectional surveys. *The Lancet*, 368, 733–43.

Asher, M.I., Stewart, A.W., Mallol, J., et al. (2010). Which population level environmental factors are associated with asthma, rhinoconjunctivitis and eczema? Review of the ecological analyses of ISAAC Phase One. *Respiratory Research*, 11, 8.

Auerbach, I., Springer, C., and Godfrey, S. (1993). Total population survey of the frequency and severity of asthma in 17 year old boys in an urban area in Israel. *Thorax*, 48, 139–41.

Badham, C. (1814). *An Essay on Bronchitis: With A Supplement Containing Remarks on Simple Pulmonary Abscess*. London: J. Callow.

Ball, T.N., Castro-Rodriguez, J.A., and Griffith, K.A. (2000). Siblings, day care attendance and the risk of asthma and wheezing during childhood. *The New England Journal of Medicine*, 343, 538–43.

Balmes, J.R. (2005). Occupational contribution to the burden of chronic obstructive pulmonary disease. *Journal of Occupational and Environmental Medicine*, 47, 154–60.

Barnes P.J. (2006). Against the Dutch hypothesis: asthma and chronic obstructive pulmonary disease are distinct diseases. *American Journal of Respiratory and Critical Care Medicine*, 174, 240–3.

Barr, R.G., Wentowski, C.C., Curhan, G.C., et al. (2004). Prospective study of acetaminophen use and newly diagnosed asthma among women. *American Journal of Respiratory and Critical Care Medicine*, 169, 836–41.

Bateman, E.D., Hurd, S.S., Barnes, P.J., et al. (2008). Global strategy for asthma management and prevention: GINA executive summary. *European Respiratory Journal*, 31, 143–78.

Beasley, R., Keil, U., Von Mutius, E., et al. (1998). Worldwide variation in prevalence of symptoms of asthma, allergic rhinoconjunctivitis and atopic eczema: ISAAC. *The Lancet*, 351, 1225–32.

Bel, E.H. (2004). Clinical phenotypes of asthma. *Current Opinion in Pulmonary Medicine*, 10, 44–50.

Berry, M., Morgan, A., Shaw, D.E., et al. (2007). Pathological features and inhaled corticosteroid response of eosinophilic and non-eosinophilic asthma. *Thorax*, 62, 1043–9.

Bierbaum, S. and Heinzmann, A. (2007). The genetics of bronchial asthma in children. *Respiratory Medicine*, 101, 1369–75.

Bjerg, A., Ekerljung, L., Middelveld, R., et al. (2011). Increased prevalence of symptoms of rhinitis but not of asthma between 1990 and 2008 in Swedish adults: comparisons of the ECRHS and GA(2)LEN surveys. *PLoS One*, 6, e16082.

Bjerg, A., Sandstrom, T., Lundback, B., et al. (2010). Time trends in asthma and wheeze in Swedish children 1996–2006: prevalence and risk factors by sex. *Allergy*, 65, 48–55.

Boezen, H.M. (2009). Genome-wide association studies: what do they teach us about asthma and chronic obstructive pulmonary disease? *Proceedings of the American Thoracic Society*, 6, 701–3.

Boezen, H.M. and Postma, D.S. (2007). Tumour necrosis factor and lymphotoxin A polymorphisms: a relationship with COPD and its progression? *European Respiratory Journal*, 29, 8–10.

Boezen, H.M., van der Zee, S.C., Postma, D.S., et al. (1999). Effects of ambient air pollution on upper and lower respiratory symptoms and peak expiratory flow in children. *The Lancet*, 353, 874–8.

Bollag, U., Capkun, G., Caesar, J., et al. (2005). Trends in primary care consultations for asthma in Switzerland, 1989–2002. *International Journal of Epidemiology*, 34, 1012–18.

Bolte, G., Bischof, W., Borte, M., et al. (2003). Early endotoxin exposure and atopy development in infants: results of a birth cohort study. *Clinical & Experimental Allergy*, 33, 770–6.

Bottcher, M.F., Bjorksten, B., Gustafson, S., et al. (2003). Endotoxin levels in Estonian and Swedish house dust and atopy in infancy. *Clinical & Experimental Allergy*, 33, 295–300.

Brauer, M., Hoek, G., Smit, H.A., et al. (2007). Air pollution and development of asthma, allergy and infections in a birth cohort. *European Respiratory Journal*, 29, 879–88.

Braun-Fahrlander, C., Riedler, J., Herz, U., et al. (2002). Environmental exposure to endotoxin and its relation to asthma in school-age children. *The New England Journal of Medicine*, 347, 869–77.

Brunekreef, B., Von Mutius, E., Wong, G.K., et al. (2012). Early life exposure to farm animals and symptoms of asthma, rhinoconjunctivitis and eczema: an ISAAC Phase Three Study. *International Journal of Epidemiology*, 41, 753–61.

Budulac, S.E., Vonk, J.M., Postma, D.S., et al. (2012). Nicotinic acetylcholine receptor variants are related to smoking habits, but not directly to COPD. *PLoS One*, 7, e33386.

Buist, A.S., McBurnie, M.A., Vollmer, W.M., et al. (2007). International variation in the prevalence of COPD (the BOLD Study): a population-based prevalence study. *The Lancet*, 370, 741–50.

Burke, H., Leonardi-Bee, J., Hashim, A., et al. (2012). Prenatal and passive smoke exposure and incidence of asthma and wheeze: systematic review and meta-analysis. *Pediatrics*, 129, 735–44.

Burney, P., Chinn, S., Luczynska, C., et al. (1996). Variations in the prevalence of respiratory symptoms, self-reported asthma attacks, and use of asthma medication in the European community respiratory health survey (ECRHS). *European Respiratory Journal*, 9, 687–95.

Burney, P.G., Chinn, S., and Rona, R.J. (1990). Has the prevalence of asthma increased in children? Evidence from the national study of health and growth 1973–86. *BMJ*, 300, 1306–10.

Burney, P.G.J., Luczynska, C., Chinn, S., et al. (1994). The European Community Respiratory Health Survey. *European Respiratory Journal*, 7, 954–60.

Burr, M.L., Limb, E.S., Maguire, M.J., et al. (1993). Infant-feeding, wheezing, and allergy—a prospective-study. *Archives of Disease in Childhood*, 68, 724–8.

Burr, M.L., Wat, D., Evans, C., et al. (2006). Asthma prevalence in 1973, 1988 and 2003. *Thorax*, 61, 296–9.

Burrows, B., Fletcher, C.M., Heard, B.E., et al. (1966). The emphysematous and bronchial types of chronic airways obstruction. A clinicopathological study of patients in London and Chicago. *The Lancet*, 1, 830–5.

Butland, B.K., Strachan, D.P., and Anderson, H.R. (1997). The home environment and asthma symptoms in childhood: two population based case-control studies 13 years apart. *Thorax*, 52, 618–24.

Calverley, P.M., Burge, P.S., Spencer, S., et al. (2003). Bronchodilator reversibility testing in chronic obstructive pulmonary disease. *Thorax*, 58, 659–64.

Camargo, C.A., Jr., Ingham, T., Wickens, K., et al. (2011). Cord-blood 25-hydroxyvitamin D levels and risk of respiratory infection, wheezing, and asthma. *Pediatrics*, 127, e180–7.

Camilli, A.E., Burrows, B., Knudson, R.J., et al. (1987). Longitudinal changes in forced expiratory volume in one second in adults. Effects of smoking and smoking cessation. *American Review of Respiratory Disease*, 135, 794–9.

Campbell, D., Ruffin, R., Mcevoy, R., et al. (1992). South Australian asthma prevalence survey. *Australian & New Zealand Journal of Medicine*, 22, A658.

Castaldi, P.J., Cho, M.H., Cohn, M., et al. (2010). The COPD genetic association compendium: a comprehensive online database of COPD genetic associations. *Human Molecular Genetics*, 19, 526–34.

Chalmers, G.W., MacLeod, K.J., Thomson, L., et al. (2001). Smoking and airway inflammation in patients with mild asthma. *Chest*, 120, 1917–22.

Chan-Yeung, M. and Malo, J.-L. (1994). Epidemiology of occupational asthma. In W. Busse and S.T. Holgate (eds.) *Asthma and Rhinitis*, pp. 44–57. Oxford: Blackwell Scientific.

Chapman, K.R., Mannino, D.M., Soriano, J.B., et al. (2006). Epidemiology and costs of chronic obstructive pulmonary disease. *European Respiratory Journal*, 27, 188–207.

Chapman, K.R., Tashkin, D.P., and Pye, D.J. (2001). Gender bias in the diagnosis of COPD. *Chest*, 119, 1691–5.

Chatzi, L. and Kogevinas, M. (2009). Prenatal and childhood Mediterranean diet and the development of asthma and allergies in children. *Public Health Nutrition*, 12, 1629–34.

Chinn, S., Jarvis, D., Burney, P., et al. (2004). Increase in diagnosed asthma but not in symptoms in the European Community Respiratory Health Survey. *Thorax*, 59, 646–51.

Cho, M.H., Castaldi, P.J., Wan, E.S., et al. (2012). A genome-wide association study of COPD identifies a susceptibility locus on chromosome 19q13. *Human Molecular Genetics*, 21, 947–57.

Chrysofakis, G., Tzanakis, N., Kyriakoy, D., et al. (2004). Perforin expression and cytotoxic activity of sputum CD8+ lymphocytes in patients with COPD. *Chest*, 125, 71–6.

Ciba Foundation Guest Symposium (1959). Ciba Foundation Guest Symposium (1959). Terminology definitions, classification of chronic pulmonary emphysema and related conditions. *Thorax*, 14, 286–99.

Ciprandi, G., Vizzaccaro, A., Cirillo, I., et al. (1996). Increase of asthma and allergic rhinitis prevalence in young Italian men. *International Archives of Allergy and Immunology*, 111, 278–83.

Committee on Diagnostic Standards for Nontuberculous Respiratory Diseases, American Thoracic Society (1962). Definitions and classification of chronic bronchitis, asthma and pulmonary emphysema. *American Review of Respiratory Disease*, 85, 762–9.

Corver, K., Kerkhof, M., Brussee, J.E., et al. (2006). House dust mite allergen reduction and allergy at 4 yr: follow up of the PIAMA-study. *Pediatric Allergy and Immunology*, 17, 329–36.

Crater, D.D., Heise, S., and Perzanowski, M. (2001). Asthma hospitalization trends in Charleston, South Carolina, 1956 to 1997: twenty-fold increase among black children during a 30-year period. *Paediatrics*, 108, E97.

Crockett, A.J., Cranston, J.M., Moss, J.R., et al. (1994). Trends in chronic obstructive pulmonary disease mortality in Australia. *Medical Journal of Australia*, 161, 600–3.

De Marco, R., Pesce, G., Marcon, A., et al. (2013). The coexistence of asthma and chronic obstructive pulmonary disease (COPD): prevalence and risk factors in young, middle-aged and elderly people from the general population. *PLoS One*, 8, e62985.

De Meer, G., Marks, G.B., and Postma, D.S. (2004a). Direct or indirect stimuli for bronchial challenge testing: what is the relevance for asthma epidemiology? *Clinical & Experimental Allergy*, 34, 9–16.

De Meer, G., Toelle, B.G., Ng, K., et al. (2004b). Presence and timing of cat ownership by age 18 and the effect on atopy and asthma at age 28. *Journal of Allergy and Clinical Immunology*, 113, 433–8.

Donohue, J.F. and Jain, N. (2013). Exhaled nitric oxide to predict corticosteroid responsiveness and reduce asthma exacerbation rates. *Respiratory Medicine*, 107(7), 943–52.

Douwes, J., Brooks, C., and Pearce, N. (2009). Protective effects of farming on allergies and asthma: have we learnt anything since 1873? *Expert Review of Clinical Immunology*, 5, 213–19.

Douwes, J., Cheng, S., Travier, N., et al. (2008). Farm exposure in utero may protect against asthma, hay fever and eczema. *European Respiratory Journal*, 32, 603–11.

Douwes, J., Gibson, P., Pekkanen, J., et al. (2002a). Non-eosinophilic asthma: importance and possible mechanisms. *Thorax*, 57, 643–8.

Douwes, J., Le Gros, G., Gibson, P., et al. (2004). Can bacterial endotoxin exposure reverse atopy and atopic disease? *Journal of Allergy and Clinical Immunology*, 114, 1051–4.

Douwes, J. and Pearce, N. (2002). Asthma and the westernization 'package'. *International Journal of Epidemiology*, 31, 1098–102.

Douwes, J. and Pearce, N. (2003). Is indoor mold exposure a risk factor for asthma? *American Journal of Epidemiology*, 158, 203–6.

Douwes, J., Pearce, N., and Heederik, D. (2002b). Does environmental endotoxin exposure prevent asthma? *Thorax*, 57, 86–90.

Douwes, J., Travier, N., Huang, K., et al. (2007). Lifelong farm exposure may strongly reduce the risk of asthma in adults. *Allergy*, 62, 1158–65.

Douwes, J., van Strien, R., Doekes, G., et al. (2006). Does early indoor microbial exposure reduce the risk of asthma? The Prevention and Incidence of Asthma and Mite Allergy birth cohort study. *Journal of Allergy and Clinical Immunology*, 117, 1067–73.

Dowse, G.K., Turner, K.J., Stewart, G.A., et al. (1985). The association between Dermatophagoides mites and the increasing prevalence of asthma in village communities within the Papua New Guinea highlands. *Journal of Allergy and Clinical Immunology*, 75, 75–83.

Eagan, T.M., Bakke, P.S., Eide, G.E., et al. (2002). Incidence of asthma and respiratory symptoms by sex, age and smoking in a community study. *European Respiratory Journal*, 19, 599–605.

Eder, W., Ege, M.J., and von Mutius, E. (2006). The asthma epidemic. *The New England Journal of Medicine*, 355, 2226–35.

Ege, M.J., Frei, R., Bieli, C., et al. (2007). Not all farming environments protect against the development of asthma and wheeze in children. *Journal of Allergy and Clinical Immunology*, 119, 1140–7.

Ellison-Loschmann, L. and Pearce, N. (2006). Improving access to health care among New Zealand's Maori population. *American Journal of Public Health*, 96, 612–17.

Ellison-Loschmann, L., Sunyer, J., Plana, E., et al. (2007). Socioeconomic status, asthma and chronic bronchitis in a large community-based study. *European Respiratory Journal*, 29, 897–905.

Ellul-Micallef, R. (1976). Asthma: a look at the past. *British Journal of Diseases of the Chest*, 70, 112–16.

Ellwood, P., Asher, M.I., Beasley, R., et al. (2005). The international study of asthma and allergies in childhood (ISAAC): phase three rationale and methods. *International Journal of Tuberculosis and Lung Disease*, 9, 10–16.

Farber, H.J., Wattigney, W., and Berenson, G. (1997). Trends in asthma prevalence: the Bogalusa Heart Study. *Annals of Allergy, Asthma & Immunology*, 78, 265–9.

Feenstra, T.L., van Genugten, M.L., Hoogenveen, R.T., et al. (2001). The impact of aging and smoking on the future burden of chronic obstructive pulmonary disease: a model analysis in the Netherlands. *American Journal of Respiratory and Critical Care Medicine*, 164, 590–6.

Fishwick, D., Pearce, N., D'Souza, W., et al. (1997). Occupational asthma in New Zealanders: a population based study. *Occupational & Environmental Medicine*, 54, 301–6.

Fleming, D.M. and Crombie, D.L. (1987). Prevalence of asthma and hay fever in England and Wales. *BMJ (Clinical Research Ed)*, 294, 279–83.

Flohr, C., Tuyen, L.N., Lewis, S., et al. (2006). Poor sanitation and helminth infection protect against skin sensitization in Vietnamese children: a cross-sectional study. *Journal of Allergy and Clinical Immunology*, 118, 1305–11.

Flohr, C., Weiland, S.K., Weinmayr, G., et al. (2008). The role of atopic sensitization in flexural eczema: findings from the International Study of Asthma and Allergies in Childhood Phase Two. *Journal of Allergy and Clinical Immunology*, 121(1), 141–7.

Friedman, N.J. and Zeiger, R.S. (2005). The role of breast-feeding in the development of allergies and asthma. *Journal of Allergy and Clinical Immunology*, 115, 1238–48.

Fuchs, O., Genuneit, J., Latzin, P., et al. (2012). Farming environments and childhood atopy, wheeze, lung function, and exhaled nitric oxide. *Journal of Allergy and Clinical Immunology*, 130, 382–8.

Gale, C.R., Robinson, S.M., Harvey, N.C., et al. (2008). Maternal vitamin D status during pregnancy and child outcomes. *European Journal of Clinical Nutrition*, 62, 68–77.

Garcia-Marcos, L., Quiros, A.B., Hernandez, G.G., et al. (2004). Stabilization of asthma prevalence among adolescents and increase among schoolchildren (ISAAC phases I and III) in Spain. *Allergy*, 59, 1301–7.

Gehring, U., Strikwold, M., Schram-Bijkerk, D., et al. (2008). Asthma and allergic symptoms in relation to house dust endotoxin: Phase Two of the International Study on Asthma and Allergies in Childhood (ISAAC II). *Clinical & Experimental Allergy*, 38, 1911–20.

Genuneit, J. (2012). Exposure to farming environments in childhood and asthma and wheeze in rural populations: a systematic review with meta-analysis. *Pediatric Allergy and Immunology*, 23, 509–18.

Gergen, P.J., Mullally, D.I., and Evans, R., 3rd (1988). National survey of prevalence of asthma among children in the United States, 1976 to 1980. *Pediatrics*, 81, 1–7.

Gibson, P.G., Saltos, N., and Borgas, T. (2000). Airway mast cells and eosinophils correlate with clinical severity and airway hyperresponsiveness in corticosteroid-treated asthma. *Journal of Allergy and Clinical Immunology*, 105, 752–9.

Gibson, P.G. and Simpson, J.L. (2009). The overlap syndrome of asthma and COPD: what are its features and how important is it? *Thorax*, 64, 728–35.

Global Initiative for Asthma (2006). *Global Strategy for Asthma Management and Prevention*. [Online] Available at: http://www.ginasthma.org/.

Global Initiative for Asthma (2013). *Global Strategy for Asthma Management and Prevention*. [Online] Available at: http://www.ginasthma.org/.

Gotzsche, P.C., Hammarquist, C., and Burr, M. (1998). House dust mite control measures in the management of asthma: meta-analysis. *BMJ*, 317, 1105–10.

Grize, L., Gassner, M., Wuthrich, B., et al. (2006). Trends in prevalence of asthma, allergic rhinitis and atopic dermatitis in 5–7-year old Swiss children from 1992 to 2001. *Allergy*, 61, 556–62.

Haahtela, T., Lindholm, H., Bjorksten, F., et al. (1990). Prevalence of asthma in Finnish young men. *BMJ*, 301, 266–8.

Halbert, R.J., Isonaka, S., George, D., et al. (2003). Interpreting COPD prevalence estimates: what is the true burden of disease? *Chest*, 123, 1684–92.

Halbert, R.J., Natoli, J.L., Gano, A., et al. (2006). Global burden of COPD: systematic review and meta-analysis. *European Respiratory Journal*, 28, 523–32.

Hancock, D.B., Eijgelsheim, M., Wilk, J.B., et al. (2010). Meta-analyses of genome-wide association studies identify multiple loci associated with pulmonary function. *Nature Genetics*, 42, 45–52.

Heederik, D. and von Mutius, E. (2012). Does diversity of environmental microbial exposure matter for the occurrence of allergy and asthma? *Journal of Allergy and Clinical Immunology*, 130, 44–50.

Hnizdo, E., Sullivan, P.A., Bang, K.M., et al. (2002). Association between chronic obstructive pulmonary disease and employment by industry and occupation in the US population: a study of data from the Third National Health and Nutrition Examination Survey. *American Journal of Epidemiology*, 156, 738–46.

Holgate, S.T. (2012). Trials and tribulations in identifying new biologic treatments for asthma. *Trends in Immunology*, 33, 238–46.

Hsieh, K.H. and Shen, J.J. (1988). Prevalence of childhood asthma in Taipei, Taiwan, and other Asian Pacific countries. *Journal of Asthma*, 25, 73–82.

Hypponen, E., Sovio, U., Wjst, M., et al. (2004). Infant vitamin d supplementation and allergic conditions in adulthood: northern Finland birth cohort 1966. *Annals of the New York Academy of Sciences*, 1037, 84–95.

Infante-Rivard, C., Esnaola Sukia, S., Roberge, D., et al. (1987). The changing frequency of childhood asthma. *Journal of Asthma*, 24, 283–8.

Isaac Steering Committee (1998). Worldwide variations in the prevalence of asthma symptoms: the International Study of Asthma and Allergies in Childhood (ISAAC). *European Respiratory Journal*, 12, 315–35.

James, A.L., Knuiman, M.W., Divitini, M.L., et al. (2010). Changes in the prevalence of asthma in adults since 1966: the Busselton health study. *European Respiratory Journal*, 35, 273–8.

Jatakanon, A., Lim, S., and Barnes, P.J. (2000). Changes in sputum eosinophils predict loss of asthma control. *American Journal of Respiratory and Critical Care Medicine*, 161, 64–72.

Johannessen, A., Omenaas, E.R., Bakke, P.S., et al. (2005). Implications of reversibility testing on prevalence and risk factors for chronic obstructive pulmonary disease: a community study. *Thorax*, 60, 842–7.

Johnston, S.L. (2007). Innate immunity in the pathogenesis of virus-induced asthma exacerbations. *Proceedings of the American Thoracic Society*, 4, 267–70.

Johnston, S.L., Pattemore, P.K., Sanderson, G., et al. (1995). Community study of role of viral-infections in exacerbations of asthma in 9–11 year-old children. *BMJ*, 310, 1225–9.

Kalvesten, L. and Braback, L. (2008). Time trend for the prevalence of asthma among school children in a Swedish district in 1985–2005. *Acta Paediatrica*, 97, 454–8.

Keeney, E.L. (1964). The history of asthma from Hippocrates to Meltzer. *Journal of Allergy & Clinical Immunology*, 35, 215–26.

Kemm, J.R. (2001). A birth cohort analysis of smoking by adults in Great Britain 1974–1998. *Journal of Public Health Medicine*, 23, 306–11.

Kharitonov, S.A. and Barnes, P.J. (2006). Exhaled biomarkers. *Chest*, 130, 1541–6.

Kimbell-Dunn, M., Pearce, N.E., and Beasley, R. (1999). Asthma. In M. Hatch (ed.) *Women and Health*, pp. 724–39. San Diego, CA: Academic Press.

King, C.S. and Moores, L.K. (2008). Clinical asthma syndromes and important asthma mimics. *Respiratory Care*, 53, 568–80.

Kirkham, P. and Rahman, I. (2006). Oxidative stress in asthma and COPD: antioxidants as a therapeutic strategy. *Pharmacology & Therapeutics*, 111, 476–94.

Kogevinas, M., Anto, J.M., Soriano, J.B., et al. (1996). The risk of asthma attributable to occupational exposures—a population-based study in Spain. *American Journal of Respiratory and Critical Care Medicine*, 154, 137–43.

Korn, S., Hubner, M., Jung, M., et al. (2013). Severe and uncontrolled adult asthma is associated with vitamin D insufficiency and deficiency. *Respiratory Research*, 14, 25.

Kraft, M. (2006). Asthma and chronic obstructive pulmonary disease exhibit common origins in any country! *American Journal of Respiratory and Critical Care Medicine*, 174, 238–40.

Kramer, M.S., Matush, L., Vanilovich, I., et al. (2007). Effect of prolonged and exclusive breast feeding on risk of allergy and asthma: cluster randomised trial. *BMJ*, 335, 815.

Laennec, R.T.H. (1821). *A Treatise on the Disease of the Chest (English translation from the French by J. Forbes)*. Preface and notes by J. Forbes. London: T. and G. Underwood.

Lau, S., Illi, S., Sommerfeld, C., et al. (2000). Early exposure to house-dust mite and cat allergens and development of childhood asthma: a cohort study. Multicentre Allergy Study Group. *The Lancet*, 356, 1392–7.

Lau, S., Nickel, R., Niggemann, B., et al. (2002). The development of childhood asthma: lessons from the German Multicentre Allergy Study (MAS). *Paediatric Respiratory Reviews*, 3, 265–72.

Lee, L., Tin, S., and Kelley, S.T. (2007). Culture-independent analysis of bacterial diversity in a child-care facility. *BMC Microbiology*, 7, 27.

Lemanske, R.F., Jr., Jackson, D.J., Gangnon, R.E., et al. (2005). Rhinovirus illnesses during infancy predict subsequent childhood wheezing. *Journal of Allergy and Clinical Immunology*, 116, 571–7.

Liard, R., Chansin, R., Neukirch, F., et al. (1988). Prevalence of asthma among teenagers attending school in Tahiti. *Journal of Epidemiology and Community Health*, 42, 149–51.

Littlejohns, P., Ebrahim, S., and Anderson, R. (1989). Prevalence and diagnosis of chronic respiratory symptoms in adults. *BMJ*, 298, 1556–60.

Littlejohns, P. and Macdonald, L.D. (1993). The relationship between severe asthma and social-class. *Respiratory Medicine*, 87, 139–43.

Liu, S., Zhou, Y., Wang, X., et al. (2007). Biomass fuels are the probable risk factor for chronic obstructive pulmonary disease in rural South China. *Thorax*, 62, 889–97.

Loerbroks, A., Apfelbacher, C.J., Amelang, M., et al. (2008). Obesity and adult asthma: potential effect modification by gender, but not by hay fever. *Annals of Epidemiology*, 18, 283–9.

Lokke, A., Lange, P., Scharling, H., et al. (2006). Developing COPD: a 25 year follow up study of the general population. *Thorax*, 61, 935–9.

Lopez, A.D., Mathers, C.D., Ezzati, M., et al. (2006a). *Global Burden of Disease and Risk Factors*. Washington, DC: The World Bank.

Lopez, A.D. and Murray, C.C. (1998). The global burden of disease, 1990–2020. *Nature Medicine*, 4, 1241–3.

Lopez, A.D., Shibuya, K., Rao, C., et al. (2006b). Chronic obstructive pulmonary disease: current burden and future projections. *European Respiratory Journal*, 27, 397–412.

Loss, G., Apprich, S., Waser, M., et al. (2011). The protective effect of farm milk consumption on childhood asthma and atopy: the GABRIELA study. *Journal of Allergy and Clinical Immunology*, 128, 766–73.

MacNee, W. (2005). Pulmonary and systemic oxidant/antioxidant imbalance in chronic obstructive pulmonary disease. *Proceedings of the American Thoracic Society*, 2, 50–60.

Magnus, P. and Jaakkola, J.J.K. (1997). Secular trend in the occurrence of asthma among children and young adults: critical appraisal of repeated cross sectional surveys. *BMJ*, 314, 1795–9.

Maier, R.M., Palmer, M.W., Andersen, G.L., et al. (2010). Environmental determinants of and impact on childhood asthma by the bacterial community in household dust. *Applied and Environmental Microbiology*, 76, 2663–7.

Majak, P., Olszowiec-Chlebna, M., Smejda, K., et al. (2011). Vitamin D supplementation in children may prevent asthma exacerbation triggered by acute respiratory infection. *Journal of Allergy and Clinical Immunology*, 127, 1294–6.

Mandhane, P.J., Sears, M.R., Poulton, R., et al. (2009). Cats and dogs and the risk of atopy in childhood and adulthood. *Journal of Allergy and Clinical Immunology*, 124, 745–50.

Manfreda, J., Becker, A.B., Wang, P.Z., et al. (1993). Trends in physician-diagnosed asthma prevalence in Manitoba between 1980 and 1990. *Chest*, 103, 151–7.

Mannino, D.M., Brown, C., and Giovino, G.A. (1997). Obstructive lung disease deaths in the United States from 1979 through 1993. An analysis using multiple-cause mortality data. *American Journal of Respiratory and Critical Care Medicine*, 156, 814–18.

Martinez, F.D. (1997). Complexities of the genetics of asthma. *American Journal of Respiratory and Critical Care Medicine*, 156, S117–22.

Martinez, F.D. and Holt, P.G. (1999). Role of microbial burden in aetiology of allergy and asthma. *The Lancet*, 354, S12–S15.

Matheson, M.C., Erbas, B., Balasuriya, A., et al. (2007). Breast-feeding and atopic disease: a cohort study from childhood to middle age. *Journal of Allergy and Clinical Immunology*, 120, 1051–7.

Matricardi, P.M., Rosmini, F., Ferrigno, L., et al. (1997). Cross sectional retrospective study of prevalence of atopy among Italian military students with antibodies against hepatitis A virus. *BMJ*, 314, 999–1003.

Matricardi, P.M., Rosmini, F., Riondino, S., et al. (2000). Exposure to food-borne and orofecal microbes versus airborne viruses in relation to atopy and allergic asthma: epidemiological study. *BMJ*, 320, 412–17.

Mazurek, J.M., Knoeller, G.E., Moorman, J.E., et al. (2013). Occupational asthma incidence: findings from the behavioral risk factor surveillance system asthma call-back survey—United States, 2006–2009. *Journal of Asthma*, 50, 390–4.

McConnell, R., Berhane, K., Gilliland, F., et al. (2002). Asthma in exercising children exposed to ozone: a cohort study. *The Lancet*, 359, 386–91.

McCormack, M.C. and Enright, P.L. (2008). Making the diagnosis of asthma. *Respiratory Care*, 53, 583–90.

McDonnell, W.F., Abbey, D.E., Nishino, N., et al. (1999). Long-term ambient ozone concentration and the incidence of asthma in nonsmoking adults: the AHSMOG Study. *Environmental Research*, 80, 110–21.

Medbo, A. and Melbye, H. (2007). Lung function testing in the elderly—can we still use $FEV_1/FVC<70\%$ as a criterion of COPD? *Respiratory Medicine*, 101, 1097–105.

Melsom, T., Brinch, L., Hessen, J. O., et al. (2001). Asthma and indoor environment in Nepal. *Thorax*, 56, 477–81.

Mendell, M.J., Mirer, A.G., Cheung, K., et al. (2011). Respiratory and allergic health effects of dampness, mold, and dampness-related agents: a review of the epidemiologic evidence. *Environmental Health Perspectives*, 119, 748–56.

Menezes, A.M., Perez-Padilla, R., Jardim, J.R., et al. (2005). Chronic obstructive pulmonary disease in five Latin American cities (the PLATINO study): a prevalence study. *The Lancet*, 366, 1875–81.

Meredith, S. and Nordman, H. (1996). Occupational asthma: measures of frequency from four countries. *Thorax*, 51, 435–40.

Meredith, S.K., Taylor, V.M., and McDonald, J.C. (1991). Occupational Respiratory-Disease in the United-Kingdom 1989—a Report to the British-Thoracic-Society and the Society-of-Occupational-Medicine by the Sword Project Group. *British Journal of Industrial Medicine*, 48, 292–8.

Miller, M.R., Hankinson, J., Brusasco, V., et al. (2005). Standardisation of spirometry. *European Respiratory Journal*, 26, 319–38.

Miravitlles, M., de la Roza, C., Naberan, K., et al. (2006). [Attitudes toward the diagnosis of chronic obstructive pulmonary disease in primary care]. *Archivos de Bronconeumología*, 42, 3–8.

Miravitlles, M., Ferrer, M., Pont, A., et al. (2005). Characteristics of a population of COPD patients identified from a population-based study. Focus on previous diagnosis and never smokers. *Respiratory Medicine*, 99, 985–95.

Mitchell, E.A. (1983). Increasing prevalence of asthma in children. *New Zealand Medical Journal*, 96, 463–4.

Mitchell, E.A., Stewart, A.W., ISAAC Phase One Study Group. International Study of Asthma and Allergy in Childhood (2002). The ecological relationship of tobacco smoking to the prevalence of symptoms of asthma and other atopic diseases in children: The International Study of Asthma and Allergies in Childhood (ISAAC). *European Journal of Epidemiology*, 17, 667–73.

Moffatt, M.F., Gut, I.G., Demenais, F., et al. (2010). A large-scale, consortium-based genomewide association study of asthma. *The New England Journal of Medicine*, 363, 1211–21.

Mommers, M., Gielkens-Sijstermans, C., Swaen, G.M., et al. (2005). Trends in the prevalence of respiratory symptoms and treatment in Dutch children over a 12 year period: results of the fourth consecutive survey. *Thorax*, 60, 97–9.

Muehleisen, B. and Gallo, R.L. (2013). Vitamin D in allergic disease: shedding light on a complex problem. *Journal of Allergy and Clinical Immunology*, 131, 324–9.

Nagel, G., Weinmayr, G., Kleiner, A., et al. (2010). Effect of diet on asthma and allergic sensitisation in the International Study on Allergies and Asthma in Childhood (ISAAC) Phase Two. *Thorax*, 65, 516–22.

Newson, R.B., Shaheen, S.O., Chinn, S., et al. (2000). Paracetamol sales and atopic disease in children and adults: an ecological analysis. *European Respiratory Journal*, 16, 817–23.

Ninan, T.K. and Russell, G. (1992). Respiratory symptoms and atopy in Aberdeen schoolchildren: evidence from two surveys 25 years apart. *BMJ*, 304, 873–5.

Nishima, S. (1993). [A study on the prevalence of bronchial asthma in school children in western districts of Japan—comparison between the studies in 1982 and in 1992 with the same methods and same districts. The Study Group of the Prevalence of Bronchial Asthma, the West Japan Study Group of Bronchial Asthma]. *Arerugi*, 42, 192–204.

Nishima, S., Chisaka, H., Fujiwara, T., et al. (2009). Surveys on the prevalence of pediatric bronchial asthma in Japan: a comparison between the 1982, 1992, and 2002 surveys conducted in the same region using the same methodology. *Allergology International*, 58, 37–53.

Noal, R.B., Menezes, A.M., Macedo, S.E., et al. (2011). Childhood body mass index and risk of asthma in adolescence: a systematic review. *Obesity Reviews*, 12, 93–104.

Notenboom, M.L., Mommers, M., Jansen, E.H., et al. (2011). Maternal fatty acid status in pregnancy and childhood atopic manifestations: KOALA Birth Cohort Study. *Clinical & Experimental Allergy*, 41, 407–16.

Ober, C. and Yao, T.C. (2011). The genetics of asthma and allergic disease: a 21st century perspective. *Immunological Reviews*, 242, 10–30.

Office of Environmental Health Hazard Assessment (1997). *Health Effects of Exposure to Environmental Tobacco Smoke*. Sacramento, CA: California Environmental Protection Agency.

Omran, M. and Russell, G. (1996). Continuing increase in respiratory symptoms and atopy in Aberdeen schoolchildren. *BMJ*, 312, 34.

Parkerson, J. and Ledford, D. (2011). Mannitol as an indirect bronchoprovocation test for the 21st century. *Annals of Allergy, Asthma & Immunology*, 106, 91–6.

Pattemore, P.K., Ellison-Loschmann, L., Asher, M.I., et al. (2004). Asthma prevalence in European, Maori, and Pacific children in New Zealand: ISAAC study. *Pediatric Pulmonology*, 37, 433–42.

Pavord, I.D., Brightling, C.E., Woltmann, G., et al. (1999). Non-eosinophilic corticosteroid unresponsive asthma. *The Lancet*, 353, 2213–14.

Pearce, N., Ait-Khaled, N., Beasley, R., et al. (2007). Worldwide trends in the prevalence of asthma symptoms: phase III of the International Study of Asthma and Allergies in Childhood (ISAAC). *Thorax*, 62, 758–66.

Pearce, N., Beasley, R., Burgess, C., et al. (1998). *Asthma Epidemiology: Principles and Methods*. New York: Oxford University Press.

Pearce, N., Beasley, R., and Pekkanen, J. (2000a). Role of bronchial responsiveness testing in asthma prevalence surveys. *Thorax*, 55, 352–4.

Pearce, N. and Douwes, J. (2005). Asthma time trends—mission accomplished? *International Journal of Epidemiology*, 34, 1018–19.

Pearce, N., Douwes, J., and Beasley, R. (2000b). The rise and rise of asthma: a new paradigm for the new millennium? *Journal of Epidemiology & Biostatistics*, 5, 5–16.

Pearce, N., Douwes, J., and Beasley, R. (2000c). Is allergen exposure the major primary cause of asthma? *Thorax*, 55, 424–31.

Pearce, N., Pekkanen, J., and Beasley, R. (1999). How much asthma is really attributable to atopy? *Thorax*, 54, 268–72.

Pearce, N., Weiland, S., Keil, U., et al. (1993). Self-reported prevalence of asthma symptoms in children in Australia, England, Germany and New Zealand: an international comparison using the ISAAC protocol. *European Respiratory Journal*, 6, 1455–61.

Peat, J.K., Tovey, E., Toelle, B.G., et al. (1996). House dust mite allergens—a major risk factor for childhood asthma in Australia. *American Journal of Respiratory and Critical Care Medicine*, 153, 141–6.

Perdrizet, S., Neukirch, F., Cooreman, J., et al. (1987). Prevalence of asthma in adolescents in various parts of France and its relationship to respiratory allergic manifestations. *Chest*, 91, 104S–106S.

Perzanowski, M.S., Miller, R.L., Thorne, P.S., et al. (2006). Endotoxin in inner-city homes: associations with wheeze and eczema in early childhood. *Journal of Allergy and Clinical Immunology*, 117, 1082–9.

Petty, T.L. (2002). COPD in perspective. *Chest*, 121, 116S–120S.

Petty, T.L. (2006). The history of COPD. *International Journal of COPD*, 1, 3–14.

Pillai, S.G., Ge, D., Zhu, G., et al. (2009). A genome-wide association study in chronic obstructive pulmonary disease (COPD): identification of two major susceptibility loci. *PLoS Genetics*, 5, e1000421.

Postma, D.S., Kerkhof, M., Boezen, H.M., et al. (2011). Asthma and chronic obstructive pulmonary disease: common genes, common environments? *American Journal of Respiratory and Critical Care Medicine*, 183, 1588–94.

Priftanji, A., Strachan, D., Burr, M., et al. (2001). Asthma and allergy in Albania and the UK. *The Lancet*, 358, 1426–7.

Rabe, K.F., Hurd, S., Anzueto, A., et al. (2007). Global strategy for the diagnosis, management, and prevention of chronic obstructive pulmonary disease: GOLD executive summary. *American Journal of Respiratory and Critical Care Medicine*, 176, 532–55.

Ramsey, C.D., Gold, D.R., Litonjua, A.A., et al. (2007). Respiratory illnesses in early life and asthma and atopy in childhood. *Journal of Allergy and Clinical Immunology*, 119, 150–6.

Redline, S. and Gold, D. (1994). Challenges in interpreting gender differences in asthma. *American Journal of Respiratory and Critical Care Medicine*, 150, 1219–21.

Rennard, S., Decramer, M., Calverley, P.M., et al. (2002). Impact of COPD in North America and Europe in 2000: subjects' perspective of Confronting COPD International Survey. *European Respiratory Journal*, 20, 799–805.

Rizwan, S., Reid, J., Kelly, Y., et al. (2004). Trends in childhood and parental asthma prevalence in Merseyside, 1991–1998. *Journal of Public Health (Oxford)*, 26, 337–42.

Robertson, C.F., Heycock, E., Bishop, J., et al. (1991). Prevalence of asthma in Melbourne schoolchildren: changes over 26 years. *BMJ*, 302, 1116–18.

Robertson, C.F., Roberts, M.F., and Kappers, J.H. (2004). Asthma prevalence in Melbourne schoolchildren: have we reached the peak? *Medical Journal of Australia*, 180, 273–6.

Ronchetti, R., Rennerova, Z., Barreto, M., et al. (2007). The prevalence of atopy in asthmatic children correlates strictly with the prevalence of atopy among nonasthmatic children. *International Archives of Allergy and Immunology*, 142, 79–85.

Ronchetti, R., Villa, M.P., Barreto, M., et al. (2001). Is the increase in childhood asthma coming to an end? Findings from three surveys of schoolchildren in Rome, Italy. *European Respiratory Journal*, 17, 881–6.

Ronmark, E., Andersson, C., Nystrom, L., et al. (2005). Obesity increases the risk of incident asthma among adults. *European Respiratory Journal*, 25, 282–8.

Salvi, S.S. and Barnes, P.J. (2009). Chronic obstructive pulmonary disease in non-smokers. *The Lancet*, 374, 733–43.

Schabussova, I., Hufnagl, K., Tang, M.L., et al. (2012). Perinatal maternal administration of Lactobacillus paracasei NCC 2461 prevents allergic inflammation in a mouse model of birch pollen allergy. *PLoS One*, 7, e40271.

Schaub, B., Liu, J., Hoppler, S., et al. (2009). Maternal farm exposure modulates neonatal immune mechanisms through regulatory T cells. *Journal of Allergy and Clinical Immunology*, 123, 774–82.

Schenker, M.B., Christiani, D., Cormier, Y., et al. (1998). Respiratory health hazards in agriculture. *American Journal of Respiratory and Critical Care Medicine*, 158, S1–S76.

Selnes, A., Nystad, W., Bolle, R., et al. (2005). Diverging prevalence trends of atopic disorders in Norwegian children. Results from three cross-sectional studies. *Allergy*, 60, 894–9.

Shaheen, S.O., Aaby, P., Hall, A.J., et al. (1996). Measles and atopy in Guinea-Bissau. *The Lancet*, 347, 1792–6.

Shaheen, S.O., Newson, R B., Henderson, A.J., et al. (2005). Prenatal paracetamol exposure and risk of asthma and elevated immunoglobulin E in childhood. *Clinical & Experimental Allergy*, 35, 18–25.

Shaheen, S.O., Newson, R.B., Sherriff, A., et al. (2002). Paracetamol use in pregnancy and wheezing in early childhood. *Thorax*, 57, 958–63.

Shaheen, S.O., Sterne, J.A., Songhurst, C.E., et al. (2000). Frequent paracetamol use and asthma in adults. *Thorax*, 55, 266–70.

Shaw, D., Green, R., Berry, M., et al. (2012). A cross-sectional study of patterns of airway dysfunction, symptoms and morbidity in primary care asthma. *Primary Care Respiratory Journal*, 21, 283–7.

Shaw, R., Woodman, K., Ayson, M., et al. (1995). Measuring the prevalence of bronchial hyper-responsiveness in children. *International Journal of Epidemiology*, 24, 597–602.

Shaw, R.A., Crane, J., O'Donnell, T.V., et al. (1990). Increasing asthma prevalence in a rural New Zealand adolescent population: 1975–89. *Archives of Disease in Childhood*, 65, 1319–23.

Sigurs, N., Gustafsson, P.M., Bjarnason, R., et al. (2005). Severe respiratory syncytial virus bronchiolitis in infancy and asthma and allergy at age 13. *American Journal of Respiratory and Critical Care Medicine*, 171, 137–41.

Silva, G.E., Sherrill, D.L., Guerra, S., et al. (2004). Asthma as a risk factor for COPD in a longitudinal study. *Chest*, 126, 59–65.

Simpson, J.L., Grissell, T.V., Douwes, J., et al. (2007). Innate immune activation in neutrophilic asthma and bronchiectasis. *Thorax*, 62, 211–18.

Simpson, J.L., McDonald, V.M., Baines, K.J., et al. (2013). Influence of age, past smoking, and disease severity on TLR2, neutrophilic inflammation, and MMP-9 levels in COPD. *Mediators of Inflammation*, 2013, 462934.

Simpson, J.L., Scott, R., Boyle, M.J., et al. (2006). Inflammatory subtypes in asthma: assessment and identification using induced sputum. *Respirology*, 11, 54–61.

Smith, A.D., Cowan, J.O., Filsell, S., et al. (2004). Diagnosing asthma: comparisons between exhaled nitric oxide measurements and conventional tests. *American Journal of Respiratory and Critical Care Medicine*, 169, 473–8.

Smith, J.M. (1976). The prevalence of asthma and wheezing in children. *British Journal of Diseases of the Chest*, 70, 73–7.

Smolonska, J., Wijmenga, C., Postma, D.S., et al. (2009). Meta-analyses on suspected chronic obstructive pulmonary disease genes: a summary of 20 years' research. *American Journal of Respiratory and Critical Care Medicine*, 180, 618–31.

Sordillo, J.E., Hoffman, E.B., Celedon, J.C., et al. (2010). Multiple microbial exposures in the home may protect against asthma or allergy in childhood. *Clinical & Experimental Allergy*, 40, 902–10.

Soriano, J.B., Davis, K.J., Coleman, B., et al. (2003). The proportional Venn diagram of obstructive lung disease: two approximations from the United States and the United Kingdom. *Chest*, 124, 474–81.

Soriano, J.B., Maier, W.C., Egger, P., et al. (2000). Recent trends in physician diagnosed COPD in women and men in the UK. *Thorax*, 55, 789–94.

Sporik, R., Holgate, S.T., Plattsmills, T.A.E., et al. (1990). Exposure to house-dust mite allergen (Der-P-I) and the development of asthma in childhood—a prospective-study. *The New England Journal of Medicine*, 323, 502–7.

State of New Jersey Department of Health (n.d.). *Industries and Asthma-Causing Agents*. [Online] Available at: http://www.state.nj.us/health/eoh/survweb/wra/agents.shtml.

Stein, R.T., Sherrill, D., Morgan, W.J., et al. (1999). Respiratory syncytial virus in early life and risk of wheeze and allergy by age 13 years. *The Lancet*, 354, 541–5.

Stewart, A.W., Mitchell, E.A., Pearce, N., et al. (2001). The relationship of per capita gross national product to the prevalence of symptoms of asthma and other atopic diseases in children (ISAAC). *International Journal of Epidemiology*, 30, 173–9.

Strachan, D.P. (1989). Hay fever, hygiene, and household size. *BMJ*, 299, 1259–60.

Strachan D.P. and Cook D.G. (1998). Parental smoking and childhood asthma: longitudinal and case-control studies. *Thorax*, 53, 204–12.

Sunyer, J., Jarvis, D., Pekkanen, J., et al. (2004). Geographic variations in the effect of atopy on asthma in the European Community Respiratory Health Study. *Journal of Allergy and Clinical Immunology*, 114, 1033–9.

Sutherland, E.R., Lehman, E.B., Teodorescu, M., et al. (2009). Body mass index and phenotype in subjects with mild-to-moderate persistent asthma. *Journal of Allergy and Clinical Immunology*, 123, 1328–34.

Tager, I.B., Segal, M.R., Speizer, F.E., et al. (1988). The natural history of forced expiratory volumes. Effect of cigarette smoking and respiratory symptoms. *American Review of Respiratory Disease*, 138, 837–49.

Tager, I.B., Weiss, S.T., Munoz, A., et al. (1983). Longitudinal study of the effects of maternal smoking on pulmonary function in children. *The New England Journal of Medicine*, 309, 699–703.

Tashkin, D.P., Detels, R., Simmons, M., et al. (1994). The UCLA population studies of chronic obstructive respiratory disease: XI. Impact of air pollution and smoking on annual change in forced expiratory volume in one second. *American Journal of Respiratory and Critical Care Medicine*, 149, 1209–17.

Taylor, D.R., Pijnenburg, M.W., Smith, A.D., et al. (2006). Exhaled nitric oxide measurements: clinical application and interpretation. *Thorax*, 61, 817–27.

Tepas, E.C., Litonjua, A.A., Celedon, J.C., et al. (2006). Sensitization to aeroallergens and airway hyperresponsiveness at 7 years of age. *Chest*, 129, 1500–8.

Thomsen, S.F., Ulrik, C.S., Larsen, K., et al. (2004). Change in prevalence of asthma in Danish children and adolescents. *Annals of Allergy, Asthma & Immunology*, 92, 506–11.

Todd, J.L., Goldstein, D.B., Ge, D., et al. (2011). The state of genome-wide association studies in pulmonary disease: a new perspective. *American Journal of Respiratory and Critical Care Medicine*, 184, 873–80.

Toelle, B.G., Peat, J.K., Salome, C.M., et al. (1992). Toward a definition of asthma for epidemiology. *American Review of Respiratory Disease*, 146, 633–7.

Trupin, L., Earnest, G., San Pedro, M., et al. (2003). The occupational burden of chronic obstructive pulmonary disease. *European Respiratory Journal*, 22, 462–9.

Turner, M.O., Hussack, P., Sears, M.R., et al. (1995). Exacerbations of asthma without sputum eosinophilia. *Thorax*, 50, 1057–61.

US DHHS (2006). The health consequences of involuntary exposure to tobacco smoke: a report of the Surgeon General. US Department of Human Health and Human Services (DHHS), Centres for Disease Control and Prevention, Coordinating Centre for Health Promotion, Office on Smoking and Health, Atlanta, GA.

US EPA (1992). Respiratory health effects of passive smoking: lung cancer and other disorders. Office of Research and Development, US Environmental Protection Agency, Washington, DC, EPA/600/6-90/006F.

Van Diemen, C.C. and Boezen, H.M. (2007). Genetic epidemiology of reduced lung function. In D.S. Postma and S.T. Weiss (eds.) *Genetics of Asthma and Chronic Obstructive Pulmonary Disease*, pp. 17–32. New York: Informa Healthcare USA.

Van Vugt, S., Broekhuizen, L., Zuithoff, N., et al. (2012). Airway obstruction and bronchodilator responsiveness in adults with acute cough. *Annals of Family Medicine*, 10, 523–9.

Vestbo, J. (2002). Epidemiology. In N.F. Voelkel and W. MacNee (eds.) *Chronic Obstructive Lung Disease*, pp. 41–55. Hamilton, BC: Decker Inc.

Vestbo, J. (2004). COPD in the ECRHS. *Thorax*, 59, 89–90.

Vestbo, J., Hurd, S.S., and Rodriguez-Roisin, R. (2012). The 2011 revision of the global strategy for the diagnosis, management and prevention of COPD (GOLD)—why and what? *Clinical Respiratory Journal*, 6, 208–14.

Vestbo, J., Prescott, E., Lange, P., et al. (1998). Vital prognosis after hospitalization for COPD: a study of a random population sample. *Respiratory Medicine*, 92, 772–6.

Visness, C.M., London, S.J., Daniels, J.L., et al. (2010). Association of childhood obesity with atopic and nonatopic asthma: results from the National Health and Nutrition Examination Survey 1999–2006. *Journal of Asthma*, 47, 822–9.

Vonk, J.M., Jongepier, H., Panhuysen, C.I., et al. (2003). Risk factors associated with the presence of irreversible airflow limitation and reduced transfer coefficient in patients with asthma after 26 years of follow up. *Thorax*, 58, 322–7.

Von Mutius, E., Weiland, S.K., Fritzsch, C., et al. (1998). Increasing prevalence of hay fever and atopy among children in Leipzig, East Germany. *The Lancet*, 351, 862–6.

Vork, K.L., Broadwin, R.L., and Blaisdell, R.J. (2007). Developing asthma in childhood from exposure to secondhand tobacco smoke: insights from a meta-regression. *Environmental Health Perspectives*, 115, 1394–400.

Wang, X., Mensinga, T.T., Schouten, J.P., et al. (2004). Determinants of maximally attained level of pulmonary function. *American Journal of Respiratory and Critical Care Medicine*, 169, 941–9.

Watson, J.P., Cowen, P., and Lewis, R.A. (1996). The relationship between asthma admission rates, routes of admission, and socioeconomic deprivation. *European Respiratory Journal*, 9, 2087–93.

Watson, L., Boezen, H.M., and Postma, D.S. (2003). Differences between males and females in the natural history of asthma and COPD. *European Respiratory Monthly*, 25, 50–73.

Weiland, S.K. and Pearce, N. (2004). Asthma prevalence in adults: good news? *Thorax*, 59, 637–8.

Weinmayr, G., Weiland, S.K., Bjorksten, B., et al. (2007). Atopic sensitization and the international variation of asthma symptom prevalence in children. *American Journal of Respiratory and Critical Care Medicine*, 176, 565–74.

Weitzman, M., Gortmaker, S.L., Sobol, A.M., et al. (1992). Recent trends in the prevalence and severity of childhood asthma. *Journal of the American Medical Association*, 268, 2673–7.

Wenzel, S.E. (2012). Asthma phenotypes: the evolution from clinical to molecular approaches. *Nature Medicine*, 18, 716–25.

Wenzel, S.E., Schwartz, L.B., Langmack, E.L., et al. (1999). Evidence that severe asthma can be divided pathologically into two inflammatory subtypes with distinct physiologic and clinical characteristics.

American Journal of Respiratory and Critical Care Medicine, 160, 1001–8.

Whincup, P.H., Cook, D.G., Strachan, D.P., et al. (1993). Time trends in respiratory symptoms in childhood over a 24 year period. *Archives of Disease in Childhood*, 68, 729–34.

Wilk, J.B., Shrine, N.R., Loehr, L.R., et al. (2012). Genome-wide association studies identify CHRNA5/3 and HTR4 in the development of airflow obstruction. *American Journal of Respiratory and Critical Care Medicine*, 186, 622–32.

Willis, T. (1678). *Practice of Physick, Pharmaceutice Rationalis or the Operations of Medicine in Humane Bodies*. London.

World Health Organization (2005). *Air Quality Guidelines, Global Update 2005. Particulate Matter, Ozone, Nitrogen Dioxide and Sulphur Dioxide*. Copenhagen: WHO Regional Office for Europe.

Xu, X., Weiss, S.T., Rijcken, B., et al. (1994). Smoking, changes in smoking habits, and rate of decline in FEV_1: new insight into gender differences. *European Respiratory Journal*, 7, 1056–61.

Yunginger, J.W., Reed, C.E., O'Connell, E.J., et al. (1992). A community-based study of the epidemiology of asthma. Incidence rates, 1964–1983. *American Review of Respiratory Disease*, 146, 888–94.

Zamel, N., McClean, P.A., Sandell, P.R., et al. (1996). Asthma on Tristan de Cunha: looking for the genetic link. *American Journal of Respiratory and Critical Care Medicine*, 153, 1902–6.

8.4

Obesity

W. Philip T. James and Tim Marsh

Introduction to obesity

The prevalence of obesity and overweight has been increasing rapidly in all regions of the world. Those countries which saw large increases in the 1980s such as the United States and the United Kingdom are now starting to see a levelling in younger age groups and there is evidence that the increase is faster in countries undergoing rapid economic development and the nutrition transition. This is of great public health concern because projections suggest that as substantial increases in obesity occur, the morbidity associated with obesity and its complications will threaten gains in life expectancy and impose unsustainable economic burdens both on society and the health services. There is therefore an urgent need to intervene to reverse the growing epidemic.

Definitions of obesity

Obesity was originally defined by analysis relating to mortality, not morbidity, undertaken by the US Metropolitan Life Insurance Company before the Second World War. A body mass index (BMI) value (kg/m^2), adjusted for clothes and shoes (James 1976), of approximately 25 defined the limit above which death rates increased. The BMI value of 30 was 20 per cent above this upper 'normal' BMI limit of 25. However, later studies showed that the mortality risk of a smoker with a BMI of 22 was roughly equivalent to that of a non-smoker who had a BMI of 30 (Royal College of Physicians 1983). In 1995, the World Health Organization (WHO 1995) accepted BMI as the method for assessing degrees of underweight and overweight and took a BMI lower limit of 18.5 for distinguishing normal from underweight. This followed a series of earlier international analyses of adults' capacity to engage in heavy agricultural work. This BMI value therefore became the next cut-off point signifying undernutrition (James et al. 1988) (Table 8.4.1).

In 1997, following the WHO Expert Consultation on obesity, the implications of overweight and obesity were accepted as a global problem (WHO 2000). In the United States, higher BMIs were preferred but in Asia a lower BMI cut-off of 23 was accepted because above this value the risks of diabetes and hypertension in particular were unacceptably high. These susceptibilities to disease are increasingly linked to epigenetics, probably nutritionally induced in pregnancy and early childhood, rather than distinct ethnic differences in the genetics of disease susceptibility (Lillycrop and Burdge 2012). There have been recurrent analyses (Flegal et al. 2007, 2013) from the United States suggesting that being overweight is advantageous from a life expectancy point of view. These findings neglect to ensure that smokers and those who have never smoked are clearly distinguished (Berrington de Gonzalez et al. 2010); observational studies are also very inappropriate as they do not take account of the well-known unintentional weight loss in those who are already ill, for example, with undiagnosed cancer who die within 1–5 years. Allowing for these factors, the data consistently suggest that non-smokers (and smokers when analysed separately) have, in a Western environment, the lowest mortality when BMIs are 22.5–25 (Lawlor et al. 2006; Keith et al. 2011). Identifying the mortality effects of overweight (BMIs of 25–29.9) require many years of follow-up with very substantial numbers of subjects (James 1976) and care to exclude other biases (Greenberg 2006). Other major studies with long follow-up periods show all-cause and ischaemic heart disease mortality rates were increased in the overweight group (Batty et al. 2006) and integrated analyses of 33 cohorts showed that the risk of non-fatal and fatal cardiovascular diseases increased progressively from a BMI of 20 whereas the impact on haemorrhagic stroke was not evident until BMIs were in the region of 30 (Asia Pacific Cohort Studies Collaboration 2004). Moreover, collaborative analyses of 57 prospective studies involving about 900,000 adults have found that in both sexes, mortality was lowest at about 22.5–25 kg/m^2 (Adams et al. 2006; Prospective Studies Collaboration 2009) and each 5 kg/m^2 BMI increase was associated with about a 30 per cent higher overall mortality. The first 3 years of follow-up had to be discarded because those who were already ill had lower BMIs and early deaths so without this adjustment the curves were J-shaped. Co-morbidities such as hypertension and diabetes in conjunction with higher body weights signify the degree of cellular and organ damage and are far more powerfully predictive of an early death than BMI alone (Padwal et al. 2011). This then can help in clarifying clinical decision-making.

Disability incurred by weight gain before death is a huge societal burden as disabilities affect younger individuals and may handicap them physically, mentally, psychologically, socially, and economically. Type 2 diabetes is now being diagnosed in overweight/obese children and adolescents (Park et al. 2012) and childhood overweight (unadjusted for adult BMI) is associated with adult cardiovascular outcomes and mortality (Reilly and Kelly 2011).

From a public health perspective the precise choice of cut-off point is arbitrary: the health hazards are progressive, age dependent, and not substantially changed at any particular cut-off point. The classic co-morbidities intrinsically linked to an excess BMI, for example, diabetes, hypertension, gall stones, and coronary heart disease are linearly related to BMI from a BMI nadir of about 19 or 20 so the choice of an upper normal value of 24.9 for individuals is very generous and ignores the issue of disability. WHO analyses use an estimated optimum population mean BMI

Table 8.4.1 The NIH and Asian adaptations of the WHO criteria for classification of overweight and obesity with their associated risks (*Mancini et al. 2011*)

Classification	BMI kg/m²	Waist circumference and associated disease risk	
Europids (NIH)		**Males/females ≤ 102 cm/≤ 88 cm**	**Males/females ≥ 102 cm/> 88 cm**
Underweight	< 18.5	None	None
Normal	18.5–24.9	None	None
Overweight	25–29.9	Increased	High
Obese class 1	≥ 30	High	Very high
Obese class 2	30–34.9	Very high	Very high
Obese class 3	≥ 35	Extremely high	Extremely high
Asians		**Males/females < 90 cm/< 80 cm**	**Males/females ≥ 90 cm/≥ 80 cm**
Underweight	< 18.5	Low (but increased risk of other clinical problems)	Average
Normal	18.5–22.9	Average	Increased
Overweight	23–24.9	Increased	Moderate
Obese class 1	25–29.9	Moderate	Severe
Obese class 2	≥ 30	Severe	Very severe

Table 8.4.2 Different waist circumference cut-off points selected by the International Diabetes Federation as part of their assessment of the metabolic syndrome

Country/ethnic group	Waist circumference (cm)	
Europids[a] In the United States, the ATP III higher values (102 cm male; 88 cm female), based on original small Dutch study of regression equivalents of BMIs 25 and 30 adopted by WHO, are likely to continue to be used for clinical purposes.	Male/female	≥ 94/ ≥ 80
South Asians Based on a Chinese, Malay, and Asian-Indian population	Male/female	≥ 90/≥ 80
Chinese	Male/female	≥ 90/≥ 80
Japanese[b]	Male/female	≥ 85/≥ 90
Ethnic South and Central Americans	Use South Asian recommendations until more specific data are available.	
Sub-Saharan Africans	Use European data until more specific data are available.	
Eastern Mediterranean and Middle East (Arab) populations	Use European data until more specific data are available.	

ATP, adult treatment panel.

[a] In future epidemiological studies of populations of Europid origin, prevalence should be given using both European and North American cut-points to allow better comparisons.

[b] Originally different values were proposed for Japanese people but new data support the use of the values shown above.

Reproduced with permission from International Diabetes Federation (IDF), The IDF consensus *worldwide definition of the metabolic syndrome*, Copyright © International Diabetes Federation, 2006, available from http://www.idf.org/webdata/docs/IDF_Meta_def_final.pdf.

of 21.0 where there was minimum risk of diseases associated with weight gain but at the same time a minimum risk of having a high proportion of adults with morbidity-related underweight, that is, BMIs lower than 17 (James et al.1988). Non-smoking individuals are likely to have an optimum life expectancy and disability-free life if their BMIs remain at about 20 throughout life.

Other criteria for classifying excess weight gain: abdominal obesity

The INTERHEART international case–control study of coronary heart disease showed that the waist–hip ratio (W/HR) was a far more sensitive measure of risk; fat deposition on the hips seems to be protective so that the risk associated with a high waist circumference (WC) is reduced by the extent to which fat is also laid down peripherally (Yusuf et al. 2005). However, WC measurement alone is also a better measure than BMI and does not require calculating a ratio; it is simple for both the public and professionals to understand and overcomes the need to measure the hip circumference, which in some societies is a culturally problematic measure to make except with female physicians taking considerable care.

The original choice of WC measurements was made so that they corresponded with the BMI cut-offs for overweight and obesity, that is, 25 and 30. These are the values which WHO then adopted (Table 8.4.1) for classifying—at least in Caucasians—excess abdominal fat. Values for the Asian population were later derived based on statistical calculations of the sensitivity and specificity of detecting hypertension or obesity at different WC levels. More recently the International

Diabetes Federation proposed new criteria for specifying the metabolic syndrome—that is, a collection of risk factors including dyslipidaemia, hypertension, diabetes, and abdominal obesity—and adopted different values for different ethnic groups despite being derived very differently (Table 8.4.2) (James 2005). Waist measurements need to be standardized with the use of a non-stretchable tape measure in the horizontal plane half way between the lower rib cage and the iliac crest in the mid-axillary line. Without these criteria the errors in measurement can be serious.

There is a strong genetic influence on fat distribution but smoking and alcohol consumption also amplify the propensity to abdominal obesity. Early nutritional and other handicaps, revealed in part by low birth weights, are also associated with later abdominal obesity when even modest weight is gained in adult life. Thus, Indian, Chinese, and Hispanic populations with a marked history of early childhood malnutrition are particularly prone to abdominal obesity with a high WC even with BMIs lower than 25.

Children's criteria for overweight and obesity

WHO developed statistical criteria for specifying both underweight and overweight in children (WHO 1995). A child who is underweight for their age, underheight for age, or underweight for height is classified as abnormal if not above the −2 standard deviations (SD) for their age and sex. Thus the greater than 2 SD for weight for height was taken as indicative of overweight with reference data from composite, meticulous US survey data but based on predominantly bottle-fed babies deemed to be healthy. The International Obesity Task Force (IOTF) group developed an international classification system for overweight and obesity in children (Cole et al. 2000) based on the BMI index (Dietz and Bellizzi 1999), and linking the childhood and adult definitions by taking, at age 18 years, those percentiles which corresponded to BMIs of 25 and 30 and using these same percentiles throughout the childhood age range for specifying overweight and obesity in childhood in girls and boys separately. Table 8.4.3 sets out the revised cut-off points to be used for this classification based on representative data from the Americas, Europe, and Asia (Cole and Lobstein 2012). It was recognized that BMI was a crude index of body fatness in children as well as adults especially in different societies with their different ages for the onset of puberty.

New definitions of 'normal' weight gain in children

The WHO has now developed a new approach for defining the normal growth of children (WHO 2007) with data from a major multinational study involving children in California, Norway, India, Oman, Ghana, and Brazil. Normal babies delivered at full term by non-smoking healthy mothers who agreed to breastfeed their babies exclusively for at least 4 months were monitored carefully with specific advice being given relating to immunization and other rearing practices. Further cohorts of pre-school children from similar environments were also chosen so that over a period of 6.5 years data on children's growth patterns were obtained. Surprisingly, whatever the ethnic background, the children's growth was almost identical and the variability in growth was far less than in the databases normally used for producing growth charts. This implies that if one takes these latest WHO ±2 SD values as the standard for children up to 5 years, then a nation's new estimates of underweight and overweight prevalences will be greater. This particularly applies to the prevalence of overweight children because in both children and adults there is an increasingly skewed distribution of weights as the average weight for age rises (Fig. 8.4.1).

The WHO then developed a reference set of growth data for children from 5 to 20 years of age still based on US data and these are accepted by governments (de Onis et al. 2012b) even if paediatricians find them unrealistic and confusing in practice (Cole and Lobstein 2012). Overweight children by the new WHO classification show a greater propensity for hypertension, higher insulin and uric acid levels, and other indices of insulin resistance (de Onis et al. 2012a).

Tracking of body fat and BMI into adult life

Children are not born obese, but are certainly becoming more obese. Most studies providing more than one measurement during childhood and adolescence show that a persistence of weight status increases with age (Singh et al. 2008). The persistence was also greater with increasing levels of overweight and perhaps more likely in girls than boys. Rolland-Cachera et al. (1987) originally focused on the issue of 'fat-rebound' in pre-pubertal school children but systematic reviews, for example, by Power et al. (1997) and Parsons et al. (1999) have found little evidence for the selective monitoring in the pre-pubertal phase for predicting the later emergence of obesity. Once children were over 5 years of age, being overweight incurred at least a 40 per cent risk of this overweight/obesity persisting into adult life and by the mid-teenage years the risk had increased to 60–75 per cent (Table 8.4.4). Barlow and Dietz (1998) advocated focusing on children over 3 years of age but there is now a very worrying increase in the prevalence of both high birth weight babies and obesity in 1–5-year-olds. The majority of 1–5-year-old children with BMIs greater than 2 SD of the new WHO limits are in lower-income countries with marked increases in these prevalences having occurred since 1990 (de Onis et al. 2010).

The predictive health significance of higher BMIs in childhood

Weight gain in children induces many early childhood problems including, in more severe degrees of overweight, developmental abnormalities of the weight-bearing joints and limbs. Metabolic problems such as insulin resistance, higher blood pressure, and dyslipidaemia are also evident in overweight and obese children even when young and higher BMIs even within the normal, that is, less than 2 SD range in 7–13-years-olds predict an early death and cardiovascular complications (Gunnell et al. 1998; Baker et al. 2007). This may simply reflect the probability of obese children remaining obese into adult life as it is difficult to disentangle an effect on mortality independent of the adult BMI achieved (Park et al. 2012). Those obese adults currently at high risk of diseases were born at a time when childhood obesity was relatively scarce so current rates of childhood obesity may prove to be more hazardous.

Genetics and obesity

Genes influence human physiology, its development, and adaptation but the rapid growth in obesity must be a consequence of environmental rather than genetic factors because the gene pool is relatively constant. Genetic factors are important in influencing the propensity to weight gain through gene–environment interactions. A genome-wide search for type 2 diabetes-susceptibility genes identified a common variant in the *FTO* (fat mass and obesity associated) and *MC4R* genes that predispose to diabetes through an effect on BMI. The 16 per cent of adults homozygous for the *FTO* risk allele weigh about 3 kg more and have a 1.67-fold increased odds of obesity. This is evident from the age of 7 years and reflects a specific increase in fat mass, perhaps expressed through increased appetite.

Neel originally proposed the 'thrifty gene' hypothesis (Neel 1962), that is, that the recurrent threat of famine and natural selection favoured genes for the highly efficient effects of insulin and the frugal use of glucose during times of little food with efficient storage of extra calories as fat during times of plenty. This hypothesis persists but if famines affected the evolution of all societies then identifying the gene clusters linked to the widespread propensity to obesity is not easy.

Table 8.4.3 Revised IOTF BMI cut-offs by age for childhood overweight and obesity

Age (years)	Boys			Girls		
	BMI 25	**BMI 30**	**BMI 35**	**BMI 25**	**BMI 30**	**BMI 35**
2	18.36	19.99	21.2	18.09	19.81	21.13
2.5	18.09	19.73	20.95	17.84	19.57	20.9
3	17.85	19.5	20.75	17.64	19.38	20.74
3.5	17.66	19.33	20.61	17.48	19.25	20.65
4	17.52	19.23	20.56	17.35	19.16	20.61
4.5	17.43	19.2	20.6	17.27	19.14	20.67
5	17.39	19.27	20.79	17.23	19.2	20.84
5.5	17.42	19.46	21.15	17.25	19.36	21.16
6	17.52	19.76	21.69	17.33	19.61	21.61
6.5	17.67	20.15	22.35	17.48	19.96	22.19
7	17.88	20.59	23.08	17.69	20.39	22.88
7.5	18.12	21.06	23.83	17.96	20.89	23.65
8	18.41	21.56	24.6	18.28	21.44	24.5
8.5	18.73	22.11	25.45	18.63	22.04	25.42
9	19.07	22.71	26.4	18.99	22.66	26.39
9.5	19.43	23.34	27.39	19.38	23.31	27.38
10	19.8	23.96	28.35	19.78	23.97	28.36
10.5	20.15	24.54	29.22	20.21	24.62	29.28
11	20.51	25.07	29.97	20.66	25.25	30.14
11.5	20.85	25.56	30.63	21.12	25.87	30.93
12	21.2	26.02	31.21	21.59	26.47	31.66
12.5	21.54	26.45	31.73	22.05	27.05	32.33
13	21.89	26.87	32.19	22.49	27.57	32.91
13.5	22.24	27.26	32.6	22.9	28.03	33.39
14	22.6	27.64	32.97	23.27	28.42	33.78
14.5	22.95	28	33.3	23.6	28.74	34.07
15	23.28	28.32	33.56	23.89	29.01	34.28
15.5	23.59	28.61	33.78	24.13	29.22	34.43
16	23.89	28.89	33.98	24.34	29.4	34.54
16.5	24.18	29.15	34.19	24.53	29.55	34.64
17	24.46	29.43	34.43	24.7	29.7	34.75
17.5	24.73	29.71	34.7	24.85	29.85	34.87
18	25	30	35	25	30	35

Reproduced from Cole TJ and Lobstein T, Extended international (IOTF) body mass index cut-offs for thinness, overweight and obesity, *Pediatric Obesity*, Volume 7, Issue 4, pp. 284–294, Copyright © 2012 The Authors. *Pediatric Obesity* © 2012 International Association for the Study of Obesity, with permission from John Wiley & Sons Ltd.

Childhood prevalence of obesity

Based on IOTF criteria, about 10 per cent of boys and 9 per cent of girls aged 5–17 years globally are overweight or obese, that is, a total of 118 million. The latest available regional prevalences using the IOTF definitions are given in Table 8.4.5.

In young children, there is emerging evidence of a flattening of the upward trends. Thus in the UK, obesity in children between the ages of 2 and 10 years increased from 10.1 per cent in 1995 to 14.6 per cent in 2010 but then was stable between 2008/2009 and 2010/2011 for 4–5-year-olds. Similarly, UK 2–15-year-olds' weights

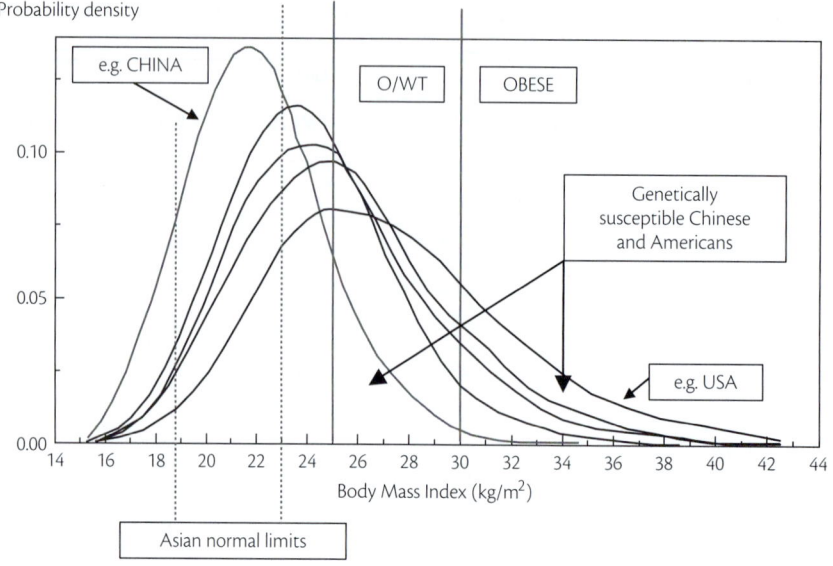

Fig. 8.4.1 The skewed distribution of BMI with increases in the average population BMI.

Source: cross-sectional data from Rose G., Population distributions of risk and disease, *Nutrition, Metabolism and Cardiovascular Diseases*, Volume 1, pp. 37–40, Copyright © 1991, illustrates the progressive marked increase in obesity rates for modest increases in mean BMI. Those in the upper BMI range for each population distribution represent the genetically susceptible individuals to weight gain. The usual Caucasian cut-offs for overweight and obesity are shown together with the Asian upper limit of 'normal' BMI.

Table 8.4.4 The likelihood of children continuing to be overweight as adults ranked by age of first measurement

Study number	Age of monitoring		% still obese as adults	
	As children	**As 'adults'**	**Males**	**Females**
3	1	20–30	36	–
5	1–5	19–26	27	–
7	7	14	90	87
7	7	16	63	62
11	7	33	43	63
6	7	35	40	20
9	1–14	10–23	42	66
8	2–14	10–24	43	–
4	9–10	31–35	57	64
11	11	33	54	64
2	9–13	42–53	63	–
1	10–13	29–34	74	72
6	13	35	40	30
4	13–14	31–35	77	70
10	13–17	27–31	58	–
11	16	33	64	78

Source: data from Power C, Lake JK, and Cole TJ., Measurement and long-term health risks of child and adolescent fatness, *International Journal of Obesity*, Volume 21, Issue 2, pp. 507–26, Copyright © 1997, with study numbers as in their analysis. The proportion of obese adults who had been originally overweight as a child was usually 3–10-fold lower than the corresponding probability of overweight children maintaining their excess weight into adulthood.

consistently increased up to 2004 but then gently declined (National Obesity Observatory 2013).

In the United States, there is also a decreasing prevalence or stabilizing of trends (Yanovski and Yanovski 2011). Obesity in 2–5-year-old children decreased from 16.7 per cent in 2003 to 14.7 per cent by 2005 and then stabilized but with an upward trend in overweight (Olds et al. 2011). Analysis across nine countries including England, United States, Sweden, China, Australia, Netherlands, and Switzerland also reported a flattening of childhood obesity for 2–19-year-old children and teenagers (Rokholm et al. 2010). These promising trends may not persist and annual monitoring of health survey data is imperative for progress to be evaluated.

The prevalence of adult overweight and obesity

Although obesity, measured as BMI, is an index of excess body fat there are a number of ways of measuring excess body fat itself, such as bio-impedance, densitometry, and plethysmography, but the last two are very expensive and have not been used for population studies. Evidence from a range of countries shows that weight tends to increase progressively as individuals age, until it reaches a peak and then begins to fall—usually after the sixth decade of life. Most data on BMI are based on self-reported heights and weights which usually underestimate the prevalence and makes comparisons difficult with measured data.

Overweight and obesity have now become a global problem and the hazards of excess weight gain are beginning to match the burden of cardiovascular diseases where the developing countries now have about 80 per cent of the world's burden for the non-communicable diseases according to 2010 WHO estimates (WHO 2011). However, only 16 per cent of global

Table 8.4.5 The prevalence and numbers of overweight and obesity in children globally. Data based on the use of the IOTF cut-off points

Region based on WHO classification	Overweight %		Obese %		Total O/W+Ob %		O/W Number (thousands)		Obese (thousands)		Total: O/W+ Ob Numbers (thousands)	
	M	F	M	F	M	F	M	F	M	F	M	F
Africa	9.2	12.2	3.4	3.7	12.6	15.9	12,667	16,222	4636	4961	17,302	21,183
Americas	18.2	17.4	9.6	10	27.9	27.3	18,727	17,165	9887	9865	28,613	27,030
Eastern Mediterranean	7.9	9.3	5	5.7	12.9	14.9	6855	7637	4330	4662	11,185	12,300
Europe	15.2	15.1	4.6	4.9	19.8	20	10,701	10,124	3245	3270	13,947	13,394
South East Asian	15.9	14.9	5.5	4.1	21.5	19	38,152	33,223	13,289	9104	51,442	42,328
Western Pacific/Oceania	10.4	6.0	6.1	4.7	16.5	10.7	18,791	9442	10,997	7301	29,789	16,743

Source: data kindly provided by Rachel Jackson Leach of the International Association for the Study of Obesity, Copyright © 2013.

health expenditure occurs in the poorer non-Organisation for Economic Cooperation and Development (OECD) countries even though they represent 82 per cent of the world's population (WHO 2012b). Table 8.4.6 shows the regional prevalences of overweight and obesity in adults. The table provides an illustration of the age-related adult changes in the prevalences in different regions of the world and shows that the main increase occurs in 20–40-year-olds.

A recent WHO report (WHO 2013) recommended the global monitoring of both overweight and obesity prevalences in adolescents (defined according to the WHO growth criteria) and adult measured BMIs.

The nutrition transition

The economic development of a country and particularly the urbanization of populations is associated with major increases in obesity prevalence (Popkin 2006). In poorer communities, middle-aged women are the first to become overweight and then, as the economy develops, women become progressively heavier with men then beginning to catch up. In developing societies, the more affluent have higher prevalences of obesity with the average BMI of the population increasing progressively as national incomes rise to a gross domestic product of about $5000 and then peaks in women at $15,000 and in men at $17,000 (Ezzati et al. 2005). Then, as societies' economies improve, there is a reversal of the socioeconomic gradient with the more affluent becoming slimmer and having lower obesity rates than the poor. With average increases in weight, the proportion of obese individuals increases markedly because of the skewing of BMI distributions (Rose 1991). Fig. 8.4.1 also highlights the fact that the most genetically sensitive members of the community are those found in the upper distributions for their society.

The hazards of excess weight in adults

Being obese significantly increases the risk of developing non-communicable diseases. Table 8.4.7 lists medical conditions associated with excess weight gain (IOTF 2010). Conditions found to be associated with high BMIs by the Institute for Health Metrics and Evaluation (IHME) 2010 global burden of disease research group are included (Lim et al.

2012). This extended set of medical conditions has not been independently validated and several of the cancer relationships were not found to be robust in the exhaustive and meticulously collated latest World Cancer Research Fund and American Institute of Cancer Research assessments (2007) of the role of weight gain in cancer development and prevention. There is evidence that obesity, particularly in mid and later life, is a major risk factor for cognitive decline (Profenno et al. 2010), both directly and indirectly because the associated hypertension and type 2 diabetes increase the speed of vascular induced changes in the brain.

The physical and other impacts of weight gain must also be considered. The impact on respiratory function is important with overweight children and adults becoming unable to engage in strenuous physical activity. Obese adults walking slowly already use up to 60 per cent of their maximum exercise capacity. Thus obese adults often do less than normal because their physical exertions are very energy consuming. Weight gain is also a marked handicap in those with any degree of respiratory impairment. Asthmatic and chronic obstructive respiratory disease patients can markedly improve their exercise tolerance and comfort if they lose weight. Weight gain also increases the risk of sleep apnoea which is associated with a large neck and a tendency to obstruct breathing. Subjects stop breathing for a quarter or half a minute before then showing marked intakes of breath as their drive to breathe takes over for perhaps a minute or two before the cycle is repeated. This feature, usually evident at night and seemingly innocuous, is a major medical handicap associated with drug-resistant hypertension because of the persistent induction of the sympathetic nervous system by the repeated episodes of anoxia. When severe it is also associated with higher mortality rates and can cause traffic accidents as abdominally obese adults with thick necks fall asleep as they drive their vehicles.

Back and joint pains are another major problem leading to greater time off work for overweight and obese patients. The mechanical force on joints and the strain on the muscular skeletal system is marked leading to frequent work absenteeism and reactive depression among many overweight and obese subjects.

Table 8.4.6 Percentage prevalence obesity or overweight (pre-obese) in adults aged 18 years+ around the world by region and gender

% obese (BMI ≥ 30 kg/m²)

		18–29	30–44	45–59	60–69	70+
Africa	Male	4.4	7.8	11.1	10.7	5.0
	Female	5.1	10.7	14.5	24.3	13.0
Americas	Male	18.8	23.8	27.8	27.5	24.7
	Female	18.6	26.1	31.7	30.3	26.9
Eastern Mediterranean Region	Male	5.2	10.2	12.7	6.5	6.6
	Female	9.7	24.3	31.5	15.9	12.3
Europe	Male	6.0	14.9	22.3	26.2	21.7
	Female	7.2	18.1	30.3	35.8	29.8
South-East Asia Region	Male	0.7	1.9	2.4	0.3	0.6
	Female	1.5	4.9	6.0	0.9	1.5
Western Pacific Region	Male	1.7	4.8	6.4	7.1	1.3
	Female	2.3	6.4	4.9	9.5	3.8

% pre-obese (BMI 25–29.9 kg/m²)

		18–29	30–44	45–59	60–69	70+
Africa	Male	18.1	23.6	29.5	27.8	14.2
	Female	13.6	18.7	20.5	30.0	15.4
Americas	Male	31.7	39.2	41.4	40.1	38.5
	Female	23.4	28.4	31.2	34.8	34.3
Eastern Mediterranean Region	Male	16.3	27.4	28.7	20.6	21.8
	Female	19.0	25.5	25.2	21.9	23.0
Europe	Male	25.1	42.0	45.6	47.2	47.6
	Female	16.6	28.0	35.2	38.8	37.8
South-East Asia Region	Male	5.1	11.8	13.6	1.7	3.4
	Female	7.0	18.9	18.2	5.0	10.3
Western Pacific Region	Male	16.4	24.4	27.1	27.3	12.7
	Female	11.7	18.3	22.5	23.2	26.0

Source: data kindly provided by Rachel Jackson Leach of the International Association for the Study of Obesity, Copyright © 2013.

The medical and other costs of excess weight

Whilst obesity is responsible for an increasingly significant burden of disease, these observations do not resonate strongly outside the health community. What does have impact with policymakers and politicians is being able to calculate the potential avoidable direct and indirect health costs of excess weight gain as in the UK Foresight *Tackling Obesities* report (Foresight 2007). The direct costs of obesity represent the monetary value of healthcare resources devoted to managing obesity-related conditions including the costs incurred by excess utilization of ambulatory care, hospitalization, medications, radiological or laboratory tests, and long-term care (including nursing home care). There is a general consensus that obesity places a significant financial burden on the healthcare system (Withrow and Alter 2011). A large proportion of the variation in cost estimates relates to the multiplicity of methods used. Finkelstein et al. (2009) found that US obese patients incur 46 per cent higher inpatient costs, 27 per cent higher physician visits and outpatient costs, and 80 per cent higher spending on prescription medications compared to normal weight individuals. The annual medical costs of obesity in the US were estimated as $75 billion in 2003; they also accounted for 4–7 per cent of total healthcare expenditure in the Netherlands (Seidell 1995) and 2 per cent in Australia (Segal et al. 1994). The European Union's combined direct and indirect costs of obesity in 2002 were approximately €33 billion a year and in 2007, the UK projected that the ongoing rise in obesity will add £5.5 billion in medical costs to the National Health Services by 2050 (Foresight 2007).

Table 8.4.7 Relative risks (RR) of health problems associated with obesity

High (RR > 3)	Diabetes, gall bladder disease, dyslipidaemia, insulin resistance, breathlessness, sleep apnoea
Moderate (RR = 2–3)	Ischaemic heart disease, stroke, hypertension, osteoarthritis, hyperuricaemia, gout
Minor (RR = 1–2)	Breast (after the age of 50), colorectal, pancreas, kidney, gall bladder cancers, reproductive hormone abnormalities, polycystic ovary syndrome, impaired fertility, low back pain due to obesity, increased risk of anaesthesia complications, fetal defects associated with maternal obesity, dementia (age 45–59)
New conditions found to be associated with high BMI[a]	Oesophageal cancer, biliary tract cancer, other urinary organ cancers, the aggregate of cardiomyopathy and myocarditis and endocarditis, the aggregate of atrial fibrillation and flutter, pulmonary vascular disease and other cardiovascular disease, chronic kidney disease

[a] New conditions based on criteria specified in *The Lancet*, Volume 380, Issue 9859, Lim S. et al., A comparative risk assessment of burden of disease and injury attributable to 67 risk factors and risk factor clusters in 21 regions, 1990–2010: a systematic analysis for the Global Burden of Disease Study 2010, pp. 2224–2260, 2012, Copyright © 2013 Elsevier Ltd All rights reserved.

There are also significant indirect costs to society from obesity due to decreased years of disability-free life, work absenteeism or reduced productivity (presenteeism), disability pensions, increased mortality before retirement, and early retirement. Although individual estimates vary, the magnitude of indirect costs is several times larger than the direct medical costs. For example, obese individuals in Sweden are 1.5–1.9 times more likely to take sick leave, and 12 per cent of obese women had disability pensions attributable to obesity, costing approximately US$300/year for every woman in the population (Narbro et al. 1996). Among US employees, annual missed workdays increased from 0.5 more days in overweight men to 5.9 more days for men with a BMI of 40 kg/m² or higher (Finkelstein et al. 2009). The annual cost from presenteeism among very obese men amounts to the equivalent of 1 month of lost productivity each year and costs employers US$3792 per year (Trogdon et al. 2008). Robroek et al. (2011) reported that up to 10 per cent of all sick leave and productivity loss could be attributed to obesity and related lifestyle behaviours.

Another approach to assessing the impact of obesity and interventions is to use utility values which relate in economic terms to the value a consumer assigns to their own condition or benefit. Both premature mortality and disability together with disability-adjusted life years (DALYs) lost or quality-adjusted life years (QALYs) are considered from national statistics of the prevalence of different medical conditions. The estimations of the DALYs as conducted by the WHO are sometimes considered unusual in that for any other risk factor the challenge was to identify the optimum value to which the average population should ideally strive. For systolic blood pressure the optimum value was estimated to be 115 mmHg and for total blood cholesterol 3.8 mmol/L. These values are very different from what one finds in clinical management guidelines but illustrate the difference between pragmatic clinical judgements and what can be considered ideal from a public health perspective. So the choice of a BMI of 21 as the optimum median population BMI was made in an analogous way based on the handicaps of a higher BMI. The completely new approach introduced by the IHME group from Seattle and Harvard and independently of the WHO (Lim et al. 2012) used huge databases and analyses of multiple studies globally together with many novel assumptions, mathematical simulations, and new dietary analyses to produce totally new results. Only mortality data, mainly from North American and European databases, were now considered in identifying optimum BMIs of 21–23 and all the risk factors were considered as independent entities even though it is well accepted that weight gain, for example, increases blood cholesterol, blood pressure, and many other risk factors. Tables 8.4.8–8.4.10 illustrate the IHME group's high body mass attributable cause-specific deaths and DALYs respectively and the changes in these indicators between 1990 and 2010. The total number of deaths and DALYs for every cause has risen substantially since 1990 and is especially marked (nearly double) for males.

Ethnic differences in susceptibility to chronic diseases on weight gain

Asian adults who gain weight have a two- to fivefold greater risk for developing type 2 diabetes and hypertension (Fig. 8.4.2) show that both type 2 diabetes and hypertension are markedly amplified by weight gain. Similar relationships have been found in analyses of Mexican national surveys who, like Asians, are more prone to selective abdominal obesity at even normal BMIs than US non-Hispanic white people (Sanchez-Castillo et al. 2005).

Whereas this ethnic difference is often assumed to be genetic, Barker and colleagues suggested a fetal nutrition hypothesis whereby environmental factors both *in utero* and early fetal life amplify the risk of abdominal obesity, diabetes, hypertension, and cardiovascular disease (Barker 2004). Systematic analyses of birth weight and future disease in aboriginal communities in North America and Australasia show a markedly increased risk of type 2 diabetes, poorer kidney function and hypertension, and with pregnancy diabetes strongly associated with metabolic abnormalities and diabetes in the offspring. The links between adverse maternal nutrition and poor infant growth with later hypertension are now evident in both poor and affluent countries (Law et al. 2001). A lower birth weight predicts a higher adult mortality rate, particularly for cardiovascular disease and diabetes with a strong relationship to later cancer in men (Risnes et al. 2011). Indian populations also have a major public health problem of vitamin B_{12} deficiency which may affect their epigenetic propensity to future non-communicable diseases; pregnant women supplemented with folic acid as well as being vitamin B_{12} deficient produce offspring which are not only small at birth but fatter, with higher levels of insulin resistance and blood pressure all of which are evident in later childhood (Yajnik et al. 2008). Poor maternal nutrition with low birth weight, maternal smoking, and maternal diabetes all

Table 8.4.8 High BMI attributable deaths by cause globally

	Males			Females		
	1990	**2010**	**Difference**	**1990**	**2010**	**Difference**
Oesophageal cancer	33,524.97	62,647.54	29,122.57	18,054.2	24,630.15	65,75.956
Breast cancer	–	–	–	26,779.96	44,528.67	17,748.71
Uterine cancer	–	–	–	15,184.55	22,477.29	7292.748
Colon and rectum cancers	27,129.16	53,868.23	26,739.07	13,164.57	21,115.17	7950.602
Gall bladder and biliary tract cancer	1401.718	3193.844	1792.126	16,249.86	26,614.04	10,364.18
Pancreatic cancer	4635.688	9720.945	5085.257	8489.134	15,236.92	6747.783
Kidney and other urinary organ cancers	7011.068	18,838.73	11,827.66	7622.154	15,888.66	8266.509
Ischaemic heart disease	457,103.5	733,943	276,839.4	446,067.2	645,124.5	199,057.4
Ischaemic stroke	120,746	197,342.5	76,596.51	209,822.2	273,904.6	64,082.34
Hypertensive heart disease	62,659.98	133,494.8	70,834.81	95,710.37	167,673.1	71,962.68
Cardiomyopathy and myocarditis	24,210.88	48,227.88	24,017	17,331.85	30,870.41	13,538.56
Atrial fibrillation and flutter	2573.11	11,450.03	8876.918	4296.871	17,539.78	13,242.91
Peripheral vascular disease	1967.884	5341.259	3373.375	2065.803	8199.166	6133.363
All causes	887,046.6	1,632,766	745,719.6	1,076,502	1,738,466	661,964

Source: data from Institute for Health Metrics and Evaluation (IHME), *Global Health Data Exchange (GHDx)*, Copyright © 2013 University of Washington, available from http://www.healthmetricsandevaluation.org/gbd/visualizations/regional. Difference = 2010 – 1990.

affect the propensity for obesity in their children, particularly if mothers are overweight/obese with or without gestational diabetes (Fall 2011). The mother's dietary fat intake may also induce a relative increase in their offspring's body fat content through epigenetic changes in the methylation of the promoter regions of the child's genes (Godfrey et al. 2011) and now women are starting pregnancy overweight and producing increasingly heavy babies with a greater propensity to persistent obesity (Gale et al. 2007). The pre-pregnancy size as well as weight gain in pregnancy play important roles in determining greater birth weight and inducing intergenerational obesity. The US Institute of Medicine (2009) has now set out guidelines advocating modest increases in weight during pregnancy.

Projections of the obesity epidemic and its consequent morbidity and costs

Monitoring the changes in the prevalence of obesity and its future occurrence and effects on chronic disease and life expectancy is essential for understanding the challenge and potential benefits of interventions. This applies particularly for children where the health impacts of being obese and overweight will not generally manifest itself until they reach later life.

Conventional analytical methods are generally unable to address satisfactorily situations in which a population's needs change over time. Simulation models combine information from different sources to provide a useful tool for examining how the effects of policies and risk factors unfold over time in complex systems and impact population health. It offers a cheaper and more pragmatic approach than many traditional methods and dynamic models particularly enable alternative scenarios and policies to be tested on specific populations to predict possible outcomes.

There are several methods for modelling the future health outcomes of obesity. Markov cohort models or second-order Markov models simulate a hypothetical cohort of people (Briggs et al. 2006). These cohorts go through a number of health states irrespective of their history. Microsimulations such as that developed for the UK Foresight *Tackling Obesities* enquiry and the OECD chronic disease model track heterogeneous individuals rather than cohorts over time, allowing individual histories to impact on their progression in the model, so microsimulations are able to simulate potential co-morbidities essential to the accurate modelling of chronic diseases. These models show that even small changes in BMI can have a significant impact on avoidable healthcare costs over the life course (Wang et al. 2011; Hollingworth et al. 2012). The OECD model has been used to analyse the most cost-effective methods to tackle obesity. Similarly the Australia Cost Effectiveness (ACE) model combines multistate life tables with Markov cohort simulations. Simulation models can provide both a framework for determining future research priorities and support policymakers to make evidence-based decisions (Carter et al. 2008).

Case study

The model developed by the National Heart Forum (UK), now UK Health Forum, for the English Foresight *Tackling Obesities* report is perhaps the most widely applied model having been used to model future trends in obesity and their future consequences for the development of non-communicable diseases in over 70 countries. The microsimulation model simulates a specified number of individuals throughout their lives and takes account of age and subgroup distributions, their probable health consequences, and the potential value of different interventions.

Table 8.4.9 Changes in high body mass attributable all-cause deaths and disability-adjusted life years (DALYs) for males by region

	Deaths			DALYs		
	1980	2010	Difference	1980	2010	Difference
Andean Latin America	3156	7333	4176.63	111,348.01	248,251.78	136,903.77
Australasia	8672.12	11,460.09	2787.97	221,855.35	288,392.92	66,537.57
Caribbean	6168.32	13,419.13	7250.81	190,326.43	409,044.01	218,717.58
Central Asia	22,535.75	42,913.61	20,377.86	676,802.43	1,284,748.1	607,945.67
Central Europe	84,899.65	102,098.41	17,198.76	2,216,833.7	2,526,365.8	309,532.1
Central Latin America	23,604.47	69,352.8	45,748.33	779,272.72	2,166,514.3	1,387,241.58
Central sub-Saharan Africa	1673.11	3816.63	2143.52	59,202.56	133,273.56	74,071
East Asia	68,866.48	218,915.32	150,048.84	2,487,876.4	7,169,331.40	4,681,455
Eastern Europe	128,048.89	217,508.3	89,459.41	3,559,015.4	5,778,140.70	2,219,125.30
Eastern sub-Saharan Africa	4838.00	16,253.71	11,415.71	176,435.17	590,483.46	414,048.29
High-income Asia Pacific	15,692.15	32,599.85	16,907.7	543,727.76	1,002,956.1	459,228.34
High-income North America	146,642.2	196,910.69	50,268.49	3,739,660.6	5,230,467	1,490,806.4
North Africa and Middle East	64,354.42	149,755.15	85,400.73	2,200,801.4	5,225,834.3	3,025,032.9
Oceania	1037.68	3606.26	2568.57	39,859.63	134,496.79	94,637.16
South Asia	33,456.55	108,325.41	74,868.86	1,264,112	3,882,620.60	2,618,508.6
Southeast Asia	11,504.95	66,623.97	55,119.02	459,916.67	2,398,952.80	1,939,036.13
Southern Latin America	20,194.3	29,930.04	9735.74	523,785.39	743,994.05	220,208.66
Southern sub-Saharan Africa	7365.59	20,408.49	13,042.9	237,466.87	659,380.76	421,913.89
Tropical Latin America	24,341.92	68,935.43	44,593.5	794,746.34	2,068,946.5	1,274,200.16
Western Europe	206,097.62	234,534.62	28437	4,938,724.9	5,638,381.2	699,656.3
Western sub-Saharan Africa	3895.9	18,065.17	14,169.26	169,311.03	728,948.34	559,637.31
Global	887,046.61	1,632,766.2	745,719.59	25,391,081	48,309,524	22,918,443

Source: data from Institute for Health Metrics and Evaluation (IHME), *Global Health Data Exchange (GHDx)*, Copyright © 2013 University of Washington, available from http://www.healthmetricsandevaluation.org/gbd/visualizations/regional. Difference = 2010 − 1990.

The Foresight report (2007) stimulated the UK government to present the first cross-government strategy to tackle obesity (Department of Health 2008) and similar analyses of all 53 countries of the WHO (Euro) region, regional analysis in Latin America (Webber et al. 2012), the Middle East (Kilpi et al. 2014), Mexico (Rtveladze et al. 2013a), Brazil (Rtveladze et al. 2013b), the Russian Federation (Rtveladze et al. 2012), and the United States (Wang et al. 2011).

These data provide the opportunity to project by non-linear regression analysis the changes in the distribution of BMI by age and sex in the years to come and the potential value of different degrees of intervention at different ages (Fig. 8.4.3). The progressive shift in the distribution of BMI seems unremitting and the magnitude of the epidemic and its consequences and costs can be predicted with some confidence.

Although the prevention of obesity in children is publicly and therefore politically appealing, it is not likely to bring rapid changes in the population's health and will do little to reduce the escalating health costs of the obesity-induced epidemic of diabetes and hypertension so has a negligible impact on the disease burden over the next 40 years. However, intervention from 18 years onwards brings much earlier and greater benefits so a focus on adults as well as children is particularly useful for several reasons (Gill 2002; Seidell et al. 2005): the obesity incidence is greatest in early adulthood with further progressive increases and is accompanied by an increasing absolute and population-attributable risk of disease. Parents as adults can also act as models for their children.

Fig. 8.4.3 shows that if the average BMI of the adult population could be reduced by 4 BMI units this would induce a major benefit but this has never been seen except perhaps in Cuba during their financial crisis when food deprivation was widespread. The co-morbidities arise particularly in overweight/obese adults over 50 years, so in terms of cost savings this group could be considered a priority but also those below 50 years who are most vulnerable to developing a co-morbidity, that is, those with pre-diabetes or incipient hypertension. The development of diabetes is particularly sensitive to weight change.

Small errors in energy balance lead to weight increases—the persistence of weight gain

The slimming industry in the United States earns well over US$100 billion yearly with women spending more than men in their attempts to benefit their health as well as feeling more attractive

Table 8.4.10 Changes in high body mass attributable all-cause deaths and disability-adjusted life years (DALYs) for females by region

	Deaths			DALYs		
	1980	2010	Difference	1980	2010	Difference
Andean Latin America	5148.021	9885.208	4737.187	174,220	323,731.7	149,511.7
Australasia	6867.192	10,806.98	3939.786	146,553.3	223,942.8	77,389.52
Caribbean	7767.224	17,963.22	10,196	236,840.4	498,643.3	261,802.8
Central Asia	28,503.85	41,637.37	13,133.52	703,823	1,065,725	361,901.5
Central Europe	103,231.9	113,528.7	10,296.77	2,181,149	2,217,842	36,693.5
Central Latin America	29,209.89	77,505.39	48,295.5	944,042.5	2,289,282	1,345,239
Central sub-Saharan Africa	1316.99	6925.107	5608.116	44,428.68	233,357.2	188,928.5
East Asia	74,780.31	162,321.7	87,541.43	2,648,171	5,652,145	3,003,974
Eastern Europe	230,328.5	291,406.3	61,077.77	4,741,909	5,731,114	989,205.7
Eastern sub-Saharan Africa	4963.361	19,768.07	14,804.71	175,397.3	698,461.1	523,063.8
High-income Asia Pacific	18,590.07	29,465.07	10,875	538,645.9	752,547.7	213,901.8
High-income North America	133,832.9	199,749.3	65,916.43	2,908,616	4,428,180	1,519,564
North Africa and Middle East	72,959.39	157,761.4	84,802.05	2,468,043	5,394,415	2,926,373
Oceania	828.5075	4243.342	3414.835	33,659.61	154,660.4	121,000.7
South Asia	25,862.95	97,587.2	71,724.25	1,007,793	3,596,099	2,588,305
Southeast Asia	15,683.01	81,327.57	65,644.57	612,422.1	2,799,747	2,187,325
Southern Latin America	17,347.76	32,621	15,273.24	396,702.9	688,535.8	291,832.9
Southern sub-Saharan Africa	14,823.8	30,555.22	15,731.42	440,299.7	906,351.1	466,051.4
Tropical Latin America	30,606.1	72,634.81	42,028.71	915,471.3	2,008,574	1,093,103
Western Europe	246,675.8	253,083.6	6407.79	4,559,679	4,572,447	12,768.2
Western sub-Saharan Africa	7174.613	27,689.51	20,514.9	296,048.9	1,064,001	767,952.2
Global	1,076,502	1,738,466	661,964	26,173,915	45,299,802	19,125,887

Source: data from Institute for Health Metrics and Evaluation (IHME), *Global Health Data Exchange (GHDx)*, Copyright © 2013 University of Washington, available from http://www.healthmetricsandevaluation.org/gbd/visualizations/regional. Difference = 2010 − 1990.

after weight loss. This concern may also explain the increase in eating disorders, bulimia, and anorexia nervosa. Yet despite this intense and, in affluent societies, nationwide effort to slim, the obesity epidemic increases with little sign of the impact of all this slimming effort.

The rate of adult weight gain, on average, is 0.5–1.0 kg per year so this amounts to a yearly accumulation of about 3500–7000 kcal. Therefore, the average discrepancy between energy intake and energy expenditure is only 10–20 kcal/day—now called the 'energy gap' and only amounts to about 0.4–0.8 per cent of normal food intake per day. This concept of only small average changes in energy storage often leads to the misleading idea that simple small changes—cutting down food a bit and going for a short walk daily—will stop this weight gain.

These small discrepancies actually show how remarkable the normal regulation of energy balance is. Thus our expenditure in all activity may vary daily by 200–300 kcal depending on how much walking or leisure time activity we undertake but the variation in food intake is much more marked and can often vary daily by 1000 kcal. So the discrepancies in energy balance with fat accumulation represent the residual effect of extremely

complex neuro-hormonal regulatory mechanisms operating on a short-, medium-, and long-term basis to preserve energy balance. Unfortunately the mechanisms which avoid weight loss are multiple and much more robust than those which limit weight gain. The bodyweight response to a change of energy intake is normally slow, with half times of about 1 year (Hall et al. 2011). Furthermore, adults with greater adiposity have a larger expected weight loss for the same lower energy intake but to reach their steady-state weight they take longer than it would for those with less initial body fat.

Physical inactivity

The obvious thermodynamic principles of energy balance require the influence of both dietary change and the reduction in physical activity (PA). Cheaper cars for personal transport and multiple mechanical and electrical aids to remove the physical demands in the home and at work have led to a significant reduction in physical exertion. The advent of computers and television mean that in many affluent societies one can earn an excellent wage and have enjoyable leisure without any physical exertion. Children's habits

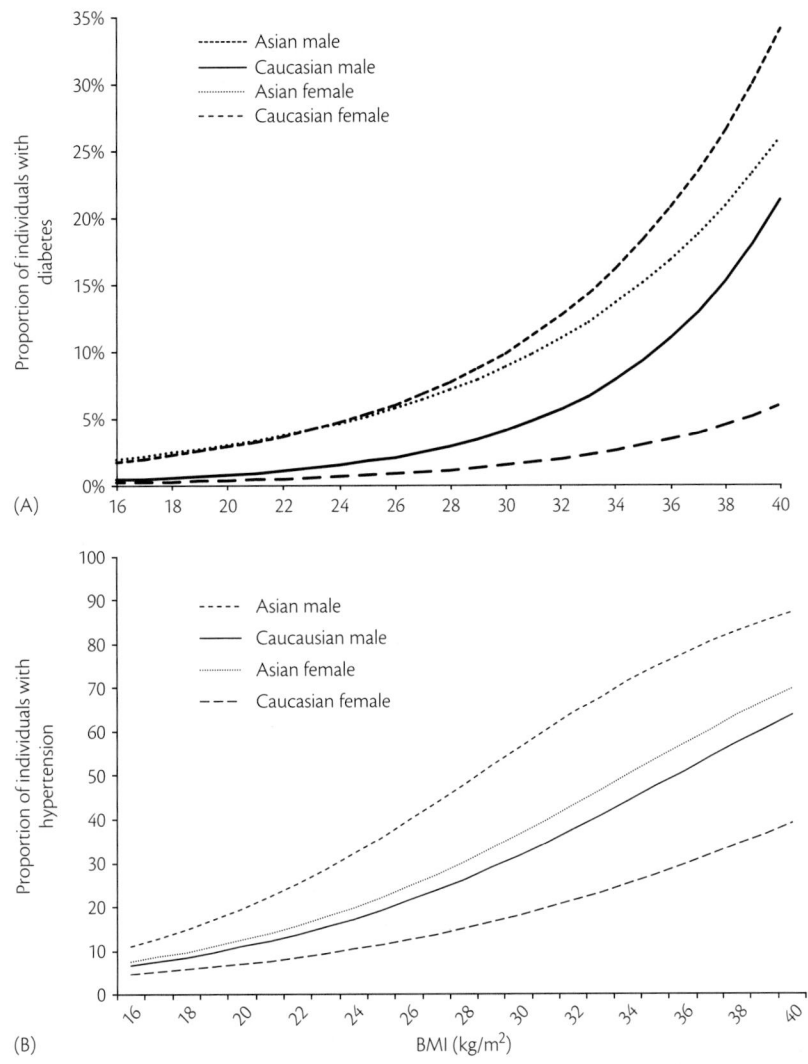

Fig. 8.4.2 The increased risk of (A) diabetes and (B) hypertension in Asian compared with Caucasian men and women in relation to their BMI.
Reproduced from Huxley R, et al., Obesity in Asia Collaboration: Ethnic comparisons of the cross-sectional relationships between measures of body size with diabetes and hypertension. *Obesity Reviews*, Volume 9, Issue Supplement s1, pp. 53–61, Copyright © 2007 The Authors, with permission from John Wiley & Sons Ltd.

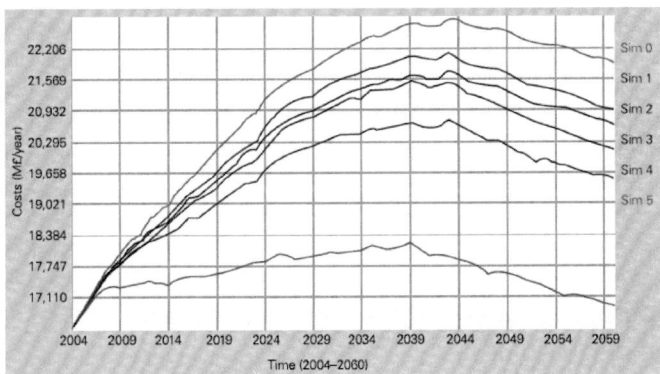

Fig. 8.4.3 The UK Foresight's modelling of the relative benefits in terms of the different effects of age-related interventions for minimizing the impact of obesity-related disease on the national health costs in England.
Reproduced from McPherson K et al., *Foresight. Tackling Obesities: Future choices—modelling future trends in obesity and the impact on health*, © Crown Copyright 2007, available from www.foresight.gov.uk. Reproduced under the Open government Licence 2.0.

are also being transformed by a remarkable secular increase in the time spent watching television or playing video games.

The evidence for current trends in PA varies, but most affluent countries have noted relatively stable rates or slight declines in leisure time physical activity (LTPA) over recent decades (Brownson et al. 2005) and in general the rates of sedentariness, defined as an absence of LTPA, have remained rather stable. Of more importance to total energy expenditure has been the decline in the other domains of PA. The number of people involved in heavy occupational activity has declined dramatically, with more than a 50 per cent reduction in 'heavy work' in Norwegian adults since the middle 1980s, this change being associated with increases in sedentary work (Anderssen et al. 2008). Other countries have noted marked increases in car usage and other motorized transport, at the expense of more active commuting through walking or cycling trips (Fox and Hillsdon 2007). One study even reported a 6 per cent increase in the risk of obesity for every hour spent commuting by car each day (Frank et al. 2004). Limited data are available on domestic settings, but with increases in technologically sophisticated labour-saving devices, and reduced time spent in preparing meals and carrying out household tasks, it seems that energy expenditure on domestic tasks and yard/garden work is likely to have reduced markedly as well.

The increase in obesity notably in the Netherlands and Scandinavia was delayed by up to a decade, perhaps related to high rates of active commuting, especially cycling, as nutritional differences are not apparent compared with several other western European countries (Select Committee on Health 2006–2007, sections 305–309). A few countries have demonstrated increasing trends in LTPA, for example, in Finland and Canada over the last 25 years and in Singapore over about 10 years (Craig et al. 2004; Barengo et al. 2006). Yet, these countries have increased obesity rates that were similar to demographically matched countries without increases in LTPA (Cutler et al. 2003; Bellanger-Ducharme and Tremblay 2005; Borodulin et al. 2007). In Finnish adults the rates of increases in obesity were also only marginally faster among the inactive and no effects of LTPA levels were evident in Norway. Therefore, the increasing obesity rates develop because of increases in energy intake, or/and from substantial reductions in energy expenditure during the working day.

Recent evidence shows that some individuals spontaneously move more readily than others with a greater increase in spontaneous activity when in positive energy balance; this accounts for about 59 per cent of the variation in fat gain on overfeeding (Levine et al. 1999). This so-called non-exercise activity thermogenesis (NEAT) in part explains the remarkable differences in a highly genetically affected different susceptibility to weight gain on overfeeding (Bouchard et al. 1990). However, the overall societal effects on physical activity are marked as shown by Levine studying rural and urban dwellers in Jamaica and in the United States (Levine et al. 2011). The urban thin adults in both countries had equivalent activity levels but walking and standing was 60 per cent greater in rural than urban Jamaicans. Obese Americans sat for almost 4 hours longer than the rural Jamaicans. Thus there are major societal effects but the genetically susceptible individuals in environments which discourage walking and activity will gain weight first.

A marked transformation of our diets has occurred but measures of energy intakes cannot discern an energy imbalance of 10–20 kcal/day, that is, less than 1 per cent of normal daily intake. Whatever the interplay of changes in intake and energy expenditure under the usual environmental conditions before 1980 children and adults on average maintained their energy balance. So there was sufficient demand for physical work both in the home and in the usual range of occupations for people's appetite regulatory centres to be repeatedly operating to ensure that sufficient but not an excess of food was eaten at that time.

With the removal of the need for physical activity to earn one's living, the biological pressure on people's brain regulatory systems has been to limit intake. In relatively sophisticated environments, the meals and portions served at home and in canteens/restaurants—at least in Europe—have become smaller, presumably in response to consumer demand. National food surveys in the United Kingdom showed a progressive fall in consumption even when allowances were made for the greater amount of food eaten outside the home. Populations have, however, become far more dependent on manufactured processed foods and snacks so energy and nutrient intakes have become dependent on the nature of the purchased food.

Three dietary features have contributed to the obesity epidemic. First is the revolution in the industrial food chain with agricultural policies and subsidies set for the last seven decades on generating ever more and cheaper food. This is now produced in marked excess to human needs in developed countries so the farming and food industries, helped by supermarket developments, have developed methods of persuading the population to purchase and therefore consume as much as possible of this produce. This need to generate profits then led to the second feature which is the intense marketing of products with the discovery that persuading people to have snacks and soft drinks increases sales, particularly if backed by price promotions, large portion sizes, and the ready availability of drinks and food throughout the day in every available location. Then there is the scientific development of food products based on the ready use of different fats, sugars, and salt combinations with additional flavours to trigger defined taste and olfactory responses linked to the pleasure-related neurochemical pathways and brain centres. These changes mean that the energy density of foods in general has increased and this, in double-blind trials, leads to unconscious overconsumption of kilocalories (Prentice and Jebb 2003). Sugar- and perhaps fat-containing foods also trigger pleasure-associated brain dopamine release with new evidence of the probable induction of reduced dopamine receptor activity with a lower dopamine release in the brain centres of those individuals who have become obese (Wang et al. 2012). This implies that more food may be needed by the obese to induce the same dopamine response as observed in lean individuals thereby contributing to the persisting high energy intake in the overweight/obese despite their desire to lose weight. In addition, some investigators now consider that sugar-containing foods trigger insulin resistance and metabolic changes which then promote overeating and even an amplified risk of diabetes (Basu et al. 2013). New meta-analyses show that dietary sugar (and particularly energy-containing sugary drinks) is associated with weight gain (Te Morenga et al. 2012) but this probably operates through an energy density effect on 'passive overconsumption'.

Some research also suggests that chronic stress acts as a risk factor for weight gain. Stress can cause changes to the parasympathetic nervous system, inhibiting satiety and stimulating hunger responses. So individuals exposed to prolonged stress (environmental or psychological) could be more likely to overindulge on so-called comfort foods.

Table 8.4.11 sets out the WHO conclusions (WHO 2003) on the causes of weight gain. WHO has recently concluded that increasing either dietary fat or sugar promote weight gain; the resulting increased energy density is amplified by starch refining and the removal of cellular wall structures which therefore reduces the water containing capacity of the food. These issues have not yet been considered.

The biological as well as societal maintenance of obesity

Unfortunately, there is now good evidence that as weight gain occurs, particularly in older adults, there is a 'resetting' of the regulatory system so weight loss is resisted. Weight gain includes 25 per cent lean tissues which require additional daily energy for their maintenance. Thus people's weight should plateau as soon as their increased weight compensates for the small discrepant intake. Unfortunately this is not as effective as we would

Table 8.4.11 Contributors to the development of obesity as set out by the WHO and categorized by the level of evidence for each contributor

Evidence	Decreases risk	No relationship	Increases risk
Convincing	Regular physical activity High-dietary NSP (fibre) intake		High intake of energy-dense nutrient-poor foods Sedentary lifestyles
Probable	Home and school environments that support healthy food choices for children[a] Promoting linear growth Breastfeeding		Heavy marketing of energy-dense foods[a] and fast-food outlets Adverse social and economic conditions (in developed countries, especially for women) Sugar-sweetened soft drinks and fruit juices
Possible	Low-glycaemic index foods	Protein content of the diet	Large portion sizes High proportion of food prepared outside the home (Western countries) 'Rigid restraint/periodic disinhibition' eating patterns
Insufficient	Increasing eating frequency		Alcohol

[a] Associated evidence and expert opinion.

Reproduced with permission from World Health Organization (WHO), *Diet, Nutrition and the Prevention of Chronic Diseases*, Report of a Joint WHO/FAO Expert Consultation, WHO Technical Report Series No. 916, Copyright © WHO 2003, available from http://whqlibdoc.who.int/trs/who_trs_916.pdf.

wish because weight gain usually continues and slowly the neuro-regulatory systems progressively adjust. In due course, the additional 10 kg extra weight then demands a permanent extra daily intake of 200–300 kcal/day. This adaptive mechanism does not occur after the acute overfeeding of young adults because they spontaneously return to their previous body weights but this is not seen when older adults are acutely overfed (Roberts et al. 1994; Roberts and Rosenberg 2006).

Putting overweight and obese individuals on a slimming diet immediately leads to the switching on of acute hormonal, hypothalamic-regulated responses involving both the thyroidal axis and the autonomic nervous system which simulate the response to semi-starvation within 2–4 days even though the obese may have 0.25–1 million extra kcal stored. The brain mechanism which increases the drive to eat is also activated immediately. Whether these mechanisms, traditionally linked to a post-leptin receptor hypothalamic change in responsiveness, are related to the cannabinoid pathways of pleasure highlighted by Volkow and her colleagues (Wang et al. 2012) is unknown. This persistent adaptive change in the brain of obese people helps to induce the regain of weight which they have taken so much trouble to lose. Those who are successful in maintaining their weight loss find that they have to fight a continuous battle for control, following daily and perhaps hourly a rigorous monitoring of their food intake and purchasing habits; they also deliberately engage in 2000–3000 kcal per week of exercise to avoid gaining weight (Wing 2004)! These adaptive problems therefore seem to explain why the obesity epidemic continues to increase despite the desire of so many adults to lose their excess weight. This means that prevention must become a high priority.

Preventive strategies: the options

The analyses presented on the impact of changes in population BMIs at different ages have emphasized the importance of tackling not just obesity but also overweight. Strategies may initially be considered on the basis of rectifying the major societal forces which currently promote the epidemic but the UK Foresight exercise displayed myriad environmental and personal factors not only affecting food intake and expenditure but where biological effects also interact to determine the propensity to obesity.

The Foresight report made clear that for both physical activity and energy intake there are very powerful environmental forces promoting weight gain that the individual does not control. So obesity was described as a 'passive' normal response of humans to the prevailing inappropriate environment. Personal responsibility plays a crucial part in weight gain but human biology is overwhelmed by the effects of today's 'obesogenic' environment, with its abundance of energy-dense food, motorized transport, and sedentary lifestyles. So the population is inexorably becoming heavier simply by living in their environment. This then means that those who successfully remain lean throughout life are either genetically fortunate or they have the advantage in educative, social, or financial terms to withstand the environmental forces and often create for themselves what is in effect a healthy 'microenvironment'.

Simply abolishing or reversing the obesogenic forces may not be useful prevention strategies. The car, mechanical aids, the computerization of so many processes, and the advent of Internet-related communications have all contributed substantially over the decades to reducing the average cost of physical activity by perhaps 750–1000 kcal/day. Nevertheless reversing these developments as a coherent public health strategy is not an option. So the challenge is how best to combine current understanding of: (1) the most effective initiatives on the basis of either coherent prevention trials or from modelling the underlying processes; (2) the most cost-efficient initiatives; (3) the most feasible initiatives on the basis of the features of the country's societal organization, cultural perceptions, and political system; and (4) whether there are other policy initiatives in the areas affecting food and physical activity which need to be integrated or, if conflicting, resolved. The currently adopted strategies are highly dependent on the political nature of the country ranging from a utilitarian regulatory approach to a more common non-interventionist personal responsibility approach. However, an increasing consensus is emerging about the types of measures needed, as set out in the US Institute of Medicine report (IOM 2012) (Box 8.4.1).

Box 8.4.1 Obesity prevention recommendations and strategies

Integrate physical activity in everyday life

◆ Enhance the physical and built environment.

◆ Provide and support community programmes designed to increase physical activity.

◆ Provide support for the science and practice of physical activity.

Market what matters for a healthy life

◆ Adopt policies and implement practices to reduce overconsumption of sugar-sweetened drinks.

◆ Increase the availability of lower-calorie and healthier food and drink options for children in restaurants.

◆ Utilize strong nutritional standards for all foods and drinks sold or provided through the government, and ensure that these healthy options are available in all places frequented by the public.

◆ Introduce, modify, and utilize health-promoting food and drink retailing and distribution policies.

◆ Broaden the examination and development of agriculture policy and research to include implications for the diet.

Make healthy foods and drinks available everywhere

◆ Develop and support a sustained, targeted physical activity and nutrition social marketing programme.

◆ Implement common standards for marketing foods and drinks to children and adolescents.

◆ Ensure consistent nutrition labelling for the front of packages, retail store shelves, and menus and menu boards that encourages healthier food choices.

◆ Adopt consistent nutrition education policies for federal programmes with nutrition education components.

Activate employers and healthcare professionals

◆ Provide standardized care and advocate for healthy community environments.

◆ Ensure coverage of, access to, and incentives for routine obesity prevention, screening, diagnosis, and treatment.

◆ Encourage active living and healthy eating at work.

◆ Encourage healthy weight gain during pregnancy and breastfeeding, and promote breastfeeding-friendly environments.

Interventions for the prevention of overweight and obesity in school children

◆ School-based multicomponent interventions addressing various aspects of diet and/or activity in the school, including the school environment (a 'whole-school approach').

◆ Removal of high-fat, high-sugar, and high-salt food and drinks from school environment.

◆ Provision of fruit and vegetables and free drinking water.

Adapted with permission from Institute of Medicine, *Accelerating Progress in Obesity Prevention: Solving the Weight of the Nation*, Recommendations May 2012, Copyright © 2012 by the National Academy of Sciences. All rights reserved, available from http://www.iom.edu/~/media/Files/Report%20 Files/2012/APOP/APOP_insert.pdf.

The WHO set a target of reducing premature mortality from non-communicable diseases by 25 per cent by the year 2025 (WHO 2012a) and for there to be no increase in adult and adolescent overweight and obesity. Oliver Du Schutter, a UN Rapporteur for Food, is more explicit (de Schutter 2012):

> Our food systems are making people sick, faced with this public health crisis, we continue to prescribe medical remedies: nutrition pills and early-life nutrition strategies for those lacking in calories; slimming pills, lifestyle advice and calorie counting for the overweight. But we must tackle the systemic problems that generate poor nutrition in all its forms by:
> ◆ taxing unhealthy products;
> ◆ regulating foods high in saturated fats, salt and sugar;
> ◆ cracking down on junk food advertising;
> ◆ overhauling misguided agricultural subsidies that make certain ingredients cheaper than other policies supporting local food

production so that consumers have access to healthy, fresh and nutritious food.

The Lancet series on obesity in 2011 concluded that (Gortmaker et al. 2011):

◆ Governments need to lead obesity prevention but few have shown leadership.

◆ Empirical evidence of how to prevent obesity is limited but growing: cost-effectiveness policy and programme analyses indicate that several are both effective and cost saving.

◆ A systems approach to obesity prevention highlights important policy needs:

  • the need for integrated interventions throughout society with measures by individuals, families, local and national governments and international policy changes

- policies that target the food and built environments

- multiple actions including non-health sectors

- investments in cross-cutting support systems

- the collection of additional data for future forecasts and evaluations of progress.

Age-related issues: childhood prevention

The current focus on childhood overweight/obesity is justified, despite the limited early economic returns (Fig. 8.4.2), on several grounds:

♦ Neither the public nor most policymakers blame the individual child for their predicament and only a few try to assign blame to their parents. This childhood focus has a politically useful place in persuading the public and politicians to recognize the importance of environmental rather than individual factors and to do something other than advocating treatment.

♦ It is readily recognized that in older children excess weight gain confers on the affected group a far higher medical burden in their lifetime and a much greater probability of an early death than if one simply is concerned about the middle aged and older person.

♦ The focus on children also chimes with the routine mantra that the key to the problem of obesity is 'education' so clearly there is merit in educating the child so that they 'do not behave' like their parents.

♦ If one is to focus on a group in society then school-aged children is a useful choice because one is guaranteed to be able to reach them in most societies through a school-mediated initiative.

Childhood prevention initiatives

These have been reviewed by Osei-Assibey et al. (2012) who suggested that reducing food promotion to young children, increasing the availability of smaller portions, and providing alternatives to sugar-sweetened soft drinks should be considered but these proposals simply set out the desirable final food changes resulting from suitable prevention schemes and one needs to consider the underlying context.

Approaches to prevention: is there a logic to the chosen initiatives?

A simpler overview than the UK's Foresight collation of different options is presented in Fig. 8.4.4 where the IOTF prevention group highlighted the different environmental systems which affect the environmental impact on both the diet and physical activity.

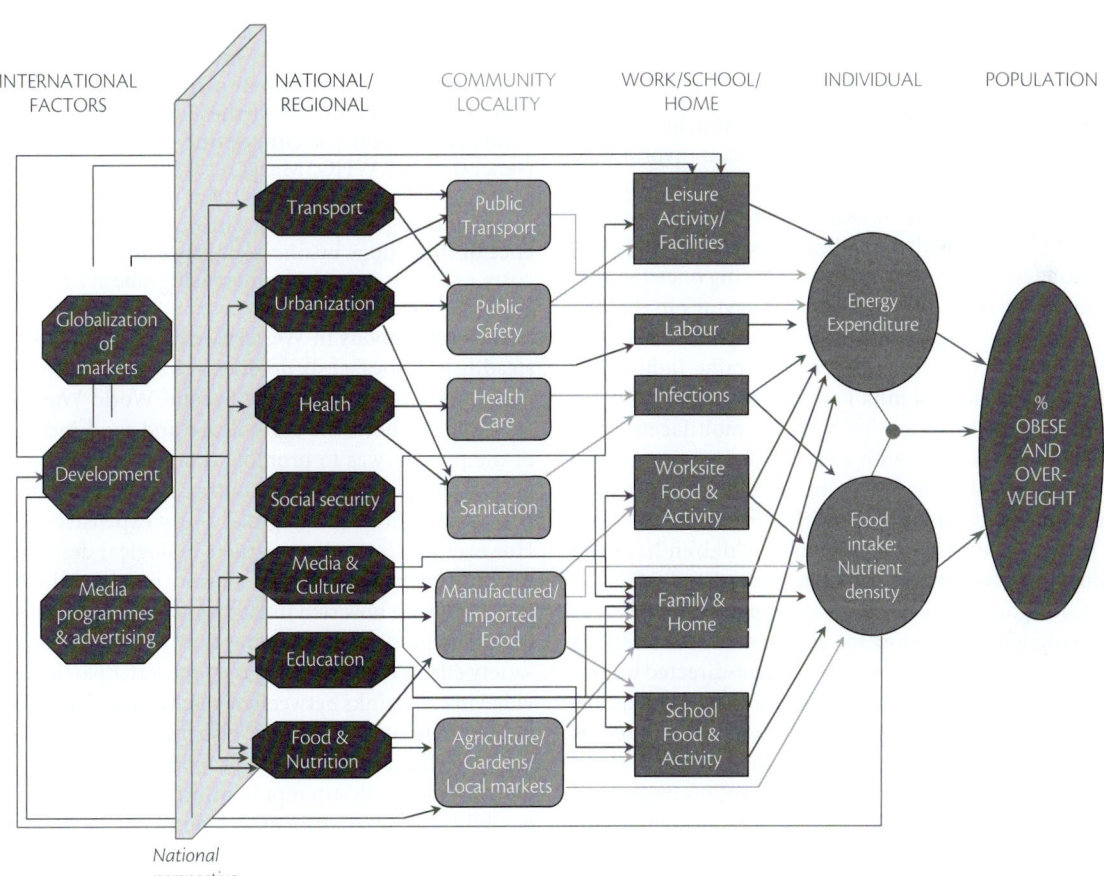

Fig. 8.4.4 Societal policies and processes influencing the population prevalence of obesity.

Adapted by permission from Macmillan Publishers Ltd: *International Journal of Obesity*, Volume 26, Issue 3, pp. 425–36, Kumanyika S. et al. Public Health Approaches to the Prevention of Obesity (PHAPO) Working Group of the International Obesity Task Force (IOTF). Obesity prevention: the case for action, Copyright © 2002.

Gortmaker et al. (2011) have summarized the prevention options and the ANGELO framework (Egger and Swinburn 1997) has helpfully defined the options both at the micro and macro level in terms of four overall areas of action:

1. Physical changes, for example, in the design of the environment for physical activity involving play areas, safe pedestrian, and cycling-friendly streets or in dietary terms the food availability in shops within easy reach of poor families.

2. Economic, which might involve incentives or taxes or other economic measures at either a local or national level.

3. Political, for example, specifying the requirement for baby-friendly hospitals to promote breastfeeding.

4. Sociocultural, for example, involving changes to the health promotion and other national or local programmes and the involvement of major cultural figures to change perceptions of what is reasonable.

On the energy expenditure side there is concordance between the need to promote physical activity and the demand to limit climate change so national transport systems, for example, trains and the use of buses, need a much higher priority than car use. This then automatically requires more routine walking by the general public. In terms of food, Table 8.4.12 illustrates how the different levels of action can be classified and then how to consider the role of different ministries of government in taking responsibility for these actions.

This approach now allows a logical analysis of the options but still does not necessarily provide a clear approach to the choice of preventive measures.

A systematic review on children's obesity prevention has emphasized the need to integrate community and parental involvement with school-based initiatives (Wang et al. 2013). Integrated analyses of appropriate cost-effective measures have then been set out by Gortmaker et al. (2011) with a number of measures being seen as not only cost-effective but likely to be cost saving once the cost of the intervention and the likely or observed savings in disability costs are compared. In order of priority they listed a 10 per cent tax on unhealthy foods and beverages, traffic light labelling, advertising restrictions of junk food and drinks to children, school-based education to reduce TV viewing, multifaceted diet and activity school initiatives with additional programmes for overweight and obese children, a focus on lowering children's soft drink intake, and family-based programmes for obese children. The intense media-wide marketing of food to children has been shown to induce confusion about nutrition, alter attitudes favouring the advertised goods, change purchasing practices in favour of the foods marketed, and distort the children's diets (Hastings et al. 2003). The additional bonus of a government-directed ban on marketing is that the initiation of these measures simply requires a government regulation which then has to be followed. There is then no cost in terms of educating schools, parents, and children. This illustrates the fact that government intervention using conventional mechanisms for adjusting societal rules or habits usually automatically involve few direct costs. Thus the more that can be undertaken by governmental processes which require industry or businesses or governmental workers to change their practices affecting food and activity, the lower the potential cost compared with individually related initiatives, for example, involving health education or personal trainers or other focused and individually based advice to individual consumers. However, it is clear that politically one needs to persuade the population through a series of accepted progressive proposals so that politicians are driven to take the progressive steps which several major food industries are lobbying intensely against.

In developing a food business it is well recognized that apart from producing a product that is attractive there are three key features which determine their increasing turnover:

1. The price of their product.

2. Its pervasive availability for consumers.

3. Promotion by intense marketing.

These three factors—price, availability, and marketing—have also been repeatedly shown to be important in the public health initiatives for the effective limiting of smoking and alcohol consumption. The same clearly now applies to the issue of obesity because even children respond to cheaper options by purchasing more, for example, of fruit in a school setting (French et al. 2001). It is also clear that the cost of foods in a Western environment is often inversely related to the nutritional quality of the product; the greater the energy density of the food, that is, in terms of kcal/g then the cheaper it is (Drewnowski and Specter 2004; Maillot et al. 2007). It is therefore not surprising that OECD analyses by health economists show that media campaigns are of no benefit in terms of reducing the disability associated with obesity (Fig. 8.4.5) or the health costs (Fig. 8.4.6). Regulatory and fiscal restrictions as well as an integrated health centre approach to treatment are beneficial rather than just media campaigns which are of little use on their own. Few governments have, however, as yet taken notice of these economic arguments but the evidence is steadily accumulating that, as the current Director General of the WHO, Margaret Chan specifies, we now have to take account not only of Big Tobacco but also of Big Alcohol, Big Food, and Big Soda (Chan 2013). Unless the power and influence of these huge business enterprises are managed, the health costs of the progressively increasing obesity rates are bound to escalate.

The cost of foods in Western environments has been changing steadily over the last six decades as a result of government policies which were set out after the Second World War and led to vast subsidies for both the agriculture and food industries. The aim of the policies was to promote the production and consumption of ever cheaper meat, milk, butter, fats, and oils so that even the poor could afford the originally very expensive meat and butter. However, in responding to their biological desire to satisfy their intrinsic energy needs the poor now purchase the cheapest products which are now rich in fat and sugars. This practice then tends to lead to 'passive overconsumption' because of the relatively poor satiety effects of fats and sugars—the latter particularly when provided in soft drinks between meals. The purchasing patterns of the poorer sections of society are also much more price sensitive; they are spending a much higher proportion of household income on food and normally attempt to minimize these costs to allow more flexibility for purchasing other household needs. Recent 2013 evidence from temporary Danish taxes on saturated fat and French taxes on soft drinks shows that population purchases fall even when there are modest increases in price.

These economic constraints require an integrated approach before satisfactory dietary changes can be supported. Putting a

Table 8.4.12 An update of an approach developed by WHO (Euro) for action by different branches of government on diet and physical activity but taking account of other issues such as food safety and environmental issues

	Dietary quality; physical activity	Food safety	Environment
(A) Ministry of Health—direct responsibilities			
Physical	Appropriately accessible health centres Promoting access to appropriate self-monitoring, e.g. weight, blood pressure	Catering in hospitals; monitoring facilities	Fluoridation systems for water Facilities for iodizing salt
Economic	Primary health payments for specific targets in management	Penalties for providing unsafe food	Subsidize iodine for iodination purposes
Policy	Baby-friendly hospitals Specifying the exclusion of unhealthy foods and drinks from all government premises, e.g. hospitals Dietary guidelines establishing fortification policies Establish policies on health claims, e.g. functional foods	Health impact of multisectoral food safety policies	Establish specific guidelines for toxicants and contaminants in soil, water, and primary food products HIA of agrochemical use
Sociocultural	Health education	Promote concept of limited clinical antibiotic use	Transform economic analyses of traffic policy to account for marked fall in disability from physical activity as well as mortality
(B) Other ministries—but driven by Health Ministry cross-government initiatives			
Physical	Ensuring playgrounds in schools, suitable cycling and road systems; urban planning; sports facilities. Designated urban areas for local food production	Provision of appropriate local abattoirs. Proper public toilet and sanitary facilities. Proper catering facilities based on stringent hygiene requirements	Urban planning: green spaces, cycle paths, parks, playgrounds, lead free Establish facilities for farmers' markets
Economic	Re-evaluate taxation and subsidy policies on food groups; regulatory policies, e.g. all government facilities should serve only healthy foods and drink choices; fast foods, soft drinks etc. excluded. Vegetable costs routinely included in meals in catering/restaurants as in Finland	Establish appropriate penalties for inappropriate hygiene	Reform Common Agricultural Policy (CAP) Finance new public transport systems Promote urban agriculture, new outlets for high-quality, affordable foods in deprived areas
Policy	Health impact assessment of agricultural policies with shift to nutrition sensitive agriculture Food labelling with appropriate, understandable, health-related information, e.g. 'traffic light' labelling Banning + taxing all fast foods and soft drinks as in France Limiting density and siting of fast food outlets in urban areas	Establish criteria for ensuring pathogen- and contaminant-free access to the food chain. Establish systematic HACCP for food chain, systematic surveillance, and mechanisms for emergency response	Reform CAP Develop soil improvement, clean water, agricultural recycling, planting, fertilizer, pesticide, water use policies
Sociocultural	Promote physical activity in the workplace Create breastfeeding time and space in the workplace with non-governmental organization help	Establish new criteria for excluding antibiotics as growth promoters and specifying veterinary use Educational initiatives for safety of fast-food outlets, and modifying nutrient composition, and limiting and ensuring appropriate food waste disposal	Change attitudes to cycle path use, pedestrian areas Educational initiatives for caterers, communal use of school recreational facilities

Adapted with permission from Robertson, A. et al., *Food and Health in Europe: a new basis of action*, WHO Regional Publications, European Series No 96, Copyright © World Health Organization 2004, available from http://www.euro.who.int/__data/assets/pdf_file/0005/74417/E82161.pdf. Inspired by the ANGELO model, Egger, G. and Swinburn, B., An 'ecological' approach to the obesity pandemic, *British Medical Journal*, Volume 315, Issue 7106, pp. 477–80, Copyright © 1997. Includes data from World Cancer Research Fund/American Institute of Cancer Research (AICR), Policy and action for Cancer prevention, *Food, physical activity: a global perspective*, AICR, Washington, DC, USA, Copyright © 2009; and WHO/IASO/IOTF, *The Asia-Pacific perspective: redefining obesity and its treatment*, February 2000, Health Communications, Australia PTY Ltd Copyright © 2000, available from http://www.idi.org.au/obesity_report.htm.

higher price on fat- and sugar-rich foods is a regressive measure, that is, poorer households will pay more as with taxes on tobacco and alcohol. An integrated economic package therefore needs to be developed so the poorer section of society obtains more financial support by other means. Then the alteration of relative food prices will still induce changes in the poorer sections of the community as well as in the middle-income group. If appropriate low-energy dense foods are also made readily available, the poorer sections of the community respond. Thus in Finland the cost of vegetables provided with main meals at

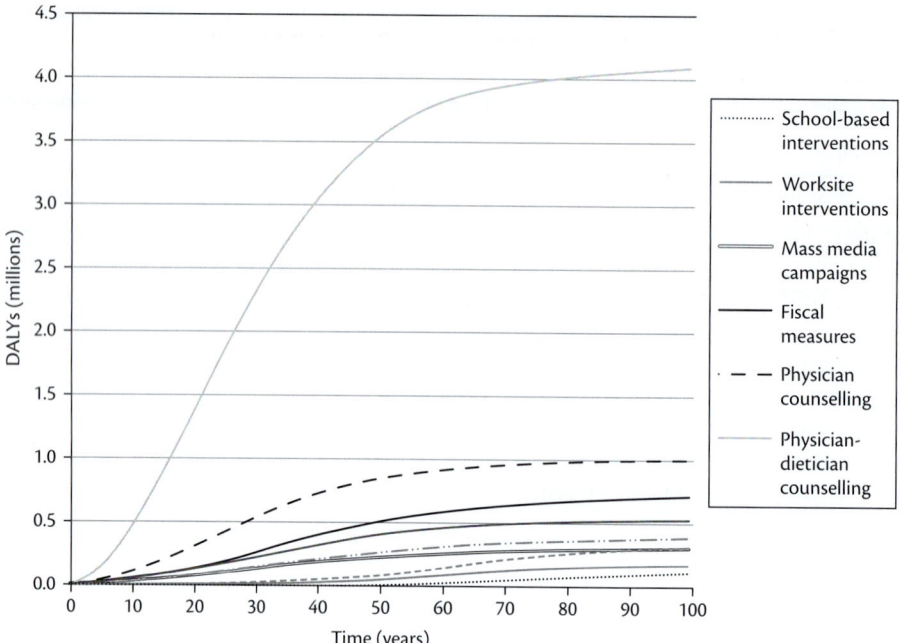

Fig. 8.4.5 Cumulative DALYs saved over time through the use of different prevention/treatment strategies. Details of models and the use of lifetime analyses provided in Sassi (2010).

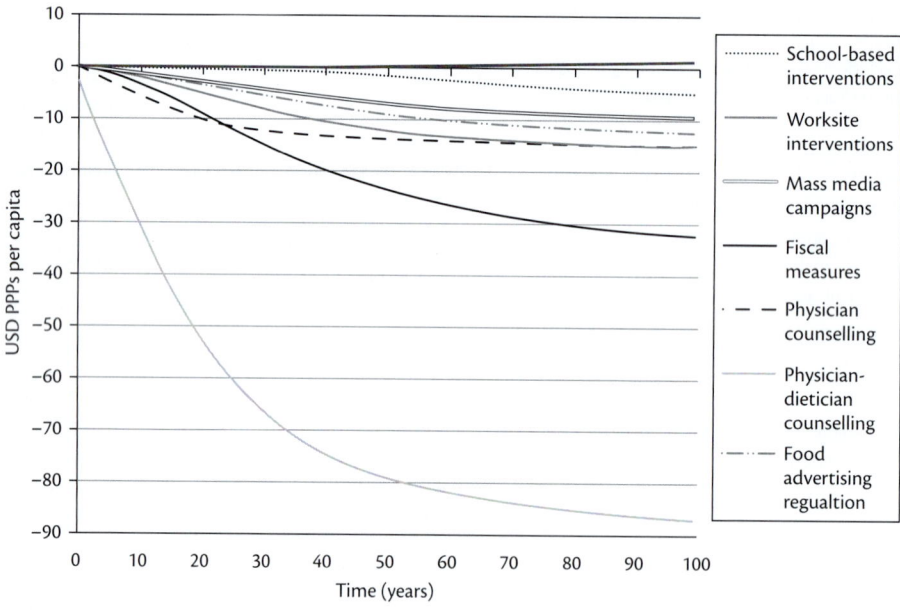

Fig. 8.4.6 Cumulative impact on health expenditure over time.

canteens and restaurants is included in the general price of the main meal. This benefited the poorer sector of the community and contributed to a trebling in the population's vegetable intake over a 15-year period with a parallel marked reduction in the prevalence of hypertension and a profound fall in cardiovascular diseases.

Conclusions

Prevention policies to reverse the prevalence of obesity are already working for children in several European countries with the most rigorous governmental action being seen in France where new Ministry of Health analyses show a 15 per cent fall in children's overweight and obesity on a national basis. France is also the country with the most stringent controls on the food and drink industries but as yet there are no studies to show a reversal in adult obesity which is a much bigger challenge. Obesity prevention will require far more rigorous integrated policies from governments who are heavily influenced by the major obesogenic industries which currently resist altering their practices.

Acknowledgements

Text extracts from United Nations, Human Rights Council, Nineteenth Session, Agenda item 3, *Report submitted by the Special Rapporteur on the right to food, Olivier De Schutter*, A/HRC/19/59, Copyright © 2012, reproduced with permission from the United Nations, available from http://www.srfood.org/images/stories/pdf/officialreports/20120306_nutrition_en.pdf.

References

Adams, K.F., Schatzkin, A., Harris, T.B., et al. (2006). Overweight, obesity, and mortality in a large prospective cohort of persons 50 to 71 years old. *The New England Journal of Medicine*, 355, 763–78.

Anderssen, S.A., Engeland, A., Sogaard, A.J., et al. (2008). Changes in physical activity behaviour and the development of body mass index during the last 30 years in Norway. *Scandinavian Journal of Medicine & Science in Sports*, 18, 309–17.

Asia Pacific Cohort Studies Collaboration (2004). Body mass index and cardiovascular disease in the Asia-Pacific Region: an overview of 33 cohorts involving 310 000 participants. *International Journal of Epidemiology*, 33, 751–8.

Baker, J.L., Olsen, L.W., and Sørensen, T.I. (2007). Childhood body-mass index and the risk of coronary heart disease in adulthood. *The New England Journal of Medicine*, 357, 2329–37.

Barengo, N.C., Nissinen, A., Pekkarinen, H., et al. (2006). Twenty-five-year trends in lifestyle and socioeconomic characteristics in Eastern Finland. *Scandinavian Journal of Public Health*, 34, 437–44.

Barker, D.J. (2004). The developmental origins of well-being. *Philosophical Transactions of the Royal Society B*, 359, 1359–66.

Barlow, S.E. and Dietz, W.H. (1998). Obesity evaluation and treatment: expert committee recommendations. *Pediatrics*, 102, 1–11.

Basu, S., Yoffe, P., Hills, N., and Lustig, R.H. (2013). The relationship of sugar to population-level diabetes prevalence: an econometric analysis of repeated cross-sectional data. *PLoS One*, 8(2), e57873.

Batty, G.D., Shipley, M.J., Jarrett, R.J., Breeze, E., Marmot, M.G., and Davey Smith, G. (2006). Obesity and overweight in relation to disease-specific mortality in men with and without existing coronary heart disease in London: the original Whitehall study. *Heart*, 92, 886–92.

Belanger-Ducharme, F. and Tremblay, A. (2005). A prevalence of obesity in Canada. *Obesity Reviews*, 6, 183–6.

Berrington de Gonzalez, A., Hartge, P., Cerhan, J.R., et al. (2010). Body-mass index and mortality among 1.46 million white adults. *The New England Journal of Medicine*, 363, 2211–19. Erratum in: *The New England Journal of Medicine* (2011); 365, 869.

Borodulin, K., Makinen, T., Fogelholm, M., et al. (2007). Trends and socioeconomic differences in overweight among physically active and inactive Finns in 1978–2002. *Preventive Medicine*, 45, 157–62.

Bouchard, C., Tremblay, A., Depres, J.P., et al. (1990). The response to long-term overfeeding in identical twins. *The New England Journal of Medicine*, 322, 1477–82.

Briggs, A., Claxton, K., and Sculpher, M. (2006). *Decision Modelling, Health Economic Evaluation*. Oxford: Oxford University Press.

Brownson, R.C., Boehmer, T.K., and Luke, D.A. (2005). Declining rates of physical activity in the United States: what are the contributors? *Annual Review of Public Health*, 26, 421–43.

Carter, C., Vos, T., Moodie, M., et al. (2008). Priority setting in health; origins, description and application of Assessing Cost Effectiveness

(ACE), Initiative. *Expert Review of Pharmacoeconomics & Outcomes Research*, 8, 593–617.

Chan, M. (2013). *Opening Address at the 8th Global Conference on Health Promotion Helsinki, Finland*. [Online] Available at: http://www.who.int/dg/speeches/2013/health_promotion_20130610/en/.

Cole, T.J., Bellizzi, M.C., Flegal, K.M., et al. (2000). Establishing a standard definition for child overweight and obesity worldwide: international survey. *British Medical Journal*, 320, 1240–3.

Cole, T.J. and Lobstein, T. (2012). Extended international (IOTF) body mass index cut-offs for thinness, overweight and obesity. *Pediatric Obesity*, 7, 284–94.

Craig, C.L., Russell, S.J., Cameron, C., et al. (2004). Twenty-year trends in physical activity among Canadian adults. *Canadian Journal of Public Health*, 95, 59–63.

Cutler, D., Glaeser, E., and Shapiro, J. (2003). Why have Americans become more obese? *Journal of Economic Perspectives*, 17(3), 93–118.

De Onis, M., Blössner, M., and Borghi, E. (2010). Global prevalence and trends of overweight and obesity among preschool children. *American Journal of Clinical Nutrition*, 92, 1257–64.

De Onis, M., Martínez-Costa, C., Núñez, F., et al. (2012a). Association between WHO cut-offs for childhood overweight and obesity and cardiometabolic risk. *Public Health Nutrition*, 16, 625–30.

De Onis, M., Onyango, A., Borghi, E., et al. (2012b). Worldwide implementation of the WHO Child Growth Standards. *Public Health Nutrition*, 12, 1–8.

Department of Health (2008). *Healthy Weight, Healthy Lives: A Cross-Government Strategy for England*. London: Department of Health. Available at: http://www.dh.gov.uk/publications.

De Schutter, O. (2012). *The Right to Food. A Report by the Special Rapporteur on the Right to Food*. Human Rights Council, 19th Session. Agenda item 3. [Online] Available at: http://www.srfood.org/images/stories/pdf/officialreports/20120306_nutrition_en.pdf.

Dietz, W.H. and Bellizzi, M.C. (1999). Assessment of childhood and adolescent obesity. *American Journal of Clinical Nutrition*, 70(Suppl.), 117–75S.

Drewnowski, A. and Specter, S.E. (2004). Poverty and obesity: the role of energy density and energy costs. *American Journal of Clinical Nutrition*, 79, 6–16.

Egger, G. and Swinburn, B. (1997). An 'ecological' approach to the obesity pandemic. *British Medical Journal*, 315, 477–80.

Ezzati, M., Hoorn, S.V., Lawes, C.M.M., et al. (2005). Rethinking the 'diseases of affluence' paradigm: economic development and global patterns of nutritional risks obesity and other cardiovascular risk factors 2005 in relation to economic development. *PLoS Medicine*, 2, 404–12.

Fall, C.H. (2011). Evidence for the intra-uterine programming of adiposity in later life. *Annals of Human Biology*, 38, 410–28.

Finkelstein, E.A., Trogdon, J.G., Cohen, J.W., et al. (2009). Annual medical spending attributable to obesity: payer- and service-specific estimates. *Health Affairs (Millwood)*, 28, 822–31.

Flegal, K.M., Graubard, B.I., Williamson, D.F., et al. (2007). Cause-specific excess deaths associated with underweight, overweight, and obesity. *Journal of the American Medical Association*, 298, 2028–37.

Flegal, K.M., Kit, B.K., Orpana, H., et al. (2013). Association of all-cause mortality with overweight and obesity using standard body mass index categories: a systematic review and meta-analysis. *Journal of the American Medical Association*, 309, 71–82.

Foresight (2007). *Tackling Obesities: Future Choices – Project Report* (2nd ed.). London: Government Office for Science. Available at: http://www.foresight.gov.uk/Obesity/Obesity.html.

Fox, K.R. and Hillsdon, M. (2007). Physical activity and obesity. *Obesity Reviews*, 8(S1), 115–21.

Frank, L.D., Andresen, M.A., and Schmid, T.L. (2004). Obesity relationships with community design, physical activity, and time spent in cars. *American Journal of Preventive Medicine*, 27, 87–96.

French, S.A., Story, M., and Jeffery, R.W. (2001). Environmental influences on eating and physical activity. *Annual Review of Public Health*, 22, 309–35.

Gale, C.R., Javaid, M.K., Robinson, S.M., et al. (2007). Maternal size in pregnancy and body composition in children. *Journal of Clinical Endocrinology & Metabolism*, 92, 3904–11.

Gill, T. (2002). The importance of preventing weight gain in adulthood. *Asia Pacific Journal of Clinical Nutrition*, 11(Suppl.), S632–6.

Godfrey, K.M., Sheppard, A., Gluckman, P.D., et al. (2011). Epigenetic gene promoter methylation at birth is associated with child's later adiposity. *Diabetes*, 60, 1528–34.

Gortmaker, S.L., Swinburn, B.A., Levy, D., et al. (2011). Changing the future of obesity: science, policy, and action. *The Lancet*, 378, 838–47.

Greenberg, J.A. (2006). Correcting biases in estimates of mortality attributable to obesity. *Obesity*, 14, 2071–9.

Gunnell, D.J., Frankel, S.J., Nanchahal, K., et al. (1998). Childhood obesity and adult cardiovascular mortality: a 57-y follow-up study based on the Boyd Orr cohort. *American Journal of Clinical Nutrition*, 67, 1111–18.

Hall, K.D., Sacks, G., Chandramohan, D., et al. (2011). Quantification of the effect of energy imbalance on bodyweight. *The Lancet*, 378, 826–37.

Hastings, G., Stead, M., McDermott, L., et al. (2003). *Review of Research on the Effects of Food Promotion to Children. Final Report Prepared for the Food Standards Agency*. [Online] Available at: http://www.food.gov.uk/multimedia/pdfs/foodpromotiontochildren1.pdf.

Hollingworth, W., Hawkins, J., Lawlor, D.A., et al. (2012). Economic evaluation of lifestyle interventions to treat overweight or obesity in children. *International Journal of Obesity*, 36, 559–66.

Huxley, R., James, W.P., Barzi, F., et al. (2008). Obesity in Asia Collaboration. Ethnic comparisons of the cross-sectional relationships between measures of body size with diabetes and hypertension. *Obesity Reviews*, 9(Suppl. 1), 53–61.

Institute of Medicine (2012). *Accelerating Progress in Obesity Prevention: Solving the Weight of the Nation*. Washington, DC: The National Academies Press.

Institute of Medicine and National Research Council (2009). *Weight Gain During Pregnancy: Reexamining the Guidelines*. Washington, DC: The National Academies Press.

International Obesity Task Force (2010). *Dynamic Modelling for Health Impact Assessment: DYNAMO HIA*. [Online] Available at: http://www.dynamo-hia.eu/News/Contentcolumn/DYNAmic_MOdel_for_Health_Impact_Assessment_DYNAMO_HIA.

James, W.P.T. (Compiler) (1976). *Research on Obesity. A Report of the DHSS/MRC Group*. London: HMSO.

James W.P.T. (2005). Assessing obesity: are ethnic differences in body mass index and waist classification criteria justified? *Obesity Reviews*, 6, 179–81.

James, W.P.T., Ferro-Luzzi, A., and Waterlow, J.C. (1988). Definition of chronic energy deficiency in adults. Report of a Working Party of the International Dietary Energy Consultative Group. *European Journal of Clinical Nutrition*, 42, 969–81.

Keith, S.W., Fontaine, K.R., Pajewski, N.M., et al. (2011). Use of self-reported height and weight biases: the body mass index–mortality association. *International Journal of Obesity*, 35, 401–8.

Kilpi, F., Webber, L., Musaiger, A., et al. (2014). Alarming predictions for obesity and non-communicable diseases in the Middle East. *Public Health Nutrition*, 17(5), 1078–86.

Kumanyika, S., Jeffery, R.W., Morabia, A., et al. (2002). Public Health Approaches to the Prevention of Obesity (PHAPO) Working Group of the International Obesity Task Force (IOTF). Obesity prevention: the case for action. *International Journal of Obesity*, 26, 425–36.

Law, C.M., Egger, P., Dada, O., et al. (2001). Body size at birth and blood pressure among children in developing countries *International Journal of Epidemiology*, 30, 52–7.

Lawlor, D.A., Hart, C.L., Hole, D.J., et al. (2006). Reverse causality and confounding and the associations of overweight and obesity with mortality. *Obesity (Silver Spring)*, 14, 2294–304.

Levine, J.A., Eberhardt, N.L., and Jensen, M.D. (1999). Role of nonexercise activity thermogenesis in resistance to fat gain in humans. *Science*, 283, 212–14.

Levine, J.A., McCrady, S.K., Boyne, S., et al. (2011). Non-exercise physical activity in agricultural and urban people. *Urban Studies*, 48, 2417–27.

Lillycrop, K.A. and Burdge, G.C. (2012). Epigenetic mechanisms linking early nutrition to longterm health. *Best Practice & Research Clinical Endocrinology & Metabolism*, 26, 667–76.

Lim, S., Vos, T., Flaxman, A., et al. (2012). A comparative risk assessment of burden of disease and injury attributable to 67 risk factors and risk factor clusters in 21 regions, 1990–2010: a systematic analysis for the Global Burden of Disease Study 2010. *The Lancet*, 380, 2224–60.

Maillot, M., Darmon, N., Vieux, F., et al. (2007). A low energy density and high nutritional quality are each associated with higher diet costs in French adults. *American Journal of Clinical Nutrition*, 86, 690–6.

Mancini, M., Ordovas, J., and Riccardi, G. (2011). *Nutritional and Metabolic Bases of Cardiovascular Disease*, Table 4.1. John Wiley & Sons.

McPherson, K., Marsh, T., and Brown, M. (2007). *Foresight. Tackling Obesities: Future Choices—Modelling Future Trends in Obesity and the Impact on Health*. London: Government Office for Science. Available at: http://www.foresight.gov.uk.

Narbro, K., Jonsson, E., Larsson, B., et al. (1996). Economic consequences of sick-leave and early retirement in obese Swedish women. *International Journal of Obesity*, 20, 895–903.

National Obesity Observatory (2013). *Statistics on Obesity, Physical Activity and Diet – England, 2012*. [Online] Available at: http://www.hscic.gov.uk/pubs/opad12.

Neel, J.V. (1962). Diabetes mellitus: a 'thrifty' genotype rendered detrimental by 'progress'? *American Journal of Human Genetics*, 14, 353–62.

Olds, T., Maher, C., Zumin, S., et al. (2011). Evidence that the prevalence of childhood overweight is plateauing: data from nine countries. *International Journal of Pediatric Obesity*, 6, 342–60.

Osei-Assibey, G., Dick, S., Macdiarmid, J., et al. (2012). The influence of the food environment on overweight and obesity in young children: a systematic review. *British Medical Journal Open*, 2, 2(6).

Padwal, R.S., Pajewski, N.M., Allison, D.B., et al. (2011). Using the Edmonton obesity staging system to predict mortality in a population-representative cohort of people with overweight and obesity. *Canadian Medical Association Journal*, 183, E1059–66.

Park, M.H., Falconer, C., Viner, R.M., et al. (2012). The impact of childhood obesity on morbidity and mortality in adulthood: a systematic review. *Obesity Reviews*, 13, 985–1000.

Parsons, T.J., Power, C., Logan, S., et al. (1999). Childhood predictors of adult obesity: a systematic review. *International Journal of Obesity*, 23(Suppl.), S1–107.

Popkin, B.M. (2006). Global nutrition dynamics: the world is shifting rapidly toward a diet linked with non-communicable diseases. *American Journal of Clinical Nutrition*, 84, 289–98.

Power, C., Lake, J.K., and Cole, T.J. (1997). Measurement and long-term health risks of child and adolescent fatness. *International Journal of Obesity*, 21, 507–26.

Prentice, A.M. and Jebb, S.A. (2003). Fast foods, energy density and obesity: a possible mechanistic link. *Obesity Reviews*, 4, 187–94.

Profenno, L.A., Porsteinsson, A.P., and Faraone, S.V. (2010). Meta-analysis of Alzheimer's disease risk with obesity, diabetes, and related disorders. *Biological Psychiatry*, 67, 505–12.

Prospective Studies Collaboration (2009). Body-mass index and cause-specific mortality in 900 000 adults: collaborative analyses of 57 prospective studies. *The Lancet*, 373, 1083–96.

Reilly, J.J. and Kelly, J. (2011). Long-term impact of overweight and obesity in childhood and adolescence on morbidity and premature mortality in adulthood: systematic review. *International Journal of Obesity*, 35, 891–8.

Risnes, K.R., Vatten, L.J., Baker, J.L., et al. (2011). Birthweight and mortality in adulthood: a systematic review and meta-analysis. *International Journal of Epidemiology*, 40, 647–61.

Roberts, S.B., Fuss, P., Heyman, M.B., et al. (1994). Control of food intake in older men. *Journal of the American Medical Association*, 272, 1601–6. Erratum in: *Journal of the American Medical Association* (1995); 273(9), 702.

Roberts, S.B. and Rosenberg, I. (2006). Nutrition and aging: changes in the regulation of energy metabolism with aging. *Physiological Reviews*, 86, 651–67.

Robertson, A., Tirado, C., Lobstein, T., et al. (2004). *Food and Health in Europe: A New Basis of Action*. European Series No 96. Geneva: WHO.

Robroek, S.J., van den Berg, T.I., Plat, J.F., and Burdorf, A. (2011). The role of obesity and lifestyle behaviours in a productive workforce. *Occupational and Environmental Medicine*, 68, 134–9.

Rokholm, B., Baker, J.L., and Sørensen, T.I. (2010). The levelling off of the obesity epidemic since the year 1999—a review of evidence and perspectives. *Obesity Reviews*, 11, 835–46.

Rolland-Cachera, M.F., Deheeger, M., Guilloud-Bataille, M., et al. (1987). Tracking the development of adiposity from one month of age to adulthood. *Annals of Human Biology*, 14, 219–29.

Rose, G. (1991). Population distributions of risk and disease. *Nutrition, Metabolism and Cardiovascular Diseases*, 1, 37–40.

Royal College of Physicians (1983). Obesity. A report of the Royal College of Physicians. *Journal of the Royal College of Physicians of London*, 17(1), 5–65.

Rtveladze, K., Marsh, T., Barquera, S., et al. (2013a). Obesity prevalence in Mexico: impact on health and economic burden. *Public Health Nutrition*, 1, 1–7.

Rtveladze, K., Marsh, T., Webber, L., et al. (2012). Obesity trends in Russia: the impact on health and healthcare costs. *Health*, 4, 1471–84.

Rtveladze, K., Marsh, T., Webber, L., et al. (2013b). Health and economic burden of obesity in Brazil. *PLoS One*, (7), e68785.

Sanchez-Castillo, C.P., Velasquez-Monroy, O., Lara-Esqueda, A., et al. (2005). Diabetes and hypertension increases in a society with abdominal obesity: results of the Mexican National Health Survey 2000. *Public Health Nutrition*, 8, 53–60.

Sassi, F. (2010). *Obesity and the Economics of Prevention. Fit Not Fat*. Paris: Organisation for Economic Co-operation and Development.

Segal, L., Carter, R., and Zimmet, P. (1994). The cost of obesity: the Australian perspective. *Pharmacoeconomics*, 5(Suppl. 1), 45–52.

Seidell, J.C. (1995). Obesity in Europe—causes, costs, and consequences. *International Journal of Risk and Safety in Medicine*, 7, 103–10.

Seidell, J.C., Nooyens, A.J., and Visscher, T.L.S. (2005). Cost-effective measures to prevent obesity: epidemiological basis and appropriate target groups. *Proceedings of The Nutrition Society*, 64, 1–5.

Select Committee on Health (2006–2007). *Third Report*. London: UK Parliament. Available at: http://www.publications.parliament.uk/pa/cm200304/cmselect/cmhealth/23/2306.htm.

Singh, A.S., Mulder, C., Twisk, J.W.R., et al. (2008). Tracking of childhood overweight into adulthood: a systematic review of the literature. *Obesity Reviews*, 9, 474–88.

Te Morenga, L., Mallard, S., and Mann, J. (2012). Dietary sugars and body weight: systematic review and meta-analyses of randomised controlled trials and cohort studies. *BMJ*, 346, e7492.

Trogdon, J.G., Finkelstein, E.A., Hylands, T., et al. (2008). Indirect costs of obesity: a review of the current literature. *Obesity Reviews*, 9, 489–500.

Wang, C.Y., McPherson, K., Marsh, T., et al. (2011). Health and economic burden of the projected obesity trends in the US and the UK. *The Lancet*, 378, 815–25.

Wang, G.-J., Volkow, N.D., and Fowler, J.A. (2012). Dopamine deficiency, eating and body weight. In K.D. Brownell and M.S. Gold (eds.) *Food and Addiction*, pp. 185–93. New York: Oxford University Press.

Wang, Y., Wu, Y., Wilson, R.F., et al. (2013). *Childhood Obesity Prevention Programs: Comparative Effectiveness Review and Meta-Analysis*. Comparative Effectiveness Review No. 115. Rockville, MD: Agency for Healthcare Research and Quality. Available at: http://www.effective-healthcare.ahrq.gov/reports/final.cfm.

Webber, L., Kilpi, F., Marsh, T., et al. (2012). High rates of obesity and non-communicable diseases predicted across Latin America. *PLoS ONE*, 7, 1–6.

Wing, R.R. (2004). Behavioural approaches to the treatment of obesity. In G.A. Bray and C. Bouchard (eds.) *Handbook of Obesity: Clinical Applications* (2nd ed.), pp. 147–67. New York: Marcel Dekker.

Withrow, D. and Alter, D.A. (2011). The economic burden of obesity worldwide: a systematic review of the direct costs of obesity. *Obesity Reviews*, 12, 131–42.

World Cancer Research Fund and American Institute of Cancer Research (2007). *Food, Nutrition, Physical Activity, and the Prevention of Cancer: A Global Perspective*. Washington, DC: AICR.

World Cancer Research Fund and American Institute of Cancer Research (2009). *Policy and Action for Cancer Prevention. Food, Physical Activity: A Global Perspective*. Washington, DC: AICR.

World Health Organization (1995). *Physical Status: The Use and Interpretation of Anthropometry*. Tech. Rep. Series 854. Geneva: WHO.

World Health Organization (2000). *Obesity: Preventing and Managing the Global Epidemic*. WHO Technical Report Series No. 894. Geneva: WHO.

World Health Organization (2003). *Diet, Nutrition and the Prevention of Chronic Diseases. Report of a Joint WHO/FAO Expert Consultation*. WHO Technical Report Series No. 916. Geneva: WHO.

World Health Organization (2007). *WHO Child Growth Standards*. Geneva: WHO.

World Health Organization (2011). *Global Atlas on Cardiovascular Disease Prevention and Control*. Geneva: WHO.

World Health Organization (2012a). *Report of the Formal Meeting of Member States to Conclude the Work of the Comprehensive Global Monitoring Framework, Including Indicators, and a Set of Voluntary Global Targets for the Prevention and Control of Non-Communicable Diseases*. A/NCD/2. [Online] Available at: http://apps.who.int/gb/NCDs/pdf/A_NCD_2-en.pdf.

World Health Organization (2012b). *WHO Global Health Expenditure Atlas*. Geneva: WHO.

World Health Organization (2013). *A Comprehensive Global Monitoring Framework Including Indicators and a Set of Voluntary Global Targets for the Prevention and Control of Non-Communicable Diseases*. Geneva: WHO.

World Health Organization, International Association for the Study of Obesity, and International Obesity Task Force (2000). *The Asia-Pacific Perspective: Redefining Obesity and its Treatment*. Balmain: Health Communications, Australia PTY Ltd. Available at: http://www.wpro.who.int/nutrition/documents/Redefining_obesity/en/.

Yajnik, C.S., Deshpande, S.S., Jackson, A.A., et al. (2008). Vitamin B12 and folate concentrations during pregnancy and insulin resistance in the offspring: the Pune Maternal Nutrition Study. *Diabetologia*, 51, 29–38.

Yanovski, S.Z. and Yanovski, J.A. (2011). Obesity prevalence in the United States,—up, down or sideways? *The New England Journal of Medicine*, 364, 987–9.

Yusuf, S., Hawken, S., Ôunpuu, S., et al. (2005). Obesity and the risk of myocardial infarction in 27 000 participants from 52 countries: a case-control study. *The Lancet*, 366, 1640–9.

8.5

Physical activity and health

Nasiha Soofie and Roger Detels

Introduction to physical activity and health

In this chapter we discuss the benefits of physical activity and conversely the harm caused by physical inactivity. We select the term physical activity because it is a behaviour involving action which benefits the individual whereas physical fitness is a condition. Physical activity is defined as any bodily movement produced by skeletal muscle that requires energy expenditure (World Health Organization (WHO) 2013a). Physical inactivity or being sedentary is associated with health risks (Bull et al. 2004). The 1996 Surgeon General's report on physical activity (Howell 1996) emphasized the health benefits of moderate intensity physical activity such as heavy yard work or gardening, brisk walking, housework, as well as leisure time exercise (Macera et al. 2005). Exercise is an important component of a healthy lifestyle, preventing chronic disease and, especially, preventing obesity (Pratt et al. 1999). Despite the well-documented benefits of physical activity, many people do not exercise on a regular basis and prefer a sedentary lifestyle (van der Aa et al. 2010). Hence, the prevalence of obesity in the developed world has substantially increased over the past two decades (Huber et al. 2011). Diabetes mellitus, hypertension, heart disease, cancer, and decreased life expectancies are all associated with obesity with a substantial impact on healthcare costs. Physical inactivity is the fourth leading cause of death worldwide (Kohl et al. 2012). It is estimated that 31 per cent of the world's population is not meeting the minimum recommendations for physical activity (Hallal et al. 2012), and that 6–10 per cent of all deaths from non-communicable diseases worldwide may be attributed to physical inactivity (Lee et al. 2012). In the case of ischaemic heart disease, that percentage increases to 30 per cent (Wen and Wu 2012). If inactivity levels were decreased by 10 per cent or 25 per cent, more than 1.3 million deaths could be averted each year. It is also estimated that the elimination of physical inactivity would increase the life expectancy of the global population by 0.68 years (Lee et al. 2012). Recommendations now generally endorse a minimum level of physical activity of 150 minutes per week (five times 30 minutes) with daily activity. Increased physical activity has been linked to behavioural, social, and physical benefits. Community-based interventions are an important strategy to promote more physical activity (Task Force on Community Preventive Services 2002). These same strategies may also enhance health promotion behaviour worldwide and contribute substantially to reduced healthcare costs and improved quality of life.

According to a WHO global health study conducted across 122 countries representing 88.9 per cent of the world's population, 31.1 per cent of adults are physically inactive (Hallal et al. 2012; Rhodes et al. 2012). The highest level of inactivity was reported for the Americas at 43.2 per cent, with the lowest level at 27.5 per cent in Africa. Women were found to be more inactive (33.9 per cent) than men (27.9 per cent) (Hallal et al. 2012). Physical activity declines with age in all of the WHO regions, resulting in a significant biological deficit (Hallal et al. 2012).

Physical activity levels are generally lower among low socioeconomic groups (Wilson et al. 2004) as a result of both psychosocial and environmental factors (De Cocker et al. 2012). Physical inactivity is also more prevalent in the lower educational groups (Gupta et al. 2012). Physical inactivity is greater in urban areas than in rural areas (Guthold et al. 2008). In summary, one out of five adults around the world is physically inactive. Physical inactivity is shown to be more prevalent among the wealthier and urban countries, as well as among women and older individuals (Dumith et al. 2011).

Definitions and measurements

Physical activity is defined as any bodily movement produced by skeletal muscle that requires energy expenditure (WHO 2013a). This includes physical activity associated with work, travel, domestic activities, and leisure/discretionary activities. While the term physical activity is easily understood, measuring the degree or amount of physical activity is difficult. Physical activity can be measured (Matthews et al. 2012) using a number of strategies or devices, including self-reports, activity diaries, telephone surveys (Mackay et al. 2007), and devices attached to various parts of the body that measure body movements and heart rate, including pedometers, accelerometers, Actiheart®, and the SenseWear® Armband Pro 3 (Bassett 2012), as well as other recently developed technologies. These devices can monitor activity up to 21 days. The International Questionnaire is a recently developed instrument used to assess total activity and time spent in sedentary activities such as watching television, films and computer/Internet activities including texting (Craig et al. 2003). The energy expended doing various activities can be measured under controlled conditions in terms of metabolic equivalents (METs). One MET is the resting metabolic rate at 3.5 mL oxygen/kg (weight)/minute. Daily METs expended can be estimated by multiplying time spent in reported activities by the METs expended as measured in controlled laboratory observations associated with each activity. However, the accuracy of the measurement ultimately depends on the accuracy of the reported time spent in each activity and the reported intensity with which the individual engaged in those activities. The accuracy of the data from the instrument attached to the body for a limited period can be extrapolated to longer-term and lifestyle estimates. However, it is difficult to establish the reliability and validity of most measures of physical activities. None of the currently available instruments provide precise measures of physical activity over the long term or for population estimates although they may provide an order of magnitude difference that can be correlated to various health outcomes.

Evidence for the benefits of physical activity

Physicians in ancient times, including Hippocrates, circa 400 BC, believed in the value of physical activity to promote health (Lee et al. 2012). Today, it is widely accepted that physical activity is essential in the prevention of chronic diseases and premature death (Inoue et al. 2008; Samitz et al. 2011; Woodcock et al. 2011). A study conducted by Warburton et al. (2006) confirmed that there is strong evidence on the effectiveness of regular physical activity in the primary and secondary prevention of several chronic diseases, including cardiovascular disease, diabetes, cancer, hypertension, obesity, depression, and osteoporosis, as well as for preventing premature death. They were also able to identify a linear relationship between physical activity and health status, such that an increase in physical activity and fitness led to additional improvements in health (Warburton et al. 2006). In addition, there is strong evidence to show that physical inactivity increases the risk of many adverse health conditions, including the major non-communicable diseases such as coronary heart disease and diabetes (Lee et al. 2012). Bull at al. (2004) used various strategies to estimate the attributable burden of disease, and estimated that 20 per cent of the burden of ischaemic heart disease, up to 15 per cent of colon cancer and type 2 diabetes, and 10 per cent of breast cancer and ischaemic stroke were due to physical inactivity (Fig. 8.5.1). Further, they estimated that 5000–7000 lost disability-adjusted life years (DALYs) were attributable to physical inactivity, resulting in ischaemic heart disease, and 1000 DALYs lost, resulting in ischaemic stroke and type 2 diabetes (Fig. 8.5.2) (Bull et al. 2004).

Cardiovascular disease

Sattelmair et al. (2011) reported that individuals who engaged in the equivalent of 150 min/week of moderate-intensity leisure-time

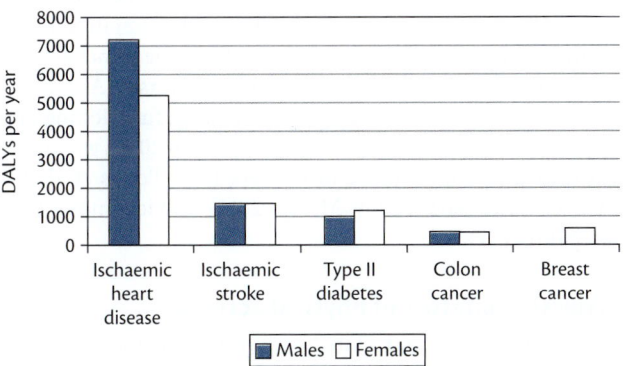

Fig. 8.5.1 Attributable DALYs due to physical inactivity for ischaemic heart disease, ischaemic stroke, type 2 diabetes, and colon and breast cancer. Reproduced with permission from Bull, F.C. et al., Physical inactivity, in *WHO Comparative Quantification of Health Risk: Global and Regional Burden of Disease Attribution to Selected Major Risk Factors, Volume 1*, World Health Organization, Geneva, Switzerland, Copyright © WHO 2004, available from http://www.who.int/publications/cra/en/.

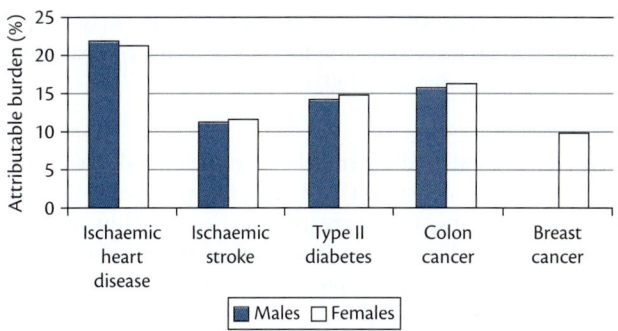

Fig. 8.5.2 Attributable burden of disease due to physical inactivity for ischaemic heart disease, ischaemic stroke, type 2 diabetes, and colon and breast cancer. Reproduced with permission from Bull, F.C. et al., Physical inactivity, in *WHO Comparative Quantification of Health Risk: Global and Regional Burden of Disease Attribution to Selected Major Risk Factors, Volume 1*, World Health Organization, Geneva, Switzerland, Copyright © WHO 2004, available from http://www.who.int/publications/cra/en/.

physical activity had a 14 per cent lower coronary heart disease risk compared with those reporting no leisure-time physical activity. Those engaging in the equivalent of 300 min/week of moderate-intensity leisure-time physical activity had a 20 per cent lower risk. At higher levels of physical activity, relative gains were modestly lower. People who were physically active at levels lower than the minimum recommended nonetheless also had significantly lower risk of coronary heart disease. There was a significant interaction by gender (P = 0.03); the association being stronger among women than men (Sattelmair et al. 2011). In another study, Sundquist et al. reported that women and men who were physically active at least twice a week had a 41 per cent lower risk of developing coronary heart disease than those who performed no physical activity at all (Sundquist et al. 2004). Li et al. reported that a high level of leisure-time physical activity and moderate level of occupational physical activity have a beneficial effect on cardiovascular health by reducing the overall relative risk of coronary heart disease and stroke among men and women by 20 to 30 per cent and 10 to 20 per cent, respectively (Li et al. 2012).

The benefits of exercise or physical activity in the prevention of cardiovascular disease may be explained from a biological perspective as a boosting of antioxidant levels, epicardial fat reduction, increases in expression of heat-shock proteins and endoplasmic reticulum stress proteins, mitochondrial adaptation, and the role of sarcolemmal and mitochondrial potassium channels. In terms of vascular benefits, the main effects are increases in exercise-induced vascular remodelling and endothelial function. Exercise-induced fibrinolytic and rheological increases also result in haematological benefits (Berlin and Colditz 1990; Golbidi and Laher 2012).

Diabetes

Epidemiological evidence suggests that individuals who maintain a physically active lifestyle are less likely to develop impaired glucose tolerance (Li et al. 2008; Gong et al. 2011; Yoon et al. 2013) and type 2 diabetes mellitus (Dowse et al. 1991; Stern 1991; Ivy 1995; Wylie-Rosett et al. 2006). Exercise also improves many other physiological and metabolic (O'Dea 1984) abnormalities that are associated with type 2 diabetes mellitus by lowering body fat, reducing blood pressure, and reducing dyslipoproteinaemia (Wallberg-Henriksson et al. 1998).

It has also been shown that physical activity may be more effective at managing the symptoms of diabetes compared with medication (Knowler et al. 2002).

Hypertension

Leading national and international professional associations recommend the consistent and long-term implementation of non-drug measures in the treatment of essential hypertension (Institute for Quality and Efficiency in Health Care 2005). So et al. (2013) reported that regular physical activity was positively associated with a lower blood pressure even in non-obese adolescents. Shahraki et al. (2012) found that physical activity reduced arterial blood pressure in female athlete students.

Cancer

Evidence that physical activity is a key modifiable lifestyle risk factor that may reduce the risk of several cancers is now accumulating (James et al. 2011; Na and Oliynyk 2011; Ulrich et al. 2012; Kuijpers et al. 2013; McClellan 2013). The risk of colon, breast (Goh et al. 2012; Guinan et al. 2013; Schmidt et al. 2013), and endometrial (John et al. 2010; Lukowski et al. 2012) cancers is reduced by 25 to 30 per cent in physically active individuals, and evidence for a beneficial effect of physical activity in reducing prostate (Rebillard et al. 2013), ovarian (Olsen et al. 2007; Leitzmann et al. 2009), lung (Emaus et al. 2011; Jones et al. 2012), and other gastrointestinal cancers (Morikawa et al. 2013; Speed-Andrews et al. 2014) is emerging (Aparicio-Ting et al. 2012). There is evidence to suggest that physical activity may alter tumour initiation events by modifying carcinogen activation, specifically by enhancing the cytochrome P450 system and selective enzymes in the carcinogen detoxification pathway. In addition, it may reduce oxidative damage by increasing a variety of antioxidant enzymes, enhancing DNA repair systems and improving intracellular protein repair systems. Physical activity may also exert a cancer-preventive effect by scavenging reactive oxygen species; altering cell proliferation, apoptosis, and differentiation; decreasing inflammation; enhancing immune function and suppressing angiogenesis (Rogers et al. 2008). Physical activity is also associated with a reduction in the psychological and physical symptoms that are associated with both the disease process and treatment (Rajarajeswaran and Vishnupriya 2009).

Osteoporosis

Osteoporosis is characterized by a decline in bone mass with a deterioration of bone tissue, enhanced bone fragility and a consequent increase in fracture risk (Anonymous 1995). As yet, we do not have a complete understanding of how physical activity impacts osteoporosis risk and development. However, there is evidence to suggest that physical activity can help with regulation of bone maintenance (Sinaki 2012), and stimulation of bone formation, as well as with accumulation of minerals, strengthening of muscles (Sinaki et al. 2010), and improving balance, thereby reducing the risk of falls and fractures (Langsetmo et al. 2012). A study by Daly et al. (2008) found that men and women who were more committed to an exercise regimen had lower levels of bone loss and better balance than their less active counterparts. Langsetmo et al. (2012) studied the impact of physical activity on body mass index (BMI) and bone mineral density (BMD) in relation to osteoporosis. The study was conducted on both men and women and found that increased physical activity was related to an increase in BMD and a decrease in BMI (Daly et al. 2008). Siegrist mentioned two types of physical activity that are important for building and maintaining bone mass and density: (1) weight-bearing exercises, in which bones and muscles work against gravity; and (2) resistance training, using muscular strength to improve muscle mass and strengthen bone (Siegrist 2008). However, further research is needed to elucidate the dose–response relationship between exercise and bone strength, the impact of high-load, high-speed, and impact-type physical training, and the risks and benefits of intensive exercise for elderly individuals with osteoporosis (Suominen 2006).

Mental health

Physical inactivity has been reported to be associated with increased risk of psychological disorders (Careket al. 2011). Conversely, physical activity has also been reported to have beneficial effects in the prevention, treatment, and management of psychiatric disorders (Wolff et al. 2011; Zschucke et al. 2013). It is known that people with depression tend to be less physically active than non-depressed individuals (Teychenne et al. 2008), whereas increasing aerobic exercise and/or strength training has been shown to significantly reduce depressive symptoms (Rimer et al. 2012). Anxiety symptoms and panic disorders also improve with regular exercise (Paluska and Schwenk 2000). Schizophrenic (Bernard and Ninot 2012; Gorczynski and Faulkner 2012; Ter Meulen and de Haan 2012) and bipolar patients (Kucyi et al. 2010) have also reported improvements in health with exercise.

Other

Additional benefits to health include fertility enhancement in reproductive-aged women (Wojtylaet al. 2011), healthier pregnancies (Downs et al. 2012), and improved neonatal outcomes (Ferraro et al. 2012). Physical activity is also associated with improved immune function (Pedersen 1991; Walsh et al. 2011a, 2011b; Wang et al. 2012; Ho et al. 2013) by promoting the activity of natural killer (NK) cells (Pedersen and Ullum 1994) and by increasing the total leucocyte, granulocyte, monocyte, and T-cell counts (Shephard and Shek 1994). Another reported benefit of physical activity involves the nervous system (Carro et al. 2001). Exercise has been reported to have neuroprotective effects to prevent neurological disorders such as multiple sclerosis (Mostert and Kesselring 2002), dementia (Laurinet al. 2001), and Alzheimer's disease (Kramer and Erickson 2007). Other reports include improvements in the health of the skin (Bates-Jensenet al. 2003), prevention of various disorders such as psoriasis (Anonymous 2012; Frankel et al 2012), and improvements in functioning of the respiratory (Menezes et al. 2012), renal (Stump 2011), gastrointestinal (Moses 1990; Brouns and Beckers 1993; Peters et al. 2001; de Oliveira and Burini 2009; Martin 2011), and locomotor (Sluka et al. 2013) systems.

Barriers/facilitators of physical activity

Despite widespread and global recognition of the significance of physical inactivity, little progress has been made in improving overall physical activity in the US population (Pratt et al. 2004) or globally. Efforts have been directed at both the individual and group levels. By targeting the community, the possibility of reaching a greater percentage of the underactive population with lower cost per person is potentially increased (King 1998).

A more comprehensive intervention strategy should include personal, interpersonal, institutional, environmental, legislative, and policy levels (King 1998). However, this comprehensive approach must also target land use, the built environment, the public health infrastructure, the safety and design of parks and facilities, and the political process in order to ensure a healthy community.

The choices we make in relation to how we use our land and how we structure our built environment impacts the way we live and move (Powell 2005). This affects the level of physical activity to which an individual is exposed at work and can achieve during leisure time. For example, an apartment block building may be built to encourage the tenants to use the stairs rather than the lift and/or it may have an in-house gym that allows tenants to conveniently engage in a healthier, more active lifestyle. Places of work such as factories, for example, should include exercise facilities which can encourage workers to engage in physical activity during their breaks. Land usage may also be designed to include safe parks equipped with outdoor gyms. These interventions require significant changes in zoning and building code regulations and the attitudes of employers (Powell 2005).

Such changes are not easily achieved, as they involve modifications and support at the community level, and should be consistent with international standards. An understanding of the population, as well as its attitudes regarding the relevance and importance of physical activity, considering age, gender ratios, ethnicity, economic status, and education should be considered prior to planning and implementing an intervention. Planners need to anticipate the need for new policies (Yancey et al. 2007). Planning strategies should include public education, school- and community-based programmes, land use policies and planning, marketing techniques, and federal funding opportunities promoting healthy and fit workplaces (Yancey et al. 2007), as well as safe facilities, particularly in high-crime areas, slums, and rural or remote areas.

Global recommendations on physical activity for health as put forward by the World Health Organization

The WHO recently published guidelines on the recommended levels of physical activity for different age groups. Specifications per age group are stated as follows (WHO 2013b):

♦ 5–17-year-olds: 60 minutes of moderate to vigorous intensity physical activity daily.

♦ 18–64-year-olds: 150 minutes of moderate intensity activity or 75 minutes of vigorous intensity physical activity per week or an equivalent combination of both.

♦ 65 years and older: 150 minutes of moderate intensity activity or 75 minutes of vigorous intensity physical activity per week or an equivalent combination of both. In addition, balance and muscle strengthening exercises are encouraged.

The relationship between diet and physical activity

An effective strategy to control weight and promote health is to adopt and adhere to a healthy eating and fitness regimen (Lloyd-Jones 2009). However, the relationship between the two is sometimes unclear.

Jago et al. studied the relationship between physical activity and diet among African American girls and found that physical activity and fat consumption were inversely related (Jago et al. 2004). Another study by Mattison et al. also found that low levels of leisure time physical activity were consistently associated with a high-fat diet (Mattison et al. 2001). A similar study on the nutritional intake of physically fit and unfit men and women published in 2001 also found that individuals with a higher level of cardiorespiratory fitness were also more likely to follow a diet that was consistent with national dietary recommendations (Brodney et al. 2001).

Sodergren et al. investigated the relationship between fruit and vegetable intake, leisure time physical activity, and sitting time in older adults. They observed that a modest increase in fruit and vegetable intake or leisure-time physical activity had a marked effect on the overall health of older adults (Sodergren et al. 2012). It is reasonable to assume that individuals committed to a fitness regimen of some sort tend to be more health conscious in terms of choice of food (Jago et al. 2004). However, further research into the determinants of lifestyle behaviours are needed (Sodergren et al. 2012).

Behaviour modifications toward a healthier lifestyle should be encouraged by educating the public about healthy food choices, proper interpretation of food labels, and strategies for self-monitoring of diet and physical activity levels. A study of healthy behaviour patterns of individuals who are more successful at adopting a healthy lifestyle may provide additional insight into potential public health strategies to improve the lifestyle of the public (Kruger et al. 2008). Kruger and colleagues reported that dietary practices, dining-out behaviour, and physical activity correlated with weight loss maintenance (Kruger et al. 2008). The study found that men were more successful than women at weight loss maintenance. Individuals who reported eating at a fast-food restaurant two or more times per week were less successful at maintaining healthy behaviour. Sedentary individuals who consumed fewer than five servings of fruit and vegetables per day were less successful in achieving a healthier diet and lifestyle (Kruger et al. 2008). The authors suggested that dining-out behaviours be reduced, and that daily consumption of fruit and vegetables, along with at least 150 minutes of physical activity per week, be encouraged in order to successfully manage weight and adopt a healthier lifestyle (Kruger et al. 2008).

Another study by Kruger et al. found that weighing oneself, keeping track of calories, planning meals, engaging in 30 minutes or more of physical activity per day, as well as leisure-time activities such as cooking and baking were more common in individuals who were successful at maintaining a healthier lifestyle (Kruger et al. 2006).

An important barrier to adopting a healthy diet in slums and for poor individuals is the lack of access to healthy food. Unhealthy foods are often cheaper and thus more affordable. Further, stores selling healthy foods are reluctant to move into high-crime areas. Public health professionals therefore must work with law enforcement agencies to assure security of businesses and residents in slum areas, which will encourage businesses selling healthy foods to operate in such areas and will assure residents that they can engage in jogging and other outdoor physical activities without being subjected to violence.

Strategies for the promotion of physical activity

Children

Health-enhancing physical activity behaviour should be established during the formative years of a child's life (Dobbins et al. 2013), that is, birth to 5 years (Bornstein et al. 2011), so as to reduce the risk of developing self-sabotaging behaviour patterns that are more difficult to address later in life. However, many studies suggest that children in care centres are inactive, with typically high levels of sedentary behaviour (Vasquez et al. 2006). With the increasing number of working women, more children will be placed in care centres. Thus, public health professionals need to target child care centres to promote (mandate) exercise and healthy eating habits. A study conducted by Sugiyama et al. proposed interventions aimed at re-structuring the daycare environment so as to promote physical activity in order to achieve healthy early childhood development and disease prevention (Sugiyama et al. 2012). Furthermore there should be public health policies in place to promote physical activity among the paediatric population, as well as to document the impact of such strategies on motor skills and development (Goldfield et al. 2012).

Adolescents

Adolescents are also known to fail in meeting the required amounts of physical activity. A study focused on enhancing physical activity levels in adolescents suggested a more contemporary approach, that is, the utilization of the Internet to inform and encourage youth to adopt an active lifestyle (Thompson et al. 2012). The rapid expansion and use of the Internet promotes a sedentary lifestyle. Countering this increasing trend promoting a sedentary lifestyle will be difficult. Because the use of the Internet and social media have become so widespread, especially among adolescents and young adults, public health professionals should consider whether the Internet itself can be used to promote a more healthy lifestyle. However, measuring the impact of strategies using the Internet will be difficult.

Neighbourhood 'walkability' has also been suggested as an important predictor of physical activity in Belgian adolescents (De Meester et al. 2012), lending credence to the importance of environment on moulding and establishing behaviour patterns. However, slums often have high crime rates, making walking in them dangerous. Communities and government must come together to make these communities safe for adopting a healthy lifestyle.

A recent school-based approach, GLAMA (Girls!Lead!Achieve! Mentor!Activate), implemented across secondary schools in Australia, was designed to develop leadership skills and school and social connectedness, in addition to a range of physical activity interventions. Activities involved running laps around the school gymnasium and promoting team effort/cooperation that did not require a very high level of motor skill or performance. This study helped highlight feasible strategies to promote physical activity at the school level and encourage students to participate (Jenkinson et al. 2012).

Adults

There have been numerous strategies aimed at increasing the level of physical activity in adults (Haskell et al. 2007). One of the longest running programmes is the 'exercise on prescription' or EoP programme (Sorensen et al. 2007) that encourages general practitioners (Sorensen et al. 2006; Orrow et al. 2013) to recommend exercise as a prevention and treatment strategy against numerous diseases and illnesses. This programme has been successfully implemented in numerous countries and populations (Gademan et al. 2012) across the world, including South Asian Muslim women (Carroll et al. 2002), Danish communities (Sorensen et al. 2011), South Africa (Dennis and Noakes 1998), and the United States. A similar intervention is the exercise referral scheme (ERS) where inactive individuals are identified within the primary care setting before being referred to a third party for prescribing and supervising an activity regimen. However, this strategy is limited in terms of cost (Anokye et al. 2011). Strategies aimed at easy access to sporting facilities or places of physical activity combined with strategies to increase adult self-efficacy and overcome perceived barriers have also been proposed (Serrano-Sanchez et al. 2012). Another study conducted by Pan et al. (2009) suggested that promotion strategies be tailored to enhance adult confidence levels, to motivate adults to be more active, to educate people on the benefits of physical activity for health, reduce barriers and target different factors appropriate for men and women and for people of different socioeconomic and demographic backgrounds.

The elderly

Although regular physical activity is critical for the promotion of health and function as people get older, they tend to adopt a more sedentary lifestyle (King et al. 1998). Home-based, group-based, and educational physical activity interventions such as telephone calls, incentives, and counselling have been explored, but resulted in physical activity changes that were small and short-lived (Van der Bij et al. 2002).

Physical activity intervention programmes are best kept simple and effective without creating a financial burden on the public health sector (Trueman and Anokye 2013).

Conclusion

Physical activity has been shown to be a key component of a healthy lifestyle that significantly reduces the risk of most non-communicable diseases, promotes mental health, and extends years of healthy, enjoyable life. The current global epidemic of diabetes and overweight is directly attributable to an increasingly sedentary lifestyle associated with the increase of labour-saving devices, passive forms of entertainment (e.g. television), and development of rapid communication modes, as exemplified by the Internet and social media to which many individuals, especially youth, are becoming addicted. The trend in lower levels of physical activity needs to be countered by a vigorous campaign targeting individuals and communities. Communities need to be designed or modified to promote physical exercise. In poor areas and slums, this means assuring the ability to exercise without fear of harm and violence. Successfully promoting a healthy lifestyle incorporating adequate physical activity will require the combined efforts of public health professionals, land use and urban planners, architects and builders, schools, and government, including law enforcement agencies. Physical activity needs to be recognized globally as an essential component of a healthy lifestyle and adopted as a daily routine by all.

References

Anokye, N.K., Trueman, P., Green, C., Pavey, T.G., Hillsdon, M., and Taylor, R.S. (2011). The cost-effectiveness of exercise referral schemes. *BMC Public Health*, 11, 954.

Anonymous (1995). American College of Sports Medicine position stand. Osteoporosis and exercise. *Medicine & Science in Sports & Exercise*, 27(4), i–vii.

Anonymous (2012). Preventing psoriasis with exercise. Your next tennis match or swim may help prevent this skin condition. *Harvard Health Letter*, 38(1), 6.

Aparicio-Ting, F.E., Friedenreich, C.M., Kopciuk, K.A., Plotnikoff, R.C., and Bryant, H.E. (2012). Prevalence of meeting physical activity guidelines for cancer prevention in Alberta. *Chronic Diseases and Injuries in Canada*, 32(4), 216–26.

Bassett, D.R. (2012). Device-based monitoring in physical activity and public health research. *Physiological Measurement*, 33(11), 1769–83.

Bates-Jensen, B.M., Alessi, C.A., Al-Samarrai, N.R., and Schnelle, J.F. (2003). The effects of an exercise and incontinence intervention on skin health outcomes in nursing home residents. *Journal of the American Geriatrics Society*, 51(3), 348–55.

Berlin, J.A. and Colditz, G.A. (1990). A meta-analysis of physical activity in the prevention of coronary heart disease. *American Journal of Epidemiology*, 132(4), 612–28.

Bernard, P. and Ninot, G. (2012). [Benefits of exercise for people with schizophrenia: a systematic review]. *Encephale*, 38(4), 280–7.

Bornstein, D.B., Beets, M.W., Byun, W., and McIver, K. (2011). Accelerometer-derived physical activity levels of preschoolers: a meta-analysis. *Journal of Science and Medicine in Sport*, 14(6), 504–11.

Brodney, S., McPherson, R.S., Carpenter, R.S., Welten, D., and Blair, S.N. (2001). Nutrient intake of physically fit and unfit men and women. *Medicine & Science in Sports & Exercise*, 33(3), 459–67.

Brouns, F. and Beckers, E. (1993). Is the gut an athletic organ? Digestion, absorption and exercise. *Sports Medicine*, 15(4), 242–57.

Bull, F.C., Armstrong, T.P., Dixon, T., Ham, S., Neiman, A., and Pratt, M. (2004) Physical inactivity. In M. Ezzati, A.D. Lopez, A. Rodgers, and C.J.L. Murray (eds.) *Comparative Quantification of Health Risks: Global and Regional Burden of Disease Attribution to Selected Major Risk Factors*, pp. 729–882. Geneva: WHO. Available at: http://www.who.int/publications/cra/en/.

Carek, P.J., Laibstain, S.E., and Carek, S.M. (2011). Exercise for the treatment of depression and anxiety. *International Journal of Psychiatry in Medicine*, 41(1), 15–28.

Carro, E., Trejo, J.L., Busiguina, S., and Torres-Aleman, I. (2001). Circulating insulin-like growth factor I mediates the protective effects of physical exercise against brain insults of different etiology and anatomy. *Journal of Neuroscience*, 21(15), 5678–84.

Carroll, R., Ali, N., and Azam, N. (2002). Promoting physical activity in South Asian Muslim women through 'exercise on prescription'. *Health Technology Assessment*, 6(8), 1–101.

Craig, C.L., Marshall, A.L., Sjöström, M., et al. (2003). International physical activity questionnaire: 12-country reliability and validity. *Medicine & Science in Sports & Exercise*, 35, 1381–95.

Daly, R.M., Ahlborg, H.G., Ringsberg, K., Gardsell, P., Sernbo, I., and Karlsson, M.K. (2008). Association between changes in habitual physical activity and changes in bone density, muscle strength, and functional performance in elderly men and women. *Journal of the American Geriatrics Society*, 56(12), 2252–60.

De Cocker, K., Artero, E.G., De Henauw, S., et al. (2012). Can differences in physical activity by socio-economic status in European adolescents be explained by differences in psychosocial correlates? A mediation analysis within the HELENA (Healthy Lifestyle in Europe by Nutrition in Adolescence) study. *Public Health Nutrition*, 15(11), 2100–9.

De Meester, F., Van Dyck, D., De Bourdeaudhuij, I., Deforche, B., Sallis, J.F., and Cardon, G. (2012). Active living neighborhoods: is neighborhood walkability a key element for Belgian adolescents? *BMC Public Health*, 12, 7.

Dennis, S.C. and Noakes, T.D. (1998). Physiological and metabolic responses to increasing work rates: relevance for exercise prescription. *Journal of Sports Science*, 16(Suppl.), S77–84.

De Oliveira, E.P. and Burini, R.C. (2009). The impact of physical exercise on the gastrointestinal tract. *Current Opinion in Clinical Nutrition and Metabolic Care*, 12(5), 533–8.

Dobbins, M., Husson, H., DeCorby, K., and LaRocca, R.L. (2013). School-based physical activity programs for promoting physical activity and fitness in children and adolescents aged 6 to 18. *Cochrane Database of Systematic Reviews*, 2, CD007651.

Downs, D.S., Chasan-Taber, L., Evenson, K.R., Leiferman, J., and Yeo, S. (2012). Physical activity and pregnancy: past and present evidence and future recommendations. *Research Quarterly for Exercise & Sport*, 83(4), 485–502.

Dowse, G.K., Zimmet, P.Z., Gareeboo, H., et al. (1991). Abdominal obesity and physical inactivity as risk factors for NIDDM and impaired glucose tolerance in Indian, Creole, and Chinese Mauritians. *Diabetes Care*, 14(4), 271–82.

Dumith, S.C., Hallal, P.C., Reis, R.S., and Kohl, H.W., 3rd (2011). Worldwide prevalence of physical inactivity and its association with human development index in 76 countries. *Preventive Medicine*, 53(1–2), 24–8.

Emaus, A. and Thune, I. (2011). Physical activity and lung cancer prevention. Recent results. *Cancer Reseseach*, 186, 101–33.

Ferraro, Z.M., Gaudet, L., and Adamo, K.B. (2012). The potential impact of physical activity during pregnancy on maternal and neonatal outcomes. *Obstetrical & Gynecological Survey*, 67(2), 99–110.

Frankel, H.C., Han, J., Li, T., and Qureshi, A.A. (2012). The association between physical activity and the risk of incident psoriasis. *Archives of Dermatology*, 148(8), 918–24.

Gademan, M.G., Deutekom, M., Hosper, K., and Stronks, K. (2012). The effect of exercise on prescription on physical activity and wellbeing in a multi-ethnic female population: a controlled trial. *BMC Public Health*, 12, 758.

Goh, J., Kirk, E.A., Lee, S.X., and Ladiges, W.C. (2012). Exercise, physical activity and breast cancer: the role of tumor-associated macrophages. *Exercise Immunology Review*, 18, 158–76.

Golbidi, S. and Laher, I. (2012). Exercise and the cardiovascular system. *Cardiology Research and Practice*, 2012, 210852.

Goldfield, G.S., Harvey, A., Grattan, K., and Adamo, K.B. (2012). Physical activity promotion in the preschool years: a critical period to intervene. *International Journal of Environmental Research and Public Health*, 9(4), 1326–42.

Gong, Q., Gregg, E.W., Wang, J., et al. (2011). Long-term effects of a randomised trial of a 6-year lifestyle intervention in impaired glucose tolerance on diabetes-related microvascular complications: the China Da Qing Diabetes Prevention Outcome Study. *Diabetologia*, 54(2), 300–7.

Gorczynski, P. and Faulkner, G. (2012). Exercise therapy for schizophrenia. *Cochrane Database of Systematic Reviews*, 5, CD004412.

Guinan, E., Hussey, J., Broderick, J.M., et al. (2013). The effect of aerobic exercise on metabolic and inflammatory markers in breast cancer survivors – a pilot study. *Supportive Care in Cancer*, 21(7), 1983–92.

Gupta, R., Deedwania, P.C., Sharma, K., et al. (2012). Association of educational, occupational and socioeconomic status with cardiovascular risk factors in Asian Indians: a cross-sectional study. *PLoS One*, 7(8), e44098.

Guthold, R., Ono, T., Strong, K.L., Chatterji, S., and Morabia, A. (2008). Worldwide variability in physical inactivity: a 51-country survey. *American Journal of Preventive Medicine*, 34(6), 486–94.

Hallal, P.C., Andersen, L.B., Bull, F.C., Guthold, R., Haskell, W., and Ekelund, U. (2012). Global physical activity levels: surveillance progress, pitfalls, and prospects. *The Lancet*, 380(9838), 247–57.

Haskell, W.L., Lee, I.M., Pate, R.R., et al. (2007). Physical activity and public health: updated recommendation for adults from the American

College of Sports Medicine and the American Heart Association. *Medicine & Science in Sports & Exercise*, 39(8), 1423–34.

Ho, R.T., Wang, C.W., Ng, S.M., et al. (2013). The effect of T'ai chi exercise on immunity and infections: a systematic review of controlled trials. *Journal of Alternative and Complementary Medicine*, 19(5), 389–96.

Howell, J. (1996). The 1996 Surgeon General's report on physical activity and health. *Nurse Practitioner Forum*, 7(3), 104.

Huber, C.A., Mohler-Kuo, M., Zellweger, U., Zoller, M., Rosemann, T., and Senn, O. (2011). Obesity management and continuing medical education in primary care: results of a Swiss survey. *BMC Family Practice*, 12, 140.

Inoue, M., Iso, H., Yamamoto, S., et al. (2008). Daily total physical activity level and premature death in men and women: results from a large-scale population-based cohort study in Japan (JPHC study). *Annals of Epidemiology*, 18(7), 522–30.

Institute for Quality and Efficiency in Health Care (2005). *Benefit Assessment of Non-Drug Treatment Strategies in Patients with Essential Hypertension: Reduction in Salt Intake. Executive Summary of Rapid Report A05-21B, Version 1.0, Executive Summaries*. Cologne: Institute for Quality and Efficiency in Health Care.

Ivy, J.L. (1997). Role of exercise training in the prevention and treatment of insulin resistance and non-insulin-dependent diabetes mellitus. *Sports Medicine*, 24(5), 321–36.

Jago, R., Baranowski, T., Yoo, S., et al. (2004). Relationship between physical activity and diet among African-American girls. *Obesity Research*, 12(Suppl.), 55S–63S.

James, E.L., Stacey, F., Chapman, K., et al. (2011). Exercise and nutrition routine improving cancer health (ENRICH): the protocol for a randomized efficacy trial of a nutrition and physical activity program for adult cancer survivors and carers. *BMC Public Health*, 11, 236.

Jenkinson, K.A., Naughton, G., and Benson, A.C. (2012). The GLAMA (Girls! Lead! Achieve! Mentor! Activate!) physical activity and peer leadership intervention pilot project: a process evaluation using the RE-AIM framework. *BMC Public Health*, 12, 55.

John, E.M., Koo, J., and Horn-Ross, P.L. (2010). Lifetime physical activity and risk of endometrial cancer. *Cancer Epidemiology, Biomarkers & Prevention*, 19(5), 1276–83.

Jones, L.W., Hornsby, W.E., Goetzinger, A., et al. (2012). Prognostic significance of functional capacity and exercise behavior in patients with metastatic non-small cell lung cancer. *Lung Cancer*, 76(2), 248–52.

King, A.C. (1998). How to promote physical activity in a community: research experiences from the US highlighting different community approaches. *Patient Education and Counseling*, 33(Suppl. 1), S3–12.

King, A.C., Rejeski, W.J., and Buchner, D.M. (1998). Physical activity interventions targeting older adults. A critical review and recommendations. *American Journal of Preventive Medicine*, 15(4), 316–33.

Knowler, W.C., Barrett-Connor, E., Fowler, S.E., et al. (2002). Reduction in the incidence of type 2 diabetes with lifestyle intervention or metformin. *The New England Journal of Medicine*, 346(6), 393–403.

Kohl, H.W. III, Craig, C.L., Lambert, E.V., et al. (2012). The pandemic of physical inactivity: global action for public health. *The Lancet*, 380(9838), 294–305.

Kramer, A.F. and Erickson, K.I. (2007). Capitalizing on cortical plasticity: influence of physical activity on cognition and brain function. *Trends in Cognitive Sciences*, 11(8), 342–8.

Kruger, J., Blanck, H.M., and Gillespie, C. (2006). Dietary and physical activity behaviors among adults successful at weight loss maintenance. *International Journal of Behavioral Nutrition and Physical Activity*, 3, 17.

Kruger, J., Blanck, H.M., and Gillespie, C. (2008). Dietary practices, dining out behavior, and physical activity correlates of weight loss maintenance. *Preventing Chronic Disease*, 5(1), A11.

Kucyi, A., Alsuwaidan, M.T., Liauw, S.S., and McIntyre, R.S. (2010). Aerobic physical exercise as a possible treatment for neurocognitive dysfunction in bipolar disorder. *Postgraduate Medicine*, 122(6), 107–16.

Kuijpers, W., Groen, W.G., Aaronson, N.K., and van Harten, W.H. (2013). A systematic review of web-based interventions for patient empowerment and physical activity in chronic diseases: relevance for cancer survivors. *Journal of Medical Internet Research*, 15(2), e37.

Langsetmo, L., Hitchcock, C.L., Kingwell, E.J.S., et al. (2012). Physical activity, body mass index and bone mineral density-associations in a prospective population-based cohort of women and men: the Canadian Multicentre Osteoporosis Study (CaMos). *Bone*, 50(1), 401–8.

Laurin, D., Verreault, R., Lindsay, J., MacPherson, K., and Rockwood, K. (2001). Physical activity and risk of cognitive impairment and dementia in elderly persons. *Archives of Neurology*, 58(3), 498–504.

Lee, I.M., Shiroma, E.J., Lobelo, F., Puska, P., Blair, S.N., and Katzmarzyk, P.T. (2012). Effect of physical inactivity on major non-communicable diseases worldwide: an analysis of burden of disease and life expectancy. *The Lancet*, 380(9838), 219–29.

Leitzmann, M.F., Koebnick, C., Moore, S.C., et al. (2009). Prospective study of physical activity and the risk of ovarian cancer. *Cancer Causes Control*, 20(5), 765–73.

Li, G., Zhang, P., Wang, J., et al. (2008). The long-term effect of lifestyle interventions to prevent diabetes in the China Da Qing Diabetes Prevention Study: a 20-year follow-up study. *The Lancet*, 371(9626), 1783–9.

Li, J. and Siegrist, J. (2012). Physical activity and risk of cardiovascular disease—a meta-analysis of prospective cohort studies. *International Journal of Environmental Research and Public Health*, 9(2), 391–407.

Lloyd-Jones, D. (2009). Diet/exercise/weight. *Circulation*, 119, e1–e161.

Lukowski, J., Gil, K.M., Jenison, E., Hopkins, M., and Basen-Engquist, K. (2012). Endometrial cancer survivors' assessment of the benefits of exercise. *Gynecologic Oncology*, 124(3), 426–30.

Macera, C.A., Ham, S.A., Yore, M.M., et al. (2005). Prevalence of physical activity in the United States: Behavioral Risk Factor Surveillance System, 2001. *Preventing Chronic Disease*, 2(2), A17.

Mackay, L.M., Schofield, G.M., and Schluter, P.J. (2007). Validation of self-report measures of physical activity: a case study using the New Zealand Physical Activity Questionnaire. *Research Quarterly for Exercise & Sport*, 78(3), 189–96.

Martin, D. (2011). Physical activity benefits and risks on the gastrointestinal system. *Southern Medical Journal*, 104(12), 831–7.

Matthews, C.E., Hagstromer, M., Pober, D.M., and Bowles, H.R. (2012). Best practices for using physical activity monitors in population-based research. *Medicine & Science in Sports & Exercise*, 44(Suppl. 1), S68–76.

Mattisson, I., Wirfalt, E., Gullberg, B., and Berglund, G. (2001). Fat intake is more strongly associated with lifestyle factors than with socio-economic characteristics, regardless of energy adjustment approach. *European Journal of Clinical Nutrition*, 55(6), 452–61.

McClellan, R. (2013). Exercise programs for patients with cancer improve physical functioning and quality of life. *Journal of Physiotherapy*, 59(1), 57.

Menezes, A.M., Wehrmeister, F.C., Muniz, L.C., et al. (2013). Physical activity and lung function in adolescents: the 1993 Pelotas (Brazil) birth cohort study. *Journal of Adolescent Health*, 51(Suppl. 6), S27–31.

Morikawa, T., Kuchiba, A., Lochhead, P., et al. (2013). Prospective analysis of body mass index, physical activity, and colorectal cancer risk associated with beta-catenin (CTNNB1) status. *Cancer Research*, 73(5), 1600–10.

Moses, F.M. (1990). The effect of exercise on the gastrointestinal tract. *Sports Medicine*, 9(3), 159–72.

Mostert, S. and Kesselring, J. (2002). Effects of a short-term exercise training program on aerobic fitness, fatigue, health perception and activity level of subjects with multiple sclerosis. *Multiple Sclerosis*, 8(2), 161–8.

Na, H.K. and Oliynyk, S. (2011). Effects of physical activity on cancer prevention. *Annals of the New York Academy of Sciences*, 1229, 176–83.

O'Dea, K. (1984). Marked improvement in carbohydrate and lipid metabolism in diabetic Australian aborigines after temporary reversion to traditional lifestyle. *Diabetes*, 33(6), 596–603.

Olsen, C.M., Bain, C.J., Jordan, S.J., et al. (2007). Recreational physical activity and epithelial ovarian cancer: a case-control study, systematic review, and meta-analysis. *Cancer Epidemiology, Biomarkers & Prevention*, 16(11), 2321–30.

Orrow, G., Kinmonth, A.L., Sanderson, S., and Sutton, S. (2013). Republished research: effectiveness of physical activity promotion based in primary care: systematic review and meta-analysis of randomised controlled trials. *British Journal of Sports Medicine*, 47(1), 27.

Paluska, S.A. and Schwenk, T.L. (2000). Physical activity and mental health: current concepts. *Sports Medicine*, 29(3), 167–80.

Pan, S.Y., Cameron, C., Desmeules, M., Morrison, H., Craig, C.L., and Jiang, X. (2009). Individual, social, environmental, and physical environmental correlates with physical activity among Canadians: a cross-sectional study. *BMC Public Health*, 9, 21.

Pedersen, B. (1991). Influence of physical activity on the cellular immune system: mechanisms of action. *International Journal of Sports Medicine*, 12, S23.

Pedersen, B.K. and Ullum, H. (1994). NK cell response to physical activity: possible mechanisms of action. *Medicine & Science in Sports & Exercise*, 26(2), 140–6.

Peters, H.P., De Vries, W.R., Vanberge-Henegouwen, G.P., and Akkermans, L.M. (2001). Potential benefits and hazards of physical activity and exercise on the gastrointestinal tract. *Gut*, 48(3), 435–9.

Powell, K.E. (2005). Land use, the built environment, and physical activity: a public health mixture; a public health solution. *American Journal of Preventive Medicine*, 28(2 Suppl 2), 216–17.

Pratt, M., Macera, C.A., and Blanton, C. (1999). Levels of physical activity and inactivity in children and adults in the United States: current evidence and research issues. *Medicine & Science in Sports & Exercise*, 31(Suppl. 11), S526–33.

Pratt, M., Macera, C.A., Sallis, J.F., O'Donnell, M., and Frank, L.D. (2004). Economic interventions to promote physical activity: application of the SLOTH model. *American Journal of Preventive Medicine*, 27(Suppl. 3), 136–45.

Rajarajeswaran, P. and Vishnupriya, R. (2009). Exercise in cancer. *Indian Journal of Medical and Paediatric Oncology*, 30(2), 61–70.

Rebillard, A., Lefeuvre-Orfila, L., Gueritat, J., and Cillard, J. (2013). Prostate cancer and physical activity: adaptive response to oxidative stress. *Free Radical Biology & Medicine*, 60, 115–24.

Rhodes, R.E., Mark, R.S., and Temmel, C.P. (2012). Adult sedentary behavior: a systematic review. *American Journal of Preventive Medicine*, 42(3), e3–28.

Rimer, J., Dwan, K., Lawlor, D.A., et al. (2012). Exercise for depression. *Cochrane Database of Systematic Reviews*, 7, CD004366.

Rogers, C.J., Colbert, L.H., Greiner, J.W., Perkins, S.N., and Hursting, S.D. (2008). Physical activity and cancer prevention: pathways and targets for intervention. *Sports Medicine*, 38(4), 271–96.

Samitz, G., Egger, M., and Zwahlen, M. (2011). Domains of physical activity and all-cause mortality: systematic review and dose–response meta-analysis of cohort studies. *International Journal of Epidemiology*, 40(5), 1382–400.

Sattelmair, J., Pertman, J., Ding, E.L., Kohl, H.W., 3rd, Haskell, W., and Lee, I.M. (2011). Dose response between physical activity and risk of coronary heart disease: a meta-analysis. *Circulation*, 124(7), 789–95.

Schmidt, M.E., Chang-Claude, J., Vrieling, A., et al. (2013). Association of pre-diagnosis physical activity with recurrence and mortality among women with breast cancer. *International Journal of Cancer*, 133(6), 1431–40.

Serrano-Sanchez, J.A., Lera-Navarro, A., Dorado-Garcia, C., Gonzalez-Henriquez, J.J., and Sanchis-Moysi, J. (2012). Contribution of individual and environmental factors to physical activity level among Spanish adults. *PLoS One*, 7(6), e38693.

Shahraki, M.R., Mirshekari, H., Shahraki, A.R., Shahraki, E., and Naroi, M. (2012). Arterial blood pressure in female students before, during and after exercise. *ARYA Atherosclerosis*, 8(1), 12–15.

Shephard, R.J. and Shek, P.N. (1994). Potential impact of physical activity and sport on the immune system—a brief review. *British Journal of Sports Medicine*, 28(4), 247–55.

Siegrist M. (2008). [Role of physical activity in the prevention of osteoporosis]. *Medizinische Monatsschrift für Pharmazeuten*, 31(7), 259–64.

Sinaki, M. (2012). Exercise for patients with osteoporosis: management of vertebral compression fractures and trunk strengthening for fall prevention. *PM & R*, 4(11), 882–8.

Sinaki, M., Pfeifer, M., Preisinger, E., et al. (2010). The role of exercise in the treatment of osteoporosis. *Current Osteoporosis Reports*, 8(3), 138–44.

Sluka, K.A., O'Donnell, J.M., Danielson, J., and Rasmussen, L.A. (2013). Regular physical activity prevents development of chronic pain and activation of central neurons. *Journal of Applied Physiology*, 114(6), 725–33.

So, H.K., Li, A.M., Choi, K.C., Sung, R.Y., and Nelson, E.A. (2013). Regular exercise and a healthy dietary pattern are associated with lower resting blood pressure in non-obese adolescents: a population-based study. *Journal of Human Hypertension*, 27(5), 304–8.

Sodergren, M., McNaughton, S.A., Salmon, J., Ball, K., and Crawford, D.A. (2012). Associations between fruit and vegetable intake, leisure-time physical activity, sitting time and self-rated health among older adults: cross-sectional data from the WELL study. *BMC Public Health*, 12, 551.

Sorensen, J., Sorensen, J.B., Skovgaard, T., Bredahl, T., and Puggaard, L. (2011). Exercise on prescription: changes in physical activity and health-related quality of life in five Danish programmes. *European Journal of Public Health*, 21(1), 56–62.

Sorensen, J.B., Kragstrup, J., Kjaer, K., and Puggaard, L. (2007). Exercise on prescription: trial protocol and evaluation of outcomes. *BMC Health Services Research*, 7, 36.

Sorensen, J.B., Skovgaard, T., and Puggaard, L. (2006). Exercise on prescription in general practice: a systematic review. *Scandinavian Journal of Primary Health Care*, 24(2), 69–74.

Speed-Andrews, A.E., McGowan, E.L., Rhodes, R.E., et al. (2014). Identification and evaluation of the salient physical activity beliefs of colorectal cancer survivors. *Cancer Nursing*, 37(1), 14–22.

Stern, M.P. (1991). Kelly West Lecture. Primary prevention of type II diabetes mellitus. *Diabetes Care*, 14(5), 399–410.

Stump, C.S. (2011). Physical activity in the prevention of chronic kidney disease. *Cardiorenal Medicine*, 1(3), 164–73.

Sugiyama, T., Okely, A.D., Masters, J.M., and Moore, G.T. (2012). Attributes of child care centers and outdoor play areas associated with pre-schoolers' physical activity and sedentary behavior. *Environment and Behavior*, 44(3), 334–49.

Sundquist, K., Qvist, J., Johansson, S.E., and Sundquist, J. (2005). The long-term effect of physical activity on incidence of coronary heart disease: a 12-year follow-up study. *Preventive Medicine*, 41(1), 219–25.

Suominen, H. (2006). Muscle training for bone strength. *Aging Clinical and Experimental Research*, 18(2), 85–93.

Task Force on Community Preventive Services (2002). Recommendations to increase physical activity in communities. *American Journal of Preventive Medicine*, 22(Suppl. 4), 67–72.

Ter Meulen, W.G. and de Haan, L. (2012). [Exercise-promoting interventions for encouraging people with schizophrenia to take physical exercise]. *Tijdschrift voor Psychiatrie*, 54(8), 741–6.

Teychenne, M., Ball, K., and Salmon, J. (2008). Physical activity and likelihood of depression in adults: a review. *Preventive Medicine*, 46(5), 397–411.

Thompson, D., Cullen, K.W., Boushey, C., and Konzelmann, K. (2012). Design of a website on nutrition and physical activity for adolescents: results from formative research. *Journal of Medical Internet Research*, 14(2), e59.

Trueman, P. and Anokye, N.K. (2013). Applying economic evaluation to public health interventions: the case of interventions to promote physical activity. *Journal of Public Health (Oxford)*, 35(1), 32–9.

Ulrich, C.M., Wiskemann, J., and Steindorf, K. (2012). [Physiologic and molecular mechanisms linking physical activity to cancer risk and progression]. Bundesgesundheitsblatt Gesundheitsforschung. *Gesundheitsschutz*, 55(1), 3–9.

Van der Aa, N., De Geus, E.J., van Beijsterveldt, T.C., Boomsma, D.I., and Bartels, M. (2010). Genetic influences on individual differences in exercise behavior during adolescence. *International Journal of Pediatrics*, 2010, 138345.

Van der Bij, A.K., Laurant, M.G., and Wensing, M. (2002). Effectiveness of physical activity interventions for older adults: a review. *American Journal of Preventive Medicine*, 22(2), 120–33.

Vasquez, F., Salazar, G., Andrade, M., Vasquez, L., and Diaz, E. (2006). Energy balance and physical activity in obese children attending day-care centres. *European Journal of Clinical Nutrition*, 60(9), 1115–21.

Wallberg-Henriksson, H., Rincon, J., and Zierath, J.R. (1998). Exercise in the management of non-insulin-dependent diabetes mellitus. *Sports Medicine*, 25(1), 25–35.

Walsh, N.P., Gleeson, M., Pyne, D.B., et al. (2011c). Position statement. Part two: Maintaining immune health. *Exercise Immunology Review*, 17, 64–103.

Walsh, N.P., Gleeson, M., Shephard, R.J., et al. (2011b). Position statement. Part one: Immune function and exercise. *Exercise Immunology Review*, 17, 6–63.

Wang, C.W., Ng, S.M., Ho, R.T., Ziea, E.T., Wong, V.C., and Chan, C.L. (2012). The effect of qigong exercise on immunity and infections: a systematic review of controlled trials. *The American Journal of Chinese Medicine*, 40(6), 1143–56.

Warburton, D.E., Nicol, C.W., and Bredin, S.S. (2006). Health benefits of physical activity: the evidence. *Canadian Medical Association Journal*, 174(6), 801–9.

Wen, C.P. and Wu, X. (2012). Stressing harms of physical inactivity to promote exercise. *The Lancet*, 380(9838), 192–3.

Wilson, D.K., Kirtland, K.A., Ainsworth, B.E., and Addy, C.L. (2004). Socioeconomic status and perceptions of access and safety for physical activity. *Annals of Behavioral Medicine*, 28(1), 20–8.

Wojtyla, A., Kapka-Skrzypczak, L., Bilinski, P., and Paprzycki, P. (2011). Physical activity among women at reproductive age and during pregnancy (Youth Behavioural Polish Survey—YBPS and Pregnancy-related Assessment Monitoring Survay—PrAMS)—epidemiological population studies in Poland during the period 2010–2011. *Annals of Agricultural and Environmental Medicine*, 18(2), 365–74.

Wolff, E., Gaudlitz, K., von Lindenberger, B.L., Plag, J., Heinz, A., and Strohle, A. (2011). Exercise and physical activity in mental disorders. *European Archives of Psychiatry and Clinical Neuroscience*, 261(Suppl. 2), S186–91.

Woodcock, J., Franco, O.H., Orsini, N., and Roberts, I. (2011). Non-vigorous physical activity and all-cause mortality: systematic review and meta-analysis of cohort studies. *International Journal of Epidemiology*, 40(1), 121–38.

World Health Organization (2013a). *Physical Activity*. [Online] Available at: http://www.who.int/topics/physical_activity/en/.

World Health Organization (2013b). *Global Recommendations on Physical Activity for Health*. [Online] Available at: http://www.who.int/dietphysicalactivity/factsheet_recommendations/en/.

Wylie-Rosett, J., Herman, W.H., and Goldberg, R.B. (2006). Lifestyle intervention to prevent diabetes: intensive and cost effective. *Current Opinion in Lipidology*, 17(1), 37–44.

Yancey, A.K., Fielding, J.E., Flores, G.R., Sallis, J.F., McCarthy, W.J., and Breslow, L. (2007). Creating a robust public health infrastructure for physical activity promotion. *American Journal of Preventive Medicine*, 32(1), 68–78.

Yoon, U., Kwok, L.L., and Magkidis, A. (2013). Efficacy of lifestyle interventions in reducing diabetes incidence in patients with impaired glucose tolerance: a systematic review of randomized controlled trials. *Metabolism*, 62(2), 303–14.

Zschucke, E., Gaudlitz, K., and Strohle, A. (2013). Exercise and physical activity in mental disorders: clinical and experimental evidence. *Journal of Preventive Medicine and Public Health*, 46(Suppl. 1), S12–21.

Diabetes mellitus

Nigel Unwin and Jonathan Shaw

Definition, classification, and diagnosis of diabetes

Diabetes is a metabolic disease characterized by hyperglycaemia (raised blood glucose) resulting from defects in insulin secretion, insulin action, or both (American Diabetes Association (ADA) 2004). Insulin, produced by the beta cells of the pancreatic islets of Langerhans, is the main hormone regulating blood glucose levels, and is released in response to rising blood glucose following eating or drinking. Insulin has wide-ranging metabolic effects, which include the stimulation of glucose uptake into skeletal muscle and liver, and key roles in lipid and protein metabolism.

Since 1979 and 1980, the ADA and the World Health Organization (WHO), respectively, have produced a series of recommendations on both classification and diagnosis of diabetes. These recommendations have changed over time to reflect the latest scientific evidence. There are small but important differences between the WHO and ADA recommendations. Most parts of the world tend to follow the recommendations of the WHO, but those of the ADA are also followed in many places outside the United States. In the description that follows, we therefore focus on the recommendations of the WHO (2006) but in appropriate places describe how those of the ADA differ.

The classification of diabetes is based on current understandings of its underlying aetiology. There are two main types of diabetes. Type 1 diabetes results from destruction of the insulin-producing cells (beta cells) in the pancreas. This is usually, but not always, associated with detectable auto-antibodies to components of the beta cell, indicating an autoimmune process. Type 2 diabetes, which accounts for 85–95 per cent of all diabetes, results from a combination of resistance to the action of insulin, particularly in skeletal muscle, liver, and fat tissue, and insufficient insulin production by the pancreas. There are several other rarer types of diabetes with specific aetiologies, such as maturity-onset diabetes of the young, associated with specific single-gene defects, and diabetes associated with toxicity to certain drugs. Gestational diabetes refers to diabetes that is diagnosed for the first time during pregnancy. Like type 2 diabetes, gestational diabetes is associated with obesity and a sedentary lifestyle, and it is typically the result of the combination of insulin resistance and insulin secretory defects. Whilst gestational diabetes typically resolves after delivery, a high proportion of women with gestational diabetes develop type 2 diabetes over the next 20 years.

A classification of diabetes is shown in Fig. 8.6.1 (WHO 2006). It is worth remembering that our current understandings of the aetiologies of diabetes remain incomplete, and the classification described here may well change in the future. The distinction between type 1 and type 2 diabetes is not always clear cut. For example, in adults, diabetes which initially appears to be type 2 diabetes, in that symptoms at presentation are minimal, and there is an adequate initial response to oral therapies, may be accompanied by auto-antibodies to the beta cells. Such cases typically follow a relatively rapid course to insulin dependency, and are essentially a subtype of auto-immune type 1 diabetes in which progression to insulin dependency occurs over months to years, instead of the days to weeks seen in classical type 1 diabetes. This type of diabetes has received various names, including latent auto-immune diabetes of adults (LADA) (Tuomi et al. 1993) and type 1.5 (Palmer and Hirsch 2003).

The relationships between the current aetiological classification and clinical stages of diabetes are shown in Fig. 8.6.1. The clinical staging includes a category called 'intermediate hyperglycaemia', in which blood glucose is considered above normal but below the diagnostic thresholds for diabetes. This category should not be considered as a clinical entity but rather as a risk category, identifying people at high risk of developing type 2 diabetes and cardiovascular disease, and providing a potential target for preventive interventions.

Diagnosis

The diagnosis of diabetes has traditionally been based on blood glucose levels, but in the last few years glycated haemoglobin (HbA1c) has been accepted as an alternative. Diagnostic thresholds, following current WHO and ADA recommendations (WHO 2006, 2011; ADA 2013), are shown in Table 8.6.1. The 'gold standard' diagnostic test or reference method has been taken to be the oral glucose tolerance test (OGTT). In brief, an OGTT involves the measurement of fasting glucose, followed by a drink containing a fixed quantity of glucose, and the measurement of blood glucose 2 hours after that drink. Undertaking an OGTT is time consuming and relatively expensive (compared to fasting glucose alone). Largely for these pragmatic reasons, the ADA recommends using fasting glucose alone as the main diagnostic test. Unfortunately, however, around one-third of individuals who have diabetes will have an abnormal result after an OGTT but fasting glucose below the diabetes threshold (Decode Study Group 1999). In other words, using fasting glucose alone misses about one-third of individuals with diabetes. Similarly, with fasting glucose, it is impossible to identify those who fall into the category of intermediate hyperglycaemia based on the post-glucose challenge result (impaired glucose tolerance (IGT)), and much of the evidence on preventing type 2 diabetes is in individuals with IGT. There is also good

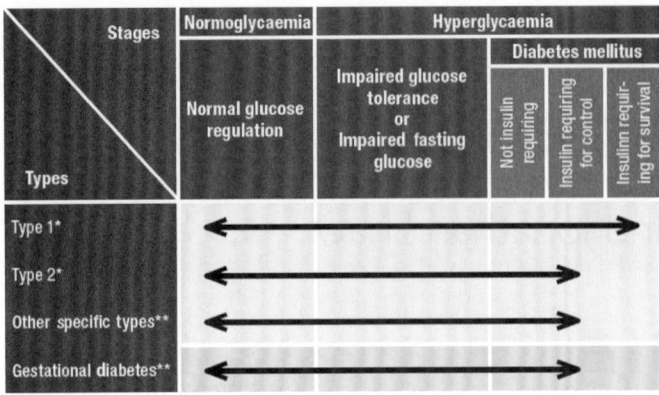

Fig. 8.6.1 The relationship between aetiological types of diabetes and clinical stages of hyperglycaemia.

* Even after presenting in an acute crisis, such as ketoacidosis, these patients can briefly return to normoglycaemia without requiring specific therapy.

** In rare instances, patients in these categories (e.g. Vacor toxicity, type 1 diabetes presenting in pregnancy) may require insulin for survival.

Reproduced with permission from World Health Organization, Definition and diagnosis of diabetes mellitus and intermediate hyperglycemia: report of a WHO/IDF consultation, Copyright © World Health Organization 2006, available from http://www.who.int/diabetes/ publications/Definition%20and%20diagnosis%20of%20diabetes_new.pdf.

evidence that the risk of cardiovascular disease associated with raised blood glucose is more strongly related to blood glucose after a glucose load than to fasting glucose (Decode Study Group 2001). It is for all these reasons that the WHO continues to recommend using an OGTT as the main diagnostic test.

The HbA1c offers a simpler approach to the diagnosis of diabetes, since it does not require fasting. HbA1c reflects glycaemic exposure over the prior 3–4 months, and so is also conceptually attractive, as it measures chronic glycaemia, rather than instantaneous blood glucose levels. However, while its place as the key indicator of glycaemic control among people with diabetes has been secure for many years, it has not been recommended for diagnostic purposes until recently (WHO 2011). The main impediment to its use for diagnosis was concern about variability between laboratories. However, this variability has now been reduced, and it is widely recommended as an alternative diagnostic test. Nevertheless, it is not without its limitations. First, laboratories and assays must be aligned to the international reference values. Second, costs of HbA1c assays are often significantly greater than for blood glucose assays. Third, certain conditions (e.g. haemoglobinopathies, iron deficiency, anaemias, liver and kidney failure) alter red cell turnover, and lead to false lowering or elevation of the HbA1c, making the HbA1c unreliable. Fourth, there is evidence that the relationship between blood glucose levels and HbA1c may be influenced by ethnicity and other factors (Hare et al. 2013), leading to concern that using HbA1c may lead to under-diagnosis or over-diagnosis of diabetes in certain subgroups of the population. It is important to recognize these limitations, and to ensure that HbA1c is only used in situations in which it is both reliable and affordable.

The thresholds for diabetes (Table 8.6.1) are based largely on epidemiological evidence that demonstrates that retinopathy only begins to occur when a certain threshold of glycaemia has been exceeded. This level, or threshold, is apparent for fasting blood glucose, for 2-hour blood glucose (as part of an OGTT) and for HbA1c, and has been taken as the diagnostic value (Colagiuri et al. 2011). It should be noted that such a threshold does not exist for renal complications of diabetes or for cardiovascular disease, partly because the simple measures of these complications (urinary albumin excretion and cardiovascular events) are not specific to diabetes.

Because there is error in laboratory measurements, and there is day-to-day variability in blood glucose levels (less so for HbA1c), the diagnosis of diabetes in someone without symptoms (such as polyuria and polydipsia) should only be made on the basis of two tests on separate occasions. In the presence of symptoms, the

Table 8.6.1 WHO and ADA criteria for the diagnosis of diabetes and intermediate hyperglycaemia in non-pregnant individuals

Diabetes	
Fasting plasma glucose	≥ 7.0 mmol/L (126 mg/dL)
or 2-hour plasma glucose[a]	or ≥ 11.1 mmol/L (200 mg/dL)
or	or
HbA1c	≥ 6.5% (48 mmol/mol)
Intermediate hyperglycaemia—impaired glucose tolerance (IGT)	
Fasting plasma glucose and	< 7.0 mmol/L (126 mg/dL) and
2-hour plasma glucose[a]	7.8–11.0 mmol/L (140–200 mg/dL)
Intermediate hyperglycaemia—impaired fasting glucose (IFG)	
Fasting plasma glucose	6.1–6.9 mmol/L (110–125 mg/dL)
and (if measured)	and (if measured)
2-hour plasma glucose[a]	<7.8 mmol/L (140 mg/dL)
Intermediate hyperglycaemia—elevated HbA1c	
HbA1c	6.0–6.4% (42–46 mmol/mol) (WHO)
	5.7–6.4% (39–46 mmol/mol) (ADA)

[a] Venous plasma glucose 2 hours after ingestion of 75 g oral glucose load (OGTT).

If 2-hour plasma glucose is not measured, status is uncertain as diabetes or IGT cannot be excluded.

Adapted with permission from World Health Organization, *Definition and diagnosis of diabetes mellitus and intermediate hyperglycemia: report of a WHO/IDF consultation*, Copyright © World Health Organization 2006, available from http://www.who.int/diabetes/publications/Definition%20and%20diagnosis%20of%20diabetes_new.pdf.

diagnosis of diabetes may be based on a single level. It is worth noting that while the diagnostic cut-points for diabetes are of necessity precisely defined (i.e. to the nearest tenth of a mmol/L) different studies suggest somewhat different cut-points often differing by at least 1 mmol/L (Tapp et al. 2006).

The rationale for the cut-points defining intermediate hyperglycaemia is less clear than that for those defining diabetes. Both fasting and 2 hours post-challenge glucose are continuously related to the future risk of diabetes and cardiovascular disease—there is no evidence for thresholds and there is a strong argument for using the actual glucose value as part of a risk score for future diabetes or cardiovascular disease (Unwin et al. 2002; WHO 2006). However, at present, this is not the case. The cut-point for IGT is based on data from the Pima Indians on the risk of incident diabetes (Bennett et al. 1982). Impaired fasting glucose (IFG) was introduced in 1997 by the ADA (The Expert Committee on the Diagnosis and Classification of Diabetes Mellitus 1997), followed by the WHO in 1999 (WHO 1999). The cut-point for IFG proposed in 1997, and still used by the WHO, was based on physiological data of the level above which first phase insulin secretion is lost in response to intravenous glucose (The Expert Committee on the Diagnosis and Classification of Diabetes Mellitus 1997). However, in 2003, the ADA recommended a lowering of the cut-point for IFG, based partly on wishing to make the prevalence of IFG more similar to IGT and partly to improve the sensitivity of IFG as a predictor of future diabetes (ADA 2004). The WHO reviewed the classification of intermediate hyperglycaemia in 2006 and decided that the evidence was not strong enough to follow the ADA and lower the IFG cut-point (WHO 2006).

Incidence, prevalence, and trends

The International Diabetes Federation (IDF) produces global estimates of the number of people with diabetes and how their numbers are expected to increase in the future (Whiting et al. 2011). These estimates are mainly based on studies in which blood glucose was tested and thus include people with diagnosed and undiagnosed diabetes. This is important because in many populations more than half the people with diabetes, sometimes as many as 80 or 90 per cent, have not been diagnosed (Whiting et al. 2011). The age-specific prevalences of diabetes from these epidemiological studies are applied to United Nations population figures and projections, applying as appropriate separate prevalences for urban and rural populations, in order to give national, regional, and global estimates. Many countries, roughly 40 per cent, have not conducted diabetes prevalence studies. For these countries prevalence estimates are based on extrapolation from studies conducted in countries considered similar (Guariguata et al. 2011).

The most recent publication estimated that in 2011 there were 366 million adults globally with diabetes, representing 8.3 per cent of all individuals aged 20–79 years (Whiting et al. 2011). Fig. 8.6.2 shows the prevalence of diabetes in adults across the world. The number of people with diabetes is projected to increase to 552 million by 2030. This estimate is highly conservative as it does not explicitly account for trends in obesity and other risk factors.

The prevalence of diabetes rises steeply with age, but tends to plateau or even fall slightly in those aged 70 years and above. Fig. 8.6.3 shows the prevalence of diabetes by age by World Bank income group. Most people with diabetes, between 85 and 95 per cent depending on the population, have type 2 diabetes. The Global Burden of Disease Study estimates for the prevalence of diabetes (Danaei et al. 2011), which uses a somewhat different methodology, are broadly similar to those of the IDF.

At the present time, it is estimated that between 70 and 80 per cent of people with diabetes live in low- and middle-income countries. This proportion will increase as a result of population growth in developing countries, ageing of their populations, and increasing exposure to risk factors for type 2 diabetes associated with mechanization and urbanization (Unwin 2007). Diabetes, particularly type 2 diabetes, is often thought of as being a disease of affluence, and thus more prevalent in richer

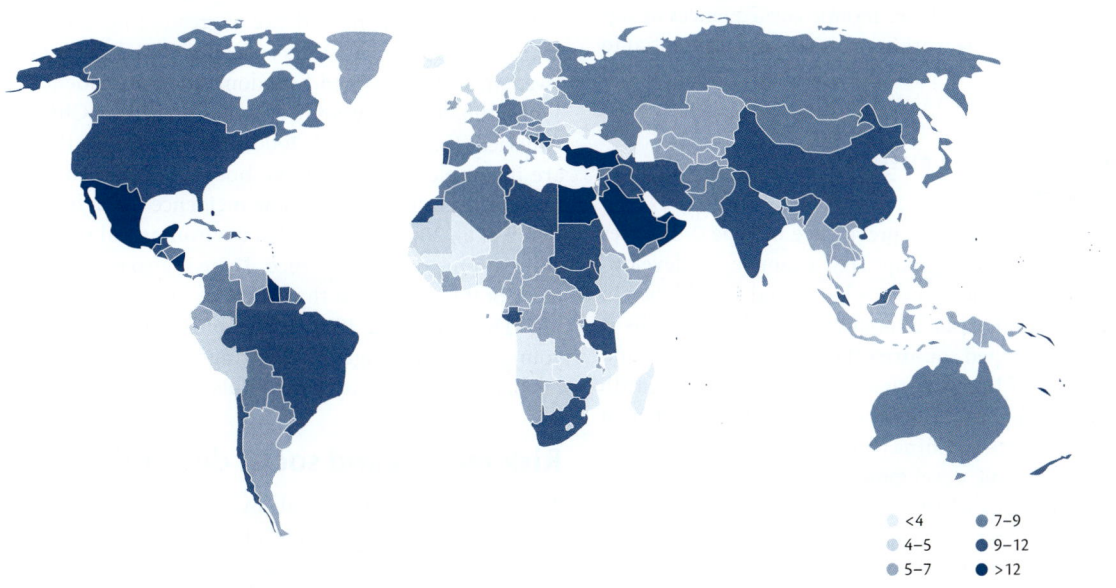

<4	7–9
4–5	9–12
5–7	>12

Fig. 8.6.2 The global prevalence (%) of diabetes in adults (20–79 years) in 2013.

Reproduced with permission from International Diabetes Federation, *Diabetes Atlas, Six Edition*, Map 2.1, International Diabetes Federation, Brussels, Copyright © 2013, available from http://www.idf.org/diabetesatlas/download-book.

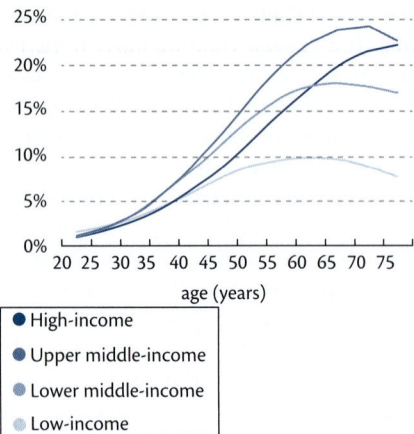

Fig. 8.6.3 Prevalence of diabetes by age and World Bank income group.
Source: data from International Diabetes Federation, *Diabetes Atlas, Six Edition*, International Diabetes Federation, Brussels, Copyright © 2013, available from http://www.idf.org/diabetesatlas/download-book.

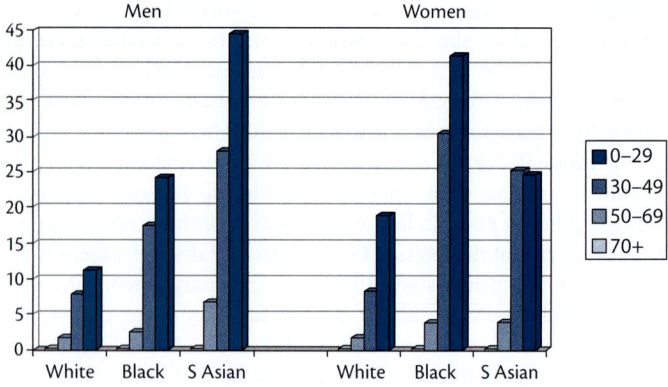

Fig. 8.6.4 Estimated prevalence (%) of diabetes by age, sex, and ethnic group in England in 2007.
Source: data from Walker, C. and Unwin, N., Estimates of the impact of diabetes on the incidence of pulmonary tuberculosis in different ethnic groups in England, *Thorax*, Volume 65, Issue 7, pp.578–581, Copyright © 2010 BMJ Publishing Group Ltd and British Thoracic Society. All rights reserved.

countries. This, however, is a misleading characterization. Upper middle-income countries now have a higher prevalence of diabetes across all adult ages than high-income countries, and lower middle-income countries a higher prevalence up to the age of 60 years (Fig. 8.6.3). Furthermore, it was recently estimated that from 1985 to 2010, the prevalence of diabetes in rural areas of developing countries had approximately quintupled (Hwang et al. 2012).

In high-income countries, the age group with the most cases of diabetes is the 60–79-year-old age group. However, in lower- and middle-income countries, the greatest numbers are aged 40–59. This difference partly reflects younger population age structures in lower- and middle-income countries, but is also partly caused by an earlier age of onset of type 2 diabetes in non-European ethnic groups. The large numbers of working-age adults with diabetes face many years of diabetes, which increases their risk of developing diabetic complications. The economic consequences of significant morbidity during the working years have the potential to cause a significant financial impact on individuals, families, and societies.

Differences in prevalence between population groups

There are large differences in the prevalence of type 2 diabetes between different population groups. For example, in developing countries, the prevalence tends to be several-fold higher in urban compared to rural areas, although as noted earlier this is changing. In most developed countries the highest prevalence and incidence is in those of lowest socioeconomic position (Agardh et al. 2011), with the opposite being described in a number of developing countries, such as China (Xu et al. 2006). It is expected that with further economic development the socioeconomic patterning of type 2 diabetes will be similar in all countries, with the poorest groups having the highest prevalence and incidence (Agardh et al. 2011).

Finally, there are marked differences in diabetes prevalence between some ethnic groups. For example, in England, most studies have found that the prevalence in people of South Asian

and African Caribbean origin is two- to fourfold higher than in people of European origin living in the same area (Oldroyd et al. 2005) (see Fig. 8.6.4, based on data from Walker and Unwin (2010)). In North America, African and Hispanic Americans (Kenny et al. 1995) have higher levels of type 2 diabetes than white Americans, with some of the highest rates of all in the indigenous peoples of North America (Gohdes 1995) and Australia (Minges et al. 2011).

Incidence of type 1 diabetes

Unlike type 2 diabetes, in which the incidence is highest in adults and rises with age, the incidence of type 1 diabetes is highest in children, and in most populations peaks between the ages of 5–14 years (IDF 2006). However, it should also be recognized that type 1 diabetes can develop at any age. Internationally there are huge differences, up to 300-fold, in the incidence of type 1 diabetes, with populations originating in Europe having the highest risk. For example, an incidence of greater than 20 per 100 000 per year (in those aged 14 years or less) is found in Finland, Norway, Sweden, and the United Kingdom, and an incidence of less than 1 per 100,000 per year in populations from China and South America (Karvonen et al. 2000). The reasons for these differences are incompletely understood, but the finding that rates tend to increase in migrants from low-incidence to high-incidence areas (Knip et al. 2005) suggests that environmental factors account for at least some of the difference. There is also evidence from several parts of the world, that the incidence of type 1 diabetes is increasing (Derraik et al. 2012; Patterson et al. 2012), particularly in younger children, again suggesting the influence of environmental factors, though the cause of this rise remains very uncertain.

Risk factors and social determinants

There are strong genetic and environmental (in its broadest sense) influences on the risk of both type 1 and type 2 diabetes, and it is the interaction between the two that results in the onset of the disease. The environmental influences on the risk of type 2 diabetes include low levels of physical activity, diets high in saturated fat, salt, and refined carbohydrate, and low in whole grains, fresh fruit, vegetables, and fibre, calorie excess and obesity, and tobacco exposure. The environmental influences on type 1 diabetes remain frustratingly elusive. In the sections that follow we use the term 'risk factor' to refer to any factor that is associated with an increased incidence of the disease, including those that are markers of early stages of the disease process.

Risk factors for type 1 diabetes

Familial and genetic

The lifetime risk of type 1 diabetes is roughly 6 per cent if a first-degree relative has the condition, such as a sibling, compared to roughly 0.4 per cent (depending on the population) if a first-degree relative is not affected. If a monozygotic twin has type 1 diabetes, the lifetime risk in the other twin is around 50 per cent (Hirschhorn 2003). There are well-established associations between combinations of human leucocyte antigen (HLA) genes and type 1 diabetes. Other genes involved in cell-mediated immunity, and therefore autoimmune disease, have also been associated with type 1 diabetes (Hirschhorn 2003; Gillespie 2006). More than 90 per cent of people with type 1 diabetes carry known genetic markers for the disease (Gillespie 2006). It is important to note, however, that while the presence of known genetic markers greatly increases the risk of the disease, the vast majority people with the genetic markers do not develop type 1 diabetes (Knip et al. 2005).

Environmental factors

The importance of environmental factors is indicated by the changing incidence of type 1 diabetes (described earlier) at a rate that is far too rapid to be due to changes in the gene pool. There is some evidence to implicate viruses, early exposure to cows' milk, and cereals, obesity, and low vitamin D levels, but for none of these is the evidence conclusive (Vehik and Dabelea 2011).

Identifying individuals at high risk of type 1 diabetes

A combination of family history, genotyping, and measurement of auto-antibodies in children aged under 5 can identify a group of individuals who are at very high risk, with 90 per cent or more going on to develop type 1 diabetes (Todd et al. 2011).

Risk factors for type 2 diabetes

It is useful to divide risk factors for type 2 diabetes into unmodifiable and modifiable.

Unmodifiable risk factors for type 2 diabetes
Age and sex

The risk of type 2 diabetes increases steeply with age. Most UK-based studies of previously diagnosed diabetes have found a slightly higher prevalence in men, whereas studies in which glucose is measured either find no sex difference or a slightly higher prevalence in women.

Familial and genetic

The strong familial clustering of type 2 diabetes, suggestive of important genetic influences, has been known for many years (Zimmet 1992). For example, the presence of type 2 diabetes in a parent or sibling approximately doubles the risk of type 2 diabetes. However, identifying genetic markers for type 2 diabetes has proved difficult, and the markers identified to date account for only a few per cent of the genetic risk (Permutt et al. 2005). The reasons for the current lack of success in accounting for the

heritability of type 2 diabetes and other chronic diseases are debated (Eichler et al. 2010). They are likely in part to reflect the (unmeasured) contribution of epigenetic changes to diabetes risk (Drong et al. 2012), discussed briefly later.

Previous gestational diabetes

Women with gestational diabetes tend to be older, more overweight, have a family history of diabetes, and be from an ethnic group with high prevalence of diabetes (Buchanan and Xiang 2005). Following delivery, glucose levels return to normal in around 90 per cent of women, but over the next 10 years, as many as 70 per cent go on to develop diabetes (Buchanan and Xiang 2005).

Ethnicity

As described previously, there are marked differences in the prevalence of type 2 diabetes by ethnic group. It remains far from clear what underlies these differences, how much is related to differences in environment (including behaviours), and how much to differences in genetic susceptibility (Oldroyd et al. 2005).

Modifiable risk factors for type 2 diabetes
Obesity, physical inactivity, aspects of diet, and alcohol

The relationship between overweight and obesity and the risk of type 2 diabetes is continuous, very strong, and is apparent below conventional cut-points for overweight (Vazquez et al. 2007). There is a large body of evidence suggesting that it is the distribution of body fat that is particularly important in determining the risk of type 2 diabetes, with the greatest risk associated with abdominal obesity (Despres 2001).

There is good evidence that physical activity lowers the risk of type 2 diabetes independently of obesity level. Regular moderate or vigorous activity has been associated with a 30–50 per cent reduction in the risk of developing type 2 diabetes (Jeon et al. 2007).

There is also evidence that the composition of the diet, over and above its calorific value, influences the risk of type 2 diabetes. Increased risk has been associated with diets low in fibre and high in saturated fat (Parillo and Riccardi 2004), and conversely intervention studies support the hypothesis that high-fibre, low-saturated-fat diets can help to prevent diabetes (Lindstrom et al. 2006b). High-glycaemic index foods have also been associated with an increased risk of type 2 diabetes (Hodge et al. 2004). Coffee consumption has been consistently associated with a lower risk of type 2 diabetes (van Dam and Hu 2005). Alcohol consumption has a U-shaped relationship with type 2 diabetes incidence, with moderate consumption (20–25 g of alcohol per day) appearing protective in both men and women (Baliunas et al. 2009).

Smoking

Smoking is associated with a dose-dependent increased risk of type 2 diabetes, with former, light, and heavy smokers having a risk of incident type 2 diabetes that is roughly 20, 30, and 60 per cent higher respectively than in those who have never smoked (Willi et al. 2007).

Birth weight, intrauterine environment, and epigenetic changes

There is a U-shaped relationship between birth weight and the risk of type 2 diabetes, and both genetic and environmental factors appear to contribute to this relationship. On the genetic side, for example, there are genetic markers associated with both low birth weight and an increased risk of diabetes as an adult (Drong et al. 2012). On the environmental side, low birth weight can be the result of poor maternal and therefore fetal nutrition, and high birth weight is linked to maternal obesity and hyperglycaemia (Drong et al. 2012). There is evidence that the impact of adverse fetal environments on the risk of type 2 diabetes carries over into the next generation, for example, the nutritional status of pregnant women can affect the risk of type 2 diabetes in their grandchildren (Drong et al. 2012).

Understanding of the mechanisms through which adverse fetal environments are able to alter gene expression in first- and second-generation offspring is increasing. This is through epigenetic modification of gene expression, which by definition is stable across cell divisions and occurs without change in the primary DNA sequence. Two mechanisms through which this occurs include methylation of DNA, and histone modification (Drong et al. 2012).

The implications of epigenetic gene modification for the future risk of type 2 diabetes are profound. It is plausible, for example, that low birth weight associated with poor fetal nutrition, particularly in rapidly modernizing countries, results in offspring with high rates of adult obesity and type 2 diabetes. This in turn leads to increased numbers of obese women, with hyperglycaemia, leading to higher birth weight offspring again at high risk of type 2 diabetes. Thus, the tendency to type 2 diabetes could become self-reinforcing.

Biological risk factors

There is a continuous positive relationship between blood glucose level (both fasting and post glucose challenge) and the risk of developing type 2 diabetes—the higher the level, the greater the risk (Unwin et al. 2002). As described previously, WHO currently defines two non-diabetic risk categories based on glucose level (see Table 8.6.1): IFG and IGT. The potential benefits of identifying and intervening in people with IGT and IFG are discussed in the section on prevention.

There is a strong tendency for several metabolic and cardiovascular risk factors to cluster within the same individuals. This clustering is strongly associated with abdominal obesity and insulin resistance, and has been labelled 'the metabolic syndrome' (Alberti et al. 2007). Core features of the metabolic syndrome include abdominal obesity; raised blood glucose, blood pressure, and triglycerides; and low high-density lipoprotein cholesterol. The presence of the metabolic syndrome in those without diabetes strongly predicts its development (Laaksonen et al. 2002).

Risk scores

Several research groups have derived 'risk scores' based on some of the risk factors described earlier in order to help predict who is at high risk of developing type 2 diabetes, and who may then benefit from preventive interventions. A recent systematic review identified ten scores that had been validated in populations external to those for whom they were developed. Overall the scores were shown to discriminate reasonably well between those who will go on to develop type 2 diabetes and those who will not (Buijsse et al. 2011).

Social determinants of diabetes

Any account of risk factors for type 2 diabetes must place the more proximal determinants within the context of the more distal, social, determinants. It is the broad economic, social, and environmental determinants (discussed in detail elsewhere in this textbook) that shape population levels of physical inactivity, tobacco exposure, alcohol consumption, and unhealthy diet, and which in turn influence the risk and distribution of type 2 diabetes (and related chronic diseases within a population) (Whiting et al. 2010). As discussed in the section on prevention, making substantial progress on reducing the incidence of type 2 diabetes at a population level will require modifying its social determinants.

Health consequences

Mortality and life expectancy

People with diabetes have a substantially higher mortality than people without diabetes, and this is found across all age groups. Overall the relative risk of death is four- to sixfold higher at ages 20–29 years, falls with age but is still 40–80 per cent higher at ages 70–79 years (Roglic and Unwin 2010). In some settings the relative risk of death may be falling, with a recent study from Canada and the United Kingdom finding that between 1996 and 2009, age-adjusted relative risk of death fell from around 2 to around 1.5 (Lind et al. 2013). This might be explained by improved care for people with diabetes, improved case finding increasing the proportion of people with diabetes who are at lower risk at diagnosis, or a combination of the two.

Most, but not all, studies have found that the relative risk of death is higher in women (i.e. compared to women without diabetes) than in men (i.e. compared to men without diabetes). It should be noted that the number of good longitudinal studies able to properly compare mortality rates in people with and without diabetes is relatively small and largely limited to wealthier countries. The relative mortality in poorer countries, where diabetes prevalence is increasing rapidly but where healthcare coverage is often wholly inadequate, may be even greater.

The higher mortality rates in people with diabetes across all age-groups leads to substantial reductions in life expectancy. A UK study estimated that type 2 diabetes at age 40 results in 8 years lost life expectancy in both men and women, and a loss of 4 years at age 60 (Roper et al. 2001). Data on loss of life expectancy in people with type 1 diabetes are harder to find. Widely quoted figures are from a review published in 1984 (Panzram 1984) which found that loss of life expectancy was at least 15 years, whatever the age of diagnosis, with some evidence that it may be over 25 years in those diagnosed under the age of 15. However, a recently published study from Pittsburgh, United States, suggests significant improvements in life expectancy over the past 40 years for people with type 1 diabetes (Miller et al. 2012), but still falling short by around 10 years compared to people without diabetes.

The proportion of deaths attributable to diabetes is not known with accuracy because diabetes is frequently not recorded on death certificates. Estimates of the number of deaths due to diabetes have been made using the relative risk of death in people with diabetes compared to those without, the known prevalence of diabetes and the underlying population mortality. These suggest that globally diabetes is responsible for around 7 per cent of all deaths. In all regions of the world, with the exception of Africa, diabetes is estimated to be responsible in adults for at least one in ten deaths (Roglic and Unwin 2010).

Diabetes-related complications

Diabetes affects multiple organ systems, and complications typically are divided into those affecting large arteries (macrovascular) including those supplying the heart, brain, and lower limbs, and those affecting small vessels (microvascular), including those of the kidney and eye and those supplying the peripheral nervous system. In addition, diabetes is associated with depression, and with liver dysfunction. As noted in later subsections there are some differences in the rate of complications by ethnic group, particularly for coronary heart disease, end-stage renal disease, and lower extremity amputation. The relative contributions to these ethnic group differences of differential healthcare access, behaviours and genetic susceptibility remains incompletely understood (Karter et al. 2002; Lanting et al. 2005).

Cardiovascular disease

The risk of cardiovascular disease in people with diabetes is two- to fourfold higher than in people without diabetes (Stamler et al. 1993; Folsom et al. 1997), and this accounts for much of the increased mortality associated with diabetes (Roglic et al. 2005). In most populations, well over 50 per cent of deaths in people with diabetes are from cardiovascular disease. For example, in people with diabetes in Teesside, England, 59 per cent of deaths in men and 74 per cent in women were due to cardiovascular disease (Roper et al. 2002).

In the United States, people with diabetes of African, Asian (Chinese and Japanese), and Hispanic origin have substantially lower rates of myocardial infarction than those of European origin, and those of the latter two groups lower rates of stroke. Similar findings exist in for people of African origin the United Kingdom (Davis 2008). People with diabetes of South Asian (Indian Asian) origin are at similar or higher risk of cardiovascular disease than those of European origin (Gholap et al. 2011). These differences are not explained by differences in conventional risk factors.

Diabetic eye disease

In developed countries, diabetes is the leading cause of blindness in people aged over 25 years (Klein and Klein 1995). Twenty years after diagnosis, virtually 100 per cent of people with type 1 diabetes have diabetic retinopathy (Klein 1997; Roy et al. 2004), and when blood pressure and blood glucose control are poor, it is estimated that 75 per cent will develop proliferative retinopathy, the most severe form. In type 2 diabetes, between 40 and 60 per cent are expected to develop retinopathy during their lifetime, with around 10 per cent developing proliferative retinopathy (Klein 1997; Eye Diseases Prevalence Research Group et al. 2004). Diabetes also increases the risk of cataracts and open-angle glaucoma (Klein and Klein 1995).

Diabetic renal disease

Diabetes is the leading cause of renal failure in developed countries, responsible for 40–50 per cent of all new patients requiring dialysis in North America, and 15–33 per cent in Europe and Australia (Atkins, 2005). In cross-sectional surveys in Europe, around one in ten people with type 1 diabetes, and one in seven with type 2 diabetes, have evidence of overt nephropathy (IDF 2006). Approximately 30 per cent of people with diabetes with overt nephropathy will progress to end-stage renal failure (Atkins

2005). There are marked differences by ethnic group in the risk of end-stage renal disease, with people of African and Asian origin in particular being at greater risk compared to those of European origin (Karter et al. 2002; Lanting et al. 2005). A high risk of diabetic renal disease has also been described from studies within Asia (Chan et al. 2009).

Neuropathy and diabetic foot problems

The nerve damage associated with diabetes can affect both peripheral and autonomic nerves. Diabetic foot problems are a result of peripheral neuropathy or peripheral vascular disease or a combination of the two (Edmonds et al. 1996). In cross-sectional studies, peripheral neuropathy is found in one in five to more than a third of people with diabetes (IDF 2006). During their lifetime, roughly 15 per cent of people with diabetes develop a foot ulcer and of these 5–15 per cent go on to amputation (Edmonds et al. 1996). In developed countries, diabetes is the single most important cause of non-traumatic lower limb amputation, accounting for 40–60 per cent of all amputations (Global Lower Extremity Amputation Study Group 2000), and people with diabetes have a 15-fold risk of amputation compared to people without diabetes (Edmonds et al. 1996). Differences exist in the risk of lower extremity amputation by ethnic group, with, for example, people of Asian origin in the United States and United Kingdom having a markedly lower risk than the European origin population (Lanting et al. 2005).

Erectile dysfunction

Diabetes increases the risk of erectile dysfunction in men. A large US cohort study (Bacon et al. 2002) found that type 1 diabetes increased the risk threefold, and type 2 diabetes increased the risk by a third. The same study found that the prevalence of erectile dysfunction in men with diabetes was around 50 per cent.

Other co-morbidities

Depressive illness is up to twice as common in people with diabetes than those without (Egede and Ellis, 2010). Depressive symptoms are also a risk factor for type 2 diabetes, associated with roughly a 50 per cent increase in risk (Demakakos et al. 2010). Depression in people with diabetes is associated with more complications and poorer self-care (Lin et al. 2004).

Non-alcoholic fatty liver disease is found in the majority of people with type 2 diabetes (Targher and Byrne, 2013). It is also a risk factor for its development, with some arguing that it is a key part of the pathogenesis (Taylor 2008). In people with diabetes it is strongly associated with the risk of complications, including macrovascular disease and, of course, chronic liver disease (Targher and Byrne 2013).

Finally, there is consistent evidence that diabetes is associated with a 30–40 per cent increased risk of several cancers including of the breast, endometrium, liver, and colon (Chan et al. 2009).

Economic impact of diabetes

Although there is a lack of robust studies into the economic impact of diabetes, it is clear that the cost of diabetes to individuals and their carers, to health services, and to national economies is substantial. On average, a person with diabetes uses more health resources than a person without diabetes—around 1.5–3 times more, depending on age and sex (Zhang et al. 2010). It was estimated that in 2010 diabetes accounted for between 5 and 15 per cent of health expenditure in over 80 per cent of countries (Zhang et al. 2010). The mean estimated expenditure varies from less than 300 ID (international dollars, adjusted for purchasing power) per person with diabetes per year in most sub-Saharan African countries, to over 3000 ID per year in most of the countries of Western Europe (Zhang et al. 2010). In sub-Saharan Africa diabetes is estimated to be responsible for 3–7 per cent of total health expenditure, and in Europe 9–12 per cent. Diabetes is a substantial cause of health expenditure in several of the poorer countries of Asia, including Bangladesh (10 per cent), India (11 per cent), Thailand (11 per cent), and Sri Lanka (16 per cent). The highest expenditure per person with diabetes by far is in the United States, with a mean expenditure of 7383 ID (Zhang et al. 2010).

At an individual level the costs of diabetes care increase dramatically with the presence of complications, being two- to three-fold higher with the presence of either micro- or macro-vascular complications, and five- to sixfold higher with the presence of both micro- and macrovascular complications than in people with diabetes without complications (Williams 2005). Diabetes, as with any other chronic illness, may limit employment and impact upon the income of people with it and the people caring for them. A study in the United Kingdom found that in people with type 2 diabetes aged less than 65 years, 7 per cent lost income because of diabetes. They lost on average £13,800 per year (at 1998 values) and their carers lost £11,000 per year (Holmes et al. 2003).

The impact of diabetes on gross domestic product (GDP) was estimated for several countries in 2007. The United Kingdom lost 0.4 per cent of GDP, the United States 1.2 per cent, and India 2.1 per cent (Economist Intelligence Unit 2007).

Prevention of diabetes and its complications

Prevention of type 1 diabetes

As noted earlier, it is possible to identify individuals based on auto-antibodies, family history, and genetic background, at very high risk of developing type 1 diabetes. This is a costly and labour-intensive exercise, but has been done as part of evaluating preventive measures in such individuals. Unfortunately none of the measures for prevention so far tested have been found to work (Gillespie 2006; Todd et al. 2011). Furthermore true primary prevention requires approaches that prevent the onset of the auto-immune process. How to prevent type 1 diabetes remains an area under active investigation (Todd et al. 2011).

Prevention of type 2 diabetes

Targeting individuals at high risk

There is excellent evidence that type 2 diabetes can be prevented, or at least its onset delayed, in individuals at high risk of type 2 diabetes, such as those with impaired glucose tolerance and/or fasting hyperglycaemia. Interventions aimed at modifying behaviours and pharmacological interventions have both been shown to be effective, and at best to reduce the incidence of type 2 diabetes by 50–60 per cent. Aspects of behavioural change that were promoted in these trials included weight loss (in those overweight and obese), increased physical activity, and a diet low in total and saturated fat and high in fibre. The more behavioural goals

that are achieved, the lower the long-term risk of type 2 diabetes (Lindstrom et al. 2006a). Based on the results of the trials, the number needed to treat to prevent one case of type 2 diabetes by behavioural interventions is around 6–7 over 3–5 years, and using oral diabetes drugs is 10–11 (Gillies et al. 2007).

While undoubtedly new approaches to the prevention of diabetes in those at high risk will be trialled, particularly additional pharmacological agents, a major challenge is how to translate the results from well-resourced trials into everyday healthcare and community settings. A recent review identified 17 translational studies, 14 of which were carried out in the United States (Johnson et al. 2013). Individuals at high risk of type 2 diabetes were identified in several ways, including the use of risk scores. The findings of the studies are encouraging in that all bar one reported greater weight loss in the intervention compared to the control arm, but there were no consistent differences in glucose or waist circumference. Clearly more work, in a greater variety of geographical settings, is required to assess the feasibility and cost-effectiveness of approaches targeting individuals at high risk of type 2 diabetes.

Population-wide approaches

Targeting individuals at high risk of diabetes is unlikely to have a large impact on the overall population incidence of type 2 diabetes, since 40–60 per cent of new cases of type 2 diabetes arise in people who had normal glucose tolerance 3–5 years earlier (Unwin et al. 2002). It is only through population-based measures aimed at reducing overweight and obesity and increasing physical activity that a large impact on the incidence of type 2 diabetes will be achieved. The potential impact of population-wide measures was illustrated in an analysis from the EPIC-Norfolk cohort. It assessed the association between the achievement of five 'diabetes healthy behaviour prevention goals' (BMI < 25 kg/m², fat intake < 30 per cent of energy intake, saturated fat intake <10 per cent of energy intake, fibre intake 15 g/1000 kcal, physical activity 4 hours/week). If the entire population were able to meet one more goal, the total incidence of diabetes would be predicted to fall by 20 per cent (Simmons et al. 2006).

As reviewed elsewhere in this textbook, achieving population-wide changes to reduce the incidence of diabetes and related chronic non-communicable diseases (NCDs) presents major challenges. The 2011 United Nations High Level Meeting on chronic NCDs strongly recognized the need for legislative, fiscal, and other policy measures. These measures need to involve all sectors of government, civic society, and, as appropriate, the private sector, in order to start to change environments from being 'obesogenic' (Egger and Swinburn 1997) towards those that promote healthier diets and physical activity. The challenge of achieving this is clear when it is appreciated that despite increasing awareness in many parts of the world amongst both policymakers and the general public on the detrimental effects of obesity, there is not yet a single population-wide example where the trend towards increasing levels of obesity has been reversed. Presumably, it is in recognition of this challenge that of the nine voluntary NCD targets adopted by the World Health Assembly in 2013, that for obesity and diabetes is for no change (a 0 per cent increase) by 2025. Even that, however, may prove overly optimistic given current trends.

Policy measures aimed at the prevention of type 2 diabetes and related NCDs will need to address the fact that these conditions tend to be socially distributed, with highest risks in the less well educated and poorer parts of the population. Interventions need to be carefully designed and evaluated to reduce inequities in outcomes between social groups.

Prevention of diabetes-related complications

While primary prevention of diabetes is the ultimate goal, there is excellent evidence that the increased morbidity and mortality in people with diabetes, compared to those without, can be significantly reduced. Some of the healthcare interventions are highly cost-effective (Table 8.6.2) (Venkat Narayan et al. 2006). Control of blood glucose, blood pressure, blood lipids, and the avoidance of smoking are core; with specific measures to reduce the incidence of sight-threatening retinopathy, morbidity and loss of the lower limbs, and progression to end-stage renal disease. The core measures overlap completely, of course, with those recommended for people at high risk of cardiovascular disease events (Mendis et al. 2011).

Given the existence of these highly effective interventions, and the fact that at diagnosis up to 50 per cent or more of people with type 2 diabetes have evidence of microvascular complications (Spijkerman et al. 2003), there is strong interest in early detection or screening. Indeed, a substantial proportion of people with type 2 diabetes are undiagnosed, particularly in low- and middle-income countries: estimated to be 50–60 per cent in the Middle East and North Africa, 50 per cent in South East Asia, and 60 per cent in the Western Pacific (Whiting et al. 2011). Although randomized controlled evidence for the benefits of the screening for type 2 diabetes is lacking, there is nonetheless a clear rationale for it, supported by studies modelling its impact on macro- and microvascular outcomes (Khunti and Davies 2012). The feasibility and cost-effectiveness of different approaches to earlier detection of type 2 diabetes will depend on the setting, and most crucially the ability of the health system to absorb and deliver effective treatment to increased numbers of people with diabetes (Glumer et al. 2006). In many situations, particularly those with limited resources, it is beneficial to target diagnostic blood glucose testing only on those individuals who are at high risk of having undiagnosed diabetes. Many risk scores, with reasonable sensitivity and specificity, have been developed to identify individuals for blood glucose testing (Brown et al. 2012). These can be used opportunistically and as part of a mass screening programme. Few of these scores, however, have been evaluated in low- or middle-income settings (Brown et al. 2012).

A detailed discussion of how to achieve reductions in morbidity and mortality in people with diabetes and the contents of good diabetes care is beyond the scope of this chapter. There are many sources of guidance on this, including the Global Guideline for Type 2 diabetes from the IDF (IDF: Clinical Guidelines Taskforce 2012). However, it is worth making the following points here. People with diabetes play the central role in managing their condition (as with most chronic conditions), and thus core to effective diabetes care is empowering people with diabetes with the knowledge and support they need to do this. Effective healthcare for diabetes, in common with many other chronic conditions (Epping-Jordan et al. 2004), requires a well-functioning healthcare system, with good communication between many different specialities and levels of care. Finally, it is an accurate generalization to state that diabetes care is currently suboptimal the world over (Venkat Narayan et al. 2006), in both rich and poor countries. In rich countries, suboptimal care includes inadequate coverage of basic preventive measures, such as regular eye and foot examinations, as well as room for much better control of glucose, blood pressure, and lipids. In poor countries, inadequate care includes no care at all for a large proportion of people with diabetes, including, in many parts of the world, lack of, or intermittent access to, insulin leading to the death of those who require it for survival (Yudkin 2000).

It is not hyperbole to state that diabetes presents one of the major public health challenges of the twenty-first century. In response to this, the United Nations General Assembly in 2006 passed a resolution calling for coordinated global action on diabetes (Unite for Diabetes 2006) and endorsing 14 November, the birthday of Frederick Banting, one of the discoverers of insulin, as World Diabetes Day.

Table 8.6.2 Examples of treatment strategies and relative reductions in morbidity and mortality in people with diabetes

Strategy	Estimated benefit
Glycaemic control in people with HbA1c > 9 per cent	Reduction of 30 per cent in microvascular disease per 1 per cent drop in HbA1c
Glycaemic control in people with HbA1c > 8 per cent	Reduction of 30 per cent in microvascular disease per 1 per cent drop in HbA1c
Blood pressure control in people whose pressure is higher than 160/95 mmHg	Reduction of 35 per cent in macrovascular and microvascular disease per 10 mmHg drop in blood pressure
Cholesterol control in people with total cholesterol < 5.2 mmol/L	Reduction of 25–55 per cent in coronary heart diseases events; 43 per cent fall in death rate
Annual screening for microalbuminuria	Reduction of 50 per cent in nephropathy using ACE inhibitors for identified cases
Annual eye examinations	Reduction of 60 to 70 per cent in serious vision loss
Foot care in people with high risk of ulcers	Reduction of 50 to 60 per cent in serious foot disease
Aspirin use in people with established cardiovascular disease	Reduction of 28 per cent in myocardial infarctions, reduction of 18 per cent in cardiovascular disease
ACE inhibitor use in all people with diabetes	Reduction of 42 per cent in nephropathy; 22 per cent reduction in cardiovascular disease

Adapted with permission from Venkat Narayan KM et al., Diabetes: The Pandemic and Potential Solutions, pp. 691–704, in Jamison DT et al., (eds.), *Disease control priorities in developing countries*, Second edition, World Bank/Oxford University Press, Washington/New York, Copyright © 2006.

References

Agardh, E., Allebeck, P., Hallqvist, J., Moradi, T., and Sidorchuk, A. (2011). Type 2 diabetes incidence and socio-economic position: a systematic review and meta-analysis. *International Journal of Epidemiology*, 40, 804–18.

Alberti, K.G.M.M., Zimmet, P., and Shaw, J. (2007). International Diabetes Federation: a consensus on type 2 diabetes prevention. *Diabetic Medicine*, 24, 451–63.

American Diabetes Association (2004). Diagnosis and classification of diabetes mellitus. *Diabetes Care*, 27, 5S–10.

American Diabetes Association (2013). Standards of medical care in diabetes—2013. *Diabetes Care*, 36, S11–S66.

Atkins, R.C. (2005). The epidemiology of chronic kidney disease. *Kidney International*, 67, S14–18.

Bacon, C.G., Hu, F.B., Giovannucci, E., Glasser, D.B., Mittleman, M.A., and Rimm, E.B. (2002). Association of type and duration of diabetes with erectile dysfunction in a large cohort of men. *Diabetes Care*, 25, 1458–63.

Baliunas, D.O., Taylor, B.J., Irving, H., et al. (2009). Alcohol as a risk factor for type 2 diabetes: a systematic review and meta-analysis. *Diabetes Care*, 32, 2123–32.

Bennett, P., Knowler, W., Pettitt, D., Carraher, M., and Vasquez, B. (1982). Longitudinal studies of the development of diabetes in the Pima Indians. In E. Eschwege (ed.) *Advances in Diabetes Epidemiology*, pp. 65–74. Amsterdam: Elsevier Biomedical Press.

Brown, N., Critchley, J., Bogowicz, P., Mayige, M., and Unwin, N. (2012). Risk scores based on self-reported or available clinical data to detect undiagnosed type 2 diabetes: a systematic review. *Diabetes Research and Clinical Practice*, 98, 369–85.

Buchanan, T.A. and Xiang, A.H. (2005). Gestational diabetes mellitus. *Journal of Clinical Investigation*, 115, 485–91.

Buijsse, B., Simmons, R.K., Griffin, S.J., and Schulze, M.B. (2011). Risk assessment tools for identifying individuals at risk of developing type 2 diabetes. *Epidemiologic Reviews*, 33(1), 46–62.

Chan, J.C., Malik, V., Jia, W., et al. (2009). Diabetes in Asia: epidemiology, risk factors, and pathophysiology. *Journal of the American Medical Association*, 301, 2129–40.

Colagiuri, S., Lee, C.M., Wong, T.Y., Balkau, B., Shaw, J.E., and Borch-Johnsen, K. (2011). Glycemic thresholds for diabetes-specific retinopathy: implications for diagnostic criteria for diabetes. *Diabetes Care*, 34, 145–50.

Danaei, G., Finucane, M.M., Lu, Y., et al. (2011). National, regional, and global trends in fasting plasma glucose and diabetes prevalence since 1980: systematic analysis of health examination surveys and epidemiological studies with 370 country-years and 2.7 million participants. *The Lancet*, 378, 31–40.

Davis, T.M. (2008). Ethnic diversity in type 2 diabetes. *Diabetic Medicine*, 25(Suppl. 2), 52–6.

Decode Study Group (1999). Is fasting glucose sufficient to define diabetes? Epidemiological data from 20 European studies. The DECODE-study group. European Diabetes Epidemiology Group. Diabetes Epidemiology: Collaborative analysis of Diagnostic Criteria in Europe. *Diabetologia*, 42, 647–54.

Decode Study Group (2001). Glucose tolerance and cardiovascular mortality: comparison of fasting and 2-hour diagnostic criteria. *Archives of Internal Medicine*, 161, 397–405.

Demakakos, P., Pierce, M.B., and Hardy, R. (2010). Depressive symptoms and risk of type 2 diabetes in a national sample of middle-aged and older adults. *Diabetes Care*, 33, 792–7.

Derraik, J.G.B., Reed, P.W., Jefferies, C., Cutfield, S.W., Hofman, P.L., and Cutfield, W.S. (2012). Increasing incidence and age at diagnosis among children with type 1 diabetes mellitus over a 20-year period in Auckland (New Zealand). *PLoS ONE*, 7, e32640.

Despres, J.P. (2001). Health consequences of visceral obesity. *Annals of Medicine*, 33, 534–41.

Drong, A.W., Lindgren, C.M., and McCarthy, M.I. (2012). The genetic and epigenetic basis of type 2 diabetes and obesity. *Clinical Pharmacology & Therapeutics*, 92, 707–15.

Economist Intelligence Unit (2007). *The Silent Epidemic: An Economic Study of Diabetes in Developed and Developing Countries*. London: Economist Intelligence Unit.

Edmonds, M., Boulton, A., Buckenham, T., et al. (1996). Report of the diabetic foot and amputation group. *Diabetic Medicine*, 13, S27–S42.

Egede, L.E. and Ellis, C. (2010). Diabetes and depression: global perspectives. *Diabetes Research and Clinical Practice*, 87, 302–12.

Egger, G. and Swinburn, B. (1997). An 'ecological' approach to the obesity pandemic. *British Medical Journal*, 315, 477–80.

Eichler, E.E., Flint, J., Gibson, G., et al. (2010). Missing heritability and strategies for finding the underlying causes of complex disease. *Nature Reviews Genetics*, 11, 446–50.

Epping-Jordan, J.E., Pruitt, S.D., Bengoa, R., and Wagner, E.H. (2004). Improving the quality of health care for chronic conditions. *Quality & Safety in Health Care*, 13, 299–305.

Eye Diseases Prevalence Research Group, Kempen, J.H., O'Colmain, B.J., et al. (2004). The prevalence of diabetic retinopathy among adults in the United States. *Archives of Ophthalmology*, 122, 552–63.

Folsom, A.R., Szklo, M., Stevens, J., Liao, F., Smith, R., and Eckfeldt, J.H. (1997). A prospective study of coronary heart disease in relation to fasting insulin, glucose, and diabetes. The Atherosclerosis Risk in Communities (ARIC) Study. *Diabetes Care*, 20, 935–42.

Gholap, N., Davies, M., Patel, K., Sattar, N., and Khunti, K. (2011). Type 2 diabetes and cardiovascular disease in South Asians. *Primary Care Diabetes*, 5, 45–56.

Gillespie, K.M. (2006). Type 1 diabetes: pathogenesis and prevention. *Canadian Medical Association Journal*, 175, 165–70.

Gillies, C.L., Abrams, K.R., Lambert, P.C., et al. (2007). Pharmacological and lifestyle interventions to prevent or delay type 2 diabetes in people with impaired glucose tolerance: systematic review and meta-analysis. *BMJ*, 334, 299.

Global Lower Extremity Amputation Study Group (2000). Epidemiology of lower extremity amputation in centres in Europe, North America and East Asia. The Global Lower Extremity Amputation Study Group. *British Journal of Surgery*, 87, 328–37.

Glumer, C., Yuyun, M., Griffin, S., et al. (2006). What determines the cost-effectiveness of diabetes screening? *Diabetologia*, 49, 1536–44.

Gohdes, D. (1995). Diabetes in North American Indians and Alaska Natives. In National Diabetes Data Group (ed.) *Diabetes in America* (2nd ed.), pp. 683–701. Washington, DC: National Institutes of Health.

Guariguata, L., Whiting, D., Weil, C., and Unwin, N. (2011). The International Diabetes Federation diabetes atlas methodology for estimating global and national prevalence of diabetes in adults. *Diabetes Research and Clinical Practice*, 94, 322–32.

Hare, M.J.L., Magliano, D.J., Zimmet, P.Z., et al. (2013). Glucose-independent ethnic differences in HbA1c in people without known diabetes. *Diabetes Care*, 36, 1534–40.

Hirschhorn, J.N. (2003). Genetic epidemiology of type 1 diabetes. *Pediatric Diabetes*, 4, 87–100.

Hodge, A.M., English, D.R., O'Dea, K., and Giles, G.G. (2004). Glycemic index and dietary fiber and the risk of type 2 diabetes. *Diabetes Care*, 27, 2701–6.

Holmes, J., Gear, E., Bottomley, J., Gillam, S., Murphy, M., and Williams, R. (2003). Do people with type 2 diabetes and their carers lose income? (T2ARDIS-4). *Health Policy*, 64, 291–6.

Hwang, C.K., Han, P.V., Zabetian, A., Ali, M.K., and Narayan, K.M. (2012). Rural diabetes prevalence quintuples over twenty-five years in low- and middle-income countries: a systematic review and meta-analysis. *Diabetes Research and Clinical Practice*, 96, 271–85.

International Diabetes Federation (2006). *Diabetes Atlas* (3rd ed.). Brussels: IDF.

International Diabetes Federation: Clinical Guidelines Taskforce (2012). *Global Guideline for Type 2 Diabetes*. Brussels: IDF. Available at: http://www.idf.org/global-guideline-type-2-diabetes-2012.

Jeon, C.Y., Lokken, R.P., Hu, F.B., and Van Dam, R.M. (2007). Physical activity of moderate intensity and risk of type 2 diabetes: a systematic review. *Diabetes Care*, 30, 744–52.

Johnson, M., Jones, R., Freeman, C., et al. (2013). Can diabetes prevention programmes be translated effectively into real-world settings and still deliver improved outcomes? A synthesis of evidence. *Diabetic Medicine*, 30, 3–15.

Karter, A.J., Ferrara, A., Liu, J.Y., Moffet, H.H., Ackerson, L.M., and Selby, J.V. (2002). Ethnic disparities in diabetic complications in an insured population. *Journal of the American Medical Association*, 287, 2519–27.

Karvonen, M., Viik-Kajander, M., Moltchanova, E., Libman, I., Laporte, R., and Tuomilehto, J. (2000). Incidence of childhood type 1 diabetes worldwide. *Diabetes Care*, 23, 1516–26.

Kenny, S., Aubert, R., and Geiss, L. (1995). Prevalence and incidence of non-insulin-dependent diabetes. In National Diabetes Data Group (ed.) *Diabetes in America* (2nd ed.), pp. 47–67. Washington, DC: National Institutes of Health.

Khunti, K. and Davies, M. (2012). Should we screen for type 2 diabetes: yes. *BMJ*, 345, e4514.

Klein, R. (1997). The epidemiology of diabetic retinopathy. In J. Pickup and G. Williams (eds.) *Textbook of Diabetes*, pp. 44.1–44.9. London: Blackwell Scientific Publications.

Klein, R. and Klein, B.E. (1995). Vision disorders in diabetes. In National Diabetes Data Group (ed.) *Diabetes in America* (2nd ed.), pp. 293–338. Bethesda, MD: National Institutes of Health.

Knip, M., Veijola, R., Virtanen, S.M., Hyoty, H., Vaarala, O., and Akerblom, H.K. (2005). Environmental triggers and determinants of type 1 diabetes. *Diabetes*, 54, S125–36.

Laaksonen, D.E., Lakka, H.-M., Niskanen, L.K., Kaplan, G.A., Salonen, J.T., and Lakka, T.A. (2002). Metabolic syndrome and development of diabetes mellitus: application and validation of recently suggested definitions of the metabolic syndrome in a prospective cohort study. *American Journal of Epidemiology*, 156, 1070–7.

Lanting, L.C., Joung, I.M., Mackenbach, J.P., Lamberts, S.W., and Bootsma, A.H. (2005). Ethnic differences in mortality, end-stage complications, and quality of care among diabetic patients: a review. *Diabetes Care*, 28, 2280–8.

Lin, E.H.B., Katon, W., Von Korff, M., et al. (2004). Relationship of depression and diabetes self-care, medication adherence, and preventive care. *Diabetes Care*, 27, 2154–60.

Lind, M., Garcia-Rodriguez, L.A., Booth, G.L., et al. (2013). Mortality trends in patients with and without diabetes in Ontario, Canada and the UK from 1996 to 2009: a population-based study. *Diabetologia*, 56(12), 2601–8.

Lindstrom, J., Ilanne-Parikka, P., Peltonen, M., et al. (2006a). Sustained reduction in the incidence of type 2 diabetes by lifestyle intervention: follow-up of the Finnish Diabetes Prevention Study. *The Lancet*, 368, 1673–9.

Lindstrom, J., Peltonen, M., Eriksson, J. G., et al. (2006b). High-fibre, low-fat diet predicts long-term weight loss and decreased type 2 diabetes risk: the Finnish Diabetes Prevention Study. *Diabetologia*, 49, 912–20.

Mendis, S., Puska, P., and Norrving, B. (eds.) (2011). *Global Atlas on Cardiovascular Disease Prevention and Control: Policies, Strategies and Interventions*, Geneva: World Health Organization.

Miller, R.G., Secrest, A.M., Sharma, R.K., Songer, T.J., and Orchard, T.J. (2012). Improvements in the life expectancy of type 1 diabetes: the Pittsburgh Epidemiology of Diabetes Complications study cohort. *Diabetes*, 61, 2987–92.

Minges, K.E., Zimmet, P., Magliano, D.J., Dunstan, D.W., Brown, A., and Shaw, J.E. (2011). Diabetes prevalence and determinants in Indigenous Australian populations: a systematic review. *Diabetes Research and Clinical Practice*, 93, 139–49.

Oldroyd, J., Banerjee, M., Heald, A., and Cruickshank, K. (2005). Diabetes and ethnic minorities. *Postgraduate Medical Journal*, 81, 486–90.

Palmer, J.P. and Hirsch, I.B. (2003). What's in a name: latent autoimmune diabetes of adults, type 1.5, adult-onset, and type 1 diabetes. *Diabetes Care*, 26, 536–8.

Panzram, G. (1984). Epidemiologic data on excess mortality and life expectancy in insulin-dependent diabetes mellitus—critical review. *Experimental & Clinical Endocrinology*, 83, 93–100.

Parillo, M. and Riccardi, G. (2004). Diet composition and the risk of type 2 diabetes: epidemiological and clinical evidence. *British Journal of Nutrition*, 92, 7–19.

Patterson, C.C., Gyurus, E., Rosenbauer, J., et al. (2012). Trends in childhood type 1 diabetes incidence in Europe during 1989–2008: evidence of non-uniformity over time in rates of increase. *Diabetologia*, 55, 2142–7.

Permutt, M.A., Wasson, J., and Cox, N. (2005). Genetic epidemiology of diabetes. *Journal of Clinical Investigation*, 115, 1431–9.

Roglic, G. and Unwin, N. (2010). Mortality attributable to diabetes: estimates for the year 2010. *Diabetes Research and Clinical Practice*, 87, 15–19.

Roglic, G., Unwin, N., Bennett, P.H., et al. (2005). The burden of mortality attributable to diabetes: realistic estimates for the year 2000. *Diabetes Care*, 28, 2130–5.

Roper, N.A., Bilous, R.W., Kelly, W.F., Unwin, N.C., and Connolly, V.M. (2001). Excess mortality in a population with diabetes and the impact of material deprivation: longitudinal, population based study. *BMJ*, 322, 1389–93.

Roper, N.A., Bilous, R.W., Kelly, W.F., Unwin, N.C., and Connolly, V.M. (2002). Cause-specific mortality in a population with diabetes: South Tees Diabetes Mortality Study. *Diabetes Care*, 25, 43–8.

Roy, M.S., Klein, R., O'Colmain, B.J., Klein, B.E.K., Moss, S.E., and Kempen, J.H. (2004). The prevalence of diabetic retinopathy among adult type 1 diabetic persons in the United States. *Archives of Ophthalmology*, 122, 546–51.

Simmons, R., Harding, A.H., Jakes, R., Welch, A., Wareham, N., and Griffin, S. (2006). How much might achievement of diabetes prevention behaviour goals reduce the incidence of diabetes if implemented at the population level? *Diabetologia*, 49, 905–11.

Spijkerman, A.M., Dekker, J.M., Nijpels, G., et al. (2003). Microvascular complications at time of diagnosis of type 2 diabetes are similar among diabetic patients detected by targeted screening and patients newly diagnosed in general practice: the Hoorn screening study. *Diabetes Care*, 26, 2604–8.

Stamler, J., Vaccaro, O., Neaton, J.D., and Wentworth, D. (1993). Diabetes, other risk factors, and 12-yr cardiovascular mortality for men screened in the Multiple Risk Factor Intervention Trial. *Diabetes Care*, 16, 434–44.

Tapp, R.J., Zimmet, P.Z., Harper, C.A., et al. (2006). Diagnostic thresholds for diabetes: the association of retinopathy and albuminuria with glycaemia. *Diabetes Research and Clinical Practice*, 73, 315–21.

Targher, G. and Byrne, C.D. (2013). Clinical review: nonalcoholic fatty liver disease: a novel cardiometabolic risk factor for type 2 diabetes and its complications. *Journal of Clinical Endocrinology and Metabolism*, 98, 483–95.

Taylor, R. (2008). Pathogenesis of type 2 diabetes: tracing the reverse route from cure to cause. *Diabetologia*, 51, 1781–9.

The Expert Committee on The Diagnosis And Classification Of Diabetes Mellitus (1997). Report of the Expert Committee on the Diagnosis and Classification of Diabetes Mellitus. *Diabetes Care*, 20, 1183–97.

Todd, J.A., Knip, M., and Mathieu, C. (2011). Strategies for the prevention of autoimmune type 1 diabetes. *Diabetic Medicine*, 28, 1141–3.

Tuomi, T., Groop, L.C., Zimmet, P.Z., Rowley, M.J., Knowles, W., and MacKay, I.R. (1993). Antibodies to glutamic acid decarboxylase reveal latent autoimmune diabetes mellitus in adults with a non-insulin-dependent onset of disease. *Diabetes*, 42, 359–62.

Unite For Diabetes (2006). *Resolution Adopted by the General Assembly: 61/225. World Diabetes Day* [Online]. Available at: http://www.unitefordiabetes.org/campaign/resolution.html.

Unwin, N. (2007). Diabetes and the good, the bad and the ugly of globalization. *International Diabetes Monitor*, 19, 5–10.

Unwin, N., Shaw, J., Zimmet, P., and Alberti, K.G. (2002). Impaired glucose tolerance and impaired fasting glycaemia: the current status on definition and intervention. *Diabetic Medicine*, 19, 708–23.

Van Dam, R.M. and Hu, F.B. (2005). Coffee consumption and risk of type 2 diabetes: a systematic review. *Journal of the American Medical Association*, 294, 97–104.

Vazquez, G., Duval, S., Jacobs, D.R., Jr., and Silventoinen, K. (2007). Comparison of body mass index, waist circumference, and waist/hip ratio in predicting incident diabetes: a meta-analysis. *Epidemiologic Reviews*, 29, 115–28.

Vehik, K. and Dabelea, D. (2011). The changing epidemiology of type 1 diabetes: why is it going through the roof? *Diabetes/Metabolism Research and Reviews*, 27, 3–13.

Venkat Narayan, K.M., Zhang, P., Kanaya, A.M., et al. (2006). Diabetes: the pandemic and potential solutions. In D.T. Jamison, J.G. Breman, A.R. Measham, et al. (eds.) *Disease Control Priorities in Developing Countries* (2nd ed.), pp. 591–604. Washington, DC: World Bank and Oxford University Press.

Walker, C. and Unwin, N. (2010). Estimates of the impact of diabetes on the incidence of pulmonary tuberculosis in different ethnic groups in England. *Thorax*, 65, 578–81.

Whiting, D., Unwin, N., and Roglic, G. (2010). Diabetes: equity and social determinants. In E. Blas and A.S. Kurup (eds.) *Equity, Social Determinants and Public Health Programmes*, pp. 77–94. Geneva: WHO.

Whiting, D.R., Guariguata, L., Weil, C., and Shaw, J. (2011). IDF Diabetes Atlas: global estimates of the prevalence of diabetes for 2011 and 2030. *Diabetes Research and Clinical Practice*, 94, 311–21.

Willi, C., Bodenmann, P., Ghali, W.A., Faris, P.D., and Cornuz, J. (2007). Active smoking and the risk of type 2 diabetes: a systematic review and meta-analysis. *Journal of the American Medical Association*, 298, 2654–64.

Williams, R. (2005). Medical and economic case for prevention of type 2 diabetes and cardiovascular disease. *European Heart Journal Supplement*, 7, D14–17.

World Health Organization (1999). *Definition, Diagnosis, and Classification of Diabetes Mellitus and its Complications. Report of a WHO Consultation. Part 1: Diagnosis and Classification of Diabetes Mellitus*. Geneva: WHO.

World Health Organization (2006). *Definition and Diagnosis of Diabetes Mellitus and Intermediate Hyperglycemia: Report of a WHO/IDF Consultation*. Geneva: WHO.

World Health Organization (2011). *Use of Glycated Haemoglobin (HbA1c) in the Diagnosis of Diabetes Mellitus: Abbreviated Report of a WHO Consultation*. Geneva: WHO.

Xu, F., Yin, X.M., Zhang, M., Leslie, E., Ware, R., and Owen, N. (2006). Family average income and diagnosed type 2 diabetes in urban and rural residents in regional mainland China. *Diabetic Medicine*, 23, 1239–46.

Yudkin, J.S. (2000). Insulin for the world's poorest countries. *The Lancet*, 355, 919–21.

Zhang, P., Zhang, X., Brown, J., et al. (2010). Global healthcare expenditure on diabetes for 2010 and 2030. *Diabetes Research and Clinical Practice*, 87, 293–301.

Zimmet, P.Z. (1992). Kelly West Lecture 1991. Challenges in diabetes epidemiology—from West to the rest. *Diabetes Care*, 15, 232–52.

Public mental health and suicide

Kristian Wahlbeck and Danuta Wasserman

Introduction to public mental health and suicide

As defined by the World Health Organization (WHO), mental health is not just the absence of illness, rather it is conceptualized as a state of well-being in which the individual realizes his or her own abilities, can cope with the normal stresses of life, can work productively and fruitfully, and is able to make a contribution to his or her community (WHO 2013). Consequently, public mental health is not just about the occurrence and prevention of mental disorders in the population, but it also concerns the promotion of mental health and well-being. Thus, public mental health can be defined as actions aimed at developing the mental health of populations and producing healthy societies.

Public mental health research encompasses research that describes collective experience, occurrence, distribution and trajectories of positive mental health, mental health problems, and their determinants; research on mental health promotion and prevention of mental disorders; research on mental health system policies and governance; service delivery; and the organization of mental health services.

Mental health is more crucial today than it has ever been, due to the societal transition into the information society era. The population's mental capital (i.e. cognitive, emotional, and social-skills resources required for role functioning) is a prerequisite for the prosperity of individuals, companies, and societies in this new era. Mental health becomes more valuable and more vulnerable, due to the many stressors in information-driven economies. At the same time, in low-income countries, poverty, discrimination, and poor mental health form a vicious circle which becomes an obstacle to economic development (Patel and Thornicroft 2009).

The huge burden and costs of impaired mental health for individuals, families, society, and the economy call for actions to prevent mental ill health and promote positive mental health and well-being. This necessitates public mental health actions, not only to treat, but also to prevent impaired mental health and promote positive mental well-being.

Magnitude and costs of mental health problems

The magnitude and costs of mental health and mental disorders is relatively neglected (Jané-Llopis et al. 2011), in spite of data showing that mental health is a growing health challenge. The share of burden attributable to mental and behavioural disorders, which is already substantial, will probably increase steadily in the future. The rising burden from mental and behavioural disorders will impose new challenges on health systems worldwide.

The recent update of the Global Burden of Diseases study (Murray et al. 2012) demonstrates the magnitude of the burden of mental health disorders. Disability-adjusted life years (DALYs) include potential years of life lost, due to premature death and equivalent years of 'healthy' life lost by virtue of being in states of poor health or disability. DALY data indicate that mental disorders constitute a growing share of the global disease burden. In 2010, mental and behavioural disorders accounted for 7.4 per cent of DALYs worldwide, which is a significant increase from 1990, when the corresponding figure was 5.4 per cent. A single major source of disability and premature death is major depressive disorder (MDD). From 1990 to 2010, MDD increased in ranking from 15th to 11th place (i.e. a 37 per cent increase) among causes of DALYs worldwide. In order of importance, other main causes of DALYs among mental disorders were anxiety disorders (1.1 per cent of DALYs worldwide), drug use disorders (0.8 per cent), alcohol use disorders (0.7 per cent), and schizophrenia (0.6 per cent) (Murray et al. 2012). Self-harm, which in 2010 ranked number 18 among worldwide causes of DALYs, adds to the total impact of mental and behavioural disorders on population health.

The distribution of DALYs varies considerably between geographical regions. The relative contribution of mental and behavioural disorders is as a rule higher in developed economies According to the Global Burden of Diseases study, mental disorders accounted for 11 per cent of the total burden of illness in high-income regions, such as Australasia, Europe, and North America. In many highly developed Western economies, up to half of the disability pensions are granted due to mental disorders, especially depression. It is, thus, foreseeable that a continued increase in the standard of living globally will contribute to a continued epidemiological transition towards increasing public health impact of mental disorders. In many of the developed economies, MDD ranks 3rd, 4th, or 5th among causes of DALYs (Murray et al. 2012). In regions with high suicide mortality rates, such as Eastern Europe, Japan, and South Korea, self-harm ranks 5th or 6th among causes of DALYs.

The disabling burden of mental and behavioural disorders is almost the same for males and females, but the major contributing causes are different. The burden of depression is 50 per cent higher for females than males. In contrast, the occurrence of alcohol and drug use disorders in males is nearly seven times higher than that for females, and accounts for almost one third of the male burden of mental and behavioural disorders. In both low- and middle-income countries, and high-income countries, alcohol use disorders are among the ten leading causes of years lived with disability (YLD). This includes only the direct burden of alcohol dependence and problem use. The total attributable burden of disability, due to alcohol use, is much larger.

The Millennium Development Goals (MDGs) primarily target childhood mortality and communicable diseases. The epidemiological shift from communicable diseases towards non-communicable psychosocial disorders constitutes a global health challenge. When setting the post-2015 development goals, promotion of population mental health is important, as mental health has vast and global well-being consequences. The WHO Action Plan 2013–2020 on mental health, approved by Member States at the WHO World Health Assembly, is a milestone in acknowledging the importance of mental health and the well-being of entire populations (WHO 2013).

Available data confirm the immense disability burden of mental disorders, not only in terms of DALYs, but also in terms of other indicators, such as loss of work days, work life productivity, and poor quality of life (Wittchen et al. 2011). This is due to the critical combination of high prevalence and high level of associated impairments and disabilities of mental disorders. Many mental disorders—anxiety, substance use, and somatoform disorders in particular—start early, which typically has adverse effects on further psychological and social development, thereby reducing school and academic achievement, social functioning, and social integration.

Compared to many somatic diseases, costs for mental disorders differ with disproportionately high indirect cost items (e.g. sick days, disability, early retirement, and deaths due to suicide) and relatively low direct costs of healthcare (i.e. low expenditures for diagnostic measures, treatment, and care). Mental disorders are dominant contributors to the global economic burden of diseases. The global cost of mental health conditions in 2010 was estimated at US$2.5 trillion, with the cost projected to surge to US$6 trillion by 2030. About two-thirds of the total cost comes from indirect costs, and the remainder from direct costs. Currently, high-income countries shoulder about 65 per cent of the burden, which is not expected to change over the next 20 years (Bloom et al. 2011).

For instance, in Europe, depressive disorder is a major cause of lost productivity (Wahlbeck 2009). In 2004, economic costs of depression were estimated to be €250 per inhabitant, or €118 billion. As mentioned earlier, direct costs account for only a minor part of the total economic burden (Sobocki et al. 2006). A majority of costs, between 65 and 85 per cent, are indirect. Data from Europe indicate that costs for depression are increasing (Sobocki et al. 2007).

People with mental disorders, including substance use disorders, are at risk of suicide. Ninety per cent of suicides are estimated to be associated with mental disorders, mostly with mood disorders, like depression, which is associated with 60 per cent of suicides (Mann et al. 2005) and also with alcohol use disorders. However, suicide is not a disease caused by well-defined pathological mechanisms,

and the occurrence of suicidal behaviour is usually an outcome of complex interactions of socioenvironmental, behavioural, and psychiatric factors. High-risk groups include those with severe somatic illness, the socially disadvantaged, those with recent loss, especially through suicide (Nordentoft 2007), and some migrant groups (Garssen et al. 2006; Westman al. 2006). People with a history of suicide attempts are especially at higher risk of dying by suicide.

According to WHO data, suicides (i.e. deaths caused from self-inflicted intentional injuries) amounted to 782,000 in 2008, which was 1.4 per cent of the total world mortality, ranging from 0.5 per cent in the African region to 1.9 per cent in the South-East Asian region (Värnik 2012). However, the WHO estimate includes neither injury deaths of undetermined intent nor deaths from unknown causes, which are generally believed to conceal unrecognized suicides. Moreover, the data from all WHO member states are not reported.

The estimated global suicide rate is 14 suicides per 100,000 inhabitants, including 18 suicides per 100,000 for males and 11 suicides per 100,000 for females. For both males and females, the highest suicide rates are found in Europe, predominantly in Eastern Europe, that is, Lithuania, the Russian Federation, Belarus and, to a lesser extent, Finland, Hungary, and Latvia: a group of countries that share similar historical and sociocultural characteristics, as well as similar alcohol use patterns. Nevertheless, some similarly high rates are found in countries that are quite distinct in relation to these characteristics, such as Cuba, Japan, Sri Lanka, and South Korea. As a whole, the lowest rates are found in Islamic countries (Bertolote and Fleischmann 2009). Due to stigmatization and legal sanctions against suicide, underreporting of suicide rates in Muslim countries may partly contribute to the low suicide mortality rates reported (Khan and Syed 2011).

The male suicide rate is higher than the rate of females, with the exception of youth suicide rates in some Asian countries, where the sex differences for suicide are reversed, and young women are more at risk for suicide than men, mainly due to impulsive attempts using pesticides as the mode of attempt (Law and Liu 2008).

Suicide in later life is a global public health problem. Those aged 65 years and above are the demographic group that constitutes the highest suicide rate in most countries reporting suicide statistics to the WHO. Non-fatal suicidal acts tend to be less common in this age group (Fässberg et al. 2012).

The epidemiology of adolescent suicide has shown striking changes over the last 100 years, with a steady decline in recent decades. One of the suggested factors explaining this trend is the growing use of antidepressants, especially selective serotonin reuptake inhibitors, in the adolescent population (Bursztein and Apter 2009). Even within countries, there is significant variability in suicidal ideation and behaviours among adolescents of different ethnic backgrounds. In the United States, American Indian/Alaska Native youth tend to have the highest rates of fatal suicidal behaviour among all ethnic groups. There are similar findings for Inuit populations in Canada, and the Ethiopian population in Israel, with regards to fatal suicide. All of these youth show a similar pattern of failure to integrate traditional cultures with a modern Western culture (Amitai and Apter 2012).

Suicide rates are higher in many disadvantaged populations groups, such as ethnic or sexual minorities. Family rejection or negative family reaction to an adolescent who is gay, lesbian, or bisexual is associated with an eightfold greater likelihood of attempting suicide compared to adolescents who experienced minimal or no family rejection (Ryan et al. 2009). The suicide risk of gay and lesbian youth is amendable; lesbian and gay youths living in areas with school anti-bullying policies that did not specifically mention sexual orientation as a protected group were nearly two times more likely to have attempted suicide in the past year compared with those living in counties where more districts had these policies (Hatzenbuehler and Keyes 2013).

A highly increased risk of suicide after a suicide attempt can be found in people with a mental disorder. To reduce risk of attempting further suicides, people with mental disorders need after-care, especially during the first 2 years after the suicide attempt (Tidemalm et al. 2008).

During the last 50 years, the epicentre of suicide mortality has moved eastwards from Western Europe to Eastern Europe and now to Asia. The biggest contributors to the number of suicides in the world are China and India, where half of the total suicides in the world occur, while South Korea has experienced enormous growth in suicide rates during the past decade (Vijayakumar 2004; Värnik 2012).

Mental health policy

In spite of their public health impact, mental health issues were largely neglected in the international public health agenda until the 1990s. In order to successfully introduce mental health issues on the political agenda during that time, a new approach has been developed in Europe. It has been stressed that mental health cannot be reduced to an issue about mental disorders. Neither the high prevalence of mental disorders, nor the need for more resources in psychiatry was used as entry points, thus, avoiding the stigma associated with mental disorders. Instead, it has been stressed that mental health is an indivisible part of public health, and that it has a significant impact on countries and their human, social and economic capital. The aim has been to raise mental health from its professional, organizational, and even political isolation to a broader sphere of public health, that is, to shift the focus from the individual level towards strengthening the mental health approach at the population level. Acknowledging the psychosocial determinants of mental health opens the door for horizontal actions to promote population mental health (Wahlbeck 2011b).

It is now widely accepted that major mental health determinants are modifiable by policy actions. During the last decades, many governments and intergovernmental organizations have developed mental health policies, as a response to increasing mental health needs in the population. Typical objectives of the policies are increased parity between mental and physical disorders, reduction of stigma, respect for human rights, a shift from hospital-based to community-based service provision and strengthening of mental healthcare capacity in primary care.

The lessons of the successful control of infectious and cardiovascular diseases indicate that the road to improved mental health among populations lies not in the investment of mental health services, but in promotion and prevention activities. Thus, lately many policy documents have taken the 'Health in All Policies' (HiAP) approach, that is, targeting determinants of mental health across policy areas in the whole population, reaching out to public policymakers to mainstream mental health promotion and prevention of mental health problems in non-health policies. HiAP is a relatively new approach to the development, implementation, and assessment of public policies across sectors that systematically take into account the health implications of decisions. It can be seen as a strategy to recognize that mental health is largely constructed in other sectors than in the health sector (Wahlbeck and Taipale 2006).

The stigma associated with mental disorders may have a negative impact on the willingness of decision-makers to commit to a high-level mental health policy. A clear public health approach, and making mental health promotion one of the core objectives, will highlight the productivity links of mental health, and offers a route to successfully avoiding the stigma and discrimination attached to mental health issues.

Mental disorders are inextricably linked to human rights issues. The stigma, discrimination, and human rights violations that individuals and families affected by mental disorders suffer are intense and pervasive. Most international mental health policy documents build on the human rights principles and stress the need for respectful treatment and empowerment of mental health service users. The United Nations Convention on the Rights of People with Disabilities (CRPD), adopted in 2006, affirms that people with mental health disabilities have the right to full participation and inclusion in society, including the right to live independently, the right to education, and the right to work. The CRPD, and related pressure from the international community, will increasingly put human and fundamental rights issues at the forefront of new regional and national mental health policies across the globe.

In May 2013, the WHO World Health Assembly approved the first WHO action plan on mental health, covering the period from 2013 to 2020 (WHO 2013). The plan's four major objectives are to: strengthen effective leadership and governance for mental health; provide comprehensive, integrated, and responsive mental health and social care services in community-based settings; implement strategies for promotion and prevention in mental health; and strengthen information systems, evidence, and research for mental health. The plan sets new directions for mental health, including a central role for provision of community-based care, and a greater emphasis on human rights. It also emphasizes the empowerment of people with mental disabilities, the need to develop strong civil society, and implement health promotion and prevention activities. The document proposes specific actions for Member States, the WHO, and partners. It also proposes indicators and targets, such as a 20 per cent increase in service coverage for severe mental disorders, and a 10 per cent reduction of the suicide rate in countries by the year 2020, which can be used to evaluate levels of implementation, progress, and impact.

Setting mental health targets in policy action plans may help focus attention and support implementation. Targets should, however, be formulated as health inequality targets to support mental health improvement and suicide reduction among the most vulnerable groups or in the most deprived areas. To be meaningful, measurement of targets should avoid masking deterioration in one segment of the population by an improvement in another segment (e.g. an increase of suicides in young people by a decrease in older people) (Wahlbeck 2009).

Stigma and public attitudes

People with mental health problems have to cope with a double problem: first, the symptoms of the mental health problem, and second, with the stigma of having a mental health problem (Rüsch et al. 2005). Stigma is a core concept in understanding the field of public mental health and provision of health services. Stigma has an in-depth influence on the status of mental health services, their resource allocation and attractiveness to the work force. It constitutes a barrier that greatly contributes to low help-seeking behaviour among people with mental health problems, and affects provision of services negatively.

Stigma and stereotypes form the public attitude towards people with mental health problems and psychiatry. Stigma related to mental health problems can be divided into: (1) perceived public stigma, that is, stereotype awareness; (2) personal stigma, that is, stereotype agreement (people's personal beliefs about mental illness); and (3) self-stigma (people's view of their own mental health problem) (Rüschet al. 2005). Discrimination of people with mental disorders is a common manifestation of stigma.

Stigma studies across the world have generally shown consistent findings. There is a lack of parity between mental and physical disorders; people with mental disorders, as well as the services they are provided, are less valued. This is extremely unfortunate, because there are clear links between popular understandings of mental illness and whether people in mental distress seek help or feel able to disclose their problems (Littlewood 1998). The core experiences of shame (to oneself or to one's family) and blame (from others) are common, although they vary between cultures. However, international studies have shown that discrimination of people with mental disorders is consistently common across cultures (Thornicroft et al. 2009; Lasalvia et al. 2013).

The stigma concept can be traced back to Goffman (1963) and social interactionists, who focused on the role of social interaction in stigma, including labelling and stereotyping. This view has been challenged by theorists who focus on structural stigma and discrimination; they argue that legislation and empowering people with mental disorders will reduce stigma. Link and Phelan reconciled these different approaches in 2001 in their modified labelling theory (Link and Phelan 2001). They identify stigma as a process involving labelling, stereotyping, separation, status loss, and discrimination. They highlight structural discrimination and disadvantage, and the fact that social, economic, and political power is necessary to stigmatize.

Unfortunately, not even large-scale and expensive anti-stigma campaigns have shown much promise in achieving changes in public attitudes (Sartorius 2010; Henderson and Thornicroft 2013). A combination of positive social contact with people with mental disorders, protest against stigmatizing messages and measures, and education seems to be most effective in fighting stigma. Social contact has shown to be the most promising evidence-based intervention method, including 'proxy' contact, for example, a narrative through a film (Quinn et al. 2011). It seems to be more productive to focus on promoting positive messages and strengths rather than dispelling negative beliefs. Programmes should offer a chance to revise stereotypes through identification with ordinary people and peers. Positive models of extraordinary people with mental disorders may not have the intended effect, because they can be dismissed as exceptions to the norm. At best, anti-stigma activities providing social contacts are mainstreamed in school curricula and training of professionals. Awareness of mental health among young Europeans in combination with role-play activities stimulating social interactions in the classroom and increasing understanding that mental health problems can be prevented are well perceived and attractive to young people (Wassermanet al. 2012).

Sensational reporting and reporting with negative undertone about mental health problems is common in the media. Many national campaigns have a network of contacts who protest against negative stories on the radio, newspapers, or television by using letters, email, and the telephone. This may be effective against reporting that people with severe mental illness are dangerous. Public protests have played a limited role in mental health campaigns compared to other civil rights movements, perhaps due to the very deeply held prejudice in society and potential for ridicule (Goldie et al. 2012).

Mental health determinants

Social, behavioural, and biological sciences have provided substantial insight into the role of risk and protective factors in the developmental pathways to mental health and mental disorders. Biological, psychological, social, and societal risk and protective factors and their interactions have been identified across the lifespan from as early as fetal life. Many of these factors are amendable and, therefore, potential targets for promotion and prevention measures. Other socioeconomic and environmental determinants for mental health problems and disorders are related to macro-issues such as poverty, lack of freedom, war, and inequity (WHO 2004).

The roots of mental health and mental disorders often lay in early life. It is well documented that poor nutrition, exposure to toxic substances such as alcohol during pregnancy, trauma during labour, maternal depression, parental neglect, sexual abuse, other forms of trauma, and lack of stimulation can impact a child's cognitive development and socioemotional status (Richteret al. 2010).

Mental health and mental illnesses are determined by multiple and interacting social, psychological, and biological factors. Individual, familial, and societal determinants of mental health often lie in non-health domains such as social policy, education, and urban planning. Promising evidence has, however, indicated that effective interventions exist (Doughty 2005): interventions in local communities (Hawkins et al. 2002), child support programmes, home visiting programmes (Olds 2002), and school programmes (Weare and Nind 2011) are some examples of effective interventions for improving mental health.

Research has, so far, mainly focused on determinants of mental ill health, largely neglecting the need to identify both risk and protective factors. Lately, there has been a heightened interest in the determinants of positive mental health and well-being. Evidence indicates that social relationships are critical for promoting well-being and buffering against mental ill health (Diener and Seligman 2002). This seems to be the case for people across all ages (Forsman et al. 2013). Although food choices are often linked to well-being in popular press, the evidence on the role of different nutritional factors is complex; thus, the direct links between eating well and feeling good remain ambiguous until more research is completed (Kirkwood et al. 2008). Not enough is known about the effects of physical exercise on mental health. Longitudinal studies provide some evidence to indicate that physical activity protects against cognitive decline in later life and the onset of depressive symptoms and anxiety (Kirkwood et al. 2008).

Mental disorders are, in the developed and developing world alike, associated with disadvantage. Many vulnerable groups are more affected by mental health problems and die more often from suicide. The greater vulnerability of disadvantaged people to mental illnesses may be explained by such factors as the experience of insecurity and hopelessness, rapid social change, and the risks of violence and physical ill health.

Major individual socioeconomic risk factors for mental health problems and suicide are poverty, poor education, unemployment, high debt, social isolation, and major life events. Socially excluded and deprived people are at a higher risk of developing mental health problems, especially depression.

On the community level, suicides are linked with socioeconomic deprivation and unemployment (Rehkopf and Buka 2005; Middleton et al. 2006). In Europe, between 1970 and 2007, a more than 3 per cent increase in national unemployment rate was linked to a 4.5 per cent increase in suicides (Stuckler et al. 2009). Suicides are also linked to social isolation, physical illness, substance abuse, family violence, and access to lethal means of suicide.

The effects of work on mental health are complex. On the one hand, work is a source of personal satisfaction and accomplishment, interpersonal contacts, and financial security. These are all prerequisites for good mental health. The workplace social capital (i.e. trusting relationships) has been shown to protect against depression (Oksanen et al. 2010). Those who become unemployed are twice as likely to have increased depressive symptoms and to be diagnosed with clinical depression compared to those who remain employed (Dooley et al. 1994). On the other hand, there is evidence indicating that a high workload, precarious work, and high emotional demand, as well as school or workplace bullying and violence, are linked with depression.

Prenatal maternal stress is a risk factor for behavioural and mental disorders, including depression. Those born small, due to fetal stressors, have an increased risk of mental disorders (Wahlbeck et al. 2001; Räikkönen et al. 2008; Lahti et al. 2010), as well as of suicide completion and attempt (Mittendorfer-Rutz et al. 2004). Hostile, unstable, and unsupportive parent–child relationships can lead to depression later in life. Corporal punishment, harsh parenting and child abuse (physical, sexual, and emotional), temporary separation (Räikkönen et al. 2011) from parents, and inter-parental conflict are associated with adverse psychological outcomes (Sarchiapone et al. 2007) and disorders in childhood (Madigan et al. 2007) and adolescence (Allen et al. 2007). Children of parents with depression are a high-risk group: six in ten will develop a mental disorder before the age of 25 (Beardslee et al. 1993). Promoting a nurturing early interaction between caregivers and the child increases resilience in the face of adverse life events and promotes life-long mental health and well-being.

Substance use is a risk factor for mental disorders. Alcohol use, for instance, causes depression (Rehm et al. 2003). Alcohol problems lead to a more serious course of depression, including earlier onset of the disorder, more episodes of depression, and more suicide attempts (Sher et al. 2008). A rise in per capita alcohol consumption has been linked to a post-war rise in suicide mortality in many European countries (e.g. Denmark, France, Hungary,

Norway, and Sweden), but not in southern Europe (Norström and Ramstedt 2005). The link seems to be more pronounced in countries where strong spirits dominate the consumption. There is strong evidence supporting the effectiveness of policies that regulate the alcohol market, for example, by taxation and restricting access, in reducing the harm done by alcohol (Anderson 2006). A natural experiment in the former USSR during the Gorbachev rule in the second half of the 1980s, characterized not only by political reforms, but also by strict limits on the sale of alcohol and restrictive attitude towards alcohol consumption, resulted in history's most effective suicide prevention programme for men (Wasserman et al. 1998). Promotion of a healthy lifestyle and avoidance of harmful drinking are cornerstones in promoting good mental health and preventing suicides.

Mental, social, and behavioural health problems interact, which may intensify their effects on behaviour and well-being. Substance abuse, violence, and abuses of women and children, on the one hand, and health problems such as heart disease, depression, and anxiety on the other, are more prevalent and more difficult to cope with in conditions of high unemployment, low income, limited education, stressful work conditions, gender discrimination, unhealthy lifestyle, and human rights violations.

Well-being and mental health promotion

In recent years, there has been a discernible shift of focus in the field of public mental health from illness to well-being. The emergence of positive psychology, and the science of well-being, has brought with it a greater interest in establishing the underlying causes of positive mental health and well-being. Standardized measures of well-being have been used in population-based surveys (Bech et al. 2003; Tennant et al. 2007) and there are several countries in Northwestern Europe (e.g. England, Iceland, and Scotland) that perform repeated measures of mental well-being in the population.

Mental health promotion aims to improve mental health of the population by strengthening well-being. It implies the creation of individual, social, and environmental conditions that are empowering and enable optimal health and development. Such initiatives involve individuals in the process of achieving positive mental health, well-being, and quality of life. Mental health promotion is an enabling process, done by, with, and for the people.

Common principles and recommendations for modern mental health promotion were laid by The Melbourne Charter in 2008. The Charter provides a framework which recognizes the influence of social and economic determinants on mental health and mental illness, and it identifies the contribution that diverse sectors (including but not exclusive to health) make in influencing those conditions that create or ameliorate positive mental health. The Charter stresses that mental health promotion is everybody's concern and responsibility; that mental well-being is best achieved in equitable, just, and non-violent societies; and that mental health is best promoted through respectful, participatory means where culture and cultural heritage and diversity are acknowledged and valued (Global Consortium for the Advancement of Promotion and Prevention in Mental Health 2009).

In many aspects, the promotion of mental health overlaps with prevention, yet both are distinct. The emphasis in mental health promotion is on positive mental health and well-being (what can be done to keep people healthy or to become even healthier), rather than illness prevention (what can be done to avoid illness).

Population-based approaches for promoting mental health and well-being utilize principles of public participation, engagement, and empowerment and are implemented in everyday contexts such as in families, schools, and workplaces. Effective mental health promotion builds on cross-sectoral collaboration with non-health sectors, including education, housing, employment and industry, transport, arts, sports, urban planning, and justice.

Disadvantaged and vulnerable populations have a significant need for mental health promotion action. Strengthening mental health adds to the human capital asset of vulnerable populations. The promotion of mental health can play an important role in breaking the intergenerational cycle of poverty and mental ill health through promoting positive mental health outcomes (Petersen et al. 2010).

The concept of well-being comprises two main elements: feeling good (hedonic well-being) and functioning well (eudaimonic well-being). Happiness and enjoyment are aspects of hedonic well-being. Resilience (the capacity to cope with adversity), sense of mastery of one's life, and sense of coherence and optimism are characteristics of eudaimonic well-being (Huppert 2008).

Being in a state known as mindfulness, 'the state of being attentive to and aware of what is taking place in the present', has also been shown to predict positive mental states, self-regulated behaviour, and heightened self-knowledge (Brown and Ryan 2003). Self-determination theory suggests that an open awareness is particularly valuable for choosing behaviours that are consistent with one's needs, values, and interests (Ryan and Deci 2000). This self-regulatory behaviour is thought to be important for well-being.

Although the intervention research-base in mental health promotion is still developing, several effective population-level interventions have been identified (Mrazek and Haggerty 1994). A large range of multifaceted outcomes from mental health promotion programmes have impacted other sectors such as education, labour and employment, and family cohesion; however, effects have often been seen after a longer follow-up time than that usually used in most standard intervention studies.

An important target for mental health promotion interventions is parenting, including early parent–child interaction and approaches to discipline in child upbringing. Programmes should address the intergenerational transition of poor parenting; abused and neglected children are more likely to become adults who are hostile, reject parenting, and display negative discipline practices towards their own children. Parenting support practices need to focus on the positive, taking an empowering approach, and enhancing positive mother–infant and father–infant interaction and enjoyment (Stewart-Brown et al. 2011).

Promoting a nurturing early interaction between caregivers and the child increases the resilience of children in the face of adverse life events and promotes life-long mental health and well-being. Home visitation programmes that provide counselling, as well as a specific intervention to strengthen parent–child interaction, have been shown to be effective when delivered by trained lay women in developing countries (Cooper et al. 2009), and by trained nurses in developed settings (Olds 2002). Such programmes have shown good effects, improving maternal sensitivity and reducing intrusiveness and improving attachment of children (Cooper et al. 2009).

The past two decades have seen a significant growth of research and good practice on mental health prevention and promotion in schools. Schools are an important setting for mental health promotion, through their role in helping to establish identity, interpersonal relationships, and other transferable skills. Across the world, an increasing number of schools are engaging in a wide range of mental health-related initiatives and policies, which, in many places, are showing promising results. Activities operate under a variety of headings, not only 'mental health', but also 'social and emotional learning', 'emotional literacy', 'emotional intelligence', 'resilience', 'life skills', and 'character education'. There is growing evidence showing the effectiveness of mental health promotion in schools. Positive impacts include the reduction of depression, aggression, impulsiveness, and antisocial behaviour, as well as the development of proficiencies that promote mental health such as cooperation, resilience, a sense of optimism, empathy, and a positive and realistic self-concept. Programmes have also been shown to help prevent and reduce early sexual experience, alcohol and drug use, violence and bullying in and outside schools, to promote pro-social behaviour and, in some cases, reduce juvenile crime (Weare and Nind 2011). Furthermore, mental health promotion programmes significantly improve academic performance. A meta-analysis summarized research on 213 social and emotional learning programmes and found that schools with effective programmes had an 11 percentile improvement in achievement tests, a 25 percentile improvement in social and emotional skills, and a 10 percentile decrease in classroom misbehaviour, anxiety and depression. Data indicates that successful school programmes include those with a sequential and integrated skills curriculum, active forms of learning to promote skills, and a focus on skill development and explicit learning goals (Durlak et al. 2011). Teacher well-being is an important component of the whole-school approach to mental well-being; results of an European study (Wasserman et al. 2010; Carli et al. 2013) showed that psychological well-being of teachers is linked to teachers' readiness to help pupils with mental health problems (Sisask et al. 2014).

For the adult population, the workplace is an important setting for mental health promotion. Actions can be implemented at both an organizational level within the workplace and targeted at specific individuals. The former can target managers and include measures to promote awareness of mental health and well-being in the workplace and improve managers' skills in risk-management of stress and poor mental health. This can be achieved by examining job content, working conditions, terms of employment, social relations at work, modifications to the physical working environment, flexible working hours, improved employer–employee communication, and opportunities for career progression. Actions targeted at individuals can include modifying workloads, providing cognitive behavioural therapy, relaxation and meditation training, time management training, exercise programmes, journaling, biofeedback and goal-setting. Structuring employment to create 'good work' brings health benefits to the individual, financial benefits to the corporation, and both direct and indirect improvements to the fabric of society. Effective programmes address work context, work content, and individual resilience. Effective management styles are those that promote organizational justice, workplace support, control possibilities of the work demand, active participation of employees, and provide clear and consistent communication. Effective work content is that which protects employees from unreasonable job demands, promotes employee control and autonomy, flexible working schedules, and job stability. For individuals, effective comprehensive programmes are those that promote training in both resilience and stress management (Czabała et al. 2011).

For older people, the most promising interventions promoting mental health include social activities. Studies have shown that associations exist between social capital in the ageing population and mental health (Forsman et al. 2011b, 2012). Crucial components of the individual-level social capital concept, such as social support and social network size, are negatively associated with depressive symptoms and depression, while loneliness is linked to depressive symptoms and depression. Research has highlighted that civic mistrust and lack of reciprocity or social participation (i.e. low individual-level social capital) are associated with depressive symptoms among older adults. Mental health of older adults can be strengthened by addressing social capital. With an increasing retirement age in many countries, work may well have a protective effect for older people, but only if it is flexible enough to take into account older people's differing capabilities and needs. Data highlight the effectiveness and subjective importance of social activities in maintaining mental health and well-being among older adults. The social activities are an important mental health resource among older adults, because of the accompanied sense of belonging to a social group, as well as feelings of purpose, with regard to everyday life and hope for the future. Psychosocial interventions aiming to increase the social contacts of older participants tend to improve mental well-being, as this reduces feelings of loneliness. In a recent systematic review and meta-analysis, social activities among older people significantly reduced depressive symptoms when compared to no-intervention controls (Forsman et al. 2011a).

Prevention of mental disorders

Prevention of mental health problems and disorders has a long history. The early ideas of the mental hygiene movement, at the beginning of the twentieth century, were first translated into experimental activities in primary healthcare, schools, and public health practices. However, the systematic development of science-based prevention programmes and controlled studies to test the effectiveness of preventive interventions did not emerge until around 1980. Since then, the multidisciplinary field of prevention science in mental health has developed at a rapid pace, facilitated by increasing knowledge on malleable risk and protective factors, generating evidence showing that preventive interventions can influence risk and protective factors and reduce the incidence and prevalence of some mental disorders (WHO 2004).

Mental disorder prevention aims at reducing occurrence, frequency and relapses, the time spent with symptoms, or the risk for a mental illness, preventing or delaying their occurrence and decreasing their impact in the affected person, their families, and society. Recently, there has been a wider acceptance and recognition of the importance of prevention in mental disorders.

Many of the effective preventive measures are harmonious with principles of social equity, equal opportunity, and care of vulnerable groups in society. Examples of these interventions include improving nutrition, ensuring primary education, access to the labour market, removing discrimination based on race and gender, and ensuring basic economic security. A particularly potent and unfortunately common threat to mental health is conflict and violence, both between individuals and between communities and countries. The resulting mental distress and disorders are substantial. Preventing violence requires larger societal efforts, but mental health professionals may be able to ameliorate the negative impact of these phenomena by implementing some specific preventive efforts and making humanitarian assistance more mental health friendly (WHO 2004).

Prevention can be categorized in a number of ways: primary prevention focuses on addressing wider determinants across whole populations. Depending on the target group, primary prevention can be universal, selective, or indicated. Selective prevention focuses on targeting groups at higher risk of developing a disorder. Indicated prevention targets high-risk people who are identified as having minimal, but detectable, signs or symptoms foreshadowing mental disorder or biological markers indicating predisposition for mental disorder, but who do not meet all diagnostic criteria for a disorder at that time. Secondary prevention involves early detection and intervention. Tertiary prevention involves working with those with an established disease in order to promote recovery and reduce the risk of relapse (Mrazek and Haggerty 1994; Campion et al. 2012).

It is increasingly accepted that prevention efforts will have a broader spectrum impact, not only on mental health, but also on employability, educational achievement, and social adjustment. This is due to common risk factors for mental disorders and possibilities in life. By acting on common risk factors, instead of trying to prevent specific disorders, a range of positive outcomes will be achieved.

The postnatal period is important for the mental health in mother and child. Research shows that the mother's depression has consequences on the cognitive development of the baby. It has been repeatedly shown that children of families with parental mental disorder have an increased risk of developing mental disorders. A range of interventions have been developed aiming to prevent trans-generational transfer by addressing risk and protective factors in children and their families. Issues addressed include the family's knowledge about mental illness, fostering psychosocial resilience in children, improving parent–child and family interactions, diminishing stigma, and increasing social network support. Some interventions target early parent–child interaction; others use a whole-family approach during childhood and early adolescence or focus on the children at risk themselves. A recent systematic review and meta-analysis indicated that the risk of mental disorders in the offspring can be reduced by 40 per cent by preventive interventions (Siegenthaler et al. 2012).

There is strong evidence showing that improving nutrition and development in socioeconomically disadvantaged children can lead to healthy cognitive development, improved educational outcomes, and reduced risk for mental ill health, especially for those at risk or who are living in impoverished communities. The most effective intervention models combine nutritional interventions (such as food supplementation) and growth charts with counselling and psychosocial care (e.g. warmth, attentive listening) (WHO 2004). In addition, iodine, which secures an adequate function of the thyroid, plays a key role in preventing mental and physical retardation and impairment in learning ability. A low to moderate iodine intake during early gestation has been linked to lower verbal IQ and poorer reading ability of offspring at age 8–9 years. Iodine supplementation programmes ensure that children obtain adequate levels of iodine through iodized salt or water. Pregnant women may in addition need targeted prevention actions to ensure sufficient iodine intake (Bath et al. 2013).

Bullying among youth is a significant public health problem; it is prevalent and frequently has detrimental effects. Being a victim of bullying is associated with being depressed or anxious, poor social and emotional adjustment, and lower academic achievement (Hertz et al. 2013). Data indicates a causal association between being a bully-victim and subsequent depression and panic disorder as well as subsequent suicide-related behaviours (Klomek et al. 2010; Copeland et al. 2013). Prevention of bullying would improve mental health outcomes for many young people, and effective anti-bullying prevention programmes have been developed. A meta-analysis of school bullying strategies concluded that whole-school approaches that included multiple disciplines and complementary components directed at different levels of school organization more often reduced victimization and bullying than the interventions that only included classroom-level curricula or social skills groups (Vreeman and Carroll 2007).

Community systems-strengthening has its roots in the action that communities have always taken to protect and support their members. Modern approaches to community healthcare are reflected in the WHO Alma Ata declaration of 1978, and in more recent WHO work on the social determinants of health (WHO n.d.). Community systems-strengthening interventions focus on developing empowering processes and building a sense of ownership and social responsibility within community members. An example of such an intervention is the *Communities that Care* (CTC) programme, which has been implemented successfully in the United States and is currently being adopted and replicated in several developed countries. The CTC intervention activates communities to implement community violence and aggression prevention systems (Hawkins et al. 2002). The strategy helps communities use local data on risk and protective factors to identify risks and develop actions. These include interventions that operate simultaneously at multiple ecological levels: the community (e.g. mobilization, media, and policy change), the school (e.g. changing school management structures, curricula, and teaching practices), the family (e.g. parent training strategies), and the individual (e.g. social competence strategies). Evaluations at various CTC sites have indicated improvements in youth outcomes such as reduction in school problems, weapons charges, burglary, drug offences, and assault charges.

There is rich evidence showing that conduct disorders, aggression, and violence of young people can be prevented. The most successful preventive interventions to reduce the risk of aggressive behaviour and conduct disorders focus on improving the social competence and pro-social behaviour of children, parents, peers, and teachers. Universal interventions that have been shown to have a successful impact on conduct problems are all school based and include classroom behaviour management, enhancing child social skills, and multimodal strategies, including the involvement of parents. Classroom behaviour management programmes (e.g. *Good Behaviour Game*) attempt to help children better meet the social demands of the classroom through the overt encouragement of desired behaviours, and the discouragement of undesired behaviours. Social skills programmes (e.g. *I Can Problem Solve* or *Promoting Alternative THinking Strategies* (PATHS)) attempt to provide children with cognitive skills that may help them cope better with difficult social situations. Skills related to listening, empathy, interpersonal problem-solving, and conflict and anger management are taught in a classroom setting. Also, selective interventions designed for a variety of settings have been found to be effective in preventing conduct problems, including prenatal and/or early childhood programmes and school or community-based programmes. Prenatal and/or early childhood programmes usually attempt to improve the skills of parents to nurture, support, and teach their children pro-social behaviour patterns and/or to develop the social skills of children. These programmes have been shown to decrease child conduct problems during adolescence, including reductions in violence and police arrests. School- or community-based programmes for selective child populations at risk have successfully targeted child social and problem-solving skills and/or parent management skills, resulting in a decrease in negative parent–child interactions and teacher ratings of conduct problems at school (Powell et al. 2007).

Recent research demonstrates that depressive episodes can be prevented in a cost-effective way and even in a cost-saving way (Cuijpers et al. 2012). Preventive interventions can reduce the incidence of new episodes of MDD by about 25 per cent. Adding a stepped-care model to the preventive intervention may reduce the number of new episodes even more (van't Veer-Tazelaar et al. 2009). Methods with proven effectiveness involve educational, psychotherapeutic, pharmacological, lifestyle, and nutritional interventions. School-based programmes targeting cognitive, problem-solving, and social skills of children and adolescents (e.g. *The Resourceful Adolescent Programme*) have reported a reduction in high depressive symptom levels of 50 per cent or more a year after the intervention. Several selective interventions targeted at coping with major life events have shown significant and long-term reduction in high levels of depressive symptoms, such as programmes for children with parental death or divorce or for unemployed adults. Indicated programmes for those with elevated levels of depressive symptoms, but no depressive disorder, have shown significant effects in reducing high levels of depressive symptoms and preventing depressive episodes. Such programmes mainly use a group format to educate people at risk in positive thinking, challenge negative thinking styles and improve problem-solving skills and have been shown to be effective in school (Clarke et al. 1995) or primary care settings.

Anxiety disorders can successfully be prevented by strengthening emotional resilience, self-confidence, and cognitive problem-solving skills in school-aged children. Cognitive behavioural programmes (e.g. the *FRIENDS* programme) have significantly reduced the first onset of anxiety disorders in school children (WHO 2004).

The evidence for the effectiveness of interventions in preventing post-traumatic stress disorder (PTSD) is limited. However, some studies show that PTSD severity can be reduced by brief preventive trauma-focused cognitive behavioural therapy (CBT). Psychological debriefing does not reduce the incidence or severity of PTSD or related psychological symptoms in civilian victims of crime, assault, or accidental trauma and should not be routinely offered (Gartlehner et al. 2013).

Several eating disorder prevention programmes have been developed and tried among children and adolescents. There is currently limited evidence in the published literature to suggest that any particular type of programme is effective in preventing eating disorders. Eating disorder prevention programmes, based on challenging the thin ideal (*The Body Project*) or promoting energy balance (the *Healthy Weight* intervention) have reduced the risk of future onset of eating disorders, but more research on their effectiveness is needed before large-scale implementation of eating disorder prevention programmes can be initiated (Stice et al. 2013).

Substance abuse disorders can be prevented by universal policy actions by reducing the availability of alcohol and drugs. Effective regulatory interventions include taxation, restrictions on availability, and total bans on all forms of direct and indirect advertising. Policy interventions aimed at reducing the harm from addictive substances have led to the prevention of substance use disorders. When applied to alcohol, education and persuasion strategies usually deal with less alcohol consumption, the hazards of driving under the influence of alcohol, and related topics. Despite their good intentions, public service announcements are considered an ineffective antidote to the high-quality pro-drinking messages that appear much more frequently through paid advertisements in the mass media.

Psychoses are severe mental disorders with a peak incidence in late adolescence and early adulthood. Universal and selective interventions are not yet viable strategies in the prevention of psychoses. The indicated prevention approach and early identification and intervention present promising possibilities to reduce the burden of schizophrenia and other psychoses. Typically, there is a delay of 1–2 years between the onset of schizophrenia and initiation of treatment, due to failure in identifying psychosis, which, in many cases, may have a slow and gradual onset. A prolonged duration of untreated psychosis has been linked to worse outcome. Several population-based preventive programmes have been developed to reduce the duration of untreated psychosis. Improving community awareness and mental health literacy of the general population reduced the delays into treatment in the Norwegian *Treatment and Identification of Psychosis Study* (TIPS) and subsequent studies in Australia. Results in the prevention and delay of transition to psychotic disorder from high-risk state, mostly involving second-generation antipsychotics and CBT, are promising, but currently still insufficient to make recommendations or to be translated into public health practice (Correll et al. 2010).

Prevention of suicides

Public health approaches to suicide prevention have to integrate societal and cultural viewpoints with medical and psychological viewpoints to develop strategies that will save most lives in an effective and measurable way.

Suicides can be prevented by public health actions and suicide prevention has consistently been shown to be highly cost-effective. Considerable evidence is available for the effectiveness of broadly applied population-level interventions, such as restriction of access to lethal means of suicide, responsible media coverage of suicide issues, and community-based multilevel interventions targeting primary care providers, gatekeepers, general populations, and patients with their relatives. The evidence for targeted interventions, which address high-risk groups, such as people who self-harm, people bereaved by suicide, and people with severe mental illness is less convincing but promising (Wasserman et al. 2012). However, selective prevention focusing on high-risk groups is important from the ethical point of view, as it diminishes suffering for the individuals and their families. Although suicide rates are higher in the high-risk groups than in the general population, universal approaches hold the potential to prevent a greater number of deaths (Pitman and Caine 2012).

Preventing suicide by restricting access to lethal methods of suicide is effective. The restriction of access to common and highly lethal suicide means, such as toxic substances and firearms, is successful in reducing suicides. Restriction of one suicide mean seems not to lead to a switch to another. The probability of individuals attempting suicide decreases when they are precluded from implementing a preferred method. Although some individuals might seek other methods, many do not; when they do, the means chosen are less lethal and are associated with fewer deaths than when more dangerous ones are available. When a lethal method is unavailable at the moment of potential action, suicide attempts might be delayed so that, in some cases, suicidal impulses will pass without fatal effects (Yip et al. 2012).

As a public health measure, means restriction has a long history; removal of the pump handle in Broad Street, London, United Kingdom, by John Snow in 1854 was an early example and a historic landmark in public health practice (Johnson 2006). Means restriction entails a community or societal action that does not depend on an individual's intention or volition. Applied to the population as a whole, it typically affects people whose suicide risk is otherwise undetected, and who do not seek therapeutic assistance to prevent their crisis or for life-saving interventions when necessary. Removal or restriction of access to a lethal method changes the context of a potential suicide by precluding potentially fatal actions or forcing the use of a less lethal method.

Application of universal measures for means restriction might be considered intrusive by the general public. The resistance to restrictions and safety measures is underpinned by the common misperception that, despite data showing powerful population level effects, a seriously suicidal person will inevitably find a way to die and that all methods have roughly equal case fatalities. In order to implement means restriction, it is important to address these misunderstandings and gain community support.

Choice of suicide mean varies according to the country and even inside one country, and by age and gender (Ajdacic-Gross et al. 2008). Suicide means used also vary over time. These patterns suggest a close link to differences in the availability and lethality of specific suicide means. Due to availability of pesticides, suicides by pesticide poisoning are common in agrarian populations in Asia (Phillips and Gunnell 2009), whereas access to high buildings and bridges make jumping from high places a common mean of suicide in urban settings (Beautrais and Gibb 2009; Chen and Yip 2009).

In times of peace, most firearm-related deaths are suicides. Enforcement of gun-control policies (e.g. purchase restrictions, waiting times for gun purchase, higher age limits, licensing of firearm owners, safe storage precautions) lowers numbers of firearm suicides (WHO 2010). Empirical data suggest that firearm regulations, which function to reduce overall gun availability, have a significant deterrent effect on male suicide, while regulations that seek to prohibit high-risk individuals from owning firearms have a lesser effect (Rodriguez Andrés and Hempstead 2011). Having a firearm in the home increases the risk of a violent death in the home; the risk of dying from a suicide in the home was tenfold greater for males in homes with guns than for males without guns in the home. Persons with guns in the home were 30-fold more likely to have died from suicide committed with a firearm than from one committed by using a different method (Dahlberg et al. 2004). Guns are highly lethal, require little preparation, and may be chosen over less lethal methods to commit suicide, particularly when the suicide is impulsive. Removal of firearms from people's homes by regulatory means is desirable and would result in a reduction of suicides, but may be difficult to achieve in countries with a strong pro-gun lobby.

Safe environments (e.g. safety doors on railway platforms, barriers on bridges, locked storage of firearms) contribute to suicide prevention. Prevention of suicide can be taken into account during the planning process or after an environment (e.g. bridges and railways) has been identified as a suicide hot-spot (Beautrais et al. 2009; Ladwig et al. 2009).

Improving the awareness and coping skills of the general public, gatekeepers (such as youth workers, police officers, and teachers), general practitioners (GPs), and other healthcare professionals to identify people at risk of suicide has been shown to be an effective way to prevent suicide (Hegerl et al. 2009; Hoven et al. 2009). Responsiveness of services to the needs of individuals with suicidal behaviours is an essential component of suicide prevention. Training of GPs and other healthcare staff to identify depression and substance use problems, and provide adequate treatment has been successful in reducing suicidality and suicides (Appleby et al. 2000). This method is especially useful for preventing suicides in females, as in a number of cultures females have a greater tendency than males to seek help from healthcare professionals (Hadlaczky and Wasserman 2009).

There is significant evidence from around the world to indicate that highly sensationalized reporting of suicides, providing detailed descriptions of the method used, can and does lead to 'copycat' suicides. Suicide contagion is a concept from the infective disease model and assumes that suicidal behaviour may facilitate the occurrence of subsequent, similar behaviours. Imitation refers to the process that explains the occurrence of contagion. Suicide contagion has been investigated primarily in adolescent populations, revealing that up to 5 per cent of all adolescent suicides may be the result of suicide clustering (Westerlund et al. 2009). On the other hand, responsible reporting on suicides reduces copycat suicide, especially among adolescents (Niederkrotenthaler and Sonneck 2007). Liaising with media as well as using the Internet-based systems has an important role in educating the public about depression, suicide preventive methods and responsible coverage of suicide (Westerlund and Wasserman 2009). Media guidelines for reporting suicides and monitoring of stigmatizing media reports have been linked with reduced stigmatization in the press and reduction of suicides. Such reporting guidelines can be based on recommendations set forth by the WHO (2000).

Mental health services

Design, management, and evaluation of mental health services are a core task of public mental health. Today, mental health service provision is in a global transition from hospital-based systems to community-based systems. The change reflects the growing evidence of what constitutes cost-effective care; it also acknowledges the failures concerning issues of social inclusion and human rights of the care systems, which were based on the old-fashioned and remote institutions (asylums).

The recent history of mental health services can be seen in terms of three periods: first, the rise of the asylum; second, the decline of the asylum; and third, balancing mental health services (Table 8.7.1).

Table 8.7.1 The key characteristics of the three periods in the historical development of mental health systems of care

Period 1: the rise of the asylum	Period 2: the decline of the asylum	Period 3: balancing mental services
Asylums built	Asylums neglected	Asylums replaced by smaller facilities
Increasing number of hospital beds	Decreasing number of hospital beds	Decrease in the number of beds slows down
Reduced role for the family	Increasing but not fully recognized role of the family	Importance of families increasingly recognized, in terms of care given, therapeutic potential, the burden carried, and as a political lobbying group
Public investment in institutions	Public disinvestment in mental health services	Increasing private investment in treatment and care and focus in public sector on cost-effectiveness and cost containment
Staff: doctors and nurses only	Clinical psychologist, occupational therapist, and social worker disciplines evolve	More community-based staff and emphasis on multidisciplinary team working
	Effective treatments emerge, beginning of treatment evaluation and of standardized diagnostic systems, growing influence of individual and group psychotherapy	Emergence of 'evidence-based' psychiatry in relation to pharmacological, social, and psychological treatments
Primacy of containment over treatment	Focus on pharmacological control and social rehabilitation, less disabled patients discharged from asylums	Emergence of concern about balance between control of patients and their independence

Adapted with permission from Thornicroft G, and Tansella M, Balancing community-based and hospital-based mental health care, *World Psychiatry*, Volume 1, Issue 2, pp. 84–90, Copyright © 2002.

A modern mental healthcare system is based on balanced care, that is, it includes both modern community-based and modern hospital-based care. In balanced care, the focus is on services that are provided in normal community settings, as close to the population served as possible, and to which admissions to psychiatric wards in a general hospital can be arranged promptly, but only when necessary (Thornicroft and Tansella 1999, 2002; Gaebel et al. 2012).

A health policy supporting the integration of health and social services, and the mainstreaming of mental health services into primary care, improves access to care. Integrating mental health services into general healthcare is the most viable way of implementing balanced care, closing the treatment gap and ensuring that people get the care they need. Because of the high prevalence of mental disorders, only complex and/or severe cases should be treated by specialized mental healthcare. To achieve this consistently, the services need to identify priority groups who should receive access to specialist care from among the 25 per cent of the whole population who suffer from a mental disorder in any given year. Well targeted services are those in which specialist care concentrates on providing direct services to people with the most severe degree of symptoms and disability. Primary care responsibility for common mental health disorders should be supported by accessible referral systems and specialist supervision (Tansella and Thornicroft 1999). Providing even minimal psychotherapy in primary care can prevent full-blown depression (Smit et al. 2006). Programmes aimed at education of primary care physicians have improved the detection of depression and even led to a decrease in suicides due to depression (Rutz 2001). The use of new media, such as e-mental health and smart phone technologies, and the use of lay health counsellors, may boost dissemination of mental health interventions, especially in low- and middle-income countries.

Another cornerstone of a balanced care system is the provision of safe and high-quality home and community-based specialist services. Any developed mental healthcare system encompasses specialized community services for children and adolescents. A modern mental health system includes crisis resolution teams, home treatment, assertive outreach and early intervention teams, day treatment facilities, and supported work. Collated evidence suggests that supported employment schemes, which consist of arranging early placement in normal work with variable support from staff, may offer better outcomes than sheltered or transitional employment approaches. People suffering from mental disorders who want to work should be offered the option of supported employment as part of their treatment package. Current evidence indicates that supported work improves clinical outcomes and supports social inclusion of people with severe mental disorders (Crowther et al. 2001).

In diversified modern mental healthcare systems, particular attention needs to be paid to maintaining high-quality communication between all parts of the care system. There is a need to address three types of interfaces: (1) those within the mental health service, between its components; (2) those within the health service, between mental health and other services (both primary and secondary care); and (3) those between health and other public services, including social services and housing departments.

Available evidence indicates that community-based and diversified mental health systems, with a wide range of services, are superior to hospital-centred mental health systems, according to a range of outcomes. For instance, community-based, well-developed and multifaceted mental health services have been linked with lower suicide rates than hospital-based traditional services (Pirkola et al. 2009). Discharged patients benefit from well-developed community care; community follow-up within 7 days of psychiatric discharge has shown a significant reduction in suicides among recently discharged psychiatric patients (While et al. 2012).

A core element of modern mental healthcare is the empowerment of service users and informal carers. Historically, people with mental health problems have lacked a voice. Empowerment translates into being treated with dignity and respect in mental health services and participation of users and carers in decisions. Data suggest that the possibility to exercise control and influence leads to positive mental health outcomes. These outcomes include increased emotional well-being, independence, motivation to participate, and more effective coping strategies. Key issues that users and carers have expressed to be important to advocate for are the rights to autonomy and self-determination, to acceptable and accessible services, user-led evaluation of services, the right for everyone to be recognized as a person before the law without discrimination, the de-stigmatization of mental disorders, and more inclusive and respectful services with user and carer involvement (WHO 2005). Increased used of peer support and 'experts by experience' in the provision of mental health services will support empowerment of service users and improve services.

Development of mental health service systems requires access to reliable data on mental health services and trends in mental health service provisions. International benchmarking, based on comparable data, is an important moving force for the development of mental health services in countries. Unfortunately, mental health information systems, in most countries, are geared towards hospital data, which are of less interest when developing a community-based mental health service provision system. Many highly relevant aspects of modern service provision, such as patient choice, service user empowerment, and respect for human rights, are hardly ever covered by health information systems (Wahlbeck 2011a).

Acknowledgements

The authors thank Daniel Ventus and Tony Durkee for assistance in preparing the text of this chapter.

References

Ajdacic-Gross, V., Weiss, M.G., Ring, M., et al. (2008). Methods of suicide: international suicide patterns derived from the WHO mortality database. *Bulletin of the World Health Organization*, 86, 726–32.

Allen, J.P., Porter, M., and McFarland, C. (2007). The relation of attachment security to adolescents' paternal and peer relationships, depression, and externalizing behavior. *Child Development*, 78, 1222–39.

Amitai, M. and Apter, A. (2012). Social aspects of suicidal behavior and prevention in early life: a review. *International Journal of Environmental Research and Public Health*, 9(3), 985–94.

Anderson, P. (2006). *Alcohol in Europe: A Public Health Perspective*. Luxembourg: European Commission.

Appleby, L., Morriss, R., Gask, L., et al. (2000). An educational intervention for front-line health professionals in the assessment and management of suicidal patients (The STORM Project). *Psychological Medicine*, 30(4), 805–12.

Bath, S.C., Steer, C.D., Golding, J., Emmett, P., and Rayman, M.P. (2013). Effect of inadequate iodine status in UK pregnant women on cognitive outcomes in their children: results from the Avon Longitudinal Study of Parents and Children (ALSPAC). *The Lancet*, 382(9889), 331–7.

Beardslee, W.R., Keller, M.B., Lavori, P.W., et al. (1993). The impact of parental affective disorder on depression in offspring: a longitudinal follow-up in a nonreferred sample. *Journal of the American Academy of Child & Adolescent Psychiatry*, 32, 723–30.

Beautrais, A. and Gibb, S. (2009). Protecting bridges and high buildings in suicide prevention. In D. Wasserman and C. Wasserman (eds.) *The Oxford Textbook of Suicidology and Suicide Prevention: A Global Perspective*, pp. 563–8. Oxford: Oxford University Press.

Bech, P., Olsen, L.R., Kjoller, M., and Rasmussen, N.K. (2003). Measuring well-being rather than the absence of distress symptoms: a comparison of the SF-36 Mental Health subscale and the WHO-Five Well-Being Scale. *International Journal of Methods in Psychiatric Research*, 12(2), 85–91.

Bertolote, J.M. and Fleischmann, A. (2009). A global perspective of the magnitude of suicide mortality. In D. Wasserman and C. Wasserman (eds.) *The Oxford Textbook of Suicidology and Suicide Prevention: A Global Perspective*, pp. 91–8. Oxford: Oxford University Press.

Bloom, D.E., Cafiero, E.T., Jané-Llopis, E., et al. (2011). *The Global Economic Burden of Noncommunicable Diseases*. Geneva: World Economic Forum.

Brown, K.W. and Ryan, R.M. (2003). The benefits of being present: mindfulness and its role in psychological well-being. *Journal of Personality and Social Psychology*, 84, 822–48.

Burzstein, C. and Apter, A. (2009). Adolescent suicide. *Current Opinion in Psychiatry*, 22, 1–6.

Campion, J., Bhui, K., and Bhugra, D. (2012). European Psychiatric Association (EPA) guidance on prevention of mental disorders. *European Psychiatry*, 27, 68–80.

Carli, V., Wasserman, C., Wasserman, D., et al. (2013). The Saving and Empowering Young Lives in Europe (SEYLE) randomized controlled trial (RCT): methodological issues and participant characteristics. *BMC Public Health*, 13(1), 479.

Chen, Y.-Y. and Yip, P. (2009). Prevention of suicide by jumping: experiences from Taipei City (Taiwan), Hong Kong and Singapore. In D. Wasserman and C. Wasserman (eds.) *The Oxford Textbook of Suicidology and Suicide Prevention: A Global Perspective*, pp. 569–72. Oxford: Oxford University Press.

Clarke, G.N., Hawkins, W., Murphy, M., et al. (1995). Targeted prevention of unipolar depressive disorder in an at-risk sample of high school adolescents: a randomized trial of group cognitive intervention. *Journal of the American Academy of Child & Adolescent Psychiatry*, 34, 312–21.

Cooper, P.J., Tomlinson, M., Swartz, L., et al. (2009). Improving the quality of the mother–infant relationship and infant attachment in a socio-economically deprived community in a South African context: a randomised controlled trial. *BMJ*, 338, b974.

Copeland, W.E., Wolke, D., Angold, A., and Costello, E.J. (2013). Adult psychiatric outcomes of bullying and being bullied by peers in childhood and adolescence. *JAMA Psychiatry*, 70, 419–26.

Correll, C.U., Hauser, M., Auther, A.M., and Cornblatt, B.A. (2010). Research in people with psychosis risk syndrome: a review of the current evidence and future directions. *Journal of Child Psychology and Psychiatry*, 51(4), 390–431.

Crowther, R., Marshall, M., Bond, G.R., and Huxley, P. (2001). Vocational rehabilitation for people with severe mental illness. *Cochrane Database of Systematic Reviews*, 2, CD003080.

Cuijpers, P., Beekman, A.T., and Reynolds, C.F. 3rd. (2012). Preventing depression: a global priority. *Journal of the American Medical Association*, 307(10), 1033–4.

Czabała, C., Charzyńska, K., and Mroziak, B. (2011). Psychosocial interventions in workplace mental health promotion: an overview. *Health Promotion International*, 26(Suppl. 1), i70–84.

Dahlberg, L.L., Ikeda, R.M., and Kresnow, M. (2004). Guns in the home and risk of a violent death in the home: findings from a national study. *American Journal of Epidemiology*, 160, 929–36.

Diener, E. and Seligman, M.E.P. (2002). Very happy people. *Psychological Science*, 13, 81–4.

Dooley, D., Catalano, R., and Wilson, G. (1994). Depression and unemployment: panel findings from the Epidemiologic Catchment Area Study. *American Journal of Community Psychology*, 22(6), 745–65.

Doughty, C. (2005). *The Effectiveness of Mental Health Promotion, Prevention and Early Intervention in Children, Adolescents and Adults. A Critical Appraisal of the Literature*. New Zealand Health Technology Assessment (NZHTA) Report, 8(2). Christchurch: NZHTA.

Durlak, J.A., Weissberg, R.P., Dymnicki, A.B., Taylor, R.D., and Schellinger, K.B. (2011). The impact of enhancing students' social and emotional learning: a meta-analysis of school-based universal interventions. *Child Development*, 82(1), 405–32.

Fässberg, M.M., van Orden, K.A., Duberstein, P., et al. (2012). A systematic review of social factors and suicidal behavior in older adulthood. *International Journal of Environmental Research and Public Health*, 9(3), 722–45.

Forsman, A.K., Nordmyr, J., and Wahlbeck, K. (2011a). Psychosocial interventions for the promotion of mental health and the prevention of depression among older adults. *Health Promotion International*, 26(Suppl. 1), i85–107.

Forsman, A., Nyqvist, F., Herberts, C., Wahlbeck, K., and Schierenbeck, I. (2013). Understanding the role of social capital for mental well-being among older adults. *Ageing & Society*, 33(5), 804–25.

Forsman, A., Nyqvist, F., Schierenbeck, I., Gustafson, Y., and Wahlbeck, K. (2012). Structural and cognitive social capital and depression among older adults in two Nordic regions. *Aging & Mental Health*, 16(6), 771–9.

Forsman, A.K., Nyqvist, F., and Wahlbeck, K. (2011b). Cognitive components of social capital and mental health status among older adults: a population-based cross-sectional study. *Scandinavian Journal of Public Health*, 39, 757–65.

Gaebel, W., Becker, T., Janssen, B., et al. (2012). EPA guidance on the quality of mental health services. *European Psychiatry*, 27(2), 87–113.

Garssen, M.J., Hoogenboezem, J., and Kerkhof, A.J. (2006). [Suicide among migrant populations and native Dutch in The Netherlands]. *Nederlands Tijdschrift voor Geneeskunde*, 150(39), 2143–9.

Gartlehner, G., Forneris, C.A., Brownley, K.A., et al. (2013). *Interventions for the Prevention of Posttraumatic Stress Disorder (PTSD) in Adults after Exposure to Psychological Trauma*. Comparative Effectiveness Review No. 109. Rockville, MD: Agency for Healthcare Research and Quality. Available at: http:// www.effectivehealthcare.ahrq.gov/reports/final.cfm.

Global Consortium for the Advancement of Promotion and Prevention in Mental Health (From Margins to Mainstream: 5th World Conference on the Promotion of Mental Health and the Prevention of Mental and Behavioural Disorders, Melbourne, 2008) (2009). The Melbourne Charter for Promoting Mental Health and Preventing Mental and Behavioural Disorders. [Online] Available at: http://www.vichealth.vic.gov.au/Publications/Mental-health-promotion/Melbourne-Charter.aspx.

Goffman, E. (1963). *Stigma: Notes on Management of Spoiled Identity*. Englewood Cliffs, NJ: Prentice-Hall.

Goldie, I., Quinn, N., and Knifton, L. (2012). *Best Practice Challenging Stigma and Discrimination Against People with Depression: Best Practice Guidelines, Values and Resources. The ASPEN Project*. [Online] Available at: http://www.antistigma.eu/sites/default/files/ASPEN_WP4_BEST_PRACTICE_TOOLKIT.pdf.

Hadlaczky, G. and Wasserman, D. (2009). Suicidality in women. In P.S. Chandra, H. Herrman, J.E. Fisher, et al. (eds.) *Contemporary Topics in Women's Mental Health: Global Perspectives in a Changing Society*, pp. 117–37. Chichester: Wiley.

Hatzenbuehler, M.L. and Keyes, K.M. (2013). Inclusive anti-bullying policies and reduced risk of suicide attempts in lesbian and gay youth. *Journal of Adolescent Health*, 53(Suppl. 1), S21.e6.

Hawkins, J.D., Catalano, R.F., and Arthur, M.W. (2002). Promoting science-based prevention in communities. *Addictive Behaviors*, 27(6), 951–76.

Hegerl, U., Dietrich, S., Pfeiffer-Gerschel, T., Wittenburg, L., and Althaus, D. (2009). Education and awareness programmes for adults: selected and multilevel approaches in suicide prevention. In D. Wasserman and C. Wasserman (eds.) *The Oxford Textbook of Suicidology and Suicide Prevention: A Global Perspective*, pp. 495–500. Oxford: Oxford University Press.

Henderson, C. and Thornicroft, G. (2013). Evaluation of the Time to Change programme in England 2008–2011. *British Journal of Psychiatry*, 202, s45–8.

Hertz, M.F., Donato, I., and Wright, J. (2013). Bullying and suicide: a public health approach. *Journal of Adolescent Health*, 53(Suppl. 1), S1–S3.

Hoven, C.W., Wasserman, D., Wasserman, C., and Mandell, D.J. (2009). Awareness in nine countries: a public health approach to suicide prevention. *Legal Medicine*, 11(Suppl. 1), S13–17.

Huppert, F. (2008). *Psychological Well-Being: Evidence Regarding its Causes and its Consequences*. London: Foresight Mental Capital and Wellbeing Project.

Jané-Llopis, E., Anderson, P., Stewart-Brown, S., et al. (2011). Reducing the silent burden of impaired mental health. *Journal of Health Communication*, 16(Suppl. 2), 59–74.

Johnson, S. (2006). *The Ghost Map: The Story of London's Most Terrifying Epidemic: And How it Changed Science, Cities and the Modern World*. London: Riverhead Books.

Khan, M.M. and Syed, E.U. (2011). Suicide in Asia: epidemiology, risk factors, and prevention. In R.C. O'Connor, S. Platt, and J. Gordon (eds.) *International Handbook of Suicide Prevention: Research, Policy and Practice*, pp. 487–506. Oxford: Wiley-Blackwell.

Kirkwood, T., Bond, J., May, C., McKeith, I., and Teh, M. (2008). *Mental Capital Through Life Challenge Report*. London: Foresight Mental Capital and Wellbeing Project.

Klomek, A.B., Sourander, A., and Gould, A. (2010). The association of suicide and bullying in childhood to young adulthood: a review of cross-sectional and longitudinal research findings. *Canadian Journal of Psychiatry*, 55, 282.e8.

Ladwig, K.-H., Ruf, E., Baumert, J., and Erazo, N. (2009). Prevention of metropolitan and railway suicide. In D. Wasserman and C. Wasserman (eds.) *The Oxford Textbook of Suicidology and Suicide Prevention: A Global Perspective*, pp. 589–94. Oxford: Oxford University Press.

Lahti, M., Räikkönen, K., Wahlbeck, K., et al. (2010). Prenatal origins of hospitalization for personality disorders: the Helsinki Birth Cohort Study. *Psychiatry Research*, 179(2), 226–30.

Lasalvia, A., Zoppei, S., Van Bortel, T., et al. (2013). Global pattern of experienced and anticipated discrimination reported by people with major depressive disorder: a cross-sectional survey. *The Lancet*, 381(9860), 55–62.

Law, S. and Liu, P. (2008). Suicide in China: unique demographic patterns and relationship to depressive disorder. *Current Psychiatry Reports*, 10, 80–6.

Link, B.G. and Phelan, J.C. (2001). Conceptualising stigma. *American Sociological Review*, 27, 363–85.

Littlewood, R. (1998). Cultural variation in the stigmatisation of mental illness. *The Lancet*, 352, 1056–7.

Madigan, S., Moran, G., and Schuengel, C. (2007). Unresolved maternal attachment representations, disrupted maternal behaviour and disorganized attachment in infancy: links to toddler behaviour problems. *Journal of Child Psychology and Psychiatry*, 48, 1042–50.

Mann, J., Apter, A., Bertolote, J., et al. (2005). Suicide prevention strategies—a systematic review. *Journal of the American Medical Association*, 294(16), 2064–74.

Middleton, N., Sterne, J.A.C., and Gunnell, D. (2006). The geography of despair among 15–44-year-old men in England and Wales: putting suicide on the map. *Journal of Epidemiology and Community Health*, 60, 1040–7.

Mittendorfer-Rutz, E., Rasmussen, F., and Wasserman, D. (2004). Restricted fetal growth and adverse maternal psychosocial and socioeconomic conditions as risk factors for suicidal behaviour of offspring: a cohort study. *The Lancet*, 364(9440), 1135–40.

Mrazek, P. and Haggerty, R. (1994). *Reducing Risks of Mental Disorder: Frontiers for Preventive Intervention Research*. Washington, DC: National Academy Press.

Murray, C.J.L., Vos, T., Lozano, R., et al. (2012). Disability-adjusted life years (DALYs) for 291 diseases and injuries in 21 regions, 1990–2010: a systematic analysis for the Global Burden of Disease Study 2010. *The Lancet*, 380, 2197–223.

Niederkrotenthaler, T. and Sonneck, G. (2007). Assessing the impact of media guidelines for reporting on suicides in Austria: interrupted time series analysis. *Australian & New Zealand Journal of Psychiatry*, 41(5), 419–28.

Nordentoft, M. (2007). Prevention of suicide and attempted suicide in Denmark. *Danish Medical Bulletin*, 54(2), 306–69.

Norström, T. and Ramstedt, M. (2005). Mortality and population drinking: a review of the literature. *Drug and Alcohol Review*, 24(6), 537–47.

Oksanen, T., Kouvonen, A., Vahtera, J., et al. (2010). Prospective study of workplace social capital and depression: are vertical and horizontal components equally important? *Journal of Epidemiology and Community Health*, 64(8), 684–9.

Olds, D.L. (2002). Prenatal and infancy home visiting by nurses: from randomized trials to community replication. *Prevention Science*, 3, 1153–72.

Patel, V. and Thornicroft, G. (2009). Packages of care for mental, neurological, and substance use disorders in low- and middle-income countries. *PLoS Medicine*, 6(10), e1000160.

Petersen, I., Swartz, L., Bhana, A., and Flisher, A.J. (2010). Mental health promotion initiatives for children and youth in contexts of poverty: the case of South Africa. *Health Promotion International*, 25(3), 331–41.

Phillips, M.R. and Gunnell, D. (2009). Restrictions of access to pesticides in suicide prevention. In D. Wasserman and C. Wasserman (eds.) *The Oxford Textbook of Suicidology and Suicide Prevention: A Global Perspective*, pp. 583–8. Oxford: Oxford University Press.

Pirkola, S., Sund, R., Sailas, E., and Wahlbeck, K. (2009). Community mental health services and suicide rate in Finland: a nationwide small area analysis. *The Lancet*, 373(9658), 147–53.

Pitman, A. and Caine, E. (2012). The role of the high-risk approach in suicide prevention. *British Journal of Psychiatry*, 201, 175–7.

Powell, N.R., Lochman, J.E., and Boxmeyer, C.L. (2007). The prevention of conduct problems. *International Review of Psychiatry*, 19(6), 597–605.

Quinn, N., Shulman, A., Knifton, L., and Byrne, P. (2011). The impact of a national mental health arts and film festival on stigma and recovery. *Acta Psychiatrica Scandinavica*, 123(1), 71–81.

Räikkönen, K., Lahti, M., Heinonen, K., et al. (2011). Risk of severe mental disorders in adults separated temporarily from their parents in childhood: the Helsinki Birth Cohort Study. *Journal of Psychiatric Research*, 45(3), 332–8.

Räikkönen, K., Pesonen, A.K., Heinonen, K., et al. (2008). Depression in young adults with very low birth weight: the Helsinki study of very low-birth-weight adults. *Archives of General Psychiatry*, 65, 290–6.

Rehkopf, D.H. and Buka, S.L. (2005). The association between suicide and the socio-economic characteristics of geographical areas: a systematic review. *Psychological Medicine*, 36(2), 145–57.

Rehm, J., Room, R., Graham, K., et al. (2003). The relationship of average volume of alcohol consumption and patterns of drinking to burden of disease: an overview. *Addiction*, 98, 1209–28.

Richter, L., Dawes, A., and de Kadt, J. (2010). Early childhood. In I. Petersen, A. Bhana, L. Swartz, A. Flisher, and L. Richter (eds.) *Mental Health Promotion and Prevention for Poorly Resourced Contexts: Emerging Evidence and Practice*, pp. 91–123. Pretoria: HSRC Press.

Rodriguez Andrés, A. and Hempstead, K. (2011). Gun control and suicide: the impact of state firearm regulations in the United States 1995–2004. *Health Policy*, 101, 95–103.

Rüsch, N., Angermeyer, M.C., and Corrigan, P.W. (2005). Mental illness stigma: concepts, consequences, and initiatives to reduce stigma. *European Psychiatry*, 20, 529–39.

Rutz, W. (2001). Preventing suicide and premature death by education and treatment. *Journal of Affective Disorders*, 62, 123–9.

Ryan C., Huebner D., Diaz R.M., and Sanchez J. (2009). Family rejection as a predictor of negative health outcomes in white and Latino lesbian, gay, and bisexual young adults. *Pediatrics*, 123, 346–52.

Ryan, R.M. and Deci, E.L. (2000). Self-determination theory and facilitation of intrinsic motivation, social development, and well-being. *American Psychologist*, 55, 68–78.

Sarchiapone, M., Carli, V., Cumo, C., et al. (2007). Childhood trauma and suicide attempts in patients with unipolar depression. *Depression and Anxiety*, 24(4), 268–72.

Sartorius, N. (2010). Short-lived campaigns are not enough. *Nature*, 468, 163–5.

Sher, L., Stanley, B.H., Harkavy-Friedman, J.M., et al. (2008). Depressed patients with co-occurring alcohol use disorders: a unique patient population. *Journal of Clinical Psychiatry*, 69(6), 907–15.

Siegenthaler, E., Munder, T., and Egger, M. (2012). Effect of preventive interventions in mentally ill parents on the mental health of the offspring: systematic review and meta-analysis. *Journal of the American Academy of Child & Adolescent Psychiatry*, 51(1), 8–17.

Sisask, M., Värnik, P., Värnik, A., et al. (2014). Teacher satisfaction with school and psychological well-being affects their readiness to help children with mental health problems. *Health Education Journal*, 73, 382–93.

Smit, F., Willemse, G., Koopmanschap, M., et al. (2006). Cost-effectiveness of preventing depression in primary care patients: randomised trial. *British Journal of Psychiatry*, 188, 330–6.

Sobocki, P., Jönsson, B., Angst, J., and Rehnberg, C. (2006). Cost of depression in Europe. *Journal of Mental Health Policy and Economics*, 9(2), 87–98.

Sobocki, P., Lekander, I., Borgström, F., et al. (2007). The economic burden of depression in Sweden from 1997 to 2005. *European Psychiatry*, 22(3), 146–52.

Stewart-Brown, S.L. and Schrader-McMillan, A. (2011). Parenting for mental health: what does the evidence say we need to do? Report of Workpackage 2 of the DataPrev project. *Health Promotion International*, 26(Suppl. 1), i10–28.

Stice, E., Becker, C.B., and Yokum, S. (2013). Eating disorder prevention: current evidence-base and future directions. *International Journal of Eating Disorders*, 46(5), 478–85.

Stuckler, D., Basu, S., Suhrcke, M., et al. (2009). The public health effect of economic crises and alternative policy responses in Europe: an empirical analysis. *The Lancet*, 374(9686), 315–23.

Tansella, M. and Thornicroft, G. (1999). *Common Mental Disorders in Primary Care*. London: Routledge.

Tennant, R., Hiller, L., Fishwick, R., et al. (2007). The Warwick–Edinburgh Mental Well-being Scale (WEMWBS): development and UK validation. *Health and Quality of Life Outcomes*, 5, 63.

Thornicroft, G., Brohan, E., Rose, D., Sartorius, N., Leese, M.; INDIGO Study Group (2009). Global pattern of experienced and anticipated discrimination against people with schizophrenia: a cross-sectional survey. *The Lancet*, 373(9661), 408–15.

Thornicroft, G. and Tansella, M. (1999). *The Mental Health Matrix. A Manual to Improve Services*. Cambridge: Cambridge University Press.

Thornicroft, G. and Tansella, M. (2002). Balancing community-based and hospital-based mental health care. *World Psychiatry*, 1(2), 84–90.

Tidemalm, D., Långström, N., Lichtenstein, P., et al. (2008). Risk of suicide after suicide attempt according to coexisting psychiatric disorder: Swedish cohort study with long term follow-up. *BMJ*, 337, 1328–30.

Van't Veer-Tazelaar, P.J., van Marwijk, H.W.J., van Oppen, P., et al. (2009). Stepped-care prevention of anxiety and depression in late life. A randomized controlled trial. *Archives of General Psychiatry*, 66(3), 297–304.

Värnik, P. (2012). Suicide in the world. *International Journal of Environmental Research and Public Health*, 9, 1.

Vijayakumar, L. (2004). Suicide prevention: the urgent need in developing countries. *World Psychiatry*, 3(3), 158–9.

Vreeman, R.C. and Carroll, A.E. (2007). A systematic review of school-based interventions to prevent bullying. *Archives of Pediatrics & Adolescent Medicine*, 161, 78–88.

Wahlbeck, K. (2009). *Background Document for the Thematic Conference on Prevention of Depression and Suicide*. Luxembourg: European Communities.

Wahlbeck, K. (2011a). European comparisons between mental health services. *Epidemiology and Psychiatric Sciences*, 20(1), 15–18.

Wahlbeck, K. (2011b). European mental health policy should target everybody. *European Journal of Public Health*, 21(5), 551–3.

Wahlbeck, K., Forsén, T., Osmond, C., et al. (2001). Association of schizophrenia with low maternal body mass index, small size at birth, and thinness during childhood. *Archives of General Psychiatry*, 58, 48–52.

Wahlbeck, K. and Taipale, V. (2006). Europe's mental health strategy. *BMJ*, 333, 210–11.

Wasserman, C., Hoven, C., Wasserman, D., et al. (2012). Suicide prevention for youth—a mental health awareness program: lessons learned from the Saving and Empowering Young Lives in Europe (SEYLE) intervention study. *BMC Public Health*, 12(1), 776.

Wasserman, D., Carli, V., Wasserman, C., et al. (2010). Saving and Empowering Young Lives in Europe (SEYLE): a randomized controlled trial. *BMC Public Health*, 10, 192.

Wasserman, D., Rihmer, Z., Rujescu, D., et al. (2012). The European Psychiatric Association (EPA) guidance on suicide treatment and prevention. *European Psychiatry*, 27(2), 129–41.

Wasserman, D., Värnik, A., Dankowicz, M., and Eklund, G. (1998). Suicide-preventive effects of perestroika in the former USSR: the role of alcohol restriction. *Acta Psychiatrica Scandinavica Supplementum*, 394, 1–44.

Weare, K. and Nind, M. (2011). Mental health promotion and problem prevention in schools: what does the evidence say? *Health Promotion International*, 26(Suppl. 1), i29–69.

Westerlund, M., Sylvia, S., and Schmidtke, A. (2009). The role of mass-media reporting and suicide prevention. In D. Wasserman and C. Wasserman (eds.) *The Oxford Textbook of Suicidology and Suicide Prevention: A Global Perspective*, pp. 515–24. Oxford: Oxford University Press.

Westerlund, M., and Wasserman, D. (2009). The role of the internet in suicide prevention. In D. Wasserman and C. Wasserman (eds.) *The Oxford Textbook of Suicidology and Suicide Prevention: A Global Perspective*, pp. 525–32. Oxford: Oxford University Press.

Westman, J., Sundquist, J., Johansson, L.M., et al. (2006). Country of birth and suicide: a follow-up study of a national cohort in Sweden. *Archives of Suicide Research*, 10(3), 239–48.

While, D., Bickley, H., Roscoe, A., et al. (2012). Implementation of mental health service recommendations in England and Wales and suicide rates, 1997–2006: a cross-sectional and before-and-after observational study. *The Lancet*, 379, 1005–12.

Wittchen, H.U., Jacobi, F., Rehm, J., et al. (2011). The size and burden of mental disorders and other disorders of the brain in Europe 2010. *European Neuropsychopharmacology*, 21, 655–79.

World Health Organization (2000). *Preventing Suicide a Resource for Media Professionals*. WHO/MNH/MBD/00.2. Geneva: Department of Mental Health, WHO. Available: http://www.who.int/mental_health/media/en/426.pdf.

World Health Organization (2004). *Prevention of Mental Disorders: Effective Interventions and Policy Options: Summary Report*. Geneva: WHO.

World Health Organization (2005). *Empowerment and Mental Health Advocacy. Briefing Paper for the WHO European Ministerial Conference on Mental Health: Facing the Challenges, Building Solutions.* Copenhagen: WHO.

World Health Organization (2010). *Guns, Knives and Pesticides: Reducing Access to Lethal Means.* Geneva: WHO. Available at: www.who.int/mental_health/prevention/suicide/vip_pesticides.pdf.

World Health Organization (2013). *Draft Comprehensive Mental Health Action Plan 2013–2020.* WHO: Geneva. Available at: http://apps.who.int/gb/ebwha/pdf_files/WHA66/A66_10Rev1-en.pdf.

World Health Organization (n.d.). *Social Determinants of Health.* [Online] Available at: http://www.who.int/hia/evidence/doh/en/index.html.

Yip, P.S.F., Caine, E., Yousuf, S., Chang, S.-S., Wu, K.C.-C., and Chen, Y.-Y. (2012). Means restriction for suicide prevention. *The Lancet*, 379, 2393–9.

Dental public health

Peter G. Robinson and Zoe Marshman

Introduction to dental public health

Poor oral health is a major public health problem. The considerable burden of oral disease at a societal level reflects the cumulative impact of many people affected to a modest degree. Oral diseases are exceedingly widespread. Their impact on individuals and the community are significant, ranging from mortality to effects on general health and quality of life, and in terms of direct costs and lost productivity.

Frequency of oral disease

Despite decreases over the last three decades, the prevalence of tooth decay is still staggering. For example, England has among the best child dental health in the developed world, yet 38 per cent of 5-year-olds have clinically significant tooth decay. Worldwide, the mean number of decayed, missing, or filled teeth among 12-year-olds is 1.67. Periodontal diseases are almost as common. More than 80 per cent of adults have inflamed gums (gingivitis) and most have evidence of destruction of the attachment between tooth and bone (periodontitis). Oral cancer is the eighth most common cancer worldwide and its incidence is increasing in some Western European countries. The highest reported incidence rates are in India and Sri Lanka where the mouth is the most common site, comprising up to 40 per cent of all cancers.

All the oral diseases of public health importance follow the same pattern of social inequality as general health conditions. In many developed countries, childhood tooth decay is a disease of poverty. For example, 5-year-olds living in the most deprived areas of England have five times the amount of decay as those living in the least deprived. Similar patterns are evident for periodontal diseases, trauma, and cancer.

Impacts of oral disease

Mortality from oral cancer is related to the site in the mouth and the timing of the diagnosis, but 5-year survival is still less than 50 per cent. In addition to mortality, oral disease affects other aspects of general health. Limited dietary choice and calorific and micronutrient intake are direct consequences of conditions such as xerostomia, poorly fitting dentures, and loss of teeth. Early childhood caries limit growth and development at the most important stage of life.

Oral diseases also directly affect quality of life. Dental pain is very common. In the United Kingdom, 29 per cent of dentate adults and 26 per cent of 12-year-olds reported oral pain in the past 12 months (Pitts and Harker 2004; Steele and O'Sullivan 2011). Even the appearance of the mouth is hugely important, affecting self-esteem and our willingness to interact with others. People with visible dental disease are judged by others to be less socially and intellectually competent and less well psychologically adjusted. Good dental appearance is regarded as a requirement for some prestigious occupations.

Considerable effort has been made to assess the extent to which oral disorders compromise aspects of daily life. This is beginning to reveal the determinants of these impacts. In turn, that information is being used to prioritize resources, to suggest avenues for action, and to evaluate interventions.

The cost of oral disease

Direct costs are incurred from the treatment of oral disease as well as the costs of other conditions caused or exacerbated by oral disease. The direct costs have been placed between 0.2 per cent and 1 per cent of the gross national product in developed countries (van Amerongen et al. 1993). The United Kingdom is at the lower end of this range yet the National Health Service (NHS) in England (population 63 million) budgets approximately £2.5 billion (US$4 billion) for dentistry. This sum is surprising since only about 50 per cent of the population are registered with an NHS dentist. The cost of treatment provided outside the NHS is not known, but may be an additional £1 billion. In the 15 member states of Europe in 2000, the estimated direct cost was US$68 billion. In Australia in 2008/2009 (population 21.5 million) the cost was US$7 billion or US$326 per person (Richardson and Richardson 2011). The cost of the Western model of dental treatment would exceed total national healthcare expenditure in many developing countries.

Indirect costs might include reduced employment or promotion expectations and opportunities, limitation of academic achievement, and the loss of economic productivity. Annually, over 20 million work days and 51 million school hours are lost in the United States alone due to oral disease and its treatment (Department of Health and Human Services 2000), equivalent to 1.5 hours for each employee annually. In Australia, 1.1 million work days and 600,000 school days are lost yearly (Richardson and Richardson 2011). Low-income families are more likely to lose time from work and school because of dental disease, hence compounding the inequalities that already exist in health, income, and educational attainment.

Prevention

Dental caries and periodontal diseases are almost entirely preventable. Clinically significant dental caries occurs only in the presence of excess dietary sugar. Its incidence is low when free sugar intake is less than 15–20 kg/year, roughly 6–10 per cent of energy intake (Moynihan and Petersen 2004). The use of fluorides, in drinking water or toothpastes, also reduces dental disease. Likewise, the presence of dental plaque is necessary for destructive periodontal disease. Targets for oral cleanliness have been calculated which appear to be compatible with freedom from periodontal disease throughout life (Burt et al. 1985). Slightly higher levels of plaque might be compatible with acceptably low levels of periodontal disease. The risk factors for oral cancer and oral trauma have also been identified and are readily modifiable at a population level.

The scope of dental public health

Dental public health is the science and art of preventing oral disease, promoting oral health, and improving the quality of life through the organized efforts of society.

Major areas of dental public health activity include:

1. Oral health surveillance.

2. Assessing the evidence on oral health and dental interventions, programmes, and services.

3. Policy and strategy development and implementation.

4. Strategic leadership and collaborative working for health.

5. Oral health improvement.

6. Health and public protection.

7. Developing and monitoring quality dental services.

8. Dental public health intelligence.

9. Academic dental public health.

10. Role within health services.

In some countries the specialty also involves provision of services to special population subgroups.

This chapter reviews the epidemiology, aetiology, and management of the four oral conditions of greatest public health importance: dental caries, periodontal diseases, oral cancer, and orofacial trauma. Approaches to oral health improvement are then outlined using the framework of the Commission on the Social Determinants of Health. Finally, we consider future developments in population oral health.

Oral diseases of public health importance

Dental caries

Dental caries and its sequelae account for 93–98 per cent of the burden of oral disease globally. It is the demineralization of tooth substance by acid metabolites of oral bacteria. In the very early stages the lesion appears as a chalky white spot on the tooth. If the lesion progresses, the surface of the tooth breaks down leading to cavitation. If the caries reaches the underlying dentine, it can spread more readily through the porous and less mineralized tissue towards the pulp. Infection of the pulp may allow the passage of bacteria along the root canals to the alveolar bone.

The direct consequences of this process are destruction of the tooth, pain, and a possible dental abscess. When dentine is exposed by cavitation, there may be transient pain associated with hot or cold drinks or sweet foods. Later, as the pulp becomes inflamed, the discomfort may be spontaneous, exquisitely painful, and of longer duration. In a dental abscess, pressure to the tooth is transmitted to the infected alveolus and the affected person avoids biting or knocking the tooth.

Four factors are necessary for caries development: dietary sugars, a susceptible tooth surface, the microflora of dental plaque, and adequate time.

The evidence implicating sugars in the aetiology of dental caries is convincing. The dental plaque that forms on the tooth surface comprises mainly bacteria, particularly *Streptococcus mutans*, which metabolize sugars to produce acids. The acids cause demineralization of the tooth structure. With each exposure to sugar, the plaque pH falls sharply and rises slowly back to normal levels over the following hour. Hence, caries incidence is related to the frequency of sugar intake.

At high pH, there is remineralization of the tooth, especially in the presence of fluoride. Saliva plays a crucial protective role against caries by simple dilution, by buffering plaque acid, and by acting as a source of minerals and chemical and immunological plaque inhibitory factors. For these reasons, dental caries is more frequent in the sites less accessible to saliva: in the pits and fissures of posterior teeth and between these teeth, and also in people with restricted salivary flow.

Epidemiology

Caries of the permanent dentition is traditionally measured by the number of decayed missing and filled teeth (the DMFT index). More precise indices record the number of surfaces affected (DMFS) and the status of the deciduous dentition (dmf). The index aggregates both disease and treatment experience, hence it is affected by treatment decisions of dentists and is less valid with increasing age. Since each of the categories is equally weighted, it is insensitive to both the severity of the disease and outcomes of treatment.

Nonetheless, the DMFT index, having been used for 75 years, will continue to be used for some time. However, historical DMF scores are not directly comparable with more recent ones as the diagnostic criterion for caries has changed. Previously, diagnosis was based on tooth cavitation detected using a sharp dental probe. Since 2001 the International Caries Detection and Assessment System (ICDAS) has been used to diagnose caries at much earlier stages before cavitation or progression into dentine. Sharp probes are no longer used, preventing damage to the tooth. If no caries is visible the tooth is now judged as having 'no obvious caries'. The lower detection thresholds reflect the emphasis on prevention. In addition to the assessment of the prevalence of caries, its impact is now routinely measured, most frequently by the use of measures of oral health-related quality of life.

Typically, the pattern has been of high caries levels in developed countries associated with exposure to sugars. In the mid 1970s, levels in many developed countries began to fall dramatically, for example, in the United Kingdom, mean DMFT of 12-year-olds decreased from 4.8 to 0.8 between 1973 and 2003 (Pitts and Harker 2004).

This fall in caries prevalence in developed countries appears to have slowed in the early to mid 1980s in the deciduous dentition. The mean DMFT of 5-year-olds in England and Wales fell from 4.0 to 1.8 between 1973 and 1983, but now appears stable at around 1.6 (Pitts and Harker 2004). Nevertheless, children and adults below the age of 50 years have better oral health than preceding generations. As these cohorts age, there will be commensurate improvements in adult oral health.

Aggregate national data on caries levels are useful, but mask important trends, particularly inequalities in oral health. When disease prevalence was high, disease was almost universal and inequalities were manifest as differences in the number of teeth affected in an individual. With lower disease prevalence, the distribution is highly skewed with typically 20–25 per cent of the population having moderate or severe caries (more than three teeth affected) and the majority having no obvious caries. This affected minority tends to be those living in the most deprived areas. Furthermore, Locker has found that dental caries has little impact on the lives of children and older adults from high-income environments but a more marked impact on those from low-income environments (Locker et al. 2007). These findings reinforce the importance of measuring both the disease impact and prevalence.

Although data are scarce, there are concerns with the rising caries levels in children in some countries undergoing economic growth and nutritional transition. For example, dental caries is very common and severe in 12-year-old children from several Asian and South American countries, but remains relatively low in most African countries where poor economic growth restricts sugar consumption. Here again, national data may mask local variations, particularly high caries levels in urban areas.

Management of dental caries

Until the nineteenth century, tooth extraction was the only useful treatment for dental caries. Treatment evolved to restorative care in which the infected parts of the tooth are removed and replaced with an inert obdurating filling, for example, dental amalgam. During the latter half of the twentieth century, in developed countries, operative treatment for adults has become increasingly complex and technology-intensive. Badly decayed teeth can now be restored with a range of adhesive tooth-coloured materials that are either formed in the mouth or prepared in laboratories and then fitted. Originally, missing teeth could only be replaced with removable dentures. Now they can be replaced with bridges that adhere to the remaining teeth or with prostheses supported by osseo-integrated implants that project out through the gingivae. Alternatives to traditional dental drills have been sought to improve the patient's experience of tooth preparation, including the use of lasers and ozone, although these are still not recommended for mainstream use.

Such treatments might reduce the social impact of dental caries on affected people, but play a very minor role in preventing the disease. Dental services accounted for 3 per cent of the caries reduction in industrialized countries during the 1970s compared to the 65 per cent contribution made by broader socioeconomic factors and fluoride toothpastes (Nadanovsky and Sheiham 1994). However, internationally, the emphasis and resources within dentistry remain focused on downstream approaches to 'cure' patients of their dental diseases, rather than evidence-based strategies to improve the oral health of populations (Baelum 2011).

In developing countries, the necessary infrastructure is often not available for complex treatment of carious teeth. In some areas, atraumatic restorative treatment (ART) is the only sustainable method because the decay is removed with hand instruments and the cavities filled with glass ionomer cements. The instruments are easily portable and treatment can be provided painlessly, at low cost, without local anaesthesia, electricity, or expensive dental equipment. Non-dentists can be trained in the technique in a matter of weeks using manuals available from the World Health Organization (WHO). The technique is most suitable for exactly the types of cavities found in many developing countries with low caries levels. Systematic reviews have confirmed the effectiveness of the ART approach (Frencken et al. 2012).

Implications of changes in caries prevalence

At the low disease prevalence in the developed world, proportionately more caries affects the accessible occlusal surfaces of the teeth. Fissure sealants can be applied to these surfaces to prevent caries and are cost-effective at low caries levels (Armfield and Spencer 2007). Only simple restorations are needed to treat existing disease at these sites. The disease also progresses more slowly, so allowing deferred operative treatment. Many lesions are detected at an earlier stage so that new dental materials can be used in minimally invasive techniques.

Increasing the intervals between dental examinations is safe and effective for children and adults with low disease incidence (National Institute for Health and Clinical Excellence 2004). There is greater scope to employ dental care professionals (DCPs), other than dentists, who can also deliver effective preventive interventions such as fluoride varnish. However, because of the skewed distribution of dental caries, there remains a minority with high levels of caries to be managed.

There are also a large cohort of people more than 50 years old who have suffered from severe dental caries and cycles of re-restoration. This so-called heavy metal generation (Fig. 8.8.1) will continue to need complex and specialized treatment for decades to come with high expectations of retaining their natural dentition into older age.

Periodontal diseases

Periodontal diseases comprise a range of inflammatory diseases of the periodontium: the attachment between gingivae and tooth. In gingivitis, the attachment remains in a healthy position whereas periodontitis is defined by migration of the epithelium which reduces the amount of periodontal ligament and bone supporting the tooth.

Gingivitis, which is exceedingly common, is an inflammatory response to plaque. Along with redness and swelling, the gums may bleed on gentle provocation such as cleaning the teeth. Pain is uncommon. Systemic involvement including hormonal changes, skin diseases, and medication use may modify these diseases or cause other gingival changes. In periodontitis, the loss of periodontal attachment is manifest by deepening of the pockets between the gingivae and teeth and by recession of the gingivae. In severe cases, the supporting structures are so depleted that the teeth become loose. The disease is rarely painful unless an acute infection complicates a periodontal pocket ('a lateral periodontal abscess') or if the exposed root surfaces are temperature sensitive.

Mild periodontal pocketing is common, being seen in approximately half of UK and 63 per cent of US adults (White et al. 2011; Eke et al. 2012). Severe periodontitis is much less frequent. Lost attachment or pockets of 6 mm or more (thought to be sufficient to threaten tooth survival) are seen in 9 per cent of UK and 25 per cent of US adults. These apparent differences between countries may be in part attributed to different survey methods. For example, the 2009–2010 US National Health and Nutrition

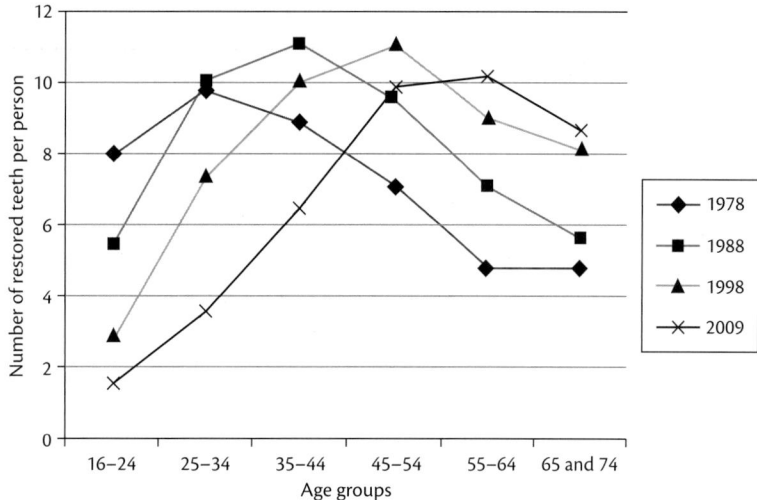

Fig. 8.8.1 The 'heavy metal' cohort

Examination Survey examined only adults over the age of 30 and examined the whole mouth. As loss of periodontal attachment is cumulative over a lifetime, restricting the sample to older adults will substantially overestimate the disease prevalence. The disease is more frequent and severe in countries where tooth cleaning practices are less sophisticated.

Periodontitis is hence a substantial problem. It has been consistently linked with psychological and social consequences on everyday life, which intervention studies indicate is reduced by treatment (Jowett et al. 2009). More severe and untreated disease results in the loss of teeth and the need for additional treatment to replace them.

Another periodontal disease of public health importance is acute necrotizing ulcerative gingivitis (ANUG; Vincent's infection or 'trenchmouth'), which causes necrosis, ulceration, soreness, and bleeding of the gingivae. The ulcerated papillae may have a grey slough and there may be a characteristic foetor. Lymphadenopathy and mild fever are variable findings. In many developed countries, ANUG is a disease of young adults. There are no good incidence data, but anecdotally, it has become less frequent among developed populations in recent years. A variant of the disease is associated with HIV infection. ANUG is also seen in children in developing countries where it can progress in the absence of treatment. In severe cases, necrosis may extend over adjacent tissues to cause gross destruction of oral and facial tissues (known as cancrum oris or noma).

Pathogenesis

The pathogenesis of periodontitis involves the interaction of plaque pathogens with the host's immune system. Considerable research is devoted to determining which, if any, specific pathogens are responsible for periodontal destruction (the 'specific plaque hypothesis'). Dental plaque is ubiquitous, but destructive disease occurs only in a minority of people. Apart from plaque, there are important determinants of periodontal disease susceptibility.

It is now clear that tobacco exerts an independent deleterious effect. Periodontal treatment is also less effective in smokers

(Reibel 2003). Stress is another risk factor: for example, greater occupational stress is associated with progression of periodontitis and ANUG has been noted among soldiers on difficult postings, students during exam terms, and people with negative life events.

Periodontitis often takes decades to become clinically detectable. While it is more common and severe with advanced years, periodontitis is not a consequence of age. It is associated with poor oral hygiene and does not progress in adults with good oral hygiene.

Treatment

For most people, the progression of periodontal destruction is compatible with the retention of a natural dentition into old age. Targets for oral cleanliness have been calculated that appear to be compatible with no or acceptably low levels of periodontal disease throughout life (Burt et al. 1985).

A significant minority of people (perhaps 5–15 per cent) may lose teeth from periodontal diseases and considerable effort is spent by dental professionals to prevent and treat them, primarily by mechanically removing plaque through regular toothbrushing and flossing of teeth. Adjunctive treatments include removal of calcified plaque (calculus), planing away the superficial layers of the roots and periodontal surgery in severe cases.

Systematic reviews are beginning to provide an evidence base for periodontal therapy although there may be considerable Hawthorne effects reflecting differences between the effectiveness of treatment provided routinely in primary care and its efficacy in clinical trials conducted in university departments. There are also few long-term studies showing effects on tooth retention.

Interventions aimed at improving oral hygiene produce short-term changes that are not sustained (Watt and Marinho 2005). Powered toothbrushes with a rotation oscillation action assist self-care although their long-term benefits on periodontal health have yet to be evaluated (Robinson et al. 2005). The most common professional procedure to prevent and treat periodontal diseases, the removal of calculus by scaling and polishing, is currently being evaluated as the available evidence was of poor quality. There is no compelling evidence of benefits from professional mechanical plaque removal alone over simple oral hygiene instruction to prevent periodontal diseases (Needleman et al. 2005a). Another common treatment, subgingival debridement, remains untested in randomized controlled trials (RCTs), but showed modest short-term reductions in pocket depths in other controlled studies (Van der Weijden and Timmerman 2002) and a systematic review of guided tissue regeneration indicated that the mean level of attachment gained is approximately 1 mm, with eight sites needing to be treated to regain 2 mm in one site (Needleman et al. 2005b).

Oral cancer

Benign oral cavity neoplasms include papillomas, polyps, and various types of granuloma. This subsection will deal principally with malignant neoplasms, of which approximately 90 per cent are squamous cell carcinomas. They may occur on the lip, tongue, gingivae, oral floor, or elsewhere in the mouth (some statistics on mouth cancer also include the pharynx). The site is often related to the aetiological factors. Lesions may present as swellings, ulcers, or red or white patches and many are painless until they become large. Five-year survival is less than 50 per cent and depends on the disease stage at presentation. Malignant change is often seen in a number of lesions which precede tumour development and present as white or red patches of unknown origin. Malignant change is also occasionally seen in oral lichen planus and hyperplastic candidiasis.

Overall, the estimated age-standardized incidence of mouth and lip cancer worldwide for males is 5.2 per 100,000 population, with dramatic variation between and within countries (Globocan 2010) (Table 8.8.1). Men are more susceptible than women in almost all populations, independent of tobacco use.

Variations in the incidence of oral malignancy are first explained by varying exposure to three risk factors. Cancer of the lower lip is strongly associated with sunlight exposure especially in fair-skinned people. Tobacco use, whether chewed or smoked, predisposes to intra-oral cancer. The high incidence of oral cancer among southern Asians is in part due to the addition of tobacco to betel quid or 'paan'. There are dose–response relationships for the duration of use and type of tobacco inhaled. Alcohol is an independent aetiological factor with additive effects with tobacco use. In some developed countries, oral cancer incidence correlates better with alcohol consumption and liver disease than with smoking and respiratory disease (Hindle et al. 2000).

Table 8.8.1 Oral cancer in males—age standardized rate per 100,000 population

	Rate per 100,000
Worldwide	5.2
India	9.8
United States	7.4
China	1.3

Source: data from Globocan, *Estimated cancer Incidence, Mortality, Prevalence and Disability-adjusted life years (DALYs) Worldwide in 2008*, International Agency for research on Cancer (IARC), World Health Organization, Copyright © IARC 2014, available from http://globocan.iarc.fr/.

In the past, oral cancer occurred mainly in older people (over 60 years). However, the incidence is increasing in developed countries because of a rising incidence in people younger than 45 years, where oral cancer may be a distinct form related to human papilloma virus (HPV) and associated with vaginal and oral sex (Conway et al. 2006; D'Souza et al. 2007). HPV-associated tumours show a predilection for the tonsils and oropharynx, and although apparently aggressive, carry a better prognosis (Fakhry et al. 2008).

Both cancer incidence and survival show distinct socioeconomic gradients. In the United Kingdom, 5-year survival for oral cancer among the most affluent was 53.9 per cent compared to 42.3 per cent in the most deprived (Cancer Research UK 2009), a difference not totally explained by smoking, alcohol drinking, and diet (Conway et al. 2010).

As early intervention improves oral cancer survival, and many cases are preceded by premalignant lesions, case finding would seem useful for disease control. However, active screening does not appear to be justified in countries with a lower prevalence and available dental services (Downer et al. 2006). Opportunistic screening as part of routine dental visits may be viable.

Trauma

Trauma to the teeth is common and frequently causes fracture of the tooth or supporting bone or bodily movement of the tooth including complete avulsion. In many cases, the long-term survival of the tooth is threatened. As the anterior and most visible teeth are most often involved, the result can be disfiguring. Worldwide, the prevalence of dentofacial trauma is approximately 10–15 per cent. Risk factors include sporting activities such as cycling and ball sports, falls, road traffic accidents, violence (including fights), and poor environments such as overcrowding. Protruding upper front teeth and inadequate lip coverage also put individuals at risk. The peak age for trauma is early adolescence with boys experiencing more injuries than girls.

Trauma to deciduous teeth is managed by monitoring, in case any consequent infection threatens the permanent tooth developing beneath it. In permanent teeth, adhesive fillings can be used to protect sensitive fractured teeth and dressings (usually calcium hydroxide) to allow continued root development in immature teeth. For permanent teeth that have been knocked out, they should be replaced in the socket as soon as possible or placed in a suitable container of milk or normal saline. Dental care should be sought immediately as tooth replantation within 30 minutes provides best long-term survival rates of avulsed teeth. The tooth should be splinted to adjacent teeth for 7–14 days and antibiotic and antitetanus treatments given. The need for urgent care means that skilled emergency dental services should ideally be available around the clock.

The cost of treating dentofacial trauma has been estimated at US$3.2–3.5 million per million subjects (Andreasen and Andreasen 1997) and in the United Kingdom, the average total cost of treating one patient with a dental traumatic injury has been estimated at US$1665 (Wong and Kolokotsa 2004).

Links with other diseases

Many associations between oral conditions and general health have been proposed in the last two decades.

Periodontal diseases have been linked to cardiovascular diseases, stroke, pre-term birth, and low birth weight. Some authors have even suggested that periodontal diseases are independent risk factors for these diseases. Epidemiological evidence supporting links between periodontal and other diseases suffers from many possible confounders, the potential for misclassification, and bias. Despite efforts to control for socioeconomic and lifestyle factors, residual confounding resulting from a failure to account fully for these variables seems inevitable. Specific cardiovascular risk factors such as tobacco use, obesity and lower serum high-density lipoprotein cholesterol are more common among people with high dental disease experience (Sanders et al. 2005). Some, such as tobacco smoking, are independent risk factors for both cardiovascular and periodontal diseases.

Systematic and narrative reviews of these associations have not yielded firm conclusions because of methodological complexity (Beck and Offenbacher 2005; Xiong et al. 2006; Persson and Persson 2008). The existing evidence suggests that interventions improving periodontal health do not modify these other health problems (Beck et al. 2008).

Epidemiological associations between other oral conditions and general health face the same methodological challenges. Poor oral hygiene predicted cardiovascular outcomes among Scottish adults, although the nature of the relationship was not determined (D'Oliveira et al. 2010). Having fewer teeth and not wearing dentures prospectively predicted the incidence of falls amongst Japanese elders, but again there may have been confounding (Yamamoto et al. 2012). Relationships between oral health and all-cause mortality were partly explained by covariates, but persisted after many of these covariates have been accounted for (Linden et al. 2012; Sabbah et al. 2013).

At present then, causal relationships between oral and general health appear putative and even if causal links are demonstrated, we cannot recommend oral health interventions to improve general health. For the time being, we assume these relationships are confounded by environmental and lifestyle factors common to both sets of diseases.

Inequalities in oral health

Inequalities occur in the distribution of almost all oral conditions, and this area of research and action has grown in parallel with the interest in health inequalities, led by the Commission for the Social Determinants of Health (CSDH 2008). The resultant formation of the Global Oral Health Inequalities Research Agenda (Sgan-Cohen et al. 2013) of the International Association of Dental Research will add impetus and, hopefully, practicable policies.

Oral health inequalities are related to socioeconomic status, ethnicity, or region, both in gradients and in fine grain (Anderson et al. 2012; Flores and Lin 2013). Whether socioeconomic status is measured by education, occupation, or income, these inequalities consistently relate to the degree of social inequality and not just the distribution of resources. For example, levels of total tooth loss across US states are related to the level of income inequality within each state and not just absolute levels of poverty (Bernabé and Marcenes 2011).

There are social gradients for oral cancer incidence in developing and developed countries (Conway et al. 2008), tooth loss (Tsakos et al. 2011), the total absence of teeth, the presence of untreated decay or the presence of a filled tooth (Elani et al. 2012), more severe periodontitis (Eke et al. 2012), worse self-rated oral health, and oral impacts (Tsakos et al. 2011). Periodontal diseases are unusual in childhood and yet have been linked to the structural determinants of health more strongly than to individual factors amongst Brazilian 12-year-olds (Jordao et al. 2012). Having brown skin colour, attending a public school, and living in an area with intermediate socioeconomic indicators were associated with higher prevalence of calculus and bleeding on probing.

The life course approach indicates how people's circumstances in early life, their experiences during childhood, with their parents and family and during preschool and formal education and beyond, accumulate to influence their health throughout life. Long-term follow-ups of birth cohorts confirm the importance of this accumulated effect. In one study, 5-year-olds of low socioeconomic status had more decay, more fillings and worse periodontitis, and were more likely to have had a tooth extracted at the age of 26 years, even after controlling for childhood oral health. Furthermore, changes in socioeconomic status throughout life were associated with differing levels of oral health in adulthood (Thomson et al. 2004).

Health improvement and reducing oral health inequalities

Three increasingly important factors are shaping approaches to improve population oral health. First, the limited effectiveness of individualized approaches to disease prevention; second, the links between oral and general health; and finally, greater concern about inequalities in health.

The limited effect of individualized approaches to disease prevention

Many of the causes of oral disease relate to individual behaviours (the consumption of sugars, ineffective oral cleaning, tobacco and alcohol use, and limited exposure to fluoride). Dentistry has traditionally adopted health education as the central thrust of prevention. As with other fields, dentists have recognized that health education cannot readily change these behaviours, which are largely determined by the social and cultural environment.

Repeated systematic reviews have investigated the effectiveness of oral health promotion practices (Sprod et al. 1996; Kay and Locker 1997; Watt and Marinho 2005; Satur et al. 2010). The most robust primary studies have tended to focus on programmes in which the intended outcome was improved knowledge or modification of the behaviours of individuals, usually involving relatively short follow-ups. The main finding from meta-analysis was the effectiveness of fluoride to prevent caries (Kay and Locker 1997). A less rigorous approach (Sprod et al. 1996) still concluded there was little evaluative literature on broader approaches to health promotion. The most recent review identified evidence supporting capacity building with non-oral healthcare providers and the use of multi-strategy community-based approaches (Satur et al. 2010).

One other consideration is that preventive strategies that focus on individuals do not appear to be suitable for dental caries, periodontal diseases, and oral cancer since there are, as yet, no effective ways of identifying which individuals are at high risk of developing the diseases (Rose 1992; Watt 2007). Whilst individuals at high risk for dental disease cannot be identified easily, it is possible to identify at-risk populations. In these situations, it can be cost-effective to target prevention at specific socioeconomic groups, particular schools or areas, with high disease incidence (Burt 1998).

Links between oral and general health

Oral health is frequently associated with general health, but only in certain circumstances is this relation causative. Instead, oral and general health conditions appear to share common risk factors that cluster in the same groups (Sanders et al. 2005), as they are distributed in the same way and follow similar socioeconomic gradients.

These epidemiological associations between oral and general health are compatible with the strategy of targeted interventions which could adopt a common risk factor approach (CRFA), tackling risk factors that are common to many conditions. The CRFA was anticipated to provide multiple benefits, reduce duplication, save resources, improve effectiveness, and reduce social inequalities. However, a recent concern with the CRFA is 'lifestyle drift' where the focus has been on behaviours rather than their upstream structural, social, and psychological determinants (Watt and Sheiham 2012). This recognition of the social context in which personal choices are made avoids the social iatrogenesis of describing oral health in individual terms (Dickson 1995).

It follows that oral health programmes should be closely integrated into programmes to improve general health for the whole population and for specific groups such as older people (Petersen et al. 2010; Satur et al. 2010). Similar observations have been made about global health policy (Dybul et al. 2012) where a focus on single diseases has ignored the problems of people experiencing multiple health problems and reinforced health inequalities.

Commission on Social Determinants of Health

Greater concern about inequalities in health has had a number of broader implications. Earlier models had seen such factors as general socioeconomic, cultural and environmental conditions and consequently people's living and working conditions as the upstream determinants of *health* (Dahlgren and Whitehead 1992). More recent models look beyond these upstream factors to consider the social determinants *of health inequalities* (Krieger 2008).

From this perspective, the social determinants of health arise and are sustained by political ecologies, power, and social relations (Krieger et al. 2012).

The CSDH adopted a conceptual framework in which a 'toxic combination of poor social policies and programmes, unfair economic arrangements and bad politics' creates a socioeconomic and political context. These structural factors shape intermediary determinants including the social position of individuals and groups (as indicated by education, occupation, income, gender, or race/ethnicity). This social position then determines the material circumstances of people, their behaviours, social cohesion, psychosocial and biological factors, and their use of the healthcare system. It is this cascade of factors that shapes the distribution of health and well-being (see Chapter 2.1).

For those concerned with improving health and reducing health inequalities, the CSDH provides a comprehensive framework for planning interventions and selecting potential entry points, which although not specific to any particular set of diseases, is directly applicable to oral health (Kwan and Petersen 2010; Marmot and Bell 2011). The commission recommended three principles of action:

1. To tackle the inequitable distribution of power, money, and resources, and create a more equitable socioeconomic and political context.

2. To improve daily living conditions so that the material circumstances, social cohesion, psychosocial and behavioural factors, and use of health services are more equitably distributed.

3. To understand the problem and assess the impact of action.

These three activities are neither discrete nor mutually exclusive. For example, action on the distribution of power and resources will improve living conditions and work at either level will involve the same actors to a greater or lesser degree. The emphasis should be to work across all levels of the model (CSDH 2008; Kwan and Petersen 2010) and hence, at all levels of society. Systematic reviews indicate that downstream, behaviourally based interventions do not appear to reduce inequalities, and may increase them (Lorenc et al. 2013). In oral health, it has long been recognized that health education carries its own dangers of disempowerment and victim-blaming and may increase inequalities in oral health (Watt 2007). Conversely, upstream approaches such as structural workplace interventions and pricing policies have the potential to reduce inequalities (Satur et al. 2010). Conway et al.'s (2008) systematic review associated oral cancer risk with low socioeconomic status but provided evidence to steer health policies which focus on lifestyles factors towards an integrated approach to tackle the root causes of disadvantage.

One refinement of the CSDH approach is the adoption of the principle of proportionate universalism. Marmot (2010) suggested that the gradient of health inequality should be reduced by working to improve the health of all portions of society, but the scale and intensity of the action should be in proportion to the level of disadvantage, for example, by targeting particular interventions at groups at greatest risk within a whole population strategy.

To public health practitioners concerned about social injustice, the growing attention given to health inequalities is exciting. However, the likelihood of reaching a consensus and prevailing upon the power imbalances that structure the social determinants of health and consequent health inequalities may be reduced during the current global economic crisis. Moreover, inequalities appear to be increasing (Thomas et al. 2010). Health inequalities may persist because the increased social mobility of recent generations has left the lower socioeconomic groups more homogeneous in terms of the individual characteristics that predispose to ill health. It may also be that the better contemporary absolute levels of health mean that the social and individual resources associated with higher socioeconomic status are more important (Mackenbach 2012). Cumulatively, these factors require substantial effort to create greater health equality.

Actions to improve health and reduce health inequality will have similar effects on oral health but some aspects are especially relevant (Box 8.8.1). Therefore, the CSDH framework and these principles will be used in the remainder of this section.

Box 8.8.1 Improving oral health and reducing inequalities within the Commission on Social Determinants of Health framework

Tackling the inequitable distribution of power, money and resources: changing the structural drivers of conditions of daily life

- Action on health and health equity at the highest level of government with coherent policies across all departments.
- Redistributive direct taxation systems.
- Publicly funded action on child development, education, working and living conditions, and healthcare.
- Market responsibility.
- Regulation of goods and services with a direct role in health.
- Political empowerment and fair representation of all.
- Oral health impact and oral health equity audit of all policies.

Improving daily living conditions: changing the circumstances in which people are born, grow, live, work, and age

- Comprehensive approaches to early life, child survival, and early life interventions.
- Comprehensive universal social protection.
- Urban planning and fairness between areas to prevent rural poverty.
- Full and fair employment with acceptable, safe work and a healthy work–life balance.
- Access to universal healthcare.
- Increasing the availability of fluoride:
  - water
  - milk
  - salt
  - tablets/drops
  - toothpastes
  - mouthrinses
  - varnishes.
- Dietary sugars.
- Oral cleaning.
- Smoking cessation.
- Prevention and management of trauma.
- Use of oral health services.

Measuring and understanding the problem and assessing the impact of action

- Routine systems with relevant measures of oral health, its determinants, and health equity.
- Dentists and dental public health specialists as advocates.

Tackle the inequitable distribution of power, money, and resources

This part of the CSDH (2008) report makes recommendations which are the most upstream and radical, to change the way that society is organized. Action on health and health equity is advocated at the highest level of government to ensure effective and coherent policies across all departments. This work will require health impact assessment and health equity audit of all policies, using the social determinants framework across all actions of ministries of health. To ensure adequate financing for publicly-funded action, the CSDH proposed redistributive direct taxation systems, which demonstrably reduce poverty.

The provision of basic human and social needs including clean water, healthcare, and education are seen as a primary role of the state rather than the market. The state also has a role in the regulation of goods and services with a direct role in health (e.g. tobacco, alcohol, and food).

The commission also proposed that health equity be made a global development goal and that the social determinants of health be placed as a guiding principle across the WHO.

Oral health can be fitted into these broad actions on health inequalities and into all health policies. Dental workers have an important role as advocates for considering the impact of policies on oral health. For example, in many countries dental caries is now a disease of poverty and particularly of children, where redistributive taxation might reduce oral health inequalities. Work with the agricultural sector, especially in relation to the production of cash crops like sugar and tobacco, has obvious applicability to oral health. Further regulation of the production, use, and marketing of tobacco, alcohol, and sugar is also feasible at all levels of influence.

Oral diseases may contribute to social stratification as they are often visible. The appearance of the mouth is used by others to form social judgements which may limit life opportunities and employment (Newton et al. 2003). Seen this way, oral health is not only a goal but a means towards greater equality. However, to reduce the social impact of oral disease, oral health services need to be organized to meet the needs of the population. Where possible there should be universal access to primary oral healthcare services.

Improve daily living conditions

The CSDH recognized that the factors that enable good health are not distributed equally throughout life and made a series of recommendations to improve daily living conditions.

The accumulation of adversity during the life course means there must be comprehensive approaches to early life for child survival and development, and comprehensive social mechanisms to support an income sufficient for healthy living. Secure and fairly paid employment and access to universal healthcare are vital.

These actions will have direct and indirect effects on oral health. Socioeconomic status at birth was found to determine tooth loss in adulthood (Thomson et al. 2004). Early childhood caries inhibits growth and development and its treatment reverses this effect (Mohammadi et al. 2009).

One well-evaluated strategy for improving daily living conditions is increasing the availability of fluoride. Other strategies focus on oral health behaviours, such as oral cleaning, smoking cessation, and trauma prevention.

Increasing the availability of fluoride

Fluoride prevents or reverses dental caries mainly through topical effects including the inhibition of demineralization of the tooth structure, enhancement of remineralization with a stronger crystal structure, and inhibition of bacterial enzymes. Consequently fluoride has been used to prevent caries by adding it to water supplies, toothpastes, foods, drinks, and in professionally applied products.

Water fluoridation

Beneficial effects of fluoride on dental health were inadvertently discovered during investigations of developmental staining of children's teeth in Colorado, United States, due to chronic ingestion of fluoride during tooth development.

An inverse relationship between dental caries and the fluoride concentration of drinking water was demonstrated in two ecological studies (now called the '21 cities studies'). The first intervention trial started in Grand Rapids in 1945 (Dean et al. 1950). Since then similar studies have taken place in many countries. Worldwide, around 435 million people now receive water from a fluoridated water supply and water fluoridation has been designated one of the ten most important public health measures currently available (Centers for Disease Control and Prevention 2010). Dean originally suggested that the optimal concentration for water fluoridation was 1 part per million (ppm) (1 mg/L), the recommended optimal range of fluoride is now 0.6–1.0 ppm F.

The effectiveness and safety of water fluoridation in caries prevention is consistently supported in authoritative narrative and systematic reviews. The most comprehensive systematic review, the York review, included the results of 88 studies (83 of which were cross-sectional) from 30 countries (McDonagh et al. 2000). The included studies were judged to be of low to moderate quality, mainly because of the lack of appropriate adjustment for the effect of confounding factors. Bearing in mind these concerns, water fluoridation was associated with a median increase of 14.6 per cent in the proportion of children without caries experience and a median reduction in DMFT of 2.25 teeth. For one extra child to be 'caries-free', six children would need to be exposed to water fluoridated at 1 ppm F. Water fluoridation was also found to have an effect over and above that of other sources of fluoride, particularly toothpaste.

A direct dose–response relationship was found between water fluoridation and dental fluorosis. At 1 ppm F the prevalence of fluorosis was estimated to be 48 per cent and for fluorosis of aesthetic concern 12.5 per cent. The numbers of additional people who would have to be exposed to water fluoridation at this level for one additional person to develop fluorosis of any level, was six. Other possible negative effects considered included bone fracture, cancer, Down syndrome, senile dementia, and goitre. No clear evidence of these potential effects was found, but interpretation of the results of these studies was difficult due to the quality of the primary data.

The cost-effectiveness of water fluoridation depends on the baseline level of caries and the capital costs of the necessary equipment. In areas where water is supplied to large numbers of people via a single source, fluoridation is most cost-effective.

Further high quality research into the safety, efficacy, cost-effectiveness (McDonagh et al. 2000), and impact of fluoridation on quality of life has been recommended (Medical Research Council 2002).

More recently, systematic reviews commissioned by the Australian National Health and Medical Research Council (2007) updated and supported the conclusions of the UK Medical Research Council review that strongly suggested that fluoridation of water supplies is effective in caries prevention. Water fluoridation appeared to be associated with mild dental fluorosis but there was no consistent evidence of increased association with cancer, bone fractures, or other adverse effects.

The introduction of water fluoridation schemes is invariably opposed by active anti-fluoridationist lobbies. Such groups tend to be small, but very vociferous, with considerable impact. The main arguments against water fluoridation include the safety concerns outlined earlier and ethical objections that fluoridation of water supplies infringes on individual freedom of choice and removes the right of adults to refuse medical treatment. Fluoridation is portrayed as 'mass medication'. The ethical objections to water fluoridation have been discussed by applying the four principles that encompass most of the moral aspects of healthcare, that is; respect for autonomy, beneficence, non-maleficence, and justice (Jones and Lennon 1997).

With regard to the claims of loss of autonomy, those proposing fluoridation suggest some reduction of individual freedom is accepted for the overall good of the community. On the argument that only dentate members of society will potentially benefit from water fluoridation, those in favour acknowledge this but fluoridation will 'do no harm' to any members of society. On the principle of justice, some claim that imposing water fluoridation is not fair on those against it. Proponents counter this argument by suggesting that the reduction in inequalities in dental health that fluoridation potentially provides is a just way of helping those least able to help themselves.

The debate about fluoridation is an interesting one. Anti-fluoridationists tend to come from relatively healthy middle-class groups. As children in these groups have the lowest caries experience, they have the least to benefit from the intervention. Unfortunately, their effect is to maintain social inequalities in health.

Water fluoridation has tended to be a sacred cow within dental public health; something to be embraced and considered immune from criticism. A more recent alternative view sees water fluoridation as modestly effective in developed countries with low caries (as demonstrated by the relatively high number needed to be treated to prevent a case), yet the political battle for new fluoridation schemes may make it very expensive to introduce.

Other vehicles for administering fluoride include the following:

- *Fluoride milk:* fluoride has been added to milk as an alternative to water since the 1950s in many countries. These schemes vary in the age at which children start drinking the milk, the number of years over which it is administered, the number of days a year the milk is consumed, and the concentration of fluoride added (Marino et al. 2006). Systematic reviews of the effectiveness of fluoridated milk for preventing caries present mixed conclusions, in part because of varied quality of the available data. The results are consistent with a caries preventive effect with cessation being associated with increasing caries incidence (Yeung et al. 2005; National Health and Medical Research Council 2007).

● *Salt fluoridation* was first used in Switzerland in the 1950s. In certain cantons and in some Latin America countries, all salt for human consumption is fluoridated. Other European countries including France only sell fluoridated salt for domestic use. The typical concentration is 250 ppm F. Several cross-sectional studies report fluoride salt to be effective at reducing caries (Jones et al. 2005).

● *Fluoride tablets/drops* use also began in the 1950s. They have been used as dietary supplements with different countries having different dosing regimens (based on child's age, weight, caries-risk, fluoride in the water). Their effectiveness has not been confirmed by any well-designed trials or systematic reviews and the available studies fail to account for confounding factors. There is some evidence that when sucked to maximize the topical dose, a preventive effect is observed in deciduous teeth. Two key problems with fluoride supplementation are adherence to dosing regimens and the risk of fluorosis. Many of the people most susceptible to caries find the dosing schedules difficult to maintain. Taken as a daily bolus, fluoride supplements increase the risk of fluorosis (Ismail and Bandekar 1999). These concerns have led to a reduction in the use of tablets/drops as a public health measure.

Topically applied fluoride

Includes delivery systems where fluoride is applied to tooth surfaces at high concentrations for a local protective effect. A series of systematic reviews of trials have investigated the effectiveness of various topical fluorides expressed as the preventive fraction (the difference in caries increments between the intervention and control groups expressed as a percentage of the increment in the control group) (Table 8.8.2).

● *Fluoride toothpaste* Toothpaste is the most widespread source of fluoride and the decline in caries experience in children in some countries has been attributed to its regular use. The fluoride compounds and concentrations found in toothpastes

Table 8.8.2 Relative effectiveness of sources of topical fluoride

Source	ppm F	Prevented fraction (%)
Toothpaste	500–1500	24
Mouthrinse	230–900	26
Varnish	7000–22,000	46 (permanent)
		33 (deciduous)
Gel	12,300	28

Source: data from Marinho, V.C.C. et al., Fluoride varnishes for preventing dental caries in children and adolescents, *Cochrane Database of Systematic Reviews*, Issue 1, Art. No.: CD002279, Copyright © 2002; Marinho, V.C.C. et al., Fluoride gels for preventing dental caries in children and adolescents, *Cochrane Database of Systematic Reviews*, Issue 1, Art. No.: CD002280, Copyright © 2002; Marinho, V.C.C. et al., Fluoride toothpastes for preventing dental caries in children and adolescents, *Cochrane Database of Systematic Reviews*, Issue 1, Art. No.: CD002278, Copyright © 2003; and Marinho, V.C.C. et al., Fluoride mouthrinses for preventing dental caries in children and adolescents, *Cochrane Database of Systematic Reviews*, Issue 3, Art. No.: CD002284, Copyright © 2003.

vary between brands and between countries. The usual concentration is 1000–1500 ppm F with higher (over 2000 ppm F) formulations available. They present a good vehicle for the frequent low-dose application of fluoride and their effectiveness in reducing caries in children has been confirmed with a prevented fraction (PF) of 24 per cent (Marinho et al. 2003a). The risk of fluorosis from toothpaste can be minimized by using a smear of paste and supervising children under 6 years of age.

Fluoride toothpaste has a distinct disadvantage over water fluoridation as a broad preventive strategy as it relies on people brushing their teeth. In developed countries infrequent brushing and high caries incidence are *associated* and so the people who have most to benefit from the use of fluoride toothpastes are less likely to use them frequently. In developing countries there may not be a tradition of tooth cleaning with toothpastes and Western proprietary brands are likely to be expensive. However, cheap locally made pastes can be profoundly effective (Yee et al. 2003).

● *Fluoride mouthrinses* Fluoride mouthrinses have been used extensively for the past 30 years. School-based programmes were common in certain countries although individual home use now predominates. Mouthrinsing is not recommended for children under 6 years of age, due to the risk of fluoride ingestion. The two main concentrations available are 0.05 per cent (230 ppm F) sodium fluoride used daily and 0.2 per cent (900 ppm F) sodium fluoride weekly. The effectiveness of mouthrinses in children has also been confirmed with a PF of 26 per cent (Marinho et al. 2003b).

● *Fluoride varnishes/gels* Topically applied fluoride varnishes and gels have been used widely for over two decades, both as part of community-based programmes and on an individual basis. Fluoride varnishes are professionally applied, with the two most commonly used varnishes containing 22,600 ppm F or 7000 ppm F. A systematic review of trials has shown the effectiveness of topical varnishes, although the included studies were of poor quality. The PF in permanent teeth was 46 per cent (Marinho et al. 2002a). However, a more recent cluster RCT of a school-based fluoride varnish programme in the United Kingdom was unable to demonstrate an effect to prevent caries in first permanent molar teeth over a 3-year period (Milsom et al. 2011).

Fluoride gels can be professionally or self-applied under supervision. The most commonly used gel is a professionally applied 12,300 ppm F acidulated phosphate fluoride. Due to the risk of excessive ingestion, this gel is not recommended for young children. The effectiveness of professionally-applied and self-applied gels have been reviewed with a PF of 28 per cent (Marinho et al. 2002b).

Behaviours

Dietary sugars

Dietary sugars are a necessary cause of clinically relevant dental decay. Unfortunately, repeated systematic reviews indicate that dietary advice neither reduces their intake nor the incidence of caries (Sprod et al. 1996; Kay and Locker 1997). Health education programmes only appear to be effective if they also involve the recommendation or prescription of fluoride vehicles.

However, the data suggest that restriction of dietary sugars by other means is preventive. For example, per capita sugar supplies and caries experience data correlate significantly in national ecological comparisons. A children's home in Australia had a dietary regimen with almost no sugar and the children had very low caries levels until they were allowed to make their own food choices at the age of 12. Likewise, caries levels fell in parallel with the availability of sugars during the Second World War (Rugg-Gunn 1993).

It is difficult for people to restrict their consumption of sugars. There are evolutionary reasons for sweet foods and drinks to be pleasant. Consequently 'hidden' sugars are used to make processed foods nicer. In addition, products used to sweeten foods may not be labelled as such, even if they carry similar risks of harm (e.g. fructose corn syrup). To add to this confusion, ecological and animal studies indicate that sugars in whole fruit (sometimes called intrinsic sugars) do not cause caries. Furthermore, intrinsic sugars have a relatively low glycaemic index and are accompanied by fibre and so are not usually associated with obesity.

A health-directed food policy focusing on the supply of products containing unhealthy sugars seems logical, and is likely to impact on dental diseases as well as broader health problems, given the growing evidence implicating them as a cause of obesity, myocardial infarction, dyslipidaemia, pancreatitis, and hepatic dysfunction (Lustig et al. 2012; Willett and Ludwig 2013). The WHO recommends countries to formulate their own specific goals to reduce the amount of free sugars, with a maximum of no more than 10 per cent of energy intake (it is approximately 15 per cent in the United States and United Kingdom). In addition, the frequency of consumption of foods containing free sugars should be limited to a maximum of four times per day

Such policies should form part of a broader strategy to reduce dietary intakes of refined grain products and potatoes. Possible strategies fall within the framework of education, substitution, regulation, pricing, or provision (Watt and Rouxel 2012). Multi-levelled fiscal policies can be used to discourage the manufacture and sale of sugar-containing products, including taxing sugar-containing foods and drinks and restricting advertising to children. Beyond approaches aimed at individuals, education can take the form of authoritative dietary guidelines to inform national policies, community initiatives, and caterers. Recommendations by the Finnish National Board of Education reduced the sale of sweet products in Finnish Schools (Kankaanpää et al. 2012). Healthcare workers can routinely ask their patients about sugar consumption (dentists do this all the time!). All of these approaches and direct consumer pressure can help convince caterers and retail outlets to provide food in a way that makes the healthy choices the easier choices.

Dietary sugars can be substituted with artificial sweeteners to reduce caries incidence. Sales of sugar-free carbonated drinks in Europe and North America demonstrate the compatibility of this measure with commercial interests. However, substitution of dietary sugars has only limited potential because the manufacture of many foodstuffs relies on other specific properties of sugars. In addition, some sweeteners have side effects and resistance to the extended use of artificial sweeteners persists.

Oral cleaning

As plaque is a necessary cause of periodontal diseases it seems logical that tooth cleaning (principally by toothbrushing) should be the cornerstone of their management and prevention. Interventions aimed at improving oral hygiene can be successful and achieve a commensurate reduction in gingival inflammation (Kay and Locker 1997; Watt and Marinho 2005). However, most studies have had short follow-up periods and the effectiveness of even the best interventions diminishes with time. Therefore few data show that attempts to improve oral hygiene to prevent destructive disease are effective. Nonetheless, the consensus is that the public health approaches to improve periodontal health should include improved oral hygiene.

The relationship between plaque removal and tooth decay is much more contentious. In a carefully designed trial, professional oral cleaning did not demonstrate any additional preventive effect above a standard preventive programme of fissure sealants and locally applied topical fluoride (Arrow 1997). Sutcliffe (1996) reviewed the effect of research methods on the observed relationship between oral cleaning and dental caries and concluded that there was 'no unequivocal evidence that good oral cleanliness reduces caries experience'. This area of research is fraught with difficulty as apart from the difficulties of measuring dental disease, studies are susceptible to selection bias, leakage of intervention, and the likely confounding effects between self-reported behaviours, diet, and oral hygiene. Studies where professional cleaning has been effective have used pastes containing fluoride. What is known is that brushing with fluoride toothpaste is effective in preventing caries. Therefore brushing as it is currently practised in most developed countries combats both caries and periodontal diseases and is to be encouraged.

The systematic reviews cited earlier demonstrated that it is difficult to achieve sustainable changes in oral hygiene behaviour. One approach has been to teach toothbrushing to both make one feel and look nice and as part of a positive and healthy lifestyle. Toothbrushing is a habit learned as a young child and is difficult to change later in life, hence interventions via healthcare workers and social agencies working with young children and their parents may be useful.

Toothbrushing often clusters with other health behaviours such as tobacco use, exercise, healthy eating, and other aspects of hygiene such as hand washing. In turn, these behaviours may relate to personal factors including greater self-efficacy, self-esteem, having confidence in one's family, life satisfaction, managing in school, and not having other health problems. Unsurprisingly then, toothbrushing is determined by structural and resource-related factors and living conditions. These factors include family structure, social support, external barriers, domestic arrangements, social norms, cultural factors, socioeconomic status, and socioeconomic development. Therefore actions across all these levels are most likely to improve periodontal health and periodontal health equity.

Smoking cessation

Cessation of smoking decreases the associated elevated risk of oral cancer within 5–10 years. Numerous other oral conditions are directly or indirectly associated with tobacco smoking. Many of these, such as stained teeth, receding gums, and altered taste are readily perceptible to the individual and may encourage or reinforce the desire to stop smoking. The dental team are also often aware of the personal and social circumstances (e.g. pregnancy or a new job) that prompt people to give up. The dental team can hence support smoking cessation by providing advice (Carr and Ebbert 2006).

Trauma: prevention and management

Maxillofacial trauma is related to environmental and structural factors such as socioeconomic status, alcohol use, and road planning and use. In children, dental trauma is closely related to area-based measures of socioeconomic status and overcrowding. Many of these factors can be alleviated by improving living conditions.

Local and individual strategies can also help reduce trauma to the face and teeth. Playground surfaces can be made of impact-absorbing materials which cushion against trauma. The use of mouthguards is compulsory for some sports in some countries. Mouthguards not only prevent dental injuries, but also prevent laceration of the facial soft tissues against the teeth, reduce the risk of mandibular fracture, and may protect the cranial cavity. The most basic type may be obtained prefabricated in a range of sizes. A more sophisticated type may be adapted to fit the mouth, typically by softening it in hot water first. Custom-made devices are the most comfortable and can be made to support the lower teeth and mandible during trauma.

Immediate first-aid for dental trauma (particularly teeth that have been knocked out) is critical to preserve the traumatized teeth. Informing athletes and their teachers and trainers of the need for immediate action can reduce the impact of the trauma.

Unfortunately orthodontic treatment of protruding front teeth is complex and prolonged, but can be justified in children of 8 or 9 years to reduce the risk of trauma.

Use of health services

The biomedical model remains the dominant approach within dental services despite the widespread recognition of the relatively small contribution of healthcare and dental care to health (Illich 1976; McKeown 1976) and oral health (Nadanovsky and Sheiham 1994, 1995). Orthodontic treatment is often advocated on the basis of social and psychological benefit. However, a 20-year follow-up study was unable to find evidence to support such a benefit (Kenealy et al. 2007). Many interventions used in dentistry (Baelum 2011) often involve cycles of placing and replacing fillings. As the quality of many fillings is not high and even the decisions to place fillings are idiosyncratic (Elderton and Nuttall 1983), the replacement of fillings several times over a lifetime leads to increasing damage to the remaining tooth.

Similar problems exist with medical and dental care. Resources are constrained and may be poorly allocated. Services still cluster around people who can afford them, while those who cannot have little control over their own health and healthcare. In every country of the world, there are people who cannot attend and/or afford dental treatment, and even in well-developed socialized systems of dental care, major inequalities exist (Watt and Sheiham 1999).

Views about the relative role of health services remain polarized. From one perspective, too narrow a focus on 'health service issues' contributes to the failure of public health to improve population health (Holland 2002; Beaglehole and Bonita 2004). The 'post-new public health' view argues that preventive and curative measures prolong life expectancy and maintain and improve the quality of life. Bunker (2001) estimated the increases in life expectancy attributable to clinical care from declines in disease-specific death rates and from specific treatments. His conclusions may have been optimistic as he generalizes results achieved in research trials to routine practice, and underestimates the role of social and other environmental factors in health (Frankel 2001; Tudor Hart 2001).

At a population level, it remains difficult to distinguish the effects of medical care from those of other health determinants. At a practical level, such a distinction may not ultimately be critical since the key is to select the interventions that can improve the health of the population (Frankel 2001).

Unfortunately, when compared to medicine, the benefits and costs of clinical dentistry at either an individual or population level are relatively unknown. However, there are some good examples of developments in the evidence base for different aspects of dental services. One such example is that of screening for dental caries in schools, an activity that is undertaken in various forms in many countries. An RCT conducted in England examined three different models of school screening and found none were effective at reducing levels of active caries and increasing attendance by children at the dentist (Milsom et al. 2006). This study led the UK screening committee to change its policy, and recommend school dental screening be stopped and the resources redirected at oral health promotion activities. Caries screening programmes that provide treatment to children directly after detection of the disease appear to be more effective.

Public health specialists can help increase the effectiveness and equity of access of services. For example, clinical dentistry can have a role in reducing the psychosocial impacts of oral disease (Awad et al. 2000; Robinson et al. 2005). For this reason, it is essential to identify more relevant measures of oral health to assess treatment need and the outcomes of care. The evidence-based approach, the use of clinical governance, and managed care should provide both the impetus and means to ensure that only effective and efficient interventions are used.

Specific changes that could be made to ensure access to dental services can still be categorized in the framework used by Penchansky and Thomas (1981). Services must be available, accessible, affordable, acceptable, and accommodating. This framework is broadly compatible with the characteristics of dental services as seen within Andersen's (1995) behavioural model of access.

Clearly people cannot use services that do not exist, so increasing their availability has a direct effect on service use. In addition, the heterogeneity of dental health in the developed world means that older people (the 'heavy metal generation') will continue to have complex dental treatment needs for decades to come, whereas the needs of younger people are likely to be more straightforward. The proportion of dental treatment that falls within this straightforward category will continue to grow. It is not cost-effective for broadly trained and highly paid dentists to undertake this less demanding and repetitive work. One approach is to delegate more straightforward treatments to other DCPs, especially in deprived communities, hence liberating dentists' time to undertake more complex treatments.

A number of countries including Australia, New Zealand, Canada, and the United Kingdom employ DCPs with a limited repertoire of treatment options (variously called school dental nurses, dental auxiliaries, and dental therapists). The scope of practice of dental therapists varies from country to country (Nash et al. 2012). In general, they may undertake diagnostic procedures and treatment planning and preventive services, place fillings in primary and permanent teeth, and extract primary teeth. They may also be permitted to extract permanent teeth. The appropriateness of these skills to the treatment needs of their populations and the relatively low cost of training and employing dental therapists means that their use is growing in some countries and being considered in others, including the United States.

Therapists can be used to increase access to care by supplementing the volume and reach of services, which enhances equity (Dyer et al. 2013). Therapists are socially acceptable where they are integrated into existing dental systems. Available data suggest that therapists offer care that is similarly effective to that provided by dentists. Substitution of dentists by therapists within small dental teams creates complexities and costs that reduce efficiency. Conversely, efficiency appears to be high if therapists work independently. However, dental organizations tend to prevent or restrict the deployment of therapists. For example, executives of the American Dental Association have advocated a free market dental system with subsidized treatment for disadvantaged families rather than a needs-based system using DCPs in areas with an undersupply of care (Bramson and Guay 2005).

In developing countries with a growing incidence of dental caries which may not be able to afford sufficient dentists to meet the needs of their populations, dental professionals may be an appropriate solution.

One particular aspect of dentistry in many countries that could be revised is the direct fee-for-service system of payment to dentists. Fee-per-item service payments encourage dentists to work quickly and may incentivize over-treatment and not prevention unless there is a specific fee for this. On the other hand, services based on capitation per patient enrolled reduce restorative treatment and increase preventive care with no evidence of 'supervised neglect' (Johansson et al. 2007).

The acceptability of dental services was highlighted in a qualitative study of people who did not go to the dentist (Gregory et al. 2007). As well as being influenced by the perceived accessibility of care, participants were swayed by their trust in dentistry and their perceptions of oral health as a commodity. For these people at least, greater marketing may have been counterproductive in encouraging use of dental services.

Dental services in middle- and low-income countries

Non-industrialized countries usually suffer from resource constraints including workforce, appropriate technology, and reliable power supplies. For example, the dentist:population ratio in many countries in Africa is less than 1:100,000 population compared to 1:1100 in many Scandinavian countries. This is exacerbated by the migration of dentists from middle- and low-income countries to more developed countries. For example, over a quarter of dentists in the United Kingdom were not UK-born and two-thirds of dental graduates from the Philippines migrate to the United States although most do not work there as dentists.

The limitations of the traditional curative approach to dental health are more extreme in the context of the developing world. The surgical approach to dentistry is technology intensive and requires the availability of continuous power and water supply. It involves expensive equipment that is difficult to use and maintain. Dentists, therefore, need to treat patients who can help them recoup their costs. These pressures limit the availability of services

and contribute to the inequalities in their provision. Large parts of the Western model of dental care may be inappropriate in developing countries, including an overemphasis of clinical surveys in healthcare planning. Services based on normative assessment limit community participation in healthcare and ignore the sociodental implications of oral disease. In one notorious example, survey data used to calculate the periodontal treatment needs of children in Kenya (Manji and Sheiham 1986) would have used the entire national dental workforce for up to 21 years. Services could concentrate on the relatively few conditions that comprise the bulk of oral health problems: toothache (not *tooth decay*), trauma, oral infections, and neoplasms (Hobdell 1993).

The primary oral healthcare approach (PHCA) is still relevant in all countries but particularly so in the developing world. It has five principles:

1. *Equitable distribution of services:* Tudor Hart's (1971) 'inverse care law' between the availability of services and the need for them also occurs in dentistry. It is particularly extreme in countries where there are wide disparities between rich and poor. In Africa, 80 per cent of the trained professional personnel live and work in affluent neighbourhoods in cities although the same proportion of the population lives in rural areas. The scope for other dental care professionals in developing countries may be greater since political lobbies of dentists may be less well established than in industrialized nations. DCPs can provide simple, but essential treatments to extend the availability of services and reduce inequalities in access. Models exist for identifying the types of personnel needed for oral healthcare in deprived communities along with training and evaluation methods (Samarawikrama 1995).

2. *Community involvement in health:* this means that people are allowed to take control of their own health and is necessary if programmes are to thrive. It is perhaps the most difficult aspect of the PHCA since it requires health professionals to relinquish their traditional hierarchical role. Individuals and communities often also regard health as beyond their control and may not consider oral health a priority. There are isolated examples of wide involvement in oral health. In Glasgow, Scotland, community-based Oral Health Action Teams (partnerships of parents, teachers, nursery nurses, health visitors, and dentists) have reduced caries levels in young children in deprived areas of the city (Blair et al. 2004).

3. *Focus on prevention:* prevention of oral diseases is universally accepted as an essential component of care, but in the past has involved people as passive recipients of information rather than active participants in health promotion. Systematic reviews suggest that programmes to optimize exposure to fluoride are the most effective.

4. *Use of appropriate technology:* 'appropriate technology' does not connote 'cheap' and 'second rate', but an approach which recognizes the needs and resources of the local community. For example, ART combines these requirements with knowledge of dental caries progression and developments in dental materials science.

5. *Multisectoral approach:* we have seen how an effective health strategy might involve a number of departments of both national and local governments, water providers, the educational system,

community members, and healthcare workers. All of this needs to be integrated coherently to go beyond just using the resources of other sectors to promote oral health. For example, if dentists simply get teachers to provide dental health education, this carries the risk of not truly involving the other sectors (Mautsch and Sheiham 1995).

Measure and understand the problem and assess the impact of action

Monitoring the social determinants of oral health requires routine systems to record relevant measures of health, its determinants, and health equity. Such data can be collected during dental treatment or through surveys.

New evidence on the role of social determinants in oral health equity and evaluations of interventions to reduce inequality should emerge from the international emphasis given to the topic. For example, WHO attention on the social determinants of health should make funding for such work a priority. One area where the global oral health inequalities research agenda can make an immediate impact is to provide a forum for sharing and interpreting new evidence.

Training on this topic is available through undergraduate and postgraduate courses for dentistry, although the extent and focus varies. The WHO Oral Health Programme provides guidance on tackling oral health inequalities, but could benefit from greater resources (Kwan and Petersen 2010).

Future developments

Several trends in oral health have been observed. First, some countries, particularly developing ones, may experience increases in dental caries due to the adoption of diets high in sugars. These trends are worrying even if they are limited to more affluent city dwellers as the increase in treatment needs is likely to place an unaffordably high burden on developing economies while this burden will be moderated by the low levels of perceived need in communities unused to receiving dental treatment. However, if disability and handicap from oral disease is to be minimized, then appropriate treatment is necessary. Numerous examples now exist of DCPs being used to provide a limited range of treatments in both the developed and developing world. DCPs can be trained quicker to provide care to similar standards to dentists, but at greatly reduced costs. Food and health policies could also be used in countries with rising caries levels to control imports and the production and sale of cariogenic foods, and drinks while encouraging the use of traditional foods, although the evidence base for the effectiveness of the use of such policies is weak.

Second, the fall in caries prevalence seen in developed countries over the past 40 years appears to have slowed, with evidence of wide inequalities between those living in the most and least deprived areas. Several studies have suggested that not only do people living in deprived areas have more dental caries, the disease has more impact on their daily lives.

Third, in many developed countries the combination of demographic changes, changed attitudes towards oral health, and the preservation of teeth produces an interesting pattern (Fig. 8.8.1). The growing number of older people who will live longer and retain many heavily restored teeth will increase the need for more care, some of it more complex, which in turn will drive more specialization.

The deprofessionalization of dentistry that has continued for the last decade appears to be gathering pace and is manifest in several different forms. In many developed countries patients are demanding 'rights' as consumers of care, even as marketing theory is being applied to dentistry, which places consumer satisfaction as being essential for business success. Similar principles are cornerstones of new public health. Health promotion takes public involvement in oral health well beyond clinical dentistry. Even within clinical care, satisfaction is an integral part of the process of care rather than just an outcome. Other agencies, such as governments and insurance companies, are increasingly involved in healthcare. Externally applied measures to minimize the costs of care and increase the accountability of healthcare organizations whilst assuring the quality of care all serve to reduce professional power within dentistry.

Gigerenzer and Gray (2011) have named the twenty-first century as the *century of the patient*. They envisage a critical mass of increasing health literate and numerate patients triggering healthcare improvements. The improvements will come about because healthcare workers will need to be better informed to keep up with their patients. They suggest widespread stakeholder participation to solve common healthcare problems using all the theoretical and practical knowledge available.

This trend of deprofessionalization is likely to continue and may help to make oral care more relevant to the needs of the people it serves. Deprofessionalization and greater lay involvement in dentistry, both at the individual and community level, will reduce the power structures and hierarchies that underpin the social determinants of health. This might be particularly important where perceived social position is a cause of health inequality independent of objective assessments of socioeconomic status (Sanders et al. 2006). Given that professions are likely to resist any tendency to undermine their power, there is an opportunity for dental public health to facilitate and manage the deprofessionalization of dentistry.

Evidence base

Only a minority of practitioners and academics appear to be contributing to the growth in the evidence base of dentistry. Those practitioners conduct a growing number of systematic reviews, but unfortunately these repeatedly conclude that there is a dearth of good primary data on which decisions can be based. Whilst a greater evidence base for individual care is needed, more research is urgently needed on the benefits of interventions at a population level, not only to improve health, but also to reduce inequalities.

Other chapters in this text will consider the evaluation of health promotion in some detail (see Chapter 2.1), but the debate about controlled trials in public health continues. Health promotion takes place in the 'real world' and other factors and time intervene between the intervention and health outcomes. For example, implementing a life course approach to reduce inequalities may take decades before its benefits are manifest. These factors have led the WHO (1998) to conclude that 'The use of RCTs to evaluate health promotion initiatives is, in most cases, inappropriate, misleading and unnecessarily expensive'. Even the keenest advocates of RCTs acknowledge that they are unsuitable for evaluating legislative and policy changes (Rosen et al. 2006). However, many of the problems often cited against conducting trials in public health can be overcome (Macintyre 2011).

Technology

Technological developments may also influence oral health and care. In developed countries, osseo-integrated implants are increasingly used to support dental prostheses. By providing a stable and retentive base for both single and multiple tooth prostheses, implants show great potential for reducing the handicap brought about by oral disease (Awad et al. 2000). At present, however, implant treatment demands considerable specialist expertise, requires regular maintenance, and is costly. Implants may therefore become a treatment limited to those who can afford them and thus contribute to inequalities in oral health. Other more long-term technological possibilities include a vaccine for dental caries, growing teeth from stem cells, the use of nanotechnology, and laser drills.

Cosmetic dentistry

As dental disease has declined in developed countries the technology that allowed restoration of damaged dentitions is now available for purely cosmetic purposes. Cosmetic dentistry procedures include bleaching teeth and the use of veneers to change their appearance. There is little evidence that dentistry to improve appearance can bring about psychological or social benefit. Therefore, cosmetic dentistry may improve appearance but not health.

Cosmetic dentistry can be seen as the medicalization of beauty and as a form of iatrogenesis. Supplier-induced demand is evident when dentists draw patients' attention to minor dental anomalies (that may have no effect on their lives) and suggest they have them corrected. Attractiveness is perhaps more important now than ever before and society is said to be suffering from a normative discontent with personal appearance. Dentistry may contribute to these problems if the availability of treatment to enhance dental appearance makes deviations from the norm less acceptable. This message is amplified in printed and broadcast media that expose us to enhanced images. Photographs in magazines have whiter and straighter teeth than would normally be encountered and exposure to these images increases our dissatisfaction with our own appearance. In addition, cosmetic dentistry will only be available to those who can afford it. It may be that the visible consumption of cosmetic dentistry will further distinguish socioeconomic groups and so contribute to the stratification of society and social inequalities. From this perspective, cosmetic dentistry might have adverse effects both on the people who receive it and on wider society and consideration may be required about whether its growth should continue unchecked.

Consumerism and the role of industry in oral health

Consumerism is widely criticized from the perspective of overconsumption, its links with media culture, and from socialist and feminist perspectives. Its role in oral health is not so clear cut. The addition of fluoride to toothpastes has been one of the most successful dental public health interventions of all time. The effectiveness of fluoridated toothpastes is demonstrated in a Cochrane systematic review of RCTs (Marinho et al. 2003a). However, the effect is cumulative and is staggering when seen over decades. The first fluoride toothpastes were introduced in the 1950s but sales rose dramatically in the United Kingdom during the 1970s (the proportion of toothpaste sales containing fluoride rose from less than 10 per cent in 1970 to more than 90 per cent in 1976). This chapter has already described the beneficial impact which continues throughout the lifetime as demonstrated by the growing cohorts of people with more sound and unfilled teeth in Fig. 8.8.1.

Although dentists were involved in the development, evaluation, and promotion of fluoridated toothpastes, it was the commercial interests of home-care product manufacturers which drove this development. There are also numerous examples of manufacturers and dental organizations working together to promote oral health that continue to this day.

The commercial marketing of dental care products has other advantages. It has raised the prominence of oral health and reinforced the idea of frequent oral cleaning as a social norm. In addition, the positive ways in which oral healthcare products are advertised has made a healthy mouth seem attainable.

Conclusions

In summary, we have argued that poor oral health is a major public health problem with a huge population burden of oral disease because of the large numbers of people affected. Whilst the incidence of dental caries has fallen in the developed world, the prevalence of the condition would be staggering when compared to any other disease. Periodontal diseases, cancer, and trauma all pose specific problems. All these diseases have significant impacts and create a considerable burden to both individuals and the community. The links between oral and general health indicate that strategies to improve both sets of problems and reduce inequalities should be integrated within the framework advocated by the CSDH. Several factors, including tighter financial pressures, trends in oral health, the deprofessionalization of dentistry, the role of consumerism in oral health, and the need for a better evidence base will modify this endeavour, as will the growth of skill mix, technology, and cosmetic dentistry.

References

Andersen, R.M. (1995). Revisiting the behavioral model and access to medical care: does it matter? *Journal of Health and Social Behavior*, 36, 1–10.

Anderson, L., Martin, N.R., Flynn, R.T., and Knight, S. (2012). The importance of substate surveillance in detection of geographic oral health inequalities in a small state. *Journal of Public Health Management and Practice*, 18, 461–8.

Andreasen, J.O. and Andreasen, F.M. (1997). *Textbook and Color Atlas of Traumatic Injuries to the Teeth*. Copenhagen: Munksgaard.

Armfield, J.M. and Spencer, A.J. (2007). Community effectiveness of fissure sealants and the effect of fluoridated water consumption. *Community Dental Health*, 24, 4–11.

Arrow, P. (1997). Control of occlusal caries in the first permanent molars by oral hygiene. *Community Dentistry and Oral Epidemiology*, 25, 278–83.

Awad, M.A., Locker, D., Korner-Bitensky, N., et al. (2000). Measuring the effect of intraoral implant rehabilitation on health related quality of life in a randomised controlled clinical trial. *Journal of Dental Research*, 79, 1659–63.

Baelum, V. (2011). Dentistry and population approaches for preventing dental diseases. *Journal of Dentistry*, 39(Suppl. 2), S9–19.

Beaglehole, R. and Bonita, R. (2004). *Public Health at the Crossroads*. Cambridge: Cambridge University Press.

Beck, J.D., Couper, D.J., Falkner, K.L., et al. (2008). The Periodontitis and Vascular Events (PAVE) pilot study: adverse events. *Journal of Periodontology*, 79, 90–6.

Beck, J.D. and Offenbacher, S. (2005). Systemic effects of periodontitis: epidemiology of periodontal disease and cardiovascular disease. *Journal of Periodontology*, 76(Suppl.), 2089–100.

Bernabé, E. and Marcenes, W. (2011). Income inequality and tooth loss in the United States. *Journal of Dental Research*, 90, 724–9.

Blair, Y., Macpherson, L.M., McCall, D.R., et al. (2004). Glasgow nursery-based caries experience, before and after a community development-based oral health programme's implementation. *Community Dental Health*, 21, 291–8.

Bramson, J.B. and Guay, A.H. (2005). Comments on the proposed pediatric oral health therapist. *Journal of Public Health Dentistry*, 65, 123–7.

Bunker, J.P. (2001). The role of medical care in contributing to health improvements within societies. *International Journal of Epidemiology*, 30, 1260–3.

Burt, B.A. (1998). Prevention policies in the light of the changed distribution of dental caries. *Acta Odontologica Scandinavia*, 56, 179–86.

Burt, B.A., Ismail, A.I., and Eklund, S.A. (1985). Periodontal disease, tooth loss, and oral hygiene among older Americans. *Community Dentistry and Oral Epidemiology*, 13, 93–6.

Cancer Research UK (2009). *Oral Cancer Survival Statistics*. [Online] Available at: http://www.cancerresearchuk.org/cancer-info/cancer-stats/types/oral/survival/oral-cancer-survival-statistics#deprivation.

Carr, A.B. and Ebbert, J.O. (2006). Interventions for tobacco cessation in the dental setting. *Cochrane Database of Systematic Reviews*, 1, CD005084.

Centers for Disease Control and Prevention. (2010). *Community Water Fluoridation*. [Online] Available at: http://www.cdc.gov/fluoridation/.

Commission on Social Determinants of Health (2008). *Closing the Gap in a Generation: Health Equity Through Action on the Social Determinants of Health. Final Report of the Commission on Social Determinants of Health*. Geneva: WHO.

Conway, D.I., McKinney, P.A., McMahon, A.D., et al. (2010). Socioeconomic factors associated with risk of upper aerodigestive tract cancer in Europe. *European Journal of Cancer*, 46, 588–98.

Conway, D.I., Petticrew, M., Marlborough, H., Berthiller, J., Hashibe, M., and Macpherson, L.M. (2008). Socioeconomic inequalities and oral cancer risk: a systematic review and meta-analysis of case-control studies. *International Journal of Cancer*, 122, 2811–19.

Conway, D.I., Stockton, D.L., Warnakulasuriya, K.A., et al. (2006). Incidence of oral and oropharyngeal cancer in United Kingdom (1990–1999)—recent trends and regional variation. *Oral Oncology*, 42, 586–92.

Dahlgren, G. and Whitehead, M. (1992). *Policies and Strategies to Promote Social Equity in Health*. Copenhagen: WHO.

Dean, H.T., Arnold, F.A. Jr., Jay, P., et al. (1950). Studies on mass control of dental caries through fluoridation of the public water supply. *Public Health Reports*, 65, 1403–8.

De Oliveira, C., Watt, R., and Hamer, M. (2010). Toothbrushing, inflammation, and risk of cardiovascular disease: results from Scottish Health Survey. *BMJ*, 340, c2451.

Department of Health and Human Services (2000). *Oral Health in America: A Report of the Surgeon General*. Washington, DC: Department of Health and Human Services.

Dickson, M. (1995). Oral health promotion. In W. Mautsch and A. Sheiham (eds.) *Promoting Oral Health in Deprived Communities*, pp. 175–86. Berlin: Deusche Stiftungfur Internationale Entwicklung.

Downer, M.C., Moles, D.R., Palmer, S., et al. (2006). A systematic review of measures of the effectiveness of screening for oral cancer and precancer. *Oral Oncology*, 42, 551–60.

D'Souza, G., Kreimer, A.R., Viscidi, R., et al. (2007). Case-control study of human papillomavirus and oropharyngeal cancer. *The New England Journal of Medicine*, 356, 1944–56.

Dybul, M., Piot, P., and Frenk J. (2012). *Reshaping Global Health*. [Online] Available at: www.hoover.org/publications/policy-review/article/118116.

Dyer, T., Owens, J., and Robinson, P.G. (2013). What matters to patients when their care is delegated to dental therapists? *British Dental Journal*, 214, E17.

Eke, P.I., Dye, B.A., Wei, L., Thornton-Evans, G.O., and Genco, R.J. (2012). Prevalence of periodontitis in adults in the United States: 2009 and 2010. *Journal of Dental Research*, 91, 914–20.

Elani, H.W., Harper, S., Allison, P.J., Bedos, C., and Kaufman, J.S. (2012). Socio-economic inequalities and oral health in Canada and the United States. *Journal of Dental Research*, 91, 865–70.

Elderton, R.J. and Nuttall, N.M. (1983). Variation among dentists in planning treatment. *British Dental Journal*, 154, 201–6.

Fakhry, C., Westra, W.H., Li, S., et al. (2008). Improved survival of patients with human papillomavirus-positive head and neck squamous cell carcinoma in a prospective clinical trial. *Journal of the National Cancer Institute*, 100, 261–9.

Flores, G. and Lin, H. (2013). Trends in racial/ethnic disparities in medical and oral health, access to care, and use of services in US children: has anything changed over the years? *International Journal of Equity in Health*, 12, 10.

Frankel, S. (2001). Commentary: medical care and the wider influences upon population health: a false dichotomy. *International Journal of Epidemiology*, 30, 1267–8.

Frencken, J.E., Leal, S.C., and Navarro, M.F. (2012). Twenty-five-year atraumatic restorative treatment (ART) approach: a comprehensive overview. *Clinical Oral Investigations*, 16, 1337–46.

Gigerenzer, G. and Gray, J.A.M. (2011). Launching the century of the patient. In G. Gigerenzer and J.A.M. Gray (eds.) *Better Doctors, Better Patients, Better Decisions*, pp. 3–29. Cambridge, MA: The MIT Press.

Globocan (2010). *Estimated Cancer Incidence, Mortality, Prevalence and Disability-adjusted Life years (DALYs) Worldwide in 2008*. Paris: International Agency for Research on Cancer, WHO. Available at: http://globocan.iarc.fr/.

Gregory, J., Gibson, B., and Robinson, P.G. (2007). The relevance of oral health for attenders and non-attenders: a qualitative study. *British Dental Journal*, 202, E18.

Hindle, I., Downer, M.C., Moles, D.R., and Speight, P.M. (2000). Is alcohol responsible for more intra-oral cancer? *Oral Oncology*, 36, 328–33.

Hobdell, M.H. (1993). Essential elements of a primary oral health care model. In S.P. Akpabio (ed.) *Promotion of Oral Health in the African Region. Proceedings of Workshop Held in Nairobi, Kenya, 2–6 August 1993*, pp. 99–108. London: Commonwealth Dental Association.

Holland, W.W. (2002). A dubious future for public health? *Journal of the Royal Society of Medicine*, 95, 182–8.

Illich, I. (1976). *Limits to Medicine*. London: Penguin.

Ismail, A.I. and Bandekar, R.R. (1999). Fluoride supplements and fluorosis: a meta-analysis. *Community Dentistry and Oral Epidemiology*, 27, 48–56.

Johansson, V., Axtelius, B., Soderfeldt, B., et al. (2007). Financial systems' impact on dental care: a review of fee-for-service and capitation systems. *Community Dental Health*, 24, 12–20.

Jones, S., Burt, B.A., Petersen, P.E., et al. (2005). The effective use of fluorides in public health. *Bulletin of the World Health Organization*, 83, 670–6.

Jones, S. and Lennon, M.A. (eds.) (1997). *Fluoridation. Community Oral Health*. Bath: Wright.

Jordao, L.M.R., Vasconcelos, D.V., da Silveira Moreira, R., and Freire, M.C.M. (2012). Individual and contextual determinants of periodontal health in 12 year old schoolchildren in a Brazilian capital city. *International Journal of Dentistry*, 2012, 325475.

Jowett, A.K., Orr, M.T.S., Rawlinson, A., and Robinson, P.G. (2009). Psychosocial impact of periodontal disease and its treatment with 24-h root surface debridement. *Journal of Clinical Periodontology*, 36, 413–18.

Kankaanpää, R., Seppänen, S., Hiiri, A., Manninen, M., Puska, P., and Lahti, S. (2012). Effect of national recommendations on the sale of sweet products in the upper level of Finnish comprehensive schools. *Community Dental Health*, 29, 149–53.

Kay, E.J. and Locker, D. (1997). *Effectiveness of Oral Health Promotion: A Review*. London: Health Education Authority.

Kenealy, P.M., Kingdon, A., Richmond, S., et al. (2007). The Cardiff dental study: a 20-year critical evaluation of the psychological health gain from orthodontic treatment. *British Psychological Society*, 12, 17–49.

Krieger, N. (2008). Ladders, pyramids and champagne: the iconography of health inequities. *Journal of Epidemiology and Community Health*, 62, 1098–104.

Krieger, N., Dorling, D., and McCartney, G. (2012). Mapping injustice, visualising equity: why theory, metaphors and images matter in tackling inequalities. *Public Health*, 126, 256–8.

Kwan, S. and Petersen, P.E. (2010). Oral health: equity and social determinants. In E. Blas and A.S. Sivasankara Kurup (eds.) *Equity, Social Determinants and Public Health Programmes*, pp. 159–76. Geneva: WHO.

Linden, G.J., Linden, K., Yarnell, J., Evans, A., Kee, F., and Patterson, C.C. (2012). All-cause mortality and periodontitis in 60–70-year-old men: a prospective cohort study. *Journal of Clinical Periodontology*, 39, 940–6.

Locker, D. (2007). Disparities in oral health-related quality of life in a population of Canadian children. *Community Dentistry and Oral Epidemiology*, 35, 348–56.

Lorenc, T., Petticrew, M., Welch, V., and Tugwell, P. (2013). What types of interventions generate inequalities? Evidence from systematic reviews. *Journal of Epidemiology and Community Health*, 67, 190–3.

Lustig, R.H., Schmidt, L.A., and Brindis, C.D. (2012). The toxic truth about sugar. *Nature*, 482, 27–9.

Macintyre, S. (2011). Good intentions and received wisdom are not good enough: the need for controlled trials in public health journal. *Journal of Epidemiology and Community Health*, 65, 564–7.

Mackenbach, J.P. (2012). The persistence of health inequalities in modern welfare states: the explanation of a paradox. *Social Science & Medicine*, 75, 761–9.

Manji, F. and Sheiham, A. (1986). CPITN findings and the manpower implications of periodontal treatment needs for Kenyan children. *Community Dental Health*, 3, 143–51.

Marinho, V.C.C., Higgins, J.P.T., Logan, S., et al. (2002a). Fluoride varnishes for preventing dental caries in children and adolescents. *Cochrane Database of Systematic Reviews*, 1, CD002279.

Marinho, V.C.C., Higgins, J.P.T., Logan, S., et al. (2002b). Fluoride gels for preventing dental caries in children and adolescents. *Cochrane Database of Systematic Reviews*, 1, CD002280.

Marinho, V.C.C., Higgins, J.P.T., Logan, S., et al. (2003a). Fluoride toothpastes for preventing dental caries in children and adolescents. *Cochrane Database of Systematic Reviews*, 1, CD002278.

Marinho, V.C.C., Higgins, J.P.T., Logan, S., et al. (2003b). Fluoride mouthrinses for preventing dental caries in children and adolescents. *Cochrane Database of Systematic Reviews*, 3, CD002284.

Marino, R., Villa A., and Weitz A. (2006). *Dental Caries Prevention using Milk as the Vehicle for Fluorides: The Chilean Experiences*. Melbourne: School of Dental Science, University of Melbourne.

Marmot, M. (2010). *Fair Society, Healthy Lives: Strategic Review of Health Inequalities in England post-2010*. London: Marmot Review.

Marmot, M. and Bell, R. (2011). Social determinants and dental health. *Advances in Dental Research*, 23(2), 201–6.

Mautsch, W. and Sheiham, A. (1995). *Promoting Oral Health in Deprived Communities*. Berlin: Zahnmedizinische Entwicklungshilfe e.V.

McDonagh, M., Whiting, P., Bradley, M., et al. (2000). *A Systematic Review of Public Water Fluoridation*. York: Publications Office, NHS Centre for Reviews and Dissemination, University of York.

McKeown, T. (1976). *The Role of Medicine: Dream, Mirage or Nemesis?* London: The Nuffield Provincial Hospitals Trust.

Medical Research Council (2002). *Water Fluoridation and Health*. London: Medical Research Council.

Milsom, K.M., Blinkhorn, A.S., Walsh, T., et al. (2011). A cluster-randomized controlled trial: fluoride varnish in school children. *Journal of Dental Research*, 90, 1306–11.

Milsom, K., Blinkhorn, A., Worthington, H., et al. (2006). The effectiveness of school dental screening: a cluster-randomized control trial. *Journal of Dental Research*, 85, 924–8.

Mohammadi, M.T., Wright, C.M., and Kay, E.J. (2009). Childhood growth and dental caries. *Community Dental Health*, 26, 38–42.

Moynihan, P. and Petersen, P.E. (2004). Diet, nutrition and the prevention of dental diseases. *Public Health Nutrition*, 7, 201–26.

Nadanovsky, P. and Sheiham, A. (1994). The relative contribution of dental services to the changes and geographical variations in caries status of 5- and 12-year-old children in England and Wales in the 1980s. *Community Dental Health*, 11, 215–23.

Nadanovsky, P. and Sheiham, A. (1995). Relative contribution of dental services to the changes in caries levels of 12-year-old children in 18 industrialized countries in the 1970s and early 1980s. *Community Dentistry and Oral Epidemiology*, 23, 331–9.

Nash, D.A., Friedman, J.W., Mathu-Muju, K.R., et al. (2012). *A Review of the Global Literature on Dental Therapists*. New York: W.J. Kellogg Foundation.

National Health and Medical Research Council (2007). *A Systematic Review of the Efficacy and Safety of Fluoridation*. Canberra: Australian Government. Available at: http://www.nhmrc.gov.au/_files_nhmrc/publications/attachments/eh41_1.pdf.

National Institute for Health and Clinical Excellence (2004). *Dental Recall-Recall Interval Between Routine Dental Examinations*. London: National Institute for Health and Clinical Excellence.

Needleman, I., Suvan, J., Moles, D.R., and Pimlott, J. (2005a). A systematic review of professional mechanical plaque removal for prevention of periodontal diseases. *Journal of Clinical Periodontology*, 32(Suppl.), 229–82.

Needleman, I., Tucker, R., Giedry-Leeper, E., et al. (2005b). Guided tissue regeneration for periodontal intrabony defects—a Cochrane Systematic Review. *Periodontology 2000*, 37, 106–23.

Newton, J.T., Prabhu, N., and Robinson, P.G. (2003). The impact of dental appearance on the appraisal of personal characteristics. *International Journal of Prosthetic Dentistry*, 16, 429–34.

Penchansky, R. and Thomas, J.W. (1981). The concept of access. Definition and relationship to consumer satisfaction. *Medical Care*, 19, 127–40.

Persson, G.R. and Persson, R.E. (2008). Cardiovascular disease and periodontitis: an update on the associations and risk. *Journal of Clinical Periodontology*, 35(Suppl. 8), 362–79.

Petersen, P.E., Kandelman, D., Arpin, S., and Ogawa, H. (2010). Global oral health of older people—call for public health action. *Community Dental Health*, 27(Suppl. 2), 257–68.

Pitts, N. and Harker, R. (2004). *Obvious Decay Experience. Children's Dental Health in the United Kingdom 2003*. [Online] Available at: http://www.statistics.gov.uk/children/dentalhealth/downloads/cdh_dentinal_decay.pdf.

Reibel, J. (2003). Tobacco and oral diseases. Update on the evidence, with recommendations. *Medical Principles and Practice*, 12(Suppl. 1), 22–32.

Richardson, B. and Richardson, J. (2011). *End the Decay: The Cost of Poor Dental Health and What Should be Done About It*. [Online] Available at: http://www.bsl.org.au/Hot-issues/End-the-decay.

Robinson, P.G., Pankhurst, C.L., and Garrett, E.J. (2005). Randomized-controlled trial: effect of a reservoir biteguard on quality of life in xerostomia. *Journal of Oral Pathology and Medicine*, 34, 193–7.

Rose, G. (1992). *The Strategy of Preventive Medicine*. Oxford: Oxford University Press.

Rosen, L., Manor, D., Engelhard, D., et al. (2006). In defense of the randomized controlled trial for health promotion research. *American Journal of Public Health*, 96, 1181–6.

Rugg-Gunn, A.J. (1993). *Nutrition and Dental Health*. Oxford: Oxford University Press.

Sabbah, W., Mortensen, L.H., Sheiham, A., and Batty, A. (2012). Oral health as a risk factor for mortality in middle-aged men: the role of socioeconomic position and health behaviours. *Journal of Epidemiology and Community Health*, 67(5), 392–7.

Samarawikrama, D.Y.D. (1995). Appropriate technology, personnel and training. In W. Mautsch and A. Sheiham (eds.) *Promoting Oral Health in Deprived Communities*, pp. 347–61. Berlin: Deusche Stiftungfur Internationale Entwicklung.

Sanders, A.E., Slade, G.D., Turrell, G., Spencer, J.A., and Marcenes, W. (2006). The shape of the socioeconomic-oral health gradient: implications for theoretical explanations. *Community Dentistry Oral Epidemiology*, 34, 310–19.

Sanders, A.E., Spencer, A.J., and Stewart, J.F. (2005). Clustering of risk behaviours for oral and general health. *Community Dental Health*, 22, 133–40.

Satur, J.G., Gussy, M., Morgan, M.V., Calache, H., and Wright, C. (2010). Review of the evidence for oral health promotion effectiveness. *Health Education Journal*, 69, 257–66.

Sgan-Cohen, H.D., Evans, R.W., Whelton, H., et al. (2013). Global Oral Health Inequalities Research Agenda (IADR-GOHIRA(R)): a call to action. *Journal of Dental Research*, 92(3), 209–11.

Sprod, A., Anderson, R., and Treasure, E.T. (1996). *Effective Oral Health Promotion: Literature Review*. Cardiff: Health Promotion Wales.

Steele, J. and O'Sullivan, I.O. (2011). *Executive Summary: Adult Dental Health Survey 2009*. London: The Health and Social Care Information Centre.

Sutcliffe, P. (1996). Oral cleanliness and dental caries. In J.J. Murray (ed.) *Prevention of Oral Disease*, pp. 68–77. Oxford: Oxford University Press.

Thomas, B., Dorling, D., and Davey Smith, G. (2010). Inequalities in premature mortality in Britain: observational study from 1921 to 2007. *BMJ*, 341, c3639.

Thomson, W.M., Poulton, R., Milne, B.J., Caspi, A., Broughton, J.R., and Ayers, K.M. (2004). Socioeconomic inequalities in oral health in childhood and adulthood in a birth cohort. *Community Dentistry Oral Epidemiology*, 32, 345–53.

Tsakos, G., Demakakos, P., Breeze, E., and Watt, R.G. (2011). Social gradients in oral health in older adults: findings from the English longitudinal survey of aging. *American Journal of Public Health*, 101, 1892–9.

Tudor Hart, J. (1971). The inverse care law. *The Lancet*, 1, 405–12.

Tudor Hart, J. (2001). Commentary: can health outputs of routine practice approach those of clinical trials? *International Journal of Epidemiology*, 30, 1263–7.

Van Amerongen B.M., Schutte G.J.B., and Alpherts W.C.J. (1993). *International Dental Key Figures: A Dynamic and Relational Data Base Analyzing Oral Health Care*. Amsterdam: Key Figure.

Van der Weijden, G.A. and Timmerman, M.F. (2002). A systematic review on the clinical efficacy of subgingival debridement in the treatment of chronic periodontitis. *Journal of Clinical Periodontology*, 29(Suppl. 3), 55–71.

Watt, R. (2007). From victim blaming to upstream action: tackling the social determinants of oral health inequalities. *Community Dentistry and Oral Epidemiology*, 35, 1–11.

Watt, R. and Marinho, V.C. (2005). Does oral health promotion improve oral hygiene and gingival health? *Periodontology 2000*, 37, 35–47.

Watt, R.G. and Rouxel, P.L. (2012). Dental caries, sugars and food policy. *Archives of Disease in Childhood*, 97, 769–72.

Watt, R. and Sheiham, A. (1999). Inequalities in oral health: a review of the evidence and recommendations for action. *British Dental Journal*, 187, 6–12.

Watt, R.G. and Sheiham, A. (2012). Integrating the common risk factor approach into a social determinants framework. *Community Dentistry Oral Epidemiology*, 40, 289–96.

White, D., Pitts, N., Steele, J., Sadler, K., and Chadwick, B. (2011). *Disease and Related Disorders—A Report from the Adult Dental Health Survey 2009*. London: The Health and Social Care Information Centre.

Willett, W.C. and Ludwig, D.S. (2013). Science souring on sugar. *BMJ*, 346, e807.

Wong, F.S. and Kolokotsa, K. (2004). The cost of treating children and adolescents with injuries to their permanent incisors at a dental hospital in the United Kingdom. *Dental Traumatology*, 20, 327–33.

World Health Organization (1998). *Health Promotion Evaluation: Recommendations to Policy Makers*. Geneva: WHO.

Xiong, X., Buekens, P., Fraser, W.D., et al. (2006). Periodontal disease and adverse pregnancy outcomes: a systematic review. *British Journal of Obstetrics and Gynaecology*, 113, 135–43.

Yamamoto, T., Kondo, K., Misawa, J., et al. (2012). Dental status and incident falls among older Japanese: a prospective cohort study. *BMJ Open*, 2(4).

Yee, R., McDonald, N., and Walker, D. (2003). An advocacy project to fluoridate toothpastes in Nepal. *International Dental Journal*, 53, 220–30.

Yeung, C.A., Hitchings, J.L., Macfarlane, T.V., et al. (2005). Fluoridated milk for preventing dental caries. *Cochrane Database of Systematic Reviews*, 3, CD003876.

8.9

Musculoskeletal disorders

Lope H. Barrero and Alberto J. Caban-Martinez

Introduction to musculoskeletal disorders

Musculoskeletal disorders (MSDs) refers to a large variety of health conditions that affect muscles, tendons, ligaments, nerves, and bones. Conditions such as osteoarthritis (OA), osteoporosis, low back pain (LBP), rheumatoid arthritis (RA), and carpal tunnel syndrome fall into this large category of health conditions.

Multiple factors related to the intrinsic characteristics of individuals, their environment, and their daily activities can contribute to the occurrence and burden of MSDs. The relative contribution of these factors can vary across populations in different parts of the world. As we learn more about the mechanisms through which these conditions occur, we have been able to improve our understanding of how multiple complex pathways can take a person from a healthy status to a disease state. This new knowledge about the diagnosis and pathogenesis of MSDs has emphasized the fact that in reality, MSDs can include several very different conditions, which in essence implies that no single pathway for diagnosis, treatment, or rehabilitation can be effective, not even in very well-defined specific populations.

The importance and major public health burden of MSDs is rooted in the fact that these conditions occur more frequently than many other conditions that can affect human health; and when they do occur, they tend to last longer than other conditions, and coexist with other, sometimes deadly conditions that are caused by the same factors or that are complications resulting from them. For example, in the United States, approximately 50 million adults have a doctor diagnosis of arthritis, yet 1.2 million, or nearly one in four adults with arthritis (24 per cent), also have heart disease (Cisternas et al. 2009). These characteristics translate directly into a large burden to society that can appear in the form of direct health services costs, reduction in opportunities for those affected, and suffering for those affected and their families. Furthermore, because of the differences in access to healthcare, the burden of these conditions may vary substantially between different latitudes, generating questions about equality and social justice.

In this chapter, we first present a brief description of some of the most important MSDs of public health importance. We then briefly describe what we know about their causes and what is already known about how to prevent them or reduce their impact to society. We will also describe the scope of the problem from a public health perspective. We present a brief account on the epidemiology of these conditions; the estimated costs to society; and the most important barriers that prevent people from obtaining some relief. Lastly, we summarize recommendations for public health policy action and for future research.

Definition and classification of musculoskeletal disorders

There is a broad scope of health conditions that comprise MSDs including inflammatory conditions such as gout and RA, age-related diseases such as OA and osteoporosis, conditions with ambiguous aetiologies such as fibromyalgia and LBP, conditions due to injuries from occupational exposures, sports injuries, as well as injuries resulting from slips, trips, and falls. While some of these conditions present with acute onset and short duration, a larger proportion of these disorders reoccur or become lifelong health conditions (Woolf et al. 2010). These conditions can substantially impair both mental (Carder et al. 2013; Holmgren et al. 2013) and physical function and therefore are a major determinant of the health of populations worldwide.

Different classifications of MSDs can be found in the scientific literature based, for example, on body part affected, whether it has a systemic origin, or based on the external causal factor (e.g. whether it is work related or not).

The International Classification of Disease, tenth revision (ICD-10) (World Health Organization (WHO) 2010, chapter XIII) provides a useful framework with which to classify diagnostic groups of MSDs and they include:

- *Arthropathies*: disorders predominantly affecting limb joints including those due to microbiological agents (e.g. RA, juvenile arthritis, gout, psoriatic spondylitis).

- *Systemic connective tissue disorders*: including autoimmune disease and collagen (vascular) disease (e.g. systemic lupus erythematosus and sicca syndrome (Sjören's syndrome)).

- *Dorsopathies*: disorders of the spine including deforming dorsopathies, spondylopathies and other dorsopathies (e.g. cevicalgia, sciatica, and LBP).

- *Soft tissue disorders*: disorders of muscles (e.g. muscle strain).

- *Osteopathies and chondropathies*: including disorders of bone density and structure (e.g. osteoporosis); and chondropathies (e.g. juvenile osteochondrosis).

- *Other disorders*: including conditions nowhere else classified including post-procedural MSDs and biomechanical lesions not elsewhere specified.

- *Additional MSDs may be found among other groups of diagnosis*: MSDs involving nerve damage (e.g. carpal tunnel syndrome) can be found among diseases of the nervous system. Also, MSDs involving sprains and strains for joints and ligaments can be found in the injury category.

Major musculoskeletal disorders: case definitions, natural history, pathophysiology, risk factors, and treatment

While there are many types of MSDs, musculoskeletal tissue degeneration in general can be initiated by systemic disease, trauma, and repeated biomechanical strain—all of which can lead to disability and pain. For example, autoimmune diseases can initiate and sustain damaging processes to body tissues including musculoskeletal tissue (Smolen and Aletaha 2008). Similarly, hormonal imbalances can generate loss of structure in bones and result in osteoporosis. On the other hand, trauma resulting, for example, from a fall at an early age, can initiate abnormal processes of gene expression or result in incomplete repair processes that end up affecting musculoskeletal tissue structures. Also, repeated loads can result in tissue micro-trauma that affects its function and eventually accumulates to major damage if recovery is not allowed.

Environmental factors (e.g. eating and physical activity habits) and individual characteristics (e.g. genetic factors and age) are determinants of MSDs (Gabriel and Michaud 2009), influencing the initiation and development of the disease process through complex relations. For example, poor eating habits can result in overweight individuals, which can affect the biomechanical loading on joints and hence lead to OA conditions (Guilak 2011; Vincent et al. 2012). Similarly, genetic factors can be involved in the onset of systemic inflammatory disease and can also influence body response at different stages of the disease process. On the other hand, ageing activates several different biochemical processes of tissue degeneration through insufficient expression of tissue components or the occurrence of other age-related diseases with the capability to influence the process of tissue degeneration.

Tissue degeneration is thought to accumulate throughout the life course, although determining the beginning of the disease process is difficult. The accumulated damage can be seen clinically based on radiographic or serologic evidence. For example, tissue tears and tissue deformation can be seen based on imaging techniques. A large body of research has been developed on new biomarkers to track the onset and development of disease (Naylor and Eastell 2012; Pisetsky et al. 2012; Rousseau and Garnero 2012). Nevertheless, such imaging findings are poor to moderate predictors of disability; and biomarkers are still in their youth and are not yet being used reliably and widely in clinical settings.

The key feature determining disability and rehabilitation from MSDs among individuals is the presence of pain (Laisné et al. 2012). Once pain occurs as a result of MSDs, most likely it will occur again intermittently throughout the individual's lifetime. If pain lasts long enough and/or is perceived as strong enough it will result in disability. How pain is managed is therefore crucial as it ultimately determines the burden of MSDs to individuals, their families, and society. The ways in which pain affects how people feel are complex and remain undetermined; however, it appears that emotional processes (e.g. depression) may be involved in how pain is perceived and, therefore, its consequences. Cognitive

(e.g. increased attention to pain), behavioural (e.g. low levels of physical activity, limitation of adaptive pain-coping behaviour, and impairment of social support), and neurophysiological factors (e.g. enhanced central nervous system pain processing and impaired neuroendocrine function) seem to mediate the pathway from emotional disturbances to final outcomes (Edwards et al. 2011).

LBP, neck pain (NP), OA, osteoporosis, and RA are some of the most common conditions among MSDs causing the largest public health burden to society worldwide.

Low back pain

Definition of LBP

LBP is characterized as pain manifesting from the anatomical area between the 12th rib and the superior aspect of the thigh either with or without radiating leg pain (Krismer et al. 2007). LBP can result from several different causes. Non-specific LBP has received the most attention from the healthcare arena because it represents more than 80 per cent of the LBP cases seen in the healthcare setting. This type of LBP can be initially classified based on whether or not it presents with pain in one or both legs, and on pain duration.

Pathophysiology of LBP

The pathophysiology of LBP can generally be classified as either mechanical or non-mechanical in origin (Biyani and Andersson 2004). Mechanical LBP can be due to disc herniation, where the annulus fibrosis around the disc tears, allowing the disc nucleus to push against nearby nerve roots and cause pain. Another possible mechanical pathway for LBP that is commonly seen in ageing populations are arthritic spurs that impinge around adjacent nerve roots in the spinal canal igniting pain. As we age, bone remodelling can cause spurs to develop at the vertebral bodies and these spurs can directly compress these nerve roots and vascular structures leading to pain, inflammation, and secondary oedema. Non-mechanical LBP can be caused by neoplastic, infectious, inflammatory arthritis, or other diseases (e.g. Paget's disease, Scheuermann's disease, Basstrup's disease, etc.); however, they are not a focus of discussion in this chapter (see Jarvik and Deyo 2002).

Natural history of LBP

Most people will feel LBP at least once in their lives independently of the root causes, although only a proportion of them is likely to seek help from healthcare services (Balagué et al. 2012). Among individuals with non-specific LPB, the frequency and duration of pain can vary considerably, with some individuals reporting multiple periods of pain with interspersed periods of less severe or no pain. This period of pain could be brief, lasting a few days, or it could be longer lasting, over a few weeks or even months, that eventually leads to disability. If the pain lasts for a significantly extended period of time beyond the normal healing period of approximately 2 months, then a chronic pain syndrome could arise (Krismer et al. 2007). Studies have also shown that when pain radiates down one or both legs there is a strong association with more significant loss of function (Hoy et al. 2010).

While a great majority of adults will experience one episode of back pain during their life, many adults will also experience new episodes of back pain (Jeffries and Grimmer-Somers 2007). In fact, recent studies have classified individuals who seek healthcare for back pain into four categories, including: those people with 'persistent mild' pain; those who start with mild pain, progressing quickly to 'recovering' with no pain; those with 'severe chronic' pain who have permanently high pain; and those with 'fluctuating' pain whose pain varied between mild and high levels (Dunn et al. 2006).

Risk factors for LBP

Risk factors for a new episode of LBP may include: poor general health, female gender, and body weight in women (Croft et al. 1999); genetics and age (incidence is higher in the third decade (Hoy et al. 2010)); occupational exposures and education (Hoy et al. 2010). Although by definition non-specific LBP has unknown causes, there are known associations between LBP and degeneration of the lumbar discs seen with clinical imaging. The scientific literature suggests that mechanical factors are associated with self-reported LBP; however, several meta-analyses and systematic reviews have suggested that mechanical factors such as awkward posture, manual material handling, pushing or pulling, and prolonged occupational sitting are not causal factors of LBP. Obesity and smoking may also play a role (Balagué et al. 2012). Genetic factors may also be implicated via disc narrowing effects on pain or via two genes (i.e. catechol-O-methyltransferase (*COMT*) and the μ-opioid receptor (*OPRM1*)) implicated in pain perception, signalling, psychological processing, and immunity. Interleukin-1 gene cluster polymorphisms are associated with modic changes and might have a pathogenic role. Genotype has also been reported to be associated with the outcome of surgery for degenerative disc disease (Balagué et al. 2012).

Treatment of LBP

In general, the recovery from acute LBP either with or without radiating pain down the legs has a favourable recovery profile. While certain interventions such as stress management, shoe inserts or insoles, back supports, ergonomics or back education, and reduced lifting programmes are not effective, exercise interventions seem to be the most effective in reducing LBP. For example, intervention studies have shown that when compared to individuals not randomized to the intervention group, those who receive specific training and advice on proper manual material handling either with or without the use of assistive devices, report less sick leave (Balagué et al. 2012).

Neck pain

Definition of NP

NP encompasses a broad range of different clinical presentations and has been defined as pain in the neck that lasts for at least 1 day either with or without radiating upper limb pain that is associated with activity limitations (Hoy et al. 2010). NP can result from different specific causes (e.g. trauma) or serious pathologies (e.g. inflammatory disorder, radiculopathy, or myelopathy), but in the majority of cases, as it was for LBP, NP is non-specific (Hoving et al. 2001).

The Bone and Joint Decade's Task Force on Neck Pain and Its Associated Disorders (Carroll et al. 2008) recommended classifying NP through the following scheme:

- Grade I NP: no signs or symptoms suggestive of major structural pathology and no or minor interference with activities of daily living; will likely respond to minimal intervention such as reassurance and pain control; does not require intensive investigations or ongoing treatment.

- Grade II NP: no signs or symptoms of major structural pathology, but major interference with activities of daily living; requires pain relief and early activation/intervention aimed at preventing long-term disability.

- Grade III NP: no signs or symptoms of major structural pathology, but presence of neurological signs such as decreased deep tendon reflexes, weakness, and/or sensory deficits; might require investigation and, occasionally, more invasive treatments.

- Grade IV NP: signs or symptoms of major structural pathology, such as fracture, myelopathy, neoplasm, or systemic disease; this grade requires prompt investigation and treatment.

Pathophysiology of NP

In a large number of individuals, NP can be a result of either muscular or ligamentous factors related to posture, poor ergonomics, stress, and/or chronic muscle fatigue. Neck muscle pain can also develop secondarily as a consequence of postural adaptations to a primary source of pain in the shoulder or other upper extremity joints (Bogduk 2011). Individuals with degenerative arthritis in the upper cervical joints can present with severe NP that transmits down into the neck or to the back of the ear.

Natural history of NP

Similar to the low back, NP is first experienced in childhood or adolescence and can manifest several times over the life course. In fact, a large proportion of individuals with NP never really experience complete resolution of their pain. Recent research studies have shown that between 50 and 85 per cent of those who experience NP at some point in their life will report NP again 1–5 years later (Haldeman et al. 2010). This NP experience appears to be similar in the general population, workers, and among individuals who experience motor vehicle crashes (Haldeman et al. 2010).

The presentation of NP among individuals who seek healthcare can vary and includes concomitant pains such as headache, shoulder, upper limb, upper and/or lower back pain (Leaver et al. 2013). However, among individuals with non-specific NP, the origin of the pain and its progression can also vary. In addition, pain arising from anatomical regions other than the neck can be explained as referred pain from innervated cervical spine structures, or as other regional conditions coexisting with NP, or as the presence of a generalized, widespread pain syndrome involving NP. Nonetheless, NP can be a complex health condition that is difficult to treat and contributes significantly to the burden of MSDs (Leaver et al. 2013).

Several factors can affect the course of NP. For example, younger age is associated with a better prognosis, whereas poor health and prior NP episodes are associated with a poorer prognosis. Poorer prognosis is also associated with poor psychological health, worrying, and becoming angry or frustrated in response to NP. Greater optimism, a coping style that involved self-assurance, and having less need to socialize, are all associated with better prognosis. Specific workplace or physical job demands are not linked with recovery from NP (Haldeman et al. 2008).

Risk factors for NP

Poor general health, smoking, higher pain, and lower Short-Form Health Survey (SF-12) mental component scores have been reported to be independently associated with higher-level disability resulting from NP (Leaver et al. 2013). Several epidemiological studies suggest that risk factors for NP have a multifactorial aetiology. For example, non-modifiable risk factors for NP include age, gender, and genetics; however, there is no evidence that common degenerative changes in the cervical spine are risk factors for NP. Research studies have also documented that additional modifiable factors for NP include smoking, exposure to environmental tobacco, and physical activity participation. Occupational health studies have also documented that high quantitative job demands, low workplace social support, sedentary work position, repetitive work, and precision work have been associated with increased risk of NP (Haldeman et al. 2008).

Treatment of NP

Generalized NP can be treated conservatively with the use of over-the-counter pain medications, ice, heat and massage, and strengthening and/or stretching exercises at home. Current strategies suggest that if the pain persists after a few weeks of conservative treatment, then further evaluation is warranted (Haldeman et al. 2010). There is a dearth of high-quality evidence elucidating the best specific treatment for NP in general. For instance, there are many reviews as there are controlled trials of therapies for NP; yet for many interventions, there is no concordance in the conclusions drawn by reviewers. Few studies have been conducted on the long-term effects of treatments for NP. As an illustration, a study conducted by Haldeman et al. (2008) suggested that compared to quality of life years with the use of standard non-steroidal anti-inflammatory drugs (NSAIDs), Cox-2 NSAIDs, exercise, manipulation, and mobilization among adults with NP, active treatments are not significantly superior to any other treatment option in the short or long term even after controlling for adverse event risks, treatment effectiveness, and patient preferences for health outcomes in their models (Linton and van Tulder 2001; Haldeman et al. 2008).

Osteoarthritis

Definition of OA

OA is a degenerative disorder of the joints that can also be termed degenerative joint disease, degenerative arthritis or osteoarthrosis. It is comprised of a group of joint conditions that involve degradation of joint tissues, including the articular cartilage and subchondral bone. Joints of the hip and knee are most frequently affected, but the joints of the hand, spine, and feet are also typically affected. Individuals with these conditions report feeling specific pain, tenderness, stiffness, and locking around the joint. Among people with chronic joint degeneration one may see muscle shrinkage and ligament loosening around the joint. Current classification schemes for OA include documentation of loss of cartilage, subchondral sclerosis, subchondral cyst formation and osteophytes on radiological imaging, and self-reported joint pain (Fransen et al. 2011).

Pathophysiology of OA

OA is said to be primary if it originated without a known cause (Punzi et al. 2010). However, OA can also be secondary to other diseases such as congenital joint disorders and diabetes. Traditionally, OA was thought to affect primarily the articular cartilage of synovial joints; however, pathophysiologic changes are also known to occur in the synovial fluid, as well as in the underlying bone structures, the overlying joint capsule, and other joint tissues (Punzi et al. 2010). During the early phases of OA, swelling of the cartilage usually occurs, because of the increased production of proteoglycans that reflects an effort by the cartilage's cellular structures to repair cartilage damage. This phase may last for several years or decades and is characterized by intense repair of the articular cartilage. As OA progresses further, however, the cartilage eventually begins to soften and lose elasticity and thereby further compromises joint surface integrity. At the microscopic level, flaking and fibrillations develop along the normally smooth articular cartilage on the surface of an osteoarthritic joint. In the long run, this loss of cartilage results in loss of joint space (Punzi et al. 2010).

Natural history of OA

OA is a joint condition that involves a slow, progressive degeneration of the joint and is the most common type of all arthritis conditions. We now know that OA develops as a result of articular cartilage damage that can be triggered by a complex interplay of genetic, metabolic, biochemical, and biomechanical factors with secondary involvement of the inflammation pathway. The overall natural process involves interactive degradation and repair processes of cartilage, bone, and synovium. Of all the cells involved in the aetiology and pathogenesis of OA, chondrocytes play a large role. Studies on animals and humans suggest that these cells exhibit numerous metabolic dysfunctions leading to OA. This pathology more than any other disease pathology can result in difficulties in daily activities such as walking, stair climbing, and other lower-extremity tasks (Gabriel and Michaud 2009).

Risk factors for OA

OA is said to be a primary disorder if it originates without a known cause, although evidence suggests that risk factors such as genetic predisposition, age, obesity, female sex, greater bone density, joint laxity, and excessive mechanical loading are associated with its aetiology (Punzi et al. 2010). Recent evidence from North American and European cohorts suggest that obesity or heavy occupational physical activity are risk factors for symptomatic knee and hip OA (Gabriel and Michaud 2009; Fransen et al. 2011). In addition, several other international studies have documented that a history of joint injury, frequent stair climbing, or frequent lifting of heavy weights is significantly associated with hip OA where the strongest association was among individuals with a history of joint injury. In a case–control study in Japan, there was an association with occupational lifting but no association with obesity (Fransen et al. 2011). In another study, OA has been associated with high obesity levels and cardiovascular disease which can cause synergistic effects (Punzi et al. 2010).

Treatment of OA

While there is no known cure for OA, certain treatments can help to reduce pain and maintain joint movement. Treatment generally includes exercise, lifestyle modification (e.g. diet), and pain relievers. If the condition is severe, joint replacement surgery is typically recommended. While specific medications designed to reduce pain (e.g. acetaminophen and opioid analgesics) are helpful, they do not have an effect on joint inflammation as do NSAIDs. In more severe cases of OA, there are two types of injections that have shown moderate evidence for pain improvement: steroid (i.e. glucocorticoid) injections and injections of a liquid known as hyaluronate, designed to mimic the natural fluid found in joint space (Iagnocco and Naredo 2012). Once these conservative and minimally invasive approaches have been exhausted, a surgical approach to rehabilitating the OA joint may be needed (Iagnocco and Naredo 2012).

Osteoporosis

Definition of osteoporosis

Osteoporosis is classified as either primary or secondary depending on what is causing the disease. The primary form of osteoporosis is a metabolic bone disease characterized by low bone mass and microarchitectural deterioration of bone tissue, leading to enhanced bone fragility and increased fracture risk (Riis 1993). Secondary osteoporosis can result from a variety of the chronic conditions that significantly contribute to bone mineral loss, or it can result from the effects of medications and nutritional deficiencies. The WHO defines osteoporosis using bone density, that is, a bone density score that is 2.5 standard deviations (SDs) or more below the young adult mean value (T-score < –2.5). However, individuals with bone density between scores 1 and 2.5 SDs below average (T-score –1 to –2.5) are said to have osteopenia (Kanis et al. 1994). In the case of the spine, decreased bone density imparts increased risk for bone fracture; for every 1 SD decrease in bone density of the spine there is an increased risk for new vertebral fractures by factor of 2.0–2.4 (Wasnich 1993).

Pathophysiology of osteoporosis

Challenges in bone mass acquisition during human growth and development and accelerated bone loss in the period after peak bone mass are both leading mechanisms for the development of osteoporosis. Studies have shown that both of these mechanisms are influenced by environmental and genetic factors (Iagnocco and Naredo 2012). In postmenopausal women, studies have attributed about two-thirds of the risk of fracture to be related to the premenopausal peak bone mass (Farmer et al. 1984). In twin and mother–daughter dyad studies, about 40–80 per cent of the variability observed in bone mass can be attributed to genetic factors. In fact, biological studies have suggested that genes regulating oestrogen receptors, transforming growth factor-β, and apolipoprotein E and collagen, influence the development of osteoporosis. Conversely, bone loss is more strongly influenced by individual-level factors such as nutritional, behavioural, and pharmacological factors yet is still associated to a lesser degree with oestrogen genetic factors (Ronis et al. 2011).

Natural history of osteoporosis

Among all metabolic bone diseases, osteoporosis is the most prevalent. In fact, in the United States alone, approximately 54 per cent of postmenopausal white women have osteopenia and 30 per cent have osteoporosis. Osteoporosis is a complex and dynamic disease of bone where there is an asymptomatic reduction in the quantity of bone mass per unit volume. When the bone mass reaches a very low threshold, the structural integrity and mechanical support provided by the bone fails, leading to fractures. The overall natural process of this disease involves a dysregulation of the homeostatic

processes between osteoclastic (bone destruction) and osteoblastic (bone growth) activity. If sufficient remodelling in one direction occurs (i.e. more bone destruction than growth), the bone becomes weakened and this could lead to fractures (Hoy et al. 2010, Huizinga and Pincus 2010).

Risk factors for osteoporosis

There are several well-known modifiable and non-modifiable risk factors for osteoporosis. Recent epidemiological studies in the United States suggest that men and non-white women at risk add approximately 30–54 million affected people. These bone diseases place individuals at higher risk for osteoporotic fractures (Hoy et al. 2010). Racial and ethnic differences in the prevalence of osteoporosis and osteoporotic fractures have been well documented. For example, among black people, hip fracture is considerably more prevalent than among white people primarily due to differences in higher peak bone mass and slower postmenopausal bone loss noted in African American women (ILO 2000). Some studies have also noted that women of Asian descent have lower bone mineral density than white women (Jarvik and Deyo 2002). In terms of age, studies have shown that decreased bone mineral density and osteoporotic fracture rates increase throughout the life course. For example, the incidence or number of new cases of hip fractures begins to increase during the seventh decade of life, vertebral fractures during the sixth decade, and wrist fractures during the fifth decade. While hip and vertebral fractures have been associated with increased mortality rates, the loss of autonomy and lower health-related quality of life remain the largest public health burden of this disease. Similarly, men also suffer from osteoporosis yet not at the same rate as women. For example the increased incidence of hip fracture in men occurs about 5–10 years later than in women (Isaacs 2010, Kanis et al. 1994). In summary, non-modifiable risk factors include age, body size, race, and family history (Drake et al. 2012; Wright and Saag 2012) while modifiable risk factors include sex hormone deficiencies, diet, certain medical conditions (e.g. anorexia nervosa) and medications, lack of physical activity, heavy alcohol consumption, and smoking (Wright and Saag 2012).

Treatment of osteoporosis

The treatment plan for osteoporosis is often multifaceted, including pharmacological and behavioural interventions to reduce risk of fracture and improve bone mineralization. For example, a treatment plan could include activities and exercise, improving nutrition, and educational training on the prevention of falls. Pharmacological interventions often complement these approaches and include drugs that modify bone reorganization, increase bone density, and subsequently reduce fracture risk. Mineral and vitamin supplementation is also paramount and includes the combined use of calcium and vitamin D (Drake et al. 2012).

Rheumatoid arthritis

Definition of RA

RA is a disease characterized by chronic inflammation of the joints; however, adjacent tissues and other body organs (i.e. such as the skin, heart, lungs, and eyes) can also be affected. In this condition, the body's immune system has turned on itself and attacks the tissues and structures within the joints. While any joint can be affected by RA, the hands and feet are most commonly affected and have the greatest potential to lead to joint destruction and functional disability (Huizinga and Pincus 2010).

Pathophysiology of RA

While the direct aetiology of RA is not well understood, several risk factors have been associated with the onset of an immune system reaction, including a joint infection, trauma, and tobacco smoke. These immune system triggers cause the tissues within the joint to enlarge and cause inflammation, particularly among individuals who have a genetic disposition for immune sensitivity. Ultimately the chronic inflammation in the joint leads to the destruction of various joint tissues, including cartilage.

Natural history of RA

The overall world prevalence of RA is approximately 1 per cent. In the United States, for example, the prevalence of RA has been documented to be approximately 0.6 per cent (1.3 million adults) of the population. Epidemiological studies have also documented geographic variations in the prevalence of RA where it is found highest among Pima (5.3 per cent) and Chippewa Indians (6.8 per cent), and lowest among individuals from Japan and China (0.2–0.3 per cent) (Helmick et al. 2008). These geographic variations in the prevalence of the disease further suggest that either a genetic or environmental component may be present (Silman and Pearson 2002). Recent population-based estimates suggest that approximately one-third of individuals with RA become work-disabled within 2 years of disease onset, and approximately 50 per cent are work-disabled after 10 years (Combe 2009; Isaccs 2010). Part of this disability and decrease in health-related quality of life is due to the physical, emotional, and social impact of the disease. While physician rating of patient pain is generally lower than pain self-reported by the patient, disease severity has been associated with the degree of pain experienced by the patient as well as their physical functioning.

Risk factors for RA

Research studies have identified both modifiable and non-modifiable risk factors that contribute to the development of RA. In fact, a large proportion of RA cases are believed to arise from the interaction between genetic (i.e. non-modifiable) and environmental (i.e. modifiable) exposures. For example, the number of new RA cases is typically two to three times higher in women than men while the onset of RA is highest among those individuals in their 60s for both men and woman (Silman and Pearson 2002). There are several modifiable risk factors that have been studied in association with RA including cigarette use, nutritional/dietary factors, infectious agents, and reproductive hormonal exposures (Pincus and Callahan 1993). Of these factors, tobacco exposure has been shown in the epidemiological literature to be the strongest and most consistent in terms of being associated with RA, particularly among people who have specific immune markers in the blood (e.g. test positive for anti-citrullinated protein/peptide antibodies) (Scott et al. 2010). Other studies have documented mixed evidence of an association between the use of oral contraceptives and a risk of RA (Brennan et al. 1997).

Treatment of RA

Treatment options for RA can vary from the newest RA drugs to inclusion of exercise and NSAIDs as well as individualized care and management tips. There are two types of drugs used in treating RA, classified as first- and second-line medications. The first-line drugs include agents such as aspirin and steroids that are commonly used to reduce the person's pain and inflammation. Second-line drugs are slow acting and include the disease-modifying antirheumatic drugs such as methotrexate (i.e. Rheumatrex® and Trexall®), and hydroxychloroquine (i.e. Plaquenil®) that thwart progressive joint disease and support remission. RA usually requires lifelong treatment, including medications, physical therapy, exercise, education, and surgical intervention depending on the disease severity (Ibrahim et al. 2012).

The scope of the problem

Hundreds of millions of people suffer from MSDs worldwide. The independence and autonomy of people to perform daily normal activities is affected by MSDs. Furthermore, epidemiological studies have documented how MSDs can affect a person's capacity to work and live independently. In fact, among individuals suffering from MSDs, the value in life that was going to be created by these sufferers can now be considered lost to society. Immeasurable suffering accompanies people with MSDs and their families. Families and society (e.g. government, industry) often contribute to social welfare and healthcare programmes that subsidize health services (Fransen et al. 2011).

Understanding and quantifying the magnitude of problem that MSDs bring to society is a difficult task (Caban-Martinez et al. 2011). Most cost estimations include only health expenditures and are available only for selected diseases and for some countries. On the other hand, measures based on disease occurrence (prevalence rates and proportion incidence) can offer a comprehensive overview of the problem in different geographical areas of the world, but not without methodological difficulties (e.g. as MSDs have a slow onset, it is frequently hard to identify the moment when the disease starts). The Global Burden of Disease (GBD) report, which uses a more elaborate measure (disability-adjusted life years (DALYs)), has recently become available. In the following subsections we present an overview of the MSD burden based on disease cost, occurrence, and years of life lost.

A few important messages can be highlighted from the information available: (1) MSDs occur very frequently, (2) MSDs are expensive, (3) the extent of the problem of MSDs is increasing over time, and (4) there are important geographical differences in the geographical distribution of MSDs.

MSDs occur very frequently

The GBD study estimated that 1700 million people suffered from MSDs in the year 2010 (Table 8.9.1). Years lived with disability (YLDs) of MSDs are not declining (Vos et al. 2012). To understand these numbers it is important to consider a few key methodological characteristics of these estimations. First and most importantly, not all MSDs were included in the study that produced these global estimations[1]; and important conditions that do fall in the MSD diagnosis categories as defined in the ICD-10 were not counted as MSDs, which highlights the fact that more people can suffer from MSDs worldwide.

In spite of the great variability found in the literature regarding case definitions (e.g. case definitions for OA can vary depending on diagnosis criteria: radiographic, symptomatic, or

Table 8.9.1 Point prevalence (P; in thousands) and prevalence rate of major musculoskeletal diseases in year 2010

MSD type	Total		Males		Females	
	P	%	P	%	P	%
Low back pain[a]	632,045	9.17	334,793	9.64	287,252	8.70
Neck pain	332,049	4.82	135,134	3.89	196,915	5.77
Knee osteoarthritis	250,785	3.64	88,885	2.56	161,900	4.74
Other MSDs	560,978	8.14	26,2779	7.56	298,199	8.73

[a] Activity-limiting low back pain (± pain referred into one or both lower limbs) that lasts for at least 1 day (Hoy et al., 2012).

Reprinted from *The Lancet*, Volume 380, Issue 9859, Vos T. et al., Years lived with disability (YLDs) for 1160 sequelae of 289 diseases and injuries 1990–2010: a systematic analysis for the Global Burden of Disease Study 2010, pp. 2163–96, Copyright © 2012, with permission from Elsevier, http://www.sciencedirect.com/science/journal/01406736.

clinical (Gabriel and Michaud 2009)), and the notable difference in information availability for different populations, the GBD study made an effort to produce case definitions that were consistent and to include some description of the impact of the condition on daily activities and loss of function (Woolf et al. 2010).

MSDs are expensive

In 2009, the world spent a total of US$5.97 trillion in health-related expenses (WHO 2012). This figure includes government expenditures and out-of-pocket expenditures in health. A large part of this cost is attributable to MSDs where among developed nations they are responsible for approximately 25 per cent of total expenses due to illness (Walsh et al. 2008). In addition, approximately 20 per cent of regular primary care visits in the vast majority of countries is due to MSDs (Walsh et al. 2008). The pain experienced by individuals with MSDs is one of the most common reasons for self-medication and for visits to a primary care setting. Among countries with ready access to medical care, MSDs account for a considerable number of healthcare visits and expenditures (Murray et al. 2012).

Most of the data available in terms of monetary expenditure on healthcare is representative of specific geographical areas and specific MSD, most frequently in developed countries. In the State of Victoria, Canada, for example, MSDs were the most frequent reason for outpatient visits to the medical centre (11.6 per cent of the total) between the years 1997 and 2000. Also, among 26 medical specialties, MSDs had the sixth highest number of inpatient episodes (6.2 per cent in years 2000/2001). In terms of cost, MSDs rank fifth in the number of bed-days away from work during the period 1997 to 2001 (Osborne et al. 2007).

These expenditures are not unique to Canada. An economic study on LBP in the United Kingdom estimated that the direct costs of LBP were £1.6 billion in 1998. When factoring the indirect costs associated with LBP, countries such as Sweden (costs per capita: US$24 direct costs versus US$266 indirect costs, 8 per cent versus 92 per cent) and the Netherlands (US$24 direct versus US$299 indirect, 7 per cent versus 93 per cent) had direct costs lower than indirect expenditures spent in the UK alone. In the United States, data from the 1988 National Health Interview Survey documented that general LBP accounted for 149 million lost work days annually while work-related LBP accounted for 102 million work days lost. In total, all cases of LBP were estimated to cost about US$1230 on average for men and US $773 on average for women with an annual productivity loss of $28 billion (Krismer et al. 2007).

The burden of MSDs is growing

In 2010, the burden of MSDs was quantified and updated using the DALY metric. This metric aims to quantify how many years are lost due to disability (YLDs) and due to mortality (years of life lost (YLLs)) for a list of 291 conditions. In simple terms, for example, if a person loses part of her capacity to perform daily activities due to a particular condition (disability weight of the condition), that person loses proportionally part of the years that she was going to live until her expected age of death. The sum of these two losses are the DALYs. For each condition 1160 sequelae were identified. For example, for the condition 'low back pain', four sequelae resulting from combining acute or subacute versus chronic pain, and pain in one or both legs versus without this pain were identified (Hoy et al. 2010). YLDs are computed as the prevalence of a sequela multiplied by the disability weight for that sequel. The YLDs arising from a disease or injury are the sum of the YLDs for each of the sequelae associated with that disease. In the study the prevalence of sequelae was estimated with uncertainty for 20 age groups, two sexes, and 21 regions of the world. The value of these estimations is based on the fact that an attempt was made to achieve comparable figures for different geographical areas for two moments in time, in the years 1990 and 2010.

A few methodological aspects need to be highlighted in order to understand DALYs: the YLLs due to mortality are generally low due to MSDs. Part of this is due to the chronic nature of these conditions, which means that their effect is exerted through the loss of quality of life rather than to the loss of years of life. However, there are exceptions. For example, the death rate is increased for all osteoporotic fractures; however, the death will not be attributed to the underlying osteoporosis, it will instead be attributed to the injury. We also see this misclassification in other MSDs such as systemic vasculitis and untreated RA, where the death certificate will likely state that the death was due to end-organ failure or other co-morbidity. As a consequence the metric does not fully capture the premature loss of life due to the individual living with the MSD. For conditions with low mortality rates such as OA, there might actually be a greater burden of death due to the condition (Woolf et al. 2010). In the case of morbidity, it is possible to estimate the YLL due to living with MSDs. It is possible to consider measuring the health state of the individual by using a set of health domains, such as overall well-being, general health, physical health, social health, mental health, and barriers to participation. In the GBD study, health loss associated with individual loss of physical and emotional function was measured rather than general welfare loss and loss of participation.

The general distribution of the burden of disease has shifted from a previously greater burden of communicable, maternal, and neonatal causes to non-communicable diseases including MSDs. In 1990, approximately 47 per cent of DALYs were caused by communicable, maternal, and neonatal causes, 43 per cent from non-communicable diseases, and 10 per cent from injuries as compared to estimates in 2010 that had shifted to 35 per cent, 54 per cent, and 11 per cent, respectively (Murray et al. 2012). In absolute terms, worldwide the DALYs due to MSDs grew from 116.6 million (116,553 thousand (88,683–147,285)) in 1990 to 169.6 million (169,621 thousand (129,768–212,730)) in 2010 (45 per cent increase); or in relative terms from 2.2 million (2198 thousand (1673–2778)) to 2.5 million (2462 thousand (1883–3088)) per 100,000 thousand people (12 per cent increase) (Table 8.9.2). These conditions would be responsible for 6.8 per cent of the DALYs, which is a much larger share compared to the 2 per cent estimated in year 2004 (Murray et al. 2012); and is particularly high in the regions with an advanced demographic and epidemiological transition, where MSDs account for 13 per cent of the DALYs.

From 1990 to 2010, the proportions of specific disease conditions in the MSDs have not changed significantly; however, LBP (49 per cent), NP (20 per cent), and OA (10 per cent) all share the largest proportion of the pie among all MSDs. Population-based survey data suggests that this observed growth in MSDs might not be due to the growth in the population alone given the relative-to-population increase of 26.5 per cent.

MSD is a larger burden for people older than 39 years old. However, it is clear that MSDs for males start being an important issue (considering all DALYs) as early as 10–14 years old in relation to other conditions at that age range, and this is pretty much maintained until the age of death; MSDs become one of the most important types of conditions in the age range from 35 to 50 years. For women, MSDs start being important at age 14 as well. However, as a proportion of all disease that women can suffer, MSDs are more important; and the age range when MSDs are most important is from 40 to 55 years (Murray et al. 2012). Considering only YLDs, for both males and females it appears that MSDs start being an important issue at the age of 10 but peak at the ages between 45 and 64 (Vos et al. 2012).

Through a geographical lens, it is clear that most world regions will have to prioritize MSDs, which went from being ranked 11th among all assessed conditions in 1990 to being ranked sixth in 2010. This is especially true for conditions such as LBP which is a problem pretty much everywhere in the world (Fig. 8.9.1). Considering only conditions capable of resulting in disability (as opposed to mortality), LBP was first in priority in the years 1990 and 2010; NP was fourth in priority in both 1990 and 2010; other MSDs went from fifth priority to sixth priority between the years 1990 and 2010. Lastly, OA went from 15th to 11th priority (Vos et al. 2012). In analysing these figures, it is important to consider that the hip and knee account for the greatest proportion of disability attributed to OA (Fransen et al. 2011).

Determinants of musculoskeletal disorders

Four risk factors can be considered major drivers of MSD occurrence worldwide: obesity (Lim et al. 2012), ageing, and the increase in trauma (particularly via road traffic collisions) (Walsh et al. 2008) and repeated mechanical loading (particularly via working conditions) (Lim et al. 2012). At another level of causation, behavioural changes related to diet and physical activity may be driving observed changes in obesity. Major determinants of these

Table 8.9.2 DALYs related to major MSDs in both sexes by age groups

Cause	50–54 years	55–59 years	60–64 years	65–69 years	70–74 years	75–79 years	80+ years
MSDs	15,257.4 (11,840–18,871.8)	14,581.2 (11434–17934.2)	12,160.5 (9634.2–14908.8)	9695.7 (7740.5–11859.0)	8292.9 (6568.1–10139.3)	5685.5 (4432.7–7000.4)	6115.7 (4791.0–7504.6)
Rheumatoid arthritis	324.2 (229–429.7)	340.9 (239.5–449.8)	325.0 (230.1–428.8)	285.2 (201.8–374.8)	274.5 (195.5–359.1)	2324.5 (159.5–292.5)	312.3 (222.3–407.0)
Osteoarthritis	2723.7 (1880–3880.6)	2698.6 (1865.8–3827.7)	2175.8 (1500–3083.3)	1690.1 (1167.1–2405.6)	1444.4 (999.5–2039.5)	1050.6 (725.9–1477.6)	1159.0 (8009–1620.3)
Low back and neck pain	9996.9 (6991.7–13351.9)	9143.0 (6389–12203.0)	7334.6 (5138–9794.0)	5673.5 (3978.6–7600.2)	4878.8 (3408.3–6503.7)	3518.5 (2453.9–4670.1)	3638.7 (2526.1–4819.1)
Low back pain	7103.3 (4859.1–9554.3)	6610.3 (4549.1–8917.0)	5424.1 (3755.8–7302.5)	4292.4 (2967–5794.7)	3779.6 (2614.8–5077.9)	2763.1 (1901.5–3707.7)	2888.2 (1988–3882.4)
Neck pain	2893.6 (2013.7–3969.6)	2532.6 (1772.6–3499.0)	1910.4 (1341–2635.8)	1381.1 (979.1–1890.8)	1099.1 (771.0–1500.7)	755.4 (525.2–1029.9)	750.5 (528.0–1.022.4)
Gout	13.3 (8.5–19.6)	14.5 (9.2–21.5)	13.9 (8.8–20.5)	11.8 (7.5–17.3)	10.6 (6.8–15.6)	8.1 (5.1–11.9)	9.3 (6.0–13.5)
Other MSDs	2199.4 (1785.9–2510.4)	2384.2 (1962.3–2690.0)	2311 (1937–2593.8)	2035.1 (1720.1–2282.0)	1684.6 (1408.4–1900.0)	883.9 (658.5–1067.1)	996.3 (762.2–1193.8)

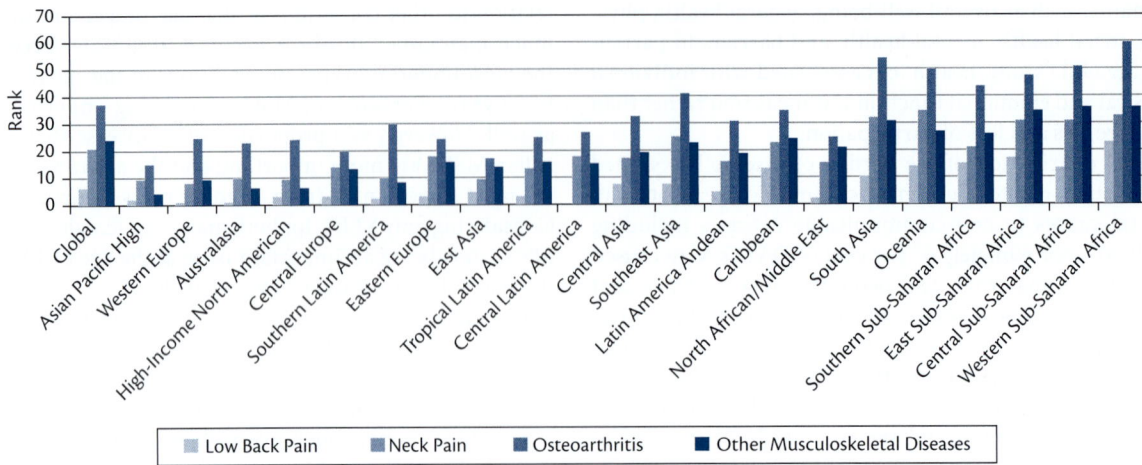

Fig. 8.9.1 Regional ranking of disability-adjusted life years due to musculoskeletal disorders ordered by global rank, 2010.

Source: data from *The Lancet*, Volume 380, Issue 9859, Vos T. et al., Years lived with disability (YLDs) for 1160 sequelae of 289 diseases and injuries 1990–2010: a systematic analysis for the Global Burden of Disease Study 2010, pp. 2163–96, Copyright © 2012, with permission from Elsevier, http://www.sciencedirect.com/science/journal/01406736.

behavioural changes include technological development, income increase, globalization, growth of mass media, and urbanization (Fig. 8.9.2).

Paradoxically, technological improvements have resulted in different consequences. On the one hand, medical advances and prevention of infant mortality (Anderson and Arias 2003) have contributed to the increase in human life expectancy (Olshansky et al. 2005) and to the ageing of the world's populations and, therefore, to the occurrence of MSDs. Also, technological advances have made possible the reduction of physical demands (Popkin et al. 1989), at least for a part of the population, which may have also contributed to obesity and therefore to the occurrence of MSDs. Lastly, the lack of permeation of such advances in many industries contributes to the existence of large, sudden physical demands or permanent low demands that are capable of promoting the occurrence of MSDs.

Other related factors include: (1) worldwide shifts in the trade of technology innovations that affect energy expenditures during leisure, transportation, and work; (2) globalization of modern food processing, marketing, and distribution techniques (most frequently linked with Westernization of the world's diet); (3) vast expansion of the global mass media; and (4) other changes that constitute the rubric of the effects resulting from an increased opening up of the world economy (Popkin et al. 1989).

Ageing

The world population is ageing. The median of the world population has gone from 23.9 years in 1950 to 29.2 years in 2010 (Fig. 8.9.3). The population above 60 worldwide has gone from roughly 204 million (8.1 per cent of the total population) in 1950 to 865 million (12.4 per cent of the total population) in 2010; and the population above 80 years old went from roughly 15 million (0.6 per cent of the total population) to roughly 210 million in 2010 (3 per cent of the total population) (United Nations 2012).

The current median age of the population in Europe, North America, and Oceania are much above the average. The growing trend in Europe is especially concerning as is the current trend in Asia, Latin America, and the Caribbean. Many countries in Asia are ageing rapidly. The number of people aged over 65 has doubled from 6.8 per cent in 2008 to 16.2 per cent in 2004. It is expected that from 2008 to 2040, the proportion of people over 65 will grow by 316 per cent in Singapore, 274 per cent in India, 269 per cent in Malaysia, 261 per cent in Bangladesh, and 256 per cent in the Philippines. In 2008, Japan had the oldest population, and in absolute terms, China and India have the largest number of people over 65 (approximately 106 and 60 million) (Fransen et al. 2011).

Obesity

A major worldwide public health concern is the increasing growth of overweight and obese individuals in both developed

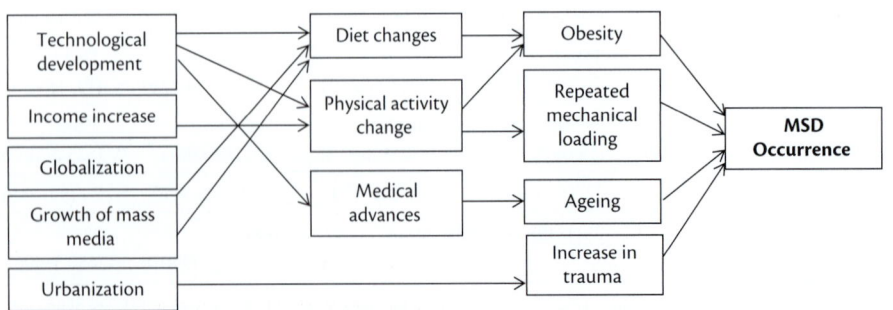

Fig. 8.9.2 Conceptual model relating the major determinants of musculoskeletal disorders.

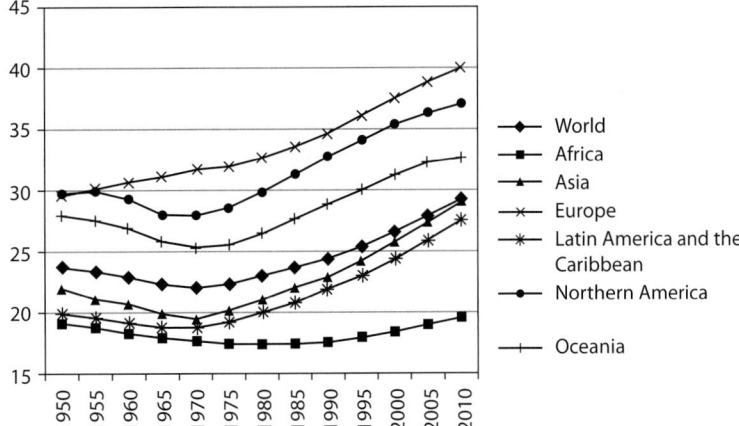

Fig. 8.9.3 Median age of the world population in the last 50 years.
Adapted from United Nations (UN), Population Estimates and Projection Section, United Nations Department of Economic and Social Affairs, Copyright © 2012, available from: http://esa.un.org/wpp/Excel-Data/population.htm.

and now developing countries. Several epidemiological studies have correlated the burden of overweight and obesity to MSDs and other health outcomes. This phenomenon is of great public health concern given that between 1980 and 2008, the mean body mass index (BMI; a proxy measurement for overweight and obese levels) worldwide increased by 0.4 kg/m² per decade for men and 0.5 kg/m² per decade for women. Gender and geographic differences in BMI status have been changing over the years. For example, male and female BMIs in 2008 were highest in specific Oceania countries, reaching 33.9 kg/m² for men and 35.0 kg/m² for women in Nauru. Female BMI was lowest in Bangladesh (20.5 kg/m²) and male BMI in the Democratic Republic of the Congo 19.9 kg/m², with BMI less than 21.5 kg/m² for both sexes in a few countries in sub-Saharan Africa, and east, south, and South East Asia. The United States had the highest BMI of high-income countries. In 2008, an estimated 1.46 billion adults worldwide had a BMI of 25 kg/m² or greater; of these, 205 million men and 297 million women were obese (Finucane et al. 2011).

Multiple factors are contributing to this trend of increasing overweight and obesity in developing countries, and are likely to have a major impact on MSDs in the future. For example, several low-income countries such as Mexico, Egypt, and South Africa have equally high levels of obesity among women as compared to higher-income countries. China also has obesity rates of 20 per cent for women and men (Popkin et al. 1989). In Asia, the population is also getting obese (Fransen et al. 2011). From 1992 to 2000, using nationally representative data for women aged 20–49 years in 36 countries, the proportion of overweight plus obese individuals exceeded underweight in most countries (Popkin et al. 1989). Small urban–rural differences in overweight, high absolute levels of overweight plus obesity, and very high ratios of overweight plus obesity to underweight have also been documented among countries with a high income and urbanization. There are even high levels of overweight individuals in rural areas of many poor countries where underweight individuals remain a public health concern. Most importantly the rates of change in the prevalence of overweight and obesity in these countries are growing. A large number of lower- and middle-income countries such as Mexico, Thailand, China, and Indonesia are experiencing an annual increase in overweight and obesity of 1 per cent (Popkin 2006). Even more concerning is the fact that the obesity problem in children matches the adult obesity, with the concomitant problems related to diabetes (Popkin et al. 1989).

Overweight and obesity can also be directly explained by the level of physical activity and diet. Although there is significant variability between countries, it is true that around the world, diet and nutritional food consumption has become increasingly energy-dense and sweeter; and that processed foods are replacing foods that are high in fibre (Popkin 2006). On the other hand, the desire to reduce physical demands has always being an objective. In the advent of the information age, where more modern technologies are used in the workplace, in the shopping arena, and at home, there is likely to be decreased levels of physical activity. The picture of overall shifts in activity, their causes, and their consequences are still incomplete. Since the beginning of time, humans have made efforts to reduce physical effort in the home and at work. In addition, the growing demand for goods that are tasteful including portions higher in fat and sugars has been growing (Popkin et al. 1989). For example, the total daily calories ingested by US children aged 2–19 years increased on average from 2065 calories in the years 2003–2004 to 2952 in the years 2005–2008; while in adults there was a slight reduction from 2170 to 2106 for the same periods (Economic Research Service 2012).

The Economic Research Service (ERS) has conducted a series of studies that have interesting conclusions about the factors that influence diet decisions. Demographic factors (i.e. lower income, younger age, and lower formal education), household characteristics (single head of the household, working parents), and acculturation (e.g. acculturated Hispanics), and misperceptions about quality of food at home, are related to lower-quality diets or bad habits regarding their diets (skipping meals, eating away from home) (ERS 2012).

The ERS found that habits such as having food away from home plays an increasing role in Americans' diets, usually with negative effects on diet quality (Guthrie et al. 2002).

Future directions

By now it should be clear that there are societal determinants of MSDs which act through several different complex pathways that give way to a significant increase in MSD occurrence, with important effects on human development and quality of life. To tackle such a complex problem, different strategies are required at different levels.

Policy level

Two actions that are non-specific to MSDs but are the platform for the health of the population are required: redressing general social inequalities, including in education, employment, housing, and food; and improving the health financing system. Such actions are typically in the range of action of governments and the platform over which other actions are built. No health system alone will be able to address health inequalities if these factors are not addressed. According to the International Labour Organization (ILO), social security benefits that include cover for lost wages in the event of illness are available to only one in five adults worldwide, and more than half of the world population lacks any form of social protection (ILO 1999, 2000). For example, approximately 5–10 per cent of adults in sub-Saharan Africa and Southern Asia as compared to 20–60 per cent of adults in middle-income countries have social security coverage. There has never been a time with as great a need for universal health coverage and strategies to finance it. Recommendations have been given by the WHO. Country governments need to make sure that if people pay at the entry level of health services, those payments should correspond to their capacity of payment on a sliding scale. They also need to improve access to and utilization of primary preventive services for the poor, despite the challenges of implementing such services in low-resource and economically constrained countries (WHO 2010b).

Efforts to finance these types of systems should include special attention to the need to better distribute available resources. Among Organisation for Economic Cooperation and Development (OECD) countries there is a known 20/80 syndrome in which they spend over 80 per cent of the world's resources on health yet make up less than 20 per cent of the world's total population. While only 6.5 per cent of the African and 3.7 per cent of South East Asian regions' gross domestic product is spent on healthcare, OECD countries spend a much larger proportion on health (12.4 per cent). Low-income countries with annual per capita income of less than US$1005 relied most heavily on out-of-pocket payments to finance healthcare. In these countries, the share of out-of-pocket payment in total health expenditure measured in US$ terms was 50 per cent compared to only 13 per cent in countries with incomes higher than US$12,276 per capita (WHO 2010b).

Other important actions that are specific to MSDs at the policy level are the creation and awareness of the scope of the MSD problem and investing in MSD research. Creating awareness is required so that action is started. Awareness moves political willingness. The recent GBD study has placed MSDs as the sixth priority worldwide among all 291 selected conditions assessed in this study. In some areas, as was already shown, MSDs are the top priority in terms of the burden of this type of condition (Vos et al. 2012). Nevertheless, the task persists; the information needs to reach and be understood by policymakers to prompt action. Efforts by the Bone and Joint Decade, a global alliance for musculoskeletal health, have focused on raising this awareness of the burden of musculoskeletal conditions by developing sustainable networks and improving access to cost-effective prevention and treatment (Global Alliance for Musculoskeletal Health 2014).

Healthcare systems are now confronted with the growing costs and increased prevalence of MSDs that will require a coherent policy for dealing with MSDs. Identifying and prioritizing the research efforts on the most effective and affordable strategies for low-resource countries to deal with these conditions is paramount (Murray et al. 2012). The revealed utmost importance of MSDs should have consequences regarding the health system's capital investments. As the expected future burden of MSDs grows, investment efforts into these cost-effective strategies will need to spread over a long-term 10-year outlook. In addition, training and educational efforts for the existing and upcoming healthcare workforce is urgently needed to adequately address the large group of individuals that will be afflicted with MSDs. Innovation in health professional education should include MSDs on a region-by-region basis, so that trends in demographic and epidemiological change are identified fast enough that a forward looking assessment of the burden can be incorporated (Murray et al. 2012).

Research in this area should follow the framework that is being proposed here. There are needs both at the policy level and at the practice level. At the policy level, there are important unresolved questions about what policies could help prevent MSDs and improve access to healthcare. At the practice level, there are needs specifically regarding best clinical practices and new treatments. An important area of research priority includes assessing the impact of modifiable risk factors through innovative treatment approaches. Public policy that addresses these risk factors may help to significantly reduce the public health burden and cost of MSDs (Haldeman et al. 2008).

Research on the specific risk factors that should be targeted in specific populations is still pending. For example, there is a dearth of epidemiological research from low- and middle-income countries in the Asian region on MSDs. Due to significant demographic and environmental differences influencing the onset and progression of various MSDs in these regions, it becomes challenging to reasonably extrapolate some of the risk factor finding from high-income countries to low- and middle-income countries. In developing countries, trends in obesity, the burden of heavy physical labour, diminished access to healthcare variations in the approach to pain treatment, and linguistic variation all contribute to differences in reported and treated MSDs (Fransen et al. 2011). Nonetheless, these observations could be lower or higher estimates of the true value, given the general lack of epidemiological data in these developing countries that could support the development of better policy (Gabriel and Michaud 2009).

Practice level

While research progresses, much is already known on what to do and it should be put into practice. We already know what the major modifiable risk factors for MSDs are and the ways to improve access to healthcare (Fig. 8.9.4). While they may require adjustments to be applied in specific contexts, the basic understanding of the problem and potential ways to tackle it have already been proposed.

For example, in the case of LBP treatment, there are several new scientific and clinical investigations underway to examine

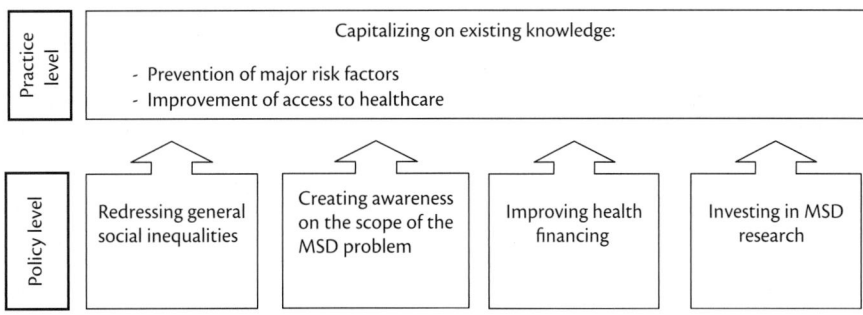

Fig. 8.9.4 Conceptual model for practice and policy levels addressing musculoskeletal disorders.

innovative technologies, new drugs, and strategic management approaches for individuals with LBP. The healthcare community should be encouraged by the fact that we already know so much about the challenges of LBP that are affected by a host of genetic, physical, psychological, environmental, cultural, and societal factors (Balagué et al. 2012). Unfortunately, individuals with MSDs are too often ignored, and their complaints often misunderstood by healthcare providers. Large population studies have shown that successful management of musculoskeletal pain must occur during the acute phase in order to hinder progression to a more chronic state. Adoption of broader standards of care for these conditions, particularly in low-resources areas, is needed (Walsh et al. 2008). This is especially the case when MSDs are co-morbid with other health conditions. For example, research has shown that MSDs are closely associated with mental health and physical disability. Among older people with MSDs, depression is common, and is associated with functional disability (Punzi et al. 2010). Studies have shown that in older adults, depression and pain are better predictors of disability than findings from radiographic imaging. These findings can inform the development of practice guidelines for screening for other co-morbid conditions that might improve the overall health of the person with MSDs (Punzi et al. 2010).

Regarding the prevention of known modifiable risk factors for MSDs, practice efforts should focus on new ways to prevent and control obesity and exposures to mechanical demands in the workplace. However, little has been done globally, nationally, or regionally to systematically address obesity (Popkin 2006). From the 1980s to 2008, trends in the mean population BMI have varied substantially between nations. Developing interventions and drafting policies that modify this observed increase in BMI by targeting these modifiable risk factors are greatly needed in most countries (Finucane et al. 2011).

Practice efforts to address MSDs should include education on diet. Two noteworthy country efforts can be seen in Finland and South Korea (Holveck et al. 2007). Finland has been reported as one of the countries that have made efforts in the direction of using intersectorial collaboration (Pietinen et al. 2010). They have developed an integrated national price and food-labelling policy coupled with educational programmes on diet and nutrition as well as advocacy efforts from select organizations. A second example is South Korea, which has long promoted the use of a traditional diet rich in vegetables and low in fat—very distinct from observed trends in other middle-income countries that have experienced a Westernized shift in dietary consumption (Lee et al. 2012). Over the years, the South Korean government has provided educational

community workshops to new brides on how to prepare traditional dishes and avoid incorporation of Western-style dishes. These efforts have resulted in lower obesity levels and lower intake of energy-dense foods that would be expected from a high-income level country.

Regarding treatment options and practice, there is a need to translate what is already known scientifically to guidelines for clinicians. In the advent of the information age, healthcare professionals can easily become bogged down with multiple sources of information from professional organizations, drug developers, and scientific journals. Data from all these sources could be combined, digested, and presented in a more systematic fashion so that the end user (i.e. healthcare professionals) can benefit from a uniform and up-to-date source of information on best practices to treat MSDs. For example, significant advances in our understanding of the evaluation of quality of life among patients with arthritis and its effect on disease progression have been studied. Translating our basic and clinical science knowledge base into real-world bedside practices should be warranted (Punzi et al. 2010). Therapeutic modalities that are currently available have been largely ineffective due to deficiencies in global MSD management.

Consider access to healthcare, where efforts need to be made so that available treatments permeate all regions. This is, of course, related to the financing aspect mentioned earlier. For example, among rural regions of the developing world, access to joint replacement surgery is scarce and likely leads to a large number of older adults living with high-grade degenerative joint disease and poor quality of life.

Despite access to new information that is made readily available to healthcare providers in developing countries, other barriers may be present (Turner 2009; Doughty et al. 2010; Vargas et al. 2010; El-Jardali et al. 2012). For example, in order to minimize the sequelae from a bout of LBP, healthcare providers in developing countries could incorporate the use of evidence-based guidelines to standardize their management approach and improve MSD treatment outcomes in their community setting. However, despite the progress made in the past two decades in developing and updating guidelines, and adapting them on a national basis, uptake by healthcare providers is not optimum (Global Alliance for Musculoskeletal Health 2014). There are challenges with implementing guidelines in low-resource setting, including the use of specific drugs or technologies that might not be readily available in those areas, as well as pressure from industry or healthcare providers who challenge changes in medical and public health practice (Balagué et al. 2012).

Note

1. From the Operations Manual of the GBD 2010 estimates: musculoskeletal diseases include M00–M85 (arthropathies, systemic connective tissue disorders, dorsopathies, soft tissue disorders, disorders of bone density and structure), M87–M99 (other osteopathies except osteomyelitis, chondropathies, and other disorders of the musculoskeletal system and connective tissue). Rheumatoid arthritis includes M05–M06 (seropositive rheumatoid arthritis and other rheumatoid arthritis). Osteoarthritis include M15–M19 (polyarthrosis, coxarthrosis (arthrosis of hip), gonarthrosis (arthrosis of knee), arthrosis of first carpometacarpal joint, other arthrosis. Back pain includes M46.9 (inflammatory spondylopathy, unspecified), M47 (spondylosis), M48 (other spondylopathies), M48.1 (ankylosing hyperostosis (Forestier)), M48.2 (kissing spine), M48.8 (other specified spondylopathies), M48.9 (spondylopathy, unspecified), M50–M54 (other dorsopathies—including cervical disc disorders, including LBP). Gout includes M10 (idiopathic gout). Other musculoskeletal disorders include M00–M02, M08, M11–M13, M20–M46 (except M46.9), M48 (except M48.0, M48.1, M48.2, M48.8, and M48.9), M60–M85, and M87–M99.

References

Anderson, R.N. and Arias, E. (2003). The effect of revised populations on mortality statistics for the United States, 2000. *National Vital Statistics Reports*, 51, 1–24.

Balagué, F., Mannion, A.F., Pellisé, F., and Cedraschi, C. (2012). Non-specific low back pain. *The Lancet*, 379, 482–91.

Biyani, A. and Andersson, G.B. (2004). Low back pain: pathophysiology and management. *Journal of the American Academy of Orthopaedic Surgeons*, 12, 106–15.

Bogduk, N. (2011). The anatomy and pathophysiology of neck pain. *Physical Medicine & Rehabilitation Clinics of North America*, 22, 367–82.

Brennan, P., Bankhead, C., Silman, A., and Symmons. D. (1997). Oral contraceptives and rheumatoid arthritis: results from a primary care-based incident case-control study. *Seminars in Arthritis and Rheumatism*, 26, 817–23.

Caban-Martinez, A.J., Lee, D.J., Fleming, L.E., et al. (2011). Arthritis, occupational class, and the aging US workforce. *American Journal of Public Health*, 101, 1729–34.

Carder, M., McNamee, R., Turner, S., Hodgson, J.T., Holland, F., and Agius, R.M. (2013). Time trends in the incidence of work-related mental ill-health and musculoskeletal disorders in the UK. *Occupational and Environmental Medicine*, 70(5), 317–24.

Carroll, L.J., Hogg-Johnson, S., Côté, P., et al. (2008). Course and prognostic factors for neck pain in workers: results of the Bone and Joint Decade 2000–2010 Task Force on Neck Pain and Its Associated Disorders. *Spine*, 33, S93–100.

Cisternas, M.G., Murphy, L.B., Yelin, E.H., Foreman, A.J., Pasta, D.J., and Helmick, C.G. (2009). Trends in medical care expenditures of US adults with arthritis and other rheumatic conditions 1997 to 2005. *Journal of Rheumatology*, 36, 2531–8.

Combe, B. (2009). Progression in early rheumatoid arthritis. *Best Practice & Research Clinical Rheumatology*, 23, 59–69.

Croft, P.R., Papageorgiou, A.C., Thomas, E., MacFarlane, G.J., and Silman, A.J. (1999) Short-term physical risk factors for new episodes of low back pain. Prospective evidence from the South Manchester Back Pain Study. *Spine*, 24, 1556–61.

Doughty, K., Rothman, L., Johnston, L., Le, K., Wu, J., and Howard, A. (2010). Low-income countries' orthopaedic information needs: challenges and opportunities. *Clinical Orthopaedics and Related Research*, 468, 2598–603.

Drake, M.T., Murad, M.H., Mauck, K.F., et al. (2012). Clinical review. Risk factors for low bone mass-related fractures in men: a systematic review and meta-analysis. *Journal of Clinical Endocrinology and Metabolism*, 97, 1861–70.

Dunn, K.M., Jordan, K., and Croft, P.R. (2006). Characterizing the course of low back pain: a latent class analysis. *American Journal of Epidemiology*, 163, 754–61.

Economic Research Service (2012). *Food Consumption and Nutrition Intakes*. [Online]. United States Department of Agriculture. Available at: http://www.ers.usda.gov/data-products/food-consumption-and-nutrient-intakes.aspx.

Edwards, R.R., Cahalan, C., Mensing, G., Smith, M., and Ja, H. (2011). Pain, catastrophizing, and depression in the rheumatic diseases. *Nature Reviews Rheumatology*, 7, 216–24.

El-Jardali, F., Lavis, J.N., Ataya, N., and Jamal, D. (2012). Use of health systems and policy research evidence in the health policymaking in eastern Mediterranean countries: views and practices of researchers. *Implementation Science*, 7, 2.

Farmer, M.E., White, L.R., Brody, J.A., and Bailey, K.R. (1984). Race and sex differences in hip fracture incidence. *American Journal of Public Health*, 74, 1374–80.

Finucane, M.M., Stevens, G.A., Cowan, M.J., et al. (2011). National, regional, and global trends in body-mass index since 1980: systematic analysis of health examination surveys and epidemiological studies with 960 country-years and 9.1 million participants. *The Lancet*, 377, 557–67.

Fransen, M., Bridgett, L., March, L., Hoy, D., Penserga, E., and Brooks, P. (2011). The epidemiology of osteoarthritis in Asia. *International Journal of Rheumatic Diseases*, 14, 113–21.

Gabriel, S.E. and Michaud, K. (2009). Epidemiological studies in incidence, prevalence, mortality, and comorbidity of the rheumatic diseases. *Arthritis Research & Therapy*, 11, 229–44.

Global Alliance For Musculoskeletal Health (2014). *The Bone and Joint Decade* [Online]. Available at: http://bjdonline.org/.

Guilak, F. (2011). Biomechanical factors in osteoarthritis. *Best Practice & Research Clinical Rheumatology*, 25, 815–23.

Guthrie, J.F., Lin, B.H., and Frazao, E. (2002). Role of food prepared away from home in the American diet, 1977–78 versus 1994–96: changes and consequences. *Journal of Nutrition Education and Behavior*, 34, 140–50.

Haldeman, S., Carroll, L., and Cassidy, J.D. (2010). Findings from the bone and joint decade 2000 to 2010 task force on neck pain and its associated disorders. *Journal of Occupational and Environmental Medicine*, 52, 424–7.

Haldeman, S., Carroll, L., Cassidy, J.D., Schubert, J., and Nygren, Å. (2008). The Bone and Joint Decade 2000–2010 Task Force on Neck Pain and Its Associated Disorders. *Spine*, 33, S5–S7.

Helmick, C.G., Felson, D.T., Lawrence, R.C., et al. (2008). Estimates of the prevalence of arthritis and other rheumatic conditions in the United States. Part I. *Arthritis & Rheumatology*, 58, 15–25.

Holmgren, K., Fjällström-Lundgren, M., and Hensing, G. (2013). Early identification of work-related stress predicted sickness absence in employed women with musculoskeletal or mental disorders: a prospective, longitudinal study in a primary health care setting. *Disability and Rehabilitation*, 35, 418–26.

Holveck, J.C., Ehrenberg, J.P., Ault, S.K., et al. (2007). Prevention, control, and elimination of neglected diseases in the Americas: pathways to integrated, inter-programmatic, inter-sectoral action for health and development. *BMC Public Health*, 7, 6.

Hoving, J.L., Gross, A.R., Gasner, D., et al. (2001). A critical appraisal of review articles on the effectiveness of conservative treatment for neck pain. *Spine*, 26, 196–205.

Hoy, D., Bain, C., Williams, G., et al. (2012). A systematic review of the global prevalence of low back pain. *Arthritis and Rheumatism*, 64, 2028–37.

Hoy, D., Brooks, P., Blythc, F., and Buchbinder, R. (2010). The epidemiology of low back pain. *Best Practice & Research Clinical Rheumatology*, 24, 769–81.

Hoy, D.G., Protani, M., Dea, R., and Buchbinder, R. (2010). The epidemiology of neck pain. *Best Practice & Research Clinical Rheumatology*, 24, 783–92.

Huizinga, T.W. and Pincus, T. (2010). In the clinic. Rheumatoid arthritis. *Annals of Internal Medicine*, 153, ITC1-1–15.

Iagnocco, A. and Naredo, E. (2012). Osteoarthritis: research update and clinical applications. *Rheumatology (Oxford)*, 51(Suppl. 7), vii2–5.

Ibrahim, I., Owen, S.A., and Barton, A. (2012). Genetics and the impact on treatment protocols in patients with rheumatoid arthritis. *Expert Review of Clinical Immunology*, 8, 509–11.

International Labour Organization (1999). *Unemployment, Social Protection and Crises: Trends and Issues*. Geneva: ILO.

International Labour Organization (2000). *Income Security and Social Protection in a Changing World. World Labour Report 2000*. Geneva: ILO.

Isaacs, J.D. (2010). The changing face of rheumatoid arthritis: sustained remission for all? *Nature Reviews Immunology*, 10, 605–11.

Jarvik, J.G. and Deyo, R.A. (2002). Diagnostic evaluation of low back pain with emphasis on imaging. *Annals of Internal Medicine*, 137, 586–97.

Jeffries, L.J. and Grimmer-Somers, K.A. (2007). Epidemiology of adolescent spinal pain: a systematic overview of the research literature. *Spine*, 32, 2630–7.

Kanis, J.A., Melton, L.J., Christiansen, C., Johnston, C.C., and Khaltaev, N. (1994). The diagnosis of osteoporosis. *Journal of Bone and Mineral Research*, 9, 1137–41.

Krismer, M., Van Tulder, M., and The Low Back Pain Group of the Bone And Joint Health Strategies for Europe Project (2007). Low back pain (non-specific). *Best Practice & Research Clinical Rheumatology*, 21, 77–91.

Laisné, F., Lecomte, C., and Corbière, M. (2012). Biopsychosocial predictors of prognosis in musculoskeletal disorders: a systematic review of the literature. *Disability and Rehabilitation*, 34, 355–82.

Leaver, A.M., Maher, C.G., McAuley, J.H., Jull, G.A., and Refshauge, K.M. (2013). Characteristics of a new episode of neck pain. *Manual Therapy*, 18(3), 254–7.

Lee, H.S., Duffey, K.J., and Popkin, B.M. (2012). South Korea's entry to the global food economy: shifts in consumption of food between 1998 and 2009. *Asia Pacific Journal of Clinical Nutrition*, 21, 618–29.

Lim, S.S., Vos, T., Flaxman, A.D., Danaei, G., Shibuya, K., and Adair-Rohani, H. (2012). A comparative risk assessment of burden of disease and injury attributable to 67 risk factors and risk factor clusters in 21 regions, 1990–2010: a systematic analysis for the Global Burden of Disease Study 2010. *The Lancet*, 380, 2224–60.

Linton, S.J. and Van Tulder, M.W. (2001). Preventive interventions for back and neck pain problems: what is the evidence? *Spine*, 26, 778–87.

Murray, C.J.L., Vos, T., Lozano, R., et al. (2012). Disability-adjusted life years (DALYs) for 291 diseases and injuries in 21 regions, 1990–2010: a systematic analysis for the Global Burden of Disease Study 2010. *The Lancet*, 380, 2197–223.

Naylor, K. and Eastell, R. (2012). Bone turnover markers: use in osteoporosis. *Nature Reviews Rheumatology*, 8, 379–89.

Olshansky, S.J., Passaro, D.J., Hershow, R.C., et al. (2005). A potential decline in life expectancy in the United States in the 21st century. *The New England Journal of Medicine*, 352, 1138–45.

Osborne, R.H., Nikpour, M., Busija, J., Sundararajan, V., and Wicks, I.P. (2007). Prevalence and cost of musculoskeletal disorders: a population-based, public hospital system healthcare consumption approach. *Journal of Rheumatology*, 34, 2466–75.

Pietinen, P., Männistö, S., Valsta, L.M., and Sarlio-Lähteenkorva, S. (2010). Nutrition policy in Finland. *Public Health Nutrition*, 13, 901–6.

Pincus, T. and Callahan, L.F. (1993). What is the natural history of rheumatoid arthritis? *Rheumatic Disease Clinics of North America*, 19, 123–51.

Pisetsky, D.S., Ullal, A.J., Gauley, J., and Ning, T.C. (2012). Microparticles as mediators and biomarkers of rheumatic disease. *Rheumatology (Oxford)*, 51, 1737–46.

Popkin, B.M. (2006). Global nutrition dynamics: the world is shifting rapidly toward a diet linked with noncommunicable diseases. *American Journal of Clinical Nutrition*, 84, 289–98.

Popkin, B.M., Haines, P.S., and Reidy, K.C. (1989). Food consumption trends of US women: patterns and determinants between 1977 and 1985. *American Journal of Clinical Nutrition*, 49, 1307–19.

Punzi, L., Oliviero, F., and Ramonda, R. (2010). New horizons in osteoarthritis. *Swiss Medical Weekly*, 140, w13098.

Riis, B.J. (1993). Biochemical markers of bone turnover II: diagnosis, prophylaxis, and treatment of osteoporosis. *The American Journal of Medicine*, 95, S17–S21.

Ronis, M.J., Mercer, K., and Chen, J.R. (2011). Effects of nutrition and alcohol consumption on bone loss. *Current Osteoporosis Reports*, 9, 53–9.

Rousseau, J. and Garnero, P. (2012). Biological markers in osteoarthritis. *Bone*, 51, 265–77.

Scott, D.L., Wolfe, F., and Huizinga, T.W. (2010). Rheumatoid arthritis. *The Lancet*, 376, 1094–108.

Silman, A.J. and Pearson, J.E. (2002). Epidemiology and genetics of rheumatoid arthritis. *Arthritis Research & Therapy*, 4, S265–72.

Smolen, J. and Aletaha, D. (2008). The burden of rheumatoid arthritis and access to treatment: a medical overview. *European Journal of Health Economics*, 8, S39–47.

Turner, T.J. (2009). Developing evidence-based clinical practice guidelines in hospitals in Australia, Indonesia, Malaysia, the Philippines and Thailand: values, requirements and barriers. *BMC Health Services Research*, 9, 235.

United Nations (2012). *Population Estimates and Projection Section*. New York: Department of Economic and Social Affairs, United Nations.

Vargas, I., Vázquez, M.L., Mogollón-Pérez, A.S., and Unger, J.P. (2010). Barriers of access to care in a managed competition model: lessons from Colombia. *BMC Health Services Research*, 10, 297.

Vincent, H.K., Raiser, S.N., and Vincent, K.R. (2012). The aging musculoskeletal system and obesity-related considerations with exercise. *Ageing Research Reviews*, 11, 361–73.

Vos, T., Flaxman, A.D., Naghavi, M., et al. (2012). Years lived with disability (YLDs) for 1160 sequelae of 289 diseases and injuries 1990–2010: a systematic analysis for the Global Burden of Disease Study 2010. *The Lancet*, 380, 2163–96.

Walsh, N.E., Brooks, P., Hazes, J.M., et al. (2008). Standards of care for acute and chronic musculoskeletal pain: the Bone and Joint Decade (2000–2010). *Archives of Physical Medicine and Rehabilitation*, 89, 1830–45.

Wasnich, R. (1993). Bone mass measurement: prediction of risk. *American Journal of Medicine*, 95, 6S–10S.

Woolf, A.D., Vos, T., and March, L. (2010). How to measure the impact of musculoskeletal conditions. *Best Practice & Research Clinical Rheumatology*, 24, 723–32.

World Health Organization (2010a). Diseases of the musculoskeletal system and connective tissue (M00-M99). In *International Statistical Classification of Diseases and Related Health Problems 10th Revision (ICD-10) Version for 2010*. [Online] Available at: http://apps.who.int/classifications/icd10/browse/2010/en#/XIII.

World Health Organization (2010b). *The World Health Report: Health Systems Financing*. Geneva: WHO.

World Health Organization (2012). *WHO Global Health Expenditure Atlas*. Geneva: WHO.

Wright, N.C. and Saag, K.G. (2012). From fracture risk prediction to evaluating fracture patterns: recent advances in the epidemiology of osteoporosis. *Current Rheumatology Reports*, 14, 205–11.

8.10

Neurological diseases, epidemiology, and public health

Walter A. Kukull and James Bowen

Introduction to neurological diseases, epidemiology, and public health

Included in this chapter are brief descriptions of headache, traumatic brain injury (TBI), epilepsy, dementia, peripheral neuropathy, parkinsonism, and multiple sclerosis (MS). Diagnosis is critical to epidemiological study but is often difficult because of long, preclinical undetectable periods. Clinical criteria rather than pathological evidence can lead to misclassification of disease and spurious inferences. To some extent biomarkers are becoming accepted as a preclinical indicator of disease or a means to add diagnostic certainty among the symptomatic.

Population-based studies are the best method to avoid spurious, biased, or non-generalizable results, but for most neurological diseases these are seldom performed. Selecting 'control' subjects from the same base that gave rise to the cases is methodologically essential but often a luxury ignored by investigators. Cohort studies must start with people free of disease but if preclinical detection of disease process is not possible, risk factor associations may be severely biased.

Determination of risk factor exposure, and estimating whether it may have occurred during a time window which had potential to result in the disease in question (and not to have resulted from the disease) is critical. In acute TBI this becomes obvious, while for Parkinson's disease (PD), which may have a 20-year preclinical period, it is cryptic. Researchers seldom have records, biological specimens, or even accurate self-report sufficient to establish historical exposure patterns. Biological markers of exposure (except for genotype) are occasionally employed in cancer studies (e.g. DNA adducts), are seldom available for neurological diseases, but may provide some hope for the future. Biopsy is seldom feasible and autopsy results reflect cross-sectional cumulative effects of disease, leaving the picture additionally confusing.

In less developed countries, the problems of diagnosis and exposure measurement grow in magnitude. Differences in available facilities and local practices are likely the easiest to overcome. Addressing political concerns and suspicions to gain cooperation necessary to begin a study may take additional time and preparation.

Headache

Clinical overview of headaches

The pathogenesis of most headaches is poorly understood. The nosology of headaches is based on the cause when known and the clinical picture when the cause is unknown. The International Classification of Headache Disorders (ICHD), second edition, is the most commonly used system of classifying headaches (Headache Classification Subcommittee of the International Headache Society 2004) (Box 8.10.1). It will soon be updated to ICHD-III. This system classifies individual headaches, so patients may have more than one type of headache. In fact, most headache patients have more than one type of headache. Headaches associated with neurological or systemic diseases are comparatively rare. Idiopathic conditions are far more common and include migraine (with or without aura), tension-type headaches, and cluster headaches. Because these idiopathic headaches are the overwhelming majority, they have the greatest impact on epidemiological studies.

Migraine without aura, previously named common migraine, is an episodic headache that may be unilateral or bilateral. Some people have throbbing pain while others have constant non-throbbing pain. Nausea, vomiting, or diarrhoea may occur. The pain often builds over a few hours. The typical length of the headache is 4–72 hours.

Migraine with aura, previously named classic migraine, has an aura consisting of an alteration of neurological function that usually precedes the headache. This commonly consists of a central area of visual loss surrounded by a rim of shimmering light (scintillating scotoma). Non-visual auras may include paraesthesias, numbness, weakness, aphasia, or vertigo. Auras usually precede the headache by about 20 minutes, though timing may vary. The headache is most commonly, though not always, unilateral, throbbing, and often associated with nausea and vomiting. It typically lasts a few hours. It may have premonitory symptoms preceding the headache and aura.

Tension-type headaches, the most common type of headache, are usually bilateral with a sensation of pressure or a tight band around the head. They are less likely to have premonitory symptoms or nausea or vomiting. They do not have auras.

Box 8.10.1 International Headache Society, abbreviated classification of headache

1. Migraine

    1.1 Migraine without aura

    1.2 Migraine with aura

2. Tension-type headache

3. Cluster headache and chronic paroxysmal hemicrania

4. Miscellaneous headaches unassociated with structural lesion

5. Headache associated with head trauma

6. Headache associated with vascular disorders

7. Headache associated with nonvascular intracranial disorder

8. Headache associated with substances or their withdrawal

9. Headache associated with noncephalic infection

10. Headache associated with metabolic disorder

11. Headache or facial pain associated with disorder of cranium, neck, eyes, ears, nose, sinuses, teeth, mouth, or other facial or cranial structures

12. Cranial neuralgias, nerve trunk pain, and deafferentation pain

13. Headache not classifiable

Adapted from International Headache Society, The International Classification of Headache Disorders: 2nd edition, *Cephalalgia*, Volume 24, Supplment 1, pp. 9–160. Copyright © International Headache Society 2004. Reprinted by permission of SAGE.

They usually last longer than migraine headaches, typically an entire or several days. They build up more slowly than migraine headaches.

Cluster headaches are named after the tendency to occur in clusters lasting weeks to months. However, other types of headaches may also occur in clusters and the diagnosis is based on the characteristics of the headache rather than the clustering. The headache develops abruptly. During a cluster, it usually occurs between one and eight times a day, often at the same time of day. The pain is more short-lived than that of other idiopathic headaches and generally subsides within 3 hours. The pain is often more severe than that seen with migraine and patients are often agitated during the attack.

In a single patient, less severe headaches tend to be tension-type while more severe headaches are migraine. Over time a patient's headaches often change from classic migraine in youth to tension-type headaches in middle age. Headache frequency may increase with age, becoming chronic daily headaches. Some term these headaches as 'transitioned migraines'. This term is not included in the ICHD and many of these cases are actually due to medication overuse.

Prevalence of headaches

Case definition, sample characteristics, methodology, and analytic designs have differed, sometimes substantially, raising questions of comparability. One-year prevalences vary from 20–90 per cent (all headaches), 3–24.6 per cent (migraine), 9.8–72.3 per cent (tension-type), and 0.5–7.3 per cent (chronic headache) (Stovner et al. 2007).

Several studies have evaluated the prevalence of migraine, reflecting the availability of validated survey instruments for this disease (Natoli et al. 2010). The 1-year prevalence of migraine is approximately 12 per cent and appears to be stable over time (Linde et al. 2011). Prevalence peaks at 30–39 years of age, and is higher in white people and those with lower incomes (Lipton et al. 2007). Less than half report their migraines to a physician and approximately 40 per cent of these did not receive a correct diagnosis (Lipton et al. 1998). Susceptibility to migraine may be affected by ethnicity since migraine appears to be more common in Caucasians compared to Africans, African Americans, or Asian Americans (Osuntokun et al. 1992; Stewart et al. 1996).

There are far fewer studies on tension-type headaches, though it is the most common type of headache. Up to 89 per cent of people suffer tension-type headaches at some time, but for most this is infrequent (Kaniecki 2012). About 25 per cent have weekly tension-type headaches and 2–3 per cent chronic tension-type headaches (Lyngberg et al. 2005a). The prevalence appears to be increasing, though the factors leading to this are not entirely clear. About half of people with tension-type headaches improve within a decade (Lyngberg et al. 2005b). Chronic daily headache from medication overuse is increasingly recognized (Tepper 2012).

Cluster headaches are the least common of the idiopathic headache disorders. Prevalence ranges from 0.056 to 0.338 per cent (Tonon et al. 2002; Katsarava et al. 2007).

Familial and genetic risks of headaches

Genetic influences on migraine have investigated principally familial aggregation and twins. Studies of single genes responsible for familial hemiplegic migraine provide insight into migraine pathophysiology (Ward 2012). The overall lifetime prevalence of migraine with aura for monozygotic (MZ) and dizygotic (DZ) twins is 7 per cent, similar to population surveys (Gervil et al. 1999; Ulrich et al. 1999). Concordance in MZ twins is 34 per cent compared to 12 per cent for DZ twins. For migraine without aura the concordance for MZ twins is 28 per cent and 18 per cent for DZ. This indicates a potential genetic contribution but modifying environmental influences must also be important. Concordance is higher for MZ than DZ twins whether raised together or apart, and about 50 per cent of the variance is explained by genetic factors with the remaining half 'non-shared environmental factors', and measurement error (Ziegler et al. 1998; Russell et al. 2007).

The relative risk (RR) of migraine in first-degree relatives of migraineurs is 1.88 compared to a control group (Stewart et al. 2006). The RR was higher in relatives of those whose headaches began before 16 years of age (RR = 2.50) than those whose headaches began later (RR = 1.44). The risk in relatives of those with severe headaches had a relative risk of 2.38 (95 per cent confidence interval (CI) 1.56–3.62) while relatives of those with less severe pain had a relative risk of 1.52 (0.99–2.34). Individual genes responsible for migraine have not been identified, though some linkages have been found in genome-wide association studies (GWAS) (Chasman et al. 2011).

Risk factors for headaches

Stress or psychological factors are often cited as contributing to tension-type headaches. However, the frequency of these factors is similar in patients with migraine and tension-type headaches. With chronicity, psychological changes increase in frequency, suggesting that psychological issues are secondary to chronic headaches rather than causative. There is an increased risk of depression in migraineurs and also an increased risk for migraine among those with prior depression, suggesting the two disorders may have mechanisms in common. The issues of migraine and depression have been reviewed (Frediani and Villani 2007).

Chronic daily headaches are more common in women, white people, and those with less education. An improvement in headache frequency after 1 year was more common in those with higher education, non-white people, and those who were married (Scher et al. 2003). However, in adolescents with a family history of migraine, migraine prevalence is the same in low- versus high-income groups suggesting that genetic factors overwhelm environmental risk factors in those genetically susceptible (Hagen et al. 2002). One of the strongest risk factors for headaches is prior headaches (RR = 4.15) (Boardman et al. 2006). Pain in other areas of the body is associated with headache (RR = 1.43).

Stroke and migraine

Migraine has been associated with stroke in a number of studies (Alhazzani and Goddeau 2013). Additional study will be needed to adequately describe the true relationship between migraine and stroke.

Costs and public health impact of headaches

The estimated 23 million people with migraines in the United States may miss 150 million workdays each year with an associated cost of up to US$17 billion (Cady 1999; Hu et al. 1999). Many more people suffer with decreased effectiveness at work than actually miss work days (Schwartz et al. 1997). In Europe, costs of headaches are substantial with mean per-person annual costs of €3561 for medication overuse, €1222 for migraine, and €303 for tension-type headaches (Linde et al. 2012). Health-related quality of life is lower in those with migraine, and this is related to the frequency of attacks (Wang et al. 2001). There are many challenges in making cost determinations due to limits on available epidemiological data (Leonardi et al. 2005). However, the best estimate suggests that migraine accounts for 1.4 per cent of all years of healthy life lost worldwide. It is the 19th leading cause of years of healthy life lost in men and 12th in women. This major public health issue deserves continued attention.

Traumatic brain injury

Clinical overview of traumatic brain injuries

TBI is commonly divided into two categories by mechanism of action: (1) penetrating or (2) closed head injuries. These also may be characterized as resulting from direct contact injuries or from concussive 'acceleration deceleration' types of injuries (Werner and Engelhard 2007). Among penetrating injuries, greater tissue damage is caused by high-velocity penetrating objects than by lower-velocity ones. Both penetrating and closed injuries may perturb or impair cerebral blood flow (CBF) leading to ischaemia

and altered cerebral metabolism. Impaired CBF resulting from cerebral vasospasm predicts poorer outcome and may occur in approximately 30 per cent of TBI cases (Werner and Engelhard 2007). Brain contusions may lead to both blood vessel and cell membrane injury resulting in vasogenic or cytotoxic oedema. Hydrocephalus may develop due to blockage of the routes of normal cerebrospinal fluid (CSF) flow. Finally, closed head injuries may lead to diffuse axonal injury. Diffuse axonal injury results in balls of axonal material occurring at axon transection sites or sites of altered axonal flow. Intracranial pressure monitoring is a concern; however, a recent trial does not support it as superior to other forms of neurological monitoring (Chesnut et al. 2012). Neurological damage due to TBI may grow after the injury because of impaired cerebral perfusion and other factors.

For mild head injuries, including skull fracture, concussion, and unspecified intracranial or head injury (Bazarian et al. 2005), the severity of the injury is usually measured by the degree of post-traumatic amnesia. More recently, concerns for chronic traumatic encephalopathy (CTE) due to repetitive mild head injuries have become a substantial concern as a cause of dementia and dysfunction years later, especially for those engaged in contact sports (Baugh et al. 2012; McKee et al. 2013). Head injury severity is usually classified by the Glasgow Coma Scale: scores of 13–15 are minor, 9–12 are moderate, 5–8 are severe, and 4 or less are very severe; and by length of coma (Jennett et al. 1976; Sherer et al. 2007).

Incidence and prevalence of traumatic brain injuries

The US Centers for Disease Control and Prevention (CDC) estimates that 1.57 million people (95 per cent CI 1.37–1.77 million) suffered a TBI in 2003 in the United States (538.2 per 100,000 population), approximately 51,000 of those resulted in death (TBI mortality 17.5 per 100,000 population) based on all reported emergency department visits, hospitalizations, and deaths. Cassidy et al. (2004) compiled a review of more than 160 published studies and found that approximately 70–90 per cent of all treated TBIs are likely to be mild which results in an expected rate for *treated* mild TBI of 100–300 per 100,000 population. Almost paradoxically, Rivara et al. found that among children with TBI the burden of disability caused by TBI was primarily due to mild TBI (Rivara et al. 2012). TBI incidence among children aged 0–4 was the highest of all age groups at 1188.5 per 100,000, while hospitalization and death rates were highest among those aged 65 and older. Falls accounted for 32 per cent of TBIs, motor vehicle traffic for 19 per cent, struck by/against events 18 per cent, and assaults 10 per cent. Men experienced about a 1.5 times greater rate of TBI than women. TBI hospitalization associated with assault was nearly six times higher for males than females across all age groups from 15 to 64. Sadly, females aged 0–4 years showed approximately twice the TBI hospitalization rate due to assault as any other female age group (Rutland-Brown et al. 2006).

Risk factors of traumatic brain injuries

Falls

Falls are perhaps the most common cause of TBI and incidence increases dramatically with advanced age. Californian 1996–1999 age-specific rates ranged from 13.6 per 100,000 in people aged less than 65 years, to 41.8 in those aged 65–74, to 104.0 in those aged 75–84, and then more than doubled to 223 per 100,000 among those aged 85 years or older (CDC 2003). Use of four or more medications may significantly increase risk of TBI from falling.

Falls are also an important cause of TBI among the very young. The 15-State CDC surveillance system allowed calculation of TBI hospitalization rates due to unintentional falls for children aged 0–11 months compared to those aged 12–23 months. Fall-related TBI hospitalizations were 71.5 per 100,000 person-years in the younger group as compared to 36.5 per 100,000 person years in the older group. Although TBI in toddlers and young children is due primarily to household or playground falls, motor vehicle accidents are the predominant cause in older children (Keenan and Bratton 2006).

Vehicle accidents

A report constructed by the US CDC based on TBIs which led to emergency department visit, hospitalization, or death in 2003, showed that overall, motor vehicle accidents (19 per cent) were second only to falls (32 per cent) as a cause of TBI based on a total overall estimate of TBI of between 1.37 million and 1.77 million events (Rutland-Brown et al. 2006). Injuries resulting from motor vehicle accidents, whether occurring to occupants or as pedestrian or cyclist versus motor vehicle, result in many of the more severe TBIs. Mandatory seat belt and child seat laws could have an effect on reducing occupant injuries, while bicycle and motorcycle helmet use may reduce the occurrence of TBI in those constituent categories.

Violence

Assaults are estimated to have accounted for approximately 10 per cent of the TBIs occurring in the United States in 2003 or roughly 160,000 TBIs (Rutland-Brown et al. 2006).

As much as 20 per cent of TBI may be the result of violence, roughly half of these are due to firearms. The age group at highest risk is 15–24 years. While males appear to be more likely to sustain an injury due to violence, women may be more likely to die as a result. The incidence of firearm-related injury or death was 42 per 100,000. The homicide rate varies dramatically by age and ethnic group. Overall it was about 14 per 100,000, but rose to 73 per 100,000 in African American males and further to 164.2 per 100,000 among 15–34-year-old African American males.

Abuse and domestic violence are important causes of TBI among women and among children (Monahan and O'Leary 1999; Valera and Berenbaum 2003; Banks 2007). Monahan estimates that about 35 per cent of the 2–3 million women battered each year by their domestic partner sustain TBI as a result. Keenan et al. (2003) found that physical abuse may be the most frequent cause of TBI in children aged less than 2 years with an estimated incidence rate of approximately 17 per 100,000 person years; infants had a higher incidence than older children and boys were at somewhat greater risk than girls.

Sports

Sports injuries account for a relatively small proportion of serious TBI. Between 2001 and 2005 approximately 208,000 emergency department visits each year in the United States were the result of sports and recreational activities (2007). The majority of these injuries occurred among children aged 10–14 years, closely followed by those aged 15–19 years. Hospital admission resulted in approximately 10 per cent of these incidents, but most such TBIs resolve spontaneously.

However chronic repetitive TBI can lead to CTE (McKee et al. 2013) resulting in long-term disability (Rivara et al. 2012).

War and sociopolitically directed violence

By the end of 2012 approximately two million US and UK men and women will have served in the wars in Iraq and Afghanistan resulting in thousands of deaths and tens of thousands of severe injuries. Injuries related to explosive blasts may account for many or most of these (Warden 2006) and effects of these types of injuries years later could have important individual and public health consequences for many years to come. Not only do blasts account for much of the observable and immediate injuries, but they may also lead to more mild or unreported TBI that can be coupled with post-traumatic stress disorder (PTSD) (Hoge et al. 2004; Holbrook et al. 2005; Okie, 2005). People who may have experienced TBI or blast-related TBI could ultimately be at higher risk for dementia as they enter ages 60–80.

Implications for public health

The potential years of productive life lost due to TBI varies with its cause, and causes are differentially age-related. The risk of seizures following TBI is increased up to 17-fold in patients with severe injuries (Annegers et al. 1998). While injuries related to motor vehicles and falls are the most common, those who are most severely affected, have the poorest outcomes, and require the most continuing care, tend to be the very young and the elderly. Sports injuries tend to be mild and resolving, but in the case of repetitive injury may result in serious sequelae years later. War-related TBIs could be the source of an unexpected public health burden because of the large numbers of soldiers serving and the high incidence of blast and other injuries coupled with the development of PTSD, psychiatric symptoms, cognitive deficits, and degenerative dementias or other neurological disorders.

Epilepsy

Clinical overview of epilepsy

The International League Against Epilepsy (ILAE) classification system is currently the most commonly used means of organizing epileptic syndromes (Box 8.10.2) (Engel 2006). Characteristics of individual seizures are divided into location-related seizures (formerly named partial or local seizures) that begin in a localized part of the brain, and generalized epilepsies that begin diffusely in the brain. The areas of brain initially involved determine the symptoms of location-related seizures. Location-related seizures may (simple partial) or may not (complex partial seizures) be associated with altered consciousness. They may secondarily generalize after a focal onset.

Generalized seizures (formerly *grand mal*) begin in widespread areas of the brain. The most common type of generalized seizure is noted for muscle stiffening followed by jerking (tonic–clonic). Absence seizures (formerly *petit mal*) consist of brief episodes of staring and lack of responsiveness. Myoclonic seizures involve brief jerks of muscles rather than repetitive clonic movements. Tonic seizures have generalized muscle stiffening. Atonic seizures involve sudden loss of muscle tone. The ILAE classification has limitations for epidemiology use because of its emphasis on syndromes and absence of aetiological factors including genetics (Camfield 2012).

Box 8.10.2 The International League Against Epilepsy classification of epileptic seizures

I. Partial (focal, local) seizures

A. Simple partial seizures
B. Complex partial seizure (with impairment of consciousness)
C. With impairment of consciousness at onset
D. Partial seizures evolving to secondarily generalized seizures

II. Generalized seizures

A. Absence seizures
B. Myoclonic seizures
C. Clonic seizures
D. Tonic seizures
E. Tonic–clonic seizures
F. Atonic seizures

III. Unclassified epileptic seizures

Adapted from Engel J, Jr., Report of the ILAE classification core group, *Epilepsia*, Volume 47, Issue 9, pp. 1558–68, Copyright © 2006, with permission from John Wiley and Sons Ltd.

Incidence and prevalence of epilepsy

Aspects of epilepsy epidemiology have been reviewed (Thurman et al. 2011). Epidemiological studies of epilepsy are challenged by the difficulty in making a correct diagnosis and the sophisticated technology required for proper diagnosis and classification. A substantial number of patients diagnosed with epilepsy do not have seizures on careful testing (Uldall et al. 2006). There is also difficulty with standardizing case ascertainment with markedly different prevalence rates using different definitions of epilepsy (Svendsen et al. 2007).

In a meta-analysis the overall incidence of epilepsy was 50.4/100,000, with 81.7 in low/median-income populations and 45.0 in high-income populations (Ngugi et al. 2011). Population-based and prospective studies had higher incidence rates than clinic-based and retrospective studies. Incidence is higher in children but both incidence and prevalence decrease with calendar time among children and increase among the elderly (Hauser et al. 1996; Hirtz et al. 2007). Others found an increased incidence in men, older people, black people, and those with pre-existing disability or co-morbid conditions (Kaiboriboon et al. 2013). A study of children in the United Kingdom found a cumulative incidence of epilepsy by age 5 to be 1 per cent in those born between 1994 and 1996 and 0.53 per cent in those born between 2003 and 2005 (Meeraus et al. 2013). The annual incidence declined by 4 per cent/year from 2001 to 2008. However, a longitudinal study from Rochester, Minnesota, United States, found a slightly higher estimate of epilepsy incidence over time (Zarrelli et al. 1999).

The prevalence of epilepsy is estimated to be 7.1/1000 (Hirtz et al. 2007). However, prevalence varies in different regions. In an African population, a greater than twofold variability was found in prevalence across regions (Ngugi et al. 2013). Younger patients more commonly had seizures attributable to trauma and older patients to infectious causes. There were similar findings between

regions of Taiwan (Chen et al. 2012). In general, poor countries have more than twice the burden of epilepsy compared to higher-income regions with much of the difference explained by preventable infections, perinatal care, and trauma (Newton and Garcia 2012). Differences in study methodology, survey methods, case definition, the availability of sophisticated medical technology in a community, and cultural differences make epilepsy prevalence studies particularly challenging.

Mortality of epilepsy

People with epilepsy may experience two to three times the risk of death as their unaffected counterparts (Sperling et al. 1999). The standardized mortality ratio for people with recurrent seizures was approximately fourfold higher than expected. A longitudinal study found a threefold excess in all-cause mortality, and a sevenfold increase among those under age 20 (Shackleton et al. 1999). Some of the risk of death in epilepsy reflects underlying diseases like brain neoplasms and cerebrovascular disease. However, there is also an increased mortality compared to the non-epileptic population due to accidents (often drowning and burns) and suicide (Lhatoo and Sander 2005). Sudden unexplained death in people with epilepsy (SUDEP) is increasingly recognized as an important cause of death in epilepsy. This increases with the duration and severity of epilepsy (Devinsky 2011). It is more common in adults. The incidence of SUDEP varies from 0.09–2.65 in community samples, 1.2–5.9 in epilepsy centres, and 6.0–9.3 among patients referred for surgery for epilepsy. In a population-based cohort of children with epilepsy who were followed for 40 years, SUDEP occurred in 9 per cent, accounting for 38 per cent of all deaths.

Infectious causes of epilepsy

In developing countries, infections are a much more important cause of epilepsy than in the United States and Europe. Parasitic, bacterial, and viral infections combine with hereditary factors, perinatal damage, head trauma, and toxic exposures to contribute to high rates of epilepsy in these countries (Newton and Garcia 2012). An example of an important infectious risk factor is *Taenia solium* cysticercosis (pork tapeworm) which causes neurocysticercosis. This is a major cause of epilepsy worldwide (Del Brutto 2012). Other infectious causes of epilepsy are various febrile illnesses, particularly encephalitis, and malaria.

Genetics of epilepsy

Genetics are increasingly recognized as a contributor to epilepsy risk. Over 200 genes are now associated with epilepsy and include monogenic, complex, mitochondrial, chromosomal, and imprinting. Screening methods have been proposed for evaluating patients with epilepsy (Lemke et al. 2012). Epigenetic factors may also influence circuit excitability and neurogenesis in epilepsy (Roopra et al. 2012). Many types of epilepsy are now recognized as genetic disorders. However, these are rare forms of epilepsy and the genetic contribution to the majority of cases remains unexplained. First-degree relatives of people with epilepsy have a two- to fourfold increase in epilepsy risk (Annegers et al. 1982). A number of epilepsies have now been shown to be due to channelopathies, mutations in ion channels (Avanzini et al. 2007). It is expected that many more genes associated with epilepsy will be identified.

Costs and public health burden of epilepsy

Only 42 per cent of those over age 18 with epilepsy are employed compared to 70 per cent of those without epilepsy (Libby et al. 2012). People with epilepsy have higher work absences. Holding other variables constant, people with epilepsy had a loss of productivity of $9504 compared to people without epilepsy. Indirect costs may account for 85 per cent of the total, and the largest share of direct costs is attributable to patients with intractable epilepsy (Begley et al. 2000). Seizure frequency is inversely associated with health-related quality of life (Leidy et al. 1999). Seizure-free individuals report a quality of life similar to the general population; however, more seizures lead to a poorer quality of life, regardless of additional co-morbidity, and irrespective of gender. Effective seizure control appears to be important in reducing costs as well as increasing patient quality of life.

Dementia

Clinical overview of dementia

Dementia presents with a progressive loss of a person's usual and customary cognitive function from any of several domains. This often begins with memory problems in Alzheimer's disease (AD) but could also begin with language deficits or disinhibition in frontotemporal lobar degeneration (FTLD), or with deficits in executive function in vascular cognitive impairment, or with sleep disorders or hallucinations in Lewy body disease. Regardless of the beginning domain, cognitive impairment associated with most dementia tends to progress and affect other cognitive domains with time. Dementia often includes behavioural changes, such as agitation, wandering, personality change, or depression, as well as sleep disturbances and psychiatric symptoms. As knowledge of specific subtypes of dementia has grown, the research community has come to rely more on specific clinical criteria for those subtypes. While the DSM (American Psychiatric Association 1994) criteria were originally constructed to provide for mutually exclusive diagnostic subgroups, it is now widely acknowledged that more than one underlying 'brain disease' may coexist and lead to the expression of dementia.

Dementia has many causes including neurodegenerative, vascular, infectious and traumatic. Among the neurodegenerative dementias that predominate with ageing are AD, Lewy body disease (aka dementia with Lewy bodies (DLB) or PD dementia) and FTLD dementias. Cerebrovascular disease may coexist with and contribute to any of these or may be a primary cause on its own as vascular dementia (VaD). Prion disease, and associated spongiform encephalopathies (e.g. Creutzfeldt–Jakob disease (CJD) and variant CJD) are rare, but potentially transmissible from ingestion of animal tissue or from contact or transplantation of human tissue. Other disorders and insults which can result in dementia include drug-induced conditions, alcoholism, Huntington's disease, subdural hematoma, brain tumours, hydrocephalus, vitamin B_{12} deficiency, multiple medical conditions, hypothyroidism, and neurosyphilis.

Criteria for the clinical diagnosis of AD dementia (McKhann et al. 2011), mild cognitive impairment due to AD (Albert et al. 2011), and preclinical AD (Sperling et al. 2011) emphasize the addition of biomarkers to characterize the underlying disease pathology. Amyloid imaging and CSF assays for amyloid-beta protein, tau, and phospho-tau proteins are of greatest importance in preclinical AD because no cognitive symptoms are present. Neuropathological criteria formerly were the clinical-pathological NIA-Reagan consensus criteria (1997) ranking the likelihood that pathological features (amyloid plaques and neurofibrillary tangles) existed in sufficient frequency to have caused the clinically observable dementia. New neuropathological criteria (Hyman et al. 2012) form a diagnosis based only on pathological features present, regardless of clinical dementia. The research community thus has taken a major step to define AD by pathology that is present (in both clinical and neuropathological criteria) and has recognized formally that asymptomatic AD occurs. This opens the door to conceptualization of secondary prevention.

Mild cognitive impairment

Clinically observable cognitive decline, not yet at the level meeting criteria for dementia, has been called mild cognitive impairment (MCI) (Petersen 2004). As a prodrome to dementia or simply an impaired state, it may have many underlying causes; MCI itself is not an aetiological diagnosis, but a characterization of affected cognition. The portion of MCI which is due to AD has now been provided with formal clinical criteria and biomarker indications (Albert et al. 2011). Recognition that the disease process in AD may have been underway for as many as 10–25 years and is potentially detectable by CSF biomarkers and/or amyloid imaging (Sperling et al. 2011; Bateman et al. 2012) changes the way epidemiologists should look at risk factor studies and the timing of exposures sufficient to cause disease onset. Pathological onset also explains in part why potential treatments given to mild or moderately impaired subjects would have little chance of success. What would a rehabilitative treatment for dementia due to AD potentially look like? Possibly in addition to slowing or stopping the formation of pathology, it would need to facilitate neuronal regeneration, branching, and connections, if recovery might happen.

Tracking and describing prognostic factors associated with cognitive decline has been the subject of many investigations. However, in the case of AD and probably other underlying causes, the timing and course of decline may be more likely to be tied to the frequency and location of damage due to pathology than it might be to education, for example. Determining and describing potentially modifiable factors which might change the course of decline in those with symptomatic disease, is one of the major challenges of AD and other dementias. The original criteria for MCI (Petersen 2007) allowed MCI to represent a variety of aetiologies in addition to AD. On the non-amnestic side, it could easily include vascular cognitive impairment as well as cognitive impairment due to FTLD or Lewy body disease. However, the amnestic side of MCI is regarded by many to represent primarily early AD (Morris et al. 2001; Morris and Cummings 2005; Morris 2006). People diagnosed with MCI also are known to recover and not go on to develop dementia. The potential progression of cognitive decline is described well by Sperling et al. (2011) as a continuum, rather than reclassification into separate categories of dementia or MCI.

Dementia and Alzheimer's disease

Prevalence and incidence of dementia and AD

Almost two decades ago, Evans and colleagues reported prevalence estimates for dementia and AD based on a community study in East Boston, Massachusetts, United States (Evans et al. 1989), placing an heuristic upper bound on estimated prevalence of dementia in United States' communities: rising from 3 per cent among those 65–74 years of age to 47 per cent in those over age 85, with over 80 per cent of the observed dementia classified as AD. Evans later projected that 10.3 million people would have AD in the year 2050. A recent meta-analysis of prevalence studies worldwide (Prince et al. 2013) shows remarkably similar age-specific prevalence and age-adjusted summary prevalence across all regions of the world, with the lowest prevalence being in sub-Saharan Africa and possibly the highest in Latin America and the Caribbean. A total of 35.6 million people worldwide were estimated to be demented in 2010; 15.94 million of those in Asia. By 2050, it is estimated that 115.38 million people will be living with dementia. An estimated $420 billion was spent on dementia care in the United States and Western Europe in 2010; worldwide $604 billion were spent (Wimo et al. 2013). An incidence rate meta-analysis (Jorm and Jolley 1998) gathered data from 23 studies. Incidence was estimated for Europe, the United States, and East Asia; dementia, AD, and VaD rates were computed. Incidence rates for clinically diagnosed dementia rose from 3.6 per 1000 person-years (aged 65–69) to 37.7 per 1000 person-years (aged 85–89) in Europe and from 2.4 to 27.5 per 1000 person years for the same age groups in the United States.

Similarly Rocca et al. (1998) re-analysed dementia and AD incidence data for 1975 through 1984 and observed that annual age-specific incidence rates have appeared to stay quite stable with time during that interval. Launer et al. (1999), combining cohorts enrolled in Denmark, France, the Netherlands, and the United Kingdom, determined that the incidence of dementia rose from 2.5 per 1000 person-years at age 65–69 to 85.6 per 1000 person-years in those aged 90 and older; while AD rose from 1.2 per 1000 person-years to 63.5 per 1000 person-years across the same age groups.

Suppose that the incidence of AD were estimated by the development of positive biomarkers including asymptomatic people. How would such a change shift the age distribution and the incidence rates?

While the tendency has been to attempt to count primary cause or pathologically 'pure' cases, dementia causing aetiologies (e.g. Alzheimer, vascular, Lewy body, FTLD) appear to commingle frequently in community dwelling cases. This commingling is consistent with the view that these diseases may exist as multiple amyloidoses resulting from aggregation of misfolded proteins (Morimoto, 2006).

Distinguishing between normal people, those with MCI and those asymptomatic people with occult dementia-related pathology, is now possible to some degree as noted in Sperling et al. (2011) based on newly developed neuroimaging techniques (Klunk et al. 2003; Mathis et al. 2003; Small 2004) and CSF biomarkers. These 'biomarkers' may provide important clues about pathological onset of disease as well as inform the study of risk factors and critical periods of exposure prior to disease onset (Mintun et al. 2006; Bacskai et al. 2007; Fagan et al. 2007; Rowe et al. 2007).

Risk (and protective) factors for AD

The attempt to identify environmental risk factors for AD has been disappointing and conflicting, for methodological as well as biological reasons. Because the pathological disease may begin from 10–25 years prior to any symptoms, the time window for exposures which could be relevant for onset is shifted even further back in time. Few observational studies were able to place any exposures except for genetic factors in this time range. Thus case–control studies were likely to be methodologically compromised by diagnostic misclassification, as well as ill-timed or missing exposure data. Cohort study designs fare only slightly better because the initial cohort would include asymptomatic people; for example, the base cohort would not effectively exclude prevalent disease, causing diagnostic misclassification. Thus, the risk or protective factors reported by epidemiological case–control or cohort studies to date must be viewed with considerable caution; the notable exception is the genetic risk factor, apolipoprotein E (APOE) e4 allele. APOE may exert independent effects or it may modify or confound the effect of environmental risk factors (Anonymous 1998; Launer et al. 1999; Mehta et al. 1999).

Higher educational level has been proposed as decreasing risk of AD, but the relationship is complex (e.g. Hendrie 1998; Geerlings et al. 1999; Koepsell et al. 2007). The idea that higher education confers greater 'cognitive reserve' to be accessed when disease strikes is tantalizing, though biologically unsubstantiated. Koepsell et al. in a clinico-pathological study found that there was 'no evidence of larger education-related differences in cognitive function when Alzheimer disease (AD) neuropathology was more advanced', concluding further that 'Higher Mini-Mental State Examination scores among more educated people with mild or no AD may reflect better test-taking skills or cognitive reserve, but these advantages may ultimately be overwhelmed by AD neuropathology' (Koepsell et al. 2007). Quality of early life environment, as measured by number of siblings and area of residence, was associated with developing AD in late life, but educational level was not significantly associated with risk of AD (Moceri et al. 2000).

Anti-inflammatory medications have been studied for their potential protective effect on AD (Breitner 1996; In t'Veld et al. 2001; Szekely et al. 2007). The Alzheimer's disease anti-inflammatory prevention trial (ADAPT) was launched in 2001. The trial enrolled 2625 subjects, aged 70 years or older, and randomized them to placebo, celecoxib, or naproxen sodium treatment arms. The trial itself was stopped early because of an excess of cardiovascular events in the treatment arms. A preliminary analysis based on data available following trial closure showed no significant effect of either celecoxib or naproxen as compared to placebo for the prevention of AD.

Oestrogen replacement therapy as a protective factor has shown a remarkably similar chequered research results history as anti-inflammatory medications, with the bulk of epidemiological evidence favouring protection and a fair amount of biological plausibility also marshalled in its support. Despite this large accumulation of epidemiological and laboratory evidence supporting the potential protective effect of oestrogen against the onset of AD, the Women's Health Initiative Memory Study (a randomized controlled trial of oestrogen and oestrogen plus progestin vs. placebo) showed a statistically significant *increased* risk of dementia among those given the active treatments (Shumaker et al. 2003, 2004). As a potential treatment for AD dementia, results also have shown no effect on AD (Henderson et al. 2000; Mulnard et al. 2000).

Factors related to cardiovascular disease and metabolic syndrome (including diabetes) may have an influence on AD and other dementias even though the exact mechanisms of interaction may not yet have been elucidated (Launer et al. 2000; Yaffe et al. 2004; Kivipelto and Solomon 2006; Laitinen et al. 2006; Li et al. 2007; Muller et al. 2007). The rationale for this approach appears to be that it is sound medical practice to treat hypertension, high cholesterol, diabetes, and obesity, and if more complete and effective treatment can be accomplished it may also, secondarily, serve to reduce the occurrence of dementia through vascular or other pathways which may or may not directly impact AD pathology.

Genetics and AD

Great progress was made regarding the genetics of AD during the late 1980s and 1990s with the discovery of presenilin-1 and -2 and amyloid precursor protein mutations as familial, autosomal dominant causes and the APOE e4 allele as a 'risk factor'. Several reviews of AD genetics describing this period of growth in greater detail include: Hardy et al. (1998), Levy-Lahad et al. (1998), St George-Hyslop (2000), and Haass (2004).

The strongest and most consistent genetic risk factor for late onset, non-autosomal dominant AD today is the APOE genotype. The association was first described from Dr Allen Roses' laboratory (Corder et al. 1993; Saunders et al. 1993; Strittmatter et al. 1993). APOE naturally occurs as three different alleles (epsilon 2, epsilon 3, and epsilon 4) which pair to form one of six genotypes for each individual. Genotypes containing the epsilon 4 allele are associated with increased risk of AD; homozygous epsilon 4 greatly increases risk (e.g. greater than eightfold). Since the initial description of increased risk associated with the epsilon 4 allele, many investigators have observed the association. Discussion of APOE genotype is now included in nearly all genetic and risk factor studies of AD, either as a focus or as a potential confounder/effect modifier of an association. Despite the huge volume of studies including the APOE genotype, relatively little is known concerning how the e2, e3, and e4 alleles actually work to influence the risk of AD.

There have been a number of GWAS of AD, using large numbers of subjects (e.g. Hollingworth et al. 2011; Naj et al. 2011), which have identified and replicated a range of new common variants. Recently two important studies have shown an increased AD risk due to TREM2 (Guerreiro et al. 2013) and in African Americans an increased risk associated with ABCA7 (Reitz et al. 2013). Because these and other current GWAS have included strong replication they are regarded as superior to most candidate gene studies that occurred between the mid 1990s and 2010. More such studies have been performed; in addition, data sharing has allowed other investigators to examine associations between these identified loci and clinical characteristics (endophenotypes) such as cognitive decline.

Vascular dementia

VaD is difficult to describe clinically and neuropathologically. The search for 'pure' cases of VaD and AD may have obstructed progress of understanding how these diseases act and interact. Vascular features commonly coexist with AD in the elderly: newer sophisticated imaging and other measures, as well as neuropathology, bear this out (Au et al. 2006). Several different criteria have been developed to diagnose VaD (Chui et al. 1992; Roman et al. 1993; American Psychiatric Association 1994). Much of the pioneering work in the clinical definition and recognition of VaD can be attributed to Hachinski and colleagues. The Hachinski

Ischaemic Score continues to be used to indicate the extent of cerebrovascular involvement in cognitive decline (Hachinski 1994).

Pathologically, VaD is an enigma, because of the lack of clear definitions for white matter damage, infarcts, and lesion location in strategic areas of the brain—VaD, in effect, lacks a pathological gold standard against which to compare the clinical diagnosis or clinical criteria and measure their effectiveness (Murray et al. 2007). Thus, the clinical diagnostic criteria have been shown to be difficult and potentially unreliable in practice, even when applied by well-experienced research investigators (Chui et al. 2000).

Lewy body disease and frontotemporal lobar degeneration

Two additional types of dementia, Lewy body disease (McKeith 2006) and FTLD (Cairns et al. 2007a), have been separated from AD based on their clinical presentations but more specifically on their pathology. Lewy body disease or DLB may be diagnosable in up to 30 per cent of dementia cases. PD is also a 'Lewy body' disease and if Parkinson's cases survive long enough they will become demented as a result (Zaccai et al. 2005; Tsuang et al. 2006). Lewy body disease or DLB often presents with fluctuating cognitive performance, visual hallucinations, REM sleep behaviour disorder, and/or parkinsonism. Memory impairment may not be as prominent in the early stages of the disease as deficits in attention, frontal subcortical skills, and visuospatial ability (Knopman et al. 2001; Korczyn and Reichmann 2006).

FTLD has undergone a revolution in classification since initial work on progranulin (Gass et al. 2006; Rademakers et al. 2007) followed by the careful study of the involvement of TDP-43 (Neumann et al. 2006; Van Deerlin et al. 2010) and the discovery of association with C9ORF72 (DeJesus-Hernandez et al. 2011) includes specific disease subtypes and may be the most frequently occurring dementia in people under the age of 65 (Mackenzie and Rademakers 2007). Behavioural variant frontotemporal dementia (bvFTD) represents a behavioural subtype with changes such as loss of personal awareness, loss of social graces, disinhibition, overactivity, restlessness, impulsivity, distractibility, hyperorality, withdrawal from social contact, apathy or inertia, and stereotyped or perseverative behaviours. The memory loss is variable and often appears to be due to lack of concern or effort. Frontal lobe impairments are notable including abstraction, planning, and self-regulation of behaviour. FTLD may also be associated with parkinsonism or motor neuron disease. Pathologically, approximately 40 per cent of FTLDs are related to mutations in the microtubule-associated protein tau (MAPT) gene on chromosome 17 and are therefore 'tauopathies'; these include Pick's disease, corticobasal degeneration, and progressive supranuclear palsy (Rademakers and Hutton 2007; Tolnay and Frank 2007). About 50 per cent of FTLDs are not tauopathies but are reactive to ubiquitin (FTLD-U) rather than mutations in MAPT (Mackenzie and Rademakers 2007). Recently, it was discovered that mutations in the progranulin gene, also on chromosome 17, were an important cause of FTLD-U disorders (Baker et al. 2006; Cruts et al. 2006; Gass et al. 2006) including primary progressive aphasia (Mesulam et al. 2007). The pathological protein involved in these disorders as well as in motor neuron disease is TDP-43 (Mackenzie et al. 2006; Neumann et al. 2006; Cairns et al. 2007b; Kwong et al. 2007). These are arguably the most exciting and important findings for dementia and FTLD in recent times. FTLD is rare compared to AD and even so is thought to be frequently misdiagnosed as a psychiatric disorder because of its early onset and unusual clinical symptoms.

Peripheral neuropathy

Clinical overview of peripheral neuropathy

Though 'peripheral neuropathy' may refer to any disease of peripheral nerves, it usually describes systemic diseases that affect peripheral nerves rather than focal diseases affecting an isolated nerve. Most of these diseases affect longer nerves first with symptoms developing first in the feet and progressing up the legs. Few peripheral neuropathies affect shorter proximal nerves first. By the time symptoms reach the knees, the hands become symptomatic followed by the anterior trunk and crown of the head. Symptoms depend on the type of nerve fibre involved. Involvement of motor fibres leads to weakness, muscle wasting, and hyporeflexia. If longstanding, motor neuropathies may lead to high arches (pes cavus) or hammer toes. Sensory nerve involvement leads to loss of sensation, distorted sensation (dysaesthesias), or spontaneous unpleasant sensations (paraesthesias). Autonomic neuropathies lead to postural hypotension, sexual dysfunction, bowel dysfunction, bladder dysfunction, and gastroparesis. The size of the affected nerve fibre can often be suggested by the history with large fibre disease causing reflex loss, vibration loss, and joint position loss. Small fibre disease often leads to autonomic dysfunction, dysaesthesias, loss of pain sensation, and loss of temperature sensation.

Electrodiagnostic testing is used to diagnose and classify peripheral neuropathies. Nerve conduction velocities can classify peripheral neuropathies into demyelinating and axonal types. Demyelinating neuropathies have disproportionate slowing and increased latencies of nerve conduction speeds. Axonal diseases cause disproportional loss of amplitude with relative preservation of conduction speed. Nerve conduction studies measure only the fast-conducting large diameter fibres. Electromyography (EMG) measures the electrical activity of muscle fibres. A loss of muscle fibre innervation by large myelinated neurons leads to increased insertional activity, positive waves, fibrillation potentials, polyphasic motor unit potentials, and decreased recruitment patterns on EMG. Occasionally, nerve or muscle biopsies are used for diagnosis of polyneuropathies.

Generally, polyneuropathies involve many peripheral nerves and result in autonomic neuropathies, sensory loss, or weakness. Mononeuropathies, as the name implies, involve a single nerve injury or entrapment, for example, carpal tunnel syndrome (CTS) or Bell's palsy. Peripheral nerve disorders are often classified as hereditary or acquired. Charcot–Marie–Tooth syndrome is a well-known hereditary form. Acquired nerve disorders are associated with trauma/compression, diabetes, alcoholism, and other nutritional and metabolic problems. They may also be related to infectious causes such as Guillian–Barré syndrome, leprosy, Lyme disease, or HIV infection; or they may be caused by toxic exposures to metals (e.g. lead, mercury), industrial chemicals, or therapeutic drugs (e.g. antineoplastic agents) (Rowland and Merritt 1995). Little is known about the epidemiology of peripheral neuropathies, though they are common. The few studies that have been conducted find prevalence rates ranging from 2.4 to 8 per cent (Martyn and Hughes 1997). Prevalence increases considerably with age to 54 per cent of those aged 85 and older (Mold et al. 2004).

Carpal tunnel syndrome

CTS is probably the most common neuropathy. Carpal tunnel release surgery is one of the most common hand surgeries. Occupational CTS from repetitive, higher-impact actions differs from non-occupational CTS by occurring nearly equally among men and women and at a lower mean age (37 vs 51 years) than non-occupational CTS (Franklin et al. 1991). Based on US workmen's compensation records, an incidence of 1.74/1000 full-time equivalent jobs was observed.

In contrast to the occupational incidence, the general population CTS incidence was 3.46/1000 person-years (Nordstrom et al. 1998). The apparent increase in incidence may reflect a true change or may be affected by popular knowledge of the condition and diagnostic suspicion. Prevalence of symptoms in relation to true disease prevalence is also a consideration (Atroshi et al. 1999). Reported CTS symptoms of tingling, pain, and numbness have a prevalence of about 14 per cent, whereas CTS was confirmed in less than 3 per cent.

CTS patients with inflammatory arthritis, diabetes, and hypothyroidism were more likely to receive CTS release surgery (Solomon et al. 1999). Heredity is the single strongest predictor of CTS with half of the risk of CTS due to genetic factors (Hakim et al. 2002). Using MZ and DZ twins, the heritability was estimated to be 0.46 (95 per cent CI 0.34–0.58). There is a bimodal age distribution with peaks at 50–54 and 75–84 years of age (Bland and Rudolfer 2003). In a case–control study, elevated body mass index was more common among cases than among control subjects (Stallings et al. 1997).

Diabetes mellitus

Diabetes is a common, yet complex cause of both mono- and polyneuropathies. Diabetic peripheral neuropathy may affect 26–47 per cent of those with diabetes (Barrett et al. 2007) though others have found lower rates of 7.8–17.4 per cent (Dyck et al. 2012). More effective glucose control could reduce the risk to some extent. The cost of diabetic peripheral neuropathy, particularly in those with pain, can be substantial (Currie et al. 1998; Barrett et al. 2007).

Microvascular disease, chronic hyperglycaemia, and type of diabetes are the most important predictors of polyneuropathy (Dyck et al. 1999). Autonomic neuropathy is strongly influenced by hyperglycaemia and is associated with increased mortality (Orchard et al. 1996). Elevated diastolic blood pressure, ketoacidosis, elevated fasting triglyceride level, and microalbuminuria are also risk factors for diabetic polyneuropathy (Tesfaye et al. 1996).

Nutritional neuropathies

Vitamin B_{12} deficiency is the most common of a number of nutritional deficiencies that can lead to peripheral neuropathy. A Cuban epidemic of peripheral neuropathy from 1992 to 1993 affected over 50,000 people with an incidence of 461 per 100,000 people (Roman 1994). Optic and peripheral forms of the disease were observed. A nutritional deficiency is suspected and treatment with multivitamins, in particular B vitamins, stopped the outbreak.

Peripheral neuropathy due to infection

HIV infection is an important cause of peripheral neuropathies including diffuse peripheral neuropathy, Guillain–Barré syndrome, mononeuropathies, neuropathies due to secondary infections, and neuropathies due to medications (Brew 2003). The incidence and prevalence vary too much between studies to allow accurate estimates.

Guillain–Barré syndrome is due to an autoimmune attack on the peripheral nerve myelin. Previously considered an idiopathic disease, it is now recognized that a significant proportion of cases are associated with prior infections (Hardy et al. 2011). Though the prevalence of leprosy is declining, it remains one of the most important causes of peripheral neuropathy in the developing world (Suzuki et al. 2012). Fortunately, early treatment can prevent many of the disabling and disfiguring effects of the disease.

Parkinsonism and Parkinson's disease

The Parkinson's research community is somewhat fragmented with regard to how idiopathic PD should be described and characterized: a) should full clinical symptomatology (e.g. cardinal signs) be required; b) should evidence of PD pathophysiology (e.g. Lewy body pathology) be sufficient to say PD exists; c) should PD be viewed as a systemic neurodegenerative disorder in contrast to focus on movement disorder (Langston 2006; Litvan et al. 2007)? The argument for expanding the view of PD continues that limiting the clinical and pathological view of the disease itself limits the potential for research progress (Langston 2006).

Clinical overview of PD

There are four cardinal features of clinical PD: tremor, rigidity, bradykinesia, and postural gait changes. The clinical diagnosis of PD usually requires two or more of these symptoms. In severe cases, patients may be unable to move (freezing) when they encounter minor obstacles such as doorways or cracks. While movement disorder specialists make the diagnosis of parkinsonism with some degree of confidence, PD usually requires histopathological confirmation. In an attempt to increase the accuracy and validity of clinical diagnosis, improvements in clinical diagnostic criteria have been proposed (Gelb et al. 1999; Jankovic et al. 2000).

Parkinsonism includes several major subclasses: idiopathic parkinsonism (PD), symptomatic parkinsonism (e.g. drug induced, toxin induced, and other specific causes), 'parkinson-plus' syndromes (e.g. multiple system atrophy (MSA), progressive supranuclear palsy), and hereditary degenerative diseases (e.g. Hallervorden–Spatz disease, Huntington disease). PD or idiopathic parkinsonism comprises approximately 80 per cent of parkinsonism.

MSA is sometimes misdiagnosed as PD; it is a relatively rare and very debilitating condition usually involving progressive autonomic failure plus poor responsiveness to levodopa or cerebellar ataxia. There is new evidence that MSA like PD and DLB is a synucleinopathy (Goedert and Spillantini 1998; Dickson et al. 1999; Armstrong et al. 2006).

Incidence and prevalence of PD

PD prevalence has been reported with dramatic inconsistency; typically prevalence has been reported in the range of about 50 per 100,000 to 200 per 100,000 of the population, with a maximum of about 350 per 100,000 people. Combined results of five European studies (de Rijk et al. 1997) included 14,636 people age 65 or older; after age adjusting to the European 1991 standard population the prevalence of PD was reported as 1.6 per 100 population (presumably age 65 or older), this translates to about 1600 per 100,000. In addition, the age-specific prevalence of PD was reported to increase from 0.6 per cent in 65–69-year-olds to 3.5 per cent in 85–89-year-olds (or 600 per 100,000 to 3500 per 100,000) (de Rijk et al. 1997).

Incidence rates for PD and parkinsonism carry many of the same caveats as for prevalence. Bower et al. (1999) studied the incidence of parkinsonism and PD in Rochester, Minnesota, United States, 1976–1990. The age-specific incidence for the 50–59 age group was 17.4 per 100,000 person-years, rising to 52.5 for ages 60–69 and peaking at 93.1 for the 70–79 age group and 79.1 for 80–99-year-olds. Parkinsonism showed an overall incidence rate of 25.6 per 100,000 person-years and rose from 26.5 at ages 50–59 to 304.8 per 100,000 person-years in those aged 80–99 (Bower et al. 1999). Age-specific incidence rates are, of course, able to be compared directly whereas summary population rates may be dependent on age structure of the population. How ageing contributes to the clinical expression or degenerative processes of PD, as well as how ageing may act with genetic and environmental risk factors, to initiate pathophysiology or onset of clinical symptoms remain key questions for the epidemiology of parkinsonism and PD.

Risk factors of PD

Researcher hopes to identify consistent environmental causes of PD were increased by the observation that 1-methyl-4-phenyl-1, 2,3,6-tetrahydropyridine (MPTP) caused acute PD shortly after ingestion (Langston and Ballard 1983; Langston et al. 1983). The structure of MPTP and its metabolism products are somewhat similar to common pesticides raising interest in such exposures as risk factors or causes of PD. The past predominance of environmental causes has at least partially given way to studies of genetic and pathophysiological aetiologies (Litvan et al. 2007; Do et al. 2011).

An excellent review of pesticide/herbicide exposure as risk factors for PD was recently published by Tanner et al. (2011). Determination of critical exposure time periods and duration of exposures is always an obstacle to overcome when studying PD risk factors because the initiation of pathophysiology may occur many years prior to any symptoms of the diagnosis of PD. Further, the time from exposure to onset of pathophysiology or clinical disease may vary dramatically. Consider the rather immediate onset of clinical symptoms following MPTP exposure compared with what may be the case with agricultural pesticides (Gorell et al. 1998; Petrovitch et al. 2002; Firestone et al. 2005). Interest in pesticide exposure as a potential cause led to a biotransformation gene approach for evaluating the occurrence of susceptible people. Specifically, some people may be more, or less, able to metabolize environmental toxins because of polymorphic genes involved in metabolism. One of the family of cytochrome P-450 biotransformation genes, $CYP2D6$, is involved in metabolism of debrisoquine (structurally similar to pesticides); some polymorphic forms are 'poor' metabolizers and others are normal or rapid metabolizers of debrisoquine. Initial studies appeared to show that poor metabolizers were at increased risk of PD but later studies and meta-analyses fail to support this conclusion

(Maraganore et al. 2000; Scordo et al. 2006). A similar approach has been taken to identify susceptibles focusing on polymorphic forms of glutathione transferases (GST) which are involved in the metabolism of pesticides and other xenobiotics (Menegon et al. 1998). Continued effort to identify gene–environment interaction in this way may eventually prove fruitful, but success is rather limited to date.

An association between exposure to metals and PD has been described by Gorell et al. (1999). And more recently an association with welding has been reported by Racette et al. (2012). Heavy metals such as iron, copper, manganese, and lead have been raised as potential risk factors in the past and Racette et al. may provide some measure of replication to those findings.

Smoking has been rather consistently associated with decreased risk of PD in reported reviews and in individual studies. Reasons for the plausibility of such an association revolve around the potential action of nicotine on neurons. Although this is one of the more consistent findings, it is not completely without alternative explanations. Most epidemiological studies of PD use 'prevalent' or existing cases in their studies. The low incidence of PD effectively precludes concentrating on only newly diagnosed cases in all but the largest of studies (or in very large cohort studies). When attempting to identify a cross-sectional sample of cases for enrolment into a case–control study, it can be shown that those patients who have had the disease the longest are the most likely to be included. The most severe, short-duration or rapidly declining cases tend to be missed. If PD cases who had a history of smoking were much more likely to die sooner than 'controls' who were smokers, then smoking would appear to be protective because of the excess of smoking 'controls'. Despite such an argument, however, the PD research community appears to be relatively confident in the potential protective effect of smoking (Ritz et al. 2007).

Dietary-related factors have been shown in some studies to affect risk of PD: fish and vegetables (Gao et al. 2007), coffee and caffeine (Ross et al. 2000), dietary folate, and vitamin B_{12} among others (de Lau et al. 2006). Body mass index has been reported to increase the risk of PD (Hu et al. 2006), while gout and hyperuricaemia has been reported to protect against it (de Lau et al. 2005; Alonso et al. 2007).

As recently as two decades ago it was commonly taught that PD was caused entirely by environmental factors. Now with the explosion of genetic knowledge and technology and an understanding of some of the proteins potentially involved in pathogenesis, Hardy states that nearly half of the disease risk has been explained by genes so far discovered (Hardy 2010). Do et al. (2011) discuss the recent GWAS and genes involved in PD risk. Glucocerebrocidase has been found to be deficient in PD brains and similarly the *GBA* gene is associated with Lewy body disease causing PD and dementia (Tsuang et al. 2012). While the list of genes involved in PD continues to grow, the acknowledged recessive gene causes appear to be *parkin* (*PARK2*), *PINK1* (*PARK6*), and *DJ-1* (*PARK7*). Autosomal dominant and genetic risk factors include *SNCA*, *UCHL1*, *LRRK2*, *GBA*, and *MAPT*. As discussed by Do and others, the list continues to grow as do the parallels with other neurodegenerative diseases such as AD and FTLD.

Public health impact of PD

PD is progressive and debilitating. While initial treatments with levodopa and similar medications effectively quell most motor symptoms, their effectiveness begins to subside in about 50 per cent of patients after 3–5 years. To date, there have been no true disease-modifying treatments available and we are only beginning to examine genetic pathways leading to pathogenesis or to drug targets that may modify the disease process prior to onset of symptoms (Siderowf et al. 2012). This aspiration is still a long way off, it appears. With increasing motor problems comes increased healthcare cost and decreased quality of life (de Boer et al. 1999); dementia is now regarded as an almost inevitable consequence of PD, assuming the patient survives long enough, leading to the need for long-term care in many instances. The overlap between PD dementia and DLB is of great interest because of the potential underlying synuclein pathology and therefore the potential genetic relationships as well (Rocca et al. 2007; Tsuang et al. 2012).

Multiple sclerosis

Clinical overview of MS

Although MS is relatively uncommon, it has a great impact on society. The impact of this disease is disproportionately large because it strikes young adults, is expensive to treat, and can cause disability. Only 21 per cent of MS patients have no work limitations and 29 per cent remain in the workforce (Minden et al. 2004). MS has substantial medical costs (Minden et al. 2004; Adelman et al. 2013). Because of lost earnings and increased healthcare costs, MS is the third leading cause of significant disability in the 20–50-year age range (LaRocca et al. 1984).

Clinically, MS is characterized by demyelinating lesions of central nervous system white matter causing motor, sensory, cerebellar, visual, brainstem, autonomic, spinal cord pathways, and other symptoms. These often occur in attacks with complete or partial recovery, with symptoms remaining stable between exacerbations (relapsing/remitting disease) (Lublin and Reingold 1996). Alternatively, symptoms may slowly progress in the absence of exacerbations (primary progressive disease). Relapsing/remitting cases may evolve into secondary progressive disease with a slow worsening of baseline function. When the disease results in death, the immediate cause is usually infectious, secondary to urinary tract involvement or pneumonia.

The length of exacerbations can be shortened by corticosteroids. There are currently nine US Food and Drug Administration-approved medications to slow the disease, with others under review. In addition to disease-modifying therapies, symptomatic treatments are often required. A multitude of new treatments are being tested, giving hope for more effective treatments in the future.

Definition of MS

The current diagnostic criteria are the revised McDonald criteria (Polman et al. 2011). These require two or more episodes of neurological deficit at different times and different locations within the nervous system. MS attacks used to fulfil the criteria must have symptoms typical of those seen with MS and have objective findings on examination or paraclinical tests. The new criteria allow diagnosis by clinical presentation alone, but also allow magnetic resonance imaging (MRI) findings to be used to demonstrate dissemination in time or location. The revised McDonald criteria allow the disease to be diagnosed at an earlier stage than previous criteria.

Case ascertainment of MS

Because of the necessity for neurological expertise and special studies to make reliable diagnoses, reported worldwide prevalence may not be completely comparable, especially where differences in the availability and quality of healthcare exist. This is especially true in light of the highly variable clinical presentation of the disease, and the variable course. The requirement for repeated attacks before a diagnosis is made and the often vague nature of the initial clinical symptoms leads to difficulties in determining exact incidence figures in a timely manner.

Prevalence of MS

MS prevalence is easier to determine than incidence, particularly considering the difficulty in determining the time of disease onset. With the new McDonald criteria, MRI availability, and increasing awareness of the disease, the time from symptom onset until diagnosis is rapidly shortening (Marrie et al. 2005). The reported prevalence of MS varies widely with latitude, from one per 100,000 or less near the equator, to over 150 per 100,000 in some high-latitude areas (Koch-Henriksen and Sorensen 2011). Migrants carry the risk of their geographic residence before their mid teens (Alter et al. 1966a, 1966b). However, prevalence and incidence relative to latitude appears to be rapidly changing, due primarily to an increase in MS in the South (Hernan et al. 1999; Wallin et al. 2004; Pugliatti et al. 2006; Koch-Henriksen and Sorensen 2011). This is less apparent in the southern hemisphere (Cristiano et al. 2012). The levelling of MS rates with latitude may partially reflect improved case ascertainment, but likely also reflects a true increase in MS in areas in which it was previously rare.

Risk factors of MS

Gender

Approximately 75 per cent of people with MS are female. However, in the first half of the twentieth century, males predominated (Kurtzke 2005). Gender rates changed to a female preponderance about mid century and the female/male ratio continues to increase by about 0.85 per cent/year (Orton et al. 2006; Wallin et al. 2012). The disease is less active during pregnancy and more active during the 3 months immediately postpartum (Confavreux et al. 1998; Langer-Gould and Beaber 2013). The changes in MS activity with hormones and pregnancy may be due to alterations in immune system function, but the temporal changes in gender ratios remain unexplained.

Ethnic background of MS

In general, MS occurs with greater frequency in white people, particularly those of northern European ancestry. Other ethnic groups have a lower incidence and prevalence of MS, but this appears to be changing. The relative risk of MS in black compared with white male veterans increased from 0.44 in the Second World War/Korean conflict to 0.67 in Vietnam to 1.16 in the Gulf War (Wallin et al. 2012). During the same time periods the relative risk among black females compared to white males increased from 1.28 to 2.86 to 3.62, catching up to white females with 1.79, 2.99, and 3.54 respectively.

Genetic susceptibility of MS

In Caucasians, some alleles of the HLA complex are associated with MS susceptibility, particularly HLA-DRB1.1501 (Haines et al. 1996). In addition, other groups of genes that influence the immune response or myelin structure have been investigated (Sadovnick et al. 1991). To date, large GWAS have identified over 60 loci associated with MS, but associations are modest, explaining less than 25 per cent of the heritability of the disease (Hafler et al. 2007; Sawcer et al. 2011; Lin et al. 2012). Nevertheless, these studies confirm the importance of genes related to immune function.

In the Danish twin study, there was concordance for MS in 24 per cent of MZ twins and 3 per cent of dizygotic twins (Hansen et al. 2005). The standardized incidence ratio for MZ twins compared to non-twins was 1.23 and 0.78 for DZ twins. There is also an increased risk of MS in other first-degree relatives of people with MS. In a Danish study, the relative risk of MS in first-degree relatives of people with MS was 7.1 (95 per cent CI 5.8–8.8) (Nielsen et al. 2005). The lifetime risk was calculated to be 2.8 per cent for male and 2.9 per cent for female first-degree relatives. Some have found that the risk of MS is higher in children of MS fathers than MS mothers (odds ratio 1.99, 95 per cent CI 1.05–3.77) (Kantarci et al. 2006). This increased rate of transmission to offspring by a subgroup in which the disease is less common (men) suggests a genetic contribution in which genes are concentrated in men with the disease. However, others have reported that the risk of MS in children whose parents have MS is similar regardless of whether the affected parent was the father or mother (Herrera et al. 2007). A Canadian study found that the age-adjusted risk of MS in siblings was 3.11 per cent (95 per cent CI 2.39–3.83) (Ebers et al. 2004). This group also found an excess of mother–daughter pairs compared to father–son pairs and suggested that epigenetic factors may contribute (Chao et al. 2010). These studies indicate that there is an important genetic contribution to the disease, but environmental factors also play a major role.

Environmental factors of MS

In the presence of inherent susceptibility, some external factors seem to be associated with MS. People with MS have a later age of exposure to common childhood exanthematous diseases, and lower birth orders though not all studies have supported this finding (Bager et al. 2006). There have been reports of clusters of disease, thought to have been related to environmental exposures, but on investigation these supposed clusters have generally not been beyond expected variability.

The strong relationship between MS and latitude has led some to postulate that areas with less sun exposure, and thus lower levels of vitamin D, may be responsible for the disease (Simon et al. 2012). Military recruits with low 25-hydroxyvitamin D (25(OH)D) levels had a subsequent increased risk of MS. Low vitamin D levels are associated with risk of MS in children. The risk of MS is lower in offspring of mothers with increased vitamin D intake. Patients with MS generally have low 25(OH)D levels. A small trial of 25(OH)D supplementation in MS patients found no difference in MRI activity (Stein et al. 2011). Other randomized treatment trials of 25(OH)D are underway.

The relationship between MS prevalence, latitude, migration, and socioeconomic factors has led some to suggest that MS is related to the degree and timing of exposure to various infectious organisms (Fleming and Cook 2006). This hygiene hypothesis states that exposure to infectious agents later in life (due to high levels of hygiene) leads to changes in the immune system that eventually lead to MS. Epstein–Barr virus (EBV) is associated with MS (Ascherio and Munger 2007; Owens and Bennett 2012). MS is extremely rare in people who have never had EBV. Furthermore, those exposed to EBV later in childhood have a two- to threefold increase in risk relative to those who acquire EBV in early childhood. Antibody titres to EBV are increased in MS, often years before recognition of the disease, but this may reflect a general upregulation of the immune system. Cytomegalovirus appears to be protective in children (Waubant et al. 2011).

Both ever-smokers and current smokers have an increased risk of MS (Jafari and Hintzen 2011). Children exposed to cigarette smoke have a higher risk of developing MS (Mikaeloff et al. 2007). Smoking is associated with increased disability, more MRI activity, and conversion to secondary progressive MS.

Overview of MS

The risk of MS appears to be due to environmental factors acting on genetically predisposed people. Eventually, these factors lead to an immune attack on the central nervous system, resulting in symptoms. The genetic factors are polygenetic. The environmental factors remain uncertain. Immunomodulating treatments have played an important role in slowing the disease, but their benefits are only partial. Much remains to be clarified about the mechanisms of the disease process, and it is hoped that a better knowledge of these mechanisms will lead to improved treatments.

Conclusion

Presenting current and useful research information on a number of neurological conditions is a difficult task. This chapter has attempted to address that challenge for some selected neurological conditions and referencing heavily to current or classic research papers. Conditions such as headache and back pain have substantial public health impact because of the age groups affected, their prevalence, and the lost productivity (or economic loss) related to them. MS, a relatively common neurological disease, can affect individuals in young adulthood, decrease their productivity, and ultimately make them dependent on others. TBI occurring in youth or young adulthood can cause years of extra medical care in addition to lost productivity among those who survive the immediate event. Epilepsy may have onset throughout the life course, it may result from trauma or may be caused by specific genes, among other causes. While there are intractable forms of epilepsy, great strides have been made in seizure control enabling patients to lead relatively full and normal lives. Neurodegenerative diseases, such as PD and AD, rob productivity, functional ability, and independence from older individuals; they also force huge increases in healthcare costs. Without question neurological diseases have substantial public health effects.

Determining the incidence and prevalence for most of the diseases and conditions in this chapter is quite an inexact science. The conditions are often difficult to define and detect in the population and for the most part they are not regarded as 'reportable' conditions. Therefore we gain insight as to disease occurrence primarily from limited but (hopefully) well-designed and conducted studies. As mentioned in the introduction to this chapter, the epidemiological study of neurological conditions is a complicated matter. Problems with diagnostic inaccuracy and insidious disease onset influence our ability to observe risk factor associations;

factors related to survival may be mistaken for risk/protective factors.

The recent work of the Human Genome Project and the HapMap Project have greatly influenced technology and have now made possible genome-wide studies that could not have been imagined a decade ago. The contribution of genes that in and of themselves cause disease may be smaller than that of genes which act together with other genes in complex ways or act to metabolize or potentiate environmental exposures. The interaction between gene and environment will be increasingly well studied in the future. Description of gene products and functions may lead to specific drug therapies never before possible. The genetic information presented in this chapter, while relatively current, may become obsolete quickly. The fields of genetics and molecular biology are moving rapidly. It is a challenge also for epidemiologists to apply the knowledge gained by the genetic researchers to the design and analysis of epidemiological studies. The diagnosis of neurological conditions may be made more accurately and earlier with genetic information. Science and the public health will benefit beyond even our current expectations.

Epidemiology must take advantage of these molecular advances. Many scholars have written on pros and cons of reductionism in science. Much of epidemiology lies in its public health context, and the same is likely to be true for genetic influences on neurological diseases. Arrays of genes may identify susceptible individuals; however, those individuals may avoid disease unless met with specific environmental or behavioural exposures. The tasks of public health and epidemiology will still involve prevention, the non-random occurrence of disease, and its environmental context—in addition to heredity. The tools to address those tasks will continue to be refined.

References

Adelman, G., Rane, S.G., and Villa, K.F. (2013). The cost burden of multiple sclerosis in the United States: a systematic review of the literature. *Journal of Medical Economics*, 16, 639–47.

Albert, M.S., Dekosky, S.T., Dickson, D., et al. (2011). The diagnosis of mild cognitive impairment due to Alzheimer's disease: recommendations from the National Institute on Aging-Alzheimer's Association workgroups on diagnostic guidelines for Alzheimer's disease. *Alzheimers Dement*, 7, 270–9.

Alhazzani, A. and Goddeau, R.P. (2013). Migraine and stroke: a continuum of association in adults. *Headache*, 53(6), 1023–7.

Alonso, A., Rodriguez, L.A., Logroscino, G., and Hernan, M.A. (2007). Gout and risk of Parkinson disease: a prospective study. *Neurology*, 69, 1696–700.

Alter, M., Leibowitz, U., and Halpern, L. (1966a). Multiple sclerosis in European & Afro-Asian populations of Israel. A clinical appraisal. *Acta Neurologica Scandinavica*, 42(Suppl. 19), 47–54.

Alter, M., Leibowitz, U., and Speer, J. (1966b). Risk of multiple sclerosis related to age at immigration to Israel. *Archives of Neurology*, 15, 234–37.

American Psychiatric Association (1994). *Diagnostic and Statistical Manual of Mental Disorders: DSM-IV*. Washington, DC: American Psychiatric Association.

Annegers, J.F., Hauser, W.A., Anderson, V.E., and Kurland, L.T. (1982). The risks of seizure disorders among relatives of patients with childhood onset epilepsy. *Neurology*, 32, 174–9.

Annegers, J.F., Hauser, W.A., Coan, S.P., and Rocca, W.A. (1998). A population-based study of seizures after traumatic brain injuries. *The New England Journal of Medicine*, 338, 20–4.

Anonymous (1997). Consensus recommendations for the postmortem diagnosis of Alzheimer's disease. The National Institute on Aging, and Reagan Institute Working Group on Diagnostic Criteria for the Neuropathological Assessment of Alzheimer's Disease. *Neurobiology of Aging*, 18, S1–2.

Anonymous (1998). Rehabilitation of persons with traumatic brain injury. *NIH Consensus Statement*, 16, 1–41.

Armstrong, R.A., Cairns, N.J., and Lantos, P.L. (2006). Multiple system atrophy (MSA): topographic distribution of the alpha-synuclein-associated pathological changes. *Parkinsonism Relat Disord*, 12, 356–62.

Ascherio, A. and Munger, K.L. (2007). Environmental risk factors for multiple sclerosis. Part I: the role of infection. *Annals of Neurology*, 61, 288–99.

Atroshi, I., Gummesson, C., Johnsson, R., Ornstein, E., Ranstam, J., and Rosen, I. (1999). Prevalence of carpal tunnel syndrome in a general population. *Journal of the American Medical Association*, 282, 153–8.

Au, R., Massaro, J.M., Wolf, P.A., et al. (2006). Association of white matter hyperintensity volume with decreased cognitive functioning: the Framingham Heart Study. *Archives of Neurology*, 63, 246–50.

Avanzini, G., Franceschetti, S., and Mantegazza, M. (2007). Epileptogenic channelopathies: experimental models of human pathologies. *Epilepsia*, 48(Suppl. 2), 51–64.

Bacskai, B.J., Frosch, M.P., Freeman, S.H., et al. (2007). Molecular imaging with Pittsburgh Compound B confirmed at autopsy: a case report. *Archives of Neurology*, 64, 431–4.

Bager, P., Nielsen, N.M., Bihrmann, K., et al. (2006). Sibship characteristics and risk of multiple sclerosis: a nationwide cohort study in Denmark. *American Journal of Epidemiology*, 163, 1112–17.

Baker, M., Mackenzie, I.R., Pickering-Brown, S.M., et al. (2006). Mutations in progranulin cause tau-negative frontotemporal dementia linked to chromosome 17. *Nature*, 442, 916–19.

Banks, M.E. (2007). Overlooked but critical: traumatic brain injury as a consequence of interpersonal violence. *Trauma, Violence & Abuse*, 8, 290–8.

Barrett, A.M., Lucero, M.A., Le, T., Robinson, R.L., Dworkin, R.H., and Chappell, A.S. (2007). Epidemiology, public health burden, and treatment of diabetic peripheral neuropathic pain: a review. *Pain Medicine*, 8(Suppl. 2), S50–62.

Bateman, R.J., Xiong, C., Benzinger, T.L., et al. (2012). Clinical and biomarker changes in dominantly inherited Alzheimer's disease. *The New England Journal of Medicine*, 367, 795–804.

Baugh, C.M., Stamm, J.M., Riley, D.O., et al. (2012). Chronic traumatic encephalopathy: neurodegeneration following repetitive concussive and subconcussive brain trauma. *Brain Imaging and Behavior*, 6, 244–54.

Bazarian, J.J., McClung, J., Shah, M.N., Cheng, Y.T., Flesher, W., and Kraus, J. (2005). Mild traumatic brain injury in the United States, 1998–2000. *Brain Injury*, 19, 85–91.

Begley, C.E., Famulari, M., Annegers, J.F., et al. (2000). The cost of epilepsy in the United States: an estimate from population-based clinical and survey data. *Epilepsia*, 41, 342–51.

Bland, J.D. and Rudolfer, S.M. (2003). Clinical surveillance of carpal tunnel syndrome in two areas of the United Kingdom, 1991–2001. *J Neurol Neurosurg Psychiatry*, 74, 1674–9.

Boardman, H.F., Thomas, E., Millson, D.S., and Croft, P.R. (2006). The natural history of headache: predictors of onset and recovery. *Cephalalgia*, 26, 1080–8.

Bower, J.H., Maraganore, D.M., McDonnell, S.K., and Rocca, W.A. (1999). Incidence and distribution of parkinsonism in Olmsted County, Minnesota, 1976–1990. *Neurology*, 52, 1214–20.

Breitner, J.C. (1996). Inflammatory processes and antiinflammatory drugs in Alzheimer's disease: a current appraisal. *Neurobiology of Aging*, 17, 789–94.

Brew, B.J. (2003). The peripheral nerve complications of human immunodeficiency virus (HIV) infection. *Muscle & Nerve*, 28, 542–52.

Cady, R.K. (1999). Focus on primary care female population with migraine. *Obstetrical & Gynecological Survey*, 54, S7–13.

Cairns, N.J., Bigio, E.H., Mackenzie, I.R., et al. (2007a). Neuropathologic diagnostic and nosologic criteria for frontotemporal lobar degeneration: consensus of the Consortium for Frontotemporal Lobar Degeneration. *Acta Neuropathologica*, 114, 5–22.

Cairns, N.J., Neumann, M., Bigio, E.H., et al. (2007b). TDP-43 in familial and sporadic frontotemporal lobar degeneration with ubiquitin inclusions. *American Journal of Pathology*, 171, 227–40.

Camfield, P. (2012). Issues in epilepsy classification for population studies. *Epilepsia*, 53(Suppl. 2), 10–13.

Cassidy, J.D., Carroll, L.J., Peloso, P.M., et al. (2004). Incidence, risk factors and prevention of mild traumatic brain injury: results of the WHO Collaborating Centre Task Force on Mild Traumatic Brain Injury. *Journal of Rehabilitation Medicine*, 43, 28–60.

Centers for Disease Control and Prevention (2003). Nonfatal fall-related traumatic brain injury among older adults—California, 1996–1999. *Morbidity and Mortality Weekly Report*, 52, 276–8.

Centers for Disease Control and Prevention (2007). Nonfatal traumatic brain injuries from sports and recreation activities—United States, 2001–2005. *Morbidity and Mortality Weekly Report*, 56, 733–7.

Chao, M.J., Herrera, B.M., Ramagopalan, S.V., et al. (2010). Parent-of-origin effects at the major histocompatibility complex in multiple sclerosis. *Human Molecular Genetics*, 19, 3679–89.

Chasman, D.I., Schurks, M., Anttila, V., et al. (2011). Genome-wide association study reveals three susceptibility loci for common migraine in the general population. *Nature Genetics*, 43, 695–8.

Chen, C.C., Chen, L.S., Yen, M.F., Chen, H.H., and Liou, H.H. (2012). Geographic variation in the age- and gender-specific prevalence and incidence of epilepsy: analysis of Taiwanese National Health Insurance-based data. *Epilepsia*, 53, 283–90.

Chesnut, R.M., Temkin, N., Carney, N., et al. (2012). A trial of intracranial-pressure monitoring in traumatic brain injury. *The New England Journal of Medicine*, 367, 2471–81.

Chui, H.C., Mack, W., Jackson, J.E., et al. (2000). Clinical criteria for the diagnosis of vascular dementia: a multicenter study of comparability and interrater reliability [see comments]. *Archives of Neurology*, 57, 191–6.

Chui, H.C., Victoroff, J.I., Margolin, D., Jagust, W., Shankle, R., and Katzman, R. (1992). Criteria for the diagnosis of ischemic vascular dementia proposed by the State of California Alzheimer's Disease Diagnostic and Treatment Centers [see comments]. *Neurology*, 42, 473–80.

Confavreux, C., Hutchinson, M., Hours, M.M., Cortinovis-Tourniaire, P., and Moreau, T. (1998). Rate of pregnancy-related relapse in multiple sclerosis. Pregnancy in Multiple Sclerosis Group. *The New England Journal of Medicine*, 339, 285–91.

Corder, E.H., Saunders, A.M., Strittmatter, W.J., et al. (1993). Gene dose of apolipoprotein E type 4 allele and the risk of Alzheimer's disease in late onset families [see comments]. *Science*, 261, 921–3.

Cristiano, E., Rojas, J., Romano, M., et al. (2012). The epidemiology of multiple sclerosis in Latin America and the Caribbean: a systematic review. *Mult Scler* 19(7), 844–54.

Cruts, M., Gijselinck, I., Van Der Zee, J., et al. (2006). Null mutations in progranulin cause ubiquitin-positive frontotemporal dementia linked to chromosome 17q21. *Nature*, 442, 920–4.

Currie, C.J., Morgan, C.L., and Peters, J.R. (1998). The epidemiology and cost of inpatient care for peripheral vascular disease, infection, neuropathy, and ulceration in diabetes. *Diabetes Care*, 21, 42–8.

De Boer, A.G., Sprangers, M.A., Speelman, H.D., and De Haes, H.C. (1999). Predictors of health care use in patients with Parkinson's disease: a longitudinal study. *Movement Disorders*, 14, 772–9.

Dejesus-Hernandez, M., Mackenzie, I.R., Boeve, B.F., et al. (2011). Expanded GGGGCC hexanucleotide repeat in noncoding region of C9ORF72 causes chromosome 9p-linked FTD and ALS. *Neuron*, 72, 245–56.

De Lau, L.M., Koudstaal, P.J., Hofman, A., and Breteler, M.M. (2005). Serum uric acid levels and the risk of Parkinson disease. *Annals of Neurology*, 58, 797–800.

De Lau, L.M., Koudstaal, P.J., Witteman, J.C., Hofman, A., and Breteler, M.M. (2006). Dietary folate, vitamin B12, and vitamin B6 and the risk of Parkinson disease. *Neurology*, 67, 315–18.

Del Brutto, O.H. (2012). Neurocysticercosis. *Continuum (Minneapolis Minn)*, 18, 1392–416.

De Rijk, M.C., Tzourio, C., Breteler, M.M., et al. (1997). Prevalence of parkinsonism and Parkinson's disease in Europe: the EUROPARKINSON Collaborative Study. European Community Concerted Action on the Epidemiology of Parkinson's disease. *J Neurol Neurosurg Psychiatry*, 62, 10–15.

Devinsky, O. (2011). Sudden, unexpected death in epilepsy. *The New England Journal of Medicine*, 365, 1801–11.

Dickson, D.W., Lin, W., Liu, W.K., and Yen, S.H. (1999). Multiple system atrophy: a sporadic synucleinopathy. *Brain Pathol*, 9, 721–32.

Do, C.B., Tung, J.Y., Dorfman, E., et al. (2011). Web-based genome-wide association study identifies two novel loci and a substantial genetic component for Parkinson's disease. *PLoS Genet*, 7, e1002141.

Dyck, P.J., Clark, V.M., Overland, C.J., et al. (2012). Impaired glycemia and diabetic polyneuropathy: the OC IG Survey. *Diabetes Care*, 35, 584–91.

Dyck, P.J., Davies, J.L., Wilson, D.M., Service, F.J., Melton, L.J., 3rd, and O'Orien, P.C. (1999). Risk factors for severity of diabetic polyneuropathy: intensive longitudinal assessment of the Rochester Diabetic Neuropathy Study cohort. *Diabetes Care*, 22, 1479–86.

Ebers, G.C., Sadovnick, A.D., Dyment, D.A., Yee, I.M., Willer, C.J., and Risch, N. (2004). Parent-of-origin effect in multiple sclerosis: observations in half-siblings. *The Lancet*, 363, 1773–4.

Engel, J., Jr. (2006). Report of the ILAE classification core group. *Epilepsia*, 47, 1558–68.

Evans, D.A., Funkenstein, H.H., Albert, M.S., et al. (1989). Prevalence of Alzheimer's disease in a community population of older persons. Higher than previously reported. *Journal of the American Medical Association*, 262, 2551–6.

Fagan, A.M., Roe, C.M., Xiong, C., Mintun, M.A., Morris, J.C., and Holtzman, D.M. (2007). Cerebrospinal fluid tau/beta-amyloid(42) ratio as a prediction of cognitive decline in nondemented older adults. *Archives of Neurology*, 64, 343–9.

Firestone, J.A., Smith-Weller, T., Franklin, G., Swanson, P., Longstreth, W.T., Jr., and Checkoway, H. (2005). Pesticides and risk of Parkinson disease: a population-based case-control study. *Archives of Neurology*, 62, 91–5.

Fleming, J.O. and Cook, T.D. (2006). Multiple sclerosis and the hygiene hypothesis. *Neurology*, 67, 2085–6.

Franklin, G.M., Haug, J., Heyer, N., Checkoway, H., and Peck, N. (1991). Occupational carpal tunnel syndrome in Washington State, 1984–1988. *American Journal of Public Health*, 81, 741–6.

Frediani, F. and Villani, V. (2007). Migraine and depression. *Neurol Sci*, 28(Suppl. 2), S161–5.

Gao, X., Chen, H., Fung, T.T., et al. (2007). Prospective study of dietary pattern and risk of Parkinson disease. *American Journal of Clinical Nutrition*, 86, 1486–94.

Gass, J., Cannon, A., Mackenzie, I.R., et al. (2006). Mutations in progranulin are a major cause of ubiquitin-positive frontotemporal lobar degeneration. *Human Molecular Genetics*, 15, 2988–3001.

Geerlings, M.I., Deeg, D.J., Penninx, B.W., et al. (1999). Cognitive reserve and mortality in dementia: the role of cognition, functional ability and depression. *Psychol Med*, 29, 1219–26.

Gelb, D.J., Oliver, E., and Gilman, S. (1999). Diagnostic criteria for Parkinson disease. *Archives of Neurology*, 56, 33–9.

Gervil, M., Ulrich, V., Kyvik, K.O., Olesen, J., and Russell, M.B. (1999). Migraine without aura: a population-based twin study. *Annals of Neurology*, 46, 606–11.

Goedert, M., and Spillantini, M.G. (1998). Lewy body diseases and multiple system atrophy as alpha- synucleinopathies. *Molecular Psychiatry*, 3, 462–5.

Gorell, J.M., Johnson, C.C., Rybicki, B.A., Peterson, E.L., and Richardson, R.J. (1998). The risk of Parkinson's disease with exposure to pesticides, farming, well water, and rural living. *Neurology*, 50, 1346–50.

Gorell, J.M., Rybicki, B.A., Cole Johnson, C., and Peterson, E.L. (1999). Occupational metal exposures and the risk of Parkinson's disease. *Neuroepidemiology*, 18, 303–8.

Guerreiro, R., Wojtas, A., Bras, J., et al. (2013). TREM2 variants in Alzheimer's disease. *The New England Journal of Medicine*, 368, 117–27.

Haass, C. (2004). Take five—BACE and the gamma-secretase quartet conduct Alzheimer's amyloid beta-peptide generation. *EMBO Journal*, 23, 483–8.

Hachinski, V. (1994). Vascular dementia: a radical redefinition. *Dementia*, 5, 130–2.

Hafler, D.A., Compston, A., Sawcer, S., et al. (2007). Risk alleles for multiple sclerosis identified by a genomewide study. *The New England Journal of Medicine*, 357, 851–62.

Hagen, K., Vatten, L., Stovner, L.J., Zwart, J.A., Krokstad, S., and Bovim, G. (2002). Low socio-economic status is associated with increased risk of frequent headache: a prospective study of 22718 adults in Norway. *Cephalalgia*, 22, 672–9.

Haines, J.L., Ter-Minassian, M., Bazyk, A., et al. (1996). A complete genomic screen for multiple sclerosis underscores a role for the major histocompatibility complex. The Multiple Sclerosis Genetics Group. *Nature Genetics*, 13, 469–71.

Hakim, A.J., Cherkas, L., El Zayat, S., MacGregor, A.J., and Spector, T. D. (2002). The genetic contribution to carpal tunnel syndrome in women: a twin study. *Arthritis Rheum*, 47, 275–9.

Hansen, T., Skytthe, A., Stenager, E., Petersen, H.C., Bronnum-Hansen, H., and Kyvik, K.O. (2005). Concordance for multiple sclerosis in Danish twins: an update of a nationwide study. *Mult Scler*, 11, 504–10.

Hardy, J. (2010). Genetic analysis of pathways to Parkinson disease. *Neuron*, 68, 201–6.

Hardy, J., Duff, K., Hardy, K.G., Perez-Tur, J., and Hutton, M. (1998). Genetic dissection of Alzheimer's disease and related dementias: amyloid and its relationship to tau [published erratum appears in *Nat Neurosci* 1998 Dec;1(8):743]. *Nature Neuroscience*, 1, 355–8.

Hardy, T.A., Blum, S., McCombe, P. A., and Reddel, S. W. (2011). Guillain–Barré syndrome: modern theories of etiology. *Current Allergy and Asthma Reports*, 11, 197–204.

Hauser, W.A., Annegers, J.F., and Rocca, W.A. (1996). Descriptive epidemiology of epilepsy: contributions of population-based studies from Rochester, Minnesota. *Mayo Clin Proc*, 71, 576–86.

Headache Classification Subcommittee of the International Headache Society (2004). The International Classification of Headache Disorders: 2nd edition. *Cephalalgia*, 24(Suppl. 1), 9–160.

Henderson, V.W., Paganini-Hill, A., Miller, B.L., et al. (2000). Estrogen for Alzheimer's disease in women: randomized, double-blind, placebo-controlled trial. *Neurology*, 54, 295–301.

Hendrie, H.C. (1998). Epidemiology of dementia and Alzheimer's disease. *Am J Geriatr Psychiatry*, 6, S3–18.

Hernan, M.A., Olek, M.J., and Ascherio, A. (1999). Geographic variation of MS incidence in two prospective studies of US women. *Neurology*, 53, 1711–18.

Herrera, B.M., Ramagopalan, S.V., Orton, S., et al. (2007). Parental transmission of MS in a population-based Canadian cohort. *Neurology*, 69, 1208–12.

Hirtz, D., Thurman, D.J., Gwinn-Hardy, K., Mohamed, M., Chaudhuri, A.R., and Zalutsky, R. (2007). How common are the 'common' neurologic disorders? *Neurology*, 68, 326–37.

Hoge, C.W., Castro, C.A., Messer, S.C., Mcgurk, D., Cotting, D.I., and Koffman, R.L. (2004). Combat duty in Iraq and Afghanistan, mental health problems, and barriers to care. *The New England Journal of Medicine*, 351, 13–22.

Holbrook, T.L., Hoyt, D.B., Coimbra, R., Potenza, B., Sise, M., and Anderson, J.P. (2005). Long-term posttraumatic stress disorder persists after major trauma in adolescents: new data on risk factors and functional outcome. *Journal of Trauma*, 58, 764–9; discussion 769–71.

Hollingworth, P., Harold, D., Sims, R., et al. (2011). Common variants at ABCA7, MS4A6A/MS4A4E, EPHA1, CD33 and CD2AP are associated with Alzheimer's disease. *Nature Genetics*, 43, 429–35.

Hu, G., Jousilahti, P., Nissinen, A., Antikainen, R., Kivipelto, M., and Tuomilehto, J. (2006). Body mass index and the risk of Parkinson disease. *Neurology*, 67, 1955–9.

Hu, X.H., Markson, L.E., Lipton, R.B., Stewart, W.F., and Berger, M.L. (1999). Burden of migraine in the United States: disability and economic costs. *Arch Intern Med*, 159, 813–18.

Hyman, B.T., Phelps, C.H., Beach, T.G., et al. (2012). National Institute on Aging-Alzheimer's Association guidelines for the neuropathologic assessment of Alzheimer's disease. *Alzheimers Dement*, 8, 1–13.

In T' Veld, B.A., Ruitenberg, A., Hofman, A., et al. (2001). Nonsteroidal antiinflammatory drugs and the risk of Alzheimer's disease. *The New England Journal of Medicine*, 345, 1515–21.

Jafari, N. and Hintzen, R.Q. (2011). The association between cigarette smoking and multiple sclerosis. *Journal of the Neurological Sciences*, 311, 78–85.

Jankovic, J., Rajput, A.H., Mcdermott, M.P., and Perl, D.P. (2000). The evolution of diagnosis in early Parkinson disease. Parkinson Study Group. *Archives of Neurology*, 57, 369–72.

Jennett, B., Teasdale, G., Braakman, R., Minderhoud, J., and Knill-Jones, R. (1976). Predicting outcome in individual patients after severe head injury. *The Lancet*, 1, 1031–4.

Jorm, A.F. and Jolley, D. (1998). The incidence of dementia: a meta-analysis. *Neurology*, 51, 728–33.

Kaiboriboon, K., Bakaki, P.M., Lhatoo, S.D., and Koroukian, S. (2013). Incidence and prevalence of treated epilepsy among poor health and low-income Americans. *Neurology*, 80, 1942–9.

Kaniecki, R.G. (2012). Tension-type headache. *Continuum (Minneapolis Minn)*, 18, 823–34.

Kantarci, O.H., Barcellos, L.F., Atkinson, E.J., et al. (2006). Men transmit MS more often to their children vs women: the Carter effect. *Neurology*, 67, 305–10.

Katsarava, Z., Obermann, M., Yoon, M.S., et al. (2007). Prevalence of cluster headache in a population-based sample in Germany. *Cephalalgia*, 27, 1014–19.

Keenan, H.T. and Bratton, S.L. (2006). Epidemiology and outcomes of pediatric traumatic brain injury. *Developmental Neuroscience*, 28, 256–63.

Keenan, H.T., Runyan, D.K., Marshall, S.W., Nocera, M.A., Merten, D.F., and Sinal, S.H. (2003). A population-based study of inflicted traumatic brain injury in young children. *Journal of the American Medical Association*, 290, 621–6.

Kivipelto, M., and Solomon, A. (2006). Cholesterol as a risk factor for Alzheimer's disease—epidemiological evidence. *Acta Neurologica Scandinavica Supplement*, 185, 50–7.

Klunk, W.E., Engler, H., Nordberg, A., et al. (2003). Imaging the pathology of Alzheimer's disease: amyloid-imaging with positron emission tomography. *Neuroimaging Clin N Am*, 13, 781–9, ix.

Knopman, D.S., Dekosky, S.T., Cummings, J.L., et al. (2001). Practice parameter: diagnosis of dementia (an evidence-based review). Report of the Quality Standards Subcommittee of the American Academy of Neurology. *Neurology*, 56, 1143–53.

Koch-Henriksen, N. and Sorensen, P.S. (2011). Why does the north–south gradient of incidence of multiple sclerosis seem to have disappeared on the northern hemisphere? *Journal of the Neurological Sciences*, 311, 58–63.

Koepsell, T.D., Kurland, B.F., Harel, O., Johnson, E.A., Zhou, X.H., and Kukull, W.A. (2007). Education, cognitive function, and severity of neuropathology in Alzheimer disease. *Neurology* 68:A169–A170.

Korczyn, A.D., and Reichmann, H. (2006). Dementia with Lewy bodies. *Journal of the Neurological Sciences*, 248, 3–8.

Kurtzke, J.F. (2005). Epidemiology and etiology of multiple sclerosis. *Physical Medicine & Rehabilitation Clinics of North America*, 16, 327–49.

Kwong, L.K., Neumann, M., Sampathu, D.M., Lee, V.M., and Trojanowski, J.Q. (2007). TDP-43 proteinopathy: the neuropathology underlying major forms of sporadic and familial frontotemporal lobar degeneration and motor neuron disease. *Acta Neuropathologica*, 114, 63–70.

Laitinen, M.H., Ngandu, T., Rovio, S., et al. (2006). Fat intake at midlife and risk of dementia and Alzheimer's disease: a population-based study. *Dementia and Geriatric Cognitive Disorders*, 22, 99–107.

Langer-Gould, A. and Beaber, B.E. (2013). Effects of pregnancy and breast-feeding on the multiple sclerosis disease course. *Clinical Immunology*, 149(2), 244–50.

Langston, J.W. (2006). The Parkinson's complex: parkinsonism is just the tip of the iceberg. *Annals of Neurology*, 59, 591–6.

Langston, J.W., and Ballard, P.A., Jr. (1983). Parkinson's disease in a chemist working with 1-methyl-4-phenyl-1,2,5,6-tetrahydropyridine. *The New England Journal of Medicine*, 309, 310.

Langston, J.W., Ballard, P., Tetrud, J.W., and Irwin, I. (1983). Chronic Parkinsonism in humans due to a product of meperidine-analog synthesis. *Science*, 219, 979–80.

Larocca, N.G., Scheinberg, L.C., Slater, R.J., et al. (1984). Field testing of a minimal record of disability in multiple sclerosis: the United States and Canada. *Acta Neurologica Scandinavica Supplement*, 101, 126–38.

Launer, L.J., Andersen, K., Dewey, M.E., et al. (1999). Rates and risk factors for dementia and Alzheimer's disease: results from EURODEM pooled analyses. EURODEM Incidence Research Group and Work Groups. European Studies of Dementia. *Neurology*, 52, 78–84.

Launer, L.J., Oudkerk, M., Nilsson, L.G., et al. (2000). CASCADE: a European collaborative study on vascular determinants of brain lesions. Study design and objectives. *Neuroepidemiology*, 19, 113–20.

Leidy, N.K., Elixhauser, A., Vickrey, B., Means, E., and Willian, M.K. (1999). Seizure frequency and the health-related quality of life of adults with epilepsy. *Neurology*, 53, 162–6.

Lemke, J.R., Riesch, E., Scheurenbrand, T., et al. (2012). Targeted next generation sequencing as a diagnostic tool in epileptic disorders. *Epilepsia*, 53, 1387–98.

Leonardi, M., Steiner, T.J., Scher, A.T., and Lipton, R.B. (2005). The global burden of migraine: measuring disability in headache disorders with WHO's Classification of Functioning, Disability and Health (ICF). *J Headache Pain*, 6, 429–40.

Levy-Lahad, E., Tsuang, D., and Bird, T.D. (1998). Recent advances in the genetics of Alzheimer's disease. *Journal of Geriatric Psychiatry and Neurology*, 11, 42–54.

Lhatoo, S.D. and Sander, J.W. (2005). Cause-specific mortality in epilepsy. *Epilepsia*, 46(Suppl. 11), 36–9.

Li, G., Rhew, I.C., Shofer, J.B., et al. (2007). Age-varying association between blood pressure and risk of dementia in those aged 65 and older: a community-based prospective cohort study. *Journal of the American Geriatrics Society*, 55, 1161–7.

Libby, A.M., Ghushchyan, V., McQueen, R.B., Slejko, J.F., Bainbridge, J.L., and Campbell, J.D. (2012). Economic differences in direct and indirect costs between people with epilepsy and without epilepsy. *Medical Care*, 50, 928–33.

Lin, R., Charlesworth, J., Van Der Mei, I., and Taylor, B.V. (2012). The genetics of multiple sclerosis. *Pract Neurol*, 12, 279–88.

Linde, M., Gustavsson, A., Stovner, L.J., et al. (2012). The cost of headache disorders in Europe: the Eurolight project. *European Journal of Neurology*, 19, 703–11.

Linde, M., Stovner, L.J., Zwart, J.A., and Hagen, K. (2011). Time trends in the prevalence of headache disorders. The Nord-Trondelag Health Studies (HUNT 2 and HUNT 3). *Cephalalgia*, 31, 585–96.

Lipton, R.B., Bigal, M.E., Diamond, M., Freitag, F., Reed, M.L., and Stewart, W.F. (2007). Migraine prevalence, disease burden, and the need for preventive therapy. *Neurology*, 68, 343–9.

Lipton, R. B., Stewart, W. F., and Simon, D. (1998). Medical consultation for migraine: results from the American Migraine Study. *Headache*, 38, 87–96.

Litvan, I., Halliday, G., Hallett, M., et al. (2007). The etiopathogenesis of Parkinson disease and suggestions for future research. Part I. *J Neuropathol Exp Neurol*, 66, 251–7.

Lublin, F.D. and Reingold, S.C. (1996). Defining the clinical course of multiple sclerosis: results of an international survey. National Multiple Sclerosis Society (USA) Advisory Committee on Clinical Trials of New Agents in Multiple Sclerosis. *Neurology*, 46, 907–11.

Lyngberg, A.C., Rasmussen, B.K., Jorgensen, T., and Jensen, R. (2005a). Has the prevalence of migraine and tension-type headache changed over a 12-year period? A Danish population survey. *Eur J Epidemiol*, 20, 243–9.

Lyngberg, A.C., Rasmussen, B.K., Jorgensen, T., and Jensen, R. (2005b). Prognosis of migraine and tension-type headache: a population-based follow-up study. *Neurology*, 65, 580–5.

Mackenzie, I.R., Baker, M., Pickering-Brown, S., et al. (2006). The neuropathology of frontotemporal lobar degeneration caused by mutations in the progranulin gene. *Brain*, 129, 3081–90.

Mackenzie, I.R. and Rademakers, R. (2007). The molecular genetics and neuropathology of frontotemporal lobar degeneration: recent developments. *Neurogenetics*, 8, 237–48.

Maraganore, D.M., Farrer, M.J., Hardy, J.A., Mcdonnell, S.K., Schaid, D.J., and Rocca, W.A. (2000). Case-control study of debrisoquine 4-hydroxylase, N-acetyltransferase 2, and apolipoprotein E gene polymorphisms in Parkinson's disease. *Mov Disord*, 15, 714–19.

Marrie, R.A., Cutter, G., Tyry, T., Hadjimichael, O., Campagnolo, D., and Vollmer, T. (2005). Changes in the ascertainment of multiple sclerosis. *Neurology*, 65, 1066–70.

Martyn, C.N. and Hughes, R.A. (1997). Epidemiology of peripheral neuropathy. *J Neurol Neurosurg Psychiatry*, 62, 310–18.

Mathis, C.A., Wang, Y., Holt, D.P., Huang, G.F., Debnath, M.L., and Klunk, W.E. (2003). Synthesis and evaluation of 11C-labeled 6-substituted 2-arylbenzothiazoles as amyloid imaging agents. *J Med Chem*, 46, 2740–54.

McKee, A.C., Stein, T.D., Nowinski, C.J., et al. (2013). The spectrum of disease in chronic traumatic encephalopathy. *Brain*, 136, 43–64.

McKeith, I.G. (2006). Consensus guidelines for the clinical and pathologic diagnosis of dementia with Lewy bodies (DLB): report of the Consortium on DLB International Workshop. *J Alzheimers Dis*, 9, 417–23.

Mckhann, G.M., Knopman, D.S., Chertkow, H., et al. (2011). The diagnosis of dementia due to Alzheimer's disease: recommendations from the National Institute on Aging-Alzheimer's Association workgroups on diagnostic guidelines for Alzheimer's disease. *Alzheimers Dement*, 7, 263–9.

Meeraus, W.H., Petersen, I., Chin, R.F., Knott, F., and Gilbert, R. (2013). Childhood epilepsy recorded in primary care in the UK. *Archives of Disease in Childhood*, 98, 195–202.

Mehta, K.M., Ott, A., Kalmijn, S., Slooter, A.J., Van Duijn, C.M., Hofman, A., and Breteler, M.M. (1999). Head trauma and risk of dementia and Alzheimer's disease: The Rotterdam Study. *Neurology*, 53, 1959–62.

Menegon, A., Board, P.G., Blackburn, A.C., Mellick, G.D., and Le Couteur, D.G. (1998). Parkinson's disease, pesticides, and glutathione transferase polymorphisms. *The Lancet*, 352, 1344–6.

Mesulam, M., Johnson, N., Krefft, T.A., et al. (2007). Progranulin mutations in primary progressive aphasia: the PPA1 and PPA3 families. *Archives of Neurology*, 64, 43–7.

Mikaeloff, Y., Caridade, G., Tardieu, M., and Suissa, S. (2007). Parental smoking at home and the risk of childhood-onset multiple sclerosis in children. *Brain*, 130, 2589–95.

Minden, K., Niewerth, M., Listing, J., Biedermann, T., Schontube, M., and Zink, A. (2004). Burden and cost of illness in patients with juvenile idiopathic arthritis. *Annals of the Rheumatic Diseases*, 63, 836–42.

Mintun, M.A., Larossa, G.N., Sheline, Y.I., et al. (2006). [11C]PIB in a non-demented population: potential antecedent marker of Alzheimer disease. *Neurology*, 67, 446–52.

Moceri, V.M., Kukull, W.A., Emanuel, I., Van Belle, G., and Larson, E.B. (2000). Early-life risk factors and the development of Alzheimer's disease. *Neurology*, 54, 415–20.

Mold, J.W., Vesely, S.K., Keyl, B.A., Schenk, J.B., and Roberts, M. (2004). The prevalence, predictors, and consequences of peripheral sensory neuropathy in older patients. *Journal of the American Board of Family Medicine*, 17, 309–18.

Monahan, K., and O'Leary, K.D. (1999). Head injury and battered women: an initial inquiry. *Health Soc Work*, 24, 269–78.

Morimoto, R.I. (2006). Stress, aging, and neurodegenerative disease. *The New England Journal of Medicine*, 355, 2254–5.

Morris, J.C. (2006). Mild cognitive impairment is early-stage Alzheimer disease: time to revise diagnostic criteria. *Archives of Neurology*, 63, 15–16.

Morris, J.C., and Cummings, J. (2005). Mild cognitive impairment (MCI) represents early-stage Alzheimer's disease. *J Alzheimers Dis*, 7, 235–9; discussion 255–62.

Morris, J.C., Storandt, M., Miller, J.P., et al. (2001). Mild cognitive impairment represents early-stage Alzheimer disease. *Archives of Neurology*, 58, 397–405.

Muller, M., Tang, M.X., Schupf, N., Manly, J.J., Mayeux, R., and Luchsinger, J.A. (2007). Metabolic syndrome and dementia risk in a multiethnic elderly cohort. *Dementia and Geriatric Cognitive Disorders*, 24, 185–92.

Mulnard, R.A., Cotman, C.W., Kawas, C., et al. (2000). Estrogen replacement therapy for treatment of mild to moderate Alzheimer disease: a randomized controlled trial. Alzheimer's Disease Cooperative Study. *Journal of the American Medical Association*, 283, 1007–15.

Murray, M.E., Knopman, D.S., and Dickson, D.W. (2007). Vascular dementia: clinical, neuroradiologic and neuropathologic aspects. *Panminerva Med*, 49, 197–207.

Naj, A.C., Jun, G., Beecham, G.W., et al. (2011). Common variants at MS4A4/MS4A6E, CD2AP, CD33 and EPHA1 are associated with late-onset Alzheimer's disease. *Nature Genetics*, 43, 436–41.

Natoli, J.L., Manack, A., Dean, B., et al. (2010). Global prevalence of chronic migraine: a systematic review. *Cephalalgia*, 30, 599–609.

Neumann, M., Sampathu, D.M., Kwong, L.K., et al. (2006). Ubiquitinated TDP-43 in frontotemporal lobar degeneration and amyotrophic lateral sclerosis. *Science*, 314, 130–3.

Newton, C.R. and Garcia, H.H. (2012). Epilepsy in poor regions of the world. *The Lancet*, 380, 1193–201.

Ngugi, A.K., Bottomley, C., Kleinschmidt, I., et al. (2013). Prevalence of active convulsive epilepsy in sub-Saharan Africa and associated risk factors: cross-sectional and case-control studies. *The Lancet Neurology*, 12, 253–63.

Ngugi, A.K., Kariuki, S.M., Bottomley, C., Kleinschmidt, I., Sander, J.W., and Newton, C.R. (2011). Incidence of epilepsy: a systematic review and meta-analysis. *Neurology*, 77, 1005–12.

Nielsen, N.M., Westergaard, T., Rostgaard, K., et al. (2005). Familial risk of multiple sclerosis: a nationwide cohort study. *American Journal of Epidemiology*, 162, 774–8.

Nordstrom, D. L., Destefano, F., Vierkant, R.A., and Layde, P.M. (1998). Incidence of diagnosed carpal tunnel syndrome in a general population. *Epidemiology*, 9, 342–5.

Okie, S. (2005). Traumatic brain injury in the war zone. *The New England Journal of Medicine*, 352, 2043–7.

Orchard, T.J., Ce, L.L., Maser, R.E., and Kuller, L.H. (1996). Why does diabetic autonomic neuropathy predict IDDM mortality? An analysis from the Pittsburgh Epidemiology of Diabetes Complications Study. *Diabetes Research and Clinical Practice*, 34(Suppl.), S165–71.

Orton, S.M., Herrera, B.M., Yee, I.M., et al. (2006). Sex ratio of multiple sclerosis in Canada: a longitudinal study. *The Lancet Neurology*, 5, 932–6.

Osuntokun, B.O., Adeuja, A.O., Nottidge, V.A., et al. (1992). Prevalence of headache and migrainous headache in Nigerian Africans: a community-based study. *East African Medical Journal*, 69, 196–9.

Owens, G.P. and Bennett, J.L. (2012). Trigger, pathogen, or bystander: the complex nexus linking Epstein-Barr virus and multiple sclerosis. *Multiple Sclerosis*, 18, 1204–8.

Petersen, R.C. (2004). Mild cognitive impairment as a diagnostic entity. *Journal of Internal Medicine*, 256, 183–94.

Petersen, R.C. (2007). Mild cognitive impairment: current research and clinical implications. *Seminars in Neurology*, 27, 22–31.

Petrovitch, H., Ross, G.W., Abbott, R.D., et al. (2002). Plantation work and risk of Parkinson disease in a population-based longitudinal study. *Archives of Neurology*, 59, 1787–92.

Polman, C.H., Reingold, S.C., Banwell, B., et al. (2011). Diagnostic criteria for multiple sclerosis: 2010 revisions to the McDonald criteria. *Annals of Neurology*, 69, 292–302.

Prince, M., Bryce, R., Albanese, E., Wimo, A., Ribeiro, W., and Ferri, C.P. (2013). The global prevalence of dementia: a systematic review and metaanalysis. *Alzheimers Dement*, 9, 63–75 e2.

Pugliatti, M., Rosati, G., Carton, H., et al. (2006). The epidemiology of multiple sclerosis in Europe. *European Journal of Neurology*, 13, 700–22.

Racette, B.A., Criswell, S.R., Lundin, J.I., et al. (2012). Increased risk of parkinsonism associated with welding exposure. *Neurotoxicology*, 33, 1356–61.

Rademakers, R., Baker, M., Gass, J., et al. (2007). Phenotypic variability associated with progranulin haploinsufficiency in patients with the common 1477C—>T (Arg493X) mutation: an international initiative. *The Lancet Neurology*, 6, 857–68.

Rademakers, R., and Hutton, M. (2007). The genetics of frontotemporal lobar degeneration. *Current Neurology and Neuroscience Reports*, 7, 434–42.

Reitz, C., Jun, G., Naj, A., et al. (2013). Variants in the ATP-binding cassette transporter (ABCA7), apolipoprotein E 4, and the risk of late-onset Alzheimer disease in African Americans. *Journal of the American Medical Association*, 309, 1483–92.

Ritz, B., Ascherio, A., Checkoway, H., et al. (2007). Pooled analysis of tobacco use and risk of Parkinson disease. *Archives of Neurology*, 64, 990–7.

Rivara, F.P., Koepsell, T.D., Wang, J., et al. (2012). Incidence of disability among children 12 months after traumatic brain injury. *Am J Public Health*, 102, 2074–9.

Rocca, W.A., Bower, J.H., Ahlskog, J.E., et al. (2007). Risk of cognitive impairment or dementia in relatives of patients with Parkinson disease. *Archives of Neurology*, 64, 1458–64.

Rocca, W.A., Cha, R.H., Waring, S.C., and Kokmen, E. (1998). Incidence of dementia and Alzheimer's disease: a reanalysis of data from Rochester, Minnesota, 1975-1984. *American Journal of Epidemiology*, 148, 51–62.

Roman, G.C. (1994). An epidemic in Cuba of optic neuropathy, sensorineural deafness, peripheral sensory neuropathy and dorsolateral myeloneuropathy. *Journal of the Neurological Sciences*, 127, 11–28.

Roman, G.C., Tatemichi, T.K., Erkinjuntti, T., et al. (1993). Vascular dementia: diagnostic criteria for research studies. Report of the NINDS-AIREN International Workshop [see comments]. *Neurology*, 43, 250–60.

Roopra, A., Dingledine, R., and Hsieh, J. (2012). Epigenetics and epilepsy. *Epilepsia*, 53(Suppl. 9), 2–10.

Ross, G.W., Abbott, R.D., Petrovitch, H., et al. (2000). Association of coffee and caffeine intake with the risk of Parkinson disease. *Journal of the American Medical Association*, 283, 2674–9.

Rowe, C.C., Ng, S., Ackermann, U., et al. (2007). Imaging beta-amyloid burden in aging and dementia. *Neurology*, 68, 1718–25.

Rowland, L.P. and Merritt, H.H. (1995). *Merritt's Textbook of Neurology*. Baltimore, MD: Williams & Wilkins.

Russell, M.B., Levi, N., and Kaprio, J. (2007). Genetics of tension-type headache: a population based twin study. *American Journal of Medical Genetics Part B*, 144, 982–6.

Rutland-Brown, W., Langlois, J.A., Thomas, K.E., and Xi, Y.L. (2006). Incidence of traumatic brain injury in the United States, 2003. *Journal of Head Trauma Rehabilitation*, 21, 544–8.

Sadovnick, A.D., Bulman, D., and Ebers, G.C. (1991). Parent-child concordance in multiple sclerosis. *Annals of Neurology*, 29, 252–5.

Saunders, A.M., Schmader, K., Breitner, J.C., et al. (1993). Apolipoprotein E epsilon 4 allele distributions in late-onset Alzheimer's disease and in other amyloid-forming diseases [see comments]. *The Lancet*, 342, 710–11.

Sawcer, S., Hellenthal, G., Pirinen, M., et al. (2011). Genetic risk and a primary role for cell-mediated immune mechanisms in multiple sclerosis. *Nature*, 476, 214–19.

Scher, A.I., Stewart, W.F., Ricci, J.A., and Lipton, R.B. (2003). Factors associated with the onset and remission of chronic daily headache in a population-based study. *Pain*, 106, 81–9.

Schwartz, B.S., Stewart, W.F., and Lipton, R.B. (1997). Lost workdays and decreased work effectiveness associated with headache in the workplace. *J Occup Environ Med*, 39, 320–7.

Scordo, M.G., Dahl, M.L., Spina, E., Cordici, F., and Arena, M.G. (2006). No association between CYP2D6 polymorphism and Alzheimer's disease in an Italian population. *Pharmacol Res*, 53, 162–5.

Shackleton, D.P., Westendorp, R.G., Trenite, D.G., and Vandenbroucke, J. P. (1999). Mortality in patients with epilepsy: 40 years of follow up in a Dutch cohort study [see comments]. *J Neurol Neurosurg Psychiatry*, 66, 636–40.

Sherer, M., Struchen, M.A., Yablon, S.A., Wang, Y., and Nick, T.G. (2007). Comparison of indices of TBI severity: Glasgow coma scale, length of coma, post-traumatic amnesia. *J Neurol Neurosurg Psychiatry*, 79(6), 678–85.

Shumaker, S.A., Legault, C., Kuller, L., et al. (2004). Conjugated equine estrogens and incidence of probable dementia and mild cognitive impairment in postmenopausal women: Women's Health Initiative Memory Study. *Journal of the American Medical Association*, 291, 2947–58.

Shumaker, S.A., Legault, C., Rapp, S.R., et al. (2003). Estrogen plus progestin and the incidence of dementia and mild cognitive impairment in postmenopausal women: the Women's Health Initiative Memory Study: a randomized controlled trial. *Journal of the American Medical Association*, 289, 2651–62.

Siderowf, A., Jennings, D., Eberly, S., et al. (2012). Impaired olfaction and other prodromal features in the Parkinson At-Risk Syndrome Study. *Mov Disord*, 27, 406–12.

Simon, K.C., Munger, K.L., and Ascherio, A. (2012). Vitamin D and multiple sclerosis: epidemiology, immunology, and genetics. *Curr Opin Neurol*, 25, 246–51.

Small, G. W. (2004). Neuroimaging as a diagnostic tool in dementia with Lewy bodies. *Dementia and Geriatric Cognitive Disorders*, 17(Suppl. 1), 25–31.

Solomon, D.H., Katz, J.N., Bohn, R., Mogun, H., and Avorn, J. (1999). Nonoccupational risk factors for carpal tunnel syndrome. *Journal of General Internal Medicine*, 14, 310–14.

Sperling, M.R., Feldman, H., Kinman, J., Liporace, J.D., and O'Connor, M.J. (1999). Seizure control and mortality in epilepsy. *Annals of Neurology*, 46, 45–50.

Sperling, R.A., Aisen, P.S., Beckett, L.A., et al. (2011). Toward defining the preclinical stages of Alzheimer's disease: recommendations from the National Institute on Aging-Alzheimer's Association workgroups on diagnostic guidelines for Alzheimer's disease. *Alzheimers Dement*, 7, 280–92.

Stallings, S.P., Kasdan, M.L., Soergel, T.M., and Corwin, H.M. (1997). A case-control study of obesity as a risk factor for carpal tunnel syndrome in a population of 600 patients presenting for independent medical examination. *Journal of Hand Surgery*, 22, 211–15.

Stein, M.S., Liu, Y., Gray, O.M., et al. (2011). A randomized trial of high-dose vitamin D2 in relapsing-remitting multiple sclerosis. *Neurology*, 77, 1611–18.

Stewart, W.F., Bigal, M.E., Kolodner, K., Dowson, A., Liberman, J.N., and Lipton, R.B. (2006). Familial risk of migraine: variation by proband age at onset and headache severity. *Neurology*, 66, 344–8.

Stewart, W.F., Lipton, R.B., and Liberman, J. (1996). Variation in migraine prevalence by race. *Neurology*, 47, 52–9.

St George-Hyslop, P.H. (2000). Molecular genetics of Alzheimer's disease. *Biological Psychiatry*, 47, 183–99.

Stovner, L., Hagen, K., Jensen, R., et al. (2007). The global burden of headache: a documentation of headache prevalence and disability worldwide. *Cephalalgia*, 27, 193–210.

Strittmatter, W.J., Saunders, A.M., Schmechel, D., et al. (1993). Apolipoprotein E: high-avidity binding to beta-amyloid and increased frequency of type 4 allele in late-onset familial Alzheimer disease. *Proceedings of the National Academy of Sciences of the United States of America*, 90, 1977–81.

Suzuki, K., Akama, T., Kawashima, A., Yoshihara, A., Yotsu, R.R., and Ishii, N. (2012). Current status of leprosy: epidemiology, basic science and clinical perspectives. *J Dermatol*, 39, 121–9.

Svendsen, T., Lossius, M., and Nakken, K.O. (2007). Age-specific prevalence of epilepsy in Oppland County, Norway. *Acta Neurologica Scandinavica*, 116, 307–11.

Szekely, C.A., Breitner, J.C., Fitzpatrick, A.L., et al. (2007). NSAID use and dementia risk in the Cardiovascular Health Study. Role of APOE and NSAID type. *Neurology*, 68, 1800–8.

Tanner, C.M., Kamel, F., Ross, G.W., et al. (2011). Rotenone, paraquat, and Parkinson's disease. *Environmental Health Perspectives*, 119, 866–72.

Tepper, S.J. (2012). Medication-overuse headache. *Continuum (Minneapolis Minn)*, 18, 807–22.

Tesfaye, S., Stevens, L.K., Stephenson, J.M., et al. (1996). Prevalence of diabetic peripheral neuropathy and its relation to glycaemic control and potential risk factors: the EURODIAB IDDM Complications Study. *Diabetologia*, 39, 1377–84.

Thurman, D.J., Beghi, E., Begley, C.E., et al. (2011). Standards for epidemiologic studies and surveillance of epilepsy. *Epilepsia*, 52 Suppl 7, 2–26.

Tolnay, M., and Frank, S. (2007). Pathology and genetics of frontotemporal lobar degeneration: an update. *Clin Neuropathol*, 26, 143–56.

Tonon, C., Guttmann, S., Volpini, M., Naccarato, S., Cortelli, P., and D'Alessandro, R. (2002). Prevalence and incidence of cluster headache in the Republic of San Marino. *Neurology*, 58, 1407–9.

Tsuang, D., Leverenz, J.B., Lopez, O.L., et al. (2012). GBA mutations increase risk for Lewy body disease with and without Alzheimer disease pathology. *Neurology*, 79, 1944–50.

Tsuang, D., Simpson, K., Larson, E.B., et al. (2006). Predicting Lewy body pathology in a community-based sample with clinical diagnosis of Alzheimer's disease. *Journal of Geriatric Psychiatry and Neurology*, 19, 195–201.

Uldall, P., Alving, J., Hansen, L.K., Kibaek, M., and Buchholt, J. (2006). The misdiagnosis of epilepsy in children admitted to a tertiary epilepsy centre with paroxysmal events. *Archives of Disease in Childhood*, 91, 219–21.

Ulrich, V., Gervil, M., Kyvik, K.O., Olesen, J., and Russell, M.B. (1999). Evidence of a genetic factor in migraine with aura: a population-based Danish twin study. *Annals of Neurology*, 45, 242–6.

Valera, E.M. and Berenbaum, H. (2003). Brain injury in battered women. *J Consult Clin Psychol*, 71, 797–804.

Van Deerlin, V.M., Sleiman, P.M., Martinez-Lage, M., et al. (2010). Common variants at 7p21 are associated with frontotemporal lobar degeneration with TDP-43 inclusions. *Nature Genetics*, 42, 234–9.

Wallin, M.T., Culpepper, W.J., Coffman, P., et al. (2012). The Gulf War era multiple sclerosis cohort: age and incidence rates by race, sex and service. *Brain*, 135, 1778–85.

Wallin, M.T., Page, W.F., and Kurtzke, J.F. (2004). Multiple sclerosis in US veterans of the Vietnam era and later military service: race, sex, and geography. *Annals of Neurology*, 55, 65–71.

Wang, S.J., Fuh, J.L., Lu, S.R., and Juang, K.D. (2001). Quality of life differs among headache diagnoses: analysis of SF-36 survey in 901 headache patients. *Pain*, 89, 285–92.

Ward, T.N. (2012). Migraine diagnosis and pathophysiology. *Continuum (Minneapolis Minn)*, 18, 753–63.

Warden, D. (2006). Military TBI during the Iraq and Afghanistan wars. *Journal of Head Trauma Rehabilitation*, 21, 398–402.

Waubant, E., Mowry, E.M., Krupp, L., et al. (2011). Common viruses associated with lower pediatric multiple sclerosis risk. *Neurology*, 76, 1989–95.

Werner, C., and Engelhard, K. (2007). Pathophysiology of traumatic brain injury. *British Journal of Anaesthesia*, 99, 4–9.

Wimo, A., Jonsson, L., Bond, J., Prince, M., Winblad, B., and Alzheimer Disease International (2013). The worldwide economic impact of dementia 2010. *Alzheimer's & Dementia*, 9, 1–11.e3.

Yaffe, K., Kanaya, A., Lindquist, K., et al. (2004). The metabolic syndrome, inflammation, and risk of cognitive decline. *Journal of the American Medical Association*, 292, 2237–42.

Zaccai, J., Mccracken, C., and Brayne, C. (2005). A systematic review of prevalence and incidence studies of dementia with Lewy bodies. *Age and Ageing*, 34, 561–6.

Zarrelli, M.M., Beghi, E., Rocca, W.A., and Hauser, W.A. (1999). Incidence of epileptic syndromes in Rochester, Minnesota: 1980–1984. *Epilepsia*, 40, 1708–14.

Ziegler, D.K., Hur, Y.M., Bouchard, T.J., Jr., Hassanein, R.S., and Barter, R. (1998). Migraine in twins raised together and apart. *Headache*, 38, 417–22.

Infectious diseases and prions

Davidson H. Hamer and Zulfiqar A. Bhutta

Introduction to infectious diseases and prions

Infectious diseases are a major cause of morbidity, disability, and mortality worldwide. During the last century, substantial gains have been made in public health interventions for the treatment, prevention, and control of infectious diseases. Nevertheless, recent decades have seen a worldwide pandemic of the human immunodeficiency virus (HIV), increasing antimicrobial resistance, and the emergence of many new viral, bacterial, fungal, and parasitic pathogens.

As a result of changes in a variety of different environmental, social, economic, and public health factors, morbidity and mortality due to infectious diseases have declined in industrialized countries during the last 150 years with the result being a gradual transition to chronic diseases including cardiovascular disease, diabetes mellitus, and cancer as major causes of mortality in these countries today. However, in contrast, in less developed countries, infectious diseases continue to contribute substantially to the overall burden of disease.

Detailed information on the definitions of infectious diseases, modes of transmission, and their control are provided in Chapter 11.3. An overview of issues related to emerging and re-emerging infections is provided in Chapter 8.17. Similarly, detailed information on diseases caused by sexually transmitted infections, HIV/acquired immunodeficiency syndrome (AIDS), tuberculosis, and malaria can be found in Chapters 8.12–8.15. This chapter will review the global burden of common infectious diseases in children and adults, determinants of the high infectious disease burden in resource-poor countries, and important aspects of the clinical manifestations, diagnosis, and treatment of the handful of infectious diseases that account for the major share of morbidity and mortality in children and adults worldwide.

Burden of infectious diseases

At the beginning of the twentieth century, infectious diseases were the leading cause of death throughout the world. At that time, three diseases—pneumonia, diarrhoea, and tuberculosis—were responsible for about 30 per cent of deaths in the United States. During the last century, there has been a decline in infectious diseases mortality in the United States from 797 deaths per 100,000 in 1900 to 36 per 100,000 in 1980. Despite substantial reductions

in all-cause mortality due to diarrhoeal disease and tuberculosis, pneumonia and influenza have continued to be major causes of mortality (Armstrong et al. 1999). Concurrent with the growth of the AIDS pandemic worldwide, there was a rise in mortality rates among persons aged 25 years and older in developed and less developed areas of the world.

In the late twentieth century, substantial reduction in child mortality occurred in low- and middle-income countries. The fall in the number of child deaths from 1960 to 1990 averaged 2.5 per cent per year and the risk of dying in the first 5 years of life halved—a major achievement in child survival. In the period from 1990 to 2001, mortality rates dropped an average of 1.1 per cent annually, mostly after the neonatal period. Deaths among children under 5 years of age dropped from nearly 12 million in 1990 to about 6.9 million in 2011. The Countdown to 2015, a multi-stakeholder group tracking progress towards the Millennium Development Goals in the 75 countries which have almost 98 per cent of the burden of maternal and child mortality, estimates that 30 countries have cut child mortality rates by half or more from 1990 to 2011, and two-thirds of the 75 Countdown countries have accelerated their progress since 2000 compared with the previous decade.

Newborn deaths, that is, deaths within the first month of life, now account for more than 40 per cent of child deaths in 35 Countdown countries, and 50 per cent or more in 12 countries. As deaths in children under the age of 5 have decreased, the proportion of these deaths that occur during the newborn period has increased. At the same time, the rate of progress in reducing newborn deaths has been far slower compared with the rate of progress in reducing deaths of older children. There has been considerable progress in the categorization and estimates for under-5 mortality through the work of the Interagency Group for child Mortality Estimation (IGME), the Child Health and Epidemiology Reference Group (CHERG), the Institute for Health Metrics and Evaluation (IHME), and the Countdown for 2015.

Neonatal causes, diarrhoea, pneumonia, and malaria account for the bulk of child deaths globally with regional variations (Liu et al. 2012). The recent distribution of these major causes of mortality in various World Health Organization (WHO) regions is presented in Fig. 8.11.1.

The South East Asian region accounts for the highest number of child deaths, over 3 million, whereas the highest mortality rates are generally seen in sub-Saharan Africa. Annually, sub-Saharan

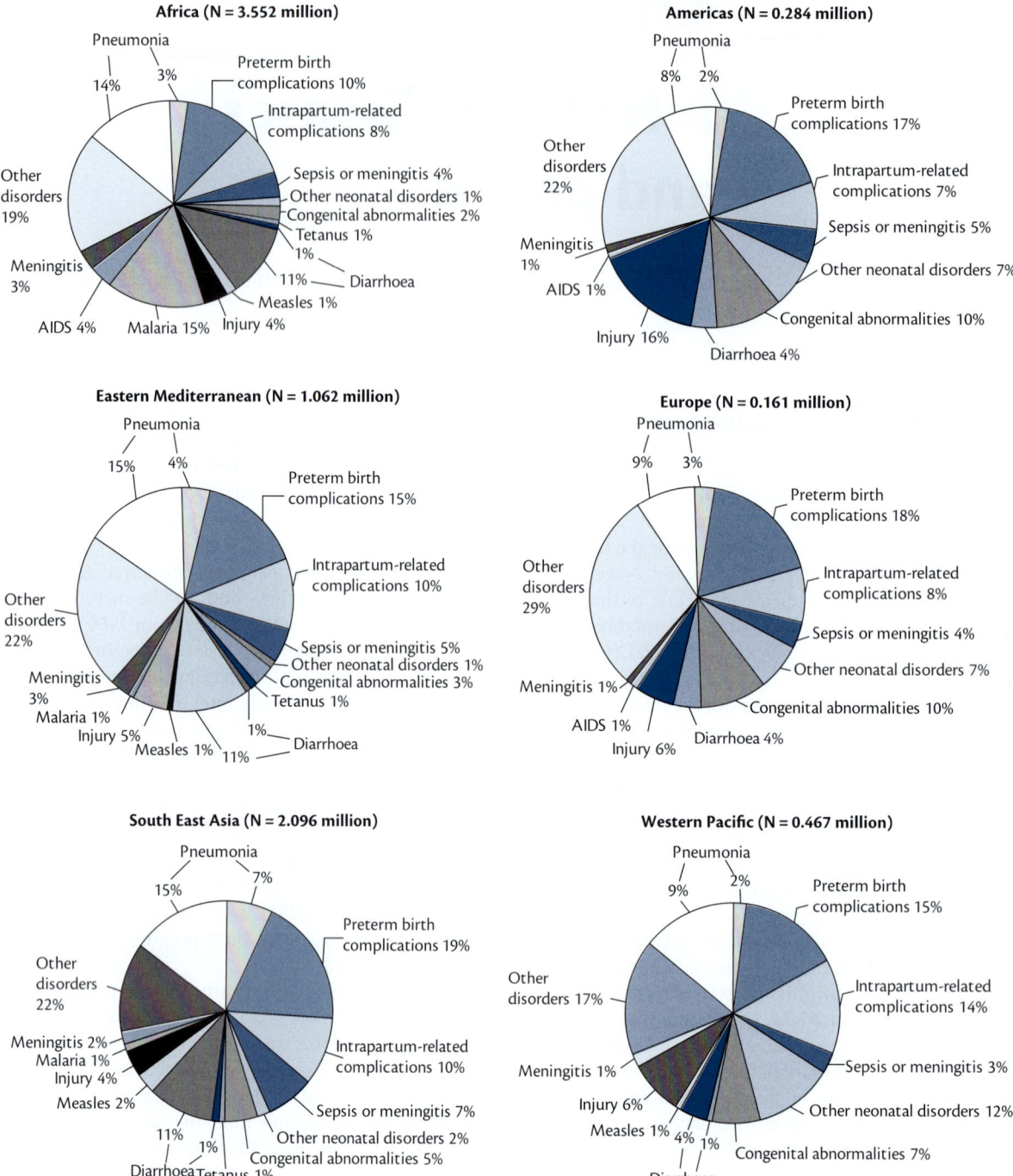

Fig. 8.11.1 Regional causes of child mortality 2010.

Reprinted from *The Lancet*, Volume 379, Issue 9832, Liu L. et al., Global, regional, and national causes of child mortality: an updated systematic analysis for 2010 with time trends since 2000, pp. 2151–61, Copyright © 2012, with permission from Elsevier, available from http://www.sciencedirect.com/science/journal/01406736.

Africa and South Asia share 41 and 34 per cent of child deaths respectively (Black et al. 2003). Only six countries account for half of worldwide deaths and 42 for 90 per cent of child deaths with the predominant causes being pneumonia, diarrhoea, and neonatal disorders, with surprisingly little contribution from malaria and AIDS (Table 8.11.1). Estimates from the 2010 Global Burden of Disease study (GBD 2010); (IHME n.d.), including a larger proportion of vital registration data, also suggested broadly comparable

figures for under-5 deaths, although some categories are clearly different, notably a higher proportion of malaria deaths among under-5 children in the GBD 2010 estimates and lower numbers for pneumonia deaths (Lozano et al. 2012).

In all, 99 per cent of neonatal deaths occur in poor countries (estimated average neonatal mortality rate (NMR) of 33/1000 live births) with the remaining divided among 39 high-income countries (estimated average NMR of 4/1000 live births) (Table 8.11.2).

Table 8.11.1 Global deaths for infectious diseases in 1990 and 2010 for all ages and both sexes combined (thousands) and age-standardized rates (per 100,000) with 95% UI and percentage change

	All ages deaths (thousands)			Age-standardized death rates (per 100,000)		
	1990	**2010**	**%Δ**	**1990**	**2010**	**%Δ**
All causes	46,511.2 (45,497.4–47,726.2)	52,769.7 (50,877.7–53 917·2)	13.5%	999.1 (979.2–1022.0)	784.5 (756.3–801.6)	−21.5
Communicable, maternal, neonatal, and nutritional disorders	15,859.2 (15,065.8–16,842.5)	13,156.4 (12,377.2–13 807.6)	−17.0%	271.1 (258.4–287.2)	189.8 (178.6–199.2)	−30.0
HIV/AIDS and tuberculosis	1770.3 (1600.2–2032.7)	2661.4 (2358.1–2895.7)	50.3%	39.3 (35.4–45.2)	39.4 (34.8–42.9)	0.2
Tuberculosis	1471.5 (1318.5–1716.1)	1196.0 (923.7–1376.8)	−18.7%	33.3 (29.8–38.7)	18.0 (13.9–20.7)	−46.0
HIV/AIDS	298.8 (242.0–378.5)	1465.4 (1334.2–1606.0)	390.4%	6.0 (4.8–7.7)	21.4 (19.4–23.5)	258.4
Disease syndromes, bacterial and viral diseases						
Sepsis and other infectious disorders of the newborn baby	534.6 (292.0–817.1)	513.7 (317.6–841.0)	−3.9%	7.4 (4.0–11.2)	7.1 (4.4–11.7)	−3.1
Diarrhoeal diseases	2487.4 (2306.8–2661.9)	1445.8 (1278.9–1607.0)	−41.9%	41.0 (38.3–43.6)	20.9 (18.5–23.3)	−49.0
Lower respiratory infections	3415.4 (3109.5–3650.9)	2814.4 (2487.8–3033.0)	−17.6%	62.3 (57.0–67.2)	41.0 (36.3–44.2)	−34.1
Upper respiratory infections	4.0 (3.6–4.2)	3.0 (2.7–3.4)	−23.6%	0.1 (0.1–0.1)	<0.05 (0.0–0.05)	−36.2
Otitis media	5.2 (0.0–61.0)	3.5 (0.0–39.8)	−33.5%	0.1 (0.0–1.0)	<0.05 (0.0–0.6)	−42.3
Meningitis	492.2 (444.1–583.3)	422.9 (360.2–471.7)	−14.1%	8.1 (7.4–9.4)	6.1 (5.1–6.7)	−25.0
Encephalitis	143.5 (126.7–168.1)	119.3 (98.0–137.1)	−16.9%	2.4 (2.1–2.8)	1.7 (1.4–2.0)	−28.3
Diphtheria	6.3 (0.0–53.0)	2.9 (0.0–24.9)	−53.5%	0.1 (0.0–0.8)	<0.05 (0.0–0.3)	−55.2
Whooping cough	166.5 (0.6–815.7)	81.4 (0.3–399.0)	−51.1%	2.3 (0.0–11.4)	1.1 (0.0–5.5)	−51.6
Tetanus	272.8 (163.4–456.1)	61.3 (31.0–114.0)	−77.5%	4.1 (2.4–7.6)	0.9 (0.4–1.6)	−78.8
Measles	631.2 (188.2–1492.6)	125.4 (41.3–295.5)	−80.1%	9.0 (2.7–21.3)	1.7 (0.6–4.1)	−80.6
Varicella	11.2 (0·0–75.0)	6.8 (0.0–46.4)	−38.9%	0.2 (0.0–1.3)	0.1 (0.0–0.7)	−50.8
Parasitic diseases and NTDs						
Malaria	975.7 (781.2–1239.5)	1169.5 (916.5–1526.9)	19.9%	16.6 (13.4–21.3)	16.7 (13.0–21.7)	0.5
Leishmaniasis	87.2 (50.6–138.4)	51.6 (33.2–76.1)	−40.9%	1.5 (0.9–2.4)	0.7 (0.5–1.1)	−51.3
Dengue	11.4 (3.7–23.5)	14.7 (6.1–24.3)	28.9%	0.2 (0.1–0.4)	0.2 (0.1–0.4)	3.2
Rabies	54.1 (32.4–103.4)	26.4 (15.2–45.2)	−51.2%	1.0 (0.6–1.9)	0.4 (0.2–0.7)	−61.7
Ascariasis	3.4 (0.0–16.4)	2.7 (0.0–13.0)	−21.7%	0.1 (0.0–0.2)	<0.05 (0.0–0.2)	−27.3
Other neglected tropical diseases	22.9 (14.3–29.5)	23.7 (16.6–30.9)	3.4%	0.5 (0.3–0.6)	0.3 (0.2–0.5)	−23.6

Data are deaths (95% uncertainty interval) or % change. %Δ, percentage change; NTDs, neglected tropical diseases.

Adapted from *The Lancet*, Volume 380, Issue 9859, Lozano, R. et al., Global and regional mortality from 235 causes of death for 20 age groups in 1990 and 2010: a systematic analysis for the Global Burden of Disease Study 2010, pp. 2095–128, Copyright © 2012, with permission from Elsevier, available from http://www.sciencedirect.com/science/journal/01406736.

As of the end of 2012, the Joint United Nations Programme on HIV/AIDS (UNAIDS) estimated that there were 34 million people living with HIV infection in 2011 (range 31.4–35.9 million) and that 2.5 million new infections occurred during 2011 along with 1.7 million deaths due to AIDS. With around 69 per cent of all people living with HIV residing in sub-Saharan Africa, the region carries the greatest burden of the epidemic. Epidemics in Asia have remained relatively stable and are still largely concentrated among high-risk groups. Conversely, the number of people living with HIV in Eastern Europe and Central Asia has more than tripled since 2000. Sadly, tuberculosis is responsible for approximately 10 per cent of HIV-associated deaths of children and adults in sub-Saharan Africa, despite substantial increases in the numbers of HIV-infected people receiving antiretroviral therapy.

Lower respiratory tract infections are the second leading cause of disability-adjusted life years (DALYs) worldwide, accounting for 4.6 per cent of the total, and diarrhoea is fourth, accounting for 3.6 per cent (Murray et al. 2012). HIV/AIDS is fifth on the list accounting for 3.3 per cent, while malaria and tuberculosis rank seventh and thirteenth, accounting for 3.3 and 2.0 per cent of

Table 8.11.2 Estimated numbers of deaths by cause in 2010

	Estimated number (millions)
Neonates aged 0–27 days	
Preterm birth complications	1.078 (0.916–1.325)
Intrapartum-related complications	0.717 (0.610–0.876)
Sepsis or meningitis	0.393 (0.252–0.552)
Pneumonia[a]	0.325 (0.209–0.470)
Congenital abnormalities	0.270 (0.207–0.366)
Other disorders	0.181 (0.115–0.284)
Tetanus	0.058 (0.020–0.276)
Diarrhoea[b]	0.050 (0.017–0.151)
Children aged 1–59 months	
Other neonatal disorders	1.356 (1.112–1.581)
Pneumonia[a]	1.071 (0.977–1.176)
Diarrhoea[b]	0.751 (0.538–1.031)
Malaria	0.564 (0.432–0.709)
Injury	0.354 (0.274–0.429)
Meningitis	0.180 (0.136–0.237)
AIDS	0.159 (0.131–0.185)
Measles	0.114 (0.092–0.176)

Uncertainty range (UR) is defined as the 2.5–97.5 percentile. Other disorders in children aged 1–59 months included congenital abnormalities, causes originated during the perinatal period, cancer, pertussis, severe malnutrition, and other specified causes. Intrapartum-related complications were formerly referred to as birth asphyxia.

[a] The estimated number of deaths in children younger than 5 years overall is 1.396 million (UR 1.189–1.642 million).

[b] The estimated number of deaths in children younger than 5 years overall is 0.801 million (UR 0.555–1.182 million).

Reprinted from *The Lancet*, Volume 379, Issue 9832, Liu L., et al., Global, regional, and national causes of child mortality: an updated systematic analysis for 2010 with time trends since 2000, pp. 2151–61, Copyright © 2012, with permission from Elsevier, available from http://www.sciencedirect.com/science/journal/01406736.

DALYs, respectively. In high-income countries, lower respiratory infections remain a leading cause of death. No communicable disease is among the top ten leading causes of DALYs in high-income countries. In contrast, pneumonia, HIV/AIDS, diarrhoea, and malaria rank among the top ten causes of death and DALYs in low- and middle-income countries.

Factors responsible for the decline in infectious diseases in industrialized nations during the last century include improved nutrition, safer food and water supplies, improved hygiene and sanitation, the introduction of antimicrobial agents, and immunizations, all of which resulted in decreased host susceptibility and reductions in disease transmission (Cohen 2000). While there have been substantial reductions in morbidity and mortality due to communicable diseases in the last century, there remain significant gaps in child and adult mortality between rich and poor countries.

Apart from the immediate causes of infections in childhood, a number of determinants contribute to the high burden of infectious diseases in developing countries. These include several distal

determinants such as income, social status, and education, which work through an intermediate level of environmental and behavioural risk factors. These risk factors, in turn, lead to the proximal causes of death (nearer in time to the terminal event), such as undernutrition, infectious diseases, and injury (Rice et al. 2000). The major social determinants affecting the mortality and morbidity of young children include poverty, crowding, poor housing conditions, indoor air pollution, malnutrition, inequity, lack of education, failure to implement breastfeeding and complementary feeding programmes, the presence of debilitating disease in addition to infections, complications of labour and low birth weight (LBW), inadequate health-related social behaviours and practices, and other social and cultural determinants of health.

Specific disease categories

As described in the previous section, a limited number of infectious diseases are responsible for a large proportion of the total global burden of morbidity and mortality, especially in resource-limited areas of the world. This section will provide an overview of the major types of infectious diseases responsible for the bulk of acute and chronic morbidity and mortality of children and adults worldwide. Detailed information on approaches for the prevention and control of these diseases is available in Chapter 11.3.

Acute respiratory infections

Acute respiratory infections (ARIs) are classified as upper or lower respiratory tract infections. Upper respiratory tract infections include the common cold, otitis media, sinusitis, and pharyngitis while lower respiratory tract infections include laryngitis, tracheitis, bronchitis, bronchiolitis, pneumonia, and any combination thereof. ARIs are not only confined to the respiratory tract, but may also have systemic effects due to extension of infection into the bloodstream, the production of microbial toxins, inflammation, and reduced lung function.

ARIs, especially bronchiolitis and pneumonia, are the most common causes of both illness and mortality in children under 5 years. In adults, pneumonia and influenza are major causes of morbidity and mortality in developed as well as less-developed nations.

Global and regional epidemiology

The annual incidence in children in Europe and North America is 34–40 cases per 1000, higher than at any other time of life, except perhaps in adults older than 75 or 80 years of age. For example, in the United States, there are about 4 million adults who develop pneumonia each year, of whom greater than 1 million are hospitalized.

Pneumonia is the most severe and largest killer of children, causing almost 20 per cent of all child deaths globally. Recent estimates indicate that there are approximately 1.4 million pneumonia deaths annually, with 75 per cent of all childhood pneumonia cases occurring in just 15 countries (Liu et al. 2012). There was a decrease in pneumonia deaths of about 0.45 million between 2000 and 2010.

Most ARI deaths are due to pneumonia. The annual incidence of pneumonia is estimated at 156 million new cases per year, of which 11–20 million (7–13 per cent) cases are severe enough to require hospitalization. Serious neonatal infections account for

30–50 per cent of neonatal mortality in different regions, and it is difficult to disentangle sepsis and deaths from pneumonia. With the inclusion of neonatal pneumonia, recent estimates indicate that pneumonia is the single largest contributor to child mortality, accounting for about 18 per cent of all under-5 deaths globally. It is also important to note that in contrast to diarrhoeal deaths where mortality rates have declined dramatically, despite the introduction of a global programme for the control of ARIs almost 15 years ago, there has been only a small reduction in the overall burden of pneumonia deaths. A recent assessment of the global burden of severe pneumonia estimated that in 2010 some 11.9 million (95 per cent confidence interval (CI) 10.3–13.9 million) episodes of severe and 3.0 million (2.1–4.2 million) episodes of very severe acute lower respiratory infections (ALRIs) resulted in hospital admissions in young children worldwide (Nair et al. 2011). Incidence was higher in boys than in girls, the sex disparity being greatest in South Asian studies. Using data from 37 hospital studies reporting case fatality ratios for severe ALRI, we estimated that roughly 265,000 (95 per cent CI 160,000–450,000) in-hospital deaths took place in young children, with 99 per cent of these deaths in developing countries. Therefore, the data suggest that although 62 per cent of children with severe ALRI were treated in hospitals, 81 per cent of deaths probably took place at home.

In terms of the overall burden of disease, upper and lower ARIs account for a major proportion of outpatient visits, antibiotic prescriptions, and healthcare costs in the United States and Western Europe. Despite gains in the availability and quality of healthcare in industrialized countries, ARIs, especially lower respiratory tract infections, remain a major cause of morbidity and mortality for adults and children. In fact, even today pneumonia and influenza together are the sixth most common cause for death among adults in the United States. Recovery from pneumonia in the elderly takes longer and complications and mortality are also more frequent than in younger populations. Pneumonia is one of the most common causes of hospitalization and decreased activities of daily living among the elderly. Risk factors for death from pneumonia in adults include advanced age, alcohol consumption, leucopenia, bacteraemia, hypoxaemia, co-morbid conditions such as diabetes mellitus, congestive heart failure, active malignancies, and immunosuppression, and certain signs and symptoms including hypothermia, hyperthermia, tachypnoea, hypotension, and altered mental status. In addition, post-obstructive pneumonia,

aspiration pneumonia, and infections due to *Staphylococcus aureus* and Gram-negative bacilli are independently associated with increased mortality risk.

Many factors such as the presence of certain co-morbid medical conditions, use of certain drugs, changes in physiochemical characteristics of the non-specific host defence system such as cilia and mucus of the respiratory tract, malnutrition, and mechanical devices contribute to an increased incidence of pneumonia among the elderly. However, an important predisposing factor to the increased incidence of infections is the age-associated decline in immune responsiveness. Changes in immune response not only decrease resistance to pathogens but also contribute to increased morbidity and mortality due to respiratory infections.

Aetiology

A wide range of different bacterial and viral pathogens is responsible for community-acquired pneumonia in children and adults. Foremost among them is *Streptococcus pneumoniae*, which accounts for up to half of all cases. Other commonly encountered bacterial pathogens include *Haemophilus influenzae*, *Chlamydia pneumoniae*, *Moraxella catarrhalis*, *Legionella pneumophila*, *Mycoplasma pneumoniae*, *Staphylococcus aureus*, and Gram-negative rods such as *Klebsiella pneumoniae* and *Escherichia coli* (Table 8.11.3). During recent years, the role of viral pathogens in the aetiology of ALRIs has been increasingly described. While influenza is well recognized as a cause of viral pneumonia, several studies have demonstrated the importance of parainfluenza virus, respiratory syncytial virus (RSV), adenovirus, and human metapneumovirus.

Issues in presentation and diagnosis

Currently, the standard WHO algorithm for ARIs defines non-severe pneumonia as cough or difficult and fast breathing (respiratory rate of 50 breaths per minute or more for children aged 2–11 months; or respiratory rate of 40 breaths per minute or more for children aged 12–59 months) and either documented fever of above 101°F or chest in-drawing. Severe pneumonia is defined as having cough or difficult breathing, with tachypnoea and in-drawing of the lower chest wall (with or without fast breathing); and very severe pneumonia—cough or difficult breathing with one or more danger signs (central cyanosis, inability to drink, or unusually sleepy). The WHO has defined pneumonia solely on

Table 8.11.3 Pathogen-specific causes of childhood and adult pneumonia

Age range	Most common causative organism
Neonates (from birth to 30 days after birth)	*Streptococcus pyogenes*, *Staphylococcus aureus*, and *Escherichia coli*
Infants (from 3 weeks to 4 months)	*S. pneumoniae*
Infants older than 4 months and preschool-aged children	Respiratory viruses and *S. pneumoniae*
Children in developing countries	*S. aureus* and *Haemophilus influenzae* including non-typable strains
Adults—outpatient	*S. pneumoniae*, *Mycoplasma pneumoniae*, *H. influenzae*, *Chlamydophila pneumoniae*, and respiratory viruses
Adults—inpatient	*S. pneumoniae*, *M. pneumoniae*, *C. pneumoniae*, *H. influenzae*, *Legionella pneumophila*, respiratory viruses, and aspiration
Adults—intensive care unit	*S. pneumoniae*, *S. aureus*, *L. pneumophila*, Gram-negative bacilli, and *H. influenzae*

the basis of clinical findings obtained by visual inspection and setting respiratory rate cut-offs. It is recognized that mortality in children due to ARIs could be reduced by one-half if early detection and appropriate treatment could be provided.

In contrast to the simple, clinical definition of pneumonia recommended by the WHO for use in developing countries, pneumonia in resource-rich countries is usually based on the presence of characteristic signs and symptoms (e.g. dry or productive cough, tachypnoea, fever, focal findings on respiratory examination), hypoxaemia, and the presence of infiltrates on chest radiograph. In general, the elderly tend to present with fewer or atypical symptoms of pneumonia than younger patients and therefore non-specific features such as fever or mental status change may be indicators of an underlying lower respiratory tract infection.

Microbiological studies can be pursued to support the diagnosis of pneumonia due to specific infectious agents and to facilitate decision-making for antibiotic management. While broad-spectrum empirical antimicrobial coverage is recommended in various guidelines, there is a potential risk for clinical failure and increased mortality if inappropriate antibiotic therapy is initiated. If available and adequate quality specimens can be obtained, blood cultures and sputum Gram stain and culture should be performed. Rapid diagnostic tests may be useful when specific diagnoses are being considered such as RSV, influenza, or *L. pneumophila*.

Clinical approaches for the management of childhood pneumonia are significantly hampered by the lack of a gold standard, as classic microbiological methods have poor sensitivity and current algorithms lack sufficient specificity. It is therefore likely that community strategies for the recognition and management of pneumonia by ancillary health workers that rely on simple clinical criteria, other than auscultation, will overdiagnose bacterial pneumonia. There are legitimate concerns that widespread use of first-line antibiotics for all ARIs will lead to loss of effectiveness.

Evidence-based interventions

Only in the early 1980s, long after immunization and diarrhoea control programmes were launched, did the international community become aware of the epidemiological magnitude of pneumonia in children. This need for action led the WHO and the United Nations Children's Fund (UNICEF) to decide that reduction of mortality from pneumonia should be the main objective of the initial ARI programme. Since early microbiological studies of lung aspirates taken from hospitalized, untreated children with pneumonia in developing countries showed that bacteria were present in more than 50 per cent of cases and it was recognized that bacterial pathogens were responsible for the most severe cases, it became apparent that prompt treatment with a full course of effective antibiotics could be life-saving.

Antibiotic treatment of pneumonia

Although recommendations for antibiotic therapy for pneumonia are based on aetiological diagnosis, identification of the causative organism in routine clinical care is very difficult and empirical antibiotic therapy is often instituted. Guidelines for the treatment of pneumonia in immunocompetent adults in industrialized nations generally recommend a macrolide or doxycycline for outpatients; an advanced macrolide such as azithromycin or clarithromycin plus a beta-lactam or a respiratory fluoroquinolone alone for less acutely ill inpatients; and a beta-lactam plus either an advanced macrolide or respiratory fluoroquinolone for adults requiring intensive care (Mandell et al. 2007).

The various modalities for antibiotic treatment in children according to disease severity are shown in Table 8.11.4.

The current WHO treatment guidelines for ARIs were developed before the rise of HIV infection in sub-Saharan Africa, and they do not include empiric treatment for *Pneumocystis jirovecii* (formerly *P. carinii*) pneumonia. Daily administration of co-trimoxazole is

Table 8.11.4 Treatment of paediatric pneumonia according to disease severity

Signs/symptoms	Classification	Treatment
Fast breathing: ≥ 60 breaths/min in child aged < 2 months ≥ 50 breaths/min in child aged 2–11 months ≥ 40 breaths/min in child aged 1–5 years	Pneumonia	Home care
		Give appropriate antibiotics for 5 days
Definite crackles on auscultations		Soothe the throat and relieve the cough with a safe remedy
		Advise the mother when to return immediately
		Follow up in 2 days
Signs of pneumonia plus chest wall in-drawing	Severe pneumonia	Admit to hospital
		Give recommended antibiotics
		Manage airway
		Treat high fever if present
Signs of severe pneumonia plus central cyanosis, severe respiratory distress, and inability to drink	Very severe pneumonia	Admit to hospital
		Give the recommended antibiotics
		Give oxygen
		Manage airway
		Antipyretics

advocated since it reduces deaths from opportunistic infections in symptomatic HIV-infected children, including pneumonia caused by *P. jirovecii*. A multicentre randomized control trial, by the APPIS Group, showed that standard empiric therapy for severe pneumonia with injectable penicillin or oral amoxicillin in severe pneumonia in infants is inadequate where HIV prevalence is high (Addo-Yobo et al. 2004). There is also concern that the current diagnostic criteria for non-severe pneumonia may be picking up non-bacterial infections as antibiotic therapy has been shown to add little in terms of improved outcomes compared to placebo. However, management of severe pneumonia in community settings by CHWs using oral amoxicillin has been shown to be both feasible and associated with improved outcomes (Bari et al. 2011; Soofi et al. 2012a). This has major implications for saving lives of children with pneumonia in difficult circumstances where referral may not be possible.

The benefits of the WHO guidelines would be enhanced if they could also be applied (with modification) throughout areas with high rates of HIV infection and where the pneumonia burden is high, even in HIV-negative children.

Integrated management of childhood infections

In the mid 1980s, the WHO initiated a control programme for ARIs that focused on cases managed by health workers. The current case management of ARIs has been incorporated into the global integrated management of childhood infections (IMCI) which train health workers to recognize fast breathing, lower chest wall in-drawing, or danger signs in children with respiratory symptoms (such as cyanosis or inability to drink).

Preventive measures

Poverty, overcrowding, air pollution, malnutrition, harmful traditional practices, and delayed and inappropriate case management are important underlying determinants for high ARI case fatality rates. Preventive strategies for pneumonia include immunizing children with the pneumococcal, measles, and *H. influenzae* type b (Hib) vaccines, hand washing, reduction of the incidence of LBW, ensuring warmth after birth and appropriate feeding, promoting adequate nutrition (including exclusive breastfeeding and zinc intake), and reducing indoor air pollution (Bhutta 2007).

Three vaccines have the potential to substantially reduce deaths in children under 5 years of age—(the Hib, measles, and pneumococcal vaccines). Two kinds of vaccines are currently available against pneumococci: a 23-valent polysaccharide vaccine (23-PSV), which is more appropriate for adults than children, and several different formulations of protein-conjugated polysaccharide vaccines (PCV), which contain 7, 10, and 13 serotypes of *S. pneumoniae*. Rates of invasive pneumococcal disease (IPD) have decreased among immunized children and non-immunized adults since the introduction of the heptavalent PCV for use in infants in the United States in 2000. Moreover, newer versions of the PCV have the potential to significantly reduce pneumonia deaths in developing countries. While the Hib vaccine is now being used in many resource-poor countries, scaling up of the PCV lags behind.

Controlled trials of hand washing promotion in child-care centres in developed countries have reported significant reduction (12–32 per cent) in rates of upper respiratory tract infections.

A community-based cluster randomized trial of hand washing promotion from Pakistan also reported that frequent hand washing (with or without soap) led to a 50 per cent reduction in pneumonia incidence and a 36 per cent lower incidence of impetigo.

About 3 billion people still rely on solid fuels, 2.4 billion on biomass, and the rest on coal, mostly in China. Globally, there is marked regional variation in solid fuel use in relation to poverty with use rates of less than 20 per cent in Europe and Central Asia and greater than 80 per cent in sub-Saharan Africa and South Asia, intricately linking to poverty. More than half of all the deaths and 83 per cent of DALYs lost attributable to solid fuel use occur as a result of lower respiratory tract infection (pneumonia) in children under 5 years of age and a systematic review of the evidence for the impact of indoor air pollution on a wide range of health outcomes including pneumonia indicates substantial benefits on pneumonia prevention.

Previously, a meta-analysis of trials of daily preventive zinc supplementation showed a significant impact on pneumonia incidence (Zinc Investigators' Collaborative Group 1999). An update of this meta-analysis reaffirms the impact on reduction in the risk of respiratory tract infections (by 8 per cent, respectively) but not on duration of disease (Aggarwal 2007).

Public health implications

Despite the introduction of a global programme for the control of ARIs almost 15 years ago, there have been limited reductions in the overall burden of deaths from pneumonia. The bulk of deaths from childhood pneumonia disproportionately affect the poor who have higher exposure rates to risk factors for developing ARIs, such as overcrowding, poor environmental conditions, malnutrition, and also limited access to curative health services. The importance of reaching the poor with pneumonia in community settings must be underscored. Such strategies involve recognizing and ambulatory management of pneumonia in community settings through community health workers, assuring transportation and access to facilities for severe pneumonia and availability of antibiotics.

Neonatal sepsis

Sepsis and meningitis are significant causes of morbidity and mortality in newborns, particularly in preterm, LBW infants. Serious infections among newborns are estimated to cause 30–40 per cent of neonatal deaths, especially in rural populations. Neonatal sepsis may be defined using clinical criteria (Table 8.11.5) and/or microbiological testing, by positive blood and/or cerebrospinal fluid (CSF) cultures. It may also be classified according to the time of disease onset: early onset (EOS) and late onset (LOS). Meningitis can occur as a part of sepsis in both the EOS and LOS time periods or as focal infection with LOS disease. The distinction has clinical relevance, as EOS disease is mainly due to bacteria acquired before and during delivery, and LOS disease to bacteria acquired after delivery (nosocomial or community sources). In the literature, however, there is little consensus as to what age limits apply, with EOS ranging from 48 hours to 6 days after delivery.

Global and regional epidemiology

The Child Health Epidemiology Reference Group (CHERG) estimated that 40.3 per cent (3.072 million) of 7.6 million under-5 deaths in 2010 occurred in neonates. Among newborn deaths,

Table 8.11.5 Clinical criteria for diagnosis of neonatal sepsis and meningitis[a]

Sepsis	Meningitis
Symptoms	*General signs*
Convulsions	Drowsiness
Inability to feed	Reduced feeding
Unconsciousness	Unconsciousness
Lethargy	Lethargy
Fever (> 37.7°C or feels hot)	High-pitched cry
Hypothermia (< 35.5°C or feels cold)	Apnoea
Signs	*Specific signs*
Severe chest in-drawing	Convulsions
Reduced movement	Bulging fontanelle
Crepitations	
Cyanosis	

[a] The more symptoms a neonate has, the higher the probability of the disease.

major causes included preterm birth complications (14.1 per cent; 1.078 million, uncertainty range (UR) 0.916–1.325), intrapartum-related complications, previously labelled as birth asphyxia, accounted for 0.717 million deaths (9.4 per cent, UR 0.610–0.876), whereas sepsis or meningitis accounted for 0.393 million (5.4 per cent, UR 0.252–0.552) neonatal deaths. The reported incidence of neonatal sepsis varies from 7.1 to 38 per 1000 live births in Asia, from 6.5 to 23 per 1000 live births in Africa, from 3.5 to 8.9 per 1000 live births in South America and the Caribbean, and from 6–9 per 1000 live births in the United States and Australia. The incidence of neonatal meningitis is 0.1–0.4/1000 live births and is higher in developing countries. Despite major advancement in neonatal care, overall case-fatality rates from sepsis range from 2 to as high as 50 per cent.

Unfortunately, hospitals in developing countries are also hot beds of infection transmission, especially multidrug-resistant nosocomial infections. Reported rates of neonatal sepsis vary from 6.5 to 38 per 1000 live hospital-born babies and the rates of bloodstream infection range from 1.7 to 33 per 1000 live births, with rates in Africa clustering around 20 and in South Asia around 15 per 1000 live births. Factors responsible for hospital-acquired neonatal sepsis include lack of aseptic technique for procedures, inadequate hand hygiene and glove use, deficient sterilization and disinfection practices, overuse of invasive devices, re-use of disposable supplies without adequate sterilization, re-use of single-use vials, overcrowded and understaffed labour and delivery rooms, unhygienic bathing and skin care, contaminated bottle feedings, inappropriate and prolonged use of antibiotics, and lack of effective infection control practices.

Aetiology

In general, Gram-negative pathogens are responsible for a substantial proportion of EOS. In contrast to industrialized countries where group B streptococci (GBS) are common causes of neonatal sepsis, *Klebsiella pneumoniae* is an important aetiology in developing countries. LOS is most commonly due to *E. coli, S. aureus,*

S. pyogenes, *S. pneumoniae*, and *Salmonella* spp. The organisms causing neonatal sepsis and meningitis in low and middle income countries are listed in Table 8.11.6.

Evidence-based interventions to address neonatal infections

Child survival and safe motherhood strategies have yet to adequately address mortality in the neonatal period. The fourth Millennium Development Goal (MDG 4) commits the international community to reducing mortality in children aged under 5 years by two-thirds from 1990 base figures by 2015. Real progress in saving newborns will depend upon provision of a good mix of preventive and therapeutic services.

Medical treatment

Reaching and treating sick newborn infants promptly is critical to survival. Normally, health workers use a combination of ampicillin and gentamicin for suspected cases of neonatal sepsis (Table 8.11.7). However, increasing antibiotic resistance among common organisms causing neonatal sepsis in both community and hospital settings presents a challenge to the selection of appropriate antibiotics. Case management of neonatal infections is mainly provided through child-health services, both in facilities and through family-community care. Scaling up of emergency obstetric care and sick neonatal care can be combined. Guidelines for integrated management of pregnancy and childbirth identify opportunities for assimilating maternal and neonatal care. Similarly IMCI has been widely implemented as the main approach for addressing child health in health systems. However, IMCI management guidelines rely on the sick child being brought to a health facility. The recent modification of IMCI to include the neonatal period (IMNCI) and expansion to community settings has now been included as a public health strategy in many countries including India. The ideal strategy would be to provide a linked strategy of care in community settings with referral to facilities in case of need or if needed, antibiotic therapy in first-level facilities.

Following the demonstration of significant reduction in neonatal mortality with the use of oral co-trimoxazole and injectable gentamicin by community health workers, this strategy could be employed in circumstances where referral is difficult. Currently in some health systems, outreach health workers, community nutrition, and child development workers are being trained to visit all mothers and neonates at home two to three times within the first 10 days, starting soon after birth, to provide home-based preventive care/health promotion and to detect neonates with sickness requiring referral. Extra contacts are proposed for LBW babies. With slight modifications, these visits can also be used to provide postpartum care to the mother.

Preventive measures

Preventive interventions need to bridge the continuum of care from pregnancy, through childbirth and the neonatal period, and beyond. Lack of positive health-related behaviour, education, and poverty are underlying causes of many neonatal deaths, either through increasing the prevalence of risk factors such as maternal infection or by reducing access to effective care.

Attempts to reduce the proportion of LBW births at the population level have had limited success. Many deaths in preterm babies and in those born at term with LBW can be prevented with

Table 8.11.6 Distribution of all isolates by age of onset

Organism isolated	N	< 7 days of life % (95% CI)	N	8–59 days of life % (95% CI)	N	60–90 days of life % (95% CI)
Staphylococcus aureus	33	11.7 (8.0–15.5)	268	15.0 (13.4–16.7)	1	2.3 (0.0–6.7)
Group A streptococci/*Streptococcus pyogenes*	4	1.4 (0.0–2.8)	50	2.8 (2.0–3.6)	8	18.2 (6.8–29.6)
Group B streptococci (GBS)	19	6.7 (3.8–9.7)	31	1.7 (1.1–2.4)	0	0.0 (–)
Group D streptococci/enterococci	4	1.4 (0.0–2.8)	13	0.7 (0.3–1.1)	0	0.0 (–)
Streptococcus pneumoniae	13	4.6 (2.1–7.1)	93	5.2 (4.2–6.3)	14	31.8 (18.1–45.6)
Other/unspecified *Streptococcus* spp.	24	8.5 (5.3–11.8)	50	2.8 (2.0–3.6)	0	0.0 (–)
Other/unspecified Gram-positives[a]	0	0.0 (–)	112	6.3 (5.2–7.4)	0	0.0 (–)
All Gram-positives	97	34.4 (28.9–39.9)	617	34.6 (32.4–36.8)	23	52.3 (37.5–67.0)
Klebsiella pneumoniae	22	7.8 (4.7–10.9)	232	13.0 (11.4–14.6)	2	4.5 (0.0–10.7)
Other/unspecified *Klebsiella* spp.	10	3.5 (1.4–5.7)	15	0.8 (0.4–1.3)	0	0.0 (–)
Escherichia coli	46	16.3 (12.0–20.6)	320	17.9 (16.2–19.7)	1	2.3 (0.0–6.7)
Pseudomonas spp.	22	7.8 (4.7–10.9)	166	9.3 (8.0–10.7)	1	2.3 (0.0–6.7)
Enterobacter spp.	10	3.5 (1.4–5.7)	59	3.3 (2.5–4.1)	0	0.0 (–)
Serratia spp.	0	0.0 (–)	40	2.2 (1.6–2.9)	1	2.3 (0.0–6.7)
Proteus spp.	6	2.1 (0.4–3.8)	7	0.4 (0.1–0.7)	0	0.0 (–)
Salmonella spp.	1	0.4 (0.0–1.0)	26	1.5 (0.9–2.0)	6	13.6 (3.5–23.8)
Haemophilus influenzae	2	0.7 (0.0–1.7)	30	1.7 (1.1–2.3)	4	9.1 (0.6–17.6)
Neisseria meningitidis	0	0.0 (–)	13	0.7 (0.3–1.1)	0	0.0 (–)
Acinetobacter spp.	19	6.7 (3.8–8.7)	113	6.3 (2.2–7.5)	3	6.8 (0.0–14.3)
Other/unspecified Gram-negatives[b]	42	14.9 (10.7–19.0)	59	3.3 (2.5–4.1)	1	2.3 (0.0–6.7)
All Gram-negatives	180	63.8 (58.2–69.4)	1080	60.5 (58.3–62.8)	19	43.2 (28.5–57.8)
Non-stated/undetermined	5	1.8 (0.2–3.3)	87	4.9 (3.9–5.9)	2	4.5 (0.0–10.7)
Total	282	100.0 (n/a)	1784	100.0 (n/a)	44	100.0 (n/a)

[a] Includes data for *Aerococcus* spp., *Bacillus* spp., and others.

[b] Includes data for *Citrobacter* spp., *Moraxella* spp., *Shigella* spp., *Aeromonas* spp. and others. Data were also extracted for coagulase-negative staphylococci: ≤ 7 days of life—3 isolates; 7–59 days of life—880 isolates; 60–90 days of life—0 isolates.

Adapted from Waters, D. et al., Aetiology of community-acquired neonatal sepsis in low- and middle-income countries, *Journal of Global Health*, Volume 1, Issue 2, pp. 154–70, Copyright © 2011, reproduced under the Creative Commons Attribution License 3.0.

extra attention to warmth, feeding, and prevention or early treatment of infections. In developing countries, 90 per cent of mothers deliver babies at home without a skilled health professional present. Simple low-cost interventions, notably tetanus toxoid vaccination, provision of clean delivery kits, exclusive breastfeeding, counselling for birth preparedness, and breastfeeding promotion through peer counsellors and women's groups, have been shown to reduce newborn morbidity and mortality (Darmstadt et al. 2005; Seward et al. 2012). Postnatally, kangaroo mother care for LBW infants, hand washing and decreased congestion in facilities, attention to environmental hygiene and sterilization, and antibiotics for neonatal infections, are additional health system measures. Alcohol-based antiseptics for hand hygiene are an appealing innovation because of their efficacy in reducing hand contamination and their ease of use, especially when sinks and supplies for hand-washing are limited. Creation of a 'step-down' neonatal care unit for very LBW

babies with mothers providing primary care also led to early discharge and reduction in hospital-acquired infection rates in another nursery in Pakistan. These interventions can be delivered through facility-based services, population outreach, and family-community strategies.

Early initiation of breastfeeding affects neonatal health outcomes through several mechanisms. Mothers who suckle their offspring shortly after birth have a greater chance of successfully establishing and sustaining breastfeeding throughout infancy, and also provide a variety of immune and non-immune components that accelerate intestinal maturation, resistance to infection, and epithelial recovery from infection. Prelacteal feeding with non-human milk antigens may disrupt normal physiological gut priming. Although the WHO currently recommends dry cord care for newborns, application of antiseptics such as chlorhexidine has been shown to be effective against both Gram-positive and Gram-negative bacteria and, in

Table 8.11.7 Antimicrobial therapy of neonatal meningitis and sepsis

Patient group	Likely aetiology	Antimicrobial choice	
		Developed countries	Developing countries
Sepsis			
Immunocompetent children	Developed countries: 　Group B streptococci, *E. coli* Developing countries: 　*Klebsiella* spp. 　*Pseudomonas* spp. 　*Salmonella* spp.	Ampicillin or penicillin plus an aminoglycoside	Ampicillin or penicillin plus gentamicin Or co-trimoxazole plus gentamicin
Meningitis			
Immunocompetent children (age < 3 months)	Developed countries: 　Group B streptococci 　*E. coli* 　*L. monocytogenes* Developing countries: 　*S. pneumoniae* 　*E. coli*	Ampicillin plus ceftriaxone or cefotaxime	Ampicillin plus gentamicin
Immunodeficient	Gram-negative bacilli *L. monocytogenes*	Ampicillin plus ceftazidime	

community studies, to reduce rates of cord infection and sepsis in newborns. Recent community-based studies evaluating the role of cord application of 4 per cent chlorhexidine suggest that this could be a very useful strategy to prevent neonatal sepsis in circumstances with high risk of infections (Mullany et al. 2006; Arifeen et al. 2012; Soofi et al. 2012b). A closely related issue is the need for general skin care. A randomized controlled trial of topical application of sunflower seed oil to preterm infants in an Egyptian neonatal intensive care unit showed that treated infants had substantially improved skin condition and half the risk of LOS infection (Darmstadt et al. 2004).

At least two doses of tetanus toxoid should be given during pregnancy so that protective antibodies can be transferred to the fetus, to protect it from neonatal tetanus. Women with a history of prolonged rupture of membranes, especially if preterm, should be given prophylactic antibiotics. This approach improves neonatal outcome by increasing the latency of pregnancy. Maternal antibiotic therapy in this situation is effective in prolonging pregnancy and reducing maternal and neonatal infection-related morbidities. A multicountry study (ORACLE I) from urban centres suggested that administration of erythromycin to women with preterm premature rupture of membranes (PPROM) was associated with significant health benefits for the newborn. A domiciliary cadre of trained birth attendants potentially can be trained to recognize PPROM and provide referral and, possibly, initial antimicrobial therapy.

An important aspect of prevention of neonatal infection in developed countries relates to GBS disease. The joint guidelines developed and implemented in the United States have led to a significant reduction in the burden of disease. The majority of newborns born to mothers with risk of GBS colonization undergo a full diagnostic evaluation and empiric therapy.

In recent years, the importance of hospital-acquired infections in newborn infants, frequently with multiresistant organisms, has been recognized. It is imperative that preventive strategies such as hand washing, reducing overcrowding and congestion, and environmental control are strictly enforced. Strategies to rotate antibiotics, reduce unnecessary hospital stay, strengthen infection prevention practices, and strict hand washing are critical to address this growing problem.

Meningitis in neonates, children, and adults

Acute meningitis is a potentially fatal infection caused by several microorganisms including bacteria, viruses, parasites, and fungi. In addition, meningitis is associated with a risk of chronic morbidity and developmental disability. Although the exact incidence of meningitis in developing countries is uncertain, case fatality rates range from 10 to 30 per cent. The recent GBD 2010 study estimated that there were 422,900 deaths from meningitis in 2010, a decrease of 14.1 per cent from 1990 (Lozano et al. 2012). Even if effective treatment is provided, between 10 and 50 per cent of survivors still develop neurological sequelae. Successful outcome of neonatal meningitis relates to several factors including age, time, and clinical stability before effective antibiotic treatment, species of microorganism, number of bacteria or quantity of active bacterial products in the CSF at the time of diagnosis, intensity of the host's inflammatory response, and time elapsed to sterilize CSF cultures. The highest rates of mortality and morbidity occur following meningitis in the neonatal period.

Aetiology

The three most common bacterial pathogens, *S. pneumoniae*, *H. influenzae*, and *N. meningitidis*, account for more than 80 per cent of cases of bacterial meningitis in the United States overall

Table 8.11.8 Aetiology and treatment of bacterial meningitis

Patient group	Common organisms	Antimicrobial therapy
Immunocompetent children (age ≥ 3 months–18 years)	*H. influenzae* *S. pneumoniae* *N. meningitidis*	Developing countries: ampicillin plus chloramphenicol Developed countries: vancomycin plus a third-generation cephalosporin (cefotaxime or ceftriaxone[a])
Immunodeficient, pregnant, and elderly (> 50 years)	*L. monocytogenes* *S. pneumoniae* *N. meningitides* Aerobic Gram-negative bacilli	Vancomycin plus ampicillin plus either cefipime or meropenem
Neurosurgical problems and head trauma	*S. aureus* *S. pneumoniae*	Vancomycin plus a third-generation cephalosporin or meropenem

[a] For resistant *S. pneumoniae*, the American Academy of Pediatrics recommends vancomycin plus cefotaxime or ceftriaxone as empiric therapy.

Source: data from Brouwer, M.C. et al., Epidemiology, diagnosis, and antimicrobial treatment of acute bacterial meningitis, *Clinical Microbiology Reviews*, Volume 23, Number 3, pp. 467–492, Copyright © 2010, American Society for Microbiology. All Rights Reserved.

(Brouwer et al. 2010), although *Listeria monocytogenes* is a greater problem for the elderly, immunocompromised, and pregnant women (Table 8.11.8). There is a relative paucity of microbiological information from developing countries, but beyond the neonatal period, the main agents of meningitis include Hib, *S. pneumoniae*, and *Neisseria meningitidis* with reported case-fatality rates of 7.7, 10, and 3.5 per cent, respectively. Table 8.11.9 shows the common bacteria causing meningitis in developing and developed countries and recommended antibiotics for treatment (van de Beek et al. Lancet 2012).

Issues in presentation and diagnosis

The clinical features that may help in diagnosing meningitis are summarized in Table 8.11.10. In general, clinicians should have a low threshold for investigating and excluding meningitis in children, as features may be non-specific. The clinical diagnosis can be confirmed by lumbar puncture and the examination of CSF. The CSF will have a cloudy appearance, elevated protein, increased leucocyte counts with a predominance of neutrophils, and the presence of pathogens on Gram stain and/or culture provide a definitive diagnosis of bacterial meningitis. The use of latex agglutination or the *S. pneumoniae* C-polysaccharide antigen test (BinaxNOW®) may help confirm the diagnosis, especially if the child has been pre-treated with antibiotics (Saha et al. 2005). A bacterial meningitis score has been shown to have an excellent negative predictive value for the presence of bacterial meningitis. If patients do not have one of the following factors—positive CSF

Gram stain, CSF absolute neutrophil count ≥1000 cells/microlitre, CSF protein ≥80 mg/dL, peripheral blood absolute neutrophil count ≥10,000 cells/microlitre, or history of seizure before or at the time of presentation—they are very unlikely to have bacterial meningitis (negative predictive value = 99.9 per cent) (Nigrovic et al. 2007). In recent years, polymerase chain reaction (PCR) techniques for diagnosis of bacterial meningitis have become available with sensitivities ranging from 80 to 100 per cent and specificities of 95 to 100 per cent (Brouwer et al. 2012).

Medical treatment

The mainstay of treatment is prompt antibiotic therapy for suspected bacterial meningitis. Antibiotics need to be started before the results of CSF culture and sensitivity are available. This requires selection of an appropriate antibiotic, known to be effective against the common bacterial pathogens prevalent locally. An increasing number of beta-lactamase-producing strains of Hib are resistant to ampicillin, and a smaller number of chloramphenicol

Table 8.11.9 Comparison of bacterial meningitis aetiology in children in the developing and developed world (prior to the widespread introduction of the Hib vaccine)

	Developing countries	Developed countries
H. influenzae	30%	65%
S. pneumoniae	23%	13%
N. meningitidis	28%	18%
Other organisms	19%	4%

Table 8.11.10 Signs and symptoms of paediatric meningitis

Symptoms or presenting history	Signs
Vomiting	Stiff neck
Inability to feed and drink	Repeated convulsions
Headache or pain in back of neck	Fontanelle bulging
Convulsions	Petechiae or purpura
Irritability	Irritability
Signs of raised intracranial pressure	
History of recent head trauma	Lethargy Evidence of head trauma
Unequal pupils	
Rigid posture or posturing	
Focal paralysis in any limbs or trunk	
Irregular breathing	

acetyltransferase-producing strains are resistant to chloramphenicol. Additionally, the proportion of CSF isolates of *S. pneumoniae* that is non-susceptible to penicillin, ceftriaxone, and cefotaxime has also increased. Currently, the drugs for suspected or confirmed bacterial meningitis include vancomycin plus an extended spectrum cephalosporin with the addition of ampicillin if *L. monocytogenes* is suspected. If these options are not available, then ampicillin + either gentamicin or chloramphenicol may be used. If sepsis is suspected, then cases should be treated with ampicillin or penicillin plus an aminoglycoside, until meningitis is confirmed. Antimicrobial therapy is described further in Table 8.11.8.

Very early parenteral administration of corticosteroids (before or with initiation of antibiotics) significantly reduces severe adverse outcomes and case fatality rates. Similarly, there is evidence to suggest that restriction of fluids in the first 48 hours may improve outcomes. A meta-analysis of randomized, controlled trials has shown the benefit of steroids in all-cause bacterial meningitis, predominantly Hib meningitis. A recent Cochrane systematic review found that corticosteroids protect against severe hearing loss and neurological sequelae, and reduce mortality among adults with community-acquired bacterial meningitis in high-income countries (van de Beek et al. 2007). While this review found evidence of a benefit for children from resource-rich countries, there was no beneficial effect of corticosteroids for children in low-income countries.

Preventive measures

Although poverty, malnutrition, overcrowding are important risk factors for disease, delayed and inappropriate case management is a common determinant of adverse outcomes. The development of effective vaccines has been a major factor in the reduction of the burden of meningitis in the developed world. These include the Hib, pneumococcal conjugate, and meningococcal vaccines.

Haemophilus influenzae type b vaccine

Currently three Hib conjugate vaccines are available for use in infants and young children with comparable efficacy (protective efficacy of Hib against development of laboratory confirmed invasive disease > 90 per cent). All industrialized countries now include Hib vaccine in their national immunization programmes, resulting in the virtual elimination of invasive Hib disease. There is comparable impressive evidence of benefit from several developing countries following introduction of Hib vaccine and many countries now include Hib vaccine in their repertoire with GAVI support.

Pneumococcal vaccine

The older 23-valent pneumococcal polysaccharide vaccine is unsuitable for use in young children. The recent development of the 7-valent protein-conjugate polysaccharide vaccine, 10-valent, and 13-valent vaccines is a major advance in the control of invasive pneumococcal disease. In the United States, the 7-PCV was included in routine vaccinations of infants and children under 2 years in 2000 and by 2001 the incidence of all invasive pneumococcal disease in this age group had declined by 69 per cent. Currently several Latin American countries are beginning to introduce pneumococcal conjugate vaccine as part of the WHO Expanded Program on Immunization (EPI) as are several countries in sub-Saharan Africa and Asia.

Meningococcal vaccine

Meningococcal polysaccharide vaccine is available for serogroups A, C, W-135, and Y. This quadrivalent vaccine is being introduced in several developed countries as part of routine vaccine schedules, especially for adolescents who will be rooming in crowded dormitories while attending university. In many developed countries this vaccine has been replaced by the quadrivalent meningococcal conjugate vaccine, which is more immunogenic and, because it induces memory cells, is likely to lead to a longer lasting protective immune response. Recent evidence of the efficacy and safety of a conjugate meningococcal B vaccine suggests that in the near future we will have highly effective vaccines for all major meningococcal serogroups (Vesikari et al. 2013).

Gastrointestinal tract infections

Diarrhoea, the most common manifestation of intestinal tract infections, is a leading cause of preventable death in most developing countries where its greatest impact is seen in infants and children. Infectious diarrhoea may be accompanied by numerous complications (Table 8.11.11). The financial burden associated with medical care and lost productivity due to infectious diarrhoea amounts to more than US$20 billion a year in the United States alone.

Invasive diarrhoea refers to diarrhoea caused by bacterial pathogens that invade the bowel mucosa, causing inflammation and tissue damage and may cause blood in stools (bloody diarrhoea). Invasive diarrhoea accounts for approximately 10 per cent of diarrhoeal episodes in children under 5 years of age and approximately 15 per cent of diarrhoea-associated deaths in this age group worldwide. Although less frequent, bloody diarrhoea generally lasts longer, is associated with higher risk of complications and case fatality rates, and is more likely to adversely affect a child's growth. The burden of disease is mainly in younger age groups; 72 per cent of deaths from diarrhoea and 81 per cent of deaths from pneumonia happen in children younger than 2 years. Pneumonia incidence falls less rapidly with age than does mortality from the disease. Diarrhoea incidence peaks at age 6–11 months and then decreases with age; proportionate mortality is highest from age 0–11 months, the ages at which the risk of disease and severe disease also peak (Fig. 8.11.2) (Fischer Walker et al. 2013).

Global and regional epidemiology

The aetiology and severity of gastrointestinal infections are determined by several epidemiological factors. Young children and the elderly are at greatest risk for more severe disease and complications. The presence of underlying medical conditions, especially those that compromise immunity, greatly enhances the risk of acquiring an infection and its ultimate severity. Poor sanitation, inadequate water supplies, and increasing globalization of food transport systems all predispose to the development of large epidemics of food- and water-borne outbreaks of gastrointestinal disease. Seasonal or cyclic weather variations also influence the epidemiology of diarrhoeal disease and food poisoning.

Several recent reviews have evaluated diarrhoea burden and mortality rates. A review carried out two decades ago estimated

Table 8.11.11 Complications of gastrointestinal infections

Complication	Causative pathogens
Dehydration	*Vibrio cholerae, Cryptosporidium parvum* (especially in immunocompromised hosts), enterotoxigenic *Escherichia coli* (ETEC), rotavirus
Severe vomiting	Staphylococcal food poisoning, norovirus, rotavirus
Haemorrhagic colitis	*Campylobacter jejuni*, enterohaemorrhagic *E. coli* (EHEC), *Salmonella, Shigella, V. parahaemolyticus*
Toxic megacolon, intestinal perforation	EHEC, *Shigella, C. jejuni* (rare), *Clostridium difficile* (rare), *Salmonella* (rare), *Yersinia* (rare)
Haemolytic uraemic syndrome (HUS), thrombotic thrombocytopenic purpura (TTP)	EHEC, *Shigella, C. jejuni* (rare)
Reactive arthritis	*C. jejuni, Shigella, Salmonella, Yersinia*
Malabsorption/malnutrition	*Cyclospora cayetanensis, Giardia lamblia, C. parvum* or *C. hominis* (especially immunocompromised hosts)
Distant metastatic infection	*Salmonella, C. jejuni* (rare), *Yersinia* (rare)
Guillain–Barré syndrome	*C. jejuni* (rare)

that 4.6 million children died annually from diarrhoea. Kosek et al. have updated these estimates by reviewing 60 studies of diarrhoea morbidity and mortality published between 1990 and 2000 (Kosek et al. 2003). They concluded that diarrhoea accounts for 21 per cent of all deaths at less than 5 years of age and causes 2.5 million deaths per year, although morbidity rates remain relatively unchanged. Despite the different methods and sources of information, each successive review of the diarrhoea burden over the past three decades has demonstrated declining mortality but relatively stable morbidity rates. Persistent high rates of diarrhoea morbidity may have significant long-term effects on linear growth and physical and cognitive function in children. Fig. 8.11.3 shows country-specific global trends for diarrhoea and pneumonia in the world from 2000 to 2010.

Aetiology

Common aetiologies of non-inflammatory diarrhoea include enterotoxigenic *E. coli* (ETEC) and other strains such as enteroaggregative (EAEC), diffusely adhering, and enteropathogenic *E. coli*, *Vibrio cholerae*; non-01 choleras such as *V. vulnificus*; parasites including *Giardia lamblia, Cryptosporidium parvum*, and microsporidia; and several different virus species including rotavirus, noroviruses, and astroviruses (Hamer and Gorbach 2010). Acute inflammatory diarrhoea is the result of infection with bacterial enteropathogens such as *Shigella, Campylobacter, Salmonella* spp., enterohaemorrhagic *E. coli* (EHEC), *V. parahaemolyticus*,

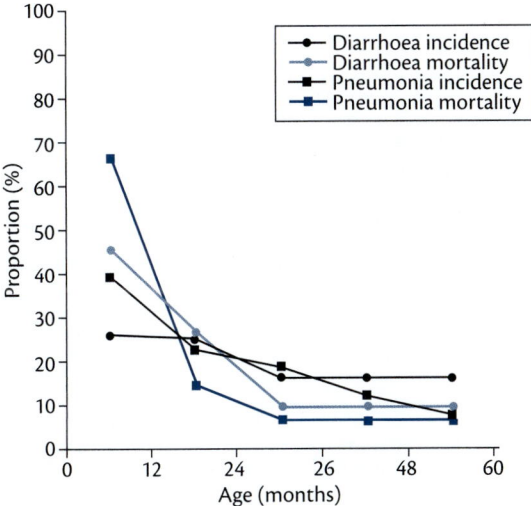

Fig. 8.11.2 Distribution of cases of, and deaths from, diarrhoea and pneumonia in children aged 0–4 years.

Reprinted from *The Lancet*, Volume 381, Issue 9875, Fischer Walker, C.L. et al., Global burden of childhood pneumonia and diarrhoea, pp. 1405–16, Copyright © 2013, with permission from Elsevier, available from http://www.sciencedirect.com/science/journal/01406736.

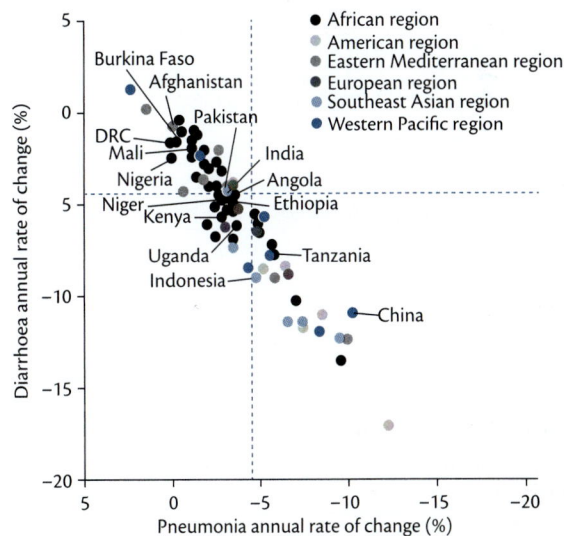

Fig. 8.11.3 Annual rates of change in diarrhoea-specific and pneumonia-specific mortality between 2000 and 2010. The 75 Countdown to 2015 countries are shown; the 15 countries with the highest burdens are labelled. Dotted lines show target annual rates of change to achieve the MDG-4. DRC, Democratic Republic of the Congo.

Reprinted from *The Lancet*, Volume 381, Issue 9875, Fischer Walker, C.L. et al., Global burden of childhood pneumonia and diarrhoea, pp. 1405–16, Copyright © 2013, with permission from Elsevier, available from http://www.sciencedirect.com/science/journal/01406736.

and *Clostridium difficile*. Among the parasites, *Entamoeba histolytica* is the most common cause of dysenteric illness although *Balantidium coli*, *Schistosoma mansoni*, *S. japonicum*, *Trichuris trichiura*, hookworms, and *Trichinella spiralis* can all cause bloody, mucoid diarrhoea.

Estimates of rotavirus and cholera as major diarrhoea aetiologies associated with increased risk of mortality are shown in Table 8.11.12 (Fischer Walker et al. 2013).

Notwithstanding these estimates from a systematic review of available literature, more robust data on diarrhoea aetiology are now available. The recent large multicountry study of diarrhoea aetiology, the Global Enterics Multi-Center Study (GEMS) (Kotloff et al. 2013), has provided much-needed insight into the aetiology of severe diarrhoea in young children. Fig. 8.11.4 provides the attributable incidence of moderate to severe diarrhoea among young children in low-income settings, stratified by age.

Infectious microorganisms in contaminated food and drink are the main source of travellers' diarrhoea. High-risk foods include uncooked vegetables, salsa, meat, and seafood. Tap water, ice, unpasteurized milk and dairy products, salads, and unpeeled fruits are also associated with an increased risk. Although many different pathogens may be responsible, the leading culprits are various forms of *E. coli*, particularly ETEC and EAEC. *C. jejuni* is encountered in a significant proportion of cases, particularly during cooler seasons. Viruses, *Shigella*, *Salmonella*, *Giardia*, *Cryptosporidium*, and *Cyclospora* spp. are responsible for a minority of travellers' diarrhoea cases.

Food poisoning is most commonly caused by the consumption of food contaminated with bacteria or bacterial toxins. Food poisoning can also be due to parasites (e.g. trichinosis), viruses (e.g. hepatitis A), and other toxins (e.g. *Amanita* mushrooms). The most well-recognized causes of bacterial food poisoning are the following: *Clostridium perfringens*, *S. aureus*, *Vibrio* spp. (including *V. cholerae* and *V. parahaemolyticus*), *Bacillus cereus*, *Salmonella* spp., *C. botulinum*, *Shigella* spp., toxigenic *E. coli* (ETEC and EHEC), and certain species of *Campylobacter*, *Yersinia*, *Listeria*, and *Aeromonas*.

Several risk factors have been demonstrated for diarrhoea-associated mortality including not breastfeeding, being underweight, stunting, wasting, vitamin A deficiency, and zinc deficiency (Fischer Walker et al. 2013).

Issues in presentation and diagnosis

Gastrointestinal infections usually result in three principal syndromes: non-inflammatory diarrhoea, inflammatory diarrhoea, and systemic disease. Non-inflammatory diarrhoea primarily involves the small intestine, whereas inflammatory diarrhoea predominantly affects the colon. The location of infection influences the clinical characteristics and certain diagnostic features of the

Table 8.11.12 Diarrhoea episodes and deaths by WHO region

Several diarrhoea episodes	African region	American region	Eastern Mediterranean region	European region	Southeast Asian region	Western Pacific region	World
Rotavirus:							
Episodes (×10³)	2557 (1901–3026)	1129 (833–1330)	1344 (990–1576)	660 (488–781)	2382 (1753–790)	1781 (1312–2090)	9853 (7277–11593)
Proportion of all severe episodes (%)	26.8%	23.4%	31.3%	25.9%	25.5%	32.6%	27.3%
Vibrio cholerae:							
Episodes (×10³)	38 (28–45)	–	–	–	416 (306–488)	2 (2–3)	456 (336–536)
Proportion of all severe episodes (%)	0.4%	–	–	–	4.5%	0.04%	1.3%
Diarrhoea deaths							
Rotavirus:							
Deaths (×10³)	95 (52.5–151.3)	2.6 (1.9–5.6)	30.2 (20.1–48.0)	1.6 (1.1–2.8)	58.1 (47.7–74.7)	5.5 (2.0–7.7)	192.7 (133.1–284.4)
Proportion of diarrhoea deaths (%)	26.8%	23.4%	31.3%	25.9%	25.5%	32.6%	27.1%
V. cholera:							
Episodes (×10³)	1.4 (0.8–2.3)	–	–	–	10.2 (8.4–13.2)	0.1 (0.02–0.1)	11.7 (7.9–16.8)
Proportion of diarrhoea deaths (%)	0.4%	–	–	–	4.5%	0.04%	1.6%

Adapted from *The Lancet*, Volume 381, Issue 9875, Fischer Walker, C.L. et al., Global burden of childhood pneumonia and diarrhoea, pp. 1405–16, Copyright © 2013, with permission from Elsevier, available from http://www.sciencedirect.com/science/journal/01406736.

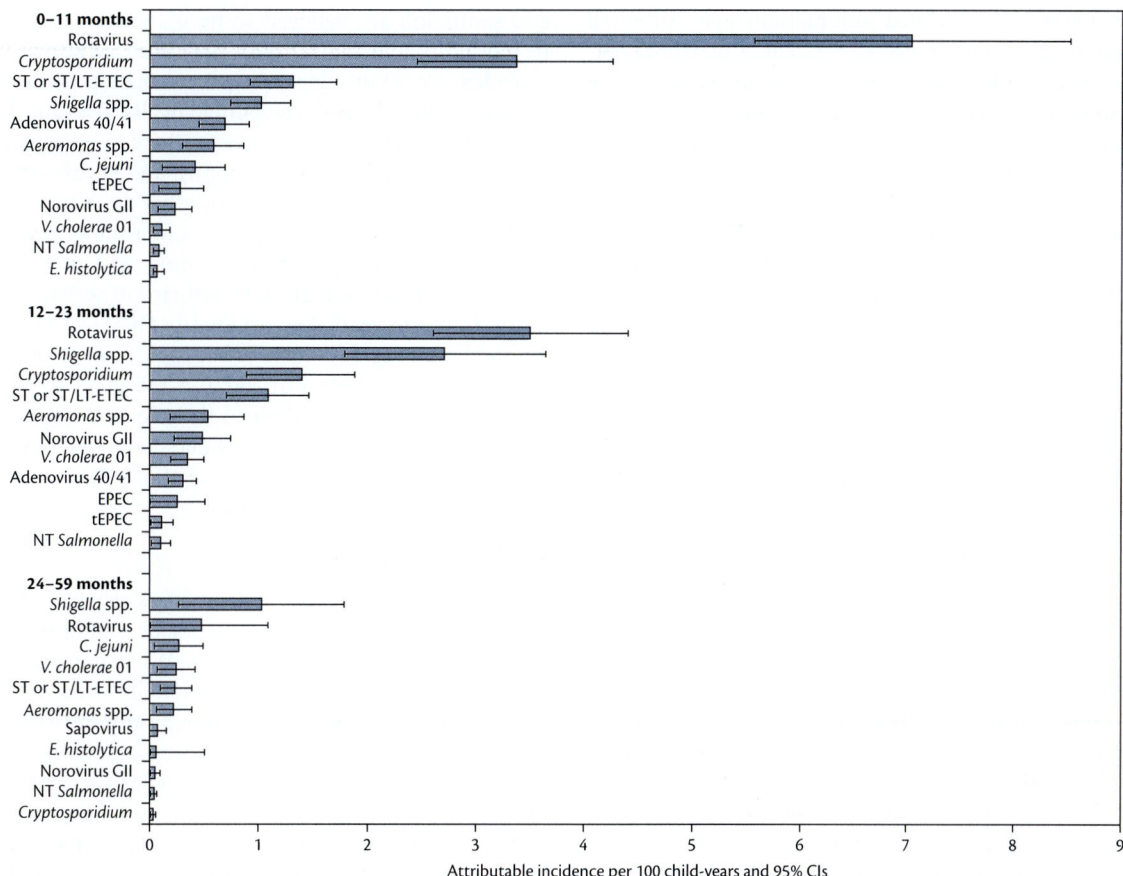

Fig. 8.11.4 Attributable incidence of pathogen-specific moderate-to-severe diarrhoea per 100 child-years by age stratum, all sites combined.
Reprinted from *The Lancet*, Volume 382, Issue 9888, Kotloff, K.L. et al., Burden and aetiology of diarrhoeal disease in infants and young children in developing countries (the Global Enteric Multicenter Study, GEMS): A prospective, case-control study, pp. 209–22, Copyright © 2013, with permission from Elsevier, available from http://www.sciencedirect.com/science/journal/01406736.

diarrhoeal disease (Table 8.11.13). Thus, organisms that target the small intestine tend to produce watery, potentially dehydrating diarrhoea, while those infecting the large intestine cause bloody mucoid diarrhoea associated with tenesmus.

Acute watery diarrhoea can be rapidly dehydrating, with stool losses of 250 mL/kg/day or more, a quantity that quickly exceeds total plasma and interstitial fluid volumes, and is incompatible with life unless aggressive fluid therapy can be provided. Such dramatic dehydration is usually due to rotavirus, ETEC, or *V. cholerae*, and it is most dangerous in the very young.

Persistent diarrhoea is defined as diarrhoea lasting 14 days or longer, is manifested by malabsorption, nutrient losses, and

Table 8.11.13 Clinical features and aetiologies of diarrhoeal diseases

Feature	Site of infection	
	Small intestine	**Large intestine**
Pathogens	*Escherichia coli* (enteropathogenic *E. coli*, enterotoxigenic *E. coli*)	*E. coli* (EIEC, EHEC)
	Cryptosporidium parvum	*Entamoeba histolytica*
	Giardia lamblia	*Shigella* spp.
	Norovirus	
	Rotavirus	
	Vibrio cholerae	
Location of pain	Mid abdomen	Lower abdomen, rectum
Volume of stool	Large	Small
Blood in stool	Rare	Common
Faecal leucocytes	Rare	Common (except in amoebiasis)
Sigmoidoscopy	Normal	Mucosal ulcers, haemorrhagic foci, friable mucosa

wasting, and is typically associated with malnutrition. Although persistent diarrhoea accounts for 8–20 per cent of diarrhoea episodes, it is associated with a disproportionately increased risk of death. Persistent diarrhoea more commonly follows an episode of bloody diarrhoea and is associated with a tenfold higher risk of mortality. HIV infection is another risk factor for persistent diarrhoea in both adults and children.

Inflammatory diarrhoea is a manifestation of invasive intestinal infection that is associated with intestinal damage and nutritional deterioration, often with systemic manifestations including fever. Although clinicians often use the term bloody diarrhoea interchangeably with dysentery, the latter is a syndrome consisting of the frequent passage of characteristic, small-volume, bloody mucoid stools, abdominal cramps, and tenesmus. Agents that cause bloody diarrhoea or dysentery can also provoke a form of diarrhoea that does not present clinically with visible blood in the stool, although mucosal damage and inflammation are present and faecal blood and white blood cells are usually detectable by microscopy.

Because of the significant morbidity and costs associated with infectious diarrhoea, making a specific laboratory diagnosis can be useful epidemiologically, diagnostically, and therapeutically. A definitive diagnosis is achieved mainly through study of faecal specimens, using bacteriological culture, viral culture, or direct electron microscopy for viral particles, and identification of microbial antigens (viruses, bacteria, parasites, or toxins). DNA probes, PCR, and immunodiagnostic tests can now be used to identify several pathogens in stool specimens. Although some diseases can be diagnosed by elevations of serum antibody titres, this method is usually retrospective and often inaccurate.

Evidence-based interventions

Increased use of oral rehydration therapy, improved nutrition, increased breastfeeding, better supplemental feeding, female education, measles immunization, and improvement in hygiene and sanitation are believed to have contributed to the decline in morbidity and mortality of diarrhoea. Syndromic diagnosis provides important clues to optimal management and is both programmatically and epidemiologically relevant. The correct treatment of diarrhoea requires mothers to recognize the problem and seek medical care promptly, and health workers to give oral rehydration solution (ORS) or other fluids to prevent or treat dehydration, dispense an appropriate antibiotic when needed, provide advice on appropriate feeding, and provide follow-up, especially for children at increased risk of serious morbidity or death. In recent years, low-osmolarity ORS and zinc supplementation (10–20 mg/day) have led to significantly improved diarrhoea outcomes (Aggarwal 2007). A recent series in *The Lancet* (Bhutta et al. 2013b) highlighted the role of 15 core interventions to address childhood pneumonia and diarrhoea, of which several are also common nutrition interventions underscored recently (Table 8.11.14) (Bhutta et al. 2013a).

Medical treatment

Since the most devastating consequences of acute infectious diarrhoea result from fluid losses, the major goal of treatment is the replacement of fluid and electrolytes. While the intravenous route of administration has been traditionally used, ORS has been shown to be equally effective physiologically and logistically more practical and less costly to administer, especially in developing countries. ORS is the treatment of choice for mild-to-moderate diarrhoea in both children and adults, as long as vomiting is not a major feature of the gastrointestinal infection. ORS can also be used in severely dehydrated patients after initial parenteral rehydration.

Although there is no doubt about the value of ORS in treating dehydrating diarrhoea, the optimal sodium concentration of the solution remains in dispute, particularly in regard to the treatment of mild-to-moderate diarrhoea in well-nourished children in industrialized countries. The high concentration of sodium

Table 8.11.14 Interventions for prevention and treatment of diarrhoea, pneumonia, and undernutrition

Diarrhoea	Pneumonia	Nutrition
Breastfeeding promotion	Breastfeeding promotion	Breastfeeding promotion
Improved water source, sanitation and hygiene	Improved water source, sanitation and hygiene	Improved water source, sanitation and hygiene
Preventive vitamin A supplementation	Preventive vitamin A supplementation	Preventive vitamin A supplementation
Preventive zinc supplementation	Preventive zinc supplementation	Preventive zinc supplementation
Rotavirus vaccine	Hib vaccine	Periconceptional folic acid supplementation or fortification
ORS	Pneumococcal vaccine	Appropriate complementary feeding
Zinc—for treatment of diarrhoea	Case management of neonatal infections	Maternal balanced energy protein supplementation
Antibiotics for dysentery	Oral antibiotics: case management of pneumonia in children	Maternal calcium supplementation
		Multiple micronutrient supplementation in pregnancy
		Management of moderate and severe acute malnutrition

(90 mmol) in the standard WHO ORS formulation may cause hypernatraemia and even seizures in children with non-cholera watery diarrhoea. Consequently, lower concentrations of sodium and a reduced osmolarity solution have been found to be effective for rehydration and not to be associated with any serious adverse clinical events (Hanh et al. 2001). The substitution of starch derived from rice or cereals for glucose in ORS has been another approach. Rice-based salt solutions produce lower stool losses, a shorter duration of diarrhoea, and greater fluid and electrolyte absorption than do glucose-based solutions in treating childhood and adult diarrhoea. ORS has major advantages over home fluids in the management of children with significant dehydration and coupled with zinc therapy (20 mg zinc sulphate daily for 10 days) is the mainstay of treatment of childhood diarrhoea.

Dietary abstinence, the traditional approach to an acute diarrhoeal illness, restricts the intake of necessary calories, fluids, and electrolytes. During an acute attack, the patient often finds it more comfortable to avoid spicy, high-fat, and high-fibre foods, all of which can increase stool volume and intestinal motility. Although giving the bowels a rest provides symptomatic relief, continued oral intake of fluids and foods is critical for both rehydration and the prevention of malnutrition. In children, it is particularly important to restart feeding as soon as the child is willing to accept oral intake.

Because certain foods and fluids can increase intestinal motility, it is wise to avoid fluids such as coffee, tea, cocoa, and alcoholic beverages. Ingestion of milk and dairy products can potentiate fluid secretion and increase stool volume. Besides the oral rehydration therapy outlined earlier, acceptable beverages for mildly dehydrated adults include fruit juices and various bottled soft drinks. Carbonated drinks should be allowed to 'de-fizz' by letting them stand in a glass before ingestion. Soft, easily digestible foods are generally acceptable to the patient with acute diarrhoea.

Since most patients with infectious diarrhoea, even those with a recognized pathogen, have a mild, self-limited course, neither a stool culture nor specific treatment is required for such cases. For more severe cases, however, empirical antimicrobial therapy should be instituted, pending the results of stool and blood cultures. Gastrointestinal infections likely to respond to antibiotic treatment include cholera, giardiasis, cyclosporiasis, shigellosis, *E. coli* diarrhoea in infants, symptomatic travellers' diarrhoea, and *C. difficile* diarrhoea. The choice of antimicrobial drug should be based on *in vitro* sensitivity patterns, which vary from region to region. A fluoroquinolone antibiotic is a good choice for empirical therapy, since these agents have broad-spectrum activity against virtually all bacterial pathogens responsible for acute infectious diarrhoea (except *C. difficile*). Resistance to fluoroquinolones in South and South East Asia is an increasing problem.

In patients with severe community-acquired diarrhoea—characterized by more than four stools per day lasting for at least 3 days or more with at least one associated symptom such as fever, abdominal pain, or vomiting—there is a high likelihood of isolating a bacterial pathogen. In this setting, a short course of a fluoroquinolone, namely 1–3 days' duration, will generally provide prompt relief with a low risk of adverse effects. Fluoroquinolones will not be effective for parasitic infections—specific antiparasitic drugs should be prescribed after identification of the offending pathogen in stool smears.

The duration of antimicrobial therapy has not been clearly defined. While courses of anywhere from 3 to 10 days of treatment have been recommended, there are several studies that included severe forms of diarrhoea which suggested that a single dose is as effective as more prolonged therapy. For example, single-dose fluoroquinolone therapy is highly effective for infections due to *V. cholerae*, *V. parahaemolyticus*, and most *Shigella* species. On the other hand, short-course treatment of salmonella gastroenteritis with fleroxacin has not been found to be clinically beneficial. When treatment is indicated, a number of studies have shown that the combination of an antimicrobial drug and an antimotility drug provides the most rapid relief of diarrhoea.

Preventive measures

Diarrhoeal disease affects rich and poor, old and young, and those in developed and developing countries alike, yet a strong relationship exists between poverty, an unhygienic environment, and the number and severity of diarrhoeal episodes—especially for children under 5 years. Poverty also restricts the ability to provide age-appropriate, nutritionally balanced diets, or to modify diets when diarrhoea develops so as to mitigate and repair nutrient losses. The impact is exacerbated by the lack of adequate, available, and affordable medical care. Thus preventive and management strategies for diarrhoea must have an equity focus.

Malnutrition is an independent predictor of the frequency and severity of diarrhoeal illness and can lead to a vicious cycle in which sequential diarrhoeal disease leads to increasing nutritional deterioration, impaired immune function, and greater susceptibility to infection.

Family knowledge about diarrhoea must be reinforced in areas such as prevention, nutrition, hand washing and hygiene, measles vaccination, preventive zinc supplements, and when and where to seek care. It is estimated that, in the 1990s, more than 1 million deaths related to diarrhoea may have been prevented each year, largely attributable to the promotion and use of these therapies.

A meta-analysis of three observational studies in developing countries shows that breastfed children under the age of 6 months are 6.1 times less likely to die of diarrhoea than infants who are not breastfed. Continued breastfeeding during the diarrhoea episode provides nutrients to the child, prevents weight loss, and improves recovery from diarrhoea. Contaminated and poor-quality complementary foods are associated with increased diarrhoea burden and stunting (Huttly et al. 1997). Ideally, complementary foods should be introduced at 6 months of age, and breastfeeding should continue for up to 2 years or even longer. Appropriate, safe, and aptly initiated complementary feeding has been shown to significantly reduce mortality in young children. Diarrhoea frequently causes fever, altering host metabolism and leading to the depletion of body stores of nutrients. These losses must be replenished during convalescence, which takes much longer than the illness does to develop. For these reasons, appropriate feeding strategies during diarrhoea episodes are a cornerstone of treatment.

Probiotics, especially *Lactobacillus rhamnosus* GG, effectively reduce the frequency and duration of diarrhoea in children and adults. Probiotics are also useful for the prevention of antibiotic-associated diarrhoea.

Various studies suggest that zinc-deficient populations are at increased risk of developing diarrhoeal diseases, respiratory tract infections, and growth retardation. A meta-analysis published in

1999 showed that continuous zinc supplementation was associated with decreased rates of childhood diarrhoea (Zinc Investigator's Collaborative Group 1999), and a meta-analysis confirms the previous findings and indicates that zinc supplementation for young children leads to reduction in diarrhoea risk (by 14 per cent), serious forms of diarrhoea, and the number of days of diarrhoea per child (Aggarwal et al. 2007).

Human faeces and contamination are the primary source of diarrhoeal pathogens. Poor sanitation, lack of access to clean water, and inadequate personal hygiene are responsible for an estimated 90 per cent of childhood diarrhoea. Promotion of hand washing reduces diarrhoea incidence by an average of 33 per cent and rigorous observational studies demonstrated a median reduction of 55 per cent in all-cause child mortality associated with improved access to sanitation facilities. Hand washing promotion strategies have also been shown to reduce diarrhoea burden with ancillary benefits in community settings.

Strict adherence to food and water precautions as already outlined will help those who travel to less developed areas of the world to decrease their risk of acquiring gastrointestinal infections. Parasitic infections, such as strongyloidiasis and hookworms, can be avoided by the use of footwear. Avoiding contact with freshwater such as rivers and lakes in endemic areas serves to prevent schistosomiasis.

Immunization represents an ideal way to prevent certain bacterial and viral diseases, but has not yet proved successful for combating many gastrointestinal pathogens. The cholera vaccine that has been available for decades suffers from low efficacy, a moderate risk of side effects, and a short duration of action. Newer oral cholera vaccines, such as the inactivated B subunit vaccine, are highly effective for prevention of severe cholera. New rotavirus vaccines have not been associated with intussusception. Measles is known to predispose to diarrhoeal disease secondary to measles-induced immunodeficiency, and it is estimated that measles vaccine at varying levels of coverage (45–90 per cent) could prevent 44–64 per cent of measles cases, 0.6–3.8 per cent of diarrhoeal episodes, and 6–26 per cent of diarrhoeal deaths among children under 5 years. Global measles immunization coverage is now approaching 80 per cent, and the disease has been eliminated from the Americas, raising hopes for global elimination in the near future, with a predictable reduction in diarrhoea as well.

Typhoid fever

Typhoid fever, a systemic disease caused by *Salmonella enterica* serovar Typhi, is an acute illness characterized by protean and non-specific symptoms, including fever and gastrointestinal infection. The systemic disease caused by *S.* Paratyphi (A, B, or C) is also clinically similar; both typhoid and paratyphoid are collectively labelled as enteric fevers. The emergence of drug-resistant strains, especially multidrug-resistant (MDR) *S.* Typhi, resistant to ampicillin, chloramphenicol, trimethoprim–sulphamethoxazole, and, more recently, fluoroquinolones, is a growing problem.

Global and regional epidemiology

The global incidence of typhoid fever in 2000 was estimated to be 21.6 million cases, with more than 200,000 deaths (Crump et al. 2004). Approximately 12.5 million cases of typhoid fever occur annually in the developing world (excluding China),

Table 8.11.15 Crude typhoid incidence rates by region, 2000

Area/region	Crude incidence[a]	Typhoid cases	Incidence classification
Global	178	10,825,487	High
Africa	50	408,837	Medium
Asia	274	10,118,879	High
Europe	3	19,144	Low
Latin America/Caribbean	53	273,518	Medium
Northern America	< 1	453	Low
Oceania	15	4656	Medium

[a] Per 100,000 persons per year.

Adapted with permission from Crump, J.A. et al., The global burden of typhoid fever, *Bulletin of the World Health Organization*, Volume 82, pp. 346–53, Copyright © World Health Organization 2004, available from http://www.who.int/rpc/TFDisBurden.pdf.

with 7.7 million cases in Asia alone. In South Asia, recent community-based studies indicate that a large proportion of cases occur in children under 5, with significant morbidity and mortality. The global case fatality rate of 1 per cent is based on conservative estimates from hospital-based fever studies; actual mortality figures may be higher in areas where referral is difficult and health services are dysfunctional. Table 8.11.15 shows the regional distribution of crude typhoid incidence rates.

There have been dramatic point-source outbreaks of typhoid related to contamination of food sources or water supply. The use of contaminated ground water, consumption of street foods, and poor personal hygiene are common risk factors for infection.

Issues in presentation and diagnosis

After ingestion in contaminated food or water, *S.* Typhi penetrates the small bowel mucosa and makes its way rapidly to the lymphatics, the mesenteric nodes, and finally the bloodstream. Following an initial bacteraemia, the organism is sequestered in cells of the reticuloendothelial system where it multiplies and re-emerges several days later in recurrent waves of bacteraemia, an event that initiates the symptomatic phase of infection. The incubation period ranges from 5 to 14 days.

Typhoid fever is a febrile illness of prolonged duration, characterized by hectic fever, delirium, persistent bacteraemia, splenomegaly, and a variety of systemic manifestations. Most children present with fever, headache, and abdominal discomfort, diarrhoea, sore throat, anorexia, dry cough, or myalgia and constipation. In the later phase of illness, more specific physical signs including hepatomegaly and splenomegaly may be observed. Rose spots may be seen in an early stage of the illness in fair-skinned children and large proportions have a centrally coated tongue (Bhan et al. 2005). Pulse–temperature dissociation is present in some patients. In approximately 50 per cent of patients, there is no change in bowel habits; in fact, constipation is more common than diarrhoea in children with typhoid fever. As a result of recurrent waves of bacteraemia, patients with typhoid fever can develop pneumonia, pyelonephritis, osteomyelitis, septic arthritis, and meningitis. Intestinal haemorrhage and perforation, the most common complications, often occur in the 3rd week of infection or during convalescence. The most serious complication, intestinal perforation, occurs in 0.5–3 per cent of the patients with typhoid, and because they occur most commonly in areas where optimal medical care is not readily available, it may be associated with case fatality rates ranging from 4.8 to 30.5 per cent. Recent elucidation of a S. Typhi specific toxin (Song et al. 2013) not only provides exciting new information on the pathogenesis of typhoid fever but also opens exciting possibilities of development of newer vaccines and interventions for this disease.

Diagnosis of typhoid and paratyphoid fever requires culture of blood, bone marrow, stools, or urine to confirm growth of S. Typhi. Laboratory findings commonly include leucopenia, thrombocytopenia, proteinurea, and elevated transaminases, but these are relatively non-specific and uncommon. In developing countries, culture facilities are expensive and mostly confined to hospitals, while most typhoid patients are diagnosed clinically and treated in outpatient settings. In other instances, serological diagnosis may be made with the Widal test. The latter, though useful, is insufficiently sensitive in endemic areas. Newer diagnostic tests have been developed, such as the Typhidot and Tubex, which detect IgM antibodies against specific S. Typhi antigens (Bhutta 2006). Since these newer assays have not proven to have adequate sensitivity and specificity for routine use in community settings, there is a need for further refinement in serological or molecular diagnosis of the disease.

Medical treatment

In the pre-antibiotic era, typhoid fever case fatality rates approached 20 per cent. Treatment with effective antimicrobial agents—ampicillin, chloramphenicol, co-trimoxazole, and later ciprofloxacin—has progressively reduced case fatality rates to less than 1 per cent, except for MDR isolates. Fluoroquinolones and third-generation cephalosporins are effective in MDR typhoid but over the last few years there have been increasing reports in Asia of S. Typhi strains with reduced fluoroquinolone susceptibility. The presence of nalidixic acid resistance *in vitro* is associated with clinical treatment failures with fluoroquinolones. Alternative therapies including azithromycin or third-generation cephalosporins are recommended in these circumstances. Given the considerable morbidity and higher mortality rates reported with MDR typhoid in children, appropriate antibiotic therapy must be instituted promptly and, when appropriate facilities are available, treatment choices should be guided by susceptibility testing.

Preventive measures

Detection of sources of infection related to recent typhoid fever in household contacts, commercial food handlers, or contaminated drinking water sources is essential to design effective preventive measures for disease containment.

Although the old whole-cell-inactivated typhoid vaccine has been withdrawn because of side effects, there are two licensed vaccines for prevention of disease: Ty21a (an attenuated strain of S. Typhi administered orally) and Vi (the purified bacterial polysaccharide vaccine, given parenterally). These two vaccines have comparable protective efficacy and while they have been largely used for travellers, recently the Vi vaccine has been used for school vaccination programmes in large public health settings in Asia. For younger children and infants the Vi conjugate vaccine has been shown to provide a high degree of protection in a series of studies in Vietnam. However, the conjugate vaccine has as yet not been produced for public health use.

Dengue fever

In recent years, dengue fever, a mosquito-borne arboviral disease, has become one of the most common and rapidly spreading vector-borne diseases (after malaria) and thus now represents a major international public health concern. Dengue virus belongs to the genus *Flavivirus* (single-stranded, non-segmented RNA viruses), which includes four serologically distinct serotypes (DEN-1, DEN-2, DEN-3, and DEN-4). Variations in virus strains within and between the four serotypes influence disease severity. There is limited protection across serotypes. Secondary infections (particularly with serotype 2) are more likely to result in severe disease and dengue haemorrhagic fever.

Global and regional epidemiology

Humans and mosquitoes are the principal hosts of dengue virus although some non-human primates can also be infected. Dengue epidemics occur during the warm, humid, rainy seasons, which favour breeding conditions for the mosquito vector, *Aedes aegypti*. More than two-fifths of the world's population (~2.5 billion) lives in areas potentially at risk for dengue, which is endemic in more than 100 countries across the globe, with tropical areas of Asia, the Western Pacific, Latin America, and the Caribbean being the most seriously affected regions.

In some case series, dengue fever has been reported as the second most frequent cause of hospitalization (after malaria) among travellers returning from the tropics. It causes an estimated 50–100 million illnesses annually, including 250,000–500,000 cases of dengue haemorrhagic fever—a severe manifestation of dengue—and 14,700–24,000 deaths (Deen et al. 2006; Lozano et al. 2012). Around 95 per cent of cases occur in children less than 15 years of age, with infants representing 5 per cent of the cases.

Issues in presentation and diagnosis

The incubation period can vary from 3 to 14 days (typically between 5 and 7 days) and viraemia can persist up to 12 days (typically 4–5 days). Fever usually lasts for 5–7 days; fevers persisting beyond 10–14 days suggest another diagnosis. The clinical features of dengue vary with patient age. Most dengue infections, especially in children, are minimally symptomatic or asymptomatic. Children may also present with atypical syndromes such as encephalopathy and fulminant liver failure.

Classic dengue fever is characterized by a high fever of abrupt onset, sometimes with two peaks (saddle back fevers), severe myalgias, arthralgia, retro-orbital pain, headaches, and any of the three types of rashes, including a petechial rash, diffuse erythematous rash with isolated patches of normal skin, and a morbilliform rash, haemorrhagic manifestations, and leucopenia. Other manifestations include flushed facies, sore throat, cough, cutaneous hyperaesthesia, and taste aberrations. Convalescence may be prolonged and complicated by profound fatigue and depression.

When the only haemorrhagic manifestation is provoked (by a tourniquet test), the case used to be categorized as grade I dengue haemorrhagic fever, but a spontaneous haemorrhage, even if mild, indicated grade II illness. Due to concerns about the widespread applicability of this grading system, it was updated by the WHO in recent years (WHO and Special Programme for Research and Training in Tropical Diseases 2009). Grades III and IV dengue haemorrhagic fever (incipient and frank circulatory failure, respectively) represent dengue shock syndrome which is characterized by sustained abdominal pain, persistent vomiting, sudden change from fever to hypothermia, alteration of consciousness, and a sudden drop in platelet count. Around 40 per cent of patients also have enlargement and tenderness of the liver. Rare presentations of infection include severe haemorrhage, severe hepatitis, rhabdomyolysis, jaundice, parotitis, cardiomyopathy, and variable neurological syndromes.

Infection with one serotype is thought to produce lifelong immunity to that serotype but only partial immunity to the others. Previous infection with a specific serotype followed by infection with a new serotype greatly increases the risk of dengue haemorrhagic fever.

Dengue virus serotypes are distinguishable by complement fixation and neutralization test. Other diagnostic tests for patients with dengue include packed cell volume, platelet count, liver function tests, prothrombin time, partial thromboplastin time, electrolytes, and blood gas analysis. Laboratory findings commonly associated with dengue include leucopenia, lymphocytosis, increased concentration of liver enzymes, and thrombocytopenia. Diagnosis can be confirmed with several laboratory tests, especially the haemagglutination inhibition test and IgG or IgM enzyme immunoassays. Platelet counts and haematocrit

determinations should be repeated at least every 24 hours to allow prompt recognition of the development of dengue haemorrhagic fever and institution of fluid replacement. Diagnostic criteria for dengue fever are provided in Fig. 8.11.5.

Evidence-based interventions

Rapid urbanization has led to an increase in the environmental factors that contribute to the proliferation of *Aedes* mosquitoes. These include uncontrolled urban development, inadequate management of water and waste, presence of a range of large water stores, and disposable, non-biodegradable containers that become habitats for the larvae. These factors can change a region from non-endemic (no virus present) to hypoendemic (one serotype present) to hyperendemic (multiple serotypes present).

Medical treatment

No specific therapeutic agents exist for dengue fever apart from analgesics and medications to reduce fever. Treatment is supportive; steroids, antivirals, or carbazochrome (which decreases capillary permeability) have no proven role. In contrast, ribavirin, interferon alpha, and 6-azauridine have shown some antiviral activity *in vitro*. Mild or classic dengue is treated with antipyretic agents such as acetaminophen, bed rest, and fluid replacement (usually administered orally and only rarely parenterally); most cases can be managed on an outpatient basis.

The management of dengue haemorrhagic fever and the dengue shock syndrome is purely supportive. Aspirin and other non-steroidal anti-inflammatory drugs should be avoided owing to the increased risk for Reye's syndrome and haemorrhage.

Preventive measures

In the absence of a vaccine, vector control is the only effective preventive measure. At a personal level, the risk of mosquito bites may be reduced by the use of protective clothing and repellents.

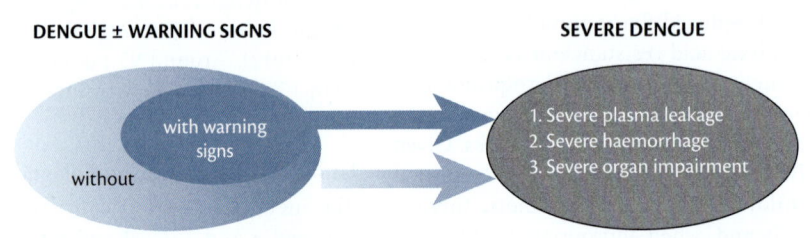

DENGUE ± WARNING SIGNS

with warning signs

without

SEVERE DENGUE

1. Severe plasma leakage
2. Severe haemorrhage
3. Severe organ impairment

CRITERIA FOR DENGUE ± WARNING SIGNS

Probable dengue

live in/travel to dengue endemic area.
Fever and 2 of the following criteria:
• Nausea, vomiting
• Rash
• Aches and pains
• Tourniquest test positive
• Leucopenia
• Any warning sign

Laboratory-confirmed dengue

(important when no sign plasma leakage)

Warning signs*

• Abdominal pain or tenderness
• Persistent vomiting
• Clinical fluid accumulation
• Mucosal bleed
• Lethargy, restlessness
• Liver enlargment >2 cm
• Laboratory: increase in HCT concurrent with rapid decrease in platelet count

*(requiring strict observation and medical intervention))

CRITERIA FOR SEVERE DENGUE

Severe plasma leakage

leading to:
• Shock (DSS)
• Fluid accumulation with respiratory distress

Severe bleeding

as evauated by clinician

Severe organ involvement

• Liver: AST or ALT >= 1000
• CNS: Impaired consciousness
• Heart and other organs

Fig. 8.11.5 Suggested dengue case classification and levels of severity.
Reproduced with permission from World Health Organization and Special Programme for Research and Training in Tropical Diseases, *Dengue Guidelines for Diagnosis, Treatment, and Prevention*, Copyright © World Health Organization 2009, available from: http://whqlibdoc.who.int/publications/2009/9789241547871_eng.pdf.

The single most effective preventive measure for travellers in areas where dengue is endemic is to avoid mosquito bites by using insect repellents containing *N, N*-diethyl-3-methyl-benzamide (DEET) or picaridin. The insect repellents should be used in the early morning and late afternoon, when *Aedes* mosquitoes are most active.

At a public health level, the risk of dengue fever outbreaks can be reduced by removing neighbourhood sources of stagnant water, especially within homes, using larvicides (especially for containers that cannot be eliminated), use of aerosolized insecticides, and introduction of predatory crustaceans.

Live attenuated tetravalent vaccines have been evaluated in phase 2 trials. Preliminary results demonstrated 80–90 per cent seroconversion rates in humans. A recently completed phase 2b trial of the recombinant, CYD tetravalent dengue vaccine in Thailand demonstrated an overall protective efficacy of 30 per cent with substantial variation among serotypes (Sabchaereon et al. 2012). While the vaccine proved to be safe, protective efficacy ranged from 9 per cent for serotype 2 to 100 per cent for serotype 4. New approaches to vaccine development being studied include infectious clone DNA and naked DNA vaccines. These vaccines offer promise in terms of immunoprotection against all serotypes as well.

Parasitic infections

A broad range of parasites plagues humans worldwide. While certain parasites, such as the *Plasmodium* species that cause malaria, are well recognized and have received intensive international support for research and programmatic control interventions, others are considered among the world's most neglected diseases. Some of the main neglected tropical parasitic diseases include the protozoan infections such as human African trypanosomiasis, visceral leishmaniasis, and American trypanosomiasis (Chagas disease) and helminthic infections such as the soil-transmitted nematodes (ascariasis, hookworms, trichuriasis), schistosomiasis, lymphatic filariasis, onchocerciasis, and dracunculiasis.

Of the 20 major helminth infections of humans, the commonest are the geohelminths. Roundworms, members of the phylum Nematoda, are responsible for an estimated 1 billion or more human infections. In many low-income countries, it is more common to be infected than not. Indeed, a child growing up in an endemic community can be infected soon after weaning, and continue to be infected and constantly re-infected for life.

Global and regional epidemiology

Recent global estimates indicate that more than a quarter of the world's population is infected with one or more helminths. The geographic distribution of roundworms in many tropical and subtropical regions closely parallels socioeconomic and sanitary conditions. In locales where several species of intestinal parasites are found, co-infection with *Ascaris lumbricoides*, *Trichuris trichiura*, and hookworms is common. In low- and middle-income countries, about 1.2 billion people are infected with the roundworm, *A. lumbricoides*, while more than 700 million are infected with hookworm (*Necator americanus* or *Ancylostoma duodenale*) or whipworm (*T. trichiura*) (Hotez et al. 2004). The GBD 2010 study estimated that 152,300 people died from neglected tropical diseases, which were predominantly parasitic infections with the

notable exception of rabies (Lozano et al. 2012). While mortality is not common, parasitic infections are responsible for substantial morbidity and indirectly contribute to death from other diseases due to their negative impact on nutritional status.

Issues in presentation

Children of school age are at greatest risk from the clinical manifestations of disease. Studies have shown associations between helminth infection and undernutrition, iron deficiency anaemia, stunted growth, poor school attendance, and poor performance in cognition tests. Some 44 million pregnancies are currently complicated by maternal hookworm infection, placing both mothers and children at higher risk of anaemia and death during pregnancy and delivery. Intense whipworm infection in children may result in trichuris dysentery syndrome, the classic signs of which include bloody diarrhoea, anaemia, growth retardation, and occasionally rectal prolapse. Heavy burdens of both roundworm and whipworm are associated with protein energy malnutrition and deficiencies of certain micronutrients such as vitamin A.

Medical treatment

The WHO recommends the use of albendazole, mebendazole, pyrantel pamoate, and levamisole (Table 8.11.16). The benzimidazoles, albendazole and mebendazole, have high efficacy against roundworm and moderate efficacy against whipworm. Single-dose mebendazole is much less effective against hookworm, with cure rates typically below 60 per cent.

Preventive measures

Better sanitation reduces soil and water transmission as transmission of geohelminths depends on transmission in environments contaminated with egg-carrying faeces. The provision of adequate sanitation is the only definitive intervention to eliminate helminthic infections, but to be effective it should cover a high percentage of the population. With high costs involved, implementing this strategy is difficult where resources are limited. Both the World Bank and the WHO promote helminth control programmes and consider it as one of the most cost-effective strategies to improve health in developing countries. These programmes emphasize mass drug administration as a major component of control.

Recommended drugs for use in public health settings include albendazole (single dose: 400 mg, reduced to 200 mg for children between 12 and 24 months), mebendazole (single dose: 500 mg), and levamisole or pyrantel palmoate. Programmes aim for mass treatment of all children in high-risk groups (communities where worms are endemic) with antihelminthic drugs every 3–6 months. A systematic review of randomized controlled trials found that deworming increases haemoglobin by 1.71 g/L (95 per cent confidence interval 0.70–2.73), which could translate into a small (5–10 per cent) reduction in the prevalence of anaemia (Gulani et al. 2007).

Home delivery of antihelminthics is problematic for several reasons and thus school-based deworming programmes are preferred. These have been shown to boost school participation and are practical as schools offer a readily available, extensive, and sustained infrastructure with a skilled workforce that can be readily trained. In Kenya, such a programme reduced school absenteeism by a quarter, with the largest gains among the youngest children. Perhaps even more importantly, this study showed that those children who had not been treated benefited

Table 8.11.16 Diagnosis and treatment of major intestinal nematode infections

Organism	Type of specimen	Specimen preparation	Size of eggs or larvae (µm)	Drug of choice	Alternative therapies
Trichuris trichiura	Stool	Direct smear or concentration	50–54 × 23	Mebendazole, 100 mg orally (PO) twice daily (bid) × 3 days	Albendazole, 400 mg PO once
Ascaris lumbricoides	Stool	Direct smear or concentration	45–70 × 35–50	Mebendazole, 100 mg PO bid × 3 days or albendazole, 400 mg PO once or pyrantel pamoate, 11 mg/kg PO once (max 1 g)	Piperazine citrate, 75 mg/kg twice daily (max. 1 g) by nasogastric tube × 2–3 days until resolution of obstruction
Ancylostoma duodenale Necator americanus	Stool	Direct smear or concentration	55–70 × 35–45	Mebendazole, 100 mg PO twice daily × 3 days	Albendazole, 400 mg PO once or pyrantel pamoate, 11 mg/kg PO × 3 days (max. 1 g)
Enterobius vermicularis	Adhesive tape preparation	Direct microscopy	50–60 × 20–30	Mebendazole, 100 mg PO once or pyrantel pamoate, 11 mg/kg PO once Repeat in 2 weeks	Albendazole, 400 mg PO once Repeat in 2 weeks
Strongyloides stercoralis	Stool, duodenal aspirate	Concentration or Baermann method	400–500 × 15	Ivermectin, 150–200 micrograms/kg PO × 1–2 days[a]	Albendazole 400 mg PO once or twice daily for 3 days

[a] Intrarectal ivermectin is an option for treatment of high-grade strongyloidiasis.

from the generally lowered transmission rate in the schools. These school-based programmes have resulted in improvements in overall nutritional status, growth, physical fitness, appetite, anaemia, and cognitive development. These measures must be coupled with community behaviour change strategies with the aim of reducing contamination of soil and water by promoting the use of latrines and hygienic behaviour. Without a change in defecation habits, periodic deworming cannot attain a stable reduction in transmission.

Prions

Prion diseases, which are also known as transmissible spongiform encephalopathies (TSEs), are responsible for rapidly progressive, fatal neurodegenerative diseases of humans and several other mammalian species. The term 'prion' is derived from *proteina-ceous* and *infectious*. An unconventional transmissible protein that lacks nucleic acid is the probable cause; this prion protein appears to consist of a modified isoform of a normal cellular prion protein (PrP^c) that is converted into PrP^{Sc}, which results in major changes in the physicochemical properties of the PrP leading to abnormal folding of normal cellular proteins. Prion diseases are associated with pathology of the brain characterized by diffuse spongiform degeneration. The transmissibility was established by intracerebral inoculation of various primate species using pas-saged prions from infected humans.

Epidemiology

Human prion diseases can be sporadic, inherited, or transmis-sible. The sporadic forms include kuru where infection occurs through ritualistic cannibalism and sporadic Creutzfeldt–Jakob disease (CJD). CJD can also occur in a familial manner due to germ-line mutations in the PrP gene or as a result of infection from bovine prions (variant CJD (vCJD)). The TSEs include bovine spongiform encephalopathy (BSE) in cattle; scra-pie in sheep; chronic wasting diseases in deer, elk, and mules; feline spongiform encephalopathy in cats (possibly secondary

to ingestion of prion-contaminated bovine tissues and bone meal); transmissible mink encephalopathy; and exotic ungu-late encephalopathy in kudu, nyala, and oryx (Ramasamy et al. 2003).

The major forms in human are sporadic CJD, vCJD, and an inherited form, the prion disease called Gerstmann–Straussler–Scheinker disease. Iatrogenic CJD can also occur as a result of infected dura mater grafts, improperly sterilized depth electrodes, transplanted corneas, and human growth hormone and gonado-trophin derived from cadaveric pituitaries.

An epidemic of BSE in the United Kingdom that began in 1986 affected nearly 200,000 cattle and was followed by human cases of vCJD starting in 1994 (Brown et al. 2001). The source of the BSE outbreak resulted from a change in the process of render-ing carcasses of livestock, which were used as a protein-rich nutritional supplement for feeding ruminants and other ani-mals. Banning the use of meat and bone meal helped to eventu-ally control the epidemic of BSE. In the mid 1990s, the United Kingdom saw a rise in human vCJD cases with 87 definite or probable case occurring there by November 2000 and a few cases identified as well in France and Ireland. Since the incubation period of vCJD is not known, it was hypothesized to be as short as 5–10 years if the BSE outbreak in the mid to late 1980s was the source. Between 2000 and 2005, the number of annual deaths due to vCJD gradually declined. In total there were 176 cases between 1995 and 2011 in the United Kingdom and 49 recorded in 11 other countries.

Clinical manifestations

Classic CJD usually presents in the elderly (median age of onset 68 years) and is characterized by dementia with the early onset of neurological signs. Death usually occurs within 4–5 months. In contrast, vCJD presents at a median age of 27 years, has an illness duration of 13–14 months, and is clinically character-ized by prominent behavioural and psychiatric symptoms, pain-ful dysaesthesias, and the delayed onset of neurological signs.

Table 8.11.17 Public health interventions and their effect on diseases

Major intervention	Disease prevented or treated
Effective antenatal care	Neonatal sepsis and meningitis, pneumonia
Skilled maternal and neonatal care	Neonatal sepsis and meningitis, neonatal tetanus
Maintenance of good personal hygiene	Neonatal sepsis and meningitis, diarrhoea, typhoid fever
Antimicrobial therapy	Neonatal sepsis, meningitis, bacteraemia, diarrhoea, pneumonia, typhoid fever, malaria, parasitic diseases
Vaccines	Pneumonia, typhoid fever, meningitis, bacteraemia
Oral rehydration therapy	Diarrhoea
Vitamin A	Diarrhoea, measles, malaria
Zinc	Diarrhoea, pneumonia, malaria
Provision of safe water, sanitation, and hygiene	Neonatal sepsis and meningitis, diarrhoea, pneumonia, typhoid fever, intestinal helminths
Breastfeeding	Neonatal sepsis and meningitis, diarrhoea, pneumonia
Complementary feeding	Neonatal sepsis, diarrhoea, pneumonia
Intermittent preventive therapy in pregnancy	Malaria
Insecticide-treated nets	Malaria
Integrated vector control	Malaria, dengue, other vector-borne diseases

In addition, vCJD cases all are homozygous for methionine at codon 129 of the PrP gene and have marked accumulation of protease-resistant PrP in brain tissue and florid plaques on neuropathology in large numbers in contrast to classic CJD where these are rare to absent.

Diagnosis and treatment

Neuropathological evaluation by Western blot or immunohistochemistry is the definitive approach for diagnosing human prion diseases. This method can also be used to monitor for vCJD and other forms of CJD. Electroencephalography (EEG) and magnetic resonance imaging (MRI) may be useful adjuncts to diagnosis in patients with CJD. Periodic sharp waves on EEG are often present in classic CJD but absent in vCJD whereas the 'pulvinar sign', an abnormal signal in the posterior thalami on T2- and diffusion-weighted MRI images, is present in the majority of patients with vCJD but is rare or absent in CJD.

There is no known therapy for any of the prion diseases. Prognosis is poor with progression to death in a median of 4–5 months for CJD and a little over a year for vCJD.

Conclusion

The global burden of infectious diseases contributing to childhood and adult morbidity and mortality is considerable. The situation is further compounded by increasing antimicrobial resistance and the emergence of new viral infections such as avian influenza (H5N1) and the coronavirus responsible for severe acute respiratory syndrome (SARS). Although the contribution of neonatal infections to overall child mortality has only recently been recognized, the persistent global burden of deaths due to diarrhoea and pneumonia underscore the need for improved public health strategies for change. There are interventions that can make a difference to childhood and adult infectious diseases (Table 8.11.17). What is needed is their implementation at scale to populations at greatest risk. This will require not only biomedical approaches but also measures to address the social determinants of disease.

Online supplementary materials

Additional online materials are available for this chapter at ℘ http://www.oxfordmedicine.com.

References

Addo-Yobo, E., Chisaka, N., Hassan, M., et al. (2004). Oral amoxicillin versus injectable penicillin for severe pneumonia in children aged 3 to 59 months: a randomised multicentre equivalency study. *The Lancet*, 364, 1141–8.

Aggarwal, R., Sentz, J., and Miller, M.A. (2007). Role of zinc administration in prevention of childhood diarrhea and respiratory illnesses: a meta-analysis. *Pediatrics*, 119, 1120–30.

Arifeen, S.E., Mullany, L.C., Shah, R., et al. (2012). The effect of cord cleansing with chlorhexidine on neonatal mortality in rural Bangladesh: a community-based, cluster-randomised trial. *The Lancet*, 379, 1022–8.

Armstrong, G.L., Conn, L.A., and Pinner, R.W. (1999). Trends in infectious disease mortality in the United States during the 20th century. *Journal of the American Medical Association*, 281, 61–6.

Bari, A., Sadruddin, S., Khan, A., et al. (2011). Community case management of severe pneumonia with oral amoxicillin in children aged 2–59 months in Haripur district, Pakistan: a cluster randomised trial. *The Lancet*, 378, 1796–803.

Bhan, M.K., Bahl, R., and Bhatnagar, S. (2005). Typhoid and paratyphoid fever. *The Lancet*, 366, 749–62.

Bhutta, Z.A. (2006). Current concepts in the diagnosis and treatment of typhoid fever. *BMJ*, 333, 78–82.

Bhutta, Z.A. (2007). Dealing with childhood pneumonia in developing countries: how can we make a difference? *Archives of Diseases of Childhood*, 92, 286–8.

Bhutta, Z.A., Das, J.K., Rizvi, A., et al. (2013a). Evidence based interventions for improvement of maternal and child nutrition: what can be done and at what cost? *The Lancet*, 382(9890), 452–77.

Bhutta, Z.A., Das, J.K., Walker, N., et al. (2013b). Interventions to address deaths from childhood pneumonia and diarrhoea equitably: what works and at what cost? *The Lancet*, 381, 1417–29.

Black, R.E., Morris, S.S., and Bryce, J. (2003). Where and why are 10 million children dying every year? *The Lancet*, 361, 2226–34.

Brouwer, M.C., Thwaites, G.E., Tunkel, A.R., and van de Beek, D. (2012). Dilemmas in the diagnosis of acute community-acquired bacterial meningitis. *The Lancet*, 380, 1684–92.

Brouwer, M.C., Tunkel, A.R., and van de Beek, D. (2010). Epidemiology, diagnosis, and antimicrobial treatment of acute bacterial meningitis. *Clinical Microbiology Reviews*, 23, 467–92.

Brown, P., Will, R.G., Bradley, R., Asher, D.M., and Detwiler, L. (2001). Bovine spongiform encephalopathy and variant Creutzfeldt-Jakob disease: background, evolution, and current concerns. *Emerging Infectious Diseases*, 7, 6–14.

Cohen, M.L. (2000). Changing patterns of infectious disease. *Nature*, 406, 762–7.

Crump, J.A., Luby, S.P., and Mintz, E.D. (2004). The global burden of typhoid fever. *Bulletin of the World Health Organization*, 82, 346–53.

Darmstadt, G.L., Badrawi, N., Law, P.A., et al. (2004). Topically applied sunflower seed oil prevents invasive bacterial infections in preterm infants in Egypt: a randomized, controlled clinical trial. *Pediatric Infectious Diseases Journal*, 23, 719–25.

Darmstadt, G.L., Bhutta, Z.A., Cousens, S., et al. (2005). Lancet Neonatal Survival Steering Team. Evidence based cost-effective interventions: how many newborn babies can we save? *The Lancet*, 365, 977–88.

Deen, J.L., Harris, E., Wills, B., et al. (2006). The WHO dengue classification and case definitions: time for a reassessment. *The Lancet*, 368, 170–3.

Fischer Walker, C.L., Rudan, I., Liu, L., et al. (2013). Global burden of childhood pneumonia and diarrhoea. *The Lancet*, 381, 1405–16.

Gulani, A., Nagpal, J., Osmond, C., et al. (2007). Effect of administration of intestinal anthelminthic drugs on haemoglobin: systematic review of randomised controlled trials. *BMJ*, 334, 1095.

Hamer, D.H. and Gorbach, S.L. (2010). Gastrointestinal infections. In D.A. Warrell, T.M. Cox, and J.D. Firth (eds.) *Oxford Textbook of Medicine* (5th ed.), pp. 2424–34. Oxford: Oxford University Press.

Hanh, S.K., Kim, Y.J., and Garner, P. (2001). Reduced osmolarity oral rehydration solution for treating dehydration due to diarrhoea in children: a systematic review. *BMJ*, 323, 81–5.

Hotez, P.J., Brooker, S., Bethony, J.M., et al. (2004). Hookworm infection. *The New England Journal of Medicine*, 351, 799–807.

Huttly, S.R., Morris, S.S., and Pisani, V. (1997). Prevention of diarrhoea in young children in developing countries. *Bulletin of the World Health Organization*, 75, 163–74.

Institute for Health Metrics and Evaluation (n.d.). *Global Burden of Disease (GBD)*. [Online] Available at: http://www.healthdata.org/gbd.

Kosek, M., Bern, C., and Guerrant, R.L. (2003). The magnitude of the global burden of diarrheal disease from studies published 1992–2000. *Bulletin of the World Health Organization*, 81, 197–204.

Kotloff, K.L., Nataro, J.P., Blackwelder, W.C., et al. (2013). Burden and aetiology of diarrhoeal disease in infants and young children in developing countries (the Global Enteric Multicenter Study, GEMS): a prospective, case-control study. *The Lancet*, 382, 209–22.

Liu, L., Johnson, H.L., Cousens, S., et al. (2012). Global, regional, and national causes of child mortality: an updated systematic analysis for 2010 with time trends since 2000. *The Lancet*, 379, 2151–61.

Lozano, R., Naghavi, M., Foreman, K., et al. (2012). Global and regional mortality from 235 causes of death for 20 age groups in 1990 and 2010: a systematic analysis for the Global Burden of Disease Study 2010. *The Lancet*, 380, 2095–128.

Mandell, L.A., Wunderink, R.G., Anzueto, A., et al. (2007). Infectious Diseases Society of America/American Thoracic Society consensus guidelines on the management of community-acquired pneumonia in adults. *Clinical Infectious Diseases*, 44, S27–S72.

Mullany, L.C., Darmstadt, G.L., Khatry, S.K., et al. (2006). Topical applications of chlorhexidine to the umbilical cord for prevention of omphalitis and neonatal mortality in southern Nepal: a community-based, cluster-randomised trial. *The Lancet*, 367, 910–18.

Murray, C.J.L., Vos, T., Lozano, R., et al. (2012). Disability–adjusted life years (DALYs) for 291 diseases and injuries in 21 regions, 1990–2010: a systematic analysis for the Global Burden of Disease Study 2010. *The Lancet*, 380, 2197–223.

Nair, H., Brooks, A.W., Katz, M., et al. (2011). Global burden of respiratory infections due to seasonal influenza in young children: a systematic review and meta-analysis. *The Lancet*, 378, 1917–30.

Nigrovic, L.E., Kupperman, N., Macias, C.G., et al. (2007). Clinical prediction rule for identifying children with cerebrospinal fluid pleocytosis at very low risk of bacterial meningitis. *Journal of the American Medical Association*, 297, 52–60.

Ramasamy, I., Law, M., Collins, S., and Brooke, F. (2003). Organ distribution of prion proteins in variant Creutzfeldt-Jakob disease. *The Lancet Infectious Diseases*, 3, 214–22.

Rice, A.L., Sacco, L., Hyder, A., et al. (2000). Malnutrition as an underlying cause of childhood deaths associated with infectious diseases in developing countries. *Bulletin of the World Health Organization*, 278, 1207–21.

Sabchareon, A., Wallace, D., Sirivichayakul, C., et al. (2012). Protective efficacy of the recombinant CYD tetravalent dengue vaccine in Thai schoolchildren: a randomised controlled phase 2b trial. *The Lancet*, 380, 1559–67.

Saha, S.K., Darmstadt, G.L., Yamanaka, N., et al. (2005). Rapid diagnosis of pneumococcal meningitis: implications for treatment and measuring disease burden. *Pediatric Infectious Disease Journal*, 24, 1093–8.

Seward, N., Osrin, D., Li, L., et al. (2012). Association between clean delivery kit use, clean deliver practices, and neonatal survival: pooled analysis of data from three sites in South Asia. *PLoS Medicine*, 9, 1–11.

Song, J., Gao, J., and Gálan, J. (2013). Structure and function of the *Salmonella* Typhi chimeric A_2B_5 typhoid toxin. *Nature*, 499, 350–4.

Soofi, S., Ahmed, S., Fox, M.P., et al. (2012a). Effectiveness of community case management of severe pneumonia with oral amoxicillin in children aged 2–59 months in Matiari district, rural Pakistan: a cluster randomised controlled trial. *The Lancet*, 379, 729–37.

Soofi, S., Cousens, S., Imdad, A., et al. (2012b). Topical application of chlorhexidine to neonatal umbilical cords for prevention of omphalitis and neonatal mortality in a rural district of Pakistan: a community-based, cluster-randomised trial. *The Lancet*, 379, 1029–36.

Van de Beek, D., Brouwer, M.C., Thwaites, G.E., and Tunkel, A.R. (2012). Advances in treatment of bacterial meningitis. *The Lancet*, 380, 1693–702.

Van de Beek, D., de Gans, J., McIntyre, P., et al. (2007). Corticosteroids for acute bacterial meningitis. *Cochrane Database of Systematic Reviews*, 1, CD004405.

Vesikari, T., Esposito, S., Prymula, R., et al. (2013). Immunogenicity and safety of an investigational multicomponent, recombinant, meningococcal serogroup B vaccine (4CMenB) administered concomitantly with routine infant and child vaccinations: results of two randomised trials. *The Lancet*, 381, 825–35.

Waters, D., Jawad, I., Ahmad, A., et al. (2011). Aetiology of community-acquired neonatal sepsis in low- and middle-income countries. *Journal of Global Health*, 1, 154–70.

World Health Organization and Special Programme for Research and Training in Tropical Diseases (2009). *Dengue Guidelines for Diagnosis, Treatment, and Prevention*. Geneva: WHO.

Zinc Investigators' Collaborative Group (1999). Prevention of diarrhea and pneumonia by zinc supplementation in children in developing countries: pooled analysis of randomized controlled trials. *Journal of Pediatrics*, 135, 689–97.

8.12

Sexually transmitted infections

Mary L. Kamb and Patricia J. Garcia

Introduction to sexually transmitted infections

Sexually transmitted infections (STIs) refer to a broad array of pathogens that are transmitted through vaginal, anal, or oral sex. More than 30 organisms and as many syndromes are recognized as transmissible through sexual contact (Table 8.12.1). However, the vast majority of STIs today are caused by a small number of pathogens, including: three bacterial STIs, chlamydia (*Chlamydia trachomatis*), gonorrhoea (*Neisseria gonorrhoeae*), and syphilis (*Treponema pallidum*); a parasitic infection causing trichomoniasis (*Trichomonas vaginalis*); several viral infections including human papillomavirus (HPV), genital herpes usually caused by herpes simplex virus type 2 (HSV-2) and less commonly HSV-1; three unrelated viruses causing hepatitis: hepatitis A virus (HAV), hepatitis B virus (HBV), and hepatitis C virus (HCV); and human immunodeficiency virus (HIV). The bacterial STIs and trichomoniasis are curable with readily available antibiotic drugs, although previous infection confers no immunity and thus exposed individuals are susceptible to reinfection. In contrast, the viral STIs are not cured with antimicrobial agents and, although symptoms can often be ameliorated with antiviral medications, tend to cause lifelong (prevalent) infections—although some infections can be transient (e.g. with HPV and HBV). Three viral infections (HPV, HBV, HAV) are preventable with vaccines.

STIs are among the world's most common contagious diseases, with the global annual incidence of curable STIs estimated by the World Health Organization (WHO) at just under 500 million cases per year (WHO 2008). Thus, in terms of global burden, curable STIs are exceeded only by diarrhoeal diseases, malaria, and lower respiratory infections. In countries with active notifiable disease surveillance systems, STIs are typically among the most common reportable conditions. For example, in the United States in 2010, laboratory-defined chlamydia and gonorrhoea were the first and second most commonly reported conditions out of more than 50 notifiable diseases, with syphilis ranking fourth (after salmonellosis) (Centers for Disease Control and Prevention (CDC) 2010). However, the burden of curable STIs is dwarfed in comparison to the viral infections. For example, an estimated 290 million women worldwide are HPV carriers (de Sanjosé et al. 2007) and available data support that roughly equal numbers of men are HPV infected (Dunne et al. 2006; Smith et al. 2011). Globally about 540 million reproductive-aged men and women are infected with HSV-2 (Looker et al. 2008). Although the majority of the world's 360 million HBV infections are transmitted vertically from mother to child, a large number of HBV infections were transmitted sexually; and while most infections are self-limited, a proportion will become chronic infections with potential to lead to severe liver disease and death (CDC 2007). Additionally, approximately 34 million people worldwide are living with HIV infections, of which about 90 per cent were transmitted sexually (Joint United Nations Programme on HIV/AIDS (UNAIDS) 2011).

The majority of STIs are asymptomatic, and thus screening asymptomatic people at risk for STI is as essential a component of effective prevention and control programmes as clinical examination and diagnostic tests in symptomatic disease. Nonetheless, many STIs are associated with disagreeable symptoms such as genital sores, discharges, or rashes that lead affected individuals to seek healthcare services. Given the high numbers of STIs that exist in almost every nation, it is not surprising to find that regardless of a nation's resources, STI symptoms can account for a large number of healthcare visits and substantial costs (Over and Piot 1996; Dallabetta et al. 2007; Owusu-Edusei et al. 2013). Highly stigmatized across all cultures, STIs may also result in psychosocial consequences such as anxiety, shame, disrupted relationships, and even intimate partner violence (Gottlieb et al. 2014). Additionally, the costs and impact of STI-associated health outcomes due to infertility, adverse pregnancy outcomes, malignancies, and HIV acquisition and transmission are increasingly recognized (Owusu-Edusei et al. 2013; Gottlieb et al. 2014). While STI case rates are highest in adolescents and young adults, the most serious health outcomes occur later in life and are disproportionately borne by women and infants. For these reasons, STI prevention and control is an important public health investment for every country.

In this chapter we summarize the global epidemiology of STIs and their associated health consequences, and report on factors affecting STI spread in the community. We also discuss STI prevention and control as a public health intervention, relying on many interrelated interventions working together to reduce STI incidence and prevalence in the community. Finally, we consider some of the most likely challenges and opportunities in STI prevention anticipated over the next few decades.

Table 8.12.1 Sexually transmitted pathogens and associated diseases or syndromes

Pathogen	Associated disease or syndrome
Bacteria	
Neisseria gonorrhoeae	*Adult*: cervicitis, urethritis, proctitis, pharyngitis, Bartholinitis, endometritis, pelvic inflammatory disease (PID), infertility, chronic pelvic pain, orchitis, epididymitis, urethral stricture, prostatitis, perihepatitis, disseminated infection, Reiter's syndrome, enhanced HIV risk, often asymptomatic (up to 2/3 women, 1/3 men) *Maternal*: ectopic pregnancy, maternal death, preterm rupture of membranes *Infant*: neonatal conjunctivitis, corneal scarring, blindness, premature birth, low birth weight (LBW)
Chlamydia trachomatis	*Adult*: cervicitis, urethritis, proctitis, pharyngitis, Bartholinitis, endometritis, PID, infertility, chronic pelvic pain, orchitis, epididymitis, urethral stricture, prostatitis, perihepatitis, disseminated infection, Reiter's syndrome, lymphogranuloma venereum (LGV)—anogenital ulcer or inguinal swelling, enhanced HIV risk, often asymptomatic (up to 2/3 women, 1/3 men) *Maternal*: ectopic pregnancy, maternal death, preterm rupture of membranes *Infant*: neonatal conjunctivitis, pneumonia, premature birth, LBW
Mycoplasma hominis	*Adult*: postpartum fever, PID
Mycoplasma genitalium	*Adult*: urethritis, cervicitis, PID, enhanced HIV risk
Ureaplasma urealyticum	*Adult*: urethritis *Maternal*: chorioamnionitis, premature delivery *Infant*: premature birth, LBW
Treponema pallidum (syphilis)	*Adult*: genital ulcer (chancre), local adenopathy, skin rashes, condyloma lata, hepatitis, arthritis, enhanced HIV risk; bone, cardiovascular (e.g. aortic disease) and central nervous system disease (e.g. meningitis, stroke, cranial nerve abnormalities, optic atrophy, tabes dorsalis, general paresis) *Maternal*: fetal loss, stillbirth, preterm delivery *Infant*: neonatal death, congenital syphilis, LBW
Gardnerella vaginalis (in association with other bacteria)	*Adult*: bacterial vaginosis, PID, enhanced HIV risk, urethral discharge *Maternal*: chorioamnionitis, prematurity, LBW
Haemophilus ducreyi (chancroid)	*Adult*: genital ulcers, inguinal adenitis, disfiguring lesions, tissue destruction, enhanced HIV risk
Calymmatobacterium granulomatis (Donovanosis)	*Adult*: Nodular swellings and ulcerative lesions of inguinal and anogenital areas (also called granuloma inguinale)
Shigella spp.	*Adult*: shigellosis in homosexual men
Salmonella spp.	*Adult*: enteritis, proctocolitis in homosexual men
Campylobacter spp.	*Adult*: enteritis, proctocolitis in homosexual men
Viruses	
Human immunodeficiency virus types 1 and 2	*Adult*: HIV-related disease, opportunistic infections, lymphomas, AIDS *Maternal*: vertical transmission to infants *Infant*: HIV infection
Herpes simplex virus types 1 and 2	*Adult*: anogenital vesicular lesions and ulcerations, recurrent genital ulcers, cold sores, cervicitis, urethritis, pharyngitis, proctitis, chronic pain, arthritis, aseptic meningitis, hepatitis, enhanced HIV risk *Maternal*: vertical transmission to infants *Infant*: ulcerations of skin, eye, mucous membranes; encephalitis, disseminated infection with hepatitis, pneumonitis, encephalitis; neurological abnormalities
Human papilloma virus (> 30 genital genotypes identified)	*Adult*: anogenital and oral warts; intraepithelial neoplasia and carcinoma of the cervix, penis, vulva, vagina, anus; oropharyngeal cancer; recurrent respiratory papillomatosis *Maternal*: vertical transmission to infant *Infant*: recurrent respiratory papillomatosis
Hepatitis B virus	*Adult*: acute hepatitis, liver cirrhosis, end-stage liver disease, hepatocellular cancer *Maternal*: vertical transmission to infant *Infant*: cirrhosis, end-stage liver disease, primary liver cancer
Hepatitis A virus	*Adult*: acute hepatitis A
Hepatitis C virus	*Adult*: acute hepatitis C, liver cirrhosis, end-stage liver disease, hepatocellular cancer

(continued)

Table 8.12.1 Continued

Pathogen	Associated disease or syndrome
Cytomegalovirus (CMV)	*Adult:* heterophil-negative infectious mononucleosis, hepatitis
	Infant: primary infection of the newborn, hepatitis, sepsis, deafness, mental retardation
Molluscum contagiosum virus	*Adult:* genital molluscum contagiosum
Human T-lymphotrophic retrovirus, type 1	*Adult:* human T-cell leukaemia or lymphoma
Human herpesvirus 8 (HHV-8)	*Adult:* Kaposi's sarcoma, primary effusion lymphoma, Castleman's disease
Protozoa	
Trichomonas vaginalis	*Adult:* vaginitis, cervicitis, urethritis, endometritis, salpingitis, enhanced HIV risk
	Maternal: chorioamnionitis, preterm delivery
	Infant: LBW, pneumonitis, fever, vaginal discharge in female infants
Entamoeba histolytica	*Adult:* amoebiasis in men who have sex with men
Giardia lamblia	*Adult:* giardiasis in men who have sex with men
Fungi	
Candida albicans	*Adult:* vulvovaginitis, balanitis
Ectoparasites	
Phthirus pubis	*Adult:* pubic lice infestation
Sarcoptes scabiei	*Adult:* scabies, Norwegian (disseminated) scabies
	Infants: Norwegian (disseminated) scabies

Global burden of sexually transmitted infections

The global burden of STIs includes overall numbers of infection, a host of short- and long-term adverse health outcomes causing morbidity and mortality in individuals, and the financial consequences (healthcare and other costs) associated with STIs and their associated health impact for both individuals and economies.

Global STI numbers

The WHO estimated that in 2008, approximately 499 million new cases of curable STIs occurred among men and women aged 15–49, including 106 million cases of chlamydia, 106 million cases of gonorrhoea, 11 million cases of syphilis, and 276 million cases of trichomoniasis (WHO 2008). New cases of STIs were common in all regions of the world, particularly the highly populated regions of the Americas (comprising the countries of North and South America and the Caribbean), East Asia and the Western Pacific, and South and Southeast Asia; however, rates were highest in the sub-Saharan Africa region (24 cases per 100 adults) and the region of the Americas (26 cases per 100 adults) (Fig. 8.12.1). Because population-based studies and active, laboratory-based reporting are limited in many countries, methodologies for estimating global STIs have been based on discrete, representative (but typically small) studies and good case-based surveillance reports contributed by countries in each region, with adjustment for unreported and undiagnosed cases (WHO 2008). The availability of such studies and reports and the methodological criteria used for including or excluding studies have varied over time, and thus assessing trends in estimates is somewhat challenging. However, comparing the 2008 global STI estimates to the most

recent prior report (2005), which used a similar methodology, suggests there has been limited if any recent improvement; in fact STI numbers are likely rising. Specifically, there was no observable change in syphilis numbers, a modest (4 per cent) increase in chlamydia cases, and larger increases in trichomonas (11 per cent) and gonorrhoea (21 per cent) cases.

All regions of the world observed increased numbers of curable STIs, supporting the case that global STI burden is indeed increasing. Increases were particularly notable in the region of the Americas and the Eastern Mediterranean region (i.e. countries of Northern Africa and the Middle East) where overall STI numbers more than doubled. While some of the increased numbers could be attributed to an increasing population, case rates of curable STI cases per 100 adults also rose in most regions—most notably in the Americas where they almost doubled between 2005 and 2008. More modest increases in case rates were observed in the Eastern Mediterranean region and in the two Asian regions; and STI case rates did not change appreciably in sub-Saharan Africa or Europe. It is possible that some of the observed increases in curable STI case numbers and rates globally were due to differences in screening practices among countries included in the report. However, reported screening practices seemed to be fairly similar across the two time periods (personal communication, WHO). Some of the increases could be attributable to broader availability of highly sensitive diagnostics (e.g. nucleic acid amplification tests (NAATs)) in some settings, as the extent to which curable STIs are asymptomatic has been relatively recently appreciated with increasingly sensitive diagnostics. However, in 2008 use of NAATs was still limited outside Europe and North America, and the vast majority of curable STIs occurred in low- and middle-income countries (WHO 2008). Additional data supporting that global

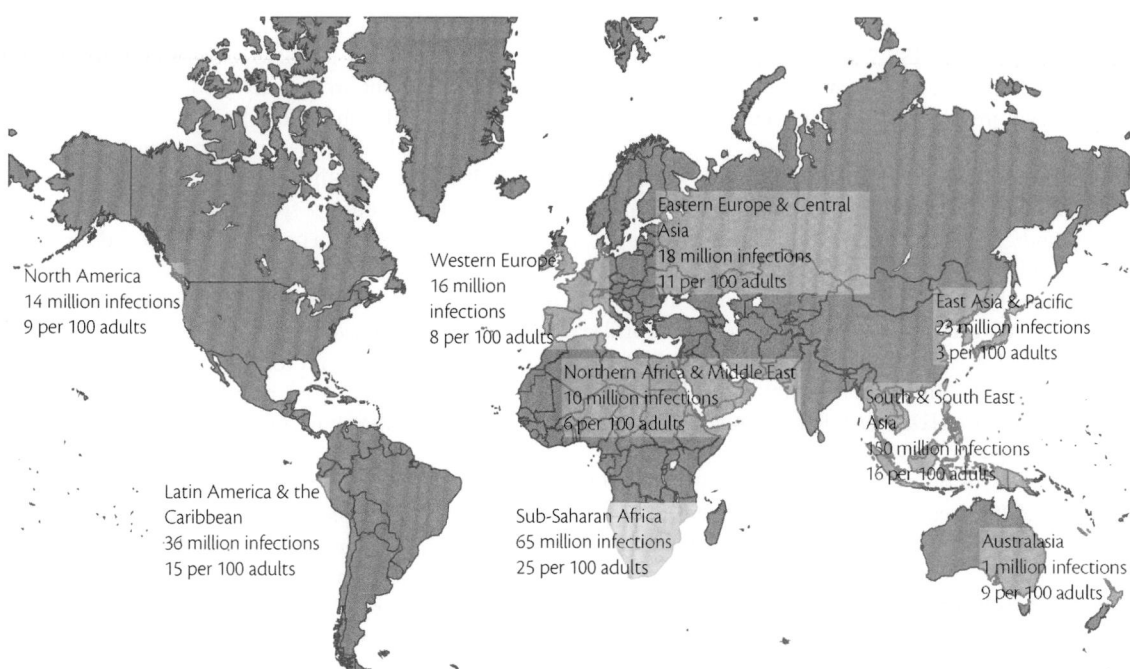

Fig. 8.12.1 Estimated annual numbers and incidence per 100 adults of curable STIs among men and women aged 15–44 years in 2008, by WHO region. Curable STIs include gonorrhoea, chlamydia, syphilis, and trichomoniasis. In 2008, approximately 499 million cases of curable STIs occurred globally among reproductive-aged adults.
Source: data from World Health Organization (WHO), Department of Reproductive Health and Research, *Global incidence and prevalence of selected curable sexually transmitted infections—2008*, Copyright © WHO 2012, available from http://apps.who.int/iris/bitstream/10665/75181/1/9789241503839_eng.pdf

burden of STIs is likely not declining comes from surveillance systems in Europe and North America, in the context of established national STI control programmes: although marked declines in syphilis and gonorrhoea case rates occurred in the past, recently trends have tended to be stable.

One problem faced by the research team conducting the 2008 estimates was identifying appropriate studies for inclusion. Many national STI reporting systems are based on syndromic management, and thus STI-specific aetiology is unknown (Gottleib et al. 2014). In some regions, such as Latin America, underreporting of STIs is common, and there is not yet consensus on which STIs to report or how to report data, resulting in burden of disease estimates that may not reflect the true situation (Garcia et al. 2011). Also notable, the authors of the most recent WHO STI estimates observed that the number of studies that met entry criteria had decreased remarkably over the 3-year interval between the 2005 and 2008 estimates, from 402 data points to 180 data points, respectively (WHO 2008). They reported that possible reasons for this included fewer studies being done in the general population, journals less interested in publishing STI surveillance data, and longer publication lead times. Public health funding focused on STIs other than HIV has also dwindled over that time interval, probably contributing to the decreasing availability of reliable STI prevalence data.

The 2008 global STI estimates evaluated curable STIs and did not attempt to estimate the extent of new and prevalent viral infections, which is difficult to estimate but easily exceeds a billion infections. For example, a 2007 review of genital HPV, arguably the most common STI, estimated that approximately 10 per cent of women worldwide had HPV infections at any point in time (de Sanjosé et al. 2007). Furthermore, US longitudinal studies

suggest that as many as 50–70 per cent of sexually active participants had evidence of an HPV infection at some point in their lives (Weinstock et al. 2004; Baseman and Koutsky 2005), and estimated that the virus accounted for about 5 million new infections annually in the United States alone (Weinstock et al. 2004; Baseman and Koutsky 2005). The vast majority of HPV infections are latent or asymptomatic and will not lead to overt disease or important health consequences. However, up to one-third of HPV infections globally are caused by oncogenic types (primarily types 16 and 18) with potential to lead to anogenital cancers, mainly occurring in low- and middle-income countries (de Sanjosé et al. 2007).

Vying with HPV in numbers is HSV-2, the agent most frequently associated with genital herpes. HSV-2 is exceedingly common, with reported population prevalences among nations ranging from 20 to 40 per cent or even higher, the vast majority of infections being asymptomatic (Smith and Robinson 2002). A 2003 systematic review estimated that worldwide, 536 million people aged 15–49 years were living with HSV-2, of whom 23.6 million were newly infected that year (Looker et al. 2008). National data are lacking in most countries. Based on 1999–2004 US national population-based surveys, about 17 per cent of reproductive-aged adults were HSV-2 infected, with prevalence increasing with advancing age (e.g. from 1.6 per cent in 14–19-year-olds up to 26.3 per cent in 40–49-year-olds) (Smith and Robinson 2002; Xu et al. 2006). In those surveys, HSV-2 prevalence varied considerably by race/ethnicity, with non-Hispanic black people having almost three times higher HSV-2 prevalence compared with other racial/ethnic groups (Xu et al. 2006). An important aspect of HSV infection is its clinical synergy with HIV; in co-infection each virus enhances shedding of the other. This phenomenon has led in turn to a population-level synergy: countries with rising HIV prevalence have reported increasing HSV-2 prevalence, suggesting that in the absence of effective prevention strategies a vicious cycle occurs with increasing prevalence of both infections (Paz-Bailey et al. 2007).

At least five distinct viruses are known to cause viral hepatitis (an acute illness characterized by nausea, malaise, abdominal symptoms, and jaundice), of which three (unrelated) viruses are common: hepatitis A, hepatitis B, and hepatitis C (CDC 2009). All three viruses are able to be transmitted sexually, although that is not their usual mode of spread. The majority of the world's 360 million chronic HBV infections were transmitted vertically from mother to child, although a substantial minority were related to injecting drug use (IDU) or other parenteral exposure including iatrogenic exposures through procedures such as haemodialysis or blood transfusion, or through sexual contact (WHO 2012a, 2014). Among US cases of HBV reported in 2007, 38 per cent had multiple sex partners, 11 per cent were men who had sex with men (MSM), and 6 per cent had sexual contact with a person known to have hepatitis B (CDC 2009). HCV, estimated at about 150 million chronic infections worldwide, is primarily transmitted through percutaneous exposures such as IDU or iatrogenic exposures, although it can also be transmitted through mucosal exposure with an infected person (e.g. through sexual activity) (WHO 2012a). Of the US cases of HCV reported in 2007 and for which risk factor information was available, IDU was the most commonly identified risk factor reported by 44 per cent of cases; 42 per cent reported multiple sex partners, 20 per cent reported having had surgery, and 10 per cent reported having sexual contact with a person known to have HCV (CDC 2009). Hepatitis A virus (HAV) is transmitted through faecal–oral contact. Among the most frequently identified risks are sexual and household contact with an HAV-infected person; accounting for about 8 per cent of reported cases in the United States (CDC 2009). The virus can be transmitted during sexual activity, and in the United States outbreaks in MSM have been linked to rectal–oral mucosal exposures during sex (CDC 2009). Risk factors for all three of the common hepatitis viruses likely vary considerably among countries depending upon prevalence of specific injecting and sexual practices, quality control of clinical procedures, and access to and availability of preventive services (e.g. vaccines against HAV and HBV, appropriately sterilized medical equipment, clean needles, condoms, education).

In addition to affecting adults, STIs can be transmitted from mother to child *in utero* or at the time of delivery. In 2011, UNAIDS estimated that 330,000 children acquired HIV infection, predominantly through perinatal transmission or contaminated breast milk (UNAIDS 2012). This represented a 43 per cent decline in new infections since the peak of the HIV pandemic in 2003, indicating effectiveness of prevention of mother-to-child transmission (MTCT) of HIV screening and treatment programmes. More than 90 per cent of perinatal HIV infections have occurred in sub-Saharan Africa (UNAIDS 2011, 2012). Less well recognized than MTCT of HIV is the contribution of maternal syphilis infection during pregnancy on global perinatal morbidity and mortality. A WHO report using a health service delivery model and universal access data for HIV and syphilis calculated that, worldwide in 2008, 1.36 million pregnant women had syphilis infections capable of transmitting *Treponema pallidum* perinatally

(Newman et al. 2013). In 2008, untreated maternal syphilis infections resulted in an estimated 521,000 adverse health outcomes in infants, ranging in severity from stillbirth or neonatal death to congenital infection in live born infants (Newman et al. 2013). Other STIs such as HSV-2 and cytomegalovirus (CMV) can be transmitted from mother-to-child *in utero*; however, global data are limited and country-specific data indicate these are substantially less common than perinatal HIV or syphilis (Xu et al. 2008).

STI-associated morbidity

Many individuals acquiring a new STI suffer disturbing physical symptoms, ranging from relatively minor discomfort or cosmetic concerns to intensely painful and recurrent conditions. Acquiring an STI may also result in psychological harm such as intense anxiety, shame, fear of disclosing to sex partners, or disrupted relationships (Cunningham et al. 2002; WHO 2007). A link between intimate partner violence and HIV has been well documented, and increasingly literature suggests that other STI diagnoses can be associated with intimate partner violence (Decker et al. 2011; Swartzendruber et al. 2012). Additionally, stigma or shame about an STI diagnosis may result in delays in health seeking and lack of full disclosure or discussion with health providers and sex partners (Cunningham et al. 2002; Fortenberry et al. 2002). This situation limits the effectiveness of both case management and partner management, and can increase likelihood of individual morbidity as well as further disease spread in the community.

In addition to short-term symptoms, many STIs are associated with long-term or chronic health problems (Table 8.12.1). Longer-term STI-associated health consequences have been broadly categorized into four areas: female reproductive health disorders (e.g. infertility, ectopic pregnancy, chronic pelvic pain); adverse pregnancy outcomes (e.g. stillbirth, neonatal death, prematurity); malignancies (e.g. anogenital cancers associated with HPV); and enhanced HIV acquisition mediated by ulceration or mucosal inflammation and increased numbers of HIV target cells associated with certain STIs. Although men are as likely, and in some settings more likely, than women to become infected with a new STI, women and infants bear the brunt of the longer-term STI-associated morbidity such as tubal factor infertility, adverse pregnancy outcomes, and cervical cancers. Exceptions to this are HBV-associated chronic liver disease and malignancy and enhanced risk for HIV infection which affect large numbers of men as well as women.

The most common of the serious STI consequences are adverse reproductive outcomes, particularly infertility, often caused by chlamydia and gonorrhoea. Chlamydia and gonorrhoea are highly prevalent infections, and from 10 to 40 per cent of women with untreated infection may develop pelvic inflammatory disease (PID)—an inflammation of the upper female tract that can manifest as endometritis, salpingitis, tubo-ovarian abscess, pelvic peritonitis, or some combination of these (CDC 2010). Up to 25 per cent of affected women are reported to experience infertility (Fortenberry et al. 2002; WHO 2007a). Tubal scarring may lead to ectopic pregnancy, associated with maternal morbidity and mortality as well as pregnancy loss. Women with a prior history of PID have been reported to be six to ten times more likely than unaffected women to develop a subsequent ectopic pregnancy; and an estimated 40–50 per cent of all ectopic pregnancies have been attributed to PID (CDC 2010). Chlamydial and gonorrhoeal infections also can lead to chronic pelvic pain in women. Trichomoniasis, the most common curable STI, primarily causes vaginal discharge in women although is typically asymptomatic in men. Vaginal discharge syndrome can be notoriously difficult to manage and may lead to multiple, costly healthcare visits, particularly in resource-poor settings without laboratory capacity to support aetiological diagnosis allowing targeted treatment with appropriate antimicrobial agents (Ryan et al. 2008).

Several STIs are associated with adverse pregnancy outcomes affecting the health or viability of infants. Perhaps the most devastating is maternal syphilis infection in pregnancy. Historical literature reported that untreated primary or secondary infections typically led to fetal death (Fiumara 1988); and that even latent infections of several years' duration could lead to complications if left untreated (Fiumara 1988). In a 2013 meta-analysis of the published literature that adjusted for other causes of poor pregnancy outcomes, untreated maternal syphilis infection resulted in seriously adverse pregnancy outcomes in over 50 per cent of cases (Gomez et al. 2013). Among untreated mothers, poor outcomes included stillbirth or fetal loss (21 per cent), neonatal death (9 per cent), prematurity or low birth weight (6 per cent), or an infected infant (15 per cent) (Gomez et al. 2013). The WHO estimated that, globally in 2008, two-thirds of syphilis-related adverse pregnancy outcomes were in women who were not tested or treated for syphilis during their pregnancies (Newman et al. 2013). Maternal infection with chlamydia during pregnancy has been associated with neonatal pneumonia and more commonly with neonatal conjunctivitis which, if left untreated, can lead to blindness. WHO estimated that in 2006, from 1000 to 4000 infants worldwide were blinded from STI-related conjunctivitis, although it is easily preventable with topical antimicrobial agents (WHO 2007a). Numerous observational studies have found an association between *T. vaginalis* infection and premature birth, although high-quality studies assessing this are limited (WHO 2007a; CDC 2010). However, some studies of *T. vaginalis* treatment during pregnancy found treatment associated with higher risks of poor pregnancy outcomes (Klebanoff et al. 2001; Kogozi et al. 2003). In addition to the well-recognized complications of HIV, other viral STIs can also cause adverse pregnancy outcomes. HSV-2 can cause neonatal herpes infection which, although unusual (estimated at one in 3000 births in the United States), is often severe or fatal when primary infection occurs during pregnancy (Brown et al. 1997; Dinh et al. 2008; Xu et al. 2008). Perinatally transmitted HPV can cause recurrent respiratory papillomatosis, a chronic condition often requiring recurrent surgical procedures. For perinatally acquired HBV, about 30 per cent will result in chronic infection, of which a portion will go on to serious complications including cirrhosis, liver failure, hepatocellular carcinoma, and death (CDC 2009).

Among the most serious complications associated with STI are certain malignancies, typically occurring after a latent period of many years or decades after the initial exposure and, therefore, often not recognized as related to an STI. STI-associated malignancies include anogenital cancers associated with oncogenic HPV types, hepatocellular carcinoma (primary liver cancer) associated with chronic HBV infection, some lymphomas associated with HIV and Kaposi's sarcomas associated with human herpes virus type 8 (HHV-8). The WHO estimates that up to 20 per cent of all cancers are related to the sexually transmitted viruses HPV

and HBV alone, and this proportion is higher in low-income nations (WHO 2013). For HPV, it has been firmly established that certain specific subtypes are the causal agents of cervical cancer, and likely of other anogenital cancers (e.g. vulvar, vaginal, penile, anal) as well (Zur Hausen 1996; Cogliano et al. 2005). Two carcinogenic HPV types, 16 and 18, are responsible for an estimated 70 per cent of all cervical cancers and 80 to 90 per cent of anal and penile cancers worldwide (Zur Hausen 1996; Munoz et al. 2003; Cogliano et al. 2005). Cervical cancer is now the second most common cancer in women worldwide, after breast cancer, but is the leading cause of cancer mortality in women in low-income countries and is estimated to account for 275,000 deaths annually worldwide (WHO 2013). The cellular changes associated with oncogenic HPV types occur slowly, presenting with dysplasia and later with localized (*in situ*) disease before proceeding to invasive cancer, a natural history which can allow early detection and treatment through cervical screening programmes (i.e. Pap test or direct cervical visualization). The great disparity in cervical cancer morbidity and mortality between high- and low-income nations has been attributed in large part to limited availability of cervical screening and treatment in poor countries lacking public health infrastructure. Additionally, a significant interaction exists between HPV and HIV which can accelerate HPV-related cellular changes and this likely further contributes to high cervical cancer incidence in poor nations with high HIV prevalence. Routine periodic cervical screening with a Pap test is the standard of care in most high-income and an increasing number of middle-income nations, with more frequent screening intervals recommended for HIV-infected women. However, in low-income nations many women have never had a Pap smear (Paz Soldan et al. 2008). Increased coverage of HPV vaccines has enormous potential to prevent cervical cancer in upcoming generations of women (Gottlieb et al. 2014) and HPV vaccines have proven to be cost-effective in different settings (Goldie et al. 2008, 2012; Campos et al. 2012).

Hepatocellular carcinoma, accounting for 695,000 deaths annually worldwide, is the third most common cause of cancer deaths in adults but ranks higher in some countries in Asia and sub-Saharan Africa (WHO 2013). Globally, just over half of hepatocellular carcinomas are attributed to chronic HBV infection, although regional estimates vary widely, ranging from 16 per cent in North America, about half of all cases in Africa and Southeast Asia, 59 per cent of cases in Eastern Mediterranean countries, and approximately 65 per cent of cases in East Asia (Perz et al. 2006). Another quarter of hepatocellular cancers globally are caused by chronic HCV infection (Perz et al. 2006). In addition to malignancies, HBV and HCV also are major contributors to cirrhosis, each estimated to account for about 30 per cent of all cases globally (Perz et al. 2006). Among the most distressing prevention failures has been the limited uptake of HBV vaccine which has been available since 1982 and has an outstanding record of safety and effectiveness (95 per cent) in preventing infection and its chronic sequelae (WHO 2012a, 2014). However, awareness of the problem and resources for increased vaccination coverage is finally increasing, and by 2011, 179 countries had included infant vaccination against hepatitis B as part of their vaccination schedules.

A fourth broad category of adverse STI-associated outcomes is related to enhanced HIV transmission and acquisition associated with certain STIs, particularly those associated with genital ulcers (e.g. syphilis, HSV-2, chancroid) or inflammation (e.g. chlamydia, gonorrhoea, trichomoniasis). Studies are clear that STIs are risk factors for both HIV transmission and acquisition (Fleming and Wasserheit 1999; Hay 2008). STI-associated genital ulcer disease was identified as a strong, independent risk factor for HIV acquisition in men (both heterosexual and homosexual) and women in early HIV research studies (Fleming and Wasserheit 1999; Hay 2008). This was also true for STIs associated with inflammation causing cervicitis or urethritis (i.e. chlamydia, gonorrhoea, trichomonas) although HIV risk was somewhat lower than that of genital ulcer disease. In HIV-uninfected people, STIs have been demonstrated to increase the numbers of HIV target cells and possibly impair natural barriers to infection, thus enhancing likelihood of HIV acquisition (CDC 2010). In HIV-infected people, co-infection with some STIs has been found to lead to periods of elevated genital viral load and increased HIV shedding, and thus co-infected individuals are more likely to transmit HIV to an uninfected partner (Cohen et al. 1997; Wang et al. 2001; Cohen 2007). Effective treatment of STI-infected people co-infected with HIV has been demonstrated to lower genital shedding of HIV-1 (Cohen et al. 1997; Ghys et al. 1997; Wang et al. 2001; Cohen 2007). Clearly, prompt detection and effective treatment of STI co-infection (especially those causing genital ulcer disease or mucosal inflammation) is an important HIV prevention intervention at the individual host level.

At the population level, the influence of STI treatment on HIV prevention is muddier. Intervention studies have demonstrated that quality STI case management (i.e. effective STI diagnosis, treatment, condom promotion) can reduce or prevent rise in HIV incidence among high-risk individuals (e.g. female sex workers) (Laga et al. 1994; Levine et al. 1998; Plummer et al. 2005). Additionally, a community randomized trial conducted in rural Tanzania in the early 1990s documented that communities receiving an improved programme of management of symptomatic STI (syndromic case management) had significantly lower HIV incidence than communities with typical STI management programmes, supporting an HIV prevention benefit at the community level (Grosskurth et al. 1995). The lack of a similar effect in subsequent community level intervention trials (i.e. Rakai study of mass treatment (Wawer et al. 1998); Masaka study of enhanced syndromic management (Korenromp et al. 2005)) evaluating various STI control strategies indicated that a community-level HIV benefit does not occur in all circumstances or for all populations. STI treatment for HIV prevention may be particularly important in settings of early (concentrated) epidemics with a high prevalence of curable STIs among 'core groups' (i.e. people with multiple partners at well-connected points in sexual networks who are responsible for continuing STI transmission) (White et al. 2004; Korenromp et al. 2005; Hay 2008). This was a characteristic of early HIV epidemics in Africa, and more recently those of Eastern Europe and Central and East Asia (Galvin and Cohen 2004). It is also a characteristic of epidemics among youth everywhere, making high-risk young people a particularly important subpopulation with whom to focus STI control strategies aimed at HIV prevention.

As noted, STI management may be particularly important in preventing transmission from people with HIV infection, underlining the importance of offering STI services to those in HIV care. The strong association of genital ulcer disease with HIV transmission, along with the earlier noted observation that high

HSV-2 prevalence often occurs in countries with high HIV prevalence, raised the question of whether treatment of genital HSV-2 might reduce the likelihood of HSV-2 or HIV shedding (or both) and thus prevent transmission or acquisition of new HIV infections (Galvin and Cohen 2004; Xu et al. 2006). Thus far this does not seem to be the case. Several large and rigorous multi-national randomized controlled trials evaluating antiviral treatment against HSV were unable to demonstrate benefit in reducing HIV acquisition or transmission (Hayes et al. 2010), perhaps because the herpes treatment provided was unable to adequately reduce inflammation. Mathematical modelling studies continue to suggest the importance of HSV-2 in HIV transmission as HIV epidemics mature (Ward and Rönn 2010), pointing out the potential impact of an effective HSV-2 vaccine should one be able to be developed (Gottleib et al. 2014).

STI costs

Given the enormous global numbers, the healthcare costs associated with acute STIs and their long-term health consequences are assumed to be substantial in every nation. However, relatively few studies have examined this well. A 1997 Guttmacher Institute brief reported that each year STIs including HIV accounted for 6 per cent of healthy years of life lost among reproductive aged women worldwide, 35 per cent higher than men of the same age (Landry and Turnbull 1998). Among women, PID accounted for 43 per cent of all healthy years lost, followed by HIV (42 per cent), syphilis and gonorrhoea (11 per cent), and chlamydial infection (4 per cent); whereas among men most (82 per cent) STI-related morbidity was due to HIV. Additionally, in 2003 the World Bank calculated that among reproductive-aged women in developing nations, STIs were the third most important cause of years of healthy productive life lost, exceeded only by pregnancy-associated maternal morbidity and HIV (World Bank 2004). An acute STI can impose substantial financial costs on individuals and economies. A 2006 review of STI treatment costs in low- and middle-income nations found the median costs for drugs alone was US$2.62, more than three times the average daily income in most low-income nations (Terris-Prestholt et al. 2006). This conservative analysis did not take into account indirect costs, such as those related to travel or missing work. A study evaluating the annual direct economic burden of STIs in the United States estimated that the direct medical costs of STIs, excluding HIV, were approximately US$3 billion in 2008. This estimate did not include direct costs related to cervical cancer screening (estimated at US$5 billion per year) or adverse pregnancy outcomes, indirect (i.e. productivity loss) or intangible (i.e. pain and suffering, deterioration in quality of life, physical impact on families) costs, or costs related to prevention (Owusu-Edusei et al. 2013).

Transmission of sexually transmitted infections

A number of risk factors have been associated with acquiring a new STI, such as age of sexual initiation, number and type (e.g. primary partner or sex worker) of sex partner, or use of barrier protection (e.g. condoms) to name just a few. In addition to studying risk factors in individuals, it is possible to study the spread of infection within populations. The spread of STIs in a population or 'community' is influenced by a limited number of proximate biological and behavioural determinants, as well as a wide range of social, economic, demographic, and cultural factors affecting individuals, communities or both (Garnet 2008).

STI transmission dynamics

An important concept in understanding both STI transmission in populations and the potential impact of various prevention strategies is the STI transmission dynamics model of May and Anderson (1987). The reproductive rate of an STI in a population (R_0), that is, the average number of new infections generated by each infected person, is based on three factors: (1) the likelihood of transmission per sexual contact between an infected person and a susceptible partner (β); (2) the average number of new sexual partnerships formed over time between infected and susceptible people (c); and (3) the average duration of infectiousness (D), where $R_0 = \beta cD$. Incidence and prevalence of a specific STI within a population will increase when $R_0 > 1$ and will decrease if $R_0 < 1$. Circumstances that reduce any of the three factors will reduce R_0 and population prevalence (Brunham 2005).

A primary focus of STI prevention programmes has been reduction in duration of infectiousness (D) by detecting and treating infected people. Measures to accomplish this goal include enhancing access to and utilization of quality healthcare, improving case finding, and improving completion of treatment after clinical contact. Prevention strategies that reduce transmission efficiency (β) and number of sexual partnerships (c) can decrease prevalence of all STIs, and could be particularly useful in preventing those that are not curable by antimicrobial therapy, such as HIV, HSV-2, and HPV. In the past most approaches to reduce transmission efficiency were behavioural (e.g. efforts to promote condom use), but an increasing number of prevention trials evaluating efficacy of biomedical interventions have shown encouraging results. For example, suppressive antiviral therapy of HSV-2 and more recently of HIV-1 have been proven to reduce transmission within discordant sexual partnerships (Corey et al. 2005; Cohen et al. 2011). Male circumcision reduces transmission of HIV and other STIs (Weiss 2007). Most importantly, effective vaccines greatly limit susceptibility, and have already substantially reduced the incidence of HBV in developed countries (WHO 2012a, 2014). Results of at least one early study of a population-wide HPV vaccination programme finding significant decreases in high-grade cervical abnormalities in young women suggests that well-implemented HPV vaccination programmes have good potential to prevent anogenital cancers as well as reduce future health costs related to screening and treatment (Brotherton et al. 2011). Finally, strategies to reduce sexual partnerships between susceptible and infected partners have potential for the broadest effects, but are difficult to implement and sustain. For example, although programmes to encourage abstinence by adolescents have been strongly encouraged in the many countries, there is growing evidence that such programmes may have limited effectiveness (Santelli et al. 2006). Encouraging a reduction in the number of sex partners, particularly among people with frequent sex partner change, may be a more plausible approach, based on experiences in several countries where HIV prevalence has fallen (Shelton et al. 2004).

Sexual networks and core groups

Networks of sexual interaction within populations also influence likelihood of contact between susceptible and infected people (Aral et al. 1996; Adimora and Schoenbach 2005). Sexual networks consist of groups or individuals who are directly or indirectly sexually connected, and the location of an individual in such networks can influence the likelihood of infection as much as or more than personal behaviour by influencing the prevalence of infection in their partners. Larger numbers of sexual linkages in a subpopulation can result in transmission of STI from core groups to the general population, especially if the sexual partnerships are formed concurrently (i.e. two or more partnerships that overlap in time) rather than sequentially, and involve dissassortative (like-with-unlike) mixing patterns (Aral et al. 1996). Sexual networks can be affected by a variety of contextual factors, such as community norms about sexual behaviour; migration and travel patterns; economic circumstances; and the societal disruptions induced by natural disasters, political conflict, and wars. As noted earlier, a related concept in STI prevention is that of the 'core group'. From the perspective of STI transmission determinants, they are defined as groups or individuals with sufficient rates of sex partner change to maintain $R_0 > 1$; and their characteristics will vary by their location in the sexual network and by specific STIs depending on duration of infection and efficiency of transmission. Targeting core groups with STI prevention efforts such as screening and condom promotion can be more efficient and cost-effective than efforts targeted more broadly (Douglas and Fenton 2008). Programmes focusing on sex workers, people living in geographic areas with a high prevalence of reported cases of sexually transmitted disease (STD), incarcerated people, or those with repeat STIs have used the core group approach (Leichliter et al. 2007; Williams and Kahn 2007).

Prevention and control of sexually transmitted infections

For communicable diseases such as STIs, effective diagnosis and treatment is an important prevention strategy. Prompt and effective treatment of curable STIs minimizes their acute symptoms and potential to develop longer term adverse sequelae in the individual patient, and also reduces further spread of the infection into the community (making STI exposure less likely). STI control is not simply STI treatment; many interrelated interventions work together to reduce STI incidence and prevalence (Steen et al. 2009). The concept that clinical management alone has serious limitations is illustrated in Fig. 8.12.2, adapted from a tuberculosis management model developed using actual data from rural women in one African nation (Waaler and Piot 1969;

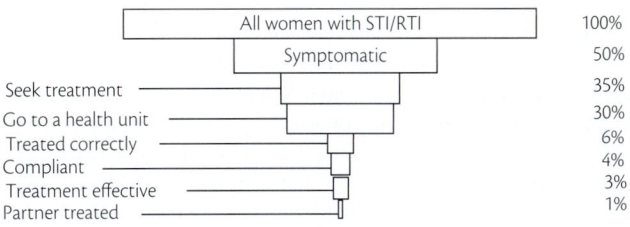

Fig. 8.12.2 Piot–Fransen model of STI prevalence and typical STI case management. The figure shows the series of steps required to ensure effective STI treatment. In typical STI case management as currently practised around the world, an increasing proportion of STI-infected individuals are missed with each succeeding step.

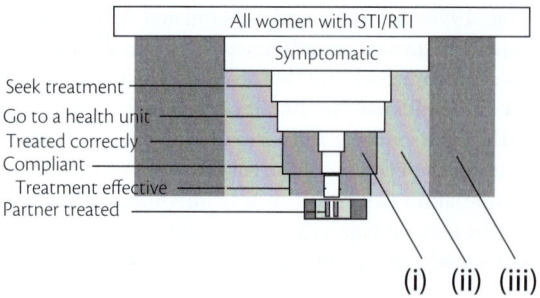

Fig. 8.12.3 Potential benefits of additional control strategies in concert with STI case management. The figure shows the potential expanded coverage of STI case management if various interventions are applied: (i) well-conducted clinic-based case management, which requires symptomatic people seek and obtain effective treatment, (ii) the addition of targeted outreach and community-based programmes that are able to identify and effectively treat most symptomatic STIs in the community, and (iii) the addition of screening of asymptomatic people.

Ryan et al. 2008). Fig. 8.12.2 describes STI prevalence in a community and a series of steps required to ensure effective STI treatment, focusing on the proportion of STIs missed (not effectively treated) at each step. The model illustrates that most people with STIs, even those with symptoms, are not effectively treated; and even fewer have sex partners who are effectively treated. However, these issues can be addressed. Fig. 8.12.3 shows the potential benefits of: (1) well-conducted clinic-based management (i.e. people coming to health facilities, whether public or private, to obtain effective STI treatment); (2) the incremental benefits that might be attained if symptomatic patients who do not come to formal health facilities could be identified and receive STI services (e.g. through pharmacies (Garcia et al. 1998, 2012), asymptomatic screening, targeted outreach programmes, community-based educational efforts and effective partner management); and (3) the incremental benefits that primary prevention might bring (e.g. through high coverage of an effective STI vaccine; or widespread community education around STI prevention, whether abstinence, delaying initiation of sex in adolescents, or promotion of safer sex practices such as correct and consistent condom use). The synergies that can occur with multiple interventions working together was demonstrated in a Peruvian study of a multicomponent intervention including well-conducted STI syndromic management provided by a network of pharmacies and physicians, a mobile-team outreach providing presumptive treatment to female sex workers, along with a condom promotion campaign directed toward young people (Garcia et al. 2012). The combination intervention was able to reduce STIs at the community level, in young adult women and in female sex workers.

From a public health perspective, a comprehensive STI prevention and control programme involves several components working together. One important component is *STI surveillance*, providing the data for programme decision making. Another component is *accessibility of healthcare*, ensuring STI infected people reach case management or other services. Perhaps the most obvious component is *STI case management*, which itself involves an integrated package of prevention and partner services supporting clinical diagnosis and treatment. Case management also includes routine screening in asymptomatic populations at risk for STI-associated adverse outcomes, typically done within clinical services. Another component of STI control is *targeted outreach for high-risk people*,

the core populations contributing disproportionately to disease spread in the community, and who often do not or cannot access facility-based healthcare. Additionally, there is a growing array of *primary prevention interventions* against STI. Last, but as important as the other components, is an *enabling environment* for STI prevention.

STI surveillance

As is true for other public health programmes, accurate STI surveillance is important in understanding the magnitude of the problem, specific STI trends over time, emergence of outbreaks or new problems (e.g. antimicrobial resistance), appropriate deployment of various prevention strategies, prioritization of resources, and monitoring of STI-related public health outcomes. There are several approaches to surveillance that can provide complementary information (WHO 2007a; Douglas and Fenton 2008). First, *case-reporting* provides a measure of new cases of STI or associated syndromes over a specified time interval and is the most common surveillance activity, especially in jurisdictions with functional reporting systems for notifiable infectious diseases. In high-income countries, gonorrhoea, chlamydia, syphilis, and congenital syphilis (i.e. fetal and infant outcomes of MTCT of syphilis) are generally nationally reportable, with reports generated by clinicians, laboratories, or both. In low-income countries where national reporting may be more difficult, reporting from sentinel clinics has proven useful. Second, *prevalence monitoring* can define the prevalence of specific STIs or related syndromes in defined populations undergoing routine assessment (e.g. patients coming for screening or diagnostic testing for infections or for examination for syndromes). Prevalence monitoring can complement case-reporting in assessing the burden of infection or disease. For example, in the United States, while notifiable cases of chlamydia have continually climbed as screening has increased, prevalence monitoring in STI and family planning clinics has shown little change, indicating that the burden of infection is unlikely to be rising (CDC 2010, 2011). Third, *sentinel surveillance* generally refers to data collection from representative 'sentinel populations' for outcomes not routinely measured, such as antimicrobial resistance or infectious aetiology of various STI-related syndromes, and is often useful for generating broader guidance about appropriate treatment regimens and national lists of essential medications. An example of sentinel surveillance is the antenatal HIV and syphilis testing from sentinel clinics done every 1 or 2 years in many countries. Fourth, *population-based surveys* involve collection of data such as prevalence of specific infections from people considered representative of the general population. Population-based surveys are costly and difficult to perform but generally provide the best assessment of population burden. In addition to these approaches for assessing morbidity, periodic surveillance of sexual behaviours, especially those linked to STI prevalence surveys as is done in integrated STI and behavioural surveys conducted in several countries, can provide information about community HIV risk and prevention needs (MacLachlan et al. 2002). Additionally, surveys of health services utilization can be useful in monitoring effectiveness of existing programmes as well as providing information on where prevention services are most needed (Douglas and Fenton 2008). Because of the large burden of disease and limited resources for collection and analysis of STI surveillance data, not to mention sufficient laboratory capacity, trained personnel and adequate reporting mechanisms, conducting effective STI surveillance can be challenging even in wealthy countries with substantial public health infrastructure. Nonetheless, surveillance is an important STI control component in every country, and especially so in low- and middle-income nations with high STI burden.

Access to STI services

Several clinic-based interventions can improve service accessibility, such as dedicated clinics, broad hours of service delivery, no-charge or low-cost services, and adequately trained and non-judgemental providers. Additionally, broader-level health marketing or social marketing can increase population awareness, attitudes, and beliefs about health services and increase health-seeking behaviour. This has been achieved through various mass media approaches (e.g. printed materials, broadcast media, and the Internet). Numerous examples of social marketing for HIV/STI prevention exist, and although these have not tended to be rigorously evaluated, many social marketing approaches appear to have important community-level effects. For example, a systematic review of the effects of social marketing on condom use in developing countries found positive trends in all studies and an overall positive effect on increasing condom use (Sweat et al. 2012). Some social marketing approaches involve public and private sector partnerships working toward a common public health goal. An example of this is the 'GYT' (Get Yourself Tested) campaign aimed at bringing attention to the growing STD epidemic in youth in the United States (McFarlane et al. in press). That campaign uses a variety of approaches including on-air and online messages, SMS promotions, informational resources, and community outreach.

STI case management

Effective STI case management involves an integrated package of services, including (where laboratory tests are available) routine STI screening in asymptomatic patients at risk for STI-associated sequelae; clinical diagnosis and treatment in symptomatic patients (whether based on laboratory-defined aetiologies or syndromic management); prevention services against new infection or reinfection (e.g. education, individualized prevention counselling, condom demonstrations and provision); and partner management. STI case management—often cited as the backbone of STI control—aims to provide prompt and effective treatment of infected patients and in so doing break the chain of infection. Case management provides individual health benefits (e.g. ameliorating symptoms and preventing complications) and can also provide overall population health benefits. From the perspective of transmission determinants, case management shortens the duration of infection (D) and thus reduces efficiency of further transmission in the community. Effective STI case management can be offered in virtually any type of clinical setting, ranging from specialty STI, HIV, and family planning clinics to primary care clinics and antenatal clinic services. However, because of the sensitive and often stigmatizing nature of STIs, particular attention must be paid to offering services that are non-judgemental and confidential, regardless of setting.

Asymptomatic screening and treatment

Routine STI screening is important in identifying asymptomatic infections in populations at risk for adverse outcomes. For example, many countries recommend annual chlamydia screening in sexually active, young women in order to identify asymptomatic infections that may result in infertility. Universal screening for syphilis and HIV in pregnant women helps prevent MTCT of these infections and subsequent adverse pregnancy outcomes. When STIs are detected, case management strategies including appropriate treatment, prevention services, and partner management should be provided in the same manner as for symptomatic patients, described in the following subsections.

Clinical management of symptoms

In an ideal world, clinical management would be guided by diagnostic tests with results available during the clinical encounter, allowing correct diagnosis and appropriate treatment. Ideal tests would be rapid, affordable, easy to use, and highly sensitive and specific. *Aetiological-based STI diagnosis* using laboratory diagnostics is the approach used in most high-income and many middle-income settings. Although results may not be available right at the clinic visit, in most cases the lab-based testing helps clarify the diagnosis and guides treatment. However, in many parts of the world laboratory capacity is limited and STI tests are generally not available, or are too costly, or results do not return sufficiently quickly and patients are lost to follow up without adequate treatment. Some promising developments have occurred in STI diagnostics in recent years. But given a lack of reliable or affordable diagnostic tests that still exists in many parts of the world, an alternative approach that is used is syndromic case management using locally validated treatment algorithms (Ryan et al. 2008).

STI syndromic case management dates from the 1970s when the WHO designed, implemented and evaluated flowcharts (algorithms) for the syndromic management of STIs, evaluating these in several sub-Saharan African nations (Mabey et al. 2010). Later in the 1990s, locally validated syndromic management approaches were promoted for care of symptomatic STI and other reproductive tract infections (RTIs) (Dallabetta et al. 2007; WHO 2007a; Ryan et al. 2008). STI management was based on the identification of a 'syndrome,' a constellation of easily elicited symptoms and recognizable clinical signs that are associated with a limited number of defined STI or RTI aetiologies. The approach was practical in that it could be carried out in almost any setting (Dallabetta et al. 2007). It did not require laboratory facilities, and patients were treated at the clinical encounter, allowing less chance for complications to develop or for further STI spread to sex partners. Costs were minimized because laboratory tests were avoided and drug regimens were simplified. The use of standardized algorithms covering the most likely conditions reduced treatment failures and the need for repeated visits or referrals to higher level centres. Standardized regimens also helped improve case-reporting for surveillance and, consequently, provide more information for programme management (Dallabetta et al. 2007; Ryan et al. 2008).

STI syndromic management had some important limitations, most critically that it did not address asymptomatic patients, who account for the majority of curable STIs (Dallabetta et al. 2007; WHO 2007a; Ryan et al. 2008). Asymptomatic women with cervical infections are at risk for serious adverse outcomes including tubal damage and infertility, but were poorly covered by this approach. Furthermore, because many genitourinary symptoms are caused by other conditions in the absence of an STI, the syndromic approach could lead to false positive diagnoses and thus to unnecessary drug use, additional costs and potential partner issues. Partner management was particularly difficult to address as many providers were hesitant to treat sex partners without a specific, laboratory-defined STI diagnosis, even though re-infection of the patient would be very likely without partner treatment. In addition, the most common presenting syndrome for women, vaginal discharge syndrome, is usually caused by non-STI-related RTIs (e.g. bacterial vaginosis, candidiasis) or by other factors. Finally, some healthcare providers, particularly physicians, were reluctant to adopt syndromic approaches because they had been trained in aetiological treatment and viewed the approach as 'unscientific' (Dallabetta et al. 2007; Ryan et al. 2008).

How well syndromic management has controlled STIs in Africa is somewhat difficult to assess. In individual patients, the approach seems most effective for management of genital ulcer syndrome in men and women, urethritis or epididymitis in men, and neonatal conjunctivitis in infants (WHO 2007a; Mabey et al. 2010). Repeated cross-sectional studies in a few nations employing syndromic management approaches suggested that bacterial causes of genital ulcer syndrome markedly declined in parts of Africa, and chancroid (a not uncommon aetiology of genital ulcer disease in the past) seemed to have almost disappeared (WHO 2007a; Paz-Bailey et al. 2005; Makasa et al. 2012). Whether this was due to efficacy of syndromic management or other prevention efforts (e.g. advocacy for 'abstinence, be faithful, use condoms' (ABC) approaches occurring during that time period), or the early deaths of those individuals most likely to develop genital ulcer disease (and thereby HIV) is difficult to ascertain. Perhaps the most compelling evidence of the value of syndromic management was the Mwanza community trial (Grosskurth et al. 1995). However, the study assessed HIV outcomes and did not focus on comparative prevalence of STI syndromes which were considered interim outcomes, and thus any supportive data are limited. Subsequent studies of high-risk men finding higher asymptomatic disease than previously realized have been a further impetus to promote improved syndromic, and ideally aetiological, management strategies (Lewis et al. 2008). Although improved laboratories and availability of point-of-care diagnostics have great potential to support better STI management, unfortunately these are still unavailable in many low- and middle-income countries with high disease burden (Garcia 2011). Thus syndromic management, for all its problems, currently remains a useful management tool as public health practitioners balance potential STI management strategies for the future with the reality of current low budgets and limited public health infrastructure.

Prevention strategies linked to STI case management

Important but sometimes overlooked aspects of STI case management are strategies aimed at preventing reinfection or new infections. Prevention of new STIs has been achieved with informational messages, prevention counselling on risk reduction, educating patients about STIs and how they are transmitted, demonstration of proper condom use and provision of condoms, and ideally a combination of these strategies. Men and women identified with an STI should be educated about the disease and counselled on means of preventing reinfection or new infections. Some individualized prevention approaches are more effective than others. For example, 'client-centred' counselling in which the provider encourages the patient to set a prevention goal and identify personalized risk reduction steps toward that goal has proven more effective than informational messages (Kamb et al. 1998). Regardless of the prevention approach used, some information should be given about completing therapy, needed follow-up examinations or testing, and preventive strategies (e.g. avoiding risky partnerships, using condoms). Also important is information about notifying sex partners in order to ensure partners are treated and to reduce the chance of reinfection or new infection in the index patient.

Partner management

Breaking the chain of infection involves treating as many sex partners of STI-infected people as possible (Steen et al. 2009). Partner management (referred to in the past as 'contact tracing') actually has many goals: reducing the chance of reinfection in the index patient, treating the partner to avoid future STI sequelae, and limiting community spread of the STI (Hogben et al. 2001; Mathews et al. 2001; Brewer 2005). Although partner management clearly has great potential to be a powerful component of STI case management, it can be difficult to carry out. Two basic approaches have been traditionally applied, *provider referral* (in which health practitioners or public health workers interview the index patient to determine names and locate partners and subsequently notify then confidentially about their exposure and need for treatment and/or testing), and *patient referral* (relying on the index patient to notify partner(s) to come for treatment and/or testing). Where laws allow, another approach that has been successfully employed in parts of the United States is *expedited partner therapy*, in which patients are provided drugs, or prescriptions for drugs, to give to exposed partners (Hogben et al. 2012).

Targeted interventions for core groups

Preventing community spread of STIs depends not on reaching *all* people but reaching the *right* people (Steen et al. 2009). Targeted interventions have a goal of identifying and treating 'core groups'—subpopulations with high STI prevalence and frequent partner change and who thus contribute disproportionately to STI spread in the community. Targeted interventions often involve specialized outreach for subpopulations that are hidden or hard to reach, but can be conducted at 'hot spots' identified through mapping exercises (e.g. bars or nightclubs), in clinical settings (e.g. dedicated clinics for MSM, sex workers, mobile men such as miners), or through peers. Depending upon the local epidemic, targeted efforts may need to address 'bridge populations', that is, those people bridging infection from a higher prevalence subgroup to the general population (e.g. clients of sex workers) (Steen et al. 2009). Effective targeted interventions have included strategies such as 100 per cent condom use campaigns, peer-driven interventions providing information or service referral, periodic presumptive treatment (e.g. for sex workers), STI screening and treatment in HIV-infected people, and supportive laws around clean needles/syringes for injecting drug users (Steen et al. 2009; WHO 2007a, 2012a; UNAIDS 2012). Targeting screening in core groups and bridge populations should not be confused with asymptomatic screening and treatment for STIs in lower-risk populations (e.g. antenatal testing). Targeted screening is aimed at preventing sustained 'upstream' epidemics that contribute to STI spread in the community while asymptomatic screening in people with low partner change is aimed at preventing STI associated health consequences. Both are important public health interventions, but with different goals.

Primary prevention

For many years primary prevention of STIs relied on 'ABCs', that is, abstinence, 'be faithful' (i.e. mutual monogamy), and condom use. In fact, substantial evidence supports the effectiveness of the male latex condom in reducing transmission of HIV and other STIs (Weller and Davis 2002; CDC 2010), as well as some serious STI-associated sequelae such as PID and precursor lesions for HPV-associated anogenital cancers (Marazzo and Cates 2011)—although condoms must be used consistently and correctly (Warner et al. 1998). Recent reviews evaluating female condom effectiveness indicate disease prevention benefits similar to male latex condoms (Minnis and Padian 2005; Vijayakuma et al. 2006). Beyond condoms, several exciting developments have occurred in the field of biomedical interventions recently: male circumcision has been proven effective in preventing HIV and other STIs; pre-exposure prophylaxis with antiviral therapy has been found to be highly effective in reducing HIV and HSV acquisition; there are strong supportive data on the benefits of periodic presumptive therapy in preventing disease in sex workers; and perhaps most importantly, there are increasing numbers of efficacious vaccines against STDs (Marazzo and Cates 2011; Gottleib et al. 2014). Safe and effective vaccines against HPV, HBV, and HAV already exist, although coverage is often inadequate in the countries with highest disease burden. The availability of more affordable vaccines could profoundly affect STI control globally (Vijayakuma et al. 2006).

Enabling environment for STI prevention

Strong programme leadership greatly supports and helps sustain effective STI prevention programmes. Such leadership includes priority setting and planning on STI control efforts, ideally using local data to guide the programme; developing and implementing partnerships that lead to productive collaborations; and ensuring ongoing programme quality. However, regardless of how effectively a programme prioritizes, collaborates and implements STI prevention programmes, it will have difficulty producing sustainable benefits without an enabling environment, that is, the political will and resources to support prevention and control efforts. An enabling environment encompasses a number of factors such as a supportive legal and regulatory milieu, the ability to secure sufficient financial and human resources for the programme and for basic science and public health evaluation research, and the ability to effectively advocate for programme priorities within the community and at the highest levels.

Some examples of laws or policies that can positively affect STI prevention programmes are the ability to provide confidential clinical services to minors without parental consent, the ability of health practitioners (e.g. nurses) responsible for STI case management to provide services and prescribe drugs, and the permissibility of expedited partner therapy (Mathews et al. 2001; Brewer 2005; WHO 2007a; CDC 2010). Securing financial resources for STI prevention is critical at many levels; examples are to ensure: sufficient programme dollars to sufficiently cover STI clinical services; availability of free (or affordable) treatment for STI-infected people; availability of prevention services; funding for ongoing monitoring and evaluation and training; and needed human resources. Such resources include an adequate workforce trained in appropriate STI clinical management, partner management, prevention services, surveillance, outreach, and evaluation. Developing an adequate public health workforce is difficult in many countries, but especially so in sub-Saharan Africa where there are grave shortages in healthcare workers in all sectors due to limited resources for educating professionals. This has been compounded by 'brain drain', when trained professionals leave to go to wealthier countries experiencing shortages or to donor agencies able to pay higher prices than governments.

Programmes are most effective when decision-makers can promote supportive laws and policies, raise political awareness about problems, and help mobilize resources around STI prevention and control. Political support from the top is especially important for conditions such as STIs because their associated stigma can makes public discussion and community involvement difficult. But when political support exists, the results can be profound. For example, in the 1990s, Thailand had a 95 per cent reduction in curable STIs following introduction of its 100 per cent condom use programme for sex workers, and Cambodia also had STI decreases after introducing a similar campaign; both were strongly supported by the governments (Steen et al. 2009). In Senegal, where sex work has been decriminalized and STI services made accessible to sex workers, STI prevalence has remained moderately low and stable, in contrast to neighbouring countries without such laws (Steen et al. 2009). In Switzerland, low HIV and hepatitis prevalence among drug users has been attributed to pragmatic policies supporting harm reduction strategies (Csete et al. 2012). The Public Health Agency of Canada's development of sexual health indicators (i.e. physical mental, emotional, and social well-being in relation to sexuality; approach to sexuality; sexual relationships; sexual experiences; and discrimination, coercion, and violence) allows measurement of trends in several dimensions of sexual health, thereby helping public health leaders to target interventions appropriately for young people (Smylie et al. 2013).

Future directions and challenges

Antimicrobial resistance has been an important factor in STI control since the development of antibiotics in the early part of the twentieth century. The recent emergence of highly resistant gonorrhoea strains in the face of a single remaining antibiotic class will prove to be an important challenge in the next decades. On the other hand, supportive global initiatives, new and improved STI diagnostics, and better information and communication technologies are already supporting improved STD control and will continue to do so in the future.

Global and regional initiatives

In May 2006, the WHO announced a new *Global Strategy for the Prevention and Control of Sexually Transmitted Infections: 2006–2015: Breaking the Chain of Transmission*, which was developed using an inclusive and broad consultative process and presented and accepted at the World Assembly (WHO 2007a). The strategy emphasized the importance of scaling up STI prevention activities, better integration of STI prevention with other public health programmes, and a focus on technical advances and advocacy. The strategy also highlighted ten actionable interventions for immediate implementation, and provided indicators and national-level targets for each: (1) scaling up services for diagnosis and treatment of STIs; (2) control of congenital syphilis as a step towards elimination; (3) scale-up of STI prevention strategies and programmes for HIV-positive people; (4) upgrading surveillance of STIs within the context of second-generation HIV surveillance; (5) control of bacterial genital ulcer disease; (6) implementation of targeted interventions in high-risk and vulnerable populations; (7) implementation of age-appropriate, comprehensive sexual health education and services; (8) promoting partner treatment and prevention of reinfection; (9) supporting roll-out of effective vaccines against HBV and HPV and, potentially, HSV-2; and (10) facilitating development and implementation of universal opt-out voluntary counselling and testing for HIV among patients with STIs. Many countries have reported progress in these areas; and perhaps the greatest measurable global progress has been in prevention of congenital syphilis.

In 2007, the WHO published *The Global Elimination of Congenital Syphilis: Rationale and Strategy for Action* outlining the estimated burden of disease, including the substantial contribution of MTCT of syphilis to infant mortality and morbidity (WHO 2007b). Subsequently the WHO, working with global partners including the US CDC, formally launched a global elimination campaign. The global congenital syphilis elimination initiative uses a four-pronged strategy of ensuring advocacy and sustained political commitment for a successful health initiative; increasing access to and quality of maternal and newborn health services; screening and treating pregnant women and partners; and establishing surveillance, monitoring and evaluation systems. The global initiative has had strong support from regions, as well as many high-burden countries (WHO 2007c). Several regional initiatives supporting congenital syphilis elimination were launched: in 2009, the Pan American Health Organization and UNICEF began the *Regional Initiative for the Elimination of Mother-to-Child Transmission of HIV and Syphilis in Latin America and the Caribbean* (Pan American Health Organization 2009), coupling two critical antenatal screening programmes and thus promoting a synergistic and, hopefully, more sustained and supportive programmatic response. In 2010, an Asia Pacific United Nations Task Force representing the regions of the Western Pacific and South East Asia adopted a similar dual elimination initiative aimed at elimination of new paediatric HIV infections and congenital syphilis in Asia-Pacific, 2011–2015 (WHO 2011). Several countries of sub-Saharan Africa developed plans for dual elimination of MTCT of HIV and syphilis.

The results of these efforts have been enhanced congenital syphilis surveillance, adoption of regional case definitions and management guidelines, and greatly improved programme monitoring of uptake of antenatal syphilis testing and appropriate treatment. The increasing use of rapid syphilis tests in antenatal clinics has further contributed to increased testing in many settings with limited laboratory capacity (Mabey et al. 2012). Rapid testing has also promoted higher treatment uptake, as treatment can be provided at the clinic visit. The WHO, working through regional offices, has encouraged countries to actively measure programme progress and work toward elimination of congenital syphilis, an important cause of preventable perinatal morbidity and mortality. Recent global estimates suggest decreases in MTCT of syphilis

have occurred since 2000 (Newman et al. 2013). In addition, at least one region (the Americas) is developing methodologies to validate elimination in countries where leaders believe elimination goals have been met. Despite these developments, progress is slow in many areas, particularly in sub-Saharan Africa where burden is high. Although integrating syphilis and HIV testing for antenatal women has been found to be a sound and cost-effective strategy (WHO 2007c; Mabey et al. 2012; Strasser et al 2012), it has been slow to be taken up in many countries—in large part due to disease-specific funding.

Antimicrobial resistance

The rapidly evolving resistance of *Neisseria gonorrhoeae*, among the world's most common curable STIs, to successive antimicrobial agents has been concerning for several decades. However, the relatively recent emergence of highly resistant strains that are increasingly less susceptible to third-generation cephalosporins—the single remaining class of antibiotics active against the pathogen—has led to some alarm around the world (Bolan et al. 2012).

N. gonorrhoeae is a highly active organism that has readily developed resistance to antimicrobial agents. Resistance to sulphanilamide was identified as early as the 1940s. Penicillinase-producing strains were isolated as early as the 1970s in South East Asia and subsequently spread widely throughout the world (Bolan et al. 2012). Resistance to other first-line therapies such as spectinomycin and tetracycline emerged in Asia in the 1980s. Fluoroquinolone-resistant gonorrhoea strains were observed in several Asian countries in the 1990s, and high levels of fluoroquinolone resistance subsequently spread throughout Asia and other parts of the world by the early 2000s (WHO 2000). With loss of the quinolone class, at present the third-generation cephalosporins are the single line of defence against gonorrhoea; and sporadic reports of resistance to cefixime are already reported (Ohnishi et al. 2011). Furthermore, increases in minimum inhibitory concentrations (MIC) of third-generation cephalosporins are now observed in laboratories around the world. Many nations have adopted steps to try to delay the emergence of cephalosporin-resistant gonorrhoea strains and reduce the public health consequences, primarily through educating clinicians and updating treatment recommendations to higher doses of intramuscular ceftriaxone, often including single-dose azithromycin or doxycycline (CDC 2013). New drugs effective against gonorrhoea are obviously important, but new drug development takes time and the organism has been highly successful in quickly developing resistance. As was the case for tuberculosis, treatment for gonorrhoea is anticipated to eventually require multiple antibiotics for cure. An effective vaccine would obviously be an ideal solution, although none is on the immediate horizon.

The WHO has initiated a *Gonococcal Antimicrobial Surveillance Programme* (GASP) to help monitor gonorrhoea resistance worldwide through a network of laboratories, WHO collaborating centres, and other international and national reference centres. Participating laboratories from each region have agreed to submit gonococcal antimicrobial susceptibility data to the regional WHO collaborating centre, where data are analysed, summarized and can be disseminated globally. Unfortunately, *N. gonorrhoeae* is a fastidious organism that has proven difficult to transport and successfully culture. Because of this, gonococcal culture and antimicrobial susceptibility testing is lacking in countries with limited laboratory capacity or trained personnel. However, even in wealthy countries, the capacity for culture (and thereby antimicrobial susceptibility testing) has been increasingly lost with the wider use of simpler molecular technologies such as NAATs. Currently most surveillance data on gonorrhoea antimicrobial resistance are available from laboratories from the Western and South East Asian Regions, Europe, and North America, although the WHO has prioritized expansion of GASP as part of their future agenda.

Antimicrobial resistance is also emerging for *Haemophilus ducreyi*, the causative agent of chancroid, although oral antibiotic therapies are still effective against this increasingly rare disease (Ryan et al. 2008). Azithromycin resistance in syphilis has been reported in a few settings, although the geographic distribution of resistant strains has not been well established, and *T. pallidum* remains exquisitely sensitive to penicillin, the first-line recommended therapy (Lukehart et al. 2004). Resistance of *T. vaginalis* to standard treatment with single-dose metronidazole occurs occasionally, requiring lengthier drug regimens or alternative treatments (Fortenberry et al. 2002). Additionally, while resistance of HSV-2 to aciclovir and related antiviral regimens is uncommon in immune-competent patients, it has been observed to occur in from 3.5 to 10 per cent of immune-compromised (e.g. HIV-infected) patients (Piret and Boivin 2011).

Information and communication technologies

Information and communication technologies (ICTs) are evolving rapidly, and nowadays the Internet, mobile devices, and cell phones and other gadgets could enable lower cost and highly engaging STI prevention and control interventions (Swendeman and Rotheram-Borus 2010). ICTs could help in diagnosing medical conditions, screening, recognizing behaviours, delivering 'just-in-time' interventions and improving surveillance systems. The Internet constitutes a potential source of information in health where patients can search for symptoms, diagnosis, or treatment, and seek out healthcare providers (Rietmeijer et al. 2003). However, the Internet has also facilitated social interactions and networking, making it easy to seek for sexual partners, and thus increasing the risk for acquiring STIs. It has been recognized that MSM are the group that more actively engaged in these practices (Ogilvie et al. 2008). Nevertheless, the Internet has proven to be an effective and low-cost tool to deliver STI prevention interventions, including partner notifications (CDC 2003; Bull et al. 2004; Levine et al. 2005; Bowen et al. 2007). Computer-based and Internet-based behavioural interventions against STIs have demonstrated efficacy comparable to face-to-face interventions (Swendeman and Rotheram-Borus 2010).

Mobile health or 'mHealth' refers to the use of mobile devices for health applications aimed at improving individuals' health and well-being through monitoring their status, improving diagnosis of medical conditions, recognizing risk behaviours, and delivering interventions—all in the user's natural mobile environment. The most common mobile devices are cellular phones; these have had incredible penetration in the population, with subscriptions globally surpassing the 5 billion mark, two-thirds of which are in low- and middle-income countries. Mobile phones have the capacity to be used to send information to patients, send reminders for appointments or medications, gather information or, with additional attachments, monitor vital signs, or even read and transmit diagnostic test results. Most of these applications are still under development; however, several ongoing mHealth pilot studies are assessing various uses of the technology. Mobile phone interventions against STIs using text-messaging or SMS are being used in several areas. Thus far, mHealth applications have been found effective in increasing adherence to antiretroviral therapies in HIV-infected patients. There is a need for high-quality research in this area aimed at STI prevention and care (Free et al. 2013).

New STI diagnostics

Great progress has been made over the past two decades in the development of rapid (i.e. point-of-care) diagnostic tests that facilitate screening and treatment of STIs, especially in settings in which it is currently difficult to provide testing (e.g. limited laboratory capacity) or in which it is difficult for patients to learn results and receive prompt treatment if results are positive (e.g. remote, hard-to-reach settings). Rapid tests are particularly useful for asymptomatic patients, but can also be useful for symptomatic patients when more sensitive and specific diagnostic tests are unaffordable. Many high-quality rapid tests exist for HIV. The use of rapid diagnostics also has the potential to improve syndromic management of STIs by increasing the specificity of the algorithms and thus reducing unnecessary treatment (e.g. for women with vaginitis).

Promotion for the development, application, and evaluation of rapid STI diagnostics appropriate for use in primary healthcare in developing countries was greatly advanced by the work of the Sexually Transmitted Diseases Diagnostics Initiative (SDI), a unit of the UNICEF/UNDP/World Bank/WHO Special Programme for Research and Training in Tropical Diseases (Peeling et al. 2006). The SDI focused on tests that met the 'ASSURED' criteria, that is, were *a*ffordable, *s*ensitive, *s*pecific, *u*ser-friendly (simple enough to perform in a few steps and with minimal training), *r*apid and robust (to enable treatment at the first visit, and not requiring refrigeration), *e*quipment-free (easy and with a non-invasive way to collect specimens), and *d*elivered to end users (Peeling et al. 2006). Development of rapid tests for syphilis has been particularly productive. Many rapid treponemal tests for syphilis exist, and at least six of these were formally evaluated by the SDI and found to meet ASSURED criteria. Although a positive treponemal test indicates lifetime exposure to syphilis, and cannot distinguish new and old infections without non-treponemal testing, treponemal tests alone can be very useful among pregnant women who would otherwise not be tested for syphilis. This is because risk for overtreatment (penicillin injection) is low compared with the risk of untreated syphilis for the infant (> 50 per cent fetal morbidity or mortality) (Mabey et al. 2012). Treponemal tests (by themselves) would be less useful in populations, such as sex workers or MSM, likely to have been treated for past syphilis infection. A rapid treponemal/non-treponemal test on a single platform has been developed, allowing screening and confirmation of syphilis. Additionally, several combined HIV and syphilis tests on a single platform have been developed and are under evaluation.

Development of sensitive and specific rapid tests for gonorrhoea or chlamydia has been less successful. However, a closed-system NAAT assay has been developed that involves a modular-cartridge-based platform that is easy to use, minimizes processing steps and contamination, and can process from one to 96 specimens in less than 2 hours. A formal evaluation of these chlamydia and gonorrhoea tests indicated solid performance when compared against laboratory-based PCR tests (Gaydos et al. 2013). Thus, although not useful in developing world settings lacking basic infrastructure, this type of user-friendly system with short turnaround times could be extremely useful in many clinical settings to accurately test patients for chlamydia and gonorrhoea at the point of care, allowing treatment to be promptly initiated.

Conclusions

At the beginning of the twenty-first century, STIs continue to be a major global health problem, accounting for substantial reproductive, perinatal, and cancer-related morbidity and mortality in addition to contributing to HIV transmission. This chapter has outlined key issues around STI transmission, prevention, and effective STI programmes. Newer strategies such as rapid point-of-care and other diagnostics with short turn-around times; simple and easy-to-use information and communication technologies; improved vaccines and therapeutics; and supportive global and regional initiatives are all anticipated to help control STIs all over the world. However, many challenges remain. In an era of increasingly available and affordable interventions and widespread HIV treatment and prevention programmes, some very basic STI control strategies (e.g. routine syphilis screening of pregnant women; gonorrhoea culture and sensitivity testing) are not yet well implemented, especially in low-income settings. New problems are also emerging in STIs, particularly the emergence of increasing gonococcal antimicrobial resistance to the final class of drugs effective against that organism. Widespread vaccine uptake against STIs has been slow. After 30 years, HBV vaccine is finally increasingly accepted; however, coverage of the recently available HPV vaccines remains spotty even in wealthy nations, and its use is low or non-existent in most middle- and low-income countries. Although there are no new vaccines against viral STIs on the immediate horizon, research in this area must continue. In the meantime, strategies that increase coverage of existing vaccines remain a priority.

STIs are stigmatizing conditions that have their greatest effects on vulnerable or marginalized populations, and thus mobilizing societal and political support for their prevention and control remains an important challenge for all nations. Given the high individual and societal costs associated with STIs, and the great potential to prevent them, efforts to sustain and scale up effective STI control programmes must remain an important global health priority.

Disclaimer

The findings and conclusions in this paper are those of the author(s) and do not necessarily represent the views of the Centers for Disease Control and Prevention.

References

Adimora, A.A. and Schoenbach, V.J. (2005). Social context, sexual networks, and racial disparities in rates of sexually transmitted infections. *Journal of Infectious Disease*, 191(Suppl. 1), S115–S122.

Aral, S.O., Holmes, K.K., Padian, N.S., et al. (1996). Overview: individual and population approaches to the epidemiology and prevention of sexually transmitted diseases and human immunodeficiency virus infection. *Journal of Infectious Disease*, 174(Suppl. 2), S127–S133.

Baseman, J.G. and Koutsky, L.A. (2005). The epidemiology of human papillomavirus infections. *Journal of Clinical Virology*, 32(Suppl. 1), S16–S24.

Bolan, G.A., Sparling, P.F., and Wasserheit, J.N. (2012). The emerging threat of untreatable gonococcal infection. *The New England Journal of Medicine*, 366(6), 485–7.

Bowen, A.M., Horvath, K., and Williams, M.L. (2007). A randomized control trial of Internet-delivered HIV prevention targeting rural MSM. *Health Education Research*, 22(1), 120–7.

Brewer, D.D. (2005). Case-finding effectiveness of partner notification and cluster investigation for sexually transmitted diseases and HIV. *Sexually Transmitted Infections*, 32(2), 78–83.

Brotherton, J.M.L., Fridman, M., May, C.L., et al. (2011). Early effect of the HPV vaccine programme on cervical abnormalities in Victoria, Australia: an ecological study. *The Lancet*, 377(9783), 2085–92

Brown, Z.A., Selke, S., Zeh, J., et al. (1997). The acquisition of herpes simplex virus during pregnancy. *The New England Journal of Medicine*, 337(8), 509–15.

Brunham, R.C. (2005). Parran Award Lecture: insights into the epidemiology of sexually transmitted diseases from Ro = βcD. *Sexually Transmitted Infections*, 32(12), 722–4.

Bull, S.S., Lloyd, L., Rietmeijer, C., and McFarlane, M. (2004). Recruitment and retention of an online sample for an HIV prevention intervention targeting men who have sex with men: the Smart Sex Quest Project. *AIDS Care*, 16(8), 931–43.

Campos, N.G., Kim, J.J., Castle, P.E., et al. (2012). Health and economic impact of HPV 16/18 vaccination and cervical cancer screening in East Africa. *International Journal of Cancer*, 130(11), 2672–84.

Centers for Disease Control and Prevention (2004). Using the Internet for partner notification of sexually transmitted diseases—Los Angeles County, California, 2003. *Morbidity and Mortality Weekly Report*, 53(6), 129–31.

Centers for Disease Control and Prevention (2009). Surveillance for acute viral hepatitis—United States, 2007. *Morbidity and Mortality Weekly Report*, 58(SS-3). Accessible at http://www.cdc.gov/hepatitis/statistics/index.htm.

Centers for Disease Control and Prevention (2010). STD treatment guidelines, 2010. *Morbidity and Mortality Weekly Report*, 59 (RR-12). Available at: http://www.cdc.gov/std/treatment/2010.

Centers for Disease Control and Prevention (2011). *Sexually Transmitted Disease Surveillance, 2011*. Atlanta, GA: US Department of Health and Services. Available at: http: //www.cdc.gov/std/stats11/.

Centers for Disease Control and Prevention (2012). Summary of Notifiable Diseases—United States, 2010. *Morbidity and Mortality Weekly Report*, 59(53), 1–116.

Centers for Disease Control and Prevention (2013). CDC Grand Rounds: the growing threat of multidrug-resistant gonorrhea. *Morbidity and Mortality Weekly Report*, 62(6), 103–6.

Cogliano, V., Baan, R., Straif, K., et al. (2005). Carcinogenicity of human papillomaviruses. *The Lancet Oncology*, 6(4), 204.

Cohen, M.S. (2007). Preventing sexual transmission of HIV. *Clinical Infectious Diseases*, 45, S287–92.

Cohen, M.S., Chen, Y.Q., McCauley, M., et al. (2011). Prevention of HIV-1 infection with early antiretroviral therapy. *The New England Journal of Medicine*, 365, 493–505.

Cohen, M.S., Hoffman, I.F., Royce, R.A., et al. (1997). Reduction of concentration of HIV-1 in semen after treatment of urethritis: implications for prevention of sexual transmission of HIV-1. AIDSCAP Malawi Research Group. *The Lancet*, 349, 1868–73.

Corey, L., Huang, M.L., Selke, S., et al. (2005). Differentiation of herpes simplex virus types 1 and 2 in clinical samples by a real-time taqman PCR assay. *Journal of Medical Virology*, 76(3), 350–5.

Csete, K. and Grob, P.J. (2012). Switzerland, HIV and the power of pragmatism: lessons for drug policy development. *International Journal on Drug Policy*, 23(1), 82–6.

Cunningham, S.D., Tschann, J., Gurvey, J.E., et al. (2002). Attitudes about sexual disclosure and perceptions of stigma and shame. *Sexually Transmitted Infections*, 78(5), 334–8.

Dallabetta, G., Field, M., Lage, M., et al. (2007). STDs: global burden and challenges for control. In G. Dallabetta, M. Laga, and P. Lamptey (eds.) *Control of Sexually Transmitted Diseases: A Handbook for the Design and Management of Programs*, pp. 23–52. Durham, NC; Family Health International/The AIDS Control and Prevention Project (AIDSCAP).

Decker, M.R., Miller, E., McCauley, H.L., et al. (2011). Intimate partner violence and partner notification of sexually transmitted infections among adolescent and young adult family planning clinic patients. *International Journal of STD & AIDS*, 22(6), 345–7.

De Sanjosé, S., Diaz, M., Castellsagué, X., et al. (2007). Worldwide prevalence and genotype distribution of cervical human papillomavirus DNA in women with normal cytology: a meta-analysis. *The Lancet Infectious Diseases*, 7(7), 453–9.

Dinh, T.H., Dunne, E.F., and Markowitz, L.E. (2008). Assessing neonatal herpes reporting in the United States, 2000–2005. *Sexually Transmitted Infections*, 35(1), 19–21.

Douglas, J.M. and Fenton, K. (2008). STD/HIV prevention programs in developed countries. In K.K. Holmes, P.F. Sparling, W.E. Stamm, et al. (eds.) *Sexually Transmitted Disease* (4th ed.), pp. 1767–86. New York: McGraw-Hill.

Dunne, E.F., Nielson, C.M., Stone, K.M., et al. (2006). Prevalence of HPV infection among men: a systematic review of the literature. *Journal of Infectious Disease*, 194(8), 1044–57.

Fiumara, N.J. (1988). Syphilis among mothers and children. *Annals of the New York Academy of Sciences*, 549(1), 187–92.

Fleming, D.T. and Wasserheit, J.N. (1999). From epidemiological synergy to public health policy and practice: the contribution of other sexually transmitted diseases to sexual transmission of HIV infection. *Sexually Transmitted Infections*, 75(1), 3–17.

Fortenberry, J.D., McFarlane, M., Bleakley, A., et al. (2002). Relationships of stigma and shame to gonorrhea and HIV screening. *American Journal of Public Health*, 92(3), 378–81.

Free, C., Phillips, G., Galli, L., et al. (2013). The effectiveness of mobile-health technology-based health behaviour change or disease management interventions for health care consumers: a systematic review. *PLoS Medicine*, 10(1), e1001362.

Galvin, S.R. and Cohen, M.S. (2004). The role of sexually transmitted diseases in HIV transmission. *Nature Reviews Microbiology*, 2(1), 33–42.

Garcia, P.J., Benzaken, A.S., Galban, E.; ALAC-ITS Members (2011). STI management and control in Latin America: where do we stand and where do we go from here? *Sexually Transmitted Infections*, 87(Suppl. 2), ii7–9.

Garcia, P.J., Cárcamo, C.P., Garnet, G.P., et al. (2012). Improved STD syndrome management by a network of clinicians and pharmacy workers in Peru: the PREVEN Network. *PLoS One*, 7(10), e47750.

Garcia, P.J., Gotuzzo, E., Hughes, J.P., et al. (1998). Syndromic management of STDs in pharmacies: evaluation and randomised intervention trial. *Sexually Transmitted Infections*, 74(Suppl. 1), S153–8.

Garcia, P.J., Holmes, K.K., Cáracamo, C.P., et al. (2012). Prevention of sexually transmitted infections in urban communities (Peru PREVEN Study), a multicomponent community-randomised controlled trial. *The Lancet*, 379(9821), 1120–1.

Garnet, G.P. (2008). The transmission dynamics of sexually transmitted infections. In K.K. Holmes, P.F. Sparling, W.E. Stamm, et al. (eds.) *Sexually Transmitted Diseases* (4th ed.), pp. 27–39. New York: McGraw Hill Medical.

Gaydos, C.A., Van Der Pol, B., Jett-Goheen, M., et al. (2013). Performance of the Cepheid CT/NG Xpert rapid PCR test for the detection of *Chlamydia trachomatis* and *Neisseria gonorrhoeae*. *Journal of Clinical Microbiology*, 51(6), 1666–72.

Ghys, P.D., Fransen, K., Diallo, M.O., et al. (1997). The associations between cervicovaginal HIV shedding, sexually transmitted diseases and immunosuppression in female sex workers in Abidjan, Côte d'Ivoire. *AIDS*, 11(12), F85–93.

Goldie, S.J., Levin, C., Mosqueira-Lovón, N.R., et al. (2012). Health and economic impact of human papillomavirus 16 and 18 vaccination of preadolescent girls and cervical cancer screening of adult women in Peru. *Revista Panamericana de Salud Pública*, 32(6), 426–34.

Goldie, S.J., O'Shea, M., Diaz, M., et al. (2008). Benefits, cost requirements and cost-effectiveness of the HPV 16,18 vaccine for cervical cancer prevention in developing countries: policy implications. *Reproductive Health Matters*, 16(32), 86–96.

Gomez, G.B., Kamb, M.L., Newman, L.M., et al. (2013). Untreated maternal syphilis and adverse outcomes of pregnancy: a systematic review and meta-analysis. *Bulletin of the World Health Organization*, 91(3), 217–26.

Gottleib, S.L., Low, N., Newman, L.M., et al. (2014). Towards global prevention of sexually transmitted infections (STIs), the case for STI vaccines. *Vaccine*, 32(14), 1527–35.

Grosskurth, H., Mosha, F., Todd, J., et al. (1995). Impact of improved treatment of sexually transmitted diseases on HIV infection in rural Tanzania: randomised controlled trial. *The Lancet*, 346(8974), 530–6.

Hay, P. (2008). HIV transmission and sexually transmitted infections. *Clinical Medicine*, 8(3), 323–6.

Hayes, R., Watson-Jones, D., and Celum, C., et al. (2010). Treatment of sexually transmitted infections for HIV prevention: end of the road or a new beginning. *AIDS*, 24(Suppl. 4), S15–26.

Hogben, M., Brewer, D.D., and Golden, M.R. (2001). Partner notification and management interventions. In S.O. Aral and J.M. Douglas (eds.) *Behavioral Interventions for Prevention and Control of Sexually Transmitted Diseases*, pp. 170–89. New York: Springer.

Hogben, M., Kidd, S., and Burstein, G.R. (2012). Expedited partner therapy for sexually transmitted infections. *Current Opinion in Obstetrics and Gynecology*, 24(5), 299–304.

Joint United Nations Programme on HIV/AIDS (2011). *Global HIV/ AIDS Response: Epidemic Update and Health Sector Progress Towards Universal Access—Progress Report 2011*. Geneva: UNAIDS. Available at: http: //www.who.int/hiv/pub/progress_report2011/ summary_en.pdf.

Joint United Nations Programme on HIV/AIDS (2012). *Global Report: UNAIDS Report on the Global AIDS Epidemic 2012*. Geneva: UNAIDS. Available at: http: //www.unaids.org/en/ media/unaids/contentassets/documents/epidemiology/2012/ gr2012/20121120_UNAIDS_Global_Report_2012_en.pdf.

Kamb, M.L., Fishbein, M.F., Douglas, J.M., et al. (1998). Efficacy of risk-reduction counseling to prevent human immunodeficiency virus and sexually transmitted diseases. *Journal of the American Medical Association*, 280, 1161–7.

Klebanoff, M.A., Carey, C., Hauth, J.C., et al. (2001). Failure of metronidazole to prevent preterm delivery among pregnant women with asymptomatic *Trichomonas vaginalis* infection. *The New England Journal of Medicine*, 345(7), 487–93.

Kogozi, G.G., Brahmbhatt, H., Wabwire-Mangen, F., et al. (2003). Treatment of trichomonas in pregnancy and adverse outcomes of pregnancy: a subanalysis of a randomized clinical trial in Rakai, Uganda. *American Journal of Obstetrics & Gynecology*, 189(5), 1398–400.

Korenromp, E.L., White, R.G., Orroth, K.K., et al. (2005). Determinants of the impact of sexually transmitted infection treatment on prevention of HIV infection: a synthesis of evidence from the Mwanza, Rakai, and Masaka intervention trials. *Journal of Infectious Disease*, 191(Suppl. 1), S168–78.

Laga, M., Alary, M., Nzila, N., et al. (1994). Condom promotion, sexually transmitted diseases treatment, and declining incidence of HIV-1 infection in female Zairian sex workers. *The Lancet*, 344(8917), 246–8.

Landry, D.J. and Turnbull, W. (1998). *Sexually Transmitted Diseases Hamper Development Efforts*. Guttmacher Institute. [Online] Available at: http: //www.guttmacher.org/pubs/ib_std.pdf.

Leichliter, J., Ellen, J., and Gunn, R. (2007). STD repeaters: implications for the individuals and STD transmission in a population. In S. Aral and J. Douglas (eds.) *Behavioral Interventions for Prevention and Control of Sexually Transmitted Diseases*, pp. 354–73. New York: Springer.

Levine, D.K., Scott, K.C., and Klausner, J.D. (2005). Online syphilis testing—confidential and convenient. *Sexually Transmitted Infections*, 32(2), 139–41.

Levine, W.C., Revollo, R., Kaune, V., et al. (1998). Decline in sexually transmitted disease prevalence in female Bolivian sex workers: impact of an HIV prevention project. *AIDS*, 12(14), 1899–906.

Lewis, D.A., Pillay, C., Mohlamonyane, O., et al. (2008). The burden of asymptomatic sexually transmitted infections among men in Carletonville South Africa: implications for syndromic management. *Sexually Transmitted Infections*, 85(5), 371–6.

Looker, K.J., Garnett, G.P., and Schmid, G.P. (2008). An estimate of the global prevalence and incidence of herpes simplex virus type 2 infection. *Bulletin of the World Health Organization*, 86(10), 805–12.

Lukehart, S.A., Godornes, C., Molini, B.J., et al. (2004). Macrolide resistance in *Treponema pallidum* in the United States and Ireland. *The New England Journal of Medicine*, 351(2), 154–8.

Mabey, D., Ndowa, F., and Latif, A. (2010). What have we learned from sexually transmitted infection research in sub-Saharan Africa? *Sexually Transmitted Infections*, 86, 488–92.

Mabey, D.C., Sollis, K.A., Kelly, H.A., et al. (2012). Point-of-care tests to strengthen health systems and save newborn lives: the case of syphilis. *PLoS Medicine*, 9(6), e1001233.

MacLachlan, E.W., Baganizi, E., Bougoudogo, F., et al. (2002). The feasibility of integrated STI prevalence and behaviour surveys in developing countries. *Sexually Transmitted Infections*, 78, 187–9.

Makasa, M., Buve, A., and Sandøy, I.F. (2012). Etiologic pattern of genital ulcers in Lusaka, Zambia: has chancroid been eliminated? *Sexually Transmitted Infections*, 39(10), 787–91.

Marazzo, J. and Cates, W. (2011). Interventions to prevent sexually transmitted infections, including HIV infection. *Clinical Infectious Diseases*, 52(Suppl. 3), S64–78.

Mathews, C., Coetzee, N., Zwarenstein, M., et al. (2001). Strategies for partner notification for sexually transmitted diseases. *Current Opinion in Obstetrics and Gynecology*, 4, CD002843.

May, R.M. and Anderson, R.M. (1987). Transmission dynamics of HIV infection. *Nature*, 326(6109), 137–42.

McFarlane, M. et al. (in press). *Normalizing Talking and Testing Among Youth Through the GYT (Get Yourself Tested) Campaign: An Integrated Approach to Sexual Health Promotion*.

Minnis, A.M. and Padian, N.S. (2005). Effectivness of female controlled barrier methods in preventing sexually transmitted infections and HIV: current evidence and future research directions. *Sexually Transmitted Infections*, 81, 193–200.

Munoz, N., Bosch, F.X., de Sanjosé, S., et al. (2003). Epidemiologic classification of human papillomavirus types associated with cervical cancer. *The New England Journal of Medicine*, 348(6), 518–27.

Newman, L., Kamb, M., Hawkes, S., et al. (2013). Global estimates of syphilis in pregnancy and associated adverse outcomes: analysis of multinational antenatal surveillance data. *PLoS Medicine*, 10(2), e1001396.

Ogilvie, G.S., Taylor, D.L., Trussler, T., et al. (2008). Seeking sexual partners on the internet: a marker for risky sexual behaviour in men who have sex with men. *Canadian Journal of Public Health*, 99(3), 185–8.

Ohnishi, M., Golparian, D., Shimuta, K., et al. (2011). Is Neisseria gonorrhoeae initiating a future era of untreatable gonorrhea?: detailed characterization of the first strain with high-level resistance to ceftriaxone. *Antimicrobial Agents and Chemotherapy*, 55, 3538–45.

Over, M. and Piot, P. (1996). Human immunodeficiency virus infection and other sexually transmitted diseases in developing countries: public health importance and priorities for resource allocation. *Journal of Infectious Disease*, 174(Suppl. 2), S162–75.

Owusu-Edusei, K. Jr., Chesson, H.W., Gift, T.L., et al. (2013). The estimated direct medical cost of selected sexually transmitted infections in the United States, 2008. *Sexually Transmitted Infections*, 40(3), 197–201.

Pan American Health Organization (2009). *Concept Paper on the Regional Initiative for the Elimination of Mother-to-Child Transmission of HIV and Congenital Syphilis in Latin America and the Caribbean*. Montevideo: CLAP/SMR.

Paz-Bailey, G., Ramaswamy, M., Hawkes, S.J., et al. (2007). Herpes simplex virus type 2: epidemiology and management options in developing countries. *Sexually Transmitted Infections*, 83(1), 16–22.

Paz-Bailey, G., Rhamna, M., Chen, C., et al. (2005). Changes in the etiology of sexually transmitted diseases in Botswana between 1993 and 2002: implications for the clinical management of genital ulcer disease. *Clinical Infectious Diseases*, 41, 1304–12.

Paz Soldan, V.A., Lee, F.H., Cárcamo, C., et al. (2008). Who is getting Pap smears in urban Peru? *International Journal of Epidemiology*, 37(4), 862–9.

Peeling, R.W., Holmes, K.K., Mabey, D., and Ronald, A. (2006). Rapid tests for sexually transmitted infections (STIs), the way forward. *Sexually Transmitted Infections*, 82(Suppl. 5), v1–6.

Perz, J.F., Armstrong, G.L., Farrington, L.A., et al. (2006). The contributions of hepatitis B virus and hepatitis C virus infections to cirrhosis and primary liver cancer worldwide. *Journal of Hepatology*, 45(4), 529–38.

Piret, J. and Boivin, G. (2011). Resistance of herpes simplex viruses to nucleoside analogues: mechanisms, prevalence and management. *Antimicrobial Agents and Chemotherapy*, 55(2), 459–72.

Plummer, F.A., Countinho, R.A., Ngugi, E.N., et al. (2005). Sex workers and their clients in the epidemiology and control of sexually transmitted diseases. In K.K. Holmes, P.F. Sparling, P.-A. Mardh, et al. (eds.) *Sexually Transmitted Diseases* (3rd ed.), pp. 143–50. New York: McGraw-Hill.

Rietmeijer, C.A., Bull, S.S., McFarlane, M., et al. (2003). Risks and benefits for Internet for populations at risk for sexually transmitted infections (STIs), results of an STI clinic survey. *Sexually Transmitted Infections*, 30(1), 15–19.

Ryan, C.A., Kamb, M., and Holmes, K.K. (2008). STI care management. In K.K. Holmes, P.F. Sparling, W.E. Stamm, et al. (eds.) *Sexually Transmitted Diseases* (4th ed.), pp. 855–76. New York: McGraw Hill Medical.

Santelli, J., Ott, M.A., Lyon, M., et al. (2006). Abstinence-only education policies and programs: a position paper of the Society for Adolescent Medicine. *Journal of Adolescent Health*, 38(1), 83–7.

Shelton, J.D., Halperin, D.T., Nantulya, V., et al. (2004). Partner reduction is crucial for balanced 'ABC' approach to HIV prevention. *BMJ*, 328(7444), 891–3.

Smith, J.S., Gilbert, P.A., Melendy, A., et al. (2011). Age-specific prevalence of human papillomavirus infection in males: a global review. *Journal of Adolescent Health*, 48(6), 540–52.

Smith, J.S. and Robinson, N.J. (2002). Age-specific prevalence of infection with herpes simplex virus types 2 and 1: a global review. *Journal of Infectious Disease*, 186(Suppl. 1), S3–28.

Smylie, L., Clarke, B., Doherty, M., et al. (2013). The development and validation of sexual health indicators of Canadians aged 16–24 years. *Public Health Reports*, 128(Suppl. 1), 53–61.

Steen, R., Wi, T.E., Kamali, A., and Ndowa, F. (2009). Control of sexually transmitted infections and prevention of HIV transmission: mending a fractured paradigm. *Bulletin of the World Health Organization*, 87, 858–65.

Strasser, S., Bitarakwate, E., Gill, M., et al. (2012). Introduction of rapid syphilis testing within prevention of mother-to-child transmission of HIV programs in Uganda and Zambia: a field acceptability and feasibility study. *Journal of Acquired Immune Deficiency Syndromes*, 61(3), 340–6.

Swartzendruber, A., Brown, J.L., Sales, J.M., et al. (2012). Sexually transmitted infections, sexual risk behavior, and intimate partner violence among African American adolescent females with a male sex partner recently released from incarceration. *Journal of Adolescent Health*, 51(2), 156–63.

Sweat, M.D., Denison, J., Kennedy, C., et al. (2012). Effects of condom social marketing on condom use in developing countries: a systematic review and meta-analysis, 1990-2010. *Bulletin of the World Health Organization*, 90(8), 613–22.

Swendeman, D. and Rotheram-Borus, M.J. (2010). Innovation in sexually transmitted disease and HIV prevention: internet and mobile phone delivery vehicles for global diffusion. *Current Opinion in Psychiatry*, 23(2), 139–44.

Terris-Prestholt, F., Vyas, S., Kumaranayake, L., Mayaud, P., and Watts, C. (2006). The costs of treating curable sexually transmitted infections in low- and middle-income countries: a systematic review. *Sexually Transmitted Diseases*, 33(Suppl.), S153–S166.

UNAIDS (2011). Global HIV/AIDS response: epidemic update and health sector progress towards Universal Access<en rule>Progress Report 2011. Available at: http://www.who.int/hiv/pub/progress_report2011/summary_en.pdf

UNAIDS (2012). Joint United Nations Programme on HIV/AIDS. Global Report: UNAIDS report on the global AIDS Epidemic 2012. ISBN 978-92-9173-592-1 Available at: http://www.unaids.org/sites/default/files/media_asset/20121120_UNAIDS_Global_Report_2012_with_annexes_en_1.pdf

Vijayakuma, G., Mabude, Z., Smit, J., et al. (2006). A review of female-condom effectiveness: patterns of use and impact on protected sex acts and STI incidence. *International Journal of STD & AIDS*, 17, 652–9.

Waaler, H.T. and Piot, M.A. (1969). The use of an epidemiological model for estimating the effectiveness of tuberculosis control measures. Sensitivity of the effectiveness of tuberculosis control measures to the coverage of the population. *Bulletin of the World Health Organization*, 41(1), 75–93.

Wang, C.C., McClelland, R.S., Reilly, M., et al. (2001). The effect of treatment of vaginal infections on shedding of human immunodeficiency virus type 1. *Journal of Infectious Disease*, 183, 1017–22.

Ward, H. and Rönn, M. (2010). Contribution of sexually transmitted infections to the sexual transmission of HIV. *Current Opinion in HIV and AIDS*, 5(4), 305–10.

Warner, L., Clay-Warner, J., Boles, J., and Williamson, J. (1998). Assessing condom use practices. Implications for evaluating method and user effectiveness. *Sexually Transmitted Infections*, 25(6), 273–7.

Wawer, M.J., Sewankambo, N.K., Serwadda, D., et al. (1999). Control of sexually transmitted diseases for AIDS prevention in Uganda: a randomised community trial. Rakai Project Study Group. *The Lancet*, 353(9152), 525–35.

Weinstock, H., Berman, S., and Cates, W., Jr. (2004). Sexually transmitted diseases among American youth: incidence and prevalence estimates, 2000. *Perspectives on Sexual and Reproductive Health*, 36(1), 6–10.

Weiss, H.A. (2007). Male circumcision as a preventive measure against HIV and other sexually transmitted diseases. *Current Opinion in Infectious Diseases*, 20(1), 66–72.

Weller, S. and Davis, K. (2002). Condom effectiveness in reducing heterosexual HIV transmission. *Cochrane Database of Systematic Reviews*, 1, CDC003255.

White, R.G., Orroth, K.K., Korenromp, E.L., et al. (2004). Can population differences explain the contrasting results of the Mwanza, Rakai, and Masaka HIV/sexually transmitted disease intervention trials?: A modeling study. *Journal of Acquired Immune Deficiency Syndromes*, 37(4), 1500–13.

Williams, S.P. and Kahn, R.H. (2007). Looking inside and affecting the outside: corrections-based interventions for STD prevention. In S. Aral and J. Douglas (eds.) *Behavioral Interventions for Prevention and Control of Sexually Transmitted Diseases*, pp. 374–96. New York: Springer.

World Bank (2004). *World Bank World Development Report 2004*. New York: Oxford University Press.

World Health Organization (2000). *Report on Infectious Diseases 2000, Overcoming Antimicrobial Resistance*. Geneva: WHO. Available at: http://www.who.int/infectious-disease-report/2000/.

World Health Organization (2007a). *Global Strategy for the Prevention and Control of Sexually Transmitted Infections: 2006–2015*. Geneva: WHO. Available at: http://www.who.int/reproductivehealth/publications/rtis/9789241563475/en/.

World Health Organization (2007b). *The Global Elimination of Congenital Syphilis: Rationale and Strategy for Action*. Geneva: WHO. Available at: http://www.who.int/reproductivehealth/publications/rtis/9789241595858/en/.

World Health Organization (2007c). *Investment Case for Eliminating Mother-to-Child Transmission of Syphilis: Promoting Better Maternal and Child Health and Stronger Health Systems*. Geneva: WHO. Available at: http://apps.who.int/iris/bitstream/10665/75480/1/9789241504348_eng.pdf.

World Health Organization (2008). *Global Incidence and Prevalence of Selected Curable Sexually Transmitted Infections—2008*. Geneva: WHO. Available at: http://www.who.int/reproductivehealth/publications/rtis/stisestimates/en/.

World Health Organization (2011). *Elimination of New Paediatric HIV Infections and Congenital Syphilis in Asia-Pacific, 2011–2015. Conceptual Framework Monitoring and Evaluation Guide*. Bangkok: UNICEF East Asia and Pacific Regional Office (EAPRO).

World Health Organization (2012a). *Prevention and Control of Viral Hepatitis Infection: Framework for Global Action*. Geneva: WHO. Available at: http://www.who.int/csr/disease/hepatitis/GHP_framework.pdf.

World Health Organization (2013). *Media Centre. Cancer Fact Sheet No. 297*. [Online] Available at http://www.who.int/mediacentre/factsheets/fs297/en/.

World Health Organization (2014). *Hepatitis B: Immunization Surveillance, Assessment, and Monitoring*. [Online] Available at: http://www.who.int/immunization_monitoring/diseases/hepatitis/en/index html.

Xu, F., Gee, J.M., Naleway, A., et al. (2008). Incidence of neonatal herpes simplex virus infections in two managed care organizations: implications for surveillance. *Sexually Transmitted Infections*, 35(6), 592–8.

Xu, F., Sternberg, M.R., Kottiri, B.J., et al. (2006). Trends in herpes simplex virus type 1 and type 2 seroprevalence in the United States. *Journal of the American Medical Association*, 296(8), 964–73.

Zur Hausen, H. (1996). Papillomavirus infections—a major cause of human cancers. *Biochimica et Biophysica Acta*, 1288(2), F55–F78.

8.13

HIV/acquired immunodeficiency syndrome

Sten H. Vermund and Suniti Solomon

Current status of the HIV/AIDS epidemic

The global pandemic of human immunodeficiency virus (HIV) infection is unprecedented in human history. While the bubonic plague in fourteenth-century Europe is estimated to have killed a quarter of the population, the epidemic of 1347–1350 was self-limited once a vast pool of susceptible humans and rodents were killed and people who recovered were immune (McEvedy 1988). Plague re-emerged periodically, but infrequently and with less intensity than the original devastating disease, and was not reported in Europe in epidemic form after the eighteenth century. In contrast, HIV emerged as a global pandemic in the 1980s and is now endemic throughout the world, declining only slightly in the first decade of the twenty-first century (Kilmarx 2009; Vermund and Leigh-Brown 2012). HIV is primarily a sexually transmitted infection (STI) and is propagated by human behaviour. Without successful control by biological and behavioural means, HIV will not be so readily controlled as was *Yersinia pestis*, the plague bacterium that was controllable with improved sanitation and rodent control well before the era of antibiotics.

An analogous global pandemic threat is that of influenza; its challenges in viral mutation and recombination and the risk of poor vaccine availability and coverage are, perhaps, as alarming as HIV as a risk to the global populace (Fedson 2009). That HIV disease, unknown until 1981, should have joined respiratory and diarrhoeal diseases, tuberculosis, malaria, and vaccine-preventable diseases like measles as the most devastating of global infectious threats reminds us of the need for vigilance in recognition and response to emerging infectious diseases (Chavers and Vermund 2007).

In countries most affected in southern Africa, HIV prevalence rates in the general adult population routinely exceed one in ten adults and rise to as high as one in two in certain age/sex groups (Karim et al. 2011). The self-perpetuating transmission cycles are facilitated by human sexual behaviours as well as the decade-long average incubation period of the virus. Rather than infecting and killing many people quickly, like plague or influenza, HIV is transmitted more gradually and kills people well after they may have infected others (Baggaley and Fraser 2010).

Advanced clinical or immunological disease has been termed the acquired immune deficiency syndrome (AIDS), a concept still useful for surveillance but imprecise for use in clinical medicine; there are many more gradations and variations of HIV disease than the binary 'AIDS' or 'no AIDS' designations. People with AIDS-defining opportunistic infections (OI) or malignancies (OM) in the pre-treatment era (before 1987) were typically severely immunologically suppressed; people with CD4+ T-lymphocyte counts under 200 cells/microlitre were ultimately included in the AIDS case definition as revised by the US Centers for Disease Control and Prevention (CDC) in 1993 (Anonymous 1992). But in the combination antiretroviral therapy (cART) era after 1996, people with AIDS could achieve levels of immunological reconstitution sufficient to permit decades of disease-free life. Hence in the era of cART, reaching a surveillance case definition of AIDS no longer suggests that an individual has current severe HIV disease, they may have partial immune reconstitution if they have received cART. This chapter will refer to HIV disease in all its levels of severity, referring to AIDS only when discussing surveillance data that use AIDS as a surrogate for advanced HIV disease.[1]

Global HIV trends

As of the end of 2011, an estimated 34 million people globally were living with HIV infection, 95–97 per cent of whom were in low- and middle-income countries (LMIC) (Joint United Nations Programme on HIV/AIDS (UNAIDS) 2011a). In 2012, UNAIDS and the World Health Organization (WHO) estimated that the pandemic would pass the 30 million cumulative HIV mortality mark; in dozens of nations, HIV is the first ranking cause of death for young adults aged 20–44 years (UNAIDS 2011b). While continuing to expand in some nations (like Pakistan) and in some subpopulations (like black men who have sex with men (MSM) in the United States), the prevalence has peaked and declined by varying degrees in a number of afflicted nations and/or population subgroups. In Thailand and Uganda, the success of control efforts predated the advent of cART and was attributed to behavioural and structural changes (Stoneburner and Low-Beer 2004; Kipp et al. 2009; Park et al. 2010). In southern sub-Saharan Africa where HIV rates are the highest, there is evidence of declining prevalence and incidence, as has been well documented in Zimbabwe (Halperin et al. 2011). Deaths may have contributed to declining prevalence (Wawer et al. 1997), though in the face of expanded cART availability, declining prevalence and incidence may well be related (Das et al. 2010).

In some parts of the world, incidence is stable and even rising, especially in selected vulnerable subgroups such as MSM in Asia, black MSM in the United States, or people who inject drugs (PWID) in Eastern Europe and central Asia (Kilmarx

2009; El-Sadr et al. 2010; Vermund et al. 2010; Beyrer et al. 2011). Successes are reported, but given that rates remain high in the general population in sub-Saharan Africa, and are persistent in most at-risk populations throughout the world, no serious observer predicts the spontaneous demise of the pandemic (Vergara et al. 2009; Larson et al. 2011; Schwartlander et al. 2011).

Children are affected in many ways by the epidemic. They may be infected through mother-to-child transmission (MTCT) *in utero*, during delivery, or post-partum via breast milk (Goldenberg et al. 2002; Fowler et al. 2010; Mofenson 2010). HIV-exposed, but uninfected infants can suffer due to the loss of one or more parents due to HIV, or due to their illness itself with its economic and social burden on the family (Newell et al. 2004). Adolescents (or abused children) can be infected sexually and may be challenging to engage in successful and sustained primary care (Ding et al. 2009). Prevention of MTCT is challenged by programmatic obstacles that are amenable to quality improvement research and intervention (Stringer et al. 2003, 2005; Bolton-Moore et al. 2007; Reithinger et al. 2007; Potter et al. 2008; Megazzini et al. 2010; Stringer et al. 2010). Prevention programmes are judged to be highly cost-effective and are the focus for intensive pregnancy screening and ART intervention (Galarraga et al. 2011). Early infant diagnosis leading to earlier cART therapy is essential to improve outcomes for HIV-infected infants (Violari et al. 2008; Ciampa et al. 2011; Ciaranello et al. 2011).

An alarming trend is one familiar to the field of STIs, namely the replenishing of the at-risk population with sexually vulnerable youth; about half of the global population is under age 25 and this corresponds to the proportion of new infections globally attributable to this age group (UNAIDS 2011b). However, since the average age of sexual debut is in the teens, this suggests the intensity of risk for adolescents and youth once they become sexually active (Underhill et al. 2007; DiClemente et al. 2008; Spiegel and Futterman 2009; Karim et al. 2011).

HIV morbidity and mortality has had a huge impact on economies of LMIC (Ferreira et al. 2011). Given the link of HIV with vulnerable populations and/or poverty, such challenges as community development, orphans, household income, and gender-power issues have been exacerbated by the HIV pandemic (Andrews et al. 2006; Hosegood et al. 2007). Disease progression and transmission of other infectious diseases, notably tuberculosis, are accelerated by HIV co-infection (Lawn and Zumla 2011; Martinson et al. 2011). Cancers such as Kaposi's sarcoma (human herpesvirus type 8 (HHV-8) co-infection) and cervical cancer (human papillomavirus (HPV) co-infection) loom large as major risks (Casper 2011; Sahasrabuddhe et al. 2012). In addition, the progression of HIV and its infectiousness is exacerbated by other co-infections (Modjarrad and Vermund 2010; Barnabas et al. 2011). Food insecurity may limit cART adherence when appetites surge with immune reconstitution and increased energy and metabolic demands (Koethe and Heimburger 2010). Hence, the global community is increasingly embracing a more holistic response to the HIV pandemic, including community development, task shifting for healthcare workers, and horizontal health system reform, while acknowledging the need for sustained emergency responses (Chopra et al. 2009). HIV may be among the most important healthcare challenges in endemic nations, but it is hardly the only one.

HIV by continent/region

Sub-Saharan Africa

Over a third of the infected people globally live in ten nations of southern Africa, by far the worst afflicted region. South Africa, for example, was the 25th most populous nation with 49 million people in mid-2009 (United States Census Bureau n.d.). Yet it ranked first for the number of people living with HIV/AIDS with an estimated 5.6 million people (range 5.4–5.9 million) in 2009 (UNAIDS n.d.). South African adults aged 15 to 49 years had an estimated 2009 prevalence rate of 17.8 per cent (range 17.2–18.3 per cent); nearly 2 million children had been orphaned by 2009. Averages mask extremes; some subpopulations in their mid 20s were over 50 per cent HIV-infected (Karim et al. 2011).

The sub-Saharan African epidemic is driven by heterosexual contact (Vermund et al. 2009). Injection drug use and male-to-male sexual contact may be increasing and represent future risk (Vlahov et al. 2010). Iatrogenic spread has also been reported through reuse of contaminated needles and use of contaminated blood products in healthcare settings (Simonsen et al. 1999; Beyrer et al. 2011). However, the overwhelming burden of transmission is, and remains of, heterosexual origin. MTCT is still common in sub-Saharan Africa due to failures to achieve high coverage of HIV testing in pregnancy and proper mother–infant coverage with ART (Stringer et al. 2003, 2005, 2010; Horwood et al. 2010). Given its large population and its low coverage rates for prevention of MTCT, Nigeria has more unmet need for HIV screening of pregnant women than any other African country.

East and South East Asia

The epidemic in South East Asia, China, Japan, Philippines, Indonesia, and other parts of the region is a complex one. While less intense than in Africa, the Asian epidemic remains intractable with persistent transmission in vulnerable populations. Countries like Japan, Korea, and Mongolia report a disproportionate number of imported HIV cases, with low indigenous transmission rates; however, high-risk populations such as MSM in Japan and STI patients in Mongolia suggest concern for future autochthonous transmission (Nemoto 2004; Davaalkham et al. 2009). In the Philippines, vulnerable populations have had surprisingly low rates of infection, but some observers believe that over time, local HIV transmission will increase (Farr and Wilson 2010). In South East Asia and Indonesia, heterosexual, MSM, and PWID transmission are all prevalent (Sharma et al. 2009; van Griensven and de Lind van Wijngaarden 2010; Vlahov et al. 2010; Couture et al. 2011). In countries like Thailand and Cambodia, successes are notable in reducing transmission among PWID and heterosexual transmission with needle exchange and universal condom advocacy, respectively (Celentano et al. 1998; Park et al. 2010). China has had some progress in addressing its serious problem of HIV among PWID, but the epidemic among MSM is rising; fortunately, heterosexual spread is not common in the world's most populous nation, even among sex workers (Wu et al. 2007; Xiao et al. 2007). An unusual outbreak of HIV in rural central China spread due to pooled red cell re-infusions to blood and plasma donors who were illegally and unethically recruited in the 1990s (Qian et al. 2005, 2006).

South Asia

India has experienced a substantial heterosexual epidemic concentrated in its southern states, with PWID-related transmission in northeastern states; the northern states have much lower incidence and prevalence (Chandrasekaran et al. 2006). Despite prevalence rates far lower than in sub-Saharan Africa, India, the second most populous nation on the globe, ranks just behind South Africa and Nigeria for the highest number of HIV-infected people (about 2.5 million in 2009) living in the nation. MSM are at risk throughout south Asia, including *hijras*, who are men who dress as women and have a long-standing cultural niche in such nations as India, Pakistan, and Bangladesh (Solomon et al. 2010; Siddiqui et al. 2011; Sahastrabuddhe et al. 2012). India faces Asia's largest unmet need for prevention of MTCT, with daunting challenges to screen vast populations of pregnant women. India's HIV rates are far higher in the south and the northeast of the nation than in the north-central or northwest. An explosive growth in HIV prevalence seen in Pakistan in 2002 underscores the fact that where risk behaviour persists, HIV is likely to spread eventually (Altaf et al. 2009; Kazi et al. 2010).

Eastern Europe and Central Asia

Although same-sex and heterosexual transmissions occur in Eastern Europe and Central Asia, most HIV transmission has been from PWID (Mathers et al. 2010). A number of countries continue to have growth in their epidemics, even as prevalence rates stabilize or even decline elsewhere in the world (Kelly and Amirkhanian 2003). While rates in Eastern Europe and Central Asia have not reached the levels elsewhere, exceedingly poor policies that have undermined risk reduction efforts among PWID have exacerbated the epidemic, most notably in Russia, a country that continues to ban any form of opiate substitution therapy (i.e. methadone or buprenorphine) (Elovich and Drucker 2008; Bridge et al. 2010). Where aggressive risk reduction has been promulgated using clean needle and syringe exchange, results have been very promising (Platt et al. 2008). All of this is sadly reminiscent of the policy blind spots in the United States that banned federal support of clean needle exchange until Congress lifted the ban in 2009; current US policies and plans are based more on prevention evidence rather than the political concerns of the past (Lurie and Drucker 1997).

Middle East and North Africa

Sexual transmission of HIV is reported in the Middle East and North Africa, particularly among MSM (Mumtaz et al. 2010). Migrant workers in the Gulf States are deported if infected, and can serve to introduce HIV in their home countries (Shah et al. 1999). Commercial sex workers have not had high rates, perhaps due to cultural and biological factors of near-universal male circumcision and lower partner exchange rates in the general population (Abu-Raddad et al. 2010). It is also true that if a foreign sex worker tests HIV-positive, she/he is deported, reducing HIV prevalence in the middle eastern nation doing the deporting. PWID has been the largest driver of transmission in this low-prevalence region (Todd et al. 2007; Sawires et al. 2009). Given its suppressive human rights policies, it is a paradox that Iran has been at the regional forefront of an assertive response to use of opiate substitution therapy to reduce drug craving and HIV risk, including services in prisons (Farnia et al. 2010).

North America and Western Europe

The HIV epidemic in North America and Western Europe has been driven by MSM, PWID, and, to a lesser extent, heterosexual transmission (Vermund and Leigh-Brown 2012). Sexual vulnerability is higher in people practising unprotected anal intercourse and using alcohol and/or illicit drugs proximate to sexual activity (Miller 2003; Shoptaw and Reback 2007). Party drugs (e.g. nitrates, amphetamines, and cocaine) have been associated with higher-risk sexual activity, an observation dating from before we even knew that HIV caused AIDS (Goedert 1984). People addicted to crack cocaine and methamphetamine may practise high-risk sex and both women and men may sell sex for drugs or money to support drug habits (Corsi and Booth 2008). Adolescents are vulnerable to peer pressures to have sex and use drugs (Fortenberry 1998). Affected subgroups have changed over time in the United States, for example, increasing numbers of MSM of black and other minority ethnic backgrounds and women, together over half the incident cases (Millett et al. 2006; El-Sadr et al. 2010). Molecular phylogenetic approaches have established historical links between HIV strains from central Africa to those in the United States and thence to Europe (Vermund and Leigh-Brown 2012). As in other high-income nations, HIV screening has virtually eliminated blood/blood product-related transmissions. MTCT has been reduced markedly since the 1980s, with peripartum ART prophylaxis in HIV-infected pregnant women and exposed newborns combined with discouragement of breastfeeding among HIV-infected mothers; MTCT of HIV is a rare public health problem in high-income nations, though some perinatal cases are still seen (Lindegren et al. 1999).

Given the value of HIV therapy in reducing infectiousness, as demonstrated by the HIV Prevention Trials Network 052 protocol (HPTN 052, discussed later in this chapter), it is disappointing that only 19–28 per cent (range of estimates from 2010) of Americans infected with HIV were on cART with successful suppression of HIV viral load (Burns et al. 2010; CDC 2011; Cohen et al. 2011; Gardner et al. 2011). High-access cities like Vancouver and San Francisco do much better and may be seeing prevention benefits from high HIV testing and cART coverage (Das et al. 2010; Montaner et al. 2010). Aggressive testing and cART use within the context of excellent primary care may also contribute to lower-than-expected HIV rates in Western European countries, though other cultural elements and aggressive prevention interventions make this hard to disentangle. Declining incidence due to wider coverage with cART has been suggested in other high-income nations as well, for example, Taiwan (Fang et al. 2004).

Central and South America

There is diversity in the south and central American epidemic, but the dominant mode of transmission seems to be anal sex among MSM (Bastos et al. 2008). PWID contributes substantially in some regions such as urban Brazil, but is a less common risk factor than in North America, Europe, or Asia (Hacker et al. 2005). Alcohol and non-injection use fuel unsafe sexual behaviours (Bastos et al. 2007; Bassols et al. 2010). Heterosexual transmission occurs and bisexual men are thought to be an important bridge population (Ramirez et al. 1994; Konda et al. 2011). Perinatal transmission is less common with most antenatal programmes in endemic areas offering HIV testing and ART, albeit imperfectly (D'Ippolito et al. 2007).

Caribbean

The second highest prevalence rates in the world, after sub-Saharan Africa, occur in the Caribbean region (Figueroa

2008). The epidemic is diverse with the worst affected nation, Haiti, experiencing a heterosexual-dominant pattern (Castro and Farmer 2005; Dorjgochoo et al. 2009). The Dominican Republic and Guyana also have substantial heterosexual transmission (Allen et al. 2006; Padilla et al. 2008; Seguy et al. 2008). MSM represent the more common afflicted group in most of the other islands (Finlinson et al. 2006; Padilla et al. 2008). Puerto Rico is a territory of the United States with close ties to major US cities like New York and Miami (connected by so-called 'air bridges' of low-cost, passport-free travel); Puerto Rico has been experiencing an substantial PWID-related transmission (Mino et al. 2011). Cuba is well-known for its mass HIV screening and quarantine approach to HIV, segregating HIV-infected people into their own communities; this has alternatively been criticized for human rights restrictions and been praised for limiting the epidemic's spread (Anderson 2009; Hsieh et al. 2010). Adolescents, as in the rest of the world, are of special concern for sexual risk behaviours (Dorjgochoo et al. 2009; Andrews 2011).

Selected mainland countries like Guyana (in South America) and Belize (in Central America) are often grouped with Caribbean countries due to proximity and socio-political synergies, even though they are not islands. Both Guyana and Belize are in the Caribbean Community and Common Market (CARICOM) and have formal public health ties with the English-speaking islands through the Caribbean Epidemiology Centre (CAREC) in Trinidad. Guyana was chosen, along with Haiti, as one of the first target countries for large US investments for HIV control and prevention, the President's Emergency Plan For AIDS Relief (PEPFAR).

Australia and Oceania

Australia has had a persistent and aggressive risk reduction programme from the early days of their epidemic (Jones et al. 2010; Kang et al. 2010; Mao et al. 2011). Their widespread and 'user-friendly' approaches to clean needle exchange and availability of opiate substitutions therapy through primary care practitioners are credited for keeping HIV rates exceedingly low in PWID (Miller et al. 2009). MSM is a principal challenge in parts of the region, though Oceania confronts pockets of heterosexual transmission (Corner et al. 2005; Vallely et al. 2010).

In summary, each global region has its specific challenges to confront in HIV control. Even at the micro-geographic level, there can be differences of just miles or even city blocks where PWID drives a micro-transmission dynamic versus sexual activity driving a local epidemic. Infection control efforts must be based in an epidemiological knowledge of the transmission drivers and sociocultural contexts of risk behaviours in a given region, or even a given neighbourhood. 'Know your epidemic' has become the adage that reminds us that a given prevention approach will not work in all settings. At the same time, there are great truths in the global pandemic: behaviour change is a vital component of any part of the effort to control transmission; high cART coverage may reduce community-level transmission; risk reduction strategies can work to reduce HIV transmissions even if the underlying challenges (e.g. PWID, sex work) are not altered markedly; risk behaviours are steeped in cultural context and traditions that are not easily changed; human rights underlie the global community's response, successful or unsuccessful, as respect for vulnerable people is the first step towards engagement and assistance.

Regional and national data are updated yearly by UNAIDS (2014) and WHO (2014).

Biological mechanisms

Unique HIV characteristics

It is unhelpful to consider HIV merely as an infectious disease; it needs also to be considered a chronic disease. Only with this merger of the infectious disease–chronic disease 'dichotomy' can one understand the challenges ahead for HIV control. The lifespan of the infected individual can vary from years to decades; this is not a classic infection paradigm of infection followed by either immunological control/recovery or death, as applies to so many other viruses. Examples of the classic infectious disease paradigm are vaccine-preventable diseases of childhood like measles and arboviruses like yellow fever; they may kill, but in people who survive, they provide lifelong immunity.

In contrast, HIV persists even in the face of the host's immunological response. Lentiviruses (i.e. slow viruses) are characterized by years and even decades of gradual pathogenic impact. The HIV-infected individual will have transient, incomplete immunological control that is overwhelmed over time by viral escape mutations and immunological collapse (Bushman et al. 2011). This is why access to cART is so vital, in order to permit the body to restore partial immunological function by suppressing viral replication and stopping the mass destruction of CD4+ T lymphocytes.

Retroviruses have ribonucleic acid (RNA) as their genetic material, requiring the virus to use a reverse transcriptase enzyme to convert RNA into deoxyribonucleic acid (DNA). The DNA can then integrate into the host cell genome with the genetic instructions hijacking the cell's protein manufacturing machinery to replicate HIV. While perhaps half of HIV-infected people with the infection have non-specific 'flu' symptoms, others may not be aware that they are ill at all (Cohen et al. 2011). Whether or not someone has experienced symptoms of acute HIV infection, in the following years, HIV-infected people do not feel ill and may transmit HIV for many years until diagnosed and treated or until illness and death.

Given that most HIV disease is asymptomatic, routine HIV testing must be promoted to identify asymptomatic disease. That screening of at-risk people is a mainstay of diagnosis and prevention is analogous to the disease control strategy for STIs and tuberculosis (Reid et al. 2004; Vermund et al. 2009). Within the pool of HIV-infected people, additional screening is essential, as for human papillomavirus-induced cervical precancerous lesions, human herpesvirus 8-induced Kaposi's sarcoma lesions, *Mycobacterium tuberculosis*, and other conditions that are far more prevalent in HIV-infected than uninfected individuals.

Viral entry and replication

HIV uses a particular protein, CD4, to recognize cells. The CD4 protein serves as a receptor for fusion, entry, and infection. CD4 is short for 'cluster of differentiation 4', a terminology used in cell cytometry and immunology, representing a surface glycoprotein on key cells that provide immunological surveillance, namely T-helper lymphocytes, macrophages, monocytes, and dendritic cells. In humans, this protein is encoded by a *CD4* gene that, if mutated, may reduce susceptibility to infection. The HIV-1 uses its protruding viral envelope protein known as gp120 to bind to CD4; gp stand for glycoprotein and 120 represents the molecular weight of this particular protein. HIV must bind to a CD4 receptor, creating a conformational shift in the gp120 that enables the virus to bind to chemokine co-receptors expressed on the host cell. Two types of co-receptors are used by HIV. One is termed CCR5 or C-C chemokine receptor type 5 that is coded by the human *CCR5* gene. The other is known as CXCR-4 or C-X-C chemokine receptor type 4 (also known as fusin), a protein encoded by the *CXCR4* gene. Once gp120-CD4 engagement has permitted viral docking with one of these two beta chemokine receptors, a structural change then occurs in viral protein gp41 (together, gp120 and gp41 make up gp160), enabling HIV to insert its fusion peptide into the CD4+ cell. HIV then fuses with the host cell membrane. CD4's primary function is a vital one, namely serving to assist T-cell receptors (TCR) on antigen-presenting cells (Wilen et al. 2012). That HIV lives in, and takes over, the machinery of the CD4+ T cell is much like the legend of the Greek soldiers within the Trojan horse, destroying the very cell that is designed to help defend against outside invaders.

Viral variation and evolution

HIV-1 has many variants, referred to as subtypes or clades, due to recombinant viruses generated through co-circulation of different viruses. High recombination and mutation rates result in the generation of circulating recombinant forms, or 'CRFs' (Kalish et al. 2004; Vermund and Leigh-Brown 2012). Over decades of viral expansion, the genetic complexity of HIV has increased globally such that over 40 CRFs have been recognized as of 2011. HIV-1 genetic diversity is greatest in west-central Africa where hunters of chimpanzees may have been infected with an HIV-precursor in the early twentieth century when they captured, killed, and skinned their primate 'bushmeat'. It is thought that chimpanzee HIV antecedents entered human populations in central Africa in the 1930s, with only indolent human-to-human transmission (Sharp and Hahn 2010). Later, conditions of migration, urbanization, loss of sexual taboos, injection-related contaminations, and global travel facilitated entry of HIV into populations practising higher-risk activities (e.g. multiple sexual partners, sex work, anal sex, injecting drugs). In central Africa, most major clades have been isolated (represented by alphabet letters A through K) (Kalish et al. 2004). Many observers suggest that there are few major biological differences among HIV clades, though there is a suggestion that C clade may be more pathogenic (Novitsky et al. 2011). Viral diversity continues to emerge and may be due to stochastic variations from founder infections with subsequent transmission within vulnerable populations (Rambaut et al. 2004; Hemelaar et al. 2011). Dating of divergence events can be estimated using 'molecular clocks' (Lewis et al. 2008). It appears that a divergence of major clades occurred in central Africa in the mid-twentieth century (Korber et al. 2000). Now that phylodynamic approaches permit estimations of sequence evolution rates, we can also use these estimates as parameters for epidemic modelling of sexual and other transmission networks (Vermund and Leigh-Brown 2012). Given that the world now confronts tremendous HIV genetic diversity, also driven by antiretroviral drug pressures, viral diversity is a principal challenge for future vaccine and antiretroviral drug development (Kalish et al. 2004; Takebe et al. 2010).

Current therapy and prognosis
Development of antiretroviral drugs

The scientific achievement represented by the discovery and development of antiretroviral drugs is among the great stories of applied scholarship in the late twentieth century (Broder 2010). The first discovered antiretroviral drug was zidovudine (ZDV) (also called azidothymidine (AZT)), a thymine analogue in the drug family of nucleoside reverse transcriptase inhibitors (NRTIs) (Mitsuya et al. 1991). When zidovudine is present, its thymine mimicry results in reverse transcriptase mistakenly adding it to the DNA strand; reverse transcription is then terminated since the zidovudine moiety does not accept the next nucleotide being added to the DNA.

Once ZDV was made available for clinical trials and then for commercial sale, there were early indications of clinical benefits in both clinical trials and also in larger population 'real-world use' conditions (Graham et al. 1992). However, viral mutation rates are high and drug-resistant strains emerged quickly, severely limiting the duration of single drug benefit (Anonymous 1994; Gardner et al. 1998). When new NRTI drugs were developed, dual therapy proved superior to monotherapy, but resistant viruses still emerged; the revolutionary change occurred with the advent of new classes of antiretroviral drugs that attacked the virus at different stages of its life cycle. Using cART, many patients who were adherent to their cART regimens could suppress HIV replication indefinitely. Current guidelines are permissive of a variety of alternative cART regimens (Thompson et al. 2010). In settings with adequate resources, nearly everyone with a detectable HIV viral load is recommended to be treated, regardless of CD4+ cell counts (Tables 8.13.1 and 8.13.2). Unfortunately for patients and for their uninfected sexual partners, low- and middle-income countries are typically limited to starting therapy at the threshold of WHO clinical status 3 or 4 and/or CD4+ cell counts <350/microlitre, or may even start at a lower threshold like <250 cells/microlitre, due to resource constraints. As this chapter goes to press, the WHO is changing its therapeutic guidelines to recommend cART for all people with CD4+ cell counts <500/microlitre, recommending consideration of treating even people with higher CD4+ cell counts, so-called universal test and treat, to benefit the patient and to reduce transmission to others.

Licensed antiretroviral therapy

There are six licensed classes of antiretroviral drugs (Table 8.13.3). Among the NRTI drugs, zidovudine, emtricitabine (FTC), lamivudine (3TC), abacavir (ABC), tenofovir disoproxil fumarate (TDF), didanosine (ddI or dideoxyinosine), and stavudine (d4T) are all in use. Stavudine has an unfavourable profile of side effects, but is still (as of early 2013) used widely in low-income countries due to its low generic cost. Non-nucleoside reverse transcriptase inhibitors (NNRTI) include efavirenz (EFV), both immediate- and extended-release forms of nevirapine (NVP), delavirdine (DLV), and newer drugs rilpivirine and etravirine.

Protease inhibitors (PIs) are often boosted with another protease inhibitor, ritonavir, to inhibit a cytochrome P450-3A4 (CYP3A4), a liver enzyme that metabolizes protease inhibitors. Ritonovir boosting both increases efficacy and reduces side effects of other PIs. PIs include amprenavir (APV), tipranavir (TPV), indinavir (IDV), saquinavir mesylate (SQV), lopinavir (LPV), ritonavir

Table 8.13.1 Preferred and alternative antiretroviral regimens for antiretroviral therapy-naive patients

Preferred regimens

Regimens with optimal and durable efficacy, favourable tolerability and toxicity profile, and ease of use.

The preferred regimens for non-pregnant patients are arranged by chronological order of FDA approval of components other than nucleosides and, thus, by duration of clinical experience.

	Comments
NNRTI-based regimen: • EFV/TDF/FTCª (AI) PI-based regimens (in alphabetical order): • ATV/r + TDF/FTCª (AI) • DRV/r (once daily) + TDF/FTCª (AI) INSTI-based regimen: • RAL + TDF/FTCª (AI)	• EFV is teratogenic in non-human primates. A regimen that does not include EFV should be strongly considered in women who are planning to become pregnant or who are sexually active and not using effective contraception. • TDF should be used with caution in patients with renal insufficiency. • ATV/r should not be used in patients who require >20 mg omeprazole equivalent per day.

Alternative regimens

Regimens that are effective and tolerable, but have potential disadvantages when compared with preferred regimens. An alternative regimen may be the preferred regimen for some patients.

	Comments
NNRTI-based regimens (in alphabetical order): • EFV + ABC/3TCª (BI) • RPV/TDF/FTCª (BI) • RPV + ABC/3TCª (BIII) PI-based regimens (in alphabetical order): • ATV/r + ABC/3TCª (BI) • DRV/r + ABC/3TCª (BII) • FPV/r (once or twice daily) + ABC/3TCª or TDF/FTCª (BI) • LPV/r (once or twice daily) + ABC/3TCª or TDF/FTCª (BI) INSTI-based regimen: • EVG/COBI/TDF/FTCª (BI) • RAL + ABC/3TCª (BIII)	• RPV is not recommended in patients with pretreatment HIV RNA >100,000 copies/mL • Higher rate of virologic failures reported in patients with pre-ART CD4 count <200 cells/mm³ who are treated with RPV + 2NRTI • Use of PPIs with RPV is contraindicated • ABC should not be used in patients who test positive for HLA-B*5701 • Use ABC with caution in patients with known high risk of CVD or with pretreatment HIV RNA >100,000 copies/mL • Once-daily LPV/r is not recommended for use in pregnant women • EVG/COBI/TDF/FTC should not be started in patients with an estimated CrCl < 70 mL/min, and should be changed to an alternative regimen if the patient's CrCl falls below 50 mL/min • COBI is a potent CYP 3A inhibitor. It can increase the concentration of other drugs metabolized by this pathway • EVG/COBI/TDF/FTC should not be used with other ARV drugs or with nephrotoxic drugs

ª 3TC may substitute for FTC or vice versa. The following combinations in the recommended list in the table are available as coformulated fixed dose combinations: ABC/3TC, EFV/TDF/FTC, EVG/COBI/TDF/FTC, LPV/r, RPV/TDF/FTC, TDF/FTC, and ZDV/3TC.

3TC = lamivudine, ABC = abacavir, ART = antiretroviral therapy, ARV = antiretroviral, ATV/r = atazanavir/ritonavir, COBI = cobicistat, CrCl = creatinine clearance, CVD = cardiovascular disease, DRV/r = darunavir/ritonavir, EFV = efavirenz, EVG = elvitegravir, FDA = Food and Drug Administration, FPV/r = fosamprenavir/ritonavir, FTC = emtricitabine, INSTI = integrase strand transfer inhibitor, LPV/r = lopinavir/ritonavir, NNRTI = non-nucleoside reverse transcriptase inhibitor, NRTI = nucleoside reverse transcriptase inhibitor, PI = protease inhibitor, PPI = proton pump inhibitor, RAL = raltegravir, RPV = rilpivirine, RTV = ritonavir, TDF = tenofovir disoproxil fumarate, ZDV = zidovudine.

Rating of recommendations: A = Strong; B = Moderate; C = Optional.

Rating of evidence: I = Data from randomized controlled trials; II = Data from well-designed non-randomized trials or observational cohort studies with long-term clinical outcomes; III = Expert opinion.

Reproduced from Panel on Antiretroviral Guidelines for Adults and Adolescents, *Guidelines for the use of antiretroviral agents in HIV-1-infected adults and adolescents*, Department of Health and Human Services, 2013 version, available at http://aidsinfo.nih.gov/ContentFiles/AdultandAdolescentGL.pdf.

(RTV), fosamprenavir calcium (FOS-APV), darunavir, atazanavir sulphate (ATV), and nelfinavir mesylate (NFV).

Three newer classes have single licensed drugs in each class, as of 2011, though more will be licensed in the future (Table 8.13.3). Raltegravir works to inhibit integrase, and is called an integrase strand transfer inhibitor. Maraviroc is a CCR5 blocker and inhibits viral entry, though it does not work against CXCR4 receptor strains of HIV. The fusion inhibitor is enfuvirtide (T-20), a costly drug given subcutaneously twice daily, used only for 'salvage therapy' of people with extensively drug-resistant HIV in high-income settings.

Some drugs are specifically formulated for paediatric use (US Food and Drug Administration 2014b). Availability of paediatric

formulations often lags, by years sometimes, the licensure of drugs suitable for adult consumption, a serious problem for the care of children with HIV infection (Dionisio et al. 2007). Antiretroviral chemotherapy principles are similar for adults and children, but the availability of paediatric formulations sometimes skews therapeutic decision making.

Many drugs are licensed generics in the US (US Food and Drug Administration 2014c). The generic market is expanding, and not all of the products have been through the FDA licensure process. The US FDA has approved a number of drugs for use in the PEPFAR in Africa, Asia, and the Caribbean (US Food and Drug Administration 2014d). The use of generics in PEPFAR has reduced costs and increased efficiency of programmes, but

Table 8.13.2 Other antiretroviral regimens for antiretroviral therapy-naive patients

Regimens that may be selected for some patients but are less satisfactory than preferred or alternative regimens listed in Table 8.13.1	
	Comments
NNRTI-based regimen: • EFV + ZDV/3TC[a] • NVP + (ABC/3TC[a] or TDF/FTC[a] or ZDV/3TC[a]) • RPV + ZDV/3TC[a] PI-based regimens: • (ATV or ATV/r or DRV/r or FPV/r or LPV/r or SQV/r) + ZDV/3TC[a] • ATV + ABC/3TC[a] • SQV/r + (ABC/3TC[a] or TDF/FTC[a]) INSTI-based regimen: • RAL + ZDV/3TC[a] CCR5 antagonist-based regimens: • MVC + (ABC/3TC or TDF/FTC or ZDV/3TC[a])	• **NVP** should not be used in patients with moderate to severe hepatic impairment (Child–Pugh B or C). • **NVP** should not be used in women with pre-ART CD4 count > 250 cells/mm[3] or in men with pre-ART CD4 count > 400 cells/mm[3] • Use **NVP** and **ABC** together with caution; both can cause HSRs within the first few weeks after initiation of therapy • **ZDV** can cause bone marrow suppression, myopathy, lipoatrophy, and rarely lactic acidosis with hepatic steatosis • **ATV/r** is generally preferred over **unboosted ATV** • Perform tropism testing before initiation of therapy with **MVC**. **MVC** may be considered in patients who have only CCR5-tropic virus • **SQV/r** was associated with PR and QT prolongation in a healthy volunteer study. Baseline ECG is recommended before initiation of **SQV/r** • **SQV/r** is not recommended in patients with: • pretreatment QT interval > 450 msec • refractory hypokalaemia or hypomagnesaemia • concomitant therapy with other drugs that prolong QT interval • complete AV block without implanted pacemaker • risk of complete AV block

[a] 3TC may be substituted with FTC or vice versa.

3TC = lamivudine, ABC = abacavir, ART = antiretroviral therapy, ATV = atazanavir, ATV/r = atazanavir/ritonavir, AV = atrioventricular, DRV/r = darunavir/ritonavir, ECG = electrocardiogram, EFV = efavirenz, FPV/r = fosamprenavir/ritonavir, FTC = emtricitabine, HSR = hypersensitivity reaction, INSTI = integrase strand transfer inhibitor, LPV/r = lopinavir/ritonavir, msec = millisecond, MVC = maraviroc, NNRTI = non-nucleoside reverse transcriptase inhibitor, NVP = nevirapine, PI = protease inhibitor, RAL = raltegravir, RPV = rilpivirine, RTV = ritonavir, SQV/r = saquinavir/ritonavir, TDF = tenofovir disoproxil fumarate, ZDV = zidovudine.

Reproduced from Panel on Antiretroviral Guidelines for Adults and Adolescents, *Guidelines for the use of antiretroviral agents in HIV-1-infected adults and adolescents*, Department of Health and Human Services, 2013 version, available at http://aidsinfo.nih.gov/ContentFiles/AdultandAdolescentGL.pdf

took a long time to negotiate, given the reluctance of Western pharmaceutical manufacturers to forgo perceived patent rights (Marques et al. 2005; Holmes et al. 2010). There are still daunting fiscal, regulatory, and operational challenges in obtaining the newest antiretroviral drugs for the global market (Waning et al. 2010).

Current recommended regimens

As of 2012, recommended components of initial antiretroviral regimens include (Thompson et al. 2010):

♦ Tenofovir (TDF)/emtricitabine (FTC), two NRTIs that are available as fixed-dose combination alone and also available with efavirenz, an NNRTI that is suitable for cART. Advantages of TDF/FTC are once-daily dosing and a high genetic barrier to resistance (TDF, not FTC). Side effects are not prominent, but include renal dysfunction and decreased bone mineral density associated with TDF.

  • An alternative is the combination of abacavir/lamivudine that is also once daily in a fixed-dose combination of two NRTI drugs. However, this combination has weaker antiviral efficacy in treatment-naive patients with baseline HIV-1 RNA greater than 100 000 copies/mL than TDF/FTC. Abacavir has cardiovascular side effects and screening for HLA-B*5701 is advisable to reduce risk of abacavir hypersensitivity.

♦ To complete the cART regimen, either TDF/FTC or abacavir/lamivudine should be complemented with the NNRTI, efavirenz. HIV can mutate easily to evade NNRTI drugs so efavirenz resistance occurs very rapidly outside the context of cART. Alternatives to efavirenz are indicated for patients with major psychiatric illness, in their first trimester of pregnancy, or for women with an intention to become pregnant.

♦ Atazanavir boosted with ritonavir (both protease inhibitors) is a once-daily alternative as the backbone of a cART regimen. It leaves open options for future regimens as it can be used with NRTIs, preserving the use of NNRTIs for a later date when they might be needed. There is less lipidogenic potential than when lopinavir boosted with ritonavir is used. Use can be complicated by hyperbilirubinaemia, need for acid-reducing agents, and risk of nephrolithiasis.

♦ Darunavir boosted with ritonavir (both protease inhibitors) is another once-daily alternative as the backbone of a cART regimen in treatment-naive patients. It is superior to lopinavir boosted with ritonavir.

♦ Raltegravir is an integrase inhibitor given twice daily. It has low potential to interact with other drugs, which is an advantage in its use. HIV can mutate quickly to evade this drug.

♦ Lopinavir boosted with ritonavir is a co-formulated pair of protease inhibitors that is heat stable and can be given once

Table 8.13.3 Antiretroviral drugs used in 2013 in the treatment of HIV infection, with licensure date at the Food and Drug Administration

Multi-class combination products		
Brand name™	**Generic name**	**Approval date**
Atripla	Efavirenz, emtricitabine and tenofovir disoproxil fumarate	2006
Complera	Emtricitabine, rilpivirine, and tenofovir disoproxil fumarate	2011
Nucleoside reverse transcriptase inhibitors (NRTIs)		
Combivir	Lamivudine and zidovudine	1997
Emtriva	Emtricitabine, FTC	2003
Epivir	Lamivudine, 3TC	1995
Epzicom	Abacavir and lamivudine	2004
Retrovir	Zidovudine, azidothymidine, AZT, ZDV	1987
Trizivir	Abacavir, zidovudine, and lamivudine	2000
Truvada	Tenofovir disoproxil fumarate and emtricitabine	2004
Videx EC	Enteric coated didanosine, ddI EC	2000
Videx	Didanosine, dideoxyinosine, ddI	1991
Viread	Tenofovir disoproxil fumarate, TDF	2001
Zerit	Stavudine, d4T	1994
Ziagen	Abacavir sulphate, ABC	1998
Non-nucleoside reverse transcriptase inhibitors (NNRTIs)		
Edurant	Rilpivirine	2011
Intelence	Etravirine	2008
Rescriptor	Delavirdine, DLV	1997
Sustiva	Efavirenz, EFV	1998
Viramune (immediate release)	Nevirapine, NVP	1996
Viramune XR (extended release)	Nevirapine, NVP	2011
Protease inhibitors (PIs)		
Agenerase	Amprenavir, APV	1999
Aptivus	Tipranavir, TPV	2005
Crixivan	Indinavir, IDV	1996
Invirase	Saquinavir mesylate, SQV	1995
Kaletra	Lopinavir and ritonavir, LPV/RTV	2000
Lexiva	Fosamprenavir calcium, FOS-APV	2003
Norvir	Ritonavir, RTV	1996
Prezista	Darunavir	2006
Reyataz	Atazanavir sulphate, ATV	2003
Viracept	Nelfinavir mesylate, NFV	1997
Fusion inhibitor		
Fuzeon	Enfuvirtide, T-20	2003
Entry inhibitor—CCR5 co-receptor antagonist		
Selzentry	Maraviroc	2007
HIV integrase strand transfer inhibitor		
Isentress	Raltegravir	2007

Adapted from U.S. Food and Drug Administration, *Antiretroviral Drugs Used in the Treatment of HIV Infection: Drugs Used in the Treatment of HIV Infection*, available from http://www.fda.gov/ForConsumers/byAudience/ForPatientAdvocates/HIVandAIDSActivities/ucm118915.htm.

daily. Side effects include hyperlipidaemia and gastrointestinal symptoms.

- Fosamprenavir boosted with ritonavir represent two protease inhibitors with a profile similar to lopinavir/ritonavir, useful when other preferred drugs are not tolerated.

- Maraviroc is a CCR5 antagonist that targets the host protein CCR5 viral co-receptor. Since one needs to ensure that CXCR4 virus is not present, one needs to perform a costly viral tropism assay before use. With limited clinical experience in treatment-naive patients, there are theoretical reasons to avoid its use in other than multiple drug failure patients who do not have CXCR4 receptor HIV strains circulating (Parra et al. 2011).

- Enfuvirtide is an HIV fusion inhibitor, used in combination therapy for 'salvage' therapy in patients with multidrug-resistant HIV. The peptide is biomimetic, that is, designed to mimic components of the HIV-1 fusion machinery, and the drug displaces normal fusion components to prevent successful virus–cell fusion. Enfuvirtide therapy is extremely costly and its inconvenient dosing (subcutaneously twice daily) regimen further limits its global relevance.

Challenges in patient care

Patient management issues are complex for HIV disease (Tables 8.13.1 and 8.13.2). Rather than the death sentence for so many in the pre-treatment era, HIV disease is now a chronic, manageable disease. It requires HIV testing, linkage to care, cART availability, national guidelines permitting cART administration, and adherence to lifelong therapeutic regimens. In the United States, only a quarter of people infected with HIV are on suppressive cART, showing how inadequate current systems are to meet the full need (Burns et al. 2010; CDC 2011; Gardner et al. 2011). In low- and middle-income countries, it is likely that fewer than 10 per cent of people infected with HIV are on cART with successful viral suppression. Special challenges exist with co-morbidities that may inhibit proper healthcare access and/or adherence to cART regimens. These include mental health problems such as depression, and substance use including opiates, stimulants, and alcohol (Altice et al. 2010; Gonzalez et al. 2011; Nel and Kagee 2011). In addition, stigmatized people who do not feel comfortable 'coming out' into the mainstream of clinical care may not reach care, or be retained in care; this is thought to be an important driver of the epidemic in black MSM in the United States, for example (Millett et al. 2006; Mimiaga et al. 2009; El-Sadr et al. 2010; Vermund et al. 2010; Millett et al. 2011; Lauby et al. 2012). Adolescents present special challenges in care and adherence rates have been suboptimal in this population (Murphy et al. 2000; Vermund et al. 2001; Murphy et al. 2002; Ding et al. 2009; Reisner et al. 2009). Children in care depend on the capabilities of their parents or guardians; many children have been orphaned and some do not know that they are HIV infected, making it difficult for them to participate in their ongoing care (Zhao et al. 2007; Vaz et al. 2011).

ART itself has an array of complications that require recognition and management (Thompson et al. 2010). PIs are associated with lipid abnormalities and cardiovascular risk. Efavirez is contraindicated in pregnancy. NRTIs can have serious, albeit rare, lactic acidosis. Stavudine can cause severe peripheral neuropathies. Beyond the scope of this chapter, these side effects require

preventive and therapeutic management from a clinician experienced in HIV drug regimens and their alternatives.

The tremendous impact on morbidity and mortality of cART in high-income countries has been well documented (Lundgren and Mocroft 2006; Walensky et al. 2006; Lauby et al. 2012). Similar benefits are seen in low- and middle-income countries, but they depend on the programmatic efficiencies, resources available from PEPFAR, the Global Fund to Fight AIDS, Tuberculosis and Malaria, local Ministries of Health, and the ability of programmes to find, recruit, and retain HIV-infected people in cART-based care (Table 8.13.4) (Rosen et al. 2005; Schwartlander et al. 2006). Scaling up of programmes has been both challenging and inspiring; new models for the management of chronic diseases in resource-limited settings are now extant, offering promise for a wide variety of diseases requiring ongoing care for their management (Stringer et al. 2006; Bolton-Moore et al. 2007; Abimiku and Institute of Human Virology 2009; Morris et al. 2009; Vergara et al. 2009; Ciampa et al. 2011; Moon et al. 2011).

Case study in prevention, care, and treatment: YRG CARE in India

While prevention, care, and treatment challenges are daunting in developing countries, there are examples of highly successful programmes that have engaged thousands of infected people and sometimes hundreds of thousands of people in prevention. One such programme is the Y.R. Gaitonde Center for AIDS Research and Education (YRG CARE) in Chennai, Tamil Nadu, India.

An Indian-owned and operated non-profit medical and research institution, the internationally recognized YRG CARE was founded in 1993 by Dr Suniti Solomon whose team identified the first case of HIV in India (Simoes et al. 1987). YRG CARE offers a wide array of HIV prevention, care, and treatment services.

YRG CARE's vision is that people with HIV and AIDS and their families live with dignity, and that there are no new infections. YRG CARE's mission is to respond to prevention, care, and research needs of the nation of India. YRG CARE offers services without judgement or discrimination, and is known for its client-centred approach, its comprehensive service portfolio, its commitment to community, and its respect for the dignity and privacy of individuals.

YRG CARE reaches out to and is committed to improving the lives of thousands of men, women, and children infected or affected by HIV in India through a wide array of prevention, education, care, and treatment services. It is also committed to conducting clinical, laboratory, and social research, building a core of young researchers, and offering training to other service providers. The centre is now focused on user-friendly clinics for MSM and PWID, adopting harm reduction approaches in community engagement (Solomon et al. 2008, 2010).

YRG CARE builds awareness about HIV infection and promotes safe behaviours in schools, colleges, STD clinics, workplaces, communities, and through helplines. As poverty, intimate partner violence, and poor perception of HIV risks make prevention especially difficult for women in India, YRG CARE promotes primary prevention amongst women through education, innovative livelihoods and sensitizing men to become change agents in the community (YRG CARE).

YRG CARE provides access to an affordable continuum of care that improves the quality of life of people living with HIV/AIDS.

Table 8.13.4 Some essential elements needed to nurture successful and complete transition of HIV care and treatment programmes to national governments and local organizations, with long-term sustainability

Essential elements	Goals
Health workforce development	Increase the numbers of healthcare providers, increasing coverage for rural care; task shifting to nurses, clinical officers, laboratory and pharmacy technicians, care partners, and community health workers
Integration of services	Enable HIV/AIDS care and treatment to be handled by sustainable primary care programmes, with key linkages to sexually transmitted infection and tuberculosis control, and family planning, for example
Physical infrastructures	Empower communities to access basic electricity, water, medical waste disposal, and clinic space for physical examinations, patient education/waiting, laboratory, and basic surgery/anaesthesia
Pharmacy logistics systems	Ensure that inventory management, shipping, and storage systems avoid stock-outs of supplies (e.g. test kits, blood draw equipment) and antiretroviral, antibiotic, and other drugs
Laboratory development	Decentralize laboratory work, as much as possible and affordable, with point-of-care diagnostic tests
Quality of care and iterative evaluation	Build sustainable quality improvement research and systems improvement efforts into HIV care programmes
Hub-and-spoke models of care	Bring primary and HIV/AIDS care closer to people who are remote from major clinical services
Data management systems	Build sustainable, affordable electronic medical record systems to harmonize systems created for the emergency HIV response
Community engagement to support programmes	Implement innovative models of outreach, retention, and adherence support in the community, using the inherent strengths of patient-to-patient and family-to-patient support as a form of task shifting
Cultural changes in the health sector	Train staff and reform procedures to protect patient confidentiality and privacy, provide more respectful, client-friendly services, and ensure that all communications are in languages spoken by patients
Management and administration	Train and capacitate health systems to use modern business practices for financial and logistical management
Long-term funding	Reset national and international priorities to emphasize health and development, rather than disparate economic development and unproductive government investments such as war and armaments

Adapted with permission from Lippincott Williams and Wilkins/Wolters Kluwer Health: Vermund SH et al., Transitioning HIV care and treatment programs in southern Africa to full local management, *AIDS*, Volume 26, Issue 10, pp. 1303–1310, Copyright © 2012 Lippincott Williams & Wilkins, Inc.

Services include HIV voluntary counselling and testing (VCT); primary healthcare; dental care; eye care; highly active antiretroviral therapy (HAART) (Solomon et al. 2013); home care; psychosocial counselling, adherence support, and nutritional counselling for clients, couples, and families; PMTCT and other ob-gyn surgical services; radiology referral services; subsidized pharmacy; matrimonial (match making) services; alternative insemination for discordant couples; and health education and treatment literacy for clients and their personal care givers. As of early 2013, over 18,000 people living with HIV have registered at its clinics for services.

YRG CARE offers state-of-the-art laboratory services, including STI investigations, OI diagnosis, and biochemical evaluations for patient services as well as for clinical trials. The laboratory is accredited by India's National Accreditation Board for Testing and Calibration Laboratories (NABL), Government of India, that adheres to international ISO/IEC standards (International Organization for Standardization and the International Electrotechnical Commission). Given YRG CARE's participation in international clinical trials, its labs are also certified by the Division of AIDS of the National Institute of Allergy and Infectious Diseases of the US National Institutes of Health. The laboratory is designated as the International Regional HIV-1 Genotyping Laboratory by the Division of AIDS (since 2006) and has been recognized as an International Regional Tuberculosis Diagnostic Laboratory for Division of AIDS clinical trials protocols. The laboratory is affiliated with the nearby University of Madras and has multiple candidates who are pursuing PhD degrees in Medical Microbiology. YRG CARE lab experts have contributed to several national and WHO (SEARO) diagnostic guidelines.

YRG CARE offers training for clinicians, obstetricians and gynaecologists, laboratory scientists and technologists, healthcare workers, social workers, and counsellors in their respective fields relating to HIV prevention and management. This includes short-term trainees from throughout India and from other Asian nations.

With a modest beginning in research in the late 1990s, YRG CARE has since emerged as a pioneer in research on HIV and related co-infections, meeting the highest standards of ethics and regulatory compliance, in partnership with global leaders (Kumarasamy et al. 2003, 2005; Solomon et al. 2009). Running across its clinic, community, and laboratory clusters, these research studies answer questions that are most important and relevant to India in the fields of epidemiology, laboratory, prevention, natural history, and treatment outcomes. The Chennai International Clinical Trials unit of YRG CARE is one of the clinical research sites for the Division of AIDS clinical trials for both therapy and prevention. YRG CARE's proactive Community Advisory Board promotes community participation in study design, implementation, literacy efforts and follow-up care.

The early days of the epidemic in India witnessed tragic consequences of the disease unchecked by effective therapy or prevention. It was a period of poor understanding of the risks of caring for someone living with HIV—both by healthcare workers and society alike. Faced with rejection, people living with HIV lived without hope and died alone. It was a period of very low prioritization of aspects of the global response that are a mainstay of intervention today—test, treat, support, and prevent. YRG CARE continues to lead the response to HIV in India in meaningful ways, introducing cutting-edge technologies in prevention, diagnosis, and care and championing compassionate advocacy to mitigate the impact of discrimination, stigma, and prejudice that is deep rooted in pockets of society. YRG CARE highlights are representative of what both non-governmental and governmental institutions have spearheaded globally in the HIV era:

◆ First voluntary counselling and testing (VCT) service in Southern India.

◆ First HIV education sessions in schools and colleges, a model now adapted and implemented by UNICEF and YRG CARE throughout Tamil Nadu state.

◆ First medical centre for people living with HIV/AIDS.

◆ Largest centre in terms of comprehensive HIV care and social support services for patients in the non-governmental sector.

◆ Extensive experience in antiretroviral therapy.

◆ A range of research projects including large population-based longitudinal trials (over 3500 participants) and Phase III clinical trials.

◆ State-of-the-art laboratory dedicated to HIV diagnosis, monitoring of HIV disease, and surveillance for antiretroviral drug resistance.

◆ Offers complete biological markers for community-based HIV field surveys.

◆ Recognized by the University of Madras as a centre for the pursuit of doctoral studies in microbiology.

YRG CARE is an organization that emerged with a new paradigm of care for Indians with a stigmatized infectious disease. Organizations throughout the world have embraced similar principles and strategies to reach out to disenfranchised groups and people who are infected or at-risk for HIV.

Elements of combination prevention

Evidence for efficacy of elements of combination prevention can come from observational data (as with male condoms or reduction in partner numbers) or from randomized clinical trials (RCTs; as with male circumcision or early treatment as prevention). Which elements might be considered essential for successful combination prevention are a matter of debate, but can be elucidated with decision-analysis and HIV transmission models (Tables 8.13.1 and 8.13.2). A consensus is emerging that combination prevention should be anchored on the use of cART given that infected people who receive and are adherent to their cART regimens can suppress HIV replication and reduce their infectiousness (Smith et al. 2012). At the time of this writing, Ministries of Health of LMIC typically limit their start of cART at the WHO recommended threshold of CD4+ cell counts less than 350/microlitre or WHO clinical status 3 or 4 (Stanecki et al. 2010). Some of the most resource-limited nations continue to authorize the start of cART at a lower threshold like less than 250 cells/microlitre, despite overwhelming evidence that this is too late for optimal clinical response (Moon et al. 2011). A large proportion of transmissions occur before patients reach the usual thresholds for ART initiation, however, a rationale for treating at earlier CD4+ cell counts (or even universal ART for all HIV-infected people).

The HIV Prevention Trials Network 052 protocol (HPTN 052) was an RCT that assessed early initiation of cART at CD4+ cell counts of up to 550/microlitre, demonstrating both reduced transmission of HIV to sexual partners as well as clinical benefits to their infected partners on cART (Cohen et al. 2011). Hence it is disappointing that only 19–28 per cent (range of estimates) of Americans infected with HIV were on cART with successful suppression of HIV viral load (Burns et al. 2010; CDC 2011; Cohen et al. 2011; Gardner et al. 2011). Even if these are overly pessimistic estimates due to some 'lost-to-follow-up' patients possibly being in therapy elsewhere, the true rates of ART coverage and viral suppression are disappointing, in both high- and low-income nations (Geng et al. 2012; Shepherd et al. 2013).

In selected venues, ecological evidence of prevention benefits from cART is emerging (Das et al. 2010; Montaner et al. 2010). Ecological analyses in San Francisco, Vancouver, China, Taiwan, and KwaZulu-Natal have suggested that higher cART coverage may correlate with lower seroincidence rates (Fang et al. 2004; Das et al. 2010; Montaner et al. 2010; Tanser et al. 2012; Jia et al. 2013). However, it is unknown whether these correlations represent success of TasP or whether other factors are contributing (Vermund 2013).

Vancouver is a case in point. Investigators and public health officials have addressed prevention of HIV with needle/syringe exchange and opiate substitution therapy among Vancouver PWID at the same time that cART was being made available (Kerr et al. 2010). Hence, it is hard to disaggregate the prevention impact of needle/syringe exchange and expanded heroin addiction therapy from cART expansion or other factors. Western Europe is also a region of interest (Vermund and Leigh-Brown 2012). It is easy to speculate that easy access to HIV testing and widespread cART use within national health systems may have resulted in lowering HIV incidence rates in Western Europe, but it is hard to know whether other sociocultural factors or prevention efforts also made impacts. However, in the United Kingdom where access to testing and treatment is facilitated by the National Health System (NHS) with free services available to all, no reduction in the incidence of new infections in MSM has been noted to date, so interpreting European experiences is not always clear-cut.

The option of moving to *immediate* offering of ART—irrespective of CD4+ cell count is being supported by public health policy in San Francisco, Vancouver, New York City, and elsewhere. If HIV testing were expanded markedly and all people were treated shortly after diagnosis and successful virally suppressed, then fewer infectious people would be transmitting to others and the epidemic might decline. Whether this is possible is the topic of intense current investigation (Burns et al. 2010; Beyrer et al. 2011; Ciampa et al. 2012; Sahasrabuddhe et al. 2012; Vermund and Hayes 2013; Vermund et al. 2013a, 2013b).

Suboptimal cART coverage and viral suppression

In the United States, current systems fail to meet the full need of HIV-infected patients, many of whom have co-morbidities that inhibit full viral suppression (Burns et al. 2010; CDC 2011; Gardner et al. 2011). These may include substance use (e.g. drugs and/or alcohol), mental health problems, financial and healthcare insurance challenges, transportation issues, and stigma/

disclosure challenges (Altice et al. 2010; Gonzalez et al. 2011; Nel and Kagee 2011). In LMICs, it is likely that fewer than 10 per cent of all infected people are successfully virally suppressed.

Stigmatized people who do not 'come out' may not reach medical care or be retained in care, as is the case with black MSM in the United States (Millett et al. 2006; Mimiaga et al. 2009; El-Sadr et al. 2010; Vermund et al. 2010; Millett et al. 2011; Lauby et al. 2012). Adolescents with HIV infection have demonstrated abysmal adherence rates in some studies, suggesting the need for services that include outreach and engagement (Murphy et al. 2000; Vermund et al. 2001; Murphy et al. 2002; Ding et al. 2009; Reisner et al. 2009). Children with HIV are dependent on their parents or guardians; many children have not had their HIV status disclosed to them and may not be participating actively in their ongoing care (Zhao et al. 2007; Vaz et al. 2011).

The gulf between current guidelines for high-income countries where all HIV-infected people are typically offered cART versus WHO and LMIC Ministries of Health that offer a smaller proportion of HIV-infected people cART (typically people under 350 CD4+ cells/microlitre) is worth highlighting. By definition, the latter policies have a larger pool of infected people who remain virally unsuppressed. If resources were obtained to treat all HIV-infected individuals (i.e. universal, immediate cART), the proportion of infectious people would decline. If a large enough pool of infectious people were made non-infectious, mathematical models suggest a decline in new infections (Baggaley and Fraser 2010; Wagner and Blower 2012; Cremin et al. 2013). It is not certain that a test-and-treat prevention strategy is feasible, acceptable, sustainable, and affordable (Shelton 2011; Vermund et al. 2013a). The most resource-limited LMICs depend on the programmatic resources available from PEPFAR and the Global Fund to Fight AIDS, Tuberculosis and Malaria; local Ministries of Health rarely have the resources to find, link, and retain HIV-infected people in cART-based care, with optimized adherence (Rosen et al. 2005; Schwartlander et al. 2006; Vermund et al. 2012). The long-term management of chronic diseases in LMICs is challenging; HIV investments may serve as a backbone for also addressing a wide variety of diseases requiring chronic management (Stringer et al. 2006; Bolton-Moore et al. 2007; Abimiku and Institute of Human Virology 2009; Morris et al. 2009; Vergara et al. 2009; Ciampa et al. 2011; Moon et al. 2011).

We also do not know whether a test-and-treat approach will have the postulated benefits in a real-world circumstance (Ciampa et al. 2012; Vermund and Hayes 2013; Vermund et al. 2013a, 2013b). Whether we can further enhance its benefits with other prevention modalities without overwhelming the public health and clinical systems is also unknown (Shelton 2011). While behaviour change is a component of all approaches, some combined interventions make sense in the context of certain epidemic circumstances, as with male circumcision in generalized epidemics and needle exchange where PWID drives transmissions.

Adapting for local epidemics

HIV is a disease based on patterns of human behaviour; hence, it is affected and modulated by stigma, discrimination, prejudice, fear, stress, depression, denial, and ignorance. Many have compared AIDS to the leprosy of the Bible when infected people were shunned and even banished. Since HIV is transmitted similarly to patterns for other sexual and blood-borne agents, it is subjected to the same societal distress surrounding other STIs. HIV transmission is more likely in the face of multiple sexual partners (i.e. high mixing rates) and failure to use condoms, so people acquiring infection are typically judged by others (Vermund et al. 2009). However, we must put stigma into its modern perspective. While a major problem in most areas, especially perhaps in concentrated epidemics in marginalized risk-groups, there are also signs of 'normalization' of HIV as a public health problem in both higher-income and LMICs, including in southern Africa. We speculate that wider access to cART has contributed to an improving social environment for many people living with HIV.

Much progress has been made in the avoidance of iatrogenic and occupational parenteral transmission by unclean syringes and needles through single use technologies, serological screening of blood or blood products, and policies to reduce inadvertent needle sticks in an occupational healthcare setting. Progress, too, has been made in offering universal screening of pregnant women and the offering, uptake, and adherence to one of a variety of antiretroviral therapy options, pre-partum, intra-partum, or post-partum, to avoid mother-to-child transmission that can take place *in utero*, during delivery, or from breastfeeding, respectively (Fowler et al. 2010; Whitmore et al. 2010). Yet too often, successful programmes are not integrated and potential synergies for combination prevention are lost. If testing/treatment successes in PMTCT, say, could be expanded into the analogous treatment as prevention cascade for adults, we might well combine components of prevention into an integrated whole, with the kind of impact on incidence not often seen in the global pandemic.

Hepatitis B virus (HBV) is spread in ways reminiscent of HIV, though HBV is typically more communicable. Our tools for HBV control include active and passive immunization, tools that are not yet available for HIV control. In addition, HIV infection is not yet curable, such that people whose viral loads are not suppressed can transmit the infection for many years. Other STIs can also be spread via blood-borne routes (e.g. syphilis, hepatitis C virus (HCV), and human T-lymphotropic virus type 1 (HTLV-1)), but sexual routes are the dominant mode of transmission for most STIs, as with HIV. Co-infections of HIV are common for both blood-borne and sexually transmitted infections. The CD4+ T-lymphocyte tropism of HIV makes it unique among the STIs and its penchant for deep lymphoid tissue invasion and quiescence are the roots of its incurability.

Stigma, discrimination, poverty, and human rights

HIV spread is steeped in gender inequality, poverty, discrimination based on sexual preference and identity, and perverse public policies that exacerbate the epidemic, rather than control it. Though over three decades have passed since the detection of AIDS, infection with HIV is still perceived as a disease of 'others'—of those living on the margins of society, whose lifestyles are considered perverse or sinful (Bos et al. 2008; Altman et al. 2012). Despite excellent advances in the area of both prevention technologies and treatment of HIV/AIDS with innovative programming and inclusive policies, such judgemental and stigmatizing values result in discrimination and marginalization of vulnerable people, especially those living with HIV and their families in communities, workplaces, and healthcare settings.

Self-stigmatization amongst people living with HIV/AIDS is also high, which in turn results in self-isolation and diminishing social relationships. This stigmatization affects prevention efforts and uptake of services. Individuals at risk will not access voluntary counselling and testing, and if tested positive will not follow up in care nor disclose to family. They often marry due to societal and cultural pressure and transmit HIV infection to their partners. This dynamic is especially apparent in communities with strong cultural pressures to have children, for example, India, where in many communities being barren is associated with greater stigma than is having HIV.

Culturally sensitive community-wide education is critical to reducing the effects of social stigma. Approaches that raise awareness about sexual identities and that raise self-esteem are also necessary to address the profound feelings of shame that marginalized communities experience.

A perspective on the role of stigma in fuelling the epidemic must recognize the fear that an HIV diagnosis still engenders among many. Yet the fact that increased HIV testing and adherence to cART-based care represents a sign of 'normalization' of HIV as a public health challenge in many countries, including some in southern Africa, where wider access to cART has probably contributed to HIV being seen more like other chronic diseases (Marum et al. 2012).

Stigma even extends to public policy and law. Perverse practices include the banning of or failing to support needle exchange for PWID in the United States before the Obama Administration (Lurie and Drucker 1997; Drucker 2012) or failing to provide ART in South Africa during the Mbeke Administration (Gow 2009). Russia's failure to legalize and promulgate clean needle distribution and opiate substitution therapy, the continued demonization of MSM in many African countries, and the insistence on ineffective 'abstinence only' educational investments in the United States are additional examples of policy gone awry (Underhill et al. 2007; Mathers et al. 2010; Burki 2012; Chin et al. 2012). In the face of the politicization of HIV/AIDS, policymakers failing to use existing tools to prevent HIV transmission are responsible for much preventable infection (Mahy et al. 2009). Failure to protect the blood supply early in the epidemic led to the infection of tens of thousands of blood and blood product recipients worldwide, especially people with haemophilia. The taboo of politicians, religious leaders, teachers, or even healthcare providers discussing sexual risk reduction frankly and clearly keeps issues of HIV prevention from being fully integrated into political, religious, and social discussions. This is unfortunate since some themes—delaying adolescent coital debut and reducing numbers of sexual partners, for example—are widely supported goals in nearly all circles and political philosophies.

While condoms are opposed by some due to a conviction that they may lead to higher risk sexual activities and/or that they may violate certain religious proscriptions against contraception, there is no strong evidence for the former view and support for the latter may be waning. For example, a major Catholic religious leader who previously opposed condom use stated in a 2010 book that 'there may be a basis in the case of some individuals, as perhaps when a male prostitute uses a condom, where this can be a first step in the direction of a moralization, a first assumption of responsibility' (Pope Benedict XVI and Seewald 2010). The religious leader later indicated that he also was referring to female prostitutes when he suggested that condom use may actually be a morally superior choice to prevent transmission to others. Such

changes in attitude can be influential in empowering at-risk people to protect themselves without going counter to religious views to which they may subscribe.

Failures in public policy have consequences. Modellers have quantified public policy failures, particularly the failure to provide clean needles and syringes for PWID in the United States from 1987 to 1995, estimating that an excess of between 4394 and 9666 infections, representing a third of incident PWID cases, was the result (Lurie and Drucker 1997). The attendant excess costs to the United States were US$244–538 million. It will be a major stride in the HIV field if public health advocacy for evidence-based prevention could be the basis for HIV control policy and investment (Mathers et al. 2010).

Behaviour change

Even in the face of biomedical interventions such as TasP or voluntary medical male circumcision, behaviour change is an essential component of prevention interventions; for example, people must agree to and adhere to the given intervention. All by itself, however, behaviour change to reduce HIV incidence has not proven robust (Wetmore et al. 2010). In studies designed to enhance adherence to ART, for example, the impact of behavioural interventions has often been very contextual or transient (Barnighausen et al. 2011). The HIVNET 015 Project EXPLORE protocol in MSM in the United States sought to lower HIV incidence with an intensive ten-visit educational programme that included reinforcement sessions (Koblin et al. 2004). Investigators were disappointed with the 18.2 per cent reduction (95 per cent CI −4.7 to 36.0 per cent) in HIV incidence in the intervention group compared to a control group receiving a short intervention (Koblin et al. 2004). However, given that the benefits were even lower in substance users and people with mental health problems, this underscored the importance of attending to these co-morbidities in order to reduce HIV transmission (Colfax et al. 2004; Salomon et al. 2009).

For TasP, willingness to test for HIV, be linked to care, and adherence to cART to reduce infectiousness all require behavioural support. Pre-exposure prophylaxis (PrEP) using cART in seronegative people to prevent infection, and increased testing and linkage to cART requires high levels of adherence to be successful. 'Serosorting' is when HIV seropositive people have sex only with other infected people, and HIV-seronegatives seek other uninfected people for sex; this obviously requires a great deal of self-efficacy and motivation. Substance abuse treatment, including needle exchange, alcohol treatment, and opiate substitution therapy, as needed, depend on motivated and able clients. Contingency cash transfers are rewards for lowering risk behaviours, and depend on behaviour change.

Classic 'ABC' approaches of *A*bstinence/*B*e faithful/*C*ondom advocacy are fully dependent upon behavioural change (Corsi and Booth 2008; Rotheram-Borus et al. 2009; Burns et al. 2010). The US CDC has published its evidence-based interventions for risk reduction in the United States; they are heavily behaviourally-based (Lyles et al. 2006; Margaret Dolcini et al. 2010). Abstinence-only education has been unsuccessful in reducing risk and was paradoxically associated with higher pregnancy rates than more comprehensive educational approaches that included STI prevention advocacy based on abstinence, partner reduction, and condom use (Underhill et al. 2007; Chin et al. 2012). It is the consensus in the HIV scientific community that 'ABC' principles are vital guides for public health intervention, but are better bundled with biomedical prevention approaches; alone behavioural change approaches are not likely to stop the global pandemic (Holmes 2004; Rotheram-Borus et al. 2009; Vermund et al. 2009, 2010, 2013b; Kurth et al. 2011; Vermund and Hayes 2013).

Linked to behaviour change, but worthy of separate consideration are the so-called structural interventions. This involves changing laws, policies, or other societal norms to reduce risk behaviour. Raising cigarette taxes to reduce tobacco use among youth or banning cigarette smoking in indoor spaces where the public has access are examples of structural interventions. If schools were improved, school fees eliminated as obstacles to full attendance, and after-school opportunities for youth were promulgated, this might be considered a structural change to seek to reduce substance abuse in higher income nations and the exchange of sexual services for money to attend school as happens in many LMICs. A law requiring all commercial transient lodgings (hotels, etc.) to provide in-room condoms would be another example of a structural intervention. Large scale programmes to offer universal testing in saturation volumes, incentives to link people with HIV to care, near-universal use of cART for all HIV-infected people, and community partnerships to maximize clinic attendance and cART adherence are the backbone of TasP programmes that, while still depending on behavioural adherence, would be enhanced considerably if a structural context could be promulgated by policymakers of routine, widespread, opt-out testing.

Packages of tools for combination prevention

'Magic bullets' have not worked to control the epidemic on their own, with the possible exceptions of needle exchange for PWID and blood screening for blood banks. Even if we had a proven, effective vaccine for HIV, vaccination would still require multiple voluntary visits to optimize immunization along with large-scale population mobilization and programme expansion for children, adolescents, and/or adults, depending on vaccine characteristics (e.g. durability of protection). Combination prevention packages must vary to target those at-risk people who are at highest risk in a given epidemiological context. If the local epidemic is being driven by PWID, then needle exchange and addiction treatment will be the best strategies, along with primary prevention of drug abuse. If sex work is a principal driver of a local epidemic, community and political mobilization of sex workers and their employers (e.g. brothel owners, pimps, madams) will be needed to ensure effective STI screening and treatment, to promote universal condom use, and perhaps to provide PrEP. Other efforts to offer sex workers a way out of the profession through protection and job retraining and job placement, as well as to control sexual trafficking, can help protect the women who are aided, and may or may not reduce prostitution or HIV incidence overall.

Some interventions have far stronger levels of evidence of efficacy to reduce HIV transmission (infectiousness) or acquisition (susceptibility) than others. Among these are voluntary medical male circumcision (VMMC) with compelling observational data supported by three definitive and remarkably consistent RCTs (Auvert et al. 2005; Bailey et al. 2007; Gray et al. 2007). ART for prevention was begun as a concept with the definitive demonstration of prevention of maternal-to-child transmission (PMTCT) with ART dating from 1994 (Connor et al. 1994). Observational data from 2000 to 2001 and an incidental finding in a clinical trial

in 2010 suggested that cART would reduce sexual transmission (Quinn et al. 2000; Fideli et al. 2001; Donnell et al. 2010). Finally, the HPTN 052 RCT, over a decade in the making, demonstrated early use of cART as a major tool to reduce infectiousness and sexual transmission to partners, while clinically benefiting the infected people as well (Cohen et al. 2011).

Other strategies are logical as adjunctive tools for HIV prevention, but are less consistently beneficial in RCTs. STI control based on syndromic management worked very well in one Tanzanian epidemic context to reduce HIV transmission, but has failed in other epidemic contexts and other treatment approaches (Korenromp et al. 2005). PrEP has had a mixed success: tenofovir-containing PrEP (cART among HIV-seronegative at-risk people) was successful in CAPRISA 004 (topical microbicide for women), iPrEx (MSM) and Partners PrEP and TDF-2 studies (heterosexual men and women), but not in the large VOICE trial (heterosexual women) or the FemPrEP studies (heterosexual women) (Abdool Karim et al. 2010; Grant et al. 2010; Celum and Baeten 2012). The Thai vaccine prime-boost strategy published in 2009 was partially effective; however, the vaccine companies did not seek licensure for marketing of either the prime or boost products, given their very modest effects (Rerks-Ngarm et al. 2009). Nonetheless, as better oral and vaginal PrEP/microbicide and vaccine products are developed, they may be added as future components to the therapeutic armamentarium. Given that PrEP is a tool for use in seronegative people and TasP a tool for use in seropositive people, work is needed to assess how these might be combined to maximize potential HIV impact at the community level.

When RCT data are not available, observational data are used to make judgements as to likely efficacy. Evidence of male condom efficacy is confirmed by effectiveness studies (Holmes 2004). Evidence for efficacy and effectiveness of female condoms is inconsistent, but they have been reported helpful in selected contexts (Gallo et al. 2012). Of certain utility, but not backed up by RCT evidence are needle exchange for drug users and opioid substitution therapy for PWID (Kerr et al. 2010). Also convincing are the use of contraception for HIV-infected women to reduce unintended pregnancies and HIV infection in infants (Rutenberg and Baek 2005; Stringer et al. 2007; Reynolds et al. 2008). A variety of behavioural and structural interventions that reduce HIV-related risk behaviours are of possible but uncertain utility, due to conflicting trial and study evidence (Gupta et al. 2008; Medley et al. 2009; Rotheram-Borus et al. 2009; Kennedy et al. 2010a, 2010b; Michielsen et al. 2010; Shepherd et al. 2010; Free et al. 2011; Johnson et al. 2011; Tan et al. 2012; Wariki et al. 2012).

Testing and linkage to care as a core strategy

The person who knows his or her own HIV serostatus is in a position to access HIV prevention or care services as they are provided in a given community; thus testing is a first gateway (Sanchez and Sullivan 2008). While people testing HIV seronegative may not change their risky behaviours, people testing HIV seropositive tend to reduce their sexual transmission risk behaviours significantly (Denison et al. 2008). People who do not know their own or their partners' serostatus are far less likely (range of 50–66 per cent) to use condoms. It is estimated that less than 20 per cent of adults in sub-Saharan Africa have been tested for HIV, yet the HPTN 043 NIMH Project ACCESS study demonstrated in a community RCT how community mobilization can increase testing rates up to tenfold (Sweat et al. 2011). The best HIV testing access includes provider-initiated, routine or opt-out testing, and voluntary home-based HIV counselling and testing (HBCT) (Marum et al. 2012). HBCT may be cost-effective for population-level scale-up in generalized epidemics, despite its higher programmatic costs.

Once a person is tested for HIV, those testing positive must be linked to cART-based care. In the HPTN 052 trial, excellence in cART care and adherence reduced viral replication and reduced HIV transmission to sexual partners by 96 per cent, termed a 'game-changer' by the director of UNAIDS (Cohen et al. 2011). HIV-infected people with 350–550 CD4+ cells/microlitre were assigned randomly to receive ART either immediately (early therapy) or after a decline in the CD4 count to 250–350 cells/microlitre or the onset of HIV-1-related symptoms (delayed therapy). Given the success of TasP in HPTN 052 when people with high CD4+ cell counts were the target, the option of immediate treatment for all HIV-diagnosed people, regardless of immunological status, is ideal, if resources are available. Still, a combination of interventions is inherently needed to make TasP a reality in public health terms: HIV testing has to be brought to scale, effective linkage to care must be a key priority for primary care programmes, and high coverage and adherence to cART must be nurtured. WHO's estimate of a 23 per cent yearly ART attrition rate in Africa illustrates the tremendous challenge faced by the public health community in this regard (Renaud-Thery et al. 2011). It is plausible that a universal testing and treatment approach (regardless of CD4+ cell count) could reduce stigma in communities where testing is common and infection is simply treated in everyone, as with other infectious diseases or chronic disease conditions.

Given this need for expanded HIV testing, accessing the service, and willingness to adhere to the prevention modality (e.g. VMMC, future HIV vaccine or microbicide, cART regimen, consistent and correct condom use), behavioural co-interventions are essential. Prevention for positives to reduce risky behaviours with counselling focused on building motivation and developing skills is promising. Interventions based on sound behavioural theory, such as the Health Belief model, can help address mental health and substance use issues, with a focus on adherence. Condom use will continue to be emphasized as an adjunctive tool for HIV/STI risk reduction (Holmes 2004; Stoneburner and Low-Beer 2004). The biomathematics of combining methods for prevention are compelling, but intimidating at the same time; substantial coverage will be needed to succeed in bringing the basic reproductive rate to less than 1 thereby offering the potential prospect of eventual elimination of HIV as a public health problem (Andrews et al. 2012; Eaton et al. 2012; Wagner and Blower 2012).

Future directions

A new construct for viewing the global HIV pandemic through the prism of MSM risk has been proposed by Beyrer et al. (2011). Based on a systematic review of published and unpublished literature from 2000 to 2009, the authors selected 133 HIV prevalence studies from 50 countries to apply an algorithmic approach for categorization. Four scenarios for LMICs were suggested: (1) settings where MSM are the predominant contributor to HIV transmission; (2) settings where HIV transmission among MSM occurs in the context of epidemics driven by PWID; (3) settings where HIV transmission among MSM occurs in the context of

well-established HIV transmission among heterosexuals; and (4) settings where both sexual and parenteral modes contribute significantly to HIV transmission. Perhaps this paradigm can serve as a model of how to guide prevention strategies by reminding policymakers and HIV control workers as to what populations are the largest drivers of local transmission dynamics.

Among the major achievements in confronting the HIV pandemic have been the development and deployment of cART that can turn a previously fatal disease into a chronic, manageable one. However, lower-income nations have huge health services challenges that must be addressed for PEPFAR achievements to be expanded and sustained (Table 8.13.4). Even in the United States and Western Europe, there is a sense of HIV fatigue such that economic downturns from 2008 onwards seem to invite cuts in HIV programmes to satisfy fiscal exigencies. However, we know from the experiences of the past that failure to prevent HIV, or to treat it early once infection has occurred, will simply cost society more in the long run, given the high direct costs of illness and indirect costs of disability or death (Walensky et al. 2006; Schwartlander et al. 2011). Prevention, including testing and early cART treatment, is a good societal and economic investment. Yet despite vast societal benefits (Walensky et al. 2006; Parham et al. 2010), HIV prevention and care are threatened in an era of fiscal constraint and global expenditure cuts in healthcare and prevention (Schneider and Garrett 2009; Holmes et al. 2012; Vermund et al. 2012).

Acknowledgements

We dedicate this chapter to our patients and friends who have died and who continue to struggle with HIV/AIDS.

Note

1. HIV/AIDS is a vast topic and within our space constraints, we have emphasized the public health aspects of this field. However, since treatment as prevention is a vital component of viral prevention, we also present a brief overview of HIV therapy.

References

Abdool Karim, Q., Abdool Karim, S.S., Frohlich, J.A., et al. (2010). Effectiveness and safety of tenofovir gel, an antiretroviral microbicide, for the prevention of HIV infection in women. *Science*, 329(5996), 1168–74.

Abimiku, A.G., Institute of Human Virology, University of Maryland School of Medicine PEPFAR Program (AIDS Care Treatment in Nigeria [ACTION]) (2009). Building laboratory infrastructure to support scale-up of HIV/AIDS treatment, care, and prevention: in-country experience. *American Journal of Clinical Pathology*, 131(6), 875–86.

Abu-Raddad, L.J., Hilmi, N., Mumtaz, G., et al. (2010). Epidemiology of HIV infection in the Middle East and North Africa. *AIDS*, 24(Suppl. 2), S5–23.

Allen, C.F., Edwards, M., Williamson, L.M., et al. (2006). Sexually transmitted infection service use and risk factors for HIV infection among female sex workers in Georgetown, Guyana. *Journal of Acquired Immune Deficiency Syndromes*, 43(1), 96–101.

Altaf, A., Saleem, N., Abbas, S., and Muzaffar, R. (2009). High prevalence of HIV infection among injection drug users (IDUs) in Hyderabad and Sukkur, Pakistan. *Journal of the Pakistan Medical Association*, 59(3), 136–40.

Altice, F.L., Kamarulzaman, A., Soriano, V.V., Schechter, M., and Friedland, G.H. (2010). Treatment of medical, psychiatric, and substance-use comorbidities in people infected with HIV who use drugs. *The Lancet*, 376(9738), 367–87.

Altman, D., Aggleton, P., Williams, M., et al. (2012). Men who have sex with men: stigma and discrimination. *The Lancet*, 380(9839), 439–45.

Anderson, T. (2009). HIV/AIDS in Cuba: lessons and challenges. *Revista Panamericana de Salud Pública*, 26(1), 78–86.

Andrews, B.E. (2011). Prevalence and correlates of HIV testing among Caribbean youth. *International Journal of STD & AIDS*, 22(12), 722–6.

Andrews, G., Skinner, D., and Zuma, K. (2006). Epidemiology of health and vulnerability among children orphaned and made vulnerable by HIV/AIDS in sub-Saharan Africa. *AIDS Care*, 18(3), 269–76.

Andrews, J.R., Wood, R., Bekker, L.G., Middelkoop, K., and Walensky, R.P. (2012). Projecting the benefits of antiretroviral therapy for HIV prevention: the impact of population mobility and linkage to care. *Journal of Infectious Diseases*, 206(4), 543–51.

Anonymous (1992). 1993 revised classification system for HIV infection and expanded surveillance case definition for AIDS among adolescents and adults. *Morbidity and Mortality Weekly Report. Recommendations and Reports*, 41(RR-17), 1–19.

Anonymous (1994). Concorde: MRC/ANRS randomised double-blind controlled trial of immediate and deferred zidovudine in symptom-free HIV infection. Concorde Coordinating Committee. *The Lancet*, 343(8902), 871–81.

Auvert, B., Taljaard, D., Lagarde, E., Sobngwi-Tambekou, J., Sitta, R., and Puren, A. (2005). Randomized, controlled intervention trial of male circumcision for reduction of HIV infection risk: the ANRS 1265 Trial. *PLoS Medicine*, 2(11), e298.

Baggaley, R.F. and Fraser, C. (2010). Modelling sexual transmission of HIV: testing the assumptions, validating the predictions. *Current Opinion in HIV and AIDS*, 5(4), 269–76.

Bailey, R.C., Moses, S., Parker, C.B., et al. (2007). Male circumcision for HIV prevention in young men in Kisumu, Kenya: a randomised controlled trial. *The Lancet*, 369(9562), 643–56.

Barnabas, R.V., Webb, E.L., Weiss, H.A., and Wasserheit, J.N. (2011). The role of coinfections in HIV epidemic trajectory and positive prevention: a systematic review and meta-analysis. *AIDS*, 25(13), 1559–73.

Barnighausen, T., Chaiyachati, K., Dabis, F., and Newell, M.L. (2011). Interventions to increase antiretroviral adherence in sub-Saharan Africa: a systematic review of evaluation studies. *The Lancet Infectious Diseases*, 11(12), 942–51.

Bassols, A.M., Boni, R., and Pechansky, F. (2010). Alcohol, drugs, and risky sexual behavior are related to HIV infection in female adolescents. *Revista Brasileira de Psiquiatria*, 32(4), 361–8.

Bastos, F.I., Caceres, C., Galvão, J., Veras, M.A., and Castilho, E.A. (2008). AIDS in Latin America: assessing the current status of the epidemic and the ongoing response. *International Journal of Epidemiology*, 37(4), 729–37.

Bastos, F.I., Caiaffa, W., Rossi, D., Vila, M., and Malta, M. (2007). The children of mama coca: coca, cocaine and the fate of harm reduction in South America. *International Journal on Drug Policy*, 18(2), 99–106.

Beyrer, C., Wirtz, A.L., Walker, D., et al. (2011). *The Global HIV Epidemics among Men Who Have Sex with Men*. Washington, DC: World Bank.

Bolton-Moore, C., Mubiana-Mbewe, M., Cantrell, R.A., et al. (2007). Clinical outcomes and CD4 cell response in children receiving antiretroviral therapy at primary health care facilities in Zambia. *Journal of the American Medical Association*, 298(16), 1888–99.

Bos, A.E., Schaalma, H.P., and Pryor, J.B. (2008). Reducing AIDS-related stigma in developing countries: the importance of theory- and evidence-based interventions. *Psychology, Health & Medicine*, 13(4), 450–60.

Bridge, J., Lazarus, J.V., and Atun, R. (2010). HIV epidemics and prevention responses in Asia and Eastern Europe: lessons to be learned? *AIDS*, 24(Suppl. 3), S86–94.

Broder, S. (2010). Twenty-five years of translational medicine in antiretroviral therapy: promises to keep. *Science Translational Medicine*, 2(39), 39ps33.

Burki, T. (2012). Russia's drug policy fuels infectious disease epidemics. *The Lancet Infectious Diseases*, 12(4), 275–6.

Burns, D.N., Dieffenbach, C.W., and Vermund, S.H. (2010). Rethinking prevention of HIV type 1 infection. *Clinical Infectious Diseases*, 51(6), 725–31.

Bushman, F.D., Nabel, G.J., and Swanstrom, R. (2011). *HIV: From Biology to Prevention and Treatment*. New York: Cold Spring Harbor Laboratory Press.

Casper, C. (2011). The increasing burden of HIV-associated malignancies in resource-limited regions. *Annual Review of Medicine*, 62, 157–70.

Castro, A. and Farmer, P. (2005). Understanding and addressing AIDS-related stigma: from anthropological theory to clinical practice in Haiti. *American Journal of Public Health*, 95(1), 53–9.

Celentano, D.D., Nelson, K.E., Lyles, C.M., et al. (1998). Decreasing incidence of HIV and sexually transmitted diseases in young Thai men: evidence for success of the HIV/AIDS control and prevention program. *AIDS*, 12(5), F29–36.

Celum, C. and Baeten, J.M. (2012). Tenofovir-based pre-exposure prophylaxis for HIV prevention: evolving evidence. *Current Opinion in Infectious Diseases*, 25(1), 51–7.

Centers for Disease Control and Prevention (2011). Vital signs: HIV prevention through care and treatment—United States. *Morbidity and Mortality Weekly Report*, 60(47), 1618–23.

Chandrasekaran, P., Dallabetta, G., Loo, V., Rao, S., Gayle, H., and Alexander, A. (2006). Containing HIV/AIDS in India: the unfinished agenda. *The Lancet Infectious Diseases*, 6(8), 508–21.

Chavers, L. S. and Vermund, S.H. (2007). An introduction to emerging and reemerging infectious diseases. In F.R. Lashley and J.D. Durham (eds.) *Emerging Infectious Diseases: Trends and Issues*, pp. 3–24. New York: Springer Publishing Company.

Chin, H.B., Sipe, T.A., Elder, R., et al. (2012). The effectiveness of group-based comprehensive risk-reduction and abstinence education interventions to prevent or reduce the risk of adolescent pregnancy, human immunodeficiency virus, and sexually transmitted infections: two systematic reviews for the Guide to Community Preventive Services. *American Journal of Preventive Medicine*, 42(3), 272–94.

Chopra, M., Lawn, J.E., Sanders, D., et al. (2009). Achieving the health Millennium Development Goals for South Africa: challenges and priorities. *The Lancet*, 374(9694), 1023–31.

Ciampa, P.J., Burlison, J.R., Blevins, M., et al. (2011). Improving retention in the early infant diagnosis of HIV program in rural Mozambique by better service integration. *Journal of Acquired Immune Deficiency Syndromes*, 58(1), 115–19.

Ciampa, P.J., Tique, J.A., Jumá, N., et al. (2012). Addressing poor retention of infants exposed to HIV: a quality improvement study in rural Mozambique. *Journal of Acquired Immune Deficiency Syndromes*, 60(2), e46–52.

Ciaranello, A.L., Park, J.E., Ramirez-Avila, L., et al. (2011). Early infant HIV-1 diagnosis programs in resource-limited settings: opportunities for improved outcomes and more cost-effective interventions. *BMC Medicine*, 9, 59.

Cohen, M.S., Chen, Y.Q., McCauley, M., et al. (2011). Prevention of HIV-1 infection with early antiretroviral therapy. *The New England Journal of Medicine*, 365(6), 493–505.

Cohen, M.S., Shaw, G.M., McMichael, A.J., and Haynes, B.F. (2011). Acute HIV-1 infection. *The New England Journal of Medicine*, 364(20), 1943–54.

Colfax, G., Vittinghoff, E., Husnik, M.J., et al. (2004). Substance use and sexual risk: a participant- and episode-level analysis among a cohort of men who have sex with men. *American Journal of Epidemiology*, 159(10), 1002–12.

Connor, E.M., Sperling, R.S., Gelber, R., et al. (1994). Reduction of maternal–infant transmission of human immunodeficiency virus type 1 with zidovudine treatment. Pediatric AIDS Clinical Trials Group

Protocol 076 Study Group. *The New England Journal of Medicine*, 331(18), 1173–80.

Corner, H., Rissel, C., Smith, B., et al. (2005). Sexual health behaviours among Pacific Island youth in Vanuatu, Tonga and the Federated States of Micronesia. *Health Promotion Journal of Australia*, 16(2), 144–50.

Corsi, K.F. and Booth, R.E. (2008). HIV sex risk behaviors among heterosexual methamphetamine users: literature review from 2000 to present. *Current Drug Abuse Reviews*, 1(3), 292–6.

Couture, M.C., Sansothy, N., Sapphon, V., et al. (2011). Young women engaged in sex work in Phnom Penh, Cambodia, have high incidence of HIV and sexually transmitted infections, and amphetamine-type stimulant use: new challenges to HIV prevention and risk. *Sexually Transmitted Diseases*, 38(1), 33–9.

Cremin, I., Alsallaq, R., Dybul, M., Piot, P., Garnett, G., and Hallett, T.B. (2013). The new role of antiretrovirals in combination HIV prevention: a mathematical modelling analysis. *AIDS*, 27(3), 447–58.

Das, M., Chu, P.L., Santos, G.M., et al. (2010). Decreases in community viral load are accompanied by reductions in new HIV infections in San Francisco. *PLoS One*, 5(6), e11068.

Davaalkham, J., Unenchimeg, P., Baigalmaa, C.H., et al. (2009). High-risk status of HIV-1 infection in the very low epidemic country, Mongolia, 2007. *International Journal of STD & AIDS*, 20(6), 391–4.

Denison, J.A., O'Reilly, K.R., Schmid, G.P., Kennedy, C.E., and Sweat, M.D. (2008). HIV voluntary counseling and testing and behavioral risk reduction in developing countries: a meta-analysis, 1990–2005. *AIDS and Behavior*, 12(3), 363–73.

DiClemente, R.J., Crittenden, C.P., Rose, E., et al. (2008). Psychosocial predictors of HIV-associated sexual behaviors and the efficacy of prevention interventions in adolescents at-risk for HIV infection: what works and what doesn't work? *Psychosomatic Medicine*, 70(5), 598–605.

Ding, H., Wilson, C.M., Modjarrad, K., et al. (2009). Predictors of suboptimal virologic response to highly active antiretroviral therapy among human immunodeficiency virus-infected adolescents: analyses of the reaching for excellence in adolescent care and health (REACH) project. *Archives of Pediatrics & Adolescent Medicine*, 163(12), 1100–5.

Dionisio, D., Gass, R., McDermott, P., et al. (2007). What strategies to boost production of affordable fixed-dose anti-retroviral drug combinations for children in the developing world? *Current HIV Research*, 5(2), 155–87.

D'Ippolito, M., Read, J.S., Korelitz, J., et al. (2007). Missed opportunities for prevention of mother-to-child transmission of human immunodeficiency virus type 1 in Latin America and the Caribbean: the NISDI perinatal study. *Pediatric Infectious Disease Journal*, 26(7), 649–53.

Donnell, D., Baeten, J.M., Kiarie, J., et al. (2010). Heterosexual HIV-1 transmission after initiation of antiretroviral therapy: a prospective cohort analysis. *The Lancet*, 375(9731), 2092–8.

Dorjgochoo, T., Noel, F., Deschamps, M.M., et al. (2009). Risk factors for HIV infection among Haitian adolescents and young adults seeking counseling and testing in Port-au-Prince. *Journal of Acquired Immune Deficiency Syndromes*, 52(4), 498–508.

Drucker, E. (2012). Failed drug policies in the United States and the future of AIDS: a perfect storm. *Journal of Public Health Policy*, 33(3), 309–16.

Eaton, J.W., Johnson, L.F., Salomon, J.A., et al. (2012). HIV treatment as prevention: systematic comparison of mathematical models of the potential impact of antiretroviral therapy on HIV incidence in South Africa. *PLoS Medicine*, 9(7), e1001245.

Elovich, R. and Drucker, E. (2008). On drug treatment and social control: Russian narcology's great leap backwards. *Harm Reduction Journal*, 5, 23.

El-Sadr, W.M., Mayer, K.H., and Hodder, S.L. (2010). AIDS in America—forgotten but not gone. *The New England Journal of Medicine*, 362(11), 967–70.

Fang, C.T., Hsu, H.M., Twu, S.J., et al. (2004). Decreased HIV transmission after a policy of providing free access to highly active antiretroviral therapy in Taiwan. *Journal of Infectious Diseases*, 190(5), 879–85.

Farnia, M., Ebrahimi, B., Shams, A., and Zamani, S. (2010). Scaling up methadone maintenance treatment for opioid-dependent prisoners in Iran. *International Journal on Drug Policy*, 21(5), 422–4.

Farr, A.C. and Wilson, D.P. (2010). An HIV epidemic is ready to emerge in the Philippines. *Journal of the International AIDS Society*, 13, 16.

Fedson, D.S. (2009). Meeting the challenge of influenza pandemic preparedness in developing countries. *Emerging Infectious Diseases*, 15(3), 365–71.

Ferreira, P.C., Pessoa, S., and Santos, M.R. (2011). The impact of AIDS on income and human capital. *Economic Inquiry*, 49(4), 1104–16.

Fideli, U.S., Allen, S.A., Musonda, R., et al. (2001). Virologic and immunologic determinants of heterosexual transmission of human immunodeficiency virus type 1 in Africa. *AIDS Research and Human Retroviruses*, 17(10), 901–10.

Figueroa, J.P. (2008). The HIV epidemic in the Caribbean: meeting the challenges of achieving universal access to prevention, treatment and care. *West Indian Medical Journal*, 57(3), 195–203.

Finlinson, H.A., Colon, H.M., Robles, R.R., and Soto, M. (2006). Sexual identity formation and AIDS prevention: an exploratory study of non-gay-identified Puerto Rican MSM from working class neighborhoods. *AIDS and Behavior*, 10(5), 531–9.

Fortenberry, J.D. (1998). Alcohol, drugs, and STD/HIV risk among adolescents. *AIDS Patient Care and STDS*, 12(10), 783–6.

Fowler, M.G., Gable, A.R., Lampe, M.A., Etima, M., and Owor, M. (2010). Perinatal HIV and its prevention: progress toward an HIV-free generation. *Clinics in Perinatology*, 37(4), 699–719, vii.

Free, C., Roberts, I.G., Abramsky, T., Fitzgerald, M., and Wensley, F. (2011). A systematic review of randomised controlled trials of interventions promoting effective condom use. *Journal of Epidemiology & Community Health*, 65(2), 100–10.

Galarraga, O., Wirtz, V.J., Figueroa-Lara, A., et al. (2011). Unit costs for delivery of antiretroviral treatment and prevention of mother-to-child transmission of HIV: a systematic review for low- and middle-income countries. *Pharmacoeconomics*, 29(7), 579–99.

Gallo, M.F., Kilbourne-Brook, M., and Coffey, P.S. (2012). A review of the effectiveness and acceptability of the female condom for dual protection. *Sexual Health*, 9(1), 18–26.

Gardner, E.M., McLees, M.P., Steiner, J.F., Del Rio, C., and Burman, W.J. (2011). The spectrum of engagement in HIV care and its relevance to test-and-treat strategies for prevention of HIV infection. *Clinical Infectious Diseases*, 52(6), 793–800.

Gardner, L.I., Harrison, S.H., Hendrix, C.W., et al. (1998). Size and duration of zidovudine benefit in 1003 HIV-infected patients: U.S. Army, Navy, and Air Force natural history data. Military Medical Consortium for Applied Retroviral Research. *Journal of Acquired Immune Deficiency Syndromes and Human Retrovirology*, 17(4), 345–53.

Geng, E.H., Glidden, D.V., Bangsberg, D.R., et al. (2012). A causal framework for understanding the effect of losses to follow-up on epidemiologic analyses in clinic-based cohorts: the case of HIV-infected patients on antiretroviral therapy in Africa. *American Journal of Epidemiology*, 175(10), 1080–7.

Goedert, J.J. (1984). Recreational drugs: relationship to AIDS. *Annals of the New York Academy of Sciences*, 437, 192–9.

Goldenberg, R.L., Stringer, J.S., Sinkala, M., and Vermund, S.H. (2002). Perinatal HIV transmission: developing country considerations. *Journal of Maternal-Fetal and Neonatal Medicine*, 12(3), 149–58.

Gonzalez, A., Barinas, J., and O'Cleirigh, C. (2011). Substance use: impact on adherence and HIV medical treatment. *Current HIV/AIDS Reports*, 8(4), 223–34.

Gow, J.A. (2009). The adequacy of policy responses to the treatment needs of South Africans living with HIV (1999–2008), a case study. *Journal of the International AIDS Society*, 12, 37.

Graham, N.M., Zeger, S.L., Park, L.P., et al. (1992). The effects on survival of early treatment of human immunodeficiency virus infection. *The New England Journal of Medicine*, 326(16), 1037–42.

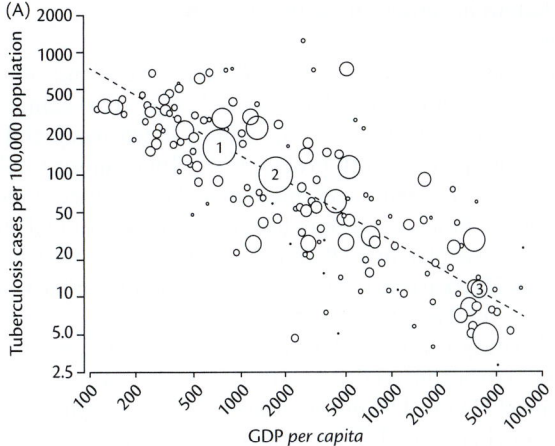

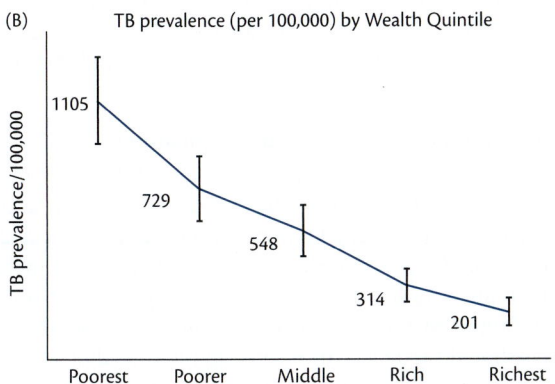

Fig. 8.14.3 Association between poverty and tuberculosis. (A) Reported tuberculosis incidence by per capita gross domestic product in 2004 (Janssens and Rieder 2008). (B) Self-reported tuberculosis prevalence in ~200,000 people in India by wealth quintile in 2008 (Oxlade and Murray 2012).

(A) Reproduced with permission from European Respiratory Society, Janssens, J.P. and Rieder, H.L., An ecological analysis of incidence of tuberculosis and per capita gross domestic product, *European Respiratory Journal*, Volume 32, Number 5, pp. 1415–1416, Copyright © 2008, doi:10.1183/09031936.00078708; and (B) Reproduced from Oxlade, O. and Murray, M., Tuberculosis and poverty: why are the poor at greater risk in India?, *PLoS One*, Volume 7, Issue 1, e47533, Copyright © 2012 Oxlade and Murray, reproduced under the Creative Common 3.0 Attribution License.

HIV infection

HIV infection profoundly alters cell-mediated immunity, the key to containment of *M. tuberculosis* infection. Individuals with HIV have a greatly increased risk of progressing from TB infection to disease. In adults with latent TB infection who acquire HIV, the risk of developing active disease doubles within a year and continually increases as cellular immunodeficiency worsens, with rates of 5 per cent to 15 per cent per year in advanced HIV disease. In individuals with HIV who become infected with *M. tuberculosis*, progression to active TB occurs rapidly, with up to 40 per cent developing clinical illness within 3 months of infection. HIV-infected individuals with successfully treated TB can be re-infected and experience high rates of disease when this occurs. Thus, in areas with a high burden of both TB and HIV infections, the co-epidemic is a function of reactivation of latent TB infection, primary infection with rapid disease progression, and re-infection.

Both low CD4 cell count and high HIV plasma viral load are associated with risk of TB in co-infected individuals. Other predictors of TB in people with HIV include positive TSTs or interferon-gamma release assays, anaemia, elevated C-reactive protein and low body mass index. Treatment of HIV infection with antiretroviral therapy substantially lowers the risk of TB, with between 50 and 80 per cent reductions in incidence rates depending on the CD4 cell count at which treatment is started. Use of isoniazid preventive therapy also reduces risk, and the combination of both antiretroviral therapy and isoniazid preventive therapy has additive effects. Nonetheless, even with use of antiretroviral therapy and isoniazid preventive therapy, the risk of TB in people with HIV remains significantly elevated compared to HIV-negative people.

The HIV epidemic has transformed the epidemiology of TB in the last 25 years, particularly in sub-Saharan Africa. HIV is the strongest commonly encountered risk factor for TB, increasing the risk of developing active TB by a factor of 14 (in high-incidence areas) (WHO 2012) to 60 (in low-incidence ones) (Corbett et al. 2003). HIV co-infection also shortens the duration of TB disease (from symptom onset to death) from years to months (Corbett et al. 2004). TB accounts for one-quarter of HIV deaths worldwide (WHO 2011a). In eight countries of southern Africa, more than half of all TB cases occur in people living with HIV, and in South Africa, the country-wide incidence of TB is over seven times the global average. Primarily as a result of the increasing prevalence of HIV infection, the incidence of TB in Africa more than doubled between 1990 and 2005, at a time when TB incidence was stable or declining in every other region of the world (except Eastern Europe) (Chaisson and Martinson 2008).

The unique characteristics of HIV-associated TB demand a tailored public health response. In areas of high HIV prevalence, the dramatic increase in TB rates over the past 25 years has overwhelmed existing TB control structures. Furthermore, TB is more difficult to diagnose and treat in the setting of HIV infection. Extrapulmonary TB, disseminated TB and negative sputum smear results are all more commonly seen in HIV infected individuals. Whereas HIV-negative individuals with smear-negative TB are at relatively low risk of death, TB is highly lethal in the setting of HIV regardless of sputum smear status. TB diagnostic strategies based on sputum smear alone are therefore destined to fail for people with HIV infection. It is now widely accepted that early initiation of antiretroviral therapy (ART) in people with HIV-associated TB can save lives (Abdool Karim et al. 2011), but TB medications (especially rifampin) interact with key antiretroviral drugs (especially nevirapine and protease inhibitors). Up to one-third of individuals who start therapy for TB and HIV concomitantly will develop symptoms of the immune reconstitution inflammatory syndrome (IRIS) (Lawn et al. 2007), but integrated TB-HIV treatment can improve survival in co-infected patients (Abdool Karim et al. 2011). Not only does HIV impair diagnosis of TB using traditional tools, but it complicates TB treatment decisions as well.

Smoking

Observational studies have suggested for more than a decade that smoking is a major risk factor for TB mortality; in 2003, a study of 43,000 adult male deaths in India suggested that over half the TB deaths could be attributed to smoking (Gajalakshmi et al. 2003). Another large study of elderly individuals in Hong Kong found that smoking increased the risk of incident pulmonary TB nearly threefold (Leung et al. 2004). A systematic review confirmed an increased risk of detectable latent TB infection, active TB disease, and TB mortality among smokers, as well as those exposed to passive smoke and indoor air pollution (Lin et al. 2007). Smoking may also be associated with an increased risk of relapse after successful cure. An epidemiological model has suggested that tobacco smoke might increase the number of TB deaths by 66 per cent (40 million deaths) by 2050, relative to the theoretical scenario of no smoking (Basu et al. 2011).

Diabetes

In the pre-insulin era, TB caused up to 50 per cent of deaths in people with diabetes. More recent observational studies suggest that diabetes increases the risk of incident TB by a factor of three (Jeon and Murray 2008). Like smoking, diabetes may also have a negative impact on TB treatment outcomes, prolonging the time to culture conversion after initiation of treatment and increasing the risk of failure and death (Dooley and Chaisson 2009). The prevalence of diabetes is projected to rise by over two-thirds in the developing world from 2010 to 2030 due primarily to population growth, ageing, and lifestyle changes including diet and obesity, making sustained reductions in global TB incidence increasingly difficult to achieve.

Silicosis

The risk of TB is greatly increased in silicosis, which develops following silica dust exposure among granite workers or gold miners (American Thoracic Society Committee of the Scientific Assembly on Environmental and Occupational Health 1997). Silicotics have an increased risk of death from TB, particularly in countries where TB is hyperendemic. In the pre-HIV era in South Africa, the risk of TB was 2.7-fold greater in gold miners compared to non-miners, with the greatest risk among those with advanced (grade 3) silicosis (Cowie 1994). Silicosis also speeds the progression of TB disease, reducing the duration of undiagnosed active TB by about 80 per cent in miners with versus without silicosis (Corbett et al. 2000).The silicosis-related TB epidemic among miners has been further exacerbated by HIV. Despite intensive control efforts such as annual screening X-rays, TB incidence in South African mines routinely exceeds 1000 per 100,000/year. A cluster randomized trial of mass screening and treatment for both active and latent TB among 80,000 gold miners did not reduce TB incidence at a community level while reducing the risk of TB by 58 per cent while individual miners were taking (but not after stopping) isoniazid preventive therapy (Churchyard et al. 2014; Fielding et al. 2012). Reducing TB transmission among silica exposed miners through combined strategies including early diagnosis and treatment, improved dust control, expanded use of antiretroviral therapy and continuous isoniazid preventive therapy is required.

Populations in congregate living settings

Prisoners

Globally, prisoners are at increased risk of TB (Baussano et al. 2010). Prisons are often characterized by overcrowding, poor ventilation, malnutrition, stress, vitamin D deficiency, and poor medical and public health programmes (Tuberculosis Coalition for Technical Assistance and International Committee of the Red Cross 2009). Prisons therefore take individuals with high epidemiological risk of active TB and expose them to conditions conducive to TB transmission (Baussano et al. 2010), and may act as a reservoir of TB with transmission to the general community. Spread of drug-resistant TB in prisons has also been described and is thought to be a major driver of the MDR-TB epidemic in the former Soviet Union. TB control in prisons can be strengthened by improving living conditions, ventilation, nutrition, and infection control. After incarceration, prisoners with untreated or ineffectively treated TB will continue to transmit TB, thus strengthening TB control in prisons benefits not only prisoners and staff but also communities.

Migrants and socially marginalized populations

As TB has declined in industrialized countries, the proportion of TB cases that are foreign-born has increased and now accounts for the majority of incident TB in many settings (Cain et al. 2008). Migrants from high TB burden settings may affect TB incidence in both high- and low-income regions; migration of southern African miners to and from their communities to South African mines is thought to have contributed to the spread of TB, including drug-resistant TB, within the Southern Africa region. Migrant populations may be at increased risk of TB due to poor nutrition, overcrowding, and poor access to healthcare; providing quality TB treatment and care in this environment is often challenging. In low-burden settings, socially marginalized populations, including homeless individuals, injecting drug users, and previously incarcerated individuals, are at increased risk of poor treatment outcomes and account for a substantial burden of TB disease. Migrant and marginalized persons require access to quality TB screening, treatment and prevention services to reduce their risk of TB and potentially interrupt transmission to the general community.

Population attributable fraction

As our understanding of the impact of various risk factors on TB incidence and mortality has deepened, quantitative projections of attributable burden have become feasible. One method for estimating the population-level burden associated with various risk factors is to calculate the population attributable fraction (PAF), defined as the proportional reduction in TB incidence that could be achieved by completely eliminating a risk factor entirely, assuming that observed epidemiological associations are completely causal. The PAF typically overestimates the fraction of disease causally resulting from a given risk factor, but it provides a useful metric for comparing the population-level burden of TB associated with diverse determinants. Such projections have led to important conclusions for shaping the future of TB control efforts.

In many locations, the strongest determinant of TB incidence is the overall economic status of a population (discussed earlier) (Dye et al. 2009). Thus, general improvement of economic conditions is likely to have substantial positive impact on TB control. Additionally, there exists a striking geographic heterogeneity in the drivers of TB epidemics worldwide. For example, HIV is associated with more than 50 per cent of TB in southern Africa, but only 1 per cent in China and 5 per cent in India, the two countries with the greatest burden of TB. Similarly, elimination of all tobacco smoking might reduce TB incidence by 20 per cent in Indonesia but only 4 per cent in Nigeria. Other settings in which specific determinants are driving country-wide epidemics of TB include alcohol abuse (PAF 35 per cent) and smoking (PAF 29 per cent) in the Russian Federation, smoking (PAF 21 per cent) in China, and undernutrition in Africa (PAF > 40 per cent in multiple countries). While HIV continues to drive the TB epidemic in sub-Saharan Africa, it is associated with only 11 per cent of TB incidence worldwide. Globally, elimination of undernutrition, smoking, and indoor air pollution would have greater impact on TB incidence than elimination of HIV, and interventions to curb alcohol misuse and diabetes would also generate substantial reductions in incidence. As our knowledge of TB risk-factor epidemiology continues to grow, it will become possible to expand these projections to TB progression, treatment outcomes, and mortality as well.

In addition to the PAF approach, epidemiological (transmission) modelling provides further insight into the potential impact of TB control interventions, by projecting the effects of those interventions on future TB transmission. For example, HIV may have greater impact on TB incidence and mortality than on transmission, since HIV-associated TB is often shorter in duration and may be less infectious. By contrast, smoking may increase TB transmission by leading to longer diagnostic delays—and thus prolonged transmission time—as cough is not initially recognized by the patient to be abnormal. Ultimately, the impact of a given epidemiological risk factor on the future burden of TB is a combination of its strength of causal association (e.g. relative risk), prevalence in the general population, and impact on transmission. Understanding each of these elements in a given epidemiological context is essential for crafting public health responses to TB that are geographically tailored and appropriate to the population-level burden of TB caused by specific determinants of disease.

Evolution of TB control

The historical cornerstones of TB control have been the detection and treatment of cases with antituberculosis chemotherapy and prevention of disease with a vaccine. In the century before the advent of antibiotics for TB, treatment consisted of bed rest, fresh air, and nutrition; these were sometimes provided in sanatoria, isolated bucolic or alpine facilities for those able to afford them. The development of antimicrobial agents, such as streptomycin in 1943, permanently altered the management of the disease; ambulatory chemotherapy for TB became widespread and sanatoria around the world closed. Strategies for finding cases in the community through mass radiography or symptom screening were employed for a number of years, referring cases found into treatment programmes. From 1974 to 1991, the WHO recommended that TB control policies focus on passive detection of cases, relying on symptomatic individuals presenting to health services for diagnosis and treatment.

Coupled with passive case detection and treatment was the widespread use of a vaccine against TB. BCG is a live, attenuated strain of *M. bovis* developed by Calmette and Guerin at the Pasteur Institute in Paris and first used in the 1920s. Early studies

of the vaccine found it highly efficacious, reducing paediatric forms of TB by as much as 83 per cent (Colditz et al. 1995), but trials over the past 30 years have not shown any consistent benefit for preventing adult TB. Currently there are multiple strains of BCG used around the world, with notable genomic differences, and the effectiveness of BCG is heterogeneous across populations. One explanation for the variable effects of BCG vaccines over time and geography is further attenuation of the immunogenicity of vaccine strains with further laboratory passage (Behr et al. 1999). Despite this inconsistent evidence of effectiveness, BCG is given at birth to the vast majority of infants around the world, with booster vaccinations given in many countries (Zwerling et al. 2011). This widespread uptake has not blunted global TB incidence or mortality.

Progression from latent TB infection to active disease can also be prevented by administration of the anti-TB drug isoniazid, with an efficacy of at least 65 per cent (Comstock 1999). Since 1998, isoniazid preventive therapy has been endorsed for people with HIV infection, and more recent guidelines have increasingly emphasized its use. Uptake of isoniazid preventive therapy, however, has played little role in global TB control for many years.

In the early 1990s, the WHO launched a new strategy for global TB control called directly observed therapy, short-course (DOTS). This strategy was supported by epidemiological models suggesting that existing tools, used appropriately, could control and eventually eliminate the disease (Styblo and Bumgarner 1991). DOTS consists of five elements: political commitment, registration and monitoring of cases, assuring a reliable supply of anti-TB drugs, case detection with bacteriology, and standardized treatment with supervision of at least the initial phase of therapy. DOTS was scaled-up from 1995 to 2010, with most countries adopting it as a TB control strategy. It has been credited with saving millions of lives since its introduction, and remains a key element of the current WHO Stop TB Strategy (2011). Although it is now widely recognized that scaling up DOTS alone will not achieve global TB control, DOTS remains one of the most successfully deployed comprehensive public health responses to a single disease.

A key historical target under DOTS was to successfully diagnose and notify 70 per cent of all cases of smear-positive TB (Dye et al. 1998). However, the sensitivity of sputum smear microscopy is relatively low, especially in children, people living with HIV and people with extrapulmonary TB. As a result, the potential for achieving worldwide TB control using sputum smear microscopy as the sole diagnostic test is limited and unrealistic. Nevertheless, rapid and accurate diagnosis of individuals with smear-positive TB remains an essential component of any TB control strategy.

Equally important to accurate and rapid diagnosis is standardized treatment. The current first-line treatment regimen for new, drug-susceptible pulmonary TB entails at least 6 months of therapy, including four drugs—isoniazid, rifampin, pyrazinamide, and ethambutol (Table 8.14.1)—during the intensive phase (usually 2 months) and two drugs—isoniazid and rifampin—during the subsequent continuation phase (usually 4 months) (WHO 2010a). For individuals without drug-resistant TB, successful completion of this course of therapy cures virtually all patients; only 2–3 per cent will relapse over long-term follow-up (Menzies et al. 2009). Unfortunately, standardized 6-month therapy also has important limitations. The treatment success rate in people who receive care outside the public health system is markedly lower

Table 8.14.1 Traditional and updated categorization of drugs for TB

Group 1: first-line oral drugs	Isoniazid
	Rifamycins: rifampin, rifabutin and rifapentine
	Ethambutol
	Pyrazinamide
Group 2: injectable drugs	Streptomycin
	Kanamycin
	Amikacin
	Capreomycin
Group 3: fluoroquinolones	Moxifloxacin
	Levofloxacin
	Ofloxacin
Group 4: oral bacteriostatic second line drugs	Ethionamide
	Prothionamide
	Cycloserine/terizidone
	Para-aminosalicylic acid
Group 5: drugs of unclear efficacy	Clofazimine
	Clarithromycin
	Amoxacillin-clavulanate
	Linezolid
	Thiocetazone
[a]Group 6: new agents with novel mechanisms of action	Bedaquiline
	Delaminid
	Linezolid/sutezolid and other oxazolidinones
	PA-824

[a] Group 6 has been added by the authors.

Adapted with permission from World Health Organization, *Guidelines for the Programmatic Management of Drug-Resistant Tuberculosis: Emergency Update 2008*, Copyright © World Health Organization 2008, available from: http://whqlibdoc.who.int/publications/2008/9789241547581_eng.pdf.

than among those treated under DOTS, existing first-line drugs have substantial toxicity and interactions with other medications (particularly antiretrovirals) (Yee et al. 2003), and an estimated 11 per cent of new TB cases are now resistant to at least one first-line drug (Wright et al. 2009).

To address limitations in the initial DOTS policy, the WHO updated its Global Plan to Stop TB in 2006 (Stop TB Partnership 2006) and again in 2011 with specific emphasis on addressing HIV-related TB and MDR-TB, strengthening health systems, engaging the private sector and empowering communities to contribute to TB control (Stop TB Partnership 2011a). In addition, the WHO strongly emphasized the importance of research into new methods to improve TB control. The revised Global Plan also included detailed budget projections and estimated that meeting the Millennium Development Goals (MDGs) for TB would cost $56 billion between 2006 and 2015, but noted that only $23 billion was available.

Implementation of the WHO DOTS/Stop TB strategy has resulted in substantial achievements in TB care and control globally. The treatment success rate among all new TB cases worldwide currently stands at 85 per cent (87 per cent for smear-positive pulmonary TB), and an estimated 20 million lives have been saved since DOTS was begun. However, in Africa and Eastern Europe,

TB incidence is only now returning to the 1990 baseline. TB prevalence has declined by 36 per cent globally since 1990, but current projections suggest that the target for halving TB prevalence will not be met globally.

To improve control of TB in the setting of high HIV prevalence, the WHO endorsed a strategy known as the '3 I's' for HIV-associated TB: *intensified* case finding, *isoniazid* preventive therapy, and *infection* control. These three elements underscore three important aspects of an appropriate public health response for HIV-associated TB. Intensified case finding is aimed at identifying HIV-infected individuals with active TB before they would be diagnosed under passive case finding, in order to reduce mortality and transmission. Isoniazid preventive therapy reduces the risk of TB in people with HIV substantially, particularly while they are taking the drug, and the combination of IPT and antiretroviral therapy can reduce TB risk by up to 90 per cent. Furthermore, people living with HIV are more likely to visit health centres and be hospitalized, where mixing of patients exquisitely susceptible to disease with others transmitting infection results in high rates of TB disease. Health centres and hospitals are frequent sites of TB outbreaks, including outbreaks of highly drug-resistant TB, among people living with HIV—often with highly fatal consequences. Infection control is therefore particularly important for prevention of TB transmission among people living with HIV.

Drug-resistant TB

Resistance to anti-TB drugs has existed since the first use of streptomycin; a large proportion of patients treated with streptomycin monotherapy in the first controlled trial of TB chemotherapy developed resistant infections (Medical Research Council 1948). Today, resistance to isoniazid is widespread and resistance to both isoniazid and rifampin, defined as MDR-TB, is increasingly prevalent.

Drug-resistant TB arises from rare, spontaneous mutations in the *M. tuberculosis* genome that renders the bacterium resistant to the action of the drug. In patients with active TB disease, a very small number of the organisms present in the body will harbour mutations to any one drug. In latent TB infection, where the number of viable organisms is even smaller and rates of division lower, the probability of even a single spontaneous drug resistance mutation is very low. The probability of simultaneous mutations to multiple drugs is small (e.g. $10^{-9} \times 10^{-9}$). Thus, combination therapy with several anti-TB drugs is effective even against a population of bacilli with small numbers of monoresistant organisms. However, improper treatment (e.g. sequential monotherapy) allows resistance to emerge with much greater probability. This process, referred to as *acquired drug resistance*, has historically been the most common means by which drug-resistant TB occurs. However, once acquired, drug-resistant TB can be transmitted to others, a situation referred to as *primary drug resistance*. In recent years, the proportion of drug resistant TB due to primary resistance has increased, but previously treated individuals are still more likely to have MDR-TB (Dalton et al. 2012).

MDR-TB is difficult to diagnose and requires treatment with second-line agents, which are more toxic, more expensive, and less efficacious. Treatment for MDR-TB typically involves five agents, a 24-month treatment course (of which 8 months require an injectable agent), and treatment costs that are at least ten times higher than for drug-susceptible TB (WHO 2010b, 2011b). Even with optimal therapy, however, fewer than 70 per cent of patients with MDR-TB are cured with current regimens (Orenstein et al. 2009). The Global Project on Anti-Tuberculosis Drug Resistance Surveillance reports that the global prevalence of MDR-TB in 2006 and 2010 was approximately 5 per cent (3 per cent in new cases and 20 per cent in previously treated cases) (Wright et al. 2009; Zignol et al. 2012). However, these data are notable for their lack of completeness (less than 2 per cent of TB patients without a prior treatment history are currently tested for drug susceptibility) and their heterogeneity. MDR-TB is a particular challenge in the countries of the former Soviet Union, where partial treatment of TB in prisons has played a key role in amplifying drug resistance. Almost 50 per cent of MDR-TB cases occur in India and China; a national survey estimated that China has over 100,000 incident cases of MDR-TB per year, the majority of which now result from primary transmission rather than acquired resistance (Zhao et al. 2012). In countries that have mounted an aggressive response to the threat of MDR-TB, notably the United States, which experienced a surge in MDR-TB prevalence in the early 1990s, the prevalence of TB drug resistance has declined (Wright et al. 2009). However, in the Tomsk Oblast of Russia, the prevalence of MDR-TB among all cases increased from 18 per cent to 28 per cent in a span of just two years (2003–2005) (Wright et al. 2009) highlighting the explosive potential of MDR-TB in the setting of insufficient public health vigilance and funding.

An effective public health response to the threat of MDR-TB involves both diagnosis and treatment (WHO 2011b). First, it is essential to scale up laboratory capacity for drug susceptibility testing (DST). As of 2008, in 27 high-MDR-TB countries, only nine had more than two quality-assured labs capable of testing for drug resistance (WHO 2011b). Second, patients with MDR-TB must have access to uninterrupted and high-quality second-line drugs. The Green Light Committee (GLC) is an international initiative to supply such drugs at a reduced price and has approved treatment for MDR-TB patients in over 70 countries; however, in 2008, it was estimated that only 1 per cent of all incident cases received second-line treatment through the GLC (WHO 2011b). Financing the MDR-TB response is particularly challenging; the cost of MDR-TB treatment alone exceeds per-capita gross national income in all 27 high-MDR countries, and many countries devote over half of their national TB control budgets to treating the less than 5 per cent of cases with MDR-TB.

The number of drugs to which TB is resistant is increasing, raising the spectre of TB that is completely untreatable. In 2006, the first cases of extensively drug-resistant (XDR)-TB, defined as MDR-TB plus resistance to a fluoroquinolone and at least one of three second-line injectable drugs, were reported as part of a nosocomial outbreak in KwaZulu-Natal, South Africa (Gandhi et al. 2006). Case-fatality in the HIV-fuelled outbreak was 98 per cent, with death occurring in a median 16 days after diagnosis. XDR-TB has subsequently been identified by routine surveillance in over 20 countries, in every region of the world (Zignol et al. 2012). In 2012, a case series highlighted four TB patients with documented resistance to all first- and second-line drugs with susceptibility tests available (Udwadia et al. 2012). This situation highlights the need to develop new drugs in the anti-TB armamentarium, but more importantly, effective public health approaches to diagnosing and treating drug-resistant TB in order to curb the emergence of such widely-resistant, potentially untreatable, organisms.

Progress in the public health response to tuberculosis

TB case finding

If TB prevalence and mortality are to be halved in a period during which TB incidence is declining by about 2 per cent per year globally, the duration of disease must be shortened, and people with active TB must be diagnosed before it is too late to avert death. Thus, passive case finding—'detecting active TB disease among symptomatic patients who present to medical services for diagnosis of symptoms'—must be augmented by more active methods (Ayles et al. 2013). Population-based TB prevalence surveys have shown that many individuals with prevalent TB are asymptomatic. Many 'asymptomatic' individuals may actually have mild symptoms, but neither patients nor clinicians regularly recognize these as indicative of TB. Thus, whereas classic symptom screening and sputum smear microscopy may be effective clinical tools for diagnosis of advanced TB disease (in the absence of HIV infection), they are far less useful as public health tools for reducing the infectious burden in the community through detection of prevalent infectious cases. The 'typical' findings of at least one of cough, fever, weight loss, or night sweats has a positive predictive value of less than 25 per cent in HIV-infected populations, though negative predictive value is generally over 90 per cent.

Without actively finding prevalent cases in the community, we cannot hope to substantially reduce the burden of TB transmission—as the majority of transmission likely occurs before individuals with active TB ever seek care. But prevalent TB is a rare disease at the population level. In a typical high-burden setting, 500 community members would need to be screened—at an estimated cost of at least US$10 per person—to identify one person with active TB. To have a 50 per cent chance of detecting that case, a method with higher sensitivity than symptom screen and sputum smear would need to be used. The most realistic method at present would be to use chest X-ray—with a sensitivity (for any abnormality) of greater than 90 per cent—as an initial screen, with culture or other high-sensitivity bacteriologic assay for confirmation. However, in most settings, the cost of this community-based case finding strategy at current prices would exceed $10,000 per case detected. Several studies in Africa have suggested that household- or community-based active case finding may reduce TB prevalence by up to 20–40 per cent over a period of a few years, but one trial (ZAMSTAR) found that an untargeted enhanced case-finding strategy had little effect on community-wide incidence or prevalence (Ayles et al. 2013). The failure to demonstrate community-level benefit of active TB screening reflects the immense logistical challenges in finding and treating early cases at a community level, not the inability of active case finding to contribute to TB control.

This reality—that the majority of TB transmission in the community is fuelled by cases that are rare on the population level and therefore resource-intensive to detect—has deepened an understanding that innovative, targeted approaches to active TB case finding are an essential component of the public health response to TB. These approaches must be targeted to the specific epidemiological situation into which they are deployed, with the aim of detecting prevalent cases more efficiently than in the community-based screening scenarios studied. Additional strategies include screening of high-risk individuals such as HIV-infected individuals, diabetics, and those in congregate settings such as prisons and mines. These initiatives provide reason for optimism that active case-finding strategies can be developed which directly reduce TB prevalence and mortality without overwhelming available TB control infrastructure and budgets.

Management of HIV-associated TB

Countries with HIV-driven TB epidemics must confront both the challenge and the opportunity afforded by the ubiquity of HIV infection among individuals with active TB. On the patient level, concomitant diagnosis, linkage to care, and effective treatment of both TB and HIV requires numerous steps to be taken and systems to be navigated. On a clinical level, the benefits of combined HIV-TB services are clear. Antiretroviral therapy (ART) reduces the risk of developing active TB by about two-thirds; initiating ART at the time of TB diagnosis (versus 8–12 weeks later) reduces mortality by up to 40 per cent in patients with severe immune compromise (Havlir et al. 2011); and dual testing for HIV and TB is an efficient method to detect and treat prevalent TB in the community. Integration of TB and HIV services has therefore been recommended for all areas with high HIV prevalence. However, successful models for such integration remain relatively uncommon. Challenges that confront integrated delivery of care for TB and HIV include clinical concerns (e.g. drug interactions, immune reconstitution), administrative barriers (e.g. different funding streams and organizational structures), and cultural differences (e.g. directly-observed therapy in TB versus patient empowerment for self-administered therapy in HIV). Nevertheless, a number of models demonstrating how HIV and TB delivery systems can be successfully integrated in high-burden settings have been published (Gandhi et al. 2009). From 2004 to 2011, the percentage of people with *diagnosed* incident TB in Africa who were tested for HIV rose from 4 per cent to 69 per cent, and the number of HIV-infected individuals screened for TB rose from under 100,000 to 3.2 million (WHO 2011a).

Dramatic progress has been made with respect to delivery of ART and isoniazid preventive therapy. In the decade from 2002 to 2011, global access to ART among people in need rose essentially from 0 per cent to 50 per cent, suggesting that the goal of universal access is attainable in a short period of time. Although ART dramatically reduces the risk of developing TB, it is currently initiated late in the HIV disease course, such that much of its potential for TB prevention is untapped. Furthermore, ART also substantially extends life expectancy while not reducing TB incidence to levels seen by HIV-uninfected people; thus, late ART may even have the paradoxical effect of increasing TB incidence at the population level. It is unlikely that ART alone, as currently delivered, will effectively turn the tide of TB in southern Africa (Lawn et al. 2011).

Attention is being paid to early initiation of ART, a so-called 'test and treat' strategy of HIV control. One admittedly optimistic epidemiological model suggests that, if ART were initiated within 1 year of HIV seroconversion among all individuals in nine African countries, HIV-associated TB incidence could be reduced by 98 per cent by 2050 (Williams et al. 2010). While such a strategy would be impossibly resource-intensive on a global scale under current financial conditions, it bears mention as a potential public health approach against both HIV and TB as HIV drug prices fall and less-toxic ART regimens are developed. Also of note, the 'test and treat' paradigm has recently been applied to TB control as well, emphasizing the importance of treating individuals with active TB on the same day that they are tested (Davis et al. 2012).

Isoniazid preventive therapy (IPT) for people living with HIV is recommended as part of the WHO '3 I's' approach. Uptake has been poor, with only 12,000 HIV-infected people worldwide registered as taking IPT by 2004. By 2010, this number had risen to 180,000, due largely to South Africa increasing its delivery of IPT from 24,000 to 124,000 people between 2009 and 2010 alone. While South Africa has demonstrated the feasibility of rapid scale-up, IPT uptake in other countries remains slow. A series of recent trials has broadened our understanding of the community-level impact of IPT among people living with HIV, and is likely to influence the global public health approach to IPT delivery in coming years. In Botswana, IPT for 36 months reduced TB incidence by over 40 per cent compared to 6 months of IPT; the effectiveness of the 6-month regimen began to wane within 6 months of completion (Samandari et al. 2011). In Brazil, where rates of ongoing TB transmission are substantially lower, a 6-month course of IPT delivered only to TST-positive individuals within HIV clinics reduced overall adjusted TB incidence rates by 27 per cent at the clinic level and by over 50 per cent among those who remained in consistent clinical care (Durovni et al. 2013). In the gold mines of South Africa, widespread use of IPT reduced TB incidence at the individual level while on therapy, but had no impact on TB rates at the population level, perhaps because of the exceedingly high rates of TB transmission and the corresponding risk of reinfection (Churchyard et al. 2012). While IPT has clear individual-level benefit for people living with HIV, its population-level impact as a public health measure depends on the logistic feasibility of delivery and the ongoing risk of TB reinfection after completing IPT. In areas where IPT can be effectively delivered, and the risk of TB reinfection is low, IPT is likely to have an important population-level impact on TB incidence. However, in areas where the annual risk of TB infection is high, IPT likely must be delivered consistently and continuously to achieve meaningful reductions in incidence. Future strategies for IPT delivery among people living with HIV in hyperendemic settings will need to balance the clear individual benefit against the less dramatic public health impact and relative logistical difficulty of implementation.

In summary, tremendous strides have been made in the public health approach to HIV-associated TB. Nevertheless, tremendous challenges remain as we begin to understand the limits of integrated care, ART, and IPT in controlling epidemics of HIV-associated TB. As ART extends life expectancy and the number of people living with HIV continues to grow, innovative public health approaches—such as those built on the models of early ART and continuous IPT—will need to be developed if we are to stem the tide of TB in areas of high HIV prevalence.

TB infection control

One area of need, and potential, for improvement in the public health response to TB is infection control especially in congregate settings such as prisons and healthcare facilities. These settings, particularly those with a high prevalence of HIV, pose tremendous risk for TB transmission and outbreak, as they introduce individuals with infectious TB into crowded settings with other immunocompromised patients. Assuming that smear-positive TB is five times more infectious than smear-negative TB and that the effective contact rate in a hospital is 40 times higher than in the community, a hospitalized smear-positive patient could generate as many TB infections in 1 week—and to patients at much greater risk of TB progression and death—as a smear-negative counterpart in the community could generate in four years. Infection control measures for TB include measures that are administrative (e.g. rapid diagnosis, isolation, and treatment of individuals with infectious TB), environmental (e.g. ventilation and reduction of crowding), and respiratory/personal protective (e.g. masks and personal respirators) (Jensen et al. 2005). When all three of these tiers are instituted, infection control measures are very effective. For example, after implementation of aggressive infection control measures following an MDR-TB outbreak at a hospital in Florida, the number of nosocomial cases of MDR-TB fell from an average of 3 per month to no new cases (other than reactivation from infections acquired prior to the intervention) over a 2-year period (Wenger et al. 1995). Similar success was seen in reducing nosocomial transmission after improving infection control measures following an outbreak of extensively drug-resistant TB in KwaZulu-Natal, South Africa (Gandhi et al. 2013). The ability of simple measures, such as improved ventilation by opening windows, to reduce household transmission of TB is of increasing interest as well, and our ability to evaluate the effectiveness of such interventions is improving with the availability of mobile household environmental monitors.

Nevertheless, despite the demonstrated efficacy of infection control measures and the need to protect healthcare workers from TB (Joshi et al. 2006), infection control remains relatively poorly implemented. As of 2008, no country had reported data on implementation of infection control measures to the WHO (WHO 2009). Solutions to difficult challenges in TB infection control (e.g. improving ventilation when outside temperatures are cold) are rarely discussed in the literature. Similarly, due to a lack of research intensity, our understanding of even basic epidemiology related to infection control remains limited. Ultimately, infection control remains a globally neglected component of the public health response to TB, requiring greater attention if we are to avert the tremendous morbidity and mortality associated with outbreaks and transmission in congregate settings.

Health systems and gender issues in TB control

National tuberculosis programmes (NTPs) are key elements to control tuberculosis, but weak and overburdened health systems have impeded progress. In addition, rapidly introduced health system reforms and poorly designed systems have adversely affected national efforts to control TB. Innovative, geographically specific health systems strengthening should complement other strategies to control TB (Atun et al. 2010; Lienhardt et al. 2012). NTPs operate within the general health system, and both impact on each other. In many high TB-burden countries, NTPs operate within weak, overburdened health systems. As a result, TB programmes are likely to benefit from the strengthening of health systems, particularly in the areas of financing, policy development, human resource management, procurement of supplies and drugs, and maintenance of health infrastructure (El-Sadr et al. 2009). Many low- and middle-income countries experience human resource

constraints, which include inadequate human resource planning, insufficient numbers of skilled and motivated staff, high turnover, and inequitable distribution of staff (e.g. urban/rural, public/private, and HIV versus TB programmes). Inadequate human resources in many high-burden countries have been identified as an important constraint in achieving TB control targets. Because healthcare worker shortages may compromise TB programmes, TB-HIV integration and task shifting has been adopted as a strategy in which less skilled community workers take on tasks such as adherence counselling, defaulter tracing and family support (Samb et al. 2007; Maher 2010).

Conversely, strengthening national TB programmes may contribute to improvements in the general health system, including areas such as human resources, laboratory infrastructure, drug forecasting, data monitoring, supervision, and quality assurance (Stop TB Partnership 2008). Examples of how the NTP may strengthen the general health system include: applying microscopes purchased for sputum smear examination to malaria smears and urinalysis; using vehicles for district supervisory support also for supervision of health posts and clinics; and adapting the TB drug procurement and distribution system to drugs for chronic diseases. The Stop TB Partnership's Global Plan to Stop TB, 2006–2015, and a Stop TB Policy Paper create a framework for using TB control activities to strengthen general health systems (Stop TB Partnership 2008, 2011a). However, implementing this policy framework in a way that achieves the desired synergy between TB programmes and general health systems remains an ongoing challenge.

Epidemiologically, women in most resource-limited settings have a risk of TB half that of men. However, among younger age strata and in settings of high HIV prevalence, women often have higher TB incidence than men. Similarly, the prevalence of undiagnosed TB (and HIV) among pregnant women is unacceptably high (Gounder et al. 2011). Women often face specific challenges in accessing TB care (e.g. travel with children for directly-observed therapy) and are more likely than men to experience TB associated stigma. On the other hand, maternal and child services are often stronger than other aspects of healthcare systems, and men may, in many cases, have poorer access to general health services (including TB care) than women. As a result, TB may go undiagnosed for longer periods of time in men than in women, a finding that is suggested by TB prevalence surveys (Corbett et al. 2009). An effective TB response should therefore not neglect the unique considerations faced by members of either gender.

Financial constraints

Tuberculosis control is threatened by four key financial factors: (1) inadequate funding, (2) poor capacity to acquire financing, (3) management of funding from numerous sources, and (4) financial constraints to patient access. It was estimated that US$56 billion would be required to achieve the MDG 6 objective for TB control and the Stop TB Partnership's goal of a 50 per cent reduction in the prevalence and mortality of TB by 2015. To address some of these challenges, global and philanthropic organizations have increased financial support for high-burden countries, new financing systems have been introduced to direct substantial funds to countries, and patient access has improved by centralizing and incorporating TB services into primary healthcare (Atun et al. 2010). Despite these interventions, escalating financial needs, drug-resistant TB and migrant populations pose further risk to the control of TB in some areas.

Social determinants

Ninety five per cent of TB cases and 98 per cent of TB deaths occur in developing countries. Since TB affects the economically active age group (15–49 years), it has a direct impact on the economy of poor countries. High TB treatment interruption rates can be attributed to competing priorities of the need to earn money versus access to care (Benatar and Upshur 2010). The impact of poverty, overcrowding, and poor living conditions on TB control efforts should not be underestimated (Lienhardt et al. 2012). Urbanization, migration, and political instability create a fertile environment for TB to flourish. This is further complicated by increasing prevalence of smoking and substance abuse. TB control is inextricably linked with multifaceted efforts to alleviate poverty and promote economic development. Overcoming these challenges requires social support which is often lacking in the communities most affected by TB (Benatar and Upshur 2010).

Engagement with civil society organizations

Civil society organizations include non-governmental, community-based, and faith-based organizations. Their main role is to champion the rights of the vulnerable. Effective partnership and meaningful engagement of civil society organizations have a pivotal role in the response to the TB epidemic (Getahun and Raviglione 2011). Such organizations can influence not only community structure but also government institutions. They are able to function in remote areas and offer a unique opportunity for scaling up of community based care for TB-HIV (Ghebreyesus et al. 2010).

New tools for tuberculosis control

New diagnostic tests

Novel diagnostics are a key emerging weapon in the global fight against TB. It has been estimated that an effective rapid diagnostic test could reduce TB incidence by 20 per cent or more (Dowdy et al. 2006; Keeler et al. 2006), and be highly cost-effective (Dowdy et al. 2008). Novel tests for active TB include liquid culture systems, molecular diagnostic platforms (e.g. Xpert MTB/RIF® assay, and urine antigen assays for lipoarabinomannan (LAM)). The microscopic observation drug susceptibility (MODS) assay was introduced as a culture technique that is similar in accuracy and speed to automated liquid-media culture (e.g. Mycobacteria Growth Indicator Tube, MGIT®), but less resource-intensive (Moore et al. 2006). The MODS assay works on the principle of identifying 'microcolonies' of TB, which are visually distinct from those of other bacteria and mycobacteria. The sensitivity and specificity of MODS for pulmonary TB has been reported at 96 per cent, with a mean time to positivity of 9 days and material/supply costs of less than US$2 per test. MODS also allows for first-line drug susceptibility testing. The primary challenges associated with microcolony culture are the requirement for a quality-assured, biosafety containment laboratory, delay in diagnosis of over a week, and difficulty in bringing non-automated, relatively labour-intensive techniques to scale. Automated liquid culture is more easily scaled up, but also substantially more expensive.

By contrast, the Xpert MTB/RIF® system is a fully-automated molecular (polymerase chain reaction (PCR)) test for active TB that provides results in 90 minutes with minimal human-resource input and similar biosafety requirements as sputum smear microscopy (Boehme et al. 2010). Recommended by the WHO for use in settings of high HIV prevalence or drug resistance, the sensitivity of Xpert MTB/RIF® for smear-positive TB is greater than 99 per cent. The specificity of Xpert MTB/RIF® is similarly high, but its sensitivity for smear-negative pulmonary TB is approximately 75 per cent in symptomatic patients (Boehme et al. 2011), and lower in prevalence surveys. Xpert MTB/RIF® can rapidly detect resistance to rifampin with sensitivity and specificity of 98 per cent or higher, thus facilitating immediate initiation of MDR-TB treatment in areas of high MDR prevalence. The primary limitations of Xpert MTB/RIF® are its requirement for climate control, stable electrical supply, and ongoing machine maintenance, and it is costlier (though more sensitive) than sputum smear. Nevertheless, a comprehensive analysis found Xpert MTB/RIF® to be cost-effective in most settings (Vassall et al. 2011).

Detection of LAM, a mycobacterial cell wall component, in urine is a novel diagnostic strategy with greatest utility in individuals with severe immune compromise. An assay is now available in a true point-of-care (lateral flow) format at a cost of US$3 per test, providing results within 30 minutes. The sensitivity of this assay has been reported as 67 per cent in patients with CD4 T-cell counts of less than 50 cells/mm^3, with specificity of greater than 98 per cent (Lawn et al. 2012). Sensitivity is unacceptably low in immunocompetent individuals, but this assay nonetheless improves markedly on the sensitivity of sputum smear microscopy in its target population, who are also the people for whom immediate diagnosis is potentially most important.

Interferon-gamma release assays (IGRAs) are blood tests that detect specific immune responses to *M. tuberculosis* (and not BCG), and have similar sensitivity to the TST but improved specificity (Pai et al. 2008). IGRAs have poor predictive value for incident active TB (Rangaka et al. 2012), and their use in serial testing (e.g. healthcare worker screening) is complicated by frequent conversions and reversions of uncertain significance. Because of their expense relative to TST, IGRAs are not recommended for use in resource-limited settings. Nevertheless, they are useful for detection of latent TB infection in some (mostly low-incidence) settings where the labour cost of placing and reading a TST is greater than the cost of the IGRA. Commercial serological antibody tests that are widely marketed for diagnosis of active TB demonstrate very poor accuracy, and the WHO issued a 'negative' recommendation against their use.

The line probe assay is a novel molecular test that uses PCR for TB drug susceptibility testing from clinical specimens and culture isolates. The most widely-used line probe assay, the Hain GenoType® MTBDRPlus assay, has a sensitivity of 98 per cent for rifampin resistance and 90 per cent for isoniazid resistance when used on smear-positive sputum specimens or culture isolates, and can provide results within a day (compared to 7–10 days for traditional phenotypic testing in culture) (Hillemann et al. 2007). This technology has recently been expanded to test for resistance to second-line drugs as well, with similar sensitivity (around 90 per cent) for amikacin/capreomycin and fluoroquinolones (Hillemann et al. 2009).

Although these novel tests add substantial value to the public health armamentarium against TB, each assay is limited in some important fashion. A true stand-alone, point-of-care test for active TB that is suitable for use in a broad population remains elusive. Ultimately, new diagnostic tests do not function in isolation, but rather serve as one component of a broader system that also consists of patient and provider preferences, treatment decisions, public health infrastructure, and linkage to care. In developing and using new diagnostics for TB control, it is important to evaluate not only their sensitivity and specificity, but also their ability to improve TB outcomes (morbidity and mortality) when functioning as part of that system.

New drugs

The current first-line treatment for TB is more than 30 years old and relies on drugs developed 40–60 years ago. It is apparent that new drugs and regimens that kill bacilli rapidly and sterilize populations of *M. tuberculosis* are urgently needed to confront the problems of TB control in the twenty-first century. The highest priority for new drugs is for agents to more effectively treat MDR and XDR-TB, as current therapies rely on toxic second-line drugs that must be taken for up to 2 years and only cure 50–70 per cent of patients (WHO 2010b). The development of more potent first-line regimens for the treatment of drug-susceptible TB will cure patients faster, reduce the duration of therapy improve adherence to therapy, improve cost-effectiveness (Owens et al. 2013), and free TB control staff to treat greater numbers of patients. More potent agents may improve the treatment of latent TB, permitting patients to take shorter courses of more potent drug/s than the 6–9 months currently required for isoniazid preventive therapy. For example, a 12-week, once-weekly course of rifapentine plus isoniazid was recently shown to be equally (if not more) effective as 9 months of isoniazid (Sterling et al. 2011).

Drugs for TB have traditionally been grouped into five categories based on their priority for use in drug-susceptible and drug-resistant TB rather than their mechanism of action (Table 8.14.1). Research into new classes of antimicrobial agents with novel mechanisms of action has led to the identification of new drugs with the potential to transform the treatment of both drug-susceptible and drug-resistant TB. Class 1 includes the current first-line drugs used for treating TB. Class 2 is the injectable agents which require intramuscular or intravenous administration, of which all except streptomycin are used in treatment of MDR TB. Class 3, the fluoroquinolones, are potent inhibitors of mycobacterial replication and may help shorten treatment of all forms of TB. Class 4 comprises older drugs that were previously used in first-line regimens but which were relegated to second-tier status because of low potency and higher toxicity. Class 5 is an assortment of unrelated drugs that are used in the treatment of some drug-resistant TB cases and have varying strengths of evidence.

We have added Class 6, a small but hopefully growing list of new agents developed to exploit novel targets in the mycobacterial life cycle, many of which are in advanced stages of clinical development. The newest approved drug for treating TB is bedaquiline, a drug that targets bacterial adenosine tri-phosphate synthase, which was shown in a phase 2 trial to double rates of culture conversion among patients with MDR-TB

(Diacon et al. 2012). Another new drug, delaminid, targets at least two steps in mycobacterial replication and metabolism and has been shown to be effective in patients with MDR-TB (Skripconoka et al. 2013). The other agents listed have all shown promising activity and are in varying stages of development for clinical use.

The promise of new TB vaccines

TB vaccines aim to reduce the risk of TB by preventing infection and reducing the risk of progression to TB disease. The current TB vaccine, BCG, the most widely used vaccine worldwide, protects children from disseminated disease but has had negligible impact on the global TB epidemic (Kaufmann 2011). The efficacy of BCG against pulmonary TB in adults is variable and ranges from –22 per cent (harmful) to +80 per cent (Rieder 2002). The efficacy of BCG varies according to vaccine strain used and geography. Environmental mycobacteria, helminths, and HIV infection (Hoft 2008) may modify vaccine-induced immune responses. The WHO recommends that BCG not be administered to HIV-infected infants as it may cause disseminated BCG disease (BCGosis) (Anonymous 2007). In order to accelerate progress towards eliminating TB as a global health threat, TB vaccines that are safe and effective in infants, adolescents, and adults are required. From a public health perspective, TB vaccines that will prevent infection as well as prevent reactivation of latent TB infection and progression to TB disease will have greatest population-level impact.

Major advances have been achieved in vaccine development making the availability of new vaccines foreseeable within the next decade. Many current vaccine strategies aim to induce TB specific T-cell immunity using disease-stage specific antigens (Lambert et al. 2009). Such 'pre-exposure' vaccines in development aim to replace BCG with a safer alternative, particularly for HIV-infected infants (McShane 2011). Strategies include recombinant BCG strains, attenuated *M. tuberculosis*, and whole-cell killed mycobacteria. All current pre-exposure vaccine candidates are designed to avert disease but will neither eradicate the pathogen nor prevent latent infection. Next-generation vaccines should attempt to both prevent TB infection and eradicate established latent TB infection (Kaufmann 2010). Another approach attempts to boost immunological memory induced by an initial priming vaccine (i.e. 'prime-boost' strategy) to improve and prolong protection. Such booster vaccines may be applied either in infancy soon after BCG vaccination, or later in adolescence when the risk of exposure to TB increases. 'Post-exposure' vaccines to prevent reactivation in latent infection target antigens and immunity pathways different from pre-exposure vaccines (Kaufmann 2011). Therapeutic vaccines administered adjunctively with treatment to shorten the duration of treatment and perhaps increase the efficacy of chemotherapy are also being clinically tested (Lambert et al. 2009; McShane 2011).

A major obstacle to vaccine development is our lack of knowledge of the immunopathogenesis of TB; better animal models that more accurately represent human disease and biomarkers indicating a protective immune response are urgently needed. Until biomarkers are available, more suitable clinical end points of TB disease and infection, particularly for paediatric and HIV-associated TB, would be invaluable assets in the effort to develop novel and effective vaccines.

The future of tuberculosis control: is elimination achievable?

TB elimination is defined as one case per million population. In order to achieve elimination, TB incidence globally will need to be reduced 1000-fold and in some high burden countries by 10,000-fold (Dye et al. 2005). Although much progress has been made under the current Stop TB plan (2006–2015), the rate of decline of TB disease globally is far from what is required to achieve TB elimination by 2050. An important milestone marking entry into the elimination phase, globally and nationally, is having fewer than ten TB deaths per million population. Encouragingly, using this definition, 35 countries and territories with populations in excess of 100,000 are already in the elimination phase, and many more could enter in the next one to two decades by simultaneously reducing TB case incidence and fatality (Dye et al. 2013). A comprehensive approach is required to achieve TB elimination by 2050 globally, particularly in high-burden countries. In New York City, TB case rates almost tripled between 1978 and 1992 and 'turning the tide' of TB was largely attributed to increased funding allowing better attention to the fundamentals of TB control (Frieden et al. 1995). These fundamentals—which can be addressed with existing technologies and should underpin all efforts to improve TB control—include health system strengthening, improved detection of persons self-presenting to health services, rapid and complete treatment initiation following diagnosis, improved cure rates, and universal access to care. These basic elements of TB control, while a necessary first step, will be inadequate to achieve elimination, however. Mathematical modelling suggests that augmenting these strategies with new TB drugs, diagnostics and vaccines may have an important impact on the global TB epidemic (Abu-Raddad 2009). The post 2015 Stop TB plan will focus on developing new tools and innovative strategies required to accelerate progress towards TB elimination by 2050. The priority areas of research to accelerate progress towards TB elimination are described in the Stop TB Research Roadmap (Stop TB Partnership 2011b). In order to maximize the population level impact, the new tools will need to be scaled up rapidly, with high coverage and combined with a range of other evidence-based interventions. The combination of intervention strategies that are likely to be effective in a given population will vary according to the relative proportion of underlying risk factors. The 'Know Your Epidemic/Know Your Response' approach requires knowledge of the TB epidemic in a country in order to select the most appropriate combination of interventions for that country.

Mathematical modelling can assist countries in assessing the relative effectiveness and cost effectiveness of different combinations of interventions. Modelling suggests that in high burden countries with high HIV prevalence, such as South Africa, preventing TB among HIV-infected persons must also be prioritized, and in high-burden countries with a low HIV prevalence, such as India and China, scaling up early case detection and treatment should be coupled simultaneously with treatment of latent TB infection in HIV-uninfected persons (Fig. 8.14.4) (Dye et al. 2013). In countries in the elimination phase, such as in Western Europe and the United States, modelling suggests that maintaining low rates of transmission while preventing reactivation TB among native populations while simultaneously preventing TB among foreign-born populations that account for the majority of cases, is required to achieve elimination of TB (Fig. 8.14.4) (Dye et al. 2013).

Conclusions

Over the past decade, for the first time in history, the number of new incident TB cases has started to decline worldwide. This momentous accomplishment can be attributed to an unprecedented scale-up of basic TB control measures, including access to diagnosis through sputum smear microscopy, use of effective drug therapy, and measures to prevent TB transmission and disease. Nevertheless, we remain far from the target of eliminating TB as a public health problem by 2050. Particular challenges include control of TB in key populations such as people living with HIV, individuals infected with drug-resistant TB, and children. Other groups at particularly high risk of TB transmission and disease include individuals living in mines, prisons, and impoverished areas; control measures in these populations are often inadequate. As TB control advances into the next decade, aggressive scale-up is needed of measures that can effectively fight TB in these populations, including active case finding in high-risk populations, antiretroviral therapy, TB preventive therapy, and infection control to prevent healthcare-associated transmission. If we are to achieve the goal of global TB elimination, existing technologies alone are likely also to be inadequate; better diagnostic tests, first- and second-line drugs, and eventually vaccines will be required. Public health leaders are beginning to envision a world free of TB—but this ambitious goal is still far from our present grasp. Only with increased funding, research, and innovation, coupled with political commitment and global attention to the fundamentals of TB control (detection, treatment, and prevention), can this vision be realized.

This chapter has outlined the epidemiology, public health approach, and future prospects for control of TB worldwide, demonstrating how existing tools have been used to turn the tide of TB incidence and bring discussion of TB elimination to the table. For the first time in more than 20 years, we also have the simultaneous promises of new first-line diagnostic tests for TB, new drugs and treatment regimens for TB, and a healthy pipeline of potential TB vaccines. Enhanced public health strategies for TB control—including active TB case finding and isoniazid preventive therapy—are finding wider use globally than ever before. Millions of people continue to die of TB every year, and we as a public health community must fulfil our obligation to continually strengthen the response to this ancient scourge until the number of TB deaths is brought to zero. To achieve this goal, however, a coordinated and comprehensive public health response will be required.

References

Abdool Karim, S.S., Naidoo, K., Grobler, A., et al. (2011). Integration of antiretroviral therapy with tuberculosis treatment. *The New England Journal of Medicine*, 365(16), 1492–501.

Abu-Raddad, L.J., Sabatelli, L., Achterberg, J.T., et al. (2009). Epidemiological benefits of more-effective tuberculosis vaccines, drugs, and diagnostics. *Proceedings of the National Academy of Sciences of the United States of America*, 106(33), 13980–5.

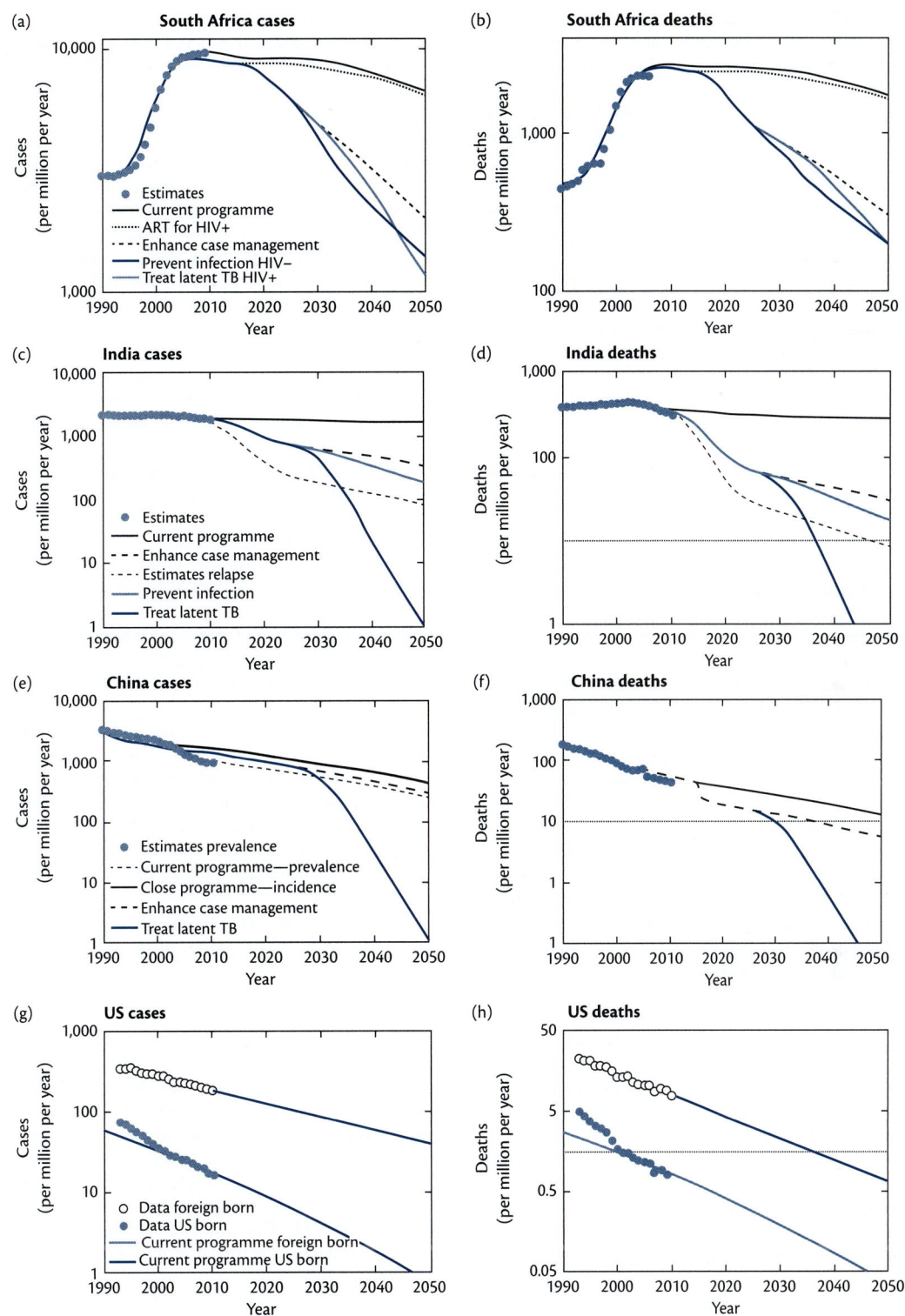

Fig. 8.14.4 Prospects for TB control in South Africa, India, China, and the United States of America.

Reprinted with permission from the *Annual Review of Public Health*, Volume 34 © 2013, pp. 271–286 by Annual Reviews www.annualreviews.org.

American Thoracic Society Committee of the Scientific Assembly on Environmental and Occupational Health (1997). Adverse effects of crystalline silica exposure. *American Journal of Respiratory and Critical Care Medicine*, 155(2), 761–8.

Andrews, J.R., Noubary, F., Walensky, R.P., Cerda, R., Losina, E., and Horsburgh, C.R. (2012). Risk of progression to active tuberculosis following reinfection with Mycobacterium tuberculosis. *Clinical Infectious Diseases*, 54(6), 784–91.

Anonymous (2007). Revised BCG vaccination guidelines for infants at risk for HIV infection. *Weekly Epidemiology Record*, 82(21), 193–6.

Atun, R., Weil, D.E., Eang, M.T., and Mwakyusa, D. (2010). Health-system strengthening and tuberculosis control. *The Lancet*, 375(9732), 2169–78.

Ayles, H., Muyoyeta, M., Du Toit, E., et al. (2013). Effect of household and community interventions on the burden of tuberculosis in southern Africa: the ZAMSTAR community-randomised trial. *The Lancet*, 382(9899), 1183–94.

Barry, C.E., 3rd, Boshoff, H.I., Dartois, V., et al. (2009). The spectrum of latent tuberculosis: rethinking the biology and intervention strategies. *Nature Reviews Microbiology*, 7(12), 845–55.

Basu, S., Stuckler, D., Bitton, A., and Glantz, S.A. (2011). Projected effects of tobacco smoking on worldwide tuberculosis control: mathematical modelling analysis. *BMJ*, 343, d5506.

Baussano, I., Williams, B.G., Nunn, P., Beggiato, M., Fedeli, U., and Scano, F. (2010). Tuberculosis incidence in prisons: a systematic review. *PLoS Medicine*, 7(12), e1000381.

Behr, M.A., Wilson, M.A., Gill, W.P., et al. (1999). Comparative genomics of BCG vaccines by whole-genome DNA microarray. *Science*, 284(5419), 1520–3.

Benatar, S.R. and Upshur, R. (2010). Tuberculosis and poverty: what could (and should) be done? *International Journal of Tuberculosis and Lung Disease*, 14(10), 1215–21.

Boehme, C.C., Nabeta, P., Hillemann, D., et al. (2010). Rapid molecular detection of tuberculosis and rifampin resistance. *The New England Journal of Medicine*, 363(11), 1005–15.

Boehme, C.C., Nicol, M.P., Nabeta, P., et al. (2011). Feasibility, diagnostic accuracy, and effectiveness of decentralised use of the Xpert MTB/RIF test for diagnosis of tuberculosis and multidrug resistance: a multicentre implementation study. *The Lancet*, 377(9776), 1495–505.

Bunyan, J. (1680). *The Life and Death of Mr. Badman*. London: Nathaniel Ponder.

Cain, K.P., Benoit, S.R., Winston, C.A., and MacKenzie, W.R. (2008). Tuberculosis among foreign-born persons in the United States. *Journal of the American Medical Association*, 300(4), 405–12.

Chaisson, R.E. and Martinson, N.A. (2008). Tuberculosis in Africa—combating an HIV-driven crisis. *The New England Journal of Medicine*, 358(11), 1089–92.

Chintu, C., Mudenda, V., Lucas, S., et al. (2002). Lung diseases at necropsy in African children dying from respiratory illnesses: a descriptive necropsy study. *The Lancet*, 360(9338), 985–90.

Churchyard, G.J., Fielding, K.L., Lewis, J.J., et al. (2014). Thibela TB Study Team. A trial of mass isoniazid preventive therapy for tuberculosis control. *New England Journal of Medicine* 2014;370:301–10. doi: 10.1056/NEJMoa1214289. PubMed PMID: 24450889.

Colditz, G.A., Berkey, C.S., Mosteller, F., et al. (1995). The efficacy of bacillus Calmette-Guerin vaccination of newborns and infants in the prevention of tuberculosis: meta-analyses of the published literature. *Pediatrics*, 96(1 Pt 1), 29–35.

Comstock, G.W. (1999). How much isoniazid is needed for prevention of tuberculosis among immunocompetent adults? *International Journal of Tuberculosis and Lung Disease*, 3(10), 847–50.

Connolly, M. and Nunn, P. (1996). Women and tuberculosis. *World Health Statistics Quarterly*, 49(2), 115–19.

Corbett, E.L., Bandason, T., Cheung, Y.B., et al. (2007). Epidemiology of tuberculosis in a high HIV prevalence population provided with enhanced diagnosis of symptomatic disease. *PLoS Medicine*, 4(1), e22.

Corbett, E.L., Bandason, T., Cheung, Y.B., et al. (2009). Prevalent infectious tuberculosis in Harare, Zimbabwe: burden, risk factors and implications for control. *International Journal of Tuberculosis and Lung Disease*, 13(10), 1231–7.

Corbett, E.L., Charalambous, S., Moloi, V.M., et al. (2004). Human immunodeficiency virus and the prevalence of undiagnosed tuberculosis in African gold miners. *American Journal of Respiratory and Critical Care Medicine*, 170(6), 673–9.

Corbett, E.L., Churchyard, G.J., Clayton, T.C., et al. (2000). HIV infection and silicosis: the impact of two potent risk factors on the incidence of mycobacterial disease in South African miners. *AIDS*, 17, 2759–68.

Corbett, E.L., Watt, C.J., Walker, N., et al. (2003). The growing burden of tuberculosis: global trends and interactions with the HIV epidemic. *Archives of Internal Medicine*, 163(9), 1009–21.

Cowie, R.L. (1994). The epidemiology of tuberculosis in gold miners with silicosis. *American Journal of Respiratory and Critical Care Medicine*, 150(5 Pt 1), 1460–2.

Dalton, T., Cegielski, P., Akksilp, S., et al. (2012). Prevalence of and risk factors for resistance to second-line drugs in people with multidrug-resistant tuberculosis in eight countries: a prospective cohort study. *The Lancet*, 380(9851), 1406–17.

Davis, J.L., Dowdy, D.W., den Boon, S., Walter, N.D., Katamba, A., and Cattamanchi, A. (2012). Test and treat: a new standard for smear-positive tuberculosis. *Journal of Acquired Immune Deficiency Syndromes*, 61(1), e6–8.

Diacon, A.H., Donald, P.R., Pym, A., et al. (2012). Randomized pilot trial of eight weeks of bedaquiline (TMC207) treatment for multidrug-resistant tuberculosis: long-term outcome, tolerability, and effect on emergence of drug resistance. *Antimicrobial Agents and Chemotherapy*, 56(6), 3271–6.

Dooley, K.E. and Chaisson, R.E. (2009). Tuberculosis and diabetes mellitus: convergence of two epidemics. *The Lancet Infectious Diseases*, 9(12), 737–46.

Dowdy, D.W., Chaisson, R.E., Moulton, L.H., and Dorman, S.E. (2006). The potential impact of enhanced diagnostic techniques for tuberculosis driven by HIV: a mathematical model. *AIDS*, 20(5), 751–62.

Dowdy, D.W., Golub, J.E., Chaisson, R.E., and Saraceni, V. (2012). Heterogeneity in tuberculosis transmission and the role of geographic hotspots in propagating epidemics. *Proceedings of the National Academy of Sciences of the United States of America*, 109(24), 9557–62.

Dowdy, D.W., O'Brien, M.A., and Bishai, D. (2008). Cost-effectiveness of novel diagnostic tools for the diagnosis of tuberculosis. *International Journal of Tuberculosis and Lung Disease*, 9, 1021–9.

Durovni, B., Saraceni, V., Moulton, L.H., et al. (2013). Effect of improved tuberculosis screening and isoniazid preventive therapy on incidence of tuberculosis and death in patients with HIV in clinics in Rio de Janeiro, Brazil: a stepped wedge, cluster-randomised trial. *The Lancet Infectious Diseases*, 13, 852–858.

Dye, C., Garnett, G.P., Sleeman, K., and Williams, B.G. (1998). Prospects for worldwide tuberculosis control under the WHO DOTS strategy. *The Lancet*, 352(9144), 1886–91.

Dye, C., Glaziou, P., Floyd, K., and Raviglione, M. (2013). Prospects for tuberculosis elimination. *Annual Review of Public Health*, 34, 271–86.

Dye, C., Lonnroth, K., Jaramillo, E., Williams, B.G., and Raviglione, M. (2009). Trends in tuberculosis incidence and their determinants in 134 countries. *Bulletin of the World Health Organization*, 87(9), 683–91.

Dye, C., Watt, C.J., Bleed, D.M., Hosseini, S.M., and Raviglione, M.C. (2005). Evolution of tuberculosis control and prospects for reducing tuberculosis incidence, prevalence, and deaths globally. *Journal of the American Medical Association*, 293(22), 2767–75.

El-Sadr, W.M. and De Cock, K.M. (2009). Health systems exist for real people. Introduction. *Journal of Acquired Immune Deficiency Syndromes*, 52(Suppl. 1), S1–2.

Fielding, K.L., Grant, A.D., Lewis, J.J., Hayes, R.J., and Churchyard, G.J. (2012). *Individual-Level Effect of Isoniazid Preventive Therapy on Risk of Tuberculosis in the Thibela TB Study*. Abstract 150bLB at 19th Conference on Retroviruses and Opportunistic Infections, Seattle, WA, March 2012.

Fox, G.J., Barry, S.E., Britton, W.J., and Marks, G.B. (2013). Contact investigation for tuberculosis: a systematic review and meta-analysis. *European Respiratory Journal*, 41(1), 140–56.

Frieden, T.R., Fujiwara, P.I., Washko, R.M., and Hamburg, M.A. (1995). Tuberculosis in New York City—turning the tide. *The New England Journal of Medicine*, 333(4), 229–33.

Gajalakshmi, V., Peto, R., Kanaka, T.S., and Jha, P. (2003). Smoking and mortality from tuberculosis and other diseases in India: retrospective study of 43000 adult male deaths and 35000 controls. *The Lancet*, 362(9383), 507–15.

Gandhi, N.R., Moll, A., Sturm, A.W., et al. (2006). Extensively drug-resistant tuberculosis as a cause of death in patients co-infected with tuberculosis and HIV in a rural area of South Africa. *The Lancet*, 368(9547), 1575–80.

Gandhi, N.R., Moll, A.P., Lalloo, U., et al. (2009). Successful integration of tuberculosis and HIV treatment in rural South Africa: the Sizonq'oba study. *Journal of Acquired Immune Deficiency Syndromes*, 50(1), 37–43.

Gandhi, N.R., Weissman, D., Moodley, P., et al. (2013). Nosocomial transmission of extensively drug-resistant tuberculosis in a rural hospital in South Africa. *Journal of Infectious Diseases*, 207(1), 9–17.

Getahun, H. and Raviglione, M. (2011). Transforming the global tuberculosis response through effective engagement of civil society organizations: the role of the World Health Organization. *Bulletin of the World Health Organization*, 89(8), 616–18.

Ghebreyesus, T.A., Kazatchkine, M., Sidibe, M., and Nakatani, H. (2010). Tuberculosis and HIV: time for an intensified response. *The Lancet*, 375(9728), 1757–8.

Golub, J.E., Mohan, C.I., Comstock, G.W., and Chaisson, R.E. (2005). Active case finding of tuberculosis: historical perspective and future prospects. *International Journal of Tuberculosis and Lung Disease*, 9(11), 1183–203.

Gounder, C.R., Wada, N.I., Kensler, C., et al. (2011). Active tuberculosis case-finding among pregnant women presenting to antenatal clinics in Soweto, South Africa. *Journal of Acquired Immune Deficiency Syndromes*, 57(4), e77–84.

Harries, A.D., Jensen, P.M., Zachariah, R., Rusen, I.D., and Enarson, D.A. (2009). How health systems in sub-Saharan Africa can benefit from tuberculosis and other infectious disease programmes. *International Journal of Tuberculosis and Lung Disease*, 13(10), 1194–9.

Havlir, D.V., Kendall, M.A., Ive, P., et al. (2011). Timing of antiretroviral therapy for HIV-1 infection and tuberculosis. *The New England Journal of Medicine*, 365(16), 1482–91.

Hillemann, D., Rusch-Gerdes, S., and Richter, E. (2007). Evaluation of the GenoType MTBDRplus assay for rifampin and isoniazid susceptibility testing of Mycobacterium tuberculosis strains and clinical specimens. *Journal of Clinical Microbiology*, 45(8), 2635–40.

Hillemann, D., Rusch-Gerdes, S., and Richter, E. (2009). Feasibility of the GenoType MTBDRsl assay for fluoroquinolone, amikacin-capreomycin, and ethambutol resistance testing of Mycobacterium tuberculosis strains and clinical specimens. *Journal of Clinical Microbiology*, 47(6), 1767–72.

Hoa, N.B., Cobelens, F.G., Sy, D.N., Nhung, N.V., Borgdorff, M.W., and Tiemersma, E.W. (2012). Yield of interview screening and chest X-ray abnormalities in a tuberculosis prevalence survey. *International Journal of Tuberculosis and Lung Disease*, 16(6), 762–7.

Hoft, D.F. (2008). Tuberculosis vaccine development: goals, immunological design, and evaluation. *The Lancet*, 372(9633), 164–75.

Janssens, J.P. and Rieder, H.L. (2008). An ecological analysis of incidence of tuberculosis and per capita gross domestic product. *European Respiratory Journal*, 32(5), 1415–16.

Jensen, P.A., Lambert, L.A., Iademarco, M.F., and Ridzon, R. (2005). Guidelines for preventing the transmission of Mycobacterium tuberculosis in health-care settings, 2005. *Morbidity and Mortality Weekly Report Recommendations and Reports*, 54(RR-17), 1–141.

Jeon, C.Y. and Murray, M.B. (2008). Diabetes mellitus increases the risk of active tuberculosis: a systematic review of 13 observational studies. *PLoS Medicine*, 5(7), e152.

Joshi, R., Reingold, A.L., Menzies, D., and Pai, M. (2006). Tuberculosis among health-care workers in low- and middle-income countries: a systematic review. *PLoS Medicine*, 3(12), e494.

Kaufmann, S.H. (2010). Future vaccination strategies against tuberculosis: thinking outside the box. *Immunity*, 33(4), 567–77.

Kaufmann, S.H. (2011). Fact and fiction in tuberculosis vaccine research: 10 years later. *The Lancet Infectious Diseases*, 11(8), 633–40.

Keeler, E., Perkins, M.D., Small, P., et al. (2006). Reducing the global burden of tuberculosis: the contribution of improved diagnostics. *Nature*, 444, 49–57.

Lambert, P.H., Hawkridge, T., and Hanekom, W.A. (2009). New vaccines against tuberculosis. *Clinics in Chest Medicine*, 30(4), 811–26.

Lawn, S.D., Harries, A.D., Williams, B.G., et al. (2011). Antiretroviral therapy and the control of HIV-associated tuberculosis. Will ART do it? *International Journal of Tuberculosis and Lung Disease*, 15(5), 571–81.

Lawn, S.D., Kerkhoff, A.D., Vogt, M., and Wood, R. (2012). Diagnostic accuracy of a low-cost, urine antigen, point-of-care screening assay for HIV-associated pulmonary tuberculosis before antiretroviral therapy: a descriptive study. *The Lancet Infectious Diseases*, 12(3), 201–9.

Lawn, S.D., Myer, L., Bekker, L.G., and Wood, R. (2007). Tuberculosis-associated immune reconstitution disease: incidence, risk factors and impact in an antiretroviral treatment service in South Africa. *AIDS*, 21(3), 335–41.

Leung, C.C., Li, T., Lam, T.H., et al. (2004). Smoking and tuberculosis among the elderly in Hong Kong. *American Journal of Respiratory and Critical Care Medicine*, 170(9), 1027–33.

Lienhardt, C., Glaziou, P., Uplekar, M., Lonnroth, K., Getahun, H., and Raviglione, M. (2012). Global tuberculosis control: lessons learnt and future prospects. *Nature Reviews Microbiology*, 10(6), 407–16.

Lin, H.H., Ezzati, M., and Murray, M. (2007). Tobacco smoke, indoor air pollution and tuberculosis: a systematic review and meta-analysis. *PLoS Medicine*, 4(1), e20.

Lonnroth, K., Jaramillo, E., Williams, B.G., Dye, C., and Raviglione, M. (2009). Drivers of tuberculosis epidemics: the role of risk factors and social determinants. *Social Science & Medicine*, 68(12), 2240–6.

Maher, D. (2010). Re-thinking global health sector efforts for HIV and tuberculosis epidemic control: promoting integration of programme activities within a strengthened health system. *BMC Public Health*, 10, 394.

Marais, B.J., Hesseling, A.C., Gie, R.P., Schaaf, H.S., and Beyers, N. (2006). The burden of childhood tuberculosis and the accuracy of community-based surveillance data. *International Journal of Tuberculosis and Lung Disease*, 10(3), 259–63.

McShane, H. (2011). Tuberculosis vaccines: beyond bacille Calmette-Guerin. *Philosophical Transactions of the Royal Society of London. Series B: Biological Sciences*, 366(1579), 2782–9.

Medical Research Council (1948). Streptomycin treatment of pulmonary tuberculosis. *British Medical Journal*, 2(4582), 769–82.

Menzies, D., Benedetti, A., Paydar, A., et al. (2009). Effect of duration and intermittency of rifampin on tuberculosis treatment outcomes: a systematic review and meta-analysis. *PLoS Medicine*, 6(9), e1000146.

Moore, D.A.J., Evans, C.A.W., Gilman, R.H., et al. (2006). Microscopic-observation drug-susceptibility assay for the diagnosis of TB. *The New England Journal of Medicine*, 355(15), 1539–50.

Orenstein, E.W., Basu, S., Shah, N.S., et al. (2009). Treatment outcomes among patients with multidrug-resistant tuberculosis: systematic review and meta-analysis. *The Lancet Infectious Diseases*, 9(3), 153–61.

Owens, J.P., Fofana, M.O., and Dowdy, D.W. (2013). Cost-effectiveness of novel first-line treatment regimens for tuberculosis. *International Journal of Tuberculosis and Lung Disease*, 17(5), 590–6.

Oxlade, O. and Murray, M. (2012). Tuberculosis and poverty: why are the poor at greater risk in India? *PLoS One*, 7(11), e47533.

Pai, M., Zwerling, A., and Menzies, D. (2008). Systematic review: T-cell-based assays for the diagnosis of latent tuberculosis infection: an update. *Annals of Internal Medicine*, 149(3), 177–84.

Rangaka, M.X., Wilkinson, K.A., Glynn, J.R., et al. (2012). Predictive value of interferon-gamma release assays for incident active tuberculosis: a systematic review and meta-analysis. *The Lancet Infectious Diseases*, 12(1), 45–55.

Rieder, H.L. (2002). *Interventions for Tuberculosis Control and Elimination.* Paris: International Union Against TB and Lung Disease.

Rieder, H.L., Cauthen, G.M., Comstock, G.W., and Snider, D.E., Jr. (1989). Epidemiology of tuberculosis in the United States. *Epidemiologic Reviews*, 11, 79–98.

Samandari, T., Agizew, T.B., Nyirenda, S., et al. (2011). 6-month versus 36-month isoniazid preventive treatment for tuberculosis in adults with HIV infection in Botswana: a randomised, double-blind, placebo-controlled trial. *The Lancet*, 377(9777), 1588–98.

Samb, B., Celletti, F., Holloway, J., Van Damme, W., De Cock, K.M., and Dybul, M. (2007). Rapid expansion of the health workforce in response to the HIV epidemic. *The New England Journal of Medicine*, 357(24), 2510–14.

Skripconoka, V., Danilovits, M., Pehme, L., et al. (2013). Delamanid improves outcomes and reduces mortality for multidrug-resistant tuberculosis. *European Respiratory Journal*, 41(6), 1393–400.

Spence, D.P., Hotchkiss, J., Williams, C.S., and Davies, P.D. (1993). Tuberculosis and poverty. *BMJ*, 307(6907), 759–61.

Sterling, T.R., Villarino, M.E., Borisov, A.S., et al. (2011). Three months of rifapentine and isoniazid for latent tuberculosis infection. *The New England Journal of Medicine*, 365(23), 2155–66.

Stop TB Partnership (2006). *The Stop TB Strategy.* Geneva: WHO.

Stop TB Partnership (2008). *Contributing to Health System Strengthening: Guiding Principles for National Tuberculosis Programmes.* Geneva: WHO.

Stop TB Partnership (2011a). *The Global Plan to Stop TB, 2011–2015. Transforming the Fight: Towards Elimination of Tuberculosis.* Geneva: WHO.

Stop TB Partnership (2011b). *An International Roadmap for Tuberculosis Research: Toward a World Free of Tuberculosis.* Geneva: WHO.

Styblo, K. and Bumgarner, R. (1991). *Tuberculosis can be Controlled with Existing Technologies: Evidence.* The Hague: Tuberculosis Surveillance Research Unit.

Swaminathan, S. and Rekha, B. (2010). Pediatric tuberculosis: global overview and challenges. *Clinical Infectious Diseases*, 50(Suppl. 3), S184–94.

Tiemersma, E.W., van der Werf, M.J., Borgdorff, M.W., Williams, B.G., and Nagelkerke, N.J. (2011). Natural history of tuberculosis: duration and fatality of untreated pulmonary tuberculosis in HIV negative patients: a systematic review. *PLoS One*, 6(4), e17601.

Trunz, B.B., Fine, P., and Dye, C. (2006). Effect of BCG vaccination on childhood tuberculous meningitis and miliary tuberculosis worldwide: a meta-analysis and assessment of cost-effectiveness. *The Lancet*, 367(9517), 1173–80.

Tuberculosis Coalition for Technical Assistance and International Committee of the Red Cross (2009). *Guidelines for Control of Tuberculosis in Prisons.* [Online] Available at: http://pdf.usaid.gov/pdf_docs/PNADP462.pdf.

Udwadia, Z.F., Amale, R.A., Ajbani, K.K., and Rodrigues, C. (2012). Totally drug-resistant tuberculosis in India. *Clinical Infectious Diseases*, 54(4), 579–81.

Van Leth, F., van der Werf, M.J., and Borgdorff, M.W. (2008). Prevalence of tuberculous infection and incidence of tuberculosis: a re-assessment of the Styblo rule. *Bulletin of the World Health Organization*, 86(1), 20–6.

Vassall, A., van Kampen, S., Sohn, H., et al. (2011). Rapid diagnosis of tuberculosis with the Xpert MTB/RIF assay in high burden countries: a cost-effectiveness analysis. *PLoS Medicine*, 8(11), e1001120.

Vynnycky, E. and Fine, P.E.M. (1997). The natural history of tuberculosis: the implications of age-dependent risks of disease and the role of reinfection. *Epidemiology & Infection*, 119(2), 183–201.

Wenger, P.N., Otten, J., Breeden, A., Orfas, D., Beck-Sague, C.M., and Jarvis, W.R. (1995). Control of nosocomial transmission of multidrug-resistant Mycobacterium tuberculosis among healthcare workers and HIV-infected patients. *The Lancet*, 345(8944), 235–40.

Williams, B.G., Granich, R., De Cock, K.M., Glaziou, P., Sharma, A., and Dye, C. (2010). Antiretroviral therapy for tuberculosis control in nine African countries. *Proceedings of the National Academy of Sciences of the United States of America*, 107(45), 19485–9.

World Health Organization (2006). *Guidance for National Tuberculosis Programmes on the Management of Tuberculosis in Children.* Geneva: WHO.

World Health Organization (2009). *WHO Policy on TB Infection Control in Health-Care Facilities, Congregate Settings and Households.* Geneva: WHO.

World Health Organization (2010a). *Treatment of Tuberculosis: Guidelines.* Geneva: WHO.

World Health Organization (2010b). *Multidrug and Extensively Drug-Resistant TB (M/XDR-TB), 2010 Global Report on Surveillance and Response.* Geneva: WHO.

World Health Organization (2011a). *Global Tuberculosis Control: WHO Report 2011.* Geneva: WHO.

World Health Organization (2011b). *Guidelines for the Programmatic Management of Drug-Resistant Tuberculosis—2011 Update.* Geneva: WHO.

World Health Organization (2012). *Global Tuberculosis Report 2012.* Geneva: WHO.

World Health Organization (n.d.). *Global Health Observatory Data Repository.* [Online] Available at: http://apps.who.int/ghodata/.

Wright, A., Zignol, M., Van Deun, A., et al. (2009). Epidemiology of antituberculosis drug resistance 2002-07: an updated analysis of the Global Project on Anti-Tuberculosis Drug Resistance Surveillance. *The Lancet*, 373(9678), 1861–73.

Yee, D., Valiquette, C., Pelletier, M., Parisien, I., Rocher, I., and Menzies, D. (2003). Incidence of serious side effects from first-line antituberculosis drugs among patients treated for active tuberculosis. *American Journal of Respiratory and Critical Care Medicine*, 167(11), 1472–7.

Zhao, Y., Xu, S., Wang, L., et al. (2012). National survey of drug-resistant tuberculosis in China. *The New England Journal of Medicine*, 366(23), 2161–70.

Zignol, M., van Gemert, W., Falzon, D., et al. (2012). Surveillance of anti-tuberculosis drug resistance in the world: an updated analysis, 2007–2010. *Bulletin of the World Health Organization*, 90(2), 111–19D.

Zwerling, A., Behr, M.A., Verma, A., Brewer, T.F., and Menzies, D., and Pai, M. (2011). The BCG World Atlas: a database of global BCG vaccination policies and practices. *PLoS Medicine*, 8(3), e1001012.

8.15

Malaria

Frank Sorvillo, Shira Shafir, and Benjamin Bristow

Introduction to malaria

Malaria remains one of the most important and intractable global public health problems. It is not hyperbole to suggest that this parasitic disease may be the most prolific killer of humans in history and its continuing impact is difficult to overstate. Currently an estimated 99 countries are affected by malaria with approximately 40 per cent of the world's population exposed to this preventable disease (World Health Organization (WHO) 2012).

Deadly periodic fevers, probably malaria, have been known since antiquity, yet it wasn't until the late nineteenth century that the cause and mechanism of transmission were elucidated (Harrison 1978). Alphonse Laveran, a French Army physician serving in North Africa, first identified the intraerythrocytic protozoan parasite, *Plasmodium*, in 1880 from the blood of a soldier with acute malaria. Seventeen years later Ronald Ross, a British physician serving in India, with painstaking effort, identified the 'dapple-winged' *Anopheles* mosquito as the vector. Both Laveran and Ross were awarded a Nobel Prize in in Physiology or Medicine for their work.

Malaria is a complex and daunting problem with an intricate life cycle and nuanced interplay of agent, host, vector, and environment that is further complicated by challenging political, economic, and social factors (Breman 2004). This chapter provides an overview of the relevant aspects of malaria focusing principally on the key public health-related issues including estimates of the current burden, description of the agent, life cycle, modes of transmission and vector aspects, discussion of epidemiological factors, basic information on clinical manifestations, diagnostic testing, treatment and chemoprophylaxis approaches, and delineation of control measures. Current challenges, controversies, and future directions are also presented.

Malaria agent

Malaria is caused by protozoal organisms of the genus *Plasmodium* (Beaver et al. 1994; Centers for Disease Control and Prevention (CDC) 2010a). While there are more than 100 species of *Plasmodium*, which can infect many animals such as reptiles, birds, and various mammals, historically, only four species of *Plasmodium* were recognized to infect humans in nature. A fifth species of malaria, the primate parasite *P. knowlesi*, though first known to cause infection in humans in 1967, has recently emerged as an important cause of zoonotic malaria in South East Asia (Antinori 2013). These five species of malaria differ in geographic distribution, clinical manifestations, and details of their life cycle. The most important species in terms of virulence and global burden is *P. falciparum*, which accounts for the vast majority of deaths. However, the impact of *P. vivax* has been increasingly recognized as considerable. *P. ovale* and *P. malariae* have more limited distribution and significance.

Life cycle

The life cycle of malaria is complex, slightly different for each species, and necessarily involves both humans and *Anopheles* mosquitoes (Aly et al. 2009; CDC 2010a). When a human host is bitten by a malaria-infected mosquito, sporozoites are inoculated (Fig. 8.15.1). The sporozoites will travel via the blood and infect liver cells where they will mature into schizonts containing large numbers of merozoites. In the case of *P. vivax* and *P. ovale*, hypnozoites, a dormant stage, can persist in the liver and, if not appropriately treated, can cause relapse by releasing merozoites into the bloodstream weeks, months, and rarely years later. The entire process of initial replication in the liver is referred to as exoerythrocytic schizogony. After this process is complete, schizonts will eventually rupture and release merozoites that will enter red blood cells (RBCs). In a process known as erythrocytic schizogony, merozoites initially form small ring stages, then larger trophozoites, and subsequently form erythrocytic schizonts via asexual replication. These schizonts rupture, releasing merozoites, which invade other erythrocytes. The cycle of rupturing merozoites will eventually synchronize, flooding the bloodstream with parasitic material, resulting in many of the clinical manifestations of infection. For *P. falciparum*, *vivax*, and *ovale*, this happens in a 2-day cycle (CDC 2010b). In the case of *P. malariae*, the cycle follows a 3-day course, while *P. knowlesi* has a 24-hour cycle. Some of the merozoites will differentiate into gametocytes (macrogametocytes and microgametocytes), the sexual erythrocytic stage, which can infect mosquitoes.

If an infected human is bitten by a susceptible *Anopheles* mosquito, the microgametocytes and macrogametocytes will be ingested and the sporogonic cycle will begin (CDC 2010a, 2010b). In the stomach of the mosquito, the microgametes will fertilize the macrogametes and a zygote will be formed. The motile, elongated zygote, known as an ookinete, will invade the midgut wall of the mosquito and develop into an oocyst. The oocyst will enlarge and eventually rupture releasing sporozoites which will migrate to the salivary glands of the mosquito and be available to infect another host. The complete cycle in the mosquito takes approximately 10–18 days, a period termed the extrinsic incubation cycle or extrinsic cycle. When the infected mosquito feeds, sporozoites will be inoculated into the human host, and the cycle will begin anew.

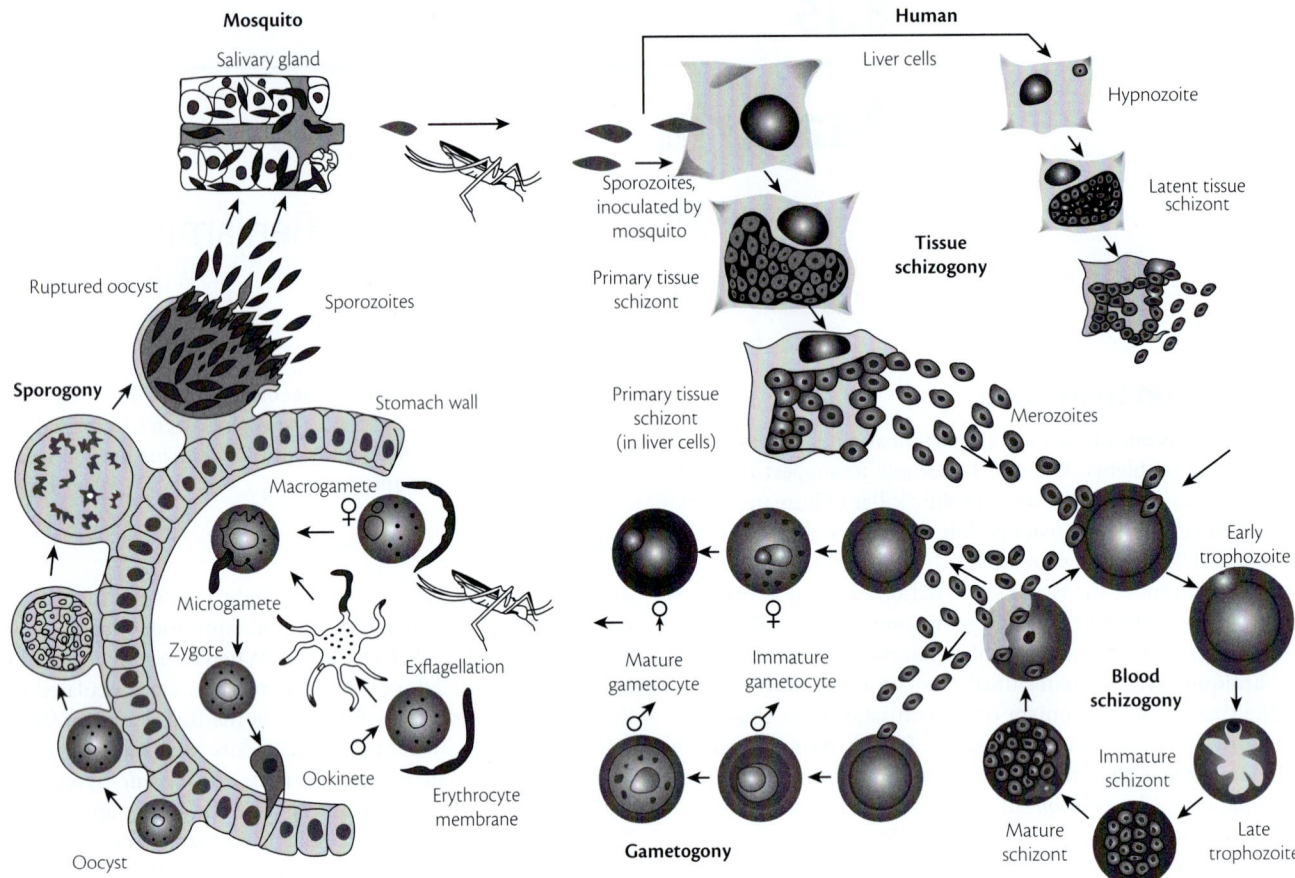

Fig. 8.15.1 Life cycle of malaria parasite.

Reproduced from Morrow, R.H., Moss, W.J., Malaria, in Detels et al. (eds.), *Oxford Textbook of Public Health*, Fifth Edition, Oxford University Press, Oxford, UK, Copyright © 2009, by permission of Oxford University Press.

Transmission

Transmission of the malaria parasite occurs through the bite of an infected female *Anopheles* mosquito (CDC 2012). Only female adult mosquitoes of the *Anopheles* genus play a role in malaria transmission as they are the only ones who take a blood meal, since they require the protein and iron from the blood for egg development. Male mosquitoes feed on nectar and other sources of sugar and therefore do not transmit malaria. Most *Anopheles* species are either nocturnal or crepuscular and consquently the highest risk of malaria transmission is from dusk until dawn. Malaria transmission can occur anywhere there are infected humans, mosquitoes that are capable of being infected, and contact between the two.

As with all mosquito species, anophelines have four stages in their life cycle which include egg, larva, pupa, which are aquatic stages, and the adult (Beaver 1984; CDC 2012). The adult female lays approximately 50–200 eggs that are deposited singly in water sources where they hatch in 2–3 days into larvae which will subsequently moult into pupae. Both larvae and pupae breathe through spiracles and must come to the surface frequently. After a few days the adult mosquito emerges. The time from egg to adult varies by species and ambient temperature but typically takes 5–14 days in tropical conditions. Anophelines can utilize diverse water sources for breeding.

The species of *Anopheles* present in an area at a given time will influence the intensity of malaria transmission (Sinka et al. 2012). Different *Anopheles* species have different capacity to serve as a malaria vector. Out of over 400 *Anopheles* species, only 30–40 are easily infected and will produce large numbers of infectious sporozoites that they can subsequently transmit when they feed on susceptible humans. Table 8.15.1 presents selected major malaria vectors by geographic regions.

Additionally, the feeding preferences and resting behaviour of the mosquito can have a significant impact on the ability to effectively transmit malaria (Beaver 1984; CDC 2012). Anthropophilic mosquitoes, species that preferentially feed on humans such as *Anopheles gambiae*, tend to be the most effective vectors. Zoophilic mosquitoes, species that preferentially feed on non-human animals, tend to be less effective. Mosquitoes that prefer to feed inside (termed endophagic) also tend to be more effective vectors than those that are exophagic, preferring to eat outside, simply because they are likely to have greater contact with humans. Resting behaviour of the mosquito is also important because of the impact that it can have on control strategies. Mosquitoes that prefer to rest inside (termed endophilic) after they have taken a blood meal will be more likely to be effectively controlled by indoor residual spraying than those that prefer to rest outside (exophilic) after their blood meal (Shiff 2002).

considered malaria until proven otherwise. Approximately one in three returned international travellers presenting to a specialized travel or tropical medicine clinic, with a systemic febrile illness, has malaria (Wilson et al. 2007). Prevention of malaria in the traveller can be accomplished via personal protective measures for mosquito bite prevention and the compliant use of an effective antimalarial chemoprophylactic agent. Most travellers who develop malaria do so because they do not adhere to an effective chemoprophylactic drug regimen; however, travellers who do adhere to an effective drug regimen can still develop malaria. Fatalities may be a result of delay in seeking medical treatment, failure to obtain an adequate travel history, delayed diagnosis, laboratory error, late initiation of treatment, and/or inappropriate therapy (Dorsey et al. 2000).

Selection of an effective chemoprophylactic drug regimen is based on assessment of malaria risk based on an individual's travel itinerary and resistance patterns, and based on the individual's medical history and preferences. The agents most commonly used for chemoprophylaxis are atovaquone/proguanil, mefloquine, doxycycline, and chloroquine. These agents are effective against the erythrocytic stages of the parasite life cycle.

For travellers to *P. vivax* and *P. ovale* endemic regions, terminal prophylaxis with primaquine directed against the liver hypnozoites should be considered at the end of travel. Primaquine can cause severe or fatal haemolysis in individuals with G6PD deficiency. G6PD deficiency must be ruled out with laboratory testing prior to administration.

Vaccine

Development of an effective malaria vaccine would be a major and important milestone in malaria control. Several approaches including subunit vaccines, whole irradiated sporozoite preparations, and transmission-blocking methods have been proposed. However, despite considerable hope, aggressive efforts, and substantial economic investment to develop an effective malaria vaccine, success has been elusive (Graves and Gelband 2006; RTS,S Clinical Trials Partnership 2012; Bejon et al. 2013). Most vaccine efficacy studies have demonstrated at best only modest protection from infection. In a recent pooled analysis of the results of phase 2 data for the most advanced candidate malaria vaccine (RTS,S/AS01 or AS02) Bejon and colleagues reported an overall vaccine efficacy of 36 per cent (95 per cent CI 24–45 per cent) that was lowest, 4 per cent (95 per cent CI –10 to 22 per cent) in high transmission areas. Moreover, no protection was observed after 3 years (0 per cent, 95 per cent CI –38 to 38 per cent). Preliminary data from the phase 3 trial have estimated modest vaccine efficacy, however the full data from this ongoing trial are not expected until 2015. A better understanding of the immunological mechanisms of malaria and second-generation vaccines may be needed before a vaccine can be effectively integrated into control efforts.

Treatment

Treatment, which can serve to reduce the reservoir of people infected with malaria, and the period of infectivity, has already been addressed in this chapter. However it should be recognized that antimalarial therapy is not directly active against gametocytes.

Challenges to malaria prevention and control

Inadequate surveillance

Current malaria surveillance activities are woefully deficient (Breman and Holloway 2007). Effective surveillance and accurate data are essential to efforts to reduce the burden of malaria. Successful targeting of interventions and pursuit of reasonable strategies for control of malaria are not possible without a clear understanding of the prevalence and incidence of malaria and where it is occurring. Importantly, surveillance also provides information that enables an evaluation of the effectiveness of ongoing interventions and enables redirecting of resources. For these reasons, strong commitments to better data and significant improvements in surveillance systems should be a priority.

Funding

Ultimately sufficient financial support may be the most important factor in the success of lasting reductions of the burden of malaria. Resource constraints have been blamed as the primary reason for the failure of the previous major mobilization against malaria (Cohen et al. 2012). Adequate funding is also key to capacity development (Greenwood et al. 2012). Despite a massive influx of resources over the past decade for malaria, increasing from about $100 million in 2003 to $1.71 billion in 2010, there has been a plateauing of funding ($1.66 billion in 2011 and $1.84 billion in 2012). Moreover, competing priorities at the global and national levels threaten continued allocation of funds. Ultimately, static funding, while admittedly considerable, may not be sufficient to realize permanent decreases in the burden of malaria.

Operational challenges

It has been suggested that the previous global effort to eradicate malaria failed, in part, as a result of requiring scientists to become field managers (Shiff 2002). Even the best tools and the most noble of goals will be destined to fail without effective implementation. Such implementation requires strong and sustained operational direction and long-term commitments with integration into national health infrastructure and participation of communities (malERA Consultative Group on Health Systems and Operational Research 2011; Najera et al. 2011).

Insecticide resistance

Sixty-four malaria-endemic countries are currently reporting mosquito resistance to at least one insecticide used for malaria control including pyrethroids (Ranson et al. 2011). In addition, selective pressure, induced by insecticides, has resulted in modified vector behaviour and emergence of new vectors being observed (Asidi et al. 2012).

Repurposing insecticides currently used for agriculture and reformulating current preparations may offer tools to combat vector resistance. Using combinations of insecticides, rotating different preparations and mosaic application are additional approaches to resistance management (malERA Consultative Group on Vector Control 2011; Alonso et al. 2013).

Drug resistance

Given the existing widespread resistance of *P. falciparum* to chloroquine and SP, the availability of highly effective artemisinin-based compounds has provided a major tool for reducing the burden of malaria. Subsidies (termed the Affordable Medicines Facility) for artemisinin-based combination therapy have led to increased availability and reduced costs (Tougheret al. 2012). However, reports of emerging artemisinin resistance on the Cambodia–Thailand and Thailand–Myanmar borders are cause for concern (Fairhurst et al. 2012). Resistance is driven by poor quality and counterfeit medication as well as the use of artemisinin monotherapy. A recent published report indicates that up to 36 per cent of antimalarial drugs collected in southeast Asia were falsified, whereas in sub-Saharan Africa, a third failed chemical assay analysis (Nayyar et al. 2012).

Resistance to SP also threatens to compromise its use for intermittent preventive therapy in pregnancy and for children and infants. Combination therapy using azithromycin and chloroquine may offer an alternative that can provide protection against sexually transmitted infections as well (Chico et al. 2011).

Testing of currently available drugs for antimalarial activity is one of the key approaches to combating drug resistance and can accelerate production of new therapies as well as reduce costs. Itraconazole, posaconazole, and atorvastatin are among such commercially available drugs that have demonstrated activity against malaria. In addition, chemical modification of available antimalarials and hybridization of existing drugs to improve their effectiveness and high-throughput screening and molecular modelling are being employed in attempts to identify new potentially effective therapies (Aguiar et al. 2012).

Summary

Malaria is a preventable disease but remains one of the world's great scourges. However, renewed resources and international resolve have resulted in progress towards reducing the burden of malaria and led to cautious optimism about the future elimination of this disease. Given the availability of proven methods for malaria control, as well as the promise offered by innovative approaches for vector control, improved diagnostics and therapy, and the potential for vaccine development, such cautious optimism is not unwarranted. The science of malaria may be reaching the point of making elimination, and even eradication, possible.

However, science alone will be insufficient to conquer malaria and both significant resources and unflagging resolve, at the international and local level, will be necessary to consolidate the recent gains made and to make additional progress. Yet, both resources and resolve are not unlimited, and areas impacted by malaria have many pressing problems such as HIV/AIDS, tuberculosis, food shortages, poverty, pollution, and other critical issues (Lozano et al. 2012). Reducing the burden of malaria will have to be part of a broader dialogue to determine priorities (De Cock et al. 2013).

References

Abeku, T. (2007). Response to malaria epidemics in Africa. *Emerging Infectious Diseases*, 13, 681–6.

Aguiar, A.C.C., da Rocja, E.M.M., de Souza, N.B., and Krettli, A. (2012). New approaches in malarial drug discovery and development—A review. *Memórias do Instituto Oswaldo Cruz*, 107, 831–45.

Alonso, P.L. and Tanner, M. (2013). Public health challenges and prospects for malaria control and elimination. *Nature Medicine*, 19, 150–5.

Aly, A.S., Vaughan, A.M., and Kappe, S.H. (2009). Malaria parasite development in the mosquito and infection of the mammalian host. *Annual Review of Microbiology*, 63, 195–221.

Antinori, S., Galimberti, L., Milazzo, L., and Corbellino, M. (2013). Plasmodium knowlesi: the emerging zoonotic malaria parasite. *Acta Tropica*, 125, 191–201.

Aponte, J.J., Schellenberg, D., Egan, A., et al. (2009). Efficacy and safety of intermittent preventive treatment with sulfadoxine-pyrimethamine for malaria in African infants: a pooled analysis of six randomised, placebo-controlled trials. *The Lancet*, 374, 1533–42.

Ash, L.R. and Orihel, T.C. (2007). *Atlas of Human Parasitology* (5th ed.). Chicago, IL: American Society for Clinical Pathology.

Asidi, A., N'Guessan, R., Akogbeto, M., Curtis, C., and Rowland, M. (2012). Loss of household protection from use of insecticide-treated nets against pyrethroid-resistant mosquitoes, Benin. *Emerging Infectious Diseases*, 18, 1101–6.

Ayi, I., Nonaka, D., Adjovu, J.K., et al. (2010). School-based participatory health education for malaria control in Ghana: engaging children as health messengers. *Malaria Journal*, 9, 98.

Baird, J.K. (2013). Evidence and implications of mortality associated with acute Plasmodium vivax malaria. *Clinical Microbiology Reviews*, 26, 36–57.

Beaver, P., Jung, R.C., and Cupp, E.W. (1984). *Clinical Parasitology* (9th ed.). Philadelphia, PA: Lea & Febiger.

Bejon, P., White, M.T., Olotu, A., et al. (2013). Efficacy of RTS,S malaria vaccines: individual-participant pooled analysis of phase 2 data. *The Lancet Infectious Diseases*, 13, 319–27.

Bian, G., Joshi, D., Dong, Y., et al. (2013). Wolbachia invades Anopheles stephensi populations and induces refractoriness to Plasmodium infection. *Science*, 340, 748–51.

Bødker, R., Akida, J., Shayo, D., et al. (2003). Relationship between altitude and intensity of malaria transmission in the Usambara Mountains, Tanzania. *Journal of Medical Entomology*, 40, 706–17.

Breman, J.G., Alilio, M.S., and Mills, A. (2004). Conquering the intolerable burden of malaria: what's new, what's needed: a summary. *American Journal of Tropical Medicine and Hygiene*, 71(Suppl. 2), 1–15.

Breman, J.G. and Holloway, C.N. (2007). Malaria surveillance counts. *American Journal of Tropical Medicine and Hygiene*, 77(Suppl. 6), 36–47.

Breman, J.G., Mills, A., Snow, R.W., et al. (eds.) (2006). *Disease Control Priorities in Developing Countries*. New York: Oxford University Press/World Bank.

Centers for Disease Control and Prevention (2010a). *Malaria: Biology*. [Online] Available at: http://www.cdc.gov/malaria/about/biology/index.html.

Centers for Disease Control and Prevention (2010b). *Malaria Parasites*. [Online] Available at: http://www.cdc.gov/malaria/about/biology/parasites.html.

Centers for Disease Control and Prevention (2010c). *Malaria Transmission in the United States*. [Online] Available at: http://www.cdc.gov/malaria/about/us_transmission.html.

Centers for Disease Control and Prevention (2010d). *Human Factors and Malaria*. [Online] Available at: http://www.cdc.gov/malaria/about/biology/human_factors.html.

Centers for Disease Control and Prevention (2010e). *Ecology of Malaria*. [Online] Available at: http://www.cdc.gov/malaria/about/biology/ecology.html.

Centers for Disease Control and Prevention (2012). *Anopheles Mosquitoes*. [Online] Available at: http://www.cdc.gov/malaria/about/biology/mosquitoes/index.html.

Centers for Disease Control and Prevention (2014). *Impact of Malaria*. [Online] Available at: www.cdc.gov/malaria/malaria_worldwide/impact.html.

Centers for Disease Control and Prevention, Filler, S.J., MacArthur, J.R., et al. (2006). Locally acquired mosquito-transmitted malaria: a guide for investigations in the United States. *Morbidity and Mortality Weekly Report. Recommendations and Reports*, 55(RR-13), 1–9.

Chico, R.M. and Chandramohan, D. (2011). Azithromycin plus chloroquine: combination therapy for protection against malaria and sexually transmitted infections in pregnancy. *Expert Opinion on Drug Metabolism & Toxicology*, 7, 1153–67.

Cirimotich, C.M., Dong, Y., Clayton, A.M., et al. (2011). Natural microbe-mediated refractoriness to Plasmodium infection in Anopheles gambiae. *Science*, 332, 855–8.

Cohen, J.M., Smith, D.L., Cotter, C., et al. (2012). Malaria resurgence: a systematic review and assessment of its causes. *Malaria Journal*, 11, 122.

Cohuet, A., Harris, C., Robert, V., and Fontenille, D. (2010). Evolutionary forces on Anopheles: what makes a malaria vector? *Trends in Parasitology*, 26, 130–6.

Das, B.S. (2008). Renal failure in malaria. *Journal of Vector Borne Diseases*, 45, 83–97.

De Cock, K.M., Simone, P.M., Davison, V., and Slutsker, L. (2013). The new global health. *Emerging Infectious Diseases*, 19, 1192–7.

Dellicour, S., Tatem, A.J., Guerra, C.A., Snow, R.W., and ter Kuile, F.O. (2010). Quantifying the number of pregnancies at risk of malaria in 2007: a demographic study. *PLoS Medicine*, 7(1), e1000221.

Desai, M., ter Kuile, F.O., Nosten, F., et al. (2007). Epidemiology and burden of malaria in pregnancy. *The Lancet Infectious Diseases*, 7, 93–104.

Devarbhavi, H., Alvares, J.F., and Kumar, K.S. (2005). Severe falciparum malaria simulating fulminant hepatic failure. *Mayo Clinic Proceedings*, 80, 355–8.

Dhingra, N., Jha, P., Sharma, V.P., et al. (2010). Adult and child malaria mortality in India: a nationally representative mortality survey. *The Lancet*, 376, 1768–74.

Doolan, D.L., Dobaño, C., and Baird, J.K. (2009). Acquired immunity to malaria. *Clinical Microbiology Reviews*, 22, 13–36.

Dorsey, G., Gandhi, M., Oyugi, J.H., and Rosenthal, P.J. (2000). Difficulties in the prevention, diagnosis, and treatment of imported malaria. *Archives of Internal Medicine*, 160, 2505–10.

Elyazar, I.R.F., Gething, P.W., Patil, A.P., et al. (2011). Plasmodium falciparum malaria endemicity in Indonesia in 2010. *PLoS One*, 6, e21315.

Fairhurst, R.M., Nayyar, G.M., Breman, J.G., et al. (2012). Artemisinin-resistant malaria: research challenges, opportunities, and public health implications. *American Journal of Tropical Medicine and Hygiene*, 87, 231–41.

Gallup, J.L. and Sachs, J.D. (2001). The economic burden of malaria. *American Journal of Tropical Medicine and Hygiene*, 64(1–2 Suppl.), 85–96.

Gamble, C.L., Ekwaru, J.P., and ter Kuile, F.O. (2006). Insecticide-treated nets for preventing malaria in pregnancy. *Cochrane Database of Systematic Reviews*, 2, CD003755.

Gething, P.W., Elyazar, I.R.F., Moyes, C.L., et al. (2012). A long neglected world malaria map: Plasmodium vivax endemicity in 2010. *PLoS Neglected Tropical Diseases*, 6, e1814.

Graves, P.M. and Gelband, H. (2006). Vaccines for preventing malaria (blood-stage). *Cochrane Database of Systematic Reviews*, 4, CD006199.

Greenwood, B., Bhasin, A., and Targett, G. (2012). The Gates Malaria Partnership: a consortium approach to malaria research and capacity development. *Tropical Medicine & International Health*, 17, 558–63.

Guyatt, H.L. and Snow, R.W. (2004). Impact of malaria during pregnancy on low birth weight in sub-Saharan Africa. *Clinical Microbiology Reviews*, 17, 760–9.

Harrison, G. (1978). *Mosquitoes Malaria and Man. A History of Hostilities Since 1880*. New York: E.P. Dutton.

Hay, S.I., Okiro, E.A., Gething, P.W., et al. (2010). Estimating the global clinical burden of Plasmodium falciparum malaria in 2007. *PLoS Medicine*, 15(7), e1000290.

Imwong, M., Snounou, G., Pukrittayakamee, S., et al. (2007). Relapses of Plasmodium vivax infection usually result from activation of heterologous hypnozoites. *Journal of Infectious Diseases*, 195, 927.

Kayentao, K., Garner, P., van Eijk, A.M., et al. (2013). Intermittent preventive therapy for malaria during pregnancy using 2 vs 3 or more doses of sulfadoxine-pyrimethamine and risk of low birth weight in Africa: systematic review and meta-analysis. *Journal of the American Medical Association*, 309, 594–604.

Keiser, J., Singer, B.H., and Utzinger, J. (2005). Reducing the burden of malaria in different eco-epidemiological settings with environmental management: a systematic review. *The Lancet Infectious Diseases*, 5, 695–708.

Kigozi, R., Baxi, S.M., Gasasira, A., et al. (2012). Indoor residual spraying of insecticide and malaria morbidity in a high transmission intensity area of Uganda. *PLoS One*, 7(8), e42857.

Lengeler, C. (2004). Insecticide-treated bed nets and curtains for preventing malaria. *Cochrane Database of Systematic Reviews*, 2, CD000363.

Lozano, R., Naghavi, M., Foreman, K., et al. (2012). Global and regional mortality from 235 causes of death for 20 age groups in 1990 and 2010: a systematic analysis for the Global Burden of Disease Study 2010. *The Lancet*, 380, 2095–128.

Malaria Atlas Project (n.d.). Website. [Online] Available at: http://www.map.ox.ac.uk/.

malERA Consultative Group on Health Systems and Operational Research (2011). A research agenda for malaria eradication: health systems and operational research. *PLoS Medicine*, 8(1), e1000397.

malERA Consultative Group on Monitoring, Evaluation, and Surveillance (2011). A research agenda for malaria eradication: monitoring, evaluation, and surveillance. *PLoS Medicine*, 8(1), e1000400.

malERA Consultative Group on Vector Control (2011). A research agenda for malaria eradication: vector control. *PLoS Medicine*, 8(1), e1000401.

Mali, S., Kachur, S.P., and Arguin, P.M. (2012). Malaria surveillance—United States, 2010. *Morbidity and Mortality Weekly Report. Surveillance Summaries*, 61, 1–22.

Marshall, J.M. and Taylor, C.E. (2009). Malaria control with transgenic mosquitoes. *PLoS Medicine*, 6(2), e20.

Munhenga, G., Brooke, B.D., Chirwa, T.F., et al. (2011). Evaluating the potential of the sterile insect technique for malaria control: relative fitness and mating compatibility between laboratory colonized and a wild population of Anopheles arabiensis from the Kruger National Park, South Africa. *Parasites & Vectors*, 4, 208.

Murray, C.J., Rosenfeld, L.C., Lim, S.S., et al. (2012). Global malaria mortality between 1980 and 2010: a systematic analysis. *The Lancet*, 379, 413–31.

Murray, C.K., Gasser, R.A. Jr., Magill, A.J., and Miller, R.S. (2008). Update on rapid diagnostic testing for malaria. *Clinical Microbiology Reviews*, 21, 97–110.

Nahlen, B.L., Korenromp, E.L., Miller, J.M., and Shibuya, K. (2005). Malaria risk: estimating clinical episodes of malaria. *Nature*, 8, 437.

Najera, J.A., Gonzalez-Silva, M., Alonso, P.L. (2011). Malaria Eradication Programme (1955–1969). *PLoS Medicine*, 8, e1000412.

Nayyar, G.M., Breman, J.G., Newton, P.N., and Herrington, J. (2012) Poor-quality antimalarial drugs in southeast Asia and sub-Saharan Africa. *The Lancet Infectious Diseases*, 12, 488–96.

Newbold, C., Craig, A., Kyes, S., et al. (1999). Cytoadherence, pathogenesis and the infected red cell surface in Plasmodium falciparum. *International Journal for Parasitology*, 29, 927–37.

Newman, R.D., Parise, M.E., Barber, A.M., and Steketee, R.W. (2004). Malaria-related deaths among U.S. travelers, 1963–2001. *Annals of Internal Medicine*, 141, 547–55.

O'Meara, W.P., Mangeni, J.N., Steketee, R., and Greenwood, B. (2010). Changes in the burden of malaria in sub-Saharan Africa. *The Lancet Infectious Diseases*, 10, 545–55.

Paaijmans, K.P., Read, A.F., and Thomas, M.B. (2009). Understanding the link between malaria risk and climate. *Proceedings of the National Academy of Sciences of the United States of America*, 106, 13844–9.

Pluess, B., Tanser, F.C., Lengeler, C., and Sharp, B.L. (2010). Indoor residual spraying for preventing malaria. *Cochrane Database of Systematic Reviews*, 4, CD006657.

Ponsford, M.J., Medana, I.M., Prapansilp, P., et al. (2012). Sequestration and microvascular congestion are associated with coma in human cerebral malaria. *Journal of Infectious Diseases*, 205, 663–71.

Pulford, J., Hetzel, M.W., Bryant, M., Siba, P.M., and Mueller, I. (2011). Reported reasons for not using a mosquito net when one is available: a review of the published literature. *Malaria Journal*, 10, 83.

Raghavendra, K., Barik, T.K., Reddy, B.P., Sharma, P., and Dash, A.P. (2011). Malaria vector control: from past to future. *Parasitology Research*, 108, 757–79.

Ranson, H., N'Guessan, R., Lines, J., et al. (2011). Pyrethroid resistance in African anopheline mosquitoes: what are the implications for malaria control? *Trends in Parasitology*, 27, 91–8.

Rogerson, S.J., Chaluluka, E., Kanjala, M., Mkundika, P., Mhango, C., and Molyneux, M.E. (2000). Intermittent sulfadoxine-pyrimethamine in pregnancy: effectiveness against malaria morbidity in Blantyre, Malawi, in 1997–99. *Transactions of the Royal Society of Tropical Medicine and Hygiene*, 94, 549–53.

Rowland, M., Downey, G., Rab, A., et al. (2004). DEET mosquito repellent provides personal protection against malaria: a household randomized trial in an Afghan refugee camp in Pakistan. *Tropical Medicine & International Health*, 9, 335–42.

RTS,S Clinical Trials Partnership, Agnandji, S.T., Lell, B., et al. (2012). A phase 3 trial of RTS,S/AS01 malaria vaccine in African infants. *The New England Journal of Medicine*, 367, 2284–95.

Shiff, C. (2002). Integrated approach to malaria control. *Clinical Microbiology Reviews*, 15, 278–93.

Sinka, M.E., Bangs, M.J., Manguin, S., et al. (2012). A global map of dominant malaria vectors. *Parasites & Vectors*, 5, 69.

Smith, T., Maire, N., Dietz, K., et al. (2006). Relationship between the entomologic inoculation rate and the force of infection for Plasmodium falciparum malaria. *American Journal of Tropical Medicine and Hygiene*, 75, 11–18.

Steketee, R.W., Nahlen, B.L., Parise, M.E., and Menendez, C. (2001). The burden of malaria in pregnancy in malaria-endemic areas. *American Journal of Tropical Medicine and Hygiene*, 64(Suppl. 1–2), 28–35.

Taylor, S.M., Parobek, C.M., and Fairhurst, R.M. (2012). Haemoglobinopathies and the clinical epidemiology of malaria: a systematic review and meta-analysis. *The Lancet Infectious Diseases*, 12, 457–68.

Taylor, W.R., Hanson, J., Turner, G.D., White, N.J., and Dondorp, A.M. (2012). Respiratory manifestations of malaria. *Chest*, 142, 492–505.

Ter Kuile, F.O., Parise, M.E., Verhoeff, F.H., et al. (2004). The burden of co-infection with human immunodeficiency virus type 1 and malaria in pregnant women in sub-Saharan Africa. *American Journal of Tropical Medicine and Hygiene*, 71(Suppl. 2), 41–54.

Thang, H.D., Elsas, R.M., and Veenstra, J. (2002). Airport malaria: report of a case and a brief review of the literature. *Netherlands Journal of Medicine*, 60, 441–3.

Tiwari, S., Ghosh, S.K., Mittal, P.K., and Dash, A.P. (2011). Effectiveness of a new granular formulation of biolarvicide Bacillus thuringiensis Var. israelensis against larvae of malaria vectors in India. *Vector-Borne and Zoonotic Diseases*, 11, 69–75.

Tougher, S., ACTwatch Group, Ye, Y., et al. (2012). Effect of the Affordable Medicines Facility—malaria (AMFm) on the availability, price, and market share of quality-assured artemisinin-based combination therapies in seven countries: a before-and-after analysis of outlet survey data. *The Lancet*, 380, 1916–26.

Tymoshenko, S., Oppenheim, R.D., Soldati-Favre, D., and Hatzimanikatis, V. (2013). Functional genomics of Plasmodium falciparum using metabolic modelling and analysis. *Briefings in Functional Genomics*, 12(4), 316–27.

Vos, T., Flaxman, A.D., Naghavi, M., et al. (2012). Years lived with disability (YLDs) for 1160 sequelae of 289 diseases and injuries 1990–2010: a systematic analysis for the Global Burden of Disease Study 2010. *The Lancet*, 380, 2163–96.

Wilson, A.L. and IPTc Taskforce (2011). A systematic review and meta-analysis of the efficacy and safety of intermittent preventive treatment of malaria in children (IPTc). *PLoS One*, 6(2), e16976.

Wilson, M.E., Weld, L.H., Boggild, A., et al. (2007). Fever in returned travelers: results from the GeoSentinel Surveillance Network. *Clinical Infectious Diseases*, 44, 1560–8.

World Health Organization (2000). *Bench Aids for the Diagnosis of Malaria Infections* (2nd ed.). Geneva: WHO. Available at: http://www.who.int/malaria/publications/atoz/9241545240/en/index.html.

World Health Organization (2010). *Guidelines for the Treatment of Malaria* (2nd ed.). Geneva: WHO. Available at: http://whqlibdoc.who.int/publications/2010/9789241547925_eng.pdf.

World Health Organization (2012a). *World Malaria Report*. Geneva: WHO. Available at: http://www.who.int/malaria/publications/world_malaria_report_2012/en/.

World Health Organization (2012b). *Malaria Rapid Diagnostic Test Performance. Results of WHO Product Testing of Malaria RDTs: Round 4*. Geneva: WHO.

Chronic hepatitis and other liver disease

Pierre Van Damme, Tinne Lernout, Koen Van Herck, Rui T. Marinho, Raymundo Paraná, and Daniel Shouval

Hepatitis B

Aetiological agent

Hepatitis B virus (HBV) is a double-stranded, enveloped virus of the *Hepadnaviridae* family. The *Hepadna* virus family has the smallest genome of all replication competent animal DNA viruses. The single most important member of the family is HBV.

The hepatitis B virion consists of a surface and a core, which contains a DNA polymerase and the e antigen. The DNA structure is double-stranded and circular with four major genes: the S (surface), the C (core), the P (polymerase), and the X (transcriptional transactivating). The S gene consists of three regions—S, pre-S1, and pre-S2—that encode the envelope protein (HBsAg). HBsAg is a lipoprotein of the viral envelope that circulates in the blood as spherical and tubular particles. The C gene is divided into two regions, the pre-core and the core, and codes for two different proteins, the core antigen (HBcAg) and the e antigen (HBeAg).

HBV strains are classified into eight genotypes designated A to H, most of which have a characteristic geographical distribution (Cao 2009; Tanwar and Dusheiko 2012). More recently, two additional genotypes, I and J, have been described in Asia (Tatematsu et al. 2009; Tran et al. 2008). Except for these newly identified genotypes, the geographic distributions of HBV genotypes are well characterized. Genotype A is highly prevalent in sub-Saharan Africa, Northern Europe, and Western Africa. Genotypes B and C are the major variants in South and South East Asia and the Pacific region. Genotype D is prevalent in Africa, Europe, the Mediterranean region and India. Genotype E is restricted to West Africa. Genotype F is found in Central and South America. Genotype G has been reported in France, Germany, and the United States and genotype H is found in Central America (Kurbanov et al. 2010; Lin and Kao 2011).

The genotypes A, B, C, D, and F have further been subdivided in up to four major subgenotypes and several minor genotypes, now identified by Arabic numerals.

The HBV infection is controlled by cellular and humoral immune responses. It can be tracked through serological detection of the virus particles or the antibodies raised by the immune system to target the virus. The presence of hepatitis B surface and/or hepatitis B core antibodies (anti-HBs and anti-HBc) in the absence of HBsAg is generally taken to indicate resolution of infection and provides evidence of previous HBV infection. Persistence of HBV infection (chronic carrier) is diagnosed by the detection of HBsAg in the blood for at least 6 months or through detection of HBV-DNA even in the absence of detectable HBsAg in patients with occult HBV infection. HBeAg is an alternatively processed protein of the pre-core gene that is only synthesized under conditions of high viral replication. HBV-DNA is used as an indicator for viral replication expressed as IU/mL or copies/mL (the value of copies/mL is approximately 5 times more than the IU units). There is a clear association between serum HBV-DNA levels (viral load) and prognosis: the cumulative incidence of cirrhosis or hepatocellular carcinoma (HCC) being 4.5 and 1.3 per cent, respectively, in persons with DNA levels less than 300 copies/mL (corresponding to 50 IU/mL), while it is 36.2 and 14.9 per cent, respectively, in persons with DNA levels of more than or equal to 10^6 copies/mL (corresponding to 2×10^5 IU/mL). This is the rationale for treating patients with high levels of HBV DNA (Chen et al. 2006; Lok and McMahon 2007).

Epidemiology

Globally, hepatitis B is one of the most common infectious diseases. Estimates indicate that about 2 billion people (i.e. about 30 per cent of the world population) have been infected with HBV worldwide, with over 240 million people being chronic carriers (World Health Organization (WHO) 2012). On the basis of sero-epidemiological surveys, the WHO has classified countries into three levels of endemicity according to the prevalence of chronic HBsAg carriage (Fig. 8.16.1): high (8 per cent or greater), intermediate (2–7 per cent), and low (less than 2 per cent) (WHO 2004).

HBV is transmitted by either percutaneous or mucous membrane contact with infected blood or other body fluid. The virus is found in highest concentrations in blood and serous exudates (up to 10^9 virions/mL). The primary routes of transmission are perinatal, early childhood exposure (often called horizontal transmission), sexual contact, and percutaneous exposure to blood or infectious body fluids (i.e. injections, needle stick, blood transfusion, tattoos).

Hepatitis B, countries or areas at risk

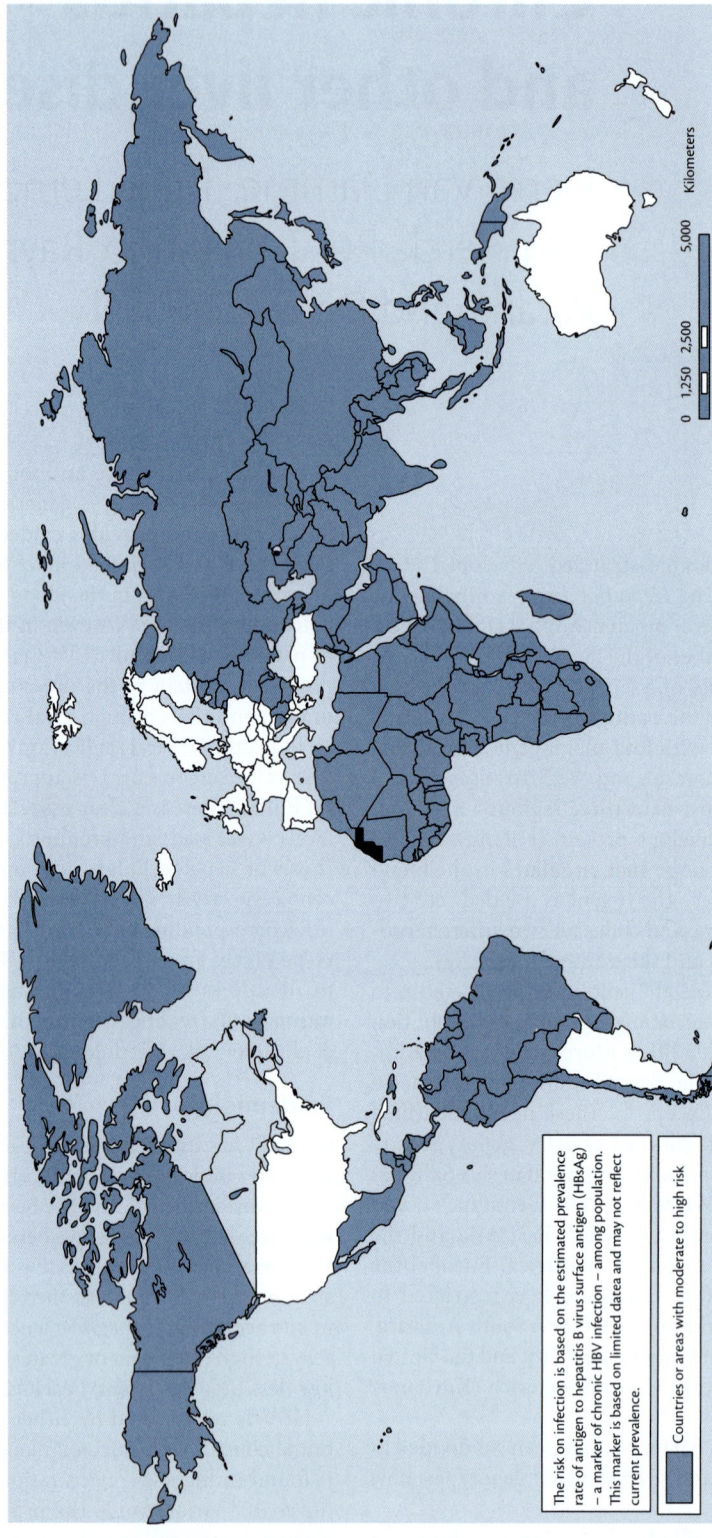

The risk on infection is based on the estimated prevalence rate of antigen to hepatitis B virus surface antigen (HBsAg) – a marker of chronic HBV infection – among population. This marker is based on limited datea and may not reflect current prevalence.

Countries or areas with moderate to high risk

0   1,250 2,500   5,000
Kilometers

Fig. 8.16.1 Map representing all countries with moderate (2–8% HBsAg positivity) and high (8% HBsAg positivity) endemicity for hepatitis B.

Reproduced with permission from World Health Organization, *Hepatitis B, Countries or Areas at Risk*, Copyright © WHO 2012, available from http://gamapserver.who.int/mapLibrary/Files/Maps/Global_HepB_ITHRiskMap.png.

Most perinatal infections occur among infants of pregnant women with chronic HBV infection. The likelihood of an infant developing chronic HBV infection is 70–90 per cent for those born to HBeAg-positive mothers (corresponding to high titres of HBV DNA) and less than 15 per cent for those born to HBeAg-negative mothers. Most early childhood infections occur in households of persons with chronic HBV infection. The most probable mechanism involves unapparent percutaneous or permucosal contact with infectious body fluids (e.g. bites, breaks in the skin, dermatological lesions, skin ulcers). Sexual transmission has been estimated to account for 50 per cent of new infections among adults in industrialized countries. The most common risk factors include multiple sex partners and history of a sexually transmitted infection. Finally, unsafe injections and other unsafe percutaneous or permucosal procedures (such as cocaine snorting) are a major source of blood-borne pathogen transmission (HBV, hepatitis C virus (HCV), human immunodeficiency virus (HIV)) in many countries. The risk of HBV infection from needle stick exposure to HBsAg-positive blood is approximately 30 per cent and worldwide unsafe injection practices account for approximately 8–16 million HBV infections each year.

In areas of high endemicity, the lifetime risk of HBV infection is more than 60 per cent, and most infections occur during the perinatal period (transmission from mother to child) or during early childhood. In areas of intermediate endemicity, the lifetime risk of HBV infection varies between 20 and 60 per cent, and infections occur in all age groups through the four modes of transmission, but primarily in infants and children. In areas of low endemicity, infection occurs primarily in adult life by sexual or parenteral transmission (e.g. through drug use). Although acute infection is more often clinically expressed in adults, infections in infants and pre-school age children are at greatest risk of becoming chronic, thereby increasing the risk of cirrhosis and primary HCC later in life. The precise mechanism by which carrier rates are influenced by age of infection is unknown but probably relates to the effect of age on the immune system's ability to clear and eliminate the infection.

Approximately 75 per cent of the world's chronic hepatitis B carriers live in Asian countries. China ranks highest, with 100 million hepatitis B carriers, and India the second highest, with a carrier pool of 35 million (Tandon and Tandon 1997). Importantly, chronic carriers of HBV are not only at risk of developing long-term progression of the infection but also represent a significant source and reservoir of infection to others.

A model developed in 2005 estimated that in the year 2000, 620,000 persons died worldwide from HBV-related causes: 580,000 (94 per cent) from chronic infection-related cirrhosis and HCC and 40,000 (6 per cent) from acute HBV infection. Infections acquired during the perinatal period, in early childhood (<5 years old), and at 5 years of age and older accounted for 21 per cent, 48 per cent, and 31 per cent of deaths, respectively (Goldstein et al. 2005).

Besides the age at which the infection is acquired, some of the variation in outcome of HBV infection may be related to the genetic heterogeneity of the virus. Progression to chronic infection appears to occur more frequently following acute infection with genotypes A and D than with the other genotypes (Tanwar and Dusheiko 2012). Chronic infection with genotype A and B appears to have a better prognosis than genotype C and D. Pre-core mutant infection is also most common in genotypes B, C, and D, which explains why pre-core mutant infection is more common in Asia and Southern Europe.

Clinical manifestations

Acute hepatitis B has a long incubation period ranging from 15 to 180 days (90 days on average) during which the individual is infectious. Individual responses to the infection vary greatly. One-third of the individuals have subclinical infection; one-third experience a mild 'flu-like' illness without jaundice; and the remaining one-third develop jaundice with dark urine, extreme fatigue, anorexia, and abdominal pain. Jaundice usually peaks within 1–2 weeks and then gradually subsides. About 95 per cent of adults recover completely, although this may require 6 months or more with persistent tiredness. A small proportion (1 per cent) of adults develop fulminant hepatitis, an exceptionally severe form of the disease which can be fatal requiring in two-thirds of cases an emergency liver transplant (Sherlock 1993). About 5–10 per cent of acutely infected adults and 50–90 per cent of newborns will become chronically infected and remain infectious.

The natural history of chronic HBV infection can vary dramatically between individuals. Risk factors which affect progression to chronic hepatitis, cirrhosis, and HCC include male gender, viral load, elevated alanine aminotransferase (ALT), genotype, and degree of fibrosis on liver biopsy. Some patients with persistent HBV infection will develop the condition commonly referred to as a chronic carrier state (HBsAg positivity in two occasions 6 months apart). These patients, who are still potentially infectious, have no symptoms and no abnormalities on laboratory testing. Some individuals with chronic HBV infection will have clinically insignificant or minimal liver disease and never develop complications. Others will have clinically apparent chronic hepatitis. Chronic infection with HBV can be either 'replicative' or 'non-replicative'. The 'replicative' phase or immune tolerance phase, characterized by positive HBeAg and high viral load (> 2 IU/mL, in particular if > 20 IU/mL), is often present in newborns and children of HBsAg-positive mothers. In 'non-replicative' infection, the rate of viral replication in the liver is low, serum HBV DNA concentration is generally low, and HBeAg is not detected. In these inactive HBsAg carriers, reactivation can occur either spontaneously or by immune suppression. Patients with chronic HBV and replicative infection generally have a worse prognosis and a greater chance of developing cirrhosis and/or HCC (Chen et al. 2006). In rare strains of HBV with mutations in the pre-core gene, replicative infection can occur in the absence of detectable serum HBeAg.

Treatment

HBV treatment depends on the phase of chronic HBV infection. Viral replication is necessary to cause liver injury, but the host immune system activation plays the main role in causing hepatocellular damage. As HBV is not directly cytopathic, if the patient is immunotolerant, he may present high viral load without necro-inflammation. When immunotolerance is lost, the host immune system causes liver injury. This is the immune clearance phase, when ALT increases and necro-inflammation and, consequently, liver fibrosis is found in the liver. A long-term immune clearance phase causes more fibrosis and compromises liver function. If the host immune system imposes immune control against the virus, viral replication dramatically drops down and liver damage almost disappears, but the HBV cannot be eliminated because its DNA is already integrated in the host cells. This is the inactive phase, which can reverse to the immunoclearance phase in case of host immune depression or viral mutations. In this case, the necro-inflammatory activity returns.

Treatment is indicated if ALT is elevated, HBV-DNA is more than 2 IU/mL (European Association for the Study of the Liver 2012) or 20 IU/mL (Lok and McMahon 2009) and if there are signs of moderate or severe liver fibrosis.

The main goal of therapy for chronic HBV infection is to significantly suppress replication of HBV, thus preventing liver disease progression to cirrhosis and its complications, and reducing secondary spread. Treatment of chronic HBV infections has some limited success. Antiviral therapy will only rarely lead to complete resolution of persistent HBV infection (negativation of HBsAg). Furthermore, residual HBV DNA in the form of intra-nuclear covalently closed circular (ccc)-DNA may still be present in patients who lost HBsAg and seroconverted to anti-HBs, a situation which leads to occult HBV infection.

In patients who are HBeAg-positive, the goal of treatment is HBeAg seroconversion with sustained suppression of HBV DNA and rarely HBsAg loss or seroconversion. In those who are HBeAg-negative, the goal of treatment is sustained suppression of HBV DNA and, consequently, reduced liver injury as measured by ALT levels as well as HBsAg loss or seroconversion (which is achieved only on rare occasions).

Recommendation for therapy is dictated by the level of HBV DNA, liver enzymes and necro-inflammatory activity in liver biopsy. More recently, non-invasive methods to define the fibrosis stage are also accepted to indicate treatment, mainly in HBeAg negative patients (European Association for the Study of the Liver 2012).

Several therapies are now licensed: nucleo(t)side analogues and interferon-based therapy. The latter is more indicated in HBeAg positive patients, but in Europe it can also be indicated in selected cases of HBeAg negative HBV carriers. Depending on the defined outcome, approximately one-third of HBeAg patients respond to a 1-year course of α-interferon therapy, taking HBeAg/Anti-HBe seroconversion as the aim of the treatment.

Currently, interferon-based therapy appears to be superior to nucleo(t)side analogues, due to the relatively higher rate of anti-HBe seroconversion, the limited duration of treatment as compared to nucleos(t)ide analogues, the potential, albeit rare, HBsAg loss after 1 year of therapy, the lower overall cost and the absence of resistance (Hoofnagle et al. 2007). On the other hand, interferon causes more adverse events and must be administered subcutaneously. Because of that, many physicians and even patients do not choose interferon as the first-line treatment.

Treatment with nucleos(t)ide analogues is very effective in suppressing viral load but the end point of treatment is undetermined and long-term treatment is required, which remains costly and unavailable to the majority of those affected. Combination therapy (interferon-based and nucleo(t)side) does not lead to a better viral response.

There are nowadays many licensed nucleo(t)side analogues: lamivudine, telbivudine, entecavir, tenofovir, and tenofovir/entricitabine. Among these, entecavir and tenofovir are usually preferred, because of the higher genetic barrier (low probability of resistance) and higher potency.

The nucleo(t)side analogue based treatment has no time definition. In the vast majority of cases, the patient needs to be treated for a long time, but they are usually safe, without significant adverse effects.

Public health impact

HBV infection is a serious global health problem. Of the approximately 2 billion people who have been infected worldwide up to 2012, more than 240 million are chronic carriers of HBV (WHO 2012). Approximately 15–40 per cent of infected patients will develop cirrhosis, liver failure or HCC. HBV infection accounts for an estimated 600,000 deaths each year, mainly due to the consequences of chronic hepatitis, such as cirrhosis and liver cancer (Goldstein et al. 2005; Lavanchy 2004; Perz et al. 2006a). Because these complications mainly occur in adults who quite often were infected with HBV as children, most of the benefits of vaccination initiated 20 years ago have yet to be realized. Table 8.16.1 summarizes the global prevalence and mortality of HBV versus the observed prevalence and mortality of HCV and human immunodeficiency virus/acquired immune deficiency syndrome (HIV/AIDS). Another consequence, often underestimated, is the stigma that HBV carries to the individual, in the family setting, as well as in social and professional life.

Prevention

All major health authorities agree that the most effective approach to reducing the burden of HBV is primary prevention through universal vaccination and control of disease transmission. Interrupting the chain of infection requires knowledge of the mode of disease transmission and modification of behaviour through individual education to practice safe sex and good personal hygiene. Screening of all donated blood and maintenance

Table 8.16.1 Global disease burden for hepatitis B, hepatitis C, and HIV/AIDS

	Hepatitis B	Hepatitis C	HIV/AIDS
Global prevalence	2 billion	150 million	34 million
Chronic infection	240 million	120 million	34 million
Number of deaths per year	600,000	350,000	1.7 million

Source: data from World Health Organization, Global Health Observatory (WHO database HIV/Aids), *Global epidemic and health care response* (PowerPoint slides), Copyright © WHO 2011, available from http://www.who.int/hiv/data/en and World Health Organization, *Prevention and Control of Viral Hepatitis Infection: Framework for Global Action*, Copyright © WHO 2012, available from http://who.int/csr/disease/hepatitis/GHP_Framework_En.pdf?ua=1.

of strict aseptic techniques with invasive health treatments have reduced the likelihood of contracting HBV.

Safe and effective HBV vaccines have been available since the 1980s, and immunization with HBV vaccine remains the most effective means of preventing HBV disease and its consequences worldwide. Although the vaccine will not cure chronic hepatitis, it is 95 per cent effective in preventing chronic infections from developing, and is the first vaccine against a major human cancer.

After the development of plasma-derived vaccines (in 1982), which continue to be used mostly in the low- and middle-income countries, recombinant DNA technology has allowed the expression of HBsAg in other organisms. As a result, different manufacturers have successfully developed recombinant DNA vaccines against HBV (commercialized in 1986).

Moreover, apart from monovalent vaccines against hepatitis B, a broad range of combination vaccines that include an HBV component exist, especially for vaccination during infancy and early childhood. Most of these simultaneously immunize against tetanus, diphtheria, and pertussis (with either a whole-cell or an acellular component); they may also include antigens for vaccination against polio and/or *Haemophilus influenzae* b. For each of these combination vaccines, it has been shown that the respective components remain sufficiently immunogenic, and that the combination vaccine is safe.

More recently, the so-called third-generation hepatitis B vaccines—based on the S-, pre-S1-, and pre-S2-antigens, or using new adjuvants—have been and are being developed. These vaccines specifically aim to enhance the immune response in immunocompromised persons and non-responders (Rendi-Wagner et al. 2006; Shouval et al. 1994).

Immunization against hepatitis B requires the intramuscular administration of three doses of vaccine given at 0, 1, and 6 months. More rapid protection (i.e. for healthcare workers exposed to HBV or the susceptible sexual partner of a patient with acute hepatitis B) can be achieved through the adoption of an alternative schedule using three doses of vaccine administered at 0, 1, and 2 months followed by a booster dose given at 12 months. The extensive use of both plasma-derived and recombinant HBV vaccines since their becoming available has confirmed their safety and excellent tolerability. However, in recent years, the safety of hepatitis B vaccine has been questioned, particularly in some countries. In 1998, several case reports from France raised concern that hepatitis B vaccination may lead to new cases or relapse of multiple sclerosis (MS) or other demyelinating diseases, including Guillain–Barré syndrome; however, no causal relation has been established (Duclos 2003). Hepatitis B vaccination is not contraindicated in pregnant or lactating women.

Seroprotection against HBV infection is defined as having an anti-HBs level 10 IU/L after complete immunization (Centers for Disease Control and Prevention 1987). Reviews on the use of HBV vaccine in neonates and infants report seroprotective levels of anti-HBs antibodies at 1 month after the last vaccine dose for all schedules in 98–100 per cent of vaccinees (Venters et al. 2004). While HBV vaccines generally induce an adequate immune response in over 95 per cent of fully vaccinated healthy persons, a huge interpersonal variability has been demonstrated in the immune response. The antibody response to hepatitis B vaccine has been shown to depend on the type, dosage and schedule of vaccination used, as well as on the age, the gender, genetic factors,

co-morbidity, and the status of the immune system of the vaccinee (Hadler and Margolis 1992; Hollinger 1989). Immunodeficient patients, such as those undergoing haemodialysis or immunosuppressant therapy, require higher doses of vaccine and more injections (at months 0, 1, 2 and 6) to achieve an adequate and sustained immune response.

Follow-up studies have shown that vaccine-induced antibodies persist over periods of at least 20 years and that duration of anti-HBs positivity is related to the antibody peak level achieved after primary vaccination (Jilg et al. 1988; Leuridan and Van Damme 2011). Follow-up of successfully vaccinated people has shown that the antibody concentrations usually decline over time, but clinically significant breakthrough infections are rare. Those who have lost antibody over time after a successful vaccination usually show a rapid anamnestic response when boosted with an additional dose of vaccine given several years after the primary course of vaccination or when exposed to the HBV. This means that the immunological memory for HBsAg can outlast the anti-HBs antibody detection, providing long-term protection against acute disease and the development of the HBsAg carrier state (Banatvala and Van Damme 2003). Hence, for immunocompetent children and adults the routine administration of booster doses of vaccine does not appear necessary to sustain long-term protection (European Consensus Group 2000). Such conclusions are based on data collected during the first 10–20 years of vaccination in countries of both high and low endemicity (Kao and Chen 2005; Zanetti et al. 2005).

Since the availability of hepatitis B vaccines in industrialized countries, strategies for HBV control have stressed immunization of high-risk groups (e.g. homosexual men, healthcare workers, patients in sexually transmitted infection clinics, sex workers, drug users, people with multiple sex partners, household contacts of chronically infected persons) and the screening of pregnant women. As observed and reported in many countries, and though it is certainly desirable to immunize these persons, it is unlikely that such a programme limited to high-risk groups will control HBV infection in the community.

In 1991, the WHO called for all children to receive the HBV vaccine. Substantial progress has been made in implementing this WHO recommendation: by the end of 2012, 179 countries had implemented or were planning to implement a universal HBV immunization programme for newborns, infants, and/or adolescents. Of these, 147 (82 per cent) countries reported HBV infant vaccination coverage over 80 per cent after the third dose; these countries are mainly situated in Europe, North and South America, Northern Africa, and Australia (UNICEF and WHO 2012).

High coverage with the primary vaccine series among infants has the greatest overall impact on the prevalence of chronic HBV infection in children (WHO 2004). According to model-based predictions, universal HBV infant immunization (without administration of a birth dose of vaccine to prevent perinatal HBV infection), would prevent up to 75 per cent of global deaths from HBV-related causes, depending on the vaccination coverage for the complete series. Adding the birth dose would increase the proportion of deaths prevented up to 84 per cent (Goldstein et al. 2005).

In countries with high or intermediate disease endemicity, the most effective strategy is to incorporate the vaccine into the routine infant immunization schedule or to start immunization at birth (< 24 hours). Countries with lower prevalence may consider immunization of children or adolescents as an addition or an alternative to infant immunization (WHO 2004, 2006).

Indeed, the effectiveness of hepatitis B newborn and infant immunization programmes has already been demonstrated in a variety of countries and settings (André and Zuckerman 1994; Lee 1997; WHO 2001). The results of effective implementation of universal hepatitis B programmes have become apparent in terms of reduction not only in the incidence of acute hepatitis B infections, but also in the carrier rate in immunized cohorts and in hepatitis-B-related mortality—two ways to measure the impact of a hepatitis B vaccination programme (Coursaget et al. 1994).

In Taiwan, the HBsAg prevalence in children under 15 years of age decreased from 9.8 per cent in 1984 to 0.7 per cent in 1999 (Chan et al. 2004). In the Gambia, childhood HBsAg prevalence decreased from 10 per cent to 0.6 per cent since the introduction of the universal infant immunization programme (Viviani et al. 1999). Data in Hawaii show a 97 per cent reduction in the prevalence of HBsAg since the start of the infant hepatitis B vaccination programme in 1991. The incidence of new acute hepatitis B infections in children and adults was reduced from 4.5/100,000 in 1990 to 0 in the period 2002–2004 (Perz et al. 2006b). In Bristol Bay, Alaska, 3.2 per cent of children were HBsAg positive before universal hepatitis B immunization; 10 years later, no child under 10 years of age was HBsAg positive (Wainwright et al. 1997). Finally, surveillance data from Italy, where a universal programme was started in 1991 in infants as well as in adolescents, have shown a clear overall decline in the incidence of acute hepatitis B cases from 11/100,000 in 1987 to 3/100,000 in 2000 (Romano et al. 2004).

Hepatitis D virus

Hepatitis D virus (HDV) is a transmissible pathogen that requires the help of a hepadnavirus like HBV for its own replication—similar to viroids or plant virus satellite RNAs. Thus, in a natural setting, HDV is only found in patients who are also infected with HBV since the HDV RNA genomes are assembled using the envelope proteins of HBV and HDV buds through the HBsAg excretory pathway.

The HDV genome is a small single-stranded RNA genome composed of approximately 1680 bases with a unique circular conformation that is replicated using a host RNA polymerase. A rolling-circle model has been developed for its RNA replication, which is unique, at least among agents that infect animals. The HDV genome contains an open reading frame translated to the small (S-HD) and large (L-HD) proteins. The L-HD amino acid sequence is identical to S-HD with the addition of a carboxy-terminal extension of 19–20 amino acids following the editing of the S-HD stop codon during the viral RNA replication cycle. The S-HD is required for viral replication and might promote RNA polymerase II elongation of nascent HDV RNA, while L-HD is essential for HDV particle assembly (Tseng and Lai 2009).

There are two types of HDV infection: co-infection and super-infection (Rizzetto and Verme 1985). HDV and HBV can infect individuals simultaneously, transmitted by the same inoculums, characterizing a co-infection. On the other hand, the HDV can infect a chronic HBV carrier, characterizing a super-infection.

A co-infection usually evolves into complete recovery, but the risk for severe acute hepatitis, even fulminant hepatitis, is higher than in the case of acute HBV mono-infection. A super-infection evolves toward chronicity in about 90 per cent of cases. Chronicity is associated with an increased risk of developing advanced chronic liver disease, early cirrhosis development, and hepatocarcinoma (Farci 2003; Smedile and Bugianesi 2005).

Eight HDV genotypes have been characterized to date on the basis of a small number of complete genome sequences with 19–38 per cent divergence at the nucleotide level of complete genomes (Hughes et al. 2011). The most frequent genotypes are: genotype I (includes the European, North American, African, and some Asian HDV isolates), genotype II (found in Japan, Taiwan, and Eastern Europe), genotype III (found exclusively in South America), genotype IV (found mainly in West-Africa) and genotype V (found in Central Africa).

The global distribution of the different genotypes of HBV and HDV is rather well known, although less is known on the types circulating among populations in remote areas and on the way the different viruses and their respective genotypes interact in multiple infected individuals. Little is also known on the viral transmission mechanisms driving the circulation of the endemic strains and epidemic outbreaks.

The prevalence of HDV infection increases in the equatorial subtropical and tropical zones, concentrating in certain population groups which are considered high endemicity models (Torres 1996). Preliminary data suggest that hepatitis delta in Brazil, endemic in the Western Amazon states, is more severe compared to other regions; however this needs further evidence (Paraná et al. 2008; Viana et al. 2005). In Western Europe, HDV is becoming rare, affecting around 5 per cent of chronic carriers (Rizzetto and Ciancio 2012).

In endemic areas, all HBV carriers should be further screened for delta hepatitis virus (which requires the availability of anti-HDV IgG and IgM serological tests).

Hepatitis C

Aetiological agent

HCV is classified in the family *Flaviviridae*. Like other flaviviruses, HCV is an enveloped RNA virus with an inner nucleoprotein core. Its envelope contains two glycoproteins, E1 and E2, which form heterodimers (to form a functional subunit) at the surface of the virion. Efforts to isolate the virus by standard immunological and virological techniques were unsuccessful and HCV was finally identified by direct cloning and sequencing of its genome. Although the virus was identified 25 years ago (in 1989) (Choo et al. 1989), its replication cycle is still not fully understood. An important feature of HCV is that the viral genome displays extensive genetic heterogeneity at the local as well as the global level. Even within a host, the HCV genome population circulates as a 'quasi-species' of closely related sequences. Worldwide, a high degree of genetic variation exists, resulting in at least six major genotypes and more than 100 distantly related subtypes (Forns and Bukh 1999). It has been reported that virus pathogenicity and sensitivity to current standards of treatment appear to vary with different subtypes (genotypes 2 and 3, responding better than genotype 1 and 4). These characteristics of HCV, much like HIV, make it a moving target for vaccine design.

Epidemiology

HCV is a major cause of acute hepatitis and chronic liver disease, including cirrhosis and HCC. Globally, an estimated 150 million persons are infected with HCV and more than 350,000 people are estimated to die from HCV-related liver diseases (Alter 2007; WHO 2012). The worldwide prevalence of HCV-infected people ranges from 1 per cent in high-income countries to around 10 per cent in low- and middle-income countries (Fig. 8.16.2). Table 8.16.1 summarizes the global prevalence and mortality of HCV versus the observed prevalence and mortality of HBV and HIV/AIDS.

The reported seroprevalence in the Nile delta ranges from 19 per cent in the 10–19-year-old age group to 60 per cent in the 30-year-old age group, and is associated with a high prevalence of liver cirrhosis in Egypt. The higher prevalence in the Nile delta is reported to be linked to parenteral anti-schistosomiasis therapy, which was carried out with inadequately sterilized injection material (Frank et al. 2000). Current estimates in the United States are that 3.9 million Americans are chronically infected with HCV, with prevalence rates as high as 8–10 per cent in African Americans. Haemodialysis patients, haemophiliacs, drug addicts, and people transfused with blood before 1990 are particularly affected by the disease. In Europe, 0.1–3.3 per cent of the population has been infected, with the highest prevalence observed in Southern Europe (Italy and Romania) (Blachier et al. 2013).

Despite infection control precautions, healthcare providers remain at risk for acquiring blood-borne viral infections due to accidental exposure. Therapeutic injections are reported as accounting for 2 million new HCV infections each year. Many of these injections are performed in less than ideal conditions, often with reuse of needles or multidose vials and mainly, but not exclusively, in low- and middle-income countries. The residual risk of transmitting HCV through blood transfusion is very low in industrialized countries but safety of blood supply remains a major source of public concern in low- and middle-income countries.

Up to 60–70 per cent of intravenous drug users living in urban areas are seropositive for HCV antibodies. The rate of infection depends on the length of drug use, with 25 per cent of infections occurring during the first year of addiction, 50 per cent after 5 years, and up to 90 per cent after more than 5 years of intravenous drug use.

Transmission

The global epidemic of HCV infection emerged in the second half of the twentieth century and has been attributed, at least in part, to the increasing use of parenteral therapies and blood transfusion during that period. In high-income countries, the rapid improvement of healthcare conditions and the introduction of anti-HCV screening for blood donors have led to a sharp decrease in the incidence of iatrogenic HCV (Prati 2006). Injectable drug use remains the main route of transmission, accounting for nearly 90 per cent of new HCV infections. Mother-to-child transmission has been widely documented. The risk of perinatal infection in children from HCV-infected mothers ranges from 3 per cent to 10 per cent in different populations. Transmission is believed to occur *in utero*, as a consequence of a high viral load in the mother (in particular, from mothers who are HIV-co-infected) (Kato et al. 1994). There is no contraindication for infected mothers to breastfeed the newborn. Sexual transmission is thought to be relatively infrequent (2–3 per cent); as such, it is not recommended in monogamic and stable couples to use condoms. However, the

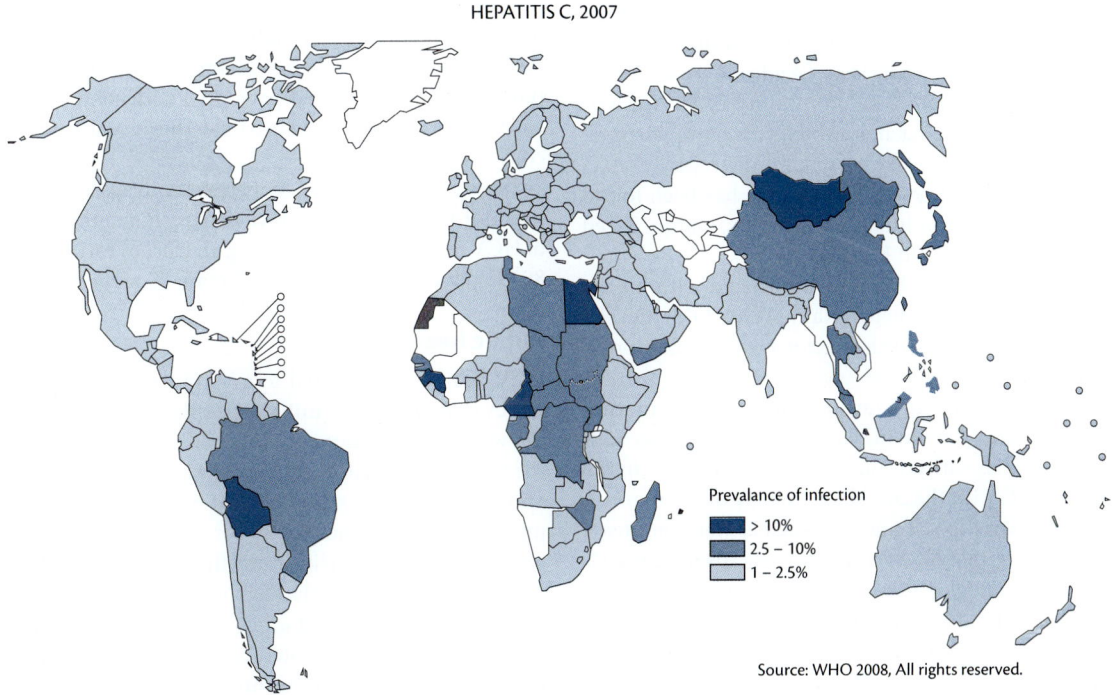

HEPATITIS C, 2007

Prevalance of infection

■ > 10%
■ 2.5 – 10%
□ 1 – 2.5%

Fig. 8.16.2 Map representing countries with low (1–2.5%), moderate (2.5–10%), and high (> 10%) hepatitis C virus prevalence.
Reproduced with permission from World Health Organization, *Hepatitis C,* Copyright © WHO 2008, available from http://www.who.int/ith/maps/hepatitisc2007.jpg.

large reservoir of HCV carriers provides multiple opportunities for exposure to potentially infected partners. Individuals with multiple sexual partners, male homosexuals, prostitutes and their clients, patients with common sexually transmitted infections, and partners of HCV and HIV co-infected persons are at the highest risk of acquiring HCV sexually.

In many cases of HCV infection, no recognizable transmission factor or route is identified (Memon and Memon 2002).

Clinical manifestations

The incubation period for hepatitis C before the onset of clinical symptoms ranges from 6 to 7 weeks on average. In acute infections, the most common symptoms are fatigue and jaundice; however, the majority of cases (between 60 and 70 per cent), even those who develop chronic infection, are asymptomatic for years. Fulminant hepatitis C forms are very rarely observed. While most patients with acute HCV infection have mild symptoms or no symptoms, 50–85 per cent of those infected develop chronic disease. Chronic disease is difficult to recognize because symptoms are mild and infection passes silently and insidiously from the acute to the chronic phase. Serological diagnosis of acute HCV infection is mainly based on recent HCV antibodies (anti-HCV) seroconversion. Persistence of HCV infection is diagnosed by the presence of HCV RNA in the blood for at least 6 months. The mechanisms of HCV persistence are currently unknown, although it is known that HCV chronicity develops despite humoral and cellular responses to HCV proteins. Factors associated with development of chronic disease appear to include older age at the time of infection, male gender, and an immunosuppressed state such as HIV infection (Lauer and Walker 2001).

Extra-hepatic manifestations of hepatitis C

Hepatitis C virus infection provokes dysfunction in B-lymphocytes with extra-hepatic manifestations of autoimmunity.

Many autoimmune and metabolic diseases have been associated with HCV infection: lichuen planus, granuloma annulare, porphyria cutanea tarda, and psoriasis (Andrade et al. 2012). The most important expression of autoimmunity in HCV carriers is HCV-related cryoglobulinaemia, which can cause purpura, vasculitis, glomerulonephritis, and peripheral neuropathy (Atta et al. 2010). A higher level of cryoglobulinaemia has been found in HCV carriers with lymph proliferative disorders, mainly B-cell non-Hodgkin lymphoma (Yu and Lin 2013).

Furthermore, HCV infection has been associated with higher risk of insulin resistance and diabetes (Naing et al. 2013). On the other side diabetes is a confirmed risk factor for the evolution to hepatocellular carcinoma.

The presence of non-organ specific autoantibodies is another expression of autoimmunity found in HCV carriers, which has been associated in some studies with advanced fibrosis and failure in the treatment of hepatitis C with the combined therapy of interferon-α plus ribavirin. Antibodies to self-antigens such as nucleoproteins (ANA), smooth muscle (SMA), liver–kidney microsomal type-1 antigen (LKM-1), immunoglobulin G (RF), neutrophil cytoplasm (ANCA), and phospholipids (APL), which are routinely used as biomarkers of autoimmune diseases, can be found in HCV-carriers with varying prevalence. Their induction seems mainly to involve immune cross-reactions caused by molecular mimicry between HCV polyprotein and human auto antigens (Atta et al. 2010).

Treatment

The primary goals for treatment of HCV infection are to reduce morbidity and mortality through complete clearance of HCV and normalization of liver enzymes, reducing disease progression, improving quality of life, and reducing the reservoir of chronic carriers, thereby controlling further transmission. In contrast with hepatitis B, chronic HCV infection is potentially curable. Virological cure or sustained viral response is defined by the persistence of negativity of HCV-RNA 6 months after ending therapy.

Treatment is recommended for patients with an increased risk of developing cirrhosis or with potential harmful extra-hepatic manifestations of HCV; most of these patients (but not all) have persistently elevated liver enzymes.

In patients with cirrhosis, the benefits of therapy will be: reduction of the risk of decompensation, reduction of the risk of evolution to hepatocellular carcinoma, and reduction of the risk of dying from a liver-related death (Veldt et al. 2007).

Effective sustained viral response has been obtained in about 50 per cent of HCV patients with genotype 1 and 80 per cent of patients with genotypes 2 or 3 who had received combined weekly pegylated interferon-based treatment with daily ribavirin for 48 weeks (Chevalier and Pawlotsky 2007; Tan and Lok 2007). This negativity of HCV-RNA 6 months after the end of therapy is maintained in 99 per cent of all patients.

More recently, the introduction of new drugs (boceprevir and telaprevir) in the HCV therapeutic schedule, increased the chance of sustained viral response (SVR) to 70 per cent in naive patients and to almost 80 per cent in patients who relapsed after the standard treatment with peginterferon + ribavirin. However, the triple therapy seems to have more adverse events, namely anaemia in boceprevir and anaemia and cutaneous rash in telaprevir (Jacobson et al. 2011; Kwo et al. 2010).

The therapy for chronic HCV is too costly for most patients in low- and middle-income countries to afford. The new drugs make the treatment cost higher, even for industrialized countries. Besides, the adverse events during treatment require multidisciplinary medical care and personnel with solid expertise to manage this treatment. Unfortunately, they are not available in most countries.

There are new oral and more specific drugs arriving, without the need for interferon or even ribavirin. They inhibit several regions of HCV (e.g. polymerase) having an efficacy estimated to be around 80–90 per cent in 12 weeks of therapy (Suzuki et al. 2012).

Public health impact

HCV has been compared to a 'viral time bomb'. The WHO estimates that about 150 million people, that is, some 2 per cent of the world's population, are infected with HCV; 75–80 per cent of them are chronic HCV carriers at risk of developing liver cirrhosis and/or HCC. It is estimated that 3–4 million persons are newly infected each year and that 20 per cent of those infected with HCV progress to cirrhosis within the first 10 years after infection (Alter 2007; Gerberding and Henderson 1992). Although the prevalence of chronic HVC reached a peak in 2001 (according to a multiple cohort model) in the United States, the prevalence of hepatitis C cirrhosis and its complications will continue to increase through the next decade (Davis et al. 2010). In Europe the prevalence of chronic hepatitis C in the last decade was 0.13–3.26 per cent. It is of great concern that about 90 per cent of people in Europe infected by viral hepatitis are unaware of their status (Blachier et al. 2013). Furthermore, chronic HCV disease is the primary indication for liver transplantation in industrialized countries (Adam et al. 2012).

Prevention

There is no vaccine against HCV. Research is in progress, but the high mutability of the HCV genome complicates vaccine development. Although 20–35 per cent of patients with acute HCV infection clear the virus spontaneously, lack of knowledge of any protective immune response following HCV infection impedes vaccine research. Although some studies have shown the presence of virus-neutralizing antibodies, it is not fully clear whether and how the immune system is able to eliminate the virus. Thus, from a global perspective, the greatest impact on HCV disease burden will likely be achieved by focusing efforts on reducing the risk of HCV transmission from nosocomial exposures (e.g. screening of blood, rigorous implementation of infection control, reducing unsafe injection practices) and high-risk behaviours (e.g. injection drug use).

Adherence to fundamental infection control principles, including safe injection practices and appropriate aseptic techniques, is essential to prevent transmission of blood-borne viruses in healthcare settings. Educational programmes aimed at the prevention of drug use and, for those already addicted, aimed at the prevention of shared needles and other equipment can decrease this source of infection. Some countries have established needle exchange programmes that provide easy access to sterile needles and syringes, accompanied by counselling and health education and instructions on the safe disposal of used syringes.

Alcoholic liver disease

Alcoholic beverages have been used in human societies since the beginning of recorded history. In 2005, a study estimated that just over 40 per cent of the world's adult population consumes alcohol

and the average consumption per drinker is 17.1 L per year (Shield et al. 2013).

It has long been known that alcohol consumption is responsible for increased illness and death. Worldwide, alcohol causes 2.5 million deaths each year, including 320,000 young people between the age of 15 and 29 (9 per cent of deaths in that age group) and 693 million (4.5 per cent of total) disability-adjusted life years (DALYs) (WHO 2011a, WHO 2011b). The burden is not equally distributed among countries. The highest disease load attributable to alcohol is found in the heavy-drinking former socialist countries of Eastern Europe and in Latin America (Fig. 8.16.3). For most diseases there is a dose–response relation to the volume of alcohol consumption, with the risk of the disease increasing with higher volume.

Alcoholic liver disease, resulting from the chronic and excessive consumption of alcoholic beverages, represents a considerable burden for the practising clinician, constituting the commonest reason for admitting patients with liver disease to a hospital. Alcohol (37 per cent), viral hepatitis (39 per cent), or both (4 per cent) are the leading indications for liver transplantation following cirrhosis, representing 57 per cent of transplants in Europe (European Liver Transplant Registry 2011) (Fig. 8.16.4), and alcohol is responsible for 50 per cent of deaths due to liver cirrhosis (WHO 2011c).

The costs to society from alcohol abuse cannot be overemphasized. In 2006, overall costs in the United States reached US$223.5 billion, out of which healthcare expenses accounted for 11 per cent. Almost three-quarters of these costs were due to binge drinking (Bouchery et al. 2011). Despite this burden, surprisingly little consensus exists on disease pathogenesis and on the factors that determine susceptibility.

Worldwide patterns of alcoholic intake and burden of disease in general and alcoholic liver disease in particular

Patterns of alcohol intake are constantly evolving as well as the prevalence and incidence of alcoholic liver disease. In 2010, 5.5

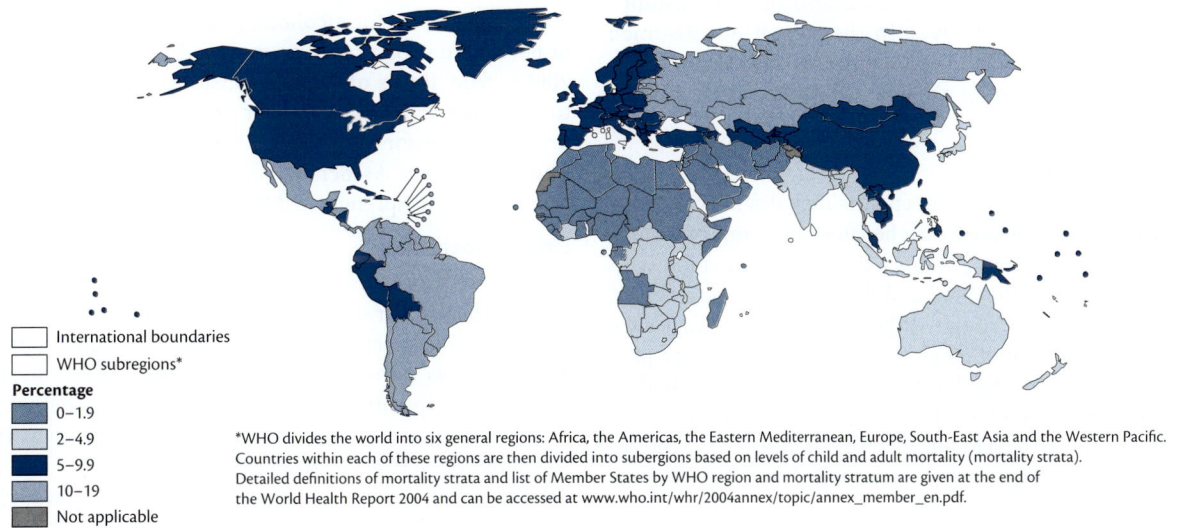

International boundaries
WHO subregions*
Percentage
- 0–1.9
- 2–4.9
- 5–9.9
- 10–19
- Not applicable

*WHO divides the world into six general regions: Africa, the Americas, the Eastern Mediterranean, Europe, South-East Asia and the Western Pacific. Countries within each of these regions are then divided into subregions based on levels of child and adult mortality (mortality strata). Detailed definitions of mortality strata and list of Member States by WHO region and mortality stratum are given at the end of the World Health Report 2004 and can be accessed at www.who.int/whr/2004annex/topic/annex_member_en.pdf.

Fig. 8.16.3 Alcohol attributable disability-adjusted life years (DALYs) as percentage of total DALYs, by WHO region, 2004.

Reproduced from World Health Organization, *Global status report on alcohol and health*, Copyright © WHO 2011, available from http://www.who.int/substance_abuse/publications/global_alcohol_report/msbgsruprofiles.pdf.

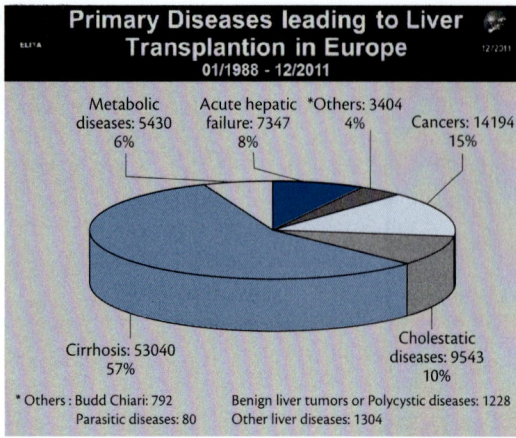

Fig. 8.16.4 Primary indications of liver transplantation in adult recipients (January 1988 to December 2011).

Reproduced with permission from European Liver Transplant Registry (ELTR), *Overall indication and results*, Copyright © ELTR 2011, available from http://www.eltr.org/spip.php?article161.

per cent of the global burden of disease was attributable to alcohol. This is almost as much as the burden of disease from tobacco (6.3 per cent) (Lim et al. 2012). Alcohol use represented the leading risk factor for global disease burden in Eastern Europe, most of Latin America, and southern sub-Saharan Africa. Given the relationship between alcohol consumption and cirrhosis (Sheron et al. 2008), it would be expected that there is a lag period between changes in per capita alcohol consumption and cirrhosis-related mortality. Data regarding this lag effect have been conflicting. In fact, a long latency time is not observed, and the usual lag period is only one year or less (Kerr et al. 2000).

Morphology and natural history of alcoholic liver disease

Fatty liver (steatosis)

The first and most predictable hepatic change attributable to alcohol is the development of large droplet (macrovesicular) steatosis. This disorder usually resolves within 2 weeks if alcohol consumption is discontinued (Diehl 1997). In the past, it was assumed that alcoholic fatty liver was a benign process. However, it is now assumed that 5–15 per cent of patients will develop cirrhosis during a 10-year follow-up period (Sorensen et al. 1984).

Alcoholic steatohepatitis

The spectrum of alcoholic steatohepatitis includes fatty infiltration of hepatocytes associated with hepatocellular injury including ballooning degeneration, Mallory bodies inflammation with neutrophils and/or lymphocytes, and fibrosis with a perivenular, perisinusoidal, and pericellular disposition. These changes are present in 10–35 per cent of all alcoholics. It is not a benign process. Some patients will develop fatal decompensation. In addition, the risk of developing cirrhosis is increased. It is estimated that the probability of developing cirrhosis is 10–20 per cent per year and 70 per cent of patients with alcoholic hepatitis will eventually develop cirrhosis (Diehl 1997).

Cirrhosis

The main causes for cirrhosis are: HBV (worldwide), HCV (in Europe), and alcohol (Cortez-Pinto et al. 2010). In 2010, more than

1 million deaths (2 per cent of all deaths) were due to liver cirrhosis. Alcoholic cirrhosis accounts for 48 per cent of cirrhosis-related deaths (Rehm et al. 2013). The long-term prognosis of alcoholic cirrhosis improves with abstinence. The 5-year survival in compensated cirrhosis patients who continue to drink is 70 per cent, but can be as high as 90 per cent if they abstain from further alcohol intake. In patients with decompensated cirrhosis, the 5-year survival drops to 30 per cent in individuals who continue to drink, but is 60 per cent in those who stay abstinent (Alexander et al. 1971; Diehl 1997).

Hepatocellular carcinoma

Alcohol can be considered both as a primary cause of HCC and as a co-factor for the development of HCC. Most of the studies on incidence of HCC in alcoholic cirrhosis date from before the identification of the HCV. As hepatitis C is relatively frequent in alcoholics, the proportional contribution of alcohol in the reported HCC incidence rates in earlier studies is likely to be overestimated. Although the exact annual incidence rate of HCC in alcoholic cirrhosis is unknown, it is estimated to be over 1.5 per cent, making it worthwhile to offer patients testing (Bruix and Sherman 2005).

Factors influencing the risk of alcoholic liver disease

Most authors agree that persons who drink heavily (50–60 g of ethanol daily) represent a population at increased risk of developing liver disease (Becker et al. 2002). However, the absolute risk of acquiring alcoholic hepatitis or cirrhosis is relatively low (6.9 per cent in the mentioned study). This suggests that genetic factors and/or environment play a role in disease risk. Many studies that address the risk factors refer to their effect on 'alcoholic liver disease' in general rather than any specific aspect of alcoholic liver disease such as steatohepatitis.

Amount of alcohol

There is a general agreement that excessive alcohol consumption is associated with an increased risk of cirrhosis. However, the exact dose or a specific dose–response relationship for cirrhosis has not been agreed on. Evidence suggests that there is an increased risk for alcoholic liver disease with the ingestion of 60–80 g/day of alcohol in men and 20 g/day in women (Day 2000). 'Safe' limits of alcohol consumption for the liver are up to one–two drinks per day for women, and up to three–four drinks per day for men, with at least three alcohol-free days per week (European Association for the Study of the Liver 2012; Michielsen and Sprengers 2003).

Drinking behaviour

Researchers from Denmark showed in a large survey of 30,630 persons that beer or spirits are more likely to promote liver disease than wine (Becker et al. 2002). At present, it is uncertain whether wine per se is responsible for this reduced risk of liver disease compared to the other alcoholic beverages, or whether it represents a surrogate for other healthy behaviours such as increased consumption of fruits/vegetables (Everhart 2003).

Binge-drinking, a mode of social behaviour nowadays, is the exaggerated form of non-mealtime drinking. It has been reported to increase the risk of alcoholic hepatitis fivefold (Barrio et al. 2005), and to increase the risk of all-cause mortality in men and women (Tolstrup et al. 2004). Also drinking multiple types of alcohol has been shown to be related to the risk of cirrhosis and non-cirrhotic liver disease (Naveau et al. 1997).

Gender

It is well recognized that women are more susceptible to alcohol-induced health disorders than men. Men and women have similar sized livers and when the rate of alcohol metabolism is normalized to liver mass, men and women have similar metabolic rates. However, blood alcohol levels after comparable doses of alcohol will usually be higher in women than in men because of their lower body volume and the higher percentage of their body mass consisting of fat. Evidence from animal models has suggested that oestrogen increases the gut permeability to endotoxin and accordingly upregulates endotoxin receptors of Kupffer cells leading to an increased production of tumour necrosis factor alpha in response to endotoxin (Enomoto et al. 1999). It is also known that the gastric alcohol dehydrogenase activity can be different in men and women (Parlesak et al. 2002).

Co-morbid conditions

Individuals with co-morbid conditions affecting the liver exhibit a greater tendency to develop liver disease in response to alcohol consumption than persons being otherwise healthy (Fattovich et al. 2004). This was clearly demonstrated in the case of hepatitis C (Corrao and Arico 1998), hepatitis B, hereditary haemochromatosis (Fletcher et al. 2002), and obesity (Naveau et al. 1997) and most probably applies to other causes of chronic hepatitis.

Genetic polymorphisms

Epidemiological evidence is strong for the existence of heritable susceptibility to alcoholic liver disease. This appears related to several gene polymorphisms, some of which impact alcohol metabolism and others that influence hepatic immune responses.

Non-alcoholic fatty liver disease and non-alcoholic steatohepatitis

Definitions

Steatosis is defined as the accumulation of fat in the liver parenchymal cells or hepatocytes. A distinction is made between macrovesicular and microvesicular steatosis. Macrovesicular steatosis implies the presence of large fat vacuoles, containing predominantly triglycerides, and occupying a large part of the cell cytoplasm, displacing the nucleus towards the cell border. The hepatocytes may be enlarged by the presence of these fat vacuoles. Macrovesicular steatosis is graded according to the percentage of hepatocytes containing fat vacuoles: less than 5 per cent is minimal or no steatosis; 5 to 30 per cent is mild steatosis; over 30 to 60 per cent is moderate; and greater than 60 per cent is considered to be severe macrovesicular steatosis (D'Allessandro et al. 1991). In microvesicular steatosis, bipolar lipids are forming micelles, which are spread over the cytoplasm, and which do not displace the nucleus. The cells usually have normal dimensions. Grading is less complex: 45 per cent is considered to be severe microvesicular steatosis (Sheiner et al. 1995). In many patients, both types of steatosis are present, called mixed type steatosis. In those cases, macrovesicular steatosis is usually predominant.

Two terms have been used interchangeably in the past two decades to describe fat accumulation in hepatocytes. These include *non-alcoholic fatty liver* (NAFL) and *non-alcoholic fatty liver*

disease (NAFLD). While NAFL has been linked to constitutional fatty infiltration of hepatocytes, which is not necessarily associated with an inflammatory response or fibrosis, NAFLD has been linked to an active hepatic injury pattern, inflammation and fibrosis. However, there is no consensus regarding the use of these two terms and the distinction between them. Regardless, in NAFL or NAFLD, steatosis is present, and alcohol is excluded as a cause of the steatosis (Harrison et al. 2004). The maximum daily alcohol consumption allowed for the definition of NAFLD is 10 g (Byrne and Wild 2010). The diagnosis of alcohol consumption relies on thorough anamnesis and hetero-anamnesis, with a detailed 7-day diary of alcohol use. Laboratory parameters are non-specific and even carboxy-deficient transferrin measurement is not very accurate in excluding significant alcohol consumption. In addition, the differential diagnosis cannot be made histologically, as the histological features of alcoholic and non-alcoholic liver disease seem to be identical. The diagnosis of the aspect of 'non-alcoholic' therefore constitutes a first problem in the interpretation of any data on the prevalence and natural history of NAFLD.

Non-alcoholic steatohepatitis (NASH) is a subgroup of NAFLD, in which liver steatosis is accompanied by signs of liver cell damage (especially ballooning of hepatocytes) and/or inflammation. In these patients, fibrous tissue may be generated, and patients can evolve to cirrhosis and its complications, including HCC. Although still debated, it is generally believed that pure steatosis does not lead to fibrogenesis, but steatosis is a sine qua non condition to NASH. NASH patients are more likely to have progressive liver disease (Angulo 2002).

Although not reflected by the name, NAFLD also implies the exclusion of other chronic liver diseases, including chronic viral hepatitis, toxic hepatitis (due to industrial toxins or solvents or to pharmacological agents), autoimmune liver disease, haemochromatosis, Wilson's disease, and some rare metabolic disorders. Hepatitis C, especially genotype 3, and Wilson's disease are two classical examples of liver diseases accompanied by steatosis, but they are not NAFLD. As will be discussed further, steatosis is no longer regarded as an innocent bystander, therefore the term NAFLD is preferred over NAFL.

Diagnosis

A first problem is the diagnosis of the aspect 'non-alcoholic'. Patients may not accurately report the quantity of alcohol they consume. Laboratory tests, including elevation of AST (aspartate transaminase) more than ALT (alanine transaminase), elevation of γ-GT (gamma-glutamyl transpeptidase) or CDT (carboxy-deficient transferrin) measurement may be helpful, but are inaccurate. Thorough anamnesis and hetero-anamnesis is the cornerstone of the diagnosis, which therefore may always remain questionable.

A second problem is the diagnosis of steatosis and steatohepatitis. Abdominal ultrasound has a sensitivity of 70–75 per cent and a specificity of 60–70 per cent in diagnosing moderate to severe steatosis (Bellentani et al. 2000). Computed tomography scanning and magnetic resonance imaging are equally specific (100 per cent) and sensitive (75 per cent) in making the same distinction (Rinella et al. 2001). These non-invasive tools are thus not very sensitive, not able to accurately grade the steatosis, and not able to diagnose the presence of inflammation or fibrosis, and hence do not distinguish between NAFLD and NASH. Magnetic resonance spectroscopy can accurately quantify the fat content of a liver sample, but the need for specific software and practical considerations limits its use to specific research centres. Scores based on laboratory parameters are not validated for the diagnosis of steatosis (Miele et al. 2007). The gold standard for the diagnosis still is liver biopsy. The invasive character of that procedure, however, limits its use on a larger scale.

The diagnosis of steatohepatitis is even more complicated. Laboratory tests, especially the elevation of aminotransferase levels, are inaccurate, although frequently regarded as a sign of liver cell damage and hence inflammation. Patients with elevated liver tests may have pure steatosis without inflammation on liver biopsy, and 50 per cent of the patients with biopsy-proven steatohepatitis have normal transaminases (Prati et al. 2002). The cut-off values for normal aminotransferase levels have recently been questioned, and lowering the upper limit of normal to 30 U/L in males and 19 U/L in females increases the sensitivity for the diagnosis of NASH from 42 per cent to 80 per cent, but specificity decreases from 80 per cent to 42 per cent (Kunde et al. 2005). Scoring systems based on laboratory parameters have been studied and need further validation. Imaging cannot distinguish steatosis from steatohepatitis. Again, liver biopsy is the gold standard. This also holds true for the diagnosis of fibrosis. Laboratory parameters are not useful, except for a stage of cirrhosis, where more specific laboratory features can be present. Imaging is not useful for the staging of fibrosis, and is only of value if signs of cirrhosis indicate advanced liver disease. Elastography, an ultrasound-based technique measuring liver stiffness (Ganne-Carrie et al. 2006), has been validated in hepatitis C, but not in NASH, and, like laboratory scoring systems, only roughly distinguishes between no or mild versus severe fibrosis and cirrhosis. Also for fibrosis, liver histology is still the gold, or at least the best, standard (Miele et al. 2007). More data are needed to approve elastography (Fibroscan®) or other non-invasive methods for clinical assessment of NASH (Friedrich-Rust et al. 2010).

Prevalence of steatosis, NAFLD, and NASH

As already mentioned, the difficulty in diagnosing non-alcoholic steatosis, and the lack of accuracy of the tools for the diagnosis of steatosis, constitute two major problems in the acquisition of precise epidemiological data. Sample selection constitutes a third problem, as some categories of patients are more at risk. In screening studies with ultrasound, prevalence varies between 16 and 23 per cent (Bellentani et al. 2000). In an autopsy series of traffic accidents, steatosis was histologically diagnosed in 24 per cent of cases. The prevalence was clearly age related: in those aged 20 years, the prevalence was 1 per cent, while in those aged 60 years the prevalence rose to 39 per cent (Hilden et al. 1997). Based on these figures, and making the distinction with alcoholic steatosis, the prevalence of non-alcoholic steatosis is estimated at 15–20 per cent in the general adult population (Angulo 2002). Exact data on the prevalence of NASH in the general population are scarce. In an autopsy series, a prevalence of 6.3 per cent was reported. The prevalence is usually estimated at 2 per cent, but this highly depends on sample selection. As a number of risk factors can be identified (see following subsections), prevalence rates may vary geographically (Neuschwander-Tetri and Caldwell 2003).

NAFLD and NASH and the metabolic syndrome

The metabolic syndrome, associating visceral overweight, dyslipidaemia, hyperinsulinaemia or diabetes mellitus, and arterial

Table 8.16.2 Diagnosis of metabolic syndrome according to ATP III

Risk factors	Limits
Central obesity (waist circumference):	
Male	> 102 cm
Female	> 88 cm
Triglycerides	≥ 150 mg/dL
High-density lipoprotein cholesterol:	
Male	< 40 mg/dL
Female	< 50 mg/dL
Arterial blood pressure	≥ 130/ ≥ 85 mmHg
Fasting glycaemia	≥ 100 mg/dL

hypertension, as defined by the Third Report of the National Cholesterol Education Expert Panel on Detection, Evaluation, and Treatment of High Blood Cholesterol in Adults (Adult Treatment Panel-ATP III) (Expert Panel 2001), seems to be closely related with NAFLD and NASH. Some authors consider NAFLD and NASH as the hepatic manifestation of the metabolic syndrome. Many epidemiological data support a close relationship between the two entities.

In patients with NAFLD, the metabolic syndrome, according to the criteria of the ATP III (Table 8.16.2), is fully present in 30 per cent of males and 60 per cent of females. Visceral adiposity is present in 40 per cent and 65 per cent of males and females, respectively, and diabetes in 10 per cent and 30 per cent, respectively. These prevalence rates are significantly higher than in the control population. The metabolic syndrome is significantly more prevalent in patients with NASH compared to patients with simple steatosis (38 per cent vs 14 per cent, $p = 0.004$) (Marchesini et al. 2003).

In patients with obesity, steatosis is present in 60–95 per cent, according to the selection of patients and the procedure used for diagnosis (e.g. ultrasound or histology in a series of patients undergoing bariatric surgery). The body mass index (BMI) is an independent predictive factor for the accumulation of fat in the liver (Marchesini et al. 2003).

Globally, the prevalence of overweight and obesity has increased since 1980, and the increase has accelerated. The global age-standardized prevalence of obesity nearly doubled from 6.4 per cent in 1980 to 12.0 per cent in 2008. Half of this rise occurred in the 8 years between 2000 and 2008 (Stevens et al. 2012). This increase of the prevalence of overweight in children and adolescents is of particular concern. The prevalence of diabetes is also increasing, and was estimated at around 9 per cent worldwide in 2008 (Danaei et al. 2011). In the United States, 22 per cent of the adult population fulfils the criteria of the metabolic syndrome (Lin and Pi-Sunyer 2007).

The natural history of NAFLD/NASH

Data on the natural history of NAFLD and NASH have the same three problems as outlined for the prevalence data. In patients with NASH, 45 per cent will exhibit fibrosis progression and 19 per cent will ultimately develop cirrhosis (Fassio et al. 2004). In patients with NAFLD, lifetime progression to cirrhosis is estimated at 2–5 per cent (Dam-Larsen et al. 2004; Ekstedt et al. 2006).

It is not clear whether only NASH patients will progress, or if pure steatosis may also lead to progressive fibrosis and ultimately cirrhosis. A long-term follow-up study (mean follow-up of 13.7 years) showed no increase in mortality in patients with elevated liver enzymes and pure steatosis on an initial biopsy. Patients with biopsy-proven NASH, on the other hand, had a higher risk of dying from cardiovascular disease (15.5 per cent vs 7.5 per cent, $p = 0.04$) and from liver-related causes (2.8 per cent vs 0.2 per cent, $p = 0.04$). Disease progression was, however, noted: 41 per cent had fibrosis progression and 5.4 per cent of patients developed cirrhosis, and this did not depend on features of inflammation on the initial biopsy (Ekstedt et al. 2006).

In patients with cryptogenic cirrhosis, more than 60 per cent have features that might have been associated with NASH and in these patients cirrhosis is believed to be an end stage of NASH (Ekstedt et al. 2006). Actually cryptogenic cirrhosis accounts for 8 per cent of the indications for liver transplantation in Europe (European Liver Transplant Registry 2011). NASH may recur after liver transplantation, further enforcing the concept of NASH as aetiology of cryptogenic cirrhosis (Maheshwari and Thuluvath 2006).

HCC has been reported in patients with NASH-associated cirrhosis. Data on prevalence and risk, however, are scarce. In the Ekstedt series (Ekstedt et al. 2006), 2.3 per cent developed HCC or 43 per cent of those with documented cirrhosis. It is thus not clear whether the risk is comparable to the 10 per cent cumulative risk usually reported in cirrhosis of any aetiology, but it might be higher (Smedile and Bugianesi 2005). HCC has not been reported without cirrhosis or extensive fibrosis. With the obesity epidemic, it is expected that HCC related to NASH will become more frequent (White et al. 2012).

Risk factors reported to be associated with an increased risk of fibrosis are: age (40 or 50 years of age), the presence of diabetes, BMI 25 or 28 or 30, hypertriglyceridaemia, elevated transaminases two times the upper limit of normal, and AST/ALT 1 (Angulo et al. 1999; Adams et al. 2005). Patients with NAFLD and diabetes have a higher probability of cirrhosis and liver-related death, compared to NAFLD patients without diabetes (Abrams et al. 2004). In the Ekstedt series (Ekstedt et al. 2006), the 41 per cent progression of fibrosis was associated with higher levels of ALT, a higher weight gain during follow-up, more severe insulin resistance and more pronounced fatty infiltration. As stated previously, patients with NASH more frequently meet the criteria of the metabolic syndrome and are more likely to have visceral obesity compared to patients with simple steatosis. As it is believed that NASH is a subgroup of NAFLD at risk for progressive fibrosis, the metabolic syndrome and its components clearly constitute a risk factor for fibrosis and cirrhosis, which will be a major burden of disease in view of the epidemic of obesity and diabetes and their related conditions.

Treatment

No specific treatment is clearly defined for NASH, but there is a consensus concerning implementation of behavioural measures as well as treating cases of advanced disease (Chuthan Sourianarayanane et al. 2013). NASH treatment is driven by the stage of the disease. In more advanced stages, drugs must be added to classical behavioural measures. Up to now, it is clear that patients with NASH benefit from physical exercise and balanced, well oriented diets, probably through weight loss and decreased insulin-resistance (Carulli et al. 2013).

Pharmacological treatment adjuvants for weight losing may be considered in some selected cases. Orlistat and sibutramine have been used, but their indication is limited due to their adverse side effects.

Bariatric surgery is recommended in patients with a BMI greater than 40 kg/m^2 or BMI greater than 35 kg/m^2 and co-morbidities. This procedure is highly effective and may be indicated even in patients with well compensated cirrhosis, but it has high risk of morbidity if the patients have portal hypertension.

For patients who evolved toward advanced liver disease or HCC, liver transplantation can be indicated, although NASH relapse post transplantation is quite frequent.

Specific pharmacotherapy includes drugs used to treat metabolic syndrome, as well as drugs with putative antioxidants effects. The most prescribed drugs are insulin-sensitizers (metformin and pioglitazone). A recent meta-analysis compared the results of the studies that involved these drugs and concluded that pioglitazone is superior compared with metformin (Musso et al. 2010), but pioglitazone has been associated with potential harmful adverse events, such as heart failure and bladder cancer.

Antioxidants are considered promising drugs for NASH, but the studies are considered preliminary. Among the putative antioxidant drugs, vitamin E has been evaluated as having the most consistent results, even with documented amelioration in liver pathology (Sanyal et al. 2010). On the other hand, prolonged use of vitamin E has been associated with adverse reactions such as risk of cerebral vascular haemorrhage, coagulation disturbance and prostatic disorders.

Despite benefits observed in the above mentioned drug therapies, the long-term use of these drugs on NASH in terms of efficacy and safety remains unknown.

Overall conclusion

In spite of the availability of safe and effective vaccines and their proven effectiveness in reducing the chronic consequences of HBV infections, the current burden of disease associated with hepatitis B remains substantial. To finally achieve the WHO goal of HBV elimination, continuous efforts will be required to keep prevention of hepatitis B on the agenda of public health officers worldwide, and to continue to improve treatment options for those already suffering chronic hepatitis B.

Even if the present burden of disease caused by hepatitis C is somewhat less impressive, the lack of an effective vaccine despite major efforts in its development, and the increased burden of chronic liver disease resulting from the high rates of HCV infection 20–30 years ago (the baby boomer generation, born 1946–1964), pose a substantial future threat to public health.

Alcoholic liver disease remains a major cause of morbidity and mortality worldwide. There is concern that, worldwide, alcoholic liver disease may increase in the next several decades. Recent data indicate that alcohol consumption is increasing in low- and middle-income countries. In addition, rates of excessive alcohol intake appear to be rising in women and binge drinking has become a common pattern of excessive alcohol use. Although alcohol-related cirrhosis mortality rates decreased in many countries during the past 30 years, rates are no longer declining in several countries and are actually increasing in low- and middle-income countries.

Although data on the prevalence and natural history of NAFLD/NASH are scarce and suffer from multiple methodological problems, it is clear that, because of their association with the metabolic syndrome and its components, which are increasing to epidemic proportions in the Western population, NAFLD and NASH will constitute a major health problem in the near future.

Key points

◆ Liver cirrhosis and primary liver cancer are important public health problems worldwide, killing more than 1 million people each year. Liver cancer is the third most common cause of deaths from cancer.

◆ Viral hepatitis B and C, and alcoholic as well as non-alcoholic fatty liver disease, represent the major causes for chronic liver diseases. All have oncogenic potential.

◆ Despite the availability and widespread use of effective hepatitis B vaccines, efforts will be required to keep the immunization programmes on the political and donor agenda.

◆ As the development of a hepatitis C vaccine has not yet resulted in success, prevention and control measures will form a major challenge to all those involved in public health. Easy and equal access to the new antiviral treatments is of the utmost importance.

◆ In low- and middle-income countries experts predict a future wave of alcohol-related liver diseases.

◆ Fatty liver disease and steatohepatitis and chronic liver diseases associated with the metabolic syndrome, may rise to epidemic proportions in the near future in Western populations.

References

Abrams, G.A., Kunde, S.S., Lazenby, A.J., et al. (2004). Portal fibrosis and hepatic steatosis in morbidly obese subjects: a spectrum of non-alcoholic fatty liver disease. *Hepatology*, 40, 475–83.

Adam, R., Karam, V., Delvart, V., et al. (2012). Evolution of indications and results of liver transplantation in Europe. A report from the European Liver Transplant Registry (ELTR). *Journal of Hepatology*, 57, 675–88.

Adams, L.A., Lymp, J.F., St Sauver, J., et al. (2005). The natural history of nonalcoholic fatty liver disease: a population-based cohort study. *Gastroenterology*, 129, 113–21.

Alexander, J.F., Lischner, M.W., and Galambos, J.T. (1971). Natural history of alcoholic hepatitis. II. The long-term prognosis. *The American Journal of Gastroenterology*, 56, 515–25.

Alter, M.J. (2007). Epidemiology of hepatitis C virus infection. *World Journal of Gastroenterology*, 13, 2436–41.

Andrade, D.L., de Oliveira, M. de F., de Souza, T.F., et al. (2012). A study about hepatitis C virus infection in patients with psoriasis in a Brazilian reference center. *Acta Gastroenterologica Latinoamericana*, 42, 285–90.

André, F.E. and Zuckerman, A.J. (1994). Review: protective efficacy of hepatitis B vaccines in neonates. *Journal of Medical Virology*, 44, 144–51.

Angulo, P. (2002). Nonalcoholic fatty liver disease. *The New England Journal of Medicine*, 346, 1221–31.

Angulo, P., Keach, J.C., Batts, K.P., et al. (1999). Independent predictors of liver fibrosis in patients with steatohepatitis. *Hepatology*, 30, 1356–62.

Atta, A.M., Oliveira, I.S., Sousa, G.M., et al. (2010). Serum cytokine profile in hepatitis C virus carriers presenting cryoglobulinaemia and non-organ-specific autoantibodies. *Microbial Pathogenesis*, 48, 53–6.

Banatvala, J.E. and Van Damme, P. (2003). Hepatitis B vaccine—do we need boosters? *Journal of Hepatology*, 10, 1–6.

Barrio, E., Tome, S., Rodriguez, I., et al. (2005). Liver disease in heavy drinkers with and without alcohol withdrawal syndrome. *Alcoholism, Clinical and Experimental Research*, 28, 131–6.

Becker, U., Gronbaek, M., Johansen, D., et al. (2002). Lower risk for alcohol-induced cirrhosis in wine drinkers. *Hepatology*, 35, 868–75.

Bellentani, S., Saccoccio, G., Masutti, F., et al. (2000). Prevalence of and risk factors for hepatic steatosis in northern Italy. *Annals of Internal Medicine*, 132, 112–17.

Blachier, M., Leleu, H., Peck-Radosavljevic, M., et al. (2013). The burden of liver disease in Europe: a review of available epidemiological data. *Journal of Hepatology*, 58, 593–608.

Bouchery, E.E., Harwood, H.J., Sacks, J.J., et al. (2011). Economic costs of excessive alcohol consumption in the U.S., 2006. *American Journal of Preventive Medicine*, 41, 516–24.

Bruix, J. and Sherman, M. (2005). AASLD Practice Guideline. Management of hepatocellular carcinoma. *Hepatology*, 42, 1208–36.

Byrne, C.D. and Wild, S.H. (2010). Body fat and increased risk of cirrhosis. *British Medical Journal*, 340, c774.

Cao, G.W. (2009). Clinical relevance and public health significance of hepatitis B virus genomic variations. *World Journal of Gastroenterology*, 15, 5761–9.

Carulli, L., Maurantonio, M., Hebbard, L., et al. (2013). Classical and innovative insulin sensitizing drugs for the prevention and treatment of NAFLD. *Current Pharmaceutical Design*, 19, 5280–96.

Centers for Disease Control and Prevention (1987). Recommendations of the Immunization Practices Advisory Committee. Update on hepatitis B prevention. *Morbidity and Mortality Weekly Report*, 36, 353–60.

Chan, C.Y., Lee, S.D., and Lo, K.J. (2004). Legend of hepatitis B vaccination: the Taiwanese experience. *Journal of Gastroenterology and Hepatology*, 19, 121–6.

Chen, C.J., Yang, H.I., Su, J., et al. (2006). Risk of HCC across a biological gradient of serum HBV-DNA levels. *Journal of the American Medical Association*, 295, 65–73.

Chevalier, S. and Pawlotsky, J.M. (2007). Hepatitis C virus: virology, diagnosis and management of antiviral therapy. *World Journal of Gastroenterology*, 7, 2461–6.

Chuthan Sourianarayanane, A., Pagadala, M.R., and Kirwan, J.P. (2013). Management of non-alcoholic fatty liver disease. *Minerva Gastroenterologica e Dietologica*, 59, 69–87.

Choo, Q.L., Kuo, G., Weiner, A.J., et al. (1989). Isolation of a cDNA clone derived from a blood-borne non-A, non-B viral hepatitis genome. *Science*, 244, 359–62.

Corrao, G. and Arico, S. (1998). Independent and combined action of hepatitis C virus infection and alcohol consumption on the risk of symptomatic liver cirrhosis. *Hepatology*, 27, 914–19.

Cortez-Pinto, H., Gouveia, M., dos Santos Pinheiro, L., et al. (2010). The burden of disease and the cost of illness attributable to alcohol drinking results of a national study. *Alcoholism: Clinical and Experimental Research*, 34, 1442–9.

Coursaget, P., Leboulleux, D., Soumare, M., et al. (1994). Twelve-year follow-up study of hepatitis B immunisation of Senegalese infants. *Journal of Hepatology*, 21, 250–4.

D'Allessandro, A., Kalayoglu, M., Sollinger, H., et al. (1991). The predictive value of donor liver biopsies for the development of primary non-function after orthotopic liver transplantation. *Transplantation*, 51, 157–63.

Dam-Larsen, S., Franzmann, M., Andersen, I.B., et al. (2004). Long term prognosis of fatty liver: risk of chronic liver disease and death. *Gut*, 53, 750–5.

Danaei, G., Finucane, M.M., Lu, Y., et al. (2011). National, regional, and global trends in fasting plasma glucose and diabetes prevalence since 1980: systematic analysis of health examination surveys and epidemiological studies with 370 country-years and 2·7 million participants. *The Lancet*, 378, 31–40.

Davis, G.L., Alter, M.J., El-Serag, H., et al. (2010). Aging of hepatitis C virus (HCV)-infected persons in the United States: a multiple cohort model of HCV prevalence and disease progression. *Gastroenterology*, 138, 513–21.e6

Day, C.P. (2000). Who gets alcoholic liver disease: nature or nurture? *Journal of the Royal College of Physicians of London*, 34, 557–62.

Diehl, A.M. (1997). Alcoholic liver disease: natural history. *Liver Transplantation and Surgery*, 3, 206–11.

Duclos, P. (2003). Safety of immunization and adverse events following vaccination against hepatitis B. *Journal of Hepatology*, 39, S83–88.

Ekstedt, M., Franzen, L.E., Mathiesen, U.L., et al. (2006). Long-term follow-up of patients with NAFLD and elevated liver enzymes. *Hepatology*, 44, 865–73.

Enomoto, N., Yamashina, S., Schemmer, P., et al. (1999). Estriol sensitizes rat Kupffer cells via gut-derived endotoxin. *American Journal of Physiology*, 277, G671–7.

European Association for the Study of the Liver (2012). Clinical practical guidelines: management of alcoholic liver disease. *Journal of Hepatology*, 57, 99–420.

European Consensus Group on Hepatitis B Immunity (2000). Are booster immunisations needed for lifelong hepatitis B immunity? *The Lancet*, 355, 561–5.

European Liver Transplant Registry (2011). *European Liver Transplant Registry*. [Online] Available at: http://www.eltr.org/publi/IMG/gif/DIA8-2.tif.

Everhart, J.E. (2003). In vino veritas? *Journal of Hepatology*, 38, 411–19.

Expert Panel on Detection, Evaluation and Treatment of High Blood Cholesterol in Adults (2001). Executive Summary of The Third Report of The National Cholesterol Education Program (NCEP) Expert Panel on Detection, Evaluation and Treatment of High Blood Cholesterol in Adults (Adult Treatment Panel III). *Journal of the American Medical Association*, 285, 2486–97.

Farci, P. (2003). Delta hepatitis: an update. *Journal of Hepatology*, 39(Suppl. 1), S212–19.

Fassio, E., Alvarez, E., Domínguez, N., et al. (2004). Natural history of non-alcoholic steatohepatitis: a longitudinal study of repeat liver biopsies. *Hepatology*, 40, 820–6.

Fattovich, G., Stroffolini, T., Zagni, I., and Donato, F. (2004). Hepatocellular carcinoma in cirrhosis: incidence and risk factors. *Gastroenterology*, 127(5 Suppl. 1), S35–50.

Fletcher, L.M., Dixon, J.L., Purdie, D.M., et al. (2002). Excess alcohol greatly increases the prevalence of cirrhosis in hereditary hemochromatosis. *Gastroenterology*, 122, 281–9.

Forns, X. and Bukh, J. (1999). The molecular biology of hepatitis C virus. Genotypes and quasispecies. *Clinical Liver Disease*, 3, 693–716.

Frank, C., Mohamed, M.K., Strickland, G.T., et al. (2000). The role of parenteral antischistosomal therapy in the spread of hepatitis C virus in Egypt. *The Lancet*, 355, 887–91.

Friedrich-Rust, M., Hadji-Hosseini, H., Kriener, S., et al. (2010). Transient elastography with a new probe for obese patients for non-invasive staging of non-alcoholic steatohepatitis. *European Radiology*, 20, 2390–6.

Ganne-Carrie, N., Ziol, M., de Ledighen, V., et al. (2006). Accuracy of liver stiffness measurements for the diagnosis of cirrhosis in patients with chronic liver diseases. *Hepatology*, 44, 1511–17.

Gerberding, J.L. and Henderson, D.K. (1992). Management of occupational exposures to bloodborne pathogens: hepatitis B virus, hepatitis C virus, and human immunodeficiency virus. *Clinical Infectious Diseases*, 14, 1179–85.

Goldstein, S.T., Zhou, F., Hadler, S.C., et al. (2005). A mathematical model to estimate global hepatitis B disease burden and vaccination impact. *International Journal of Epidemiology*, 34, 1329–39.

Hadler, S.C. and Margolis, H.S. (1992). Hepatitis B immunization: vaccine types, efficacy, and indications for immunization. In J.S. Remington and M.N. Swartz (eds.) *Current Topics in Infectious Diseases* (Vol. 12), pp. 282–308. Boston, MA: Blackwell Scientific Publications.

Harrison, S.A. and Neuschwander-Tetri, B.A. (2004). Nonalcoholic fatty liver disease and non-alcoholic steatohepatitis. *Clinics in Liver Disease*, 8, 861–79.

Hilden, M., Christoffersen, P., Juhl, E., et al. (1997). Liver histology in a 'normal' population–examination of 503 consecutive fatal traffic casualties. *Scandinavian Journal of Gastroenterology*, 12, 593–8.

Hollinger, F.B. (1989). Factors influencing the immune response to hepatitis B vaccine, booster dose guidelines and vaccine protocol recommendations. *American Journal of Medicine*, 87(Suppl. 3A), 36–40.

Hoofnagle, J.H., Doo, E., Liang, T.J., et al. (2007). Management of hepatitis B: summary of a clinical research workshop. *Hepatology*, 45, 1056–75.

Hughes, S.A., Wedemeyer, H., and Harrison, P.M. (2011). Hepatitis delta virus. *The Lancet*, 378, 73–85.

Jacobson, I.M., McHutchison, J.G., Dusheiko, G., et al. (2011). Telaprevir for previously untreated chronic hepatitis C virus infection. *The New England Journal of Medicine*, 364, 2405–16.

Jilg, W., Schmidt, M. and Deinhardt, F. (1988). Persistence of specific antibodies after hepatitis B vaccination. *Journal of Hepatology*, 6, 201–7.

Kao, J.H. and Chen, D.S. (2005). Hepatitis B vaccination: to boost or not to boost? *The Lancet*, 366, 1337–8.

Kato, N., Ootsuyama, Y., Nakazawa, T., et al. (1994). Genetic drift in hypervariable region I of the viral genome in persistent hepatitis C virus infection. *Journal of Virology*, 68, 4776–84.

Kerr, W.C., Fillmore, K.M., and Marvy, P. (2000). Beverage-specific alcohol consumption and cirrhosis mortality in a group of English-speaking beer-drinking countries. *Addiction*, 95, 339–46.

Kunde, S.S., Lazenby, A.J., Clements, R.H., et al. (2005). Spectrum of NAFLD and diagnostic implications of the proposed new normal range for serum ALT in obese women. *Hepatology*, 42, 650–6.

Kurbanov, F., Tanaka, Y., and Mizokami, M. (2010). Geographical and genetic diversity of the human hepatitis B virus. *Hepatology Research*, 40, 14–30.

Kwo, P.Y., Lawitz, E.J., McCone, J., et al. (2010). Efficacy of boceprevir, an NS3 protease inhibitor, in combination with peginterferon alfa-2b and ribavirin in treatment-naive patients with genotype 1 hepatitis C infection (SPRINT-1): an open-label, randomised, multicentre phase 2 trial. *The Lancet*, 376, 705–16.

Lauer, G.M. and Walker, B.D. (2001). Hepatitis C virus infection. *The New England Journal of Medicine*, 345, 41–52.

Lavanchy, D. (2004). Hepatitis B virus epidemiology, disease burden, treatment, and current and emerging prevention and control measures. *Journal of Viral Hepatitis*, 11, 97–107.

Lee, W.M. (1997). Hepatitis B virus infection. *The New England Journal of Medicine*, 337, 1733–45.

Leuridan, E. and Van Damme, P. (2011). Hepatitis B and the need for a booster dose. *Clinical Infectious Diseases*, 53, 68–75.

Lim, S.S., Vos, T., Flaxman, A.D., et al. (2012). A comparative risk assessment of burden of disease and injury attributable to 67 risk factors and risk factor clusters in 21 regions, 1990–2010: a systematic analysis for the Global Burden of Disease Study 2010. *The Lancet*, 380, 2224–60.

Lin, C.L. and Kao, J.H. (2011). The clinical implications of hepatitis B virus genotype: recent advances. *Journal of Gastroenterology and Hepatology*, 26(Suppl. 1), 123–30.

Lin, S.X. and Pi-Sunyer, E.X. (2007). Prevalence of the metabolic syndrome among US middle-aged and older adults with and without diabetes: a preliminary analysis of the NHANES 1999–2002 data. *Ethnicity & Disease*, 17, 35–9.

Lok, A.S. and McMahon, J. (2007). Chronic hepatitis B: AASLD Practice Guidelines. *Hepatology*, 45, 507–39.

Lok, A.S. and McMahon, J. (2009). Chronic hepatitis B: update 2009. *Hepatology*, 50, 661–2.

Maheshwari, A. and Thuluvath, P.J. (2006). Cryptogenic cirrhosis and NAFLD: are they related? *American Journal of Gastroenterology*, 101, 664–8.

Marchesini, G., Bugianesi, E., Forlani, G., et al. (2003). Nonalcoholic fatty liver, steatohepatitis, and the metabolic syndrome. *Hepatology*, 37, 917–23.

Memon, M.I. and Memon, M.A. (2002). Hepatitis C: an epidemiological review. *Journal of Viral Hepatitis*, 9, 84–100.

Michielsen, P.P. and Sprengers, D. (2003). Who gets alcoholic liver disease: nature or nurture? (summary of the discussion). *Acta Gastroenterologica Belgica*, 66, 292–3.

Miele, L., Forgione, A., Gasbarrini, G., et al. (2007). Noninvasive assessment of liver fibrosis in non-alcoholic fatty liver disease (NAFLD) and non-alcoholic steatohepatitis (NASH). *Translational Research*, 149, 114–25.

Musso, G., Gambino, R., Cassader, M., et al. (2010). A meta-analysis of randomized trials for the treatment of nonalcoholic fatty liver disease. *Hepatology*, 52, 79–104.

Naing, C., Mak, J.W., Wai, N., and Maung, M. (2013). Diabetes and infections–hepatitis c: is there type 2 diabetes excess in hepatitis C infection? *Current Diabetes Reports*, 13, 428–34.

Naveau, S., Giraud, V., Borotto, E., et al. (1997). Excess weight risk factor for alcoholic liver disease. *Hepatology*, 25, 108–11.

Neuschwander-Tetri, B.A. and Caldwell, S.H. (2003). Nonalcoholic fatty liver disease: summary of an AASLD Single Topic Conference. *Hepatology*, 37, 1202–19.

Paraná, R., Vitvitski, L., and Pereira, J.E. (2008). Hepatotropic viruses in the Brazilian Amazon: a health threat. *Brazilian Journal of Infectious Diseases*, 12, 253–6.

Parlesak, A., Billinger, M.H., Bode, C., and Bode, J.C. (2002). Gastric alcohol dehydrogenase activity in man: influence of gender, age, alcohol consumption and smoking in a Caucasian population. *Alcohol and Alcoholism*, 37, 388–93.

Perz, J.F., Armstrong, G.L., Farrington, L.A., et al. (2006a). The contributions of hepatitis B virus and hepatitis C virus infections to cirrhosis and primary liver cancer worldwide. *Journal of Hepatology*, 45, 529–38.

Perz, J.F., Elm, J.L. Jr., Fiore, A.E., et al. (2006b). Near elimination of hepatitis B infections among Hawaii elementary school children universal infant hepatitis B vaccination. *Pediatrics*, 118, 1403–8.

Prati, D. (2006). Transmission of hepatitis C virus by blood transfusions and other medical procedures: a global review. *Journal of Hepatology*, 45, 607–16.

Prati, D., Taioli, E., Zanella, A., et al. (2002). Updated definitions of healthy ranges for serum alanine aminotransferase levels. *Annals of Internal Medicine*, 137, 1–10.

Rehm, J., Samokhvalov, A.V., and Shield, K.D. (2013). Global burden of alcoholic liver diseases. *Journal of Hepatology*, 59, 160–8.

Rendi-Wagner P., Shouval D., Genton B., et al. (2006). Comparative immunogenicity of a PreS/S hepatitis B vaccine in non- and low responders to conventional vaccine. *Vaccine*, 24, 2781–9.

Rinella, M., Alonso, E., Rao, S., et al. (2001). Body mass index as a predictor of hepatic steatosis in living liver donors. *Liver Transplant*, 7, 409–13.

Rizzetto, M. and Ciancio, A. (2012). Epidemiology of hepatitis D. *Seminars in Liver Disease*, 32, 211–19.

Rizzetto, M. and Verme, G. (1985). Delta hepatitis—present status. *Journal of Hepatology*, 1,187–93.

Romano, L., Mele, A., Pariani, E., et al. (2004). Update in the universal vaccination against hepatitis B in Italy: 12 years after its implementation. *European Journal of Public Health*, 14(Suppl.), S19.

Sanyal, A.J., Chalasani, N., Kowdley, K.V., et al. (2010). Pioglitazone, vitamin E, or placebo for nonalcoholic steatohepatitis. *The New England Journal of Medicine*, 362, 1675–85.

Sheiner, P., Emre, S., Cubukcu, O., et al. (1995). Use of donor livers with moderate-to-severe macrovesicular fat. *Hepatology*, 22, 205A.

Sherlock, S. (1993). Clinical features of hepatitis. In A.J. Zuckerman and H.S. Thomas (eds.) *Viral Hepatitis*, pp. 1–11. London: Churchill Livingstone.

Sheron, N., Olsen, N., and Gilmore, I. (2008). An evidence-based alcohol policy. *Gut*, 57, 1341–4.

Shield, K.D., Rylett, M., Gmel, G., et al. (2013). Global alcohol exposure estimates by country, territory and region for 2005–a contribution to the Comparative Risk Assessment for the 2010 Global Burden of Disease Study. *Addiction*, 108(5), 912–22.

Shouval, D., Ilan, Y., Adler, R., et al. (1994). Improved immunogenicity in mice of a mammalian cell-derived recombinant hepatitis B vaccine containing pre-S1 and pre-S2 antigens as compared with conventional yeast-derived vaccines. *Vaccine*, 12, 1453–9.

Smedile, A. and Bugianesi, E. (2005). Steatosis and hepatocellular carcinoma risk. *European Review for Medical and Pharmacological Sciences*, 9, 291–3.

Sorensen, T.I., Orholm, M., Bentsen, K.D., et al. (1984). Prospective evaluation of alcohol abuse and alcoholic liver injury in men as predictors of development of cirrhosis. *The Lancet*, 2, 241–4.

Stevens, G.A., Singh, G.M., Lu, Y., et al. (2012). National, regional, and global trends in adult overweight and obesity prevalences. *Population Health Metrics*, 10, 22.

Suzuki, Y., Ikeda, K., Suzuki, F., et al. (2012). Dual oral therapy with daclatasvir and asunaprevir for patients with HCV genotype 1b infection and limited treatment options. *Journal of Hepatology*, 58, 655–62.

Tan, J. and Lok, A. (2007). Update on viral hepatitis: 2006. *Gastroenterology*, 23, 263–7.

Tandon, B.N. and Tandon, A. (1997). Epidemiological trends of viral hepatitis in Asia. In M. Rizzetto, R.H. Purcell, J.L. Gerin, and G. Verme (eds.) *Viral Hepatitis and Liver Disease*, pp. 559–61. Turin: Edizioni Minerva Medica.

Tanwar, S. and Dusheiko, G. (2012). Is there any value to hepatitis B virus genotype analysis? *Current Gastroenterology Reports*, 14, 37–46.

Tatematsu, K., Tanaka, Y., Kurbanov, F., et al. (2009). A genetic variant of hepatitis B virus divergent from known human and ape genotypes isolated from a Japanese patient and provisionally assigned to new genotype J. *Journal of Virology*, 83, 10538–47.

Tolstrup, J.S., Jensen, M.K., Tjonneland, A., et al. (2004). Drinking pattern and mortality in middle-aged men and women. *Addiction*, 99, 323–30.

Torres, J.R. (1996). Hepatitis B and hepatitis delta virus infection in South America. *Gut*, 38 (Suppl. 2), S48–55.

Tran, T.T., Trinh, T.N. and Abe, K. (2008). New complex recombinant genotype of hepatitis B virus identified in Vietnam. *Journal of Virology*, 82, 5657–63.

Tseng, C.H. and Lai, M.M. (2009). Hepatitis delta virus RNA replication. *Viruses*, 1, 818–31.

UNICEF and WHO (2012). *Immunization Summary. A Statistical Reference Containing Data Through 2010*. New York: UNICEF.

Veldt, B.J., Heathcote, E.J., Wedemeyer, H., et al. (2007). Sustained virologic response and clinical outcomes in patients with chronic hepatitis C and advanced fibrosis. *Annals of Internal Medicine*, 147, 677–84.

Venters, C., Graham, W., and Cassidy, W. (2004). Recombivax-HB: perspectives past, present and future. *Expert Review of Vaccines*, 3, 119–29.

Viana, S., Paraná, R., Moreira, R.C., et al. (2005). High prevalence of hepatitis B virus and hepatitis D virus in the western Brazilian Amazon. *American Journal of Tropical Medicine and Hygiene*, 73, 808–14.

Viviani, S., Jack, A., Hall, A.J., et al. (1999). Hepatitis B vaccination in infancy in the Gambia: protection against carriage at 9 years of age. *Vaccine*, 17, 2946–50.

Wainwright, R., Bulkow, L.R., Parkinson, A.J., et al. (1997). Protection provided by hepatitis B vaccine in a Yupik Eskimo Population: results of a 10 year study. *Journal of Infectious Diseases*, 175, 674–7.

White, D.L., Kanwal, F., and El-Serag, H.B. (2012). Association between nonalcoholic fatty liver disease and risk for hepatocellular cancer, based on systematic review. *Clinical Gastroenterology and Hepatology*, 10, 1342–59.

World Health Organization (2001). *Expanded Programme on Immunization. Introduction of Hepatitis B Vaccination into Childhood Immunization*

Services: Management Guidelines, Including Information for Health Workers and Parents (WHO/V&B/01.31). Geneva: WHO. Available at http://www.who.int/vaccines-documents/DocsPDF01/www613.pdf.

World Health Organization (2004). Hepatitis B vaccines (WHO position paper). *Weekly Epidemiological Record*, 79, 255–63.

World Health Organization (2006). *Vaccines and Biologicals. WHO Vaccine Preventable Disease Monitoring System. Global Summary 2006 (Data up to 2005)*. Available at: http://www.who.int/vaccines-documents/GlobalSummary.pdf.

World Health Organization (2011a). *Alcohol.* [Fact sheet on the harmful use of alcohol] Geneva: WHO. Available at: http://www.who.int/mediacentre/factsheets/fs349/en/index.html.

World Health Organization (2011b). *Global Status Report on Alcohol and Health*. Geneva: WHO. Available at: http://www.who.int/substance_abuse/publications/global_alcohol_report/msbgsruprofiles.pdf.

World Health Organization (2012). *Prevention and Control of Viral Hepatitis Infection: Framework for Global Action*. Geneva: WHO.

Yu, S.C. and Lin, C.W. (2013). Early-stage splenic diffuse large B-cell lymphoma is highly associated with hepatitis C virus infection. *Kaohsiung Journal of Medical Sciences*, 29, 150–6.

Zanetti, A.R., Mariano, A., Romanò, L., et al. (2005). Long-term immunogenicity of hepatitis B vaccination and policy for booster: an Italian multicentre study. *The Lancet*, 366, 1379–84.

Emerging and re-emerging infections

David L. Heymann and Vernon J. M. Lee

Introduction to emerging and re-emerging infections

The microbial world is complex, dynamic, and constantly evolving. Infectious organisms reproduce rapidly, mutate frequently, cross the species barrier between animal hosts and humans, and adapt with relative ease to their new environments. Because of these characteristics, infectious organisms are able to alter their epidemiology, their virulence, and their susceptibility to anti-infective drugs.

When disease is caused by an organism that is newly identified and not known previously to infect humans or has changed in susceptibility to an anti-infectious drug, it is commonly called an emerging infectious disease, or simply an emerging infection. When disease is caused by an infectious organism previously known to infect humans that has re-entered human populations or changed in epidemiology, it is called a re-emerging infection. A report published by the United States Institute of Medicine in 1992 first called attention to emerging and re-emerging infectious diseases as evidence that the fight against infectious diseases was far from won, despite great advances in the development of anti-infective drugs and vaccines (Lederberg et al. 1992).

All forms of infectious organisms—bacteria, viruses, parasites, and prions—are able to emerge or re-emerge in human populations, and it is estimated that up to 70 per cent or more of all emerging infections have a source in animals (zoonotic infections). When a new infectious organism enters human populations there are several potential outcomes. Infected humans may become ill or remain asymptomatic. Once humans are infected, human-to-human transmission may or may not occur. If it occurs, it may be limited to one, two, or more generations, or it may be sustained indefinitely. Among those infectious organisms that cause disease, some maintain their virulence, while others appear to attenuate over time. Changes in the epidemiological characteristics of infectious organisms may occur gradually through a process of adaptation, or they may occur abruptly as the result of a sudden genetic exchange during reproduction and/or replication.

Epidemiology of emerging and re-emerging infections

Many factors influence the transmission of an infectious organism to and among humans including the type of organism, the incubation period (time from exposure to the infectious organism to clinical disease and infectiousness), clinical outcomes, mutations, and human genetics.

Infections of limited human-to-human transmission

Rabies is a zoonotic infection that commonly occurs after the bite of a rabid animal, and variant Creutzfeldt–Jakob disease (vCJD) is a zoonotic infection associated with beef and bovine spongiform encephalopathy (BSE) or 'mad cow disease'. These infections cause illness in humans but cannot transmit from one human to another unless there is iatrogenic transmission through non-sterile medical procedures, blood transfusion, or organ transplant. In several instances, corneal transplantation from a person who died with undiagnosed rabies infection has caused rabies in transplant recipients. The recent identification of several humans with vCJD associated with blood transfusion demonstrates its potential to spread iatrogenically within the human population.

Other zoonotic infections in humans are able to initially transmit from person to person, but then are unable to sustain transmissibility. Thought to have a rodent reservoir in the sub-Saharan rain forest, the monkeypox virus infects humans who come in contact with an infected animal. Transmission is sustained through one or two generations and then ceases. In the first generation of cases, the case fatality rate can approach 10 per cent, but with passage through human populations the virulence and case fatality of human monkeypox appear to decrease as its transmissibility declines. The monkeypox virus caused a limited, multistate outbreak in the United States in 2003, linked to Gambian giant rats imported from West Africa and distributed to pet shops as exotic pets. In the pet shops, prairie dogs, thought to have been the source of the outbreak, appear to have been infected with the monkeypox virus by the Gambian giant rats, and they then transmitted the virus onwards to humans (Guarner et al. 2004).

Another zoonotic infectious organism with limited human-to-human transmission is the Ebola virus. With a relatively short incubation period, infection leads to rapid progression to disease with a severe and often fatal outcome that limits the potential for contact of infected humans with others. The potential for attenuation of the Ebola virus with passage is unknown, though in its present form it is generally agreed that it is unlikely that it will be able to sustain transmission. The Ebola outbreak in 2014 in West Africa spread more widely than previous outbreaks due to the lack of a robust response when it was first identified. The same time-proven response measures can stop outbreaks: hospital infection control and protection of health workers, contact tracing with contacts placed under surveillance and isolation if Ebola symptoms develop, and community health education on transmission, burial practices, and prevention. The 2014 outbreak spread in an area where health systems were being rebuilt after years of civil strife and there was thus inadequate infection control, low access to healthcare, and great movement of populations. This led to the WHO declaration of a Public Health Emergency of International Concern and control remains possible with adequate resources.

Infections with sustained transmission

Infection with the human immunodeficiency virus (HIV), thought to have emerged from a non-human primate sometime in the late nineteenth or early twentieth century, has a long incubation (latent) period during which it is difficult to detect clinically. Though amplification of transmission is thought to have begun during the 1970s through risky sexual behaviour, HIV escaped detection until the early 1980s by which time it had already spread throughout the world and caused a series of epidemics that led to its endemicity. During 2010, HIV was estimated to have caused 2.7 million human infections and 1.8 million deaths worldwide, placing it high on the list of causes of human morbidity and mortality (UNAIDS 2011).

One common infectious organism that is able to sustain transmission—the influenza virus—demonstrates the great diversity of infectious organisms. The RNA viruses that cause seasonal human epidemics of influenza are highly unstable genetically and mutate frequently during replication. Mutation, or genetic drift, results in susceptibility of individuals regardless of their exposure to the viruses before drift, requiring annual antigenic modifications in seasonal influenza vaccines to ensure protection. The short incubation period, and the mild illness caused by the majority of infections, especially among school aged children, result in rapid transmission potential that leads to seasonal influenza epidemics.

At the same time, different subtypes of influenza viruses are found across a variety of avian species, and these occasionally infect humans directly from birds, or from intermediary animal populations that have been infected by birds. The H5N1 avian influenza virus that was first identified in Hong Kong as the cause of human illness in 1997 continues to cause occasional severe infections in humans but remains a zoonotic human infection and does not transmit easily from person to person. This virus, however, like many other avian influenza viruses has the potential to mutate and gain the epidemiological characteristics that would permit it to spread easily among humans to cause an epidemic or a pandemic. Pandemics are, by definition, infectious disease outbreaks that spread across the world, and they are the result of the lack of immunity to a new infectious organism to which there has been no previous human exposure. The highly fatal 1918 influenza pandemic is thought to have originated from an avian influenza virus that may have undergone adaptive mutation in non-human mammals over time, attaining human transmissibility characteristics before

crossing the animal/human species (Taubenberger and Morens 2006).

Other influenza pandemics in 1957, 1968, and 2009 are thought to have been caused by genetic reassortments during the intracellular replication process in an animal dually infected with viruses containing human and avian influenza genetic components (Guan et al. 2010; York and Donis 2013). The 2009 H1N1 pandemic influenza virus showed genes from swine, avian, and human influenza. Though the 2009 pandemic virus is thought to have its origins in the Americas, risk factors for emergence of influenza viruses in humans are thought to be highest in areas such as South China and South East Asia where there are large populations of aquatic birds (the hosts of many different types of avian influenza viruses) and where humans live in close proximity to animals such as pigs that may be easily infected by these aquatic birds.

Geographic distribution of emerging and re-emerging infections

Emerging infections have the potential to occur in every country and on every continent (Fig. 8.17.1). Though the term emerging infections was introduced in the early 1990s, the previous 40 years had seen a panoply of newly identified infections in humans on every continent. The year 1976 was especially illustrative of this phenomenon with the identification of the 1976 swine flu virus (H1N1), thought to be a direct descendant of the virus that caused the pandemic of 1918, at a military base in Fort Dix (United States) (Sencer 2011); the identification of *Legionella pneumophila* as the cause of an outbreak of severe respiratory illness among a group of veterans staying at a hotel in downtown Philadelphia (United States), initially feared to be a human outbreak of swine influenza (H1N1) (Centers for Disease Control and Prevention (CDC) 2012a); and the identification of the Ebola virus as the cause of simultaneous outbreaks of haemorrhagic fever in Sudan and the Democratic Republic of Congo (then called Zaire) (CDC 2012b).

Nine years earlier, in 1967, the Marburg virus had been identified for the first time in an outbreak in Germany that caused 25 primary infections and seven deaths among laboratory workers who were infected by handling monkeys from Uganda, and six secondary cases in health workers who took care of primary cases, with subsequent spread to family members (Slenczka and Klenk 2007). A member of the same filovirus family as Ebola, the Marburg virus has caused sporadic small outbreaks in Africa during the 1970s and 1980s, and larger outbreaks in 1998 in the Democratic Republic of Congo and 2005 in Angola. Since the Marburg virus was first identified in 1967 there have been over 40 other newly identified infectious organisms in humans, an average of one per year.

Economic impact of emerging and re-emerging infections

Outbreaks caused by emerging and re-emerging infections are costly (Fig. 8.17.2). They consume healthcare resources and divert them from endemic disease problems, result in productivity loss, and decrease trade and tourism revenue. At times they economically devastate entire sectors. This has occurred after major

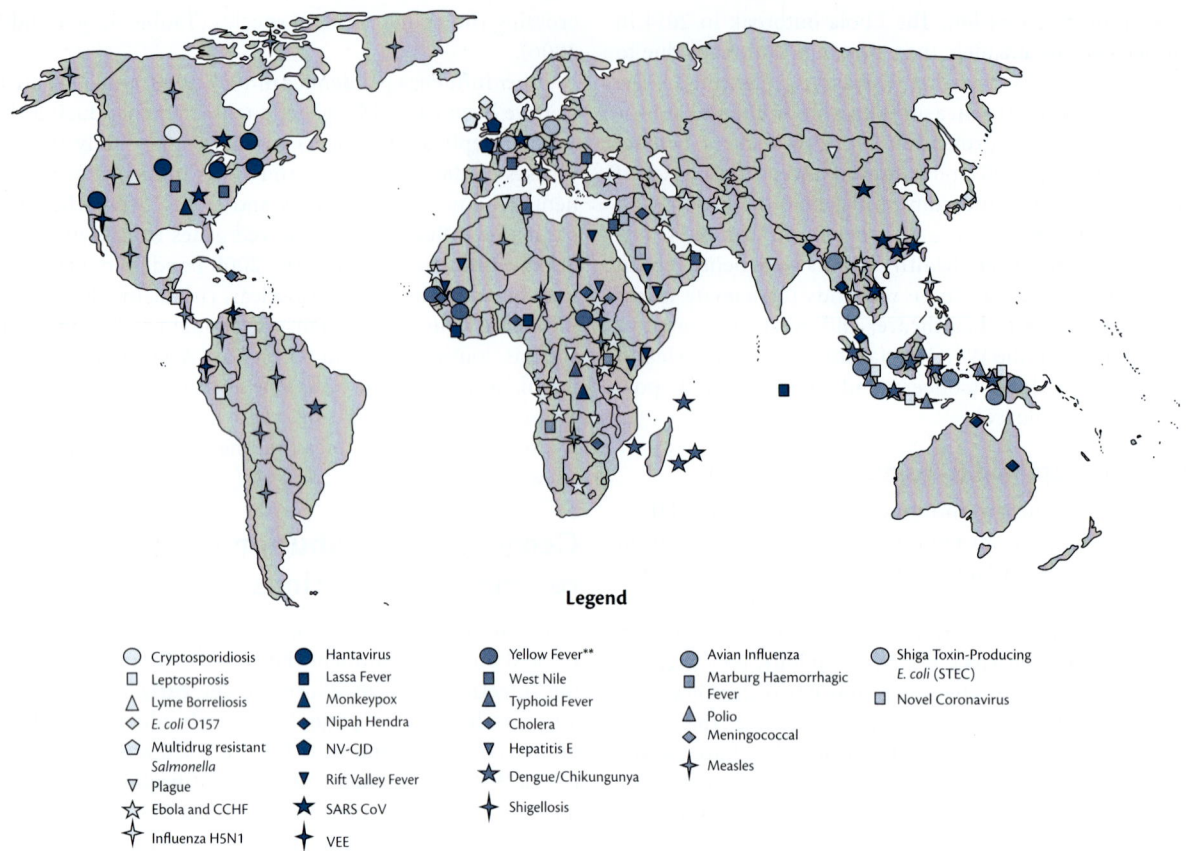

Legend

○ Cryptosporidiosis	● Hantavirus	● Yellow Fever**	● Avian Influenza	● Shiga Toxin-Producing
□ Leptospirosis	■ Lassa Fever	■ West Nile	■ Marburg Haemorrhagic	E. coli (STEC)
△ Lyme Borreliosis	▲ Monkeypox	▲ Typhoid Fever	Fever	□ Novel Coronavirus
◇ E. coli O157	◆ Nipah Hendra	◆ Cholera	▲ Polio	
⬠ Multidrug resistant	⬟ NV-CJD	▽ Hepatitis E	◆ Meningococcal	
Salmonella	▼ Rift Valley Fever	☆ Dengue/Chikungunya	✛ Measles	
▽ Plague	★ SARS CoV			
☆ Ebola and CCHF		✛ Shigellosis		
✴ Influenza H5N1	✚ VEE			

Fig. 8.17.1 Selected emerging and re-emerging infectious diseases, 1996–2012.
Source: data from World Health Organization (WHO), Global Alert and Response (GAR), *Disease Outbreaks by Year*, Copyright © WHO 2014, available from http://www.who.int/csr/don/archive/year/en/.

outbreaks of emerging or re-emerging infections during the past 20 years, with economic losses ranging from an estimated US$36 million after the re-emergence of cholera in Tanzania in 1998 (World Health Organization (WHO) 2007a), to approximately US$39 billion after the emergence of BSE in the United Kingdom during the period 1990–1998 (WHO 2007a). During 2009, after the pandemic of H1N1 had been identified, the Mexican economy lost an estimated US$2 billion, mainly due to decreased trade and tourism.

Costs from outbreaks can be direct, indirect, or intangible. The most apparent direct costs are those associated with medical care of patients. Indirect costs arise at the individual level from loss of work and caregiving by relatives, and through interventions aimed at reducing the impact of the outbreak such as quarantining of contacts or closure of schools. Indirect costs also arise at the macro-economic level because of their impact on travel, tourism, trade, and consumer confidence. Fear of transmission causes international tourists to choose alternative holiday locations, and local populations to avoid any perceived source of infection such as foods from animals that may have been implicated in the outbreak, restaurants, and other public leisure venues—sectors of the economy that are significant contributors to the gross domestic product (GDP) of many countries. Misinformed consumers avoided purchasing pork during the 2009 pandemic of H1N1 influenza even though it was not a continued source of human infection,

and avoided fresh vegetables during the 2011 outbreak of *Escherichia coli* O104 in Europe when speculation occurred as to its cause. Finally, there are intangible costs such as the loss of life. Economists have attempted to estimate the economic cost of death, but fail to capture other non-economic and socio-cultural changes that can be a consequence of a highly lethal outbreak.

The severe acute respiratory syndrome (SARS) was a good example of an emerging infection with severe indirect costs, as it was responsible for sizeable economic losses and insecurity in financial markets across Asia and worldwide. With fewer than 9000 cases, the outbreak was estimated by the Asian Development Bank to have cost Asian countries an estimated US$18 billion in GDP terms for 2003, and up to US$60 billion of gross expenditure and business losses (Asian Development Bank 2003).

In 2008, the World Bank estimated that the cost of a severe influenza pandemic (which would apply to other pandemics of similar severity) could be up to US$2–3 trillion taking into account healthcare costs and impact on the economy (Burns et al. 2008). It is therefore important to prepare for and respond to infectious disease outbreaks in order to minimize their healthcare and economic impact. Though the economic impact of the 2009 pandemic of H1N1 did not reach these proportions, the H5N1 virus continues to circulate among poultry in Asia with potential to cause a highly lethal and costly pandemic.

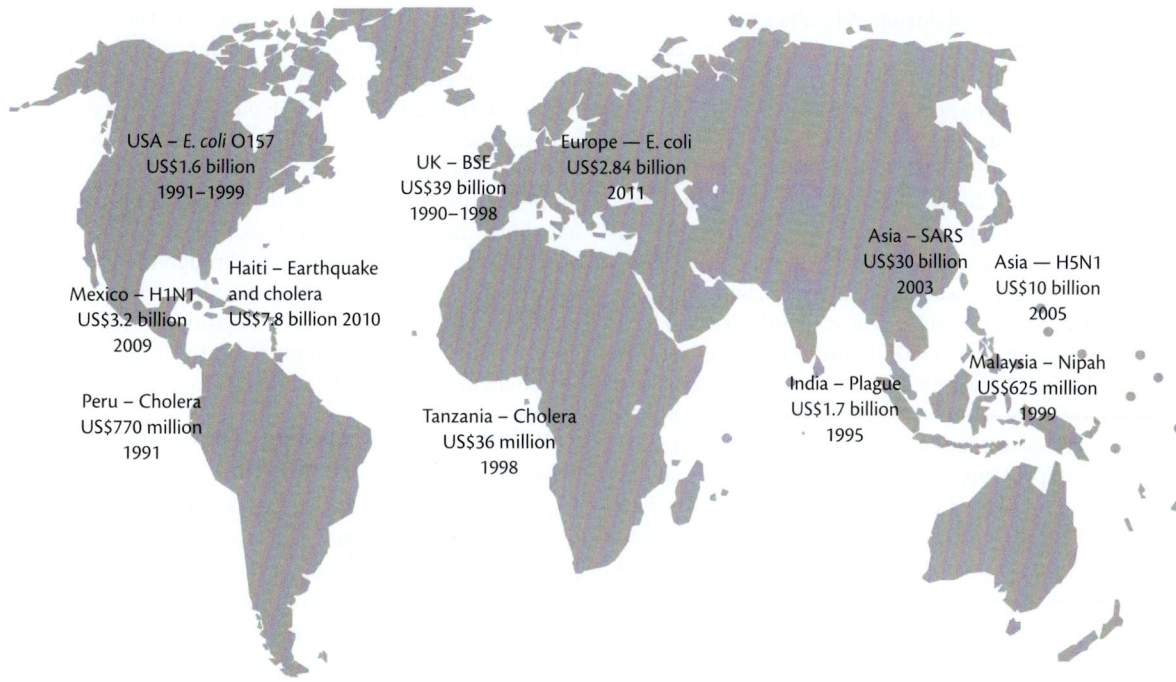

ᵃExcludes economic impact of human sickness and death.

Fig. 8.17.2 Direct economic impact of selected infectious disease outbreaks, 1990–2011.

Source: data from *Food Poison Journal*, German E. coli O104:H4 Outbreak—$2.84 Billion in Human Damage, June 2011, Copyright © 2011 Marler Clark, LLP, available from http://www.foodpoisonjournal.com/foodborne-illness-outbreaks/german-e-coli-o104h4-outbreak—284-billion-in-human-damage/#.UPi_IB2R89U; European Commission, *Factsheet Haiti Two Years on: European Commission's Actions to Help Rebuild the Country*, 2012, Copyright © European Union, 1995–2014, available from http://ec.europa.eu/europeaid/news/documents/factsheet_haiti_en.pdf; Marc P. Girarda et al., The 2009 A (H1N1) influenza virus pandemic: A review, *Vaccine*, Volume 28, Issue 31, pp. 4895–4902, Copyright © 2010 Published by Elsevier Ltd; and WHO (2006, 2007a).

Factors influencing emergence and re-emergence

Many external factors may align in such a manner as to provide opportunities for the emergence or re-emergence of infectious diseases. They range from weakened public health infrastructure and failure of safety procedures/regulations to increases in population, anthropogenic activities or climate change, civil disturbance/human displacement, and human behaviour that varies from misperceptions about the seriousness of the risks that cause emerging infections and the use of anti-infective drugs, to the safety of public health interventions and the desire to deliberately cause terror and harm.

Weakened public health infrastructure

Weakening of public health infrastructure resulted in part from decreased investment in public health during the second half of the twentieth century. This is compounded by poverty in lower-resourced countries where there are competing priorities for development, and suboptimal access to healthcare and sanitation. Deficient infrastructure also leads to a lack of the robust public health practices that could prevent the emergence of infectious diseases, or prepare communities to respond to them should they emerge.

Aedes aegypti has now become well established in many large cities worldwide following the deterioration of mosquito control

campaigns during the 1970s. The resurgence of the *Aedes* species has been confounded by the adoption of modern consumer habits in urban areas where discarded household appliances, tyres, plastic food containers, and jars create abundant mosquito breeding sites. With the increase in *Aedes* species there has been an increased risk of dengue outbreaks. Prior to 1970, nine countries, mainly in Latin America, reported outbreaks of dengue. In 1983, 13 countries in Latin America and Asia reported dengue outbreaks, and by 1998, 1.2 million cases were reported from 56 countries. During 2001, 69 countries reported dengue outbreaks, and it is now endemic in more than 100 countries in Africa, the Americas, the Eastern Mediterranean, South East Asia, and the Western Pacific. By 2010, reported dengue infections exceeded 2.2 million annually with more than 20,000 deaths, and estimates place the actual number of infections worldwide at between 50–100 million (WHO 2012a). Major dengue outbreaks have occurred during the past decade in Brazil, Indonesia, Thailand, Vietnam, Bangladesh, India, Pakistan, and Cape Verde. During 2012, an outbreak of dengue occurred in Portugal with 191 probable cases reported (WHO 2012b).

In 2005, the Chikungunya virus, likewise transmitted by *Aedes* species, emerged and spread throughout several southern Pacific islands. A total of 3100 human infections were reported by a sentinel network on La Réunion within the first 6 months of the outbreak, leading to an estimate of over 204,000 human infections by March 2006. In 2007, the Chikungunya virus spread north to Europe, where it caused an outbreak with 292 suspected human infections in northern Italy, and during 2010–2011 Chikungunya epidemics occurred throughout southern India (WHO 2012c).

Lapses in childhood immunization coverage due to weakened childhood immunization programmes in Russia resulted in the re-emergence of diphtheria, with major epidemics in the early 1990s. Reported cases of diphtheria in the Russian Federation increased from just over 1200 in 1990 to over 5000 in 1993. Likewise, lapses in yellow fever vaccination programmes in sub-Saharan Africa since the 1950s have left large susceptible populations in both rural and urban areas of the region, with sporadic urban outbreaks in cities in Côte d'Ivoire (2001), Senegal and Guinea (2002), and Burkina Faso (2004) (Jamison et al. 2006). This is in contrast to the successful smallpox eradication programme that achieved sustained investment and close links between policy and political support, research, and field programmes that contributed to its success; progress in the eradication of polio that has decreased the annual number of children paralyzed to fewer than 700 in 2011 (WHO 2012d); and the decrease in measles mortality by 74 per cent (2007) since intensified efforts at measles mortality reduction were begun during 2000 (WHO 2008a).

Surveillance systems are critical in the early detection of outbreaks and during their containment, and to monitor progress. Setting up of surveillance systems requires substantial investment in infrastructure and manpower, and the commitment to sustain these systems in the long term. Most epidemiologists recognize that it was in part because of substandard surveillance systems in developing countries that HIV rapidly spread during the late 1970s, and was not detected until it was first identified in the United States in the early 1980s.

Failure of safety procedures/regulations

Substandard universal precautions and hospital regulations during the 1980s led to breaches in sterile injection practices and nosocomial infections of HIV in the former USSR and Romania, together infecting over 250 children, accompanied by high levels of hepatitis B in both patients and health workers (Matic et al. 2006). Likewise substandard universal precautions led to nosocomial outbreaks of Ebola haemorrhagic fever in the Democratic Republic of Congo in 1976 and 1995, where syringes and/or failed barrier nursing amplified the transmission to patients, health workers, and the community (CDC 2012b). Continued lapses in universal precautions led to the amplification of recent outbreaks of Ebola infection in the Democratic Republic of Congo and Uganda, and contributed to nosocomial transmission of SARS in hospitals in China, Hong Kong, Taiwan, Singapore, Vietnam, and Canada where outbreaks then spread to communities.

Blood transfusions are another potential source of infection, especially for emerging infections which are not yet known and therefore impossible to detect by screening. A substantial proportion of HIV cases in the early phases of the epidemic were transmitted by blood transfusion (Curran et al. 1984). Although most countries now test banked blood for HIV and many other known infectious organisms, many resource-poor countries struggle to bank blood and ensure that transfusions are safe (Goodnough et al. 2003).

Changes in the process of rendering the carcasses of ruminant animals for the preparation of bone meal which was fed to other ruminant animals, are thought to have been the cause of the outbreak of BSE in cattle that also led, in May 1995, to the death of a 19-year-male in the United Kingdom, the first human death from what is now known to be variant vCJD or human bovine spongiform encephalopathy (hBSE) (Prusiner 1997; Trevitt and Singh 2003). The BSE and hBSE outbreaks demonstrate the health consequences of regulations for rendering that had changed over a 10-year period prior to 1995, inadvertently permitting rendered parts of cattle infected with the BSE-causing prion to contaminate bone meal used for livestock feed. The most likely source of human infection is thought to be through the preparation or consumption of contaminated meat and/or beef products. The BSE and hBSE outbreaks led to the recognition of the need for stronger government intervention along the entire 'feed to food' continuum to better ensure the safety of foodstuffs for human consumption.

Population shifts including rapid increase and uncontrolled urbanization

Population shifts can lead to the emergence, re-emergence, and transmission of infectious diseases. Classic examples are the plague epidemics in Europe in the fourteenth century thought to have originated in Asia and spread first along the Silk Road, then by trade on merchant ships sailing the Mediterranean; and smallpox that is thought to have arrived in the Americas from Europe during the years of exploration and colonization that began in the fifteenth century. These epidemics incited fear and killed many who became infected, threatening to bring down entire civilizations. The world is much more easily travelled and interconnected since then, with large numbers of people moving from continent to continent every day. This has facilitated the international spread of emerging diseases as illustrated by the SARS epidemic that spread from a medical doctor who had treated patients with a severe atypical pneumonia in Guangdong Province, China. He became ill, but travelled to Hong Kong for a wedding and spent a night in a hotel where he somehow passed the infection to tourists and other travellers who then seeded outbreaks in Vietnam, Singapore, Canada, and other parts of the world within days.

Population growth can result in increased disease transmission, especially where the infrastructure is unable to cope. The world's population more than doubled in the second half of the twentieth century, accelerating most rapidly in the developing countries of the tropics and subtropics. Rural–urban migration has resulted in crowded living conditions, and inadequacy of water and sanitation systems, and other basic infrastructure. In 1950, there were two urban areas in the world with populations greater than 7 million; by 1990, this number had risen to 23. In 2012, as urban migration continues, there are 25 megacities, each with more than 10 million people.

Population increases in Latin America resulted in breakdowns in sanitation and water systems in large coastal cities. In 1991, when cholera re-emerged in Peru after having been quiescent for approximately 100 years, it rapidly spread throughout other urban areas in Latin America. Thought to have originated from contaminated seafood on the Peruvian coast, the disease caused nearly 400,000 reported cases and over 4000 deaths in 16 South American countries that year. By 1995, there were more than 700,000 reported cases and just over 6000 deaths in the Americas, and in 2012, cholera remains endemic in many areas (Delgado et al. 2011).

Uncontrolled urbanization, with overcrowding and substandard living conditions in slum areas of Asia and Africa, has likewise contributed to the re-emergence of tuberculosis (TB) and plague. HIV infection, also concentrated in urban areas, has facilitated the re-emergence of TB, showing the sometimes dynamic interaction among infectious agents. The most recent serious outbreak of plague occurred in five states in India in 1994, where almost 700 suspected bubonic or pneumonic plague cases and 56 deaths were reported; a smaller outbreak of 16 persons with pneumonic plague was reported from northern India in 2002 (Gupta and Sharma, 2007).

Anthropogenic activities or climate change

Deforestation that disrupts natural habitats of animals, and forces animals, searching for food, into closer contact with humans has been linked to the emergence and re-emergence of Lassa Fever in West Africa, and sine nombre virus in North America. First identified in 1969 when two nurses died with a haemorrhagic fever syndrome in Nigeria, the Lassa Fever virus is now known to be transmitted to humans from human food supplies and/or the household environment contaminated by urine and/or other excreta of infected rodents (Fichet-Calvet and Rogers 2009; Senior 2009). In many instances, rats invade human living spaces in search of food because rainforests, a natural habitat, have been destroyed. Sin nombre virus is a hantavirus, first identified in an outbreak in the southwestern United States in 1993. It is now known to spread from infected rodents to humans through aerosolized excreta found in dust of homes that have been invaded by rodents (CDC 2012c).

The Nipah virus outbreaks in Malaysia and Singapore in 1998–1999 are another example where evidence suggests that anthropogenic activities, including clearing of forests for agricultural purposes, encroached on the natural reservoir for the Nipah virus, the fruit bat. The virus, excreted in bat guano, is thought to have infected pigs that were farmed in areas that had penetrated the forests. The virus subsequently spread to humans in close contact with the infected pigs, and resulted in outbreaks with approximately 250 human infections and 100 deaths from Nipah-caused viral encephalitis. Additional outbreaks of the Nipah virus from 2001 to 2009 in Bangladesh suggested indirect transmission from bats to humans through palm wine collected from palm trees where fruit bats are known to feed, and direct human-to-human transmission in hospitals (Epstein et al. 2006). Another virus thought to be carried by bats, the Ebola Reston virus, infected pigs in the Philippines in 2009, and the virus spread from pigs to pig farmers and workers in slaughterhouses causing asymptomatic infection (Miranda and Miranda 2011).

In Latin America, Chagas disease re-emerged as an important human disease after deforestation caused triatomine populations to move from their wild natural hosts to involve humans and domestic animals in the transmission cycle, eventually transforming the disease into an urban infection that can also be transmitted by blood transfusion. Other emerging infections influenced by changing habitats of animals include Lyme borreliosis in Europe and North America, transmitted to humans who come into contact with ticks that normally feed on rodents and deer, the natural reservoir of *Borrelia burgdorferi*.

Climatic changes, both anthropogenic and from natural variations, also influence the development of epidemics. The narrow band of desert in sub-Saharan Arica, in which epidemic *Neisseria meningitides* infections traditionally occur, has enlarged as

drought spread south to involve Uganda and Tanzania. Climate extremes, whether involving excessive rainfall or drought, can likewise displace animal species and bring them into closer contact with human settlements, or increase vector breeding sites. A 1998 outbreak of Japanese encephalitis in Papua New Guinea has been linked to extensive drought, which led to increased breeding sites for the *Culex* mosquito as rivers dried into stagnant pools (Erlanger et al. 2009). It is thought that mosquitoes then transmitted the Japanese encephalitis virus from infected pigs and/or wild birds to humans. The Japanese encephalitis virus is now widespread in Southern Asia from India and Thailand to Malaysia, and as far north as Korea and Japan.

Above-normal rainfall associated with the occurrence of the warm phase of the El Niño Southern Oscillation phenomenon is thought to have been the cause of extensive flooding in East Africa from December 1997 to March 1998, increasing the breeding sites for *Aedes* mosquitoes. Mosquitoes then facilitated the transfer of the Rift Valley fever (RVF) virus from infected cattle, sheep, and/or goats to humans who had been forced to live in close proximity to animals on islands of dry land surrounded by flood water. During this period, the largest RVF outbreak ever reported in East Africa occurred in Kenya, Somalia, and Tanzania. The total number of human infections in northern Kenya and southern Somalia alone was estimated at 89,000 with an estimated 478 deaths. During 2006 and 2007, RVF caused outbreaks with approximately 250 human infections and 130 deaths in Kenya, Somalia and Sudan; and an outbreak of 172 cases and 15 deaths occurred in 2010 in South Africa (Hightower et al. 2012).

Public health consequences of civil disturbance, human displacement, and natural disasters

Human population movements on a large scale as a result of war, conflict, or natural catastrophe often result in crowded, unhygienic, and impoverished living conditions. This in turn heightens the risk of emergence and re-emergence of infectious diseases. In the aftermath of civil disturbance in Rwanda in 1994, over 48,000 cases of cholera and 23,800 deaths were reported within 1 month among Rwandans who had been displaced to refugee camps in Goma, Democratic Republic of Congo (Goma Epidemiology Group, 1995).

A collateral impact of war, conflict, or natural catastrophe such as earthquakes is the destruction or weakening of health systems with diminished capacity to detect, prevent, and respond to infectious disease outbreaks. One consequence of the 27-year civil war in Angola was the outbreak of Marburg haemorrhagic fever in 2004 that spread to more than 200 humans, 90 per cent of whom died. Emergence of the Marburg virus was detected late and transmission was amplified in overcrowded and understaffed health facilities where lack of investment during the war had resulted in substandard infection control. Another large outbreak of Marburg virus infection was identified in late 1998 in the Democratic Republic of Congo, also a conflict-ravaged country. This emergence resulted in sporadic cases with small chains of transmission over a 2-year period in a remote area where civil war had interrupted supply lines and communication to health facilities in the region (Bausch et al. 2006).

Natural disasters can also create conditions that facilitate the direct or indirect spread of infectious disease. Flooding commonly disrupts clean water supplies, and in 2009 in the Philippines, where leptospirosis is endemic, more than 2000 reported human infections, with an estimated case fatality rate of 10 per cent, were associated with flooding caused by a major typhoon (Amilasan et al. 2012). The deterioration of clean water supplies and health services in Haiti after a major earthquake in 2010 served as fertile ground for a cholera importation that led to an outbreak of approximately 600,000 infections and 7500 deaths, approximately 6 per cent of the entire post-earthquake population (CDC 2012d; Piarroux and Faucher 2012).

Human behaviour

Occupation

Throughout history, some human occupations have been associated with infectious disease. Anthrax has been called wool-sorters' disease because of transmission of its spores from infected animals to humans who shear sheep and other wool-producing animals, or whose occupation leads to exposure to their hides. It has also been associated with butchers who come into contact with infected animals at the time of slaughter or during preparation of meat for markets. Anthrax spores infect humans either intra-dermally, causing cutaneous anthrax, or by ingestion or inhalation, causing enteric or pulmonary/inhalation anthrax.

Though intensive research has failed to confirm the origins of Ebola haemorrhagic fever outbreaks, infection is thought to occur as humans encounter animal sources, possibly infected bats and/or non-human primates infected by bats, somewhere in the transmission cycle. An outbreak of Ebola haemorrhagic fever in humans in 1995 was linked to a woodsman, who worked deep within the tropical rainforest making charcoal, where he was believed to have become infected with the Ebola virus that he then carried back to his home village. An outbreak of Ebola in Gabon in 1996 is thought to have had a point source in a chimpanzee that was killed and butchered by a group of young hunters; and in 1994 a Swiss researcher infected with the Ebola virus in a forest reserve in West Africa is thought to have become infected while conducting chimpanzee autopsies in search of the cause of a major die-out of the animals (Daszak 2006). A more recent outbreak of Ebola in Uganda has been associated with exposure to bat guano in gold mines in 2008 (Food and Agricultural Organisation 2011).

In 2003, a veterinarian in the Netherlands became infected with the influenza A (H7N7) virus during an investigation of influenza outbreaks in poultry and later died from acute respiratory failure. A total of 89 humans, including the veterinarian, were confirmed to have H7N7 influenza virus infection linked to this poultry outbreak and no further deaths occurred. The majority of human infections are thought to have occurred as a result of direct contact with infected poultry; but there were three possible instances of transmission of infection from poultry workers to family members (Jong et al. 2009). The H5N1 influenza virus has caused major lethal epidemics of influenza among poultry in many Asian countries, and exposure of children or adults to infected poultry being raised in backyards or industrial poultry farms has resulted in periodic human infections. By August 2012, a total of 608 sporadic infections had been reported to the WHO with an estimated case fatality rate of approximately 59 per cent (WHO 2012e). Several countries have reported small clusters of persons infected with H5N1 infection that do not sustain transmission, usually occurring in family members or others who have close contact with an infected person.

Healthcare workers are exposed to emerging and re-emerging infections on two fronts. Laboratory and health workers are at especially high risk of emerging and re-emerging infections, and can themselves be conduits of transmission. In the 1995 outbreak of Ebola haemorrhagic fever in Kikwit (Democratic Republic of Congo), almost one-third of those infected were health workers, and in the 2003 SARS outbreak in Singapore, ten health workers were thought to have been infected while treating an infected health worker colleague who is also thought to have infected her husband, three other patients, and seven visitors to the hospital (Wilder-Smith et al. 2005). These examples show the potential for health workers to become infected, and in some instances to sustain and amplify transmission in hospitals, and through their patients and family members, to the community. Laboratory workers are also at risk of infection: the last human case of smallpox was caused by a laboratory accident in the United Kingdom, and the last-known human cases of SARS occurred in laboratory accidents in Singapore and China.

Mistrust and misinformation

During 2003, unsubstantiated rumours circulated in northern Nigeria that the oral polio vaccine (OPV) was unsafe and vaccination of young children could cause infertility. Mistrust and misinformation that followed led to the government-ordered suspension of polio immunization in two northern states and substantial reductions in polio immunization coverage in those states, and a large number of others (Larson and Heymann 2010). The result was a polio outbreak across northern Nigeria that then spread to, and re-emerged in, previously polio-free areas in sub-Saharan Africa, the Middle East, and as far as Indonesia. Over 70 per cent of all children worldwide who were paralysed by polio during the following year, 2004, were living in Nigeria—or in other parts of sub-Saharan Africa that had been re-infected by polio virus genetically linked to viruses that had a Nigerian origin (United Nations Children's Fund 2006; Modlin 2010).

Misinformation about the safety of vaccines against pertussis, measles, and hepatitis B has likewise led to decreases in vaccine uptake among children, and in some instances industrialized country outbreaks of pertussis and measles. An example is a decrease in uptake of the measles, mumps and rubella (MMR) vaccine in the United Kingdom from a coverage of 92 per cent at the time of a falsified publication in 1998 that suggested a link between MMR and autism, to a low of 79 per cent during 2003 (Pearce et al. 2008). To ensure vaccine uptake is maximized, public confidence in the benefit, safety, and effectiveness of vaccines must be upheld, which in turn, relies on a comprehensive evidence base underpinning vaccination strategies (Larson et al. 2011).

Deliberate use to cause terror and harm

Infectious organisms have been deliberately used to cause terror and harm throughout history, with accounts of the use of highly infectious and lethal organisms such as smallpox to kill or weaken the opposition during wars in the eighteenth century (Riedel 2005), and this has continued into the twenty-first century. It was graphically illustrated in 1979 in an outbreak of inhalation anthrax in Sverdlovsk, 1400 km east of Moscow, in the then Soviet Union. Attributed at first by government officials to the consumption of contaminated meat, it was later shown to have been caused by the unintentional release of anthrax spores from a Soviet military microbiology facility. It is estimated that up to 358 humans were infected and that between 45 and 199 died (Meselson et al. 1994) (see Chapter 8.18).

In the United States in late September 2001, the deliberate dissemination of anthrax spores in four known letters sent through the United States Postal Service caused massive disruption of postal services in the United States, and in many other countries around the world. The anthrax letters—dated 11 September 2001, and postmarked 7 days later—caused huge public alarm and prompted a massive public health response. A total of 22 persons are thought to have been infected by anthrax spores sent through the postal system; 11 developed cutaneous anthrax and the remaining 11 developed inhalation anthrax, of whom five died. Twenty of the 22 patients were exposed to work sites that were found to be contaminated with anthrax spores. Nine of them had worked in mail processing facilities through which the anthrax letters had passed (Bouzianas 2009).

Other bacteria, viruses, mycotic organisms, and biological toxins are also considered to have the potential for deliberate use to cause harm to humans. Great concern has been expressed by many countries about the potential health consequences that could be caused by the deliberate introduction of infectious organisms such as the variola virus into a human population where smallpox vaccination is no longer practised, or the plague bacillus that could potentially cause an outbreak of pneumonic plague. Stockpiles for vaccines against infections such as smallpox and anthrax are currently being maintained, at great expense, as part of emergency contingency planning in some countries.

In addition to the deliberate use of existing infectious agents, new laboratory research can result in the creation of novel agents that have the potential for human spread. One example is the laboratory research on H5N1 influenza viruses to determine the mutations that will facilitate human spread. While the research was performed to understand the determinants of transmission in an academic setting, if these more transmissible viruses were to fall into the wrong hands, it could result in a pandemic of unprecedented proportions. This has resulted in much debate among the scientific and regulatory communities on the merits of research with potential dual uses.

Antimicrobial drug resistance—susceptibility of infectious organisms to anti-infective drugs

Bacteria, viruses, and parasites all have the potential to develop resistance to anti-infective drugs by spontaneous mutation and natural selection, or through the exchange of genetic material between strains and species. These resistant organisms can then transmit from human to human, replacing more susceptible organisms with resistant strains. Soon after development of the first antibiotics, warning signs of microbial resilience began to appear. By the end of the 1940s, resistance of hospital strains of *Staphylococcus aureus* to penicillin emerged in the United Kingdom with levels as high as 14 per cent, and by the end of the 1990s, levels had risen to of 95 per cent or greater. Resistance has also developed to semi-synthetic penicillin derivatives as *S. aureus* has acquired genes encoding resistance to methicillin and other narrow-spectrum beta-lactamase-resistant antibiotics. Methicillin-resistant *S. aureus* (MRSA), first identified

in the United Kingdom in 1961 within a year of the introduction of methicillin, is now widespread in hospital-acquired infections in the United Kingdom and throughout the world (Johnson 2011).

The bacterial and viral infections that contribute most to human disease are also those in which antimicrobial resistance is rapidly emerging: diarrhoeal diseases such as dysentery; respiratory tract infections, including pneumococcal pneumonia and TB; sexually transmitted infections such as gonorrhoea and HIV; and infectious organisms that have now accumulated resistance genes to virtually all currently available anti-infective drugs such as extremely drug-resistant TB (XDR-TB).

Since 2008, Gram-negative Enterobacteriaceae have been shown to be resistant to a broad range of beta-lactam antibiotics including carbapenems that are widely used for their treatment. Carbapenem-resistant bacterial infections have been identified in many countries across the world with emergence thought to have occurred somewhere in Asia (Kumarasamy et al. 2010).

The causes of antimicrobial drug resistance (AMR) are complex, and involve both the human and animal health sectors, and others such as plant and fish agriculture. AMR is a major global public health issue because it threatens the effectiveness of antimicrobials in combating infection, which has been one of the most important advances in clinical medicine. A lack of effective antimicrobials could lead the world back to the pre-antimicrobial era where simple infections often led to severe outcomes, and where effective measures to control the spread of disease, especially those for which there are no vaccines, would be lost. AMR also increases healthcare and other indirect costs as more expensive treatments are required, and illnesses may be prolonged.

Use of anti-infective drugs in human health

Behaviours such as over- or under-prescribing of antibiotics by health workers, excessive demand for antibiotics by the general population, or the use of substandard drugs with inferior anti-infective drug content, have had a remarkable impact on the selection and survival of resistant microbes, rapidly increasing levels of microbial resistance.

In Thailand, among 307 hospitalized patients in the late 1980s, 36 per cent of persons who were treated with anti-infective drugs did not have an infectious disease (Aswapokee 1990). Over-prescribing of anti-infective drugs occurs in most other countries as well. In Canada, it has been estimated of the more than 26 million people treated with anti-infective drugs, up to 50 per cent were treated inappropriately (Kondro 1997). This has also led to community-based resistance where otherwise healthy individuals may be carrying resistant microbes which can result in transmission or infection. Findings from community surveys of *Escherichia coli* in the stool samples of healthy children in China, Venezuela, and the United States suggest that although multiresistant strains were present in each country, they were more widespread in Venezuela and China, countries where less control is maintained over antibiotic prescribing and sales (Lester et al. 1990).

The availability of multiple drugs to treat TB since the 1940s has reduced death rates from TB substantially. Resistant organisms have emerged, however, facilitated by inappropriate prescribing and poor adherence to treatment regimes. Multi-drug resistant TB (MDR-TB) has now become widespread, especially in prison settings in Eastern Europe, and resistant organisms are now being transmitted to healthy populations throughout the world. In 2006, an outbreak of extremely drug-resistant TB (XDR-TB), against which almost all TB drugs are ineffective, occurred in South Africa (WHO 2012f), and all XDR-TB cases that were tested for HIV were found to be HIV-positive as well. To date, more than 60 countries have reported XDR-TB (WHO 2011), and with HIV infection endemic, the world provides continued fertile ground for the transmission of all forms of TB, including MDR- and XDR-TB.

Malaria is another major infection with high mortality that has been reduced substantially with the introduction of antimalarial drugs. By 1976, however, chloroquine-resistant *Plasmodium falciparum* malaria had developed and was highly prevalent in South East Asia. Ten years later, chloroquine-resistant malaria was found worldwide, as was high-level resistance to two second-line drugs, sulphadoxine/pyrimethamine and mefloquine. Subsequently, use of artemisinin combination therapy is now recommended by the WHO to ensure effective treatment, but since 2009 there are reports of artemisinin resistance in South East Asia, threatening to derail efforts to control malaria in Asia, and worldwide (Nayyar et al. 2012).

Prevention and control of resistant infections such as MRSA and *Clostridium difficile* in healthcare facilities is an important key to reducing the spread of AMR, and control of such hospital-acquired infections must be a priority.

Use of anti-infective drugs in animal husbandry and agriculture

Large quantities of anti-infective drugs are indiscriminately added to animal feed in some countries to promote animal growth, resulting in the selection of resistant bacterial strains in animals. Antibiotics are also used in agriculture for spraying of fruit trees, rice paddies, and flowers to avoid bacterial blights.

Some of the organisms that infect animals freely circulate between animals and humans, providing opportunities for zoonotic infection with resistant organisms, and for swapping or exchanging resistant genes, thus increasing the speed with which anti-infective resistance evolves in both agriculture and human populations. Alternative approaches can reduce such antibiotic use as in Norway, where the introduction of effective vaccines in farmed salmon and trout, and improved health management, reduced the annual anti-infective use in farmed fish by 98 per cent from 1987 to 2004 (WHO 2012g). During the 1990s, Norway and other countries throughout Europe banned the non-discriminate use of antibiotics for growth promotion in animal feed.

The weakness of surveillance and monitoring systems for antimicrobial resistance, partially the result of the lack of easy-to-use surveillance tools, makes it difficult to understand the extent and evolution of the AMR problem globally. The lack of financial investment for research into new antimicrobials and vaccines is also a major global problem. Many of the anti-infective drugs currently in use were developed decades ago and the lack of drugs that target non-similar areas on microbes limits treatment modalities available to combat infections.

The WHO has proposed a five-pronged containment strategy for AMR (Fig. 8.17.3), the implementation of which is being promoted worldwide through activities set up around a World Health Day in 2011, and a report on AMR in 2012. Underpinning

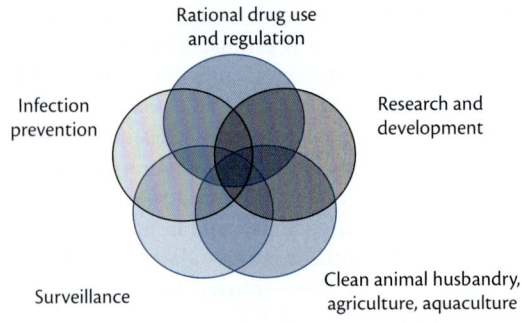

Fig. 8.17.3 The five key areas for containment of antimicrobial resistance.
Source: data from World Health Organization (WHO), *Model based on the WHO Global Strategy for Containment of Antimicrobial Resistance*, Copyright © WHO 2001, available from http://www.who.int/csr/resources/publications/drugresist/en/EGlobal_Strat.pdf.

this strategy is the need for national commitments for sufficient and sustainable resources to be made available to combat AMR (WHO 2012h).

Public health security: globalization and emerging/re-emerging infectious disease organisms

Our world of increased human mobility and interdependence facilitates the transfer of infectious organisms from country to country, and across continents. Infectious organisms efficiently travel in humans, insects, food, and animals, and can spread around the globe and emerge in new geographic areas with ease and speed. Some are transported by migratory birds. Others, such as disease-carrying mosquitoes, travel in the passenger cabin or luggage hold of jets, to cause tropical infections in temperate countries when they feed on airport workers or those who live nearby. They thus threaten public health security—our collective vulnerability to acute infectious disease outbreaks across international borders (Heymann 2003).

In 2000, among 312 athletes participating in an international triathlon held in Malaysia, 33 became infected with leptospirosis and returned to their home countries during the incubation period. While leptospirosis lacks human transmissibility and therefore did not set up local foci or transmission, the outbreak of SARS in 2003 clearly did, and demonstrates the full potential of emerging infectious organisms to spread internationally. From a medical doctor infected in Guangdong Province of China, who unknowingly carried the new infectious organism to a Hong Kong hotel, SARS spread in individual chains of transmission from infected hotel guests to 8422 reported cases in North and South America, the Middle East, Europe, and Asia with a case-fatality rate of approximately 11 per cent (WHO 2003).

During the years 1969–2003, 18 instances of airport malaria were reported to the WHO—malaria infections in workers at airports or in persons who live nearby who had not travelled to malaria-endemic countries (WHO 2007b). Their infection originated from malaria-infected *Anopheles* mosquitoes that had travelled from countries with endemic malaria and took a blood meal from airport workers or other persons upon landing. In 2003, a seven-person outbreak of malaria among persons in Florida who had not previously travelled to malarious areas demonstrated the potential for imported malaria to set up local foci of transmission if the *Anopheles* mosquito is present (Morbidity and Mortality Weekly Report 2004).

Livestock, animal products, and food can also carry infectious organisms that emerge or re-emerge in non-endemic countries. VCJD, identified in persons in 11 countries, most of whom had not previously travelled to the United Kingdom (Diack et al. 2012), clearly demonstrates the ability of infections to travel in animals or animal products. RVF emerged in humans in Yemen and Saudi Arabia in 2000, 2 years after a major outbreak of RVF in East Africa. Infection has since become endemic in livestock in the Arabian Peninsula, and is thought to have been imported from East Africa in livestock traded across the Red Sea (Balkhy and Memish 2003). In 2000, imported raspberries contaminated with *Cyclospora* caused an outbreak in the United States. It is hypothesized that the raspberries imported from Guatemala were contaminated when surface water was used to spray them with fungicide before harvest (Ho et al. 2002). In 2011, an outbreak caused by *Escherichia coli* O104 linked to sprouts grown from imported beans resulted in over 3000 infections and 31 deaths from haemolytic uramic syndrome (European Food Safety Authority 2012).

Concerns about the international spread of emerging and re-emerging infections and the need for strong public health security are not new. By the fourteenth century, governments had recognized the capacity for international disease transmission and legislated preventive measures, as reflected in the establishment of quarantine in the city state of Venice. Arriving ships were not permitted to dock for 40 days, and people at land borders were held in isolation for 40 days in the hope of keeping plague from entering.

Many European leaders of the mid-nineteenth century, worried by the cholera pandemic of the time, threats of plague, and the weakness of quarantine measures, began to recognize that controlling the spread of infectious diseases from one nation to another required cooperation between those nations. International conventions were organized and draft covenants signed, almost all of which related to some type of quarantine regulations.

From 1851 to 1897, ten international sanitary conferences were held among a group of 12 European countries, focusing exclusively on the containment of epidemics in their territories. The inaugural 1851 conference in Paris lasted 6 months and was followed in 1892 by the first International Sanitary Convention that dealt with cholera. Five years later, at the 10th International Sanitary Conference, a similar convention that focused on plague was signed.

New policies then emerged in the late nineteenth century, such as the obligatory telegraphic notification of first cases of cholera and plague, a model that a small group of South American nations followed when they signed the first set of international public health agreements in the Americas during the 1880s. In addition to cholera and plague, often carried by immigrants arriving from Europe, the agreements in the Americas covered yellow fever that was endemic in much of the American region at that time, and that from time to time caused major urban epidemics.

During the following decade, 12 countries attended the First International Sanitary Convention of the American Republics in Washington, DC, leading to the creation of the Pan American Sanitary Bureau (now called the Pan American Health Organization) in 1902. Its counterpart in Europe was the Office International d'Hygiène Publique (OIHP), established in 1907, and based in Paris.

In 1951, 3 years after its founding, the WHO adopted a revised version of the International Sanitary Regulations (1892) that remained focused on the control of cholera, plague, and yellow fever and was rooted firmly in the preceding agreements of the nineteenth and twentieth centuries.

The International Health Regulations

In 1969, the Member States of the WHO agreed to a new set of international sanitary regulations—the International Health Regulations (IHR)—aimed at better ensuring public health security with minimal interruption in travel and trade. In addition to requiring reporting of four infectious diseases—cholera, plague, yellow fever, and smallpox—the IHR were aimed at stopping the spread of disease by pre-established control measures at international borders. They included reporting requirements for these four diseases, and described appropriate responses such as yellow fever and smallpox vaccination for passengers arriving from countries where yellow fever or smallpox outbreaks had been reported. The IHR provided a legal framework for global surveillance and control of spread of infectious diseases.

By 1996, it had become clear, however, that the IHR were not able to ensure public health security as had been envisioned. Over the previous 30 years, border posts proved inadequate to stopping the international spread of infectious diseases which often crossed borders while still in the incubation period in humans, or silently in non-human hosts—insects, animals, food, and agriculture goods. At the same time, countries reported the occurrence of cholera, plague, and yellow fever late or not at all because of fear of stigmatization and economic repercussions (smallpox had been removed from the list when it was certified eradicated in 1980). The IHR also did not meet the challenges caused by other emerging and re-emerging infectious disease and their rapid transit round the globe.

From 1996 until 2005, WHO Member States therefore undertook a process to examine and revise the IHR. The result—the IHR (2005) (WHO 2008b)—provided a more up-to-date legal framework requiring reporting of any public health emergency of international concern (PHEIC), and the use of real-time evidence to recommend measures to stop their international spread. A PHEIC is defined as an extraordinary event that could spread internationally or might require a coordinated international response (WHO 2012i). Under the IHR (2005) an event is evaluated for its potential to become a PHEIC by the country in which it is occurring even though reporting might legitimately come from elsewhere, using a decision tree instrument developed for this purpose (Fig. 8.17.4). If the criteria for a PHEIC are met, an official notification must be provided to the WHO. Notification is also required for even a single occurrence of a disease that would always threaten global public health security—smallpox, poliomyelitis caused by a wild-type poliovirus, human influenza caused by a new virus subtype, and SARS. In addition, there is a second list that includes diseases of documented—but not inevitable—international impact. An event involving a disease on this second list, which includes cholera, pneumonic plague, yellow fever, Ebola, and the other haemorrhagic fevers, still requires the use of the decision tree instrument to determine if it is a PHEIC. Thus, two safeguards create a baseline

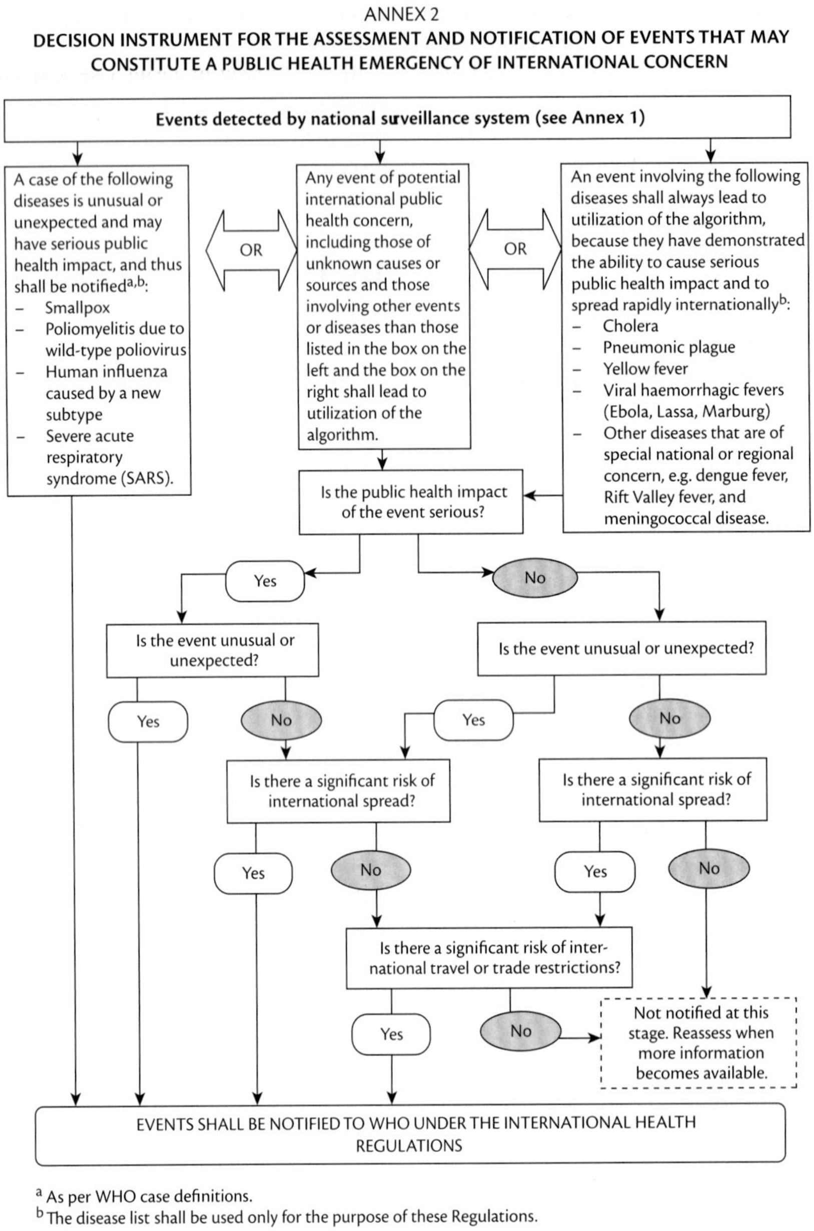

ANNEX 2
**DECISION INSTRUMENT FOR THE ASSESSMENT AND NOTIFICATION OF EVENTS THAT MAY
CONSTITUTE A PUBLIC HEALTH EMERGENCY OF INTERNATIONAL CONCERN**

Fig. 8.17.4 Decision tree for assessment of a potential public health event of international concern.
Reproduced with permission from World Health Organization (WHO), *International Health Regulations*, Second edition, Copyright © WHO 2005, available from: http://www.who.int/ihr/publications/9789241596664/en/.

of public health security by requiring countries to respond, in designated ways, to well-known threats.

In contrast to previous regulations, the IHR (2005) introduced a set of core capacity requirements for surveillance and response. All countries were to meet these requirements during the first 5 years of implementation of the IHR (2005) in order to rapidly detect, assess, notify, report, and contain the events covered by the regulations so that their potential for international spread and negative economic impact would be minimized. The IHR (2005) likewise require collective action by all WHO Member States in the event that an emerging or re-emerging infectious disease threatens to spread internationally, and the free sharing of information pertaining to this threat. They thus provide a safety net against

the international spread of emerging or re-emerging infections, requiring collaboration between all states to ensure the timely availability of surveillance information and technical resources that better guarantee international public health security.

Other international frameworks have also been developed to contain and curtail the international spread of emerging infections. Among them are the WHO Global Strategy for the Containment of Antimicrobial Resistance (WHO 2001a) described earlier in this chapter (see 'Use of anti-infective drugs in animal husbandry and agriculture'). Though not legally binding, this framework calls on countries to work across the human health, animal health, agricultural, and trade sectors to ensure more rational use of anti-infective drugs in order to limit the factors that accelerate the selection and proliferation of anti-infective drug-resistant microbes.

Recommendations for the future

National and international systems for addressing the threat of infectious diseases

To enable the world to deal effectively with the threat of emerging and re-emerging diseases, there is the need for countries to follow the international frameworks laid out by such agreements as the International Health Regulations (2005) and the WHO Global Strategy for the Containment of Antimicrobial Resistance (2001a); and also by the United Nations Framework Convention on Climate Change, still under negotiation. These international agreements call for action at the global, national, and subnational levels that will decrease the risks factors that influence emergence and re-emergence of infectious diseases. At the same time, if followed they will result in better detection and response where and when emerging and re-emerging public health events occur, be they at the animal/human interface or in other situations where a series of risk factors align in such a way as to permit their occurrence. Effectively preventing, or rapidly detecting, assessing, and responding to infectious disease outbreaks will save lives and protect economies.

The link between health and overall human development is also important, as many factors such as poverty, lack of education, and basic community infrastructure play a role in emergence and re-emergence. As concluded by the WHO Commission on Macroeconomics and Health (2001b), health considerations must be placed squarely at the centre of economic development, and all sectors of society must work together to achieve this goal, as it is not the sole purview of the health sector alone.

A better understanding of our ecosystem and causative factors will enable preventive actions that reduce the likelihood of disease emergence, especially infections at the animal/human interface. One example is safe and healthy market programmes to encourage proper handling and distribution of livestock and maintenance of strict sanitation in markets where animals or animal products are sold that could be a source of infection.

For emerging and re-emerging infections that are able to transmit from person to person, the window of opportunity for effective intervention often closes quickly. The most important defence against their international spread is robust surveillance and preparedness, response protocols, and mitigation systems. This includes highly sensitive national surveillance systems, public health laboratories that can rapidly detect such outbreaks, and mechanisms for timely outbreak containment and mitigation. It also necessitates good communications systems, and risk communication and health education programmes, to enable coordinated preparedness and response by all stakeholders. These are the core capacities required by the IHR (2005), and it is clear that the same systems that detect and contain naturally occurring outbreaks also permit detection and initial response to deliberately caused outbreaks of infectious disease.

The collaborative action required by IHR (2005) when emerging or re-emerging infections threaten to spread internationally likewise provides a framework for global surveillance and response that is a departure from previous international conventions and regulations. The IHR (2005) explicitly acknowledge that non-state sources of information about outbreaks often precede official notification, especially when countries may be reluctant to reveal an event in their territories. Collaboration among countries for public health security in the face of emerging and re-emerging infections is vital. If an outbreak of emerging or re-emerging infectious disease occurs in a country that requires international assistance to help in containment activities, as agreed by the WHO and the affected country after confidential and pro-active consultation, other countries are obligated to provide the technical expertise required to the country through WHO or bilaterally. To this end, global databases of professionals with expertise in specific diseases or epidemiological techniques are maintained as part of the requirement of the IHR (2005), together with non-governmental organizations present in countries and in a position to reach remote areas. Such mechanisms, which are further supported by the WHO network of Collaborating Centres (national laboratories and institutes throughout the world serving as international reference centres), help optimize the use of global expertise and resources. The IHR (2005) were instrumental in the coordination of the international response to the H1N1 influenza pandemic in 2009. Upon the recommendation of the IHR Emergency Committee set up by the Director General of the WHO, the pandemic was declared within weeks of its onset, and triggered a series of obligations for collaboration among countries under the IHR (2005). Operational protocols that had been developed as part of pandemic planning and preparedness activities in countries around the world were implemented, together with coordinated actions under the IHR (2005).

The future

The vision embraced by the IHR (2005) is of a world alert and ready to respond collectively to the threat of emerging and re-emerging infections that represent an acute threat to public health security. This requires an unbroken line of defence within countries and globally, using the most up-to-date technologies of surveillance and response.

The IHR (2005) require adherence to new norms and standards for reporting and responding to emerging and re-emerging infections despite the economic consequences that may result. Their full achievement will provide the highest level of public health security possible. National core capacities as described in the IHR (2005) must be put in place within the national public health system that can detect, investigate, communicate, and contain events that threaten public health security as soon as they appear. An interconnected system must be operating at the national and international levels, engaged in specific threat and risk assessment and management activities that minimize collective vulnerability to public health events.

These two goals are interdependent and must be sustained. They involve measures that the international community must continually invest in, strive to achieve, and assess for progress. In today's mobile, interdependent, and interconnected world, threats arising from emerging and epidemic-prone diseases affect all countries. Such threats reinforce the need for shared responsibility and collective action in the face of universal vulnerability, in sectors that go well beyond health.

References

Amilasan, A.-S., Ujiie, M., Suzuki, M., et al. (2012). Outbreak of leptospirosis after flood, the Philippines, 2009. *Emerging Infectious Diseases*, 18(1), 91–4.

Asian Development Bank (2003). *SARS: Economic Impacts and Implications*. [Online] Available at: http://www.adb.org/publications/sars-economic-impacts-and-implications.

Aswapokee, N., Vaithayapichet, S., and Heller, R.F. (1990). Pattern of antibiotic use in medical wards of a university hospital, Bangkok, Thailand. *Reviews of Infectious Diseases*, 12(1), 136–41.

Balkhy, H.H. and Memish, Z.A. (2003). Rift Valley fever: an uninvited zoonosis in the Arabian Peninsula. *International Journal of Antimicrobial Agents*, 21(2), 153–7.

Bausch, D.G., Nichol, S.T., Muyembe-Tamfum, J.J., et al. (2006). Marburg hemorrhagic fever associated with multiple genetic lineages of virus. *The New England Journal of Medicine*, 355(9), 909–19.

Bouzianas, D.G. (2009). Medical countermeasures to protect humans from anthrax bioterrorism. *Trends in Microbiology*, 17(11), 522–8.

Burns, A., Mensbrugghe van der, D., and Timmer, H. (2008). *Evaluating the Economic Consequences of Avian Influenza*. [Online] Available at: http://siteresources.worldbank.org/EXTAVIANFLU/Resources/EvaluatingAHIeconomics_2008.pdf.

Centers for Disease Control and Prevention (2012a). *Legionella Topic Home*. [Online] Available at: http://www.cdc.gov/legionella/index.htm.

Centers for Disease Control and Prevention (2012b). *Questions and Answers about Ebola Hemorrhagic Fever*. [Online] Available at: http://www.cdc.gov/ncidod/dvrd/spb/mnpages/dispages/ebola/qa.htm.

Centers for Disease Control and Prevention (2012c). *Tracking a Mystery Disease: The Detailed Story of Hantavirus Pulmonary Syndrome (HPS)*. [Online] Available at: http://www.cdc.gov/hantavirus/hps/history.html.

Centers for Disease Control and Prevention (2012d). *Haiti Cholera Outbreak*. [Online] Available at: http://www.cdc.gov/haiticholera/.

Curran, J.W., Lawrence, D.N., Jaffe, H., et al. (1984). Acquired immunodeficiency syndrome (AIDS) associated with transfusions. *The New England Journal of Medicine*, 310(2), 69–75.

Daszak, P. (2006). Risky behavior in the Ebola zone. *Animal Conservation*, 9(4), 366–7.

Delgado, G., Morales, R., Mendez, J.L., and Cravioto, A. (2011). The re-emergence of cholera in the Americas. In T. Ramamurthy and S.K. Bhattacharya (eds.) *Epidemiological and Molecular Aspects on Cholera*, pp. 79–95. New York: Springer.

Diack, A.B., Ritchie, D., Bishop, M., et al. (2012). Constant transmission properties of variant Creutzfeldt–Jakob disease in 5 countries. *Emerging Infectious Diseases*, 18(10), 1574–9.

Epstein, J., Field, H., and Luby, S. (2006). Nipah virus: impact, origins, and causes of emergence. *Current Infectious Disease Reports*, 8(1), 59–65.

Erlanger, T.E., Weiss, S., Keiser, J., Utzinger, J., and Wiedenmayer, K. (2009). Past, present, and future of Japanese encephalitis. *Emerging Infectious Diseases*, 15(1), 1–7.

European Food Safety Authority (2012). *Shiga Toxin-Producing E. coli Outbreak(s)*. [Online] Available at: http://www.efsa.europa.eu/en/topics/topic/ecolioutbreak2011.htm.

Fichet-Calvet, E. and Rogers, D.J. (2009). Risk maps of Lassa fever in West Africa. *PLoS Neglected Tropical Diseases*, 3(3), e388.

Food and Agricultural Organisation (2011). *Investigating the Role of Bats on Emerging Zoonoses*. Rome: FAO. Available at: http://aitoolkit.org/site/DefaultSite/filesystem/documents/BATS ZOONOSES.pdf.

Goma Epidemiology Group (1995). Public health impact of Rwandan refugee crisis: what happened in Goma, Zaire, in July, 1994? *The Lancet*, 345(8946), 339–44.

Goodnough, L., Shander, A., and Brecher, M.E. (2003). Transfusion medicine: looking to the future. *The Lancet*, 361(9352), 161–9.

Guan, Y., Vijaykrishna, D., Bahl, J., Zhu, H., Wang, J., and Smith, G.J.D. (2010). The emergence of pandemic influenza viruses. *Protein & Cell*, 1(1), 9–13.

Guarner, J., Johnson, B.J., Paddock, C.D., et al. (2004). Monkeypox transmission and pathogenesis in prairie dogs. *Emerging Infectious Diseases*, 10(3), 426–31.

Gupta, M.L. and Sharma, A. (2007). Pneumonic plague, northern India, 2002. *Emerging Infectious Diseases*, 13(4), 664–6.

Heymann, D.L. (2003). The evolving infectious disease threat: implications for national and global security. Harvard University/Commission on Human Security for Global Health. *Journal of Human Development*, 4, 191–207.

Hightower, A., Kinkade, C., Nguku, P.M., et al. (2012). Relationship of climate, geography, and geology to the incidence of Rift Valley Fever in Kenya during the 2006–2007 outbreak. *American Journal of Tropical Medicine and Hygiene*, 86(2), 373–80.

Ho, A.Y., Lopez, A.S., Eberhart, M.G., et al. (2002). Outbreak of cyclosporiasis associated with imported raspberries, Philadelphia, Pennsylvania, 2000. *Emerging Infectious Diseases*, 8(8), 783–8.

Jamison, D., Feachem, R., Makgoba, M., et al. (2006). *Vaccine-Preventable Diseases*. Washington, DC: World Bank. Available at: http://www.ncbi.nlm.nih.gov/books/NBK2284/.

Johnson, A.P. (2011). Methicillin-resistant Staphylococcus aureus: the European landscape. *The Journal of Antimicrobial Chemotherapy*, 66(Suppl. 4), iv43–iv48.

Jong, M.C.M.D., Stegeman, A., Goot, J.V.D., and Koch, G. (2009). Intra- and interspecies transmission of H7N7 highly pathogenic avian influenza virus during the avian influenza epidemic in the Netherlands in 2003. Interspecies transmission of H7N7 low pathogenic avian influenza virus to poultry. *Revue Scientifique et Technique*, 28(1), 333–40.

Kondro, W. (1997). Study reveals extent of Canada's overprescribing. *The Lancet*, 349(9059), 1156.

Kumarasamy, K., Toleman, M., Walsh, T., et al. (2010). Emergence of a new antibiotic resistance mechanism in India, Pakistan and the UK: a molecular, biological and epidemiological study. *The Lancet Infectious Diseases*, 10(9), 597–602.

Larson, H.J., Cooper, L.Z., Eskola, J., Katz, S.L., and Ratzan, S. (2011). Addressing the vaccine confidence gap. *The Lancet*, 378(9790), 526–35.

Larson, H.J. and Heymann, D.L. (2010). Public health response to influenza A(H1N1) as an opportunity to build public trust. *Journal of the American Medical Association*, 303(3), 271–2.

Lederberg, J., Shope, R., and Oaks, S.C.J. (1992). *Emerging Infections: Microbial Threats to Health in the United States*. Washington, DC: National Academy Press.

Lester, S., del Pilar, P.M., Wang, F., Perez Schael, I., Jiang, H., and O'Brien, T. (1990). The carriage of Escherichia coli resistant to antimicrobial agents by healthy children in Boston, in Caracas, Venezuela, and in Qin Pu, China. *The New England Journal of Medicine*, 323(5), 285–9.

Matic, S., Lazarus, J.V., and Donoghoe, M.C. (2006). *HIV/AIDS in Europe: Moving from Death Sentence to Chronic Disease Management*. Geneva: WHO.

Meselson, M., Guillemin, J., Hugh-Jones, M., et al. (1994). The Sverdlovsk anthrax outbreak of 1979. *Science*, 266(5188), 1202–8.

Miranda, M.E.G. and Miranda, N.L.J. (2011). Reston ebolavirus in humans and animals in the Philippines: a review. *The Journal of Infectious Diseases*, 204(Suppl. 3), S757–60.

Modlin, J.F. (2010). The bumpy road to polio eradication. *The New England Journal of Medicine*, 362(25), 2346–9.

Morbidity and Mortality Weekly Report (2004). Multifocal autochthonous transmission of malaria—Florida, 2003. *Journal of American Medical Association*, 292(3), 324–5.

Nayyar, G.M.L., Breman, J.G., Newton, P.N., and Herrington, J. (2012). Poor-quality antimalarial drugs in southeast Asia and sub-Saharan Africa. *The Lancet Infectious Diseases*, 12(6), 488–96.

Pearce, A., Law, C., Elliman, D., Cole, T.J., and Bedford, H. (2008). Factors associated with uptake of measles, mumps, and rubella vaccine (MMR) and use of single antigen vaccines in a contemporary

UK cohort: prospective cohort study. *BMJ (Clinical Research ed.)*, 336(7647), 754–7.

Piarroux, R. and Faucher, B. (2012). Cholera epidemics in 2010: respective roles of environment, strain changes, and human-driven dissemination. *Clinical Microbiology and Infection*, 18(3), 231–8.

Prusiner, S.B. (1997). Prion diseases and the BSE crisis. *Science*, 278(5336), 245–51.

Riedel, S. (2005). Edward Jenner and the history of smallpox and vaccination. Proceedings (Baylor University, Medical Center), 18(1), 21–5.

Sencer, D.J. (2011). Perspective: swine-origin influenza: 1976 and 2009. *Clinical Infectious Diseases*, 52(Suppl. 1), S4–7.

Senior, K. (2009). Lassa fever: current and future control options. *The Lancet Infectious Diseases*, 9(9), 532.

Slenczka, W. and Klenk, H. D. (2007). Forty years of marburg virus. *The Journal of Infectious Diseases*, 196(Suppl.), S131–5.

Taubenberger, J.K. and Morens, D.M. (2006). 1918 Influenza: the mother of all pandemics. *Emerging Infectious Diseases*, 12(1), 15–22.

Trevitt, C.R. and Singh, P.N. (2003). Variant Creutzfeldt–Jakob disease: pathology, epidemiology, and public health implications. *American Journal of Clinical Nutrition*, 78(3), 651S–656.

UNAIDS (2011). *World AIDS Day Report*. Geneva: UNAIDS.

United Nations Children's Fund (2006). *Japanese Support for Polio Eradication and Malaria Prevention in Nigeria*. [Online] Available at: http://www.unicef.org/media/media_35425.html.

Wilder-Smith, A., Teleman, M.D., Heng, B.H., Earnest, A., Ling, A.E., and Leo, Y.S. (2005). Asymptomatic SARS coronavirus infection among healthcare workers, Singapore. *Emerging Infectious Diseases*, 11(7), 9–12.

World Health Organization (2001a). *WHO Global Strategy for Containment of Antimicrobial Resistance*. Geneva: WHO. Available at: http://whqlibdoc.who.int/hq/2001/WHO_CDS_CSR_DRS_2001.2.pdf.

World Health Organization (2001b). *Macroeconomics and Health: Investing in Health for Economic Development* (Vol. 8). Geneva: WHO.

World Health Organization (2003). *Summary of Probable SARS Cases with Onset of Illness from 1 November 2002 to 31 July 2003*. [Online] Available at: http://www.who.int/csr/sars/country/table2004_04_21/en/index.html.

World Health Organization (2006). International Food Safety Authorities Network (INFOSAN), Successful strategies in controlling avian influenza. [Online] Available at: http://www.who.int/foodsafety/fs-management/No-04-Avianinfluenza-Aug06-en.pdf.

World Health Organization (2007a). *The World Health Report 2007. A Safer Future: Global Public Health Security in the 21st Century*. Geneva: WHO.

World Health Organization (2007b). *Infectious Disease Threats to Our Public Health Security: From SARS to Avian Influenza*. [Online] Available at: http://www.ama-assn.org/resources/doc/cphpdr/david_heymann.pdf.

World Health Organization (2008a). *Global Measles Deaths Drop by 74%*. [Online] Available at: http://www.who.int/mediacentre/news/releases/2008/pr47/en/index.html.

World Health Organization (2008b). *International Health Regulations (2005)* (2nd ed.). Geneva: WHO.

World Health Organization (2011). *Tuberculosis: MDR-TB & XDR-TB 2011 Progress Report*. [Online] Available at: http://www.who.int/tb/challenges/mdr/factsheet_mdr_progress_march2011.pdf.

World Health Organization (2012a). *Impact of Dengue*. [Online] Available at: http://www.who.int/csr/disease/dengue/impact/en/.

World Health Organization (2012b). *Dengue Fever in Madeira, Portugal*. [Online] Available at: http://www.who.int/csr/don/2012_10_17/en/index.html.

World Health Organization (2012c). *Chikungunya*. [Online] Available at: http://www.who.int/mediacentre/factsheets/fs327/en/.

World Health Organization (2012d). *Poliomyelitis*. [Online] Available at: http://www.who.int/mediacentre/factsheets/fs114/en/index.html.

World Health Organization (2012e). *Cumulative Number of Confirmed Human Cases of Avian Influenza A(H5N1) Reported to WHO*. [Online] Available at: http://www.who.int/influenza/human_animal_interface/H5N1_cumulative_table_archives/en/index.html.

World Health Organization (2012f). *Drug-Resistant Tuberculosis*. [Online] Available at: http://www.who.int/tb/challenges/mdr/tdrfaqs/en/index.html.

World Health Organization (2012g). *New WHO Book Showcases Ways to Safeguard Medications: The Evolving Threat of Antimicrobial Resistance—Options for Action*. [Online] Available at: http://www.who.int/mediacentre/news/notes/2012/amr_20120308/en/index.html.

World Health Organization (2012h). *The Evolving Threat of Antimicrobial Resistance Options for Action*. [Online] Available at: http://whqlibdoc.who.int/publications/2012/9789241503181_eng.pdf?ua=1.

World Health Organization (2012i). *International Health Regulations (2005)*. [Online] Available at: http://www.who.int/ihr/en/.

World Health Organization (2013). *Global Alert and Response (GAR), Disease Outbreaks by Year*. [Online] Available at: http://www.who.int/csr/don/archive/year/en/.

York, I. and Donis, R.O. (2012). The 2009 pandemic influenza virus: where did it come from, where is it now, and where is it going? *Current Topics in Microbiology and Immunology*, 370, 241–57.

8.18

Bioterrorism

Nicholas S. Kelley and Michael T. Osterholm

History of biological warfare and terrorism

Since antiquity, those in conflict have sought ways to increase their chance of victory. As early as 1320 BC, infectious diseases were used as weapons during wars (Trevisanato 2007). Plague-infested bodies were catapulted over the fortified walls of Caffa (now Feodosiya, Ukraine) by the Tartar army in 1346 (Wheelis 2002). Clothing and blankets contaminated with variola virus, the causative agent of smallpox, were provided to native Indian populations in North and South America from the sixteenth to the eighteenth centuries. While in most cases these devastating infections were not intentionally transmitted, their occurrence made resistance to hostile troops difficult. The Delaware Indians, in contrast, were deliberately infected with variola, which resulted in a smallpox outbreak that allowed the British to take a contested fort due to the reduced numbers of Delaware defending the fort. The Continental Army, fighting for independence from the British, were variolated (an early version of smallpox vaccination) in 1777 to help protect the troops from outbreaks of smallpox that had devastated the army and to minimize the impact of intentional spread of smallpox by loyal colonists (Dembek 2011).

The First World War saw limited use of biological warfare agents. Biological warfare is defined as the intentional release of a biological agent(s) or toxin(s) to incapacitate or kill humans, animals, or plants to provide an advantage in combat. After the First World War, many nations began to develop biological warfare programmes, but none were as large as Japan's. From 1931 to 1945, unit 731, based in Manchuria, killed more than 20,000 individuals, including prisoners, allied prisoners of war, and civilians during their testing and trials of biological agents (Riedel 2004). After the Second World War ended, the United States, United Kingdom, Soviet Union, and other countries significantly expanded their biological weapons programmes. After years of refinement, it was clear to many nations the devastation these weapons could cause, how indiscriminate they were, and the limited response strategies available if they were used. In 1969, the United States stopped its offensive biological weapons programme, and in 1972 the Biological Weapons Convention Treaty (BWCT) was ratified. As of July 2013, 170 countries have ratified this treaty, which explicitly prohibits the development, stockpiling, and use of biological weapons (United Nations 2013).

While it was suspected that the Soviet Union, a signer of the BWCT, had continued work after an unusual anthrax outbreak in 1979, it was not until 1992 that it was confirmed that *Bacillus anthracis*, which causes anthrax, was accidentally released at a military facility in Sverdlovsk, infecting at least 77 people and killing 66 (Dembek 2011). After the collapse of the Soviet Union, evidence was found that described the massive nature of its biological weapons programme. It has since been dismantled.

In 1991, the United Nations confirmed that Iraq also had an extensive biological weapons programme, which eventually was dismantled and destroyed. While it is suspected that other nations such as North Korea have biological weapons programmes, this information has not been confirmed. The BWCT does not allow for verification that countries are following the treaty, and the inability to independently verify the dismantling of biological weapons programmes has posed challenges.

While it is possible that a nation could still use a biological weapon, the biggest threat today comes from terrorists using biological agents. Biological terrorism is the intentional release of a biological agent(s) or toxin(s) to incapacitate or kill humans, animals, or plants. While biological terrorism can result in a substantial disease impact, the psychological impact can be profound; this makes biological agents attractive to terrorists. Many organizations have threatened to use biological agents, but to date there has been limited use of them for terrorism purposes. In the autumn of 1984, a Bhagwan Shree Rajneesh sect based in Oregon contaminated multiple salad bars with *Salmonella typhimurium* in an effort to change the outcome of an election by reducing the number of people healthy enough to vote (Torok et al. 1997). In July 1993, the Aum Shinrikyo cult released aerosolized *B. anthracis* from the roof of its building in downtown Tokyo (Takahashi et al. 2004). Several technical failures prevented this release over several days from having human health impacts. In the autumn of 2001, the US government concluded that Dr Bruce Ivins had mailed five letters that contained *B. anthracis* to the media and politicians. These letters resulted in 22 people becoming infected with anthrax and five of them dying (Jernigan et al. 2002; Rasko et al. 2011). This limited attack using the US postal system almost stopped mail delivery across the country, and the decontamination of contaminated facilities cost approximately $320 million (Schmitt and Zacchia 2012). These events and the continued desire of terrorist groups like Al Qaeda and their affiliates to acquire or develop biological weapons serve as a reminder of the need for preparedness against biological terrorism.

Agents of concern

Numerous infectious diseases harm humans, but only a select number are considered to be agents of concern for biological warfare or terrorism. These agents have characteristics that make them

Table 8.18.1 US government classification of biological agents that could be used as a weapon

Category A	
Definition	Highest priority agents that pose significant risk to public health and national security
Characteristics	• Can be easily disseminated or transmitted from person to person • Result in high mortality rates and have the potential for major public health impact • Might cause public panic and social disruption • Require special action for public health preparedness

Examples of diseases (agents)	• Anthrax (*Bacillus anthracis*)
	• Plague (*Yersinia pestis*)
	• Smallpox (variola)
	• Tularaemia (*Francisella tularensis*)
	• Viral haemorrhagic fevers:
	  • Filoviruses:
	    • Ebola
	    • Marburg
	  • Arenaviruses:
	    • Lassa
	    • Machupo
	    • Toxins
	    • Botulism (*Clostridium botulinum*)

Category B	
Definition	Second-highest priority agents
Characteristics	• Are moderately easy to disseminate • Result in moderate morbidity rates and low mortality rates • Require specific enhancements of CDC's diagnostic capacity and enhanced disease surveillance

Examples of diseases (agents)	• Brucellosis (*Brucella* species)
	• Glanders (*Burkholderia mallei*)
	• Melioidosis (*Burkholderia pseudomallei*)
	• Psittacosis (*Chlamydia psittaci*)
	• Q fever (*Coxiella burnetii*)
	• Typhus fever (*Rickettsia prowazekii*)
	• Food safety threats:
	  • *Salmonella* species
	  • *Escherichia coli* O157:H7
	  • *Shigella*
	• Water safety threats:
	  • *Vibrio cholera*
	  • *Cryptosporidium parvum*
	• Toxins:
	  • Epsilon (*Clostridium perfringens*)
	  • Ricin (*Ricinus communis* [castor beans])
	  • Staphylococcal enterotoxin B

Category C	
Definition	Third-highest priority agents including emerging pathogens that could be engineered for mass dissemination in the future
Characteristics	• Availability • Ease of production and dissemination • Potential for high morbidity and mortality rates and major health impact
Examples of agents	• Nipah virus • Hantavirus

Adapted from Centers for Disease Control and Prevention, Emergency Preparedness and Response, *Bioterrorism agents/disease*, available from http://www.bt.cdc.gov/agent/agentlist-category.asp

more likely to be used in biological warfare or terrorism. The US Centers for Disease Control and Prevention (CDC) has grouped these characteristics into risk categories A, B, and C (Table 8.18.1). Most preparedness for bioterrorism is focused around category A agents. These agents can be easily disseminated, cause severe disease and high mortality rates if not treated properly, and can pose significant challenges for management and response, which could give rise to public panic.

In 2002, the Public Health Security and Bioterrorism Preparedness and Response Act was passed and signed into law. The US Department of Health and Human Services (DHHS) and the US Department of Agriculture (USDA) were required by this law to identify biological agents or toxins that could have significant human and/or agricultural health impacts. These agents became known as select agents. Those using, possessing, or transferring these agents must follow stringent guidelines, biosafety standards, and protocols (42 CFR Part 73; 9 CFR Part 121; 7 CFR Part 331). The list of select agents is periodically updated, with the last update in October 2012. Several of the select agents are denoted as Tier 1 agents, which require additional security measures to be in place. Tier 1 agents are listed in Box 8.18.1. All category A agents and two category B agents have been identified as Tier 1 select agents.

Dispersal of agents

To be used in biological warfare or terrorism, these agents need to be distributed to their intended targets while remaining infectious. Large-scale distribution would require either of two primary routes: aerosols and products.

The aerosol route requires the agent to be propagated and treated in a manner that allows for small particles (1–5 μm) to be inhaled. Aerosolized agents can be widely distributed either as a slurry using a nozzle that generates an aerosol or as a fine powder. The liquid-based aerosols can be used to attack large areas by using a crop-dusting plane or confined spaces by releasing aerosols into ventilation systems. Fine powders can contaminate large indoor areas and pose risks for re-aerosolization, as noted during the 2001 anthrax letter attacks.

The other possible route of attack is using products that are consumed or used in daily life. Food is the product of most concern. Given the global distribution of the food supply chain, an agent could be introduced anywhere along the chain. While it is likely that treatment steps, such as cooking food or sanitizing water, will kill the agent or reduce its concentration to below infectious levels, infection through this route cannot be ruled out.

While all Tier 1 agents are infectious, only smallpox, plague, and the viral haemorrhagic fevers (Ebola and Marburg) are of concern with regard to subsequent person-to-person transmission. These agents can be responsible for amplified outbreaks due to secondary and tertiary transmission after the initial attack. They also raise the risk of an individual deliberately infecting him- or herself or others as a means of attack—in essence, becoming a biological suicide bomber.

Characteristics of agents

Bacterial

Anthrax

The causative agent of anthrax (Center for Infectious Disease Research and Policy (CIDRAP) 2013a) is the large Gram-positive bacillus *Bacillus anthracis* (American Society for Microbiology (ASM) 2013a). It is a rapidly growing, non-motile, catalase-positive, aerobic/facultative anaerobic organism. Vegetative bacilli are not environmentally stable and readily form spores in the presence of oxygen or when nutrients are exhausted. These spores are extremely environmentally stable and can remain viable for decades.

Anthrax spores are found in soil around the world. Most mammals are susceptible to anthrax, and infections are common in grazing animals. Human infections primarily stem from contact with contaminated animal products. There are four clinical forms of anthrax in humans: cutaneous, inhalation, gastrointestinal, and injection. Cutaneous and inhalation are the two forms most likely to result from a bioterrorism event. During an aerosol event, inhalation and cutaneous anthrax would be common routes of infection initially for those in the plume of anthrax spores. Once they settle out of the air, they can be re-aerosolized, allowing for additional rounds of infections.

Inhalation anthrax

When small particles (1–5 μm) of *B. anthracis* are inhaled, the particles end up in the alveoli of the lungs (ASM 2013a). The minimum infectious dose for inhalation anthrax has been estimated to be between 10 and 8000 spores, with an uncertain dose–response association (Franz et al. 1997; Fennelly et al. 2004; Coleman et al. 2008). In the lungs, macrophages ingest the spores, transporting them to the lymph nodes (Russell et al. 2008). At this point the spores germinate and multiply, enabling a systemic infection to occur. During the initial stage of infection, symptoms include fever, fatigue, cough, chills, and malaise (Jernigan et al. 2001). These non-specific symptoms make it hard to initially diagnose anthrax without laboratory testing. If this initial phase of infection is not treated, the infection enters the final phase, with a rapidly progressing fever signalling the onset of respiratory and cardiac collapse. Without prompt treatment, the case-fatality rate for inhalation anthrax approaches 80 per cent (Holty et al. 2005), but early, aggressive treatment can cut that rate in half. Inhalation anthrax is treated with ciprofloxacin or doxycycline plus two additional antibiotics (Malecki et al. 2001). Post-exposure prophylaxis involves ciprofloxacin, doxycycline, or levofloxacin. An anthrax vaccine is available under emergency use authorization for use in adults in combination with antibiotics after a widespread airborne release of anthrax (Wright et al. 2010). The incubation period for inhalation anthrax ranges from 1 to 6 days.

Cutaneous anthrax

Abrasions or cuts on the skin provide an opportunity for anthrax spores to germinate at the site, creating a papule. As spores begin to multiply, the vegetative cells end up in the regional lymph nodes. This results in painful oedema and ulcerations around the original papule. After a few days a black eschar forms over the ulcerated papule. In most people these infections resolve without complications with proper antibiotic treatment (Inglesby et al. 2002). Cutaneous anthrax is treated with ciprofloxacin or doxycycline.

Plague

The causative agent of plague is a Gram-negative bacillus, *Yersinia pestis* (CIDRAP 2013b). It is a slow-growing, non-motile, catalase-positive, facultative anaerobic organism (ASM 2013b). *Y. pestis* is not considered environmentally stable and will die within a few hours. Wild rodents are the primary reservoir for *Y. pestis*, although many mammals can become incidental hosts (Perry and Fetherston 1997). The flea is the vector sustaining transmission of plague. Plague is endemic in many regions of the world, particularly Africa, Asia, and the Americas. Most human cases are the result of contact with infected mammals or fleas.

There are three primary forms of plague: bubonic, pneumonic, and septicaemic (Perry and Fetherston 1997; Inglesby et al. 2000). Without proper treatment, bubonic and pneumonic plague generally turn into septicaemic plague and are fatal. Pneumonic plague is the form most likely to result from a bioterrorism event. Pneumonic plague can be spread person to person through respiratory droplets, but most naturally occurring cases do not result in secondary transmission, although it is possible that super-spreading events can occur (Hinckley et al. 2011).

During an aerosol event, *Y. pestis* would be inhaled; as few as 100 organisms can cause an infection. The incubation period is typically 1–4 days but is dose-dependent, with symptoms possible in less than 24 hours after a significant exposure. Initial symptoms include nausea, vomiting, diarrhoea, and abdominal pain, without evidence of a respiratory infection. A fever, productive coughs (with evidence of blood), chest pain, and cyanosis typically follow (Inglesby et al. 2000). A key indicator of pneumonic plague is the rapid development of severe pneumonia symptoms after gastrointestinal symptoms (Babin 2010). Disease progression is rapid, septicaemia is common, and prompt treatment is critical. Without proper treatment within 24 hours of symptom onset, the case-fatality rate approaches 100 per cent, with death typically occurring within 5 days (Gage et al. 2000; Inglesby et al. 2000). Streptomycin or gentamicin are the primary treatment options for pneumonic plague (Inglesby et al. 2000), while doxycycline or ciprofloxacin are the primary antibiotics for post-exposure prophylaxis. A vaccine for plague is not currently available (Food and Drug Administration 2014).

Tularaemia

The causative agent of tularaemia (CIDRAP 2013c) is the small Gram-negative coccobacillus *Francisella tularensis* (ASM 2013c).

It is a slow growing, non-motile, weakly catalase-positive aerobic organism. *F. tularensis* can survive for prolonged periods in moist environments, such as brackish water (Berrada and Telford 2011). Environmental amoebae can also ingest *F. tularensis*, thereby increasing its survival in the environment. Small mammals are the primary reservoirs for *F. tularensis*. Ticks, mosquitoes, and biting flies are all known vectors. There are four subspecies of *F. tularensis*: *tularensis* (type A), *holarctica* (type B), *mediasiatica*, and *novicida* (Sandström et al. 1992; Farlow et al. 2005; Huber et al. 2010). All four subspecies can cause human disease, with subspecies *tularensis* (type A) causing the most severe disease. Type A is found primarily in the United States and contains two distinct clades: 1 and 2. Type B is found around the world and is the primary source of *F. tularensis* infections outside the United States.

Tularaemia symptoms range from acute-onset pneumonia to painful lesions that can take weeks to resolve. Ulceroglandular, glandular, and pneumonic tularaemias are the most common clinical syndromes (Dennis et al. 2001). Pneumonic tularaemia is the most likely form to result from a bioterrorism event in which the agent is released into the air. Tularaemia is not contagious.

During an aerosol event, *F. tularensis* could be inhaled, and as few as ten organisms can cause an infection (Franz et al. 1997). The incubation period is typically 3–5 days. Initial symptoms include nausea, a non-productive cough, sudden onset of fever, and myalgia, with pneumonia that doesn't respond to typical treatment (Dennis et al. 2001). Without proper antibiotic treatment, the case-fatality rate approaches 80 per cent but drops to less than 10 per cent with proper treatment. Streptomycin or gentamicin is the primary treatment choice for pneumonic tularaemia, while doxycycline or ciprofloxacin is the primary option for postexposure prophylaxis (Dennis et al. 2001). No vaccine for tularaemia is currently licensed for use.

Glanders

The causative agent of glanders (CIDRAP 2012a) is a Gram-negative coccobacillus, *Burkholderia mallei*. It is a slow-growing, non-motile, catalase-positive, aerobic/facultative anaerobic organism (ASM 2013d). It is an obligate mammalian pathogen without an environmental reservoir. In most environments it is quickly inactivated, but it can remain viable in warm and moist environments for 2–3 weeks.

The primary mammalian reservoir for *B. mallei* are equids (Dvorak and Spickler 2008). Glanders is a rare human disease, with most human infections occurring from exposure to infected horses or laboratory exposures. There are three primary routes of exposure: inoculation, ingestion, and inhalation (Gilad et al. 2007; Dembek 2011). It is assumed that the infectious dose for *B. mallei* is low. The clinical course of glanders is varied and characterized by four types of infection: localized, pulmonary, septicaemic, and chronic. Pulmonary infections are the likeliest to stem from bioterrorism, as they result from an airborne release of *B. mallei*. Without proper treatment, pulmonary infections typically result in septicaemic glanders as early as a week after symptom onset and may become chronic. Treatment of glanders consists of two phases: intensive therapy with ceftazidime or meropenem, then eradication with TMP/SMX or amoxicillin/clavulanic acid (Lipsitz et al. 2012). Because of the risk of relapse, treatment typically lasts 14 weeks, and follow-up can last for years (Dembek

2011). There is no vaccine for glanders. Without proper treatment, the septicaemic form of glanders is normally fatal, but with proper treatment the case-fatality rate drops to 50 per cent. The incubation period for the pulmonary form is from 1 to 14 days. Although there have been rare cases of human-to-human transmission of glanders, it is generally not considered contagious.

Melioidosis

The causative agent of melioidosis (CIDRAP 2012a), *Burkholderia pseudomallei*, is a Gram-negative, slow-growing, motile, catalase-positive, aerobic/facultative anaerobic bacillus (ASM 2013d). *B. pseudomallei* is a saprophyte and remains viable in the soil and water, its reservoir, for years. It is endemic in South East Asia and northern Australia. Human infections are most common after significant rainfall and primarily affect soldiers, agriculture workers, or those with compromised immune systems who have exposure to contaminated soil or water (Baker et al. 2011; Dembek 2011; Vidyalakshmi et al. 2012).

Melioidosis can have a wide variety of clinical presentations, making diagnosis challenging, especially when cases occur outside of endemic regions. Clinical presentations can be grouped into four types: localized, pulmonary, septicaemic, and disseminated (Dembek 2011). Again, pulmonary infections are the greatest concern for bioterrorism, as they result from an airborne release of *B. pseudomallei*. These infections can be mild to severe, with pulmonary abscesses and productive cough. Pulmonary infections may lead to septicaemic infections, which are often fatal without proper treatment and fatal half the time with proper treatment. Treatment of melioidosis is identical to glanders (Lipsitz et al. 2012) and lasts as long (Dembek 2011). *B. pseudomallei* is naturally resistant to aminoglycosides and macrolides. There is no vaccine for melioidosis. The incubation period for *B. pseudomallei* is wide-ranging; cases can involve clinical symptoms within days of exposure or years after exposure. Although there have been rare cases of human-to-human transmission of melioidosis, it is generally not considered contagious.

Viral

Smallpox

The causative agent of smallpox (CIDRAP 2013d) is brick-shaped DNA virion, variola virus (ASM 2013e). It is assumed that environmental survival for variola would be similar to the vaccinia virus, which is quickly destroyed in high temperature and humidity (Henderson et al. 1999). Variola is stable in smallpox scabs for up to 4 months (MacCallum and McDonald 1957). Humans are the only host for smallpox; there are no animal or environmental reservoirs. Smallpox was officially declared eradicated in December 1979; therefore, any case would likely be associated with a laboratory accident (stocks of the virus are officially stored in high-security labs in the United States and Russia) or terrorism (Fenner et al. 1988; Henderson et al. 1999). Most of the world's population is susceptible to smallpox now, as vaccination has not routinely occurred for decades.

The variola virus has been classified as variola major or minor, primarily based on severity of symptoms. Variola minor typically produces a less severe infection. There are five clinical types of smallpox, with over 90 per cent of cases being ordinary (classic) smallpox (Fenner et al. 1988). The incubation period for ordinary smallpox is typically 12 days but can range from 7 to 19 days. The initial stage of infection consists of fever, headache, backache, chills, and vomiting. Around day 5 a rash begins near the mouth (Fenner et al. 1988; Henderson 1999). The rash spreads from the face to the trunk and then the extremities. The lesions are maculopapular for the first 2 days, then vesicular for the next 3 days, then pustular for a week. Eventually these pustular lesions scab over and fall off. The pustules are hard and slightly raised and appear as confluent, semiconfluent, or discrete.

Smallpox is primarily transmitted by respiratory droplets or aerosols (Fenner et al. 1988; Milton 2012). The infectious dose is fewer than 100 virions, and the disease is highly contagious (Franz et al. 1997). Individuals are most contagious during the first week after rash onset and typically infect three to six other people. Treatment for smallpox typically consists of supportive care. A vaccine is available in large quantities and is the primary means of controlling an outbreak. If the vaccine is provided within 4 days of exposure, it significantly reduces morbidity and mortality (Dixon 1948; Henderson et al. 1999). The overall case-fatality rate for ordinary smallpox is 30 per cent in an unvaccinated population (Rao 1972). Other forms of smallpox, like the flat-type and haemorrhagic, have case-fatality rates of over 90 per cent. These rates, however, may be significantly different with modern medicine, which includes investigational antiviral drugs against the variola virus and critical care medicine.

Viral haemorrhagic fevers

The diseases caused by several RNA viruses from, for example, the families Arenaviridae (Lassa), Bunyaviridae (hantavirus), Filoviridae (Ebola), and Flaviviridae (dengue) are known as viral haemorrhagic fevers (Marty et al. 2006; King et al. 2011; CIDRAP 2012b). These viruses are all capable of causing haemorrhagic symptoms to varying degrees. The Ebola and Marburg viruses will be reviewed in more detail, as they are listed as Tier 1 agents (Animal and Plant Health Inspection Service 2014).

Four of the five Ebola subtypes are found in sub-Saharan Africa, including Zaire, Sudan, Côte d'Ivoire, and Bundibugyo (Leroy et al. 2011). The fifth subtype, Reston, is found in the Philippines and so far has not been associated with human disease (Miranda et al. 1999). The case-fatality rates for the four strains of Ebola in Africa are varied and can reach 90 per cent for the Zaire subtype (Feldmann and Geisbert 2011). Ebola is assumed to be primarily transmitted by body fluids of infected humans or animals. It can theoretically be transmitted by aerosol, which is of concern for bioterrorism (Borio et al. 2002). The incubation period ranges from 2 to 21 days. Symptoms include fever, headache, myalgia, maculopapular rash, prostration, diarrhoea, vomiting, and jaundice (Feldmann and Geisbert 2011; Kortepeter et al. 2011). Evidence of haemorrhages may occur toward the end of the disease progression.

Marburg is also found in sub-Saharan Africa. It is very similar clinically to Ebola but typically not as deadly. Supportive care is the only treatment available for Ebola and Marburg (Borio et al. 2002; Feldmann and Geisbert 2011). No antivirals have been shown to be effective for either disease, and a vaccine is not available. Outbreaks are controlled by strict contact precautions and contact tracing.

Toxins

Botulism

The causative agent of botulism (CIDRAP 2012c) is a toxin produced by *Clostridium botulinum*. It is a Gram-positive, anaerobic, spore-forming, motile bacillus (ASM 2013f). It is commonly found in soil. Spores are extremely environmentally stable, and their germination produces botulinum toxin. Eight different botulism toxins have been identified: A through H (Franz et al. 1997; Barash and Arnon 2014), with type A, B, and E toxins the most common causes of human disease (CDC 1998; Shapiro et al. 1998). The botulism toxin is the most lethal toxin known and can be ingested, inhaled, or injected (Franz et al. 1997). The ingestion and inhalation routes are the most concerning from a bioterrorism standpoint. The incubation time for ingestion of the toxin can be as short as 2 hours and up to 8 days (Arnon et al. 2001). The incubation time for inhalation botulism is unknown. Botulism is characterized by an acute, afebrile, descending flaccid paralysis (Shapiro et al. 1998; Arnon et al. 2001). Supportive care and treatment with the botulinum antitoxin are the primary response strategies. The case-fatality rate for ingestion botulism is under 10 per cent, while the case-fatality rate for inhalation botulism is unknown. Treatment of botulism typically requires intensive care, such as mechanical ventilation, which likely would be in short supply during an attack, thus increasing the case-fatality rate.

Public health surveillance and preparedness for bioterrorism

Surveillance

A robust public health surveillance system is the primary vehicle through which an unusual emerging infectious disease or bioterrorism event will be detected. These surveillance systems comprise three main components: laboratory (including routine reportable disease surveillance), syndromic, and environmental surveillance (Kman and Bachmann 2012). Laboratories around the world that process clinical samples are typically required to alert public health authorities if they detect an agent of concern for bioterrorism. Regulations regarding the agents to be reported and the time frame for reporting vary by jurisdiction. Laboratory-based surveillance takes time and can require several hours to days after a sample is collected before results are available, but it provides evidence of a specific organism, which is key for initiating the appropriate public health response.

Syndromic surveillance involves the collection of data from cases with defined and common symptoms within a defined population. The number of physicians reporting patients with influenza-like illness (ILI) every winter is a common form of syndromic surveillance. With the appropriate background information about symptoms in a defined population, a baseline syndromic surveillance measurement can be useful for identifying unusual increases in patients with similar symptoms. For example, if hospitals started reporting an increase in patients presenting with ILI in June that was above the June baseline, this finding would be cause for concern. An investigation should be initiated to determine the cause of the sudden increase in ILI. The CDC has a national programme called BioSense that is based on the timely review of aggregated syndromic surveillance data. Many countries and some large cities have similar programmes. There are also several Internet-based tools useful for syndromic surveillance and analysis (Salathe et al. 2013). Syndromic surveillance can be critical for identifying unusual events that could be the result of a covert biological attack.

Environmental surveillance consists of environmental monitoring for biological agents. The US military and other militaries have developed environmental monitoring systems that can alert them to biological, chemical, or radiological attack from a distance. Civilian detection capabilities typically rely on environmental monitoring in fixed locations. The BioWatch programme currently in use in the United States is a fixed-location environmental monitoring system for select biological agents (Kman and Bachmann 2012). These systems can provide an early warning that a biological agent was present at the location having a positive detection. This allows for public health and law enforcement authorities to conduct an investigation of the cause of the positive result, in theory before any individuals become sick. If it is determined that a bioterrorism attack has occurred, the appropriate public health response can be initiated before syndromic surveillance is able to detect unusual illness patterns. This finding can potentially prevent significant morbidity and mortality if immediate public health action occurs, including the widespread distribution of appropriate antibiotics and vaccines.

Preparedness for bioterrorism

Even a limited bioterrorism event will likely overwhelm public health and medical authorities. The anthrax mailings in 2001, for example, strained national, state, and local public health response capabilities. While there have been major advances in preparedness since 2001, the current climate of fiscal austerity has stalled or started to reverse most of these gains (Gursky and Bice 2012). The location or region responding to the bioterrorism event will likely need to alter its standards of care owing to the number of patients, limited staff availability (due to illness, exhaustion, or other reasons), and shortages of supplies necessary for treating patients as well as individuals needing routine or emergency medical care.

The public health and medical communities have done extensive work on altering the standards of care to meet surges in medical care needs during disasters, and handbooks are available on how to manage these large-scale events (Barbera and Macintyre 2007, 2009). The US Institute of Medicine has extensively reviewed the guidelines for establishing crisis standards of care, frameworks for responding to these disasters, and triggers for implementing these standards (Altevogt et al. 2009; Hanfling et al. 2012; Hanfling et al. 2013). These guidelines help ensure that the care meets legal, ethical, and medical standards during a crisis. Basic medical care, such as supportive care and rapid access to the right medical countermeasures, is paramount during a crisis, as it will help the greatest number of people.

In the United States, staffing support during a large-scale response such as a bioterrorism attack would come from a variety of federal and volunteer sources. At the federal level there are rapidly deployable teams of medical and public health professionals within the DHHS that could respond, such as the Disaster Medical Assistance Teams (DMATs) (Frasca 2010). The Department of Defense has similar support capacity that could be used under certain conditions. A cadre of volunteers from the Red Cross and other disaster relief agencies and the Medical Reserve Corps are also available (Frasca 2010).

The quantity of medical countermeasures necessary for treating a large population is unlikely to be present in the location of a bioterrorism event. Some national governments maintain strategic national stockpiles (SNS) with medical countermeasures available for rapid deployment. In the United States, the CDC maintains the SNS and there are plans in each state and many cities for how to rapidly distribute its resources to the public and first responders in the event of a bioterrorism attack. The SNS contain enough treatment or prophylactic doses of antibiotics, vaccines, and other medical products such as personal protective equipment and ventilators to support a response in several US cities simultaneously.

The development of medical countermeasures to respond to bioterrorism has been a challenge. To date the greatest success in medical countermeasure enhancement has been against smallpox, with a new vaccine and new treatment options available and stockpiled. Medical countermeasure development globally has been supported primarily by the US government, specifically through the Biomedical Advanced Research and Development Authority. While work has been done on developing vaccines and other medical countermeasures, primarily antibiotics, the work has met with limited success; several regulatory, procedural, and financial challenges must be overcome (Russell and Gronvall 2012).

Challenges for the future

Dual-use research of concern

Scientific advances have enabled countless benefits to society; however, the tools used to arrive at these benefits may also cause harm. Some dual-use research raises significant potential for misuse, known as dual-use research of concern (DURC). A virus engineered to be more transmittable in an effort to understand the risk it possesses to public health would be considered as DURC, for example. The work can be done by a scientist with altruistic motivations or it could be done by a terrorist. If there were a laboratory accident that released the new agent from the lab or if it were intentionally released, the public health impact could be the same. In 2004, the National Research Council identified seven types of experiments that raised concern regarding their potential for misuse (Committee on Research Standards and Practices to Prevent the Destructive Application of Biotechnology 2004). These types of experiments are supposed to be reviewed for additional biosecurity information at the institution conducting the research, and oversight is primarily a local issue (Epstein 2012). The National Institutes of Health has created requirements for Institutional Biosafety Committees, which would be the groups responsible for reviewing these experiments at the institutional level.

The National Science Advisory Board for Biosecurity (NSABB) was created as an advisory body to the US Government on dual-use and DURC issues. NSABB has, among its guidance documents, proposed a strategy for minimizing misuse of research information, a code of conduct for responsible research, and guidance for educating amateur biologists on dual-use issues (NSABB on Biosecurity 2007, 2011, 2012). These guidelines only apply for US Government-funded research. The World Health Organization published guidelines for responsible life science research in 2010 (World Health Organization 2010). The publication and dissemination of research with DURC potential is a controversial issue, largely left to the decision of journal editors who don't necessarily have clear guidelines or experience with this topic (Patrone et al. 2012). This became very clear recently with the controversy surrounding and subsequent publication of two studies on highly pathogenic influenza A/H5N1 virus in which the viruses were modified to be more transmittable among mammals (Osterholm et al. 2012).

Conclusion

History shows us that individuals have tried and will continue to try to use biological agents for terror. A large-scale bioterrorism event would be unprecedented, straining and challenging every facet of medical and public health response. In our globally connected economy with its just-in-time supply chains, any large-scale bioterrorism event would quickly become a global event because of both the potential risk of infection and the shock to the global economy. A robust public health and medical workforce is necessary to respond effectively and efficiently to these types of events.

References

Altevogt, B.M., Stroud, C., Hanson, S., Hanfling, D., and Gostin, L. (eds.) (2009). *Committee on Guidance for Establishing Standards of Care for Use in Disaster Situations. Guidance for Establishing Crisis Standards of Care for Use in Disaster Situations.* Washington, DC: National Academies Press.

American Society for Microbiology (2013a). *Sentinel Level Clinical Microbiology Laboratory Guidelines for Suspected Agents of Bioterrorism and Emerging Infectious Diseases: Bacillus anthracis.* [Online] Available at: http://www.asm.org/images/PSAB/Anthrax_July23_2013.pdf.

American Society for Microbiology (2013b). *Sentinel Level Clinical Microbiology Laboratory Guidelines for Suspected Agents of Bioterrorism and Emerging Infectious Diseases: Yersinia pestis.* [Online] Available at: http://www.asm.org/images/PSAB/Plague_July_23_2013.pdf.

American Society for Microbiology (2013c). *Sentinel Level Clinical Microbiology Laboratory Guidelines for Suspected Agents of Bioterrorism and Emerging Infectious Diseases: Francisella tularensis.* [Online] Available at: http://www.asm.org/images/PSAB/TularemiaJuly242013.pdf.

American Society for Microbiology (2013d). *Sentinel Level Clinical Microbiology Laboratory Guidelines for Suspected Agents of Bioterrorism and Emerging Infectious Diseases: Glanders: Burkholderia mallei and Melioidosis: Burkholderia pseudomallei.* [Online] Available at: http://www.asm.org/images/PSAB/Burkholderia_July2013.pdf.

American Society for Microbiology (2013e). *Sentinel Level Clinical Microbiology Laboratory Guidelines for Suspected Agents of Bioterrorism and Emerging Infectious Diseases: Smallpox.* [Online] Available at: http://www.asm.org/images/PSAB/Smallpox_July2013.pdf.

American Society for Microbiology (2013f). *Sentinel Level Clinical Microbiology Laboratory Guidelines for Suspected Agents of Bioterrorism and Emerging Infectious Diseases: Botulinum Toxin.* [Online]. Available at: http://www.asm.org/images/PSAB/Botulism_July2013.pdf.

Animal and Plant Health Inspection Service (2014). *Centers for Disease Control and Prevention. Select Agents and Toxins List.* [Online] Available at: http://www.selectagents.gov/Select Agents and Toxins List.html.

Arnon, S.S., Schechter, R., Inglesby, T.V., et al. (2001). Botulinum toxin as a biological weapon. *Journal of the American Medical Association*, 285(8), 1059–70.

Babin, S.M. (2010). Using syndromic surveillance systems to detect pneumonic plague. *Epidemiology and Infection*, 138(1), 1–8.

Baker, A., Tahani, D., Gardiner, C., Bristow, K.L., Greenhill, A.R., and Warner, J. (2011). Groundwater seeps facilitate exposure to Burkholderia pseudomallei. *Applied and Environmental Microbiology*, 77(20), 7243–6.

Barash, J.R. and Arnon, S.H. (2014). A novel strain of Clostridium botulinum that produces type B and type H botulinum toxins. *Journal of Infectious Diseases*, 209(2), 183–91.

Barbera, J. and Macintyre, A. (2007). *Medical Surge Capacity and Capability: A Management System for Integrating Medical and Health Resources During Large-Scale Emergencies* (2nd ed.). Washington, DC: US Department of Health and Human Services. Available at: http://www.phe.gov/Preparedness/planning/mscc/handbook/Documents/mscc080626.pdf.

Barbera, J. and Macintyre, A. (2009). *Medical Surge Capacity and Capability: The Healthcare Coalition in Emergency Response and Recovery*. Washington DC: US Department of Health and Human Services. Available at: http://www.phe.gov/Preparedness/planning/mscc/Documents/mscctier2jan2010.pdf.

Berrada, Z.L. and Telford, S.R. III (2011). Survival of Francisella tularensis Type A in brackish-water. *Archives of Microbiology*, 193(3), 223–6.

Borio, L., Schmaljohn, A.L., James, M., et al. (2002). Hemorrhagic fever viruses as biological weapons. *Journal of the American Medical Association*, 287(18), 2391–405.

Centers for Disease Control and Prevention (1998). *Botulism in the United States, 1899–1996. Handbook for Epidemiologists, Clinicians, and Laboratory Workers* [Online] 1998. Available at: http://www.cdc.gov/ncidod/dbmd/diseaseinfo/files/botulism.pdf.

Centers for Disease Control and Prevention (n.d.). *Bioterrorism Agents/Disease* [Online] Available at: http://www.bt.cdc.gov/agent/agentlist-category.asp.

Center for Infectious Disease Research and Policy (2012a). *Glanders And Melioidosis Agent Overview*. [Online] Available at: http://www.cidrap.umn.edu/infectious-disease-topics/glanders-melioidosis.

Center for Infectious Disease Research and Policy (2012b). *Viral Hemorrhagic Fever Agent Overview*. [Online] Available at: http://www.cidrap.umn.edu/infectious-disease-topics/vhf.

Center for Infectious Disease Research and Policy (2012c). *Botulism Agent Overview*. [Online] Available at: http://www.cidrap.umn.edu/infectious-disease-topics/botulism.

Center for Infectious Disease Research and Policy (2013a). *Anthrax Agent Overivew*. [Online] Available at: http://www.cidrap.umn.edu/infectious-disease-topics/anthrax.

Center for Infectious Disease Research and Policy (2013b). *Plague Agent Overview*. [Online] Available at: http://www.cidrap.umn.edu/infectious-disease-topics/plague.

Center for Infectious Disease Research and Policy (2013c). *Tularemia Agent Overview*. [Online] Available at: http://www.cidrap.umn.edu/infectious-disease-topics/tularemia.

Center for Infectious Disease Research and Policy (2013d). *Smallpox Agent Overview*. [Online] Available at: http://www.cidrap.umn.edu/infectious-disease-topics/smallpox.

Coleman, M.E., Thran, B., Morse, S.S., Hugh-Jones, M., and Massulik, S. (2008). Inhalation anthrax: dose response and risk analysis. *Biosecurity and Bioterrorism*, 6(2), 147–60.

Committee on Research Standards and Practices to Prevent the Destructive Application of Biotechnology (2004). *Biotechnology Research in an Age of Terrorism*. Washington, DC: The National Academies Press.

Dembek, Z.F. (ed.) (2011). *Medical Managment of Biological Casualties Handbook* (7th ed.). Washington, DC: US Government Printing Office.

Dennis, D.T., Inglesby, T.V., Henderson, D.A., et al. (2001). Tularemia as a biological weapon: medical and public health management. *Journal of the American Medical Association*, 285(21), 2763–73.

Dixon, C.W. (1948). Smallpox in Tripolitania, 1946; an epidemiological and clinical study of 500 cases, including trials of penicillin treatment. *Journal of Hygiene (London)*, 46(4), 351–77.

Dvorak, G.D. and Spickler, A.R. (2008). Zoonosis update: glanders. *Journal of the American Veterinary Medical Association*, 233(4), 570–7.

Epstein, G.L. (2012). Preventing biological weapon development through the governance of life science research. *Biosecurity and Bioterrorism*, 10(1), 17–37.

Farlow, J., Wagner, D.M., Dukerich, M., et al. (2005). Francisella tularensis in the United States. *Emerging Infectious Diseases*, 11(12), 1835–41.

Feldmann, H. and Geisbert, T.W. (2011). Ebola haemorrhagic fever. *The Lancet*, 377(9768), 849–62.

Fennelly, K.P., Davidow, A.L., Miller, S.L., Connell, N., and Ellner, J.J. (2004). Airborne infection with Bacillus anthracis from mills to mail. *Emerging Infectious Diseases*, 10(6), 996–1002.

Fenner, F., Henderson, D., Arita, I., Jezek, Z., and Ladyni, I. (1988). *Smallpox and its Eradication*. Geneva: WHO.

Food and Drug Administration (2014). *Complete List of Vaccines Licensed for Immunization and Distribution in the US*. [Online] Available at: http://www.fda.gov/BiologicsBloodVaccines/Vaccines/ApprovedProducts/UCM093833.

Franz, D.R., Jahrling, P.B., McClain, D.J., et al. (1997). Clinical recognition and management of patients exposed to biological warfare agents. *Journal of the American Medical Association*, 278(5), 399–411.

Frasca, D.R. (2010). The Medical Reserve Corps as part of the federal medical and public health response in disaster settings. *Biosecurity and Bioterrorism*, 8(3), 265–71.

Gage, K.L., Dennis, D.T., Orloski, K.A., et al. (2000). Cases of cat-associated human plague in the Western US, 1977–1998. *Clinical Infectious Diseases*, 30(6), 893–900.

Gilad, J., Harary, I., Dushnitsky, T., Schwartz, D., and Amsalem, Y. (2007). Burkholderia mallei and Burkholderia pseudomallei as bioterrorism agents: national aspects of emergency preparedness. *Israel Medical Association Journal*, 9(7), 499–503.

Gursky, E.A. and Bice, G. (2012). Assessing a decade of public health preparedness: progress on the precipice? *Biosecurity and Bioterrorism*, 10(1), 55–65.

Hanfling, D., Altevogt, B., Viswanathan, K., and Gostin, L. (eds.) (2012). *Committee on Guidance for Establishing Standards of Care for Use in Disaster Situations. Crisis Standards of Care: As Systems Framework for Catastrophic Disaster Response*. Washington, DC: National Academies Press.

Hanfling, D., Hick, J., and Stroud, C. (eds.) (2013). *Crisis Standards of Care: A Toolkit for Indicators and Triggers*. Washington, DC: National Academies Press.

Henderson, D.A. (1999). Smallpox: clinical and epidemiologic features. *Emerging Infectious Diseases*, 5(4), 537–9.

Henderson, D.A., Inglesby, T.V., Bartlett, J.G., et al. (1999). Smallpox as a biological weapon. *Journal of the American Medical Association*, 281(22), 2127–37.

Hinckley, F., Biggerstaff, B.J., Griffith, K.S., and Mead, P.S. (2011). Transmission dynamics of primary pneumonic plague in the USA. *Epidemiology and Infection*, 140(3), 554–60.

Holty, J.C., Bravata, D.M., Liu, H., Olshen, R.A., and Mcdonald, K.M. (2005). Systematic review: a century of inhalational anthrax cases from 1900 to 2005. *Annals of Internal Medicine*, 144(4), 270–80.

Huber, B., Escudero, R., Busse, H.-J., et al. (2010). Description of Francisella hispaniensis sp. nov., isolated from human blood, reclassification of Francisella novicida (Larson et al. 1955) Olsufiev et al. 1959 as Francisella tularensis subsp. novicida comb. nov. and emended description of the genus Franc. *International Journal of Systematic and Evolutionary Microbiology*, 60(Pt 8), 1887–96.

Inglesby, T.V., Dennis, D.T., Henderson, D.A., et al. (2002). Plague as a biological weapon. *Journal of the American Medical Association*, 283(17), 2281–90.

Inglesby, T.V., Toole, T.O., Henderson, D.A., et al. (2013). Anthrax as a biological weapon, 2002. *Journal of the American Medical Association*, 288(17), 2236–52.

Jernigan, D.B., Raghunathan, P.L., Bell, B.P., et al. (2002). Investigation of bioterrorism-related anthrax, United States, 2001: epidemiologic findings. *Emerging Infectious Diseases*, 8(10), 1019–28.

Jernigan, J., Stephens, D.S., Ashford, D.A., et al. (2001). Bioterrorism-related inhalational anthrax: the first 10 cases reported in the United States. *Emerging Infectious Diseases*, 7(6), 933–44.

King, A., Lefkowitz, E., Adams, M.J., and Carstens, E.B. (eds.) (2011). *Viral Taxonomy*. Amsterdam: Elsevier.

Kman, N.E. and Bachmann, D.J. (2012). Biosurveillance: a review and update. *Advances in Preventive Medicine*, 2012, 301408.

Kortepeter, M.G., Bausch, D.G., and Bray, M. (2011). Basic clinical and laboratory features of filoviral hemorrhagic fever. *Journal of Infectious Diseases*, 204(Suppl. 3), S810–16.

Leroy, E.M., Gonzalez, J.P., and Baize, S. (2011). Ebola and Marburg haemorrhagic fever viruses: major scientific advances, but a relatively minor public health threat for Africa. *Clinical Microbiology and Infection*, 17(7), 964–76.

Lipsitz, R., Garges, S., Aurigemma, R., Baccam, P., and Blaney, D. (2012). Workshop on treatment of and postexposure prophylaxis for Burkholderia pseudomallei and B. mallei infection, 2010. [Online] *Emerging Infectious Diseases*, 18(12), e2.

MacCallum, F.O. and McDonald, J.R. (1957). Effect of temperatures of up to 45 degrees C on survival of variola virus in human material in relation to laboratory diagnosis. *Bulletin of the World Health Organization*, 16(2), 441–3.

Malecki, J., Wiersma, S., Cahill, K., Grossman, M., and Hochman, H. (2001). Update: Investigation of bioterrorism-related anthrax and interim guidelines for exposure management and antimicrobial therapy, October 2001. *Morbidity and Mortality Weekly Report*, 50(42), 909–19.

Marty, A., Jahrling, P.B., and Geisbert, T.W. (2006). Viral hemorrhagic fevers. *Clinics in Laboratory Medicine*, 26(2), 345–86.

Milton, D.K. (2012). What was the primary mode of smallpox transmission? Implications for biodefense. *Frontiers in Cellular and Infection Microbiology*, 2, 150.

Miranda, M.E., Ksiazek, T.G., Retuya, T.J., et al. (1999). Epidemiology of Ebola (subtype Reston) virus in the Philippines, 1996. *Journal of Infectious Diseases*, 179(Suppl. 1), S115–19.

National Science Advisory Board on Biosecurity (2007). *Proposed Framework for the Oversight of Dual Use Life Sciences Research: Strategies for Minimizing the Potential Misuse of Research Information* [Online] Available at: http://oba.od.nih.gov/biosecurity/pdf/Framework for transmittal 0807_Sept07.pdf.

National Science Advisory Board on Biosecurity (2011). *Strategies to Educate Amateur Biologists and Scientists in Non-life Science Disciplines About Dual Use Research in the Life Sciences*. [Online] 2011. Available at: http://oba.od.nih.gov/biosecurity/pdf/FinalNSABBReport-AmateurBiologist-NonlifeScientists_June-2011.pdf.

National Science Advisory Board on Biosecurity (2012). *Enhancing Responsible Science: Considerations for the Development and Dissemination of Codes of Conduct for Dual Use Research*. [Online] Available at: http://oba.od.nih.gov/oba/biosecurity/documents/COMBINED_Codes_PDFs.pdf.

Osterholm, M.T. and Relman, D.A. (2012). Creating a mammalian-transmissible A/H5N1 influenza virus: social contracts, prudence, and alternative perspectives. *Journal of Infectious Diseases*, 205(11), 1636–8.

Patrone, D., Resnik, D., and Chin, L. (2012). Biosecurity and the review and publication of dual-use research of concern. *Biosecurity and Bioterrorism*, 10(3), 290–8.

Perry, R.D. and Fetherston, J.D. (1997). Yersinia pestis—etiologic agent of plague. *Clinical Microbiology Reviews*, 10(1), 35–66.

Rao, A. (1972). *Smallpox*. Bombay: Korhari Book Depot.

Rasko, D.A., Worsham, P.L., Abshire, T.G., et al. (2011). Bacillus anthracis comparative genome analysis in support of the Amerithrax investigation. *Proceedings of the National Academy of Sciences of the United States of America*, 108(12), 5027–32.

Riedel S. (2004). Biological warfare and bioterrorism: a historical review. *Proceedings (Baylor University Medical Center)*, 17(4), 400–6.

Russell, B.H., Liu, Q., Jenkins, S.A., Tuvim, M.J., Dickey, B.F., and Xu, Y. (2008). In vivo demonstration and quantification of intracellular Bacillus anthracis in lung epithelial cells. *Infection and Immunity*, 9, 3975–83.

Russell, P.K. and Gronvall, G.K. (2012). U.S. medical countermeasure development since 2001: a long way yet to go. *Biosecurity and Bioterrorism*, 10(1), 66–76.

Salathe, M., Freifeld, C., Mekaru, S., Tomasulo, A., and Brownstein, J.S. (2013). Influenza A (H7N9) and the importance of digital epidemiology. *The New England Journal of Medicine*, 369(5), 401–4.

Sandström, G., Sjöstedt, A., Forsman, M., Pavlovich, N.V., and Mishankin, B.N. (1992). Characterization and classification of strains of Francisella tularensis isolated in the central Asian focus of the Soviet Union and in Japan. *Journal of Clinical Microbiology*, 30(1), 172–5.

Schmitt, K. and Zacchia, N.A. (2012). Total decontamination cost of the anthrax letter attacks. *Biosecurity and Bioterrorism*, 10(1), 98–107.

Shapiro, R.L., Hatheway, C., and Swerdlow, D.L. (1998). Botulism in the United States: a clinical and epidemiologic review. *Annals of Internal Medicine*, 129(3), 221–8.

Takahashi, H., Keim, P., Kaufmann, A.F., Keys, C., and Smith, K.L. (2004). Bacillus anthracis incident, Kameido, Tokyo, 1993. *Emerging Infectious Diseases*, 10(1), 117–20.

Torok, T.J., Tauxe, R.V., Wise, R.P., et al. (1997). A large community outbreak of salmonellosis caused by intentional contamination of restaurant salad bars. *Journal of the American Medical Association*, 278(5), 389–95.

Trevisanato, S.I. (2007). The 'Hittite plague', an epidemic of tularemia and the first record of biological warfare. *Medical Hypotheses*, 69(6), 1371–4.

United Nations (2013). *Membership of the Biological Weapons Convention*. [Online] Available at: http://www.unog.ch/__80256ee600585943.nsf/(httpPages)/7be6cbbea0477b52c12571860035fd5c?OpenDocument#_Section2.

Vidyalakshmi, K., Lipika, S., Vishal, S., Damodar, S., and Chakrapani, M. (2012). Emerging clinico-epidemiological trends in melioidosis: analysis of 95 cases from western coastal India. *International Journal of Infectious Diseases*, 16(7), e491–7.

Wheelis, M. (2002). Biological warfare at the 1346 siege of Caffa. *Emerging Infectious Diseases*, 8(9), 971–5.

World Health Organization (2010). *Responsible Life Sciences Research for Global Health Security: A Guidance Document*. [Online] Available at: http://www.who.int/csr/resources/publications/HSE_GAR_BDP_2010_2/en/index.html.

Wright, J.G., Quinn, C.P., Shadomy, S., and Messonnier, N. (2010). Use of anthrax vaccine in the United States. *Morbidity and Mortality Weekly Report*, 59(rr06), 1–30.

SECTION 9

Prevention and control of public health hazards

Tobacco

Tai Hing Lam and Sai Yin Ho

Introduction to tobacco use

Please respond to the following statements before reading further:

1. About one out of 20 smokers (i.e. 5 per cent or less), if they continue to smoke, will eventually be killed by smoking.

2. To reduce deaths caused by smoking, preventing young people from smoking is the most important action.

Response: strongly agree/agree/disagree/strongly disagree.

Most people will choose agree or strongly agree for these two statements. However, in fact, smoking kills one in two smokers and quitting smoking prevents more deaths more quickly.

Tobacco is the world's most important and most avoidable public health problem. Tobacco killed 100 million people in the last century, mostly in developed countries, and could kill 1 billion this century, mostly in low- and middle-income countries (LMICs) especially China. Currently, tobacco kills 5.4 million people every year. Unless urgent action is taken, tobacco will kill 8 million per year by 2030, 80 per cent of whom will be in developing countries. 'Of the more than 1 billion smokers alive today, around 500 million will be killed by tobacco' (World Health Organization (WHO) 2008). But millions of lives have been saved since the 1960s, mostly in developed countries (notably the United States and United Kingdom) which have progressively and successfully implemented effective tobacco control policies.

Tobacco control is the most remarkable example of global public health actions against non-communicable diseases (NCDs). It is unique in having an international public health treaty, the WHO Framework Convention on Tobacco Control (FCTC), which has been ratified by 176 parties covering 88 per cent of the world's population (as of 30 November 2012). It is one of the most rapidly ratified United Nations (UN) treaties of all time but two of the world's largest countries have not ratified the FCTC, namely the United States and Indonesia (WHO 2012a).

In the September 2011 Political Declaration of the UN on NCDs, tobacco use tops the list of four major risk factors that also include the harmful use of alcohol, unhealthy diet, and physical inactivity (UN 2011).

Globally, the epidemic of tobacco-induced diseases, mortality, and related social and economic burden is still expanding. Using the host–agent–vector model of infectious diseases, the tobacco epidemic is an epidemic of the agent, that is, tobacco. It is sometimes also described as an epidemic of smoking and its harms to others. These two descriptions tend to blame the agent (tobacco) and the host (smokers) or focus on the victims (passive smokers).

However, some might also consider that the tobacco epidemic is really a tobacco industry epidemic. The agent is produced massively, its use by the host is heavily promoted, and control measures are aggressively obstructed by the vector, the tobacco industry. There will be no tobacco epidemic without the tobacco industry. Tobacco control must therefore target the vector. Helping the hosts, that is, smokers, to quit smoking and preventing non-smokers, especially young people and women, from starting smoking are also important, but the impact will be limited to those who can be and are being helped effectively. Smoking cessation campaigns and services cannot produce substantial public health benefits when the tobacco industry is not under strict control. The success of tobacco industry control and other control measures will lead to more quitting, less relapse, and less uptake of smoking.

Effective control measures are stated in the FCTC and translated into six policies of WHO's MPOWER package as follows (WHO 2008):

◆ *Monitor* tobacco use and prevention policies.

◆ *Protect* people from tobacco smoke.

◆ *Offer* help to quit tobacco use.

◆ *Warn* about the dangers of tobacco use.

◆ *Enforce* comprehensive restrictions on tobacco advertising, promotion, and sponsorship.

◆ *Raise* taxes on tobacco.

Note that these six policies are not ranked, and all six are needed as a comprehensive approach against the tobacco industry and tobacco use. However, their implementation varies greatly even among countries that have ratified and are parties of the FCTC. WHO evaluates the progress and publishes global status reports regularly, which is part of the M ('monitor') under MPOWER.

Tobacco kills up to two in three smokers

At least one in two smokers killed

It is important to understand and warn about the dangers of tobacco use: first, the absolute risk of death from all causes combined, and second, the large number of resultant deaths globally, regionally, and locally. This absolute risk, that a smoker will have a 50 per cent chance of being killed by tobacco, is easy to understand and more relevant to individuals than relative risks (RRs) or number of deaths. RRs only tell the exposed people that they

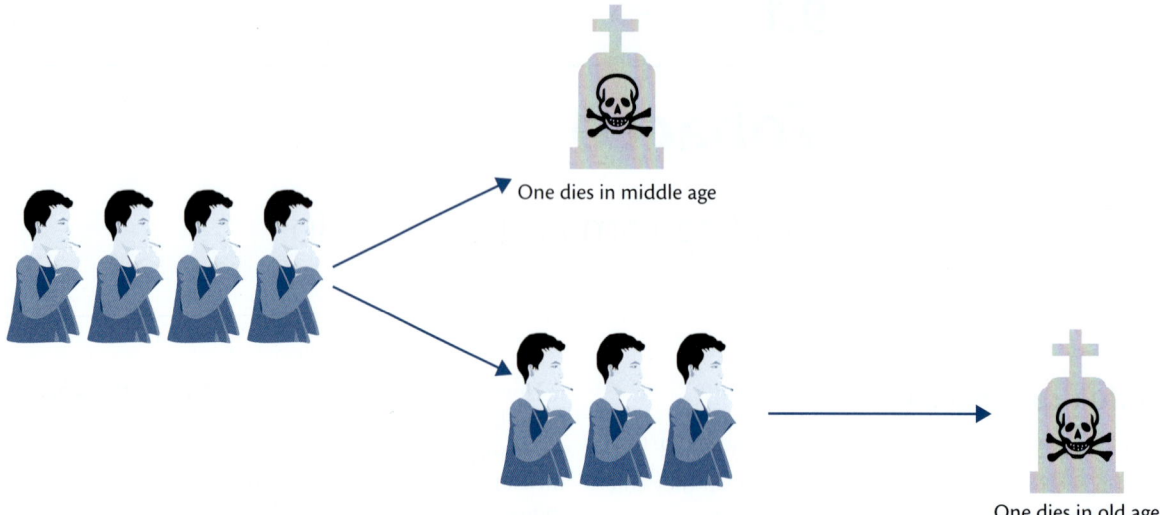

One dies in middle age

One dies in old age

Fig. 9.1.1 One in two smokers will be killed by smoking.

have higher risks than those who are unexposed, but not the exact probability of harm, the absolute risk. Large RRs do not mean large absolute risks if the incidence rate in the unexposed is low. Telling smokers that millions have died from tobacco elsewhere might be alarming to some, but difficult to comprehend to others.

The WHO statement 'Tobacco kills up to one in every two users' (WHO 2008) is derived from Peto, who stated 'about half of teenagers who keep smoking steadily will eventually be killed by tobacco (about a quarter in old age plus a quarter in middle age)' (Peto 1994) (see Fig. 9.1.1). This was based on the translation of the RR of two in the prospective British Doctors Study by Doll and Peto with 40 years of follow-up (Doll et al. 1994). This is a unique example of how an RR can be translated into absolute risk for public health actions and communication of risks.

From relative risk to absolute risk

The RR is the absolute risk of disease or mortality in the exposed group (smokers) divided by that in the unexposed (non-smokers). Translating the RR into an absolute risk in the exposed without knowing the absolute risk in the unexposed is only feasible for total or all-cause mortality. This is based on the attributable fraction (AF) in the exposed (AF = (RR − 1)/RR). With an RR of two for total mortality in smokers compared with non-smokers, the AF in smokers is (2 − 1)/2 = 0.5. That means of all smokers who died, half were due to smoking. Because all smokers will eventually die, the denominator of all smoker deaths can be turned into all current smokers who are alive, and hence of all current smokers, 50 per cent or one in two will eventually be killed by smoking (Lam 2012).

Up to two in three smokers killed

Previously reported RRs could have been underestimated. The RR is based on a comparison of mortality rates of current smokers and non-smokers after some years of follow-up. Current smokers recruited at baseline are survivors as their weaker counterparts might have died. Non-smokers can be either never smokers or former smokers. The latter could have quit smoking while still being healthy (healthy quitters), or they had to quit because of ill health

(ill quitters). Hence, RR can be underestimated as current smokers tend to be healthier (lower mortality rate in the numerator), and non-smokers can include some ill quitters (greater mortality rate in the denominator). This bias is particularly strong when a cohort includes older people.

Another bias could be due to insufficient duration of follow-up, especially for diseases that take many years to develop. A longer follow-up would yield more deaths and allow subgroup analysis. The results from Doll and Peto's study, after 50 years of follow-up, showed that if smoking started at a young age, two in three smokers (RR of 3) will be killed by smoking (Doll et al. 2004). That two in three very young smokers will be killed by smoking is particularly relevant for controlling smoking in children and youth, but this statement has not yet been publicized widely. Latest findings based on large contemporary cohorts in the United States and United Kingdom also revealed all-cause mortality RRs approaching 3 in male and female current smokers compared with never smokers (Jha et al. 2013; Pirie et al. 2013; Thun et al. 2013).

Not many cohort studies, especially those from LMICs, have been followed up for as long as the British doctor cohort studies and hence, their RRs of mortality due to smoking tend to be underestimated. In a small cohort of 1696 people followed up for 20 years, Lam et al. (1997) found an RR of about 2, which is similar to that from Doll and Peto but greater than those of earlier (Yuan et al. 1996) and more recent cohort studies from China (Elliott et al. 2009) with shorter duration of follow-up.

The total exposure to tobacco in smokers varies by countries and cohort studies. Another explanation for the smaller RRs of cohort studies in China and other LMICs at an earlier stage of the tobacco epidemic is that their exposure to tobacco could be lower. Smokers in these cohort studies tended to have started smoking at an older age and could not afford to smoke as much as those in high-income countries.

A recent meta-analysis by Gellert et al. (2012) on smoking and all-cause mortality focused on elderly people (aged 60 or above). Based on 17 cohort studies from seven countries, the RR was 1.85 in current smokers. This means that the one in two deaths is still applicable to older smokers.

Public health applications

Such epidemiological findings can be used for more effective public health advocacy, education, and publicity campaigns. The AF of 50 per cent can be translated into the number of people in a specific population who will be killed by smoking. If there are 4 million adults, and the prevalence of smoking is 50 per cent, the number of people to be killed is 4 million × 0.5 × 0.5 = 1 million. The same can be applied to children and young people. A statement that among today's 4 million children in our country/city/district, about 1 million will be killed by tobacco, if the current prevalence of smoking is not reduced, is more striking. On the other hand, such figures can be used positively, saying that prevention of smoking and promotion of quitting can save millions of lives. As there is a trend of increased smoking in children and youth in many LMICs, if the RR of 3 is used, the estimates will be even more alarming.

For unknown reasons, the 'one in two deaths' message is not used in many websites that help smokers quit, including the US Centers for Disease Control and Prevention (CDC) website. The US Surgeon General's (USSG's) report (US Department of Health and Human Services (2004) does not include total mortality. Existing pictorial warnings in cigarette packs of more than 50 jurisdictions also do not show or highlight this risk. Even recent warnings in Canada and Australia in plain packaging do not have it (Physicians for a Smoke-Free Canada n.d.). The 'one in two risk' has seldom been used as a key campaign message until recently. In 2011, Ireland was the first country to use it for a major social marketing campaign resulting in wide media coverage and great increases in calls to the quitline and demand for smoking cessation services (Howell and HSE Social Marketing Working Group on Tobacco 2012). The Hong Kong Council on Smoking and Health launched a campaign on 'one in two' with a video for TV in October 2012. For public health information and education, the mortality risk of 'one in two' to 'two in three' should be highlighted consistently and widely (Lam 2012). For randomized controlled trials on smoking cessation advice or counselling, there is also no report about using such absolute risk warning, and new trials are warranted.

Clinical applications

The AF of 50 per cent can also be used to motivate clinicians or other healthcare professionals (HCPs) to be more active in helping smokers to quit. If they can help two smokers to quit, they would have saved one life. However, the AF does not tell when the smokers will be killed by smoking. The message to the smokers can be simple: 'If you and your good friend continue to smoke, one of you will be killed by smoking prematurely. We cannot predict who and when, but the premature death can come quickly and suddenly, and when it comes, it will be too late. Quit smoking now.'

Note that AF in the exposed can be used in clinical epidemiology for individuals with a disease and is exposed to the risk (causal) factor of the disease. If the RR of lung cancer due to smoking is 20 (Aubin et al. 2011), AF in the exposed is (20 − 1)/20 = 95 per cent. Clinically, one can tell the smoker who has lung cancer that the probability that his lung cancer is due to his smoking is about 95 per cent. This probability will be greater if the smoker has smoked heavily for a long duration, as the RR refers to an 'average'

smoker, and there is a dose–response relation between RR and the amount of exposure (i.e. pack-years).

Specific harms of tobacco: active smoking

Causation versus association

Of the four major risk factors, tobacco use is the one confirmed to be a causal factor of the largest number of diseases. Hence, the term 'cause' or 'causal factor' should be used for smoking instead of risk factor, which implies association rather than causation. Similarly, the terms 'tobacco-induced diseases' or 'tobacco-caused diseases' are clearer than terms such as 'tobacco-related' or 'smoking-related' diseases. The USSG reports are the longest and most comprehensive series of reviews, with the latest on active smoking published in 2004 (US Department of Health and Human Services 2004). Updated reports are published regularly often with new harms added to the previous lists. Globally, different review panels use quite similar criteria for causal inference. Despite the remarkable consensus on many diseases, disagreements remain as to whether the evidence is sufficient (or only suggestive) to reach a conclusion on causation for some diseases. More evidence to prove or confirm causation of additional diseases is of scientific interest and can add to the total disease burden estimates, but is not essential for tobacco control.

International Agency for Research on Cancer

The International Agency for Research on Cancer (IARC), a WHO agency, is the world authority in the evaluation of carcinogenic risks to humans. The 1986 and 2002 IARC monographs classify tobacco smoking and tobacco smoke as a Group 1 carcinogen, meaning that there is sufficient evidence that it can cause cancer in human. The most updated and comprehensive reviews released by IARC in 2009 conclude that tobacco smoking is the single largest cause of cancer worldwide, and 'Tobacco smoking causes cancers of the lung, oral cavity, naso-, oro- and hypopharynx, nasal cavity and accessory sinuses, larynx, oesophagus, stomach, pancreas, colorectum, liver, kidney (body and pelvis), ureter, urinary bladder, uterine cervix and ovary (mucinous), and myeloid leukaemia. Also, a positive association has been observed between tobacco smoking and cancer of the female breast. For cancers of the endometrium (post-menopausal) and of the thyroid, there is evidence suggesting lack of carcinogenicity' (IARC 2012). Note that two important cancers are added, that is, cancer of the colon and ovary, for which the evidence is now considered sufficient, but that for breast cancer is still limited (Secretan et al. 2009; IARC 2012). The report also concludes that bidi (hand-rolled cigarette commonly used in South Asia) smoking increases the risk for cancers of the oral cavity, oropharynx, hypopharynx, larynx, lung, oesophagus, and stomach, and smokeless tobacco causes cancer of the oral cavity, oesophagus, and pancreas.

The 2010 USSG report

The 2010 USSG report focused on mechanisms rather than causal inference. The major conclusions are: (1) no risk-free exposure level; (2) tobacco smoke causes adverse health outcomes through DNA damage, inflammation, and oxidative stress; (3) risk is related to the duration and level of exposure; (4) exposures are due to powerful nicotine addiction in the brain; (5) low levels of exposure, including second-hand smoking, lead to rapid and sharp increases in endothelial dysfunction and inflammation, which are implicated in acute cardiovascular events and thrombosis; and (6) evidence is insufficient that modifications in tobacco production can reduce risks. Moreover, it has important new conclusions that cigarette smoking produces insulin resistance and chronic inflammation, which can accelerate macro- and micro-vascular complications. Hence, for diabetes: (1) smoking increases the risk of type 2 diabetes; (2) people with diabetes need more insulin; and (3) smokers with diabetes have more complications including heart and kidney disease, amputation, retinopathy, and peripheral neuropathy. The report has a very readable booklet for the public that is highly recommended (Centers for Disease Control and Prevention 2010).

Discrepancies and potential confusions

The conclusions on causal relations for cancers from the IARC are mostly similar to the 2004 USSG report. The most notable exceptions are that the 2002 IARC publication has included liver, nasal cavities and nasal sinuses, and nasopharyngeal cancer as causally related to smoking and cancers of the *tongue and lip* are specifically stated under oral cavity. The 2004 USSG report, which appeared later, does not. The 2012 IARC report has now added that smoking causes colon and ovarian cancer. Another notable discrepancy is that although the statement that smoking can cause erectile dysfunction (ED) is often shown in pictorial or other health warnings on cigarette packs, the 2004 USSG report considers that the evidence for causation is only suggestive but not sufficient.

Important new results

Since the 2004 USSG report, there has been no new meta-analysis or systematic review on ED. New results based on cross-sectional surveys have shown a consistent association between smoking and ED in Australia (Millett et al. 2006), Boston (Kupelian et al. 2007), Hong Kong (Lam et al. 2006), and China (He et al. 2007), and a Swiss survey showed that smoking was associated directly with premature ejaculation and indirectly with ED in young men (Mialon et al. 2012). Results from a randomized controlled trial showed that quitting smoking improved ED (Chan et al. 2010). A smoking cessation clinic study showed that quitters had better erectile function than those who relapsed (Harte and Meston 2012). All three meta-analyses in 2007 concluded that smoking is associated with an increased risk of active tuberculosis (TB) disease and mortality (mostly due to reactivation of previous TB infection) and the evidence is strong and consistent (Bates et al. 2007; Lin et al. 2007; Slama et al. 2007). A mathematical model predicted that 'smoking would produce an excess of 18 million tuberculosis cases and 40 million deaths from tuberculosis between 2010 and 2050, if smoking trends continued along current trajectories. The effect of smoking was anticipated to increase the number of tuberculosis cases by 7 percent (274 million v 256 million) and deaths by 66 percent (101 million v 61 million), compared with model predictions that did not account for smoking' (Basu et al. 2011). The causal relation also suggests that tobacco control must be integrated with TB control in TB endemic countries. Public health advocacy has to be based on precise and sometimes conservative estimates of disease burden. With new results, systematic reviews by different authorities will come up with revised or updated conclusions. Public health professionals need to keep updated and critically appraise the original sources of information.

Specific harms of tobacco: passive smoking

Numerous reviews

No other substance like second-hand smoke (SHS) has been subject to so many systematic reviews within such a short period since the first two reports of an association with lung cancer were published in 1981 (Hirayama 1981; Trichopoulos et al. 1981). The massive and aggressive criticisms from the tobacco industry and its scientists were also unprecedented.

The 2006 USSG report

The 2006 USSG report is the most comprehensive review focusing on SHS (US Department of Health and Human Services 2006). It concludes that the evidence is sufficient that SHS causes: (1) premature death and disease in children and adults who do not smoke; (2) sudden infant death syndrome, acute respiratory infections, ear problems and more severe asthma in children, and smoking by parents causes respiratory symptoms and slows lung growth in their children; and (3) immediate adverse effects on the cardiovascular system, coronary heart disease (CHD) (25–30 per cent increased risk) and lung cancer (20–30 per cent increased risk) in adults. The conclusions that have great public health implications are: (1) there is no risk-free level of exposure to SHS; (2) many millions of children and adults are still exposed; and (3) eliminating smoking in indoor spaces fully protects non-smokers from SHS, but separating smokers from non-smokers and cleaning the air and ventilating buildings cannot eliminate exposure. The list of diseases with suggestive but insufficient evidence is much longer, and most notably includes childhood cancer (leukaemia, lymphoma, and brain tumour), onset of childhood asthma, and adult-onset asthma, breast cancer, nasal sinus cancer, stroke, atherosclerosis, and chronic obstructive pulmonary disease (COPD).

The 2002 IARC monograph

The 2002 IARC monograph concludes that involuntary smoking is a Group 1 carcinogen based on more than 50 studies in many countries, causing lung cancer with excess risk from spousal exposure of 20 per cent for women and 30 per cent for men (Aubin et al. 2011). Excess risk from workplace exposure is 16–19 per cent. The US Cal/EPA 2006 report concludes that SHS can induce asthma and can cause premenopausal breast cancer with an excess risk of 80–120 per cent and these are different from the 2006 USSG report. The 2009 IARC report has added that parental smoking can cause hepatoblastoma in offspring, that there is limited evidence for cancer of larynx and pharynx, and the evidence for female breast cancer remains inconclusive.

The estimation of deaths from SHS is less straightforward. It depends on what diseases are to be included, and what criteria (sufficient or suggestive evidence for causation) or reviews or meta-analyses are being used. Reliable SHS exposure data are not available in many places, and definitions of exposure vary in different surveys, which may not be based on a sample representative of a whole country. The WHO Global Burden of Disease Study estimates that SHS has caused 603,000 premature deaths in never smokers in 2004, including 166,000 from lower respiratory infections, 1100 from asthma in children, 35,800 from asthma, 21,000 from lung cancer, and 379,000 from ischaemic heart disease in adults. Of all deaths from SHS, 28 per cent occur in children and 47 per cent in women. The report notes that current smokers may be especially susceptible because of high and close exposure or existing smoking-caused diseases (Oberg et al. 2011).

National or local estimates of mortality in non-smokers due to SHS are critically important for advocacy for legislation to ban smoking completely. The 2006 USSG report estimates that in 2005, SHS killed over 3000 Americans from lung cancer, 46,000 from CHD, and 430 newborns from sudden infant death syndrome. The 2007 China Tobacco Control report estimates that SHS killed more than 100,000 Chinese non-smokers. In Hong Kong, the results that SHS killed 150 catering workers from lung cancer and CHD (Hedley et al. 2006), and 1324 people (from stroke, heart disease, chronic lung disease, and lung cancer) each year (McGhee et al. 2005), had been used successfully in campaigns leading to the 2006 law amendments extending the total ban of smoking to all indoor workplaces, restaurants and bars, and many other public places. New results on SHS will contribute important new evidence for causal inference for asthma in children (Burke et al. 2012), stroke (Oono et al. 2011), TB disease (Lin et al. 2007; Slama et al. 2007; Leung et al. 2010), COPD (Yin et al. 2007; He et al. 2012), and acute respiratory symptoms (Monto and Ross 1978). The uncertainty about SHS and breast cancer remains (Pirie et al. 2008).

Adverse effects of SHS in current smokers

There is a paucity of data on the adverse effects from SHS in current smokers, mainly because of the exclusion of current smokers in most, if not all, studies on SHS. In Hong Kong, SHS exposure was reported to be strongly associated with increased acute respiratory symptoms and recent outpatient service use in adult current smokers (Lam et al. 2005) and to be associated with increased risks for persistent respiratory symptoms among adolescent current smokers (Lai et al. 2009). The main purpose of banning smoking completely in indoor workplaces is to protect workers, which is an occupational health issue. Opponents and the tobacco industry have advocated for smoking areas or smoking rooms, but workers who need to serve or clean inside smoking rooms are heavily exposed to SHS. A further argument is that smoker-employees can be deployed to work in smoking areas. Results on additional harms of SHS to active smokers can be used as a counter-argument. Also, both adult and youth smokers should be warned to avoid SHS, which may motivate some to support a totally smoke-free legislation and to quit smoking.

Chemicals and carcinogens

Tobacco smoke

Tobacco smoke is a very complex mixture containing more than 7000 chemical compounds (Rodgman and Perfetti 2009). Hundreds of these compounds are toxic and at least 69 are carcinogens. The list is expected to further increase. Also new additives have been and will continue to be added to cigarettes by the tobacco industry. These include various flavours (including menthol and fruits), and herbs or herbal medicine to attract special groups of smokers, such as children and youth, and people who believe in herbal medicine (Eriksen et al. 2012). The effectiveness

of using such information to warn about the harm of smoking needs to be evaluated. The main problem is that smokers do not feel any acute toxic effects from such chemicals because the level of exposure to each compound is low.

Second-hand smoke

SHS is a complex mixture of mainstream smoke (smoke inhaled and exhaled by the smoker) and side-stream smoke (from the burning end of the cigarette). Many of the toxic substances have a higher concentration in side-stream smoke than mainstream smoke, and it has often been mistakenly publicized that SHS is more harmful than active smoking. In terms of toxicity, this is not true because the toxic substances in SHS are greatly diluted by the ambient air before inhalation by the non-smokers. Hence, the exposure level of various compounds from SHS in a non-smoker is much lower than that in a smoker. In terms of the number of people affected to varying extents from mild irritation to deaths due to lung cancer or CHD, this statement can be true because of the widespread SHS exposure in non-smokers, and the absolute number of non-smokers, including children, is always greater than the number of smokers. Public health professionals should be mindful that messages are based on strong evidence and are effective.

Third-hand smoke

Third-hand smoke (THS) refers to the residual tobacco smoke pollutants on dust, surfaces, clothes, and human body after SHS has cleared. It can be re-emitted as gases as well as react with other pollutants such as nitrous acid to form tobacco-specific nitrosamines, some of which are carcinogenic (Burton 2011). Although the phenomenon of smelling residual smoke is not new, the coining of THS (Winickoff et al. 2009) has triggered much research and public interest. THS is accumulated with each cigarette smoked and remains for weeks. Young children are particularly at risk of exposure as they explore their home environment. However, no studies have linked THS exposure to physical harm and more studies on the chemistry and health risk of THS are warranted (Matt et al. 2011).

Risk perception of the public

The risk perception and tolerance of the public is often irrational and their resulting actions are not proportional to the magnitude of risks. Most people have zero tolerance to less toxic contaminants in foods, such as malachite green in fish, but relatively few are aware of the chemicals and carcinogens in tobacco smoke. More awareness of the harms of SHS has led to the rapid decline in tolerance to SHS. Non-smokers take various actions to avoid exposure and to complain about smokers who smoke near them. The past few decades have witnessed a change from total acceptance of smoking to zero tolerance among many non-smokers, especially in countries with comprehensive smoking bans.

The protection of innocent non-smokers, including children and women and employees, has been the major driver for smoke-free legislation. In China and many LMICs, awareness is low and even non-smoking physicians are not concerned about their own exposure to SHS (Lam et al. 2011). Tobacco control advocates need to learn from successful experiences in using SHS and in comparing the risk of tobacco smoke with other toxic compounds to change risk perception and motivate actions from non-smokers.

Although the harm of THS has yet to be shown, parents who are aware of that potential risk are more likely to adopt home smoking bans (Winickoff et al. 2009). This represents an opportunity to promote a totally smoke-free environment in the private home, the last frontier in the battle of tobacco control.

Warn about the dangers

Numerous surveys reveal that the knowledge about tobacco harms is often superficial. The earliest health warning required by governments or law was mostly a small and inconspicuous statement that smoking is harmful to health on tobacco advertisements (started in 1971 in the United States) or cigarette packs. Unfortunately, this is still the situation in many countries such as China.

Canada was the first country to require pictorial health warnings by law on cigarette packs in 2001. Its success has spurred many countries to follow suit. The Canadian Cancer Society 2012 report showed that 63 countries or jurisdictions and territories, covering 40 per cent of the world's population, require pictorial warnings (Canadian Cancer Society 2012).

The FCTC Article 11 requires that health warnings 'should be 50 percent or more of the principal display areas but shall be no less than 30 percent' (WHO 2003) and may be in the form of, or include, picture warnings. Many countries have done more than this minimum, with Australia having some of the largest warnings in the world at 75 per cent of the package front and 90 per cent of the back. From December 2012, Australia has also implemented plain packaging (Fig. 9.1.2) to prohibit tobacco company colours, logos, and design elements on the brand part of the package, and to standardize the shape and format of the package. The Constitutional challenges launched by the tobacco companies against the Australian Government have been rejected by the High Court of Australia. Several countries (such as Canada, Norway, India, New Zealand, Turkey, and the United Kingdom) are planning to follow and these will be accompanied by legal challenges from the tobacco industry. Not all governments have the political will or the legal and other resources to defend against these. Nevertheless, the Australian success has served as a role model and the Australian court ruling will help governments, at least in common law countries, to defend and fight against new legal challenges.

Strong and increasing evidence shows that pictorial warnings are highly cost-effective in raising awareness and reducing tobacco use. The bigger the size of the warnings, the more effective they are. Some countries have also switched to the use of shocking images of diseased or damaged organs or dead bodies, including dead fetuses or babies. It is also important to start using the most striking pictures, have a set of more warnings (Australia has now a set of fourteen for plain packaging), and to require frequent rotations, with the printing costs totally borne by the tobacco companies and with minimal delay (as tobacco companies will produce many more packs before the law is passed and argue that they need many months or years to print new packs). The law should provide the health ministry the authority to change or update the pictures and warnings without having to amend the law. The warnings must be based on evidence that is considered sufficient for causation by most authorities. Information on pictorial warnings from all countries can be obtained from the Tobacco Labelling Resource Centre (n.d.) and the WHO warnings database (n.d.).

The tobacco industry has been fighting strongly in every country against such warnings, citing comments from smokers that they will take no notice of such warnings, and argues that printing such warnings increases production costs and affects the tobacco companies' rights to use their intellectual property to

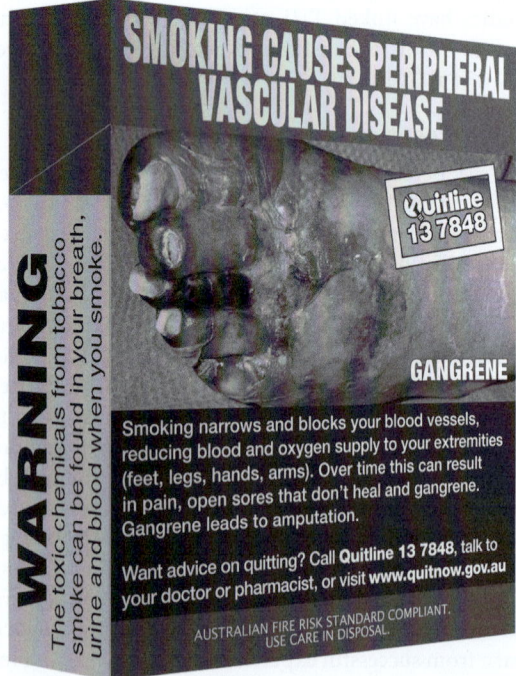
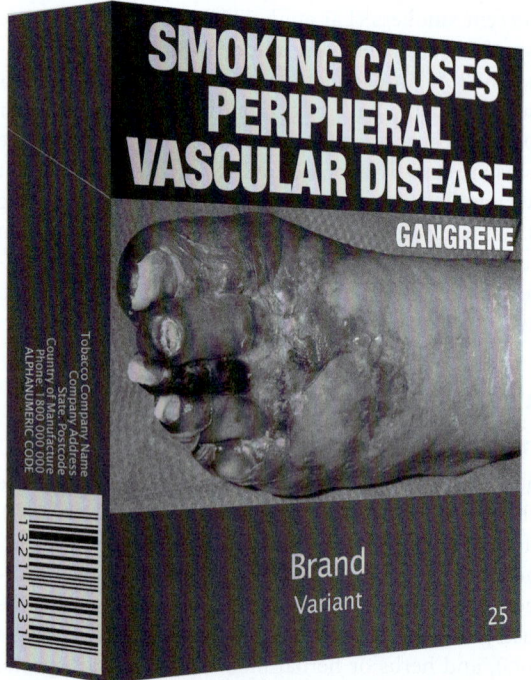

Fig. 9.1.2 Plain packaging and pictorial health warnings on Australian cigarette packs.

show their brand names and logos, jeopardizing freedom of trade and expression. In the United States, despite the Food and Drug Administration Rule in June 2011 requiring pictorial warnings to cover 50 per cent of the package front and back as from September 2012, the implementation is on hold due to the successful legal challenge of the tobacco industry. The outcome of future legal proceedings is uncertain.

FCTC Article 11 (a) requires parties to ensure that 'tobacco product packaging and labelling do not promote a tobacco product by any means that are false, misleading, deceptive or likely to create an erroneous impression. . .', and that 'These may include terms such as "low tar," "light," "ultra-light," or "mild"' (WHO 2003). Many countries still have tobacco products not complying with this article. The development and promotion of Chinese-style cigarettes as safer and healthier by the Chinese tobacco industry is particularly objectionable.

Although research has shown clearly that there is no completely safe form of tobacco, the tobacco industry continues to promote 'safer' cigarettes. There is evidence to show that such efforts have gained traction. The Global Adult Tobacco Survey in China (Chinese Center for Diseases Control and Prevention 2012) shows that more professionals and those with higher education believe that 'light' or 'low tar' cigarettes are safer. Because of the traditional belief in herbal medicine, adding such substances into cigarettes has been a major new effort by the Chinese tobacco industry to promote safer Chinese-style cigarettes.

Media campaigns

Mass media campaigns can be highly effective to raise awareness, motivate smokers to quit, and prevent young people from starting smoking. The effectiveness increases with the intensity of the campaigns, as well as the content and messages. Well-planned and sustained TV campaigns can reach most people, resulting in behavioural changes. Many antismoking videos have been systematically evaluated and confirmed to be effective in developed countries. However, the *WHO Report on the Global Tobacco Epidemic, 2011* showed a paucity of mass media campaigns against tobacco in many countries, especially in LMICs (Eriksen et al. 2012). The high costs of producing videos and broadcasting them on TV may be a factor, but could be overcome through global sharing of videos that have been shown to be effective, and by using alternative media such as YouTube and mobile phones. Further research, development, and evaluation are warranted.

Media campaigns are also needed to solicit public support for legislation and other government actions. Even when there is majority support for tax increases and smoke-free areas, objections from a small percentage of the population, sometimes leveraged on by the tobacco industry, can put great pressures on governments and legislators. Media campaigns to solicit public support need to be justified strongly by warnings that emphasize how many people, especially young people, will be killed by smoking, and such justification can further raise awareness.

Alternative ways to collaborate with the media should also be explored. Press conferences on local study results usually attract much media coverage, free of charge. The WHO's World No Tobacco Day is an annual event that can be linked to other broad-based activities that can garner substantial media reporting and commentaries. International news, for example, on important findings from medical journals, or on resolutions from the WHO or the FCTC can trigger the interest of local mass media. Public health advocates need to learn what the media want and how to work with them. For sustained effects, media campaigns need to be well planned and repeated, with updated results and new activities.

Monitoring tobacco use and prevention
Prevalence of smoking

Globally, about 20 per cent of all adults smoke cigarettes, consuming 5.9 trillion cigarettes in 2009. Even if smoking prevalence remains the same, tobacco consumption as a whole will increase due to the rising world population, especially in LMICs. China is the world's largest producer and consumer of cigarettes, accounting for 38 per cent of global consumption. Because of its huge population and high smoking prevalence, China has the largest number of smokers (adults and youth) and smoking-induced deaths. The second to fifth highest cigarette-consuming countries are the Russian Federation, United States, Indonesia, and Japan.

Monitoring tobacco use is fundamental to our understanding of the extent of the epidemic, assessing the current and projecting the future burden of disease, and evaluating the effectiveness of prevention polices. The *Tobacco Atlas*, 4th edition (Eriksen et al. 2012), shows comprehensive world tables including prevalence in men and women, and in boys and girls. Sex-specific data are important since males and females have great differences in tobacco use. Time-trend data will become available for more countries. Interpretation of trend data where available should take into account variations in survey methods over time, and sampling errors.

In 1998, the WHO, US CDC, and Canadian Public Health Association initiated the Global Tobacco Surveillance System (GTSS) (Warren et al. 2009a) to help countries monitor tobacco use, using standardized methods in school-based and household surveys. The Global Youth Tobacco Survey (GYTS), Global School Personnel Survey (GSPS), Global Health Professions Student Survey (GHPSS), and Global Adult Tobacco Survey (GATS) started in 1999, 2000, 2007, and 2007 respectively (Warren et al. 2009b). The surveys are in progress, with greatest coverage for the GYTS as it started early. The GATS is a nationally representative household survey of men and women aged 15 or older. It includes: (1) tobacco use, (2) knowledge attitudes and perceptions, (3) cessation, (4) SHS exposure, (5) economics, (6) media, and (7) background characteristics. These surveys also provide essential data for monitoring prevention policies.

Other tobacco use

The tobacco epidemic started in the United Kingdom and United States with the invention of machines (in 1881 in the United States) for mass production of cigarettes, and the aggressive advertising and promotion of cigarettes by the tobacco companies, before the serious health hazards were widely known. Tobacco use, however, also includes kreteks (Indonesia), roll-your-own cigarettes (Europe and New Zealand), bidis (South Asia, mainly India), pipes (worldwide), sticks (Papua New Guinea), water pipes (North Africa, the Mediterranean region, and parts of Asia), cigars (worldwide), and various forms of smokeless tobacco, including chewing tobacco (worldwide), moist snuff (Scandinavia and United States), dissolvable smokeless tobacco products (high-income countries), and dry snuff (Europe) (Eriksen et al. 2012).

The International Tobacco Control Policy Evaluation Project

The ITC Project is the first international cohort study on the psychosocial and behavioural impact of key national level policies of the FCTC (International Tobacco Control Policy Evaluation Project n.d.). ITC includes 20 countries with 50 per cent of the world's population and 70 per cent of the world's tobacco users and covers:

◆ Health warning labels and package descriptors

◆ Smoke-free legislation

◆ Pricing and taxation of tobacco products

◆ Communication and education

◆ Cessation

◆ Tobacco advertising and promotion.

Stages of tobacco epidemic

The patterns of smoking and tobacco-induced diseases, particularly lung cancer, vary greatly in different countries. Lopez et al. (1994) defined four stages of the tobacco epidemic, based on developed countries like the United Kingdom, United States, and Australia. Smoking prevalence rose rapidly since the 1900s, first in men peaking in the 1950s, followed by women about two decades later reaching a lower peak, and then declined since the 1960–1970s, after large numbers of smokers stopped. Tobacco deaths in men lagged this, peaking about three decades later in the 1980s and then declined as a result of increased cessation, whereas in women, tobacco deaths continued to increase or plateau into the present century. This four-stage model highlights the long delay (about three decades) between widespread smoking and its full effects on mortality. It has been applied to other countries or regions, with sub-Saharan Africa in Stage 1, Latin America in Stage 2, Eastern Europe in Stage 3, and the United Kingdom in Stage 4.

A recent review of the model after two decades showed that in developed countries, the prevalence of smoking has continued to decline in both sexes and the proportion of deaths due to smoking has declined in men and continues to increase or plateau in women (Thun et al. 2012). Latest findings also support that tobacco deaths in the United States have plateaued in men but continue to rise in women (Thun et al. 2013). The model generally applies to men in developing countries but cannot predict when (or if) women will begin smoking in large numbers. Thus, modified criteria and separate models are needed to describe the epidemic entirely for men and women in developing countries. The long lag between peak tobacco deaths and peak tobacco consumption is a key reason for the lack of urgent action among governments and politicians.

Smoking in women

A limitation of this model is that it does not take into account the history and timing of tobacco control measures. Data from Hong Kong (Lai 2012) show that its downward male smoking trend (from 39.7 per cent in 1982 to 19.9 per cent in 2010) appears to be similar to Australia and the United States, but its female trend from 5.6 per cent to 3.0 per cent does not follow the model. About three decades ago, tobacco control advocates in Hong Kong predicted a great rise in female smoking prevalence, which did not happen. This could be due, at least partly, to the early introduction of tobacco control measures including a 300 per cent increase in tobacco tax in 1983 (and 100 per cent in 1991), and legislation restricting (1982, 1990, 1992, 1998, 1999, and 2007) and eventually banning tobacco advertising (2008).

Enforce bans on tobacco advertising

It is recognized that a comprehensive ban on advertising, promotion, and sponsorship would reduce the consumption of tobacco products. Before restrictions on tobacco advertising in the mid 1960s, many high-income countries, such as the United Kingdom and United States, witnessed aggressive advertising especially targeting women. Now, 103 countries have some restrictions on tobacco marketing, but only 24 countries (10 per cent of the world population) have banned all forms of direct and indirect advertising (WHO 2013a).

Partial restrictions are ineffective as the tobacco industry has many ways to bypass them. In Hong Kong, where all forms of tobacco advertising are banned but the display of cigarettes at retailing shops and newspaper stands is allowed, the tobacco companies pay large sums of money to expand the display area with spotlights on individual cigarette packs. The government has difficulty prosecuting this as newspaper stand and shop owners will protest such actions. LMICs should aim to move directly to a total ban. Some African countries have done so before the multinational tobacco companies have gained a foothold. Other countries like Thailand have banned the display of cigarettes.

Banning of indirect advertising is very difficult as some cigarettes share the same brand as non-tobacco products (brand stretching). In China, a famous and very expensive cigarette brand from Shanghai was named, many decades ago, 'Zhong Hua' meaning China. The tobacco company launched a campaign of 'I love Zhong Hua', featuring two Chinese characters in the same format as the cigarette logo. Some Chinese brands are named after a famous place or an animal (such as Panda). Bypassing advertising bans in this manner is increasing, but many governments have no experience or resources to prosecute them or the confidence that they will win in court.

Banning of sponsorship is the most difficult of all. The FCTC defines this as 'any form of contribution to any event, activity or individual with the aim, effect or likely effect of promoting a tobacco product or tobacco use either directly or indirectly' (WHO 2003). Victoria in Australia was the first to use tobacco tax proceeds to establish a health foundation in 1987 to replace tobacco sponsorship. This successful example has been cited by tobacco control advocates in many countries, but few have succeeded (such as Thailand). Many organizations' events and activities, politicians, legislators, researchers, and other individuals are receiving tobacco sponsorships/money. They are unlikely to support stringent tobacco control measures, and may join the tobacco alliance directly or indirectly. Governments need to ban offering and receipt of all forms of tobacco sponsorships. Interim measures could include legislation requiring disclosure and policies forbidding such sponsorships. To help implement and enforce comprehensive bans on tobacco advertising, promotion, and sponsorship, the WHO has developed a 3-day training workshop for LMICs (World Health Organization and International Union Against Tuberculosis and Lung Disease 2011).

Protect people from tobacco smoke

A major breakthrough in tobacco control was the designation of smoke-free areas to protect people from SHS, and the related non-smokers' rights movement starting in the 1980s in the United States. Banning of smoking in public places by law has been introduced, often progressively from a partial to total ban, and is expanding to include all public places (from indoor to outdoor) and all indoor workplaces (public and private). Further bans were introduced in outdoor areas in some countries, such as busy streets in Japan. With overwhelming public support, Singapore has recently extended the smoking bans to the common areas of residential buildings, covered walkways, pedestrian bridges, a 5-metre radius from the edge of bus stops, and outdoor compounds of hospitals. The number of people protected by comprehensive smoke-free laws has doubled from 2008 to 2010, but 89 per cent of the world's population remain unprotected (Eriksen et al. 2012).

Public support is strong only in countries where awareness of the harms of SHS is high together with strong political will of governments. The tobacco industry has worked to oppose this, building alliances with smokers' rights groups and others who may be adversely affected, such as the hotel and catering industry. Some restaurant workers or their unions are mobilized by their employers, with support from tobacco companies, to protest. The tobacco industry will lobby governments and legislators and repeatedly argue that banning smoking in restaurants and bars will result in loss of customers, revenue, and jobs. However, in all jurisdictions, implementation of smoke-free laws has mostly resulted in no changes or increased restaurant sales, and savings in cleaning costs and reduction of fire risks.

A total ban is needed to eliminate SHS exposure. However, the tobacco industry is often successful in exploiting loopholes in such laws (such as no legal liability or penalty for venue owners or managers if they allow smoking in their statutory smoke-free areas in Hong Kong). Many restaurant owners still believe that their business will suffer from total smoking bans, particularly in LMICs. Public health advocates must distinguish between the tobacco companies and venue owners even when they form an alliance. Mass media and other campaigns, such as motivating students and other non-smokers to demand smoke-free dining areas, are effective ways to change the minds of some restaurant owners and workers. Some will never be convinced but all will want a level playing field such that any new laws should equally apply to all venues; allowing some restaurants to have smoking areas but not others will not work.

A national smoke-free law is needed but in China, only some major cities have started to introduce local smoke-free legislation. However, enforcement is weak, penalties for violation low, and compliance is expectedly unsatisfactory. Mass media campaigns are needed before the implementation of the new law. Initial law enforcement with substantial penalties is essential to convince the public and venue owners about the government's seriousness. Effective enforcement of comprehensive smoke-free legislation saves lives by reducing heart attacks, increasing quitting in the population, and reducing smoking among employees (Glasgow et al. 1997).

Raise taxes on tobacco

Raising taxes is the most effective way to reduce tobacco consumption quickly. Repeated and sufficiently high increases in tax drove the decline in consumption especially in high-income countries a few decades ago. On the other hand, with economic development and increasing incomes in LMICs such as China, the reduction in real tobacco prices has substantially contributed to increasing consumption. High prices are particularly effective in preventing the uptake of smoking in the young and reducing consumption among low-income people, with more quitting in both groups. Strong evidence has come from both high- and LMICs, such as the United Kingdom, South Africa, Morocco, and Israel (Eriksen et al. 2012). A more recent example is from France, where tripling the price of cigarettes has halved consumption and doubled government revenue in 2003–2004 (Gallus et al. 2006).

The seminal World Bank report in 1999 states that all evidence from high- and LMICs shows that price increases are highly effective in reducing demand. The statement that 'On average, a price rise of 10 percent on a pack of cigarettes would be expected to reduce demand for cigarettes by about 4 percent in high-income countries and by about 8 percent in low- and middle-income countries' (World Bank 1999) has been widely cited. The *Tobacco Atlas*, 4th edition (Eriksen et al. 2012) shows different degrees of reduction, 2–6 per cent in high- and 2–8 per cent in LMICs. The model in the World Bank report shows that raising prices by 10 per cent worldwide would result in 40 million smokers quitting in 1995 and preventing at least 10 million deaths. This estimate is conservative because if one in two smokers will be killed by tobacco, 40 million current smokers quitting would prevent about 20 million deaths. As price increases will also reduce uptake of smoking in young people, there will be further reduction of deaths in the more distant future.

Big variations in the excise tax as a percentage of cigarette prices are shown in the *Tobacco Atlas*. The WHO recommends that excise tax should reach at least 70 per cent of the retail price but only five nations have achieved this standard (Eriksen et al. 2012). The World Bank proposes that taxes should account for two-thirds to four-fifths of the retail price (Mackay et al. 2006). Tobacco tax increase can also generate additional income for governments. As of 2010, at least 166 WHO Member States have imposed a tobacco excise tax, and at least 27 of them used a portion of the tobacco tax revenue for health purposes. Numerous economic analyses have shown that the economic costs of tobacco, including lost productivity and health and other expenditures from tobacco-induced disease burden, are greater than tobacco tax income. The 2012 Asian Development Bank report estimated that in China, India, Philippines, Thailand, and Vietnam, a 50 per cent price increase would reduce tobacco deaths by over 27 million, and generate over $27 billion additional revenue annually (Asian Development Bank 2012).

Given these data, it is not clear why most governments have not implemented the WHO recommendation of at least 70 per cent, even after they have ratified the FCTC. Collusion between the tobacco industry and government officials, the loss of tobacco tax revenue if consumption falls sharply, or inadequate funding allocation for tobacco control in LMICs are possible reasons. More research is needed to find the root causes for this, and effective ways to convince governments to do so.

Any tax increase is not welcomed in general by the public and may lead to dissatisfaction towards governments, which could result in protests and unrest. The economic argument that reduction of tobacco use can save healthcare expenditures has little direct immediate impact because such savings are only realized in the future. A very strong argument from opponents is that high taxes will result in increased smuggling, making cheaper illicit cigarettes more available to many low-income smokers especially youth. However, a recent report showed that tax increases in the United Kingdom have not led to increased smuggling.

Tobacco industry

In celebrating the fifth anniversary of the FCTC, WHO Director General Dr Margaret Chan said, 'the tobacco industry is ruthless, devious, rich and powerful. As we all know, neither WHO nor public health is rich, but with the Framework Convention now in place, we are indeed powerful' (WHO 2010). It is the only industry that has been openly and repeatedly discredited, condemned, and shamed by WHO.

The tobacco industry is dominated by several multinational tobacco companies. The China National Tobacco Corporation is the largest state-owned enterprise producing the greatest number of cigarettes in the world. Despite the progress in tobacco control in some countries, and the FCTC, the tobacco companies remain some of the most profitable in the world (Eriksen et al. 2012).

Tobacco company documents

Research and numerous reports have exposed the tobacco industry's various anti-public health measures. Most of the findings are based on the analysis of millions of pages of internal tobacco company documents exposed since 1994 and during litigation proceedings against the tobacco companies in the 1994 seminal judgement in the United States, now deposited in Minnesota, United States and Guildford, United Kingdom (Mackay et al. 2006; Shafey et al. 2009). These documents are still under-researched but are now easily accessible for public health professionals and researchers, particularly those interested in what the tobacco industry had said about their countries or regions and strategies including the targeting of children or women. They provide insights into the varied strategies employed by the tobacco industry to promote the continued use of tobacco among different communities and population segments (Mackay et al. 2006; Shafey et al. 2009; Eriksen et al. 2012; World Health Organization 2013b).

Tobacco corporate social responsibility

The tobacco companies spend huge sums of money in funding smokers' groups, tobacco associations and institutes, and other alliances to oppose tobacco control measures; funding researchers to challenge the evidence of tobacco harms particularly from SHS; funding research but suppressing or distorting unfavourable results; and funding government and non-government organizations and various events or programmes on education, arts, culture and sports, environmental protection, and medical, health, or rehabilitation programmes to promote cigarette brands and corporate image and to buy in supporters or silence potential opponents (World Health Organization 2013b).

Youth Smoking Prevention (YSP) programmes, funded by the tobacco industry, are particularly deceptive and troubling. These are ineffective as they focus on young people only and portray smoking as an adult habit thus making it more appealing for adolescents. YSP programmes have attracted NGOs interested in adolescent health, community leaders, and schools who do not understand their motivation. This has created much confusion and frustration for tobacco control advocates, who need to be extremely cautious about how to expose the tobacco connections and ineffectiveness of YSP programmes, yet not to alienate those who have been deceived. The WHO booklet from Western Pacific Regional Office on YSP is an invaluable resource (WHO 2003). How should youth programmes be organized that can be distinguished from YSP? In Hong Kong, the strategy is to promote the WHO booklet (Ho et al. 2010) and to launch youth quitting programmes instead of smoking prevention programmes. It is useful to bear in mind and emphasize that the great majority of young people do not smoke. Over-emphasis on youth smoking may result in over-estimation of peer smoking in adolescents, which can increase adolescent smoking (Ho et al. 2010).

The tobacco industry has not changed, as evidenced by their current efforts to use litigation and legal threats against governments that are planning or have introduced new control measures. The *Tobacco Atlas*, 4th edition, lists legal challenges against tobacco control measures by the tobacco industry in 18 countries (Eriksen et al. 2012). The tobacco companies will launch more of these in more countries. Some tobacco control advocates in the West have called for government to buy the tobacco companies to control them. However, the example of China's national tobacco monopoly indicates that the result could be even worse. Some tobacco control advocates in China have called for the separation of the administration arm, which can then monitor and control the enterprise arm more independently.

Should governments sue the tobacco industry? A major landmark was the success of the US government's 1999 lawsuit which resulted in the major tobacco companies paying settlements of US$206 billion over 25 years to 46 states to compensate for government spending on smoking-related healthcare (Gruber 2001). The number of anti-tobacco legal cases has been increasing but only slowly. The ultimate legal defeat of the tobacco industry would be to make tobacco illegal.

WHO FCTC

The FCTC is an evidence-based treaty and a paradigm shift in developing a regulatory strategy on demand reduction and supply issues (WHO 2003). The success of the FCTC has prompted and inspired public health advocates to call for similar treaties, such as a framework convention on alcohol control (FCAC) (Casswell and Thamarangsi 2009; Lam and Chim 2010). The FCTC is a readable, action-oriented document that can be used by governments, public health professionals, and the public. It has led to a global movement and is a strong lobbying document to pressurize governments to comply with the international treaty that they have ratified. The FCTC only stipulates the minimum that governments must do, and Australia's plain packaging in 2012 clearly shows that more can be done.

Countries that have not ratified the FCTC are under great pressure to ratify. Many governments have not yet fulfilled their obligations to comply fully with the FCTC, and these are reported regularly in WHO MPOWER reports.

The FCTC is governed by the Conference of the Parties (COP), which comprises all Parties (countries or jurisdictions) to the Convention. It reviews and makes decisions to promote its effective implementation, and adopts protocols, annexes, and amendments to the Convention. Starting from COP3, the regular sessions of COP are held biennially.

The Protocol to Eliminate Illicit Trade in Tobacco Products, in pursuance of FCTC Article 15, is the first protocol adopted by the COP as effective, appropriate, and comprehensive domestic and international responses to eliminate all forms of illicit trade (World Health Organization Framework Convention on Tobacco Research 2012).

Framework Convention Alliance

The FCTC is not just for health ministries or governments. NGOs have played key roles from the beginning of its negotiation, and their influence is expanding. The Framework Convention Alliance (FCA) created in 1999 has over 350 organizations from more than 100 countries. It is a civic society alliance whose mission is to help develop and implement the FCTC as the basis for effective global tobacco control (FCA n.d.). The FCTC has become the benchmark for the evaluation of the performance and effectiveness of tobacco control measures of parties, countries, or regions. For example, those who have been performing badly are being shamed by The Dirty Ashtray Award by civil society; China received one such award for making excuses not to print warning pictures on cigarette packing at COP3 in 2008.

FCTC and UN Political Declaration on NCDs

The FCTC has laid the foundation for the 2011 UN Political Declaration for the control of NCDs, and now the reverse is happening. As a follow-up to the UN Political Declaration, WHO is consulting on the development of the NCD Global Monitoring Framework (WHO 2012b) and the Global Action Plan on NCDs (2013–2020) (WHO 2012c). After lobbying by the FCA, the draft Global Action Plan on NCDs (10 October 2012) now explicitly promotes the FCTC and urges all WHO Member States to accelerate its implementation. While the NCD Global Monitoring Framework includes a tobacco smoking target (voluntary, to be determined), FCA further advocates to monitor specific process and impact indicators on the implementation of FCTC policy measures. There will be rapid and major developments on all these fronts.

Research and evaluation

The FCTC is based on solid research conducted mostly in high-income countries. Evidence from LMICs is inadequate. Progress in policies and implementation in some countries has been rapid and great, and previous experiences and evidence can become outdated while the impact of new measures need to be rapidly evaluated to guide further action. In countries with slow progress, the lack of funding and research is very serious. Their needs for local data and evidence are more urgent and should be most relevant for local policies and implementation. Further and relevant research is needed for all countries to support and evaluate the implementation of the FCTC. The Global Network of the Society for Research on Nicotine and Tobacco (SRNT) has published a series of papers in a themed issue of *Nicotine & Tobacco Research* on the research requirements and needs for all the FCTC articles to support specific policies and practices (Leischow et al. 2012). This is a most thorough analysis of the state of science to provide new directions and priorities for research. A commentary

by Mackay emphasizes that 'advocates and activities MUST keep their feet firmly based in science, and never stray from that science' but 'The need to bridge the existing gaps between research, policy, and practice appears to be a global phenomenon' (Mackay 2013).

Offer help to quit tobacco use

Quitting smoking saves lives and the earlier the better. In cancer patients, increasing evidence shows that quitting smoking can improve the effectiveness of treatment and survival and more successful trials are needed to motivate HCPs to help such patients to quit (McBride and Ostroff 2003; Parsons et al. 2010).

Most successful former smokers quit without pharmaceutical therapy or professional services ('cold turkey'). They do have different experiences including past failures that deserve further study. On the other hand, effective treatments are available which have helped many to quit. The pursuit for more effective pharmaceutical treatments, including nicotine vaccination will go on, as the existing treatments are expensive and failures common.

The 1990 USSG report on smoking cessation was the first comprehensive review about the benefits of quitting (US Department of Health and Human Services 1990). The excess risk of ischaemic heart disease is reduced by half after stopping for 1 year, but it takes 10 years of quitting for lung cancer risk to reduce to 30–50 per cent of continuing smokers. The 2007 IARC report on risk reversal, the most recent comprehensive review, concludes that the evidence is adequate for: (1) lower risk in former smokers and (2) lower risk with prolonged abstinence for lung, laryngeal, oral, oesophageal (squamous cell), pancreatic, bladder, and cervical cancer (seven items), and CHD incidence and death in subjects with or without the disease, cerebrovascular incidence and death in those without established disease (three items), and cough and phlegm, decline in forced expiratory volume in 1 second in healthy subjects and those with mild to severe disease and COPD mortality (five items). For overall mortality, those 'stopping at 60, 50, 40 or 30 years of age gain, respectively, about 3, 6, 9 or almost the full 10 years of life expectancy, in comparison with those who continue to smoke' (IARC 2007). Those who stopped smoking before middle age, at about 20–30, avoid nearly all of the future mortality risks from tobacco (Doll et al. 2004; Pirie et al. 2013).

Quitting or preventing uptake?

Uptake prevention and quitting have different target subjects and need different strategies. Most people intuitively support very strongly the prevention of smoking in children and young people and believe that this is the *most* important measure. They want more health education against youth smoking and consider health education in schools the most important action. Such a belief is exploited by the tobacco industry's YSP programme.

The 1999 World Bank report states that if quitting results in reducing adult cigarette consumption by half by the 2020s, about one-third of tobacco-related deaths in the 2020s would be prevented and almost half would be prevented thereafter, preventing 20 or 30 million tobacco deaths in the first quarter and 100 million in the second quarter of this century. If young smokers are reduced by half by the 2020s, hundreds of millions of tobacco deaths would be prevented after 2050. This would prevent none of the 150 million tobacco deaths in the 2020s, about 10–20 million out of 300 million in the second quarter of the century. Hence, quitting will prevent more deaths more quickly in the first half of this century than that from preventing young people from starting, although the latter is also important for preventing deaths in the second half of the century.

Nicotine dependence or habit

Smoking is often wrongly described as a habit or a personal choice. Nicotine is strongly addictive and most smokers are both nicotine and psychosocially dependent. The Fagerstrom test is the most commonly used test to measure nicotine dependence (Heatherton et al. 1991). But the term 'nicotine addict' is seldom used to describe heavily nicotine-dependent smokers and the term 'treatment of nicotine dependence' is much less frequently used than 'smoking cessation therapy'. HCPs need to understand why smokers frequently fail in their attempts to quit, or relapse after a short time.

Smoking cessation interventions include smoking cessation clinics (which vary from simple counselling to specialized in-hospital treatment) or telephone quitlines, smoking cessation advice and counselling during routine consultation, and pharmacological aids and therapies. Most of these have been confirmed by numerous trials to be effective and more cost effective than other medical treatments. The Cochrane Library should be consulted for updated reviews and conclusions (Cochrane Review Groups n.d.). Effectiveness means greater quit rates after interventions than no interventions, but failures occur more often than successes.

The seminal randomized controlled trial by Russell (1979) that brief advice by general practitioners in the United Kingdom increased the quit rate from 0.3 per cent to 3.3 per cent has led to a strong argument that if all physicians can spare a little time advising patients to quit, even though the absolute quit rate is low, many smokers will benefit, resulting in major community impact. Thirty years later, the review by Aveyard and Foulds (2009) showed that a brief intervention of at least 1 minute is effective (versus no intervention). However, most clinicians are too busy to spare even 1 minute and many feel incompetent. They also do not have any incentive, support, or pressure to do so. Such barriers are still common in both high- and LMICs. To address these issues, a simple 30-second pilot intervention emphasizing 'one in two risk' was recently conducted in China with promising results (Lin et al. 2013).

Do most smokers want to quit?

The 2008 MPOWER report states 'Among smokers who are aware of the dangers of tobacco, three out of four want to quit' (WHO 2008) without specifying the country. But the reference (Jones 2006) indicates that this statement is based on a survey of US adults in 2006 and it should be noted that the denominator is *not* all smokers. While this may be true in countries at the late stage of the tobacco epidemic, the Global Adult Tobacco Use Surveys in China and other LMICs show that most smokers do not intend to quit (Cooper et al. 2010; Chinese Center for Diseases Control and Prevention 2012). A deeper understanding of the smoker's intention and the strength of their motivation or determination to quit or reduce smoking can guide public health policies and planning on cessation services. Social support from family, friends, co-workers, and employers is needed.

Clinical or public health approaches?

During the early years of tobacco control, the emphasis was mostly on public health measures such as legislation and taxation. These measures were deemed more effective than clinical services that target individual smokers, especially since few physicians or HCPs were prepared to act. The high costs of clinical services also rendered them less cost-effective. The controversy over these two approaches has become more complex as effective pharmaceutical treatments have become available (Chapman and MacKenzie, 2010; West et al. 2010). While the Bloomberg Initiative to Reduce Tobacco Use does not support smoking cessation services for individuals, these services are rapidly developing elsewhere, such as in the United Kingdom. More quitlines and international quitting campaigns such as Quit and Win have also been developed. The WHO has provided detailed guidelines for setting up and running national quitlines especially in LMICs (WHO 2011).

Quit rates for all the existing nicotine replacement therapies and drugs are not high as most users fail to quit after receiving treatment. The costs are high and adherence is low. The high failure rate is demoralizing. The 5As in the United States (ask, advise, assess, assist, arrange) has been one of the most referenced guidelines (Cornuz and Willi 2008) but these are too demanding for busy HCPs. Simpler guidelines or methods are recommended such as ABC in New Zealand (McRobbie et al. 2008). Development and randomized controlled trials of shorter advice of less than 1 minute are needed (Lam 2012; Lam et al. 2012).

Public health professionals need to understand that the clinician's job is primarily treatment. If clinicians are frustrated by failures of smokers to quit despite their efforts, they should be made more aware and become more motivated to support or join in public health advocacy campaigns. Clinicians and their professional organizations are strong allies for public health in general and tobacco control in particular. Public health professionals should collaborate with clinicians to develop more effective measures to increase cessation in individual smokers and in the population.

Pilot cessation clinics

In LMICs, many physicians are smokers, and they seldom advise their patients to quit smoking. Some smoke quite openly, if smoking is allowed in the healthcare settings, such as hospitals. Even non-smoking HCPs are mostly inactive (Lam et al. 2011). In recent years in China, smoking cessation clinics have been established in many hospitals as a requirement for designation as smoke-free hospitals. This was also done to comply with the FCTC. But most clinics have attracted few smokers, from the hospitals and the community. Opening a clinic without strong support from top management, including adequate funding, capacity building, and incentives for HCPs, will not work. Lacking strong tobacco control measures in the greater environment, and funding to promote the cessation clinics, the wait for smokers to come will be in vain.

As a first step, introducing a pilot smoking cessation clinic with provision of training and support can motivate a hospital and its management and some HCPs to become interested, firstly in treatment, and then in tobacco control in general. The pilot can act as a springboard, bringing tobacco control advocates into a hospital to train interested HCPs in both smoking cessation intervention and tobacco control advocacy. With a core of trained HCPs, the clinic can become a focal point for further actions, such as implementation of smoke-free hospital policy, and extending beyond the clinic and the hospital into the community, such as supporting smoke-free workplaces and tobacco tax increases or public education campaigns in the neighbourhood. The clinic can also motivate the smoking HCPs to quit smoking, or to discourage smoking within the hospital, and become a training site for other staff and medical and other students.

On the other hand, public health professionals should work closely with clinicians to set up strategies for proactive approaches to help smokers outside the clinic, such as in the wards and outpatient departments and to promote quitting and tobacco control within and beyond the hospital to develop the cessation clinics into tobacco control advocacy centres. Systematic evaluation of the impacts and sharing of experiences are essential for further improvements and development.

Smoking cessation can also act as the 'carrot' for the 'stick' of government proposed policies to expand smoke-free places and increase tobacco tax. Tobacco control opponents often argue that the policies are unfair to smokers and unkind to the poor, leaving the smokers nowhere to smoke and depriving the poor of their only affordable pleasure. Many government officers have difficulty responding to such allegations. If government-subsidized free smoking cessation services are offered, the simple answer is that smokers are encouraged to quit using the pilot clinics. If they quit, they will not need to find permissible places to smoke and will save a lot of money for more healthy and pleasurable commodities for the whole family.

Some government officers also feel that because there are so many smokers, they will not have the resources or capacity to open an adequate number of cessation clinics to cope with the demand. Some even feel that smokers should pay for the services, using the money saved from buying cigarettes. In reality, only a small percentage of smokers will visit cessation clinics, and many more will quit by themselves, often with social support from the family and others. A few cessation clinics or a quitline should therefore be sufficient and the sudden increase in visits and calls serves as an indicator of the effectiveness of the new control measures. Furthermore, if all or even a small percentage of the excess revenue arising from the increase in tobacco tax is used to support smokers to quit and to promote quitting, governments will have a strong justification that part of the money obtained from smokers will be used to benefit the smokers.

Quitting or smoking reduction?

Many smokers who claim that they have reduced smoking may not be reporting the truth, and total abstinence is the only proven way for the benefits to be realized. Smoking reduction may be a distraction from total abstinence. Evidence for the benefits of smoking reduction and organized or regular services or campaigns focusing only on smoking reduction are scarce. But there are many smokers who do not want to quit completely but are willing to reduce smoking. New evidence has shown that helping such smokers can increase quit rate and reduction (Chan et al. 2011). Smoking cessation campaigns and services will not attract such smokers. New approaches are needed to assess the needs of smokers who are not willing to quit and to recruit and help them to reduce, and to follow up and evaluate further whether such approaches are effective in eventually helping the smokers to quit.

Controversies of harm reduction

Evidence, mainly from Sweden, that smokeless tobacco users have a lower risk of lung cancer and other diseases than cigarette smokers, has triggered debates about switching from cigarettes to smokeless tobacco as a harm reduction measure (WHO 2003). Opponents to such switching argue that it does not reduce the harm substantially, and promotion of switching can be seen as promotion of smokeless tobacco use resulting in reduced motivation to quit. It may also increase uptake of smokeless tobacco use in young people. More broadly, such strategies effectively entail the replacement of nicotine from tobacco use with nicotine-containing products (Foulds and Branstetter 2012). The debate is continuing, but the tobacco companies are moving fast to promote smokeless tobacco and develop other nicotine products. The UK National Institute for Health and Care Excellence (NICE) has released draft guidance for consultation, which includes NRT and e-cigarettes but excludes smokeless tobacco (NICE 2013).

Endgame or endless war?

The rapid reduction of smoking prevalence in some countries, the increasing impact of the FCTC, and strong political will of some governments have led to optimism and aspirations that a smoke-free country has become reachable within 20 years. The Bhutanese 2004 law aims to end tobacco sale, the 2010 Finland Tobacco Act aims to end tobacco use, and the US government has the 'vision of a society free from tobacco-related death and disease' (US Department of Health and Human Services 2012). In March 2011, the New Zealand government committed to become an essentially smoke-free nation by 2025 and the website has much information on policies and actions (Smokefree New Zealand 2025 n.d.).

On the other hand, the war against tobacco and the tobacco industry has just begun in many LMICs, where political will is lacking to fight wholeheartedly. For the pessimists, new tobacco control advocates and younger public health professionals, this appears to be an endless war, sometimes with more battles lost than won. However, a careful review of past battles, globally and in many countries with more advanced tobacco control measures, indicates many more victories, every one of which had been fought initially by only a few dedicated and courageous people (Lam 2013). Fighting a battle today anywhere is much easier than it was a few decades ago. We now have the FCTC and another new international treaty under the FCTC (COP5) and more will be forthcoming. We also have the UN Declaration against NCDs (and tobacco). When we are facing the aggressive challenges from the tobacco industry including suing governments, we know Big Tobacco is desperate and that eventually, the public health goals will prevail, despite occasional loss, compromises, and setbacks. For public health professionals, our experiences in tobacco control will guide us to tackle the other three risk factors. If tobacco cannot be controlled successfully, the chances for success in controlling the other risk factors will be slim. Fighting against the risk factors and NCDs will be an endless war, as promoting health and well-being of all people will be our never-ending mission.

Acknowledgements

We thank Dr L. Xu for her help in literature search, referencing, and preparing the figures. Our sincere gratitude goes to Professors

J. Mackay and R. Peto, who have been inspirational and supportive to our research and public health advocacy on tobacco control.

Text extracts from *British Medical Journal*, Projected effects of tobacco smoking on worldwide tuberculosis control: mathematical modelling analysis, Basu, S. et al. Volume 343, D5506, Copyright © 2011, reproduced with permission from British Medical Journal Publishing Group Ltd.

Text extracts from World Health Organization (WHO), *WHO Report on the Global Tobacco Epidemic*, WHO, Geneva, Switzerland, Copyright © 2008, reproduced with permission of the World Health Organization, available from http://www.who.int/tobacco/mpower/mpower_report_full_2008.pdf.

Text extracts from International Agency for Research on Cancer (IARC) Handbooks Of Cancer Prevention, *Evaluating the Effectiveness of Smoke-free Policies*, IARC, Lyon, France, Copyright © 2009, reproduced with permission of the World Health Organization, available from http://www.iarc.fr/en/publications/pdfs-online/prev/handbook13/handbook13.pdf.

Text extracts from *WHO Tobacco Framework*, World Health Organization, Geneva, Switzerland, Copyright © 2003, reproduced with permission of the World Health Organization, available from http://www.who.int/tobacco/framework/WHO_FCTC_english.pdf.

References

Asian Development Bank (2012). *Tobacco Taxes: A Win–Win Measure for Fiscal Space and Health*. Mandaluyong City, Philippines: Asian Development Bank.

Aubin, H.J., Benyamina, A., Karila, L., Luquiens, A., and Reynaud, M. (2011). [Current strategies for treatment of alcohol problems]. *La Revue du Praticien*, 61, 1373–7.

Aveyard, P. and Foulds, J. (2009). *The 2008 US Clinical Practice Guideline: The Key Recommendations and a Commentary*. Ask the Experts. Available at: http://www.treatobacco.net.

Basu, S., Stuckler, D., Bitton, A., and Glantz, S.A. (2011). Projected effects of tobacco smoking on worldwide tuberculosis control: mathematical modelling analysis. *British Medical Journal*, 343, d5506.

Bates, M.N., Khalakdina, A., Pai, M., Chang, L., Lessa, F., and Smith, K.R. (2007). Risk of tuberculosis from exposure to tobacco smoke: a systematic review and meta-analysis. *Archives of Internal Medicine*, 167, 335–42.

Burke, H., Leonardi-Bee, J., Hashim, A., et al. (2012). Prenatal and passive smoke exposure and incidence of asthma and wheeze: systematic review and meta-analysis. *Pediatrics*, 129, 735–44.

Burton, A. (2011). Does the smoke ever really clear? Thirdhand smoke exposure raises new concerns. *Environmental Health Perspectives*, 119, A70–4.

Canadian Cancer Society (2012). *Cigarette Package Health Warnings: International Status Report* (3rd ed.). Canadian Cancer Society. Available at: http://www.tobaccolabels.ca/wp/wp-content/uploads/2014/04/Cigarette-Package-Health-Warnings-International-Status-Report-English-CCS-Oct-2012.pdf.

Casswell., S. and Thamarangsi., T. (2009). Reducing harm from alcohol: call to action. *The Lancet*, 373, 2247–57.

Centers for Disease Control and Prevention (2010). *A Report of the Surgeon General: How Tobacco Smoke Causes Disease…And What it Means to You*. Available at: http://www.cdc.gov/tobacco/data_statistics/sgr/2010/consumer_booklet/pdfs/consumer.pdf.

Chan, S.S., Leung, D.Y., Abdullah, A.S., et al. (2010). Smoking-cessation and adherence intervention among Chinese patients with erectile dysfunction. *American Journal of Preventive Medicine*, 39, 251–8.

Chan, S.S., Leung, D.Y., Abdullah, A.S., Wong, V.T., Hedley, A.J., and Lam, T.H. (2011). A randomized controlled trial of a smoking reduction plus nicotine replacement therapy intervention for smokers not willing to quit smoking. *Addiction*, 106, 1155–63.

Chapman, S. and MacKenzie, R. (2010). The global research neglect of unassisted smoking cessation: causes and consequences. *PLoS Medicine*, 7, e1000216.

Chinese Center for Diseases Control and Prevention (2012). *Global Adult Tobacco Survey (GATS): China 2010 Country Report*. Beijing: Chinese Center for Diseases Control and Prevention.

Cochrane Review Groups (n.d.). *Cochrane Tobacco Addiction Group*. Available at: http://onlinelibrary.wiley.com/o/cochrane/clabout/articles/TOBACCO/frame.html.

Cooper, J., Borland, R., Yong, H.H., et al. (2010). To what extent do smokers make spontaneous quit attempts and what are the implications for smoking cessation maintenance? Findings from the International Tobacco Control Four Country Survey. *Nicotine & Tobacco Research*, 12, S51–7.

Cornuz, J. and Willi, C. (2008). Nonpharmacological smoking cessation interventions in clinical practice. *European Respiratory Review*, 17, 187–91.

Doll, R., Peto, R., Boreham, J., and Sutherland, I. (2004). Mortality in relation to smoking: 50 years' observations on male British doctors. *British Medical Journal*, 328, 1519.

Doll, R., Peto, R., Wheatley, K., Gray, R., and Sutherland, I. (1994). Mortality in relation to smoking: 40 years' observations on male British doctors. *British Medical Journal*, 309, 901–11.

Elliott, P., Chambers, J.C., Zhang, W., et al. (2009). Genetic loci associated with C-reactive protein levels and risk of coronary heart disease. *Journal of the American Medical Association*, 302, 37–48.

Eriksen, M., Mackay, J., and Ross, H. (2012). *Tobacco Atlas* (4th ed.). Atlanta, GA: American Cancer Society; New York: World Lung Foundation. Available at: http://www.TobaccoAtlas.org.

Foulds, J. and Branstetter, S. (2012). Tobacco harm reduction. In D. Riley and R. Pates (eds.) *Drugs and Harm Reduction*, pp. 213–28. West Sussex: Wiley-Blackwell Publisher.

Framework Convention Alliance (n.d.). Website. [Online] Available at: http://www.fctc.org.

Gallus, S., Schiaffino, A., La Vecchia, C., Townsend, J., and Fernandez, E. (2006). Price and cigarette consumption in Europe. *Tobacco Control*, 15, 114–9.

Gellert, C., Schottker, B., and Brenner, H. (2012). Smoking and all-cause mortality in older people: systematic review and meta-analysis. *Archives of Internal Medicine*, 172, 837–44.

Glasgow, R.E., Cummings, K.M., and Hyland, A. (1997). Relationship of worksite smoking policy to changes in employee tobacco use: findings from COMMIT. Community Intervention Trial for Smoking Cessation. *Tobacco Control*, 6(Suppl. 2), S44–8.

Gruber, J. (2001). Tobacco at the crossroads: the past and future of smoking regulation in the United States. *The Journal of Economic Perspectives*, 15, 193–212.

Harte, C.B. and Meston, C.M. (2012). Recreational use of erectile dysfunction medications and its adverse effects on erectile function in young healthy men: the mediating role of confidence in erectile ability. *Journal of Sexual Medicine*, 9, 1852–9.

He, J., Reynolds, K., Chen, J., et al. (2007). Cigarette smoking and erectile dysfunction among Chinese men without clinical vascular disease. *American Journal of Epidemiology*, 166, 803–9.

He, Y., Jiang, B., Li, L.S., et al. (2012). Secondhand smoke exposure predicted chronic obstructive pulmonary disease and other tobacco related mortality in a 17-years cohort study in China. *Chest*, 142(4), 909–18.

Heatherton, T.F., Kozlowski, L.T., Frecker, R.C., and Fagerstrom, K.O. (1991). The Fagerstrom Test for Nicotine Dependence: a revision of the

Fagerstrom Tolerance Questionnaire. *British Journal of Addiction*, 86, 1119–27.

Hedley, A.J., Mcghee, S.M., Repace, J.L., et al. (2006). Risks for heart disease and lung cancer from passive smoking by workers in the catering industry. *Toxicological Sciences*, 90, 539–48.

Hirayama, T. (1981). Non-smoking wives of heavy smokers have a higher risk of lung cancer: a study from Japan. *British Medical Journal (Clinical Research Ed.)*, 282, 183–5.

Ho, S.Y., Wang, M.P., Lo, W.S., et al. (2010). Comprehensive smoke-free legislation and displacement of smoking into the homes of young children in Hong Kong. *Tobacco Control*, 19, 129–33.

Howell, F. and HSE Social Marketing Working Group On Tobacco (2012). 1 in every 2 smokers will die of a tobacco related disease: can you live with that? In *15th World Conference on Tobacco or Health*, Singapore.

International Agency for Research on Cancer (2007). *Tobacco Control: Reversal of Risk after Quitting Smoking*. IARC Handbooks of Cancer Prevention, Volume 11. Lyon: IARC.

International Agency for Research on Cancer (2009). *Evaluating the Effectiveness of Smoke-free Policies*. Lyon: IARC. Available at: http://www.iarc.fr/en/publications/pdfs-online/prev/handbook13/handbook13.pdf.

International Agency for Research on Cancer (2012). *A Review of Human Carcinogens. Part E: Personal Habits and Indoor Combustions*. IARC Monographs on the Evaluation of Carcinogenic Risks to Humans. Volume 100E. A Review of Human Carcinogens. Lyon: IARC. Available at: http://monographs.iarc.fr/ENG/Monographs/vol100E/mono100E.pdf.

International Tobacco Control Policy Evaluation Project (n.d.). *About ITC*. [Online] Available at: http://www.itcproject.org/about.

Jha, P., Ramasundarahettige, C., Landsman, V., et al. (2013). 21st-century hazards of smoking and benefits of cessation in the United States. *The New England Journal of Medicine*, 368, 341–50.

Jones, J.M. (2006). *Smoking Habits Stable; Most Would Like to Quit*. [Online] Available at: http://www.gallup.com/poll/23791/Smoking-Habits-Stable-Most-Would-Like-Quit.aspx.

Kupelian, V., Link, C.L., and McKinlay, J.B. (2007). Association between smoking, passive smoking, and erectile dysfunction: results from the Boston Area Community Health (BACH) Survey. *European Urology*, 52, 416–22.

Lai, H.K., Ho, S.Y., Wang, M.P., and Lam, T.H. (2009). Secondhand smoke and respiratory symptoms among adolescent current smokers. *Pediatrics*, 124, 1306–10.

Lai, V.W. (2012). Stages of the cigarette epidemic on entering its second century. Invited commentary. *Tobacco Control*, 21, 101–2.

Lam, T.H. (2012). Absolute risk of tobacco deaths: one in two smokers will be killed by smoking: comment on 'Smoking and all-cause mortality in older people'. *Archives of Internal Medicine*, 172, 845–6.

Lam, T.H. (2013). Conversation with Judith Mackay. *Addiction*, 108, 1897–904.

Lam, T.H., Abdullah, A.S., Ho, L.M., Yip, A.W., and Fan, S. (2006). Smoking and sexual dysfunction in Chinese males: findings from men's health survey. *International Journal of Impotence Research*, 18, 364–9.

Lam, T.H., Chan, S.S., Abdullah, A.S., Wong, V.T., Chan, A.Y., and Hedley, A.J. (2012). Smoking reduction intervention for smokers not willing to quit smoking: a randomised controlled trial. *Hong Kong Medical Journal*, 18(Suppl. 3), 4–8.

Lam, T.H. and Chim, D. (2010). Controlling alcohol-related global health problems. *Asia-Pacific Journal of Public Health*, 22, 203–8S.

Lam, T.H., He, Y., Li, L.S., He, S.F., and Liang, B.Q. (1997). Mortality attributable to cigarette smoking in China. *Journal of the American Medical Association*, 278, 1505–8.

Lam, T.H., Ho, L.M., Hedley, A.J., et al. (2005). Secondhand smoke and respiratory ill health in current smokers. *Tobacco Control*, 14, 307–14.

Lam, T.H., Jiang, C., Chan, Y.F., and Chan, S.S. (2011). Smoking cessation intervention practices in Chinese physicians: do gender and smoking status matter? *Health and Social Care in the Community*, 19, 126–37.

Leischow, S.J., Ayo-Yusuf, O., and Backinger, C.L. (2012). Converging research needs across framework convention on tobacco control articles: making research relevant to global tobacco control practice and policy. *Nicotine & Tobacco Research*, 15(4), 761–6.

Leung, C.C., Lam, T.H., Ho, K.S., et al. (2010). Passive smoking and tuberculosis. *Archives of Internal Medicine*, 170, 287–92.

Lin, H.H., Ezzati, M., and Murray, M. (2007). Tobacco smoke, indoor air pollution and tuberculosis: a systematic review and meta-analysis. *PLoS Medicne*, 4, e20.

Lin, P.R., Zhao, Z.W., Cheng, K.K., and Lam, T.H. (2013). The effect of physician's 30 s smoking cessation intervention for male medical outpatients: a pilot randomized controlled trial. *Journal of Public Health*, 35, 375–83.

Lopez, A.D., Collishaw, N.E., and Piha, T. (1994). A descriptive model of the cigarette epidemic in developed countries. *Tobacco Control*, 3, 242–7.

Mackay, J. (2013). The role of research on the development and implementation of policy. *Nicotine & Tobacco Research*, 15(4), 757–60.

Mackay, J., Eriksen, M., and Shafey, O. (2006). *Tobacco Atlas* (2nd ed.). New York: American Cancer Society.

Matt, G.E., Quintana, P.J., Destaillats, H., et al. (2011). Thirdhand tobacco smoke: emerging evidence and arguments for a multidisciplinary research agenda. *Environmental Health Perspectives*, 119, 1218–26.

McBride, C.M. and Ostroff, J.S. (2003). Teachable moments for promoting smoking cessation: the context of cancer care and survivorship. *Cancer Control*, 10, 325–33.

McGhee, S.M., Ho, S.Y., Schooling, M., et al. (2005). Mortality associated with passive smoking in Hong Kong. *British Medical Journal*, 330, 287–8.

McRobbie, H., Bullen, C., Glover, M., et al. (2008). New Zealand smoking cessation guidelines. *New Zealand Medical Journal*, 121, 57–70.

Mialon, A., Berchtold, A., Michaud, P.A., Gmel, G., and Suris, J.C. (2012). Sexual dysfunctions among young men: prevalence and associated factors. *Journal of Adolescent Health*, 51, 25–31.

Millett, C., Wen, L.M., Rissel, C., et al. (2006). Smoking and erectile dysfunction: findings from a representative sample of Australian men. *Tobacco Control*, 15, 136–9.

Monto, A.S. and Ross, H.W. (1978). The Tecumseh study of respiratory illness. X. Relation of acute infections to smoking, lung function and chronic symptoms. *American Journal of Epidemiology*, 107, 57–64.

National Institute for Health and Care Excellence (2013). *Tobacco: Harm-Reduction Approaches to Smoking*. NICE. Available at: http://www.nice.org.uk/nicemedia/live/14178/63996/63996.pdf.

Oberg, M., Jaakkola, M.S., Woodward, A., Peruga, A., and Pruss-Ustun, A. (2011). Worldwide burden of disease from exposure to second-hand smoke: a retrospective analysis of data from 192 countries. *The Lancet*, 377, 139–46.

Oono, I.P., MacKay, D.F., and Pell, J.P. (2011). Meta-analysis of the association between secondhand smoke exposure and stroke. *Journal of Public Health*, 33, 496–502.

Parsons, A., Daley, A., Begh, R., and Aveyard, P. (2010). Influence of smoking cessation after diagnosis of early stage lung cancer on prognosis: systematic review of observational studies with meta-analysis. *British Medical Journal*, 340, b5569.

Peto, R. (1994). Smoking and death: the past 40 years and the next 40. *British Medical Journal*, 309, 937–9.

Physicians for a Smoke-Free Canada (n.d.). *Picture Based Cigarette Warnings*. [Online] Available at: http://www.smoke-free.ca/warnings.

Pirie, K., Beral, V., Peto, R., Roddam, A., Reeves, G., and Green, J. (2008). Passive smoking and breast cancer in never smokers: prospective study and meta-analysis. *International Journal of Epidemiology*, 37, 1069–79.

Pirie, K., Peto, R., Reeves, G.K., Green, J., Beral, V., and Million Women Study Collaborators (2013). The 21st century hazards of smoking and benefits of stopping: a prospective study of one million women in the UK. *The Lancet*, 381, 133–41.

Rodgman, A. and Perfetti, T.A. (2009). *The Chemical Components of Tobacco and Tobacco Smoke*. Boca Raton, FL: CRC Press.

Russell, M.A. (1979). Tobacco dependence: is nicotine rewarding or aversive? *NIDA Research Monograph*, 100–22.

Secretan, B., Straif, K., Baan, R., et al. (2009). A review of human carcinogens—Part E: tobacco, areca nut, alcohol, coal smoke, and salted fish. *Lancet Oncology*, 10, 1033–4.

Shafey, O., Eriksen, M., Ross, H., and MacKay, J. (2009). *Tobacco Atlas* (3rd ed.). Atlanta, GA: American Cancer Society.

Slama, K., Chiang, C.Y., Enarson, D.A., et al. (2007). Tobacco and tuberculosis: a qualitative systematic review and meta-analysis. *International Journal of Tuberculosis and Lung Disease*, 11, 1049–61.

Smokefree New Zealand 2025 (n.d.) *SMOKEFREE 2025*. [Online] Available at: http://smokefree.org.nz/smokefree-2025.

Thun, M., Peto, R., Boreham, J., and Lopez, A.D. (2012). Stages of the cigarette epidemic on entering its second century. *Tobacco Control*, 21, 96–101.

Thun, M.J., Carter, B.D., Feskanich, D., et al. (2013). 50-year trends in smoking-related mortality in the United States. *The New England Journal of Medicine*, 368, 351–64.

Tobacco Labelling Resource Centre (n.d.) *Health Warnings*. [Online] Available at: http://www.tobaccolabels.ca/healthwarningsinfo.

Trichopoulos, D., Kalandidi, A., Sparros, L., and MacMahon, B. (1981). Lung cancer and passive smoking. *International Journal of Cancer*, 27, 1–4.

United Nations (2011). *Resolution 66/2. Political Declaration of the High-level Meeting of the General Assembly on the Prevention and Control of Non-communicable Diseases*. New York: United Nations. Available at: http://www.who.int/nmh/events/un_ncd_summit2011/political_declaration_en.pdf.

US Department of Health and Human Services (1990). *The Health Benefits of Smoking Cessation: A Report of the Surgeon General*. Available at: http://www.surgeongeneral.gov/library/reports/.

US Department of Health and Human Services (2004). *The Health Consequences of Smoking: A Report of the Surgeon General*. Available at: http://www.cdc.gov/tobacco/data_statistics/sgr/2004/complete_report/index.htm.

US Department of Health and Human Services (2006). *The Health Consequences of Involuntary Exposure to Tobacco Smoke: A Report of the Surgeon General*. Available at: http://www.surgeongeneral.gov/library/reports/secondhandsmoke/index.html.

US Department of Health and Human Services (2012). *Ending the Tobacco Epidemic: Progress Toward a Healthier Nation*. Washington, DC: US Department of Health and Human Services.

Warren, C.W., Asma, S., Lee, J., Lea, V., and Mackay, J. (2009a). *Global Tobacco Surveillance System: The GTSS Atlas*. Atlanta, GA: CDC Foundation. Available at: http://www.cdc.gov/tobacco/global/gtss/tobacco_atlas/.

Warren, C.W., Lee, J., Lea, V., et al. (2009b). Evolution of the Global Tobacco Surveillance System (GTSS) 1998–2008. *Global Health Promotion*, 16, 4–37.

West, R., Mcneill, A., Britton, J., et al. (2010). Should smokers be offered assistance with stopping? *Addiction*, 105, 1867–9.

Winickoff, J.P., Friebely, J., Tanski, S.E., et al. (2009). Beliefs about the health effects of 'thirdhand' smoke and home smoking bans. *Pediatrics*, 123, e74–9.

World Bank (1999). *Curbing the Epidemic—Governments and the Economics of Tobacco Control*. Washington, DC: World Bank. Available at: http://documents.worldbank.org/curated/en/1999/05/437174/curbing-epidemic-governments-economics-tobacco-control.

World Health Organization (2003). *WHO Framework Convention on Tobacco Control*. Geneva: WHO. Available at: http://www.who.int/tobacco/framework/WHO_FCTC_english.pdf.

World Health Organization (2008). *WHO Report on the Global Tobacco Epidemic, 2008: The MPOWER Package*. Geneva: WHO. Available at: http://www.who.int/tobacco/mpower/mpower_report_full_2008.pdf.

World Health Organization (2010). Opening remarks on the fifth anniversary of the WHO Framework Convention on Tobacco Control. *In Convention on Tobacco Control: A Triumph for Public Health*. Geneva, Switzerland, 26 February 2010.

World Health Organization (2011). *Developing and Improving National Toll-Free Tobacco Quit Line Services. A World Health Organization Manual*. Geneva: WHO. Available at: http://www.who.int/tobacco/publications/smoking_cessation/quit_lines_services/en/index.html.

World Health Organization (2012a). *Status of the WHO Framework Convention on Tobacco Control (FCTC)*. [Online] Available at: http://www.fctc.org/images/stories/FCTC_ratification_latest_010612.pdf.

World Health Organization (2012b). *A Comprehensive Global Monitoring Framework, Including Indicators, and a Set of Voluntary Global Targets for the Prevention and Control of Noncommunicabale Diseases*. [Online] Available at: http://www.who.int/nmh/events/2012/discussion_paper3.pdf.

World Health Organization (2012c). *Development of an Updated Action Plan for the Global Strategy for the Prevention and Control of Noncommunicable Diseases*. [Online] Available at: http://www.who.int/nmh/events/2012/action_plan_20120726.pdf.

World Health Organization (2013a). *WHO Report on the Global Tobacco Epidemic. Enforcing Bans on Tobacco Advertising, Promotion and Sponsorship*. [Online] Available at: http://www.who.int/tobacco/global_report/2013/en/.

World Health Organization (2013b). *Tobacco Industry and Corporate Responsibility*. Geneva: WHO. Available at: http://www.who.int/tobacco/publications/industry/CSR_report.pdf.

World Health Organization (n.d.) *Tobacco Free Initiative (TFI): WHO FCTC Health Warnings Database*. [Online] Available at: http://www.who.int/tobacco/healthwarningsdatabase/en/index.html.

World Health Organization and International Union Against Tuberculosis And Lung Disease (2011). *Tobacco Advertising, Promotion and Sponsorship: Enforcing Comprehensive Bans*. Geneva: WHO. Available at: http://www.who.int/tobacco/publications/building_capacity/training_package/adv_promotion_sponsorship.

World Health Organization Framework Convention on Tobacco Research (2012). *Conference of the Parties to the WHO Framework Convention on Tobacco Control*. Fifth session. Seoul, Republic of Korea, 12–17 November 2012. Available at: http://apps.who.int/gb/fctc/PDF/cop5/FCTC_COP5(1)-en.pdf.

Yin, P., Jiang, C.Q., Cheng, K.K., et al. (2007). Passive smoking exposure and risk of COPD among adults in China: the Guangzhou Biobank Cohort Study. *The Lancet*, 370, 751–7.

Yuan, J.M., Ross, R.K., Wang, X.L., Gao, Y.T., Henderson, B.E., and Yu, M.C. (1996). Morbidity and mortality in relation to cigarette smoking in Shanghai, China. A prospective male cohort study. *Journal of the American Medical Association*, 275, 1646–50.

Public health aspects of illicit psychoactive drug use

Don Des Jarlais, Jonathan Feelemyer, and Deborah Hassin

Illicit psychoactive drug use and public health: an introduction

The misuse of psychoactive drugs is a major public health problem in many countries throughout the world. Nicotine (in the form of tobacco products) and alcohol are the most commonly used and misused psychoactive drugs, and account for the greatest mortality and morbidity related to psychoactive drug use. Since nicotine and alcohol are discussed in Chapters 9.1 and 9.3, this chapter focuses on illicit psychoactive drugs, in particular opiates such as heroin, cocaine, and amphetamine-type stimulants (ATS), which cause major public health problems even if they are not of the magnitude of the problems caused by nicotine and alcohol.

The United Nations Office on Drugs and Crime (UNODC) compiles annual estimates of the prevalence of the use of various illicit psychoactive drugs (UNODC 2012) and assesses trends over time. In the most recent *World Drug Report* published in 2012, the UNODC estimated that in 2010, between 3.4 and 6.6 per cent of the adult population (persons aged 15–64) used an illicit drug in the previous year. Of these, some 10–13 per cent of drug users were considered to be problem users with drug dependence and/or drug-use disorders.

With respect to the use of specific illicit drugs, the UNODC (2012) estimated that cannabis was by far the most commonly used drug, with 2.6–6.0 per cent of adults (120–420 million adults) having used it in the previous year, followed by opioids, cocaine, and ATS that were each used by approximately 0.5 per cent of adults (35 million). These estimates have been relatively stable over the previous 5 years.

The Global Burden of Disease project recently estimated the numbers of deaths and of disability-adjusted life years (DALYs) lost attributable to illicit drug use for 1990 and 2010. Attributable deaths increased from 68,577 in 1990 to 157,805 in 2010 (Lim et al. 2012). DALYs also increased substantially during the same period, from 15,171,000 to 23,810,000. Men suffered much greater effects than women; in 2010, there were 109,420 deaths attributable to drug use among men and 48,365 deaths among women.

Deaths and DALYs attributable to drug use were quite modest compared to deaths and DALYs attributable to tobacco smoking and alcohol use. For the 2010 analysis, there were 5,695,349 deaths attributable to tobacco smoking and 4,860,168 deaths attributable to alcohol use. Similar to the effects of drug use, the effects of tobacco smoking and alcohol use were much greater among men than women.

Despite the modest numbers of adults who use illicit drugs, they generate many costs to society, including lost productivity, increased disability and deaths, disruption of family and other social relationships, and costs of increased law enforcement and incarceration. This chapter will focus on health-related aspects of illicit drug use. Approximately 0.5–1.3 per cent of all deaths among adults in the world are related to illicit drug use and 4 per cent of adult deaths in Europe (European Monitoring Centre for Drugs and Drug Addiction 2011; UNODC 2012).

Basic biological and psychological research over the last two decades has led to a greatly increased understanding of the mechanisms of drug use. A review of this research is beyond the scope of this chapter, but it may help to state a few general summary statements as a background: (1) there is great individual variation in reactions to different drugs; (2) repeated drug use does lead to observable changes in brain systems, particularly in those systems related to reward or reinforcement of behaviours; (3) the major problem in treating substance use disorders (SUDs) is not the initial ceasing to use drugs, but avoiding relapse back to use; (4) while it is not yet appropriate to think in terms of a 'cure' for SUDs, there are effective treatments to manage the condition; (5) there are very important differences in the effects of different drugs but also very important similarities in the compulsive use of different drugs; and (6) increased knowledge of the effects of various drugs has uncovered great complexity rather than uncovering any simple methods for ameliorating the harmful effects of drugs on the brain and behaviour. Thus, while knowledge of drug effects and their mechanisms is likely to continue to increase rapidly, it is unrealistic to expect that there will be any 'magic bullet' breakthroughs for either the prevention or treatment of SUDs in the near future.

Current global patterns in drug use

Geography is not necessarily destiny with respect to what drugs a person might use, but there are strong geographical patterns in the use of different drugs. The information on geographic differences in use of specific drugs that follows is summarized from the

World Drug Report (UNODC 2012). The *World Drug Report* is based on reports from various participating countries, so that the data can vary in quality and should be interpreted as estimates. Law enforcement information, particularly on seizures of drugs, is also used in assessing trends in international drug use. However, the *World Drug Report* is the best available information on the trends in the global use of different illicit drugs.

Cannabis

Cannabis is the most prevalent of illicit substances used globally; it is estimated that there are between 120 and 224 million users of cannabis worldwide. Cannabis cultivation has increased in recent years, although many of the increases are small-scale growing operations. While the cannabis herb is prevalent in most countries, cannabis resin, or 'hashish', is more heavily utilized in locations including Afghanistan, the Middle East, and small pockets of Western Europe and northern Africa. The highest level of cannabis use is reported in Australia and Oceania, with annual prevalence of use among adults of 9.1–14.6 per cent, followed by North America (10.8 per cent of adults), Western and Central Europe (7 per cent of adults), and West Central Africa (5.2–13.5 per cent of adults). The prevalence of cannabis use in Asia is low (1–3.4 per cent of adults), however given the very large population of the region, it remains the largest population of cannabis users worldwide.

Opioids

Opioid consumption has remained stable recently, with annual prevalence rates ranging from 0.6 per cent to 0.8 per cent among adults. The highest levels of opioid use were in North America (3.8–4.2 per cent of adults), Oceania (2.3–3.4 per cent of adults), and Eastern Europe and South Eastern Europe (1.2–1.3 per cent of adults), all of which reported higher than global average use. It is important to note that prescription opioid users outnumber heroin users in North America and Australia while in Eastern Europe and South Eastern Europe heroin is the main opioid of use. Increase in heroin use was observed in 2010 in South Asia and South East Asia as well as several African countries, while in Europe, synthetic opioids including fentanyl and buprenorphine have replaced much of the heroin use in countries such as Estonia and Finland. In Russia, as a result of a recent shortage in heroin, increases in desomorphine, acetyl opium and fentanyl have been reported.

Cocaine

Prevalence of cocaine consumption among 15–64-year-olds has remained recently relatively stable, ranging from 0.3 per cent to 0.4 per cent. While there have been slight decreases in cocaine consumption in the United States between 2006 and 2010, the same decreases were not observed in Europe, where cocaine use continues to remain stable, and in Australia, where cocaine use has seen a slight increase. Emerging trafficking routes for cocaine, especially in Africa, may have led to a spillover of use in that region.

Cocaine use is most prevalent in North America (1.6 per cent of adults), Western and Central Europe (1.3 per cent of adults), and Oceania (1.5–1.9 per cent of adults). There were decreases noted between 2009 and 2010 in North America (1.9–1.6 per cent of adults) and South America (0.9–0.7 per cent of adults), while

increases were noted in Oceania (1.4–1.7 per cent to 1.5–1.9 per cent of adults), reflecting increases in Australia specifically. While limited data exist in Africa and parts of Asia, there are indications that there is an increasing and emerging use of cocaine in those regions; this may reflect the increased trafficking of cocaine through these areas.

Amphetamine-type stimulants

The illicit use of ATS, which includes methamphetamine, ecstasy, and amphetamine, is more difficult to measure globally due to the small-scale operations that are used to produce these illicit drugs, but has been estimated to be between 0.3 and 1.2 per cent of the global population. Based on seizures of amphetamine, use has decreased in recent years and has been surpassed by methamphetamine use. Seizures of ecstasy have increased in recent years, especially in the European market, doubling from 2009 to 2010; the availability of this drug has also increased in other regions including the United States, South East Asia, and Oceania. New trade routes that often are used for cocaine trafficking are increasingly being used for ATS trafficking, with evidence of spillover into West Africa.

ATS (excluding ecstasy) is most prevalent in Oceania, North America, and Central America, while there is evidence of increasing use in Asia, especially with the increased seizure of methamphetamine in the region. Ecstasy use globally is comparable to prevalence rates of cocaine use (0.2–0.6 per cent of the population aged 15–64), but higher rates were observed in regions including Oceania (2.9 per cent of population aged 15–64), North America (0.9 per cent of population aged 15–64), and Western and Central Europe (0.8 per cent of population aged 15–64). Ecstasy in particular tends to be much more prevalent in young people; of the estimated 2.6 million users in 2010 in the United States, 2.5 million were between the ages of 15 and 34, while in Europe, of the estimated 2.5 million users in 2010, 2 million were between 15 and 34 years of age. As a whole, this group of drugs remains the second most used drug globally (behind cannabis).

Historical interpretation and implications for public health

Even with the imprecision in the global data, there are identifiable patterns in drug use in different regions of the world. Some of these patterns reflect cultural differences, as the illicit use of different drugs has been incorporated to varying degrees into different cultures and different national societies. The primary factor in the geographical distribution of the use of different drugs, however, involves production, distribution networks and markets. Various drugs are produced in specific geographic areas and then transported through complex networks to established markets. Once production has become established in a geographic area and once a market for a drug has been established in an area, it is very difficult to fundamentally change these factors. The reinforcing nature of drug use leads many persons to continue using drugs and often paying very high prices for the drugs. (At least very high prices compared to the costs of producing the drugs.) Once production capabilities have become established in a geographic area, it can be quite difficult to dislodge them. The production usually becomes integrated into the local culture, including corruption of local authorities.

This is not to say that drug production areas, distribution routes, and drug markets cannot change. Two types of changes are of particular relevance to public health. First, over the last several decades globalization has transformed the illicit drug business just as it has transformed licit businesses. The improvements and cost reductions in communication, transportation, and the ability to transfer capital, have greatly increased the diffusion of illicit drug use to many new countries.

Second, while law enforcement efforts have generally not been able to stop international drug distribution, law enforcement efforts have led to rerouting of distribution routes. As a result local drug markets and drug problems typically develop along the new distribution routes. For example, new routes and new drug problems have developed most recently in Africa (UNODC 2012).

The implications of these changes in drug production, distribution, and marketing for public health are both clear and of considerable concern. Illicit drug use is likely to continue in areas where it is currently established and is likely to diffuse to new areas. Public health officials need to plan for continued—and perhaps increased—use of illicit drugs and implement programmes to reduce the health and social problems associated with illicit drug use.

Epidemiological methods for studying illicit drug use

As illicit drug use is, by definition, illegal there are many difficulties in collecting rigorous data on the topic. The difficulties include: (1) social desirability responding (Pauls and Stemmler 2003) in which persons who use drugs may deny (or minimize) their drug use in order to present a desirable image to the researchers and/or to themselves; (2) locating subjects, as many persons who use drugs at high levels may be homeless or unstably housed; and (3) the effects of drugs on memory (though greatest memory problems may be associated with alcohol use). Various techniques have been developed to reduce these problems including: (1) audio-computer assisted self-interviewing (ACASI) (Des Jarlais et al. 1999), in which questionnaires are programmed into computers so that the research subject listens to the questions over headphones and responds to the questions using either the keyboard or a touch screen. ASCSI does not require the subjects to be literate and the questions can be presented identically to all subjects; (2) respondent-driven sampling (Heckathorn 1997), in which subjects are reimbursed for recruiting other subjects. Restrictions are placed on the numbers of subjects that any individual subject can recruit, and additional data is collected in order to increase generalizability to the underlying population; and (3) timeline follow back (Sobell and Sobell 1992), a method in which major events in a subject's life are used to anchor to the recall of events over long time periods.

There are several major methods for studying the epidemiology of illicit drug use. These include household surveys of the general population, school surveys of drug abuse among young adults, administrative data from the Treatment Episode Data Set, and special studies aimed at examining drug use among particular groups, such as those who use drugs at high frequencies.

Household surveys of the general population

Surveys of random samples of household members provide what is usually considered to be the best estimates of the use of different drugs in a country. Such surveys are quite expensive but provide data that cannot be obtained through any other method. The US National Survey of Drug Use and Health (Substance Abuse & Mental Health Services Administration 2012) is conducted annually with a sample of over 67,500 respondents age 12 years or older. The findings from the most recent year (2011) indicate that 9.4 per cent reported any illicit drug use in the previous year, and 8.7 per cent reported illicit drug use in the previous month. The most commonly used illicit drug was marijuana, with psychotherapeutics the second most commonly used illicit drug. Additionally, there were an estimated 1.9 million people with non-medical use of pain relievers in 2011; this figure remained unchanged from 2010.

School surveys

Surveys can also be conducted in schools. School-age youth are of particular interest because illicit drug use typically begins during adolescence, and trends in the use of different drugs are often much more pronounced in this age group. Thus, school surveys may be particularly useful for generating predictions about future drug use. 'Monitoring the Future' is the largest and longest running school survey in the United States (Johnston et al. 2011). In the 2011 survey, of the 46,700 students who were interviewed, 34.7 per cent of US high school students reported using illicit drugs in the previous year, with marijuana, used by 31 per cent, being the most commonly used illicit drug and inhalants being the second most commonly used illicit drug.

Administrative data

Persons with SUDs frequently come into contact with both law enforcement and health agencies. They may be arrested for possession of drugs and/or they may seek treatment for both their substance abuse disorder and for related health problems, such as overdose and infections. According to the Treatment Episode Data Set (TEDS) (Department of Health and Human Services 2008), there were 1.8 million admissions to licensed drug and alcohol treatment programmes in 2007, a slight decrease from the nearly 1.9 million admissions in 2006. Among those seeking treatment, five substances accounted for 96 per cent of TEDS admissions: alcohol (40 per cent), opiates (19 per cent, primarily heroin), marijuana/hashish (16 per cent), cocaine (13 per cent), and stimulants (8 per cent, primarily methamphetamine). The number of admissions for these five illicit substances decreased slightly from 2006 to 2007.

Special studies

While surveys can provide data about the breadth of drug use in the general and school populations, and administrative data can provide useful information about problems associated with illicit drug use, these types of studies do not provide the depth of information needed to understand the problems associated with specific forms of illicit drug use. Special studies usually recruit persons who use drugs at high frequencies. Injecting drug users with or at risk for HIV infection are an example. Special studies may also recruit subjects from clinical (drug treatment programme) settings from the community. They may be cross-sectional (one-time data collection) or cohort studies (with the same subjects followed over time).

Public health consequences of drug use

There are many different adverse consequences of drug use, both for individuals, their families, and for society as a whole. These include the disruption of psychological and social functioning due to drug use itself, the spread of infectious diseases associated with drug use, particularly injecting drug use, and drug-induced fatal overdoses.

Dependence/addiction/disorder

Differentiation between substance use and substance use disorders

In theory, individuals can use psychoactive substances without experiencing problems, symptoms, or impairments from the substances. In the case of alcohol, light or moderate use is associated with a number of health benefits (e.g. decreased cardiovascular mortality) compared to abstainers, in what has been called the 'J-shaped curve' (Costanzo et al. 2010). However, progression from non-problem to problem use appears to be much more likely for illegal psychoactive substances, particularly cocaine and opioids (Lev-Ran et al. 2013). Clinical and research experts distinguish between substance use and problem SUDs through the diagnostic criteria for SUDs. These are most often assessed through the criteria provided to the mental health and substance abuse fields in the *Diagnostic and Statistical Manual of Mental Disorders* (DSM) of the American Psychiatric Association. The first two editions of the DSM did not include specific criteria, but based on research conducted in the 1970s, such criteria were first presented in the third edition, DSM-III (American Psychiatric Association 1980), in 1980. The criteria for SUDs have undergone considerable evolution since this first presentation.

DSM-III

DSM-III was the first to divide SUDs into abuse and dependence. Abuse (pathological use, consequences, e.g. impaired functioning) was considered to be the milder condition (Rounsaville et al. 1986), while dependence, characterized by physiological components (i.e. tolerance and/or withdrawal), was assumed to be more severe. However, a rationale for the actual selection and organization of the criteria was never published. The approach was criticized and a better approach sought (Rounsaville et al. 1986).

The Dependence Syndrome

Developed separately from DSM-III, the 'Dependence Syndrome' (Edwards and Gross 1976; Edwards et al. 1981) posited a 'bi-axial' SUD concept (Edwards and Gross 1976; Edwards et al. 1981): (1) broader *dependence* concept (inability to control use, indicated by tolerance, withdrawal, other criteria), and (2) *consequences* of use (social, legal, medical).

DSM-III-R, ICD-10, and DSM-IV

The Dependence Syndrome was the basis of the definition of dependence in DSM-III-R (Rounsaville et al. 1986), published in 1987, the 10th edition of the International Classification of Diseases (ICD-10) published in 1992, and DSM-IV, published in 1994. Initially, only dependence was proposed for DSM-III-R (Rounsaville et al. 1986), but concerns that lack of a secondary diagnosis would leave individuals without treatment led to the addition of abuse (Hasin et al. 2013). The initial presentation of the Dependence Syndrome included an assumption that dependence and its consequences were related, but DSM-III-R and DSM-IV defined abuse hierarchically to dependence, that is, abuse was not to be diagnosed if dependence was present (Hasin et al. 2006a).

DSM-IV dependence: valid, reliable

The seven criteria for DSM-IV dependence include: (1) withdrawal, (2) tolerance, (3) using in larger amounts or for longer periods than intended, (4) repeated efforts to stop or control use, (5) much time spent using, (6) physical or psychological problems related to use, and (7) important activities given up in order to use. DSM-IV dependence is diagnosed if at least three criteria are present within a 12-month period. A review (Hasin et al. 2006a) from one of the NIH planning conferences showed that DSM-IV substance dependence, diagnosed with three or more criteria, was highly reliable in a number of test–retest studies in varied populations, as were continuous measures of the dependence criteria. DSM-IV dependence also showed strong validity in cross-sectional and prospective US and international studies. Consequently, dependence has been the diagnosis routinely used as an inclusion criterion in trials of pharmacological interventions, is often studied in controlled experiments oriented to treatment development, and is a common phenotype in molecular genetic studies.

DSM-IV abuse: a category with many problems

The four criteria for DSM-IV abuse include: (1) hazardous use, (2) social or interpersonal problems related to use, (3) neglect of major roles in order to use, and (4) legal problems related to use. DSM-IV abuse is diagnosed only in the absence of dependence. Abuse is diagnosed if one or more of the criteria are present. A number of problems were identified with DSM-IV *abuse* and its hierarchical relationship to dependence. (1) *Lack of a justifiable concept.* Abuse diagnosed with one criterion may be normative in some groups, for example, driving after drinking. While this is risky behaviour, it is arguably not sufficient grounds for a psychiatric diagnosis. (2) *Inconsistent reliability.* The test–retest reliability of abuse is often much lower than dependence (Hasin et al. 2006a). (3) *Validity of assumptions about abuse and dependence.* Researchers and clinicians alike have assumed that abuse is the mild diagnosis and dependence is more severe. This has led to several incorrect assumptions about their relationship that are not supported by empirical findings. For example, abuse is not necessarily a prodromal stage of dependence (Hasin et al. 1990, 1997; Schuckit et al. 2000; Grant et al. 2001; Schuckit and Smith 2001). In addition, not all dependence cases have abuse criteria (Hasin et al. 1990, 1997, 2005; Schuckit et al. 2000; Grant et al. 2001, 2007; Schuckit and Smith 2001; Hasin and Grant 2004). Further (as is apparent on inspection of the face validity of the criteria), the criteria defining abuse are not all mild relative to dependence.

Diagnostic 'orphans'

Undiagnosed 'orphans' with two dependence and no abuse criteria may be more serious than single-criterion abuse cases (Hasin and Paykin 1998; Pollock and Martin 1999).

DSM-5

DSM-5 was published in May 2013. Changes in DSM are intended to implement new knowledge, improve validity, reduce clinician burden, and correct problems identified in previous versions. In 2007, the American Psychiatric Association convened the

Substance Disorders Workgroup to identify DSM-IV strengths and weaknesses and recommend improvements. Correcting problems with DSM-IV abuse was a major issue faced by the Workgroup (Schuckit and Saunders 2006; Hasin et al. 2013). Other issues included adding or dropping criteria, and setting a diagnostic threshold.

Relationship of DSM-IV abuse and dependence

Factor analyses of dependence and abuse criteria showed either a single factor or two factors whose high correlations often led to interpretation that a single dimension was warranted (Hasin et al. 2006a; Hasin et al. 2013). Item response theory (IRT) was a method used by workgroup members and other investigators to provide more information about the relationship of criteria to each other than factor analytic studies. Results from 39 IRT studies with over 200,000 subjects (e.g. Hasin et al. 2013) had two very consistent findings. First, DSM-IV dependence and abuse criteria (except legal problems) were always *unidimensional*, indicating a single condition (Hasin et al. 2013). Second, abuse and dependence criteria were always *intermixed across the severity spectrum* (Hasin et al. 2013), indicating that abuse criteria are not necessarily milder than dependence. These findings supported adding abuse to dependence to create a single DSM-5 SUD, solving some of the problems with abuse.

Specific criteria

The Workgroup focused on legal problems (abuse) and craving. Reasons to drop *legal problems* included low prevalence, little added information, poor discrimination and fit with other criteria (Hasin et al. 2013). In secondary analysis of clinical data (Hasin et al. 2012), no patient 'lost' a diagnosis without this criterion. Addition of *craving* was suggested by behavioural and biological studies (O'Brien et al. 1998; Miller and Goldsmith 2001; Waters et al. 2004; O'Brien 2005; Weiss 2005; Foroud et al. 2007; Heinz et al. 2009). IRT shows that craving is unidimensional with the other criteria, but may be redundant (Mewton et al. 2011; Casey et al. 2012). Results comparing IRT total information curves for SUD criteria with and without craving were inconsistent. Some though not all consider craving to be central to diagnosis and treatment (Hasin et al. 2013).

Workgroup recommendation: DSM-5 SUD

DSM-IV dependence was reliable and valid. An enormous amount of evidence indicated that dependence and three of the abuse criteria were indicators of the same single underlying condition, with available evidence showing that craving also fit within this latent trait. Therefore, the Workgroup recommended adding the abuse criteria and craving to dependence to define a single DSM-5 SUD (Hasin et al. 2013). These recommendations were implemented as the new DSM-5 SUD (Hasin et al. 2013).

Threshold

In inherently dimensional conditions such as SUD, identifying a threshold for multiple purposes (e.g. treatment; research) is challenging (Kendler and Gardner 1998; Hasin et al. 2006b, 2013). In the absence of a strong empirical basis for defining a diagnostic threshold (i.e. minimum number of criteria necessary to make a diagnosis), the Workgroup sought a threshold maximizing agreement with the prevalence and with DSM-IV abuse *or* dependence to avoid unduly affecting prevalence rates. In secondary analyses of existing epidemiological and clinical data (Hasin et al. 2012; Peer et al. 2013), two or more criteria accomplished this (Hasin et al. 2013).

Severity levels

All DSM-5 workgroups were asked to create mild, moderate, and severe severity indicators. The Workgroup preferred a simple unweighted criterion count as evidence-based (Hasin et al. 2006b, 2013; Hasin and Beseler 2009; Beseler and Hasin 2010; Dawson et al. 2010), but busy clinicians find rating dimensions 'burdensome' (Frances 2009). Therefore, the Workgroup defined mild, moderate and severe as two to three, four to five, and six or more SUD criteria, respectively.

Name of the DSM-5 disorder and chapter

Each version of DSM includes a chapter on substance-related conditions that defines not only the disorders just discussed, but also such conditions as substance-specific intoxication and withdrawal syndromes, and substance-related mental disorders (e.g. substance-induced mood disorder). For DSM-5, the Workgroup was asked by the American Psychiatric Association Board of Trustees to accept Gambling Disorder as a related disorder in the chapter. To accommodate this change, a change in the title was necessary. The Board of Trustees assigned the title, 'Substance-Related and Addictive Disorders', despite the DSM-5 SUD Workgroup having previously approved a title (by majority but not consensus) not including the term 'addiction'. This lack of agreement over the title reflects an overall tension in the field over the terms 'addiction' and 'dependence', as seen in editorials (O'Brien et al. 2006; O'Brien 2011) advocating 'addiction' as a general term, reserving 'dependence' specifically for tolerance and/or withdrawal, and the more than 80 comments on these editorials that debated the pros and cons of these terms. Issues with the terms 'dependence' and 'addiction' involve the stigma associated with each, and with assumed confusion on the part of general medical practitioners about whether dependence involves only tolerance and withdrawal, or indicates a wider phenomenon. Resolving these issues empirically appears difficult, and therefore some continued debate appears likely. However, the term 'substance use disorder' avoids this debate and can be used generally.

Future directions

The logic underlying the changes made to DSM-5 SUD was based on extensive evidence that DSM-IV dependence was valid and that the eleven criteria defining DSM-5 SUD were all indicators of the same underlying trait. Therefore, the Workgroup reasoned that the condition defined by the eleven criteria would also be valid. However, collecting and analysing empirical data supporting this reasoning was beyond the mandate of the Workgroup, and beyond the time and resources available for its work. (Similar conditions limited DSM-IV SUD validity studies prior to the publication of DSM-IV in 1994, leaving issues for subsequent research.) The combination of abuse and dependence into a single disorder solves many of the problems that were identified with abuse in DSM-IV. After the publication of DSM-5 in 2013, studies of the antecedent, concurrent, and predictive validity of DSM-5 SUD compared to DSM-IV dependence would provide needed information about additional benefits of the changed criteria for SUDs in DSM-5.

Infectious diseases

Infectious diseases have become one of the most important adverse consequences of illicit drug use. This is particularly true for the injection of illicit drugs, as the multiperson use (sharing) of the needles and syringes for injecting is a relatively efficient method for transmitting blood-borne viruses. Drug use can also affect sexual behaviour—drug users may exchange sex for drugs or money to purchase drugs, sexual decision-making may be impaired under the influence of drugs, and some drugs may increase the perceived pleasure of sex, leading to more frequent or prolonged sexual activities. Thus, drug users often have elevated rates of sexually transmitted infections compared to demographically similar persons who do not use drugs (Zenilman and Shahmanesh 2011). Of course, high rates of drug use can also impair sexual functioning or reduce sexual desire (Smith 2007), leading to lower rates of sexual activity among drug users.

HIV/AIDS

HIV/AIDS has been an extremely dramatic development in the field of psychoactive drug use. The use of psychoactive drugs (both licit and illicit) always carried some risk of death, but HIV/ AIDS increased the risk of death by several orders of magnitude. AIDS was first observed among persons who inject drugs in 1981 (Centers for Disease Control and Prevention 1981), and the development of the HIV antibody test provided good information on the size of the problem, and confirmed that sharing needles and syringes was the dominant mode of HIV transmission among persons who injected drugs (PWID) (see Chapter 8.13).

The initial studies in cities such as New York showed approximately half of the drug injectors in the city were infected with the virus (Des Jarlais et al. 1989). It also rapidly became clear that the virus could be transmitted to newborn children and to non-drug injecting sexual partners (Padian et al. 1987; Barzilai et al. 1990; Morgan et al. 1990; Kane 1991; Moschese et al. 1991). At the time, there was no effective treatment for HIV infection, and AIDS was almost uniformly fatal. AIDS thus suddenly became a severe threat to the lives of very large numbers of PWID, their sexual partners and their newborn children. The emergence of this new threat to the lives of drug users and their communities generated a great deal of public attention. In some areas, such as the Netherlands (Buning et al. 1988), the United Kingdom (Stimson et al. 1988), and Australia (Lowe et al. 1990), this led to rapid pilot testing and implementation of effective programmes for reducing HIV transmission. In other areas, the stigmatization of drug users and the fear of doing anything that might 'condone' or 'encourage' drug use, prevented implementation of effective prevention programmes (Anderson 1991). As noted later, this political will problem continues to this day.

Another disturbing factor that emerged from the early research on HIV among PWID was the potential for extremely rapid transmission of the virus among some groups of drug users. HIV can spread very rapidly among PWID, with increases in HIV prevalence from 10 per cent to 50 per cent per year (Des Jarlais et al. 2012). The city of Bangkok, Thailand, experienced a well-documented example of extremely rapid transmission,

with HIV prevalence increasing by approximately 4 per cent per month during a period in 1989 (Vanichseni and Sakuntanaga 1990). There appear to be several factors that facilitate situations of very rapid transmission (Nyindo 2005), including: (1) the local population of drug injectors is not aware of the threat of HIV/AIDS and thus do not reduce their risk behaviour, (2) effective restrictions on access to sterile needles and syringes, and (3) mechanisms that generate rapid injecting partner change, in which drug users may share needles and syringes with large numbers of other drug users over a short time period. These mechanisms include shooting galleries, where drug users come to rent needles and syringes, return the used equipment to the persons operating the gallery, who then rent the used needle and syringe to other drug users; 'dealer's works', where a person selling drugs may have a needle and syringe to lend to customers, who use and then return the needle and syringe for use by the next customer, 'hit doctors', who for a small fee will inject drug users who have difficulties injecting themselves, and the same needle and syringe may be used for many of the hit doctors' customers; and semi-public injecting sites such as abandoned buildings where large numbers often congregate to inject with a very limited number of needles and syringes. Homeless drug users are particularly likely to use such semi-public injecting sites.

HIV is highly infectious during the acute infection stage (Brenner et al. 2007) so that these mechanisms that generate sharing needles and syringes among large groups of injectors may be a critical component of very rapid transmission of HIV. The mechanisms may also develop rather quickly, with changes in law enforcement activities, drug distribution patterns, the frequencies of drug injection, and the economic circumstances in the local population of PWID. A situation in which HIV does not appear to be a threat among PWID can rapidly change to a situation in which a high seroprevalence epidemic has already occurred.

While there are clear difficulties in monitoring the evolving situation with respect to HIV among PWID, injecting drug use and HIV infection among PWID continues to spread globally. In 2004 there were 130 countries with injecting drug use and 78 countries with HIV among PWID (Aceijas et al. 2004). In 2008 there were 148 countries with injecting drug use and 120 countries with HIV among PWID (Mathers et al. 2008). The study in *The Lancet* (Mathers et al. 2008) shows HIV prevalence in different countries throughout the world. There are five countries where HIV prevalence has exceeded 20 per cent and nine countries where HIV prevalence has exceeded 40 per cent. The same factors that have led to great increases in global trade overall—improvements in transportation, communication, fewer restrictions on the flow of capital—have also led to increased trade in illicit drugs. Given these factors and the tremendous profits to be made in the distribution of illicit drugs, there would not appear to be any immediate likelihood of reducing the illicit supply of psychoactive drugs. We will therefore need to continually address the many health problems associated with the injection of psychoactive drugs.

In stark contrast to the potential for extremely rapid transmission of HIV among PWID discussed earlier, it is also well established that it is possible to avert HIV epidemics among PWID. Large-scale implementation of HIV prevention programmes, particularly needle/syringe access programmes, when HIV prevalence is very low in a population of PWID can keep the prevalence low (under 5 per cent) indefinitely (Des Jarlais et al. 1995;

Stimson 1995; Wodak and Maher 2010; Iverson et al. 2012). It is important to note, however, that there have been instances of outbreaks of HIV when it appeared that HIV was under control in the local PWID population. The most famous of these is probably the Vancouver outbreak (Strathdee et al. 1997), and the most recent outbreak of HIV among PWID that occurred in Greece (Paraskevis et al. 2011).

One important aspect of successful HIV prevention in many countries has been the active involvement of drug users and former drug users themselves (Kerr et al. 2006). They have often served as front line, community outreach prevention workers and have formed user groups and networks to represent their interests in policy decision-making. The contributions of these groups have often been critical for the on-the-ground effectiveness of HIV prevention programmes (Wood et al. 2003).

The above examples of highly successful HIV prevention programming are all from high-income countries. Most—but certainly not all—of current HIV transmission is occurring in low- and middle-income countries (Mathers et al. 2008) and we do not yet have sufficient long-term data from HIV prevention programming in resource-limited settings to draw any firm conclusions with respect to effectiveness. There are multiple reasons for the lack of long-term data on the effectiveness of HIV prevention for PWID in low- and middle-income countries: HIV epidemics among PWID in low- and middle-income countries generally occurred more recently than HIV epidemics among PWID in high-income countries, implementation of HIV prevention in low- and middle-income countries is generally at very low levels (Mathers et al. 2010), and there have often been insufficient resources for conducting long-term outcome studies.

There are several concerns for why prevention programming may not be as effective in low- and middle-income countries as in high-income countries. First, there is the simple scarcity of resources for prevention programmes. Some types of HIV prevention programmes, particularly long-term drug treatment programmes and antiretroviral treatment for HIV, are comparatively expensive, and it may not be possible to provide these on a public health scale in many low- and middle-income countries. This is not simply a matter of financial resources, but also a matter of appropriately trained health workers.

Second, while PWID are stigmatized in almost all countries, the stigmatization may be particularly severe in many low- and middle-income countries. This may lead political leaders to be less willing to allocate resources to HIV prevention and treatment for PWID. In particular, to the extent that injecting drug use is seen as a practice associated with degenerate Western culture, nationalism in low- and middle-income countries may lead political leaders to fail to implement evidence-based HIV prevention programmes for PWID (Rhodes et al. 2003; Cohen 2010). The stigmatization of injecting drugs may compound the stigmatization of having (or simply being at risk for) HIV, leading PWID to avoid using the programmes that are available.

Third, effective HIV prevention programmes require at least passive cooperation from law enforcement, and relationships between drug users and law enforcement may be particularly problematic in many low- and middle-income countries. In some countries, drug addiction may be a status offence (simply being an addict is sufficient basis for incarceration, without having to be found in possession of drugs). Many low- and middle-income

countries also have official registries of persons known to be addicted, and persons on these registries may lose important civil rights. Addicts may also be subject to police brutality (Booth et al. 2003; Wolfe et al. 2010). Thus, drug users may be very reluctant to participate in HIV prevention activities if such participation risks exposure to law enforcement activities. Carrying clean needles and syringes, in particular, may be risky for drug users in such settings.

Fourth, and of critical importance, political leaders in some transitional, low- and middle-income countries have viewed injecting drug use as a foreign, 'decadent' behaviour from the West that must be resisted in order to protect cultural traditions. Thus, interventions that appear to accept continuing drug use (such as syringe exchange) or appear to merely substitute the use of one narcotic drug for another (methadone maintenance treatment) are strongly resisted regardless of scientific evidence. One of the most important examples of this cultural resistance is the Russian opposition to methadone maintenance treatment (Wolfe 2007; Burki 2012).

Sexual transmission of HIV among drug users

As noted earlier, HIV is transmitted among drug users not only through the sharing of injecting equipment but also sexually. Both injecting and non-injecting drug use may facilitate sexual transmission of HIV through multiple mechanisms, including: exchange of sex for drugs or money to obtain drugs, impaired decision-making regarding safer sex (use of condoms, restricting the number of partners) when under the influence of drugs, and, for some drugs, perceived increases in sexual pleasure when combining drug use with sexual activity.

There have been a number of interventions developed to reduce unsafe sexual activity among injecting and non-injecting drug users (Meader et al. 2013). These interventions typically provide information about sexual transmission of HIV, the effectiveness of condoms in reducing sexual transmission, and may include skills training in topics such as correct condom use and negotiating safer sex. These interventions do have evidence of efficacy in changing sexual behaviour, but with only modest effect sizes. Thus, the most effective method of reducing sexual transmission of HIV among PWID may be to avert epidemics of injecting-related transmission in the first place.

Since the mid-1990s, various types of antiretroviral treatment (ART) medications have been developed to treat HIV infection. When used in combination, these medications can arrest the damaging effects of HIV on the immune system and restore health. Combination ART does not cure HIV infection but can significantly reduce viral loads among persons with the infection and is literally life-saving. Drug users, however, have generally benefited less than others from these medications. Drug users are often diagnosed late with HIV and have higher mortality rates from the virus (Grigoryan et al. 2009). Adherence to ART regimens can be difficult for many patients, but particularly for persons who are actively using drugs. With appropriate support services, however, drug users do as well as others on ART (Wisaksana et al. 2010).

The discovery of HIV/AIDS among persons who inject drugs forced a re-examination of public policies towards drug use. AIDS greatly increased mortality among persons who inject and the virus was transmitted to non-injecting sexual partners and newborn children. The activist and scientific responses have been impressive. We now have a consensus on the elements of 'comprehensive prevention, care and treatment of HIV' for persons who inject drugs (World Health Organization (WHO) 2009), including needle and syringe programmes, opiate substitution treatment, HIV testing and counselling, ART, prevention and treatment of sexually transmitted infections, condom programmes for PWID and their sexual partners, targeted information, education and communication for PWID and their sexual partners, and vaccination, diagnosis, and treatment of viral hepatitis infection. Implementation of these components at sufficient scale can avert HIV epidemics and reverse epidemics that have developed. However, implementation is inadequate in many countries (Mathers et al. 2010). Whether adequate implementation will occur is partially a matter of scarce resources, but primarily a matter of the stigmatization of drug users and the lack of political will to commit resources to the problem (Des Jarlais et al. 2010).

HCV among persons who inject drugs

Both HIV and hepatitis C virus (HCV) are transmitted through sharing of drug injection equipment. HIV co-infection increases HCV disease progression, and the great majority of HIV seropositive PWID are also infected with HCV.

HCV is much more transmissible through shared injection equipment than HIV, and can be effectively transmitted through the sharing of drug preparation equipment (cookers, filters) (Hagan et al. 2001), so that HCV prevalence is usually much higher than HIV prevalence among PWID. A recent systematic review found reports on HCV antibody prevalence in PWID in 77 countries (Nelson et al. 2011). Using midpoint estimates, country-specific prevalence ranged from 10 to 90 per cent, although in 25 countries prevalence was between 60 and 80 per cent, and in 12 it exceeded 80 per cent. The total number of anti-HCV positive PWID worldwide was estimated to be 10 million. A systematic review and meta-regression of time to acquisition of HCV infection in PWID also showed that, in high-income countries, HCV prevalence declined after 1995, corresponding to a period when harm reduction services expanded in these regions of the world (Hagan et al. 2008). Other recent studies have shown that combination prevention strategies—substance use treatment and access to sterile injecting equipment—are also associated with reduced likelihood of HCV seroconversion at the individual level (Hagan et al. 2011; Turner et al. 2011). However, there are currently no areas, even in high-income countries, where combined prevention has limited HCV incidence among PWID to less than 1/100 person-years at risk, as has been achieved by combined prevention for HIV among PWID.

Treatment of chronic HCV infection benefits individual patients and will also remove a source of infectiousness in the local PWID population. When treated with the new direct-acting antivirals (Food and Drug Administration 2012), up to 75 per cent of patients with genotype 1 infection may achieve a sustained virological response (SVR), in comparison to 40 per cent SVR in those treated with the previous regimen of pegylated interferon and ribavirin (Manns et al. 2001; Fried 2002; McHutchison et al. 2009; Kwo et al. 2010). (SVR involves eradication of the HCV in the body. It can be considered a cure, and lifelong treatment is *not* required in contrast to antiretroviral treatment for HIV.) Interferon can cause relatively severe side effects, including depression, so that new treatment regimens that do not require interferon could greatly increase the numbers of persons who would seek treatment and successfully complete treatment for HCV infection. Clinical trials of such new treatment regimens are currently underway.

Access to HCV treatment is currently extremely limited, and it is estimated that fewer than 5 per cent of HCV-infected PWID in the United States and Australia receive HCV treatment (Stoove et al. 2005; Paterson et al. 2007). New programmes to encourage PWID to enter treatment and provide support during treatment are also needed. Concurrent treatment for SUDs does improve completion rates for HCV treatment (Dimova et al. 2013).

Drug-induced (overdose) deaths

Drug-induced deaths (from drug overdoses) are another major adverse consequence of drug use. Narcotics are the most frequent cause of fatal overdoses because of their ability to depress respiration, but many fatal overdoses involve combinations of narcotics and other drugs such as alcohol or benzodiazepines. Data on fatal overdoses are typically obtained from toxicology studies conducted by medical examiners. Stimulant drugs such as cocaine can also induce deaths, usually by interfering with the functioning of the heart, but such cases are much less common than narcotic induced respiratory depression.

Interpreting overdose statistics as a measure of a country's drug problem can be quite difficult, as the number of recorded overdoses can depend upon a wide variety of factors including drug use patterns, injecting versus non-injecting routes of drug administration, the availability of emergency health services (and drug users' trust in calling for emergency assistance), as well as the quality of data collection and reporting.

Nevertheless, there is great variation in the numbers of fatal overdoses per capita across different countries, and these data undoubtedly reflect an important aspect of the drug problem in each country. Fig. 9.2.1 shows the reported per capita drug-induced deaths for the European Union (EU) countries for 2011.

The EU average was 21 fatal overdoses per million in the population and this has been stable for several years, but with a wide range; from under 5 per million in Romania to almost 150 per million in Estonia (European Monitoring Centre for Drugs and Drug Addiction 2011). The reasons for this great variation are not well understood, but there are undoubtedly multiple causal factors.

In the United States, drug overdose deaths have increased steadily over the last decade, primarily due to overdoses from pharmaceutical analgesics and not 'street' drugs such as heroin. In 2010, of the 38,329 overdose deaths in the United States, there were an estimated 16,651 overdose deaths due to opioid analgesics; over 75 per cent of these overdose deaths were unintentional. Opioids were also frequently implicated in overdose deaths involving other pharmaceutical drugs including benzodiazepines (77.2 per cent), antiepileptic and antiparkinsonism drugs (65.5 per cent), antipsychotic and neuroleptic drugs (58 per cent), antidepressants (57.6 per cent), other analgesics, antipyretics, and antirheumatics (56.5 per cent), and other psychotropic drugs (64.2 per cent). These data highlight the frequent involvement of drugs to treat mental health disorders in overdose deaths, such as benzodiazepines, antidepressants, and antipsychotics (Jones et al. 2013).

Reducing the numbers of persons using opioid drugs through effective substance use treatment would reduce the chances of

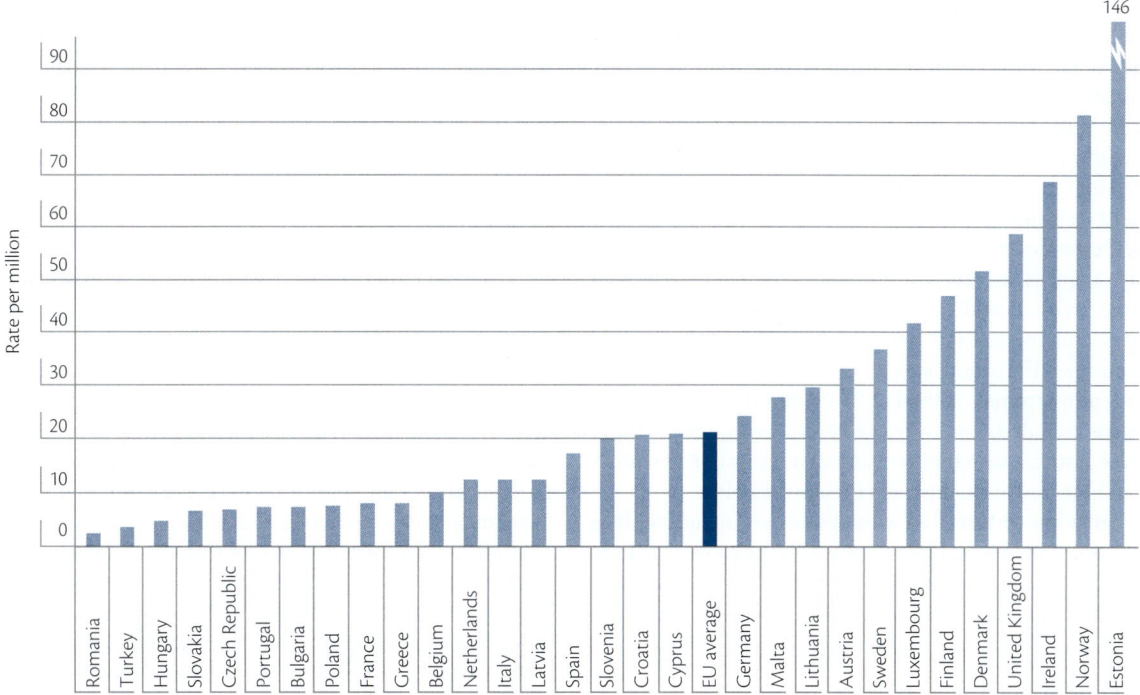

Fig. 9.2.1 European Monitoring Centre for Drugs and Drug Addiction (EMCDDA) 2011 estimated mortality rates among all adults (15–64 years) due to drug-induced deaths.

Reproduced from European Monitoring Centre for Drugs and Drug Addiction (EMCDDA), Drug-related infectious diseases and drug-related deaths, in EMCDDA (ed.), *Annual Report 2011: The State of the Drugs Problem in Europe*, Publications Office of the European Union, Luxembourg, Copyright © 2011.

overdose deaths. This can be a slow process, however, and the period just after a person has left treatment can be a high-risk period for overdose. The person will have lost tolerance so that his or her usual dose may precipitate an overdose. There are also methods for reducing overdose deaths without reducing drug use itself. Many syringe exchange programmes distribute naloxone to their participants and have trained participants in how to administer naloxone to a fellow user experiencing an overdose (Guardino et al. 2010). Naloxone is a very potent narcotic antagonist and can reverse an overdose within minutes. The US state of North Carolina has implemented a naloxone distribution programme specifically designed to provide naloxone for reversing pharmaceutical analgesic overdoses (Centers for Disease Control and Prevention 2012).

Treatment of substance use disorders

While there are effective methods for reducing transmission of infectious pathogens and for reducing overdoses among persons who use drugs, the ideal method for addressing these problems would be to eliminate drug use among persons with SUDs. We are very far from having treatments that produce permanent abstinence among persons with SUDs. Indeed, SUDs are best considered as 'chronic, relapsing conditions', for which treatment may reduce drug use but that return to drug use should be expected for the great majority of those who receive treatment.

The WHO, UNODC, and the Joint United Nations Programme on HIV/AIDS (UNAIDS) technical guide outlines a comprehensive package for prevention and treatment for PWID (WHO et al. 2012). Included in this package are needle and syringe programmes, opiate substitution treatment (OST), HIV testing and counselling, antiretroviral treatment, prevention and treatment of sexually transmitted infections, condom programmes for PWID and their sexual partners, targeted information, education, and communication for PWID and their sexual partners, prevention, vaccination and treatment of viral hepatitis, and prevention, diagnosis, and treatment of tuberculosis. This comprehensive package has been endorsed by the WHO, UNAIDS, UNODS, the UN General Assembly, the Economic and Social Council, the UN Commission on Narcotic Drugs, the Global Fund, and PEPFAR (WHO et al. 2012). According to their guidelines, a 'moderate' level coverage for these services should include at least 100 to 200 syringes per PWID per NSP, at least 20–40 per cent of PWID in opiate substitution treatment, and 25–75 per cent of PWID who are HIV positive receiving ART medication.

Opiate substitution treatment/medication assisted treatment

OST has been implemented for nearly 50 years, and has gained wider acceptance, especially among developing countries, in the last 5–10 years. Opiate use continues to be problematic globally, with an estimated 12.8–21.9 million people using heroin, or illicit opiates, in the last 12 months (UNODC 2012); nearly 50 per cent of these users are in Asia (Mathers et al. 2008).

There are two primary types of pharmacological medication used to treat opiate use: methadone, which has been used for decades, and more recently, buprenorphine. These two substances are approved as essential medicines for treatment of opiate abuse by the WHO (Farrell et al. 2012).

Public and private clinics throughout the world manage opiate addiction with opiate substitution therapy, and the results of these programmes over the years have generally been quite positive. Studies evaluating OST programmes have shown very substantial reductions in both drug use, and the associated risk behaviours associated with opiate use such as drug injection and sharing of injection-related equipment (Gowing et al. 2011). Additionally, measurements examining the quality of life of drug users in OST programmes have shown positive changes in drug users' lives, with more positive changes seen the longer patients remain in treatment (Padaiga et al. 2007; Lua and Talib 2012; Wang et al. 2012).

A review completed in 2013 among low- and middle-income countries examined the overall success of retention among participants in OST programmes. A total of 58 studies from 12 different countries were included, and overall retention was above 50 per cent after 12 months, and retention values were similar to studies conducted in high-income countries (Feelemyer 2014).

As many behaviours associated with opiate use, including drug injection, are associated with blood-borne infections such as hepatitis C and HIV, OST programmes act not only as a means to reduce drug use, but also to reduce the transmission of disease among PWID and their sexual partners (Mark et al. 2006).

Cognitive behavioural therapy

Cognitive behavioural therapy (CBT) is used in many clinical settings to treat symptoms of addiction, neurosis, and personality disorders. Applied in Marlatt and Gordon's model of relapse prevention (Marlatt and Donovan 2005), CBT for drug addiction targets cognitive, affective, and situation triggers for substance use while at the same time providing necessary skills and training needed for coping alternatives.

CBT for substance dependence targets five main strategies: identifying triggers for relapse, coping skills training, drug refusal skills training, functional analysis of substance use, and increasing non-use related activities (Kadden et al. 1992). One of the main goals of this therapy is to see drug users 'dis-associate' certain internal and external triggers that are associated with drug use and associated risk behaviours (Kadden 2001).

Studies examining the relationship between CBT treatment and substance use have shown that integrating CBT is associated with better treatment outcomes compared to treatment programmes that do not utilize CBT among participants (Hester and Miller 2003). A more recent systematic review of studies evaluating a wide range of drugs documented statistically significant changes across all substance use related behaviours along with reductions in drug use and continued abstinence from drug use over time among those involved in CBT treatment (Magill and Ray 2009).

The most noticeable changes in behaviour are observed in the first few months of treatment, indicating that CBT treatment can influence large changes among drug users in short periods of time (Magill and Ray 2009). Clinicians generally agree that CBT treatment for drug use should be used in conjunction with other treatments including psychosocial interventions or pharmacological treatment in order to increase a participant's self-efficacy to quit using drugs (Yen et al. 2004).

Contingency management

Contingency management (CM) interventions that aim to treat those using psychoactive and illicit substances are based on extensive literature and empirical science that looks at drug use and addiction as forms of operant behaviour conditioning, by which behaviour is in some way shaped, or controlled, by its consequences (Higgins and Silverman 1999). The CM approach seeks to use alternative non-drug reinforcers with the aim of decreasing substance use if these reinforcers are prevalent and incompatible with continued drug use and abuse (Carroll et al. 1989; Higgins et al. 1994).

One of the most important aspects of the CM approach is to retain participants in drug treatment programmes (such as detoxification, counselling or opiate substitution treatment), which is associated with greater changes in drug abstinence and associated risk behaviours (Elk et al. 1998). Most models have built upon the premise of retention as one of several incentives (money, vouchers, prizes, etc.), with increasing incentives given to participants the longer they successfully attend drug treatment. When a participant misses an appointment, the incentives are returned to a baseline level (Ledgerwood et al. 2008).

Studies examining the use of CM as a supplementary tool for drug treatment have shown that under treatment, participants significantly reduce drug use, and document increased retention compared to participants who were not offered CM (Rawson et al. 2006). Addiction severity has also been shown to decrease, over time, when CM is incorporated into drug treatment (McLellan et al. 1992). Additionally, the use of CM in methadone maintenance programmes has been associated with longer treatment follow-up periods, higher levels of drug-free urine screens among participants, and better adherence to methadone prescriptions (Griffith et al. 2000).

Short-term contingency management has the potential for dramatic results in short periods of time. However, CM should not be considered a long-term treatment for substance use, as there is evidence of diminishing return as CM is offered over longer periods of time.

Motivational interviewing

Motivational interviewing (MI) is used in clinical settings to motivate change among individuals (Miller and Rollnick 2002), and is used in a wide range of treatment settings for drug users. Treatment for drug users focuses on MI tools including helping clients explore and resolve their ambivalence regarding drug use, and its associated risk behaviours (Miller et al. 2003). Characteristics of MI may include participants expressing commitment, desire, ability, need, readiness, or reasons to change or maintain their drug use habits.

Through a dialogue among drug users and clinicians, MI seeks to extend verbal commitments to change in participants' everyday lives, such that permanent and long-term changes in drug use can be achieved. As motivation for change increases, the focus of MI shifts from commitment toward a development plan for participants. This development plan is put together based on the dialogue collected by clinicians over different MI sessions (Amrhein et al. 2003). Minimizing resistance to change is an important factor in the plan and ensuring participant success (Miller and Rollnick 2002).

Studies evaluating the practice of MI in drug treatment settings have shown that integrating this approach into conventional drug treatment settings is associated with positive changes in drug use and drug use behaviour. A meta-analysis of studies that used MI for treatment of substance abuse among adolescents found that nearly 70 per cent of included studies documented a positive change when integrating this treatment method (Barnett et al. 2012).

The utilization of MI among participants with substance abuse who are co-infected with HIV has also been evaluated. Participants who were given MI treatment showed significant reduction in their primary illicit drug use after 30 days, and results extended to 60 days after implementation of treatment. Additionally, more significant changes in overall drug use were noted among those who underwent MI along with conventional treatment, compared to those that were not offered supplementary MI sessions (Aharonovich et al. 2012).

Motivational interviewing has become more widely used in many practice settings, and the overall outcome of integrating MI into existing programmes has been positive. By discussing issues related to drug use with participants, along with continued commitments to change, MI has the potential to dramatically reduce drug use when integrated into, or used as a standalone treatment regimen for, drug dependence and other psychological issues.

Residential treatment and detoxification

Detoxification programmes for drug use have been a chosen form of treatment used in a number of countries, and have been used for decades to enable participants to discontinue drug use and associated high-risk behaviour. By placing participants in a programme that does not allow exposure to illicit substances while allowing for treatment of withdrawal symptoms, detoxification programmes have the potential to reduce drug use while also reducing needle use, HIV infection, and seroconversion (Metzger et al. 1993).

Detoxification alone may not be sufficient for participants who are severely dependent on certain substances that cause severe withdrawal symptoms (such as heroin and alcohol) (Mattick and Hall 1996), but is still the chosen first treatment step in the majority of those seeking long-term drug treatment (Kleber and Riordan 1982). In many countries, detoxification now includes the utilization of pharmacological substances to treat withdrawal symptoms, such as methadone or buprenorphine for heroin users, particularly adolescent drug users (Kaminer 1995); this is essential to reducing craving and relapse among participants. However, it is important to continually monitor those in detoxification treatment, especially those who are in outpatient treatment, to ensure continued participation along with abstinence from drug use.

Studies over time have reported positive results when participants are engaged in detoxification, especially when treatment includes medication to treat withdrawal. A systematic review among adolescent substance users reported a higher level of retention along with significant reduction in drug use, after 1 year, when detoxification was initiated in conjunction with pharmacological substance treatment (Minozzi et al. 2009). Even greater reductions in drug use, and greater compliance, were achieved when psychosocial components were integrated into treatment.

However, in detoxification programmes where pharmacological substances are not offered, high rates of relapse and dropout still occur. In Russia, for example, pharmacological treatment is still illegal and as a result high rates of relapse and continued drug use occur among a high percentage of participants who initiate detoxification (Elovich and Drucker 2008). For this reason,

detoxification programmes in most countries now include multidimensional treatment options, to handle not only drug withdrawal and relapse, but also drug cues and triggers related to drug use (Amato et al. 2008).

Early detoxification programmes documented high levels of relapse due to the lack of intervention options for those who need continued treatment. However, as new models for detoxification now include medications, psychosocial components, and other treatment options, higher levels of retention, and significant reductions in drug use, can now be achieved over a long period of time. As a result, social as well as environmental changes can be addressed to reduce the chances of relapse. The earlier someone begins detoxification treatment, the greater chance that permanent change in drug use can be achieved (Kaminer 1995).

Self-help and 12-step programmes for drug use

Self-help, including the 12-step programmes, has been used by many to work through the issues of their drug-taking behaviours through social support and peer discussion. The most common of these programmes for drug users include Narcotics Anonymous (NA) and Cocaine Anonymous (CA) (National Institute on Drug Abuse 2011). All self-help programmes stem from the original 12-step recovery programme of Alcoholics Anonymous set forth in the *Big Book* and the *Twelve Steps and Twelve Traditions* (Alcoholics Anonymous World Services 2002). These programmes help to reduce relapse and drug use through community oriented, 12-step mutual help groups among participants with similar substance abuse problems (Kelly and Myers 2007).

One of the distinctions in self-help programmes is the lack of systematic clinician involvement in treatment. Often, groups are formed among adults, exclusive of formal treatment, although many of the participants in these programmes have come from long-term drug treatment programmes or detoxification centres (Timko et al. 2000). More recently, as adolescent drug use has increased, these programmes have evolved to include adolescent and younger drug users as well.

Twelve-step and self-help programmes offer many positive benefits for drug users. These groups offer unique approaches and ideas for abstinence related behaviours for those that are dealing with drug triggers or cues in their everyday lives. They are also offered at little to no cost, and do not require revealing of personal information to doctors or clinicians. Finally, 12-step and self-help programmes often lead to participants developing a network of fellow ex-users, which can be very helpful as many drug users' previous networks included other drug users, and avoiding these previous networks is an important factor in avoiding relapse (Baer et al. 1993).

Studies among drug users in self-help and 12-step programmes have shown positive results. A recent 3-year study of drug users in self-help programmes showed that over time, many former drug users maintained continuous abstinence from drug use while participating in the programme, and abstinence was greater the more sessions that were attended (Laudet 2007). A study among adolescents in inpatient treatment followed by participation in self-help programmes found that abstinence was greater the more sessions that were attended (Kelly et al. 2004).

Self-help programmes have evolved over time from the original programmes focused on alcohol to encompass many different drugs of abuse. Along with complementary treatment including detoxification and pharmacological therapy, self-help programmes have the potential to bring together users while keeping them in networks of other users who are also trying to stop using drugs. By attending these meetings and avoiding cues and triggers that may lead to drug use and associated risk behaviours, longer periods of treatment success can be achieved.

Harm reduction and human rights

Harm reduction

The emergence of HIV/AIDS among injecting drug users has been a profound challenge to public health systems. In some areas, there was a rapid response, and potential HIV epidemics among IDUs were averted. In other areas, HIV epidemics occurred before effective public health responses, but the responses eventually brought the epidemics under control, and in still other areas, HIV epidemics are occurring among PWID without any effective public health response. The HIV/AIDS crisis has furthered the development of a policy framework that provides a new perspective on the use of psychoactive drugs (both licit and illicit). This perspective has generally come to be known as 'harm reduction' (Buning 1991; Berridge 1999).

One of the most well-known harm reduction programmes, needle and syringe exchange programmes (NSP), has been in operation for many years in high-income locations and has begun to emerge in low- and middle-income countries in recent years. A systematic review of structural level NSP (structural NSP distribute at least ten needles/syringes per PWID per year) in low- and middle-income countries completed in 2013 documented noticeable reductions in both HIV and HCV infections among PWID in conjunction with the implementation and scale up of NSP. More noticeable changes were especially noticeable when more needles were made available per PWID in a particular location (Des Jarlais et al. 2013).

It may be best to present harm reduction in the words of its practitioners (Harm Reduction Coalition (n.d.): 'Harm reduction is a set of practical strategies that reduce negative consequences of drug use, incorporating a spectrum of strategies from safer use, to managed use, to abstinence. Harm reduction strategies meet drug users "where they're at," addressing conditions of use along with the use itself'.

Because harm reduction demands that interventions and policies designed to serve drug users reflect specific individual and community needs, there is no universal definition of or formula for implementing harm reduction. However, the Harm Reduction Coalition considers the following principles central to harm reduction practice (Harm Reduction Coalition 2007):

Accepts, for better and for worse, that licit and illicit drug use is part of our world and chooses to work to minimize its harmful effects rather than simply ignore or condemn them.

Understands drug use as a complex, multi-faceted phenomenon that encompasses a continuum of behaviors from severe abuse to total abstinence, and acknowledges that some ways of using drugs are clearly safer than others.

Establishes quality of individual and community life and well-being—not necessarily cessation of all drug use—as the criteria for successful interventions and policies.

Calls for the non-judgmental, non-coercive provision of services and resources to people who use drugs and the communities in which they live in order to assist them in reducing attendant harm.

Ensures that drug users and those with a history of drug use routinely have a real voice in the creation of programs and policies designed to serve them.

Affirms drugs users themselves as the primary agents of reducing the harms of their drug use, and seeks to empower users to share information and support each other in strategies which meet their actual conditions of use.

Recognizes that the realities of poverty, class, racism, social isolation, past trauma, sex-based discrimination and other social inequalities affect both peoples' vulnerability to and capacity for effectively dealing with drug-related harm.

Does not attempt to minimize or ignore the real and tragic harm and danger associated with licit and illicit drug use.

The two basic components of harm reduction are utilizing evidence-based interventions to reduce the adverse individual and societal consequences of drug use and respecting the civil rights of drug users (Des Jarlais 1995; Gilmore 1996; Elliott 2004; Wolfe and Malinowska-Sempruch 2004). An important insight of harm reduction is that many of the adverse consequence of drug use can be addressed among persons who continue to use drugs. This is critical because while there are effective treatments to reduce drug use among persons with SUDs, our ability to achieve permanent abstinence among persons who use drugs is quite limited and likely to remain so for the indefinite future.

Harm reduction has a moral component in addition to its evidence-based component. Health should be considered a fundamental human right of persons who use drugs (Wood et al. 2010). Given the structure of the human nervous system, it is very unlikely that we will ever have a world without problems associated with drug use. Denying the human rights of drug users, however, will only make the problems worse.

References

Aceijas, C., Stimson, G.V., Hickman, M., et al. (2004). Global overview of injecting drug use and HIV infection among injecting drug users. *AIDS*, 18(17), 2295–303.

Aharonovich, E., Greenstein, E., O'Leary, A., Johnston, B., Seol, S.G., and Hasin, D.S. (2012). HealthCall: technology-based extension of motivational interviewing to reduce non-injection drug use in HIV primary care patients—a pilot study. *AIDS Care*, 24(12), 1461–9.

Alcoholics Anonymous World Services, et al. (2002). *Twelve Steps and Twelve Traditions*. New York: Alcoholics Anonymous World Services.

Amato, L., Minozzi, S., Davoli, M., Vecchi, S., Ferri, M.M., and Mayet, S. (2008). Psychosocial and pharmacological treatments versus pharmacological treatments for opioid detoxification. *Cochrane Database of Systematic Reviews*, 3, CD005031.

American Psychiatric Association (1980). *Diagnostic and Statistical Manual of Mental Disorders* (3rd ed.). Washington DC: American Psychiatric Press.

Amrhein, P.C., Miller, W.R., Yahne, C.E., Palmer, M., and Fulcher, L. (2003). Client commitment language during motivational interviewing predicts drug use outcomes. *Journal of Consulting and Clinical Psychology*, 71(5), 862–78.

Anderson, W. (1991). The New York needle trial: the politics of public health in the age of AIDS. *American Journal of Public Health*, 81, 1506–17.

Baer, J.S., Marlatt, G.A., and McMahon, R.J. (1993). *Addictive Behaviors Across the Life Span*. Newbury Park, CA: Sage.

Barnett, E., Sussman, S., Smith, C., Rohrbach, L.A., and Spruijt-Metz, D. (2012). Motivational interviewing for adolescent substance use: a review of the literature. *Addictive Behaviors*, 37(12), 1325–34.

Barzilai, A., Sperling, R.S., Hyatt, A.C., Wedgwood, J.F., Reidenberg, B.E., and Hodes, D.S. (1990). Mother to child transmission of human immunodeficiency virus 1 infection despite zidovudine therapy from 18 weeks of gestation. *Pediatric Infectious Disease Journal*, 9(12), 931–3.

Berridge, V. (1999). Histories of harm reduction: illicit drugs, tobacco, and nicotine. *Substance Use & Misuse*, 34(1), 35–47.

Beseler, C.L. and Hasin, D.S. (2010). Cannabis dimensionality: dependence, abuse and consumption. *Addictive Behaviors*, 35(11), 961–9.

Booth, R.E., Kennedy, J., Brewster, T., and Semerik, O. (2003). Drug injectors and dealers in Odessa, Ukraine. *Journal of Psychoactive Drugs*, 35(4), 419–26.

Brenner, B.G., Roger, M., Routy, J.P., et al. (2007). High rates of forward transmission events after acute/early HIV-1 infection. *Journal of Infectious Diseases*, 195(7), 951–9.

Buning, E.C. (1991). Effects of Amsterdam needle and syringe exchange. *International Journal of the Addictions*, 26(12), 1303–11.

Buning, E.C., van Brussel, G.H.A., et al. (eds.) (1988). *Amsterdam's Drug Policy and its Implications for Controlling Needle Sharing. Needle Sharing Among Intravenous Drug Abusers: National and International Drug Perspectives*. Research Monograph. Rockville, MD: National Institute on Drug Abuse.

Burki, T. (2012). Russia's drug policy fuels infectious disease epidemics. *The Lancet Infectious Diseases*, 12(4), 275–6.

Carroll, M.E., Lac, S.T., and Nygaard, S.L. (1989). A concurrently available nondrug reinforcer prevents the acquisition or decreases the maintenance of cocaine-reinforced behavior. *Psychopharmacology (Berlin)*, 97(1), 23–9.

Casey, M., Casey, M., Adamson, G., Shevlin, M., and McKinney, A. (2012). The role of craving in AUDs: dimensionality and differential functioning in the DSM-5. *Drug and Alcohol Dependence*, 125(1–2), 75–80.

Centers for Disease Control and Prevention (1981). First report of AIDS. *Morbidity and Mortality Weekly Report*, 50(21), 429.

Centers for Disease Control and Prevention (2012). Community-based opioid overdose prevention programs providing naloxone—United States, 2010. *Journal of the American Medical Association*, 307(13), 1358–64.

Cohen, J. (2010). No opiate substitutes for the masses of IDUs. *Science*, 329(5988), 165–7.

Costanzo, S., Di Castelnuovo, A., Donati, M.B., Iacoviello, L., and de Gaetano, G. (2010). Alcohol consumption and mortality in patients with cardiovascular disease: a meta-analysis. *Journal of the American College of Cardiology*, 55(13), 1339–47.

Dawson, D.A., Saha, T.D., and Grant, B.F. (2010). A multidimensional assessment of the validity and utility of alcohol use disorder severity as determined by item response theory models. *Drug and Alcohol Dependence*, 107(1), 31–8.

Department of Health and Human Services (2008). *Treatment Episode Data Set (TEDS) Highlights—2007*. Rockville MD: Substance and Mental Health Services Administration.

Des Jarlais, D.C. (1995). Editorial: harm reduction – a framework for incorporating science into drug policy. *American Journal of Public Health*, 85(1), 10–12.

Des Jarlais, D.C., Arasteh, K., and Gwadz, M. (2010). Increasing HIV prevention and care for injecting drug users. *The Lancet*, 375 (9719), 961–3.

Des Jarlais, D.C., Feelemyer, J.P., Modi, S.N., Abdul-Quader, A., and Hagan, H. (2013). High coverage needle/syringe programs for people who inject drugs in low and middle income countries: a systematic review. *BMC Public Health*, 13, 53.

Des Jarlais, D.C., Feelemyer, J.P., Modi, S.N., et al. (2012). Transitions from injection-drug-use-concentrated to self-sustaining heterosexual HIV epidemics: a systematic review. *PLoS One*, 7 (3), e31227.

Des Jarlais, D.C., Friedman, S.R., Novick, D.M., et al. (1989). HIV-1 infection among intravenous drug users in Manhattan, New York City, from 1977 through 1987. *Journal of the American Medical Association*, 261, 1008–12.

Des Jarlais, D.C., Hagan, H., Friedman, S.R., et al. (1995). Maintaining low HIV seroprevalence in populations of injecting drug users. *Journal of the American Medical Association*, 274(15), 1226–31.

Des Jarlais, D.C., Paone, D., Milliken, J., et al. (1999). Audio-computer interviewing to measure risk behaviour for HIV among injecting drug users: a quasi-randomised trial. *The Lancet*, 353(9165), 1657–61.

Dimova, R.B., Zeremski, M., Jacobson, I.M., Hagan, H., Des Jarlais, D.C., and Talal, A.H. (2013). Determinants of hepatitis C virus treatment completion and efficacy in drug users assessed by meta-analysis. *Clinical Infectious Diseases*, 56(6), 806–16.

Edwards, G., Arif, A., and Hadgson, R. (1981). Nomenclature and classification of drug- and alcohol-related problems: a WHO Memorandum. *Bulletin of the World Health Organization*, 59(2), 225–42.

Edwards, G. and Gross, M.M. (1976). Alcohol dependence: provisional description of a clinical syndrome. *British Medical Journal*, 1(6017), 1058–61.

Elk, R., Mangus, L., Rhoades, H., Andres, R., and Grabowski, J. (1998). Cessation of cocaine use during pregnancy: effects of contingency management interventions on maintaining abstinence and complying with prenatal care. *Addictive Behaviors*, 23(1), 57–64.

Elliott, R. (2004). Drug control, human rights, and harm reduction in the age of AIDS. *HIV/AIDS Policy & Law Review*, 9(3), 86–90.

Elovich, R. and Drucker, E. (2008). On drug treatment and social control: Russian narcology's great leap backwards. *Harm Reduction Journal*, 5, 23.

European Monitoring Centre for Drugs and Drug Addiction (2011). Drug-related infectious diseases and drug-related deaths. In EMCDDA (ed.) *Annual Report 2011: The State of the Drugs Problem in Europe*. Luxembourg: Publications Office of the European Union. Available at: http://www.emcdda.europa.eu/online/annual-report/2011.

Farrell, M., Wodak, A., and Gowing, L. (2012). Maintenance drugs to treat opioid dependence. *British Medical Journal*, 344, e2823.

Feelemyer, J., Des Jarlais, D., Arasteh, K., Abdul-Quader, A., and Hagan, H. (2014). Retention of participants in opiate substitution programs in low and middle-income countries: an international systematic review. *Addiction*, 109(1), 20–32.

Food and Drug Administration (2012). *Approval of Incivek (telaprevir), a Direct Acting Antiviral Drug (DAA) to Treat Hepatitis C (HCV)*. [Online] Available at: http://www.fda.gov/ForConsumers/ByAudience/ForPatientAdvocates/ucm256328.htm.

Foroud, T., Wetherill, L.F., Liang, T., et al. (2007). Association of alcohol craving with alpha-synuclein (SNCA). *Alcoholism: Clinical and Experimental Research*, 31(4), 537–45.

Frances, A. (2009). Whither DSM-V? *British Journal of Psychiatry*, 195(5), 391–2.

Fried, M.W. (2002). Side effects of therapy of hepatitis C and their management. *Hepatology*, 36(5 Suppl. 1), S237–44.

Gilmore, N. (1996). Drug use and human rights: privacy, vulnerability, disability, and human rights infringements. *Journal of Drug Policy*, 14, 155–69.

Gowing, L., Farrell, M.F., Bornemann, R., Sullivan, L.E., and Ali, R. (2011). Oral substitution treatment of injecting opioid users for prevention of HIV infection. *Cochrane Database of Systematic Reviews*, 8, CD004145.

Grant, B.F., Compton, W.M., Crowley, T.J., et al. (2007). Errors in assessing DSM-IV substance use disorders. *Archives of General Psychiatry*, 64(3), 379–80; author reply 81–2.

Grant, B.F., Stinson, F.S., and Harford, T.C. (2001). Age at onset of alcohol use and DSM-IV alcohol abuse and dependence: a 12-year follow-up. *Journal of Substance Abuse*, 13(4), 493–504.

Griffith, J.D., Rowan-Szal, G.A., Roark, R.R., and Simpson, D.D. (2000). Contingency management in outpatient methadone treatment: a meta-analysis. *Drug and Alcohol Dependence*, 58(1–2), 55–66.

Grigoryan, A., Hall, H.I., Durant, T., and Wei, X. (2009). Late HIV diagnosis and determinants of progression to AIDS or death after HIV diagnosis among injection drug users, 33 US States, 1996–2004. *PLoS ONE*, 4(2), e4445.

Guardino, V., Des Jarlais, D.C., Arasteh, K., et al. (2010). Syringe exchange programs—United States, 2008. *Morbidity and Mortality Weekly Report*, 59(45), 1488–91.

Hagan, H., Pouget, E.R., and Des Jarlais, D.C. (2011). A systematic review and meta-analysis of interventions to prevent hepatitis C virus infection in people who inject drugs. *Journal of Infectious Disease*, 204(1), 74–83.

Hagan, H., Pouget, E.R., Des Jarlais, D.C., and Lelutiu-Weinberger, C. (2008). Meta-regression of hepatitis C virus infection in relation to time since onset of illicit drug injection: the influence of time and place. *American Journal of Epidemiology*, 168(10), 1099–109.

Hagan, H., Thiede, H., Weiss, N.S., Hopkins, S.G., Duchin, J.S., and Alexander, E.R. (2001). Sharing of drug preparation equipment as a risk factor for hepatitis C. *American Journal of Public Health*, 91(1), 42–6.

Harm Reduction Coalition (n.d.). *Principles of Harm Reduction*. [Online] Available at: http://harmreduction.org/about-us/principles-of-harm-reduction/

Hasin, D.S. and Beseler, C. L. (2009). Dimensionality of lifetime alcohol abuse, dependence and binge drinking. *Drug and Alcohol Dependence*, 101(1–2), 53–61.

Hasin, D.S., Fenton, M.C., Beseler, C., Park, J.Y., and Wall, M.M. (2012). Analyses related to the development of DSM-5 criteria for substance use related disorders: 2. Proposed DSM-5 criteria for alcohol, cannabis, cocaine and heroin disorders in 663 substance abuse patients. *Drug and Alcohol Dependence*, 122(1–2), 28–37.

Hasin, D.S. and Grant, B.F. (2004). The co-occurrence of DSM-IV alcohol abuse in DSM-IV alcohol dependence: results of the National Epidemiologic Survey on Alcohol and Related Conditions on heterogeneity that differ by population subgroup. *Archives of General Psychiatry*, 61(9), 891–6.

Hasin, D.S., Grant, B., and Endicott, J. (1990). The natural history of alcohol abuse: implications for definitions of alcohol use disorders. *American Journal of Psychiatry*, 147(11), 1537–41.

Hasin, D., Hatzenbuehler, M.L., Keyes, K., and Ogburn, E. (2006a). Substance use disorders: Diagnostic and Statistical Manual of Mental Disorders, fourth edition (DSM-IV) and International Classification of Diseases, tenth edition (ICD-10). *Addiction*, 101(Suppl. 1), 59–75.

Hasin, D.S., Hatzenbuehler, M., Smith, S., and Grant, B.F. (2005). Co-occurring DSM-IV drug abuse in DSM-IV drug dependence: results from the National Epidemiologic Survey on Alcohol and Related Conditions. *Drug and Alcohol Dependence*, 80(1), 117–23.

Hasin, D.S., Liu, X., Alderson, D., and Grant, B.F. (2006b). DSM-IV alcohol dependence: a categorical or dimensional phenotype? *Psychological Medicine*, 36(12), 1695–705.

Hasin, D.S., O'Brien, C., Auriacombe, M., et al. (2013). DSM-5 criteria for substance use disorders: recommendations and rationale. *The American Journal of Psychiatry*, 170(8), 834–51.

Hasin, D. and Paykin, A. (1998). Dependence symptoms but no diagnosis: diagnostic 'orphans' in a community sample. *Drug and Alcohol Dependence*, 50(1), 19–26.

Hasin, D.S., Van Rossem, R., McCloud, S., and Endicott, J. (1997). Differentiating DSM-IV alcohol dependence and abuse by course: community heavy drinkers. *Journal of Substance Abuse*, 9, 127–35.

Heckathorn, D.D. (1997). Respondent-driven sampling: a new approach to the study of hidden populations. *Social Problems*, 44(2), 174–99.

Heinz, A., Beck, A., Grüsser, S.M., Grace, A.A., and Wrase, J. (2009). Identifying the neural circuitry of alcohol craving and relapse vulnerability. *Addiction Biology*, 14(1), 108–18.

Hester, R.K. and Miller, W.R. (2003), *Handbook of Alcoholism Treatment Approaches: Effective Alternatives*. Boston, MA: Allyn and Bacon.

Higgins, S.T., Bickel, W.K., and Hughes, J.R. (1994). Influence of an alternative reinforcer on human cocaine self-administration. *Life Sciences*, 55(3), 179–87.

Higgins, S.T. and Silverman, K. (1999). *Motivating Behavior Change Among Illicit Drug Abusers: Research on Contingency Management Interventions*. Washington, DC: American Psychological Association.

Iverson, J., Topp, L., Wand, H., Kaldor, J., and Maher, L. (2012). Low incidence of HIV among people who inject drugs over two decades in Australia. In *International AIDS Conference*, Washington, DC.

Johnston, L., O'Malley, P., Bachman, J., and Schulenberg, J. (2011). *Monitoring the Future: National Results on Adolescent Drug Use*. Ann Arbor. MI: The University of Michigan Institute for Social Research.

Jones, C.M., Mack, K.A., and Paulozzi, L.J. (2013). Pharmaceutical overdose deaths, United States, 2010. *Journal of the American Medical Association*, 309(7), 657–9.

Kadden, R.M. (2001). *Cognitive-Behaviour Therapy for Substance Dependence: Coping Skills Training*. Storrs, CT: University of Connecticut.

Kadden, R., Carroll, K., Donovan, D., et al. (1992). *Cognitive-Behavioral Coping Skills Therapy Manual: A Clinical Research Guide for Therapists Treatment Individuals with Alcohol Abuse and Dependence. NIAAA Project MATCH Monograph Series 3*. Washington, DC: Government Printing Office.

Kaminer, Y. (1995). Pharmacotherapy for adolescents with psychoactive substance use disorders. *NIDA Research Monograph*, 156, 291–324.

Kane, S. (1991). HIV, heroin and heterosexual relations. *Social Science & Medicine*, 32(9), 1037–50.

Kelly, J.F., Abrantes, A., and Brown, S.A. (2004). An 8-year follow-up of adolescent AA/NA involvement following inpatient treatment. In *Annual Meeting of the Research Society on Alcoholism*, July, Vancouver, Canada.

Kelly, J.F. and Myers, M.G. (2007). Adolescents' participation in Alcoholics Anonymous and Narcotics Anonymous: review, implications and future directions. *Journal of Psychoactive Drugs*, 39(3), 259–69.

Kendler, K.S. and Gardner, C.O., Jr. (1998). Boundaries of major depression: an evaluation of DSM-IV criteria. *American Journal of Psychiatry*, 155(2), 172–7.

Kerr, T., Kerr, T., Spittal, P.M., et al. (2006). Harm reduction by a 'user-run' organization: a case study of the Vancouver Area Network of Drug Users (VANDU). *International Journal of Drug Policy*, 17(2), 61–9.

Kleber, H.D. and Riordan, C.E. (1982). The treatment of narcotic withdrawal: a historical review. *Journal of Clinical Psychiatry*, 43(6 Pt. 2), 30–4.

Kwo, P.Y., Lawitz, E.J., McCone, J., et al. (2010). Efficacy of boceprevir, an NS3 protease inhibitor, in combination with peginterferon alfa-2b and ribavirin in treatment-naive patients with genotype 1 hepatitis C infection (SPRINT-1): an open-label, randomised, multicentre phase 2 trial. *The Lancet*, 376(9742), 705–16.

Laudet, A. and White, W. (2007). Predicting sustained remission from poly substance use: a three-year follow-up study. In *69th Annual Scientific Meeting of the College on Problems of Drug Dependence (CPDD)*, Quebec City, Canada.

Ledgerwood, D.M., Alessi, S.M., Hanson, T., Godley, M.D., and Petry, N.M. (2008). Contingency management for attendance to group substance abuse treatment administered by clinicians in community clinics. *Journal of Applied Behavior Analysis*, 41(4), 517–26.

Lev-Ran, S., Le Strat, Y., Imtiaz, S., Rehm, J., and Le Foll, B. (2013). Gender differences in prevalence of substance use disorders among individuals with lifetime exposure to substances: results from a large representative sample. *American Journal on Addictions*, 22(1), 7–13.

Lim, S.S., Vos, T., Flaxman, A.D., et al. (2012). A comparative risk assessment of burden of disease and injury attributable to 67 risk factors and risk factor clusters in 21 regions, 1990–2010: a systematic analysis for the Global Burden of Disease Study 2010. *The Lancet*, 380(9859), 2224–60.

Lowe, D., Milechman, B., Cotton, R., et al. (1990). Maximizing return rates and safe disposal of injection equipment in Australian needle & syringe exchange programs. In *6th International Conference on AIDS*, June, San Francisco, CA.

Lua, P.L. and Talib, N.S. (2012). A 12-month evaluation of health-related quality of life outcomes of methadone maintenance program in a rural Malaysian sample. *Substance Use & Misuse*, 47(10), 1100–5.

Magill, M. and Ray, L.A. (2009). Cognitive-behavioral treatment with adult alcohol and illicit drug users: a meta-analysis of randomized controlled trials. *Journal of Studies on Alcohol and Drugs*, 70(4), 516–27.

Manns, M.P., McHutchison, J.G., Gordon, S.C., et al. (2001). Peginterferon alfa-2b plus ribavirin compared with interferon alfa-2b plus ribavirin for initial treatment of chronic hepatitis C: a randomised trial. *The Lancet*, 358(9286), 958–65.

Mark, H.D., Nanda, J., Davis-Vogel, A., et al. (2006). Profiles of self-reported HIV-risk behaviors among injection drug users in methadone maintenance treatment, detoxification, and needle exchange programs. *Public Health Nursing*, 23(1), 11–19.

Marlatt, G.A. and Donovan, D.M. (2005). *Relapse Prevention: Maintenance Strategies in the Treatment of Addictive Behaviors*. New York: Guilford Press.

Mathers, B.M., Degenhardt, L., Ali, H., et al. (2010). HIV prevention, treatment, and care services for people who inject drugs: a systematic review of global, regional, and national coverage. *The Lancet*, 375(9719), 1014–28.

Mathers, B.M., Degenhardt, L., Phillips, B., et al. (2008). Global epidemiology of injecting drug use and HIV among people who inject drugs: a systematic review. *The Lancet*, 372(9651), 1733–45.

Mattick, R.P. and Hall, W. (1996). Are detoxification programmes effective? *The Lancet*, 347(8994), 97–100.

McHutchison, J.G., Everson, G.T., Gordon, S.C., et al. (2009). Telaprevir with peginterferon and ribavirin for chronic HCV genotype 1 infection. *The New England Journal of Medicine*, 360(18), 1827–38.

McLellan, A.T., Kushner, H., Metzger, D., et al. (1992). The Fifth Edition of the Addiction Severity Index. *Journal of Substance Abuse Treatment*, 9(3), 199–213.

Meader, N., Semaan, S., Halton, M., et al. (2013). An international systematic review and meta-analysis of multisession psychosocial interventions compared with educational or minimal interventions on the HIV sex risk behaviors of people who use drugs. *AIDS and Behavior*, 17(6), 1963–78.

Metzger, D.S., Woody, G.E., McLellan, A.T., et al. (1993). Human immunodeficiency virus seroconversion among intravenous drug users in- and out-of-treatment: an 18-month prospective follow-up. *Journal of Acquired Immune Deficiency Syndromes*, 6(9), 1049–56.

Mewton, L., Slade, T., McBride, O., Grove, R., and Teesson, M. (2011). An evaluation of the proposed DSM-5 alcohol use disorder criteria using Australian national data. *Addiction*, 106(5), 941–50.

Miller, N.S. and Goldsmith, R.J. (2001). Craving for alcohol and drugs in animals and humans: biology and behavior. *Journal of Addictive Diseases*, 20(3), 87–104.

Miller, W.R. and Rollnick, S. (2002). *Motivational Interviewing: Preparing People for Change*. New York: Guilford Press.

Miller, W.R., Yahne, C.E., and Tonigan, J.S. (2003). Motivational interviewing in drug abuse services: a randomized trial. *Journal of Consulting and Clinical Psychology*, 71(4), 754–63.

Minozzi, S., Amato, L., and Davoli, M. (2009). Detoxification treatments for opiate dependent adolescents. *Cochrane Database of Systematic Reviews*, 2, CD006749.

Morgan, G., Wilkins, H.A., Pepin, J., Jobe, O., Brewster, D., and Whittle, H. (1990). AIDS following mother-to-child transmission of HIV-2. *AIDS*, 4(9), 879–82.

Moschese, V., Lombardi, V., Alimandi, M., Galli, E., and Rossi, P. (1991). Mother-to-child transmission of HIV-1 infection. Epidemiological and experimental studies. *Allergologia et Immunopathologia*, 19(1), 1–5.

National Institute on Drug Abuse (2011). *Seeking Drug Abuse Treatment: Know What to Ask*. Washington DC: US Department of Health and Human Services, National Institutes of Health.

Nelson, P.K., Mathers, B.M., Cowie, B., et al. (2011). Global epidemiology of hepatitis B and hepatitis C in people who inject drugs: results of systematic reviews. *The Lancet*, 378(9791), 571–83.

Nyindo, M. (2005). Complementary factors contributing to the rapid spread of HIV-I in sub-Saharan Africa: a review. *East African Medical Journal*, 82(1), 40–6.

O'Brien, C. (2011). Addiction and dependence in DSM-V. *Addiction*, 106(5), 866–7.

O'Brien, C.P. (2005). Anticraving medications for relapse prevention: a possible new class of psychoactive medications. *American Journal of Psychiatry*, 162(8), 1423–31.

O'Brien, C.P., Childress, A.R., Ehrman, R., and Robbins, S.J. (1998). Conditioning factors in drug abuse: can they explain compulsion? *Journal of Psychopharmacology*, 12(1), 15–22.

O'Brien, C.P., Volkow, N., and Li, T.K. (2006). What's in a word? Addiction versus dependence in DSM-V. *American Journal of Psychiatry*, 163(5), 764–5.

Padaiga, Z., Subata, E., and Vanagas, G. (2007). Outpatient methadone maintenance treatment program. Quality of life and health of opioid-dependent persons in Lithuania. *Medicina (Kaunas)*, 43(3), 235–41.

Padian, N., Marquis, L., Francis, D.P., et al. (1987). Male-to-female transmission of human immunodeficiency virus. *Journal of the American Medical Association*, 258(6), 788–90.

Paraskevis, D., Nikolopoulos, G., Tsiara, C., et al. (2011). HIV-1 outbreak among injecting drug users in Greece, 2011: a preliminary report. *Euro Surveillance*, 16, 36.

Paterson, B.L., Backmund, M., Hirsch, G., and Yim, C. (2007). The depiction of stigmatization in research about hepatitis C. *International Journal of Drug Policy*, 18(5), 364–73.

Pauls, C.A. and Stemmler, G. (2003). Substance and bias in social desirability responding. *Personality and Individual Differences*, 35(2), 263–75.

Peer, K., Rennert, L., Lynch, K.G., Farrer, L., Gelernter, J., and Kranzler, H.R. (2013). Prevalence of DSM-IV and DSM-5 alcohol, cocaine, opioid, and cannabis use disorders in a largely substance dependent sample. *Drug and Alcohol Dependence*, 127(1–3), 215–19.

Pollock, N.K. and Martin, C.S. (1999). Diagnostic orphans: adolescents with alcohol symptom who do not qualify for DSM-IV abuse or dependence diagnoses. *American Journal of Psychiatry*, 156(6), 897–901.

Rawson, R.A., McCann, M.J., Flammino, F., et al. (2006). A comparison of contingency management and cognitive-behavioral approaches for stimulant-dependent individuals. *Addiction*, 101(2), 267–74.

Rhodes, T., Mikhailova, L., Sarang, A., et al. (2003). Situational factors influencing drug injecting, risk reduction and syringe exchange in Togliatti City, Russian Federation: a qualitative study of micro risk environment. *Social Science & Medicine*, 57(1), 39–54.

Rounsaville, B.J., Spitzer, R L., and Williams, J.B. (1986). Proposed changes in DSM-III substance use disorders: description and rationale. *American Journal of Psychiatry*, 143(4), 463–8.

Schuckit, M.A. and Saunders, J.B. (2006). The empirical basis of substance use disorders diagnosis: research recommendations for the Diagnostic and Statistical Manual of Mental Disorders, fifth edition (DSM-V). *Addiction*, 101(Suppl. 1), 170–3.

Schuckit, M.A. and Smith, T.L. (2001). A comparison of correlates of DSM-IV alcohol abuse or dependence among more than 400 sons of alcoholics and controls. *Alcoholism: Clinical and Experimental Research*, 25(1), 1–8.

Schuckit, M.A., Smith, T.L., and Landi, N.A. (2000). The 5-year clinical course of high-functioning men with DSM-IV alcohol abuse or dependence. *American Journal of Psychiatry*, 157(12), 2028–35.

Smith, S. (2007). Drugs that cause sexual dysfunction. *Psychiatry*, 6(3), 111–14.

Sobell, L.C and Sobell, M.B (1992). Timeline follow-back. In R.Z. Litten and J.P. Allen (eds.) *Measuring Alcohol Consumption*, pp. 41–72. New York: Humana Press.

Stimson, G.V. (1995). AIDS and injecting drug use in the United Kingdom, 1987–1993: the policy response and the prevention of the epidemic. *Social Science & Medicine*, 41(5), 699–716.

Stimson, GV., Alldritt, L.J., Dolan, K.A., Donoghoe, M.C., and Lart, R.A. (1988). *Injecting Equipment Exchange Schemes: Final Report.* London: Monitoring Research Group, Goldsmith's College.

Stoove, M.A., Gifford, S.M., and Dore, G.J. (2005). The impact of injecting drug use status on hepatitis C-related referral and treatment. *Drug and Alcohol Dependence*, 77(1), 81–6.

Strathdee, S., Patrick, D.M., Currie, S.L., et al. (1997). Needle exchange is not enough: lessons from the Vancouver injection drug use study. *AIDS*, 11, F59–F65.

Substance Abuse & Mental Health Services Administration (2012). *National Survey of Drug Use and Health: 2010–2011 NSDUH State Estimates of Substance Use and Mental Disorders.* Rockville, MD: Substance Abuse & Mental Health Services Administration.

Timko, C., Moos, R.H., Finney, J.W., and Lesar, M.D. (2000). Long-term outcomes of alcohol use disorders: comparing untreated individuals with those in Alcoholics Anonymous and formal treatment. *Journal of Studies on Alcohol*, 61(4), 529–40.

Turner, K.M., Hutchinson, S., Vickerman, P., et al. (2011). The impact of needle and syringe provision and opiate substitution therapy on the incidence of hepatitis C virus in injecting drug users: pooling of UK evidence. *Addiction*, 106(11), 1978–88.

United Nations Office on Drugs and Crime (2012). *World Drug Report.* Vienna: United Nations.

Vanichseni, S. and Sakuntanaga, P. (1990). Results of three seroprevalence surveys for HIV and IVDU in Bangkok. In *Sixth International Conference on AIDS*, June, San Francisco, CA.

Wang, P.W., Wu, H.C., Yen, C.N., et al. (2012). Change in quality of life and its predictors in heroin users receiving methadone maintenance treatment in Taiwan: an 18-month follow-up study. *American Journal of Drug and Alcohol Abuse*, 38(3), 213–19.

Waters, A.J., Shiffman, S., Sayette, M.A., et al. (2004). Cue-provoked craving and nicotine replacement therapy in smoking cessation. *Journal of Consulting and Clinical Psychology*, 72(6), 1136–43.

Weiss, F. (2005). Neurobiology of craving, conditioned reward and relapse. *Current Opinion in Pharmacology*, 5(1), 9–19.

Wisaksana, R., Indrati, A.K., Fibriani, A., et al. (2010). Response to first-line antiretroviral treatment among human immunodeficiency virus-infected patients with and without a history of injecting drug use in Indonesia. *Addiction*, 105(6), 1055–61.

Wodak, A. and Maher, L. (2010). The effectiveness of harm reduction in preventing HIV among injecting drug users. *New South Wales Public Health Bulletin*, 21(3–4), 69–73.

Wolfe, D. (2007). Paradoxes in antiretroviral treatment for injecting drug users: access, adherence and structural barriers in Asia and the former Soviet Union. *International Journal of Drug Policy*, 18(4), 246–54.

Wolfe, D., Carrieri, M.P., and Shepard, D. (2010). Treatment and care for injecting drug users with HIV infection: a review of barriers and ways forward. *The Lancet*, 376(9738), 355–66.

Wolfe, D. and Malinowska-Sempruch, K. (2004). *Illicit Drug Policies and the Global HIV Epidemic: Effects of UN and National Government Approaches.* New York: International Harm Reduction Development, Open Society Institute.

Wood, E., Kerr, T., Spittal, P.M., et al. (2003). An external evaluation of a peer-run 'unsanctioned' syringe exchange program. *Journal of Urban Health*, 80(3), 455–64.

Wood, E., Werb, D., Kazatchkine, M., et al. (2010). Vienna Declaration: a call for evidence-based drug policies. *The Lancet*, 376(9738), 310–12.

World Health Organization, United Nations Office on Drugs and Crime, and Joint United Nations Programme on HIV/AIDS (2012). *Technical Guide for Countries to Set Targets for Universal Access to HIV Prevention, Treatment and Care for Injecting Drug Users, 2012 Revision.* Geneva: WHO. Available at: <http://www.who.int/hiv/pub/idu/targets_universal_access/en/>.

Yen, C.F., Wu, H.Y., Yen, J.Y., and Ko, C.H. (2004). Effects of brief cognitive-behavioral interventions on confidence to resist the urges to use heroin and methamphetamine in relapse-related situations. *Journal of Nervous and Mental Disease*, 192(11), 788–91.

Zenilman, J. and Shahmanesh, M. (2011). *Sexually Transmitted Infections: Diagnosis, Management, and Treatment.* Sudbury, MA: Jones & Bartlett.

9.3

Alcohol

Robin Room

Alcohol and its effects

Alcoholic beverages have been consumed in most, if not all, human societies since the beginning of recorded history. Beverages containing ethanol (C_2H_5OH) can be fermented from a large number of organic materials that comprise carbohydrates, and in one part of the world or another, these products are prepared from fruits, berries, various grains, plants, honey, or milk. Under most circumstances, such fermented beverages can contain up to 14 per cent ethanol. The most widely commercialized fermented beverages are beer prepared from barley or other grains (usually 3–7 per cent ethanol), apple and other fruit ciders (usually 3–7 per cent ethanol), and grape wine (usually 8–14 per cent ethanol). Other fermented beverages are also common in particular cultures, often from home production or in commercial form: for example, sorghum or millet beers in Eastern and Southern Africa, palm wine toddy in West Africa and the Indian subcontinent, pulque (prepared from the maguey cactus) in Mexico, and rice wine (sake) in Eastern Asia.

Distilled beverages, in which ethanol is concentrated by evaporation and condensation from a fermented liquid, came to Europe from Arabia in the Middle Ages. In Europe, at first, their use was primarily medicinal, but by the 1600s, popular use as a social beverage spread rapidly. Distilled beverages can be made up of almost-pure ethanol, but those sold for drinking usually contain between 25 per cent and 50 per cent ethanol. Distilled alcohol is also added to wine, producing 'fortified wines' with about 20 per cent ethanol. Because distilled beverages and fortified wines do not readily spoil, they could be shipped over long distances, even before refrigeration and airtight packaging became available, and played a particularly important part in commerce and exploitation in the age of the European empires. Different cultures consume varying strengths of alcoholic beverages, often with water or a 'mixer' being added to distilled beverages and, in some cultures, also to wine and other fermented beverages.

Use-values of alcohol

Ethanol has many uses in human life. These include non-beverage uses as a fuel and as a solvent. Important beverage-related use-values include use as a medicine, as a religious sacrament, as a foodstuff, and as a thirst-quencher (Mäkelä 1983). But, alcoholic beverages have received special attention as a public health hazard because of their psychoactive properties. These properties carry with them another set of use-values: in terms of psychopharmacology, ethanol is a depressant, and alcoholic beverages have long been used to affect mood and feelings. With enough consumption, alcohol becomes an anodyne and, indeed, an anaesthetic; distilled spirits were used as an anaesthetic in surgical practice before the mid-nineteenth century. Many drinkers seek and appreciate the levels of intoxication which lie between mild mood alteration at one end of the spectrum and being comatose at the other.

The decisions to drink and how much to drink are, however, often not made by the individual in isolation. Drinking is usually a social act, and the pace and level of drinking are frequently subject to collective influence, with drinking together being seen as an expression of solidarity and community. Although drunkenness may be sought to relieve misery or loneliness, it is more commonly associated with sociable celebration.

Adverse effects

Alcohol consumption can have a variety of adverse effects, some of which are acute effects associated with the particular drinking event. Drinking progressively impairs physical coordination, cognition, and attention, resulting in an increased risk of accidents and injury. Above a threshold level, drinking can also affect intention and judgement, so intoxication potentially plays a causal role in violent behaviour and crime (Graham et al. 1998). This relation appears to be culturally mediated, because there is a substantial variation between cultures in the association of intoxication with violence and crime (Room 2001). A sufficient amount of alcohol may result in a potentially fatal overdose, by interrupting various autonomic bodily functions.

Other adverse effects of alcohol consumption are chronic effects related to a repeated pattern of drinking. Alcohol consumption can adversely affect nearly every organ of the body, although some effects are not common. Chronic conditions in which alcohol is implicated as an important cause include liver cirrhosis; cancers of the upper digestive tract, liver, and breast; cardiomyopathy; and gastritis and pancreatitis (Rehm et al. 2010). Through a variety of mechanisms, alcohol is also implicated in the incidence and course of infectious diseases (Parry et al. 2009).

Repeated heavy drinking can also adversely affect mental health; specific neurological disorders are associated with sustained heavy drinking. More common concomitants include depression and affective disorders. Alcoholism—the experience of loss of control over drinking, along with other psychological and physical sequelae—has also been considered a mental disorder in modern times. In current nosologies, alcoholism has been replaced by the terms *alcohol use disorder* (in *Diagnostic and Statistical Manual of Mental Disorders*, 5th edition (DSM5) terminology) and the *alcohol dependence syndrome* (in the *International Classification of Diseases*, 10th edition (ICD-10)).

The impairment of coordination and judgement produced by drinking potentially affects bystanders and the drinkers' acquaintances, friends, and family, as well as themselves: the effects can be through impairment of coordination or judgement during the drinking event, resulting in injury or distress, or through impairment of performance in family, friendship, work, and other social roles as a result of recurring drinking episodes (Laslett et al. 2011). The actual and potential adverse effects on others have historically been the primary justification for alcohol controls and other societal responses to problematic drinking (Room 1996); the effects on the adult drinker's own health have been of much less importance in determining public policy on alcohol.

Positive effects

For the drinker, and sometimes for those around, alcohol consumption can have positive effects. We have already mentioned the different use-values of alcohol—which mean that drinkers are usually willing to pay more than just the cost of production and distribution of the beverage. Apart from its valued effects on mental state, alcohol use has some positive outcomes on health. By far the most important of these, in terms of public health, is its potential for preventing cardiovascular disease (CVD). A fairly consistent finding in studies in several societies is that drinking at moderate levels protects against CVD (Klatsky 1999), although controversy about the existence and extent of this effect remains (e.g. Fillmore et al. 2006). The findings on the upper limit of drinking for such protection vary. Taken together, it appears that most of the protective effect can be gained with as little as one drink of an alcoholic beverage every second day (Maclure 1993). About half of this effect seems to come from inhibiting the build-up of plaque in arteries, whereas the other half seems to result from a relatively immediate effect of diminishing the likelihood of blood clots. To the extent this is true, irregular or occasional drinking is likely to have less protective effect.

Although it has been argued that this protection comes primarily from red wine constituents (particularly resveratrol) rather than from the ethanol, the balance of evidence favours an ethanol effect (Klatsky 1999). However, relatively little is known about how this effect interacts with or overlaps other risk and protective factors for chronic heart disease (CHD), such as regular exercise, diet, or taking aspirin (acetylsalicylic acid) or other pharmaceuticals (Criqui et al. 1998). The protective effect of alcohol appears to be higher for cigarette smokers than for non-smokers (Kozlowski et al. 1994).

Drinking is also often bad for the heart (Chadwick and Goode 1998; Poikolainen 1999). Studies have found that a pattern of intermittent heavy drinking, such as getting drunk every weekend, is associated with an elevated rate of coronary death (Kauhanen et al. 1997; Bagnardi et al. 2008), probably through mechanisms such as heart arrhythmias (Kupari and Koskinen 1998; McKee and Britton 1998). Data from countries in the former Soviet Union, where a pattern of intermittent intoxication is common, support the strong adverse effect of binge drinking on heart disease mortality (Rehm and Room 2009; Zaridze et al. 2011). During a period of deliberate restriction of alcohol supplies, the estimated per capita consumption in Russia, including the illicit alcohol market, fell from 14.2 L in 1984 to 10.7 L in 1987 (Shkolnikov and Nemtsov 1997)—a fall of 25 per cent. The death rate from ischaemic heart disease among males fell by 10 per cent

in the same period (Leon et al. 1997). This rate rose again when the restrictions lapsed, although this time, unlike between 1985 and 1988, other risk factors also changed.

Research on cumulative effects of alcohol
Effects on the drinker's health

In most studies, the relationship between amount of drinking and overall mortality is a J-shaped curve, with abstainers, and often, very light drinkers showing a higher mortality than those drinking a little more. This may be because, in these findings, a substantial part of the study population were older adults, and thus were at risk of mortality from CVD. Studies limited to younger cohorts typically found a monotonic relationship between amount of drinking and mortality (Andréasson et al. 1991; Rehm and Sempos 1995). Such an association might also be expected in any population, such as in some developing countries, that has a low rate of CVD.

The pattern of drinking is also a potentially important factor in mortality due to alcohol. Although this has long been obvious in casualty deaths, there is growing recognition of its significance in other causes of death, as implied by the earlier-mentioned Russian data. However, until recently, there have been only few measurements of this pattern in studies on alcohol and overall mortality. Variations among cultures in drinking habits may partly explain why the J-curve relation of volume of drinking to mortality shows different low-points in different cultures.

The risks and potential benefits associated with a given level of drinking, thus, vary with the age and sex of the drinker, and possibly with other sociocultural characteristics, as well as with the pattern and circumstances related to drinking. This variation has posed a considerable challenge because of political demand in a number of countries for advice on 'low-risk drinking' or 'safe drinking' guidelines. Whereas earlier guidelines were inclined to be stated only in terms of the volume of drinking, in line with the measurement methods of medical epidemiology literature, more recent guidelines have also emphasized limits on the amount consumed on a given occasion or day (Stockwell and Room 2012).

Current literature on the cumulative effects of drinking on health relies substantially on summations of prospective epidemiological literature, following the tradition set up by English et al. (1995). Using meta-analysis on studies of the relationship between volume of drinking and specific causes of death in which alcohol was either a risk or protective factor, the studies following this tradition derive attributable fractions for different levels of the volume of drinking and apply these fractions to segments of the population at each level in order to arrive at estimates on total lives and life-years lost and gained, subtracting the projected protective effects of alcohol from the negative burden. In addition to life-years lost, the study's most comprehensive indicator, disability-adjusted life years (DALYs), includes a projection of the burden of disability attributable to alcohol.

According to estimates for 2010, 3.9 per cent of the total burden of disease globally (as measured in DALYs) is attributable to alcohol (Lim et al. 2012). This compares with 6.3 per cent for tobacco and 1.0 per cent for illegal drugs. As earlier estimates showed (Ezzati et al. 2002), the alcohol share of the burden is highest in high-income societies, including Eastern Europe and Northern Asia, as well as in Latin America. The relative position of alcohol among risk factors is actually highest in middle-income countries, where it ranks first; although the alcohol share of all DALYs is lower in other developing regions, this fraction is calculated on the basis of a higher total burden of disease and disability in these countries.

Effects at the population level

So far, we have dealt with estimates of alcohol's effects at the individual level. The methodological difficulties in the studies underlying these estimates extend beyond those we have already discussed (Edwards et al. 1994). The estimates rely primarily on prospective epidemiological studies in which alcohol consumption is measured at one point in time; such a measurement is, at best, a poor surrogate for either of the main aspects of alcohol consumption as a risk factor—chronic effects of cumulated alcohol consumption or acute effects of intoxication at a specific event. In these studies, the effects of possible confounders are dealt with by statistically controlling for them in the analysis. But this can be problematic if drinking and the potential confounder are causally intertwined, as is true in the case of hypertension or tobacco smoking. Consider, for instance, a person who only smokes when under the influence of alcohol; controlling for that person's smoking behaviour potentially obscures some of the alcohol effect.

From a public health perspective, it is the effects at the population level, rather than the individual level, that are the main concern. If drinking was entirely a matter of individual choice and behaviour, and if the effects of drinking happened only to the drinker, then effects at the population level would be a simple aggregation of the effects at the individual level. But neither of these conditions is applicable. Drinking is by and large a social activity, and the drinking behaviour of a person is likely to influence and be influenced by those around that person. In a given population, the amounts drunk by infrequent or light drinkers and by heavy drinkers tend to move up and down in concert. Thus, if there is some health gain when those at the lower end of the spectrum increase their consumption, there will also be health losses from an increase in consumption for those at the top end of the spectrum. In view of this, it has been argued that the level of per-drinker consumption where the balance of health benefits and losses is optimized in a population is likely to be considerably lower than the optimum level of consumption for the individual drinker (Skog 1996). For instance, Skog (1996) argued that the optimum level of alcohol consumption with respect to mortality was likely to be lower than the present-day per-capita consumption of any nation in Western Europe. His argument is supported by findings of a generally positive relationship of the level of alcohol consumption with total mortality in time-series analysis of differenced data in a number of high-income countries (Norström and Ramstedt 2005).

By their design, the prospective studies typically used for investigations of alcohol's effects on mortality or morbidity do not measure the effects of drinking on others. Other types of individual-level studies, such as studies of the effects of drinking–driving (Perrine et al. 1989) or studies of homicide and other crimes (Wolfgang 1958), document the importance of such effects in terms of death or injury. But the strongest evidence of the magnitude of these effects comes from aggregate-level studies of the covariation of changes over time in a given society or place. Differenced time-series analyses in European societies

have suggested that a 1 L change in per capita alcohol consumption produces about a 1 per cent change in the overall mortality rate (Her and Rehm 1998; Norström 1996). Here again, however, drinking patterns and social circumstances are likely to make a difference. For instance, the drop in Russian total mortality during the alcohol restrictions of 1985–1988 implies a decline of about 2.7 per cent in age-standardized mortality for each 1 L drop in per capita consumption (calculated from Shkolnikov and Nemtsov (1997) and Leon et al. (1997)). Even specifically for heart disease, any protective effects from changes in low-level drinking seem to be outbalanced in the population as a whole by negative effects from changes at high-consumption levels, levels of consumption typical in high-income societies. Thus, time-series analyses of differenced data on alcohol consumption and on CHD mortality in 14 European countries found no evidence of net protective effects and some evidence of net adverse effect (Hemström 2001; Ramstedt 2006).

Alcohol as an issue in public health
Shifting societal responses to problematic drinking

Efforts to control problematic drinking date back to the beginning of recorded history. These efforts have been many-sided, including informal responses in the family and community, as well as governmental controls. Religious teachings and movements have often been directed against drinking or intoxication: Moslems are forbidden by their faith to drink at all, and drinking is also discouraged or forbidden in at least some branches of all the major world religions.

In the last few centuries, European and Europe-derived societies have been hosts to conflicting trends in terms of alcohol issues. The production of alcoholic beverages became an important part of European economies and of imperial domination and trade in the age of European colonization. Alcohol production and exports took on political importance not only in the wine cultures of Southern Europe, but also in such countries as the Netherlands and Britain. In America, in the late-eighteenth century, distilled spirits was the only profitable way to get grain to market (Rorabaugh 1979). In recent decades, alcohol beverage industries have become increasingly internationalized and concentrated (Jernigan 2010), and multinational companies, mostly based in Europe or North America, have pressed with considerable success to open up global markets for alcohol.

Starting in the early 1800s, there were substantial waves of popular, and eventually, governmental response to the problems that were resulting from the very heavy consumption of alcoholic beverages in English-speaking and Northern European societies (Blocker 1989; Levine 1991). As a culmination of decades of popular temperance movements, in the early twentieth century, alcohol prohibition was adopted in 13 countries (Schrad 2010) and imposed on indigenous people in colonial territories, and stringent controls were placed on the availability of alcohol in some other countries. Although alcohol's impact on public order and morals and on family life were more central to the temperance movement thinking than the public health issues, mainstream thought in medicine and public health acknowledged the substantial adverse impacts of alcohol on health (Emerson 1932), and prohibition or an alternative, stringent controls on the availability of alcohol (Catlin 1931), were often identified with the public health interest.

In the United States, and some other societies which had prohibited or greatly restricted alcohol availability, there was a strong reaction against it by the early 1930s, with middle-class youth in the lead (Room 1984a, 1984b). In this cultural–political context, as the new generation moved into professional and research positions, adverse effects of alcohol were downplayed or denied (Herd 1992; Katcher 1993), and alcohol issues almost disappeared from public health textbooks and discourse. Any problems with drinking were seen as attributable to a relatively small cadre of alcoholics, unable to control their drinking because of a mysterious predisposing factor. As late as 1968, the main emphasis of the American Public Health Association was on building treatment capacity for alcoholism (Cross 1968).

The 'new public health' approach

The last three decades of the twentieth century saw the rise of what has been termed in the alcohol literature the 'new public health' approach (Beauchamp 1976; Tigerstedt 1999) to alcohol issues. This approach brought together several strands of research and philosophy. In contrast to a concept in terms of 'alcoholism', the approach was premised on a disaggregated approach: there was a diversity of alcohol-related problems, fairly widely distributed among the drinking population (Knupfer 1967; World Health Organization (WHO), Expert Committee on Problems Related to Alcohol Consumption 1980). It was noted that for many problems, the heaviest drinkers accounted for only a minority, because there were so many more drinking at somewhat lower levels (Moore and Gerstein 1981); picking up Rose's (1981) phrase, Kreitman (1986) termed this the 'preventive paradox'. Attention was, therefore, paid not only to the heaviest drinkers, but also to the whole range of drinking levels, and indeed, to the distribution of consumption in the population (Ledermann 1956; De Lint and Schmidt 1968). What happens with moderate drinkers, it was argued, influences the social climate for heavy drinking, because drinking is largely a social activity, marked by mutual influences and norms of reciprocity (Bruun et al. 1975a; Skog 1985). In a given population, it was found that rates of alcohol-related problems tend to rise and fall with changes in the level of consumption (Seeley 1960). Controls on the availability of alcohol, including taxes, affect the level of consumption, and thus, also the rates of alcohol-related problems (Seeley 1960; Terris 1967; Popham et al. 1976). The level of alcohol consumption in a population, and controls on alcohol availability, is thus seen as a public health concern, and part of a society's overall 'alcohol policy' (Bruun et al. 1975a).

In enumerating the elements of the new public health approach, we have given references for early statements of each element. It will be seen that the strands of this approach were woven together gradually over a period of some years. A 1975 report by an international group of researchers (Bruun et al. 1975a) became a pivotal document for the approach. A few years later, the approach was given an authoritative endorsement in the United States by a committee of the National Academy of Sciences (Moore and Gerstein 1981). The most recent restatement of the approach by an international group of scholars appeared in 2010 (Babor et al. 2010), with a somewhat parallel analysis oriented to the developing world (Room et al. 2002).

The approach has had considerable influence on WHO programmes in the field of alcohol (Room 2005; WHO 2007). For instance, action on the availability and marketing of alcohol and on pricing policies are key elements of WHO's Global Strategy to Reduce the Harmful Effects of Alcohol, adopted in 2010 (WHO 2010). At national levels, there has been a considerable variation in its influence on policy. In Sweden, where it is known as the Total Consumption Model, it attained dominance as the basis for official policy (Sutton 1998). However, policies based on this approach have been eroded as a consequence of Sweden's accession to the European Union (Holder et al. 1998). The approach also has had considerable backing in other Nordic countries.

In English-speaking countries, it has encountered substantial resistance in the cultural–political realm. Those allied with the alcoholic beverage industry have strongly attacked the approach, both in analyses and polemics (e.g. Mott 1991; Grant and Litvak 1998) and through direct political action to remove official proponents (Room 1984c). An approach that contemplates government regulation and influencing of private consumer choices is also unwelcome to those committed to consumer sovereignty and the primacy of individual choice (e.g. Peele 1987). Often, proponents of approaches seeking to 'domesticate' drinking—to reduce problems from drinking by integrating it into everyday life—have portrayed the new public health approach as antithetical to this (Olsson 1990), although some researchers have noted that there is no necessary antithesis (Whitehead 1979).

In terms of its influence on policy, the approach has undoubtedly had some effect in strengthening the defence of existing control structures and regulations. But efforts to get the approach adopted as the practical base for policy have met with resistance and failure in a number of countries (Hawks 1993; Room 2004). One response to this resistance has been some calls for an alternative approach (Stockwell et al. 1997), arguing that policy measures directed at heavy and problematic drinkers are more politically acceptable than measures directed at all drinkers.

The policy approach offered as an alternative is a focus on harm reduction, primarily by reducing instances of intoxication or insulating the drinkers from harm (Plant et al. 1997; Stimson et al. 2007). However, there is in fact usually no conflict between approaches aimed at total consumption and approaches aiming to reduce harm from heavy drinking. As Stockwell et al. (1997) noted, 'aggregate consumption levels are in fact likely to fall if effective [harm reduction] strategies are introduced' (p. 6). Conversely, many measures that affect the whole drinking population—taxation being a good example—are especially hard on heavier drinkers. Nor are targeted harm reduction measures necessarily more politically acceptable than measures that affect all drinkers. Old systems of rationing and individual buyer surveillance (Järvinen 1991), which were directed specifically at restraining heavy drinking, are now politically unacceptable in any high-income society, although rationing, at least, was highly effective as a targeted prevention measure (Norström 1987). Thus the first act of a new government elected in Australia's Northern Territory was to dismantle a new system requiring electronic identification to purchase alcohol, which had put into effect a ban on alcohol purchases by specific problematic drinkers (Room 2013).

Beyond its specific features, the controversy over the new public health approach replicates familiar patterns of controversy over public health approaches in general, particularly when those approaches impinge on familiar and valued patterns of behaviour, with substantial economic interests at stake. At the level of the knowledge base, the approach has had considerable success: The empirical evidence underlying the approach has considerably strengthened since the approach was first put forward. At a political level, however, the approach has had only limited success, and primarily in areas peripheral to its main focus—that is, in drinking–driving and minimum-age limits for drinkers.

Strategies of prevention and control and their effectiveness

Simplifying them, there are seven main strategies to minimize alcohol problems. One strategy is to educate or persuade people not to use alcohol or about ways to use it so as to limit harm. A second strategy, a kind of negative persuasion, is to deter drinking-related behaviour with the threat of penalties. A third strategy, in the positive direction, is to provide alternatives to drinking or to drink-related activities. A fourth strategy is in one way or another to insulate the user from harm. A fifth strategy is to regulate availability of alcohol or the conditions of its use; prohibition of supply may be regarded as a special case of such regulation. A sixth strategy is to work with social or religious movements oriented to reducing alcohol problems. And, a seventh strategy is to treat or otherwise help people who have trouble with their drinking habits. We will consider, in turn, these strategies and the evidence on their effectiveness.

Education and persuasion

In principle, education can be offered to any segment of the population in a variety of venues, but it is usually education of youth in schools that first comes to mind in the prevention of alcohol problems. Community-based prevention programmes, which are often also directed at adults, also may include an educational component.

Education offers new information or ways of thinking and leaves it to the listener to draw conclusions concerning beliefs and behaviour. However, most alcohol education programmes go beyond this. A common theme in North American evaluative literature on alcohol education is that 'knowledge-only' approaches do not result in changes in behaviour (Botvin 1995). School-based alcohol education has, thus, usually had a persuasional element, aiming to influence students in a particular direction.

Persuasion is directly concerned with changing beliefs or behaviours, and may or may not also offer information. Mass media campaigns aimed at persuasion have been a very common component of prevention programmes for alcohol-related problems, but this can also be pursued through other media and modalities.

In most societies, public health-oriented persuasion about alcohol must compete with a variety of other persuasive messages, including those intended to sell alcoholic beverages. The evidence that alcohol advertising influences teenagers and young adults towards increased drinking and problematic drinking is becoming stronger (Casswell et al. 2002). Even where alcohol advertising is not allowed in the mass media, these messages are often conveyed to consumers and potential consumers in a variety of other ways.

Evidence on effectiveness

The literature on effectiveness of educational approaches is dominated by studies on school-based education from the United States. This means that alcohol education has usually been in the context of drug and tobacco education and that the emphasis has been on abstention (Beck 1998) or at least on delaying the start of drinking, in cultural circumstances where the median age of actually starting to drink is about 13 years although the minimum legal drinking age is 21 years. In general, despite the best efforts of a generation of researchers, this literature has had difficulty showing substantial and lasting effects (Foxcroft et al. 2003; Gorman et al. 2007). There is a good argument from general principles for alcohol education in the context of consumer and health, but there is little evidence from the formal evaluation literature at this point of its effectiveness beyond the short term (Babor et al. 2010).

Persuasive media campaigns have also been a favourite modality in many places in recent decades. In general, evaluations of such campaigns have been able to demonstrate impacts on knowledge and awareness about substance use problems, but show little success in affecting attitudes and behaviours (Babor et al. 2010). As with school education approaches, there are hints in literature that more success may come from influencing the community around the drinker—in terms of attitudes of significant others or popular support for alcohol policy measures—than from directly persuading the drinker himself or herself. Thus, media messages can be effective as agenda-setting mechanisms in the community, increasing or sustaining public support for other preventive strategies (Casswell et al. 1989).

Deterrence

In its broadest sense, deterrence means simply the threat of negative sanctions or disincentives for behaviour—a form of negative persuasion. Criminal laws deter in two ways: by general deterrence, which is the effect of the law in preventing a prohibited behaviour in the population as a whole; and specific deterrence, which is the effect of the law in discouraging those who have been caught from doing it again (Ross 1982). A law will have a greater preventive effect and be cheaper to administer to the extent it has a strong general deterrence effect.

Prohibitions on driving after drinking more than a specified amount are now in effect in most nations (WHO 2004). In many societies, there have also been laws against drinking in public places, against public drunkenness (being in a public place while intoxicated) and against obnoxious behaviour while intoxicated. Other common prohibitions are concerned with producing or selling alcoholic beverages outside state-regulated channels and with aspects of drinking under a specified minimum age.

Evidence on effectiveness

Drinking–driving legislation, such as 'per se' laws outlawing driving while at or above a defined blood-alcohol level, has been shown to be effective in changing behaviour and reducing rates of alcohol-related problems (Ross 1982; Hingson 1996; Babor et al. 2010). The effect is through both general and specific deterrence. The quickness and certainty of punishment as well as its severity are important in the deterrent value (too much severity tends to undercut the quickness and certainty). Drinking–driving is an ideal area for applying general deterrence, as the gains from breaking the law are limited and automobile drivers typically have something to lose by being caught.

Many English-speaking and Scandinavian countries have had a tradition of criminalizing drinking in public places or public drunkenness as such. The trend in the 1970s and following was to decriminalize public drunkenness, although in many places it remains illegal. In the 1990s and following, there has been some trend to criminalize drinking in specific public places (Pennay and Room 2012). Criminalization of such behaviours has some effect in moving behaviour around, but is not very effective in changing the behaviour of marginalized heavy drinkers who have little to lose.

Providing and encouraging alternative activities

Another strategy, in principle involving positive incentives, is to provide and seek to encourage activities that are an alternative to drinking or to activities closely associated with drinking. This includes initiatives such as making soft drinks available as an alternative to alcoholic beverages, providing locations for sociability as an alternative to taverns, and providing and encouraging recreational activities as an alternative to leisure activities involving drinking. Job creation and skill development programmes are other examples.

Evidence on effectiveness

'Boredom' and 'because there's nothing else to do' are certainly among the reasons given by some for drinking. And, there are often good reasons of general social policy for providing and encouraging alternative activities. But as has been noted, the problem with alternatives to drinking is that drinking combines so well with many of them. Soft drinks are indeed an alternative to alcoholic beverages for quenching thirst, but they may also serve as a mixer in an alcoholic drink. Involvement in sports may go along with drinking as well as replace it. The few evaluation studies of providing alternative activities, again from a restricted number of societies, have generally not shown lasting effects on drinking behaviour (Moskowitz et al. 1983; Norman et al. 1997), although they undoubtedly often serve a general social purpose in broadening opportunities for the disadvantaged (Carmona and Stewart 1996).

Insulating use from harm

A major social strategy for reducing alcohol-related problems in many societies has been measures to separate the drinker, and particularly heavy drinkers, from potential harm. This separation can be physical (in terms of distance or walls), it can be temporal, or it can be cultural (e.g. defining the drinking occasion as 'time out' from normal responsibilities). These 'harm-reduction' strategies, as they are called in the context of illicit drugs, are often built into cultural arrangements around drinking, but can also be the object of purposive programmes and policies (Moore and Gerstein 1981), such as promotion of 'designated drivers', where one person in a social group is chosen to abstain and drive in the particular social situation (DeJong and Hingson 1998).

A variety of modifications to the driving environment positively affect casualties associated with drinking and driving, along with other casualties. These include mandatory use of seat belts, airbags, and improvements in the safety of vehicles and roads. Many other practical measures to separate intoxication episodes from casualties and other adverse consequences have been put into practice, although usually without formal evaluation.

Evidence on effectiveness

Drinking–driving countermeasures are a prime example of an approach in terms of insulating drinking behaviour from harm, as they seek to reduce alcohol-related traffic casualties without necessarily stopping or reducing alcohol use (Evans 1991). There is substantial evidence on the success of a range of such countermeasures, including environmental change approaches as well as deterrence (DeJong and Hingson 1998; Babor et al. 2010). Some environmental measures that reduce traffic casualties in general—such as requiring the wearing of seat belts in cars or providing sidewalks separated from the road—may prevent casualties associated with intoxication even more than other casualties.

Regulating the availability and conditions of use

In terms of the substantial harm to health and public order they can cause, alcoholic beverages are not ordinary commodities. Governments have, thus, often actively intervened in the markets for such beverages, far beyond usual levels of state intervention in markets for commodities.

Total prohibition can be viewed as an extreme form of regulation of the market. In this circumstance, where no one is licensed to sell alcohol, the state has no formal control over the conditions of the sales that occur nevertheless, and there are no legal sales interests, controlled through licensing, to cooperate with the state in market regulation.

With a general prohibition, typically, the consumption of alcohol does fall in the population, and there are also declines in the rates of the direct consequences of drinking such as cirrhosis or alcohol-related mental disorders (Moore and Gerstein 1981; Teasley 1992). But prohibition also brings with it characteristic negative consequences, including the emergence and growth of an illicit market and the crime associated with this. Partly for this reason, alcohol prohibition at a national level is now a live option only in Islamic societies, where the law reflects religious belief, which helps to sustain compliance. Local-area alcohol prohibitions are more widespread.

The features of alcohol control regimes that regulate the legal market in alcohol vary greatly. Special taxes on alcohol are very common, imposed often as much for revenue as for public health considerations. Most societies have minimum-age limits forbidding sales to underage customers and many have regulations forbidding sales to the already intoxicated. Often, the regulations include limiting the number of sales outlets, restricting hours and days of sale, and limiting sales to special stores or drinking places. Rationing of alcohol purchases— limiting the amount individuals can buy in a given time period—has also been used as a means of regulating availability. Regulations restricting or forbidding advertising of alcoholic beverages attempt to limit or channel efforts by private interests to increase demand for particular alcoholic beverages. Such regulations potentially complement education and persuasion efforts. State monopolization on sales of some or all alcoholic beverages at the retail and/or wholesale level has also been commonly been used as a mechanism to minimize alcohol-related harm (Room 1993).

Effectiveness of specific types of regulation on availability

The decades since the 1970s have seen the development of a burgeoning literature on the effects of alcohol control measures.

Reference guides for communities, summarizing the research evidence and attuned to particular national or regional conditions, are becoming available (e.g. Neves et al. 1998; Grover 1999). Specific types of regulation of the alcohol market, and the evidence on their effectiveness, are discussed as follows:

Minimum-age limits

A minimum-age limit is a partial prohibition, applied to one segment of the population. There is a strong evaluation literature showing the effectiveness of establishing and enforcing minimum-age limits in reducing alcohol-related problems (Babor et al. 2010). However, this literature is mostly based on North America, focusing mostly on youthful driving casualties and evaluating reduction from and increases to age 21 years as the limit, a minimum-age limit higher than in most societies. There is limited evidence on the applicability of the literature's findings in other societies and where youth cultures may be less automobile-focused (but see Møller 2002; Kypri et al. 2006).

Taxes and other price increases

Generally, consumers show some response on the price of alcoholic beverages, as on all other commodities. If the price goes up, the drinker will drink less; data from high-income societies suggests this is at least as true of the heavy drinker as of the occasional drinker (Babor et al. 2010). Studies have found that alcohol tax increases reduce the rates of traffic casualties, of cirrhosis mortality, and of incidents of violence (Cook 2007).

Limiting sales outlets and hours and conditions of sale

A substantial body of literature shows that levels and patterns of alcohol consumption, and rates of alcohol-related casualties and other problems, are influenced by such sales restrictions, which typically make the purchase of alcoholic beverages slightly inconvenient or influence the setting of and after drinking (Babor et al. 2010; Livingston 2013). Enforced rules influencing 'house policies' in drinking places on not serving intoxicated customers, for example, have also been shown to have some effect (Saltz 1997).

Monopolizing production or sale

Studies of the effects of privatizing retail alcohol monopolies have often shown some increase in levels of alcohol consumption and problems, in part because the number of outlets and hours of sale typically increase with privatization (Her et al. 1999) and partly also because the new private interests typically exert political influence for further increases in availability. From a public health perspective, it is the retail level that is important, although monopolization of the production or wholesale level may facilitate revenue collection and effective control of the market.

Rationing sales

Rationing the amount of alcohol sold to an individual potentially directly impacts on heavy drinkers and has been shown to reduce levels both of intoxication-related problems such as violence and of drinking-history-related problems such as cirrhosis mortality (Schechter 1986; Norström 1987). But, although a form of rationing—the medical prescription system—is well accepted in most societies for psychoactive medications, it has proved politically unacceptable nowadays for alcoholic beverages in high-income societies.

Advertising and promotion restrictions

Many societies have regulations on advertising and other promotion of sales of alcoholic beverages (WHO 2004). Although it is well accepted that advertising can strongly affect consumer choices on products in the market, it has proved difficult to measure the effects of advertising on demand for alcoholic beverages as a whole, partly because the effects are likely to be cumulative and long-term, making them difficult to measure. However, the evidence on the effects of advertising and promotion on overall demand has become somewhat stronger in recent literature (Casswell 1995; Casswell and Zhang 1998; Babor et al. 2010).

Social and religious movements and community action

Substantial reductions in alcohol-related problems have often been the result of spontaneous social and religious movements, which put a major emphasis on quitting intoxication or drinking. In recent decades, efforts have also been made to form partnerships between state organizations and non-governmental groups to work on alcohol problems, often at the level of the local community. There has been an active tradition of community action projects on alcohol problems, often using a range of prevention strategies (Giesbrecht et al. 1990; Greenfield and Zimmerman 1993; Holmila 1997; Holder 1998). School-based prevention efforts have also moved increasingly to try to involve the community, in line with general perceptions that such multifaceted strategies will be more effective (Paglia and Room 1999).

Although some of the biggest historical reductions in alcohol problem rates have resulted from spontaneous and autonomous social or religious movements, support or collaboration from a government can easily be perceived as official co-optation or manipulation (Room 1997). Thus, there is considerable question about the extent to which such movements can or should become an instrument of government prevention policies.

Evidence on effectiveness

In the short term, movements of religious or cultural revival can be highly effective in reducing levels of drinking and of alcohol-related problems. Alcohol consumption in the United States fell by about half in the first flush of temperance enthusiasm in 1830–1845 (Moore and Gerstein 1981). Rates of serious crime are reported to have fallen for a while to a fraction of their previous level in Ireland in the wake of Father Mathew's temperance crusade (Room 1983). The enthusiasm that sustains such movements tends to decay over time, although they often leave behind new customs and institutions of much longer duration. For instance, although the days when the historic temperance movement in English-speaking societies was strong are long gone, the movement had the long-lasting effect of largely removing drinking from the workplace in these societies.

Particularly in the developing world, religious or cultural renewal movements oriented to reducing or prohibiting drinking are often a strong avenue of preventive action (Room et al. 2002). A reform movement among poor indigenous people in a region of Ecuador touched off in 1987 by religious renewal movements and an earthquake appears to have had lasting effects on popular sobriety (Butler 2006).

Treatment and other help

Providing effective treatment or other help for drinkers who find they cannot control their drinking can be regarded as an obligation of a just and humane society. The help can take several forms: a specific treatment system for alcohol problems, professional help in general health or welfare systems, or non-professional assistance in mutual-help movements. To the extent such help is effective, it is also a means of preventing or reducing future alcohol-related problems in the person helped, although its effectiveness at a population level is less clear.

Treatments for alcohol problems need not be complex or expensive. The evaluation literature suggests that brief outpatient interventions aimed at changing cognitions and behaviour around drinking are as effective in most circumstances as longer and more intensive treatment (Finney and Monahan 1998; Long et al. 1998). Positive results from such interventions in primary healthcare settings were shown in a WHO study that included a number of countries (Babor et al. 1994).

Evidence on effectiveness

In terms of the effects of treatment on those who come for it, there is good evidence on the effectiveness of treatment for alcohol problems. Typically, the improvement rate from a single episode of treatment is about 20 per cent higher than the no-treatment condition: further treatment episodes are often needed. Brief treatment interventions or mutual-help approaches usually result in net savings in social and health costs associated with the heavy drinker (at least where healthcare is not self-paid), as well as improving the quality of life (Holder and Cunningham 1992; Holder et al. 1992).

The effectiveness of providing treatment as a strategy for reducing rates of alcohol problems in a society is more equivocal. In a North American context, it has been argued that the steep increase in alcohol problems treatment provision and mutual-help group membership in recent decades contributed to reducing alcohol problems rates (Smart and Mann 1990). But the strength of the evidence for this contention is disputed (Holder 1997; Smart and Mann 1997). A treatment system for alcohol problems is an important part of an integrated national alcohol policy, but as an instrument of prevention—of reducing societal rates of alcohol problems—it is unlikely to be very cost-effective (Chisholm et al. 2004).

Building integrated alcohol policies

Alcohol policy at a community or societal level

Often, the different strategies for preventing alcohol problems appear to be synergistic in their effects (DeJong and Hingson 1998). For instance, controls on availability are more likely to be adopted, continued, and respected when the public has been successfully persuaded of their effects and effectiveness. But strategies can also work at cross-purposes: a prohibition policy, for instance, makes it difficult to pursue measures that insulate drinking from harm.

In a society where alcohol is a regular item of consumption, in view of the resulting rates of alcohol-related social and health problems, there is a strong justification for adopting a comprehensive policy concerning alcohol, taking into account production, marketing, and consumption, and the prevention and treatment of alcohol-related problems. In recent years, the idea that there

should be an integrated alcohol policy at community or national levels, reaching across the many sectors of government and civil society that deal with alcohol issues, has become a common public health aim, although accomplishing this has often proved difficult (Smart and Mann 1997; Crombie et al. 2007; WHO 2011).

In terms of strategies we have reviewed for managing and reducing the rates of alcohol problems in the society, there is a clear evidence for effectiveness and cost-effectiveness of measures regulating the availability and conditions of use, and for some of the measures which insulate use from harm. With respect to some aspects of alcohol problems, notably drinking–driving, deterrence measures also fall in the same category. Despite their perennial popularity, evidence of the effectiveness of education or persuasion and treatment strategies in reducing societal rates of problems is limited at best. Education and treatment are good things for a society and a government to be doing about alcohol problems, but they do not constitute in themselves a public health policy on alcohol (Babor et al. 2010). These strategies will nevertheless be pursued in most societies, and they can best be pursued with attention to using relatively cost-effective methods, and to integrating targets and messages with other aspects of alcohol policy.

Alcohol policy in a global perspective

Apart from lapsed agreements made a century ago among the European colonial powers about control of the spirits trade in Africa (Bruun et al. 1975b), there is little tradition of collaboration on alcohol policy at the international level. It has been largely up to each nation to cope on its own with the serious social and health problems associated with drinking. Although alcohol smuggling has a long history, the nation-state could usually rely on distances and traditional trade barriers to keep alcohol issues largely a matter within its borders, in terms of the supply as well as of the problems.

Since the 1980s, an accelerated rate of economic globalization has been seen, which has increasingly rendered obsolete the assumption that alcohol issues are local issues. This globalization affects alcohol issues in three main ways. The first of these is the influence of a global ideology of free markets. In its sweep, this ideology has caught up and dismantled a variety of market arrangements that served to hold down and to structure alcohol consumption. State and provincial alcohol monopolies in North America were weakened or dismantled (Her et al. 1999). In Eastern Europe and the countries in transition, alcohol monopolies were swept away along with most other governmental intrusions in the market (Moskalewicz 1993). Many of the municipally-run beer halls in Southern African countries were privatized (Jernigan 1997). In line with the general ideology, privatization of alcohol production and distribution has been often suggested, abetted or imposed on developing countries by international development agencies (White and Batia 1998). Where the market is organized in a state licensing system for private interests, free-market ideology has often overridden any concerns about public health risks or community need (Room 2004).

Second, trade agreements, trade dispute mechanisms, and the growth of new sales media have effectively reduced the ability of national and subnational governments to control their local alcohol markets. The influence of trade agreements and trade dispute decisions in breaking down alcohol controls, including control of price through taxation, has been most fully documented for North America (Room et al. 2006) and Europe (Tigerstedt 1990; Holder et al. 1998), but these mechanisms also operate in the developing world. For instance, average taxes on alcoholic beverages in South Korea were lowered in 2000 as a result of complaints to the World Trade Organization by the European Union and the United States (Kim 2000). In 2010–2012, the European Union and United States, joined by Australia, Canada, and five other countries, have argued that Thailand's proposed warning labels on alcohol bottles would violate trade agreements, a first step towards seeking a trade court judgement (O'Brien 2013).

Third, alcohol production, distribution, and marketing became increasingly globalized (Room et al. 2002; Jernigan 2010). Transnational alcohol companies expanded rapidly into low- and middle-income countries in search of new markets, benefiting from weak policy environments and the sweeping tide of market liberalization. Although most alcoholic beverages are still produced in the country in which they are sold, industrially produced beverages were increasingly produced in plants owned, co-owned, or licensed by multinational firms. To promote increased sales, these firms have been able to transform and step up the marketing techniques used in the national market, bringing to bear all the marketing resources and expertise they have developed in other markets.

In light of these converging trends, there is a growing need for mechanisms to express public health interests in alcohol issues at the international level, both in trade agreements and settlements of trade disputes, and in creating mutual obligations for one nation to back up rather than subvert the alcohol regulations and policies of another.

Ways forward for the public health interest

At international levels

The comparative risk analysis in the WHO's estimation of the global burden of disease (GBD) has underlined the substantial role of alcohol in death and disability, particularly in middle- and high-income countries. There are also substantial harms from drinking to others, and these harms are mostly not included in the GBD frame (Laslett et al. 2011). The high rates of harm reflect not only the levels of use and heavy use of alcohol, but also that current expert evaluations rate it as intrinsically among the most harmful of psychoactive substances that humans use (Nutt et al. 2010).

These findings contrast with the current omission of alcohol from international systems of control of psychoactive substances. International markets in most commonly used psychoactive substances are under strict control under the three drug treaties of 1961, 1971, and 1988. International markets in tobacco are also controlled, though more lightly, under a 2003 Framework Convention. Alcohol is thus unique as a commonly used and problematic psychoactive substance on which there is no current international control agreement. As noted, this has left the path open for international limits to be placed on national and local control policies through trade agreements and disputes (Ziegler, 2009; O'Brien 2013).

Apart from any specific treaty provisions, the lack of a treaty status for alcohol has also had implications for resources devoted to alcohol issues in intergovernmental agencies. In 2013, the number of posts at such agencies devoted to alcohol issues, almost all at the WHO, was in the single digits. In contrast, the number of posts in intergovernmental agencies devoted to tobacco was in the dozens, and to drugs in the hundreds. The treaty processes also mean that, both for drugs and for tobacco, there are regular meetings of parties to the treaties to review progress and consider further actions.

Symbolically, in the early 2010s there was increased recognition at the international level of the importance of alcohol control in public health. In 2010, The World Health Assembly (WHA) adopted a Global Strategy for the Reduction of Harmful Use of Alcohol (WHO 2010). In 2013, implementing United Nations decisions to put a global focus on preventing and controlling non-communicable diseases, the WHA acted to support a draft action plan (WHO 2013a) and a global monitoring framework (WHO 2013b) which included specific attention to alcohol as one of four main risk factors, although the targets and actions specified for alcohol were much less specific and ambitious than those for other risk factors such as tobacco. However, these actions were not accompanied by increases in resources for implementation concerning alcohol issues.

To remedy the deficit in alcohol control at the international level, there are growing calls for a framework convention on alcohol control to be negotiated under the WHO auspices or otherwise, on the model of the tobacco convention (Anonymous 2007; Room et al. 2008), although the advisability of this path has been contested (Taylor and Dhillon 2013, and commentaries). Another option was briefly discussed at the 2012 WHO Expert Committee on Drug Dependence: scheduling alcohol under one of the United Nations drug conventions. This was referred for consideration at a future Expert Committee meeting (WHO 2012, p. 16). It is clear that alcohol would qualify for scheduling under the treaties' criteria. Scheduling alcohol under a drug treaty would provide de-facto insulation from trade treaty restrictions on control, and indeed provide mechanisms for countries to control imports. Such a step would presumably require amending at least one of the drug treaties to allow for regulated domestic markets for non-medical use of at least some scheduled drugs, but moves in the 2010s towards regulated cannabis markets point anyway toward such a development.

Apart from the sphere of intergovernmental action and agencies, there has also been a deficit in international activity in the sphere of non-governmental organizations (NGOs). At a global level, the main NGOs active have been the Global Alcohol Policy Alliance, the International Council on Alcohol and Addictions and the World Medical Association; at regional levels, there are such bodies as Eurocare and Forut. While the global alcohol industry is well organized to oppose effective alcohol policies, through such organs as the International Center on Alcohol Policy (Bakke and Endal 2010; Casswell 2013), the alcohol area lacks the dense networks of public health-oriented international NGO activity found in fields such as tobacco and drugs.

At national and subnational levels

As outlined earlier, over the last 40 years, a substantial literature has emerged which allows a differentiation of prevention strategies and policies in terms of their effectiveness. Some strategies—for example, school education, public information campaigns, and provision of alternatives—are often politically popular but have limited or no effect. A few strategies that have proved effective—notably, drinking–driving countermeasures—have been applied in a number of countries. Other effective strategies—especially controls on price and availability—have been widely resisted in the political process, and undercut by trade agreements. Ironically, our knowledge of the effectiveness of availability and price controls has often come from studies made possible by the fact that the stricter controls of the past were being dismantled (Olsson et al. 2002).

From the perspective of promoting public health, the lessons of this literature need to be applied. We now have much better evidence than formerly of the scope and distribution of the problems. We have a literature on policy impacts with good information on cost-effectiveness. The need is to focus policy attention, and to build public support for action. A wide range of government departments are responsible for the diversity of problems due to drinking. Police and justice agencies deal with drink-driving and with alcohol-related violence; welfare departments and agencies deal with family problems and immiseration when a parent drinks heavily; hospitals and health services deal with sickness and injury due to drinking. Typically, different levels of government each have some responsibility: for instance, taxes may be a national responsibility, hospitals a state or provincial task, welfare a local government task. Efforts to coordinate across departments and levels of government also run up against the issue that the State has mixed interests with respect to alcohol sales (Mäkelä and Viikari 1977), and are often impeded by alcohol not being a major priority for any of the players. Both at national and subnational levels, effective action will require that priorities be set in a situation where responsibilities are often divided and dispersed.

It is clear that, with sufficient political will, the difficulties can be transcended. For instance, in Victoria, Australia, the commitment to drive down the loss of lives—particularly young lives—from traffic crashes drove effective cross-department coordination and a series of policy and enforcement measures—some involving alcohol. Between 1989 and 2004, traffic deaths were halved (Johnston 2006), and they have since fallen further. The steady success of efforts to decrease the proportion of the population smoking cigarettes is another example of a good public health result with concerted action. Just such focused and coordinated attention and action will be required to drive down rates of alcohol-related problems.

Acknowledgements

'Strategies of prevention and control and their effectiveness' and 'Building integrated alcohol policies' sections have been adapted from Robin Room, 'Prevention of alcohol-related problems' pp. 467–471, in Michael Gelder et al. (eds.) *New Oxford Textbook of Psychiatry*, Oxford University Press, Oxford, UK, Copyright © 2012, by permission of Oxford University Press, http://www.oup.com.

References

Andréasson, S., Romelsjö, A., and Allebeck, P. (1991). Alcohol, social factors, and mortality among young men. *British Journal of Addiction*, 86, 877–87.

Anonymous (2007). A framework convention on alcohol control [editorial]. *The Lancet*, 370(9593), 1102.

Babor, T., Caetano, R., Casswell, S., et al. (2010). *Alcohol: No Ordinary Commodity—Research and Public Policy* (2nd ed.). Oxford: Oxford University Press.

Babor, T.F., Grant, M., Acuda, W., et al. (1994). Randomized clinical trial of brief interventions in primary health care: summary of a WHO project (with commentaries and a response). *Addiction*, 89, 657–78.

Bagnardi, V., Zatonski, W., Scotti, L., La Vecchia, C., and Corrao, G. (2008). Does drinking pattern modify the effect of alcohol on the risk of coronary heart disease? Evidence from a meta-analysis. *Journal of Epidemiology and Community Health*, 62, 615–19.

Bakke, Ø. and Endal, D. (2010). Vested interests in addiction research and policy alcohol policies out of context: drinks industry supplanting government role in alcohol policies in sub-Saharan Africa. *Addiction*, 105, 22–8.

Beauchamp, D. (1976). Exploring new ethics for public health: developing a fair alcohol policy. *Journal of Health Politics, Policy, and Law*, 1, 338–54.

Beck, J. (1998). 100 years of 'just say no' versus 'just say know'. *Evaluation Review*, 22, 15–45.

Blocker, J. (1989). *American Temperance Movements: Cycles of Reform*. Boston, MA: Twayne Publishers.

Botvin, G.J. (1995). Principles of prevention. In R.H. Coombs and D. Ziedonis (eds.) *Handbook on Drug Abuse Prevention: A Comprehensive Strategy to Prevent the Abuse of Alcohol and Other Drugs*, pp. 19–44. Boston, MA: Allyn and Bacon.

Bruun, K., Edwards, G., Lumio, M., et al. (1975a). *Alcohol Control Policies in Public Health Perspective*. Volume 25. Helsinki: Finnish Foundation for Alcohol Studies.

Bruun, K., Rexed, I., and Pan, L. (1975b). *The Gentlemen's Club*. Chicago, IL: University of Chicago Press.

Butler, B.Y. (2006). *Holy Intoxication to Drunken Dissipation: Alcohol Among Quichua Speakers in Otavalo, Ecuador*. Albuquerque, NM: University of New Mexico Press.

Carmona, M. and Stewart, K. (1996). *Review of Alternative Activities and Alternatives Programs in Youth-Oriented Prevention*. CSAP Technical Report 13. Rockville, MD: Center for Substance Abuse Prevention.

Casswell, S. (1995). Does alcohol advertising have an impact on public health? *Drug and Alcohol Review*, 14, 395–404.

Casswell, S. (2013). Vested interests in addiction research and policy. Why do we not see the corporate interests of the alcohol industry as clearly as we see those of the tobacco industry? *Addiction*, 108, 680–5.

Casswell, S., Gilmore, L., Maguire, V., et al. (1989). Changes in public support for alcohol policies following a community-based campaign. *British Journal of Addiction*, 84, 515–22.

Casswell, S., Pledger, M., and Pratap, S. (2002). Trajectories of drinking from 18 to 26 years: identification and prediction. *Addiction*, 97(11), 1427–37.

Casswell, S. and Zhang, J.F. (1998). Impact of liking for advertising and brand allegiance on drinking and alcohol-related aggression: a longitudinal study. *Addiction*, 93, 1209–17.

Catlin, G.E.G. (1931). *Liquor Control*. London: Thornton Butterworth.

Chadwick, D.J. and Goode, J.A. (eds.) (1998). *Alcohol and Cardiovascular Diseases*. Chichester: John Wiley & Sons.

Chisholm, D., Rehm, J., van Ommeren, M., and Monteiro, M. (2004). Reducing the global burden of hazardous alcohol use: a comparative cost-effectiveness analysis, *Journal of Studies on Alcohol*, 65(6), 782–93.

Cook, P.J. (2007). *Paying the Tab: The Costs and Benefits of Alcohol Control*. Princeton, NJ: Princeton University Press.

Criqui, M. (1998). Discussion. In D.J. Chadwick and J.A. Goode (eds.) *Alcohol and Cardiovascular Diseases*, pp. 122–4. Chichester: John Wiley & Sons.

Crombie, I.K., Irvine, L., Elliott, L., et al. (2007). How do public health policies tackle alcohol-related harm? A review of 12 developed countries. *Alcohol and Alcoholism*, 42(5), 492–9.

Cross, J.N. (1968). *Guide to the Community Control of Alcoholism*. New York: American Public Health Association.

DeJong, W. and Hingson, R. (1998). Strategies to reduce driving under the influence of alcohol. *Annual Review of Public Health*, 19, 359–78.

De Lint, J. and Schmidt, W. (1968). The distribution of alcohol consumption in Ontario. *Quarterly Journal of Studies on Alcohol*, 29, 968–73.

Edwards, G., Anderson, P., Babor, T.F., et al. (1994). *Alcohol Policy and the Public Good*. Oxford: Oxford University Press.

Emerson, H. (ed.) (1932). *Alcohol and Man: The Effects of Alcohol on Man in Health and Disease*. New York: Macmillan.

English, D.R., Holman, C.D.J., Milne, E., et al. (1995). *The Quantification of Drug Caused Morbidity and Mortality in Australia*. Canberra: Australian Government Publishing Service.

Evans, L. (1991). *Traffic Safety and the Driver*. New York: Van Nostrand Reinhold.

Ezzati, M., Lopez, A.D., Rodgers, A., et al. and The Comparative Risk Assessment Collaborating Group (2002). Selected major risk factors and global and regional burden of disease. *The Lancet*, 360, 1347–60.

Fillmore, K.M., Kerr, W.C., Stockwell, T., et al. (2006). Moderate alcohol use and reduced mortality risk: systematic error in prospective studies. *Addiction Research and Theory*, 14(2), 101–32.

Finney, J.W. and Monahan, S.C. (1998). Cost-effectiveness of treatment for alcoholism: a second approximation. *Journal of Studies on Alcohol*, 57, 229–43.

Foxcroft, D.R., Ireland, D., Lister-Sharp, F.J., et al. (2003). Longer-term primary prevention for alcohol misuse in young people: a systematic review. *Addiction*, 98(Suppl. 4), 397–411.

Giesbrecht, N., Conley, P., Denniston, R., et al. (eds.) (1990). *Research, Action and the Community: Experiences in the Prevention of Alcohol and Other Drug Problems*. DHHS Publication No. (ADM) 89–1651. Rockville, MD: Office of Substance Abuse Prevention.

Gorman, D.M., Conde, E., Huber, J.C. Jr. (2007). The creation of evidence in 'evidence-based' drug prevention: a critique of the Strengthening Families Program Plus Life Skills Training evaluation. *Drug and Alcohol Review*, 26(6), 585–93.

Graham, K., Leonard, K.E., Room, R., et al. (1998). Current directions in research on understanding and preventing intoxicated aggression. *Addiction*, 93, 659–76.

Grant, M. and Litvak, J. (1998). Introduction: beyond per capita consumption. In M. Grant and J. Litvak (eds.) *Drinking Patterns and their Consequences*, pp. 1–4. Washington, DC: Taylor and Francis.

Greenfield, T. and Zimmerman, R. (eds.) (1993). *Experiences with Community Action Projects: New Research in the Prevention of Alcohol and Other Drug Problems*. DHHS Publication No. (ADM) 93–1976. Rockville, MD: Center for Substance Abuse Prevention.

Grover, P.T. (ed.) (1999). *Preventing Problems Related to Alcohol Availability—Environmental Approaches: Reference Guide*. Washington, DC: Center for Substance Abuse Prevention. DHHS Publication No. SMA 99–3298. Available at: http://text.nlm.nih.gov/ftrs/dbaccess/csap.

Hawks, D. (1993). The formulation of Australia's National Health Policy on Alcohol. *Addiction*, 88(Suppl.), 19S–26S.

Hemström, Ö. (2001). Per capita alcohol consumption and ischaemic heart disease mortality. *Addiction*, 96(Suppl. 1), 93–112.

Her, M., Giesbrecht, N., Room, R., et al. (1999). Privatizing alcohol sales and alcohol consumption: evidence and implications. *Addiction*, 94, 1125–39.

Her, M. and Rehm, J. (1998). Alcohol and all-cause mortality in Europe 1982–1990: a pooled cross-section time-series analysis. *Addiction*, 93, 1335–40.

Herd, D. (1992). Ideology, history, and changing models of liver cirrhosis epidemiology. *British Journal of Addiction*, 87, 179–92.

Hingson, R. (1996). Prevention of drinking and driving. *Alcohol Health and Research World*, 20, 219–26.

Holder, H. (1997). Can individually directed interventions reduce population-level alcohol-involved problems? *Addiction*, 92, 5–7.

Holder, H.D. (1998). *Alcohol and the Community: A Systems Approach to Prevention*. Cambridge: Cambridge University Press.

Holder, H.D. and Cunningham, D.W. (1992). Alcoholism treatment for employees and family members: its effect on health care costs. *Alcohol Health and Research World*, 16, 149–53.

Holder, H.D., Kühlhorn, E., Nordlund, S., et al. (1998). *European Integration and Nordic Alcohol Policies*. Aldershot: Ashgate.

Holder, H.D., Lennox, R.D.L., and Blose, J.O. (1992). Economic benefits of alcoholism treatment: a summary of twenty years of research. *Journal of Employee Assistance Research*, 1, 63–82.

Holmila, M. (ed.) (1997). *Community Prevention of Alcohol Problems*. Basingstoke: Macmillan.

Järvinen, M. (1991). The controlled controllers: women, men, and alcohol. *Contemporary Drug Problems*, 18, 389–406.

Jernigan, D.H. (1997). *Thirsting for Markets: The Global Impact of Corporate Alcohol*. San Rafael, CA: Marin Institute for the Prevention of Alcohol and Other Drug Problems.

Jernigan, D.H. (2010). The extent of global alcohol marketing and its impact on youth. *Contemporary Drug Problems*, 37, 57–89.

Johnston, I. (2006). *Halving Roadway Fatalities: A Case Study from Victoria, Australia 1989–2004*. Washington, DC: International Technology Scanning Program, Federal Highway Administration. Available at: http://international.fhwa.dot.gov/halving_fatalities/halving_fatal ities.pdf.

Katcher, B.S. (1993). The post-repeal eclipse in knowledge about the harmful effects of alcohol. *Addiction*, 88, 729–44.

Kauhanen, J., Kaplan, G.A., Goldberg, D.E., et al. (1997). Beer bingeing and mortality: results from the Kuopio ischaemic heart disease risk factor study, a prospective population-based study. *British Medical Journal*, 315, 846–51.

Kim, H.-R. (2000). Revised liquor taxes leave soju makers in lurch. *Korea Herald*. 13 March.

Klatsky, A.L. (1999). Moderate drinking and reduced risk of heart disease. *Alcohol Research and Health*, 23(1), 15–23.

Knupfer, G. (1967). The epidemiology of problem drinking. *American Journal of Public Health*, 57, 973–86.

Kozlowski, L.T., Heller, D.A., Pillitteri, J.L., et al. (1994). Tobacco use, the health effects of moderate alcohol drinking, and the assessment of their interaction. *Contemporary Drug Problems*, 21, 81–9.

Kreitman, N. (1986). Alcohol consumption and the preventive paradox. *British Journal of Addiction*, 81, 353–63.

Kupari, M. and Koskinen, P. (1998). Alcohol, cardiac arrhythmias and sudden death. In D.J. Chadwick and J.A. Goode (eds.) *Alcohol and Cardiovascular Diseases*, pp. 68–79. Chichester: John Wiley & Sons.

Kypri, K., Voas, R.B., Langley, J.D., et al. (2006). Minimum purchasing age for alcohol and traffic crash injuries among 15- to 19-year-olds in New Zealand. *American Journal of Public Health*, 96(1), 126–31.

Laslett, A.-M., Room, R., Ferris, J., Wilkinson, C., Livingston, M., and Mugavin, J. (2011) Surveying the range and magnitude of alcohol's harm to others in Australia. *Addiction*, 106(9), 1603–11.

Ledermann, S. (1956). *Alcool, Alcoolisme, Alcoolisation*. INED Cahier No. 29. Paris: Presses Universitaires de France.

Leon, D.A., Chenet, L., Shkolnikov, V.M., et al. (1997). Huge variation in Russian mortality rates 1984–94: artefact, alcohol, or what? *The Lancet*, 350, 383–8.

Levine, H.G. (1991). Temperance cultures: concern about alcohol problems in Nordic and English-speaking cultures. In M. Lader, G. Edwards, and D.C. Drummond (eds.) *The Nature of Alcohol and Drug Related Problems*, pp. 15–36. Oxford: Oxford University Press.

Lim, S.S., Vos, T., Flaxman, A.D., et al. (2012). A comparative risk assessment of burden of disease and injury attributable to 67 risk factors and risk factor clusters in 21 regions, 1990–2010: a systematic analysis for the Global Burden of Disease Study 2010, *The Lancet*, 380, 2224–60.

Livingston, M. (2013). To reduce alcohol-related harm we need to look beyond pubs and nightclubs. *Drug & Alcohol Review*, 32, 113–14.

Long, C.G., Williams, M., and Hollin, C.R. (1998) Treating alcohol problems: a study of program effectiveness and cost-effectiveness according to length and delivery of treatment. *Addiction*, 93, 561–71.

Maclure, M. (1993). Demonstration of deductive meta-analysis: ethanol intake and risk of myocardial infarction. *Epidemiologic Reviews*, 15, 328–51.

Mäkelä, K. (1983). The uses of alcohol and their cultural regulation. *Acta Sociologica*, 26, 21–31.

Mäkelä, K. and Viikari, M. (1977). Notes on alcohol and the state. *Acta Sociologica*, 20, 155–79.

McKee, M. and Britton, A. (1998). The positive relationship between alcohol and heart disease in Eastern Europe: potential physiological mechanisms. *Journal of the Royal Society of Medicine*, 91, 402–7.

Møller, L. (2002). Legal restrictions resulted in a reduction of alcohol consumption among young people in Denmark. In R. Room (ed.) *The Effects of Nordic Alcohol Policies: What Happens to Drinking When Alcohol Controls Change?*, pp. 93–100. NAD Publication 42. Helsinki: Nordic Council for Alcohol and Drug Research. Available at: http://www.drugslibrary.stir.ac.uk/documents/nad42.pdf.

Moore, M.H. and Gerstein, D.R. (eds.) (1981). *Alcohol and Public Policy: Beyond the Shadow of Prohibition*. Washington, DC: National Academy Press.

Moskalewicz, J. (1993). Privatization of the alcohol arena in Poland. *Contemporary Drug Problems*, 20, 263–75.

Moskowitz, J.M., Mailvin, J., Schaeffer, G.A., et al. (1983). Evaluation of a junior high school primary prevention program. *Addictive Behaviors*, 8, 393–401.

Mott, G. (1991). The anti-alcohol network. *Moderation Reader*, 5(5), 6–20.

Neves, P., de Pape, D., Giesbrecht, N., et al. (1998). *Communities Take Action! A Practical Guide for Municipalities, Enforcement Agencies, Community Groups, and Others Concerned about the Impact of Alcohol on Public Health and Safety*. Toronto: Addiction Research Foundation.

Norman, E., Turner, S., Zunz, S.J., et al. (1997). Prevention programs reviewed: what works? In E. Norman (ed.) *Drug-Free Youth: A Compendium for Prevention Specialists*, pp. 22–45. New York: Garland Publishing.

Norström, T. (1987). Abolition of the Swedish rationing system: effects on consumption distribution and cirrhosis mortality. *British Journal of Addiction*, 82, 633–41.

Norström, T. (1996). Per capita consumption and total mortality: an analysis of historical data. *Addiction*, 91, 339–44.

Norström, T. and Ramstedt, M. (2005). Mortality and population drinking: a review of the literature. *Drug and Alcohol Review*, 24(6), 537–47.

Nutt, D.J., King, L.A., and Phillips, L.D. (2010). Drug harms in the UK: a multicriteria decision analysis. *The Lancet*, 376, 1588–65.

O'Brien, P. (2013). Australia's double standard on Thailand's alcohol warning labels. *Drug & Alcohol Review*, 32(1), 5–10.

Olsson, B. (1990). Alkoholpolitik och alkoholens fenomenologi: uppfattningar som artikulerats i pressen [Alcohol policy and the phenomenology of alcohol: concepts articulated in the press]. *Alkoholpolitik*, 7, 184–95.

Olsson, B., Ólafsdóttir, H., and Room, R. (2002). Introduction: Nordic traditions of studying the impact of alcohol policies. In R. Room (ed.) *The Effects of Nordic Alcohol Policies: What Happens to Drinking when Alcohol Controls Change?* pp. 5–16. NAD Publication 42. Helsinki: Nordic Council for Alcohol and Drug Research.

Paglia, A. and Room, R. (1999). Preventing substance use problems among youth: a literature review and recommendations. *Journal of Primary Prevention*, 20, 3–50.

Parry, C., Rehm, J., Poznyak, V., and Room, R. (2009). Alcohol and infectious disease: an overlooked causal linkage? *Addiction*, 104(3), 331–2.

Peele, S. (1987). The limitations of control-of-supply models for explaining and preventing alcoholism and drug addiction. *Journal of Studies on Alcohol*, 48, 61–77.

Pennay, A. and Room, R. (2012). Prohibiting public drinking in urban public spaces: a review of the evidence. *Drugs: Education, Prevention and Policy*, 19(2), 91–101.

Perrine, M.W., Peck, R.C., and Fell, J.C. (1989). Epidemiologic perspectives on drunk driving. In *Surgeon General's Workshop on Drunk Driving: Background Papers*, pp. 35–76. Washington, DC: US Department of Health and Human Services.

Plant, M., Single, E., and Stockwell, T. (eds.) (1997). *Alcohol: Minimizing the Harm—What Works?* London: Free Association Books.

Poikolainen, K. (1999). It can be bad for the heart, too—drinking patterns and coronary heart disease. *Addiction*, 93, 1757–9.

Popham, R., Schmidt, W., and de Lint, J. (1976). The effects of legal restraint on drinking. In B. Kissin and H. Begleiter (eds.) *The Biology of Alcoholism: vol. 4. Social Aspects of Alcoholism*, pp. 579–625. New York: Plenum.

Ramstedt, M. (2006). Is alcohol good or bad for Canadian hearts? A time-series analysis of the link between alcohol consumption and IHD mortality. *Drug and Alcohol Review*, 25(4), 315–20.

Rehm, J., Baliunas, D., Borges, G.L.G., et al. (2010). The relation between different dimensions of alcohol consumption and burden of disease—an overview. *Addiction*, 105(5), 817–43.

Rehm, J. and Room, R. (2009). A case study in how harmful alcohol consumption can be. *The Lancet*, 373, 2176–7.

Rehm, J. and Sempos, C.T. (1995). Alcohol consumption and all-cause mortality. *Addiction*, 90, 471–80.

Room, R. (1983). Alcohol and crime: behavioral aspects. In S. Kadish (ed.) *Encyclopedia of Crime and Justice* (Vol. 1), pp. 35–44. New York: Free Press.

Room, R. (1984a). Alcohol control and public health. *Annual Review of Public Health*, 5, 293–317.

Room, R. (1984b). A 'reverence for strong drink': the lost generation and the elevation of alcohol in American culture. *Journal of Studies on Alcohol*, 45, 540–6.

Room, R. (1984c). Former NIAAA directors look back: policy makers on the role of research. *Drinking and Drug Practices Surveyor*, 19, 38–42.

Room, R. (1993). The evolution of alcohol monopolies and their relevance for public health. *Contemporary Drug Problems*, 20, 169–87.

Room, R. (1996). Alcohol consumption and social harm—conceptual issues and historical perspectives. *Contemporary Drug Problems*, 23, 373–88.

Room, R. (1997). Voluntary organizations and the state in the prevention of alcohol problems. *Drugs and Society*, 11, 11–23.

Room, R. (1999). The idea of alcohol policy. *Nordic Studies on Alcohol and Drugs*, 16 (English Suppl.), 7–20.

Room, R. (2001). Intoxication and bad behaviour: understanding cultural differences in the link. *Social Science & Medicine*, 53, 189–98.

Room, R. (2004). Disabling the public interest: alcohol policies and strategies for England. *Addiction*, 99, 1083–9.

Room, R. (2005). Alcohol and the World Health Organization: the ups and downs of two decades. *Nordic Studies on Alcohol and Drugs*, 22 (English suppl.), 146–62.

Room, R. (2013). Healthy is as healthy does: where will a voluntary code get us on international alcohol control? *Addiction*, 108(3), 456–7.

Room, R., Giesbrecht, N., and Stoduto, G. (2006). Trade agreements and disputes. In N. Giesbrecht, A. Demers, A. Ogborne, et al. (eds.) *Sober Reflections: Commerce, Public Health, and the Evolution of Alcohol Policy in Canada, 1980–2000*, pp. 74–9. Montreal and Kingston: McGill-Queen's University Press.

Room, R., Jernigan, D., Carlini-Marlatt, B., et al. (2002). *Alcohol and Developing Societies: A Public Health Approach*. Helsinki: Finnish Foundation for Alcohol Studies.

Room, R., Schmidt, L., Rehm, J., and Mäkelä, P. (2008). International regulation of alcohol. *British Medical Journal*, 337, a2364.

Rorabaugh, W.J. (1979). *The Alcoholic Republic*. New York: Oxford University Press.

Rose, G. (1981). Strategy of prevention: lessons from cardiovascular disease. *British Medical Journal*, 282, 1847–51.

Ross, H.L. (1982). *Deterring the Drinking Driver: Legal Policy and Social Control*. Lexington, MA: Lexington Books.

Saltz, R.F. (1997). Prevention where alcohol is sold and consumed: server intervention and responsible beverage service. In M. Plant, E. Single, and T. Stockwell (eds.) *Alcohol: Minimizing the Harm—What Works?*, pp. 72–84. New York: Free Association Books.

Schechter, E.J. (1986). Alcohol rationing and control systems in Greenland. *Contemporary Drug Problems*, 13, 587–620.

Schrad, M. (2010). *The Political Power of Bad Ideas: Networks, Institutions, and the Global Prohibition Wave*. Oxford: Oxford University Press.

Seeley, J.R. (1960). Death by liver cirrhosis and the price of beverage alcohol. *Canadian Medical Association Journal*, 83, 1361–6.

Shkolnikov, V.M. and Nemtsov, A. (1997). The anti-alcohol campaign and variations in Russian mortality. In J.L. Bobadilla, C.A. Costello, and F. Mitchell (eds.) *Premature Death in the New Independent States*, pp. 239–61. Washington, DC: National Academy Press.

Skog, O.-J. (1985). The collectivity of drinking cultures: a theory of the distribution of alcohol consumption. *British Journal of Addiction*, 80, 83–99.

Skog, O.-J. (1996). Public health consequences of the J-curve hypothesis of alcohol problems. *Addiction*, 91, 325–37.

Smart, R.G. and Mann, R.E. (1990). Are increased levels of treatment and Alcoholics Anonymous large enough to create the recent reduction in liver cirrhosis? *British Journal of Addiction*, 85, 1385–7.

Smart, R.G. and Mann, R.E. (1997). Interventions into alcohol problems: what works? *Addiction*, 92, 9–13.

Stimson, G., Grant, M., Choquet, M., et al. (eds.) (2007). *Drinking in Context: Patterns, Interventions, and Partnerships*. New York: Routledge.

Stockwell, T. and Room, R. (2012). Constructing and responding to low-risk drinking guidelines: conceptualisation, evidence and reception. *Drug and Alcohol Review*, 31(2), 121–5.

Stockwell, T., Single, E., Hawks, D., et al. (1997). Sharpening the focus of alcohol policy from aggregate consumption to harm and risk reduction. *Addiction Research*, 5, 1–9.

Sutton, C. (1998). Swedish alcohol discourse: constructions of a social problem. Uppsala: *Acta Universitatis Upsaliensis, Studia Sociologica Upsaliensia*, 45.

Taylor, A.L. and Dhillon, I.S. (2013). Alternative legal strategies for alcohol control: not a framework convention—at least not right now. *Addiction*, 108, 450–5.

Teasley, D.L. (1992). Drug legalization and the 'lessons' of Prohibition. *Contemporary Drug Problems*, 19, 27–52.

Terris, M. (1967). Epidemiology of cirrhosis of the liver: national mortality data. *American Journal of Public Health*, 57, 2076–88.

Tigerstedt, C. (1990). The European Community and the alcohol policy dimension. *Contemporary Drug Problems*, 17, 461–79.

Tigerstedt, C. (1999). Alcohol policy, public health, and Kettil Bruun. *Contemporary Drug Problems*, 26, 209–35.

White, O.C. and Batia, A. (1998). *Privatization in Africa*. Washington, DC: World Bank.

Whitehead, P.C. (1979). Prevention of alcoholism. In D. Robinson (ed.) *Alcohol Problems*, pp. 162–71. New York: Holmes and Meier.

Wolfgang, M.E. (1958). *Patterns in Criminal Homicide*. Philadelphia, PA: University of Pennsylvania Press.

World Health Organization (2004). *Global Status Report: Alcohol Policy*. Geneva: WHO.

World Health Organization (2012). *Global Strategy to Reduce the Harmful Effects of Alcohol*. Geneva: WHO. Available at: http://www.who.int/substance_abuse/activities/gsrhua/en/index.html.

World Health Organization (2012). *WHO Expert Committee on Drug Dependence: Thirty-fifth Report*. Geneva: WHO. Available at: http://apps.who.int/iris/bitstream/10665/77747/1/WHO_trs_973_eng.pdf.

World Health Organization (2013a). *Draft Action Plan for the Prevention and Control of Noncommunicable diseases 2013–2020: Report by the Secretariat*. Geneva: WHO. Available at: http://apps.who.int/gb/ebwha/pdf_files/WHA66/A66_9-en.pdf.

World Health Organization (2013b). *Draft Comprehensive Global Monitoring Framework and Targets for the Prevention and Control of Noncommunicable Diseases*. Report by the Director-General. Geneva: WHO. Available at: http://apps.who.int/gb/ebwha/pdf_files/WHA66/A66_8-en.pdf.

World Health Organization, Expert Committee on Problems Related to Alcohol Consumption (1980). *Problems Related to Alcohol Consumption*. Technical Report Series 650. Geneva: WHO.

World Health Organization, Expert Committee on Problems Related to Alcohol Consumption (2007). *Second Report*. Technical Report Series 944. Geneva: WHO. Available at: http://www.who.int/substance_abuse/activities/expert_comm_alcohol_2nd_report.pdf.

Zaridze, D., Brennan, P., and Boreham, J., et al. (2009). Alcohol and cause-specific mortality in Russia: a retrospective case-control study of 48,557 adult deaths. *The Lancet*, 373, 2201–14.

Ziegler, D.W. (2009). The alcohol industry and trade agreements: a preliminary assessment. *Addiction*, 104(Suppl.), 13–26.

Injury prevention and control: the public health approach

Corinne Peek-Asa and Adnan Hyder

Introduction to injury prevention and control

Injuries contribute significantly to premature life lost and years lived with disability for all countries, all regions of the world, and all age groups. According to analyses of the 2010 Global Burden of Disease data, injuries cause over 5 million deaths per year, accounting for nearly 10 per cent of all deaths and more than 11 per cent of disability-adjusted life years (DALYs) (Global Burden of Disease Study 2012). For children under 14 years of age, road traffic crashes, drowning, fires, poisoning, interpersonal violence, and war are all in the leading ten causes of death. Deaths represent just a small proportion of the many injuries that cause serious injury and potentially life-long disability, and injuries also cause significant psychological trauma and financial loss. The burden of traumatic injuries necessitates that injury prevention be considered an international public health priority.

Because the majority of us will suffer multiple minor injuries throughout our lives, most of which cause only minor discomfort or inconvenience, we may be lulled into believing that injuries are just part of life. However, a serious injury or the traumatic death of a loved one can completely change the course of the lives of those affected. The toll of these injuries is also extremely deleterious to families, communities, and societies.

Many injuries can be prevented, and global investment in traumatic injury prevention will have significant long-term health and financial benefits. For developed countries, progress has been made in reducing the toll of traumatic injuries. In the United States, for example, road traffic crashes per million vehicle miles travelled decreased nearly 90 per cent from the 1930s into the twenty-first century (Institute of Medicine 1999). Mortality rates have decreased for deaths from drowning, residential fires, homicide, and poisoning, among others. However, these rates remain unacceptably high knowing that many effective prevention strategies have not yet been widely implemented.

The burden of traumatic injury worldwide is disproportionately concentrated in lower-income countries. The World Health Organization (WHO) anticipates that, if current trends continue, road traffic injuries, interpersonal violence, war, and self-inflicted injuries will all be among the leading 15 causes of DALYs lost by the year 2020. Road traffic crashes, which in 1990 ranked as the ninth leading cause of DALYs lost, is predicted to reach the rank of three in 2020 (Peden et al. 2002). Operations of war will rise from the rank of 16 in 1990 to eight by 2020, and interpersonal violence will rise from rank 19 to 12. Despite some successes in many areas of injury prevention, new risks, changing environments, and increasing population size constantly challenge injury control efforts.

Effective injury prevention strategies will require organization of the public health response and increased integration of professionals from many backgrounds. Modern injury control research combines ideas and skills from public health, biomechanics, engineering, behavioural sciences, law, law enforcement, medicine, and urban planning, among others. Research that identifies how effective interventions in high-income countries (HICs) can be translated in low- and middle-income settings is a priority, but injury prevention strategies will need to be appropriate for local environments. Injury prevention activities that integrate multiple approaches within an organized public health response have a stronger chance of success.

This chapter will present the current state of knowledge regarding the burden of injuries and will introduce the basic concepts of building injury prevention infrastructure and capacity.

Causal model of injuries

Injuries are generally divided into the two broad categories of intentional and unintentional. Intentional injuries are those in which there was an intent to commit harm, either to oneself or someone else. Unintentional injuries occur without a direct intent to commit harm, even if gross negligence was involved. For example, a motor vehicle occupant death caused by a drunk driver would be considered an unintentional injury even though in many countries the driver could be prosecuted for a crime.

Injuries are further classified by their cause, such as motor vehicle occupant injuries, drowning, suicide/attempted suicide, homicide/assault, or residential fire injuries. Until the late 1990s, cause and intent were coded together, so that, for example, a poisoning death would not be distinguished as intentional or unintentional. In the 1990s, collaboration between the US Centers for

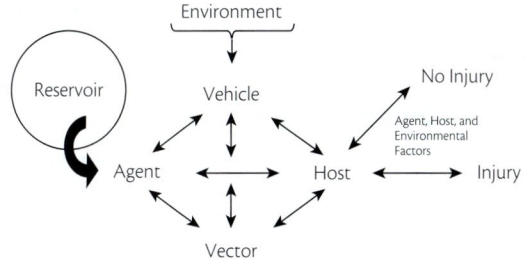

Fig. 9.4.1 Causal model for injuries.

Disease Control and Prevention and the American Public Health Association recommended that cause and intent be considered as separate components of describing an injury, and most data are now coded accordingly (Centers for Disease Control and Prevention 1997). Through this collaboration, a matrix to code injuries by intent and cause using the International Classification of Diseases, 9th revision, was developed. This matrix served as a template to create codes for injury cause and intent that are now included in the 10th revision of this coding system.

Injury causes are very broad and represent a diverse range of physical harm, and thus can be difficult to tie together conceptually. The traditional epidemiological model for infectious diseases provides a framework for the epidemiological study of traumatic injury (Fig. 9.4.1). At the centre of the causal pathway for injuries is the agent–host interaction. The agent, which in the case of injuries is energy, is absorbed by the host to cause injury. Energy can take many forms, such as mechanical, electrical, chemical, radiation, and thermal. An example of an agent–host relationship is a motor vehicle crash, in which the energy exerted on the individual is mechanical. The reservoir is the place in the environment where the agent is found. The potential for energy transfer exists everywhere, but its potential to cause injury is limited to specific conditions. For instance, the potential energy in a motor vehicle exists only when the car is being driven, and causes injury only when the vehicle crashes.

Vehicles and vectors are mechanisms which transport energy from the reservoir to the host. A vehicle is an inanimate object, such as a motor vehicle; a vector is animate, such as a dog biting a child. For many injury causes, vehicles and vectors are both involved in energy transfer, such as when one individual (vector) stabs another with a knife (vehicle). The injury outcome is the trauma or injury sustained by the individual, and is influenced by host responses to the energy. Only energy transmitted beyond a host's tolerance causes an injury, and therefore not all exposures to energy result in noticeable injury. A human has some resistance to energy which can be increased through exercise or protective devices, or reduced through changes in intrinsic factors such as existing medical conditions or age and through extrinsic factors such as fatigue and alcohol.

This causal model is important when considering injury prevention strategies. Injury prevention aims to prevent energy transfer or to reduce the amount of energy that is transferred. Prevention activities can focus on the host, on the environment, on vehicles or vectors, or combine all of these components. A theoretical approach to injury prevention based on this model is presented later in this chapter (see 'Theoretical basis for injury prevention').

Injury data sources

Globally, improved data infrastructures and increased access to data has aided in the rising awareness of the burden of injury and violence as a health problem. Data that provide information related to injuries can be found from a wide variety of sources, both within and outside of the health sector (Institute of Medicine, 1999; Hyder and Morrow 2006). Mortality data, most frequently collected through vital statistics reporting, is the most commonly used source for measuring the burden of injury. Most countries have some structure for death reporting that includes the cause of death, although the quality of these data varies markedly around the world.

Efforts to combine global mortality data to compare incidence, years of potential life lost, and DALYs have improved our knowledge of the burden of injury. The Global Burden of Disease study attempted to collect consistent and internationally comparable data (Murray and Lopez 1996; WHO 2002) and is one of the most comprehensive sources of injury mortality data. The data, however, have limitations in reporting and in coding injury types, and thus are an underestimate of overall injuries. The recent Global Burden of Diseases, Injuries, and Risk Factors study is the most comprehensive effort to compare incidence and risk factors for injuries and diseases (Murray et al. 2013). This effort made several key advances in global data comparisons which included expanded and clarified definitions of causes of death, the integration of risk factors and risk behaviours, and improved estimates to reduce uncertainty.

Although these global estimates are extremely valuable for comparisons, they provide little detail about risk factors and circumstances for injuries. Detailed surveillance systems that focus on specific types of fatal injuries have been very helpful to identify and prioritize prevention approaches. For example, the Fatal Accident Reporting System of the US Department of Transportation provides details of road traffic deaths and has helped improve car and road design and has assisted in development and implementation of safety policies. The Census of Fatal Occupational Injuries maintained by the US Bureau of Labor Statistics has helped compare workplace fatalities by occupation and industry and prioritized workplace hazards.

In comparison with mortality data, population-based data of non-fatal injuries and their outcomes are more challenging to collect and far less available, especially in the developing world. In HICs, population-based data describing non-fatal injuries can be found within hospital reporting data, often used to monitor national health indicators. Sources that include injuries as one of many health outcomes often lack detail to inform injury prevention approaches. Other sources are specific to injuries, such as trauma registries. Efforts to pool trauma data, such as the US National Trauma Data Bank or Canadian National Trauma Registry, are helpful in describing larger patient samples, but trauma registries can rarely be tied to a population base. Many data sources outside the health sector cover a wide spectrum of injury-related events, such as data from law enforcement, the transportation sector, criminal and justice sectors, and insurance companies. This diversity of data sources makes the field of injuries and violence unique in terms of the inter-sectoral nature of the information (Norton et al. 2006).

In many instances, data sources can to be linked together to provide a more complete description of the injury. Motor vehicle crash injuries, for example, often require data from traffic enforcement to describe the cause and nature of the crash and data from the health sector to describe the injuries and their severity. Linking these data sources can be impeded by issues of privacy and access to identifying information for linkage, as well as data quality issues. In low- and middle-income countries these data systems, if they exist at all, are often not computerized and have never been evaluated for quality, making such linkages even more challenging. However, information from multiple sources is often necessary to examine causal hypotheses about injuries.

A growing emphasis on improving health behaviour has led to global efforts to collect data on risk behaviours. Many countries conduct surveys of health behaviours, such as the US Youth Risk Behavior Survey (Eaton et al. 2012). More recently, multicountry surveys have been launched to compare risk behaviours across countries. One example is the Health Behaviour in School-aged Children study, which surveys adolescents in more than 40 countries (Roberts et al. 2009). These surveys help establish ties between the prevalence of risk behaviours and experiences with injury and violence.

Despite improvements in data infrastructures that have been possible with technological advances, access to high-quality and detailed data on injury and violence remains an important limitation in most countries. Data limitations are particularly problematic in low-income countries. In many low-income countries, death reporting is the only major source of information about the burden of injuries, and these data can have gaps in reporting and coding. The public health infrastructure and routine collection of health information in the developing world has been fragile, especially in regions such as sub-Saharan Africa and South Asia. It is thus not surprising that there has been little tradition of developing specific information sources for injuries. Population-based studies from low- and middle-income countries, though, consistently conclude that the injury burden is higher than reported in national official statistics and that injuries are significantly under-reported in these regions.

Global burden of injury

According to the 2010 Global Burden of Disease study, over 5 million deaths occur as a result of injuries around the world each year (Table 9.4.1) (Global Burden of Disease Study 2012). More than 25 per cent of these deaths are caused by road traffic injuries (RTIs), with self-inflicted injuries (self-harm) and falls comprising a further 17 and 11 per cent respectively. Likewise, injury death rates are highest for RTIs, followed by self-inflicted injuries and falls; similar patterns are observed for non-fatal health outcomes using DALY rates per 100,000 population (Fig. 9.4.2). Unintentional injuries, including RTIs, falls, drowning, fire burns and poisoning, together result in more than 3.7 million deaths.

RTIs alone kill over 1 million people every year. In 2010, RTIs became the 8th leading cause of death worldwide, up from 10th in 1990—a per cent change of 47 per cent. Males account for more than two-thirds of these deaths. According to the WHO's *Global Status Report on Road Safety*, the majority of those killed are from low- or middle-income countries (LMICs) (WHO 2009). The absolute number of fatalities and the mortality rate resulting from RTIs vary considerably across countries, and although all age groups are affected, young adults, particularly males, are most at risk of loss of life. Since this age group corresponds to the most economically productive segment of the population, RTIs have serious implications for national economies and account for more than 75 million DALYs—some 33 DALYs per 100,000 population.

Falls are the second leading cause of unintentional injury deaths and there were over 540,000 fall-related deaths in 2010. This constitutes a mortality rate of 8 per 100,000 population. More males die from falls than females (approximately 59 per cent and 41 per cent respectively). In addition, falls account for approximately 35 million DALYs or 514 DALYs per 100,000 population.

Table 9.4.1 Deaths from injuries worldwide, 2010

	Total	Females	Males
All injuries	5,073,321 (100%)	1,614,521 (100%)	3,458,800 (100%)
Unintentional injuries	3,715,668 (65.1%)	1,215,865 (75.3%)	2,499,803 (72.3%)
Road traffic injuries	1,328,535 (26.2%)	331,436 (20.5%)	997,100 (28.8%)
Falls	540,499 (9.5%)	221,762 (13.7%)	318,738 (9.2%)
Drowning	349,120 (6.9%)	103,135 (6.4%)	245,986 (7.1%)
(Fire) Burns	337,590 (6.7%)	177,328 (11.0%)	160,262 (4.6%)
Poisoning	180,443 (3.6%)	62,023 (3.8%)	118,420 (3.4%)
Other unintentional injuries	979,481 (19.3%)	320,181 (19.8%)	659,297 (19.1%)
Intentional injuries	1,357,653 (26.8%)	398,656 (24.7%)	958,997 (27.7%)
Self-harm	883,715 (17.4%)	304,634 (18.9%)	579,081 (16.7%)
Interpersonal violence	456,268 (9.0%)	87,828 (5.4%)	368,440 (10.7%)
Other intentional injuries	17,670 (0.3%)	6194 (0.4%)	11,476 (0.3%)

Source: data from *Global Burden of Disease Study 2010 (GBD 2010) Results by Cause 1990–2010*, Institute for Health Metrics and Evaluation (IHME), Seattle, USA, Copyright © 2012.

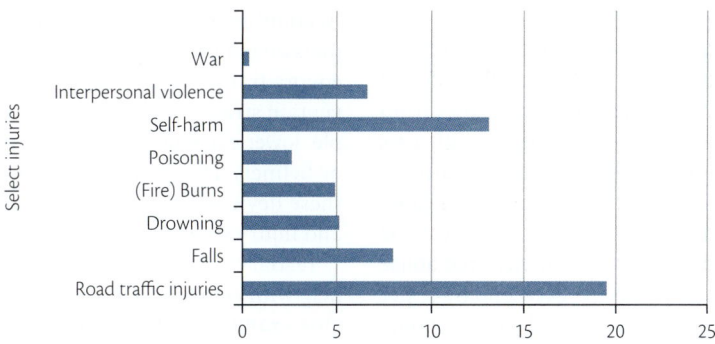

Fig. 9.4.2 Distribution of disability-adjusted life years (000) worldwide per 100,000 population, 2010.
Source: data from *Global Burden of Disease Study 2010 (GBD 2010) Results by Cause 1990–2010*, Institute for Health Metrics and Evaluation (IHME), Seattle, USA, Copyright © 2012.

Drowning and fire burns are also significant causes of fatal injury—contributing 9.3 per cent and 9.1 per cent to the global burden of unintentional injury deaths respectively. Drowning accounts for nearly 350,000 deaths in 2010—more than 64,000 of these drowning deaths were among children aged 1–4 years old. Males comprise the majority (70 per cent) of drowning deaths irrespective of age group. The mortality rate from drowning is approximately 5 per 100,000. Non-fatal drowning events result in more than 19 million DALYs lost per year.

Well over 330,000 deaths in 2010 were caused by fire burns, which result in more than 19 million DALYs—287 DALYs per 100,000. However, unlike other injuries, more females than males die from fire burns (compare 53 per cent and 47 per cent respectively). In 2010, more than 180,000 fatal poisonings were estimated, which correlates to a mortality rate of nearly 3 per 100,000 population. Other unintentional injuries including unintentional exposure to firearms, and non-venomous animal contact, that is, bites or attack, among others contributed 19 per cent of the global burden of injuries and result in nearly 980,000 deaths worldwide.

In 1990 self-harm ranked 14th in the top 25 causes of worldwide deaths; and in 2010, it also ranked 13th and is the second leading cause of injury death after RTIs, and the leading cause of intentional injury deaths. Self-inflicted injuries, including suicides, attempted suicide, self-destructive behaviours, and self-mutilation, cause the deaths of over 880,000 people globally, resulting in more than 36 million DALYs lost. Self-harm or self-inflicted injury deaths peak in the 20–24 age group and more than 65 per cent of self-inflicted injury deaths in 2010 were among males. Although self-harm ranks 21st on the top 25 causes of death among females, it ranks 9th in the Caribbean and 10th in East Asian regions. On the other hand, self-harm mortality rates among females are highest in South Asia and Asia Pacific (16.5 and 15.3 per 100,000 population respectively).

Interpersonal violence, including assault by firearm, sharp objects or other means, causes more than 450,000 deaths worldwide; and females account for less than 20 per cent of these deaths. The mortality rate due to interpersonal violence among both sexes is approximately 7 per 100,000 population. However, the extent to which intimate partner violence (IPV) is accurately reported as interpersonal violence is unknown given varying cultural norms and reporting tendencies around the world. For example, a case of apparent self-immolation may in fact be domestic violence involving fire. Women in countries who have conducted programmes to screen and respond to intimate partner violence, including victim's assistance programmes and social marketing campaigns against intimate partner violence, may be less inhibited to divulge their experiences with violence. Thus the use of country or regionally specific demographic surveys as a supplement to global aggregate data is essential to determine the actual burden.

War or 'collective violence and legal intervention', was estimated to cause more than 17,000 deaths worldwide in 2010, almost two-thirds of which are males (65 per cent). War results in some 960,000 DALYs lost.

Economic and societal burden

The average annual cost of road traffic crashes has been estimated at about 1 per cent of the gross national product in developing countries, 1.5 per cent in countries in economic transition, and 2 per cent in highly motorized countries. The annual economic cost of road traffic injuries globally is about US$518 billion (Jacobs et al. 2000). In low- and middle-income countries, the annual cost of road traffic crashes is about US$65 billion, exceeding the total annual amount received by these countries in development assistance. Policies that reduce deaths and injuries from RTIs can save millions of dollars regardless of the income or development level of the country.

Studies exploring the economic and social costs of road traffic injuries in low-income countries show that males who provided the majority of the household income in India and Bangladesh were the most common victims of road traffic fatalities and the consequences included reduced household income and reduced food consumption for the victim's family (Aeron-Thomas et al. 2004). In addition, the poor were found to spend a much greater proportion of their income on funeral and/or medical costs than the non-poor. A recent qualitative study of the intangible costs of RTIs in Mexico acknowledges similar findings but also emphasizes the loss of a family member to RTI can impact not only a family's household economy, but the very stability of the familial unit—in whichever form—as well as the individual family member's sense of her or his life's purpose (Pérez-Núñez et al. 2012).

Estimates of the cost of violence in the United States reach over 3 per cent of the gross domestic product. In England and Wales, the total costs from violence amount to an estimated US$40 billion annually. The economic effects of interpersonal violence are expected to be more severe in poorer countries, and yet, there is a scarcity of studies on the costs of violence in low- and middle-income countries (WHO 2004). However, estimates from low- and middle-income countries indicate that the overall costs of violence are substantial, ranging up to 25 per cent of annual gross domestic product. Comparisons with HICs are complicated by the fact that economic losses related to productivity tend to be undervalued in lower-income countries. For example, child abuse results in US$94 billion in annual costs to the US economy (1 per cent of GDP) and intimate partner violence costs the US economy nearly US$13 billion (0.1 per cent of GDP); this can be compared to 1.6 per cent of GDP in Nicaragua and 2 per cent of GDP in Chile. The cost of gun violence also has been calculated at US$155 billion annually in the United States.

Theoretical basis for injury prevention

The causal model for injuries allows the injury process to be categorized into distinct phases which are important for prevention (Haddon 1970, 1972). The *pre-injury* phase is the period prior to the energy transfer, the *injury* phase is the often millisecond period in which the energy is transferred to the host, and the *post-injury* phase is the period of recovery and rehabilitation. Prevention approaches affect the injury process in one of these three injury phases.

Primary injury prevention includes prevention strategies that aim to prevent the transfer of injury to the host, and thus act in the pre-injury phase. Examples of successful primary prevention strategies include roadway designs that reduce motor vehicle collisions, child-resistant caps on medication bottles to prevent ingestion and poisoning, and pool fences to prevent submersion and drowning (Graham 1993; Thompson and Rivara 2000).

Secondary injury prevention includes strategies that reduce the amount of energy that is transferred to the host. While these strategies are often put in place long before the injury event, their function acts to reduce energy transferred during the injury phase. Examples of secondary prevention strategies include seat belts and air bags (Evans 1995), motorcycle and bicycle helmets (US General

Accounting Office 1991; Thomas et al. 1994). Seat belts and helmets do not prevent the crash itself, but they reduce the amount of energy transmitted to the host during the crash. Secondary prevention strategies might not prevent injury completely. For example, lower extremity injuries are not prevented by either seat belts or helmets. However, studies have consistently shown that when these devices are present, the risk for mortal injury is much less and injury severity is reduced.

Tertiary prevention strategies act in the post-injury phase to help with recovery and rehabilitation once an injury has occurred. One example is the development of trauma systems, which help with triage and transport of an injured individual to reduce the time between injury and definitive medical care (Mann et al. 1999; Nathens et al. 2000). Optimizing resources to enable recovery and rehabilitation does not prevent the injury or reduce the amount of energy transfer, but tertiary prevention strategies can have enormous impact on improving survival, function and quality of life following an injury.

The Haddon matrix is a framework that combines these injury phases with the major components of the injury causal model to help identify prevention approaches (Table 9.4.2). This matrix, developed by Dr William Haddon in the United States, was the foundation for the study of motor vehicle crashes and countermeasures for highway safety and continues to be an applicable theoretical framework for injury prevention (Haddon 1972). Using the three injury phases, Haddon categorized prevention approaches into those that affect the host, vehicles and vectors, the physical environment, and the sociocultural environment. An example of the Haddon matrix with examples from motor vehicle occupant protection is included in Table 9.4.2.

The Haddon matrix provides a framework for identifying individual approaches to injury prevention. However, one single intervention strategy is unlikely to be highly effective. Multiple collaborative approaches need to be combined to maximize success. For example, the success of seat belt use in reducing motor vehicle occupant fatalities in the United States required a combination of engineering, education, policy, and enforcement that led to the current use rate of 80 per cent (National Highway Traffic Safety Administration 2007). Although seat belts were developed

Table 9.4.2 The Haddon matrix (illustrative)

Phases	Factors			
	Human	**Vehicle**	**Physical environment**	**Sociocultural environment**
Pre-injury	Reduce alcohol intoxication, programmes to increase defensive driving and decrease road rage	Increase vehicle stability, increased visibility	Improvements in road structure and traffic controls, traffic calming measures	Support safety programmes and increase consumer awareness of safety issues
Injury	Use of seat belts and car seats, proper placement of car seats, booster seats	Increase energy absorbed by the vehicle frame, safety features such as air bags, head rests, shatterproof windshields, and collapsible steering columns	Install energy-absorbing guard rails	Programmes to provide car seats, educational programmes about car seat installation and placement
Post-injury	Stabilize serious injuries, reduce bleeding and other complications	Design for easier extrication	Enhanced emergency medical systems and field care	Support infrastructure of trauma care, including 911 system, emergency and trauma care, and rehabilitation services

and available from the early 1900s, they were not required to be a standard feature on passenger cars in the United States until 1968. The steps to getting seat belts installed as a regular feature in passenger cars required considerable advocacy and policy initiatives. However, once the seat belts were installed, use rates without any occupant incentive or education were about 11 per cent. Efforts in the areas of legislation, enforcement, and public education were necessary to achieve the high use rates currently observed. Stricter legislation, for example, is associated with higher use, as evidenced by the higher use rates consistently observed among states with primary (not wearing a seat belt is by itself a citable offence) compared with secondary (not wearing a seat belt can be cited only along with another citation) laws in the United States (National Highway Traffic Safety Administration 2007).

Risk factors for injuries

The social–ecological model is helpful in conceptualizing the relationship of injury risk factors and also the level at which different types of prevention strategies work. The most common social–ecological model used in injury prevention includes four levels: individual, relationship, community, and societal (Fig. 9.4.3) (Dahlberg and Krug 2002; Centers for Disease Control and Prevention 2009). This model posits that individual behaviour is largely determined by the influence of interpersonal relationships, community norms, and societal factors such as culture and political influence.

Individual-level variables that influence injury risk include age, gender, socioeconomic status, health status, and personality characteristics such as risk tolerance and the practice of safety behaviours. Many examples of the influence of individual-level characteristics on injury risk have been documented. For example, men have higher rates of injury than women for almost all causes of injury, and this difference is found consistently across the world. However, women appear to be at greater risk of fire-related burn injuries compared with men, and burn-related injuries account for a much higher proportion of injuries in young children when compared with other age groups (Jie and Ren 1992; Liu et al. 1998). Individual characteristics have been widely

documented to influence the risk for motor vehicle-related deaths. Driver speeding, drinking, distraction, and drowsiness have been identified almost universally around the world as risk factors (Liu et al. 2003; WHO 2004). Declining resiliency and poor health status is an important individual risk factor for injuries among the elderly, particularly falls (Carpenter et al. 2009). Low bone density, poor nutritional status, low body mass index, low calcium intake, co-morbid conditions (hypertension, diabetes), poor performance in activities of daily living, poor cognitive function, poor vision, environmental factors affecting balance, family history of hip fracture, and alcohol consumption have all been identified as individual characteristics associated with increased fall risk (Cummings et al. 1995; Dargent-Molina et al. 1996; Clark et al. 1998; Boonyaratavej et al. 2001). Individual-level interventions often focus on increasing knowledge and encouraging behaviour change.

Relationship-level factors that predict injury include family and interpersonal relationship influences, including the environment in which these relationships occur. Interpersonal relationship factors can increase or decrease risk for injury. For children, parents are a key factor in safety. Limited adult supervision has been associated with pedestrian, drowning and poisoning injury risk in young children (Azizi et al. 1993; Soori, 2001; Brenner 2003; Chadbunchachai et al. 2012). Parent communication style has been tied to risky driving attitudes of teens, and parent driving may influence the driving behaviour of their children (Yang et al. 2013). As we mature, peers and long-term partners become strong influences. The home environment can also influence injury risk. Low socioeconomic status, poor home conditions, and failure to remove home hazards are all factors associated with high and differential rates of home injury (Edelman 2007; Nyberg et al. 2012). Relationship-level interventions often focus on influential communication or changes in the home environment.

Community factors include schools, workplaces, neighbourhoods, all of which are influenced by community social norms and environments. Globally, community factors and characteristics vary more than individual characteristics. For example, the majority of drowning incidents in HICs are associated with recreational or occupational activities, while in most low- and middle-income countries they are associated with everyday activities near natural bodies of water (Kobusingye et al. 2001; Brenner 2003; Hyder et al. 2008). Rural and urban environments also have distinct and different patterns of injury, with injury rates from such causes as road traffic, drowning, poisoning, and occupational-related causes higher in rural communities (Peek-Asa et al. 2004). Prevention strategies usually are designed to impact the climate, processes, and policies in a given local community.

Societal factors encompass the cultural norms and sociopolitical characteristics that influence safety specifically, such as the safety culture. Broad social factors such as population health, socioeconomic status, and political stability also influence injury risk (Centers for Disease Control and Prevention 2009). For example, injury death rates are far higher in low-income countries when compared to HICs. For road traffic deaths, motorization rates rise with income (Kopits and Cropper 2003). In HICs, high motorization rates are not strongly correlated with road traffic deaths (Graham 1993). However, a growing number of LMICs that are experiencing very rapid increases in motorization have had a disproportionate increase in road traffic fatality rates

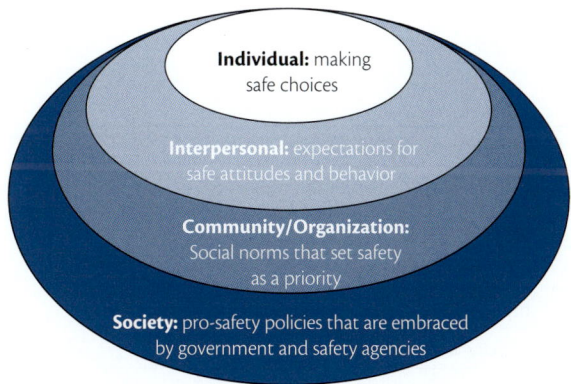

Fig. 9.4.3 The social–ecological model.
Adapted with permission from Dahlberg, L. L., and Krug, E. G., Violence: A global public health problem, in Krug, E. et al. (Eds.), *World Report on Violence and Health*, World Health Organization, Geneva, Switzerland, Copyright © 2002, available from http://www.who.int/violence_injury_prevention/violence/world_report/en/.

(Ghaffar et al. 1999). Much of this increase is due to the lack of an organized safety culture, lack of road traffic safety laws and their enforcement, and governing agencies not prioritizing road safety. Prevention strategies at the societal level often focus on policy implementation and enforcement as well as efforts to change social norms.

Successful injury prevention strategies

Reducing the burden of injury requires multifaceted and comprehensive efforts. As demonstrated through the Haddon matrix and the social–ecological model, injuries occur as a complex interplay between individuals and their physical and sociocultural environments. Injury rates have very clear patterns and determinants that are affected by individual, family, community, geographic, and sociocultural factors. These factors and their interplay must be understood for effective intervention and prevention. Although individual, one-time programmes can have impact by increasing knowledge, encouraging behaviour change, or modifying an environment, long-term and sustainable reductions in injury usually require changes at the sociocultural level.

As the evidence base of successful injury prevention and intervention strategies increases, so do opportunities to translate these programmes to new populations. Translational research, both at the clinic and community level, is a promising priority for injury prevention. Considerations for translation of programmes to new populations include the priority of the injury problem in the new population; human and economic resources to implement and sustain the programme; and cultural relevance of the programme (Woolf 2008). Injury prevention research, which tends to have a relatively short period between action and measurable impact, will likely gain in priority as nations realign research investments to focus on high-impact projects (Zerhouni 2005).

Resources to identify successful injury prevention programmes

A growing evidence base helps guide decisions on the most effective injury prevention strategies. In addition to information to measure the scope, burden, and cost of injuries, several good resources are available to identify evidence-based injury prevention approaches (see Table 9.4.3).

Cochrane Collaboration

The Cochrane Collaboration provides scientific evidence-based reviews of healthcare interventions through the Cochrane Library (Bero and Rennie 1995; Higgins and Green 2011). The Cochrane Library now houses more than 6,000 systematic reviews and more than 8,500 study protocols. This includes more than 500 reviews on injury prevention topics. Abstracts are available free of charge and full reviews are available by subscription, with most major libraries holding subscriptions (see Table 9.4.3). Cochrane reviews are highly weighted towards evidence from randomized controlled trials, which excludes many of the observational evaluations conducted for injury interventions. The search strategy protocol requires inclusion of international findings as well as unpublished data, and when sufficient data are present meta-analyses are conducted. Thus, these reviews are meant to be applicable to an international audience. Recent additions on injury prevention include home safety education, alcohol interventions, and a synthesis of evaluations of the WHO Safe Communities programme (Spinks et al., 2009; Kendrick et al. 2012; Muckle et al. 2012).

Campbell Collaboration

The Campbell Collaboration, begun in 1999, includes systematic reviews of social intervention, divided into the categories of education, crime and justice, international development, and social welfare (Davies and Boruch 2001). The goal of the collaboration is to provide evidence for policy decisions regarding social issues. While the majority of injury prevention-related reviews are found within the crime and justice reviews, many reviews in the other categories are strongly related to injury and violence prevention. The Campbell Collaboration includes evidence from all types of study designs, and has methods groups to ensure systematic interpretation of findings. Recent injury-related reviews address court-mandated interventions for domestic violence, interventions to reduce distress among victims of violence, and school-based bullying prevention programmes (Farrington et al. 2008; Feder et al. 2008; Regehr et al. 2013).

Table 9.4.3 Injury prevention strategies web resources

Cochrane Reviews	http://www.cochrane.org/reviews/index.htm
Campbell Collaboration	http://www.campbellcollaboration.org/
Society for the Advancement of Violence and Injury Research	http://www.savirweb.org/
The Safe States Alliance	http://www.safestates.org/
The Road Traffic Injuries Research Network	http://www.rtirn.net
The International Society for Child and Adolescent Injury Prevention	http://www.iscaip.net
Department of Violence and Injuries Prevention (WHO)	http://www.who.int
Centers for Disease Control and Prevention:	
Injury Prevention and Control	http://www.cdc.gov/injury/
WISQARS, an injury and violence data query tool	http://www.cdc.gov/injury/wisqars/index.html

The Guide to Community Preventive Services: Systematic Reviews and Evidence-Based Recommendations (the *Guide*) was developed by the Task Force on Community Preventive Services, established by the United States Centers for Disease Control and Prevention (Pappaioanou and Evans 1998). The *Guide's* recommendations are primarily based on evidence of effectiveness, including the suitability of the study design, but they also assess the applicability of the intervention to other populations or settings, the economic impact, barriers observed in implementing the interventions, and if the intervention had other beneficial or harmful effects (Briss et al. 2000). The *Guide* then provides a recommendation as to whether the approach is 'strongly recommended', 'recommended', has 'insufficient evidence', or is 'discouraged'. The *Guide* has injury-related reviews in the categories of alcohol, motor vehicle, physical activity, substance abuse, worksite, mental health, social environment, and violence (see Table 9.4.3).

Many global sources of information provide guidance on a variety of injury issues. The National Center for Injury Prevention and Control in the United States provides information about many injury prevention programmes and includes WISQARS, an injury and violence data query tool (see Table 9.4.3). The Department of Violence and Injuries Prevention of the WHO offers a diversity of guidelines and manuals that provide assistance in implementing programmes or conducting research. Examples include guidelines for establishing injury surveillance systems, conducting community based surveys and evaluating pre-hospital care. International non-governmental organizations also offer a variety of assistance and expert members on specific issues (see Table 9.4.3). Examples include the Society for the Advancement of Violence and Injury Research, the Safe States Alliance, the International Society for Child and Adolescent Injury Prevention, the Road Traffic Injuries Research Network, and the International Society for Violence and Injuries Prevention (for website details see Table 9.4.3).

Examples of injury prevention approaches

Successful injury prevention strategies: road traffic injuries

With increased knowledge about the burden of road traffic injuries globally there is growing attention to making roadways safer. Over the last several decades, many high-income countries have experienced decreases in motor vehicle occupant death rates, even while the total miles driven, and thus exposure to the roadway, have increased. In contrast, middle- and low-income countries have experienced large increases in road traffic fatality rates. Nearly 90 per cent of road traffic deaths now occur in low- or middle-income countries, although these countries have only 48 per cent of the world's registered vehicles (WHO 2009). Worldwide, almost half of road traffic deaths are among pedestrians, cyclists, and riders of two-wheeled vehicles. As the fleet of vehicles on these roadways gets more complicated, especially with a growing number of passenger and industrial vehicles, there is potential for continued increases in fatality rates. Efforts to reduce road traffic injuries throughout the world are a good case study of how an integrated approach can lead to successful prevention.

The main reason for success in HICs has been a comprehensive approach to intervention that has included integration of environmental, engineering, legislative, and educational approaches. These changes have evolved over decades, leading to

the development of a safety culture around road traffic. A 'culture of safety' exists when safety is embraced as a fundamental goal at multiple levels: government, community, and individual. The paradigm shift to a traffic safety culture was first formalized in 1997 by the Swedish government with their Vision Zero Initiative (n.d.). Since then, many other countries have adopted similar initiatives which include a traffic safety culture as the foundation.

Historically, as the number of passenger vehicles increased with industrialization, many high-income countries focused efforts on protecting vehicle occupants, and these efforts have shown many successes. In the United States, The National Highway Traffic Safety Administration and the Federal Highway Safety Administration estimate that 243,000 lives were saved between 1966 and 1990 as a result of highway, traffic, and motor vehicle safety programmes (Institute of Medicine 1999). Road modifications mandated by the Federal Highway Traffic Safety Act of 1966 led to safer roadway infrastructures which allowed more cars to travel at higher speeds while reducing crash risk (Graham 1993). At the same time, changes to the motor vehicle itself increased the likelihood of survival in a crash. In addition to the implementation of seat belts and then air bags, legislation required modifications that improved vehicle crash worthiness. Some examples of these modifications include shatter-resistant windshields, collapsible steering columns, crash-friendly dashboard surfaces, frames that are resistant to passenger space intrusion, increased strength of the vehicle frame, seat, and doors, lap and shoulder belts, and air bags (Haddon and Baker 1981). Studies have found that these safety improvements to the motor vehicle led to a 24–40 per cent decrease in fatal crashes and saved over 9000 lives each year (Robertson 1981; Institute of Medicine 1999).

Most of these changes were due in part to legislative efforts, and these efforts were themselves multifaceted in nature. For example, the implementation of many of these laws required a successful engineering development as a foundation—improved crash worthiness of cars was based on concentrated research to identify the most successful design features, which were then required legislatively. Other legislative approaches are more behavioural in nature, such as laws that require seat belt use, driver training, speed limits, and laws that aim to reduce drunk driving. Implementation of these laws requires successful advocacy and education of legislators. However, their effectiveness varies dramatically. For example, most countries have laws against drinking and driving, yet countries have wide variation in the rate of alcohol-involved crashes as well as the number of drinking drivers, drivers cited for drinking and driving, and punished for drinking and driving. While this variation has much to do with factors associated with patterns of alcohol consumption, access to transportation, and the driving culture, this variation is also due to factors associated with the laws themselves. The effectiveness of legislative approaches depends on the level of enforcement that accompanies them and on the perception that the legislated consequences will actually occur (Mann et al. 2003). For example, the effectiveness of drinking and driving laws is influenced by the level of enforcement, the ability of courts to impose penalties, and that the nature of the penalties serves as a deterrent.

The focus on motor vehicle occupants without concomitant integration of urban planning, sustainable transportation, and pedestrian and bicycle safety may be problematic in the long run. More recently, countries throughout Europe as well as Australia and the United States have introduced an approach called 'traffic calming' that aims to control motor vehicle traffic and speed in neighbourhoods, and thus increase safety and walkability in communities (Ewing 1999). The concept of traffic calming dates back to the Dutch city of Delft in the 1960s, when residents angry with fast-moving cars cutting through their local streets blocked them with gardens, social areas, and playgrounds (Ewing 1999). Modern traffic calming involves a variety of approaches to reduce traffic volume and speed in residential areas using visually appealing strategies.

Success in reducing road traffic deaths has depended on the development of an infrastructure that can identify and respond to road hazards, and a wide variety of approaches to address these hazards. In some developed and many developing countries, the car culture is growing without concomitant safety cultures (Bishai et al. 2003; WHO 2007). Highway design standards are often outdated or translated too directly from an industrialized country, and insufficient resources for roadway maintenance are available (Transport and Road Research Laboratory 1991). Poorly designed and maintained roadways are even further stressed by an ever-increased number and variety of vehicles. In addition to a growing number of passenger cars and a high proportion of commercial vehicles and buses, developing countries' roadways include animal-powered vehicles, small engine vehicles (such as scooters and motorcycles) that carry multiple people, bicycles, human-powered transport vehicles (such as rickshaws), and pedestrians. This complex mix of vehicles contributes to increased deaths on the road.

In order to avert the growing toll of road traffic deaths, the WHO has called for a 'systems approach' in which the interaction between vehicles, roads, road users and their physical, social, and economic environments form the basis for a multisectoral response (WHO 2004). The implementation of comprehensive traffic safety laws has been identified as one of the most important actions to reduce global road traffic injuries, and these laws must include enforcement with appropriate penalties and concomitant public awareness campaigns. The WHO has also called on governments to identify lead agencies in traffic safety, and to give these agencies a clear mission and authority for creating safer roads. Governments must also encourage multisectoral collaboration and support ongoing collection of data. These steps all fit within defined models of creating a global traffic safety culture.

Successful injury prevention strategies: drowning

Drowning prevention efforts often focus on three types of strategies: (1) remove, reduce, or change the water hazard; (2) change behaviour in risk-taking, supervision, or skills around water; and (3) prevent contact between people and the water environment (Wilson and Rogmans 2006). While these strategies remain relevant in all settings, drowning is experienced differently in HIC and LMIC settings. In HICs drowning events are often associated with recreational swimming, in swimming pools or along the coast; while drowning in LMICs often occurs as a result of everyday activities near open bodies of water, ditches, or uncovered wells (Hyder et al. 2008). Therefore, successful drowning prevention strategies are often not transferable from HICs to LMICs.

Since the 1970s, HICs have implemented well-established preventive measures to prevent drowning events including: mandating fencing and self-closing or self-latching gates around domestic and public swimming pools; requiring supervision by certified lifeguards at public pools and swimming beaches; and recommending the use of personal flotation devices for boaters and novice swimmers (Thompson and Rivara 1998; Pearn et al. 2008; Centers for Disease Control and Prevention, 2012). For adults, basic swimming instruction is an important skill, and deters the likelihood of drowning particularly in domestic or public swimming pools. A recent evaluation of a rip current related intervention in Australia revealed intervention area respondents were more likely to report they would never swim at an unguarded beach, and if caught in a rip would: signal a guard, not swim directly to the beach against the rip, and float and drift with the rip (Hatfield et al. 2011). The knowledge of basic life support or resuscitative measures, that is, cardiopulmonary resuscitation, among non-medical personnel is also crucial to treat drowning victims. Likewise, alcohol is an important risk factor for drowning that ought to be avoided whether at swimming pools, at swimming beaches or on watercrafts including recreational boats.

Many of these drowning prevention strategies are applicable to children though swim instruction thus far has been understudied and has yielded limited effectiveness (Asher et al. 1995). Attentive supervision of children in and around domestic swimming pools, swimming beaches and around the home is crucial. And yet, a recent Cochrane review of home interventions found there was a lack of evidence that home safety interventions were effective in preventing children being left alone in the bath, which is a common cause of drowning among children (Kendrick et al. 2012).

In LMICs, the epidemiology of drowning is quite different as children comprise the largest burden. In Bangladesh, for example, drowning is one of the most common causes of death in children aged 1–4 years (Borse et al. 2011). More importantly, the critical risk factor—water—abounds; a single district alone might have 50,000 or more ditches and ponds. Obviously, fencing off these bodies of water is not feasible in this context; however, other barrier-based interventions for drowning prevention in children younger than 5 years have been piloted in rural Bangladesh (Callaghan et al. 2010). Door barriers (which prevent young children from leaving the home) and playpens (which limit movement of young children) appear to work in pilot settings, especially for children aged 1–3 years at high risk of drowning when their mothers are busy performing their daily household tasks. In addition, crèches (day care centres) have also shown promise by removing children from high-risk contexts during the highest risk time of day in similar settings (Rahman et al. 2010). These interventions might be effective ways to reduce the number of drowning events and to ease the burden of supervision on mothers. Producing such barriers in the community or making them available at little or no cost to low-income families in LMICs, particularly in regions where drowning is most endemic, is an important agenda for global public health. However, large-scale studies are needed to determining the true effectiveness of these interventions before they can be widely recommended.

Successful injury prevention strategies: burns

There are sufficient data available from HICs to support the claim that burns can be successfully prevented using education, engineering changes, enforcement of legislative protection, and environmental modifications (Peck et al. 2009). A range of successful burn prevention strategies such as smoke detectors, regulating hot water heater temperatures, mandating flame-resistant children's sleepwear, and enforcing safe and proper electrical wiring of residences and businesses have been implemented across HICs (Mock et al. 2008). Installing smoke detectors in the United States, for example, has been associated with a 61 per cent reduction in the risk of death from residential house fires (Marshall et al. 1998). This reduction has been made possible by programmes such as the Smoke Alarm Installation and Fire Safety Education of the National Center for Injury Prevention and Control (part of the Centers for Disease Control and Prevention) which has targeted low-income households since 1998 and has installed approximately 553,000 smoke alarms with 3755 lives potentially saved (Kress et al. 2012). Further, should someone in a HIC suffer a burn, she or he is likely to be transported to a dedicated burn centre in a timely fashion to receive specialized care necessary to reduce damage and restore functioning.

Many of these strategies are impractical for LMICs given certain institutional and environmental challenges and a different epidemiology of burns. For example, childhood burns risk factors include: use of kerosene, cooking in open spaces, overcrowding, and lack of parental supervision (Dissanaike and Rahimi 2009; Mashreky et al. 2010; Van Niekerk et al. 2010). Interventions that have been proposed include separating the cooking area from the living area, increasing the height of cooking surfaces, making separate cooking stations outside the house, reducing the amount of flammable substances available in the household, and enhancing child supervision (WHO 2008).

Two vulnerable groups can be identified in LMICs—young infants and children and adolescent/adult females (Golan et al. in press). For younger children, a partitioned area imposed during cooking hours, shelves at appropriate heights, and supervision to avoid young children carrying hot objects are being suggested. In addition, timely outpatient assessment and treatment is vital to mitigating the impact of such burns, and creation of social awareness has been used for mothers and caretakers (Mukerji et al. 2001). Interventions for the second risk group (young women) include safe, inexpensive and efficient kerosene lamps and stoves placed above the floor level (McLoughlin 1995). Other efforts at encouraging women (through grassroots education and multi-media) to wear appropriate clothing to reduce clothes catching fire and using flame-resistant materials in the manufacturing of local dresses are being explored (Jayaraman et al. 1993).

Some of these interventions have been reiterated by the WHO's world report on child injury prevention which also promotes the use of safe kerosene lamps, separating cooking areas from living areas, raising cooking facilities off the ground, banning of fireworks, and wearing flame-retardant clothing materials (WHO 2008). In LMIC households, cookstoves are commonly used for cooking and heating and unfortunately, poor manufacturing standards, low quality control, and a lack of safety features have made this a key risk factor for burns (Peck et al. 2008). In response, the Global Alliance for Clean Cookstoves, led by the United Nations Foundation, seeks to encourage 100 million homes in LMICs to adopt clean and safe cookstoves by 2020 as well as support a clean and innovative cookstove industry. Such cookstoves will dramatically reduce fuel consumption, exposure to harmful emissions and smoke, and the risk of fire burns (Global Alliance for Clean Cookstoves n.d.).

Successful injury prevention strategies: acute care

Many injuries lead to death because of inadequate emergency and trauma care, and pre-hospital deaths are disproportionately large in LMICs. In low-income countries, pre-hospital mortality is extremely high. For example, one study found that 81 per cent of trauma deaths occurred in the pre-hospital setting in Ghana, a low-income country, compared with 72 per cent for Mexico, a middle-income country, and 59 per cent in the United States (Mock et al. 1998).

Improvements in emergency medical response and trauma care have had a major impact in preventing deaths from injuries. Reducing the time between injury and definitive treatment leads to improved outcomes (Institute of Medicine 1999). The most effective way to reduce time to treatment is through the implementation of a trauma system, with changes in the social environment to include better coordination between agencies, triage and transport protocols, assignment of treatment levels to trauma centres, and improved training and certification at all levels of emergency care delivery.

Early evaluations of trauma systems conducted in high-income countries focused on the number of deaths that could be prevented, and estimates were in the range of 20 per cent to 40 per cent (Shackford et al. 1986; Mackenzie et al. 1992; Mullins et al. 1994). One meta-analysis of the effectiveness of pre-hospital trauma systems in LMICs concluded that injury mortality could be reduced by approximately a quarter (Henry and Reingold 2012). Effects were strongest for middle-income countries, largely because they had stronger health infrastructures on which to build trauma systems. One study estimated that if injury case fatality rates in LMICs could be reduced to the same level as those in HICs, more than 1.7 million deaths, over a third of all injury deaths, could be reduced globally (Mock et al. 2012).

Developing systems for coordinated care, especially when out-of-hospital coordination is involved, is a challenge. In many countries, no organized system to identify and transport patients to the hospital exist (Nielsen et al. 2012). In low-income countries and in rural areas, patients are more likely to arrive at the hospital in private vehicles than in an ambulance (Young et al. 2003; Nielsen et al. 2012). The private citizens who provide emergency transport are also the most likely to provide first aid in the absence of trained emergency response personnel. Because building emergency transportation infrastructures would be expensive, experts have proposed formalizing relationships with commercial vehicles and local citizens to create an organized approach (Mock et al. 2012).

Lack of trained specialists in emergency care, both in the field and in hospitals, is another barrier to reducing trauma death. Many countries lack trained medical personnel, equipment, and infrastructure (Kobusingye et al. 2005). An evaluation of trauma care capabilities in Mexico, Vietnam, India, and Ghana indicated that even when a sufficient number of healthcare professionals were trained, 'brain drain' from rural to urban and from low- to higher-income communities led to widespread provider shortages (Mock et al. 2006). In order to develop a stronger trauma response system, improvements must be made in the areas of increased human resources, physical resources, security for healthcare personnel, transportation systems to get patients to definitive treatment, and administrative infrastructure (Kobusingye 2005; Mock et al. 2006).

Although many of these improvements require new resources, system-wide changes are possible through effective planning even in the absence of significantly increased resources. For example, several low-cost trauma training programmes have been developed and used effectively in low-income countries, and these have contributed to decreased injury mortality (Kobusingye 2005). Administrative changes, such as making necessary diagnostic equipment available for critical trauma cases, are also low cost. However, identifying and implementing low-cost strategies cycles back to the need for data. Finding the low-cost strategies that will work in a healthcare facility will be enhanced by data systems that can track trends in patient treatment and be used for quality assurance. These systems are lacking in many healthcare organizations throughout the world.

Improving emergency medical systems and trauma treatment capacity could greatly reduce injury mortality worldwide, and also reduce the physical, emotional, and financial consequences of severe injuries. These efforts need to be in collaboration with general worldwide efforts to improve access to public health and medical services. Over the past few years, the WHO has released guidelines for pre-hospital and trauma care with a special focus on LMICs, and approaches to improved acute care are increasingly evaluated in different countries.

Building capacity for injury prevention

In order to identify and implement successful injury prevention strategies, countries, states, and local communities need to develop necessary infrastructure and capacity to conduct the essential activities of an injury prevention programme. Infrastructure includes the designation or creation of agencies and leadership to oversee and integrate essential injury control activities within an inter-sectoral strategic framework. Capacity includes the availability of human, financial, relational, and structural resources. Both components are vital to the sustainability of any injury prevention and control programme. Since there is a lack of trained injury prevention professionals in many LMICs, capacity development efforts are critical in the developing world to address their high burden of injuries and unique challenges.

The WHO Department of Violence and Injury Prevention and Disability has recently responded to this need by outlining three key domains for such efforts in *Capacity Building for Preventing Injury and Violence: Strategic Plan 2009–2013* (WHO Department of Violence and Injury Prevention and Disability 2009). These domains include:

◆ Human resources: people and the knowledge and skills they require.

◆ Institutional and infrastructural capacity: the systems and structures necessary to allow for effective human resources.

◆ Networks and partnerships: a means by which capacities can be strengthened within and across settings (WHO Department of Violence and Injury Prevention and Disability 2009).

In order to facilitate such efforts, the WHO has developed two training programmes, Teach Violence and Injury Prevention (TEACH-VIP) and Mentor Violence and Injury Prevention

(MENTOR-VIP). TEACH-VIP, now in its second iteration, is a comprehensive injury prevention and control curriculum which is delivered via PowerPoint presentations and supplementary information structured around 67 lessons—22 'core' and 45 advanced' (WHO n.d. a). Whereas the TEACH-VIP training curriculum focuses on the transfer of knowledge, MENTOR-VIP offers an opportunity for junior investigators and injury prevention professionals to further develop key skills. MENTOR-VIP is a 12-month mentorship programme which matches mentees with leading injury prevention experts to accomplish specific goals (WHO n.d. b). In addition to training materials developed by the World Health Organization, many new online training modules are available. One example is the Road Traffic Injury Prevention and Control in Low- and Middle-Income Countries, which provides seven modules to introduce a non-expert audience to road traffic safety principles (http://www.jhsph.edu/research/centers-and-institutes/johns-hopkins-international-injury-research-unit/training/courses-in-injury-prevention/free-online-training/). The CDC National Center of Injury Control and Prevention offers several online training programs focused on topics such as the principles of prevention (http://www.cdc.gov/violenceprevention/POP.html) and concussion management (http://www.cdc.gov/violenceprevention/POP.html).

The development of a critical mass of trained injury professionals within a country or region to understand the local environment, develop, implement, and evaluate appropriate prevention programmes is a crucial step. The Fogarty International Center of the National Institutes of Health in the United States has provided opportunities for twinning between US-based and developing country institutions for capacity development which targets all three WHO domains (Fogarty International Center n.d.). These programmes cover collaborations in countries such as China, Columbia, and Pakistan; topics from traumatic brain injuries, violence, to emergency care; and promote sustainable research and dissemination of results to influence policy and investments in each country.

Conclusion

Despite the high burden of injuries throughout the world, investment in safety and injury prevention infrastructure has been low. In low-income countries such as Pakistan and Uganda, approximately US$0.07 per capita was devoted to safety. In every country, the amount invested in prevention is far surpassed by the amount spent on the treatment of traumatic injuries, and thus studies that focus on cost benefits are badly needed. International assistance has also not prioritized safety or injury prevention. External assistance to the health sectors of low-income countries was US$2–3 per DALY lost to infectious diseases, but only US$0.06 per DALY lost to injuries (Mock et al. 2004).

Since 90 per cent of the world's population lives in LMICs, and the burden of injuries is predicted to increase in these countries, it is imperative that future research and development activities focus especially on their needs. Basic research to describe the existing burden, causes, and distribution of injuries is still needed in LMICs. Trials of injury interventions have largely not been conducted in LMICs, and there is a great need to modify, adapt and test existing, as well as new interventions in these specific settings. Work is also required to assess barriers to implementation of such interventions globally.

The role of international organizations (such as the WHO and the World Bank) and national agencies (such as ministries of health or medical research councils) needs to be emphasized in moving ahead the injury prevention agenda. The international movements currently underway for violence prevention and road traffic injuries prevention as promulgated through the two WHO world reports are examples of how joint global–national partnerships are needed for making change.

Progress will also be supported if a growing number of professionals become advocates for safety. Professionals from public health, medicine, engineering, social services, urban planning, law and law enforcement, among others, can all have a strong voice in raising awareness for safety programmes and to encourage individuals to make safe choices.

Key points

◆ Injuries and violence are a leading cause of mortality and morbidity worldwide.

◆ Injuries disproportionately affect young and vulnerable populations, and injury rates are disproportionately high among LMICs.

◆ Prevention of injuries is very feasible and works best with a multidisciplinary and integrated approach.

◆ A growing body of research and resources can help identify potentially effective approaches to prevent and reduce the consequences of injury.

◆ Building capacity for injury prevention should be a priority for all countries, but is an urgent need for LMICs.

References

Aeron-Thomas, A., Jacobs, G.D., Stexton, B., Gururaj, G., and Rahmann, F. (2004). *The Involvement and Impact of Road Crashes on the Poor: Bangladesh and India Case Studies*. Published Project Report PRP 010. Crowthorne: Transport Research Laboratory LTD.

Asher, K.N., Rivara, F.P., Feliz, D., Vance, L., and Dunne, R. (1995). Water safety training as a potential means of reducing risk of young children's drowning. *Injury Prevention*, 1, 228–33.

Azizi, B.H., Zulkifli, H.I., and Kasim, M.S. (1993). Risk factors for accidental poisoning in urban Malaysian children. *Annals of Tropical Paediatrics*, 13(2), 183–8.

Bero, L. and Rennie, D. (1995). The Cochrane Collaboration. Preparing, maintaining, and disseminating systematic reviews of the effects of health care. *Journal of the American Medical Association*, 274, 1935–8.

Bishai, D., Hyder, A.A., Ghaffar, A., Morrow, R.H., and Kobusingye, O. (2003). Rates of public investment for road safety in developing countries: case studies of Uganda and Pakistan. *Health Policy and Planning*, 18(2), 232–5.

Boonyaratavej, N., Suriyawongpaisal, P., Takkinsatien, A., Wanvarie, S., Rajatanavin, R., and Apiyasawat, P. (2001). Physical activity and risk factors for hip fractures in Thai women. *Osteoporosis International*, 12(3), 244–8.

Borse, N., Hyder, A.A., Streatfield, P.K., Arifeen, S.E., and Bishai, D. (2011). Childhood drowning and traditional rescue measures: case study from Matlab, Bangladesh. *Archives of Disease in Childhood*, 96(7), 675–80.

Brenner, R.A. (2003). Prevention of drowning in infants, children and adolescents. *Pediatrics*, 112(2), 440–5.

Briss, P.A., Zaza, S., Pappaioanou, M., et al. (2000). Developing an evidence based guide to community preventive services-methods. *American Journal of Preventive Medicine*, 19(1S), 35–43.

Callaghan, J.A., Hyder, A.A., Khan, R., Blum, L.S., Arifeen, S., and Bacqui, A.H. (2010). Child supervision practices for drowning prevention in rural Bangladesh: a pilot study of supervision tools. *Journal of Epidemiology and Community Health*, 64(7), 645–7.

Carpenter, C.R., Scheatzle, M.D., D'Antonio, J.A., Ricci, P.T., and Coben, J.H. (2009) Identification of fall risk factors in older adult emergency department patients. *Academic Emergency Medicine*, 16(3), 211–19.

Centers for Disease Control and Prevention (2009). *Violence Prevention: The Social-Ecological Model: A Framework for Violence Prevention*. [Online] Available at: http://www.cdc.gov/ViolencePrevention/overview/social-ecologicalmodel.html.

Centers for Disease Control and Prevention (2012). Drowning—United States, 2005–2009. *Morbidity and Mortality Weekly Report*, 61(19), 344–7.

Centers for Disease Control and Prevention and the Injury Control and Emergency Health Services Section of the American Public Health Association (1997). Recommended framework for presenting injury mortality data. *Morbidity and Mortality Weekly Report Recommendations and Reports*, 46(RR-14), 1–30. Available at: http://www.cdc.gov/mmwr/preview/mmwrhtml/00049162.htm.

Chadbunchachai, W., Suphanchaimaj, W., Settasatien, A., and Jinwong, T. (2012). Road traffic injuries in Thailand: current situation. *Journal of the Medical Association of Thailand*, 95(Suppl. 7), S274–81.

Clark, P., de la Pena, F., Gomez Garcia, F., Orozco, J.A., and Tugwell, P. (1998). Risk factors for osteoporotic hip fractures in Mexicans. *Archives of Medical Research*, 29(3), 253–7.

Cummings, S.R., Nevitt, M.C., Browner, W.S., et al. (1995). Risk factors for hip fracture in white women. *The New England Journal of Medicine*, 332(12), 767–73.

Dahlberg, L.L. and Krug, E.G. 2002). Violence: a global public health problem. In E. Krug, L.L. Dahlberg, J.A. Mercy, A.B. Zwi, and R. Lozano, (eds.) *World Report on Violence and Health*, pp. 1–56. Geneva: WHO.

Dargent-Molina, P., Favier, F., Grandjean, H., et al. (1996). Fall-related factors and risk of hip fracture: the EPIDOS Prospective Study. *The Lancet*, 348(9021), 145–9.

Davies, P. and Boruch, R. (2001). The Campbell Collaboration does for public policy what Cochrane does for health. *British Medical Journal*, 323(7308), 294–5.

Dissanaike, S. and Rahimi, M. (2009). Epidemiology of burn injuries: highlighting cultural and socio-demographic aspects. *International Review of Psychiatry*, 21(6), 505–11.

Eaton, D.K., Kann, L., Kinchen, S., et al. (2012). Youth risk behavior surveillance—United States. *Morbidity and Mortality Weekly Report*, 61(4), 1–162.

Edelman, L.S. (2007). Social and economic factors associated with the risk of burn injury. *Burns*, 33(8), 958–65.

Evans, L. (1995). Restraint effectiveness, occupant ejection from cars, and fatality reductions. *Accident Analysis & Prevention*, 22, 167–75.

Ewing, R.H. (1999). *Traffic Calming: State of the Practice*. FHWA-RD-99-135. Washington DC: Federal Highway Administration.

Farrington, D., Baldrey, A.C., Kyvsgaard, B., and Ttofi, M. (2008). Effectiveness of programs to prevent school bullying. *Campbell Collaboration Library of Systematic Reviews*, 5, 6. Available at: http://campbellcollaboration.org/lib/project/77/.

Feder, L., Wilson, D.B., and Austin, S. (2008). Court-mandated interventions for individuals convicted of domestic violence. *The Campbell Collaboration*, Cambridge, UK.

Fogarty International Center (n.d.). *Fogarty International Collaborative Trauma and Injury Research Training Program (TRAUMA)*. [Online] Available at: http://www.fic.nih.gov/Programs/Pages/trauma-injury.aspx.

Ghaffar, A., Hyder, A.A., Mastoor, M.I., and Shaikh, I. (1999). Injuries in Pakistan: directions for future health policy. *Health Policy and Planning*, 14(1), 11–17.

Global Alliance for Clean Cookstoves (n.d.). Website. [Online] Available at: http://www.cleancookstoves.org.

Global Burden of Disease Study (2012). *Global Burden of Disease Study 2010 (GBD 2010) Results by Cause 1990–2010*. Seattle, WA: Institute for Health Metrics and Evaluation.

Golshan, A., Patel, C., and Hyder, A.A. (2013). A systematic review of the epidemiology of unintentional burn injuries in South Asia. *Journal of Public Health*, 35(3), 384–96.

Graham, J.D. (1993). Injuries from traffic crashes: meeting the challenge. *Annual Review of Public Health*, 14, 515–43.

Haddon, W., Jr. (1970). On the escape of tigers: an ecologic note. *American Journal of Public Health*, 60, 2229–34.

Haddon, W., Jr. (1972). A logical framework for categorizing highway safety phenomena and activity. *Journal of Trauma*, 12, 193–207.

Haddon, W. and Baker, S.P. (1981). Injury control. In D.W. Clark and B. McMahaon (eds.) *Preventive and Community Medicine* (2nd ed.), pp. 109–40. Boston, MA: Little, Brown, and Company.

Hatfield, J., Williamson, A., Sherker, S., Brander, R., and Hayen, A. (2011). Development and evaluation of an intervention to reduce rip current related beach drowning. *Accident Analysis & Prevention*, 46, 45–51.

Henry, J.A. and Reingold, A.L. (2012). Prehospital trauma systems reduce mortality in developing countries: a systematic review and meta-analysis. *Journal of Trauma and Acute Care Surgery*, 73(1), 261–8.

Higgins, J.P.T. and Green, S. (eds.) (2011). *Cochrane Handbook for Systematic Reviews of Interventions Version 5.1.0* [updated March 2011]. The Cochrane Collaboration. Available at: http://www.cochrane-handbook.org.

Hyder, A.A., Borse, N.N., Blum, L., Khan, R., El Arifeen, S., and Baqui, A.H. (2008). Childhood drowning in low- and middle-income countries: urgent need for intervention trials. *Journal of Paediatrics and Child Health*, 44(4), 221–7.

Hyder, A.A. and Morrow, R.H. (2006) *Measures of Health and Disease in Populations*. In R.B. Black, M. Merson, and A. Mills (eds.) *International Public Health: Diseases, Programs, Systems and Policies* (2nd ed.), pp. 1–42. Boston, MA: Jones & Bartlett Publishers.

Institute of Medicine (1999). *Reducing the Burden of Injury: Advancing Prevention and Treatment*. Washington, DC: National Academy Press.

Jacobs, G., Aeron-Thomas, A., and Astrop, A. (2000). *Economic Cost of Road Traffic Injuries*. London: Transport Research Laboratories.

Jayaraman, V., Mathangi Ramakrishnan, K., and Davies, M.R. (1993). Burns in Madras, India: an analysis of 1368 patients in 1 year., *Burns*, 19, 339–44.

Jie, X. and Ren, C.B. 1992). Burn injuries in the Dong Bei area of China: a study of 12,606 cases. *Burns*, 18(3), 228–32.

Kendrick, D., Young, B., Mason-Jones, A.J., et al. (2012). Home safety education and provision of safety equipment for injury prevention. *Cochrane Database of Systematic Reviews*, 12, CD005014.

Kobusingye, O., Guwatudde, D., and Lett, R. (2001). Injury patterns in rural and urban Uganda. *Injury Prevention*, 7(1), 46–50.

Kobusingye, O.C., Hyder, A.A., Bishai, D., Hicks, E.R., Mock, C., and Joshipura, M. (2005). Emergency medical systems in low- and middle-income countries: recommendations for action. *Bulletin of the World Health Organization*, 83(8), 626–31.

Kopits, E. and Cropper, M. (2003). *Traffic Fatalities and Economic Growth*. Policy Research Working Paper 3035. Washington, DC: World Bank.

Kress, H.C., Noonan, R., Freire, K., Marr, A., and Olson, A. (2012). Top 20 violence and injury practice innovations since 1992. *Journal of Safety Research*, 43(4), 257–63.

Liu, E.H., Khatri, B., Shakya, Y.M., and Richard, B.M. (1998). A 3 year prospective audit of burn patients treated at the Western Regional Hospital of Nepal. *Burns*, 24(2), 129–33.

Liu, G.F., Han, S., Liang, D.H., et al. (2003). Driver sleepiness and risk of car crashes in Shenyang, a Chinese Northeastern city: population-based case-control study. *Biomedical and Environmental Sciences*, 16(3), 219–26.

MacKenzie, E., Steinwachs, D., and Bone, L. (1992). Inter-rater reliability of preventable death judgments. The Preventable Death Study Group. *Journal of Trauma*, 33(2), 292–302.

Mann, N.C., Mullins, R.J., MacKenzie, E.J, Jurkovich, G.J., and Mock, C.N. (1999). A systematic review of published evidence regarding trauma system effectiveness. *Journal of Trauma*, 47, S25–33.

Mann, R.E., Smart, R.G., Stoduto, G., et al. (2003). The effects of drinking-driving laws: a test of the differential deterrence hypothesis. *Addiction*, 98(11), 1531–6.

Marshall, S.W., Runyan, C.W., Bangdiwala, S.I., Linzer, M.A., Sacks, J.J., and Butts, J. D. (1998). Fatal residential fires: who dies and who survives? *Journal of the American Medical Association*, 279(20), 1633–7.

Mashreky, S.R., Rahman, A., Khan, T.F., Svanström, L., and Rahman, F. (2010). Determinants of childhood burns in rural Bangladesh: a nested case-control study. *Health Policy*, 96(3), 226–30.

McLoughlin, E. (1995). A simple guide to burn prevention. *Burns*, 21, 226–9.

Mock, C., Joshipura, M., Arreola-Risa, C., Quansah, R. (2012). An estimate of the number of lives that could be saved through improvements in trauma care globally. *World Journal of Surgery*, 36, 959–63.

Mock, C.N., Jurkovich, G.J., nii-Amon-Kotei, D., Arreola-Risa, C., and Maier, R.V. (1998). Trauma mortality patterns in three nations at different economic levels: implications for global trauma system development. *Journal of Trauma*, 44(5), 804–12.

Mock, C., Nguyen, S., Quansah, R., Arreola-Risa, C., Viradia, R., and Joshipura, M. 2006). Evaluation of trauma care capabilities in four countries using the WHO-IATSIC Guidelines for Essential Trauma Care. *World Journal of Surgery*, 30(6), 946–56.

Mock, C., Peck, M., Peden, M., and Krug, E. (eds.) (2008). *A WHO Plan for Burn Prevention and Care*. Geneva: WHO.

Mock, C., Quansah, R., Krishnan, R., Arreola-Risa, C., and Rivara, F. (2004). Strengthening the prevention and care of injuries worldwide. *The Lancet*, 363(9427), 2172–9.

Muckle, W., Muckle, J., Welch, V., and Tugwell, P. (2012). Managed alcohol as a harm reduction intervention for alcohol addiction in populations at high risk for substance abuse. *Cochrane Database of Systematic Reviews*, 12, CD006747.

Mukerji, G., Chamania, S., Patidar, G.P., and Gupta, S. (2001). Epidemiology of paediatric burns in Indore, India. *Burns*, 27(1), 33–8.

Mullins, R. J., Veum-Stone, J., Helfand, M., et al. (1994). Outcome of hospitalized injured patients after institution of a trauma system in an urban area. *Journal of the American Medical Association*, 271(24), 1919–24.

Murray, C. and Lopez, A. (1996). *Global Burden of Disease and Injuries*. Cambridge, MA: Harvard University Press.

Murray, C.J., Ezzati, M., Flaxman, A.D., et al. (2013). GBD 2010: design, definitions, and metrics. *The Lancet*, 380(9859), 2063–6.

Nathens, A., Jurkovich, G., Cummings, P., Rivara, F., and Maier, R. (2000). The effect of organized systems of trauma care on motor vehicle crash mortality. *Journal of the American Medical Association*, 283(15), 1990–4.

National Highway Traffic Safety Administration (2007). Seat belt use in 2006–use rates in states and territories. *Traffic Safety Facts*, DOT-HS-810-960. Available at: http://www-nrd.nhtsa.dot.gov/pdf/nrd-30/NCSA/RNotes/2007/810690.pdf.

Nielsen, K., Mock, C., Joshipura, M., Rubiano, A.M., Zakariah, A., Rivara, F. (2012). Assessment of the status of prehospital care in 13 low- and middle-income countries. *Prehospital Emergency Care*, 16(3), 381–9.

Norton, R., Hyder, A.A., and Gururaj, G. (2006). Unintentional injuries and violence. In R.B. Black, M. Merson, and A. Mills (eds.) *International Public Health: Diseases, Programs, Systems and Policies* (2nd ed.), pp. 323–54. Silver Boston, MA: Jones & Bartlett Publishers.

Nyberg, C., Schyllander, J., Stark Ekman, D., and Janson, S. (2012). Socio-economic risk factors for injuries in Swedish children and adolescents: a national study over 15 years. *Global Public Health*, 7(10), 1170–84.

Pappaioanou, M. and Evans, C., Jr. (1998). Development of the Guide to Community Preventive Services: a U.S. Public Health Service initiative. *Journal of Public Health Management & Practice*, 4(S2), 48–54.

Pearn, J.H., Nixon, J.W., Franklin, R.C., and Wallis, B. (2008). Safety legislation, public health policy and drowning prevention. *International Journal of Injury Control and Safety Promotion*, 15(2), 122–3.

Peck, M., Molnar, J., and Swart, D. (2009). A global plan for burn prevention and care. *Bulletin of the World Health Organization*, 87(10), 802–3.

Peck, M.D., Kruger, G.E., van der Merwe, A.E., Godkaumbura, W., and Ahuja, R.B. (2008). Burns and fires from non-electric domestic appliances in low and middle income countries Part I. The scope of the problem. *Burns*, 34(3), 303–11.

Peden, M., McGee, K., and Sharma, G. (2002). *The Injury Chart Book: A Graphical Overview of the Global Burden of Injuries*. Geneva: WHO.

Peek-Asa, C., Zwerling, C., and Stallones, L. (2004). Acute traumatic injuries in rural populations. *Am J Public Health*, 94(10), 1689–93.

Pérez-Núñez, R., Pelcastre-Villafuerte, B., Híjar, M., Avila-Burgos, L., and Celis, A. (2012). A qualitative approach to the intangible cost of road traffic injuries. *International Journal of Injury Control and Safety Promotion*, 19(1), 69–79.

Rahman, A., Miah, A.H., Mashreky, S.R., Shafinaz, S., Linnan, M., and Rahman, F. (2010). Initial community response to a childhood drowning prevention programme in a rural setting in Bangladesh. *Injury Prevention*, 16(1), 21–5.

Regehr, C., Alaggia, R., Dennis, J., Pitts, A., and Saini, M. (2013). Interventions to reduce distress in adult victims of sexual violence and rape: A systematic review. *The Campbell Collaboration*, Cambridge, UK.

Roberts, C., Freeman, C., Samdal, O., et al. (2009). The Health Behaviour in School-aged Children (HBSC) study: methodological developments and current tensions. *Int J Public Health*, 54(Suppl. 2), 140–50.

Robertson, L.S. (1981). Automobile safety regulations and death reductions in the United States. *American Journal of Public Health*, 71(8), 818–22.

Shackford, S.R., Hollingworth-Fridlund, P., Cooper, G.F., and Eastman, A.B. (1986). The effect of regionalization upon quality of trauma care as assessed by concurrent audit before and after institution of a trauma system: a preliminary report. *Journal of Trauma*, 26(9), 812–20.

Soori, H. (2001). Developmental risk factors for unintentional childhood poisoning. *Saudi Medical Journal*, 22(3), 227–30.

Spinks, A., Turner, C., Nixon, J., and McClure, R.J. (2009). The 'WHO Safe Communities' model for the prevention of injury in whole populations. *Cochrane Database of Systematic Reviews*, 8, CD004445.

Thomas, S., Acton, C., Nixon, J., Battistutta, D., Pitt, W.R., and Clark, R. (1994). Effectiveness of bicycle helmets in preventing head injury in children: case-control study. *British Medical Journal*, 308, 173–7.

Thompson, D.C. and Rivara, F.P. (2000). Pool fencing for preventing drowning in children. *Cochrane Database of Systematic Reviews*, 2, CD001047.

Transport and Road Research Laboratory (1991). *Towards Safer Roads in Developing Countries: A Guide for Engineers and Planners, Overseas Development Administration*. Berkshire: Transport and Road Research Laboratory.

US General Accounting Office (1991). *Motorcycle Helmet Laws Save Lives and Reduce Costs to Society*. GAO/RCED-91-170. Washington, DC: US General Accounting Office.

Van Niekerk, A., Menckel, E., and Laflamme, L. (2010). Barriers and enablers to the use of measures to prevent pediatric scalding in Cape Town, South Africa. *Public Health Nursing*, 27(3), 203–20.

Vision Zero Initiative (n.d.). Website. [Online] Available at: http://www.visionzeroinitiative.com/.

Wilson, J. and Rogmans, M. (2006). Purposes and scope of prevention of drowning. In J.J.L.M. Bierens (ed.) *Handbook on Drowning: Prevention, Rescue, Treatment*, pp. 87–92. Berlin: Springer.

Woolf, S.H. (2008). The meaning of translational research and why it matters. *Journal of the American Medical Association*, 299(2), 211–13.

World Health Organization (2002). *The World Health Report 2002: Reducing Risks, Promoting Health Life*. Geneva: WHO.

World Health Organization (2004). *The Economic Dimensions of Interpersonal Violence*. Geneva: WHO.

World Health Organization (2008). *World Report on Child Injury Prevention*. Geneva: WHO.

World Health Organization (2009). *Global Status Report on Road Safety: Time for Action*. Geneva: WHO.

World Health Organization (n.d. a). TEACH-VIP 2. [Online] Available at: http://www.who.int/violence_injury_ prevention/capacity building/teachvip/en/print.html.

World Health Organization (n.d. b). MENTOR-VIP. [Online] Available at: http://www.who.int/violence_injury_prevention/capacitybuilding/mentor_vip/en/.

World Health Organization Department of Violence and Injury Prevention and Disability (2009). *Capacity Building for Preventing Injury and Violence: Strategic Plan 2009–2013*. Geneva: WHO. Available at: http://www.who.int/violence_injury_prevention/capacitybuilding/strategic_plan/Strategic_plan.pdf

Yang, J., Campo, S., Ramirez, M., Krapfl, J.R., Cheng, G., and Peek-Asa, C. (2012). Family communication patterns and teen drivers' attitudes toward driving safety. *Journal of Pediatric Health Care*, 27(5), 334–41.

Young, T., Torner, J., Sihler, K., Hansen, F., Peek-Asa, C., and Zwerling, C. (2003). Factors associated with mode of transport to acute care hospitals in rural communities. *Journal of Emergency Medicine*, 24(2), 189–98.

Zerhouni, E.A. (2005). Translational and clinical science—time for a new vision. *The New England Journal of Medicine*, 353(15), 1621–3.

Interpersonal violence: a recent public health mandate

Rachel Jewkes

Introduction to interpersonal violence

Violence is inherently a human rights violation that has a profound impact on the physical and mental health and social functioning of its victims and survivors. It is increasingly recognized to be a highly prevalent global problem, with wide-ranging health and social consequences, and a huge economic burden on countries. Interpersonal violence is, however, a social construct that is inherently preventable.

The *World Health Report on Violence and Health* described interpersonal violence as encompassing child maltreatment, youth violence, intimate partner violence, sexual violence, and elder abuse (Krug et al. 2002). This is a fairly robust categorization but it is important to recognize that interpersonal violence is not necessarily age or gender related. In settings where there is a pronounced culture of violence, adults of all ages may use violence to resolve conflict or assert dominance in a range of other settings including conflict between neighbours, in contexts of crime, in prisons, in the workplace, and between health professionals and patients.

Interpersonal violence is experienced and perpetrated by millions of people worldwide each year and the health and social impact is huge. In 2004, interpersonal violence was the 22nd leading cause of death, and 600,000 deaths worldwide were attributed to it, that is, 1 per cent of the global burden of mortality. In the age group of 15–44 years, however, interpersonal violence is among the leading cause of mortality. Future projections suggest that the contribution of interpersonal violence to global mortality over the next 15 years is expected to rise sharply, unless there is effective public health action to prevent it.

Commensurate with this scale of violence is a massive economic impact. A report published in 2004 estimated the cost of violence in the United States to be 3.3 per cent of the gross domestic product, and in England and Wales, the total costs from violence were estimated to amount to $40.2 billion annually (Waters et al. 2004). A costing study of intimate partner violence estimated that in 2009 it was more than £15 billion in England and Wales alone (Walby 2010).

Magnitude of interpersonal violence

One of the most common forms of interpersonal violence is intimate partner violence. This encompasses physical, sexual, emotional and economic abuse, and a range of acts from threats of violence, social isolation, intimidation, insults, through to rape, beatings and at the most extreme end of the spectrum, forms of torture. A recent systematic review concluded that globally 30 per cent of women aged 15 and over have ever experienced physical or sexual intimate partner violence (Devries et al. 2013). There is considerable variation in prevalence between global regions and settings. In the Eastern Mediterranean, Africa, and South East Asia the prevalence was 37 per cent, compared to 23–25 per cent in high-income countries, the Western Pacific, and European regions (World Health Organization (WHO) 2013). In some countries of the world, like South Africa, intimate partner violence is the most common cause of female homicide (Abrahams et al. 2013), and globally intimate partner violence is estimated to account for 36 per cent of female homicides (WHO 2013).

The global estimate for the proportion of women who have experienced non-partner sexual violence is 7.2 per cent (95 per cent confidence interval = 5.3 per cent to 9.1 per cent), with the prevalence ranging from 5 per cent in South East Asia to 12 per cent in Africa (Devries et al. 2013). Research with men on perpetration has shown that in some settings, including South Africa and Papua New Guinea, 20–40 per cent of men have ever raped a female non-partner (Abrahams et al. 2011; Jewkes et al. 2013).

Child abuse can be physical, sexual, or emotional and may also encompass physical and emotional neglect. Research has often used very different definitions and these often reflect cultural differences in normative child rearing practices. Comparability across settings can thus be hard, but one estimate from Gilbert was that in high-income countries each year 4–16 per cent of children are physically abused and one in ten is neglected or psychologically abused. Further during the whole of childhood, between 5 per cent and 10 per cent of girls and up to 5 per cent of boys are exposed to penetrative sexual abuse, and 15–40 per cent are exposed to any type of sexual abuse (Reza et al. 2007; Gilbert et al. 2009).

It was estimated in 2000 that 565 young people aged 10–29 die every day across the world from violence and that for each death 20–40 require hospitalization (Krug et al. 2002). The global youth homicide rate estimate was 9.2 per 100,000 people, but regional variations were substantial. This rate varied from 0.9 per 100,000 in high-income countries to 17.6 in Africa and 36.4 in Latin America (Krug et al. 2002). Youth violence is highly gendered, with the overwhelming majority of perpetrators and victims being male. Recent research for South Africa, for example, has shown that the rate of homicide (21.7/100,000) for teenage boys (15–17 years) was nearly five times the teenage girls' rate (4.6/100,000) (Mathews et al. 2013).

Elder abuse is a much less researched form of interpersonal violence. Its subcategories generally include physical, psychological, sexual, financial, and discriminatory abuse and neglect. It is generally measured as exposure to people aged over 65 or over 60 (Cooper et al. 2008). The category is often measured in a way that fails to distinguish between other forms of violence experienced by older people (e.g. intimate partner violence) from violence that is a result of the constrained power of older people (i.e. because a person is elderly). This is an area that is growing in recognition, especially for elderly people with cognitive impairment. The main perpetrators are family members and care-givers. In some parts of sub-Saharan Africa a particularly horrific dimension of elderly abuse is seen in witchcraft-related violence and murders (Meel 2009). Understanding and preventing abuse of the elderly is an area that requires considerable further research.

Health consequences

The health impact of interpersonal violence extends well beyond the most immediate injuries and mortality. One area that has been the subject of considerable research is the intersections between HIV and gender-based violence. There is substantial evidence of the importance of gender inequity and intimate partner violence exposure in women's risk of acquiring HIV (Jewkes 2010; Jewkes et al. 2010b). Research from South Africa and Uganda shows that exposure to intimate partner violence raises HIV risk by about 50 per cent and that nearly one in four new HIV infections could be prevented if women were not subjected to intimate partner violence and relationship power inequalities (Jewkes et al. 2010b; Kouyoumdjian et al. 2013). Furthermore young women who have experienced sexual abuse in childhood are also at two-thirds greater risk of incident HIV infections (Jewkes et al. 2010b). Jewkes et al. argue that the evidence points to four key dimensions to the interface between gender inequity, violence, and HIV (Jewkes et al. 2010b).

First, women may become directly infected with HIV through rape. This is biologically inarguable and has been seen in clinical practice, yet population-based research suggests that the risks of HIV acquisition from rape are not great (Dunkle et al. 2004; Jewkes et al. 2010b). This is because the act is usually a single act of intercourse and the risks entailed in this are not very great. Further fears that rapists may be more likely than other men to have HIV, at least in South Africa have been shown to be unfounded (Jewkes et al. 2011b). None the less there is the potential for HIV acquisition during rape, in high prevalence sub-Saharan African countries many men who rape will be infected, and so it is vitally important that the violation of the rape is not compounded by preventable infection with HIV.

Secondly, women who experience more gender inequity and violence are less able to protect themselves from HIV, for example, they have sex more frequently and use condoms less often. The former may reflect a lesser ability to gain respect for their right not to have sex when they don't want it, but in some settings it may also reflect a practice of taking another partner for an emotionally more fulfilling relationship when trapped with a violent partner. Women who have more equitable relationships are much more able to use condoms consistently with their partner (Jama Shai

et al. 2010). This may be explained by women's ability to negotiate in such situations, but qualitative research points strongly to the acquiescence of women to male dominance in relationships and suggests that more commonly women who submit to unequal relationships are more likely to submit to an agenda of male control and so their own wants are not even considered (Jewkes and Morrell 2012).

Thirdly, childhood sexual abuse increases the risk of a range of risky sexual practices, including having multiple and concurrent partners, transactional sex, and substance abuse. All of these increase the risk of HIV acquisition as well as rendering women vulnerable to further partner violence or rape. Women who have experienced sexual abuse thus have a sustained elevated risk of HIV (Jewkes et al. 2010b). The mechanisms of increased risk are partly though the long-term mental health impact of child sexual abuse and often co-occurring emotional neglect, including an increased risk of post-traumatic stress disorder (PTSD) and substance abuse, as well as insecure adult attachment which is associated with increased rate of partner change and greater difficulties in emotional relationships. In this way abuse risks intersect with cycles of risk of violence and HIV.

Fourthly, ideals of marked gender hierarchy generally legitimize the use of violence in making and sustaining it, and often co-occur with ideals of masculinity that emphasize heterosexual performance, particularly toughness, strength, and having many partners (discussed later) (Jewkes and Morrell 2010). As a consequence, men who are violent towards women often engage in a range of sexually risky practices and some research has shown that they are more likely to be HIV infected (Decker et al. 2009; Jewkes et al. 2011b). If these research findings pertain more broadly, women partners of violent men are at higher risk of HIV acquisition per sexual act.

Interpersonal violence has a major impact on women's reproductive health. Childhood sexual abuse and child marriage increase the risk of early pregnancy and child bearing with higher maternal and infant mortality. Intimate partner violence also increases the risk of having had an induced abortion by more than twofold, young teenage pregnancy, and for those who have children the risk of a low birth rate baby is increased by 16 per cent (WHO 2013).

Child abuse has an important impact on mental health for boys and girls. Although there has been a strong emphasis in research on sexual and physical violence, the impact of emotional abuse and neglect is increasingly recognized. South African research shows that adolescent women who have experienced emotional neglect are at greater risk of depression, suicidality and alcohol abuse, and adolescent men were at greater risk of depression and drug abuse (Jewkes et al. 2010a). The same study found sexual abuse associated with alcohol abuse and depression in the men and alcohol abuse in the women. The impact of child abuse is discussed further later in this chapter. Mental health is also impacted by experience of intimate partner violence and non-partner rape. Women so exposed are at more than twice the risk of depression, and the latter group also have more than twice the risk of alcohol abuse (WHO 2013). Rape is also particularly likely to result in PTSD, and in fact is more likely to cause PTSD than any other violence exposure (Tolin and Foa 2006).

Interpersonal violence also has a range of social consequences including a greater risk of school dropout due to pregnancy, which impacts on future employment and lifetime earnings. Violence results in more time off due to injury and its other health effects, and even women not working may experience social incapacity, impacting on childcare and homemaking.

Understanding its roots

On first reflection the category of interpersonal violence appears to consist of a disparate range of acts that share most acutely the use of physical force to cause hurt or injury. However, a deeper understanding of the roots of the different forms of violence awakens a realization that these are very profoundly interconnected. Firstly, in many cases the same people perpetrate different forms of interpersonal violence. For example, the aggressive young boy who bullies at school may later engage in violent fights with other youths, be sexually violent, violent to his partner, beat his children, and engage in group violence against an elderly woman accused of witchcraft. Whilst it's important to recognize that many people are violent in one context and not in others, violent behaviours are strongly patterned and a propensity to the use of violence in one situation does increase the likelihood of its use in others.

The second interconnection arises from the observation that many of the perpetrators of violence have themselves been victims. The most formative violence exposures in this regard are those of children to emotional or physical maltreatment, the trauma of witnessing intimate partner violence between parents, sexual abuse, and bullying. All of these are common exposures among those who perpetrate interpersonal violence and are risk factors for their doing so. Research with a nationally representative sample of US adolescents has shown that in its relationship with intimate partner sexual violence perpetration, experience of physical abuse in childhood is completely mediated by involvement in delinquent behaviour (Casey et al. 2009).

Except in the context of evenly matched gang fights, victims of interpersonal violence do not bring the violence on themselves, yet victimization is by no means random. For all forms of interpersonal violence there are factors that increase the likelihood of victimization and here again, an interconnectedness of forms of violence becomes visible. So women who have experienced sexual abuse as children are more likely to be re-victimized sexually as adults, and to experience intimate partner violence.

So how is the interconnectedness explained? There are three explanations of importance here. First, the different forms of violence have largely overlapping root causes and risk factors, which are discussed in more detail later. Second, the use of violence in conflict, to punish or otherwise assert dominance is a learned behaviour, and thus is part of culture. Violence's use has transferability between contexts, notwithstanding the differences between these. Social learning encompasses how violence is used and what forms it may take, who are appropriate victims, what are acceptable or required triggers for its use, what meanings will be attached to its use, and what patterns of reward or punishment can be expected to follow. In this way violence needs to be understood as inherently part of culture. For example, Wood et al. (2007) researching intimate partner violence in South Africa's Eastern Cape Province have shown that it is widely regarded as a normal part of gender relations and will be interpreted by the community, family, and victims as unexceptional providing the victim is not injured by the violence, indeed it is commonly interpreted as deserved, good for teaching the partner right from wrong, and is

socially rewarded to the extent that it may result in acquiescence. Whilst interpersonal violence is always culturally patterned, a further cultural dimension, which is often referred to as 'the' culture of violence, relates to the threshold that triggers its use. Essentially there is marked cultural difference in the general level of triggers, with some societies, such as Papua New Guinea, having very low thresholds for the use of many forms of interpersonal violence. In other cultural settings, thresholds are very much higher, or the use of violence in general in interpersonal relations is viewed as inappropriate. Third, interpersonal violence is most commonly socially rewarded, at least at some level in the short term. There may also be very pronounced social rewards in contexts where 'men of violence' are revered, their physical power viewed with awe, and political power and economic rewards may flow from this. At a more micro-level, when violence is used to assert dominance and win submission this may be rewarded with the desired behaviour. Consequences for perpetrators may be quite different in the longer term, but in the short term it is often rewarded.

The fourth explanation lies in the nature and impact of victimization itself. Victims are often selected because they are vulnerable. Thus children who are disabled, mentally or physically less able, or very poor are more likely to be victimized. Victimization increases such vulnerability by causing disempowerment to be more acutely perceived, as well as often actually increasing disempowerment. Furthermore negative coping strategies after victimization, including problem drinking, may create vulnerability to further violence of other forms. In this way interpersonal violence creates cycles of vulnerability across different types of violence.

Risk factors for interpersonal violence

Risk factors for violence perpetration have been described as operating at a range of different ecological levels. This has been presented in an ecological model that highlights how some of these pertain and exert effects at an individual level, others at a family, peer or relationship level, others at a community level and still others at a societal level.

Individual level

Genotype

There is evidence that genes may be important in the development of aggression. Research points towards a general heritable tendency to antisocial behaviour, of which sexual coercion is one form. There may be important gene × environment interactions, particularly with the expression of aggression in genetically susceptible individuals after exposure to a harsh environment, or else a person with antisocial tendencies might be more likely to be drawn to situations and settings where antisocial behaviour is more common or more possible (Johansson et al. 2008). The evidence is predominantly focused on non-sexual aggression. However both sexual aggression and general aggression are heritable in mice (Canastar and Maxson 2003) and one study of twins concluded that over a quarter of sexual coercion was explained by genetic factors, but the genetic element in psychopathy was higher (Johansson et al. 2008).

The monoamine oxidase A gene (*MAOA*) has been described as impacting on a heritable tendency for antisocial behaviour. This encodes the MAOA enzyme, which metabolizes neurotransmitters such as norepinephrine (NE), serotonin (5-HT) and dopamine

(DA) and thus inactivates them (Shih et al. 1999). It is very rare for the gene encoding MAOA to have been deleted, although this is found associated with heritable aggression in humans and mice (Rowe 2001). More common are functional polymorphisms that result in lower activity of the MAOA enzyme (Caspi et al. 2002). A prospective study conducted in New Zealand has shown that child maltreatment has a much stronger association with subsequent antisocial behaviour in males with low MAOA enzyme activity, than those with higher activity (Caspi et al. 2002). In this study 11 per cent of violent convictions were attributable to the gene. Findings of research on exposure to physical punishment in early childhood, having the *MAOA* gene and likelihood of subsequent delinquency are inconsistent (Reif et al. 2007; Prichard et al. 2008; Edwards et al. 2010). The role of genetics in interpersonal violence, including sexual aggression, is clearly an important area for further work.

Other biological influences: androgens and neurological deficits and sexual offending

The role of androgens in interpersonal violence is questionable. A positive relationship between testosterone and self-reported aggressiveness has been reported for men and women (Christiansen and Knussmann 1987), but this has not been confirmed by all authors (Campbell et al. 1997). Several researchers have investigated links between blood testosterone levels and sexual or other aggression in prison populations, but found no evidence that testosterone levels influence the likelihood of sex offending, any more than general violent offending (Giotakis et al. 2003).

The role of brain damage in sexual offending has been the subject of research but the overall conclusion of a recent review of the literature is that the evidence is extremely weak (Fabian 2012). One of the few controlled studies with paedophiles found no differences on neuropsychological measures or positron emission tomography scans (Cohen et al. 2002). Whilst brain trauma may be important in some individuals, there is currently no evidence that brain damage makes an important contribution at a population level.

Early years' exposures

Irrespective of genotype, there is evidence that an individual's risk of perpetrating interpersonal violence can be shaped in the first days, months, and years of life. There is considerable evidence that perpetrators of interpersonal violence, including sexual violence, are more likely to have failed to form secure attachment bonds in childhood. This is linked to exposure to emotional, physical, and sexual abuse as well as to domestic violence, removal from the family, family disruption, and parental loss due to death or divorce may be risk factors for perpetration (Maniglio 2010).

Attachment

There is considerable evidence that the use of interpersonal violence is linked to a failure to form secure attachment bonds in childhood. One of the critical pathways through which the childhood home environment, particularly in early childhood, impacts upon psychological development is through attachment to primary caregivers, usually mothers (Bowlby 1969, 1973, 1980). If attachment bonds between the child and their primary caregiver are secure, children acquire the necessary skills to establish close relationships and grow to desire the intimacy of others. If these bonds are insecure, children do not acquire the necessary skills to establish close relationships, and may grow to fear intimacy with other individuals, exhibit hostility or aggression within their relationships, or to seek intimacy in maladaptive ways (Bowlby 1969, 1973). The failure to form secure attachment bonds is due to poor socialization experiences, such as violent parenting, and disordered attachment has in particular been described as consequent of parenting that combines harsh punishment and expressions of affection (Fonagy and Target 2003; Marshall and Barbaree 1990). A failure to form secure attachment bonds in childhood results in a failure to learn interpersonal and other skills necessary to achieve intimacy as adults. Insecure attachments are marked by an expectation that what is needed will not be given, and as a result coercion, whether through physical violence, emotional manipulation or sexual violence, is often used to get it (Bowlby 1969, 1973, 1980). In the arena of relationships, insecurity may result in more dismissive and hostile attitudes towards others and a tendency to perceive others negatively and distrustfully. This has been shown in sex offenders, but is also likely to increase propensity to intimate partner violence, youth violence and interpersonal violence in the community (Marshall 1989; Stirpe et al. 2006; Whitaker et al. 2008). Individuals with disorganized attachment are much more aggressive, distrustful, and less empathetic when older and have a propensity to general interpersonal violence (Fonagy and Target 2003).

Dysfunctional parenting and disturbed family histories, with unstable caregiving often due to maternal post-natal depression, or parental intimate partner violence, have been shown to be associated with interpersonal violence and various categories of offending among children, including sexual offending (Lightfoot and Evans 2000; Seto and Lalumiere 2010).

Child abuse victimization

Physical and emotional abuse and neglect in childhood are exposures that result in a failure to form secure attachments. Emotional abuse and neglect has been subject to much less research than physical abuse, but a multicountry study on men's violence in Asia and the Pacific has shown that men who rape non-partners and those who have been violent to intimate partners are more likely to have been exposed to all of these in childhood, and these findings support the research from South Africa (Fulu et al. 2013; Jewkes et al. 2011a). In contrast to this, a large national study of adolescents from the United States found that those who had been sexually violent to a partner were significantly more likely to have experienced physical abuse themselves, but not emotional neglect (Casey et al. 2009) and another did not find sexually violent youth to be more likely to have experienced physical violence (Borowsky et al. 1997).

The evidence of childhood sexual abuse as a risk factor for subsequent perpetration is very extensive and probably has been the most comprehensively investigated of all risk factors for perpetration. In a meta-analysis, a history of child sexual abuse was five times more common among adolescent sexual offenders than among adolescent non-sexual offenders (Seto and Lalumiere 2010). Further, sexual offenders against children are much more likely to have sexual abuse victimization histories than non-offenders or non-sexual offenders (Whitaker et al. 2008). Several large national studies of US adolescents and men in college have found that those who had sexually assaulted a partner were significantly more likely to have experienced sexual abuse themselves (Borowsky et al. 1997; Casey et al. 2009; Malamuth et al. 1991, 1995).

Witnessing intimate partner violence in the home is both extremely traumatic for children and may be part of social learning about intimate relations. Both of these may explain the consistent finding that men who have been so exposed in childhood are more likely to be physically or sexually violent towards their intimate partners (and girls so exposed to experience violence themselves) (Malamuth et al. 1991, 1995; Borowsky et al. 1997; Fulu et al. 2013). South African research has also shown that men who have been exposed in childhood are more likely to get involved in fights at work and in the community, and have been arrested for having an illegal firearm (Abrahams and Jewkes 2005).

Personality

These early years of exposure have a profound impact on personality when older. Psychopathy has been the most extensively discussed in relation to perpetration of interpersonal violence. Psychopathy is a constellation of personality traits and socially deviant behaviours, spanning affective, interpersonal, and behavioural traits. Hare has proposed that the characteristics of psychopathy include egocentricity, lack of remorse and empathy, pathological lying, manipulativeness, and the persistent violation of social norms (Hare 1996). These traits enable psychopaths to treat others as objects and feel no guilt or remorse. They are thus much more likely to perpetrate interpersonal violence, particularly severe physical violence, emotional violence, and rape.

In the US general population the prevalence of psychopathy is usually estimated at 1 per cent, but the prevalence of psychopathic traits without a full clinical diagnosis is higher (Lilienfield 2005). Individuals with heightened levels of some of the characteristics of psychopathy have been described as subclinical and non-clinical psychopaths (LeBreton et al. 2006). The prevalence of psychopathy as a diagnosis is dependent on assessment measure scores. Research on Canadian incarcerated sex offenders shows that a relatively small difference in cut point (25 versus 30) on the PCL-R (Hare Psychopathy Checklist—Revised) (Hare 2003) resulted in twice as many offenders being diagnosed as psychopathic (29 per cent vs. 13 per cent) (Olver and Wong 2006). This suggests that the presence of psychopathic traits may be important in understanding interpersonal violence at subclinical levels and indeed this has been suggested by research in South Africa where two traits were measured, Machiavellian egocentricity and blame externalization, and were significantly higher among men who had raped in both the past year and their lifetime (Jewkes et al. 2011a). There are similar findings from US college students, among whom subclinical scores on psychopathic traits have been associated with rape perpetration (Abbey et al. 2011; DeGue and DiLillo 2004; Ouimette 1997). Psychopaths have been described as having an inability to connect sexual behaviour with emotional feelings, such as warmth and tenderness, and a hedonistically orientated lack of impulse control and are thus more likely to be sexually as well as physically violent (Cleckley 1988).

Personality disorders of offenders

Research on personality disorders in populations of offenders shows that sex offenders against children and adults show significantly more Cluster A, Cluster B and antisocial personality disorders than non-offenders (Whitaker et al. 2008). Psychopathy is common among more violent child sex offenders (Rosenberg et al. 2005). Schizoid personality features include social detachment and restricted emotionality, and avoidant features include social inhibition and inadequacy. Both of these interfere with the development of normal peer relationships, including intimate relationships with women, and are more prevalent among sex offenders, particularly against children (Fazel et al. 2002; Whitaker et al. 2008). Men who sexually molest children are socially and emotionally immature, have poor social skills, low levels of self-esteem, poor impulse control, and more signs of psychotic thinking (Finkelhor and Araji 1986). Relating to children provides a sense of power and control and opportunity for dominance not available to them in adult relationships (Finkelhor and Araji 1986).

Substance abuse

Alcohol abuse is strongly associated with use of interpersonal violence. There are physiological effects, but also complex cultural beliefs about and meanings given to the relationship between alcohol and violent, including sexually violent, behaviour. Alcohol has a physiological effect of reducing inhibitions, reasoning, and, in men who were more irritable, prone to anger and have low levels of anger control, can result in ready use of violence (Finkelhor and Araji 1986). Research on intimate partner violence and rape in particular commonly finds that men who are violent are more likely to have heavy alcohol use (Koss and Dinero 1988; Jewkes et al. 2006, 2011a; Tsai et al. 2011; Fulu et al. 2013). Many cultures (or subcultures) link alcohol consumption to disinhibition, sexual desire, and performance, and perceive it to give courage to make advances that men may be reticent to make when sober, and as mitigating antisocial or aggressive behaviour (Lightfoot and Evans 2000; Seto and Lalumiere 2010). Alcohol abuse also has an economic impact on families, leading to greater financial strain, and may be a trigger for conflict over finances.

A further question is whether violence associated with alcohol more often results in serious injury or mortality. There is some evidence that shows that when a perpetrator is drunk and the victim sober there was a greater likelihood of rape completion and victim injury than when they had both been drinking (Brecklin and Ullman 2002). In the case of youth homicide, alcohol is estimated to be responsible for 26 per cent and 16 per cent of years of life lost by men and women respectively, with the proportion lower in high-income countries and as high as 40 per cent in low-income countries (WHO 2004).

Drug use

Drug use is also intimately connected with youth violence and homicide, most directly because the trade in drugs in many settings is associated with violence and turf wars between dealing gangs (Blumstein et al. 2000). Research on rape has shown that men who have raped are more likely to use drugs, indeed a prospective study from South Africa concluded that 24 per cent of all rapes would have been prevented if drug use had not occurred (Jewkes et al. 2012). The great majority of the drug use reported was marijuana use, but the authors argued that drug use was most likely an indicator of engagement in a subcultural peer context where both drug use and rape was seen as 'normal' (Jewkes et al. 2012). This conclusion is supported by findings of a multicountry study that drug use was associated with having ever engaged in multiple perpetrator rape (sometimes referred to as gang rape), but not single perpetrator rape (Jewkes et al. 2013).

Depression

There is evidence that men who use violence against intimate partners are more likely to be depressed (Nduna et al. 2010; Fulu et al. 2013). It is not clear whether depression causes men to become violent, or is an emotional response to having used violence and the negative impact that this has on a relationship. It is possible that, as with alcohol abuse, depression and feelings of hopelessness may exaggerate irritability in men who are inherently more irritable and prone to anger, and as a result they may more readily use violence.

Propensity to use violence

The use of interpersonal violence in one context is closely related to its use in others. This has particularly been highlighted in the relationship between perpetration of violence against children and sexual violence against non-partners by men who have been physically or sexually violent to an intimate partner. Rape of non-partners has been found to be more common among men who are physically violent towards partners (Malamuth et al. 1991, 1995; Jewkes et al. 2006, 2011a, 2013). It seems likely that a system of patriarchy and gender hierarchy that legitimates the use of physical violence by men to assert dominance in a relationship and 'correct' behaviour of wives and girlfriends would also find expression in sexual violence, as well as other forms of violence, such as verbal violence. There is also some evidence that verbal violence against women is more common among sexually coercive men in US colleges and among South African working men (Malamuth et al. 1991, 1995; Abrahams et al. 2004).

Relationship, peer, or micro-social level

Conflict

The dynamics of particular relationships are also important influences of the propensity for use of violence. Intimate partner violence is more common in relationships that are more conflictual, and experimental evidence suggests that interventions that build communications skills and reduce relationship conflict are impactful in reducing intimate partner violence (Jewkes et al. 2008). Poor communication skills of either partner may result in conflicts escalating readily to violence. Conflict escalating to violence is also more common in relationships where one partner is more irritable and prone to outbursts of anger. Perceived challenges to men's 'right' to what they perceive as traditional gender privileges and their non-fulfilment of expected provider roles are often causes of conflict.

Social learning around violence acceptability

In teenage peer relationships, it has been observed that friends are similar in their characteristics in a wide range of domains and aggression is no exception (McPherson et al. 2001). There has been considerable debate about whether aggressive young people choose each other as friends or whether as friends they become more similar in regard to aggression (Snyder et al. 1997; Steglich et al. 2010). There has been limited longitudinal research, but one study from Chile suggests that children do not select friends based on their levels of aggression, rather that similarity among friends is a product of the friendship, although it is also possible that aggressive male youth may be forced together if non-aggressive peers

reject them (Steglich et al. 2010). This partly explains the strong connection between gang membership and violence perpetration that has been described in many settings (Bourgois 1996; Jewkes et al. 2006, 2011a). The importance of perceived social acceptability of violence was also highlighted by a study that found the parents of violence perpetrators, when compared with parents of non-perpetrators, were much more likely to have encouraged gang membership (Morris et al. 2002).

Social learning about sexual violence as normative, is demonstrated in research with incarcerated American adolescents that has shown that sexual assault perpetrators were nearly four times as likely as non-perpetrators to know a perpetrator of sexual assault (Morris et al. 2002). Among a community-based sample of men, perceived peer approval of coercing sex was much higher among men who rape (Abbey et al. 2007). A further aspect of social learning is reflected in the perpetration of sexual abuse by those who have themselves been sexually abused in childhood. Research from New Zealand provides an additional perspective on this as sexually abusive adolescents and children were found to have been more likely to have had contact with adults who were known paedophiles or suspected to have engaged in sexual abuse of other children, even when they did not have confirmed sexual abuse victimization themselves (Lightfoot and Evans 2000). These children may have experienced abnormal sexualization through exposure to inappropriate sexual experiences (e.g. pornography exposure or verbal experiences) (Lightfoot and Evans 2000).

There is also a social learning element in the use of violence in child rearing practices, particularly physical punishment. Physical violence is generally used to punish or gain control over a child and is used more readily by parents raising children in contexts where beating is more common and where there is less role modelling of non-violent parenting and discipline practices.

Delinquent behaviour

The use of interpersonal violence, including rape, among adolescents is strongly associated with other antisocial behaviour (Ageton 1983; Calhoun et al. 1997; Malamuth et al. 1991; Knight and Sims-Knight 2003). Delinquency is an area where multiple risk factors and violent behaviour intersect. There may be genetic roots in some young men, as research has shown that men with genetically determined low MAOA enzyme activity and exposure to harsh punishment in early childhood are more likely to become delinquent (Edwards et al. 2010). Further it is strongly related to personality traits of psychopathy, which themselves may be genetically determined (Abbey et al. 2011). Delinquency is also socially modelled and much more common among youth who have themselves experienced physical aggression in childhood, and are more susceptible to peer pressure (Malamuth et al. 1995; Casey et al. 2009).

Multicountry research on both intimate partner violence perpetration and rape perpetration has shown that these are associated with having currently or previously been in a gang (Borowsky et al. 1997; Jewkes et al. 2011a; Fulu et al. 2013). They are also associated with having been involved in other interpersonal crime or theft, having a weapon, and having had an illegal gun (Jewkes et al. 2011a; Fulu et al. 2013). School bullying is one manifestation of delinquent behaviour, and often a precursor of antisocial behaviour in adulthood (Bender and Lösel 2011). South African research has shown perpetration of school sexual bullying to be strongly associated with subsequent rape perpetration (Jewkes et al. 2011a).

One of the important avenues in the prevention of delinquency is health and education sector interventions for children with conduct disorders. Children with conduct disorders may go on to develop personality disorders as adults, particularly antisocial personality disorders. Conduct disorders are treatable in children, but they require parents to be trained in managing problem behaviour, or out-of-home placements with staff or foster parents appropriately trained. Treatment is most effective when provided to younger children (pre-adolescent); this has been part of the theoretical basis for the Incredible Years programme of Webster-Stratton and colleagues.

Masculinities and delinquent peers

Gang or otherwise delinquent peer contexts are also ones in which the masculinities of involved boys are shaped. Negative early childhood influences that generate feelings of insecurity greatly increase the likelihood that as boys grow into men they will adopt masculinities that emphasize strength, toughness, and demonstrate control over others. Such masculinities are familiar within a gang, or otherwise pugilistic peer context, where there is a readiness to show toughness among gang members, between them and potential rivals, dominance over women and to display power over others (e.g. in the context of crime).

Within any social setting there are multiple ways of, and aspirations for, being a man or boy. Some subcultural masculinities are particularly violent, and emphasize dominance over women, with a heightened sense of male sexual entitlement, which readily translates into rape (Bourgois 1996). This is particularly commonly found associated with gangs and among men positioned on the antisocial fringes.

Community level

Many of the structural drivers of interpersonal violence operate at a community level. These include poverty, patriarchy, and structural influences on these such as race or ethnicity. In a profound way these impact on the culture of the local context.

Poverty

Poverty, low educational attainment, and social disadvantage are structural drivers of interpersonal violence. Gangs, which are archetypically associated with many forms of violence, are very largely confined to life in low-income areas. In conditions of poverty, gangs provide young men access to experiences of power when other routes of attainment of power and status are unattainable, such as through working or fulfilling provider roles (Bourgois 1996; Wood and Jewkes 2001; Wood et al. 2007). Poverty increases the risk of intimate partner violence and child maltreatment both because it increases economic strains on families and relationships, and also because it generates feelings of inadequacy and powerlessness that may be expressed through the use of violence. Poverty further traps women within violent relationships and can reduce their options for taking action to protect themselves, or to get the violence to stop. Economic empowerment interventions for women have been shown to be a very fruitful avenue for enabling women to protect themselves from intimate partner violence (Pronyk et al. 2006).

The relationship between rape and poverty is complex. Multiple perpetrator (gang) rape is most clearly linked to poverty because

this is important in the context of gangs (Jewkes et al. 2013). The role of social disadvantage in single perpetrator rape is less clear because perceptions of sexual entitlement are a very powerful part of the context of rape and these may stem from social advantage rather than disadvantage. South African research has shown that among the less well off, it is the slightly less poor or less disadvantaged who are more likely to have raped (Jewkes et al. 2006, 2011a). Authors have argued that a sense of entitlement stemming from relative advantage, within a context of general disadvantage, is played out in a perverse way in a context in which few or none would be able to attain objectively high levels of material 'success' (Jewkes et al. 2011a).

Social norms: the cultural scaffolding for interpersonal violence

For all forms of interpersonal violence, social learning around the acceptability of the use of violence, and for gender-based violence, the acceptability of directing it to women, within subcultural contexts is important in perpetration. The importance of social norms on the use of violence in partner violence perpetration was first made visible by anthropological work looking at factors associated with violence across a wide range of cultural settings (Levinson 1989). More recently research on intimate partner violence has increasingly explored the importance of community level norms on the use of violence, for example indicated by community murder rates, as a risk factor for intimate partner violence and found it to be highly associated (Koenig et al. 2006).

Social norms on gender relations and violence are also very important. The phrase 'cultural scaffolding' was coined by Gavey to describe the protective social context that enables the reproduction of sexual violence through allowing men to reconfigure sexually coercive behaviour, especially with dates, girlfriends, or wives as 'not rape' (Gavey 2005). The scaffolding includes an array of rape myths that place the blame for rape at the feet of women and enable a cognitive justification for coercive behaviour, ideas of sexual entitlement within marriage (conjugal rights), and the positioning of women as worthy objects of male sexual conquest. This scaffolding is argued to stem from a framework of patriarchy whereby men are positioned as hierarchically superior to women and accorded greater social value. This ideological scaffolding provides the cultural space for men to perpetrate rape without embracing an identity as 'a rapist' or 'a perpetrator'. Similarly youth violence and bullying are often seen as being normal for the age group and is seen as 'not violence' but more the rough and tumble of growing up (Wood and Jewkes 2001).

In some settings the use of interpersonal violence is integrally related to culturally constructed notions of legitimate entertainment. This is very clearly seen in research on rape where men have been asked about their motivations. For example, in a six-country study on men's use of violence in Asia and the Pacific 59 per cent of men who had raped a non-partner indicated that one of the reasons they did it was for entertainment (Jewkes et al. 2013). In South Africa, seeking 'fun' motivated nearly half of South African men who had raped (Jewkes et al. 2011a). Quite similar findings pertain in youth violence, where research in the United Kingdom has shown that fights in bars are very often started for fun (Graham and Wells 2003).

The cultural scaffolding around child abuse is such that physical violence used by caregivers against children is often described as being 'necessary' in order to teach children how to behave and instil discipline, and is thus seen as 'not violence'. In many cultures the use of violence in child-rearing is so ubiquitous that many parents and teachers cannot imagine that there is any other way to properly raise children. Further settings such as in sub-Saharan Africa, societies are characterized by a very pronounced age hierarchy (as well as gender hierarchy) and children are raised to be obedient to adults in all ways, including to relative strangers. This can lead to children being placed in positions of vulnerability, especially to sexual abuse (Jewkes et al. 2005).

Masculinities

The most pervasive ways in which culture influences interpersonal violence is in the arena of gender. Gender attitudes held at an individual level are usually rooted in cultural models of gender relations, but within these there is considerable individual variation. Sexually aggressive men from diverse settings have greater hostility towards women, stronger sexual dominance desires, and more traditional attitudes towards gender roles and sexual relationships (Koss and Dinero 1988; Malamuth et al. 1991, 1995; Abbey et al. 2011; Jewkes et al. 2011a). Intimate partner violence is much more common among men who hold more gender inequitable views as well as those who engage in more controlling behaviours (Fulu et al. 2013). However, individually held attitudes and social norms theory do not on their own explain the social structure of gender. R.W. Connell (1987), a highly influential gender theorist, describes the existence of multiple, mutable masculine positions and identities, that are produced against a backdrop of history, cultural, and material circumstances, arranged hierarchically with respect to each other (some are viewed as legitimate whilst others are censored), and superior to women. Recognizing the global dominance of patriarchy, Connell argues that all masculine positions are constructed within a gender value system that values men over women and within which men are more powerful. Connell emphasizes that gender identities are socially constructed and integrally linked to hierarchies of power. Her analysis is critical to understanding both gender relations (i.e. between men and women) as well as the interrelationships among men. Connell argues for the existence in a particular setting of a hegemonic masculinity, which is a cultural ideal of manhood that gains its legitimacy from acceptance that is shared between those who embody and benefit from the ideal and those subordinated through it (after Gramsci (1971)). Hegemony connotes the existence of agreed values and practices, not necessarily associated with repression and violence. However, in many contexts, being dominant and in control of women are important aspects of hegemonic masculinity, and violent behaviours are justified in pursuit and demonstration of this (e.g. Wood and Jewkes 2001).

The different masculine positions that are adopted by men in a given setting vary, but there are global commonalities that have been observed. The first is that in any given setting there are normally masculinities that are notably violent and combine practices of violence between men with violent domination over others, particularly women. Men who adopt these masculine positions often are involved in illegal and antisocial behaviour. Further their dominance over women encompasses both the use of violence against women and demonstrations of power through (hetero)sexual success with or dominance over women, for example, in paying for sex, having many sexual partners, and so forth. These masculinities are sometimes referred to as hyper- or emphasized masculinities and are very closely associated with violence between men as well as sexual and physical violence against women.

The hegemonic masculinity within a given setting is much more moderate than this. It may not be numerically the most common position, but has the greatest cultural power, in that it is a masculinity that generally embodies a recognized cultural ideal of how men 'should' be, even if some men are unable to occupy the position due to economic circumstances. Hegemonic masculinities vary considerably globally, particularly in their relationship with men's violence. In some settings, such as South Africa, showing toughness and strength is absolutely integral to a hegemonic position. Men may be expected to be head of a household, a provider, and for women to be obedient. The cultural legitimacy accorded to a hegemonic masculine position results in men being able to exercise power over women without the use of violence, rather through women's acquiescence to men's dominance, but violence may be used. In some countries, such as Sweden, hegemonic masculinities are much more gender equitable and not expected to entail violence (Hearn et al. 2012). The relationship between hegemonic masculinity and the use of violence is extremely important in understanding the prevalence of interpersonal violence within a given cultural setting.

There are of course other masculinities and some are much more gender equitable and less violent, even in contexts of very patriarchal hegemonic masculinities. Some are constructed as resistance masculinities and may strive to be different, as is the case with gay masculine identities. Hegemonic masculinities often emphasize heterosexuality and are constructed very consciously in opposition to the feminine or homosexual, and indeed men may be identified as victims of male violence because they are perceived as being 'unmanly'.

The importance of masculinities in interpersonal violence should not mask the role of women. Women are responsible for perpetration of much violence against children, but for other forms of interpersonal violence the majority of perpetrators are men. Women do use violence against intimate partners, but much of it is retaliatory violence and where they initiate it their violence differs in meaning with the violence of men because it is not perpetrated within an overall context of gender power inequity. They also may engage in youth violence with other women. In a given setting women also adopt multiple feminine positions, some of which are highly acquiescent to dominant positions of men. These positions may render women vulnerable to violence but they may also provide some protection. Femininities which are constructed as resistance femininities may be viewed by men as threats and make women deliberate targets of violence, for example, in attacks on lesbians. There is an increasing literature from high-income countries and some settings with rapid social change, such as South Africa, on 'modern' femininities. These are characterized by women adopting many of the practices of men, without necessarily challenging the dominance of men in the gender order. They may be associated with particularly risky behaviour such as fighting among women, binge drinking, and having many sexual partners (Jewkes and Morrell 2012).

The importance of understanding gender identities in relation to interpersonal violence is that they provide a unifying framework for understanding both male dominance over women and the use of violence between men and between women. Other connected practices such as alcohol bingeing very often stem from links between alcohol excess and control and toughness, or alcohol and resistance (e.g. in conservative settings), which is highly gendered. It also connects interpersonal violence with some of its associated sexual practices and associated health risks. First, by linking gun or weapon ownership, or carrying, with manhood. Secondly, sexual assault and rape perpetrators from a range of countries, including the United States, South Africa, Botswana, and Swaziland, have more dating and consensual partners and more casual sex than other men, although they may not have more frequent sex as they have less emotionally engaged relationships with partners (Koss and Dinero 1988; Malamuth et al. 1991, 1995; Abbey et al. 2006; Jewkes et al. 2006, 2011a, 2011b; Kalichman et al. 2007; DeGue et al. 2010; Tsai et al. 2011). Changing the values upon which gender identities are constructed is an important avenue for intervention in interpersonal violence reduction.

Stigma

Gender values of a society are also expressed in perceptions of blame in cases of gender-based violence and in social responses to victims. Rape stigma is particularly powerful as it may be expressed in perceptions that women and girls who have been raped are sullied, and to blame for what happened, and this can lead to their ostracism. In some settings the rape is seen as a mark against the family's honour and not just a woman's own, and they may even be killed. Children born of rape may be rejected by families and communities too. Rape stigma is a very substantial barrier to access to services and legal redress after rape, and thus creates impunity for those who perpetrate.

Societal level

At a societal level it is important to understand that the dominant social values, especially gender values, are expressed in laws, policies, and through social institutions such as the police and courts. Thus in very patriarchal societies, except in settings with deliberate initiatives to build human rights (such as South Africa), laws very often restrict women's autonomy and may increase their vulnerability to violence and reduce their ability to bargain with, or leave, violent partners. Examples of such laws are those that make divorce hard to access, allow parents to marry very young girls, fail to criminalize rape in marriage, restrict married women's access to property and inheritance, or render women as legal minors.

Dominant values are also reflected in legal systems even where laws are more progressive. The police may refuse to open cases if they believe an act not to be a crime, this has particularly been reported in cases of rape and domestic violence. Courts may have a low threshold for declining to prosecute and where women are viewed with suspicion their evidence in court may be insufficient for a conviction (Jewkes and Abrahams 2002). If women cannot get legal redress for acts of intimate partner violence or rape or child abuse, perpetrators are sent a powerful message that they may anticipate impunity and that their acts are not viewed as serious.

At a societal level, laws may influence access to risk and protective factors including alcohol. In some countries alcohol is very cheap, easily accessible at all hours, and poorly regulated. These factors result in considerably higher alcohol consumption patterns, especially by young people, and so to a stronger link between interpersonal violence and heavy drinking. Similarly firearms are very effectively controlled by laws in some settings. South Africa is an example of a country where tighter gun control translated into a substantial reduction in gun-related homicides, these accounted for 17 per cent of female homicides in 2009, a reduction of nearly 50 per cent from one decade earlier (Abrahams et al. 2013). In comparison in the United States, with its very liberal gun laws, 67.5 per cent of homicide is perpetrated with a firearm.

Summarizing the prevention challenge

There have been a number of systematic reviews that have sought to summarize the evidence for what works in interpersonal violence prevention and the field in many areas is growing rapidly. A key review of interventions evaluated with randomized controlled trials for preventing sexual and intimate partner violence was published by the WHO (WHO and London School of Hygiene and Tropical Medicine 2010). The challenge in interpersonal violence prevention can be summarized as one that requires three avenues of intervention. The first are interventions to reduce the risk of the perpetration of interpersonal violence. Here the task, starting from the start of life, is to build a supportive home environment, with interventions to strengthen parenting, reduce exposure of children to all forms of violence, and provide treatment for depression and substance abuse, as well as increasing understanding of good parenting practices. There are a range of interventions that have been shown to be effective in high-income, as well as low- and middle-income settings in this regard. There have also been a series of key systematic reviews showing that interventions are effective in reducing child maltreatment and strengthening positive parenting (McCloskey 2011; Knerr et al. 2013).

Prevention requires changes to constructions of masculinity that emphasize dominance over women and legitimize the use of violence between men. Interventions, such as Stepping Stones and Program H, have been shown to be effective in changing masculinities, as well as some school-based programmes (Welbourn, 1995; Wolfe et al. 2009; Ricardo et al. 2012). The key challenge is to scale up interventions that are known to be effective and overcome the vested interests of patriarchy that resist prioritization of this endeavour. Addressing and acknowledging the context of poverty, low school achievement, and underemployment of men and teenage boys which provides the backdrop for interpersonal violence is also important, but research shows that change can occur within this context. Interventions that empower and build relationship skills, particular communication skills, and conflict skills are also very important in reducing all forms of interpersonal violence.

Interventions to address social norms on the use of violence are important and creating violence-free environments, especially schools with zero tolerance for bullying and violence, is very important. Abolishing the use of corporal punishment in schools, as well as homes, is also an important part of the agenda. In settings where it is entrenched, evidence suggests that outlawing it has a contribution but teaching positive discipline to teachers is critical to ensure its eradication.

The second broad intervention focus aims to socially and economically empower women and girls, to protect themselves from victimization, and to support themselves if they do want to leave a violent relationship; and to change societal norms and expectations about gender roles and relationships, including the acceptability of different forms of gender-based violence, which provide a self-perpetuating learning environment in which boys may grow up to expect to be able to use violence against girls and to normalize its use against them. There has been a recent burgeoning of research into the role of economic empowerment of women in intimate partner violence prevention, following the success of the Image study (Pronyk et al. 2006). Understanding the role of economic empowerment within the broader basket of interventions and the contexts in which it is most effective is critical.

The third intervention is to strengthen formal and informal legal, health, and social support structures and prevention. These interventions aim to increase accountability for violence and prevent further violence from occurring, as well as trying to break the intergenerational cycles of violence that are commonly seen. Interventions include strengthening laws, child protection systems, improving the functioning of police and courts in cases of interpersonal violence, and adopting and enforcing a range of other legislation and policies to reduce risk including those focused on gun control and the prevention of problem drinking.

This prevention agenda is an ambitious programme, but we do know that interpersonal violence can be prevented. The best confirmatory evidence of this comes from the United States, where the prevalence of all forms of interpersonal violence has very substantially declined over the last 20 years. For example child maltreatment and victimization is believed to have declined by 40–70 per cent (Finkelhor and Jones 2006), intimate partner violence has declined by 49 per cent, and figures from the Federal Bureau of Investigation show that the homicide rate declined from 9.8 to 4.7 per 100,000 from 1990 to 2010, making the current homicide rate comparable to that of 1960. Unfortunately it is much less clear which interventions worked. Criminologists and public health researchers have extensively debated the causes of the decline, because of the importance of understanding this for its replication in other settings, but unfortunately they only agree that they do not know how to attribute it. However, it was a period when there was much more public health intervention to raise awareness of, and the prevention of, child maltreatment. There was a 24 per cent reduction in families living in poverty and there were increasing policing interventions and crime reduction activities, as well as a range of other social changes including changes to build gender equity (Finkelhor and Jones 2006). The clustering of reduction in all forms of interpersonal violence (except child neglect, but this may be an artefact of case identification) strongly supports an argument that they are all closely interconnected and the need for a multipronged approach to prevention.

Conclusions

Interpersonal violence is a problem of huge global magnitude, responsible for a very substantial global burden of disease and with considerable economic impact. It is largely preventable and this chapter has sought to argue that although forms of interpersonal violence differ, prevention can substantially be unified as there are a common set of risk factors. Further when interpersonal violence does decline, as in the United States, a decline across all forms is seen to occur. Social norms around gender and the use of violence are extremely important in all forms of interpersonal violence and need to be a key focus for intervention. The prevention agenda in interpersonal violence, especially gender-based violence and child maltreatment, has historically been dominated by secondary prevention, with responses from child protection

and the criminal justice system and the provision of services to victims. This is very important, but it is only a small part of the prevention agenda. First prize for the future will go to developing robust multisectoral primary prevention interventions that have an impact on multiple risk factors and change the social context within which interpersonal violence occurs.

References

Abbey, A., Jacques-Tiura, A.J., and Lebreton, J. (2011). Risk factors for sexual aggression in young men: an expansion of the confluence model. *Aggressive Behaviour*, 37, 450–64.

Abbey, A., Parkhill, M.R., Beshears, R., Clinton-Sherrod, A.M., and Zawacki, T. (2006). Cross-sectional predictors of sexual assault perpetration in a community sample of single African American and Caucasian Men. *Aggressive Behaviour*, 32, 54–67.

Abbey, A., Parkhill, M.R., Clinton-Sherrod, M., and Zawacki, T. (2007). A comparison of men who committed different types of sexual assault in a community sample. *Journal of Interpersonal Violence*, 22, 1567–80.

Abrahams, N. and Jewkes, R. (2005). Effects of South African men's having witnessed abuse of their mothers during childhood on their levels of violence in adulthood. *American Journal of Public Health*, 95, 1811–16.

Abrahams, N., Jewkes, R., Hoffman, M., and Laubsher, R. (2004). Sexual violence against intimate partners in Cape Town: prevalence and risk factors reported by men. *Bulletin of the World Health Organization*, 82, 330–7.

Abrahams, N., Jewkes, R., Martin, L.J., and Mathews, S. (2011). Forensic medicine in South Africa: associations between medical practice and legal case progression and outcomes in female murders. *PLoS ONE*, 6, e28620.

Abrahams, N., Mathews, S., Martin, L.J., Lombard, C., and Jewkes, R. (2013). Intimate partner femicide in South Africa in 1999 and 2009. *PLoS Medicine*, 10, e1001412.

Ageton, S. (1983). *Sexual Assault Among Adolescents*. Lexington, MA: Lexington Books.

Bender, D. and Lösel, F. (2011). Bullying at school as a predictor of delinquency, violence and other anti-social behaviour in adulthood. *Criminal Behaviour and Mental Health*, 21(2), 99–106.

Blumstein, A., Rivara, F.P., and Rosenfeld, R. (2000). The rise and decline of homicide—and why. *Annual Review of Public Health*, 21, 505–41.

Borowsky, I.W., Hogan, M., and Ireland, M. (1997). Adolescent sexual aggression: risk and protective factors. *Pediatrics*, 100, e7.

Bourgois, P. (1996). In search of masculinity—violence, respect and sexuality among Puerto Rican crack dealers in East Harlem. *British Journal of Criminology*, 36, 412–27.

Bowlby, J. (1969). *Attachment and Loss. Vol. 1: Attachment*. New York: Basic Books.

Bowlby, J. (1973). *Attachment and Loss. Vol. 2: Separation*. New York: Basic Books.

Bowlby, J. (1980). *Attachment and Loss. Vol. 3: Loss, Sadness and Depression*. New York: Basic Books.

Brecklin, L.R. and Ullman, S.E. (2002). The roles of victim and offender alcohol use in sexual assaults: results of a National Violence Against Women Survey. *Journal of Studies on Alcohol*, 63, 57–63.

Calhoun, K.S., Bernat, J.A., Clum, G.A., and Frame, C. (1997). Sexual coercion and attraction to sexual aggression in a community sample of young men. *Journal of Interpersonal Violence*, 12, 392–406.

Campbell, A., Muncer, S., and Odber, J. (1997). Aggression and testosterone: testing a bio-social model. *Aggressive Behaviour*, 23, 229–38.

Canastar, A. and Maxson, S. (2003). Sexual aggression in mice: effects of male strain and female estrous state. *Behavioural Genetics*, 33, 521–8.

Casey, E.A., Beadnell, B., and Lindhorst, T.P. (2009). Predictors of sexually coercive behaviour in a nationally representative sample of adolescent males. *Journal of Interpersonal Violence*, 24, 1129–47.

Caspi, A., McClay, J., Moffitt, T.E., et al. (2002). Role of genotype in the cycle of violence in maltreated children. *Science*, 297, 851–4.

Christiansen, K. and Knussmann, R. (1987). Androgen levels and components of aggression in men. *Hormone Behaviour*, 21, 170–80.

Cleckley, H. (1988). *The Mask of Sanity*. St Louis, MO: Mosby Press.

Cohen, L.J., Nikiforov, K., Gans, S., et al. (2002). Heterosexual male perpetrators of childhood sexual abuse: a preliminary neuropsychiatric model. *Psychiatric Quarterly*, 73, 313–35.

Connell, R. (1987). *Gender and Power: Society, the Person and Sexual Politics*. Palo Alta, CA: University of California Press.

Cooper, C., Selwood, A., and Livingston, G. (2008). The prevalence of elder abuse and neglect: a systematic review. *Age and Ageing*, 37, 151–60.

Decker, M.R., Seage, G.R. 3rd, Hemenway, D., et al. (2009). Intimate partner violence functions as both a risk marker and risk factor for women's HIV infection: findings from Indian husband–wife dyads. *Journal of Acquired Immune Deficiency Syndromes*, 51, 593–600.

Degue, S. and Dilillo, D. (2004). Understanding perpetrators of non-physical sexual coercion: characteristics of those who cross the line. *Violence and Victims*, 19, 673–88.

Degue, S., Dilillo, D., and Scalora, M. (2010). Are all perpetrators alike? Comparing risk factors for sexual coercion and aggression. *Sexual Abuse*, 22, 402–26.

Devries, K.M., Mak, J.Y., Garcia-Moreno, C., et al. (2013). Global health. The global prevalence of intimate partner violence against women. *Science*, 340, 1527–8.

Dunkle, K.L., Jewkes, R.K., Brown, H.C., Gray, G.E., Mcintryre, J.A., and Harlow, S.D. (2004). Gender-based violence, relationship power, and risk of HIV infection in women attending antenatal clinics in South Africa. *The Lancet*, 363, 1415–21.

Edwards, A.C., Dodge, K.A., Latendresse, S.J., et al. (2010). MAOA-uVNTR and early physical discipline interact to influence delinquent behavior. *Journal of Child Psychology and Psychiatry*, 51, 679–87.

Fabian, J. (2012). Neuropsychology, neuroscience, volitional impairment and sexually violent predators: a review of the literature and law and their application to civil commitment proceedings. *Aggression and Violent Behaviour*, 17, 1–15.

Fazel, S., Hope, T., O'Donnell, I., and Jacoby, R. (2002). Psychiatric, demographic and personality characteristics of elderly sex offenders. *Psychological Medicine*, 32, 219–26.

Finkelhor, D. and Araji, S. (1986). Explanations of pedophilia: a four factor model. *Journal of Sex Research*, 22, 145–61.

Finkelhor, D. and Jones, L. (2006). Why have child maltreatment and child victimisation declined? *Journal of Social Issues*, 62, 685–716.

Fonagy, P. and Target, M. (2003). *Psychoanalytic Theories: Perspectives from Developmental Psychopathology*. New York: Routledge.

Fulu, E., Jewkes, R., Roselli, T., and Garcia-Moreno, C. (2013). Prevalence and risk factors for male perpetration of intimate partner violence: findings from the UN Multi-country Study on Men and Violence in Asia and the Pacific. *The Lancet Global Health*, 1(4), e187–207.

Gavey, N. (2005). *Just Sex? The Cultural Scaffolding of Rape*. Hove: Routledge.

Gilbert, R., Widom, C.S., Browne, K., Fergusson, D., Webb, E., and Janson, S. (2009). Burden and consequences of child maltreatment in high-income countries. *The Lancet*, 373, 68–81.

Giotakis, O., Markianos, M., Vaidakis, N., and Christodoulou, G. (2003). Aggression, impulsivity, plasma sex hormones and biogenic amine turnover in a forensic population of rapists. *Journal of Sex & Marital Therapy*, 29, 215–25.

Graham, K. and Wells, S. (2003). 'Somebody's gonna get their head kicked in tonight!' aggression among young males in bars—a question of values. *British Journal of Criminology*, 43, 546–66.

Gramsci, A. (1971). *Selections from a Prison Notebook*. London: Lawrence & Wishart.

Hare, R. (1996). Psychopathy: a clinical construct whose time has come. *Criminal Justice and Behaviour*, 23, 25–54.

Hare, R. (2003). *Psychopathy Checklist—Revised*. Toronto: Multi-health Systems.

Hearn, J., Nordberg, M., Andersson, K., et al. (2012). Hegemonic masculinity and beyond: 40 years of research in Sweden. *Men and Masculinities*, 15, 31–55.

Jama Shai, N., Jewkes, R., Levin, J., Dunkle, K., and Nduna, M. (2010). Factors associated with consistent condom use among rural young women in South Africa. *AIDS Care*, 22, 1379–85.

Jewkes, R. (2010). Gender inequities must be addressed in HIV prevention. *Science*, 329, 145–7.

Jewkes, R. and Abrahams, N. (2002). The epidemiology of rape and sexual coercion in South Africa: an overview. *Social Science & Medicine*, 55, 1231–44.

Jewkes, R., Dunkle, K., Koss, M.P., et al. (2006). Rape perpetration by young, rural South African men: prevalence, patterns and risk factors. *Social Science & Medicin*, 63, 2949–61.

Jewkes, R., Dunkle, K., Nduna, M., Jama, N., and Puren, A. (2010a). Associations between childhood adversity and depression, substance abuse & HIV & HSV2 in rural South African youth. *Child Abuse and Neglect*, 34, 833–41.

Jewkes, R., Dunkle, K., Nduna, M., and Shai, N. (2010b). Intimate partner violence, relationship gender power inequity, and incidence of HIV infection in young women in South Africa: a cohort study. *The Lancet*, 367, 41–8.

Jewkes, R., Fulu, E., Roselli, T., and Garcia-Moreno, C. (2013). Prevalence and risk factors for non-partner rape perpetration: findings from the UN Multi-country Cross-sectional Study on Men and Violence in Asia and the Pacific. *The Lancet Global Health*, 1(4), e208–18.

Jewkes, R. and Morrell, R. (2010). Gender and sexuality: emerging perspectives from the heterosexual epidemic in South Africa and implications for HIV risk and prevention. *Journal of the International AIDS Society*, 13, 6.

Jewkes, R. and Morrell, R. (2012). Sexuality and the limits of agency among South African teenage women: theorising femininities and their connections to HIV risk practices. *Social Science & Medicine*, 74, 1729–37.

Jewkes, R., Nduna, M., Levin, J., et al. (2008). Impact of Stepping Stones on incidence of HIV, HSV-2 and sexual behaviour in rural South Africa: cluster randomised controlled trial. *British Medical Journal* 337, a506.

Jewkes, R., Nduna, M., Jama-Shai, N., and Dunkle, K. (2012). Prospective study of rape perpetration by young South African men: incidence & risk factors for rape perpetration. *PLoS ONE*, 7, e38210.

Jewkes, R., Penn-Kekana, L., and Rose-Junius, H. (2005). 'If they rape me, I can't blame them': reflections on the social context of child sexual abuse in South Africa and Namibia. *Social Science & Medicine*, 61, 1809–20.

Jewkes, R., Sikweyiya, Y., Morrell, R., and Dunkle, K. (2011a). Gender inequitable masculinity and sexual entitlement in rape perpetration South Africa: findings of a cross-sectional study. *PloS ONE*, 6, e29590.

Jewkes, R., Sikweyiya, Y., Morrell, R., and Dunkle, K. (2011b). The relationship between intimate partner violence, rape and HIV amongst South African men: a cross-sectional study. *PLoS ONE*, 6, e24256.

Johansson, A., Santtila, P., Harlaar, N., et al. (2008). Genetic effects on male sexual coercion. *Aggressive Behaviour*, 34, 190–202.

Kalichman, S., Simbayi, L.C., Cain, D., Cherry, C., Henda, N., and Cloete, A. (2007). Sexual assault, sexual risks and gender attitudes in a community sample of South African men. *AIDS Care*, 19, 20–7.

Knerr, W., Gardner, F., and Cluver, L. (2013). Improving positive parenting skills and reducing harsh and abusive parenting in low- and middle-income countries: a systematic review. *Prevention Science*, 14, 352–63.

Knight, R.A. and Sims-Knight, J.E. (2003). The developmental antecedents of sexual coercion against women: testing alternative hypotheses with structural equation modelling. *Annals of the New York Academy of Sciences*, 989, 72–85.

Koenig, M.A., Stephenson, R., Ahmed, S., Jejeebhoy, S.J., and Campbell, J. (2006). Individual and contextual determinants of domestic violence in North India. *American Journal of Public Health*, 96, 132–8.

Koss, M.P. and Dinero, T.E. (1988). Predictors of sexual aggression among a national sample of male college students. *Annals of the New York Academy of Sciences*, 528, 133–47.

Kouyoumdjian, F.G., Calzavara, L.M., Bondy, S.J., et al. (2013). Intimate partner violence is associated with incident HIV infection in women in Uganda. *AIDS*, 27, 1331–8.

Krug, E., Dahlsberg, L., Mercy, J.A., Zwi, A.B., and Lozano, R. (2002). *World Health Report on Violence and Health*. Geneva: WHO.

LeBreton, J.M., Binning, J.F., and Adorno, A. (2006). Subclinical psychopaths. In J.C. Thomas and D. Segal (eds.) *Comprehensive Handbook of Personality and Psychopathology, Vol. 1, Personality and Everyday Functioning*, pp. 388–411. New York: Wiley.

Levinson, D. (1989). *Family Violence in Cross-Cultural Perpective*. Newbury Park, CA: Sage.

Lightfoot, S. and Evans, I. (2000). Risk factors for a New Zealand sample of sexually abusive children and adolescents. *Child Abuse and Neglect*, 24, 1185–98.

Lilienfeld, S. (2005). *Psychopathic Personality Inventory – Revised*. Lutz, FL: Psychological Assessment Resources, Inc.

Malamuth, N., Linz, D., Heavey, C.L., Barnes, G., and Acker, M. (1995). Using the confluence model of sexual aggression to predict men's conflict with women: a 10 year follow up study. *Journal of Personality & Social Psychology* 69, 353–69.

Malamuth, N.M., Sockloskie, R.J., Koss, M.P., and Tanaka, J.S. (1991). Characteristics of aggressors against women: testing a model using a national sample of college students. *Journal of Consulting and Clinical Psychology*, 59, 670–81.

Maniglio, R. (2010). The role of deviant sexual fantasy in the ethiopathogenesis of sexual homicide: a systematic review. *Aggression and Violent Behaviour*, 15, 294–302.

Marshall, W. (1989). Invited essay: intimacy, loneliness and sexual offenders. *Behaviour Research and Therapy*, 27, 491–503.

Marshall, W.l. and Barbaree, H. (1990). An integrated theory of the etiology of sexual offending. In W. Marshall, D. Laws., and H. Barbaree (eds.) *Handbook of Sexual Assault: Issues, Theories and Treatment of Offenders*, pp. 257–75. New York: Plenum.

Mathews, S., Abrahams, N., Jewkes, R., Martin, L., and Lombard, C. (2013). The epidemiology of child homicides in South Africa. *Bulletin of the World Health Organization*, 91(8), 562–8.

McCloskey, L. (2011). *Systematic Review of Parenting Interventions to Prevent Child Abuse Tested with Randomised Control Trial (RCT) Designs in High Income Countries*. Pretoria: Sexual Violence Research Initiative.

McPherson, M., Smith-Lovin, L., and Cook, J. (2001). Birds of a feather: homophily in social networks. *Annual Review of Sociology*, 27, 415–44.

Meel, B.L. (2009). Witchcraft in Transkei Region of South African: case report. *African Health Sciences*, 9, 61–4.

Morris, R.E., Anderson, M.M., and Knox, G. (2002). Incarcerated adolescents' experiences as perpetrators of sexual assualt. *Achives of Pediatric and Adolescent Medicine*, 156, 831–5.

Nduna, M., Jewkes, R.K., Dunkle, K.L., Shai, N.P., and Colman, I. (2010). Associations between depressive symptoms, sexual behaviour and relationship characteristics: a prospective cohort study of young women and men in the Eastern Cape, South Africa. *Journal of the International AIDS Society*, 13, 44.

Olver, M.E. and Wong, S. (2006). Psychopathy, sexual deviance and recidivism among sex offenders. *Sexual Abuse*, 18, 65–82.

Ouimette, P. (1997). Psychopathology and sexual aggression in nonincarcerated men. *Violence and Victims*, 12, 389–95.

Prichard, Z., Mackinnon, A., Jorm, A.F., and Easteal, S. (2008). No evidence for interaction between MAOA and childhood adversity for antisocial behavior. *American Journal of Medical Genetics Part B*, 147B, 228–32.

Pronyk, P., Hargreaves, J.R., Kim, J.C., and Al, E. (2006). Effect of a structural intervention for the prevention of intimate partner violence and HIV in rural South Africa: a cluster randomised trial. *The Lancet*, 368, 1973–83.

Reif, A., Rosler, M., Freitag, C.M., et al. (2007). Nature and nurture predispose to violent behavior: serotonergic genes and adverse childhood environment. *Neuropsychopharmacology*, 32, 2375–83.

Reza, A., Breiding, M., Blanton, C., et al. (2007). *Violence Against Children in Swaziland: Findings from a National Survey on Violence Against Children in Swaziland May 15–June 16, 2007*. UNICEF. Available at: http://www.unicef.org/swaziland/sz_publications_2007violenceagainstchildren.pdf.

Ricardo, C., Eads, M., and Barker, G. (2012). *Engaging Boys and Young Men in the Prevention of Sexual Violence: A Systematic and Global Review of Evaluated Interventions*. Pretoria: Sexual Violence Research Initiative.

Rosenberg, A.D., Abell, S.C., and Kanitz Mackie, J. (2005). An examination of the relationship between child sexual offending and psychopathy. *Journal of Child Sexual Abuse*, 14, 49–66.

Rowe, D. (2001). *Biology and Crime*. Los Angeles, CA: Roxbury.

Seto, M.C. and Lalumiere, M. (2010). What is so special about male adolescent sexual offending? A review and test of explanations through meta-analysis. *Psychological Bulletin*, 136, 526–75.

Shih, J.C., Chen, M., and Ridd, J. (1999). Monoamine oxidase: from genes to behaviour. *Annual Review of Neurosciences*, 22, 197–217.

Snyder, J., Horsch, E., and Childs, J. (1997). Peer relationships of young children: affiliative choice and the shaping of aggressive behaviour. *Journal of Clinical Child Psychology*, 26, 145–56.

Steglich, C.E.G., Snijders, T.A.B., and Pearson, M. (2010). Dynamic networks and behaviour: separating selection from influence. *Sociological Methodology*, 40, 329–93.

Stirpe, T., Abracen, J., Stermac, L., and Wilson, R. (2006). Sexual offenders' state-of-mind regarding childhood attachment: a controlled investigation. *Sexual Abuse*, 18, 289–302.

Tolin, D.F. and Foa, E.B. (2006). Sex differences in trauma and posttraumatic stress disorder: a quantitative review of 25 years of research. *Psychological Bulletin*, 132, 959–92.

Tsai, A.C., Leiter, K., Heisler, M., et al. (2011). Prevalence and correlates of forced sex perpetrtaion and victimisation in Botswana and Swaziland. *American Journal of Public Health*, 101, 1068–74.

Walby, S. (2010). *The Cost of Domestic Violence: Up-date 2009*. Lancaster: Lancaster University.

Waters, H., Hyder, A., Rajkotia, Y., Basu, S., Rehwinkel, J.A., and Butchardt, A. (2004). *Economic Dimensions of Interpersonal Violence*. Geneva: WHO.

Welbourn, A. (1995). *Stepping Stones*. Oxford: Strategies For Hope.

Whitaker, D.J., Le, B., Hanson, R.K., et al. (2008). Risk factors for perpetration of child sexual abuse: a review and meta-analysis. *Child Abuse and Neglect*, 32, 529–48.

Wolfe, D.A., Crooks, C., Jaffe, P., et al. (2009). A school-based program to prevent adolescent dating violence: a cluster randomized trial. *Archives of Pediatrics & Adolescent Medicine*, 163, 692–9.

Wood, K. and Jewkes, R. (2001). 'Dangerous' love: reflections on violence among Xhosa township youth. In R. Morrell (ed.) *Changing Men in Southern Africa*, pp. 317–36. Pietermaritzburg: University of Natal Press, Zed Press.

Wood, K., Lambert, H., and Jewkes, R. (2007). 'Showing roughness in a beautiful way': talk about love, coercion, and rape in South African youth sexual culture. *Medical Anthropology Quarterly*, 21, 277–300.

World Health Organization (2004). *Global Status Report on Alcohol 2004*. Geneva: WHO.

World Health Organization (2013). *Global and Regional Estimates of Violence Against Women: Prevalence and Health Effects of Intimate Partner Violence and Non-Partner Sexual Violence*. Geneva: WHO.

World Health Organization/London School of Hygiene and Tropical Medicine (2010). *Preventing Intimate Partner and Sexual Violence Against Women: Taking Action and Generating Evidence*. Geneva: WHO.

Collective violence: war

Barry S. Levy and Victor W. Sidel

Collective violence as threat to public health

In 1966, the World Health Assembly declared violence 'a major and growing public health problem across the world' (World Health Assembly 1996). The *World Report on Violence and Health*, published by the World Health Organization (WHO) in 2002, was the first comprehensive report by the WHO on violence as a public health problem (Krug et al. 2002). The WHO report presented a typology of violence that defines three broad categories based on the characteristics of those committing the violent acts: self-directed violence, interpersonal violence, and collective violence. Other chapters in the textbook cover the first two categories of violence (see Chapters 8.7 and 9.5), and this chapter will deal primarily with war, an important component of collective violence.

Collective violence has been characterized as 'the instrumental use of violence by people who identify themselves as members of a group—whether this group is transitory or has a more permanent identity—against another group or set of individuals in order to achieve political, economic, ideological, or social objectives' (Krug et al. 2002, p. 215). Collective violence includes armed conflict (such as war), state-sponsored violence (such as genocide, repression, disappearances, and torture), and organized violent crime (such as gang warfare and banditry).

The *World Report* gives examples of collective violence: 'Violent conflicts between nations and groups, state and group terrorism, rape as a weapon of war, the movement of large numbers of people displaced from their homes, and gang warfare' (Krug et al. 2002, p. 215). As the *World Report* notes, 'all of these occur on a daily basis in many parts if the world' and 'the effects of these different types of events on health in terms of deaths, physical illness, disabilities, and mental anguish are vast' (Krug et al. 2002, p. 215). Also included in this chapter is limited information on what has been termed *terrorism* and the *war on terror*, as Chapter 8.18 covers *bioterrorism*. This chapter will not cover the topic of *gang warfare*, which is covered in Chapter 9.5.

The health impacts of collective violence

Direct consequences of war and military operations

Armed conflicts in the twenty-first century largely consist of the civil wars (conflicts within countries, to which other countries sometimes contribute military troops). In the 2001–2010 period, there were 69 armed conflicts globally; in 2010, 30 of these armed conflicts were still active. Of these armed conflicts, those that result in 1000 battle-related deaths within a year are classified as wars. In 2001, there were ten wars; in 2010, there were four wars, including the Iraq War (Stockholm International Peace Research Institute 2012; Levy and Sidel 2013a). During the 2001–2010 period, there were 221 non-state conflicts (the use of armed force between two organized groups, neither of which is the government of a state, that results in at least 25 battle-related deaths in a year); the number of non-state conflicts per year decreased during this period, with 26 non-state conflicts active during 2010 (Stockholm International Peace Research Institute 2012).

Some of the impacts of war on public health are obvious, whereas others are not. The direct impact of war on mortality and morbidity is apparent. Many people, including an increasing percentage of civilians, are killed or injured during war. An estimated 191 million people died directly or indirectly as a result of conflict during the twentieth century, more than half of whom were civilians (Rummel 1994). The exact figures are unknowable because of the generally poor recordkeeping in many countries and its disruption in time of conflict.

War has direct, immediate, and deadly effects on human life and health. The 'body counts' and the data on those with war-caused injuries and disabilities, both physical and psychological, although woefully incomplete, document the many people tragically killed and wounded as a direct result of military activities. Through the early twentieth century up to the start of the Second World War, the vast preponderance of the direct casualties of war were uniformed combatants, usually members of national armed forces. Although non-combatants suffered social, economic, and environmental consequences of war and may have been the victims of what is now termed *collateral damage* of military operations, 'civilians' were generally not directly targeted and were largely spared direct death and disability resulting from war (Levy and Sidel 2008).

However, since 1937, when Nazi forces bombed the city of Guernica, a non-military target in the Basque region of Spain, military operations have increasingly killed and maimed civilians through purposeful targeting of non-military targets. The use of 'carpet bombing' and the collateral damage of heavy attacks on military targets have caused many civilian casualties. The percentage of civilian deaths as a proportion of all deaths directly caused by war has therefore increased dramatically. Many of these civilian deaths may have been indirectly rather than directly caused by war.

Since September 11, 2001, there has been increasing concern in the United States and other countries about violence conducted by individuals and groups to create fear and advance a political agenda—a form of violence commonly called *terrorism*. We believe that there needs to be a balanced approach to strengthening systems and protecting people in response to the threat of terrorism, an approach that strengthens a broad range of public health capacities and preserves civil liberties (Levy and Sidel 2012). Terrorism is often defined in a partisan fashion: those called *terrorists* by one side in a conflict may be viewed as 'patriots', 'freedom fighters', or 'servants of God' by the other. We have defined terrorism as, 'politically motivated violence or the threat of violence, especially against civilians, with the intent to instil fear'. This definition includes violent acts conducted by nation-states against civilians with the intent to instil fear as well as acts committed by individuals and subnational groups. The term *terrorism* has considerable overlap with the term *war* and many actions conducted during war fit our definition of terrorism. The 'war on terror' of the George W. Bush administration in the United States, in contrast to use of education, law enforcement, economic aid, and other methods to prevent terrorism, led some analysts to include this war on terror as an example of collective violence.

Indirect effects of war and other military activities

Along with the direct impacts of war and other military activities on health, collective violence may also cause serious health consequences through its impact on the physical, economic, social, and biological environments in which people live. The environmental damage may affect people not only in nations directly engaged in collective violence, but also in all nations. Much of the morbidity and mortality during war, especially among civilians, has been the result of damage to the societal infrastructure, including destruction of food and water supply systems, healthcare facilities and public health services, sewage disposal systems, power plants and electrical grids, and transportation and communication systems. Destruction of infrastructure has led to food shortages and consequent malnutrition, contamination of food and drinking water and resultant food-borne and waterborne illness, and healthcare and public health deficiencies and resultant disease (Levy and Sidel 2008).

Preparation for war can also adversely affect human health. Some of the impacts are direct, such as injuries and deaths during training exercises, and others are indirect. As with war itself, preparation for war can divert human, financial, and other resources that otherwise might be used for health and human services.

Damage to the physical environment—water, land, and air—and extensive use of non-renewable resources may be the result of preparation for war as well as war itself. Lakes, rivers, streams and aquifers, land masses, and the atmosphere may be polluted through testing and use of weapons. Non-renewable resources are extensively consumed in weapons production, testing, and use.

The economic environment may also be adversely affected by the diversion of resources from education, housing, nutrition, and other human and health services to military activities and through an increase in national debt and/or taxation. These economic impacts affect both developed and developing countries. In our globalized world, armed conflict in one part of the world may have substantial impacts globally, such as in increases in oil and food prices.

Governmental and societal preoccupation with preparation for wars—often known as *militarism*—may lead to massive diversion of resources away from the promotion of human welfare. This preoccupation may lead to policies that promote 'pre-emptive war' (when an attack is allegedly imminent) and to 'preventive war' (when an attack may be feared sometime in the future). Diversion of resources towards war-related activities is a problem worldwide, but is especially important in developing countries. Many developing countries spend substantially more on military expenditures than on health-related expenditures; for example, in recent years, Angola spent US\$196 per capita for military expenditures (in 2010) and US\$183 per capita for health (in 2008).

The social environment may be affected by increasing militarism, by encouragement of violence as a means for settling disputes, and violation of human rights and restriction of civil liberties. Preparation for war can also promote violence.

Another important indirect impact of war is the creation of many refugees and internally displaced persons: Many of the world's 10.5 million refugees have left their native countries as a result of war. Refugees often flee to neighbouring less-developed countries, which are often already facing significant challenges in addressing the public health needs of their own populations. In addition, the vast majority of the 27.5 million internally displaced persons worldwide have left their homes to escape war. These internally displaced persons are often worse off than refugees who have left their countries because they frequently do not have easy access to food, safe water, healthcare, shelter, and other necessities.

Approximately 9.9 million of these internally displaced persons are in five countries: the Democratic Republic of Congo, Iraq, Somalia, Sudan, and Syria. Refugees and internally displaced persons experience much higher rates of mortality and morbidity, much of it due to malnutrition and infectious diseases. The vast majority of refugees and internally displaced persons as a result of war are women, children, and elderly people who may be highly vulnerable not only to disease and malnutrition, but also to threats to their security.

The environment may be disrupted during war or the preparation for war. Conventional weapons may damage the environment such that the health-supporting infrastructure—systems of food and water supply, sewage disposal, medical care and public health, power generation and supply, transportation, and communication—is severely disrupted or destroyed. Malnutrition of the affected population may increase the frequency and severity of infectious diseases. The biological environment may also be disrupted by the production, testing, and use of biological weapons. Ionizing radiation from the production, testing, use, and disposal of nuclear weapons and radioactive materials, such as depleted uranium, may also contaminate and damage the environment. So may the release of hazardous and toxic substances from damaged industrial facilities or from the production, testing, use, and unsafe disposal of chemical weapons.

Hazardous wastes from military operations represent potential contaminants of air, water, and soil. For example, groundwater was contaminated with trichloroethylene (TCE), a probable human carcinogen, and other toxins at the Otis Air Force Base in Massachusetts; 125 chemicals were dumped over a period of 30 years at the Rocky Mountain Arsenal in Colorado; and benzene, a human carcinogen, was found in extremely high concentrations at the McChord Air Force Base in the State of Washington (Westing 2008).

Both during war and the preparation for war, military forces consume huge amounts of fossil fuels and other non-renewable materials. Energy consumption by military equipment can be substantial. For example, an armoured division of 348 battle tanks operating for 1 day consumes more than 2.2 million L of fuel and a carrier battle group operating for 1 day consumes more than 1.5 million L of fuel. The US military annually consumes millions of tons of fuel and emits huge amounts of carbon monoxide, oxides of nitrogen, hydrocarbons, and sulphur dioxide (Westing 2008).

Weapons systems

Conventional weapons

Conventional weapons consist of explosives, incendiaries, and weapons of various sizes, ranging from 'small arms and light weapons' to heavy artillery and bombs. Small arms and light weapons (SALW), which include pistols, rifles, machine guns, and other hand-held or easily transportable weapons, are the weapons most often used in wars. Although some restrictions have been placed on their use in war, such as the outlawing of the use of 'dum-dum bullets' (which cause extensive injuries when striking a human), there has been little effective effort to prohibit their use. In the Millennium Report of the United Nations (UN) Secretary-General to the General Assembly, Kofi Annan stated that small arms could be described as weapons of mass destruction because the fatalities they produce 'dwarf that of all other weapons systems—and in most years greatly exceed the toll of the atomic bombs that devastated Hiroshima and Nagasaki' (Annan 2000).

Conventional weapons have accounted for the overwhelming majority of adverse environmental consequences due to war. During the Second World War, for example, extensive carpet bombing of cities in Europe and Japan accounted not only for many deaths and injuries, but also for widespread devastation of urban environments. During the Persian Gulf War, the more than 600 oil fires in Kuwait accounted for widespread environmental devastation and respiratory ailments among people who were exposed to the smoke from these fires. The bombing of mangrove forests during the Vietnam War led to destruction of these forests, and the resultant bomb craters have remained several decades afterwards, often filling with stagnant water that serves as a breeding ground for mosquitoes transmitting malaria and other mosquito-borne diseases.

The international trade in small arms and light weapons fuels much collective violence, especially in developing countries. The UN General Assembly, in 2013, took a major step towards regulating the international trade in these conventional weapons by overwhelmingly approving the Arms Trade Treaty, which links purchases of arms to the human-rights records of the purchasing countries. The Treaty is designed to prevent exported weapons from contributing to human rights violations, terrorism, or organized crime, and to prohibit arms shipments that are deemed to be harmful to women or children.

Armed drones

Unarmed drone aircraft have been used for many years to conduct surveillance. Since 2004, the United States has been conducting armed drone strikes over Pakistan in an effort to kill people that it suspects of being terrorists. The US Central Intelligence Agency contends that its drone strikes have killed more than 600 militants in Pakistan since May 2010, but no non-combatant civilians.

However, the Bureau of Investigative Journalism at the City University in London has reported that most of the 1842 people who have been killed in more than 230 armed drone strikes in Pakistan since 2008 have been militants, but at least 218 of them may have been non-combatant civilians. In late 2011, a US citizen was killed by a targeted armed drone attack in Yemen. In early 2012, the US Attorney General asserted a right to kill US citizens in other countries who are plotting attacks against the United States.

Nuclear weapons

Nuclear weapons have become increasingly widespread since their development in the 1940s. There are now an estimated 19,000 nuclear warheads in at least nine nations—the United States, Russia, the United Kingdom, France, China, Israel, India, Pakistan, and North Korea (Stockholm International Peace Research Institute 2012). The United States currently has approximately 1000 nuclear war heads on alert on land-based intercontinental ballistic missiles (ICBMs) and submarine-launched ballistic missiles; Russia currently maintains 1200 war heads on alert, nearly all of which are on ICBMs.

The historic high in the explosive capacity of the global nuclear weapons stockpiles was reached in 1960 with an explosive capacity equivalent to 20,000 megatons (20 billion tons or 40 trillion pounds) of trinitrotoulene, or equivalent to that of 1.4 million of the nuclear bombs dropped on Hiroshima (Sutton and Gould 2008). In the United States in 1967, the nuclear stockpile had reached approximately 32,000 nuclear warheads of 30 different types. In 2012, the US stockpile was about 9400 warheads. Five thousand of the nuclear weapons in the United States, Russia, and possibly other countries are on 'hair-trigger' alert, ready to fire on a few minutes' notice.

The detonation of nuclear bombs over Hiroshima and Nagasaki in August 1945 during the Second World War led to the immediate deaths of approximately 200,000 people, primarily civilians, as well as to lasting injury and later death of many others, together with massive devastation—and widespread radioactive contamination—of the environment in these two cities (Sutton and Gould 2008). Atmospheric testing of nuclear weapons by the United States, the Soviet Union, and other countries also led to environmental contamination, with increased rates of leukaemia and other cancers among populations who were downwind from these tests. The effects of exposure to iodine-131 (a radioactive isotope of iodine produced by the testing) on children has been well documented (Institute of Medicine and National Research Council 1999). In addition to the potential for use of nuclear weapons by national armed forces, there is an increasing threat of their use by non-state actors.

From 1945 to 1990, the United States produced approximately 70,000 nuclear weapons; other nations also produced many of these weapons. Production of nuclear weapons has led to major environmental contamination (Levy and Sidel 2005). For example, the area around Chelyabinsk in Russia has been heavily contaminated with radioactive materials from the nuclear weapons production facility in that area. The level of ambient radiation in and near the Techa River in the area has been documented to be as high as 28 times the normal background radiation level (Burmistrov et al. 2006). Another example is the leakage of radioactive materials from the storage of wastes from nuclear weapons production at Hanford, along the Columbia River in Washington State, leading to extensive radioactive contamination (Westing 2008).

The dismantling and disposal of nuclear weapons has also led to environmental contamination. The primary site for the disassembly of US nuclear weapons is the Pantex Plant, located 17 miles northeast of Amarillo in the Texas panhandle (Levy and Sidel 2005). Overall, the United States has dismantled more than 60,000 nuclear war heads since the 1940s; during the 1990s, 11,751 war heads were dismantled. Approximately 14,000 plutonium pits (hollow shells of plutonium encased in steel or another metal that are essential components of nuclear weapons) are in interim staging at Pantex (Levy and Sidel 2005). Plutonium, an element first produced in the Manhattan Project in 1942, has a half-life of 24,000 years. Plans to increase production capacity to 50 to 80 pits per year have been delayed because of budgetary reasons.

Radiological weapons

'Dirty bombs', consisting of conventional explosive devices mixed with radioactive materials, or attacks on nuclear power plants with explosive weapons could widely scatter highly radioactive materials. Another example of a radioactive substance used in weapons is depleted uranium (DU), uranium from which the uranium isotope usable for nuclear weapons or as fuel rods for nuclear power plants has been removed (Depleted Uranium Education Project 1997). DU is used militarily as a casing for armour-penetrating shells. An extremely dense material, uranium used as a casing increases the ability of the shell to penetrate the armour of tanks; uranium is also pyrophoric and bursts into flames on impact. DU-encased shells were used by the United States during the Persian Gulf War, the Iraq War, and the war in Kosovo; similar shells were used by the United Kingdom in the Iraq War. DU, which is both radioactive and extremely toxic, has been demonstrated to cause contamination of the soil and groundwater. Use of DU is considered legal by the nations that have used it, but its use is considered by other nations to be illegal under the Geneva Conventions and other international treaties.

Chemicals

A variety of chemical weapons and related materials have the potential for direct health effects during collective violence and also for contaminating the physical environment during war and the preparation for war. The potential for exposure exists not only for military and civilian populations, who may be exposed during the use of chemical weapons in wartime, but also for workers involved in the development, production, transport, and storage of these weapons and for community residents living near facilities where these weapons are developed, produced, transported, and stored. In addition, disposal of these weapons, including their disassembly and incineration, can be hazardous.

During the Vietnam War, the US military used defoliants on mangrove forests and other vegetation, which not only defoliated and killed trees and other plants, but may also have led to excessive numbers of birth defects and cases of cancer among nearby residents (Levy and Sidel 2005). In addition, development and production of conventional weapons involve the use of many chemicals that are toxic and can contaminate the environment. Furthermore, there is now a plausible threat of non-state agents using chemical weapons; a Japanese cult, Aum Shinrikyo, used

sarin in the subway system of two Japanese cities in the mid 1990s, accounting for the deaths of 19 people and injuries to thousands (Lee et al. 2012).

The Chemical Weapons Convention (CWC), which came into force in 1997, prohibits all development, production, acquisition, stockpiling, transfer, and use of chemical weapons. It requires each state party to destroy its chemical weapons and chemical weapons production facilities, as well as any chemical weapons it may have abandoned on the territory of another state party. The verification provisions of the CWC affect not only the military sector but also the civilian chemical industry worldwide through certain restrictions and obligations regarding the production, processing, and consumption of chemicals that are considered relevant to the objectives of the convention. These provisions are to be verified through a combination of reporting requirements, routine onsite inspection of declared sites, and short-notice challenge inspections. The Organization for the Prohibition of Chemical Weapons (OPCW) in The Hague, established by the CWC, ensures implementation of the provisions of the CWC. The disposal of chemical weapons required by the CWC has raised controversy about the safety of two different methods of disposal: incineration and chemical neutralization. The controversy about safety and protection of the environment has delayed completion of the disposal by the date required by the CWC.

Biological agents

These consist of bacteria, viruses, other microorganisms, and their toxins, which can not only directly produce illness in humans, but can also be used against other animals or plants, thereby adversely affecting human food supplies or agricultural resources and indirectly affecting human health. Biological agents have been used relatively infrequently during warfare, but there has long been a potential for their use. These agents have been used as weapons, albeit sporadically, since ancient times. In the sixth century BC, Persia, Greece, and Rome tried to contaminate drinking water sources with diseased corpses. In AD 1346, Mongols besieging the Crimean seaport of Kaffa placed cadavers of plague victims on hurling machines and threw them into Kaffa. In the mid-eighteenth century, during the French and Indian War, a British commander sent blankets infected with smallpox to Native Americans. During the First World War, Germany dropped bombs containing plague bacteria over British positions and used cholera in Italy. During the 1930s, Japan contaminated the food and water supplies of several cities and sprayed the cities with cultures of microorganisms.

Gruinard Island, off the coast of Scotland, was contaminated in 1942 by a test use of anthrax spores by the United Kingdom and the United States (Harris and Paxman 1962). During the 1950s and 1960s, secret large-scale open-air tests at the US Army Dugway Proving Ground may have introduced the microorganisms that cause Q fever and Venezuelan equine encephalitis into the deserts of Western Utah (Cole 1988). In 1979, the accidental release of anthrax spores near Sverdlovsk in the Soviet Union resulted in at least 77 cases of inhalation anthrax and at least 66 deaths (Meselson et al. 1994).

There is concern that biological agents could be used as terrorist weapons. In the autumn of 2001, anthrax spores were disseminated through the US mail, causing 23 cases of inhalational and skin anthrax, five of which were fatal. The Centers for Disease

Control and Prevention has identified three categories of diseases caused by biological agents, according to its level of concern that they may be used as terrorist weapons. Category A consists of the agents that cause anthrax, botulism, plague, smallpox, tularaemia, and viral haemorrhagic fevers. Category B consists of the agents that cause brucellosis, glanders, melioidosis, psittacosis, Q fever, typhus fever, viral encephalitis, water safety threats, and food safety threats (such as *Salmonella* and *Shigella* species, and *Escherichia coli* O157:H7), as well as epsilon toxin of *Clostridium perfringens*, ricin toxin from castor beans, and staphylococcal enterotoxin B. Category C consists of the agents that cause emerging infectious diseases such as Nipah virus and hantavirus (Centers for Disease Control and Prevention 2012).

Antipersonnel landmines

Tens of millions of antipersonnel landmines are still deployed in 72 countries and seven disputed areas. These landmines have been termed 'weapons of mass destruction, one person at a time'. They have mostly been placed in rural areas, posing a threat to residents of these areas and often disrupting farming and other activities. Civilians are the most likely to be injured or killed by landmines, which injure or kill approximately 4000 people annually; the vast majority of landmine victims are civilians, primarily poor people living in rural areas. About one-quarter of landmine victims are children. It is estimated that half of all landmine victims die of their injuries before they reach appropriate medical care. Although a mine may cost only a few dollars to produce, it may cost more than US$1000 to remove. And its adverse economic impact on human health and well-being is substantially higher. Mines, in addition to maiming and killing people, make large areas of land uninhabitable. Remaining in place for many years, they pose long-term threats to people, including refugees and internally displaced persons returning to their homes after long periods of war. Since the entry into force of the Anti-Personnel Landmine Convention in 1997, production of landmines has been markedly reduced, although 12 countries continue to produce antipersonnel landmines, including China, India, Pakistan, Russia, and the United States. Since 1997, millions of landmines that had been implanted in the ground have been removed (International Campaign to Ban Landmines n.d.). Many of the mines are still buried and additional resources will be required to continue unearthing and destroying them, tasks that pose inherent risks to demining personnel (Sirkin et al. 2008).

Weapons in space

The deployment of weapons in space represents another risk of weapons systems igniting armed conflict or adding to its potential health consequences. Attempts by the United Nations to limit weapons in space have thus far failed. In 2008, Russian and Chinese delegates to a UN conference presented a draft treaty banning weapons in space, but the United States opposed such a treaty. The risk of an arms race of weapons in space continues.

The role of public health in addressing war

War and the preparation for war have enormous adverse impact on humans and their environment. Public health workers have an important part to play in response to war. As the World Health Assembly declared in 1981, 'the role of health workers in promoting and preserving peace is a significant factor for achieving health for all' (World Health Assembly 1981).

Prevention of war

The health and environmental problems created by collective violence can appear to be overwhelming. However, standard public health principles and implementation measures can be successfully applied in addressing these problems. The following subsection of this chapter highlights three standard public health approaches that can be developed and implemented in addressing these environmental problems: (1) surveillance and documentation, (2) education and raising awareness, and (3) advocacy for sound policies and programmes.

Surveillance and documentation

Much can be accomplished by undertaking surveillance and other activities to document the problems caused by war. Although the numbers of deaths, injuries, and diseases among uniformed combatants are generally well documented, deaths, injuries, and diseases among civilians are more difficult to document. Household cluster surveys have been used during the Iraq War to estimate the civilian casualties. Technical approaches to surveillance can include environmental monitoring as well as biological monitoring, the latter to document and assess the human burden of environmental contaminants and their adverse health consequences. Non-technical approaches can include information from physician reports, reports in the mass media, and assessments by government agencies.

Education and raising awareness

Much can also be accomplished by educating and raising the awareness of health professionals, policymakers, and the general public about the problems caused by war. A multifaceted approach that incorporates publications by citizens' groups and professional organizations, information in the mass media, and personal communication is often valuable. In addition, public health workers can assist people in distinguishing between accurate and inaccurate information and in setting priorities.

Advocacy for sound policies and programmes

Finally, much can also be accomplished by advocating for improved policies and programmes that help prevent collective violence and minimize its public health impact.

Levels of prevention

Those concerned with the promotion and protection of health classify preventive measures into four basic categories: pre-primary (primordial) prevention, primary prevention, secondary prevention, and tertiary prevention. Pre-primary prevention consists of measures to prevent adverse health consequences by removing the conditions that lead to them. Primary prevention consists of measures to prevent the health consequences of a specific illness or injury by preventing its occurrence in a specific individual or among members of a specific group. Secondary prevention consists of measures to prevent or limit the health consequences of an illness or injury, or to limit the spread of an infectious disease to others, after the disease process has begun. Tertiary prevention consists of efforts to rehabilitate those injured and to reintegrate them into society or, in the case of prevention of collective violence, to prevent the resumption of violence.

Pre-primary prevention

In general, pre-primary (primordial) prevention requires political and social will. Pre-primary and primary prevention may be difficult to accomplish because the causes of the disease or injury may be unknown and, when they are known, the preventive methods may be difficult to implement technically or politically. As measures for pre-primary or primary prevention are usually more effective and rarely have negative consequences, they are generally considered preferable to secondary prevention, even when implementation is difficult or expensive. Secondary prevention is usually easier to implement politically and technically but, because such methods are often ineffective or only partially effective, they may create a false sense of security and encourage risk taking, can be more expensive than primary prevention, and many measures are more likely than pre-primary or primary prevention methods to have adverse consequences. The health consequences of war and the aftermath of war can be prevented or reduced through pre-primary prevention. This generally requires cooperation among civil society (non-governmental) organizations, governmental agencies, and organizations of health professionals.

The underlying causes of collective violence include poverty, socioeconomic inequalities, adverse effects of globalization, and shame and humiliation. Some of the underlying causes of war and militarism are becoming more prevalent or worsening.

Persistence of socioeconomic disparities and other forms of social injustice are among the leading underlying causes of war. The rich–poor divide is growing. In 1960, in the 20 richest countries, the per-capita gross domestic product (GDP) was 18 times that of the 20 poorest countries; by 1995, this gap had increased to 37 times. Inequality is not restricted to personal income, but includes other important areas of life, such as health status, access to healthcare, education, and employment opportunities. In addition, abundant national resources, such as oil, minerals, metals, gemstones, drug crops, and timber, have fuelled many wars in developing countries.

Globalization is similarly a two-edged sword. Insofar as globalization leads to good relations among nation-states and reductions in poverty and disparities within and among nations, it may play a powerful role in prevention of collective violence. Conversely, if globalization leads to exploitation of people, the environment, and other resources, it may cause war.

The Carnegie Commission on Preventing Deadly Conflict has identified the following factors that put nations at risk of violent conflict, including:

- Lack of democratic processes and unequal access to power, especially in situations where power arises from religious or ethnic identity and leaders are repressive or abusive of human rights.
- Social inequality characterized by markedly unequal distribution of resources and access to these resources, especially where the economy is in decline and there is, as a result, more social inequality and more competition for resources.
- Control by one group of valuable natural resources, such as oil, timber, drugs, or gems.

- Demographic changes that are so rapid that they outstrip the capability of a nation to provide basic necessary services and opportunities for employment (Carnegie Commission on Preventing Deadly Conflict 1998).

The United States and other developed nations must increase funding for humanitarian and sustainable development programmes that address the root causes of collective violence, such as hunger, illiteracy, and unemployment.

Promoting multilateralism

Since its founding in 1946, the UN has attempted to live up to the goal stated in its charter: 'To save succeeding generations from the scourge of war' (United Nations, 1945). Its mandate, along with preventing war, includes protecting human rights, promoting international justice, and helping the people of the world to achieve a sustainable standard of living. Its affiliated programmes and specialized agencies include, among many others, the United Nations Children's Fund (UNICEF), the WHO, the Food and Agriculture Organization (FAO), the International Labour Organization (ILO), the United Nations Development Programme (UNDP), and the Office of the UN High Commissioner for Refugees (UNHCR). These UN-related organizations, and the UN itself, have made an enormous difference in the lives of people.

The UN spends about US$5 billion a year. By comparison, annual global military expenditures—more than US$2 trillion— would pay for the entire UN system for about 400 years.

The UN has no army and no police. It relies on the voluntary contribution of troops and other personnel to halt conflicts that threaten peace and security. The United States and other member states on the Security Council decide when and where to deploy peacekeeping troops. Long-term conflicts fester while conflicting national priorities deadlock the UN's ability to act. In fact, if stymied by the veto, the UN has little power beyond the bully pulpit.

Ending poverty and social injustice

Poverty and other manifestations of social injustice contribute to conditions that lead to collective violence (Levy and Sidel 2013b). Growing socioeconomic and other disparities between the rich and the poor within countries, and between rich and poor nations, also contribute to the likelihood of armed conflict. By addressing these underlying conditions through policies and programmes that redistribute wealth within nations and among nations, and by providing financial and technical assistance to less-developed nations, countries such as the United States can minimize poverty and other forms of social injustice that lead to collective violence.

Creating a culture of peace

Public health workers can do much to promote a culture of peace, in which non-violent means are utilized to settle conflicts. A culture of peace is based on the values, attitudes, and behaviours that form the deep roots of peace. They are in some ways the opposite of the values, attitudes, and behaviours that promote collective violence, but should not be equated with just the absence of war. A culture of peace can exist at the level of the family, workplace, school, community, state, and the world. Public health workers and others can play important roles in encouraging the development of a culture of peace at all these levels.

The Hague Appeal for Peace Civil Society Conference was held in 1999 on the 100th anniversary of the 1899 Hague Peace Conference. The 1899 conference, attended by governmental representatives, was devoted to finding methods for making war more humane. The 1999 conference, attended by 1000 individuals and representatives of civil society organizations, was devoted to finding methods to prevent war and to establish a 'culture of peace'. The document adopted at the 1999 conference, the Hague Appeal for Peace and Justice for the twenty-first century, has been translated by the UN into all its official languages and distributed widely around the world. Its ten-point action agenda addressed education for peace, human rights, and democracy; the adverse effects of globalization; sustainable and equitable use of environmental resources; elimination of racial, ethnic, religious, and gender intolerance; protection of children; reduction of violence; and other issues.

Primary prevention

Primary prevention includes preventing specific elements of collective violence and sharply reducing preparation for war, as follows.

Strengthening nuclear weapons treaties

Unlike the implementation of treaties banning chemical weapons and biological weapons, there is no comprehensive treaty banning the use or mandating the destruction of nuclear weapons. Instead, a series of overlapping incomplete treaties has been negotiated. The Partial Test Ban Treaty (PTBT) of 1963, promoted in part by concerns about radioactive environmental contamination, banned nuclear tests in the atmosphere, under water, and in outer space. The expansion of the PTBT, the Comprehensive Nuclear-Test-Ban-Treaty (CTBT), a key step towards nuclear disarmament and preventing proliferation, was opened for signature in 1996 but has not yet received sufficient signatures or ratifications to enter into force. It bans nuclear explosions, for either military or civilian purposes, but does not ban computer simulations and subcritical tests, which some nations rely on to maintain the option of developing new nuclear weapons. As of late 2012, the CTBT had been signed by 183 nations and ratified by 157. Entry into force requires ratification by the 44 nuclear-capable nations, of which 36 had ratified it by late 2012. The following nuclear-capable nations had not ratified it: China, Egypt, India, Iran, Israel, North Korea, Pakistan, and the United States.

The Treaty on the Non-Proliferation of Nuclear Weapons (the 'Nuclear Non-Proliferation Treaty', or NPT) was opened for signature in 1968 and entered into force in 1970. By late 2012, a total of 189 states parties (nations) had ratified the treaty. The five nuclear weapon states recognized under the NPT—China, France, Russia, the United Kingdom, and the United States—are parties to the treaty. The NPT attempts to prevent the spread of nuclear weapons by restricting transfer of certain technologies. It relies on a control system carried out by the International Atomic Energy Agency (IAEA), which also promotes nuclear energy. In exchange for the non-nuclear weapons states' commitment not to develop or otherwise acquire nuclear weapons, the NPT commits the nuclear weapon states to good-faith negotiations on nuclear disarmament.

Every 5 years since 1970 the states parties have held a review conference to assess implementation of the treaty. The International Court of Justice (the World Court) in 1996 in an advisory opinion urged that the nations possessing nuclear weapons move expeditiously towards nuclear disarmament, as is required by Article VI of the NPT.

The United States should help stop the spread of nuclear weapons by actively supporting and adhering to these treaties, and by setting an example for the rest of the world by renouncing the first use of nuclear weapons and the development of new nuclear weapons. It should work with Russia to dismantle nuclear war heads and increase funding for programmes to secure nuclear materials so that they will not fall into the hands of non-state actors.

Increasing attention is being focused on the elimination of nuclear weapons. Policymakers, such as former US Secretaries of State Henry Kissinger and George Shultz and former military leaders, have called for measures towards the elimination of these weapons (Shultz et al. 2007). One measure that may accomplish this is a nuclear weapons convention comparable to the Chemical Weapons Convention, the Biological and Toxin Weapons Convention, and the Anti-Personnel Landmine Convention. In 2007, Costa Rica and Malaysia submitted to the UN an updated draft of a nuclear weapon convention, modelled after the Convention on Chemical and Biological Weapons as well as the International Treaty on Anti-Personnel Landmines. The proposed convention which supplements existing international treaties, such as the NPT and CTBT, if adopted, would prohibit nations from pursuing or participating in the development, testing, production, stockpiling, transfer, use, and threat of use of nuclear weapons. Nations possessing nuclear weapons would need to destroy their nuclear arsenals, vehicles to deliver nuclear weapons would also be destroyed or converted to non-nuclear weapon uses, and production of weapons-usable fissile material would be prohibited.

Strengthening the Chemical Weapons Convention

The CWC is the strongest of the arms control treaties outlawing a single class of weapons. Inspection and verification of compliance with its provisions lies in the hands of the Organization for the Prohibition of Chemical Weapons (OPCW) in The Hague, established by the CWC (Lee et al. 2012). Controversies about safety and protection of the environment during the disposal of chemical weapons required by the CWC have delayed completion of the disposal, and large stockpiles still remain in a number of the world's nations that pose a continuing threat to health and to the environment.

Strengthening the Biological and Toxin Weapons Convention

Although the development, production, transfer, or use of biological weapons was prohibited by the 1975 Biological and Toxin Weapons Convention (BWC), several nations are believed to retain stockpiles of such weapons. The verification measures included in the BWC are weak and attempts to strengthen them have been unsuccessful. The United States has blocked attempts to strengthen the verification measures of the BWC, announcing that such measures might lead to exposure of US industrial or military secrets. All nations should support strengthening of the BWC and should refrain from secret activities, often termed *defensive* that may fuel a biological arms race.

Perhaps even more important, global public health capacity to deal with all infectious disease must be strengthened. Significant vulnerabilities to persistent global reservoirs of endemic illness in impoverished and underserved populations could lead to future pandemics. The best individual and collective efforts at diagnosing and treating disease outbreaks can be overwhelmed by any natural or intentionally induced epidemic. Consequently, support for strong global preventive public health capabilities provides the best ultimate defence against infectious disease threats.

Promoting the support of the Anti-Personnel Mine Ban Convention (the Ottawa Treaty)

As of late 2012, a total of 160 nations were parties to this 1997 convention. Thirty-six nations had neither signed nor ratified it, including China, India, Iran, Israel, Russia, and the United States. Resources are needed to clear the millions of landmines that are deployed.

Secondary prevention

The consequences of collective violence can also be prevented or diminished by secondary prevention if war occurs, by preventing deaths and injuries among military personnel and civilians, by preventing environmental destruction, and by seeking an end to the war. Secondary prevention methods include strengthening adherence to the Geneva Convention and other treaties that lessen the effects of war; reducing military activities, including preparation for war; and negotiating effective treaties to lessen environmental damage.

Tertiary prevention

Critical measures after an armed conflict include rehabilitating and reintegrating those living with disabilities due to the conflict; repairing the damage to the physical, social, cultural, and economic environments; and preventing further conflicts. Tertiary prevention methods include programmes for physical and social rehabilitation for individuals, groups, and communities; provision of appropriate aid to communities and nations damaged by collective violence, such as the Marshall Plan after the Second World War; environmental remediation; and the establishment of truth and reconciliation commissions, such as in South Africa after Apartheid.

The role of non-governmental organizations

Non-governmental organizations (NGOs) can be potentially important partners for public health workers in preventing and alleviating the consequences of collective violence. These *civil society organizations* focus on war from a medical and public health perspective by:

◆ Intervening to mitigate the consequences of armed conflict.

◆ Researching the effects of war.

◆ Educating the public and decision-makers about the impact of war on health and the environment.

◆ Advocating for changes in global attitudes and policies concerning war and for changes concerning the most dangerous weapons and practices of war (Loretz 2008).

Some NGOs provide direct humanitarian assistance to the victims of collective violence. These organizations generally participate in secondary and tertiary prevention, but some, such as the International Committee of the Red Cross, have also begun to play a role in primary prevention. Humanitarian assistance organizations may also play a role in primary prevention of violence. They may be strong advocates for civilian populations among whom they live and to whom they provide humanitarian assistance (Waldman 2008).

Acknowledgements

The authors acknowledge the helpful information on several subjects provided by Robert Gould, MD, which was included in the manuscript.

Text extracts from Krug E.G. et al. (ed.), 2002 *World Report on Violence and Health*, World Health Organization, Geneva, Switzerland, Copyright © 2002, reproduced with permission of the World Health Organization, available from http://www.who.int/violence_injury_prevention/violence/world_report/en/full_ en.pdf.

Text extract from *Demography*, Gender scripts and age at marriage in India, Volume 47, Issue 3, 2010, pp. 667–687, Copyright © Springer 2010, reproduced with kind permission from Springer Science+Business Media

References

Annan, K.A. (2000). *We The Peoples: The Role of the United Nations in the 21st Century*. New York: United Nations. Available at: http://www.un.org/en/events/pastevents/pdfs/We_The_Peoples.pdf.

Burmistrov D., Kossenko M., and Wilson R. (2006). *Radioactive Contamination of the Techa River and its Effects*. Cambridge, MA: Harvard University. Available from: http://phys4.harvard.edu/~wilson/publications/pp747/techa_cor.htm.

Carnegie Commission on Preventing Deadly Conflict (1998). *Preventing Deadly Conflict: Final Report*. New York: Carnegie Corporation of New York.

Centers for Disease Control and Prevention (2012). *Bioterrorism Agents/Diseases*. [Online] Centers for Disease Control and Prevention. Available at: http://www.bt.cdc.gov/agent/agentlist-category.asp.

Cole L.A. (1988). *Clouds of Secrecy: The Army's Germ Warfare Tests Over Populated Areas*. Totowa, NJ: Rowman & Littlefield.

Depleted Uranium Education Project (1997). *Metal of Dishonor: Depleted Uranium*. New York: International Action Center.

Harris, R. and Paxman, J. (1962). *A Higher Form of Killing: The Secret Story of Chemical and Biological Weapons*. New York: Hill and Wang.

Institute of Medicine and National Research Council (1999). *Exposure of the American People to Iodine-131 from Nevada Nuclear-Test: Review of the National Cancer Institute Report and Public Health Implications*. Washington, DC: National Academy Press.

International Campaign to Ban Landmines (n.d.). *Why The Ban*. [Online]. Available at: http://www.icbl.org.

Krug, E.G., Dahlberg, L.L., Mercy, J.A., Zwi, A.B., and Lozano, R. (eds.) (2002). *World Report on Violence and Health*. Geneva: World Health Organization. Available at: http://www.who.int/violence_injury_prevention/violence/world_report/en/full_en.pdf.

Lee, E.C., Bleek, P.C., and Kales, S.N. (2012). Chemical weapons. In B.S. Levy and V.W. Sidel (eds.) *Terrorism and Public Health: A Balanced Approach to Strengthening Systems and Protecting People* (2nd ed.), pp. 183–202. New York: Oxford University Press.

Levy, B.S. and Sidel, V.W. (2005). War. In H. Frumkin (ed.) *Environmental Health: From Local to Global*, pp. 269–87. New York: Jossey-Bass.

Levy B.S. and Sidel V.W. (eds.) (2008). *War and Public Health* (2nd ed.). New York: Oxford University Press.

Levy, B.S. and Sidel, V.W. (eds.) (2012). *Terrorism and Public Health: A Balanced Approach to Strengthening Systems and Protecting People* (2nd ed.). New York: Oxford University Press.

Levy, B.S. and Sidel, V.W. (2013a). Adverse health consequences of the Iraq War. *The Lancet*, 381, 949–58.

Levy, B.S. and Sidel V.W. (eds.) (2013b). *Social Injustice and Public Health* (2nd ed.). New York: Oxford University Press.

Loretz, J. (2008). The role of nongovernmental organizations. In B.S. Levy and V.W. Sidel (eds.) *War and Public Health* (2nd ed.), pp. 381–92. New York: Oxford University Press.

Meselson, M., Guillemin, J., Hugh-Jones, M., et al. (1994). The Sverdlovsk anthrax outbreak of 1979. *Science*, 266, 1202–8.

Rummel, R.J. (1994). *Death by Government: Genocide and Mass Murder Since 1900*. New Brunswick, NJ: Transaction Publications.

Shultz, G.P., Perry, W.J., Kissinger, H.A., et al. (2007). A world free of nuclear weapons. *Wall Street Journal*, 4 January, Sect. A:15.

Sirkin, S., Cobey, J.C., and Stover, E. (2008). Landmines. In B.S. Levy and V.W. Sidel (eds.) *War and Public Health* (2nd ed.), pp. 102–16. New York: Oxford University Press.

Smith, D. (2007). World at war. *The Defense Monitor*, 36(1), 1–9.

Stockholm International Peace Research Institute (2012). *SIPRI Yearbook 2012: Armaments, Disarmament, and International Security*. New York: Oxford University Press.

Sutton P.M. and Gould R.M. (2008). Nuclear weapons. In B.S. Levy and V.W. Sidel (eds.) *War and Public Health* (2nd ed.), pp. 152–76. New York: Oxford University Press.

United Nations (1945). *The Charter of the United Nations*. New York: United Nations. Available at: https://www.un.org/en/documents/charter/pre amble.shtml.

Waldman, R. (2008). The roles of humanitarian assistance. In B.S. Levy and V.W. Sidel (eds.) *War and Public Health*, (2nd ed.), pp. 369–80. New York: Oxford University Press.

Westing, A.H. (2008). The impact of war on the environment. In B.S. Levy and V.W. Sidel (eds.) *War and Public Health* (2nd ed.), pp. 69–84. New York: Oxford University Press.

World Health Assembly (1981). *Resolution WHA34.38*. Geneva: World Health Organization.

World Health Assembly (1996). *Resolution WHA49.25 on Prevention of Violence: A Public Health Priority*. Geneva: World Health Organization.

9.7

Urban health in low- and middle-income countries

Mark R. Montgomery

Introduction to urban health in low- and middle-income countries

Sometime in the next 30 years, if projections from the United Nations (UN) prove to be on the mark, the populations of poor countries will cross an historic threshold, becoming for the first time more urban than rural (United Nations 2012). In public health, as in other fields, the full implications of this urban transition are only beginning to be appreciated. Part of the difficulty is that the term 'urban' refers to a bewildering variety of environments. The health circumstances of small cities and towns differ in many ways from those of larger cities. Within any given city, some residents live in secure, gated communities having all the amenities of Europe or the United States, whereas others—especially those who live in slums—exist in grim Dickensian settings lacking the most basic of human needs in water supply, sanitation, and housing. The health systems of these cities are also astonishingly varied. An urban system will often present the full array of health providers, ranging from traditional healers, purveyors of drugs in street markets, ill-equipped pharmacists and chemists operating from ramshackle storefronts, and so on up the scale to the most highly-trained of surgeons. Among all urban providers, a high percentage are likely to be engaged in private practice, whether on a full-time or part-time basis, and for this reason urban healthcare is more monetized than rural care. In urban areas, unlike rural, it is not so much the distance to services that presents a barrier to their use, but rather the social, informational, and economic costs of access.

To be sure, the urban–rural contrast should not be overdrawn. Many residents of the developing world live on the peripheries of cities in locations that are arguably neither urban nor rural; circular migration and other social linkages have long connected the two sectors; and the multiplicity of contacts provides opportunities for communicable diseases to pass between them. Although urban health cannot be separated out and studied apart from rural, it may nevertheless be useful to consider the features of urban health environments and behaviour that have a distinctive quality. To draw out these distinctions with proper care and nuance would of course require a book-length treatment. Those seeking more comprehensive accounts of urban health than can be provided here, could refer to the recent US National Research Council report (Panel on Urban Population Dynamics 2003) and to Montgomery and Ezeh (2005a, 2005b) and especially Harpham (2007) and Mercado et al. (2007) for reviews.

To convey the scale of the urban health challenge that lies ahead, we provide in the first section of the chapter a sketch of the demographic forces that are reshaping the landscape of low- and middle-income countries (see 'The demographic context'). We then go on to summarize the urban health differentials that can be identified in data from internationally comparable sample surveys (see 'The urban burden of disease: overview'). Here we begin by documenting urban–rural differences and proceed to give closer attention to the within-urban inequalities in health. The next section draws out the salient features of the supply side of urban health, with particular emphasis on the money costs and quality of healthcare (see 'The urban health system'). In the final section of the chapter, we turn to a description of urban health risks that have not been sufficiently appreciated, or which, to be effectively addressed, would require an expansive conception of the role of the public health system (see 'Urban health risks and risk factors'). Extreme-weather events, such as the damaging storms that are expected to increase in severity as global warming proceeds, are a leading example of such risks.

The demographic context

The urban population of the developing world, estimated by the United Nations Population Division to have been 2.67 billion persons in the year 2011, is projected to increase to 3.92 billion by 2030 and further to 5.12 billion by 2050 (United Nations 2012). These additions to the cities and towns of poor countries will account for nearly 90 per cent of all world population growth over the period. By 2050, according to the projections, almost two-thirds of the inhabitants of poor countries will live in urban areas, with the number of large cities in these countries reaching historically unprecedented levels. As late as 1970 there were only two metropolitan areas in the world—the Tokyo and the New York–Newark agglomerations—with populations of 10 million or more. (Cities of this size are commonly called *mega-cities*.) By 2025, according to the UN forecasts, the low- and middle-income countries alone will contain 29 cities of this size. Even more striking is the number of cities in the 1–5 million range. In 1970 only 73 such cities were found in the developing world, whereas by 2025 the UN projects a total of no fewer than 454 cities in this range.

Forecasts such as these seem to have fostered the impression that most urban dwellers in poor countries live in huge urban agglomerations. This is simply not the case. As Fig. 9.7.1 shows,

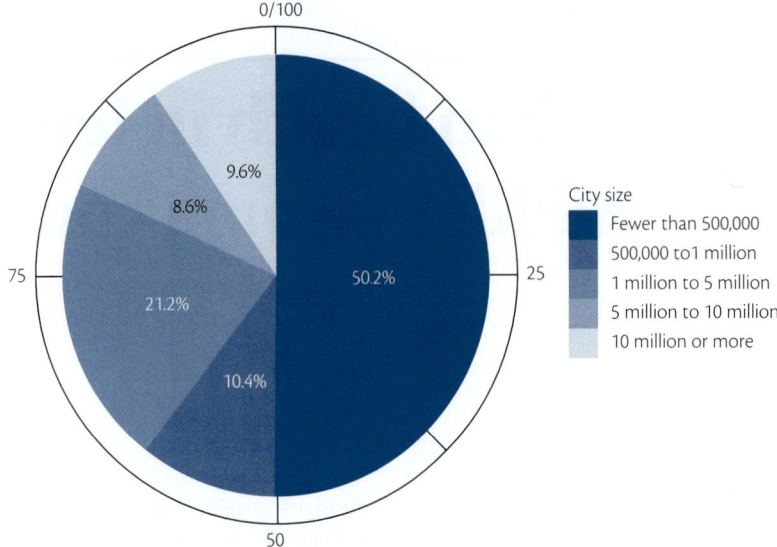

Fig. 9.7.1 Distribution of urban population by city size, low- and middle-income countries in 2011.
Source: data from United Nations, *World Urbanization Prospects, The 2011 Revision*, Department of Economic and Social Affairs, Population Division, United Nations, New York, USA, Copyright © 2012.

among all developing-country urbanites, only 9.6 per cent live in mega-cities. By contrast, over five times that number live in the small cities ranging up to a half-million in size. As the Panel on Urban Population Dynamics (2003) has argued, such smaller cities warrant much more attention than they have been given.

These cities are generally less well-provisioned than larger places with basic services such as improved sanitation and adequate supplies of drinking water. Rates of malnutrition and the risks of infant and child mortality can be little different in small cities from what is seen in the countryside. Yet the municipal governments of such cities seldom possess the range of health expertise and managerial talent that can be found in the governments of larger places. As low- and middle-income countries continue to decentralize their political and administrative systems, transferring more responsibilities for service delivery and revenue-raising from national governments and health ministries to the local tiers of government and the local ministry offices, the thinner resources and weaker capabilities of smaller cities will need careful attention (Panel on Urban Population Dynamics 2003). The preoccupation with the largest of developing-country cities in health policy discussions, and the general neglect of small cities, has left unaddressed a wide array of important health concerns.

The urban burden of disease: overview

Because very few low- and middle-income countries maintain reliable vital statistics systems, sample surveys provide much of what is known of urban health in these countries.[1] The two major ongoing survey programmes are the Demographic and Health Surveys (DHS), which has fielded and put into the public domain over 250 surveys since the mid 1980s, and the Multiple Indicator Cluster Surveys (MICS), for which some 100 surveys are now available.[2] The DHS and MICS surveys are nationally representative, and are designed to provide reliable estimates for the urban sector as a whole. However, the sample sizes are too small to yield reliable

health estimates at the level of individual cities. The DHS and MICS programmes have broad data-collection agendas in which health is only one among many areas of inquiry. This breadth is both a weakness and a strength: while limiting inquiry into specific conditions, it enables health measures to be linked to household economic and social variables, allowing some investigation of the social determinants of health (Marmot 2005; Marmot and Wilkinson 2005).

The survey programmes have focused mainly on women of reproductive age and their children. Men are not always interviewed, and even when they are, it is uncommon for a man to be sought out unless he is the partner of an interviewed woman of reproductive age. Nor are the elderly eligible to be interviewed. As a result, cross-national comparisons of the health of the urban elderly are not yet possible (but see Zimmer and Kwong 2004; Kaneda et al. 2005; Hu et al. 2007; Wong et al. 2006; World Health Organization (WHO) 2007a).

Table 9.7.1 summarizes the health data that are routinely gathered in the course of a DHS and MICS survey. This table presents only the core measures that are almost always collected; a number of surveys have been far more ambitious than the list in the table would suggest. Of course there are limits on what can be learned about health in a survey interview. When they are led through their reproductive histories by a skilled interviewer, women can supply reliable information on infant and child survival, but they are unlikely to give medically meaningful accounts of the causes of death. Adult mortality also presents difficulties for the DHS and MICS survey instruments, given that the women who are the primary respondents are generally no older than 50 years of age themselves. Ingenious attempts have been made to measure maternal mortality via the 'sisterhood' method (Graham et al. 1989), and the DHS and MICS surveys could, in theory, do more along these lines. Obviously, asymptomatic conditions cannot be identified in the course of an interview unless blood or tissue samples are collected or the interviewee undergoes a

Table 9.7.1 Health data routinely collected in the Demographic and Health Surveys and the Multiple Indicator Cluster Surveys

Demographic group	Health data	Gaps
Infants and children	Survival, approximate age at death; vaccination status; recent experience of fever, cough, diarrhoea; height and weight for age (in many surveys)	No reliable cause-of-death information; no detailed account of health-seeking behaviour
Adolescents and women of reproductive age	Knowledge of reproduction, contraception, HIV/AIDS, and sources of contraception and healthcare; detailed data on use of contraception; for recent births, nature and timing of prenatal care, place of delivery and attendance	Induced abortion and aftermath not studied; maternal mortality examined indirectly via 'sisterhood' methods; no exploration of asymptomatic health conditions unless biomarkers are collected
Sources of care	Knowledge of sources of contraception and healthcare; in some cases supplemented with an urban 'community questionnaire'	No systematic inventory of health providers; not obvious whether geographic boundaries effectively define urban accessible care

physical examination. (Collection of biomarker data is becoming more common in the DHS programme, but is not yet the norm.) Even reports on symptomatic morbidities and conditions may be clouded by local understandings of what constitutes disease. The measurement of health-seeking behaviour is also difficult to do well via general-purpose surveys. Although instruments can be designed to retrace the steps leading from problem recognition to treatment, relatively few such surveys of this type have been fielded.

Averages and inequalities

It is commonly believed that in modern-day populations, rural levels of health are worse than urban, and this belief is supported by good scientific evidence. In its analysis of 90 surveys from the DHS programme, the Panel on Urban Population Dynamics (2003) found that on average, the urban populations of poor countries exhibit lower levels of child mortality than rural populations, and similar urban–rural differences were evident across a range of health indicators. HIV/AIDS presents the large exception to the general rule of urban health advantage. As will be discussed later, although the epidemic is penetrating rural areas and may be driving up incidence rates there, prevalence continues to be higher in urban areas, often substantially so. Apart from HIV/AIDS, however, in most low- and middle-income countries the urban advantage in terms of average health levels is too well documented to dispute.

But averages can be a misleading basis upon which to set health priorities. Upon disaggregation, urban health averages can be shown to mask wide within-city differentials, and when these are examined, the urban poor are often discovered to face health risks that are nearly as bad as those of rural villagers and are sometimes decidedly worse. To see the urban situation clearly, two types of disaggregation are needed at a minimum: the urban poor must be distinguished from other urban residents; and among the poor, those living in communities of concentrated deprivation—slums, in the usual shorthand—need to be considered separately from the poor who live elsewhere (Montgomery and Hewett 2005). It is also important to distinguish cities from each other on the basis of their health institutions and personnel, and in terms of the strength of oversight and management that is exercised by municipal and other tiers of government.

The data needed to explore these distinctions are not always available. Demographic surveys will usually allow a country's urban poor to be studied as a group, but seldom provide reliable estimates of health among the poor in any given city, to say nothing of the subgroup of poor residents who live in a city's slums. Although there is good reason to expect deficiencies of health personnel and services in the smaller and less-advantaged cities, the empirical evidence on this point is still very thin. The comprehensive review provided by Dussault and Franceschini (2006) emphasizes urban–rural imbalances in health personnel, but does not differentiate among types of urban areas.

The urban poor

Intra-urban health inequalities—which are all too often overlooked by health and development agencies—are readily apparent in household survey data. Using the DHS surveys mentioned earlier, the Panel on Urban Population Dynamics (2003) estimated all-cause infant mortality for the urban poor, other urban households, and all rural households. The results are summarized in Table 9.7.2. As can be seen, the urban poor face significantly greater mortality risks than other urban residents, although as a rule, rural-dwellers face even higher levels of risk. In a

Table 9.7.2 Infant mortality estimates for urban poor, urban non-poor, and rural, by region (rates expressed per 1000 births).

DHS surveys (in region)	Rural	Urban poor	Urban non-poor
North Africa	81	60	43
Sub-Saharan Africa	103	89	74
South East Asia	59	53	27
South, Central, West Asia	74	69	49
Latin America	69	62	39
Total	86	75	56

Source: data from Panel on Urban Population Dynamics and Mark R. Montgomery et al. (eds.), *Cities Transformed: Demographic Change and Its Implications in the Developing World*, National Academies Press, Washington, DC, USA, Copyright © 2003.

Table 9.7.3 Height for age Z-scores among children 3–36 months of age, by residence and poverty status

DHS surveys (in region)	All rural	Urban poor	Urban non-poor
North Africa	−155.00	−122.35	−86.53
Sub-Saharan Africa	−184.60	−153.64	−125.86
South East Asia	−139.01	−106.46	−48.18
South, Central, West Asia	−176.78	−157.95	−120.31
Latin America	−157.09	−130.28	−80.61
Total	−173.51	−145.43	−109.37

Source: data from Panel on Urban Population Dynamics and Mark R. Montgomery et al. (eds.), *Cities Transformed: Demographic Change and Its Implications in the Developing World*, National Academies Press, Washington, DC, USA, Copyright © 2003.

survey-by-survey comparison of the poor urban and rural infants, this study found that the risks facing the urban poor were significantly lower in about two-thirds of the surveys. However, in 29 per cent of the surveys, poor urban infants faced significantly higher mortality risks than their rural counterparts. (In the remaining surveys, no significant difference existed between poor urban and rural infants.) Hence, even the generalization that urban infant mortality is lower than rural needs to be carefully qualified; much depends on whether the urban poor are separated out in the urban–rural comparisons.

The evidence available does not yet permit broad pronouncements to be made about the relative risks of the urban poor and rural-dwellers that apply irrespective of health measure. The National Research Council study analysed children's height for age—an indicator that summarizes a child's history of nutrition and disease—obtaining the results shown in Table 9.7.3 for children in the age range of 3–36 months. Table 9.7.3's entries are Z-scores, with a value of −100 indicating that a child is one standard deviation shorter, given its age and sex, than the median height of an international reference population. The urban poor are again seen to exhibit worse health than other urban children. When the heights of poor urban and rural children were compared, in almost all surveys (60 of the 67 examined) the poor urban children were found to be significantly taller for their age than were rural children. In the height-for-age measure, evidence of an urban advantage persists even for the urban poor.

As is well known, poor urban dwellers are exposed to substantial risks when their neighbourhoods lack the public health infrastructure needed to safeguard water supply and assure sanitary disposal of waste (UN-Habitat 2003a, 2003b). WHO (2002) estimates that in 2001, diarrhoeal diseases accounted for some 2 million deaths, almost all of which took place in low- and middle-income countries, with unsafe water, inadequate sanitation, and poor hygiene likely implicated in a large percentage of these. In its examination of data from the Demographic and Health Surveys, the Panel on Urban Population Dynamics (2003) demonstrated that urban poverty is associated with a lack of access to piped drinking water and with inadequate sanitation. Table 9.7.4 presents selected findings from this study, again comparing poor urban households with other urban and also rural households. As the table shows, the urban poor are markedly ill-served by comparison with other urban households. Rural households

receive even less than poor urban households by way of water and sanitation services, although they benefit to an extent from lower population densities, which offer a form of natural protection against some communicable diseases.

Investments in public health infrastructure require the mobilization of substantial funds, and although public health authorities can help publicize needs and exert pressure, the key decision-makers are generally located elsewhere in the political-bureaucratic system.[3] There are, however, complementary initiatives that lie squarely within the purview of public health. As McGranahan (2007) argues, citing Cairncross and Valdmanis (2006) among others, the literature on water and sanitation has tended to give too little attention to the hygienic and storage behaviours that cause water to be contaminated after it has been drawn from the pipes. Important faecal–oral routes for contamination can be addressed through domestic hygiene interventions, including an emphasis on hand washing especially after defecation, control of flies, and encouragement of safer practices in food preparation and water storage. Cairncross and Valdmanis (2006) assembled evidence showing that behavioural interventions in these areas can achieve substantial reductions in diarrhoeal diseases.

Other important health risks also arise in or near the homes of the poor, with the risks presented by indoor air pollution being increasingly recognized. Recent estimates suggest that worldwide, more than 2 billion people rely on solid fuels, traditional stoves, and open fires for their cooking, lighting, and heating needs (Larson and Rosen 2002). These fuels generate hazardous pollutants—including suspended particulate matter, carbon monoxide, nitrogen dioxide, and other harmful gases—that are believed to substantially raise the risks of acute respiratory infections and chronic obstructive pulmonary disorders. Such fuels are often used by the urban poor, who must cook in enclosed or inadequately ventilated spaces. The health burdens associated with indoor air pollution are likely to fall heavily upon women, who spend much of their time cooking and tending fires, and also afflict the children who accompany them.

The spatially concentrated urban poor

It is not surprising that when poor city-dwellers live in close proximity to each other without the benefit of safe drinking water and adequate sanitation, they face elevated risks from water-, air-, and food-borne diseases. This much has been known since the eighteenth century in the West, well before the mechanisms of disease transmission were understood (Woods 2003). It remains difficult, however, to divide the overall risks facing slum-dwellers into the risks attributable to household poverty, and the additional risks produced by the spatial concentration of poverty in slum neighbourhoods and communities.

Although not definitive on this score, Fig. 9.7.2 is suggestive of the impact of concentrated poverty on child mortality in Nairobi, Kenya. In the slums of Nairobi, child mortality rates, at 150 per thousand births, are substantially above the rates seen elsewhere in that city; slum mortality rates are high enough even to exceed rural Kenyan mortality. The magnification of risk evident in the Nairobi slums may be due to multiple factors: the poor quality and quantity of water and sanitation in these communities; inadequate hygienic practices; poor ventilation and dependence on hazardous cooking fuels; the city's highly monetized health system, which

Table 9.7.4 Percentages of poor urban households with access to services, compared with rural households and the urban non-poor

DHS countries (in region)		Piped water on premises	Water in neighbourhood	Flush toilet	Pit toilet
North Africa	Rural	41.6	37.3	41.3	17.5
	Urban poor	67.3	27.8	83.7	8.5
	Urban non-poor	90.8	7.8	96.3	2.6
Sub-Saharan Africa	Rural	7.8	55.7	1.1	47.6
	Urban poor	26.9	61.6	13.0	65.9
	Urban non-poor	47.6	45.8	27.4	67.2
South East Asia	Rural	18.6	53.7	55.5	24.3
	Urban poor	34.0	53.7	61.8	22.9
	Urban non-poor	55.8	40.1	89.0	9.4
South, Central, West Asia	Rural	28.1	53.6	4.3	55.4
	Urban poor	58.0	36.3	39.8	34.1
	Urban non-poor	80.2	17.7	64.0	23.2
Latin America	Rural	31.4	36.4	12.6	44.0
	Urban poor	58.7	35.2	33.6	47.0
	Urban non-poor	72.7	24.9	63.7	31.6
Total	Rural	18.5	50.7	7.5	46.6
	Urban poor	41.5	49.4	28.3	51.7
	Urban non-poor	61.5	34.0	48.4	46.5

Source: data from Panel on Urban Population Dynamics and Mark R. Montgomery et al. (eds.), *Cities Transformed: Demographic Change and Its Implications in the Developing World*, National Academies Press, Washington, DC, USA, Copyright © 2003.

for the poor delays or prevents access to Nairobi's modern health services; and the transmission of disease among densely settled slum-dwellers.

There are additional factors of a social epidemiological character that are worth considering. Facing health threats from their unprotected physical environments—with the lack of services being a constant reminder of social exclusion—and lacking the incomes needed to counteract these daily threats, the urban poor may well feel unable to take effective action to safeguard their health. Poor individuals and families may thus lack the sense of

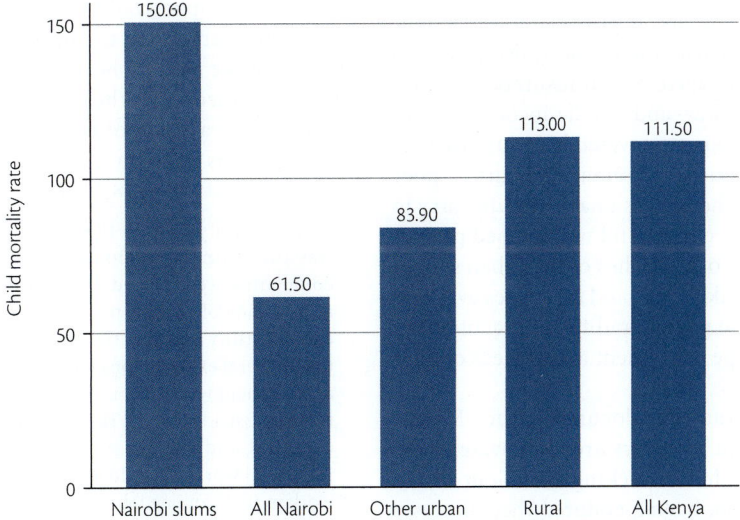

Fig. 9.7.2 Comparison of child mortality rates ($_5q_0$) in the Nairobi slums sample with rates for Nairobi, other cities, rural areas, and Kenya as a whole.

Source: data from African Population and Health Research Center, *Population and Health Dynamics in Nairobi's Informal Settlements: Report of the Nairobi Cross-Sectional Slums Survey (NCSS) 2000*, African Population and Health Research Center, Nairobi, Copyright © 2002.

self-efficacy needed to energize their health-seeking behaviour in such difficult environments. Poor communities may be reminded by the absence of basic services that the community as a whole is socially excluded and lacks the political voice needed to bring attention to its plight. At the individual and family level, as we will discuss, social exclusion combined with the daily stresses of poverty may bring on paralyzing fatigue, anxiety, low-level depression, and other expressions of mental ill health. At the community level, the symptoms may be expressed in the weaknesses and fragilities of local community organizations, that is, in the lack of what has been termed 'bonding' social capital.

The urban health system

The concept of 'health system' is a very broad one and bringing definition to it is especially difficult in urban areas, within which a disparate set of health providers serves what is typically a highly diverse population, with core health needs arising in part from the many ways in which the population's subgroups come into contact. The urban health system is itself situated within larger political-economic frames at the country level. In the structural adjustment era of the 1980s and early 1990s, a number of low- and middle-income countries introduced user fees into public-sector care as they undertook broad health sector reforms (Harpham 2007). As discussed earlier, in many of these countries the process of decentralization—a transformation of governance that accelerated in the mid 1990s, and which is in its way as profound as the urban transformation—is reshaping relationships between national, regional, and local governments, with important implications for health service planning, finance, and service delivery. These developments provide the context for our discussion of urban health systems.

A distinguishing feature of urban health systems is the prominence of the private sector. Not surprisingly given the higher average levels of income in urban populations and the income diversity that establishes market niches, private services tend to be much more developed in cities than in rural areas, especially in the larger cities (Dussault and Franceschini 2006). Fee-for-service arrangements are generally characteristic of urban healthcare, whereas rural services are often ostensibly provided free of money cost (or made available for nominal fees) at public health-posts and clinics. Even in Latin America, where health insurance systems are more inclusive than in other low- and middle-income regions, only 20 per cent of the urban poor are covered by insurance (Fay 2005). In the more monetized urban economy, the urban poor without cash on hand can find themselves unable to gain entry to the modern system of hospitals, clinics, and well-trained providers. They may then seek care in other niches of the urban system where less-trained providers make drugs and diagnoses available for affordable fees, and may also pursue traditional practitioners, who can adjust the level and type of payment to the needs of their poor clients.

As the Islam et al. (2006) study has documented for Manila and Indore, India, urban health providers are well aware of the effects of monetization on the health-seeking behaviour of the poor. They see poor clients who, having endured their illnesses until care cannot be put off any longer, finally present themselves in a more debilitated condition than they would otherwise have been. Health providers realize that the poor are likely to abandon

courses of prescribed medication to save on the costs of purchasing medicines, or may economize by buying less than what was prescribed. They are not really surprised when the poor fail to return as requested for follow-ups and assessments of progress.

In very few low- and middle-income countries is it possible for the urban poor to receive subsidized care from for-profit private providers, and generally such subsidies are available only through the private non-profit and public-sector clinics and hospitals. Manila's public-sector subsidy programme provides one instructive example. In this health system, subsidies are made available for the purchase of medicines but supplies are not similarly covered. As one physician said in exasperation,

> Sometimes, they say they can ask for discounts or even for free medicines, depending on the [income] class. But in supplies, they cannot. So for instance, they get antibiotics for free [but] if you do not have syringe, how can you provide it? We still ask them to buy syringe to provide for the vaccines. (Islam et al. 2006, p. 52)

As this quotation suggests, stock-outs of medicines and basic supplies such as syringes occur frequently in Manila's public-sector facilities. When they occur, it is left to the patient to find the funds to seek out prescribed medicines and supplies at private pharmacies or other sources. In the Manila case, the lowest tier of the public health system—the *barangay* health centre—is a vital component of the system for the poor, because for various reasons the *barangay* centres are more likely to hold small stocks of some of the subsidized medicines.

As the Manila example illustrates, subsidies for the urban poor often depend on an unsystematic set of arrangements, requiring poor patients and their families to spend time searching and negotiating with what must be a bewildering variety of personnel at scattered locations. As they engage in this form of health-seeking behaviour, the poor can be discouraged by the difficulties of finding affordable transport, inconvenient hours of operation at clinics or health centres, the frequent absence of key staff, and long waits to receive care. In effect, the poor are being asked to invest their own time in the hope of securing reduced money costs of medicines. In a full-cost sense, a subsidy for the poor that exists in theory may prove to be no subsidy at all.

We have emphasized the money costs of healthcare, which clearly discourage the urban poor, but they can also be driven away from the modern health system by the indifference or abuse that they anticipate at the hands of formal sector health workers. For example, a study of urban Zimbabwe described the nature of interactions between nurses and women from the community (Bassett et al. 1997, p. 185) thus:

> To community women, the expectation of abrupt or rude treatment was the main complaint about the health services. Community complaints were voiced most strongly in the urban areas, where accusations of patient neglect and even abuse suggested a heightened hostility between the clinic and community in the urban setting. Several explanations for nurse behavior were put forward, chief among them was elitism. . . it is in urban areas that class differentiation is most advanced. [The perspective of nurses differed. For them] overwork and low pay promote the adoption of the attitude of an industrial worker—to do what is required and no more. Most nurses work more than one job, not to get rich but to survive.

As this quotation suggests, much of the literature emphasizes the social distance between providers and their patients, the formal language that providers can use to reinforce their own status, and the possibilities for rude or abusive behaviour on the part of staff towards poor patients. But the literature has not much stressed how difficult it is, even for the most well-intentioned and diplomatic health provider, to get basic information across to poor, illiterate, and possibly intimidated patients. As a Manila obstetrician-gynaecologist explained (Islam et al. 2006, p. 54):

I guess for 90% of our patients, it is us who tell them things. Although there are some who are really inquisitive especially those who have had some education. [But among the urban poor?] They just accept everything we tell them. They rarely ask questions. And sometimes it is difficult to relate to them. They have a hard time understanding what we are saying, even if we use the most basic words or terms. Like for instance, sometimes, we tell them, this is the right way to take the medicine, to make sure that they understand us, we ask them to demonstrate. [Are they receptive to that?] Some, yes. But the others just don't care. They don't know anything, they don't even know when was their last period, family history, nothing. It's really frustrating.

When the poor do succeed in receiving formal healthcare, is that care likely to be of sufficient quality to make an effective difference to their health? An urban quality-of- care study in New Delhi raises serious doubts on this score (Das and Hammer 2007a, 2007b). The study was set in both slum and non-slum neighbourhoods, covering a range of income levels. A full inventory was made of the health providers who serve these neighbourhoods; it revealed that a 15-minute walk would bring a typical neighbourhood resident within reach of 70 health providers of some sort. Even for the poor, access in the sense of geographic distance was not the problem in this case; and if anything, the Delhi poor tended to seek care for illness at least as often as the non-poor. The study assessed the quality of healthcare provision in two ways: via a series of vignettes measuring provider knowledge of the steps to take in making a diagnosis and prescribing treatment or referral (rating the provider responses in relation to examination protocols); and by a follow-up in which many of the same providers were observed as they interacted with patients.

The study found that the quality of care available in the poor neighbourhoods was so low that the authors could fairly describe it as 'money for nothing'. Both public-sector and private providers serve the poor neighbourhoods of Delhi, and both know less about appropriate care than the providers who practise in better-off neighbourhoods. (Levels of health provider knowledge were low across all study neighbourhoods, but were especially low in the poor neighbourhoods.) Evidently, the Indian public sector does not see to it that its more competent providers are allocated to the poor neighbourhoods where they are needed most. When later observed as they interacted with patients, healthcare providers generally asked even fewer questions and exerted even less effort in examinations than their vignettes had suggested they would. In short, it would seem that even strenuous health-seeking efforts on the part of the New Delhi poor would bring them no assurance of reasonable quality healthcare.

Mayank et al. (2001), who studied poor urban women in Dakshinpuri, another New Delhi slum, found that local antenatal clinics did little to provide pregnant women with information about the risks of pregnancy and childbirth. A number of pregnant women suffered from potentially serious ailments—over two-thirds were clinically diagnosed as anaemic, and 12 per cent were found to be seriously anaemic. Yet relatively few understood

that high fevers and swelling of the face, hands, or feet might be symptoms of conditions that could endanger their pregnancy. Fewer than 10 per cent of women attending the local clinic were given any advice about the danger signs of pregnancy. Perhaps it is not altogether surprising that the maternal mortality rate in this urban sample was estimated at 645 deaths per 100,000, a rate not much different from that prevailing in rural India.

Fig. 9.7.3 shows that low quality of care is generally characteristic of urban India (Fig. 9.7A) and is also a concern in the urban areas of the Philippines (Fig. 9.7B). The figure depicts the percentage of women who, in one or more prenatal care visits, were warned of the complications of pregnancy. Among poor urban Indian women, not even 40 per cent are told during prenatal visits of the danger signs of pregnancy. Although the percentages are somewhat higher in the urban Philippines, less than half of poor

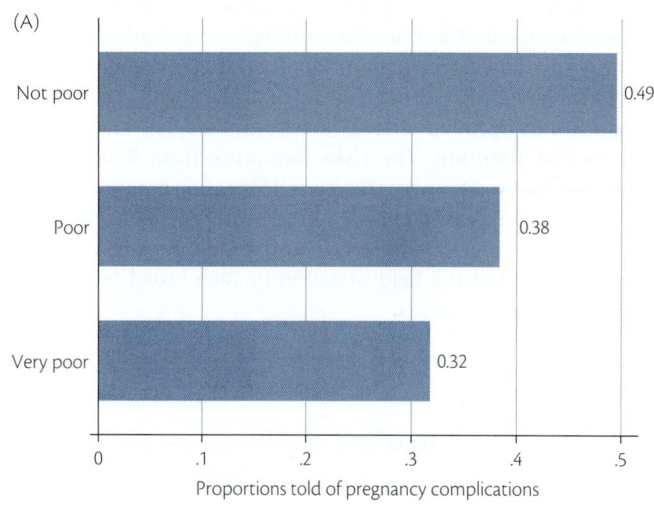

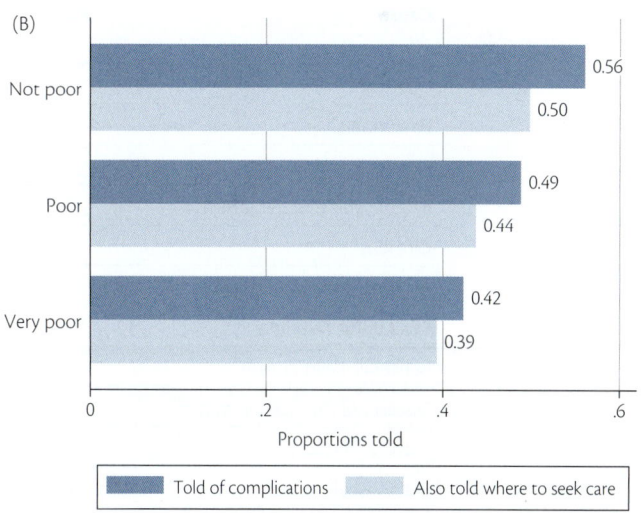

Fig. 9.7.3 Information on pregnancy complications given during prenatal care, by relative poverty. Women with one or more visits, urban India and urban Philippines. (A) Women informed of complications and their danger signs during pregnancy, urban India. (B) Women informed of complications and danger signs during pregnancy, and told where to seek care if these appear, urban Philippines. Reproduced from Islam, M., Montgomery, M.R., and Taneja, S., *Urban Health and Care-Seeking Behavior: A Case Study of Slums in India and the Philippines*, PHRPlus Program, Abt Associates, Bethesda, MD, USA, 2006.

women are informed of the risks and fewer still are told where to seek care if signs of danger surface.

Urban health risks and risk factors

In this section we turn attention to specific urban risks and causes of mortality and morbidity. Several themes unite this material. First among them is the importance of disaggregation of urban health conditions and risk factors by poverty and place. A second and closely-related theme is that of urban social epidemiology, with emphasis on the concepts of individual and collective efficacy in health-seeking. A third theme in the discussion concerns health conditions or risks that are sometimes overlooked, or which are not as well integrated as they might be in urban public health policies. Mental health is perhaps the leading example of such a condition. It is closely associated with poverty and with the health threats that arise from violence and alcohol abuse, which place disproportionate burdens on women. Other examples include the burdens of illness and death stemming from road traffic accidents and outdoor air pollution. In many countries HIV/AIDS already occupies a prominent place on the urban health agenda, whereas urban tuberculosis and malaria receive less attention. The risks stemming from flooding and other extreme-weather events also call for action across a range of actors in government and civil society. Only the most expansive public health programmes in low- and middle-income countries have conceived of the field of action in such broad terms as to encompass all these areas.

To bring some order to a wide-ranging discussion, we begin with an overview of urban causes of death and disability, drawing upon data from Mexico, one of the few low- and middle-income countries that can provide reliable information. With this as background, we then present a series of remarks on the specific features of urban health that warrant closer study.

The urban burden of disease

Table 9.7.5 shows the 15 leading causes of disability-adjusted life years (DALYs) lost in rural and urban areas for Mexico. Several lessons can be extracted from this table. First, urban areas do not necessarily present health profiles that are wholly distinct from those of rural areas. In Mexico, the causes of DALYs lost are much the same in urban and rural areas, although they follow a different rank order. Of the top five causes in Mexico's urban areas, three (deaths related to motor vehicles, homicide and violence, and cirrhosis) are also found among the top five in rural areas. Second, interventions to address two of the most important causes of death and disability in urban Mexico—traffic-related deaths and injuries—would in many countries be considered outside the scope of the public health system. Third, the table reminds us that even in a middle-income country such as Mexico, diarrhoeal disease and pneumonia continue to be important causes of urban death and disability—here as elsewhere, an epidemiological transition is underway whereby the burden of disease is tilting towards non-communicable causes, but this transition is evidently far from being complete.

Table 9.7.5 Disability-adjusted years of life lost in Mexico by cause and residence (1991 estimates, expressed per 1000 population)

Cause	Rural	Rural rank	Urban	Urban rank	Rural/ urban
Diarrhoea	12.0	1	2.8	9	4.28
Pneumonia	9.3	2	3.9	7	2.39
Homicide and violence	9.2	3	7.4	2	1.23
Motor vehicle-related deaths	7.9	4	8.3	1	0.95
Cirrhosis	7.5	5	6.3	4	1.19
Anaemia and malnutrition	6.8	6	2.4	11	2.86
Road traffic accidents	5.5	7	6.8	3	0.81
Ischaemic heart disease	5.1	8	5.3	6	0.96
Diseases of the digestive system	4.7	9	1.7	15	2.74
Diabetes mellitus	4.1	10	5.7	5	0.72
Brain vascular disease	3.0	11	3.0	8	1.02
Alcoholic dependence	3.0	11	1.9	13	1.56
Accidents (falls)	2.8	13	2.6	10	1.09
Chronic lung disease	2.6	14	1.9	13	1.39
Nephritis	2.2	15	2.2	12	1.01

Source: data from Lozano, R. et al., El peso de las enfermedades en Mexico, in K. Hill et al. (eds.), *Las Consecuencias de las Transiciones Demografica y Epidemiological en Ame´rica Latina*, El Colegio de Mexico, Mexico City, Mexico, Copyright © 1999.

Mental health

Mental health as such does not appear in Table 9.7.5, but it is arguably a central factor in the health of the urban poor, and one whose contribution to the urban burden of disease has been under-appreciated. Over the past decade, the WHO has issued a series of reports emphasizing the importance of mental health in developing as well as developed countries (WHO 1996, 2001, 2005a). In a recent review, Prince et al. (2007, table 1) summarized the WHO burden-of-disease estimates for mental health in low-income and middle-income countries. In these countries, mental ill health accounts for roughly 24 per cent of all DALYs lost to non-communicable diseases. For reasons to be described shortly, this figure is likely to understate the full impacts of mental health. Yet, as the authors noted, 'Despite these new insights, ten years after the first WHO report on the global burden of disease, mental health remains a low priority in most low-income and middle-income countries' (Prince et al. 2007, p. 860).

Community-based studies of mental health in low- and middle-income countries suggest that 12–51 per cent of urban adults suffer from some form of depression (see 16 studies reviewed by Blue (1999)). Anxiety and depression are typically found to be more prevalent among urban women than men and are believed to be more prevalent in poor than in non-poor urban neighbourhoods (Almeida-Filho et al. 2004). In a study of Mumbai, Parkar et al. (2003) give an evocative account of the stresses that affect men and women in a slum community just north of the city. Men in this community are deeply frustrated by the lack of work, and this is reflected in a high incidence of alcoholism and violence directed at their wives. Although less is known about mental health among adolescents in low- and middle-income countries, recent studies indicate that this age group also warrants attention. Harpham et al. (2004) made use of the WHO's short-form, self-reporting questionnaire—a bank of 20 items designed to detect depression and anxiety—to study the mental health of adolescents in Cali, Columbia. Girls were found to be three times more likely than boys to exhibit signs of ill health (as Prince et al. (2007) note, among adults the female–male ratio is typically 1.5–2.0) and further multivariate analysis showed that low levels of schooling, within-family violence, and perceptions that violence afflicts the community were all significantly associated with mental ill health among adolescents.

There are two avenues by which an individual's mental ill health might affect other dimensions of health. First, it has been hypothesized that socioeconomic stress undermines the physiological systems that sustain health. Prince et al. (2007, panel 2) emphasized the effects of depression on serotonin metabolism, cortisol metabolism, inflammatory processes, and cell-mediated immunity; they also note that mental disorders are implicated in a range of behaviours (e.g. smoking, poor diet, obesity) that raise the risks of other diseases. Boardman (2004), McEwen (1998), Steptoe and Marmot (2002), and Cohen et al. (2006) provide supportive evidence, although Hu et al. (2007) were sceptical of the hypothesized link from poverty to socioeconomic stress to cortisol metabolism, finding little evidence for it in their large sample of Taiwanese elderly. The possibility of such adverse spill-over effects from an individual's mental ill health to other areas of health, and the need for a full accounting of these effects in calculating the disease burden stemming from

mental disorders, is the principal theme of the comprehensive review by Prince et al. (2007).

The second avenue needing exploration also involves spill-over effects, but in this case the posited linkage would connect women's mental health to the health-seeking energies they can deploy on behalf of their children and other family members. To judge from the review by Prince et al. (2007, p. 867), very little research has been conducted on how mental health affects women's health-seeking behaviour. A few studies have linked mental ill health to the difficulties that individuals face in adhering to their own treatment regimens, especially the demanding protocols required in antiretroviral therapies for HIV/AIDS and directly-observed treatments, short-course (DOTS) for tuberculosis. A bit more attention has been given to the associations between a woman's mental health and her reproductive health, and between the health status of pregnant women and their children's birth weights, with the latter possibly involving health-seeking behaviour. But almost nothing seems to have been written on whether and how mental ill health undermines the sense of self-efficacy that motivates a woman to seek healthcare for others in her family. This is a surprising gap in the literature, especially in view of the well-documented role that women play in protecting the health of their families and the equally common finding that mental ill health is more common among women than men.[4]

Intimate partner violence and alcohol abuse

Violence in urban areas takes a variety of forms, ranging from political and extra-judicial violence to gang violence, local violent crime, and abuse taking place within the home. Moser (2004, tables 1 and 2) developed a framework within which these complex forms of violence can be analysed and described the points of intervention within the judicial, public health, and other urban systems (also see Winton 2004). Garrett and Ahmed (2004) have developed a module for measuring aspects of crime, violence, and physical insecurity that could be adapted for use in surveys, so that these problems can be better documented than they are at present. Our discussion will mainly be concerned with intimate partner violence and its links to alcohol abuse and women's mental health. Heise et al. (1994) reviewed community-based data for eight urban areas from different regions of the developing world, finding that mental and physical abuse of women by their partners was common, with damaging consequences for women's physical and psychological well-being. Using data collected from a module included in several DHSs, Kishor and Johnson (2004) examined whether women had ever been beaten by a spouse or partner. In Cambodia, 18 per cent of women had been beaten, and the percentages in the other study countries were also high: Columbia (44 per cent), Dominican Republic (22 per cent), Egypt (34 per cent), Haiti (29 per cent), India (19 per cent), Nicaragua (30 per cent), Peru (42 per cent), and Zambia (48 per cent). In seeking to understand why women who were the victims of violence did not seek help from the authorities or others outside the home, this study found that embarrassment was a major reason given by women, as well as the belief that it would be futile to seek care or that partner violence was simply a part of life. In some countries (but not in all), poor women were more likely than other women to have experienced violence at the hands of their spouses or partners. Where the connection could be explored, strong links were also found between spousal alcohol abuse and violence.

These findings were echoed in the WHO (2005b) study summarized in Fig. 9.7.4, which covered both urban and rural study sites. The WHO analysis also documented a close association between the experience of violence and women's mental health. Among the women in this study's Bangladeshi urban site who had been abused by their partner, some 21 per cent had had thoughts of suicide, as against only 7 per cent of women who had not been abused. In all but one of the sites in the study (Brazil, Namibia, Peru, Tanzania, and Thailand), the difference in this measure of mental health was statistically significant, and the ratios are on the order of 2:1 or higher.

Other forms of urban violence also merit attention. Crime is particularly prevalent in Latin America's large cities, where it disproportionately victimizes men living in low-income neighbourhoods (Barata et al. 1998; Grant 1999; Heinemann and Verner 2006). Data collected between 1991 and 1993 in São Paulo suggested that men aged 15–24 in low-income areas were over five times likelier to fall victim to homicide than were men of the same age in higher-income areas (Soares et al., cited in Grant 1999). South African cities also exhibit extraordinarily high rates of violent crime (Stone 2006).

A need exists for systems that can provide women and the poor with some protection from the varied forms of urban violence to which they are vulnerable within and outside the home. To create such systems will require new partnerships linking agencies across urban sectors. In the transport sector, for example, there is a need to make safe the areas where the poor wait for buses and jeepneys; the health sector also has a role to play in security, in that public latrines can be places of risk especially for women; and the authorities responsible for electrification and road construction need to attend to the unlit paths and lanes within slums, a concern for the poor who must commute in the early morning hours or late at night. Effective partnerships against crime and violence involve the formulation of community-driven violence-prevention strategies and the initiation of dialogue between community groups

and the police. (The police may initially resist efforts to involve them in this way, complaining of having to be 'social workers' as well as policemen.) Creation of safe spaces is especially high on the policy agenda for adolescent girls and boys (Erulkar and Matheka 2007).

Reproductive health

The Panel on Urban Population Dynamics (2003) provides a lengthy discussion of reproductive health among urban women, and here we select only a few points for emphasis. Among all urban women, those who are poor are significantly less likely to use modern contraception to achieve control over their family-building (see Table 9.7.6). They are generally more likely to use contraception than rural women, but in some regions of the developing world there is little to separate the two groups. The unmet need for modern contraception—this is measured by the proportion of women in a reproductive union who say that they want to prevent or delay their next birth, believe themselves to be capable of conceiving, and yet do not make use of modern contraception to achieve their stated aims—is markedly higher among poor urban than other urban women.

As the Panel on Urban Population Dynamics (2003) discusses, it is not clear that even when they use modern contraception to prevent conception, urban women do so in an effective manner. Although quantitative estimates are limited to selected case studies, unintended pregnancy and induced abortion are evidently not uncommon for urban women.[5] To cite a few examples: women in three squatter settlements in Karachi, Pakistan, were estimated to have a lifetime rate of 3.6 abortions per woman (Jamil and Fikree 2002). Another study found abortion to be widespread in Abidjan, Côte d'Ivoire, where abortion is illegal yet nearly one-third of the women surveyed who had ever been pregnant had had one (Desgrées du Loû et al. 2000). A recent study of Ouagadougou, Burkina Faso by Rossier (2007) estimated an annual abortion rate of 4 per cent among women aged 15–49 years, suggesting that over a reproductive lifetime, a woman would have 1.4 abortions on average. Calvés (2002) studied women in their 20s living in

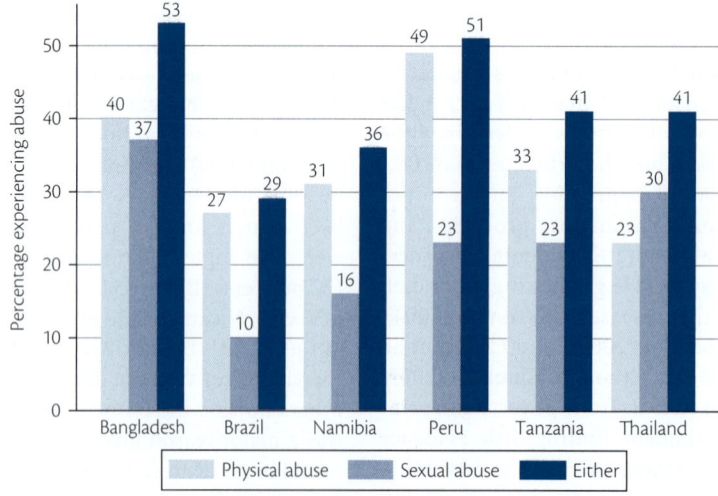

Fig. 9.7.4 Experience of physical or sexual violence by an intimate partner since age 15, among ever-partnered urban women.
Reproduced with permission from World Health Organization, *WHO Multi-Country Study on Women's Health and Domestic Violence Against Women: Summary Report of Initial Results on Prevalence, Health Outcomes and Women's Responses,* Copyright © World Health Organization 2005, available from http://www.who.int/gender/violence/who_multicountry_study/en.

Table 9.7.6 Contraceptive use for women aged 25–29 by residence and, for urban areas, poverty status

DHS surveys in region	All rural	Urban poor	Urban non-poor
North Africa	0.26	0.37	0.48
Sub-Saharan Africa	0.08	0.13	0.22
South East Asia	0.44	0.40	0.47
South, Central, West Asia	0.33	0.35	0.44
Latin America	0.32	0.37	0.47
Total	0.22	0.26	0.35

Source: data from Panel on Urban Population Dynamics and Mark R. Montgomery et al. (eds.), *Cities Transformed: Demographic Change and Its Implications in the Developing World*, National Academies Press, Washington, DC, USA, Copyright © 2003.

Yaoundé, Cameroon. Of these young women, 21 per cent reported having had an abortion; just over 8 per cent had had more than one. Once again, the fact that modern contraceptive services are available in urban areas does not imply that women, especially poor women, have the knowledge and the social and economic wherewithal to make effective use of the methods.

Maternal mortality risks offer another revealing view of urban reproductive health. Because it is difficult to predict whether life-threatening problems will emerge in the course of a woman's pregnancy, delivery, and the aftermath, the prevention of maternal mortality depends crucially on fast access to emergency care. It might be thought that cities, which offer many more transport options than do rural areas, would exhibit much lower levels of maternal mortality. The cases in which the expected urban advantage does not emerge are therefore instructive about the circumstances of the urban poor. Fikree et al. (1997) compared maternal mortality rates in the low-income communities of Karachi with rates in six rural districts elsewhere in Pakistan. While the estimate of maternal mortality ratios for Karachi was the lowest among all these sites, the rural estimates are significantly higher than Karachi's only for the remote districts of Loralai and Khuzdar. It appears that Karachi's poor suffer from maternal health disadvantages not unlike those that afflict Pakistan's rural dwellers.

Why did the urban health advantage not prove greater in this case? In the poor communities of Karachi, some 68 per cent of births are delivered at home and 59 per cent are attended by traditional birth attendants (TBAs). Yet rural women are even more likely to deliver at home and to have family members or TBAs in attendance. Another study of Karachi slums (Fikree et al. 1994) identified the core of the problem: when acute pregnancy and delivery complications arise in these communities, there can be critical delays in locating male decision-makers and obtaining their consent to hospital care. (It has not been customary for husbands or other men to be present at the time of childbirth.) Delays in initiating the search for care are compounded by the tendency for poor Karachi families to pursue local care first, going from place to place in the neighbourhood before making an effort to reach the modern health facilities located outside the neighbourhood. Fikree et al. (2004) has illustrated similar care-seeking patterns in a study of postpartum morbidities in the Karachi slums.

HIV/AIDS

An enormous literature is now available on the social epidemiology of HIV/AIDS in both developing and developed countries. Despite the quantities of research underway on HIV/AIDS, much remains to be learned about its social components. Indeed, although HIV/AIDS is commonly thought to be more prevalent in urban than rural areas, until recently the scientific basis for this belief has been thin (UNAIDS 2004, p. 31). In only a few low- and middle-income countries are community-based studies of prevalence now available that can quantify the urban–rural differences.[6] For example, findings from several nationally representative community-based studies in which prevalence is estimated from blood samples taken in connection with a DHS survey, show that for Mali, Kenya, and Zambia, urban prevalence rates are clearly much higher than rural rates. The estimated percentage with HIV in urban and rural areas in Mali was 2.20 and 1.50 respectively; for Kenya 10.00 and 5.60 respectively; and for Zambia 23.10 and 10.80 respectively.[7] Where HIV/AIDS is concerned, there is little evidence of the 'urban advantage' that is seen in other domains of health. However, circular and urban-to-rural migration is contributing to the spread of disease in rural areas (UNAIDS 2004, p. 33), and many observers foresee an era of rising rural incidence and prevalence.

Because the community-based studies are relatively recent, the role played by urban poverty in the risks of HIV/AIDS in low- and middle-income countries is only beginning to be studied. Using the community surveys conducted under the DHS programme, Mishra et al. (2007) found that contrary to expectation, HIV prevalence is higher among the better-off families. These families were more likely to live in urban areas, which accounts for a part of the association, and other risk factors (including sexual risk-taking, use of condoms, and male circumcision) tended to mask the association between living standards and prevalence. Even with statistical controls for such factors in place, a positive association between living standards and HIV prevalence persisted. In studies of urban adolescents and other selected socioeconomic groups, however, poverty has been linked to higher HIV prevalence as well as to a number of contributing risk factors, including earlier sexual initiation and more reported forced or traded sex, which would seem to place poor women at higher risk of contracting the virus (Hallman 2004). In short, the association with living standards is still a matter of dispute.

Tuberculosis

Tuberculosis is even today among the leading causes of death for adults in low- and middle-income countries, killing an estimated 1.6 million people worldwide in 2005 (WHO 2007b). Much as in the nineteenth century, urban crowding increases the risk of contracting tuberculosis (van Rie et al. 1999), and high-density, low-income urban communities may face elevated levels of risk. The interactions between HIV/AIDS and tuberculosis, and the spread of multidrug-resistant strains of the disease, have generated fears of a global resurgence of tuberculosis and have caused WHO to expand its programme beyond DOTS as such.

The concept of urban collective efficacy is directly relevant to the DOTS strategy, the core of WHO's treatment strategy. In a study of tuberculosis in urban Ethiopia, Sagbakken et al. (2003) showed how the local social resources of urban communities (organized in 'TB clubs') can be marshalled to reduce the stigma associated with the disease and encourage patients to adhere to the demanding short-course regimen of treatment. Similar interventions have been fielded in urban India, as described by Barua and Singh (2003), using community health volunteers to identify local residents with symptoms of tuberculosis and referring them to hospitals for diagnosis; local health workers attached to the hospitals then provide follow-up care and lend support during treatment. An elaborate system of care, involving multiple urban community and health service associations in Lima, Peru, is described by Shin et al. (2004). As reported by the WHO (2007b, p. 78), Bangladesh has made urban DOTS a focus in a programme that links non-governmental organizations (NGOs), private practitioners, medical colleges, and the corporate sector. As the country profiles presented in WHO (2007b) make clear, a number of countries have yet to reach WHO's treatment success rate target of 85 per cent of identified patients, and although data are scarce, it is very likely that detection rates of tuberculosis among the urban poor are well below rates for other urban residents.

Urban malaria

Although malaria has often been regarded as a problem afflicting rural populations, and rural rates of transmission are known to be markedly higher than urban rates, there is clear evidence that malaria vectors have adapted to urban conditions in sub-Saharan Africa (Modiano et al. 1999) and some evidence suggestive of urban risks has emerged for parts of Asia as well. As Hay et al. (2004) argue, urban population growth in South East Asia, as well as sub-Saharan Africa, may be contributing substantially to the global burden of malaria morbidity. Keiser et al. (2004) calculate that in urban sub-Saharan Africa, some 200 million city dwellers face appreciable risks of malaria, and they estimate that 25–100 million clinical episodes of the disease occur annually in this region's cities and towns. Indirect estimates suggest wide variations in prevalence by site, even within small geographic areas, with higher prevalence in the suburbs and city peripheries (especially when these are adjacent to wetlands) than in city centres.[8]

Pictet et al. (2004) describe a recent urban intervention programme mounted in Ouagadougou, Burkina Faso's capital, which aimed to make use of the social resources of urban communities to provide care in uncomplicated cases of child malaria. Inspired by a rural programme that yielded good results, this urban programme enlisted local community residents ('health agents'), gave them training in the recognition of malarial symptoms in young children, and supplied the agents with packets of chloroquine and paracetamol in age-appropriate doses. (In Ouagadougou, a high fraction of malaria cases still respond to chloroquine, although the parasite's resistance is evidently growing.) In cases of childhood fevers, it has been common practice for residents of the Ouagadougou slums to buy chloroquine tablets (or drugs that have a similar appearance) in local markets, using these to medicate their ill children. Preliminary research showed, however, that the residents had little knowledge of the dosages or lengths of treatment appropriate for children. Hence, when judged against the medication practices that were already prevalent in these communities, the programme intervention was expected to improve the standard of malaria care.

When pilot-tested in two communities in Ouagadougou, the malaria intervention showed the expected positive results in the lower-income community, which was located on the fringes of the city and somewhat isolated from sources of modern healthcare. Of the two study communities, this was the more homogeneous in social and economic terms, and it exhibited evidence of greater 'neighbourliness' and other forms of social interaction through which information about the intervention might have circulated. In the other pilot community, however, easier access was already available to modern health clinics and reputable pharmacies, and more residents could afford to pay for their own care. In this middle-income site it proved difficult to sustain community interest in the intervention. As this Ouagadougou example shows, urban health interventions can be designed so as to tap the social energies and social organization of local neighbourhoods and communities, but the design may need to be tailored to fit the specific circumstances of each such community.

Traffic-related injuries and deaths

We now broaden the discussion to encompass sectors that have not always been linked to or carefully integrated with urban public health programmes, yet which have significant implications for health. Injuries and deaths from traffic accidents are a prominent case in point. Table 9.7.5 for Mexico shows just how important these are among all urban causes of death and disability, but the great range of factors involved—touching on engineering concerns and urban planning and land-use policies as well as individual behaviour—seem in many countries to have inhibited the public health sector from taking action. The scale of this public health problem is enormous: the WHO (2004) estimates that road traffic injuries lead to 1.2 million deaths annually and an additional 20–50 million non-fatal injuries, the majority of which occur in low- and middle-income countries. Two recent discussions—World Bank (2009) and Marquez and Farrington (2013)—highlight the importance of road traffic injuries among all urban non-communicable risks.

To elucidate the factors involved, Híjar et al. (2003) conducted a detailed analysis of pedestrian injuries in Mexico City, where pedestrian death rates are estimated at three times those of Los Angeles. Using a mix of spatially-coded quantitative data and qualitative methods, these authors developed portraits of drivers and victims that underscore the importance of several mutually reinforcing risk factors: poverty, a lack of understanding of how drivers are apt to react to pedestrians, inattention by drivers and pedestrians alike to risky conditions, insufficient public investment in traffic lights and road lighting, and dangerous mixes of industrial, commercial, and private traffic. Bartlett (2002) draws on hospital- and community-based studies to show how poverty and gender affect the risks, and how the time pressures on urban parents limit the effort they can devote to closely supervising their children.

In seeking to raise the public health profile of these important causes, the WHO (2004, 2007d) has given particular emphasis to the risks that are faced by adolescents and young adults, among whom road traffic injuries rank (worldwide) in the top three causes of death in the ages of 5 to 25 years (WHO 2007d, p. 3). In the WHO's Africa region, it is pedestrians (especially children aged 5–9) who face the greatest risks, whereas in South East Asia, the deaths occur disproportionately to riders of bicycles and motorized two-wheelers, who are aged 15–24 years. Fig. 9.7.5 shows how in poor countries of Asia, it is the vulnerable road users—pedestrians,

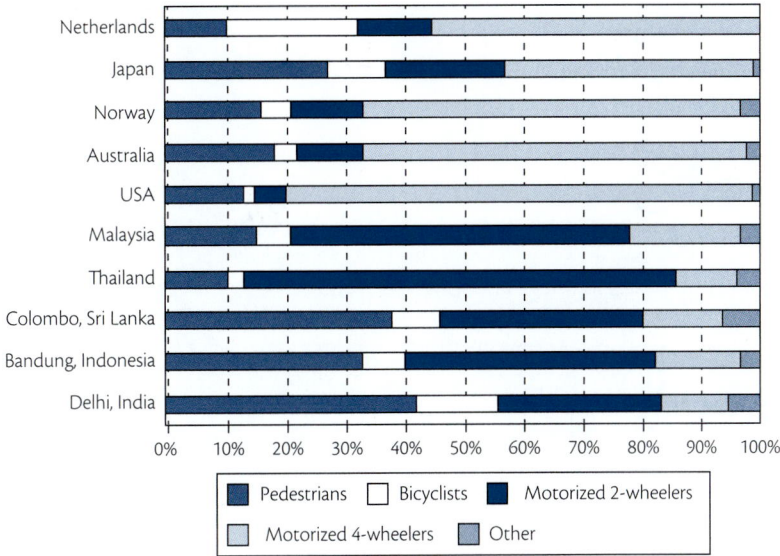

Fig. 9.7.5 Composition of road traffic injuries by type, selected developed countries and Asian low- and middle-income countries.
Reproduced with permission from World Health Organization, *World report on road traffic injury prevention*, Copyright © World Health Organization 2004, available from http://whqlibdoc. who.int/publications/2004/9241562609.pdf.

bicyclists, and operators of motorized two-wheelers—who bear a greater share of the injury burden than the occupants of cars, vans, and buses. For adolescents, young adults, and children alike, males face greater risks than females.

The full package of interventions known to be effective in high-income countries has typically not been implemented in low-income countries (World Bank 2009; Marquez and Farrington 2013). The interventions include behavioural interventions—the promotion through media campaigns and other public health communication outlets of seat-belt use for adolescents and adults and appropriate restraints for infant and child passengers, and encouragement for bicycle and motorcycle riders to wear helmets—as well as traffic engineering concerns, such as the need to remove 'unforgiving' roadside objects, properly maintain existing roads, and situate new ones so that high-speed traffic is not routed through densely settled communities or placed near busy markets, schools, and children's play-spaces. In many low- and middle-income countries, only meagre resources are allotted to traffic control and enforcement of speed and road safety laws. Public health planners will also need to assess the priority that has been given to emergency rescue services (which may involve connections between the health system and the police) and the availability of pre-hospital care and in-hospital trauma centres.

Outdoor air pollution

Traffic and vehicular regulation are also key factors in outdoor air pollution. The Latin American literature is especially rich in scientific analyses of outdoor urban air pollution and its effects on respiratory illness via the intake of airborne particulates and other pollutants emitted by industry and vehicles. Ribeiro and Alves Cardoso (2003) provide a thorough review of such studies for São Paulo; for Mexico City, Santos-Burgoa and Riojas-Rodríguez (2000) have assembled and reviewed a great range of studies. There is increasing interest in the problem in India, China, and other rapidly-developing countries of Asia, where the effects of

economic growth are readily apparent in levels and severity of outdoor air pollution.[9] In Delhi, a crucial public health intervention was recently made by the Supreme Court in a decision that mandated conversion to compressed natural gas for bus, taxi, and other fleets of vehicles. There is reason to think that on a per-vehicle basis, this intervention has been effective; however, because the total volume of traffic has increased in Delhi, it is not yet obvious that the total volume of particulates and other pollutants has decreased (Kumar 2007; Narain and Krupnick 2007).

Extreme weather events and climate change

Among the extreme weather-related events that put the health of urban dwellers at risk, two deserve particular mention here: the problem of flooding and, at the other end of the spectrum, the problem of water scarcity. Flooding can be characterized as a sudden-onset extreme event; it has afflicted both coastal and inland cities, with many cities inundated on a seasonal or periodic basis. As global warming proceeds, increases in sea level, rising sea surface temperatures, and the mounting likelihood of heavy precipitation will combine to put large urban populations at greater risk. The risks are already readily apparent in Asia, many of whose largest cities are located in the flood-plains of major rivers (the Ganges–Brahmaputra, Mekong, and Yangtze rivers) and in coastal areas that have long been cyclone-prone. Mumbai saw massive floods in 2005, as did Karachi in 2007 and again in 2010. Fig. 9.7.6 depicts Asian cities at risk of both inland and coastal flooding. Flooding and storm surges also present a threat in coastal African cities (e.g. Port Harcourt, Nigeria, and Mombasa, Kenya) and in Latin America (e.g. Caracas, Venezuela).

Excellent accounts of the health consequences of flooding include Portier et al. (2010), Ahern et al. (2005), Shultz et al. (2005), ActionAid International (2006), and Kovats and Akhtar (2008), with an authoritative summing-up in a recent Intergovernmental Panel on Climate Change report (2012). Urban flooding risks in poor countries stem from a number of

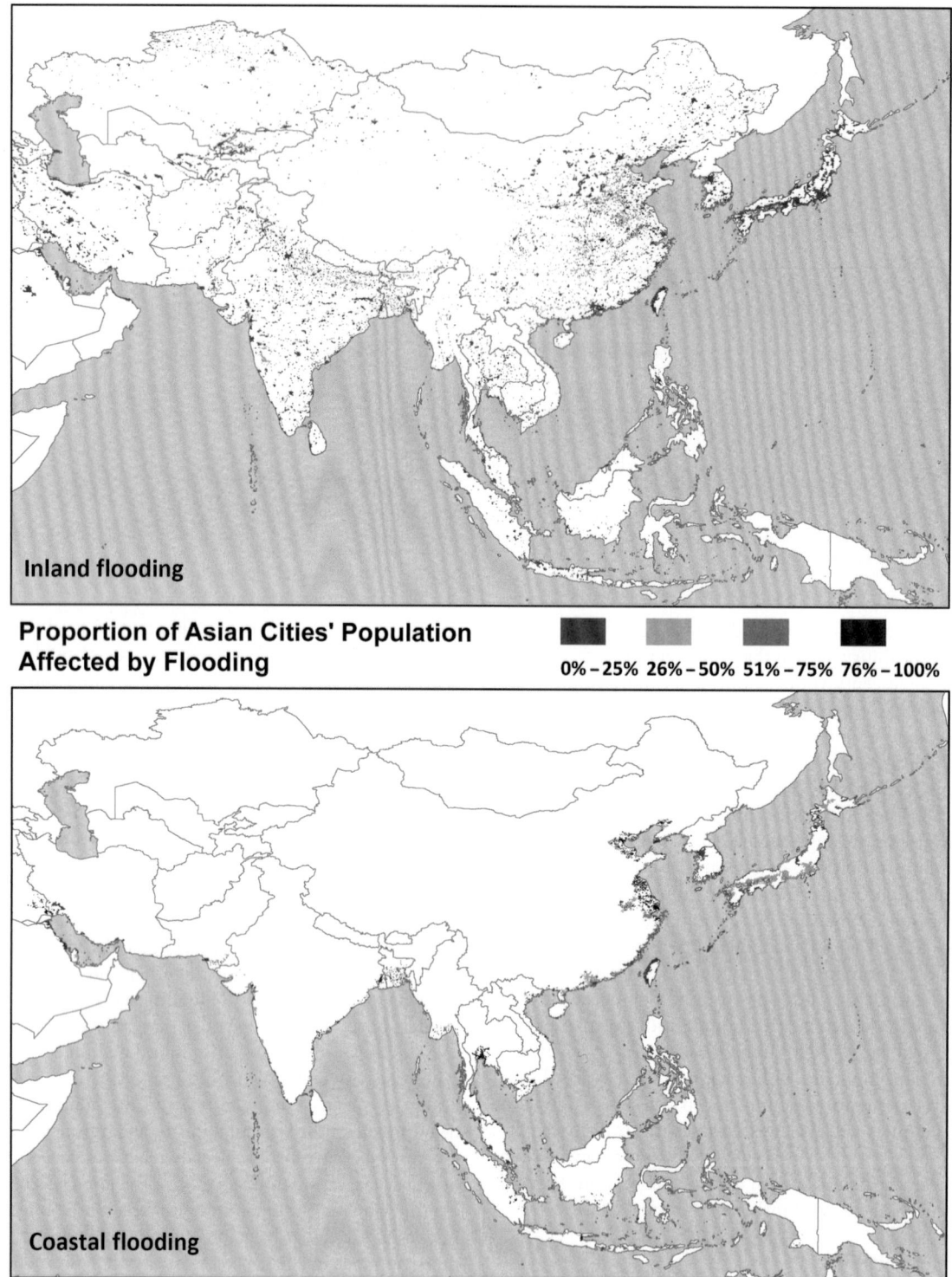

Fig. 9.7.6 For Asian cities, percentage of population at risk of coastal or inland flooding. Calculations by author with Deborah Balk and Zhen Liu.

Source: data from Balk, D., et al., Mapping urban settlements and the risks of climate change in Africa, Asia, and South America, pp. 80–103, in J.M. Guzman et al. (eds.), *Population Dynamics and Climate Change*, United Nations Fund for Population Activities (UNFPA) and International Institute for Environment and Development (IIED), New York, USA, Copyright © 2009.

factors: the predominance of impermeable surfaces that cause water run-off; the general scarcity of parks and other green spaces to absorb these flows; rudimentary drainage systems that are often clogged by waste and which in any case are quickly overloaded with water; and the ill-advised development of marshlands and other natural buffers. When urban flooding takes place, faecal and other hazardous materials contaminate flood waters and spill into open wells, elevating the risks of water-borne disease. Urban floods are thus well-described as 'complex emergencies'. The urban poor are often more exposed than others to these hazards, because the housing they can afford tends to be located in the riskier areas.

The international community is marshalling its response to such looming threats under the Hyogo Framework for Action (HFA) 2005–2015, an initiative which aims to fully integrate disaster planning, early warning, preparedness, and vulnerability reduction into economic development strategies, and which strives to ensure that multiple units and levels of government are well coordinated and linked with NGOs, community-based organizations, and other elements of civil society (International Strategy for Disaster Reduction 2009; United Nations 2007). While giving due consideration to needs for coordination at the international, regional, and national levels, the Hyogo Framework returns repeatedly to the theme of integration at the level of the community, as for example in the development of early warning systems that are people-centred, whose warnings are timely and intelligible to those at risk, and which tell people how and why they should respond to imminent threats (Red Cross/Red Crescent 2007; International Federation of Red Cross and Red Crescent Societies 2009). Urban adaptation strategies will need to be devised that are spatially specific and sensitive to the great variation across city neighbourhoods in the socioeconomic factors that determine exposure to risk, vulnerability, and recovery-resilience.

The risks posed by water scarcity are slower-developing, but arguably just as important to public health over the long term. As shown in Balk et al. (2009), nearly 1 billion city dwellers in poor countries live in arid zones, where they face shortfalls in drinking water on a seasonal or perennial basis that leave them with too little to meet basic daily needs. As global warming causes already-dry areas to become drier still, more city residents will be placed at risk. In the next two to three decades, however, the proximate cause of increases in exposure is not likely to be climate change as such, but rather the continued population growth of cities in arid zones. McDonald et al. (2011) examined the relative importance of demographic and climate change factors up to 2040, and found that over this period, population growth will be by some measure the dominant factor in increasing the numbers of people lacking adequate access to water.

Enough is already known to sketch the elements of an urban disaster risk reduction strategy for poor countries (Satterthwaite et al. 2007). But in moving from broad descriptions of such risks to focused, prioritized interventions, it is essential to document the specific cities and neighbourhoods that are repeatedly beset by excesses of water (that is, by flooding) as well as water insufficiencies. Internationally-accessible data repositories, the most prominent being the EM-DAT (http://www.emdat.be) database, record only the large-scale floods and droughts and do not pinpoint their locations. A promising alternative approach, which was pioneered in Latin America, is that of the DesInventar (http://www.desinventar.net) initiative. Its distinguishing feature is the effort to collect reliable information on a spatially specific basis for both small-scale and large-scale events. As more countries adopt this approach, an empirical record will accumulate that can help in setting intervention programmes on a firm grounding of evidence.

Local governments can be held politically accountable for their responses to local floods and similar disasters (Roberts 2008) and local political leaders would therefore seem to have a keen interest in addressing these risks. But in poor countries, and especially outside the largest cities and national capitals, municipal governments are often severely constrained in terms of authority, budgets, and both technical and managerial expertise (Tanner et al. 2009; World Bank 2011; Jha et al. 2012). They are already overwhelmed with day-to-day management and generally lack the capacity to foresee and properly prepare for emergencies. If their needs have not been anticipated in the design of a decentralized system, smaller cities will likely face a yawning gulf between what they should do in the event of an emergency and what they are prepared for and able to do. To plan adequately for the upcoming era of climate change, the urban public health system must engage with partners across a broad range of urban agencies. Many of the priority areas needing attention are already areas of concern on other counts—for instance, improvements in water and sanitation systems for the urban poor—but the prospect of climate change adds a new element of urgency to them.

Conclusions

The sketch of urban health in low- and middle-income countries provided here is no substitute for the full treatment that the issues deserve, but it may at least suggest where further basic scientific and programme intervention research is most needed. A theme running through the discussion is the need for concerted action, with the public health sector working in tandem with other local government agencies. Public health professionals cannot by themselves mandate the provision of safe water and adequate sanitation for the urban poor, with all the attendant financial costs; nor can they, acting alone, rise to meet the challenges of mitigating urban air pollution, reorganizing traffic and pedestrian activities to reduce deaths and injuries, and readying cities to adapt to the threats that will be posed by climate change. What is needed is what Harpham (2007) terms 'joined-up government,' whereby public health agencies join with concerned actors in other sectors of municipal, regional, and national governments. Because the urban health system is dauntingly complex, with private for-profit and private non-profit care being a significant presence in most cities, effective partnerships are also likely to require engagement with the private sector. With political and administrative decentralization now well underway in many low- and middle-income countries, the arena in which creative partnerships are forged will increasingly be the local and municipal level. Much remains to be learned about how health expertise that is now situated in national ministries of health, and the international funding and technical assistance that has also been directed to national ministries, can be redeployed effectively to meet the many health needs of cities and their neighbourhoods.

Acknowledgements

Text extracts from *Social Science & Medicine*, Volume 45, Issue 14, Bassett, M.T. et al., Professionalism, patient satisfaction and quality of healthcare: Experience during Zimbabwe's structural adjustment programme, pp. 1845–1852, Copyright © 1997, reprinted with permission from Elsevier, available from http://www.sciencedirect.com/science/journal/02779536.

Notes

1. See WHO (2007c, p. 14), which indicates that of the 115 countries reporting to WHO on the quality of cause-of-death statistics, only 29 (representing a mere 13 per cent of world population) were judged to have adequate records.

2. For more information, see http://www.measuredhs.com/aboutdhs for the DHS programme and http://www.childinfo.org/index.htm for the MICS.

3. See Evans (2007) on recent innovations in financing for improvements in urban water supply, sanitation, and housing.

4. See Montgomery and Ezeh (2005b) for further discussion with attention to social capital and collective efficacy.

5. The Alan Guttmacher Institute (1999) provides an excellent overview of induced abortion, a generally hidden and difficult-to-study area of health. See International Family Planning Perspectives, which is a good source of information on this topic; the publication archive is http://www.guttmacher.org/pubs. The journal Studies in Family Planning is another helpful source: http://www.blackwell-synergy.com/loi/sifp.

6. See Dyson (2003). Country profiles are available at http://www.census.gov/ipc/www/hivaidsn.html, but these profiles are worked up from the reports of selected clinics and various sentinel sites, which do not necessarily yield statistically representative portraits for urban or rural populations.

7. Estimates of urban and rural prevalence of HIV from the Demographic and Health Surveys: Mali, 2001; Kenya, 2003; and Zambia, 2001–2002. Sources: Mali Ministère de la Santé (2002), Kenya Central Bureau of Statistics (2003), Zambia Central Statistical Office (2003).

8. A detailed, time-series study of Dar es Salaam, Tanzania (Caldas de Castro et al. 2004), which relies on an unusual combination of high-resolution aerial photography and extensive ground validation, depicts the micro-zones of high malaria risk within this city.

9. For an overview of air pollution issues in Asia, see http://www.healtheffects.org/Asia/papasan-overview.htm.

References

ActionAid International (2006). *Unjust Waters: Climate Change, Flooding and the Protection of Poor Urban Communities: Experiences from Six African Cities*. London: Action AID International Report.

African Population and Health Research Center (2002). *Population and Health Dynamics in Nairobi's Informal Settlements: Report of the Nairobi Cross-Sectional Slums Survey (NCSS) 2000*. Nairobi: African Population and Health Research Center.

Ahern, M.R., Kovats, S., Wilkinson, P., Few, R., and Matthies, F. (2005). Global health impacts of floods: epidemiological evidence. *Epidemiologic Reviews*, 27, 36–45.

Alan Guttmacher Institute (1999). *Sharing Responsibility: Women, Society, and Abortion Worldwide*. New York: Alan Guttmacher Institute.

Almeida-Filho, N., Lessa, I., Magalhães, L., et al. (2004). Social inequality and depressive disorders in Bahia, Brazil: interactions of gender, ethnicity, and social class. *Social Science & Medicine*, 59, 1339–53.

Balk, D., Montgomery, M.R., McGranahan, G., et al. (2009). Mapping urban settlements and the risks of climate change in Africa, Asia, and South America. In J.M. Guzmán, G. Martine, G. McGranahan, D. Schensul, and C. Tacoli (eds.) *Population Dynamics and Climate Change*, pp. 80–103. New York: United Nations Fund for Population Activities (UNFPA) and International Institute for Environment and Development (IIED).

Barata, R.B., Ribeiro, M.C., Guedes, M.B., and Moraes, J.C. (1998). Intra-urban differentials in death rates from homicide in the city of São Paulo, Brazil, 1988–1994. *Social Science & Medicine*, 47, 19–23.

Bartlett, S.N. (2002). The problem of children's injuries in low-income countries: a review. *Health Policy and Planning*, 17, 1–13.

Barua, N. and Singh, S. (2003). *Representation for the Marginalized—Linking the Poor and the Health Care System. Lessons from Case Studies in Urban India*. Draft paper. New Delhi: World Bank.

Bassett, M.T., Bijlmakers, L., and Sanders, D.M. (1997). Professionalism, patient satisfaction and quality of health care: experience during Zimbabwe's structural adjustment programme. *Social Science & Medicine*, 45, 1845–52.

Blue, I. (1999). *Intra-Urban Differentials in Mental Health in São Paulo, Brazil*. Ph.D. thesis, South Bank University, London.

Boardman, J.D. (2004). Stress and physical health: the role of neighborhoods as mediating and moderating mechanisms. *Social Science & Medicine*, 58, 2473–83.

Cairncross, S. and Valdmanis, V. (2006). Water supply, sanitation, and hygiene promotion. In D.T. Jamison, J.G. Bremen, A.R. Measham, et al. (eds.) *Disease Control Priorities in Developing Countries* (2nd ed.), pp. 771–92. Washington, DC: World Bank and Oxford University Press.

Caldas de Castro, M., Yamagata, Y., Mtasiwa, D., et al. (2004). *Integrated urban malaria control: a case study in Dar es Salaam, Tanzania*. Working Paper. Princeton, NJ: Office of Population Research, Princeton University.

Calvés, A.E. (2002). Abortion risk and decision making among young people in urban Cameroon. *Studies in Family Planning*, 33, 249–60.

Cohen, S., Doyle, W.J., and Baum, A. (2006). Socioeconomic status is associated with stress hormones. *Psychosomatic Medicine*, 68, 414–20.

Das, J. and Hammer, J. (2007a). Location, location, location: residence, wealth, and the quality of medical care in Delhi, India. *Health Affairs*, 26, 338–51.

Das, J. and Hammer, J. (2007b). Money for nothing: the dire straits of medical practice in Delhi, India. *Journal of Development Economics*, 83, 1–36.

Desgrées du Loû, A., Msellati, P., Viho, I., and Welffens-Ekra, C. (2000). The use of induced abortion in Abidjan: a possible cause of the fertility decline. *Population*, 12, 197–214.

Dussault, G. and Franceschini, M.C. (2006). Not enough there, too many here: understanding geographic imbalances in the distribution of the health workforce. *Human Resources for Health*, 4, 1–16.

Dyson, T. (2003). HIV/AIDS and urbanization. *Population and Development Review*, 29, 427–42.

Erulkar, A.S. and Matheka, J.K. (2007). *Adolescence in the Kibera slums of Nairobi, Kenya*. New York: Population Council.

Evans, B. (2007). Understanding the urban poor's vulnerabilities in sanitation and water supply. Paper presented at *Innovations for an Urban World*, the Rockefeller Foundation's Urban Summit, Bellagio, Italy.

Fay, M. (ed.) (2005). *The Urban Poor in Latin America*. Washington, DC: The World Bank.

Fikree, F.F., Gray, R.H., Berendes, H.W., and Karim, M.S. (1994). A community-based nested case-control study of maternal mortality. *International Journal of Gynecology & Obstetrics*, 47, 247–55.

Fikree, F.F., Midhet, F., Sadruddin, S., and Berendes, H.W. (1997). Maternal mortality in different Pakistani sites: ratios, clinical causes and determinants. *Acta Obstetricia et Gynecologica Scandinavica*, 76, 637–45.

Fikree, F.R., Ali, T., Durocher, J.M., and Rahbar, M.H. (2004). Health service utilization for perceived postpartum morbidity among poor women living in Karachi. *Social Science & Medicine*, 59, 681–94.

Garrett, J. and Ahmed, A. (2004). Incorporating crime in household surveys: a research note. *Environment and Urbanization*, 16, 139–52.

Graham, W., Brass, W., and Snow, R.W. (1989). Estimating maternal mortality: the sisterhood method. *Studies in Family Planning*, 20, 125–35.

Grant, E. (1999). *State of the Art of Urban Health in Latin America. European Commission Funded Concerted Action: 'Health and Human Settlements in Latin America'*. London: South Bank University.

Hallman, K. (2004). *Socioeconomic Disadvantage and Unsafe Sexual Behaviors Among Young Women and Men in South Africa*. Policy Research Division Working Papers, No. 190. New York: Population Council.

Harpham, T. (2007). Background paper on improving urban population health. Paper presented at *Innovations for an Urban World*, the Rockefeller Foundation's Urban Summit, Bellagio, Italy.

Harpham, T., Grant, E., and Rodriguez, C. (2004). Mental health and social capital in Cali, Colombia. *Social Science & Medicine*, 58, 2267–77.

Hay, S.I., Guerra, C.A., Tatem, A.J., Noor, A.M., and Snow, R.W. (2004). The global distribution and population at risk of malaria: past, present, and future. *The Lancet Infectious Diseases*, 4, 327–36.

Heinemann, A. and Verner, D. (2006). *Crime and Violence in Development: A Literature Review of Latin America and the Caribbean.* World Bank Policy Research Working Paper, No. 4041. Washington, DC: World Bank.

Heise, L.L., Raikes, A., Watts, C.H., and Zwi, A.B. (1994). Violence against women: a neglected public health issue in less developed countries. *Social Science & Medicine*, 39, 1165–79.

Híjar, M., Trostle, J., and Bronfman, M. (2003). Pedestrian injuries in Mexico: a multi-method approach. *Social Science & Medicine*, 57, 2149–59.

Hu, P., Wagle, N., Goldman, N., Weinstein, M., and Seeman, T. (2007). The associations between socioeconomic status, allostatic load, and measures of health in older Taiwanese persons: Taiwan Social Environment and Biomarkers of Aging study. *Journal of Biosocial Science*, 39, 545–56.

Intergovernmental Panel on Climate Change (2012). *Managing the Risks of Extreme Events and Disasters to Advance Climate Change Adaptation. A Special Report of Working Groups I and II of the Intergovernmental Panel on Climate Change.* Cambridge: Cambridge University Press.

International Federation of Red Cross and Red Crescent Societies (2009). *World Disasters Report 2009: Focus on Early Warning, Early Action.* Geneva: International Federation of Red Cross and Red Crescent Societies.

International Strategy for Disaster Reduction (2009). *Global Assessment Report on Disaster Risk Reduction: Risk and Poverty in a Changing Climate.* Geneva: International Strategy for Disaster Reduction, United Nations.

Islam, M., Montgomery, M.R., and Taneja, S. (2006). *Urban Health and Care-Seeking Behavior: A Case Study of Slums in India and the Philippines.* Bethesda, MD: PHRPlus Program, Abt Associates.

Jamil, S. and Fikree, F.F. (2002). *Determinants of Unsafe Abortion in Three Squatter Settle-Ments of Karachi.* Karachi: Department of Community Health Sciences.

Jha, A.K., Bloch, R., and Lamond, J. (2012). *Cities and Flooding: A Guide to Integrated Urban Flood Risk Management for the 21st Century.* Washington, DC: World Bank.

Kaneda, T., Zimmer, Z., and Tang, Z. (2005). Socioeconomic status differentials in life and active life expectancy among older adults in Beijing. *Disability and Rehabilitation*, 27, 241–51.

Keiser, J., Utzinger, J., Caldas de Castro, M., Smith, T.A., Tanner, M., and Singer, B.H. (2004). *Urbanization in Sub-Saharan Africa and Implications for Malaria Control.* Working Paper. Princeton, NJ: Office of Population Research, Princeton University, and Swiss Tropical Institute.

Kenya Central Bureau of Statistics (2003). *Kenya Demographic and Health Survey 2003: Preliminary Report.* Nairobi; Central Bureau of Statistics.

Kishor, S. and Johnson, K. (2004). *Profiling Domestic Violence: A Multi-Country Study.* Calverton, MD: Measure DHS+, ORC/Macro.

Kovats, R.S. and Akhtar, R. (2008). Climate, climate change and human health in Asian cities. *Environment and Urbanization*, 20, 165–75.

Kumar, N. (2007). *Spatial Sampling for Demography and Health Survey.* Paper presented at the 2007 Annual Meetings of the Population Association of America, New York, NY, Department of Geography, University of Iowa.

Larson, B.A. and Rosen, S. (2002). Understanding household demand for indoor air pollution control in developing countries. *Social Science & Medicine*, 55, 571–84.

Lozano, R., Murray, C., and Frenk, J. (1999). El peso de las enfermedades en Mexico. In K. Hill, J.B. Morelos, and R. Wong (eds.) *Las Consecuencias de las Transiciones Demografica y Epidemiological en América Latina*, pp. 39–53. Mexico City: El Colegio de México.

Mali Ministère de la Santé (2002). *Enquête Démographique et de Santé Mali 2001.* Calverton, MD: Ministère de la Santé (Mali) and ORC Macro.

Marmot, M.G. (2005). Social determinants of health inequalities. *The Lancet*, 365, 1099–104.

Marmot, M.G. and Wilkinson, R.G. (eds.) (2005). *Social Determinants of Health* (2nd ed.). Oxford: Oxford University Press.

Marquez, P.V. and Farrington, J.L. (2013). *The Challenge of Non-Communicable Diseases and Road Traffic Injuries in Sub-Saharan Africa: An Overview.* Washington, DC: World Bank.

Mayank, S., Bahl, R., Rattan, A., and Bhandari, N. (2001). Prevalence and correlates of morbidity in pregnant women in an urban slum of New Delhi. *Asia-Pacific Population Journal*, 16, 29–44.

McDonald, R.I., Green, P., Balk, D., et al. (2011). Urban growth, climate change, and freshwater availability. *Proceedings of the National Academy of Sciences of the United States of America*, 108(15), 6312–17.

McEwen, B.S. (1998). Protecting and damaging effects of stress mediators. *The New England Journal of Medicine*, 338, 171–9.

McGranahan, G. (2007). *Urban Environments, Wealth and Health: Shifting Burdens and Possible Responses in Low and Middle-Income Nations.* Human Settlements Discussion Paper Series, Urban Environment-1. London: International Institute for Environment and Development (IIED). Available at: http://www.iied.org/pubs.

Mercado, S., Havemann, K., Nakamura, K., et al. (2007). Responding to the health vulnerabilities of the urban poor in the 'new urban settings' of Asia. WHO Centre for Health Development, Alliance for Healthy Cities, and Southeast Asian Press Alliance. Paper presented at *Innovations for an Urban World*, the Rockefeller Foundation's Urban Summit, Bellagio, Italy.

Mishra, V., Bignami, S., Greener, R., et al. (2007). *A Study of the Association of HIV Infection and Wealth in Sub-Saharan Africa.* DHS Working Papers, No. 31. Calverton, MD: Macro International.

Modiano, D., Sirima, B., Sawadogo, A., Sanou, I., and Paré, J. (1999). Severe malaria in Burkina Faso: urban and rural environment. *Parassitologia*, 41, 251–4.

Montgomery, M.R. and Ezeh, A.C. (2005a). The health of urban populations in developing countries: an overview. In S. Galea and D. Vlahov (eds.) *Handbook of Urban Health: Populations, Methods, and Practice*, pp. 201–22. New York: Springer.

Montgomery, M.R. and Ezeh, A.C. (2005b). Urban health in developing countries: insights from demographic theory and practice. In S. Galea and D. Vlahov (eds.) *Handbook of Urban Health: Populations, Methods, and Practice*, pp. 317–60. New York: Springer.

Montgomery, M.R. and Hewett, P.C. (2005). Urban poverty and health in developing countries: household and neighborhood effects. *Demography*, 42, 397–425.

Moser, C.O.N. (2004). Urban violence and insecurity: an introductory roadmap. *Environment and Urbanization*, 16, 3–16.

Narain, U. and Krupnick, A. (2007). *The Impact of Delhi's CNG Program on Air Quality.* Discussion Paper 07-08. Washington, DC: Resources for the Future.

Panel on Urban Population Dynamics (2003). *Cities Transformed: Demographic Change and Its Implications in the Developing World.* Washington, DC: National Academies Press.

Parkar, S.R., Fernandes, J., and Weiss, M.G. (2003). Contextualizing mental health: gendered experiences in a Mumbai slum. *Anthropology & Medicine*, 10, 291–308.

Pictet, G., Kouanda, S., Sirima, S., and Pond, R. (2004). *Struggling with Population Heterogeneity in African Cities: The Urban Health and Equity Puzzle.* Paper presented to the 2004 annual meetings of the Population Association of America, Boston MA.

Portier, C.J., Thigpen, T.K., Carter, S.R., et al. (2010). *A Human Health Perspective on Climate Change: A Report Outlining the Research Needs on the Human Health Effects of Climate Change.* Research Triangle Park, NC: Environmental Health Perspectives/National Institute of Environmental Health Sciences.

Prince, M., Patel, V., Saxena, S., et al. (2007). No health without mental health. *The Lancet*, 370, 859–77.

Red Cross/Red Crescent (2007). *Red Cross/Red Crescent Climate Guide*. Geneva: Red Cross/Red Crescent.

Ribeiro, H. and Alves Cardoso, M.R. (2003). Air pollution and children's health in São Paulo (1986–1998). *Social Science & Medicine*, 57, 2013–22.

Roberts, D. (2008). Thinking globally, acting locally: institutionalizing climate change at the local government level in Durban, South Africa. *Environment and Urbanization*, 20, 521–37.

Rossier, C. (2007). *Attitudes Towards Abortion and Contraception in Rural and Urban Burkina Faso*. Paris: Institut National d'Etudes Démographique.

Sagbakken, M., Bjune, G., Frich, J., and Aseffa, A. (2003). From the user's perspective—a qualitative study of factors influencing patients' adherence to medical treatment in an urban community, Ethiopia. Paper presented at the conference *Urban Poverty and Health in Sub-Saharan Africa*, African Population and Health Research Centre, Nairobi.

Santos-Burgoa, C. and Riojas-Rodríguez, H. (2000). *Health and Pollution in Mexico City Metropolitan Area: A General Overview of Air Pollution Exposure and Health Studies*. Presentation to the Panel on Urban Population Dynamics, U.S. National Research Council, Mexico City.

Satterthwaite, D., Huq, S., Reid, H., Pelling, M., and Romero-Lankao, P. (2007). *Adapting to Climate Change in Urban Areas: The Possibilities and Constraints in Low- and Middle-Income Nations*. Human Settlements Discussion Paper Series, Climate Change and Cities, No. 1. London: International Institute for Environment and Development.

Shin, S., Furin, J., Bayona, J., Mate, K., Kim, J.Y., and Farmer, P. (2004). Community-based treatment of multidrug-resistant tuberculosis in Lima, Peru: 7 years of experience. *Social Science & Medicine*, 59, 1529–39.

Shultz, J.M., Russell, J., and Espinel, Z. (2005). Epidemiology of tropical cyclones: the dynamics of disaster, disease, and development. *Epidemiologic Reviews*, 27, 21–35.

Steptoe, A. and Marmot, M. (2002). The role of psychobiological pathways in socio-economic inequalities in cardiovascular disease risk. *European Heart Journal*, 23, 13–25.

Stone, C. (2006). *Crime, Justice, and Growth in South Africa: Toward a Plausible Contribution from Criminal Justice to Economic Growth*. Center for International Development Working Paper No. 131. Cambridge, MA: Harvard University.

Tanner, T.M., Mitchell, T., Polack, E., and Guenther, B. (2009). Urban governance for adaptation: assessing climate change resilience in ten Asian cities. IDS Working Paper 315. Brighton: Institute for Development Studies at the University of Sussex.

UNAIDS (2004). *2004 Report on the Global AIDS Epidemic*. New York: UNAIDS.

UN-Habitat (2003a). *The Challenge of Slums: Global Report on Human Settlements 2003*. London: Earthscan.

UN-Habitat (2003b). *Water and Sanitation in the World's Cities: Local Action for Global Goals*. London: Earthscan.

United Nations (2007). *Words Into Action: A Guide for Implementing the Hyogo Framework*. New York: United Nations.

United Nations (2012). *World Urbanization Prospects, The 2011 Revision*. New York: Department of Economic and Social Affairs, Population Division, United Nations.

Van Rie, A., Beyers, N., Gie, R.P., Kunneke, M., Zietsman, L., and Donald, P.R. (1999). Childhood tuberculosis in an urban population in South Africa: burden and risk factor. *Archives of Disability in Children*, 80, 433–7.

Winton, A. (2004). Urban violence: a guide to the literature. *Environment and Urbanization*, 16, 165–84.

Wong, R., Peláez, M., Palloni, A., and Markides, K. (2006). Survey data for the study of aging in Latin America and the Caribbean. *Journal of Aging and Health*, 18, 157–79.

Woods, R. (2003). Urban–rural mortality differentials: an unresolved debate. *Population and Development Review*, 29, 29–46.

World Bank (2009). *Confronting 'Death on Wheels': Making Roads Safe in Europe and Central Asia*. Washington, DC: World Bank.

World Bank (2011). *Migration and Remittances Factbook 2011* (2nd ed.). Washington, DC: World Bank.

World Health Organization (1996). *Investing in Health Research and Development: Report of the Ad Hoc Committee on Health Research Relating to Future Intervention Options*. Geneva: WHO.

World Health Organization (2001). *The World Health Report 2001. Mental Health: New Understanding, New Hope*. Geneva: WHO.

World Health Organization (2002). *The World Health Report 2002. Reducing Risk, Promoting Healthy Life*. Geneva: WHO.

World Health Organization (2004). *World Report on Road Traffic Injury Prevention*. Geneva: WHO. Available at: http://whqlibdoc.who.int/publications/2004/9241562609.pdf.

World Health Organization (2005a). *Mental Health: Facing the Challenges, Building Solutions*. Report from the WHO European Ministerial Conference, Copenhagen, Denmark. Copenhagen: WHO.

World Health Organization (2005b). *WHO Multi-Country Study on Women's Health and Domestic Violence Against Women: Summary Report of Initial Results on Prevalence, Health Outcomes and Women's Responses*. Geneva: WHO.

World Health Organization (2007a). *Global Age-Friendly Cities: A Guide*. Geneva: WHO.

World Health Organization (2007b). *Global Tuberculosis Control: Surveillance, Planning, Financing*. Geneva: WHO.

World Health Organization (2007c). *World Health Statistics 2007*. Geneva: WHO.

World Health Organization (2007d). *Youth and Road Safety*. Geneva: WHO.

Zambia Central Statistical Office (2003). *Zambia Demographic and Health Survey 2001–2002*. Calverton, MD: Central Statistical Office (Zambia), Central Board of Health (Zambia), and ORC Macro.

Zimmer, Z. and Kwong, J. (2004). Socioeconomic status and health among older adults in urban and rural China. *Journal of Aging and Health*, 16, 44–70.

SECTION 10

Public health needs of population groups

10.1

The changing family

Gavin W. Jones

Family change across the world: kinship, family structure, and effect of socioeconomic and ideational change

The doyen of family sociologists, William Goode, argued that the differences between non-Western and Western family systems extended far back in time (Goode 1963, p. 22). Nevertheless, he went on to propose that there would in future be a convergence towards some form of nuclear, or conjugal, family system. In this, he was mistaken (McDonald 1992; Cherlin, 2009, p. 578). His key point that family systems in different regions have to be studied in their own right, however, holds: 'No useful analysis of African family systems can be undertaken using European concepts of marriage, household, parenthood, kinship' (Oppong 1992, p. 82). There is also no doubt that almost everywhere, family systems are changing in response to pervasive and far-reaching technological, socioeconomic and ideational forces. One of the best-known family sociologists in the United States recently wrote:

> that the Western family 'changed more dramatically in the latter half of the twentieth century than in any comparable span of time in our history'. (Furstenberg 2011, p. 192)

Is the same generalization true for the rest of the world? Though conditions differ so greatly that it is difficult to generalize, Furstenberg's comment is certainly equally applicable to the East and South East Asian family, including China, and to the family in Latin America, though arguably not to the South Asian family.

What are some of the socioeconomic changes that have been impinging on family life? Firstly, the rapid pace of urbanization and rapid economic development in many parts of the world that were once characterized as 'less developed countries' has dramatically changed the options and the imperatives for family members. Latin America and East Asia are now heavily urbanized regions, and although urbanization is not as advanced in the rest of Asia or in Africa, even there some countries that were once predominantly rural, such as Indonesia, have passed the 50% urban population threshold. With more of the population drawn into the cities, and rising levels of education, particularly for women, the forces of globalization and neo-liberal economic structures have both drawn more women into the workforce and lessened job security. Then there have been remarkable technological developments in such fields as high-speed transportation, thus cutting travel times, and in social media, enabling a wider net of contacts to be maintained and providing instantaneous access to knowledge of all kinds. Technological developments in the medical field have widened the options in extending life and in avoiding conception and birth, options which bring with them not only benefits but also a range of ethical issues.

In Asia, the world's most populous continent, trends in family change differ greatly between subregions and countries. Common elements in most cases are rising levels of female education and labour force participation, fertility decline, and a trend towards later age at childbearing (partly resulting from postponement of marriage), and rising rates of divorce. Both rising levels of education and economic (and advertising) pressures to maintain or increase consumption worked to propel women into the labour force. Ideological changes led to increased demands for equality in the workplace and in the home. Improved contraception has both loosened the tight connection between sexual gratification and marriage and enabled married women to postpone childbearing.

Family structures differ markedly between Asian countries, but it is possible to detect general patterns which differentiate South East Asia from the other main regions of Asia. Rigidly patrilineal kinship systems characterize northwest India, China and Korea, with patrilocal residence. In such systems, 'daughters were effectively lost to their parents when they married' (Das Gupta 2010, p. 128); women had no role as sister and daughter, but only as wife and mother. In the Indian system, there was resistance to enabling husbands and wives to be too emotionally attached, as this could threaten the unity of the patriarchal family (Caldwell et al. 1982). In contrast, the South East Asian region is characterized by bilateral kinship, which provides flexibility in post-marital residence, and continuing close relations between a woman and her natal family. In this region, there is a desire for children of both sexes; it is noteworthy that the only part of South East Asia that suffers from distorted sex ratios at birth due to misuse of pre-natal diagnostic techniques for non-medical purposes is northern Vietnam, which is the one area of South East Asia where most of the population does not follow a bilateral kinship system (Jones 2009, p. 13; Guilmoto 2012a). South East Asian kinship systems also facilitate the option of divorce if a marriage turns out unsatisfactorily.

These family systems have major health implications, for example, through the distribution of resources within and across generations. How resources are allocated depends on relationships of authority within families. Those in the family whose status is relatively low (typically based on sex, age, or birth order) tend to receive fewer resources. In societies where there is a strong preference for male children, infant mortality is higher among girls than boys (for India, see Das Gupta 1987; for Egypt, see Yount 2003; for China, see Coale and Banister 1994; Croll 2000), though in recent years the son preference has been manifested more in sex-selective abortion, as a result of the ability to detect the sex of the fetus at an early stage (Guilmoto 2012b).

Accepted gender roles within families determine how much time women spend in the paid labour force as compared with childrearing and housework. There are complex implications for resource allocation and health. In Western countries, working women's greater earnings and increased status have given them more control over resources, but have probably contributed to increases in divorce rates and in rates of non-marital childbearing, both of which have resulted in increased poverty among women and children. Also, the dual responsibilities of market work and childrearing and housework responsibilities (see Hochschild and Machung 1989) can take a toll on women's physical and mental health, and potentially have adverse effects on other members of the family.

Smaller families

The size and composition of households is a dynamic process, changing over the life cycle as children are born, grow up, and leave the family. Migration affects household composition, as does the decreasing prevalence of extended family forms where these were once more prominent. Smaller nuclear, or conjugal, families do not necessarily mean fewer family relationships; as in many parts of the world, including Western countries, families tend to be 'residentially nuclear but functionally extended', in the words of a Filipino sociologist (Castillo 1979), and engage in 'intimacy at a distance'. The web of contacts, in other words, can be quite dense although members of the extended family may be living far apart, even in different countries. Revolutionary developments in communications have made such contacts easier to maintain.

Household composition, of course, is not the same as family composition. Solitary living has increased enormously in Western societies. Whereas in 1950, just 10 per cent of households in Europe were one-person households, five decades later, they accounted for 30 per cent of British and 40 per cent of Swedish households (Coontz 2004, p. 975). But solitary residence does not necessarily mean lack of family contact; nor are absent members necessarily uninvolved in family matters. Indeed, maintenance of the role of absent members—including those who live overseas for lengthy periods—both in household functioning and decision-making, is increasingly observed and accepted as part of the reality of a globalizing world with mobile populations (see, e.g. Parrenas 2008; Douglass 2011).

Whether we focus on the residential household or the family, however, the declines in fertility that have taken place almost universally except in parts of sub-Saharan Africa, clearly make for smaller family size. As measured by the total fertility rate (TFR)— the number of children a woman would bear by the end of her reproductive period if she followed the currently prevailing age specific fertility rates throughout her childbearing ages—fertility over the past three decades remained very low in Europe, declining from 1.9 to 1.6 children per woman; it declined from 2.6 to 1.6 in East Asia, from 4.5 to 2.2 in South East Asia, from 5.0 to 2.7 in South Asia, and from 4.2 to 2.2 in Latin America. Only in sub-Saharan Africa did fertility remain really high, still at about 5.0 children per woman in 2010. Fewer children being born into families directly lowers the number of family members living together, though more complex factors also affect family size. In particular, different family types—whether nuclear or some kind of extended family, have different implications for family size. Nuclear families are the norm in Western countries and in a wider range of non-Western countries than was often recognized.

Average household size has been falling almost everywhere. For example, in Indonesia, average household size decreased from 4.87 people in 1971 to 4.27 in 1995 and 3.84 in 2010. In Thailand, it declined from 5.8 in 1970 to 4.6 in 1990, and was expected to continue falling steadily to 3.3 in 2015 (Mason et al. 1993, p. 70). Extended family contacts will, of course, widen the network of interaction, but not to anything like the extent in the past, when an average individual in Thailand had five siblings, six children, ten uncles and aunts, 30 nieces and nephews, 60 first cousins, 120 first cousins of his parents, and 720 second cousins.

When fertility falls to very low levels, there are fewer close relatives for an individual to interact with. An extreme example is the one-child family in China, resulting from a policy that requires over one-third of the population to have only one child, and over another half to have '1.5 children' (i.e. those whose first child is a girl can have a second child); in other words, more than 60 per cent of all Chinese couples are required to have only one child (Gu 2009, pp. 76–80). Where each family has only one child, that child has no siblings, and while he/she may have a number of uncles and aunts, because the parent generation was not yet subject to the one-child family rule, there will be very few cousins. Once the second generation of one-child families emerges, the web of close relatives shrinks further. If two only children, who are themselves the children of only children, marry, between them they will have eight grandparents (living or deceased) and four parents, but no cousins, aunts or uncles at all. Hence extended family relationships disappear in this context. Not only this, but the family responsibility to care for the elderly falls squarely on the young couple.

Many countries have even lower fertility rates than China. Where fertility has fallen to really low levels—TFR below 1.5— half of all women have at most one child (Le Bras 1979). This does not necessarily mean that most children are growing up as only children. For one thing, children are born to a cohort of women whose average number of children is currently higher than suggested by the cross-sectional snapshot provided by period fertility rates. But this aside, many women are not having children at all. The proportion of women not marrying before reaching the end of their reproductive period is now around 15 per cent in Singapore and Myanmar, well above 10 per cent in Japan and Thailand, and considerably higher than this for the tertiary educated in these and some other Asian countries. Having children outside of marriage is rare in these countries. Moreover, some of those who marry are not having children. In European countries, though having children outside of marriage is now common, an increasing proportion of adults are remaining childless; in Western Europe, around 10–20 per cent of the cohort of women born in 1965 remained childless at the end of their reproductive period. However, the situation appears rather different when viewed from the perspective of the child; no children, of course, grow up in no-children families. Among women who have children, many are having just one, but many are having two or more. Taking into account childless women, this can still average out at just above one per woman. As Preston (1976, p. 105) and Le Bras (1979) noted, women with large families contribute disproportionately to the average family size of children.

Comparing the families of five or six children typical of earlier generations and those averaging two children, there are significant differences in the way children are raised and the social dynamics within the family. Typically, in large families, the older children play a role from a young age in assisting with the raising of their younger siblings, and perhaps later in financing their education. With low fertility, parents' attention is focused on just one or two children. This has positive implications for human capital; the investment of money and time by the parents will no doubt assist their one or two children to achieve better results in school and in career-related activities. The trade-off between quantity and quality of children has been resoundingly resolved in favour of quality in the East Asian countries (Montgomery et al. 2000), in Western countries, and more recently in countries as varied in background as Brazil and Iran, and this is a major reason for the very low fertility they are now experiencing. The smaller cohorts of children should also enable government investment in education to achieve more per child.

What are the downsides to small family size? In China, both parents and the government fear the so-called 4–2–1 syndrome. This can be interpreted in two alternative ways: a great deal of attention focused on the one child by two parents and four grandparents, or as a weighty responsibility placed on the one child for the care of two parents and four grandparents as they age. When two only children marry, they will be responsible for four parents and eight grandparents. The young couple can only live with one set of parents, which means that the other half of their parent and grandparent families will be 'empty nesters'. What proportion of families are in this situation? It has certainly risen substantially, though exactly how much needs to be carefully studied. The issue is not unique to China. There are many single-child families throughout East Asia, despite the absence of a one-child policy, though in the other East Asian countries ultra-low fertility is due to a much larger extent than in China to non-marriage, and therefore to a larger proportion of potential couples with no children at all (Frejka et al. 2010, figures 4 and 5).

The issue of 'self-centredness' of only children is also frequently raised—the 'little emperor' syndrome. It is frequently speculated in China that divorce rates will rise with the clash of wills and personalities when two 'little emperors' marry each other. Inherently plausible as these speculations may be, they require evidence and research to back them up.

Delayed marriage and the rise of cohabitation

In Western countries, the 'golden age' of marriage from the 1950s to the 1970s (Festy 1980) has given way to an age of delayed marriage and increased cohabitation. Even though the rise of cohabitation has meant that delays in marriage do not accurately reflect the delay in forming relatively stable unions, overall, union formation and childbearing has been delayed (Mathews and Hamilton 2009). There are large differences between Western countries in the extent of the rise in cohabitation. Three broad groupings are evident. Cohabitation is very common in the Nordic countries, France, the United Kingdom, and the Netherlands (where among those aged 20–34 who are either married or cohabiting, 40 to over 50 per cent are cohabiting); there is an intermediate group of Germanic and Eastern European countries, the United States, and

Australia, where the proportion is around 20 to 30 per cent; and the Southern European countries and Poland, where cohabitation is less common (around 5 to 15 per cent) (OECD 2014).

The United States differs from the countries of Europe in significant ways in matters affecting cohabitation patterns; for example, Americans are more religious than other Westerners, though this religiosity is adapted to a culture of expressive individualism (Cherlin 2009, pp. 103–104, 113). Americans begin to have partners (whether married or cohabiting) at a relatively younger age than most Europeans, and to become parents at a younger age. Marriages and cohabiting relationships in the United States, and to some extent in Great Britain (Kiernan 2003, p. 32; Beaujouan and Ní Bhrolcháin 2011), are far more fragile than in most of Europe. American women are much more likely to spend time as lone parents in their teens or twenties than are women in Western Europe (Cherlin 2009, pp. 16–18). Overall, in the United States, about 41 per cent of births were non-marital in 2010—in other words being borne by single mothers or those in cohabiting relationships (Martin et al. 2012). The widening interval between sexual debut and marriage has exposed many more teenagers to the risk of pregnancy and childbirth outside marriage (Furstenberg 1990, p. 150), although the rate of teenage childbearing has declined considerably over the past decade.

In developing countries, very early marriage has long characterized most of sub-Saharan Africa and South Asia, as well as parts of South East Asia, the Caribbean, and Central America. In recent decades, average age at marriage has risen almost universally, but substantial proportions of women are still marrying very early. Comparable data from surveys conducted in the 1990–2001 period show that across the developing world, more than a third of women currently aged 20–24 had married prior to the age of 18 (Mensch et al. 2005, p. 137).

Unlike Western countries or Latin America, cohabitation does not feature importantly in Asian patterns of partnering. Asia does, however, show remarkable diversity in marriage systems and marriage patterns. While in general, average age at marriage is rising for both males and females throughout Asia, this rise is from a base that varies greatly. It is in East and South East Asia that truly remarkable changes in marriage patterns have taken place. In recent decades, the traditional universal marriage norms have been abandoned and the average age at marriage and proportions not marrying at all have risen sharply (Fig. 10.1.1; for more detail, see Jones 2007; Jones and Gubhaju 2012). However, there are wide differences between countries, and even between different ethnic groups within one country, such as Malays, Chinese, and Indians in Malaysia.

Broadly comparing East Asia, South East Asia, and South Asia, the changes in South East Asia as a whole are not as great as those in East Asia (excluding China), while most of South Asia remains firmly locked in an entirely different pattern of universal, arranged marriage. South Asian marriage systems have turned out to be remarkably enduring. While in East and South East Asia the location of most marriages on the continuum from parent-arranged to self-arranged marriage has shifted decisively towards the self-arranged end, very little such change has occurred in South Asia.

Socioeconomic change is undoubtedly responsible for much of the change in marriage patterns, but it is hard to explain the very high singlehood in Myanmar and the lack of change in Vietnam

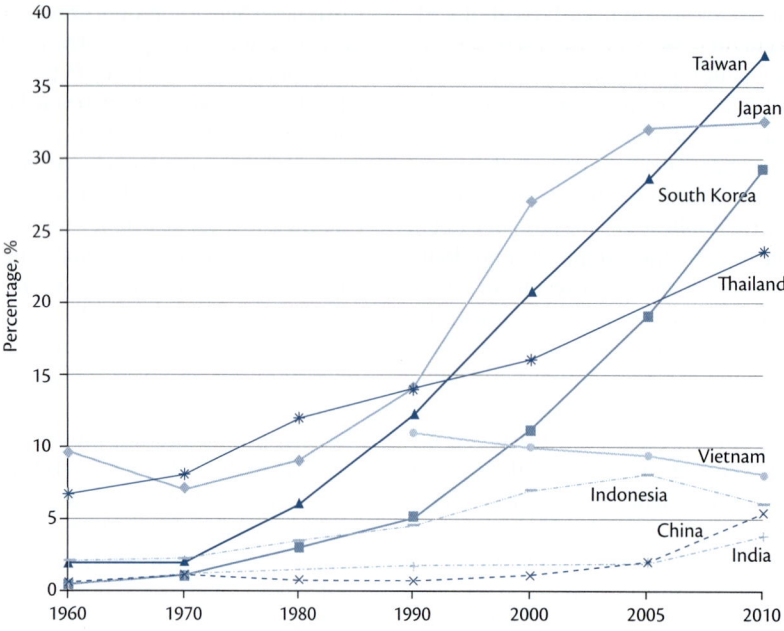

Fig. 10.1.1 Proportion single among females aged 30–34, 1960–2010.
Source: data compiled by the author from population census reports for various years for the countries included.

in these terms. Within East Asia, Chinese marriage patterns differ widely from elsewhere; though average age at marriage for women is rising in China, marriage is 'concertinaed' at ages in the 20s, and by age 30, only a tiny proportion of Chinese women remain single. By contrast, in Japan, Korea, Thailand, Myanmar, Singapore, and among the Chinese population of Malaysia, delays in marriage have been such that substantial proportions of women remain single in their late 30s, an age beyond which not much childbearing takes place. Indonesia has seen gradually rising age at marriage but this has reversed according to the recent 2010 Population Census.

Turning attention to South Asia and South West Asia, The Islamic Republic of Iran shows a strong shift towards a delayed marriage pattern, with the proportion of women single at ages 35–39 not much below that in the Republic of Korea. However, in the Indian subcontinent, the lack of change in arranged marriage patterns in the face of very considerable socioeconomic change is striking. Evidence from a large survey in India (the India Human Development Survey 2005) indicates that:

> Marriage decisions remain within the purview of the family, and less than 5% of the IHDS respondents had a primary role in choosing their husbands. However, nearly 62% of the respondents felt that they were consulted in this decision. (Desai and Andrist 2010, p. 675)

'Consultation' clearly did not go to the extent of arranging for the spouses-to-be to meet; among the respondents who felt they had a choice in partner selection, around 55% met their husbands on or around the day of the wedding. The persistence of early and arranged marriage in India is seen by Desai and Andrist (2010, p. 681) as 'part of a script in which gender is performed by women through a symbolic display of segregation, modesty and chastity, and early marriage is part and parcel of culture in action'.

In Latin America, as in Europe, the key trend in union formation is the rise in cohabitation, which appears to have been just as marked as in Europe, though from a more complex starting point. Latin America was marked by patterns of 'old cohabitation' (characterizing countries with mixed indio, mestizo, and European populations, and those with a history of slavery) and 'new cohabitation' (characterizing countries with more dominant European populations, notably Argentina, Chile, Brazil, Mexico, and Columbia). Cohabitation has increased sharply throughout Latin America in recent decades, though to varying degrees in different countries (Fussell and Palloni 2004; Esteve et al. 2012), and the long-standing educational gradient, whereby the better educated cohabited less and married more, has been attenuated. The factors lying behind these trends are complex, but ideational change in the direction of greater secularization and tolerance of non-conformist behaviour appears to be strongly implicated, except perhaps in Brazil (Esteve et al. 2012).

Late marriage, delayed transition to adulthood, and the role of singles

A trend affecting most of the world is the tendency for children to be dependants for a longer period of time, and to remain in the natal home until a later age. In agrarian and early industrial societies, children frequently began to work at quite a young age. Though age at marriage was young in many such societies, young marrieds frequently continued to live in the home of one or other set of parents until they had the resources to form their own household. The rise of universal schooling tended to delay both entry into the workforce and marriage, to a marked degree in countries where most children continue through secondary education and substantial proportions pursue tertiary education.

In the United States, 50 years ago, the vast majority of women and most men had completed schooling, left home, entered the workforce, and begun families of their own by the time they reached their early 20s (Furstenberg 2010). These transitions have now been considerably delayed (Arnett 2004). Likewise, in much of Asia, extended education and delayed marriage are leading to later home leaving and in general a delay in reaching the milestones that signify adulthood and independence (Xenos et al. 2006). If adolescence is defined as the period between attaining sexual maturity and marriage, then it is a lengthening period in most young Asians' lives, though in South Asia, with the exception of Sri Lanka and to some extent Pakistan, early marriage remains the norm. In most of Asia, unlike in most Western countries (though the 'family-centric' Mediterranean countries share characteristics with Asian countries in this respect), there is a continued tradition of living at home until married, and in many countries, the need to do so is strongly reinforced by the high cost of owning or renting housing, and the convenience of living at home without paying board (on Japan, see Retherford and Ogawa 2006, pp. 17–19; on Singapore, see Jones 2012). Therefore, young people are living longer at home, in an unmarried state.

Many issues have to be negotiated between parents and children in this evolving situation. In East and South East Asian countries, only in the last few decades has extended singlehood become really common, so those who are remaining single into their 30s are a pioneering group, whose roles in family and society are still being negotiated (Situmorang 2007, 2011; Maeda 2008; Ibrahim and Hassan 2009; Tan 2010). Thailand, Singapore, and Myanmar are somewhat different in that over a fairly long period, substantial proportions of men and women have been remaining single, and this has led to adjustments of societal expectations, such that most singles do not feel much pressure to marry from family and friends. Little is known about the role of such singles beyond their immediate family, for example, whether working singles are contributing financially to education of cousins, nephews, and nieces.

In societies where girls were formerly married off on reaching puberty, or shortly thereafter, the transition to adulthood was abrupt and, for many, traumatic. This remains the case in much of Africa and South Asia. But elsewhere in Asia, delayed marriage has led to an extended period of adolescence between puberty and marriage, raising issues about sexuality and relationships with the opposite sex that simply did not arise in times of early, parent-arranged marriage (Lloyd et al. 2005). In Indonesia, for example, extended education for girls, long past the age at which their grandmothers were already married and having children, and widened employment opportunities, has brought them out of the household and into daily contact, not only with a range of men, but also with the stimulus of sexually explicit material through movies, videos, magazines, books, and the Internet. Premarital sexual activity is taken for granted in many of these information sources, but the material is designed to stimulate and titillate rather than to educate. Very little sex education is provided in schools or other contexts (Utomo and McDonald 2009, p. 137). At the same time, influences deriving from religion and ethnicity are still strong, and in some ways growing stronger. 'Faced with the conservative forces of idealized morality portrayed through religion, on the one hand, and Western influences promoting a more liberal approach on the other, it is little wonder that many teenagers are confused' (Jones 2002, p. 232).

There are other aspects of delayed marriage to keep in mind. One has to do with the maturity of the marriage partners. Five decades ago, when half of Malay girls in Malaysia were married before they reached age 17, they were unlikely to be emotionally mature at the time they married. But at least co-residence with

one or other set of parents—most commonly the bride's parents—meant a period of 'apprenticeship' into many aspects of married life. Age at marriage has now increased dramatically, and the age at which Malay women are bearing their first child is 4 years older than for their mother's generation and 7 years older than their grandmother's generation; some of them are having their first child in their mid to late 30s. There are a number of possible implications of later childbearing in both Asian and Western countries. Women are no doubt emotionally more mature when they are bearing their children, but they and their husbands may be more settled in 'child-free' ways, requiring a greater adjustment when the first child comes along than for couples who married at a younger age. The window of opportunity for having a second child is also very small when childbearing is postponed to these ages. Furthermore, there is a somewhat greater risk of birth abnormalities occurring when the mother and/or father are older. The greater availability of *in vitro* fertilization and assisted reproductive technologies enables more older mothers to have babies, but the risks of multiple pregnancies and premature births could contribute to chronic health problems in the children.

Divorce

In the second half of the twentieth century, divorce rates were on the whole higher in Western countries, particularly the United States and Russia, than in most of Asia (Dommaraju and Jones 2012, table 1). In South Asian countries, divorce is a rare event; divorce is not a feasible way out of a disharmonious marriage, because the options of returning to the natal family, or of earning an independent income, are not generally open to a divorced woman. However, the gap between Western and East Asian countries has narrowed because divorce rates stopped rising in many Western countries around the 1980s, while in East Asian countries, divorce rates have been rising steadily since 1980, particularly in the period since 1990 in the case of Japan, Republic of Korea, and Hong Kong. The rise in Republic of Korea was particularly sharp between 1995 and 2000—the period in which the Asian financial crisis occurred. In China, freeing up of divorce regulations in 2001 and 2003 may have contributed to the sharp rise in divorce rates in the 2000–2005 period. In Taiwan, as in other East Asian societies, increase in divorce has taken place in a context of decreased prevalence of marriage. The chance of re-marriage after divorce has declined (Yang and Tsai 2009), indicating a growing acceptance of and perhaps preference for singlehood.

Japanese divorce rates have risen to such an extent that Japan can no longer be considered as a society characterized by low levels of marital dissolution. About one-third of Japanese marriages are now likely to end in divorce (Raymo et al. 2004). Traditional marriage stability in Japan, while it did not necessarily have much to do with whether a marriage was happy, at least gave some assurance that children would be cared for, and that wives could expect economic security. With the awareness of increasing fragility of marriage, decisions about whether to marry and about whether to raise children when single motherhood is a possibility, come more into play (Bumpass et al. 2009, p. 223).

Trends in divorce in East Asia appear, then, to be going the way of the West, and partly for the same reasons (Dommaraju and Jones 2012). Substantial increases in divorce rates in East Asian countries signify a significant change in circumstances and attitudes to divorce, because in the past divorce carried a considerable stigma, and the pressure to remain in a disharmonious marriage for 'the sake of the children' and also for the sake of appearances and family honour, was very strong. It would appear that factors such as increasing economic independence of women, and the pressures (and widened range of personal contacts) in the big city environments in which an increasing proportion of East Asians live, are influencing divorce trends.

In Western countries, divorce rates no longer reflect very accurately trends in the breakdown of long-term relationships, because of the rise of cohabitation. It is impossible for couples who are not officially married to divorce. Understanding the relationship of cohabitation to breakdown of unions requires analysis of the proportion of cohabiting relationships that are dissolved; the proportion that are converted to marriages; and the proportion of such marriages that are dissolved. In Europe, around one-third of cohabiting unions are dissolved within 5 years (Kiernan 2003, table 1), considerably higher than the proportion of marriages that are dissolved within the same length of time; of cohabiting relationships that are converted to marriages, divorce rates also tend to be higher than for marriages that did not commence with a cohabiting relationship, though 'when the pre-existing characteristics of those who cohabit are taken into account, the risk of marriage breakdown is no different from and may be lower among those cohabiting before marriage than among those who marry directly' (Beaujouan and Ní Bhrolcháin 2011, p. 19). In any case, official figures on divorce trends clearly do not fully reflect the breakdown of long-term relationships, many of which, both marital and cohabiting relationships, involve children. It might be noted that in Japan, while divorce rates do not fully reflect relationship breakdown because cohabitation is increasing, the breakdown of cohabiting relationships rarely involves children, because very few children are born to cohabiting couples.

Non-marital childbearing, divorce, and effects on children

In Europe, 'sexual activity, childbearing and marriage have become disconnected so that increasingly it is socially acceptable to have one without either of the other two. But this has happened in different ways in different parts of Europe' (Pritchett and Viarengo 2012, p. 67). Notably, in northwest Europe, childbearing remains reasonably robust, much of it in non-marital relationships; in many countries of Eastern and southern Europe, though, marriage rates remain high and extramarital births are rare but fertility is very low.

Changing conventions about marriage and divorce in the West and in East Asian countries have multiple causes. In the West, 'family relations have become more discretionary; a greater premium is placed on emotional gratification and a lower value on obligation and authority' (Furstenberg 1990, p. 153). Such factors, stressed in 'second demographic transition' theory (van de Kaa 1987; Lesthaeghe 2010), have explanatory power for Western countries and perhaps for Japan; for East Asia more generally, however, more important than individualism may be women's willingness to break from the shackles of patriarchal structures in a context of widened economic opportunities. Moreover, some weakening in these countries of community perceptions of divorce as a

disgraceful event has undoubtedly lowered the bar to the decision to divorce.

In all these contexts, however, the effect of divorce on children needs to be considered. As Carlson and England (2011, p. 2) put it: 'The freedom to leave unhappy relationships might be counted as a victory for adults, but the same cannot be said for children'. Multiple studies suggest that children whose parents divorce have a greater risk during late childhood and early adolescence of experiencing 'school failure, delinquency, precocious sexual behavior, and substance abuse' (Furstenberg 1990, pp. 161–162). Nevertheless, the effect of divorce on children is a complex subject. Many studies suffer from methodological shortcomings, and assessments differ, particularly with regard to whether family conflict produces more adverse effects on children than divorce itself (Cherlin 2009, pp. 19–24, 192–197).

The effect of marital disruption (and more generally, in the era of cohabitation, relationship disruption) on children is a controversial and emotional issue. Many studies show that children raised by solo mothers or by a mother in unstable relationships are more likely to experience emotional and behavioural problems than children growing up in stable married families. For example, in Britain, 'children born into cohabiting families where the parents had separated and solo mothers who had not married the natural father. … were around three times more likely than children in stable married families to be exhibiting behavioural problems' (Kiernan and Mensah 2009). However, careful control for factors lying behind the differences in the family situation in which children grow up is necessary before attributing the behaviour to the family situation itself. In the British study under discussion, controls for various factors—notably the mental well-being of mothers and family poverty—attenuated the differences, though they did not eliminate them entirely (Kiernan and Mensah 2009). On the other hand, when the child's emotional well-being was the dependent variable, it appeared that the parental socioeconomic circumstance and mother's mental well-being may fully account for differences between children living in different family trajectories.

In sub-Saharan Africa, patterns whereby many fathers do not continue to live with their children are common (Adepoju and Mbugua 1997; Therborn 2004, pp. 177–181). In parts of Africa characterized by polygyny, the mother–son bond tends to be strong. In South Africa, among the African population, in 2007 only 29 per cent of children aged 17 years or younger were living with both parents, while 43 per cent were living with mother only, and 26 per cent were living with neither parent (Republic of South Africa 2012, table 2.6). Almost half of children whose father was alive had no contact with him; unfortunately, in South Africa, 'family instability in childhood plays a major role in setting young people on pathways to adulthood that potentially compromise their life chances' (Goldberg 2013, p. 246).

Ageing and the family

The trend towards an older population is an inexorable one in most parts of the world. Japan has the oldest age structure of any country in the world (23 per cent of the population aged 65+), followed by Europe as a whole (16 per cent). Some Asian countries—Republic of Korea, China, Singapore, and Thailand—are well along in the ageing process, with between 8 per cent and 11 per cent elderly. But many of the higher-fertility countries in South Asia and Africa have only around 3 or 4 per cent in the over-65 age groups. Everywhere, however, the percentage of elderly is rising, and by 2030 it is expected to reach 30 per cent in Japan, 22 per cent in Europe, and 17 per cent in China and Thailand.

There is little doubt that issues related to population ageing will be central, not only to national policy reactions to ultra-low fertility, but also to family level adjustments needed to cope with radically altered population structures. At an aggregate level, the issues can be well illustrated by trends in ageing support ratios—that is, the ratio of the population aged 20–64 to the population aged 65+. Admittedly, the age limits used for this calculation do not accurately reflect the actual dependency situation, which depends on the ages at which people actually enter and withdraw from the labour force, and on the proportion of the elderly requiring various kinds of support (in the case of physical support, usually quite small). But as a general indicator, the ageing support ratio does give a sense of the trends which are so dramatic that modification of these ages will not alter the picture greatly.

The ageing support ratios were vastly different in different world regions in 1980 (see Fig. 10.1.2). Since then, they have fallen sharply in East Asia and South America, and this sharp decline is expected to continue until 2050. South Asia is 35 years behind East Asia in reaching an ageing support ratio as low as 8. In the 40 years between 2010 and 2050, the ageing support ratio will halve in Japan, and will fall to less than one-third its current level in countries such as China, Thailand, and Brazil. Leaving aside Africa, where the decline in the ageing support ratio will be very

slow, and South Asia, where it will be relatively slow, there will be a marked convergence in ageing support ratios in the different regions at very low levels—around 2 to 3. Such declines will require major adjustments of policies with regard to income support programmes, orientation of health services to give much more weight to gerontology, and labour market policy, including retirement ages.

It should be noted that living arrangements of the elderly differ considerably in Asia from those in Western countries, with a much higher proportion living with a child or grandchild (United Nations 2005). And although the percentage of elderly Japanese and Koreans living with a child or grandchild has been gradually declining, it does not appear likely to reach levels as low as in France or the United States. Demographic trends do, however, raise issues about whether the family can be relied on as in the past to provide care for those elderly who need it. There are a number of aspects to the problem. The first is the sharply declining ratio of potential carers to numbers of elderly, as crudely indicated by trends in the support ratios. The number of living children of older persons has been declining through movement of smaller birth cohorts into the main 'caring ages'. And as documented by Schroder-Butterfill and Kreager (2005) in a study in East Java, de facto childlessness may differentially affect the poorest and most vulnerable groups. The second is that a high proportion of the potential carers (usually women) are now drawn into the paid workforce (consistent with government policy in these countries), and are therefore not available for full-time caring work. Moreover, many of these potential carers are in the so-called

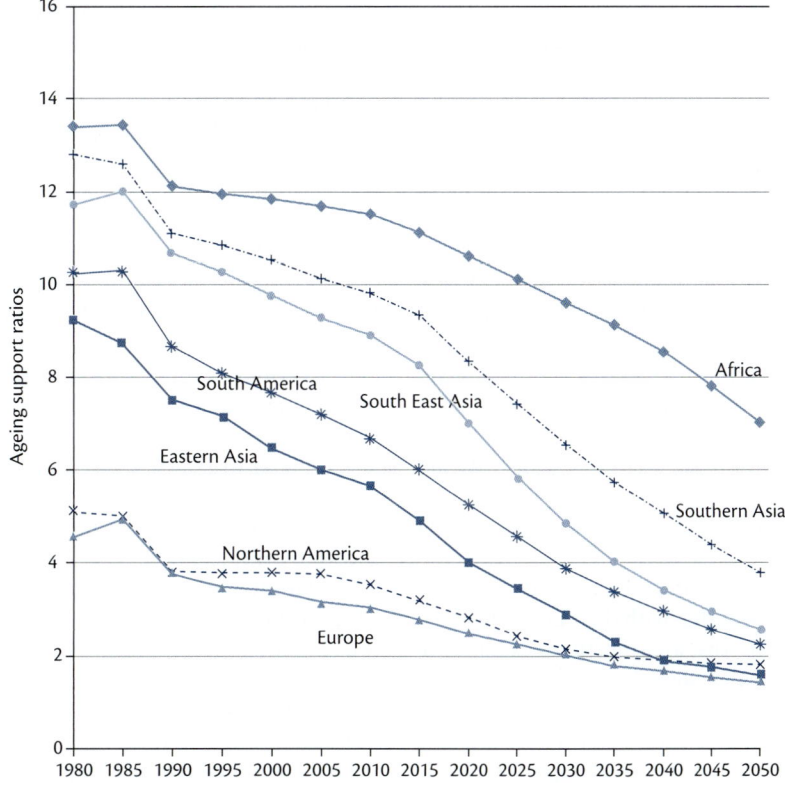

Fig. 10.1.2 Ageing support ratios (population aged 20–64/65+) by region.

Source: data from the detailed indicators in United Nations Population Division, *World Population Prospects: The 2012 Revision*, Copyright © 2014 United Nations, available from http://esa.un.org/unpd/wpp/unpp/panel_indicators.htm.

sandwich generation, required to support not only the grandparent generation but also their own children who are spending a longer time living with (and depending on) their parents. The third is that, despite the general improvement in health status of the elderly at any given age, the rising proportion of the elderly and the rising proportion of the elderly who are 'old-old' (i.e. 75 years and above) will inevitably mean a rising load of frail and disabled elderly, who need full-time care. The ratio of elderly population who suffer from senile dementia to non-working women at various ages is projected to rise substantially over the coming two decades in Japan (Ogawa 2006, figure 11). This suggests that Japan will not be able to rely on the traditional family support network to care for the infirm elderly; the rise in the burden placed on middle-aged Japanese women providing in-home nursing care will simply be too great.

There will be less possibility of the family providing intensive care for the increasing number of disabled or frail elderly in Asian countries, for three reasons: the lowered proportion of children per elderly person, the increased labour force participation of women (the traditional carers), and the movement of children of the elderly to other localities. These trends have major implications for policy on elder care. Despite the tradition in Asian families of caring for family members in various kinds of need, and official rhetoric about the key support role of the Asian family as a fundamental (and by implication, unchanging) characteristic of Asian societies, this traditional reliance on family will be subjected to intensive pressures. Governments will almost inevitably be forced to step in.

We need to bear in mind that co-residence is not the only indicator of close caring relationships. Assistance can notionally be divided into three categories: financial assistance, emotional support, and physical support. The first two of these do not require co-residence, particularly in the age of the mobile phone. In Thailand, there has been an extraordinary rise in the proportion of the elderly living in houses with a telephone—from 15 per cent in 1994 to 76 per cent in 2007. Moreover, while the proportion of elderly living in the same house as a child is slowly declining in Thailand, the proportion is considerably higher if those living in close proximity are included (Knodel and Chayovan 2008, p. 41).

The care needs of the elderly should not be exaggerated. The great majority of the elderly do not need care; for example, in Thailand, more than 80 per cent of those in their 70s and even 65 per cent of those aged over 80, say that they can care for themselves (Knodel and Chayovan 2011, table 1). The positive contributions made by the elderly in society and family, for example through taking care of grandchildren and through serving as mentors and confidants of their grandchildren as they enter adolescence, need to be recognized and supported (Hamid and Yahaya 2008; Ananta and Ariffin 2009).

The challenge, of course, in harnessing the capacities of grandparents to develop a special relationship with their grandchildren, is to avoid burdening them with what are sometimes exploitative child-minding arrangements. In all societies, the role of grandparents in childcare appears to be greatly valued, as opposed to the alternatives of formal childcare arrangements or, in some countries, reliance on domestic servants. 'Grandparent care is commonly viewed as the "next best thing" to parental care, and is highly valued for its supposed intrinsic benefits: the fostering of closer inter-generational relationships, the quality of grandparent care in contrast with the formal market, and the satisfaction that grandparents apparently derive from the caregiving role' (Jenkins 2010, p. 6; see also Wheelock and Jones 2002). However, grandparents are not always so positive about the role, which can be very stressful, especially when they feel that they lack the choice to determine the parameters of their caregiving.

The family, development, and health

Being born into the wrong family can almost guarantee a difficult life. 'The family has long been a mechanism by which advantage—and disadvantage—is transferred across generations' (Carlson and England 2011, p. 9). In the American context, Lareau and Cox argue that class differences in parents' cultural resources (e.g. knowledge necessary to help their children interact with institutions—such as gaining access to college-prep courses in high school and navigating the college admission process) serve to exacerbate inequality in the life chances of youth from different classes, especially in getting a college education (see Carlson and England 2011, p. 14). In Indonesia, only 2 per cent of the children of the poorest 20 per cent of the population continue to tertiary education, compared with 40 per cent of children of the richest 20 per cent.

From a public health perspective, issues abound in relation to conventional family structures as well as to rapid changes in these structures. Many examples could be given, but one will be chosen here: reproductive health issues arising from two contrasting situations—patterns of early marriage and childbearing in Africa and South Asia, and delays in marriage in other developing countries.

In many sub-Saharan African countries, as well as in Bangladesh and parts of India, data from the 1980s and 1990s showed that more than 10 per cent of women in their early 20s had had a child by age 15, and between a quarter and a half had a child by age 18 (Singh 1998, table 2). In conditions of high mortality, 'socialization processes that support and encourage early marriage and childbearing are often deeply entrenched' (Singh 1998, p. 133), and these socialization processes do not change rapidly in the face of declining mortality. The dangers of early childbearing to the health of mother and child are well known. But other dangers emerge when marriage is delayed and young people are exposed to the risks of premarital intercourse for longer periods of time: a greater risk of unintended pregnancies, induced abortion and sexually transmitted diseases. Increased levels of infection by sexually transmitted diseases and HIV can affect young women's health and indeed survival, the outcome of their pregnancies, as well as their future fertility. Yet policies in many countries make it difficult for the unmarried to obtain access to contraception.

The family is seen in most countries as the key institution on which a stable society is built. Thus changes in family form and function are normally suspected of threatening the social order. One concern tends to be about ageing, and whether the family will continue to have the capacity to provide the necessary physical, social, and emotional support for the elderly as their share of the population increases. Delayed marriage also leads to disquiet, though not, in most countries, to specific policies to encourage marriage. But it raises important issues about the role of singles in society, as well as practical issues such as their access to contraception, which proves to be divisive in many countries.

Family policy in many countries tends to be conservative in promoting the generally accepted family values. The model of universal heterosexual marriage in which children are raised in an intact family until they marry and leave home is the norm. In Asian countries, this of course remains overwhelmingly the main family form, and there is a great deal to be done to enhance the quality of life for mainstream families of this kind. One key need is to develop policies that will facilitate marriage and enable women and men to combine work with childrearing—to avoid the low fertility trap that East Asian countries have perhaps entered into, but also to enable women to realize the potential resulting from their higher levels of education, without succumbing to the exhaustion of the 'double shift'. At the same time, in countries such as India, Bangladesh, and Indonesia, stricter enforcement of legal minimum ages at marriage is needed, to lower the proportion of girls being married below this age.

But there are also other family forms in all societies, including childless couples, those cohabiting without entering formal marriage, blended families following re-marriage, the various kinds of lesbian/gay/bisexual/transgender (LGBT) pairings (Blasius 2001), single parents post divorce raising a child or children, and singles continuing to live with parents until into their 30s. The reality of considerable pluralism in family types and functions needs to be recognized. It is important that those who are not in mainstream family relationships are not made to feel ostracized and discriminated against by policy.

On elder care, increased strain will be placed on families whose characteristics and circumstances are changing in ways that will make it increasingly harder to deal with these strains. For example, in India, the percentage of elderly people is expected to double in 27 years after 2010, to 10.5 per cent. In Thailand, this percentage is expected to increase by 2.5 times over the same period, to 20.5 per cent. Although the percentage of elderly in India in 2037 will be only half that in Thailand and only a third that in Japan, even the smaller increase that India faces poses significant challenges. The policy emphasis in all countries must be on active ageing, financial independence, and a positive attitude towards the contribution the elderly make within families. Nonetheless, an increasing role of government in elder care cannot be avoided. The retirement age in many countries also needs to be increased, as it reflects the life expectancy situation decades ago, and will be increasingly untenable in terms of providing income maintenance for the rapidly increasing number of retirees. The extent to which government needs to replace the role of family in elder care, and its capability of doing so, will vary across regions.

Acknowledgements

Text extracts from Desai, Sonalde and Lester Andrist, Gender scripts and age at marriage in India, *Demography*, Volume 47, Issue 3, pp. 667–687, Copyright © 2010, reproduced with kind permission from Springer Science+Business Media.

References

Adepoju, A. and Mbugua, W. (1997). The African family: an overview of changing forms. In A. Adepoju (ed.) *Family, Population and Development in Africa*, pp. 41–59. London: Zed Books.

Ananta, A. and Ariffin, E.N. (2009). *Older Persons in Southeast Asia: An Emerging Asset*. Singapore: Institute of Southeast Asian Studies.

Arnett, J.J. (2004). *Emerging Adulthood: The Winding Road from the Late Teens through the Twenties*. New York: Oxford University Press.

Beaujouan, É. and Ní Bhrolcháin, M. (2011). Cohabitation and marriage in Britain since the 1970s. *Population Trends*, 145, 35–59.

Blasius, M. (2001). *Sexual Identities, Queer Politics: Lesbian, Gay, Bisexual and Transgender Politics*. Princeton, NJ: Princeton University Press.

Bumpass, L.L., Rindfuss, R.R., Choe, M.K., and Tsuya, N.O. (2009). The institutional context of low fertility: the case of Japan. *Asian Population Studies*, 5(3), 215–35.

Caldwell, J.C., Reddy, P.H., and Caldwell, P. (1982). The causes of demographic change in rural South India: a micro-approach. *Population and Development Review*, 8(4), 689–728.

Carlson, M.J. and England, P. (eds.) (2011). *Social Class and Changing Families in an Unequal America*. Stanford, CA: Stanford University Press.

Castillo, G. (1979). *Beyond Manila: Philippine Rural Problems in Perspective*. Ottawa: International Development Research Center.

Cherlin, A.J. (2009). *The Marriage-Go-Round: The State of Marriage and the Family in America Today*. New York: Alfred A. Knopf.

Coale, A.J. and Banister, J. (1994). Five decades of missing females in China. *Demography*, 31(3), 459–79.

Coontz, S. (2004). The world historical transformation of marriage. *Journal of Marriage and Family*, 66(4), 974–9.

Croll, E.J. (2000). *Endangered Daughters: Discrimination and Development in Asia*. London: Routledge.

Das Gupta, M. (1987). Selective discrimination against female children in rural Punjab, India. *Population and Development Review*, 13(1), 77–100.

Das Gupta, M. (2010). Family systems, political systems and Asia's 'missing girls': the construction of son preference and its unravelling. *Asian Population Studies*, 6(2), 123–52.

Desai, S. and Andrist, L. (2010). Gender scripts and age at marriage in India. *Demography*, 47(3), 667–87.

Dommaraju, P. and Jones, G. (2012). Divorce trends in Asia. *Asian Journal of Social Science*, 39(6), 725–50.

Douglass, M. (2011). *Global Householding and International Migration Research—Paradigms, Emerging Dynamics and Public Policy in East and Southeast Asia*. Paper presented at Workshop on Householding in Transition: Emerging Dynamics in 'Developing' East and Southeast Asia, National University of Singapore, 25–26 July.

Esteve, A., Lesthaeghe, R., and Lopez-Gay, A. (2012). The Latin American cohabitation boom. 1970–2007. *Population and Development Review*, 38(1), 55–81.

Festy, P. (1980). On the new context of marriage in Western Europe. *Population and Development Review*, 6(2), 311–15.

Frejka, T., Jones, G., and Sardon, J.-P. (2010). East Asian childbearing patterns and policy developments. *Population and Development Review*, 36(3), 579–606.

Furstenberg, F.F. (1990). Coming of age in a changing family system. In S.S. Feldman and G.R. Elliott (eds.) *At the Threshold: The Developing Adolescent*, pp. 147–70. Cambridge: Harvard University Press.

Furstenberg, F.F. (2010). On a new schedule: transitions to adulthood and family change. *Future of the Child*, 20, 67–87.

Furstenberg, F.F. (2011). The recent transformation of the American family: witnessing and exploring social change. In M.J. Carlson and P. England (eds.) *Social Class and Changing Families in an Unequal America*, pp. 192–220. Stanford, CA: Stanford University Press.

Fussell, E. and Palloni, A. (2004). Persistent marriage regimes in changing times. *Journal of Marriage and Family*, 66(5), 1201–13.

Goldberg, R.E. (2013). Family instability and pathways to adulthood in Cape Town, South Africa. *Population and Development Review*, 39, 231–56.

Goode, W.J. (1963). *World Revolution and Family Patterns*. New York: The Free Press.

Gu, B. (2009). The arrival of low fertility in China. In G. Jones, P.T. Straughan, and A. Chan (eds.) *Ultra-low Fertility in Pacific Asia: Trends, Causes and Policy Issues*, pp. 73–95. London: Routledge.

Guilmoto, C. (2012a). *Sex Imbalances at Birth: Trends, Differentials and Policy Implications*. Bangkok: UNFPA.

Guilmoto, C. (2012b). Son preference, sex selection and kinship in Vietnam. *Population and Development Review*, 38(1), 31–54.

Hamid, T.A. and Yahaya, N. (2008). National policy for the elderly in Malaysia: achievements and challenges. In H.G. Lee (ed.) *Ageing in Southeast and East Asia: Family, Social Protection and Policy Challenges*, pp. 108–33. Singapore: Institute of Southeast Asian Studies.

Hochschild, A. and Machung, A. (1989, *The Second Shift: Working Parents and the Revolution at Home*. New York: Viking Penguin.

Ibrahim, R. and Hassan, Z. (2009). Understanding singlehood from the experiences of never-married Malay Muslim women in Malaysia: some preliminary findings. *European Journal of Social Sciences*, 8(3), 395–405.

Jenkins, B. (2010). Grandparent childcare in Australia: a literature review. *Elder Law Review*, 6, 1–19.

Jones, G.W. (2002). The changing Indonesian household. In K. Robinson and S. Bessell (eds.) *Women in Indonesia: Gender, Equity and Development*, pp. 291–34. Singapore: Institute of Southeast Asian Studies.

Jones, G.W. (2007). Delayed marriage and very low fertility in Pacific Asia. *Population and Development Review*, 33(3), 453–78.

Jones, G.W. (2009). Women, marriage and family in Southeast Asia. In T. Devasahayam (ed.) *Gender Trends in Southeast Asia: Women Now, Women in the Future*, pp. 12–30. Singapore: Institute of Southeast Asian Studies.

Jones, G.W. (2012). Population policy in a prosperous city-state: dilemmas for Singapore. *Population and Development Review*, 38(2), 311–36.

Jones, G.W. and Gubhaju, B. (2012). Marriage trends in Southeast Asia. In L. Williams and P. Guest (eds.) *Southeast Asian Demography*, pp. 65–91. Ithaca, NY: Southeast Asia Program, Cornell University.

Kiernan, K. (2003). *Cohabitation and Divorce Across Nations and Generations*. CASE paper 65, Centre for Analysis of Social Exclusion. London: London School of Economics.

Kiernan, K.E. and Mensah, F.K. (2009). Unmarried parenthood, family trajectories, parent and child well being. In K. Hansen, H. Joshi, and S. Dex (eds.) *Children of the 21st Century: From Birth to Age 5*, pp. 77–94. Bristol: Policy Press.

Knodel, J. and Chayovan, N. (2008). *Population Ageing and the Well-Being of Older Persons in Thailand: Past Trends, Current Situation, and Future Challenges*. Papers in Population Ageing Series, Number 5. Bangkok: UNFPA Thailand and Asia and the Pacific Regional Office.

Knodel, J. and Chayovan, N. (2011). *Intergenerational Family Care for and by Older People in Thailand*. Paper presented in Conference on Shifting Boundaries of Care Provision in Asia: Policy and Practice Changes, Asia Research Institute, National University of Singapore, 14–15 March.

Le Bras, H. (1979). *Child and Family*. Paris: OECD.

Lesthaeghe, R. (2010). The unfolding story of the second demographic transition. *Population and Development Review*, 36(2), 211–51.

Lloyd, C., Behrman, J., Stromquist, N., and Cohen, B. (eds.) (2005). *The Changing Transitions to Adulthood in Developing Countries: Selected Studies*. Washington, DC: National Academies Press.

Maeda, E. (2008). Relational identities of always-single Japanese women. *Journal of Social and Personal Relationships*, 25(6), 967–87.

Martin, J.A., Hamilton, B.E., Ventura, S.J., Osterman, M.J., Wilson, E.C., and Mathews, T.J. (2012). Births: final data for 2010. *National Vital Statistics Reports*, 61(1), 1–72.

Mason, A., Phananiramai, M., and Poapongsakorn, N. (1993). Households and their characteristics. In B.O. Campbell, A. Mason, and E.M. Pernia (eds.) *The Economic Impact of Demographic Change in Thailand, 1980–2015*, pp. 219–28. Honolulu, HI: University of Hawaii Press.

Mathews, T.J. and Hamilton, B.E. (2009). *Delayed Childbearing: More Women are Having Their First Child Later in Life*. NCHS Data Brief, No. 21, Atlanta, GA: Centers for Disease Control and Prevention.

McDonald, P. (1992). Convergence or compromise in historical family change? In E. Berquo and P. Xenos (eds.) *Family Systems and Cultural Change*, pp. 15–30. Oxford: Clarendon Press.

Mensch, B.S., Singh, S., and Casterline, J.B. (2005). Trends in the timing of first marriage among men and women in the developing world. In C. Lloyd, J. Behrman, N. Stromquist, and B. Cohen (eds.) *The Changing Transitions to Adulthood in Developing Countries: Selected Studies*, pp. 118–71. Washington, DC: National Academies Press.

Montgomery, M.R., Arends-Kuenning, M., and Mete, C. (2000). The quantity–quality transition in Asia. *Population and Development Review*, 26(Supp.), 223–56.

OECD (2014). *OECD Family Database*. Paris: OECD. Available at: http://www.oecd.org/els/social/family/database.

Ogawa, N. (2006). Population aging and policy options for a sustainable future: the case of Japan. *Genus*, LX1(3–4), 369–410.

Oppong, C. (1992). Traditional family systems in rural settings in Africa. In E. Berquo and P. Xenos (eds.) *Family Systems and Cultural Change*, pp. 69–86. Oxford: Clarendon Press.

Parrenas, R.S. (2008). *The Force of Domesticity: Filipina Migrants and Globalization*. New York: New York University Press.

Preston, S.H. (1976). Family sizes of children and family sizes of women. *Demography*, 13(1), 105–14.

Pritchett, L. and Viarengo, M. (2012). Why demographic suicide? The puzzles of European fertility. *Population and Development Review*, 38(Suppl.), 55–71.

Raymo, J., Iwasawa, M., and Bumpass, L. (2004). Marital dissolution in Japan: recent trends and differentials. *Demographic Research*, 11(14), 395–419.

Republic of South Africa (2012). *White Paper on Families in South Africa*. Pretoria: Department of Social Development.

Retherford, R.D. and Ogawa, N. (2006). Japan's baby bust: causes, implications and policy responses. In F.R. Harris (ed.) *The Baby Bust: Who Will Do the Work? Who Will Pay the Taxes?*, pp. 5–47. Lanham, MD: Rowman and Littlefield Publishers.

Schroder-Butterfill, E. and Kreager, P. (2005). Actual and de facto childlessness in old age: evidence from East Java, Indonesia. *Population and Development Review*, 31(1), 19–55.

Singh, S. (1998). Adolescent childbearing in developing countries: a global review. *Studies in Family Planning*, 29(2), 117–36.

Situmorang, A. (2007). Staying single in a married world: never-married women in Yogyakarta and Medan. *Asian Population Studies*, 3(3), 287–304.

Situmorang, A. (2011). Delayed marriage among lower socio-economic groups in an Indonesian industrial city. In G.W. Jones, T.H. Hull, and M. Mohamad (eds.) *Changing Marriage Patterns in Southeast Asia: Economic and Socio-Cultural Dimensions*, pp. 83–99. London: Routledge.

Tan J.E. (2010). Social relationships in the modern age: never-married women in Bangkok, Jakarta and Manila. *Journal of Comparative Family Studies*, 41(5), 749–65.

Therborn, G. (2004). *Between Sex and Power: Family in the World, 1900–2000*. London: Routledge.

United Nations (2005, *Living Arrangements of Older Persons around the World*. New York: United Nations.

United Nations Population Division (2012). *World Population Prospects: The 2012 Revision*. Available at: http://esa.un.org/unpd/wpp/unpp/panel_indicators.htm.

Utomo, I.D. and McDonald, P. (2009). Adolescent reproductive health in Indonesia: contested values and policy inaction. *Studies in Family Planning*, 40(2), 133–46.

Van de Kaa, D.J. (1987). Europe's second demographic transition. *Population Bulletin*, 42(1), 1–59.

Wheelock, J. and Jones, K. (2002). Grandparents are the next best thing: informal childcare for working parents in urban Britain. *Journal of Social Policy*, 441, 451–52.

Xenos, P., Achmad, S., Lin, H.S., et al. (2006). Delayed Asian transitions to adulthood: a perspective from national youth surveys. *Asian Population Studies*, 2(2), 149–86.

Yang, C.-I. and Tsai, H.-J. (2009). Changes in fertility and marriage rates in Taiwan. In Ya-Chen Chen (ed.) *Women in Taiwan: Sociocultural Perspectives*, pp. 61–82. Indianapolis, IN: University of Indianapolis Press.

Yount, K.M. (2003). Gender bias in the allocation of curative health care in Minia, Egypt. *Population Research and Policy Review*, 22(3), 267–99.

Women, men, and health

Sarah Payne and Lesley Doyal

Women, men, and health: an introduction

This chapter focuses on sex and gender influences on the health of men and women. In recent decades health professionals and policymakers have taken an increased interest in the ways in which the risks of early mortality, and the causes of death and poor health, vary for men and women. At the same time research in the medical and social sciences has helped to identify more closely the significance of sex and gender influences on health and also the complexity of such influences.

Although we focus here specifically on sex and gender, it is important to note from the outset that differences between women and men across the life course need to be seen in the context of other influences. Socioeconomic status, ethnicity, age, and sexuality are especially important although more research is needed on the nature of these intersectional influences on health (Iyer et al. 2008). In addition the health gap between women and men varies globally, reflecting levels of development within countries, cultural influences, and health system factors including access to care.

In the following sections we explore some of the explanations for these differences between women and men in their experiences of health and healthcare and their likelihood of developing specific diseases. We begin with an overview of data on male and female mortality and morbidity, before looking at the part played by sex and gender in shaping these variations. The picture which emerges from this exploration suggests quite complex factors are involved and various directions of causality. The next section will therefore look in more detail at the ways in which sex and gender, alongside other determinants of heath such as geographical location, poverty, and socioeconomic status, can influence health. This will be done through examining specific conditions, including coronary heart disease (CHD) and HIV/AIDS. We finish this chapter with a discussion of gender differences in the appropriateness and availability of healthcare.

Men, women, and mortality

Mortality data are widely available on a global basis, are relatively reliable compared with some other measurements of health, and begin to suggest how health differs between women and men—although of course mortality is inevitably a very crude measurement of absence of health. Figures for life expectancy at birth show that women can expect to live longer than their male counterparts in virtually every country (see Table 10.2.1). In 2009, for example, there were only three countries worldwide where men might expect to outlive women: Tonga, Tuvalu, and the Central African Republic (World Health Organization (WHO) 2012a). There were three further countries where men and women had the same life expectancy, while in the remaining 187 countries women could expect to live longer than men.

Many of the countries with a narrow gap between women and men have low levels of life expectancy overall, particularly those in the sub-Saharan region of Africa. For example, in Nigeria, women had only 1 year's advantage over men, while in Sierra Leone, women's life expectancy was 2 years higher than that of men (WHO 2009). These low levels of life expectancy reflect a number of social determinants of health, in particular poverty, poor nutrition, and weak health systems, while for women they also reflect rates high maternal mortality.

The countries where the mortality gap between women and men is narrow also include some with higher average life expectancy. For example, women have only a 2-year advantage over men in Bangladesh and in Pakistan, where life expectancy is in the low 60s, and only a 3-year advantage in Algeria, where overall life expectancy is 72 (WHO 2009).

Where there is a wide gap between women and men, overall life expectancy is higher, although these countries are diverse in terms of economic status, level of development, and culture: Brazil, Malawi, France, and Kyrgyzstan, for example, all have a female advantage of 7 years (WHO 2012a). Countries in Eastern Europe have some of the greatest advantages in female life expectancy. Seven countries with a gap between female and male life expectancy of 10 years or more were formed following the breakup of the USSR, including the Russian Federation where in 2009 the female advantage was 12 years, reflecting a deterioration in men's health prior to the dissolution of the USSR which was followed by further increases in male mortality during social changes experienced in the post-communist era (Pietilä and Rytkönen 2008). One of the most important features of life expectancy, in recent years, has been a trend in richer countries towards a narrowing gap between women and men, reflecting primarily improvements in male health (Organisation for Economic Cooperation and Development (OECD) 2011).

These variations in the gap in life expectancy between women and men across different cultures, time periods, locations, and levels of development indicate that the underlying reasons for such differences do not simply reflect economic factors or specific cultural factors but are explained by quite complex influences involving both biological and social causes, as we shall see.

Mortality can also be explored across the life course, revealing further patterns of difference between males and females.

Table 10.2.1 Differences in male and female life expectancy, 2009—selected countries

Country	Male life expectancy at birth 2009	Female life expectancy at birth 2009	Difference in years (negative = female advantage)	Difference in years in 2004
Russian Federation	62	74	−12	−13
Sri Lanka	65	76	−11	−7
Estonia	70	80	−10	−12
Cambodia	57	65	−8	−7
Republic of Korea	77	83	−6	−8
Finland	77	83	−6	−7
Czech Republic	74	80	−6	−6
United States of America	76	81	−5	−5
Australia	80	84	−4	−5
United Kingdom	78	82	−4	−5
China	72	76	−4	−4
Egypt	69	73	−4	−4
Samoa	68	72	−4	−4
Nepal	65	69	−4	0
Kenya	58	62	−4	+1
Côte D'Ivoire	49	52	−3	−6
Iceland	80	83	−3	−4
India	63	66	−3	−2
Angola	51	53	−2	−4
Sierra Leone	48	50	−2	−3
Pakistan	62	64	−2	−1
South Africa	54	55	−1	−2
Niger	57	58	−1	+1
Somalia	51	51	0	−2
Cameroon	51	51	0	−1

Reproduced with permission from World Health Organization, *Global Health Repository*, Copyright © World Health Organization 2014, available from http://apps.who.int/gho/data/node.main.

In 2011, for example, there were only two countries where girls under 5 years had a higher mortality risk than boys: India and the Solomon Islands (WHO 2012d). In 14 countries, under-5 mortality rates were the same for both, including Bahrain and Sweden, while in the majority of countries, boys under the age of 5 die more frequently than girls. The greatest excess risks for boys are found in sub-Saharan Africa: the under-5 mortality rate for boys is around 174 per 1000 live births in Guinea Bissau compared with a rate of 147 for girls (WHO 2012d). Thinking through the explanations for this range of differences in under-5 mortality rates starts to open up the way in which both sex and gender impact on health chances. The variations in how many girls and boys die before their fifth birthday reflect biological influences, alongside social, economic, and cultural factors, including gender differences which affect the treatment of girl and boy children (Ravindran 2000).

There are also differences in life expectancy at the other end of the life course, although the gap between women and men is often less extreme. For example, although there is a 12-year female advantage in overall life expectancy in Russia, by the age of 65 this advantage has narrowed to 5 years, and is only slighter higher than other countries including Japan, France, and South Africa (OECD 2011; United Nations (UN) 2012).

There are further variations between women and men in what they die from, and again exploring these helps to illustrate the importance of both sex and gender in health chances. Globally, similar proportions of men and women (26 per cent and 29 per cent) die from communicable diseases such as respiratory infections, tuberculosis, or HIV and AIDS (WHO 2011a). A further 62 per cent of men and 65 per cent of women die from non-communicable diseases. However, there are wider differences between men and women in accidental and non-accidental injury, which accounts for twice as many male as female deaths (WHO 2011a). Within this category, men are more likely than women to die as a result of homicide, particularly among younger age groups, with four times as many deaths among men from violence (WHO 2012f). There are also gender differences in the perpetrators of such violence: women are more at risk of being killed by close family, particularly partners, while more men are killed by people outside their circle of family and acquaintances (Hemmenway et al. 2002).

Men are similarly much more likely than women to die or be injured as a result of conflict, and more than 90 per cent of deaths in conflict situations are among men (WHO 2011a). This reflects the ratio of men to women both in formal military organizations and in informal or paramilitary organizations, as well as the roles played by men and women in such organizations. However, conflict situations also increase the risk of poor health for women, including, for example, infectious diseases, accidental death, and sexual violence (WHO and London School of Hygiene and Tropical Medicine (LSHTM) 2010). In addition, displacement among civilian populations due to conflict combined with the loss of employment, land, or source of income creates economic insecurity and poverty, leading to high risks of poor mental health and malnutrition among displaced populations, the majority of whom are female.

There are also differences between men and women in other injury-related deaths. For example, in Mauritius the male road traffic mortality rate is six times greater than the female rate, while in Egypt and the United States, male mortality is twice as high as female road accident mortality (WHO 2011a).

One important cause of female deaths in many countries is maternal mortality. Although this accounts for less than 1 per cent of all female deaths worldwide (WHO 2011a), it is a particularly modifiable cause of death, in that improved healthcare before conception, during pregnancy, and in childbirth can dramatically reduce the risk of death. As such, maternal mortality is also important in explanations of the ways in which the ratio of male:female deaths varies over time and between countries.

More than 280,000 women died in 2010 as a result of complications following pregnancy and childbirth, including problems arising from miscarriage and terminations, and deaths due to women's reduced immunity to some diseases during pregnancy or deterioration in a pre-existing illness as a result of pregnancy or childbirth (WHO 2012f). The risk of maternal mortality varies widely: the majority of deaths occur in less economically developed countries and there has been a significant decline in the number of maternal deaths worldwide in recent years (WHO 2012f). However, the decrease is less than is needed to meet the Millennium Development Goal on maternal mortality, and in some countries rates have increased. For example, the maternal mortality ratio in Chad in 2010 was 1100 maternal deaths per 100,000 live births (up from 920 in 1990) and in Somalia the rate was 1000 per 100,00 live births (an increase from 890 in 1990) (WHO 2012f). These rates compare with very low ones in high-income countries such as Australia, where the rate was 7 per 100,000 live births, and Sweden where the maternal mortality rate was 4.

Variations in the relative risk of dying as a result of pregnancy and childbirth reflect the importance of social determinants of health, particularly poverty, nutrition, the availability of care, as well as maternal age and number of previous pregnancies. In Sierra Leone, for example, three-fifths of births are not attended by skilled health personnel. Similarly, in Niger, a country with a maternal mortality rate of 1600 per 100,000 live births in 2000,

only 11 per cent of women received skilled healthcare during childbirth (WHO 2012f).

Overall, then, women have longer life expectancy than men, although the gap varies between countries and there are differences between women and men for some causes of death. The next section explores alternative indicators of the differences between women and men, focusing on measures of morbidity or illness.

Men, women, and morbidity

Figures for death are useful for broad comparisons between women and men but they also have limitations. Most importantly, they do not accurately capture health experience across the life course. Some causes of death are not usually associated with a period of ill health beforehand—accidental injury, for example—while others may be associated with poor health and low quality of life for some years before death occurs. And of course there are many illnesses which are serious and debilitating but not life-threatening. This is important when exploring health differences between women and men as it is possible that excess male mortality does not equate to a similar disadvantage in terms of health enjoyed during a lifetime.

In the past some writers argued that despite their advantage in life expectancy, women experience poorer health during their lives in comparison with men—the suggestion that 'women get sicker but men die quicker' (Lorber 1997). However, growing evidence on patterns of health across the life course reveal a more complex reality. The gap between women and men widens or narrows at different stages reflecting different age-related patterns of health (Payne 2006). In addition more women are diagnosed with some illnesses—osteoarthritis, for example—while men are more at risk of others, including respiratory diseases (Zandman-Goddard et al. 2012).

One of the reasons why there is no simple story to tell in terms of the burden of ill health among women and men is that morbidity can be measured in a range of ways, and each measure is potentially different in terms of how well it captures the experiences of men and women. The main indicators include self-reported health, based on individuals' judgements of their own health; data on use of healthcare services, including inpatient and community services; and composite indicators of health at population level, such as measures of healthy-adjusted life expectancy (HALE) and measures of disability-adjusted life years (DALYs). Each of these shows a range of differences between women and men which vary across the life course as well as between different demographic groups and between countries.

Self-reported health

There are variations between countries in whether women or men are more likely to report their health as poor. The WHO's *World Health Survey* from 2005, for example, showed that in China, France, India, Malawi, Pakistan, and Portugal more women reported their health as either bad or very bad, while more men reported their health as either good or very good (WHO 2005).

The size of the gap between women and men varied in this survey, with particularly wide differences in the Russian Federation where nearly a quarter of women reported their health as either bad or very bad, compared with 13 per cent of men (WHO 2005)—a finding which contrasts to the much higher mortality among men and highlights the complexity of these measurements and what they mean.

More recent figures (OECD 2011) reveal greater proportions of men who report their health as good or excellent, compared with women, across a range of different countries, including Denmark, France, Poland, and Japan. The gap between women and men is similar despite country-level variations in levels of health overall. For example, in France, 71 per cent of men compared with 66 per cent of women described their health as good or excellent, and while overall levels of good health were much lower in Japan, a similar difference exists between men and women with 31 per cent of men and 28 per cent of women reporting their health as good or excellent.

However, women do not always report poorer health than men. In the OECD data more women (70 per cent) than men (66 per cent) reported their health as good or excellent in Finland in 2011 (OECD 2011). In Australia, national data for 2011–2012 showed that similar proportions of women and men reported their health as either very good or excellent (Australian Bureau of Statistics 2012). Recent data from both the United States and England also reveals little difference between women and men in how they report their health status (Craig and Mindell 2012; Sondik et al. 2012). The range of variations between countries is difficult to interpret. They might reflect variations in the wording of survey questions and some are also influenced by whether or not the data are age-standardized. They might also reflect class or income differences as poorer health is reported by those in lower-income groups, which may include a greater proportion of women in some countries, especially less affluent ones (World Bank 2012). As these differences are based on a subjective measure it is likely that cultural differences are also important in shaping perceptions of health status.

However, the variations, particularly the relatively narrow gap between women and men in richer countries compared with the wider gap found in poorer countries, might also reflect the fact that men in some societies do enjoy better health than women.

One indication of the limitations of self-reported measures comes from studies showing that men who report poor health are more likely to die prematurely than those reporting themselves as being in good health. However, there is less evidence of such an association for women (Benjamins et al. 2004; Jylhä 2009). This may mean that self-report surveys are measuring different things for women and men. One factor that affects self-reported health is the extent to which there are gender differences in knowledge about how some behaviours affect health risks, including smoking and diet, for example, and in how this knowledge is drawn upon in self-assessments of current health status.

Use of health services

Health differences between women and men can also be explored using data on consultation with health professionals. Again these figures are likely to be influenced by more than health status and symptoms alone. A number of considerations affect the use of healthcare, including: economic factors such as whether an individual has health insurance or the means to pay user fees in countries where access to healthcare requires payment; the ability to take time off from either paid employment or caring responsibilities to visit health facilities; and the availability of appropriate services and transport to reach them.

Of course these factors are themselves influenced by gender. For example, women are more often responsible for the care of children and vulnerable dependants and this can limit their ability to seek help when faced with health symptoms. Women are also less likely to be able to finance health consultations—where they do not have command over household expenditure, for example, or where they earn less than men and are less able to afford user fees and charges. In some countries women also need to be accompanied when using services and are therefore dependent on someone being available and willing to take them (Baghdadi 2005; Simkhada et al. 2008).

Again the *World Health Survey 2005* is useful in that it provides data on the same measurement for a number of different countries. These surveys show various patterns of difference between women and men in their use of healthcare. For example, in France, India, the Russian Federation, and China more men than women reported using primary care from general practitioners, community services, and outpatient care in the past 12 months. More women than men reported receiving inpatient treatment in Portugal, Malawi, and China, but in France and the United Kingdom more men reported such treatment. However, in all of these countries more men than women reported not using any form of healthcare in the previous 12 months.

More recent national survey data on use of care is not available for all countries. However figures for the United Kingdom reveal that women consult more often than men throughout the healthcare system and also take more prescribed medication. Similar gendered patterns of consultation are also found in the United States and Australia (Wilkins et al. 2008; Sondik et al. 2012).

There are further differences between women and men in terms of what they are treated for. For example, in general practice in the United Kingdom more women than men are treated for hypertension, depression, and anxiety while men are more often treated for CHD and diabetes (Wilkins et al. 2008). The difference in treatment for depression is particularly wide, with more than twice as many women as men diagnosed with this illness. However, men are more frequently hospitalized for mental health problems, particularly in younger age groups.

Overall, data on consultation suggests that women do consult more often than men, and are more likely to use healthcare although patterns vary between countries and also in response to other factors including age. However, gender-linked influences, including financial or cultural constraints, for example, limit their use of services in some countries and may help explain variations in the gap between women and men.

Composite health indicators

The third way in which we can assess the health differences between women and men is through composite indicators of health at population level. One of the best known of these is the estimate of HALE produced by the WHO (see Table 10.2.2). HALE is a measure which begins with life expectancy at birth and is then adjusted downwards to reflect an estimate of time spent during the life course in poor health (Salomon et al. 2012). This estimate is carried out for each of WHO's member countries, using a range of survey statistics and other measures to calculate the adjustment separately for men and women.

Figures for 2010 revealed that global HALE at birth for men was lower than for women (58 years compared with 62 years)

Table 10.2.2 Differences in male and female healthy life expectancy (HALE), 2010—selected countries

Country	Male HALE	Female HALE	Difference in years (negative = female advantage)
Russian Federation	55	64	−9
Estonia	61	67	−6
Sri Lanka	62	67	−5
Côte D'Ivoire	45	50	−5
Republic of Korea	60	64	−4
China	65	69	−4
Angola	49	53	−4
Czech Republic	64	68	−4
Egypt	57	60	−3
Sierra Leone	47	50	−3
Cambodia	56	59	−3
South Africa	49	52	−3
Finland	64	67	−3
Samoa	59	62	−3
India	55	57	−2
Nepal	57	59	−2
Pakistan	55	57	−2
Cameroon	49	51	−2
United States of America	65	67	−2
Australia	67	69	−2
Kenya	54	56	−2
United Kingdom	66	68	−2
Iceland	65	67	−2
Somalia	47	48	−1
Niger	48	49	−1

Source: data from *The Lancet*, Volume 380, Issue 9859, Salomon, J.A. et al., Healthy Life Expectancy for 187 Countries, 1990–2010: a systematic analysis for the Global Burden Disease Study 2010, pp. 2144–62, Copyright © 2012 Elsevier Ltd. All rights reserved.

(Salomon et al. 2012). Women, however, lose a greater proportion of their healthy years to disability, due to their longer life expectancy. Trends in recent years show that women have gained more than men in both life expectancy and healthy life expectancy (Salomon et al. 2012). However, as with mortality and life expectancy, the extent of female advantage varies. In the Russian Federation, for example, female HALE at birth in 2012 was more than 8 years greater than male HALE, with similarly wide gaps in other East European countries. In France, Germany, and the United Kingdom women had only 2 or 3 years' advantage, while in countries such as Mali, Nigeria, and Somalia, with lower levels of life expectancy, the female advantage in terms of HALE was also low. Again, it is interesting to compare these figures with self-reported health—particularly those which show that women in the Russian Federation are less likely than men to describe themselves as having good health.

An alternative measure of health, using DALYs, highlights the distribution of the burden of disease and combines data on death with data on poor health and disability. DALYs are based on calculations of the value of years of disability-free life which are lost as a result of either premature death or the onset of disability (Murray et al. 2012). DALYs can be used in relation to specific conditions as well as overall health and indicate the value of particular interventions which reduce mortality or disability, such as health promotion or clean water policies. Worldwide, an estimated 2.5 billion DALYs are lost annually due to various health conditions (Murray et al. 2012). Nearly 35 per cent of these are due to infectious and parasitic diseases, including HIV/AIDS and tuberculosis which account for nearly 5 per cent of the total, and diarrhoeal diseases which account for 4 per cent (Murray et al. 2012). Heart disease contributes 11 per cent of lost DALYs, injuries a further 11 per cent, and mental health problems account for around 7.5 per cent of the total number of DALYs lost each year.

Overall, there is a narrow gap between women and men in their experience of morbidity using this measure: men make up 55 per cent of total DALYs lost per annum while women make up 45 per cent (Murray et al. 2012). However, men are much more likely than women to experience illness or disability, as well as premature death as a consequence of accidental and non-accidental injury, and have higher numbers of DALYs lost due to heart disease, alcohol and drug use disorders, and cancer. Males also have higher numbers of DALYs lost for neonatal disabilities. Healthy years lost by women are especially likely to result from complications of pregnancy and childbirth, depression and anxiety, and nutritional deficiencies. DALYs related to reproductive health including maternal disorder, disability arising from pregnancy and childbirth, sexually transmitted infections, gynaecological disorders, and cancers of the reproductive organs, account for around 5 per cent of the female burden of ill health but only 1 per cent of male DALYs (Murray et al. 2012).

DALYs have been criticized for various reasons which have a gendered dimension. The mental health aspects of rape and sexual violence, for example, are not counted by the DALYs approach and they focus on economic rather than social costs of disease and poor health—the loss of income or the costs of care, for example, rather than suffering, stigma, and individual well-being (Sen and Bonita 2000). This needs to be borne in mind when using DALYs to assess the gender gap in health, as there may well be variations between women and men in the social impact of different diseases.

Summary—differences between women and men in morbidity

The various ways of counting morbidity or ill health among women and men suggest a complex relationship between sex, gender, and health, which is mediated by age. Other factors such as socioeconomic status, for example, also play a part. While the picture for mortality is relatively straightforward, with most countries showing poorer life expectancy and higher death rates among men, morbidity data suggest that patterns for ill health vary for men and women around the world. On the whole women report poorer health, use services more, particularly where healthcare is relatively accessible, and experience more of some conditions especially those associated with chronic ill health. However, men experience higher levels of illness and disability from those conditions which also contribute to their higher mortality rates.

Sex and gender influences on health are central to explanations of these differences. The next section discusses what is meant by these terms and how they might affect health, before considering their contribution to specific diseases.

Sex, gender, and health

In order to understand sex- and gender-linked influences on health, it is important to clarify what we mean by sex and gender. Despite increasing recognition of the various ways in which sex and gender can impact on the health of men and women, the terms are still sometimes used wrongly. In particular, while 'gender' is now found more often than in the past in biomedical literature, it is often used interchangeably for 'sex' rather than as a distinct concept with a very different meaning (Doyal 2001; Krieger 2003).

Sex and health

'Sex' refers to biological influences including not only differences between women and men based on the reproductive system, but also those reflecting genetic and hormonal factors. For many years reproductive differences between women and men were seen as the most significant sex-linked influence on health. However, research in the past two decades has widened our understanding of the complexity of sex-linked factors on men's and women's health.

The Committee on Understanding the Biology of Sex and Gender Differences, set up by the Institute of Medicine in the United States in 1999, produced an important review of the evidence relating to biological factors and their effects on health. The final report concluded that 'sex matters' (Wizeman and Pardue 2001). That is to say, the health of men and women is influenced in important ways by 'genetic, biochemical, physiological, physical' elements, as well as those which are social in origin (Wizeman and Pardue 2001). While hormonal and reproductive factors play a part in patterns of health and in vulnerability to different conditions, this review also highlighted the significance of genetic and molecular factors, and important differences between men and women in gene expression. The report concluded with a number of recommendations for further research in the field, stressing that genetic factors are not fully understood as yet.

The range of sex-linked influences on health

Sex-linked factors play a key part in human health throughout the life course. Males are more vulnerable to mortality than females at every age, from conception onwards (Waldron 1985). For example, studies of fetal mortality—deaths in the womb at any gestational age—reveal higher mortality among males than females (MacDorman et al. 2007). Indeed the higher rate of male deaths prior to birth is an important indication of the part played by biological factors in male excess mortality.

Hormones play a key role in differences in health experience between women and men. Female sex hormones appear to protect women against a range of conditions including, for example, ischaemic heart disease (Waldron 1985). One explanation for this advantage is that oestrogen increases the flexibility of the female circulatory system, and that high blood pressure is less damaging for premenopausal women (Bird and Rieker 2008). Similarly, oestrogen affects cholesterol, increasing high-density lipoprotein cholesterol levels and decreasing low-density lipoprotein cholesterol, and improves the functioning of the heart (Wizeman and Pardue 2001). However, evidence on the role of biology is mixed and inconclusive (Vaidya et al. 2011).

Hormones are also implicated in irritable bowel syndrome, another condition where there is a female excess. Women are up to four times as likely to suffer from this chronic painful condition. While this reflects gender-linked factors such as stress and anxiety, there is also evidence that men may receive protection from testosterone while female hormones may increase the severity of the symptoms experienced (Cain et al. 2009).

Hormonal changes across the menstrual cycle also appear to affect health outcomes for women in the context of interventions as diverse as smoking cessation and surgery for breast cancer (Kucuk and Atalay 2012). Further evidence of biological influences comes from research on alcohol-related damage. Women and men have different patterns of risk from alcohol consumption. Women suffer the adverse effects of alcohol in terms of brain and liver damage more quickly than men do and are more likely to suffer health damage at the same level of consumption as men. These variations are partly due to differences in metabolism and hormonal factors, which mean that women's bodies process alcohol differently (Redgrave et al. 2003).

There are also differences in male and female immune systems, which are related to reproductive factors, particularly the capacity of women to conceive and carry a child. These differences mean that women's immune systems are more at risk from auto-immune disorders (Zandman-Goddard et al. 2012). Changes in the immune system of pregnant women put them at higher risk of some communicable diseases ranging from measles to malaria (Wizeman and Pardue 2001; Rieker et al. 2010). However, other pregnancy-related changes such as the tendency for auto-immune diseases such as rheumatoid arthritis to go into remission highlight the complexity of the relationship between sex and the immune system (Rieker et al. 2010).

Recent research has also suggested important sex differences in gene expression, contributing to women's higher risks for some forms of cancer. For example, among smokers, women appear to be more at risk of lung cancer than men at the same level of smoking, and lung cancer is also more common among non-smoking women than non-smoking men (Paggi et al. 2010). This has been related to gene expression, simplistically defined as a process that allows a particular gene to come into play or not. Expression of genes related to lung cancer may be greater among women than men due to the location of the expressed gene on the X chromosome, leading to an increased risk of this cancer as well as shaping the type of lung cancer which women develop (Payne 2006; Paggi et al. 2010).

In addition, there is increasing evidence of sex differences in the way the brain is organized, including the use of language and verbal abilities (Wallentin 2009). For example, some studies report that women recover more language ability than men following a left-hemisphere stroke (Wizeman and Pardue 2001) but this is not a universal finding (Wallentin 2009). There are also differences between women and men in the way the brain responds to noxious stimuli, which in turn affect experiences of symptoms such as pain. Women have higher prevalence rates for what are often described as 'pain conditions', including headache, abdominal pain, and facial pain (Popescu et al. 2010). While this reflects the fact that the expression of pain is culturally more sanctioned for women than men, biological factors also play a part, especially differences between women and men in particular neurological pathways (Popescu et al. 2010).

However, we must be wary of attributing too much to biology. For example, research on the relationship between parity and some health conditions, especially non-reproductive carcinomas such as colorectal cancer, has suggested that there might be a relationship for women between pregnancy and subsequent health risks. But recent studies have also revealed a similar relationship between parity and mortality for men, implying that social factors such as stress, access to resources, and expectations associated with having children may be more significant than biological factors in this association (Jaffe et al. 2011).

Wizeman and Pardue (2001) point out the limitations in this area of knowledge. Despite many years of research on the ways in which biology impacts on health, conclusive evidence and clear understanding of the pathways concerned remains scarce. There are various reasons for this, including a lack of research which is disaggregated for men and women and the fact that research findings which fail to find a difference between women and men are often not published, despite the fact that such results also advance our understanding.

We should also note that some writers have challenged the way in which biology, in particular, has been used in an overly simplistic way. Springer et al. (2012) for example, take issue with Wizeman and Pardue's statement that 'every cell has a sex', arguing that biological sex has been 'reified' as a dichotomous variable, separate from gender influences, and is often treated as more important in the health of both women and men. However, biology or sex-linked factors interact with environmental factors, including gender differences.

Gender and health

'Gender' refers to socially constructed differences between women and men, that is, the conventions, roles and expectations of men and women which are culturally ascribed (Krieger 2003). Gendered influences on health include access to health-promoting resources, exposure to health damaging and health promoting factors in daily life, and different expectations of behaviour such as drinking alcohol, risk-taking, and the use of healthcare. In addition, gender impacts on health through the ways in which health services are organized and delivered, particularly when such services operate in gender insensitive ways.

One of the key differences between sex and gender is the extent to which they are fixed, or can change over time. Sex—male or female—is assigned to a child at birth on the basis of external genitalia, and is fixed other than for a minority of people undergoing medical sex reassignment. Gender is generally ascribed on the basis of biological sex, although what is meant in any one society or culture by gender may vary over the years and between social or other groupings. Thus a child is identified at birth as either male or female and this in turn leads to the categorizations embedded in masculinity or femininity in that society.

Gender is also an important influence on the health of men and women through what is described by Springer et al. (2012) as the 'entanglement' between biology and gender. Krieger and Zierler (1995) describe such interactions in terms of *the biological expression of gender* and the *gendered expression of biology*. The biological expression of gender refers to the ways in which gender becomes embodied. For example, in many societies gender is constructed to mean that women see themselves, and are seen by others, as weaker than men. This can result in women taking less exercise, or choosing less strenuous forms of activity, which in turn affect the female body. The gendered expression of biology refers to the ways in which biological understandings of women and men lead to gendered differentiations, which often take the form of discrimination. So, for example, women's reproductive capacity is used to justify their exclusion from some forms of paid work on the basis that it is unsafe. Similarly their exclusion from medical research is said to be justified on the basis that it may cause harm to an unborn child. This then strengthens social constructions of gender in which women are seen as less able to undertake some forms of paid work, or less vulnerable to some forms of disease.

For many writers, gender is seen as something that is 'performed' in various ways, in exchange with other people. That is, we 'do' gender in our daily lives—in our paid work, in relationships, in leisure activities, and so on (Courtenay and Messerschmidt 2011). This view of gender allows us to see how it changes over time and across societies, and also how individuals might 'do' gender differently at different times and in different settings. In addition, it highlights the fact that what is appropriate gendered behaviour for one group may not be so for another—gender roles vary according to class and ethnicity for example. Finally it allows for the possibility that individuals might choose to adopt gender roles which are not commensurate with their biological sex. But while various gender roles may be available, it is also the case that in all societies some forms of masculinity and femininity are more sanctioned than others and this may impact on health in negative or positive ways.

Many writers have observed that in most if not all cultures, masculinity is privileged over femininity, but it is also true that not all men are equally advantaged. The term 'hegemonic masculinity' refers to the most privileged form of masculinity, typically occupied by white middle-class men (Connell and Messerschmidt 2005; Connell 2012). Men occupying different class positions may experience masculinity in a range of ways, with associated health benefits and/or risks. Similarly, women's experiences of gender interact with other positions or social practices, again with varying health consequences.

Gender affects the health of both men and women in a number of interlocking ways. Firstly, gender mediates the effect of physical and psychological risks encountered in daily life. There is substantial evidence, for example, that material factors such as poverty and social exclusion, socioeconomic status, poor housing and environmental disadvantage, occupation, and unpaid work all impact on health in varying ways and to varying degrees (WHO 2008). And men and women may face differential risks of experiencing these adverse effects, because of their gender. Secondly, gender roles and expectations are closely associated with individual behaviour which in turn may impact on the health of women and men.

Socioeconomic determinants of health and gender

Material factors influence the health of women and men in complex ways through aspects of daily life such as paid work and employment status, household work and domestic labour, income, caring responsibilities, living arrangements, and experiences of conflict, stress, and violence. The extent to which men and women are exposed to these risk factors, and how they impact on their health, varies in relation to geographical location, socioeconomic status, and cultural differences (WHO 2008).

Paid employment exerts numerous effects on health. There are a range of hazards associated with particular jobs, including exposure to unsafe chemicals, hazardous work environments, and dangers inherent in the nature of the work itself. The gender division of labour, which sees men more often employed in certain sectors and in certain occupations within sectors, creates a gendered division of occupational risk. Men typically work in industries and in jobs with a higher mortality risk—including construction, transport, and the emergency services, for example.

However, in recent years the occupational injury gap between women and men has narrowed, following a rise in the numbers of women in the labour force, and there has been a corresponding increase in some forms of injury-related mortality among women (WHO 2008; Forastieri 2010). Other work-related hazards affect the risk of poor health—repetitive strain injury, for example, from keyboard work and some production processes in manufacturing. Such injuries are more common among women partly as a result of the jobs they occupy, and partly because the design of workstations is often based on male rather than female physiology (Forastieri 2010).

Gender differences in occupational risk are compounded by differences outside the workplace and in particular by gender differences in domestic work. Women still carry out most household chores. For example in the United Kingdom despite their increasing participation in paid work, women still spend on average twice as many hours per day as men in housework and childcare (Lader et al. 2006). In addition, even where men take on some of the work, women retain overall responsibility for domestic labour—for planning, organizing, and ensuring it is done. Domestic labour carries further implications for health including the stress of managing responsibilities, loneliness, and isolation, as well as the lack of an independent income and low status for those women who are not also employed. Women working at home are particularly vulnerable to mental health problems in comparison with those who have paid work but the strain of juggling two roles and the dual burden of paid work and domestic labour also puts women who enter the labour market at risk of poor mental health (Harryson et al. 2012).

Poverty and social exclusion also carry pronounced health risks for both men and women. However, there are gender differences in the risk of such poverty, with women in most parts of the world being more likely to be poor (WHO 2008). This is due to lower wages, working in the informal sector, reduced access to paid work as a result of caring responsibilities, and, in some countries, cultural restrictions, and also reflects that fact that women may not always share equally in household resources. Poverty is often especially severe among older women whose health is already frail (WHO 2003).

Exposure to violence creates further risks including poor mental health, post-traumatic stress disorders, and physical injuries. Violence is one of the most important causes of death for younger age groups (WHO and LSHTM 2010) but there are marked gender differences not only in the level of risk from violence but also in the source. Although both women and men are at risk from interpersonal violence, violence against men is more common in the public domain, and they are more at risk from strangers. However, women are more likely to be exposed to violence in the home—from partners and members of their family (WHO and LSHTM 2010). Women are at particular risk from sexual violence both in the home and elsewhere, and the consequences for their health can include pregnancy and sexually transmitted infections as well as mental health problems. Although sexual violence against men is less common, and in the past there has been too little research on this, it may be especially damaging for mental health due to feelings of stigma and shame (Sivakumaran 2010).

Taken together these material aspects of daily life can create particular health stresses which are often different for men and women. To these health risks, we can add those associated with 'doing gender'—the ways in which social constructions of masculinity and femininity are associated with the increased risk of particular behaviours which further impact on health.

'Doing gender'—masculinity, femininity, and health

Behaviour has long been seen as the leading gendered explanation for men's poorer health and premature mortality. In the seventeenth century, John Graunt suggested that women lived longer than men despite their experiences of illness because, 'Men, being more intemperate than Women, die as much by reason of their Vices, as Women do by the Infirmity of their Sex' (Graunt, cited in Ciocco 1940, p. 61). There are still important differences between women and men in behaviours such as smoking, alcohol and substance use, physical activity, diet, risk-taking, and the use of healthcare services including preventive care and screening. These differences taken together are a key part of the explanation for men's higher mortality; a number of writers in this area have highlighted the extent to which masculinity, in particular, accounts for the greater mortality risks experienced by men across a range of cultural settings (Courtenay and Messerschmidt 2011).

One of the most damaging behaviours—smoking and tobacco use—has a strongly gendered history. More men than women die each year from smoking-related diseases: lung cancer, for example, killed twice as many men as women worldwide in 2002 (WHO 2009). This reflects the gender ratio in smokers: throughout the world more men than women smoke and in countries where the epidemic is relatively new the great majority of those using tobacco are male (Erikson et al. 2012). In Malaysia, for example, 53 per cent of men smoke compared with less than 3 per cent of women; in Malawi 26 per cent of men and 4 per cent of women smoke, while in Bangladesh the figures are 46 per cent and 2 per cent (Erikson et al. 2012).

However, more developed regions where smoking has a longer history have seen increasing numbers of women using tobacco, to the point where in some countries similar proportions of women and men are smokers: in Norway and Sweden, for example (Erikson et al. 2012). Alcohol and substance use also have gendered profiles. Excessive consumption of alcohol on a regular basis is associated with an increased risk of a number of diseases, including cirrhosis of the liver and other liver disease, some forms of CHD and mouth cancers (WHO 2011c). Other forms of alcohol consumption, including what is sometimes referred to as 'binge drinking' where high levels of alcohol are consumed over a short period of time, also lead to an increased risk of violence and accidental injury, as well as self-harm and suicide (WHO 2011c).

National and international data show that more women than men can be described as 'abstainers', that is, as non-drinkers. The extent of the gender gap varies: in the Philippines, for example, women are three times more likely than men to be lifelong abstainers, while in Iceland the ratio of female to male abstainers is nearly 2:1 (WHO 2011c). When we look at men and women who are defined as drinkers, men usually consume more units of alcohol on a weekly basis and/or have a high daily intake. Per capita consumption is higher for women than men in only one country, Ecuador, while in all other countries men drink more than women (WHO 2011b). In Bosnia and Herzegovina, for example, male per capita consumption was twice as high as female consumption, and in South Africa it is 1.6 times higher.

If we look at heavy episodic drinking, defined as drinking heavily on at least one occasion in a 7-day period, this is also more common among men than women around the world. Nearly half of men in Ireland, for example, report such levels of consumption compared with 14 per cent of women, while other countries with high levels of male binge drinking include the Czech Republic, Botswana, and Paraguay (WHO 2012c). In England, in 2011, more than 39 per cent of men, compared with 28 per cent of women, reported drinking more than the daily recommended units on at least 1 day in the previous week (Craig and Mindell 2012) and in Australia, men were three times as likely to drink more than daily or weekly recommended limits (Australian Bureau of Statistics 2012).

Among young people, heavy episodic drinking is also more common among men (WHO 2011c) and while increases in binge drinking among young women in some high-income countries have led to concern, it remains the case that this behaviour is more frequent for males (Emslie et al. 2009).

Diet is also an important, modifiable, contributor to health risks. The influence of diet on health is becoming increasingly clear, with growing evidence suggesting that a diet which is rich in fruit, vegetables, and fibre and low in fat may reduce the risk of various health problems including cancer and heart disease (World Cancer Research Fund and American Institute for Cancer Research 2007). Gender differences in what we eat may therefore play an important role in explaining different patterns of health for men and women. Men are more likely than women to die from colorectal cancer, for example, and part of the explanation for this seems to stem from differences in diet (Payne 2007).

On the whole, men's diets are less healthy than those of women, particularly in high-income countries, where men are more likely to consume inadequate amounts of vegetables and fruit and also to eat higher than recommended amounts of red meat (Payne 2006; Craig and Mindell 2012). More women than men in Australia, for example, report meeting recommended levels of fruit and vegetable intake (Australian Bureau of Statistics 2012). However, in low- and middle-income countries, particularly those where food is scarce, women and girls are less likely than men to be eating adequate levels of fruit and vegetables. In Malawi, for example, 42 per cent of women and 37 per cent of men have diets with less than the recommended amount of fruit and vegetables. In other low-income countries, including Pakistan, Swaziland, and Kenya, a large majority of both men and women report diets insufficient in fruit and vegetables and the differences between them are slight (WHO 2005). In these countries, where there is a high risk of food insecurity, there are important gender differences in the distribution of food within households, in expectations about what men and women will eat, and also in what will be given to male and female children.

However, food intake and diet also need to be set against energy requirements and again there are important gender differences both in levels of physical activity and in kinds of activity. In high-income countries lack of physical activity is a health concern which has increased in prominence in recent years. Physical activity can have a positive effect on health. It helps to protect against heart disease and may play a part in reducing vulnerability to other conditions, including some cancers and mental health problems (WHO 2009). The WHO estimates that physical inactivity is the fourth leading risk factor for global mortality, associated with 27 per cent of diabetes DALYs, 25 per cent of breast and colon cancer DALYs, and 30 per cent of cardiovascular DALYs (WHO 2010). Physical activity levels in most communities are different for men and women, although the size of the gap varies in relation to other factors including employment-related activity and available leisure time.

Data on activity are complex, and not always comparable. Some surveys refer to total physical activity including that associated with work and travel—cycling and walking, for example—as well as leisure activities such as sport. One of the problems with this data is that physical domestic work, mainly carried out by women, is often not included in such measures (O'Brien Cousins and Gillis 2005). This means that some figures, particularly those in low- and middle-income countries, based on total activity, overestimate the extent to which women are leading sedentary lives. Data based on sports leisure activity, however, might also miss out some activities which are more frequent among women—dancing, for example (O'Brien Cousins and Gillis 2005).

Data in high-income countries often focuses on leisure activity rather than total activity, making it difficult to compare findings with poorer countries. Such data show a gap between men and women in time spent in physical activity, with men tending to be more active. In the United States, for example, a higher proportion of men participate regularly in physical activity and women are more likely to be insufficiently active (Sondik et al. 2012). Similarly, in England, more men than women achieve 'recommended' levels of physical activity, with the widest gap in young adults between 16 and 24 years of age (Craig and Mindell 2012).

Figures for total physical activity in low- and middle-income countries suggest that men might be more likely than women to have active lifestyles, although this is likely to reflect a failure to count some aspects of women's activities. In Kenya, for example, while less than 10 per cent of adults report physical activity levels which are too low, women are slightly more likely than men to report insufficient time spent in physical activity (WHO 2005). Similarly in Malawi, few people have low levels of activity, but activity levels are lower among women than men. Activity levels are slightly lower in Pakistan, where women are twice as likely as men to report insufficient activity; and in India and China women are also less likely than men to report sufficient levels of activity.

However, in these countries it is also important to consider activity, or energy expenditure, alongside diet and calorie intake. In the poorest countries women, in particular, experience health risks because of activity levels that are high in the context of too little food. These problems are especially severe for pregnant and breastfeeding women and carry long-term implications both for their health and that of their child. Jackson and Palmer-Jones (1998), for example, talk of an 'energy trap' resulting from development policies which aim to increase various kinds of work in order to reduce poverty but which fail to take account of the increased need for food created by increased levels of activity. Gender differences in food allocation and access to calories, as well as in work carried out, mean this is a particularly acute problem for women (Patel 2012).

Diet and activity levels in high-income countries are also connected to a further health risk: obesity. Obesity is associated with various diseases including CHD, some forms of cancer, and diabetes. Obesity, defined as a body mass index (BMI) over 30, is generally more common among women than men, although this varies between countries, and more men than women are defined as overweight (with a BMI of between 25 and 30) (WHO 2012b).

In England, in 2011, 65 per cent of men were overweight or obese compared with 61 per cent of women (Craig and Mindell 2012), while in Australia 70 per cent of men were overweight or obese in 2011–2012 compared with 55 per cent of women (Australian Bureau of Statistics 2012). Similarly, in the United States, 69 per cent of men compared with 55 per cent of women were overweight or obese (Sondik et al. 2012). In older age groups and in lower-income groups in particular, women are more likely than men to be defined as obese (Zaninotto et al. 2006).

A final gendered aspect of behaviour which affects health and mortality risk is the use of preventive services and healthcare. We have already discussed gender differences in consultation as a measure of morbidity, and highlighted the role of economic factors in the use of healthcare, but it is also important to consider the ways in which men and women differ in help-seeking behaviour. A number of studies have suggested that men are reluctant to seek medical help and attend services less readily than women. As one man put it, 'I don't go to the doctor unless something scares the hell out of me' (Stibbe 2004, p. 36). Men describe themselves as unwilling to make a fuss or waste the time of health professionals (Courtenay and Messerschmidt 2011).

Although there are a number of variations in data on health service use, reflecting age and socioeconomic differences, for example, overall men do appear less willing to see themselves as in need of healthcare. Men are more difficult to engage in health promotion activities including screening, leading some healthcare providers to devise various gender-sensitive strategies to increase take-up among men, such as placing clinics and information points in workplaces and bars (Wilkins et al. 2008; Courtenay and Messerschmidt 2011).

Overall, gender differences in roles, expectations, and behaviour combine to increase the risk for men of premature mortality and the risk for women of chronic health problems (Snow 2008). Masculinity, insofar as it involves risk-taking and unhealthy behaviours, increases risks of accidental and non-accidental injury, non-communicable diseases associated with smoking, alcohol, and substance use. Masculine practices also increase some health risks for women, particularly the risks associated with male violence and sexually transmitted infections.

Female gender roles and expectations may lead to reduced risks for some conditions, due to lower rates of smoking, alcohol and substance use, better diets, and less risk-taking, although the lower rates of physical activity more common among women will also affect their health risks. In poorer countries however, women have different problems associated with insufficient food for the work they are expected to carry out. There are also pressures on both men and women arising from the stress of gender role expectations, particularly in relation to failure to meet expectations.

In order to illustrate these different influences and the complex associations between sex and gender we turn now to look at specific health problems: cardiovascular diseases, cancer, mental health difficulties, HIV/AIDS, and malaria.

The impact of sex and gender on specific health problems

Cardiovascular diseases

Cardiovascular diseases include CHD and stroke. Taken together, cardiovascular diseases account for around one-tenth of the global burden of disease, with more men than women affected. CHD is the major contributor to this burden, particularly among men, while strokes account for similar levels of illness among men and women. These conditions are also important in overall mortality: more men than women die as a result of CHD but women are more likely to die from a stroke (WHO 2012f). One of the key differences between women and men in these illnesses is the age at which risk increases: men are more likely than women to die prematurely from CHD and the male to female ratio is greatest in mid-life. Women with CHD die on average 10 years later than men (Wizeman and Pardue 2001). In the United Kingdom, for example, the male mortality rate for CHD among those aged 45–54 is nearly five times higher than the female rate, but by the age of 75 female deaths outnumber those of men (Scarborough et al. 2010). Men's greater risk of premature death and illness for CHD is found throughout the world (Riska 2010).

Why do men have higher risks than women for CHD at an early stage in the life course? In the aetiology of CHD, raised blood pressure and blood cholesterol are significant risk factors, and behaviours which are more common among men than women—particularly poor diet and smoking—are important underlying explanations. While women gain protection from heart disease due to female hormones, men increase their risks through their adoption of risky behaviours. The later age at which women appear to be at risk of CHD has led to speculation that until the menopause female hormones might offer women some degree of protection. However, most recent research has failed to support this suggestion. For example, women's CHD risk does not increase immediately following the menopause but some years later, suggesting that other factors may be important instead of, or alongside, female hormones. In addition hormone replacement therapy does not appear to offer women protection from CHD, indeed it might actually increase their risk (Riska 2010).

However, there are also concerns over possible differences between women and men in the recognition and treatment of CHD. Because heart disease is seen as primarily a male condition, women may be less likely to have their illness diagnosed or to be offered appropriate treatment (Riska 2010). This is dealt with further later in this chapter.

Cancer

Overall mortality from cancer is higher among men, and while both men and women are vulnerable to reproductive-related cancers, men are also more likely than women to die from cancers related to particular lifestyles and behaviours (WHO 2011a).

Although cancers of the female reproductive organs lead to more deaths among women than male reproductive cancers do among men, the difference does not compensate for the male excess cancer mortality stemming from factors such as tobacco use, dietary influences, and alcohol consumption.

Lung cancer in particular accounts for more than twice as many deaths among men as among women (WHO 2011a). The main cause of lung cancer for both men and women is tobacco use and in countries where tobacco use remains a predominantly male habit, the male to female ratio is especially high (Erikson et al. 2012). In Thailand, for example, the ratio of men to women for lung cancer mortality is around 2.3:1, while in Denmark, where equal numbers of men and women now smoke, the ratio has reduced to 1.4:1 in recent years (WHO 2012e).

However, research suggests that the risk of lung cancer is different for women and men irrespective of absolute levels of tobacco use. These differences stem from both gendered differences in patterns of tobacco use—the type of cigarettes smoked, for example, and the depth of inhalation—and also biological factors. Women appear to have a greater biological vulnerability to lung cancer due to genetic factors while their greater use of low-tar cigarettes leads to an increased risk of one form of lung cancer—adenocarcinoma (Kiyohara and Ohno 2010). However, while lung cancer is a particularly fatal form of cancer with very low 1-year and 5-year survival rates, women also appear to have better prospects for survival in comparison with men and this too is related to biological differences between women and men.

Thus sex and gender-linked factors interact to produce different risks of cancer for women and men, reflecting both hormonal and genetic influences and the impact of certain behaviours.

Mental health and illness

Among chronic and debilitating conditions, the most significant in terms of numbers affected and the impact on daily living are those associated with mental illness. Mental health problems, including depression, anxiety, substance use, and schizophrenia, account for 11 per cent of the global burden of disease (WHO 2012f). Around 450 million people worldwide experience mental illness of one kind or another at any one time. There are important differences between women and men in their risks of various mental health problems. In particular more women are diagnosed as suffering from depression and anxiety-related conditions, and in community-based surveys more women are found to be suffering from symptoms of these illnesses (Payne 2006; Snow 2008). Figures for DALYs lost in 2010 due to mental illness show the total burden evenly divided between males and females. However, within that overall figure, women experience much more ill health due to depression and anxiety, in comparison with men.

Men on the other hand are more frequently treated for mental health difficulties associated with alcohol and substance use, including harmful use, dependence, and psychosis. Male DALYs for drug use disorders are more than twice as high as female DALYs, while those for alcohol related disorders are more than four times higher for men than for women (Courtenay and Messerschmidt 2011; Murray et al. 2012). Men are also more likely to commit suicide than women in virtually every country in the world, with deaths from suicide in 2008 twice as high among men as women (WHO 2011a). In contrast, more women than men carry out acts of deliberate self-harm.

While there is some evidence that biological influences play a part in shaping mental health—particularly in relation to conditions such as postnatal depression—most research suggests that gendered factors play the more significant role. These include stress-linked factors such as those associated with poverty, parenting, employment, exposure to the threat of violence and gendered expectations, as well as the extent to which gender stereotyping in mental health services affects the delivery of care by increasing diagnoses of depression among women. Under-diagnosis of depression among men may help to explain their higher rates of alcohol and drug use disorders, and higher rates of suicide (Wilkins et al. 2008; Courtenay and Messerschmidt 2011).

HIV/AIDS

In many parts of the world HIV/AIDS is one of the most significant threats to the health of both women and men. It is transmitted either through unprotected vaginal or anal sex, as a result of contaminated needles in the context of injecting drug use or from mother to child *in utero* or during breastfeeding. There were 2.7 million new infections and nearly 1.8 million deaths in 2010 (UNAIDS 2011). About 68 per cent of those who were HIV positive were living in sub-Saharan Africa, and around half of all AIDS-related deaths occurred in the same region (UNAIDS 2011).

The overall number of deaths has decreased markedly since the spread of antiretroviral drugs in the mid 1990s. Similarly, the number of new infections is declining in many parts of the world including 22 sub-Saharan countries. Nevertheless, there has been a marked increase in the number of people living with HIV which has risen by 17 per cent from 2001 to 2010 and is now estimated to be around 34 million (United Nations Development Programme 2012). This is due to the fact that levels of new infection continue to be high combined with the extended lifespan that accompanies greater access to HIV treatment.

Globally, the proportion of women living with HIV has now stabilized at around 50 per cent though they make up 60 per cent of those affected in sub-Saharan Africa. Young women are at particular risk: in South Africa, for example, 21 per cent of girls and young women aged 15–24 were HIV positive in 2010 compared with 7 per cent of men of the same age (UNAIDS 2011). This has led to high rates of mother-to-child transmission with about 90 per cent of all HIV-positive children in the world living in Africa. Women are making up an increasing proportion of the positive population in some parts of Asia, Eastern Europe, and South America.

Women are biologically more vulnerable than men to HIV infection. In unprotected vaginal intercourse, women are at greater risk than men because the vaginal wall is exposed to seminal fluid for a longer period of time. This is especially dangerous in the presence of traumatic injury or existing genital infections which are more likely to be found in women (Dunkle et al. 2004). The risk of transmission from a single heterosexual act is estimated to be around 0.04 per cent for females to males and around 0.8 per cent from males to females (Boily et al. 2009). However, it is important to note that anal sex is riskiest of all and this is most likely to affect men who have sex with men (MSM).

Turning to gender, women again have a particular vulnerability due to the fact that they are less able to negotiate sexual relationships—to demand protection, for example—and may be forced or coerced into unprotected sex, especially at young ages. This is exacerbated by their lack of access to women-initiated or -controlled prevention methods. The example of the Asian region highlights this with particular clarity. In 1990, women made up some 17 per cent of the total HIV-positive population but by 2007 this had doubled to 35 per cent (UNAIDS 2009). Most had only ever had one sexual partner so that sex with their husbands can be a major threat to the health of many. This reflects the high rates of extra-marital sex among married men with both male and female sex workers who themselves are at very high risk of infection.

While men do not have the heightened physiological vulnerability we have noted in the case of women, the social construction of masculine gender may lead them to risk their health. While this can take many different forms it will usually include the social expectation that 'real' (heterosexual) men will 'perform' their masculinity through having frequent (often unprotected) sex with different women. A similar social pressure towards sexual performance is often found among those men who are active in gay 'communities'.

HIV and AIDS have severe consequences for the well-being of both women and men. The initial stage of HIV involves a gradual decline in the capacity of the body to fight off opportunistic infections. Those who are positive are said to have acquired immune deficiency syndrome (AIDS) when their immune system has weakened to the point when they have one or several of what are called AIDS defining illnesses. These include *Pneumocystis* pneumonia and the virus-induced cancer Kaposi's sarcoma. In women, cervical cancer is also regarded as an AIDS-defining condition when it occurs along with HIV infection. Without treatment, infections and malignancies increase in frequency, severity, and duration until death intervenes.

Relatively little is known about the differences between women and men in the biological development of HIV and AIDS. However, the evidence indicates that for men, the first opportunistic illnesses are more likely to be cytomegalovirus, Kaposi's sarcoma, or oral hairy leucoplakia while for women they are more likely to be oesophageal candidiasis or toxoplasmosis (Women's Health Research 2009).

Untreated HIV infection also poses a particular threat to women during pregnancy. In sub-Saharan Africa, seropositive status is becoming increasingly important as a cause of maternal morbidity and mortality (Black et al. 2009). Since 1998, HIV has been the leading indirect cause of maternal deaths in South Africa, reversing a previous decline in mortality rates. A recent study showed that HIV-positive women in Johannesburg were around six times more likely to die from maternal causes than their negative counterparts (Black et al. 2009).

In most parts of the world there are also marked gender differences in use of HIV services. As the pandemic became increasingly 'feminized' it was widely assumed that women were missing out on treatment compared with men. However, recent studies have shown that in many settings it is actually (heterosexual) men who have least access to services relative to their needs (Natrass 2006). This reflects both women's greater likelihood of diagnosis in the context of maternity care and also men's reluctance to engage in medical encounters which appears to be especially significant in the context of HIV (Skovdal et al. 2011).

Thus sex and gender again intertwine both in terms of men's and women's vulnerability to infection and in the consequences of the disease. However, in the case of HIV the intersections between sex and gender need to be understood in the context of sexual identities and practices.

Malaria

In 2010, there were between 150 and 290 million cases of malaria, and around 660,000 people—mainly children—died from this disease (WHO 2012g). These figures are falling in comparison with earlier years. The global impact of malaria on the burden of illness is calculated at more than 1 million DALYs per annum (Murray et al. 2012). The vast majority of those affected by malaria live in sub-Saharan Africa.

Reducing the incidence of malaria (along with HIV/AIDS and tuberculosis) was part of the eight Millennium Development Goals and has been a key focus of the work of the WHO. Malaria incidence reflects a range of factors—increasing resistance to the drugs used to treat the disease and to insecticides used to prevent transmission, lack of access to necessary medicine and to preventive measures particularly in poorer countries, and deforestation in some areas creating wider vectors of transmission. However, figures in the first decade of the twenty-first century suggest the efforts of global organizations such as the WHO and The Global Fund have met with some success as prevalence and deaths have fallen, despite a slowing down in the rate of improvement more recently (WHO 2012g).

There are important differences between women and men in the risk of malaria and these have changed in the last few years. In comparison with earlier periods when there was an excess of female deaths, in 2008 20,000 more males than females died of malaria (WHO 2012g). This is due to 24,000 more male deaths compared with female deaths among children under 5—in every other age group more females die of malaria. This pattern reflects both sex- and gender-based influences. For example, women's risk of contracting malaria increases in pregnancy, due to temporary changes in the immune system and this biological risk factor is reflected in the slight over-representation of female deaths worldwide during reproductive years. Gender factors can also play a part where women have less access than men to preventive measures such as bednets treated with insecticide, due to household division of resources. In addition, women's responsibility for work, such as water collection and some agricultural labour, increases their exposure to mosquitoes and their risk of being bitten. Studies have also found women to be less well informed than men about the risks of malaria and about means of protection, while women in some cultures are less able to access healthcare when infected because they have less control over household resources and because they may need to be chaperoned when attending health services (Tanner and Vlassoff 1998).

Gender and the delivery of healthcare

The final way in which gender impacts on health is through the delivery of healthcare. In addition to material circumstances and behaviour, the health of both men and women is also associated with the way in which healthcare is provided and we need to ask if health services are equally available for women and men, if they are accessible and if they are appropriate.

Gender differences in availability and access

There are a number of ways in which gender affects access to healthcare. Most importantly perhaps, gender affects the resources that are necessary in order to use health services. Around the world women earn less than men, and, where health insurance is related to paid work, are more often in jobs without insurance cover (Payne 2006). In the United States, more men than women do not have a 'usual place' of healthcare, and more men use hospital emergency rooms; while women make more visits to healthcare than men (Sondik et al. 2012).

In many low- and middle-income countries, while both men and women experience difficulty in obtaining healthcare due to the location of services and the need to meet the costs of user fees, women are particularly disadvantaged due to lack of independent income or say in how household resources are used (Baghdadi 2005; Sen and Ostlin 2007).

In addition to access, there may be further differences in availability. Where services are only open during the day they are less available to those with paid work who cannot take time off, or to those whose caring responsibilities prevent attendance. While more men are prevented from using daytime services due to employment, they are also more often in jobs where time off for medical appointments is sanctioned. For women juggling full-time or part-time work with childcare, seeking medical help may be particularly difficult.

Similarly some cultures require women to consult with female health professionals who may not always be available. Even where it is not culturally prescribed, women are more likely to report a preference for a female clinician, particularly when consulting about intimate health problems. For example, women are more likely to prefer a female colonoscopist when being screened for bowel cancer, but the lack of women in this profession means their preferences are often not met, potentially delaying detection of bowel cancer among women (Menees et al. 2003; Chong 2012).

Gender differences in the quality of care

The second way in which gender impinges on healthcare is through differences in the quality of care offered to men and women. One important factor affecting this is medical knowledge. Medical research has for some time been criticized for failing to disaggregate findings for women and men and for failing to include women in studies of health problems affecting both sexes (Doyal 1998). This focus on male subjects is problematic when it is assumed that findings can be extended to female populations as though there is no difference. Both symptom recognition and treatment which is based on men may fail women—women metabolize pharmaceuticals differently to men, for example, and prescribed drugs may be more or less effective, or carry different risks for women when research was conducted on men (Wizeman and Pardue 2001). Similarly, risk factors affecting women's health tend to have been less intensively studied: health risks associated with housework, for example, rather than the question of role strain, have only been explored relatively recently compared with the health risks of traditionally male occupations (Artazcoz et al. 2007).

In the United States, research funded by the National Institutes of Health has been required since 1994 both to include sufficient numbers of men and women, and members of minority ethnic groups, and to provide separate analyses and reporting of results.

Despite this there is evidence that there are still a number of studies either focusing on men alone or failing to disaggregate findings for men and women and there is still room for improvement (Vidaver et al. 2000; Geller et al. 2011). In countries without such guidelines the bias is even greater.

Studies have also explored the different ways in which services respond to women and men. Women are less likely to have heart conditions recognized by their primary physician, for example, because they often present with atypical symptoms including fatigue, shortness of breath, or cold sweats. Men on the other hand are seen as candidates for heart complaints by themselves, by their families and by healthcare workers, and the symptoms men typically present with have become the norm (Riska 2010). In addition, chest pain, a key symptom of heart disease, is more likely to have other causes for women than men which can lead to under-diagnosis of heart disease. Not surprisingly, perhaps, women are less often referred both for tests and for treatment, and tend to be at a more advanced stage of illness when they are treated, with the risk this implies (Governder and Penn-Kekana 2008).

Equally, men are less likely than women to have mental health problems such as depression recognized (Wilkins et al. 2008). Under-diagnosis and under-treatment of depression in men contribute to higher rates of male suicide mortality; where there have been increases in prescriptions of antidepressants among men, suicide rates have fallen (Gunnell et al. 2003).

In addition, healthcare may not be sensitive to more subtle gender differences in health needs. Some services are gender blind and unknowingly discriminate against men or women by failing to identify their specific needs. For example, most smoking cessation interventions do not highlight gender differences in successful strategies, including the fact that women and men appear to smoke for different reasons and may take up smoking again in response to different stress factors (Samet and Yoon 2010). In addition, women metabolize nicotine differently to men, and have more adverse reactions to withdrawal in comparison with men (Perkins 2001). Women and men also may need different kinds of support, both from friends or family and from health services (Samet and Yoon 2010).

Conclusion

What we have seen in this chapter is that both sex and gender play an important part in shaping the health of men and women, alongside other forms of diversity. Sex, or biology, is more than reproduction. The health of both men and women is also affected by hormonal differences, and by genetic factors, which impact on vulnerability to different diseases as well as the chances of recovery and survival. Gender, or socially constructed difference, also affects health—by increasing the chances of exposure to specific risk factors, such as poverty, or by helping to shape the behavioural choices made by men and women—the way we 'do' masculinity or femininity. Gender is also important in the way health services are delivered—from how research is conducted and how medical knowledge is constructed and disseminated, to health policy and planning which shapes the availability of medical care, access to care, and how appropriately it meets the needs of men and women. All of these factors combine at the level of the individual to shape their health experience and their need for care, while that care itself needs to be planned and delivered in such a way that both men and women are able to benefit.

Key messages

◆ Both sex and gender play a part in women's and men's health.

◆ Sex or biological factors affect incidence and also survival for various diseases.

◆ Gender is socially constructed and affects exposure to risk factors as well as influencing health behaviours.

◆ Gender also affects the delivery of healthcare, access to care, and how well care meets the needs of women and men.

References

Artazcoz, L., Borrell, C., Cortès, I., et al. (2007). Occupational epidemiology and work related inequalities in health: a gender perspective for two complementary approaches to work and health research. *Journal of Epidemiology and Community Health*, 61, ii39–45.

Australian Bureau of Statistics (2012). *Australian Health Survey: First Results, 2011–12*. Canberra: Australian Bureau of Statistics.

Baghdadi, G. (2005). Gender and medicines: an international public health perspective. *Journal of Women's Health*, 14, 82–6.

Benjamins, M., Hummer, R., Eberstein, I., et al. (2004). Self-reported health and adult mortality risk. *Social Science & Medicine*, 59, 1297–306.

Bird, C. and Rieker, P. (2008). *Gender and Health: The Effects of Constrained Choices and Social Policies*. Cambridge: Cambridge University Press.

Black, V., Brooke, S., and Chersich, M. (2009). Effect of human immunodeficiency virus treatment on maternal mortality at a tertiary center in South Africa: a five-year audit. *Obstetrics and Gynecology*, 114, 292–9.

Boily, M., Baggaley, R., Wang, L., et al. (2009). Heterosexual risk of HIV-1 infection per sexual act: systematic review and meta-analysis of observational studies. *The Lancet Infectious Diseases*, 9, 118–29.

Cain, K., Jarrett, M., Burr, R., et al. (2009). Gender differences in gastrointestinal, psychological, and somatic symptoms in irritable bowel syndrome. *Digestive Diseases and Sciences*, 54, 1542–9.

Chong, V. (2012). Gender preference and implications for screening colonoscopy: impact of endoscopy nurses. *World Journal of Gastroenterology*, 18, 3590–4.

Ciocco, A. (1940). Sex differences in morbidity and mortality. *The Quarterly Review of Biology*, 15, 59–73.

Connell, R. (2012). Gender, health and theory: conceptualizing the issue, in local and world perspective. *Social Science & Medicine*, 74, 1675–83.

Connell, R. and Messerschmidt, J.W. (2005). Hegemonic masculinity: rethinking the concept. *Gender and Society*, 19, 829–59.

Courtenay, W. and Messerschmidt, J.W. (2011). *Dying to be Men: Psychosocial, Environmental and Biobehavioural Directions in Promoting the Health of Men and Boys*. New York: Routledge.

Craig, R. and Mindell, J. (2012). *Health Survey for England 2011 Volume 1: Health, Social Care and Lifestyles*. Leeds: Health and Social Care Information Centre.

Doyal, L. (1998). *Gender and Health*. Technical paper WHO/FRH/WHD/98.16. Geneva: World Health Organization.

Doyal, L. (2001). Sex, gender and health: the need for a new approach. *British Medical Journal*, 323, 1061–3.

Dunkle, K., Jewkes, R., Heather, C., et al. (2004). Gender-based violence, relationship power and the risk of HIV infection in women attending antenatal clinics in South Africa. *The Lancet*, 363, 1415–21.

Emslie, C., Lewars, H., Batty, G.D., et al. (2009). Are there gender differences in levels of heavy, binge and problem drinking? Evidence from three generations in the west of Scotland. *Public Health*, 123, 12–14.

Erikson, M., Mackay, J., and Ross, H. (2012). *Tobacco Atlas* (4th ed.). Atlanta, GA: American Cancer Society.

Forastieri, V. (2010). *Women Workers and Gender Issues on Occupational Safety and Health*. Geneva: International Labour Office.

Geller, S., Koch, A., Pellettieri, B., et al. (2011). Inclusion, analysis and reporting of sex and race/ethnicity in clinical trials: have we made progress? *Journal of Women's Health*, 20, 315–20.

Governder, V. and Penn-Kekana, L. (2008). Gender biases and discrimination in care: interpersonal interactions. *Global Public Health*, 3(Suppl. 1), 90–103.

Gunnell, D., Middleton, N., Whitley, E., et al. (2003). Why are suicide rates rising in young men but falling in the elderly? A time-series analysis of trends in England and Wales 1950–1998. *Social Science & Medicine*, 57, 595–611.

Harryson, L., Novo, M., and Hammarström, A. (2012). Is gender inequality in the domestic sphere associated with psychological distress among women and men? Results from the Northern Swedish Cohort. *Journal of Epidemiology and Community Health*, 66, 271–6.

Hemmenway, D., Sihinoda-Tagawa, T., and Miller, M. (2002). Firearm availability and female homicide victimisation rates among 25 high-populous countries. *Journal of American Women's Medical Association*, 57, 100–4.

Iyer, A., Sen, G., and Ostlin, P. (2008). The intersections of gender and class in health status and health care. *Global Public Health*, 3, 13–24.

Jackson, C. and Palmer-Jones, R. (1998). *Work Intensity, Gender and Well-Being*. Discussion Paper No 96. New York: United Nations Research Institute for Social Development.

Jaffe, D., Eisenbach, Z., and Manor, O. (2011). The effect of parity on cause-specific mortality among married men and women. *Maternal and Child Health Journal*, 15, 376–85.

Jylhä, M. (2009). What is self-rated health and why does it predict mortality? Towards a unified conceptual model. *Social Science & Medicine*, 69, 307–16.

Kiyohara, C. and Ohno, Y. (2010). Sex differences in lung cancer susceptibility: a review. *Gender Medicine*, 7, 381–401.

Krieger, N. (2003). Genders, sexes and health: what are the connections—and why does it matter? *International Journal of Epidemiology*, 32, 652–7.

Krieger, N. and Zierler, S. (1995). Accounting for the health of women. *Current Issues in Public Health*, 1, 251–6.

Kucuk, A.I. and Atalay, C. (2012). The relationship between surgery and phase of the menstrual cycle affects survival in breast cancer. *Journal of Breast Cancer*, 15, 434–40.

Lader, D., Short, S., and Gershuny, J. (2006). *Time Use Survey 2005*. London: Office for National Statistics.

Lorber, J. (1997). *Gender and the Construction of Illness*. London: Sage.

MacDorman, M., Hoyert, D., Martin, J., et al. (2007). Fetal and perinatal mortality. *National and Vital Statistics Reports*, 55, 1–18.

Menees, S., Inadomi, J., Korsnes, S., et al. (2003). Women patients' preference for women physicians is barrier to colon cancer screening. *Gastrointestinal Endoscopy*, 62, 219–23.

Murray, C., Vos, T., and Lozano, R. (2012). Disability-adjusted life years (DALYs) for 291 diseases and injuries in 21 regions, 1990–2010: a systematic analysis for the Global Burden of Disease Study 2010. *The Lancet*, 380, 2197–223.

Natrass, N. (2006). *AIDS, Gender and Access to Antiretroviral Treatment in South Africa*. CSSR Working Paper No 178. Cape Town: UCT.

O'Brien Cousins, S. and Gillis, M. (2005). 'Just do it…before you talk yourself out of it': the self-talk of adults thinking about physical activity. *Psychology of Sport and Exercise*, 6, 313–34.

Organisation for Economic Cooperation and Development (2011). *Health at a Glance 2011: OECD Indicators*. Paris: OECD.

Paggi, M.G., Vona, R., Abbruzzese, C., et al. (2010). Gender-related disparities in non-small cell lung cancer. *Cancer Letters*, 298, 1–8.

Patel, R.C. (2012). Food sovereignty: power, gender, and the right to food. *PLoS Medicine*, 9, e1001223.

Payne, S. (2006). *The Health of Men and Women*. Cambridge: Polity.

Payne, S. (2007). Not an equal opportunity disease—a sex and gender-based review of colorectal cancer in men and women, part 1. *The Journal of Men's Health and Gender*, 42, 131–9.

Perkins, K. (2001). Smoking cessation in women: special considerations. *CNS Drugs*, 15, 391–411.

Pietilä, I. and Rytkönen, M. (2008). 'Health is not a man's domain': lay accounts of gender difference in life-expectancy in Russia. *Sociology of Health & Illness*, 30, 1070–85.

Popescu, A., LeResche, L., Truelove, E.L., et al. (2010). Gender differences in pain modulation by diffuse noxious inhibitory controls: a systematic review. *Pain*, 150, 309–18.

Ravindran, S. (2000). *Engendering Health*. Seminar 489 May 2000. [Online] Available at: http://www.india-seminar.com/2000/489/489%20ravindran.htm.

Redgrave, G., Swartz, K., and Romanoski, A. (2003). Alcohol misuse by women. *International Review of Psychiatry*, 15, 256–68.

Rieker, P., Bird, C., and Lang, M. (2010). Understanding gender and health: old patterns, new trends and future directions. In C. Bird, P. Conrad, A. Freemont, and S. Timmermans (eds.) *Handbook of Medical Sociology*, pp. 52–73. Nashville, TN: Vanderbilt University Press.

Riska, E. (2010). Coronary heart disease: gendered public health discourses. In E. Kuhlmann and E. Annandale (eds.) *The Palgrave Handbook of Gender and Health Care*, pp. 158–71. Basingstoke: Palgrave Macmillan.

Salomon, J.A., Wang, H., Freeman, M., et al. (2012). Healthy life expectancy for 187 countries, 1990–2010: a systematic analysis for the Global Burden Disease Study 2010. *The Lancet*, 380, 2144–62.

Samet, J. and Yoon, S. (2010). *Gender, Women and the Tobacco Epidemic*. Geneva: World Health Organization.

Scarborough, P., Bhatnagar, P., Wickramasinghe, K., et al. (2010). *Coronary Heart Disease Statistics: 2010 Edition*. London: British Heart Foundation Health Promotion Research Group.

Sen, G. and Bonita, R. (2000). Global health status: two steps forward, one step back. *The Lancet*, 356, 577–82.

Sen, G. and Ostlin, P. (2007). *Unequal, Unfair, Ineffective and Inefficient: Gender Inequality in Health: Why It Exists and How We Can Change It. Final Report to the WHO Commission on Social Determinants of Health*. Geneva: World Health Organization.

Simkhada, B., Teijlingen, E.R., Porter, M., et al. (2008). Factors affecting the utilization of antenatal care in developing countries: systematic review of the literature. *Journal of Advanced Nursing*, 61, 244–60.

Sivakumaran, S. (2010). Lost in translation: UN responses to sexual violence against men and boys in situations of armed conflict. *International Review of the Red Cross*, 92, 259–77.

Skovdal, M., Campbell, C., Madanhure, C., et al. (2011). Masculinity as a barrier to men's use of HIV services in Zimbabwe. *Globalization and Health*, 15, 1–14.

Snow, R.C. (2008). Sex, gender, and vulnerability. *Global Public Health*, 3, 58–74.

Sondik, E., Madans, J., and Gentleman, K. (2012). *Vital and Health Statistics Series 10 Number 256: Summary Health Statistics for US Adults: National Health Interview Survey 2011*. Hyattsville, MD: National Center for Health Statistics.

Springer, K., Stellman, J., and Jordan-Young, R. (2012). Beyond a catalogue of differences: a theoretical frame and good practice guidelines for researching sex/gender in human health. *Social Science & Medicine*, 74, 1817–24.

Stibbe, A. (2004). Health and the social construction of masculinity in Men's Health magazine. *Men and Masculinities*, 7, 31–51.

Tanner, M. and Vlassoff, C. (1998). Treatment seeking behaviour for malaria: a typology based on endemicity and gender. *Social Science & Medicine*, 46, 523–32.

UNAIDS (2009). *Transmission in Intimate Personal Relationships in Asia*. Geneva: UNAIDS.

UNAIDS (2011). *World AIDS Day Report 2011*. Geneva: UNAIDS.

United Nations (2012). *UN Data: Life Expectancy as Age X*. [Online] Available at: <http://data.un.org/Data.aspx?d=GenderStat&f=inID%3A36>

United Nations Development Programme (2012). *Strategy Note: HIV, Health and Development*. New York: United Nations Development Programme.

Vaidya, D., Becker, D., Bittner, V., et al. (2011). Ageing, menopause, and ischaemic heart disease mortality in England, Wales, and the United States: modelling study of national mortality data. *British Medical Journal*, 343, 1–10.

Vidaver, R., Lafleur, B., Tong, C., et al. (2000). Women subjects in NIH-funded clinical research literature: lack of progress in both representation and analysis by sex. *Journal of Women's Health and Gender-based Medicine*, 9, 495–504.

Waldron, I. (1985). What do we know about the causes of sex differences in mortality? *Population Bulletin of United Nations*, 18, 59–76.

Wallentin, M. (2009). Putative sex differences in verbal abilities and language cortex: a critical review. *Brain and Language*, 108, 175–83.

Wilkins, D., Payne, S., Granville, G., et al. (2008). *The Gender and Access to Health Services Study: Final Report*. London: Department of Health.

Wizeman, T. and Pardue, M. (2001). *Exploring the Biological Contributions to Health: Does Sex Matter?* Washington, DC: National Academy Press.

Women's Health Research (2009). *Fact Sheet: Sex Differences in HIV/AIDS*. Society for Women's Health Research. [Online] Available at: http://www.womenshealthresearch.org/site/PageServer?pagename=hs_healthfacts_hiv.

World Bank (2012). *World Development Report 2012: Gender Equality and Development*. Washington, DC: World Bank.

World Cancer Research Fund and American Institute for Cancer Research (2007). *Food, Nutrition, Physical Activity and the Prevention of Cancer: A Global Perspective*. Washington, DC: World Cancer Research Fund/American Institute for Cancer Research.

World Health Organization (2003). *Gender, Health and Ageing*. Geneva: WHO.

World Health Organization (2005). *World Health Surveys*. Geneva: WHO. Available at: http://www.who.int/healthinfo/survey/en.

World Health Organization (2008). *Closing the Gap in a Generation: Health Equity through Action on the Social Determinants of Health: Final Report of the Commission on Social Determinants of Health*. Geneva: WHO.

World Health Organization (2009). *Global Health Risks: Mortality and the Burden of Disease Attributable to Selected Major Risks*. Geneva: WHO.

World Health Organization (2010). *Global Recommendations on Physical Activity and Health*. Geneva: WHO.

World Health Organization (2011a). *Causes of Death 2008: Summary Tables*. [Online] Available at: http://www.who.int/evidence/bod.

World Health Organization (2011b). *Global Status Report on Alcohol and Health*. Geneva: WHO.

World Health Organization (2011c). *Management of Substance Abuse: Country Profiles*. Geneva: WHO.

World Health Organization (2012a). *Life Expectancy: Global Health Repository*. Geneva: WHO. Available at: http://apps.who.int/gho/data/?vid=710

World Health Organization (2012b). *Obesity and Overweight*. Geneva: World Health Organization.

World Health Organization (2012c). *Patterns of Consumption: Heavy Episodic Drinking by Country. Global Health Repository*. Geneva: WHO. Available at: http://apps.who.int/gho/data/?vid=2250#.

World Health Organization (2012d). *Under-Five Mortality Rate (Probability of Dying by Age 5 per 1000 Live Births)*. [Online] Available at: http://apps.who.int/gho/data/?theme=main&node=102#.

World Health Organization (2012e). *WHO Mortality Database: Tables*. [Online] Available at: http://www.who.int/healthinfo/morttables/en/index.html.

World Health Organization (2012f). *World Health Statistics*. Geneva: WHO.

World Health Organization (2012g). *World Malaria Report*. Geneva: WHO.

World Health Organization and London School of Hygiene and Tropical Medicine (2010). *Preventing Intimate Partner and Sexual Violence Against Women: Taking Action and Generating Evidence*. Geneva: WHO and London School of Hygiene and Tropical Medicine.

Zandman-Goddard, G., Peeva, E., Rozman, Z., et al. (2012). Sex and gender differences in autoimmune diseases. In S. Oertelt-Prigione and V. Regitz-Zagrosek (eds.) *Sex and Gender Aspects in Clinical Medicine*, pp. 104–24. London: Springer.

Zaninotto, P., Wardle, H., Stamatakis, E., et al. (2006). *Forecasting Obesity to 2010*. London: Department of Health.

Child health

Cynthia Boschi-Pinto, Nigel Rollins,
Bernadette Daelmans, Rajiv Bahl,
Jose Martines, and Elizabeth Mason

The situation of children in the world

Within the life course, the period of life before attaining adulthood is divided into three age subgroups based on epidemiology and healthcare needs: the first 5 years (*under-5 children*), the next 5 years (*older children*), and the second decade of life (*adolescents*). The first 5 years of life are further subdivided into the neonatal period (the first 28 days of life), infancy (the first year of life), and pre-school years (from 1 to 5 years). This chapter focuses on the health of under-5 children.

The most important indicators of health status of under-5 children relate to their mortality, morbidity, nutrition, growth, and development. Poor health and survival are linked to social and economic development and child mortality is one of the most sensitive barometers of this relationship. An overview of the health situation and inequalities among children in the world is presented in this section.

Mortality in under-5 children

Every year 139 million babies are born in the world, of which nearly 5 million will die before their first birthday and an additional 1.7 million before reaching age 5. The first 12 years of the twenty-first century witnessed a 36 per cent decline in under-5 mortality rates (U5MRs)—from 75 in the year 2000 to 48 per 1000 live births in 2012. Despite the progress made in recent decades, 6.6 million children less than 5 years of age continue to die in a year (United Nations Children's Fund (UNICEF) et al. 2013). This figure is more than twice the number of all individuals dying in the same period from HIV infection or AIDS, malaria, and tuberculosis combined. Over 70 per cent of under-5 deaths occur within the first year of life, but the risk of death is the highest closest to birth; it then decreases over the subsequent days, months, and years.

More than 80 per cent of all under-5 deaths are clustered in just two regions of the world: sub-Saharan Africa and South Asia (Fig. 10.3.1) (World Health Organization (WHO) n.d.). Although the African continent has only 25 per cent of the world's under-5 population, it accounts for 51 per cent of the global under-5 deaths; in contrast, less than 1 per cent of under-5 deaths take place in Europe. It is noteworthy that 50 per cent of all these deaths are concentrated in five countries: India, Nigeria, Democratic Republic of Congo, Pakistan, and China (UNICEF et al. 2013).

Most children eventually die from only a small number of diseases and conditions. Globally, the single most important cause of death among newborn babies is complications due to preterm birth, which claims one-third of newborn lives. Birth asphyxia and sepsis are the second and third major causes of death in this early period of life. Among older children (1–59 months), pneumonia, diarrhoeal disease, and malaria are the leading causes of mortality, accounting together for about 50 per cent of the 3.7 million postneonatal deaths (Liu et al. 2012; World Health Organization 2013).

The so-called epidemiological transition has a complex, dynamic course which reflects changes in demographic, socioeconomic, cultural, biological, technological, and environmental domains. As a result, important modifications are seen in the patterns of causes of death that usually shift from acute infectious diseases and deficiency-related conditions to non-communicable diseases (NCDs), leading to a relative increase in conditions such as perinatal causes (prematurity, birth asphyxia, and trauma), congenital abnormalities, and injuries. Of the overall 2.7 million fewer under-5 deaths in 2010, as compared to the year 2000, nearly 60 per cent were due to reductions in deaths caused by pneumonia, measles, and diarrhoeal diseases.

Poverty, low levels of maternal education, and poor quality healthcare are underlying determinants of most under-5 deaths. Levels, trends, and progress in both infant and under-5 mortality are unequally distributed between and within regions and countries. Children in low-income countries are nearly 14 times more likely to die before the age of 5 than children in high-income countries (UNICEF et al. 2013). Sub-Saharan Africa has, in general, the highest burden of global child mortality, accounting for 97 per cent of all under-5 deaths attributable to malaria in the world, 91 per cent of all deaths due to HIV and AIDS, 56 per cent due to diarrhoeal diseases, and more than 47 per cent of deaths due to pneumonia. Further critical inequities are present within countries, where children from the poorest families, living in rural areas, and whose mothers are less educated are those more likely to die.

Morbidity in under-5 children

Because the measurement of morbidity is more complex than that of mortality, information on the distribution of morbidity burden among under-5s is scarce. Despite the limitations of

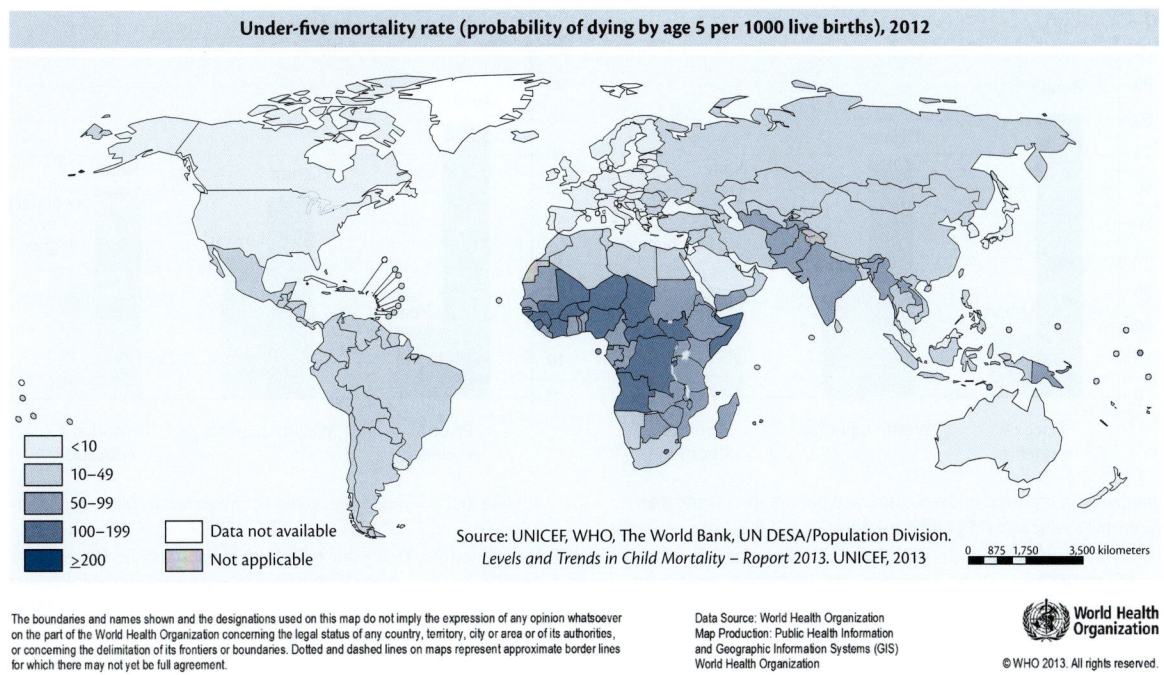

Fig. 10.3.1 World distribution of under-5 mortality rates, 2012.
Reproduced with permission from WHO Global Health Observatory, World Health Organization, Geneva, Switzerland, Copyright © WHO 2013, available from: http://gamapserver.who.int/mapLibrary/Files/Maps/global_underfivemortality_2012.png.

data, it is known that the main causes of morbidity highly correlate with the major causes of death in under-5 children. In 2010, 120 million episodes of pneumonia occurred in children less than 5 years of age, of which 14 million progressed to severe illness (Fischer Walker et al. 2013). An overall 5.5 per cent risk of long-term major respiratory sequelae from childhood pneumonia in non-hospitalized children has been reported, with a threefold higher risk in hospitalized children (Edmond et al. 2012).

Recent estimates of diarrhoeal disease burden show a median of 2.9 episodes per child per year, with the highest number of annual episodes recorded in the African (449 million annual episodes) and South East Asia (437 million annual episodes) regions (Fischer Walker et al. 2012). An important consequence of persistently high rates of diarrhoea morbidity is a negative effect on child growth and development.

Incidence of both pneumonia and diarrhoea are closely associated with poor home environments, undernutrition, and lack of access to health services. The prevalence of pneumonia and diarrhoea can be more than twice as high among the poorest children as among the richest ones. These differences in reported morbidity within countries are illustrated in Fig. 10.3.2.

Nutrition, growth, and development in under-5 children

The nutritional status of under-5 children is usually assessed through three standard indicators: stunting, wasting, and underweight. A stunted child is a child who falls below minus two standard deviations (−2 SD) from the median height-for-age of the WHO Child Growth Standards (World Health Organization 2006a). Stunting is usually a result of chronic undernutrition or nutritional deprivation over a lengthy period of time. A child is

considered wasted when he/she falls below −2 SD from the median weight-for-height of the WHO Standards. Wasting usually reflects an acute nutritional deficiency, due either to reduced food consumption or acute weight loss during an illness. Finally, a child is said to be underweight if his/her weight falls below −2 SD from the median weight-for-age of the WHO Standards, which can be a result of stunting, wasting or both.

Globally, there were 165 million children under-5 stunted, 52 million wasted, and 101 million underweight in 2011 (UNICEF et al. 2012). The proportion of under-5s who are underweight declined by 36 per cent between 1990 and 2011, bringing the world closer to the target of halving the proportion of underweight children between 1990 and 2015. Poor nutritional status of a child is strongly correlated to his/her vulnerability to diseases, to delayed physical and mental development, and to an increased risk of mortality. As described for morbidity and mortality, underweight is usually associated with inadequate maternal education and low levels in other indicators of well-being.

In contrast, almost 43 million under-5 children in the world are overweight (weight-for-height above 2 SD), a 54 per cent increase from an estimated 28 million in 1990 (UNICEF et al. 2012). Prevalence is highest in high- (8.4 per cent) and upper-middle- (6.4 per cent) income countries, where nearly 17 million children are overweight. Obese children have increased risks of adult obesity, diabetes, liver disease, and poor social and economic performance in later life.

The first years of life provide the greatest opportunities for development. Young children have maximum plasticity of neuronal systems and thus benefit the most from interventions. Nonetheless, they are highly vulnerable to negative effects of poor environments such as increased morbidity, undernutrition, and delays in development. Annually, over 200 million children under 5 years of age have

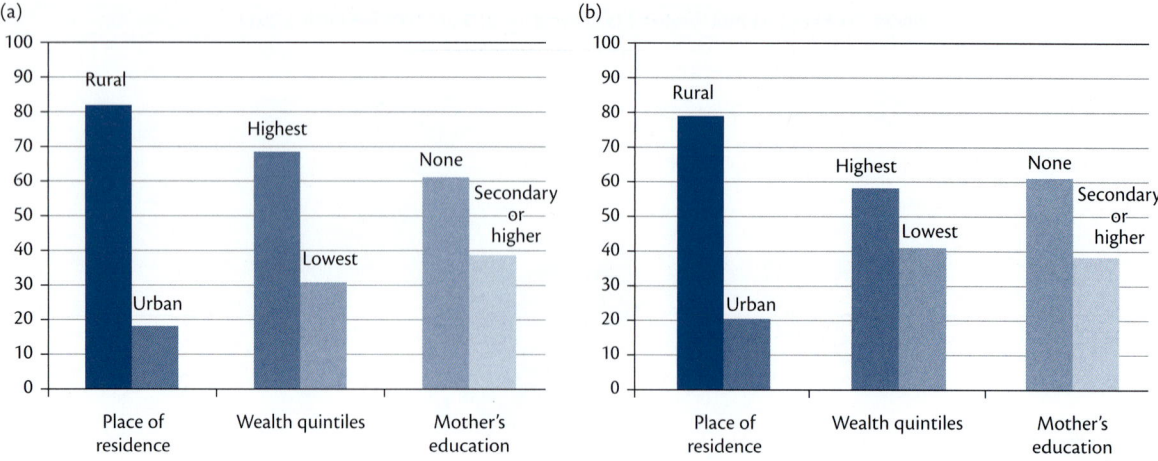

Fig. 10.3.2 Inequities in reported under-5 suspected pneumonia (a) and diarrhoea (b) morbidity in the 2 weeks preceding the interview by place of residence, wealth quintiles, and mother's education in 11 African countries and five Asian countries.
Source: data from Ghana Statistical Service et al. (2009), National Population Commission et al. (2009), National Statistics Directorate et al. (2010), National Statistics Office et al. (2009), Statistics Sierra Leone and ICF Macro (2009), Institut National de la Statistique et al. (2010), Instituto Nacional de Estatística et al. (2010), Kenya National Bureau of Statistics et al. (2010), Ministry of Health and Family et al. (2010), National Bureau of Statistics et al. (2011), National Institute of Statistics et al. (2011), National Statistical Office and ICF Macro (2011), Central Statistical Agency and ICF International (2012), Edmond (2012), Fischer Walker (2012, 2013), Liu et al. (2012), Ministry of Health and Population et al. (2012), National Institute of Statistics of Rwanda et al. (2012), Zimbabwe National Statistics Agency et al. (2012), World Health Organization (2013).

significantly impaired growth and development, most of whom live in south Asia (Grantham-McGregor et al. 2007).

A child's environment and activities while growing shape their cognitive abilities and general development. Optimal child development is a result of adequate nutrition, prevention, and timely management of illness, care, and stimulation. Malnourished, sick, and disabled children are at particular risk of a poor development. They have more difficulty learning, are less active, and may be less able to receive the attention needed from those who care for them. Effective interventions that impact on child development are available along the life course. They aim to improve maternal health and fetal outcomes, caregiver–child interactions, responsiveness and stimulation through play and communication. Through stimulation and interactions, these interventions intend to enhance the child's ability to learn socially and intellectually and grow physically.

The frequent contact of mothers, their babies, and young infants with health services provides a unique opportunity for these services to actively promote and support early child development.

Addressing health needs of the child in low- and middle-income countries

Children whose environments have limited resources need interventions to protect them against the major causes of mortality and morbidity summarized in the previous section. There are two main types of interventions. The first promote health and prevent specific disease conditions. The second are case management interventions which help reduce severity of illness thereby improving health and survival. Key interventions are reviewed in the following text for each of the major causes of under-5 mortality and summarized in Table 10.3.1.

Newborn conditions

The proportion of under-5 deaths that occur within the first month of life has increased 19 per cent since 1990, because declines in the

neonatal mortality rate have been slower than those in the mortality rate for older children. Improving newborn health and survival requires a continuum of care from pregnancy, childbirth, and the newborn period, into childhood and adolescence. Newborn health interventions can be classified into those relevant for all mothers and newborns, and those relevant only for newborns with conditions that require additional care.

Care for all mothers and newborns

Newborn health and survival requires empowerment (particularly of girls and women) and health promotion through life, which includes nutrition and education, prevention of harmful practices such as female genital mutilation, delay in sexual debut, prevention and treatment of sexually transmitted infections, and support for optimal timing and spacing of pregnancies. Care during pregnancy is important for newborn survival. Interventions of proven benefit for newborn health provided during antenatal care include tetanus immunization, screening for and treatment of syphilis and HIV, prevention and treatment of malaria and calcium supplementation in populations with low dietary calcium intake. Antenatal care provides the basis for continued care during and after childbirth by planning for birth with a skilled attendant and preparing for unforeseen complications, and by helping the family prepare for maternal and newborn care practices, such as early initiation of and exclusive breastfeeding.

Skilled care at childbirth is needed for all women and babies without exception because the complications that may occur during and immediately following childbirth (for both mothers and babies) cannot be predicted and may very rapidly become fatal. This means that skilled childbirth care in first-level health facilities, with the backup of a hospital that can manage complications, should be available 24 hours a day, every day. For a home birth, it is crucial to have access to a skilled attendant and a companion who can stay with the mother and baby for the first 12–24 hours. For a woman and her family who cannot have access to a skilled attendant in a home birth, it is essential to ensure that they have

Table 10.3.1 Summary of key interventions to address major causes of child mortality and morbidity

Important causes of under-5 mortality and morbidity	Preventive interventions	Case management interventions
Newborn conditions: • Preterm birth • Perinatal asphyxia • Neonatal sepsis	• Antenatal care • Skilled care during labour and birth • Care at the time of birth (warmth, cord care, and early initiation of breastfeeding) • Care during the first days and weeks after birth (exclusive breastfeeding, warmth, hygienic skin and cord care, and prompt care-seeking for illness)	• Tocolytics and antenatal corticosteroids for preterm labour • Antibiotics for preterm premature rupture of membranes • Additional care of preterm and LBW infants (addressing feeding, warmth, and breathing problems) • Caesarean section or assisted vaginal delivery in case of fetal distress • Resuscitation if unable to breathe after birth • Diagnosis and treatment of neonatal sepsis and local infections
Pneumonia	• Immunization against pneumococcus, *Haemophilus influenzae*, pertussis, diphtheria, and measles • Exclusive breastfeeding up to 6 months; continued breastfeeding with safe and appropriate complementary feeding at least up to 2 years • Reduction in environmental risk factors—e.g. indoor air pollution	• Treatment of pneumonia with amoxicillin • Treatment of severe pneumonia with parenteral antibiotics, oxygen, and other supportive treatment
Diarrhoea	• Early and exclusive breastfeeding up to 6 months; continued breastfeeding with safe and appropriate complementary feeding at least up to 2 years • Vitamin A supplementation • Immunization against rotavirus and measles • Water and sanitation, hand washing with soap	• Fluid replacement to prevent dehydration • Zinc treatment for 10–14 days during diarrhoea • Antibiotics for dysentery
Malaria	• Vector control • Use of ITNs	• Treatment of non-severe malaria with oral antimalarial drugs recommended for the area • Treatment of severe malaria with parenteral antimalarial drugs
HIV/AIDS	• Primary prevention of HIV and of unintended pregnancies in HIV-infected women • ARVs—treatment of pregnant women when indicated, prophylaxis for others • Exclusive breastfeeding with ARVs or replacement feeding for HIV-positive mother • Co-trimoxazole prophylaxis for HIV-exposed and HIV-infected children	• ART for children who are eligible for it
Malnutrition	• Early initiation of breastfeeding • Exclusive breastfeeding up to 6 months of age • Continued breastfeeding with safe and appropriate complementary foods up to at least 2 years • Preventing vitamin A, iron, iodine, and zinc deficiency through supplementation, food fortification, or dietary diversification • Community-based screening for severe acute malnutrition using mid-upper arm circumference (MUAC) measurements	• Community-based management of children with severe malnutrition without complications • Hospital management of severely malnourished children with complications

knowledge of maternal and newborn danger signs, and a plan for a clean delivery and early care-seeking if problems arise.

Care for all newborns at the time of birth and during the days and weeks that follow includes several relatively simple and effective interventions that do not require advanced technology (Box 10.3.1). The most critical time to deliver these interventions is immediately after birth. Another important time period is the first 24 hours after birth as a large proportion of maternal and

neonatal deaths occur during this window. Thereafter, at least one additional contact with a health provider within the first week, preferably on the second or third day of life, is required.

Management and care of newborn conditions

Fifteen million premature babies are born every year of which nearly 1 million die due to complications of *preterm birth* (WHO 2012a). Appropriate management of preterm labour can reduce

Box 10.3.1 Basic newborn care at the time of birth and in the days and weeks after birth

Care at the time of birth

- Birth in a warm room.
- Drying the baby thoroughly immediately after birth.
- Keeping the baby in skin-to-skin contact with the mother.
- Hygienic cord care.
- Eye care.
- Early initiation of breastfeeding as soon as the mother and the baby are ready (usually within the first hour of birth).

Care during the first days and weeks

- Exclusive breastfeeding.
    - Keeping the newborn warm.
    - Hygienic cord and eye care.
    - Vaccination.
- Prompt recognition of danger signs (not feeding well, reduced activity, fast or difficult breathing, fever or low body temperature, or convulsions) and care seeking by the family.

mortality and morbidity in neonates. Key interventions include tocolytics to delay birth, and corticosteroids given to the mother during preterm labour to promote lung maturation of the baby. In addition, if there is preterm pre-labour rupture of membranes antibiotics should be given.

Additional care of preterm and low birth weight (LBW) infants is critical for improving newborn survival. Identification of LBW infants within the first hours after birth should be a part of the basic newborn-care package. In settings where birth weight measurement is not feasible, such as for home births, all newborns perceived to be 'small' should receive additional care. These may include one additional contact in the first week and weekly contacts thereafter until the infant is feeding and growing well.

In addition to basic newborn care, LBW infants need more attention for warmth, feeding, hygiene, early detection of infections, and growth monitoring. Kangaroo mother care or skin-to-skin care is the best way to keep them warm and to encourage breastfeeding. Mothers who cannot breastfeed directly should be taught to express breast milk and to feed from a cup. Much of this additional care can be provided at home and in first-level health facilities. However, care for babies weighing less than 1500 g, who have difficulty feeding or breathing due to lung immaturity, is best provided in a hospital.

Perinatal asphyxia is responsible for 10 per cent of all under-5 deaths. The most important intervention for preventing deaths and severe morbidity due to perinatal asphyxia is monitoring of progress in labour and maternal and fetal well-being during labour using a partograph. Fetal monitoring should be conducted during labour, and should be associated with prompt and appropriate action if fetal distress is detected. When fetal distress is suspected, assisted vaginal or Caesarean birth may be needed which requires functional referral mechanisms. The second key intervention for prevention of asphyxia-related mortality and

morbidity is neonatal resuscitation. Given the likelihood/possibility of this, all birth attendants should be skilled and equipped to perform neonatal resuscitation, which includes positive pressure ventilation with a self-inflating bag and mask using room air, in addition to thorough drying and stimulation.

Management of *newborn infections* in a swift and appropriate manner can substantially reduce neonatal mortality. It is therefore important to have community- and health-facility-based activities which support families in identifying the danger signs and seeking timely and appropriate care. Newborns with severe infections should receive parenteral antibiotics, along with intravenous fluids or alternative feeding methods and other supportive therapy such as oxygen in a hospital. Research studies are currently underway to determine if a proportion of these children can be safely managed at home using intramuscular or oral antibiotics.

Acute respiratory infections

Acute respiratory infections (ARIs), particularly pneumonia, are the leading cause of under-5 mortality as they are responsible for 18 per cent of all child deaths worldwide. Interventions to control ARIs can be divided into preventive interventions such as immunization against specific pathogens, improvements in nutrition, safer environments, and case management interventions.

Widespread use of vaccines against pneumococcus, *Haemophilus influenzae* (Hib), pertussis, diphtheria, influenza, and measles has the potential to substantially reduce the incidence of ARIs in children in low- and middle-income countries. Two particularly important vaccines are those against *Pneumococcus* and Hib, pathogens responsible for about half of all cases of pneumonia.

Two types of pneumococcal vaccines are currently licensed for use: a polysaccharide vaccine effective against 23 different strains of *Pneumococcus* and two different formulations of protein-conjugated vaccines (PCVs) effective against ten or 13 serotypes of pneumococcus, respectively. The serotypes included in these vaccines account for the majority of serious pneumococcal disease in children worldwide (Johnson et al. 2010). Use of these vaccines in countries in North America and Europe has seen declines in rates of invasive pneumococcal disease in children and also in pneumonia hospitalization (Grijalva et al. 2007; Jardine et al. 2010; Pilishvili et al. 2010; Miller et al. 2011). Studies to document the impact of PCVs in low-income countries are ongoing. PCVs are increasingly available in low-income, high-mortality countries, but gaps in vaccine uptake within countries could reduce their impact.

The use of Hib conjugate vaccines in developed countries has resulted in the virtual elimination of invasive Hib disease (meningitis and bacteraemic pneumonia) because of immunity in vaccinated children and a herd effect in those not vaccinated. There are several Hib conjugate vaccines available, all of which are effective when given in early infancy and have virtually no side effects. The success of these vaccines is seen in most low-income countries which have introduced Hib vaccines.

Vaccination should be seen as complementary to other strategies for pneumonia control, such as improved care-seeking and case management, better nutrition (including exclusive breastfeeding for the first 6 months of life), and measures to reduce indoor air pollution. Results from two meta-analyses of published studies showed that young children exposed to smoke from use of household biomass fuel had a rate of acute lower respiratory infection twice that of children not exposed (Smith et al. 2004; Dherani et al. 2008). In a trial in Guatemala, environmental interventions to reduce exposure to indoor air pollution have been shown to reduce the incidence of severe respiratory infections in children (Smith et al. 2011).

Clinical guidelines for ARI case management rely on two simple clinical signs: fast breathing and lower chest wall in-drawing to identify children with ARI who need antibiotic therapy (WHO 2012b). Fast breathing detects about 85 per cent of pneumonia patients. The specificity of fast breathing is 70–80 per cent, which means that 20–30 per cent of children with ARI who do not need antibiotics will receive them. However, the use of this sign renders decision-making by first-level health workers simple thereby increasing the proportion of children with pneumonia who receive antibiotics. Chest in-drawing is the inward movement of the lower chest wall when a child breathes in. Children with chest wall in-drawing who do not have any of the danger signs can be successfully treated with oral amoxicillin (Hazir et al. 2008; Addo-Yobo et al. 2011; Bari et al. 2011; Soofi et al. 2012).

Children with audible stridor when calm and any general danger signs such as lethargy or unconsciousness and inability to feed should be managed in a hospital with parenteral antibiotics and supportive care. Oxygen should be used in children who are unable to feed or drink, are drowsy or lethargic, or have central cyanosis, head nodding, respiratory rate of 70 breaths/minute or more, or severe chest wall in-drawing. Pulse oximetry should preferably be used to assess hypoxaemia (WHO 2012b).

Diarrhoea

Diarrhoea remains one of the leading causes of death among under-5 children in low- and middle-income countries. Strategies for the control of diarrhoeal diseases have remained substantially unchanged since the early 1980s. A package of proven prevention and treatment measures is available that, if taken to scale, will lead to a significant reduction in the burden of diarrhoeal disease. It consists of a seven-point plan for diarrhoea control and includes promotion of early and exclusive breastfeeding, vitamin A supplementation, rotavirus and measles vaccination, promotion of hand washing with soap and improved water supply, promotion of community-wide sanitation, fluid replacement to prevent rehydration, and zinc treatment (UNICEF and WHO 2009).

Exclusively breastfed children under 6 months of age are ten times less likely to die of diarrhoea than non-breastfed infants (Lamberti et al. 2011). This is because breast milk contains antimicrobial factors in addition to eliminating the intake of potentially contaminated food and water. Safe and appropriate complementary foods introduced at 6 months of age and continued breastfeeding for at least up to 2 years can improve nutritional status of infants and young children helping to prevent nutritional deterioration, impaired immune function, and greater susceptibility to infection sometimes caused by sequential episodes of diarrhoea.

Rotavirus is the most common cause of diarrhoea worldwide, accounting for at least one-third of severe and potentially fatal watery diarrhoea episodes, primarily in low- and middle-income countries where an estimated 450,000 vaccine-preventable rotavirus deaths occurred in 2008 (Tate et al. 2012). Two licensed rotavirus vaccines (85–98 per cent protective efficacy against severe diarrhoea in high- and middle-income and 50–70 per cent in

low-income countries), derived from human or bovine rotavirus (Armah et al. 2010; Zaman et al. 2010), have been introduced into national immunization programmes in over 35 countries worldwide. Candidate vaccines are undergoing field trials in low- and middle-income countries. In countries where diarrhoeal deaths account for at least 10 per cent of mortality among children aged less than 5 years, the introduction of the vaccine is strongly recommended (WHO 2009).

Human faeces are the primary source of diarrhoeal pathogens. Poor sanitation, lack of accessible clean water, and inadequate personal and domestic hygiene are responsible for an estimated 88 per cent of diarrhoeal cases everywhere (WHO 2007). Hand washing with soap reduces the risk of diarrhoea by an average of 48 per cent (Munos et al. 2010), and is best when undertaken as part of a package of behaviour-change interventions such as treating and safely storing drinking water at the point of use. However, the required behaviour change is complex and often difficult to sustain. Thus, significant resources should also be directed towards extending and sustaining water, sanitation, and hygiene services at community level.

Most deaths from diarrhoea occur because of dehydration associated with acute diarrhoea, and because of dysentery (bloody diarrhoea). Management of diarrhoea includes:

◆ Treating dehydration with oral rehydration salts (ORS) solution, or with an intravenous electrolyte solution in cases of severe dehydration.

◆ Providing children with 20 mg per day of zinc for 10–14 days.

◆ Continuing or increasing breastfeeding during and increasing feeding after the diarrhoeal episode.

◆ Using antibiotics only when appropriate (i.e. bloody diarrhoea) and not administering antidiarrhoeal drugs

Use of oral rehydration solution reduces diarrhoea-specific mortality by 69 per cent (Munos et al. 2010). Two noteworthy advances in the management of acute diarrhoea are: newly formulated ORS containing lower concentrations of glucose and salts, and zinc supplementation. ORS formulation has proved safe and effective in the prevention and treatment of dehydration. However, mothers' and health workers' acceptance of standard ORS has been suboptimal because watery stools persist and the duration of diarrhoea is not reduced. Efforts over the past decades have led to the development of a new ORS formulation. Compared with standard ORS, this lower sodium and glucose ORS reduces stool output, vomiting, and the need for intravenous fluids. The new ORS is safe and effective in both non-cholera diarrhoea and cholera in children and adults. WHO and UNICEF now recommend the use of ORS containing 75 meq of sodium and 75 mmol of glucose per litre (total osmolarity of 245 milliosmol per litre) everywhere (WHO 2005a). In addition to fluid replacement, children with diarrhoea should continue to be fed during the episode. Food intake supports fluid absorption and helps maintain nutritional status and ability to fight infection.

A recent review of relevant clinical trials indicates that zinc supplements given during an episode of acute diarrhoea reduce the duration, the risk of hospitalization, and the incidence of future episodes of diarrhoea (Fischer Walker and Black 2010). Studies from India show that including zinc in the management of acute diarrhoea has some programmatically important effects such as the reduction of hospital admissions for diarrhoeal disease (Mazumder et al. 2010). The addition of zinc to ORS in the treatment of diarrhoea has also increased the use-rates of ORS and reduced prescription of drugs of unknown identity and antibiotics (Bhandari et al. 2008). All children with acute diarrhoea should be given zinc supplements for 10–14 days during and after diarrhoea (10 mg per day for infants younger than 6 months of age and 20 mg per day for those over 6 months).

Dysentery—an inflammatory disorder of the lower intestinal tract, resulting in pain, fever, and severe diarrhoea, often accompanied by the passage of blood and mucus—is a major cause of diarrhoeal morbidity and mortality. *Shigella* is the most common and severe cause of bloody diarrhoea. The primary treatment for shigellosis is the use of antimicrobials which can decrease mortality attributable to dysentery by more than 99 per cent (Traa et al. 2010). The choice of effective, safe, oral, and inexpensive drugs for use in low- and middle-income countries has become problematic because of the increasing prevalence of antimicrobial drug resistance to several commonly used antibiotics. Ciprofloxacin is the current treatment drug of choice due to its effectiveness, safety, ease of administration by the oral route, short course, and low cost. However, ciprofloxacin-resistant strains are already appearing and this has made development of a vaccine for *Shigella* a high priority. For severe cholera cases, WHO recommends the use of oral antibiotics to which strains of *Vibrio cholerae* in the area are known to be sensitive; possible choices are: tetracycline, doxycycline, co-trimoxazole, erythromycin, and chloramphenicol. Antibiotic management of cholera results in a 63 per cent reduction in rates of clinical failure and a 75 per cent reduction in rates of bacteriological failure (Das et al. 2013).

Malaria

Malaria accounts for 7 per cent of child deaths worldwide. Nearly 500,000 children under age 5 are killed by malaria every year, 97 per cent of them in sub-Saharan Africa. Together with pneumonia and diarrhoea, malaria claimed the most lives among children 1–59 months of age (Liu et al. 2012). Chapter 8.15 on malaria describes malaria interventions in greater detail.

Vector control remains the most generally effective measure to prevent malaria transmission in all ages. For example insecticide-treated nets (ITNs) have been shown to be particularly effective in reducing uncomplicated malaria incidence and parasite infection prevalence in young children (Eisele et al. 2010).

Prompt parasitological confirmation by microscopy or alternatively by rapid diagnostic tests in all patients suspected of malaria should happen before treatment is started. Treatment solely on the basis of clinical suspicion should only be considered when a parasitological diagnosis is inaccessible. Once diagnosed, the child should be treated early with a safe and effective antimalarial medicine as delaying treatment could result in progression to severe disease, which is associated with a high case-fatality rate.

Malaria case management has been greatly affected by the emergence and spread of chloroquine and sulfadoxine/pyrimethamine resistance. To counter the threat of drug resistance of *Plasmodium falciparum* to monotherapies and to improve treatment outcomes, use of artemisinin-based combination antimalarials is recommended for treatment of uncomplicated malaria (WHO 2010a). In areas with poor access to health facilities, early recognition, prompt, and appropriate treatment require treatment in the home or community.

HIV and AIDS

In 2011, 3.4 million children under the age of 15 were living with HIV, 92 per cent of them in sub-Saharan Africa. Every day about 900 children are newly infected. While HIV/AIDS accounts for about 2 per cent of under-5 deaths globally (Liu et al. 2012; WHO 2013), in southern Africa it is responsible for about 26 per cent of these child deaths. In countries such as South Africa, where general HIV prevalence is among the highest in the world, the estimated proportion of child death due to HIV/AIDS reached 28 per cent in 2010. Although the proportional mortality due to HIV/AIDS among under-5s remains unacceptably high in some African countries, it has declined significantly in the last decade due to scaling-up of interventions to prevent infections in children. Diagnosis of HIV-infection in children less than 18 months is based on demonstrating the presence of HIV DNA through polymerase chain reaction testing and beyond this age by detecting antibodies to HIV through an enzyme-linked immunosorbent assay. This is because maternal antibodies to HIV can pass through the placenta and remain present in HIV-exposed but uninfected children until the age of 18 months.

Over 90 per cent of HIV-infected children are infected through mother-to-child transmission (MTCT), which may occur during pregnancy, birth, or through breastfeeding. Without any interventions, the risk of transmission is between 20 and 45 per cent, but this can be reduced to less than 2 per cent with a package of evidence-based interventions (WHO 2010b). Antiretroviral (ARV) drug interventions given to pregnant HIV-infected women are very effective at preventing peripartum MTCT and also protect the health and survival of mothers (WHO 2010b).

Postnatal ARV interventions are now recommended to reduce the risk of HIV transmission through breastfeeding. These can be given either to the mother (Shapiro et al. 2010; Kesho Bora Study Group 2011) or to the infant (Coovadia et al. 2012). The effectiveness of these interventions has transformed the landscape in which programmatic and individual decisions about feeding practices in the context of HIV can be made. Based on the strength of this evidence and programmatic considerations, national authorities are advised to promote and support one infant feeding practice for HIV-infected mothers, namely, either breastfeeding with ARVs or to avoid all breastfeeding and use replacement feeds (WHO 2010b). Achieving high coverage of these interventions in resource-limited countries has, however, been challenging. Access to CD4 counts to establish which pregnant women are eligible for lifelong ARV treatment and who should receive prophylaxis has been a barrier in many settings to effective scaling up. It is also recognized that women in high-prevalence countries are likely to have repeated pregnancies that would each involve ARV interventions, either prophylaxis or treatment. For these reasons, and also to protect the health of mothers, several national programmes have opted to start all pregnant HIV-infected women on lifelong treatment (Centers for Disease Control and Prevention 2013). Whether all HIV-infected pregnant women will want to start lifelong treatment and how best to support women to remain in care and achieve high rates of adherence remain important unanswered questions.

In settings where diarrhoea, pneumonia, and malnutrition continue to be significant causes of child mortality, breastfeeding is likely to give HIV-exposed infants the greatest chance of HIV-free survival (Kagaayi et al. 2008; Peltier et al. 2009). To achieve this, mothers known to be HIV-infected should be provided with either lifelong ARV therapy or ARV prophylaxis interventions to reduce HIV transmission through breastfeeding. These mothers should therefore exclusively breastfeed their infants for the first 6 months of life, introducing appropriate complementary foods thereafter, and continue breastfeeding for the first 12 months of life. Breastfeeding should then only stop once a nutritionally adequate and safe diet without breast milk can be provided.

In countries where infectious diseases and malnutrition do not contribute significantly to child mortality, mothers known to be HIV-infected may be advised to give their infants replacement feeds and avoid all breastfeeding. Commercial infant formula milk should be given as the replacement feed to these HIV-uninfected infants only when the following specific conditions are met:

♦ Safe water and sanitation are assured at the household level and in the community, and

♦ The mother or other caregiver can reliably provide sufficient infant formula milk to support normal growth and development of the infant; and

♦ The mother or caregiver can prepare it cleanly and frequently enough so that it is safe and carries a low risk of diarrhoea and malnutrition; and

♦ The mother or caregiver can, in the first 6 months, exclusively give infant formula milk; and

♦ The family is supportive of this practice; and

♦ The mother or caregiver can access healthcare that offers comprehensive child health services.

Irrespective of the common causes of death, when infants and young children are known to be HIV-infected, mothers are strongly encouraged to exclusively breastfeed for the first 6 months of life and continue breastfeeding as per the recommendations for the general population that is up to 2 years or beyond.

HIV-exposed or HIV-infected children may acquire a serious life-threatening form of pneumonia caused by *Pneumocystis jirovecii* (previously known as *carinii*), which often occurs before their HIV status has been confirmed. Co-trimoxazole, a fixed-dose combination of sulfamethoxazole and trimethoprim, is a broad-spectrum antimicrobial agent that targets a range of aerobic Gram-positive and Gram-negative organisms, fungi, and protozoa. The drug is widely available in both syrup and solid formulations at low cost in most places, including resource-limited settings. Regular prophylaxis with trimethoprim-sulfamethoxazole (co-trimoxazole) provides a simple, inexpensive, and effective strategy to reduce the risk of this infection, and has been shown to reduce mortality of HIV-infected children by up to 40 per cent even in the absence of ART (Chintu et al. 2004). Co-trimoxazole prophylaxis may also reduce the risk of malaria-related mortality in both HIV-infected and exposed children (Sandison et al. 2011) while it is unclear whether this would be effective in other children as well. Because of difficulty in diagnosing HIV infection in infants, co-trimoxazole prophylaxis is recommended for all HIV-exposed children born to mothers living with HIV starting at 4–6 weeks after birth and continuing until HIV infection has been excluded and the infant is no longer at risk of acquiring HIV through breastfeeding (Newell et al. 2004).

HIV-exposed and HIV-infected children should receive all vaccines as early in life as possible, except Bacillus Calmette–Guérin (BCG) and yellow fever vaccines. In asymptomatic children, the decision to give late BCG should be based on the local risk of tuberculosis. Infants with symptomatic HIV infection should not receive yellow fever vaccines.

Antiretroviral therapy (ART), which means ARV drugs given in the correct way and with adherence, can substantially improve survival of HIV-infected children as without treatment 50 per cent of infected children die before the age of 2 (WHO 2006c). The availability of simple fixed-dose combinations of ARV drugs and other formulations such as 'sprinkles' make earlier initiation and adherence to treatment by children more feasible. Understanding, however, the particular needs of adolescents infected with HIV such as access to adolescent-friendly sexual and reproductive health services are increasingly recognized as priorities. 'Treatment 2.0' is a WHO/UNAIDS initiative that aims to catalyse the next phase of HIV treatment scale-up through promoting innovation and efficiency gains (WHO 2011a). It will help countries to reach and sustain universal access to treatment, and capitalize on the preventive benefit of ART through focused work in five priority areas: optimize drug regimens, provide point of care diagnosis, reduce costs, adapt delivery systems, and mobilize communities.

Malnutrition

Malnourished children have substantially higher risks of death from common childhood illness such as diarrhoea, pneumonia, and malaria. Nutrition-related factors directly or indirectly contribute to 45 per cent of deaths in children under 5 years of age (Black et al. 2013).

Interventions to prevent malnutrition include promotion of optimal feeding of infants and young children, prevention and treatment of illness, and amelioration of micronutrient deficiencies in the diet. Early initiation of breastfeeding, exclusive breastfeeding up to 6 months of age, and continued breastfeeding along with complementary foods up to at least 2 years of age are key interventions to combat undernutrition. Early initiation of breastfeeding, ideally within the first hour after birth, is associated with a reduced risk of neonatal mortality (Edmond et al. 2006) and exclusive breastfeeding during the first 6 months of life is associated with about a tenfold lower risk of death due to any cause than not breastfeeding at all, and a two- to threefold lower risk of death than partial breastfeeding (Bahl et al. 2003). Continued breastfeeding into the second year of life also reduces the risk of child mortality and malnutrition. Multiple approaches exist to promote breastfeeding through health facility and community programmes, including health education, professional support, lay support, and mass media campaigns. Safe and appropriate complementary feeding started at 6 months of age can reduce the prevalence of malnutrition and contribute to reduced mortality. Promotion of safe and appropriate complementary feeding improved weight-for-age and height-for-age gains by 0.24–0.87 SD in pilot studies (WHO 1998). Effects of this magnitude if reproduced on a large scale could translate into tangible reductions in rates of malnutrition and the mortality attributable to it.

To improve the nutritional status of children and prevent them from becoming severely malnourished, the dietary management of moderate malnutrition should be based on optimal use of locally available nutrient-dense foods. Intake of nutrients present in inadequate amounts in the habitual diet can be increased through a number of approaches, including dietary diversification and fortification of certain staple foods with vitamins and minerals. In situations of food shortage, or where some nutrients are not sufficiently available through local foods, specially formulated supplementary foods are usually required to complement the regular diet; these supplementary foods are not intended for prevention of malnutrition (WHO 2012d).

Common micronutrient deficiencies such as those of vitamin A, iron, iodine, and zinc, both at clinical and subclinical levels, contribute to illness and mortality in children. Approaches to prevent these deficiencies include supplementation (WHO 2011c, 2011c, 2011d), food fortification, and dietary diversification (Pan American Health Organization and WHO 2003; WHO 2005b).

Severe acute malnutrition in children 6–59 months of age is defined as weight-for-height criterion less than –3 SD of the WHO Growth Standards median, or mid-upper-arm circumference (MUAC) less than 115 mm, or the presence of bilateral oedema. For infants less than 6 months, there is no agreed cut-off value for MUAC.

Children with severe malnutrition should first be assessed with a full clinical examination to confirm whether they have medical complications and whether they have an appetite. Children who pass the appetite test and are clinically well and alert should be treated as outpatients whilst those with medical complications or who fail the appetite test should be treated as inpatients. Young infants less than 6 months with severe acute malnutrition who are found to have recent weight loss or ineffective feeding should always be admitted.

Case management is generally organized in two phases: the stabilization phase (usually 3–5 days) when children with severe acute malnutrition who have complications require careful evaluation and treatment of infections, electrolyte imbalance, hypoglycaemia, and hypothermia; and the rehabilitation phase (usually 4–6 weeks) consisting of the provision of nutritional and psychosocial support to achieve full nutritional recovery. Therapeutic feeding should start early in the stabilization phase and include giving a low-protein milk-based formula diet with additional vitamins and minerals such as the WHO-recommended F-75 (75 kcal/100 mL). In the rehabilitation phase, a milk formula with higher protein and energy content such as F-100 should be given and additional iron is needed to address deficiencies. Ready-to-use therapeutic foods (RUTFs) have replaced liquid F-100 in a variety of settings because they do not contain free water and can therefore be used without risk of bacterial contamination. Most RUTFs are lipid-based pastes combining milk powder, electrolytes, and micronutrients to meet recommended nutritional values and offer the malnourished child the same nutrient intake as F-100 when consumed in isoenergetic amounts. RUTFs also contain 10–14 mg/100 g of iron, therefore no additional intake of iron is necessary.

In combination with community-based screening, RUTFs are highly effective in the treatment of severe acute malnutrition in children 6–59 months of age without complications (Collins et al.

2006; WHO et al. 2007). These children can be managed in the community without the risks of nosocomial infections or any other disruptions regarding hospital care to the family.

In children less than 6 months of age who have severe acute malnutrition, care should focus on managing sepsis and other underlying complications and on re-establishing breastfeeding where this has been ineffective. They need milk-based diets and should generally be managed in a hospital, where their mothers can obtain additional support.

Strengthening of child health services

It is not possible to scale-up child health interventions effectively without dealing with the challenges that affect health systems in many low-income countries. Programmes to address newborn and child health are implemented through 'complex public and private organizations that rely on systems to provide medicines, finance health services, assure quality and efficiency of care, manage the health workforce, and generate information needed for effective operational decisions' (Countdown Working Group on Health Policy and Health Systems et al. 2008).

Key input components to the health system (Fig. 10.3.3) include evidence-based policies, adequate and skilled health workforce, and sufficient health financing—critical determinants of access, quality, and demand for effective interventions. Service delivery, together with medical products and technologies, reflect the immediate outputs of the health system, that is, the availability and distribution of care (WHO 2010c).

Governance

Supportive laws and policies are a prerequisite for strengthening the health sector's capacity to respond to the needs of the population. Examples of evidence-based policies that have a specific bearing on child health and that are currently being promoted in countries to tackle the burden of ill health and excess mortality are (WHO 2012c):

- Maternity protection in accordance with the International Labour Organization Convention 183.
- Policy on midwives authorized to administer a core set of life-saving interventions.
- Policy on postnatal home visits in the first week of life.
- The International Code of Marketing of Breast-milk Substitutes.
- Policy on community treatment of pneumonia with antibiotics.
- Policy on low osmolarity ORS and zinc.
- Policy on rotavirus and pneumococcal vaccines.

In order to facilitate the adoption of these policies in countries, advocacy and policy dialogue with a wide range of stakeholders is usually required. Some policies gain wide adherence rapidly while others lag behind. For example, among the 75 countries with the highest burden of maternal and child deaths, the number of those with a policy allowing community health workers to treat pneumonia has more than doubled from 18 to 38 between 2008 and 2012. In contrast, only 23 of these high-burden countries have adopted legislation on the International Code of Marketing of Breast-milk Substitutes, which was almost unanimously endorsed by the member states of the WHO in 1981.

Monitoring and evaluation of health systems strengthening

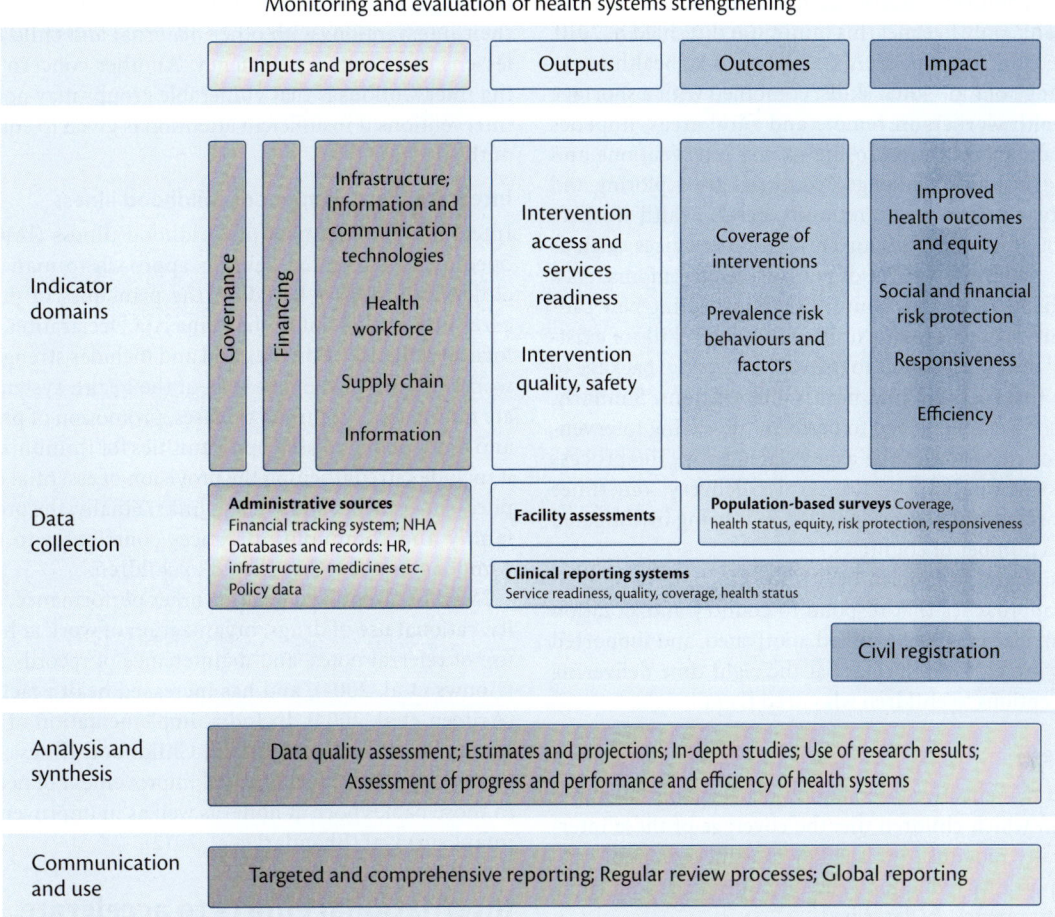

Fig. 10.3.3 Health system building blocks.
Reproduced with permission from *Monitoring and evaluation of health systems strengthening: An operational framework*, Paper prepared by World Health Organization (WHO), World Bank, Global Alliance on Vaccines Initiative (GAVI) and Global Fund to Fight AIDS, Tuberculosis and Malaria (GFATM), Copyright © WHO 2010, available from http://www.who.int/healthinfo/HSS_MandE_framework_Nov_2009.pdf.

Critical subsystems

Economic hardship and financial crises have eroded the health sector in many countries over the past two decades. Many national health systems are in disarray, with a deteriorating infrastructure and a public health sector subject to the resource restrictions consequent to structural adjustment and macroeconomic ceilings. As a result, human resources working in the health sector have been destabilized and undermined. In many countries, households spend considerable amounts on healthcare and out-of-pocket expenditures for health services can be between two and three times greater than the total health expenditure by governments and donors.

The higher the proportion of user payments in the total finance for heath, the greater the relative share of financial burden on the poor and thus they are unable to afford necessary healthcare. Household expenditure surveys suggest that more than 150 million individuals globally face severe financial hardship each year due to healthcare costs. Prepayment systems involve advance collection of funds through tax-based insurance or social health insurance schemes and should be used to promote fair access to health services. Both provide financial risk protection and promote equity through prepayment of healthcare costs and pooling of health risks. Out-of-pocket expenditures should be gradually converted into prepayment schemes, including community finance programmes. Unfortunately, rectifying the current state of healthcare services could take many years.

Health workers are 'all people engaged in actions whose primary intent is to enhance health'. This includes health service providers such as doctors, nurses, midwives, pharmacists and community health workers. It also includes health management and support workers who dedicate all or part of their time to improving health' (WHO 2006d). The availability of a competent workforce is key to successfully delivering child healthcare and services. Critical shortages, inadequate skill mix, and uneven geographical distribution of the health workforce are major barriers to achieving globally set child health goals and targets. The minimum threshold necessary to deliver essential maternal and child health services is estimated as 23 doctors, nurses, and midwives per 10,000 population. Countries that fall below this threshold struggle to provide skilled care at birth to significant numbers of pregnant women, as well as emergency and specialized services for newborns and young children, impacting the burden of women and children mortality directly. Among countries categorized as low-income economies by the World Bank, only five met this minimum threshold in 2010.

In almost all countries, a poor mix of the types of health workers and their range of individual skills, combined with a shortage of qualified health workers in remote and rural areas, impedes access by women and children to life-saving interventions and services. To address these challenges, countries are exploring and applying different solutions. Community-based health workers can provide a number of life-saving child health services, such as immunizations and management of non-severe pneumonia. As a result, governments in various countries are instituting new cadres of community health workers or upgrading the skills of existing community resource persons to deliver an essential package of health services that include child health interventions. Similarly, midwifery personnel are enabled to perform life-saving interventions such as resuscitation of the asphyxiated baby. The process of sharing tasks at various levels of service delivery sometimes referred to as task-shifting or task delegation is being investigated and applied in a number of countries.

Comprehensive and long-term health workforce development strategies and approaches that respond to country and situation needs must be in place to ensure skilled, motivated, and supported health workers are at the right place at the right time delivering the right interventions to children who need them.

Service delivery

Despite the fact that effective interventions exist against all major conditions from which children die, the coverage of these interventions generally remains low. The key to achievement of substantial child mortality reduction is quality universal coverage of the interventions previously described.

Before the mid 1990s, child health programmes in low- and middle-income countries focused on immunization, control of diarrhoeal diseases, ARIs, and nutrition. Their implementation led to reduction in under-5 mortality in many countries, but this approach encountered limitations. The narrow focus on single interventions has failed to consider the child in a holistic manner, leading to many missed opportunities for care in contacts with a health practitioner. It was also difficult to resolve upstream health-system constraints such as management or human resource policies using this approach. Solving these problems involves ensuring access to an integrated package of interventions that are organized around the continuum of care. It also means that care should span across the home, community, health centre, and hospital. The advantages of delivering interventions as packages include the following:

* Many interventions go naturally together because they are delivered by the same person at the same time.

* Packaging is more cost-effective in terms of training, implementation, and supervision.

* Packaging meets the needs of the individual caregiver and the child much better than isolated and uncoordinated single-intervention delivery, thus reinforcing the continuum of care.

Potential obstacles to packaging of interventions may be related to policy, programmes, and the organizational structure of ministries and health services. For example, managers responsible for single issue-focused programmes may feel that packaging their interventions with other maternal and child health services lessens their delivery efficiency. Another concern about packaging interventions is that vulnerable groups may not get any of the interventions if insufficient attention is given to equitable delivery of the package.

Integrated management of childhood illness

Integrated management of childhood illness (IMCI) was developed as an integrated delivery approach to managing common childhood diseases based on the principles of primary healthcare (PHC) as set out in the Alma Ata Declaration. This approach focuses holistically on the child and includes strengthening health workers' skills at the first level of the health system for appropriate treatment of common diseases, promotion of proper nutrition, and reduction of missed opportunities for immunization. Further, it includes strengthening the provision of essential drugs and supplies, supervision, and referral links. Finally, the promotion of key family and community practices contributes to the remaining components of PHC as related to children.

IMCI has improved health worker performance, drug availability, rational use of drugs, organization of work at health facilities, use of referral notes, and maintenance of records at district level (Gouws et al. 2004), and has increased health facility utilization (Arifeen et al. 2004). In India, implementation of the Integrated Management of Neonatal and Childhood Illness (IMNCI) programme resulted in substantial improvement of neonatal survival in those babies born at home as well as in improvement of general infant survival (Bhandari et al. 2012).

International efforts to accelerate progress in child survival

In September 2000, at the United Nations (UN) Millennium Summit, 189 national leaders endorsed 'The Millennium Declaration', aimed at promoting poverty elimination, which includes the development of education, promotion of and respect for human rights and equality, and improvement of the environment. The declaration was a commitment to attain eight specific goals by 2015 and to accomplish the aims established. While all the *Millennium Development Goals* (MDGs) are relevant to child health, MDGs 1, 4, 5, and 6 are directly related to child survival (see Box 10.3.2). The fourth MDG has the explicit target of 'reducing by two-thirds, between 1990 and 2015, the under-5 mortality rate' (UN 2000). Based on an U5MR of 90 per 1000 live births in 1990, the global target is to reach a mortality rate of 30 per 1000 live births by 2015.

Overall, substantial progress has been made towards achieving MDG 4. Reductions in under-5 mortality in many regions and countries have diminished the global number of under-5 deaths by more than 47 per cent, from 12.6 million in 1990 to an estimated 6.6 million in 2012. The most pronounced falls in U5MRs have occurred in four regions: Latin America and the Caribbean; East Asia and the Pacific; Central and Eastern Europe and the Commonwealth of Independent States (CEE/CIS); and the Middle East and North Africa. All have more than halved their regional rates of under-5 mortality since 1990. The corresponding decline for South Asia was 53 per cent, which in absolute terms translates into 2.6 million fewer under-5 deaths in 2012 than in 1990 — by far the highest absolute reduction among all regions. Sub-Saharan Africa, though lagging behind the other regions, has registered a 45 per cent decline in the U5MR (UNICEF et al. 2013).

Countries that have rapidly increased coverage for multiple interventions across the continuum of care have accelerated child survival. Their success can mainly be attributed to improvements in service quality—bringing them closer to home and expanding access to essential care.

In September 2010, the Secretary-General of the UN launched the *Global Strategy for Women's and Children's Health* (Partnership for Maternal, Newborn & Child Health 2010). The main goal of the 'Global Strategy' is to save the lives of 16 million women and children by 2015 and accelerate progress to achieve MDGs 4 and 5. The strategy has helped catalyse new attention and investment to some of the most frequent causes of women's and children's mortality. In response to the UN Global Strategy, WHO co-chaired the Commission on Information and Accountability, which delivered a report (WHO 2011e) with ten recommendations on accountability towards the 'Global Strategy'. The ten recommendations are categorized under the headings: better information for better results, better tracking of resources, and better oversight of results and resources—nationally and globally.

Other recent global initiatives and events are tackling different aspects of implementing the 'Global Strategy', including the Child Survival Call to Action, The Family Planning Summit, and the UN Commission on Life-Saving Commodities for Women and Children. To accelerate progress and achieve improved health outcomes for all children, it is important to ensure universal access to good-quality basic care, clean water, sanitation, and other social sector services such as education. This also includes creating the national legal, policy, and budget frameworks to promote the realization of children's rights to these services.

Child rights

Efforts to ensure effective accountability for children's health are further enhanced by the recognition that availability of and access to health information and services for children and their caregivers are basic human rights. Recognition of need for legal entitlements of every child, regardless of his/her status or situation, elevates associated responsibilities and political commitments to legal obligations. This paradigm shift thus enables the establishment of not merely a normative but indeed legal foundation for addressing the health needs of children.

The UN Convention on the Rights of the Child (CRC), adopted in 1989 and ratified by all but two UN Member States, is the principal legal instrument for the protection of children's well-being, and outlines the core obligations of States in relation to children's health. Article 24 directly addresses the child's right to health and healthcare (Box 10.3.3), while other provisions refer to the many underlying determinants of children's health. The CRC thus provides a valuable holistic blueprint of all essential needs and legal entitlements of children needed to ensure their survival, health, and optimal development.

Conclusion

ARIs, diarrhoea, malaria, measles, and HIV are the main causes of illness and death in children aged 28 days to 5 years. Among newborn babies, most deaths are due to prematurity, birth asphyxia, and infections. Undernutrition is associated with 45 per cent of all under-5 deaths. Despite the substantial progress made in reducing under-5 mortality, 6.6 million children under 5 still die each year.

Poor health and survival are linked to social and economic disadvantages. Child deaths are unequally distributed in the world. Within countries, child morbidity and mortality tend to be higher in the rural areas and within the poorer and least educated families. Poorly nourished, LBW, sick, and disabled children all are at particular risk of adverse outcomes and have special needs for care. Global progress in child health is attributable to a broad range of factors that include high coverage of good quality effective interventions, development programming, and strategic delivery of health services, along with improvements in education, child protection, respect for human rights, and economic gains in developing countries.

Key points

◆ Approximately two-thirds of under-5 deaths could be prevented by universal coverage of a small set of existing interventions that do not require expensive technology. Among these interventions, the promotion of breastfeeding, management and prevention of neonatal conditions, ARIs, diarrhoea, malaria, and HIV infection, in addition to improved feeding have the highest impact in reducing child mortality.

◆ Reduction in neonatal mortality requires increased effective coverage of interventions during pregnancy, childbirth, and in the postnatal period.

◆ Coverage with the key earlier-mentioned interventions remains low. Integrating the interventions into packages of care that are organized along a continuum from pregnancy, birth, neonatal period, and childhood, and delivered at all levels—from the home and community through the first-level facility and hospital—would contribute to improved efficiency in intervention delivery and to the achievement of high coverage.

◆ Strengthening the health system will be key for increasing the coverage and quality of health interventions.

◆ The development of an operational plan to which programmes can be held accountable, along with a good financing and human resource strategy, will yield long-term benefits for the child and the health system at large and is an essential element to follow the development of a child survival strategy.

References

Addo-Yobo, E., Anh, D.D., El-Sayed, H.F., et al. for the Multicenter Amoxicillin Severe pneumonia Study (MASS) Group (2011). Outpatient treatment of children with severe pneumonia with oral amoxicillin in four countries: the MASS study. *Tropical Medicine & International Health*, 16, 995–1006.

Arifeen, S.E., Blum, L.S., Hoque, D.M.E., et al. (2004). Integrated management of childhood illness (IMCI) in Bangladesh: early findings from a cluster randomized study. *The Lancet*, 364, 1595–602.

Armah, G.E., Sow, S.O., Breiman, R.F., et al. (2010). Efficacy of pentavalent rotavirus vaccine against severe rotavirus gastroenteritis in infants in developing countries in sub-Saharan Africa: a randomised, double-blind, placebo-controlled trial. *The Lancet*, 376, 606–14.

Bahl, R., Frost, C., Kirkwood, B.R., et al. (2003). Infant feeding patterns and risks of death and hospitalization in the first half of infancy: multicentre cohort study. *Bulletin of the World Health Organization*, 83, 418–26.

Bari, A., Sadruddin, S., Khan, A., et al. (2011). Community case management of severe pneumonia with oral amoxicillin in children aged 2–59 months in Haripur district, Pakistan: a cluster randomised trial. *The Lancet*, 378, 1796–803.

Bhandari, N., Mazumder, S., Taneja, S., et al. (2008). Effectiveness of zinc supplementation plus oral rehydration salts compared with oral rehydration salts alone as a treatment for acute diarrhea in a primary care setting: a cluster randomized trial. *Pediatrics*, 121, e1279–85.

Bhandari, N., Mazumder, S., Taneja, S., Sommerfelt, H., Strand, T.A.; IMNCI Evaluation Study Group (2012). Effect of implementation of Integrated Management of Neonatal and Childhood Illness (IMNCI) programme on neonatal and infant mortality: cluster randomised controlled trial. *British Medical Journal*, 344, e1634.

Black, R.E., Victora, C.G., Walker, S.P., et al. (2013). Maternal and child undernutrition and overweight in low-income and middle-income countries. *The Lancet*, 382, 427–51.

Cairncross, S., Hunt, C., Boisson, S., et al. (2010). Water, sanitation and hygiene for the prevention of diarrhoea. *International Journal of Epidemiology*, 39, i193–205.

Centers for Disease Control and Prevention (2013). Impact of an innovative approach to prevent mother-to-child transmission of HIV—Malawi, July 2011–September 2012. *Morbidity and Mortality Weekly Report*, 62, 148–51.

Central Statistical Agency [Ethiopia] and ICF International (2012). *Ethiopia Demographic and Health Survey 2011*. Addis Ababa, Ethiopia and Calverton, MD: Central Statistical Agency and ICF International.

Chintu, C., Bhat, G.J., Walker, A.S., et al. (2000). Co-trimoxazole as prophylaxis against opportunistic infections in HIV-infected Zambian children (CHAP): a double-blind randomized placebo-controlled trial. *The Lancet*, 364, 1865–71.

Collins, S., Dent, N., Binns, P., et al. (2006). Management of severe acute malnutrition in children. *The Lancet*, 368, 1992–2000.

Coovadia, H.M., Brown, E.R., Fowler, M.G., et al. (2012). Efficacy and safety of an extended nevirapine regimen in infant children of breastfeeding mothers with HIV-1 infection for prevention of postnatal HIV-1 transmission (HPTN 046): a randomised, double-blind, placebo-controlled trial. *The Lancet*, 379, 221–8.

Countdown Working Group on Health Policy and Health Systems, Cavagnero, E., Daelmans, B., et al. (2008). Assessment of the health system and policy environment as a critical complement to tracking intervention coverage for maternal newborn and child health. *The Lancet*, 371, 1284–93.

Das, J.K., Ali, A., Salam, R.A., and Bhutta, Z.A. (2013). Antibiotics for the treatment of *Cholera, Shigella* and *Cryptosporidium* in children. *BMC Public Health*, 13(Suppl. 3), S10.

Dherani, M., Pope, D., Mascarenhas, M., et al. (2008). Indoor air pollution from unprocessed solid fuel use and pneumonia risk in children aged five years : a systematic review and meta-analysis. *Bulletin of the World Health Organization*, 86, 390–8.

Edmond, K., Scott, S., Korczak, V., et al. (2012). Long term sequelae from childhood pneumonia; systematic review and meta-analysis. *PLoS One*, 7, e31239.

Edmond, K.M., Zandoh, C., Quigley, M.A., et al. (2006). Delayed breastfeeding initiation increases risk of neonatal mortality. *Paediatrics*, 117, 380–6.

Eisele, T.P., Larsen, D., and Steketee, R.W. (2010). Protective efficacy of interventions for preventing malaria mortality in children in *Plasmodium falciparum* endemic areas. *International Journal of Epidemiology*, 39, i88–101.

Fischer Walker, C. and Black, R.E. (2010). Zinc for the treatment of diarrhoea: effect on diarrhoea morbidity, mortality and incidence of future episodes. *International Journal of Epidemiology*, 39(Suppl. 1), i63–9.

Fischer Walker, C.L., Perin, J., Aryee, M.J., Boschi-Pinto, C., and Black, R.E. (2012). Diarrhea incidence in low- and middle-income countries in 1990 and 2010: a systematic review. *BMC Public Health*, 12, 220.

Fischer Walker, C.L., Rudan, I., Liu, L., et al. (2013). Global burden of childhood pneumonia and diarrhoea. *The Lancet*, 381, 1405–16.

Ghana Statistical Service (GSS), Ghana Health Service (GHS), and ICF Macro (2009). *Ghana Demographic and Health Survey 2008*. Accra, Ghana: GSS, GHS, and ICF Macro.

Gouws, E., Bryce, J., Habicht, J.P., et al. (2004). Improving antimicrobial use among health workers in first-level facilities: results from the multicountry evaluation of the integrated management of childhood illness strategy. *Bulletin of the World Health Organization*, 82, 509–15.

Grantham-McGregor, S., Cheung, Y.B., Cueto, S., et al. on behalf of the International Child Development Steering Group (2007). Developmental potential in the first 5 years for children in developing countries. *The Lancet*, 369, 60–70.

Grijalva, C.G., Nuorti, J.P., Arbogast, P.G., Martin, S.W., Edwards, K.M., and Griffin, M.R. (2007). Decline in pneumonia admissions after routine childhood immunisation with pneumococcal conjugate vaccine in the USA: a time-series analysis. *The Lancet*, 369, 1179–86.

Hazir, T., Fox, L.M., Nisar, Y.B., et al. (2008). New Outpatient Short-Course Home Oral Therapy for Severe Pneumonia Study Group. Ambulatory short-course high-dose oral amoxicillin for treatment of severe pneumonia in children: a randomised equivalency trial. *The Lancet*, 371, 49–56.

Institut National de la Statistique and ICF Macro (2010). *Enquête Démographique et de Santé de Madagascar 2008–2009*. Antananarivo, Madagascar: Institut National de la Statistique and ICF Macro.

Instituto Nacional de Estatística [São Tomé e Príncipe], Ministério da Saúde, and ICF Macro (2010). *Inquérito Demográfico e Sanitário, São Tomé e Príncipe, IDS STP, 2008–2009*. Calverton, MD: Instituto Nacional de Estatística.

Jardine, A., Menzies, R.I., and McIntyre, P.B. (2010). Reduction in hospitalizations for pneumonia associated with the introduction of a pneumococcal conjugate vaccination schedule without a booster dose in Australia. *Pediatric Infectious Disease Journal*, 29, 607–12.

Johnson, H.L., Deloria-Knoll, M., Levine, O.S., et al. (2010). Systematic evaluation of serotypes causing invasive pneumococcal disease among children under five: the pneumococcal global serotype project. *PLoS Medicine*, 7(10), e1000348.

Kagaayi, J., Gray, R.H., Brahmbhatt, H., et al. (2008). Survival of infants born to HIV-positive mothers, by feeding modality, in Rakai, Uganda. *PLoS ONE*, 3(12), e3877.

Kenya National Bureau of Statistics and ICF Macro (2010). *Kenya Demographic and Health Survey 2008–09*. Calverton, MD: Kenya National Bureau of Statistics and ICF Macro.

Kesho Bora Study Group (2011). Triple antiretroviral compared with zidovudine and single-dose nevirapine prophylaxis during pregnancy and breastfeeding for prevention of mother-to-child transmission of HIV-1 (Kesho Bora study): a randomised controlled trial. *The Lancet Infectious Diseases*, 11, 171–80.

Lamberti, L., Fischer Walker, C.L., Noiman, A., Victora, C., and Black, R.E. (2011). Breastfeeding and the risk for diarrhoea morbidity and mortality. *BMC Public Health*, 11(Suppl. 3), S15.

Liu, L., Johnson, H., Cousens, S., et al. (2012). Global, regional, and national causes of child mortality: an updated systematic analysis for 2010 with time trends since 2000. *The Lancet*, 379, 2151–61.

Mazumder, S., Taneja, S., Bhandari, N., et al. (2010). Effectiveness of zinc supplementation plus oral rehydration salts compared with oral rehydration salts alone for diarrhoea in infants aged less than 6 months in Haryana state, India. *Bulletin of the World Health Organization*, 88, 754–60.

Miller, E., Andrews, N.J., Waight, P.A., Slack, M.P., and George, R.C. (2011). Herd immunity and serotype replacement 4 years after seven-valent pneumococcal conjugate vaccination in England and Wales: an observational cohort study. *The Lancet Infectious Diseases*, 11, 760–8.

Ministry of Health and Family [Maldives] and ICF Macro (2010). *Maldives Demographic and Health Survey 2009*. Calverton, MD: Ministry of Health and Family and ICF Macro.

Ministry of Health and Population [Nepal], New ERA, and ICF International Inc. (2012). *Nepal Demographic and Health Survey 2011*. Kathmandu, Nepal: Ministry of Health and Population, New ERA, and ICF International.

Munos, M.K., Walker, C.L., and Black, R.E. (2010). The effect of oral rehydration solution and recommended home fluids on diarrhoea mortality. *International Journal of Epidemiology*, 39(Suppl. 1), i75–87.

National Bureau of Statistics [Tanzania] and ICF Macro (2011). *Tanzania Demographic and Health Survey 2010*. Dar es Salaam, Tanzania: National Bureau of Statistics and ICF Macro.

National Institute of Statistics, Directorate General for Health, and ICF Macro (2011). *Cambodia Demographic and Health Survey 2010*. Phnom Penh, Cambodia and Calverton, MD: National Institute of Statistics, Directorate General for Health, and ICF Macro.

National Institute of Statistics of Rwanda [Rwanda], Ministry of Health [Rwanda], and ICF International (2012). *Rwanda Demographic and Health Survey 2010*. Calverton, MD: National Institute of Statistics of Rwanda, Ministry of Health, and ICF International.

National Population Commission [Nigeria] and ICF Macro (2009). *Nigeria Demographic and Health Survey 2008*. Abuja, Nigeria: National Population Commission and ICF Macro.

National Statistical Office and ICF Macro (2011). *Malawi Demographic and Health Survey 2010*. Zomba, Malawi, and Calverton, MD: National Statistical Office and ICF Macro.

National Statistics Directorate [Timor-Leste], Ministry of Finance [Timor-Leste], and ICF Macro (2010). *Timor-Leste Demographic and Health Survey 2009–10*. Dili, Timor-Leste: National Statistics Directorate [Timor-Leste] and ICF Macro.

National Statistics Office [Philippines], and ICF Macro (2009). *National Demographic and Health Survey 2008*. Calverton, MD: National Statistics Office and ICF Macro.

Newell, M.L., Coovadia, H., Cortina-Borja, M. et al.; Ghent International AIDS Society (IAS) Working Group on HIV Infection in Women and Children (2004). Mortality of infected and uninfected infants born to HIV-infected mothers in Africa: a pooled analysis. *The Lancet*, 364, 1236–43.

Pan American Health Organization and World Health Organization (2003). *Guiding Principles for Complementary Feeding of the Breastfed Child*. Washington, DC: Pan American Health Organization.

Partnership for Maternal, Newborn & Child Health (2010). *Global Strategy for Women's and Children's Health*. [Online] Available at: http://www.who.int/pmnch/activities/jointactionplan/en/.

Peltier, C.A., Ndayisaba, G.F., Lepage, P., et al. (2009). Breastfeeding with maternal antiretroviral therapy or formula feeding to prevent HIV postnatal mother-to-child transmission in Rwanda. *AIDS*, 23, 2415–23.

Pilishvili, T., Lexau, C., Farley, M.M., et al. (2010). Sustained reductions in invasive pneumococcal disease in the era of conjugate vaccine. *Journal of Infectious Diseases*, 201, 32–41.

Sandison, T.G., Homsy, J., Arinaitwe, E., et al. (2011). Protective efficacy of co-trimoxazole prophylaxis against malaria in HIV exposed children in rural Uganda: a randomised clinical trial. *British Medical Journal*, 342, d1617.

Shapiro, R.L., Hughes, M.D., Ogwu, A., et al. (2010). Antiretroviral regimens in pregnancy and breast-feeding in Botswana. *The New England Journal of Medicine*, 362, 2282–94.

Smith, K.R., McCracken, J.P., Weber, M.W., et al. (2011). Effect of reduction in household air pollution on childhood pneumonia in Guatemala (RESPIRE): a randomised controlled trial. *The Lancet*, 378, 1717–26.

Smith, K.R., Mehta, S., and Maeusezahl-Feuz, F. (2004). Indoor smoke from household solid fuels. In M.R. Ezzati, A. Lopez, and C. Murray (eds.) *Comparative Quantification of Health Risks: Global and Regional Burden of Disease Due to Selected Major Risk Factors*, pp. 1435–93. Geneva: WHO.

Soofi, S., Ahmed, S., Fox, M.P., et al. (2012). Effectiveness of community case management of severe pneumonia with oral amoxicillin in children aged 2–59 months in Matiari district, rural Pakistan: a cluster-randomised controlled trial. *The Lancet*, 379, 729–37.

Statistics Sierra Leone and ICF Macro (2009). *Sierra Leone Demographic and Health Survey 2008*. Calverton, MD: Statistics Sierra Leone and ICF Macro.

Tate, J.E., Burton, A.H., Boschi-Pinto, C., Steele, A.D., Duque, J., and Parashar, U.D. (2012). WHO-coordinated Global Rotavirus Surveillance Network. *The Lancet Infectious Diseases*, 12, 136–41.

Traa, B.S., Walker, C.L., Munos, M., and Black, R.E. (2010). Antibiotics for the treatment of dysentery in children. *International Journal of Epidemiology*, 39(Suppl. 1), i70–4.

United Nations (2000). *United Nations Millennium Declaration*. New York: UN. Available at: http://www.un.org/millennium/declaration/ares552e.htm.

United Nations Children's Fund and World Health Organization (2009). *Diarrhoea: Why Children Are Still Dying and What Can Be Done*. Geneva: WHO; New York: UNICEF. Available at: http://www.who.int/maternal_child_adolescent/documents/9789241598415/en/index.html.

United Nations Children's Fund, World Health Organization, and the World Bank (2012). *Levels and Trends in Child Malnutrition. Report 2012. UNICEF-WHO-World Bank Joint Child Malnutrition Estimates*. New York: UNICEF. Available at: http://www.who.int/nutgrowthdb/estimates.

United Nations Children's Fund, World Health Organization, World Bank, and United Nations DESA/Population Division (2013). *Levels and Trends in Child Mortality. Report 2013. Estimates Developed by the UN Inter-agency Group for Child Mortality Estimation*. New York: UNICEF. Available at: http://www.who.int/maternal_child_adolescent/documents/levels_trends_child_mortality_2013/en/index.html.

World Health Organization (1998). *Complementary Feeding of Young Children in Developing Countries: A Review of Current Scientific Knowledge*. WHO/NUT/98.1. Geneva: WHO.

World Health Organization (2005a). *Diarrhoea Treatment Guidelines for Clinic Based Health Care Workers*. Geneva: WHO. Available at: http://www.who.int/maternal_child_adolescent/documents/a85500/en/index.html.

World Health Organization (2005b). *Guiding Principles for Feeding Non-Breastfed Children 6–24 Months of Age*. Geneva: WHO.

World Health Organization (2006a). *Multicentre Growth Reference Study Group. WHO Child Growth Standards: Length/Height-for-Age, Weight-for-Age, Weight-for-Length, Weight-for-Height and Body Mass Index-for-Age: Methods and Development*. Geneva: WHO.

World Health Organization (2006b). *The Role of the Health Sector in Strengthening Systems to Support Children's Health Development in Communities Affected by HIV/AIDS: A Review*. Geneva: WHO. Available at: http://www.who.int/maternal_child_adolescent/documents/9241594624/en/index.html.

World Health Organization (2006c). *Guidelines on Co-Trimoxazole Prophylaxis for HIV-Related Infections Among Children, Adolescents and Adults. Recommendations for a Public Health Approach*. Geneva: WHO. Available at: http://www.who.int/hiv/pub/guidelines/ctx/en/index.html.

World Health Organization (2006d). *World Health Report 2006: Working Together for Health*. Geneva: WHO.

World Health Organization (2007). *Combating Waterborne Disease at the Household Level*. Geneva: WHO. Available at: http://www.who.int/water_sanitation_health/publications/combating_disease/en/.

World Health Organization (2009). WHO position paper on rotavirus vaccines, 2009. *Weekly Epidemiological Record*, 84(51–52), 533–40. Available at: http://www.who.int/wer/2009/wer8451_52/en/index.html.

World Health Organization (2010a). *Guidelines for the Treatment of Malaria* (2nd ed.). Available at: http://whqlibdoc.who.int/publications/2010/9789241547925_eng.pdf.

World Health Organization (2010b). *Antiretroviral Drugs for Treating Pregnant Women and Preventing HIV Infection in Infants*. Geneva: WHO. Available at: http://www.who.int/hiv/pub/mtct/antiretroviral2010/en/index.html.

World Health Organization (2010c). *Monitoring the Building Blocks of the Health System: A Handbook of Indicators and their Measurement Strategies*. Geneva: WHO. Available at: http://www.who.int/healthinfo/systems/monitoring/en/index.html.

World Health Organization (2011a). *Global Health Sector Strategy on HIV/AIDS 2011–2015*. Geneva: WHO. Available at: http://www.who.int/hiv/pub/hiv_strategy/en/index.html

World Health Organization (2011b). *Guideline: Intermittent Iron Supplementation in Preschool and School-Age Children*. Geneva: WHO. http://whqlibdoc.who.int/publications/2011/9789241502009_eng.pdf.

World Health Organization (2011c). *Guideline: Use of Multiple Micronutrient Powders for Home Fortification of Foods Consumed by Infants and Children 6–23 Months of Age*. Geneva: WHO.

World Health Organization (2011d). *Guideline: Vitamin A Supplementation in Infants and Children 6–59 Months of Age*. Geneva: WHO. http://whqlibdoc.who.int/publications/2011/9789241501767_eng.pdf.

World Health Organization (2011e). *Keeping Promises, Measuring Results: Commission on Information and Accountability for Women's and Children's Health*. Geneva: WHO. Available at: http://www.who.int/topics/mille.

World Health Organization (2012a). *Born Too Soon. The Global Action Report on Preterm Birth*. Geneva: WHO.

World Health Organization (2012b). *Recommendations for Management of Common Childhood Conditions. Evidence for Technical Update of Pocket Book Recommendations* Geneva: WHO. Available at: http://www.who.int/maternal_child_adolescent/documents/management_childhood_conditions/en/index.html.

World Health Organization (2012c). *Countdown to 2015. Accountability for Maternal, Newborn & Child Survival. An Update on Progress in Priority Countries*. Geneva: WHO. Available at: http://countdown2015mnch.org/documents/countdown-news/count_complete_small.pdf.

World Health Organization (2012d). *Technical Note: Supplementary Foods for the Management of Moderate Acute Malnutrition in Infants and Children 6–59 Months of Age*. Geneva: WHO.

World Health Organization (2013). *World Health Statistics 2013*. Geneva: WHO. Available at: http://www.who.int/gho/publications/world_health_statistics/2013/en/.

World Health Organization (n.d.). *Global Health Observatory*. [Online] Available at: http://www.who.int/gho/map_gallery/en/.

World Health Organization, World Food Programme, United Nations Standing Committee on Nutrition, and United Nations Children's Fund (2007). *Community-Based Management of Severe Acute Malnutrition. Joint UN Statement 2007*. Geneva: WHO.

Zaman, K., Dang, D.A., Victor, J.C., et al. (2010). Efficacy of pentavalent rotavirus vaccine against severe rotavirus gastroenteritis in infants in developing countries in Asia: a randomised, double-blind, placebo-controlled trial. *The Lancet*, 376, 615–23.

Zimbabwe National Statistics Agency and ICF International (2012). *Zimbabwe Demographic and Health Survey 2010–11*. Calverton, MD: Zimbabwe National Statistics Agency and ICF International Inc.

10.4

Adolescent health

Pierre-André Michaud, Anne-Emmanuelle Ambresin, Richard F. Catalano, Judith Diers, and George C. Patton

Adolescence and youth: definition, biopsychosocial development, and demography

The terms 'youth', 'adolescents', and 'young people' are used to describe people in the transition from childhood to adulthood. The World Health Organization (WHO) defines 'adolescents' as people aged 10–19, 'youth' as those aged 15–24, and 'young people' as those aged 10–24 (WHO 1989; Sawyer et al. 2012). Defining this life phase by age has some value in both measurement of health and programming but in reality adolescence is better viewed as a life phase that varies in timing between individuals and cultures. In this chapter, we will interchangeably use the words 'adolescents' and 'young people', as the categories are arbitrary and the health problems faced are similar.

In most cultures and individuals, adolescence begins with the appearance of overt physical signs of puberty and ends with the acquisition of the statute of adulthood and/or parenthood, the whole process leading to greater emotional and social autonomy (Patton and Viner 2007). Adolescence is largely shaped by biological and socioeconomic factors. At an individual level, there is a 4–5-year variation in the onset of puberty ('pubertal timing') even where living conditions are similar for all members of a group. The age at which the physical changes linked with puberty occur does, to some extent, shape the psychosocial development of the individual and the adoption of health risk behaviours (Michaud et al. 2006): young people whose puberty begins earlier tend to engage in exploratory or risky behaviours at an earlier age than those who mature later. In Western countries, pubertal timing has decreased by 4–5 years over the past 150 years so that the mean age for menarche, a late pubertal event in females, is now 12–13 years in most high-income countries (Ong et al. 2006; Patton and Viner 2007) whereas it was around 16–17 years two centuries ago. The secular trends in the timing of puberty are in part related to improved nutrition.

Brain development is active throughout adolescence and actually continues to the end of the third decade of life (Giedd 2008; Sawyer et al. 2012). Puberty and its hormonal surge triggers the development of subcortical structures involved in the arousal of emotions and sensations (Dahl 2004). In contrast, the development of the prefrontal cortex, which is implicated in planning complex cognitive behaviour, personality expression, decision making, and moderation of social behaviour, is not complete until young adulthood. This gap in the pace of the maturation of different parts of the brain may account for adolescence being a period of heightened impulsivity and emotional responses as well as of vulnerability to problems related to emotional control (United Nations Children's Fund (UNICEF) 2011).

In pre-industrial societies, the adolescent transition from puberty to adult roles, as defined by the onset of sexual activity, marriage, and parenthood, ranged from around 2 years in girls to 4 years in boys. In today's developed economies, longer periods of education and the availability of effective contraception means that adolescence commonly persists for well over a decade. The lengthening of adolescence has thus been accompanied by a later acquisition of professional capabilities and independence that are the hallmarks of an adult status (Patton and Viner 2007; UNICEF 2012) yet allowing a more sophisticated level of professional skills. Finally, with the emergence of new electronic media, young people around the world have access to information that was not previously available (UNICEF 2012). The spreading of the Internet and information and communication technologies represents an opportunity for adolescents in low- and middle-income countries (LMICs) to gain unprecedented skills and capabilities. It has also created a new means of socialization in which young people can engage with others across the globe.

There are considerable variations between individuals in both biological and psychosocial aspects of development. Yet a division of adolescence into three phases has retained its heuristic value:

◆ Early adolescence is characterized by puberty and rapid physical growth, with a marked interest in one's self-image.

◆ Middle adolescence represents a period of experimentation potentially associated with risky behaviours such as unprotected sexual intercourse, and the use of legal and illegal psychoactive substances. Many risk behaviours are transitory and it should be kept in mind that exploration intrinsically belongs to child and adolescent development (Dahl 2004). However, some can lead to long-term morbidity, such as tobacco use or unsafe sex resulting in an HIV infection.

◆ Late adolescence is a period of progressive stabilization during which young people tend to form more stable relationships and acquire long-term perspectives, a developmental process which extends into early adulthood.

Health of adolescents in the global public health context

Today's generation of young people is, relative to other age groups, the largest in history. With a population of 1.8 billion, 10–24-year-olds now comprise over a quarter of the global population. This large increase in the youth population arises from improved infant and child survival following dramatic improvements over the past 50 years in maternal antenatal care, acute childhood illness, and malnutrition. Nearly 90 per cent live in LMICs where they may comprise more than a third of the population.

Adolescents have been a major focus in recent global approaches to sexual and reproductive health. A life-course perspective also places adolescents centrally in other health agendas including the prevention of non-communicable diseases, mental disorders, and injuries (Innocenti Research Centre 2007; Temin and Levine 2009). A cluster of health risk behaviours and states that largely start in adolescence (tobacco, alcohol, obesity, physical inactivity) are potential drivers of future non-communicable diseases in adults (Beaglehole et al. 2011). This adolescent contribution to disease burden in those over 60 years old includes high blood pressure, cholesterol, and glucose (29 per cent); tobacco use (10 per cent); physical inactivity (7 per cent); and overweight and obesity (7 per cent) (Gore et al. 2011). A range of global factors has come into play in shaping the health of young people. Perhaps the most immediate effect is the widespread dissemination of values and lifestyles that are potentially damaging to health. Tobacco use, alcohol and other substance use, physical inactivity, and obesity have spread rapidly to many LMICs in the last two decades. Indeed rates of adolescent tobacco use have diminished in many high-income countries whereas elsewhere rates are escalating rapidly.

In comparison to younger children, adolescents have seen fewer health gains. In a study of 50 countries with longitudinal data, the mortality of children had declined by over 80 per cent in the last 50 years. In contrast, mortality among adolescents had improved only marginally and there has been a reversal of historical mortality patterns in which early childhood mortality exceeds adolescent deaths. Over that time causes of death in adolescents have changed with a fall in infectious deaths in most high- and middle-income countries and a rise in deaths due to injuries, that now account for around 40 per cent of all adolescent deaths globally. Causes of injury death include suicide, motor vehicle injury, and homicide, with a major difference in patterns and rates of death in different parts of the world. In contrast, in low-income countries in sub-Saharan Africa and southern Asia infectious diseases, including HIV, tuberculosis, malaria, and maternal causes remain major contributors to death in young people. Moreover, as recently stated by Capua et al. (2013), 'Coverage rates for the adolescent vaccinations continue to lag behind those of the childhood vaccinations, despite their importance', even in high-income countries. Adolescents need both boosters and new vaccines such as the one against human papilloma virus (HPV) (see 'Sexual and reproductive health' section).

Young people bear a substantial disease burden in all regions of the world, both in terms of years of life lost (YLL) and years of life lost due to disability (YLD). Overall they account for over 15 per cent of the total disability-adjusted life year (DALY) toll for all age groups and are the only age group where disease burden is higher in women than men. Africa has the highest regional rate of disease burden for those aged 10–24, 2.5 times greater than in high-income countries that have the lowest. The major global causes of disease for those aged 10–24 are neuropsychiatric conditions for both sexes, injuries in males, and maternal conditions in females.

We now also recognize ways in which the health of adolescent girls affects the health of the next generation. The influences range from viral infections such as rubella and HIV, maternal malnutrition and micronutrient deficiency, obesity and gestational diabetes, and health risks associated with alcohol, tobacco, and illicit and psychotropic drugs use (Bhutta et al. 2011).

Health-specific issues

Injuries and inflicted violence against and among adolescents

Injuries among young people include sports and traffic accidents, interpersonal violence, war, and suicide (see 'Mental health' section). Injuries account for substantial mortality and morbidity during adolescence (WHO 2002b, 2008; Patton et al. 2009; Gore et al. 2011). Apart from sub-Saharan Africa, where HIV leads to a large proportion of deaths, in the rest of the world, injuries among adolescents make up almost half of deaths in males. Worldwide, the death rates among males aged 10–24 years are around 14 per cent from road traffic injuries, 9 per cent from interpersonal violence, 6 per cent from self-inflicted injuries, 5 per cent from drowning, and 3 per cent linked with war; among females, the respective rates are 6 per cent from self-inflicted injuries, 5 per cent for road traffic injuries, and 2.5 per cent from drowning. Consequently, for males aged 10–24 years, traffic accidents, violence, and self-inflicted injuries account for 14 per cent of DALYs (197/100,000), while among females, they represent 5.6 per cent (66/100,000) (Gore et al. 2011).

The road traffic accident rate has increased alarmingly in some LMICs and now accounts for 90 per cent of the world's road traffic fatalities. Among explanations is the growth of motorized transport, the lack of education in driving skills, and, perhaps more importantly, poor roads and other infrastructure, lack of car safety, lack of legislation around seat belts, and the use of alcohol. WHO predicts that the road traffic injuries rate will rise to become the fifth leading cause of death by 2030 (WHO 2009). Most traffic injuries occur among 'vulnerable' individuals, that is, pedestrians, cyclists, or users of two-wheelers. Four main types of strategies can be developed to address traffic injuries (Munro et al. 1995): modifying the road environment, increasing the safety of vehicles, providing guidance and support, and reducing the exposure of young people to traffic.

Many adolescents are involved in physical fights: during early adolescence these are often linked with various types of conflicts, while during later adolescence they are linked with involvement in the drug trade and other forms of illegal activities. Unemployment is probably the single most important risk factor for such behaviour. The percentages of interpersonal violence vary from one country to another; for example, in Malawi, 24 per cent of males and 21 per cent of females report such events, while the percentages are 68 per cent and 74 per cent respectively in Djibouti. Among males, interpersonal violence is the second most common cause of violent deaths: in South America, it is the most frequent cause of death as well as the leading cause of DALYs, both among males and females: in Salvador for instance, the death rate for males due to homicide is 157/100,000, a rate that is higher than the one due to road traffic accidents (UNICEF 2012). In the United States, the rate of death from homicide is as high as 18/100,000 (3/100,000 among girls).

Among factors playing a role in the occurrence of violence is the economic and political situation of the country. For example, countries which have the largest gap between richer and poorer inhabitants (as measured by the Gini index[1]) have higher rates of violence among adolescents overall (Viner et al. 2012). Violence prevention needs to address risk factors at the individual, family, community, and societal levels (Dahlberg and Potter 2001) as outlined in the section 'Prevention and health promotion'.

Mental health

Mental disorders are estimated to be the leading cause of disease burden for young people across the globe. In countries where mortality from infectious disease and maternal causes is low, mental disorders and substance abuse account for over half the disease burden arising in adolescents. Globally, major depression accounts for the highest proportion (8.2 per cent) of disease burden in 10–24-year-olds. Schizophrenia (4.1 per cent), bipolar disorder (3.8 per cent), alcohol use disorders (3.0 per cent), and self-inflicted injuries (2.8 per cent) are also in the ten leading causes of disease burden in young people.

A question of whether there have been secular trends towards higher adolescent rates and earlier onset of common mental disorders and substance abuse has attracted a good deal of attention. There are some conflicting reports, in part related to limited available survey data before 1980, with some of the rise likely to have occurred prior to this (Rutter and Smith 1995; Costello et al. 2006). In industrialized countries, the clearest increases have been documented in the areas of substance use, eating disorders, and conduct disorders ('antisocial behaviour') (Hagell 2012). There have been sharp recent rises in the visits to doctors by adolescents for depression reported in high-income countries (Ma et al. 2005), higher rates of depression and anxiety disorder in later cohorts in retrospective studies of adults (Kessler et al. 2005), and data from recent surveys in the United Kingdom and Europe to suggest that rates of adolescent emotional problems have increased (Collishaw et al. 2004). Changes in the social context of development and lifestyles adopted by adolescents are commonly cited as reasons for the shift but there remains a lack a clarity about which specific changes may be responsible.

There are challenges in providing clinical care for adolescent mental disorders. Adolescents are often reluctant to seek help or communicate around mental health problems in a way which is readily identifiable by family, teachers, or other adults (Tylee et al. 2007). For this reason the adoption of youth-friendly practice (also see 'Youth suicide and self-harm' section) is particularly relevant in the management of mental disorders (Sanci et al. 2010). Secondly, it may be difficult to distinguish more transient emotional problems from disorders that become debilitating and persistent. It seems clear that many adolescents can fulfil criteria for a DSM-IV mental disorder but that many do not persist in this form into adulthood (Copeland et al. 2011). This may be particularly true of more serious mental disorders such as bipolar disorder and schizophrenia where the early symptoms may be non-specific and not diagnostic. Most mental disorders in adolescents will be managed in primary care, where key competencies for health workers include being able to communicate well with young people, screen for mental health problems, and to provide treatments which include counselling, brief psychotherapy, and appropriate psychotropic medication.

Youth suicide and self-harm

Suicide and self-harm become prominent during the adolescent and young adult years in many countries and globally constitute the second leading cause of death in young people. Worldwide, it is estimated that there are at least 160,000 deaths from suicide in young people aged 15–24 years each year. In high- and middle-income countries with low rates of death due to infectious and maternal causes, it accounts for an even larger proportion of deaths. Typically rates are higher in males than females but with exceptions such as rural China and rural India where female rates are as high (Patton et al. 2009; Bergen et al. 2012).

By comparison with suicide, self-harm is relatively common. Around one in 20 young people in their mid-teens in high-income countries report some self-harm, typically self-laceration or self-poisoning, in the previous 12 months (Hawton and James 2005). Typically self-harm is a transient phenomenon with most self-harmers ceasing within a few months (Moran et al. 2012). Even so, self-harm is an important risk factor for premature death, with a minority of these deaths due to suicide. Self-harmers have high rates of death due to accidental injury and in later life from non-communicable diseases including cancer and cardiovascular disease (Bergen et al. 2012). In part this is likely to be mediated through high rates of health risk behaviours that include substance use and abuse.

Both suicide and self-harm in young people are commonly accompanied by mental disorders that include depression, substance abuse, and personality characteristics that include impulsivity and poor social problem-solving skills (Bergen et al. 2012). In addition, dysfunctional social networks such as being disconnected from community and family ties, parental separation, experience of bullying, and a history of sexual or physical abuse are common in the background of young suicide victims and self-harmers.

Approaches to prevention of suicide have commonly relied on population-based strategies that limit access to lethal means such as guns, lethal poisons, agricultural chemicals, pharmaceutical products that have high fatality rates (paracetamol), or preventing jumping from popular suicide destinations. Screening programmes to identify high-risk youth have had some attention and can increase mental health service use but do place a substantial burden on schools and have high false negative rates (Gould et al. 2009). Treatment studies have been few, but smaller-scale studies raise the possibility of brief psychological therapies being effective in adolescent self-harm (Donaldson et al. 2005).

Substance use and misuse

Substance use disorders including those related to alcohol use become prominent in the later adolescent and young adult years and represent the leading risk factor for disease burden in this population. Alcohol misuse in this age group accounts for a similar burden of disease as HIV. However, substance misuse is also a major contributor to mortality and disease-related disability later in life. Tobacco use commonly begins during the adolescent years but is a major contributor to disease burden later in life.

The global epidemiology of substance use in adolescence is changing rapidly with increases in use being clear in many LMICs. A recent report on the health of the world's adolescents found comparable data on tobacco use across six countries, representing 45 per cent of the worldwide population of young people (Patton et al. 2012). Rates of early tobacco use were high in Austria, Chile, Malta, and Namibia in both boys and girls. European regions, Latin America, North America, and many sub-Saharan African countries also show rates of tobacco use similar for boys and girls. Indonesia, Jamaica, Jordan, most Asian regions, the Caribbean, and the eastern Mediterranean have higher rates of tobacco use among boys.

Data on binge drinking were available for 50 countries and 18 per cent of the worldwide population. Estimates for binge drinking from high-income countries were somewhat higher than those derived from LMICs, with the exception of some Latin American countries. Austria, Ireland, and the United States had the highest rates with close to a third of children aged 15 years reporting binge drinking in the past month. Data on cannabis misuse in the past 30 days were available in 40 countries representing 12 per cent of the worldwide population, with the best data available for the European regions and North America. There were substantial variations in rates of use, with the highest in Canada, France, the Netherlands, Spain, and the United States. Intravenous drug users constitute a very vulnerable population, with a high degree of malnutrition, chronic skin infections, unplanned pregnancy, and a high rate of sexually transmitted infections (STIs), including hepatitis B and C and HIV. Adolescents who start using drugs at an earlier age are at higher risk of becoming injecting drug users (Trenz et al. 2012); this is also true for young people who drop out of education or experience homelessness, this holds true for both the United States as well as countries undergoing huge societal change such as Russia (Niccolai et al. 2011).

There is a range of reasons to take adolescent substance misuse seriously. Heavy adolescent use (e.g. misuse) may have profound adverse physical (e.g. blood-borne transmissible disease including HIV and hepatitis C) and psychological effects (e.g. psychotic and anxiety disorders related to cannabis use), as well as impairing social development (e.g. school failure and unemployment). Secondly, heavy use of alcohol and other psychoactive substances increases the likelihood of unprotected sex, unwanted pregnancies, dangerous driving, and interpersonal violence. Finally, the early initiation of substance use increases the likelihood of heavy and dependent use extending into adulthood, with many negative health and social consequences for users and their families (Patton et al. 2007).

Sexual and reproductive health

There is no area that has been more influenced by the biological and societal shifts reviewed at the beginning of this chapter, as has the sexual and reproductive health of young people. Both societal transformation (including cultural and social norms) and behavioural patterns create a situation of unique vulnerabilities as well as unique opportunities to build on young people's sexual and reproductive health assets such as the knowledge and skills to avoid unplanned and/or early pregnancy, STIs

including HIV, and sexual violence and abuse. An important issue during adolescence is the acquisition of a stable sexual orientation. LGBT (lesbian/gay/bisexual/transsexual) youth often endure difficulties in their coming out process, especially in certain cultural contexts that condemn homosexuality. It has been repeatedly shown that LGBT adolescents have a higher rate of mental difficulties and of suicidal conduct (Society for Adolescent Health and Medicine 2013). Another issue is the one of 'intergenerational cycle', a concept which stresses the fact that some behaviour patterns such as unintended pregnancy and fatherhood among adolescents tend to persist from one generation to another: multidimensional approaches including education represent an effective way to overcome this phenomenon (de Almeida Mda and Aquino 2009).

In almost all countries regardless of development status, the gap between the first sexual intercourse and marriage is widening, which means that most early sexual experiences occur among unmarried young women and men. However, an estimated 100 million adolescent girls in this decade will have their first sexual intercourse while married (nearly one in every four girls) and most likely with an older partner, with the consequence that they do not have the power to influence contraceptive or condom use (Wellings et al. 2006). The age at which adolescents tend to engage in sexual experiences varies, depending on contextual and cultural factors. In Latin America, 17 per cent of adolescent girls aged 15–19 years have had sex before age 15, in sub-Saharan Africa this figure is 14 per cent, and in South Asia the proportion is 8 per cent (UNICEF 2012).

The use of effective contraception among 15–24-year-olds has increased considerably since the early 1990s (Lloyd 2005). According to the most recent data available, contraceptive use was around 12 per cent in Africa, between 42 and 68 per cent in Latin America, between 13 and 47 per cent in Asia, and between 21 and 38 per cent in the Middle East among married and unmarried adolescents aged 15–19 years (Blanc et al. 2009). By contrast, 82 per cent of sexually active 15-year-olds in Europe and Canada reported having used condoms or contraceptive pills at last intercourse (Godeau et al. 2008). In countries with high rates of HIV, the proportion of adolescents using male condoms has also improved. For example, the rates of boys aged 15–19 years using male condoms vary between 40 (e.g. in United Republic of Tanzania, Uganda, and Malawi) and above 70 per cent (e.g. in South Africa, Namibia, and Swaziland) (UNICEF 2012). Early pregnancy represents a risk factor for poor reproductive outcomes. A recent review from the WHO stresses various preventive strategies such as increasing education and sexual education, the introduction of social support programmes, or prevention of unsafe abortion (Chandra-Mouli et al. 2013).

STIs, including HIV and HPV, constitute another important threat to health, as adolescents (especially young inexperienced individuals) are particularly vulnerable to acquiring such infections. Prevention strategies include individual screening, sexual education, and large-scale information campaigns (Berlan and Holland-Hall 2010). Among all potential approaches to improve safe sexual behaviour, retention in school seems to be effective. For instance, Baird and colleagues have recently shown a decrease in HIV infection rates among women receiving cash to stay in school (Baird et al. 2012). Finally, the introduction of HPV vaccine, even if it has been slow in low-income countries, is another effective preventive strategy in the area of STIs (Markowitz et al. 2012).

Chronic conditions, including malnutrition and obesity

As the importance of infections is decreasing around the world, thanks to vaccination, pharmacological treatments, and the improvement of hygiene, non-communicable diseases more and more constitute a real challenge. As stated by Proimos et al. obesity, childhood cancer, congenital defects and use of tobacco, alcohol, and drugs are and will be on the increase in the coming years. Indeed, around 10 per cent of adolescents suffer from some type of chronic condition broadly defined as conditions necessitating some care for at least 6 months (Suris et al. 2004), most of them belonging to the so-called 'non communicable diseases'. Chronic conditions encompass wide-ranging conditions, going from a mere myopia to cancer, cystic fibrosis, or myopathies and dystrophies. Among chronic conditions, mental disorder is a leading cause of DALYs among adolescents and includes unipolar depressive disorders, alcohol use disorders, self-inflicted injuries, schizophrenia, and bipolar affective disorders (see 'Mental health' section) (Patel et al. 2007). Given the improvement in medical care of many severe conditions, many individuals currently survive into adolescence and adulthood, where formerly they would not have survived past infancy. The increase in survival rate is thus directly associated with an increase in prevalence of chronic conditions.

Most chronic conditions affect the adolescent's biopsychosocial development and well-being. The extent of this impact depends on age of onset, duration, whether they are visible or not, congenital or acquired, expected survival, mobility, physiological functioning, cognition, emotional/social impairment, sensory functioning, communication impairment, course, and uncertainty (Suris et al. 2004). Areas affected may include growth and puberty, self-esteem, isolation from peers or overprotection by parents, and lack of school or professional achievement. Thus these issues will have to be dealt with more and more by the healthcare system. Its challenge will be to develop adequate and efficient ambulatory or inpatient care, thus improving the efficacy of treatments and therapeutic adherence of these youngsters in the short and long term (WHO 2002a; Narring et al. 2004).

Chronic malnutrition in earlier years is responsible for widespread stunting and adverse health and social consequences throughout the lifespan, including underweight. For instance, in Bangladesh, Senegal, and Niger, a third of female adolescents are underweight (UNICEF 2012). This is best prevented in childhood but actions to improve access to food could benefit adolescents as well. Anaemia is one of the key nutritional problems in adolescent girls, and in many African countries, more than half of female adolescents are anaemic (UNICEF 2012). Preventing teenage pregnancy and improving the nutritional status of girls before they enter pregnancy could reduce maternal and infant morbidity and mortality, and contribute to breaking the cycle of intergenerational malnutrition.

Over the past decade WHO has recognized that overweight and obesity represent a major public health challenge, reaching pandemic proportions among adults as well as among children and adolescents (Wang et al. 2002; UNICEF 2012). This pandemic was first observed and is still prominent in the United States and Western Europe, but has also occurred in middle-income countries such as Eastern Europe, South America, and East Asia. For instance, in Maldives, Bolivia, and Brazil, around a quarter of adolescent girls are overweight (UNICEF 2012). The prevalence of overweight and obesity has increased markedly in the last two decades in most high- and middle-income countries (Wang et al. 2002). This trend has arisen as a result of obesogenic environments, more sedentary time with diminished physical activity, and increasing calorie consumption. Urbanization encourages the use of automobiles and other motorized vehicles; in many high-income countries, suburbs lack shops, entertainment, or other destinations within walking distance.

Service delivery and early clinical interventions

There are sound reasons for offering effective healthcare and early individualized preventive service for adolescents. These years coincide with major shifts in disease burden and the adoption of lifestyle and health risk behaviours that have substantial effects on later health (see 'Health-specific issues' section). Moreover, healthcare through service delivery is one of the fundamental rights relevant to youth among others like gender equality and the right to education (United Nations 2003).

There is growing recognition that health service delivery should be tailored to the particular developmental needs of youth as well as the preventive orientation necessary for this age group. In 2002, the WHO called for the development of adolescent-friendly health services (AFHS) worldwide (WHO 2002a). The five themes underpinning AFHS are equity, effectiveness, accessibility, acceptability, and appropriateness of care. Although initially focused on primary healthcare in low-income countries, this framework has the potential to promote best practice healthcare for adolescents in high-income countries and within specialist health services as well (Tylee et al. 2007; Viner 2007).

Accessibility and acceptability of services remain key barriers to effective service delivery (Tylee et al. 2007). The reasons adolescents don't use services when they are available are: cost, lack of convenience (e.g. health facilities might be located a long distance from where young people live or have inconvenient opening hours), or lack of publicity and visibility. In some parts of the world, services are not provided due to geographic, financial, or attitudinal restrictions. Fear of a lack of confidentiality is a further major reason for young people's reluctance to seek help. When young people do seek help, they are often unhappy with the style of consultation and then don't return for follow-up (Tylee et al. 2007).

Professional organizations such as the American Medical Association have provided guidelines for adolescent preventive services (Elster and Kuznets 1994) that allow for the early detection of health problems that would potentially benefit from early intervention. Among these recommendations is the importance of screening young people for psychosocial issues and health risk behaviours. 'HEEADSSS' is a simple mnemonic screening tool, designed to cover the main risk areas among young people (see Table 10.4.1) (Goldenring and Rosen 2004).

These screening guidelines are based on the assumption that once a problematic behaviour is identified, the delivery of an intervention will contribute to modify the natural course of such

Table 10.4.1 HEEADSSS

HEEADSSS mnemonic	Examples of questions to assess the HEEADSSS
Home	Who lives with you? Where do you live? Do you have your own room?
	What are relationships like at home?
Education/employment	How are your grades? Any recent changes? Any dramatic changes in the past? What are your future education/employment plans/goals?
Eating	Have you dieted in the last year? How? How often?
	Have you done anything else to try to manage your weight?
	How much exercise do you get in an average day? Week?
Activities	What do you and your *friends* do for fun? (with whom, where, and when?)
	What do you and your *family* do for fun? (with whom, where, and when?)
Drugs	Do any of your friends use tobacco? Alcohol? Other drugs?
	Does anyone in your family use tobacco? Alcohol? Other drugs?
	Do you use tobacco? Alcohol? Other drugs?
	Is there any history of alcohol or drug problems in your family? Does anyone at home use tobacco?
Sexual activity	Have you ever been in a romantic relationship?
	Tell me about the people that you've dated. *OR* Tell me about your sex life.
	Have any of your relationships ever been sexual relationships?
	Are your sexual activities enjoyable?
	What does the term 'safer sex' mean to you?
Suicide and depression	Do you feel sad or down more than usual? Do you find yourself crying more than usual?
	Are you 'bored' all the time?
	Are you having trouble getting to sleep?
	Have you thought a lot about hurting yourself or someone else?
Safety	Have you ever been seriously injured? (How?) How about anyone else you know?
	Do you always wear a seat belt in the car?
	Have you ever ridden with a driver who was drunk or high? When? How often?
	Is there any violence in your home? Does the violence ever get physical?
	Have you ever been physically or sexually abused? Have you ever been raped, on a date or at any other time? (If not asked previously)

behaviour, be it substance misuse, an eating disorder, or unsafe sex. In other words, early intervention refers to interventions targeting adolescents displaying the early signs and symptoms of a health problem or experiencing a first episode of illness such as a mental disorder, for example. Ideally, these interventions should occur shortly after a need has arisen, aiming to reduce distress, shorten the episode of care, enhance protective factors, and minimize the level of intervention required.

As discussed previously, the shifting patterns of disease among adolescents have driven interventions to be more focused on non-communicable and non-fatal causes of disease both in adolescence and into adult life in order to respond to this shift and have a greater impact on public health outcomes. Current early intervention efforts have focused on ten main areas: physical activity, nutrition, tobacco, alcohol and other drugs, family planning, mental health, violent and abusive behaviours, unintentional injuries, sexually transmitted diseases, and clinical preventive services. For example, clinical intervention in an emergency room to reduce unintentional injuries showed that adolescents receiving counselling in a single risk area increased the use of seat belts and

bicycle helmets compared to the controls (Ketvertis et al. 2003). Other examples showing effectiveness of early intervention are programmes of tobacco cessation combining a variety of approaches, including taking into account the young person's preparation for quitting, supporting behavioural changing and enhancing motivation (Grimshaw and Stanton 2006). Early brief interventions using motivational interviewing and counselling help in the reduction of consumption of drugs and alcohol (Jensen et al. 2011).

Prevention and health promotion

Adolescent-onset behavioural problems implicated in non-communicable diseases include unsafe driving, mental health, violence, alcohol, tobacco and drug misuse, as well as unsafe sex and teen pregnancy (Patton et al. 2009). These health risks are all largely preventable. Over the last 40 years the integration of life course research with prevention trials and community epidemiology has offered a new way forwards in adolescent health (O'Connell et al. 2009). This prevention science framework posits that to prevent the onset of a problem, one must change the factors

Table 10.4.2 Risk factors affect multiple behaviour problems

Risk factors	Substance use	Delinquency	Teen pregnancy	School dropout	Violence	Depression and anxiety
Community						
Availability of drugs	✓				✓	
Availability of firearms		✓			✓	
Community laws and norms favourable towards drug use, firearms, and crime	✓	✓			✓	
Media portrayals	✓				✓	
Transitions and mobility	✓	✓		✓	✓	✓
Low neighbourhood attachment and community disorganization	✓	✓			✓	
Extreme economic deprivation	✓	✓	✓	✓	✓	
Family						
Family history of the problem behaviour	✓	✓	✓	✓	✓	✓
Family management problems	✓	✓	✓	✓	✓	✓
Family conflict	✓	✓	✓	✓	✓	✓
Favourable parental attitudes and involvement in the problem behaviour	✓	✓			✓	
School						
Academic failure beginning in late elementary school	✓	✓	✓	✓	✓	✓
Lack of commitment to school	✓	✓	✓	✓	✓	
Individual/peer						
Early and persistent antisocial behaviour	✓	✓	✓	✓	✓	✓
Rebelliousness	✓	✓		✓	✓	
Friends who engage in the problem behaviour	✓	✓	✓	✓	✓	
Favourable attitudes toward the problem behaviour	✓	✓	✓	✓	✓	
Early initiation of the problem behaviour	✓	✓	✓	✓	✓	
Constitutional factors	✓	✓			✓	✓

A tick at the intersection of a row and a column on this table indicates that there are at least two longitudinal studies that demonstrate that the risk factor measured earlier in an adolescent's life predicts the behaviour problem during adolescence. Reprinted with permission from the *Clinical Manual of Adolescent Substance Abuse Treatment*, (Copyright © 2011). American Psychiatric Publishing. All rights reserved.

that predict it (Coie et al. 1993; O'Connell et al. 2009). Such factors are commonly termed risk and protective factors and include those from an individual's family, school, and peer contexts as well as individual factors. Risk factors increase the likelihood of problems, and protective factors either directly decrease the likelihood of problems or mediate or moderate exposure to risk (O'Connell et al. 2009).

Table 10.4.2 lists risk factors for multiple problem behaviours. There is a good deal of commonality in risk factors across problem behaviours, suggesting that prevention programmes that seek to reduce, for example, family management problems or academic failure are likely to prevent multiple problems despite the fact that the programmes themselves may be focused on single problems such as conduct problems or academic success.

Although there has been less research on protective factors, longitudinal, prospective studies have identified seven factors that promote positive social development and reduce behaviour problems, including individual factors: high intelligence; resilient temperament; social, emotional, and cognitive competence; and environmental factors: opportunities for prosocial involvement; recognition for positive involvement; bonding; and healthy beliefs and standards for behaviour (Catalano et al. 2011).

Prevention science has utilized this knowledge about risk and protective factors to design preventive interventions to reduce risk and enhance protection. A growing number and diverse array of preventive interventions have been tested in controlled trials and found to be efficacious in preventing adolescent health problems (O'Connell et al. 2009). In a recent review of prevention programmes, Catalano and colleagues (2012) examined the evidence from controlled trials across multiple behaviour problems including obesity, violence, mental health, substance use, traffic crashes, pregnancy, and STIs by examining recent reviews and conducting targeted searches for controlled preventive trials. While only presenting illustrative examples in their article,

Table 10.4.3 Types of approaches that have controlled trials demonstrating efficacy

Prevention programmes/policies	Violence	Drug use	HIV STI	Unintended pregnancy	Vehicle crashes	Obesity	Mental health
1. Prenatal and infancy programmes (e.g. NFP)		✓		✓			
2. Early childhood education	✓	✓					
3. Parent training	✓	✓			✓		✓
4. After-school recreation	✓						
5. Mentoring with contingent reinforcement		✓					
6. Cognitive behaviour therapy							✓
7. Classroom organization, management, and instructional strategies	✓	✓		✓			✓
8. Classroom curricula	✓	✓		✓		✓	✓
9. Community-based training/motivational Interviewing			✓	✓			
10. Cash transfer for school fees/stipend				✓			
11. Multicomponent positive youth development	✓			✓			
12. Policies (e.g. MLDA, access to contraceptives)		✓		✓	✓		
13. Community mobilization	✓	✓					
14. Medical intervention			✓	✓			
15. Law enforcement					✓		
16. Family planning clinic				✓			

Table 10.4.3 provides the results of the more comprehensive programme review across multiple problems. A check at the intersection of a row and a column indicates that there is at least one controlled prevention trial of the approach with evidence of impact post intervention on an indicator of the behaviour problem in the column. While most of these studies were conducted in high-income countries, a number have been conducted in LMICs. The reader is referred to high-quality reviews of controlled prevention trials available from the Center for the Study and Prevention of Violence (n.d.), The Cochrane Collaboration (n.d.), and The Campbell Collaboration (n.d.) for reviews of specific programmes. Many behaviour problems have common risk and protective factors, and there is evidence that interventions that address these common risk factors have affected multiple problems despite the prevention programme focus on only a single behaviour problem (Flay et al. 2004; Schweinhart et al. 2005; Hawkins et al. 2008).

Table 10.4.3 suggests that wide-ranging prevention strategies are effective from pre- and postnatal home visiting programmes; early childhood education; primary and secondary school programmes to improve instruction, classroom management, and attendance; and school curricula that provide skills and norms that support avoiding problem behaviour, from risky sex, to drugs, to violence. A few illustrative examples follow.

The Gatehouse Project is a primary prevention programme which includes both institutional and individual-focused components to promote the emotional and behavioural well-being of young people in secondary schools. Using a school-based cluster randomized controlled trial, it has shown effectiveness on behaviours such as substance use by young people, with a 3–5 per cent risk difference between intervention and control students for any drinking, any and regular smoking, and friends' alcohol and tobacco use across the three waves of follow-up (Bond et al. 2004).

Nurse–Family Partnership (NFP) is a programme in which trained, registered nurses provide low-income, single, first-time mothers with biweekly structured visits during pregnancy and for 2 years post birth. Nurses share information on how mothers can reduce their use of alcohol, tobacco, and other drugs during pregnancy; improve their prenatal health and diet; sensitively and responsibly care for their infants; achieve their own education and occupational goals; avoid unwanted future pregnancies; and access community services. The programme has been demonstrated in controlled trials to reduce the mother's reliance on public welfare (157 fewer days over 2 years), the number of subsequent births were reduced by 43 per cent, verified reports of child abuse and neglect (32 vs. 65 per cent) decreased, and mothers increased their workforce participation (82 per cent increase in months worked). Children at age 15 have been shown to have fewer arrests (20 vs. 45 per cent), and less alcohol use (1.09 vs. 2.49 days' drinking in past 6 months), and fewer lifetime sexual partners (0.92 vs. 2.48) compared to those not receiving services (Olds et al. 1998).

Strengthening Families Programme for Parents and Youth 10–14 is a 7-week universal parent training programme offered to parents and adolescents in weekly 2-hour sessions. The programme targets family, peer, and individual risk and protective factors, including parent communication and child management skills; children's social skills, stress management, and ability to refuse peer drug offers; and parent/child conflict resolution and bonding. Across multiple studies conducted in rural communities in the United States the programme has been shown to reduce substance use (24 per cent less alcohol use; 40.1 per cent less drunkness) and delinquency (37–77 per cent less depending on the behaviour) up to 5 years post intervention for participants versus control group members (Spoth et al. 2001).

Conditional Cash Transfer (CCT) Programmes provide payments that come with conditions. Examples include payment of school fees and supplemental cash to poor parents with the condition that they send their child to school. Trials in Malawi and Kenya found reduced self-reported sexual activity (13 per cent less likely to ever have sex), pregnancy (31 per cent less likely), and marriage (41 per cent less likely) in one or both countries, and girls and young women who received the CCTs were 15 per cent less likely to drop out of school compared to controls (Duflo et al. 2006; Baird et al. 2010). Preliminary findings from the study in Malawi showed a 60 per cent reduction in HIV prevalence and a 75 per cent reduction in herpes simplex virus-2 prevalence (2010).

Unplugged is a 12-hour, teacher-led alcohol, tobacco, and other drug use prevention programme for early secondary school students. Lessons target peer influence and societal risks and aim to improve students' goal-setting, decision-making, and drug refusal skills. In a study of students in seven European countries, programme benefits included reduced any (odds ratio (OR) = 0.80) and frequent drunkenness (OR = 0.62) and frequent past-month marijuana use (OR = 0.74) (Faggiano et al. 2010).

Prevention approaches also include community policies and laws ranging from access to contraceptives for those under age 18 to graduated driving laws in which new drivers have restrictions on conditions under which they may drive, and raising the legal drinking age to 21 (Catalano et al. 2012). Two examples relate to health policy for mature minors and the use of taxation.

Policies that ensure minors' right to obtain contraception without parental notification or consent and provide contraception at no cost to minors have been associated with an 8.5 per cent decreased adolescent birth rate. Youth who were provided with contraception combined with sexuality education in school-based clinics were more likely to delay initiation of sexual intercourse (79 vs 90 per cent at age 17) and have lower pregnancy rates (pregnancy rate in intervention schools declined by 30.1 per cent versus an increase of 57.6 per cent in control schools) compared to youth not exposed to the intervention (Zabin et al. 1986).

Systematic reviews of multiple studies have shown that price and tax increases on alcoholic beverages have been associated with reduction in alcohol use by adolescents and young adults (aggregate-level $r = -0.17$ for beer, -0.30 for wine, -0.29 for spirits, and -0.44 for total alcohol), including excessive drinking and alcohol-related health problems (mean reported elasticity = -0.28, individual-level $r = -0.01$, $p < 0.01$) (Wagenaar and Toomey 2002).

There is also growing evidence that these programmes can be cost effective. In the United States, Aos and colleagues estimated cost effectiveness of diverse prevention programmes (Aos et al. 2004). Their work demonstrated that, while not all prevention programmes realize monetary benefits, many do, returning between $2 and 42 for every dollar invested (Catalano et al. 2012).

Community monitoring systems are an essential element of effective prevention programmes. These assess behaviour problems, as well as risk and protective factors, and can help communities apply prevention strategies relevant for that setting (Mrazek et al. 2004). Several local surveys exist that have been tested in multiple countries, including the Communities That Care (CTC) Youth Survey (Arthur et al. 2002) which measures risk, protection, and substance use, delinquency, violence, and depression, and the European School Survey Project on Alcohol and Other Drugs (ESPAD) (Hibell et al. 2009) which focuses on assessing adolescent drug use and risks. The school-based Global Student Health Survey (GSHS) assesses nine problem behaviours and some predictors among young people aged 13–15 years (WHO 2004).

In the field of adolescent sexual and reproductive health and specifically of HIV prevention, a large review conducted by the WHO has drawn attention to the potential for effective interventions within the media or within schools settings (WHO et al. 2006). There are also a number of initiatives and programmes which have proven effective in preventing unplanned pregnancies among adolescents (Kirby 2007).

Also, several avenues have proven effective to address child and adolescent obesity, from primary to tertiary care. These include the involvement of the family, the schools, and the community in the care of overweight and obese adolescents, but also the development of strategies and policies which aim at improving the nutritional supply and environment of young people (Hassink et al. 2011). Indeed, adolescence is a timely period to shape healthy eating and exercise habits that can contribute to physical and psychological benefits during the adolescent period and to reducing the likelihood of nutrition-related chronic diseases in adulthood.

Finally, the prevention of injuries is mainly improved through environmental and legislative measures such as enforced control of firearms, mandatory use of helmets or seat belts, or improvement of roads (WHO 2008).

Despite the growing evidence that prevention can be effective, most preventive interventions have been developed in high-income countries (Catalano et al. 2012). Even in high-income countries like the United States, prevention approaches that are not effective or have not been evaluated are more widely used than prevention programmes that have been tested and found to be effective (Ringwalt et al. 2009). The underutilization of effective programmes in LMICs is even greater, where fewer prevention programmes have been tested (Catalano et al. 2012). One current challenge is how the use of tested, efficacious prevention policies and programmes can be extended globally while recognizing that communities and nations are different from one another, and need to decide locally what policies and programmes they use, because risk and protection factors as well as the cultural and the political context vary by community. Catalano and colleagues (Catalano et al. 2012) suggest three solutions to meet this challenge.

First, the marketplace (government, public health agencies, schools, and parents) must recognize that: (1) adolescent health is a priority, (2) behaviour problems are implicated in poor health outcomes in adolescence and adulthood, and (3) there are effective policies and programmes that can prevent behaviour problems. A shift of 10 per cent of the total funds spent on adolescent health and education to effective prevention policies and programmes could make a big difference in adolescent and adult morbidity and mortality worldwide.

Second, more research is needed on the impact of translating these efficacious approaches to a range of communities and across nations. Translation of effective approaches must recognize differences in local conditions, but also recognize that the policy or programme has active ingredients that need to be preserved in order for the programme to work. Some interventions created in high-income countries can be translated to and be effective in LMICs (Kirby 2007).

Third, using surveys to understand country and community epidemiology can help assess and address local needs with efficacious prevention programmes. By regularly assessing local risk and protective factors and behaviour problems in youth, communities and nations can understand and prioritize their need for specific prevention approaches.

Conclusion

The knowledge on global adolescent health has made rapid progress in recent years, demonstrating the substantial mortality and disease burden arising in this age group. It is a rapidly changing picture in which many countries are making a transition from high mortality and disability in infancy and younger childhood to one where the adolescent years are dominating the picture of mortality and disease burden in the developmental years.

There is now recognition that adolescence is central to major global health agendas beyond sexual and reproductive health. In injury, mental health, and risks for later life non-communicable diseases, it is difficult to conceive a successful strategy that does not address the onset of these problems in the adolescent years. In addition, there are major social and economic challenges that will continue to drive adolescent health and disease in the years to come. These include the ongoing economic difficulties in many countries, with resultant high youth unemployment, the rapid urbanization of many countries and loss of traditional communities, the growth in migration both within and between countries, and ongoing civil unrest and military conflict in many parts of the globe.

There are no simple answers to these considerable challenges. Rather, responses will need to be made at multiple levels and in the different settings in which young people are growing up. They include the provision of youth-friendly healthcare, the development, implementation, and evaluation of strategies at school and community levels for promoting the health development of the young, the implementation of legislative and environmental policies that take into account local culture and history, and the engagement of public health professionals with fields well beyond health in the implementation of these strategies.

Note

1. The Gini index/coefficient is a measure of the equality or inequality in incomes (or other indicators) which can be assessed across countries. Income Gini index is considered as an indicator of equity in a given country.

References

Aos, S., Lieb, R., Mayfield, J., Miller, M., and Pennucci, A. (2004). *Benefits and Costs of Prevention and Early Intervention Programs for Youth*. Olympia, WA: Washington State Institute for Public Policy.

Arthur, M.W., Hawkins, J.D., Pollard, J.A., Catalano, R.F., and Baglioni, A.J., Jr. (2002). Measuring risk and protective factors for substance use, delinquency, and other adolescent problem behaviors: the Communities That Care Youth Survey. *Evaluation Review*, 26, 575–601.

Baird, S., Chirwa, E., Mcintosh, C., and Ozler, B. (2010). The short-term impacts of a schooling conditional cash transfer program on the sexual behavior of young women. *Health Economics*, 19(Suppl.), 55–68.

Baird, S.J., Garfein, R.S., Mcintosh, C.T., and Ozler, B. (2012). Effect of a cash transfer programme for schooling on prevalence of HIV and herpes simplex type 2 in Malawi: a cluster randomised trial. *The Lancet*, 379, 1320–9.

Beaglehole, R., Bonita, R., Horton, R., et al. (2011). Priority actions for the non-communicable disease crisis. *The Lancet*, 377, 1438–47.

Bergen, H., Hawton, K., Waters, K., et al. (2012). Premature death after self-harm: a multicentre cohort study. *The Lancet*, 380, 1568–74.

Berlan, E.D. and Holland-Hall, C. (2010). Sexually transmitted infections in adolescents: advances in epidemiology, screening, and diagnosis. *Adolescent Medicine: State of the Art Reviews*, 21, 332–46, x.

Bhutta, Z., Dean, S.V., and Imam, S. (2011). *Systematic Review of Preconception Health Risk and Interventions*. Geneva: WHO.

Blanc, A.K., Tsui, A.O., Croft, T.N., and Trevitt, J.L. (2009). Patterns and trends in adolescents' contraceptive use and discontinuation in developing countries and comparisons with adult women. *International Perspectives on Sexual and Reproductive Health*, 35, 63–71.

Bond, L., Patton, G., Glover, S., et al. (2004). The Gatehouse Project: can a multilevel school intervention affect emotional wellbeing and health risk behaviours? *Journal of Epidemiology and Community Health*, 58, 997–1003.

Capua, T., Katz, J.A., and Bocchini, J.A.J. (2013). Update on adolescent immunizations: selected review of US recommendations and literature. *Current Opinion in Pediatrics*, 25, 397–406.

Catalano, R.F., Fagan, A.A., Gavin, L.E., et al. (2012). Worldwide application of the prevention science research base in adolescent health. *The Lancet*, 379, 1653–64.

Catalano, R.F., Haggerty, K.P., Hawkins, J.D., and Elgin, J. (2011). Prevention of substance use and substance use disorders: the role of risk and protective factors. In Y. Kaminer and K.C. Winters (eds.) *Clinical Manual of Adolescent Substance Abuse Treatment*, pp. 25–63. Washington, DC: American Psychiatric Publishing.

Center for the Study and Prevention of Violence (n.d.). *Blueprints Project*. [Online] Available at: http://www.colorado.edu/cspv/blueprints.

Chandra-Mouli, V., Camacho, A.V., and Michaud, P.A. (2013). WHO guidelines on preventing early pregnancy and poor reproductive outcomes among adolescents in developing countries. *Journal of Adolescent Health*, 52, 517–22.

Coie, J.D., Watt, N.F., West, S.G., et al. (1993). The science of prevention. A conceptual framework and some directions for a national research program. *American Psychologist*, 48, 1013–22.

Collishaw, S., Maughan, B., Goodman, R., and Pickles, A. (2004). Time trends in adolescent mental health. *Journal of Child Psychology and Psychiatry*, 45, 1350–62.

Copeland, W., Shanahan, L., Costello, E.J., and Angold, A. (2011). Cumulative prevalence of psychiatric disorders by young adulthood: a prospective cohort analysis from the Great Smoky Mountains Study. *Journal of the American Academy of Child and Adolescent Psychiatry*, 50, 252–61.

Costello, E.J., Erkanli, A., and Angold, A. (2006). Is there an epidemic of child or adolescent depression? *Journal of Child Psychology and Psychiatry*, 47, 1263–71.

Dahl, R.E. (2004). Adolescent brain development: a period of vulnerabilities and opportunities. Keynote address. *Annals of the New York Academy of Sciences*, 1021, 1–22.

Dahlberg, L.L. and Potter, L.B. (2001). Youth violence. Developmental pathways and prevention challenges. *American Journal of Preventive Medicine*, 20, 3–14.

De Almeida Mda, C., and Aquino, E.M. (2009). The role of education level in the intergenerational pattern of adolescent pregnancy in Brazil. *International Perspectives on Sexual and Reproductive Health*, 35, 139–46.

Donaldson, D., Spirito, A., and Esposito-Smythers, C. (2005). Treatment for adolescents following a suicide attempt: results of a pilot trial. *Journal of the American Academy of Child and Adolescent Psychiatry*, 44, 113–20.

Duflo, E., Dupas, P., Kremer, M., and Sinei, S. (2006). *Education and HIV/AIDS Prevention: Evidence from a Randomized Evaluation in*

Western Kenya. World Bank Policy Research Working Paper 4024. Washington, DC: World Bank.

Elster, A. and Kuznets, N. (eds.) (1994). *AMA Guidelines for Adolescent Preventive Services (GAPS): Recommendations and Rationale*. Baltimore, MD: Williams & Wilkins.

Faggiano, F., Vigna-Taglianti, F., Burkhart, G., et al. (2010). The effectiveness of a school-based substance abuse prevention program: 18-month follow-up of the EU-Dap cluster randomized controlled trial. *Drug and Alcohol Dependence*, 108, 56–64.

Flay, B.R., Graumlich, S., Segawa, E., Burns, J.L., and Holliday, M.Y. (2004). Effects of 2 prevention programs on high-risk behaviors among African American youth: a randomized trial. *Archives of Pediatrics & Adolescent Medicine*, 158, 377–84.

Giedd, J.N. (2008). The teen brain: insights from neuroimaging. *Journal of Adolescent Health*, 42, 335–43.

Godeau, E., Nic Gabhainn, S., Vignes, C., Ross, J., Boyce, W., and Todd, J. (2008). Contraceptive use by 15-year-old students at their last sexual intercourse: results from 24 countries. *Archives of Pediatrics & Adolescent Medicine*, 162, 66–73.

Goldenring, J.M. and Rosen, D.S. (2004). Getting into adolescent heads: an essential update. *Contemporary Pediatrics*, 21, 64–80.

Gore, F.M., Bloem, P.J., Patton, G.C., et al. (2011). Global burden of disease in young people aged 10–24 years: a systematic analysis. *The Lancet*, 377, 2093–102.

Gould, M.S., Marrocco, F.A., Hoagwood, K., Kleinman, M., Amakawa, L., and Altschuler, E. (2009). Service use by at-risk youths after school-based suicide screening. *Journal of the American Academy of Child and Adolescent Psychiatry*, 48, 1193–201.

Grimshaw, G. and Stanton, A. (2006). Tobacco cessation interventions for young people. *Cochrane Database of Systematic Reviews*, 4, CD003289.

Hagell, A. (ed.) (2012). *Changing Adolescence: Social Trends and Mental Health*. Bristol: The Policy Press.

Hassink, S.G., Hill, K.S., and Biddinger, S. (2011). Pediatric obesity: practical applications and strategies from primary to tertiary care. *Pediatrics*, 128(Suppl.), 845–90.

Hawkins, J.D., Kosterman, R., Catalano, R.F., Hill, K.G., and Abbott, R.D. (2008). Effects of social development intervention in childhood fifteen years later. *Archives of Pediatrics and Adolescent Medicine*, 162, 1133–41.

Hawton, K. and James, A. (2005). Suicide and deliberate self-harm in young people. *British Medical Journal*, 330, 891–4.

Hibell, B., Guttormsson, U., Ahlström, S., et al. (2009). *The 2007 ESPAD Report: Substance Use Among Students in 35 European Countries*. Stockholm: Swedish Council for Information on Alcohol and Other Drugs.

Innocenti Research Centre (2007). *An Overview of Child Well-being in Rich Countries*. Geneva: UNICEF.

Jensen, C.D., Cushing, C.C., Aylward, B.S., Craig, J.T., Sorell, D.M., and Steele, R.G. (2011). Effectiveness of motivational interviewing interventions for adolescent substance use behavior change: a meta-analytic review. *Journal of Consulting and Clinical Psychology*, 79, 433–40.

Kessler, R.C., Berglund, P., Demler, O., Jin, R., and Merikangas, K.R. (2005). Lifetime prevalence and age-of-onset distributions of DSM-IV disorders in the National Comorbidity Survey replication. *Archives of General Psychiatry*, 62, 593–602.

Ketvertis, K.M., Johnston, B.D., and Rivara, F.P. (2003). Behavior change counseling in the emergency department to reduce injury risk: a randomized, controlled trial. *Pediatrics*, 111, 1125.

Kirby, D. (2007). *Emerging Answers 2007*. Washington, DC: National Campaign to Prevent Teen Pregnancy. Available at: http://www.thenationalcampaign.org/EA2007/EA2007_full.pdf.

Lloyd, C. (2005). *Growing Up Global: The Changing Transitions to Adulthood in Developing Countries*. Washington, DC: National Research Council and Institute of Medicine, National Academies Press.

Ma, J., Lee, K.V., and Staffod, R.S. (2005). Depression treatment during outpatient visits by US children and adolescents. *Journal of Adolescent Health*, 37, 434–42.

Markowitz, L.E., Tsu, V., Deeks, S.L., et al. (2012). Human papillomavirus vaccine introduction—the first five years. *Vaccine*, 30(Suppl. 5), F139–48.

Michaud, P.A., Suris, J.C., and Deppen, A. (2006). Gender-related psychological and behavioural correlates of pubertal timing in a national sample of Swiss adolescents. *Molecular and Cellular Endocrinology*, 254–5, 172–8.

Moran, P., Coffey, C., Romaniuk, H., et al. (2012). The natural history of self-harm from adolescence to young adulthood: a population-based cohort study. *The Lancet*, 379, 236–43.

Mrazek, P.J., Biglan, A., and Hawkins, J.D. (2004). *Community-Monitoring Systems: Tracking and Improving the Well-Being of America's Children and Adolescents*. Falls Church, VA: Society for Prevention Research. Available at: http://www.preventionresearch.org/CMSbook.pdf.

Munro, J., Coleman, P., Nicholl, J., Harper, R., Kent, G., and Wild, D. (1995). Can we prevent accidental injury to adolescents? A systematic review of the evidence. *Injury Prevention*, 1, 249–55.

Narring, F., Tschumper, A., Inderwildi Bonivento, L., et al. (2004). *Santé et styles de vie des adolescents agés de 16 à 20 ans en Suisse (2002)*. *Raisons de santé*. Lausanne: Institut Universitaire de Médecine Sociale et Préventive.

Niccolai, L.M., Verevochkin, S.V., Toussova, O.V., et al. (2011). Estimates of HIV incidence among drug users in St. Petersburg, Russia: continued growth of a rapidly expanding epidemic. *European Journal of Public Health*, 21, 613–19.

O'Connell, M.E., Boat, T., and Warner, K.E. (eds.) (2009). *Preventing Mental, Emotional, and Behavioral Disorders Among Young People: Progress and Possibilities*. Washington, DC: The National Academies Press.

Olds, D.L., Henderson, C.R., Jr., Cole, R., et al. (1998). Long-term effects of nurse home visitation on children's criminal and antisocial behavior: 15-year follow-up of a randomized controlled trial. *Journal of the American Medical Association*, 280, 1238–44.

Ong, K.K., Ahmed, M.L., and Dunger, D.B. (2006). Lessons from large population studies on timing and tempo of puberty (secular trends and relation to body size): the European trend. *Molecular and Cellular Endocrinology*, 254–5, 8–12.

Patel, V., Flisher, A.J., Hetrick, S., and McGorry, P. (2007). Mental health of young people: a global public health challenge. *The Lancet*, 369, 29–40.

Patton, G.C., Coffey, C., Cappa, C., et al. (2012). Health of the world's adolescents: a synthesis of internationally comparable data. *The Lancet*, 379, 1665–75.

Patton, G.C., Coffey, C., Lynskey, M.T., et al. (2007). Trajectories of adolescent alcohol and cannabis use into young adulthood. *Addiction*, 102, 607–15.

Patton, G.C., Coffey, C., Sawyer, S.M., et al. (2009). Global patterns of mortality in young people: a systematic analysis of population health data. *The Lancet*, 374, 881–92.

Patton, G.C. and Viner, R. (2007). Pubertal transitions in health. *The Lancet*, 369, 1130–9.

Ringwalt, C., Vincus, A.A., Hanley, S., et al. (2009). The prevalence of evidence-based drug use prevention curricula in U.S. middle schools in 2005. *Prevention Science*, 10, 33–40.

Rutter, M. and Smith, D. (1995). *Psychosocial Disorders in Young People: Time Trends and their Causes*. Chichester: Wiley & Sons.

Sanci, L., Lewis, D., and Patton, G. (2010). Detecting emotional disorder in young people in primary care. *Current Opinion in Psychiatry*, 23, 318–23.

Sawyer, S.M., Afifi, R.A., Bearinger, L.H., et al. (2012). Adolescence: a foundation for future health. *The Lancet*, 379, 1630–40.

Schweinhart, L.J., Montie, J., Xiang, Z., Barnett, W.S., Belfield, C.R., and Nores, M. (2005). *Lifetime effects: The High/Scope Perry Preschool study through age 40*. Monographs of the High/Scope Educational Research Foundation, 14. Ypsilanti, MI: High/Scope Press.

Society for Adolescent Health and Medicine (2013). Recommendations for promoting the health and well-being of lesbian, gay, bisexual, and transgender adolescents: a position paper of the Society for Adolescent Health and Medicine. *Journal of Adolescent Health*, 52, 506–10.

Spoth, R.L., Redmond, C., and Shin, C. (2001). Randomized trial of brief family interventions for general populations: adolescent substance use outcomes 4 years following baseline. *Journal of Consulting and Clinical Psychology*, 69, 627–42.

Suris, J.C., Michaud, P.A., and Viner, R. (2004). The adolescent with a chronic condition. Part I: developmental issues. *Archives of Disease in Childhood*, 89, 938–42.

Temin, M. and Levine, R. (2009). *Start With a Girl: A New Agenda for Global Health*. Washington, DC: Centre for Global Development.

The Campbell Collaboration (n.d.). Website. [Online] Available at: http://www.campbellcollaboration.org.

The Cochrane Collaboration (n.d.). Website. [Online] Available at: http://www.cochrane.org.

Trenz, R.C., Scherer, M., Harrell, P., Zur, J., Sinha, A., and Latimer, W. (2012). Early onset of drug and polysubstance use as predictors of injection drug use among adult drug users. *Addictive Behaviors*, 37, 367–72.

Tylee, A., Haller, D.M., Graham, T., Churchill, R., and Sanci, L.A. (2007). Youth-friendly primary-care services: how are we doing and what more needs to be done? *The Lancet*, 369, 1565–73.

United Nations (2003). *State of the World Population 2003: Making 1 Billion Count: Investing in Adolescents' Health and Rights*. Maryland, MD: UNFPA.

United Nations Children's Fund (2011). *The State of the World's Children 2011: Adolescence, An Age of Opportunity*. New York: UNICEF.

United Nations Children's Fund (2012). *A Report Card on Adolescence. Progress for Children*. New York: UNICEF.

Viner, R.M. (2007). Do adolescent inpatient wards make a difference? Findings from a national young patient survey. *Pediatrics*, 120, 749–55.

Viner, R.M., Ozer, E.M., Denny, S., et al. (2012). Adolescence and the social determinants of health. *The Lancet*, 379, 1641–52.

Wagenaar, A.C. and Toomey, T.L. (2002). Effects of minimum drinking age laws: review and analyses of the literature from 1960 to 2000. *Journal of Studies on Alcohol Supplement*, 14, 206–25.

Wang, Y., Monteiro, C., and Popkin, B.M. (2002). Trends of obesity and underweight in older children and adolescents in the United States, Brazil, China, and Russia. *American Journal of Clinical Nutrition*, 75, 971–7.

Wellings, K., Collumbien, M., Slaymaker, E., et al. (2006). Sexual behaviour in context: a global perspective. *The Lancet*, 368, 1706–28.

World Health Organization (1989). *The Health of Youth*. Geneva: WHO.

World Health Organization (2002a). *Adolescent Friendly Health Services: An Agenda for Change*. Geneva: WHO.

World Health Organization (2002b). *World Report on Violence and Health*. Geneva: WHO.

World Health Organization (2004). *Global School-Based Student Health Survey (GSHS)* [Online]. Available at: http://www.who.int/chp/gshs/en/.

World Health Organization (2008). *World Report on Child Injury Prevention*. Geneva: WHO.

World Health Organization (2009). *Global Status Report on Road Safety: Time for Action*. Geneva: WHO.

World Health Organization, Ross, D.A., Dick, B., and Ferguson, J. (2006). *Preventing HIV/AIDS in Young People: A Systematic Review of the Evidence from Developing Countries*. Geneva: WHO.

Zabin, L.S., Hirsch, M.B., Smith, E.A., Streett, R., and Hardy, J.B. (1986). Evaluation of a pregnancy prevention program for urban teenagers. *Family Planning Perspectives*, 18, 119–26.

Ethnicity, race, epidemiology, and public health

Raj Bhopal

Introduction to ethnicity in relation to race and related variables

Humans comprise one biological species and their similarities, both genetically and behaviourally, are remarkable. Nonetheless, humans show differences between individuals and between groups (Bhopal 2014). Amongst the important concepts that help them differentiate themselves, ethnicity and race are particularly relevant to medical sciences, reflected in increasing numbers of publications (Afshari and Bhopal 2010). Remarkably, humans are mentally equipped to differentiate between individuals and groups, including by race-related physical features, from early infancy (Anzures et al. 2013; Xiao et al. 2013).

Race and ethnicity are complex, intertwining, and important concepts that are used by societies to identify and evaluate social groups and individuals. As epidemiology is based on variables that differentiate the health experiences of populations, race and ethnicity are central to the discipline, and to public health (Bhopal 2008). Table 10.5.1 sets out some criteria for a good epidemiological variable in relation to ethnicity, race, and their commonly used proxy of country of birth. Even though race has come under attack because of its historical harms (Kohn 1995), it remains important in public health, not least to help redress historical harms (Krieger 2003). Increasing international migration (see Chapter 10.9) has made these concepts of great contemporary importance (Segal et al. 2010) and the International Organization of Migration and the World Health Organization (WHO) are leading efforts to catalyse work in this field globally (WHO Regional Office for Europe 2010; WHO 2010).

Traditionally, race focused around subgrouping human populations based upon biological factors such as skin colour, facial shape, and hair type. Your race, based on this concept, is the group you belong to, or are perceived to belong to, in the light of such factors (Bhopal 2014). Racial classifications based solely on biology have proven of modest scientific value and questionable validity, and have been open to abuse socially, for example, the Nazi 'final solution' (Bhopal 2014). This concept of race is changing to incorporate social factors, and a shared history, and hence it is converging with ethnicity and in this renewed form remains important, especially in the United States (Satcher 2001). The new genetic technologies and genome analysis techniques are, however, leading to a reappraisal, and worryingly to a potential resurgence, of the biological race concept (Fujimura and Rajagopalan 2011).

Ethnicity is a concept that, in principle, uses cultural and social factors such as family origins, language, diet, and religion to subgroup humans. Your ethnicity, based on this concept, is the group you belong to, or are perceived to belong to, in the light of such factors (Bhopal 2014). Family origin is based in ancestry and in this respect ethnicity is akin to race. Ethnicity is in vogue, particularly in Europe, partly due to the abuse of the race concept politically (Bhopal 2007). In practice, race and ethnicity are often used synonymously, with the compound word race/ethnicity (or race-ethnicity) appearing, especially in the United States (Afshari and Bhopal 2010).

Race and ethnicity are related to but separate from nationality (the nation you belong to, as identified by citizenship and/or passport) and country of birth (Bhopal 2007). It is not only race but also other related characteristics such as ethnicity, religion, and migration status that are relevant to racism. Racism is the product of the view, and its expression through individual, institutional and social attitudes, conventions, and behaviours that some groups are superior to others on the basis of their race or related characteristics as above. Racism is then used to provide advantage to these ostensibly, but not in reality, superior groups.

Race and ethnicity are especially important to identity where people of different racial and ethnic groups mix, that is, multiethnic, multiracial, multicultural societies, themselves resulting from rapid immigration (Bhopal 2014; Segal et al. 2010; also see Chapter 10.9). Scientific disciplines have utilized race and ethnicity to advance both understanding and applications of research. The sheer complexity of the concepts has made this task difficult, and the misapplication of race and ethnicity has often done more harm than good (Kohn 1995; Bhopal 2007). Nonetheless, migration status, race, and ethnicity are excellent in differentiating the health and healthcare status of subpopulations, and this property gives them central status in quantitative health sciences, public health and clinical care (Table 10.5.1). Building on evolutionary thinking extended to modern times, I have created a model (Fig. 10.5.1). The left half of the figure shows how migration from and indeed within Africa some 60,000–70,000 years ago over several millennia led to differentiation among human populations. The genetic differences arising have been closely aligned in modern times with the concept of race, and cultural ones to ethnicity, but as we have seen these are merely issues of emphasis. There would have been differentiation in many other ways but I have limited these to socioeconomic and technological. The time period of 60,000–70,000 years was enough to cause

Table 10.5.1 Ethnicity (or race or country of birth) as an epidemiological variable

Criteria for a good epidemiological variable	Criteria in relation to ethnicity (or race or country of birth)
Impacts on health in individuals and populations	Ethnicity is a powerful associated influence on health
Accurately measurable	In most populations ethnicity is difficult to assess (not true for country of birth)
Differentiates populations in their experience of disease or health	Huge differences by ethnicity are seen for many diseases, health problems and for factors which cause health problems
Differentiates populations in some underlying characteristic relevant to health, e.g. income, childhood circumstance, hormonal status, genetic inheritance, or behaviour relevant to health	Differences in disease patterns in different ethnic groups reflect a rich mix of environmental factors and may also reflect population changes in genetic factors, particularly in populations where migration has been high
Generates testable aetiological hypotheses, and/or helps in developing health policy, and/or helps plan and deliver healthcare and/or helps prevent and control disease	It is hard to test specific hypotheses because there are so many underlying differences between populations of different ethnicity Ethnic differences in disease patterns profoundly affect health policy Knowing the ethnic structure of a population is critical to good decision-making By understanding the ethnic distribution of diseases and risk, preventative and control programmes can be targeted at appropriate ethnic groups

Reproduced from Raj. S Bhopal, *Ethnicity, Race, and Health in Multicultural Societies*, Second Edition, Table 1.3, p. 8, Oxford University Press, Oxford, UK, Copyright © 2014 Raj. S Bhopal, by permission of Oxford University Press.

differentiation but not enough to create new human species. In modern times, especially in the last 1000 years or so, new migrations have created multicultural societies. In these new societies immigrants come with the health status variations from their place of origin (whether effectively permanent as in genetic ones or highly changeable, e.g. low blood pressure). The effects of the migration process (e.g. selection effects), the journey, the new life circumstances, and discrimination at the new settlement influence the health status. The complexity of the process is self-evident.

Race and ethnicity are important in health and healthcare, particularly in demonstrating inequalities (differences) and inequities (differences where there is a presumed or demonstrated element of injustice, called disparities in the United States) (WHO 2010). The analysis of such inequalities can lead to insights into the forces causing them and hence point to the actions required

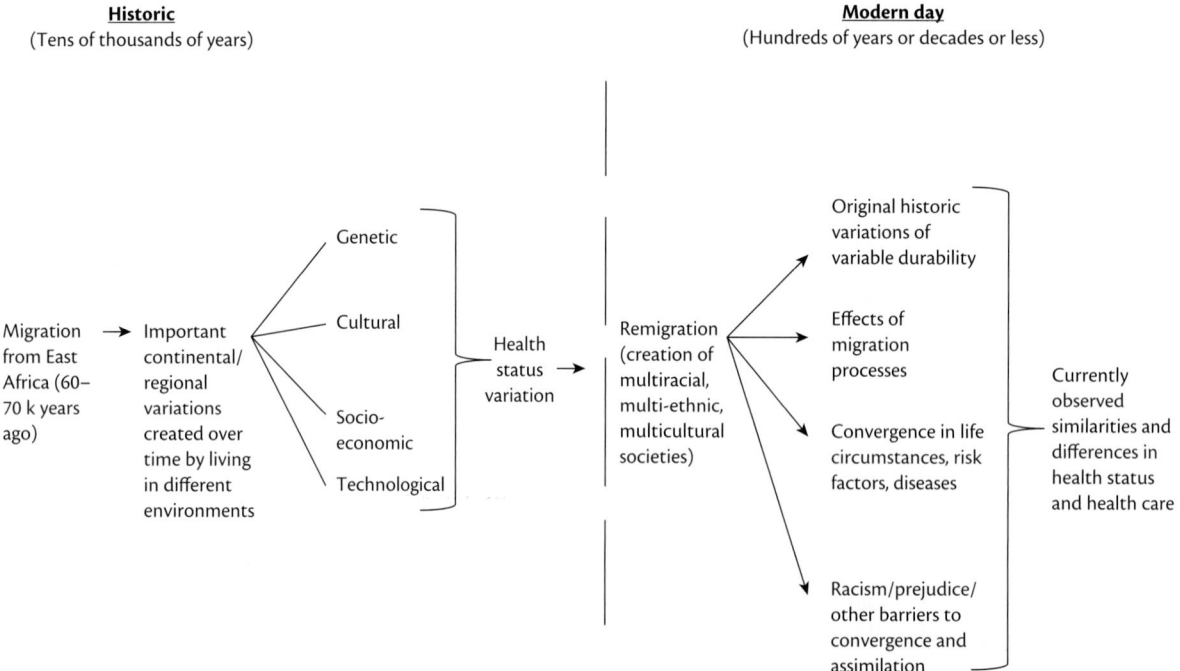

Fig. 10.5.1 Model linking evolutionary and current-day forces to produce variations in health status and healthcare by migration status, race, and ethnicity.
Reproduced from Raj. S Bhopal, *Ethnicity, Race, and Health in Multicultural Societies*, Second Edition, Figure 10.1, p. 339, Oxford University Press, Oxford, UK, Copyright © 2014 Raj. S Bhopal, by permission of Oxford University Press.

Table 10.5.2 Potential problems and benefits of ethnicity and race in health sciences

Issue	Potential problems	Potential benefits
Credibility	Gives backing to scientifically difficult concepts that have been abused previously	Utilizing concepts in health sciences will lead to their development and improvement and to health improvement
Division of society	Reducing social cohesion, by an emphasis on differences, and the creation of a sense of inferiority and superiority	Helping heal existing social divisions by acknowledging and working on differences, as well as demonstrating similarities
Racism	Provides information that can be abused by those who wish to demonstrate inferiority and superiority of particular groups	Information can combat past injustices, and guide future actions to prevent such racism
Ethnocentricity	Sets a standard usually based on the majority population that may be inappropriate for a particular ethnic group	By demonstrating that in some respects ethnic minority populations have better health, more challenging standards can be set for the population, including the majority, e.g. the standard is the population with the best health
Emphasis on problems	Stigmatizing and stereotyping minority populations by focusing on conditions where their health is worst	By showing that in some respects their health is better or no worse than the majority's research can counteract existing stigmas and stereotypes about minorities
Scientific advances	As in the past, science might be led into unsound inferences, and unethical practices	If the causal dividend of studying race and ethnicity can be realized, important advances in population health could be achieved
Development of health services	Either as a result of faulty information or interpretation, health services may veer away from true needs	With the appropriate data services might adapt to meet needs better
Individual clinical care	Clinicians might be misled by generalities, stereotypes, and misleading research and scholarship	Armed with an understanding of ethnicity and race clinical care might become more effective
Attitudes to immigration	Adverse data on health status or health case utilization may create/perpetuate negative attitudes to immigration	By showing immigrants' contributions to healthcare delivery or the health of the nation the benefits of immigration may be clearer

Reproduced from Raj. S Bhopal, *Ethnicity, Race, and Health in Multicultural Societies*, Second Edition, Table 1.5, p. 23, Oxford University Press, Oxford, UK, Copyright © 2014 Raj. S Bhopal, by permission of Oxford University Press.

to counter them. Such insights can stimulate research. While race and ethnicity are of value in clinical care, they can also lead to stereotyping, stigma, and racism. The potential value of ethnicity and race will be achieved only if understanding and application of these concepts is advanced. Some potential problems and benefits are in Table 10.5.2.

Applying the concepts of race and ethnicity: terminology and classifications to underpin data collection

Creating ethnic and racial labels, as in national censuses, is the first step to assessing a person's ethnicity, and the remaining steps depend upon the purposes of data collection. Whatever the purpose, understanding the terminology we are using, and its origins, is vital to collecting and interpreting the data. Concepts need to be simplified. In simplification, and especially in implementation, the original meaning and intent of the concepts may be unwittingly altered. To utilize the concepts of race and ethnicity as variables in population health we create population classifications. This process is pragmatic and, in the absence of firm theoretical underpinnings, it is subjective, malleable, and designed to meet perceived needs in particular populations, places, and times. The process used to devise the ethnic group question in the UK census has been particularly clearly described and provides insights that

are relevant even now (Sillitoe 1978). The process will utilize only one or a few of the facets of complex concepts. Each population subgroup needs to have a label that is both meaningful and acceptable, both to those creating and using the classification and those who are so classified. Presently, most classifications are designed for self-report of race or ethnicity, whereas in the past usually race was assigned by an official, professional, or researcher.

The value of the classification achieved, as opposed to the alternatives, should be judged by whether it serves the stated purposes. In quantitative health sciences the purpose is to establish and explain differences in health status of populations, in public health it is to improve health through prevention and control of disease, and in clinical medicine it is to make diagnosis and treatment easier. Other purposes including maintaining segregation, as in apartheid, or to perpetuate racism, though repugnant in the modern world have been important and could return, but are not pertinent to contemporary public health.

Classifications vary across times and places, reflecting both the pragmatic nature of the process of their creation and the varying purposes for which they were designed. Many complex classifications of race have been proposed. Only those relating to broad continental groupings continue to hold influence. The classification process is, inevitably, arbitrary, subjective, context specific, purpose driven, and imprecise. The process is atheoretical in that there is no coherent, valid genetic or social theory that underpins classifications. The prime value of such classifications is in social, rather than biological, contexts and in service applications. Nonetheless, such classifications allow analysis of differences and similarities that have importance in population sciences (US Department of Health and Human Services 1985; Davey Smith et al. 2000; Bhopal 2007; WHO 2010).

As societies are becoming more racially and ethnically diverse, such classifications, despite their limitations, are in increasing use. At any one place and time, though numerous classifications are possible, one tends to dominate, with minor variants. Usually, this is the classification used in the census, or equivalent national or regional population registries in places where a census is not conducted (Sillitoe 1978; US Office of Management and Budget 1997; Bhopal 2007; Stronks et al. 2009).

The variable terminology supporting both concepts and classifications is problematic for international collaborative work. These challenges of classification, terminology, and agreement on concepts are similar to those for other complex variables such as social class and educational status—race and ethnicity are not uniquely problematic. Despite their difficulties, most classifications do work in the sense that they add to our capacity for analysis of similarities and differences in the health of populations and to take actions to improve health (WHO 2010).

Challenges of collecting and interpreting data using the concepts of ethnicity and race

The ethical justification for collecting data by race, ethnicity, and health is health improvement either directly through more informed evidence-based law, policy, or practice, or through better understanding of disease causation achieved through research. People setting up health databases and research studies need to make choices on which aspects of migration status (so often a proxy for ethnicity), race, and ethnicity are to be captured and on the method of data collection. The interpretation and utilization of the data are dependent on these choices.

Collecting data by migration status, race, or ethnicity is difficult, and requires agreement on concepts and terminology, excellent information systems, excellent communications, and understanding between data providers and data holders. There are three main approaches to assigning ethnicity and race: self-assessment, assessment by another on the basis of relevant data, and assessment by another on the basis of observation (see Box 10.5.1). The

Box 10.5.1 Main methods of assigning migration status, race, and ethnicity

Skin colour/physical feature
Country of birth of self or parents/grandparents
Name analysis
Family origin, and ancestry or pedigree analysis
Self-assessed ethnic or racial group
Self-reported migration status details—length of residence, country of birth or origin, whether asylum seeker, refugee, or undocumented

Adapted with permission from Raj. S Bhopal, *Ethnicity, Race, and Health in Multicultural Societies*, Second Edition, Table 3.3, p. 76, Oxford University Press, Oxford, UK, Copyright © 2014 Raj. S Bhopal, by permission of Oxford University Press.

last is not recommended. Major sources of data important to public health, which often do not have complete or valid information on race or ethnicity, include censuses, population registers, death and birth certificates, healthcare records, and disease registries. Data linkage holds great promise as a means of enriching such data sets, including the addition of race and ethnicity codes where they are absent (Johnman et al. 2012).

Data systems for monitoring the health and healthcare of multiethnic, multiracial populations need to be designed to record, retrieve, and analyse data on relevant variables including racial and/or ethnic group, language preference, religion, and dietary needs. The documentation for such systems should include information on the concepts underlying such variables and methods whereby the variables were collected, to allow proper interpretation by data users. The users need to interpret the data and come to valid explanations for differences and similarities, or at least valid questions that guide interpretation. A conceptual framework for interpretation of differences includes: data and system error; random error; bias in data collection; and differences in socioeconomic, lifestyle, and other cultural and genetic factors. Misinterpretation, particularly reaching unsubstantiated conclusions that differences arise from genetic factors, needs to be avoided. Definitive explanations for population subgroup differences are unlikely to be achieved, but the findings will raise questions that focus attention on priorities.

Societal responses to variations in health status by migrant status, race, and ethnicity

Generally, socially diverse societies are conscious that the health status and healthcare needs of their populations vary by migrant status, or racial or ethnic group. Once noted, such variations are not easily ignored. The responses range from merely studying the differences, blaming the minority population for their health problems and even excluding them from services, setting up special initiatives, adapting services to meet needs, and creating a general policy of equality and equity of service to meet need (Johnson 1984). The response depends on the social context and political and public views on migrants, race and ethnicity as illustrated here for the United Kingdom, United States, Australia, South Africa, the Netherlands, and Hungary.

In the United Kingdom, the health focus has been on immigrants and their descendants utilizing, primarily, the concept of ethnicity. Each group of immigrants, whether Irish, Jewish, or Indian, has been associated, rightly or wrongly, with raising the risk to the wider society of infectious diseases and environmental hazards and that kind of perception is harmful to the group. Since the 1970s there has been an appreciation of the potential value of studying variations in disease patterns, which has increased attention on ethnic minority groups. This has been followed by a policy response, backed by strong legislation, to tackle health problems seen in excess in minority groups (Johnson 1984). The 1990s and early twenty-first century have seen the rise of a social justice agenda accompanied by powerful antidiscriminatory legislation to promote equality in Britain's multiethnic society. For legal purposes, race in its broadest sense (including ethnicity, religion, migration status etc.) has been firmly embedded within the wider equality agenda, being one of nine legally protected characteristics in the Equality Act 2010.

Race and ethnicity classifications in the United States have been designed to help redress historical discrimination (US Office of Management and Budget 1997), and this goal remains a top political priority. In the United States attention in the field has focused on African (black) and Native American origin populations and more recently on Hispanic populations. The concept of race still dominates. Until the latter half of the twentieth century the response to racial inequality and racial discrimination was generally unsupportive or openly discriminatory. Following the civil rights movement and the Civil Rights Act 1964 the aim of narrowing the gap between the health of African Americans and white Americans has come to the fore, especially since a landmark report in 1985 (US Department of Health and Human Services 1985). This objective has not been achieved and, despite much policy analysis and interventions, inequalities have been difficult to eliminate, though this remains the goal (Sloan et al. 2010). More recently, attention has turned to a wider range of minority populations.

Australia is a country of immigrants but, surprisingly, immigrant health, ethnicity and race have not loomed large in the health response. Rather, the focus has been on the indigenous populations, especially the Aborigines (Hill et al. 2007). The late twentieth century saw an awakening to the appalling health and health services they have and a resolve to improve matters. Efforts to date have paid little dividend in terms of narrowing inequality. However, the rising population size of Aborigines following a near catastrophic decline in the nineteenth century signals improvement, that is, that death rates are reducing, which is true in absolute terms though not relative to the whole population, and are lower than birth rates. This challenge has implications for the worldwide indigenous populations (see Chapter 10.6).

South Africa under apartheid (1948–1994) exemplified the damaging effects of promoting separate development for different racial groups, the results being excellent health, well-being and service for the country's white population compared to the other groups, especially the black African majority. Vigorous efforts are being made to redress these injustices in post-apartheid South Africa but there is ambivalence about the continued value of using race and ethnicity in this context. As in the United States, however, it is problematic to resolve problems caused by racism, without using the concept to tackle the resulting problems, although the whole area is embroiled in controversy (Ellison and de Wet 1997).

The Netherlands became one of the world's most diverse multiethnic societies in the late twentieth century. It institutionalized the use of country of birth as the primary, proxy measure of ethnicity (Stronks et al. 2009). Its policy response has been unstable in the light of political change. The current attitude is that while special efforts may be required for the foreign-born, rapid integration and assimilation should occur such that the descendants of migrants ought to require no special services. Research in the Netherlands is advanced, including the development of major cohort studies (Dekker et al. 2011).

Hungary is a country that has had a tumultuous history, and is currently transforming itself into a modern European state. One of its great challenges is to translate the ideal of equality— enshrined in its constitution and laws—in relation to its sizeable Roma (Gypsy) population (Ministry of Foreign Affairs Budapest 2004). This ethnic minority group, though nomadic by tradition, has been settled in Hungary for centuries, some people tracing their roots in and around Hungary back to the fourteenth or fifteenth century. The Roma population is, comparative to the population as a whole, very poor, with low levels of education and employment, and a multiplicity of health challenges, including a life expectancy 10 years lower than non-Roma. The vision in Hungary is a grand one and the result is of the greatest significance for Europe as a multi-ethnic continent.

The variety of responses in these countries is striking. Nonetheless, some pattern is discernible: first comes an awareness of health problems and especially of a risk of infectious disease harming society as a whole; second comes the formal study of health status and healthcare by migrant status, ethnic or racial group; third there is articulation of policy and plans sometimes backed by legislation; fourth we see a move from policies of exclusion of minorities to the promotion of the welfare of minorities; fifth there are specific actions to redress inequities; and, finally, there is an attempt to adapt general services to meet needs. The scale of the public health challenge is great and none of the six countries considered here has yet achieved the goal of substantially and sustainably narrowing health inequalities or achieving equity of service.

Spurred by rising global and national movements for universal human rights in the late twentieth century, and a realization that immigration is vital to their economic and demographic health, many countries are changing their stance, with equity of health status and healthcare being a central focus (WHO 2010).

Data on race and ethnic group have both harmed and benefited minority populations, and will continue to do so, yet without the data the need for services cannot be established. Data need to be collected within international ethical and legal frameworks that safeguard the human rights of minority and majority populations alike (International Organization for Migration (IOM) 2009). The goals of equality and equity, and monitoring of progress towards the goals, cannot be achieved without data on migration status, race, or ethnicity, as recognized by the WHO in 1983 (Colledge et al. 1983) and re-emphasized in the WHO's and IOM's global consultation (WHO 2010).

Assessing health and healthcare needs of racial and ethnic minorities using quantitative and qualitative data

A health needs assessment is an overview of quantitative and qualitative data on a population or subgroup of the population (see Chapter 11.1). Its purpose is to help improve population health and healthcare. Health needs assessment in racial and ethnic minority groups is sometimes problematic for lack of comparable and high-quality data, particularly at local and international levels, and at the level of subgroup detail required (Rafnsson and Bhopal 2009). At the local level it is often limited to qualitative studies or consultations. For national studies data from administrative databases utilizing broad racial or ethnic categories or proxies such as country of birth may need to be used (Stronks et al. 2009). The limitations of such data need to be understood to reduce the risk of making poor decisions.

Needs assessment for minority populations starts by examining the health status, disease patterns, and healthcare utilization within each group. This is the absolute risk approach (Bhopal 2007, 2008).

The findings are then compared with other minority and majority groups. In most instances the standard comparison is with the white (European origin) population as a whole, even although this may contain within it subgroups that may be as disadvantaged as the non-white groups under study. This is done either for ease, habit, ethnocentrism, limited availability of data, the policy and political leverage of the approach, or statistical power (Bhopal 2007). An alternative approach, but rarely used, is to set the comparison against the group with the most desirable level of the health indicator under study. These comparative approaches comprise the relative risk approach (Bhopal 2008). Qualitative data enrich and help validate the quantitative analysis by giving needs assessors access to opinions, perceptions, beliefs, attitudes, self-reported behaviour, and case histories (Bandesha and Litva 2005; Bhopal 2007).

Health needs assessments (Gill et al. 2007) have shown that commonly held views on the needs of minorities are often erroneous, for example, levels of immunization are sometimes high not low (Baker et al. 2011), life expectancy may be greater than in the population as a whole, and health education materials may bear little relation to disease patterns and so on (Bhopal 1988). Some generalizations hold: health needs vary substantially by group; minority groups are better off in health status and even healthcare in some respects and worse off in others; service quality, including for preventive health issues and face-to-face communications, is usually worse for minority groups; and needs as articulated by minority groups in consultations and qualitative research mostly focus on communication, information, religious requirements, dietary preferences, and informed consent (Gill et al. 2007). Since health needs assessment is an intensive and costly process, and not always achievable, some principles are important as follows (Bhopal 2007):

1. Avoid the piecemeal approach to tackling minority health needs whereby so-called race- or ethnic-specific topics are tackled one by one. A balanced overview is needed (Gill et al. 2007).

2. Base the needs assessment on ranks of causes using case numbers and disease rates (Table 10.5.3).

3. Refine understanding by looking at comparative indices, which will focus attention on inequalities and inequities (Table 10.5.3).

4. Interpret the quantitative data in the light of the qualitative findings.

5. Draw with care, and with due emphasis on social and economic deprivation as explanatory factors, causal hypotheses based on differences.

6. Beware that inferences of biological differences between groups may be particularly prone to error and misinterpretation, and may harm the standing of minority groups.

7. Make a judgement, preferably in consultation with minority populations concerned, on how the data can be best used to improve the health and healthcare of the population, majority and minority groups alike.

8. Minority ethnic groups must not be excluded from, or inhibited from, using major public health and healthcare initiatives, even if segregated or special services are set up. There is an important but unanswered question of whether people who do not belong to particular ethnic groups can be excluded from special services set up for a particular group. I believe this could be indefensible in law and on ethical grounds, especially if a person from another ethnic group could demonstrate an equal need for such services.

9. The needs of minority groups should be met simultaneously with the rest of the population, not deferred until some later date to be handled as a separate matter.

10. All public health policies and plans should make explicit how the needs of minority groups are to be met.

Inequalities, inequities, and disparities in health and healthcare by race and ethnicity

Health status, disease occurrence, and mortality patterns in populations are sculpted by factors such as wealth, environmental quality, diet, behaviour, and genetic inheritance (Box 10.5.2) (Nazroo 1998; Davey Smith et al. 2000; Krieger 2002). Most of these factors are directly or indirectly related to ethnicity and/or race, therefore, it is unsurprising that there are stark health inequalities by race and ethnicity. The questions of interest are why they occur and what needs to be done to narrow them. Specific health inequalities are likely to have their own causes. For example, ethnic inequalities in risk of skin cancers such as melanoma are likely to have a biological basis relating to skin pigmentation, while inequalities in stroke need to take account of many factors, including healthcare, cultural, economic, and biological matters over the life course.

The concept of inequity, as opposed to inequality, is central to policy and strategy. Inequity implies an inequality that is unfair or unjust (disparity is the equivalent word in the US context), for example, those arising from inadequate access to knowledge or services, and these form a primary target for action, particularly if effective interventions are available. Other inequalities, for example, the differences in the rate of skin cancer, are not unjust. They pose, nonetheless, a major challenge to understanding and a focus for both science and services.

Inequalities are demonstrable using virtually all classifications of migration status (see Chapter 10.9), race, and ethnicity, and are usually sharpened by taking account of population heterogeneity and examining men and women separately. The differences between such groups are often large, particularly for specific conditions, for example, diabetes, stroke, and bowel cancer, and less so for general measures of health, for example, life expectancy. Even where such inequalities have been carefully studied and actions to reverse them are proposed, mostly they have not

Table 10.5.3 The standard table for assessment of the pattern of disease, particularly for needs assessment purposes

Disease or condition	Number of cases	Rate	Rank position on number of cases or rate	SMR/relative risk	Rank on SMR

been greatly narrowed and sometimes they have widened. Ethnic group inequalities could help set new more demanding targets, for example, in many countries in Europe, North America, and Australia the target for coronary heart disease mortality could be set as the low rate in the Chinese population (Nijjar et al. 2010), and that for bowel cancer as the South Asian population's low rate (Bhopal et al. 2012). One of the dilemmas is the choice of which of the many inequalities to tackle, and this requires principles.

Principles for setting priorities for the health and healthcare of racial and ethnic minority populations

Priority setting is a process for making rational choices from multiple alternatives (see Chapter 3.5). The public health sciences, particularly epidemiology, can underpin priority setting, which follows from the process of health needs assessment. Quantitative and qualitative data on health status and service utilization are often available (though they may be crude). In contrast, relevant information on cost and effectiveness of interventions is rarely available, posing a formidable challenge (Bhopal 2007).

Priority setting benefits from principles, for example, that the priorities are those actions that maximally benefit the health of a population or subpopulation. Another principle is that because similarities between human populations tend to outweigh differences, the priorities of general society are of great importance to racial and ethnic minority groups. These general priorities, however, are necessary but not sufficient. They need adjustment on the

basis of health needs assessment. For long-settled communities, and minorities born or raised in the country, the adjustments may be modest or even minor. For others, such as those who do not speak the local language, or those suffering racial discrimination, the adjustments needed may be substantial. Reductions of inequalities and inequities (disparities), however, can only be achieved if health improvement occurs fastest in the most disadvantaged population—and getting the priorities wrong can widen inequalities (Bhopal 2007).

All healthcare and public health policies and plans should make explicit what the priorities are, whether they are different for different groups, and how the needs of minority groups are to be met. Evaluation of services and audit of quality of care providing evidence that the quality of care for minority populations is not equitable is particularly effective in bringing about change, as it goes against international and national policies and laws promoting equality.

Policy and strategy to improve health and healthcare for racial and ethnic minority groups

Health services for minority groups are usually set within the policies and strategies for the population as a whole, in practice the majority (or most powerful) population. Ideally, policies for the whole population would address the needs of minority groups in an integrated way. This concept is known as mainstreaming (Bhopal 2007). In practice this may not happen for reasons including absence of understanding or agreement that this is important, the complexity of the issues raised and lack of expertise, time, and publication space within policy and strategy documents. Mostly, minority populations are expected to adapt themselves to benefit from the available services. Professionals delivering the service tend to make some adjustments on an ad hoc basis. Increasingly, we see two further policy responses—setting up specialist services for minority groups but within the main service, and the development of strategies to help re-shape existing services to meet needs. The complete separation of services for minorities is currently not in favour. Here, I consider briefly the policy response in the United Kingdom and the United States.

The UK policy response until about 1990 was intermittent and fragmented, with a mixture of stand-alone projects and modifications to mainline services. Progress has been made on key requirements such as interpretation services and dietary needs in hospital (Gill et al. 2007). The Race Relations Amendment Act 2000 building on the 1976 Act, coupled with explicit or implicit policies from the government health departments, drove more widespread changes based on a positive duty to promote racial equality (The Home Office 2001). These national initiatives affect everyone and are being translated, often with great difficulty, into local action plans and ultimately service changes. The work on race and ethnicity was incorporated within the wider equality agenda in the Equality Act 2010.

The United States has had a long-standing programme for affirmative action based on human rights principles that aims to redress historical wrongs (US Department of Health and Human Services 1985). Its racial and ethnic classification is explicitly designed to help achieve this goal (US Office of Management and

Budget 1997). The pluralistic nature of the healthcare system of the United States, based on private healthcare principles, makes a cohesive strategy impossible to enact nationally but huge progress is being made, with global leadership, especially in research (National Institutes of Health and US Department of Health and Human Services 2012).

While many policies, strategies, and action projects exist, health services internationally have struggled with the challenge of equitable healthcare in multicultural societies. These struggles are especially seen in relation to undocumented migrants (see Chapter 10.9), indigenous populations (see Chapter 10.6), and long-established but still culturally and socially distinct populations such as Roma. Current opinion favours mainstreaming with adaptation of general existing services, and incorporation of minorities' needs into the design of new services. These ideals are constrained by lack of funds, expertise, data, and the ongoing political controversies around immigration, asylum, race equality, and human rights. While policy, strategy, and action is highly dependent on local context, some of the principles, experience, and lessons are transferable internationally.

To date the challenges have been tackled mostly at the level of structure and process—what systems might work and what should we do? Equity in service delivery is increasingly the central focus, with outcomes in terms of healthcare delivery and its quality as the benchmark. The achievement of outcomes measured in terms of health status is seldom the centrepiece of discussion, although the United States has recently moved to this (Warnecke et al. 2008). This is currently too great a challenge for most countries, not least because the causes of health status differences are often not clear. Even conceptually, it is difficult to set a benchmark. What would be the goal? Racial and ethnic inequalities and inequities in health and healthcare are far more complex than socioeconomic inequalities, not least because socioeconomic factors are part of them. Racial and ethnic inequalities are very hard to predict and vary by cause of ill health and by risk factor and are rapidly changing. The importance of the wider determinants of health such as wealth, housing, employment, and education for minority groups is, however, clear. Policies and strategies to achieve better health for minorities are strengthened and sustained by their incorporation within a broader agenda for social justice and civil rights, and within wider policies to reduce inequalities.

Race equality impact assessment methods are being developed. These are being applied to a wide range of policies, for example, transport, health and safety, and employment practices. In this way there is an interconnection, and synergy, across the different sectors of social life. Effective responses are constrained by lack of funds, expertise, data (particularly on what works and why), and the ongoing political controversies (usually negative in tone) around immigration, asylum, race equality, and human rights. Policies are most powerful and effective when they are supported by a coherent legal and ethical framework. The framework, of necessity, reflects the values of the society and particularly those of politicians.

Research on and with racial and ethnic minority groups

Research utilizing race and ethnicity influences society and will be interpreted to meet social goals. Just as modern-day work is mostly used to further current goals of social equality and justice, so it was that much research in the past was used to further previous social and political goals such as the continuation of slavery, the justification of Empire, the maintenance of social and material inequality (including apartheid), anti-immigration policies focused on those who were not Northern Europeans, eugenics, and the Nazi genocides (Bhopal 2007). The most important lesson from this history is that this research on racial and ethnic minorities needs to be done within an ethical framework emphasizing benefit to the population studied primarily, and to wider society secondarily. Researchers are developing consensus statements on how to achieve this (Mir et al. 2013).

The full range of health sciences and their methodological approaches—literature review, qualitative studies, case-histories, case series, laboratory research, analysis of routine statistics, case–control studies, cohort studies, trials—are potentially applicable to race, ethnicity, and health research. An explosion of research on the genetic and environmental basis of ethnic/racial variations is underway as virtually all societies become multi-ethnic ones through migration (Afshari and Bhopal 2010).

Researchers need to make explicit how they are using ethnicity and race for, and adapting their classifications and methods to, the research questions under study. Researchers should not always be constrained by available classifications designed for administrative purposes though veering from them should be done thoughtfully. Researchers who are knowledgeable about the minority groups under study are more likely to be trusted and more likely to achieve the high response rates and informed consent that are essential, and also to interpret data with minimal error and bias. In writing up and publishing their work, researchers should minimize the danger of harm to the groups studied, particularly, the stigma which can ensue from associating them with problems for healthcare systems. Overemphasis of health problems, especially when imbalanced, can lead to stereotyping and fuel racism.

The ideal population research study would be inclusive of all minority groups, have uniformly high response rates, provide data that are comparable across all groups, collect information on all relevant facets of race and ethnicity, include data on all potential confounding variables, and be analysed and interpreted in a way that advances science, improves health status, and develops better healthcare. In practice, many ideals are sacrificed to make studies feasible. In making pragmatic choices, researchers should make themselves and others aware of the limitations of the work.

The challenge of race, ethnicity, and health research includes demonstrating tangible health benefits in addition to satisfying curiosity and extending the boundaries of knowledge. Minority health is a beguiling research theme for it often focuses on underprivileged groups; it is interesting and often unearths unusual results; differences between groups can be demonstrated with ease; and even small studies can yield robust, significant and relevant results.

There are numerous challenges in epidemiology of race and ethnicity—see Box 10.5.3. There are others relating to other social, population, and medical sciences. One of the greatest overall challenges is doing good work in the light of inherent complexity and amidst criticism. Researchers are left with the decision to either avoid the controversy and difficulty associated with race and ethnicity variables (an action which may be socially, politically,

Box 10.5.3 Some challenges for epidemiological research on ethnicity, race, and health

- Inclusion of minorities in research and analysis of data by migrant status, race, or ethnicity.
- Clarification of the purpose of the research.
- Definitions of concepts relating to migration status, ethnicity, and race that are internationally agreed.
- Definition and precision of terms, and migrant group/ethnic/racial classifications and clarification on how they have been used.
- Recognition of heterogeneity within minority and majority groups alike.
- Identification of representative populations.
- Ensuring comparability of populations that are to be compared, requiring especially socioeconomic data over the life course to show this.
- Avoiding misinterpretation of differences that are due to confounding variables.
- Accurate measurement of the denominators and numerators in calculating rates.
- Ensuring the quality of data, particularly in cross-cultural comparability.
- Maximizing completeness of data collection.
- Pinpointing specific genetic basis of genetic hypotheses.
- Properly argued interpretation of associations as causal or non-causal.
- Maximizing validity and generalizability of the research.
- Presentation of research to achieve benefits for the population studied, and avoid stigmatization and racism.
- Appropriate action to follow the research that, ideally, benefits the entire population.

Reproduced from Raj S. Bhopal, Glossary of terms relating to ethnicity and race for reflection and debate, *Journal of Epidemiological Community Health*, Volume 58, Issue 6, pp. 441–45, Copyright © 2004, with permission from the BMJ Publishing Group Ltd.

legally, and scientifically unacceptable) or to do their best, with the express intention of continually improving their work.

There is still massive potential for causal understanding through the in-depth investigation and explanation of racial and ethnic variations—see Table 10.5.4 for an example of the approach needed. The huge potential of research on racial and ethnic minorities for service planning and delivery also needs good design and a clear focus, better data, and experience of putting research to use. Improvements will come from conceptual openness, explicit and defined terminology, and imaginative solutions

Table 10.5.4 Categorizing and analysing the factors which may underlie an epidemiological variable: the example of stroke

Category of potential explanatory underlying difference	Example of possible specific differences by migrant status, race or ethnic group	Implications for data collection
Biological	Unique variants of human genes, or varying frequencies of such variants (polymorphisms) lead to different biochemistry or physiology	Collect biological data including DNA, blood, and other tissues
Co-existing diseases	One group may have more or less of another disease which raises or reduces the risk of stroke disease, e.g. diabetes	Collect clinical data, including appropriate diagnostic tests
Behavioural	One group may eat more fruits, vegetable, and salads than another, and perhaps smoke less	Collect data on behaviours relating to health
Social	Members of a group may spend less time with friends and family, and other social networks, so increasing psychosocial strain	Collect psychosocial data as potential explanations
Occupational	The pattern of working, including likelihood of employment, the hours worked, and the type of occupations is substantially different	Collect data on employment histories
Economic	Members of a group may earn less than the average or have varying amounts of accumulated family wealth	Collect data on differences in income and wealth and their effect on lifestyles and stress
Healthcare	Members of a group may be treated differently from the expected standard by healthcare professionals	Collect data on quality, quantity and timing of healthcare interventions

Reproduced from Raj. S Bhopal, *Ethnicity, Race, and Health in Multicultural Societies*, Second Edition, Table 9.2, p. 288, Oxford University Press, Oxford, UK, Copyright © 2014 Raj. S Bhopal, by permission of Oxford University Press.

to the fundamental issues such as matching denominators and numerators, representativeness of the population, comparability of subgroups, and validity of the measurement tools.

For many causes, morbidity and mortality rates are lower in minorities but these gain little attention. The perception that the health of minority groups is poor can augment the belief that immigrants and racial or ethnic minorities are a burden. The perception of poorer health arises from a focus on those differences where the excess of disease is in the minority population. It is naïve to believe that the mere demonstration of inequalities by migration status, race, or ethnicity will narrow them and it is plausible that such studies can perpetuate and even augment inequalities. The study of racism is important but relatively neglected (Afshari and Bhopal 2010). Racism, undoubtedly, is a difficult subject to study in the health arena, but there is also a reluctance to take it on, though less so in the United States than in other places including Europe (Parker 1997; Krieger et al. 2010).

The promise of causal understanding has meant a focus on variation in diseases, as opposed to the quality of services. So there is a gap in the research record on the quality of care received by minority groups, to the detriment of the services and populations served. Minority populations are seriously under-represented in major studies, especially cohort studies (Ranganathan and Bhopal 2006) and trials (Geller et al. 2011).

Conclusions: theoretical, ethical, and future-orientated perspectives on health, race, and ethnicity

Used responsibly, race and ethnicity have the potential to improve public health, healthcare, clinical care, and medical science (Gill et al. 2007; Tobias et al. 2009) but used unwisely they can do immense damage (Kohn 1995). Stringent attention to underlying theory and the principles of ethics and justice is essential as the primary safeguard against harm. There is no single theory (or group of theories) on race and ethnicity and health that is widely accepted or applied. Biological theories based on species and sub-species have not withstood testing and social theories have not yet been articulated in a way that has made a major impact in medical sciences. Advances in the science of genetics are reopening old debates on the biological underpinnings of racial and ethnic differences. Articulating coherent and useful theories on migration, race, and ethnicity in the health domain is a continuing challenge. Migration status, race, and ethnicity conform, and contribute, to the general epidemiological theories on the forces that shape population differences in health status and hence they are important in public health and healthcare.

A rational, analytic approach to the interpretation of data, set within broader epidemiological theories of health, is needed. Interventions utilizing race and ethnicity need to be carefully evaluated to judge the likely balance of benefits to costs. In a political environment where anti-immigration sentiment is high and encouraged, the use of race and ethnicity indicators may be counterproductive. There is an imperative to achieve benefits in terms of health improvement and to demonstrate this unequivocally.

Public health and medical care are humanitarian disciplines that are focused on the most needy (the at-risk or already sick) who are often also the most economically disadvantaged. The key

to doing good is a social and cultural milieu of equality/equity/non-discrimination. Given this, the thoughtful application of the approaches of the social and population health sciences to race and ethnicity should yield workable classifications and data that can be interpreted using epidemiological frameworks for analysis. The analysis arising can feed into needs assessment, priority setting, the inequalities debate, policy- and strategy-making, and scholarship and research. There is a virtuous cycle around data—the more it is used the more the enthusiasm for its collection and for improvement in data systems. Data also improves services both directly (through better decisions) and through the motivating effects of monitoring and evaluation in improving performance. Race and ethnicity are important concepts and variables in epidemiology and public health.

Acknowledgements

This chapter is a summary and synthesis of Raj S. Bhopal, *Migration, Ethnicity, Race, and Health in Multicultural Societies*, Second Edition, Oxford University Press, Oxford, UK, Copyright © 2014 Raj. S Bhopal, by permission of Oxford University Press. I am grateful to OUP and the editors of the *Oxford Textbook of Public Health* for agreement to do this. I thank Anne Houghton for secretarial support in the preparation of this chapter and Prof. Sean Valles for thoughtful feedback.

References

Afshari, R. and Bhopal, R.S. (2010). Ethnicity has overtaken race in medical science: MEDLINE-based comparison of trends in the USA and the rest of the world, 1965–2005. *International Journal of Epidemiology*, 39(6), 1682–3.

Anzures, G., Quinn, P.C., Pascalis, O., Slater, A.M., Tanaka, J.W., and Lee, K. (2013). Developmental origins of the other-race effect. *Current Directions in Psychological Science*, 22(3), 173–8.

Baker, D., Garrow, A., and Shiels, C. (2011). Inequalities in immunisation and breast feeding in an ethnically diverse urban area: cross-sectional study in Manchester, UK. *Journal of Epidemiology and Community Health*, 65(4), 346–52.

Bandesha, G. and Litva, A. (2005). Perceptions of community participation and health gain in a community project for the South Asian population: a qualitative study. *Journal of Public Health*, 27(3), 241–5.

Bhopal, R. (2008). *Concepts of Epidemiology: Integrating the Ideas, Theories, Principles and Methods of Epidemiology* (2nd ed.). Oxford: Oxford University Press.

Bhopal, R., Bansal, N., Steiner, M., Brewster, D.H., and on behalf of the Scottish Health and Ethnicity Linkage Study (2012). Does the 'Scottish effect' apply to all ethnic groups? All cancer, lung, colorectal, breast and prostate cancer in the Scottish Health and Ethnicity Linkage Cohort Study. *BMJ Open*, 2, e001957.

Bhopal, R.S. (1988). Health education for ethnic minorities—current provision and future directions. *Health Education Journal*, 47(4), 137–40.

Bhopal, R.S. (2014). *Migration, Ethnicity, Race, and Health in Multicultural Societies* (2nd ed.). Oxford: Oxford University Press.

Colledge, M., Van Geuns, H.A., and Svensson, P.G. (1983). *Migration and Health: Towards an Understanding of the Health Care Needs of Ethnic Minorities*. Copenhagen: WHO.

Davey Smith, G., Chaturvedi, N., Harding, S., Nazroo, J., and Williams, R. (2000). Ethnic inequalities in health: a review of UK epidemiological evidence. *Critical Public Health*, 10(4), 377–408.

Dekker, L.H., Snijder, M.B., Beukers, M.H., et al. (2011). A prospective cohort study of dietary patterns of non-western migrants in the Netherlands in relation to risk factors for cardiovascular diseases: HELIUS-Dietary Patterns. *BMC Public Health*, 11, 441.

Ellison, G. and de Wet, T. (1997). *Towards Rational Debate of 'Race', 'Population Group', Ethnicity and Culture in South African Health Research*. Cape Town: IDASA and International Sociological Association's Research Group on Ethnic, Race and Minority Relations.

Fujimura, J.H. and Rajagopalan, R. (2011). Different differences: the use of 'genetic ancestry' versus race in biomedical human genetic research. *Social Studies of Science*, 41(1), 5–30.

Geller, S.E., Koch, A., Pellettieri, B., and Carnes, M. (2011). Inclusion, analysis, and reporting of sex and race/ethnicity in clinical trials: have we made progress? *Journal of Women's Health*, 20(3), 315–20.

Gill, P.S., Kai, J., Bhopal, R.S., and Wild, S. (2007). Health care needs assessment: black and minority ethnic groups. In R.J. Abingdon (ed.) *Health Care Needs Assessment. The Epidemiologically Based Needs Assessment Reviews*, pp. 227–389. Abingdon: Radcliffe Medical Press Ltd.

Hill, K., Barker, B., and Vos, T. (2007). Excess indigenous mortality: are indigenous Australians more severely disadvantaged than other indigenous populations? *International Journal of Epidemiology*, 36(3), 580–9.

International Organization for Migration (2009). *International Migration Law N°19—Migration and the Right to Health: A Review of International Law*. Geneva: IOM.

Johnman, C., Blakely, T., Bansal, N., Agyemang, C., and Ward, H. (2012). Linkage of data in the study of ethnic inequalities and inequities in health outcomes in Scotland, New Zealand and the Netherlands: insights for global study of ethnicity and health. *Public Health*, 126(3), 245–7.

Johnson, M.R. (1984). Ethnic minorities and health. *Journal of the Royal College of Physicians of London*, 18, 228–30.

Kohn, M. (1995). *The Race Gallery: The Return of Racial Science*. London: Jonathan Cape.

Krieger, N. (2002). Shades of difference theoretical underpinnings of the medical controversy on black–white differences in the United States, 1830–1870. In T.A. La Veist (ed.) *Race, Ethnicity and Health*, pp. 11–33. San Francisco, CA: Jossey-Bass.

Krieger, N. (2003). Does racism harm health? Did child abuse exist before 1962? On explicit questions, critical science, and current controversies: an ecosocial perspective. *American Journal of Public Health*, 93(2), 194–9.

Krieger, N., Carney, D., Lancaster, K., Waterman, P.D., Kosheleva, A., and Banaji, M. (2010). Combining explicit and implicit measures of racial discrimination in health research. *American Journal of Public Health*, 100(8), 1485–92.

Ministry of Foreign Affairs Budapest (2004). *Fact Sheets on Hungary: Gypsies/Roma in Hungary*. Budapest: Ministry of Foreign Affairs.

Mir, G., Salway, S., Kai, J., et al. (2013). Principles for research on ethnicity and health: the Leeds Consensus Statement. *European Journal of Public Health*, 23(3), 504–10.

National Institutes of Health and US Department of Health and Human Services (2012). *NIH Health Disparities Strategic Plan and Budget and Budget Fiscal Years 2009–2013*. Bethesda, MD: US Department of Health and Human Services.

Nazroo, J.Y. (1998). Genetic, cultural or socio-economic vulnerability? Explaining ethnic inequalities in health. *Sociology of Health & Illness*, 20, 710–30.

Nijjar, A.P., Wang, H., Quan, H., and Khan, N.A. (2010). Ethnic and sex differences in the incidence of hospitalized acute myocardial infarction: British Columbia, Canada 1995–2002. *BMC Cardiovascular Disorders*, 10, 38.

Parker, H. (1997). Beyond ethnic categories: why racism should be a variable in ethnicity and health research. *Journal of Health Service Research and Policy*, 2(4), 256–9.

Rafnsson, S.B. and Bhopal, R.S. (2009). Large-scale epidemiological data on cardiovascular diseases and diabetes in migrant and ethnic minority groups in Europe. *European Journal of Public Health*, 19(5), 484–91.

Ranganathan, M. and Bhopal, R. (2006). Exclusion and inclusion of non-white ethnic minority groups in 72 North American and European Cardiovascular Cohort Studies. *PLoS Medicine*, 3(3), e44.

Satcher, D. (2001). Our commitment to eliminate racial and ethnic health disparities. *Yale Journal of Health Policy, Law, and Ethics*, 1, 1–14.

Segal, U.A., Elliott, D., and Mayadas, N.S. (2010). *Immigration Worldwide Policies, Practices, and Trends*. Oxford: Oxford University Press.

Sillitoe, K. (1978). Ethnic origin: the search for a question. *Population Trends*, 13, 25–30.

Sloan, F.A., Ayyagari, P., Salm, M., and Grossman, D. (2010). The longevity gap between black and white men in the United States at the beginning and end of the 20th century. *American Journal of Public Health*, 100(2), 357–63.

Stronks, K., Kulu-Glasgow, I., and Agyemang, C. (2009). The utility of 'country of birth' for the classification of ethnic groups in health research: the Dutch experience. *Ethnicity & Health*, 14(3), 1–14.

The Home Office (2001). *Race Relations (Amendment) Act 2000: New Laws for a Successful Multi-Racial Britain* London: Home Office Communication Directorate.

Tobias, M., Blakely, T., Matheson, D., Rasanathan, K., and Atkinson, J. (2009). Changing trends in indigenous inequalities in mortality: lessons from New Zealand. *International Journal of Epidemiology*, 38(6), 1711–22.

US Department of Health and Human Services (1985). *Report of the Secretary's Task Force on Black and Minority Health*. Washington, DC: US Government Printing Office.

US Office of Management and Budget (1997). Standards for maintaining, collecting, and presenting federal data on race and ethnicity. *Federal Register*, 62, 58788–90.

Warnecke, R.B., Oh, A., Breen, N., et al. (2008). Approaching health disparities from a population perspective: the National Institutes of Health Centers for Population Health and Health Disparities. *American Journal of Public Health*, 98(9), 1608–15.

WHO Regional Office for Europe (2010). *How Health Systems can Address Health Inequities Linked to Migration and Ethnicity*. Copenhagen: WHO.

World Health Organization (2010). Health of Migrants—The Way Forward: Report of a Global Consultation. Geneva: WHO.

Xiao, W.S., Xiao, N., Quinn, P., Anzures, G., and Lee, K. (2013). Development of face scanning for own- and other-race faces in infancy. *International Journal of Behavioral Development*, 37(2), 100–5.

The health of indigenous peoples

Ian Anderson and Sue Crengle

Indigenous peoples: a contested concept

People who are described as indigenous, or who describe themselves as such, are found in nearly all regions of the world. They include San and Pygmy peoples in Africa; Australian Aboriginal, Māori, and other Polynesian peoples of the Pacific; and distinct peoples across Asia and the Indian subcontinent, circumpolar regions, and the Americas. They have a range of social, cultural, and political characteristics, and nearly all contemporary commentators note the difficulty in developing a definition of 'indigenous' that satisfactorily embraces the full range of these contexts (Stamatopoulou 1994; Kingsbury 1998; Niezen 2003; Coates 2004; Stephens et al. 2005). This debate is not just academic. The contested nature of indigenous identities has significance within and between indigenous communities—where it is often a marker of insider and outsider status (Weaver 2001). Further, legal and political ramifications of these definitions impact on access to resources, land title, and recognition of rights.

Who decides these matters? There is tension between the rights of people to represent themselves (self-identification) and international bodies (which are entangled in these debates, have distinct interests, and may ascribe a social identity not acceptable to the peoples in question). However, debates that have occurred as nation states or international bodies have engaged with this problem demonstrate both the challenge of agreeing on a definition and the cultural, intercultural, political, geographic, and historical dimensions of this concept.

Arguably, the ambiguity is less where there has been a distinct population, such as the first-recorded human inhabitants of regions such as Australia, New Zealand, and the Americas, and a defined historical moment in which external powers colonized these regions, dispossessed peoples, developed legal original inhabitants, and maintain political and social distinction between native peoples and settlers (Stephens et al. 2006). In other contexts, such as Asia, Africa, and the Middle East, distinctions are less clear with multilayered histories of colonization between and within countries. In India, for example, social hierarchies created categories in which social position is established at birth with some groups designated as tribal or indigenous on a sociocultural basis (Stephens et al. 2006). In Africa the idea of indigenous is highly contested. Many would claim all Africans are indigenous in relation to European colonization. However, groups such as the San or Pygmy people claim indigenous status notwithstanding this colonial history, having a history of colonization by African peoples prior to Europeans (Stephens et al. 2006).

These definitional debates echo through public health. *The Lancet* published a series of papers in 2006 on indigenous health across the globe. A year earlier, it published an introductory commentary to the series, which argued that, despite the aims of the United Nations International Decade of the World's Indigenous Peoples, 'little had been achieved [in] strengthening international cooperation for the solution of problems faced by indigenous people in such areas as human rights, the environment, development, education, and health' (Stephens et al. 2005). Anthropologist Adam Kuper wrote to the journal arguing that it should not proceed with the proposed series, as 'indigenous' is commonly used as a euphemism for 'primitive', and not only was the term difficult to define, it was also difficult to identify who is indigenous given the complex historical layers of migration, intermarriage, and linguistic and cultural change. These problems, Kuper argued, become even more 'acute and embarrassing, when it comes to determining who should be accepted as being a genuinely indigenous person' (Kuper 2005, p. 983). Following the publication of the series, he argued that it was dangerous to presume that health problems were inherent to peoples' indigenous status, nor were health inequalities limited to populations labelled as indigenous (Kuper 2007). Some papers in the series engaged with the definitional challenges (Kingsbury 1998; Niezen 2003; Stephens et al. 2005, 2006; Anderson et al. 2006; Montenegro and Stephens 2006; Ohenjo et al. 2006), but also documented patterns of poorer health and health inequalities compared to benchmark non-indigenous populations. The inference that health inequalities are inherent to indigenous status is arguably not the focus of public health thinking on indigenous health. The dominant paradigm today is much more closely aligned to public health models that have emerged out of thinking in relation to the social determinants of health, which have been used in the analysis of patterns of health inequality in other populations (Carson et al. 2007; Mowbray 2007).

Despite these debates, since the 1970s the concept of indigenous peoples has attained a significant status and has been 'a basis for group mobilization, international standard setting, transnational networks and programmatic activity of intergovernmental and nongovernmental organizations' (Kingsbury 1998, p. 414).

Cultural and political frameworks

There are two broad approaches to the academic construction of indigeneity: one is cultural, the other political (Coates 2004). The cultural framework emphasizes cultural characteristics of indigenous people and contrasts them with urban capitalist societies. The political model emphasizes political characteristics and political and social relationships with settler societies. Although this definitional debate presents a challenge, Niezen argues that 'a rigorous definition…would be premature and, ultimately, futile…there are multiple approaches to the term "indigenous" each with its own political origins and implications' (Niezen 2003, p. 19).

The classic cultural model of indigenous peoples is described as a small-scale society, who live by more traditional local modes of economic productions such as hunting and gathering, herding or non-intensive forms of subsistence agriculture. In the culture of these societies there is a strong emphasis on kinship relationship and local forms of political organization (O'Neil 2009). Perhaps some archetypal examples can easily be characterized as small scale—Aboriginal Australians and southern African San peoples—but this approach has inherent problems. Although it may be historically accurate to characterize social circumstances of some indigenous peoples as small scale, this is not so for peoples such as descendants of the Mayan and Incan civilizations in central and South America. It also fails to account for historical transformations of indigenous populations that are, no matter how remote, increasingly connected to global cultural and economic processes. Many indigenous populations are urbanized and integrated within capitalist economies—even though they may maintain traditional economic practices and occupy relatively marginal positions within the broader economy. For some, such as Australian Aboriginal people in remote central and northern regions, the transition has been from a subsistence economy to the welfare economy. In Guyana, indigenous peoples (Amerindians) constitute 9.2% of the population, are mainly outside the cash economy, and are disproportionately among the poorest people in the country, which ranked 104 of 177 countries in the Human Development Index (HDI) (Hartley 2008; Nogkynrih 2008).

San is a collective name for indigenous peoples of southern Africa with a connection to the region dating back 27,000 years. They lived a hunter-gather lifestyle until the late twentieth century, but most now live sedentary lifestyles. Although they maintain a social and cultural distinctiveness, their culture and economic mode of production has changed. Cultural change notwithstanding, indigenous peoples may respond to social trends and cultural change in a distinct way from the dominant society. This includes the adoption or transformation of cultural forms such as musical styles or particular responses to cash economies. Some cultural change may be resisted, but indigenous peoples may also readily engage with forms of development such as mining or farming. Many retain distinct identities and cultural practices in the face of dispossession and social marginalization, and a sense of connection to a pre-colonial past.

The political framework commonly emphasizes minority status. This is true for indigenous populations such as the Ainu of Japan and Canadian Aboriginal and Native America communities. Contemporary political circumstances of indigenous peoples are shaped by their dispossession from traditional lands and natural resources and incorporation within institutional and political structures of settler states. The management of indigenous peoples by settler states has often involved legal frameworks, policies, and administrative structures, and the rights of indigenous peoples and those of settler majorities are frequently differentiated. This pattern of political disempowerment is reflected in other forms of social and cultural marginalization.

The minority status of indigenous peoples figures prominently in how they are framed within some jurisdictions. In the Russian federation, for instance, people recognized officially as indigenous are the 'numerically small indigenous peoples of the North, Siberia and the Far-East' (Donato n.d.). There are 44 such groups with a total population of 250,000 people, and their cultural, territorial, and political rights are enshrined through the constitution and national legislation. But not all indigenous populations are demographic minorities. The indigenous people of Fiji have a dominant political status, and the indigenous population of Bolivia is also in the majority (Montenegro and Stephens 2006).

Debates about the cultural construction of indigeneity echo debates about ethnicity as a construct in health analysis. Ethnicity has, for example, been defined as 'voluntaristic self-identification with a group culture' (Bradby 2012, p. 955). In the North American literature—where racial categories are prominent in official discourse and frequently used in administrative data collections—the conceptual distinction between ethnicity and race is particularly germane. Although race is generally now recognized as socially constructed categories 'established hundreds of years ago to divide humans into five major subpopulations' (Ford and Harawa 2010, p. 252) (largely on the basis of differences in appearance), there is still a tendency to slip into the biological essentialism that locates the social characteristics of distinct populations. Perhaps the distinction to be made is that indigeneity implies a social stratification that has emerged historically in relation to colonial processes resulting in a differentiation of the civic status of indigenous peoples compared with settler populations. Ford and Harawa propose a definition of ethnicity that encompasses this formulation: ethnicity is a 'two-dimensional, context-specific, social construct with an attributional dimension that describes group characteristics…and a relationship dimension that indexes a group's location within a social hierarchy' (Ford and Harawa 2010, p. 251). This approach integrates cultural and political frameworks without falling into the pitfalls of a cultural essentialism that disallows either cultural diversity or change. However, it only works if colonialism—and responses to it—is conceptualized as a significant process in the production of social stratification.

Policy and law

Over the past few decades, debates on the rights of indigenous peoples have focused on recognition of indigenous peoples and the consequent rights that flow from this. This has been influenced by the broader human rights movement, as well as by indigenous-led political movements. Local political movements that resulted in indigenous land rights in nation states such as Australia, Canada, Norway, and Sweden have been in turn influenced by transnational politics.

These developments have had a long genesis. The International Labour Organization (ILO) started working on indigenous issues when it operated within the League of Nations prior to the Second World War. However, it was unable to draw attention to these issues until, under the League's successor, the United Nations, it developed a draft protocol, which later formed the basis of the 1957 ILO Convention 107, which offered directives to governments responsible for indigenous populations. Article 1, ILO Convention 169, ratified in 1989, defined indigenous peoples as:

(a) Tribal people in independent countries whose social, cultural and economic conditions distinguish them from other sections of the national community and whose status is regulated wholly or partially by their own customs or traditions or by special laws or regulations

(b) Peoples in independent countries who are regarded as indigenous on account of their descent from the populations which inhabited the country, or a geographical region to which the country belongs, at the time of conquest or colonization or the establishment of present state boundaries and who irrespective of their legal status, retain some or all of their own social, economic, cultural and political institutions. (Department of Economic and Social Affairs 2004)

The development of an agreed definition of indigenous peoples with global application has been a significant focus of international processes (Department of Economic and Social Affairs 2004). The ILO definition is commonly cited, as is the working definition developed in 1972 by a United Nations study:

Indigenous communities, peoples and nations are those which, having a historical continuity with pre-invasion and pre-colonial societies that developed on their territories, consider themselves distinct from other sectors of the societies now prevailing in those territories, or parts of them. (Coates 2004, p. 6).

The substantive focus of these global movements coalesced around issues of rights. In 1985 the United Nations Working Group on Indigenous Populations began drafting the United Nations Declaration on the Rights of Indigenous Peoples (UNDRIP), often described as the most comprehensive statement of the rights of indigenous peoples. On 13 September 2007 the United Nations Assembly adopted the UNDRIP with an overwhelming majority of 143 votes (with only four negative votes (Canada, Australia, New Zealand, and the United States) and 11 abstentions) (International Work Group for Indigenous Affairs 2007). Those nation states that voted in the negative subsequently reversed their opposition. The United States was the last to do so, when, in 2010, President Obama announced his government's intention to support the Declaration, noting that 'What matters far more than words—what matters far more than any resolution or declaration—are actions to match those words' (White House Tribal Nations Conference 2011). Les Malzer, Chair of the Global International Indigenous Peoples' Caucus, noted that:

The Declaration does not represent solely the viewpoint of the United Nations, nor does it represent solely the viewpoint of the Indigenous Peoples. It is a Declaration which combines our views and interests and which sets the framework for the future. It is a tool for peace and justice, based upon mutual recognition and mutual respect. (Malezer 2007)

The UNDRIP also has indigenous critics. Some argue it is framed by colonial and gendered assumptions and question its potential as a tool for addressing indigenous disadvantage (Watson 2011). Protracted arguments during its development included a dispute about whether the appropriate terminology should be 'indigenous peoples', 'indigenous people', or 'indigenous populations'. The contestation of such apparently trivial distinctions was pursued by some governments which opposed the use of the first construct

on the basis that it inferred collective rights (Niezen 2003). Other governments denied the existence of indigenous peoples within their jurisdictions (despite, in some cases, strong support for indigenous rights in other contexts), as seen in comments sent in 1995 from the People's Republic of China to a working group of the United Nations Commission on Human Rights:

Although there is no indigenous peoples' question in China, the Chinese Government and people have every sympathy with indigenous peoples' historical woes and historical plight. (Kingsbury 1998, pp. 417–418)

In Myanmar, which has a population of 50 million with 68% coming from one ethnic group, the other 'ethnic nationalities' are usually considered Myanmar's indigenous peoples in international fora (Hartley 2008). In Thailand, indigenous peoples are commonly referred to as tribal peoples or ethnic minorities. There are fisher peoples to the south and highland peoples spread across 20 provinces in the north and north-west, and nine groups ('hill tribes') in the highlands are recognized by the government. Some reluctance, by some Asian nations, to recognize indigenous populations has shifted over time. In 2008 the Japanese parliament recognized the Ainu as the indigenous people of northern Japan and noted that Japan was not culturally homogeneous and that Ainu have a distinct language, religion, and culture (United Nations Permanent Forum on Indigenous Issues n.d.).

The ways in which indigenous peoples have been treated within constitutional and legislative structures of nation states reflect colonial history, the cultural legacy of settler peoples, and the further development of political structures and institutions in these nation states. Legal and policy definitions applied to indigenous peoples have impacted on the allocation of resources, access to services, and the realization of rights. Some jurisdictions have treaties between settler and indigenous peoples (Kunitz 1994). Others, such as Australia, have constitutional and legislative frameworks that define and regulate indigenous peoples (Anderson and Whyte 2006). Others do not formally recognize indigenous peoples. These contexts are important in understanding the development of policy and programme responses to indigenous health needs.

The original Australian constitution had two 'race' clauses. Their interpretation is contested, but after a 1967 referendum resulted in their deletion, the Commonwealth government began to become directly involved in indigenous policy and programme development (Chesterman and Galligan 1997). In 1981, the Constitutional Section of the Department of Aboriginal Affairs proposed that 'An Aboriginal or Torres Strait Islander is a person of Aboriginal or Torres Strait Islander descent who identifies as an Aboriginal or Torres Strait Islander and is accepted as such by the community in which he (she) lives' (Gardiner-Garden 2000, p. 4). This became the basis of the 'working definition' of Aboriginality and has been used in determining eligibility in administrative processes.

In Canada, by contrast, the 1982 Constitution Act recognizes three politically distinct groups of Aboriginal peoples: Indians (First Nations), Inuit, and Métis. In the British North America Act of 1867 the federal government was given responsibility for 'Indian and lands reserve Indians' and the provincial governments the responsibility for off-reserve services. The situation is complicated: First Nations people are distinguished as Status or Non-Status indigenous, with a Status Indian being accorded rights under the federal Indian Act, while a Non-Status Indian identifies as First Nations but without formal recognition (Clark et al. 2010).

A significant ongoing debate about the potential benefit or harm to people who are indigenous flows from the application of these constitutional, legal, and policy frameworks. In some jurisdictions, such as Canada, there are issues in relation to the regulation of access to services, or funding of services. Potential benefits could flow from legislative and policy programmes that target resources or recognize title to land. Some argue this inevitably produces (or recognizes) a form of differentiated citizenship that has a potential for both benefits or harms (Mercer 2002, 2003).

Health and social data

Health and social outcomes for indigenous peoples are frequently observed as poor. Indigenous health status varies, reflecting in part broader social characteristics of the dominant society. There are, for example, apparent differences in health outcomes between indigenous populations in resource-rich and resource-poor societies. Although these outcomes and inequalities appear to be persistent, in a number of instances health outcomes have been shown to improve, and there are some circumstances and measures where inequalities do not exist. This section illustrates some of these patterns.

Indigenous health status data is fragmented and incomplete, and the quality varies according to the capacity, and willingness, of nations to develop information systems that monitor indigenous health outcomes, and technical and social factors shape the quality of data. Technical factors include the inclusion of data items on indigenous status within administrative data sets and health surveys, definitions of indigenous people, and the development of systems for collation, analysis, and communication of indigenous health information. Social factors include the willingness of institutions and people involved in collection and collation of health information to commit to strategies to ensure high-quality data. Even within a technically robust indigenous health system, data quality can be undermined when questions about indigenous status are not systematically asked, or if indigenous people feel unsafe to answer such questions. Another challenge is the extent to which data measurement reflects indigenous peoples' values and priorities. While it is not necessarily true that indigenous people do not value aspects of health measurement framed by the biomedicine of public health standards, these measures may only partly capture different indigenous understanding and conceptions of health. Some jurisdictions are devoting resources to the development of strategies to improve the quality of indigenous health-related data. Transnational processes have also been established to provide mechanisms to ideas, resources, and best practice (Australian Institute of Health and Welfare (AIHW) 2006).

American Indians and Alaska Natives constituted approximately 1.6% of the US population in 2008 (Chino and Lavery 2010). Chino and Lavery argue that a number of demographic characteristics of these populations impact on the availability and collection of data, including their small population size, geographic dispersion, and concentration within rural and often remote areas. This is further impacted by misclassification or inconsistent collection of racial data, culturally inadequate survey methods, investigator

bias, the failure of investigators to establish rapport or trust, and factors such as community perception about use of data and the mistrust of institutions.

Data issues are even more complex across Latin American and the Caribbean (with an estimated 400 indigenous groups). In some countries health problems remain undocumented due to absence of data or publication bias. Further, the 'political nature of indigeneity' also determines availability of data—in many countries indigeneity... might or might not be recognised. Even if indigeneity is measured, data are not always disaggregated by ethnicity' (Montenegro and Stephens 2006, p. 1859). The authors of a regional survey of indigenous health in Latin America and the Caribbean noted a pattern of poor health and social outcomes characterized by higher infant and maternal mortality, infectious diseases such as tuberculosis and gastroenteritis in children, and environmental contamination, as well as an increasing problem with chronic diseases such as obesity, diabetes, and heart disease (Montenegro and Stephens 2006).

In international reporting on indigenous health, regional data are sometimes used as a proxy where disaggregated data are unavailable for regions (usually rural or remote) in which indigenous people form a significant proportion of the population. The indigenous people of Cambodia, for example, constitute 1% of the total population, and, in the north-east, in particular, have a distinct economy (Donato n.d.). Although explicit reference is made to indigenous peoples in the 2007 Human Development Report from Cambodia, disaggregated data for indigenous peoples are not presented. Rather, the report shows provinces in the north-east with the highest concentrations of indigenous people have the lowest reported HDI for Cambodia (Donato n.d.). In India there are about 532 scheduled tribes (indigenous peoples regarded as socially disadvantaged). In 1991, they constituted about 8% of the total population, concentrated in five states. A lack of disaggregated health data does not allow a comprehensive analysis of health status. However, childhood mortality rates for 0–5 years were 136/1000 in Bihar and 167/1000 in Madhya Pradesh. In rural India, Scheduled Tribes have the highest proportion of the poor (54%) of any social group. Of those states with the highest rate of poverty, Bihar ranks first at 66% (Food and Agriculture Organization Investment Centre 1998).

Headline indicators

In some jurisdictions it is well documented that indigenous peoples fare worse on the sentinel headline indicators compared with non-indigenous populations. Although gaps are closing or have closed in some jurisdictions, there are no known cases in which indigenous populations exceed non-indigenous outcomes on key headline indicators. In Australia for 2005–2007, life expectancy at birth was estimated at 67 years for indigenous males and 73 years for indigenous females, representing gaps of 11.5 and 9.7 years, respectively, compared with all Australians (AIHW 2011a). Differences in estimations of life expectancy are documented across jurisdictions, although headline estimates such as this require sophisticated data systems. Even then, differences in the conceptual approach to measurement, method, and the quality of indigenous data make direct comparisons of life expectancy problematic (AIHW 2011b).

In some jurisdictions change has been documented. In the Northern Territory of Australia, indigenous life expectancy at birth rose during 1967–2004 from 52 years for males and 54 years for females to 60 years for males and 68 years for females. Māori, the indigenous people of New Zealand, accounted for about 15% of the usually resident population in the 2006 census (Ministry of Health 2010). In 1951 the difference in Māori life expectancy at birth was about 16 years for women and 14 years for men compared with the non-indigenous population. By 2006 life expectancy for both Māori and non-Māori had increased and the inequality had narrowed to around 8 years for both women and men. Life expectancy projections for the Canadian Aboriginal population show an average increase of 1–2 years from those recorded in 2001. By 2017, life expectancy for the total Canadian population is projected to be 79 years for men and 83 years for women: for the Inuit, projected life expectancy in 2017 is 64 years for men and 73 years for women, while for Métis and First Nations populations it is 73–74 years for men and 78–80 years for women (Statistics Canada 2010). Trends are mixed for the HDI (a single measure that combines life expectancy, educational attainment, and income) over the period 1990–2000 for indigenous peoples in Australia, Canada, New Zealand, and the United States. For this period, HDI scores for indigenous peoples in North America and New Zealand increased at a faster rate relative to benchmark non-indigenous populations, closing the HDI gap, whereas in Australia the HDI scores of indigenous peoples decreased, resulting in a widened gap in this context (Cooke et al. 2007).

Child mortality rates provide a useful insight into patterns of indigenous health. An analysis of global indigenous health patterns highlighted persistent inequality in infant mortality for indigenous peoples compared with non-indigenous benchmark populations. Data from distinct sources over different time periods show that inequalities were greater, and infant mortality outcomes significantly worse, for indigenous peoples in poorer countries, relative to resource-rich countries (Stephens et al. 2006). In Australia, infant mortality rates for indigenous peoples have declined over recent decades; based on these trends it is estimated that the infant mortality gap will close over the next decade (National Indigenous Health Equality Council 2010). There is evidence that this gap has closed for some indigenous populations such as native Hawaiians (Anderson et al. 2006).

Improvements in indigenous health outcomes must be interpreted within the context of broader population trends. In New Zealand improvements for Māori have not matched those of the non-Māori population, resulting in an increase in the inequalities between Māori and non-Māori in many areas (Blakely et al. 2007). All-cause mortality rates for both Māori and non-Māori have decreased over time (Blakely et al. 2007) but relative differences in all-cause mortality have increased. The standardized mortality rate ratio (Māori versus European) in 1981 was 1.83 for males and 2.30 for females. In 2004 the rate ratios had increased to 2.37 and 2.74 respectively. Similarly, cardiovascular disease mortality in all ethnic groups fell between 1981 and 2004, but rates did not decline as quickly in the Māori population as the European population. As a result, between 1981 and 2004 the Māori versus European standardized mortality rate ratios increased from 1.79 to 2.99 (males) and 2.62 to 4.04 (females) (Blakely et al. 2007).

Patterns of morbidity

Indigenous morbidity patterns should be understood within country or regional contexts. Here, infectious disease and chronic disease issues, including mental health and substance use, are briefly touched upon.

The relative importance of infectious disease partly reflects regional patterns of morbidity. Globally significant infectious diseases—tuberculosis, malaria, and HIV/AIDS—impact on distinct indigenous populations but vary according to context (Montenegro and Stephens 2006; Ohenjo et al. 2006; Gracey and King 2009). The HIV/AIDS impact, for example, is shaped by factors such as poverty, homelessness, substance misuse, and access to healthcare, and high rates have been documented in communities such as American Indians and Alaskan Natives, Canadian Aboriginal peoples, and indigenous peoples of Africa and the Asia Pacific (Gracey and King 2009). However, although a major cause of death in Namibia and Botswana (with a mortality rate in Botswana of 28/1000 population in 2004), the prevalence rate for the San people in Ganzi was lower (at 21.4%) than the national average of 35.4% (Ohenjo et al. 2006). While Latin American and Caribbean countries are experiencing rapid and complex epidemiological transition, non-communicable diseases and injuries continue to have a significant impact across the region (De Maio 2011). A survey of the disease burden caused by neglected tropical diseases in Latin America and the Caribbean noted that hookworm infection, other soil-transmitted helminth infections, and Chagas disease were the most significant group of these infectious diseases in the region followed by dengue, schistosomiasis, leishmaniasis, trachoma, leprosy, and lymphatic filariasis. This group of infections is associated with extreme poverty, and in this region is noted as prevalent among selected vulnerable populations, including indigenous populations and communities of African descent (Hotez et al. 2008). In wealthier nations, indigenous peoples have been shown to be at higher risk of infectious diseases, although their impact appears to be declining in some contexts. For example, mortality rates due to infectious diseases have significantly declined over the period 1977–2004 for indigenous Australians in the Northern Territory (Thomas et al. 2006). Similarly, since the early 1900s incidences of infectious diseases have fallen among Māori and non-Māori populations. However, the incidence of rheumatic fever is high among Māori and Pacific children and young people (40–100/100,000) when compared to the non-Māori, non-Pacific population whose rate (1/100,000) is consistent with that of other 'developed' nations (Craig et al. 2007; Lennon 2009; Milne et al. 2012). Furthermore, despite the overall decline in infectious disease mortality, inequalities in infectious disease risk have actually increased over the past 20 years in New Zealand for Māori and Pacific peoples (Baker et al. 2012).

The health of indigenous peoples is increasingly impacted by the global epidemic of chronic non-communicable diseases manifest in physiological, biochemical, and disease syndromes, and has been documented in indigenous populations in the Americas, Australia, and across the Pacific (Montenegro and Stephens 2006; Ohenjo et al. 2006; Gracey and King 2009). In Australia, a burden of disease analysis demonstrated that non-communicable diseases (including mental health) accounted for 70% of the difference in indigenous disease burden (as measured by disability-adjusted life years) compared with the total Australian population (Vos et al.

2007, 2008). Disease management strategies have consequently focused on lifestyle interventions or strategies to reduce behavioural risks, in conjunction with broader strategies that address the social determinants of health. These patterns of change can be multifaceted. For example, in the Northern Territory, mortality rates due to ischaemic heart disease and diabetes mellitus increased between 1977 and 2001, but this increase slowed after 1990. By comparison, death rates from chronic obstructive pulmonary disease rose before 1990, but fell thereafter. There were non-significant declines in death rates from cardiovascular diseases and rheumatic heart disease. Mortality rates from renal failure rose in those aged 50 years. The ratios of mortality rates from these chronic diseases for Northern Territory indigenous people compared to the total Australian population increased throughout the period (Thomas et al. 2006).

There is also the emerging significance of cancer morbidity and mortality. In New Zealand, the incidence of melanoma was lower among Māori than non-Māori (Robson et al. 2010), and the incidence of bowel cancer among the Māori population was lower than that of non-Māori but has risen steadily since the early 1980s and is now similar to that of non-Māori (Blakely et al. 2007). Despite the similar incidence, Māori have higher rates of mortality than non-Māori (Blakely et al. 2007; Robson et al. 2010). One study examined the role of demographics, disease characteristics, patient co-morbidity, treatment, and healthcare factors on colon cancer survival and found that Māori had significantly poorer cancer survival rates than non-Māori, which was not explained by demographic or disease characteristics (Hill et al. 2010). The most important factors were healthcare access and patient co-morbidities. Trends in indigenous cancer mortality in the Northern Territory also showed a mixed pattern—the indigenous cancer mortality rate was higher than the total Australian rate for cancers of the liver, lungs, uterus, cervix, and thyroid, and, in younger people only, for cancers of the oropharynx, oesophagus, and pancreas, but mortality rates were lower for melanoma, renal cancer, and, in older people, cancers of the prostrate and bowel. Significantly increased mortality was noted for a number of preventable cancers (Condon et al. 2004; Cunningham et al. 2008). In a matched cohort study of 815 indigenous patients and 810 non-indigenous patients, after adjusting for stage at diagnosis, treatment, and co-morbidities, non-indigenous patients had better survival relative to indigenous patients (Valery et al. 2006).

Indigenous peoples have been shown to be at increased risk of mental health and substance misuse issues; for example, increasing harmful consumption of alcohol has been noted over the past two decades in San settlements and has been associated with increased reports of domestic violence (Ohenjo et al. 2006). A study of mortality for the indigenous peoples of Kamatchatka in the Russian north estimated that 'alcohol poisoning' accounted for 26% of violent deaths from 1958 to 1993. Further, improvements in health status and mortality over this period, which resulted from social and economic development, were eliminated by increased trauma-related mortalities (Bogoyavlensky 1997). In the Australian indigenous burden of disease study, mental health disorders (including substance use) were shown to account for 6% of the difference relative to the total Australian population, with substance use disorders accounting for 50% of this amount. Intentional harm (through suicide, homicide, and violence) accounted for a further 4% of the gap (Vos et al. 2008).

Strategies for improving health

The development of domestic health strategy of indigenous peoples reflects, in part, the characteristics of the relationships between indigenous peoples and nation states, as well as the characteristics of the broader health policy and institutional landscape. Some nation states have a relatively long history of development of indigenous health policy—in other contexts there is still little evidence of indigenous health development in national policy. National policy and planning framework components potentially include:

◆ A strategy to ensure healthcare resources are available on an equitable basis.

◆ A workforce strategy to enhance indigenous participation in the health workforce and the cultural competence of the broader health workforce.

◆ Mechanisms for indigenous community participation in policy and programme delivery.

◆ Health promotion, and disease prevention programmes.

◆ Consideration of relationships between western and traditional health systems (Mignone et al. 2007).

◆ Indigenous health information, monitoring, and evaluation systems.

The United Nations programme of action for the second International Decade of the World's Indigenous People recommends:

◆ Access free of discrimination to community-based and culturally appropriate healthcare services, health education, adequate nutrition, and housing.

◆ Systems for collection and disaggregation of data on indigenous peoples.

◆ Consultation to integrate indigenous healers and health concepts into policies, programmes, and projects.

◆ Access, especially for women, to medical treatment information, ensuring prior and informed consent.

◆ National monitoring systems to report abuses and neglect within health systems.

◆ Programmes that address priorities including HIV/AIDS, malaria, and tuberculosis; cultural practices with negative health impacts; environmental degradation; and health problems connected to forced relocation, armed conflict, migration, trafficking, and prostitution.

The key strategies of the Pan American Health Organization align with the United Nations programme (Pan American Health Organization n.d.).

Improved access to quality, effective healthcare, based on need, is a common element to indigenous health strategy, often with a focus on development of primary healthcare systems. In New Zealand, for example, access is similar among Māori and non-Māori in absolute terms, but the excess burden of disease carried by the Māori population suggests poorer access to primary care (Ministry of Health 2010). Furthermore, a higher proportion of Māori report unmet need for primary care compared to non-Māori, and Māori experience a higher rate of admission to hospital for ambulatory sensitive conditions. This suggests current access to primary care is not meeting health needs. Increasing access has been shown to reduce ambulatory sensitive hospitalizations among Māori and other 'high-needs' groups (Tan et al. 2012).

Additionally, indigenous health strategies have a preventive or health promotion focus. Increasingly, strategies for improving indigenous health outcomes have drawn upon frameworks, theories, and empirical research emerging from the fields of social epidemiology and the social determinants of health (Anderson et al. 2007; Carson et al. 2007; Mowbray 2007). This provides a lens through which indigenous health strategy can be developed in relation to programmes to address poverty, education, housing strategies, or antiracism strategies. Although social factors play a pivotal role in the production of indigenous health outcomes and inequalities, there is debate about how these relationships are mediated. The social gradient in health has been useful in explaining the relationship between health outcomes and social position for other populations—in which health outcomes decline with declining social position—and some have argued that it can be extended to indigenous populations (Marmot 2011). However, one review of empirical research found a less universal and less consistent social economic status patterning for indigenous Australians (Shepherd et al. 2012).

Similarly, socioeconomic status and deprivation play an important role. However, such differences play a role in shaping Māori outcomes but do not fully account for ethnic inequalities in health outcomes (Blakely et al. 2007). (Contributing factors include differences in access to health programmes and services, and ethnic differences in the quality of care.) The body of evidence examining these issues for indigenous health more generally remains incomplete but is expanding.

An international symposium on the social determinants of indigenous health reached a consensus that action in this field should take into account: the diversity of indigenous peoples; the effect of colonization; human rights; self-determination; poverty and economic development; data gaps and quality; indigenous culture and worldviews; reform of institutions and services; racism; and family and community health (Mowbray 2007).

Cultural development and strategies for improving health

Issues of cultural development and racism are frequently raised in discussions on indigenous health and well-being and often within the context of addressing the impacts of colonialism (Mowbray 2007). There are a number of plausible positive associations between the promotion and protection of indigenous languages and culture and indigenous health and its social determinants such as education and employment. Strategies to strengthen culture have the potential to enhance self-worth, improve social capital and strengthen engagement with mainstream service providers. Indigenous cultures and their protection are also afforded a central place within indigenous rights discourse. There are, for example, a number of references to culture in the *United Nations Declaration on the Rights of Indigenous Peoples* (United Nations 2008). For example:

Article 5
Indigenous peoples have the right to maintain and strengthen their distinct political, legal, economic, social and cultural

institutions, while retaining their right to participate fully, if they so choose, in the political, economic, social and cultural life of the State.
Article 8
1. Indigenous peoples and individuals have the right not to be subjected to forced assimilation or destruction of their culture.
Article 11
1. Indigenous peoples have the right to practise and revitalize their cultural traditions and customs. This includes the right to maintain, protect and develop the past, present and future manifestations of their cultures, such as archaeological and historical sites, artefacts, designs, ceremonies, technologies and visual and performing arts and literature.

Indigenous cultures continue to be distinct in relation to dominant cultures so the discussion about the link with health development is important. It should be expected that health values, behaviours, and practices of indigenous peoples are in some way culturally shaped. This may also include the ongoing application of traditional knowledge to health experiences and the ongoing utilization of traditional healing practices and traditional healers, although it should be noted that indigenous peoples may use both traditional healers as well as biomedically trained health practitioners. Culture can influence the decisions of indigenous peoples about when and why they should seek health services, their acceptance of treatment, the likelihood of adherence to treatment and follow up and the likely success of prevention and health promotion strategies. However, there is cultural diversity within indigenous populations and ongoing evidence of cultural development and dynamism. Indigenous people as with people of all cultures, respond to cultural issues in ways that demonstrate agency. Individual experiences and preferences can significantly shape choice and patterns of healthcare behaviour. Culture is not in any simple way a determinant of values and behaviour.

This is an important context when it comes to addressing questions about the potential harmful impact of some aspects of culture. For example, in some contexts it has been pointed out that indigenous cultural norms in relation to violence or gender have reinforced behaviours, which have significant negative consequences on the health and well-being of indigenous communities. Culture may impact on poor food choice or risky health behaviour. Health development may require change in values and behaviours. However, we should assume that it is quite likely that there already exists a diversity of views on issues of concern. The need to change in values and behaviours is true of all cultures, not just that of indigenous peoples. Supporting indigenous people to lead change is important to ensure that such issues can be addressed in a way that is meaningful, effective and ultimately culturally enriching.

A discussion on the relationship between culture and health would be incomplete without reference to the potential harms caused by aspects of inter-cultural relationships and racism in particular. There is a growing international literature that points to the impact of the exposure of racism on health outcomes more generally (Paradies 2006) and in relation to indigenous peoples (Larson et al. 2007; Paradies et al. 2008; Priest et al. 2011). There are a number of possible pathways through which exposure to racism could impact on health outcomes, indirectly mediated through chronic stress pathways or more directly through the impact on health-seeking behaviours, health risk behaviours, or through other determinants of health such as education or work. Cultural change within dominant cultural groups is likely to be important for longer-term indigenous health gain perhaps through the development of effective antiracism strategies.

Recognizing success

It would be difficult to identify a contemporary indigenous population in which all health inequalities with respect to the dominant colonizing population have been eradicated. It is not, however, as we have demonstrated earlier in this chapter, difficult to find examples of indigenous peoples whose health has improved or in which some inequalities have lessened. It is important to document positive change as it can provide insights into strategies that have some potential to be more generally applied. It also moderates the view that indigenous health problems are intractable.

In order to document positive change a system needs to be in place to produce disaggregated population level data over time. The jurisdictions in which this is the case are still a small minority—such as Canada, United States, Australia, and New Zealand. Even so, measurement systems are patchy and often unable to adequately account for regional differences. There is a growing interest in the complexity of the relationship between statistical data and indigenous identifies and on the development of strategies to improve the quality of national data systems (Axelsson and Skold 2011). A further challenge is that health change is complex in that some gains may be masked by emergent problems. For example, in jurisdictions in which there is evidence of improved infant health outcomes and improvements in infectious disease mortality (such as Australia and New Zealand), this has been offset by the rising impact of chronic diseases such as diabetes, ischaemic heart disease, renal disease, stroke, and cancers. It is also possible that improved longevity may have given rise to the expression of other diseases such as some cancers. Finally, it should also be noted that it is possible that some health outcomes may be improving while inequalities remain static or even worsen when outcomes are improving within the dominant populations at the same or greater rates. Importantly we need to not only document changes, but we also need to be able to attribute it so that we are able to make sure that strategies are effective or change direction when they are not.

Indigenous health inequality is a challenging issue globally. However, a number of the case studies cited in this chapter demonstrate that change is possible and these problems are not insoluble. A global perspective is very useful in that it does help to bring a broader perspective to these issues and assists in the development of effective strategies for health gain. However, as has been illustrated a number of times throughout this chapter, it also points to the significant differences in context that need to be taken into account when building local strategies and capacity.

Acknowledgements

Text extracts from Department of Economic and Social Affairs, *The Concept of Indigenous Peoples*, United Nations, New York, USA, Copyright © 2004, reproduced with permission of the United Nations.

Text extracts from Malezer, L., *Statement by the Chairman, Global Indigenous Caucus*, United Nations, New York, USA, Copyright © 2007, reproduced with permission of the United Nations.

Text extracts from *United Nations Declaration on the Rights of Indigenous Peoples*, Copyright © United Nations, reproduced with permission of the United Nations, available from http://www.un.org/esa/socdev/unpfii/documents/DRIPS_en.pdf.

References

Anderson, I., Baum, F., and Bentley, M. (2007). *Beyond Bandaids: Exploring the Underlying Social Determinants of Aboriginal Health*. Darwin: Cooperative Research Centre for Aboriginal Health.

Anderson, I., Crengle, S., Leialoha Kamaka, M., Chen, T.-H., Palafox, N., and Jackson-Pulver, L. (2006). Indigenous health in Australia, New Zealand, and the Pacific. *The Lancet*, 367(9524), 1775–85.

Anderson, I. and Whyte, J.D. (2006). Australian federalism and Aboriginal health. *Australian Aboriginal Studies*, 2006(2), 5–12.

Australian Institute of Health and Welfare (2006). *International Group for Indigenous Health Measurement Vancouver 2005*. Canberra: AIHW.

Australian Institute of Health and Welfare (2011a). *The Health and Welfare of Australia's Aboriginal and Torres Strait Islander People: An Overview*. Canberra: AIHW.

Australian Institute of Health and Welfare (2011b). *Comparing Life Expectancy of Indigenous People in Australia, New Zealand, Canada and the United States: Conceptual, Methodological and Data Issues*. Canberra: AIHW.

Axelsson, P. and Skold, P. (eds.) (2011). *Indigenous Peoples and Demography: The Complex Relation between Identity and Statistics*. New York: Berghahn Books.

Baker, M.G., Barnard, L.T., Kvalsvig, A., et al. (2012). Increasing incidence of serious infectious diseases and inequalities in New Zealand: a national epidemiological study. *The Lancet*, 379(9821), 1112–19.

Blakely, T., Tobias, M., Atkinson, J., Yeh, L.-C., and Huang, K. (2007). *Tracking Disparity: Trends in Ethnic and Socioeconomic Inequalities in Mortality, 1981–2004*. Wellington: Ministry of Health.

Bogoyavlensky, D.D. (1997). Native peoples of Kamchatka: epidemiological transition and violent death. *Arctic Anthropology*, 34(1), 56–67.

Bradby, H. (2012). Race, ethnicity and health: the costs and benefits of conceptualising racism and ethnicity. *Social Science & Medicine*, 75, 955–8.

Carson, B., Dunbar, T., Chenhall, R., and Bailie, R.S. (2007). *Social Determinants of Indigenous Health*. Sydney: Allen & Unwin.

Chesterman, J. and Galligan, B. (1997). *Citizens Without Rights: Aborigines and Australian Citizenship*. Cambridge: Cambridge University Press.

Chino, M. and Lavery, J. (2010). United States of America. In L.J. Pulver, M. Haswell, I. Ring, et al. (eds.) *Indigenous Health—Australia, Canada, Aotearoa New Zealand and the United States—Laying Claim to a Future that Embraces Health for Us All*, pp. 67–85. Geneva: World Health Organization.

Clark, W., Whetung, V., Kinnon, D., and Graham, C. (2010). Canada. In L.J. Pulver, M. Haswell, I. Ring, et al. (eds.) *Indigenous Health—Australia, Canada, Aotearoa New Zealand and the United States—Laying Claim to a Future that Embraces Health for Us All*, pp. 44–56. Geneva: World Health Organization.

Coates, K.S. (2004). *A Global History of Indigenous Peoples: Struggle and Survival*. New York: Palgrave Macmillan.

Condon, J.R., Barnes, T., Cunningham, J., and Armstrong, B.K. (2004). Long-term trends in cancer mortality for indigenous Australians in the Northern Territory. *Medical Journal of Australia*, 504, 504–7.

Cooke, M., Mitrou, F., Lawrence, D., Guimond, E., and Beavon, D. (2007). Indigenous well-being in four countries: an application of the UNDP'S Human Development Index to indigenous peoples in Australia, Canada, New Zealand, and the United States. *BMC International Health and Human Rights*, 7(1), 9.

Craig, E., Jackson, C., and Han, D. (2007). *Monitoring the Health of New Zealand Children and Young People: Indicator Handbook.* Auckland: Paediatric Society of New Zealand and New Zealand Child and Youth Epidemiology Service.

Cunningham, J., Rumbold, A., Zhang, X., and Condon, J.R. (2008). Incidence, aetiology, and outcomes of cancer in indigenous peoples in Australia. *The Lancet Oncology,* 9(6), 585–95.

De Maio, F.G. (2011). Understanding chronic non-communicable diseases in Latin America: towards an equity-based research agenda. *Globalization and Health,* 7, 36.

Department of Economic and Social Affairs (2004). *The Concept of Indigenous Peoples.* New York: United Nations.

Donato, J. (n.d.). *Human Development Reports and Indigenous Peoples.* New York: United Nations Permanent Forum on Indigenous Issues.

Food and Agriculture Organization Investment Centre (1998). *India: Overview of Socio-Economic Situation of the Tribal Communities and Livelihoods in Madhya Pradesh and Bihar.* Rome: FAO.

Ford, C.L. and Harawa, N.T. (2010). A new conceptualization of ethnicity for social epidemiologic and health equity research. *Social Science & Medicine,* 71, 251–8.

Gardiner-Garden, J. (2000). *The Definition of Aboriginality.* Canberra: Parliament of Australia. Available at: http://www.aph.gov.au/LIBRARY/pubs/rn/2000-01/01RN18.htm.

Gracey, M. and King, M. (2009). Indigenous health part 1: determinants and disease patterns. *The Lancet,* 374(9683), 65–75.

Hartley, B. (2008). *MDG Reports and Indigenous Peoples: A Desk Review.* New York: United Nations Permanent Forum on Indigenous Issues.

Hill, S., Sarfati, D., Blakely, T., et al. (2010). Ethnicity and management of colon cancer in New Zealand: do indigenous patients get a worse deal? *Cancer,* 116(13), 3205–14.

Hotez, P.J., Bottazzi, M.E., Franco-Paredes, C., Ault, S.K., and Periago, M.R. (2008). The neglected tropical diseases of Latin America and the Caribbean: a review of disease burden and distribution and a roadmap for control and elimination. *PLoS Neglected Tropical Diseases,* 2(9), e300.

International Work Group for Indigenous Affairs (2007). *Declaration on the Rights of Indigenous Peoples.* Available at: http://www.iwgia.org/sw248.asp.

Kingsbury, B. (1998). 'Indigenous peoples' in international law: a constructivist approach to the Asian controversy. *American Journal of International Law,* 92(3), 414–57.

Kunitz, S.J. (1994). *Disease and Social Diversity: The European Impact on the Health of Non-Europeans.* New York: Oxford University Press.

Kuper, A. (2005). Indigenous people: an unhealthy category. *The Lancet,* 366, 983.

Kuper, A. (2007). Misguided medicine. *Foreign Policy,* 158, 96–8.

Larson, A., Gillies, M., Howard, P., and Coffin, J. (2007). It's enough to make you sick: the impact of racism on the health of Aboriginal Australians. *Australian and New Zealand Journal of Public Health,* 31(4), 322–9.

Lennon, D. (2009). Acute rheumatic fever. In R.D. Feigin, J.D. Cherry, G.J. Demmler-Harrison, and S.L. Kaplan (eds.) *Feigin & Cherry Textbook of Pediatric Infectious Diseases,* pp. 419–34. Philadelphia, PA: Saunders.

Malezer, L. (2007). *Statement by the Chairman, Global Indigenous Caucas.* New York: United Nations.

Marmot, M. (2011). Social determinants and the health of indigenous Australians. *Medical Journal of Australia,* 194(10), 512–13.

Mercer, D. (2002). Theorizing citizenship in British settler societies. *Ethnic Racial Studies,* 25(6), 989–1012.

Mercer, D. (2003). 'Citizen minus'?: indigenous Australians and the citizenship question. *Citizenship Studies,* 7(4), 421–45.

Mignone, J., Bartlett, J., O'Neil, J., and Orchard, T. (2007). Best practices in intercultural health: five case studies in Latin America. *Journal of Ethnobiology and Ethnomedicine,* 3, 31.

Milne, R.J., Lennon, D., Stewart, J.M., Vander Hoorn, S., and Scuffham, P.A. (2012). Mortality and hospitalisation costs of rheumatic fever and rheumatic heart disease in New Zealand. *Journal of Paediatrics and Child Health,* 48(8), 692–7.

Ministry of Health (2010). *Tatau Kahukura: Māori Health Chart Book 2010.* Wellington: Ministry of Health.

Montenegro, R.A. and Stephens, C. (2006). Indigenous health in Latin America and the Caribbean. *The Lancet,* 367, 1859–69.

Mowbray, M. (2007). *The Social Determinants of Indigenous Health: The International Experience and its Policy Implications.* Adelaide: Commission on Social Determinants of Health.

National Indigenous Health Equality Council (2010). *Child Mortality Target: Analysis and Recommendations.* Canberra: National Aboriginal and Torres Strait Islander Health Equality Council.

Niezen, R. (2003). *The Origins of Indigenism: Human Rights and the Politics of Identity.* Berkeley, CA: University of California Press.

Nogkynrih, A.K. (2008). *Integration of Indigenous People's Perspective in Country Development Processes: Review of Selected CCAs and UNDAFs.* New York: Secretariat of the United Nations Permanent Forum on Indigenous Issues.

Ohenjo, N.O., Willis, R., Jackson, D., Nettleton, C., Good, K., and Mugarura, B. (2006). Health of indigenous people in Africa (Indigenous Health 3). *The Lancet,* 367, 1937–46.

O'Neil, D. (2009). *Social Organisation: Glossary of Terms.* San Marcos, CA: Palomar College. Available at: http://anthro.palomar.edu/status/glossary.htm.

Pan American Health Organization (n.d.). *Strategic Directions and Plan of Action 2003–2007.* Geneva: World Health Organization.

Paradies, Y. (2006). A systematic research of empirical research on self-reported racism and health. *International Journal of Epidemiology,* 35, 888–901.

Paradies, Y., Harris, R., and Anderson, I. (2008). *The Impact of Racism on Indigenous Health in Australia and Aotearohea: Towards a Research Agenda.* Discussion Paper Series Number 4. Darwin: Cooperative Research Centre for Aboriginal Health.

Priest, N., Paradies, Y., Steward, P., and Luke, J. (2011). Racism and health among urban young Aboriginal people. *BMC Public Health,* 11, 568.

Robson, B., Purdie, G., and Cormack, D. (2010). *Unequal Impact II: Māori and Non-Māori Cancer Statistics by Deprivation and Rural–Urban Status, 2002–2006.* Wellington: Ministry of Health.

Shepherd, C., Jianghon, L., and Zubrick, S. (2012). Social gradients in the health of indigenous Australians. *American Journal of Public Health,* 102(1), 107–17.

Stamatopoulou, E. (1994). Indigenous peoples and the United Nations: human rights as a developing dynamic. *Human Rights Quarterly,* 16(1), 58–81.

Statistics Canada (2010). *Aboriginal Statistics at a Glance: Life Expectancy.* [Online] Available at: http://www.statcan.gc.ca/pub/89-645-x/2010001/life-expectancy-esperance-vie-eng.htm.

Stephens, C., Nettleton, C., Porter, J., Willis, R., and Clark, S. (2005). Indigenous peoples' health—why are they behind everyone, everywhere? *Lancet,* 366(9479), 10–13.

Stephens, C., Porter, J., Nettleton, C., and Willis, R. (2006). Disappearing, displaced, and undervalued: a call to action for indigenous health worldwide. *The Lancet,* 367, 2019–28.

Tan, L., Carr, J., and Reidy, J. (2012). New Zealand evidence for the impact of primary healthcare investment in Capital and Coast District Health Board. *New Zealand Medical Journal,* 125(1352), 7–27.

Thomas, D.P., Condon, J.R., Anderson, I.P., et al. (2006). Long-term trends in indigenous deaths from chronic diseases in the Northern Territory: a foot on the brake, a foot on the accelerator. *Medical Journal of Australia,* 185(3), 145–9.

United Nations (2008). *United Nations Declaration on the Rights of Indigenous Peoples, 13 September 2007.* New York: UN.

United Nations Permanent Forum on Indigenous Issues (n.d.). *Indigenous Peoples Voices Fact Sheet.* New York: United Nations.

Valery, P., Coory, M., Stirling, J., and Green, A. (2006). Cancer diagnosis, treatment, and survival in indigenous and non-indigenous Australians: a matched cohort study. *The Lancet*, 367(9525), 1842–8.

Vos, T., Barker, B., Begg, S., Stanley, L., and Lopez, A.D. (2008). Burden of disease and injury in Aboriginal and Torres Strait Islander peoples: the indigenous health gap. *International Journal of Epidemiology*, 38, 470–7.

Vos, T., Barker, B., Stanley, L., and Lopez, A. (2007). *The Burden of Disease and Injury in Aboriginal and Torres Strait Islander Peoples 2003*. Brisbane: School of Population Health, University of Queensland.

Watson, I. (2011). The 2007 declaration on the rights of indigenous peoples. Indigenous survival—where to from here? *Griffith Law Review*, 20(3), 507–14.

Weaver, H.N. (2001). Indigenous identity: what is it, and who really has it? *American Indian Quarterly*, 25(2), 240–55.

White House Tribal Nations Conference (2011). *Achieving a Brighter Future for Tribal Nations: Progress Report*. Washington, DC: White House.

10.7

People with disabilities

Donald J. Lollar and Elena M. Andresen

Introduction to people with disabilities

Public health has traditionally identified disability alongside morbidity and mortality as negative public health outcomes. Preventing disabilities, therefore, has been a goal of public health activities. The programmes created to prevent conditions associated with disability are, indeed, a crucial aspect of public health work in the areas of birth defects (e.g. encouraging women of child-bearing age not to drink alcohol or smoke), injuries (e.g. preventing falls or automotive crashes), chronic illnesses (reducing obesity and increasing physical activity), and promoting health while ageing. This primary prevention emphasis begs the question that asks what happens to those who become disabled in spite of our best primary prevention efforts. Individuals who fall through the public health prevention net by experiencing disabling conditions have been regarded as best served by medical and rehabilitation systems and services, thus outside the purview of public health. Medical and rehabilitative services are, indeed, crucial to those living with disabilities, but in fact do not take the place of public health emphasis on health promotion and prevention for this population or for the prevention of secondary conditions.

In recent years public health practitioners have begun to re-think this traditional stance, acknowledging that people with disabilities as a population are at greater risk for additional health and health-related problems (that is, secondary conditions), and are, therefore, worthy of appropriate public health intervention. The basic premise of this chapter, however, is that people with disabilities can and should experience a health status comparable to their peers without disabling conditions. People with disabilities can live healthy lives.

Public health's basic mission is to promote the health of populations through primary prevention activities. As applied to people with disabling conditions, this would include preventing secondary conditions, that is, those conditions for which people with disabilities are at greater risk because of their primary disabling condition. Reducing or preventing secondary conditions promotes health and reduces health expenditures. In some countries, medical care and rehabilitation services are the primary societal intervention for disability. These targeted services are rarely identified with public health activities which are focused on the general population.

This chapter will describe current issues surrounding the inclusion of disability as an evolving public health concept and people with disabilities as an emerging population in public health. The three core public health functions—assessment, policy development, and assurance—will be used to amplify our understanding of and responsibility to this portion of the population (Institute of Medicine 1988). Specific emphasis will be placed on dimensions of disability, issues of disability across the lifespan, descriptions of international disability and public health activities, and the role of environmental factors that interact with these three public health functions. This chapter is meant to redefine disability and its conceptual and scientific relationship to public health.

As a preface, however, recent history must be understood in order to provide a context for how public health and disability are evolving towards one another. Public health, while concerned with the population as whole, has become progressively more concerned about certain populations at greater risk for disease, injury, and other aetiological agents. Health disparities have become a greater emphasis for public health in the past decade. This trend has focused primarily on ethnic minorities and other excluded groups who are more susceptible to diseases or other health conditions by virtue of being poor and marginalized with less access to healthcare. Disability, however, has not been usually included as a focus of health disparity science, policy, or programmes—but should be. Simultaneously, an international civil rights movement developed among people with disabilities over the past 25 years, culminating in the adoption by the United Nations (UN) of a Convention on the Rights of Persons with Disabilities (CRPD) in 2006 (UN 2006a). While public health has evolved from a medically based orientation, the disability rights movement has focused on disability as a human rights issue. While these two models have vastly different emphases, there is growing awareness among public health professionals that people with disabilities can be viewed as a large minority population who are more vulnerable to various co-morbid conditions or secondary conditions that are more probable due to a primary disabling condition. Table 10.7.1 provides an overview of basic differences between the perspectives.

While the medical model locates the problem within the individual and their condition, the social/rights model places the problem within society, marginalizing individuals on the basis of their medical condition. Change in the medical approach focuses on the individual while the social model focuses on the need to change societal attitudes and the environment. Intervention moves from individual treatment in the medical model to social action in the social model. Policy emphasis therefore is on health and medical care in the medical model rather than human rights policy and social action. In response to these differences, the World Health Organization (WHO) invested almost 10 years of work by international experts to refine a model that would incorporate both perspectives.

Table 10.7.1 Medical and social model perspectives

Area of concern	Medical model	Social model
Locus of problem	Individual	Society
Focus of change	Individual behaviour	Societal attitudes/culture
Changes needed	Personal adjustment	Environmental changes
Intervention strategy	Individual treatment	Social action
Policy issues	Medical/healthcare	Human rights/access to care

Conceptual model and framework

The WHO's model is becoming both the conceptual and scientific framework for integrating public health and disability.

During the past 40 years, several paradigms of disability had developed with some connection to public health. These models evolved somewhat but the WHO model currently best represents disability in the context of public health and this model was approved by the World Health Assembly in 2001. The WHO's International Classification of Functioning, Disability and Health (ICF) (WHO 2001) combines the medical and social models into what is described as a biopsychosocial model of disability. Fig. 10.7.1 depicts the ICF model. The model includes both biological and social elements in its presentation.

The WHO began work to revise its previous disability classification in the early 1990s. Over the course of almost a decade, over 800 individuals, including individuals living with disabling conditions, representing more than 60 countries participated in the revision process. The resulting product emerged as a member of the WHO family of international classifications, the most notable member being the International Classification of Diseases (ICD) (WHO 1992). The ICF took a different conceptual approach, addressing components of health rather than consequences of disease—the focus of the earlier edition. In addition, a most crucial conceptual and coding component was added to ICF—environmental factors. The importance of the environment as it interacts with health and functioning is explicit in this system. Environmental elements for the ICF interact with every other component.

The ICF does not address causes or aetiologies, but rather addresses function and health. From the beginning, then, the emphasis was to provide a complement to the ICD. In addition, the purpose of the classification is to provide a foundation for the scientific study of function, health, and disability, as well as providing a common language to be used across populations, sectors, age groups, and users. The coding system outlined in the ICF allows public health professionals to collect data for population use, in addition to its use in clinical work to assess individual needs, plan interventions, and assess outcomes.

The components of the framework provided in Fig. 10.7.1 include functioning across all spheres—body structures and functions, personal activities, and societal participation. Body functions and structures, respectively, refer to the physiological functions of body systems and the anatomical parts of the body. A problem with body functions or structures is referred to as 'impairment'. A personal task or action undertaken by an individual is defined as an 'activity', and a difficulty in this area is called an 'activity limitation'. Likewise, functioning in society in a life situation is defined as 'participation', with a problem in this functioning called a 'participation restriction'. Finally, an 'environmental factor' includes any physical, social/attitudinal, and systemic element that affects the functioning of the individual, potentially in all components of body, person, and society (WHO 2001). Table 10.7.2 provides an outline of the one-level, two-character codes for each of the components of the ICF. The full coding system of the ICF allows coding up to six characters, allowing functional descriptions at both broad and granular levels. The functional codes can be used in both public health surveillance and in epidemiological studies. Of particular importance for epidemiological studies is the inclusion of qualifier codes that can be attached after the functional dimension. Qualifiers range from zero to four for severity, and encompass a spectrum from 'no problem' to 'complete problem'. In addition, qualifiers can be used clinically to show changes in limitation and participation due to interventions and can be used to monitor change over time (WHO 2001).

This framework provides the most coherent system for common understanding of disability concepts, definitions, and specific functional codes to be used in public health assessment, policy development, and assurance across countries, age groups, and sectors.

Assessment and measurement of disability

Public health assessment is defined as the regular, systematic collection and analysis of information on the health of a community or population. It should include data on health status, health needs of the population, and epidemiological and other studies of health problems. Assessment begins with a most basic tenet—one must define what health issue is to be assessed. Case definitions are crucial to appropriate identification of a health issue and are the basis for surveillance, epidemiology, and potential intervention strategies. Historically, definitions of disability and identification of those experiencing disability have varied greatly in public health or other sectors such as education, work, and economics. Definitions for the purpose of identification of those with disabilities usually fall into one of six categories.

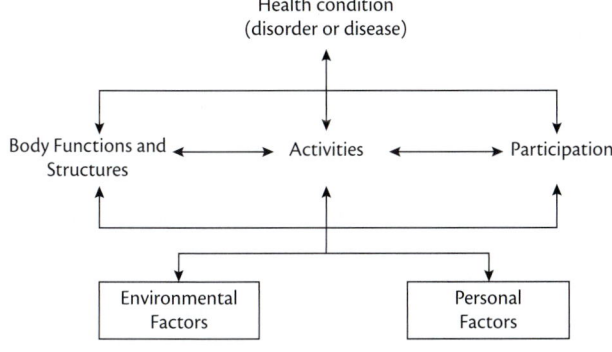

Fig. 10.7.1 International Classification of Functioning, Disability and Health Interactions among the ICF components.

Reproduced with permission from World Health Organization, *International Classification of Functioning, Disability and Health for Children and Youth*, World Health Organization, Geneva, Switzerland, Copyright © WHO 2007.

Table 10.7.2 International Classification of Functioning, Disability and Health, ICF One-level Classifications

Body functions	Body structures
b1 Mental functions	s1 Structures of the nervous system
b2 Sensory functions and pain	s2 Eye, ear and related structures
b3 Voice and speech functions	s3 Structures for voice and speech
b4 Cardiovascular, haematological, immunological, and respiratory	s4 Cardiovascular, immunological, and respiratory structures
b5 Digestive, metabolic and endocrine	s5 Digestive, metabolic, and functions endocrine structures
b6 Genitourinary and reproductive functions	s6 Genitourinary and reproductive structure
b7 Neuromusculoskeletal and movement-related functions	s7 Structures related to movement
b8 Functions of the skin and related functions	s8 Skin and related structures
Activities and participation	**Environmental factors**
d1 Learning and applying knowledge	e1 Products and technology
d2 General tasks and demands	e2 Natural environment and human-made changes to environment
d3 Communication	e3 Support and relationships
d4 Mobility	e4 Attitudes
d5 Self-care	e5 Services, systems, and policies
d6 Domestic life	
d7 Interpersonal interactions and relationships	
d8 Major life areas	
d9 Community, social and civic life	

Reproduced with permission from World Health Organization, *International Classification of Functioning, Disability and Health*, World Health Organization, Geneva, Switzerland, Copyright © WHO 2001.

Traditional approaches to defining disability for public health have focused on equating a particular diagnosis with having a disability. An individual with a diagnosis of cerebral palsy or autism, for example, would be assumed to have a disability. A second definitional approach has been to focus on the impairment, that is, if someone cannot hear in one ear or has intellectual or learning difficulty, s/he would be considered to have a disability. Thirdly, limitations in particular activities, such as self-care or mobility, have been defined as disabilities. Still another approach has been to identify those with life role problems such as working or going to school due to a health problem as having a disability. Yet another approach to definition is to identify those who need special programmes, such as special education or vocational rehabilitation or therapies such as physical, occupational, or speech therapy as, thereby, having a disability. Finally, another approach to identification is to ask individuals if they or others would identify themselves as having a disability (self-identification). Using one or several of these six different definitions in surveys or a census will produce different estimates of prevalence. For example, countries trying to assess disability using a question, such as 'Is anyone in the household deaf, blind, or mute?' will find a prevalence of disability in the 1–2 per cent range. On the other hand an activity-oriented question or set of questions, asking, for example, 'Does anyone in your household have difficulty seeing a friend across the street?' or 'Does anyone in your household have difficulty taking care of themselves in eating, drinking, toileting, or dressing?', the prevalence of disability reaches double digits, and in some countries might approach 20 per cent (UN 1990).

In more developed countries, several of the six approaches to defining disability can be used according to the government agency, survey, or purpose for the definition. For example, definitions to address civil rights issues for people with disabilities will be intended to be broad to ensure rights for all identified in the population, while an agency providing compensation related to work injuries will define disability eligibility more stringently (Lollar and Crews 2003). Crews et al. (2012) compared the approaches to measuring vision loss in 12 federally funded surveys in the United States using nearly 100 vision measures. The varied questions created widely divergent prevalence estimates for vision loss, due to different questions addressing impairment, activity limitations, and/or societal participation. Authors concluded that decisions at the beginning of survey planning regarding the specific functional outcome one is wishing to measure would allow for more comparability among disability measures. At a minimum, describing the ICF dimension being measured will allow researchers to understand, if not explain, differences in prevalence figures.

Table 10.7.3 provides prevalence of disability in selected countries by source, across low-, middle-, and high-income countries. These figures highlight the different rates outlined by the various definitions described. In addition, this table highlights the trend towards higher rates of disability being found in surveys than in censuses. Censuses, however, need to be used for comparisons

Table 10.7.3 Prevalence of disability in selected countries by source[a]

Censuses			Surveys		
Country	Year	% with disability	Country	Year	% with disability
United States	2000	19.3	New Zealand	2001	25.6
Canada	2001	18.5	Australia	2003	20.0
Brazil	2000	14.9	Uruguay	2004	7.6
United Kingdom	2001	17.6	Spain	2008	8.5
Poland	2002	14.3	Austria	2002	12.8
Ethiopia	1984	3.8	Zambia	2006	11.0
Uganda	2002	3.5	Sweden	2002	19.9
Mali	1987	2.7	Ecuador	2005	12.1
Mexico	2000	1.8	Netherlands	2002	25.6
Botswana	2001	3.5	Nicaragua	2003	10.3
Chile	2002	2.2	Germany	2007	8.4
India	2001	2.1	China	2006	6.4
Columbia	2005	6.4	Italy	2002	6.6
Bangladesh	2005	2.5	Egypt	2006	1.2
Kenya	1989	0.7			

[a] Rates vary according to type of disability identifier questions used, and are explained in the text.

Adapted with permission from World Health Organization and World Bank, *World Report on Disability*—Technical Appendix A, Copyright © World Health Organization/World Bank, Geneva, 2011, available from: http://whqlibdoc.who.int/publications/2011/9789240685215_eng.pdf.

because poorer countries often have no other mechanism for data collection (Mont 2007a). Approaches that more accurately describe the population's disability prevalence are important in all countries, not just those with fewer resources.

The United Nations Statistics Division (UNSD) published the first compendium of disability statistics in 1990 (UN 1990) that included data from 55 countries, and provided prevalence estimates and differing case definitions. A major goal of the volume was to begin to set international standards for disability statistics. Since that initial effort, the UNSD has published the Guidelines and Principles for the Development of Disability Statistics (UN 2001). This document was much clearer about how national statistical offices could improve the questions used, collection methods employed, and overall approach to dissemination of data. The UN guidelines used the ICF framework to assist countries as they work towards harmonization and comparability in disability data.

In 2001, the UNSD convened a group of disability experts from around the world to address the need for disability measures to be more standardized. From this conference emerged the Washington City Group on Disability Measurement (city groups are a mechanism used by the UN to focus on specific topics and are named after the city in which they meet first.) This international group developed a short set of questions that continue to be field-tested internationally (UNSD 2012). After intensive discussion and analysis of questions used in numerous countries, a set of six questions focusing on personal activities is being tested. The questions currently cover difficulty seeing, hearing, walking, or climbing stairs, remembering or concentrating, washing oneself, and communicating (Centers for Disease Control and Prevention

(CDC) 2006a). Zambia, for example, in the 2000 Census asked 'Are you disabled in any way?' asking for a yes/no response. This was followed by a list of 'disabilities', including blind, deaf/dumb, mentally ill, mentally retarded or physically handicapped, also asking for a yes/no response. This approach produced a disability prevalence of 2.7 per cent. Using the Washington Group's six-question approach, prevalence was measured at 8.5 per cent (Madans 2012).

In nations with very limited resources, collecting systematic and ongoing data on disability may be virtually impossible. However, exceptional efforts are sometimes possible, for example, the 2005 National Disability Survey in Afghanistan (Handicap International 2006). This project developed surveys measuring the frequency of disability and characteristics of the population, for example, inclusion in education. For many poorer nations, however, data are developed with few direct internal efforts, and with the need to apply some estimating procedures.

The conclusion has been that in surveys and censuses respondents can more reliably and validly report person-level activities than diagnoses or impairments. Therefore, across settings and countries, comparable data on disabilities can be generated. There is continuing discussion about how to ensure inclusion of those with intellectual or mental health problems in sets of disability questions.

As definitions are clarified, there are then several kinds of questions that can be asked by public health about a subpopulation, such as: 'What characterizes this group, beyond its disability status?', 'What conditions are most associated with disability?', and 'Are there disparities between this group and the general population on specific health measures such as obesity, physical activity, or smoking?'.

In a recent publication from the United States, selected chronic health conditions contributing to a limitation of activity ('disability') indicated that arthritis and other musculoskeletal conditions were most frequently associated with limitations among working age adults, aged 18–44 years. Mental illness was the second condition most associated with activity limitations. After those two came fractures or joint injuries. With increasing age, 45–64 years, arthritis was still the most frequently cited condition associated with activity limitation, but was followed by heart and circulatory conditions. Mental illness and diabetes were also mentioned often. The same conditions were associated with activity limitations in people aged 65–74, but in the 75 years and over age group, cognitive impairment and vision or hearing problems were substantially increased. Throughout, however, arthritis and heart problems were most related to causing activity limitations (CDC 2006b).

In Australia, data have indicated that 20 per cent of people are living with a disability, also defined as limitation of activity, but also including impairments, and participation restrictions. Among the population, 6.3 per cent have experienced a profound or severe core activity limitation, indicating a need for help with self-care, mobility, or communication. Australia uses a four-factor approach to the kind of disability reported—physical or diverse, sensory or speech, psychiatric, and intellectual or learning. Fifteen per cent of the population have reported physical/diverse category as the disability most affecting their everyday life. Approximately 2 per cent of the population reported psychiatric and sensory/speech while the intellectual category contributed just under 1 per cent. As with the United States, older age groups experience more disabling conditions, but prevalence of severe disability is rather stable (Australian Institute of Health and Welfare 2006).

The Canadian Participation and Activity Limitation Survey from 2001 indicated that 12.4 per cent of individuals reported some degree of disability, defined as limitations in daily living due to a physical, psychological, or health condition. Among adults, the most common limitation was mobility, defined as having problems walking, climbing stairs, or moving from one room to another. Working-aged adults reported the next most common form of disability was from pain (69.5 per cent) (Statistics Canada 2002).

Data from the United Kingdom used 'limiting long-term illness' as the disability approach, and reported 16 per cent of the population in that category. As in Canada, the most common limitation was mobility, followed by lifting, carrying, and dexterity. Musculoskeletal problems were most commonly reported as the cause of limitations, then heart and circulatory difficulties, followed by respiratory disorders (Department of Health 1991).

All of these high-income countries have the ability to collect disability data from several sources (e.g. census and varied national surveys) and using several definitions (e.g. from reported impairments, activity limitations, and participation restrictions). Population-based interventions are better able to be tailored to a particular group when the characteristics of the population are more clearly understood. Low-income countries, on the other hand, are usually able to collect disability data only during a decennial census and, thus, have substantially less information for the purpose of policy or programme development or assurance of services, whether rehabilitation or public health.

An example of characterizing those identified as having a disability, regardless of the definition, is the data from the United States. The public health agenda for the country has been established every 10 years since the 1980s. The current 'Healthy People 2020' includes 'disability status' as a demographic variable for many of the health objectives. One objective is to reduce the number of adults with disabilities who feel sad, depressed, or unhappy. The disparity between those with and those without disabilities in the general population at baseline was 21 per cent (28 per cent adults with disabilities versus 7 per cent of the general population). Likewise, a 9 per cent disparity was reported on life satisfaction between adults with and those without disabilities (United States Department of Health and Human Services 2010). In the United States, 31.2 per cent of people with disabilities report obesity, while those without disability reported 19.6 per cent. Physical inactivity was also twice as prevalent among people with disabilities as those without disabilities (22.4 per cent versus 11.9 per cent) (CDC 2006c).

In a report from the Special Rapporteur on Disability of the UN Commission for Social Development in 2006, results of a UN survey were presented. The survey included questions related to national monitoring of disability. Of the 73 countries responding, about 50 per cent had adopted an official definition of disability and 48 per cent had worked on collecting disability data. In terms of the range of data, 43 per cent were collecting data on the prevalence of disability, while 55 per cent include types of disabilities. Fifty-six per cent reported using data to develop policy (UN 2006b).

Using the ICF framework, and given the importance of the environment on the health and well-being of individuals with disabilities, assessment of environmental factors is also emerging. Satariano (1997) noted the importance of environment in the ageing process and indicated that public health professionals need to understand and conceptualize the role of the physical environment so as to enhance the independence and mobility of this population. Altman et al. (2003), using data from the National Health Interview Survey in the United States, concluded that people with disabilities are more likely to report environmental barriers to their participation in life. The type of functional or activity limitation appears to be related to which barriers are most reported, and respondents in this study emphasized physical barriers rather than attitudinal or policy barriers. This element of assessment is continuing to develop as shown by the emphasis being placed on extended sets of questions to assess environmental factors by the Washington City Group (Madans 2012).

Child disability measurement

Child disability prevalence around the world has been estimated for both the overall population of children under 18 with any disability (150,000,000 worldwide) as well as those with moderate or severe disabling conditions (93,000,000) (WHO and World Bank 2011). Assessing children and youth can be just as or more difficult than assessing adults. First, a child or youth is not usually asked to respond to questions, but rather a parent or other proxy. Second, if activity limitations are the approach used to assess, at early ages the inability to complete the tasks must be developmentally appropriate—that is, the child is not supposed to be able to complete a task, such as dressing or toileting. Also, developmental stages make interpretation of limitations more problematic. Because of these differences, WHO empowered a working group of international consultants in childhood disability to revise the ICF so that unique aspects of child and youth development and function would be captured (Lollar and Simeonsson, 2005). The ICF-CY (Children and Youth) was approved by the WHO in 2006, and published in 2007 (WHO 2007b).

In a 2006 report from the Australian Institute of Health and Welfare, 8.3 per cent of Australian children were reported to have a disability. The report indicated the most prevalent disabling conditions related to intellectual or learning (4.3 per cent) and physical or diverse (4.2 per cent). Sensory or speech accounted for 3.4 per cent, while psychiatric conditions were reported for 1.2 per cent of the children and youth.

A 2003 study from the United States used the ICF as a framework and the National Health Interview Survey Disability Supplement from 1994–1995 to show limitations in activities among children and youth (Fedeyko and Lollar 2003). The prevalence was 12 per cent using this approach. Learning limitations were more than twice as prevalent as the next highest contributors—communication and social/emotional difficulties. Sensory limitation (vision and hearing) was a distant fourth in prevalence. The *Chartbook on Trends in the Health of Americans* (CDC 2006b) indicated that according to age, different health conditions undermine function more often. Pre-schoolers have a higher prevalence of speech problems, breathing difficulties related to asthma, and learning or other developmental problem. Learning problems and attention-deficit hyperactivity disorder were the major contributors to activity limitations among school-age children. Among older children, emotional and behavioural problems were additional important aetiologies. Stein and Silver (2002) compared four different definitions of chronic conditions and disabilities among children. The children and youth ranged in age from birth to 17 years. Using a common data set, the National Health Interview Survey from the United States, operational definitions identified between 13.7 to 17 per cent. Differing definitions including those using specific diagnoses associated with developmental disabilities, those using consequences of conditions, such as limitations, need for therapies or medication, and the use of compensatory equipment or assistive technology. They concluded that there was significant overlap in the characteristics and prevalence figures, even using different conceptual definitions.

Durkin et al. (1995) employed an activity limitation approach to develop a screener of ten questions for childhood disability. It has been used in several countries, included Bangladesh, Jamaica, and Pakistan with 15.6 per cent, 14.7 per cent, and 8.2 per cent, respectively, of children identified as having disabilities (Durkin et al. 1994). The method used to identify the children was different, however, in that the studies are not usually population-based. The Multiple Indicator Cluster Surveys (MICS) used the ten-question screener, called the Disability Module, in 20 countries and published a compendium of results (United Nations Children's Fund (UNICEF) 2008). The positive aspect is that children identified by the screener can be evaluated more thoroughly, if resources are available. The Washington City Group is currently developing another set of screener questions in collaboration with the Durkin effort.

In addition, UNICEF has begun a project to enhance collection of data on child disability with the convening of a panel to develop a second-stage assessment to more clearly identify the specific limitations of children screened as more likely to experience disabling conditions (Cappa 2012). This assessment is based on the assumption that many countries will not have professional resources for completing a complete developmental evaluation, so the assessment will focus on community workers as interviewers with parents as primary respondents. This project will use the MICS currently used for broad health issues.

The US National Survey of Children with Special Health Care Needs has just been completed and uses a similar activity-oriented approach more explicitly following the ICF-CY model: it includes 13 questions and questions related to social and emotional limitations (Maternal and Child Health Bureau 2005). An analysis by Lollar et al. (2012) found that children with special health-care needs present clinically with various functional difficulties across an array of health conditions. The data demonstrate that functional difficulties contribute significantly to outcomes, such as emergency room visits, parental work patterns, and limitations in daily activities. Including functional difficulties alongside diagnostic/health conditions provides opportunities to provide richer characterization of children with disabilities for public health practice, training, policy, and research.

Ageing and disability

Disability is not an obligatory consequence of ageing, however some changes in function are typical, and life-long experiences or environmental influences, or personal characteristics of one's phenotype, contribute to increasing disability. The major reasons for disability at older ages are chronic conditions, and Chapter 10.8 provides an excellent overview of health conditions that lead to disability for adults (e.g. heart disease contributes the largest group of disability-adjusted life years (DALYs) among adults aged 60 and older). Gerontological research and clinical care have been slow to embrace the ICF as a framework to assess and study aetiology or outcomes of disability in older ages. Existing systems (e.g. based on the Nagi model) prevail, and assessment tools often use various types of activities of daily living (ADLs) and instrumental ADLs (see Chapter 10.8). However, disability can be assessed and measured using the function-based ICF.

At present, while some rehabilitation research and clinical assessment may be ICF-based (e.g. occupational therapy, where environment is a key aspect of assessment and intervention), the more promising avenue to have ICF-based measurement data comes from work that maps existing clinical and rehabilitation function measures to the ICF. Stroke assessment is one such group of patients (Moriello et al. 2008; Stucki and Cieza 2008; Quintas et al. 2012). When these measures are used, it is important to explicitly also include environmental measurements, because traditional ADL/IADL measures include items that rate disability directly involving a combined measurement of function with supports, and not function separately from elements like assistive technology or personal assistance.

The advantage of having good environmental evidence is demonstrated by examining US data. Trends on older adult disability have demonstrated decreasing disability among older adults in countries like the United States (Freedman 2006). Because the measures used to examine disability do not have environmental details, speculation about the trends includes the possibility that older adults in economically advantaged countries might have gradually embraced technologies to compensate for decreasing function. An example might be that meal preparations are easier when an older adult uses a microwave and more processed foods (Freedman 2006).

Summary measures of health and disability

Public health statistics sometimes move beyond descriptive epidemiology, and further into evaluating the impact and costs of disability. Some nations use statistics that are particularly focused on evaluating the relative effectiveness of public health interventions, among which are the years of healthy life (YHL), quality-adjusted life years (QALYs), and DALYs. Each of these measures incorporates the premise that living with less than optimal health is discounted in some way. This assumes that general populations place higher value on better health. All of the measurement techniques incorporate disabilities along with health states. In practice, these measures provide a common metric in which to examine how the cost of various interventions may result in increased quality/health/disability-adjusted years of life. When examined directly, there is evidence that 'values' for different disability and health states may be different between general population members and people with disability or serious health conditions (e.g. Patrick et al. 1994; Hays et al. 1996; Kannisto and Sintonen 1997).

The DALYs indicator was developed with support from the World Bank (Murray and Lopez 1996), and has been used in numerous reports to assess public health priorities and to set a future public health agenda. Because DALYs incorporate the term disability, and because they are employed so frequently to set public health priorities, it is important that public health professionals understand the relationship between DALYs and the 'current' definitions of disability.

DALYs are based on a definition of disability that correlates with individual disease states. This emphasis on disease assumes that all disease states translate into similar activity limitations and participation restrictions, and assumes no influence of, equal influence of, or only random influence of environmental factors. Over several years, public health professionals, economists, and the disability community have questioned several of the core terms, methods, and implications of the use of DALYs, including using the term disability to describe the statistics. Chamie (1995) suggested that DALYs misrepresent the concept of disability, and it would be better using a term such as *morbidity-adjusted* or *illness-adjusted*, given the method used to generate the measure.

The method requires health professionals (not the general public) to assess the burden of 22 disease-related conditions using preference weighting—the person trade-off (PTO) method. Healthcare professional ratings, not population-based data, are used to characterize disability. The largely medical-model methodology used to generate DALYs, the lack of a functional definition of disability in most countries to identify people with disabilities, and the exclusion of people with disabilities in the development process makes the outcomes of this utility suspect (Grosse et al. 2009). Mont (2007b) suggested that DALYs were a poor indicator of how public health interventions affect or improve the lives of people with disabilities. He reported that the primary objective in the development of this indicator was to implement a metric that could help national policymakers in allocating resources to reduce poor health. Given the competing needs of people and the minimal resources available, governments have to make difficult

decisions regarding public health improvement. Mont concluded that 'an indicator that does not properly embody the intended goals can build in systematic bias against achieving them' (Mont 2007b). The use of DALYs to inform public health policy is questionable, and methods incorporating increased levels of participation by people with disabilities compared to people without disabilities should be developed. Mont and Loeb (2008) have developed a protocol for addressing impact of activity limitations and impairments on participation using population-based data from Zambia. This approach provides a more scientific and generalizable approach to measuring the impact of disabling conditions on people with disabilities. In addition, it allows monitoring of changes in participation across the population and for comparisons across populations.

In summary, whatever the source (e.g. survey, census, or administrative data), public health data should be both periodic and predictable in timing. Ideally, definitions and measures of disability can be applied across the age span, and have a common underlying functional framework that incorporates how people interact with their environment. Different depths of data, and level of specificity of disability definitions, can be useful; however, to fully understand disability at a population level, some common data standards are required. It is important that disability definitions be separated from health and social outcomes so that analyses can compare groups with and without disabilities. Finally, if disability data are to be accepted for the purpose of policy development, people with disabilities should be included at each point in the development, collection, and analysis of data. The disability community dictum of 'nothing about us without us' is particularly important as public health assesses, characterizes, and compares this population with the general population (Charlton 1998; Meyers and Andresen 2000).

Carers/caregivers/personal assistance services

Beyond obtaining the data to determine the prevalence of people with disabilities, public health should also address the needs of those who provide assistance or care to individuals with disabilities. In ICF terms, these supportive functions and relationships are an important part of the environmental influences that contribute to improved health and participation of people with disabilities. Most often, these supportive roles are filled by family members, but also may include paid caregivers or carers in societies where this is socially acceptable and among people with financial means. Because disability increases with age, global ageing (see Chapter 10.8) generates some of the increasing size of the caregiver population. Other factors include improved survival of infants and children who grow up with disability, improved survival of people following physical trauma, and changing health conditions, like obesity, that influence disability prevalence among adults (Field and Jette 2007).

Care provided by informal and paid caregivers commonly includes assistance with functions (e.g. mobility, communication) and personal care, but can extend to helping with roles such as work and parenting, or school, and includes interpersonal support from companionship. Carers UK suggests that approximately 3 million carers work in the United Kingdom and that 60 per cent of people will be a carer at some point in their life (ACE National Action for Carers and Employment 2007; Carers UK 2007). Australian data (Australian Institute of Health and

Welfare 2006) indicates that 202,000 persons are the primary carers of individuals under 65 years of age and live with the person for whom they care. Data from Canada indicate that parents of children with disabling conditions report substantial tension as a result of trying to coordinate work, family, and child-care duties, compromising the quality of life (Canadian Institute of Child Health 2000). Data from 2009 on family caregivers of older adults in the United States estimated there were over 42 million at any one time: accounting for those who provided care at some time during the year, the figure was over 61 million Americans (Feinberg et al. 2011). The economic value of this unpaid care in the United States was estimated to have increased from $375 billion in 2007, to $450 billion in 2009. Poorer health and increased stress are often seen to increase among those who have greater intensity and hours of caregiving (Talley and Crews 2007; DeFries and Andresen 2010; Kusano et al. 2011). Public health associations in high-income countries are only beginning to address this subject, and low-income countries are even less able to address this important health issue.

The Asian countries of Singapore and Japan are both models of successful ageing, and have two of the oldest populations in the world (UN Department of Economic and Social Affairs, Population Division 2007). However, in Japan the projected dementia estimates associated with this demographic are that 2.6 million people will experience dementia by 2015 (Yamamoto et al. 1997), a figure that suggests the large future need of caregivers. In both Japan and Singapore, this changing demographic and the accompanying need for supportive services is preceded by an historical change in women's roles. Women's increasing education and employment is accompanied by decreasing time that can be committed to traditionally expected roles in caregiving for parents (Yamamoto et al. 1997; Yeoh et al. 2009; Yeoh and Huang 2010). In Singapore, the role of caring for older adults has shifted to a national reliance on foreign domestic workers to perform the live-in work of personal assistance for both ageing adults and others with disability. These foreign women workers often have limited formal training in providing personal assistance (Yeoh et al. 2009; Yeoh and Huang 2010). Nations like Singapore and Japan will continue to consider how to approach caregiving and personal assistance for people with disabilities. The relative economic wealth of Western and other developed nations does not provide models for how less advantaged nations, with even more rapidly growing ageing populations, will deal with the needs of people with disability, and the underlying commitment to their independence and inclusion.

Policy development for disability

Data by themselves do not make a difference in public health or the lives of people with disabilities. Policy development addresses the need for public health policies using scientific knowledge in public decision-making. Integral to the development of a more consistent approach to public health data collection on disability is the uses made of those data. Since 1982 when the World Programme of Action was adopted by the UN General Assembly, disability policy has been a global mandate (UN 1982). The Standard Rules on the Equalization of Opportunities for Persons with Disabilities (UN 1993) were developed by the UN to operationalize the World Programme of Action, and were the basis for policy directions

globally. While the Standard Rules were not created to address health of people with disabilities or public health, they do impact the health of this portion of the public.

The Standard Rules are divided into three groups: preconditions for equal participation (rules 1–4), target areas for equal participation (rules 5–12), and implementation measures (rules 13–22). The end product of these rules is that people with disabilities have an opportunity to participate in society equal to that of people without disabilities. It is a step beyond traditional public health and moves beyond the emphasis on preventing disease, injury, and disability to embrace the higher-order outcome of participation. However, this is the move made when the WHO adopted as its mission to 'improve health and well-being around the globe'. This broader interpretation is the result of an ongoing interaction between public health professionals and the disability community.

It is noteworthy that Rules 2 and 3 concerning medical care and rehabilitation are the traditional roles acknowledged by public health. The emphasis in Rule 2 on Medical care is on early detection, assessment, and treatment of *impairment* that can 'prevent, reduce or eliminate disabling effects' (UN 1993). States are also encouraged to provide regular treatment and medication needed for people with disabilities to maintain or improve functioning. Rule 3 recommends that national rehabilitation programmes for all people with disabilities should be developed. Programmes should focus on the lived needs of the individuals with the goal of full participation and equality. Recommendations are that individuals be involved in their own rehabilitation, that services be available in the local community, and that advocacy groups be included in national programme planning.

Implementation measures are, in fact, the processes that must be in place for the preconditions and target areas to be addressed. Most of the target areas are really the specific outcome areas in which opportunities should arise, for example, in education, employment, recreation and sports, culture, and religion. Throughout the document, the term 'health' is rarely found. The notion of health promotion is also absent, and can only be found by a generous reading of early detection, assessment, and treatment of impairment or the provision of healthcare and related services to all people to reduce or prevent the 'disability effects of impairment' (UN 1993). An emerging area for public health intervention focuses specifically on promoting health and preventing secondary conditions often associated with primary disabilities, such as decubitus ulcers or skin sores among persons with spinal injuries. Physical activity and nutrition, smoking, and alcohol abuse, for example, are clear areas for public health policy and assurance in many countries. People with disabilities, however, are often not seen as a vulnerable population for public health messages. Formulation of policy addressing not only rehabilitation and medical services, but also health promotion and secondary condition prevention are important areas to be addressed among people with disabilities.

South Africa provided arguably the most complete national strategy interpreting the UN Standard Rules (Office of the Deputy President 1997). The White Paper on an Integrated National Disability Strategy includes policy guidelines for the major areas of the Standard Rules, including prevention, healthcare, and rehabilitation. Secondary prevention is included and suggests that the results might be the prevention of complications, such as contractures for those with cerebral palsy. Inclusion of secondary prevention is a critical element in health policy relative to disability.

A national database is being developed to provide an array of medical- and disability-related services, as well as to collect information on health-related needs and incidence of impairments. The policy objectives for data and research focus on the gaps between physical and/or mental conditions and their resources, including the environmental factors influencing their lives.

Since 2007, 137 countries have signed the first UN convention of the new century, a convention establishing the rights of people with disabilities, indicating their intent to ratify (UN 2007). The UN CRPD provides a roadmap to end discrimination and marginalization of people with physical or mental conditions and has as a goal to eliminate exploitation and abuse of this population. Its premise is that people with disabilities have an inherent right to life equal to that of people living without disabilities, and will receive equal protection and rights, including controlling their own financial affairs and the right to privacy. A shift in perspective is explicit in the CRPD. People with disabilities are not objects of pity or charity, but rather are citizens with rights and dignity, with the capacity to contribute to their society.

Health is addressed by the UN establishing both a right to health and ensuring the access to healthcare for persons with disabilities (UN 2007, Article 25). Article 25 addresses equal opportunity to the same quality and range of services for people with disabilities as for the general population. Services to identify disabling conditions early followed by appropriate intervention are mandated. This includes the prevention of secondary conditions for this population across the lifespan. Ethical decisions such as preventing the withholding of food or fluids or basic healthcare and services are also addressed in Article 25. Training of health professionals to provide clinical or public health services equally across the population is another tenet of Article 25 of the CRPD. Consistent with CRPD is the move by countries to include disability as part of their national health agenda. Countries have begun to formulate public health policy by setting national health goals.

Healthy People 2020 is the national public health agenda for the United States. The inclusion of a chapter in this volume focusing on improving the health and well-being of people with disabilities was a major step forward for public health policy in the United States (Box 10.7.1). As a foundation for setting these objectives, DATA2010 was used to identify specific health disparities for this population. The disparities of greatest concern included not getting needed healthcare, participating less in activities to encourage physical fitness, using tobacco more, having a higher percentage of overweight or obesity, receiving less social-emotional support, and having more emotional distress. In addition, annual dental visits are fewer for people with disability, and fewer women with disabilities have mammograms and Pap tests when appropriate (United States Department of Health and Human Services 2010).

Regional reports from selected countries in Asia and the Americas have been completed by the International Disability Rights Monitor Reports (Center for International Rehabilitation 2003, 2004, 2005). These reports include information from 33 countries and reflect policy data on disability measures, as well as health, rehabilitation, and medical issues. Completed most often by disability advocates in their home countries, these data reflect substantial difficulties in most areas of health, rehabilitation, and medicine.

The most recent international policy-focused project was mandated by the World Health Assembly of the WHO. A directive was initiated to develop a world report on disability. The *World Report on Disability* (WPD) was published in 2011 and provides the most comprehensive compendium of international disability information (WHO 2011). The WPD frames prevention of health conditions as a development issue, with the assumption that environmental factors, such as unsafe water and sanitation, poor roads, and unsafe workplaces, often contribute to the incidence of disabling conditions. A chapter is devoted to health among people with disabilities with the most important premise that people with disabilities are not, by definition, sick or ill. Rather, people with disabilities may live healthy lives. While certain conditions are associated with poor health, the common assumption of disability equalling illness undermines public health emphases to improve and maintain the health of this population. The WPD goes on to address secondary conditions, general health needs, as well as the need for specialty care.

Specific emphasis is given to ensuring that people with disabilities benefit equally from public health programmes as do the general population. This is the most important policy document thus far that addresses health and disability, alongside disability and well-being. The report continues to generate important and more detailed global studies. For example, a follow-up report in 2012 highlighted the issue of community inclusion for people living with intellectual disability drawing from contributing evidence in 95 countries and from over 40 detailed national profiles (Inclusion International 2012).

Child disability policy

As with public health assessment, policy issues are different for children with disabling conditions. The 1989 UN Convention on the Rights of the Child specifically addresses children with disabilities in Article 23 (UN 1989). It is committed to the notion that these children should enjoy a full life under conditions that allow them to live with dignity, self-determination, and participation in the life of their community. It indicates the right to special care and assistance for them and their families or caregivers. Finally, any such help should come without cost and should include education, training, healthcare, rehabilitation, and services with the goal of individual development and social integration. This convention has been signed by virtually all countries in the world, and provides the foundation for national policies addressing the needs of children with disabilities. Healthcare and rehabilitation are included in those rights.

Assessment can identify the magnitude of problem and the population to be targeted. Policies can be developed that indicate attention to those needing such. The final core function of public health, however, is most crucial to those individuals living with a disability—assurance.

Assurance and the health of people with disability

Assurance focuses on the certitude that needed services will be provided to individuals and communities so that health goals can be reached. Assurance also suggests that services must not only be present, but also maintained so that goals can be met. Implicit in these assertions is the notion that there are challenges or barriers

---

Box 10.7.1 Healthy People 2020: disability and health objectives

Systems and policies

DH-1 Include in the core of Healthy People 2020 population data systems a standardized set of questions that identify 'disabilities'.
DH-2 Increase the number of Tribes, States, and the District of Columbia that have public health surveillance and health programs for people with disabilities and caregivers.
DH-3 Increase the proportion of U.S. master of public health (M.P.H.) programs that offer graduate-level disability and health.

Barriers to health care

DH-4 Reduce the proportion of people with disabilities who report delays in receiving primary and periodic care due to specific barriers.
DH-5 Increase the proportion of youth with special health care needs whose health care provider has discussed transition from pediatric to adult health care.
DH-6 Increase the proportion of people with epilepsy and uncontrolled seizures who receive appropriate medical care.
DH-7 Reduce the proportion of older adults with disabilities who use inappropriate medications.

Environment

DH-8 Reduce the proportion of people with disabilities who report physical or program barriers to local wellness programs.
DH-9 Reduce the proportion of people with disabilities who encounter barriers to participating in home community activities.
DH-10 Reduce the proportion of people with disabilities who report barriers to obtaining the assistive devices, service animals, technology services, and accessible technologies that they need.
DH-11 Increase the proportion of newly constructed and retrofitted U.S. homes and residential buildings that have visitable features.
DH-12 Reduce the number of people with disabilities living in congregate care residencies.

Activities and participation

DH-13 Increase the proportion of people with disabilities who participate in social, spiritual, recreational, community and civic activities to the degree that they wish.
DH-14 Increase the proportion of children and youth with disabilities who spend at least 80 percent of their time in regular education programs.
DH-15 Reduce unemployment among people with disabilities.
DH-16 Increase employment among people with disabilities.
DH-17 Increase the proportion of adults with disabilities who report sufficient social and emotional support.
DH-18 Reduce the proportion of people with disabilities who report serious psychological distress.
DH-19 Reduce the proportion of people with disabilities who experience nonfatal, unintentional injuries that require medical care.
DH-20 Increase the proportion of children with disabilities, birth through age 2 years, who receive early intervention services in home or community-based settings.

Reproduced from US Department of Health and Human Services, Disability and Health, in *Healthy People 2020*, US Department of Health and Human Services, Washington, DC, USA, 2010, available from http://www.healthypeople.gov/2020/topics-objectives/topic/disabilityandhealth/objectives.

---

to the provision and use of services which must be addressed. Assurance suggests, when needed, the use of authority may be required so that services will be provided and that they will not be too costly to access (Institute of Medicine 1988).

Assurance of services includes not only the presence of services but also the access to those services. Access includes physical proximity or transport to reasonably travel to the services, physical accessibility to the services, policies and systems that allow financial access, and attitudes that encourage participation in the services. The services include clinical preventive services usually set as a baseline for everyone in any particular country, health promotion activities, and prevention of secondary conditions, in addition to basic medical care and rehabilitation.

Poverty and disability

A basic barrier to assurance of public health services and attention is poverty. Poverty not only contributes to acquiring a disability, but the presence of a disability contributes to poverty, particularly in low-income countries. Braithwaite and Mont (2008) surveyed poverty assessments and disability for the World Bank and concluded that the poor data on disability status keeps us from accurately estimating the relationship that 'common sense and anecdotal evidence would suggest'. Data that indirectly suggests this relationship however is available. Employment rates among people with disabilities are substantially lower for this group (in the United States, 75 per cent versus 37 per cent for individuals with and without disabilities, respectively) (United States Department of Health and Human Services 2010). In lower resource countries, we can assume the proportion of people with disabilities working is even lower.

Primary prevention programmes are extremely important in public health across the life span. However, even with intense efforts to prevent birth defects, developmental disabilities, injuries, and chronic illnesses, for the foreseeable future, children and adults will continue to live with disabling conditions.

Children and adults will be affected by poor nutrition, prenatal exposures and events, poorly controlled diseases, conflicts, and environmental factors. A Canadian report reflected that 'among those experiencing the worst income inequity are children with disabilities or children with parents who have disabilities' (CICH 2000). The relationship between poverty and disability has long been established, alongside the general relationship between health status and poverty (Fujiura and Kiyoshi 2000; Park et al. 2002; United Kingdom Public Health Association 2007). Yeo and Moore (2003) in discussing the relationship between poverty and disability and health status, concluded that people with disabilities are among the poorest of the poor and are not represented in international development organizations and activities. People with disabilities, for reasons such as stigma, few resources, or transport may be unable to access appropriate health, medical, or rehabilitation services. In many countries public health activities are difficult to implement for the population in general, precluding any focus on those with disability. However, societies are judged by the way they relate to the most vulnerable of their citizens. In 2004, the World Bank held a conference on development and disability. James D. Wolfensohn, then World Bank Group President, reported that the Millennium Development Goals set by the UN and World Bank could not be achieved without the inclusion of people with disabilities (Wolfensohn 2004). Increasing development and improving economic standards cannot be successful without all populations being included.

Public health services

Equal access to care and equal access to public health prevention is as important for people with disabilities as it is for the general public. Disparities in access to preventive healthcare are documented in some countries, although as we descried above, data for monitoring disparities is not universal or consistent. Violence against women and children with disabling conditions is a prime example of the need for equal access to prevention and care. Ortoleva and Lewis (2012) reported on the international problem of violence towards women with disabilities, addressing both the commonalities with women in general who experience violence, while also highlighting the unique forms, causes, and results for this population of women. Services for women experiencing violence are seen as a public health issue, and women with disabilities must be included for screening, services, and programmes addressing this major problem. Likewise, children with disabilities are at greater risk of being victims of violence according to a systematic review of international studies (Jones et al. 2012). The analysis reported odds ratios of 3.68 for combined violence measures, 3.56 for physical violence, and 2.88 for sexual violence for children with disabilities using children without disabilities as the comparison. Any violence against children is unacceptable, but this disparity is appalling, and contrary to the UN conventions focusing on the rights of children and people with disabilities. Public health programmes and services should be a top priority for national efforts on behalf of this vulnerable population.

Primary prevention messages can be of equal importance for all segments of the population, including persons with disabilities. People with disabilities, for example, might be just as vulnerable, or more so, to heart problems than the general population. Public health messages are not generally tailored so that those living with disabilities feel included. People with disabilities are sometimes even included in messages as potential outcomes of inappropriate behaviour, such as showing someone in a wheelchair in a message that promotes safe driving. Public health prevention messages should be developed to acknowledge that people with disabilities are potential recipients as well. Public health messages should also be tailored to reach individuals with disabilities. People who have limited mobility are at greater risk for weight gain than the general population because of reduced physical activity (United States Department of Health and Human Services 2006). It is also necessary to be aware that some in the disability community might interpret primary prevention activities related to injuries or screening for birth defects as inimical to their existence, and thus feel suspicious, if not angry, about public health prevention activities. Communication between public health professionals and the disability community is critical so that important public health education can be developed with participation from people living with disabilities, but without losing poignant public health messages.

Perhaps the most important public health message for individuals with disabilities is consistent with that for the general population. Encouraging children, youth, and adults to be responsible for their own health is a powerful message that is particularly cogent for people with disabilities. For anyone who experiences multiple medical interventions, there can develop a sense of losing control over one's body, and equating that loss of control over medical procedures with a loss of control over one's health. At both individual and population levels, self-efficacy, a belief in one's ability to have control over one's life and health, is an important mediating variable for positive health outcomes.

Beyond public health education are the clinical services that all countries, whether well or less developed, attempt to provide their citizens (US Preventive Services Task Force 1996). These services include immunization, cancer screening, and cardiovascular disease prevention for both men and women, health guidance regarding nutrition and physical activity, sexuality and pregnancy education, as needed, drug use education including alcohol, smoking, and other important health information. In more developed countries, medical care and rehabilitation are emphasized, while clinical preventive services are not. Often, rehabilitation becomes equated with medical rehabilitation and providers focus on the disabling condition and its medical complications. Primary care should be emphasized in the care of people with disability, so as to provide the immunizations, health screenings, education, and other primary care activities. Specialists might not be familiar with or sensitive to the need for these services in this population. Many individuals with disabilities, if they have specialized care, do not use primary care and, therefore, might not receive appropriate services. Jones and Kerr (1997) reported that individuals with cognitive impairments did not receive annual health screenings. Austin (2003) found that people with disabilities in the US state of Oregon using services funded through public mechanisms are at greater risk of developing smoking-related cancers, were more likely to be diagnosed at a later stage of cancer and, therefore, not receive timely screening for cancer. In addition, treatment was more often delayed among this population. A public health responsibility is to ensure that people with disabilities are not lost to the provision of clinical preventive services.

Secondary conditions prevention

The term 'secondary conditions' is new and evolving in the vocabulary and objectives of public health. Introduced in the early 1990s into public health in the United States, the term has come to denote those conditions that are preventable but are present because of a pre-established primary disabling condition. A secondary condition is one to which an individual is more susceptible by virtue of living with a disability. The term 'secondary' does not reflect level of importance but rather that it comes temporally after the primary condition (Lollar 1999). 'Conditions' was chosen to indicate that this secondary problem could have characteristics beyond the medical or even physical ones. Thus, depression could be a primary disabling condition, but could also be a secondary condition associated with a physical impairment. Social isolation is another common secondary condition not physical in nature, but certainly related to the presence of and vulnerability associated with a disabling condition. Of course, more common examples are physical fatigue from the exertion of moving a wheelchair or urinary tract infections associated with but not a required co-morbid diagnosis of spinal cord injury or spina bifida. To reiterate, an important characteristic of a secondary condition is that it can be prevented. Thus, medical, rehabilitative, and public health professionals are involved with activities to prevent secondary conditions at the individual and the population level. Given that Disabled Persons International has affiliates in more than 120 countries (Disabled Persons International n.d.), it is clear that people live with disabilities around the globe. To reiterate, medical care and rehabilitative services are crucial functions that might be closely associated with public health. The health of people with disabilities, however, should not be assumed to be poor by virtue of having a disabling condition. Health is also a right for people with disabilities.

Ravesloot et al. (1997) completed a study of adults with disabilities across several diagnoses. The authors indicated that their results were surprising because they had assumed that each diagnostic group would report different secondary conditions. Instead, the results indicated common secondary conditions across all diagnoses. Traci et al. (2002) used a survey of common secondary conditions in a study of individuals with developmental disabilities. Physical fitness and conditioning problems were the most prevalent (59 per cent), followed by communication and mobility difficulties (57 per cent and 50 per cent, respectively). Low frustration tolerance and weight problems were next in prevalence. The authors concluded that these difficulties included major behavioural and lifestyle limitations, while more medically oriented conditions, such as bowel problems or respiratory difficulties, were reported substantially less.

This topic cannot be completed without a mention of 'secondary benefits'. Disabling conditions usually challenge the individual and family's functioning and participation, and often lead to secondary conditions. There are, however, benefits that may come as a result of living with a disability or being a family member. Benefits often include openness to and acceptance of differences in other human beings and seeing the humanity beyond the difference. Creative problem-solving is also often required in adapting to a world that is not often accommodating. Strength of will is also often developed by living with a disabling condition due to increased physical and emotional energy required to complete tasks (Lollar 2006). Friendships based on the shared experience of disability provide both social and emotional support, and the identifications created are often long-lasting. These benefits may become protective factors for future adjustment and participation for both children and adults, and should be included in public health evaluation, policy, and assurance. Prevention of secondary conditions should be an integral part of any nation's public health agenda for people with disabilities, regardless of the healthcare financing system.

Public health interventions

Interventions must be provided at both an individual and a population level. Using a self-efficacy conceptual model, several programmes have been developed to improve the health and well-being of people with disabilities. Seekins et al. (1991) have developed *Living Well with a Disability*, an eight-session workshop co-led by people with disabilities and a professional that helps participants learn to set health goals and find ways to meet them. This approach has reduced secondary conditions and medical visits among the participants. Some 15 US states among the 50 have implemented the programme. In addition, state programmes have also been instituted that educate healthcare providers about how to make their physical office space and medical staff attitudes more accessible to those with disabilities (e.g. North Carolina Office on Disability and Health 1999) and US national associations have followed suit (e.g. Chun 2011).

The WHO begins with the notion that many countries with low incomes have medical care and rehabilitation consistent with those poor resources. These services subsequently are equated with public health. This translation of medicine and rehabilitation into public health is a necessary, but not sufficient, approach to improving the health and well-being of people with disabilities. Medical care is important, even critical, for all citizens regardless of disability status. Rehabilitation services, whether medical, educational, vocational, or social, are specific services focused on outcomes related to the designated area—for example, work or school. The lived experience of individuals with disabilities is much broader than just medicine or rehabilitation, even defined broadly. Public health must encompass these services, as needed, but must also include those services discussed in previous sections—health education, preventive services, prevention of secondary conditions, and environmental facilitators of health and well-being.

Towards this end, WHO community-based rehabilitation (CBR) activities have been developed in more than 90 countries and strive to provide comprehensive strategies to include people with disabilities in the life of their communities (WHO 2007a). This emphasis, sponsored by the WHO, focuses on providing equal access to medical and rehabilitation services, but also to education, employment, participation in sport and numerous other community activities. Public health professionals, in conjunction with CBR staff, can collaborate to provide the expertise from both public health and the disability community that will improve the health of people with disabilities. The *World Report on Disability* provides a strong case for the utility of CBR throughout the world (WHO and World Bank 2011).

Major directions

Communication, cooperation, coordination

The most pressing need is for public health and disability communities to acknowledge their respective perspectives of the other.

Public health professionals do not easily acknowledge that people with disabilities are a legitimate population, and a minority, that deserves public health attention. The disability community must accept that health is a core issue for all people, and particularly for themselves, because they are often more vulnerable to additional health problems. The public health community can be a strong partner towards improving health and well-being among people with disabilities. Likewise, the disability community can assist the public health community in achieving these goals.

There is a growing interaction between public health professionals and members of the disability community. A prime example of this communication and cooperation was a leader in Disabled Persons International co-chairing the WHO Environmental Task Force to complete the ICF. On the Disabled Persons International website there is support for use of the ICF to conceptualize disability and to collect data using ICF definitions (Disabled Persons International n.d.). In the United Kingdom, a report on the 'Life Chances of Disabled People' has been completed by disability researchers and addresses inclusion of people with disabilities (Prime Minister's Strategy Unit 2005). The Office on Disability Issues has created an advisory body of 23 people with disabilities called Equality 2025, whose responsibility it is to advise government on disability issues, including health and well-being. Likewise, in 2006 the UN Department of Social and Economic Affairs commissioned an audit to evaluate the accessibility of the Internet for people with disabilities (Nomensa 2006). Five sectors from the CRPD were selected for assessment—travel, finance, media, politics, and retail. Importantly, health was not included. The evaluation concluded that only three sites among the 100 audited from 20 countries achieved appropriate accessibility ratings, and that there was a failure around the world to provide basic levels of Internet accessibility for those living with disabilities. As noted above, community inclusion of people with intellectual disability also has been evaluated (Inclusion International 2012).

In 2001 and 2002, the UN sponsored two workshops on measuring disability. The groups were composed equally of disability advocates and national statistical office representatives from the same countries. English-speaking countries in eastern Africa met in Kampala in 2001, and the ESCWAR region, including Arab-speaking countries and Israel met in Cairo, Egypt in 2002 (UN Statistics Division 2001, 2002). During each of the 2 weeks, the groups interacted to come to a better understanding of how disability statistics and disability policy were connected and the advocates and statisticians developed pilot questions to be used in censuses or surveys in their countries. Participation and involvement of service users and carers have not been the norm, but should become part of every nation's public health efforts to achieve valid disability data and pragmatic disability policy.

Currently, the joint project between the Washington City Group and UNICEF relative to disability measures for children is a prime example of coordination of effort on behalf of children with disabling conditions.

Disability framework and measurement

The WHO disability framework approved in 2001, along with the children's version approved in 2006, provide the foundation for public health functions to be achieved. The ICF is finding more traction in countries around the world. Clinical use of ICF codes is found in Germany with the work of Stucki et al. (2002a, 2002b).

Physicians throughout Italy are being trained to use ICF coding alongside ICD codes in clinical work (Disability Italian Network 2005). The Measuring Health and Disability in Europe (MHADIE) project of the European Union is implementing an ICF approach in addressing a standardized approach to data collection on disability in its 25 member states (MHADIE 2005).

Surveys have been incorporating the ICF framework in Qatar (R.J. Simeonsson, personal communication) and in the United States (Maternal and Child Health Bureau 2005). As noted earlier, the Washington Group on disability measurement includes some 75 countries in its early efforts to develop a short set of ICF-based functional questions to identify people living with some of the most prevalent activity limitations associated with disability (CDC 2006a). There is still the challenge of identifying individuals with mental health problems or with cognitive impairments, but the process has begun. Because the WHO process for revision of both the ICD and the ICF is under the auspices of the committee on Family of International Classifications (WHO-FIC), there will be growing congruence in the use of these complementary classifications in both clinical and public health settings.

Public health education and training

Public health education is expanding around the world. A study by Tanehaus et al. (2000) indicated that schools of public health in the United States were including some disability-related coursework. As an outgrowth of this study, two products were developed. Courses have been inserted into the curriculum of several schools of public health in the United States, including Georgia State University in Atlanta, Georgia, the University of Texas/Dallas, Texas, and Oregon Health & Science University in Portland, Oregon. Second, two books addressing disability and public health have been published. One volume encompasses all major public health core areas—epidemiology, health services, global health, environmental health, and ethics (Lollar and Andresen 2010). Public health experts in these fields have contributed chapters that provide a link between public health and disability in their particular specialty and provide references and case studies for each area. Using this approach, any discipline within public health could integrate disability into its courses (Allen and Garberson 2007). A second book focuses on disability as it intersects public health (Drum et al. 2009). Finally, a specific objective in the health agenda for the US (DH-3) is to increase the proportion of US master of public health programmes that offer graduate-level courses in disability and health. Efforts will be made to address this academic goal during the next 10 years (United States Department of Health and Human Services 2010).

Conclusions

People living with disabilities have traditionally not been included in public health activities. As more people with disabilities live longer because of better nutrition, medical interventions, and public health interventions such as immunizations, there will be a greater need for this population to be included in public health interventions, to be a target for specific public health messages, and to be acknowledged as a population worthy of attention when public health planning is being instituted. This 'epidemic of survival' provides an opportunity for public health to address a minority population around the world.

People with disabilities need to be encouraged to take responsibility for their health behaviours, but also to challenge the health, social, economic, and political systems that undermine progress towards health and well-being. Public health workers and people with disability can jointly address environmental barriers to health, including non-health issues, such as access to healthcare and education, societal attitudes towards those with disabling conditions, and policies and systems, for example, health and education. Training of public health professionals in disability issues is emerging, and this education of young people can lead to long-term changes in public health perceptions and practice.

References

ACE National Action for Carers and Employment (2007). *Work and Families Act: 2006*. [Online] Available at: http://www.acecarers.org.uk.

Allen, D. and Garberson, W. (eds.) (2007). *One in Five: Disability in the Public Health Curriculum*. Unpublished manuscript.

Altman, B., Lollar, D.J., and Rasche, E. (2003). *The Experience of Environmental Barriers Among Persons with Disabilities*. Presentation to the American Sociological Association.

Austin, D. (2003). *Disabilities are Risk Factors for Late Stage or Poor Prognosis Cancers*. Paper presented at Changing Concepts of Health and Disability: Science and Policy Conference, Oregon Health and Science University, Portland.

Australian Institute of Health and Welfare (2006). *Disability and Disability Services in Australia*. Canberra: Australian Institute of Health and Welfare.

Braithwaite, J. and Mont, D. (2008). *Disability and Poverty: A Survey of World Bank Poverty Assessment and Implications*. Social Protection Discussion Paper, No. 0805. New York: World Bank.

Canadian Institute of Child Health (2000). *The Health of Canada's Children*. Ottawa: Canadian Institute of Child Health.

Cappa, C. (2012). *Second-Stage Assessment: Rationale, Objectives, and Challenges*. Presentation at the Expert Consultation on the Measurement of Child Disability, 6 June UNICEF, New York.

Carers UK (2007). *The Voice of Carers*. [Online] Available at: http://www.carersuk.org.

Center for International Rehabilitation (2003). *International Disability Rights Compendium*. Washington, DC: Center for International Rehabilitation.

Center for International Rehabilitation (2004). *International Disability Rights Monitor: Regional Report of the Americas 2004*. Chicago: International Disability Network.

Center for International Rehabilitation (2005). *International Disability Rights Monitor: Regional Report of Asia 2005*. Chicago: International Disability Network.

Centers for Disease Control and Prevention (2006a). *Washington City Group Report on Disability Measurement*. Washington, DC: CDC.

Centers for Disease Control and Prevention (2006b). *Chartbook on Trends in the Health of Americans*. Washington, DC: CDC.

Centers for Disease Control and Prevention (2006c). *Disability and Health State Chartbook*. Atlanta, GA: CDC.

Chamie, M (1995). What does morbidity have to do with disability? *Disability and Rehabilitation*, 17(7), 323–7.

Charlton, J.I. (1998). *Nothing About Us Without Us: Disability Oppression & Empowerment*. Berkeley, CA: University of California Press.

Chun, A. (ed.) (2011). *Geriatric Care by Design. A Clinician's Handbook to Meet the Needs of Older Adults Through Environmental and Practice Redesign*. Chicago, IL: American Medical Association.

Crews, J.E., Lollar, D.J., Kemper, A.R., et al. (2012). The variability of vision loss assessment in federally sponsored surveys: seeking conceptual clarity and comparability. *American Journal of Ophthalmology*,154(Suppl. 6), S31–44.e1.

DeFries, E.L. and Andresen, E.M. (2010). Caregiver health. In J.C. Cavanaugh and D.K. Cavanaugh (eds.) *Aging in America: Vol. 2. Psychological, Physical, & Social Issues*, pp. 81–99. Westport, CT: Greenwood Publishing Group.

Department of Health (1991). *The Health of the Nation*. London: HMSO.

Disability Italian Network (2005). *ICF: Basic and Advanced Course*. Gardolo: DIN.

Disabled Persons International (n.d.). Website. [Online] Available at: http://www.dpi.org/.

Drum, C.E., Krahn, G.L., and Bersani, H. (eds.) (2009). *Disability and Public Health*. Washington, DC: American Public Health Association.

Durkin, M.S., Islan, S., Hasan, Z.M., and Zaman, S.S. (1994). Measures of socioeconomic status for child health research: comparative results from Bangladesh and Pakistan. *Social Science & Medicine*, 38, 1289–97.

Durkin, M.S., Wang, W., Shrout, P.E., et al. (1995). Evaluating a ten questions screen for childhood disability: reliability and internal structure in different cultures. *Journal of Clinical Epidemiology*, 48(5), 657–66.

Fedeyko, H.J. and Lollar, D.J. (2003). Classifying disability data. Using survey data to study disability: results from the National Health Interview Survey on Disability. *Social Science and Disability*, 3, 55–72.

Feinberg, L., Reinhard, S.C., Houser, A., and Choula, R. (2011). *Valuing the Invaluable: 2011 Update. The Growing Contributions and Costs of Family Caregiving*. Washington, DC: AARP Public Policy Institute.

Field, M.J. and Jette, A.M. (eds.) (2007). *The Future of Disability in America*. Washington, DC: National Academies Press.

Freedman, V.A. (2006). Late-life disability trends: an overview of current evidence. In M.J. Field, A.M. Jette, and L. Martin (eds.) *Workshop on Disability in America*, pp. 101–12. Washington, DC: National Academies Press. Available at: http://www.nap.edu/catalog.php?record_id=11579.

Fujiura, G.T. and Kiyoshi, Y. (2000). Trends in demography of childhood poverty and disability. *Exceptional Children*, 66(2), 187–99.

Grosse S., Lollar D.J., Campbell V.A., and Chamie M. (2009). *Disability and Disability-Adjusted Life Years (DALYs): Not the Same. Public Health Reports*, 124, 197–202.

Handicap International (2006). *Conducting Surveys on Disability: A Comprehensive Toolkit*. Bakhashi, P., Trani, J-F., Rolland, C. Lyon, France: Handicap International.

Hays, R.D., Siu, A.L., Keeler, E., et al. (1996). Long-term care residents' preferences for health states on the quality of well-being scale. *Medical Decision Making*, 16, 254–61.

Inclusion International (2012). *Inclusive Communities = Stronger Communities. Global Report on Article 19: The Right to Live and be Included in the Community*. London: Inclusion International. Available at: http://www.inclusion-international.org/wp-content/uploads/Global-Report-Living-Colour-dr2-2.pdf.

Institute of Medicine (1988). *The Future of Public Health*. Washington, DC: National Academy Press.

Jones, L., Bellis, M.A., Wood, S., et al. (2012). Prevalence and risk of violence against children with disabilities: a systematic review and meta-analysis of observational studies. *The Lancet*, 380, 899–907.

Jones, R.G. and Kerr, M.P. (1997). A randomized control trial of an opportunistic health screening tool in primary care for people with intellectual disability. *Journal of Intellectual Disability Research*, 41, 409–15.

Kannisto, M. and Sintonen, H. (1997). Later health-related quality of life in adults who have sustained spinal cord injury in childhood. *Spinal Cord*, 35, 747–51.

Kusano, C., Bouldin, E.D., Anderson, L.A., et al. (2011). Adult informal caregivers reporting financial burden in Hawaii, Kansas, & Washington: results from the 2007 BRFSS. *Disability and Health Journal*, 4(4), 229–37.

Lollar, D.J. (1999). Clinical dimensions of secondary conditions. In R.J. Simeonsson and L.N. McDevitt (eds.) *Issues in Disability and Health: The Role of Secondary Conditions and Quality of Life*, pp. 41–50. Chapel Hill, NC: University of North Carolina.

Lollar D.J. (2006). Preventing secondary conditions and promoting health. In I.L. Rubin and A.C. Crocker (eds.) *Medical Care for Children and Adults with Developmental Disabilities*, pp. 33–42. Baltimore, MD: Paul H. Brookes Publishing.

Lollar, D.J. and Andresen, E.M. (eds.) (2010). *Public Health Perspectives on Disability: Epidemiology to Ethics & Beyond*. New York: Springer.

Lollar, D.J. and Crews, J.E. (2003). Redefining the role of public health in disability. *Annual Review of Public Health*, 24, 195–208.

Lollar, D.J., Hartzell, M.S., and Evans, M.A. (2012). Functional difficulties and health conditions among children with special health needs. *Pediatrics*, 129(3), 714–22.

Lollar, D.J. and Simeonsson, R.J. (2005). Diagnosis to function: classification for children and youths. *Developmental and Behavioral Pediatrics*, 26(4), 323–30.

Madans, J.H. (2012). *The Washington Group on Disability Statistics*. Presentation to the Expert Consultation on the Measurement of Child Disability, 6 June, UNICEF, New York.

Maternal and Child Health Bureau (2005). *Survey of Children with Special Healthcare Needs*. Washington, DC: Maternal and Child Health Bureau.

Measuring Health and Disability in Europe (2005). *MHADI Press Release*. [Online] Available at: http://www.mhadie.it/aboutus.aspx.

Meyers, A.R. and Andresen, E.M. (2000). Enabling our instruments: accommodation, universal design, & assured access to participation in research. *Archives of Physical Medicine and Rehabilitation*, 81(12 Suppl. 2), S5–S9.

Mont, D. (2007a). *Measuring Disability Prevalence*. Social Protection Discussion Paper. New York: World Bank.

Mont, D. (2007b). Measuring health and disability. *The Lancet*, 369, 1658–63.

Mont, D. and Loeb, M. (2008). *Beyond DALYs: Developing Indicators to Assess the Impact of Public Health Interventions on the Lives of People with Disabilities*. Social Protection Discussion Paper, No. 0815. New York: World Bank.

Moriello, C., Byrne, K., Cieza, A., Nash, C., Stolee, P., and Mayo, N. (2008). Mapping the Stroke Impact Scale (SIS-16) to the International Classification of Functioning, Disability and Health. *Journal of Rehabilitation Medicine*, 40(2), 102–6.

Murray, C.J.L. and Lopez, A.D. (eds.) (1996). *The Global Burden of Disease: A Comprehensive Assessment of Mortality and Disability from Diseases, Injuries and Risk Factors in 1990 and Projected to 2000*. Cambridge, MA: Harvard University Press.

Nomensa (2006). *United Nations Global Audit of Web Accessibility*. [Online] Available at: http://www.nomensa.com/resources/research/united-nations-global-audit-of-accessibility.html.

North Carolina Office on Disability and Health (1999). *Removing Barriers: Tips and Strategies to Promote Accessibility*. Chapel Hill, NC: North Carolina Office on Disability and Health.

Office of the Deputy President (1997). *Integrated National Disability Strategy: A White Paper*. Ndabeni, South Africa: Office of the Deputy President.

Ortoleva, S. and Lewis, H. (2012). *Forgotten Sisters: A Report on Violence Against Women with Disability: An Overview of its Nature, Scope, Causes, and Consequences*. Northeastern University School of Law Research Report, No. 104. Boston, MA: Northeastern University School of Law.

Park, J., Turnbull, A.P., and Turnbull, H.R. (2002). Impacts of poverty on quality of life in families of children with disabilities. *Exceptional Children*, 68(2), 151–70

Patrick, D.L., Starks, H.E., Cain, K.C., Uhlmann, R.F., and Pearlman, R.A. (1994). Measuring preferences for health states worse than death. *Medical Decision Making*, 14, 9–18.

Prime Minister's Strategy Unit (2005). *Improving the Life Chances of Disabled People: Final Report*. London: Department of Health.

Available at: http://webarchive.nationalarchives.gov.uk/+/http://www.cabinetoffice.gov.uk/media/cabinetoffice/strategy/assets/disability.pdf.

Quintas, R., Cerniauskaite, M., Ajovalasit, D., et al. (2012). Describing functioning, disability, and health with the International Classification of Functioning, Disability, and Health Brief Core Set for Stroke. *American Journal of Physical Medicine & Rehabilitation*, 1(13 Suppl. 1), S14–21.

Ravesloot, C., Seekins, T., and Walsh, J. (1997). A structural analysis of secondary conditions experienced by people with physical disabilities. *Rehabilitation Psychology*, 42(1), 3–16.

Satariano, W.E. (1997). The disabilities of aging—looking to the physical environment. *American Journal of Public Health*, 87(3), 331–2.

Seekins, T., Clay, J., Kirchmyer, S., Ali, O., Murphy, K., and Ravesloot, C. (1991). *Developing and Implementing a Program for Preventing and Managing Secondary Conditions Experienced by Adults with Physical Disabilities*. Missoula, MT: RTC on Rural Rehabilitation.

Statistics Canada (2002). *Participation and Activity Limitation Survey: A Profile of Disability in Canada*. Ottawa: Statistics Canada.

Stein, R.E.K. and Silver, E.J. (2002). Comparing different definitions of chronic conditions in a national data set. *Ambulatory Pediatrics*, 2, 63–70.

Stucki, G. and Cieza, A. (2008). The International Classification of Functioning, Disability and Health (ICF) in physical and rehabilitation medicine. *European Journal of Physical and Rehabilitation Medicine*, 44(3), 299–302.

Stucki, G., Cieza, A., Ewert, T., Kostanjsek, N., Chatterji, S., and Ustun, B. (2002a). Application of the International Classification of Functioning, Disability and Health in clinical practice. *Disability and Rehabilitation*, 24, 281–2.

Stucki, G., Ewert, T., and Cieza, A. (2002b). Value and application of the ICF in rehabilitation medicine. *Disability and Rehabilitation*, 24, 932–8.

Talley, R.C. and Crews, J.E. (2007). Framing the public health of caregiving. *American Journal of Public Health*, 97(2), 224–8.

Tanehaus, R.H., Meyers, A.R., and Harbsion, L.A. (2000). Disability and the curriculum in US graduate schools of public health. *American Journal of Public Health*, 90, 1315.

Traci, M.I., Seekins, T., Szalda-Petree, A., and Ravesloot, C. (2002). Assessing secondary conditions among adults with developmental disabilities: a preliminary study. *Mental Retardation*, 40(2), 119–31.

United Kingdom Public Health Association (2012). *The State of Britain's Health: Poverty and Inequality*. [Online] Available at: http://www.ukpha.org.uk/default.asp?action=article&ID=71&KeyWords=poverty%2Cand%2Cinequality.

United Nations (1982). *World Programme of Action. Resolution 37/52*. New York: UN.

United Nations (1989). *Convention on the Rights of the Child*. New York: UN.

United Nations (1990). *Disability Statistics Compendium*. New York: UN.

United Nations (1993). *Standard Rules on Equalization of Opportunities for Disabled Persons*. New York: UN.

United Nations (2001). *Guidelines and Principles for the Development of Disability Statistics*. Series Y, No. 10. New York: UN.

United Nations (2006a). *Convention on the Rights of Persons with Disabilities*. New York: UN.

United Nations (2006b). *Global Survey on Government Action on the Implementation of the Standard Rules on the Equalization of Opportunities for Persons with Disabilities*. New York: UN.

United Nations (2007). *Convention on the Rights of People with Disabilities*. New York: UN.

United Nations Children's Fund (2008). *Monitoring Child Disability in Developing Countries: Results from the Multiple Indicator Cluster Surveys*. New York: UNICEF.

United Nations Department of Economic and Social Affairs, Population Division (2007). *World Population Ageing 2007*. New York: United Nations Publications.

United Nations Statistics Division (2001). *Workshop Report on Disability Statistics for Africa: Kampala, September 10–14*. New York: UN.

United Nations Statistics Division (2002). Workshop Report on Disability Measurement for ESCWA Countries: Cairo, June 1–5. New York: UN.

United Nations Statistics Division (2012). *Washington Group on Disability Statistics*. [Online] Available at: http://unstats.un.org/unsd/methods/citygroup/washington.htm.

United States Department of Health and Human Services (2006). *Midcourse Review, Healthy People 2010: Disability and Secondary Conditions*. Washington, DC: Department of Health and Human Services.

United States Department of Health and Human Services (2010). Disability and health. In *Healthy People 2020*, Section 6-1. Washington, DC: Department of Health and Human Services.

US Preventive Services Task Force (1996). *Guide to Clinical Preventive Services* (2nd ed.). Alexandria, VA: International Medical Publishing.

Wolfensohn, J.D. (2004). *Disability and Inclusive Development*. Keynote presentation at World Bank Conference, 1 December, Washington, DC.

World Health Organization (1992). *International Classification of Diseases (10th revision)*. Geneva: WHO.

World Health Organization (2001). *International Classification of Functioning, Disability and Health*. Geneva: WHO.

World Health Organization (2007a). *Disability and Rehabilitation Team*. [Online] Available at: http://www.who.int/disabilities/cbr/en.

World Health Organization (2007b). *International Classification of Functioning, Disability and Health—Children and Youth*. Geneva: WHO.

World Health Organization and World Bank (2011). *World Report on Disability*. Geneva: WHO/World Bank.

Yamamoto, N. and Wallhagen, M. (1997). The continuation of family caregiving in Japan. *Journal of Health and Social Behavior*, 38(2), 164–76.

Yeo, R. and Moore, K (2003). Including disabled people in poverty reduction work: 'nothing about us, without us'. *World Development*, 31(3), 571–90.

Yeoh, B.S. and Huang, S. (2010). Foreign domestic workers and home-based care for elders in Singapore. *Journal of Aging & Social Policy*, 22(1), 69–88.

Yeoh, B.S., Huang, S., and Gonzalez, J. (1999). Migrant female domestic workers: debating the economic, social and political impacts in Singapore. *International Migration Review*, 33(1), 114–36.

Health of older people

Julie E. Byles and Meredith A. Tavener

Introduction to health of older people

This chapter considers the phenomenon of population ageing, health needs of older people, and approaches to health and social care. Ageing reflects biological and social processes that occur across the life course, and that affect individuals at different rates. These processes are associated with ageing, but are not synonymous with chronological age. They vary between individuals and according to characteristics such as gender, geographic location, lifestyle, and socioeconomic and ethnic background.

The definition of 'old age' varies across settings, over time, and from person to person. In the past, the United Nations (UN) and other international agencies used 60 years or older (60+) to define 'the elderly', but more recently there is a growing consensus that 65+, or even older ages, should be used. However, people over 65 years of age are not one homogenous group. Indeed, people become more different from one another as they get older. Some people will continue to work well into older age, others will retire early to enjoy leisure activities or work in voluntary capacities, some will cease work to care for frail and dependent relatives or friends, and some will stop working due to their own ill health and disability. As people age, some will age well and with little disability while others will become frail and dependent. It is essential to recognize this heterogeneity in defining needs, designing and evaluating interventions, and planning for the future for this diverse segment of the population.

Older people are sometimes categorized as 'young old' aged 60–69 years, 'old old' aged 70–79 years, and 'oldest old' aged 80 years and over. Further, as more and more people reach older ages, there is increasing interest in studying the needs and characteristics of centenarians and 'super-centenarians' (110+). Alternatively, older people have been considered as being in the 'third age', a period of personal achievement following working life; or being in the 'fourth age', defined as a time of frailty and dependency. At any age there is great variance of experience, capacity, and health status between individuals. The process of ageing is universal but not uniform.

Demographics and projections

The age of the world's population is increasing both structurally and numerically. By 2050, the number of people aged 60 years or older worldwide will exceed the number of people aged 15 years or younger. Worldwide, population ageing is 'unprecedented, without parallel in the history of humanity' (UN Department of Economic and Social Affairs (DESA), Population Division, 2001).

In 2010, there were an estimated 524 million people who were aged 65 years or older worldwide, representing 8 per cent of the total population. This population proportion is projected to rise to 21 per cent in 2050. Also in 2010, the median age of the world population was estimated to be 26 years. The country with the youngest population was Yemen (median 15 years of age), and the country with the oldest population was Japan (median 41 years). By 2050, it is anticipated that the world median age will increase to 36 years, with Spain projected to reach a median age of 55 years (UN DESA, Population Division 2001).

The rapid increase in numbers of people at older ages is shown in Fig. 10.8.1.

Older populations in many low-income countries are growing more rapidly than those in more industrialized countries. Between 2007 and 2009, 81 per cent of the world's net gain of older individuals took place in low-income countries (Kinsella and He 2009). Between now and 2050, the number of older adults in high-income countries is expected to increase by 71 per cent, which is much less than the 250 per cent increase expected for low-income countries (World Health Organization (WHO) et al. 2011). The more developed a country is, the more likely it is that ageing will occur within an affluent environment, with higher levels of overall health resources and healthcare infrastructure. Ageing in lower-income countries can also occur in the context of higher rates of infectious disease, alongside the emergent burden of chronic illness.

Figs. 10.8.2 and 10.8.3 illustrate the age and sex structure of the populations of countries at different stages of development: India and Japan. Japan's population projection is for negative growth, with greater proportions of older women, and a decreasing proportion of the working-age segment. In contrast, India is moving from a very young population profile, towards an older population, although in much lower proportions than in the United States and Japan. The UN Population Division anticipates that India's oldest age group (80 years and older) will triple from 1 to 3 per cent of the overall population (Bloom 2011). It is also projected that India's 60+ population will encompass 323 million people by 2050, which is greater than the current total US population (Bloom 2011). In the United States, by 2050, the 'oldest old' (80+) will include the youngest of the post-war baby boomers, and will represent 7.4 per cent of the entire US population (Kinsella and He 2009).

Determinants of population ageing

The process of population ageing can be considered a major success story, coming largely as a result of reductions in fertility, gains in infant and child survival, and, more recently, to gains in

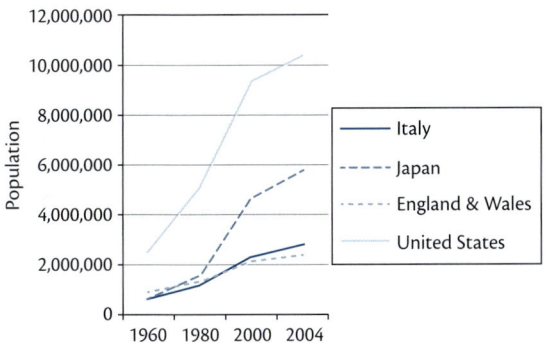

Fig. 10.8.1 Population at advanced ages 80–99 years, as at 1 January, 1960, 1980, 2000 and 2004 for selected countries.

Source: data from Rau, R. et al., Continued reductions in mortality at advanced ages, *Population and Development Review*, Volume 34, Issue 4, pp. 747–68, Copyright © 2008 The Population Council, Inc., with permission from John Wiley & Sons, Inc.

life expectancy at older ages. The earliest observed influence of population ageing occurred in Europe as a result of declines in fertility and childhood mortality. In the United Kingdom, reductions in infant and childhood mortality began in the nineteenth century, and accelerated in the twentieth century initially due to improved living conditions and sanitation, and then to better nutrition, immunization, antitoxins, immune sera, and antibiotics. From the middle of the twentieth century reductions in deaths from heart disease and stroke further extended adult life expectancy. Recently, there have been further mortality declines among advantaged groups (UN DESA, Population Division 2009; WHO et al. 2011). In low-income countries, successful infant and child health programmes (such as growth chart monitoring, oral rehydration for diarrhoea, breastfeeding promotion, and immunization for common infections) are probably responsible for rapid rates of mortality decline at younger ages (UN 2012).

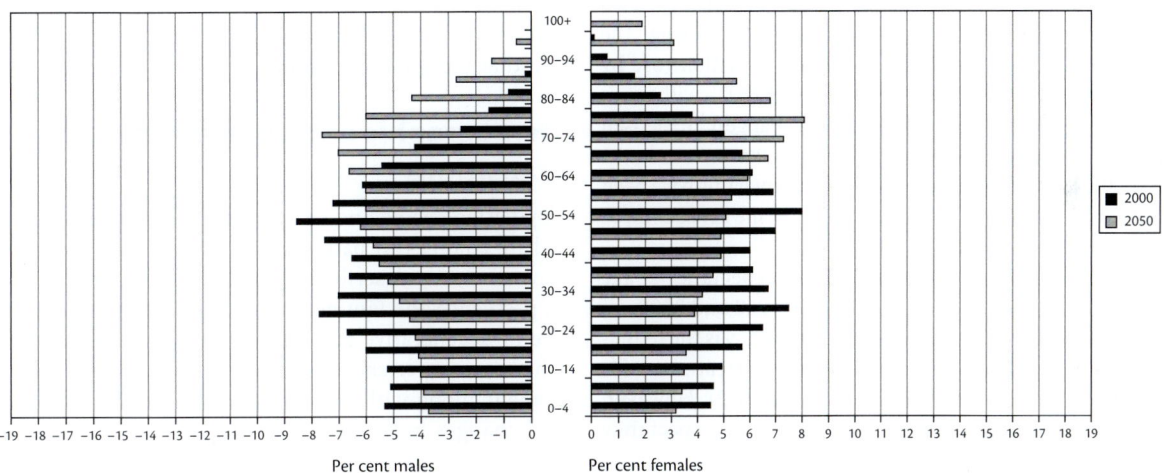

Fig. 10.8.2 Population pyramid for India, showing age and sex structure in 2000 and 2050 projection.

Source: data from United States Census Bureau, *International Data Base*, available from http://www.census.gov/population/international/data/idb/informationGateway.php.

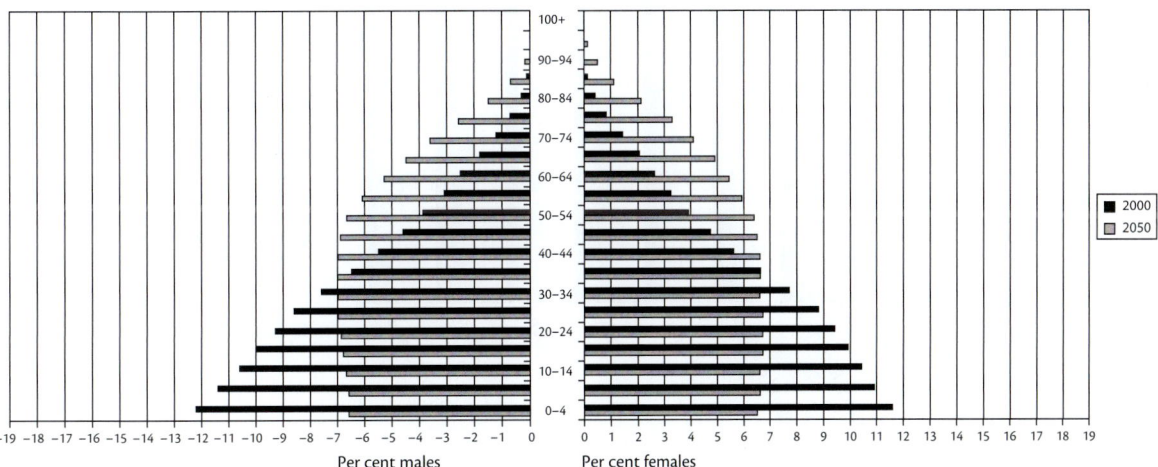

Fig. 10.8.3 Population pyramid for Japan, showing age and sex structure in 2000 and 2050 projection.

Source: data from United States Census Bureau, *International Data Base*, available from http://www.census.gov/population/international/data/idb/informationGateway.php.

Fertility rates have declined dramatically across the world (UN DESA, Population Division 2011). Currently, at least 50 per cent of the world's people live in a region in which fertility rates are below replacement level. In high-income countries with low mortality rates, the replacement rate is based on an average of 2.1 children per woman in the population (UN DESA, Population Division 2011). In 2012, fertility rates were 2.06 in the United States, 1.91 in the United Kingdom, and 1.39 in Japan. The country with the highest fertility rate was Niger (7.16) and the lowest was in Singapore (0.78) (Central Intelligence Agency 2012).

Declines in fertility are attributed to urbanization, industrialization, and social mobility which have all had an influence on family structures (Kinsella and He 2009). In addition, the emancipation of women, their greater chances for education, later age at marriage, and access to contraception have all played a part (Kinsella and He 2009). China's one-child policy has had a dramatic impact on fertility, and has contributed to China's rate of population ageing (Riley 2004).

As fertility rates decline, life expectancy begins to have a greater impact on population ageing. Human life expectancy has increased dramatically over the twentieth century and is still increasing. The highest life expectancy recorded in a national population rose by 3 months per year since 1840 (Oeppen and Vaupel 2002), with more recent data showing no deceleration in this rate of change (Christensen et al. 2009). Also, while early increases in life expectancy were due to reductions in infant and child mortality, more recent gains have been due to better survival in adult life, with increases in life expectancy at age 60 and at age 80 years (Rau et al. 2008).

Fig. 10.8.4 shows the dramatic change in life expectancy at age 80 for men and women in selected countries in 1960 and 2000.

A main influence on improved adult life expectancy is the reduction in smoking, combined with improvements in treatments for cardiovascular disease (Murphy and Di Cesare 2012). However, there is evidence that these trends in increasing life expectancy may not continue, partly because many of the gains from smoking reduction have already been observed (Christensen et al. 2009), and partly because of increases in obesity (Olshansky et al. 2005).

Increases in life expectancy have also not been uniform across the world. Declines in life expectancy have been seen in sub-Saharan Africa, largely due to the impact of AIDS and due to political upheaval (Moser et al. 2005). The impact of HIV/AIDS has been felt strongly in regions such as sub-Saharan Africa, where there has been a decrease in life expectancy from 62 years in 1990–1995 to 49 years in 2005–2010 (UN Joint United Nations Programme on HIV/AIDS, 2002). Countries of Central and Eastern Europe (CEE) (such as the Czech Republic, Hungary, and Poland) demonstrated reduced life expectancies during the 1970s and 1980s; however, life expectancies in these countries improved in the 1990s (Leon 2011). This difference in change in life expectancy reflects the dramatic effects of social, economic, and political upheaval at a societal level, and has also been attributed to high-risk consumption of alcohol, smoking, and poor diet, particularly among males (Leon 2011).

In some populations, international migration has also had a role in changing age (and gender) distributions, but generally migration has had less of an impact than fertility and mortality (Lesthaeghe and Moors 2000).

Demographic and epidemiological transitions

Population ageing and changes in life expectancy are accompanied by changes in patterns of prevalent and incident diseases. Omran (1971) described epidemiological transitions as the age of pestilence and famine, the age of receding pandemics, and the age of degenerative and man-made diseases. Countries such as China are experiencing substantial changes in economic development, along with increasing urbanization, population ageing, and changes in the health profile. Non-communicable diseases,

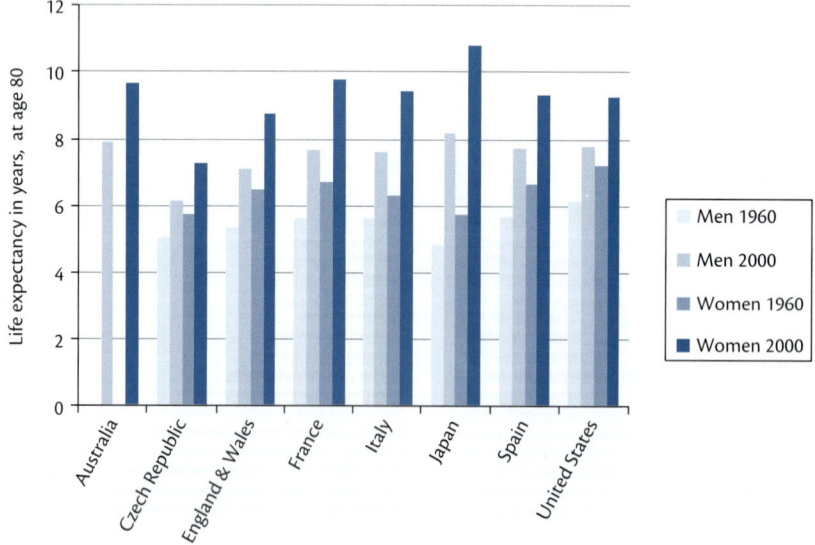

Fig. 10.8.4 Life expectancy at age 80 for men and women, for the years 1960 and 2000, selected countries.
#note: no data available for Australia, 1960.
Source: data from Rau, R. et al., Continued reductions in mortality at advanced ages, *Population and Development Review*, Volume 34, Issue 4, pp. 747–68, Copyright © 2008 The Population Council, Inc., with permission from John Wiley & Sons, Inc.

particularly cardiovascular diseases and cancers, are currently leading causes of morbidity and mortality. Prevailing risk factors include unhealthy diet, physical inactivity, obesity, hypertension, and tobacco use (Li et al. 2012). Similar epidemiological trends have been observed in India and Latin America, and in parts of Africa (WHO 2011). On a global scale, these epidemiological changes are substantial. For example, it is estimated that nearly 15 per cent of the global burden of diabetes is accounted for by 35 million people with diabetes in India (Siegel et al. 2008).

In addition to the rise of non-communicable disease, many rapidly ageing low-income countries are also experiencing high levels of infectious diseases including childhood infections and HIV/AIDS (WHO 2011). HIV infection predominantly affects people aged 15–49 years, but also affects people aged over 50 years. In 2007, an estimated 14 per cent of adults living with HIV in sub-Saharan Africa were aged 50 years and over (Negin and Cumming 2010). HIV also has significant implications for older grandparents and their role as caretakers of children orphaned as a result of parental HIV infection (WHO 2011).

Mortality rates and life expectancy

Mortality rates tend to increase at older ages; however, in recent decades the rate of death has slowed at all ages. Also, at advanced ages (after age 70 or 80), 'old-age mortality deceleration' takes place. The mortality rates of a population can be summarized in a life table which can be used to calculate life expectancy of people at different ages. Life expectancy is the average number of additional years of life that a person at a given age could expect to live, providing age-specific mortality levels remain constant (UN DESA, Population Division 2009).

Table 10.8.1 shows life expectancy at birth and age 60 for males and females in different regions of the world, and for example countries within those regions. In 2009 the highest life expectancy at birth was 86 years among females in Japan, and the lowest was 44 years among males in Malawi (WHO 2012b, table 1). However, for people who achieve 'old age', their life expectancy is greater than life expectancy at birth. In Malawi in 2009, a male who had already lived to 60 could expect to live to 72 years.

Inequalities in life expectancy

Life expectancy varies between countries, and between different population groups within countries. Between-country differences reduced between 1950 and 1990, largely associated with improved access to safe water and sanitation, childhood immunization, improved childhood nutrition, and declining fertility (Hosseinpoor et al. 2012). However, large inequalities in life expectancy still exist. Across low-income group countries, life expectancy remains low at 57 years (WHO 2012b, table 1).

Hosseinpoor et al. (2012) assessed country-specific deviations in life expectancy from the highest attained life expectancy at that time. This measure of inequality showed a shortfall in men's life expectancy of around 19 years during 1950–1955, falling to and around 12 years since 1975–1980. Women tended to have a greater shortfall in life expectancy than men, and shortfalls were greatest in countries with lower incomes. Women in the low-income countries had the biggest difference in life expectancy, with a current shortfall of around 26.7 years (Hosseinpoor et al. 2012).

Table 10.8.1 Life expectancy (LE) at birth and age 60 years, for male and female, selected countries and regions

WHO region	LE at birth, 2009		LE at age 60, 2009	
Country	Male	Female	Male	Female
African Region	**52**	**56**	**14**	**16**
Botswana	59	62	16	18
Malawi	44	51	12	16
South Africa	54	55	15	18
Region of the Americas	**73**	**79**	**21**	**24**
United States of America	76	81	22	25
Brazil	70	77	19	22
South East Asia Region	**64**	**67**	**16**	**18**
Bangladesh	64	66	16	17
Korea (Democratic Republic of)	67	72	16	19
India	63	66	15	17
European Region	**71**	**79**	**19**	**23**
Belgium	77	83	21	25
Czech Republic	74	80	19	23
United Kingdom	78	82	22	25
Eastern Mediterranean Region	**64**	**67**	**16**	**18**
Islamic Republic of Iran	70	75	18	20
Pakistan	63	64	16	17
United Arab Emirates	77	80	20	22
Western Pacific Region	**72**	**77**	**19**	**22**
Australia	80	84	23	26
Cambodia	57	65	14	17
China	72	76	18	21
Japan	80	86	23	29
Papua New Guinea	62	65	15	17

Reproduced with permission from World Health Organization, *World Health Statistics 2012*, pp. 52–61, WHO Library Cataloguing-in-Publication Data (NLM classification: WA 900.1), Copyright © World Health Organization 2012, available from http://www.who.int/gho/publications/world_health_statistics/2012/en/.

Within-country differences in life expectancy are observed according to gender, socioeconomic disadvantage, area of residence, occupation, and cultural groups. For example, Australian Aboriginal and Torres Strait Islander people have a life expectancy approximately 10–14 years less than the overall Australian population (Australian Bureau of Statistics (ABS) 2011). In Canada, men at age 25 have a remaining life expectancy of 55.3 years if they are in the highest income quintile, compared with 48.2 years if they are in the lowest quintile. Life expectancy at age 25 is also shorter among men reporting indigenous ancestry, with remaining life expectancy at age 25 estimated at 46.9 years for Registered Indians, 48.1 years for non-Status Indians, and 48.5 years for Métis (Tjepkema and Wilkins 2011).

Life expectancy is different to maximum life span which is the longest an individual member of a species or group has survived.

While the maximum life span that humans can achieve is widely debated, it is unlikely that we have reached it yet (Vaupel 2010). We are seeing people living longer and longer, and it is expected that many children born since 2000 in countries with high life expectancies will live to at least 100 years (Christensen et al. 2009). On current evidence, it is considered that genetic factors have a modest role in determining how long individuals live, and that most of the increase in human lifespan is due to advances in medicine and public health (Vaupel 2010). Longer lifespans will have great impact on health services and social structures, requiring radical changes to how people learn, work, and care for each other across their lives.

Causes of death at older ages

Table 10.8.2 shows the most common causes of death among people aged 60 years or over. Globally, the most common causes of death for people in this age group are cardiovascular diseases, cancers, and chronic obstructive pulmonary disease. Cardiovascular causes of death include mostly ischaemic heart disease and cerebrovascular disease. Deaths from neuropsychiatric conditions are mostly due to Alzheimer's and other dementias. The majority of accidental deaths among people aged 65 years or over are due to falls (Rubenstein 2006).

In higher-income countries over 90 per cent of deaths among people aged 60 years or over are due to non-communicable diseases (group II), whereas in low-income countries almost 20 per cent in this age group are due to communicable diseases (group I) with most of the remainder due to diseases in group II.

Morbidity and disability

Healthy life expectancy

As the WHO has argued, as well as adding years to life, it is also important to add life to years (WHO 2012a). Healthy life expectancy (or health-adjusted life expectancy (HALE)) estimates

Table 10.8.2 Common causes of death at age 60 years or over for men and women, 2004

Cause of death	% of all male deaths	% of all female deaths
Cardiovascular	42	49
Malignant neoplasms	19	15
Respiratory	12	10
Respiratory infection	6	5
Infectious and parasitic	5	4
Injuries	4	3
Digestive	4	3
Neuropsychiatric	2	3
Genitourinary	2	2
Diabetes and other endocrine	2	4

Reproduced with permission from World Health Organization, *The Global Burden of Disease: 2004 update* (NLM classification: W 74), Copyright © World Health Organization 2008, available from http://www.who.int/healthinfo/global_burden_disease/2004_report_update/en/.

life expectancy, but with adjustment for time spent with a disability and/or other impairment to good health, based on severity-adjusted prevalence by age and sex. Within the context of population ageing, age-associated limitations in performing everyday activities can have substantive effects on demands and costs of healthcare and services. Healthy life expectancy estimations can help answer questions raised regarding whether extra years of life are being spent in poor or good health.

Fig. 10.8.5 presents inequalities in HALE at birth across selected countries. The best HALE is seen in low-mortality countries such as Japan where healthy life expectancy is estimated to be 75 years at birth.

A study of inequalities in life expectancies and healthy life expectancy at 50 years of age for the 25 countries in the European Union found that, on average, a 50-year-old man could expect to live until 67.3 years free of activity limitation (and a woman to 68.1 years). However, there was a great variation in healthy life expectancy between countries, ranging from 9.1 years for men in Estonia to 23.6 years for men in Denmark. There was also a greater variation in healthy life expectancy than for life expectancy. Higher healthy life expectancies were associated with higher gross domestic product, lower unemployment, and with life-long learning (Jagger et al. 2008).

If healthy life expectancy increases relative to life expectancy, then people will spend a greater proportion of their life in good health and 'compression of morbidity' will operate (Fries et al. 1989). If people live longer due to reduction in fatal illness, but with disability due to chronic disease then there will be 'expansion of morbidity'. A third scenario, 'dynamic equilibrium', could occur if the population prevalence of some chronic diseases increases with ageing, but the progression of some degenerative diseases reduces.

Compression of morbidity may be prevailing in some populations. However, data to test this hypothesis are difficult to find and hard to interpret. Very few countries are capable of making reliable assessments over time, between geographic regions or socioeconomic groups. In some settings, there is evidence that the prevalence of disability at older ages may be decreasing, but other studies find an increase in disability (Vaupel 2010). In Denmark, it has been possible to compare the health of centenarians born in 1895–1896 with that of centenarians born in 1905, showing that among women, those in the more recent cohort had slightly better health (Engberg et al. 2008).

In the United Kingdom, both life expectancy and healthy life expectancy have increased over time (Le Grand et al. 2010). Over a 20-year period, life expectancy increased more than healthy life expectancy. Males were expected to live in poor health for an extra 2.2 years, and females for an extra 1.5 years. In contrast, the US Health and Retirement Study has found that successive cohorts of people aged 51–56 are in relatively poorer health, reporting more difficulty with daily tasks, more pain, more chronic conditions, more psychiatric problems, and higher use of alcohol (Soldo et al. 2006).

A recent study which assessed disability trends in 12 Organization for Economic Cooperation and Development (OECD) countries among individuals aged 65 years and over, reported mixed results (Lafortune et al. 2007). Disability declined among elderly people in five out of the 12 countries (Denmark, Finland, the Netherlands, the United States, and Italy). At the same time three countries demonstrated increased rates of severe

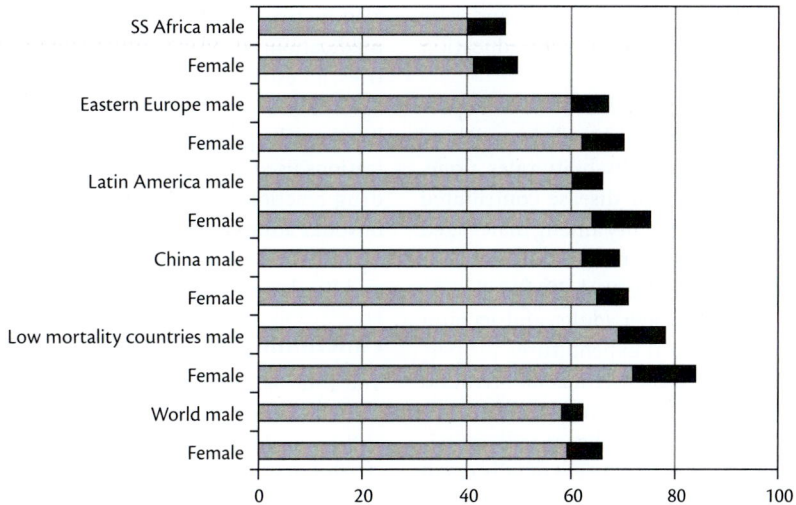

Fig. 10.8.5 Life expectancy and health-adjusted life expectancy at birth, for selected countries.

Adapted from Mathers, C.D. et al., Global patterns of healthy life expectancy in the year 2002, *BMC Public Health*, Volume 4, Issue, pp. 66, Copyright © 2004 Mathers et al.; licensee BioMed Central Ltd. Reproduced under the Creative Commons Attribution 2.0 Generic Licence.

disability (Belgium, Sweden, and Japan), indicating that increased longevity can still lead to increased numbers of older people in poor health and in need of long-term care.

If compression of morbidity is to occur at a population level, greater health promotion and risk reduction activities will be needed for disadvantaged groups that have high levels of health risks. Van Baal et al. (2006) have attempted to estimate HALE for cohorts with different risk factors. Men who were aged 65 years, healthy weight and non-smokers, were likely to live a further 21 years with 16.5 of these years in good health. In contrast, smokers were expected to live 15.4 years with 9.4 years in good health. Preventing smoking is likely to result not only in more years of life, but also more years in good health. Similar effects were also observed for prevention of obesity although the absolute compression of morbidity is small. It is expected that, even if preventive activities were highly successful in reducing or postponing disability, increasing numbers of people living to very old ages means that there will also be greater numbers of people with disabling conditions. At a population level, even if compression of morbidity dominates, there will be increasing needs for health and other care as populations age.

Major causes of morbidity and disability

Worldwide, ischaemic heart disease and cerebrovascular disease and cancers are the leading cause of disability and death combined among people aged 60 years and over (measured by disability-adjusted life years (DALYs)) (see Table 10.8.3).

Other major causes of DALYs include chronic obstructive lung disease, dementias, and cataract (and other vision disorders). Older people are also susceptible to respiratory infections such as pneumonia. In regions where tuberculosis is endemic, older people are particularly vulnerable.

Alzheimer's Disease International (2013) estimate that there are more than 35 million people with dementia worldwide, and that this figure will nearly double every 20 years, passing 115 million in 2005, particularly in developing countries. Women are more

Table 10.8.3 DALYs for males and females aged 60 years and over, 2004

	Males (%)	Females (%)
Cardiovascular	33	34
Cancers	16	12
Sense organ	10	12
Respiratory	10	8
Neuropsychiatric	6	9
Infectious and parasitic	5	4
Respiratory infection	4	3
Digestive	4	3
Injuries	4	3
Diabetes	3	4
Musculoskeletal diseases	2	4
Genitourinary	2	1
Endocrine	1	1
Oral	1	1
Nutritional deficiencies	0	1
Other neoplasm	0	0
Skin diseases	0	0
Congenital	0	0

Reproduced with permission from World Health Organization, *The Global Burden of Disease: 2004 update* (NLM classification: W 74), Copyright © World Health Organization 2008, available from http://www.who.int/healthinfo/global_burden_disease/2004_report_update/en/.

likely to develop dementia than men are, due to their greater longevity. A study of dementia incidence in seven countries (Cuba, the Dominican Republic, Venezuela, Mexico, Peru, China, and India) found an incidence rate of dementia of around 20–30 cases per 1000 person-years. Dementia rates increased with age and were higher in women, and were inversely associated with education levels (Prince et al. 2012).

Musculoskeletal conditions (such as osteoarthritis and osteoporosis) are also common among older people, and tend to contribute to disability more than death. Considering disability rates alone, musculoskeletal disease and cardiovascular disease contributed equally as the most common causes of disability among males aged 65 or over, and musculoskeletal is the single most important contributor to disability burden for women (Klijs et al. 2011).

Falls are a major cause of disability in older adults, and account for an estimated 6 per cent of all medical expenditures for persons aged over 65 in the United States (Rubenstein 2006). Around 30 per cent of older people living in the community will fall each year, and on average, people in residential aged care will experience around two falls per year. Around 5–10 per cent of falls result in serious injuries, and both the risk of falls and the risk of injury from falls increase with age and frailty.

The prevalence of diseases and morbid disorders among older people has increased over time, partly due to earlier diagnosis of diseases such as diabetes and hypertension, but also due to rise of disabling non-fatal conditions such as arthritis (Christensen et al. 2009). Older people are also likely to have more than one condition. Most older adults have a range of active health problems that interact with each other and complicate approaches to treatments. Figures vary from study to study, with prevalence of multimorbidity at age 75 ranging from 3.5 to 98.5 per cent in studies conducted in primary care, from 13.1 to 71.8 per cent in general population samples (Fortin et al. 2012). In one Australian study of men and women aged 70 years and over, the median number of conditions per person was 7.0 (Byles et al. 2005). This state (called multimorbidity or co-morbidity) is important because it is associated with many important health outcomes such as quality of life, activities of daily living, health service utilization, and mortality.

Population statistics often do not recognize the prevalence of co-morbidity among older people. For instance, deaths and DALYs are enumerated according to the underlying cause and contributing causes are often not counted. However, while the recorded cause may be quite specific, the reality is that a number of co-morbid conditions could have caused or contributed to death or disability.

Common conditions affecting older people are associated with a range of functional limitations such as cognitive impairment, mobility restrictions, and urinary incontinence. Urinary incontinence affects 10–30 per cent of older people, and women are affected twice as often as men (Chiarelli et al. 2005). Undernutrition is another problem that commonly underlies and exacerbates many conditions affecting older people, even in countries where food supplies are reliable and plentiful.

Iatrogenic disease

Iatrogenic disease is common in older people, particularly in those taking multiple medications. While medications can be beneficial in management of multiple health problems of older people, they also have the potential to cause serious adverse effects. Older people have reduced volume of distribution for drugs, and slower rates of drug metabolism and elimination, and so are vulnerable to overdose. Reduced physiological reserve renders older people more susceptible to drug toxicity. Also, multiple medications increase the risk of drug–drug interaction. Multiple medicines

also increase medication complexity which can increase risk of medication error and reduce adherence. In high-income countries, an estimated 60–90 per cent of community-dwelling people aged 65 years and over take medications. Over 50 per cent use at least one drug on a regular basis with the average number of medications used ranging from two to five (Byles et al. 2003). Adverse drug reactions have been associated with around 30 per cent of hospital admissions among older people and it is estimated that up to half these adverse reactions could be prevented (Simonson and Feinberg 2005).

Functioning, disability, and health

The International Classification of Functioning, Disability and Health (known as the ICF) recognizes that functioning and disability occur in personal, environmental, and social contexts (Üstun et al. 2003). Using this model, successful ageing includes not only absence of disease, but also capacities in terms of mobility, self-care, and social activities and participation.

Activities of daily living (ADLs) and instrumental activities of daily living (IADLs) describe functional limitations. ADLs are the basic functions of feeding, bathing, dressing, grooming, toileting, bladder control, bowel control, transfer from bed to chair, walking and stair climbing. IADLs are higher-order activities needed to function independently in modern life, including using the telephone, going shopping, cooking meals, housekeeping, doing laundry, using transport, using medications, and managing finances. Disability on ADLs and IADLs increases with age, and is greater in women than in men. Studies of prevalence of disability on ADLs have been undertaken around the world and in different population settings. A study in Malaysia found that around 25 per cent of adults aged 65 years or over reported needing help in at least one ADL item (Hairi et al. 2010). Note, however, that older adults will experience multiple transitions moving in and out of periods of disability and recovery of function (Hardy et al. 2005).

Frailty

Frailty is a term that is commonly used to describe older people who are at risk of poor outcomes due to diminished adaptive reserve. Fried et al. (2001) have developed an operational definition of frailty (frailty phenotype) that includes decreased resiliency and reserve, cycles of decline across multiple systems, negative energy balance, sarcopenia, and decreased strength and exercise tolerance. Symptoms and signs include exhaustion, weight loss, weak grip strength, slow walking pace, and low energy expenditure. Other definitions of frailty, such as the frailty index, include the accumulation of a broader range of limitations and deficits (Lacas and Rockwood 2012). Studies have shown that deficits on the frailty index accumulate exponentially with age, and at any given age, women on average have more deficits than do men. However, women tolerate functional deficits better than men do, and have a lower risk of adverse outcomes in association with scores on the frailty index (Rockwood and Mitnisky 2011).

Mental health in older age

There are a number of reasons to expect that people experience poorer mental health in late life, due partly to psychosocial stressors and loss, but also due to increasing frailty and physical illness. Psychosocial stressors can include bereavement, as well as financial stress, loneliness, isolation, and lack of social support. There is also a theory of terminal decline whereby people with relatively stable mental health throughout life experience sudden onset of psychological morbidity towards the end of life (Gerstorf et al. 2010).

There is a strong correlation between depression and co-morbid physical conditions, and as populations age and chronic disease rates increase, mental health conditions will also rise. Consequently, it is projected that depression will be the second leading cause of global disease burden by the year 2020 (Moussavi et al. 2007).

Perceptions of ageing

Images and stereotypes

'Ageism' was defined in 1969 by US gerontologist Robert Butler as a combination of prejudicial attitudes towards ageing and older people, discriminatory practices against older people, and institutional practices and policies that perpetuate older age stereotypes (Butler 1969). A report by the American Association of Retired Persons concluded that many Americans had misconceptions about ageing and older people, including that they are senile, asexual, and miserable (Abramson and Silverstein 2006). Although some changes have occurred for the better in terms of depictions of ageing, older adults are still generally viewed less favourably than the young.

'Middle age' and 'old age' are subjective concepts based on attributes ascribed by individuals and/or society. Such concepts can influence at which age youth ceases, and the age at which men and women are considered to be 'old'. Age UK reports that 'people aged over 70 are more likely to be seen as stereotypically warm (or friendly) rather than competent' (Abrams et al. 2011). Musaiger and D'Souza (2009) found that women were viewed as 'elderly' when aged in their 40s, but men were viewed more favourably, and were only 'elderly' when aged in their 70s (Musaiger and D'Souza 2009). Across European Social Survey countries, there was a gap of 22 years between when youth was perceived to end, and old age began. The greatest differences in perceived age occurred in Norway where youthful years ended at 33.7 years; and in Greece at 51.7 years. In comparison, old age is perceived to begin at 55.1 in Turkey, and 68.2 years in Greece (Abrams et al. 2011).

Older people's own perceptions

The Growing Old in America report (Taylor et al. 2009) explored 'markers of old age'. The study reported that 'turning 85' was the most commonly endorsed marker of what it meant to be old, with the second and third markers being 'can't live independently' and 'can't drive a car' respectively. Other markers included 'has trouble walking up stairs', 'retires from work', and 'has grey hair'. The English Longitudinal Study of Ageing found that self-assessed health was strongly related to how old individuals felt, with study participants reporting better health, and also feeling younger than their actual age (Demakakos et al. 2007).

Interviews with older adults in Australia reflected acceptance of ageist stereotypes. Participants aged 65 and 89 years described oldness as 'not trying, withdrawn, isolated, irritating, self-oriented, living outside the mainstream, unattractive, uninteresting, frail, senile, silly, over the hill, narrow-minded, a burden, lonely, vulnerable, dowdy, and unproductive' (Minichiello et al. 2000). Such

internalized ageism can be dangerous in that older adults may experience worse functional health and even reduced will to live (Levy et al. 2000). Levy et al. (2002) also found that older individuals who held more positive self-perceptions of ageing (measured over 20 years earlier) lived 7.5 years longer than individuals with less positive self-perceptions of ageing. This advantage remained after accounting for age, gender, socioeconomic status, feeling lonely, and level of functional health.

Within the context of Western societies, where older age is portrayed as negative, individuals born after the Second World War (referred to as 'baby boomers') are said to be challenging old age stereotypes. Popularly portrayed images of baby boomers have them prolonging a lifestyle plateau that involves spending their children's inheritance, enjoying empty nest 'me time' and taking a 'sea change' in retirement. These descriptions fail to account for diversity in the health and social circumstances of these birth cohorts.

Productivity and social contribution

Older people do not need to take part in paid employment to be said to contribute to a community, however, with societal emphasis pointed towards the anticipated demands that the ageing population will make, significant contributions as volunteers, carers and mentors are easily overlooked. Psychologist Erik Erikson warned that later life would consist of a period of unproductive ageing that would last for many years' duration (Erikson et al. 1986). In odds with this are the ageing baby boomers who are predicted to shift the focus away from dependency to an image of active, productive ageing. But what constitutes being productive in older age?

Too often, the use of old-age dependency ratios (whereby the number of persons aged 14 or under and persons aged 65 years or over are contrasted against the number of persons aged 15–64 years) (UN DESA, Population Division 2009), can depict anyone aged 65 years or older as unproductive. Yet, 'many older people continue to make substantial social, economic, and cultural contributions' (Lloyd-Sherlock et al. 2012). In Australia, for example, almost 30 per cent of older people participate in voluntary work (ABS 2007), contributing $2 billion to the economy (National Seniors Productive Ageing Centre 2009). Older people are more likely than younger people to be involved in religious organizations (23 per cent), arts groups (6 per cent) and health organizations (12 per cent), often bearing substantial out-of-pockets costs themselves such as transportation to and from their volunteering activities (Council on the Aged 2008). Warburton and colleagues (2007) report that volunteering is positively associated with good health and well-being in later life, can provide feelings of being productive for those no longer in paid employment, but often goes unrecognized unless it can be quantified and counted.

Childcare is pivotal to the social and economic well-being of families, and grandparents are the largest providers of informal care. Keeping within an Australian context, the contribution of grandparents' care giving labours for grandchildren to the national economy has been estimated at approximately $74.5 billion (Women's Health Australia 2006), with almost one in five children aged 0–11 years (19 per cent) cared for by grandparents (ABS 2005). In addition to providing temporary childcare, some grandparents are also legal guardians of their grandchildren: due to a parent's drug or alcohol problem, relationship breakdown, trauma of some kind, mental or physical illness, or death (ABS 2005). According to the US Census 2000 Supplementary Survey, between 2.3 and 2.4 million grandparents have primary responsibility for raising 4.5 grandchildren (Hayslip and Patrick 2003; US Census Bureau 2003). In Britain, more women aged over 75 years are grandmothers in 2009 than in 1998, and higher levels of childcare are provided by grandmothers than grandfathers.

Contributing to community-based organizations through active membership can benefit both older people and the places where they live. Older people can represent a powerful force for cohesion within a neighbourhood, participating in community councils, local church groups and sports organizations. According to the UK charity organization WRVS, more time is spent by older people in leadership roles (an average of 5 hours a month) than any other age group (WRVS 2011).

Community-based organizations can play a particularly important role in older men's ageing experience, enhancing well-being and social connection beyond paid work. Projects such as *Men's Sheds*, a concept originally developed in Australia, provides space, tools and equipment to men in later life, so that they can feel involved in productive activity. Age UK has piloted its own series of Men's Sheds projects, from 2010 to 2012, evaluating older men's learning as a well-being phenomenon. Later life mentoring and learning can address concerns about older men's poor social participation, particularly in rural areas (Golding et al. 2008), and for Indigenous men, men with limited education, and men from disadvantaged socioeconomic backgrounds (Misan and Sergeant 2009).

Ageing in specific populations

Age and gender

While conditions which affect people at older ages are similar among men and women (except for breast cancer and reproductive cancers), there are differences in the incidence of these conditions and the peak age of onset. For instance, men experience peak incidence of coronary artery disease earlier than women. Lung cancer is more common among men who have had higher rates of smoking, although lung cancer is now the second most common cancer among women, reflecting their increasing smoking habits. Also, while there are few differences on self-rated health, older women have higher rates of functional disability than men: reporting a higher prevalence of arthritis, asthma, depression and cognitive loss.

Women also tend to live longer than men and so are more likely to experience disease and disability associated with advanced age. In 2009, a newborn girl could expect to live to 71 years of age (global average), while a newborn boy could expect to live up to age 66 years (WHO 2012b). Differences in male life expectancy have been partially attributed to health behaviours including a high incidence of alcohol abuse and smoking, leading to high rates of accidents, violence, and cardiovascular disease (Mathers et al. 2004; Leon 2011).

Historical adherence to a male model of health meant that many findings from clinical research were generalized from men to women. For example, protocols for diagnosing and treating heart disease were based upon research with middle-aged, white, male patients. As a result, women were diagnosed later with more advanced disease and had poorer treatment outcomes (Miller 2001).

Women's longevity also means that they are more likely to experience the death of their spouse and to spend a proportion

Table 10.8.4 Older women are far more likely than older men to be widowed

Percentage of those aged 60+ who are widowed, 1985–1997		
Region	Women %	Men %
Africa		
Northern Africa	59	8
Sub-Saharan Africa	44	7
Latin America and the Caribbean		
Caribbean	34	12
Central America	36	12
South America	37	13
Asia		
Eastern Asia	49	14
South Eastern Asia	49	14
Southern Asia	51	11
Central Asia	58	13
Western Asia	48	8
Oceania	44	15
Developed Regions		
Eastern Europe	48	14
Western Europe	40	12
Other developed regions	39	11

Reproduced with permission from, United Nations, Widowhood: Invisible women, secluded or excluded, *Women2000 and Beyond*, December 2001, The World's Women 2000: Trends and Statistics, Copyright © United Nations 2001, available from http://www.un.org/womenwatch/daw/public/wom_Dec%2001%20single%20pg.pdf.

of their older age widowed (see Table 10.8.4), very often with an accompanying loss of social status and reduced economic circumstances. For women aged 60 years or over in Northern Africa, widowhood has been as high as 59 per cent (UN DESA 2001). In parts of Africa, a woman who has been widowed has no rights to owning her late husband's land, leaving her in poverty. Older women are also especially vulnerable in the event of crises such as war, natural disaster, and famine, partly because they generally control fewer economic resources than older men, and also because much of the care of children and other vulnerable people falls to older women.

Gender differences in terms of social roles and human rights will have significant effects on the experience of ageing. For example, during the life course women may be excluded from schooling, receive lower quantities of nutritious food, have no control over household decisions, and receive no health insurance from an employer.

Ageing in rural areas

The majority of the world's population lives in rural areas. As young people leave rural areas to find work, and as older people move into rural areas in retirement, the proportion of older people in rural populations increases; and rural populations can age faster than urban populations. Social infrastructure is also changing in rural areas, with fewer local facilities. Living in rural areas has been associated with economic hardship, poorer quality housing, less access to services, and higher commodity prices (Phillipson and Scharf 2005). However, people in these areas do also report greater social cohesion and higher levels of neighbourhood safety, when compared to people in urban areas.

Ethnic minority elders

Ethnic minority groups can be particularly vulnerable as they age. Within the WHO European Region there are approximately 75 million migrants (8.4 per cent of the total population and 29 per cent of all migrants worldwide) (WHO 2010). Inequities exist in both health of these individuals, and their access to health services. With ethnic minority groups in populations rapidly increasing, health disparities between minority and non-minority older adults have become a significant concern.

In the United Kingdom, for example, data from the Black and Minority Ethnic Elders Study demonstrated that older adults from ethnic minority groups were more likely to report worse health than the white population, particularly those of African/Caribbean or South Asian ethnicity (PRIAE Policy Research Institute on Ageing and Ethnicity 2005). Many older people in these ethnic groups are first-generation immigrants and may have particular issues as they age that relate to migration stress, their reasons for having to leave their country of birth, language limitations, and separation from family members in their country of origin. Within the Netherlands, immigrant elderly are a rapidly growing segment of Dutch society, and have poorer health, potentially due to assimilation to a new living environment, and particularly difficulties in speaking the local language (Denktaş et al. 2009).

Vulnerable older people and elder abuse

The growth of an ageing population worldwide has brought with it the possibility of an increase in the incidence of older people who will experience abuse. Difficulties in identifying abuse persist due to unclear definitions and perceptions of social and cultural contexts in which abuse can occur. The International Network for the Prevention of Elder Abuse and Neglect (INPEA) says that 'Elder abuse is a single, or repeated act, or lack of appropriate action, occurring within any relationship where there is an expectation of trust which causes harm or distress to an older person' (WHO and INPEA 2002).

Elder abuse can take various forms: physical, verbal, psychological/emotional, sexual, and financial. It can also simply reflect intentional or unintentional neglect (Biggs et al. 2009; Sev'er 2009; Acierno et al. 2010). Estimates of the prevalence of elder abuse range from 2 per cent to 27 per cent (Yan and Tang 2004; Naughton et al. 2012). Older women are more likely to be abused than older men (Laumann et al. 2008; Sev'er 2009). Moreover, elder abuse can have serious consequences for the health and well-being of older people, such as depression and being admitted to an aged care home (Lachs et al. 2002), and death.

A longitudinal study conducted by Lachs et al. (1998) found that older persons who were mistreated were three times more likely to die during a 3-year period, compared with those who did not experience abuse (taking into account adjustment for co-morbidity and other factors associated with mortality). At completion of 13-years follow-up, the authors reported that only 9 per cent of those with mistreatment were alive, compared with 41 per cent without mistreatment.

Health and social care for older people

Healthcare planners are often challenged by concerns about increasing demands and rising costs of healthcare in the face of population ageing. People aged 65 years and over tend to have more admissions to hospital than younger people, and they have longer lengths of hospital stay. They also have more visits to doctors and use more medications. However, people aged 65 years and older contribute only modestly to time trends in per capita costs of healthcare compared with the rest of the population, and it has been estimated that population ageing accounts for only a 0.5 per cent annual growth rate of healthcare expenditure (Breyer et al. 2010). It has also been noted that costs of healthcare increase more with proximity to death than with age (Palangkaraya and Yong 2009). Restricting acute and tertiary level services for older people overlooks important benefits that even very old people can gain from appropriate healthcare.

Health promotion for old age

Three stages in promoting healthy old age have been described (Kalachea and Kickbusch 1997). The first is increasing capacity for health in early life and includes good maternal nutrition, and optimizing the development of vital organs such as brain, muscle, bone, and blood vessels during childhood and early adulthood to build resources that may affect later capacity (such as increasing peak bone density to protect against osteoporosis). The second stage occurs in adult life and involves strategies to reduce damage (such as avoiding smoking), to protect against damage (balanced fruit and vegetable focused diet) or to prevent loss through lack of use (such as physical activity). The third stage is in late life and involves minimizing the progression of disease and disability, protecting against increased environmental demands or stresses, and compensating for lost capacity. Examples of these approaches to health promotion include secondary prevention of stroke, rehabilitation, exercise and strength training, social support, correction of deficits in vision and hearing, and modifications to domestic and outdoor environments.

Several key health behaviours are associated with diseases that are common in older age. These associations would suggest that primary prevention approaches are likely to be effective in reducing the incidence of disease at older ages. For example, smoking is a risk factor for cardiovascular disease, stroke, respiratory disease, and many cancers, and smoking prevention is important in reducing the incidence of these conditions, even at older ages. The British Doctors' Study shows that over 7 years of life expectancy are gained by avoiding smoking after the age of 35 years (Doll et al. 2004).

Physical activity is strongly associated with lower rates of cardiovascular disease, depression, and osteoporosis in many observational studies, and some small trials have demonstrated short-term health benefits among older participants. However, older people may find it difficult to maintain high levels of exercise, and encouragement of exercise requires attention to physical environments as well as education of the individual. Neighbourhood factors such as the availability of transport, housing density, pedestrian oriented urban design, and diversity of land use can increase physical activity (Saelens et al. 2003).

Observational studies suggest a clear association between nutrition and health at older ages. For example, the Baltimore Study of Ageing found that men who consumed at least five servings of fruits and vegetables per day and who obtained 12 per cent energy or less from saturated fat had 31 per cent lower all-cause mortality (P < 0.05), and were 76 per cent less likely to die from CHD (P < 0.001) than other men in the study (Tucker et al. 2005). However, dietary intervention studies and studies of vitamin supplementation have not demonstrated significant health benefits (Davey Smith and Ebrahim 2005; Bengmark 2006).

Obesity and overweight are increasing in prevalence and are associated with increased risk of stroke, coronary artery disease, diabetes, arthritis, and some cancers (Popkin 2011). In a review of observational studies, long-term weight loss was also associated with reduced risk of developing diabetes and cardiovascular disease (Avenell et al. 2004).

Social determinants of health

Social inequity is also a major determinant of ill health at all ages (Marmot 2005). Poor circumstances have their first impact during pregnancy, when deficiencies in nutrition, maternal stress, smoking and misuse of drugs and alcohol, insufficient exercise, and inadequate prenatal care can inhibit optimal fetal development. Taking a life course approach to health promotion, poor fetal development is a risk for health in later life. The impact of disadvantage continues throughout childhood and adult life and is manifest in terms of psychosocial stress (which can have both physical and mental health impacts), poor education, poor nutrition, social exclusion, underemployment and poor job security, and work-related stress and injury. Smoking, alcohol, and drug use are higher among people in disadvantaged circumstances. Disadvantaged people also tend to live in poorer neighbourhoods with high rates of violence and crime, in overcrowded circumstances, and potentially in areas with high levels of environmental hazards. Thus while it is useful to highlight behaviours of individuals as risk factors for ill health at later ages, addressing these problems requires that the social circumstances that underpin these behaviours are also understood and improved where possible.

A number of studies have demonstrated an association between social support and improved survival, reduced disability and healthcare use, and improved quality of life (Golden et al. 2009). It is thought that these health effects are mediated through the influence of social support on health behaviour, improved access to care, and possibly through physiological pathways. A systematic review of 30 studies of social support interventions for older people identified some evidence that educational and social activity group interventions that target specific groups can alleviate social isolation and loneliness among older people (Cattan et al. 2005). However, the methods and generalizability of the reported studies varied and more work is required to develop both theoretically sound social support interventions and better methods for evaluating the outcomes of these approaches.

Prevention of specific conditions affecting older people

Cardiovascular diseases, diabetes, and dementia

Many clinical trials provide evidence in support of the effectiveness of drug therapy in primary and secondary prevention of cardiovascular disease (O'Keefe et al. 2009). It has been estimated that the combined effects of six preventative drugs in combination (three low-dose antihypertensives, a statin to lower cholesterol, aspirin, and folic acid) could prevent up to 88 per cent of coronary heart disease and 80 per cent of stroke (Wald and Law 2003a, 2003b). This therapy has been proposed for all people over the age of 55 regardless of cardiovascular risk, but may be more beneficial among older people and people with pre-existing disease among whom the risk:benefit ratio is greater. However, there are many cost and safety issues to consider before universal multi-chemoprophylaxis becomes common practice. Furthermore, a recent review of randomized trials of folate supplementation shows that the anticipated reductions in cardiovascular disease risk have not been achieved, although there is a modest reduction in stroke risk (Durso 2006).

Treatment of diabetes in elderly patients must consider not only the importance of glucose control, but also other health risks and priorities and patient preferences. Life expectancy should also be considered. Control of other risk factors such as lipids and hypertension, as well as glucose control, is also important and may have considerable short-term advantages. For people with shorter life expectancy, long-term control of hyperglycaemia may be less important than in younger patients (Durso 2006). As for many conditions affecting older people, randomized controlled trial evidence is lacking. Observational evidence suggests that intensive control of diabetes mellitus can have favourable effects on microangiopathy (Katakura et al. 2007). Physical activity in people with impaired glucose tolerance has been associated with reduced likelihood of developing diabetes (Bethel and Califf 2007).

There have been many epidemiological studies and randomized clinical trials assessing risk factors for dementia. Most of these identified risk factors are also risk factors for cardiovascular disease and stroke. However, there is currently no evidence that modifying these risk factors, or other interventions, will reduce the onset of dementia, although they will have benefits in reducing overall vascular disease risk (Román et al. 2012), and may have a small effect on cognitive decline (Dehnel 2013).

Falls and fractures

Numerous modifiable risk factors for falls and osteoporosis have been identified. However, reduction of fall-related injury at a population level requires that preventive activities become embedded within everyday social functions and physical structures (McClure et al. 2005). A number of interventions have been shown to reduce the risk of falls, including health/environment risk factor screening/intervention programmes, muscle strengthening and balance retraining, and home hazard assessment and modification (Gillespie et al. 2012). Multifactorial falls prevention programmes have been shown to be effective in reducing falls in community-dwelling older people, and for older people with a history of falling. Important components include group or home-based exercise (including t'ai chi), individual risk assessment, home safety assessment and modification

Vitamin D has not been shown to reduce falls among community-dwelling people, but may be important among people with lower vitamin D levels, and may prevent falls and fractures (including hip fracture) among people living in institutional care (Avenell et al. 2009). There is evidence that bisphosphonates improve bone density and reduce osteoporotic fractures (Cranney et al. 2002). Hormone replacement therapy (HRT) may also reduce fractures; however, recent studies show increased risk of cardiovascular disease and breast cancer and so HRT is not currently recommended for fracture prevention (Writing Group for the Women's Health Initiative 2002).

Preventive activities in primary care

Immunization

Vaccination of community-dwelling older people may be a cost-effective way to prevent hospitalization for influenza or pneumonia and deaths. However, much of the evidence for vaccination in the elderly comes from observational studies and may reflect other differences between vaccinated and non-vaccinated groups (Jefferson et al. 2010).

Medication review

Some studies have shown medication review to be beneficial for older people living in the community, for example, Zermansky et al. (2002), but other studies did not find any effect of medication review on medicines use (Allard et al. 2001; Sellors et al. 2003). One large Australian randomized controlled trial demonstrated a positive effect on medication use and a reduced incidence of falls 12 months after medication review (Pit et al. 2007).

Health assessments, case finding, and screening

Reviews of evidence for prevention-based assessment programmes for older people have come to varying conclusions, but a recent review indicates that assessments have some positive effects to reduce disability burden among older adults when based on multidimensional assessment with clinical examination (Huss et al. 2008). This review also found differences between studies in content and duration of assessments and length of follow-up. The effectiveness of assessments may depend on multiple follow-ups, and benefits may be most pronounced for the 'young-old' (under 78 years) and for those with a low risk of death (Huss et al. 2008).

Many cancer screening programmes for younger people are not promoted for older people. For instance, breast cancer screening is encouraged for women aged 40–70 (US Preventive Services Task Force 2010). Evidence for ceasing screening after age 70 is not clear since few mammography screening trials enrolled women older than 69 and no trials enrolled women older than 74. The incidence of breast cancer increases with age, but the benefits of screening may be outweighed by competing morbidities among older women. Screening for cervical cancer is not recommended for women over the age of 70 years if they have had three normal Pap smears in the past 10 years (US Preventive Services Task Force 2012). The incidence of cervical cancer decreases at older ages, and so screening older women has low yield. Also, in Western countries, many women have had a hysterectomy and do not require cervical screening. Screening for colorectal cancer is recommended for adults over the age of 50 and up to the age of 80 years depending on the person's health and co-morbidities (US Preventive Services Task Force 2009). While there is limited evidence of benefit of screening for oral cancer, assessment of the mouth, teeth, and gums is helpful for older people with cognitive impairment and who may have conditions that limit chewing, swallowing and communication (National Guideline Clearinghouse 2011).

Reablement

Even among frail older people with chronic illness, it is possible to improve independence and health status through restorative approaches to care that help people re-learn or develop new skills to manage illness and participate in daily activities. These approaches not only benefit the older person and their families, but are seen as the main strategy for addressing increasing demands for aged care. Available evidence suggests that a restorative approach to home care can be cost-effective in reducing demand for ongoing services (Ryburn et al. 2009).

Systems of care

There are many strategies that enable people to successfully manage existing specific conditions and live a normal life. Quality care for chronic diseases to prevent complications and to compensate for functional impairment is essential for optimizing health and quality of life for older people. Further, since the health needs of older people are complex, their care should be multidisciplinary and include older people as partners in their own health management. New healthcare technologies such as e-health systems provide opportunity for wider involvement of health professionals, families, and individuals.

Primary care

Primary care is considered to be of great importance in reducing healthcare inequalities and in improving the quality and outcomes of healthcare among older people. However, care for older people is central to the prevailing medical model. It is essential that the needs of growing numbers of older people are reflected in healthcare provision by examining common health problems seen among older people in primary care and matching provider training to meeting these needs. There is a risk that older people will simply receive an increasing number of medications for each of their symptoms with increasing risk of an adverse reaction, and potentially diagnosable and treatable problems will be missed.

Hospital services

Older people presenting to hospital tend to be sicker, present with more urgent conditions, and have more co-morbid diseases and medications, than young people (Bridges et al. 2004). Cardiopulmonary disorders are among the most common medical reasons for presentation, and fall-related injury is the most common surgical emergency among older people presenting to emergency departments. Adverse drug-related events (unfavourable medical events related to medication use or misuse) account for around 10 per cent of emergency department visits, the most frequently implicated medications being non-steroidal anti-inflammatory drugs, antibiotics, anticoagulants, diuretics, hypoglycaemics, beta blockers, calcium channel blockers, and chemotherapeutic agents.

Older patients tend to have complex health problems and longer length of stay than younger patients. The discipline of geriatric medicine has evolved to meet these needs, and specialist geriatric units now exist within major hospitals. A systematic review shows positive effects of hospital geriatric evaluation and management units on mortality, place of discharge, and change in functional status (Ellis et al. 2011).

Disease-specific services

Specialist services for patients suffering stroke have been evaluated in randomized controlled trials and meta-analysis, and appear to reduce mortality, disability, and institutionalization by about 20 per cent at 12 months. These units have been adopted in high-income countries, but also have the potential to substantively improve stroke outcome in low- and middle-income countries. Similar models have also been applied for management of diabetes, respiratory disease, and cardiovascular disease (Gentles and Potter 2001). Specialist services for fractured neck of femur patients (orthogeriatric services) have also been examined in small randomized controlled trials with pooled effects showing a non-significant trend towards improved survival and less dependence (Langhorne et al. 2012).

Health services for people with dementia have followed a trend of moving out of institutional care and into the community (Hilton and Jolley 2012). Multidisciplinary specialist care includes integration of specialist medical approaches with psychosocial care and support for informal caregivers.

Hospital at home and day services, rehabilitation, and transitional care

'Hospital at home' and early discharge schemes have been promoted in efforts to reduce demand on acute hospital services. A review of 22 trials evaluating early-discharge hospital at home schemes found little evidence of benefit or costs savings. However, early discharge schemes for older patients may reduce the pressure on acute hospital beds (Shepperd et al. 2009).

There is an increasing demand for rehabilitation for older people. Traditionally this process has occurred in hospital or other institutional settings, but more recently community-based rehabilitation options have been explored. Where countries lack investment in hospital services for elderly people, community-based rehabilitation offers an alternative model that requires evaluation. Many studies have been undertaken to evaluate this approach to rehabilitation, but these studies have not been considered adequate to provide evidence of its effectiveness (Ward et al. 2008).

Long-term care

A common approach to population ageing has been to establish institutional care, despite its costs and very limited accessibility for a majority of elderly people. In Egypt, for example, the number of aged care institutions has more than doubled over the past 20 years (Boggatz and Dassen 2005).

At any one time, the majority of older people will not live in institutions, but many will require some form of long-term care during the course of their life. In high-income countries there is a trend towards care being increasingly provided in community settings. Care in the community is now the preferred and most common care arrangement and there has been a reduction in the numbers of people in institutional care, despite the ageing of the population.

Future need for long-term care will be determined by demographic trends, the relationship between age and disability, the extent to which community care permits people to stay at home, and the willingness of relatives to provide continued unpaid help. Most of these factors will result in more rather than less need for long-term institutional care. In many countries, current levels of provision will be inadequate to meet future needs, placing increasing demands on other health services such as acute hospitals.

Informal care and social support

Within the context of an ageing population, the role of informal carer is paramount, but may be socially and politically invisible. Within the United States, the contributions of informal carers represent an important component of the US economy, with an estimated annual economic value of approximately $350 billion, which is more than four times the total amount spent on formal (paid) care services (Gibson and Houser 2007). A report released by Carers Australia in 2010 showed that the value of informal care rose by 33 per cent, between 2005 and 2010, to exceed $40 billion per annum (Access Economics 2010).

Many people providing care for older people will themselves be old. UK census data show that females provide more hours of informal care than males. People aged over 65 years provide more informal care than young carers and the number of hours of care provided is similar for those elders in good, fair, or poorer health (Doran et al. 2003).

While both caregivers and care recipients generally regard home-based care as preferable to institutionalization, caregiving can be physically and emotionally taxing (Schultz and Matire 2004). Lee and Porteous (2002) found that middle-aged women providing care were less likely to be in full-time employment and they had worse physical and mental health and higher levels of stress than other women. They were less likely to be within a healthy weight range, were more likely to use medications for sleeping difficulty or depression, and had lower life satisfaction scores and higher depression scores. When women gave up their caring roles, they reported fewer visits to their general practitioner and less use of medications for nerves than current caregivers. In many cases, people who took on caring were already in poor health themselves. Legg et al. (2013) analysed data from 44,465,833 individuals free from permanent sickness or disability, of whom 5,451,902 (12.3 per cent) reported providing informal care. They reported an association between provision of care and self-reported poor health, after accounting for age, sex, ethnicity, marital status, economic activity, and education. The association also increased with the amount of care provided (Legg et al. 2013).

The tradition of family support for older people is changing in many countries as a result of economic and political conditions, women's increased participation in paid work, and where diseases such as AIDS have affected middle-aged adults leaving older people and children without support. In China, where filial piety is a traditional value, family responsibility for older people is made explicit in policy and is incorporated into the marriage contract (Zavoretti 2006). Even so, economic development, urbanization, and demographic transition are having an impact on intergenerational support. We must ensure that the important role of unpaid care is recognized as a high priority, and that the needs of informal carers are taken into account in planning and allocating resources.

Age-friendly cities

The WHO promotes the goal of age-friendly cities that support older people, by optimizing opportunities for health, participation, and security. By 2030, two-thirds of the world's population will live in cities, and in these cities around one in every four people will be aged 60 years or over. Environments for older people need to consider not only design and physical features, but also infrastructure, policies, and service provision. Aspects to be addressed include housing, transport, pedestrian safety, safety from violence and crime, opportunities for employment, and social involvement of older people. Many older people may not drive a motor vehicle, or may lose their ability to drive. Older people also have more difficulty with public transport and are vulnerable as pedestrians. In Manhattan, United States, for example, almost 50 per cent of pedestrian fatalities occurred among the 17 per cent of the city aged 60 and over. Older people are also particularly vulnerable to environmental changes including heat waves, which are increasingly common in urban environments (Buffel et al. 2012).

Public health implications of population ageing

As seen in this chapter, population ageing is a global phenomenon that will have a major impact on disease and disability patterns and on health service use. A coordinated and appropriate public health response is essential if this phenomenon is to translate into an opportunity for longevity and healthy ageing, rather than a threat to global health and resources. Public health is important in monitoring trends and transition in risk factors, disease and disability, encouraging effective health promotion practices, and in setting policy for equitable and efficient use of healthcare resources for this growing population. Health promotion for older age begins in early life and continues throughout life to the oldest age. Much more knowledge is needed as to how we can optimize the conditions and experiences of ageing. Recognition of the contributions made by older people themselves to their families and communities and national wealth is also of fundamental importance in meeting the challenges of an ageing population and in meeting the health needs of increasing numbers of older people.

Summary

◆ Ageing is universal, but not uniform.

◆ Population ageing is occurring at far greater rates in low- and middle-income countries than in high-income countries, and will place considerable strains on health and social care sectors.

◆ Increased longevity has not been experienced uniformly across socioeconomic groups or in different countries.

◆ Severe disability is becoming less common in successive cohorts of older people indicating that a compression of morbidity and disability is occurring.

◆ Health services for older people have had dramatic effects in improving survival and reducing disability associated with the inevitable increases in chronic diseases at older ages.

◆ Families in all countries provide a major part of the care needed by older people but do require knowledge and support of formal health and social services.

◆ Public health has major roles in surveillance, prevention, and development of services for older people.

References

Abrams, D., Russell, P., Vauclair, C.-M., and Swift, H. (2011). *Ageism in Europe. Findings from the European Social Survey. A Report from EURAGE (European Research Group on Attitudes to Age)*. London: Age UK.

Abramson, A. and Silverstein, M. (2006). *AARP Images of Aging in America, 2004*. Washington, DC: AARP and the University of Southern California.

Access Economics (2010). *The Economic Value of Informal Care in 2010. Report for Carers Australia, October 2010*. Canberra: Access Economics.

Acierno, R., Hernandez, M.A., Amstadter, A.B., et al. (2010). Prevalence and correlates of emotional, physical, sexual, and financial abuse and potential neglect in the United States: The National Elder Mistreatment Study. *American Journal of Public Health*, 100(2), 292–7.

Allard, J., Hébert, R., Rioux, M., Asselin, J., and Voyer, L. (2001). Efficacy of a clinical medication review on the number of potentially inappropriate prescriptions prescribed for community-dwelling elderly people. *Canadian Medical Association Journal*, 164(9), 1291–6.

Alzheimer's Disease International (2013). *Dementia Statistics*. [Online] Available at: http://www.alz.co.uk/research/statistics.

Australian Bureau of Statistics (2005). *Australian Social Trends, 2005. 4102.0*. Canberra: ABS.

Australian Bureau of Statistics (2007). *Voluntary Work, Australia, 2006. 4441.0*. Canberra: ABS.

Australian Bureau of Statistics (2011). *Deaths, Australia, 2010*. Canberra: ABS.

Avenell, A., Broom, J., Brown, T., et al. (2004). Systematic review of the long-term effects and economic consequences of treatments for obesity and implications for health improvement. *Health Technology Assessment*, 8(21), 1–182.

Avenell, A., Gillespie, W., Gillespie, L., and O'Connell, D. (2009). Vitamin D and vitamin D analogues for preventing fractures associated with involutional and post-menopausal osteoporosis. *Cochrane Database of Systematic Reviews*, 2, CD000227.

Bengmark, S. (2006). Curcumin an atoxic antioxidant and natural NF-κB, COX-2, LOX and iNOS inhibitor—a shield against acute and chronic diseases. *Journal of Parenteral & Enteral Nutrition*, 30, 45–51.

Bethel, M.A. and Califf, R.M. (2007). Role of lifestyle and oral anti-diabetic agents to prevent type 2 diabetes mellitus and cardiovascular disease. *The American Journal of Cardiology*, 99(5), 726–31.

Biggs, S., Manthorpe, J., Tinker, A., Doyle, M., and Erens, B. (2009). Mistreatment of older people in the United Kingdom: findings from the First National Prevalence Study. *Journal of Elder Abuse & Neglect*, 21(1), 1–14.

Bloom, D.E. (2011). *Population Dynamics in India and Implications for Economic Growth*. Boston, MA: Program for the Global Demography for Aging (PGDA), Harvard School of Public Health.

Boggatz, T. and Dassen, T. (2005). Ageing, care dependency, and care for older people in Egypt: a review of the literature. *Journal of Clinical Nursing*, 14, 56–63.

Breyer, F., Costa-Font, J., and Felder, S. (2010). Ageing, health, and health care. *Oxford Review of Economic Policy*, 26(4), 674–90.

Bridges, J., Meyer, J., Dethick, L., and Griffiths, P. (2004). Older people in accident and emergency: implications for UK policy and practice. *Reviews in Clinical Gerontology*, 14(01), 15–24.

Buffel, T., Phillipson, C., and Scharf, T. (2012). Ageing in urban environments: developing 'age-friendly' cities. *Critical Social Policy*, 32, 597–619.

Butler, R. (1969). Age-ism: another form of bigotry. *The Gerontologist*, 9, 243–6.

Byles, J., Heinze, R., Balakrishnan, R., and Parkinson, L. (2003). Medication use among older Australian veterans and war widows. *Internal Medicine Journal*, 33, 388–91.

Byles, J.E., D'Este, C., Parkinson, L., O'Connell, R., and Treloar, C. (2005). Single index of multimorbidity did not predict multiple outcomes. *Journal of Clinical Epidemiology*, 58(10), 997–1005.

Cattan, M., White, M., Bond, J., and Learmouth, A. (2005). Preventing social isolation and loneliness among older people: a systematic review of health promotion interventions. *Ageing & Society*, 25(1), 41–67.

Central Intelligence Agency (CIA) (2012). *The World Factbook. Country Comparisons, Total Fertility Rate* [Online]. Available at: https://www.cia.gov/library/publications/the-world-factbook/rankorder/2127rank.html.

Chiarelli, P., Bower, W., Attia, J., Sibbritt, D., and Wilson, A. (2005). The prevalence of urinary and faecal incontinence in the community: a systematic review. *Australasian Journal on Ageing*, 24, 19–27.

Christensen, K., Doblhammer, G., Rau, R., and Vaupel, J.W. (2009). Ageing populations: the challenges ahead. *The Lancet*, 374, 1196–208.

Council on the Aged (2008). *COTA Over 50s, The Voice of Older Australians, Policy Compendium, August 2008*. Adelaide: National Policy Office, COTA.

Cranney, A., Wells, G., Willan, A., et al. (2002). II. Meta-analysis of alendronate for the treatment of postmenopausal women. *Endocrine Reviews*, 23(4), 508–16.

Davey Smith, G. and Ebrahim, S. (2005). Folate supplementation and cardiovascular disease. *The Lancet*, 366(9498), 1679–81.

Dehnel, T. (2013). The European Dementia Prevention Initiative. *The Lancet Neurology*, 12(3), 227–8.

Demakakos, P., Gjonca, E., and Nazroo, J. (2007). Age identity, age perceptions and health. *Annals of the New York Academy*, 1114, 279–87.

Denktaş, S., Koopmans, G., Birnie, E., Foets, M., and Bonsel, G. (2009). Ethnic background and differences in health care use: a national cross-sectional study of native Dutch and immigrant elderly in the Netherlands. *International Journal for Equity in Health*, 8, 35.

Doll, R., Peto, R., Boreham, J., and Sutherland, I. (2004). Mortality in relation to smoking: 50 years' observations on male British doctors. *British Medical Journal*, 328(7455), 1519.

Doran, T., Drever, F., and Whitehead, M. (2003). Health of young and elderly informal carers: analysis of UK census data. *British Medical Journal*, 327(7428), 1388.

Durso, S. (2006). Using clinical guidelines designed for older adults with diabetes mellitus and complex health status. *Journal of the American Medical Association*, 295(16), 1935–40.

Ellis, G., Whitehead, M.A., Robinson, D., O'Neill, D., and Langhorne, P. (2011). Comprehensive geriatric assessment for older adults admitted to hospital: meta-analysis of randomised controlled trials. *British Medical Journal*, 343, d6553.

Engberg, H., Christensen, K., Andersen-Ranberg, K., Vaupel, J.W., and Jeune, B. (2008). Improving activities of daily living in Danish centenarians – but only in women: a comparative study of two birth cohorts born in 1895 and 1905. *The Journals of Gerontology*, 63A(11), 1186–92.

Erikson, E.H., Erikson, J.M., and Kivnick, H.Q. (1986). *Vital Involvement in Old Age*. New York: WW Norton & Company.

Fortin, M., Stewart, M., Poitras, M.-E., Almirall, J., and Maddocks, H. (2012). A systematic review of prevalence studies on multimorbidity: toward a more uniform methodology. *The Annals of Family Medicine*, 10(2), 142–51.

Fried, L.P., Tangen, C.M., Walston, J., et al. (2001). Frailty in older adults: evidence for a phenotype. *The Journals of Gerontology*, 56A(3), M146–56.

Fries, J., Green, L., and Levine, S. (1989). Health promotion and the compression of morbidity. *The Lancet*, 333(8636), 481–3.

Gentles, H. and Potter, J. (2001). Alternatives to acute hospital care. *Reviews in Clinical Gerontology*, 11(4), 373–8.

Gerstorf, D., Ram, N., Mayraz, G., et al. (2010). Late-life decline in well-being across adulthood in Germany, the United Kingdom, and the United States: something is seriously wrong at the end of life. *Psychology and Ageing*, 25(2), 477–85.

Gibson, M. and Houser, A. (2007). *Valuing the Invaluable: A New Look at the Economic Value of Family Caregiving*. Issue Brief June 2007, IB-82. Washington, DC: AARP Public Policy Institute.

Gillespie, L., Robertson, M., Gillespie, W., et al. (2012). Interventions for preventing falls in older people living in the community. *Cochrane Database of Systematic Reviews*, 9, CD007146.

Golden, J., Conroy, R.M., and Lawlor, B.A. (2009). Social support network structure in older people: underlying dimensions and association with psychological and physical health. *Psychology, Health & Medicine*, 14(3), 280–90.

Golding, B., Kimberley, H., Foley, A., and Brown, M. (2008). Houses and sheds in Australia: an exploration of the genesis and growth of neighbourhood houses and men's sheds in community settings. *Australian Journal of Adult Learning*, 48(2), 237–62.

Hairi, N.N., Bulgiba, A., Cumming, R., Naganathan, V., and Mudla, I. (2010). Prevalence and correlates of physical disability and functional limitation among community dwelling older people in rural Malaysia, a middle income country. *BMC Public Health*, 10, 492.

Hardy, S.E., Dubin, J.A., Holford, T.R., and Gill, T.M. (2005). Transitions between states of disability and independence among older persons. *American Journal of Epidemiology*, 161(6), 575–84.

Hayslip, B. and Patrick, J. (eds.). (2003). *Working with Custodial Grandparents*. New York: Springer.

Hilton, C. and Jolley, D. (2012). Coming of age: reflections on old age psychiatry as a specialty in the National Health Service, 1989–2010. *International Psychogeriatrics*, 24(07), 1023–5.

Hosseinpoor, A., Harper, S., Lee, J., Lynch, J., Mathers, C., and Abou-Zahr, C. (2012). International shortfall inequality in life expectancy in women and men, 1950–2010. *Bulletin of the World Health Organization*, 90, 588–94.

Huss, A., Stuck, A.E., Rubenstein, L.Z., Egger, M., and Clough-Gorr, K.M. (2008). Multidimensional geriatric assessment: back to the future multidimensional preventive home visit programs for community-dwelling older adults: a systematic review and meta-analysis of randomized controlled trials. *The Journals of Gerontology Series A: Biological Sciences and Medical Sciences*, 63(3), 298–307.

Jagger, C., Gillies, C., Moscone, F., et al. (2008). Inequalities in healthy life years in the 25 countries of the European Union in 2005: a cross-national meta-regression analysis. *The Lancet*, 372(9656), 2124–31.

Jefferson, T., Di Pietrantonj, C., Al-Ansary, L.A., Ferroni, E., Thorning, S., and Thomas, R.E. (2010). Vaccines for preventing influenza in the elderly. *Cochrane Database of Systematic Reviews*, 2, CD004876.

Kalachea, A. and Kickbusch, I. (1997). A global strategy for healthy ageing. *World Health*, 50(4), 4–5.

Katakura, M., Naka, M., Kondo, T., et al. (2007). Development, worsening, and improvement of diabetic microangiopathy in older people: six-year prospective study of patients under intensive diabetes control. *Journal of the American Geriatrics Society*, 55(4), 541–7.

Kinsella, K. and He, W. (2009). *US Census International Population Reports. An Ageing World: 2008*. Washington, DC: US Census Bureau.

Klijs, B., Nusselder, W., Looman, C., and Mackenbach, J. (2011). Contribution of chronic disease to the burden of disability. *PLoS ONE*, 6(9), e25325.

Lacas, A. and Rockwood, K. (2012). Frailty in primary care: a review of its conceptualization and implications for practice. *BMC Medicine*, 10, 4.

Lachs, M., Williams, C., O'Brien, S., Pillemer, K., and Charlson, M. (1998). The mortality of elder mistreatment. *Journal of the American Medical Association*, 280(5), 428–32.

Lachs, M.S., Williams, C.S., O'Brien, S., and Pillemer, K.A. (2002). Adult protective service use and nursing home placement. *Gerontologist*, 42(6), 734–9.

Lafortune, G., Balestat, G., and the Disability Study Expert Group Members (2007). *Trends in Severe Disability Among Elderly People: Assessing Evidence in 12 OECD Countries and Future Implications*. Paris: OECD.

Langhorne, P., de Villiers, L., and Pandian, J.D. (2012). Applicability of stroke-unit care to low-income and middle-income countries. *The Lancet*, 11(4), 341–8.

Laumann, E., Leitsch, S., and Waite, L. (2008). Elder mistreatment in the United States: prevalence estimates from a nationally representative study. *The Journals of Gerontology B: Psychological Sciences and Social Sciences*, 63(4), S248–54.

Lee, C. and Porteous, J. (2002). Experiences of family caregiving among middle-aged Australian women. *Feminism & Psychology*, 12(1), 79–96.

Legg, L., Weir, C.J., Langhorne, P., Smith, L.N., and Stott, D.J. (2013). Is informal caregiving independently associated with poor health? A population-based study. *Journal of Epidemiology and Community Health*, 67, 95–7.

Le Grand, J., Sherriff, R., Griffin, M., Srivastava, D., and Sinclair, D. (2010). *HALE One Hundred: Towards 100 Healthy and Active Years*. A Report for Health England, No.6, 2010. Oxford: Health England.

Leon, D.A. (2011). Trends in European life expectancy: a salutary view. *International Journal of Epidemiology*, 40(2), 271–7.

Lesthaeghe, R. and Moors, G. (2000). Recent trends in fertility and household formation in the Industrialised World. *Review of Population and Social Policy*, 9, 121–70.

Levy, B., Ashman, O., and Dror, I. (2000). To be or not to be: the effects of aging stereotypes on the will to live. *Omega: Journal of Death and Dying*, 40, 409–20.

Levy, B., Slade, M., Kunkel, S., and Kasl, S. (2002). Longevity increased by positive self-perceptions of aging. *Journal of Personality and Social Psychology*, 83(2), 261–70.

Li, L., Guo, Y., Chen, Z., Chen, J., and Peto, R. (2012). Epidemiology and the control of disease in China, with emphasis on the Chinese Biobank Study. *Public Health*, 126(3), 210–13.

Lloyd-Sherlock, P., McKee, M., Ebrahim, S., et al. (2012). Population ageing and health. *The Lancet*, 379(9823), 1295–6.

Marmot, M. (2005). Social determinants of health inequalities. *The Lancet*, 365, 1099–104.

Mathers, C.D., Iburg, K.M., Salomon, J.A., et al. (2004). Global patterns of healthy life expectancy in the year 2002. *BMC Public Health*, 4, 66.

McClure, R., Turner, C., Peel, N., Spinks, A., Eakin, E., and Hughes, K. (2005). Population-based interventions for the prevention of fall-related injuries in older people. *Cochrane Database of Systematic Reviews*, 1, CD004441.

Miller, M.A. (2001). Gender-based differences in the toxicity of pharmaceuticals – the Food and Drug Administration's perspective. *International Journal of Toxicology*, 20, 149–52.

Minichiello, V., Browne, J., and Kendig, H. (2000). Perceptions and consequences of ageism: views of older people. *Ageing and Society*, 20, 253–78.

Misan, G. and Sergeant, P. (2009). *Men's Sheds – A Strategy to Improve Men's Health*. Paper presented at the 10th National Rural Health Conference, 17–20 May 2009, Cairns, Queensland, Australia.

Moser, K., Shkolnikov, V., and Leon, D.A. (2005). World mortality 1950–2000: divergence replaces convergence from the late 1980s. *Bulletin of the World Health Organization*, 83, 202–9.

Moussavi, S., Chatterji, S., Verdes, E., Tandon, A., Patel, V., and Ustun, B. (2007). Depression, chronic diseases, and decrements in health: results from the World Health Surveys. *The Lancet*, 370(9590), 851–8.

Murphy, M. and Di Cesare, M. (2012). Use of an age-period-cohort model to reveal the impact of cigarette smoking on trends in twentieth-century adult cohort mortality in England and Wales. *Population Studies*, 66, 259–77.

Musaiger, A. and D'Souza, R. (2009). Role of age and gender in the perception of aging: a community-based survey in Kuwait. *Archives of Gerontology and Geriatrics*, 48(1), 50–7.

National Guideline Clearinghouse (2011). *Oral Hygiene Care for Functionally Dependent and Cognitively Impaired Older Adults. Update*. [Online] Available at: http://guidelines.gov/content.aspx?id=34447.

National Seniors Productive Ageing Centre (2009). *Still Putting In: Measuring the Economic and Social Contributions of Older Australians*. Canberra: NSPAC.

Naughton, C., Drennan, J., Lyons, I., et al. (2012). Elder abuse and neglect in Ireland: results from a national prevalence survey. *Age and Ageing*, 41(1), 98–103.

Negin, J. and Cumming, R. (2010). HIV infection in older adults in Sub-Saharan Africa: extrapolating prevalence from existing data. *Bulletin of the World Health Organization*, 88, 847–52.

Oeppen, J. and Vaupel, J. (2002). Broken limits to life expectancy. *Science*, 296, 1029–31.

O'Keefe, J., Carter, M., and Laviev, C. (2009). Primary and secondary prevention of cardiovascular diseases: a practical evidence-based approach. *Mayo Clinic Proceedings*, 84(8), 741–57.

Olshansky, S., Passaro, D., Hershow, R., et al. (2005). A potential decline in life expectancy in the United States in the 21st century. *New England Journal of Medicine*, 352, 1138–45.

Omran, A.R. (1971). The epidemiologic transition: a theory of the epidemiology of population change. *The Milbank Memorial Fund Quarterly*, 49(4), 509–38.

Palangkaraya, A. and Yong, J. (2009). Population ageing and its implications on aggregate health care demand: empirical evidence from 22 OECD countries. *International Journal of Health Care Finance and Economics*, 9(4), 391–402.

Phillipson, C. and Scharf, T. (2005). Rural and urban perspectives on growing old: developing a new research agenda. *European Journal of Ageing*, 2(2), 67–75.

Pit, S., Byles, J., Henry, D., Holt, L., Hansen, V., and Bowman, D. (2007). A quality use of medicines program for general practitioners and older people: a cluster randomised controlled trial. *Medical Journal of Australia*, 187(1), 23–30.

Popkin, B.M. (2011). Does global obesity represent a global public health challenge? *American Journal of Clinical Nutrition*, 93(2), 232–3.

PRIAE Policy Research Institute on Ageing and Ethnicity (2005). *Black and Minority Ethnic Elders' in the UK: Health and Social Care Research Findings*. Leeds: PRIAE.

Prince, M., Acosta, D., Ferri, C. P., et al. (2012). Dementia incidence and mortality in middle-income countries, and associations with indicators of cognitive reserve: a 10/66 Dementia Research Group population-based cohort study. *The Lancet*, 380(9836), 50–8.

Rau, R., Soroko, E., Jasilionis, D., and Vaupel, J.W. (2008). Continued reductions in mortality at advanced ages. *Population and Development Review*, 34(4), 747–68.

Riley, N. E. (2004). China's population: new trends and challenges. *Population Bulletin*, 59(2), 1–36.

Rockwood, K. and Mitnisky, A. (2011). Frailty defined by deficit accumulation and geriatric medicine defined by frailty. *Clinics in Geriatric Medicine*, 27, 17–26.

Román, G.C., Nash, D.T., and Fillit, H. (2012). Translating current knowledge into dementia prevention. *Alzheimer Disease & Associated Disorders*, 26(4), 295–9.

Rubenstein, L.Z. (2006). Falls in older people: epidemiology, risk factors and strategies for prevention. *Age and Ageing*, 35(Suppl. 2), ii37–41.

Ryburn, B., Wells, Y., and Foreman, P. (2009). Enabling independence: restorative approaches to home care provision for frail older adults. *Health & Social Care in the Community*, 17(3), 225–34.

Saelens, B., Sallis, J., Black, J., and Chen, D. (2003). Neighbourhood-based differences in physical activity: an environment scale evaluation. *American Journal of Public Health*, 93(9), 1552–8.

Schultz, R. and Matire, L. (2004). Family caregiving of persons with dementia: prevalence, health effects, and support strategies. *American Journal of Geriatric Psychiatry*, 12(3), 240–9.

Sellors, J., Kaczorowski, J., Sellors, J., et al. (2003). A randomized controlled trial of a pharmacist consultation program for family physicians and their elderly patients. *Canadian Medical Association Journal*, 169(1), 17–22.

Sev'er, A. (2009). More than wife abuse that has gone old: a conceptual model for violence against the aged in Canada and the US. *Journal of Comparative Family Studies*, 40(2), 279–92.

Shepperd, S., Doll, H., Broad, J., Gladman, J., et al. (2009). Early discharge hospital at home. *Cochrane Database of Systematic Reviews*, 1, CD000356.

Siegel, K., Narayan, K.M.V., and Kinra, S. (2008). Finding a policy solution to India's diabetes epidemic. *Health Affairs*, 27(4), 1077–90.

Simonson, W. and Feinberg, J. (2005). Medication-related problems in the elderly: defining the issues and identifying solutions. *Drugs Aging*, 22(7), 559–69.

Soldo, B., Mitchell, O., Tfaily, R., and McCabe, J. (2006). *Cross-Cohort Differences in Health on the Verge of Retirement*. NBER Working Paper no. 12762, December 2006. Cambridge, MA: National Bureau of Economic Research (NBER).

Taylor, P., Parker, K., Wang, W., Morin, R., and Cohn, D.V. (2009). *Growing Old in America: Expectations vs. Reality*. Washington, DC: PEW Research Center.

Tjepkema, M. and Wilkins, R. (2011). *Remaining Life Expectancy at Age 25 and Probability of Survival to age 75, by Socio-Economic Status and Aboriginal Ancestry*. No. 82-003-X. Ottawa: Statistics Canada.

Tucker, K.L., Hallfrisch, J., Qiao, N., Muller, D., Andres, R., and Fleg, J.L. (2005). The combination of high fruit and vegetable and low saturated fat intakes is more protective against mortality in aging men than is either alone: the Baltimore Longitudinal Study of Aging. *The Journal of Nutrition*, 135(3), 556–61.

UNAIDS Joint United Nations Programme on HIV/AIDS (2002). *Report on the Global HIV/AIDS Epidemic, July 2002*. Geneva: UNAIDS.

United Nations (2012). *The Millennium Development Goals Report 2012*. New York: UN.

United Nations Department of Economic and Social Affairs (2001). *The World's Women 2000: Trends and Statistics*. New York: UN DESA.

United Nations Department of Economic and Social Affairs, Population Division (2001). *World Population Ageing: 1950–2050*. New York: UN DESA.

United Nations Department of Economic and Social Affairs, Population Division (2009). *World Population Ageing 2009*. New York: UN DESA.

United Nations Department of Economic and Social Affairs, Population Division (2011). *World Fertility Report 2009*. New York: UN DESA.

US Census Bureau (2003). *Brief Report. Grandparents Living with Grandchildren: 2000*. Washington: US Census Bureau.

US Preventive Services Task Force (2009). *Screening for Colorectal Cancer, Topic Page. Summary of Recommendations* [Online]. Available at: http://www.uspreventiveservicestaskforce.org/uspstf/uspscolo.htm.

US Preventive Services Task Force (2010). *Screening for Breast Cancer, Topic Page. Summary of Recommendations*. [Online]. Available at: http://www.uspreventiveservicestaskforce.org/uspstf/uspsbrca.htm.

US Preventive Services Task Force (2012). *Screening for Cervical Cancer, Topic Page. Summary of Recommendations* [Online]. Available at: http://www.uspreventiveservicestaskforce.org/uspstf/uspscerv.htm.

Üstun, T.B., Chatterji, S., Bickenbach, J., Kostanjsek, N., and Schneider, M. (2003). The International Classification of Functioning, Disability and Health: a new tool for understanding disability and health. *Disability and Rehabilitation*, 25(11–12), 565–71.

van Baal, P.H., Hoogenveen, R., de Wit, G.A., and Boshuizen, H. (2006). Estimating health-adjusted life expectancy conditional on risk factors: results for smoking and obesity. *Population Health Metrics*, 4(14).

Vaupel, J.W. (2010). Biodemography of human ageing. *Nature*, 464, 536–42.

Wald, N. and Law, M. (2003a). Correction: a strategy to reduce cardiovascular disease by more than 80%. *British Medical Journal*, 327(7415), 586.

Wald, N. and Law, M. (2003b). A strategy to reduce cardiovascular disease by more than 80%. *British Medical Journal*, 326(7404), 1419.

Warburton, J., Paynter, J., and Petriwskyj, A. (2007). Volunteering as a productive ageing activity: incentives and barriers to volunteering by Australian Seniors. *Journal of Applied Gerontology*, 26, 333–54.

Ward, D., Drahota, A., Gal, D., Severs, M., and Dean, T. (2008). *Care home versus hospital and own home environments for rehabilitation of older people. Cochrane Database of Systematic Reviews*, 4, CD003164.

Women's Health Australia (2006). *Women's Health Australia. The Australian Longitudinal Study on Women's Health, June 2006*. Technical Report 26. Newcastle: University of Newcastle in association with The University of Queensland, Australia.

World Health Organization (2010). *How Health Systems Can Address Health Inequities Linked to Migration and Ethnicity*. Copenhagen: WHO Regional Office for Europe.

World Health Organization (2011). *Global Status Report on Noncommunicable Diseases, 2010*. Geneva: WHO.

World Health Organization (2012a). *Good Health Adds Life to Years: Global Brief for World Health Day, 2012*. Geneva: WHO.

World Health Organization (2012b). *World Health Statistics, 2012*. Geneva: WHO.

World Health Organization and International Network for the Prevention of Elder Abuse (INPEA) (2002). *Missing Voices: Views of Older Persons on Elder Abuse*. Geneva: WHO.

World Health Organization, US National Institute of Aging, and US National Institutes of Health (2011). *Global Health and Aging*. Washington, DC: National Institute on Aging, National Institutes of Health.

Writing Group for the Women's Health Initiative Investigators (2002). Risks and benefits of estrogen plus progestin in healthy postmenopausal women: principal results from the Women's Health Initiative randomized controlled trial. *Journal of the American Medical Association*, 288(3), 321–33.

WRVS (2011). *Gold Age Pensioners. Valuing the Socio-Economic Contribution of Older People in the UK*. Cardiff: WRVS.

Yan, E.-W. and Tang, C.-K. (2004). Elder abuse by caregivers: a study of prevalence and risk factors in Hong Kong Chinese families. *Journal of Family Violence*, 19(5), 269–77.

Zavoretti, R. (2006). Family-based care for China's ageing population. A social research perspective. *Asia Europe Journal*, 4, 211–28.

Zermansky, A., Petty, D., Raynor, D., Lowe, C., Freemantle, N., and Vail, A. (2002). Clinical medication review by a pharmacist of patients on repeat prescriptions in general practice: a randomised controlled trial. *Health Technology Assessment*, 6(20), 1–86.

Forced migrants and other displaced populations

Catherine R. Bateman Steel and Anthony B. Zwi

Introduction to forced migrants and other displaced populations

Migration and displacement have always been features of human life but the intensification of globalization, and increased ease of travel and interconnectedness, has seen the effects of displacement reaching far beyond the immediate contexts in which they occur. Forced migration is displacement that involves coercion and the implication that those involved have moved against their will. The previous few decades with the end of the cold war, rapid globalization, increasing inequality between and within nations, ongoing wars, and conflict (United Nations High Commissioner for Refugees (UNHCR) 2006), have created a landscape where forced migration affects all populations to some extent, whether as displaced or as hosts to the displaced. Health professionals will undoubtedly be confronted with the effects of forced migration and called upon to engage in responses for those affected regardless of where they practice. This chapter aims to provide a global overview of forced migration and the public health challenges facing populations forced to move from their usual homes, in order to assist the public health professional in framing their own responses. It begins by presenting a brief history of forced migration and the legal definition of 'refugee'. We describe the emergence of categories of forced migrants that do not meet the legal definition of 'refugee', describe how these groups are treated by states, and the implications for people's lives and health. The chapter then explores the social and political factors that have influenced the treatment of refugees by states. We lay out some of the major health issues that refugees face in both developing and developed countries. The wide variety of actors involved in both protecting forced migrants and providing health services is presented, along with a discussion of the contextual conditions that have an impact, often detrimental, on the health of forced migrants. As well as describing the structural factors that create and limit health outcomes, this analysis seeks to highlight the agency and voice of forced migrants, exploring the importance of understanding and projecting these, and of appreciating the rationales for how forced migrants may act in the often chaotic situations in which they find themselves. We consider how interactions with other actors, within the complex social, political, and legal context of forced migration, may lead to seemingly unhealthy choices, and at times, barriers to engaging with services. Yet, forced migrants make choices, when possible, seeking to protect their well-being and fight for better, and healthier, outcomes.

Causes of displacement

The global context

Forced migration reached record levels in 2011 with more people becoming refugees in that year than in any year since the start of the new millennium. Humanitarian crises in countries such as Sudan, Libya, Somalia, and Côte d'Ivoire, as well as ongoing instability in Afghanistan and Iraq amongst others, contributed to a staggering 4.3 million people being newly displaced from their homes (UNHCR 2011). Whilst war, violence, and natural disaster are major contributors, and the causes most commonly associated with forced migration, it is important to consider the broader global dynamics that shape and create the forced migration situation.

Globalization, inequality, and perceptions of crisis

Forced migration cannot be fully understood without considering the global context and the shifting global forces that shape the form and patterns of migration. Globalization and its role in shaping the dynamics of forced migration need to be considered. Although globalization is a contested concept with disputed definitions, most people accept it as a global process of integration which affects sociocultural, economic, and political domains (see Chapter 1.5). The increased ease of travel, and the cultural interconnectedness that projects visions of opportunities in distant lands, provides a context which may facilitate migration amongst those with powerful forces driving them from their homes.

The economic implications of the globalized landscape are also worthy of mention in any analysis of forced migration. There is a polarized debate over the effects of globalization on human development and health. Some commentators argue, like Feachem (2001), that the forces of economic globalization may be beneficial to the poor, increasing wealth and therefore health; while others (Baum 2001; MacDonald 2007) highlight the poor health situation in many developing countries and the vast inequities present, and suggest that globalization plays a part in generating these conditions by creating an uneven playing field and weighting the economic benefits towards those that already have power and wealth. They argue that globalization cannot be separated from economic policies that serve the interests of the wealthy, reinforcing or exacerbating inequalities, fuelling conflicts, and contributing to public health crises in developing countries. This analysis suggests that the only way to improve health is to seriously restructure the dominant international financial institutions. Taking the middle ground, Lee (2004) suggests that rigorous, ongoing analysis is required to assess the positive and negative impacts on health within the overall conceptual domain of globalization. Zwi and Alvarez-Castillo (2003) argue that globalization has often led to poor health outcomes for vast populations and that this in turn is responsible for fuelling forced migration. Regardless of our standpoint on globalization, what it is, how it impacts on health, and its influence, what is clear is that global inequities exist and are dramatic, the impact of such inequities cannot be ignored as major contributors to forced migration, whether or not associated with violence.

Castles (2004) provides an analysis that calls for careful examination of the global context when describing forced migration dynamics. He argues that the current perception of a global 'asylum crisis' should be seen more as a crisis of North–South relationships, within which 'asylum' is but one aspect. The current picture of forced migration, he argues, is a result of disparities between 'North' and 'South'. Although the North–South conceptualization does not perhaps accurately represent the divisions we see today, we can see the dynamics he describes as 'North–South' as being between the wealthy and less-wealthy nations. While disparities exist and people search for a better life, or simply for survival, forced migration will continue. The disparity is also reflected in how the effects of forced migration are absorbed globally, further deepening the crisis in North–South relations. He shows that while there has repeatedly been a perception of impending asylum crises ever since the 1800s, which largely do not fully emerge as feared, there are some new features. He cites the increase in endemic violence and human rights violations as a feature that has increased the volume of forced migration in recent times. Castles (2004) shows, however, that for the North, there is no significant economic or social crisis resulting from forced migration and contrary to popular belief, the North has not had to absorb large influxes of people. The situation is nonetheless construed by those in the North as a crisis because it highlights the 'erosion of nation-state sovereignty'. The South, however, has absorbed the vast majority of forced migrants from neighbouring countries (Allotey and Reidpath 2003). This combined with increasingly restrictive policies of wealthy countries that seek to limit refugee absorption from the South, leads to a tension in North–South relations, and opens space for people smuggling and trafficking, further threatening the sense of control over borders that the North is seeking to maintain, and therefore deepening the sense of crisis perceived by the North. Hence the burden has been left largely with the South, while in the North, incomplete pictures of fear that exclude vulnerable people have been painted and promoted (Grove and Zwi 2006). In their review of globalization, forced migration, and health, Zwi and Alvarez Castillo (2003) suggest that public health professionals have a responsibility to examine the context and whole picture, and in so doing, to break down these 'incomplete pictures of fear' and advocate for a more humane globalization that has a chance of decreasing the poor health outcomes associated with forced migration.

Immediate drivers of displacement

There is general agreement on the range of factors that contribute to displacement and forced migration. However, the importance of particular factors, and the linkages between them, varies in different contexts. Identification of specific causes has implications for both the states involved and the migrants themselves, given that the perceived cause of displacement has an impact on the international response, the level of funding support provided, and the attitudes of host populations to those seeking protection. The health consequences of forced migration will be shaped by not only the causes of displacement, but also by the perceptions of all actors regarding these causes and their relationship to them. In this respect, the terms and context within which forced migrants are described and 'presented' greatly affects the societal response and opportunities, or constraints, operating.

Forced migration has traditionally been associated with war and violence. The conception of a refugee as defined by the United Nations (UN) Convention, fleeing from persecution to a place of safety in another country, was clear-cut and well understood. As Moore and Shellman (2004) describe, the central model was one of:

Violence in = Forced migration out.

However, whilst the main causes of involuntary displacement remain armed conflict, repression, and war, other factors such as natural disasters and development projects are also important, as are the more complex set of economic, social, and political circumstances that may lead to trafficking and people smuggling.

Martin (2002) focuses attention on natural and man-made disasters and border changes leading to statelessness, as factors which lead to forced migration, alongside the well-recognized factors related to persecution, human rights violations, repression, and conflict. Environmental factors, such as rising sea levels and extreme weather conditions, are also increasingly recognized as important. Some argue that these causes may, over time, supersede conflict as a primary cause of forced migration (Myers and Kent 1995). Resource constraints, including depleted access to land and water, and conflict over precious minerals, are likely to become increasingly important, especially as the global population increases from around 6 billion people at present to nearly 9 billion by 2050.

While all these factors are important, quantifying their effects is difficult. Data are available regarding numbers of 'Convention' refugees (see 'Categories of forced migrants' section) and also, more recently, regarding internally displaced persons (IDPs). These data may give some indication of the level of displacement produced by conflicts and violence, alongside immediate natural disasters such as tsunamis and earthquakes. However, more insidious environmental and economic effects are far harder to quantify.

The increased complexity of recent times in describing and understanding factors that cause displacement raise new concerns that go beyond the simple 'violence migration' model therefore calls for new approaches. Major challenges include an increased focus on economic migrants and those who are forced to move as a result of environmental and climate changes; there is also a rise in 'mixed migration', a term which recognizes that many migrants fall somewhere on the spectrum between forced and voluntary migration and are hard to categorize as one or the other.

Particularly important is a call for a shift in policies of protection for host countries to developing policies which address the root causes within countries from which people are forced to migrate; and a growing recognition that understanding causes may allow predictions of impending displacement as well as the identification of the means to avert large-scale displacement. Some analyses continue to support the primacy of violent conflict, or threat of conflict as the major predictor of populations leaving their homes. Moore and Shellman (2004) analysed a global sample of 40 countries and using a model that incorporated a wide range of indicators (government threat, dissident threat, government-dissent interaction, ethnic or non-ethnic civil wars, war on territory, income opportunity, political freedom and the rule of law, and cultural and family ties), they found that the first three were the primary determinants of forced migration flows. These were more important than other factors such as size of economy or type of political institution. Apodaca (1998) analysed a variety of models developed to predict forced migration and concluded that human rights violations are one of the most important predictors.

Economic migration has often been portrayed in the media as freely chosen migration that should not confer a responsibility to protect on accepting states. However, analysts such as Castles (2003) argue that forced migration is linked to economic migration and that the two are 'closely related (and indeed often indistinguishable) forms of expression of global inequalities and societal crises'. These inequities have intensified since the end of the cold war. He argues that studies of the causes of forced migration have neglected the over-arching economic and social structures which should be seen in relation to 'US political and military domination, economic globalization, North–South inequality and transnationalism' (Castles 2003).

Debates regarding causes of displacement have particular salience in relation to the protection offered to forced migrants. As subsequent sections of this chapter describe, the nature and extent of protection is often determined by perceived cause. Therefore, understanding these debates is crucial as they may have effects on what and how protection, if any, is offered to forced migrant populations.

Categories of forced migrants

Definitions of forced migration have been debated for more than 50 years, dating back to the first UN Convention on Refugees in 1951. The legal framework that emerged under the Convention centred on 'refugees' as a specially defined group and is based upon the 1951 Convention and a subsequent 1967 protocol. According to these, a refugee is a person who:

> owing to a well-founded fear of being persecuted for reasons of race, religion, nationality membership of a particular social group, or political opinion, is outside the country of his nationality, and is unable to or, owing to such fear, is unwilling to avail himself of the protection of that country. (UNHCR 2009)

This definition has been modified by regional instruments in Africa and Latin America, as described in a later section. The International Association for the Study of Forced Migration (IASFM), however, defines forced migration much more widely as:

> a general term that refers to the movements of refugees and internally displaced people (those displaced by conflicts) as well as people displaced by natural or environmental disasters, chemical or nuclear disasters, famine, or development projects. (Forced Migration Online 2008)

This definition encompasses a wide range of forced migrants, and these can be distinguished into several distinct groups (Table 10.9.1).

The definitions of other forced migrant groups, and their sources, are outlined in the following subsections. They highlight the increased attention devoted to describing, as well as defining, the many forms of forced migration that exist. The discourse and narratives presented have a marked impact on how people see, and respond to, those forced to leave their usual homes and livelihoods.

Internally displaced persons

Unlike refugees, there is no legal definition of an IDP. It is generally accepted that if a person meets the definition of a refugee, but their displacement does not take them across an international border, then they are internally displaced. The Secretary General of the UN has appointed a representative to deal with IDPs and the Office of the United Nations High Commissioner for Human Rights (OHCHR) has produced a set of Guiding Principles to address the specific needs of IDPs who are described as:

> persons or groups of persons who have been forced or obliged to flee or to leave their homes or places of habitual residence, in particular as a result of, or in order to avoid the effects of, armed conflict, situations of generalized violence, violations of human rights or natural or human-made disasters, and who have not crossed an internationally recognized State border. (Deng 1998)

Asylum seekers

Asylum seekers are those who are fleeing persecution and are seeking refugee status in another country. According to the UNHCR, an asylum seeker is:

> Someone who has made a claim that he or she is a refugee, and is waiting for that claim to be accepted or rejected. The term contains no presumption either way—it simply describes the fact that someone has lodged the claim. Some asylum seekers will be judged to be refugees and others will not. (UNHCR 2009)

The application referred to relates to being recognized under the 1951 Convention as a refugee and therefore being entitled to the protection and support stipulated by the Convention. They may or may not arrive in a country with authorization, nevertheless, they have a legal right to claim asylum and are therefore not 'illegal'.

Trafficked persons

The 2003 Protocol to Prevent, Suppress and Punish Trafficking in Persons, especially Women and Children, describes trafficking as:

> recruitment, transportation, transfer, harbouring, or receipt of persons, by means of the threat or use of force or other forms of coercion, of abduction, of fraud, of deception, of the abuse of power or of a position of vulnerability or of the giving or receiving of payments or benefits to achieve the consent of a person having control over another person, for the purpose of exploitation. Exploitation shall include, at a minimum, the exploitation of the prostitution of others or other forms of sexual exploitation, forced labour or services, slavery or practices similar to slavery, servitude or the removal of organs. (UN 2003, Resolution 25)

Table 10.9.1 Categories of forced migrants

Refugee	A person who 'owing to a well-founded fear of being persecuted for reasons of race, religion, nationality, membership of a particular social group, or political opinion, is outside the country of his nationality, and is unable to or, owing to such fear, is unwilling to avail himself of the protection of that country' (UNHCR 2009)
Internally displaced persons	'Persons or groups of persons who have been forced or obliged to flee or to leave their homes' (Deng 1998). Or places of habitual residence, in particular as a result of, or in order to, avoid the effects of armed conflict, situations of generalized violence, violations of human rights or natural or human-made disasters, and who have not crossed an internationally recognized State border
Asylum seeker	'Someone who has made a claim that he or she is a refugee, and is waiting for that claim to be accepted or rejected. The term contains no presumption either way—it simply describes the fact that someone has lodged the claim. Some asylum seekers will be judged to be refugees and others will not' (UNHCR 2009)
Trafficking in persons	'Recruitment, transportation, transfer, harbouring or receipt of persons, by means of the threat or use of force or other forms of coercion, of abduction, of fraud, of deception, of the abuse of power or of a position of vulnerability or of the giving or receiving of payments or benefits to achieve the consent of a person having control over another person, for the purpose of exploitation' (United Nations 2003)
Smuggling in persons	'The procurement, in order to obtain, directly or indirectly, a financial or other material benefit, of illegal entry of a person into a state, party of which the person is not a national or permanent resident' (United Nations 2000) [Article 3 (a)]
Environmentally displaced person	'A person displaced owing to environmental causes, notably land loss and degradation, and natural disaster' (Deng 1998)
Development displacees	'People who are compelled to move as a result of policies and projects implemented to supposedly enhance "development"' (Forced Migration Online 2008)

Text extracts from United Nations High Commissioner for Refugees (UNHCR), *Protecting refugees and the role of UNHCR*, Copyright © UNHCR 2009, available from http://unhcr.org.au/unhcr/images/protecting%20refugees.pdf, reproduced with permission from the United Nations.

Text extracts from Deng, F., *The Guiding Principles on Internal Displacement*, United Nations, New York, Copyright © United Nations 1998, reproduced with permission from the United Nations.

Text extract from United Nations, *Protocol to Prevent, Suppress and Punish Trafficking in Persons, Especially Women and Children, Supplementing the United Nations Convention Against Transnational Organized Crime*, G.A. Res. 25, Annex II, U.N. GAOR, 55th Session, Copyright © United Nations 2003, reproduced with permission from the United Nations.

Text extract from United Nations, *Protocol Against The Smuggling Of Migrants By Land, Sea And Air*, Copyright © United Nations 2000, reproduced with permission from the United Nations.

Text extracts from United Nations, *Glossary of Environment Statistics, Studies in Methods, Series F*, United Nations, New York, USA, Copyright © United Nations 1998, reproduced with permission from the United Nations.

Text extracts from Forced Migration Online, *What is Forced Migration?*, Copyright © 2010 Forced Migration Online and Contributors, available from http://www.forcedmigration.org/whatisfm.htm, reproduced with permission from Forced Migration Online.

Smuggled persons

Smuggling of aliens or 'illegal migrant smuggling' is defined by the UN 2000 Protocol Against Smuggling of Migrants by Land, Sea and Air, which supplemented the UN Convention Against Transnational Organized Crime, to mean:

> the procurement, in order to obtain, directly or indirectly, a financial or other material benefit, of illegal entry of a person into a state, party of which the person is not a national or permanent resident. (UN 2000, Article 3(a))

Environmentally displaced persons

The Organisation for Economic Cooperation and Development's online *Glossary of Statistical Terms* describes an environmental refugee as 'a person displaced owing to environmental causes, notably land loss and degradation, and natural disaster' (United Nations 1997). However, the term was first described by El-Hinnawi (1985), a researcher from the United Nations Environment Programme (UNEP) in 1985, who defined environmental refugees as:

> those people who have been forced to leave their traditional habitat, temporarily or permanently, because of a marked environmental disruption (natural and/or triggered by people) that jeopardized their existence and/or seriously affected the quality of their life.

'Environmental disruption' in this definition is taken to mean any physical, chemical, and/or biological changes in the ecosystem (or resource base) that render it, temporarily or permanently, unsuitable to support human life. The validity of the term 'environmental refugees' has been debated greatly since that time. Actors emerge from a realm of perspectives including environmentalists, economists, and refugee advocates, each with a different interpretation of the term. Some prefer to use the term 'environmental migrant' or 'environmental displacee'; different terms establish different implications for both the individuals and states involved.

Development displacees

There is no legal definition for development displacees; however, Forced Migration Online suggests they are:

> people who are compelled to move as a result of policies and projects implemented to supposedly enhance 'development'. These include large-scale infrastructure projects such as dams, roads, ports, airports; urban clearance initiatives; mining and deforestation; and the introduction of conservation parks/reserves and biosphere projects. Affected people usually remain within the borders of their country. People displaced in this way are sometimes also referred to as 'oustees', 'involuntarily displaced' or 'involuntarily resettled'. (Forced Migration Online 2008)

Interestingly, large-scale agricultural projects do not seem to be specifically mentioned.

Forced migration statistics

Assessing the volume of global flows of forced migrants is valuable in identifying trends and the patterns of distribution with respect to where the burden for providing assistance and care lies. In specific countries and contexts, where people are forced to migrate from their place of origin, the first step in addressing public health and other more general concerns is often to define the size of the population at risk. Donors, governments, aid agencies, and community organizations require basic demographic and related data to inform planning and service delivery. The collection of data is complicated and surrounded by controversy, having the potential to immediately reframe what looks like a technical issue into a political one.

The two main sources of statistics on forced migrants are the United Nations High Commissioner for Refugees (UNHCR) and the US Committee for Refugees and Immigrants (USCRI). These organizations produce differing estimates for different types of forced migrants in different geographical contexts. The logistic difficulties of collecting reliable data from shifting forced migrant populations leaves space for political interests to enter, and seek to shape, the field. This is compounded by disagreement over definitions of forced migrants and which groups to include in which categories, as mentioned earlier, with significant implications for the rights and entitlements of such groups, as well as for who bears the responsibilities for addressing their needs. Despite contested data, available sources provide valuable information on trends and distribution.

UNHCR forced migration statistics

The UNHCR provides data based on 'persons of concern', an increasingly wide-ranging term. 'Persons of concern' includes refugees (as defined by the 1951 Convention or the 1969 Organisation of African Unity (OAU) Convention); persons granted complementary protection (alternative forms of protection for those that fall outside of the terms of the 1951 Convention) and those with forms of temporary protection; asylum seekers who in the year of data collection are still pending a final decision on an application for protection; stateless persons; refugees who returned to their country of origin in the year of data collection; and IDPs (see Table 10.9.2). For the purposes of UNHCR the latter are limited to conflict-generated IDPs to whom UNHCR protection or assistance is extended, but does not include all IDPs.

UNHCR reported that in 2011 the number of forcibly displaced persons exceeded 42 million for the fifth consecutive year (UNHCR 2011). This figure included refugees, IDPs, and asylum seekers. It was estimated that 4.3 million people were newly displaced in 2011 due to conflict or persecution, with 800,000 of these displaced across international borders. This was a 20 per cent increase since 2010 of new displacement. There was also an increase of 700,000 in refugees and IDPs protected by the UNHCR and 7.1 million, three quarters of the UNHCR refugee population, were reported to be in a protracted refugee situation. Developing countries hosted four-fifths of the world's refugees (UNHCR 2011). The countries of origin for refugees are shown in Fig. 10.9.1. Afghanistan produced the greatest number of refugees followed by Iraq and Somalia. UNHCR statistics demonstrate that the majority of refugees remain within their region of origin.

Table 10.9.2 Persons of concern to United Nations High Commissioner for Refugees (UNHCR 2011)

	2011
Newly displaced	4.3 million
Refugees	10.4 million
IDPs	15.5 million
Asylum seekers	876,100
Stateless	12 million
Resettlement	79,800[a]
Unaccompanied children	17,700
Protected by UNHCR	25.9 million[b]
Forcibly displaced people worldwide	42.5 million

[a] Resettlement—with or without UNHCR assistance—by 22 countries.
[b] Protected by UNHCR—refugees and IDPs.
Source: data from United Nations High Commissioner for Refugees (UNHCR), A Year of Crises: *UNHCR Global Trends 2011*, UNHCR, Geneva, Switzerland, Copyright © UNHCR 2012, available from http://www.unhcr.org/4fd6f87f9.html.

Pakistan was the country that hosted the most refugees in 2011, followed by Iran and Syria. Almost half of the world's refugees falling under the UNHCR mandate were hosted in countries with a GDP per capita of less than $3000.

It is important to note that Palestinian refugees falling under the mandate of the United Nations Relief and Works Agency for Palestinian Refugees in the Near East (UNRWA) are not included in the UNHCR refugee figures, but are included in the 42 million forced migrants. The Palestinian community has been one of the largest groups of refugees that has remained without being fully resettled or absorbed into host-nations; a reflection of how community members on the ground suffer while local, national, regional, and global powers resolve, or fail to resolve, higher-level strategic and political issues.

Given the importance of these numbers, they are invariably contested and debated; with key actors seeking to shape what data are collected and presented, who are counted, and what the implications are for future activities. Indeed each 'player' in the system, whether they be a UN or non-governmental agency, a recipient or state of origin, a local community or professional group, and many others, has their own rationale for inflating or deflating the numbers of people whether they be refugees or IDPs, in or outside of camps, dependant or free of other major influences.

Internally displaced persons

The global number of IDPs at the end of 2011 was estimated by the UNHCR to be 26.4 million, with 15.5 million benefiting from UNHCR assistance. The figure for 2011 was the second highest on record, according to the UNHCR this was partly due to displacement from Afghanistan, Côte d'Ivoire, Libya, South Sudan, Sudan, and Yemen (UNHCR 2011). Fig. 10.9.2 shows the distribution of IDPs globally.

Asylum seekers

In 2011, 876,100 applications for asylum or refugee status were submitted to UNHCR offices or governments. One-tenth of all

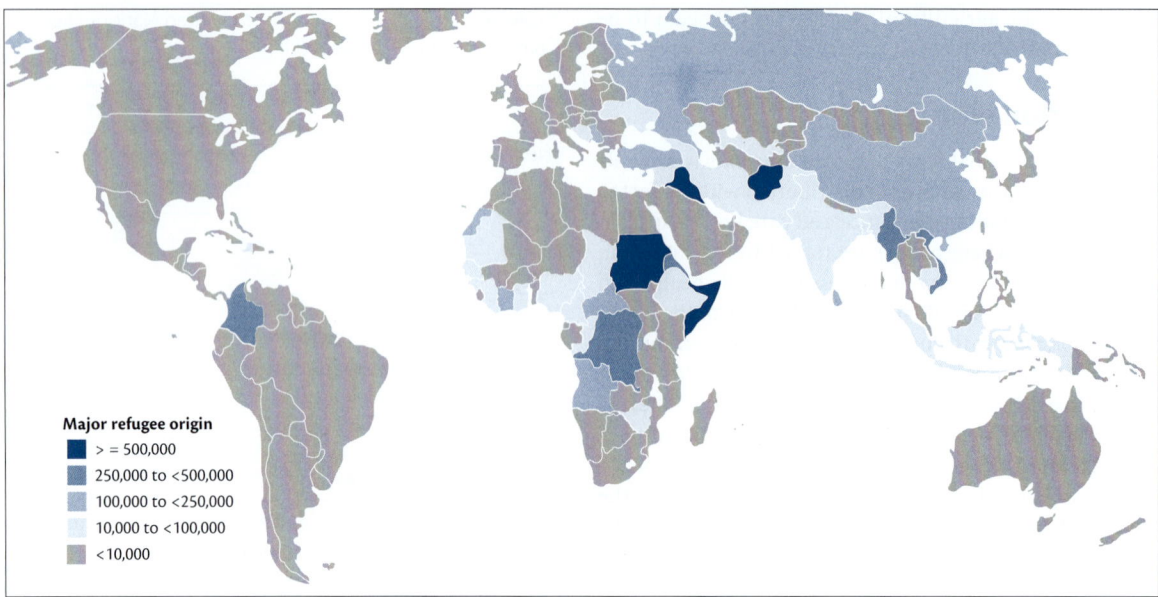

Fig. 10.9.1 Country of origin for refugees under UNHCR mandate 2011.
Reproduced from United Nations High Commissioner for Refugees (UNHCR), *A Year of Crises: UNHCR Global Trends 2011*, UNHCR, Geneva, Switzerland, Copyright © United Nations High Commissioner for Refugees 2012, available from http://www.unhcr.org/4fd6f87f9.html.

these applications were registered in South Africa, making it the top asylum destination by a clear margin, more than half these claims were from Zimbabwean nationals. The United States was the next highest receiver of asylum applications with almost half coming from China, Mexico and El Salvador. The UNHCR noted significant differences between countries in recognition rates suggesting differences in how asylum seekers are treated. For example, between eight European countries the recognition rate for Afghan asylum seekers ranged from 3 to 33 per cent (UNHCR 2011).

Legal framework

Refugees

The 1951 Convention, which forms the basis of all international refugee law, was drafted in the aftermath of the Second World War in response to the large numbers of displaced people caused by the war. The Convention included restrictions on who would be classified as a 'refugee' based on geographical and temporal factors that were specific to the European context. As a result, the 1967 Protocol relating to the Status of Refugees was adopted which removed these restrictions and allowed for more general application of the Convention. The Convention and Protocol laid out not only the definition of a refugee but also the scope of protection to which refugees were entitled. The most fundamental of these is *non-refoulement*, the right to remain rather than be returned to a place where their lives or freedoms would be at risk. Debate has raged over the continuing relevance of the Convention definition, given that it excludes large numbers of people in need of international protection, notably internally displaced persons and those that have migrated as a result of generalized (as opposed to individualized) violence, civil war, and widespread human rights abuses.

Africa and Latin America responded to the limitations of the Convention and Protocol by adopting their own regional laws and standards. The Organisation of African Unity (OAU) (now known as the African Union) adopted the 1967 Convention Governing the Specific Aspects of Refugee Problems in Africa (Barnett 2002). This is the only legally binding regional instrument and has a refugee definition similar to that of the Convention but includes those who flee due to 'external aggression, occupation, foreign domination or events seriously disturbing public order in either part or the whole of his country of origin or nationality' (OAU 1969).

In Latin America, the Cartagena Declaration, adopted in 1984, included a definition of refugee similar to that of the OAU Convention but which also included reference to 'massive violation of human rights' (Regional Refugee Instruments & Related 1984). The latter is not legally binding but has been adopted by many states and incorporated into some national legislation in the region.

Persons who have participated in war crimes and violations of humanitarian and human rights law, including the crime of terrorism, are specifically excluded from the Convention and cannot be recognized as refugees.

The UNHCR has been given a mandate to provide international protection to refugees and seek permanent solutions to their problems through its Statute, adopted by the UN General Assembly (UNGA) in December 1950. Over the years, the UNGA has allowed UNHCR to extend its responsibilities and is increasingly focused not only on refugee protection but also on managing refugees in the field.

Internally displaced persons

Whilst IDPs do not have the same legal framework of protection, they have become included in the UNHCR's 'people of concern' and are therefore often covered by its mandate. The United Nations Office for Coordination of Humanitarian Affairs (OCHA) has produced a set of Guiding Principles to address the specific needs of internally displaced persons (Deng 1998). The guidelines

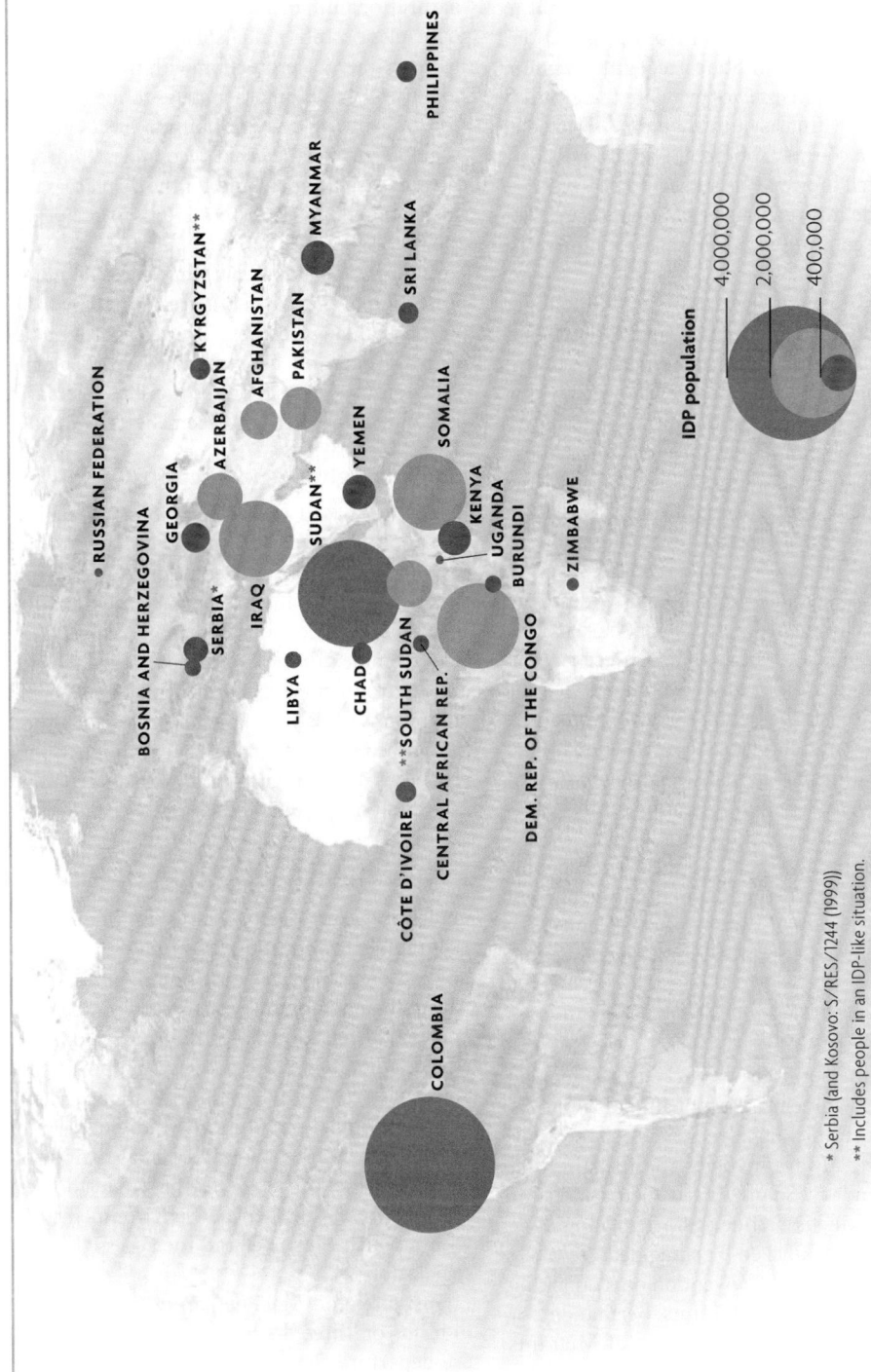

Fig. 10.9.2 Distribution of IDP populations globally 2011.
Reproduced from United Nations High Commissioner for Refugees (UNHCR), A Year of Crises: UNHCR Global Trends 2011, UNHCR, Geneva, Switzerland, Copyright © United Nations High Commissioner for Refugees 2012, available from http://www.unhcr.org/4fd6f879.html.

* Serbia (and Kosovo: S/RES/1244 (1999))
** Includes people in an IDP-like situation.

identify rights and guarantees that should be afforded to IDPs although they are not legally binding.

Asylum seekers

The Declaration of Territorial Asylum (DTA) adopted by the UNGA in 1967 is based on article 14 of the Universal Declaration of Human Rights, which declares that 'everyone has the right to seek and to enjoy in other countries asylum from persecution'. The principles of the DTA are that all States recognize asylum granted by one State, that States themselves evaluate the grounds for asylum, and that no one seeking asylum should be rejected at borders or if already within a country should not be compulsorily returned to any State in which they may be subject to persecution. Exceptions can only be made in situations of national security or for asylum seekers that have committed a crime against humanity, against peace or a war crime.

Asylum may be granted by States on the basis of the 1951 Refugee Convention, in which an individual has been deemed a 'refugee' as defined by the Convention. However, given the restrictions of this definition and the increasing numbers of people who are seeking protection but do not fit the Convention definition, alternative forms of protection have developed. Often termed 'complementary' or 'subsidiary' protection, McAdam (2006) describes the plethora of alternative forms of protection for 'non-Convention refugees' that previously had been treated much the same as Convention refugees by states.

'Non-Convention' refugees, such as those fleeing widespread violence rather than targeted individual persecution, have to look to instruments of human rights law, rather than refugee law, for protection. However, human rights instruments do not attach the same clear rights and standards as the Refugee Convention and it has also been argued that human rights law can be weak on implementation (McAdam 2006). This has led many to argue that complementary protection is a lesser form of protection, and there is a danger of States using these forms of protection to decrease the numbers of Convention refugees and therefore their level of commitment. Debate continues as to whether expanding the current Convention definition, or expanding systems of complementary protection, will weaken or broaden protection to those seeking asylum.

Trafficking and smuggled persons

Although the reasons for a person to be trafficked or smuggled are very similar, international agreements and national laws treat them quite differently. Unlike trafficking, which may occur internally in a country, smuggling always involves the illegal crossing of an international boundary. Smuggling is seen as a crime against a *state* whereas trafficking is a crime against an *individual*. Consequently persons that are trafficked or smuggled are likely to be treated quite differently. The UN Convention on Trafficking mandates states to consider granting victims permanent or temporary resident status, whereas the Smuggling of Migrants Protocol calls on states to facilitate the return of smuggled persons to the country from which they came.

Environmental and developmental displacees

The concept of environmental refugees or displacees is particularly contentious and the subject of much current debate. There

is little agreement on whether environmental factors can be seen as primary causes of displacement and equally no consensus on a definition for those displaced from their homes by these factors. As a result the legal protection available is marginal. The current legal regime has no specific mandate to protect environmental displacees, if they are displaced across international borders; however, 'natural or human-made disasters' are covered by the Guiding Principles on Internal Displacement (Deng 1998). These place the primary duty for protection with the national authority; however, no duty is placed on other states to recognize the need for protection. A growing body of opinion has begun calling for a system of global governance that recognizes environmental factors as a cause of displacement and for the displacees to be protected under international law (Courtland Robinson 2003; Biermann and Boas 2007).

Similarly, developmental displacees do not have frameworks of protection of their own but are covered by the Guiding Principles on Internal Displacement. There is a need to recognize the needs of this group and for research on displacement not to fall into a dichotomy that separates conflict-related displacement from development-related displacement (Cernea 2007).

Evolving rights of protection

Protection based on a definition of refugees fleeing from the effects of violent conflict has been the prevailing paradigm, and whilst the centrality of conflict-related displacement has been debated, conflict and violence clearly remain significant causes of forced migration and suffering. Analysis reflecting the increasingly complex drivers of forced migration, including economic and environmental concerns, whilst vital, should be careful not to compromise existing rights of protection. These rights of protection, based on conflict as the central tenet, should not be further eroded by the recognition that there are other causes of forced migration that need to be seriously considered.

Public health situation of forced migrants

Forced migrants live in a range of different social, political, and geographical conditions. They may form distinct populations or be dispersed amongst host populations; they may be displaced within their own country, to a nearby or distant country of asylum; and may dwell anywhere from a developing country experiencing conflict, to a more peaceful but poverty-stricken developing country, to a wealthy developed nation. The health of each forced migrant population, and each individual within the group, will be shaped by these factors, as well as their prior health and social condition, the journeys they have had to take, the stability and security present in their new environments, the social structures within which they live, and the access they have to services and social support.

Gushulak and MacPherson (2000) describe migration health in terms of 'three distinct but interdependent undertakings: The pre-departure phase, the migratory journey itself, and the arrival at destination', each of which influences health. Factors such as social networks, assets, language, knowledge, information or access to services, food security issues, poor shelter, sanitation, and availability of safe water will influence health outcomes.

In this section we describe the major health challenges facing forced migrant populations. This is followed by an overview of the public health responses and an indication of where more detailed technical advice may be found.

Refugees in developing countries

Developing countries continue to absorb the vast majority of forced migrants, in particular as developed nations have become more restrictive. Within developing countries, people who are forcibly displaced either within or across borders may find themselves in a variety of possible contexts, settling short or long term either in a camp situation or dispersed within a host population. Each presents threats and opportunities.

The type of settlement formed has implications for health and well-being. The typical refugee camp setting has presented a range of problems, although improvements in public health knowledge and experience, and informing policy and practice with evidence, have led to better outcomes.

The impact of forced migration falls heavily on developing nations, and within these countries, on host populations. This is particularly so where forced migrants reside in non-camp situations.

Camps and non-camp settlements

Camps, whilst constructed with the intention of providing protection, safety, and access to services, may also pose risks. Poorly planned refugee settlements may have inadequate infrastructure, may pose risks to safety, or set up new inequalities. The combination of overcrowding, poor hygiene and sanitation, lack of water, poor nutrition, and inadequate shelter provides conditions for spread of many diseases, particularly communicable disease. Refugees may arrive in a poor condition, suffering from malnutrition, and with poor immunity, reflecting limited access to immunization services. Disrupted social structures decrease the capacity to deal with sickness. Communicable disease spreads quickly and may be particularly severe. Psychological distress is also a major issue due to the insecure, restricted environment and lack of resources.

Debates over the utility of camps are highlighted by Harrell-Bond (2000) who argues that as a concept they have failed. Originally based on modernization theory, the premise was that camp settlements would become new agricultural centres and eventually be integrated with host populations to the benefit of all. However, this was abandoned as the theory became discredited and was replaced by a view that refugees should be seen as temporary. Harrell-Bond suggests that those in camps are in 'prison-like' settlements with poor conditions, increased vulnerability to disease and often poor nutrition. She also argues that camps do not help host populations, as large sums of money are diverted to camps which may be demolished if refugees do move on, as well as diverting scarce human and material resources from the host population. She suggests that it would be far more appropriate and cheaper to help integrate refugees into host populations and invest in the country and strengthening existing social structures, as a whole.

In many situations of forced migration, for example, when the Kosovar Albanians fled from Kosovo over the border into Albania, integration with host populations there was the norm. Following political instability and violence in Timor-Leste in 2006, 4 years after independence, makeshift camps were established within Dili, the capital city, for IDPs, while many also fled and were integrated with host communities in the districts. The latter necessarily absorbed a portion of the social and economic costs associated with accommodating those who fled.

However, Salama et al. (2004) show that, despite the problems associated with camps, there are also benefits. The increased knowledge base and coordination of humanitarian interventions have led to improvements in health, with better nutrition, sanitation, and health services. The burden of ill health may shift from displaced populations who are relatively well serviced, especially if they cross international borders and become refugees, relative to host populations and IDPs whose needs may be greater and who have less access to assistance.

Mortality

Crude mortality rates (CMRs) are often used as an indicator of the immediate impact of complex emergencies. Toole and Waldman (1990) proposed a definition of the acute phase of a complex emergency as greater than one death per 10,000 people per day, based on a doubling of the baseline mortality rate in sub-Saharan African countries. Surveillance systems to monitor the impact of emergencies have been established in the past 15 years based on this definition. In recent decades, it has not been unusual to see CMRs in refugee populations of 30 times the baseline in the country of origin (Toole and Waldman 1997); some of the highest recorded were amongst Rwandan refugees who flooded into North Kivu in 1994 where average crude mortality rates were 20–35 deaths per 10,000 (Salama et al. 2004). In refugee camps, CMRs of 2 per 10,000 are now rarely seen; however, the situation in non-camp situations has deteriorated (Salama et al. 2004). Refugees are usually at greatest risk in early days of displacement, with mortality rates subsequently diminishing. The highest risk group is young children with most deaths occurring in the under-5 age group, demonstrated dramatically in one Somali camp in which 70 per cent of children under 5 appear to have died over an 8-month period (Moore et al. 1993; Toole and Waldman 1997).

Causes of death

The main causes of death in developing country refugee situations are similar to those of developing country populations in general. The most common causes of death in Africa are diarrhoeal disease, measles, acute respiratory infections, and malaria (where endemic), exacerbated by a high prevalence of acute malnutrition (Toole and Waldman 1997). These diseases typically account for the vast majority of reported deaths in refugee populations, at times up to 95 per cent thereof. This is in contrast to European countries affected by war, where the most common causes of death are injuries, as well as communicable diseases, neonatal problems, and nutritional deficiencies. Recent analyses suggest that chronic diseases require attention, given the ageing population, and violence, instability, and forced migration in populations in which communicable diseases have been relatively well controlled and chronic diseases have emerged as problems (Chan and Sondorp 2007).

The conditions affecting refugees may have been brought with them from the country of origin, may be acquired in the host country (with refugees susceptible due to lack of sufficient immunity), or may result from the camp conditions themselves.

Diarrhoeal disease

Possibly the greatest threat to life amongst refugees is diarrhoeal disease. The main pathogens of concern are usually cholera and shigella. In some refugee camps, more than 40 per cent of deaths in the acute phase of an emergency can be attributed to diarrhoeal disease, and over 80 per cent of these deaths are in children under the age of 2 years (Salama et al. 2004). Outbreaks are exacerbated by factors such as the sharing and contamination of water sources and food, the scarcity of soap, and inadequate sanitation.

Amongst Rwandan refugees in camps in North Kivu, 85 per cent of the 50,000 deaths amongst the 800,000 people that flooded into the area in early July 1994 were caused by diarrhoea, with 40 per cent from shigella dysentery and 60 per cent from cholera (Salama et al. 2004). The primary drinking source, which was lake water, became rapidly contaminated, and as water was also scarce, infection spread swiftly through the refugees. Deaths in Goma were associated with a number of preventable causes (Siddique et al. 1995). Among Kurdish refugees, 70 per cent of deaths were a result of diarrhoea (Toole and Waldman 1997). In the elderly and young children, dysentery case-fatality rates can be as high as 10 per cent. Important public health interventions include the need to supply sufficient water, control excreta and hygiene, and increase public awareness of basic rules of hygiene. Evidence-informed case management is necessary to avoid unnecessary deaths.

Measles

Another of the most feared diseases in camps is measles—a particularly large problem in refugee situations in the 1970s and 1980s until it was recognized that vaccination should be accorded priority. The risk of death from measles is exacerbated in the presence of malnutrition, a common occurrence amongst refugee populations, as are secondary complications. Globally, measles kills hundreds of thousands of people each year. In 2000 there were 562,000 measles deaths but with improved surveillance and vaccination rates this was reduced to 122,000 deaths in 2012 (WHO 2012). While it is less of a problem in previously well-vaccinated populations, in developing countries, measles death rates can range from 1 to 5 per cent, and in refugee settings among malnourished children, the death rate may reach 10–30 per cent.

In 1985, 53 and 42 per cent of refugee deaths in eastern Sudan and Somalia, respectively, were caused by measles (Salama et al. 2004). The situation has improved in refugee camps due to mass vaccination, but IDPs still suffer as they have less access to vaccinations and, since 1990, it is more common to find high rates of measles in IDPs than in refugees. Measles is included in the Expanded Program on Immunisation but there is often low coverage in young children especially where human resources for health are limited or conflict affects normal service delivery. Increasing attention is being devoted to ensuring that services can continue to be supplied in fragile states.

Malaria

In areas where malaria is endemic, it can cause high rates of mortality and morbidity amongst refugees. This is particularly the case when people are displaced from an area of low endemicity to one of high endemicity. Drug resistance also plays a large part with chloroquine resistance and more recent resistance to fansidar reported in Rwandan refugees in Zaire. Local communities in low endemic areas may be placed at risk by refugees arriving from high endemic areas, especially if local conditions favour the mosquito. In Africa, 30 per cent of annual malarial deaths occur in complex emergency settings. This is because in complex emergencies (CEs) overcrowding increases the frequency of bites and also delays intervention thereby increasing the time that the parasite is in the blood (Salama et al. 2004). An example is Burundi which had a major epidemic in 2000–2001 when the population of 7 million reported 2.8 million cases of malaria, the war in 1993 caused control efforts to break down, populations were moving, and there was widespread resistance to chloroquine.

Acute respiratory infections

Refugee camp conditions facilitate the spread of acute respiratory infections (ARIs) and rank amongst the leading causes of death in displaced populations. The lack of shelter, overcrowding with poor ventilation, and exposure that characterize the refugee existence contribute to the susceptibility to ARIs with poor outcomes. Young children are particularly affected. In Kabul, in 1993, 30 per cent of under-5 deaths and 23 per cent of deaths in displaced persons were a result of ARIs (Salama et al. 2004). Vaccinations against malaria, diphtheria, and pertussis have led to decreased mortality from ARIs. It is not just that these pathogens cause ARIs but they also render hosts less able to defend themselves from bacterial infection.

Tuberculosis

Tuberculosis (TB) is becoming increasingly important in complex emergencies and situations of forced migration—in part as a result of disrupted therapy (Connolly et al. 2004). TB can become a major problem, leading to a large numbers of deaths. Poor nutrition and over-crowding exacerbate the risk of TB, as may underlying HIV in some populations. A recent study of instability and internal displacement in Timor-Leste revealed a number of problems in maintaining continuity of treatment for those with TB. As a result, many may have incomplete or inadequate treatment.

Meningococcal disease

Meningococcal disease is a potentially major problem for refugees when they are in overcrowded settlements in an endemic area, such as the 'meningitis belt' of sub-Saharan Africa that stretches from Senegal to Ethiopia. In Africa, a threshold incidence of 15 cases per 100,000 population per week is used to define the presence of an 'epidemic'. In CEs, large epidemics have also been reported outside the traditional malaria belt. The Democratic Republic of the Congo had six epidemics in 6 months in 2002 and epidemics have also occurred in Uganda, Rwanda, and Tanzania (Salama et al. 2004). Immunization has proved to be an effective control measure but is only effective in epidemics, routine immunization is not effective as the current vaccines only produce immunity for 3–5 years and may not be used in children under 2 years. Therefore, the World Health Organization (WHO) only recommends mass immunization in areas where epidemic proportions have been reached, and they estimate that this can reduce deaths by up to 70 per cent.

Hepatitis

Outbreaks of hepatitis E have occurred in African refugee camps. It is transmitted by the entero-faecal route, and therefore water supplies are often involved. Case-fatality rates vary from 1–4 per cent but there have been particularly high attack rates and case-fatality rates (up to 20 per cent) reported amongst pregnant women. The high level of previous exposure to hepatitis A and B in developing countries makes it likely that any hepatitis epidemic with high attack rates in adults is likely to be caused by hepatitis E.

HIV/AIDS and other sexually transmitted infections

The pattern of HIV/AIDS and sexually transmitted infections (STIs) amongst refugee populations in developing countries will depend on many factors, including the level of infection prior to displacement (Dualeh and Shears 2002). Speigel (2004), working at the UNHCR, has highlighted the key preventive and other responses to HIV/AIDS. Conflict situations and camp conditions have often been thought to exacerbate the spread of STIs, due to breakdown of social structures, behavioural change, sexual violence, and lack of access to services and testing (Zwi and Cabral 1991). However, Speigel (2004) describes other factors inherent in refugee situations that may retard the spread of these diseases, such as decreased mobility, and the possibility of a host country having increased services in comparison to the country from which people have fled. He argues that each situation should be examined independently and that the spread of STIs is most likely to be determined by the complex interactions between a number of groups: refugees and their hosts, the original conflict-affected population, IDP populations in the country of origin, and host communities in country of origin. He argues for public health responses to be broad and focus not only on camps but the entire situation, including host populations.

Other communicable diseases

Outbreaks of other less common communicable diseases have been reported in some refugee camps, as highlighted by Dualeh and Shears (2002). Typhoid fever is endemic in many tropical areas and may occur sporadically in refugee situations. Leishmaniasis and trypanosomiasis have also been reported in epidemic proportions amongst displaced populations in Uganda and Sudan. Viral haemorrhagic fevers occur in selected areas and may place refugee communities at risk. Rift Valley fever has been documented among Somali refugees in Kenya, yellow fever occurred amongst displaced populations from Ethiopia to Sudan, and dengue fever affects refugees in endemic areas of South East Asia.

Connolly et al. (2004) provide an excellent overview of the literature on communicable diseases and complex emergencies.

Malnutrition—protein energy deficiencies

Moderate to severe acute malnutrition is a common occurrence in refugee settings. Children are particularly affected, with some deteriorating in terms of nutritional status after arrival in camps, due to inadequate nutrition or diarrhoeal disease. Surveys undertaken between 1988 and 1995 documented a range of 11–81 per cent of children under 5 years suffering acute malnutrition in conflict affected populations (Toole and Waldman 1990). Acute malnutrition can be both the cause and effect of other illnesses, and

contributes to mortality both directly and indirectly. Malnutrition and measles are particularly linked with malnutrition exacerbating measles, and measles itself contributing to high malnutrition rates in those that survive it (Toole and Waldman 1990). This 'synergistic relationship' that malnutrition has with communicable disease requires an integrated response aimed at improving nutrition combined with efforts to improve public health services.

Micronutrient deficiencies

As a result of inadequate food rations micronutrient deficiencies occur frequently in refugee populations. The most common diseases seen are iron and vitamin A deficiencies but other diseases include scurvy (vitamin C deficiency), pellagra (niacin and/or tryptophan deficiency), and beriberi (thiamine deficiency). As Prinzo and Benoist (2002) discuss, the solutions are not simple and each setting may require a different approach, including providing fortified blended cereal and finding ways to exchange rations for locally produced fresh fruit and vegetables.

Food and nutritional interventions need to be responsive to cultural as well as economic issues.

Reproductive health

The reproductive health needs of refugees have gained recognition since the mid 1990s. The burden is undeniably greater for women as a result of insecurity in their social situations and gender-based violence. Women lack basic necessities such as sanitary napkins and condoms, and pregnancy itself can be a serious health threat in settings in which services are lacking or overwhelmed (Krause et al. 2000). Referral services are often non-existent and birthing or abortion may be undertaken in unsafe situations. Women may have no, or limited, access or means to carry out family planning, rape and sexual coercion are typically increased, and there may be pressures on women to rebuild the population. Female genital mutilation may occur and STIs, including HIV, may be relatively common (Krause et al. 2000). A particularly important set of risks relate to sexual and other forms of gender-based violence, common in all societies and increased where societal norms are less able to be enforced or reinforced, and in which men with guns can demand whatever they like in return for precious resources such as safety, food, and onward passage. Intense efforts have focused on improving all aspects of reproductive health for women affected by complex emergencies and forced migration—and a Minimum Initial Services Package has been produced to address these needs. A study by Hynes et al. (2002) showed that due to the strength of the response there have actually now been better reproductive health outcomes in refugee camps than in host population or origin countries. However, the lessons learned require expansion across settings.

Mental health and psychosocial needs

Mental health problems are recognized as an important source of morbidity globally (Prince et al. 2007) and are likely to be even greater amongst displaced populations. Epidemiological assessments have documented high rates of mental illness in these populations. Studies have tended to focus on trauma-related conditions, although low prevalence conditions such as psychosis have also proven significant in post-conflict and refugee settings. There is much debate about the validity of Western-derived measurement and about the trauma focus, with further development of relevant culturally valid ways to measure psychiatric morbidity still required. Despite the measurement debate, there is clearly a substantial burden of mental distress in these settings, and support for vulnerable people is vital in situations of social breakdown, especially where usual systems of social support and healing are disrupted (Silove et al. 2000a). It may be of value to identify and respond to the needs of three different groups of people who experience psychosocial and mental distress in these situations: those who are mentally ill, who need treatment; those who have had particularly horrific experiences and need care and support in order to recover; and what tends to be the majority who need a more stable social and political environment in which they can resume their normal day-to-day activities necessary to promote mental health.

Internally displaced persons

While IDPs in developing countries have very similar health problems to refugees, they also have particular vulnerabilities. Some of these result from falling through gaps in a system geared to protect a particular group of forced migrants (i.e. 'Convention refugees'). Particularly in developing countries, but also in more developed states, the limited data available suggest higher morbidity and mortality in IDPs compared with refugees (Salama et al. 2001). With limited protection granted by the international community, the responsibility for protection and assistance often lies with their own governments. Yet, it is these governments themselves that have often contributed to the displacement experienced. Governments may not even officially recognize the existence of IDPs for fear of international scrutiny or interference. A growing number of countries have developed laws and policies to govern responses to IDP populations but not all make concerted attempts to implement these policies, and even when there is political will the states involved are often the poorest countries of the world, limiting their ability to respond. There is no mandated international body although UNHCR may include them amongst their persons of concern and they are increasingly supported by agencies which follow the UN's Guiding Principles on Internal Displacement (Deng 1998).

IDP populations rarely experience access to health services at the same standard as offered to other citizens and are likely to be markedly poorer than those available to refugees. Recent efforts to improve quality and responsiveness of interventions in humanitarian crises and complex emergencies have contributed to better health outcomes. IDPs, however, have poor access to these improved systems of protection and assistance.

Collection of data is more difficult amongst IDP populations and relatively few studies focus specifically on IDPs. However, the IDP-specific health data that are available suggest that access to healthcare for IDPs is often extremely limited. Salama et al. (2001) show how some of highest mortality rates in humanitarian emergencies have been found in IDP populations; Sudan and Somali, for example, reached 8 per 10,000/day and 17 per 10,000/day respectively (Salama et al. 2001). In Ethiopia and the Democratic Republic of the Congo, delays in vaccinations led to measles outbreaks. In Ajiep (southern Sudan), severe acute malnutrition amongst IDPS reached 36 per cent during a famine in 1998.

Although international humanitarian law applies to all civilians affected by armed conflict and therefore IDPs should be afforded the same protection and assistance as the un-displaced host population, there may be multiple reasons why IDPs face discrimination and therefore do not receive the help they need.

Even in developed countries IDPs may have poor health outcomes. They are often subject to the discrimination and exclusion experienced by their developing country counterparts. The Internal Displacement Monitoring Centre (IDMC) describes the situation for a number of IDP groups in developed nations:

> While IDPs in the Balkans generally have satisfactory access to water, sanitation and healthcare, they are more likely than the local population to suffer from trauma-related problems. Roma IDPs usually live in informal settlements with very poor sanitary conditions. IDPs in Azerbaijan and the Russian Federation access healthcare less easily than the local population in some areas, due to administrative inconsistencies, lack of healthcare facilities and the demand for informal payments for medical treatment. (IDMC 2008)

IDPs, whether in developing or developed countries, are clearly living with a higher burden of illness and mortality than many other forced migrant groups. Initiatives are emerging that aim to support this extremely vulnerable population, but they are yet to be supported by any legal framework.

Refugees and asylum seekers in developed countries

Refugees and asylum seekers often reach destinations in developed countries after long, precarious journeys. Prior to the journey, they will have faced many of the routine health problems that present themselves in disrupted developing country settings. The journey itself will have produced health challenges; people may have been detained at points along the way or experienced significant anxiety and distress through difficult and dangerous journeys and experiences. On arrival, the range of situations they find themselves in will further shape their health condition. Those who have applied for refugee status prior to arrival may have undergone health checks already in the country of origin, as is the practice of many developed countries; therefore, certain health conditions may have been picked up. Depending on the country they arrive in, they will then have a different range of options available to address their health problems. However, those applying for refugee status on arrival have an even more complicated journey; they may be detained for short or long periods, they may have extensive periods on temporary visas or they may find themselves living illegally without authorization from the host country. Typically asylum seekers are often isolated with difficulty in communication, in a situation of poverty, discrimination, and a lack of social structure, causing many to suffer from trauma-related problems and many general health problems, exacerbated by poor provision of health information and barriers to accessing to services.

Biggs and Skull (2003) discuss the specific medical conditions that may be present amongst refugees in developed countries. These include communicable disease such as TB, HIV, STIs, hepatitis B and C, and parasitic diseases, all compounded by incomplete immunization. In addition, nutritional deficiencies (vitamin D in particular), mental health problems, and other non-communicable diseases such as diabetes and reproductive health issues are common.

Screening for health problems among newly 'arrived' refugees, or prior to arrival for those applying for refugee status overseas, is common practice. Biggs and Skull (2003) point out that there is little evidence demonstrating that screening has proved effective as many people have limited contact with services and many are lost to follow up. Refugees seeking asylum in the United States are screened before arrival to identify 'inadmissible conditions' such as HIV, TB, and leprosy. They may also be screened for diseases that are known to be prevalent and targets of public health intervention. For example, Somali refugees were mass treated for malaria and intestinal parasites. The types of health problems sought and treated in newly arrived immigrants also reflect particular areas of concern for asylum seekers, including infectious disease, gynaecological health (rape, genital surgery, STIs), and mental health (torture, trauma) (Adams et al. 2007).

Burnett and Peel (2001) evaluated the health needs of asylum seekers and refugees in Britain. They point out that these groups are subject to 'poverty, dependence, and lack of cohesive social support' as well as racial discrimination. They consider a range of studies examining the health status of refugees and found, for example, that 21 per cent of migrants to Spain from sub-Saharan Africa were chronic carriers of hepatitis B, and 3.4 per cent of refugees arriving in the United States in 1988 had TB. They highlight the lack of screening programmes available and how the focus has tended to be on protecting hosts rather than a responsibility to provide healthcare to all.

One specific refugee and asylum health condition that has been investigated somewhat more extensively than other health issues is mental health (see Chapter 8.7). Gerritsen et al. (2004) describe how early research focused on those who used services, or victims of trauma, followed by early population-based studies in Western settings which have tended to focus on psychiatric disorders such as post-traumatic stress disorder (PTSD), anxiety, and depression. In a review of the literature, Fazel et al. (2005) show documented rates of PTSD of 4–70 per cent, depression 3–88 per cent, and anxiety 2–80 per cent. Their meta-analysis suggests that one in ten refugees in Western countries have PTSD, one in 20 has major depression, and one in 25 has a generalized anxiety disorder. Although lower than some estimates, this is still ten times higher than rates of PTSD in the general population in the United States. Data for asylum seekers alone is sparse but there are reasons to believe they have even higher rates due to their vulnerability because of disruption, separation from family members, increased levels of torture and trauma, lack of language skills, and the often hostile reception from host population fuelled by media perceptions. The current trend towards detention, and temporary rather than permanent protection have added extra stress, as evidenced by studies of asylum seekers in detention centres and on temporary protection visas showing very high rates of mental illness (Silove et al. 2000b, 2007).

Problems that asylum seekers in particular face, rather than refugees, relate to issues of having a temporary and often contested legal status, and in some cases being considered illegal, with implications (real or perceived) for access to health services. Many countries such as the United Kingdom and Australia have fluctuating policies with regards to what asylum seekers, of differing categories, may be entitled to in terms of healthcare. This can act as a barrier to health for many asylum seekers. The increased use of detention for asylum seekers, whilst claims are processed, has been challenged heavily by health professionals as a result of evidence that it is detrimental to health. The other popular policy of extending only temporary protection to some asylum seekers,

therefore also causing confusion with regards to health entitlements, and long-term insecurity with associated health risks, has also caused concern to health professionals (Silove et al. 2000b). Australia has passed legislation to allow off-shore processing for asylum seekers. A policy of this kind raises more complex questions in terms of entitlement and availability of healthcare. Health professionals have called for screening to ensure those with the most severe mental and physical health problems are identified and if necessary processed on the mainland.

Healthcare for asylum seekers may be difficult to access on many levels: policies of active deterrent of asylum seekers may mean they are not entitled to care, or there may be lack of prioritizing refugees; health professionals often misunderstand what the policies are and may refuse to register asylum seekers, they also fear the burden of vulnerable groups; those that do offer treatment may lack understanding of the refugee health situation; temporary registration with GPs may be offered rather than permanent (limiting access to immunizations and screening); and language problems are also a great barrier, with many practitioners having inadequate access to interpreting services.

Harris and Telfer (2001) estimated that in 1999–2000 there were over 10,000 asylum seekers living in the community in Australia. Many had to survive for many months or years with no right to work and no medical cover through the national Medicare scheme, resulting in untreated medical conditions. A study in Sydney suggested that most presenting to an Asylum Seeker Centre providing health services had fairly serious psychological or physical symptoms. Some related to trauma and torture, others were infectious diseases, musculoskeletal complaints, and gynaecological problems. Up to 40 per cent of the asylum seekers were denied Medicare. A few are picked up by the Asylum Seeker Assistance Scheme and the Red Cross assists others. Hospital fees are particularly high and case studies have shown that some people are denied hospital treatment until assurance of payment is provided.

Trafficked and smuggled people

People that are trafficked or smuggled are not an entirely distinct group from other types of forced migrants already described. Trafficked people have been coerced or tricked into allowing another person to organize their passage to another country; also smuggled across borders are those who 'voluntarily' migrate for a vast range of reasons but feel unable to do so through legal channels. Although these groups may appear distinct from refugee populations they may include Convention refugees and others whose circumstances are very close to those of refugees. Resorting to illegal and clandestine methods of migrating to another country, either through being coerced and misled or through having such limited choices as to choose this route, is often a result of many of the factors behind the forced migration of refugees and internally displaced people.

Gushulak and MacPherson (2000) describe some of the reasons why people may fall into a trafficking situation. Poverty, exposure to violence, restrictive barriers—for example, screening for certain diseases or security barriers, slow processing of routine immigration applications which may cause delay to family reunification—all may encourage people to take alternative routes—especially when traffickers may offer what appear to be attractive possibilities. They state that the reasons why someone is more likely to migrate through these illegal methods are also reasons that place a person at higher risk of having poor health prior to migration. The journeys faced by trafficked and smuggled people are often extremely precarious, with high levels of morbidity and mortality attached as a result: unseaworthy and overcrowded boats on long journeys, stowed in containers, attached to carriers, attempts to cross inhospitable land with extremes of temperature, drowning from swimming attempts, violence from traffickers, and illegal activities such as smuggling drugs with people. On arrival people are then subject to many of the difficulties already outlined that face asylum seekers. Some trafficked and smuggled people may seek asylum and depending on the policies of the countries may incur some health benefits; however, many will be forced into illegal employment and be either too scared to make or prevented from making an approach to health services. Disease prevention and control in this population will be extremely poor—leading to increased prevalence of disease in the trafficked community as a whole.

Busza et al. (2004) examine the need for careful understanding of trafficking situations and to unravel the local dynamics. They state that even when intermediaries are involved, and even when they are taking people into exploitative arenas such as sex work, these situations remain a complex mixture of voluntary and forced migration. Whilst economic disadvantage may fuel the choice, there is still a choice being made in some contexts and organizations seeking to stem the flow or break up these systems may compromise the health or the individuals involved more than they help. Attempts to 'save' people may make them even more vulnerable—for example, the raiding of brothels and other such moves can force vulnerable people to go underground making engagement with health services difficult.

The health of trafficked and smuggled people is affected by the fact that they cannot easily be separated out from each other or from other types of 'voluntary' migration that are not truly voluntary but have strong forces pushing people on. The policies developed by states towards any of these groups are likely to impact on the capacity of other groups to access healthcare. Displaced people are more vulnerable to trafficking and may in desperation turn to smugglers. This should be kept in mind by health professionals to avoid vulnerable people missing out on essential services and support.

Public health solutions and interventions

Forced migration clearly has major impacts on public health. Specific solutions and interventions need to be sensitive to culture and context, and include a critical assessment of the political dynamics that may affect how assistance is actually received and impacts on the lives of forced migrants. Harrell-Bond et al. (1992), the doyens of analysts examining forced migration, along with other key commentators such as Crisp (1999) and Bakewell (n.d.), demonstrate how resources to deal with forced migration are structured by broader ideological, political, and economic decisions. Harrell-Bond et al. (1992) argue that refugee camps and many of the structures and organizations set up are part of a system of control of those in need. She argues that the allocation of resources (whether aid, political or military resources) is a 'central component in an ideology of control'. The granting of aid often legitimizes a group and their struggles; politics influences the status and visibility accorded to different groups. Even where humanitarian and development assistance are well targeted

at forced migrants in need, the impact of services, systems, and funds, may be both positive and negative. While the forced migrants in great need may be able to access resources, these are not distributed equitably, and local populations, which often bear the brunt of providing for such community members, frequently are marginalized and unable to access new resources or services.

A valuable compilation of insights (Essed et al. 2004) highlights how forced migrants interact with agencies and the implications for ethics, policies, and politics. A case study by Turner (2004) in the same volume, for example, demonstrates how UNHCR effectively displaces older men as providers in their families and in so doing creates new dependencies. UNHCR becomes 'a better husband'—at the same time undermining and transforming traditional household and family relationships. These political complexities are vital to keep in mind when planning and implementing a public health response with vulnerable communities.

Key actors and organizations in refugee health

There is an extensive range of organizations involved in addressing forced migration. The UN has designated the UNHCR as the key multilateral agency for identifying and dealing with refugee issues. More recently, the mandate of UNHCR, as described earlier, has been extended to include other 'people of concern' including IDPs and asylum seekers. Other agencies with a specific mandate for dealing with forced migrants include the International Organisation on Migration, the International Centre for Migration and Health, the American Refugee Committee International, the US Committee on Refugees, and the Global IDP Project.

A wide range of multilateral agencies including the WHO, UN Population Fund (UNFPA), UNICEF, International Committee of the Red Cross (ICRC), International Federation of Red Cross and Red Crescent Societies (IFRC), and UNAIDS has some concern with forced migrants. Key non-governmental organizations (NGOs) include Merlin, Médecins Sans Frontières (MSF), International Medical Corps (IMC), International Rescue Committee (IRC), OXFAM, Save the Children Fund, CARE, Caritas, CONCERN, and the Norwegian Refugee Council. Academic bodies include the Oxford University Refugee Studies Program, the Centers for Disease Control and Prevention (CDC), and the Refugee Studies Program in Cairo. A number of important journals, notably the *Journal of Refugee Studies, Disasters* and *Conflict and Health*, and the website of Forced Migration Online, provide avenues for academic debate.

Developing countries and complex emergency settings

The principles of public health and epidemiology only began to be systematically applied to complex emergency situations from the early 1970s (Salama et al. 2004). Since then, new academic and practitioner fields have developed, including emergency public health and public health nutrition. With the introduction of an indicator to measure the impact of a complex emergency through CMRs, alongside the development of simplified measurements of malnutrition, and threshold rates for epidemics, it has become increasingly possible to draw meaningful inferences from data collected.

An understanding of the dynamics of disease and related mortality in CEs has grown, and practice improved on the basis of experience and research evidence. Guidelines and technical manuals have been produced and efforts enhanced to promote organizational learning and enhanced service delivery, building on a growing evidence base. The call for evidence with which to inform policy and practice (Banatvala and Zwi 2000) reinforced what was already happening in the field where practitioners and academics were drawing lessons from experiences and enhancing the quality of their responses.

Mortality rates are now much lower than previously seen, malnutrition is declining in many settings, and measles, a major killer in the past, is less catastrophic following efforts to ensure early immunization of children. Enhanced understanding of risks of communicable diseases has decreased risks, although failures to apply evidence, such as in Goma following the Rwandan genocide, still lead to tens of thousands of preventable deaths. Epidemics of some communicable diseases are better controlled and may be less serious and last for shorter periods given improved surveillance and earlier detection of outbreaks. The pattern seen is often similar to the baseline in developing countries, in terms of the major killers. However, the shift has been to seeing many of the highest mortality rates outside of camps, where the public health response has not been as well developed.

Toole and Waldman (1997) describe the need for primary, secondary, and tertiary prevention. In primary prevention, they argue that political and diplomatic mechanisms should be developed to prevent conflicts evolving to the point of mass displacement, and that epidemiology may be able to add value in studying some of the dynamics that indicate conflict developing on a large scale. Secondary prevention comprises early detection of population movements, contingency planning so that relevant actors are prepared for the scale and nature of likely public health crises, having well-trained personnel with knowledge and experience in dealing with the health problems associated with refugee situations and able to rapidly assess and intervene in partnership with local organizations, along with the capacity to monitor and evaluate programmes swiftly and effectively. Tertiary prevention involves channelling resources into combating the sources of morbidity and mortality already outlined. This involves providing shelter and protection, adequate food rations, adequate clean water and sanitation facilities, programmes for preventing specific communicable diseases, preparing for epidemics, specific programmes such as maternal and child health or mental health, managing diarrhoeal disease, and setting up health information systems.

The social, cultural, and political challenges of instituting these levels of prevention, alongside the practical implications of working in such settings, are substantial. Salama et al. (2004) describe how the field has been growing over 30 years, with increasing attention by humanitarian actors since the 1990s to codify technical guidelines. In the early 1990s, there was a growing disappointment and recognition amongst the actors attempting to engage with these complexities, and provide emergency assistance to refugees, that the field was uncoordinated and lacking in technical direction. Research, adverse publicity, and heightened calls for accountability around standards of service delivery and to the supposed beneficiaries of humanitarian interventions, all pointed to the need for significant improvements.

Initiatives were beginning to emerge that were investigating ways to address these issues, but the field was ultimately galvanized by events in 1994 in Goma, Zaire. The unprecedented rapid influx of refugees and the resulting massive cholera epidemic, producing one of the highest mortality rates recorded, led to a serious reappraisal of humanitarian work in these settings. The Joint Evaluation of Emergency Assistance to Rwanda was an impressive, multiagency, multidonor-funded initiative, paving the way to a deep review of the humanitarian and relief field and the standards of care and conduct.

In terms of future public health directions, Salama et al. (2004) describe the need to move beyond the current refugee and IDP paradigms, as non-camp populations affected by conflict are now often greater in number and burden, and mechanisms to deliver services to such populations are less clear. There is a need for enhanced coverage in all settings of known effective public health interventions, and for the more upstream causes of CEs to be addressed. The technical needs identified include the development of more context-specific methods for assessing mortality rates as an indicator based on surrounding baseline CMRs, and considering which other indicators may point to a deteriorating situation such as fluctuations in disease incidence, levels of displacement, and decreasing food security. They suggest that implementation of control measures should be early, not when mortality and malnutrition are already high, and that whilst communicable disease control should continue to be prioritized along with nutrition and food security, that enhanced efforts at addressing mental health, reproductive health, and neonatal health should also be incorporated. Important policy issues include better means of determining direction and coordination of public health interventions, early identification of a lead agency, and greater effort to support fledgling governments to take the lead with the support of a coherent international system. They suggest that the skills of relief workers should be strengthened and broadened to include knowledge of assessment and prevention of disease, monitoring and evaluation, and international systems, policies, and regulatory bodies.

Ensuring equity in the response and equity in access to services and resources made available remains a considerable and under-emphasized challenge.

Developed countries

In developed countries, the complex political arena and the increasingly restrictive views of host populations towards asylum seekers and refugees complicates the task of addressing the public health of forced migrants. Whilst an array of motivated and effective actors plays a number of different roles in this field, there are few central bodies charged with overseeing the public health of forced migrants as a whole. The policies of the host nations themselves are likely to shape the public health landscape and in situations where these policies seem to be detrimental to the health of this population, public health professionals may find themselves having to take increasingly political roles to fulfil their public health duties.

Advocacy groups and health professional organizations have set up refugee and asylum seeker health networks and centres through which to provide services and support and advocate for more inclusive social and health policies.

The Health of London Project established a health centre in 1999 to provide access to good-quality primary care for forced migrants. The service aims to provide a thorough initial health assessment, along with effective responses to issues such as mental health problems and communicable diseases. In Europe, Médecins du Monde, an NGO, has stepped in to provide care for groups with restricted access to healthcare, particularly failed asylum seekers.

The best way in which to organize healthcare for resettled refugees, and for asylum seekers, remains contentious. A key issue point of debate is whether they should be integrated within mainstream services, or offered separately through distinct services for these marginalized groups (Finney Lamb and Cunningham 2003). Such centres are often voluntarily run and unable to cover the full extent of need. Hull and Boomla (2006) discuss the implications of such NGO provision, including some of the unanticipated negative aspects.

Another potential theoretical divide that can emerge with health approaches to asylum seekers and refugees is that between public health and human rights frameworks. Governments are more responsive to public health arguments whereby health problems of forced migrant populations may be addressed for the benefit of the wider population, often highlighting the risk brought with incoming refugees and forced migrants of communicable diseases. However, these approaches focus more on protecting the host than the forced migrants' right to receive healthcare (Burnett and Peel 2001) and may reinforce discrimination and marginalization of the migrants who are seen as posing a risk to the general community and demanding excessive use of public services (Grove and Zwi 2006). Tarantola et al. (2008) argue for much closer links between public health, human rights, and development—all equally relevant to forced migration.

Hull and Boomla (2006) describe recent UK government proposals to deny general practitioners the discretion of registering overseas visitors including failed asylum seekers, and to provide care to them. They highlight the possibility that such a policy will inadvertently increase costs through more emergency admissions, and they stress that such a policy is a breach of human rights, ethically unsupportable, and may place clinicians in conflict with their professional duties.

Ashcroft (2005) describes the language of the UK and Australian governments as 'Orwellian' in an overview of their approaches to asylum seekers and health. In discussing the UK government's move to make failed asylum seekers pay for all non-emergency care, despite not having the right to work, he states that the treatment of asylum seekers is an ethical issue and that denial of medical treatment should not be used as a lever to exclude people or get them to leave the country. In some cases, the presence of HIV seropositivity has been used to exclude refugees from the opportunity to resettle in a third country; this is of particular concern given the heightened risk of violence and infection that may characterize the lives of many refugees. Using this against such vulnerable community members is a double victimization.

As Silove et al. (2000b) stated:

the medical profession has a legitimate role in commenting on the general and mental health risks of imposing restrictive and discriminatory measures on asylum seekers, especially when some of these administrative procedures threaten one of the fundamental principles underpinning the practice of medicine: primum non nocere [do no harm].

In response to current debates in Australia, the Australian Medical Association issued a position statement on the Health Care of Asylum Seekers and Refugees (Australian Medical Association 2011). This lays out not only the health vulnerabilities of these populations but also that medical practitioners should insist on the rights of their patients being respected and lays out certain competencies necessary for treating asylum seekers. These include identifying victims of torture, assessing and managing trauma, identifying suicide risk and recognizing health conditions specific to these groups such as TB.

Further study is required to document the patterns of disease, the links to the asylum experience, and impact of policies, not only on forced migrant health but also the implications for host populations are required. Given the more restrictive policy environment, health professionals require a strong evidence base from which to lobby for improved access to services as a first step in improving the health of refugees and asylum seekers in developed countries.

Emerging issues for public health professionals

Many of the issues raised in earlier sections have a technical focus, even if their links with broader sociopolitical issues have been acknowledged. In this concluding section of the chapter, we highlight some of the many issues which challenge professionals and societies, not only on a technical level, but in terms of the values underpinning how we, individually and collectively, whether as citizens or professionals, see and respond to others, especially those who have been forced to flee.

This section seeks to highlight, briefly, a number of key themes: globalization and poverty, quality and accountability, ethics and researching with forced migrants, voice, visibility, and agency. They are central to understanding the context within which forced migration arises and health needs should be understood and addressed.

Globalization and poverty

There is increasing evidence of widening gaps in income and basic needs between the well-off and the impoverished in many settings. Labonte and Schrecker (2005) identify the key links between current patterns of globalization and the influence these have on the social determinants of health. The challenges are evident in the failure to address the Millennium Development Goal (MDG) targets, while extreme wealth continues to be generated and monopolized by small fractions of the world's population. Resource constraints are likely to increase; countries engaging actively with global economic and political opportunities may do well but not all their citizens will necessarily benefit.

Evidence of gaps is widespread; and it is apparent that the MDGs, a major driving force at present in international development, do not adequately address issues of equity (Attaran 2005). Such concerns are likely to be amplified in relation to especially vulnerable and socially excluded communities such as forced migrants, data on whom may be unavailable and systems of response to which will be fragmented, uncoordinated, and inadequately monitored. Colson (2007) argues cogently that much greater emphasis should be placed on understanding the 'factors that provide the impetus to leave' and not focusing only on the aftermath of such forced migrations.

Quality and accountability

A key challenge in engaging with situations of violence, social exclusion, and disempowerment is in ensuring that work undertaken to assist those affected does no harm, or at least strives to limit the potential harm and maximize the potential value. The international community, through the UN, other multilateral and bilateral agencies, and international NGOs, all ostensibly seek to assist those forced to flee or migrate.

One way in which evidence improvements are underway is in relation to enhancing and seeking to assure the quality of humanitarian and relief work. Major Quality and Accountability initiatives such as SPHERE, the Humanitarian Code of Conduct, the Humanitarian Accountability Partnership, and many others contribute to enhanced practice. There remains a need to facilitate self-reflection and open review, transparency of difficulties limitations and failures, and promotion and funding for the search to do better.

The vast majority of incentives currently in place, however, encourage the hiding, rather than the declaration, of weaknesses, so as to elicit the next tranche of funding. This is counterproductive when seeking to reflect and improve services and their responsiveness to need. New thinking is required: how do we develop systems of trust and collegiality, mutual support between affected communities, services providers, and agencies, to ensure that all incentives operate to maximize the gain for those at greatest risk?

New initiatives in the humanitarian and relief areas of activity seek to enhance practice and open out debate and public scrutiny. In so doing, weaknesses are identified, guidelines and lessons for better practice formulated, and processes which seek to engage and creatively respond to problems, developed. Taking forward such action requires promoting an ability to report and record limitations and inadequacies, and to carefully and systematically document strengths and limitations, weaknesses and potentials, to address real problems. Services are never ideal and always have constraints and limits; it is crucial to establish ways of examining them such that opportunities to change, to experiment, to creatively engage with solving problems are established.

New and enhanced knowledge management systems would be most valuable if they assisted in finding innovative means of conceptualizing problems, sharing information and insights of what works in different contexts, and developing systems to ensure accountability to the intended beneficiaries, the forced migrants themselves.

Ethics and researching with forced migrants

Ethical issues require considerable attention especially given the power imbalances present and in relation to research. Forced migrants may be especially vulnerable and risk being abused, either through their stories and survival strategies being exposed and used by their opponents to undermine them; the very practice of talking with an outsider or sharing information may heighten risk, vulnerability, and the attention of those seeking further to undermine and disempower. Real risks may result from security lapses, confidentiality lapses, exposure of coping strategies and adaptations; as well as stigma and reinforcement of difference and of 'otherness'.

A major challenge in research with refugees and other forced migrants is to assist them in documenting their experiences of forced migration (Mackenzie et al. 2007). In so doing, the locus of power in the research relationship has the potential to shift from the researcher him or herself, to the communities being researched. The project may shift from research *on* refugees to research *with* refugees and research *by* refugees for action and change.

While this may be conceptually and morally attractive, the practicalities of achieving this are impeded at multiple levels, not least of which is establishing a trusting relationship between the researcher and the communities with whom they research. Engaging with forced migrants is itself a major challenge: Such communities are often highly dependent on others, and may be reliant on outside agencies with expertise and resources and/or on local power-brokers in control of the basic necessities of life and survival—food, water, shelter, and security.

Zwi et al. (2006) have highlighted the importance of reconceptualizing such research to consider the potential to ensure benefit and reciprocity for the subjects of research and to shift the locus of decision-making in their direction. They offer a model to describe this process, while Mackenzie et al. (2007) present a case study of applying many of these considerations to work with forced migrants on the Thai–Burmese border. Of note is the transfer of power to community organizations, with women's groups from the Thai–Burmese border having control over the stories and narratives collected from them and academics being required to obtain permission from them to publish and distribute and write up such material.

Innovative approaches to research are emerging and warrant support. Youth-focused research highlights the importance of young people in exploring and documenting their own lives and experiences. Young people play a central role in refining and redefining the issues, identifying the challenges and the potential approaches to solving them through new models of participatory action research. Such collaboration needs to build skills, resilience, and opportunities to shape the future.

Voice, visibility, and agency

There is increasing recognition of the importance of hearing from those most affected by any public health condition and ensuring that their voices are heard; empowering them to help shape the proposed solutions. Black (2003) emphasizes the importance of advocacy as a central component of work with marginalized and disempowered groups and reinforces the centrality of ensuring that the voices of those affected, and of the range of stakeholders engaged, is heard.

The voices of forced migrants may be silenced while those of powerful agencies and governments are privileged in shaping our understanding both of the problems and of the solutions which surround forced migration (Harrell-Bond and Voutira 2007). Power imbalances, vulnerability, and cultural and linguistic differences are among the many barriers to creating an environment in which refugees and IDPs are able to take an active part in shaping solutions. As with the youth, truly participatory models of action and research require sensitivity to the challenges of the context and understanding of the conditions that usually deny refugees a voice.

It is crucial that we hear the voices of those most affected by forced migration if we are to recognize the range of experiences, and the positive and negative change and transformation which results. As Eastmond (2007) states eloquently: 'while transformation and change are part of the refugee experience, not all change is perceived as loss or defined as problematic or unwelcome by all individuals involved. Nor are refugees necessarily helpless victims, but rather likely to be people with agency and voice' (p. 253). Learning and recognizing how agency, transformation, resilience, adaptation and change are shaped, notably, but not only, in relation to gender and power, would not be possible without hearing from and learning with, those most affected.

Conclusion

Forced migrant populations frequently suffer vast health challenges. Their experiences need to be understood within the context of accelerating globalization, with its positive and negative features transforming the lives of millions of people.

The role of public health professionals in working alongside forced migrants to bring about improvements in their health is demanding and complex. A comprehensive understanding of the dynamics of forced migration and sensitivity to the constraints placed on individuals and populations is vital to gain trust and provide opportunities for transforming health outcomes. Particularly, given the increasingly restrictive environments that forced migrants find themselves in, public health professionals can have a crucial role in advocating for forced migrant health, enabling forced migrants to speak and be heard, and to bring about improvements in their own health.

Improving knowledge and understanding is central to affirming the rights and the agency of those affected. Public health can play an important role, and indeed has done so, in improving technical quality of service delivery. Key gaps remain, however, in understanding, appreciating, and responding to the varied ways in which those forced to move seek to shape, transform, and better their own lives and experiences.

Acknowledgements

Text extracts from United Nations High Commissioner for Refugees (UNHCR), *Protecting Refugees and the Role of UNHCR*, Copyright © UNHCR 2009, available from http://unhcr.org.au/unhcr/images/protecting%20refugees.pdf, reproduced with permission from the United Nations.

Text extracts from Deng, F., *The Guiding Principles on Internal Displacement*, United Nations, New York, Copyright © United Nations 1998, reproduced with permission from the United Nations.

Text extract from United Nations, *Protocol to Prevent, Suppress and Punish Trafficking in Persons, Especially Women and Children, Supplementing the United Nations Convention Against Transnational Organized Crime*, G.A. Res. 25, Annex II, U.N. GAOR, 55th Session, Copyright © United Nations 2003, reproduced with permission from the United Nations.

Text extract from United Nations, *Protocol Against The Smuggling Of Migrants By Land, Sea And Air*, Copyright © United Nations 2000, reproduced with permission from the United Nations.

Text extract from United Nations, *Glossary of Environment Statistics, Studies in Methods, Series F*, United Nations, New York, USA, Copyright © United Nations 1998, reproduced with permission from the United Nations.

Text extracts from Forced Migration Online, *What is Forced Migration?*, Copyright © 2010 Forced Migration Online and Contributors, available from http://www.forcedmigration. org/whatisfm.htm, reproduced with permission from Forced Migration Online.

Further reading

The following manuals give technical advice in managing public health aspects of forced migration:

Médecins Sans Frontières (MSF) (1997). *Refugee Health: An Approach to Emergency Situations*. London: Macmillan. Available at: http://www.refbooks.msf.org/msf_docs/en/Refugee_Health/RH1.pdf.

World Health Organization (2006). *Communicable Disease Control in Emergencies. A Field Manual*. Available at http://www.who.int/infectious-disease-news/IDdocs/whocds200527/whocds200527chapters/.

Relevant websites

ALNAP—'learning, accountability, performance in humanitarian action' http://www.alnap.org.

Forced Migration Online—http://www.forcedmigration.org.

SPHERE—http://www.sphereproject.org.

The Humanitarian Accountability Partnership—http://www.hapinternational.org.

United Nations High Commissioner for Refugees—http://www.unhcr.org.

References

Adams, K., Gardiner, L., and Assefi, N. (2007). Healthcare challenges from the developing world: post-immigration refugee medicine. *British Medical Journal*, 328, 1548–52.

Allotey, P.A. and Reidpath, D.D. (2003). Refugee intake: reflections on inequality. *Australian and New Zealand Journal of Public Health*, 27, 12–16.

Apodaca, C. (1998). Human rights abuses: precursor to refugee flight? *Journal of Refugee Studies*, 11, 80–93.

Ashcroft, R. (2005). Standing up for the medical rights of asylum seekers. *Journal of Medical Ethics*, 31, 125–6.

Attaran, A. (2005). An immeasurable crisis? A criticism of the millennium development goals and why they cannot be measured. *PLoS Medicine*, 2, e318.

Australian Medical Association (2011). *Health Care of Asylum Seekers and Refugees—2011* [Online]. Available at: https://ama.com.au/position-statement/health-care-asylum-seekers-and-refugees-2011.

Bakewell, O. (n.d.). *Can we Ever Rely on Refugee Statistics?* [Online]. Available at: http://www.radstats.org.uk/no072/article1.htm.

Banatvala, N. and Zwi, A.B. (2000). Public health and humanitarian interventions: developing the evidence base. *British Medical Journal*, 321, 101–5.

Barnett, L. (2002). Global governance and the evolution of the international refugee regime. *International Journal of Refugee Law*, 14, 238–62.

Baum, F. (2001). Health equity justice and globalisation: some lessons from the People's Health Assembly. *Journal of Epidemiology and Community Health*, 55, 613–16.

Biermann, F. and Boas, I. (2007). *Preparing for a Warmer World—Towards a Global Governance System to Protect Climate Refugees*. Global Governance Working Paper. Amsterdam: Global Governance Project.

Biggs, B. and Skull, S. (2003). Refugee health: clinical issues. In P. Allotey (ed.) *The Health of Refugees: Public Health Perspectives from Crisis to Settlement*, pp. 54–67. Melbourne: Oxford University Press.

Black, R. (2003). Ethical codes in humanitarian emergencies: from practice to research? *Disasters*, 27, 95–108.

Burnett, A. and Peel, M. (2001). Asylum seekers and refugees in Britain: health needs of asylum seekers and refugees. *British Medical Journal*, 322, 544–7.

Busza, J., Castle, S., and Diarra, A. (2004). Trafficking and health. *British Medical Journal*, 328, 1369–71.

Castles, S. (2003). Toward a sociology of forced migration and social transformation. *Sociology*, 37, 13–34.

Castles, S. (2004). *Confronting the Realities of Forced Migration*. [Online] Available at: http://www.migrationinformation.org/Feature/print cfm?ID=22.

Cernea, M. (2007). Development-induced and conflict-induced IDPs: bridging the research divide. *Forced Migration Review*, Special Issue, 25–7.

Chan, E.Y. and Sondorp, E. (2007). Medical interventions following natural disasters: missing out on chronic medical needs. *Asia Pacific Journal of Public Health*, 19, 45–51.

Colson, E. (2007). Linkage methodology: no man is an island. *Journal of Refugee Studies*, 20, 321–33.

Connolly, M.A., Gayer, M., Ryan, M.J., Speigel, P., Salama, P., and Heymann, D.L. (2004). Communicable diseases in complex emergencies: impact and challenges. *The Lancet*, 364, 1974–83.

Courtland Robinson, W. (2003). *Risks and Rights:The Causes, Consequences, and Challenges of Development-Induced Displacement*. Washington, DC: The Brookings Institution-SAIS Project on Internal Displacement.

Crisp, J. (1999). *'Who has Counted the Refugees?' UNHCR and the Politics of Numbers. New Issues in Refugee Research*. Geneva: UNHCR.

Deng, F. (1998). *Guiding Principles on Internal Displacement*. New York: OCHA.

Dualeh, M. and Shears, P. (2002). Refugees and other displaced populations. In R. Detels, J. McEwen, R. Beaglehole, and H. Tanaka (eds.) *Oxford Textbook of Public Health* (4th ed.), pp. 1737–56. Oxford: Oxford University Press.

Eastmond, M. (2007). Stories as lived experience: narratives in forced migration research. *Journal of Refugee Studies*, 20, 248–64.

El-Hinnawi, E. (1985). *Environmental Refugees*. Nairobi, Kenya: United Nations Environment Programme.

Essed, P., Frerks, G., and Schrijvers, J.E. (eds.) (2004). *Refugees and the Transformation of Societies. Agency, Policies, Ethics and Politics*. New York: Berghahn Books.

Fazel, M., Wheeler, J., and Danesh, J. (2005). Prevalence of serious mental disorder in 7000 refugees resettled in western countries: a systematic review. *The Lancet*, 365, 1309–14.

Feachem, R. (2001). Globalisation is good for your health, mostly. *British Medical Journal*, 323, 504–6.

Finney Lamb, C. and Cunningham, M. (2003). Dichotomy or decision-making: specialization and mainstreaming in health service design for refugees. In P. Allotey (ed.) *The Health of Refugees. Public Health Perspectives from Crisis to Settlement*, pp. 156–68. Melbourne: Oxford University Press.

Forced Migration Online (2008). *What is Forced Migration?* [Online]. Available at: http://www.forcedmigration.org/whatisfm.htm.

Gerritsen, A., Bramsen, I., Deville, W., Van Willigen, L., Hovens, J., and Van Derploeg, H. (2004). Health and health care utilisation among asylum seekers and refugees in the Netherlands: design of a study. *BMC Public Health*, 4, 1–10.

Grove, N. and Zwi, A.B. (2006). Our health and theirs: forced migration, othering and public health. *Social Science & Medicine*, 62, 1931–42.

Gushulak, B. and MacPherson, D. (2000). Health issues associated with the smuggling and trafficking of migrants. *Journal of Immigrant Health*, 2, 67–78.

Harrell-Bond, B. (2000). *'Are Refugee Camps Good for Children?' New Issues in Refugee Research*. New York: UNHCR.

Harrell-Bond, B. and Voutira, E. (2007). In search of 'invisible actors': barriers to access in refugee research. *Journal of Refugee Studies*, 20(2), 282–98.

Harrell-Bond, B., Voutira, E., and Leopold, M. (1992). Counting the refugees: gifts, givers, patrons and clients. *Journal of Refugee Studies*, 5(3/4), 205–25.

Harris, M.F. and Telfer, B.L. (2001). The health needs of asylum seekers living in the community. *Medical Journal of Australia*, 175, 589–92.

Hull, S. and Boomla, K. (2006). Primary care for refugees and asylum seekers. *British Medical Journal*, 332, 62–3.

Hynes, M., Sheik, M., Wilson, H.G., and Spiegel, P. (2002). Reproductive health indicators and outcomes among refugee and internally displaced persons in postemergency phase camps. *Journal of the American Medical Association*, 288, 595–603.

Internal Displacement Monitoring Centre (2008). *Internal Displacement: Global Overview of Trends and Developments in 2007*. Geneva: Internal Displacement Monitoring Centre.

Krause, S.K., Jones, R.K., and Purdin, S.J. (2000). Programmatic responses to refugees' reproductive health needs. *International Family Planning Perspectives*, 26, 181–7.

Labonte, R. and Schrecker, T. (2005). Globalization and social determinants of health: promoting health equity in global governance *Globalization and Health*, 3, 7.

Lee, K. (2004). Globalisation: what is it and how does it affect health? *Medical Journal of Australia*, 180, 156–8.

MacDonald, T.H. (2007). *The Global Human Right to Health: Dream or Possibility?* Oxford: Radcliffe Publishing.

MacKenzie, C., McDowell, C., and Pittaway, E. (2007). Beyond 'do no harm': the challenge of constructing ethical relationships in refugee research. *Journal of Refugee Studies*, 20, 299–319.

Martin, S. (2002). Averting forced migration in countries in transition. *International Migration*, 40, 25–40.

McAdam, J. (2006). *The Refugee Convention as a Rights Blueprint for Persons in Need of International Protection. New Issues in Refugee Research*. New York: UNHCR.

Moore, P.S., Marfin, A.A., Quenemoen, L.E., Gessner, B.D., Ayub, Y.S., and Sullivan, K.M. (1993). Mortality rates in displaced and resident populations of Central Somalia during the famine of 1992. *The Lancet*, 341, 935–8.

Moore, W. and Shellman, S. (2004). Fear of persecution: forced migration 1952–1995. *Journal of Conflict Resolution*, 48, 723–45.

Myers, N. and Kent, J. (1995). *Environmental Exodus: An Emergent Crisis in the Global Arena*. Washington, DC: Climate Institute.

Organisation of African Unity (1969). *OAU Convention Governing the Specific Aspects of the Refugee Problems in Africa*. Addis-Ababa: OAU.

Prince, M., Patel, V., Saxena, S., et al. (2007). No health without mental health. *The Lancet*, 370, 859–77.

Prinzo, W. and Benoist, B. (2002). Meeting the challenges of micronutrient deficiencies in emergency affected populations. *Nutritional Society*, 2002, 251–7.

Regional Refugee Instruments & Related (1984). *Cartagena Declaration on Refugees. Colloquium on the International Protection of Refugees in Central America, Mexico and Panama*. [Online]. Available at: http://www.oas.org/dil/1984_Cartagena_Declaration_on_Refugees.pdf.

Salama, P., Spiegel, P., and Brennan, R. (2001). No less vulnerable: the internally displaced in humanitarian emergencies. *The Lancet*, 357, 1430–2.

Salama, P., Spiegel, P., Talley, L., and Waldman, R. (2004). Lessons learned from complex emergencies over past decade. *The Lancet*, 364, 1801–13.

Siddique, A.K., Salam, A., Islam, M.S., et al. (1995). Why treatment centres failed to prevent cholera deaths among Rwandan refugees in Goma, Zaire. *The Lancet*, 345, 359.

Silove, D., Austin, P., and Steel, Z. (2007). No refuge from terror: the impact of detention on the mental health of trauma-affected refugees seeking asylum in Australia. *Transcultural Psychiatry*, 44, 359–93.

Silove, D., Ekblad, S., and Mollica, R. (2000a). The rights of the severely mentally ill in post-conflict societies. *The Lancet*, 355, 1448–549.

Silove, D., Steel, Z., and Watters, C. (2000b). Policies of deterrence and the mental health of asylum seekers. *Journal of the American Medical Association*, 284, 604–11.

Spiegel, P. (2004). HIV/AIDS among conflict-affected and displaced populations: dispelling myths and taking action. *Disasters*, 28, 322–39.

Tarantola, D., Byrnes, A., Johnson, M., Kemp, L., Zwi, A.B., and Gruskin, S. (2008). Human rights, health and development. *Australian Journal of Human Rights*, 13, 2.

Toole, M. and Waldman, R. (1990). Preventing excess mortality in refugee and displaced populations in developing countries. *Journal of the American Medical Association*, 263, 3296–302.

Toole, M. and Waldman, R. (1997). The public health aspects of complex emergencies and refugee situations. *Annual Review of Public Health*, 18, 283–312.

Turner, S. (2004). New opportunities: angry young men in a Tanzanian refugee camp. In P. Essed, G. Frerks, and J. Schrijvers (eds.) *Refugees and the Transformation of Societies. Agency, Policies, Ethics and Politics*, pp. 94–106. New York: Berghahn Books.

United Nations (1997). *Glossary of Environment Statistics, Studies in Methods. Series F.* New York: UN.

United Nations (2000). *Protocol Against The Smuggling Of Migrants By Land, Sea And Air.* New York: UN.

United Nations (2003). *Protocol to Prevent, Suppress and Punish Trafficking in Persons, Especially Women and Children, Supplementing the United Nations Convention Against Transnational Organized Crime, G.A. Res. 25, annex II, U.N. GAOR, 55th Sess.* New York: UN.

United Nations High Commissioner for Refugees (2006). *Looking to the Future. The State of The World's Refugees 2006: Human Displacement in the New Millennium.* Geneva: UNHCR.

United Nations High Commissioner for Refugees (2009). *Protecting Refugees and the Role of UNHCR* [Online]. Available at: http://unhcr.org.au/unhcr/images/protecting%20refugees.pdf.

United Nations High Commissioner for Refugees (2011). *UNHCR Global Trends.* Geneva: UNHCR.

World Health Organisation (2014). Measles deaths reach record lows with fragile gains towards global elimination. [Online]. Available at http://www.who.int/mediacentre/news/notes/2014/measles-20140206/en/.

Zwi, A.B. and Alvarez-Castillo, F. (2003). Forced migration globalization and public health: getting the big picture into focus. In P. Allotey (ed.) *The Health of Refugees*, pp. 14–34. Melbourne: Oxford University Press.

Zwi, A.B. and Cabral, A.J. (1991). Identifying 'high risk situations' for preventing AIDS. *British Medical Journal*, 303, 1527–9.

Zwi, A.B., Grove, N.J., Mackenzie, C., et al. (2006). Placing ethics in the centre: negotiating new spaces for ethical research in conflict situations. *Global Public Health*, 1, 264–77.

Prisons: from punishment to public health

Ernest Drucker

Introduction to prisons: from punishment to public health

The premise of this chapter is that the work of public health should now include consideration of criminal justice systems and incarceration, assessing their specific and changeable effects on population health. Our goal is to determine and measure the outcomes (both intended and unintended) of our varied attempts to use criminal justice systems for public safety and social control. To accomplish this goal we must examine immediate effects and long-term health and social consequences of various forms of punishment, assessing their impacts on individuals and populations both during and after incarceration. This will involve using common public health metrics and methods to determine the collective impacts that systems of criminal justice and their application may play as *social determinants of health* in any society. This work is largely based on the author's experiences and research within the US system—admittedly an extreme case, but one that can serve as a cautionary tale for applying a set of epidemiological principles to the data of criminal justice to demonstrate just how consequential criminal justice policies can be for a nation's public health. This chapter uses epidemiological principles and data to create a basic template—a framework for the public health analysis of imprisonment. It considers the consequences of incarceration for individual inmates, their families, communities, and societies at large. As a first such attempt, it is necessarily a thin slice of a vast body of material and concepts about both prisons and public health, but my hope is that it still may serve as a useful primer and a map for future explorations.

The appearance of a chapter on prisons in a public health textbook is a landmark in the development of our contemporary appreciation of the actual and potential significance of both crime and its punishment in human affairs. The rationale and conceptual framework for examining modern criminal justice systems as a public health phenomenon are a consequence of the large scale and potency of state systems of punishment. As these grow in size and importance, they play an increasingly significant role in determining the health of entire populations. In this chapter, I examine the basis of these systems' functioning and the forms and levels of the punishment they mete out—viewed as health determinants. While my own experience and much of my understanding of these relationships derives from US data, my aim here is to provide a template for public health analysis of other societies and their contemporary systems of criminal justice. I will interrogate the stated intentions and document the concrete behaviours of these systems and their demonstrable outcomes affecting individual and collective health outcomes.

Viewing these systems through a public health lens provides us with some new models for gauging their significance and expands the assessment of their many impacts that extend beyond the administration of criminal justice, including effects upon population morbidity, mortality, social justice, family and community health, and human rights. In examining the public health consequences of criminal justice methods and their application to specific populations, we are drawn first to the examples of the large-scale use of incarceration as punishment (*mass or hyper-incarceration*) and the range of important health and social consequences that occur as a function of its large scale and concentration of the use of imprisonment, that is, its 'dosage effects' upon populations (Drucker 2013).

Prisons have many health effects—upon morbidity, mortality, and the life course of individual prisoners and upon their children—suggesting an intergenerational impact. International imprisonment data, employing uniform measures that allow clear comparisons of the prevalence and population characteristics of imprisonment worldwide, are still often incomplete or unreliable. Even so, these data do enable us to make basic comparisons and link the data to public health. This is most evident for the developed nations—especially the United States, the nation with the largest number of prisoners and the highest rate of imprisonment in the world—whose data density makes it a case study of mass incarceration and of the wealth of data that are possible to study (Christie 1997).

Another major goal of this analysis is methodological—to demonstrate how well criminal justice data lends itself to the methods of public health analyses, to observe important patterns of contemporary population health issues (such as HIV and addiction), and to see evidence of incarceration as a contemporary driver of population health. Using a 'public health lens' (Drucker 2013) to examine criminal justice and incarceration provides a much-needed model to approach this important but often overlooked determinant of population health. It includes a model of prevention, the scientific methodologies needed to identify risk and protective factors, as well demonstrating the value of multidisciplinary collaboration characteristic of all effective public health interventions. Other chapters in this text cover some of the same territory (e.g. drugs, violence, mental health) under different rubrics, but my hope is that this exposition will allow the public health professional and student to see the scope and location of many of the field's most important features relative to public health and encourage their own further exploration.

Prisons and society

What is there to say about prisons as discussed here for the first time in a venerable textbook of public health? First off, while medicine and public health are themselves certainly also venerable, crime and punishment are even more so. The trope of crime and punishment, established early in human history, is arguably a foundational constant of human social development and the organization of the modern state. Differences in systems of governance based on the *rule of law* are a defining characteristic of most organized societies. But so is the frequent transgression of these rules and, with that basic fact, the need to address these violations—the criminology of everyday life. If the social contract is about anything it is about meshing individuals to the contours of their social order—and that order is ultimately defined by its rules and restrictions—including the responses to their violation, as much as by their benefits and opportunities.

Historically most of the theory, scholarship, and research about criminal justice systems and the populations they affect most directly (offenders and their victims), have drawn their core conceptions and research questions from the fields of criminal law and sociology/criminology. The social sciences have traditionally concerned themselves with prisons as the social and political end points of crime and its punishment (Garland 1991; Morris and Rothman 1995). These fields appropriately emphasize the objectives and methods of crime control, that is, their desired impacts on public safety, while examining the characteristics and behaviours of the affected populations (both criminals and victims) and the workings of the systems of enforcement that accompany them.

The framework of criminal justice theories and policies have focused on response to transgressions and attitudes towards deviance: including the importance of social order (Durkheim), the structural aspects of social justice and the inequities of class (Marx), and the exercise of state power and its attempts to use criminal justice systems to exert political control over individual and group behaviour (Foucault).

This body of thought constitutes the conceptual foundation and basis of the legal structures and practices of criminal justice. These criminal justice concepts and models concern themselves with core societal issues, for example, assuring social order, supporting the conditions for secure and peaceful communities, protection of family life, providing safety from violence, and providing for the administration of justice under law. These experiences and the data they yield have heretofore (understandably) been almost entirely discussed in terms of their success or failure in the establishment and maintenance of law and order—with a focus on public safety and crime control. In this public health analysis of criminal justice systems and their consequences we take a different perspective—examining the full range of effects of the workings of criminal justice systems—not just effect on crime but on the overall health and well-being of entire populations, which includes, but is by no means limited to, crime and its victims.

Criminal justice systems apply punishment to individuals in response to real or perceived offences against other individuals and the common good. But it is *punishment itself*, not just the formal rules under which it operates, that is the essential variable for public health. Both for individuals and in the aggregate, it is the forms and severity of punishment that are the measurable exposures that drive the public health impact of imprisonment. The human experience and responses to punishment form the basis of any therapeutic or pathogenic agency that the criminal justice system may have. Nils Christie, the great Norwegian criminologist, has put it very clearly: 'punishment is pain' and 'imposing punishment within the institution of law means the inflicting of pain, intended as pain' (Christie 1981).

Punishment by incarceration involves extended suffering and deprivation of freedom (perhaps the greatest pain of all), administered for the reasons of exercising control. But this pain has a wider audience than the offender and many collateral consequences, among them it has the added purpose of deterring others, who may learn from the example and desist from transgressing. In public health terms, the consequences of punishment depend on the scale and methods of its application in practice. All systems of law enforcement expose the offender to life-altering effects—ranging in severity from disapproval and stigma, to often brutal and humiliating treatment, long periods (up to a lifetime) of misery in prison, or (in the ultimate punishment) to loss of life itself, by execution. In the forms and levels of punishment that each society metes out, we may see ample evidence of its limitations. Increasingly these include the inevitability of significant collateral consequences on populations other than the offender, particularly their families, which also defines the system's larger impacts on society, and its powerful tendencies and abilities to replicate and sustain itself.

Individual and population data

Just as individual cases are the foundations of clinical medicine (upon which public health is built), it is the individual cases of 'crime and punishment' that form the data of the criminological sciences. This primacy of the individual case in law (as in clinical medicine) has great historical power and authority, framed as it is in deeply rooted (and wholly understandable) moral precepts of ethics and justice, right and wrong, and the conditions of each individual's implicit and explicit social contracts with authorities and government—where we routinely sacrifice some of our autonomy (individual freedom) in exchange for the many benefits of organized society and the fundamental protection of those rights—for example, of our property and personal safety, as well as protection of the weak from the strong.

The aggregation of individual case data (on both crimes and punishment) comprises the units of analysis in analytic criminology and jurisprudence, these aggregations are only a summary of the individual cases—as much an expression of the system's ever changing definitions and rules as determined by each society's systems of making and enforcing laws in practice, and played out as criminal justice procedures and outcomes. While many crimes are violations of 'natural law' (e.g. violence, theft), criminal offences are determined by legal statutes, and laws always subject to change, sometimes arbitrarily so.

The legal doctrines that govern criminal justice theory and practice demonstrate that the *individual case* is the core unit of analysis, and the target of intervention. In clinical medicine, the individual case is also the basis of practice, but public health data and clinical epidemiology are recognized as the key to understanding the overall impact and burden of disease, in the distribution and determinants of population health. Similarly, while the aggregate data of criminology are essential for shaping beliefs, expectations, and the many questions that occupy criminal justice theory and scholarship, the actual models of legal practice in courts of law, steadfastly remain based solely on the individual case and its precedents.

However, the 'case definition' of a particular instance of criminal offence may not be as rigorously defined as we are accustomed to in medicine and public health. The categorization of criminal acts as criminal justice data are ultimately determined by very subjective criteria—the interpretations of legal statutes by the police, prosecutors, judges, and juries—always negotiable in legal practice and adjudication. This inherent vagueness of criminal justice cases sets limits on their reliable use in scientific analysis. Aggregate or population research (which might be used to validate case data) is generally *not* admissible as evidence in criminal court cases, except for forensic findings of fact, used as evidence in the determination of guilt or innocence on a case-by-case basis. Such variability in legal case definitions still leaves us with individual criminal cases as the basic unit of analysis, both for practice and for the scientific analysis of crime and punishment data—compromising our ability to ascertain clear and replicable findings of complex relationships that determine population health outcomes.

But, while *individual* crime and its punishment may be the foundational unit of all theories and practices of criminal justice and its enforcement systems (Garland and Duff 1994), the public health lens allows us to step back and recognize the wider social and population significance of the individual circumstances of punishment and the workings of our criminal justice system itself. We therefore seek near universal or paradigmatic models of the relationships between individuals with their governments and each other (i.e. the social contract). In public health we are challenged to see criminal justice systems anew, as an important factor in the larger framework for any population's health and well-being. We are therefore obliged to undertake the task of assessing the health and social consequences of our systems of criminal justice as a determinant of population health—an obligation that feeds back to the accountabilities of any system of governance for all of the diverse, often damaging, collective consequences of its actions—and not just the simple sum of an array of individual criminal acts and their punishment. Despite these limitations we may still understand criminal justice phenomena in public health terms—one of the many systems in complex modern societies that makes substantial contributions (for better or worse) to the general health and well-being of the people. More specifically, we may examine the relationship of different systems of criminal justice and their methods of punishment to the population's health.

Prisons and public health: the epidemiology of punishment

Systems of criminal justice and the modes and levels of punishment meted out are a defining feature of different societies. We are now learning that these may affect population health in many ways—first off (as in all epidemics) by their scale. As our systems of criminal justice and the uses of incarceration reach new levels (with over 9 million prisoners worldwide and growing (Walmsley 2012)), we must learn to better understand the nature and significance of these systems and the collective consequences of their common modes and levels of punishment and examine evidence of their effects on populations. We start with the fundamentals of epidemiology—prevalence and incidence levels and trends; patterns of risk by time, place, and person; and models of primary, secondary, and tertiary prevention.

The prevalence of imprisonment at the national level worldwide, ranges by a full order of magnitude from less than 50 to over 700 per 100,000 population (Fig. 10.10.1). The application of such dramatically different rates of punishment by imprisonment is the first metric of its public heath significance. With this understanding of the reality and significance of such wide variations in the magnitude and methods of punishment by imprisonment between societies, we may embark upon a closer examination of their specific consequences and population impacts. And we must remain mindful of the fact that any system of punishment, has powerful influences on the larger population beyond the individual offender—effects that may extend far beyond the individual cases of crime and its punishment which are its intended targets.

Criminal justice systems as a determinant of health

As we consider the public health significance of our systems of crime and punishment we are drawn to the special role of imprisonment and its effects on health outcomes for prisoners and others close to them. To accomplish this goal we must examine criminal justice systems closely—using the traditional epidemiological tools, metrics, and analytic methods and models of public health (i.e. morbidity and mortality; the traditional statistical analysis of population health data by risk factors and population variables). We wish to fully understand the health outcomes of particular methods employed in systems of punishment, and the consequences of that system for population health.

As systems of criminal justice grow in scale globally, they are emerging as a new form of social influence that emulates the role of the many other biological risks and social pathogens to which we are all 'exposed'—such as environmental factors (pollution and effects of climate change), poverty, inequality and social injustice, violence, and wars. And, just as we consider the effects of the application of various modes of punishment to individuals who transgress laws as a means of crime control (i.e. imprisonment as incapacitation of offenders by their temporary removal from society and as a deterrent for others) we are now realizing that the effects of widespread punishment are already evident in many nations (Waquant 2009), and thus may already be appreciated as significant determinants of public health when applied to an entire society—particularly as *hyper-incarceration* or *mass incarceration* of particular racial or ethnic groups.

Just as the rule of law reflects the political and social realities of its time and place in any society, we must now also be aware of how these systems can impact public health. Amidst the many other developments of a rapidly changing world we are now beginning to understand the important role of international crime and corruption as phenomena that have powerful effects on *global health*, for example, the illicit drug trade, human trafficking, civil wars, child

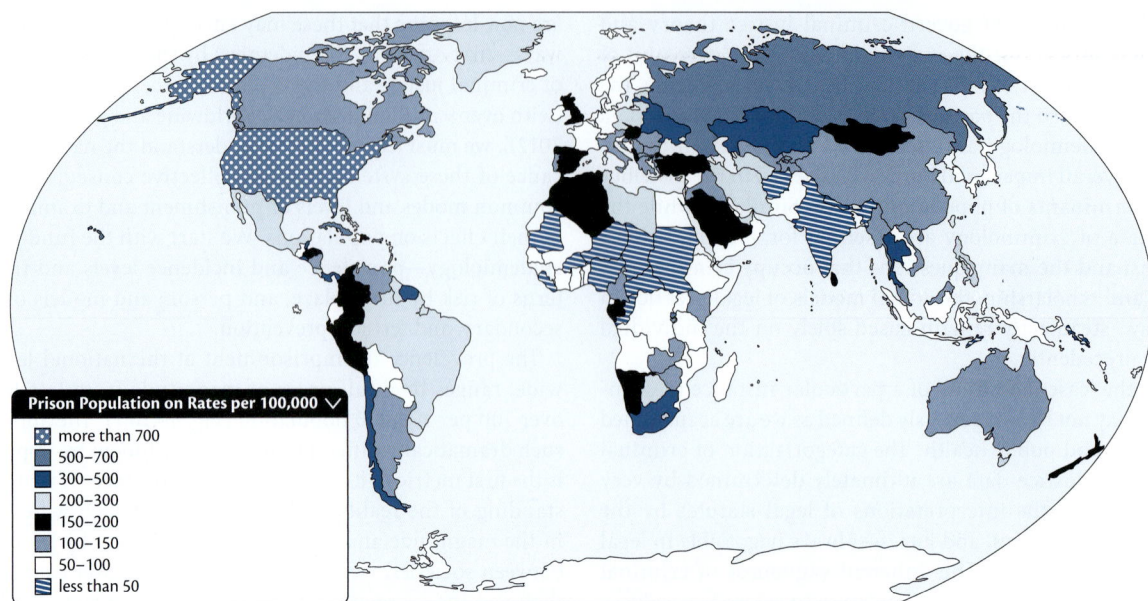

Fig. 10.10.1 Global rates of imprisonment.

Reproduced with permission from ChartsBin statistics collector team 2010, *World Prison Population Rates per 100,000 of the national population*, Copyright 2011 ChartsBin.com, available from http://chartsbin.com/view/eqq.

soldiers, terrorism, as well as many environmental risks where violations of protective laws endanger and degrade the atmosphere, the seas, and the fertile landscape on which we all depend. In these ways the successes and failures of our attempts at crime control emerge as one of the most potent new determinants of population health and the prosperity and social welfare of nations.

Effects of incarceration on crime

The impact that imprisonment has upon individuals typically focuses on its role in controlling crime, not on its health consequences for offenders and their families—although crime reduction (certainly the prevention of violent crime) can be seen as a positive population health effect of incarceration. The conventional wisdom in criminology is that incarceration controls crime in two ways: deterrence and incapacitation. For deterrence it is held that the example of the punishment of offenders builds the fear of punishment into others who might be caught committing a crime. The other intended role of imprisonment in crime prevention is through 'incapacitation', that is, removing the individual from society for some length of time limits his or her ability to commit new crimes while behind bars.

The literature of criminology is full of studies debating the effectiveness of incarceration as a deterrent (something that is very difficult to prove or disprove), but there is a general consensus about the role of incarceration in incapacitation—imprisonments clearly does limit the harms that any individual might do while free. By this logic, the greater the number of criminals who are incarcerated the more crime is prevented overall—at the very least by the incapacitation effect. This is a common claim used to support high imprisonment rates and long sentences (without parole) as a guarantor of public safety. These arguments have intuitive appeal, but the data on the incapacitation effects of mass incarceration are often equivocal (Drago et al. 2009), in part because so many other factors determine the variations in crime rates in any

society. In addition, of course, the vast majority of prison inmates have not committed a violent crime.

Yet the notion persists that by taking criminals off the street, imprisonment prevents them from committing new crimes, an idea that remains a cornerstone of the justification for high rates of imprisonment. Getting the 'bad guys off the street' has a pragmatic intuitive appeal, aside from satisfying some more retributive impulses. What these criminological models do not generally acknowledge, however, are the long-term adverse individual health and social consequences of incarceration itself—that is, the effects of systematic punishment on human beings. This is where a public health model can be most useful.

Both acute and chronic problems are important effects of exposure to the systematic punishments that are routinely associated with incarceration—that is, the many daily humiliations, experiences of personal helplessness in the face of the arbitrary exercise of power (often sadistic) by the prison authorities, brutality and cruel treatment by other prisoners and guards, and significant dangers of traumatizing personal assaults—including sexual assault by both other inmates and guards. Attempts to prevent such cruelty and violence in prisons runs throughout their history—and is the subject of the efforts of many national and international organizations struggling to establish and enforce standards that assure humane prison conditions (van Zyl Smit and Snacken 2009) and to promote the fair and humane treatment of all incarcerated persons in detention and prisons, meeting contemporary ethical, legal, and human rights standards (John Howard of London and District n.d.).

The prisons revolving door: re-entry and recidivism

Most of those who are incarcerated are only 'incapacitated' temporarily, and most return to the communities from which they came—albeit the worse for the experience (Travis 2005). Recidivism (readmission to prison) due to new offences or failures to meet the conditions of parole (e.g. relapse to drug use) is taken as a failure of the rehabilitation potential associated with arrest and imprisonment. An analysis of US recidivism patterns of 40,000 offenders released from state prisons in 1994, discovered that 56.2 per cent resumed their pre-incarceration offending trajectories after release, with no apparent effect of imprisonment on future risk of re-incarceration (Loughran et al. 2009; see also Pathways to Desistence 2014), controlling for age and other characteristics. Another meta-analysis (Cullen et al. 2011) concluded that the absolute impact of incarceration is, 'at best, marginal and at worst, iatrogenic' in predicting recidivism. In a series of studies, Clear and Rose and others (Clear 1996, 2009; Rose and Clear 1998; Fagan et al. 2003) have found that higher rates of arrest and incarceration in a community often lead to higher community rates of incarceration. In sum, most studies have found either no change or decreased rates of recidivism associated with shorter sentences or early release, while also finding little effect of increases in 'dosage' (sentence length) on a wide array of offenders.

Aside from these studies of prevalence, there is an important body of research by Belfast criminologist Shadd Maruna (2011) that examines re-entry as an opportunity to stop the recurrent cycles of recidivism by addressing it with the same degree of seriousness and formal institutions (even rituals) that accompanies one's entrance into the criminal justice system in the first place (e.g. re-entry courts aimed at reducing recidivism through specific structures and procedures that are instituted with all the thoughtfulness and ritual that accompanies the process of accusation of a crime, adjudication, and sentencing leading up to admissions to prison).

Morbidity and mortality

The rates of mortality in prison populations include all the usual causes of death seen in comparable populations. But the incidence and prevalence of mortality data also reflect the selective nature of prison and jail populations and reflect these environments and their unique risks—and (in some cases) protections, for example, higher rates of suicides but lower rates of homicide in prisons and jails, with important differences to be seen between jails (short-term detention facilities) and prisons—where inmates may spend the rest of their natural lives growing old behind prison bars (Fellner 2012; Williams et al. 2012). See Table 10.10.1.

Prevalence

The current US prison rate of 720 per 100,000 members of the population is both the highest rate and greatest number of prisoners of any nation in the world: with 5 per cent of the world's population, the United States now accounts for 25 per cent of the world's prisoners. If this population of current and former prisoners inhabited their own city, it would be the largest in America. The US prison system now represents the extreme of epidemic incarceration—between 1975 and 2010 about 10 million Americans were in state and federal prisons and local jails.

The significance of prevalence measures of incarceration

Incarceration systematically damages key elements of the psychological and physical health of prison inmates, causing or exacerbating conditions including addiction, mental illness, and chronic infectious or metabolic diseases. Restrictions placed on ex-felons

Table 10.10.1 Mortality rate per 100,000 US state prisoners, by cause of death, 2001–2009

Cause of death	2001	2002	2003	2004	2005	2006	2007[a]	2008	2009
All causes	242	245	258	252	253	250	257	260	257
Illness	217	218	232	225	225	218	226	228	227
Heart disease	63	67	67	68	68	67	54	65	66
Cancer	53	54	63	57	61	59	46	65	69
Liver disease	19	17	20	18	19	19	14	18	19
AIDS-related	23	20	17	12	12	10	9	7	7
All other illness[b]	59	60	64	71	65	64	103	74	66
Suicide	14	14	16	16	17	17	16	15	15
Homicide	3	4	4	4	4	4	4	3	4
Drug/alcohol intoxication	3	3	2	2	3	4	3	4	4
Accident	2	3	2	3	2	3	2	2	2
Other/unknown	3	3	2	3	1	3	5	8	4

Note: data are from the *Prisoners at Midyear* series. Data may have been revised from previously published statistics to reflect updated information. State prison mortality rates are per 100,000 inmates held in state custody (including private facilities) on 30 June of each year. The mortality rates presented are not adjusted for age sex, race, geographic location, or any other characteristic. Executions are not included; for data on executions, see *Capital Punishment, 2009 – Statistical Tables*.

[a] In 2007, a high number of cases were missing cause of death information. These cases were classified as all other illnesses.

[b] Includes other specified (such as cerebrovascular disease, influenza, cirrhosis, and other non-leading natural causes of death) as well as unspecified illnesses. See *Methodology* for details on illness classifications.

Sources: Bureau of Justice Statistics, Deaths in Custody Reporting Program (DCRP), National Prisoner Statistics (NPS).

Reproduced from Noonan, M.E. and Carson, E. A., *Prison and Jail Deaths in Custody, 2000–2009—Statistical Tables*, US Department of Justice, Office of Justice Programs, Bureau of Justice Statistics, 2011, available online: http://www.bjs.gov/content/pub/pdf/pjdc0009st.pdf.

after they have left prison extend many of the elements of punishment that occur within prisons—including restrictions on access to employment, decent housing, public benefits for education, and civic participation (voting), as well as the stigma of being an ex-felon, which disables their ability to function effectively in the outside world, incapacitating their attempts to regain a foothold in noncriminal life and to re-establish a place in their families and home communities, for example, in Russia every prisoner has a large red stamp in their passport. These serve to extend the damages of a prison sentence to 'life on the outside' (Gonnerman 2004).

Potential years of life lost and DALYs associated with imprisonment for drug offences in the United States: 1975–2010

Assessing the relative significance of incarceration for population health can usefully employ the public health measures of potential years of life lost (PYLLs) and disability-adjusted life years (DALYs). With large-scale systems of incarceration, such as the US one, the years of life 'lost' to imprisonment are now comparable to those for many diseases, world wars, and very large-scale natural disasters. Over the last 35 years, the United States has incarcerated 8–10 million individuals, mostly young adult males in the age range 18–34, often for drug offences during the stages of its most rapid growth. The result of incarcerating this many young men can be understood as representing a minimum of 14 million PYLLs. Given the average lifespan of this population, 14 million PYLLs translates to 350,000 deaths in a population of a similar age—more than the number of US soldiers killed in combat in the Second World War (Drucker 2002).

Disabilities imposed by time spent within prisons

None of the rationales for imprisonment (in the United States or most democracies) includes the concept that this form of punishment should cause long-term hardship or permanent harm to individuals and their families. While some societies still defend the most lurid responses to crimes (including flogging, amputations, stoning, and executions), most developed Western democracies show a long and clear trend away from those sorts of punishments. In developed nations (formerly including the United States) there has been a steady movement since the Second World War towards better prison conditions, shorter prison sentences, and more genuine and effective efforts at rehabilitation.

In part this has come about as a result of recognition of the eventual re-entry of most prisoners into the communities from which they came. In the United States, of the 700,000 prisoners who now leave prison each year, over 60 per cent return directly to their home communities. Most are seeking to re-establish the family and social ties that constitute their only social capital—the networks of support so necessary to the prospect of their resuming normal lives. But most do not stay outside very long: recidivism is massive, with about one-third of released prisoners rearrested within the first 12 months, and two-thirds of released prisoners returning within 3 years. This is the most powerful factor that now defines incarceration as a chronic condition—the 'revolving prison door' that has become the hallmark of America's brand of mass incarceration.

In addition to PYLLs, the impact of incarceration can also be measured by DALYs—defined by the World Health Organization

(n.d.) as 'the sum of years of productive life lost due to disability'—DALYs represent the 'burden of disease'. While one effect of incapacitation is to prevent continued criminal behaviour while incarcerated, prison also incapacitates these individuals in quite another way, that is, by making them far less capable of returning to a productive life on the outside once their prison term ends. For the United States as a whole (in 2004), there were 12,844 DALYs per 100,000 general population. At any time about 13 per cent of the nation's population was disabled due to the usual problems of illness, disabling injuries, and ageing. Of the 700,000 individuals released from US prisons in 2009, about 30 per cent were sufficiently 'disabled' to fail at re-entry and be incarcerated in the first year after their release, yielding a DALY rate of 30,000 per 100,000 (or 30 per cent). Thus the DALY figure in the first year after release from incarceration is more than double that due to all other disabilities in the general population.

Incarceration as a population exposure

The consequences of involvement with the criminal justice system can now be viewed as we would the long-term effects of *toxic exposure to punishment*. The US data for lifetime risks of imprisonment (Table 10.10.2) clearly show the wide disparities in this exposure by race and its powerful association with educational attainment—a marker for future economic and social outcomes (such as marriage) and for life expectancy itself.

The graphic representation of these same data (Fig. 10.10.2) illustrates the exposure history of the entire US population to imprisonment—showing a tripling over successive birth cohorts.

While a primary intent of incarceration is to punish (by depriving the prisoner of the benefits of freedom for a finite period of time), the long-term effects of incarceration on physical and mental health extend punishment far beyond the period of the sentence itself. Viewed in these terms, incarceration imposes a substantial 'burden of disease' for individuals and populations of prisoners.

Table 10.10.2 Lifetime imprisonment rates for US birth cohorts by race and age

Risk of imprisonment by age 30–34: men born 1945–1949, 1970–1974		
	Born 1945–1949 (%)	Born 1970–1974 (%)
All white men	1.2	2.8
All non-college	1.8	5.1
High school dropout	4.2	14.8
High school only	0.7	3.8
Some college	0.7	0.9
All black men	9.0	22.8
All non-college	12.1	30.9
High school dropout	14.7	62.5
High school only	10.2	20.3
Some college	4.9	8.5

Adapted from Western, B. and Wildeman, C., *Annals of the American Academy of Political and Social Science*, Volume 621, Number 1, pp. 221–242, Copyright © 2009 American Academy of Political and Social Science. Reprinted by Permission of SAGE Publications.

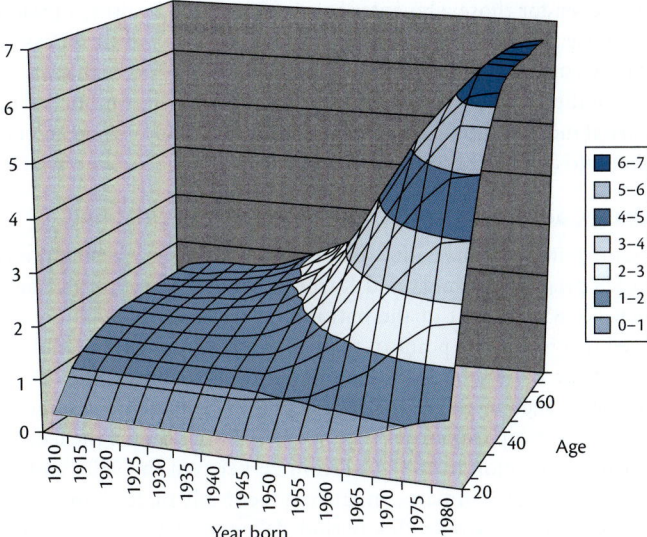

Fig. 10.10.2 Percentage of adults ever incarcerated in state or federal prison, by year of birth and age.

Source: data from Bonczar, T.P. and Beck, A.J., *Lifetime Likelihood of Going to State or Federal Prison*, Bureau of Justice Statistics Special Report, US Department of Justice, Office of Justice Programs, 1997, available from http://www.bjs.gov/index.cfm?ty=pbdetail&iid=1042.

It is difficult to reconcile these data with the basic rights granted by democratic constitutions and human rights standards. Yet in the United States every year, hundreds of thousands of prisoners become afflicted with physical and mental diseases in prison that do not go away at the end of their sentences, and have their lives disabled by the punitive ways our society treats ex-felons.

The conditions within prisons have powerful effects, many of which stay with the individual for life. The adverse effects of incarceration on individual prisoners include the ongoing consequences of poor healthcare services in prisons; failure of prison security to provide a safe environment (the ensuing rape, violence, and gang activity that have become a routine part of prison life); serious and persistent mental health problems and inadequate mental healthcare in prisons; and a paucity of addiction treatment and the absence of effective drug rehabilitation. All this is in addition to the immediate and longer-term psychological implications of trauma associated with overcrowding, poor prison conditions, and many severe disciplinary methods, including isolation and solitary confinement.

Individual healthcare and imprisonment: a sentinel population for vulnerability

The populations of prisons are an important sentinel population of the most vulnerable sectors of any society. A former Medical Director of Corrections in New York State, calls prisons 'a window on our society' arguing that inmates are 'public health sentinels' for the most vulnerable populations suffering from all the physical and mental illnesses, communicable diseases, and consequences of alcohol and substance abuse (Greifinger 2002, 2005). Greifinger also notes that the morbidity of American prisoners is higher than virtually any other group (Glaser and Greifinger 1993) for diabetes, asthma, hypertension, and heart disease. In the United Kingdom, recent disclosures reveal that poor food, bad healthcare, and stress are responsible for many deaths in British prisons—with

'self-inflicted' causes accounting for more than half of all deaths over the last decade (Thompson 2010). Deaths in custody (including community corrections) are increasing: 'almost 230 people died in prison or other forms of custody in England and Wales during 2011–12', representing a 15 per cent rise on the previous year (Anonymous 2012; Prisons and Probation Ombudsman for England and Wales 2013; Inquests n.d.).

There are many serious health problems already prevalent among the populations most likely to be incarcerated—they do not begin with arrest and imprisonment. Overwhelmingly, prisoners in most countries come from the poor communities—often immigrants or ethnic and racial minorities. Their ills in prison faithfully mirror those that these same populations suffer at home—where they have generally gone untreated, for example, mental illness, drug addiction and alcoholism, infectious diseases—especially sexually transmitted diseases (STDs)—viral hepatitis, and HIV/AIDS are at very high levels in this population and demand significant care in prison as well.

Many of the chronic illnesses seen in prisoners—addiction, mental illnesses, diabetes, hypertension, asthma, heart disease—were poorly controlled at the time of admission to the prison system as a result of poverty and long histories of poor access to healthcare. In some cases, such as those involving court-ordered care for prisoners with HIV/AIDS, for example, prisoners may receive better medical care in prison than they would receive outside. But the norm is inadequate healthcare for the incarcerated. This tends to worsen the pre-existing condition, especially in the case of addiction and mental illness, which figure so prominently in the reasons for arrest and incarceration in the first place.

More than 80 per cent of US prison inmates enter prison with histories of, or current, problems with drug abuse or dependency, and drug use often continues throughout prison stays—typically at lower levels, but often with more dangerous practices associated with clandestine injecting via unsterile needles and syringes shared by many inmates. Drug users are generally distrusted when it comes to receiving routine medical care (both in prisons and outside), with many medical providers discounting their demands for pain medications—even in cases involving bone fractures.

Healthcare services are a constant flash point for correctional institutions in America and elsewhere. A study of New York State prison health services found that medical care complaints represented the most frequent inmate grievance—about 20 per cent of all complaints filed by inmates (Correctional Association of New York 2009).

These medical grievances include:

◆ Denials of and delays in access to healthcare.
◆ Inadequate examinations by nurses and physicians.
◆ Failures to treat chronic medical problems expeditiously.
◆ Delays in access to specialists and inadequate follow-up by prison providers on specialists' recommendations.
◆ Problems with receiving medications and the health education needed to comply with complex medication regimens. (Correctional Association of New York 2009)

In addition to the neglect of pre-existing medical conditions and major lapses in consistent medical care, the deprivations and stresses of prison life and the poor quality of prison diet increase the severity of chronic diseases. Ironically, imprisonment is often the occasion for these individuals to receive medical care for the first time. In the United States, prisoners are the only civilian population with a 'right to healthcare' under the US Constitution's Eighth Amendment, which bars 'cruel and unusual punishment', leading to legal support for prisoners' unique entitlement to decent medical care in America. But, despite frequent court mandates to provide this care, extremely poor inmate health services persist in many of the nation's prison systems. This is also true of the continuity of care in prisons and aftercare upon release. Adult inmates are regularly transferred from one prison to another, with disruptive effects on any healthcare that they do get. Prisoners often assert (and a recent New York study confirms) that they are not promptly seen and evaluated when transferred to a new facility. Records often fail to follow them in a timely fashion. Many inmates being discharged from custody leave without adequate documentation of their medical status and without appropriate medication or a medical discharge plan. In the United States there are new plans for extending access to healthcare for prisoners after release under the terms of the Affordable Care Act (ACA), going into effect in 2014 (Phillips 2013).

Increased potential for contracting an infectious disease such as AIDS, hepatitis, tuberculosis, or a STD is another feature of prison life. Inmates face a heightened risk of acquiring blood-borne infectious diseases, due in large part to the sharing of contraband drug-injecting equipment with others in prison. The risk of acquiring STDs is increased through consensual but unprotected sex, and by rape in prison. In the United States an estimated 60,500 inmates—4.5 per cent of the nation's prisoners—report experiencing sexual violence ranging from unwanted touching to non-consensual sex, according to a recent Bureau of Justice Statistics survey of federal and state inmates (Mazza 2012). Yet few inmates see any point in seeking the protection of prison authorities; a separate Bureau of Justice Statistics survey found that only about 6500 official allegations of prison sexual violence (by staff or inmates) were reported to correctional officials in 2006—about 11 per cent of the cases. The report found a number of methodological problems that are common to studies of sex offences in prisons: that is, low response rates from victims due to embarrassment or fear of reprisal, difficulties verifying victims' self-reports, and the lack of common terms to describe sexual abuse (Mazza 2012). Recent reports of sexual offences by staff in juvenile detention centres in the United States have launched a new federal investigation of sexual violence faced by close to 3 million juveniles arrested each year (Travis 2009).

Ageing prison populations

Another effect of mass incarceration and longer sentences is that prison inmates are now an ageing population. According to the most recent report of the Bureau of Justice Statistics (2010), 4.3 per cent of all inmates in the United States in state or federal prisons were over the age of 55 as of mid-year 2008, compared with 3.5 per cent at mid-year 2004, a 23 per cent increase. It costs $70,000 per year to house older prisoners, two to three times the cost of housing younger prisoners. This situation will only worsen in the years to come as longer sentences intersect with shorter life expectancies. As previously noted, many of today's prison inmates will die in prison because their sentences exceed their life expectancies. Of the 5200 men at Louisiana's infamous Angola penitentiary, an 18,000-acre former plantation, journalist Mary Foster estimates that approximately 90 per cent of inmates will die in prison, due to the length of their sentences. These health issues collectively mean

that, even for those who enter prison young and healthy, a prison sentence is tantamount to being afflicted with a chronic illness or long-term disability. The deplorable state of prison healthcare is one of the prime reasons a prison term leads to a lifetime of full or partial incapacitation, transforming a finite sentence of incarceration into a lifelong disabling condition.

Drugs, addiction, and their treatment in prisons

Significant problems with drug use and alcoholism are ubiquitous in US prisons (Mumola and Karberg 2006). US studies estimate that 60–83 per cent of the nation's correctional population has used drugs at some point in their lives, twice the estimated drug use of the total US population (40 per cent) (Fellner 2012). Drug offenders accounted for 21 per cent of the US state prison population in 1998 (up from 6 per cent in 1980), 59 per cent of the federal prison population in 1998 (up from 25 per cent in 1980), and 26 per cent of all jail inmates, mirroring the steady increase in arrests for drug offences over this period. Women in US prisons were more likely than men to report using drugs in the month before their offence (62 vs. 56 per cent) and were also more likely than male inmates to have committed their offence under the influence of drugs or while engaging in petty theft or prostitution to get cash for drugs.

A programme recently instituted in Baltimore, Maryland, United States, provided methadone maintenance for prisoners who were soon to be transferred to community-based methadone programmes at release. These prisoners had significantly better outcomes than a control population provided with only 'counselling and passive referral' after discharge. Results included more time spent in treatment during the 12-month post-release period, and far fewer positive urine tests for heroin and cocaine (Prisons and Probation Ombudsman for England and Wales 2013). But because of hostility towards the use of methadone in correctional settings in the United States (it is also barred in almost all drug courts), such programmes are rare.

Accordingly, the first thing many released prisoners do on getting out is seek relief by injecting heroin—often with lethal results. Over 25 per cent of drug fatalities due to overdose are now thought to stem from this phenomenon. The failure to address addictions in the criminal justice system is the single most significant reason for re-arrest and recidivism once released. This amounts to a systemic failure that diminishes each individual's chances of successful re-entry at the end of a prison term. Instead, re-entry becomes associated with a resumption of drug use that, while not altogether absent, had been greatly reduced during imprisonment. But this is a clear case of incarceration heightening a disabling condition with lethal effects on the outside.

Internationally many other countries now also have large proportions of drug users in prison, but many now also offer a wide range of treatments (including methadone) to incarcerated drug users (United Nations Office on Drugs and Crime 2013). Many also have employed harm reduction strategies to reduce HIV and hepatitis C virus transmission in prisons (e.g. methadone substitution treatment and access to clean injecting equipment) and now also seek to avoid imprisonment for those with addictions (Dolan et al. 1996, 2003).

Most US prisons have been resistant to this approach. While there are many very dedicated peer drug counsellors in prisons, their efforts to rebuild self-esteem and equip inmates to deal with the dependency and high risk of relapse are thwarted in these anti-therapeutic environments dominated by punishment. There is little incentive to offer effective drug treatment in modern American prisons—a neglect framed as part of the prison ideology in which inmates must assume 'personal responsibility' for their present circumstances. Building on this seemingly reasonable conception, most drug treatment in prisons is moralistic in tone, depicting addiction as evidence of personal weakness (confirmed by the great personal failure that incarceration has come to represent) and often seen by inmates themselves as ample justification for their current punishment.

In consequence, the way the United States treats drug addiction in prison has become an extension of the moral crusades of America's war on drugs— where legitimate questions of how best to minimize the harm from drugs are subordinated to the goals of zero tolerance—even for therapeutic drugs that soften the pains of withdrawal. Drug problems of prisoners have now become the basis of a virulent ideology of condemnation and demonization, undermining any personal strengths they may bring with them into prison and creating further, lifelong problems for inmates— problems that may result in their rapid return to drug use after release.

Evidence for this failure can be seen in the high rates of drug overdose that occur in the period immediately following discharge of drug users from prisons. Multiple studies have confirmed that overdose deaths among people who used heroin prior to incarceration are increased tenfold in the 2 weeks after release from prison, as compared to the usual overdose rate (Binswanger et al. 2007).

This result has been seen in the United Kingdom, Canada, and Australia, which all have drug problems similar to that in the United States but incarceration rates of drug users that are only about one-quarter of US rates. Opiate overdoses are thought to be due to the loss of tolerance associated with the greatly reduced use of opiates in prison. In the United States, the most significant reason for this can be found in the failure to treat opiate dependency adequately in prisons. More specifically, it can be attributed to the failure to allow known opiate-dependent individuals to use methadone in prisons. When there *is* drug treatment (consisting mostly of prisoners talking in groups), the most common philosophy is modelled after the drug-free therapeutic communities that philosophically dominate American drug treatment—generally to the exclusion of approaches that employ medications such as methadone or buprenorphine, known to be the most effective methods available to treat opiate addiction.

The high rate of drug incarcerations ensures that drug problems will be very common in prison populations worldwide. In the United States, state corrections officials estimate that between 70 and 85 per cent of inmates need some level of substance abuse treatment. But sustained, professional, supervised drug and alcohol treatment is currently available in fewer than half of federal, state, and local adult detention facilities. Juvenile correctional facilities are also staffed to serve only a fraction of those who need treatment services. In approximately 7600 correctional facilities surveyed, 172,851 inmates were in drug treatment programmes in 1997, less than 11 per cent of the inmate population and less than 20 per cent of those with addiction histories (Mumola and Karberg 2006). While some state prison systems expanded drug treatment programmes in the 1990s, these have now been cut

severely in most systems—another consequence of the recent state budget crises including, for example, a 40 per cent reduction in California in 2009 alone (Rothfeld 2009).

The injection of heroin within correctional facilities has been documented in many prisons worldwide and continues to exist, notwithstanding vigorous attempts to deter and detect the importation of drugs and injecting equipment into these facilities. Although episodes of drug injecting inside these facilities are generally far less frequent than in the community, adverse consequences (including HIV infection) are well documented. While the use of methadone or buprenorphine maintenance for addiction treatment is prohibited in state and federal prisons throughout the United States, a small number of local jails do offer brief detoxification programmes using these medications. In the past decade, some jail facilities have begun to offer methadone maintenance treatment as well.

A large-scale methadone maintenance treatment programme, serving 2000 patients per year, was established in New York City's Riker's Island jail in the 1970s—operated by the Montefiore health service—the first jail programme to offer this treatment in the United States. The Riker's Island approach continued methadone for all new admissions already in maintenance at the time of arrest (mostly detainees) and initiated methadone treatment for those with sentences of less than a year. This programme paved the way for several small pilot methadone programmes in prisons and jails in Maryland, Puerto Rico, and New Mexico. But all such programmes face formidable struggles to maintain their modest gains in the face of widespread correctional hostility to this approach to drug treatment, despite the powerful evidence of its benefits elsewhere in the world.

By contrast, as of January 2008, methadone maintenance has been implemented in prisons in at least 29 other countries or territories, with the proportion of all prisoners in care ranging from less than 1 per cent to over 14 per cent (Dolan et al. 2003; Binswanger et al. 2007). In Canada, any methadone maintenance patient who is incarcerated is maintained on methadone throughout his or her time in custody, and many heroin users are started on methadone during a period of federal incarceration. Even in Eastern Europe and Central Asia, some prisons now offer methadone maintenance or a short course of methadone-to-detoxification in some pre-trial detention facilities.

Tobacco and smoking bans in prisons

While smoking bans have a clear role in many public settings such as restaurants, hospitals, and workplaces, prisons have their own idiosyncratic problems associated with smoking prohibition, such as smuggling, trading, and black markets. Recent bans of smoking in prisons in many countries, easily understood as a public health measure on the outside, clash with the important and unique place of tobacco in circumstances of confinement. The important role of smoking tobacco in prisons relates to it providing some relief from the boredom and many stresses of imprisonment—similar to the role it plays in war. Of course, in prisons, smoking also plays a central role in contraband economies—part of the black market for many drugs within prisons. Tobacco can be exchanged for goods, buy protection, and be used to pay debts for gambling.

Smoking cessation programmes therefore face the formidable 'enmeshment of tobacco in prison life' (Proescholdbell et al. 2008) as staff seek to rein it in with nicotine patches, bupropion, and quitlines. Earlier experiences had examined the feasibility of psychiatric and chemical dependency units becoming smoke free. They noted the need for interventions directed at staff and patients and commented 'we are observing a tremendous amount of self-reported anger, depression and other "emotional" symptoms as most (90 per cent) of the patients are smokers and highly addicted to nicotine' (Patten et al. 1996).

Environmental issues of indoor air quality are also significant for this captive population, calling for provision of non-smoking cells and areas within prisons and environment protections which in enclosed and poorly ventilated areas are costly and may compromise security arrangements (Proescholdbell et al. 2008). In Australia, attempts to introduce smoking bans in prison have been delayed 'by legal arguments that a prisoner's cell constitutes their "home" and thus supports their right to smoke' (Butler et al. 2007). Some jurisdictions have a policy of not accommodating smoker and non-smoker inmates together, but a 2001 survey of prisoners found that one-third of non-smokers shared a cell with a smoker. The authors comment that these 'arguments need to be balanced against the human right for conditions leading to good health for smoking and non-smoking prison inmates and staff' (Butler et al. 2007). Prisoners discussing a future smoking ban in focus groups in New South Wales, Australia, spoke of 'turning the jail system on its ear' if they were prevented from smoking—there was a prison riot in Queensland, Australia, attributed in part to a prison 'non-smoking' ban. 'Concerns about adverse effects of smoking bans need to be balanced against the rights of prisoners wishing to be in a smoke-free environment' (Butler et al. 2007).

AIDS and incarceration

The global HIV epidemic now directly implicates national criminal justice policies and imprisonment—especially those related to substance abuse and illicit drug markets. Policies which involve large-scale arrests and the disproportionate incarceration of impoverished marginal populations drive HIV before them—including some of the most vulnerable populations for HIV, that is, economic and political migrants and displaced refugee populations (Spiegel 2004). Case incidence patterns are shifting rapidly as HIV enters new human populations and selects for access to new channels of transmission.

While sexual transmission remains the principal mode of transmission worldwide, injecting drug use continues to spread to new regions (most recently sub-Saharan Africa) (Mathers et al. 2010) and remains a major vector of infection as do the economic pressures and opportunities associated with large illicit drug markets in impoverished regions. These factors are allied to increased imprisonment of these populations—particularly in those nations addressing burgeoning drug markets with harsh punitive criminal justice responses. Once again the United States is an unhappy poster child for this modern plague—in large part because of its criminal justice policies and practices associated with its 35-year 'war on drugs'. In 2008, the US Centers for Disease Control and Prevention estimated that approximately 56,300 Americans are newly infected with HIV annually (Hall et al. 2008).

There is now growing evidence that mass incarceration is contributing to the continued high incidence of HIV in the United States. This relationship is particularly powerful for US racial minorities. While constituting 12 per cent of the US population, African Americans account for 45 per cent of all new AIDS diagnoses and are now estimated to have an incidence rate eight times that of white Americans. For African American women, the magnitude of these racial disparities is even more pronounced— their HIV rates are nearly 23 times the rate for white women. Discovering the causes of such dramatic disparities in HIV rates is a very high public health priority and crucial for efforts to control the US AIDS epidemic.

Although a great deal of research already exists on US racial and ethnic disparities in HIV, much of it remains focused on individual risk behaviours while neglecting more collective phenomena, including effects related to involvement with the criminal justice system. But the US association of incarceration and the AIDS epidemic is now very strong: between 17 and 25 per cent of all people in the United States who are estimated to be infected with HIV disease will pass through a correctional facility each year, roughly 190,000–250,000 of the country's estimated total of 1 million HIV-positive individuals (Spaulding et al. 2006). Research on HIV risk is now examining the social conditions and structure of this group's community networks, especially within African American populations. Focusing on the role of the criminal justice system as an important factor driving the AIDS epidemic, these data suggest a strong correlation between the circumstances of high arrest and incarceration rates and high HIV prevalence within many African American subpopulations and their communities (Peterman et al. 2005).

The care of HIV-infected inmates is a major issue (and expense) in the prisons of nations with high rates of AIDS. Thus New York State (with over 53,000 prisoners in 2010) has about 1700 HIV-infected inmates receiving medical care using antiretroviral drugs, at an annual cost of more than $25 million. But best estimates are that these 1700 individuals are only about one-third of the New York State prisoners infected with HIV—most of whom do not know they are infected (there is no routine testing of inmates). These HIV-positive individuals have a great need for testing programmes to identify them and to initiate their treatment as early as possible— both for their own benefit and for reducing transmission risk in the prison and, on re-entry, in their communities.

HIV rates among African Americans in New York State prisons are estimated at 5–7 per cent among men and 7–9 per cent among women, and the risk appears to carry over to their sexual partners in their home communities (Adimora and Schoenbach 2005). Recent evidence also suggests that cyclical patterns of release and re-incarceration may foster instability in sexual and social networks involving drug use, leading to broader social disorganization that increases AIDS transmission risk. In conjunction with unstable housing, untreated drug addiction, and recurrent imprisonment, a 'churn' in social networks occurs that is now typical of these communities. These destabilizing effects act within the social networks established in the prison feeder communities of many cities to produce increases in risk for HIV transmission both by sex and by drug use. Two-thirds of prisoners return to incarceration within 3 years of release and subsequently re-enter their home communities a few years later. This pattern of serial disruption spreads risk across these communities, affecting even those not directly linked to ex-prisoners. 'Risk networks' can include drug use and sexual partners of ex-prisoners, who may form a bridge between this population's periodic exposure to the criminal justice system and the surrounding population. This connection between the widespread incarceration of African American males and high rates of HIV in many urban communities dramatically demonstrates an important long-term community health impact of the criminal justice system.

Mental health

Mental health problems are another hallmark of prison populations in the United States and elsewhere—and another source of the mounting toll of lifelong disabilities that incarceration imposes. In the United States, 400,000 to 600,000 prison inmates (15–20 per cent of all prisoners) have a major acute or chronic psychiatric disorder, and serious psychiatric cases are now recurrent in the prison system. In addition to failing to treat many pre-existing mental health problems experienced by prisoners, incarceration itself, and especially many of the increasingly punitive practices employed to control prisoners through the massive use of isolation and solitary confinement, often creates new mental health issues, that stay with and handicap individuals long past the end of their prison sentences.

Following the United States' 'deinstitutionalization' from psychiatric hospitals for the chronically mentally ill (from the 1950s through the 1970s) the strong association of drug use, addiction, and mental illness has led the US criminal justice system to become the default response for these former hospital patients—most dramatically among the poor and homeless (see Fig. 10.10.3). Chicago political scientist Bernard Harcourt notes that a growing number of individuals who were previously monitored due to mental health issues, are now being sent to jail (Harcourt 2007a, 2007b). A US Justice Department study released in September 2006 (James and Glaze 2006) found that 56 per cent of those in state prisons (and a higher proportion of those in local jails) reported mental health problems within the past year. Harcourt states that

one reason for the increase in the number of mentally ill inmates may be a trend away from institutionalizing these individuals in mental hospitals and asylums. Harcourt writes that, 'over the past 40 years, the United States dismantled a colossal mental health complex and rebuilt—bed by bed—an enormous prison' (2007b). However there is a growing movement in the United States and elsewhere to establish mental health courts to deflect these cases (often with dual diagnosis of substance abuse) to alternatives to prisons, with some positive results now being seen (Hiday et al. 2013). But this system is also very limited due to severe shortages of properly trained and supervised mental health personnel and inadequate budgets.

Homicide and suicide in prisons and jails

While in the most extreme cases, the experience of prison or jail leads to homicide or suicide, in some respects prisons are safer than many of the communities from which many inmates come. In 2002, the US homicide rate in state prisons was 4 per 100,000, and in local jails 3 per 100,000, versus 6 per 100,000 in the general, non-incarcerated population. On the other hand, the rate of suicide in US prisons (14 per 100,000) is significantly higher than in the general US resident population (11 per 100,000). And, in local jails, the suicide rate is over four times higher (47 per 100,000) than outside. These data suggest that the stresses associated with the harrowing process of recurrent arrest, police handling at booking and arraignment, and pre-trial confinement—and even brief detention in chaotic and crowded jails—are particularly traumatic, and can often prove fatal. Over 40 per cent of those in solitary confinement, a widely used disciplinary measure in US jails and prisons, develop major psychiatric disorders. Not surprisingly, while those placed in solitary represent only 5 per cent of the prison population, they account for almost half of the suicides (Mumola 2005).

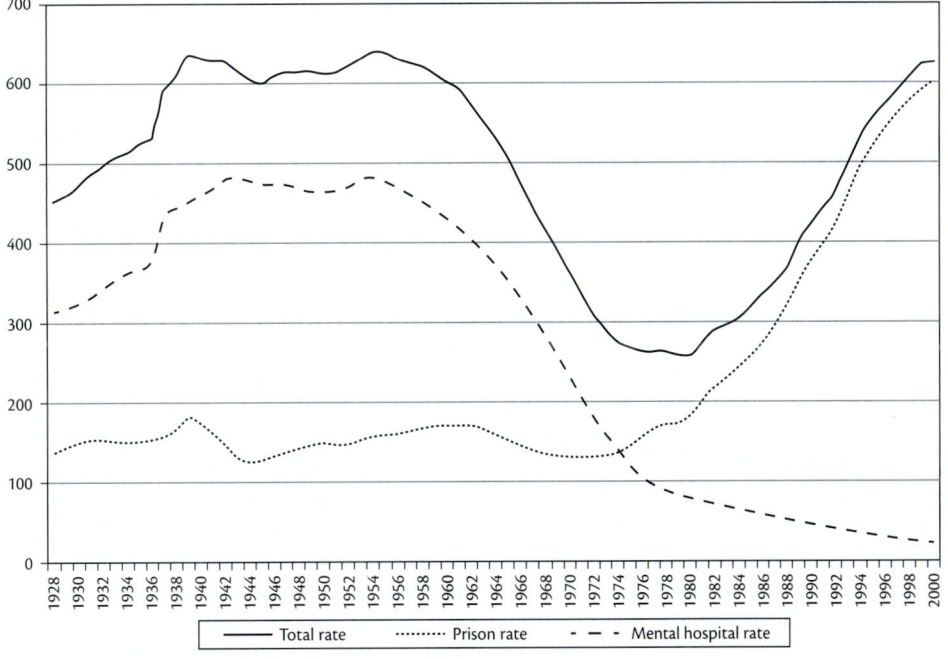

Fig. 10.10.3 Institutionalization in the United States (per 100,000 adults).

UK data from a 2001 Home Office research study shows that the rates and causes of death among prisoners and offenders under community supervision were above that of the general population (Sattar 2001). Figures released by the Ministry of Justice in a report called Safety in Custody show that in 2011, out of a population of 85,851 prisoners, 57 killed themselves, which is 0.66 per 1,000 prisoners. In the general population of the UK, from 2006 to 2010, the registered yearly suicide rate has been stable; around 0.00017 per 1,000 population according to the Office for National Statistics' latest release (http://www.theguardian.com/news/datablog/2012/sep/17/prison-probation-suicide-mapped). A majority of those convicted who committed suicide in 2012 were male (96.5%), white (87%) and aged between 21 and 49 (79%). Most of them were on remand (35%) or sentenced prisoners (59%). In terms of nationality, 22.8% of the prisoners who committed suicide were non-UK nationals.

Punitive isolation and solitary confinement

The United States, with only 5 per cent of the world's population (and 25 per cent of its prisoners) now has over half of all the world's prisoners who are in long-term solitary confinement. More than 25,000 inmates are permanently in isolation in 'supermax' (short for 'super-maximum security') prisons in the United States, where they may spend years locked in small, often windowless cells with solid steel doors, let out for showers and solitary exercise in a small, enclosed space once or twice each week. A report by Human Rights Watch (2000) found that supermax prisoners have almost no access to educational or recreational activities and are usually handcuffed, shackled, and escorted by two or three correctional officers every time they leave their cells.

Supermax prisons describe 'control-unit' prisons which represent the most secure levels of custody in the prison systems of certain countries which were ostensibly designed to house the most violent or dangerous inmates—'the worst of the worst'. But many of the prisoners there do not meet these criteria. Instead, supermax prisons are a response to the rapid growth of prison populations and shrunken state budgets, which have overwhelmed the ability of corrections professionals to operate safe, secure, and humane facilities. Lacking funds to recruit, properly train, and retain adequate staff, or to provide programmes and productive activities for those in existing congregate prisons, these thinly staffed, overcrowded, and impoverished facilities breed more tension and violence. An additional 50,000–80,000 prisoners are housed in 'restrictive segregation units', many of them in isolation.

In the United States, the trend towards more long-term solitary confinement is inseparable from the explosive growth of mass incarceration. In 2009, Harvard surgeon Atul Gawande published a startling article about the use of solitary confinement in American prisons, noting that almost exclusively in the United States over the past 20 years there has been a wide-scale increase in the use of isolation (Gawande 2009). Indeed, sustained isolation has now become institutionalized as a cornerstone of America's criminal justice system and its requirement for extreme sanctions to handle the huge population of prisoners (Cloud et al. in press).

In 1995, a California federal court reviewed the state's first supermax prison, with the presiding judge noting that the conditions 'hover on the edge of what is humanly tolerable for those with normal resilience' (King 2007). This echoes an 1890 observation by a US Supreme Court inquiry on the effects of isolation: noting that many prisoners became insane or committed suicide (Diamond et al. 2001; Hatton and Fisher 2009). Clearly the practice of locking away tens of thousands of prisoners in solitary confinement for long stretches of time has a profoundly deleterious effect on the long-term mental health of these inmates. The massive use of punitive isolation in American prisons has also become the basis for significant unrest and rebellion by inmates. In the summer of 2013 over 20,000 California inmates began a hunger strike as protest of the massive use of solitary at the Pelican Bay supermax prison and throughout the 110,000-inmate California system.

Women and prisons

Women's healthcare needs, always more prominent than those of young males, are also typically inadequately addressed in prisons. In addition to facing all the routine gynaecological, reproductive, and nutritional issues of women who are not incarcerated, the overwhelming majority of women in prisons are survivors of violence and trauma (Diamond et al. 2001; Hatton and Fisher 2009). And more than 60 per cent of incarcerated women are parents, who must deal as best they can with separation from their children and families, along with the depression, anxiety, and low self-esteem that this entails. Not surprisingly, incarcerated women suffer from serious mental illnesses at much higher rates than male inmates.

In the United States, over the last 25 years the number of women and girls caught in the criminal justice system has risen dramatically—with more than 200,000 women behind bars and more than 1 million on probation and parole. The percentage of women behind bars increased by 757 per cent between 1977 and 2004, double the increase in the incarcerated male population during the same period. The number of women in prison—along with the number of women giving birth in prison—continues to rise each year. Few get the services they need. Many of these women struggle with substance abuse, mental illness, and histories of physical and sexual abuse. Notably, despite the persistence of racial disparities, white women are now among the US groups with the fastest growth rate in US prison systems.

The increased incarceration of women for drug offences has, in some states, become a proxy for America's resurgent battles to ban abortions, a new line of challenge to the nation's Supreme Court support of abortions in the 1973 case of Roe v. Wade (Paltrow 2013). Legal scholar and reproductive rights advocate Lynn Paltrow notes that 'while all pregnant women have benefited from Roe v. Wade, today's system of mass incarceration makes it likely that if Roe is overturned women who have abortions will go to jail' (Paltrow 2013). Paltrow shows that many of the state increases in female imprisonment are intended to establish separate legal 'personhood' for fertilized eggs, embryos, and fetuses—as the basis for arrests and detentions of pregnant women involved in drug use and, for those who seek to go to term, seizure of their newborns under child protection laws.

Paltrow emphasizes that these cases reveal that both pregnant women who have abortions (and those who do not) are already being arrested and incarcerated at high rates (driven by the overall patterns of drug use related to larger racial disparities built into the American criminal justice system), 'creating a Jane Crow system of law that disproportionately punishes African American women' (Paltrow and Flavan 2013). Paltrow and Flavin have identified and detailed 417 cases of arrests and forced interventions on pregnant women in the United States between 1973 and 2005, where the pregnancy was the basis of arrest and prosecution because drugs were involved (Paltrow and Flavan 2013).

Of the more than 200,000 women found in US prisons or jails each year, about 12,000 are pregnant at the time they are incarcerated. And these women and girls are subjected to harsh treatment, even when pregnant. Women, including the thousands who will deliver their babies while incarcerated, are routinely subjected to the risks of shackling—still a common degrading practice in the United States.

The privatization of correctional services

The use of privately contracted security corporations is growing worldwide. The development of private prisons in the United Kingdom, Australia, and several European and Asian nations has followed a similar pattern (Department of Justice 2006). The United Kingdom was the first country in Europe to use prisons run by the private sector, with 14 prisons today holding 13,500 inmates in England and Wales—just under 15 per cent of the total UK prison population (Panchamia 2012).

In the United States, federal and state government had long contracted out specific prison services for medical services, food preparation, vocational training, inmate transportation—as well as construction and maintenance services—amounting to tens of billions of dollars. Beginning in the 1980s, rapid growth in prison populations (resulting from the war on drugs), prison overcrowding, and rising costs, private-sector firms in the security business took the opportunity to expand massively into prisons.

The United States led the movement to employ private firms to operate state prisons and with the world's largest prison system, now leads in the proportion of its facilities contracted to private firms. While 50 per cent of the US state prison systems (with a total of 1.2 million inmates) currently use no privately operated prison services, the 25 states that do now rely on private services for over 25 per cent of the operations of their state are located mainly in Southern and Western states. As of December 2000, there were 153 private correctional facilities (prisons, jails, and detention centres) operating in the United States with a capacity of over 119,000 (Corrections Corporation of America 2012).

Several large private sector correctional service companies are publicly traded—with the Corrections Corporation of America (2013) now 'the nation's largest owner and operator of privatized correctional and detention facilities and one of the largest prison operators in the United States—behind only the federal government and three states.' The Corrections Corporation of America currently operates 66 correctional and detention facilities, including 46 facilities that it owns, with a total capacity over 92,000 beds in 20 states and the District of Columbia. Prison privatization is an aggressively entrepreneurial business—working to increase its market and buying entire prisons from cash-strapped states in exchange for 20-year management contracts and a guaranteed occupancy rate of 90 per cent (Corrections Corporation of America 2012; Kirkham 2012). Community organizations have criticized the proposals. Critics argue that the contractual obligations of states to fill the prisons to 90 per cent occupancy are poor public policy and end up costing taxpayers more than state-run prisons would.

Immigration detention

The detention of foreign immigrants who have not been admitted through legal channels has become a major job of prison systems in many countries. Asylum seekers, political and economic refugees, and victims of human trafficking now are filling prisons, increasingly used as holding areas while these populations await disposition of their cases (Venters et al. 2009).

In the United States, more people are convicted of immigration offences than of any other type of federal crime with illegal re-entry into the United States the most common charge. As a surge of new immigration offenders flow into the US federal prison system, they are being held primarily in private prisons operated by multibillion-dollar corporations that contract with the government. Privately run prisons and immigration detention centres in the United States and elsewhere often violate basic human rights of these populations. 'These are basically second-class prisoners' (Greene 2012), '[and governments are] not putting dollars into the things that keep prisoners relatively content: medical care and food, with complaints and rebellions now common due to poor conditions and inadequate medical care' (Grant 2012).

Last year the United States deported at least 400,000 illegal immigrants, a new record (Grant 2012). Arresting undocumented immigrants has become a new focus of the otherwise shrinking prison industrial complex, driving the growth of both the federal system and the use of private security firms to assume an increased role (and increased profits) from our widely contested and highly punitive immigration policies. An integral part of the increased criminalization of immigration is the expansion of prison privatization—now also becoming widespread in the many ancillary institutions that support mass incarceration—for example, youth services and half-way houses used post release, all have been found to have very high rates of violence and abuse, as well as corrupt ties to local government.

As immigration debates rage across the political landscape, the use of mass incarceration also plays a major role in the immigration debate and is responsible for vast suffering of immigrant populations. One inevitable result of the outsourcing of these operations to private providers is increased violence throughout the privately operated for-profit facilities established for immigrant detention, where detainees are granted little or no protection from the violation of their most fundamental human rights—and have scant access to legal services. There have been many uprisings at low-security private prisons housing undocumented immigrants, following complaints from prisoners about food, medical conditions, and staff members, according to a federal court affidavit filed by the Federal Bureau of Investigation (Shed 2011). A recent US press article reported on a privately operated federal prison in Mississippi holding many undocumented immigrants from Mexico where inmates attacked guards, set fires, and took hostages—with the death of one correctional officer (Shed 2011). This Mississippi prison and other private facilities also hold inmates who are *not* awaiting deportation but are in prison for illegally crossing the border, a federal offence.

In Italy, the Identification and Expulsion Center is a detention complex on the outskirts of Rome where illegal immigrants are held for months before deportation (Povoledo 2013). These detention centres throughout Europe equate immigration with criminality, overlook the economic benefits that immigrants can bring, and fail to take account of the increasingly multicultural nature of European society.

Conclusions: the future of public health and criminal justice

The rapid rise in incarceration in the United States and several other countries from the 1970s through the 2000s has had broad effects, affecting not only those imprisoned but also their families, communities, and international politics. The expansive reach of 'mass incarceration' and its collateral effects has been accompanied in many cities by increased contact between citizens and law enforcement, increases in the time and financial impositions on individuals awaiting trial, a decline in the quality of correctional healthcare, and a reduction in available services for formerly incarcerated individuals. These complex and inter-related patterns show the ways in which imprisonment, human rights, and public health are now intimately related. With their growing concentration of vulnerable populations and their relationship to drug markets, immigration, human trafficking, border security, and global pandemics associated with sex and drugs (HIV), the international public health significance of criminal justice systems and prisons grows apace.

This examination of prisons through the lens of public health has documented the long- and short-term implications of criminal justice involvement, particularly incarceration, for public safety as well as their economic, social, and health effects on society. With this new public health basis of concern, there is renewed professional interest on the possibilities for families, schools, and neighbourhood institutions to divert individuals from criminal offending, recidivism, and the risks of jail and prison. The fiscal burdens of incarceration in the United States and elsewhere have also animated new efforts to develop and strengthen community-based sanctions as alternatives to custodial ones. These challenges, their individual and collective effects, and their concentration within the most vulnerable racial and ethnic minority communities in many nations, have motivated an intense re-examination of the 'carceral continuum' (Shedd 2011), now viewed across the multiple domains of public health, healthcare, and social services.

As a preventive discipline, public health has much to contribute to addressing the contemporary problems of criminal justice—indeed it may prove to be the most salient perspective available to us. From a preventive perspective, public health goals must now include reforms of sentencing laws (especially for drug offences) and re-examine and challenge all the basic structures of punitive patterns of incarceration from the perspective of the toxic effects of many of the forms of punishment now in effect, for example, solitary confinement. If public health can establish its legitimacy in this arena it can make very important contributions not only to health, but to fundamental human rights and help to resolve some of the greatest conflicts of modern life in our complex and ever more inter-related global culture.

References

Adimora, A.A. and Schoenbach, V.J. (2005). Social context, sexual networks, and racial disparities in rates of sexually transmitted infections. *Journal of Infectious* Diseases, 191(Suppl. 1), S115–22.

Anonymous (2012). Rise in custody deaths in England and Wales. *BBC News UK*, 14 September. [Online] Available at: http://www.bbc.co.uk/news/uk-19604024.

Binswanger, I.A., Stern, M.F., and Elmore, J.G. (2007). Release from prison—a high risk of death for former inmates. *The New England Journal of Medicine*, 356, 157–65.

Bureau of Justice Statistics (2010). *Prison Inmate Characteristics*. [Online] Available at: http://www.bjs.gov/index.cfm?ty=tp&tid=132.

Butler, T., Richmond, R., Belcher, J., Wilhelm, K., and Wodak, A. (2007). Should smoking be banned in prisons? *Tobacco Control*, 16, 291–3.

Christie, N. (1981). *Limits to Pain*. [Online] Available at: http://www.prisonpolicy.org/scans/limits_to_pain/.

Christie, N. (1997). *Crime Control as Industry*. New York: Routledge.

Clear, T.R. (1996). Backfire: when incarceration increases crime. *Journal of the Oklahoma Criminal Justice Research Consortium*, 3(2), 1–10.

Clear, T.R. (2009). *Imprisoning Communities: How Mass Incarceration Makes Disadvantaged Neighborhoods Worse*. New York: Oxford University Press.

Cloud, D., et al. (in press). Solitary confinement and public health in the United States. *American Journal of Public Health*.

Correctional Association of New York (2009). *Healthcare in New York Prisons 2004–2007*. New York: Correctional Association of New York.

Corrections Corporation of America (2012). Solicitation Letter. Available at: http://big.assets.huffingtonpost.com/ccaletter.pdf.

Corrections Corporation of America (2013). *Annual Report 2012*. [Online] Available at: http://thomson.mobular.net/thomson/7/3368/4799/.

Cullen, F.T., Lero-Jonson, C., and Nagin, D.S. (2011). Prisons do not reduce recidivism: the high cost of ignoring science. *The Prison Journal*, 91(Suppl. 3), 48S–65S.

Department of Justice (2006). https://www.gov.uk/government/uploads/system/uploads/attachment_data/file/340833/MCG_2006_report.pdf.

Diamond, P.M., Wang, E.W., Holzer, C.E., III, et al. (2001). The prevalence of mental illness in prison. *Administration and Policy in Mental Health and Mental Health Services Research*, 29(1), 21–40.

Dolan, K., Hall, W., and Wodak, A. (1996). Methadone maintenance reduces injecting in prison. *British Medical Journal*, 312(7039), 1162.

Dolan, K., Rutter, S., and Wodak, A.D. (2003). Prison-based syringe exchange programmes: a review of international research and development. *Addiction*, 98(2), 153–8.

Drago, F., Galbiati, R., and Vertova, P. (2009). The deterrent effects of prison: evidence from a natural experiment. *Journal of Political Economy*, 117(2), 257–80.

Drucker, E. (2002). Population impact of mass incarceration under New York's Rockefeller drug laws: an analysis of years of life lost. *Journal of Urban Health*, 79(3), 434–5.

Drucker, E. (2013). *A Plague of Prisons: The Epidemiology of Mass Incarceration in America*. New York: The New Press.

Fagan, J., West, V., and Holland, J. (2003). Reciprocal effects of crime and incarceration in New York City neighborhoods. *Fordham Urban Law Journal*, 30, 1551–602.

Fellner, J. (2012). *Old Behind Bars: The Aging Prison Population in the United States*. New York: Report of Human Rights Watch.

Garland, D. (1991). *Punishment and Modern Society: A Study in Social Theory*. Chicago, IL: University of Chicago Press.

Garland, D. and Duff, A. (eds.) (1994). *Criminology and Social Theory—The Culture of Control: Crime and Social Order in Contemporary Society, A Reader on Punishment*. Oxford: Oxford University Press.

Gawande, A. (2009). Annals of human rights: hellhole. *The New Yorker*, 30 March.

Glaser, J.B. and Greifinger, R.B. (1993). Correctional health care: a public health opportunity. *Annals of Internal Medicine*, 118(2), 139–45.

Gonnerman, J. (2004). *Life on the Outside*. New York: Farrar, Strauss and Giroux.

Grant, D. (2012). Deportations of illegal immigrants in 2012 reach new US record. *Christian Science Monitor*, 24 December. Available at: http://www.csmonitor.com/USA/2012/1224/Deportations-of-illegal-immigrants-in-2012-reach-new-US-record.

Greene, J. (2012). *Privately Operated Federal Prisons for Immigrants: Expensive. Unsafe. Unnecessary. Report on Federal Prisons for Undocumented Immigrants*. [Online] Available at: http://www.justicestrategies.org.

Greifinger, R. (2002). National Commission on Correctional Health Care. Executive Summary. In *The Health Status of Soon-To-Be-Released Inmates, A Report to Congress*. Unpublished report, on file with the National Commission of Correctional Health Care. Available at: http://www.ncchc.org/pubs/pubs_stbr.vol2.html.

Greifinger, R.B. (2005). Inmates as public health sentinels. *Washington University Journal of Law & Policy*, 22, 253–64.

Hall H.I., Song, R., Rhodes, P., et al. (2008). Estimation of HIV incidence in the United States. *Journal of the American Medical Association*, 300(5), 520–9.

Harcourt, B.E. (2007a). Cruel and unusual punishment. In L. Levy, K. Karst, and A. Winkler (eds.) *Encyclopedia of the American Constitution, Supplement II*. New York: Macmillan.

Harcourt, B.E. (2007b). The mentally ill, behind bars. *The New York Times*, 15 January.

Hatton, D.C. and Fisher, A.A. (eds.) (2009). *Women Prisoners and Health Justice: Perspectives, Issues, and Advocacy for an International Hidden Population*. Oxford: Radcliffe.

Hiday, V.A., Wales, H.W., and Ray, B. (2013). Effectiveness of a short-term mental health court: criminal recidivism one year postexit. *Law and Human Behavior*, 37, 401–11.

Human Rights Watch (2000). *Out of Sight: Super-Maximum Security Confinement in the United States*. [Online] Available at: http://www.hrw.org/reports/2000/supermax/index.htm#TopOfPage.

Inquests (n.d.). *Deaths in Prison*. [Online] Available at: http://inquest.gn.apc.org/website/statistics/deaths-in-prison.

James, D.J. and Glaze, L.E. (2006). Mental health problems of prison and jail inmates. *Bureau of Justice Statistics*, September, NCJ 213600. Available at: http://www.bjs.gov/content/pub/pdf/mhppji.pdf.

John Howard of London and District (n.d.). *About Us*. [Online] Available at: http://www.jhslondon.on.ca/about/mandate/.

King, R.D. (2007). Security, control and the problems of containment. In Y. Jewkes, B. Crewe, and J. Bennett (eds.) *The Handbook on Prisons*, pp. 329–55. Portland, OR: Willan Publishing.

Kirkham, C. (2012). With states facing shortfalls, private corporation offers cash for prisons. *Huffington Post*, 14 February. http://www.huffingtonpost.com/2012/02/14/private-prisons-buying-state-prisons_n_1272143.html.

Loughran, T., Mulvey, E.P., Schubert, C.A., Fagan, J., Losoya, S.H., and Piquero, A.R. (2009). Estimating a dose–response relationship between length of stay and future recidivism in serious juvenile offenders. *Criminology*, 47(3), 699–740.

Maruna, S. (2011). Re-entry as a rite of passage. *Punishment & Society*, 13(1), 3–28.

Mathers, B.M., Degenhardt, L., Ali, H., et al. for the 2009 Reference Group to the UN on HIV and Injecting Drug Use (2010). HIV prevention, treatment, and care services for people who inject drugs: a systematic review of global, regional, and national coverage. *The Lancet*, 375, 1014–28.

Mazza, G.J. (ed.) (2012). *Review Panel on Prison Rape: Report on Sexual Victimization in Prisons and Jails*. Washington, DC: US Department of Justice. Available at: http://ojp.gov/reviewpanel/pdfs/prea_final-report_2012.pdf.

Morris, N. and Rothman, D. (1995). *Oxford History of Prisons: The Practice of Punishment in Western Societies*. Oxford: Oxford University Press.

Mumola, C.J. (2005). Suicide and homicide in state prisons and local jails. *Bureau of Justice Statistics*, August, NCJ 210036.

Mumola, C.J. and Karberg, J.C. (2006). Drug use and dependence, state and federal prisoners, 2004. *Bureau of Justice Statistics*, October, NCJ 213530.

Paltrow, L. and Flavan, J. (2013). The policy and politics of reproductive health arrests of and forced interventions on pregnant women in the United States, 1973–2005: implications for women's legal status and public health. *Journal of Health Politics, Policy and Law*, 38(2), 299–343.

Paltrow, L.M. (2013). *Roe v Wade* and the new Jane Crow: reproductive rights in the age of mass incarceration. *American Journal of Public Health*, 103(1), 17–21.

Panchamia, N. (2012). *Competition in Prisons*. Institute for Government. Available at: http://www.instituteforgovernment.org.uk/sites/default/files/publications/Prisons%20briefing%20final.pdf.

Pathways to Desistence (2014). *Pathways to Desistence Study. Articles published and in press June, 2014*. [Online] Available at: http://www.pathwaysstudy.pitt.edu/publications.html

Patten, C.A., Martin, J.E., and Owen, N. (1996). Can psychiatric and chemical dependency treatment units be smoke free? *Journal of Substance Abuse Treatment*, 13(2), 107–18.

Peterman, T.A., Lindsey, C.A., and Selik, R.M. (2005). This place is killing me: a comparison of counties where the incidence rates of AIDS increased the most and the least. *Journal of Infectious Diseases*, 191(Suppl. 1), S123–6.

Phillips, S.D. (2013). *The Affordable Care Act: Implications For Public Safety And Corrections Populations*. Washington, DC: Sentencing Project.

Povoledo, E. (2013). Italy's migrant detention centers are cruel, rights groups say. *The New York Times*, 5 June.

Prisons and Probation Ombudsman for England and Wales (2013). *Annual Report 2012–2013*. [Online] http://www.ppo.gov.uk/docs/ppo-annual-report-2012-13.pdf.

Proescholdbell, S.K., Foley, K.L., Johnson, J., and Malek, S.H. (2008). Indoor air quality in prisons before and after implementation of a smoking ban law. *Tobacco Control*, 17, 123–7.

Rose, D.R. and Clear, T.R. (1998). Incarceration, social capital and crime: examining the unintended consequences of incarceration. *Criminology*, 36(3), 441–5.

Rothfeld, M. (2009). State to eliminate 40% of funding designed to turn prisoners' lives around. *Los Angeles Times*, 17 October.

Sattar, G. (2001). *Rates and Causes of Death Among Prisoners and Offenders under Community Supervision*. Home Office Research Study No. 231. London: Home Office.

Shedd, C. (2011). Countering the carceral continuum. The legacy of mass incarceration. *Criminology & Public Policy*, 10(3), 865–71.

Spaulding, A.C., Seals, R.M., Page, M.J., Brzozowski, A.K., Rhodes, W., and Hammett, T.M. (2009). HIV/AIDS among inmates of and releasees from US correctional facilities, 2006: declining share of epidemic but persistent public health opportunity. *PLoS ONE*, 4(11), e7558.

Spiegel, P. (2004). HIV/AIDS among conflict-affected and displaced populations: dispelling myths and taking action. *Disasters*, 28(3), 322–39.

Thompson, T. (2010). Poor food and stress 'responsible for rising number of deaths in UK prisons'. *The Observer*, 8 August.

Travis, J. (2005). *But They All Come Back: Facing the Challenges of Prisoner Reentry*. Washington, DC: The Urban Institute Press.

Travis, J. (2009). *Charting a New Course: A Blueprint for Transforming Juvenile Justice in New York State*. Report of Governor David Paterson's Task Force on Transforming Juvenile Justice. New York: Task Force on Transforming Juvenile Justice.

United Nations Office on Drugs and Crime (2013). *Drug Treatment and Rehabilitation in Prison Settings*. [Online] Available at: http://www.unodc.org/docs/treatment/111_PRISON.pdf.

Van Zyl Smit, D. and Snacken, S. (2009). *Principles of European Prison Law and Policy: Penology and Human Rights*. Oxford: Oxford University Press.

Venters, H., Dasch-Goldberg, D., Rasmussen, A., and Keller, A.S. (2009). Into the abyss: mortality and morbidity among detained immigrants. *Human Rights Quarterly*, 31(2), 474–95.

Walmsley, R. (2012). *World Prison Population List* (9th ed). London: International Centre for Prison Studies, University College London.

Available at: http://www.idcr.org.uk/wp-content/uploads/2010/09/WPPL-9-22.pdf.

Waquant, L. (2009). *Punishing the Poor: The Neoliberal Government of Social Insecurity*. Durham, NC: Duke University Press.

Williams, B.A., Stern, M.F., Mellow, J., Safer, M., and Greifinger, R.B. (2012). Aging in correctional custody: setting a policy agenda for older prisoner health care. *American Journal of Public Health*, 102(8), 1475–81.

World Health Organization (n.d.). *Mental Health: DALYs/YLDs Definition*. [Online] Available at: http://www.who.int/mental_health/management/depression/daly/en/

SECTION 11

Public health functions

Health needs assessment

Michael P. Kelly, Jane E. Powell, and Natalie Bartle

Introduction to health needs assessment

The idea of health needs assessment is, on the face of it, straightforward. In theory it ought to and could inform the planning and provision of health services in any jurisdiction. It is a simple formula: measure health, assess need, and orient services accordingly. In an uncomplicated world the assessment of health need and healthcare need would be a tool for tackling inequalities, a prerequisite for the allocation of resources and the first step in planning and evaluating care (Stevens and Raftery 1997).

In practice, however, as we will show, this neat and tidy formula raises some fundamental problems about the appraisal of, and the response to, health needs. The apparently straightforward approach requires us to confront some of the most vexing problems of definition and measurement in health and public health. Terms like health, healthcare, need, equity, equality, fairness, and justice, among others, have to be considered in detail (Gillam et al. 2012). They turn out to be far from simple or straightforward.

Needs assessment has been defined as a process which takes 'a population-based, epidemiological and public health approach to the planning of health interventions' (Clarke et al. 2009). That means using data about population patterns of health to do rational planning in order to meet the particular needs of all, or parts, of the community, taking account of equity, efficiency, and affordability. In principle, this approach to needs assessment might be used as the basis for planning in any health system (Clarke et al. 2009). It aspires to 'maximize the appropriate delivery of effective health interventions or care...in an evidence based way...[to] maximize equity' (Powell 2006).

However, 'need' is a slippery idea, which is not easily defined. Two broad approaches to assessing need will be outlined. The first is a very practical approach, which emphasizes measurement and tends to focus on the needs of subsets of populations and rarely tries to assess need in whole populations except in emergency situations (Clarke et al. 2009). In this view there are several levels of need: subsets in the population, groups of people with specific conditions, or a population using a particular service, for example. Both individuals and families will each generate different profiles of need. The second, broader, and more political and philosophical approach to need operates mostly at the level of total populations or whole societies and is concerned with broader questions of justice, fairness, and equity. We explore both of these approaches and identify some of the tensions between them in this chapter.

Epidemiological health needs assessment

We begin by focusing on the more practical approaches. In this view, assessment of need must include an assessment of the effectiveness of interventions to meet identified health needs (Mooney 1992; Pencheon et al. 2001). The assumption is that the relative total need can be measured sufficiently by just a few factors such as standardized mortality or morbidity rates. It emphasizes quantification and objective comparative measurement. This type of needs assessment is usually dependent on existing or available data, it seldom involves generating new information from primary research because this would be too expensive and take too long. Health needs assessment tends therefore to be based pragmatically on the routine data sources that are there already (Clarke et al. 2009).

There are a number of distinct steps. It begins with clear problem definition. To do this, two questions need to be considered. What do we want to find out about the population, and how can we go about finding it out? A series of further questions can then be asked to help clarify the process: why is this assessment needed now, who will be affected, what would the consequences be of doing nothing, how much time is available, how can the results and the recommendations be presented to maximal effect, are sufficient resources available, and how will the needs assessment be itself assessed and evaluated (Clarke et al. 2009)?

A detailed project plan identifying the component parts of the exercise should be prepared. Central to the exercise will be an epidemiological assessment which will determine how many people in the population need care and at what level and what services are available for them. It is important to identify the denominator population, that is, the total population or relevant subpopulation because otherwise it is very difficult to interpret prevalence (total number of cases) and incidence (new cases in a given time period) (Clarke et al. 2009). Collecting data like this tends to be more straightforward in developed countries. In less developed countries data systems tend not to be so reliable, although where data systems are less than optimal other options may be available (Bonnefoy et al. 2007).

Details of the structure of the population need to be built into needs assessment; the age, ethnic, occupational, and geographical contours of the local population and the patterns of health inequalities will need to be assessed and described (Kelly 2010a). The level and severity of the diseases of interest need to be examined at this stage too, along with an assessment of the prevalence of relevant risk factors—for example, levels of smoking, physical activity, and alcohol consumption. In a population with a significant number of Afro-Caribbean people an assessment of sickle cell disease might be a particular focus of interest; in a mining community chest disease might command attention. The absolute number of people suffering from the condition, and the degree of severity can then be calculated (Clarke et al. 2009). If assumptions have to be made in the absence of data and proxy variables are used, these must be made explicit.

The next stage is to develop an assessment of the clinical effectiveness of interventions for the condition or conditions of interest. There are a variety of ways of assessing effectiveness. However, if we are concerned to determine the clinical effectiveness of a medicine, or some other kind of intervention, we will get a more accurate assessment if we use evidence in which a control is used and potential biases are minimized. If this is so, we can be reasonably sure that the observed size of the effect is a consequence of the intervention and not some other biasing factor. Some commentators suggest that using only evidence drawn from the top of the evidence hierarchy to assess clinical effectiveness is the way to do this (Clarke et al. 2009). The evidence hierarchy is a device which categorizes studies according to the methods they have used and the degree of bias which is associated with the methods. Randomized controlled trials (RCTs) and the meta-analyses of such trials rest at the top of the hierarchy as these methods are deliberately designed to eliminate bias and offer the greatest certainty that the observed relationship between the independent and the dependent variable is the consequence of that relationship, and not some other factor.

It is possible to make an assessment of the effectiveness of interventions by examining clinical trial data for its quality or bias. So it would be quite appropriate, but very time-consuming, for someone conducting a needs assessment, who is interested in the effectiveness of particular treatments, to examine RCT findings directly. An easier route is to use the evidence of effectiveness which has already been appraised for its quality in Cochrane reviews. These are produced by The Cochrane Collaboration, a worldwide network of reviewers conducting quality appraisal of primary intervention studies. Alternatively, data examined by the National Institute for Health and Care Excellence (NICE) who conduct clinical and cost-effectiveness analyses of new technologies, treatment pathways, and preventive interventions in the United Kingdom can also be consulted. The assessment of effectiveness is based on a set of principles which collectively are known as health technology assessment (Kelly and Moore 2012).

After the effectiveness analysis is complete, a synthesis of the evidence is then undertaken of the epidemiology in the local population, incidence and prevalence, underlying risk factors, treatments, and interventions ranked according to effectiveness, along with evidence of cost-effectiveness and actual costs (see later). These will, of necessity, be imprecise, but if assumptions are made explicit they will suffice as a starting point for needs assessment (Clarke et al. 2009).

Once data have been collected on the local population of interest, the next stage is to compare locally derived data with data from other places in a *comparative* needs assessment. This allows an appraisal of the degree to which local provision is consistent with what might be expected on the basis of the comparisons. This is sometimes difficult because rates of interventions vary both within and between countries, but the process is about putative

differences between the observed and the expected values rather than exactness. It is important to consult with stakeholders at this point and genuine community participation is important. Rapid needs assessment may come into play where statistical and other data are unavailable (Clarke et al. 2009). All of this is brought together in a 'case for change document' which will outline what is in place, what ought to be done, what stakeholders believe should be done, and what the community want done. Costed options are essential to inform redistribution of resources. The final step is to act on the needs assessment and implement a plan.

Health systems are complex socio-technical arrangements consisting of people, cultures, and practices, organizational structures, equipment, and technologies. Health systems are constrained, because whatever the system, the resources to fund them are finite. Because of finite resources it is not possible to do everything, to fulfil every need, or to adopt every new drug, procedure, or device. At the same time demand for health services rises because expectations of what medicine can achieve increase. People, especially in advanced societies, frequently think that they deserve or have some entitlement to—that they *need*—the best and most up-to-date medicines and procedures. The availability of a medicine therefore often creates the demand *and* the need for it—patients want it and doctors want to use it. All of this adds to the demands on the resources in the system.

Health systems have to adapt to constantly evolving sets of inputs in the form of new medicines, medical technologies, and approaches to medical and surgical interventions. Decisions have to be made about the adoption and use of these new things. In addition, the health needs of populations are complex and change. For example, the age and ethnicity distributions of populations alter. Not only do populations change, but health systems themselves also evolve. Needs assessment is one means of deciding how to allocate scarce resources to prioritize and tackle need in the face of these complexities. A needs assessment provides a basis for decision-making, which will include local knowledge and understanding of the nature of communities, their socio-demographics, and physical environment. Health needs assessment consists of a range of techniques to assess and meet need in a rational and systematic way against this background of complex and changing systems, population diversity, evolution, and increasing expectations and demand. An understanding of the social environment and the social relationships within those environments is essential to successful implementation of needs assessment.

Later in this chapter we explore some of the difficulties attached to this approach. However, it is very important to remember that applying rational principles in this way arose from an understanding that the operation of an unmanaged system in which historical patterns of supply, the generosity of benefactors, the preference of medical practitioners to live in attractive areas, and their wish to provide services that were consistent with *their* interests led to very unequal and inefficient distribution of resources. So whatever the imperfections of the rational approach, it was born out of a desire to do things better and more fairly.

Health economics and needs assessment

Over the last several decades, two important techniques have come into general use to assist the allocation of resources in the face of scarcity in health systems: health technology assessment which helps to assess effectiveness of interventions and cost utility analysis in health economics, to help assess cost-effectiveness (Kelly et al. 2010). We have already discussed health technology assessment earlier in the context of assessments of effectiveness. We now turn our attention to the contribution of health economics.

The discipline of health economics has been profoundly influential in the approach to health needs assessment outlined in the previous section. It is possible to trace a link between the ethics that govern economic thinking and the techniques and tools that economists develop and apply. Trends and momentum for change in advanced health systems are also important because health economics has over the years operated with changing concepts of need, and approaches to, and techniques for measurement, assessment and evaluation of health programmes and interventions. There have also been some important new ideas to challenge conventional orthodoxies (Sassi et al. 2001; Coast et al. 2008).

As a starting point we look to utilitarianism—which is the ethical basis of the discipline of economics. It is a theory that holds that the proper course of action is the one that maximizes utility, specifically defined as maximizing happiness and reducing suffering. Utilitarian ideas grew out of the writings of Jeremy Bentham. Bentham had legal training and wrote on a wide range of subjects connected with creating conditions for common or social good and living in harmony. He spent much of his time travelling and tried to interest various heads of European states in his ideas. One Bentham idea that illustrates his thinking related to prisons. He suggested a surveillance system called the 'panopticon'. The theory of 'panopticon' is that prisoners behave appropriately in a prison setting if they believe that someone they could see in a watch tower holding a gun, could see them at all times. This idea seems at first rather odd as a model for social good. But Bentham theorized that the armed guard would only need to make their presence felt for a short time, and after that prisoners would behave as if the armed guard was there, and would not know if in reality the guard had disappeared. He argued the 'panopticon' principle of surveillance of behaviour that conforms to social norms could be applied successfully to engender harmonious living among social groups and communities in society as a whole—the threat of the use of force, rather than the actual use of force.

Utilitarian ideas, theories, and techniques are concerned with the common good or the greatest happiness of the greatest number (Bentham 1834). Utilitarianism in allocation of resources for the common good of society has much to commend it. But the tools and techniques do tend to favour the status quo. They do not challenge or on the whole try to amend existing resource allocations that might be considered to be unfair or unequal. Utilitarian tools and techniques if applied without critical reflection implicitly approve existing resource allocation and aim to improve social welfare starting from that point. They make what might be viewed as conservative changes to reallocate resources, so that at least one person is made better off and nobody else worse off (Pareto 1935).

Utilitarianism, or the greatest utility of the greatest number, is the ethic that still guides economic thinking, tools, and techniques and is also central to the ethic of health needs assessment. However, at the end of the nineteenth century, the future direction of economics as a discipline was influenced by the introduction into mainstream economic theories of mathematical thinking from the physical sciences and engineering. The concerns and

subject matter of economics moved from a focus on questions of political economy, for example, generating free trade between countries for maximizing the common good and how the growing population would feed itself, to more narrowly focused, 'scientific' questions, for example, how to maximize utility in buying goods and services and how to maximize profits (Ormerod 1994).

Economics moved away from broad questions of how resources should best be applied for the good of society—a mix of value judgement on social welfare and observation of facts, to empirical testing of hypotheses using data—more akin to a version of laboratory experiments. For example, economists became very interested in the relationship between unemployment and inflation and used empirical testing of data to test hypotheses concerning these variables.

A new more scientific language and a range of tools and techniques emerged from economic theories which tended to distance itself from the messy details of complex behaviour. The legacy of these changes still survives within economics. A quick perusal of the main economics journals today reveals numerous articles containing strings of equations to test hypotheses, as well as outlining the intricacies and new derivatives of different economic techniques and tools and how to apply them rigorously. In addition, the need within the economics discipline to find mathematical solutions to applied problems has guaranteed survival of the basic assumptions of the economic way of thinking, that is, people, firms, and institutions are perfectly rational and behave predictably, as if they have perfect information and control over environment and events. In economics, people are assumed to be equal and social/cultural and environmental/place variations between them are not acknowledged explicitly. So when health needs assessment is defined as rational this is the underlying rationality.

Health economics has developed particular techniques and tools, in particular the quality-adjusted life year (QALY) (Cohen and Henderson 1988; Powell 2007). This is steeped in utilitarianism—allocating resources efficiently for the common good—in this instance fair allocation of health technologies and other interventions in the face of finite resources. Economic thinking is predicated on the notion that most resources are scarce and have limits, but demand on those resources is potentially infinite. This creates choice and opportunity cost meaning that once resources have been allocated and used they cannot be reallocated and used again in another way (Powell 2007). Health has been characterized as a multidimensional, dynamic concept subject to changing human expectations and revision over time (McGuire et al. 1988). The economics of health has therefore also developed over time to reflect these changes. Since the Second World War, successive generations of theorists have sought to embrace new ideas about health. For example, economic, social, and psychological aspects of health have been included to reflect changing expectations, the nature of health systems, stage of economic development, and passing time (World Health Organization (WHO) 1947, 1948, 1952). From the late 1980s in developed countries, definitions of health broadened considerably to reflect the notion that well-being is inseparable from and crucial to health, and in turn, both are influenced by society as a whole (Bowling 2001).

An important idea that has been used in health economics in this regard is quality of life (QoL) (Bowling 2001). Various instruments have been developed to measure QoL (McIntyre et al. 2008). The best QoL measures detect the cultural factors that influence health perceptions, including the health of others in the individual's community or group, the nature and severity of illness, demographic characteristics, and social environment (Locker 1981). Debates about QoL measures have ranged over whether QoL should be measured at all (Hunt 1999), how it should be measured if it has to be (Walker and Rosser 1993; Bowling 2001), and how QoL measures might be applied (Fitzpatrick et al. 1992; Fletcher et al. 1992; Sassi et al. 2001). QoL is a hotly contested concept. However, it has been applied successfully to measure the outcome of health interventions and very importantly in units of common currency using the QALY. A distinction is made between the concepts of QoL and health status. QoL measures try to capture current broad definitions of 'health' (Walker and Rosser 1993), while health status measures include socioeconomic dimensions as well as physical factors. QoL relates in addition 'to how a person feels and functions in his or her everyday life' (Bowling 2001).

The QALY itself is used to assess cost-effectiveness of interventions. A QALY is a number indicating the size of health gain from an intervention. QALYs are conceptualized by first imagining years of life lived in perfect health with a perfect QoL. The QALY is constructed by combining estimates of life years saved (life years) by the intervention with values for utility of different health states (quality adjustment). It is created by combining quantitative information of length of survival with 'softer' information of patient perceptions of QoL (Bush et al. 1972; Weinstein and Stason 1975). The essence of the QALY is that people will trade-off length of life for QoL—they would rather live shorter lives with full QoL than longer lives in which QoL is poor. QALYs are the outcome measure used in cost utility economic evaluation. Cost utility analysis provides a standardized form of economic evaluation that focuses particular attention on the quality of the outcome produced or averted by investment in health programmes.

Cost utility analysis and the QALY have been widely used around the world in the assessment of the cost-effectiveness of new drugs and of other types of clinical interventions. But it has proved less well suited to assessing preventive public health type interventions. The literature identifies a number of conceptual, methodological, and practical difficulties in evaluating the effectiveness and cost-effectiveness of primary prevention interventions (Lorgelly et al. 2010). There are difficulties of producing evidence of cost-effectiveness for public health guidance and methodological difficulties associated with applying health economic techniques to public health interventions (Kelly et al. 2005; Chalkidou et al. 2008; Weatherly et al. 2009). These difficulties and issues spring from the focus on efficiency within economic evaluation techniques to the exclusion of the determinants of health and inequalities in health, which are central preoccupations in public health (Barendregt 2006; Lorgelly et al. 2010; Ogilvie et al. 2011). This is important because as we will show, health needs assessment is itself premised on principles of economic efficiency as well as the principle of equity. And so the same problem that applies to the application of simple cost utility analyses to preventive interventions also applies more broadly to health needs assessment.

Equity, efficiency, and health economics

Health systems may be characterized by the way they organize, finance, and deliver resources to attempt to balance competing health and well-being objectives. Equity in the distribution of resources is the main objective of a health system where citizens have *entitlement* and equal access to the means of achieving good health and well-being according to health *need*. Efficiency in the allocation of resources—where the cost of good health and well-being is minimized and the benefits maximized—is often prioritized by governments over equity in order that the overall *cost* of a health system as a proportion of gross domestic product, is controlled. Efficiency and equity are generally viewed as competing objectives that most health systems fail to reconcile because both objectives cannot be optimized at the same time—creating an equity–efficiency trade-off. This in turn raises concerns about justice and generates philosophical arguments about where the balance between efficient resource allocation and equitable distribution of health resources to meet health need, should lie. Early forms of health needs assessment and similar approaches—social audit and rapid appraisal—attempted to establish the size of different health needs and to prioritize and allocate resources pro rata on that basis.

Health economists were critical of the early needs assessment approaches for a number of reasons. They argued that the allocation of resources according to the size of a problem can be very misleading; not all needs can be met and resources are finite. Therefore measuring need gives no guidance concerning resource allocation to meet those needs and offers no rules by which resources can be allocated across programmes and interventions. Specifically, no attention is given to costs and benefits of treatments, only to the size of problems (Mooney 1992). The practice of needs assessment changed in response to these arguments (Wright 2001). During the early 1980s, the way of thinking in health economics gathered momentum in relation to the wholesale recasting of 'need' as a concept—seeing the fulfilment of the size and volume of health needs as in direct opposition to the objective of maximizing health status through the efficient allocation of healthcare resources.

Economists argue that the size of a health need—how many people have a certain disease at levels of severity—says nothing about how to maximize efficiency in the allocation of resources, so that the ratio of marginal benefit to marginal cost is equal across all interventions (Mooney 1992; Drummond et al. 2005). Health economic techniques and tools were directed at inefficiencies in the allocation of healthcare resources and 'the need for healthcare' defined as 'capacity to benefit' from healthcare became recognized as a key aspect of health status. As a consequence, the health intervention needed in any given circumstance is a function of factors such as the level of prevailing resources, the availability and effectiveness of health interventions, and the perspective and values of those making the assessment. Over time, notions of health need have come to be defined as a result of momentum in economic discourse and debates and the development and proliferation of common currency QoL measures that reflect the outcome and efficiency of interventions to improve health and well-being.

Health economics, it is argued, provides a way of thinking logically through the problems of setting priorities for health improvement as well as offering the techniques of programme budgeting and marginal analysis to support decision-making in resource allocation. Programme budgeting can be used as an information framework to allow health services to be disaggregated into programmes which have relatively homogeneous outputs (Cohen and Henderson 1988). The information in any programme budget will include cost or expenditure data together with an indicator of output from a programme. Services are ranked on the basis of ratio of marginal benefit to marginal cost. Marginal analysis provides rules for deciding how resources should be moved between subcategories of a programme. In terms of allocative efficiency, the concept of opportunity cost figures prominently in these techniques, where the benefit foregone is in health status.

Health systems and the equity–efficiency trade-off

We next examine the relationship between equity, efficiency, and cost, describing debates about resource allocation in Beveridge and Bismarckian health systems. These systems take their names respectively from William Beveridge whose report was used as the basis for the policies which helped establish the welfare state in Britain (Ross 1952) and Prince Otto von Bismarck who set up the first schemes of national insurance in Germany in the 1880s (Taylor 1955; Thomson 1957). We outline the ways theories of justice underpin equity–efficiency trade-offs, explaining the background to the emergence of new policy concepts and techniques of assessing, measuring, evaluating, and prioritizing efficient and equitable allocation of resources. The nature of the determinants of health and the role of physical and social environment in the improvement of community health outcomes are considered with respect to equity, need, and efficiency.

Healthcare is financed and provided free at the point of use by government through taxation in Beveridge-type health systems. Beveridge health systems differ from Bismarck-type systems in which healthcare is financed by multiple employer-based insurance schemes and taxation in which providers are privately rather than publicly owned. Both types of system, however, face the same problem of increasing demand in the face of finite resources to fund the systems. In recent decades, some reformers of health systems and health policies have attempted to create market incentives within the system to control overall healthcare expenditure, increase quality, bring down prices, and increase choice (Bevan et al. 2010)—for example, providing a choice of provider for healthcare treatments and services as a way of taking some people off waiting lists. However, the economic and social trade-off is that this comes at a price—leaving those who cannot afford to move to languish on the longer waiting list.

Alternatively, other systems that prioritize access and provide universal coverage to meet health need provide a narrower range of healthcare services because price signals to reallocate resources within the system are absent. An equity–efficiency trade-off occurs and this can create a dash from central decision-making to localism where the allocation of resources is determined by local decision-makers. Much of the tension in the balance between efficiency and equity, however, can be traced to expectations and changes over time in the common understanding of what constitutes good health and well-being in communities and countries. Inevitably, these understandings are related to stage of economic development, economic performance, and historical gross national product.

The political and philosophical approach

At the heart of the approach to needs assessment outlined so far is a relatively one-dimensional idea of need. There is an altogether different approach in the philosophical literature which defines

need as a dynamic, politically and ideologically value-laden idea. In the political and philosophical view the starting point is *unmet* health needs. It is argued that unmet need creates unfair deficits in the distribution of health and well-being among communities and populations—deficits that society should take steps to address. In this view, need is described as something that is likely to be dynamic over time as technologies, expectations, and availability of services change. Measurement of need will therefore vary in different contexts, such as in the clinical setting and at the population level. Needs assessment planning would therefore involve considerations of allocative efficiency along with social values (McIntyre et al. 2009).

But here the argument changes gear because morbidity turns out not to be a good guide to unmet need! We may posit that one person's need is greater than another's because there is a greater degree of morbidity—they are sicker. This in turn implies that one health state is more deserving than another because of the extent of the disease. It also assumes we can accurately measure the differences in disease states. This, however, may be a false premise because degrees of illness in a strictly biological or pathological sense, even if they can be measured accurately and meaningfully compared, tell us nothing about an individual's QoL with different degrees of morbidity and therefore their needs in a social or psychological sense. Some people cope extremely well with illness and have a relatively good QoL while others seem to be rendered incapable of normal social functioning with relatively minor ailments. The subjective experience of illness and an individual's response to it significantly affects their expression of need. It is difficult to measure need solely by assessing biological morbidity in any absolute sense (Locker 1981; Anderson and Bury 1988).

There is a still more difficult issue relating to health differences in populations. All health systems, and by definition all health needs assessment, have to confront the systematic differences in the pattern of health in populations. The health of individuals varies, and the health of groups of individuals also varies; so men and women, age groups, and ethnic groups show *average* differences in life expectancy and patterns of disease. The health of one country varies compared to other countries; within countries there are differences between individuals and groups. These variations occur because of biological inheritance, because of differential exposure to factors which cause disease, and because health services are not uniformly or equally spread between individuals and populations. In any case, individuals make widely different use of available services, especially preventive ones. Some people die relatively young, while others live to a ripe old age. Some people live life with multitudes of health problems and disabilities, others lead lives of a good quality and die peacefully in their beds in their 90s. So as a starting point the demands placed on health systems of these different individuals and groups vary. If we are trying in some way to meet the health needs or demands of various individuals and populations on what basis should we do it?

A straightforward answer is that we should seek to measure the needs of individuals or populations and we should allocate provision to meet the need accordingly, as that would be the fairest way to do it. But that in turn raises several questions—how exactly would we measure need? Could we do it in a way that was accurate and precise and more importantly could we do it in a way that was fair? And fair exactly to whom? To the people in need or to the people who are not in need and whom we might call upon to fund the needs of others in greater need than them? But why should those not in need, subsidize those who are in need? Is that fair? The answer as to whether one thinks it is fair will be dictated by a political preference as well as general ideas about fairness which would in turn be influenced by other ideas about ethics, morality, duty, responsibility, and liberty for example. Is it fair to have one's income taken away to fund the needs of others? Not forgetting that some people's health needs are generated by the choices that they themselves have made in how they have lived their lives, whether they have chosen to smoke, to excessively consume alcohol and food, and to take drugs or engage in sexual practices which might expose them to risk of infection. These people have health needs, but whose responsibility is it to meet those needs? Again the answer will be influenced by other value positions.

Patterning of health differences

There is another very important dimension at play here which we have not so far explored; this is the *patterning* of health differences, which removes the discussion from the level of the individual to the level of the social or population. The differences in health experience and health outcomes, the differences in access to services, the differences in exposures to risks, and even the differences in behaviours which are health damaging are not distributed randomly or evenly in the population. Health experience and health outcomes are strongly patterned by social position. In short, on whatever measure used to assess health status, be it mortality, morbidity, or self-defined health state, the measures follow a strict social gradient. Those who are better off *on average* enjoy better health, live longer, make better and more appropriate use of services, and generally get a better deal out of health systems. Moreover, this applies under whatever arrangements for the funding of services operate. It holds true in market systems like the United States, it holds true in social insurance systems as found in much of Western Europe, and it holds true in societies where care is free at the point of use like the United Kingdom. This is called the health gradient—and is one of the most enduring and vexatious characteristics of contemporary health systems (Graham and Kelly 2004).

Comparative data for the United Kingdom and the United States illustrate the gradient. They show similar patterns of graded health differences measured by income for, among other things, self-assessed health, diabetes, heart disease, and lung disease (Banks et al. 2006). The gradient is described in many texts, reports, and papers (Mackenbach 2005; Commission on Social Determinants of Health 2008; Wilkinson and Pickett 2009; Marmot 2010; Bleich et al. 2012). The shape of the gradient varies; it tends to be steeper in societies with very heterogeneous populations and rather gentler in societies which are more socially homogeneous, but only by degree. Health differences linked to social position remain an enduring and structural feature of contemporary developed societies. In both developing and low-income countries the same features of health inequities apply although the shape of the gradient tends to be more curvilinear. In some developing and low-income countries a small affluent elite enjoy good health outcomes and the majority of the population are in a less desirable situation (Bonnefoy et al. 2007).

In broad terms the state of the contemporary world is one where health differences, however measured, prevail across all societies and also between societies. There are absolute health differences between rich and poor societies and between rich and poor people and those not so poor, in all societies (Kelly and Doohan 2012). So here we encounter a major problem with the apparently rational calculus of health needs assessment. Whether health need is expressed in terms of health status or outcome, need (including subjective expression of need) varies systematically across the population and there are considerable health inequalities. It can be, and often is, argued that the needs of the most or the relatively disadvantaged are paramount and therefore resources should be deployed in such a way that they meet those needs first. All that would remain to be done would be to find a technical solution to the measurement of need.

In addition to the health gradient there are two other ways of looking at health differences called health disadvantage and health gaps (Graham and Kelly 2004). Health disadvantage simply focuses on differences, acknowledging that there are differences between individuals, distinct segments of the population, or between societies. It is a descriptive and non-judgemental approach. The health gaps approach, in contrast, focuses on the differences between the worst off and everybody else, often inviting the conclusion that those who are not the worst off enjoy uniformly good health. The gap approach also invites the conclusion that this state of affairs is wrong or unfair.

A gap approach and a gradient approach lead to rather different solutions. Conceptually, narrowing health gaps look to actions which will improve the health of the poorest regardless of the rest of society. Such an approach would be one which achieved both an absolute and a relative improvement in the health of the poorest groups. The health gradient approach takes, as its starting point in contrast, the acknowledgement that the penalties of inequities in health affect the whole social hierarchy even though they increase from the top to the bottom.

Gaps and gradient approaches lead to quite different assessment of need and how to meet those needs. It may seem counterintuitive, but if policies or actions only attempt to target the needs of the neediest at the bottom of the social hierarchy, there will be little or no impact on health inequalities across the rest of society (Rose 1985, 1992). This is because inequities in health will still exist, the social determinants continue to exert their malign influence, and the health needs of the majority of the population remain unattended to. The alternative approach advocated by the Marmot reviews, for example, and the WHO (Bonnefoy et al. 2007) involves a consideration of the whole gradient in health inequities rather than only focusing on the health of the most disadvantaged. An effective policy is one that meets two criteria. It is associated with: (1) improvements in health (or a positive change in its underlying determinants) for all socioeconomic groups up to the highest, and (2) a rate of improvement which increases at each step down the socioeconomic ladder. In other words, a differential rate of improvement is required: greatest for the poorest groups, with the rate of gain progressively decreasing for higher socioeconomic groups. It locates the causes of health inequity, not in the disadvantaged circumstances and health-damaging behaviours of the poorest groups, but in the systematic differences in life chances, living standards, and lifestyles associated with people's unequal positions in the socioeconomic hierarchy (Graham 2004a, 2004b, 2006; Graham and Kelly 2004). The significant caveat is that where the health gap is both large and the population numbers in the extreme circumstances are high, a process of prioritizing action by beginning with the most disadvantaged would be the immediate concern.

From health inequality to health equity

The gradient leads to some other questions. Does it matter that there are patterns of inequalities in health? Why should we seek to remedy this state of affairs? Why use the instruments of health service provision to deal with this problem? Why conduct needs assessment to try to change the gradient? After all, all societies demonstrate a gradient to some extent. Even though health differences are clear, a case can be made that over the last century and a half, things have improved for nearly everyone—at least in the developed West. Rates of infant mortality are at an historic low and life expectancy has never been greater. Furthermore, while *average* patterns of morbidity and mortality in different social groups and populations may be clear, there are wide variations between individuals. In short, not all well-to-do people live to a healthy ripe old age, and not everyone who is disadvantaged dies young. To be human is to know that we will eventually die and that the manner and timing of our death is in almost all circumstances beyond our control whether we are rich or poor. So is it the case that patterned average differences in *early* and largely *preventable* death and suffering are unfair and unjust just because they are theoretically preventable—particularly when there is no necessary inevitability that relatively disadvantaged people should die earlier than anyone else? There is no straightforward answer.

A number of writers have explored the theme of injustice in this context. The WHO has had a long-standing interest in the matter. The WHO's Commission on the Social Determinants of Health used a series of definitions to clarify things which were based on the work of Whitehead (Whitehead 1992; Whitehead and Dahlgren 2006) and Solar and Irwin (2010). A distinction is made between health inequality and health inequity. Health inequality is defined as *health differences which are not avoidable or preventable, are not the consequence of human actions and activities, but are based on genetic or constitutional individual differences, age or biological sex.* These are sometimes also referred to as variations (Kelly et al. 2007). Health inequity, in contrast, is defined as *unfair and avoidable or remediable differences.* Health equity in turn is defined as *the absence of unfair and avoidable or remediable differences in health among social groups* (Solar and Irwin 2010). The italics highlight the difference in definitions. It is particularly important to note that the difference in definition between inequity and inequality is not used universally and many writers and commentators use the two terms as synonyms. Also the distinctions between individual differences which are based on human biology and differences arising from interaction between an organism and an external man-made hazard are in reality difficult to draw in anything other than an analytic sense. Empirically the divides are much fuzzier than these definitions suggest. However, as a way of beginning to find some clarity the distinction is helpful. Equity and inequity are not products of nature; they are the products of human actions and, as they are socially, economically, and/or politically produced they are, theoretically at least, modifiable. The defining characteristics of equity are fairness and justice; the defining characteristics of inequity are unfairness and injustice (Whitehead and Dahlgren 2006).

Fairness and unfairness can be conceptualized as absolutes; something or some state of affairs is either fair or unfair—it cannot be both at the same time. But thinking like this in absolute terms misses the point that fairness and unfairness are not properties, things or states of affairs, but are about *relationships* between people. Fairness and unfairness arise as a consequence of the nature of the *relationships* between people and the ebb and flow of human affairs. So too justice is not a simple measure of equitable distribution of resources according to need, but is about the nature of relationships in society.

Justice may be understood in terms of the properties of people, their conduct, the rules that govern their affairs, and the characteristics of institutions—an absolute definition. The alternative is a *relational* concept of justice which concerns itself with the 'justness' of relations between people—X is unjust to Y (Pogge 2003). Such relations involve human agency, purpose, and motive. From a relational point of view justice should not be about fair distribution; it should be about seeking to identify the agents responsible for the social arrangements that determine the shape of human relationships (Pogge 2003).

Health equity may be conceptualized in distributional or relational terms in the same way that justice can be. The distributional approach is focused on the goal of equalizing good health across society—which is really the underlying value position of most health needs assessment and much of the discourse about health inequity. The relational view is about the balance between the harms inflicted and harms mitigated or prevented. In the relational view, social institutions and those responsible for them should have more concern to prevent and mitigate those things they cause themselves and for which they are responsible, rather than those things which are outside of their control (Pogge 2003). So the real issue in relational terms, with which equity should be concerned, is not the fact that health is differentially distributed, but that social systems contribute to the differential distribution of health and disease. Poverty is the greatest contributor of all to ill health. Organizing economic arrangements so that they do not generate the conditions of poverty which generate ill health is thus, it may be argued, a moral duty. Therefore focusing on assessing need without looking at the wider determinants of the causes of inequity in the first place, is misguided. The global economic order is responsible for the generation of ill health and health inequities (Pogge 2003), and social arrangements that have negative effects on health are unjust (Venkatapuram 2011).

In a celebrated paper called 'What is the point of equality?' Anderson (1999) outlined a number of the problems associated with the distributional concept of equality. She warns against the notion that we can construct institutions to make them more equal and fair, not least because this tends towards greater and greater state interference in the lives of the citizenry. She notes that one of the dangers associated with egalitarianism and the distributional approach is that it pushes the limits of the state further into the lives of ordinary people. This is a particular danger if states become concerned with equities of health rather than oppressions of the powerful against the powerless. In other words, focusing on rearranging healthcare resources to make the patterning of health more equitable is rather like moving deck chairs around on the deck of the Titanic after she hit the iceberg—largely irrelevant and pointless when the ship is sinking. 'Recent egalitarian writing has become dominated by the view that the fundamental aim of equality is to compensate people for undeserved bad luck—being born with poor native endowments, bad parents and disagreeable personalities, [and] suffering from accidents and illnesses' (Anderson 1999). This, she says, is not really the issue. We should instead be preoccupied with ending oppression (which is a relationship) rather than trying to ensure that everyone gets what they morally deserve. It is about creating a community in which people have equality in relationships with one another (Anderson 1999). She argues for democratic equality which means that all law abiding citizens are allowed effective access to the social conditions of their freedom. Anderson criticizes the view that the purpose of distributive justice is to compensate people for their misfortune. Her argument strikes at the heart of the idea that health inequities are simply unfair; her position is that while life may be unfair, bad luck is not at the heart of it—it is the relations between people and the way that they treat each other that is much more fundamental.

Anderson draws our attention to the fact that the concept of equality can mean a number of different things depending on the underlying political value position and the epistemological assumptions of the theory. So a utilitarian seeking to maximize the greatest happiness of the greatest number would see things differently to a Marxist seeking absolute parity in access to wealth, for example. She demonstrates that equality is a rationalist rather than an empiricist concept, meaning that the discourse about distributional equality and health equity is premised on the manipulation of ideas and the contest between different ideas and political philosophies, rather than being something that can be demonstrated by empirical methods (Millican 2007). True, protagonists will appeal to empirical evidence about poverty and about wealth to justify their arguments, but in the end, much of the discussion about equality is grounded in ideal discussions of future desired states and institutions and the manipulation of ideas to justify that view, rather than the case being made that empirically things could be changed by doing x, y, or z. Where x, y, or z are suggested, they are selected on the basis of ideological preference, not empirical science.

Bernard Williams argued that the proper grounds for the distribution of healthcare are health need (Williams 1962). This he saw as a fundamental truth (Wolff 2007). Others have argued that this is not a fundamental truth at all. Nozick has argued that the focus on need, common among egalitarian thinkers, is to define people quintessentially as consumers. The task then becomes one of finding the best way to ensure the fair distribution of available goods to consumers (Nozick 1974). The problem of course with this approach, is that this casts humanity into a fundamentally passive role and it doesn't consider individuals as active producers (Wolff 2007). Williams also argued that there is nothing about need itself intrinsically that should motivate action on equity (Williams 1962). What society decides to do for people, particularly in health need, depends upon a moral and ethical stance.

Another argument is that the goal of fair distribution should be treating the worst off as well as possible rather than flat equity (Wolff 2007). John Rawls argued that difference in the distribution of primary goods such as health is tolerable, so long as the welfare of the most disadvantaged is looked after (Rawls 1971). Dworkin takes this argument a stage further. He suggests that we need to determine why the worst off are in that position. Dworkin asserts that some may not be able to work because they are unable to find work; but others may decide they do not want to work. Dworkin

also notes that some people's needs are greater than others (someone who is severely disabled has greater need than someone who is able bodied for example—although as we noted above this is a highly questionable first premise). But needs, Dworkin notes, are compounded by taste. Some people's needs are determined by expensive tastes say for drugs or wine or jewellery. Dworkin therefore distinguishes between brute bad luck and circumstance from optional bad luck involving some degree of culpability for being in need. For Dworkin, this distinction is all important, as it is his view that the state has a duty to deal with the former, but not the latter (Dworkin 2000; Wolff 2007).

Some philosophical reflections

Health needs assessment is not value neutral, it is premised on a number of philosophical and political concepts. It is helpful to explore the arguments relating to these ideas not least because although they are fundamental to health needs assessment the conventional literature about health needs assessment seldom considers the underlying assumptions and issues in detail. This is particularly so with respect to the central importance of utilitarianism and its contested place in the philosophical canon. The discussion is made all the more confusing because many of the relevant ideas like justice, equality, fairness, and so on are in common as well as technical philosophical usage and the meanings attached to common sense understanding of the words and the technical vocabulary usage are seldom commensurate.

Another very intriguing characteristic of the literature—a literature after all which readily uses terms like justice, fairness, equality, is that with the exception of Sen (more of whom later), the origins of the arguments about justice and need are conducted entirely without reference to their antecedents in Christian or Islamic teachings or the teachings of the other major world religions. The secular attempts to define the equal society, justice, and fairness struggle in this regard to find a moral or ethical point of reference. The other very odd thing is that conventional political philosophy has, down the years, actually paid scant attention to health and health inequalities and issues of distribution of healthcare resources (Venkatapuram 2011).

At the heart of the debates about equity and health inequity in contemporary society is, as we saw earlier, social justice. Health inequities are considered by many commentators to be unjust and unfair and this is advanced as a reason for allocating resources following needs assessment, more fairly. Just as utilitarianism is central to health needs assessment, it has also been central to theories of justice too viz. what produced the greatest happiness in the greatest number was considered to be socially just (Venkatapuram and Marmot 2009). This absolute or distributional approach to justice was based on a highly individualistic model and was premised in turn on the individual as the unit of analysis and not the alternative which is the relational conception of social life. The solution in the utilitarian view of the world is fair distribution and systems which can efficiently distribute resources, a principle at the very heart of health needs assessment. The utilitarian argument overlooks, by virtue of its basis in the maximization of utility, not only the fact that humans are motivated by a variety of things, not just maximizing utility, but also love, social conflict, human venality, and sheer and utter evil, and it doesn't seem to have a concept of the social. In other words, individual utility maximizing motivated agents are the focus of the argument, not social relations between people. This individualistic approach chimes with medicine.

Medicine has as its principal focus, pathology in the individual human body. This means that, with only a few historical exceptions, the intellectual interests have been oriented to phenomena located in individual human bodies or minds with pathology measurable in ways that reflect the individual and individual variation from some notion of what is normal or healthy (Antonovsky 1985, 1987; Carter 2003). This approach received an enormous boost with the rise of germ theory and with the fantastic successes of the isolation of pathogenic microbes and then antibiotics to combat them. Of course medicine has other foci too; especially body systems, but the variables and phenomena of particular interests are individual. The pathogenic paradigm, in which the fundamental rationale is isolating the specific cause (pathogens) of specific outcomes (pathologies), reinforces the individualistic approach. Psychology has likewise made its main focus the individual so measures of intelligence, personality, quality of life, all reside in the individual or are characteristics or properties of individuals. The approach is about the degree to which things go wrong in individual bodies and minds and the preceding causes of the pathology. Need as an individual property is an obvious next step in this way of thinking.

Economics and especially health economics has bought into this individualistic paradigm in a big way. The QALY and the application of cost utility analysis and health technology assessment are deeply infused with an individualistic orientation. The greatest happiness of the greatest number is the utilitarian philosophical view which sits very comfortably with the individualistic paradigm because it conceptualizes the notion of the good as the aggregate of lots of different individual utilities. The ontological consequence of this—that is, the assumptions made about what constitutes human life and how and why it is the way that it is—is the idea that the essence and meaning of human existence can be captured by isolating these individual characteristics and seeing how they connect to each other. So individual characteristics as different as height, weight, blood pressure, bone density, hair colour, IQ, biological sex, and size of tumour, for example, can each in turn be linked to the presence of other characteristics in the individual like health of mother *in utero*, poor nutritional status in childhood, genetic coding, parental heredity, age, chromosome structure, and exposure to tobacco smoke. The causal link is from one individual characteristic to another.

Now all of this is intuitively meaningful—in the modern Western world the individual and the individuated self are touchstones of the way we live our lives and the way the state regulates our lives—we have, for example, individual national insurance numbers, passport numbers, birth certificates, tax codes, and genomic structures. Individual variables seem natural. Further in medical terms there have been some remarkable successes in isolating disease mechanisms and offering curative technologies using the individual approach—although far less than the popular imagination often supposes—using these principles.

However, there are two fundamental objections which suggest that another way of viewing things might be helpful. First the individualist approaches dehumanize people—people are reduced to some subhuman characteristic—a number, a genetic code, a pathological organism, a utility. But second, and more importantly,

and notwithstanding the advances that have followed in the wake of some of the individualistic connections which have been made, above all it ignores or relegates the fact that humans live in groups and that those groups are in relations with each other and that membership of those groups is a defining characteristic of identity and of profound importance to most people—one's family, class, tribe, caste, gender, ethnicity, and nationality are all paramount social markers in life. Moreover, the relationships within which we live our lives, the relations with other people and the relationships within and between different groups, shape the nature of our human selves, our experiences, and our behaviour. The defining characteristic of human life is belonging—to be a member of multiple groups and communities. We live our lives in a network of interlinked and overlapping relations with others. Knowingly or not, the desire to belong has far-reaching consequences on the types of behaviours that we adopt and the choices that we make. Not surprisingly, therefore, the effects of social exclusion or isolation from social groups are of paramount importance when trying to explain the health of an individual.

What this makes us pause and reflect on is not that the individual understanding of human affairs is unimportant—that would clearly be an absurd position to adopt. Rather it is that a full understanding of the human condition requires additionally another set of concepts—which capture human relationships—relational concepts—in order to develop a rounded account of human life. And moreover inequity and injustice are best understood in relational not individualistic terms.

Social theorists have grasped the idea of a well-rounded approach very neatly in the conception of the dynamic interaction between agency and structure. The idea of agency is that we are all unique biological, psychological, and physical individuals. We all engage in individually motivated actions and behaviours which are in part the results of our unique individuality. But the sum of all human behaviours is social structure which is the consequence of the millions and billions of human relationships that are the medium for individual actions. Those structures or webs of human relationships are relational and in turn they constrain, drive, and facilitate individual human behaviour. So we have individual behaviour, the medium for its expression which are human relationships, and social structures, which are the sum of all those relationships, which in turn impinge on and delimit the possibilities of individual behaviour (Giddens 1979, 1984; Elder-Vass 2010).

This rather abstract approach allows us in turn to consider some of the thorny problems at the heart of health needs assessment. Thinking of the dynamic interaction between agency and structure moves us beyond the methodological individualism of traditional epidemiology and therefore of health needs assessment and provides an escape from the individual level of explanation (Frohlich et al. 2001). This in turn allows for a fuller understanding of the dynamics of the development of health inequalities (Abel and Frohlich 2012).

This way of thinking has been linked to what is called capability theory (Sen 2009). The core characteristic of capability theory is its focus on what people are effectively able to do within relationships with each other (Abel and Frohlich 2012). Individuals being able to engage effectively in what they really want to do, is the core idea. These engagements include being active, healthy, and being able to work but the list is not limited to these activities. In the capability approach, resources and their fair distribution to individuals (the focus of the traditional utilitarian approach) are not the central interest. Resources are not ends in themselves they are means to ends. And neither are resources reducible to monetary utilities. People's abilities to realize their life goals and plans are the focal point. In the capability approach, the issue of justice, fairness, and need does not apply to resources per se but to the range of options for agency—the capabilities (Abel and Frohlich 2012).

Sen is a seminal thinker in relation to these arguments. He makes the case for a dynamic approach to social justice. He has argued that to think about justice in terms of fairness is a major shift away from the traditional ways that philosophers have thought about justice. This is because they were locked into the utilitarian/distributional tradition (Sen 2009). This is important in the context of needs assessment which is fundamentally utilitarian and implies that through its rationality and market allocative efficiency it will be possible to deliver fairness by market redistribution. This follows a tradition which goes back, according to Sen, to the Enlightenment. The utilitarian position is a rationalist position writ large, that is, a position which is about the manipulation of ideas, rather than the observation of empirical facts (Millican 2007). The ideas about social justice which are being manipulated are that it is possible to design institutional arrangements that will deliver justice and this will be the basis of a perfect society. For Sen, justice is a relative concept and is about relations between people. Justice is a process, an aspiration; it is about advancing justice or reducing injustice. It is not about finding or describing the perfectly just society. Because social structures and their properties emerge out of human relationships, it means that to try to legislate to change social systems to make them more just or fair can only ever be partially effective. In a sociological sense justice and injustice are properties of social systems not abstract transcendental things that can be made by social actors. Sen's approach is comparative, plural, iterative, dynamic, and acknowledging of alternatives.

Justice in this view is not a given—a rationally derived static universal principle. It is about relations between people and arises as a consequence of social action and social structure. Therefore injustice will also arise socially in social interaction and is decided upon morally or metaphysically. The judgement about whether the relations between people, such as differences in health, are just or unjust is a value judgement. In short, seeking to bring about equality in relation to health by the utilitarian redistribution of resources is never likely to work, or to produce fairness and justice because justice is not a quality of individuals or institutions. Equality is about human relationships and the utilitarian approach at the heart of health needs assessment is based on an alternative individualistic ontology.

Sen's argument is that theories of justice major on something; it could be happiness as in the case of classical utilitarianism, and it could be resources or income. Sen argues that in contrast to these utility-based or resource-based lines of thinking, individual advantage is judged in the capability approach by a person's capability to do things they have a reason to value. A person's advantage in terms of opportunities is judged to be lower than that of another if they have less capability—less real opportunity—to achieve those things that they have reason to value. The focus is on the freedom that a person actually has to do this or be that— things that they value doing or being (Sen 2009). Sen's approach is about human life and the opportunities for living—living as against just existing. Justice for Sen cannot be created by social institutions. Justice should aim to reduce injustice, that is, change the nature of the relationships between people, rather than aiming to produce a perfectly just society.

Conclusion

Health needs assessment can be seen as a highly rationalist, straightforward means of identifying health needs, of linking needs to patterns of health inequities, of marshalling appropriate resources to match those needs, and then deploying resources accordingly. And of course that is what it aspires to do. But that aspiration is based on the traditional rationalist approach of utilitarianism and in turn on an individualist ontology. Need, as we have shown, is not a static, objective thing. It is therefore intrinsically difficult to measure and as soon as one starts to try to capture the idea fundamental questions about fairness and justice are raised.

The objective and measurable concept of need is located in an individualist ontology. When we think instead in relational terms about equity, justice, and human capabilities a different perspective is possible. Capabilities theory captures the idea of equity in a far more nuanced way than individualistic utilitarian accounts. It also offers a more complete way of understanding how we might rethink health needs assessment.

So rather than seeking to measure individualistic objective variables and then seeking to apply resources accordingly, the relational capabilities approach bids us to think about the relations between service providers and users in a much more novel way. It requires us to not try to match resources to a completely slippery and spuriously objective concept of need, but instead makes us consider the nature of the relationships between people and services.

Maximizing health outcomes, a utilitarian fundamental principle, may not be what social justice requires and alleviating injustice may require more than maximizing efficiency (Venkatapuram 2011). The argument then hinges on several fundamental things: the degree to which the structure and organization of services permits people to meet their own capabilities, the degree to which it allows human potentials to be realized, and the degree to which the relationships with services do not distort or alienate people from themselves or from others. The capability approach privileges human functioning, not maximizing utility or achieving an idealized and biologically improbable disease-free state (Venkatapuram 2011).

This means that service design should reflect and respect human dignity; this means respect for an individual person, but at the same time acknowledging the limitations which disease and disability genuinely impose on people while recognizing that there is not a direct cause and effect linear relationship between disease state and social functioning. It should acknowledge the fact that illness and disease by their very nature tend to exacerbate disconnectedness between the person and their normal role responsibilities, their primary social attachments, and their desired capabilities. The experience of disease and disability can also produce a profound separation of the individual from their sense of self or their sense of who and what they want to be. The capability approach therefore requires us to respect the lifeworlds of ordinary people and work with them to build their skills, assets, and capabilities (rather than focusing on their deficits and trying to correct them via redistributional activities). These skills, assets, and capabilities allow them to manage their lifeworlds with minimal interference. The kinds of skills which enhance capabilities include interpersonal relationships, technical skills to manage the routine aspects of social and economic and domestic life, skills to develop emotional and psychological resistance (often referred to as coping or resilience mechanisms), and an ability to make life seem meaningful. These skills enable people to manage the routine travails of ordinary living as well as the more significant life events which engulf everybody from time to time (Kelly 2010b). It also allows people to manage the material lifeworld they inhabit. This is important because the material and psychological lifeworlds mediate the stressors—physical, psychological, and biological—which assault the human body periodically. The greater the ability people have to control their lifeworlds, the greater the resilience they will have. Skills to control the lifeworld are quintessentially capabilities. The inability to exert that control forms the basis of the patterning of health inequities because the ability to exert control is not spread uniformly through the population. Following Sen's prescription, we should seek not to measure need in a potentially spuriously scientific way, but rather acknowledge that the *total* population, all of us, are in need of strengthening our capabilities. Further it is relatively easy to predict where the need to develop more capabilities and skills is greatest and that is among the poor, the disadvantaged, subgroups and minorities, and people with disabilities. Efforts to develop and build the skills and capabilities should be proportionately, but not exclusively, focused on these groups. The level of self-empowerment to help to realize these capabilities needs to be appropriate for the individual. This is an important consideration when deciding where to deploy resources.

Moreover, upstream efforts need to embrace a public health preventive approach; an education in basic skills for living, appropriate role modelling as the basis of the most appropriate skills for human interaction, appropriate deportment, manners, respect for others, management of emotions, and the development of an appropriate sense of self and identity are the basics of human socialization. This means that the early years are particularly important and that taking the edge off encounters between people that are destructive and harmful is paramount.

While all of this plays out on life's grand stage, it must also apply to the way health services are provided and delivered. If services are organized around allocative efficiency alone and neglect the sense of self, the identity, the skills required to negotiate the system, and they alienate patients and public from and systematically deskill the recipients of care, they meet no one's needs at all, and serve only to make the patterns of inequities worse. They become, in other words, a contributor to the problem, rather than a solution to the problem. Unfortunately, the utilitarian approach with its individualistic ontology, and its emphasis on ideal rationality, is focused on a question, which on the face of it is not unreasonable, of how to match resource deployment to need. This is in fact the wrong question, so it often ends up doing exactly the opposite of what it is trying to do and making matters worse.

None of this should be taken to be a yet another Utopian recipe for the perfect society. Human venality, greed, jealousy, laziness, prejudice, incompetence and even evil will always be part of the human condition, resources will always be scarce and groups will compete, sometimes viciously, for those resources. But the development of human capabilities allows the harder edge of human existence to be ameliorated. It does mean though that the temptation to try to find purely rationalist solutions which can only ever work in theory, or indeed in Utopia—nowhere—rather like transcendent theories of justice, must be resisted. It must be acknowledged that it is about human relationships and allowing those relationships to be as humanly meaningful and fulfilling and permitting of enhancing human capabilities as possible. The most important task in a good and just society is to prevent the erosion of those things which protect and maintain human capabilities. It is to protect the virtuous and the virtues and to enhance them where possible and to protect them by supporting social arrangements which facilitate that. Relationships cannot be legislated for, nor made to happen by complex processes of resource allocation. Justice and the social arrangements that maintain relationships are in the end the emergent properties of social relations. Those relations must be cultivated in a humane, and as far as possible, just way that protects and enhances people's capabilities. This must be the prerequisite for any state wanting to deploy its healthcare resources in a way that is both effective and meaningful. Building capability into service design is a fundamental prerequisite.

References

Abel, T. and Frohlich, K.L. (2012). Capitals and capabilities: linking structure and agency to reduce health inequalities. *Social Science & Medicine*, 74, 236–44.

Anderson, E.S. (1999). What is the point of equality? *Ethics*, 109, 287–337.

Anderson, R. and Bury, M. (eds.) (1988). *Living With Chronic Illness: The Experience of Patients and their Families*. London: Unwin Hyman.

Antonovsky, A. (1985). *Health Stress and Coping*. San Francisco, CA: Jossey Bass.

Antonovsky, A. (1987). *Unravelling the Mystery of Health: How People Manage Stress and Stay Well*. San Francisco, CA: Jossey Bass.

Banks, J., Marmot, M., Oldfield, Z., and Smith, J.P. (2006). *The SES Health Gradient on Both Sides of the Atlantic*. Cambridge, MA: National Bureau of Economic Research.

Barendregt, J. (2006). Economics and public health: an arranged marriage. *European Journal of Public Health*, 17(2), 124.

Bentham, J. (1834). *Deontology or the Science of Morality*. London: Longman.

Bevan G., Helderman J., and Wilsford D. (2010). Changing choices in healthcare: implications for equity, efficiency and cost. *Health Economics Policy and Law*, 5, 251–67.

Bleich, S.N., Jarlenski, M.P., Bell, C.N., and LaVeist, T.A. (2012). Health inequalities: trends, progress and policy. *Annual Review of Public Health*, 33, 7–40.

Bonnefoy, J., Morgan, A., Kelly, M.P., et al. (2007). *Constructing the Evidence Base on the Social Determinants of Health*. Report to the World Health Organization Commission on the Social Determinants of Health. Available at: http://www.who.int/social_determinants/knowledge_networks/add_documents/mekn_final_guide_112007.pdf.

Bowling, A. (2001). *Measuring Disease* (2nd ed.). Buckingham: Open University Press.

Bush, J., Fanshel, S., and Chen, M. (1972). Analysis of a tuberculin testing program using a health status index. *Socio-Economic Planning in Science*, 6, 49–68.

Carter, K.C. (2003). *The Rise of Causal Concepts of Disease: Case Histories*. Aldershot: Ashgate.

Chalkidou, K., Culyer, A., Naidoo, B., and Littlejohns, P. (2008). Cost-effective public health guidance: asking questions from the decision-maker's viewpoint. *Health Economics*, 17(3), 441–8.

Clarke, A., Powell, J., and Lansang, M.A. (2009). Needs assessment: a practical approach. In R. Detels, R. Beaglehole, M.A. Lansang, and M. Gulliford (eds.) *Oxford Textbook of Public Health* (5th ed.), pp. 1549–61. Oxford: Oxford University Press.

Coast, J., Smith, R., and Lorgelly, P. (2008). Should the capability approach be applied in health economics? *Health Economics*, 17, 667–70.

Cohen, D.R. and Henderson, J.B. (1988). *Health Prevention and Economics*. Oxford: Oxford Medical Publications.

Commission on Social Determinants of Health (2008). *Closing the Gap in a Generation: Health Equity Through Action on the Social Determinants of Health*. Geneva: WHO.

Drummond, M., Sculpher, M., Torrance, G., O'Brien, B., and Stoddart, G. (2005). *Methods for the Economic Evaluation of Health Care Programmes* (3rd ed.). Oxford: Oxford University Press.

Dworkin, R. (2000). *Sovereign Virtue*. Cambridge MA: Harvard University Press.

Elder-Vass, D. (2010). *The Causal Power of Social Structures: Emergence, Structure and Agency*. Cambridge: Cambridge University Press.

Fitzpatrick, R., Fletcher, A., Gore, S., Jones, D., Spiegelhalter, D., and Cox, D. (1992). Quality of life measures in health care I: applications and issues in assessment. *BMJ*, 305, 1074–7.

Fletcher, A., Gore, S., Jones, D., Fittzpatrick, R., Spiegelhalter, D., and Cox, D. (1992). Quality of life measures in health care II: design, analysis and interpretation. *BMJ*, 305, 1145–8.

Frohlich, K.L., Corin, H., and Potvin, L. (2001). A theoretical proposal for the relationship between context and disease. *Sociology of Health & Illness*, 23(6), 776–97.

Giddens, A. (1979). *Central Problems in Social Theory: Action, Structure and Contradiction in Social Analysis*. Berkeley, CA: University of California Press.

Giddens, A. (1984). *The Constitution of Society: Outline of the Theory of Structuration*. Berkeley, CA: University of California Press.

Gillam, S., Yates, J., and Badrinath, P. (2012). *Essential Public Health: Theory and Practice*. Cambridge: Cambridge University Press.

Graham, H. (2004a). Social determinants and their unequal distribution: clarifying policy understandings. *Milbank Quarterly*, 82, 101–24.

Graham, H. (2004b). Tackling health inequalities in England: remedying health disadvantages, narrowing gaps or reducing health gradients. *Journal of Social Policy*, 33, 115–31.

Graham, H. (2006). Socioeconomic inequalities in health: evidence on patterns and determinants. *Benefits*, 14, 77–90.

Graham, H. and Kelly, M.P. (2004). *Health Inequalities: Concepts, Frameworks and Policy*. London: Health Development Agency. Available at: http://www.nice.org.uk/page.aspx?o=502453.

Hunt, S.M. (1999). The researcher's tale: a story of virtue lost and regained. In C.R.B. Joyce, C.A. O'Boyle, and H. McGee (eds.) *Individual Quality of Life Approaches to Conceptualisation and Assessment*, pp. 225–32. Amsterdam: Harwood Academic Publishers.

Kelly, M.P. (2010a). The axes of social differentiation and the evidence base on health equity. *Journal of the Royal Society of Medicine*, 103, 266–72.

Kelly, M.P. (2010b). A theoretical model of assets: the link between biology and the social structure. In A. Morgan and E. Ziglio (eds.) *International Health and Development: Investing in the Assets of Individuals, Communities and Organisations*, pp. 41–58. New York: Springer.

Kelly, M.P. and Doohan, E. (2012). The social determinants of health. In M.H. Merson, R.E. Black, and A.J. Mills (eds.) *Global Health: Diseases, Programs, Systems and Policies* (3rd ed.), pp. 75–113. Burlington, MA: Jones & Bartlett.

Kelly, M.P., McDaid, D., Ludbrook, A., and Powell, J. (2005). *Economic Appraisal of Public Health Interventions*. London: Health Development Agency. Available at: http://www.cawt.com/Site/11/Documents/Publications/Population%20Health/Economics%20of%20Health%20Improvement/Economic_appraisal_of_public_health_interventions.pdf.

Kelly, M.P. and Moore, T.A. (2012). The judgement process in evidence based medicine and health technology assessment. *Social Theory and Health*, 10, 1–19.

Kelly, M.P., Morgan, A., Bonnefoy, J., et al. (2007). *The Social Determinants of Health: Developing an Evidence Base for Political Action*. Final Report to the World Health Organization Commission on the Social Determinants of Health. Available at: http://www.who.int/social_determinants/resources/mekn_report_10oct07.pdf.

Kelly, M.P., Morgan, A., Ellis, S., Younger, T., Huntley, J., and Swann, C. (2010). Evidence based public health: a review of the experience of the National Institute of Health and Clinical Excellence (NICE) of developing public health guidance in England. *Social Science & Medicine*, 71, 1056–62.

Locker, D. (1981). *Symptoms and Illness: The Cognitive Organisation of Disorder*. London: Tavistock.

Lorgelly, P., Lawson, K., Fenwick, E., and Briggs, A. (2010). Outcome measures in economic evaluations of public health interventions: a role for the capacity approach? *International Journal of Environmental Research and Public Health*, 7(5), 2274–89.

Mackenbach, J. (2005). *Health Inequalities: Europe in Profile*. London: COI for the UK Presidency of the EU.

Marmot, M. (2010). *Fair Society, Healthy Lives: Strategic Review of Health Inequalities in England post 2010*. London: UCL. Available at: http://www.ucl.ac.uk/gheg/marmotreview/Documents/finalreport.

McGuire, A., Henderson, J., and Mooney, G. (1988). *The Economics of Healthcare*. London: Routledge.

McIntyre, D., Mooney, G., and Jan, S. (2009). What is need and how do we measure it? In R. Detels, R. Beaglehole, M.A. Lansang, and M. Gulliford (eds.) *Oxford Textbook of Public Health* (5th ed.), pp. 1535–48. Oxford: Oxford University Press.

Millican, P. (2007). Introduction. In D. Hume, *An Enquiry Concerning Human Understanding* (P. Millican ed.), pp. 1–42. Oxford: Oxford University Press.

Mooney, G.H. (1992). *Economics Medicine and Healthcare* (2nd ed.). Brighton: Wheatsheaf.

Nozick, R. (1974). *Anarchy, State and Utopia*. Oxford: Blackwell.

Ogilvie, D., Bull, F., Powell, J.E., et al. (2011). An applied ecological framework for evaluating infrastructure to promote walking and cycling: the iConnect study. *American Journal of Public Health*, 101, 473–81.

Ormerod, P. (1994). *The Death of Economics*. London: Faber and Faber.

Pareto, V. (1935). *Mind and Society*. New York: Harcourt Brace Jovanovich.

Pencheon, D., Guest, C., Melzer, D., and Muir Gray, J.A. (eds.) (2001). *Oxford Handbook of Public Health Practice*. Oxford: Oxford University Press.

Pogge, T.W. (2003). Relational conceptions of justice: responsibilities for health outcomes. In S. Anand, P. Fabienne, and A. Sen (eds.) *Health, Ethics and Equity*, pp. 8–33. Oxford: Clarendon.

Powell, J. (2006). *Health Needs Assessment: A Systematic Approach*. National Library for Health: Health Management Specialist Library.

Powell, J.E. (2007). Health economics in public health. In J. Orme, J. Powell, P. Taylor, and M. Grey (eds.) *Public Health in the 21st Century: New Perspectives on Policy Participation & Practice*, pp. 287–301. Maidenhead: Open University Press.

Rawls, J. (1971). *A Theory of Justice*. Cambridge MA: Harvard University Press.

Rose, G. (1985). Sick individuals and sick populations. *International Journal of Epidemiology*, 14, 32–8.

Rose, G. (1992). *The Strategy of Preventive Medicine*. Oxford: Oxford University Press.

Ross, J.R. (1952). *The National Health Service in Great Britain: An Historical and Descriptive Study*. London: Oxford University Press.

Sassi, F., Archard, L., and Le Grand, J. (2001). Equity and health care economic evaluation. *Health Technology Assessment*, 5(3), 1–138.

Sen, A. (2009). *The Idea of Justice*. London: Allen Lane.

Solar, O. and Irwin, A. (2010). *A Conceptual Framework for Action on the Social Determinants of Health*. Social Determinants of Health Discussion Paper 2, Policy and Practice. WHO: Geneva.

Stevens, A. and Raftery, J. (eds.) (1997). *Health Needs Assessment: The Epidemiologically Needs Based Reviews*. Oxford: Radcliffe.

Taylor, A.J.P. (1955). *Bismarck: The Man and the Statesman*. London: Hamish Hamilton.

Thomson, D. (1957). *Europe Since Napoleon*. London: Longman.

Venkatapuram, S. (2011). *Health Justice: An Argument from the Capabilities Approach*. Cambridge: Polity.

Venkatapuram, S. and Marmot, M. (2009). Epidemiology and social justice in the light of social determinants of health research. *Bioethics*, 23, 79–89.

Walker, S.R. and Rosser, R.M. (1993). *Quality of Life Assessment: Key Issues in the 1990s*. Lancaster: Kluwer Academic Publishers.

Weatherly, H., Drummond, M., Claxton, K., et al. (2009). Methods for assessing the cost-effectiveness of public health interventions: key challenges and recommendations. *Health Policy*, 93(2–3), 85–92.

Weinstein, M. and Stason, W. (1977). Foundations of cost-effectiveness analysis for health and medical practices. *The New England Journal of Medicine*, 296(13), 716–21.

Whitehead, M. (1992). Perspectives in health inequity. *International Journal of Health Services*, 22, 429–45.

Whitehead, M. and Dahlgren, G. (2006). *Levelling Up. Part 1. A Discussion Paper on Concepts and Principles for Tackling Inequities in Health*. Copenhagen: WHO.

Wilkinson, R. and Pickett, K. (2009). *The Spirit Level*. London: Allen Lane.

Williams, B. (1962). *The Idea of Equality, Philosophy, Politics and Society*. Oxford: Blackwell.

Wolff, J. (2007). Equality: the recent history of an idea. *Journal of Moral Philosophy*, 4, 125–36.

World Health Organization (1947). *Constitution of the World Health Organization*. Geneva: WHO.

World Health Organization (1948). *Official Records of the World Health Organization*. Geneva: WHO.

World Health Organization (1958). *The First Ten Years: The World Health Organization*. Geneva: WHO.

Wright, J. (2001). Assessing health needs. In D. Pencheon, C. Guest, D. Melzer, and J.A. Muir Gray (eds.) *Oxford Handbook of Public Health Practice*, pp. 38–47. Oxford: Oxford University Press.

Prevention and control of non-communicable diseases

K. Srinath Reddy

Introduction to prevention and control of non-communicable diseases

In September 2011, the United Nations (UN) held a High-Level Meeting on Non-Communicable Diseases (NCDs), involving heads of state and other senior government functionaries from across the world. The only prior occasion that the UN had convened such a meeting on a health-related issue was in 2001, when a concerted global response to the HIV/AIDS epidemic was framed. It was clear from the political resolution adopted at the 2011 summit that the NCDs were being recognized as a similar grave threat to global health and development, warranting concerted global action for prevention and control (UN General Assembly 2011).

The transition between 2000 and 2015, in the framing of global development goals, also illustrates how NCDs have finally emerged on the radar screen of global health priorities. Action on NCDs, including tobacco control, did not feature in the Millennium Development Goals of 2000. This was despite the fact that NCDs had already become the leading cause of death globally towards the end of the twentieth century and tobacco had claimed about 100 million lives in that century. However, all of the groups working to draft the post-2015 Sustainable Development Goals (SDGs) have acknowledged the need to incorporate the prevention and control of NCDs within the ambit of any health goal proposed for inclusion among the SDGs (International Institute for Sustainable Development 2013; Leadership Council of the Sustainable Development Solutions Network 2013; UN 2013).

What are non-communicable diseases?

Despite all this attention, most people, many policymakers, and even some health professionals do not know what the term 'NCDs' means and includes. The descriptor emerged initially to indicate diseases which were considered to be non-infectious in origin and spread, at a time when global health was mainly concerned about infectious diseases. For the purpose of the UN high-level meeting, the World Health Organization (WHO) proposed to restrict the term to four major disease groups: cardiovascular diseases (CVDs, which include stroke), diabetes, cancers, and chronic respiratory diseases (such as asthma, emphysema, and chronic bronchitis). These four groups of disorders, though very different in their clinical profile, are linked by four common risk factors: tobacco, unhealthy diet, physical inactivity, and alcohol.

Many find the term 'NCDs' unsatisfactory for several reasons. First, some of the cancers (e.g. cervix, liver, and stomach) and some forms of heart disease (e.g. rheumatic heart disease) are linked to viral or bacterial infections. Second, in the socio-epidemiological understanding of disease causation, disease-causing agents like tobacco, alcohol, and unhealthy foods are marketed aggressively across countries and can be considered 'communicable'. Behaviours too are vulnerable to change under the influence of cultural and commercial messages that are communicated to people. Third, where do mental illness, vision and hearing disorders, haemoglobinopathies like thalassaemia, musculoskeletal and gynaecological disorders, and some renal diseases fit in, if the term is restricted to four groups of diseases?

Other terms which have been used to describe NCDs are 'chronic diseases' and 'lifestyle-related diseases'. These too are unsatisfactory. There is nothing 'chronic' in the clinical picture of acute myocardial infarction (heart attack), stroke (brain attack), or sudden cardiac death, even if the underlying pathology may have had an insidious growth. Labelling NCDs as 'lifestyle-related diseases' places the blame on individuals, without taking into account the social and economic factors that operate at the population level, influencing personal behaviours and often overriding informed choice as the main determinant.

Would it be better to choose a descriptor that is more directly linked to the common risk factors than to a disparate group of diseases? A term like 'diet, inactivity, tobacco, and alcohol-related disorders' (DITA disorders) will clearly spell out the causes that need to be countered to reduce the NCD burden and may shape the attitude of health professionals, policymakers, and people to emphasize prevention instead of focusing mainly on disease management as at present.

However, it must be recognized that the UN summit has now legitimized the term NCDs in the global health parlance. The nomenclature has finally been registered on the consciousness of national policymakers across the world and, therefore, has come to stay. Global public health must accept the term as indicative of four major disease groups which are partly but not wholly linked by four risk factors and their determinants, and not quibble about which diseases are in or out. Conditions like mental illness will surely need attention and action, as will injuries and disabilities, but the ambit of NCDs is now defined by the criteria set by the WHO and UN.

Global burden of non-communicable diseases

The WHO estimated that NCDs accounted for 36 million deaths in 2008, contributing to 63 per cent of the 57 million deaths from all causes worldwide (WHO 2011a). About 80 per cent of the NCD-related deaths occurred in the low- and middle-income countries (LMICs) which also accounted for 90 per cent of the 9 million NCD-attributable deaths that occurred below the age of 60 years (WHO 2011b). Even when deaths under 70 years of age are considered, 48 per cent of the NCD related deaths in LMICs occurred below that age in 2008, in comparison to 26 per cent in high-income countries (HICs). The Global Burden of Diseases study 2010 (GBD 2010) estimated that mortality due to NCDs increased from 57 per cent of total mortality in 1990 to 65 per cent in 2010, with a continued high burden of deaths in middle age in the LMICs (Lozano et al. 2013).

Comparisons of NCD mortality, across countries or regions, provide varying profiles, depending on which statistical measure is used. When absolute numbers of NCD-attributable deaths are considered, the LMICs account for the largest fraction because of their cumulative population size. The HICs presently have higher proportional mortality rates (NCD deaths as a percentage of all deaths, within countries) but these too are rising in the LMICs. The highest proportional mortality rates due to NCDs are presently seen in Eastern and Central Europe. Due to the large proportion of deaths occurring at a young age, LMICs have higher age-standardized mortality rates for NCDs, when compared to countries like the United States, Australia, or New Zealand. In every region of the world, other than sub-Saharan Africa, NCDs account for a higher proportion of deaths than the combined contribution of communicable diseases, pregnancy-related events, and nutritional deficiency. Even in sub-Saharan Africa, the age-standardized mortality rates of CVDs are higher than those in HICs but that burden is obscured by the overwhelming effect of HIV/AIDS, malaria, and tuberculosis on proportional mortality. Indeed, the highest rate of rise in NCD related mortality over the next two decades is projected for Africa (WHO 2011c).

Among the NCDs, CVDs are the most prominent, accounting for 48 per cent of all NCD-related deaths in 2008. This group features two dominant disorders, coronary heart disease (CHD) and cerebrovascular disease (stroke). In addition, there are several other cardiovascular disorders like rheumatic heart disease, cardiomyopathies, hypertensive heart disease, and peripheral vascular disease. Cancers contributed to 21 per cent of NCD deaths, chronic respiratory diseases to 12 per cent, and diabetes to 3.5 per cent. Since deaths in people with diabetes are often due to CHD or stroke, its contribution to NCD mortality is larger than the directly attributed fraction suggests.

Apart from mortality, disease burdens are also estimated in terms of disability-adjusted life years (DALYs). This is a summated measure of years of life lost due to death from a disease and a measure of 'life years lost' to years of disability accruing from the disease, weighted for the extent of disability. In 2010, NCDs contributed to 54 per cent of total DALYs lost globally due to all health disorders combined. This represents a substantial increase from the 43 per cent of DALY loss attributed to NCDs in 1990. In the two decades between 1990 and 2010, DALY loss from CVD rose by 22.6 per cent, cancer by 27.3 per cent, and diabetes by 69 per cent, while the DALY loss due to chronic respiratory diseases decreased by 2 per cent (Murray et al. 2013).

There are considerable variations across the world in the profile of NCDs. In Africa, China, Japan, South East Asia, and some countries of South America, stroke is the dominant form of CVD. In others like the United States, United Kingdom, Europe, and Australia, CHD is the dominant form of CVD. In others, both forms are co-dominant. In general, the early stages of the CVD epidemic are marked by haemorrhagic stroke and hypertensive heart disease as the major manifestations of high blood pressure. As societies move to high-fat diets and increased rates of smoking, thrombotic CVDs (CHD and thrombotic stroke) become prominent. In cancer too, there is considerable geographic variation in the types of cancers that are most frequent. This is related to variations in patterns of diet, tobacco consumption, alcohol use, and exposure to cancer-causing viruses.

Based on models of demographic and developmental transitions expected to occur over the coming two decades, the WHO estimates that the number of deaths attributable to NCDs would rise to 55 million by 2030, if urgent measures are not taken to contain the threat of these diseases. This will amount to 70 per cent of all global deaths that year. Action would be needed not only on timely diagnosis and treatment of manifest disease but, more importantly, on the prevention and control of risk factors before they result in disease.

NCDs also have an adverse impact on the economy, at national and global levels. This is due to the combined burden of healthcare costs and productivity losses resulting from deaths in working age and disease-related disability that curtails the ability to engage in fully productive work. A study conducted by the World Economic Forum and the Harvard School of Public Health estimated that the world would lose $47 trillion, during 2011–2030, due to NCDs and mental illness (Bloom et al. 2011). About $30 million of this would be due to CVD, cancers, diabetes, and chronic respiratory diseases. NCDs also result in catastrophic health expenditure and can push families into poverty because of unaffordable costs of technology-intensive medical care (Heeley et al. 2009).

Risk factors and determinants

Among the several risk factors associated with NCDs, three categories can be identified: biological, behavioural, and socioeconomic. Of these, the four behavioural risk factors identified by the WHO (unhealthy diet, physical inactivity, tobacco consumption, and harmful use of alcohol) are positioned centrally. They are influenced upstream by socioeconomic determinants like education and income that operate at the individual level, and societal factors like trade policies, urban design and transport, media and cultural influences that operate at the population level. Behaviours in turn have a substantial impact on biological risk factors like blood pressure, body weight, body shape (central obesity), blood lipids, and blood sugar which are the downstream mediators of risk.

While the four behavioural risk factors are indeed the main contributors to NCDs, becoming the critical link between social determinants and biological causes, there are other risk factors too which contribute to NCDs. These vary from viruses causing cancer, to indoor and outdoor air pollution causing respiratory diseases and CVDs. Family history plays a role too, but the focus of a public health strategy must be on modifiable risk factors.

The role that genetic factors play has not been sufficiently well defined to predict risk in many NCDs. Disorders like CHD and maturity-onset diabetes are polygenic and the variability explained by the identified genes so far is low. Study of gene–environmental interactions in NCDs suggests that the environment is the dominant determinant in the development of these conditions (Florez et al. 2006). However, genetic markers are more prominently associated with some cancers and help in risk prediction and targeted therapy. The role of epigenetics, wherein gene expression is altered by environmental exposures such as tobacco, diet, and chemical pollutants, is now coming to the fore. Similarly, the role of early life influences, of fetal and childhood nutrition and growth, is being invoked to explain adult susceptibility to NCDs (Barker et al. 2002). Further research in these areas may help to better identify population groups and individuals at a high risk of one or more of the NCDs.

The GBD 2010 supports this approach by revealing that the four major behavioural risk factors and high blood pressure account for the largest fraction of global deaths and disability (Lim et al. 2012). Global trends reveal that while tobacco consumption is declining in HICs, it is rising in LMICs. Similarly the population mean of systolic blood pressure has declined or stabilized in HICs but has risen and is now the highest in LMICs (Danaei et al. 2011). Overweight and obesity are continuing to rise in prevalence across all regions of the world. Diabetes too is escalating as a global epidemic, with LMICs dominating the league table of countries with the largest numbers of people with diabetes (International Diabetes Federation 2012).

Alongside the global transition, where NCD mortality rates are stabilizing or declining in HICs but rising in LMICs, there is also evidence of a progressive reversal of the social gradient as the epidemics mature. In the early stages of the NCD epidemics, harmful behaviours are more often associated with the higher disposable incomes of the rich, placing them in the high-risk category. However, as the epidemics advance, mediators of risk are mass produced for mass consumption and the ubiquitous presence of tobacco, alcohol, processed foods, labour saving devices, and motorized transport systems writes the prescription for mass epidemics. At a later stage, the affluent and educated sections benefit from their greater access to information, health services, healthy foods, and leisure time exercise to avoid or reduce the risk of NCDs. On the other hand, the poor and less educated sections have inadequate knowledge of NCDs and their risk factors, cannot afford regular purchase and consumption of fruit, vegetables, healthy oils, and fish, which are often costlier than unhealthy processed foods, and usually lead more stressful lives. In such a mature epidemic, the poor will be the most vulnerable victims and experience the highest burden of NCDs (Reddy et al. 2007). Across the world, different stages of this transition are evident in different regions, based on the level of economic and social development.

A comprehensive response

Health services are frequently confronted by the challenge of balancing a broad public health response focusing on the determinants which operate at the population level and a medical response which places emphasis on providing clinical care to individuals with manifest disease or at a high risk of developing it. This challenge is often exacerbated by the limited resources available to the health system, especially in LMICs.

However, the strategic approach is best guided by understanding how 'risk' operates even in individuals, with respect to risk factors like elevated blood pressure or blood cholesterol or smoking. For example, abundant evidence, gathered from both observational epidemiology and clinical trials, enables us to state the following principles of risk for CVD:

1. Risk operates in a continuous manner, and not across arbitrary thresholds. This is true of biological variables like blood pressure, blood cholesterol, blood sugar, body mass index, and even to the number of cigarettes smoked per day.

2. Most adverse events arise in a population in people in the mid-range of a risk factor distribution—while high levels of any risk factor place individuals at higher relative risk, the majority of people in a population have risk factor levels in the mid-range and, therefore, contribute to the largest number of events.

3. When multiple risk factors coexist, the overall risk is additive.

4. In all populations, the majority of the CVD events arise in people with concurrent elevation of many risk factors rather than in individuals with a high level of a single risk factor.

Based on this, we can derive the principles of prevention:

1. Small reductions in risk factor levels, when achieved across the whole population, result in a large reduction of CVD events.

2. Non-drug measures prevent risk across the whole population and reduce it in people who have already acquired a high-risk profile.

3. Drug therapy to reduce risk is most cost-effective in people who are at high risk of adverse events in the next 10 years.

4. Best results are achieved through a combination of population-based prevention and high-risk individual management approaches.

For example, half of all blood pressure-related deaths occur below the clinical threshold of 140/90 mmHg which defines hypertension. Since the risk of CVD rises progressively at levels above 110/70 mmHg in adults, it is inconceivable that a majority of the population should be treated with drugs. Healthy diet, regular physical activity, and avoiding harm from alcohol can not only help individuals to lower blood pressure, but can shift the population distribution of blood pressure to the left, with a lower mean. This will substantially reduce the burden of CHD and stroke in that population. Among those with 'clinical hypertension', the combination of risk factors will determine the overall 'absolute risk' of CVD and define the threshold for intervention with drug therapy. For further discussion, see Chapter 8.1.

While these principles are derived from CVD epidemiology, they are also applicable to other NCDs where behavioural risk factors translate into biological risk. They would hold true for the relationship of body mass index, central obesity, and physical inactivity to diabetes or the relationship of air pollution to chronic respiratory diseases. Similarly, the risk of cancer with tobacco exposure has a continuous relationship. This makes a strong case for population-based strategies to reduce risk exposure across a wide range, rather than focusing only on those at the highest level of exposure.

The fact that many biological risk factors are driven by a clustering of behaviours also provides the rationale for a strategy that focuses on the four behavioural risk factors identified by the WHO. Blood lipids, blood sugar, blood pressure, and obesity are influenced by diet, physical activity, and alcohol. Tobacco interactively amplifies the risk of each of these biological risk factors for NCDs. Action on these risk behaviours, therefore, will provide great benefits to populations as well as individuals by reducing the levels and effects of several biological risk factors.

In relation to the risk factors for NCDs, changing the behaviours of individuals is essential but is difficult and will take a concerted effort over a long time. More research is also required to ascertain the most effective ways in which this could be achieved, especially in the current global context where so much health-related information, and misinformation, is transmitted and shared through the Internet and social media networks, often on a peer-to-peer basis. It is critical, in parallel, to change environmental factors so as to create settings and environments that actively promote healthy behaviours and activities.

A comprehensive and integrated strategy should therefore encompass effective public health interventions to minimize risk factor exposure in the whole population and to reduce the risk of disease-related events in individuals at high risk. As this combination of the population approach and the high-risk approach is synergistically complementary, cost-effective, and sustainable, such an approach provides the strategic basis for early, medium-term, and long-term impact on NCDs.

The response to NCDs, therefore, requires concerted action at the level of policy, health systems, community action, and individual behaviours. Since the determinants of risk are driven by many social forces, including social inequalities that expose vulnerable segments of society to greater risks and reduced access to health promoting programmes, screening, and medical care, a comprehensive policy response is necessary, involving several sectors such as agriculture, food processing, urban design and transport, commerce, education, and communication. Tobacco control, for example, requires higher taxes on all tobacco products, a ban on tobacco advertising, effective health warnings, and smoke-free public and work places. Promotion of healthy diets would need availability of fruit, vegetables, and healthy oils at affordable prices and reduction of salt, sugar, and trans and saturated fats, in processed foods. Promotion of physical activity would require provision of safe pedestrian pathways, protected cycling lanes, community recreational facilities, green spaces, and mass transport systems that encourage walking to and from stations.

Health services must gear up capacity for early detection and treatment of NCDs and risk factors in primary healthcare, so that NCDs and their complications can be prevented and early therapy can be initiated when they do occur. At higher levels of care, more advanced diagnostic tests and treatments must become available at affordable cost.

Community level action, to promote good health and prevent disease, should involve schools, work sites, residential districts, associations of women, and young people. Apart from increasing health literacy, health-promoting environments must be created through smoke-free and exercise-friendly physical spaces, cafeterias serving healthy food, and group activities that reduce stress and engender well-being. Individuals too must learn to exercise healthy choices related to tobacco, diet, physical activity, and alcohol.

The World Health Organization's global action plan

The UN meeting in 2011 identified a target of 25 per cent reduction in mortality due to NCDs, between the ages of 30 and 70 years, to be achieved globally by 2030. The World Health Assembly, in May 2013, approved a global action plan for prevention and control of NCDs, along with a set of voluntary targets and indicators linked to actions which will enable this goal to be achieved (WHO 2013).

This plan lists nine voluntary targets which are connected to 25 indicators (Table 11.2.1). To achieve these targets, WHO recommends the following actions.

Tobacco use

- Implement the Framework Convention on Tobacco Control (FCTC).
- Reduce affordability of tobacco products by increasing tobacco excise taxes.
- Create, by law, completely smoke-free environments in all indoor workplaces, public places, and public transport.
- Warn people of the dangers of tobacco and tobacco smoke through effective health warnings and mass media campaigns.
- Ban all forms of tobacco advertising, promotion, and sponsorship.

Harmful alcohol use

- Excise tax increases on alcoholic beverages.
- Comprehensive restrictions and bans on alcohol advertising and promotion.
- Restrictions on the availability of retailed alcohol.
- Implement the WHO global strategy to reduce harmful use of alcohol.

Unhealthy diet and physical inactivity

- Salt reduction through mass media campaigns/reduced salt content in processed foods.
- Replacement of trans fats with polyunsaturated fats.
- Public awareness programme about diet and physical activity.

Health system

- Integrate highly cost-effective NCD interventions into the basic primary healthcare package to advance the universal health coverage (UHC) agenda.
- Explore viable health financing mechanisms and innovative financing approaches, like tobacco and alcohol taxation, to generate resources to expand health coverage.
- Improve availability of affordable basic technologies and essential medicines, including generics, required to treat major NCDs in both public and private facilities.

Table 11.2.1 Voluntary global targets from the Action Plan for the Prevention and Control of Non-communicable Diseases 2013–2020

Mortality and morbidity	
1.	Premature mortality from non-communicable disease	A 25% relative reduction in risk of premature mortality from cardiovascular diseases, cancer, diabetes, or chronic respiratory diseases
Behavioural risk factors	
2.	Harmful use of alcohol	At least 10% relative reduction in the harmful use of alcohol, as appropriate, within the national context
3.	Physical inactivity	A 10% relative reduction in prevalence of insufficient physical inactivity
4.	Salt/sodium intake	A 30% relative reduction in mean population intake of salt/sodium
5.	Tobacco use	A 30% relative reduction in prevalence of current tobacco use in people aged 15+ years
Biological risk factors	
6.	Raised blood pressure	A 25% relative reduction in the prevalence of raised blood pressure or contain the prevalence of raised blood pressure, according to national circumstances
7.	Diabetes and obesity	Halt the rise in diabetes and obesity
National system response	
8.	Drug therapy to prevent heart attacks and strokes	At least 50% of eligible people receive drug therapy and counselling (including glycaemic control) to prevent heart attacks and strokes
9.	Essential non-communicable disease medicines and basic technologies to treat major non-communicable diseases	An 80% availability of the affordable basic technologies and essential medicines, including generics, required to treat major non-communicable diseases in both public and private facilities

Adapted with permission from World Health Organization, *Sixty Sixth World Health Assembly; Follow-up to the Political Declaration of the High-level Meeting of the General Assembly on the Prevention and Control of Non-communicable Diseases*, Copyright © World Health Organization 2013, available from http://apps.who.int/gb/ebwha/pdf_files/WHA66/A66_R10-en.pdf.

◆ Scale-up early detection and coverage starting with very cost-effective, high-impact interventions.

◆ Strengthen and reorient health systems to address NCDs and risk factors through people-centred primary healthcare and UHC.

Cardiovascular disease and diabetes

◆ Multidrug therapy (including glycaemic control for diabetes mellitus and control of hypertension through a total risk management approach) to individuals who have had a heart attack or stroke, and to people with high risk (≥ 30 per cent) of a fatal and non-fatal cardiovascular event in the next 10 years.

◆ Acetylsalicylic acid for acute myocardial infarction.

◆ Multidrug therapy (including glycaemic control for diabetes mellitus and control of hypertension through total risk approach) to individuals who have had a heart attack or stroke, and to people with moderate risk (≥ 20 per cent) of a fatal and non-fatal cardiovascular event in the next 10 years.

◆ Acetylsalicylic acid, atenolol, and thrombolytic therapy (e.g. streptokinase) for acute myocardial infarction.

◆ Treat congestive cardiac failure with an angiotensin-converting enzyme inhibitor, beta-blocker, and diuretic.

◆ Cardiac rehabilitation post myocardial infarction.

◆ Secondary prevention of rheumatic fever and rheumatic heart disease.

◆ Anticoagulation for medium- and high-risk non-valvular atrial fibrillation and for mitral stenosis and atrial fibrillation.

◆ Low-dose acetylsalicylic acid for ischaemic stroke.

◆ Care of acute stroke and rehabilitation in stroke units.

◆ Interventions for foot care; educational programmes, access to appropriate footwear; and multidisciplinary clinics.

Diabetes

◆ Lifestyle interventions for preventing type 2 diabetes.

◆ Influenza vaccination.

◆ Preconception care among women of reproductive age (includes patient education and intensive glucose management for gestational diabetes).

◆ The early detection of diabetic retinopathy by regular dilated eye examination followed by appropriate laser photocoagulation therapy to prevent blindness.

◆ Enalapril to prevent progression of renal disease.

Cancer

◆ Prevention of liver cancer through hepatitis B immunization.

◆ Prevention of cervical cancer through screening (visual inspection with acetic acid) linked with timely treatment of pre-cancerous lesions.

◆ Vaccination against human papillomavirus, as appropriate if cost-effective and affordable, according to national programmes and policies.

◆ Population-based cervical cancer screening linked with timely treatment.

◆ Population-based breast cancer mammography screening (50–70 years) linked with timely treatment.

◆ Population-based colorectal cancer screening at ages over 50 years, linked with timely treatment.

◆ Oral cancer screening in high-risk groups (e.g. tobacco users) linked with timely treatment.

◆ Palliative care; using cost-effective treatment modalities including opioid analgesics for pain relief.

Chronic respiratory disease

◆ Access to improved stoves and cleaner fuels to reduce indoor air pollution.

◆ Cost-effective interventions to prevent occupational lung diseases, that is, exposure to silica, asbestos.

◆ Treatment of asthma based on WHO guidelines.

◆ Influenza vaccination for patients with chronic obstructive pulmonary disease.

Research and surveillance

◆ Develop and implement a prioritized national research agenda for NCDs.

◆ Strengthen research capacity through cooperation with research institutes.

◆ Implement other policy options to promote and support national capacity for high-quality research and development.

◆ Develop national targets and indicators based on global monitoring framework.

◆ Establish/strengthen a comprehensive NCD surveillance system, including reliable registration of deaths by cause, cancer registration, periodic data collection on risk factors, and monitoring national response.

◆ Integrate NCD surveillance/monitoring into national health information systems.

◆ Monitor trends and determinants of NCDs and evaluate progress in their prevention and control.

These recommendations for national and global actions are based on evidence of high impact on population-attributable risk and cost-effectiveness of the interventions (Beaglehole et al. 2011; WHO 2011d; Bonita et al. 2013). They combine policy and community level interventions which impact on behaviours across the population and health service interventions which enable risk reduction in individuals at high risk of NCD-related death or disability. While many of these are steered by the health system, they will require multi-sectoral actions to influence the determinants of NCDs. Together, they provide a comprehensive framework for prevention and control of NCDs.

Health system challenges

Implementation of the various measures proposed in the WHO's Global NCD Action Plan (as discussed earlier) will pose several challenges to national health systems, especially those in the LMICs. These include: health financing; human resources for health; access to essential drugs and technologies and information systems, apart from infrastructure and governance.

Even as escalating costs of healthcare are straining health systems across the world, there is the imminent danger of the expanding NCD epidemics loading unaffordable costs on health budgets. Most LMICs have to contend with competing priorities, with continued commitment to funding programmes for maternal and child health, control of infectious diseases, and nutrition along with fresh commitments to programmes for NCD prevention and control. It should be noted that some key policy measures such as for the control of tobacco and alcohol use will not demand many resources.

Indeed, higher taxes on tobacco and alcohol will yield additional revenues which can be allocated to NCD-related health programmes. Each measure like downward regulation of salt, sugar, and saturated and trans fats in processed foods would not incur expenditure for the government.

However, programmes for clinical care will entail substantial additional costs to the health budget. This can be contained by integrating NCD prevention into existing health programmes (like tobacco control, maternal and child health, and HIV/AIDS programmes) and investing more in primary care than in tertiary care.

As many countries move towards implementation of UHC, NCD-related services should be included so that essential healthcare is provided in an accessible, affordable, and equitable manner to all who need it. The growing global momentum for UHC coincides with the increasing recognition of NCDs as a major health priority, indicative of a convergence that accommodates NCDs in UHC (Frenk and de Ferranti 2012).

Most LMICs have severe shortages in their healthcare workforce, at various levels (specialist doctors, primary physicians, nurses, allied health professionals, and community health workers). Even as capacity is progressively scaled up at each of these levels, 'task shifting' and 'task sharing' can enhance the outreach and effectiveness of NCD programme delivery. Non-physician healthcare providers like nurses and community health workers have been shown to detect and manage diabetes, hypertension, and asthma efficiently with good health outcomes (Coleman et al. 1998; Abegunde et al. 2007; Farzadfar et al. 2012). Health workers in different health programmes can be multiskilled to perform some functions related to NCD prevention and control, in addition to their primary functions. Specific programmes for NCD prevention and control would also need a multilayered work force with competencies attuned to the programme. Training programmes need to be developed for this purpose. Public health education too must be strengthened to increase public health expertise for policy and programme design, delivery, and evaluation.

Provision of essential drugs and access to needed technologies are also priorities which the health system must address. Since NCDs usually require long-term and often lifelong care for chronic conditions, the availability and affordability of drugs becomes a major concern to affected individuals and families. This is true of drugs for the treatment of hypertension and diabetes, where the cost of drugs in several LMICs amounts to a large fraction of the average monthly wage (Van Mourik et al. 2010). With respect to cancer, treatment for curable cancers is often out of reach, because of the prohibitive cost of drugs. In several countries, palliative pain-relief therapy is unavailable to cancer patients. Even inhalers for asthma therapy are not universally available.

There is a great need for increasing the production and availability of generic drugs. Countries with high manufacturing capacity for such drugs (such as China, India, and Brazil) must supply not only their domestic markets but also other needy markets. Pooled procurement, at national and global levels, will help keep costs under control. The WHO is examining mechanisms for such global procurement and distribution of essential NCD-related drugs. At the national level, it must ensure that frequently needed NCD drugs of proven efficacy should be entered into the Essential Drug List (EDL). Measures to ensure affordability and access, including price control and public provision of life-saving cancer drugs, should also be considered by governments.

Access to technologies is also vital for NCD prevention and control. While high-cost technologies should be judiciously used, based on rational guidelines, low-cost technologies can greatly advance primary care. Point-of-care diagnostics need to be promoted, to enable early detection of risk factors. Use of information technology and mobile phones offer a potentially powerful health system innovation that can transform primary care for NCDs (Krishna et al. 2009). They can also help in strengthening surveillance systems, enabling programme managers to acquire real-time data from sentinel sites across the country and provide a rapid response.

Health services too must be reconfigured to provide chronic care and emergency care for NCDs. Presently, the health systems of most LMICs are designed to deliver acute episodic care, rather than continuous care involving periodic reviews and monitoring. Integration of primary with secondary and tertiary services, with clearly defined and dependable systems for bi-directional referral and follow-up, is also a requirement of NCD-related care. Emergency care services too need to be geared up, to save lives through early intervention in cases of acute coronary or cerebrovascular events.

Conclusion

Prevention and control of NCDs will be the dominant health challenge of the twenty-first century. While it would be unrealistic to expect that all NCDs can be prevented, a large fraction of them can be prevented from occurring or affecting people in young and middle ages. Prevention of premature mortality and reduction of NCD-related morbidity and disability are goals that every national health system must pursue and all global partnerships must support. That these are achievable has been demonstrated in many HICs. Success does not derive only from costly clinical care. Prevention, through policies which create conducive environments in which people can make and maintain healthy living choices without formidable barriers, has contributed to most of the decline in NCDs that has been observed in HICs. Tobacco control is a prime example of how NCD mortality rates decline in response to policy and community-led initiatives (Unal et al. 2004). Countries like Finland and Poland have demonstrated how policies and community-based programmes influencing dietary choices can put brakes on the CVD epidemic (Zatonski and Willett 2005; Puska 2013).

The decline of cervical cancer, with organized screening and treatment (Mathew and George 2009), and the decline in lung cancer mortality, due to falling smoking rates in HICs, offer lessons for LMICs. It has also been observed that risk factor reduction explains 44–76 per cent of declining mortality in the United States, with improvements in clinical care contributing to the rest (Ford and Capewell 2011). LMICs can learn from the global experience of countries which have already experienced the NCD epidemics in full tide. At the same time, they will have to prioritize prevention and primary care over high-cost tertiary and terminal care, if their health systems are to successfully cope with the demands of multiple health burdens in a resource-constrained situation. Fortunately, knowledge related to effective prevention and lifesaving clinical care is available. It is now time to translate that abundant knowledge into effective action, if the ambitious but achievable goal of '25 by 25' is to be realized.

References

Abegunde, D.O., Shengelia, B., Luyten, A., et al. (2007). Can non-physician health-care workers assess and manage cardiovascular risk in primary care? *Bulletin of the World Health Organization*, 85(6), 432–40.

Barker, D.J.P., Eriksson, J.G., Forsén, T., and Osmond, C. (2002). Fetal origins of adult disease: strength of effects and biological basis. *International Journal of Epidemiology*, 31(6), 1235–9.

Beaglehole, R., Bonita, R., Horton, R., et al. (2011). Priority actions for the non-communicable disease crisis. *The Lancet*, 377(9775), 1438–47.

Bloom, D.E., Cafiero, E.T., Jané-Llopis, E., et al. (2011). *The Global Economic Burden of Non-Communicable Diseases*. Geneva: World Economic Forum. Available at: http://www.weforum.org/reports/global-economic-burden-non-communicable-diseases.

Bonita, R., Magnusson, R., Bovet, P., et al. (2013). Country actions to meet UN commitments on non-communicable diseases: a stepwise approach. *The Lancet*, 381(9866), 575–84.

Coleman, R., Gill, G., and Wilkinson, D. (1998). Noncommunicable disease management in resource-poor settings: a primary care model from rural South Africa. *Bulletin of the World Health Organization*, 76(6), 633–40.

Danaei, G., Finucane, M.M., Lin, J.K., et al. (2011).National, regional, and global trends in systolic blood pressure since 1980: systematic analysis of health examination surveys and epidemiological studies with 786 country-years and 5.4 million participants. *The Lancet*, 377, 568–77.

Farzadfar, F., Murray, C.J.L., Gakidou, E., et al. (2012). Effectiveness of diabetes and hypertension management by rural primary health-care workers (Behvarz workers) in Iran: a nationally representative observational study. *The Lancet*, 379(9810), 47–54.

Florez, J.C., Jablonski, K.A., Bayley, N., et al. (2006). TCF7L2 polymorphisms and progression to diabetes in the Diabetes Prevention Program. *The New England Journal of Medicine*, 355(3), 241–50.

Ford, E.S. and Capewell, S. (2011). Proportion of the decline in cardiovascular mortality disease due to prevention versus treatment: public health versus clinical care. *Annual Review of Public Health*, 32, 5–22.

Frenk, J. and de Ferranti, D. (2012). Universal health coverage: good health, good economics. *The Lancet*, 380(9845), 862–4.

Heeley, E., Anderson, C.S., Huang, Y., et al. (2009). Role of health insurance in averting economic hardship in families after acute stroke in China. *Stroke*, 40(6), 2149–56.

International Diabetes Federation (2012). *Global Diabetes Plan: 2011–2021*. Brussels: International Diabetes Federation. Available at: https://docs.google.com/viewer?url=http%3A%2F%2Fwww.idf.org%2Fsites%2Fdefault%2Ffiles%2FGlobal_Diabetes_Plan_Final.pdf.

International Institute for Sustainable Development (2013). *Post-2015 Consultation on Health Culminates in High-level Dialogue*. [Online] Available at: http://post2015.iisd.org/news/post-2015-consultation-on-health-culminates-in-high-level-dialogue/.

Krishna, S., Boren, S.A., and Balas, E.A. (2009). Healthcare via cell phones: a systematic review. *Telemedicine and e-Health*, 15(3), 231–40.

Leadership Council of the Sustainable Development Solutions Network (2013). *An Action Agenda for Sustainable Development: Report for the UN Secretary General*. New York: Sustainable Development Solutions Network. Available at: http://unsdsn.org/resources/publications/an-action-agenda-for-sustainable-development/.

Lim, S.S., Vos, T., Flaxman, A.D., et al. (2012). A comparative risk assessment of burden of disease and injury attributable to 67 risk factors and risk factor clusters in 21 regions, 1990–2010: a systematic analysis for the Global Burden of Disease Study 2010. *The Lancet*, 380(9859), 2224–60.

Lozano, R., Naghavi, M., Foreman, K., et al. (2013). Global and regional mortality from 235 causes of death for 20 age groups in 1990 and 2010: a systematic analysis for the Global Burden of Disease Study 2010. *The Lancet*, 380(9859), 2095–128.

Mathew, A. and George, P.S. (2009). Trends in incidence and mortality rates of squamous cell carcinoma and adenocarcinoma of cervix—worldwide. *Asian Pacific Journal of Cancer Prevention*, 10(4), 645–50.

Murray, C.J., Vos, T., Lozano, R., et al. (2013). Disability-adjusted life years (DALYs) for 291 diseases and injuries in 21 regions, 1990–2010: a systematic analysis for the Global Burden of Disease Study 2010. *The Lancet*, 380(9859), 2197–223.

Puska, P. (2013). Community-based cardiovascular prevention programs: theory and practice. *Archives of Iranian Medicine*, 16(1), 2–3.

Reddy, K.S., Prabhakaran, D., Jeemon, P., et al. (2007). Educational status and cardiovascular risk profile in Indians. *Proceedings of the National Academy of Sciences of the United States of America*, 104, 16263–8.

Unal, B., Critchley, J.A., and Capewell, S. (2004). Explaining the decline in coronary heart disease mortality in England and Wales between 1981 and 2000. *Circulation*, 109(9), 1101–7.

UN General Assembly (2011). *Political Declaration of the High-Level Meeting of the General Assembly on the Prevention and Control of Non-communicable Diseases*. New York: United Nations.

United Nations (2013). *A New Global Partnership: Eradicate Poverty and Transform Economies Through Sustainable Development*. New York: United Nations Publications. Available at: http://www.un.org/sg/management/pdf/HLP_P2015_Report.pdf.

Van Mourik, M.S.M., Cameron, A., Ewen, M., and Laing, R.O. (2010). Availability, price and affordability of cardiovascular medicines: a comparison across 36 countries using WHO/HAI data. *BMC Cardiovascular Disorders*, 10, 25.

World Health Organization (2011a). *Causes of Death 2008. Summary Tables*. [Online]. Available at: http://www.who.int/evidence/bod.

World Health Organization (2011b). *Noncommunicable Diseases Country Profile 2011*. Geneva: WHO. Available at: http://whqlibdoc.who.int/publications/2011/9789241502283_eng.pdf.

World Health Organization (2011c). *Global Status Report on Non-Communicable Diseases 2010*. Geneva: WHO.

World Health Organization (2011d). *From Burden to 'Best Buys': Reducing the Economic Impact of Non-Communicable Diseases in Low- and Middle-Income Countries. Health Promotion*. [Online] Available at: http://ideas.repec.org/p/gdm/wpaper/7511.html.

World Health Organization (2013). *Sixty Sixth World Health Assembly; Follow-up to the Political Declaration of the High-level Meeting of the General Assembly on the Prevention and Control of Non-communicable Diseases*. Geneva: WHO. Available at: http://apps.who.int/gb/ebwha/pdf_files/WHA66/A66_R10-en.pdf.

Zatonski, W.A. and Willett, W. (2005). Changes in dietary fat and declining coronary heart disease in Poland: population based study. *BMJ*, 331, 187–8.

Principles of infectious disease control

Robert J. Kim-Farley

Principles of infectious disease control: overview

Infectious diseases remain a leading cause of morbidity, disability, and mortality worldwide. Lower respiratory infections are the third leading causes of death worldwide (World Health Organization (WHO) 2008). Their control is a constant challenge that faces health workers and public health officials in both industrialized and developing countries. Only one infectious disease, smallpox, was eradicated and stands as a landmark in the history of the control of infectious diseases. The international community is now well down the path towards eradication of poliomyelitis and dracunculiasis (Guinea worm infection). Other infectious diseases, like malaria and tuberculosis, foiled eradication attempts or control efforts and are re-emerging as increasing threats in many countries, including both developing and developed countries. Some infectious diseases, such as tetanus, will always be a threat if control measures are not maintained. Newer infectious diseases, like AIDS, demonstrate the truth of McNeill's statement that infectious disease will remain 'one of the fundamental parameters and determinants of human history'. The history of infectious diseases is an exciting story in itself and readers interested in the subject are referred to McNeill (1976) or the comprehensive work on the history of human diseases (Kiple 1993).

This chapter provides a global and comprehensive view of infectious disease control through examination of the magnitude of disease burden, the chain of infection (agent, transmission, and host) of infectious diseases, the varied approaches to their prevention and control, and the factors conducive to their eradication as well as emergence and re-emergence. Although this chapter provides many examples of infectious diseases that illustrate modes of transmission and approaches to infectious disease control, this chapter does not attempt to be comprehensive in listing all infectious diseases. Detailed recommendations on control measures for any specific disease are outlined periodically in the updated reports of the American Public Health Association, *Control of Communicable Diseases Manual* (Heymann 2010), the comprehensive two-volume work *Mandell, Douglas and Bennett's Principles and Practice of Infectious Diseases* (Mandell et al. 2009), and the textbook *Infectious Diseases* (Gorbach et al. 2004). For readers specifically interested in paediatric infectious diseases there is the comprehensive two-volume *Feigin and Cherry's Textbook of Pediatric Infectious Diseases* (Feigin et al. 2009); for

infectious diseases in emergency medicine settings there is the textbook *Infectious Diseases: Emergency Department Diagnosis & Management* (Red and White Emergency Medicine Series) (Slaven et al. 2006); and for tropical infectious diseases there is *Tropical Infectious Diseases: Principles, Pathogens, and Practice* (Guerrant et al. 2011). A comprehensive treatment of the worldwide distribution of infectious diseases is provided in *Atlas of Human Infectious Diseases* (Wertheim et al. 2012). The Centers for Disease Control and Prevention (CDC) publishes up-to-date disease surveillance information for the United States and recommendations for control measures in the *Morbidity and Mortality Weekly Reports* and provides annual summaries of notifiable infectious diseases in the *Summary of Notifiable Diseases, United States* (CDC 2011). Many other countries have similar types of publications. The WHO publishes worldwide surveillance information and recommendations for control measures in the *Weekly Epidemiological Record*. A more detailed background on infectious agents as determinants of health and disease is provided in Chapters 8.11–8.15.

Definitions of infectious diseases and their control

Infection occurs when an infectious agent enters a body and develops or multiplies. *Infectious agents* are organisms capable of producing inapparent infection or clinically manifest disease and include bacteria, rickettsia, chlamydiae, fungi, parasites, viruses, and prions. An *infectious disease*, or communicable disease, is an infection that results in clinically manifest disease. Infectious disease may also be due to the toxic product of an infectious agent, such as the toxin produced by *Clostridium botulinum* causing classical botulism. As this is a textbook of public health, the infectious diseases considered are those that manifest in human hosts and are a result of the interaction of people, animals, and their environment. Infectious diseases may be due to infectious agents exclusively found in human hosts such as rubella virus, in the environment such as *Legionella pneumophila*, or primarily in animals such as *Brucella abortus*.

Control of infectious diseases refers to the actions and programmes directed towards reducing disease incidence (new infections), reducing disease prevalence (infections in the community at any given point in time), or completely eradicating the disease. Control aimed at reducing the incidence of infectious disease or their risk factors can be considered as *primary prevention* of infectious disease. Primary prevention protects health through individual and community-wide measures, including such actions as maintaining good nutritional status, keeping physically fit, immunizing against infectious diseases, providing safe water, and ensuring the proper disposal of faeces.

Control aimed at reducing the prevalence by shortening the duration of infectious disease can be considered as *secondary prevention* of infectious disease. Secondary prevention corrects departures from good health through individual and community-wide measures, including such actions as screening that result in early detection of disease, prompt antibiotic treatment, and ensuring adequate nutrition. It should be noted that such control efforts in secondary prevention in a group of infected individuals may also result in primary prevention in uninfected people. For example, prompt and specific drug therapy for tuberculosis patients resulting in sputum conversion to culture-negative status renders them no longer a source of infection to others and treatment of HIV-positive pregnant women reduces transmission of HIV to their newborns.

Control aimed at reducing or even eliminating long-term impairments of infectious disease can be considered as *tertiary prevention* of infectious disease. Tertiary prevention reduces or eliminates disabilities, minimizes suffering, and promotes adjustment to permanent disabilities through such actions as providing orthopaedic appliances and its associated rehabilitation for victims of poliomyelitis, counselling and vocational training, and prevention of opportunistic infections. For example, the prevention of opportunistic infections in HIV infection can be considered as tertiary prevention (Osterholm and Hedberg 2005).

Global burden of infectious diseases

A WHO analysis of the global burden of disease estimates that infectious diseases caused 12.3 million deaths, accounting for 21 per cent of total global mortality of 56.8 million deaths in 2008 (WHO 2008). Five diseases—lower respiratory infections, AIDS, diarrhoeal diseases, tuberculosis, and malaria—account for some 81 per cent of the total infectious disease burden. Most infectious disease (some 97 per cent) deaths occur in the economically developing group of countries where approximately a quarter of deaths are due to an infectious cause (WHO 2008). However, infectious diseases are also of importance in more developed countries. In the United States, for example, influenza still ranks as an important cause of death.

The current magnitude of morbidity and mortality due to infectious diseases worldwide is highlighted by the WHO as follows (WHO 2012a):

- *Acute lower respiratory infections*, including pneumonia and influenza, cause some 447 million episodes of illness each year and result in 3.5 million deaths annually. These infections are the highest cause of infant and child mortality in developing countries.

- *HIV* newly infects about 2.7 million people each year and causes an estimated 1.8 million AIDS-related deaths annually, down from a peak of 2.2 million that occurred in the mid 2000s. There are now about 34 million people living with HIV as of the end of 2011 (Joint United Nations Programme on HIV/AIDS 2011).

- *Diarrhoeal diseases* are also a major cause of morbidity and mortality in infants and children in developing countries. Each year there are some 4.6 billion episodes with 2.5 million deaths

due to diarrhoeal disease, of which the vast majority are among children under 5 years of age.

- *Tuberculosis,* caused by *Mycobacterium tuberculosis,* infects about one-third of the world's population. It is estimated that there are approximately 8.8 million people who develop clinical disease and 1.1 million who die of tuberculosis each year.

- *Malaria* is estimated to cause some 241 million cases of acute illness. An estimated 827,000 deaths per year worldwide are attributable to malaria, mainly in children under the age of 5 years.

- *Influenza* epidemics, caused by influenza A and B viruses, are estimated to kill from 500,000 to 1 million people worldwide each year. Influenza pandemics, of which there were 3 in the last century, have killed as many as 40–50 million people (as occurred during the 1918–1919 'Spanish flu' pandemic) and, as with the current concerns regarding avian influenza (H5N1), continue to threaten to re-emerge as a major public health emergency.

Chain of infection: agent, transmission, and host

The chain of infection is the relationship between an infectious agent, its routes of transmission, and a susceptible host. The prevention and control of infectious diseases depend upon the interaction of these three factors that may result in the human host clinically manifesting disease.

Agent

The infectious agent is the first link in the chain of infection and is any microorganism whose presence or excessive presence is essential for the occurrence of an infectious disease. Examples of infectious agents include the following:

- *Bacteria:* for example, spirochetes and curved bacteria such as *Borrelia burgdorferi* causing Lyme disease; Gram-negative rods such as *Yersinia pestis* causing plague; Gram-positive cocci such as *Streptococcus pyogenes*, group A causing erysipelas; and Gram-positive rods such as *Mycobacterium tuberculosis* causing tuberculosis.

- *Rickettsiae:* for example, *Rickettsia rickettsii* causing Rocky Mountain spotted fever, and *Rickettsia prowazekii* causing epidemic louse-borne typhus fever.

- *Chlamydiae:* for example, *Chlamydia psittaci* causing psittacosis (ornithosis), and *Chlamydia trachomatis* causing trachoma and genital infections.

- *Fungi*: for example, *Trichophyton schoenleinii* and *Microsporum canis* causing tinea capitis (ringworm of the scalp), and *Trichophyton rubrum, Trichophyton mentagrophytes*, and *Epidermophyton floccosum* causing tinea pedis (ringworm of the foot, or athlete's foot).

- *Parasites:* for example, helminths such as *Trichinella spiralis* causing trichinosis, filaria such as *Brugia malayi* causing filariasis (which may lead to the symptom of elephantiasis), nematodes such as *Enterobius vermicularis* causing enterobiasis (pinworm disease), trematodes such as *Clonorchis sinensis* causing clonorchiasis (oriental liver fluke disease), cestodes such as *Taenia solium* causing taeniasis (beef tapeworm disease), and protozoa such as *Trypanosoma cruzi* causing American trypanosomiasis (Chagas' disease).

- *Viruses*: for example, Paramyxoviridae such as measles virus which causes measles, Togaviridae such as rubella virus which causes rubella, Picornaviridae such as the hepatovirus which causes hepatitis A, and arthropod-borne viruses (arboviruses) such as dengue viruses which cause dengue fever.

- *Prions*: small proteinaceous infectious particles which cause such diseases as kuru, Creutzfeldt–Jakob disease (and its variant associated with exposure of humans to the bovine spongiform encephalopathy, or 'mad cow', agent), and the Gerstmann–Straussler–Scheinker syndrome.

There is increasing evidence that some infectious agents, often with cofactors, are associated with human tumours. Examples include: *Schistosoma haematobium* with bladder cancer, *Schistosoma japonicum* with colorectal cancer, *Clonorchis sinensis* with cholangiocarcinoma, hepatitis B and C viruses with hepatocellular carcinoma, *Helicobacter pylori* with gastric cancer, and human papillomaviruses with cervical cancer. Cancers attributed by the International Agency for Research on Cancer (IARC) to infectious agents are considered to account for some 22 per cent of cancer deaths in the developing world and 6 per cent in industrialized countries (WHO 2003).

Agents can be described by their ability to infect (infectivity), be transmitted (infectiousness), and cause disease (pathogenicity) as well as their ability to cause serious disease (virulence). The *infectivity* of an infectious agent is the extent to which the agent can enter, survive, and multiply in a host and is measured by the ratio of the number of people who become infected to the total number exposed to the agent. Rhinoviruses that can cause the common cold are examples of infectious agents with high infectivity.

The *infectiousness*, or transmissibility, of an infectious agent is the extent to which the agent can be transmitted from one host to another. It is measured by the basic reproduction number (known as R_0) which is determined by the number of secondary infections in a susceptible population that result from a primary infection. Epidemic-prone diseases such as measles and pertussis caused by measles virus and *Bordatella pertussis* bacteria, respectively, are examples of diseases due to highly infectious agents with an R_0 of 10 or greater.

The *pathogenicity* of an infectious agent is the extent to which clinically manifest disease is produced in an infected population and is measured by the ratio of the number of people developing clinical illness to the total number infected. Examples of highly pathogenic infectious agents are the measles virus and the human (α) herpesvirus 3 (varicella-zoster) causing measles and chickenpox, respectively, in which most infected susceptible people will manifest disease.

The *virulence* of an infectious agent is the extent to which severe disease is produced in a population with clinically manifest disease. It is the ratio of the number of people with severe and fatal disease to the total number of people with disease. An example of a highly virulent infectious agent is HIV whereby nearly all untreated people with AIDS will die.

Characteristics of infectious agents that affect pathogenicity include their ability to invade tissues (invasiveness), produce toxins (intoxication), cause damaging hypersensitivity (allergic) reactions, undergo antigenic variation, and develop antibiotic resistance. An example of an infectious agent with high *invasiveness* is the *Shigella* organism which can invade the submucosal tissue of the intestine and cause clinically manifest shigellosis (bacillary dysentery). An example of an infectious agent that has a high degree of ability to *produce toxins* is the *Clostridium botulinum* organism which can elaborate toxins in inadequately prepared food and cause classical botulism. An example of an infectious agent that is highly *allergenic* is the *Mycobacterium tuberculosis* organism which can cause tuberculosis. An example of an infectious agent that has a high degree of *antigenic variation* is the type A influenza virus which frequently experiences minor antigenic changes—antigenic 'drift'. Influenza A viruses, on an irregular basis, may also undergo a major antigenic change creating an entirely new subtype—antigenic 'shift'. Antigenic shifts that have the characteristic of high transmissibility between people may result in an influenza pandemic when large numbers of individuals are exposed to the new subtype for which they have no prior immunity. An example of an infectious agent that can develop *antibiotic resistance* that challenges control efforts is *Neisseria gonorrhoeae* that has both chromosomally mediated and resistance transfer plasmid-mediated genetic factors for antibiotic resistance.

The *infective dose* of an infectious agent is the number of organisms needed to cause an infection. The infective dose may vary depending upon the route of transmission and host susceptibility. An example of an infectious agent that needs only a very low infective dose (as few as ten organisms) is *Escherichia coli* O157:H7 which causes enterohaemorrhagic diarrhoea. An example of an infectious agent that needs a relatively higher infective dose is *Vibrio cholerae* which requires around 100 million bacteria to be ingested to cause cholera disease in a healthy adult.

Control measures for infectious diseases directed at inactivating the agent are designed according to the type of agent and its reservoirs and sources. For example, an agent like *Vibrio cholerae* can be inactivated through adequate chlorination of the water supply. This is a chemical method for provision of safe water to control cholera. An agent like hepatitis B virus can be inactivated through adequate autoclaving of injection and surgical equipment. This is a sterilization method to control hepatitis B. Details of these and other methods of control directed at the agent are provided in the sections in this chapter on control measures applied to the agent and the environment.

Routes of transmission

Control efforts are often designed to break the routes of transmission, the mechanisms by which infectious agents are spread from reservoirs or sources to human hosts. A *reservoir* of an infectious agent is any person, other living organism, or inanimate material in which the infectious agent normally lives and grows. The *source* of infection for a host is the person, other living organism or inanimate material from which the infectious agent came. *Horizontal transmission* refers to transmission between individuals whereas *vertical transmission* refers to the specific situation of transmission between parent to offspring (e.g. transplacentally *in utero*, during passage through the birth canal, or through breast milk). The routes of transmission have been summarized in the *Control of Communicable Diseases Manual* (Heymann 2010) as follows:

Direct transmission

Direct and essentially immediate transfer of infectious agents to a receptive portal of entry through which human or animal infection may take place. This may be by direct contact such as touching, biting, kissing or sexual intercourse, or through direct projections (droplet spread) of droplet spray onto the conjunctiva or onto the mucous membranes of the eye, nose or mouth during sneezing, coughing, spitting, singing or talking (risk of transmission in this manner is usually limited to a distance of about 1 meter or less from the source of infection). Direct transmission may also occur through direct exposure of susceptible tissue to an agent in soil, through the bite of a rabid animal, or trans-placentally. (Heymann 2010)

Indirect transmission

Vehicle-borne

Contaminated inanimate materials or objects (fomites) such as toys, handkerchiefs, soiled clothes, bedding, cooking or eating utensils, surgical instruments or dressings; water, food, milk, and biological products including blood, serum, plasma, tissues or organs; or any substance serving as an intermediate means by which an infectious agent is transported and introduced into a susceptible host though a suitable portal of entry. The agent may or may not have multiplied or developed in or on the vehicle before being transmitted. (Heymann 2010)

Vector-borne

Mechanical: includes simple mechanical carriage by a crawling or flying insect through soiling of its feet or proboscis, or by passage of organisms through its gastrointestinal tract. This does not require multiplication or development of the organism.

Biological: propagation (multiplication), cyclic development, or a combination of these (cyclopropagative) is required before the arthropod can transmit the infective form of the agent to humans. An incubation period (extrinsic) is required following infection before the arthropod becomes infective. The infectious agent may be passed vertically to succeeding generations (*transovarian transmission*); *trans-stadial transmission* indicates its passage from one stage of the life cycle to another, as from nymph to adult. Transmission may be by injection of salivary gland fluid during biting, or by regurgitation or deposition on the skin of feces or other material capable of penetrating through the bite wound or through an area of trauma, often created by scratching or rubbing. This transmission is by an infected nonvertebrate host and not simple mechanical carriage by a vector as a vehicle. An arthropod in either role is termed a vector. (Heymann 2010)

Airborne transmission

The dissemination of microbial aerosols to a suitable portal of entry, usually the respiratory tract. Microbial aerosols are suspensions of particles in the air consisting partially or wholly of microorganisms. They may remain suspended in the air for long periods of time, some retaining and others losing infectivity or virulence. Particles in the 1- to 5-micrometer range are easily drawn into the alveoli of the lungs and may be retained there. Not considered as airborne are droplets and other large particles that promptly settle out (see 'Direct transmission').

Droplet nuclei: usually the small residues that result from evaporation of fluid from droplets emitted by an infected host (see above). They also may be created purposely by a variety of atomizing devices, or accidentally as in microbiology laboratories, abattoirs, rendering plants or autopsy rooms. They usually remain suspended in the air for long periods.

Dust: the small particles of widely varying size that may arise from soil (e.g., fungus spores), clothes, bedding, or contaminated floors. (Heymann 2010)

Control measures for infectious diseases directed at interrupting transmission are designed according to the type of transmission for the agent. Direct transmission of an agent like *Neisseria gonorrhoeae*, for example, can be reduced by using condoms as a barrier method of control of gonorrhoea. Vector-borne transmission of an agent like *Plasmodium falciparum* can be reduced by using a residual insecticide against *Anopheles* mosquitoes as a chemical vector control method for malaria. Airborne transmission of an agent like *Mycobacterium tuberculosis* from sputum-positive pulmonary tuberculosis patients in hospital can be reduced by the use of special ventilation in the patient's room as an environmental method of control of tuberculosis. It should be recognized that some infectious agents may have more than one route of transmission. Poliovirus, for example, can be spread via direct transmission through the faecal–oral route and pharyngeal spread, or indirect transmission through contaminated food or other materials. Details of these and other methods of control directed at interrupting transmission are provided in the section on 'Tools for control of infectious diseases' in this chapter.

Host

The human host is the final link in the chain of infection. The infectious agent may enter the host through the following portals of entry.

- *Respiratory tract*: infectious agents can be inhaled into the respiratory tract and will be deposited at different levels of the pulmonary tree according to the size of the aerosol, droplet nuclei, or dust particles. For example, *Mycobacterium tuberculosis* in airborne droplet nuclei, 1–5 μm in diameter, may be inhaled into the alveoli of the lungs of a vulnerable host and result in tuberculosis.

- *Intact skin*: some infectious agents, such as *Necator americanus* which causes hookworm disease, can penetrate the intact skin.

- *Gastrointestinal tract*: an infectious agent, such as *Vibrio cholerae* which causes cholera, may enter via the gastrointestinal tract. People who have a compromised gastric function, such as gastric achlorhydria, may be at increased risk of disease.

- *Mucous membranes*: infectious agents, such as measles viruses, may be deposited on mucous membranes, including the conjunctiva of the eye, by droplet spread or by direct contact with infected people or contaminated objects.

- *Genitourinary system*: some infectious agents, such as *Escherichia coli* which causes urinary tract infections, can enter the urinary tract via an ascending route from the urethra colonized with the organism. Structural abnormalities of the urinary tract and procedures such as urinary catheterization may predispose the host to disease. Sexually transmitted infectious agents, such as *Neisseria gonorrhoeae* which causes gonorrhoea, may enter the male or female genital orifices.

- *Placenta*: certain infectious agents, such as rubella virus which causes congenital rubella syndrome, can cross the placenta resulting in transplacental transmission, a direct route of transmission from the mother to the fetus that is a form of vertical transmission.

Infectious agents also enter the host though *mechanisms that get past the body's natural barriers*, including wounds that break the integrity of the skin or mucous membranes; invasive procedures, parenteral injections, parenteral infusions, blood transfusions, or organ transplants that may introduce an agent into the body; or insect vectors that may inject agents through the skin.

The most important *host factors* regarding developing clinically manifest disease and the severity of disease are immune status and age. Infants, young children, and the elderly are at generally higher risk from more severe disease due to immaturity or deterioration of their immune systems, respectively. Host co-infections or other health conditions that diminish the immune status, for example, HIV infection or malnutrition, respectively, are also risk factors.

Many *host defence mechanisms* help prevent infection or disease. *Non-specific* host defence mechanisms include the intact skin (by providing a natural barrier), sinus and nasal cilia (by moving mucus and particles towards the nasal cavity), tears, saliva, and mucus (by preventing drying and containing lysozymes and other components with antimicrobial properties), and gastric acid (by the antimicrobial and antiparasitic properties of hydrochloric acid). *Specific* host defence mechanisms include naturally acquired immunity from previous infection, transplacentally acquired passive immunity in the newborn from the mother, artificially acquired active immunity from immunization, and artificially acquired passive immunity from immunoglobulins and antitoxins.

Host responses to infection that prevent or reduce the severity of infectious disease include: (1) polymorphonuclear leucocytosis stimulated by some bacterial infections that increases the number of phagocytic white blood cells, (2) fever that may slow the multiplication of some infectious agents, (3) antibody production that may neutralize some infectious agents or their toxins, (4) interferon production that may block intracellular replication of viruses, and (5) cytotoxic immune cell responses that kill cells infected with viruses

The *manifestation of infection* in the host may vary from inapparent (subclinical) infection to severe disease that may even result in death. The interaction between an infectious agent, routes of transmission, and host factors determines the spectrum of signs and symptoms. Sometimes the host may become an asymptomatic carrier of the infectious agent and be a source of infection for others.

Control measures for infectious diseases directed at the host are designed according to the immune status of the host and the likelihood of host exposure to certain infectious agents. For example, measles disease can be prevented by active immunization with measles vaccine to develop host immunity. Pneumonic plague can be prevented in those in close contact with patients with plague pneumonia by chemoprophylaxis using tetracycline or sulphonamide. Details of these and other methods of control directed at the host are provided in the section on control measures applied to the host in this chapter.

Tools for control of infectious diseases

The primary concern of infectious disease control in public health, whether in developing or industrialized countries, is the reduction, elimination, or even eradication of infectious disease. This is accomplished by directing control measures to the agent, the routes of transmission, or the host. Such control measures include: (1) identifying and then reducing or eliminating infectious agents at their sources and reservoirs, (2) breaking or interfering with the routes of transmission of infectious agents, and (3) identifying susceptible populations and then reducing or eliminating their susceptibility.

The tools for control of infectious diseases are related to recognition and evaluation of the patterns of diseases and the results of interventions to control them. In infectious disease control, the most important tool for recognition and evaluation is *surveillance* of disease defined as:

the process of systematic collection, orderly consolidation and analysis, and evaluation of pertinent data with prompt dissemination of the results to those who need to know them, and particularly those who are in a position to take action. It includes the systematic collection and evaluation of:
1. Morbidity and mortality reports
2. Special reports of field investigations of epidemics and of individual cases
3. Isolation and identification of infectious agents by laboratories
4. Data concerning the availability, use and untoward effects of vaccines and toxoids, immune globulins, insecticides and other substances used in control
5. Information regarding immunity levels in segments of the population
6. Other relevant epidemiologic data
A report summarizing the above data should be prepared and distributed to all cooperating persons and others with a need to know the results of the surveillance activities. The procedure applies to all jurisdictional levels of public health from local to international. (Heymann 2010)

Surveillance, therefore, is 'information for action'. More detailed information on surveillance or on field investigations is given in Chapter 5.19.

Tools for control related to *interventions* include:

♦ *Control measures applied to the host*: active immunization, passive immunization, chemoprophylaxis, behavioural change, reverse isolation, barriers, and improving host resistance.

♦ *Control measures applied to vectors*: chemical, environmental, and biological.

♦ *Control measures applied to infected humans*: chemotherapy, isolation, quarantine, restriction of activities, and behavioural change.

♦ *Control measures applied to animals*: active immunization, isolation, quarantine, restriction or reduction, chemoprophylaxis, and chemotherapy.

♦ *Control measures applied to the environment*: provision of safe water, proper disposal of faeces, food and milk sanitation, and design of facilities and equipment.

♦ *Control measures applied to infectious agents:* cleaning, cooling, pasteurization, disinfection, and sterilization.

Achieving maximum impact on control of a specific infectious disease may involve more than one of these interventions. For example, the control of hepatitis A infection can be achieved through interventions that may include: active immunization, passive immunization, food preparation and hand-washing behaviours, provision of safe water, food sanitation, and proper disposal of faeces.

The tools for control can also be considered according to the level at which they are applied: individual, institutional, or community based. At the *individual level*, control measures, usually initiated by a clinician, are directed towards the specific infectious disease threats to the particular individual. Examples include chemoprophylaxis to prevent wound infection, pre-exposure prophylactic immunization against rabies for a veterinarian, and use of diphtheria antitoxin in a patient with diphtheria.

At the *institutional level*, control measures, usually initiated by the officials of the institution, are directed to a group of people who are in close contact with each other, such as people in day-care centres, schools, military barracks, hospital wards, nursing homes, and correctional facilities. Examples include: (1) administering amantadine hydrochloride or rimantadine for chemoprophylaxis or chemotherapy of influenza A in a high-risk institutional population, (2) quarantining institutionalized young children during a measles outbreak, and (3) hepatitis B immunization of staff and clients of institutions for the developmentally disabled.

At the *community level*, control measures, usually initiated by local, state or national public health agencies, are directed to the community at large. Examples include childhood immunization programmes, provision of safe water, regulation of food supplies, and recall of contaminated food products.

It should be noted that some control measures, such as immunization, may take place at all levels while others, such as the provision of safe water to a community, are more specifically applied at a particular level.

The tools for the control of infectious diseases and their relationship to the chain of infection are the main focus of the remainder of this chapter.

Control measures applied to the host

Control measures applied to the host range from relatively easily administered immunization to behavioural changes that may be extremely difficult for an individual to accept and practise. This section details the types of control measures applied to susceptible hosts and gives examples of their application in the control of selected infectious diseases.

Active immunization

One of the most efficient control measures applied to a host is one that renders the host immune from infectious disease by an infectious agent. Active immunization is a cornerstone of public health measures for the control of many infectious diseases and is considered one of the most cost-effective methods of individual, institutional, and community protection for vaccine-preventable infectious diseases. The most powerful example of the potential impact of active immunization against an infectious disease is that of smallpox vaccination. Mobilization of political will on a worldwide basis, coupled with full application of the strategies of active surveillance and containment immunization against smallpox, ultimately resulted in the complete global eradication of the disease and cessation of transmission of the infectious agent, variola virus.

Active immunization is usually considered synonymous with the term vaccination, and is the process of administration of an antigen that can induce a specific immune response that protects a susceptible host from an infectious disease. Some draw a distinction between the two terms. Narrowly defined, *vaccination* is the process of administration of an antigen and *immunization* is the development of a specific immune response. Administering an antigen without evoking an immune response is possible, since no vaccine is 100 per cent effective. Conversely, someone can become immunized even if they were not administered an antigen. For example, the live, attenuated oral polio vaccine viruses can be transmitted from the recipient to other close contacts.

Active immunization can be accomplished through different types of antigens, including the following:

- *Inactivated toxins:* diphtheria toxoid is an example of a formaldehyde-inactivated preparation of diphtheria toxin that protects against clinically manifest disease, although the immunized person may still become infected with toxin-producing strains of *Corynebacterium diphtheria*. Tetanus toxoid and *Clostridium perfringens* toxoid (pig bel vaccine) are other examples of inactivated toxin preparations.

- *Inactivated complex antigens:* whole-cell pertussis vaccine is an example of a heat or chemically treated preparation of killed whole pertussis bacteria that protects against clinically manifest disease, although the immunized person may still become infected with *Bordetella pertussis*. Inactivated polio vaccine and inactivated influenza vaccine are other examples of inactivated vaccines.

- *Purified antigens:* acellular pertussis vaccine is an example of a vaccine composed of isolated and purified immunogenic pertussis antigens. Other vaccines with purified components include polyvalent capsular polysaccharide pneumococcal, polysaccharide meningococcal, protein-polysaccharide conjugate *Haemophilus influenzae* type b, and plasma-derived hepatitis B vaccines.

- *Recombinant antigens:* hepatitis B recombinant vaccine is an example of a vaccine composed of hepatitis B surface antigen subunits made through recombinant DNA technology. Human papillomavirus vaccine is another example of a DNA recombinant vaccine.

- *Live, attenuated vaccines:* measles vaccine is an example of a vaccine containing live infectious agents that are of reduced virulence, but induce protective antibodies against measles viruses. Other live, attenuated vaccines include oral polio, mumps, rubella, yellow fever, and bacille Calmette–Guérin (BCG) vaccines.

Protective *antibody responses* usually take 7–21 days to develop. Although most vaccines must be given before exposure to be effective, some vaccines may protect even if administered after exposure to an infectious agent. For example, measles vaccine may provide protection against measles disease if given within 72 hours of exposure. This occurs since the percutaneous route of administration of the antigen evokes an immune response faster than the measles virus results in disease through the respiratory route of natural exposure.

Duration of protection varies from only months, such as with killed whole-cell cholera vaccine, to years or even life with some live attenuated vaccines, such as measles vaccine. Some inactivated toxoids and vaccines, such as tetanus toxoid, may require a priming series of doses to be optimally effective and additional booster doses to maintain protective antibodies. Many new technologies are being explored that may increase the number and efficacy of vaccines available against infectious disease, including immune stimulating complexes, live viral or bacterial vector vaccines, and timed-release vaccines.

It should be recognized that vaccines vary in their efficacy and no vaccine is 100 per cent effective. *Vaccine efficacies* vary with type of vaccine, manufacturing techniques, storage and handling conditions, skill of administration, age of vaccination, and other host factors. Vaccines for routine use are safe. However, no vaccine is 100 per cent safe. Potential vaccinees, or their parents or guardians, should be screened for contraindications and be informed of potential side effects.

Immunization schedules for the routine control of infectious diseases preventable by immunization vary between countries and are usually based on expert advice to governments and physicians. For example, recommended policies for immunization in the United States are provided by the Advisory Committee on Immunization Practices (ACIP) and are published in the *Morbidity and Mortality Weekly Report* (ACIP 2012). In addition, the American Academy of Pediatrics periodically publishes comprehensive immunization recommendations in its *Report of the Committee on Infectious Diseases* (Committee on Infectious Diseases 2012). At the global level, the WHO publishes recommended immunization schedules and control strategies for vaccine-preventable diseases that are periodically updated by expert advisory groups in the WHO *Weekly Epidemiological Record*.

In *outbreak settings*, immunization schedules may be modified. For example, the age of immunization for measles may be lowered to 6 months of age during a measles outbreak. In such situations, people receiving vaccine before the routinely recommended age of immunization should be immunized again at the recommended age since immunization at the earlier age may not have been optimally effective.

Immunization programmes include vaccines for routine child, routine adult, travel, selected high-risk populations, and occupational settings. For example, tetanus toxoid is universally recommended; yellow fever vaccine is only recommended in geographic areas of epidemiological risk (i.e. in certain areas of Africa and South America); typhoid fever vaccine is only recommended for individuals subject to unusual exposure to typhoid, including people living in the same household as known carriers; and anthrax vaccine is only recommended for veterinarians and people occupationally exposed to possibly contaminated industrial raw materials.

Beyond protection of the individual, vaccination may also provide a degree of community protection. This phenomenon is known as herd immunity. *Herd immunity* is the relative protection of a population group achieved by reducing or breaking the chains of transmission of an infectious agent because a sufficient percentage of the population is immune, that is, resistant to infection through immunization or prior natural infection. When the immunity level in a population becomes such that the effective reproduction number of the disease in that population, R, is less than 1, the disease will eventually die out. Herd immunity is a complex phenomenon and varies according to the infectious agent, its routes of transmission, the degree to which immunization protects against infection versus only clinically manifest disease, and the distribution of immunization in the population. Typically, for childhood vaccine-preventable diseases, the immunity levels in the population to achieve herd immunity range from

around 84 per cent (for rubella) to over 90 per cent (for pertussis). The mechanisms of herd immunity are several, including 'direct protection of vaccinees against disease or transmissible infection and indirect protection of non-recipients by virtue of surreptitious vaccination, passive antibody, or just reduced sources of transmission and, hence, risks of infection in the community' (Fine 1993).

A particularly difficult problem for vaccine-preventable infectious disease control programmes is complacency by the population that can result from the very successes of the programmes and highlights the continuing need to educate the public and decision-makers. Low rates of vaccine-preventable infectious disease may mistakenly lead parents to consider that vaccination is no longer important for maintaining their children's health and may result in political leaders reducing funding for immunization programmes. Low disease rates may also focus undue attention on the relatively rare serious side effects of vaccination in relation to current rates of disease. Such side effects should only be compared in relation to rates of disease and its complications that would occur without immunization programmes.

A comprehensive treatment of active immunization is given by Plotkin et al. (2008).

Passive immunization

Passive immunization is a temporary immunity in a host due to the protection afforded by antibody produced in another host. Passive immunity may be acquired either naturally or artificially.

Naturally acquired passive immunity is achieved through transfer of maternal antibodies via the placenta. It is the way that newborn infants are provided with a temporary immunity against many infectious diseases for which the mother is immune. This immunity wanes over time and eventually leaves the infant susceptible to these diseases.

An important use of transplacental immunity as a control measure is in the prevention of tetanus neonatorum (neonatal tetanus) by immunization of women before or during pregnancy with tetanus toxoid. This is especially important in developing countries where the disease typically occurs when the umbilical cord is cut with an unclean instrument contaminated with tetanus spores or when substances contaminated with tetanus spores are placed on the umbilical stump after delivery. Control by active immunization of the infant cannot be achieved in sufficient time since the average incubation period is only 6 days (with a range from 3 to 28 days). An adequately immunized mother, however, will usually effectively transfer maternal antibodies against tetanus across the placenta to her newborn and prevent tetanus neonatorum.

Another example of naturally acquired passive immunity is the relative protection against measles disease in a young infant born to a mother who previously had the disease. Typically, such infants are immune for approximately 6–9 months or more after birth, depending upon how many residual maternal antibodies are present at the time of pregnancy. Other diseases for which there is usually an effective transplacental immunity in infants, for variable amounts of time, include diphtheria, mumps, poliomyelitis, rubella, and varicella (chickenpox). It should be noted that if the mother is not immune, or if residual maternal antibodies have significantly waned, then the infant may be susceptible to disease.

Research is ongoing as to other infectious diseases that may be preventable in the neonate or infant through immunization of the mother before or during pregnancy. Examples include

Haemophilus influenzae type b and group B streptococcal and meningococcal diseases (Insel et al. 1994). Many diseases, however, are not prevented by transplacental immunity.

Breastfeeding is a form of naturally acquired passive antibody transfer to neonates and infants. Breast milk and colostrum contain secretory immunoglobulin A (IgA) antibodies that may play a protective role in the prevention of infections with such agents as respiratory syncytial virus, rotavirus, and *Haemophilus influenzae* type b.

Artificially acquired passive immunity is acquired through administration of an antibody-containing preparation, antiserum, or immune globulin. It has a place in the control of certain infectious diseases in special situations. This immunity also wanes over a relatively short period of time.

Examples of the use of artificially acquired passive immunity to control infectious disease include the following:

- *Rabies*: natural immunity to rabies in humans does not exist. Susceptible individuals bitten by an animal known or suspected to be rabid should receive rabies immune globulin to neutralize the rabies virus in the wound. It should be noted that, besides passive immunization with rabies immune globulin, such individuals should also receive active immunization with rabies vaccine.

- *Hepatitis A*: in areas where sanitation is poor, hepatitis A infection commonly occurs at an early age and therefore most adults in developing countries are already immune. However, epidemics may occur in industrialized countries. Passive immunization with immune globulin may be given to: (1) all household and sexual contacts of patients with hepatitis A, (2) other food handlers in an establishment where hepatitis A has occurred in a food handler, (3) all individuals in an institution where a focal outbreak of hepatitis A has occurred, and (4) people from industrialized countries travelling to highly endemic areas. It should be noted that vaccines for active immunization for hepatitis A are now available.

- *Diphtheria*: treatment of this disease is an example of the use of an antibody containing product (diphtheria antitoxin) produced in an animal (only diphtheria antitoxin from horses is available) administered as part of the treatment regimen for secondary prevention of disease. In suspected cases of diphtheria, the antitoxin must be given as soon as possible because it is only effective in neutralizing diphtheria toxins not yet bound to cells.

- *Other important infectious diseases, including hepatitis B, measles, tetanus, varicella*: depending upon the circumstances of exposure, susceptibility of the host, and status of the host's general immune system there are circumstances under which hepatitis B immune globulin, tetanus immune globulin, varicella-zoster immune globulin, or immune globulin may be warranted.

Chemoprophylaxis

Chemoprophylaxis is the prevention of infection or its progression to clinically manifest disease through the administration of chemical substances, including antibiotics. Chemoprophylaxis can also consist of the treatment of a disease to prevent complications of that disease. Chemoprophylaxis may be specifically directed against a particular infectious agent or it may be non-specifically directed against many infectious agents. The use of antibiotics before surgical procedures is an example of non-specific chemoprophylaxis to prevent wound infections in the postoperative period. Examples of specific chemoprophylaxis are given below.

The use of chemoprophylaxis to *prevent development of infection* is illustrated by using chloroquine to prevent malarial parasitaemia caused by *Plasmodium vivax, Plasmodium ovale, Plasmodium malariae*, and chloroquine-sensitive strains of *Plasmodium falciparum*. For some chloroquine-resistant strains of *Plasmodium falciparum*, alternative regimens include mefloquine alone, doxycycline alone, primaquine alone, or an atovaquone/proguanil combination primaquine may be given to reduce the risk of a relapse from intrahepatic forms of *Plasmodium vivax* and *Plasmodium ovale* after discontinuation of chemoprophylaxis with any chemosuppressive drugs other than primaquine. Determination of a specific malaria chemoprophylactic regimen is complex. It must take into account the geographic area, the possibility of pregnancy, the weight of an individual (dose size for children is determined by body weight), and the risks of adverse reactions to the chemoprophylactic regimen.

Other examples of prevention of development of infection include the following:

- The use of silver nitrate, erythromycin, or tetracycline instilled into the eyes of a newborn to prevent gonococcal ophthalmia by transmission of *Neisseria gonorrhoeae* from an infected mother during birth.

- The use of tetracycline, sulphonamides (including sulfadiazine and trimethoprim-sulfamethoxazole), chloramphenicol, or streptomycin in close contacts of confirmed or suspected cases of plague pneumonia to prevent plague pneumonia by transmission of *Yersinia pestis*.

- The use of benzathine penicillin in those in sexual contact with confirmed cases of early syphilis to prevent syphilis by transmission of *Treponema pallidum*.

An example of the use of chemoprophylaxis to *prevent the progression of an infection to active manifest disease* is the use of isoniazid (INH) to prevent the progression of latent infection with *Mycobacterium tuberculosis* to clinical tuberculosis. People less than 35 years of age who are tuberculosis test positive should receive INH to prevent clinical tuberculosis. The decision to use INH, especially in individuals more than 35 years of age (who are at higher risk of clinical hepatitis from the use of the drug), must be determined based on such information as length of infection, closeness of association with a current case, status of the immune system, presence of acute liver disease, possibilities of pregnancy, and risks of adverse reactions.

Other examples of prevention of progression of an infection to active manifest disease through the use of chemoprophylaxis include the following:

- Co-trimoxazole or pentamidine to prevent subclinical latent infection with *Pneumocystis jirovecii* (formerly *carinii*) from progressing to clinically manifest *Pneumocystis* pneumonia in immunosuppressed people such as HIV-infected individuals.

- Mebendazole, albendazole, or pyrantel pamoate to prevent infection with *Necator americanus, Ancylostoma duodenale,* and *Ancylostoma ceylanicum* from progressing to the clinically manifest anaemia of hookworm disease.

- Pyrimethamine combined with sulfadiazine and folinic acid (to avoid possible bone marrow depression) to prevent asymptomatic infants congenitally infected with *Toxoplasma gondii* from progressing to clinically manifest chorioretinitis and other sequelae of congenital toxoplasmosis.

In some situations, establishing *screening* programmes to detect and treat asymptomatic infections or unrecognized disease in defined populations is useful. An example is the screening for *Chlamydia trachomatis* in sexual partners of people infected with *Chlamydia trachomatis,* women with mucopurulent cervicitis, sexually active women 25 years of age or younger, and women older than 25 years of age with risk factors for chlamydia. A more detailed background on screening as a public health function is given in Chapter 11.4.

An example of the use of chemoprophylaxis to *treat an infectious disease to prevent complications of the disease* is the use of penicillin (or erythromycin in penicillin-sensitive patients) to treat streptococcal sore throats caused by *Streptococcus pyogenes* group A to prevent acute rheumatic fever.

Other examples of prevention of complications of an infectious disease through the use of chemoprophylaxis include the following:

- Tetracycline for adults, or penicillin for children, for treatment of Lyme disease caused by *Borrelia burgdorferi* in the erythema chronicum migrans stage to prevent or reduce the severity of late cardiac, arthritic, or neurological complications.

- Benzathine penicillin for treatment of syphilis in its primary, secondary, or early latency period to prevent late manifestations of the disease such as cardiovascular syphilis.

- Ketoconazole for treatment of blastomycosis caused by *Blastomyces dermatitidis* in its early stages to prevent progression of chronic pulmonary or disseminated blastomycosis that may lead to death.

Potential problems with the use of chemoprophylaxis may include compromise of the host's own non-specific defence mechanisms, other replacement infectious agents causing disease by growing in the place of the infectious agent affected by the specific chemoprophylactic regimen (e.g. severe diarrhoea from intestinal infections with *Clostridium difficile* may occur when the normal bacteria flora in the intestines have been lost due to antibiotics), and emergence of resistant strains of the infectious agent. The development of antibiotic resistance can be reduced by using antibiotics only when needed, selecting the proper antibiotic (or, in some situations, the appropriate multidrug therapy) for the infectious agent, and ensuring compliance with the appropriate regimen for the duration of treatment.

Behavioural change

Perhaps the most challenging tool for the control of infectious diseases, and sometimes one of the most powerful and cost-effective, is behaviour change in the host that reduces or eliminates risk of exposure to an agent. Everyone has developed habits of living (lifestyles) that are not easily changed. Some of these behaviours are protective against infectious diseases. Others render the individual at higher risk of infection.

Examples of higher risk of exposure to infectious agents through behaviour, and behaviour changes that can have an impact on the chain of transmission, include the following.

Sexual behaviour

Many infectious agents are transmitted by the direct transmission route through sexual contact, including *Chlamydia trachomatis* causing chlamydial genital infections, *Neisseria gonorrhoeae* causing gonorrhoea, *Treponema pallidum* causing venereal syphilis, *Calymmatobacterium granulomatis* causing granuloma inguinale, *Haemophilus ducreyi* causing chancroid, herpes simplex virus causing herpes simplex, *Trichomonas vaginalis* causing trichomoniasis, human papillomaviruses causing condyloma acuminate, and HIV causing AIDS.

Abstinence behaviour, that is, refraining from sexual activity with other people, eliminates the risk of transmission of these agents through sexual contact. The delaying of age of first sexual activity avoids the risk of transmission of these agents at an early age. Restricting sexual contact to only between two uninfected people who do not have sexual activity with any other people virtually eliminates the risk of transmission of these agents through sexual behaviours. The exceptions are due to other routes of transmission of some of these agents (e.g. HIV acquired through intravenous drug use in one partner being transmitted through sexual contact to the other partner). Limiting the number of sexual partners, and limiting those sexual partners to people who also have few sexual partners, reduces the risk of exposure. However, at the individual level, if one of these sexual partners has an infectious agent transmissible by sexual contact, the risk of transmission may still be high. Finally, condom use during sexual activity in high-risk situations will markedly reduce, but not eliminate, transmission. A more detailed background on sexually transmitted diseases is provided in Chapter 8.12.

Intravenous drug use behaviour

Injection of drugs using non-sterile needles or syringes previously used by other intravenous drug users may transmit infectious agents in blood through the vehicle-borne route of indirect transmission, including HIV causing AIDS; hepatitis B virus causing viral hepatitis B; and *Plasmodium vivax, Plasmodium malariae,* and *Plasmodium ovale* causing malaria.

Abstinence behaviour, that is, refraining from intravenous drug use, eliminates the risk of transmission of such agents through contaminated needles and syringes. Using a sterile needle and sterile syringe for intravenous drug use will break the chain of transmission of these infectious agents through this route. Some community public health programmes, in addition to promoting drug abstinence and drug rehabilitation, conduct needle and syringe exchanges and education regarding methods of decontamination to help promote the use of sterile injection equipment among intravenous drug users (see Chapter 9.2).

Eating behaviour

Eating certain foods may result in exposure to infectious agents through the vehicle-borne route of indirect transmission. These behaviours include consuming raw molluscs by which an infectious agent like the hepatitis A virus can cause viral hepatitis A, eating raw eggs by which an infectious agent like a *Salmonella* serotype can cause salmonellosis, and consuming raw beef by which an infectious agent like *Taenia saginata* can cause beef tapeworm infection.

Although food and diet are strongly ingrained behaviours, modification of dietary patterns is possible. Cooking foods like beef, pork, and eggs can markedly reduce risk of transmission of infectious agents. In addition, reducing risks by elimination of infectious agents from the food may be possible (see the section on control methods applied to the environment). Eating shortly after cooking so that foods are not left standing at ambient temperatures for extended times and paying attention to food recalls are also important behaviours. Hand washing before eating also reduces risk of transmission of many infectious agents that are spread through direct or indirect routes of faecal–oral transmission, such as *Shigella dysenteriae*, *Shigella flexneri*, *Shigella boydii*, and *Shigella sonnei* which may cause shigellosis (bacillary dysentery), which is estimated to cause 600,000 deaths per year with two-thirds of the cases in children under 10 years of age (Heymann 2010).

Working behaviour

In certain occupations, many behaviours may result in exposure to infectious agents and should be targets for control programmes in occupational safety and health settings. Specific examples include the following:

- Dental workers performing procedures with bare hands may result in exposure to hepatitis B viruses from infected patients.
- Health workers improperly handling used needles may result in needle-stick injuries leading to exposure to HIV from infected patients.
- Hospital laboratory workers improperly processing specimens containing infectious agents without appropriate glove or eyewear protection may result in exposure to these agents.
- Veterinarians who do not properly handle animals may result in brucellosis (undulant fever) due to exposure to *Brucella abortus*, *Brucella melitensis*, *Brucella suis*, or *Brucella canis*.

Occupational hazards related to non-infectious materials may predispose an individual to increased risk of infectious diseases. For example, working conditions and behaviours in industrial plants and mines that lead to silicosis due to long-term inhalation of free crystalline silica dust will greatly increase the risk of developing tuberculosis.

Working behaviours appropriate for the particular occupational setting may include wearing protective clothing, eyewear, and gloves; hand washing and changing clothes after work; receiving appropriate vaccinations for the working environment; meticulous adherence to needle disposal and equipment sterilization procedures; and using hooded laboratory benches when handling infectious specimens that can become aerosolized.

Other behaviours

Other behaviours that may reduce the transmission of infectious agents include the following:

- Scheduling outdoor activities at periods of low vector activity, applying insect repellents and sleeping under bednets reduce the indirect transmission of vector-borne agents of infectious diseases like malaria.
- Searching oneself for attached ticks every 3 to 4 hours when playing or working in tick-infested areas reduces the indirect transmission of vector-borne agents of infectious diseases like Rocky Mountain spotted fever.
- Avoiding sharing of utensils, cups, toothbrushes, or towels reduces the indirect transmission of vehicle-borne agents of infectious diseases like mononucleosis.
- Wearing of shoes reduces the direct transmission of infectious agents like those causing hookworm disease.
- Frequently bathing and regular washing of clothes in hot soapy water controls body lice.
- Breastfeeding reduces diarrhoeal diseases in the infant, although it may transmit HIV from HIV-infected mothers.
- Hand washing after defecation or touching potentially contaminated surfaces, people, or animals (including those found in petting zoos) prior to preparing food or touching one's own eyes, mucous membranes, or mouth reduces the risk of direct or indirect transmission of a wide variety of infectious agents.
- Large family sizes and crowding may facilitate airborne transmission of infectious agents in droplet nuclei for infectious diseases like tuberculosis.

Some of these other behaviours, like crowding, are conditioned by circumstances such as poverty that are not easily or directly amenable to programmes promoting behavioural change.

Reverse isolation

Certain rare circumstances exist where a means of avoiding transmission of an infectious disease to a highly susceptible host is to provide reverse, or protective, isolation. Such isolation attempts to protect infection-prone patients from potentially harmful infectious agents. Reverse isolation procedures range from provision of a private room with the use of masks, gloves and gowns by all people entering the room, to elaborate facilities with laminar airflow rooms and sterilization of all food. Protective isolation is usually conducted for a limited time until the normal immune system recovers, a regimen of passive immunization is begun, or a bone marrow transplant is successful.

Examples of people who may need periods of reverse isolation include those who have such diseases as X-linked agammaglobulinaemia, DiGeorge's syndrome, and severe combined immunodeficiency; or those who have received therapies, such as some forms of cancer chemotherapy, that have severely compromised the person's immune system in combating many infectious diseases.

Barriers

One tool of control that can be applied to the host is the use of barriers between the host and the infectious agent. The effectiveness of such barriers, however, may be dependent on the behaviour of the host to use them consistently and education to use them correctly. Examples of barriers include the following:

- Screens, bednets (including bednets impregnated with pyrethroid insecticides such as permethrin), long-sleeved shirts and trousers (with the cuffs tucked into boots as a mechanical barrier), and repellents (such as N,N-diethyl-meta-toluamide known as DEET) to prevent transmission of malaria through the bite of infected female *Anopheles* mosquitoes or West Nile virus through *Culix* mosquitoes.

• Condoms to prevent transmission of HIV and other sexually transmitted infectious agents through sexual intercourse.

• Masks (air-purifying respirators) to prevent transmission of tuberculosis through airborne droplet nuclei from patients with sputum-positive pulmonary tuberculosis.

General improvement in host resistance

Improving host resistance though general improvement of the immune system is a non-specific approach, but may be important in certain settings. Kwashiorkor, marasmus, and other forms of malnutrition debilitate the host's immune system and may make an individual more susceptible to infectious diseases. Moreover, people who are malnourished and succumb to an infectious disease are at higher risk of the disease being of greater severity and leading to other complications.

Malnutrition also encompasses micronutrient deficiencies. Vitamin A deficiency, for example, has been linked to higher rates of mortality associated with measles disease. Correcting vitamin A deficiency, through programmes of supplementation, fortification and dietary modification in high-risk populations, can reduce mortality rates due to measles.

A complex interaction exists between infectious diseases, such as diarrhoeal diseases, and malnutrition. A downward spiral of infection may lead to malnutrition that, in turn, leads to more infections, and so on. If unchecked, especially in developing countries, this downward spiral can ultimately result in death.

International travel

The special situation of international travel combines many control measures applied to the host already mentioned. The increase in the numbers of travellers, the speed of travel, and the ability to reach areas previously infrequently visited have reduced the effectiveness of surveillance for infectious diseases at ports of arrival and increased infectious disease risks. Advice for prevention against infectious diseases must be both general and specific.

General advice includes such issues as avoidance of eating and drinking potentially contaminated food or drink (including ice) and swimming or bathing in polluted water. Specific advice provided by health professionals should be provided based on information about the area to be visited and may include such measures as active immunization against yellow fever, active or passive immunization against hepatitis A, chemoprophylaxis against malaria, repellents against potentially infected mosquitoes, and not walking barefoot in areas of risk for infection with hookworms *Strongyloides stercoralis* and *Strongyloides fuelleborni*. A more detailed background on international travel and health is provided in the annually updated WHO publication on *International Travel and Health* (WHO 2012b).

Control measures applied to vectors

Vector-borne transmission is the only or main route of transmission for many infectious diseases. There exist more than 100 arthropod-borne viruses that may produce clinically manifest diseases in humans. Control of vector-borne diseases includes measures to: (1) change behaviour and create barriers to the susceptible host, (2) reduce or break the chain of transmission of the infectious agent from an infected host to the vector, and (3) directly control the vector population itself. Chemical, environmental, and biological controls are the primary means of directly controlling the vector population.

Chemical control

Chemicals used in the control of vectors that act as digestive poisons, contact poisons, or fumigants include minerals, natural plant products (botanicals), chlorinated hydrocarbons, organophosphates, carbamates, and fumigants. Chemical control measures include the following public health interventions:

• Spraying chemical insecticides such as organochlorine insecticides (e.g. dichlorodiphenyltrichlorothane, or DDT, and dieldrin), organophosphorus insecticides (e.g. malathion and fenitrothion), and carbonate insecticides (e.g. propoxur and carbaryl) to prevent malaria through control of mosquitoes.

• Spraying chemical biodegradable insecticides such as temephos (Abate®) to prevent onchocerciasis through control of *Simulium* fly vectors.

• Using traps impregnated with decamethrin to prevent African trypanosomiasis (sleeping sickness) through reduction of the population of infective species of *Glossina* (tsetse fly) vectors.

• Treating snail breeding places with chemical molluscicides to prevent schistosomiasis due to the free-swimming cercariae (larval forms) of *Schistosoma mansoni, Schistosoma haematobium, and Schistosoma japonicum* that develop in snails.

• Treating step-wells and ponds with chemical insecticides such as temephos (Abate®) to prevent dracunculiasis due to infected cyclops (a crustacean copepod).

• Suppressing rat populations by poisoning, preceded or accompanied by measures to control fleas, as an additional measure to supplement environmental sanitation to control rodent populations to prevent human plague.

The use of spraying for control of mosquitoes is complicated due to concerns about environmental contamination by chemicals such as DDT and dieldrin which have led to them being banned in many countries. In addition, the emergence of mosquito vectors resistant to the insecticides diminishes their effectiveness in many areas. New methods of application, such as ultra-low-volume spraying of malathion, reduce the amounts of insecticide used.

Environmental control

Environmental control of vectors includes the following public health interventions:

• Eliminating breeding sites of mosquito larvae by filling and draining areas of stagnant water and removing objects around houses that may collect water.

• Destroying the habitats of the tsetse fly vector.

• Properly implementing landfill procedures, placing lids on rubbish bins, covering food for human consumption, screening privies, cleaning up spilled food, and appropriately storing food.

- Placing roach and fly traps.
- Constructing rat-proof houses.
- Eliminating rodent habitats.

It is also important to note that certain development projects may have an impact on the environment that facilitates the growth of vector or intermediate-host populations and results in increased infectious diseases. Construction of artificial waterways may serve as breeding sites for *Simulium* fly vectors that can transmit *Onchocerca volvulus* resulting in onchocerciasis. Irrigation schemes can foster the growth of snail intermediate hosts required for the transmission of species of *Schistosoma* resulting in schistosomiasis. Carefully conducted environmental and health impact studies that consider the impact of a construction project on the vector and intermediate host populations, and ways to modify the project to reduce such populations, are important environmental control measures.

Biological control

Biological control of vectors includes the following public health interventions:

- *Introduction of predators and parasites:* the introductions of *Gambusia affinis*, a small fish that feeds on mosquito larvae, and of *Coelomomyces*, a fungal parasite, are examples of control measures that are effective against *Aëdes* mosquitoes.
- *Insect growth regulators:* the use of such regulators may result in death or sterility of vectors by interfering with normal insect development. An example is the use of methoprene (Altosid®) to control flood water mosquitoes.
- *Genetic modification:* although still at an experimental phase, researchers have developed transgenic, or genetically modified, mosquitoes that are malaria resistant with higher survival rates that could eventually replace mosquitoes that carry malaria parasites.

Control measures applied to infected humans

Control measures may be applied to infected people at the individual level, in the institutional or hospital setting, and at the community level.

Hospital infection control

The hospital setting is a unique situation that requires special efforts to prevent and control nosocomial infections, or healthcare-associated infections (HAIs), which are infections that originate or occur in a hospital or other healthcare setting. HAIs are a major problem worldwide. In the United States alone, some 2 million HAIs occur annually resulting in an estimated 90,000 deaths (McKibben et al. 2005). It has been estimated that HAIs result in some US$35.7–45 billion in annual direct medical hospital patient costs based on using the Consumer Price Index for inpatient hospital services (Scott 2009).

Infection control programmes for hospitals should ideally include the following elements:

- An infection control committee responsible for overall coordination of infection control activities.
- One or more infection control practitioners responsible for nosocomial disease surveillance, analysis of data, consultation, and training of hospital staff.
- A hospital epidemiologist to supervise the infection control practitioners, oversee data collection and analysis, and implement any needed emergency infection control measures.
- An engineer to direct engineering and preventive maintenance operations, especially ventilation equipment.
- A sanitarian to develop procedures for proper disposal of liquid and solid wastes; and sanitation of water, ice, and food.
- Effective guidelines for patient care practices.
- Surveillance of patient care practices, patient infections, and environmental contamination by infectious agents.
- Coordination with other departments (microbiology laboratory, central services, housekeeping, food service, and laundry).
- Vector control.
- Thorough investigation of problems.

Examples of specific control measures that may be applied to infected humans at the individual, institutional and community levels are detailed as follows.

Chemotherapy

Treatment of people with infectious diseases or subclinical infections may be a control tool for some infectious diseases. Such treatment may or may not have an impact on disease progression in the patient. It should be noted that rapid case detection and prompt application of appropriate chemotherapeutic agents are needed to limit infectivity.

Some important examples of control by chemotherapy include the following:

- Treatment of patients with sputum-positive pulmonary *tuberculosis* with appropriate multidrug therapy will usually result in sputum conversion rendering them non-infectious to others within a few weeks. Recommended treatment regimens include isoniazid (INH) combined with one or more of the following antibiotics: rifampin, streptomycin, ethambutol, and pyrazinamide. The WHO has recommended that adherence to a complete course of multidrug therapy be directly observed by another responsible person as part of the DOTS (directly observed treatment, short-course) global strategy for the control of tuberculosis.
- Patients with *leprosy* treated with appropriate multidrug therapy are considered no longer infectious within 3 months of regular and continued treatment. Recommended treatment regimens for multibacillary leprosy include the following antibiotics: rifampicin, dapsone, and clofazimine.
- Treatment of patients with *streptococcal sore throats* with penicillin (or erythromycin for penicillin-sensitive patients) will usually render them no longer infectious after 24–48 hours.
- Patients with *pertussis* treated with antibiotics such as erythromycin or trimethoprim-sulfamethoxazole, although they may not affect the patient's symptoms, will usually result in the patient no longer being infectious after 5–7 days.

Of special note is the situation of treatment of people who are carriers:

> A person or animal that harbors a specific infectious agent without discernible clinical disease, and which serves as a potential source of infection. The carrier state may exist in an individual with an infection that is unapparent throughout its course (such an individual is commonly known as *healthy or asymptomatic carrier*), or during the incubation period, convalescence, and post-convalescence of a person with a clinically recognizable disease (commonly known as *incubatory or convalescent carrier*). Under either circumstance the carrier state may be of short or long duration (*temporary or transient carrier, or chronic carrier*). (Heymann 2010)

A chronic carrier of diphtheria, for example, may shed the infectious agent *Corynebacterium diphtheriae* for 6 months or more, but appropriate antibiotic therapy will usually promptly stop the carrier state. Another example is that of untreated patients with typhoid fever due to *Salmonella typhi*. Between 2 to 5 per cent of such patients will become permanent carriers. Treatment with appropriate antibiotics may be effective in ending the carrier state.

Antibiotic treatment may not always eliminate a carrier state for some infectious agents. For example, the treatment of people with salmonellosis with an antibiotic may not terminate the period of communicability and can even result in emergence of antibiotic-resistant strains. However, antibiotic therapy may be still warranted under certain circumstances.

In some situations, establishing screening programmes in defined target populations for identification of asymptomatic or unrecognized infections that could be transmitted to others may be appropriate. Such screening should include the necessary follow-up with appropriate chemotherapy and counselling. An example would be screening close contacts of diphtheria patients with nose and throat cultures for the presence of *Corynebacterium diphtheriae*. Identified carriers with positive cultures should be treated with appropriate antibiotic therapy.

Isolation

Isolation is the 'separation, for a period at least equal to the *period of communicability*, of infected persons or animals from others, in such places and under such conditions as to prevent or limit the direct or indirect transmission of the infectious agent from those infected to those who are susceptible to infection or who may spread the agent to others' (Heymann 2010).

The US CDC and the Hospital Infection Control Practices Advisory Committee (HICPAC) have provided guidelines for isolation precautions in hospital settings (Siegel et al. 2007). There are two levels of isolation precautions, namely: (1) a standard precautions level designed for the care of all hospitalized patients, and (2) a transmission-based precautions level designed for the care of hospitalized patients that are suspected or confirmed to be infected by agents spread by contact, droplet, or airborne routes of transmission. These are summarized from guidelines as follows.

Standard precautions are universally applied precautions designed to reduce the risk of transmission by infectious agents from blood; body fluids, secretions, and excretions; non-intact skin; and mucous membranes. The essential elements of standard precautions include handwashing; personal protective equipment (use of gloves, appropriate application of mask and eye protection or a face shield, and utilization of gowns); proper handling of patient-care equipment; adequate environmental control measures for routine care, cleaning, and disinfection of frequently touched surfaces; appropriate handling, transporting, and processing of used linen; proper handling and disposal of needles, scalpels, and other sharp instruments; adequate protection when undertaking patient resuscitation; respiratory hygiene/cough etiquette; and placement of patients who contaminate the environment in private rooms.

Airborne precautions are used, in addition to standard precautions, in settings where patients are suspected or confirmed to be infected by agents transmitted by airborne droplet nuclei. The essential elements of airborne precautions include preferably placing patients in an airborne infection isolation room (AIIR) that has monitored negative air pressure (if necessary, it is possible to use cohorting of patients with the same active infections); use of mask respirators (N-95 air-purifying respirators); and limiting patient movement and transport from the room (placing a surgical mask on the patient if they are being moved for an essential purpose). An example of an infectious disease for which patients are recommended to be placed under airborne precautions is a patient in hospital with measles through the fourth day of rash. Although isolation of patients with measles not in hospital is not practical in the general population, schoolchildren should remain out of school until at least the fourth day of rash.

Droplet precautions are used, in addition to standard precautions, in settings where patients are suspected or confirmed to be infected by agents transmitted by droplets. The essential elements of droplet precautions include placement of patients in a private room (if necessary, it is possible to use cohorting of patients with the same active infections or maintaining a spatial separation of at least 3 feet between the infected patient and other patients and visitors); use of a mask when working within 3 feet of the patient; and limiting patient movement and transport from the room (placing a surgical mask on the patient if they are being moved for an essential purpose). Examples of infectious diseases for which patients are recommended to be placed under droplet precautions include pharyngeal diphtheria caused by *Corynebacterium diphtheriae* and pneumonic plague caused by *Yersinia pestis*.

Contact precautions are used, in addition to standard precautions, in settings where patients are suspected or confirmed to be infected or colonized by agents transmitted by direct or indirect contact. The essential elements of contact precautions include placement of the patient in a private room (if necessary, it is possible to use cohorting of patients with the same active infections); use of gloves when entering the patient's room and removing them before leaving the room; wearing a gown when entering the patient's room and removing the gown before leaving the room; limiting patient movement and transport to essential purposes only; and, when possible, dedicate the use of patient-care equipment to a single patient (if necessary, it is possible to use such equipment on a cohort of patients with the same active or colonized infections). Examples of infectious diseases for which patients are recommended to be placed under contact isolation precautions include cutaneous diphtheria caused by *Corynebacterium diphtheriae*, rubella, and disseminated herpes simplex caused by herpes simplex virus.

Quarantine of potentially infected persons

Quarantine is the 'Restriction of activities for well persons or animals who have been exposed (or are considered to be at high risk of exposure) to a case of communicable disease during its period of communicability (i.e., *contacts*) to prevent disease transmission during the incubation period if infection should occur' (Heymann 2010).

Two categories of quarantine are as follows (Heymann 2010):

Absolute or complete quarantine: the limitation of freedom of movement of those exposed to a communicable disease for a period of time not longer than the longest usual incubation period of that disease, in such a manner as to prevent effective contact with those not so exposed.

Modified quarantine: a selective, partial limitation of freedom of movement of contacts, commonly on the basis of known or presumed differences in susceptibility and related to the assessed risk of disease transmission. It may be designed to accommodate particular situations. Examples are exclusion of children from school, exemption of immune persons from provisions applicable to susceptible persons, or restriction of military populations to the post or to quarters. Modified quarantine includes: *personal surveillance*, the practice of close medical or other supervision of contacts to permit prompt recognition of infection or illness but without restricting their movements; and *segregation*, the separation of some part of a group of persons or domestic animals from the others for special consideration, control or observation; removal of susceptible children to homes of immune persons; or establishment of a sanitary boundary to protect uninfected from infected portions of a population. (Heymann 2010)

Examples of diseases where quarantine may be considered include the following.

- *Pneumonic plague*: people who have been in the same household or in face-to-face contact with patients with pneumonic plague and who do not accept chemoprophylaxis should be placed under *absolute quarantine* with strict isolation, including careful surveillance, for 7 days.
- *Measles*: although absolute quarantine is impractical, a *modified quarantine* is recommended in settings where young children are living in dormitories, wards, or institutions. When measles occurs in such institutional settings, strict *segregation* of infants is recommended.
- *Lassa fever*: close *personal surveillance* of all close contacts is recommended. Such people include those who live or are in close contact with Lassa fever patients as well as laboratory personnel testing specimens from such patients.

Restriction of activities

Controlling infectious disease transmission by restriction of the activities of people in the community who are potentially infectious to others may be appropriate in certain circumstances. Examples include the following:

- Individuals with a diarrhoeal disease should be excluded from handling food and caring for patients in hospital, children, and elderly people.
- Known carriers of *Salmonella typhi* should be excluded from food handling and care of patients.
- People with staphylococcal disease should avoid contact with debilitated people and infants.
- People with rubella should be excluded from school or work for 7 days after the onset of rash and from contact with pregnant women.

Behavioural change

Behaviour change in an infected person to protect others may be difficult to accomplish and often requires continuing education and counselling. However, this should be considered in preventing the transmission of infectious agents in the following situations.

Sexual behaviour

Examples of infectious agents transmitted through sexual activities are discussed in the earlier section on control measures applied to the host and in more detail in Chapter 8.12. Individuals who suspect that they may have a sexually transmitted disease should be encouraged to have health-seeking behaviours. People with a sexually transmissible infectious agent should be treated and asked to cooperate with health officials to trace their sexual contacts. Patients with diseases such as lymphogranuloma venereum and syphilis, for example, should refrain from sexual contact until all lesions are healed. HIV-infected individuals should be counselled to treat genital ulcer disease promptly since such disease may increase transmissibility of HIV. Also, HIV-infected people should avoid sexual intercourse with HIV-negative individuals or, if having sexual intercourse with HIV-negative individuals, use methods such as condoms to reduce the risk of transmission. For a more detailed overview of HIV and AIDS see Chapter 8.13.

Intravenous drug use behaviour

In addition to counselling to abstain from intravenous drug use and establishing drug rehabilitation programmes to help individuals who wish to abstain, promoting behaviour change in the use of injection equipment is important. Discouraging the sharing of injection equipment and education on methods for the decontamination of needles and syringes for intravenous drug use reduce risks of transmission of infectious agents through contaminated injection equipment.

Food preparation behaviour

Individuals who should be restricted from handling food (e.g. carriers of *Salmonella typhi*) should be counselled regarding their condition and potential to infect others if they handle food. Food handlers who have an infectious disease that is potentially transmissible through the vehicle-borne means of food should be discouraged from handling food for others. The importance of hand washing, especially after defecation and before handling food, should be stressed.

Other behaviours

Other behaviours that may reduce risk of transmission of infectious agents to other people include the following:

- *Cough and sneeze behaviour*: patients with infectious diseases directly transmitted by droplet spread or airborne transmitted by droplet nuclei (e.g. patients with sputum-positive tuberculosis) should cover their mouth and nose when coughing or sneezing.
- *Avoidance of contaminated drinking water*: people suffering from dracunculiasis should avoid entering a source of drinking water if they have an active ulcer or blister.
- *Avoidance of vector bites*: patients with the vector-borne disease of African trypanosomiasis (sleeping sickness) with trypanosomes in their blood should prevent tsetse flies from biting.

◆ *Avoidance of donating organs or bodily fluid by certain people:* individuals who are infected with HIV or who have sexual and other behaviours that have placed them at increased risk for HIV infection should not donate blood, plasma, tissues, cells, semen for artificial insemination, or organs for transplantation.

Control measures applied to animals

A zoonosis is any infectious agent or infectious disease that may be transmitted under natural conditions from vertebrate animals, both wild and domestic, to humans. A detailed approach to zoonoses is given in the comprehensive work *CRC Handbook Series in Zoonoses* (Beran and Steele 1994). In the control of zoonoses many approaches are used that are applied to animals, including the following.

Active immunization

Active immunization, or vaccination, of selected animals may protect susceptible animal hosts from certain infectious diseases. This protection of animals, in turn, prevents susceptible humans from exposure to the infectious agent of those diseases from animals. An example of an infectious disease in animals in which some control can be achieved through immunization in selected animal populations is rabies. The reservoir of the rabies virus is varied and includes dogs, foxes, wolves, skunks, raccoons, and bats. Preventive measures include efforts to vaccinate all dogs.

Other examples of immunization of animals under certain conditions include: (1) immunization of young goats and sheep using a live attenuated strain of *Brucella melitensis* and calves using a strain of *Brucella abortus* in areas of high endemicity for brucellosis; and (2) immunization of animals at risk for acquiring infection with *Bacillus anthracis* that could be transmitted to man causing anthrax.

Restriction or reduction

Restriction is the limiting of the movement of animals and includes isolation and quarantine. Reduction is the killing, known as culling, of selected animals. Selective use of restriction of animals or reduction of animal populations that are infected, or potentially infected, with a zoonotic infectious agent are methods used to decrease or eliminate the opportunity of exposure of susceptible humans, or other animals, to such animals.

The example of rabies can also be used to illustrate the use of restriction or reduction of an animal population to help control an infectious disease. Heymann (2010) recommends the following measures:

Preventive measures

1. Register, license, and vaccinate all owned dogs, and other pets when feasible, in enzootic countries; control ownerless animals and strays. Educate pet owners and the public on the importance of local community responsibilities (e.g. pets should be leashed in congested areas when not confined on the owner's premises; strange-acting or sick animals of any species,—domestic or wild—should be avoided and not handled; animals that have bitten a person or another animal should be reported to relevant authorities, such as the police/local health departments; if possible, such animals should be confined and observed as a preventive measure; and wildlife should be appreciated in nature and not be kept as pets). Where animal population reduction is impractical, animal contraception and repetitive vaccination campaigns may prove effective.

2. Detain and observe for 10 days any healthy-appearing dog or cat known to have bitten a person (stray or ownerless dogs and cats may be euthanized and examined for rabies by fluorescent microscopy); dogs and cats showing suspicious clinical signs of rabies should be euthanized and tested for rabies.

3. Euthanize unvaccinated domestic animals bitten by known rabid animals; if detention is elected, hold the animal in a secure facility for at least 6 months under veterinary supervision, and vaccinate against rabies 30 days before release. If previously vaccinated, booster immediately with rabies vaccine, and detain for at least 45 days.

4. Cooperate with wildlife conservation authorities in programs to reduce the carrying capacity of wildlife hosts of sylvatic rabies, and to reduce exposures to domestic animals and human populations—such as in circumscribed enzootic areas near campsites, and in areas of dense human habitation. (Heymann 2010)

Epidemic (epizootic) measures

In urban areas of industrialized countries, strict enforcement of regulations requiring collection, detention and euthanasia of ownerless and stray dogs, and of non-immunized dogs found off owners' premises; control of the dog population by castration, spaying or drugs have been effective in breaking transmission cycles. (Heymann 2000)

Other measures

Other examples of restricting or reducing of animal populations include the following:

◆ Rat-proofing dwellings and reduction of the rat population to prevent rat bites that may transmit the infectious agents *Streptobacillus moniliformis* and *Spirillum minus* causing the rat-bite fevers of streptobacillosis and spirillosis, respectively.

◆ Rat suppression by poisoning (after achieving flea control) in rodent populations with a high potential for epizootic plague.

◆ Elimination of animals infected with *Brucella abortus*, *Brucella melitensis*, *Brucella suis*, and *Brucella canis* by segregation or slaughter to prevent brucellosis.

◆ Slaughtering dairy cattle that test positive for infection with *Mycobacterium bovis*, the infectious agent of bovine tuberculosis.

Chemoprophylaxis and chemotherapy

Chemoprophylaxis of an animal is using chemical substances (e.g. antibiotics) that prevent infection or its progression to clinically manifest infectious disease in the animal. Chemotherapy of an animal is using these chemical substances to treat an infectious disease in an animal. Both chemoprophylaxis and chemotherapy are control measures that may be used to reduce or prevent the opportunity of an infectious agent from being transmitted from an animal to susceptible humans. However, caution should be applied in the routine use of chemoprophylaxis in cattle, feed lots, and poultry farms that can promote the emerging of drug resistance and its associated problems in humans as well.

Psittacosis is an example of a zoonosis controlled by chemoprophylaxis or chemotherapy in selected animal populations. The infectious agent, *Chlamydia psittaci*, may be directly transmitted to humans from infected birds when the dried droppings, secretions, or dust from the feathers of such infected birds are inhaled. Imported psittacine species of birds should be placed under quarantine and receive an appropriate antibiotic chemotherapeutic regimen such as chlortetracycline administered in their feed for 30 days.

Another example is chemoprophylaxis in selected dogs at high risk of infection with *Echinococcus granulosus*. This infectious agent can be transmitted to humans through hand-to-mouth transmission of the tapeworm eggs from dog faeces causing echinococcosis due to *Echinoccus granulosus*, or cystic hydatid disease. Such high-risk dogs should periodically receive antihelminth treatment with a chemotherapeutic agent such as praziquantel (Biltricide®).

Control measures applied to the environment

Control measures applied to the environment are designed to interrupt the routes of transmission by which an infectious agent may be spread through the environment. Just as the routes of transmission are varied, so, too, are the control methods that can be applied. Control measures that affect transmission that can be applied to the host, agents, vectors, infected humans, and other animals are reviewed elsewhere in this chapter. Environmental factors may also have a direct impact on the host, agent, or vector. For example, low humidity may predispose to certain infections due to a greater permeability of mucous membranes in the host; cold, dry climates inhibit development of the infective larvae agent of hookworm disease; and higher altitudes and colder climates limit the mosquito vector.

The recognition of the relationship between disease and filth led to a sanitary revolution in industrialized countries that markedly reduced infectious diseases even before the arrival of the antibiotic era. Improved methods for storing and preserving food, better housing, and smaller families with a resultant decrease in the risk of infections at an early age all contributed to reductions in infant and child mortality rates.

This section focuses on general environmental control measures not mentioned elsewhere. Some of these methods, such as provision of safe water, have the potential to prevent several different infectious diseases and significantly reduce rates of disease in the community.

Provision of safe water

It has been estimated that some 783 million still lack safe drinking water in 2010 (WHO and United Nations Children's Fund 2012). Contaminated drinking water, sometimes the result of poorly designed or maintained systems of sewerage, may lead to the water-borne indirect transmission of such infectious agents as *Giardia lamblia* causing giardiasis, pathogenic serotypes of *Salmonella* causing salmonellosis, and *Cryptosporidium* species causing cryptosporidiosis.

Purification of water can occur though natural methods or human intervention. Examples of natural methods that contribute to water purification include the processes of evaporation and condensation, filtration through the earth, plant growth, aeration, and reduction and oxidation of organic material by bacteria. Purification of water for public consumption is conventionally done through such processes as coagulation of colloids by aluminium salts or with other techniques; filtration through such materials as coal, sand, or diatomaceous earth; and disinfection with such chemicals as chlorine derivatives. In special situations, boiling and distillation can be used for purification (Solomon et al. 2009).

Proper disposal of faeces

It has been estimated that some 2.5 billion people in the developing world do not have an adequate system for proper disposal of faeces with some 1.1 billion people practising open defecation (WHO and United Nations Children's Fund 2012). Infectious agents in faeces that may result in infectious diseases include poliovirus causing poliomyelitis; *Shigella dysenteriae*, *Shigella flexneri*, *Shigella boydii*, and *Shigella sonnei* causing shigellosis; and *Entamoeba histolytica* causing amoebiasis.

Infectious agents in faeces may be transmitted by the direct transmission route (including the faecal–oral mode), the vehicle-borne route (including water as noted in the previous section), and the vector-borne route (including the simple mechanism of flies carrying infected faeces on their feet). Public health environmental control measures to interrupt these routes of transmission by ensuring the proper disposal of faeces include the following:

- Appropriate on-site disposal through such means as properly constructed sanitary privies in rural areas with no sewerage systems.

- On-site disposal of domestic wastewater (such as use of septic tanks or cesspools).

- Sewerage systems with treatment of wastewater. Such treatment may include preliminary treatment, sedimentation, chemical coagulation and flocculation, biological treatment (such as activated sludge units and trickling filters), stabilization ponds, sludge management, and disinfection (usually with chlorine) of effluents discharged into drinking, bathing or shellfish-growing waters.

The importance of personal health-promoting behaviours of using toilets, keeping toilets clean, and hand washing after defecation are a part of control efforts aimed at the proper disposal of faeces.

Food sanitation

Food-borne infectious diseases remain a problem in both industrialized and developing countries. In the United States in 2011 alone, it is estimated that some 48 million people became ill, 128,000 were hospitalized, and 3000 died of foodborne-related diseases (CDC 2012a). Significant food-borne outbreaks and sporadic cases continue to occur due to such factors as the following:

- Contamination of meat, poultry, and eggs with infectious agents, including pathogenic serotypes of *Salmonella*, *Yersinia pseudotuberculosis* and *Yersinia entercolitica*, and *Listeria monocytogenes*.

- Contamination of vegetables, especially lettuce and leafy green vegetables, with the infectious enterohaemorrhagic strain of *Escherichia coli* O157:H7. Other outbreaks in fruits, juices, and vegetables have been due to contamination with hepatitis A and pathogenic serotypes of salmonella.

- Problems in food storage, handling, and preparation in commercial eating places and in homes.

- Larger and more centralized production and processing facilities, coupled with increasingly extensive distribution networks, which may result in transmission of infectious agents to many people if a commercial product becomes contaminated.

Industrialized countries have significantly reduced the transmission of some infectious agents through major public health programmes in food sanitation, including: (1) inspecting eating and drinking establishments, (2) inspecting meat and poultry, (3) improving shellfish sanitation, and (4) promoting adequate cooking, canning, and refrigeration methods. Some cities and counties have instituted restaurant grading systems based on inspection reports, including required public display of the restaurant's grade as a guide for consumers.

Examples of vehicle-borne indirect transmission of infectious agents through food that can be controlled though a comprehensive public health food sanitation programme include the following:

- Pathogenic serotypes of *Salmonella* transmitted by ingesting food made from infected animals or contaminated by the infectious agent in faeces that may cause salmonellosis. Methods of control—preventive measures: 'a) handwashing before, during and after food preparation; b) refrigerating prepared foods in small containers; c) thoroughly cooking all foodstuffs derived from animal sources, particularly poultry, pork, egg products and meat dishes; d) avoiding recontamination within the kitchen after cooking is completed; and e) maintaining a sanitary kitchen and protecting prepared foods against rodent and insect contamination' (Heymann 2010).

- *Staphylococcus aureus* causing staphylococcal food intoxication by ingesting food containing the staphylococcal enterotoxin. Methods of control—preventive measures: 'Reduce food-handling time (from initial preparation to service) to a minimum, no more than 4 hours at ambient temperature. If foods are to be stored for more than 2 hours, keep those that are perishable hot (above 60°C/140°F) or cold (below 5°C/41°F), in shallow containers, and covered.' 'Temporarily exclude people with boils, abscesses and other purulent lesions of hands, face or nose from food handling.' (Heymann 2010).

- *Trichinella spiralis* transmitted by ingesting raw or improperly cooked meat or meat products, mainly pork, containing infectious encysted larvae that may cause trichinosis. Methods of control—preventive measures:

1. Educate the public on the need to cook all fresh pork and pork products and meat from wild animals at a temperature and for a time sufficient to allow all parts to reach at least 71°C (160°F), or until meat changes from pink to grey, which allows a sufficient margin of safety. This should be done unless it has been established that these meat products have been processed either by heating, curing, freezing or irradiation adequate to kill trichinae.

2. Grind pork in a separate grinder, or clean the grinder thoroughly before and after processing other meats.

3. Adopt regulations to encourage commercial irradiation processing of pork products. Testing carcasses for infection with a digestion technique is useful, as is immunodiagnosis of pigs with an approved ELISA test.

4. Adopt and enforce regulations that allow only certified trichinea-free pork to be used in raw pork products that have a cooked appearance, or in products that are traditionally not heated sufficiently in final preparation to kill trichinae.

5. Adopt laws and regulations to require and enforce the cooking of garbage and offal before feeding to swine. (Heymann 2010).

Milk sanitation

Milk may be a vehicle for indirect transmission of such infectious agents as: *Mycobacterium bovis* causing tuberculosis, *Corynebacterium diphtheriae* causing diphtheria, *Listeria monocytogenes* causing listeriosis, and *Campylobacter jejuni* and *Campylobacter coli* causing *Campylobacter* enteritis.

Public health control measures to break the chain of transmission of infectious agents through milk include:

- Mechanization and sanitization of milking processes.

- Refrigeration of milk to inhibit bacterial growth.

- Pasteurization of milk through high-temperature short-time, batch, ultra-pasteurization, or ultra-high-temperature methods that help to kill any bacteria from the cow or others that may have come into direct contact with milk during the milking and handling process.

- Monitoring milk quality by testing for bacteria using a standard bacterial plate count, by testing for density of coliform organisms, and by use of the phosphatase test to assay for pasteurization.

- Periodically testing cows for tuberculosis and brucellosis.

The use of raw milk for human consumption may result in outbreaks. A study showed that some 60 per cent of dairy-related outbreaks reported to the CDC between 1993 and 2006 were associated with raw milk products (CDC 2012b). It should be noted that post-pasteurization contamination of milk may also result in outbreaks of milk-borne diseases.

Design of facilities and equipment

The design and proper maintenance of buildings, rooms, and equipment can help break the chain of transmission of infectious agents. Laminar airflow hoods in laboratory workbenches, ventilation systems in hospitals, and disposable intravenous equipment are examples of systems designed to reduce risk of transmission. Routine maintenance needed to retain the original design standards for control of transmission of infectious agents include: (1) replacement of air filters, (2) cleaning of cooling towers, (3) monitoring of positive pressure rooms and airlocks, and (4) replacement of in-dwelling peripheral venous catheters.

Examples of infectious agents whose transmission can be reduced through proper design and maintenance include the following:

- *Legionella* species, the infectious agents responsible for legionellosis, are usually transmitted through airborne transmission via aerosol production. Transmission of the agent from cooling towers can be reduced by periodically cleaning off any scale or sediment, routinely using biocides to kill slime-forming organisms, and draining such towers when not in use.

- *Staphylococcus aureus*, the infectious agent responsible for staphylococcal disease in medical and surgical wards of hospitals, can be controlled by enforcing strict aseptic technique, including procedures to change intravenous infusion sites at least every 48 hours and replace indwelling peripheral venous catheters every 72 hours.

- *Bacillus anthracis*, the infectious agent responsible for anthrax, can be transmitted, among other ways, through inhalation of anthrax spores. Proper design of industrial plants that handle raw animal fibres include providing facilities for adequate ventilation and control of dust, washing and changing clothes after work, and eating away from the places of work.

Other methods

In addition to the environmental methods of control of transmission of infectious agents already mentioned, the following are other methods, some specific and some general, that should also be noted.

- Improvement of housing conditions to *reduce crowding* (as measured by the number of people per room and not total population density). Reduction in crowding is a general measure that can reduce the transmission of infectious agents, especially direct transmission from direct contact or direct projection (droplet spray).

- *Improvement in working conditions* can affect the risk of infectious disease. For example, control of particulate matter by proper ventilation in occupations such as textile mill workers, metal grinders, and pottery factory workers can reduce inflammation of the lungs and thus decrease the risk of developing tuberculosis. Excessive physical exertion and the stress of exhausting work can also increase the risk of tuberculosis.

- Improved *irrigation* and agricultural practices and *removing vegetation* or *draining and filling* of snail-breeding sites can reduce or eliminate the freshwater snail hosts of such infectious agents as *Schistosoma mansoni*, *Schistosoma haematobium* and *Schistosoma japonicum* that cause schistosomiasis in humans.

- *Adequate screening* of blood, serum, plasma, tissues, or organs can break the chain of vehicle-borne transmission from such biological products. Examples include screening for hepatitis B surface antigen and HIV antibodies in donated blood to prevent transmission of hepatitis B and HIV, respectively.

- Installation of *screened living and sleeping quarters* and use of *bednets*, including bednets impregnated with a synthetic pyrethroid such as permethrin, can reduce exposure to mosquitoes infected with the infectious agents of malaria.

Control measures applied to the agent

Control of some infectious diseases can be achieved through means that remove the infectious agents from the environment or inactivate the agents. Physical measures (such as heat, cold, ultraviolet light, and ionizing radiation) and chemical measures (such as liquid disinfectants and antiseptics, gases, and chlorination) can be used. Examples of control measures applied to infectious agents include the following:

- *Cleaning* is the removing of infectious agents from surfaces through such physical actions as vacuum cleaning or washing and scrubbing using soap or detergent and hot water. Cleaning also helps remove organic materials that might support the growth or survival of infectious agents.

- *Cooling* may inhibit bacterial multiplication and some infectious agents, such as *Trichinella* cysts and *Taenia solium* larvae (cysticerci), can be killed by freezing temperatures.

- *Pasteurization* is heating to a temperature of 75°C/167°F for 30 minutes to kill pathogenic vegetative bacteria. It does not inactivate bacterial spores. Pasteurization is a commonly used process to help ensure safety of milk and to prolong its storage quality.

- *Disinfection* is the reduction or killing of vegetative harmful bacterial infectious agents outside the body or on objects. Disinfection may not inactivate all bacterial spores and viruses. *Disinfectants* are used to eliminate pathogenic bacteria from the skin surface and from contaminated inanimate surfaces and include: (1) alcohols, (2) halogens such as iodine and chlorine, (3) surface active compounds such as the quaternary ammonium compound benzalkonium chloride, (4) phenolics, and (5) alkylating agents such as glutaraldehyde and formaldehyde. *Antiseptics* are a class of disinfectant that can be applied on body surfaces; they have a lower toxicity than environmental disinfectants and are usually less effective in killing microorganisms.

- *Sterilization* is the complete removal or killing of all infectious agents in, or on, an object. Sterilization of equipment for surgery and wound dressings; parenteral administration of drugs, vaccines or nutrients; catheterization; and dental work are all important means of controlling infectious diseases by killing infectious agents. Sterilization can be accomplished through use of fire, steam (such as in an autoclave), heated air, certain gases (such as ethylene oxide), ultraviolet light, ionizing radiation, liquid chemicals, and filtration. The method of sterilization chosen depends on the type of equipment to be sterilized.

The use of sterilized *disposable equipment*, such as disposable needles, syringes, and catheters, has the potential to reduce the risk of transmission of infectious agents. However, it must be assured that such equipment is disposed of properly and is not reused. For example, disposable syringes cannot be properly resterilized because the plastic from which they are made cannot withstand the heat necessary for sterilization. Technologies, such as the single-use disposable needle and syringe developed for immunization programmes, help assure such disposable equipment is not reused.

Control and prevention programmes

The preceding sections have considered the issues and given examples of control measures for infectious diseases at individual, institutional, and community levels and the tools for control directed at the host, routes of transmission, and the agent. Control and prevention programmes using these tools must be developed according to a number of factors including: (1) the risk of disease; (2) the magnitude of disease burden (as measured by mortality, degree of disability, morbidity, and economic costs); (3) the feasibility of control strategies; (4) the cost of control measures; (5) the effectiveness of such measures (on current levels of disease and impact on future cases or outbreaks); (6) the adverse effects or complications of the control measures; and (7) the availability of resources. Public health planning for the control of infectious diseases must consider these issues to design optimal, evidence-based control and prevention programmes.

The tools of disease surveillance for recognition and evaluation of the patterns of disease can provide information on the risk and magnitude of disease burden to individuals, people in institutions, subgroups of populations, and the community at large. Establishment and maintenance of the infrastructure for surveillance, including a system for the reporting of notifiable infectious diseases and unusual events, must be a high priority.

Feasibility of possible control and prevention strategies must be assessed through operational research, pilot projects, or from field experience. The fact that a particular measure can help control a disease does not mean it can be applied on a sufficient scale to have the desired impact. The cost of control activities (in both human and material resources) can be assessed through costing studies that can also provide the data needed to conduct more rigorous cost–benefit and cost-effectiveness analyses. A costly measure, even if it provides a high degree of control for an infectious disease, may not be affordable to the society or reasonable to apply in the light of other less expensive alternative strategies. For example, use of sterile, disposable products may be more costly than reusable, sterilizable products. Effectiveness of control measures may be assessed through epidemiological studies to find out their impact on reduction in the incidence or prevalence of disease.

The availability of resources for prevention and control programmes forces public health planners to set priorities by taking into account all these factors and then designing programmes that have maximum impact within available resources. Planners have a responsibility to mobilize additional necessary resources by raising public awareness and generating political will. Effective communication of disease burden and the results achievable through well-managed and effective control programmes can be a powerful tool for advocacy. Ideally, communities or their representatives should actively participate in the planning, execution, and evaluation of public health programmes.

Prevention effectiveness is 'the measure of the impact on health (including effectiveness, safety and cost) of prevention policies, programmes, and practices. The assessment of prevention effectiveness is the ongoing process of applying evaluation tools to prevention practices' (CDC 1995). Recognizing that systems for assessing the effectiveness of prevention strategies (including prevention strategies for infectious diseases) are weak or non-existent in both developing and industrialized countries alike, the CDC has suggested the following objectives for prevention effectiveness activities: 'evaluate the impact of prevention, use results of evaluation research to establish programme priorities, and establish or apply standardized methods to compare the benefits and effectiveness of alternative prevention strategies' (CDC 1995).

The current situation of *international migration* of many people worldwide presents an additional complexity to the design of programmes for the control of infectious diseases. Pertinent issues include refugee camps, legal status of migrants in recipient countries, and temporary return migration. Public health officials must consider the most effective mix of combined control measures applied to the host, agent, and routes of transmission when designing suitable control and prevention programmes (Gellert 1993).

International commerce and transportation are important areas of concern for public health infectious disease control programmes, especially as the speed of travel has increased. The tools of control include such measures as:

◆ Spraying insecticides effective against mosquito vectors of malaria in aircraft before departure, in transit, or on arrival.

◆ Rat-proofing or periodic fumigation to control rats on ships, docks, and warehouses to prevent plague.

Specific international control measures relating to aircraft, ships, and land transportation for infectious diseases are detailed in the *International Health Regulations (2005)* (WHO 2005).

The challenge facing infectious disease control programmes is to design an optimal set of interventions at local, institutional, community, national, and international levels supported and accepted by the political leadership and the people to whom these measures are applied.

Eradication

A unique end point in the control of infectious diseases is that of eradication. Eradication is the cessation of all transmission of an infectious agent by extermination of that agent. To date, only one human infectious disease, *smallpox*, and one animal infectious disease, rinderpest, have been eradicated. The WHO World Health Assembly in May 1980 confirmed its global eradication some 3 years after the last naturally acquired case of smallpox in October 1977 (Fenner et al. 1988). The magnitude of this accomplishment is appreciated when one realizes that, in the early 1950s, it was estimated that 50 million cases of smallpox still occurred each year in the world, some 150 years after Edward Jenner had performed the first vaccination and wrote: 'it now becomes too manifest to admit of controversy, that the annihilation of the Small Pox, the most dreadful scourge of the human species, must be the final result of this practice' (Fenner et al. 1988). Rinderpest (known as cattle plague or steppe murrain) was an infectious viral disease of cattle and some other even-toed ungulates, that was associated with a high mortality rate. In 2011, after widespread vaccination campaigns, the United Nations declared the disease eradicated.

The goal of global eradication has been set by the World Health Assembly for two other infectious diseases, poliomyelitis caused by wild poliovirus and dracunculiasis (Guinea worm infection), the latter caused by the infectious agent *Dracunculus medinensis*. A high level of sustained political will, aggressively applied disease surveillance, and effective control measures are the required elements to achieve eradication of the infectious agents for these diseases.

Impressive progress has been made towards the global *eradication of poliomyelitis* since the 1988 World Health Assembly set the goal for its eradication. Polio cases have decreased by over 99 per cent since that date, from some 350,000 cases in over 125 countries to only 650 reported cases in 2011. In 2012, only parts of three countries in the world (Nigeria, Pakistan, and Afghanistan) remain endemic for the disease (WHO 2012c). Poliomyelitis control measures that will lead to eradication include the following:

♦ Achieving and maintaining high levels of routine coverage of infants with at least three doses of oral polio vaccine.

♦ Mass application of oral polio vaccine in countries where poliomyelitis is endemic through national immunization days, usually by providing oral polio vaccine to every child less than 5 years of age twice each year, separated by 4–6 weeks, and conducted during the low season of poliovirus transmission.

♦ 'Mopping-up' operations after the use of national immunization days has reduced transmission of disease to defined focal geographic areas, usually by providing oral polio vaccine house-to-house to all children less than 5 years of age on two occasions separated by 4–6 weeks.

♦ Aggressive action-oriented surveillance for acute flaccid paralysis. Such surveillance includes: (1) case investigation, (2) a laboratory network for isolation and characterization of polioviruses in suspect cases of poliomyelitis and people in close contact with them, and (3) limited outbreak response immunization providing one house-to-house round of oral polio vaccine to children less than 5 years of age living in the same village or neighbourhood of the patient.

Significant strides in the *eradication of dracunculiasis* have also been made. Over the last decade the total number of dracunculiasis cases has declined by more than 95 per cent. In 2010, fewer than 1800 cases were reported and, by 2011, the disease was limited to only certain areas of sub-Saharan Africa. Dracunculiasis control measures that are leading to its ultimate eradication include the following:

♦ Establishing a national programme office, conducting baseline surveys, and preparing and refining a national plan of action.

♦ Educating the population in endemic areas that the source of Guinea worm comes from their drinking water.

♦ Ensuring that people with blisters or emerging worms do not enter sources of drinking water through behaviour changes and by converting step-wells into draw-wells.

♦ Promoting the boiling or filtering of water through a fine mesh cloth to remove copepods. Treating drinking water with chlorine or iodine will also kill the copepods and infective larvae.

♦ Providing non-infected water through construction of wells or rainwater catchments.

♦ In selected endemic villages, controlling copepod populations with temephos (Abate®) insecticide placed in reservoirs, tanks, ponds, and step-wells.

♦ Implementing an intensified surveillance and aggressive case-containment strategy as programmes get close to achieving eradication.

The eradication of a disease requires a unique set of conditions, including the following: (1) a defined, accessible reservoir of the infectious agent; (2) affordable and effective control measures that can interrupt the chain of infection directed at the host, agent, or route of transmission; and (3) a surveillance mechanism adequate to monitor and ultimately certify the disappearance of the infectious agent.

It is likely that measles may be targeted for global eradication in the future. Some countries and geographic regions have already targeted measles for elimination—a term sometimes used to describe the eradication of a disease from a large geographic area. Other diseases that may potentially be targeted for eradication in the future include: mumps, rubella, hepatitis B, leprosy, and diphtheria.

Emerging infectious diseases

New, emerging and re-emerging infectious diseases have become a focus for the attention of public health prevention and control programmes in both industrialized and developing countries. Such infectious diseases have thwarted any expectation that infectious diseases will soon be eliminated as public health problems and resulted in a widening spectrum of diseases, many of which were once thought to be almost conquered. Krause has reflected on this as follows:

> Bacteria reproduce every 30 minutes. For them, a millennium is compressed into a fortnight. They are fleet afoot, and the pace of our research must keep up with them, or they will overtake us. (Krause 1998)

Many factors contribute to the emergence of new or re-emergence of those previously known (Lederberg et al. 1992; CDC 1994; Murphy 1994), including the following:

♦ Human *demographic change* by which people begin to live in previously uninhabited remote areas of the world and are exposed to new environmental sources of infectious agents, insects, and animals.

♦ *Breakdowns of sanitary and other public health measures* in overcrowded cities and in situations of civil unrest and war.

♦ *Economic development and changes in the use of land*, including deforestation, reforestation, and urbanization.

♦ *Climate change*, including global warming, which may extend the favourable habitats for vectors such as mosquitoes.

♦ Other *human behaviours*, such as increased use of child-care facilities, sexual and drug use behaviours, and patterns of outdoor recreation.

♦ *International travel and commerce* that quickly transport people and goods vast distances.

♦ *Changes in food processing and handling*, including foods prepared from many different individual animals and transported great distances.

♦ *Evolution of pathogenic infectious agents* by which they may infect new hosts, produce toxins, or adapt by responding to changes in the host immunity.

♦ *Development of resistance of infectious agents* such as *Mycobacterium tuberculosis* and *Neisseria gonorrhoeae* to chemoprophylactic or chemotherapeutic medicines.

♦ *Resistance of the vectors* of vector-borne infectious diseases to pesticides.

♦ *Immunosuppression of people* due to medical treatments or new diseases that result in infectious diseases caused by agents not usually pathogenic in healthy hosts.

♦ *Deterioration in surveillance systems* for infectious diseases, including laboratory support, to detect new or emerging disease problems at an early stage.

Examples of emerging infectious disease threats include the following:

- Toxic shock syndrome, due to the infectious toxin-producing strains of *Staphylococcus aureus*, illustrates how a new technology yielding a new product, super-absorbent tampons, can create the circumstances favouring the emergence of a new infectious disease threat.

- Lyme disease, due to the infectious spirochete *Borrelia burgdorferi*, illustrates how changes in the ecology, including reforestation, increasing deer populations, and suburban migration of the population, can result in the emergence of a new microbial threat that has now become one of the most prevalent vector-borne disease in the United States.

- Shigellosis, giardiasis, and hepatitis A are examples of emerging diseases that have become threats to staff and children in child-care centres as the use of such centres has increased due to changes in the work patterns of societies.

- Opportunistic infections, such as pneumocystis pneumonia caused by *Pneumocystis jirovecii* (formerly *carinii*), chronic cryptosporidiosis caused by *Cryptosporidium* species, and disseminated cytomegalovirus infections, illustrate emerging disease threats to the increasing number of people who are immunosuppressed because of cancer chemotherapy, organ transplantation, or HIV infection.

- Foodborne infections such as diarrhoea caused by the enterohaemorrhagic strain O157:H7 of *Escherichia coli* and waterborne infections such as gastrointestinal disease due to *Cryptosporidium* species are examples of emerging disease threats that have arisen due to such factors as changes in diet, food processing, globalization of the food supply, and contamination of municipal water supplies.

- Hantavirus pulmonary syndrome first detected in the United States in 1993 and caused by a previously unrecognized hantavirus illustrates how exposure to certain kinds of infected rodents can result in an emerging infectious disease.

- Nipah virus disease first detected in Malaysia in 1999 and caused by a previously unrecognized Hendra-like virus demonstrates how close contact with fruit bats and pigs can result in an emerging infectious disease.

- Severe acute respiratory syndrome (SARS), a viral respiratory illness caused by the SARS-associated coronavirus (SARS-CoV) that was first reported in Asia in February 2003 and spread to more than 20 countries in North America, South America, Europe, and Asia affecting over 8000 people and killing over 700 before the SARS global outbreak was contained in 2004, shows the need for continued vigilance in surveillance and outbreak response capacity.

- The emergence of the novel influenza A virus in birds, highly pathogenic avian influenza (H5N1), that has occasionally infected humans is an example of an antigenic shift in an influenza virus that, should it develop into a form easily transmissible from human to human, could potentially lead to a pandemic.

Antimicrobial drug resistance as a major factor in the emergence and re-emergence of infectious diseases deserves special attention. Although significant reductions in infectious disease mortality have occurred since the introduction of antimicrobials for general use in the 1940s, antimicrobial drug resistance has emerged because of their widespread use in humans.

Drugs that once seemed invincible are losing their effectiveness for a wide range of community-acquired infections, including tuberculosis, gonorrhoea, pneumococcal infections (a leading cause of otitis media, pneumonia, and meningitis), and for hospital-acquired enterococcal and staphylococcal infections. Resistance to antiviral (e.g. amantadine-resistant influenza virus and aciclovir-resistant herpes simplex), antifungal (e.g. azole-resistant *Candida* species), and antiprotozoal (e.g. metronidazole-resistant *Trichomonas vaginalis*) drugs is also emerging. Drug-resistant malaria has spread to nearly all areas of the world where malaria occurs. Concern has also arisen over strains of HIV resistant to antiviral drugs. Increased microbial resistance has resulted in prolonged hospitalizations and higher death rates from infections; has required much more expensive, and often more toxic, drugs or drug combinations (even for common infections); and has resulted in higher health care costs (CDC 1994).

Antimicrobial drug resistance has also emerged because of the use of antimicrobials in domesticated animals. For example, the use of fluoroquinolones in poultry has created a reservoir of quinolone-resistant *Campylobacter jejuni* that has now been isolated in humans.

An aggressive public health response to these new, emerging and re-emerging infectious disease threats must be made to characterize them better and to mount an effective response for their control. For example, the 1999 outbreak of West Nile fever in New York City and surrounding areas that, within a 4-year period, spread throughout the United States demonstrates how a viral encephalitis, initially classified as Saint Louis encephalitis and later confirmed to be due to West Nile virus, can reach far beyond its normal setting.

The WHO has outlined the following high-priority areas (WHO 1995):

- Strengthen global surveillance of infectious diseases.

- Establish national and international infrastructures to recognize, report, and respond to new disease threats.

- Further develop applied research on diagnosis, epidemiology, and control of emerging infectious diseases.

- Strengthen the international capacity for infectious disease prevention and control.

Emerging infectious diseases are addressed in detail in Chapter 8.17.

Bioterrorism: the deliberate use of biological agents to cause harm

Another unfortunate source of an infectious disease threat is the spectre of biological warfare or bioterrorism, especially in an age where terrorist acts are frequent events (Christopher et al. 1997). The 2002 World Health Assembly resolution urges member states 'to treat any deliberate use, including local, of biological and chemical agents and radionuclear attack to cause harm also as a global public health threat, and to respond to such a threat in other countries by sharing expertise, supplies and resources in order rapidly to contain the event and mitigate its effects' (WHO 2002).

The WHO recommends the following (WHO 2004):

◆ Public health authorities, in close cooperation with other government bodies, should draw up contingency plans for dealing with a deliberate release of biological or chemical agents intended to harm civilian populations. These plans should be consistent or integral with existing plans for outbreaks of disease, natural disasters, large-scale industrial or transportation accidents, and terrorist incidents.

◆ Preparedness for deliberate releases of biological or chemical agents should be based on standard risk-analysis principles, starting with risk and threat assessment in order to determine the relative priority that should be accorded to such releases in comparison with other dangers to public health in the country concerned. Considerations for deliberate releases should be incorporated into existing public health infrastructures, rather than developing separate infrastructures.

◆ Preparedness for deliberate releases of biological or chemical agents can be markedly increased in most countries by strengthening the public health infrastructure, and particularly public health surveillance and response, and measures should be taken to this end.

◆ Managing the consequences of a deliberate release of biological or chemical agents may demand more resources than are available, and international assistance would then be essential.

Many countries are developing rapid response capability to deal with such contingencies, especially in the light of the 2001 bioterrorist attack using anthrax in the United States.

Conclusion

Only through worldwide concerted action will the effort to control infectious disease be effective. We are now in an era where, as Nobel Laureate Dr Joshua Lederberg has stated, 'The microbe that felled one child in a distant continent yesterday can reach yours today and seed a global pandemic tomorrow' (quoted in CDC 1994). As Hans Zinsser stated over 60 years ago:

> Infectious disease is one of the few genuine adventures left in the world. The dragons are all dead and the lance grows rusty in the chimney corner… About the only sporting proposition that remains unimpaired by the relentless domestication of a once free-living human species is the war against those ferocious little fellow creatures, which lurk in the dark corners and stalk us in the bodies of rats, mice and all kinds of domestic animals; which fly and crawl with the insects, and waylay us in our food and drink and even in our love. (Hans Zinsser 1934, quoted in Murphy 1994)

Acknowledgements

Text extracts from Heymann, D.L. (ed.), *Control of Communicable Diseases Manual*, Nineteenth Edition, American Public Health Association, Washington, USA, Copyright © American Public Health Association 2008, with permission from American Public Health Association.

Text extracts from World Health Organization (WHO), *Public Health Response to Biological and Chemical Weapons: WHO Guidance*, Second edition of Health aspects of chemical and biological weapons: report of a WHO Group of Consultants, WHO, Geneva, Switzerland, Copyright © 2004, reproduced with permission from the World Health Organization, available from http://whqlibdoc.who.int/publications/2004/9241546158.pdf.

References

Beran, G.W. and Steele, J.H. (eds.) (1994). *Handbook Series of Zoonoses*. Boca Raton, FL: CRC Press.

Centers for Disease Control and Prevention (1994). *Addressing Emerging Infectious Disease Threats: A Prevention Strategy for the United States*. Atlanta, GA: CDC.

Centers for Disease Control and Prevention (1995). *Prevention Effectiveness: Making Prevention a Practical Reality*. Atlanta, GA: CDC.

Centers for Disease Control and Prevention (2011). Summary of notifiable diseases, United States, 2009. *Morbidity and Mortality Weekly Report*, 58(53), 1–100.

Centers for Disease Control and Prevention (2012a). *Estimates of Foodborne Illness in the United States*. Atlanta, GA: CDC. Available at: http://www.cdc.gov/foodborneburden/index.html.

Centers for Disease Control and Prevention (2012b). *Feature: Raw (Unpasteurized) Milk*. Atlanta, GA. Available at: http://www.cdc.gov/Features/RawMilk.

Christopher, G.W., Cieslak, T.J., Pavlin, J.A, et al. (1997). Biological warfare: a historical perspective. *Journal of the American Medical Association*, 278, 412–17.

Committee on Infectious Diseases (2012). *American Academy of Pediatrics: Red Book: 2012 Report of the Committee on Infectious Diseases* (29th ed.). Elk Grove Village, IL: American Academy of Pediatrics.

Feigin, R.D., Cherry, J., Demmler-Harrison, G.J., and Kaplan, S.L. (ed.) (2009). *Feigin and Cherry's Textbook of Pediatric Infectious Diseases* (6th ed.). Philadelphia, PA: W.B. Saunders.

Fenner, F., Henderson, D.A., Arita, I., Jecek, Z., and Ladnyi, I.D. (1988). *Smallpox and its Eradication*. Geneva: WHO.

Fine, P.E. (1993). Herd immunity: history, theory, practice. *Epidemiologic Reviews*, 15, 265–302.

Gellert, G.A. (1993). International migration and control of communicable diseases. *Social Science & Medicine*, 37, 1489–99.

Gorbach, S.L., Bartlett, J.G., and Blacklow, N.R. (eds.) (2004). *Infectious Diseases* (3rd ed). Philadelphia, PA: Lippincott Williams and Wilkins.

Guerrant, R.L., Walker, D.H., and Weller, P.F. (eds.) (2011). *Tropical Infectious Diseases: Principles, Pathogens, and Practice* (3rd ed.). Philadelphia, PA: W.B. Saunders.

Heymann, D.L. (ed.) (2008). *Control of Communicable Diseases Manual* (19th ed.). Washington, DC: American Public Health Association.

Immunization Practices Advisory Committee (2006). General recommendations on immunization. *Morbidity and Mortality Weekly Report*, 55, RR 15.

Insel, R.A., Amstey, M., Woodin, K., and Pichichero, M. (1994). Maternal immunization to prevent infectious diseases in the neonate or infant. *International Journal of Technology Assessment in Health Care*, 10, 143–53.

Joint United Nations Programme on HIV/AIDS (2011). *UNAIDS World AIDS Day Report*. Geneva: UNAIDS.

Kiple, K.F. (ed.) (1993). *The Cambridge World History of Human Disease*. Cambridge: Cambridge University Press.

Krause, R.M. (ed.) (1998). *Emerging Infections: Biomedical Research Reports*. New York: Academic Press.

Lederberg, J., Shope, R.E., and Oaks, S.C. Jr. (eds.) (1992). *Emerging Infections: Microbial Threats to Health in the United States*. Washington, DC: National Academy Press.

Mandell, G.L., Bennett J.E., and Dolin, R. (eds.) (2009). *Mandell, Douglas and Bennett's Principles and Practice of Infectious Diseases* (7th ed.). New York: Elsevier Churchill Livingstone.

McKibben, L., Horan, T., Tokars, J.I., et al. (2005). Guidance on public reporting of healthcare-associated infections: recommendations of the Hospital Infection Control Practices Advisory Committee. *American Journal of Infection Control*, 33, 217–26.

McNeill, W.H. (1976). *Plagues and Peoples*. Garden City, NY: Anchor Press/Doubleday.

Murphy, F.A. (1994). New, emerging, and reemerging infectious diseases. *Advances in Virus Research*, 43, 1–52.

Osterholm, M.T. and Hedberg C.W. (2005). Epidemiololologic principles. In G.L. Mandell, J.E. Bennett, and R. Dolin (eds.) *Mandell, Douglas and Bennett's Principles and Practice of Infectious Diseases* (6th ed.), pp. 158–68. New York: Elsevier Churchill Livingstone.

Plotkin, S.A., Orenstein, W.A., and Offit P.A. (ed.) (2008). *Vaccines* (5th ed.). Philadelphia, PA: W.B Saunders.

Scott, R.D., II (2009). *The Direct Medical Costs of Healthcare-Associated Infections in U.S. Hospitals*. Atlanta, GA: Division of Healthcare Quality Promotion, National Center for Preparedness, Detection, and Control of Infectious Diseases, CDC.

Siegel, J.D., Rhinehart, E., Jackson, M., Chiarello, L., and the Healthcare Infection Control Practices Advisory Committee (2007). *2007 Guideline for Isolation Precautions: Preventing Transmission of Infectious Agents in Healthcare Settings*. [Online] Available at: http://www.cdc.gov/niosh/docket/archive/pdfs/NIOSH-219/0219-010107-siegel.pdf.

Slaven, E.M., Stone, S.C., and Lopez, F.A. (ed.) (2006). *Infectious Diseases: Emergency Department Diagnosis & Management*. Red and White Emergency Medicine Series. New York: McGraw-Hill.

Solomon, S.L., Fraser, D.W., and Kaplan, S.L. (2009). Public health considerations. In R.D. Feigin, J.D. Cherry, G.J. Demmler-Harrison, and S.L. Kaplan (eds.) *Textbook of Pediatric Infectious Diseases* (5th ed.), pp. 3221–44. Philadelphia, PA: W.B. Saunders.

Wertheim, H.F.L., Horby, P., and Woodall, J. (ed.) (2012). *Atlas of Human Infectious Diseases*. Oxford: Wiley-Blackwell.

World Health Organization (1995). *Communicable Disease Prevention and Control: New, Emerging, and Re-Emerging Infectious Diseases*. No. A48/15. Geneva: WHO.

World Health Organization (2002). *Global Public Health Response to Natural Occurrence, Accidental Release or Deliberate Use of Biological and Chemical Agents or Radionuclear Material That Affect Health*. World Health Assembly Resolution, WHA55.16, Geneva: WHO.

World Health Organization (2003). *Communicable Disease 2002: Global Defence Against the Infectious Disease Threat*. WHO/CDS/2003.15. Geneva: WHO.

World Health Organization (2004). *Public Health Response to Biological and Chemical Weapons*. Geneva: WHO.

World Health Organization (2005). *International Health Regulations* (2005). Geneva: WHO.

World Health Organization (2008). *The Global Burden of Disease: 2004 Update*. Geneva: WHO.

World Health Organization (2012a). *Global Health Observatory Data Repository*. Geneva: WHO.

World Health Organization (2012b). *International Travel and Health*. Geneva: WHO.

World Health Organization (2012c). *Poliomyelitis. Fact Sheet No. 114*. Geneva: WHO. Available at: http://www.who.int/mediacentre/factsheets/fs114/en.

World Health Organization and United Nations Children's Fund (2012). *Progress on Drinking Water and Sanitation 2012 Update*. Geneva: WHO.

11.4

Population screening and public health

Allison Streetly and Lars Elhers

Introduction to population screening and public health

The concept of screening, with the active identification of a disease or pre-disease condition in individuals who presume themselves to be healthy but may benefit from early treatment, sounds easy and attractive. The presumption is that if this is done, the clinical course of the disease will be altered and prognosis improved. Unfortunately, the reality of screening is more difficult and screening programmes, like other healthcare interventions, may do harm (Raffle and Gray 2007). Unlike most other healthcare interventions, screening programmes are offered to individuals who consider themselves to be healthy and the harms caused by screening programmes are therefore particularly difficult to accept. Consequently, it is important to appreciate what the potential benefits and harms of screening may be, the conditions required for a cost-effective programme, and why the public may favour screening whilst policymakers may not. Public health scientists and practitioners contribute by providing and appraising evidence concerning the benefits and harms of screening, managing screening programmes, and informing the expectations of the public and other stakeholders. This chapter outlines the principles that underpin the development and implementation of screening programmes. It also provides a brief summary of screening applications at different stages of life.

Development of screening as a concept

Historical development

The potential benefits of screening were first demonstrated by the use of mass miniature radiography (MMR) for the identification of individuals with tuberculosis (TB), and became common in many countries after effective TB treatment became available from 1946. Subsequently, screening was considered for other chronic conditions especially in the United States, where a law on the control of chronic diseases and the availability of screening was passed in the late 1950s. Wilson from the United Kingdom worked with Jungner, a Swedish biochemist, to develop suggested criteria which should be met before a screening programme is adopted (Wilson and Jungner 1968).

In the past 50 years, professional attitudes towards screening have changed by the appreciation that screening also has disadvantages and should only be introduced for certain defined conditions and in carefully controlled circumstances (Holland and Stewart 1990, 2005). By contrast, despite widely quoted mishaps, screening has become much more popular with the general public. In recent years, especially in high-income countries, the population has become more health conscious and, with the growth of the Internet, knowledgeable about health matters. This has increased the demand for health interventions. A firm belief has developed that the earlier a diagnosis is made, the better will be the outcome. This belief in the efficacy of screening is fuelled through the advocacy of charities concerned with individual diseases, by private clinics and providers who may have good intentions but also a profit motive, and by some doctors and politicians anxious to publicize their belief in the value of prevention. Screening has become a commercial enterprise, in terms of the promoting as well as the supply of reagents and equipment. It has in some cases become driven by financial incentives to promote unproven tests and services, for example, in the form of mobile screening units in supermarkets. Governments are often willing to 'invest' in screening services, even at relatively high cost and with relatively small benefits, as, for example, in screening for breast cancer, in order to show that they care. Critics who advocate caution in particular instances have been undermined or attacked (Holland and Stewart 1990, 2005).

Concepts in screening

Definitions of screening

McKeown (1968) defined screening as 'medical investigation which does not arise from a patient's request for advice for a specific complaint'. This definition of screening may encompass: (1) research for the validation of a procedure; or (2) tests done for public health reasons, for example, to identify the source of infection in a food outbreak; or (3) as a direct contribution to the health of the individual. It is this last, prescriptive screening, which is now the most common objective. There have been a number of modifications of this definition since 1968. The UK National Screening Committee (2000) (now part of Public Health England) defined screening as 'a public health service in which members of a defined population, who do not necessarily perceive that they are at risk of, or are already affected by, a disease or its complications are asked a question or offered a test to identify those individuals who are more likely to be helped than harmed by further tests or treatment to reduce the risk of disease or its complications'.

Clinical practitioners commonly misuse use the term 'screening' when they systematically apply tests to their existing patients to detect evidence of elevated risks or early-stage complications as, for example, when diabetic patients are examined annually for signs of retinal disease or peripheral nerve damage. The term 'screening' is also used inappropriately when individuals are offered tests non-systematically, as when they are tested for infectious diseases. These approaches are more correctly termed 'testing' (Gostin 2000) or 'opportunistic screening' or 'case finding'. The term 'screening' should only be used when populations, or groups of people who are thought to be at risk, are systematically offered screening tests as in national programmes for cancer of the breast and cervix.

Benefits and disadvantages

It is essential to recognize both the benefits and possible harms of screening for individuals and populations (Table 11.4.1) (Chamberlain 1984; Raffle and Gray 2007). Questions of over-diagnosis and/or overtreatment are relevant to most population screening programmes. If thousands of tests are done, 'errors' are bound to occur and some individuals incorrectly labelled, particularly if programmes are not subjected to stringent continuing quality control. Such individuals may become stigmatized and anxious, while others are falsely reassured. Thus the ethics of screening are important. Cochrane and Holland (1971) emphasized that screening differs from most other forms of healthcare in that it is the healthcare provider who offers the intervention (often a test) with the implicit promise that undergoing this test may provide benefit. Hence, prevention programmes such as screening should only be introduced if they are likely on balance to do more good than harm to the particular population if the relevant principles and criteria are met. In many countries, national and professional bodies have published the tests and conditions for which screening must be justified, often with appropriate reviews. The United Kingdom provides a model approach in the form of the UK National Screening Committee, which is responsible for the review and ongoing assessment of screening. Equally important, but often done in a less structured way, is the evaluation and review of screening programmes throughout their life which may include the decision to stop an existing programme, for example, when the prevalence of a condition declines or alternative approaches to prevention are developed (e.g. human papilloma virus (HPV) vaccine for cervical cancer).

Considerations when implementing a screening programme

The criteria for introducing a screening programme provide a framework for ensuring that all the key issues are considered and appropriately evidenced. Many of the criteria are self-evident such as 'the condition being an important health problem' although there is an inevitable subjectivity to such criteria in terms of what is considered 'important'. Test performance and cost-effectiveness are two of the key criteria and these are discussed further in the following subsections.

Criteria for introducing a screening programme

Before the introduction of screening for a condition, certain basic criteria should be fulfilled. The widely accepted criteria proposed by Wilson and Jungner (1968) served as the basis for a more elaborate set listed in the UK National Screening Committee's Second Report (2000) (Box 11.4.1). Similar lists have been proposed by other countries and the World Health Organization (Andermann et al. 2008). These criteria require continuing review with advances in knowledge. For example, in the United Kingdom, recent amendments were made to take account of genetic screening (UK National Screening Committee 2000, n.d.) and there is currently a proposal to consider very rare conditions that might be detected in the newborn period, where the requirement to obtain strong evidence from randomized controlled trials (RCTs) is not considered ethical or feasible.

Consideration of the performance of a screening test

A key consideration listed in the earlier-mentioned criteria is the performance of the test. There are specific ways in which the performance of tests should be assessed before a decision to introduce screening is made. These are described in the following subsections.

Properties of screening tests

Screening tests must be applied to large numbers of healthy individuals, most of whom will be identified as screen negative. This means that screening tests must be evaluated in low-prevalence settings and not just in the high-prevalence settings, like hospitals,

Table 11.4.1 Potential benefits and disadvantages of screening programmes

Benefits	Disadvantages
Improved prognosis for some cases detected	Longer morbidity for cases whose prognosis is not altered
Less radical treatment which cures some early treated cases	Over-treatment of questionable abnormalities
Resource savings	Resource costs
Reassurance for those with negative test results	False reassurance for those with false negative results
	Anxiety and sometimes morbidity for those with false positive results
	Hazards of screening test itself, for example exposure to radiation

Box 11.4.1 UK National Screening Committee (2000) criteria for adopting a screening programme

Ideally, all the following criteria should be met before screening for a condition is initiated:

1. The condition should be an important health problem.

2. The epidemiology and natural history of the condition, including development from latent to declared disease, should be adequately understood, and there should be a detectable risk factor, disease marker, latent period, or early symptomatic stage.

3. All the cost-effective primary prevention interventions should have been implemented as far as practicable.

4. If the carriers of a mutation are identified as a result of screening, the natural history of people with this status should be understood, including the psychological implications.

5. There should be a simple, safe, precise, and validated screening test.

6. The distribution of test values in the target population should be known, and a suitable cut-off level defined and agreed.

7. The test should be acceptable to the population.

8. There should be an agreed policy on the further diagnostic investigation of individuals with a positive test result and on the choices available to those individuals.

9. If the test is for mutations, the criteria used to select the subset of mutations to be covered by screening, if all possible mutations are not being tested, should be clearly set out.

The treatment

10. There should be an effective treatment or intervention for patients identified through early detection, with evidence of early treatment leading to better outcomes than late treatment.

11. There should be agreed evidence-based policies covering which individuals should be offered treatment and the appropriate treatment to be offered.

12. Clinical management of the condition and patient outcomes should be optimized in all healthcare providers prior to participation in a screening programme.

The screening programme

13. There should be evidence from high-quality randomized controlled trials that the screening programme is effective in reducing mortality or morbidity.

14. There should be evidence that the complete screening programme (test, diagnostic procedures, treatment/intervention) is clinically, socially, and ethically acceptable to health professionals and the public.

15. The benefit from the screening programme should outweigh the physical and psychological harm.

16. The opportunity cost of the screening programme should be economically balanced in relation to expenditure on medical care as a whole (i.e. value for money).

17. There should be a plan for managing and monitoring the screening programme and an agreed set of quality assurance standards.

18. Adequate staffing and facilities for testing, diagnosis, treatment and programme management should be available prior to the commencement of the screening programme.

19. All other options for managing the condition should have been considered (e.g. improving treatment, providing other services).

20. Evidence-based information, explaining the consequences of testing, investigation, and treatment, should be made available to potential participants to assist them in making an informed choice.

21. Public pressure for widening the eligibility criteria for reducing the screening interval, and for increasing the sensitivity of the testing process, should be anticipated.

22. If screening is for a mutation, the programme should be acceptable to people identified as carriers and to other family members.

Reproduced from the National Screening Committee, *Second Report of the National Screening Committee*, Department of Health, London, UK, © Crown Copyright 2000, licensed under the Open Government Licence v2.0, available from http://www.screening.nhs.uk/criteria.

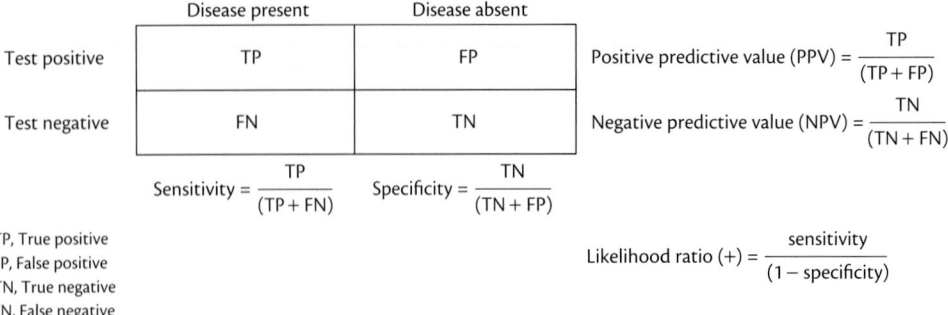

Fig. 11.4.1 Properties of a screening test.

where tests are often developed. Cochrane and Holland (1971) listed some desirable characteristics of screening tests including the requirement that they should be acceptable to screened subjects, safe, rapidly and easily applied, and not too costly.

The classification of individuals by screening test may be compared with the true disease status by a reference method or 'gold standard' (Fig. 11.4.1). Important characteristics to be assessed before any screening test can be considered for use in a screening programme include specificity and sensitivity. Specificity is defined as the proportion of disease-free subjects who are classified as true negatives by the test. Sensitivity is defined as the proportion of subjects with the condition of interest who are classified as true positives by the test. Ideally, both measures should be high. Clinicians commonly misperceive that high sensitivity is more important than specificity, in other words, a case must not be 'missed'. In reality, all screening programmes will 'miss' some true positive cases and specificity is as, if not more, important for an effective and acceptable programme because high false-positive rates can outweigh the benefits to the few true positives identified, with negative consequences for individuals who test false positive. In particular, if the prevalence of the condition to be identified is low, it is important to realize that if the tests were developed in a high-prevalence setting, such tests are often not piloted on large enough numbers of unaffected individuals to be certain of the specificity with the degree of accuracy (sensitivity) required.

The positive predictive value of a test is the proportion of subjects with a positive test result who have the condition of interest. The positive predictive value is determined by the relative proportions of true positives and false positives and, with sensitivity and specificity remaining constant, the positive predictive value depends on the prevalence of the condition of interest. When the condition is common, true positives will be frequent but if the condition is rare, true positives will be infrequent. Conditions that are sought by screening programmes commonly have a prevalence lower than 1 per cent, consequently the positive predictive value of a screening test will be low unless both sensitivity and specificity are extremely high (Table 11.4.2). In practical terms, this means that false positive results may outnumber true positive results, and the impact of screening on those who do not have the condition of interest is an important concern, as has been the case in the debates concerning breast cancer screening.

As an example, a mean cell haemoglobin (MCH) of 27 pg is used as the cut-off in the detection of beta thalassaemia. This was shown to have a sensitivity of 100 per cent in a sample of 6314 results with 104 carriers from two London hospitals that serve a

Table 11.4.2 Positive predictive values (PPV) at different values for sensitivity and specificity and disease prevalence

Prevalence	PPV (%) if sensitivity = 75% and specificity = 75%	PPV (%) if sensitivity = 95% and specificity = 95%
10%	25.0	67.9
1%	2.94	16.1
0.1%	0.30	1.9
0.01%	0.03	0.2

high-prevalence population (Wald and Leck 2000). At this prevalence, the positive predictive value in this sample is approximately 77.4 per cent. In lower-prevalence areas, the predictive value of the same cut-point was estimated to range from 1.3 to 30 per cent depending on prevalence (National Health Service Sickle Cell and Thalassaemia Screening Programme n.d.). Using HbA2 estimation, in combination with the MCH result, to increase the specificity of the testing procedure, resulted in important reductions in the workload associated with follow-up of screen positives without compromising detection rate. Another example is the detection of maternal alpha zero carriers (who could be at risk of a hydrops fetus), where use of a MCH cut-off point of 25 pg gives a positive predictive value, in a research setting with results validated against DNA analysis, of 1:424 with 100 per cent sensitivity. Use of the MCH cut-point in combination with a question about family origins to increase specificity gives an estimated predictive value of 1:3 or 33 per cent (12/36) (Sorour et al. 2007). Applying this approach in practice reduces partner recall from 1:61 requiring follow up to 1:1497 requiring partner follow-up (a 96 per cent reduction in partner recall). These examples show how important the predictive value is as a measure of the impact of screening test on programme workload. They also demonstrate that when conditions are of low prevalence attending to the specificity of a test is extremely important if staff and public commitment to a programme are to be maintained.

When screening tests, such as biochemical markers, are quantitative, rather than a binary classification, the cut-off point used to separate 'normal' from 'abnormal' may be varied. A low cut-off point will give a high sensitivity but low specificity. As the cut-off point is increased the sensitivity decreases and specificity increases. Thus, there is a reciprocal relationship between sensitivity and specificity. The area under the receiver operating characteristic (ROC) curve is used as a summary measure of test performance with the larger the area under the curve the better the test performance.

In general, the performance of a screening procedure may be improved by modifications that increase both sensitivity and specificity. This can sometimes be achieved by combining several tests together. Wald et al. (2003) compared combinations of two, three, or four biochemical measures in the antenatal detection of Down's syndrome. They reported that the 'double', 'triple', or 'quadruple' tests gave detection rates of 57, 62, and 70 per cent, respectively, while the odds of being affected given a positive result were 1:56, 1:52, and 1:45, respectively.

The likelihood ratio of a positive test provides another measure for assessing test performance. The post-test odds of disease are given by the product of the likelihood ratio of a positive test and the pre-test odds of disease. The likelihood ratio provides a measure of the relative increase in frequency of the disease in subjects who test positive compared with the untested population. The likelihood ratio of a positive test is given by sensitivity divided by (1 – specificity) (Fig. 11.4.1).

In summary, a screening test is not a diagnostic test. Instead, screening tests separate individuals into groups who have either a low or a high probability of disease being present. This is commonly misunderstood by members of the public who assume that a positive result is 'bad news' and a negative result means that 'all is clear'. This can result in considerable anxiety for the individuals who subsequently turn out to have a 'false positive result' if these perceptions are not addressed appropriately. A positive screening test result must usually be followed up by appropriate confirmatory tests to establish whether the screening result was a true positive, confirming the diagnosis and need for treatment, or more commonly that the result was a 'false positive' and the individual can be reassured. In addition, a good screening test will inevitably 'miss' some cases and this is difficult to communicate to the public and politicians and a challenge for committed professionals who often find this lack of perfection difficult to live with.

Cost-effectiveness and opportunity costs of screening

Screening programmes vary widely in purpose, process, and scope. Some population screening programmes are very costly, while others are relatively inexpensive. By definition, the implementation of any new population screening programme will require the allocation of scarce health resources—people, time, facilities, equipment, and knowledge—that could have been used for other purposes. The opportunity costs of implementing a new healthcare programme are the amount of health outcome forgone, for example, the quality-adjusted life years (QALYs) or disability-adjusted life years (DALYs) that could be gained by using the same resources on other healthcare activities instead. For this reason, explicit choices and prioritizations may be necessary. Evaluation, particularly health economic evaluation, seeks to inform decisions about the use of scarce resources in healthcare by estimating the 'value for money' of a programme (Drummond et al. 2007).

Different countries may apply slightly different criteria to evaluate the pros and cons of a population screening programme but it is generally accepted that screening should be cost-effective (Andermann et al. 2008). Therefore, the decision to fund and implement a new screening programme should be informed by a pre-assessment of the marginal costs and effects of the programme compared to the best alternative(s).

The assessment for the introduction of a new population screening programme is, however, perhaps the most difficult type of health economic evaluation for multiple reasons. Firstly, the evaluation typically needs to be over a very long time horizon in order to capture the full clinical benefits of the programme. Because screening and early detection of illness may change the clinical course of the disease in the future, it is often necessary to include clinical evidence with a long follow-up period and lifetime modelling. Differences in timing raise a number of methodological questions such as discounting and extrapolation which add to the uncertainty (see Chapter 6.6). Studies with such a long follow-up may also be planned and conducted in a time and place that is very different from the situation in which the population screening is eventually introduced. For example, the RCTs of screening for abdominal aortic aneurysm (AAA) were planned and conducted in a time when there was less international focus and action on reducing smoking rates, and changes in societal values and norms over time, which made it difficult to predict whether or not the same results from RCTs of population screening would be obtainable several years later. In the case of AAA screening, the United Kingdom's recent experience has been that AAA prevalence rates are much lower than expected and therefore the pre-evaluation assumptions informing the cost-effectiveness modelling were based on out-of-date and high assumptions about prevalence (Choke et al. 2012).

Secondly, a broad societal perspective of the economic evaluation of population screening programmes is often needed. This increases the cost of collecting data for the economic evaluation and may increase uncertainty. Screening is not just a test but a whole system of activities needed to achieve risk reduction. Depending on the circumstances, this may involve elective treatment, recovery and rehabilitation, and an increased need for health and social care which may not be in place either. The entire chain of activities may include several providers in primary, secondary, and social care. Analysts should also be aware of 'hidden' costs, that is, where the association between participation and costs in other sectors are not obvious. For example, an invitation to participate in a screening programme or a test result could make people anxious, and some may stay home from work or go to their general practitioner (GP) for advice or request for an extra health check.

Thirdly, the full costs of providing screening programmes are usually underestimated at the planning stages (Raffle and Gray 2007). For example, Ehlers et al. (2008) concluded in a review of health economic evaluations of screening for AAAs that most studies considered only short-term hospital costs at the cardiovascular department and employed a number of 'optimistic' assumptions in favour of AAA screening. Pre-assessments of cost-effectiveness of population screening programmes seldom include the costs of the quality assurance work needed including definitions of new standards, preparation of reports, inspections and external assurance schemes, coordinating bodies, and education. It is easier to assure quality of screening if the number of people involved is relatively small, and it is an exceedingly difficult task if tens of thousands of nurses and doctors need to have an up-to-date understanding of the programme, the technology, and the standard procedures. The requirements of the IT system, the procurement of equipment, and the maintenance agreements may also be very difficult to assess from scratch especially if the people involved in the implementation and pre-evaluation of the screening programme do not possess any prior experience in organizing population screening. Consequently, the costs of national screening programmes often turn out to be much higher than anticipated, especially if new care services require implementation or re-organization as well, or service gaps are highlighted which limit the benefits of screening. This was the case in newborn hearing screening in England which though effective in identifying screen positive infants, has struggled to achieve timely enrolment in care (Raffle and Gray 2007).

Fourthly, there are often strong beliefs in the value of screening. Researchers may have strong personal interests in starting new screening programmes and a systematic review of cost-effectiveness may additionally be affected by publication bias where only positive outcomes of screening are published.

Fifthly, results of cost-effectiveness studies cannot easily be transferred from one country to another. Whereas the evidence for the clinical efficacy may be transferable between countries with similar population characteristics, this is seldom the case with cost data. This is because of differences in the availability of healthcare resources, clinical practice patterns, and relative input prices. Disease prevalence and acceptability of tests may vary as well. Consequently, while a screening programme may be cost-effective in one country, this may not apply to another.

Finally, many cost-effectiveness analyses only compare hospital-based screening interventions with 'doing nothing', but this may not be the best alternative to population screening. There may be other approaches that represent a cost-effective way of addressing the same risk, or different ways of delivering an intervention. Furthermore, improvement science has shown that a 'knowing–doing gap' in current practice may be improved significantly through better health services management. Thus, an alternative to the implementation of a new screening programme may be improved case-finding or improvements in the healthcare pathway in the present system of care. If the randomized controlled screening trial is old, which it often is, then the comparator in the trial may not represent the best present alternative to a new population screening programme. In such cases, researchers should look for other ways to estimate cost-effectiveness. If costs and effects of screening are in fact compared to an inefficient organization, the calculated incremental cost-effectiveness ratio will be biased.

Despite the difficulties in performing pre-assessments of cost-effectiveness of screening programmes, a health economic evaluation can provide important inputs to local decision-makers on the expected 'value for money' of the programme and whether it should be started. This is preferable to not making a systematic attempt to quantify costs and consequences.

Ethics of screening

Lawrence Gostin (2000) observed that 'screening is far from a neutral scientific pursuit. Rather, screening is political . . . fraught with complex choices and weighing values—cost, efficiency,

autonomy, and justice' (p. 201). In view of this, screening must be viewed within its social and ethical context. However, the ethical framework for screening can be considered at more than one level. The traditional biomedical ethical approach, which primarily concerns the individual, is arguably not the most relevant one. Instead a multilevel approach is necessary to ensure that introduction of a screening programme is as consistent as possible with a given society's values. This section outlines some key ethical questions that must be negotiated if a screening programme is to be introduced.

At the *health system* or *societal* level, the implementation of screening raises questions concerning resource allocation and prioritization. Funding of any screening programme involves an opportunity cost of other healthcare services forgone. The criteria used to justify screening are generally oriented towards increasing efficiency, a utilitarian value of ensuring the greatest good for the greatest number, given available resources. However, the valuation of different outcomes may present difficult problems. For example, in Down's syndrome screening, it may be feasible to estimate the cost per affected birth prevented but it is difficult, and in some societies unacceptable, to weigh this cost against the cost of treatment and care of affected individuals.

There are also questions of equity because the proposed health benefits of screening may be differentially distributed to certain groups in the population. Some men's groups argue that since screening programmes are implemented to detect women's cancers, including breast and cervical cancer screening, fairness requires that screening programmes should also be implemented to detect cancers that affect men, including cancer of the prostate, even if considerations of efficiency do not support this. More generally, screening programmes may be used more by higher socioeconomic groups than lower-income groups and minorities. Screening, thus, has the potential to increase inequalities in health while improving the overall health of the total population. Screening outcomes, and inequalities in outcomes, should be important measures for quality assurance of screening programmes.

At the level of the *screening programme*, the selection of population groups to be screened, the choice of screening procedures, the value attached to different screening outcomes and the nature of available treatment services might appear to be purely technical issues, but these processes also raise ethical questions. A screening programme may be either universal or targeted. If a targeted strategy is chosen, there is a risk of stigmatizing the target population as being particularly associated with an undesirable health outcome, such as a sexually transmitted disease. If the target population is defined on grounds of age, as is done for breast cancer screening, then this raises questions concerning the 'right to health' of women who are either younger or older than the proposed age cut-off points. While efficiency arguments may favour a more focused strategy, considerations of equity favour a more universal approach (Sassi et al. 2001).

As discussed earlier, screening tests often have low positive predictive values and this means that there may be large numbers of subjects with false positive results and a smaller number of subjects with true positive results. Major benefits from screening are shared by a few true positives and these benefits must be balanced against potential harm to many false positives. As a minimum, this indicates an ethical requirement for adequate quality assurance to ensure the reliability and validity of testing procedures, the safety of diagnostic services, and the adequacy of information communication to screened subjects.

The selection of screening outcomes also requires careful consideration. This is especially true for screening processes that may impact on reproductive outcomes. The possibility of making a diagnosis before birth and giving parents an informed choice over reproductive outcomes appear to be positive developments. However, these processes may be viewed as related to the concept of 'eugenics' which literally means 'well-born'. It is often used to refer to movements and social policies influential during the early twentieth century and in a historical and broader sense, it can also be a study of 'improving human genetic qualities'. It is a social philosophy which advocates the improvement of human hereditary traits through various forms of intervention (Osborn 1937; Wikipedia 2013). Although introduced with good intentions, the concept of eugenics now has negative connotations that mainly date from the Nazi period from 1933 to 1945. Contemporary developments in genetics have increased the potential for genetic screening and testing.

Finally, it is ethically unjustified to initiate screening unless adequate treatment services are available to provide treatment and care for subjects identified through the screening programme. Hence those advocating for screening programmes must also advocate for investment in appropriate treatment services.

There are also ethical issues relating to the autonomy of the individual. Most screening programmes are voluntary and should be offered to individuals, enabling them to make an informed choice to participate in screening or not. In reality, as Gostin (2000) describes, voluntary population screening programmes are offered as routine interventions with limited opportunities for individuals to opt-out of participation. Family practices in the United Kingdom are performance managed against a nationally agreed target for uptake of cervical cancer screening and this target implies limited recognition of the scope for individual discretion in participation. Consequently, there has been increasing interest in the meaning, measurement, and value of 'informed choice'. Marteau and colleagues (2001) identified two components of informed choice which are incorporated into their proposed definition of informed choice as one 'that is based on relevant knowledge, consistent with the decision-maker's values and behaviourally implemented' (p. 100). According to this definition, choices are uninformed if subjects either lack good quality information or their attitudes are not reflected in their behaviour (Marteau et al. 2001).

What kind of information do individuals need to make an informed choice? The answer varies for different screening programmes. In antenatal screening programmes which may have consequences for reproductive choices and outcomes, it is particularly important that the potential implications of undergoing a screening test should be fully understood. In newborn-screening programmes, there is a move to expand the screening tests offered to include a wider range of conditions but the significance of information provided by screening varies for different conditions, making informed choice more difficult and impractical (Nijsingh 2007).

In the context of cancer screening, the potential benefit of screening may be communicated in terms of the 'number needed to screen', which is the inverse of the absolute risk reduction (Welch 2001). Rembold (1998) estimated that the 'number needed to screen' to prevent one death from colon cancer was 1374 over 5 years and for mammography, to prevent one death from breast cancer was 2451 over 5 years for women aged 50–59 years. From the individual's perspective, these statistics are not encouraging, however, understanding the limitations and the potential for harm from screening are equally, important (Welch 2001). More aggressive cancers are most likely not to be detected as they develop rapidly and so are often diagnosed by clinical services as 'interval' cancers between screening rounds. As screening tests typically have a low positive predictive value, a positive screening test may lead to more invasive procedures with potential negative consequences. Screening may identify abnormalities that might never have caused clinical disease, leading to unnecessary treatment, as exemplified by prostate cancer screening (Welch 2001).

The information required to inform an individual's choice to participate in screening is technically complex and wide-ranging. Consequently, there may be limited opportunities for truly informed choice in routine screening programmes. In democratic societies, it may be legitimate for the state to make decisions on the implementation of screening programmes through what the Nuffield Council on Bioethics (2007) terms the state's 'stewardship' role. It is through the stewardship role that states discharge their obligation to protect and fulfil their citizens' right to health. However, this should also include promoting citizens' capacity to make informed choices through better public education about screening. Helping individuals, who may have little understanding of the issues, to make decisions at difficult times in their lives should not be the sole or even main approach (Nijsingh 2007). It is usually more helpful to increase awareness of relevant screening issues before they plan families or are offered screening tests. Much more needs to be done to develop an educated public who understand screening programmes, and in particular more communication and understanding of the broader social perspectives relevant to screening rather than simply the technical issues of test performance if screening is to be successfully incorporated and accepted widely by communities.

Organization and operation of screening programmes

Challenges in implementing screening programmes

Introducing and sustaining screening programmes

The first step in implementing a screening programme should be a formal review of the evidence to evaluate whether this supports its introduction (Box 11.4.1). If this step is omitted, screening may be introduced by enthusiasts with testing diffusing into routine practice without formal evaluation. This is particularly likely to occur with tests that are not costly and have broad public support, for example, ultrasound in pregnancy. Even when there is good evidence to support such a programme, converting existing variable local practices into a standard programme across a region or country may be more difficult than introducing a new planned programme *de novo*. In general, a decision to implement a new population screening programme should be made at the national level to make sure that only the right programmes are introduced, properly implemented, and with consistent and coherent public and professional communications. It is important to avoid having a screening programme start on its own without coordination, standardization, and quality assurance as sorting out the resultant mess may be far more expensive and challenging than setting a national programme up correctly from the beginning (Raffle and Gray 2007). Furthermore, once a programme is in routine use, it can be very difficult to adjust or stop even if there is no evidence on effectiveness and strong indications of harm (Gray 2009).

The decision to introduce a programme must be viewed in the context of a particular time and place. This is illustrated by international differences in approach. For example, screening for toxoplasmosis in pregnancy is recommended in France but not in the United Kingdom because of the different prevalence and epidemiology of the condition in these two countries. Likewise, a screening programme that is considered cost-effective in a high-income country may often be unaffordable in a middle- or low-income country.

Temporal variations in the need for screening are illustrated by the example of antenatal syphilis screening in the United Kingdom. Syphilis declined dramatically after the Second World War, following the introduction of antibiotics to treat the disease. By the 1990s, there were calls for the antenatal screening programme for syphilis to be stopped. However, a 1999 review argued against this because of recent outbreaks of the disease. On the basis of this review, the decision was made to continue screening and rates of syphilis have increased since that time, albeit mostly in men who have sex with men and the cost-effectiveness is now arguably not supported (Connor et al. 2000).

Clarifying objectives of the programme

Clarifying the aims and objectives of the screening programme represents another important step, which should involve professionals, users, and the voluntary sector. A classic example of a well-meaning approach to introducing screening that miscarried was the US Sickle Cell Act of 1970. This was intended to help identify those with sickle cell disease and provide care for them. However, the programme was introduced without adequate public education or planning. As a result, carriers identified by the programme were stigmatized, sometimes being refused jobs or losing employment due to misunderstanding of the differences between the disease and carrier states. Ultimately, the public refused to be tested because of the negative impacts of testing (Anionwu 2001). An important lesson from this experience is that the public need to be well informed, educated, and continuously engaged if the implementation of screening programmes is to achieve the potential benefit and be well accepted with sustained support.

Defining the scope of the programme

Defining the scope of a screening programme should be considered prior to more detailed planning as otherwise some aspects of required service development may be omitted, causing difficulties later. In the United Kingdom, the term 'screening programme' is defined as 'the whole system of activities needed to deliver high-quality screening. This encompasses identifying and informing those to be offered screening through to the treatment and follow-up of those found to have an abnormality, as well as support for those who develop disease despite screening' (UK National Screening Committee 2000). A key criterion for the introduction of a screening programme is that 'clinical management of the conditions and patient outcomes should be optimized

by all healthcare providers prior to participation in a screening programme' (UK National Screening Committee 2000). For example, the introduction of a newborn hearing programme requires planning and development of a service of adequate capacity and quality in tertiary specialist centres. These aspirations have seldom been achieved by the time screening is introduced.

Planning implementation

Planning and implementing the programme should cover a range of aspects such as education and training and standardization of testing procedures. These processes require project planning skills and the overall coordination and sequencing of programme implementation is important. Clinical services may be overwhelmed if a screening programme were to suddenly start which placed significantly increased demands on them. Conversely, if services are set up and referrals do not occur relatively quickly, there may be disillusionment and disinvestment. It may be optimal if services experience some increase in demand early on but without overwhelming them. Professional and public education need time to implement and should precede public awareness campaigns in order to avoid difficulties for frontline professionals. The United Kingdom experience and approach to planning and implementation are discussed in detail by Raffle and Gray (2007).

Information systems

Adequate information and information systems should not be neglected in the planning and budgeting for a screening programme. Information systems are needed to manage the process of screening, provide fail-safe systems, and monitor and assist evaluation of the outcomes of screening programme.

A characteristic of an effectively delivered screening programme is that population-orientated fail-safe systems operate independently of the individual practitioners responsible for patient care. These systems should ensure that all those eligible are offered screening, that those with inconclusive, missing, or screen-positive results are followed up and managed appropriately. Problems with these processes should be rapidly identified and addressed. In the cervical screening programme a series of fail-safe actions are identified at the level of the call–recall system, the general practice, the cytology laboratory, and the colposcopy clinic that follows up cases requiring further management (National Health Service Cancer Screening Programme 2004). Screening programmes that do not operate such systems are unsafe and risk high-level failures of process with loss of population support.

Data derived from information systems are also important for quality assurance and in monitoring programmes' success against specified objectives in terms of population outcomes. Failures of process may be less visible in the early stages of the programme but may cause problems later on. In addition, without adequate information, it may be difficult to demonstrate the benefits of the programme and hence to maintain investment.

Quality assurance/improvement in screening programmes

Importance of quality assurance

Quality assurance and performance management should be integral parts of any organized screening programme, with the overall aim of ensuring that the programme achieves the potential health benefits while minimizing associated risks and harms.

The process of quality assurance

The term 'quality assurance' refers to the process by which the quality of a screening programme, in all its key dimensions, can be evaluated and improved. Variations in quality should be identified so as to actively correct problems or implement improvements. According to Donabedian (2003), a narrow definition of quality assurance requires the collection and interpretation of information, followed by making adjustments to the system. A wider definition includes processes of system design or redesign, linked to resource allocation so as to address problems, as well as including educational and motivational activities to modify the behaviour of health professionals. Quality assurance should be cyclical: moving from assessment of performance, to action, followed by review. Quality assurance has little meaning if it operates only as a monitoring and reporting cycle, in isolation from those able to make real changes and allocate resources to address problems. A well-developed quality management system should specify when and how any task is to be undertaken and by whom (Balmer et al. 2000). A named individual should be identified as responsible for the quality of each component of the screening process, with involvement of the whole organization to plan, deliver, and evaluate quality of services (Moullin 2002). Strong user involvement in the process is recommended. Service quality is dynamic and standards should be continually reviewed and tightened so that quality is maintained and progressively increased, particularly in response to rising expectations from patients. Communication is a key aspect of maintaining quality and good partnerships between service providers are required (Moullin 2002).

Dimensions of quality

The processes of quality assurance should address several dimensions (Donabedian 2003). *Effectiveness* should be enhanced so as to optimize the benefits or health gains from screening. *Efficiency* is required to ensure that the maximal benefits are obtained from available resources. The *equity* of screening uptake and screening outcomes should be evaluated to ensure that screening is accessible to all eligible groups and benefits are fairly distributed. The *safety* of screening programmes is important to ensure that errors are avoided and harms are minimized. The *acceptability* of the screening programme to the public and service users should be ensured. Standards for any programme should encompass each relevant dimension of quality.

Measuring and monitoring quality: developing criteria and standards

To successfully monitor the quality of a programme first requires determination of what to monitor. Clarifying the agreed objectives for a programme should be the first step, using the evidence that supports the introduction of the programme as a starting point. Following this, key priorities for monitoring should be identified including structures, processes, and outcomes (UK National Screening Committee 2003).

Raffle and Gray (2007) recommend defining the objectives of a programme to encapsulate what a 'good' programme should look like. Box 11.4.2 gives an example from the sickle cell and thalassaemia screening programme in England. A similar approach has been used in the United Kingdom for other programmes including

---

Box 11.4.2 Example of screening programme aims and objectives—NHS newborn sickle cell screening programme

Programme aims

- To achieve the lowest possible childhood death rate and to minimize childhood morbidity from sickle cell disorders.

Overall outcome to be achieved at national level

- Mortality rate in children with sickle cell disorders under 5 years of less than 4 per 1000 person years of life (two deaths per 100 affected infants) by 2010.
- To identify with specific sensitivity babies born with conditions where early intervention is likely to be beneficial.

Programme objectives

- To offer screening for sickle cell diseases to all infants.
- To process tests and report results in a timely manner.
- To identify and arrange timely follow-up of infants identified as needing further investigation.
- To ensure effective and acceptable follow-up, care, and support for affected infants and their carers.
- To ensure treatment is offered and parental education is started in a timely manner.
- To minimize the adverse effects of screening—including failure to follow up screen-positive infants, inaccurate or inadequate information, unnecessary investigation and follow-up, inappropriate disclosure of information and failure to communicate results to parents (normal and carrier).
- To ensure that responsibility, accountability, and performance management for all aspects of the programme are clear and that these link together from local to national level and between the newborn and antenatal programme.

Reproduced from the National Health Service Sickle Cell and Thalassaemia Screening Programme, *Standards for the Linked Antenatal and Newborn Screening Programmes*, Second Edition, NHS Sickle Cell and Thalassaemia Screening Programme, London, UK, © Crown Copyright 2011, licence under the Open Government Licence v.2.0, available from http://sct.screening.nhs.uk/standardsandguidelines.

the breast screening and diabetic retinopathy programmes. Once objectives are defined, ways of measuring their attainment should be identified, with specific criteria and standards developed for each. A criterion is defined 'as an attribute of structure, process, or outcome that is used to draw an inference about quality' (Donabedian 2003, p. 60). A standard is defined as 'a specified quantitative measure of magnitude or frequency that specified what is good or less so' (Donabedian 2003, p. 60). Criteria, therefore, cover the key dimensions of quality to be assured, while standards specify exactly what is to be expected for each.

Ideally, a baseline assessment of performance should precede and inform the setting of the screening programme standards. Standards may include both minimum acceptable standards to be achieved by all, and achievable standards that might be reached by the top quartile of programmes. Achievable or developmental standards target attainment in an environment of increasing expectations. The process of setting standards is iterative and continuous, requiring regular review, particularly in the early years of a programme. Once set, it is necessary to identify the interventions required to meet the standards, to monitor service delivery against standards, and for continuous improvement of services. Standards should also be based on an understanding of patients' requirements and expectations. Moullin (2002) recommends that standards should be realistic and achievable within available resources; service users should contribute to the development process.

The measurement of outcomes of screening programmes can be very challenging but is essential. Outcomes of a programme are generally assessed at national- or state-wide level, in contrast to the quality assurance process which is more useful for assessing the operation of a programme at a local or unit level. Table 11.4.3 gives an example of the outcome standards set for the newborn screening programme for sickle cell disease in England (National Health Service Sickle Cell and Thalassaemia Screening Programme 2011).

Different types of programmes and the different challenges in their organization

The challenges of screening are typically presented in relation to screening for cancer, although screening also covers infections, genetic conditions, and vascular conditions.

Infections
Examples include pre-conception syphilis screening as recommended in the United States; hepatitis B, rubella susceptibility, and HIV screening in pregnancy in the United Kingdom; and toxoplasmosis screening in pregnancy in France. The purpose of screening should be clarified as different actions and subsequent monitoring may be required. Screening for infection may identify susceptibility, as in the case of rubella screening that may indicate a need for immunization. Screening may identify past infection and sero-conversion, as in the case of hepatitis B and HIV, with potential benefits of intervention for the infant (hepatitis B) or both mother and infant (HIV) (Department of Health 1998). In pregnancy, there may be benefits either for the mother and/or the baby. Most of the benefits to the infant will be gained if infections, such as syphilis, are identified before pregnancy.

A specific problem of infection screening, such as HIV in pregnancy, is that a non-immune individual can subsequently become infected after a negative screening test. The same applies, for example, to screening of migrants for TB who are at high risk of reinfection due to environmental conditions. Screening may also fail to detect very recently infected individuals if the test is for sero-conversion. Screening may, if inappropriately applied as in the case of a meningitis outbreak, identify asymptomatic carriers of a particular organism.

Genetic screening as distinct from genetic testing
Developments in genetics have opened up many new possibilities for the diagnosis of a variety of diseases, but the same principles apply as for other forms of screening despite the historical tendency to 'genetic exceptionalism'. If genetic tests are offered, either there must be an effective intervention available for individuals found to be affected, or the information provided by the result must help the individual or other family members to make better decisions than if the information was not available. This section specifically considers the application of genetic tests to populations, that is, screening (for genetic testing see Chapter 2.5).

Genetic tests may be used in a variety of settings for differing purposes, including diagnostic testing, to confirm or exclude a genetic disorder in an asymptomatic individual, and predictive testing in asymptomatic individuals who have a family history. In most situations, genetic tests are applied to individuals known to be at high risk and hence, these are not defined as 'screening'. Examples of genetic screening at different stages of the life course include firstly newborn screening to identify *affected individuals* and start treatment as early as possible, for example, cystic fibrosis and sickle cell disease; and secondly, *carrier identification* to assist reproductive choice before birth of an affected individual and to identify couples at risk. Worldwide, carrier tests are

Table 11.4.3 Outcome measures for a newborn sickle cell screening programme in England

Outcome	Criteria	Minimum standard	Achievable standard
Best possible survival for affected infants detected by the programme	Mortality rates expressed in person years	Mortality rate in children under 5 of less than four per 1000 person-years of life (two deaths per 100 affected children)	Mortality rate in children under 5 of less than two per 1000 person years of life (one death per 100 affected children)
Accurate detection of all infants born with major clinically significant abnormalities	Sensitivity of the screening programme	99% for HbSS, 98% for HbSC, 95% for other variants	99.5% for HbSS, 99% for HbSC, 97% for other variants

usually offered preconception but they can be offered at any time up to early pregnancy and in high-risk groups to enable individuals to make informed choices. Well-known examples include carrier screening for thalassaemia (Bozkurt 2007; Cousens et al. 2010) or Tay–Sachs disease (Amato et al. 2009). For autosomal recessive conditions, if both partners are carriers, there is a one-in-four risk in each pregnancy of an affected infant and testing pre-conception offers a wider range of choices than testing in pregnancy.

Other ongoing developments in screening and testing which are likely to become more debated include non-invasive genetic tests of maternal blood (cell-free fetal DNA testing) (American College of Obstetricians and Gynecologists 2012). In some common conditions, preventive genetic testing may contribute to the identification of individuals at high risk; for example, *BRCA1* and *BRCA2* gene mutations, which can identify women at particular risk for developing breast cancer. Testing for *BRCA1* and *BRCA2* does not meet the criteria for a screening programme in populations at low risk of the condition.

Challenges of genetic screening

The Human Genome Project has raised public expectations of genetic screening but it is essential to appreciate the associated problems. The human genome has several million single nucleotide polymorphisms, and thus, the 'number of possible genetic associations is limited only by the rate at which laboratories are able to type these polymorphisms' (Colhoun et al. 2003). These difficulties are often neglected as is the fact that *associations* of a gene with a condition should be subjected to the same rigorous assessment as the findings of an environmental risk factor associated with a disease.

As with all screening tests, genetic screening may have psychological consequences, thus adequate counselling services must be provided. For common conditions, genetic screening is unlikely to be of great use in view of the complex interaction between environmental, behavioural, biological, and genetic factors. Its use is likely to be greatest in screening populations for a few clearly defined single-gene conditions. For example, its application has been followed by a reduction of rates of thalassaemia in a high-risk population in Iran, where treatment costs for those affected are considered unaffordable to the society and individual families who hence wish to have the option of prenatal diagnosis and termination (Samavat and and Modell 2004).

An issue arising with newborn screening programmes for both cystic fibrosis and sickle cell disease is that the methods currently used by programmes aiming to detect disease cases also detect the carrier state. In England and the United States, there has been a debate as to the merits of revealing carrier status to parents of infants at a stage where the child cannot make such a decision. In both, the view that has prevailed is that if the condition is identified as part of screening 'carriers should be reported to parents and follow-up counselling is offered to ensure understanding of the difference between carrier state and disease and also the genetic significance of the carrier state' (Human Genetics Commission 2006, 2011; Lin and Barton 2007). The UK Human Genetics Commission (2006) emphasizes that such decisions must at their core reflect societal views and not the views of technical experts. This is particularly relevant if preconception screening is not available especially now that preimplantation genetic diagnosis is more routinely available (Gøtzsche 2012). A second common problem, particularly relevant to newborn screening and carrier testing to identify couples at risk, is the potential to identify non-paternity. This underscores the importance of public education and awareness about such programmes starting with secondary school-aged children.

Governance of screening programmes

Population screening programmes should generally adhere to the principles of good governance described in Chapter 6.8, such as the rule of law, transparency, responsiveness, consensus orientation, equity and inclusiveness, effectiveness and efficacy, and accountability. There are, however, a number of inherent dilemmas and conflicts of interests in the governance of population screening that necessitate separation of responsibilities and authority between the national level, the regional/local level, and third-party inspection roles.

Public expectations of screening (including the media) are usually very high and there is a poor understanding that screening cannot detect all cases of illness and may cause harm. Examples of lawsuits against responsible physicians and 'scandals' reported in the media threaten to reduce transparency and accountability because health workers also have a need to protect themselves against wrongful accusations. Handling of the media and communication of evidence about what a screening programme should and should not be expected to deliver are better performed at the national than the local level. Inspections of the quality are more likely to establish trust if they are done by a third party than by those doing the screening. In cases where the public and media threaten to drive increases in sensitivity to avoid missed cases, external controls may be a more efficient way to guard against overdiagnosis and overtreatment.

Conflicts of interest may also arise in decisions to start, expand, contract, or stop a screening programme. Local physicians may have personal interests in starting and expanding programmes for research, financial, or other private reasons. Local agencies may be seeking to maximize their budgets or enlarge their staffing, and these conflict with the principles of effectiveness and efficacy. Companies with a market interest and other interest groups such as patient organizations cannot be expected to provide a truly balanced view and may threaten the consensus-oriented principle of doing the most beneficial thing with scarce resources. Even scientific societies may be biased towards screening because they also represent local interests in the matter. For these reasons, a decision to start screening should be taken at a national level and definition of standards, clinical guidelines, and quality assurance should not solely be a local matter.

Evaluating, restricting, and stopping existing programmes

Evaluation of ongoing screening programmes should be part of their oversight. It should be performed regularly using the same stringent framework to ensure that the programme is performing and delivering the outcomes expected of it, and that it still represents the best use of scarce healthcare resources. This requires a commitment to the collation of data and external independent review.

National health authorities may over time wish to restrict or stop existing screening programmes for a number of different reasons: some screening programmes may have started haphazardly without a national decision based on solid evidence. In a for-profit health system there is a market for all kinds of tests even without proven effect. Private insurance companies selling whole-body computed tomography scans or routine periodic health examinations are examples. In public healthcare systems, the use of inexpensive and easily accessible tests may also turn into de facto screening programmes driven by public demand, commercial, or private interests. If, later on, new research evidence show a lack of benefits and/or serious adverse events it will be necessary to restrict or stop the screening activities.

The balance between the good and harm may also change over time. Even if the introduction of a screening programme was initially based on a national decision supported by solid evidence, and even if the programme was carefully designed and piloted and nationally coordinated the programme may eventually grow beyond its optimal size. If programme activities are over-resourced, screening may be performed too often or in too many subgroups. As more resources are invested in a screening programme the law of diminishing returns prevails. The extra benefits obtained from screening decrease disproportionately with increased harm, and after a certain point of time, the net health gain starts to decline. Thus, overinvestments need to be withdrawn and the scope of the programme reduced to its optimal size (Donabedian 2003; Gray 2009).

Other factors such as changes in epidemiology or costs, technological developments, new research findings, or knowledge of alternative ways of preventing disease (or reducing risks) may change the opportunity costs of the programme. Funding shortages may also call for restricting or stopping existing activities. Once a screening programme is implemented, however, it may be extremely difficult to stop or restrict the scope even if it bears no provable health benefits and does harm (Raffle and Gray 2007). For example, in Denmark, it took 20 years after TB was eradicated before TB stations were closed down and before a large company like the Carlsberg breweries stopped mandatory chest X-rays for all newly employed personnel. In all those years, the screening activities were more harmful than beneficial as X-rays carry a small risk of inducing cancer (Gøtzsche 2012).

Experience shows that it may take years to stop harmful screening practices (Raffle and Gray 2007). Many politicians support screening because they feel the need for 'doing something', and screening may intuitively seem worthwhile to most people. Screening programmes can be strongly supported by advocacy groups, interest groups, or commercial interests. Raffle and Gray (2007) describe what they call the popularity paradox that the greater the harm through overdiagnosis and overtreatment from screening, the more people there are who believe they owe their health, or even their life, to the programme. Reducing or stopping screening activities can only be done through governmental intervention and only if there is an organizational and political governance structure that enables and facilitates such decisions. For example, the Japanese child neuroblastoma screening programme started in 1985. After an international panel in 1990 concluded that screening did not reduce mortality but resulted in harm, a national committee under the Ministry of Health, Labour and Welfare reviewed the policy and stopped the programme in 2004.

The Japanese media was generally supportive of the Government's recommendation. There was widespread public awareness about the pitfalls of cancer screening. There was little demand among parents (due to limited knowledge of neuroblastoma) and, perhaps most importantly, no advocacy groups in favour of screening (Raffle and Gray 2007).

Formal evaluations of existing screening programmes are a key tool for stopping or restricting screening programmes and for continuous improvements in their operations. A clear distinction should be made, however, between regular evaluations of the operation of a programme and independent (external) critical and research-based evaluation of a screening programme suspected of producing more harm than good. The first is part of an ongoing process of review and quality improvement while the latter serves as an input to deciding whether or not to restrict or stop an activity. Both types of evaluations are costly but necessary. The costs of not doing both types of evaluations are the human and financial costs of potential harmful and ineffective screening.

Formal evaluations of the operation of ongoing screening programmes should be performed regularly. A stringent framework should be applied to ensure that the programme is performing and delivering the outcomes expected cost-effectively. The same criteria that should be met before screening is initiated should also be met when the programme is up and running. The programme should adopt the principles of good governance and performance according to the highest possible quality standards. It is also important to ensure that relevant data on the epidemiology, test performance, and outcomes are collected from the outset. Evaluation of ongoing programmes should be seen as an important supplement to short-term performance reporting of process measures as they may provide important information that lead to changes in the policies or practices, or uncover problems that require more research. This type of evaluation, however, can probably never lead to programmes being closed down.

There should be an independent national body to commission and/or grant new research to secure formal independent external evaluation of existing programmes whenever needed. Depending on the circumstances this may be done on a regular basis, for example, every fifth year or on an ad hoc basis. Such independent evaluations should be performed with the explicit aim to investigate whether or not the programme should be restricted, expanded, or stopped. Research-based evaluations are able to provide good input to a decision whether or not to stop or restrict a programme only if researchers are truly independent, unbiased, and professional. For example, Gøtzsche (2012) describes the need for independent reviews of national breast screening programmes (especially in woman aged over 40) and explains how, in an environment dominated by powerful people in favour of screening, it may be almost impossible to establish truly independent evaluation committees. Furthermore, where professionals are convinced of the benefits from screening, this may hinder necessary research. Quality assurance and regular formal evaluations will not automatically ensure that harmful screening programmes will be stopped. While continuous quality assurance can reveal that certain policies or activities within the programme should be changed, these are performed by the professionals working in the programme and who are all, presumably, convinced of the net benefits of screening. Stopping the programme will probably never be considered a real option.

Healthcare systems should therefore have the capacity for independent critical evaluations performed by unbiased research units. Such evaluations can be done anonymously to avoid legal accusations and other reprisals from those who strongly favour screening. However, it is important for independent researchers to be engaged directly with policymakers (and advocacy coalitions) to influence agenda setting and prepare a way for changing current practices (Gibson 2003; Buse et al. 2009).

An example where evaluation of an ongoing screening programme is crucial is cervical cancer screening, where new HPV immunization programmes are predicted to reduce the number of screen-detected cases. If the immunization programme is effective, it will gradually reduce the need for screening and, at some point, decisions will need to be made about scaling down or perhaps even stopping population screening.

Screening at different stages of life

This section provides a brief summary of debates concerning screening at different stages of life.

Antenatal and newborn screening

One of the most comprehensive reviews on appropriate procedures in the antenatal and neonatal period was published by Wald and Leck (2000). Screening during this period has been shown to be of particular importance and been used longest. Even so, many questions remain. Recommendations in the United Kingdom for antenatal screening include Down's and fetal anomalies, thalassaemia and sickle cell disease, infectious disease (HIV, hepatitis B, syphilis). Conditions not recommended for antenatal screening include: group B *Streptococcus*, *Cytomegalovirus*, *Chlamydia*, hepatitis B, HTLV1 toxoplasmosis, domestic violence, and pre-eclampsia.

Newborn screening

Screening of newborn infants consists of routine biochemical tests on an infant's blood spot and physical examination including testing for hearing impairment. In the United Kingdom, current recommendations are for testing for phenylketonuria, congenital hypothyroidism, cystic fibrosis, sickle cell disease, and medium chain acyl-CoA dehydrogenase deficiency with a proposal to introduce three more conditions. Physical examination is usually performed in the first year of life, seeking signs of congenital heart disease, congenital cataract, cryptorchidism, congenital dislocation or developmental dysplasia of the hip, as well as other congenital malformations. The latter has been controversial, but evidence of the effectiveness of ultrasound screening is now accumulating. A national screening programme for hearing impairment has been implemented in the United Kingdom.

Screening in childhood

Screening in childhood is important, both to follow up findings from the neonatal period and to identify remediable defects or problems. A large number of bodies recommend a variety of procedures at different stages. Screening for hearing, visual impairment, and congenital hip displacement is straightforward, but there is also a need to identify children from disadvantaged households who are at particular risk of developing both physical and behavioural impairments which are often neglected.

Screening in adolescence

The major need at this stage is to build on the findings of the schoolchild examinations and provide confidential accessible health services to aid the adolescent to confront and deal with such problems as fertility and sex, drugs, and alcohol use. All opportunities should be taken to educate the adolescent on healthy living, personal safety, nutrition, exercise, and so on. Only opportunistic testing (rather than screening) is recommended for *Chlamydia trachomatis*, a common, curable sexually transmitted infection which is often asymptomatic but can lead to life-threatening ectopic pregnancy, pelvic inflammatory disease, and infertility. Some areas such as Montreal, Australia, and Rome, have introduced school education followed by the offer of carrier testing for relatively common recessively inherited conditions. Due to the burden of disease, many countries also offer various forms of pre-marital testing, most notably in Cyprus for thalassaemia major (Bozkurt 2007; Cousens et al. 2010).

Screening in adults

Screening in adults is big business. Media interest in health is insatiable and politicians have capitalized on public expectations and beliefs that 'prevention is better than cure'. It is therefore essential to critically consider the benefits and disadvantages of screening procedures.

Cancer

As the second largest cause of mortality in high-income countries, cancer is potentially an important area of health benefit. Specific problems for cancer screening are 'length-time' and 'lead-time' biases. Length-time bias refers to the fact that screening is most effective at detecting slow developing cancers which are less likely to be the cause of an individual's death but by detection can cause considerable anxiety. More aggressive tumours are likely to develop rapidly in the intervals between screening rounds. Lead-time bias refers to the problem for evaluation of programmes that detect cancers earlier than would have been the case with symptomatic screening and may thus appear to lengthen the time from diagnosis to survival when there is no true change in natural course or treatments which may even shorten life expectancy.

Breast cancer

The major trials of breast cancer screening have been done in the United States (Shapiro et al. 1982) and Sweden (Taban et al. 1985, 1989). Other trials were done in the United Kingdom, which before introducing a national scheme of breast cancer screening, had a major public enquiry (Forrest 1987). Screening for breast cancer is a highly emotive subject which has been the subject of very critical analysis (Gøtzsche et al. 2012). Under research conditions, as in the two original studies, there is a reduction in breast cancer mortality following mammographic screening. The reduction in total mortality in the test group is not so marked and the benefits in practice are smaller. There are arguments about which age range of women should be included in the scheme, the methods of mammography, the interval between repeat screening, and the interpretation of mammograms. There is no doubt that for the scheme to be effective, there needs to be good organization, careful quality control of both mammography and the subsequent breast biopsy, as well as good specialized treatment services including surgery, radiotherapy, and chemotherapy. The scheme, if properly executed, is costly, and critics suggest that the resources could be better used on clinical breast cancer treatment services. The major problems with the services are poor information to participants, increased anxiety in those screened, particularly the false positives, side effects from the biopsy, and the risks of radiation exposure. The most recent UK review (The Independent UK Panel of Breast Cancer Screening 2012) continues to recommend screening 50–70-year-old women every 3 years. In view of the popularity of breast cancer screening, it would be a daring policymaker who would suggest that the scheme should cease.

Cervical cancer

A programme of screening was first proposed in the mid 1960s. The original scheme was wasteful, including any woman attending any gynaecological service or family planning. In the United Kingdom, since 1998, the service has been re-launched on the basis of a call–recall system based on the GP patient register. Women are first invited at the age of 25 years and then recalled every 3 years until age 50 when the interval is increased to 5 years. About 80 per cent of the eligible women are screened, comparable to breast cancer screening coverage. Although mortality from cervical cancer has fallen considerably, it required an enormous effort. Raffle (2004), in an analysis of screening records of 348,419 women in Bristol, calculated that 1000 women need to be screened for 35 years to prevent one death, over 80 per cent of women with high-grade cervical intra-epithelial neoplasia will not develop invasive cancer but all will need to be treated, and for each death that is prevented, over 150 women have an abnormal result, over 80 women are referred for investigation, and over 50 women receive treatment.

The original test method of cytological examination has been superseded by liquid-based cytological examination and now by HPV culture which allows automation. In future, cervical cancer prevention through screening may be superseded by the HPV vaccination which is now introduced for girls aged 13 years in the United Kingdom and for boys and girls in Australia.

Colorectal cancer

A number of studies have shown that early detection by screening can reduce mortality (Hardcastle et al. 1996; Kronborg et al. 1996). As a result, screening for individuals aged over 50 years has now been introduced in the United Kingdom. Individuals are mailed a filter paper to be returned to the centre for faecal occult blood testing (FOBT). If the screening test is positive, then a colonoscopy and/or double-contrast barium enema is performed. Some advocate flexible sigmoidoscopy as an alternative before these procedures. It is suggested that the screening tests are done at 5-yearly intervals. Some authorities advocate screening by colonoscopy.

Prostate cancer

Although a biochemical screening test—prostate specific antigen (PSA)—and digital rectal examination and transrectal ultrasound are available, confirmation by biopsy is essential.

Prostate cancer is one of the commonest cancers in men, particularly the elderly. It has therefore become a 'cause celebre' in screening arguments advocated strongly by many groups, particularly prostate charities, male advocacy groups, and commerce. It has been the subject of intense argument and review. Although it is common, many more men die with the cancer than of it (Martin 2007). Many studies have not shown any evidence that mortality is reduced or postponed if screening is undertaken in asymptomatic individuals. With present knowledge, there is no case for screening well individuals but those with prostate symptoms of frequency nocturia, inadequate voiding, etc. should be investigated and it should be noted that this is an area of very active research.

Type 2 diabetes and diabetic retinopathy

Type 2 diabetes is common but there are divided views about the usefulness of screening for it. Wareham and Griffin (2001) do not advocate universal screening. The UK National Screening Committee also does not consider population screening worthwhile. Diabetic eye disease is the most common cause of preventable visual loss in the UK working population. Different methods of screening for diabetic retinopathy are available and have been evaluated (Squirrel and Talbot 2003). These use retinal photography and screening by optometrists. They are certainly worthwhile, but must be subject to stringent quality control and audit. They are quite difficult to establish satisfactorily although a successful programme has been implemented in the United Kingdom, but there remain challenges reaching those most likely to benefit from screening (Forster et al. 2013).

Cardiovascular disease

There is an ongoing debate regarding the merits of screening for cardiovascular disease (this includes coronary heart, disease, stroke, and AAA). The main risk factors for these conditions (smoking, raised cholesterol, lack of exercise, overweight, and hypertension) are very common in Western populations. Approaches to risk reduction in the whole population have been advocated instead of screening as being the most cost-effective. In the United Kingdom, a whole-population systematic approach to case finding has been introduced. This aims to help prevent heart disease, stroke, diabetes, kidney disease, and certain types of dementia by offering a check to assess the individual's risk of heart disease, stroke, kidney disease, and diabetes and to give support and advice to help them reduce or manage that risk (NHS Health Check 2014). Evidence of the benefits of AAA screening is demonstrated for areas with higher prevalence of the condition (Elhers et al. 2008).

Mental illness

Depression is the third commonest reason for consultation in general practice in England. A variety of questionnaires have been proposed for screening for this condition but none have met the criteria for an effective instrument. Arrol et al. (2003) in New Zealand found two questions—'During the past month, have you often been bothered by feeling down, depressed or hopeless?' and 'During the past month, have you often been bothered by little interest or pleasure in doing things?'—detected most cases of depression. There is a case for opportunistic screening for depression using such a simple questionnaire in general practice. There do not appear to be appropriate indications for screening for other mental conditions or personality disorders, alcohol misuse, or domestic violence.

Screening in the elderly

This is an important issue in view of the increasing proportion of the elderly in many societies. Scientific evidence of the benefits of screening in this age group is sparse.

In a randomized controlled 3-year trial in Denmark, Hendricksen et al. (1984, 1989) showed reduced mortality resulting from a programme of 3-monthly home visits that improved the provision of home help, equipment, and modifications to the home. The costs incurred were offset by savings, which were twice as great, from reductions in hospital nursing home care.

Since elderly persons have more contact with primary care services than any other age group, these contacts should be used for opportunistic case finding of common conditions such as hypertension, hearing loss, and visual impairment, as well as symptomatic conditions like bacteriuria, incontinence, and foot problems. Behavioural concerns such as inappropriate medication, lack of physical exercise, depression, dementia, alcohol problems, and social isolation should also be considered. Home visits to those aged over 75 years may not only identify inappropriate housing, hazards in the home which may cause falls, but also social isolation, undernutrition, and elder abuse. Thus, screening in this age group is concerned with case finding and improving quality of life.

Conclusion

The concept of screening for disease offers the possibility of bringing beneficial health interventions to apparently healthy subjects, free from known disease. This chapter has discussed some of the difficulties associated with this approach. These problems must be analysed from several different disciplinary perspectives. The epidemiological approach is required to analyse problems of screening-test performance, as well as questions of the effectiveness of intervention through screening. Applying screening techniques raises important ethical questions concerning the relationships between individuals, screening programmes, and the wider society. These reflect uncertainty and disagreement as to how the benefits and harms from intervening through screening should be valued and distributed. Developing a screening programme represents a complex technical challenge, and sound planning and project management strategies should be employed for implementation. Ongoing screening programmes should be continuously improved through application of quality assurance and the implementation of systems to minimize errors and harm. They should also be evaluated from time to time to ensure that the benefits expected in terms of effectiveness and cost-effectiveness are achieved and this requires ongoing systems of data collection and evaluation. Application of these principles to different screening programmes in the main areas of infections, genetic conditions, vascular disease, and cancer, and at different stages of life, requires detailed and specialized knowledge.

Further reading

Holland, W.W. and Stewart, S. (1990). *Screening in Healthcare*. London: The Nuffield Provincial Hospitals Trust.

Holland, W.W. and Stewart, S. (2005). *Screening in Disease Prevention: What Works?* Oxford: Radcliffe Publishing.

Holland, W.W., Stewart, S., and Masseria, C. (2006). *Screening in Europe*. Copenhagen: European Observatory on Health Systems and Policy.

Raffle, A.E. and Gray, J.A.M. (2007). *Screening: Evidence and Practice*. Oxford: Oxford University Press.

Wald, N. and Leck, I. (eds.) (2000). *Antenatal and Neonatal Screening* (2nd ed.). Oxford: Oxford University Press.

References

Amato, A., Gridanti, M., Lerone, M., et al. (2009). Prevention strategies for severe haemoglobinopathies in endemic and non-endemic countries: the Latium example. *Prenatal Diagnosis*, 29, 1171–4.

American College of Obstetricians and Gynecologists (2012). Noninvasive prenatal testing for fetal aneuploidy. *Obstetrics and Gynecology*, 120, 1532–4.

Andermann, A., Blancquaert, I., Beauchamp, S., and Déry, V. (2008). Revisiting Wilson and Jungner in the genomic age: a review of screening criteria over the past 40 years. *Bulletin of the World Health Organization*, 86(4), 241–320.

Anionwu, E. (2001). *The Politics of Sickle Cell and Thalassaemia*. Milton Keynes: Open University Press.

Arrol, B., Khin, N., and Kerse, N. (2003). Screening for depression in primary care with two verbally asked questions: cross sectional study. *British Medical Journal*, 327, 1144–6.

Balmer, S., Bowens, A., Bruce, E., Farrar, H., Jenkins, C., and Williams, R. (2000). *Quality Management for Screening*. Leeds: University of Leeds. Available at: http://www.leeds.ac.uk/hsphr/nuffield_publications/documents/screening.pdf. Available at: http://www.nsc.nhs.uk/uk_nsc/uk_nsc_ind.htm.

Bozkurt, G. (2007). Results from the north Cyprus thalassaemia prevention programme. *Haemoglobin*, 31, 257–64.

Buse, K., Mays, N., and Walt, G. (2009). *Making Health Policy*. London: Open University Press.

Chamberlain, J.M. (1984). Which prescriptive screening programmes are worthwhile? *Journal of Epidemiology and Community Health*, 38, 270–7.

Choke, E., Vijaynagar, B., Thompson, J., Nasim, A., Bown, M.J., and Sayers, R.D. (2012). Changing epidemiology of abdominal aortic aneurysms in England and Wales: older and more benign? *Circulation*, 125(13), 1617–25.

Cochrane, A.L. and Holland, W.W. (1971). Validation of screening procedures. *British Medical Bulletin*, 27, 3–8.

Colhoun, H.M., McKeigue, P.M., and Davey Smith, G. (2003). Problems of reporting genetic associations with complex outcomes. *The Lancet*, 361, 865–72.

Connor, N., Roberts, J., and Nicoll, A. (2000). Strategic options for antenatal screening for syphilis in the United Kingdom: a cost effectiveness analysis. *Journal of Medical Screening*, 7, 7–13.

Cosford, P.A. and Leng, G.C. (2007). Screening for abdominal aortic aneurysm. *Cochrane Database of Systematic Reviews*, 2, CD002945.

Cousens, N.E., Gaff, C.L., Metcalfe, S.A., and Delatycki, M.B. (2010). Carrier screening for beta-thalassaemia: a review of international practice. *European Journal of Human Genetics*, 18(10), 1077–83.

Department of Health (1998). *Screening of Pregnant Women for Hepatitis B and Immunisation of Babies at* Risk. Health Service Circular: HSC 1998/127. London: Department of Health.

Donabedian, A. (2003). *An Introduction to Quality Assurance in Healthcare*. Oxford: Oxford University Press.

Drummond, M.F., Schulper, M., Torrance, G.W., O'Brien, B.J., and Stoddart, G.L. (2007). *Methods for the Economic Evaluation of Health Care Programmes*. Oxford: Oxford University Press.

Elhers, L., Sørensen, J., Jensen, L.G., Bech, M., and Kjølby, M. (2008). Is population screening for abdominal aortic aneurysm cost-effective? *BMC Cardiovascular Disorders*, 8(8), 32.

Forrest, A.P.M. (1987). *Breast Cancer Screening. Report to the Health Ministries of England Wales Scotland and Northern Ireland by a Working Group Chaired by Sir Patrick Forrest*. London: HMSO.

Forster, A.S., Forbes, A., Dodhia, H., et al. (2013). Non-attendance at diabetic eye screening and risk of sight-threatening diabetic retinopathy: a population-based cohort study. *Diabetologia*, 56(10), 2187–93.

Gibson, B. (2003). Beyond 'Two Communities'. In V. Lin and B. Gibson (eds.) *Evidence-Based Health Policy: Problems and Possibilities*, pp. 18–32. Melbourne: Oxford University Press.

Gostin, L.O. (2000). *Public Health Law. Power, Duty, Restraint*. Berkeley and Los Angeles, CA: University of California Press.

Gøtzsche, P.C. (2012). *Mammography Screening. Truth, Lies and Controversy*. London: Radcliffe Publishing.

Gøtzsche, P.C., et al. (2012). Why mammography screening has not lived up to expectations from the randomised trials. *Cancer Care Control*, 23(10), 15–21.

Gray, M. (2009). *Evidence-Based Healthcare and Public Health*. London: Churchill Livingstone Elsevier.

Hardcastle, J.D., Chamberlain, J.O., Robinson, M.H., et al. (1996). Randomised controlled trial of faecal-occult-blood screening for colorectal cancer. *The Lancet*, 348, 1472–7.

Hendricksen, C., Lund, E., and Stromgaard, E. (1989). Hospitalisation of elderly people: a three year controlled trial. *Journal American Geriatric Society*, 37, 119–22.

Hendriksen, C., Lund, E., and Tromgaard, E. (1984). Consequences of assessment and intervention among elderly people a three year randomised controlled trial. *British Medical Journal*, 289, 1522–4.

Holland, W.W. and Stewart, S. (1990). *Screening in Healthcare*. London: The Nuffield Provincial Hospitals Trust.

Holland, W.W. and Stewart, S. (2005). *Screening in Disease Prevention: What Works?* Oxford: Radcliffe Publishing.

Human Genetics Commission (2006). *Making Babies: Reproductive Decisions and Genetic Technologies*. London: Human Genetics Commission. Available at: http://www.hgc.gov.uk/UploadDocs/DocPub/Document/Making%20Babies%20Report%20-%20final%20pdf.pdf.

Human Genetics Commission (2011). *Increasing Options, Informing Choice: A Report on Preconception Genetic Testing and Screening*. London: Human Genetics Commission.

Kronborg, O., Fenger, C., Olsen, J., Jørgensen, O.D., and Søndergaard, O. (1996). Randomised study of screening for colorectal cancer with faecal-occult-blood test. *The Lancet*, 348, 1467–71.

Lin, K. and Barton, M. (2007). *Screening for Haemoglobinopathies in Newborns. Reaffirmation Update for the US Preventive Services Taskforce*. Evidence synthesis No. 52. Rockville, MD: Agency for Healthcare Research and Quality, US Department of Health and Human Services.

Marteau, T.M., Dormandy, E., and Michie, S. (2001). A measure of informed choice. *Health Expectations*, 4, 99–108.

Martin, R.M. (2007). Commentary: prostate cancer is omnipresent, but should we screen for it? *International Journal of Epidemiology*, 36, 278–81.

McKeown, T. (ed.) (1968). *Screening in Medical Care: Reviewing the Evidence*. Oxford: Oxford University Press for Nuffield Provincials Hospital Trust.

Moullin, M. (2002). *Delivering Excellence in Health and Social Care*. Buckingham: Open University Press.

National Health Service Cancer Screening Programme (2004). *Guidelines on Failsafe Actions for the Follow-Up of Cervical Cytology Reports*. Sheffield: NHS Cancer Screening Programmes. http://www.cancerscreening.nhs.uk/cervical/publications/nhscsp21.html.

National Health Service Sickle Cell and Thalassaemia Screening Programme (2011). *Standards for the Linked Antenatal and Newborn Screening Programmes* (2nd ed). London: NHS Sickle Cell and Thalassaemia Screening Programme. Available at: http://sct.screening.nhs.uk/standardsandguidelines.

National Health Service Sickle Cell and Thalassaemia Screening Programme (n.d.). *UPDATE (Outline of Policy for Implementation of Antenatal Screening)*. Available at: http://sct.screening.nhs.uk/cms.php?folder=2424.

NHS Health Check (2014). *Free HNS Health Check*. [Online] Available at: http://www.healthcheck.nhs.uk.

Nijsingh, N. (2007). Informed consent and the expansion of newborn screening. In A. Dawson and M. Verweij (eds.) *Ethics, Prevention and Public Health*, pp. 198–212. Oxford: Oxford University Press.

Nuffield Council on Bioethics (2007). *Public Health: Ethical Issues*. London: Nuffield Council on Bioethics.

Osborn, F. (1937). Development of a eugenic philosophy. *American Sociological Review*, 2, 389–97.

Raffle, A. (2004). Cervical screening. *British Medical Journal*, 328, 1272–3.

Raffle, A.E. and Gray, J.A.M. (2007). *Screening: Evidence and Practice*. Oxford: Oxford University Press.

Rembold, C.M. (1998). Number needed to screen: development of a statistic for disease screening. *British Medical Journal*, 317, 307–12.

Samavat, A. and Modell, B. (2004). Iranian national thalassaemia screening programme. *British Medical Journal*, 329, 1134–7.

Sassi, F., Le Grand, J., and Archard, L. (2001). Equity versus efficiency: a dilemma for the NHS. *British Medical Journal*, 323, 762–3.

Shapiro, S., Venet, W., Strox, P., et al. (1982). Ten to fourteen year effect of screening on breast cancer mortality. *Journal of the National Cancer Institute*, 69, 349–55.

Sorour, Y., Heppinstall, S., Porter, N., et al. (2007). Is routine molecular screening for common a-thalassaemia deletions necessary as part of antenatal screening programme? *Journal of Medical Screening*, 14, 60–1.

Squirrel, D.M. and Talbot, J.F. (2003). Screening for diabetic retinopathy. *Journal of the Royal Society of Medicine*, 96, 273–6.

Taban, L., Fagerberg, G., Gunman, D., et al. (1989). The Swedish two county trial of mammographic screening for breast cancer: recent results and calculation of benefit. *Journal of Epidemiology and Community Health*, 43, 107–14.

Taban, L., Gad, A., Holmberg, L.H., et al. (1985). Reduction in mortality for breast cancer after mass screening with mammography. *The Lancet*, ii, 829–32.

The Independent UK Panel of Breast Cancer Screening (2012). *The Benefits and Harms of Breast Cancer Screening: An Independent Review*. [Online] Available at: http://www.screening.nhs.uk/breastcancer.

Thompson, I.M., Ankerst, D.P., Chi, C., et al. (2005). Operating characteristics of prostate-specific antigen in men with an initial PSA level of 3.0 ng/mL or lower. *Journal of the American Medical Association*, 294, 66–70.

UK National Screening Committee (2000). *Second Report of the National Screening Committee*. London: Department of Health. Available at: http://www.screening.nhs.uk/criteria.

UK National Screening Committee (2003). *New World Symphony— Screening and Quality Management in the Reorganised NHS in England*. Available at: http://www.nsc.nhs.uk.

UK National Screening Committee (n.d.). *Programme Appraisal Criteria*. [Online] Available at: http://www.screening.nhs.uk/criteria.

Wald, N.J., Huttly, W.J., and Hackshaw, A.K. (2003). Antenatal screening for Down's syndrome with the quadruple test. *The Lancet*, 361, 835–6.

Wald, N. and Leck, I. (eds.) (2000). *Antenatal and Neonatal Screening* (2nd ed.). Oxford: Oxford University Press.

Wareham, N.J. and Griffin, S.J. (2001). Should we screen for type 2 diabetes? Evaluation against national screening committee criteria. *British Medical Journal*, 322, 986–8.

Welch, H.G. (2001). Informed choice in cancer screening. *Journal of the American Medical Association*, 285, 2776–8.

Wikipedia (2013). *Eugenics*. [Online] Available at: http://en.wikipedia.org/wiki/Eugenics.

Wilson, J.M.G. and Jungner, G. (1968). *Principles and Practice of Screening for Disease*. Paper Number 34. Geneva: World Health Organization.

11.5

Environmental health practice

Yasmin E.R. von Schirnding

Introduction to environmental health practice

Concept and scope of environmental health

In considering the practice of environmental health, it is necessary firstly to have an understanding of the concept of environmental health, which can be defined in various ways. In its broadest context, environmental health is concerned with the health effects associated with the environment. This includes both the physical (natural and man-made or 'built') as well as the social environment. It is less concerned with the health of the environment per se as it is with its impacts on human health. In this respect, environmental health is an integral part of the discipline of public health, with strong links to the environmental sciences.

The World Health Organization (WHO) has defined environmental health in various ways to include 'Those aspects of human health and disease that are determined by factors in the environment. It also refers to the theory and practice of assessing and controlling factors in the environment that can potentially affect health' (WHO 1989). While *health* has been defined by the WHO as 'A state of complete physical, mental and social well-being and not merely the absence of disease or infirmity' (WHO 1946), environmental health has tended to focus mainly on the physical environment, with less emphasis on the social environment and on social and mental well-being. Nevertheless, both the physical as well as the social aspects of the environment are important aspects of the realm of environmental health.

An updated definition of environmental health by the WHO gives added emphasis to this social component and describes environmental health as comprising 'those aspects of human health, including quality of life, that are determined by physical, chemical, biological, social and psychosocial factors in the environment. It also refers to the theory and practice of assessing, correcting, controlling, and preventing those factors in the environment that can potentially affect adversely the health of present and future generations' (WHO 2004).

Virtually any aspect of the environment can affect human health—either positively or negatively. Typical environmental health concerns addressed by environmental health practitioners include ambient and indoor air quality, food safety, water quality, sanitation, waste management, housing quality, noise pollution, electromagnetic radiation, occupational and industrial hygiene, vector control, and toxic chemical exposures.

In recent years, increasing attention has been given to the health effects associated with natural ecosystems and to global (climate) change, addressing health issues in the context of complex (eco) systems analysis (McMichael et al. 2006; Patz et al. 2008; McMichael 2013). With growing appreciation of the links between ecology and health, the integrity of natural ecosystems, and the transdisciplinary and intersectoral nature of environmental health, there have been calls for new approaches to dealing with environmental health hazards (Soskolne et al. 2007). With the global spotlight on sustainable development, practitioners have begun to look at environmental health risks more holistically from the viewpoint of various economic sectors like housing, transport, or energy, and settings or systems like the city at large.

In this respect, it is interesting to note how the discipline of environmental health has evolved, from its roots in the sanitation movement of the 1800s in the United Kingdom (Hamlin 1998) with a fairly narrow focus on sanitation, environmental hygiene, inspection, and control, to an increasingly broader approach addressing health and environment concerns in the context of sustainable development (von Schirnding 2002a) and with more focus on ecosystems and ecology in general (Rapport et al. 2009).

It was back in 1848, with the passage of the Public Health Act in the United Kingdom (Calman 1998), that provision was made for the appointment of Inspectors of Nuisances—the predecessors of today's environmental health officers. This resulted from an enquiry by Edwin Chadwick, a Poor Law Commissioner, who, in 1842, published a major report on sanitary conditions in England (Chadwick 1842). Chadwick's investigation into the causes of poverty concluded that people often became poor as a result of ill health from an adverse environment. That situation prevails today.

A high prevalence of ill health and disease in a population make poverty eradication and economic development elusive goals. People who are poor are more likely to get sick—however, people who are sick are more likely to become poor. Poverty eradication, economic development, and a healthy environment are inextricably linked and are fundamental to ensuring human health. A responsive health system, a healthy environment, and an intact life support system are vital to sustaining the health of the population. In the following subsections, we look briefly at some of the major trends in health, environment, and development in recent years, before highlighting environmental health issues and the burden of environmentally related disease.

Global trends

Of overriding significance is the fact that on a global scale there has been unprecedented wealth creation and economic development in the past decades, coupled with intensified global efforts targeting major causes of death and disease throughout the world. This has been accelerated in part due to initiatives such as the Millennium Development Goals (MDGs) process which set in motion an ambitious programme of goals and targets to eradicate poverty by the year 2015 (United Nations (UN) 2000).

Life expectancies for men and women are increasing. For example, from 1970 to 2010, life expectancy at birth for males increased from 56.4 years to 67.5 years, and for females from 61.2 years to 73.3 years (Wang et al. 2013). A greater proportion of total deaths now occur among people over the age of 70 years, compared with 20 years ago. There have been significant declines in infectious disease mortality, and burdens of HIV and malaria are falling. Far fewer children under the age of 5 years are dying (Wang et al. 2013) with deaths in this age group having declined by almost 60 per cent since 1970.

Nevertheless, despite huge progress in human development over the past decades, today, one out of five people live on US$1.25 per day or less, and big gaps in progress remain in some regions of the world. The most afflicted continent is Africa. Moreover, the distribution of income at the country level has worsened in much of the world, despite narrowing in gaps in health and education (United Nations Development Programme (UNDP) 2011).

Human population growth continues apace, increasing by 75–80 million people a year (Sachs 2012) and projected to reach a total of 9 billion by the middle of the twenty-first century and 10 billion by the end of this century. It is estimated that 3.4 billion people (around half the world's population) currently live in urban areas, and by 2050 this number may rise to 6.3 billion. Sixty per cent of the global population will be living in cities by 2030. Urban growth will be greatest in Africa and Asia, followed by Latin America and Oceania. While currently it is estimated that about 1 billion people live in slum-like conditions, by 2030 this number could double (Satterthwaite 2007).

With rapid economic development and urbanization in developing countries, air and water pollution levels have been increasing, as has the generation of municipal and hazardous waste. In the last 30 years, however, in many industrialized nations stronger environmental laws have resulted in cleaner and safer drinking and recreational water as well as in improved air quality. On a global basis nevertheless, the trend for pollution of air and drinking water supplies is upward (McMichael et al. 2006; Goldman and Torres 2009). Growth in incomes has been associated with deterioration in key environmental indicators such as carbon dioxide emissions, soil and water quality, and forest cover (UNDP 2011).

Environmental health issues

Environmental health practitioners face a growing diversity of environmental hazards to deal with, in many different settings, in developed and developing countries alike. Often it is difficult to distinguish the traditional risks associated with poverty from new and emerging ('modern') ones associated with urbanization and industrialization, agriculture, and land-use practices. Developing countries frequently must deal simultaneously with the impact on health of both. For example, pesticides and faeces may contaminate the same water supplies, and air pollution may stem simultaneously from burning dirty household fuels and the use of industrial fossil fuels (World Resources Institute et al. 1998).

Problems may have to be dealt with simultaneously at the global, national, and local levels. For example while water supply and sanitation, waste disposal, or toxic chemicals are often of special relevance at the local or micro level, other problems are more important at the regional or global level (global climate change, or long-range transport of air pollution). Health impacts associated with global change and disturbances to natural ecosystems (disruption of bio-geophysical systems such as the climate system and associated rising temperatures, declining rainfall, extreme weather events, degradation of land and water, depletion of resources, and other effects) (McMichael 2013) have to be dealt with at all levels, and may impact severely on poor countries and on the poor in general. While poor countries have contributed least to global climate change they have experienced the greatest loss in rainfall and the greatest increase in its variability, with implications for agricultural productivity and livelihoods (UNDP 2011).

While problems may differ in urban and rural environments, increasingly the divide between urban and rural is becoming blurred. Cities have provided numerous positive benefits associated with increased job opportunities and provision of essential services and facilities, but environment and health problems may nevertheless be profound, especially in cities that are not economically homogeneous. In informal settlement areas in particular, infectious diseases associated with inadequate water and sanitation, and dirty household fuels may be prevalent. Rich and poor people live in very different epidemiological worlds, even within the same city, and this situation occurs in both high-income as well as low-income countries (WHO and UN-Habitat 2010). Infant mortality rates are often higher among poor segments of urban populations in developed countries.

Lead poisoning illustrates very well the unequal burden of risk borne by poor inner-city children who are not only more exposed to sources of lead in and around the home environment (from flaking lead-based paint, for example, or contaminated air and dust), but are also more vulnerable to the toxic effects of lead, being often nutritionally deprived and having inadequate access to healthcare facilities. This is true even of children living in such countries as the United States and parts of Europe (Tong et al. 2000). Within inner-city areas, studies from South Africa have shown substantial socioeconomic differentials in blood lead burden among inner-city children (von Schirnding et al. 1991).

Poorer countries also have higher levels of household deprivation as evidenced by such factors as indoor air pollution, and inadequate access to clean water and sanitation. The environmental burdens of poverty fall directly on poor populations. As income levels rise, however, and with increased affluence and associated lifestyles and consumption patterns, these burdens tend to lessen, concomitant with environmental burdens which are more diffuse, indirect, and delayed, and affect a more temporally and spatially displaced public (UNDP 2011). Risks associated with community urban air pollution are an example.

With further economic development, these more localized burdens tend eventually to lessen too (or be displaced elsewhere), while environmental risks associated with global effects—for example, greenhouse gas emissions—tend to rise with high levels of materials and energy consumption and waste generation (UNDP 2011). The most disadvantaged people carry a double (or triple) burden of deprivation—they are more vulnerable to the global effects of environmental degradation, have often to cope with new and emerging risks associated with rapid industrialization and urbanization, but also have to deal with threats to their immediate environment like indoor air pollution, dirty water, and poor sanitation.

Burden of disease

It has been previously estimated that at least a quarter of the global burden of disease may be attributable to poor environmental conditions (25 per cent of all deaths in developing regions and 17 per cent of all deaths in developed regions) (WHO 1996). This, however, was thought to be a conservative estimate due to the lack of evidence for many diseases, and the fact that the causal pathway between disease outcome and exposure is complex.

Among children aged 0–14 years it was estimated that 36 per cent of the disease burden may be caused by environmental factors (WHO 1996), with the highest burdens occurring in sub-Saharan Africa and South Asia, and with respiratory infections and diarrhoeal disease being the largest contributors to the environmental burden and mortality. In developing countries, the environmental fraction of diarrhoea, respiratory infections, and malaria accounted for 26 per cent of deaths in children under 5 years.

The global burden of disease estimates have recently been updated (Murray et al. 2012) and the latest findings indicate a predominance of non-communicable disease risks in 2010 compared with 1990. Nevertheless, still today, pneumonia and diarrhoea are the leading killers of young children, accounting for 29 per cent of deaths among children under the age of 5 years. Nearly 90 per cent of these deaths occur in sub-Saharan Africa and South Asia, reflecting uneven progress in reducing child mortality (United Nations Children's Fund (UNICEF) 2012). Further information

on the relevance of global burden of risk estimates for environmental health practice is provided in Box 11.5.1 and Table 11.5.1.

Without substantially more progress, declines in major childhood deaths will not occur. The MDGs remain unfulfilled for many of these countries. At the same time, rapid industrialization and urbanization associated with increased vehicle and industrial emissions is reflected in extremely high levels of air pollution from multiple sources. This is against a backdrop of continued dependence in many multi-million people crowded cities on dirty fuels for heating and cooking that place human health at risk.

The 2010 global burden of disease estimates provide a sense of where environmental health practice could make a big impact in future. Continued support to improve access to water and sanitation services and a transition to cleaner household fuels is a high priority in much of sub-Saharan Africa and Asia.

It remains a travesty that in 2013, 783 million people still do not use an improved drinking water source, and 2.5 billion do not use an improved sanitation facility, mostly in the poorest households and rural areas; 1.1 billion people (949 million people in rural areas, and 105 million people in urban areas), practice open defecation (UNICEF 2012).

Nearly 90 per cent of the deaths due to diarrhoea worldwide have been attributed to unsafe water, inadequate sanitation, and poor hygiene. In addition, around 3 billion people worldwide use solid fuels as their main cooking fuel (UNICEF 2012). (In 2004, it was estimated that solid fuel use contributed to nearly 2 million premature deaths, nearly half of them childhood pneumonia.) It is to be hoped that the integrated Global Action Plan for the Prevention and Control of Pneumonia and Diarrhoea (GAPPD) will impact significantly on ending these preventable deaths (UNICEF and WHO 2013).

From this it is evident that health, environment, and development problems differ in various parts of the world, as do priorities with respect to their management. There is, however, a need in all situations for decision-makers and the public to have ready

---

Box 11.5.1 Global burden of risk estimates highlight priorities for environmental health practice

The recent global comparative risk assessment of burden of disease and injury attributable to risks published as part of the update of the global burden of disease study 2010 (Lim et al. 2012) provides new data on major environmental risks. The proportion of deaths or disease burden caused by risk factors was calculated, holding other independent factors constant.

Of the 67 risk factors and risk clusters, several related directly to environmental factors. These include: unimproved water and sanitation (separately for water source and sanitation), air pollution (ambient particulate matter pollution, household air pollution from solid fuels and ambient ozone pollution), residential radon, and lead exposure. On a global basis, there have been shifts in these risks since 1990 suggesting some decline in traditional risks such as unimproved water and sanitation, but increases in ambient particulate matter pollution, ozone pollution, and lead exposure, with declines in household air pollution (Table 11.5.1).

In 1990, household air pollution accounted for 7 per cent of global DALYs and ranked second in leading risk factors. In 2010, household air pollution ranked fourth, accounting for 4.5 per cent of global DALYs. The burden attributable to ambient particulate matter pollution has remained largely unchanged (3.2 per cent of global DALYs in 1990 compared with 3 per cent in 2010). Unimproved water and sanitation together accounted for 0.9 per cent of DALYs in 2010 compared with 2.1 per cent in 1990.

These global trends, however, mask major regional differences. Thus household air pollution ranked fourth globally across all risks but ranked first in South Asia, second in sub-Saharan Africa, and fourth in East Asia. Ambient air pollution ranked ninth globally but fourth in East Asia. While unimproved sanitation and water have dropped relative to other risks at a global level (to ranks of 25 and 34 respectively), in sub-Saharan African countries and many Asian countries both still rank around the top ten.

Source: data from *The Lancet*, Lim, S.S. et al., Volume 380, Issue 9859, A comparative risk assessment of burden of disease and injury attributable to 67 risk factors and risk factor clusters in 21 regions, 1990–2010: a systematic analysis for the global burden of disease study 2010, pp. 2224–60, Copyright © 2012.

Table 11.5.1 Disability-adjusted life years (1000s) attributable to environmental risk factors

Risk factor	1990	2010
Unimproved water and sanitation	52,169	21,187
Water	21,172	7775
Sanitation	36,050	14,927
Air pollution		
Ambient particulate matter	81,699	76,163
Household air pollution from solid fuels	175,909	110,962
Ambient ozone pollution	2534	2456
Residential radon	—	2114
Lead exposure	5365	13,936

Reprinted from *The Lancet*, Lim, S.S. et al., Volume 380, Issue 9859, A comparative risk assessment of burden of disease and injury attributable to 67 risk factors and risk factor clusters in 21 regions, 1990–2010: a systematic analysis for the global burden of disease study 2010, pp. 2224–60, Copyright © 2012, with permission from Elsevier, http://www.sciencedirect.com/science/journal/01406736.

access to accurate information on health hazards associated with environmental risk factors. In the following section we discuss the nature of environmental health effects and factors influencing exposure, and then go on to discuss how environmental health practitioners proceed to assess these.

Environmental health assessment

Nature of environmental health effects

Environmental health practitioners must concern themselves not only with addressing known exposures and disease outcomes associated with these but also, importantly, diseases of unknown cause, with potential environmental links. In addition, still today, for many substances, it is not known whether or not there are safety thresholds for an adverse effect, and, if so, what those levels are.

Certain cancers and 'subtle' diseases and conditions related to environmental factors (e.g. lead in relation to intelligence, moderate hearing loss, or raised blood pressure) may not be recognized as such. Thus, the situation remains that much environmental disease goes unrecognized. With regard to chemicals, typically exposures to complex mixtures occur, which have not been well characterized.

Health outcomes

Environmental health effects result from a complex set of genetic, environmental, social, and other factors. Health effects may arise directly from a specific chemical, physical, or biological agent, or indirectly from the broader physical and social environment (e.g. housing, land-use, transport, agriculture, or industry). While as indicated earlier, infectious agents resulting in such illnesses as diarrhoea and respiratory infections may be associated with inadequate water and sanitation and indoor air pollution, non-infectious agents are associated with non-communicable (chronic) illnesses. These include cancers, respiratory conditions like asthma, birth defects, and other illnesses.

Environmental health effects may include minor, temporary ill-health conditions, as well as acute illness and chronic disease. Relatively resistant and susceptible persons may exist at either extreme of the distribution. Effects are frequently irreversible. Acute ill-health effects may follow relatively shortly after an exposure (e.g. poisoning by pesticides, or following a chemical spill), whereas chronic exposure may occur as a result of an individual cumulative exposure over extended periods of time. A long time period may occur between the exposure and the health effect. An example would be asbestos exposure and mesothelioma (Selikoff et al. 1965). Dispersal of the population at risk over time and the long incubation period make it difficult to reconstruct exposures. Some persistent pollutants like PCBs and heavy metals like lead and mercury can accumulate in the environment for years, and may affect people over large distances, causing health effects long after their use has been discontinued. Acute health effects are usually easier to detect than chronic effects, which are difficult to relate to specific hazards or sources.

Multifactorial exposure

In addition, as indicated, many environmental diseases are multifactorial as far as the causal factors are concerned and it may be difficult to determine the effects of one exposure in the light of existence of effects of simultaneous exposure to other factors. Prevention has tended to focus on exposures associated with a single agent or medium (e.g. air or water); however, people are often exposed simultaneously to a wide variety of physical, biological, and chemical agents and may be exposed via several pathways (air, water, food) from one source. As indicated earlier, in developing countries people may be exposed both to hazards associated with poverty (unsafe drinking water and inadequate sanitation), pollution, unsafe agricultural and land-use practices, etc. Relatively little is known, however, of the effects of cumulative exposures and how various risk factors might interact (Tickner 2005).

Also, in dealing with low-level exposures one may deal with factors which play a contributory rather than a primary role, and the co-action of other factors may be needed for an effect to occur. Exposures may be interactive, sometimes resulting in an additive or even synergistic (multiplicative) effect. The risk of health impacts associated with exposure to asbestos, for example, may be significantly increased (multiplied many times) in smokers (Selikoff et al. 1968).

Vulnerable groups

The poor, the elderly, women, and young children may be particularly affected.

The elderly, for example, may be especially vulnerable to some toxic substances which may take longer to eliminate from the body. They may also be more vulnerable to respiratory illnesses associated with air pollution, for example. During pregnancy, women may have altered physiologies and metabolize toxic substances differently, while, during menopause, women may be especially vulnerable, for example, to the release of toxic substances such as lead from bones.

Children are particularly vulnerable to environmental insults (Goldman and Torres 2009). Children are not merely 'little adults'. They are more exposed than adults, as, due to their rapid metabolism, growth, and development, they drink, eat, and breathe in more of a contaminant relative to their bodyweight than do adults. Children also have enhanced hand-to-mouth activity and they play close to the ground, increasing their exposures still further. In addition, they have immature, and therefore vulnerable, physiologies. The unborn fetus may be especially vulnerable to toxic chemicals.

Thus different groups have differing vulnerabilities and susceptibilities, including genetic dispositions, nutritional status, health, and physiological status which may influence their exposure (and response). Gene–environment interactions are known to be of importance and different subsets in the population may have different exposure–effect relationships. People may be more or less vulnerable at various stages of their lives.

To intervene on the causes of disease thus requires a good understanding of the health risks and their causes, as well as the susceptible individuals/population, so that surveillance and monitoring systems can be developed to identify in advance potential problems, thereby enabling effective interventions to be designed and implemented.

Role of epidemiology and toxicology

An important part of the work of the environmental health practitioner involves assessing the risks to which people may be exposed in the environment. While there is less uncertainty today about the extent of both direct and indirect risks to human health which are associated with factors in the environment, nevertheless there is still much to be learned about the way in which the environment influences human health.

In conducting health assessments, it is necessary to establish the nature of exposure and health outcome relationships, and to assess causality. Of the various fields that contribute to environmental health (e.g. environmental science, chemistry, physics, engineering, medicine, and many others) of key importance are epidemiology and toxicology, as well as exposure assessment.

Environmental epidemiology is concerned with the distribution and determinants of ill health effects in human populations at risk from environmental exposures. As workplace exposures have decreased over time, and environmental exposures have increased, an appreciation of the multiple causation of disease has grown. Various types of study design have been used in environmental epidemiology to assess the nature of the relationship between an exposure and health outcome(s) in a particular setting or population group. These include ecological studies, cross-sectional studies, case–control studies, cohort or follow-up studies, and intervention studies. They can be challenging to conduct due to the complexity of the health risks and exposures involved, and the need to take into account all the potential sources of confounding (extraneous factors associated with the outcome of interest) and bias.

No matter how well designed and executed, however, epidemiological studies disclose health risks only after exposures have occurred. Also, it is sometimes the case that there is too narrow a range of exposure for epidemiological studies to detect health effects in populations. In addition, it is difficult to measure exposure at the individual level (air pollution is an example) and exposure measurements made at an area or neighbourhood level may sometimes be (incorrectly) presumed to relate at an individual level, leading to what in epidemiological terms is referred to as the 'ecological fallacy'. This is where inferences about individuals are based on inferences about groups. Thus within an 'exposed' area, owing to micro-variations in exposure and other factors

affecting people's exposure (e.g. behaviour patterns), people may not be homogeneously affected, but be assumed to be so.

Toxicological studies, which are experimental studies of the effect of pollutants on human beings or animals under controlled conditions, are also needed in order to identify in advance any adverse effects of substances under investigation. These have the benefit of allowing for a wider range of exposures to be assessed and can take account of the problem of confounding factors in epidemiological studies. However, extrapolation from laboratory animals to humans, at high to low doses, is complex with many assumptions involved. And it is not usually possible to reproduce all the contributing factors in the laboratory.

While there exist internationally harmonized guidelines for toxicity testing such as those established by the Organisation for Economic Cooperation and Development (OECD), specific testing for toxicity varies by country and depends on the type of substance and the statute under which it is covered. In the United States, for example, pesticides in food require tests of acute and chronic toxicity, neurotoxicity tests, cancer bioassays, tests of reproductive and developmental toxicity, and others (Goldman and Torres 2009).

Making causal inferences

The concept of risk is linked to that of causation. From the previous discussions it is evident that the relationship between many environmental exposures and health outcomes is complex. Even under optimal conditions and with the best study designs, it is difficult to make definitive assertions regarding causality.

Bradford Hill (1965) listed the criteria shown in Box 11.5.2 as being key to assessing whether an observed association is likely to be causal or not.

Risk assessment

While epidemiology and toxicology are used to generate new evidence on health effects, risk assessment too relies on science-based information but synthesizes *existing* information and weighs it up with the aim usually of addressing a particular regulatory or policy issue aimed at reducing or eliminating the risk (Bartel 2005). In this respect the National Research Council (NRC) has referred to it as a mixture of 'science and judgment' (NRC 1994).

Risk assessment is used in many fields, including environmental health. It is concerned with the process of estimating, usually in quantitative terms, the harm that will result from exposure to an environmental hazard (Fiorino 1995). Risk assessors might, for example, want to analyse the risks associated with being exposed to an indicator like indoor air pollution, to a specific agent like lead in paint, or to a suspected contaminant in food or drinking water.

The conceptual framework for risk assessment was set out by the NRC in 1983 (NRC 1983) and divided the process into four key elements: hazard identification, dose–response assessment, exposure assessment, and risk characterization. Risk is a function of hazard and dose. *Hazard identification* concerns the identification of environmental agents and health effects for assessment, based on evidence for causality from epidemiological and toxicological studies (see Chapter 7.5). *Dose–response* assessment describes the quantitative relationship between exposure and disease based on models that predict the level of response from any dose. *Exposure assessment* involves estimating or measuring the magnitude,

---

Box 11.5.2 Criteria for causality

The strength of the association refers to how large the effect or the size of the association is—a strong association (as measured by a relative risk or odds ratio) is more likely to have a causal component than is a modest association. Absence of a strong association does not, however, rule out a causal association. In environmental epidemiology frequently one is dealing with relative risks in the range of 1–2—since they often apply to the general population, however, the attributable risk or public health impact in terms of the absolute number of cases can be large.

Consistency refers to a relationship that is observed repeatedly in different settings using different methods—for example, in differing groups, places, circumstances, time—by others. Finding an association consistently using different study designs, methods, and so on reduces the probability that an association is due to an error in the study design.

Specificity refers to an association that is specific for an outcome or group of individuals—that is, altering only the cause would alter the effect. An example would be mesothelioma in relation to asbestos exposure. Due to the multifactorial nature of many environmental diseases, this is not normally the case, however.

Temporality implies that the factor must precede the outcome it is assumed to affect. This is a critical factor in assessing causality.

Biological gradient refers to a dose–response relationship between the exposure and the disease. An increasing amount of exposure increases the risk.

Biological plausibility is concerned with the extent to which the association is consistent with what is already known about the response to the exposure and/or disease—that is, does it make sense?

Coherence of evidence implies that the causal association should not fundamentally contradict present substantive knowledge.

Experimental evidence stresses that causation is more likely if evidence is based on randomized experiments.

Reasoning by analogy implies that for analogous exposures and outcomes an effect has already been shown. For example, is the observed association supported by a similar association?

Source: data from Hill, A.B., The environment and disease: association or causation?, *Proceedings of the Royal Society of Medicine*, Volume 58, Issue 5, pp. 295–300, Copyright © 1965.

---

duration, and timing of human exposure to the agent of concern. It necessitates defining the exposed population and the routes of exposure. The final step is *risk characterization*. Information from the previous three steps is combined and the level of response for the identified health effect(s) at the particular level of exposure to the agent(s) in the defined population is estimated.

Tools to aid decision-making

While obtaining knowledge on various risks is fundamental to the practice of environmental health, it is equally necessary to put in place adequate health and environment surveillance and monitoring systems to assess environmental health conditions. In the following sections we deal with the need to develop indicators for health and environment, and with health impact assessment procedures, which have become critical tools to aid decision-making in environmental health.

Indicators

Monitoring systems

Surveillance and monitoring systems of potential hazards, exposures, and diseases exist in various settings, and have been used for differing purposes. Examples include air and water pollution monitoring, blood lead monitoring programmes, poison centre surveillance, and birth defect registries. The blood lead monitoring programme conducted by the US Centers for Disease Control and Prevention (CDC) played an important role in assessing how blood lead levels in the US population fell in association with reductions in the lead content of petrol during the 1980s at a time in which there was much scepticism in many quarters about the role that lead in petrol played in influencing blood lead levels (Goldman and Torres 2009). This shows how essential it is that

information systems are developed that are supportive of policy and decision-making.

From the perspective of environmental health, of key importance is that the exposure information collected is relevant to health concerns, and not merely to monitor the effectiveness of environmental control measures. Frequently it is the case that exposure information is based on data from high-exposure areas obtained for the purpose of assessing compliance with legislated exposure limits. Such compliance-oriented methods are not optimal for accurate estimation of likely exposure levels of the population.

For many pollutants there is a sharp decrease in concentration levels as one moves away from a source. Similarly, significant vertical variations may occur in the concentration level of a pollutant. Knowledge of spatial and temporal variability of concentrations of exposure may therefore be important from a health point of view, and it may also be necessary to take into account that the exposure may be mediated by more than one environmental pathway. Also of relevance is that health and environmental data from monitoring programmes are frequently available at differing levels of resolution, making it difficult to determine any associations. The complexity and intersectoral nature of environmental health surveillance can thus prove very challenging, and few routine monitoring systems are set up to assess exposure to potential contaminants comprehensively.

Role of indicators

Increasingly, however, communities are demanding access to relevant information on the state of the environment and its influence on health, sometimes as part of their 'right to know' (pollutant release and transfer registries exist in many parts of the world). With an increasing array of information available (of varying quality and usefulness), there is a growing need for scientifically sound and useful information to be obtained and made accessible to decision-makers and the public alike. The development of indicators is of importance in this regard, and environmental health practitioners have an important role to play in their design and use.

The Oxford Dictionary defines an indicator as 'providing specific information on the state or condition of something' (Oxford Dictionaries n.d.) They are a way of 'seeing the big picture by looking at a small piece of it' (Plan Canada 1999). While much information may be available from existing monitoring systems (notwithstanding their shortcomings), if useful indicators are determined in advance, it may be possible to incorporate their data requirements into the information system. As the raw data may not always be in a form which is useful from the point of view of decision-making, indicators can play a key role in turning it into useful information, thereby giving it added value, and also, importantly, in simplifying it. They can give a snapshot (synthesis) view of environment and health trends and can be used to track progress, to help build the evidence base for effective policies, to identify issues and priority problems, provide data for the development of interventions, and for their evaluation.

Indicators have been used in many different fields, at the global, regional, national, local, and sectoral levels. The UN system has been actively involved in indicator development for many years, and there exist numerous data sets on indicators of health, environmental health, environment, sustainable development, poverty, housing, urban development, and others (von Schirnding 2002b, 2007). Indicators have also been applied and developed in various settings and sectors, and have been used in different ways for various purposes, including in ecosystem health, health promotion, healthy cities, and countless other ways (Cheadle et al. 1992; Takano and Nakamura 2001; von Schirnding 2002b).

Types of indicators

Descriptive indicators may be used to highlight what is happening to the environment or to human health, in order to assess trends, and to obtain baseline information on which to formulate subsequent policy options and plans. Examples would be 'ambient concentration levels of sulphur dioxide in an area', 'infant mortality rate', 'percentage of the population using biomass for cooking or heating', 'incidence of acute respiratory infections in children under five' or 'proportion of the population living in informal settlement areas'.

They may be of use at a local level (pollution concentration levels), at a national level (mortality rates, incidence of food poisoning), or at a global level (temperature increases in relation to climate change). A performance indicator on the other hand is one that is linked to a reference value or policy target, illustrating how far the indicator is from the desired level. Examples would be 'the proportion of the population living in electrified areas', 'the number of children immunized against infectious diseases' or 'the proportion of food outlets inspected in an area'.

Composite indicators may be developed, which condense a wide range of information on different but related phenomena into a single measure or index. In the field of health, the disability-adjusted life year (DALY) is an example of a composite measure of the burden of disease which combines the years of healthy life lost due to premature death, disability or disease. Gross national product (GNP) is another example of a composite indicator, as

is the Human Development Index (HDI) which combines information on life expectancy at birth, education level, and income level. These demand high levels of statistical and measurement competence in weighting and combining various variables, and may be difficult to interpret depending on how the components are chosen and weighted, which might be somewhat subjective. They are nevertheless useful for summarizing data and for drawing comparisons between countries.

Indicators have an especially important role to play in the context of the planning process (Plan Canada 1999) and setting goals and targets, which need to be measureable.

There are many examples of goal setting in the area of environmental health at all levels—global to local. One example at the global level would be the MDGs (Sachs and McArthur 2005). For example, Goal 7 of the MDGs is: 'Ensure environmental sustainability'. The target is: 'To halve, by 2015, the proportion of people without sustainable access to safe drinking water and basic sanitation'. Associated indicators are: 'Proportion of population using an improved water source', and 'Proportion of population using an improved sanitation facility'. Indicators have also been used in health and environment planning processes at the national and local level. In this respect it is important to emphasize that even the best set of well-developed indicators can fail to meet their objectives if they are unrelated to a methodical planning process (Brugman 1997). Indicators should be applicable to the users, rather than being merely technically relevant to data providers. In fact indicators may be derived by community groups and used for community-based monitoring.

Indicator development

The process of indicator development includes defining the characteristics to be measured, identifying the target audience and the purpose of the indicator, choosing a suitable framework, defining criteria for selecting the indicator, identifying and evaluating the indicator, pilot testing, and choosing the final indicator or indicator set (Plan Canada 1999). Criteria which have been developed to guide the development, selection, and evaluation of indicators include such factors as their general relevance, scientific soundness, and their applicability to users. Ideally they should be credible, unbiased, and representative of the condition of interest, as well as be consistent, comparable in different settings in time and space, and readily understandable, based on information that is easily accessible. The definitions used for the indicators should be clear, and the data sources and methods used for their collection should be specified (Kjellstrom and Corvalan 1995).

All potential major sources of information relevant to the chosen indicator should be identified. In many countries, despite inevitable problems related to data quality and coverage, and the limitations of routine monitoring systems, it is nevertheless usually possible to find some basic data of use, even if rudimentary or incomplete. If data on health outcomes and exposures is truly unavailable/unusable/inaccessible, it may be prudent to focus instead on action indicators. It may also be possible to use proxy measures of actual exposure (e.g. in relation to air pollution) like traffic volume, distance from a road, proximity to industry, and so on.

Many sources of information can be consulted, including routine data collected and published by government departments and agencies, universities, research organizations, community-based organizations, monitoring groups, industry, and the private sector. On a global (and national) basis, data collected by international organizations, and the UN system, including the WHO, the United Nations Environment Programme (UNEP), the UNDP, and UNICEF, can be useful.

Sometimes it may be necessary to focus on sentinel diseases, that is, diseases that may be indicative of an environmental problem (e.g. diarrhoeal disease, acute respiratory infections, acute poisonings, rare cancers). One data source on environmental health effects is the WHO's Environmental Health Criteria series. These documents provide critical reviews of the effects of chemicals, or combinations of chemicals, and physical and biological agents on human health and the environment. Two series are available, one on chemicals, and one on risk assessment methodology (WHO n.d. a) There is also the UNEP's International Register of Potentially Toxic Chemicals (UNEP n.d.), the WHO's guidelines on air and water quality (WHO n.d. b), the International Agency for Research on Cancer's (IARC's) monographs on evaluation of carcinogenic risks of chemical substances (IARC n.d.), and many others.

Indicator frameworks

Several indicator frameworks have been developed for presenting the various linkages between factors under consideration. One of the earliest of these, upon which many others have been subsequently based, is the OECD Pressure-State-Response (P-S-R) Framework (OECD 2001) which looked at the various pressures which impacted on the state of the environment and necessitated various policy responses.

Modifications to this model such as the D-P-S-I-R (driving forces, pressure, state, impact, response) model adopted by the European Environment Agency made provision for broader driving forces to be taken account of, as well as impacts (including on health) deriving from changes to the state of the environment. The WHO's 'DPSEEA' model (driving force, pressure, state, exposure, effect, action) divides the 'impact' component further into exposure and health effects separately (Kjellstrom and Corvalan 1995; von Schirnding 2002b).

Thus, for example, if applied in environmental health, one can think of 'driving forces' as including such indicators as the population growth rate, or the level of economic development, while the resulting 'pressures' which may be exerted on the environment may be in the form of indicators like pollutant emissions. This may in turn cause the 'state' (quality) of the environment to be degraded through the dispersal and accumulation of pollutants in various environmental media like air, soil, water, and food (indicators might include pollutant concentration levels in media). People may then become 'exposed' to these hazards in the environment (an indicator might be people exposed to air pollution levels above standards) and a variety of 'health effects' may subsequently occur (indicators like air pollution-related morbidity and mortality could be useful). Various 'actions' can then be implemented at different points in the framework (indicators might include clean air policies, technical control measures, treatment regimens or education measures).

While this may be considered a somewhat linear and simplistic model of what is in reality a complex web of circular feedback loops, it can nevertheless be useful for presenting data in a way that shows the linkages between exposures, health effects, and policy actions in a straightforward and readily understandable, actionable way. The form in which the information is conveyed may have considerable impact on how it is used and interpreted. Nevertheless when it comes to dealing with complex ecosystems, for example, deciding what to measure, and how to measure it, and present it, can be very challenging (Cole et al. 1998). In the realm of climate change, development of indicators of vulnerability and preparedness to inform public health adaptation strategies and project the impact of climate change on human health, is an example (English et al. 2009).

Environmental health impact assessment

It is critical to conduct research on specific hazards, carry out epidemiological studies, conduct risk assessments, do environmental monitoring and surveillance of risks, and develop indicators. Most importantly, it is necessary to prevent risks to human health occurring from the outset. In many countries relatively little attention has been paid to the health impacts of planned developments. This, however, is a critical aspect of the practice of environmental health. Impact assessment provides a powerful (yet under-utilized) tool to institutionalize a holistic, cross-sectoral approach to addressing health in public policy (Bhatia and Wernham 2008).

Key steps

In line with the principle of sustainability, development should minimize negative health impacts and maximize health benefits. Health impact assessment (HIA) is a decision-support tool aimed at adding value to the decision-making process by analysing potential effects of planned policies, programmes, or projects on health (Davenport et al. 2006). It aims to identify and predict the impacts of proposed developments on environmental parameters that have a strong health significance. Using information from epidemiological and toxicological studies, researchers attempt to identify, predict, and evaluate possible changes in health which could occur as a result of the development under consideration. A risk assessment is then undertaken (see Chapter 7.5).

HIA is to an extent based on the environmental impact assessment (EIA) process, with a number of procedural steps accompanied by opportunities for stakeholder involvement. Steps to conduct an HIA include *screening* to identify projects or policies for which an HIA would be useful; *scoping* to identify which health impacts should be assessed and which populations are affected; *assessing* the magnitude, direction, and certainty of health impacts; *reporting* results to decision-makers; and *evaluating* the impact of HIA on the decision-making process. Some HIAs focus on biomedical outcomes (e.g. respiratory disease), while some define health holistically to include social, environmental, and economic conditions. Others focus on equity impacts (Dannenberg et al. 2006).

HIA approaches

Some approaches consider HIA independently of EIA while in other cases HIA is integrated with EIA. For example, in some European countries HIA has evolved independently of EIA and is applied in a wide range of public policy decisions not subject to EIA (Kemm et al. 2004). Despite much work done over the past years however, in a majority of countries, health impacts are all too infrequently incorporated into the impact assessment process.

In comparison with EIA, HIA is still, in many ways, in a rudimentary phase. This is somewhat surprising given the substantial growth in HIA activity in recent years, as evidenced by the number of publications, training courses, and guidance materials developed (Davenport et al. 2006).

Indeed it is interesting to note that even in the country where EIA originated (namely the United States with the promulgation of the National Environmental Policy Act of 1969 (NEPA 1969), and which established the foundation for environmental policy in the United States)—health impacts are still infrequently incorporated into the EIA process, although this is gradually changing. While the objectives and regulations of NEPA do indeed provide for the protection of human health and welfare, in practice where health impacts have been considered, these have been narrowly focused on chemicals and toxic exposures. A comprehensive and systematic approach to addressing human health impacts in impact assessment procedures has yet to evolve. A range of institutional, organizational, and disciplinary factors may account for this (Rattle and Kwiatkowski 2003).

It is also a consequence of the complexity of relationships between exposures and health outcomes as discussed earlier. Sometimes there may be inadequate evidence and methodological challenges involved in predicting health outcomes and it is necessary to make decisions at the pace required by political or economic priorities, which may be based on existing evidence, albeit flawed or inadequate, and professional opinion.

Some have contended that a voluntary approach to HIA is preferable to a regulatory approach, where there is more procedural rigidity and stricter rules of evidence required (Cole et al. 2004). That said, it is often the case that causal certainty and quantitative precision are unrealistic and unnecessary standards for impact assessment. What seems likely is that HIA linked to EIA will conform to the limits of EIA, rather than HIA expanding the scope of the EIA (Cole and Fielding 2007), although there is some evidence in Canada that there has been some success with expanding the traditional EIA approach.

Need for capacity building

Whatever the case may be, HIA methodology has been criticized for the lack of rigour in its use of evidence, and guidance is needed on the kinds of public health effects to be included in an impact assessment, as well as on the methods for analysing health effects. New analytical tools are needed to translate the impacts presented in an EIA into valid health impact predictions. The scope of health issues that could be addressed is broad, and includes conditions as diverse as traffic injuries, social cohesion, traditional diets, domestic violence, psychological problems, and so on (Bhatia and Wernham 2008).

Impact assessment training for environmental health practitioners should be included in the curricula of schools of public health as well as in continuing education courses. There is only one university graduate school course on HIA in the United States (Bhatia and Wernham 2008). Countries should advocate for formal guidance on incorporating health into EIA. Examples exist in Australia and Canada, where guidance for social impact assessment contributed to institutionalizing these issues as routine considerations within EIA.

A guide to reviewing available evidence for use in HIA has recently been developed by the WHO (Mindell et al. 2010). However, in order for HIA to be more effective, environmental health practitioners need to familiarize themselves with the EIA process and they need also to be more involved in community collaboration (Bhatia and Wernham 2008). In practice, there often exists a tension between the need to involve communities in the HIA process but at the same time to give priority to expert- and research-generated evidence (Wright et al. 2005).

Intersectoral action and partnerships

The previous subsections on indicators for decision-making, and on HIA processes, have highlighted the possibilities for these tools to help institutionalize intersectoral approaches to policy and decision-making. In this section, we discuss the nature of the intersectoral planning process in addressing health and environment concerns at various levels, which is a key aspect of the practice of environmental health.

The intersectoral nature of environmental health is recognized in the WHO's Constitution (WHO 1948), which states that the Organization shall 'promote, in cooperation with other specialized agencies, where necessary, the improvement of nutrition, housing, sanitation, recreation, economic or working conditions and other aspects of environmental hygiene'.

Intersectoral action for health (IAH) has been identified as an important component for achieving the goal of 'Health for All' (HFA) by the year 2000 (WHO 1981). The concept has been developed in a number of international fora, including the Alma Ata conference in 1978 (WHO 1978), the World Health Assembly (WHA) Technical Discussion on Intersectoral Action (WHO 1986a), the Ottawa Charter on Health Promotion (WHO 1986b), the Sundsvall meeting on Supportive Environments for Health (Haglund et al. 1996), in the WHO Commission on Environment and Health (WHO 1992), and at the international conference on 'Intersectoral Action for Health—A Cornerstone for Health-for-All in the 21st Century', held in Canada in 1997 (WHO 1997; Kreisel and von Schirnding 1998).

At this last meeting IAH was defined as 'a recognized relationship between part or parts of the health sector with part or parts of another sector which has been formed to take action on an issue to achieve health outcomes…in a way that is more effective…than could be achieved by the health sector acting alone'.

Addressing the underlying determinants of health is essential in order to ensure long-term health improvements which are sustainable. By addressing health, environment, and development concerns in an intersectoral way a win–win situation occurs: the health sector gains because disease prevention can move upstream and take advantage of the intersectoral approach to development and environmental improvements. The environmental sector gains because environmental issues can become grounded in matters of local and direct concern to people.

Global initiatives

Rachel Carson's book *Silent Spring*, published in 1962 (Carson 1962), was one of the early and most powerful warnings to humanity about the consequences of its actions on the environment. About a decade later the UN Conference on the Human Environment was held in Stockholm, Sweden (UN 1972), which was followed in 1983 by the World Commission on Environment and Development headed by former Norwegian Prime Minister Gro Harlem Brundtland (World Commission on Environment and Development 1987). This linked the issue of environmental protection to economic growth and development. The Commission's report 'Our Common Future' (World Commission on Environment and Development 1987) launched the concept of sustainable development into the mainstream of world debate.

Sustainable development was defined in the report as 'Development that meets the needs of the present without compromising the ability of future generations to meet their own needs' (World Commission on Environment and Development 1987). It essentially meant meeting people's development needs in such a way as not to exceed the earth's carrying capacity in the longer term. Although specific definitions for sustainable development vary, broadly speaking, the concept is concerned with balancing environmental, social and economic objectives in order to maximize societal well-being, both now and in the future. This has been referred to as the triple-bottom-line approach to human well-being (Sachs 2012).

While subsequent environmental conferences built on this growing recognition of the links between environment and development, the awareness of the links between environment and development is also evident in the public health movement, especially, for example, as highlighted in WHOs 'Health-for-All' strategy in 1977 (WHO 1977) and renewed in 1998 (Yach 1996; WHO 1998) which aimed to achieve for all people of the world a level of health which would enable them to lead 'socially and economically productive lives'.

A key milestone was the Ottawa Charter on Health Promotion in 1986 (WHO 1986b) which addressed the need for a broader understanding of public health beyond primary healthcare and which stressed the necessity to take a more holistic view of health and, among other factors, to develop healthy public policy and create environments which were supportive of health. Strong emphasis was placed on the environmental component of health and to see health in ecological terms.

Significantly, the Ottawa Charter emphasized the importance of actions both outside of, as well as within, the health sector. It also emphasized the need to look at the settings where people lived, worked, and recreated. This was followed up on in a subsequent conference held in 1991 in Sundsvall, Sweden on Supportive Environments for Health (Haglund et al. 1996), which looked at the role of various sectors in influencing health outcomes, serving as inputs for the subsequent UN Conference on Environment and Development held in 1992 (UN 1992).

In parallel with the progressive greening of the public health movement (emphasizing more of a socio-ecological approach), more emphasis has been placed on the human element in recent environmental (sustainable development) conferences. These have been key in fostering intersectoral partnerships to reduce environmental hazards in line with sustainable development objectives.

United Nations Conference on Environment and Development

The UN Conference on Environment and Development (UNCED) (UN 1992)—a watershed event popularly referred to as the 'Earth Summit'—resulted in the adoption of Agenda 21—a global action plan with concrete goals, targets, and outputs for measures needed to achieve environmentally sustainable development into the twenty-first century. It also resulted in the 'Rio Declaration' which encompassed important agreements on 27 principles adopted by 178 nations (including the Precautionary Principle, and the Polluter Pays Principle), and several key conventions such as those on Climate Change (including the Kyoto Protocol) and on Biological Diversity (and the Cartagena Protocol).

The Rio Declaration, in its preamble, alluded to the central role of health in sustainable development by stating that 'Human beings are at the center of concerns for sustainable development. They are entitled to a healthy and productive life in harmony with nature'. This concept was further developed during the planning process for the World Summit on Sustainable Development (WSSD) (UN 2002) which took place in Johannesburg, 10 years after UNCED.

World Summit on Sustainable Development

At WSSD, health was singled out as one of the five priority issues to be addressed, along with water, energy, agriculture, and biodiversity (Annan 2002; WEHAB Working Group 2002). In the Johannesburg Plan of Implementation (JPOI) which emerged from this conference, particular emphasis was placed on health issues in relation to environment and poverty concerns. Improving access to safe water, sanitation, clean air, improved waste management, and sound management of chemicals were among the key environmental health issues that received special attention in Johannesburg (von Schirnding 2005).

Of particular note was the call to increase access to sanitation to improve health and reduce infant and child mortality, prioritizing water and sanitation in national sustainable development strategies and poverty reduction strategies where they exist. A new target was agreed, namely to halve by the year 2015 the proportion of people who do not have access to basic sanitation. This target complemented the MDG target on access to safe drinking water. Other agreements concerned the safer use of chemicals, reduction of risks associated with heavy metals, reduction of air pollution exposures and related health impacts (through the use of cleaner fuels, modern pollution control techniques, and reduced dependence on traditional fuel sources for cooking and heating), and to increase the global share of renewable energy sources.

There was also a call for capacity building in health to better assess health and environment linkages. Other aspects emphasized in the JPOI included the need to integrate health concerns within strategies, policies, and programmes for sustainable development. Many of the MDGs and targets agreed by world leaders in 2000 were confirmed at WSSD. WSSD was thus an important milestone for health (von Schirnding 2005) which took concerted effort by key players including many countries and the UN system, most notably the WHO (WEHAB Working Group 2002; WHO 2002a, 2002b, 2002c).

United Nations Conference on Sustainable Development (Rio+20)

This momentum was somewhat lost in the subsequent run-up to the twentieth anniversary of UNCED. In June 2012, the world's leaders and 50,000 delegates from 193 countries gathered in Rio to seek a new consensus on global actions to safeguard the future of the planet. 'Rio+20' (UN 2012) aimed to review progress over the past 20 years and to renew political commitments to sustainable development. According to some, however, an important opportunity for a paradigm shift in international policy was lost (Barbier 2012).

While many new green economy policies were endorsed in the final document 'The Future We Want', no new international commitments nor legally binding agreements were made, albeit voluntary agreements were made by countries to meet their own sustainable development targets. Key global health outcomes related to global environmental change were omitted from the outcome document, and in the view of some observers, health was inadequately highlighted as a cross-sectoral priority for sustainable development, with many important linkages to other sectors like energy, biodiversity, land and water management, and climate change largely absent (Langlois et al. 2012). Coming out of WSSD where health made a strong showing, and out of the MDG process where health had a central position, at the very least, the Rio+20 experience confirmed the importance of the health community remaining actively engaged in the sustainable development agenda (Singh et al. 2012).

It should also be pointed out that all three conferences (UNCED with its focus on environment, WSSD with its focus on the social dimension—poverty, and Rio+20 with its focus on the economy) failed to ensure the integration of the three pillars of sustainable development. In addition, the trade-offs and synergies across the economic, environmental, and social objectives have not yet been agreed (Sachs 2012). The process of setting sustainable development goals in the follow-up process to Rio+20 is a way to remedy this, providing the three pillars of sustainable development are not considered separately from each other. Health can be used as a tool to integrate across the three dimensions of sustainable development. Measurable targets are needed to ensure health remains a prerequisite for, and an outcome of, sustainable development—in all its dimensions.

The Commission on Global Governance for Health which was created in 2012 will now emphasize the need to ensure that health is protected and promoted in global policy arenas outside the health sector (Ottersen et al. 2011). As German Chancellor Angela Merkel said in her welcome message to the 2012 World Health Summit held in Berlin (quoting Arthur Schopenhauer) 'Health is not everything, but without health, everything is nothing' (Kleinert et al. 2012).

National and local initiatives

Global concerns about the environment have led to common approaches to environmental health planning and policy development and international cooperation in controlling some environmental hazards. While governments share the main responsibility for ensuring healthy living environments, they can do so only by working in collaboration and partnership with other groups. Involving stakeholders in all stages of the decision-making process is an important part of the practice of environmental health. Over recent years there has been an increasing trend towards decentralized government services and more emphasis on health and environmental actions by NGOs and the community itself. Intersectoral, participatory planning has become more central to the way governments do business in the field of environmental health.

Most health and environment action plans that have been developed in countries, involve articulation of a common vision, identification of key issues and their ranking/prioritization,

collection and analysis of data and information, development of a plan of action with goals and targets (and indicators), a resource mobilization plan, and, following implementation, a process of monitoring, evaluation, and follow-up. Sometimes a rational and comprehensive process will have been put in place while in others planning will have been done in a more incremental way.

Where partners have been involved in the definition of problems as well as in their solution, there has been a better chance of commitments being met in the long term. Identifying the right partners has proved to be a critical step, as this plays a key role in determining the legitimacy or otherwise of the planning initiative. In general, success has been achieved in situations where all partners have an interest in the problem and are interdependent in reaching solutions (Box 11.5.3). Service users and providers are normally represented, as well as other interested and affected parties and parties with particular knowledge and expertise. Groups such as business and industry, local, national, and regional government, trade unions, community groups and residents, women's groups, youth groups, and the media might commonly be represented.

There have been a number of collaborative planning initiatives at various levels of government which involve partnerships with NGOs and local communities, whereby health authorities have been able to address problems more effectively. For example, there have been the national environment and health action plans at the national level and local health and environment planning initiatives such as local Agenda 21 initiatives, and initiatives like the WHO healthy cities movement, the UN Human Settlements programme, and UNEP's sustainable cities movement (von Schirnding 1997a).

These have led to a better understanding of the importance of environment and development issues within health ministries, as

---

Box 11.5.3 Ingredients for successful partnerships

Among the key ingredients for a successful partnership are the following:

◆ The contributions of all partners should be understood and valued.

◆ The core interests of individual organizations should be protected.

◆ Partners should be able to gain resources and/or legitimacy.

◆ There should be opportunities for action and capacity for action.

◆ There should be a clear mandate and authorization from the government body concerned.

◆ Agreement should be reached on how results will be acted on.

◆ There should be a clearly defined decision-making process.

Reproduced with permission from von Schirnding, Y.E.R., *Intersectoral Action for Health: Addressing Health and Environment Concerns in Sustainable Development*, WHO/PPE/PAC/97.1, World Health Organization (WHO), Geneva, Switzerland, Copyright © WHO 1997, available from http://apps.who.int/iris/bitstream/10665/63359/1/WHO_PPE_PAC_97.1.pdf?ua=1.

Box 11.5.4 United Kingdom National Environmental Health Action Plan

The UK National Environmental Health Action Plan, intended to improve environmental health in the United Kingdom, set out ways in which improvements could be made and identified the sectors responsible. It contained more than 160 actions with a checklist against which progress could be measured. In drawing up the plan the views of a wide range of people and organizations were taken into account. Five areas were set out in the plan, namely institutional framework, environmental health management tools, specific environmental hazards, living and working environments, and economic sectors. The objectives, bases for action, and actions were set out for each of the areas covered by the plan. These were divided into three types according to their urgency, namely basic requirements, prevention and control of medium- and long-term hazards, and promotion of well-being and mental health. The plan gave both an overview of the provision of environmental health and a detailed analysis of the main factors contributing to it, setting out a range of specific actions which may be needed to improve it. In this way the means of achieving the objectives of the plan were established.

Source: data from United Kingdom Department of the Environment, *The UK National Environmental Health Action Plan*, The Stationery Office, London, UK, Copyright © 1996.

well as a better understanding of health issues within environment ministries. In many cases successful intersectoral committees or commissions and fora have been set up, and in the process alliances and linkages formed with various sectors. Linkages with the finance and planning sectors, however, have frequently been among the weakest of these.

On a global basis, approaches to incorporate health and environment issues in national plans and programmes have varied from country to country depending upon priorities and planning mechanisms and the way in which responsibilities are divided. This has led to a wide variety of approaches being adopted (Box 11.5.4).

Sometimes health and environment plans have been included in the national plans for sustainable development or for economic and social development. Sectoral plans might include health and environment issues or health considerations might be included in national environmental action plans and so forth.

Healthy cities

The healthy cities project has been instrumental in helping to address health and environment issues at the local level in many countries and settings. What started as a small-scale initiative of the WHO arising from the Beyond Healthcare conference held in Toronto, Canada in 1984, became a major movement involving thousands of cities throughout the world.

The healthy cities concept and approach has been translated in different ways according to different priorities and emphases of different localities: healthy cities in Europe and Africa, healthy islands in the Western Pacific region, healthy municipalities and communities in North America, healthy villages in the eastern Mediterranean, as well as healthy settings which encompassed schools, homes, and other settings where people live, work, and recreate (von Schirnding 1997b).

Importantly, the healthy cities movement emphasizes process—in particular the building of political commitment and a common vision locally to push health higher up the urban policy agenda. Secondly, there is involvement of a wide range of stakeholders including local communities, and emphasizing community empowerment and participation rather than an expert-led health agenda. Thirdly, strategy development within local government, in the form of a city health plan based on intersectoral partnerships and the necessary stakeholder engagement, is important. This goes along with the development of health information systems, the integration of health into other urban policy and planning processes, and the use of tools to assess health effects (Rydin et al. 2012).

In a review of the healthy cities project in Europe (WHO Regional Office for Europe 2008) a majority of cities were found to be implementing collaborative plans, projects, or programmes with greater cross-sector involvement. Most had developed city health plans and city health profiles, although health-effects assessments were often lacking. Implementation of these intersectoral policies, however, has proven more difficult than expected. According to the commission by *The Lancet*, most cities evaluated are still struggling with the holistic approach in which health is fully integrated into urban planning. This is no doubt in part due to lack of adequate understanding of the complexity of systems at work in these urban settings, prompting utilization of a systems approach to the analysis of healthy cities in the future (Rydin et al. 2012).

Of key importance though, is that the health sector fit in with planning processes in other sectors rather than the other way around. This is especially true of the healthy cities movement if it is to be more than merely a health promotion, awareness-raising initiative. As we have seen in other areas like HIA, the health sector is also frequently lacking the expertise and capacity needed to measure or estimate the health impacts associated with proposed projects or policies. Until it has developed that capacity its ability to meaningfully participate in intersectoral work may be limited. What is needed is to be able to better characterize the health burden from the perspective of the sector, rather than the specific vehicle of exposure—for example, air or water.

While the national and local intersectoral health and environment planning processes have been useful in obtaining a better understanding of the nature and causes of environmental health problems in various countries, problems and weaknesses have been identified including: gaps in data availability and quality, difficulties in detecting trends (geographical and temporal), difficulty in disaggregating data, poor linkages of health and environmental data, and sectoral data, emphasis on symptoms rather than on causes of problems, little focus on analysis of management structures and capacity, and lack of clarity in priority-setting processes. Many of these issues have been discussed in earlier sections. Environmental health management issues are further elaborated on in the following section.

Environmental health management and policy

While there is more acceptance now of the links between health status and the determinants of health, especially those that arise from the activities of sectors other than health, there are still problems acting on this knowledge. Greater attention needs to be paid to developing institutional, managerial, administrative, and financial capacities to address problems. Definitions of environmental health aside, it has become increasingly complex to define roles and responsibilities in environmental health in light of its inherent intersectoral nature.

The Institute of Medicine (IOM) report *Investing in a Healthier Future* (2012) came up with the recommendation that it is of critical importance to develop a detailed description of a basic set of public health services that must be made available in all jurisdictions. They developed the concept of a minimum package of public health services which includes foundational capabilities and basic programmes which no health department can be without. These apply regardless of the specific area of control—for example, whether it be infectious disease control or environmental health. They are capabilities that are needed across all programmes.

Some of these foundational public health capabilities defined by the committee include the following:

◆ Information systems and resources, including surveillance and epidemiology.

◆ Health planning (including community health improvement planning).

◆ Partnership development and community mobilization.

◆ Policy development, analysis, and decision support.

◆ Communication (including health literacy and cultural competence).

◆ Public health research, evaluation, and quality improvement.

The committee also made recommendations on basic programmes which are activities that no well-run public health department can be without. High-level categories of basic programmes include maternal and child health promotion, injury control, communicable disease control, chronic disease prevention, environmental health, and mental health and substance abuse.

When it comes to managing environmental health issues which are intersectoral and whose determinants frequently lie outside the control of the health sector, or outside of jurisdictional boundaries, with different organizations and agencies having differing roles and responsibilities, things become complicated. In addition, systems of organization in many government authorities worldwide may be based on concepts of bureaucracy, hierarchy, professional authority, disciplinary specialization, and sectoral analysis (von Schirnding 1997a). To facilitate implementation of intersectoral plans there may be a need for institutional restructuring and readjustment.

This may include internal reforms within government departments. Issues that may need to be addressed might include mechanisms for interjurisdictional cooperation in implementing policies and plans, decentralization of structures to facilitate community involvement of sectors, and better coordination between and within governance structures. Various types of jurisdictional reform can take place, which might include the transfer of powers and functions from one department to another or from one tier of government to another, or changing geographical boundaries, consolidating multiple jurisdictions, forming various coordinating mechanisms, and so on. Thus many barriers and obstacles need to be overcome in coordinating action between sectors. Sharing power, information, and financial resources are all important.

Environmental health services

While there is no universal understanding of what precisely constitutes an environmental health service, it is essentially concerned with developing and implementing environment and health policies, largely through monitoring and control activities, but also increasingly through environmental health promotion efforts. Environmental health services worldwide have been established and developed within a complex framework of policies, institutions and legislation. The concept of environmental health, the problems to be addressed, the way in which services are delivered, and the way in which governments are organized differ considerably throughout the world.

Environmental health activities are carried out in many different settings at various tiers of government, in the private sector, the workplace, healthcare facilities, and so on. In most countries a range of different agencies have responsibility for various aspects of environment and human health at different levels of government. Normally there are separate regulatory agencies dealing with the environment, health, food safety, agriculture, and so on, which have various environmental health responsibilities. Different tiers of government have different responsibilities. Thus, for example, regulatory frameworks and standards (e.g. for air, drinking water, etc.) may be set at a national level, while implementation and enforcement may occur at a state, regional, or local level. Inspection of food preparation premises, food hygiene, sanitation, vector control, and so on, are normally done at the local level. This requires strong monitoring and enforcement abilities which are sometimes in short supply, especially in some developing countries (see Table 11.5.2).

Internationally a shift has occurred towards organizational diversification regarding environmental health services. In the context of the development of primary healthcare services and district health systems in many developing countries, and parallel development outside of the health sector of environmental management systems, the placement of environmental health services is a fundamental issue in need of addressing. Despite the fact that environmental health is recognized as a major and core function of a public health department, it is also the case that the public health sector has gradually lost organizational responsibility for many aspects of environmental health.

This includes, increasingly, such aspects as air quality, waste management, chemical safety, meat inspection, and many other areas. While it would be unmanageable for the full ambit of environmental health services to be located centrally in one department, in light of its intersectoral nature, what is needed is to

Table 11.5.2 Examples of environmental health concerns at local, national, and global levels

Local	Regional/national	Global
Dust control	Hazardous waste	Climate change
Noise control	Air quality standards	Transboundary pollution
Solid waste	Water quality standards	Ozone depletion
Sanitation	Regulation of toxic chemicals	Marine pollution
Vector control	Food safety policy	

Box 11.5.5 Organizational responsibility for environmental health in the United States

In the first part of the twentieth century in the United States, a typical scenario was a health department headed by a physician, with nurses responsible for immunization programmes and sanitarians/sanitary engineers responsible for sanitary inspection, water and sanitation, food safety, vector control, and so on. Sanitarians were generalists trained to respond to a broad array of environmental health issues.

With increasing industrialization and growing public awareness about the widespread contamination of the environment in the 1960s, a number of environmental laws dealing with water and air quality, toxic substances, and other issues were passed and the US EPA was established. Separate state-level environmental agencies were also established, with responsibility for enforcement of these new environmental laws. At this time many of the traditional environmental health functions falling under health departments were transferred to environmental departments with positive (increased funding and visibility) but also negative (schism in environment and health actions) repercussions. Separate data systems, uncoordinated planning, and loss of oversight of community health and environment issues resulted. With the new environmental 'medium-specific' laws, and the emergence of environmental health specialists in particular areas like water or air quality, environmental health professionals became increasingly disconnected from their public health roots and counterparts in health departments at state or local level and the agencies grew apart too.

Subsequently in the 1970s and 1980s there was a growing public awareness and involvement in environmental health issues and a demand for more accountability and transparency in decision-making. With the advent of environmental impact assessment legislation and requirements for public involvement, watchdog groups and advocacy organizations were formed with a strong focus on environmental justice, human rights, and equity concerns. Increasing initiatives to reconnect environmental and public health sprang up out of a sense of growing dissatisfaction over the inability of accountable agencies to address these in a coordinated and integrated way.

Source: data from Kotchian S., The practice of environmental health, pp. 895–925, in Frumkin H., (Ed), *Environmental Health: From Global to Local*, Jossey-Bass, San Francisco, USA, Copyright © 2005.

---

develop organizational structures that facilitate the movement of professionals across different departments, sectors, and organizations. Box 11.5.5 gives a case study from the United States, which is typical of the situation in many countries around the world, who face similar challenges in regard to the placement of environmental health functions subsequent to the establishment of environmental departments and new environmental regulations.

Environmental health practitioners

In general, environmental health practitioners and professionals have as their main responsibilities the identification, assessment, management, communication, and remediation of health risks resulting from environmental factors. They include people working in a wide range of professions and specialties and include environmental health officers (EHOs), sanitarians, health inspectors, clinicians, epidemiologists, toxicologists, environmental scientists, environmental engineers, veterinarians, and many others.

Environmental health officers

As stated at the beginning of this chapter, the roots of the environmental health profession today can be found in the sanitary and public health movement of the United Kingdom during the 1800s. The role of the health inspector has steadily changed over the years and has evolved from a focus on inspection and control to a role associated as well with education, health promotion, and community development. Commensurate with the changing role of the health inspector has been a change in title—variously referred to over time and in different settings as sanitarian, inspector of nuisances, sanitary inspector, health inspector/technician/assistant, public health officer, environmental health officer, environmental health practitioner/specialist/professional.

Notwithstanding changing roles and titles, the theory and conceptual basis of environmental health is firmly based in public health, and the practice of environmental health, as embodied in the day to day work of EHOs and others, is closely associated with

inspection and environmental control, with EHOs being responsible for administering and enforcing legislation related to environmental health.

Nonetheless, with the increasing involvement in environmental health of professionals and specialists from a wide variety of fields including environmental chemistry, physics, environmental science, geography, environmental engineering, public health, medicine, and others, the role of the EHO outside of its traditional ambit of inspection, monitoring and control, will continue to evolve. This also has a bearing on their role inside of, and outside of, the health service, and the challenges and constraints faced while working on the broader determinants of health, within the principles of sustainable development, but remaining firmly public health based.

Normally an EHO would be a public employee in a health department in local government or at regional/provincial/state level who investigates environmental hazards and public health nuisances with the view to mitigating or eliminating these. EHOs are involved in inspection of housing, food establishments, schools, daycare centres, nursing homes, and many other premises, and are also involved in vector control, pollution control, and health promotion activities. They may also be employed by the military and by the private sector.

Qualifications and training

Environmental health requires, in many countries, a university degree, with field training and professional certification needed for environmental health officers/practitioners. In the United Kingdom, a degree in environmental health is required, as well as certification and registration with the Chartered Institute of Environmental Health. Fourteen universities in the United Kingdom offer accredited environmental health degrees, including undergraduate and post-graduate degrees. A post-graduate environmental health qualification is required for graduates from other scientific disciplines (Chartered

Institute of Environmental Health n.d.). The Chartered Institute of Environmental Health offers training modules in specialized areas of environmental health as does the Environmental Health Registration Board (n.d.).

In Canada, environmental health officers require a bachelor's degree in environmental health or a related field as well as a certificate in public health inspection. Five universities in Canada offer degree programmes approved by the Canadian Institute of Public Health Inspectors (n.d.). A bachelor's degree and professional licence is also a requirement in parts of the United States and there exists the National Environmental Health Association (NEHA) offering environmental health credentials and registration/certification for practitioners. Interestingly, the premier NEHA credential is referred to as the Registered Environmental Health Specialist/Registered Sanitarian (REHS/RS) (NEHA n.d.).

There exists too the International Federation of Environmental Health (n.d.) to promote cooperation between countries where environmental health issues are cross-boundary. Regional groups exist in Africa, the Americas, Asia and the Pacific, Europe, and the Middle East. Member countries in turn have their own professional institutes and associations of environmental health. These include such bodies as the Environmental Health Workers Association of Uganda, the Public Health Inspectors Union of Sri Lanka, the Malta Association of Environmental Health Officers, the Kenya Association of Public Health Officers, and numerous others, reflecting the variety of names given to those practising environmental health around the world.

In a developing country such as South Africa, degree courses in environmental science or health are offered at universities and diploma courses (e.g. the National Diploma in Environmental Health) at technical institutions. Degrees in technology in environmental health are also offered. Environmental health practitioners require practical training and registration with the Health Professions Council of South Africa (n.d.).

Training programmes have been updated to accommodate the changing role of the environmental health officer in South Africa from law enforcer to community facilitator, in line with changing political and economic realities which make legislation difficult to enforce, especially in the context of rapid urbanization, informal settlements, and a large informal sector.

Clinicians

Clinicians are becoming increasingly involved in the practice of environmental health. The diagnosis of illnesses that are associated with environmental exposures is an important clinical function that expanded from the field of occupational medicine, to a focus on the broader environment outside of the workplace (Laumbach and Kipen 2005). Treating environmentally related diseases is often the same as treating these illnesses from other causes, although in some cases (e.g. lead poisoning), specialized treatments may be required. Clinicians need to be alert to the role that environmental factors may play and adopt a high 'index of suspicion' in assessing underlying signs, symptoms and diseases in patients—whether adults or children (Laumbach and Kipen 2005).

If an environmental cause is suspected, an environmental history would need to be taken in order to obtain information on potential sources and pathways of exposure (both current and past), and the age and development stage of children, should they be assessed. In the case of infants, for example, breastfeeding could be a source of exposure to be considered, and the hand-to-mouth pathway could be of special significance.

Examples of environmental health problems dealt with by clinicians include lead poisoning, asthma associated with air pollution, poisoning by pesticides, hearing loss caused by noise, cancer associated with excessive radiation, and many others. Apart from diagnosing and treating environmental diseases, clinicians also have an important role to play in prevention, including advocacy for protective standards, and patient education.

Children's environmental health issues have become of increasing importance to paediatricians. In 1997, an Executive Order on Children's Environmental Health and Safety was signed in the United States and a cabinet-level oversight committee was formed between the US EPA and the Department of Health and Human Services. Since then, children's environmental health has become an increasingly important part of paediatric practice. Improved exposure and risk assessment and toxicity testing is needed to more adequately address children's environmental health issues, however (Galvez et al. 2005). As part of the WHO's contribution to the follow-up to the WSSD held in 2002, an international alliance on 'Healthy Environments for Children' (HECA) was formed to help advocate for worldwide action on environmental health issues affecting children (WHO n.d. c).

Environmental health policy

Environmental health policy is concerned with selecting actions to reduce or eliminate harmful effects of environmental exposures. Some measures may be short term and remedial while others may be preventive and longer term. Actions can take many forms and involve such factors as regulations and standards, technological control measures, product design, personal or community protection measures, health and environment action plans, housing or transport policies, awareness raising, and education measures and so on. They can take the form of standards that directly regulate the amount of a contaminant in an environmental media, for example, an air pollution standard or drinking water standard. Other policies can benefit health more indirectly, for example, an environmental protection measure that safeguards biodiversity, or a policy in a sector like energy which may determine which fuels are used, and hence their impact on air quality and health.

By better aligning the policies of sectors with the potential to affect health we can maximize opportunities for health. Thus health professionals need constantly to motivate for policies that are beneficial to health—for example, food and agricultural policies that promote integrated vector control over use of toxic chemicals, that encourage substitution of crops that harm health, and that promote consumption of diets balanced in fruits and vegetables. Similarly energy policies need to support clean energy sources, cleaner and more energy efficient transport, and energy efficient buildings while transport policies need to encourage use of bicycles and public transport, and so forth.

The overall cumulative impact of such policies can be substantial. This would also help ensure that health does not become sacrificed for short-term sectoral or economic gain. That is not to imply that health and environmental goals always coincide—frequently they do not. DDT is one example where the immediate health gains were used to lobby for its continued use in sub-Saharan

Africa despite its longer-term insidious negative impact on the environment.

Some laws and regulations may in turn contain policies embedded in them. For example, NEPA in the United States states that 'Congress recognizes that…each person should enjoy a healthful environment and that each person has a responsibility to contribute to the preservation and enhancement of the environment' (Johnson 2005).

Federal laws form much of the environmental framework in the United States and are emulated in many other countries. Examples of such laws include the Safe Drinking Water Act, and the Clean Air Act. A strong science base is normally required for setting standards, and a science-based risk assessment process undertaken to inform risk management policies and strategies, which of necessity also take into account social, economic, and political considerations.

Policies may also span the spectre of government—from global to local. In general they tend to become more specific and targeted as they go from national to state/provincial/regional to local. In the United States, for example, federal statutes and regulations may be issued and states and local governments will issue statutes or ordinances needed to comply with these, or they may develop their own regulations. Policies may be preventive and aim to reduce hazards directly in a prospective manner (e.g. air pollution regulations) or they may be retrospective and require, for example, clean-up of a toxic waste site. Other types of policies may be aimed at awareness raising and education of the public rather than regulatory control (Johnson 2005).

International policy principles have been adopted as well, for example, coming out of UNCED the Precautionary Principle was adopted, which states 'where there are threats of serious or irreversible damage, lack of full scientific certainty shall not be used as a reason for postponing cost-effective measures to prevent environmental degradation' (Johnson 2005). Another principle adopted was the Polluter Pays Principle—that is, those who cause pollution should pay the price to clean it up. Economic instruments such as pollutant trading systems are also in use which shift the societal cost of pollution to the polluter (Goldman and Torres 2009).

Impacts originating from a multitude of small sectors rather than from one large obvious source such as a major polluting factory, for example, are often more difficult to control. Smaller enterprises usually have fewer resources at their disposal and are more resistant to change, or may be less knowledgeable about standards which may apply, than large-scale industry. In developing countries, fewer controls are generally applied and control technology may be less well developed. In the absence of local standards (which demand relevant epidemiological and exposure data, which may often not be available), international standards are often applied but may not be appropriate (Goldman and Torres 2009) due to the differing prevailing lifestyles, cultures, climate, demographic attributes, institutional and policy framework, level of economic development, and so on, which differ from country to country.

Environmental standards may be risk based (i.e. based on assessments of environmental or health risks) or technology based (i.e. based on the best available technology) or a combination of both (Goldman and Torres 2009). Pollution prevention is key. Increasingly it has been recognized that controlling pollutants one medium at a time can result in transferring pollutants from one medium to another, for example, from air to water to land. Multimedia approaches are thus preferable. Reduction of pollution at source is optimal, but other strategies include waste minimization, reuse, recycling, emissions control, and, finally, clean-up. Environmental monitoring has an important role to play in evaluating the success or otherwise of the various control measures adopted, and the public may have an important role in advocacy, monitoring, and enforcement of environmental policies.

Financial incentives

As environmental health protection measures inevitably involve costs, cost–benefit analyses may be undertaken to weigh costs and benefits of an action, while cost-effectiveness analyses might be performed to look at alternative solutions to a problem. Attempts may also be made to assess economic inequities in impacts, taking into consideration issues of environmental justice. Economic and fiscal policies can influence the potential for health gains and their distribution in society. Financial incentives can be set up so that they can contribute to a healthier lifestyle and discourage the use of harmful products and substances. When combined with appropriate legislation and health education programmes many of the negative health trends could be retarded or even reversed.

International regulations

When pollutants cross boundaries, or where there are global impacts and concerns, international agreements and standards come into play. In parallel with the role that international conferences have played in galvanizing action on health and environment issues, so too do international environmental treaties offer the prospect of further advances in public health. Due in part to the WHO's and others' increasing involvement in international conferences and treaty-making processes in recent years, health issues have received increasing recognition and attention. Mechanisms in international environmental law can be used to provide motivations for research aimed at further strengthening the evidence base related to health, and to achieve improved surveillance and monitoring systems concerned with ill health. Increased efforts are needed to more fully realize the potential of international law to promote global environmental health (von Schirnding et al. 2002).

Many multilateral environmental agreements have health implications, for example, the Montreal Protocol on Protection of the Ozone Layer (1987), the Basel Convention on the Control of Transboundary Movements of Hazardous Wastes and their Disposal (1989), the Convention on Biological Diversity adopted in 1992 (including the Cartagena Protocol on Biosafety), the Kyoto Protocol of the UN Framework on Climate Change (1997), the Rotterdam Convention on the Prior Informed Consent Procedure for Certain Hazardous Chemicals and Pesticides in International Trade (1998), and the Stockholm Convention on Persistent Organic Pollutants (2001).

Environmental agreements in existence today, however, recognize the sovereign right and responsibility of nations to set their own standards. So, for example, the Basel Convention does not cover handling and disposal of wastes within a country, and the Rotterdam Convention does not require prior consent for chemicals manufactured and produced within a country (Goldman and Torres 2009).

Conclusion

This chapter has highlighted a number of key issues relating to the nature and practice of environmental health, which is a complex, dynamic, and evolving multidisciplinary field. It is increasingly evident that environmental health practitioners face numerous challenges in addressing the myriad factors influencing health-and-environment relationships in differing contexts and settings.

The multiplicity and interaction of chemical, physical, and biological risks in the environment, the various media and pathways of exposure, the differing vulnerabilities and susceptibilities of diverse groups, and the changing priorities and capacities for the management of environmental health risks in various parts of the world, all need to be addressed by practitioners of environmental health.

Despite dramatic advances in the recognition and amelioration of environmental health risks worldwide in recent decades, there nevertheless remain significant gaps in knowledge of new and emerging risks, and in approaches needed to more effectively address them. Improved indicators which are reflective of complex health-and-environment interactions, and health impact and risk assessment procedures which can better predict impacts associated with differing environment and development parameters and scenarios, are needed.

So too are systems approaches needed for addressing the complexity of issues associated with ecosystems, global change, urbanization, and sectors like energy, housing, and transport. Economic development, the environment, and human health are closely intertwined and interconnected, and need to be addressed as such.

As evidenced by the intersectoral health and sustainable development planning processes which have been underway in recent years at all levels—global to local—there will be more of a need for practitioners to work proactively with communities and other stakeholders and partners in addressing the complexity of health and environment issues. While increasing capacity is needed to assess and address intersectoral impacts, the causes of which frequently lie outside the domain of the health sector, tools like health impact assessment can help to institutionalize intersectoral processes in policymaking and decision-making.

With the continuing development of improved risk assessment procedures and environmental health management tools and policy instruments, and ongoing capacity development of environmental health practitioners and professionals in various settings and tiers of government worldwide, excellence in the practice of environmental health will culminate in increasingly healthier environments for current and future generations to come.

References

Annan, K. (2002). *Towards a Sustainable Future. American Museum of Natural History's Annual Environmental Lecture.* New York: American Museum of Natural History.

Barbier, E.B. (2012). The green economy post Rio+20. *Science*, 338(6109), 887–8.

Bartel, S. (2005). Risk assessment. In H. Frumkin (ed.) *Environmental Health: From Global to Local*, pp. 940–60. San Francisco, CA: Jossey-Bass.

Bhatia, R. and Wernham, A. (2008). Integrating human health into environmental impact assessment: an unrealized opportunity for environmental health and justice. *Environmental Health Perspectives*, 116(8), 991–1000.

Brugman, J. (1997). Is there a method in our measurement? The use of indicators in local sustainable development planning. *Local Environment*, 2(1), 59–72.

Calman, K. (1998). The 1848 Public Health Act and its relevance to improving health in England now. *BMJ*, 317, 596–8.

Canadian Institute of Public Health Inspectors (n.d.). Website. [Online] Available at: http://www.ciphi.on.ca/.

Carson, R.L. (1962). *Silent Spring.* Cambridge: Riverside Press.

Chadwick, E. (1842). *Report of the Sanitary Condition of the Labouring Population and on the Means of its Improvement.* London: Printed by R. Clowes & Sons, for Her Majesty's Stationery Office.

Chartered Institute of Environmental Health (n.d.). Website. [Online] Available at: http://www.cieh.org.

Cheadle, A., Wagner, E., Koepsell, E., et al. (1992). Environmental indicators: a tool for evaluating community-based health promotion programs. *American Journal of Preventive Medicine*, 8, 345–50.

Cole, B. and Fielding, J. (2007). Health impact assessment: a tool to help policy makers understand health beyond healthcare. *Annual Review of Public Health*, 28, 393–412.

Cole, B., Wilhelm, M., Long, P., Fielding, J., Kominski, G., and Morgenstern, H. (2004). Prospects for health impact assessment in the United States: new and improved environmental impact assessment of something different? *Journal of Health Politics, Policy and Law*, 29, 1153–86.

Cole, D.C., Eyles, J., and Gibson, B.L. (1998). Indicators of human health in ecosystems – what do we measure? *Science of the Total Environment*, 224(1–3), 201–13.

Dannenberg, A.L., Bhatia, R., Cole, B.L., et al. (2006). Growing the field of health impact assessment in the United States: an agenda for research and practice. *American Journal of Public Health*, 96(2), 262–70.

Davenport, C., Mathers, J., and Parry, J. (2006). Use of health impact assessment in incorporating health considerations in decision-making. *Journal of Epidemiology and Community Health*, 60(3), 196–201.

Department of the Environment (1996). *The UK National Environmental Health Action Plan.* London: Department of the Environment.

English, P.B., Sinclair, A.H., Ross, Z., et al. (2009). Environmental health indicators of climate change for the United States: findings from the state environmental health indicator collaborative. *Environmental Health Perspectives*, 117(11), 1673–81.

Environmental Health Registration Board (n.d.). *Welcome.* [Online] Available at: http://www.ehrb.co.uk.

Fiorino, D.J. (1995). *Making Environmental Policy.* Los Angeles, CA: University of California Press.

Galvez, M., Forman, J., and Landrigan, P.J. (2005). Children. In H. Frumkin (ed.) *Environmental Health: From Global to Local*, pp. 805–45. San Francisco, CA: Jossey-Bass.

Goldman, L. and Torres, E.B. (2009). Environmental health practice. In R. Detels, R. Beaglehole, M.A. Lansang, and M. Gulliford (eds.) *Oxford Textbook of Public Health* (5th ed.), pp. 1639–52. Oxford: Oxford University Press.

Haglund, B., Pettersson, B., Finer, D., and Tillgren, P. (eds.) (1996). *Creating Supportive Environments for Health: Stories from the Third International Conference on Health Promotion, Sundsvall, Sweden.* Geneva: WHO.

Hamlin, C. (1998). *Public Health and Social Justice in the Age of Chadwick: Britain, 1800–1854.* Cambridge: Cambridge University Press.

Health Professions Council of South Africa (n.d.). Website. [Online] Available at: http://www.hpcsa.co.za.

Hill, A.B. (1965). The environment and disease: association or causation? *Proceedings of the Royal Society of Medicine*, 58, 295–300.

Institute of Medicine (2012). *For the Public's Health: Investing in a Healthier Future.* Washington, DC: The National Academies Press.

International Agency for Research on Cancer (n.d.). *IARC Monographs on Evaluation of Carcinogenic Risks to Humans*. [Online] Available at: http://monographs.iarc.fr/.

International Federation of Environmental Health (n.d.). Website. [Online] Available at: http://www.ifeh.org/.

Johnson, B.L. (2005). Environmental health policy. In H. Frumkin (ed.) *Environmental Health: From Global to Local*, pp. 961–87. San Francisco, CA: Jossey-Bass.

Kemm, J., Parry, J., and Palmer, S. (2004). *Health Impact Assessment: Concepts, Techniques and Applications*. Oxford: Oxford University Press.

Kjellstrom, T. and Corvalan, C. (1995). Framework for the development of environmental health indicators. *World Health Statistics Quarterly*, 48(2), 144–54.

Kleinert, S., Bonk, M., and Horton, R. (2012). New voices in global health and sustainable development. *The Lancet*, 382, S1–2.

Kotchian, S. (2005). The practice of environmental health. In H. Frumkin (ed.) *Environmental Health: From Global to Local*, pp. 895–925. San Francisco, CA: Jossey-Bass.

Kreisel, W. and von Schirnding, Y.E.R. (1998). Intersectoral action for health: a cornerstone for health for all in the 21st century. *World Health Statistics Quarterly*, 51(1), 75–8.

Langlois, E.V., Campbell, K., Prieur-Richard, A., Karesh, W.B., and Daszak, P. (2012). Towards a better integration of global health and biodiversity in the new sustainable development goals beyond Rio+20. *Ecohealth*, 9(4), 381–5.

Laumbach, R. and Kipen, H.M. (2005). Health care services. In H. Frumkin (ed.) *Environmental Health: From Global to Local*, pp. 1010–31. San Francisco, CA: Jossey-Bass.

Lim, S.S., Vos, T., Flaxman, A.D., et al. (2012). A comparative risk assessment of burden of disease and injury attributable to 67 risk factors and risk factor clusters in 21 regions, 1990–2010: a systematic analysis for the global burden of disease study 2010. *The Lancet*, 380, 2224–60.

McMichael, A.J. (2013). Globalization, climate change, and human health. *The New England Journal of Medicine*, 368, 1335–43.

McMichael, A.J., Woodruff, R.E., and Hales, S. (2006). Climate change and human health: present and future risks. *The Lancet*, 367(9513), 859–69.

Mindell, J., Biddulph, J., Taylor, L., et al. (2010). Improving the use of evidence in health impact assessment. *Bulletin of the World Health Organization*, 88(7), 543–50.

Murray, C.J.L., Ezzati, M., Flaxman, A.D., et al. (2012). GBD 2010: a multi-investigator collaboration for global comparative descriptive epidemiology. *The Lancet*, 380, 2055–8.

National Environmental Health Association (n.d.). *Registered Environmental Health Specialist/Registered Sanitarian (REHS/RS)*. [Online] Available at: http://www.neha.org/credential/REHS.html.

National Environmental Policy Act (1969). *U.S.C. 4321-4347 Public Law 91–190, 42*.

National Research Council (1983). *Risk Assessment in the Federal Government: Managing the Process*. Washington, DC: National Academies Press.

National Research Council (1994). *Science and Judgment in Risk Assessment*. Washington, DC: National Academies Press.

Organisation for Economic Co-operation and Development (2001). *Environmental Indicators*. Paris: OECD.

Ottersen, O.P., Frenk, J., and Horton, R. (2011). University of Oslo Commission on global governance for health, in collaboration with the Harvard Global Health Institute. *The Lancet*, 378, 1612–13.

Oxford Dictionaries (n.d.). *Indicator*. Oxford University Press. [Online] Available at: http://www.oxforddictionaries.com/definition/english/indicator?q=indicator.

Patz, J., Campbell-Lendrum, D., Gibbs, H., and Woodruff, R. (2008). Health impact assessment of global climate change: expanding on comparative risk assessment approaches for policy making. *Annual Review of Public Health*, 29, 27–39.

Plan Canada (1999). *Sustainable Communities Indicator Program* (Vol. 39, No. 5). Toronto: Plan Canada.

Rapport, D.J., Gaudet, C.L., Constanza, R., Epstein, P.R., and Levin, R. (2009). *Ecosystem Health: Principles and Practice*. Chichester: John Wiley and Sons.

Rattle, R. and Kwiatkowski, R.E. (2003). Integrating health and social impact assessment. In H.A. Becker and F. Vanclay (eds.) *The International Handbook of Social Impact Assessment*, pp. 92–107. Cheltenham: Edward Elgar.

Rydin, Y., Bleahu, A., Davies, M., et al. (2012). Shaping cities for health: complexity and the planning of urban environments in the 21st century. *The Lancet*, 379, 2079–108.

Sachs, J.D. (2012). From Millennium Development Goals to sustainable development goals. *The Lancet*, 379, 2206–11.

Sachs, J.D. and McArthur, J. (2005). The Millennium Project: a plan for meeting the millennium development goals. *The Lancet*, 365, 347–53.

Satterthwaite, D. (2007). *The Transition to a Predominantly Urban World and its Underpinnings*. Human Settlements Discussion Paper Series – Urban Change. London: International Institute for Environment and Development.

Selikoff, I.J., Churg, J., and Hammond, E.C. (1965). Relation between exposure to asbestos and mesothelioma. *Journal of Occupational Medicine*, 7(10), 542.

Selikoff, I.J., Hammond, E.C., and Churg, J. (1968). Asbestos exposure, smoking and neoplasia. *Journal of the American Medical Journal*, 204(2), 106–12.

Singh, S., Kalmus-Eliasz, M., and Yore, D. (2012). Health at the Rio+20 negotiations. *The Lancet*, 380(9846), e5–6.

Soskolne, C.L., Butler, C.D., Ijsselmuiden, C., London, L., and von Schirnding, Y.E.R. (2007). Toward a global agenda for research in environmental epidemiology. *Epidemiology*, 18(1), 162–6.

Takano, T. and Nakamura, K. (2001). An analysis of health levels and various indicators of urban environments for healthy cities projects. *Journal of Epidemiology and Community Health*, 55, 263–70.

Tickner, J.A. (2005). Prevention. In H. Frumkin (ed.) *Environmental Health: From Global to Local*, pp. 849–94. San Francisco, CA: Jossey-Bass.

Tong, S., von Schirnding, Y.E.R., and Prapamontol, T. (2000). Environmental lead exposure: a public health problem of global dimensions. *Bulletin of the World Health Organization*, 78(9), 1068–77.

United Nations (1972). *United Nations Conference on the Human Environment*, Stockholm, Sweden, 5–16 June.

United Nations (1992). *United Nations Conference on Environment and Development (UNCED)*, Rio de Janeiro, 3–14 June.

United Nations (2000). *United Nations Millennium Assembly. 55th Session of the United Nations*. New York: UN.

United Nations (2002). *World Summit on Sustainable Development (WSSD)*, Johannesburg, 26 August–4 September.

United Nations (2012). *The Future We Want: Rio +20 Outcome Document, 20–22 June, Rio de Janeiro, Brazil*. New York: UN.

United Nations Children's Fund (2012). *Pneumonia and Diarrhoea: Tackling the Deadliest Diseases for the World's Poorest Children*. New York: UNICEF.

United Nations Children's Fund and World Health Organization (2013). *Integrated Global Action Plan for the Prevention and Control of Pneumonia and Diarrhoea (GAPPD)*. New York: UNICEF.

United Nations Development Programme (2011). *Human Development Report*. New York: UNDP.

United Nations Environment Programme (n.d.). *International Register of Potentially Toxic Chemicals*. [Online] Available at: http://www.unep.ch/.

Von Schirnding, Y.E.R. (1997a). *Intersectoral Action for Health: Addressing Health and Environment Concerns in Sustainable Development*. WHO/PPE/PAC/97.1. Geneva: WHO.

Von Schirnding, Y.E.R. (1997b). Addressing health and environment concerns in sustainable development with special reference to participatory planning initiatives such as healthy cities. *Ecosystem Health*, 3(4), 220–8.

Von Schirnding, Y.E.R. (2002a). Health and sustainable development: can we rise to the challenge? *The Lancet*, 360, 632–7.

Von Schirnding, Y.E.R. (2002b). *Health in Sustainable Development Planning: The Role of Indicators*. Geneva: WHO.

Von Schirnding, Y.E.R. (2005). The world summit on sustainable development: reaffirming the centrality of health. *Globalisation and Health*, 1, 8.

Von Schirnding, Y.E.R. (2007). Sustainable development and the use of health and environment indicators. In T. Hak, B. Moldan, and A. Dahl (eds.) *Sustainability Indicators: A Scientific Assessment* (SCOPE 67), pp. 237–48. Washington, DC: Island Press.

Von Schirnding, Y.E.R., Bradshaw, D., Fuggle, R.F., and Stokol, M. (1991). Blood lead levels in South African inner-city children. Blood lead levels in inner city Cape Town children. *Environmental Health Perspectives*, 94, 125–30.

Von Schirnding, Y.E.R., Onzivu, W., and Adede, A.O. (2002). International environmental law and global public health. *Bulletin of the World Health Organization*, 80(12), 970–4.

Wang, H., Dwer-Lindgren, L., Lofgren, K.T., et al. (2013). Age-specific and sex-specific mortality in 187 countries, 1970–2010: a systematic analysis for the global burden of disease study 2010. *The Lancet*, 380, 2071–94.

WEHAB Working Group (2002). *A Framework for Action on Health and the Environment*. New York: UN.

World Commission on Environment and Development (1987). *Our Common Future*. Oxford: Oxford University Press.

World Health Organization (1946). *Preamble to the Constitution of the World Health Organization as adopted by the International Health Conference, New York. June 19–22, 1946*. New York: WHO.

World Health Organization (1948). *Constitution*. Geneva: WHO.

World Health Organization (1977). *Health-for-All by the Year 2000*. Geneva: WHO.

World Health Organization (1978). *Alma Ata Primary Healthcare Conference*. Geneva: WHO.

World Health Organization (1981). *Global Strategy for Health-for-All by the Year 2000*. Geneva: WHO.

World Health Organization (1986a). *Intersectoral Action for Health. The Role of Intersectoral Cooperation in National Strategies of Health-for-All*. Geneva: WHO.

World Health Organization (1986b). *Ottawa Charter for Health Promotion. First International Conference on Health Promotion, Ottawa, Canada, 17–21 November*. Geneva: WHO.

World Health Organization (1998). *Health-for-All in the 21st Century*. A/51. Geneva: WHO.

World Health Organization (1989). *Environment and Health. The European Charter and Commentary. First European Conference on Environment and Health, Frankfurt, Germany, 7–8 December*. Geneva: WHO.

World Health Organization (1992). *Commission on Environment and Health: Our Planet, Our Health*. Geneva: WHO.

World Health Organization (1996). *Preventing Disease Through Healthy Environments: Towards an Estimate of the Environmental Burden of Disease*. Geneva: WHO.

World Health Organization (1997). *Intersectoral Action for Health: A Cornerstone for Health-for-All in the 21st Century. Report of the International Conference*. WHO/PPE/PAC/97.6. Geneva: WHO.

World Health Organization (2002a). *Health and Sustainable Development: Addressing the Issues and Challenges. Background Paper for the World Summit on Sustainable Development*. WHO/HDE/HID/02.12. Geneva: WHO.

World Health Organization (2002b). *Making Health Central to Sustainable Development. Planning the Health Agenda for the World Summit on Sustainable Development. Report of a WHO Meeting, 29 November–1 December 2001. Oslo, Norway*. WHO/HDE/HID/02.5. Geneva: WHO.

World Health Organization (2002c). *Health and Sustainable Development. Summary Report of Meeting of Senior Officials and Ministers of Health. 19–22 January 2002. Johannesburg, South Africa*. WHO/SDE/HDE/02.7. Geneva: WHO.

World Health Organization (2004). *Public Health, Social and Environmental Determinants of Health (PHE), Air Quality Deteriorating in Many of the World's Cities*. [Online] Available at: http://www.who.int/phe/en 2004.

World Health Organization (n.d. a). *International Programme on Chemical Safety*. [Online] Available at: http://www.who.int/ipcs/en.

World Health Organization (n.d. b). *WHO News*. [Online] Available at: http://www.who.int/mediacentre/.

World Health Organization (n.d. c). *Healthy Environments for Children Alliance*. [Online] Available at: http://www.who.int/heca/.

World Health Organization and UN-Habitat (2010). *Hidden Cities: Unmasking and Overcoming Health Inequities in Urban Settings*. Geneva: The WHO Centre for Health Development, Kobe, and United Nations Human Settlements Programme.

World Health Organization Regional Office for Europe (2008). *City Leadership for Health: Summary Evaluation of Phase 4 of the WHO European Healthy Cities Network*. Geneva: WHO.

World Resources Institute, United Nations Environment Program, United Nations Development Program, and World Bank (1998). *1998–99 World Resources: A Guide to the Global Environment*. New York: Oxford University Press.

Wright, J., Parry, J., and Mathers, J. (2005). Participation in health impact assessment: objectives, methods and core values. *Bulletin of the World Health Organization*, 83(1), 58–63.

Yach, D. (1996). Renewal of the Health-for-All strategy. *World Health Forum*, 17, 321–31.

Strategies and structures for public health intervention

Sian Griffiths

Introduction to strategies and structures for public health intervention

The mantra that public health is everybody's business can be two edged. On the one hand, it implies wide support for interventions which would improve health. On the other, it implies such wide responsibility that no one makes public health interventions their priority. Thus, strategies for improving public health and structures for their implementation are complex and situation dependent. It is not always possible to translate a successful programme in city A to one in city B, country C to country D, or urban area E to rural area F. However, the knowledge base for effective interventions is growing and the appreciation of the critical role of cross-sectoral and multilevel approaches is deepening.

In 2012, the American Heart Association published its report on effective interventions with the strongest evidence for improving dietary habits, increasing physical activity, and reducing smoking. Economic incentives to make healthier foods more affordable; improved sidewalk, street, and land-use design to encourage physical activity; and smoking bans were among the 43 most effective interventions identified (American Heart Association 2012).

Thus, public health interventions require a wide range of strategies to translate policies into effective action plans (Kickbusch and Buckett 2010) and structures for their implementation if they are to be effective at producing population-level improvements in health. Strategies may be global agreements, national plans, or local government or community agreements for action. To be implemented, they require structures which are both directly and indirectly concerned with health outcomes, evidence-based processes, and outcome measures of their effectiveness. Strategies may directly involve the health services which make contributions both to improving health, as well as to managing disease, but more often than not, strategies are multisectoral, address the broader determinants of health, and involve an ecological perspective which engages politicians, the corporate sector, civil society, local communities, and the public. This chapter will discuss the concept of strategic approaches for improving the public's health and give examples of health-promoting strategies at global, national, local, and individual levels.

Why a strategic approach?

Health is created by a complex variety of interacting influences. The World Health Organization's (WHO's) definition of health highlights not only the physical and psychological aspects of good health, but also its socioeconomic and environmental dimensions (WHO 1948). The growing awareness of this broader perspective is currently reflected at many levels, for example, in the growing popularity of the discipline of global health in universities across the United States (Merson and Page 2009), in the emphasis by public health leaders in China on the need for a new curriculum with a biopsychosocial basis for training future public health specialists (Li et al. 2011), and by the repositioning of the public health workforce in England from the health service to work within local governments (Department of Health 2011a).

Increasing awareness of the influence of work on health (WHO Regional Office for the Western Pacific 1999) and the need for positive strategies to promote productivity (Department for Work and Pensions 2008), as well as of the links between education of women (United Nations Population Fund n.d.) and healthier birth outcomes (The Lancet 2013a), are further examples, as is the need to respond to the increasing numbers of food scares and scandals (Dai and Jiang 2013), the challenges of food security (WHO n.d. a), and to the growing concerns about the impact of climate change on health (The Lancet 2010). Strategies and structures are therefore continually evolving in attempts to meet the impact of these and other changing influences on the public's health.

Strategic development is dynamic and linked to policy. For example, in China, amongst the first challenges faced by the new People's Republic of China in 1949 was the need to improve the general health and hygiene of the population. Strategies for tackling inadequate sanitation, communicable diseases, and providing basic care at the community level for mothers and children led to the creation of the 'barefoot doctor system', a forerunner for many current models of community-based primary care. In the latter part of the twentieth century, China became one of the largest forces in the world economy but during the 'opening up', the lack of strategy for the health services meant that market forces dominated, resulting in greater inequity in health and decimation of the public health system. Health was not a priority and economic strategies held sway. As a consequence, the first decade of the twenty-first century brought the urgent need to bridge the gap between China's world-class economy and its poor health service provision in which many people were unable to afford basic care. The inequities between the affluent East Coast and urban areas were growing and China now faces not only the problems of an increasingly ageing population and growing challenge from non-communicable diseases (NCDs), but the poorer, less-developed parts of the country remain in greater need of infectious disease surveillance, improvements in maternal health, and implementation of basic primary care programmes, whilst at the same time also facing a growing burden of NCDs. The massive movements of migrants from rural to urban communities, estimated to be around 200 million in 2012, add extra challenges for public health (Jin et al. 2013). At the national level, in addition to hospital service reform, new policies placing greater emphasis on prevention, a stronger public health system, and new strategies to improve primary care are in development to reduce the growing health burdens resulting from rapid urbanization, growing consumption of tobacco, and the increasing rates of lifestyle-related NCDs (The NCD Alliance 2013a).

The experience of China demonstrates the need for national strategy to be interpreted at local levels according to the needs of the population and the resources available. The wide variations in health status, as well as access to care, underline that the delivery of strategy relies not only on national strategic intent, but on appropriate infrastructures and resources at the local level. This was demonstrated in 2003 by the severe acute respiratory syndrome (SARS) epidemic in Hong Kong.

The need for strategy: lessons from SARS in Hong Kong

Amongst the global lessons learned from the experience of SARS in 2003 was that better strategies and structures were needed across all sectors of the health and political systems to respond to the threat of new emerging infectious diseases and to the possibility of a pandemic. When SARS hit Hong Kong in 2003, its surveillance systems were focused on the possibility of an H5N1 (avian flu) pandemic and influenza-like illnesses, and were monitoring in the hospital system. Activity on the Hong Kong borders, where shop shelves were emptied of white vinegar to be boiled by local residents as protection from a serious unknown disease, was not detected and there was no formal accurate information about the atypical pneumonia outbreak in the Guangdong Province available to Hong Kong or to the international community at the time. Only when a group of healthcare workers and medical students in Hong Kong were admitted to one of the largest teaching hospitals within a few days in early March with an unidentified respiratory illness was alarm triggered in the healthcare community.

Whilst the story of the spread of the disease to the local community and to the rest of the world is now well known, the Independent Inquiry commissioned by the Hong Kong government (Hong Kong Special Administrative Region Government 2003) provided the opportunity to review what strategies had been in place and how well they had worked. The Inquiry found that whilst the healthcare staff could be commended for the care they gave the patients, the healthcare system itself had structural deficits and the strategy for action was inadequate. The ability to rapidly legislate to designate the new disease as notifiable was not in place, and interventions were hindered by outdated legislation. The organization of health protection functions, hospital management, and the relationships with central government all needed review. Better collaboration and communication outside Hong Kong, within Hong Kong, and within the healthcare sector was also needed, and it was recognized that to manage workforce capacity for future epidemics, training and research were all

needed. These findings had much in common with the Canadian experience (the country hardest hit by SARS outside of Asia), where it was found that amid the commendable response by public health and healthcare workers to contain SARS, there were still many systematic deficiencies to adequately address outbreak containment, surveillance, information management, and infection control (Naylor et al. 2004).

Since 2003, policy changes in both jurisdictions amongst others, including China, Canada, and Singapore, have resulted in significant progress in strengthening their structures and strategies to combat emerging infectious diseases. In Hong Kong, as in many other countries, surveillance information is now available through a real-time system of reporting of data not only across the Pearl River Delta but globally through the network coordinated by the WHO. Active networks not only of government officials responsible for resilience, but also of researchers, are in regular communication. Communication between the hospital and the community has been improved by streamlined systems and the creation of geographical coterminosity between catchment areas. Extensive plans are now in place for all sectors and staff to be trained through 'drills' which are intersectoral, and which have clear leadership and chains of command and control. The public and the media are better informed about communicable diseases and about preventive measures, such as hand washing. Efforts are continually being made to ensure that communication is open and transparent with press releases and letters to medical staff to keep them abreast of emergent diseases.

The new improved infrastructure was put to the test in 2008 with the threat of the H1N1 pandemic (Cowling 2010). Unlike the SARS experience of 2003, the media and politicians worked together to ensure public health messages about H1N1 were clear and well communicated to the public, based on up-to-date information regularly provided by the Centre for Health Protection (CHP). The CHP, which was established post SARS, was able to play its part in the global network of surveillance for communicable diseases acting as the central structure to coordinate local responses, and ensuing global collaboration and communication (Hong Kong Government n.d.).

The experiences of SARS and H1N1, and more recently H7N9 in Asia and the Middle East respiratory syndrome coronavirus (MERS-CoV), have demonstrated the need for cross-sectoral strategy, a clear plan for proposed implementation, as well as identified structures to support its implementation. The experience of H1N1 demonstrated that both strategy and structures had improved with the lessons learned from SARS and, in 2013, the flow of information about H7N9 to the press, various professions, and the public is significantly better, as is the support from the global scientific community.

Defining strategy

Strategies are, therefore, a necessary step in the translation of policies into plans and action. They create the bridge between policy and practice. Mintzberg (1987) has described five aspects of strategies:

1. Plan—with purposeful intended action.

2. Ploy—competitive manoeuvring.

3. Pattern—signalling a plan in a series of actions.

4. Position—relevant to the outside world.

5. Perspective—an organizational personality.

Translating the aspects of strategy into public health practice requires certain features:

1. Focus on populations rather than individuals.

2. Address the social determinants of health and their impact on poverty.

3. Be based on values of social justice and equity.

4. Reflect a global perspective.

5. Be aware of the dynamic relationship between the environment and health.

6. Place priority on prevention rather than curative care.

7. Understand the importance of systems and structures.

8. Take a transdisciplinary and multisectoral approach.

9. Ensure decision making is based on:

  a. vital statistics (population-based data)
  b. data, scientific evidence, and good research
  c. surveillance and outbreak investigation.

10. Be committed to advocacy and in tune with politics.

Strategic plans may relate to the health status or needs of a defined group of people or of the population as a whole, and may take various forms, such as laws, rules and regulations, guidelines, recommendations, and mandates (Kawamoto 2004).

Health strategy and health service strategy are both important for delivering better public health interventions. Health services are responsible for dealing with disease, and they do not control the major forces which cause disease. They can, however, play a significant role in prevention both at institutional and individual levels through the services they provide and the institutional influences they exert. Health strategy is, however, conceptually broader and requires engagement at different population levels with a wide variety of forces which impact on health—social, economic, political—and with a wide range of multisectoral stakeholders. Strategies for health are underpinned by values, such as those supporting the Millennium Development Goals (MDGs), a strategy to eliminate world poverty (UN n.d. a, n.d. b), which is based on the unacceptability of poverty and disadvantage, and committed to promoting equity and greater opportunity for the 20.6 per cent of the world's population still living on less than $US1.25 a day. Improving public health is a key component of the MDGs—both directly, in the aspirations to improve child health and maternal health and to combat HIV/AIDS, and also indirectly through strategies for raising educational standards, promoting gender equality, and seeking environmental sustainability—all of which will improve the health of populations.

The 2010 MDG Summit concluded with the adoption of a global action plan, 'Keeping the Promise: United to Achieve the Millennium Development Goals', and the announcement of a number of initiatives against poverty, hunger, and disease. In a major push to accelerate progress on women's and children's health, a number of heads of states and governments from developed and developing countries, along with the private sector, foundations, international organizations, civil society, and

research organizations, pledged over $40 billion in resources over the next 5 years (UN n.d. b).

As the timeline for achievement of the MDGs approaches, the next phase of the post-2015 agenda is being considered, with many advocating for issues such as a greater focus on both overnutrition with its impacts on the increasing burden of NCDs and also on undernutrition.

'For mothers, this means less strength and energy for the vitally important activities of daily life. It also means increased risk of death or giving birth to a pre-term, underweight, or malnourished infant. For young children, poor nutrition in the early years often means irreversible damage to bodies and minds during the time when both are developing rapidly. And for 2.6 million children each year, hunger kills, with malnutrition leading to death' (Save the Children 2012).

Undernutrition is the single greatest cause of child deaths in most low- and middle-income countries (World Bank 2013) with the most effective preventive public health strategies including promoting breastfeeding, supplementing diets with micronutrients, immunization, and hygiene.

Levels of health strategy: global, national, local, and individual

Overview

Strategies may be at multiple population levels and be influenced not only by local factors, but also by global policies, linking both vertically and horizontally. Vertical strategies may be concerned with single programmes, such as those addressing HIV/AIDS in sub-Saharan Africa, whereas horizontal strategies may focus on addressing a wider range of influences such as those creating or alleviating poverty.

Poverty and poor health are inextricably linked and strategies to reduce poverty are essential for improving health opportunity. Addressing the root causes of poverty whilst promoting greater equity are key strategic objectives underpinning the work of the WHO Commission on Social Determinants of Health (2008), an influential global think tank which has raised the profile of the debate on the need for strategic action across four main dimensions—political, economic, social, and cultural.

Health is a universal aspiration and a basic human need. The development of society, rich or poor, can be judged by the quality of its population's health, how fairly distributed across the social spectrum and the degree of protection provided from disadvantage due to ill-health. Health equity is central to this premise. (Commission on Social Determinants of Health 2008, p. 7)

Proposed strategies to reduce health inequity include:

1. Improving the conditions of daily life at home and at work, for women and men, in rural and urban settings, and for all ages.

2. Addressing the inequitable distribution of power and money, forces that shape the conditions of daily life.

3. Acting based on knowledge, a professional workforce, alliances with civil society, and evaluation.

The Commission did not stop with making these strategic statements, but has backed them up with a series of papers which provide examples of good practice to support their implementation.

The work of the Commission can be contextualized within a framework of strategic declarations from the WHO, particularly from the Declaration of Alma Ata (WHO 1978). This declaration, and subsequent iterations, echo public health's historic roots by reflecting the importance of the socio-environmental conditions in which people live and the need for community-based action to improve health. Emphasis is placed on the importance of interactive roles of government, communities, and individuals alongside the healthcare sector to promote good health and prevent disease. Whilst the health sector has a role in promoting health through the services it provides, its role beyond acute medical care is significant with potential for involvement with upstream activity to prevent ill health in the entire population. This was proposed in the Declaration of Alma Ata, which called for 'a comprehensive health strategy that not only provided health services but also addressed the underlying social economic and political causes of poor health'. De facto effective prevention would rely on working with, and across, other sectors and, in particular, promoting joined-up government at all its levels including greater community engagement through better primary care.

The conceptual framework of Alma Ata was further developed by the Ottawa Charter (WHO 1986), which promoted the concept of healthy public policy rather than focusing only on health policy, extending consideration of health to all policy environments, including the concept of health impact assessment.

The *Ottawa Charter* defined five key areas for strategic public health action:

1. Building healthy public policy.

2. Creating supportive environments.

3. Strengthening community action.

4. Developing personal skills.

5. Reorienting health services towards prevention and a holistic approach (WHO 1986).

The Ottawa Charter stated unequivocally that health is created in the context of everyday life where people live, love, work, and play. It expanded the concept of health determinants to include environmental challenges and people's empowerment. It included not only the basic well-described determinants but broadened the strategic thinking to the need to combine diverse but complementary approaches in order to promote lifestyles conducive to health. These now include, in particular, legislation, fiscal measures, taxation, and organizational change

Subsequently, in 2005, the *Bangkok Charter* (WHO 2005) further broadened the notion of 'Health in All Policies' (HiAP) by highlighting the need to work across the corporate sector and at a global level, stating that the promotion of health was:

1. Central to the global development agenda.

2. A core responsibility for all governments.

3. A key focus of communities and civil society.

4. A requirement for good corporate practice.

Underpinning concepts included those of social justice, stressing the importance of the values of gender and health equity, respect for diversity and human dignity, and the search for peace and security.

A further iteration has been the move to ensure HiAP (European Portal for Action on Health Inequalities n.d.) and to develop public health policy from the starting point of the crucial role that health plays in the economic life of a society. The central concern of this approach is that the health impacts of policy affect all sectors, and thus governments should adopt a systematic approach to addressing the key determinants of health by considering the impact on health of all their policies. Better health is both a fundamental human right and a sound social investment. Thus within healthy public policy, there needs to be an explicit concern for health and equity in all areas of policy and an accountability for the health impact of these policies. The development of healthy public policy requires not only an investment of resources by government—linking economic, social, and health policies—but also a foundation built on the basic principles of social justice to ensure health promotion and healthy lives. In their review of HiAP, Leppo et al. stress that, in practice, it is usually also necessary to prioritize efforts and to seek synergies to enhance health and other important societal goals (Leppo et al. 2013). HiAP stresses a whole of government approach. As demonstrated by the Pan American Health Organization (PAHO) series of case studies (Etienne et al. 2013), working together and across sectors is not only more effective, but also a prerequisite to further improve the health and well-being of communities at the national, regional, and global level. In selecting the case studies the PAHO team used the criteria that the project included demonstration of political support at a high level, had formal intersectoral structures and a specific budget with explicit commitment from other sectors if they were to be included as part of this initiative, and that the project would reduce health inequity. Scientific evidence of the impact of the programme and mechanisms for participation and community empowerment were also essential.

The implementation of the HiAP approach relies on resources and skills, good information, and a supportive context with political will and governance structures and processes for intersectoral communication and implementation (Pitcher et al. 2010).

Example of HiAP: South Australia's Strategic Plan

Adopting the HiAP's approach, South Australia's Strategic Plan (SASP) expresses the values, priorities, and actions for the future direction of the state. It provides a reference point for the activities of the government through each of its agencies, and describes a whole-of-state plan with 98 targets that can be achieved only through cooperation within and between government, industry, and the community. Its objectives are to:

◆ Grow prosperity.

◆ Improve well-being (which contains a number of health-specific targets).

◆ Attain sustainability.

◆ Foster creativity and innovation.

◆ Build communities.

◆ Expand opportunity.

An important feature of SASP is that neither the objectives nor any individual targets stand alone—they are all part of a larger, interrelated framework and achieving one does not come at the expense of another. The aim is to encourage collaborative behaviour and innovative thinking to address some of the most complex issues facing Southern Australia (Pitcher et al. 2010).

HiAP has also been adopted by the European Union (EU) as part of its strategic approach seeking to complement national action on health. The EU health policies aim to:

◆ Protect people from health threats and disease.

◆ Promote healthy lifestyles.

◆ Help national authorities in the EU cooperate on health issues (European Commission 2007).

HiAP is one of the four principles adopted by the EU. The three further principles are:

◆ *A strategy based on shared health values*: this principle places particular emphasis on reducing poverty and inequities and on the importance of indicators of comparable health data at all levels. Further work on how to reduce inequities in health and how to promote health literacy programmes for different age groups is part of the strategic approach.

◆ *Health is the greatest wealth*: highlights that spending on health is not just a cost, it is an investment and that although health expenditure may be regarded as an economic burden, the real costs to society are the direct and indirect costs linked to ill health. The report estimates that the annual economic burden of coronary heart disease can amount to 1 per cent of the gross domestic product (GDP), and the costs of mental disorders to 3–4 per cent of the GDP. It emphasizes that with 97 per cent of spending going on acute care healthcare and treatment, there is an underinvestment in prevention and improving of the population's overall physical and mental health.

◆ *Strengthening the EU's voice in global health*: the EU's contribution to global health requires interaction of policy areas, such as health, development cooperation, external action, research, and trade linking with the WHO and other relevant United Nations (UN) agencies, the World Bank, the International Labour Organization, the Organisation for Economic Cooperation (OECD), and the Council of Europe, as well as other strategic partners and countries.

The strategy has three objectives related to its policy priorities, which together culminate in an overarching framework for action at all levels across the population:

1. *Fostering good health in an ageing Europe*: promoting health and preventing disease requires efforts throughout the lifespan to tackle key issues including poor nutrition; physical activity; alcohol, drugs, and tobacco consumption; environmental risks; traffic accidents; and accidents in the home. Improving the health of children, adults of working age, and older people will help create a healthy, productive population and support healthy ageing now and in the future.

2. *Protecting citizens from health threats*: emphasizing the need for surveillance and mechanisms to respond to health threats, including emerging infections, as well as adaptation to climate change.

3. *Supporting dynamic health systems and new technologies*: e-health, genomics, and biotechnologies can improve prevention of illness, delivery of treatment, and support a shift from hospital care to prevention and primary care. New technologies must be evaluated properly, including for cost-effectiveness and equity, and health professionals' training and capacity implications must be considered.

The EU health strategy creates a framework within which jurisdictions take forward their own strategies tailored to national needs. It raises not only the aspirations but also the need for effective implementation and for monitoring progress.

Another example of a continent-wide strategy addressing different health needs comes from Africa where significant numbers of low-income countries face different challenges associated with poverty and infectious diseases. The strategy produced by the African Union Ministers of Health is structured using the framework of *Vision and Mission, Principles, Goals, and Objectives*.

Its goal is to contribute to Africa's socioeconomic development by improving the health of its people and by ensuring access to essential healthcare for all Africans, especially the poorest and most marginalized, by 2015. The vision is expressed as working towards 'an integrated and prosperous Africa free of its heavy burden of disease, disability and premature death', and the mission is to build an effective, African-driven response to reduce the burden of disease and disability through strengthened health systems, scaled-up health interventions, intersectoral action, and empowered communities. The strategic principles include health as a human right and a developmental concern requiring a multisectoral response, equity in healthcare as a foundation for all health systems, and effectiveness and efficiency as central to realizing the maximum benefits from available resources. Evidence is proposed as the basis for sound public health policy and practice and more of the same is not enough: 'new initiatives will endeavour to set standards that go beyond those set previously' (NEPAD n.d.).

Global-level action

Whilst the previous examples have been concerned with strategic aspirations for their own geographical location, other strategies focus more globally. For example, the US Centers for Disease Control and Prevention's (CDC's) Global Health Strategy 2012–2015 (CDC 2012) outlines how the CDC will leverage its core strengths to advance four overarching global health goals: improving the health and well-being of people around the world, improving capabilities for preparing and responding to infectious diseases and emerging health threats, building country public health capacity, and maximizing organizational capacity. The US Department of Health and Human Services (HHS) has also produced a Global Health Strategy based on the underlying principles of:

◆ Using evidence-based knowledge to inform decisions.

◆ Leveraging strengths through partnership and coordination.

◆ Responding to local needs.

◆ Building local capacities.

◆ Ensuring a lasting, measurable impact.

◆ Emphasizing prevention.

◆ Improving the equity of health.

Three fundamental goals and ten key objectives contribute to achieving HHS's global health vision of a healthier, safer world.

This strategy is another example of the acceptance of the important links between health, politics, and economics, as well as of health and security with broad objectives, such as leadership and technical expertise in science; policy, programmes, and practice to improve global health; advancing US interests in international diplomacy; development and security through global health action; and increasing the safety and integrity of global manufacturing and supply chains and advancing health diplomacy (United States Global Health n.d.).

Whilst the HHS strategy for global health demonstrates the importance of the global conditions needed to generate health, other strategies will focus on diseases, conditions, age groups, or predeterminants. Strategies may be produced by governments at a local or national level, by interest groups or NGOs, or by other institutions with an interest in health. For example, governments in Australia, Canada, and the United Kingdom, as well as others, are producing strategies for mental health. The aims of the Australian national mental health strategy, for instance, are to:

◆ Promote the mental health of the Australian community.

◆ Where possible, prevent the development of mental disorders.

◆ Reduce the impact of mental disorders on individuals, families, and the community.

◆ Assure the rights of people with mental illness.

Produced in 2002, it remains under constant revision and includes the:

◆ National mental health policy.

◆ National mental health plan.

◆ Mental health statement of rights and responsibilities (Australian Government Department of Health and Ageing 2012).

Changing Directions, Changing Lives is the first Canadian mental health strategy and was published in 2012. The strategy was produced 'to help to ensure that people who experience mental health problems and illnesses—especially those with the most severe and complex ones—are treated with respect and dignity, and enjoy the same rights as all Canadians'. The strategy provides six strategic directions for change to improve mental healthcare (Box 11.6.1).

Change will not be possible without a whole-of-government approach to mental health policy (Mental Health Commission of Canada 2012).

In England, the mental health strategy published in 2011 follows many of the same themes. *No Health Without Mental Health: A Cross-Government Mental Health Outcomes Strategy for People of All Ages* sets shared objectives to improve people's mental health and well-being, and plans to improve services for people with mental health problems. The strategy sets out the policy for how the government, working with all sectors of the community and taking a life course approach, will improve the mental health and well-being of the population and provide people with high-quality services that are equally accessible to all (Department of Health 2011b).

The strategy incorporates the key elements of defining a policy, setting out aims and objectives, and proposing goals and how they will be monitored. The key elements of the English national policy are expressed as:

> Putting people who use services at the heart of everything we do: 'No decision about me without me' is the governing principle. Care should be personalized to reflect people's needs, not those of the profession or the system. People should have access to the information and support they need to exercise choice of provider and treatment; focusing on measurable outcomes and the NICE Quality Standards that deliver them rather than top-down process targets; and empowering local organizations and practitioners to have the freedom to innovate and to drive improvements in services that deliver support of the highest quality for people of all ages, and all backgrounds and cultures. (HM Government 2011)

Strategies may also be focused on specific diseases, for example, NCDs. Globally, the overall economic and social costs of NCDs are vastly in excess of their direct medical costs. In addition to their burden on health systems, NCDs impact on economies, households and individuals, and result in poverty, inequity, and opportunity loss. The burden of NCDs continues to grow not only in affluent countries, but in low- and middle-income countries as

---

Box 11.6.1 Six strategic directions for changes to improve mental health and the mental health care system

1. To promote mental health across the lifespan in homes, schools, and workplaces, and prevent mental illness and suicide wherever possible.

2. To foster recovery and wellbeing for people of all ages living with mental health problems and illnesses, and uphold their rights.

3. To provide access to the right combination of services, treatments and supports, when and where people need them. A full range of services, treatments and supports includes primary health care, community-based and specialized mental health services, peer support, and supported housing, education and employment.

4. To reduce disparities in risk factors and access to mental health services, and strengthen the response to the needs of diverse communities and Northerners.

5. To work with First Nations, Inuit, and Métis to address their mental health needs, acknowledging their distinct circumstances, rights, and cultures.

6. To mobilize leadership, improve knowledge, and foster collaboration at all levels.

Reproduced with permission from Mental Health Commission of Canada, *Changing Directions, Changing Lives: The Mental Health Strategy for Canada*, Copyright © 2012, available from http://strategy.mentalhealthcommission.ca/pdf/strategy-summary-en.pdf.

well, where 80 per cent of NCD deaths occur (Mohammed n.d.). For example, in China, reducing cardiovascular mortality by 1 per cent per year between 2010 and 2040 could generate an economic value equivalent of 68 per cent of China's real GDP in 2010 or over US$10.7 trillion (World Bank 2011). In Egypt, NCDs could be leading to an overall production loss of 12 per cent of Egypt's GDP (Rocco et al. 2011) and, in Brazil, the cost of NCDs between 2005 and 2009 was predicted to equal 10 per cent of Brazil's 2003 GDP (World Bank 2005). In India, eliminating NCDs could have, in theory, increased India's 2004 GDP by 4–10 per cent (Mahal et al. 2009).

Thus, NCDs are a long-standing, progressive, and costly threat to healthy populations. Diseases such as diabetes are associated not only with the problems of diminished functional capacity, increased physical and psychosocial morbidity, co-morbidities, and complications, but also lead to higher utilization of health services and higher medical costs, as well as opportunity costs that are associated with self-care and disability and shorter life expectancy than those without diabetes.

The global concern with NCDs is reflected by their strategic priority on the agenda not only of the WHO, but also of the UN. In 2011, the Secretary General of the UN, Ban Ki-Moon, in remarks to the General Assembly meeting on the Prevention and Control of Non-Communicable Diseases, stated that 'addressing NCDs is critical for global public health, but it will also be good for the economy, for the environment, for the global public good in the broadest sense. If we come together to tackle NCDs, we can do more than heal individuals—we can safeguard our very future' (UN News Centre 2011).

Senior scientists and clinical academics have also added their voices, for example, in the grand challenges to address the threat by:

- Raising public awareness.
- Enhancing economic, legal, and environmental policies.
- Modifying risk factors.
- Engaging businesses and the community.
- Mitigating health impacts of poverty and urbanization.
- Reorienting health systems (Daar et al. 2007).

The WHO continues to build on the Global Strategy for the Prevention and Control of NCDs (WHO 2013a), which was first adopted in 2000, and has been followed by strategies to address tobacco control, and lifestyle factors such as diet, exercise, and alcohol consumption. These have so far materialized into the Physical Activity and Health campaign (WHO 2004), the Reduction of Harmful Use of Alcohol campaign (WHO n.d. b), as well as an Action Plan for the Global Strategy for the Prevention and Control of NCDs for 2008–2013 (WHO 2009a). This set of actions also called for high-level political commitment and the concerted involvement of governments, communities, and healthcare providers for successful implementation. The 66th World Health Assembly (WHA) in 2013 concluded with Member States adopting an 'omnibus resolution' on NCDs. This resolution combined major decisions and recommendations in a single, comprehensive resolution, including:

- Adopting the global monitoring framework (GMF), including nine targets and 25 indicators.

- Endorsing the Global NCD Action Plan 2013–2020 (GAP).
- Agreeing to establish a global coordination mechanism (GCM) for NCDs, and to develop terms of reference by November 2013.
- Agreeing to establish a set of indicators to measure the implementation of the GAP (The NCD Alliance 2013b).

The GAP lays out the vision of a world free of the avoidable burden of NCDs with the goal of reducing the preventable and avoidable burden of morbidity, mortality, and disability due to non-communicable diseases. The means of achievement will be through multisectoral collaboration and cooperation at national, regional, and global levels. The objective is for populations to reach the highest attainable standards of health and productivity at every age so that NCDs are no longer a barrier to well-being or socioeconomic development (WHO 2013b).

The principles adopted should be:

- 'Life-course approach
- Empowerment of people and communities
- Evidence-based strategies
- Universal health coverage
- Management of real, perceived or potential conflicts of interest
- Human rights approach
- Equity-based approach
- National action and international cooperation and solidarity
- Multisectoral action.' (WHO 2013b)

The objectives of the plan are to raise the priority given to the prevention and control of NCDs at all levels, through strengthened international cooperation and advocacy; to strengthen national capacity, leadership, governance, multisectoral action, and partnerships to reduce modifiable risk factors and underlying social determinants through creation of health-promoting environments; and to strengthen and orient health systems to people-centred primary healthcare and universal health coverage. This should be underpinned by promoting and supporting national capacity for high-quality research and development as well as monitoring the trends and determinants of NCDs to evaluate progress in their prevention and control.

Progress can be measured by adopting voluntary global targets (Box 11.6.2).

By creating a framework and setting targets, emphasis is shifting from analysis of the problem to implementing changes that can make a difference, monitored through a set of measurable outcomes.

National-level action

Whilst at a *global level* the WHO produces strategies to provide direction for change, action to implement change is needed at a national population level. Examples of national strategies for mental health were given earlier in this chapter—each being country specific. Another approach is the proposal for a common framework for national action, an example of which is the Framework Convention on Tobacco Control (FCTC) (WHO n.d. c), which was the first international treaty negotiated under the auspices of the WHO, adopted by the WHA on 21 May 2003 and entered into force on 27 February 2005. It was developed in response to the threats posed by the globalization of the tobacco epidemic and is an evidence-based treaty that reaffirms the right of all people to the highest standard of health. By mid 2013, 176 jurisdictions had signed up to the Convention, including 90 per cent of the world's population.

Box 11.6.2 Voluntary global targets

1. A 25 per cent relative reduction in risk of premature mortality from cardiovascular diseases, cancer, diabetes, or chronic respiratory diseases.

2. At least 10 per cent relative reduction in the harmful use of alcohol, as appropriate, within the national context.

3. A 10 per cent relative reduction in prevalence of insufficient physical activity.

4. A 30 per cent relative reduction in mean population intake of salt/sodium.

5. A 30 per cent relative reduction in prevalence of current tobacco use in persons aged 15+ years.

6. A 25 per cent relative reduction in the prevalence of raised blood pressure or contain the prevalence of raised blood pressure, according to national circumstances.

7. Halt the rise in diabetes and obesity.

8. At least 50 per cent of eligible people receive drug therapy and counselling (including glycaemic control) to prevent heart attacks and strokes.

9. An 80 per cent availability of the affordable basic technologies and essential medicines, including generics, required to treat major noncommunicable diseases in both public and private facilities.

Reproduced with permission from World Health Organization (WHO), *Noncommunicable diseases and mental health: about 9 voluntary global targets*, Copyright © WHO 2014, available from: http://www.who.int/nmh/ncd-tools/definition-targets/en/ www.who.int/nmh/ncd-tools/definition-targets/en/.

Support for *national-level* implementation has been provided by the *WHO MPOWER package* (WHO n.d. d), which gives strategic advice on six proven evidence-based policies to reduce tobacco-related harm (see also Chapter 9.1). This is a vertical strategic approach, focusing specifically on one risk factor, tobacco smoking. The recommended headline actions are:

Monitor tobacco use and prevention policies
Protect people from tobacco smoke
Offer help to quit tobacco use
Warn about the dangers of tobacco
Enforce bans on tobacco advertising, promotion, and sponsorship
Raise taxes on tobacco. (WHO n.d. d)

Importantly, MPOWER provides examples of successful initiatives which have reduced the burden of tobacco-related harm. For example, legislation is a key element to achieving the MPOWER measures and many countries have actively legislated to stop smoking in public places through the banning of tobacco smoking indoors in environments such as workplaces, shops, restaurants, bars, and residential care homes. In 2013, additional steps have been taken in Australia to introduce plain packaging of cigarettes and are now being studied by other countries who are deciding whether to follow suit (*The Lancet* 2013b).

But, whilst national legislation can provide environments in which tobacco harm is reduced, local strategies are also necessary particularly to engage the health sector.

Local-level action

Engagement of health services at a *local level* has been shown to be essential for the translation of the objectives of the FCTC. Whilst health promotion in schools about the harms of tobacco in schools plays an important role in raising awareness, local services also need to provide support such as smoking cessation services in special clinics and within routine services in both public and private sectors. Non-government organizations (NGOs), for example, the

Action on Smoking and Health (ASH) in the United Kingdom (ASH UK n.d.) and Australia (ASH Australia n.d.), and the Hong Kong Council on Smoking and Health (COSH) (n.d.) provide invaluable support in both leading and assisting the implementation of strategies. In Hong Kong, COSH advocates with government and also provides additional services and support for smokers who wish to quit, such as manning quitlines, organizing local campaigns, and providing smoking cessation information. Smoking cessation community clinics, such as the Hong Kong's Hospital Authorities' Smoking Cessation and Counselling Centres, are supported by other NGOs, as well as the government, and increase the effectiveness of smoking cessation services by providing nicotine replacement therapy and continuity of care. Among smokers who are aware of the dangers of tobacco, three out of four want to quit. Like people dependent on any addictive drug, it is difficult for most tobacco users to quit on their own, and they benefit from help and support to overcome their dependence from a variety of sources including local clinics, support groups, and advice from helplines.

Whilst MPOWER seeks to provide global guidance that can be translated into local action, other strategies will be jurisdiction specific. Typically such strategies describe the epidemiology of the target population, its demography, the distribution of mortality and morbidity, its health needs, and local characteristics. Since the purpose of a strategy is to bring about change, plans for implementation will be included, as well as a framework for monitoring and evaluation, often promoting targets or objectives to be achieved. Many countries have produced strategies for tackling major health priorities, including strategies for addressing the epidemic of NCDs.

Typically, development of a strategic framework at a *local level* will analyse needs, priorities, and plans for implementation of a policy and engage stakeholders in its implementation. One example of this approach comes from Hong Kong where, in line with

WHO and the Western Pacific Regional Action Plan (WPRO) NCD strategies, the Hong Kong Department of Health has developed a strategic framework for NCDs (Hong Kong Government 2013). This framework was produced following a series of processes engaging not only with the health sector but more widely, particularly with the NGO sector which plays a significant role in health promotion and service delivery.

The first step was to review international literature as well as local epidemiology and health service information. The plan was then drawn up using a set of strategic principles (Box 11.6.3).

To flesh out the framework, the strategy group engaged other arms of government, professional groups, non-government agencies, representatives of the business sector, and the community to agree on a work programme based on promoting the need for prevention and early intervention, and to ensure that any action was to be evidence based, outcome focused, and addressing broader health determinants to reduce the burden of disease related to NCDs. Particular emphasis was placed on informing the population to promote responsibility for their own health, engagement of public and private sectors, engaged professionals, and a sustainable health system (Hong Kong Government 2013).

Implementing strategy

With frameworks and principles for strategy in place, action to address specific health behaviours and challenges needs to be planned and monitored. In Hong Kong, for example, a government-level committee to review progress on strategy implementation, chaired by the health minister, was established. Task forces were then established to develop action plans for the four

---

Box 11.6.3 Principles for strategy development

1. *Viewing health from a public health perspective:* the patterns of NCDs in the whole population were considered.

2. *Understanding health determinants:* taking account of the general socioeconomic and cultural environments and their impact on communities, as well as health behaviours.

3. *Considering health disparity/inequity:* diseases are unfairly distributed and poorer communities have higher rates of disease, seek health services later, and often have less access to healthcare.

4. *Clustering of risk factors in the community:* many NCDs share common behavioural risk factors and many people have more than one chronic disease leading to multi-morbidity. For example, four of the most important NCDs—diseases of the circulatory system, cancer, chronic respiratory diseases, and diabetes mellitus—share three major behavioural risk factors, namely smoking, physical inactivity, and unhealthy diet, and are mediated through common biomedical risk factors, notably excess weight, hypertension, and an adverse lipid profile. Local information about disease patterns, such as mortality from cancer, behaviours such as smoking rates, and hospital admission rates for cardiovascular disease, all helped to provide the scale and distribution of the burden of NCDs in the community.

5. *Adopting the life course approach:* the life course approach acknowledges the interactive and cumulative impact of social and biological influences throughout life, particularly the importance of predisposing factors in early life.

6. *Identifying a preventive strategy:* three levels of prevention are recognized as essential considerations for the strategy: primary, secondary, and tertiary. Primary prevention is concerned with measures that prevent the onset of disease, for example, health education and immunization. Secondary prevention inhibits the progression of a disease after its occurrence by early detection and diagnosis followed by prompt and effective treatment. Screening programmes for cancers or hypertension are examples of secondary prevention. Tertiary prevention refers to the rehabilitation of patients with an established disease with the objective of minimizing residual disabilities and complications, and maximizing potential years of life.

7. *Balancing population-wide versus individual-based approaches:* population-wide approaches seek to achieve an overall lowering of the risk in the whole population. Individual-based approaches identify the high-risk individuals.

8. *Recognizing the importance of health literacy and social marketing:* health literacy (WHO n.d. e) is the ability to read, understand, and act on healthcare information. Poor health status is associated with low health literacy. Social marketing (Lefebvre and Flora 1988) is an approach which focuses on motivating people to use health information and change behaviour in ways that promote and maintain good health. Effective social marketing, which may be promoted by different sectors, such as healthcare providers, local health departments, NGOs, or national government offices use different communication channels like mass media, message placement in clinics, and community-level outreach to influence health behaviour among target populations and audiences (Evans 2006) of varying levels of health literacy and health behaviours.

9. *Setting health priorities:* priority setting is necessary for the rational utilization of resources for public health programmes in a community.

10. *Establishing a framework for monitoring and evaluation.*

Source: data from Hong Kong Government, Department of Health, *Promoting Health in Hong Kong: A Strategic Framework for Prevention and Control of Non-communicable Diseases,* available from http://www.change4health.gov.hk/filemanager/common/image/strategic_framework/promoting_health/promoting_health_e.pdf.

Box 11.6.4 Example of strategy implementation: reducing alcohol harm in Hong Kong

Having identified reducing alcohol harm as a priority for implementing the NCD strategy, the HK Working Group on Injuries and Alcohol Misuse proposed ten recommendations to address alcohol related harm (Hong Kong Government 2011):

1. Strengthen surveillance of alcohol consumption through collecting data from all sectors.

2. Strengthen surveillance of alcohol-related harm by collecting data from the healthcare sector.

3. Promote research to understand drinking patterns, particularly among the young, and assessment of impact of measures taken.

4. Involve all health professionals through education and practice.

5. Encourage healthcare professionals to identify at-risk drinkers and explore the development of tools to enable this to happen.

6. Provide secondary, tertiary, and mental health services for those identified with needs.

7. Working together of government, NGOs, schools, and employers in partnership to maximize efforts.

8. Develop evidence-based and culture-relevant advice and information that can be disseminated in all sectors.

9. Strengthen community awareness and actions through publicity, media, and other means.

10. Review legislation and consider age restrictions for selling alcohol.

  The recommendations were then used to establish process measures for monitoring implementation and various partners, such as NGOs and community groups, were involved in promoting the strategy. Healthcare providers were also included to provide health education and care for individuals and to engage with professional groups.

Source: data from Hong Kong Government, Department of Health, *Promoting Health in Hong Kong: A Strategic Framework for Prevention and Control of Non-communicable Diseases*, available from http://www.change4health.gov.hk/filemanager/common/image/strategic_framework/promoting_health/promoting_health_e.pdf.

---

priority areas: diet, physical activity, alcohol (see Box 11.6.4), and injury. Other established groups developed action plans including those for reducing tobacco smoking, better primary care, and cancer prevention. Cross-referencing and shared initiatives were coordinated through the strategy's steering group.

Action aimed to be population based and outcome focused, and included developing health education materials for educators and healthcare professionals, and developing guidelines for screening and brief interventions to identify and manage at-risk drinkers. Emphasis is placed on increasing an individual's ability to make informed choices about alcohol consumption. It was also important that the steering groups represented their organizations and that the plans were derived with their input and shared with their colleagues, including top management in their institutions.

As in many cases, agreeing on the plan was relatively straightforward, but its implementation has been less so. At a territory-wide level, implementation has been complicated by the aspirations not only of the alcohol industry but also the government itself to promote alcohol sales. When the financial secretary announced a tax reduction for wine and beer, the health sector was caught unawares. This tax reduction was solely for financial reasons—to stimulate the economy and to make Hong Kong a centre for wine trading. The health consequences of cheaper alcohol were not a consideration for this policy change despite the clear evidence from other countries showing that unit price increase for alcoholic drinks is one of the most effective ways to reduce alcohol-related harm, and it is therefore not surprising that early indications are that alcohol sales have dramatically increased (Kim et al. 2013).

This example demonstrates the difficulties often faced by public health interventions in which gaining consensus is easier than implementing the recommendations.

Putting strategy into action at a local level

The process of strategy development uses the whole range of public health tools and skills. Much of the focus of the work will be on the process of gaining commitment from partners, patients, and the public, and overcoming the barriers they perceive. Successful implementation relies on clarity of the health challenge, key aims and objectives, as well as structures which support engaging the right people in the community to create change, and ensure that proposed changes are implemented and sustainable. Some key questions guiding local-level action are shown in Table 11.6.1.

Structures for implementing strategy: the PEOPLE framework:

The acronym PEOPLE (Hong Kong Government 2013, pp. xiii–xiv) can be used as a tool to review the structural support for strategy implementation:

1. **P**artnership.

2. **E**nvironment.

3. **O**utcome-focused.

4. **P**opulation-based interventions.

5. **L**ife course approach.

6. **E**mpowerment.

1. Partnership

Partnerships between different sectors of society and at different population levels are essential to maximize the strengths of different knowledge bases and skills.

Table 11.6.1 Questions guiding local-level action

How do we make the case?	By doing a local needs assessment, and taking into account local and national strategies
What are we aiming to do?	Expressed by clear aims and objectives with indicators and targets
How do we involve patients and the public?	Be clear about why patients and public need to be involved and how to engage them at all stages of the strategy identifying the barriers to change
How do we engage/communicate with partners?	Make sure all those who are affected by the strategy are involved including clinicians and partner organizations. Identifying who will support and who will oppose and how to deal with this; communicate with all involved as the work is taken forward
How can we make change happen?	Securing change is the core of the work and needs to be addressed in the planning stage. This stage should include a description of the actions that are required, and an assessment of the resource implications, securing adequate resources in order for implementation to be possible and appropriate
How do we know we have done what we wanted to do?	Evaluate the impact to demonstrate achievement against the standards and targets
How can we make change stick?	Change needs to be sustained to ensure that it becomes routine practice. This may requires a change in work environment with a process of ongoing monitoring and audit to stop people reverting to old patterns of working

Adapted from Hill, A. et al., *Public Health and Primary Care: Partners in Population Health*, Volume 1, Oxford University Press, New York, USA, Copyright © 2007, by permission of Oxford University Press USA.

Case study: creation of Public Health England—emphasis on partnership

As part of the healthcare reform process in England, in 2013, the public health system has been restructured by the creation of Public Health England (PHE) to reflect the need for strong central and local partnerships. The main drive for this reform is the recognition that public health is not the product of health service activity, and that addressing upstream broader social and economic determinants are key to promoting better health.

At a central level, the PHE strategy directorate will be responsible for 'a coherent, credible and internationally recognized strategy for the transformation of the public's health' (PHE n.d.) providing 'the leadership for a widely-owned strategic direction for public health that is strongly supported by local authorities, the National Health Service (NHS) and other partners'. Key to its implementation is the repositioning of local Directors of Public Health from the NHS to local government authorities that will have new duties and powers for Health and Wellbeing Boards which will use processes, such as the production of Joint Strategic Needs Assessments (JSNAs) and Joint Health and Wellbeing Strategies (JHWSs), to promulgate local plans for improving health and well-being and reducing inequalities in their local communities. It is envisaged that there will be a continuous process of strategic assessment and planning involving all sectors to 'develop local evidence-based priorities to improve the public's health and reduce inequalities', and helping determine what actions local authorities, the local NHS and other partners will need to take to meet health and social care needs, and to address the wider determinants that impact on health and well-being (Department of Health 2013a).

How well these structural changes work in delivering their objectives of reducing inequalities and addressing local health needs through joint strategies will need monitoring and evaluation.

2. Environment

Environmental influences play a key role in effective intervention. At a broad level, they may be economic, social, political, and physical.

Case study: healthy settings

The healthy settings approach, which considers health promotion and disease prevention in the context of broader settings, provides an example of structuring environments to be health promoting. The WHO defines a *setting for health* as the place or social context in which people engage in daily activities in which environmental, organization, and personal factors interact to affect health and well-being. Settings are characterized by physical boundaries, a range of people with defined roles, and an organizational structure (WHO n.d. f). Examples of settings are:

◆ Schools.

◆ Hospitals.

◆ Cities/villages.

◆ Workplaces.

In healthy settings, people can create and solve problems related to health, and actively use and shape the environment. Different settings provide diverse ways to implement health strategies.

Schools have an integral responsibility and role in encouraging health promotion as part of a larger social health model. The healthy schools movement, promoted by the WHO, has played a key role in developing and sharing experiences across many countries. For example, in India, the school fostering health programme has been emphasizing that a balanced diet, regular physical activity, and lifestyle management play a key role in the prevention and control of many diseases. One of its key programmes has been to work with schools to promote the 'Mid day Meal Program', which encourages healthy eating and hygiene (Healthy India n.d.). The School Health Foundation of India has established a scheme for 'Healthy School' Certification based on the achievement of ten points of criteria (School Health Foundation of India n.d.). In Mississippi, United States, the state's Department of Education has established an Office of Healthy Schools committed to offering technical assistance and services to enable schools and communities to create programmes, based on CDC guidance, which encourage lifelong healthy behaviours (Mississippi Office of Healthy Schools n.d.).

In England, the aims of the National Healthy Schools Programme (NHSP) are to:

♦ Support children and young people in developing healthy behaviours.

♦ Help to raise pupil achievement.

♦ Help to reduce health inequalities.

♦ Help promote social inclusion.

Health promoting schools have been characterized as having six domains for action: the formal curriculum, the school ethos, school policies and practices, school health services, school–home–community interactions, and organizational structures. National Healthy Schools also provide education and support of young peoples' personal and social health (including sex and relationship education), healthy eating, physical activity, and emotional health and well-being. The evidence regarding interventions to improve children's health indicates the value of intersectoral, comprehensive programmes, and these can be developed and implemented through the structure of health-promoting school programmes (Department of Health n.d.).

Hospitals are another example of a setting in which to promote health, as well as provide health services. The promotion of healthy hospitals can be described from two perspectives—through the care they give and through the lens of environmental sustainability. The initial declarations on health promoting hospitals focused on the former with statements that hospitals should:

1. Promote human dignity, equity and solidarity, and professional ethics, acknowledging differences in the needs, values and cultures of different population groups.

2. Be oriented towards quality improvement, the wellbeing of patients, relatives and staff, protection of the environment and a realisation of the potential to become learning organisations.

3. Focus on health with a holistic approach and not only on curative services.

4. Be centred on people providing health services in the best way possible to patients and their relatives to facilitate the healing process and contribute to the empowerment of patients.

5. Use resources efficiently and cost-effectively, and allocate resources on the basis of contribution to health improvement, forming as close links as possible with other levels of the healthcare system and the community. (WHO Health Promoting Hospitals Network 1997)

The US CDC on Healthy Hospital Choices strategies suggests that hospitals could engage to promote better health where recommended—promoting healthy hospital food, physical activity, breastfeeding and lactation support, and tobacco-free choices (National Center for Chronic Disease Prevention and Health Promotion 2010). However, over recent years, the responsibility of hospitals to contribute to sustainability has been a growing theme.

The NGO 'Healthier Hospital Initiative' has created a network of hospitals committed to improving not only the health of patients and staff, but also to promoting the role hospitals can play in creating a sustainable environment through engaging leadership, healthier food, cleaner energy, less waste, safer chemicals, and smarter purchasing (Healthier Hospitals Initiative 2013).

In England, the NHS has created a Sustainable Development Unit which works across health, public health, and social care to help health and care organizations to fulfil their potential as leading environmentally sustainable and low-carbon organizations (NHS n.d.).

These roles of hospitals and healthcare facilities in civil society as providers of care, as providers of employment, and as influencers of the local environment and the local community are often forgotten.

Cities/villages are also important healthy settings as they encompass the overarching areas where people live. The WHO healthy cities project (WHO n.d. g) is a global movement established to create health-supportive environments, which will enable the achievement of good quality life. They focus on ensuring basic sanitation and hygiene needs are met, as well as ensuring access to healthcare. In Europe, the primary aim is to put health high on the social, economic, and political agenda of city governments, and engage all sectors to provide policies and plans to address inequality and urban poverty, and address the needs of vulnerable groups and the social, economic, and environmental determinants of health (WHO Europe Office n.d.).

Workplaces are other important settings where health should be promoted. Just as the younger population spends most of their day at schools, adults usually spend more time at their workplaces than in any other setting. Workplaces can support programmes aimed at improving the health conditions and awareness amongst workers/employees for mental, as well as physical, well-being:

Providing a psychologically safe workplace is no longer something that is simply nice to do, it is increasingly becoming a legal imperative. (Mental Health Commission of Canada 2013)

The WHO healthy workplace model suggests a comprehensive way of thinking and acting that addresses:

♦ Work-related physical and psychosocial risks.

♦ Promotion and support of healthy behaviours.

♦ Broader social and environmental determinants (WHO n.d. h).

The programme for Health at Work seeks to ensure a positive approach to health and work which includes training managers to be aware and communicate about well-being and mental ill health, as well as encouraging a culture of health (mental and physical) at work. This approach highlights the mutual benefits of health and productivity, linking traditional health and safety with well-being initiatives (Healthy Workplaces 2011).

This positive approach to health is demonstrated by the replacement of sick certificates with 'fit notes' in the United Kingdom. Introduced in April 2010, fit notes are issued to individuals by doctors to provide evidence that they 'may be fit for work' or 'not fit for work' (Department for Work and Pensions n.d.).

3. Outcome-focused

A strategy that is *outcome-focused* ensures an optimal investment of available resources with the greatest health gains through the monitoring of health outcomes. Focusing on outcomes can help programmes measure the successes and failures of what has already been implemented, and allow room for evaluation, adjustment, and improvement.

Case study: public health outcomes in England

An example of outcome-focused strategies is the use of health inequality targets in England. These targets and headline indicators were initially promulgated in 2006 as part of a national strategy to promote health, and identified 14 areas for measurement

(Department of Health 2006). Two health inequalities targets on infant mortality and life expectancy in addition to 12 headline indicators for areas in which evidence suggested actions could lead to a greater emphasis on prevention were proposed. These have subsequently been refined and published as the *Public Health Outcomes Framework for England 2013 to 2016* (Department of Health 2013b), which has the outcome targets of increased healthy life expectancy and reduced differences in life expectancy and healthy life expectancy between communities, as well as indicators in four domains: improving the wider determinants of health, health improvement, health protection and healthcare public health, and preventing premature mortality (Fig. 11.6.1).

This framework will guide public health action at the local level and regular monitoring will take place, allowing progress to be tracked and performance to be compared between different geographical areas based on local authority boundaries.

4. Population-based interventions

Preventive strategies can target individuals or target populations as a whole. Placing emphasis on the whole population produces collective health benefits and can change the patterns of behaviours and disease prevalence by having a small impact on many people.

Case study: Less Salt, More Life campaign in Argentina

In 2011, bread makers in Argentina voluntarily reduced the salt in bread by 40 per cent and restaurants in Buenos Aries removed salt from their tables as part of a campaign to reduce hypertension and reduce heart disease. Discussions also took place with the

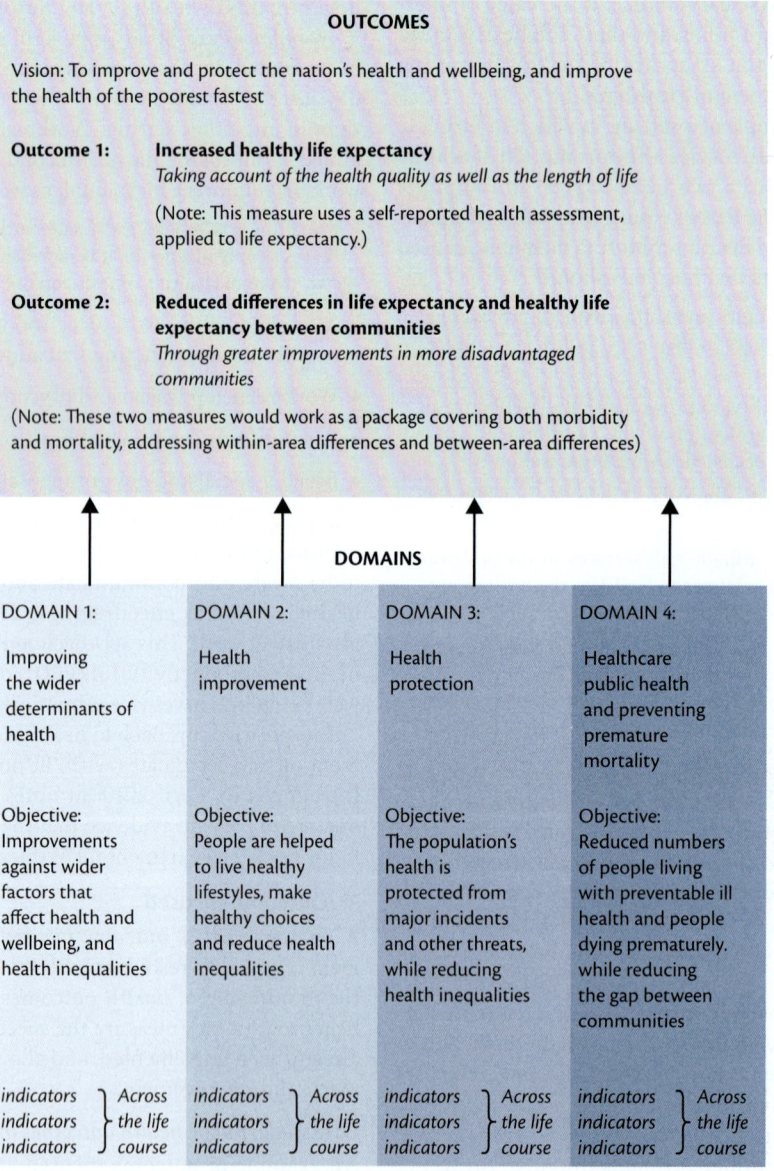

Public Health Outcomes Framework

OUTCOMES

Vision: To improve and protect the nation's health and wellbeing, and improve the health of the poorest fastest

Outcome 1: **Increased healthy life expectancy**
Taking account of the health quality as well as the length of life

(Note: This measure uses a self-reported health assessment, applied to life expectancy.)

Outcome 2: **Reduced differences in life expectancy and healthy life expectancy between communities**
Through greater improvements in more disadvantaged communities

(Note: These two measures would work as a package covering both morbidity and mortality, addressing within-area differences and between-area differences)

DOMAINS

DOMAIN 1:	DOMAIN 2:	DOMAIN 3:	DOMAIN 4:
Improving the wider determinants of health	Health improvement	Health protection	Healthcare public health and preventing premature mortality
Objective: Improvements against wider factors that affect health and wellbeing, and health inequalities	Objective: People are helped to live healthy lifestyles, make healthy choices and reduce health inequalities	Objective: The population's health is protected from major incidents and other threats, while reducing health inequalities	Objective: Reduced numbers of people living with preventable ill health and people dying prematurely, while reducing the gap between communities
indicators indicators indicators } Across the life course	indicators indicators indicators } Across the life course	indicators indicators indicators } Across the life course	indicators indicators indicators } Across the life course

Fig. 11.6.1 Example of strategic domains.

Reproduced from Department of Health, *Public Health Outcomes Framework 2013 to 2016 and technical updates 2013*, Crown Copyright 2013, licensed under the Open Government License v.2.0, available from https://www.gov.uk/government/publications/healthy-lives-healthy-people-improving-outcomes-and-supporting-transparency.

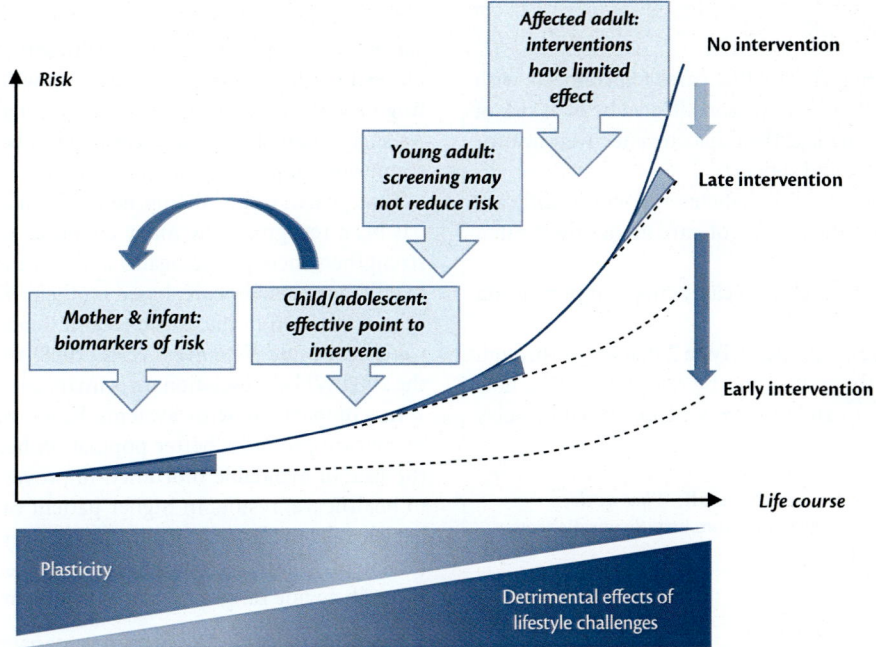

Fig. 11.6.2 Life course view of NCD.
Reprinted from *Progress in Biophysics and Molecular Biology*, Volume 106, Issue 1, Hanson, M. et al., *Developmental plasticity and developmental origins of non-communicable disease: Theoretical considerations and epigenetic mechanisms*, pp. 272–280. Copyright © 2011, with permission from Elsevier, http://www.sciencedirect.com/science/journal/00796107.

food industry on reducing the salt content of processed food. Prior to the campaign, the daily salt consumption was estimated to be two to three times that of recommended levels. Population-level salt reduction is considered to be one of the most cost-effective strategies to reduce hypertension and its consequences (He and MacGragor 2009). The government established a national committee with cross-government representation, working with the big food companies and unions to come to voluntary agreements. The coordinated monitoring plan will evaluate progress. It is estimated that with a 3 g salt reduction in each individual's diet, 6000 cardiovascular deaths, 13,000 myocardial infarctions, and 13,000 strokes could be avoided overall (Laspiur 2012).

5. Life course approach

A life course approach addresses cumulative adverse effects on people's lives by fostering health from gestation through to old age. The risks of developing disease and disability accumulate with age and are influenced by social and physical factors at all stages of life (Fig. 11.6.2).

There are critical periods, such as gestation and early childhood and also adolescence, when environmental exposures do more harm to health and its potential, as well as sensitive developmental stages when social and cognitive factors are more easily acquired, than at other times. Thus, social behavioural and environmental factors impact on the potential for a healthy future and continue to do so throughout the life course to old age (Kuh Ben-Shlomo 1997; WHO n.d. i).

Understanding the importance of the life course has led to different initiatives to develop strategies to promote preconception care, promote optimum care in pregnancy, efforts to ensure safe delivery, a focus on vulnerable children and adolescents, and interventions tailored to promoting and maintaining health in middle and older age.

6. Empowerment structures for local action—community based initiatives

Empowerment gives everyone in the community the opportunity to achieve their full potential by gaining control over decisions and actions that influence health. There are many levels of involvement when empowering people and their communities (Box 11.6.5).

Box 11.6.5 Principles for involving the public in public health strategy implementation

- The community must be seen as being part of the solution, not the problem.
- Community representatives need mechanisms to link to the wider community.
- Community input must be accountable to the local community. Any strategy has to take into account marginalized minority groups.
- To ensure the public can truly benefit, financial support is necessary.
- The community should raise issues that are of concern to them.
- The community needs to see concrete outcomes from their voluntary involvement, otherwise, they might lose interest.
- Meetings involving the community must avoid jargon.

Source: data from Crowley, P., Community development and primary care groups, pp. 41–42, in *Communities Developing for Health*, UK Health for All Network, Liverpool, UK, Copyright © 2000.

Box 11.6.6 Role of Diabetes UK

Diabetes UK is the leading charity that cares for, connects with and campaigns on behalf of every person affected by or at risk of diabetes. We help people manage their diabetes effectively by providing information, advice and support.

We campaign with people with diabetes and with healthcare professionals to improve the quality of care across the United Kingdom's health services.

We fund pioneering research into care, cure and prevention for all types of diabetes.

We work to stem the rising tide of Type 2 diabetes—through risk assessment, early diagnosis, and by communicating how healthy lifestyle c hoices can help many people avoid or delay its onset.

Reproduced with permission from Diabetes UK, *What we do*, Copyright © Diabetes UK 2014, available from http://www.diabetes.org.uk/About_us/What-we-do/.

Case study: Partners for Mental Health

The Canadian Mental Health strategy emphasizes the need to engage patients and their carers in determining what they want from health services:

> The mobilization of the Canadian public to take action on mental health issues is essential in order to ensure that mental health remains a high priority. (Mental Health Commission of Canada n.d.)
>
> Partners for Mental Health 'has one focused goal…to catalyze a social movement that will empower individuals and organizations to take action to improve mental health' and in particular to engage with the general public to increase engagement in and advocacy for mental health issues. (Mental Health Commission of Canada n.d.97)

Effective strategy implementation also relies on community engagement and the conciliation of top-down directives with bottom-up initiatives. As such, it is important to engage the public and patient groups in implementation as their lack of engagement will result in a failing strategy. Ways of engagement may be through minimum participation, where people are merely passive receivers of information, for example, receiving health education materials or through active partnership, in which patient groups or the public are partners, empowered to play expanded roles and to take responsibility. For example, Diabetes UK plays a pivotal role in providing advocacy and advice for diabetic patients at national and local levels (Box 11.6.6).

The PEOPLE framework provides a useful conceptual framework for strategic planners.

Delivering public health strategy

Health service contribution: the role of primary care

How public health services are delivered is obviously key to their effectiveness not only in dealing with disease, but in promoting better public health. We have already referred to the structural changes in England which are based on enabling a greater focus on the determinants of health. At the same time, the role of health services and of public health within health services is important for delivering better health outcomes. For example, providing antenatal care, well-baby checks, postnatal support, and immunizations are all part of a public health service delivered in different places by different systems including within a primary care setting or within a government-run maternal or child health clinic. As such, public health services need to be considered within the framework of primary care provision.

That primary care should be the foundation of health services has been recognized by many countries who strive to develop or strengthen their public health and healthcare systems. The need to enhance primary care, based on the principles of Alma Ata, has been reaffirmed in the World Health Report 2008, *Primary Health Care: Now More Than Ever* (WHO 2008) and further highlighted in the 2009 WHA's resolution on primary care policies (WHO 2009b).

In comparison with systems based on specialist care, primary care produces better population health outcomes, reduces the rate of avoidable mortality, improves continuity and access to healthcare, results in higher patient satisfaction, and reduces health-related disparities at a lower overall cost for healthcare (Starfield 1998). It contributes to the health of the population through a wide range of services, which include:

1. Health promotion and proactive management of diseases:
   - Immunization.
   - Promotion of healthy lifestyles.
   - Risk assessment and reversal.
   - Screening of health-related problems and diseases.
   - Appropriate treatment and prevention of disease complications.
   - Enabling management of illness and disability.
   - Supportive and palliative care for end-stage disease.

2. Ambulatory treatment of acute diseases.

3. Supporting health protection and promotion within the community.

4. Planning and coordinating care of individuals at all levels and across different healthcare professionals.

Primary care health services provide ongoing care at a community level and, as such, they are often closely interrelated with public health services. In many situations, primary care clinicians are indeed the main providers of public health services and increasing attention is being paid to effective and efficient models for integrating personal healthcare and public health, and organizing primary care on the principle of care for individuals in the context of an identified population over time. To quote Van Weel et al. (2008):

> The future of primary care, and health care in general, will depend on how effectively primary practices achieve this community-oriented primary care approach and contribute to equity and social cohesion. Current efforts to revitalise primary health care worldwide should go hand in hand with attention to the social determinants of health. Just as the social determinants' approach to improving health equity must involve health care so must programmes to control priority public health conditions include attention to the social determinants of health.

Now More Than Ever (WHO 2008) emphasizes yet again how implementing primary care strategies needs to be context specific, in particular with reference to income and resources. For example, the Chinese healthcare system is investing significantly in community health centres and community-based systems to provide universal access to primary care, to emphasize prevention, to enable choice between Western and traditional medicines, and to strengthen programmes within local communities.

The primary care strategy of the reforms in China aims to strengthen the establishment of the public health service system by:

* Building sound public health networks of disease prevention, health education, maternal and child healthcare, mental health, first aid, blood collection and supply, health supervision, and family planning.

* Improving the public health functions of the medical services system based on a basic medical services network.

* Setting up an information-sharing and resources-sharing public health services system.

* Enhancing the capacity of public health services.

* Enhancing the capacity to respond to public health emergencies.

* Decreasing the urban–rural inequity in utilization of public health services. (Government of China 2009)

Another example of the promotion of the strategic focus for healthcare reform through developing primary care services to deliver public health comes from Chile. In Chile, the health policy has defined a detailed benefit package, which is well publicized among the population as an enforceable right. People are being informed about the kind of services, including access to specialized care, which they can claim from their primary-care teams. In combination with sustained investment, such unambiguous entitlements create a powerful dynamic for the development of primary care (WHO 2008, chapter 6).

The public health workforce

Improving public health requires the combined efforts of people from many professions and disciplinary backgrounds (Sim et al. 2007).

For example, voluntary NGOs frequently have greater insights into the health needs of disadvantaged groups within communities than do statutory organizations. As such, it is not enough to focus on any one sector or any one activity but to recognize the interactions and different levels at which these influences are working. In the United Kingdom, public health practice is recognized as having three overlapping domains of health protection, health improvement, and health services (HM Government 2010). This structural framework recognizes the interactions between the different aspects of practice and that practice needs to be underpinned by an understanding not only of epidemiology and biostatistics, but of ethical issues within a global context.

The workforce in public health is multidisciplinary. The formal definition of a public health professional is a person educated in public health or a related discipline who is employed to *improve health* through a *population focus* (Institute of Medicine 1988). A useful way of considering the workforce, adopted in the United Kingdom, is that there are three main groupings: (1) specialists; (2) those who practise public health as part of their role, such as primary care workers; and (3) those with an interest whose work impinges on the public's health. In the United Kingdom, specialists are those who have demonstrated a high level of competence in proscribed areas and public health specialist training is defined

by competency acquisition through work-based placements. This approach is based on the historical origins of the public health specialty which derives from the role of the nineteenth-century Medical Officers of Health, instituted as key players in the sanitary reforms which accompanied the Industrial Revolution. Incorporated into the NHS in 1974 and recently again relocated in local authority government, their descendants need no longer be doctors but need to have acquired competence in nine levels of public health practice:

1. Surveillance and assessment of the population's health and well-being.

2. Assessing the evidence of effectiveness of health and healthcare interventions, programmes and services.

3. Policy and strategy development and implementation.

4. Strategic leadership and collaborative working for health.

5. Health improvement.

6. Health protection.

7. Health and social service quality.

8. Public health intelligence.

9. Academic public health.

Standards of specialist practice are maintained through a professional body, the Faculty of Public Health (n.d.), which oversees:

* The quality of specialist training.

* Professional development of public health specialists in the United Kingdom.

* Maintenance of the professional standards in the discipline.

Some overseas countries adopt a similar approach and standards including the Hong Kong College of Community Medicine (n.d.), which is part of the Hong Kong Academy of Medicine. The Academy is an overarching medical body representing the professional groups in medicine (Hong Kong Academy of Medicine n.d.). The Colleges within the Academy are professionally led and independent of government or licensing bodies. Their remit is to set professional medical standards and curricula from postgraduate to specialist levels. Licensing bodies, such as the UK General Medical Council (n.d.) or the Hong Kong Medical Council (n.d.), act as professional regulators and issue the licences to practise.

In the United Kingdom, where senior public health specialists may come from a variety of professional backgrounds, a voluntary register was created using equivalent standards of competence to medical counterparts. With the many changes in the United Kingdom, public health specialist regulation is currently under review.

Defining specialist professional training and standards is a less daunting challenge than harnessing the contribution of the wider workforce because it is enormous, diverse, diffused, and often ignorant of its own potential for improving health. An attempt was made by the English Department of Health to establish regional Teaching Public Health Networks to enhance communication and coordinate wider training. The networks were intrinsically collaborative and sought to break down historical boundaries between the further and higher education sectors, and barriers between education, health, and other sectors (Sim et al. 2007). However, the current English reorganization of public health means that the complex future challenges will require the re-engagement of many people, from specialists and practitioners to a wider workforce, in new organizational arrangements currently being developed by PHE.

In the United Kingdom, further education has traditionally focused on acquisition of practical job skills and this has been the basis of public health training. In other countries, greater emphasis has been placed on academic training and qualifications, particularly acquisition of Master degrees in Public Health, often provided by academics working in Schools of Public Health. In the United States, there is an active system of accreditation of Schools of Public Health through the Council on Education for Public Health (CEPH) (n.d.) and a set of agreed competencies for MPH programmes (Association of Schools & Programs of Public Health (ASPPH) n.d.). However, since public health is a dynamic and constantly developing field, it is always under review and the ASPPH's 'Framing the Future' Task Force has launched a Master of Public Health (MPH) Expert Panel to update the MPH for the twenty-first century (ASPPH 2012). In addition, greater focus has been placed on defining learning objectives for the growing field of undergraduate education, often to be found in Liberal Arts Colleges thus underlining the multidisciplinary approach to public health practice.

Public health education in China

In contrast to the humanities-based courses of the United States, public health education in China remains embedded in medical education and the initiation of MPH degrees is a recent and rapidly developing movement. The origins of public health practice lie in the Sanitary Departments established in 1905, but many public health functions were implemented by police and other interdisciplinary groups. Municipality public health administrations followed German models and early public health campaigns were organized by interdisciplinary working groups rather than individuals with specialized public health education. In 1928, the National Ministry of Health had four foci, which included training health personnel including a focus on public health skills.

A blueprint for establishing provincial health bureaus that included an education and propaganda department was established and Ministry field stations started postgraduate training programmes for public health-oriented jobs, such as public health officers, sanitary inspectors, and public health teachers for schools.

After 1949, the public health education system, like all the educational structures, was substantially transformed. Patriotic health campaigns focused on mass mobilization, balanced preventive and curative strategies, and incorporated elements of traditional Chinese and Western medicine. A mainly biomedical model of public health emerged in line with the Soviet model with five major disciplines, namely, school hygiene, occupational hygiene, food hygiene, environmental hygiene, and radiation hygiene.

China's 'barefoot doctor system' was instituted in the late 1960s, producing a cadre which was a hybrid between clinical physician and public health practitioner who provided vaccines, created water and sanitation systems, improved stoves and toilets, provided basic medical care, assisted in family planning policies, and collected information about epidemics. Structures of undergraduate- and graduate-level public health training re-emerged in 1978 in China, with much of the curricula and format deriving from international models.

Public health and pre-clinical medical students now take a common-stem curriculum during the first several years of training. Four years of basic science and clinical requirements are generally followed by 1 year focused on various aspects of public health. Chinese CDCs are the major employer of graduates but increasingly strong links are being forged with local academic departments.

Traditional Chinese medical school curricula are being restructured at many institutions, providing an important opportunity to expand the role of public health education. Within China, there are regular meetings among School of Public Health deans to share ideas and experiences for improving public health education as well as international meetings with counterparts from the United States (Bangdiwala et al. 2011).

Research

As discussed in earlier chapters, public health research remains underfunded in most jurisdictions despite the importance of the evidence base to guide effective policies and professional practices. High-tech medical proposals with quick returns are often more attractive to funders.

Earlier in the chapter we have stressed the importance of evaluation and monitoring health interventions as key components of the strategic approach. Increasingly, strategies are developed which recognize the inter-relationship between health and health services. For example, in the United Kingdom when launching *Investing in Research, Improving Health*, the responsible Minister wrote:

> We are committed to tackling disease prevention wherever possible and are excited by the emerging understanding of the biological links between inequalities and health. The benefits to health and healthcare are explicit but we are also alert to the potential for economic benefits. The life sciences have a key part to play and a tradition of excellence on which to build. (Chief Scientist Office, NHS Scotland 2009)

In England, the National Institute for Health Research has an arm which focuses on public health. The Public Health Research (PHR) programme commissions research to provide new knowledge on the benefits, costs, acceptability, and wider impact of non-NHS interventions (NHS 2013) (Fig. 11.6.3).

However, as in other countries such as Australia, the lion's share of available funding goes to basic sciences and clinical research, with allocations to public health and health services research in single-digit figures (Australian Government National Health and Medical Research Council 2008).

Barriers to implementing strategy

Whilst many organizations produce strategies, many do not achieve their goals. To some extent this is because they are aspirational and at times unrealistic. Management literature suggests that there are four main barriers to effective strategy implementation. These are:

1. *The vision barrier*: in the age of the knowledge-based economy, the workforce needs to understand the strategy.

2. *The people barrier*: personal incentives need to be tied to the long-term initiatives supporting the strategy, not to short-term (financial) results.

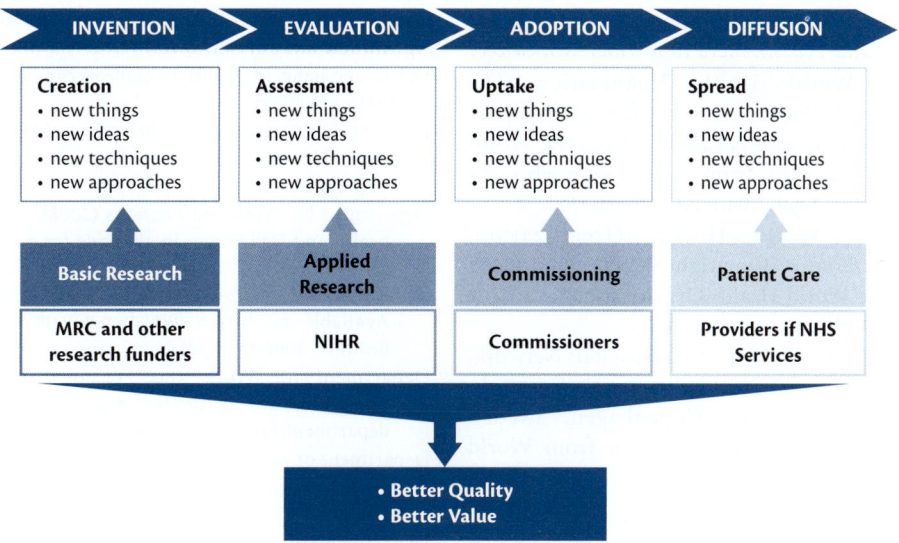

Fig. 11.6.3 The research pathway.
Reproduced with permission from The National Institute for Health Research (NIHR), *NIHR Briefing Note 1.1*, Version 9, Copyright © 2014, available from http://www.nihr.ac.uk/files/pdfs/Briefing%20documents/1.1%20The%20National%20Institute%20for%20Health%20Research.pdf.

3. *The resource barrier:* strategies need to be linked to budgets.

4. *The management barrier:* managers need to discuss strategies but often focus on budgets (Kaplan and Norton 2001).

Thus, there may be over-attention being paid to the day-to-day duties rather than tackling the projects that have been identified as key to organizational sustainability and success. Important strategies may be perceived as overwhelming and too difficult to tackle. Lack of teamwork can inhibit cooperation across organizational divisions and different players have different priorities. Recommendations for successful implementation of strategic plans include:

◆ *Focus:* having too many priorities means no action and not everything can be or is a priority, so agree on what the top two to three goals are.

◆ *Communicate clearly and often*, and understand each other's language and contextual background.

◆ *Emphasize and reward teamwork* which may involve trade-offs, negotiation, and difficult conversations about resource allocation and expectations.

◆ *Regular review of progress:* provide a framework for ensuring that all stakeholders reach their objectives.

◆ *Accountability needs to be clearly defined.*

◆ *Emphasize implementation of* the strategic plan is the most important aspect of planning.

Identifying the barriers to implementation and overcoming them is a key success factor for any organization. Teamwork, accountability, and resolution of conflicting priorities, or hidden agendas, will help ensure the implementation of the top two to three goals (Dane 2010).

Conclusion

This chapter has focused on strategies for promoting public health and structures for their implementation. As the scope of public health broadens and more consideration is given to the wider determinants of health and to the challenges of the future—the NCD epidemic, changing patterns of demography and disease, and climate change and its impact on health—more partners will need to be involved in signing up to strategies to tackle the threats they pose to public health. The example of SARS in 2003 demonstrated the problems that can occur when a strategy is missing. The experiences of China during its economic opening up demonstrate the need to constantly review the impact of broader determinants on equity in health and health services. Different examples of evidence-based and value strategies have been discussed with reference to examples and experiences in different countries and settings. The need for fit-for-purpose structures in the health systems, public health workforce, and research community has been highlighted and barriers to achieving the strategic goals described. All too often strategies remain merely fine words. The fundamental challenge is their implementation and continuous refinement in the light of delivery.

Acknowledgements

This chapter contains public sector information licensed under the Open Government Licence v2.0.

Text extracts from Save the Children, *State of the World's Mothers 2012: Nutrition in the First 1,000 Days*, Westport, Connecticut, USA, p.3, Copyright © 2012, reproduced with permission from Save the Children.

Text extracts reprinted from *The Lancet*, Volume 372, Issue 9642, van Weel, C., et al., Integration of Personal and community health care, pp. 871–2, Copyright © 2008, with permission from Elsevier, http://www.sciencedirect.com/science/journal/01406736.

Text extracts from World Health Organization, *The Ottawa Charter for Health Promotion: First International Conference on Health Promotion*, Ottawa, 21 November 1986, Copyright © 1986, reproduced with permission from the World Health Organization, available from http://www.who.int/healthpromotion/conferences/previous/ottawa/en/.

Text extracts from World Health Organization, *The Bangkok Charter for Health Promotion in a Globalized World*, Copyright © 2005, reproduced with permission from the World Health Organization, available from http://www.who.int/healthpromotion/conferences/6gchp/bangkok_charter/en.

Text extracts from World Health Organization, *MPOWER: Tobacco Free Initiative*, Copyright © 2014, reproduced with permission from the World Health Organization, available from http://www.who.int/tobacco/mpower/en/.

Text extracts from WHO Health Promoting Hospitals Network, *The Vienna Recommendations on Health Promoting Hospitals*, WHO Regional Office for Europe, Copenhagen, Sweden Copyright © 1997, reproduced with permission from World Health Organization.

References

Action on Smoking and Health Australia (n.d.). *The Tobacco Problem and Our Aims*. [Online] Available at: http://www.ashaust.org.au/.

Action on Smoking and Health UK (n.d.). *About ASH*. [Online] Available at: http://www.ash.org.uk/about-ash.

American Heart Association (2012). *Researchers Identify Evidence-Based Public Health Interventions for Policy Makers*. [Online] Available at: http://newsroom.heart.org/news/researchers-identify-evidence-237575.

Association of Schools & Programs of Public Health (n.d.). *MPH Core Competency Model*. [Online] Available at: http://www.aspph.org/educate/models/mph-competency-model/.

Association of Schools and Programs of Public Health (2012). *MPH Expert Panel*. [Online] Available at: http://www.asph.org/document.cfm?page=1218.

Australian Government Department of Health and Ageing (2012). *National Mental Health Strategy*. [Online] Available at: http://www.health.gov.au/internet/main/publishing.nsf/Content/mental-strat.

Australian Government National Health and Medical Research Council (2008). *Report of the Review of Public Health Research Funding in Australia*. [Online] Available at: http://www.nhmrc.gov.au/_files_nhmrc/file/research/phr/Nutbeam.pdf.

Bangdiwala, S.I., Tucker, J.D., Zodpey, S., et al. (2011). Public health education in India and China: history, opportunities, and challenges. *Public Health Reviews*, 33(1), 204–24.

Centers for Disease Control and Prevention (2012). *CDC Global Health Strategy 2012–2015*. [Online] Available at: http://www.cdc.gov/globalhealth/strategy/.

Chief Scientist Office, NHS Scotland (2009). *Investing in Research, Improving Health*. 2009. [Online] Available at: http://www.cso.scot.nhs.uk/Publications/research.pdf.

Commission on Social Determinants of Health (2008). *Closing the Gap in a Generation: Health Equity Through Action on the Social Determinants of Health*. Geneva: WHO. Available at: http://whqlibdoc.who.int/publications/2008/9789241563703_eng.pdf.

Council on Education for Public Health (n.d.). *About*. [Online] Available at: http://ceph.org/about/#.

Council On Smoking and Health (n.d.). *About COSH*. [Online] Available at: http://www.smokefree.hk/en/content/web.do?page=ChairmanMessage.

Cowling, B.J., Ng, D.M.W., Ip, D.K.M., et al. (2010). Community psychological and behavioral responses through the first wave of 2009 pandemic (H1N1) in Hong Kong. *Journal of Infectious Disease*, 202(6), 867–76.

Crowley, P. (2000). Community development and primary care groups. In A. Hobbs (ed.) *Communities Developing for Health*, pp. 41–2. Liverpool: UK Health for All Network.

Daar, A.S., Singer, P.A., Persad, D.L., et al. (2007). Grand challenges in chronic non-communicable diseases. *Nature*, 450, 494–6.

Dai, C. and Jiang, M. (2013). Fake meat scandals add to Chinese food fears. *BMJ*, 346, f3385.

Dane, M. (2010). *Overcoming Barriers to Plan Implementation*. [Online] Available at: http://suite101.com/article/overcoming-barriers-to-plan-implementation-a213233.

Department for Work and Pensions (2008). The role of the workplace in health and well-being. In *Working for a Healthier Tomorrow: Dame Carol Black's Review of the Health of Britain's Working Age Population*, pp. 51–60. London: Department for Work and Pensions. Available at: http://www.dwp.gov.uk/docs/hwwb-working-for-a-healthier-tomorrow.pdf.

Department for Work and Pensions (n.d.). *Fit Note*. [Online] Available at: https://www.gov.uk/government/organisations/department-for-work-pensions/series/fit-note.

Department of Health (2006). *Tackling Health Inequalities: Status Report on the Program for Action 2006. Update on Headline Indicators*. London: DOH.

Department of Health (2011a). *Public Health in Local Government*. [Online] Available at: https://www.gov.uk/government/uploads/system/uploads/attachment_data/file/216708/dh_131904.pdf.

Department of Health (2011b). *The Mental Health Strategy for England*. [Online] Available at: https://www.gov.uk/government/publications/the-mental-health-strategy-for-england.

Department of Health (2013a). *Statutory Guidance on Joint Strategic Needs Assessments and Joint Health and Wellbeing Strategies 2013*. [Online] Available at: https://s3-eu-west-1.amazonaws.com/media.dh.gov.uk/network/18/files/2013/03/Statutory-Guidance-on-Joint-Strategic-Needs-Assessments-and-Joint-Health-and-Wellbeing-Strategies-March-20131.pdf.

Department of Health (2013b). *Public Health Outcomes Framework 2013 to 2016*. [Online] Available at: https://www.gov.uk/government/publications/healthy-lives-healthy-people-improving-outcomes-and-supporting-transparency.

Department of Health (n.d.). *National Healthy School Status: A Guide for Schools*. [Online] Available at: http://www.salisbury.anglican.org/resources-library/schools/schools-every-child-matters/be-healthy.

Diabetes UK (n.d.). *What we do*. [Online] Available at: http://www.diabetes.org.uk/About_us/What-we-do/.

Etienne, C., Teruel, J., Galvao, L.A., Garza, S.M., and Martinelli, R. (2013). *Health in All Policies: Experiences from the Americas*. Washington, DC: Pan American Health Organization. Available at: http://www.paho.org/saludyuniversidades/.

European Commission (2007). *Together for Health: A Strategic Approach for the EU 2008–13*. White Paper. [Online] Available at: http://ec.europa.eu/health-eu/doc/whitepaper_en.pdf.

European Portal for Action on Health Inequalities (n.d.). *Health in All Policies (HiAP)*. [Online] Available at: http://www.health-inequalities.eu/HEALTHEQUITY/EN/policies/health_in_all_policies/.

Evans, W.D. (2006). How social marketing works in health care. *BMJ*, 332, 1207.

Faculty of Public Health (n.d.). *About Us*. [Online] Available at: http://www.fph.org.uk/about_us.

General Medical Council (n.d.). *About Us*. [Online] Available at: http://www.gmc-uk.org/.

Government of China (2009). *Opinions of the CPC Central Committee and the State Council on Deepening the Health Care System Reform*. [Online] Available at: http://www.china.org.cn/government/scio-press-conferences/2009-04/09/content_17575378.htm.

Hanson, M., Godfrey, K.M., Lillycrop, K.A., Burdge, G.C., and Cluckman, P.D. (2011). Developmental plasticity and developmental origins of non-communicable disease: theoretical considerations and epigenetic mechanisms. *Progress in Biophysics and Molecular Biology*, 106(1), 272–80.

He, F. and MacGragor, G. (2009). A comprehensive review on salt and health and current experience of worldwide salt reduction programmes. *Journal of Human Hypertension*, 23, 363–84.

Healthier Hospitals Initiative (2013). *About*. 2013. [Online] Available at: http://healthierhospitals.org/about-hhi.

Healthy India (n.d.). *Mid-day Meals*. [Online] Available at: http://healthy-india.org/healthy-spaces/schools/mid-day-meals.html.

Healthy Workplaces (2011). *Healthy Workplace Guide: Ten Steps to Implementing A Workplace Health Program* [Online] Available at: http://www.healthyworkplaces.info/wp-content/uploads/2012/11/Healthy-Workplace-Guide_Ten-steps.pdf.

Hill, A., Griffiths, S., and Gillam, S. (2007). *Public Health and Primary Care: Partners in Population Health, Volume 1*. Oxford: Oxford University Press.

HM Government (2010). *Healthy Lives, Healthy People: Our Strategy for Public Health in England*. London: The Stationery Office. Available at: http://www.official-documents.gov.uk/document/cm79/7985/7985.pdf.

HM Government (2011). *No Health Without Mental Health: A Cross-Government Mental Health Outcomes Strategy for People of All Ages*. [Online] Available at: https://www.gov.uk/government/uploads/system/uploads/attachment_data/file/135457/dh_124058.pdf.pdf.

Hong Kong Academy of Medicine (n.d.). *Overview*. [Online] Available at: http://www.hkam.org.hk/.

Hong Kong College of Community Medicine (n.d.). *Background*. [Online] Available at: http://www.hkccm.org.hk/.

Hong Kong Government (2011). Department of Health. *Action Plan to Reduce Alcohol-Related Harm in Hong Kong*. [Online] Available at: http://www.dh.gov.hk/english/pub_rec/pub_rec_ar/pdf/ncd_ap2/action_plan_whole_document_e.pdf.

Hong Kong Government (2013). Department of Health. *Promoting Health in Hong Kong: A Strategic Framework for Prevention and Control of Non-communicable Diseases*. [Online] Available at: http://www.change4health.gov.hk/filemanager/common/image/strategic_framework/promoting_health/promoting_health_e.pdf.

Hong Kong Government (n.d.). *Department of Health. Centre for Health Protection*. Available at: http://www.chp.gov.hk/en/index.html.

Hong Kong Special Administrative Region Government (2003). *SARS in Hong Kong: From Experience to Action. Report of the SARS Expert Committee*. [Online] Available at: http://www.sars-expertcom.gov.hk/english/reports/reports.html.

Institute of Medicine (1988). *The Future of Public Health*. Washington, DC: Committee for the Study of the Future of Public Health.

Jin, M., Griffiths, S.M., Fong, H., and Dawes, M.G. (2013). Health of China's rural–urban migrants and their families: a review of literature from 2000–2012. *British Medical Bulletin*, 106, 19–43.

Kaplan, R.S. and Norton, D.P. (2001). *The Strategy-Focused Organization*. Boston, MA: HBS Press.

Kawamoto, K. (2004). Learning about health care policy: part 1. *The Journal of Education, Community, and Values*, 2004, 4(5).

Kickbusch, I. and Buckett, K. (eds.) (2010). *Implementing Health in All Policies, Adelaide 2010*. Adelaide: Government of South Australia, Department of Health. Available at: http://www.who.int/sdhconference/resources/implementinghiapadel-sahealth-100622.pdf.

Kim, J.H., Wong, A.H., Goggins, W.B., Lau, J., and Griffiths, S.M. (2013). Drink driving in Hong Kong: the competing effects of random breath testing and alcohol tax reduction. *Addiction*, 108(7), 1217–28.

Kuh, D. and Ben-Shlomo, Y. (1997). *A Life-course Approach to Chronic Disease Epidemiology*. Oxford: Oxford University Press.

Laspiur, S. (2012). *Argentine Initiative: To Reduce Sodium Consumption 'Less Salt, More Life'*. [Online] Available at: http://new.paho.org/panamericanforum/wp-content/uploads/2012/08/less-salt-more-life_PAHO-consortium_ARG.pdf.

Lefebvre, R.C. and Flora, J.A. (1988). Social marketing and public health intervention. *Health Education & Behavior*, 15(3), 299–315.

Leppo, K., Ollila, E., Peña, S., Wismar, W., and Cook, S. (eds.) (2013). *Health in All Policies, Seizing Opportunities, Implementing Policies*. Finland: Ministry of Social Affairs and Health. Available at: http://www.euro.who.int/__data/assets/pdf_file/0007/188809/Health-in-All-Policies-final.pdf.

Li, L.M., Tang, J.L., Lv, J., Jiang, Y., and Griffiths, S. (2011). The need for integration in health sciences sets the future direction for public health education. *Public Health*, 125(1), 20–4.

Mahal, A., Karan, A., and Engelgau, M. (2009). *The Economic Implications of Non-Communicable Disease for India. The International Bank for Reconstruction and Development*. Washington, DC: World Bank.

Mental Health Commission of Canada (2012). *Changing Directions, Changing Lives: The Mental Health Strategy for Canada*. [Online] Available at: http://strategy.mentalhealthcommission.ca/pdf/strategy-summary-en.pdf.

Mental Health Commission of Canada (2013). National Standard of Canada. January 2013.

Mental Health Commission of Canada (n.d.). *Call to Action*. [Online] Available at: http://strategy.mentalhealthcommission.ca/strategy/call-to-action/.

Merson, M.H. and Page, K.C. (2009). *The Dramatic Expansion of University Engagement in Global Health. Implications for US Policy: A Report of the CSIS Global Health Policy Center*. Washington, DC: Center for Strategic & International Studies. Available at: http://dspace.cigilibrary.org/jspui/bitstream/123456789/26577/1/The%20Dramatic%20Expansion%20of%20University%20Engagement%20in%20Global%20Health.pdf?1.

Mintzberg, H. (1987). The strategy concept i: five Ps for strategy. *California Management Review*, 30(1), 11–24.

Mississippi Office of Healthy Schools (n.d.). *Health Education Services*. [Online] Available at: http://healthyschoolsms.org/health_education/index.html.

Mohammed, A. (n.d.). *The Global Burden of NCDs*. [Online] Available at: http://ncdaction.org/page/the-global-burden-of-ncds.

National Center for Chronic Disease Prevention and Health Promotion (2010). *Healthy Hospital Choices*. [Online] Available at: http://www.cdc.gov/nccdphp/dnpao/hwi/docs/HealthyHospBkWeb.pdf.

National Health Service (2013). *The National Institute for Health Research Report*. [Online] Available at: http://www.nihr.ac.uk/files/pdfs/Briefing%20documents/1.1%20The%20National%20Institute%20for%20Health%20Research.pdf.

National Health Service (n.d.). *Sustainable Development Strategy Consultation*. [Online] Available at: http://www.sdu.nhs.uk/.

Naylor, C.D., Chantler, C., and Griffiths, S. (2004). Learning from SARS in Hong Kong and Toronto. *Journal of the American Medical Association*, 291(20), 2483–7.

NEPAD (n.d.). *Africa Health Strategy 2005–2007*. [Online] Available at: http://www.nepad.org/system/files/AFRICA_HEALTH_STRATEGY(health).pdf.

Pitcher, S., Jordan, D., and Buckett, K. (2010). South Australia's strategic plan and health in all policies. In I. Kickbusch and K. Buckett (eds.) *Implementing Health in All Policies Adelaide 2010*, pp. 87–92. Adelaide: Government of South Australia, Department of Health. Available at: http://www.who.int/sdhconference/resources/implementinghiapadel-sahealth-100622.pdf.

Public Health England (n.d.). *What We Do*. [Online] Available at: https://www.gov.uk/government/organisations/public-health-england.

Rao, M., Prasad, S., Adshead, F., and Tissera, H. (2007). The built environment and health. *The Lancet*, 370(9593), 1111–13.

Rocco, L., Kimie, T., Suhrcke, M., and Fumagalli, E. (2011). *Chronic Diseases and Labor Market Outcomes in Egypt*. World Bank Policy Research Working Paper No. 5575. Washington, DC: World Bank.

Save the Children (2012). *State of the World's Mothers 2012: Nutrition in the First 1,000 Days*. [Online] Available at: http://www.savethechildren.org/atf/cf/%7B9def2ebe-10ae-432c-9bd0-df91d2eba74a%7D/STATEOFTHEWORLDSMOTHERSREPORT2012.PDF.

School Health Foundation of India (n.d.). *Healthy School Certification*. [Online] Available at: http://schoolhealth.in/uncategorized/healthy-school-certification/.

Sim, F., Lock, K., and McKee, M. (2007). Maximizing the contribution of the public health workforce: the English experience. *Bulletin of the World Health Organization*, 85(12), 901–80.

Starfield, B. (1998). *Primary Care: Balancing Health Needs, Services and Technology*. New York: Oxford University Press.

The Lancet (2010). *Climate Change Series*. [Online] Available at: http://www.thelancet.com/series/health-and-climate-change.

The Lancet (2013a). *Women Deliver. Interview with Ana Langer, Director of the Women and Health Initiative at the Harvard School of Public Health*. [Online video] Available at: http://www.lancet.com/themed/women-deliver-2013.

The Lancet (2013b). Tobacco control—political will needed. *The Lancet*, 381(9877), 1511.

The Medical Council of Hong Kong (n.d.). *Homepage*. [Online] Available at: http://www.mchk.org.hk/.

The NCD Alliance (2013a). *NCD Alliance Report 2012–2013: Putting Non-Communicable Diseases on the Global Agenda*. [Online] Available at: http://ncdalliance.org/sites/default/files/resource_files/NCD%20Alliance%20Report%202012-2013.pdf.

The NCD Alliance (2013b). *66th World Health Assembly – May 2013*. [Online] Available at: http://www.ncdalliance.org/wha66.

United Nations (n.d. a). *Millennium Development Goals*. [Online] Available at: http://www.un.org/millenniumgoals/.

United Nations (n.d. b). *2010 Summit on the Millennium Development Goals*. [Online] Available at: http://www.un.org/millenniumgoals/bkgd.shtml.

United Nations News Centre (2011). *Remarks to General Assembly meeting on the Prevention and Control of Non-Communicable Diseases*. Secretary-General Ban Ki-moon General Assembly. [Online] Available at: http://www.un.org/apps/news/infocus/sgspeeches/search_full.asp?statID=1299.

United Nations Population Fund (n.d.). *Empowering Women through Education*. [Online] Available at: http://www.unfpa.org/gender/empowerment2.htm.

United States Global Health (n.d.). *Strategy Objectives of the HHS Global Health Strategy*. [Online] Available at: http://www.global-health.gov/global-programs-and-initiatives/global-health-strategy/strategy-objectives/.

van Weel, C., de Maeseneer, J., and Roberts, R. (2008). Integration of personal and community health care. *The Lancet*, 372, 871–2.

WHO Health Promoting Hospitals Network (1997). *The Vienna Recommendations on Health Promoting Hospitals*. Copenhagen: WHO Europe.

World Bank (2005). *Brail: Addressing the Challenge of Non-communicable Diseases in Brazil*. Washington, DC: World Bank.

World Bank (2011). *Toward a Healthy and Harmonious Life in China: Stemming the Rising Tide of Non-communicable Diseases*. [Online] Available at: http://www.worldbank.org/en/news/feature/2011/07/26/toward-health-harmonious-life-china-stemming-rising-tide-of-non-communicable-diseases.

World Bank (2013). *Improving Nutrition Through Multisectoral Approaches*. [Online] Available at: http://www-wds.worldbank.org/external/default/WDSContentServer/WDSP/IB/2013/02/05/000356161_20130205130807/Rendered/PDF/751020WP0Impro00Box374299B00PUBLIC0.pdf.

World Health Organization (1948). *WHO Definition of Health*. [Online] Available at: http://www.who.int/about/definition/en/print.html.

World Health Organization (1978). *Declaration of Alma-Ata. International Conference on Primary Health Care, Alma-Ata, USSR, 6–12 September 1978*. [Online] Available at: http://www.who.int/publications/almaata_declaration_en.pdf.

World Health Organization (1986). *The Ottawa Charter for Health Promotion. First International Conference on Health Promotion, Ottawa, 21 November 1986*. [Online] Available at: http://www.who.int/healthpromotion/conferences/previous/ottawa/en/.

World Health Organization (2004). *Global Strategy on Diet, Physical Activity and Health. Strategy Documents. May 2004: Final Strategy Document and Resolution*. [Online] Available at: http://www.who.int/dietphysicalactivity/strategy/eb11344/en/.

World Health Organization (2005). *The Bangkok Charter for Health Promotion in a Globalized World*. [Online] Available at: http://www.who.int/healthpromotion/conferences/6gchp/bangkok_charter/en/.

World Health Organization (2008). *The World Health Report 2008—Primary Health Care: Now More Than Ever*. [Online] Available at: http://www.who.int/whr/2008/en/.

World Health Organization (2009a). *Noncommunicable Diseases and Mental Health. 2008–2013 Action Plan for the Global Strategy for the Prevention and Control of Noncommunicable Diseases*. [Online] Available at: http://www.who.int/nmh/publications/9789241597418/en/.

World Health Organization (2009b). *62nd World Health Assembly: Daily Notes on Proceedings*. [Online] Available at: http://www.who.int/mediacentre/events/2009/wha62/journal/en/index.html.

World Health Organization (2013a). *Global Action Plan for the Prevention and Control of Noncommunicable Diseases 2013–2020. Revised Draft*. [Online] Available at: http://www.who.int/nmh/events/2013/revised_draft_ncd_action_plan.pdf.

World Health Organization (2013b). *Draft Action Plan for the Prevention and Control of Noncommunicable Diseases 2013–2020*. [Online] Available at: http://www.who.int/nmh/publications/ncd_action_plan2013.pdf.

World Health Organization (2014). *Noncommunicable Diseases and Mental Health: About 9 Voluntary Global Targets*, Copyright © WHO 2014, available from: http://www.who.int/nmh/ncd-tools/definition-targets/en/ www.who.int/nmh/ncd-tools/definition-targets/en/.

World Health Organization (n.d. a). *Food Security*. [Online] Available at: http://www.who.int/trade/glossary/story028/en/.

World Health Organization (n.d. b). *Global Strategy to Reduce Harmful Use of Alcohol*. [Online] Available at: http://www.who.int/substance_abuse/activities/gsrhua/en/.

World Health Organization (n.d. c). *WHO Framework Convention on Tobacco Control*. [Online] Available at: http://www.who.int/fctc/en/.

World Health Organization (n.d. d). *MPOWER. Tobacco Free Initiative*. [Online] Available at: http://www.who.int/tobacco/mpower/en/.

World Health Organization (n.d. e). *Track 2: Health Literacy and Health Behaviour. 7th Global Conference on Health Promotion: Track Themes*. [Online] Available at: http://www.who.int/healthpromotion/conferences/7gchp/track2/en/index.html.

World Health Organization (n.d. f). *Introduction to Healthy Settings*. [Online] Available at: http://www.who.int/healthy_settings/about/en/.

World Health Organization (n.d. g). *Healthy Settings*. [Online] Available at: http://www.who.int/healthy_settings/en/.

World Health Organization (n.d. h). *Healthy Workplaces: A WHO Global Model for Action*. [Online] Available at: http://www.who.int/occupational_health/healthy_workplaces/en/.

World Health Organization (n.d. i). *Ageing and Life-Course. Care and Independence in Older Age*. [Online] Available at: http://www.who.int/ageing/en/.

World Health Organization Europe Office (n.d.). *Environment and Health*. [Online] Available at: http://www.euro.who.int/en/what-we-do/health-topics/environment-and-health.

World Health Organization Regional Office for the Western Pacific (1999). *Regional Guidelines for the Development of Healthy Workplaces*. [Online] Available at: http://www.who.int/occupational_health/regions/en/oehwproguidelines.pdf.

Strategies for health services

Chien Earn Lee

Introduction to strategies for health services

The previous edition of this chapter started with two questions. Firstly, why public health professionals should be interested in health services, which led to the second question: do health services actually make a meaningful contribution to population health?

Writers such as McKeown (1979) contended that the main drivers of improvements in health had been nutrition, environment, and behaviour rather than healthcare. He showed that three-quarters of the decline in mortality in England and Wales between 1841 and 1971 had been due to a reduction in deaths from infectious disease and that three-quarters of this reduction had preceded the widespread introduction of immunization or antibiotics.

Others such as Illich (1976) argued that instead of improving health, healthcare has a direct and adverse effect on health, for example, side effects of prescribed drugs, hospital-acquired infections, poorly performed surgery, and the consequences of following up spurious abnormalities from the increasing numbers of laboratory investigations.

However, as several commentators have noted, McKeown was describing a period in which healthcare still had relatively little to offer. It was only in the 1960s and 1970s that safe and effective drugs for many chronic diseases became widely available (Nolte and McKee 2004). Contrary to the situation before the 1960s, health services are now making an important contribution to overall improvements in life expectancies in industrialized countries. Many new treatments have been introduced that have been shown, in high-quality evaluative research, to prolong life. Examples include effective treatment for hypertension and heart failure, secondary prevention following myocardial infarction, and chemotherapy for many childhood cancers.

International differences provide many natural experiments to examine this issue further (McKee and Bojan 1998). For example, prior to 1990 the death rates from causes amenable to medical care (i.e. deaths from causes that are potentially preventable with timely and effective healthcare) were higher in former communist countries of Central and Eastern Europe than in the West (Bojan et al. 1991; Boys et al. 1991). Excluding early neonatal deaths, for which only incomplete data are available, Velkova et al. (1997) estimated that amenable causes accounted for 24 per cent of the East–West gap in male life expectancy between birth and the age of 75 years in 1988. The corresponding figure for females was 39 per cent.

There is now considerable evidence that, unlike the situation prior to the 1970s, health services, although only one of the determinants of health, others being genetic predisposition, individual behaviour and lifestyle, and environmental circumstances, can make a substantial difference to population health (McKee and Figueras 2009).

The Ottawa Charter for Health Promotion (World Health Organization 1986) recommended the reorientation of health services and their resources, beyond its responsibility for providing clinical and curative services, towards the promotion of health. The Charter also emphasized the need to work towards enhancing life skills to increase the options available for people to exercise more control over their own health and over their environments and to make choices conducive to health.

Public health professionals have a key advocacy role to ensure that resources in hospitals (which invariably receive the lion's share of the healthcare budget) are used effectively, efficiently, and equitably to optimize outcomes, and that community-based services which are less urgent but no less important than acute services are not neglected. The capabilities of public health professionals in developing systems-based solutions and mobilizing intersectoral action will need to grow to improve population health

The remainder of this chapter explores the changing context of healthcare services, the emerging themes in healthcare services, and strategies for delivering and improving healthcare services

The context for healthcare services

Healthcare services do not exist in a vacuum. While this statement seems self-evident, it has often not been adequately taken into account in developing and evolving healthcare strategies. As a result, strategies have either not taken root (especially those related to 'transplanted' best practices from other systems) or like the proverbial frog being slowly boiled alive, failed to respond in a timely manner to meet new challenges. Contextual factors that need to be considered include societal and professional norms and values as they influence the central principles of the system as well as the desire for reform. Economic factors such as the level of economic development would affect the level of disposable resources available for health services (Maxwell 1981), while the upward pressure on healthcare expenditures has been the key driver for healthcare reforms around the world. Healthcare systems must also be able to respond proactively to factors affecting population health needs such as the changing demographics and patterns of disease as well as the impact of technological change. The role of education in producing sufficient professional and managerial capability will also influence the health system's capacity for serious and sustainable action. These contextual factors are discussed here under the headings of defining norms and values, the reality of macroeconomics, demographic pressures, changing disease patterns, technological changes, the quest for quality and reducing waste, and rising patient expectations.

Norms and beliefs

Healthcare systems act as mirrors that reflect deeply rooted social and cultural expectations of the population that they serve (Contandriopoulos et al. 1998). Although these norms and beliefs are generated outside the formal structure of the healthcare system, they play a major role in defining the system's overall characteristics.

Societies have dominant belief systems where the daily tensions between differing values and beliefs in a society are held in relative stability (Benson 1975). A useful approach to understanding belief systems sees these tensions as grouped around four poles (Habermas 1987): values, understanding of phenomena, definition of jurisdictions and allocation of resources, and logic of regulation.

In this framework, values include the tensions and trade-offs between equity, individual autonomy, and efficiency (Clark 1988). Understanding of phenomena relates to how concepts such as life, death, sickness, health, and pain are interpreted and thus viewed as relating to the objectives of a healthcare system (Gillett 1995). Definition of jurisdictions and allocation of resources comprise the perceptions of the role and functions of those working in the healthcare sector, as well as the allocation of resources between prevention and cure and between healthcare and broader determinants of health. The logic of regulation relates to how society chooses to regulate the delivery of healthcare. This may be technocratic with trained experts guiding the system on the basis of their knowledge and position within the hierarchy; professional self-regulation which has the physician (as the best agent of the patient) at the centre of the system; the market-based model in which regulations reflect supply and demand in a competitive market; or the democratic model, in which the population, either directly or, more often, through elected or appointed representatives, is responsible for setting out the framework for delivery of healthcare.

An understanding of the dominant belief system in a society is important for public health professionals as it contributes to knowledge of why systems are as they are, how they have changed, and the objectives that individuals within the healthcare system are pursuing. It will also influence the choice of strategies that should be adopted to bring about meaningful and sustained change (McKee and Figueras 2009). For example, some societies view healthcare as predominantly a social and collective good. Such societies would more readily accept policies designed to create intentional cross subsidies, from young to old, rich to poor, and from healthy to sick, than societies that view healthcare as a commodity that can be bought and sold in the market.

Norms and beliefs can and do evolve over time. For example, years of spectacular growth have seen more people pulled from abject poverty in modern Asia than at any other time in history. But as they become more affluent, the region's citizens want more from their governments. Across the continent, pressure is growing for public pensions, national health insurance, unemployment benefits, and other hallmarks of social protection. As a result, the world's most vibrant economies are shifting gear, away from simply building wealth towards building states with better and more comprehensive welfare provisions (*The Economist* 2012). While such changes increase the demands on healthcare systems, they also provide opportunities to introduce changes and strategies that may not have been acceptable based on previous norms and beliefs.

Macroeconomic factors

The historically high rates of economic growth seen during the 1960s and 1970s have not been sustained in the 1990s. This has been compounded by economic volatility with shorter boom and bust cycles with globalization. With economies across the world becoming more and more connected to one another, adverse economic conditions in one country can rapidly spread to other countries and escalate to global proportions, as was seen in the global financial crisis in the late 2000s.

At the same time, the expansion of healthcare coverage both in terms of scope of services and population covered is adding significantly to the upward pressures on healthcare expediture. There are already concerns that the current level of expenditure on healthcare is not sustainable and is adversely affecting other sectors of the economy. For example, the United States spent more than 17 per cent of its gross domestic product on health, raising concerns about the heavy burden placed on companies doing business in the United States which can put them at a substantial competitive disadvantage in the international marketplace.

The macroeconomic environment influences the political decision-making process, in particular, the allocation of resources to competing sectors. The growth in health spending slowed or fell in real terms in 2010 in almost all Organisation for Economic Cooperation and Development (OECD) countries, reversing a long-term trend of rapid increases. Overall, health spending grew by nearly 5 per cent per year in real terms in OECD countries over the period 2000–2009, but this was followed by zero growth in 2010. Preliminary figures for a limited number of countries suggest little or no growth in 2011. Countries like the United Kingdom that invested heavily in healthcare in 1990s are having to scale back in the face of the tightening economic situation. The UK government aims to deliver £20 billion (4 per cent) efficiency savings in the National Health Service (NHS) by the end of 2014–2015. The challenge at present is how to balance increased demand from patients with the requirement for productivity and efficiency, whilst maintaining excellent, quality care.

Demographic pressures

Dr Gro Harlem Brundtland, former Director-General of the World Health Organization, called ageing one of humanity's great achievements and also one of its greatest challenges. In rich countries, the number of people over 65 who will require medical care, is expected to increase by between 50 per cent and 120 per cent from 1995 to 2025 and the elderly incur disproprotionately more healthcare cost than the young. For example, in the United States, the elderly account for less than 15 per cent of the total population but incur more than one-third of healthcare spending (and this is before taking into account social or long-term care costs).

The greatest challenge lies in the developing countries. While developed countries grew affluent before they became old, developing countries are growing old before they get affluent. The demographic shift towards an older population that took place gradually in Europe over a century, is taking place in the developing countries at a pace which far outstrips these countries' socioeconomic development. The impact of ageing on demand for healthcare is often compounded by falling birth rates, leading to an increasing dependency ratio.

It is, however, necessary to enter three caveats. Firstly a study of American Medicare data showed that while estimated lifetime cost increases with age, the cost associated with an additional year of life and the average annual cost over a person's lifetime both decreased as the age at death increased (Lubitz et al. 1995). This could be due to less intensive treatment the older the patients are in their respective last year of life (Scitovsky 1988). This suggests that healthcare cost will be more substantially affected by the expected increase in the absolute number of elderly people than increased longevity beyond the age of 65.

Secondly, the health and social profile of the elderly of the future may be different from current elderly. They are likely to be better educated and would have benefited from a lifetime of better nutrition. On the other hand, they are also likely to have adopted a more sedentary lifestyle and have higher expectations of healthcare. For these reasons, we should not make simplistic extrapolations of demand based on current data of the elderly to a future population.

The final caveat is that pessimistic predictions of the costs of ageing are based on the assumption that health services will continue to expand in their current form which is highly hospital centric. The impact of ageing on disease burden and costs can be moderated by greater emphasis on prevention of disease and disability and transforming models of care for the elderly.

Changing healthcare workforce

Specialization in the pursuit of greater knowledge and expertise has characterized scientific progress in medicine for nearly two centuries (Cassel and Reuben 2011). A more recent development is the creation of subspecialties, recognizing that there are some specific populations of patients who would benefit from the highly focused knowledge and skills obtained by additional training and certification beyond that of a 'general' specialist. As these tertiary subspecialists require high patient volume to maintain proficiency in their skills, they are usually based at referral centres.

Many new and emerging subspecialties are cross-disciplinary. In the United States, sleep medicine crosses six different specialties, and palliative medicine is a subspecialty option for ten different primary specialties. The proliferation of specialties has led to concerns that medical care would become increasingly fragmented with the concomitant loss or undervaluing of the generalist physician with decreased attractiveness as a career choice for young doctors.

As trade barriers come down, the forces of globalization have increased the movement of all types of professionals throughout the world, and healthcare is no exception. Richer countries are increasingly relying on immigration as a means of coping with domestic shortages of healthcare professionals. This trend has led to concerns that the outflow of healthcare professionals is adversely affecting the healthcare system in many of these source countries. Insufficient human resources for health in developing countries have been identified as one of the main constraints

limiting progress on such initiatives as 3by51 and the Millennium Development Goals (MDGs) (Institute of Medicine (IOM) 2004). Recipient countries on the other hand need to develop the means to effectively assimilate the influx of healthcare professionals from diverse backgrounds and cultures.

Countries are also exploring expanded scope of practice for healthcare professionals as a means of addressing access-to-care problems. Nurse practitioners, physical and occupational therapists, and other allied healthcare professionals are growing in independence from physicians' oversight. For example, several states in the United States have passed legislation allowing pharmacists limited ability to evaluate and manage drug regimens as well as dispense drugs.

Changing burden of disease

The term 'epidemiological transition' refers to the complex changes in patterns of health and disease as societies develop. It describes the interactions between these patterns and their demographic, economic, and sociological determinants and consequences.

In the classical (Western) model, Omran (1971) described the transition from the Age of Pestilence and Famine with its high mortality and low average life expectancy (20–40 years), through the Age of Receding Pandemics, to the Age of Degenerative and Man-Made Diseases with its relatively low levels of mortality (average life expectancy of more than 50 years) and morbidity overshadowing mortality as an index of health.

Although the classical model assumes linear unidirectional change, counter transitions have also been observed where age-specific mortality rates rise rather than fall over time due to causes such as the HIV/AIDS pandemic in sub-Saharan Africa (Gaylin and Kates 1997). There is also an emerging awareness of old problems that never went away resulting in an overlap of eras, often with large disparities emerging between and within countries. On the other hand, although chronic diseases such as diabetes have usually been considered as diseases of affluence, four out of five people with diabetes now live in low- and middle-income countries (International Diabetes Federation 2012). In short, health systems in these countries must continue to grapple with the unfinished agenda of communicable diseases while addressing the new agenda of non-communicable ones in an ageing population.

As the burden of disease is dynamic (Murray and Lopez 1996), the configuration of health services must evolve accordingly to meet the changing health needs of the population. Health services cannot remain trapped in structures designed for a time when disease patterns were different. For example, the increasing incidence and prevalence of chronic diseases requires health systems to organize health services with greater emphasis on prevention and community-based services instead of the current hospital-centric model which is more suited for acute episodic care.

Current care delivery models are, however, often overly complex and uncoordinated, requiring many steps and patient 'hand-offs' that slow down care delivery and decrease safety. Healthcare organizations, hospitals, and physician groups also typically operate as separate 'silos', acting without the benefit of complete information about the patient's condition, medical history, services provided in other settings, or medications provided by other clinicians (IOM 2001).

Public health professionals have a central role in tracking and explaining trends in diseases (including predicting emerging trends), designing mechanisms to address them, supporting the changes in service delivery that are required, and monitoring responses to these changes. With appropriate interventions, Olshansky (1986) has postulated the 'Age of Delayed Degenerative Diseases' as the fourth stage of the epidemiological transition.

Technological changes

The pace of change in healthcare is steadily accelerating. Hip replacements have been joined by knees, shoulders, and finger joint replacements. Transplant surgeons have added heart, liver, and pancreas transplants to their initial successes with kidneys. AIDS has been transformed from a rapidly progressive fatal disease to one in which increasing numbers of patients are keeping the disease under control with complex cocktails of antiviral therapy. The list is almost endless.

The growth of healthcare technology is widely held to have contributed substantially to the upward pressure on healthcare expenditure. For example, the rapid growth in cardiology services throughout the developed world is driven more by angioplasty and other technological advances in care than by changes in the prevalence of heart disease (Dash et al. 2009). Although its precise contribution is controversial (Mossialos and Le Grand 1999), a study by the Health Care Financing Administration estimated that approximately half of the growth in real per capita healthcare costs in the United States is attributable to the introduction and diffusion of new medical technology for the 1940–1990 period, within an estimated probable range of 38–62 per cent of growth (Smith et al. 2000).

There are various reasons for this increase. New technologies are often more expensive than the ones they replaced. Even where the actual technology is less expensive, it may lead to increased costs as other aspects of the service are reorganized to reflect changing patterns of treatment. For example, the introduction of new treatments may lead to an expansion in the number of individuals with indications for treatment, either because a previously untreatable condition becomes treatable or, as side effects or contraindications are reduced, the threshold for treatment falls. Finally, the diffusion of technology from tertiary centres, in some cases into primary care, can markedly reduce barriers to access and thus increase uptake.

Since the 1980s, there has also been an unparalleled revolution in the pace and volume of communication. The development of new ways of storing and delivering knowledge has transformed the way healthcare services are delivered and used, bringing benefits but also risks. It enables the separation of assessment from service provision allowing healthcare professionals to seek and provide advice without the need for face-to-face consultation. Telemedicine has led to the expansion of roles and the need for new competencies in healthcare workers. It also provides opportunities to optimize the value of highly trained subspecialists by making their expertise accessible to a wider patient population through physician-to-physician telemedicine approaches.

Quest for quality and reduction of waste

In tandem with the rapid growth in medical science and technology, healthcare is becoming more complex with more to know, more to do, more to manage, more to watch, and more people involved than ever before (IOM 2001). Healthcare systems have, however, struggled to translate knowledge into practice. For

example, it takes an average of 17 years for research evidence to reach clinical practice (Green et al. 2009). Small-area variation studies by Wennberg (1984) showed that decisions by clinicians in different areas regarding patients presenting with identical complaints could vary by as much as 40 per cent.

Geographical variation of expenditure has also been identified. For example, in 2004, per capita spending on health ranged from roughly $4000 in Utah to $6700 in Massachusetts in the United States (Congressional Budget Office 2008). Higher spending does not necessarily mean better outcomes. The primary reason for such variations has been previously cited as clinical uncertainty about the most appropriate treatment in any given circumstance (Anderson and Mooney 1990). This position is, however, becoming increasingly untenable as medical knowledge advances and evidence-based practice guidelines are developed for many conditions.

Healthcare systems are also grappling with the consequences of unsafe care. A study in *The New England Journal of Medicine* (Landrigan et al. 2010) reported that 25 per cent of hospitalized patients are harmed by medical errors. IOM's landmark study 'To Err is Human' (1989) estimated that there were 98,000 annual deaths from medical errors in the United States. The IOM's follow-up publication 'Crossing the Quality Chasm' has identified six dimensions where healthcare needs to improve:

◆ Safe—reducing harm to patients.

◆ Effective—providing appropriate care based on scientific knowledge to avoid underuse or overuse of services.

◆ Patient-centred—providing care that is based on what matters to patients taking into account their preferences, needs, and values.

◆ Timely—reducing unnecessary delays that may compromise care outcomes.

◆ Efficient—avoiding waste not just of material resources but also ideas and energy.

◆ Equitable—providing consistent quality of care regardless of personal characteristics such as gender, ethnicity, geographic location, and socioeconomic status.

Inappropriate care and errors waste precious resources. Waste occurs not just at the individual clinician–patient interface but as a result of poor coordination between providers and across subsectors, inadequate management of capital resources, and operational budgets. The IOM committee that produced the report 'Best Care at Lower Cost: The Path to Continuously Learning Health Care in America' estimated that there was $750 billion in unnecessary health spending in 2009 in the United States alone. The IOM Committee recommended a more nimble healthcare system that is consistently reliable and that constantly, systematically, and seamlessly improves. Healthcare systems must learn by avoiding past mistakes and adopt newfound successes.

The International Cochrane Collaboration has played a major role in providing evidence of what healthcare interventions can (and cannot) achieve by undertaking systematic reviews of available evidence in the literature using standardized methods, and disseminating the information (Chalmers and Altman 1995). Unfortunately such information is not always translated into daily practice as it challenges traditional models based on clinical autonomy.

Increasing patient expectations

The development of new and more expensive technologies coupled with the ready access to information, particularly with the growth of the Internet, has led to higher and growing public expectations which may be difficult to meet.

Increasingly people are also taking over responsibility for their own care aided by online advice and other sources of information. The public increasingly expects healthcare systems to be responsive at all times (24 hours a day, every day) and that access to care should be provided over multiple channels such as the Internet, by telephone, and by other means in addition to face-to-face visits. Patients expect healthcare services to make information available to patients and their families that allow them to make informed decisions when selecting a health plan, hospital, or clinical practice, or choosing among alternative treatments.

Through the Internet, patients draw on the perspectives not only of physicians but also other sufferers from their condition. However, it comes with risks too. Those searching the web must be aware of its unregulated nature, with posts of views ranging from Nobel laureates to quacks (Eysenbach et al. 1998; Sandvik 1999). Internet prescribing may offer price savings for some, but it may also circumvent regulatory safeguards designed to reduce risks to patients.

Emerging themes in health services

This section explores some of the themes that are emerging in response to the changing context of health services. The evolving macroeconomic environment coupled with the demand for health services brought about by changing demographics, epidemiology, and patient expectations have led to a reassessment of the relationship between the state and the market as well as the way health services are organized and financed. Developments in technology underpinned by changes in norms and beliefs are challenging traditional hierarchies and stimulating new ways of delivering health services with greater involvement of patients in their own care. These themes will be considered in turn.

State and market

During the 1980s and 1990s, many countries began to re-examine the role of the state in the regulation, funding, and delivery of health services. Countries where the state has played a central role are exploring new pluralistic solutions with involvement of a range of actors at varying distances from the state. Some functions are being devolved to local government or to statutory agencies at arm's length from government or transferred altogether to private ownership. Conversely, countries in which the state has traditionally played a less central role, acting only as a source of regulation between competing private interests, are now reassessing the need to expand their role and intervene more actively (Saltman and Figueras 1997).

It would be quite wrong, however, to see these developments as a process of convergence to some ideal model of a health system. Instead, the situation in each country represents the complex interplay of the economic, social, demographic, epidemiological, managerial, and technological forces described earlier and deep-seated cultural beliefs. The debate is often characterized as a dichotomy between the state and the market but this is a gross oversimplification (Saltman and von Otter 1995). In some instances elements of both have been combined albeit in differing proportions to allow an increased use of market-style incentives with continued ownership and operation of facilities by the public sector in quasi- or internal markets.

The introduction of market mechanisms into the health sector creates a series of conceptual and practical challenges. Conceptually, healthcare is considered in many societies as a social good, in which the provision of services to each individual is also valuable to the community as a whole, whether because of ideas of self-interest, as in the treatment of dangerous mental illness or contagious disease, or altruism. Such principles have led to the creation of systems to ensure universal coverage and solidarity. In contrast, market incentives are intrinsically based on the assumption that services provided are a commodity, with demand driven by individual preference (McKee and Figueras 2009).

Another difficulty is that the neoclassical concept of a market is based on the relationship between a buyer and a seller. However, healthcare systems typically comprise a more complex set of relationships involving the patient, various health professionals, a provider institution, and a payer, with health professionals acting as both suppliers of services and agents for the patient (Young and Saltman 1985). Finally, the assumption in neoclassical economic theory that cross-subsidies between different patients are inefficient is incompatible with the social function of the healthcare system where there are substantial cross-subsidies between young and old, rich and poor, and healthy and sick.

The key practical challenge in introducing market mechanisms into healthcare is the development of real prices. This is a tedious and expensive process which requires a robust costing system to compute the real cost (including overheads) at the service as well as patient level. Some attempts to implement market mechanisms have floundered as the transaction costs and the costly duplication of facilities to secure a competitive advantage (Saltman and von Otter 1995) outweighed the improvements in operational efficiency. Another reason for the failure of market mechanisms in healthcare is that competition operates at the wrong level. Porter and Teisberg (2006) argue that currently competition is both too broad and too narrow. Competition is too broad because much of the competition now takes place at the level of health plans, networks, hospital groups, physician groups, and clinics. Instead, it should occur in addressing particular medical conditions. Competition is too narrow because it now takes place at the level of discrete interventions or services. Instead it should take place at the patient level, addressing medical conditions over the full cycle of care, including monitoring and prevention, diagnosis, treatment, and the ongoing management of the condition.

Some other attempts have, however, been more successful. In these systems, the introduction of market principles does not mean that the government intervenes less but it intervenes differently. Even as we are familiar with market failures in healthcare, there can be government failure too—which can occur in a state- or market-based system. The manner of government intervention matters more than the fact of intervention. The purported failure of market mechanisms may at times be due more to poor implementation than the mechanism itself. Oftentimes markets fail in healthcare, because they are allowed to fail. For markets to work, government intervention such as setting the ground rules for competition and providing clear standards for market participants with tight monitoring and evaluation as well as making prices transparent is needed.

A related issue is the changing approach to regulation. Governments need to find the appropriate balance between regulatory and competitive measures—which will change with time—depending on the context in which they are implemented. Regulation is becoming more sophisticated with greater recognition that traditional 'command and control' measures need to be complemented by a more extensive regulatory toolkit (which includes 'softer' tools such as education and community engagement). Governments also need to be cognizant of the risk of perverse incentives with poorly drafted regulations.

Many countries are beginning to question whether self-regulation of healthcare professionals can retain credibility as a system that serves the best interests of the public. Self-interest of the profession plays out in various ways, at times negatively. For example, one professional group may use the regulatory structure to exercise control and influence over another group, or to keep hold of their monopoly on very profitable services. The key question for policymakers, then, is one of governance: to what extent are healthcare professional regulators sufficiently independent of the groups they regulate—and to what extent do they act in the best interests of patients and the public? Several countries have moved to 'shared regulation' whereby the government and other credible experts from outside the regulated profession sit with members of the profession around the table. The proportion of places around the table is a matter for each country to determine, based on local context (Dzau et al. 2012).

Governments that have successfully incorporated market principles rely on competition and market forces to improve service delivery and efficiency, while retaining the prerogative of the state to intervene directly when the market failed to keep healthcare costs down (Atwal 2010). Markets are necessary to help government work better, and good government is necessary to help markets work better (Menon 2010). In fact some researchers have concluded that governments have to be more competent to supervise contracting and other market-style arrangements than to run services directly (Kettl 1993).

Reorganizing the system: decentralization, recentralization, and privatization

Decentralization has been defined as the transfer of authority from a high, or national, level to a lower, or subnational, level (Rondinelli 1981). Decentralization has multiple meanings, interpretations, and implementation in different countries and different contexts. The common essence of decentralization lies in strengthening local authorities through transfer of power and resources from the central government.

Decentralization has become attractive because of disillusionment with the perceived failings of large centralized, bureaucratic institutions. These include inefficiency, lack of responsiveness, and failure to innovate. Decentralized institutions are seen to have several advantages. Those working in them are better equipped to identify changing circumstances and needs, and thus can respond more flexibly. They can be more innovative than centralized institutions and they can generate higher morale, more commitment, and greater productivity. Decentralization can also facilitate enhanced partnerships with the local population, thus increasing the democratic input into policymaking.

The experience of many countries in recent years demonstrates that there are certain areas where decision-making power should not be decentralized. Four such areas include:

- Basic framework for health policy, strategic decisions on the development of health resources such as capital, personnel, expensive equipment.

- Research and development as they shape the future of the entire system.

- Regulations concerning public safety.

- Monitoring, assessment, and analysis of the health of the population and healthcare provision (as these are tools for influencing the behaviour of decentralized units).

Borgenhammer (1993) has also identified certain social and cultural conditions that are necessary for successful decentralization. These include adequate local administrative and managerial capacity, ideological certainty in the implementation of tasks, and readiness to accept several interpretations of a particular problem. Organizations undertaking decentralization must engage in a process of articulation of their mission, create internal cultures around core values, and establish mechanisms to monitor results (Osborne and Gaebler 1993).

With respect to health services, decentralization enables better access with people benefiting from the convenience of having core health services close to where they live. However, decentralization can have negative effects (Collins and Green 1994). These include fragmentation of services, loss of critical mass in services, and unacceptable variations in practice (Borgenhammer 1993). For health services there is substantial clinical evidence that centralizing certain complex conditions and procedures, specialization with co-location of specialist staff and services in facilities to generate a critical volume of cases has led to better clinical outcomes and higher productivity. The aim then is to 'decentralize where possible, centralize where necessary' (NHS 2007). This entails the creation of a primary and community care infrastructure that is able to deliver integrated services close to patients' homes with consolidation of centres that perform only a small number of procedures (Dash et al. 2009).

Privatization requires separate consideration as it is fundamentally different, in several important aspects, from other types of decentralization. Its advocates argue that it brings benefits from the introduction of economic incentives for greater efficiency and higher quality in the management of healthcare (Cabinet Office 1999). It is also attractive to some governments as a means of attracting private capital into the health sector, thus reducing demands on scarce public funds.

These benefits, however, come with considerable risks. Private management and capital investment require financial returns that are consistent with those obtainable in other private markets. The pressures involved in achieving these returns can result in adverse selection (e.g. practices that intentionally discriminate against the poor and other vulnerable groups). Activities that do not generate immediate returns such as primary and secondary prevention activities are likely to be relegated to lower priority (Himmelstein et al. 1999). If privatization is not to undermine wider health policies, privatization must be accompanied by strengthened central regulatory controls. This increases administrative cost for both regulators and providers.

Two broad findings emerge from the debate on decentralization. The first is whether the advantages of decentralization outweigh the disadvantages, such as fragmented and duplicated services and high transaction costs, an issue that must be resolved on a case-by-case basis (Saltman and Figueras 1997). Secondly, a policy of decentralization requires a series of measures to create an appropriate framework, including development of a shared vision and a means of monitoring outcomes.

Ecosystem approach to healthcare

Health status is largely determined by the interaction of four linked factors: genetic susceptibility, behaviour and lifestyle, socioeconomic status, and environmental conditions (Lalonde 1974). Addressing these factors requires the concerted effort of partners outside of the traditional health sector such as in housing, agriculture and education, as well as improved coordination and continuity of care between hospital and community based services (including primary healthcare).

Healthcare systems are moving, albeit at different speeds, from an illness to a wellness/health model, shifting the allocation of funds from curative to preventive care. This is, however, a delicate balancing exercise due to the need to maintain current services while preparing for the future. The Institute for Healthcare Improvement in America has developed a framework that seeks to optimize health system performance by simultaneously pursuing three dimensions, the 'Triple Aim' of improving the patient experience of care (including quality and satisfaction), improving the health of populations, and reducing the per capita cost of healthcare (Berwick et al. 2008).

The components of the Triple Aim are not independent of each other. The pursuit of any one goal can result in changes that affect the other two, sometimes negatively and sometimes positively. For example, improving care for individuals can raise costs if the improvements are associated with new, effective, but costly technologies or drugs. Conversely, eliminating overuse or misuse of therapies or diagnostic tests can lead to both reduced costs and improved outcomes.

The balanced pursuit of the Triple Aim is unfortunately not congruent with the current business models of any but a small number of healthcare organizations. Payment dynamics often lead hospitals to focus only on care within their walls, viewing readmissions for chronic diseases such as congestive heart failure as the result of defects outside the hospital and not as their responsibility to avert (Bisognano and Kenney 2012). For hospitals paid based on number of patients treated, averting readmission incurs costs from additional effort such as patient education and post-discharge follow-up (which may not be reimbursed as these occur outside the hospital) and reduces revenue by decreasing the number of patients being admitted. In such instances, rational common interests and rational individual interests are in conflict. Lack of system knowledge among clinicians and organizations leads them to optimize the components of the system with which they are most familiar, at the expense of the whole

Movement between the various care levels (primary, secondary, tertiary, and community care) typically involves passage across an interface that is governed by rules of varying degrees of formality. Examples include referral to hospital by a primary care physician or discharge from an acute hospital to a long-stay facility. However, these movements are often not seamless, thus hampering efforts to enable patients to be treated in the most cost-effective settings.

The pursuit of the Triple Aim requires health services to move from the current silo-based approach to a more systematic and integrated model of care. Integrated care brings together inputs, delivery, management and organization of services related to diagnosis, treatment, care, rehabilitation, and health promotion as a means to improve the services in relation to access, quality, user satisfaction, and efficiency (Gröne and Garcia-Barbero 2001).

Measurement drives behaviour. As such, the move towards better integration of care has been accompanied by efforts to measure health status rather than just healthcare. The proposed framework shown in Fig. 11.7.1 (Arah et al. 2006) illustrates a measurement system that takes into account non-healthcare determinants of health, health system performance across the various care sectors, and embeds healthcare within the broader economic, social, and political context of a country. A framework that is unduly narrow and clinical in its focus will miss this big-picture perspective.

Patient engagement and empowerment

Very few healthcare-delivery models currently view the patient as a resource who can help improve healthcare delivery for themselves and each other. Patients are either viewed as liabilities who consume scarce resources, or as passive vessels into which treatments are poured (Dzau et al. 2012). At times, healthcare services not only fail to take advantage of the patient's capabilities, they also diminish them: studies have shown that during hospitalization, older people actually lose the ability to function independently (Creditor 1993; Sager et al. 1996).

Patients with chronic diseases can profoundly change the development and progression of their conditions through effective self-care, goal-setting, and adherence to prescribed medication, exercise, and nutrition regimes. A survey by the Commonwealth Fund (Schoen et al. 2011), however, suggests that this opportunity is being lost in many healthcare systems, owing to the professionals' failure to prepare patients for this role by discussing treatment goals/priorities, making treatment plans that patients can carry out in daily life, and giving clear instructions on symptoms and when to seek care.

On the other hand, we have the positive example in Jönköping, Sweden, where patients with kidney failure have been trained to use hospital dialysis machines themselves, thereby improving the efficiency, productivity, convenience, and safety of care delivery. These patients have also been empowered to provide advice to one another on ways of managing their illness (Dzau et al. 2012).

Several important issues need to be addressed in increasing patient participation in healthcare systems (Saltman and Figueras 1997). One is whether choice is equally important in all healthcare decisions. Another is, given the special characteristics of healthcare, do users have access to enough information and are they able to understand it sufficiently to make an informed choice? Several countries have sought to inform the public by means of publication of rankings of outcomes by hospital or physician. However, these are subject to substantial methodological limitations and also provide scope for opportunistic behaviour by providers, either to exclude patients with higher risks or to manipulate the data that are presented. Finally, enhancing choice risks increasing health inequalities as those with most resources (time, money

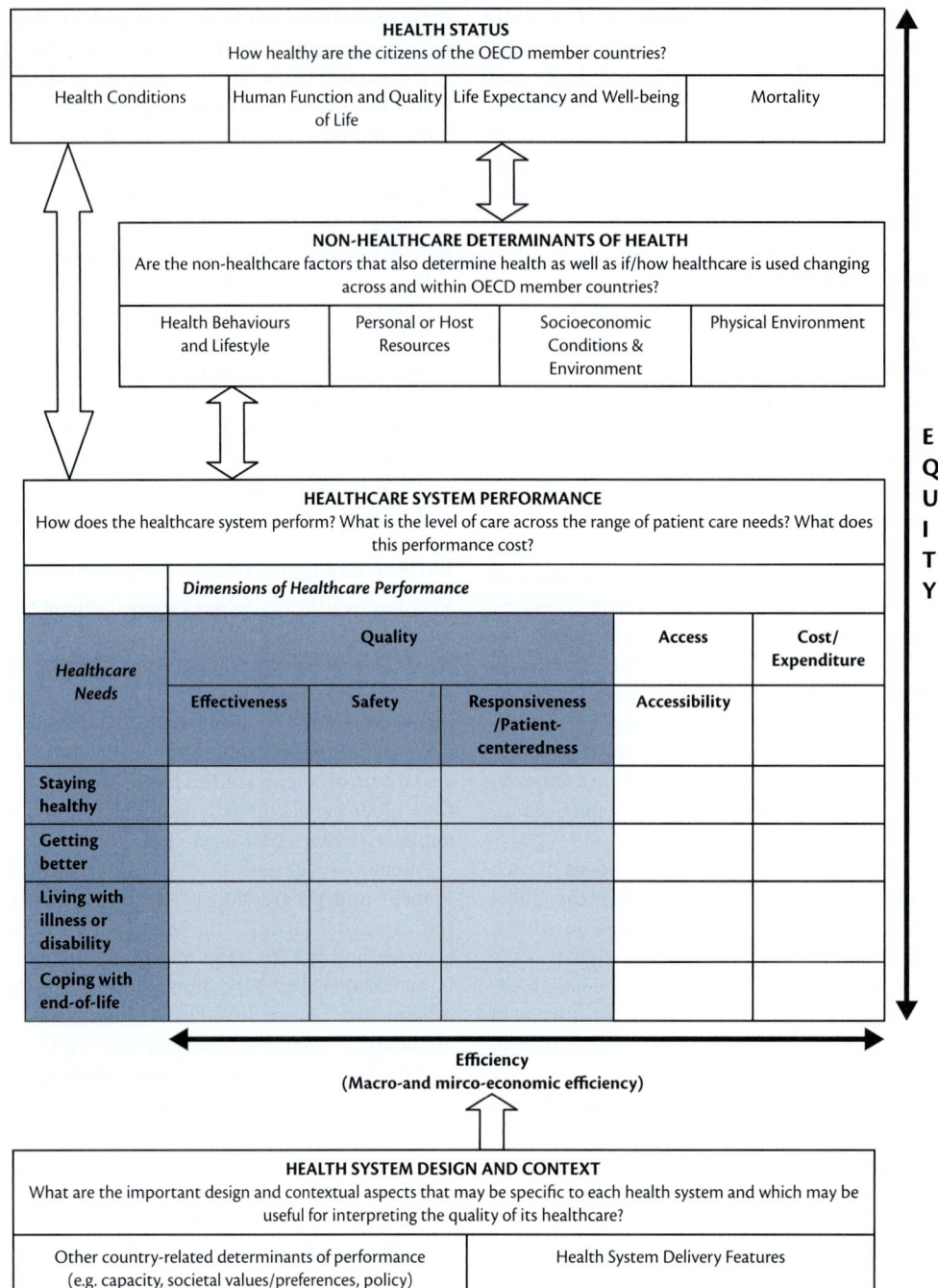

Fig. 11.7.1 Conceptual framework for OECD Health Care Quality Indicator (HCQI) Project.

Reproduced from Arah, O.A. et al., A conceptual framework for the OECD Health Care Quality Indicators Project, *International Journal for Quality in Health Care*, Volume 18, Issue Supplement 1, pp. 5–13, Copyright © 2006 International Society for Quality in Health Care and Oxford University Press, by permission of Oxford University Press.

and energy) are likely to have the greatest opportunity to make choices.

Cost sharing

Increasingly, the debate about healthcare costs is no longer about 'who pays?' but about the optimal formula for cost sharing, bearing in mind the need to balance efficiency goals against equity concerns (Lim 2004). Proponents of this approach argue that there is 'no free lunch'. Health insurance premiums have to be paid by

the insured, employee medical benefits form part of wage costs, and public expenditures on healthcare are ultimately paid for by taxpayers. The key question is how best to structure the healthcare system, and the means of financing it, in order to keep it efficient, while making it accessible to all at rates that are affordable to them (Ministry of Health 1993).

People with the most control over what drugs get prescribed and what procedures get done have little incentive to lower these costs (indeed, to the extent that they get paid for the procedure, their incentives are often quite the opposite). Furthermore in a fee for service system, it is not in the economic interest of doctors and hospitals to put themselves out of business by promoting disease prevention. Likewise, patients often feel little need to control the costs of their own medical care if it is fully covered by insurance or the state. These approaches fuel overconsumption of healthcare services, hence contributing to rising healthcare costs. Some healthcare systems have thus tried to structure their financing system to give the individual maximum incentive to stay healthy, save for his or her medical expenses, and avoid using more medical services than is absolutely required.

Cost sharing for health services can help limit overconsumption of healthcare and could instil greater personal responsibility for health. On the other hand, cost sharing (or patient co-payment) can and has led to access and equity problems in some countries. Hence, cost sharing or co-payment should be one component of a multifaceted, multilayered healthcare financing system (Lim 2004). It is important to achieve an appropriate balance between personal responsibility with sufficient incentives for people to be prudent and to look after their own health, and risk pooling to provide a comprehensive safety net should they fall sick.

Cost sharing also allows governments to target their social spending more carefully. For example, greater subsidies could be directed at financially needier patients through financial means-testing. Social provision should be about protecting the poor more than subsidizing the rich. At the same time, in fast-ageing societies, especially, increased expenditures on the elderly must not squeeze out healthcare investments in the young (*The Economist* 2012).

These emerging themes bring new opportunities for public health practitioners to reorient health services towards the maximization of health gains. The next section will explore strategies for health services to translate these opportunities into reality.

Strategies for health services

In devising strategies for health services, we need to take into account the complex nature of healthcare where reductionist, mechanical, and linear methods of problem-solving tend to flounder against the laws of unforeseen consequences and incomplete information. It is also important to differentiate the means from the ends. For example, while healthcare systems aim for universal coverage to ensure that no one is denied healthcare that they need because of inability to pay, the means they have employed to achieve this can markedly differ.

Another consideration in developing strategies for health services is the mismatch between the lifecycles of different elements in the healthcare system such as major infrastructure (e.g. hospitals), technological advances (including information technology), service models, and government/regulatory policies. This can pose a major problem for planning and coordination, in particular to ensure alignment and timeliness in response to a constantly changing environment.

It is impossible in the space available to provide a comprehensive overview of every strategy that might be employed to enhance health services. Instead, this section focuses on key steps in the strategic planning process for health services where public health professionals have a potentially vital role to play. It starts by looking at the needs assessment and priority setting process to ensure that the health services provided reflect the health needs of the population that they serve. Following that, it reviews the design and organization of health services to enhance the efficiency with which services are delivered. It concludes by discussing the enablers that are necessary to implement, sustain, and enhance these services.

Needs assessment and priority setting

'Need' may best be defined as the ability to benefit from 'healthcare', which depends both on morbidity and on the effectiveness of care. Need should not be confused with supply or demand. The relationship between need and demand is mediated by differing illness behaviours. Demand is what people would be willing to pay for in a market or might wish to use in a system of free healthcare, and supply is what is actually provided. It is misleading to measure existing service provision as though it were an indicator for need. Similarly, the measurement of waiting lists, reflecting as they do demand mediated by doctor as agent, is also misleading (Stevens and Gabbay 1991).

Healthcare needs are those that can benefit from healthcare (health education, disease prevention, diagnosis, treatment, rehabilitation, terminal care). Health needs incorporate the wider social and environmental determinants of health, such as deprivation, housing, diet, education, and employment. This wider definition allows us to look beyond the confines of the medical model based on health services, to the wider influences on health. Health needs of a population will be constantly changing, and many will not be amenable to medical intervention (Wright et al. 1998).

Fig. 11.7.2 illustrates how need, demand, and supply might overlap or differ. It shows seven fields of services divided into (E) those

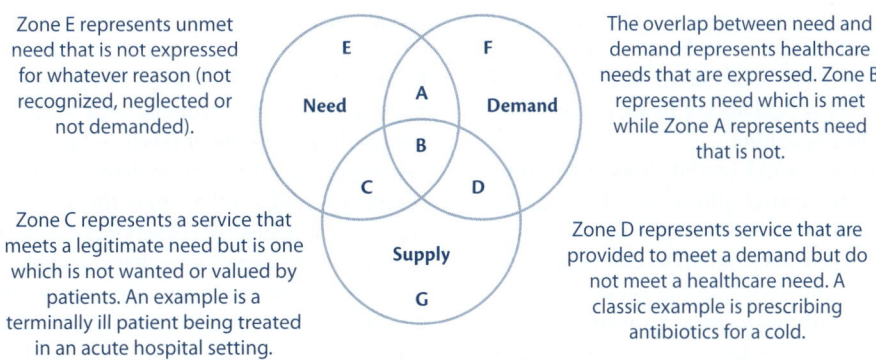

Zone E represents unmet need that is not expressed for whatever reason (not recognized, neglected or not demanded).

The overlap between need and demand represents healthcare needs that are expressed. Zone B represents need which is met while Zone A represents need that is not.

Zone C represents a service that meets a legitimate need but is one which is not wanted or valued by patients. An example is a terminally ill patient being treated in an acute hospital setting.

Zone D represents service that are provided to meet a demand but do not meet a healthcare need. A classic example is prescribing antibiotics for a cold.

Fig. 11.7.2 Need, demand, and supply of healthcare.
Reproduced with permission from NHS Confederation, *Priority Setting—Strategic Planning*, The NHS Confederation, London, UK, Copyright © The NHS Confederation 2008.

for which there is a need but no demand and supply, (F) those for which there is a demand but no need or supply, (G) those for which there is a supply but no need or demand, and then (A–D) the various degrees of overlap (NHS Confederation 2008).

The key challenge is to make the three circles of need, demand, and supply more congruent. This includes demand management and changing supply as well as better definition of need. Demand management may involve curtailing it where it is inappropriate (areas F and D in Fig. 11.7.2) or stimulating it (areas A and B). Varied mechanisms through which demand can be influenced include: the accessibility and organization of services, the provision of health information, education, and financial incentives. Demand can also be induced by supply: geographical variation in hospital admission rates is explained more by the supply of hospital beds than by indicators of mortality (Feldstein 1964); referral rates of general practitioners owe more to the characteristics of individual doctors than to the health of their populations (Wilkin 1992).

Strategies that act on supply of health services include reducing the number of healthcare professionals or facilities, setting global budgets for providers (Schwartz et al. 1996), giving professionals incentives to reduce the amount of care provided, and reducing access to care (Abel-Smith et al. 1995). Even need can be shifted somewhat, with new findings on disease pathology and new treatments that are effective.

Distinguishing between individual needs and the wider needs of the community is important in the planning and provision of local health services. Without a proper need assessment process, the pattern of health services will frequently reflect only what a few people perceive to be the needs of the population rather than what they actually are and often those whose needs are greatest will receive the least (Hart 1971).

Assessment of health needs is a systematic method of identifying unmet health and healthcare needs of a population and making changes to meet these unmet needs (Wright et al. 1998). The principal activities involved in healthcare needs assessment are the assessment of incidence and prevalence (how many people need the service/intervention), the effectiveness and cost-effectiveness of services (do they confer any benefit, and if so at what cost, i.e. what is the relative benefit?) and baseline services. Changing the provision of healthcare services for the better necessitates knowledge of existing services, both to know which services ought to change and to identify opportunities for the release of resources to enable the change to happen.

Health needs assessment should not just measure ill health, as this assumes that something can be done to tackle it. It should incorporate the concept of a capacity to benefit which requires an assessment of the effectiveness of health interventions and attempts to make explicit what benefits are being pursued, at the level of individuals and the population.

Health needs assessment should include two other objectives. Firstly to improve the spatial allocation of resources so that broadly equal populations receive broadly equal resources. Secondly the accurate targeting of resources so that those who get a service need it, and those who need a service get it.

As the capacity to benefit is always going to be greater than available resources, health needs assessment should also incorporate questions of priority setting (Donaldson and Mooney 1991). Some commentators have argued that rationing should not be necessary if either sufficient funding was made available, typically by redirecting it from other areas of public expenditure or raising taxes, or by ensuring that available resources are used more efficiently.

In reality, some form of rationing has always taken place in all healthcare systems although, in most cases, this was implicit, inextricably linked to clinical judgement. Priority setting or rationing in healthcare continues to be a politically charged topic, but recently its necessity has gained wider recognition as it is impossible to provide everyone with every effective intervention they might need or want (Sabik and Lie 2008). Explicitly addressing priority setting is necessary to develop fairer methods to allocate scarce healthcare resources (Fleck 1994) through a transparent process that balances clinical, ethical, and economic considerations (Black 1994).

Priority-setting approaches can be broadly grouped into two categories: outlining principles and defining practices. Countries such as Norway, the Netherlands, Sweden, and Denmark decided to develop principles that would guide prioritization efforts. In the Netherlands, the Dunning Committee (Committee on Choices in Health Care 1992) proposed four criteria that any intervention to be funded from social insurance should meet: necessity, effectiveness, efficiency, and individual responsibility. They described these principles as forming a sieve for sifting out services that should not be publicly funded ('Dunning's funnel'). The idea was that one should apply these successively beginning with the principle of necessity, and then limiting the number of services provided. The Committee excluded services that could easily be paid for by the individuals themselves. One example the committee gave was routine adult dental care. Although such dental care is necessary, effective, and efficient, adults can easily pay for such services out of pocket, and it is therefore best left to an individual's responsibility. The drawback of this approach is that because of their abstractness, government commissions that outlined principles have had little direct impact on their countries' policies.

Other countries, such as the United Kingdom, Israel, New Zealand, and the state of Oregon in the United States established bodies that would actually recommend what services should be provided within the system. Decisions may lead to blanket exclusions of interventions or of condition–intervention combinations, as in the approach taken in Oregon, or production of guidelines, as has been done in New Zealand (The National Advisory Committee on Health and Disability) and by the National Institute of Health and Care Excellence in the United Kingdom. The experience of Oregon has been especially interesting because of the technical and ethical issues it has raised. It was designed to create a list of condition–intervention pairs, ranked on the basis of cost–benefit, with a cut-off point based on available resources below which combinations would not be funded. This initial method was, however, abandoned because of a public outcry over the resulting ranking of services, for example: appendectomy was rated lower than cosmetic dentistry. In response to this public reaction as well as criticism of the methodology, the Commission set out to rank healthcare services based on more broadly defined criteria, where expert knowledge and intuitive judgements by the Commissioners about appropriateness played a much larger role. The process also raised important ethical questions as the exercise was confined to poor women and children in the Medicaid programme and services denied to them would remain available to others (Rosenbaum 1992).

In the United Kingdom, the National Institute for Clinical Excellence (now the National Institute for Health and Care Excellence (NICE)) was established in 1999 to: appraise new health technologies, develop clinical guidelines, and assess interventional procedures (Rawlins 1999). In conducting these activities, NICE addresses questions including what constitutes necessary and appropriate care, how to incorporate cost-effectiveness considerations, and what interventions should be publicly funded.

The challenge of healthcare prioritization is to identify an appropriate balance between an expert-led process and a process that emphasizes public involvement in decision-making to ensure that decisions reached are legitimate. Ultimately, while public health professionals have an important role in providing the evidence on which any debate on priority setting must be based, priority setting in a publicly funded system is the responsibility of politicians. Decision-making inevitably involves trade-offs between objectives as a balance is sought among universal coverage, comprehensiveness of services, equity, efficiency, cost containment, and broader social values (Sabik and Lie 2008).

Design and organization of health services to ensure efficient service delivery

Conventional service delivery is often based on institutional hospital care and a supply of trained health professionals—all relatively expensive with inpatient care typically consuming 45–75 per cent of resources dedicated to healthcare (Saltman and Figueras 1997). Moreover, different professionals often work in organizational silos, and fail to integrate services to achieve best value and best care. New technologies in fields such as genetics, imaging, miniaturization, pharmaceuticals, and information are changing the mix of preventive, diagnostic, and treatment practices, enabling services to be delivered less expensively to wider populations in their own homes or communities instead of hospitals.

Health systems have adopted several strategies to meet these challenges. They include organizing the network of hospital services to achieve a more efficient and effective configuration through decentralization and centralization initiatives (see 'Reorganizing the system: decentralization, recentralization, and privatization'). Three other strategies are described in the following subsections: improved targeting of interventions, substitution, and integration of services in the hospital and community.

Improved targeting of interventions

Bohmer (2011) identified specification and planning as a common habit of high-value healthcare organization. These organizations specify decisions and activities in advance. Whenever possible, both operational decisions, such as those related to patient flow (admission, discharge, and transfer criteria), and core clinical decisions, such as diagnosis, tests, or treatment selection, are based on explicit criteria. Criteria-based decision-making is manifested in the use of clinical decision support systems and treatment algorithms, severity and risk scores, criteria for initiating a call to a rapid-response team, or triggering the commitment of a future resource (e.g. a discharge planner, pre-procedure checklists, and standardized patient assessments). Specification also applies to separating heterogeneous patient populations into clinically meaningful subgroups—by disease subtype, severity, or risk of complications—each with its own distinct pathway. For example, genomic testing has allowed oncology units to divide patients into separate groups according to their probable response to specific therapies (for instance, Kirsten RNA-associated rat sarcoma 2 virus (*KRAS*) gene testing for cetuximab therapy). And at Intermountain Healthcare in Utah and Idaho, the needs of psychiatric patients are divided into mild (routine care by a primary care physician), moderate (team care), and severe (specialist referral), using a scoring system based on published guidelines (Rathod et al. 2010).

To promote such standardization, we need to accelerate the healthcare evidence base and support the rapid sharing of clinical protocols, best practices, and outcomes data. There is concurrently a need to make effective use of information technologies to automate clinical information and make it readily accessible to patients and all members of the care team (IOM 2001). Excellent information infrastructure and well-thought out and implemented modes of ongoing communication can reduce the need to craft laborious, case-by-case strategies for coordinating patient care.

A second common characteristic of high value organizations is infrastructure design. They deliberately design microsystems (Nelson et al. 2011)—including staff, information and clinical technology, physical space, business processes, and policies and procedures that support patient care—to match their defined subpopulations and pathways. Thus, different conditions or patient groups have different microsystem designs. The various tasks of care are allocated to different members of a clinical team (including the patient), with the skills and training of each staff member matched to the work.

Substitution

Substitution refers to the process of regrouping resources (staff, equipment, information, facilities, etc.) across and within care settings to exploit the best and least costly solutions to achieve better clinical, financial, and patient-related outcomes. A useful typology differentiates substitution into three categories: moving the location at which care is delivered, introducing new technologies, and changing the mix of staff and skills. There may be other substitution types according to different combinations of these three (Warner 1996). For example, moving care from the hospital to community based care may involve:

- Location only such as for physiotherapy.

- Location and technology such as for point-of-care laboratory testing and telemedicine that allows remote consultations.

- Location and staff and/or skills such as nurse-led home care.

- All substitution types such as home dialysis services.

In addition to substitution, the weightage of services across the spectrum of care is also changing with greater emphasis being placed on prevention and self-management to reduce the demand for care. Prevention programmes have historically focused on younger or working-age adults, but there is increasing recognition of the value of prevention programmes aimed at older people with services focused on increasing functionality. These health promotion and primary prevention strategies should ultimately reduce the total demand for healthcare services and healthcare costs. However, the difficulties in measuring health promotion in terms of cost-effectiveness so that it can be compared with other health services interventions, has meant that health promotion's role has tended to be undervalued. Public health professionals have to develop more and better ways to evaluate health promotion that satisfy the needs of policymakers, managers, and clinicians so the full potential of health promotion can be realized (McKee and Bojan 1998).

Health services should be reoriented from a hospital-centric model to a model with primary healthcare at the core of the healthcare system, and secondary and tertiary care serving as supporting, referral levels. Healthcare systems configured around primary care produce healthier populations at lower cost. In the United States, for example, overall health is better in regions with more primary care physicians and where primary care functions well. By contrast, overall health is worse where specialists predominate (Starfield et al. 2005). An effective primary care system has the following virtues (Oldham 2012):

◆ It can coordinate the care of the many people with multiple, complex health needs, in a way that individual specialists cannot.

◆ It can deliver care closer to people, increasing convenience, especially in areas remote from hospitals.

◆ As a first point of contact for patients it facilitates the early detection of illness, and thereby improves outcomes.

In addition to substitution within healthcare, substitution should also occur between healthcare and other sectors, recognizing the importance of lifestyle and social determinants in improving health outcomes. For example, the 'actual' causes of mortality in the United States and other developed countries include behaviour such as smoking, violence, physical inactivity, poor nutrition, and unsafe choices (McGinnis and Foege 1993). The health and social sectors in some countries are thus pooling resources particularly in the provision of services to the elderly to tackle social isolation, engage communities more widely, adapt or develop homes, and make cities more age-friendly places.

Integration of care

The involvement of increasingly more parties in the delivery of healthcare accentuates the need to adopt a systems perspective to foster evolution of care delivery as a whole rather than focusing on single elements. Care processes need to be redesigned to enable coordinated, seamless care across patient conditions, disciplines/specialties, settings and clinicians, and over time. The key challenge is to match evidence-based, appropriate, and responsive care to patients according to their needs (such as various chronic diseases) across the various stages of their life. Capital investments and operating expenses should encourage thinking across boundaries. As an illustration, questions to be asked might include, 'Might two additional home outreach nurses be better for heart failure patients than another cardiologist?' (Berwick 2008).

One way of achieving this is by designing distinct integrated care platforms (Leape 2009) for conditions that share common work and support requirements, such as chronic disease care, complex acute care, palliative, and end of-life care. Every care platform must have the following characteristics:

◆ Patient centredness: personnel, facilities, and services are organized to meet all patients' needs efficiently and responsively; to be available when and where needed, and to include the patient and family as partners in care.

◆ Work assignment: work is assigned to the individuals who are responsible for its completion. Assignments strive to maximize the performance capability of each individual while ensuring that work is done by the least expensive qualified caregiver or multidisciplinary team at the location most accessible to the patient. The physician participates when his/her special expertise is required and when patient expectations permit no alternative.

◆ Support: the support framework—people, systems, and tools (e.g. technologies, IT, telecommunications)—is defined by the work and patient participation.

◆ Community linkage: linkages to community advocacy, support, and education groups (especially health literacy) are incorporated into the design as appropriate (e.g. for patients with chronic conditions).

◆ Variation management: ensuring quality and efficiency requires determining whether variations in process are appropriate. Process and outcome measures should thus be incorporated into daily work. Use of such measures makes it possible to understand the degree to which performance is consistent with best practices, and the extent to which patients are being helped. Exception analysis assesses whether variations result from: (1) adaptations to a specific patient requirement, (2) evolution of new evidence (good), (3) lack of training in appropriate care, or (4) poorly defined care pathways (bad).

◆ Transparency: the results of the delivery process and outcomes of care should be shared with all concerned, including patients. This would enable patients, caregivers, organizations, and managers to know the 'state of the system' with respect to its reliability, adherence to evidence, cost, and progress in improvement.

For the integrated platform to work we need an 'integrator' which accepts responsibility for the Triple Aim of improving the patient experience of care, improving the health of populations, and reducing the per capita cost of healthcare for a specified population. The simplest such form, such as Kaiser Permanente, has fully integrated financing and either full ownership of or exclusive relationships with delivery structures which enables it to use those structures to good advantage. A unified financing or a single delivery system is not, however, necessarily a prerequisite for an integrator. That role might be within the reach of a powerful, visionary insurer; a large primary care group in partnership with payers; or a regional health system that will link healthcare organizations (as well as public health and social service organizations) whose missions overlap across the spectrum of delivery (Berwick 2008). At the patient level, the integrator ensures that members of the population, especially those with chronic illnesses, have someone who can work with them to establish a plan for their ongoing care, guide them through the jungle of health services, and be their advocate.

The integrator has to segment the population according to need such as health status, level of support from family or others, and socioeconomic status, to facilitate efficient and equitable resource allocation (Lynn et al. 2007). In most cases, the integrator would not be a direct provider of all necessary services. Instead, it would need to commission some services from suppliers through business relationships consciously designed to facilitate pursuit of the desired outcomes.

Enablers

Three key enablers are needed to translate strategies into reality: intelligent purchasing, a workforce with the appropriate capacity and capability, and a robust information and knowledge management system.

Intelligent purchasing

All health systems exercise some form of purchasing but the prevailing approach to paying for healthcare, based predominantly on individual services and products, encourages wasteful and ineffective care (IOM 2012). Payment systems that are based on workload tend to disincentivize providers from coordinating care for patients across settings and over time as the benefits of investments (and cost) made by one group of providers are realized by a different group of providers. For example, investments in primary care preventative efforts tend to reduce demand for hospital services rather than primary care services. Hospitals may not be keen on these systems-level savings since their own reimbursement may decline with the decreased workload.

Health systems need to move from passive forms of purchasing—the mere reimbursement of providers—to more proactive and strategic forms of purchasing that consider which interventions should be purchased, how they should be purchased and from whom (Figueras 2005). In an increasing number of countries intelligent purchasing is seen as an alternative to a traditional command-and-control approach to implement health policy objectives, including as a means of reorienting the focus of health services, to ensure that they reflect health needs and provide cost-effective care. Its essential characteristic is that it separates purchasers from providers but binds each party by means of contracts to explicit commitments, with creation of the economic motivation to fulfil these commitments (McKee and Figueras 2009).

Payers/purchasers should adopt outcome- and value-oriented payment models where payment systems align financial incentives with the implementation of care processes based on best practices and the achievement of better patient outcomes. Payment systems should also reduce fragmentation of care by supporting high-quality, team-based care focused on patients' needs. Contracts can be used to develop intersectoral responses to health problems and to reorient healthcare providers so that they integrate prevention with curative care.

Contracts should also provide an opportunity for providers to share in the benefits of quality improvement. Substantial improvements in quality are most likely to be obtained when providers are highly motivated and rewarded for carefully designing and fine-tuning care processes to achieve increasingly higher levels of quality and safety. Rewards should thus be located close to the level at which the reengineering and process redesign needed to improve quality are likely to take place (IOM 2001).

Purchasers represent the interests of their populations, in particular the vulnerable and disadvantaged groups as well as underserved communities, by allocating resources and purchasing services in accordance with their needs. There is, however, a need to guard against the risk of providers underemphasizing or phasing out services that are less profitable. Contracts should thus provide fair payment for good clinical management of the types of patients seen. Clinicians should be adequately compensated for taking good care of all types of patients, neither gaining nor losing financially for caring for sicker patients or those with more complicated conditions. The risk of random incidence of disease in the population should reside with a larger risk pool, whether that is large groups of providers, health plans, or insurance companies (IOM 2001).

Purchasing also offers a means for enhancing participation by the population in the organization of healthcare by providing the opportunity for consumers and purchasers to recognize quality differences in healthcare and direct their decisions accordingly. To do this, consumers need to have good information on quality and the ability to use that information as they see fit to meet their needs.

Implementation of an intelligent purchasing system is a complex process requiring a high level of skills and well-developed information systems. At a minimum, information is required on patient flow, cost, and utilization across specialties or diagnostic groups and demographic and risk groups. Purchasing decisions also need to take into account the reality that medical care is extremely complex. Diagnostic labels are often imprecise and clouded by a degree of legitimate uncertainty. Decisions on clinical management also incorporate values and beliefs relating to factors such as attitude to risk and the utility placed on different health states. It is thus important that expectations of what can be achieved are realistic (McKee and Clarke 1995). Contracts must incorporate sufficient flexibility and reflect the views of all those concerned if they are to retain any credibility. It should also be recognized that purchasing may not be the best option for some services especially where clear specifications in terms of the desired product/service cannot be defined clearly.

While the focus of purchasing should ideally be on outcomes, outcomes are typically more difficult to measure and may only become apparent long after the intervention took place. Some outcomes may also be rare and the sample size required to detect a deviation from what is expected may be very large. For example, Mant and Hicks (1995) have shown, on the basis of knowledge of effective treatment for myocardial infarction, that, in a comparison of two typical hospitals, it would take 73 years of data to detect a significant 3 per cent reduction in mortality whereas the corresponding difference in process measures, relating to uptake of treatments, would emerge after only 4 months. Where process or structure measures are used there should be evidence that they correlate with a good outcome. Measures based on structure can be of some value, based on the assumption that high-quality care cannot be provided in the absence of basic prerequisites, such as adequately trained staff, but this is a necessary rather than a sufficient measure and should normally be supplemented by measures of either process or outcome.

All these activities (e.g. needs assessment, performance analysis, negotiating, and monitoring) incur transaction costs. A substantial increase in quality and efficiency is required to justify these additional costs. Increasingly, purchasers and providers are entering into long-term contractual relationships that reduce transaction costs (Rosen and McKee 1995). If transaction costs can be minimized without compromising the pursuit of the objectives of equity and health gain, intelligent purchasing can provide a formidable instrument to promote population health.

Workforce

A major challenge in transitioning to the desired models of care described previously is preparing the workforce to acquire new skills and adopt new ways of relating to patients and each other. At least three approaches can be taken to support the workforce in this transition:

• *Redesign the way health professionals are trained.* Healthcare professionals should be taught evidence-based practice and equipped with the skills and tools to access and apply the expanding knowledge base. They should also have sufficient communication and behavioural skills to work effectively with patients, not least in helping to promote treatment adherence and health-enhancing lifestyle changes. In addition they need to acquire the skills to improve the processes and systems of care through proven methods and actions. Furthermore as effective health services will increasingly be delivered by collaborative teams of clinicians, with each member playing a vital role, the training should adopt a multidisciplinary approach and continually advance the effectiveness of teams instead of training health professionals purely by discipline. As almost every country wants more patients to be treated in the community rather than in hospitals, we need to ensure that healthcare professionals spend considerable time during training in the community, not just in hospitals. We also need to review the necessity for the expensive additional years of education for an increasing number of doctors and nurses to be trained in very narrow subspecialties (Emanuel and Fuchs 2012) and its alignment with the wider interests and needs of the population.

• *Modify the ways in which health professionals are regulated.* Regulation of healthcare professionals is designed to protect the public and ensure that patients are kept safe, but providing such protection needs to be balanced against the regulatory burden and the need to retain sufficient freedom for innovators to succeed. Regulation should be focused on the patient and should be independent of professional interests. Scope-of-practice laws and other workforce regulations need to allow for innovation in the use of all types of clinicians to meet patient needs in the most effective and efficient way possible. Statutory regulation should be used to protect the public in areas of high risk, but other processes should be used when the risk is low. Ongoing licensure and certification requirements should also reflect the need for lifelong learning and evaluation of competencies to ensure that healthcare professionals have the specific skills for the time and contexts in which they work (Dzau et al. 2012).

• Examine how the *liability system* can constructively support changes in care delivery while remaining part of an overall approach to accountability for healthcare professionals and organizations.

In addition to the professional workforce, it is also important to work on securing the supply of informal care. Care provided by families is the backbone of long-term care. But it is difficult to maintain or increase it in the face of falling support ratios, urbanization and migration, and changing work patterns. One option is to direct cash and services to support carers. Another is to use technological innovations to provide information and support. Governments can also innovatively incentivize or reinforce traditional family caring responsibilities through the tax system and other regulatory measures (Hope et al. 2012).

Information and knowledge management

The knowledge of how to configure structures and processes to attain the best possible clinical outcomes will become one of the health service's most important assets. Healthcare organizations must thus create, maintain, and disseminate the institutional knowledge required to realize good outcomes.

As healthcare is complex and constantly changing, we need to build healthcare systems that continually learn, in real time and with new tools, how to better manage problems. Data generated in healthcare delivery—whether clinical, delivery process, or financial—should be collected in digital formats, compiled, and protected as resources for managing care, capturing results, improving processes, strengthening public health, and generating new insights. Decision support tools and knowledge management systems can be included routinely in healthcare delivery to ensure that decisions are informed by the best evidence. The characteristics of a continuous learning healthcare system are summarized in Table 11.7.1 (IOM 2012).

Regulators have a key role in facilitating this learning process by clarifying and improving rules governing the collection and use of clinical data to safeguard patient privacy while promoting the seamless use of such data for better care coordination and management, improved care, and enhanced knowledge. Legal protections should be put in place to shield individuals from improper use of de-anonymized health data and educational campaigns

Table 11.7.1 Characteristics of a continuously learning healthcare system

Science and informatics

Real-time access to knowledge—a learning healthcare system continuously and reliably captures, curates, and delivers the best available evidence to guide, support, tailor, and improve clinical decision-making and care safety and quality.

Digital capture of the care experience—a learning healthcare system captures the care experience on digital platforms for real-time generation and application of knowledge for care improvement.

Patient–clinician partnerships

Engaged, empowered patients—a learning healthcare system is anchored on patient needs and perspectives and promotes the inclusion of patients, families, and other caregivers as vital members of the continuously learning care team.

Incentives

Incentives aligned for value—in a learning healthcare system, incentives are actively aligned to encourage continuous improvement, identify and reduce waste, and reward high-value care.

Full transparency—a learning healthcare system systematically monitors the safety, quality, processes, prices, costs, and outcomes of care, and makes information available for care improvement and informed choices and decision-making by clinicians, patients and their families.

Culture

Leadership-instilled culture of learning—a learning healthcare system is stewarded by leadership committed to a culture of teamwork, collaboration, and adaptability in support of continuous learning as a core aim.

Supportive system competencies—in a learning healthcare system, complex care operations and processes are constantly refined through ongoing team training and skill building, systems analysis and information development, and creation of the feedback loops for continuous learning and system improvement.

Reprinted with permission from National Academy of Sciences, *Best Care at Lower Cost: The Path to Continuously Learning Healthcare in America*, Copyright © 2013, courtesy of the National Academies Press, Washington, D.C., USA.

should be conducted, aimed at providers and public alike, to raise awareness of the rights, responsibilities, risks and benefits related to health data.

Conclusion

Health services have an important role to play in improving the health status of populations. This chapter has identified mechanisms through which public health can play a major role in maximizing the health gain obtained from health services, in particular in the design of systems that ensure that patients are managed at the level of the healthcare system that is most appropriate, the creation of mechanisms that identify and promote high-quality clinical care, and the reorientation of curative services towards prevention.

Public health professionals, with their emphasis on improving population health, have a key role in ensuring that the pursuit of health gain becomes a central objective of healthcare services, whatever other objectives are being pursued by others (McKee and Figueras 2009). To do so, they must promote the equitable use of interventions that are effective and appropriate for the population in question, reduce interventions that are ineffective or harmful, and maximize the health gains obtained with the available funding. Much will depend on the ability of the public health profession to adapt and bring its portfolio of tools and skills to bear on rapidly changing health services.

References

Abel-Smith, B., Figueras, J., Holland, W., McKee, M., and Mossialos, E. (1995). *Choices in Health Policy: An Agenda for the European Union*. Aldershot: Dartmouth Press/Office for Official Publications of the European Communities.

Anderson, T.F. and Mooney, G. (eds.) (1990). *The Challenges of Medical Care Variations*. Basingstoke: Macmillan.

Arah, O.A., Westert, G.P., Hurst, J., and Klazinga, N.S. (2006). A conceptual framework for the OECD Health Care Quality Indicators Project. *International Journal for Quality in Health Care*, 2006, 5–13.

Atwal, P. (2010). *How Do You Solve A Problem Like Health Reform: Has Singapore Got It Right?* [Online] Available at: http://healthaffairs.org/blog/2010/11/12/how-do-you-solve-a-problem-like-health-reform-has-singapore-got-it-right/.

Benson, J.K. (1975). The interorganisational network as a political economy. *Administrative Science Quarterly*, 20, 229–49.

Berwick, D.M., Nolan, T.W., and Whittington, J. (2008). The triple aim: care, health, and cost. *Health Affairs*, 27, 759–69.

Bisognano, M.A. and Kenney, C. (2012). *Pursuing the Triple Aim: Seven Innovators Show the Way to Better Care, Better Health, and Lower Costs*. San Francisco, CA: Jossey-Bass.

Black, D. (1994). *A Doctor Looks at Health Economics*. Office of Health Economics annual lecture. London: Office of Health Economics.

Bohmer, R.M.J. (2011). The four habits of high-value health care organizations. *The New England Journal of Medicine*, 365, 22.

Bojan, F., Hajdu, P., and Belicza, E. (1991). Avoidable mortality. Is it an indicator of quality of medical care in Eastern European countries? *Quality Assurance of Health Care*, 3, 191–203.

Borgenhammer, E. (1993). At vårda liv: orgnisation, etik, kvalitet. [Looking after life: organisation, ethics, quality.] Stockholm: SNS Förlag.

Boys, R.J., Forster, D.P., and Jozan, P. (1991). Mortality from causes amenable and non-amenable to medical care: the experience of Eastern Europe. *British Medical Journal*, 303, 879–83.

Cabinet Office (1999). *Modernising Government*. London: HMSO.

Cassel, C.K. and Reuben, D.B. (2011). Specialization, subspecialization, and subsubspecialization in internal medicine. *The New England Journal of Medicine*, 364, 1169–73.

Chalmers, I. and Altman, D.G. (1995). *Systematic Reviews*. London: BMJ Publications.

Clark, D.G. (1988). Autonomy, personal empowerment and quality of life in long-term care. *Journal of Applied Gerontology*, 7, 279–97.

Collins, C.D. and Green, A.T. (1994). Decentralisation and primary health care: some negative implications in developing countries. *International Journal of Health Services*, 24, 459–75.

Committee on Choices in Health Care (1992). *Choices in Health Care*. Rijswijk: Ministry of Welfare HCA.

Congressional Budget Office (2008). *Geographic Variation in Health Care Spending*. Washington, DC: Congressional Budget Office.

Contandriopoulos, A.P., Lauristin, M., and Leibovich, E. (1998). Values, norms, and the reform of health care systems. In R. Saltman, J. Figueras, and C. Sakallarides (eds.) *Critical Challenges for Health Care Reform in Europe*, pp. 339–62. Buckingham: Open University Press.

Creditor, M. (1993). Hazards of hospitalization in the elderly. *Annals of Internal Medicine*, 118, 219–23.

Dash, P., Llewellyn, C., and Richardson, B. (2009). Developing a regional health system strategy. *Health International*, 8, 26–35.

Donaldson, C. and Mooney, G. (1991). Needs assessment, priority setting, and contracts for health care: an economic view. *British Medical Journal*, 303, 1529–30.

Dzau, V., Grazin, N., Bartlett, R., et al. (2012). *A Neglected Resource: Transforming Healthcare through Human Capital. Report of the Innovative Delivery Models Working Group*. London: Imperial College.

Emanuel, E. and Fuchs, V. (2012), Shortening Medical Training by 30%. *Journal of the American Medical Association*, 307(11), 1143–4.

Eysenbach, G., Diepgen, T.L., Muir Gray, J.A., et al. (1998). Towards quality management of medical information on the Internet: evaluation, labelling, and filtering of information. *British Medical Journal*, 317, 1496–502.

Feldstein, M.S. (1964). Effects of differences in hospital bed scarcity on type of use. *British Medical Journal*, ii, 562–5.

Figueras, J., Jakubowski, E., and Robinson, R. (eds.) (2005). *Purchasing to Improve Health Systems Performance*. Maidenhead: Open University Press.

Fleck, L.M. (1994). Just caring: health reform and health care rationing. *Journal of Medicine and Philosophy*, 19, 435–43.

Gaylin, D.S. and Kates, J. (1997). Refocusing the lens: epidemiologic transition theory, mortality differentials, and the AIDS pandemic. *Social Science & Medicine*, 44(5), 609–21.

Gillett, G. (1995). Virtue and truth in clinical science. *Journal of Medical Philosophy*, 20, 285–98.

Green, L., Ottoson, J., García, C., and Hiatt, R. (2009). Diffusion theory and knowledge dissemination, utilization, and integration in public health. *Annual Review of Public Health*, 30, 151–74.

Gröne, O. and Garcia-Barbero, M. (2001). Integrated care: a position paper of the WHO European Office for Integrated Health Services. *International Journal of Integrated Care*, 1, e21.

Habermas, J. (1987). *Théorie de l'agir communicationnel*. Paris: Fayard.

Hart, J.T. (1971). The inverse care law. *The Lancet*, i, 405–12.

Himmelstein, D.U., Woolhandler, S., Hellander, I., et al. (1999). Quality of care in investor-owned vs not for profit HMOs. *Journal of the American Medical Association*, 282, 159–63.

Hope, P., Bamford, S., Kneale, D., et al. (2012). *Creating Sustainable Health and Care Systems in Ageing Societies. Ageing Societies Working Group 2012*. London: Imperial College.

Illich, I. (1976). *Limits to Medicine*. London: Marion Boyars.

Institute of Medicine (1989). *To Err is Human: Building A Safer Health System*. Washington, DC: National Academy Press.

Institute of Medicine (2001). *Crossing the Quality Chasm: A New Health System for the 21st century*. Washington, DC: National Academy Press.

Institute of Medicine (2004). *The Migration of Health Care Workers: Creative Solutions to Manage Health Workforce Migration*. Washington, DC: National Academy Press.

Institute of Medicine (2012). *Best Care at Lower Cost The Path to Continuously Learning Health Care in America*. Washington, DC: National Academy Press.

International Diabetes Federation (2012). *IDF Diabetes Atlas* (5th ed.). Brussels: International Diabetes Federation.

Kettl, D.F. (1993). *Sharing Power: Public Governance and Private Markets*. Washington, DC: Brookings Institution.

Lalonde, M. (1974). *A New Perspective on Health of Canadians: A Working Document*. Ottawa: Information Canada.

Landrigan, C.P., Parry, G.J., Bones, C.B., Hackbarth, A.D., Goldmann, D.A., and Sharek, P.J. (2010). Temporal trends in rates of patient harm resulting from medical care. *The New England Journal of Medicine*, 363(22), 2124–34.

Leape, L., Berwick, D., Clancy, C., et al. (2009). Transforming healthcare: a safety imperative. *Quality and Safety in Health Care*, 18, 424–8.

Lim, M.K. (2004). Shifting the burden of health care finance: a case study of public–private partnership in Singapore. *Health Policy*, 69, 83–92.

Lubitz, J., Beebe, J., and Baker, C. (1995). Longevity and medical care expenditures. *The New England Journal of Medicine*, 332, 999–1003.

Lynn, J., Straube, B.M., Bell, K.M., Jencks, S.F., and Kambic, R.T. (2007). Using population segmentation to provide better health care for all: the 'bridges to health' model. *Milbank Quarterly*, 85, 185–208.

Mant, J. and Hicks, N. (1995). Detecting differences in quality of care: the sensitivity of measures of process and outcome in treating acute myocardial infarction. *British Medical Journal*, 311, 793–6.

Maxwell, R.J. (1981). *Health and Wealth: An International Study of Health Spending*. Cambridge, MA: Lexington Books.

McGinnis, J.M. and Foege, W.H. (1993). Actual causes of death in the United States. *Journal of the American Medical Association*, 270, 2207–12.

McKee, M. and Bojan, F. (1998). Reforming public health services. In J. Figueras, R. Saltman, and C. Sakallarides (eds.) *Critical Challenges for Health Care Reform*, pp. 135–54. Buckingham: Open University Press.

McKee, M. and Clarke, A. (1995). Guidelines, enthusiasms, uncertainty and the limits to purchasing. *British Medical Journal*, 310, 101–4.

McKee, M. and Figueras, J. (2009). Strategies for health services. In R. Detels, R. Beaglehole, M.A. Lansang, and M. Gulliford (eds.) *Oxford Textbook of Public Health* (5th ed.), pp. 1668–81. Oxford: Oxford University Press.

McKeown, T. (1979). *The Role of Medicine: Dream, Mirage or Nemesis?* Oxford: Blackwell Scientific.

Menon, R. (2010). *Markets and Government: Striking a Balance in Singapore*. Singapore: Economic Policy Forum.

Ministry of Health (1993). *Affordable Healthcare: A White Paper*. Singapore: Ministry of Health.

Mossialos, E. and Le Grand, J. (1999). Cost containment in the EU: an overview. In E. Mossialos and J. Le Grand (eds.) *Health Care and Cost Containment in the European Union*, pp. 1–154. Ashgate: Aldershot.

Murray, C.J.L. and Lopez, A. (1996). *The Global Burden of Disease*. Cambridge, MA: Harvard University Press.

National Health Service (2007). *Healthcare for London: A Framework for Action*. [Online] Available at: http://www.londonprogrammes.nhs.uk/publications/a-framework-for-action/.

Nelson, E.C., Batalden, P.B., Godfrey, M.M., and Lazar, J.S. (2011). *Value by Design: Developing Clinical Microsystems to Achieve Organizational Excellence*. San Francisco, CA: Jossey-Bass.

NHS Confederation (2008). *Priority Setting—Strategic Planning*. [Online] Available at: http://www.nhsconfed.org/Publications/Pages/Prioritysettingstrategicplanning.aspx.

Nolte, E. and McKee, M. (2004). *Does Health Care Save Lives? Avoidable Mortality Revisited*. London: The Nuffield Trust.

Oldham, J., Richardson, B., Dorling, G., and Howitt, P. (2012). *Primary Care—The Central Function and Main Focus Report Of The Primary Care Working Group 2012*. London: Imperial College.

Olshansky, S.J. and Ault, A.B. (1986). The fourth stage of the epidemiologic transition: the age of delayed degenerative diseases. *The Milbank Quarterly*, 64, 355–91.

Omran, A.R. (1971). The epidemiologic transition: a theory of the epidemiology of population change. *The Milbank Memorial Fund Quarterly*, 49, 509–38.

Osborne, D. and Gaebler, T. (1993). *Reinventing Government*. Reading, MA: Addison-Wesley.

Porter, M. and Teisberg, E.O. (2006). *Redefining Healthcare: Creating Value-Based Competition on Results*. Boston, MA: Harvard Business School Press.

Rathod, R.H., Farias, M., Friedman, K.G., et al. (2010). A novel approach to gathering and acting on relevant clinical information: SCAMPs. *Congenital Heart Disease*, 5, 343–53.

Rawlins, M. (1999). In pursuit of quality: the National Institute for Clinical Excellence. *The Lancet*, 353, 1079–83.

Rondinelli, D. (1981). Government decentralisation in comparative theory and practice in developing countries. *International Review of Administrative Sciences*, 47, 133–45.

Rosen, R. and McKee, M. (1995). Short termism in the NHS. *British Medical Journal*, 311, 703–4.

Rosenbaum, S. (1992). Poor women, poor children, poor policy: the Oregon Medicaid experiment. In M. Strosberg, J. Wiener, R. Baker, and I.A. Fein (eds.) *Rationing America's Medical Care: The Oregon Plan and Beyond*, pp. 103–4. Washington, DC: Brookings Institution.

Sabik, L.M. and Lie, R.K. (2008). Priority setting in health care: lessons from the experiences of eight countries. *International Journal for Equity in Health*, 7, 4.

Sager, M.A., Francke, T., Inouye, S.K., et al. (1996). Functional outcomes of acute medical illness and hospitalization in older persons. *Archives of Internal Medicine*, 156, 645–52.

Saltman, R.B. and Figueras, J. (1997). *European Health Care Reform: Analysis of Current Strategies*. Copenhagen: World Health Organization.

Saltman, R.B. and von Otter, C. (eds.) (1995). *Implementing Planned Markets in Health Care*. Buckingham: Open University Press.

Sandvik, H. (1999). Health information and interaction on the Internet: a survey of female urinary incontinence. *British Medical Journal*, 319, 29–32.

Schoen, C., Osborn, R., Squires, D., et al. (2011). New 2011 survey of patients with complex care needs in eleven countries finds that care is often poorly coordinated. *Health Affairs*, 30, 2437–48.

Schwartz, F.W., Glennerster, H., and Saltman, R.B. (eds.). (1996). *Fixing Health Budgets—Experience from Europe and North America*. Chichester: Wiley.

Scitovsky, A.A. (1988). Medical care in the last twelve months of life: the relation between age, functional status, and medical care expenditures. *The Milbank Memorial Fund Quarterly: Health and Society*, 66, 640–60.

Smith, S.D., Heffler, S.K., and Freeland, M.S. (2000). *The Impact of Technological Change on Healthcare Cost Spending: An Evaluation of the Literature*. Health Care Financing Administration Working Paper. Available at: http://www.cms.gov/Research-Statistics-Data-and-Systems/Statistics-Trends-and-Reports/NationalHealthExpendData/downloads/tech_2000_0810.pdf.

Starfield, B., Shi, L., Grover, A., et al. (2005). The effects of specialist supply on populations' health: assessing the evidence. *Health Affairs*, Suppl. Web Exclusives: W5-97–W5-107.

Starfield, B., Shi, L., and Macinko, J. (2005). Contribution of primary care to health systems and health. *The Milbank Quarterly*, 83, 457–502.

Stevens, A. and Gabbay, J. (1991). Needs assessment needs assessment. *Health Trends*, 23, 20–2.

The Economist (2012). Rethinking the welfare state: Asia's next revolution. *The Economist*, 8 September.

Velkova, A., Wolleswinkel-van den Bosch, J.H., and Mackenbach, J.P. (1997). The east–west life expectancy gap: differences in mortality from conditions amenable to medical intervention. *International Journal of Epidemiology*, 26, 75–84.

Warner, M. (1996). *Implementing Healthcare Reforms Through Substitution*. Cardiff: Welsh Institute for Health and Social Care.

Wennberg, J.E. (1984). Dealing with medical practice variations: a proposal for action. *Health Affairs*, 3(2), 6–31.

Wilkin, D. (1992). Patterns of referral: explaining variation. In M. Roland and A. Coulter (eds.) *Hospital Referrals*, pp. 76–91. Oxford: Oxford University Press.

World Health Organization (1986). *Ottawa Charter for Health Promotion: First International Conference on Health Promotion*. Geneva: World Health Organization.

Wright, J., Williams, R., and Wilkinson, J.R. (1998). Development and importance of health needs assessment. *British Medical Journal*, 316, 1310–13.

Young, D.W. and Saltman, R.B. (1985). *The Hospital Power Equilibrium—Physician Behaviour and Cost Control*. Baltimore, MD: Johns Hopkins University Press.

11.8

Training of public health professionals in developing countries

Vonthanak Saphonn, San Hone, and Roger Detels

Introduction to training of public health professionals in developing countries

Public health and medical structures, systems, and training are essential for the health of a country (Heller et al. 2007; Bangdiwala et al. 2010). This is particularly true for developing countries, which have great disparities in wealth and limited funds to invest in the health of their citizens. In developing countries, as well as in developed countries, public health services and medical resources must be made available at the national, provincial, sub-provincial, and local district levels. The skills and requirements of public health and medical professionals at each of these levels differ and are unique within each level. The mandate of public health is broad, and therefore requires some level of specialization within the profession. Thus, various public health professionals are responsible for assuring access to healthcare, maternal/child health services, protection of the environment, including provision of adequate and safe levels of water and safe disposal of human and other waste, implementation of community health programmes such as immunization coverage, prevention and control of endemic and epidemic health threats from microbial agencies, addressing the current chronic disease epidemic, and administration/management of the broad and diverse public health workforce at each level. Thus, public health training requires providing training not only in medical sciences, but also in technical fields such as microbiology, chemistry and the physical sciences, management sciences and behavioural, social, and political sciences, statistics, epidemiology, and research methodologies.

The public health workforce draws individuals from a variety of backgrounds relevant to their intended public health role, including medicine, nursing, and the behavioural, management, and biological/physical sciences (Beaglehole and Dal Poz 2003). Generally, health training programmes provide training at the certificate level primarily for health professionals and others serving at the local level, which may include health volunteers (who are the core of many health systems and provide service at the village level), specialized training (e.g. nurse midwife), as well as training at the master's level (usually requiring 1–3 years of graduate study) and the doctoral level (requiring 4–6 years of graduate study) for those who become leaders of public programmes and researchers. Training at the graduate level also includes specialized training in specific fields for those who focus on environmental, social, and healthcare aspects of public health, as well as in the broad mandate of public health. Although most public health training programmes provide basic initial training in public health, there is also an important need to provide postgraduate and refresher training to ensure that the public health workforce continues to utilize the most modern strategies and resources.

In the opinion of some public health professionals, including the authors, there is too often a mismatch between the role and responsibilities of public health professionals at each level and the training that they receive. Too often, public health curricula in developing countries were developed by the European colonialists based on the European system, and do not adequately address current health problems of the country. This mismatch reflects both the content of the training programmes and the strategies/content of the country's public health system itself. Public health planners, managers, and administrators are confronted by a range of barriers to achieving optimal public health, including funding constraints, politics, and the scarcity of qualified personnel and public health leaders. It is the responsibility of public health trainers to develop strategies and curricula to overcome these barriers and to ensure that the training of public health professionals is appropriate and has the flexibility to provide trainees with the ability to devise new strategies to address constantly changing public health issues and problems. In some instances, this requires reconsideration of the current public health structure to ensure maximum effectiveness. Public health programmes need to ensure that health professionals in training see a clear career path for themselves, that there is an optimal distribution of health professionals, particularly to rural and remote areas, and that the system provides both monetary and non-monetary incentives to motivate them. In this chapter, we address each of these issues in greater depth and make suggestions for improvement and enhancement of health training in developing countries.

Typical public health structures in developing countries—health system structure in developing countries

Typically, government health systems in developing countries have a tiered system for providing health, comprising the national, provincial, sub-provincial, and local levels. In addition, in most developing countries there is also a private healthcare system which provides services primarily to the wealthy. Further non-governmental and national and international organizations may provide clinical services. Sometimes these operate outside the purview of the government-sponsored public health system which can create problems. In this chapter we will focus on training relevant for the government-sponsored public health system.

The highest number of health personnel work at the lowest level, with decreasing numbers at the sub-provincial, provincial, and national levels. Duration and intensity of training for health workers at the local, sub-provincial, provincial, and national levels increases, with the highest levels of training and responsibility focused on the national level.

The public health systems in developing countries are usually divided into three levels: (1) the central administrative level, which develops and recommends health policies for the entire country and administers national programmes, national training institutions, and national hospitals that provide complicated tertiary care; (2) the provincial health departments, which are responsible for implementing national policies and programmes, and provincial hospitals, which often see referrals from the local healthcare facilities and for conducting regional training programmes for local health professionals and volunteer health workers; and (3) the local or district level, which implements national and provincial programmes, such as maternal/child health programmes and vaccination campaigns (Fig. 11.8.1).

The district level (health centre or health post) usually provides a minimum package of activities and healthcare to a population of approximately 5000–10,000 each, and a referral hospital for a complementary package of activities. The health force at the village or commune level includes volunteer health workers who are selected from the local population and provide minimal first aid and referral to the district health centre or hospital. They also help organize immunization sessions, give oral vaccinations (e.g. polio) and high-dose vitamin A to children, but are not allowed to give injections. In addition they promote health education activities, including promoting environmental sanitation. The position carries with it a level of prestige that is its main reward. Volunteer health workers usually receive training for several weeks. Nurses and/or nurse midwives, who also operate at the district level, receive training for 1 or more years and are responsible for childhood immunizations, family planning, maternal and child healthcare, and delivery of treatment for tuberculosis and HIV which require daily observed treatment.

Responsibilities/roles of public health professionals at each level in developing countries

Levels of training and duration vary, depending on the role that the graduate is expected to play in the health system. At the highest level, usually for bachelor's or master's programmes, the trainee will receive instruction in administration of health programmes (although care is usually taught through the medical education system), content and strategies for health education, and behaviour modification to achieve a healthy lifestyle, the strategies for assuring a safe water supply, appropriate disposal of human and other waste products, oral health, systems of health financing, control strategies for the major infectious diseases affecting the country (which usually include tuberculosis, malaria, parasite infections,

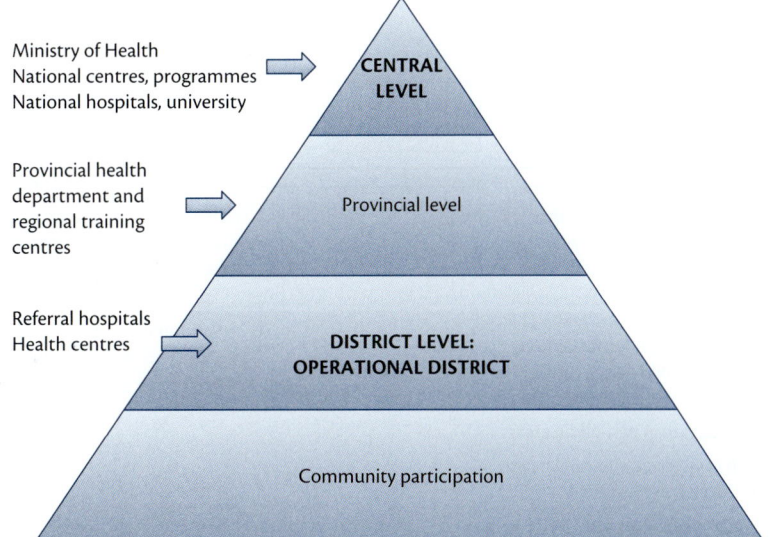

Fig. 11.8.1 The health system.
Reproduced by kind permission of Dr Lo Veasnakiry.

and HIV, plus any locally endemic diseases), and administration and strategies for immunization programmes. Some developing countries require a medical degree or other health science or a technical degree as a prerequisite for entering into a Master of Public Health (MPH) programme. Graduates of these programmes are expected to lead public health programmes. Programmes at this level usually require the trainee to complete an internship in the field at the local or rural level to ensure their understanding of the system and the culture of the populace at the point of delivery. Research methodologies, if available, are usually taught in the relatively few PhD/doctoral programmes in medical and public health institutions. However, many developing countries are only recently investing in schools of public health and in most research is not conducted. Recently there has been a movement to use the Internet to provide distance learning for public health at the MPH level and for postgraduate/refresher courses that target developing countries, which are offered through various universities and government agencies (Mokwena et al. 2007). Although these programmes are probably quite useful for teaching methodology and public health strategies, they may have difficulties in training relevant to practice at the local level in different countries, as they cannot offer hands-on field experience. One strategy to overcome this difficulty is to have discussion sessions on specific topics through the web, which include practitioners at the local level. Because most developing countries do not have the resources to invest in research programmes most public health programmes are not evidence based.

At the village level, many countries employ volunteer health workers who have had only a few weeks of training and perform very routine functions, such as tending to minor wounds, routine first aid, and encouraging villagers to take their medications as recommended by physicians and allied health workers at the district or higher levels. They usually have the best knowledge of the village and the villagers in terms of health status and needs, and assist more highly trained health professionals. They may receive some remuneration from the villages, but are not usually paid by the ministries of health.

A typical health structure at the district/township level is presented in Fig. 11.8.2.

Health professionals at the lower levels also include nurse midwives and allied health personnel who usually have 1–3 years of training. Nurse midwives are responsible for pregnant women in the district, encouraging enrolment in prenatal programmes, staffing the antenatal clinics, delivering babies, and providing postnatal guidance. They need to be able to recognize difficult pregnancies that will require more highly trained medical personnel to ensure safe delivery. These problem pregnancies are usually referred to the station or higher-level hospital. Transportation to the hospital, particularly in emergency and complicated deliveries, can be a problem. Allied health personnel in districts with nurse midwives usually perform the other medical, sanitation, and health education roles, and direct and facilitate health campaigns such as the polio immunizations days. In some countries, nurse midwives perform both roles, although they may be assisted by assistant nurse midwives who have had less but some training. Nurse midwives may be responsible for as many as 10–15 villages. The rural and urban health centres may have facilities for care of patients, including injuries requiring more than simple first aid. Patients with complicated illnesses, however, are referred to station or provincial-level hospitals, and are diagnosed and treated by physicians. The station hospitals may have a laboratory to perform routine procedures, but are usually not able to do more sophisticated biochemical and microbiological assays, which are usually done at the provincial level.

One problem with the laboratories at each of the different levels is that quality control procedures are often not implemented and standardized. Few of these laboratories participate in quality control programmes, although some wealthier developing countries (e.g. China) have implemented quality control programmes at the county and provincial levels. Thus, there is a problem with quality control and safety in many of these laboratories (Callaway 2012). A second problem is staffing these laboratories with well-trained, competent technicians who are periodically required to update their laboratory skills to ensure valid results and safe procedures.

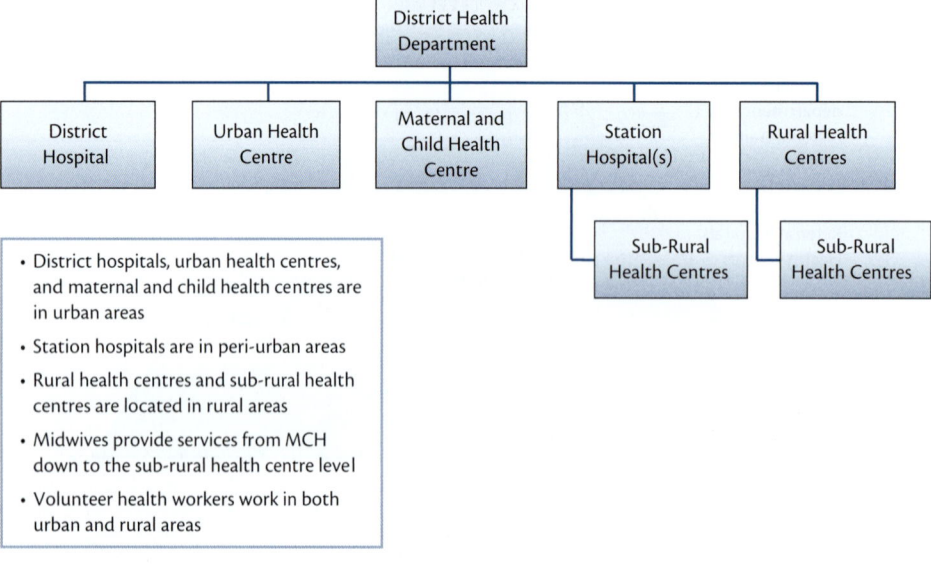

Fig. 11.8.2 Health structure/system at the district level.

Complicated surgical procedures and medical management of serious health problems are usually performed only at the provincial and national/tertiary levels. A serious problem in developing countries with limited resources and populations in remote areas is diagnosis and transport of patients to tertiary care facilities with sufficient speed to ensure successful treatment.

Training of health workers may occur at each of the levels of the public health system, although training of higher levels of health professionals is usually limited to universities, medical schools, and schools of public health, dentistry, health sciences, and nursing.

Education for health professionals in developing countries

In all developing countries, completion of medical school is required for healthcare professionals working in the various healthcare facilities at the national and provincial levels and district-level hospitals. Many developing countries require graduating physicians to work a minimum number of years at the district level as a strategy for providing healthcare at the peripheral levels of the health system. A medical degree is often also required at the national and provincial levels for staff responsible for administering national programmes. Specialized medical training is usually only required at the national-level healthcare facilities, and sometimes at provincial-level health facilities. Specialized training is usually required for health professionals conducting dental care and pharmaceutical services.

Advanced training is required for health professionals who will design and direct health information systems such as disease surveillance, and who will design and conduct health research to inform policy decisions and evaluate health programmes. These activities are usually directed at the national level, although they may involve staff at the provincial, district, and local levels.

Nurses usually require bachelor's degree-level training. However, midwives who work at the district level may receive an associate midwife degree, which may require only 1–3 years of certificate-level training, depending on the country. Some countries also have midwife assistants who receive shorter training. Staff providing lower-level nursing, medical imaging, sanitary services, low-level laboratory services, and physical therapy usually have limited training.

Problems with providing public health training in developing countries

Health professionals at the district level, who often have had only 1–3 years of training, are expected to assist in planning and management of public health programmes, recognition of the need for and initial conduct of outbreak investigations, implementation and monitoring of immunization programmes, prevention, treatment, and monitoring of tuberculosis and HIV programmes (e.g. directly observed therapy), programmes to prevent malaria (e.g. bednet distribution and mosquito control programmes), and basic health education in strategies to prevent disease and promote healthy lifestyles. Their training may not include training in the various skills and knowledge required to carry out these responsibilities, including the need for collection of accurate data that can be used to plan and support effective health systems (International Institute for Viral Registration and Statistics 1989). Thus, there is a need for congruency in the training of public health professionals and the responsibilities they will assume (Sudhinaraset et al. 2013). A major barrier to achieving proper training at all levels of public health training is the scarcity of qualified faculties in these programmes. Refresher training for health workers is important to ensure that they keep up with current and changing strategies and policies. The training of health professionals at the local level is often not integrated, so that staff members know only their own responsibilities but do not have a holistic understanding of where their efforts fit into the broad public health system.

Funding for public health programmes and training is often a low priority for political leaders and decision-makers. The majority of health programmes in developing countries are subsidized by international donors who have their own health agendas, and which may differ from those of the country.

Clear public health career tracks are often not apparent for qualified individuals who wish to choose a career in public health. Further, public health professionals at every level are usually not paid well. Often physicians who are willing to work in public health must also have private practices to generate enough income to support their families (Chomitz et al. 1998; Ferrinho et al. 2004). Thus, they are not able to dedicate their full efforts to their public health responsibilities. Physicians are often reluctant to work in remote rural areas (WHO 2010a). Public health workers at the peripheral level are usually paid low wages or are expected to volunteer their services. In these situations, other reward structures must be created to motivate volunteers and low-level workers (Henderson and Tulloch 2008; Mangham and Hanson 2008).

Strategies to overcome barriers to optimal public health training

The fundamental principles for designing public health training involve both academic and practical components. For training programmes to be responsive to needs, the needs must be clearly delineated. It is important that the tasks and responsibilities of health professionals at every level of the public health system be designed to meet the needs of the constituency and the level of responsibility expected at that level. A first step is to conduct needs assessments at each level, from the local and provincial levels to the national level, and from the village health worker to the researcher and the policymaker (Bangdiwala et al. 2010). The assessment should involve members of the community or constituency at that level. Formulation of the responsibilities and tasks at each level can then be clearly defined, and documentation of formal job descriptions provided so that an appropriate training curriculum may be developed for health workers expected to perform the required tasks at that level of the system. Training resources should then be identified and/or developed for the required training at each level of the public health system. At each level, the curriculum should be designed and evaluated for responsiveness to the job descriptions of the positions that graduates are intended to fill. The faculty of the training programmes at each level should include individuals who have had experience in delivering services at that level. The training should include providing an understanding of where the responsibilities of the health professional being trained fit into the public health system of the country.

It is important for those designing public health systems to delineate clear career paths for health professionals at each level. Defining these career paths will inform and, if done well, attract potential students to pursue those careers. An important component of defining career paths is to include incentives for individuals in these career paths (Calcutta Declaration, 1999). A problem in many developing countries is the high attrition rate of trained health volunteers, in part due to a lack of monetary incentive. In some developing countries, training, especially for nurses, may better prepare trainees for work in developed countries. Thus, migration of health professionals, particularly doctors and nurses, to better working conditions and pay in developed countries reduces the potential workforce, whose training was funded by the developing countries (Stilwell et al. 2004; Naicker et al. 2009; WHO 2010b). In these situations, developing countries may be considered to be subsidizing healthcare in developed countries!

Incentives for health workers should include monetary rewards, but it is important that they also include recognition of the importance of the health professionals at every level in the entire system in advancing the health of their constituencies. This recognition is particularly important at the lowest and least financially rewarding levels. Prestige and recognition of worth are powerful incentives!

Assuring that the public health system remains responsive to changing needs

Finally, it is important to monitor and periodically evaluate the performance of the health system at each level. Over time, specific needs change, due to a range of factors; therefore, training programmes may no longer prepare trainees for the changing needs of the constituency at that level, and must adapt their training to current needs. In addition, previously trained workers need to update their skills. Thus, it is important to also include postgraduate training at all levels for health workers that will recognize and retrain health professionals to meet the changing demands on the health system.

Summary

A well-designed, responsive public health system is essential for the well-being of citizens of developing (as well as developed) countries, and must be a government priority. The effectiveness of the health system ultimately depends on the quality, ability, and performance of the people who work in the system. Appropriate and competent training for health workers at each level is therefore essential to the effectiveness of the health system and, ultimately, the health of a country's citizens, and must include postgraduate/ refresher training to ensure the continued competency of the public health workforce.

References

Bangdiwala, S.I., Fonn, S., Okoye, O., et al. (2010). Workforce resources for health in developing countries. *Public Health Reviews*, 32, 296–318.

Beaglehole, R. and Dal Poz, M.R. (2003). Public health workforce: challenges and policy issues. *Human Resources for Health*, 1, 4.

Calcutta Declaration on Public Health (1999). Regional Conference on Public Health in South East Asia in the 21st Century, Calcutta, 22–24 November 1999. *J Epidemiol Community Health*, 54, 749.

Callaway, E. (2012). Biosafety concerns for laboratories in the developing world. *Nature*, 485, 425.

Chomitz, K., Setiadi, G., Azwar, A., et al. (1998). *What Do Doctors Want? Developing Incentives for Doctors to Serve in Indonesia's Rural and Remote Areas*. Unpublished World Bank Policy Research Working Paper 1888.

Ferrinho, P., van Lerberghe, W., Fronteira, I., et al. (2004). Dual practice in the health sector: a review of the evidence. *Human Resources for Health*, 2, 14.

Heller, R. F., Chongsuvivatwong, V., Hailegeorgios, S., et al. (2007). Capacity-building for public health. *Bulletin of the World Health Organization*, 85, 901–80.

Henderson, L.N. and Tulloch, J. (2008). Incentives for retaining and motivating health workers in Pacific and Asian countries. *Human Resources for Health*, 6, 18.

Institute for Viral Registration and Statistics (1989). *Health Data Issues for Primary Health Care Delivery Systems in Developing Countries*. Bethesda, MD: International Institute for Viral Registration and Statistics.

Mangham, I.J. and Hanson, K. (2008). Employment preferences of public sector nurses in Malawi: results from a discrete choice experiment. *Tropical Medicine & International Health*, 13, 1–9.

Mokwena, K., Mokgatle-Nthabu, M., Madiba, S., et al. (2007). Training of public health workforce at the National School of Public Health: meeting Africa's needs. *Bulletin of the World Health Organization*, 85, 949–54.

Naicker, S., Plange-Rhule, J., Tutt, R., et al. (2009). Shortage of health care workers in developing countries—Africa. *Ethnicity & Disease*, 19(Suppl. 1), S1–60–4.

Stilwell, B., Diallo, K., Zurn, P., et al. (2004). Migration of health-care workers from developing countries: strategic approaches to its management. *Bulletin of the World Health Organization*, 82, 595–600.

Sudhinaraset, M., Ingram, M., Lofthouse, H. K., et al. (2013). What is the role of informal healthcare providers in developing countries? *PLoS ONE*, 8, e54978.

World Health Organization (2010a). *Increasing Access to Health Workers in Remote and Rural Areas Through Improved Retention. Global Policy Recommendations; Executive Summary*. Geneva: WHO.

World Health Organization (2010b). *Migration of Health Workers*. Fact Sheet No. 301. Geneva: WHO.

11.9

Training of local health workers to meet public health needs

Piya Hanvoravongchai and
Suwit Wibulpolprasert

Introduction to training of local health workers to meet public health needs

People are living longer. Globally, life expectancy at birth has increased substantially over the past 40 years (Wang et al. 2012) with fewer premature deaths and a shift of disease burden from communicable, maternal, neonatal, and nutritional causes to non-communicable diseases (NCDs) (Murray et al. 2012). However, longer life does not necessarily mean better health or less healthcare needs. While world populations are ageing, there are also more people living with diseases and disabilities. Promoting health and preventing disease burden is a priority, especially in the fight against NCDs and the unfinished agenda of the Millennium Development Goals. The global commitment to reduce relative mortality from NCDs by 25 per cent by 2025 (World Health Organization (WHO) 2012a) requires additional financing, health workforce, and social and legislative measures, through various strategies, such as enforcing tobacco control, reducing population salt consumption, improving diets and increasing physical activity, reducing harmful consumption of alcohol, ensuring access to essential drugs and technologies, and providing appropriate medical care to those with high risk of cardiovascular diseases (Beaglehole et al. 2011; Bonita et al. 2013). The increasing threats of emerging diseases and re-emerging infectious diseases and the possible negative health consequences from climate changes also require health systems preparedness and active responses from the healthcare sector and its health workforce.

'Health workers', as defined in *the World Health Report 2006*, includes 'all people engaged in actions whose primary intent is to enhance health' (WHO 2006). Health workers are one of the six crucial building blocks of health systems. They are key for improving health service delivery with regards to equity, quality, efficiency, and accessibility. They also manage all other financial and non-financial resources in the health system. Moreover, investing in health workers accounts for a large share of public health spending in most countries. Nevertheless, there are a number of challenges for health workforce systems globally, including shortages and inappropriate distribution of key health professionals,

as well as poor workforce performance and weak management (Chen et al. 2004; Haines and Cassels 2004). The current weakness of health workforce systems in many countries is a major obstacle to providing necessary health services to achieve national health targets and internationally agreed-upon health-related development goals (Chen et al. 2004; Haines and Cassels; 2004, Travis et al. 2004; WHO 2006; Kanchanachitra et al. 2011).

One of the strategies being proposed to address these challenges is the 'task shifting' concept, whereby some specific tasks are assigned or delegated to health staff or workers who have less training (Hanvoravongchai 2007; McPake and Mensah 2008). Evidence, especially from low- and middle-income countries, indicates that task shifting is an important policy option and the results can be as effective as when professionals carry out those tasks (Huicho et al. 2008; Callaghan et al. 2010; De Brouwere et al. 2009; Fulton et al. 2011). Using human capital effectively through adequately trained but not over-qualified staff is considered one of the key principles driving healthcare delivery innovations for the next century, together with more active involvement of patients and communities in health service delivery (Dzau et al. 2012). Non-professional health workers, such as community and local health workers, are being recognized as valuable assets for implementing effective health system interventions (Singh and Sachs 2013; Tulenko et al. 2013).

Who are the local and community health workers?

Local and community health workers (L/CHWs) are terms that have been used interchangeably to refer to non-professional health staff who work in local communities. The WHO defined community health workers as 'people with limited education who are trained in a short time to carry out either a wide range or restricted aspects of healthcare services' (WHO 1978, 1987). They include: 'men and women chosen by the community, and trained to deal with the health problems of individuals and the community, and to work in close relationship with the health services'.

L/CHWs may vary in terms of labels in different countries and in different situations, their basic education and training periods, and their responsibilities. For example, they may be called community health workers, village health volunteers (VHVs), village health communicators (VHCs), health guides (HGs), sanitation monitors, barefoot doctors, feldschers, health guides, lady health workers, community health advisors, or health extension workers. In many countries, there are multiple categories of L/CHWs in a community.

Countries use L/CHWs to fulfil many public health-related roles, and they constitute a major workforce for public health in many developing countries. The statistics on the numbers of local and community health workers are limited. The *World Health Statistics 2012* (WHO 2012b) reported that between 2005 to 2010, for the countries where data was available, there were over 1 million L/CHWs in China, approximately 50,000 each in both Bangladesh and India, 25,000 in Ethiopia, almost 20,000 in Nigeria, 10,000 each in both Malawi and Pakistan, and smaller numbers in several other African countries. In Thailand, it is estimated that there are approximately 1 million village health volunteers serving the country's population of 65 million. Although they prominently serve in low-income developing countries, L/CHWs also serve in higher-income countries. For example, in the United States, the American Public Health Association (2009) defines community health workers as 'the frontline public health workers who are trusted members of and/or have an unusually close understanding of the community served'. They may be called Promotores de Salud, community health representatives, community health advisors, etc. The US Centers for Disease Control and Prevention maintains a database of local and community health workers that contains information on over 10,000 workers in more than 200 programmes (Rosenthal 2000).

L/CHWs are usually recruited from the community, with involvement of the local community in identifying suitable candidates (Bhutta et al. 2010). Some are tested for their literacy and numeracy, and interviewed by judges to explore their motivation and willingness. Given the necessary role as a link between the local community and local healthcare providers, both sides usually have influence in the final selection. The World Health Organization (1989) proposed that L/CHWs should be:

◆ Members of the communities in which they work.

◆ Selected by the communities.

◆ Answerable to the communities for their activities.

◆ Supported by the health system but not necessarily a part of its organization.

◆ Less trained than professional workers.

Frontline workers, such as community health workers and village health volunteers, have improved healthcare coverage and increased health equity. The linkage to both the community and local healthcare providers enables local and community health workers to serve as intermediaries who promote trust and facilitate access to healthcare services and delivery of public health interventions (Bhattacharyya et al. 2001). They play essential roles in bridging the gap between the community people and healthcare professionals. They also help with community mobilization and capacity-building processes.

After several decades of development, ample evidence has been published regarding the L/CHW role as a key agent in improving health. In Africa, the use of community health workers has been found to improve health development (World Bank 1994; Gericke et al. 2003; Lehmann et al. 2004; Perry et al. 2014). In certain communities, they can satisfy basic healthcare needs that cannot realistically be met by other means (WHO 1989). L/CHWs are generally better distributed geographically (Berman et al. 1987; Chapman et al. 2005) and there is little or no 'external brain drain' of this workforce. They are also more accessible and acceptable to communities, resulting in an increase in health service utilization, especially among poorer households (Berman 1984; Berman et al. 1987). Extending services through L/CHWs is seen as a way to reduce inequity in child healthcare (Victora et al. 2003; Masanja et al. 2005; Haines et al. 2007). A systematic review of the interventions carried out by community health workers found that health interventions such as tuberculosis treatment, immunization, promoting breastfeeding, and interventions reducing other agents of child morbidity and mortality are as effective when delivered by L/CHWs as by professionals (Lewin et al. 2010).

Roles and responsibilities of L/CHWs

To respond to public health needs, L/CHWs have many roles and responsibilities (Box 11.9.1). They are usually regarded as health leaders and health advisors in the community in which they work. They work as educators, communicators, detectors of problems, and problem-solvers. They provide information that promotes individual and family self-care and responsibility as integral components of everyday life. They sometimes play an important role in stimulating communities for action as community organizers.

Other than roles as educators and motivators, most L/CHWs, especially those in developing countries, are also engaged in delivering first-aid treatment and dispensing basic medications (WHO 1987). Some L/CHWs support delivery of general basic health services; for example, village health volunteers in Bangladesh, Bhutan, and Thailand. L/CHWs in Botswana, Sudan, and Yemen provide regular school health activities, and L/CHWs in Botswana, Jamaica, China, and Papua New Guinea assist in health centre clinic activities. More specific or sophisticated service is conducted only by L/CHWs in some countries. For example, in Columbia and Papua New Guinea, L/CHWs also give injections, particularly for immunization (WHO 1987).

In some countries, local or community health workers are assigned specifically defined tasks that require special trained skills. For example, in Pakistan, lady health workers are women recruited from the same community for which they serve, to provide reproductive health services and to promote positive health behaviours. In Bangladesh, the Shasthyo Sebika is trained to deliver directly observed treatment for tuberculosis and sell essential medications. The increasing interest in 'task shifting' to enable rapid scale-up of key health interventions and increase productivity of health professionals means more skilled tasks may be allocated to paraprofessionals and local health workers (Lehmann et al. 2009). For example, local health workers may be assigned to deliver specific health or medical interventions, such as vaccinations, malaria control, assisting pharmacists, or implementing HIV/AIDS screening, testing, and adherence monitoring (Bhutta et al. 2010; Callaghan et al. 2010).

Box 11.9.1 Various roles and responsibilities of local and community health workers reported in earlier studies

- Provide first aid to accident victims and treat simple illnesses.
- Dispense basic essential drugs.
- Give pre- and post-natal advice and motivation.
- Deliver babies.
- Provide childcare advice and motivation.
- Perform school health activities.
- Stimulate nutrition motivation and give demonstrations.
- Implement nutrition actions (weigh children, maintain charts, and distribute food supplements).
- Promote immunization and give injections.
- Promote family planning and distribute supplies.
- Promote environmental sanitation, personal hygiene, and general health habit motivation.
- Implement communicable disease actions including surveillance, screening, referral, prevention, motivation, and follow-up.
- Conduct non-communicable disease screening, referral, prevention, motivation, and follow-up.
- Assist health centre's clinical activities (i.e. not in village).
- Refer difficult cases to health centre or hospital.
- Collect vital statistics, maintain records, report community health status and problems.
- Visit homes of disabled, elderly, and community members with health needs on a regular basis.
- Inform, educate, and empower community members about public health issues.
- Provide informal counselling and social support.
- Advocate individual and community needs.
- Mobilize support and partnership between the community and local health facility.
- Perform tasks outside the health sector (e.g. agriculture).
- Participate in community meetings and community campaigns.

Source: data from World Health Organization (WHO), *The Community Health Worker*, WHO, Geneva, Switzerland, Copyright © 1987; Bhutta, Z.A. et al., *Global Experience of Community Health Workers for Delivery of Health Related Millennium Development Goals: A Systematic Review, Country Case Studies, and Recommendations for Integration into National Health Systems*, Global Health Workforce Alliance, Geneva, Switzerland, Copyright © 2012; Wibulpolprasert, S., *Community Financing: Thailand's Experiences*, Health Policy Planning, Volume 4, pp. 354–360, Copyright © 1991; Lehmann, U., and Sanders, D., *Community Health Workers: What Do We Know About Them? The State of the Evidence on Programmes, Activities, Costs and Impact on Health Outcomes of Using Community Health Workers*, World Health Organization (WHO), Geneva, Switzerland, Copyright © 2007.

As a trusted member (and leader) of the community, L/CHWs can integrate health issues into other community development activities, a role that could be difficult for health professionals. In many countries, L/CHWs combine service and developmental functions that are not confined to the field of health. The relative importance of these two functions varies according to socioeconomic situations and the availability and accessibility of local health services. The service function is less important where there is ready access to healthcare facilities. The developmental function is useful in all circumstances, and is crucial in less developed communities. Walt (1990) concluded that L/CHWs not only provide basic health services, but also promote the key principles of primary healthcare; that is, equity, intersectoral collaboration, community involvement, and use of appropriate technology.

Competency-based training

Because L/CHWs are recruited from the community where they reside, there can be enormous variations in their background knowledge and skills. Training is necessary, and must be designed to be appropriate for the local community health problems, the existing capacity, and the roles and responsibilities they are expected to assume. The prerequisite of any training programme is a full understanding of the expected competency of L/CHWs.

Training programmes should be designed to address the local needs, and designs of the programmes may vary according to the health system context and the roles of L/CHWs. 'Competency-based' training or education is an approach frequently advocated to ensure that the teaching and learning processes lead to the expected outcomes.

'Competence' or 'competency' is defined by the WHO as 'the acquisition of sufficient knowledge, psychomotor, communication and decision-making skills and attitudes to enable performance of actions and specific tasks to a defined level of proficiency' (WHO 2011). Competency-based training therefore focuses on ensuring that all trainees will acquire necessary knowledge, skills, and attitudes to fulfil their roles. This differs from the previous paradigm of top-down teaching and being trainer-oriented.

In practice, the training programmes for L/CHWs vary greatly across countries and regions. Most L/CHWs are volunteers and receive short but systematic training. Some L/CHWs receive longer-term training and may have appointments as government officers, for example, auxiliary midwives in Myanmar and community health aides in Jamaica. The major determinants of the training programme tend to be the underlying characteristics of the individuals recruited for training, the roles and responsibilities they will have, and the nature of health problems they will encounter. Designing a competency-based training programme for L/CHWs therefore requires an understanding of the existing health problems in the community, the roles and responsibilities that they will take in relation to other health professionals and staff, and the tools and support that will be available to them.

Competency-based training requires the learning process to be problem and practice based so that relevant skills and attitudes can be developed and fostered. An excellent L/CHW training programme should lead to 'transformative learning', whereby trainees acquire knowledge, skills, and attitudes that change their perspectives and mindset and enable them to be active leaders or 'change agents' for better health and well-being of the populations in their communities (Frenk et al. 2010). Training assessment at the end of the training programme should also be designed to evaluate the competency sets that the trainees are expected to have. Following up their activities in the community can also yield additional input to further revise the training programme or to determine whether additional 'on the job' training is required.

Desired competency sets of L/CHWs

Competency sets that are expected to be learning outcomes of the training programme should include both *general competency* and certain *specific competency* sets. The level of competency in each set can also range from simply being aware, being knowledgeable, or being proficient. For example, L/CHWs should have good communication skills, but need only be knowledgeable about disease symptoms and complications and aware of specific treatment options for diseases prevalent in the community. Moreover, the discipline-specific competency sets can differ based on the expected functions and responsibilities of each workforce. For example, some types of local health workers may require broader knowledge of a disease that they will encounter, such as HIV/AIDS or malaria. The overall competency sets need to be designed based on the context and the roles these local health workers will have.

General or cross-cutting competencies should include general skills in communication, advocacy, and teaching. Health workers should have the attitudes of public altruistic mindset, empathy, equity, etc. They should be culturally sensitive and have good interpersonal skills. Moreover, each L/CHW should have general work skills such as literacy and numeracy, computer literacy, and presentation, writing, and basic analytical skills. Leadership, time management, and

financial management skills would also be necessary for L/CHWs who are expected to become local leaders for positive changes. Burns (2002) proposed the following seven areas of generic competency for any workers, which are also relevant for L/CHWs:

1. Knowing how to learn.

2. Reading, writing, and computation skills.

3. Communication skills: effective speaking and listening.

4. Adaptability, problem-solving skills, and creative thinking.

5. Personal management for personal and professional growth.

6. Group-related competency: interpersonal skills, teamwork, and negotiation.

7. Leadership and organizational effectiveness skills.

Specific competencies may include knowledge about health and diseases, including dental and mental health. Community health workers should have knowledge and basic skills related to common infections and health risks, as well as basic epidemiology. Non-health disciplines such as law may also be useful. In addition to discipline-specific competency, the desired competency may be subject-specific such as maternal and child health, HIV and sexually transmitted diseases, vaccine-preventable diseases, disease surveillance, NCDs, health promotion, education for behavioural change, and long-term care. For specific tasks, function-specific competency would be necessary, such as community leadership and capacity-building, population and community assessment and problem-solving, clinical care coordination, home visits and outreach strategies, and health insurance enrolment. L/CHWs who are expected to work with specific populations in their community, such as vulnerable populations or populations at risk, underserved populations, and hard-to-reach populations, may need additional skill sets and cultural sensitivity. The combination of general and specific competency areas to be included in the desired competency sets needs to be designed and agreed upon by the organizers of training programmes. Expected competencies can vary within and across countries and regions.

In South East Asia, the WHO proposed a framework for the core competencies of local health volunteers based on the community and home-based health development model to be adopted and adapted by the countries (WHO 2004). Their proposed core competencies cover three key areas: basic medical care, health promotion, and disease prevention. For basic medical care, the volunteers are required to have skills for interviewing, observing, assessing mental health, and other basic skills for laboratory test interpretation and decision-making for referrals and emergency management. For health promotion, the trainees should acquire necessary knowledge and skills for counselling and to assess growth and development of children. For successful disease prevention, certain skills are required, such as giving injections, detecting emerging diseases, and additional knowledge and skills for community health assessment and problem detection, such as family violence, drug use, and community mental health.

Designing an effective L/CHWs training programme

As mentioned earlier, an effective training programme needs to be designed carefully to address local health problems, inform about the local health system context, and train for expected competencies. Designing a good training programme therefore requires good preparation, starting with appropriate local workers or candidates being recruited, through later steps of training programme evaluation and post-training support. These can be summarized into six key steps as following:

1. Recruitment and needs assessment.

2. Curriculum preparation.

3. Selecting training period and timing.

4. Selecting learning methods.

5. Monitoring progress and evaluating training results.

6. Post-training support.

Recruitment and needs assessment

Recruitment of L/CHWs is an important step in the training programme design. Selection of the workers is generally based on their linkage to the community with community involvement in identifying potential L/CHWs. However, additional entry criteria are also required. Willingness to work for the community and to gain new knowledge and skills is a very important precondition for an effective local health workforce. This can be assessed through an interview by community leaders and representatives from local health centres. In addition, for countries with low achievement in basic education, it is important to screen for literacy and numeracy, which are necessary for the training processes. Such skills cannot be expected to be developed by the L/CHW training programme.

After recruitment, trainees should be assessed for their basic knowledge and skills. Their level of existing competencies will give an understanding of the training needs, based on current gaps. The scope and content of training programmes can then be appropriately designed.

Curriculum preparation

The training curriculum can be likened to a map to guide a traveller to the correct destination. The local health worker training curriculum should be prepared to accommodate the training needs and the practicality of its implementation. The training curriculum should include the scope and the content of the training, how it is organized, the learning activities, information on the roles of the trainers and the trainees, the training materials that will be used, and the type of evaluation that will be implemented to assess the progress and achievement of the trainees. Many training programmes develop customized curricula to match specific groups of trainees. They use common core resources and incorporate additional lessons and best practices from the community or region they are working with. An example of the key components of rural health workers' training curricula proposed by the US Rural Assistance Center is provided in Box 11.9.2 (Rural Assistance Center 2012).

The training curricula may cover broad skills and competency training for general local health workforces or specific programmes/skills training for specialized health workers. The design of the curriculum must recognize that its implementation may require flexibility especially when carried out in the field. A national curriculum should provide room for local adaptation, as it may need to be adjusted to take into account the diversity in

---

Box 11.9.2 The curriculum for a rural health workers training programme

The US Rural Assistance Center, in its community health workers toolkit, proposes that the rural health workers' training curriculum should include, but is not limited to, the following components:

♦ Training on accessing healthcare and social services systems.

♦ Translating, interpreting, and facilitating client–provider communications.

♦ Gathering information for medical providers.

♦ Delivering services as part of a medical home team.

♦ Educating social services providers on community/population needs.

♦ Teaching concepts of disease prevention and health promotion to lay populations.

♦ Managing chronic conditions.

♦ Home visiting.

♦ Understanding community prejudices.

♦ Patient privacy.

♦ Safety.

Reproduced with permission from Rural Assistance Center, *Community Health Workers Toolkit*, Copyright © 2012, available from http://www.raconline.org/communityhealth/chw/.

---

the context, the situation, and the participants. In certain situations, participatory curriculum design is needed when the course contents and methods are shaped by the interactions between the trainers and trainees.

Training period and timing

As part of the curriculum, the training period and timing should be specified. An effective L/CHWs training programme should cover both pre-service and in-service training. *Pre-service* training refers to the training that the L/CHWs receive after their recruitment to prepare them for their service. It usually includes teaching of basic theories and preparation of knowledge and skills for their practice. *In-service* training is the training provided to active L/CHWs who are already working in the community. It is as important as initial training, and can be either *refresher training* to remind the workers of the previous curriculum or training of *new knowledge or skills* to carry out additional services, or both.

The period of training may vary according to the level of training requirements, which reflects different roles and training needs across countries and programmes. Table 11.9.1 shows the training periods of various L/CHW programmes in sub-Saharan African countries (Funes et al. 2012). The formal or informal role the trainees will play in the system influences the length of the initial training. Training of volunteer or informal health workers is generally shorter than a week, while training of other community health workers with formal roles could take longer. Training of health extension workers in Ethiopia and Nigeria lasts longer than

Table 11.9.1 A summary of pre-service training programmes in some sub-Saharan African countries

Length of training	Illustrative names	Roles in health system	Minimum education	Example countries
< 1 week	Village health worker/volunteer	Informal	None	Senegal, Nigeria, Ghana, Tanzania, Mali
1–2 weeks	Village health worker	Formal	Primary school	Uganda, Rwanda
2 months–1 year	Community health workers	Formal	High school	Zambia, Ghana, Kenya, Malawi, Mozambique
> 1 year	Health extension workers	Formal	High school	Nigeria, Ethiopia

Reproduced with permission from Funes et al., *Preparing the next generation of community health workers: The power of technology for training*, Dalberg Global Development Advisors, Washington DC, USA, Copyright © 2012, available from http://www.dalberg.com/documents/Technology_and_CHWs.pdf. Source: data from Singh P and Sullivan S, *One Million Community Health Workers; Technical Task Workers Report*, The Earth Institute, Copyright © 2011; Bhutta ZA et al., *Global Experience of Community Health Workers for Delivery of Health Related Millennium Development Goals: A Systematic Review, Country Case Studies, and Recommendations for Integration into National Health Systems*, Global Health World Alliance (GHWA) and World Health Organization (WHO), Copyright © 2010; and Conway, MD et al., Addressing Africa's health workforce crisis, *McKinsey Quarterly*, November 2007, Copyright © 2007.

1 year (Funes et al. 2012). The period of refresher training and new skills training is generally short.

In Thailand, the Village Health Volunteer (VHV) Training Curriculum is compulsory for all new recruits or those serving more than 5 years. The training experience covers two courses, main and elective. At the end of the training programme, the participants are expected to have taken the following eight subjects: primary healthcare, village health volunteer, laws related to VHVs, staying healthy and having a happy life, necessary public health services, communication in primary healthcare, planning of community projects, and management. Trainees can also take additional 6-hour elective courses, such as communicable or NCDs.

Bhutta et al. (2010) compiled a review of community health worker programmes for the Global Health Workforce Alliance. They proposed a recommended framework for training that includes 6 months of pre-service or initial training, another 6 months for on-the-job training, and monthly training for new knowledge and skills. Refresher training can be taken every 6 months.

Timing of training is also a very important factor for both pre-service and in-service training plans. The design of the training programme should carefully explore the most suitable timing for training that may vary across communities. L/CHWs, especially health volunteers, usually have other daily activities that may require most of their time. They may also be involved in other community actions that make demands on their free time. In some agrarian-based societies, villagers may not be able to attend any training activities during the busy seasons of farming or harvesting crops.

It is also important to coordinate the training schedule and harmonize the training curriculum across programmes or projects to avoid duplication and improve efficiency. One study in sub-Saharan Africa found that, in addition to the ministries of health and government agencies, there were more than 20 organizations that train community health workers in the region. In many countries, there were more than ten organizations providing health worker training, and some were in the same location but without coordination, leading to duplication (Funes et al. 2012).

Selecting learning methods and learning experience

L/CHWs are adults who are recruited from the community. Their levels of knowledge, skills, and life experiences may greatly vary. Understanding adult learning theories and practices can be useful

for effective design of the training programme experience. The learning processes must be an important consideration when designing teaching for adults. According to Malcolm Knowles, who is sometimes referred to as the father of adult education, adult learning is different in many ways from child learning. He proposes five common characteristics of adult learners as shown in Box 11.9.3 (Merriam 2001). As summarized by James Clawson (2006), 'Adults don't learn like children. Adults are more discerning in what they are willing to learn, more questioning, and more resentful of being told what to learn'.

Therefore, teaching adults should not be didactic, but emphasize learning approaches that are problem-based and collaborative. The interactions between teacher and learner should also be based on a more equal relationship. Based on the adult learning theory, adult training should be 'student-centred, experience-based, problem-oriented and collaborative' (Burns 2002).

Training methods for L/CHWs in the past emphasized lecture-based learning and focused on the theories and knowledge that may be complicated and not interesting for adult students (Gilson et al. 1989). Classroom-style teaching is also not conducive for skills development, especially for general public

---

Box 11.9.3 Five principles of adult learning according to Malcolm Knowles

1. Adults have an independent self-concept and can be self-directed in their learning.

2. Adults bring life experiences and knowledge to learning.

3. Adults are goal oriented with their learning needs closely related to their roles.

4. Adults are problem oriented and interested in practical applications of knowledge.

5. Adult learners are internally motivated to learn and want to be respected.

Source: data from Merriam, S.B., Andragogy and Self-Directed Learning: Pillars of Adult Learning Theory, in Merriam, S.B., (ed.), *The New Update on Adult Learning Theory: New Directions for Adult and Continuing Education*, Number 89, Spring 2001, Jossey-Bass Higher and Adult Education Series, Copyright © 2001 John Wiley & Sons Ltd.

health competency. Several other learning approaches may be more favourable to adult learning, such as action learning, experiential learning or learning by doing, project-based learning, and self-directed learning (Conlan et al. 2010).

Post-training support

Supervision and support are commonly acknowledged as key functions to the success of L/CHWs. Because they work mainly in the field or in the community, 'regular supervision and support will help maintain the interest and motivation of these workers to carry out their assigned tasks' (Curtale et al. 1995). Despite its importance, supervision and support are often among 'the weakest links in L/CHW programs' (Lehmann and Sanders 2007). Inadequate supervision was found to be one of the main factors limiting the effectiveness of L/CHW programmes (Bhutta et al. 2010). An effective training programme should not end at the conclusion of the training period, but prepare and plan for supervision and support for the trainees over the long term to promote success and sustainability of the programme (Baker et al. 2007).

Distance training and the use of new technologies to provide L/CHW training and support are increasingly mentioned as the trend forwards. With the increased availability of mobile phones and the Internet, effective use of information technology can be employed for training purposes. Digital training materials are also cheaper to transfer and easier to customize and localize. The Dalberg Global Development Advisors (Funes et al. 2012) proposed several reasons to support their prediction that distance learning will play an important role in the future (Box 11.9.4).

Motivation and incentives

L/CHWs are like other health workers who require appropriate motivation and incentives to foster their efficiency and effectiveness. Motivations are mainly internal drive that encourages L/CHWs to carry out their tasks with happiness. Incentives are usually an external force that drives them to work more effectively. Motivation can be generated through role models, inside understanding of the importance of their works, and realization of the successes and achievements. Incentives may be physical, like financial incentives and some fringe benefits including health benefits, and non-financial ones like the social recognition, opportunity for continuing education, permanent job opportunity, and career development.

Those that are volunteers should focus on using motivation and non-financial incentives. L/CHWs who receive longer training and carrying out formal or more permanent jobs, such as the health extension workers, require adequate financial incentives. Thus each L/CHW programme should properly design an appropriate package for motivation and incentives to ensure long-term sustainable successes. The training programme can also serve as an initial venue to drive the motivation of L/CHWs and to promote an understanding of incentives available for them.

Conclusion

L/CHWs are an important component of health workforce systems. They can be trained to carry out basic tasks and specific functions to support health professionals and other types of health workers in delivering health services. They also have closer links to the community and generate more trust.

To ensure that local health workers have adequate competency to fulfil their roles, effective training programmes are needed. Training can be both pre-service and in-service and include new knowledge and skills or refresher training. Training can be about core public health knowledge and disciplines, as well as general work competency, such as communication and leadership skills. The training curriculum should be well designed to accommodate the needs and the practicality of its implementation and take into account the adult learning theory in the choices of training methods and learning experience.

Designing an effective training programme should start from the recruitment process and must ensure that the system of support and recognition is in place after training is completed. This requires strong political support for the local health worker programme, intersectoral approaches to training and functions of these workers, and active community participation in recruitment and support. In addition, an effective incentive package should be incorporated in the L/CHW programme to build up motivation of the L/CHWs as well as to provide appropriate financial and non-financial incentives to ensure long-term sustainable success of the L/CHW programme.

Box 11.9.4 Five reasons why distance learning could play an important role in L/CHW training

1. Implementers can more easily reach L/CHWs who live in remote, difficult-to-access areas.

2. By permitting L/CHWs to learn within their communities, distance learning can support continuity of care.

3. Distance learning would obviate the burdens of travel for L/CHWs and reduce time spent away from household management or employment.

4. L/CHWs could learn at a flexible pace, refresh their knowledge in short modules, and learn continuously.

5. By relying on communication technology, supervisor support and peer networks can be facilitated.

Reproduced with permission from Funes et al., *Preparing the next generation of community health workers: The power of technology for training*, Dalberg Global Development Advisors, Washington DC, USA, Copyright © 2012, available from http://www.dalberg.com/documents/Technology_and_CHWs.pdf.

References

American Public Health Association (2009). *Support for Community Health Workers to Increase Health Access and to Reduce Health Inequities*. Washington, DC: American Public Health Association.

Baker, B., Benton, D., Friedman, E., and Russell, A. (2007). *Systems Support for Task Shifting to Community Health Workers*. Geneva: The Global Health Alliance.

Beaglehole, R., Bonita, R., Horton, R., et al. (2011). Priority actions for the non-communicable disease crisis. *The Lancet*, 377, 1438–47.

Berman, P.A. (1984). Village health workers in Java, Indonesia: coverage and equity. *Social Science & Medicine*, 19, 411–22.

Berman, P.A., Gwatkin, D.R., and Burger, S.E. (1987). Community-based health workers: head start or false start towards health for all? *Social Science & Medicine*, 25, 443–59.

Bhattacharyya, K., Winch, P., Leban, K., et al. (2001). Community health worker incentives and disincentives: how they affect motivation retention and sustainability. *BMC Health Services Research*, 1, 4.

Bhutta, Z.A., Lassi, Z.S., Pariyo, G., and Huicho, L. (2010). *Global Experience of Community Health Workers for Delivery of Health Related Millennium Development Goals: A Systematic Review, Country Case Studies, and Recommendations for Integration into National Health Systems*. Geneva: Global Health Workforce Alliance.

Bonita, R., Magnusson, R., Bovet, P., et al. (2013). Country actions to meet UN commitments on non-communicable diseases: a stepwise approach. *The Lancet*, 381, 575–84.

Burns, R. (2002). *The Adult Learner at Work: A Comprehensive Guide to the Context, Psychology and Methods of Learning for the Workplace*. Sydney: Allen & Unwin.

Callaghan, M., Ford, N., and Schneider, H. (2010). A systematic review of task-shifting for HIV treatment and care in Africa. *Human Resources for Health*, 8, 8.

Chapman, J., Congdon, P., Shaw, S., and Carter, Y.H. (2005). The geographical distribution of specialists in public health in the United Kingdom: is capacity related to need? *Public Health*, 119, 639–46.

Chen, L., Evans, T., Anand, S., et al. (2004). Human resources for health: overcoming the crisis. *The Lancet*, 364, 1984–90.

Clawson, J. (2006). Adult learning theory: it matters. In J. Clawson and M.E. Haskins (eds.) *Teaching Management*, pp. 34–48. Cambridge: Cambridge University Press.

Conlan, J., Grabowski, S., and Smith, K. (2010). Adult learning. In M. Orey (ed.) *Emerging Perspectives on Learning, Teaching, and Technology*. [Online] Athens, GA: Department of Educational Psychology and Instructional Technology, University of Georgia. Available at: http://epltt.coe.uga.edu/index.php?title=Adult_Learning.

Curtale, F., Siwakoti, B., Lagrosa, C., Laraja, M., and Guerra, R. (1995). Improving skills and utilization of community health volunteers in Nepal. *Social Science & Medicine*, 40, 1117–25.

De Brouwere, V., Dieng, T., Diadhiou, M., Witter, S., and Denerville, E. (2009). Task shifting for emergency obstetric surgery in district hospitals in Senegal. *Reproductive Health Matters*, 17, 32–44.

Dzau, V.J., Grazin, N., Bartlett, R., et al. (2012). *A Neglected Resource: Transforming Healthcare Through Human Capital. Report of the Innovative Delivery Models Working Group*. London: Imperial College.

Frenk, J., Chen, L., Bhutta, Z.A., et al. (2010). Health professionals for a new century: transforming education to strengthen health systems in an interdependent world. *The Lancet*, 376, 1923–58.

Fulton, B.D., Scheffler, R.M., Sparkes, S.P., Auh, E.Y., Vujicic, M., and Soucat, A. (2011). Health workforce skill mix and task shifting in low income countries: a review of recent evidence. *Human Resources for Health*, 9, 1.

Funes, R., Hausman, V., and Rastegar, A. (2012). *Preparing the Next Generation of Community Health Workers: The Power of Technology for Training*. Washington, DC: Dalberg Global Development Advisors.

Gericke, C., Kurowski, C., Ranson, M., and Mills, A. (2003). *Feasibility of Scaling-Up Interventions: The Role of Intervention Design*. Disease Control Priorities Project Working Paper No. 13. London: London School of Hygiene and Tropical Medicine.

Gilson, L., Walt, G., Heggenhougen, K., et al. (1989). National community health worker programs: how can they be strengthened? *Journal of Public Health Policy*, 10, 518–32.

Haines, A. and Cassels, A. (2004). Can the millennium development goals be attained? *British Medical Journal*, 329, 394–7.

Haines, A., Sanders, D., Lehmann, U., et al. (2007). Achieving child survival goals: potential contribution of community health workers. *The Lancet*, 369, 2121–31.

Hanvoravongchai, P. (2007). Scaling up health workforces in response to critical shortages. *The Lancet*, 370, 2080–1.

Huicho, L., Scherpbier, R.W., Nkowane, A.M., Victora, C.G., and Multi-Country Evaluation of IMCI Study Group (2008). How much does quality of child care vary between health workers with differing durations of training? An observational multicountry study. *The Lancet*, 372, 910–16.

Kanchanachitra, C., Lindelow, M., Johnston, T., et al. (2011). Health in Southeast Asia 5 Human resources for health in southeast Asia: shortages, distributional challenges, and international trade in health services. *The Lancet*, 377, 769–81.

Lehmann, U., Friedman, I., and Sanders, D. (2004). *Review of the Utilisation and Effectiveness of Community-Based Health Workers in Africa*. JLI Working Paper. Boston, MA: Global Health Trust, Joint Learning Initiative on Human Resources for Health and Development (JLI).

Lehmann, U. and Sanders, D. (2007). *Community Health Workers: What Do We Know About Them? The State of the Evidence on Programmes, Activities, Costs and Impact on Health Outcomes of Using Community Health Workers*. Geneva: World Health Organization.

Lehmann, U., Van Damme, W., Barten, F., and Sanders, D. (2009). Task shifting: the answer to the human resources crisis in Africa? *Human Resources for Health*, 7, 49.

Lewin, S., Munabi-Babigumira, S., Glenton, C., et al. (2010). The effect of lay health workers on mother and child health and infectious diseases. *Cochrane Database of Systematic Reviews*, 3, CD004015.

Masanja, H., Schellenberg, J.A., De Savigny, D., Mshinda, H., and Victora, C.G. (2005). Impact of Integrated Management of Childhood Illness on inequalities in child health in rural Tanzania. *Health Policy and Planning*, 20(Suppl. 1), i77–i184.

McPake, B. and Mensah, K. (2008). Task shifting in health care in resource-poor countries. *The Lancet*, 372, 870–1.

Merriam, S.B. (2001). Andragogy and self-directed learning: pillars of adult learning theory. *New Directions for Adult and Continuing Education*, 2001, 3–14.

Murray, C.J., Vos, T., Lozano, R., et al. (2012). Disability-adjusted life years (DALYs) for 291 diseases and injuries in 21 regions, 1990–2010: a systematic analysis for the Global Burden of Disease Study 2010. *The Lancet*, 380, 2197–223.

Perry, H.B., Zulliger, R., and Rogers, M.M. (2014). Community health workers in low-, middle-, and high-income countries: an overview of their history, recent evolution, and current effectiveness. *Annual Review of Public Health*, 35, 399–421.

Rosenthal, E. (2000). *A Summary of the National Community Health Advisor Study*. Washington, DC: Georgetown University Law Center.

Rural Assistance Center (2012). *Community Health Workers Toolkit*. [Online] Available at: http://www.raconline.org/communityhealth/chw/.

Singh, P. and Sachs, J.D. (2013). 1 million community health workers in sub-Saharan Africa by 2015. *The Lancet*, 382, 363–5.

Travis, P., Bennett, S., Haines, A., et al. (2004). Overcoming health-systems constraints to achieve the Millennium Development Goals. *The Lancet*, 364, 900–6.

Tulenko, K., Mogedal, S., Afzal, M.M., et al. (2013). Community health workers for universal health-care coverage: from fragmentation to synergy. *Bulletin of the World Health Organization*, 91, 847–52.

Victora, C.G., Wagstaff, A., Schellenberg, J.A., Gwatkin, D., Claeson, M., and Habicht, J.P. (2003). Applying an equity lens to child health and mortality: more of the same is not enough. *The Lancet*, 362, 233–41.

Walt, G. (1990). *Community Health Workers in National Health Programmes. Just Another Pair of Hands?* Oxford: Oxford University Press.

Wang, H., Dwyer-Lindgren, L., Lofgren, K.T., et al. (2012). Age-specific and sex-specific mortality in 187 countries, 1970–2010: a systematic analysis for the Global Burden of Disease Study 2010. *The Lancet*, 380, 2071–94.

Wibulpolprasert, S. (1991). Community financing: Thailand's experience. *Health Policy and Planning*, 6, 354–60.

World Bank (1994). *Better Health in Africa: Experience and Lessons Learned*. Washington, DC: World Bank.

World Health Organization (1978). *Primary Health Care.* Geneva: WHO.

World Health Organization (1987). *The Community Health Worker.* Geneva: WHO.

World Health Organization (1989). *Strengthening the Performance of Community Health Workers in Primary Health Care. Report of a WHO Study Group.* World Health Organization Technical Report Series. Geneva: WHO.

World Health Organization (2004). *Comprehensive Community- and Home-Based Health Care Model.* New Delhi: WHO Regional Office for South-East Asia.

World Health Organization (2006). *The World Health Report 2006: Working Together for Health.* Geneva: WHO.

World Health Organization (2011). *Sexual and Reproductive Health: Core Competencies in Primary Care.* Geneva: WHO.

World Health Organization (2012a). *Second Report of Committee A. 65th World Health Assembly.* Geneva: WHO.

World Health Organization (2012b). *World Health Statistics 2012.* Geneva: World Health Organization.

Emergency public health and humanitarian assistance in the twenty-first century

Les Roberts and Richard Brennan

Introduction to emergency public health and humanitarian assistance

Examples of humanitarian actions likely precede recorded history. Zakah, a pillar of Islam, the New Testament story of the Good Samaritan, the central theme of mercy in Buddhism, and similar concepts in almost all religions suggest that the systemization of compassion towards those in crisis may be an inevitable manifestation of social organization. Thus, it may be surprising that the science, and in particular the health science, associated with responding to natural and man-made crises has mostly developed in the past half century.

During the Biafran War (1967–1970) perhaps half of the 2,000,000 population inside the shrinking breakaway enclave died of malnutrition and disease by the end of the conflict (Western 1972). During this crisis, profound advances in modern humanitarian relief arose. Unable to determine which children were starving and which children were just skinny or small, the Friends Overseas Service Committee triggered the development of the Quaker Upper Arm Circumference (QUAC) Stick, the first scheme for assessing nutritional anthropometry. The Centers for Disease Control and Prevention (CDC) tested the universally accepted theory that malnourished children could not produce an immunological response to being vaccinated by using intervention and control groups. They vaccinated some very malnourished children and followed up weeks later by drawing blood from the study children to see if immunity had developed. In this first known controlled trial in an emergency, it turned out that malnourished children could indeed be effectively vaccinated (Ifekwunigwe et al. 1980). Other developments included the first known public health adaptation of capture–recapture methodologies from wildlife biology in order to estimate the number of deaths (and thus the first real-time conflict mortality measurement), the first guidelines for such things as running feeding centres, and the creation of the medical relief organization Médecins Sans Frontières (MSF).

In the crises that followed, more and more central insights into the science of keeping vulnerable people alive and healthy accumulated at an ever increasing rate. The East Pakistan Crisis, by chance arising where an international diarrhoeal research centre was based, brought the advent of oral rehydration therapy (ORT) (Sack et al. 1970). Relief for Cambodians on the Thai border demonstrated the value of surveillance and rapid assessments (Glass et al. 1980). The famine and conflict in the Horn of Africa in the early 1980s provided the rationale for the caloric content of rations, a two-stage measles vaccination strategy for children less than 9 months, and a variety of other 'best practices' (Toole et al. 1988, 1989). By the 1990s, comprehensive outlines of priorities and best practices were in place based on the accumulation of these various lessons learned and documented (Toole 1990; CDC 1992; MSF 1997).

Most of these guidelines were developed based on experiences in settings of extreme poverty and high mortality, where the excess (above the normal) mortality profiles were dominated by infectious diseases, primarily diarrhoea, respiratory infections, and malaria. These cold war era crises often continued for many years with large numbers of people displaced and supported in camps for a variety of geo-political and economic reasons. The world of humanitarian response today has little in common with the Biafran era. Today, most of the world's displaced have not crossed a border and are displaced within their own country. Many, perhaps most of the world's most vulnerable displaced are in urban settings. And finally, likely as a result of the developments of the relief community and greater global wealth, few crises in the twenty-first century to date have been associated with extended periods of high mortality, as were seen in Cambodia, Mozambique, Sudan, Somalia, Biafra, the Democratic Republic of Congo (DR Congo), and elsewhere in the last century. Expanding humanitarian efforts have evolved to focus more on issues of suffering, often from chronic or mental health related disorders.

To address these new realities, this chapter will look at four areas where the twenty-first-century humanitarian endeavour is likely to differ dramatically from the twentieth century: preparedness and planning, changing institutional structures and architecture, the evolving public health profile of emergency relief needs, and the role of new and innovative technologies. The role of emergency planning and relief workers has grown, professionalized, and become politicized at a dramatic rate in recent years and we attempt here to create a framework for understanding these transitions.

Definitions and classification

There is currently no universally accepted definition of the term 'disaster'. This lack of standardization can be attributed in part to the broad range of disciplines involved in disaster management. Nonetheless, common to most definitions is the concept of large-scale loss that exceeds a community's own capacity to respond effectively, requiring some form of external assistance.

The United Nations International Strategy for Disaster Reduction (UNISDR) defines a disaster as 'a serious disruption of the functioning of a community or a society involving widespread human, material, economic or environmental losses and impacts, which exceeds the ability of the affected community or society to cope using its own resources' (UNISDR 2010). This definition is also one of several recognized by the World Health Organization (WHO).

Similarly, there is no standard classification system for disasters, although numerous have been proposed. Generally, disasters are associated with the hazards that cause them. They can be classified as either natural or human generated, with subclassifications of each (Table 11.10.1). Natural disasters are often subclassified according to whether they are acute onset or slow/gradual onset, human-generated disasters as intentional or non-intentional.

Epidemiology

According to the Centre for Research on the Epidemiology of Disasters, during the 10 years between 2002 and 2011, on average approximately 700 natural and technological disasters occurred globally each year. These disasters affected around 270 million people annually and resulted in an average of 123,000 deaths (International Federation of Red Cross and Red Crescent Societies

Table 11.10.1 Classification of disasters

Natural	Human generated
Acute onset	Technological
◆ Geophysical:	◆ Industrial accident:
◆ Earthquake	◆ Explosion
◆ Tsunami	◆ Fire
◆ Volcanic eruption	◆ Hazardous material release
◆ Avalanche	◆ Structural collapse
◆ Hydrometerological:	◆ Transportation crash
◆ Flood	Societal
◆ Windstorm	◆ Civil strife
◆ Tornado	◆ Mass gathering
◆ Winter storm	◆ Terrorism
◆ Extreme temperature	War/complex emergencies
◆ Forest fire	
◆ Landslide	
◆ Biological:	
◆ Epidemic, pandemic	
Gradual/chronic onset	
◆ Drought, food insecurity	
◆ Desertification	
◆ Insect/pest infestation (e.g. locusts)	

2012). The most severely affected region was Asia, followed by Africa and the Americas. According to a study by the WHO in 2007, most countries had experienced a major disaster over the preceding 5 years.

Those most vulnerable to the public health impacts of disasters are the poor. While 27 per cent of disasters occurred in countries categorized as having low human development, they accounted for 47 per cent of deaths, because of their limited capacities to mitigate, prepare for, and respond to disasters. Moreover, the economic costs run into billions of dollars and a single disaster can set back development many years, with obvious implications for public health programming and health outcomes.

These figures do not include conflict-related disasters, the impacts of which are more difficult to quantify. The World Bank estimated that 1.5 billion people live in countries affected by repeated cycles of political and criminal violence, and fragility (World Bank 2011). Most modern-day conflicts are protracted civil wars, in which civilians are often deliberately targeted and frequently displaced from their communities. Often called 'complex emergencies', they are associated with high rates of morbidity and mortality.

In such conflicts, large numbers of deaths can result from violent injury, as in the Rwandan genocide, the Balkan conflicts of the 1990s, and the recent war in Syria. But in many instances, most deaths are due to the so-called indirect health consequences of conflict—increased rates of infectious diseases, acute malnutrition, and complications of chronic diseases that arise due to societal disruption, population displacement, and breakdown in health services. This has been well described in crises in DR Congo, Ethiopia, Somalia, and Sudan (Toole 1997; Coghlan et al. 2006).

Globally, the most frequent types of disasters are transport accidents, followed by floods, windstorms, industrial accidents, earthquakes, and droughts/food insecurity (Table 11.10.2). Climate change is expected to affect the frequency and severity of floods, windstorms, and droughts, with their associated public health impacts (World Health Organization and World Meteorological Organization 2012). For example, severe droughts and associated food insecurity have occurred at more frequent intervals over the past decade in the Sahel and Horn of Africa. Monsoon-associated floods in Pakistan in 2010 and 2012 were among the most severe ever recorded.

The number of ongoing conflicts is more difficult to quantify, as definitions vary. The Uppsala Conflict Database defines a conflict as a 'contested incompatibility that concerns government or territory or both where the use of armed force between two parties results in at least 25 battle-related deaths in a year. Of these two parties, at least one has to be the government of a state'. Based on this definition there were 37 ongoing conflicts in 2011, of which 27 were intra-state, one inter-state, and nine internationalized (Uppsala Conflict Data Program n.d.).

The highest death tolls from natural and technological disasters have been associated with earthquakes/tsunamis, windstorms, extreme temperatures, and droughts/food insecurity (Table 11.10.2). Total death tolls from conflict have been difficult to estimate and can be politicized. The Uppsala database records only battlefield deaths and omits the indirect deaths referenced earlier. But as has been documented in DR Congo, Sudan, Iraq, and elsewhere, total conflict-related deaths (battlefield and indirect) can be enormous and may exceed those due to all other

Table 11.10.2 Frequency, impact, and geographic distribution of major types of disasters, 2002–2011

Disaster	Frequency per year	Average deaths per year	Average number of people affected	Average cost of damage (millions of dollars)	Region with highest frequency	Region with highest deaths
Droughts/food insecurity	24	7732	93,132,500	3328	Africa	Asia
Earthquakes/tsunamis	29	67,974	7,905,700	46,153	Asia	Asia
Extreme temperatures	24	14,598	9,050,800	4222	Europe	Europe
Floods	179	5733	117,584,900	27,804	Asia	Asia
Forest fires	11	70	214,600	2757	Americas	Europe
Insect infestation	1	n.a.	50,000	n.a.	Africa	n.a.
Landslides	19	955	396,100	190	Asia	Asia
Volcanic eruptions	6	56	143,900	18	Americas	Asia
Windstorms	102	17,355	39,801,100	58,0178	Asia	Asia
Industrial accidents	52	1366	100,800	3728	Asia	Asia
Transport accidents	200	6162	9,000	49	Africa	Africa
Conflict[a]	37	n.a.	n.a.	n.a.	Africa	Africa

n.a.: not available.

[a] Conflict data from The Uppsala Conflict Data Program (UCDP), Uppsala University, Copyright © 2014, available from http://www.pcr.uu.se/research/ucdp/.

Source: data from International Federation of Red Cross (IFRC) and Red Crescent Societies, *World Disasters Report, 2012*, IFRC, Geneva, Switzerland, Copyright © 2012 The International Federation of Red Cross and Red Crescent Societies. All rights reserved.

disasters combined (Burnham et al. 2006; Uppsala Conflict Data Program n.d.).

Moreover, elevations in mortality rates can persist for years after the formal end of conflict, as documented in Angola, DR Congo, and South Sudan. Women and children are almost always the most vulnerable in these contexts. Of the 20 countries with the highest child mortality rates, 15 have experienced conflict over the past two decades. Similarly, of the ten countries with the highest maternal mortality, nine have recently endured conflict. According to the World Bank, no low-income fragile or conflict-affected country has achieved even one of the eight Millennium Development Goals—three of which are health related.

An important aspect of disasters that can expose the affected populations to increased public health risks is forced displacement. According to the *World Development Report 2012*, there were an estimated 72.7 million people forcibly displaced worldwide in 2011—and this number is growing annually. An estimated 14.9 million are refugees, 26.4 million are internally displaced persons (mostly due to violence), 16.4 million are displaced due to natural disasters, and a further 15.2 million displaced due to development projects and activities.

The process of displacement can increase the risk of infectious diseases (e.g. through housing in unsanitary conditions or exposure to disease-carrying vectors), food scarcity and malnutrition, physical violence, sexual abuse, and psychological trauma. Access to health services is often limited and ongoing health programmes (e.g. vaccinations) disrupted. Higher disease rates are often documented among internally displaced persons (IDPs), as the well-developed mechanisms to provide protection and humanitarian assistance to refugees do not always apply directly in IDP settings (Salama et al. 2001).

Different types of disasters are associated with reasonably predictable public health risks and associated patterns of morbidity and mortality (Pan American Health Organization 2000) (Table 11.10.3). Earthquakes are often associated with large numbers of deaths and injuries, but infrequently with major population displacements, food scarcity, or increased risks of communicable diseases. Flash floods are often associated with many deaths, few injuries, damage to water systems, and food shortages. Conflicts are associated with a large number of public health risks and consequences. This type of information can assist with the planning and coordination of clinical and public health services.

In addition to climate change, there are other important global trends that threaten to increase the frequency and impact of disasters. Increasing urbanization, poor urban planning, poor land use, unregulated industrialization, new and emerging infectious diseases, and terrorism, all have the potential to expose greater numbers of people to hazards (United Nations International Strategy for Disaster Reduction 2010; WHO 2011a; Bhui et al. 2012). The Christchurch earthquake of 2011, Bangkok floods of 2011, and Superstorm Sandy in New York City in 2012, all demonstrated that disasters that strike densely populated urban areas have the potential for substantial public health and economic impact. The Nigeria floods of 2012 have brought attention to the issues of settlements in flood-prone zones. The severe acute respiratory syndrome epidemic of 2003 and the H1N1 pandemic of 2009 have demonstrated the need for stronger public health surveillance and response mechanisms. Terrorist attacks across a range of countries have revealed security threats that need to be addressed in disaster planning and mass casualty response plans (WHO 2007).

Table 11.10.3 Short-term effects of major disasters

Effect	Conflict	Earthquakes	High winds (without flooding)	Tsunamis/flash floods	Slow-onset floods	Landslides	Volcanoes	Droughts
Deaths[a]	Many	Many	Few	Many	Few	Many	Many	Varies—many with famine
Severe injuries	Many	Many	Moderate	Few	Few	Few	Few	Rare
Increased risk of communicable diseases	High	Potential risk following all major natural disasters. Probability rising with displacement, overcrowding, and deteriorating sanitation						
Damage to health facilities	Varies. May be specifically targeted and looted	Severe (structure and equipment)	Severe	Severe but localized	Severe (mainly equipment)	Severe but localized	Severe (structure and equipment)	Rare
Damage to water systems	Severe	Severe	Light	Severe	Light	Severe but localized	Severe	Varies
Food shortage	Common	Rare (may occur due to economic and logistic factors)	Common	Common	Rare	Rare		Common
Major population displacements	Common	Rare (may occur in heavily damaged urban areas)	Common (generally limited)					Common

[a] Potential lethal impact in absence of preventive measures.

Adapted with permission from Pan American Health Organization (PAHO), *Natural Disasters: Protecting the Public Health*, PAHO, Washington DC, USA, Copyright © 2000, available from http://www.preventionweb.net/files/1913_VL206114.pdf.

Preparing for disasters—health emergency risk management

The most effective means of reducing the public health risks and impacts of disasters is to employ a comprehensive emergency risk management approach. Emergency risk management (ERM)[1] consists of a continuum of synergistic steps that can reduce the risks and consequences of disasters, including prevention (risk reduction and mitigation), preparedness, response, and recovery. These steps are so closely interconnected that for all practical purposes they should not be considered in isolation from each other. Risk assessments and risk reduction activities directly inform disaster preparedness and response, for example. Moreover, the manner by which agencies respond to an emergency will directly impact the recovery process (WHO 2011b).

ERM for health draws on the disciplines of risk management, disaster management, and health systems. The approach emphasizes managing the risks prior to a disaster occurring so that potential public health consequences may be prevented or minimized. Specifically, ERM entails identifying and reducing hazards and associated vulnerabilities, preparing for and responding effectively to disasters, and recovering, rehabilitating, and reconstructing after a disaster has occurred. Experience has demonstrated that countries and communities that have invested sufficient resources in ERM have responded more effectively and have been more resilient to the effects of disasters. Strengthened ERM also has the potential to contribute to sustainable development.

Bangladesh is one of the most natural-disaster prone countries on the planet. Large numbers of people live on a low, flat alluvial delta vulnerable to floodwater coming from the Brahmaputra basin to the north and the typhoon-prone Indian Ocean to the south. A typhoon in 1970 resulted in approximately a quarter of a million deaths (Bern et al. 1993). Over the next decades, the people of Bangladesh built 311 elevated typhoon and flood shelters that could hold 350,000 people and implemented community-based response strategies. A similar 1991 typhoon affecting a far larger population resulted in 138,000 deaths (Mallick et al. 2005). During the 1991 storm, seeking a storm shelter early and being in an official shelter were highly protective against death although only 17 per cent of the affected populations sought shelter in response to the storm warning sirens. Since then, advances in storm warning, public communications and community response have resulted in Southern Bangladesh being held up as an example of disaster preparedness (United Nations Development Programme 2010).

Guiding principles

In addition to the emphasis on managing risks, ERM is guided by the following key principles Brennan et al. 2009):

◆ *All-hazards.* Many of the key functions required to manage risks are common across all hazards, for example, assessments, communications, logistics, etc. Moreover, it is neither efficient nor cost-effective to develop separate plans, procedures, trainings, rosters, and response mechanisms for each individual hazard. While some hazard-specific considerations will rarely be required (e.g. radio-nuclear), an all-hazards approach allows for more efficient management of risks and responses.

◆ *Multisectoral approach.* Many activities required to protect and preserve health are managed primarily by other sectors, for example, water and sanitation, shelter, food security, law and order, etc. Effective mechanisms for multisectoral collaboration and coordination are therefore necessary to ensure optimized emergency risk management in the health sector. These should be established at national and local levels, wherever possible.

◆ *Prepared community.* Communities are always the first to respond to disasters and can play a critical role in meeting emergent health needs. Community resilience can be strengthened by building their capacity to prevent, mitigate, prepare for, respond to, and recover from disasters. Local governments, civil society organizations, and individual citizens all have the potential of contributing to ERM.

Key components of emergency risk management

Prevention, risk reduction, and mitigation

There are few measures taken by the health sector alone that can actually prevent a disaster from occurring. The main example is effective vaccination programmes to prevent outbreaks of diseases, such as measles and yellow fever. Most disaster prevention and risk reduction depend largely on the efforts of other sectors (e.g. structural engineers, urban planners), as well as appropriate government policies, plans, and legislation. The application of effective industry standards and government regulations, for example, can minimize the risk of chemical releases from industrial sites. Adherence to building codes will reduce the risks of structural damage and subsequent deaths and injuries following an earthquake. Appropriate land use can reduce the risks of floods and landslides, while improved residential zoning can minimize the exposure of populations to floodwaters.

The area of conflict prevention is more complex and requires consideration of a broad range of political, social, cultural, economic, and security issues. It is likely that many brewing interstate tensions are prevented from escalating into open conflict, such as Eritrea and Ethiopia over the past decade. Such successes almost always involve multiple players and a variety of factors going well again and again over time. Thus, there is little capacity to weigh the relative importance of each factor and thus develop a precise science of conflict prevention (International Crisis Group 2005).

Disaster risk assessment

Collaboration with other sectors in disaster risk assessment is essential to identifying risks in advance and developing clear strategies to manage them (International Federation of the Red Cross 2006). The health component of a multisectoral risk assessment aims to determine the likelihood and potential public health impact of future disasters. Possible health consequences include direct impacts on people (e.g. injury, disease) or health facilities, and/or secondary effects due to damaged infrastructure (e.g. water and sanitation systems), population displacement, environmental damage, etc.

Classically, risk is considered as a result of the interaction of potential hazards, level of exposure to those hazards, existing community/societal vulnerabilities, and local capacities. This interaction is well represented by the following illustrative formulation:

$$\text{Risk} = \text{hazard} \times \text{exposure} \times \text{vulnerability/capacities.}$$

The first step in the risk assessment is hazard identification and analysis. This includes describing the full range of possible hazards (e.g. natural, technological, biological, and societal), their potential scale, population likely to be exposed, geographic location, and historical record, including their previous health impacts.

Vulnerability analysis attempts to determine the exposure and susceptibility that a given community may have to the identified hazards. For example, a coastal community will have greater vulnerabilities to hurricanes than communities located at a distance from the shoreline. Issues to consider include baseline health and nutritional status, socioeconomic status, physical location and environment, access to healthcare, health knowledge and behaviours, availability of other services and infrastructure (e.g. water, sanitation, transportation), marginalized groups, etc. A review of health infrastructure and programmes should be considered within the analysis, as damage to health facilities can have substantial implications for the community.

An associated assessment of national and local capacities to manage the identified risks is also required. This will allow health professionals, disaster managers and other stakeholders to determine their strengths and weaknesses, and provide an indication of what may be required for capacity development.

Strategies and programmes

Information from the risk and capacity assessments is then used to develop strategies and programmes to reduce the potential impact on public health by the identified hazards. These may include general health system strengthening measures to improve the coverage and effectiveness of existing health services (e.g. vaccinations, training and supervision of staff, improved drug management). They may also include specific health sector interventions that can mitigate the effects of disasters, such as the successful safe hospital programme in Latin America (Pan American Health Organization 2002) and early warning alert and response systems for outbreak control.

The International Health Regulations (IHR) is an international legal instrument that outline obligations and rights of 194 countries to prevent and respond to acute public health risks that have the potential for international spread (WHO 2005). These mostly include epidemics, chemical spills, or nuclear incidents. The IHR aims to limit disturbances to international travel and trade while protecting public health by preventing disease spread. Countries have obligations to report any potential events to the WHO, as well as to strengthen their surveillance and response capacities. The WHO, in turn, provides technical assistance to countries for response and for capacity building, as well as working with its Member States more broadly to ensure global public health security.

Preparedness

The UNISDR definition of preparedness is 'the knowledge and capacities developed by governments, professional response and recovery organizations, communities and individuals to effectively anticipate, respond to, and recover from, the impacts of likely, imminent or current hazard events or conditions' (UNISDR 2010). Many emergency organizations also use the related term 'readiness' to describe their ability to rapidly and appropriately respond to a disaster.

Sound preparedness clearly arises from an effective risk assessment and is linked to early warning systems. It should ensure that the required resources and capacities can be rapidly deployed following the onset of a disaster. Clear emergency functions should have been specified in advance and rosters of qualified and experienced staff developed. Stockpiles of essential drugs, equipment, and supplies should be established and maintained, including strong logistics procedures. All emergency staff should be trained in the relevant technical standards, performance standards, and response procedures (Sphere Project 2011). Standard operating procedures should address key administrative, financial, procurement, and communications functions. Coordination mechanisms should be developed in advance, both for improved health sector and intersectoral functioning. Contingency planning may take into account possible scenarios and triggers for response, and further strengthen coordination.

While most preparedness plans will follow an all-hazards approach, some hazard-specific planning may also be required. This is especially relevant for radio-nuclear and chemical incidents, as well as epidemics and pandemics. When planning for conflict-related crises, issues related to protection become especially relevant and should be anticipated and prepared for.

Preparedness and readiness require strong institutional commitments and dedicated budgetary support. Regular exercises and simulations are necessary to test plans and to inform adjustments to procedures. Lessons learned from actual disaster responses should also be fed back into the preparedness plans to ensure that they are better placed to address field realities.

Response

Timely and effective response has the potential to save lives, reduce disability, prevent disease, and contribute positively to the recovery process. The success of the response will clearly be directly related to the effectiveness of preparedness and the associated response plans. Strengthening and reinforcement of both public health (e.g. vaccinations, environmental health) and clinical (e.g. trauma care) services will be required.

Coordination mechanisms should ideally be in existence prior to the disaster, as noted earlier. But in some instances, these mechanisms may be either weak or rudimentary. Wherever possible, existing national coordination mechanisms should be supported and strengthened, with the Ministry of Health taking the lead in the health sector. For disasters requiring an international response, operational agencies may come together under the 'cluster system', which provides a process for joint assessments, planning, promotion of standards, and monitoring and evaluation (Interagency Standing Committee 2013). The WHO is the lead agency for the Global Health Cluster and usually leads the health cluster at country level as well.

Monitoring and evaluating (M&E) the response is a critical step, but is often not well managed. Many factors conspire to make M&E challenging—the acuteness and scale of the disaster, remote and/or austere sites for operations, insecurity, lack of capacity, etc. It is not always possible to document the impact of the response in terms of mortality and morbidity rates, or prevalence of malnutrition. But responding agencies should be able to, at the minimum, document the coverage of the services that they provide, demonstrate that they are meeting the needs of the most vulnerable, and document that they are effectively filling gaps. The requirements of accountability to the affected population(s) demand this attention to M&E.

Recovery

Effective response should lead to more timely and efficient recovery, which should, in turn, lead to improved risk reduction and preparedness, and greater resilience of communities and the health sector. This is central to the so-called build back better approach. Recovery programmes are increasingly informed by post-disaster needs assessments (PDNAs), which provide a measure of loss within each sector and a prioritized plan for recovery and reconstruction (World Bank Global Facility for Disaster Reduction and Recovery 2011).

Following protracted conflicts and disasters, time-limited national transitional health plans may be adopted. These can help the country's health system evolve from a humanitarian model, in which services are designed mainly to provide life-saving services and are provided largely by non-governmental organizations (NGOs) to a developmental model. Liberia provides an impressive example of how a well-designed transitional national health policy and plan can support the gradual expansion of health services over time, following a period of protracted health system dysfunction due to years of conflict.

Organizing disaster and emergency risk management

National and regional levels

Many countries have established National Disaster Management Authorities (NDMAs) to oversee the design and implementation of disaster and emergency risk management efforts. These authorities usually have responsibility for leading risk assessments, developing disaster risk reduction and mitigation strategies, strengthening preparedness, and leading response and recovery efforts. In some high-profile disasters, other government ministries or departments may assume the lead role in managing the response, for example, the Prime Minister's office. A number of countries, such as Pakistan, have also extended disaster management authorities to provincial and district levels.

The capacities of and resources available to such agencies vary considerably. Countries such as Indonesia have invested substantially in developing national systems, while others have been far less proactive or successful. Nonetheless, it is important for Ministries of Health to engage vigorously with NDMAs to ensure that health is well positioned within national disaster management policies, plans, and arrangements. The impact of disasters is perhaps best defined by their effects on the public's health, although this may not always be obvious to some disaster managers. Ministries of Health should establish their own national programmes for health emergency risk management and ensure that health is well represented in national dialogues and initiatives.

Because the effects of disasters often span borders (e.g. the 2004 Asian tsunami), regional bodies and initiatives have also been established to promote coordination and collaboration on ERM. ASEAN has established a coordinating centre for humanitarian assistance and disaster management, the League of Arab States has developed an Arab Strategy for Disaster Risk Reduction 2020 (ASDRR), and the Organization of American States and League of Arab States have developed programmes to plan for, prepare for, and coordinate responses to crises.

International level

There is a broad range of bodies involved in ERM and disaster response at the international level, including UN agencies, the Red Cross and Red Crescent Movement, NGOs, donors, governments, and, increasingly, the military and private sector. The UN's Office for the Coordination of Humanitarian Affairs (OCHA) plays an important role in convening the major relief agencies and coordinating international humanitarian policy, planning, and relief efforts. The UN Interagency Standing Committee (IASC), chaired by OCHA, is the main international body representing the major relief agencies and plays a central role in setting global policies and establishing procedures for international response. The WHO is the main health agency on the IASC.

Following suboptimal responses to major disasters in Haiti and Pakistan in 2010, an IASC-led process of humanitarian reform was initiated in 2011 to improve the leadership, predictability, coordination, and effectiveness of emergency response. Known as the Transformative Agenda, this process also emphasizes accountability to affected populations as one of the key principles guiding humanitarian action.

The medical relief agency MSF plays a special role in international emergency response. Although it stands outside some of the formal coordination mechanisms at international level, it has the largest operational field presence of any such agency. It has resources and capacities that are matched by no other medical NGO.

Public health needs

Oxygen, water, and food remain the essential priority human needs in almost all settings including the most acute of hardships. The initial handbooks overviewing the public health priorities in high-mortality, low-resource settings remain as relevant today as when they were written (CDC 1992; MSF 1997). Most were lacking in some areas now better appreciated, with obstetric care being perhaps the most dramatic example. Usually those handbooks defined an emergency in terms of a doubling or quadrupling of the baseline mortality rate. In settings of extreme hardship, those displaced and whose livelihoods and social order are disrupted will generally continue to die and suffer from the same ailments they experienced before the crisis but at a higher rate. In some categories of disasters such as natural disasters like earthquakes and floods, death profiles are briefly but dramatically altered but prolonged elevated mortality is rare. Thus, in the most typical disruption and displacement scenarios, acute respiratory infections, diarrhoea, and in some places malaria, dominate the prevention and treatment priorities. Yet, these kinds of crises, with mortality rates elevated fourfold or more, are accounting for a smaller and smaller fraction of all humanitarian aid. Most aid workers today can work an entire lifetime and never see the dramatically elevated mortality of ten or 20 times the baseline rates seen repeatedly in the 1960s through the Rwandan Crisis of 1994. For example, if we use the threshold of 2 per cent of the population dying each month (ten times the highest of baselines) in a population over 100,000 people to define a humanitarian catastrophe, a review of both published and unpublished mortality reports suggests that from 1979 to 1994, there was such a catastrophe on average every 2 years, but none have been reported since that time (Roberts 2013). The camp-based relief setting has also become rare, forcing relief agencies to work in cities and with existing government institutions.

This change away from relief typified by water and food delivery and lifesaving primary healthcare approaches is being driven by four forces: the global transition from a disease burden profile typified by acute infectious illness to one dominated by chronic diseases, more aid funding and fewer acute wars inducing a lower threshold of what is considered a humanitarian crisis, changing motivations, and the rise of the rights-based framework within humanitarian relief.

Transition from acute infectious diseases to chronic conditions

The epidemiological transition occurring in developing countries has been well documented. For example, Lopez et al. contrast the causes of death among adults in various regions based on 1990 and 2001 data respectively (Fig. 11.10.1) (Lopez et al. 2006). Over those 11 years, the non-HIV infectious disease adult death rates declined markedly in Latin America and the Caribbean, the Middle East and North Africa, East Asia and the Pacific, and South Asia. In each locality, this reduction in infectious disease death rates corresponded with lower overall adult mortality. Only in the post-Soviet Europe and Central Asia region and Africa did adult mortality rise over this period; in the former, primarily from cardiovascular diseases and unintentional injuries, and in Africa primarily from HIV. In Africa, overall mortality still decreased over this period because of dramatic reductions in infant and child mortality.

The impact of this epidemiological transition was evident in recent crises in Bosnia, Kosovo, and Iraq, where Ministries of Health and aid agencies were confronted with morbidity profiles dominated by non-infectious diseases. For example, among Kosovar refugees in Macedonia treated by the Red Cross in emergency clinics, hypertension, diabetes-related issues, and dialysis were dominant needs (Gardemann 2002).

Similar experiences were noted in recent crises in Northern Africa (e.g. Libya), the Middle East (e.g. Syria), and Asia (e.g. Indonesia).

Adding to this need to transition medical preparedness for emergencies is the growing appreciation of HIV as a non-fatal chronic condition. An estimated 5 million Africans regularly received antiretroviral drugs (ARVs) in 2011 (WHO et al. 2011), a fraction of the total number of Africans who are HIV positive. As most of the world's protracted conflicts are in Africa and a disproportionate number of humanitarian operations occur there, planning for the chronic disease support aspects of HIV needs to be part of the humanitarian public health portfolio (O'Brien et al. 2010).

For the 2010 presidential elections in Côte D'Ivoire, the agency ICAP anticipated political unrest and provided 3 months of advance supplies of ARVs to almost everyone in the country on the therapy. Widespread violence did rock the country after the elections and in some areas government health facilities were closed for weeks. A non-random but widespread assessment after the crisis suggested that people appropriately managed their personal drug supplies and there were almost no ARV supply ruptures from the crisis (Twyman 2012). This kind of new chronic disease programme planning will undoubtedly become more widespread within the relief community.

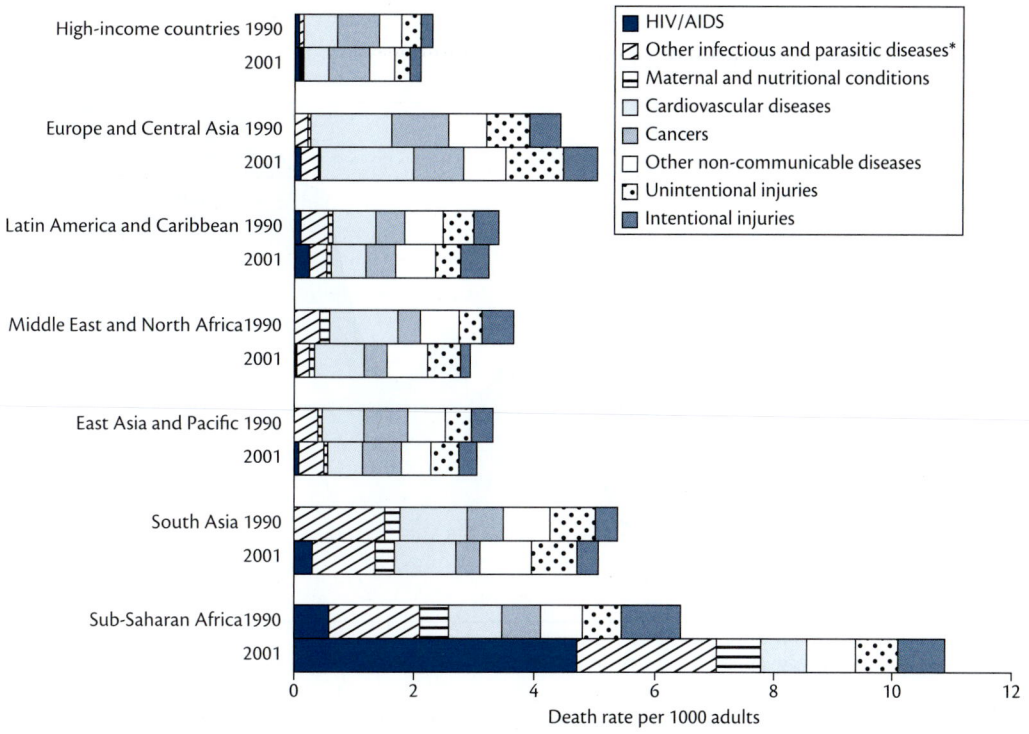

Fig. 11.10.1 Death rates by disease group and region in 1990 and 2001 for adults aged 15–59 years. *Includes respiratory infections. Cause-specific death rates for 1990 (estimated from Murray, C.J.L., Lopez, A.D. (eds.) *The Global Burden of Disease: A Comprehensive Assessment of Mortality and Disability from Diseases, Injuries and Risk Factors in 1990 and Projected to 2020.* Cambridge: Harvard University Press, 1996) might not be completely comparable to those for 2001 because of changes in data availability and methods, plus some approximations in mapping 1990 estimates to the 2001 regions East Asia and Pacific, South Asia, and Europe and Central Asia. For all geographical regions, high-income countries excluded and shown as single group at top of graph. The geographical regions therefore refer to low-and-middle-income countries only.
Reprinted from *The Lancet*, Volume 367, Issue 9524, Lopez, A.D. et al., Global and regional burden of disease and risk factors, 2001: systematic analysis of population health data, pp. 1747–57, Copyright © 2006, with permission from Elsevier. http://www.sciencedirect.com/science/journal/01406736.

More aid and fewer high-intensity conflicts

Spending on humanitarian assistance has increased dramatically in recent decades. The 2011 Arab Spring aside, there has been a dramatic downward trend in the numbers of conflicts since the end of the cold war. The number of ongoing conflicts is estimated to have declined by over 50 per cent since the collapse of the Soviet Union (Gleditsch et al. 2002). Garfield estimated the global populations affected by conflict over time, disaggregated by levels of conflict intensity (Fig. 11.10.2) (Garfield et al. 2012). While the numbers of people living in the two highest levels of conflict intensity have reduced dramatically over the past 10–15 years, the numbers living in post-conflict environments have dramatically increased. Nonetheless, worsening violence and major population displacements over the past 1–2 years in Syria, the Central African Republic, and South Sudan call into question the certainty that this positive trend of diminishing violent crises will continue in the years to come.

According to Global Humanitarian Assistance, formal humanitarian assistance spending increased fourfold from 1990 to 2010 (United Nations Children's Fund 2013). Thus, the world is spending more money and delivering more humanitarian programming to fewer people in the most acute settings. Unfortunately, however, more aid is being taken up by the increasing numbers of people requiring relief after natural disasters, and to a lesser extent, technological disasters such as the Fukushima nuclear

meltdown in 2011. This has the effect of lowering the mortality prioritization with regard to what is considered a humanitarian crisis. It also means since much if not most humanitarian spending is in post-conflict settings, that humanitarian assistance is now inseparable from development work.

Changing motivations and the rights-based framework

Aid meant to induce development may be different in nature from humanitarian aid designed to prevent deaths and suffering in the short term. Donors are continuing to place increasing emphasis on sustainability of humanitarian interventions and demanding local participation and empowerment. These are natural changes in perspective that match a transition from death aversion to development priorities. A few NGOs such as MSF maintain a philosophy that they work primarily to reduce death and suffering but most others now hold long-term impact and sustainability as central objectives. This creates several new conditions for relief work. Many relief efforts in the 1980s and 1990s defined success by the lowering of the crude mortality rate (CDC 1992). This is rare today. Sustainability efforts usually require training and supporting local officials and institutions, committing to multi-year engagements, and monitoring changes in behaviours. These require different skills from those prevalent in relief agencies in the twentieth century. Reconstruction activities following

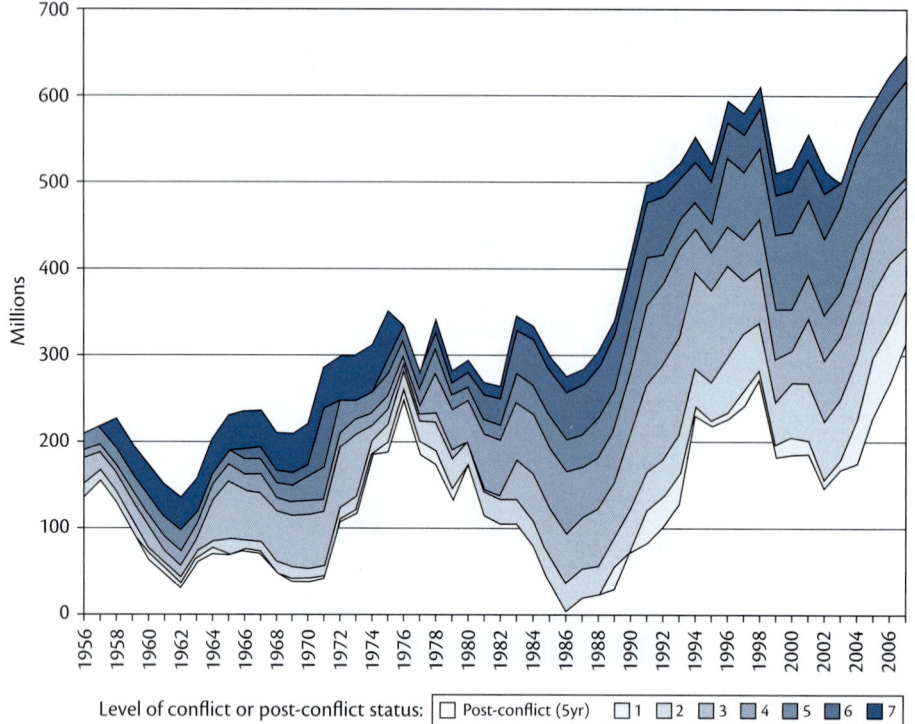

Fig. 11.10.2 Populations living in areas of conflict or post-conflict areas, 1956–2007.

Reproduced from Garfield, R.M. et al., Changes in size of populations and level of conflict since World War II: implications for health and health services. *Disaster Medicine and Public Health Preparedness*, Volume 6, Issue 3, pp. 241–6, Copyright © 2012, by permission of Cambridge University Press.

earthquakes and tsunamis often employ many times more construction and economic experts than health professionals and epidemiologists.

In tandem with this shift in focus from just averting deaths, has been the rise of a rights-based approach to programing. UNICEF defines a human rights-based approach as 'a conceptual framework for the process of human development that is normatively based on international human rights standards and operationally directed to promoting and protecting human rights' (UNICEF 2013). This framework, while not fundamentally contradictory, is very different in focus and in programme implications from the 'public health' approach of the last century's relief operations (CDC 1992; MSF 1997). This public health approach concentrated on how the relief community could reduce the most deaths and suffering with the assets available. This manifested in specific interventions like measles immunization, latrine construction, or primary healthcare clinics which brought broader benefits at low costs.

The rights-based approach has the advantage that it more readily encompasses issues like psychological suffering which are harder to measure, and values such as that girls should have equal chances for advancement as boys. But, the term 'normatively based' in the UNICEF definition is not well defined or constant. For example, UN resolutions or agency position statements often stress the need to have child re-unification programmes where benefit is difficult to demonstrate (Ager and Metzler 2012). In the public health approach the benefits and the cost-effectiveness of programmes are more readily established, and new ideas can be compared with established programmes. Rights-based programming, in contrast, has no equivalent incentive to demonstrate

cost-effectiveness and in fact is more driven by the strength of resolutions or declarations. Thus, if one wants to advocate for the value of counselling rape victims, in a rights-based framework it would be more efficient to attempt to pass a UN resolution than to evaluate the effectiveness of programmes in the field. With the public health approach, the opposite would be true.

In summary, humanitarian public health needs have broadened as the clientele served has begun to span a broader range of development levels, as the need to support people with chronic conditions including HIV has become more important. This may be an indication that the humanitarian endeavour has worked over the past half century. A Biafra-like scenario, where half the population died in a 4-year period, is rare today. Thus, the world's growing sources of compassion and aid can serve more than just those on the verge of death.

New developments for the twenty-first century

A host of new developments make it likely that relief work in the middle of the twenty-first century will look little like efforts in Biafra and South East Asia the century before. The advances of the past decades that will likely expand in the future can be considered in three broad categories: political trends, new approaches, and new technical advances. These categories interact with and influence each other, with technical advances often creating the potential for new orderings of social organization. While not comprehensive, this section seeks to imagine the likely changes to come in the field of humanitarian response.

Political trends

The melding of political and humanitarian agendas

National governmental political agendas and humanitarian relief have never been completely independent. In 1919, the US Congress formed the American Relief Administration (ARA), supposedly an independent NGO-like entity, headed by future President Herbert Hoover, to act as an independent famine relief mechanism in Europe in the years following the First World War (Fisher 1927). Oxfam, among the most famous of NGOs for its politically neutral funding sources, was formed in large part to lobby the British government to loosen the Allied blockade of occupied Europe (Oxfam n.d.). MSF co-founder Bernard Kouchner later became the French Minister of Humanitarian Affairs and the Foreign Minister, allotting funding for his creation, MSF. That humanitarian and political interests overlap is not completely unhealthy if in a democracy the populace is privately choosing to fund humanitarian ventures while simultaneously influencing the priorities of their government to do the same. On the other hand, countries are often in open competition with each other, and the linking of aid to enhance economic, military, or political competitiveness would be antithetical to the humanitarian endeavour. Two documents have attempted to keep humanitarian aid 'neutral' in the eyes of combatants and beneficiaries over the last part of the twentieth century.

Both the Third Geneva Convention of 1949 and the Red Cross Code of Conduct, to which most NGOs and the UN aspire to adhere, actively encourage the separation of humanitarian endeavours and self-interested agendas of individual states. The fourth tenet of the non-binding Red Cross Code of Conduct explicitly states, 'We shall endeavour not to act as instruments of government foreign policy' (International Federation of Red Cross and Red Crescent Societies n.d.). The ICRC and MSF are particularly famous for keeping political and military forces at arm's length even during the acute phases of crises. For example, during the 1992 crisis when Kurds fled northern Iraq but were not allowed into Turkey, the MSF refused to move in public or cooperate with any military personnel carrying a weapon. Many military personnel, including the British and American forces who had just invaded Iraq and were thus belligerents in this conflict, operated within the displaced community without weapons so as to work with MSF and other NGO personnel. Thus, until 2001, while funding influenced where relief went and what kinds of relief efforts were funded, an honest effort was made on the part of most donors and most international NGOs to not undertake patently political activities to advance the agenda of one country.

Nonetheless, a remarkable change in the landscape of humanitarian assistance has been the melding of political and humanitarian agendas after the terrorist attacks on New York City on 11 September 2001. Beginning with the invasion of Afghanistan, this narrowing separation of political and humanitarian ventures was often ignored or blurred. In October 2001, US Secretary of State Colin Powell addressed leaders of the American NGO community referring to their organizations as 'force multipliers' (International Federation of Red Cross and Red Crescent Societies n.d.). In Afghanistan, US humanitarian aid was openly discussed as a military tool for winning hearts and minds. In May of 2003, USAID Administrator Andrew Ntasios told the American NGOs that they needed to do a better job of advertising that the goods and services they provide to the Afghan people were coming from the US government. He told the American NGOs that they were an 'arm of the US government' (Klien 2003). Military activities such as distributions and school construction often made it unclear what was being done by combatants and what was being done by NGOs (Falconer 2009). MSF, who had been working in Afghanistan for 33 years, was forced to pull out there and in Iraq after their aid workers were targeted for assassination (Katz and Wright 2004). This blurring of aid and political agendas was again demonstrated when the Central Intelligence Agency hired a physician to conduct a sham vaccination campaign in Pakistan as part of the hunt for Osama Bin Laden in 2011 (Roberts and VanRooyen 2013; Rubenstein 2013).

The responses to natural disasters are not devoid of political overtones or agendas either. Following the 2005 tsunami in a largely Muslim area of the Pacific, the US Secretary of State called the disaster a 'wonderful opportunity' for the United States (Anonymous 2005). Preferential responses to former colonies and near neighbours appear to be an inevitable aspect of bilateral giving following natural calamities.

Since 2003, the number of annual incidents of violence against aid workers has doubled globally (Jackson 2012). It is not yet clear how the active blurring of humanitarian endeavours and military and political strategizing will play out in other non-conflict settings. There is little doubt that the humanitarian space available in politically tense settings will continue to diminish. New overt military and humanitarian blending during the Arab Spring of 2011, particularly in Libya, may create models of humanitarian and military blending less concerning than those seen in Afghanistan and Iraq and more acceptable to the affected populations. While the 1999 NATO bombing of Kosovo, and to a lesser extent, conflicts in Bosnia, Somalia, and Cambodia, set the stage for such transparent coordination between specific national agendas and humanitarian actors, that coordination has reached a new level of openness and complexity in recent years.

Humanitarian accountability

While aid agencies and the Red Cross Code of Conduct have always purported to support local empowerment and accountability of aid deliverers to beneficiaries and donors alike, many new developments have made that aspiration more common. The third edition of the Sphere Standards (Sphere Project 2011), perhaps the most widely followed guidelines for humanitarian practice, has an expanded emphasis on local participation and accountability to beneficiaries. In 2010, the UN passed an 'Accountability Framework' which may or may not result in more cost-efficient services on the ground, but certainly contributes to an international focus on recording transparently what is achieved by aid efforts and at what cost (UN 2010). Likewise, in 2011, the IASC developed an operational framework on how to ensure accountability to affected populations in humanitarian emergencies which is widely cited among humanitarian players (IASC 2011). Thirdly, the rise of wealthy, highly functional governments in all regions of the world raises the expectations of aid delivery procedures. For example, in 2003, India became a net creditor to the IMF and the WFP (Bijoy 2011). The rise of local NGOs as a primary international delivery mechanism, the prevalence of social networking, and the economic downturn in post-2008 Europe and North America all point toward a future where local and more players have a larger role in what aid is provided and how it will be disbursed.

New approaches

The growing appreciation of local capacities to provide exacting technical services combined with technical advances and greater emphasis on accountability, have paved the way in the past decade for exciting new ways of delivering aid. Among these are the following.

Home-based treatments

In the 1980s, the promotion of ORT was championed aggressively by the UN and aligned agencies because it was seen as a way to overcome the primary barrier to successful treatment of acute illness, namely early detection and treatment. The logic was that if people did not have to go through the effort of transporting the patient and their things to a medical facility, far more people would get treated. This was partially the logic behind the barefoot doctors programme in post-revolution China and a variety of other initiatives such as mobile clinics (Gish and Walker 1977).

Over the past decade, ambitions to provide antiretroviral treatments in areas of modest medical infrastructure and limited resources have resulted in a variety of models for drug distribution and patient monitoring using community or patient volunteers, or paid community health workers. The evidence suggests that patient management and monitoring schemes that are not physician based, where the monitoring occurs closer to the community level, are associated with better patient retention and survival (Callaghan et al. 2010). In focused settings of high malaria transmission, home-based treatment of fever has been shown to be an effective life-saving approach (Kidane and Morrow 2000).

In emergency settings, no home treatment strategies have received more attention or inspired as much enthusiasm as home therapeutic feeding. Home therapeutic feeding usually involves training and equipping mothers of malnourished children to cure the child at home with a nutritious ready-to-use food such as eeZeePaste NUT® or Plumpy'Nut® which come precooked and are resistant to bacterial growth. These ready-to-use home treatment products cut down on attrition in feeding centres, are a less expensive means for treating moderately malnourished children, and have been shown to be highly effective in field trials (Patel et al. 2005).

Crowd sourcing and mobile phones

The widespread availability of mobile phones and social media has made it possible to have the whole population participate in the monitoring of crises. One of the most well known of these efforts is the Ushahidi platform, formed during the violent period following the 2008 Kenyan elections (Ushahidi n.d.).

Perhaps the most dramatic application of the Ushahidi platform was in the February 2010 Chilean earthquake. The 8.8 magnitude quake was followed by a series of aftershocks that damaged thousands of buildings and ultimately killed an estimated 521 people. Within 48 hours of the initial quake, an Ushihidi–Chile platform was established and a team of graduate students in New York began mapping press reports and text messages to create a picture of damage and where people were trapped. One hundred 'incidents' were mapped in the first day of operation and 700 were mapped by the end of 3 days. In the weeks that followed, the Ushihidi platform updated local press members and the general public about food distributions, dangerous buildings, the occurrence of looting, and the progress of children re-attending school (Carlsen et al. 2011). Crowd sourcing strategies have also been used to inform Chinese authorities about acute situations in the aftermath of the Szechuan earthquake, to map the occurrence of sexual violence in Syria, and to map unsafe areas following the Japanese tsunami of 2011.

Mobile phones by themselves are allowing for some exciting innovations. Somalis affected by conflict have received humanitarian aid in the form of phone credits which can be used to purchase goods in local shops (Global Communities n.d.). Mobile phones have been given out in DR Congo with solar chargers to enable communities to call local authorities, the UN, or human rights workers when human rights abuses are taking place (Guinote 2012). Many of these initiatives are exploratory and controlled trials will be needed to establish such procedures as effective protective investments. One particularly interesting application of mobile phone use took place in the weeks following the 2010 earthquake in Haiti. The largest mobile-phone carrier sent out a signal detecting active SIM cards every day in relation to the nearest mobile-phone tower. They were thus able to record the position of 1.9 million active phones for 42 days before and 158 days after the earthquake. They estimated that 630,000 people in Port-au-Prince left the capital in the 19 days following the earthquake (Bengtsson et al. 2011). It is likely such mobile-phone tracking will become increasingly utilized in the years to come.

Monetary aid

As part of the promotion of local and beneficiary empowerment, providing aid that allows beneficiaries to set their own priorities has become increasingly popular. The example of giving displaced Somalis mobile-phone credit was discussed earlier. But, giving cash directly to beneficiaries in lieu of rations or material goods has several advantages. People are more likely to end up with what they want and the transfer costs are far lower. It has the potential to support the local economy including creating incentives for future increased local food production. It potentially has downsides such as driving local inflationary pressures and exposing people to increased risks of exploitation and extortion. A recent comprehensive review generally weighs the upsides as being greater than the downsides but suggests that implementers will need to choose the contexts carefully and develop methods for monitoring the success of direct cash assistance (Harvey 2007).

Closely related to monetary aid is the distribution of credit vouchers or coupons. Sometimes these have a specific purpose such as paying for school fees or uniforms. The most common flexible distribution is non-food item (NFI) or food item fairs where a select collection of vendors selling at predetermined prices gather in one place and beneficiaries with coupons spend their coupons at this one place and time. This system has the advantages of giving beneficiaries choice over the aid items they receive, it supports local markets, and leaves beneficiaries less open to local extortion. A recent analysis of such a NFI fair aimed at recently displaced populations in South Kivu Province, DR Congo found that local authorities missed most IDPs when constructing vulnerable lists and included many locals. At the end of the NFI distribution process, the NFI 'vulnerability score' as defined by UNICEF was unchanged by the distributions (O'Keeffe and Zadravecz 2012). As with so many new practices, implementation and evaluation procedures will need to be developed locally to match each context in order to maximize the efficiency of distributions via fairs and similar voucher systems.

New technical advances

A host of new technical advances or tools also create the potential for transformative advances in humanitarian relief in this century. Some technologies, such as the Global Positioning System (GPS), are so essential to relief efforts at present that it is hard to realize that the technology was almost non-existent 20 years ago. It is likely to evolve as a tracking tool for people, goods, and vehicles. One-dollar GPS transmitters will likely result in the tracking of individual cases of vaccines and drugs, and curb looting of warehouses by armed groups. Eye and fingerprint scanning technologies are reducing ration theft and false registrations across the globe. Advances in medicine, in diagnostic techniques, or protective devices such as long-lasting impregnated bednets, are constantly changing the practice of humanitarian relief. Some of the more promising new technical and medical breakthroughs are highlighted here.

Satellite imagery and remote sensing has already changed humanitarian practice. UNHCR has used satellite images to count people moving from Darfur into Chad. For years, remote sensing has been used to predict crop failure and crop yields. The destruction of villages in Darfur and DRC has been documented with before and after remote images. But lately, satellite imagery has been used to undermine the impunity brought by national sovereignty. For example, in 2006, the government of Zimbabwe cleared the major cities of people living on land for which they did not have deeds. It is estimated that 700,000 people had their homes destroyed (Tibaijuka 2005). Satellite images from before and after were the primary evidence of governmental wrongdoing and of the magnitude of the forced displacement. At the time, almost no international press was permitted to operate in Zimbabwe.

Cloud computing and Internet collaboration hold potential for a host of new ideas and innovations that may assist those responding to emergencies. Groups like Hackers for Humanity attempt to channel the efforts of Internet talents to charities (Hackers for Humanity n.d.). A variety of efforts to solve 'humanitarian problems' have been addressed by crowdsourcing for a solution. The degree to which these efforts change the lives of people affected by crises is difficult to assess. Some more focused software or cloud-based advances are now widely used and are filling specific niches. For example, Martus is a free online resource that allows human rights NGOs to store, access, and process data via a cloud mechanism that leaves no data on the computer used for entry. All data is encrypted and it is advertised that only users with their own passcode can access the data stored on multiple servers on multiple continents (Martus n.d.). Niche tools such as Martus are likely to increase the efficacy and safety of human rights and humanitarian work in the decades to come.

Internet accountability mechanisms: Google Earth and the Internet are allowing for greater accountability of aid from the perspective of small private donors. A model held up as innovative but already being reproduced is that of Charity Water. Charity Water does not directly implement water supply and sanitation projects, but instead subcontracts with local operational partners to turn Western private donations into water and sanitation infrastructure (Charity Water n.d.). Charity Water provides donors with the latitude and longitude of the specific things people have paid to have built so that over time they can see if indeed a well was built or public tap installed, and they can monitor if it continues to be used over time. They even install monitors so that donors to a specific project can see at any given moment if water is flowing from it. While not all aid is remotely visible, this process of linking donors to beneficiaries visually or by social media will likely grow over time and the process of humanitarian assistance will be better for it.

Conclusion

The twenty-first century is likely to see an ever growing humanitarian movement that will become more focused on economic, emergency preparedness, and developmental issues. Aid will be more politicized, while simultaneously more locally controlled and with greater accountability for implementation. The post-Biafra humanitarian endeavour has been associated with a dramatic decline in extreme episodes of excess deaths associated with crises and the new face of humanitarian relief, which often looks a lot like development work of old, has largely been built on the successes of twentieth-century humanitarian relief.

Acknowledgement

The author is a staff member of the World Health Organization. The author alone is responsible for the views expressed in this publication and they do not necessarily represent the decisions or policies of the World Health Organization.

Note

1. The term 'disaster risk management' can also be used, but ERM is the more common. While definitions vary, for the purposes of this chapter the terms 'disaster' and 'emergency' are used interchangeably.

References

Ager, A. and Metzler, J. (2012). *Child Friendly Spaces: A Structured Review of the Current Evidence-Base*. World Vision. [Online] Available at: http://reliefweb.int/sites/reliefweb.int/files/resources/CFS_Literature_Review_final_Aug_2012.pdf.

Anonymous (2005). Condi Rice: tsunami provided 'wonderful opportunity' for US. *Agence France Presse*, 18 January. Available at: http://www.commondreams.org/headlines05/0118-08.htm.

Bengtsson, L., Lu, X., Thorson, A., et al. (2011). Improved response to disasters and outbreaks by tracking population movements with mobile phone network data: a post-earthquake geospatial study in Haiti. *PLoS Medicine*, 8, 8.

Bern, C., Sniezek, J., Mathbor, G.M., et al. (1993). Risk factors for mortality in the Bangladesh cyclone of 1991. *Bulletin of the World Health Organization*, 71(1), 73–8.

Bhui, K.S., Hicks, M.H., Lahley, M., and Jones, E. (2012). A public health approach to understanding and preventing violent radicalization. *BMC Medicine*, 10, 16.

Bijoy, C.R. (2011). India: transiting to a global donor. In Reality of Aid Management Committee (eds.) *South-South Development Cooperation: A Challenge to the Aid System?* [Online] Available at: http://www.realityofaid.org/userfiles/roareports/roareport_3ce2522270.pdf.

Brennan, R.J., Bradt, D.A., and Abrahams, J. (2009). Medical issues in disasters. In P. Cameron, G.A. Jelinek, A.M. Kelly, et al. (eds.) *Textbook of Adult Emergency Medicine* (3rd ed.), pp. 785–92. London: Churchill Livingstone.

Burnham, G., Lafta, R., Doocy, S., and Roberts, L. (2006). Mortality after the 2003 invasion of Iraq: a cross-sectional cluster sample survey. *The Lancet*, 368, 1421–8.

Callaghan, M., Ford, N., and Schneider, H. (2010). A systematic review of task- shifting for HIV treatment and care in Africa. *Human Resources for Health*, 8, 8.

Carlsen, J., Dougherty, J., Iacucci, A.A., et al. (2011). *Grant Report for Mozilla Corporation*. [Online] Available at http://newmediatask force.files.wordpress.com/2011/02/ushahidi-chile-grant-report-16-jan-2011.pdf.

Centers for Disease Control (1992). Famine-affected, refugee, and displaced populations: recommendations for public health issues. *Morbidity and Mortality Weekly Report*, 2441(13), 1–76.

Charity Water (n.d.). Website. [Online] Available at: https://www.charity-water.org.

Coghlan, B., Brennan, R.J., Ngoy, P., et al. (2006). Mortality in the Democratic Republic of Congo: a nationwide survey. *The Lancet*, 367, 44–51.

Falconer, B. (2009). Military hijacking aid effort in Afghanistan, say NGOs. *Mother Jones*, 3 April.

Fisher, H.H. (1927). *The Famine in Soviet Russia, 1919–1923: The Operations of the American Relief Administration*. New York: Macmillan.

Gardemann, J. (2002). Primary health care in complex humanitarian emergencies: Rwanda and Kosovo experiences and their implications for public health training. *Croatian Medical Journal*, 43(2), 148–55.

Garfield, R.M., Polonsky, J., and Burkle, F.M. (2012). Changes in size of populations and level of conflict since World War II: implications for health and health services. *Disaster Medicine and Public Health Preparedness*, 6(3), 241–6.

Gish, O. and Walker, G. (1977). *Mobile Health Services*. London: Tri-Med Books Ltd.

Glass, R., Nieburg, P., Cates, W., et al. (1980). Rapid assessment of health status and preventive-medicine needs in newly arrived Kampuchean refugees, Sa Kaeo, Thailand. *The Lancet*, 315, 868–72.

Gleditsch, N.P., Wallensteen, P., Eriksson, M., et al. (2002). Armed conflict 1946–2001: a new dataset. *Journal of Peace Research*, 39(5), 615–37.

Global Communities (n.d.). http://www.chfinternational.org/node/36995.

Guinote, F. (2012). *Calling for Help: How Cell Phones Help Protect Children's Rights in the DRC*. Available at: http://womensrefugeecommission.org/blog/1292-calling-for-help-how-cell-phones-help-protect-childrens-rights-in-the-drc

Hackers for Humanity (n.d.). Website. [Online] Available at: http://www.hackersforhumanity.com/.

Harvey, P. (2007). *Cash-Based Responses in Emergencies*. Overseas Development Group (ODI), Humanitarian Policy Group Briefing Paper 25. London: Overseas Development Group.

Ifekwunigwe, A.E., Grasset, N., Glass, R., and Foster, S. (1980). Immune response to measles and smallpox vaccinations in malnourished children. *American Journal of Clinical Nutrition*, 33(3), 621–4.

Interagency Standing Committee (2011). *End Discrimination and End Discrimination and Ensure Equitable Outcomes for All Outcomes for All. 2010–2011 Accountability Frameworks for AGDM and Targeted Actions*. Geneva: UN.

Interagency Standing Committee (2013). *Transformative Agenda Protocols*. [Online] Available at: http://www.humanitarianinfo.org/iasc/pageloader.aspx?page=content-documents-default&publish=0.

International Crisis Group (2005). *Ethiopia and Eritrea: Preventing War*. Africa Report No. 101, 22 December 2005. [Online] Available at: http://www.crisisgroup.org/~/media/Files/africa/horn-of-africa/ethiopia-eritrea/Ethiopia%20and%20Eritrea%20Preventing%20War.

International Federation of Red Cross and Red Crescent Societies (2012). *World Disasters Report, 2012*. Geneva: IFRC.

International Federation of Red Cross and Red Crescent Societies (n.d.). *Red Cross Code of Conduct*. [Online] Available at: http://www.ifrc.org/en/publications-and-reports/code-of-conduct/.

International Federation of the Red Cross (2006). *What is VCA? An Introduction to Vulnerability and Capacity Assessment*. Geneva: IFRC.

International Strategy for Disaster Reduction (2009). *2009 UNISDR Terminology on Disaster Risk Reduction*. Geneva: UNISDR.

Jackson, A. (2012). Remembering the humanitarians. *Aljazeera*, 16 August. [Online] Available at: http://www.aljazeera.com/indepth/opinion/2012/08/201281213836229581.html.

Katz, I.T. and Wright, A.A. (2004). Collateral damage – Médecins sans Frontières leaves Afghanistan and Iraq. *The New England Journal of Medicine*, 351, 2571–3.

Kidane, G. and Morrow, R.H. (2000). Teaching mothers to provide home treatment of malaria in Tigray, Ethiopia: a randomised trial. *The Lancet*, 356, 550–5.

Klien, N. (2003). Bush to NGOs: watch your mouths. *The Globe and Mail (Canada)*, 30 June.

Lopez, A.D., Mathers, C.D., Ezzati, M., et al. (2006). Global and regional burden of disease and risk factors, 2001: systematic analysis of population health data. *The Lancet*, 379, 1747–57.

Mallick, D.K., Rahman, A., Alam, M., et al. (2005). Case study 3: Bangladesh floods in Bangladesh: a shift from disaster management towards disaster preparedness. *IDS Bulletin*, 36(4), 53–70.

Martus (n.d.). Website. [Online] Available at: https://www.martus.org/.

Médecins Sans Frontières (1997). *Refugee Health*. London: Macmillan Education Ltd.

O'Brien, D.P., Venis, S., Greig, J., et al. (2010). Provision of antiretroviral treatment in conflict settings: the experience of Médecins Sans Frontières. *Conflict and Health*, 4, 12.

O'Keeffe, J. and Zadravecz, F. (2012). *Bunyakiri NFI Post-Fair Evaluation*. Unpublished Report for RHA. Columbia Mailman School of Public Health.

Oxfam (n.d.). *History of Oxfam*. [Online] Available at: http://www.oxfam.org.uk/what-we-do/about-us/history-of-oxfam.

Pan American Health Organization (2000). *Natural Disasters: Protecting the Public Health*. Washington, DC: PAHO.

Pan American Health Organization (2002). *Guidelines for Vulnerability Reduction in the Design of New Health Facilities*. Washington, DC: PAHO.

Patel, M.P., Sandige, H.L., Ndekha, M.J., et al. (2005). Supplemental feeding with ready-to-use therapeutic food in Malawian children at risk of malnutrition. *Journal of Health, Population and Nutrition*, 23(4), 351–7.

Roberts, L. (2013). *The Lack of an Evidence Base for Humanitarian Interventions*. Paper presented at Evidence Live, Oxford, UK 24 March. Abstract available at: http://www.evidencelive.org/2013/programme.

Roberts, L. and VanRooyen, M.J. (2013). Ensuring public health neutrality. *The New England Journal of Medicine*, 368, 1073–5.

Rubenstein, L. (2013). Unhealthy practice. *Foreign Affairs*, 24 April. Available at: http://www.foreignaffairs.com/articles/139344/leonard-s-rubenstein/unhealthy-practice.

Sack, R.B., Cassels, J., Mitra, R., et al. (1970). The use of oral replacement solutions in the treatment of cholera and other severe diarrhea. *Bulletin of the World Health Organization*, 43, 351–60.

Salama, P., Spiegel, P., and Brennan, R. (2001). No less vulnerable: the internally displaced in humanitarian emergencies. *The Lancet*, 357, 1430–1.

Sphere Project (2011). *The Sphere Project: Humanitarian Charter and Minimum Standards for Humanitarian Response*. Rugby: Practical Action Publishing.

Tibaijuka, A.K. (2005). *Report of the Fact-Finding Mission to Zimbabwe to Assess the Scope and Impact of Operation Murambatsvina by the UN Special Envoy on Human Settlements Issues in Zimbabwe July 2005*. [Online] Available at: http://ww2.unhabitat.org/documents/ZimbabweReport.pdf.

Toole, M.J., Nieberg, P., and Waldman, R.J. (1988). The association between inadequate rations, undernutrition prevalence, and mortality in refugee camps: case studies of refugee populations in Eastern Thailand,

1979–1980, and Eastern Sudan, 1984–1985. *Journal of Tropical Pediatrics*, 34(5), 218–24.

Toole, M.J. Steketee, R.W., Waldman, R.J., Nieburg, P. (1989). Measles prevention and control in emergency settings. *Bulletin of the World Health Organization*, 67, 381–8.

Toole, M.J. and Waldman, R.J. (1990). Prevention of excess mortality in refugee and displaced populations in developing countries. *Journal of the American Medical Association*, 263(24), 3296–302.

Toole, M.J. and Waldman, R.J. (1997). The public health aspects of complex emergencies and refugee situations. *Annual Review of Public Health*, 18, 283–312.

Twyman, P. (2012). Presentation at 'Health in Times of Crisis: Preparing and Responding Effectively'. Mailman School of Public Health, New York, 30 April.

United Nations (2010). *Agenda Item 130: Review of the Efficiency of the Administrative and Financial Functioning of the United Nations*. 29 January 2010. [Online] Available at: http://www.un.org/en/strengtheningtheun/pdf/A-64-640.pdf.

United Nations Children's Fund (2013). *Human Rights-based Approach to Programming*. Global Humanitarian Assistance. [Online] Available at: http://www.unicef.org/policyanalysis/rights/index.html. See data at: https://docs.google.com/spreadsheet/ccc?key=0AvGCmVxSBN08dFJ2cGRKRkhpYTdWU0liNXgtTy1odlE#gid=24.

United Nations Development Programme (2010). *Success Story Leads. Bangladesh: Comprehensive Disaster Management Programme*. [Online] Available at: http://web.undp.org/comtoolkit/success-stories/ASIA-Bangladesh-crisisprev.shtml.

United Nations International Strategy for Disaster Reduction (2010). *Emerging Challenges for Early Warning Systems in Context of Climate Change and Urbanization*. Coppet: Humanitarian & Development Network.

Uppsala Conflict Data Program (n.d.). *Uppsala Conflict Data Program*. [Online] Available at: http://www.pcr.uu.se/research/ucdp/.

Ushahidi (n.d.). Website. [Online] Available at: http://www.ushahidi.com/about-us.

Western, K.A. (1972). *The Epidemiology of Natural and Manmade Disasters: The Present State of the Art*. Dissertation for D.T.P.H., University of London.

World Bank (2011). *World Development Report 2011: Conflict, Security and Development*. Washington, DC: World Bank.

World Bank Global Facility for Disaster Reduction and Recovery (2011). *Analysing the Social Impacts of Disasters. Volume 1: Methodology*. Washington, DC: World Bank.

World Health Organization (2005). *International Health Regulations (2005)* (2nd ed.). Geneva: WHO.

World Health Organization (2007). *Mass Casualty Management Systems*. Geneva: WHO.

World Health Organization (2011a). *Strengthening Response to Pandemics and other Public-Health Emergencies*. Geneva: WHO.

World Health Organization (2011b). *Disaster Risk Management for Health: Fact Sheets*. [Online] Available at: http://www.who.int/hac/techguidance/preparedness/factsheets/en/index.html.

World Health Organization, UNAIDS, and United Nations Children's Fund (2011). *Global HIV/AIDS Response: Epidemic Update and Health Sector Progress towards Universal Access*. Geneva: WHO. Available at: http://www.who.int/hiv/pub/progress_report2011/en/index.html.

World Health Organization and World Meteorological Organization (2012). *Atlas of Health and Climate*. Geneva: WHO.

11.11

Principles of public health emergency response for acute environmental, chemical, and radiation incidents

Naima Bradley, Jill Meara, and Virginia Murray

Introduction to principles of public health emergency response

Acute environmental, chemical, and radiation incidents and emergencies can have significant effects on people's health, including loss of life. New threats reveal new challenges for managing the health risks and effects of emergencies. Deaths, injuries, diseases, disabilities, psychosocial problems, and other health impacts can be avoided or reduced by skilled disaster management involving health and other sectors.

Incident and emergency risk management for health refers to the systematic analysis and management of health risks, posed by incidents and emergencies, through a combination of:

◆ Hazard and vulnerability reduction to prevent and mitigate risks.

◆ Preparedness.

◆ Response.

◆ Recovery measures.

This is summarized in Fig. 11.11.1. Public health services and expertise have a vital role in reducing harm and saving life at every stage in this cycle.

The traditional focus of the health sector has been on emergency response. The challenge is to broaden the focus of incident and emergency risk management to a more proactive approach which emphasizes prevention and mitigation, and the development of community and country capacities to provide timely and effective response and recovery. Resilient health systems based on primary healthcare at community level can reduce underlying vulnerability, protect health facilities and services, and help to scale-up the response to meet the wide-ranging health needs.

Examples of natural, biological, technological and societal hazards that can put the health of vulnerable people at risk and cause significant harm to public health include:

◆ Natural: earthquake, landslide, tsunami, cyclone, flood or drought.

◆ Biological: epidemic disease, infestations of pests.

◆ Technological: chemical or radiological releases or contamination, transport crashes.

◆ Societal: conflict, stampedes, acts of terrorism.

Emergencies and other crises may cause ill health directly or through the disruption of health services, leaving people without access to healthcare in times of emergency. They also affect basic infrastructure such as water supplies and safe shelter which are essential for public health.

International consensus views disasters as barriers to progress on the health-related Millennium Development Goals (MDGs), as they often set back hard-earned development gains in health and other sectors. One United Nations instrument that takes forward the emergency and disaster agenda is the *Hyogo Framework for Action 2005–2015: Building the Resilience of Nations and Communities to Disasters* (United Nations Office for Disaster Risk Reduction 2007). This 10-year plan, which will be extended in 2015 for the next 20–30 years, focuses on making the world safer from natural hazards and other emergencies. It identifies five priorities for action which are:

◆ Governance: organizational, legal, and policy frameworks.

◆ Risk identification, assessment, monitoring, and early warning.

◆ Knowledge management and education.

◆ Reducing underlying risk factors.

◆ Preparedness for effective response and recovery.

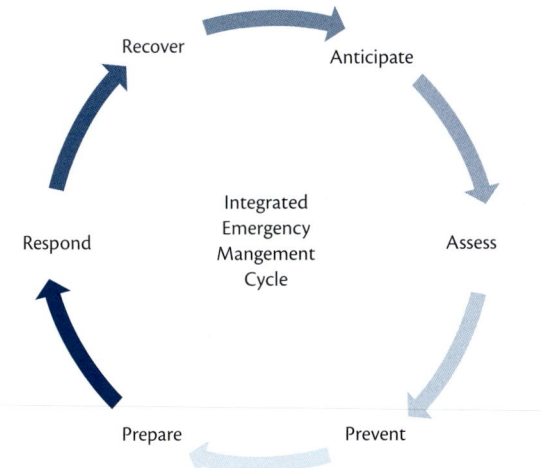

Fig. 11.11.1 The integrated emergency management cycle.
Reproduced with permission from National Health Service (NHS), *NHS Commissioning Board Emergency Preparedness Framework 2013*, Copyright © 2013, available from http://www.england.nhs.uk/wp-content/uploads/ 2013/03/eprr-framework.pdf.

Progress has been made at global, regional, national, and community levels, but countries' capacity for risk reduction, emergency preparedness, response, and recovery remains extremely variable. The 2007 World Health Organization (WHO) global assessment found that less than 50 per cent of national health sectors had a specified budget for emergency preparedness and response (United Nations Office for Disaster Risk Reduction 2007). Factors affecting capacity included:

◆ Weak health and disaster management systems.

◆ Lack of access to resources and know-how.

◆ Continuing insecurity due to conflict.

A number of high-risk countries have strengthened their disaster prevention, preparedness, and response systems; in some countries, the health sector has led initiatives developing multisectoral approaches to emergency risk management. Multisectoral working is needed to protect the health of the population during and after a major incident or emergency. Wider determinants of health such as water, sanitation, nutrition, and security also need to be adequately addressed. Essential infrastructure such as communications, logistics, energy and water supplies, emergency services, and banking facilities need to be protected through multisectoral working to ensure the continuity of health services.

This chapter, following from Chapter 11.10 in this volume, considers the various stages of an emergency response and the role of public health at each stage. Case studies are used to illustrate the principles described. Of note is the importance of emergency responders at the scene to save life and protect people (including the emergency responders).

This chapter addresses the following:

◆ *Local command and control management arrangements for emergency response:* including the local emergency response arrangements and how they interact with international obligations such as the International Health Regulations from the WHO (see Chapter 11.10).

◆ *Exposure and risk assessment:* in any incident response it is essential to assess exposure, as soon as possible, to members of the public, workers, and responders using biological or environmental monitoring or modelling. This will allow assessment of health risks to exposed people and define further environmental and people sampling and modelling to refine risk assessments. There are significant differences in exposure assessment methods between chemical and radiation incidents.

◆ *Countermeasures for public health protection:* countermeasures are important to ensure that advice that is given early enough to be effective to reduce exposure, even at the early stages of an incident when little is known. Countermeasures are usually advised by public health professionals in conjunction with their partners in response. Countermeasures are broadly similar for all hazards and include decontamination, sheltering, evacuation, specific antidotes, and medical treatments. The chapter touches on mechanisms of recovery and return to normal.

◆ *Public reassurance in emergencies and incidents:* it is essential to have clear messages for information and reassurance to cover both affected and unaffected members of the public. These need to build trust in the systems that have been invoked to protect the public.

◆ *Follow-up of affected populations* is often essential. Approaches on how to undertake appropriate follow-up of affected populations including ongoing care and epidemiological follow up are discussed in the context of the Public Health England health registers protocol.

◆ *Identify and publish the lessons learned* and examine the importance of sharing learning to decrease the chance of an incident reoccurring and to identify lessons to improve emergency preparedness, response, and recovery.

◆ *Conclusion:* including evidence and research gaps and future challenges.

◆ *Additional sources of information.*

Planning for an effective response: legislative background

Developing and testing local, regional, and national emergency plans is key to an effective emergency response. These plans should be tailored to address the most important risks to health from natural disasters, man-made accidents, and malicious attacks. At national level, the UK government monitors the most significant potential threats through its National Risk Assessment (NRA). This is a confidential assessment conducted every year, covering a 5-year time horizon. In 2013, the National Risk Register (NRR), the public version of the NRA, which identifies the highest priority emergency risks taking into account both likelihood and impact, added a new risk to the register, the risk from wildfires (Cabinet Office 2013).

The NRR and relevant local risk registers will identify the impact of emergencies (e.g. fires, explosions, and major releases) from major industrial sites as a significant risk. The European Union (EU) Seveso Directive's main aim is to prevent and mitigate the effects of emergencies at approximately 10,000 sites across Europe. A new Directive on the control of major accident hazards involving dangerous substances (known as 'Seveso III'), published in 2012, to be implemented in the United Kingdom by 2015 amends the scope of the legislation and has new requirements for public participation and better access to information about risks from activities at certain industrial sites.

Case study: the UK Civil Contingencies Act and Control of Major Accident Hazards Regulations

A key piece of emergency planning legislation is the Civil Contingencies Act 2004 (CCA); its principal objective is to ensure consistency across all government departments and agencies, whilst setting clear responsibilities for frontline responders at a local level. The CCA defines two categories of organizations: category 1 responders such as emergency services, local authorities, health bodies, and government departments are subject to the full set of civil protection duties. The primary role for category 2 organizations is to cooperate and share relevant information with category 1 responders. Examples of category 2 responders are utility companies and transport providers. Local Health Resilience Partnerships (LHRPs) have been created to provide strategic forums for joint planning for emergencies in the new health system. They will support the health sector's contribution to multi-agency planning through Local Resilience Forums (LRFs).

Three elements are identified in the definition of civil emergency under the CCA: serious damage to human welfare, the environment, and national security.

Local risk registers and plans are needed to reflect unique local characteristics; for example, coastal flooding will only affect certain areas of the country. Most local risks need to be considered in a multi-agency setting; this is done through LRFs which include representatives from local emergency responders as well as public, private, and voluntary organizations. LRFs publish local risk registers and develop and exercise local emergency plans.

In the United Kingdom, the Control of Major Accident Hazards Regulations 1999 (COMAH), as amended in 2005, and the Control of Major Accident Hazard Regulations (Northern Ireland) 2000 implement the requirements of the Seveso Directive (currently Seveso II). They aim to prevent and mitigate the effects of major incidents involving dangerous substances, therefore they cover high-risk sites such as those in the chemical and petro-chemical sectors. COMAH defines two types of sites called 'top tier' and 'lower tier'. For the higher-risk 'top tier' sites, local authorities will prepare and test emergency plans addressing the consequences of foreseeable major accidents from these sites.

Case study: Seveso accident

In 1976, there was a major incident at a chemical plant manufacturing pesticides and herbicides near the town of Seveso, Italy (Pesatori et al. 2003). The resulting cloud covered an 18-square kilometre area. Ten days after the accident, 2,3,7,8-tetrachlorodibenzo-p-dioxin (TCDD) was confirmed as one of the main components of the toxic cloud. TCDD, the most toxic dioxin, is toxic by ingestion and inhalation. The International Agency for Research on Cancer classifies TCDD as a chemical which can cause cancer in humans.

The dispersal of TCDD resulted in widespread contamination of land and vegetation. Although no fatalities were reported,

193 cases of chloracne were observed, mainly in children who were exposed outdoors in the immediate aftermath. Several hundred people were evacuated and approximately 2000 were treated. Studies of the long-term impacts of this exposure are still under way.

This accident prompted the adoption of legislation aimed at the prevention and control of such accidents.

Nuclear licensed sites

Many countries have separate arrangements for regulation of ionizing radiations and the nuclear industry. For example, in the United Kingdom, emergency preparedness duties with respect to nuclear sites are described in the Radiation (Emergency Preparedness and Public Information) Regulations (REPPIR) 2001. As for the COMAH regulations, the REPPIR regulations take precedence over the CCA in relation to specialized emergency preparedness and response but CCA guidance applies in areas not covered by these regulations.

The Office for Nuclear Regulation identifies the emergency planning zones (DEPZ) for sites where there could be an off-site radioactive release. There is a legal requirement for local authorities to prepare plans for responding to an off-site nuclear emergency, including within the DEPZ.

International Health Regulations

The International Health Regulations (IHR), agreed by the World Health Assembly in 2005 and revised in 2007 (WHO 2008), were introduced to protect the world from global health threats. The need for such an internationally binding instrument was identified following the emergence of severe acute respiratory syndrome in 2003, which demonstrated how quickly a new disease could spread. As a result, 196 countries acknowledged a responsibility for collective action against infectious diseases, and food and environmental contamination, deemed to be public health emergencies of international concern. Member states are responsible for developing, strengthening, and maintaining the capacity to detect, assess the risks of, and respond to public health emergencies. Furthermore, countries are required to notify the WHO of these threats through their designated National IHR Focal Point within 24 hours.

The European Commission identified a need to ensure consistent and coordinated implementation of the IHR by the EU Member States and address gaps in emergency planning, response, risk assessment and management, and risk communication identified during cross-border emergencies such as the pandemic influenza (H1N1) in 2009/2010. The Commission also acknowledged that cross-border arrangements needed to be strengthened to deal with environmental incidents such as the volcanic ash cloud in 2010. As a result, the EU Decision on serious cross-border threats to health was published to strengthen the EU's capabilities to deal with threats of biological, chemical, and unknown origin (European Commission 2013). Extreme weather and other natural events such as heat waves and cold spells are included in the scope of the EU Decision but radiological or nuclear health threats are not as they are already dealt with by the Euratom Treaty establishing the European Atomic Energy Community.

Emergency response framework

Rapid implementation of collaborative arrangements described in the emergency plans, coordination, and communication are the key to successful management of an emergency. Most emergencies are handled at the local level by emergency services and local responders. Established local early alerting mechanisms will notify other agencies and provide support and advice. For major incidents, the multi-agency coordination mechanism is managed through a 'command and control' flexible framework involving strategic, tactical, and operational levels. The gold command will develop the strategy to manage the many aspects of an incident, the silver level will identify how to implement the strategy, direct the operations, and monitor progress, and the bronze level will carry out the tactical decisions and involve the physical deployment of resources. In the initial phase of an incident, the local ambulance service, fire service, and/or police will usually be the first blue-light services on the scene. They provide the bronze level management of the incident including setting up cordons, fighting fires, and treating casualties.

The multi-agency coordination groups will be led by the most appropriate emergency responder. For example, the police may lead in cases where a crime or threat to public safety is involved (e.g. deliberate release of a toxic chemical). For large accidental fires, the response may be led by the fire and rescue services. In the event of an incident with significant health and environmental impact, a Strategic Co-ordinating Group can request the establishment of a Science and Technical Advice Cell (STAC) to coordinate the scientific and technical advice, including health advice during the response to an emergency.

Case study: levels of national emergency response in the United Kingdom

At national level, the UK government defines three levels of response: significant (level 1), (e.g. severe weather), serious (level 2) (e.g. pandemic influenza), and catastrophic (level 3). Level 1 emergencies require the involvement of a lead government department or a Devolved Administration. Level 2 and level 3 emergencies require a response coordinated by the Cabinet Office Briefing Rooms (COBR). The 7 July London bombings provide an example of a level 2 emergency. The Prime Minister would lead a level 3 emergency with very high and widespread impact (e.g. Chernobyl-type accident).

Once activated, COBR coordinates and monitors the national response, supported by a number of cells providing authoritative advice on, for example, intelligence, recovery, impact management, response, and public information. Specialist scientific and technical advice will be coordinated by the Science Advisory Group for Emergencies (SAGE). The SAGE membership will depend on the type of incident but will include national specialist advisors and, if necessary, the wider scientific and technical community. For example, a major release from an industrial site in England would involve the site operator for site-specific information; the Department of Health and Public Health England for scientific and technical advice on the health effects of the release; the health service to coordinate the NHS response; the health and safety, environmental, and food regulators to provide advice on relevant areas; and the national meteorological agency to provide weather information, for example, dispersion modelling of the release.

Situation reports (Sit Reps) will be required from government departments, agencies, and regional and local responders to build an up-to-date and accurate picture of the incident, its impacts, and what is being done to manage them. The output will be the 'Common Recognised Information Picture' or CRIP shared with all responders.

Fig. 11.11.2 shows the link between local, regional, and national interactions in the UK emergency response depending on the geographical spread and severity of the impacts.

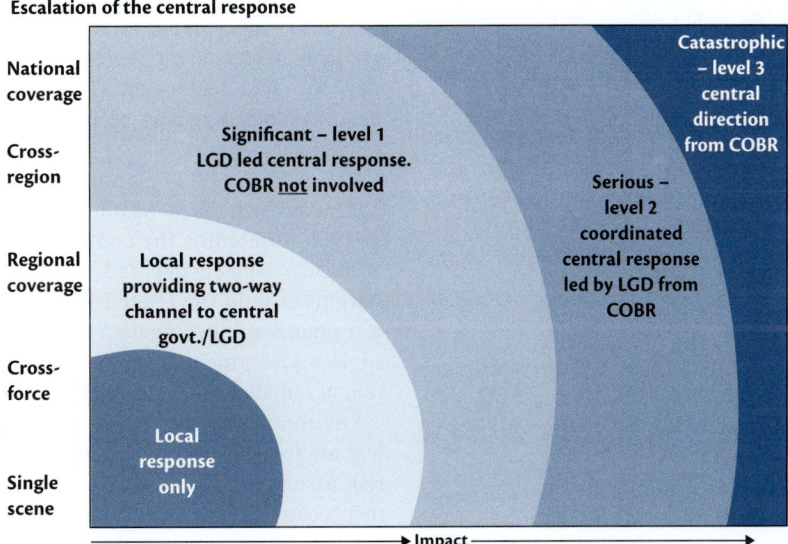

Escalation of the central response

Fig. 11.11.2 Local, regional, and national interactions in the UK emergency response depending on the geographical spread and severity of the impacts.
Reproduced from Cabinet Office Civil Contingencies Secretariat, *Emergency Response and Recovery: Non statutory guidance accompanying the Civil Contingencies Act 2004* © Crown Copyright 2013, licence under the Open Government Licence v.2.0, available from https://www.gov.uk/government/uploads/system/ uploads/attachment_data/file/253488/ Emergency_Response_and_ Recovery_5th_ edition_October_2013.pdf.

Exposure and risk assessment

Problem formulation

Immediate risks to health should be addressed by precautionary advice given at an early stage. This will usually be in line with pre-prepared advice contained in the emergency plans (e.g. sheltering or evacuation to reduce or eliminate exposures, depending on the scenario).

A clear description of the problem assists in selecting the level or type of risk assessment required (e.g. qualitative/quantitative) and ensuring that risk management decisions are as robust as possible. Basic information is required at an early stage such as:

◆ What time did the incident occur (and how long is it likely to last)?

◆ What is the location of the incident?

◆ What is the hazard, that is, the chemical or radiological agent that may cause adverse health effects?

◆ Who is potentially affected?

Communication with partner agencies is a vital aspect of the emergency response which will allow rapid access to the good quality scientific and technical information needed for effective public health risk assessment and response. Additional information gathered through these channels will fill in the information gaps and refine the risk assessment. It is important to record and update all the information received, noting the uncertainties and assumptions.

A very basic conceptual model can be used at this stage. For emergencies, this is presented in the form of the 'source–pathway–receptor' model (Box 11.11.1). Without a source–pathway–receptor linkage, harm will not occur.

Risk assessment

Risk assessment is one component of the risk management process. The risk assessment stage will take into account the probability of an event occurring and the magnitude of the consequences of the event. In the early stages of an incident, the risk assessment will be subjective but will be refined and quantified as more information is gathered.

The generic risk assessment process involves four stages: hazard identification, assessing the consequences, assessing their probabilities, and characterizing the risks and uncertainties (Gormley et al. 2011). In an emergency situation, the public health risk assessment can be done through a combination of qualitative and quantitative methods.

The source

Information about the source can be obtained from the site operator for industrial accidents. In the United Kingdom, if the incident is the result of a road traffic accident involving radioactive

---

Box 11.11.1 Example of source–pathway–receptor model

Source: chemical release due to road traffic accident involving a tanker.
Pathway: dispersion of the chemical through the air.
Receptor: residents (children and adults).

---

materials, information is available from RADSAFE whose remit is to provide advice and assistance to its members. The specialized fire and rescue's hazardous materials and environmental protection officers will provide invaluable, on-the-scene information in the early phase of a chemical incident. The key requirement is to identify the chemical(s) released and its/their physical form. The chemical's physico-chemical properties will provide information on its ease of spread throughout the environment. Understanding its toxicological properties and the quantities released is also key to successful risk assessment.

Most incidents involving chemicals and radiation will require access to specialist advice to interpret the information gathered. It is important to remember that the substances contained in a product inventory are not always those of most public health concern. For example, a fire may break chemicals down to form complex molecules and other hazards depending on the temperature and oxygen availability.

The pathway

The pathway describes how the pollutant spreads in the environment. If it is a gas, the main pathway will be through the air and dispersion modelling can be used to predict how it will move spatially and temporally. Liquids, depending on their volatility, may disperse through the soil, water, and air. Solids will disperse more slowly; however, fine solids will form dusts that can disperse quickly in the right conditions. Food can also be part of a complex exposure pathway, for example, some chemicals travelling in the air can be deposited on crops which are later ingested leading to exposure.

Exposure to a substance can be assessed through a combination of methods: by sampling or monitoring the external environment, by modelling the external environment, or by measuring the substance in the body.

Timely information on the type, concentration, and environmental distribution of the pollutants is needed for public health risk assessment. The concentration of a substance in the environment can be monitored and/or modelled with varying degrees of accuracy and precision depending on the time and resources available. Unless arrangements have been made at the planning stage for rapid deployment of sampling and measurement equipment, information may be received too late to inform the risk assessment.

An example of a planned monitoring system is the UK Radioactive Incident Monitoring Network (RIMNET), set up in 1988 to monitor the consequences for the United Kingdom of nuclear incidents abroad. RIMNET comprises 96 monitoring stations around the United Kingdom. A range of organizations can submit monitoring data to RIMNET. Public Health England advises government departments on the public health interpretation of radiation monitoring data.

Environmental matrices containing the substance of interest (e.g. air, food, water, dust, or soils) can be used to aid public health risk assessment. In certain circumstances, real-time measurements can be made, for example, for chemicals in air or monitoring of levels of radiation. Monitoring should be planned as soon as possible. The monitoring strategy should ensure that the samples taken are representative of the general bulk material as substances are rarely homogeneously dispersed in the environmental media. The methods used to take and store the samples should not degrade the substance of interest. The analytical techniques used must be appropriately sensitive, accurate, and reproducible. For direct measurements, monitoring over the right time interval allows comparison with any predefined health based standards.

Modelling external exposure involves computer simulation to estimate the pollutants' concentration and predict their behaviour through one or more environmental media. Air dispersion models are often used during large-scale incidents. A number of data sources are required, depending on the sophistication of the model, for example, source term, weather data, and topography.

Monitoring and modelling should be considered together in a multi-agency group attended by specialist scientific staff as information gained from monitoring could be used to inform the model and model outputs can predict areas to monitor for effective exposure assessments. The uncertainties for this type of external exposure assessment include the accuracy, completeness, and relevance of the data.

The receptors

For the purpose of a health risk assessment, the receptors are the people potentially exposed. Some population groups exhibit adverse health effects when exposed to lower pollutant levels or react more quickly than the general population. These are called 'sensitive receptors'. Children, the elderly, people with pre-existing diseases, and pregnant women may be sensitive receptors, depending on the hazard involved.

The primary exposure routes for chemicals are absorption (contact between the chemical and the skin or eyes), inhalation (breathed into the lungs), ingestion (through contaminated food and/or water), and injection (through breaks in the skin). For radioactive materials, an additional exposure route is external irradiation, where gamma and/or beta radiation particles emitted by materials outside the body penetrate the skin and deposit their energy inside. Alpha particles are a risk to human health only when taken into the body by inhalation, ingestion, or through open wounds as they are easily stopped by the dead layers of the skin.

The duration of exposure is important to assess and estimate health risks. Single or short-term exposures to some chemicals at a sufficient concentration can trigger adverse health effects (e.g. carbon monoxide). Other chemicals require exposure for days and months to cause lasting health effects (e.g. some respiratory irritants).

Once inside the body, chemicals move through the metabolic pathways, are transformed, and either stored or eliminated. Biological markers of exposure can be used to enhance the risk assessment and measure the internal dose. However, the right study design, including the choice of the most appropriate body fluid or tissue to be tested, collection, storage, processing, and analytical protocols require a thorough understanding of the exposure route, absorption, and metabolism of the chemical of interest. Specialist scientific advice should be sought before considering human bio-monitoring to assess exposure.

Risk characterization

This step of the risk assessment is usually a quantitative assessment involving a comparison of the concentrations measured against health-based values, where they exist. These values are different for different chemicals and for the same chemicals in different environmental matrices. For example, health guidelines have been set for lead in air, water, and in blood. Health-based values

are derived at levels below which adverse health effects are considered unlikely for so-called threshold chemicals. Exposure to some chemicals can lead to health effects at any level of exposure, these chemicals are called 'non-threshold chemicals' and health-based concentrations are set for tolerable risks.

For some airborne chemicals, the use of Acute Exposure Guideline Levels (AEGLs) can be useful. Three vales are identified, the level of the chemical in air at or above which the general population could experience notable discomfort (AEGL1), the level of the chemical in air at or above which there may be irreversible or other serious long-lasting effects or impaired ability to escape (AEGL2), and the level of the chemical in air at or above which the general population could experience life-threatening health effects or death (AEGL3).

Radiation has both threshold and non-threshold effects. Acute injuries occur above a threshold high dose. At lower doses there are stochastic risks, mainly of cancer induction that are assumed to have a linear no-threshold dose–response function. Public and occupational exposures to radiation aim to be as low as reasonably achievable (ALARA) within the context of specific dose limits to aid emergency planning. Strenuous efforts should be made to avoid acute radiation injuries in emergency situations.

Case study: the Goiânia accident

On 13 September 1987, two people entered an abandoned private radiotherapy institute and removed a caesium-137 teletherapy unit in the city of Goiânia, Brazil (International Atomic Energy Agency 1998). They took the source home and dismantled the source assembly. The source capsule ruptured and dispersed some of the radioactive caesium chloride salt it contained. The items were sold for scrap.

Over the next few days, people noticed that the material glowed blue in the dark. Friends and relatives came to see it and took some of the material to show their families; this led to the widespread contamination of people and the environment. Some decorated their skin and ingested the caesium present on their hands. A number of people suffered from gastrointestinal symptoms and skin injuries and sought medical attention. Eleven people were hospitalized but were diagnosed as suffering from food poisoning and other skin diseases.

The scale of the problem was assessed by monitoring and several areas were evacuated. Medical triage was carried out in a local stadium where people were decontaminated. Medical examinations and interviews were carried out. The more seriously exposed persons were found to be suffering from acute local radiation injury to the skin from beta irradiation and to deeper lying tissue damage from penetrating gamma radiation.

Over time, 112,000 persons were monitored, of whom 249 were found to be contaminated either internally or externally. Inhalation was not considered to be a major route of exposure; this was confirmed by ambient air monitoring. After their initial whole-body external exposures, patients who had also been exposed internally suffered subsequent chronic, low-dose, whole-body exposure. Urine and faecal samples were used to screen for internal contamination. More than 4000 urine and faecal samples from a total of 80 persons were analysed in the period from October 1987 to January 1988. Prussian blue was given to patients to treat internal contamination by increasing the excretion of caesium isotopes and thus reducing the dose.

Four people died within 4 weeks of being admitted to hospital.

From an environmental point of view, aerial and foot surveys covered 67 square kilometres of urban areas and over 2000 kilometres of road. The worst contamination was confirmed to be within a 1-square kilometre area including the scrap yards and residences where the source was dismantled and caesium chloride handled. Eighty-five houses were found to have been significantly contaminated; most were decontaminated by vacuum cleaning and high-pressure water jets. Four houses had to be demolished. Countermeasures related to soil and fruit were only necessary, however, for soil and fruit within a 50-metre radius of the main contamination centre. Drinking water contamination was found to be low and groundwater was free of contamination.

This incident generated large quantities of low-level radioactive wastes (3500 cubic metres). This waste is now buried in a near-surface repository on the outskirts of the city, where it must be isolated for the next 300 years.

The United Kingdom introduced the High-Activity Sealed Radioactive Sources and Orphan Sources (HASS) Regulations 2005 to reduce the opportunity for accidents involving radioactive sources such as the one in Goiânia.

Countermeasures and risk management techniques for public health protection

The next stage of the process considers the options available to prevent or control the risks. It is likely that more than one possible risk management strategy will be available.

Countermeasures fall into two categories, preventative countermeasures to avoid or reduce people's exposure (decontamination, sheltering, and evacuation) and those used to treat casualties once exposure has occurred (antidotes and medical treatment). It is important to stress that lifesaving treatment should always take priority. Health plans should include arrangements for ambulance transport of contaminated casualties with serious injuries, without exposing ambulance crews to significant risk.

A combination of countermeasures can be used depending on the type, scale, and severity of the incident. This should be continuously re-evaluated as the incident evolves and more information is collated to inform the risk assessment. For all of this to happen effectively, multi-agency plans need to be developed and exercised so that organizations understand their roles, how they will communicate with each other and members of the public, and the pros and cons of specific countermeasures. The plans should allow responders to scale the response up or down depending on the severity of the release and the outcome of the risk assessment.

For high-risk fixed industrial sites and nuclear installations, plans usually include local sheltering and evacuation strategies based on maps dividing a geographical area into zones, taking into account local infrastructure (e.g. availability of local transport systems, location of rest centres) and effective warning and informing of residents within a certain emergency zone (e.g. using sirens).

For all countermeasures, vulnerable sections of the community need to be identified early as they may require assistance (people with special educational needs/disabilities, requiring medical support, the elderly, the frail, and children) or not be able to understand the messages. Some population groups may be particularly sensitive to the substance released; for example, consideration should be given to minimize the exposure of pregnant women in a radiation incident.

Case study: Graniteville train crash 2005

On 6 January 2005, at 2.40 a.m., a freight train collided with a parked train, derailing a number of cars in the centre of Graniteville, a small community just outside Aiken in South Carolina (Mitchell et al. 2005).

Approximately 60 tonnes of liquefied chlorine gas was quickly released. Residents called the emergency services within a minute of the crash and reported a bleach smell and smoke on the ground. The fire department issued a shelter in place message at 6.30 a.m. The evacuation message was not issued until 2.30 p.m. Delays in advising evacuation resulted in a large number of sheltering people experiencing adverse health effects.

Approximately 5400 people were evacuated, 554 sought treatment in hospitals, and 75 were admitted. Nine people died.

Lessons identified from this incident were that better emergency response planning for chemical incidents was needed and that emergency plans for local risks needed to be developed and exercised with the local community. Emergencies from fixed sites are often used in emergency planning; however, transport risks need to also be planned for.

Sheltering, shelter in place

Shelter in place (also called shelter *in situ*) is invoked when the safest place to take refuge or cover from an actual or perceived danger is indoors (e.g. in a house, business place, or school). Most buildings can provide significant protection against short-lived chemical and radiation releases. In the United Kingdom, the message used by the emergency services, usually through the local media, is 'go in, stay in, and tune in' and was developed by an independent National Steering Committee on Warning and Informing the Public (HM Government 2004).

Vehicles, boats, and caravans offer a lower level of protection than residential building, so sheltering in these conditions should be a last resort and for short periods. Closing windows, air conditioning, and vents will help reduce airborne exposures.

Evacuation

Evacuation can range from small-scale, locally managed and coordinated evacuation (one or two streets) to mass (or wide-area) evacuations requiring national coordination (e.g. for wide-area flooding) (HM Government 2014). Evacuation should be conducted in a controlled, systematic way to minimize potential exposure and other risks. Mass evacuation is a complex undertaking as transport, support for vulnerable groups, and the availability of shelter in a designated local authority rest centre (e.g. a school or leisure centre) will be necessary. Longer-term psychological impacts of unscheduled evacuations amongst vulnerable populations must not be underestimated.

Evacuation may be preferred for longer-lived incidents, especially when it can be implemented before people are exposed (e.g. before a release reaches a community), or before an incident happens.

The fire and rescue services will activate pre-existing plans for evacuation of members of the public and non-essential personnel to a safe distance for defined scenarios, for example, where there is an explosive risk.

Decontamination

Decontamination usually refers to external decontamination of people to reduce further exposure or avoid secondary contamination. In the United Kingdom, the management of public mass decontamination is the joint responsibility of the fire and rescue services and the Department of Health. The fire and rescue services are equipped with mobile mass decontamination units including disrobe and re-robe packs. Following the terrorist attacks in the United States on 11 September 2001, new equipment and training procedures, particularly focusing on mass decontamination (Health Protection Agency 2009) in public places in the event of a chemical, biological, radiological or nuclear (CBRN) attack, have been provided to the UK fire and rescue services. Ambulance services and hospitals also have access to decontamination pods or facilities.

Contaminated casualties should be evacuated to a safe environment and individual or mass decontamination should be carried out as soon as possible, preferably within 15 minutes of exposure for maximum benefit. Casualties are usually asked to remove their clothes from head to foot to reduce the risk of inhalation of any contaminant. Recent research in decontamination techniques shows that, in the initial phase of an incident involving non-caustic chemicals, the blotting and rubbing of exposed skin surfaces with dry absorbent material, that is, dry decontamination, is most effective unless the use of water is recommended by expert advisors.

The water decontamination method is the rinse–wipe–rinse method. After removal of contaminated clothing, casualties are asked to drench themselves under a lukewarm shower to remove water soluble material and dusts (rinse), apply a detergent solution using a soft brush to remove organic matter (wipe), and drench again to remove the detergent (rinse).

Non-ambulant casualties and those with open wounds should be decontaminated by trained personnel.

People monitoring for radioactive contamination

Non-invasive screening of the public for radioactive contamination can be used to triage large numbers of people and assess the need for medication intervention, decontamination, and/or further contamination monitoring. Depending on the radionuclides, walk-through portals and hand-held equipment can be used to detect internal or external contamination. Portable or transportable whole-body monitors should be used to detect the presence of internal contamination and for dose assessment following decontamination.

Antidotes

Treatment for chemical and radiation exposure is mostly symptomatic and supportive. Very few antidotes for individual toxins exist and where they do, they should be administered under medical supervision.

For nuclear reactor accidents where iodine usually forms a significant part of the release, the administration of stable iodine before or in the few hours after exposure, in conjunction with sheltering can form a very effective countermeasure strategy.

Depending on the chemical, antidotes can be used to form an inert complex with the poison, speed up detoxification, reduce the rate of conversion to a more toxic compound, and so on. For example, chelating agents such as dicobalt edetate are recommended to treat moderate to severe cyanide poisoning in adults and 2,3 dimercaptosuccinic acid (DMSA) has been recommended for lead poisoning. Prussian blue (ferric hexacyanoferrate) is used to increase the faecal excretion of caesium and thallium from the body, thus reducing the internal dose.

In the United Kingdom, health professionals seek advice from the National Poisons Information Centre (Public Health England 2013).

Recovery

Recovery is the process of restoring and rebuilding the community in the aftermath of an incident; this can take years or decades for the most serious events. Most successful recovery strategies begin during the emergency phase of the incident and begin to address the environmental, health, infrastructure, and economic impact of the incident as soon as possible. Recovery roles and responsibilities should be planned and rehearsed in a multi-agency setting. Local authorities will usually lead the recovery phase of the incident and comprehensive guidance and toolkits have been developed to support evidence-based decision-making (Public Health England 2009, 2012).

Public reassurance in emergencies and incidents

The scientific basis of accurate public risk communication is mature. There is also a considerable literature on the need to build trust in the systems that will be used in an emergency to protect casualties, the public, and emergency responders. More recently, papers considering emergency incident response communication as a contributory factor in public concern have been published (Drury et al. 2012; House of Commons Science and Technology Committee 2012; Pearce et al. 2013a, 2013b).

Radiation and chemical exposures can provoke all of the 'fright factors' that are known to be most feared by the public (Slovic 1987; Meara 2002). There is an extensive literature and a lot of guidance to help risk communicators in emergency situations (Department of Health 1998; Cabinet Office Strategy Unit 2002; Calman 2002; HM Treasury and Government Information and Communication Service 2003; Wessely et al. 2005).

Regulators and organizations with responsibilities for health protection have been criticized for taking a low media profile during emergencies (House of Commons Science and Technology Committee 2012). Scientific organizations can find it difficult to communicate in high-pressure situations where the facts are not known and the uncertainties about what may occur are extensive.

Basic principles of good public communication in incidents include:

◆ Decide who are the best organizations and people to deliver the public messages.

◆ Begin communicating as soon as possible, acknowledging inevitable uncertainties.

◆ Use national helplines that have a large capacity to deliver the essential health protection messages.

◆ Take account of people's desire to find out about the safety of their loved ones.

◆ Comparing familiar risks with unfamiliar ones can help put risks into context, but care must be taken to ensure that elective risks are not used as the comparison for unavoidable risks. In general, people declare a lower tolerance for unavoidable risks.

◆ Always tell the truth or give the reason(s) why the truth cannot be given. There may be unknown factors or facts that cannot be shared for security purposes; if this is the case, explain why and what these are.

◆ Develop public generic information materials in 'peacetime' that can be adapted quickly during an incident to speed up delivery of public health advice. These should include information about the mechanisms of harm, locations where harm may occur, the things people can do to protect themselves, and how effective these will be. Accurate information is likely to improve compliance with public health advice.

◆ Develop experience in using modern communication methods, such as social media to deliver important health messages.

◆ Remember that the emergency responders may need information and support as well as members of the public.

◆ One session of psychological debriefing after recent trauma does not reduce psychological distress or prevent the development of post-traumatic stress disorder (Rose et al. 2002).

Case study: public risk communication during the polonium contamination in London 2006

In 2006, following enquiries relating to an unexpected death, radioactive polonium was found to have contaminated many public places in London (Rubin et al. 2007; Morgan et al. 2008). Detailed investigation eventually revealed that the public health risks were low, but this was not known at the start of the incident. The investigation needed clear objectives and a prioritized approach to make best use of the environmental and people-monitoring facilities that were available.

There was potential for significant public concern, disruption, and economic impact, which did not happen. A British Airways press release stimulated a disproportionate response and for a brief period there was radiation screening of passengers coming from the United Kingdom at an airport in the United States.

While the emergency response was still going on, researchers carried out a random telephone survey of 1000 Londoners and more than 100 potentially exposed people who had visited contaminated venues at the relevant times. The random survey showed that the health protection communications, which included significant media interviews and a daily press release, were generally successful as only 11.7 per cent of those who replied perceived their health to be at risk because of the incident. The number of visitors to London did not decrease.

The daily health protection press releases were considered important to keep people informed. Seventy-one per cent of responders understood that they could not be contaminated if they had not been in the relevant venues. Fifty-eight per cent of responders understood that polonium is only dangerous if it enters the body.

The authors suggested that the factors contributing to this effective public communication were:

◆ The incident was linked to espionage rather than terrorism in the public consciousness. People who thought the motive was terrorism (15 per cent of the sample) were significantly more likely to feel that their health was at risk than the people who attributed the incident to espionage, criminal activity, or spying.

◆ The public perception was that one person had been targeted. People who thought the incident was intended to harm the general public (14 per cent of the sample) were significantly more likely to feel that their health was at risk than those who thought that it was intended to harm one person only.

◆ The people who had been in the contaminated venues were significantly less deprived than average. Lower earners were more than four times more likely to feel that their personal health was at risk.

◆ It was not possible to investigate the impact of the low-key way in which venue monitoring was conducted (i.e. without the use of sophisticated personal protective equipment). However, the appearance of 'suited and booted' staff in public places where the mass media were present could have caused alarm.

Despite these positive outcomes, people who had been in contaminated areas and had been offered urine testing tended not to be happy with the information they received. Some of this displeasure was inevitable because they wanted details related to the criminal investigation that could not be made public. Other people wanted more numerical information about their test results. Uniquely for polonium in urine testing, this was difficult to provide because the same amount of urinary excretion can be associated with a radiation dose that varies by a factor of ten, depending on the assumptions made. For the lowest category of risk, there were insufficient resources to undertake detailed dose assessments, using individual-specific assumptions so people were only told that their results were 'of no concern'. These complexities are not easy to put across in the midst of an emergency incident.

A small number of people (seven out of 3837) who contacted the telephone helpline that was set up for the incident failed to be reassured by direct discussion with specialist health protection staff, even if they had not been at any of the contaminated venues (Morgan et al. 2008). Of these, four were contacted by a psychiatrist who found evidence of pre-existing psychological stressors and a history of health-related anxiety. The authors concluded that access to psychiatric help may be useful in incidents such as the polonium contamination in London.

Follow-up of affected populations

There are two main reasons to undertake follow-up of populations affected by chemical, radiological, or environmental incidents: part of the long-term response to help and provide services for affected people, and to gather scientific information about the health effects of the exposures that they may have received. In most cases, the decision to set up a follow-up study is done for elements of both reasons.

The former may be particularly useful if there is to be ongoing treatment of or compensation for affected people. Compensation usually takes many years to organize, by which time the affected people may have moved away from the local area or died.

Follow-up of affected cohorts provides a unique way to study the health effects of toxins on the general population and much useful information can be gained. One of the key recommendations of a UK government Committee on Toxicity inquiry into the

Lowermoor aluminium water pollution incident was that 'it is vital to identify populations which may need to be monitored in any later epidemiology studies as early as possible after the incident. If identification of these populations is delayed, exposed individuals may move out of the area and be lost to follow up' (Committee on Toxicology of Chemicals in Food, Consumer Products and the Environment 2013).

There are two major problems with emergency response follow-up studies that distinguish them from other epidemiological research. Firstly, the decision to set up the study may need to be taken very early on in the incident, in order to capture, as fully as possible, the cohort of participants for the study. Secondly, it may be more difficult than in a planned study to determine each individual's exposure to the noxious agent.

It is not straightforward to decide if a follow-up study is needed in each incident. Done properly, the work will be resource intensive in all but the smallest of incidents. If the cohort does not accurately reflect all those who may have been harmed, then its scientific power and usefulness as a tool to help patient care may be limited in the long term. Paranthaman et al. (2012) have proposed a decision framework to help responders decide if a follow-up health register study is indicated based on a Delphi consensus study of emergency responders and epidemiologists (Box 11.11.2). The study presented participants with four scenarios and asked responders whether a follow-up study should be set up and why. Although there was a spectrum of views from the range of responders, 11 factors were defined by the participants as important in making the decision about setting up a health register. The factors are not mutually exclusive and their relevance needs to be debated by the team setting up the follow-up study.

Measuring individual or group 'doses' to noxious agents may be difficult in emergency situations as resources are rightly focused on more urgent aspects of the response. For some agents, for example, intakes of radionuclides, there are accurate biodosimetry methods that can be used in the weeks and months following an incident to retrospectively assess exposure. However, for other agents there is no measurable signal after the event, or the signal decays very quickly. This poses real logistical problems if large numbers of people need to be measured and may well swamp national capability to perform such measurements. Triage arrangements may be needed to ensure that people with the highest clinical need for testing have priority.

In other situations, environmental measurements, combined with information about where people were at the time of the incident, what they were doing, and what injuries they may have suffered allow post hoc assessment of likely 'doses'. These can be calibrated by actual measurements taken in smaller numbers of people with similar locations and behaviours at the time of the release.

Some of the work to set up a follow-up study is needed in the acute phase of the incident. Therefore emergency plans need to specify how the decision to set up a follow-up study will be taken and plan for the resource and practical implications of this work. Exercising these plans will help to spot rate-limiting steps and identify actions that can be done in advance, for example, detailed understanding of how to collect patient data from hospitals, community services, and rest centres, developing generic data collection, and patient information forms that can be adapted when an incident occurs.

There are ethical and data protection concerns whenever new follow-up studies are started. The objectives of follow-up studies

---

Box 11.11.2 Important factors to consider when setting up a health register after a major incident

- There is exposure to an agent with potential to harm public health but there is little prior experience, or exposure to a well-known agent but the incident has novel characteristics.

- There is insufficient knowledge of the type and latency of health effects, but reasonable grounds to suspect that they will occur.

- The incident is likely to lead to significant political/public/media interest that may increase societal concern.

- The register will be used in the clinical management of affected patients, especially in the long term.

- There is a reasonable possibility of short- or long-term physical and/or psychological sequelae from the incident.

- There is potential for specific adverse effects in vulnerable groups, for example, pregnant women, potential for teratogenicity.

- Follow-up studies have the potential to produce significant new knowledge about health effects of exposures and benefit the wider population as well as affected individuals.

- Follow-up studies have the potential to enable interventions to reduce the impact of exposures.

- It will be possible to identify the population at risk including detailed demographic data (though not necessarily collected at the time of the incident).

- It will be possible to identify, measure, or estimate exposures of individuals or groups (though not necessarily at the time of the incident).

- There are sufficient data on the spatial distribution of the contamination or exposure (though not necessarily measured at the time of the incident).

Adapted from Paranthaman, K. et al., Development of a decision framework for establishing a health register following a major incident, *Prehospital Disaster Medicine*, Volume 27, Issue 6, pp. 524–30, Copyright © World Association for Disaster and Emergency Medicine 2012, reproduced by permission of Cambridge University Press.

must be clear at the start and data protection and other ethical aspects considered at the emergency planning stage. This will minimize workload and delay when setting up the most complete possible register of affected individuals in an emergency situation. It is not ethical to collect and store information 'just in case' without explicit consideration of how these data can help the individuals concerned or contribute to an adequately powered scientific study.

A pragmatic approach at the early stages of any incident, before the decision about a follow-up study has been taken, is to ensure that basic contact details are logged by all members of the public interacting with emergency responders. If a follow-up study is advised, these people can be contacted again for more information and advice.

Patient questionnaire and other data collection techniques need to be developed with care to ensure that all the relevant information is obtained in the most efficient manner. Detailed, timed information about where the person was, what they were doing, and other aspects of 'exposure' is usually needed as well as information about symptoms and health status, including mental health status. The objectives of the study should be at the heart of the data collected by that study.

Identify and publish the lessons learned

Reporting incidents is vital to share learning, decrease the chance of the incident reoccurring, and to improve emergency response. However, many incidents and emergencies are very poorly documented. Incident reports may also be useful for members of the public who have been placed at risk, colleagues who are responding to similar incidents, and public health professionals who are called to give evidence in public or legislative inquiries into the incident. Only with detailed documentation can lessons be identified that can then change policy and practice.

A process to ensure consensus on what information will be gathered and how data collection will be organized during and after an incident or emergency should have been established as part of the pre-incident emergency planning. Collation of data for reporting should start as soon as possible during the crisis event with plans for continuous updating as more data become available from the multidisciplinary (or potentially international) response.

Organizations, including public health partners, performing incident or emergency responses should jointly develop and document how the quality and validity of information are assured. This needs documented procedures and training for incident responders, including administrative staff, in the methods for information gathering, analysis, and quality assurance.

Kulling et al. (2011) set out a summary of the requirements for reports on health crises and critical health events and recommended issues that should be managed actively at an early stage in a response. These include:

- The mandate for the emergency report and that of the respective authority/organization.
- Early identification of the authors and their responsibilities.
- Ethical approval and quality assurance statements for the report if required.
- A summary of the pre-event status if needed, such as baseline disease patterns and user patterns of hospitals and health

facilities as well as other relevant previous incidents or disasters described as well as preparedness plans.

- A summary of the incident or emergency.
- A method statement to include descriptions of hazard and exposure assessments, decision flow, and information management.
- A description of the interventions and how they were evaluated in terms of effects, outcomes, and impacts balanced against the goal(s) and objectives of the interventions. It may be useful to distinguish between immediate-, medium- and long-term impacts.
- Coordination and collaboration between organizations from health and other sectors.
- Adverse health effects in the responders.
- Identify interventions that restore normality to the pre-event level, including how responding organizations intervened to provide resilience and reduce vulnerability in people at risk.
- Consider summarizing the lessons identified by describing:
  - What went well.
  - What went badly.
  - What could be done better.

The final task is to publish the report in an appropriate peer-review publication for all to share and learn from.

Conclusion

This chapter has explained the stages of response to radiation, chemical, and environmental emergencies using a generic 'all hazards' framework and a 'source–pathway–receptor' risk assessment model which is adaptable to any situation and conforms with international obligations.

In recent years there have been many chemical, radiation, and environmental disasters that have challenged the emergency preparedness of countries around the globe. Adequate resources for response and pre-planning are vital to deliver a slick, professional, and proportionate response and to define the important factors to consider when setting up a health register after a major incident. The knowledge gained by careful evaluation of emergency responses can greatly improve the efficiency of emergency preparedness (Lurie et al. 2013). However, there are great challenges in doing research under such circumstances. There remain a significant number of evidence gaps and so detailed documentation and follow-up of future incidents will continue to be needed to fill those gaps and improve emergency preparedness and response in the future.

Further reading

Baker, D., Karalliedde, L., Murray, V., Maynard, R., and Parkinson, N.H.T. (eds.) (2012). *Essentials of Toxicology for Health Protection: A Handbook for Field Professionals* (2nd ed.). Oxford: Oxford University Press.

Bradley, N., Harrison, H., Hodgson, G., Kamanyire, R., Kibble, A., and Murray, V. (eds.) (2014). *Essentials of Environmental Public Health: A Handbook for Field Professionals*. Oxford: Oxford University Press.

Department of Energy & Climate Change (2013). *Nuclear Emergency Planning: Consolidated Guidance*. London: Department of Energy &

Climate Change. Available at: https://www.gov.uk/government/publications/nuclear-emergency-planning-consolidated-guidance.

Department of Health (2013). *Health Emergency Preparedness, Resilience and Response from April 2013: Summary of the Principal Roles of Health Sector Organisations*. London: Department of Health. Available at: https://www.gov.uk/government/uploads/system/uploads/attachment_data/file/156099/EPRR-Summary-of-the-principal-roles-of-health-sector-organisations.pdf.pdf.

HM Government (2012). *Enhanced SAGE Guidance. A strategic framework for the Scientific Advisory Group for Emergencies (SAGE)*. [Online] Available at: https://www.gov.uk/government/uploads/system/uploads/attachment_data/file/80087/sage-guidance.pdf.

Kreis, I.A., Busby, A., Leonardi, G., Meara, J., and Murray, V. (eds.) (2012). *Essentials of Environmental Epidemiology for Health Protection: A Handbook for Field Professionals*. Oxford: Oxford University Press.

Rojas-Palmer, C., Liland, A., Jerstad, A.N., et al. (2009). *TMT Handbook: Triage, Monitoring and Treatment of People Exposed to Ionising Radiation Following a Malevolent Act*. Østerås: Norwegian Radiation Protection Authority. Available at: http://www.tmthandbook.org/index.php?option=com_content&task=view&id=42&Itemid=1.

World Health Organization (2011). *Disaster Risk Management for Health Fact Sheets*. [Online] Available at: http://www.unisdr.org/we/inform/publications/19966.

References

Cabinet Office (2013). *National Risk Register of Civil Emergencies*. London: HMSO. Available at: https://www.gov.uk/government/publications/national-risk-register-for-civil-emergencies-2013-edition.

Cabinet Office Strategy Unit (2002). *Risk: Improving Government's Capability to Handle Risk and Uncertainty Summary Report*. London: HMSO.

Calman, K.C. (2002). Communication of risk: choice, consent, and trust. *The Lancet*, 360, 166–8.

Committee on Toxicology of Chemicals in Food, Consumer Products and the Environment (2013). *Report of the COT Subgroup Report on the Lowermoor Water Pollution Incident*. [Online] Available at: http://cot.food.gov.uk/pdfs/lwpiapp811.pdf.

Department of Health (1998). *Communicating about Risks to Public Health: Pointers to Good Practice*. London: HMSO.

Drury, J., Kemp, V., Newman, J., et al. (2012). Psychosocial care for persons affected by emergencies and major incidents: a Delphi study to determine the needs of professional first responders for education, training and support. *Emergency Medical Journal*, 30(10), 831–6.

European Commission (2013). *European Parliament Legislative Resolution of 3 July 2013 on the Proposal for a Decision of the European Parliament and of the Council on Serious Cross-Border Threats to Health (COM(2011)0866—C7-0488/2011—2011/0421(COD))*. [Online] Available at: http://www.europarl.europa.eu/sides/getDoc.do?type=TA&language=EN&reference=P7-TA-2013-311.

Gormley, A., Pollard, S., and Rocks, S. (2011). *Guidelines for Environmental Risk Assessment and Management. Green Leaves III*. [Online] Available at: https://www.gov.uk/government/uploads/system/uploads/attachment_data/file/69450/pb13670-green-leaves-iii-1111071.pdf.

Health Protection Agency (2009). *Centre for Radiation, Chemical and Environmental Hazards Chemical Surveillance Report 1st January–31st December 2009*. [Online] Available at: http://www.hpa.org.uk/webc/HPAwebFile/HPAweb_C/1284475648621.

HM Government (2004). *Preparing for Emergencies: What You Need to Know*. London: HMSO. Available at: http://www.direct.gov.uk/prod_consum_dg/groups/dg_digitalassets/@dg/@en/documents/digitalasset/dg_176618.pdf.

HM Government (2014). *Evacuation and Shelter Guidance. Non-Statutory Guidance to Complement Emergency Preparedness and Emergency Response and Recovery*. London: HMSO. Available at: https://www.gov.uk/government/uploads/system/uploads/attachment_data/file/274615/Evacuation_and_Shelter_Guidance_2014.pdf.

HM Treasury and Government Information and Communication Service (2003). *Communicating Risk*. London: HMSO.

House of Commons Science and Technology Committee (2012). *Devil's Bargain? Energy Risks and the Public First Report of Session 2012–13 HC 428 [Incorporating HC 1742-i to -iv, Session 2010–12]*. London: HMSO. Available at: http://www.publications.parliament.uk/pa/cm201213/cmselect/cmsctech/428/42802.htm.

International Atomic Energy Agency (1988). *The Radiological Incident in Goiânia*. [Online] Available at: http://www-pub.iaea.org/MTCD/publications/PDF/Pub815_web.pdf.

Kulling, P., Birnbaum, M., Murray, V., and Rockenschaub, G. (2011). (A48) Guidelines for reports on health crises and critical health events—a tool for the development of disaster medicine research. *Prehospital and Disaster Medicine*, 26, s17.

Lurie, N., Manolio, T., Patterson, A.P., Collins, F., and Frieden, T. (2013). Research as a part of public health emergency response. *The New England Journal of Medicine*, 368, 1251–5.

Meara, J.R. (2002). Getting the message across: is communicating risk to the public worth it? *Journal of Radiological Protection*, 22, 79–85.

Mitchell, J.T., Edmonds, A.S., Cutter, S.L., et al. (2005). *Evacuation Behavior in Response to the Graniteville, South Carolina, Chlorine Spill*. [Online] Available at: http://www.colorado.edu/hazards/research/qr/qr178/qr178.pdf.

Morgan, O.W., Page, L., Forrester, S., and Maguire, H. (2008). Polonium-210 poisoning in London: hypochondriasis and public health. *Prehospital and Disaster Medicine*, 23(1), 96–7.

Paranthaman, K., Catchpole, M., Simpson, J., Morris, J., Muirhead, C.R., and Leonardi, G.S. (2012). Development of a decision framework for establishing a health register following a major incident. *Prehospital and Disaster Medicine*, 27(6), 524–30.

Pearce, J.M., Rubin, G.J., Amlôt, R., Wessely, S., and Brooke Rogers, M.B. (2013a). Communicating public health advice after a chemical spill: results from national surveys in the United Kingdom and Poland. *Disaster Medicine and Public Health Preparedness*, 7, 65–74.

Pearce, J.M., Rubin, G.J., Selke, P., et al. (2013b). Communicating with the public following radiological terrorism: results from a series of focus groups and national surveys in Britain and Germany. *Prehospital and Disaster Medicine*, 28(2), 1–10.

Pesatori, A.C., Consonni, D., Bachetti, S., et al. (2003). Short- and long-term morbidity and mortality in the population exposed to dioxin after the 'Seveso accident'. *Industrial Health*, 41, 127–38.

Public Health England (2009). *UK Recovery Handbook for Radiation Incidents*. [Online] Available at: https://www.gov.uk/government/publications/uk-recovery-handbook-for-radiation-incidents-and-associated-publications.

Public Health England (2012). *UK Recovery Handbook for Chemical Incidents*. [Online] Available at: https://www.gov.uk/government/publications/uk-recovery-handbook-for-chemical-incidents-and-associated-publications.

Public Health England (2013). *The National Poisons Information Service (NPIS)*. [Online] Available at: http://www.hpa.org.uk/ProductsServices/ChemicalsPoisons/PoisonsInformationService/NationalPoisonsInformationService/.

Rose, S.C., Bisson, J., Churchill, R., and Wessely, S. (2009). Psychological debriefing for preventing post traumatic stress disorder (PTSD) (Review). *Cochrane Database of Systematic Reviews*, 2, CD000560.

Rubin, G.J., Page, L., Morgan, O., et al. (2007). Public information needs after the poisoning of Alexander Litvinenko with polonium-210 in London: cross sectional telephone survey and qualitative analysis. *BMJ*, 335(7630), 1143.

Slovic, P. (1987). Perception of risk. *Science*, 236, 280–5.

United Nations Office for Disaster Risk Reduction (2007). *Hyogo Framework for Action 2005–2015: Building the Resilience of Nations and Communities to Disasters*. A/CONF.206/6. New York: United Nations. Available at: http://www.unisdr.org/we/inform/publications/1037.

Wessely, S., Fischhoff, B., and Krasnov, V.N. (2005). Guidelines for communicating the risk of chemical, biological, or nuclear terrorism: how to inform the public, improve resilience, and not generate panic. In S. Wessely and V.N. Krasnov (eds.) *Psychological Responses to the New Terrorism: A NATO-Russia Dialogue* (NATO Security Through Science Series—E: Human and Societal Dynamics, Vol. 3), pp. 233–41. Amsterdam: IOS Press.

World Health Organization (2008). *International Health Regulations 2005* (2nd ed.). Geneva: WHO. Available at: http://whqlibdoc.who.int/publications/2008/9789241580410_eng.pdf.

Private support of public health

Quarraisha Abdool Karim and Roger Detels

Introduction to private support of public health

Private support for public good may be understood as the cooperation between private individuals and/or the commercial sector and the public sector in order to more effectively meet the needs of society locally or globally (Buse and Waxman 2001). This relationship is not necessarily unidirectional, and in several instances, also benefits the giver through increase in turnover from positive product or company branding through media coverage that accompanies giving (Broadbent and Laughlin 2003). The World Health Organization (WHO) defines public–private partnerships (PPPs) in the health sector as the bringing together of a set of actors for the common goal of improving the health of populations based on mutually agreed roles and principles (Kickbusch and Quick 1998). While these principles are based on the founding ideas and values of human ethics such as beneficence, non-maleficence, autonomy, and equity (Buse and Walt 2000a) the reality is that the relationship between giver and recipient is not an equal one.

Over time, while anonymous individual giving has continued, some of these ad hoc institutional contributions have evolved into more defined and legally recognized structures also referred to as philanthropic organizations and includes giving by more wealthy individuals and families as well as corporate institutions. Giving, particularly by North Americans, dates back to the formation of 'foundations' in the earliest years of the twentieth century as a result of wealth acquired through industrialization. In the United States, this idea was catalysed by a 'tax break' provided by the US government to private companies and citizens who donated a certain proportion of their wealth to federal or state government projects or priority initiatives (Butler 2001). Private entities had autonomy to choose which government or global projects or priorities they would support, and the extent thereof, while deriving the benefit of reduced taxation.

This type of charitable tax deduction by the US government, has allowed foundations to reduce their tax burden by as much as 25 per cent (Strom 2007). *The New York Times* has estimated that charitable deductions cost the US government US$40 billion in lost tax revenue in 2006 (Strom 2007). In effect, this substantial private philanthropic support means that the foundations, and not the US government, are determining where significant public funds are spent. Philanthropists and foundations take pride in their autonomy in determining what to invest in and traditionally

have identified areas that minimize overlap and define their giving identity. Eli Broad, one of the major donors, summarizes the essence and impetus for private giving by asserting that smart philanthropists get more for their money than governments because they know how to invest wisely (Strom 2007).

However, it is important to recognize that foundations often determine their targets and objectives on personally identified and defined priorities rather than an objective assessment of international and national need. Foundations are likely to invest in areas that governments may be reluctant to for political or moral reasons, for example, sexuality education, gender-based violence, fertility control, and harm reduction programmes.

History of giving

One of the earliest known foundations in the United States was the Russell Sage Foundation that was founded in 1906 with a focus on working women and poverty-related illnesses (Hammack and Wheeler 1994). The establishment of larger and more encompassing foundations began with the founding of the Carnegie Foundation by Andrew Carnegie in 1911 'to do real and permanent good in this world' (Carnegie Corporation of New York n.d.) followed by The Rockefeller Foundation in 1913 (Menasha and Hsig 1915).

These early gifts had a significant impact on institution creation to support and build public health capacity. Public health provided the optimal mechanism through which Rockefeller philanthropy was able to apply their scientific findings for the public good (Birn and Fee 2013). The Rockefeller Foundation established the International Health Commission in its first year (The Rockefeller Foundation 2013). This was the first allocation of funds from private sources for international public health activities and had a wide sphere of influence—52 countries on six continents and 29 islands to improve their public health systems. The Rockefeller Foundation simultaneously initiated a 20-year programme to support the Bureau of Social Hygiene which focused on research and education on fertility control, maternal health, and sex education. This foundation played a key role in founding the world's first schools of public health, first at Johns Hopkins, then at Harvard, and later in other parts of the United States, as well as in 21 other countries that includes the establishment of the London School of Tropical Medicine and Hygiene in 1921, the China Medical Board in 1914, and the Peking Union Medical College in 1921. The last two institutions have played a pivotal role in the development of public health in China (The Rockefeller Foundation 2013b).

The Wellcome Trust which was established in 1936 in the United Kingdom is dedicated to supporting research to improve human and animal health. It is the largest non-governmental research funder in the UK and among the largest such providers in the world (Wellcome Trust n.d.).

A hallmark of this type of giving was the insightfulness of individuals in anticipating, prioritizing, and filling an important gap and creating a strong foundation for others, including governments, to build on. This type of nimble, risk-taking investment is in keeping with the business model based on entrepreneurship that sees and seizes opportunities. These are the principles on which the foundation wealth was created—unfettered by ponderous, risk-averse decision-making, never-ending procedures and systems that are the hallmark of most government or public sector bureaucracies.

Current giving

Since those early years of giving, private support for public health has increased in magnitude and scale, particularly in the past decade. Today, the Bill & Melinda Gates Foundation is the largest private grant-making foundation in the world (McCoy et al. 2009) supporting three major programmes worldwide that include a US-based programme to enhance secondary and post-secondary education, a global development programme which focuses on the alleviation of hunger and poverty, and a global health programme that includes increasing access to childhood immunization programmes and research in neglected diseases such as tuberculosis (TB), malaria, and HIV (McCoy et al. 2009). In 2007, 61 per cent of their US$2.01 billion budget was allocated to health (McCoy et al. 2009). This foundation has single-handedly redefined the concept of individual social responsibility and has inspired similar giving trends across the globe including among wealthy individuals in developing countries. In South Africa, for example, the Motsepe Foundation established in 2013 by Patrice Motsepe, one of the country's wealthiest individuals and listed on the Fortune 500's top ten wealthiest people, has committed 50 per cent of his family wealth to philanthropy and $US10 million over the next 5 years towards several health, education, and job creation efforts (Morvaridi 2012).

Globally, there are now over 40 major foundations, as well as countless smaller ones (Foundation Center 2014). This increase can be attributed in part to at least three phenomena: substantial growth in personal wealth among a few, global solidarity around the AIDS epidemic and other health threats, and the rise in citizen pressure for corporate accountability/social responsibility. Corporate social responsibility programmes are a new form of giving that adopt a more entrepreneurial approach for product branding, creating brand loyalty and increasing product sales and are not the focus of this chapter.

Globalization of health threats, global solidarity, and the emergence of public–private partnerships

The global burden of disease, especially infectious diseases, disproportionately affects populations in developing countries due to poverty, weak healthcare delivery systems, inadequate investment in health, and inadequate access to pharmaceuticals, vaccines, and drugs (Widdus 2001). Post-industrial revolution eradication of these diseases in developed countries and the growth of a for-profit pharmaceutical industry have resulted in neglect of research and development in drugs and other medical products for 'diseases of poverty', since such products are perceived as being not likely to generate significant return on their investment.

The rise of multi- and extremely drug-resistant strains of TB (MDR- and XDR-TB), outbreaks of severe acute respiratory syndrome, swine flu, and avian flu, and growing antibiotic resistance have served as sharp reminders of the continuing threat posed by these neglected tropical diseases as well as emerging and re-emerging infectious diseases to everyone regardless of geographical location, in our increasingly globalized world.

Interventions that reduce cost, provide market incentives, and create infrastructure that will allow for product access (Widdus 2001) require the private sector such as pharmaceutical companies to collaborate and work with public and not-for-profit entities to ensure a fast and efficient response (Widdus 2001, 2005). The proliferation of global PPPs (Croft 2005) reflects this approach and is rapidly reconfiguring the global public health landscape (Buse and Walt 2000a).

The substantial investments made by the Doris Duke Medical Research Institute and the Howard Hughes Medical Institute in creating state-of-the-art research facilities and laboratories in KwaZulu-Natal at the epicentre of the HIV epidemic and MDR- and XDR-TB are examples of contemporary US philanthropy in resource-constrained settings to address health challenges that are of local and global importance.

Other examples of private support

Private support of public health, given by foundations, industry, pharmaceutical companies, and professional organizations, has been directed towards disease control and treatment, poverty alleviation, education, training of health workers, infrastructure development, research, improved agricultural practices, health information dissemination, and sponsorship of the many global health alliances.

Specific examples include the provision of drugs and the reduction of drug prices for developing countries, the earliest example being the Mectizan Donation Program by Merck & Co. Inc. for treatment for onchocerciasis (river blindness) in West Africa in 1988. In 1998, GlaxoSmithKline provided albendazole for treatment of lymphatic filariasis as part of the mectizan programme. To date, this ongoing programme has reached more than 80 million people (Mectizan Donation Program 2012).

Another major contribution has been the establishment of special training programmes and scholarships/fellowships for training health personnel. Many foundations are set up for this purpose alone or as part of a broader portfolio. For example, the Robert Wood Johnson Foundation has a clinical scholars programme for US students (Robert Wood Johnson Foundation 2012). Additionally, foundations may provide gifts to schools, which may include equipment or teaching resources.

Another important contribution of private agencies has been to research. The Howard Hughes Medical Institute, for example, was established by Hughes Aviation to conduct research into human illness (Howard Hughes Medical Institute n.d.) and has established and funded research centres (Howard Hughes Research Institutions) within major academic medical centres in the United States. The Gates Foundation currently supports a large number of research projects targeting a broad range of global health problems. The Wellcome Trust funds a broad portfolio of research in health which includes a long-standing commitment to supporting tropical medicine and public health research. There are also the very significant contributions made by pharmaceutical companies to the research and development of vaccines and treatments, both independently and in PPPs. Increasingly, these efforts are focusing on the so-called neglected diseases that disproportionately affect the world's poorest nations.

HIV/AIDS and tuberculosis: catalysing a new category of giving

The role of activism in advancing the scientific agenda and public access to product advances is most apparent in HIV/AIDS. Since the first reported cases of AIDS in the early 1980s in the United States and the discovery of the causative organism, HIV has spread rapidly across the globe resulting in several million deaths prior to the discovery of effective antiretroviral therapy (Curran and Jaffe 2011; Sharp and Hahn 2011). The transformation of AIDS from a uniformly lethal disease to a chronic, manageable condition has resulted in rapid and phenomenal declines in mortality rates in industrialized countries. This outcome, however, has as yet remained elusive in developing countries that bear a disproportionate burden of the disease.

The hosting of the XIIIth International AIDS Conference in Durban, South Africa in 2000 was the first time that many in industrialized countries came face to face with the plight of the millions of people infected with HIV in developing countries, who were continuing to die because they were unable to access antiretroviral treatment, with high costs posing a major barrier. While the inequities and disparities in terms of access to life-saving drugs and healthcare between industrialized and developing countries were not new, this conference was a sharp reminder and catalysed a whole new approach to public giving in healthcare provision and novel partnerships.

The creation of the Global Fund for AIDS, Tuberculosis and Malaria (GFATM) in 2007 was the quintessential PPP in modern history with respect to harmonizing of resources from multiple sources to address three diseases that in combination are the major contributors to high rates of morbidity and mortality in resource-constrained settings and which contribute disproportionately to the global burden of disease (Vitoria et al. 2009). Funding from the Bill & Melinda Gates Foundation, which by 2012 had provided over US\$26 billion in grants (equal to the total budget of the WHO), stimulated additional large donations by Warren Buffett and the William Clinton Foundation.

The GFATM model builds on the emergence of formalized PPPs to address specific public health challenges, including product development catalysed by The Rockefeller Foundation in the late 1990s with their investment in HIV vaccine development through support for the International AIDS Vaccine Initiative (IAVI) at a time when most had given up on a vaccine. The funds from the Rockefeller Foundation were used by IAVI to leverage funds from other foundations and governments and changed the HIV vaccine development landscape initially through advocacy efforts and subsequently through investments in product development and clinical trial infrastructure. IAVI energized the quest for a HIV vaccine through its intra-mural programme, expansion of the number of academic institutions engaged in this quest, and even encouraged some pharmaceutical companies to invest in vaccine development.

This model was used subsequently by The Rockefeller Foundation to leverage and harmonize resources to increase access to drugs to reduce mother-to-child transmission (MTCT) of HIV through the MTCT+ initiative coordinated by the Elizabeth Glaser Foundation, and access to antiretroviral treatment for AIDS patients in resource-constrained settings (Barr 2007). The disease- and/or product-specific PPP approach builds on the Bayh-Dole Act that was passed by the US Congress in 1980 (Barr 2007) to promote collaboration in the United States between the federal government, universities, and private pharmaceutical companies in the development and marketing of new pharmaceutical products.

Public–private partnerships

PPPs may be classified or described according to purpose, organizational structure, scope of activity, or approach. Three categories are described as follows (Buse and Walt 2000b):

- Product-based partnerships that enable access: this includes drug or product donation programmes; bulk purchase of products for low-income countries, for example, the albendazole donation programme; and childhood immunization programme vaccine purchases.

- Product-development partnerships that enable and incentivize partnerships for discovery and/or commercialization, for example, the Malaria Vaccine Initiative (MVI) established in 1999, the International AIDS Vaccine Initiative described earlier, the International Partnership for Microbicides, and the Tuberculosis Vaccine Initiative.

- Systems-based partnerships that support government efforts to strengthen health service delivery through health systems strengthening.

A PPP could involve financing from various sources such as equity contributions, debt contributions, bank guarantees/letter of credit/performance guarantees, bond/capital markets financing, mezzanine/subordinated contributions, and inter-creditor agreements in some combination of equity and debt (World Bank Group 2011). Sources may include governments, private foundations, individuals, and the business/corporate sector (McCoy et al. 2009). Some of the wealthiest non-profit charitable foundations globally are the Bill & Melinda Gates Foundation (Vogel 2006), the Stichting INGKA Foundation, the Wellcome Trust, and the Howard Hughes Medical Institute to mention a few. Whilst in previous years giving was largely unregulated, in the light of the post-2009 global financial and economic crisis, a lot has changed. Countries like the United States have called for more strict regulations regarding tax credits for charitable giving by private companies. This would cover federal taxes, but the individual states have their own regulations regarding state-controlled taxes. The increase in the extent of giving to resource-constrained settings by both the US government and private donors has elevated health to diplomatic status wherein good health is viewed as essential for economic development and social stability at a country level. This goal of ensuring good governance and sustainable societies free of need that is facilitated through bi- and multilateral partnerships between those who have and those who do not through the establishment of a global civil society (Vogel 2006) redefines the meaning of globalization.

Since the inception of PPPs in the United Kingdom (Spackman 2002), almost £56 billion have been attributed to over 800 projects spanning car parks, schools, tolled highways, and power plants (Garvin and Bosso 2008). Globally, a lot of attention has also been given to healthcare, education, social housing (Flinders 2005), and disaster control. Healthcare in particular remains one of the major recipients of PPP funding (Howard 1983, 1991; Novignon et al. 2012). PPP initiatives in health include infectious disease control (Ardian et al. 2007; Kane et al. 2010; Sinanovic and Kumaranayake 2010; Lal et al. 2011; Sturchio and Cohen 2012), drug or vaccine development (Wheeler and Berkley 2001; Nwaka and Ridley 2003; Nwaka 2005; Sanhai et al. 2008), management of hospitals (Goldman et al. 1992; DeVol et al. 2007; Lester 2012), and the building of hospitals (Weiner and Alexander 1998; McKee et al. 2006) or institutes of health.

PPPs can function at a global or country level and imply a mutually beneficial, synergistic alliance between the private and public sectors towards a common goal that is shaped by good governance, equity, and efficiency (Goldman et al. 1992). Whilst benefits of PPPs include the mobilization of funds, technology transfer, strengthened delivery systems (Kraak et al. 2012), greater efficiency in terms of time, scope, and improved options, there are also risks involved. PPPs are not the solution to all health challenges and may not be the most effective or efficient approach in several instances (UK Parliament 2011). For example, the UK Parliament's Treasury Select Committee's review of the PFI scheme in August 2011 concluded that: 'Private Finance Initiative (PFI) funding for new infrastructure, such as schools and hospitals, does not provide taxpayers with good value for money and stricter criteria should be introduced to govern its use'. Careful thought and planning needs to be given to evaluate its appropriateness in each instance to ensure it is not counterproductive.

In the health sector, the most significant PPP exists between the WHO and the corporate sector (Buse and Waxman 2001). This partnership builds on the United Nations (UN) idea of a 'Global Compact' (Williams 2008) that encourages corporate responsibility in the areas of labour, human rights, and the environment in response to globalization (Buse and Waxman 2001). What is distinctive in the case of the WHO is its commitment to health and the principles inculcated in its mission and accountability to its constituency, namely its member states (Buse and Waxman 2001). The corporate partnership with WHO has been met with mixed reactions. Some board members have expressed concerns that commercial interests would mean compromising the integrity of the WHO in terms of subordination of its values, re-orientation of its mission, weakened capacity to promote and monitor international regulations, displacement of priorities, and self-censorship (Buse and Waxman 2001). A number of examples cited of this threat of 'institutional capture' include: (1) the guidelines for the management of hypertension which were unduly influenced by a pharmaceutical

company that had stood to benefit from the drugs prescribed, and (2) deliberations on breastfeeding which were considered to have been censored in favour of the WHO's new set of commercial constituencies (Buse and Waxman 2001).

At a country level, delays in procurement processes or changing needs of communities (Fussel and Beresford 2009) can reduce the efficiency and nimbleness of private partners (Hodge 2004; Fussel and Beresford 2009) or rigid commitments could undermine existing government policies and infrastructure resulting in coexisting government projects being jeopardized and the worsening of the very many issues facing human society in the developing world.

There were more than 90 international partnerships in health in 2004 (Nishtar 2004). The majority addressed infectious diseases, notably AIDS, TB, and malaria. Some involved individual governments, non-governmental organizations, or both forming an alliance with the for-profit sector. For example, Sanofi-Aventis has an extensive international programme of humanitarian sponsorship, including a partnership with the Nelson Mandela Foundation and the South African Department of Health to provide free TB treatment in severely affected areas within South Africa (Sanofi-Aventis 2007).

Other notable partnerships are the global health alliances, such as the Global Alliance for Vaccines and Immunizations, Roll Back Malaria, the Stop TB Partnership, and the Global Polio Eradication Program. They may be principally driven by a company, be legally independent, or hosted by a civil society organization (Nishtar 2004). The Stop TB Partnership, for example, comprises a network of more than 500 partners, including governments of both developed and developing countries, research and technical health institutes, multilateral organizations, civil society, pharmaceutical companies and other industry partners, and is housed within the WHO (Stop TB Partnership n.d.).

Prioritization of need: competing candidates

One of the major issues facing PPPs is the correct distribution of funds based on the degree of need. Depending on the period in question as well as the global climate in terms of crisis management, funds are generally distributed according to urgency and magnitude of need. In the healthcare sector, a lot of attention has been given to the global HIV/AIDS pandemic but recent literature cites a need for a more balanced and better-rounded approach (Bygbjerg 2012). Furthermore, over and above the current agenda of infectious disease particularly in the low- and middle-income countries, there are issues of development, industrialization, urbanization, investment, and ageing, which in turn drive the rising prevalence of non-communicable diseases (NCDs), the majority of which now occur in developing countries (Bygbjerg 2012). Malnutrition and infection in early life tend to increase the incidence of NCDs in later life (Bygbjerg 2012). In addition, the presence of infectious diseases and NCDs together (Boutayeb 2006) can result in adverse interactions (Bygbjerg 2012). Therefore, attempts to fund each health initiative separately are likely to exacerbate the overall situation and distort the countries' health priorities (Bygbjerg 2012). Rather, joint approaches that target improving the healthcare system as a whole are preferable (Bygbjerg 2012).

Challenges

Whilst the concept of PPPs might be conceptually appealing, they are associated with many challenges (Hodge and Greve 2005; Asante and Zwi 2007) such as sustainability; collaboration between donors, governments, health departments and civil society; corruption; and numerous ethical and moral dilemmas. Other challenges which exist include balancing private commercial interests with public health interests, managing conflicts of interest, assessing partnership compatibility, and evaluating partnership outcomes (Kraak et al. 2012). In addition, money borrowed from the private sector is often more expensive than money borrowed by governments and these costs are passed along to the public although the private sector would assert that they can save money in the end because they can operate with greater efficiency. Others argue that the initial capital outlay required may counter the efficiencies gained. Moreover, these expenditures need to be translated into the correct and most effective set of approaches, strategies, and investments for improving the health of the poor (McCoy et al. 2009). There are also issues of transparency and government oversight (Fussel and Beresford 2009). Commercial considerations may limit public oversight during procurement (Fussel and Beresford 2009). Contract provisions may limit changes that are necessary later on in the project in order to safeguard public interests as new public policies which may evolve (Fussel and Beresford 2009).

Private investments and global health—at a crossroads?

Private giving in all its forms, has benefited individuals, institutions in the United States and outside, the recipient countries, and global health enormously and has achieved goals which otherwise would have been impossible to attain and importantly within a relatively short timeline. There is no question that the recent surge in giving has reduced health disparities and changed the global landscape in select diseases and is at an important crossroads. In contrast to private giving in public health in the early twentieth century that was modest, catalytic, and individually determined, the giver today is much more visible, contributions much more substantial, and there is active involvement in shaping the global agenda and in decision-making on priority setting and resource allocation in international bodies and at a country level. The magnitude of the budgets of a few foundations has in some instances overshadowed the work of smaller philanthropic organizations and created uncertainty as to their added value. On the other hand, the skewing by philanthropic giving of the priority setting and investment process globally and nationally, has associated costs that may sometimes outweigh the benefits. For example, some perceive a conflict of interests when a foundation or industry plays a pivotal role at this level of decision-making, particularly where there may be some vested interest in the products used or in determining what proportion of the budget goes to which country. Other concerns include the imposition of unduly onerous conditions on the disbursement and use of the funds. While there is a need for accountability in use of funds for their intended purposes, that accountability should enable the desired outcomes to be reached effectively and efficiently while respecting national sovereignty and avoiding excessive micro-management.

Corporate social responsibility programmes have a different set of issues compared to foundations (Shah 2011). For example, while Rio Tinto, one of the largest global mining firms, is justifiably proud of its success in confronting malaria in Equatorial Africa, it has at the same time, dumped billions of tons of toxic waste in Papua New Guinea. Similarly, Coca Cola's global distribution system has enabled more effective distribution of oral rehydration salts for diarrhoea, a major killer of children, particularly in Africa, but on the other hand, Coca Cola and other producers of modified, unhealthy fast foods are also contributing to the burgeoning NCD epidemic in developing countries.

Foundations have always based their giving on personal perspectives of their founders and subsequent leaders. They rarely consult public health leaders in determining these goals. With the influx of large sums of money by a few foundations, this approach can very easily distort the public health agenda globally and nationally as well as the role of smaller foundations.

Large donations by private industry to international organizations like the WHO create an inherent dilemma for the latter. With over 80 per cent of its budget coming from industry, the WHO has limited flexibility to focus funds on its own priorities. In 2004–2005, WHO ended up spending 61 per cent of its budget on illnesses that accounted for only 11 per cent of global mortality because that was where the funds that were being donated were requested to be directed.

At a national level, large donations can dwarf the total budget of the recipient country and cannot be matched by the local government in many resource-constrained settings. The concern is that the local public health agenda could end up being determined by external agencies which is a particular problem when the donor's agenda is not aligned with the country's priorities, and diverts scarce resources such as trained personnel and infrastructure to lower priorities. Donor programmes often offer higher salaries which draw staff out of the public sector, leaving fewer staff within government to work on other health priorities resulting in deterioration of other important public health programmes and exacerbating the existing public health human resource crisis extant in most developing countries. For example, in Haiti, the dramatically improved HIV/AIDS situation, facilitated by private funding, has been associated with a parallel decline in other measures of the population's health, including infant mortality rates (Farmer and Garrett 2007).

Notably in these settings local government funding typically is less than 5 per cent of total government expenditures. External funding can therefore perpetuate underfunding of health and undermine the responsibility that the government takes for healthcare delivery in their country. In countries with entrenched non-functioning bureaucracies and corruption, donor funds could exacerbate corruption as funds are diverted from their intended purpose to benefit some government officials.

There are clear advantages to private funding being directed at specific public health challenges and emergencies. This has enabled eradication of smallpox, substantial increases in childhood immunization coverage, and catalysed improved responses in natural disasters or emergency situations. This type of funding works well when there are mutually agreed priorities among the various stakeholders, and involve quick and nimble investments for a short duration while the parties responsible work on plans and systems to address longer-term sustainability issues.

In relation to long-term sustainability in this context, there are at least four inter-related concerns.

Firstly, when private donations are not synchronized with global or local priority setting and are targeted at chronic conditions which require a long-term investment such as AIDS, withdrawal of funding could result in a sharp worsening of the situation. In the case of AIDS, for example, an interruption in drug supplies could lead to treatment interruptions and promote the emergence of drug-resistant strains of HIV.

Hence, significant private funding initiatives with a specific long-term focus, for example, eradication of poliomyelitis or development of a new drug or vaccine, need to be sustained until the goal is achieved for such investments to be effective.

A second area where issues of sustainability are a concern with private funding relates to a foundation having a diverse portfolio. Specifically, the concern here relates to the withdrawal of funding before the goal is achieved or the shifting of funds from one incomplete initiative to a new one. While in the corporate world, this type of prioritization and re-prioritization is typical, such an approach could be counterproductive when addressing a multitude of public health challenges. As an illustration, the Gates Foundation provides 17 per cent of the global budget (US$86 million) to eradicate poliomyelitis, support childhood immunization programmes, develop an AIDS vaccine and microbicides, and pre-exposure prophylaxis studies. In addition, its funds support the Grameen Foundation that uses microfinance loans to empower women in Bangladesh. In partnership with The Rockefeller Foundation, the Gates Foundation supports novel agricultural practices in developing countries to enhance food security. All of these initiatives are important long-term projects with uncertain outcomes. When and how decisions will be made to continue or stop investments will have a critical and wide-ranging impact.

A third area of concern relates to who and how priorities are identified, particularly in settings with multiple challenges. For example, some express concern that the substantial funding in AIDS treatment is at the expense of HIV prevention or other health priorities. Others view it as an opportunity to concurrently strengthen healthcare delivery systems and integrate services notably for TB, maternal health, and infant health, resulting in an overall benefit to all health services. As AIDS funding focuses disproportionately on infant, maternal, and adult morbidity and mortality patterns, any gains will immediately translate to better disease burden outcomes in these settings and less to building essential health infrastructures.

With the global efforts to treat AIDS patients a new and major partner has been the pharmaceutical industry. The unprecedented price cuts and negotiation of intellectual property rights have been laudable and quoted as an example for extension to other diseases and products. Capacity building and technology transfer to less developed economies is viewed as a major opportunity to enable national governments in developing countries to meet the needs of their populations, as opposed to drug donations that meet short-term needs but create longer-term dependence.

A fourth level of concern is the lack of harmonization among donors at a country level.

In some countries, there are so many donors, each with their own agenda, that coordination and alignment to national priorities becomes very difficult. The disparity is further exacerbated if corruption is rife. A more critical issue relates to the diversion of critical human resource capacity away from government-identified priorities to donor priorities. The duplication of services by multiple funders also creates redundancy and inefficiencies.

External investment in a country's health should prioritize partnering with improving and supporting existing public infrastructure, and should recognize that a country's government would generally be in a better position to judge its health priorities than an external organization based in a rich country (Widdus 2003). This of course assumes that the national government is well functioning and capable of determining its priorities.

In some developing countries, in the absence of local acceptable leadership, the UN agencies have assumed a leadership role and private funding and bilateral donor aid gets channelled through these structures at a country level, bypassing the appropriate governmental agencies and thus creating a situation where the government may block access to the target of these charitable organizations.

HIV/AIDS provides another example of harmonization at a country level. All the UN agencies have been part of the 'Three Ones' agreement: *one* agreed-upon HIV/AIDS action framework that provides the basis for coordinating the work of all partners; *one* national AIDS coordinating authority, with a broad based multisector mandate; and *one* consensus for country-level monitoring and evaluation system (WHO 2004). Similar agreements are needed for donor-supported health projects in general.

China provides a unique example of how government authoritarianism has helped achieve this kind of coordination. Although it was motivated by a different purpose, China insists that large donor agencies have government approval before being allowed to work in-country, and thus, the relevant officials have been able to have a direct role in deciding where and how donor money should be channelled. In South Africa, in contrast, during the Mbeki AIDS denialist era, it was private and donor funding channelled through non-governmental and academic institutions that ensured access to antiretroviral treatment for the millions dying from AIDS.

Moving forward

The generous giving of the foundations, industry, and private donors has benefited public health greatly. They have sometimes also had unintended negative consequences. How can the positive impact of private giving be maximized? A few suggestions for strategies that may contribute to this goal include:

◆ Objective assessment of priorities against defined and objective criteria.

◆ Transparency and communication with key stakeholders on priority setting.

◆ Consideration should be given to the short- and long-term impact of investments.

◆ Investment should build capacity at a national level for sustainability of investments.

◆ Ongoing internal monitoring of progress and periodic evaluation of the impact of the programme by an external group.

◆ Establishment of advisory committees that include both international and local experts.

◆ Partnering with key stakeholders to ensure harmonization and synergy if there are multiple investors.

◆ Development of transparent governance mechanisms, policies, and procedural frameworks.

◆ Sustained funding commitment for long-term issues.

Many of these recommendations have already been incorporated in the GFATM. As we move forward and the role of private funding continues to grow, it is important that the strengths of private giving such as focus, nimbleness, innovation, risk-taking, and efficiencies do not get lost in massive, ineffective, and paralysing bureaucratic structures. To achieve the full potential of private giving, it is critical that it is structured to produce the maximum good with the fewest negative consequences.

References

Ardian, M., Meokbun, E., Siburian, L., et al. (2007). A public–private partnership for TB control in Timika, Papua Province, Indonesia. *International Journal of Tuberculosis and Lung Disease*, 11, 1101–7.

Asante, A.D. and Zwi, A.B. (2007). Public–private partnerships and global health equity: prospects and challenges. *Indian Journal of Medical Ethics*, 4, 176–80.

Barr, D.A. (2007). Ethics in public health research: a research protocol to evaluate the effectiveness of public–private partnerships as a means to improve health and welfare systems worldwide. *American Journal of Public Health*, 97, 19–25.

Birn, A.-E. and Fee, E. (2013). The Rockefeller Foundation and the international health agenda. *The Lancet*, 381, 1618–19.

Boutayeb, A. (2006). The double burden of communicable and non-communicable diseases in developing countries. *Transactions of the Royal Society of Tropical Medicine and Hygiene*, 100, 191–9.

Broadbent, J. and Laughlin, R. (2003). Public–private partnerships: an introduction. *Accounting, Auditing & Accountability Journal*, 16, 332–41.

Buse, K. and Walt, G. (2000a). Global public–private partnerships: part I—a new development in health? *Bulletin of the World Health Organization*, 78, 549–61.

Buse, K. and Walt, G. (2000b). Global public–private partnerships: part II—What are the health issues for global governance? *Bulletin of the World Health Organization*, 78, 699–709.

Buse, K. and Waxman, A. (2001). Public–private health partnerships: a strategy for WHO. *Bulletin of the World Health Organization*, 79, 748–54.

Butler, S.M. (2001). *Why the Bush Tax Cuts Are No Threat To Philanthropy*. [Online] Available at: http://www.heritage.org/research/reports/2001/03/why-the-bush-tax-cuts-are-no-threat-to-philanthropy.

Bygbjerg, I.C. (2012). Double burden of noncommunicable and infectious diseases in developing countries. *Science*, 337, 1499–501.

Carnegie Corporation of New York (n.d.). Website. [Online] Available at: http://www.carnegie.org.

Croft, S.L. (2005). Public–private partnership: from there to here. *Transactions of the Royal Society of Tropical Medicine and Hygiene*, 99, S9–14.

Curran, J.W. and Jaffe, H.W. (2011). AIDS: the early years and CDC's response. *Morbidity and Mortality Weekly Report Surveillance Summaries*, 60, 64–9.

DeVol, R., Bedroussian, A., and Charuworn, A. (2007). *An Unhealthy America: The Economic Burden of Chronic Disease*. Santa Monica, CA: Milken Institute.

Farmer, P. and Garrett, L. (2007). *From 'Marvelous Momentum' to Health Care for All: Success Is Possible With the Right Programs*. [Online] Available at: http://www.foreignaffairs.com/articles/62458/paul-farmer-and-laurie-garrett/from-marvelous-momentum-to-health-care-for-all-success-is-possible.

Flinders, M. (2005). The politics of public–private partnerships. *The British Journal of Politics & International Relations*, 7, 215–39.

Foundation Center (2013). *Top Funders* [Online] Available at: http://www.foundationcenter.org.

Fussel, H. and Beresford, C. (2009). *Public Private Partnerships: Understanding the Challenge* (2nd ed.). Vancouver: Center for Civic Governance, Columbia Institute.

Garvin, M.J. and Bosso, D. (2008). Assessing the effectiveness of infrastructure public–private partnership programs and projects. *Public Works Management & Policy*, 13, 162–78.

Goldman, H.H., Morrissey, J.P., Ridgely, M.S., Frank, R.G., Newman, S.J., and Kennedy, C. (1992). Lessons from the program on chronic mental illness. *Health Affairs*, 11, 51–68.

Hammack, D.C. and Wheeler, S. (1994). *Social Science in the Making: Essays on the Russell Sage Foundation, 1907–1972*. New York: Russell Sage Foundation.

Hodge, G.A. (2004). The risky business of public–private partnerships. *Australian Journal of Public Administration*, 63, 37–49.

Hodge, G.A. and Greve, C. (2005). *The Challenge of Public–Private Partnerships: Learning from International Experience*. Cheltenham: Edward Elgar Publishing.

Howard, L.M. (1983). International sources of financial cooperation for health in developing countries. *Bulletin of the Pan American Health Organization*, 17, 142–57.

Howard, L.M. (1991). Public and private donor financing for health in developing countries. *Infectious Disease Clinics of North America*, 5, 221–34.

Howard Hughes Medical Institute (n.d.). *Origins: 1905–1953*. [Online] Available at: http://www.hhmi.org/about/origins.html.

Kane, S., Dewan, P.K., Gupta, D., et al. (2010). Large-scale public–private partnership for improving TB-HIV services for high-risk groups in India. *International Journal of Tuberculosis and Lung Disease*, 14, 1066–8.

Kickbusch, I. and Quick, J. (1998). Partnerships for health in the 21st century. *World Health Statistics Quarterly*, 51, 68–74.

Kraak, V.I., Harrigan, P.B., Lawrence, M., Harrison, P.J., Jackson, M.A., and Swinburn, B. (2012). Balancing the benefits and risks of public–private partnerships to address the global double burden of malnutrition. *Public Health Nutrition*, 15, 503–17.

Lal, S.S., Uplekar, M., Katz, I., et al. (2011). Global Fund financing of public–private mix approaches for delivery of tuberculosis care. *Tropical Medicine & International Health*, 16, 685–92.

Lester, G. (2012). The osteoarthritis initiative: a NIH public–private partnership. *HSS Journal*, 8, 62–3.

McCoy, D., Chand, S., and Sridhar, D. (2009). Global health funding: how much, where it comes from and where it goes. *Health Policy and Planning*, 24, 407–17.

McCoy, D., Kembhavi, G., Patel, J., and Luintel, A. (2009). The Bill & Melinda Gates Foundation's grant-making programme for global health. *The Lancet*, 373, 1645–53.

McKee, M., Edwards, N., and Atun, R. (2006). Public–private partnerships for hospitals. *Bulletin of the World Health Organization*, 84, 890–6.

Mectizan Donation Program (2012). *25 Years of the Mectizan Donation Program*. [Online] Available at: http://www.mectizan.org/news/25-years-of-the-mectizan-donation-program.

Menasha, M.C.E. and Hsig, R.M. (1915). *The Rockefeller Foundation, Annual Report, 1913–1914*. New York: The Rockefeller Foundation.

Morvaridi, B. (2012). Capitalist philanthropy and hegemonic partnerships. *Third World Quarterly*, 33, 1191–210.

Nishtar, S. (2004). Public–private 'partnerships' in health—a global call to action. *Health Research Policy and Systems*, 2, 5.

Novignon, J., Olakojo, S.A., and Nonvignon, J. (2012). The effects of public and private health care expenditure on health status in sub-Saharan Africa: new evidence from panel data analysis. *Health Economics Review*, 2, 22.

Nwaka, S. (2005). Drug discovery and beyond: the role of public–private partnerships in improving access to new malaria medicines. *Transactions of the Royal Society of Tropical Medicine and Hygiene*, 99, 20–9.

Nwaka, S. and Ridley, R.G. (2003). Virtual drug discovery and development for neglected diseases through public–private partnerships. *Nature Reviews Drug Discovery*, 2, 919–28.

Robert Wood Johnson Foundation (2012). *Grants: Robert Wood Johnson Foundation Clinical Scholars*. [Online] Available from: http://www.rwjf.org/en/grants/national-program-offices/R/robert-wood-johnson-foundation-clinical-scholars.html.

Sanhai, W.R., Sakamoto, J.H., Canady, R., and Ferrari, M. (2008). Seven challenges for nanomedicine. *Nature Nanotechnology*, 3, 242–4.

Sanofi-Aventis (2007). *Sanofi-Aventis Joins the Fight Against Tuberculosis in South Africa*. [Online] Available at: http://en.sanofi.com/Images/15299_brochure_aam_en.pdf.

Shah, S. (2011). How private companies are transforming the global public health agenda. *Foreign Affairs*, 9 November.

Sharp, P.M. and Hahn, B.H. (2011). Origins of HIV and the AIDS pandemic. *Cold Spring Harbor Perspectives in Medicine*, 1, a006841.

Sinanovic, E. and Kumaranayake, L. (2010). The motivations for participation in public–private partnerships for the provision of tuberculosis treatment in South Africa. *Global Public Health*, 5, 479–92.

Spackman, M. (2002). Public–private partnerships: lessons from the British approach. *Economic Systems*, 26, 283–301.

Stop TB Partnership (n.d.). *Global Laboratory Initiative (GLI)*. Available at: http://www.stoptb.org/wg/gli/default.asp.

Strom, S. (2007). Big gifts, tax breaks and a debate on charity. *The New York Times*, 6 September. Available at: http://www.nytimes.com/2007/09/06/business/06giving.html?pagewanted=all&_r=0.

Sturchio, J.L. and Cohen, G.M. (2012). How PEPFAR's public–private partnerships achieved ambitious goals, from improving labs to strengthening supply chains. *Health Affairs*, 31, 1450–8.

The Rockefeller Foundation (2013a). *Our History. Moments in Time: 1913–1919*. [Online] Available at: http://www.rockefellerfoundation.org/about-us/our-history/1913-1919.

The Rockefeller Foundation (2013b). *Medicine in China*. [Online] Available at: http://rockefeller100.org/exhibits/show/education/china-medical-board.

UK Parliament (2011). *Committee Publishes Report on Private Finance Initiative Funding*. Available at: http://www.parliament.uk/business/committees/committees-a-z/commons-select/treasury-committee/news/pfi-report/.

Vitoria, M., Granich, R., Gilks, C.F., et al. (2009). The global fight against HIV/AIDS, tuberculosis, and malaria current status and future perspectives. *American Journal of Clinical Pathology*, 131, 844–8.

Vogel, A. (2006). Who's making global civil society: philanthropy and US empire in world society. *The British Journal of Sociology*, 57, 635–55.

Weiner, B.J. and Alexander, J.A. (1998). The challenges of governing public–private community health partnerships. *Health Care Management Review*, 23, 39–55.

Wellcome Trust (n.d.). Website. [Online] Available at: http://www.wellcome.ac.uk/.

Wheeler, C. and Berkley, S. (2001). Initial lessons from public–private partnerships in drug and vaccine development. *Bulletin of the World Health Organization*, 79, 728–34.

Widdus, R. (2001). Public–private partnerships for health: their main targets, their diversity, and their future directions. *Bulletin of the World Health Organization*, 79, 713–20.

Widdus, R. (2003). Public–private partnerships for health require thoughtful evaluation. *Bulletin of the World Health Organization*, 81, 235.

Widdus, R. (2005). Public–private partnerships: an overview. *Royal Society of Tropical Medicine and Hygiene*, 99, S1–8.

Williams, O.F. (2008). The UN Global Compact: the challenge and the promise. *Leadership and Business Ethics*, 2008, 229–49.

World Bank Group (2011). *PPP in Infrastructure Resource Center for Contracts, Laws and Regulations*. New York: World Bank.

World Health Organization (2004). *WHO: 'Three Ones' Agreed by Donors and Developing Countries*. [Online] Available at: http://www.who.int/3by5/newsitem9/en/.

11.13

The future of international public health in an era of austerity

Margaret Chan and Mary Kay Kindhauser

Introduction to the future of international public health

Since the twenty-first century began, the drive to improve health has experienced unprecedented commitments, opportunities, innovations, successes, setbacks, and surprises. Health also faces new threats arising from the radically increased interdependence of nations and policy spheres. The forces driving these changes are powerful, virtually universal, and almost certain to shape the public health agenda for years to come.

This chapter provides an overview of the remarkable progress of public health during the first decade of the twenty-first century, despite setbacks from global crises. It explores complex threats to health and emphasizes public health solutions that are either already under way or that need urgently to be pursued. The chapter concludes with a description of trends in the way public health is conceived, organized, and delivered, as reflected in new approaches to health development and new instruments for global health governance. These recent developments are cause for optimism that the momentum for better health that marked the start of this century will continue.

A decade of remarkable progress

The twenty-first century began well for public health. Leaders of 191 nations signed the Millennium Declaration in 2000 and committed themselves to reaching its eight goals by 2015 (United Nations (UN) 2000). With poverty reduction as an overarching objective, the Millennium Development Goals (MDGs) represent an ambitious attack on human misery, including that caused by disease and poor health. Three of the goals aim to reduce the mortality caused: by AIDS, malaria, tuberculosis, and other infectious diseases; by diseases of childhood; and by complications of pregnancy and childbirth. Other goals, for nutrition, education, gender equality, and the environment, including water supply and sanitation, tackle some of the most important determinants of ill health and premature death, especially in low-income settings. The final goal calls for the development of partnerships, including cooperation with pharmaceutical companies, to provide affordable access to essential drugs in developing countries.

The results have been remarkable (World Health Organization (WHO) 2012a). The incidence of new HIV infections has declined, as have deaths from malaria and tuberculosis (UN 2013). Mortality in children under the age of 5 dropped by more than 40 per cent from 1990 to 2011, and continued to decline year after year at accelerated rates (United Nations Children's Fund 2012). After decades of stagnation, maternal mortality rates dropped by 47 per cent from 1990 to 2010 (WHO 2012b). Although many countries will not reach the health-related MDGs by the target date of 2015, the overall achievements to date support the conclusion that aid for health development is working. They show the value of concentrating development efforts on a limited number of time-bound objectives that can be monitored and measured.

The MDGs are not, however, the only public health achievements of recent years. Life expectancy has risen globally for both men and women, a gain of more than 10 years since 1970, to a global average of 70 years in 2011 (The Lancet 2012; UN Department of Economic and Social Affairs 2012a). The WHO South East Asian region has seen a gain of more than 8 years in only the past two decades. By the next century, global life expectancy is projected to be above 80 years. Furthermore, rates of illness and death caused by infectious diseases are decreasing, as are rates of maternal illness and child mortality (WHO n.d. a).

Recent challenges

Improvements in global health are nevertheless fragile. Progress against infectious diseases is constantly threatened by antimicrobial resistance, as illustrated by the growing problem of multidrug-resistant (MDR) and extensively drug-resistant (XDR) tuberculosis. Long-standing public health challenges continue to persist particularly in low- and medium-income countries. These include the inadequate provision of safe water and safe waste disposal which contribute to childhood mortality, the burden of occupational diseases which constitute a major cause of morbidity in developing countries, environmental pollution and its acute and long-term health consequences especially in heavily-polluted cities, and violence, both interpersonal and armed conflict, which continues to be a major cause of mortality and morbidity particularly among the young in developed and developing countries.

More broadly, new dangers arise from a world of radically increased interdependence. A crisis in one part of the world can spread quickly and have profoundly inequitable consequences, adversely affecting countries that had nothing to do with the causes of the crisis. The international systems that govern trade, financial markets, and business relations can have a larger effect on the lives and opportunities of citizens, including the chances they have to enjoy a healthy life expectancy, than the policies of their governments.

The financial crisis of 2008 was a jolt, changing the global economic outlook from prosperity to austerity. The consequences on national health budgets and international aid for health development are still being felt. The drive to improve health, especially of the poor, has been severely tested. Some resource-intensive health initiatives have suffered funding shortfalls. For example, in its June 2012 report, the Independent Monitoring Board of the Global Polio Eradication Initiative concluded that the primary risk to the initiative was its precarious financial position (Independent Monitoring Board of the Global Polio Eradication Initiative 2012).

Since the global financial crisis began, many traditional donors of development assistance have come under increasing pressure to demonstrate that investments in health development elsewhere bring measurable results at home. Nevertheless, the momentum for better health has continued, including an emphasis on greater efficiency in the delivery of health services and frugal innovations that aim for simplicity, ease of use, and affordability; and the development of new initiatives, such as the UN Strategy for Women's and Children's Health, an accountability framework for tracking resources and measuring results.

In recent years the world has also woken up to the profound challenges posed by chronic non-communicable diseases (NCDs), including heart disease, stroke, diabetes, cancers, chronic respiratory disease, and mental health issues. Although NCDs were not recognized as a major threat to development when the MDGs were conceptualized, they have rapidly increased in prevalence and prominence.

Responding to the challenge of these diseases, particularly through prevention, will require major changes in the public health mind set and in the organization of health services, which, in most parts of the developing world, are geared towards the control of infectious diseases. These trends are moving public health into a new political space that deals with transnational threats to health and addresses determinants that lie well beyond the traditional concerns of the health sector.

Potential opportunities

Although the financial crisis will likely have an impact on health for some time to come, new initiatives, continuing innovations, and a quest for new sources of funding, show that the drive to improve health is still strong. Other signals come from the ethical principles embodied in some of the most successful global health initiatives and public–private partnerships formed to develop new methods of prevention and treatment for diseases of the poor. The GAVI Alliance, for example, works on the basis that every child deserves the best vaccines available, regardless of where the child was born or the income status of their parents. Product-development partnerships, such as the Medicines for Malaria Venture and the Meningitis Vaccine Project, seek to address the lack of incentives to develop new products for diseases

that mainly affect the poor by pioneering ways to bring such badly needed yet unprofitable drugs to market. In the largest sense, all of these initiatives represent a striving for greater fairness in access to the benefits of medical progress.

The international public health community has also increasingly agreed on treaties, regulations, codes of practice, and political declarations as instruments of global health governance, even in areas where public health policies are perceived as threats to powerful economic interests. The ability to reach agreement on these instruments, some of which are legally binding, such as the International Health Regulations (IHR), demonstrates the high priority given to health matters. They also reflect appreciation for the transnational nature of many of today's most important health challenges, and the need for collective action against common threats.

Public health has not always endured adverse world events with such resilience. The Declaration of Alma Ata, which launched the Health for All movement in 1978, was followed almost immediately by an oil crisis, a global recession, and the introduction of structural adjustment programmes that shifted government budgets away from social services, including health (Chan 2008). Largely as a result of these events, the 1980s became known as the 'lost decade for development'. Against this backdrop, the current determination to maintain the momentum for better health in an era of almost universal austerity appears all the more remarkable.

A health landscape of unprecedented complexity

Public health in the twenty-first century faces challenges of unprecedented complexity, with causes and consequences that extend well beyond the health sector. Foremost among these challenges is the rise of chronic NCDs, which have overtaken infectious diseases as the leading cause of mortality worldwide (WHO 2011a). This shift has its roots in demographic ageing; rapid urban growth; industrialization of food production; globalized marketing and the ready availability of highly processed foods, sugary beverages, and tobacco products; and the revolution in information technology, which contributes to increasingly sedentary lifestyles.

In addition, phenomenal increases in the speed and volume of international travel and trade have made emerging and epidemic-prone diseases a much larger threat. The demand for healthcare is rising rapidly at a time when the training and retention of doctors and nurses has stagnated, resulting in a shortage of more than 4 million healthcare workers worldwide, especially in Asia and Africa (WHO 2006). Globalization has contributed to the exodus of large numbers of health workers from the countries that invested in their training. The complex landscape of public health is also overcrowded. The proliferation of global health initiatives has created new challenges for distributive efficiency and the overall effectiveness of aid. This is particularly apparent in the added burden that multiple agencies, implementing health programmes within countries, place on already weak infrastructures and capacities.

These new challenges are superimposed upon traditional and long-standing barriers to better health—weak health systems, enduring poverty, and endemic infectious diseases closely associated with poverty.

Health in a world of growing inequalities

Health in its own right is of fundamental importance and, like education, is among the basic capabilities that give value to human life (Sen 1999). It is also a central driver of poverty reduction and socioeconomic development. The promotion of health-related human rights is a core value within the UN and WHO, and endorsed in many human rights instruments. These rights depend on the provision of social and economic human rights, such as the right to food, housing, work, and education. Health-related human rights underscore all efforts to ensure fair access to health-care for all.

Health is also a central element of human security. As the WHO Constitution notes, 'Unequal development in different countries in the promotion of health and the control of disease, especially communicable disease, is a common danger' (WHO 2005). Humanitarian emergencies, including natural and human-made disasters, infectious disease outbreaks, environmental hazards, conflicts, and the deliberate use of biological agents to incite terror, are traditionally considered the main threats to health security worldwide. However, wider considerations of human security, with the individual as a focus, also encompass issues of safe food and water, adequate shelter, clean air, poverty-related threats, violence, and the adverse effects of climate change on health (Ogata and Sen 2009). The Commission on Social Determinants of Health issued recommendations for addressing these and other threats to health that arise from the way societies are organized and governed (WHO 2008a).

Evidence is mounting that gaps, within and between countries, in income levels, in opportunities, and in health outcomes, life expectancy, and access to care, are now wider than at any time in recent history. The difference in life expectancy between the richest and poorest countries exceeds 40 years. Women in Afghanistan have a lifetime risk of maternal death of one in eight compared with one in 47,600 in Ireland. In Mali, one in five children die before the age of 5, whereas in Japan, the corresponding figure is three per 1000 live births (WHO 2012c). Annual government expenditures on health range from as little as $1 per person to nearly $7000 (WHO 2010a). In the decades before the 2008 financial crisis, in the Organisation for Economic Cooperation and Development (OECD) countries, the average income of the richest 10 per cent was about nine times that of the poorest 10 per cent, the largest gap in 50 years (OECD 2011a). These findings counter the assumption that the benefits of economic growth will automatically trickle down to the disadvantaged. They also suggest that the social contract is unravelling in many countries (Gurria 2011).

Decades of experience have shown that the world will not become a fair place for health by itself. Health systems will not automatically gravitate towards greater equality or naturally evolve towards universal coverage. Decisions aimed at increasing a country's economic growth will not automatically protect the poor or promote their health. International trade agreements will not, by themselves, guarantee food security, job security, health security, or access to affordable medicines. All of these outcomes require deliberate policy decisions that place equity at the forefront (Blas and Sivasankara Kurup 2010).

Social inequalities, including inequalities in health outcomes and in access to services, matter in ways that go beyond issues of human rights and social justice. Equality contributes to social cohesion and stability. Societies with the greatest equality have the best health outcomes, irrespective of the level of government expenditure on health. Equity-focused policies for improving child survival, health, and nutrition not only accelerate progress but also do so in a cost-effective way (Carrera et al. 2012).

Demographic change: an older world population concentrated in cities

Populations around the world are experiencing unprecedented demographic change. With the world population now standing at 7.2 billion, another 2.4 billion could be added by 2050 (UN Department of Economic and Social Affairs 2012b). Behind these numbers lie other important demographic trends common to many countries. Overall, women are bearing fewer children, people are living longer and healthier lives, populations are ageing, and increasing numbers of migrants are moving from rural areas to cities and from one country to another in search of better opportunities (UN Department of Economic and Social Affairs 2012c). A sharp contrast exists between the poorest nations—with their rapidly growing and young populations, and the richer nations, with their near-zero population growth and large numbers of elderly who have chronic diseases associated with ageing.

The trend towards ever-older populations is now universal. Worldwide, the proportion of older people in the total population is increasing at more than three times the overall population growth rate. Populations are ageing fastest in low- and middle-income countries. A transition towards an older society, which took place over more than a century in Europe, is now taking place in less than 25 years in countries like Brazil, China, and Thailand. By 2017, for the first time in history, the population of people aged 65 and older is expected to outnumber children under the age of 5 (WHO 2012d). These trends have major implications for healthcare, including its costs, especially as most elderly people will eventually develop multiple co-morbidities.

Rapid urbanization is another universal trend. By 2030, an estimated six out of every ten people will be living in towns or cities, with the most explosive growth expected in Asia and Africa. For a growing proportion of the world's population, prospects for a healthy life are tied to living conditions in cities. When cities are planned, managed, and governed well, life flourishes and health outcomes are better than those seen in rural areas. However, cities also concentrate risks and hazards for health, magnifying some long-standing threats to health and introducing others. When large numbers of people are linked together in space and connected by shared services, the consequences of adverse events—contamination of the food or water supply, high levels of air or noise pollution, a chemical spill, a disease outbreak, or a natural disaster—are vastly amplified.

Cities also tend to promote unhealthy lifestyles, such as 'convenient' diets that depend on inexpensive and readily available processed foods, sedentary behaviour, tobacco use, and the harmful use of alcohol and other substances. Many of these lifestyle choices contribute to obesity and the growing prevalence of NCDs, conditions that are increasingly concentrated among the urban poor. Poverty, which in previous centuries was greatest in scattered rural areas, is now heavily concentrated in cities.

In many countries, urbanization has outpaced the ability of governments to build essential infrastructures, and to enact and enforce legislation that makes life in cities safe, rewarding, and healthy. More than 800 million people worldwide, or one in three urban residents, live in slum conditions with inherent health problems resulting from rapid unplanned urbanization (WHO Centre for Health Development n.d.). Although more than 90 per cent of urban slums are located in the developing world, nearly every city everywhere has pockets of extreme deprivation side by side with areas of extreme wealth. In every part of the world, certain city dwellers suffer disproportionately from poor health, and these inequalities can be traced back to differences in their social and living conditions. Effective urban governance is needed to deal with these problems. In developing countries, the best urban governance can help produce 75 years or more of life expectancy. With poor urban governance, life expectancy can be as low as 35 years (WHO 2010b).

The rise of chronic non-communicable diseases

Long associated with affluent societies, today NCDs disproportionately affect the poor. The WHO estimates that 36 million deaths worldwide in 2008 were caused by NCDs, primarily cardiovascular diseases, cancers, diabetes, and chronic respiratory diseases. Of these deaths, nearly 80 per cent occurred in developing countries. Nine million occurred before the age of 60, countering the belief that these are diseases of 'old age' (WHO 2013a).

The health impacts of NCDs affect all countries, but are most severe in the developing world, where health services are ill-prepared to deal with the demands of chronic care; health budgets are already overstretched; systems for financial protection are weak or non-existent; and the costs of care, usually paid out-of-pocket, tend to delay patients from seeking treatment until the disease has reached an advanced stage that is more difficult and costly to manage. For diabetes, which has reached epidemic proportions in urban parts of Asia, studies show that patients there develop the disease sooner, are more seriously ill, and die earlier than their counterparts in Europe and North America (Yoon et al. 2006).

Four shared risk factors are responsible for a considerable proportion of the burden of chronic diseases: energy-dense, nutrient-poor diets that rely on the low price and convenience of highly processed foods; tobacco use; the harmful use of alcohol; and inadequate physical activity. An intervention that modifies one of these risk factors can reduce the risk for several diseases

The long time lag between the development of high population levels of risk and the emergence of population-wide disease further supports the importance of early intervention to reduce risk factors, especially in poorer countries where they tend to be neglected in the face of competing health needs. The exceptionally high costs of these diseases to national economies over a sustained period of time provide yet another compelling reason to focus on prevention. In some countries, the costs of caring for diabetes alone consume nearly 15 per cent of the national health budget (Zhang et al. 2010). The costs to individual households are equally devastating. The WHO estimates that, in most low- and middle-income countries, patients with diabetes, who live on US$1 or US$2 per day respectively, would need to spend between 25 per cent and 50 per cent of their monthly income to buy one vial of insulin from a private pharmacy (Barceló et al. 2003).

The WHO stresses the importance of taking a life-course approach to prevention, starting at the very beginning of life. Evidence is mounting that undernutrition during gestation and early childhood increases the risk of NCDs, especially cardiovascular disease and diabetes, later in life (Boekelheide et al. 2012).

Early detection and management are equally important as a strategy for reducing both the disease burden and the costs to economies. In 2011, the WHO and the World Economic Forum identified a core set of 'best buy' interventions for the prevention and control of NCDs, ranging from counselling and drug therapy for cardiovascular disease to measures to prevent cervical cancer. These are interventions that have significant public health impact, and are highly cost-effective, inexpensive, and feasible to implement (WHO and the World Economic Forum 2011).

Threats from the constantly evolving microbial world

Infectious diseases cause two main categories of threats to public health. The first category occurs in populations at risk from endemic infectious diseases, including AIDS, tuberculosis, malaria, pneumonia, diarrhoeal diseases, the neglected tropical diseases, and sexually transmitted diseases. These diseases cause high morbidity, disability, and mortality, and their control has been given high priority by national governments and the international community. Most have effective, often low-cost interventions for prevention or treatment, and many now benefit from global health initiatives established to deliver these interventions. With the sole exception of disease eradication, gains against infectious diseases are always fragile. Recent gains against nearly all of these diseases, but most especially those targeted by the MDGs, can be undone by complacency that leads to diminished control efforts or lapses in vigilance, or by the development of antimicrobial resistance.

The second category of threats, which is of more direct concern to global health security, arises from emerging and re-emerging epidemic-prone diseases, especially those that travel efficiently internationally and result in pandemics. Factors that may enhance the transmission of such diseases include increased population movements through international travel or migration or in response to disasters; growth in international trade in food and biological products; social and environmental changes linked with urbanization, deforestation, and a changing climate; the development of sophisticated new medical procedures; and changes in animal husbandry and the industrialization of food production (Ong and Heymann 2007). Many of the diseases in the first category of threats can become epidemic-prone if they are not comprehensively addressed. The development of antimicrobial resistance may result in 'super-bugs' that can quickly spread and result in epidemics. For example, bacteria containing the New Delhi metallo-β-lactamase-1 (NDM-1) enzyme are resistant to nearly all antibiotics. Common infections caused by bacteria with NDM-1 may therefore become life-threatening (Nordmann et al. 2011).

The 2003 outbreak of severe acute respiratory syndrome (SARS) demonstrated how much the world has changed in terms of its vulnerability to emerging diseases. SARS spread rapidly along the routes of international air travel and caused significant economic losses and social disruption well beyond the outbreak zones. As the emergence of diseases is tied to fundamental changes in the way humanity inhabits the planet, more novel infectious diseases can be anticipated. Two recent examples of new infectious diseases include avian influenza A (H7N9) (Gao et al. 2013) and the Middle East respiratory syndrome coronavirus (MERS-CoV) (Bermingham et al. 2012).

A crisis in human resources for health

The WHO estimates that the world faces a shortage of 4.2 million doctors, nurses, and other healthcare staff, with 1.5 million needed in Africa alone. Of the 57 countries with the most critical shortages, 36 are in sub-Saharan Africa. This part of the world accounts for 11 per cent of the global population and 24 per cent of the global burden of disease, but has only 3 per cent of the world's health workforce (WHO 2006) (Fig. 11.13.1). The shortage is felt by nearly all countries, but has its most severe impact in the developing world, where it jeopardizes the delivery of essential, life-saving health services, including childhood immunization, care during pregnancy and childbirth, and access to treatment for AIDS, tuberculosis, and malaria. The inadequacy of human resources for health significantly correlates with higher rates of maternal mortality, infant mortality, under five mortality (Anand and Barnighausen 2004), and poorer childhood vaccination coverage (Anand and Barnighausen 2007). Survival declines proportionately as the number of health workers declines. The effect is even more acute in the growing number of countries that face a double burden of infectious and NCDs.

The causes of these shortages are manifold. Years of underinvestment have left many developing countries with limited capacity to train healthcare workers. Decades of economic and sectoral reform capped expenditures, froze recruitment and salaries, and restricted public budgets, resulting in unattractive work conditions with poor facilities, frequent drug stock-outs, inadequate equipment and supplies, shortages of support personnel, large numbers of patients with little capacity to pay, and few opportunities for career advancement (Narasimhan et al. 2004).

In Africa, medical graduates in several countries decline to work in rural areas because of lack of clinical support (Mullan et al. 2011). Moreover, the orientation of training, based on Western medicine, is often poorly aligned with the health needs of populations in the developing world.

'Push and pull' forces operate to encourage health workers to leave rural and lower-resourced areas to work under the more favourable conditions of urban employment or to seek employment abroad, a trend accelerated by the globalization of labour markets. Within countries, the discrepancy in salaries between regular public sector jobs and comparable jobs with the private sector or better-funded global health initiatives has exacerbated the human resource crisis (Vujicic et al. 2004; Atun et al. 2008). In sub-Saharan Africa, which has few opportunities for postgraduate medical education, many graduates seeking advanced training travel to Europe and North America, and many do not return (Mullan et al. 2011). The relative shortage of health workers is also exacerbated by rising demand for healthcare in many countries. The Global Health Workforce Alliance was established by the World Health Assembly in 2006 to provide a common platform for action to address these problems (Global Health Workforce Alliance n.d.).

International migration of the health workforce is a multifaceted public health challenge that has elicited intense debate. Some view the recruitment of foreign health workers as the only way for wealthy countries to cope with rising demand for healthcare. Some stress the right of health workers to migrate to countries that offer better conditions of work and pay and better opportunities to use their skills and advance their careers. Others point to the need to balance the rights of individual health workers to migrate with the right of people in the developing world to receive essential healthcare. In addition, widespread concerns have been raised about unethical and unfair recruitment practices. In response to this crisis, the World Health Assembly adopted a *Global Code of*

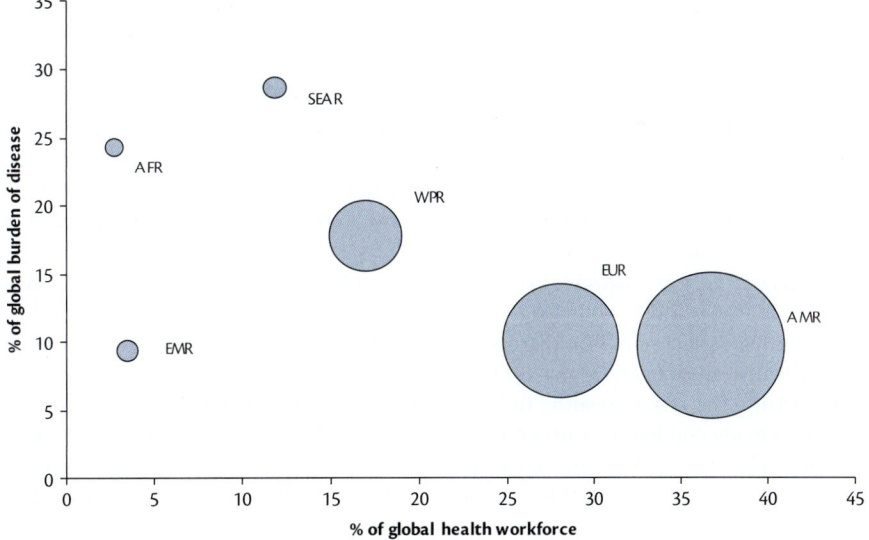

Fig. 11.13.1 Healthcare worker distribution by level of health expenditure and burden of disease, WHO regions.

Key: AFR, Regional Office for Africa; AMR, Regional Office for the Americas; EMR, Regional Office for the Eastern Mediterranean; EUR, Regional Office for Europe; SEAR, Regional Office for South-East Asia; WPR, Regional Office for the Western Pacific.

Reproduced with permission from World Health Organization, *Working Together for Health: The World Health Report 2006*, World Health Organization, Geneva, Switzerland, Copyright © WHO 2006, available from http://www.who.int/whr/2006/whr06_en.pdf.

Practice for the International Recruitment of Health Personnel in 2010, after nearly 6 years of debate (WHO 2010c). Compliance with the code is, however, voluntary; monitoring is under way to assess its effectiveness.

A shrinking arsenal of safe and effective medicines

The overuse, underuse, and misuse of antibiotics, in both human and veterinary medicine, have accelerated the emergence and international spread of drug-resistant pathogens. The speed with which the therapeutic arsenal of antimicrobials is shrinking far outpaces the development of replacement drugs, which are regarded by the pharmaceutical industry as less lucrative than medicines for chronic conditions, and less likely to have a long market life owing to the rapid emergence of resistance. These trends raise the spectre of a post-antibiotic era in which many common infections will no longer have a cure and, once again, kill unabated. The implications extend to many other life-saving and life-prolonging interventions. Some sophisticated interventions, such as joint replacements, organ transplants, cancer chemotherapy, and care of preterm infants, would become far more difficult or even too dangerous to undertake without effective antibiotics.

Replacement treatments for first-line antimicrobials that have lost their effectiveness are more costly and more toxic and require much longer durations of treatment, including hospital-based treatment. Studies have documented higher mortality among patients infected with drug-resistant pathogens. Among the world's 12 million tuberculosis cases in 2010, the WHO estimates that 650,000 involved MDR tuberculosis strains. Treatment of MDR tuberculosis is challenging, typically requiring 2 years of medication with toxic and expensive medicines, some of which are constantly in short supply. Even with the best of care, only slightly more than 50 per cent of these patients will be cured (WHO 2012e). The emergence of malaria parasites resistant to artemisinins, the last remaining class of effective drugs for the treatment of malaria, counts among the greatest fears of public health today. Evidence of resistance to artemisinins on the Cambodia–Thailand border, the historical epicentre for the emergence of drug-resistant malaria parasites, was confirmed in 2009. In 2011, the WHO launched an ambitious global plan to stop the further emergence of artemisinin-resistance at its source, and thus prevent, or at least significantly delay, further international spread.

Many other pathogens are developing resistance to multiple drugs—some pathogens like gonorrhoea and typhoid fever to nearly all drugs. Hospitals have become the breeding ground for highly resistant pathogens, such as methicillin-resistant *Staphylococcus aureus* (MRSA), extended spectrum beta-lactamase-producing (ESBL) bacteria, and carbapenemase-producing Enterobacteriaceae (CPE), increasing the risk that hospitalization kills instead of heals. Many are now found in the community, increasing the risk to health. To raise awareness and action, the WHO made combating antimicrobial resistance a priority at World Health Day 2011, and has since strengthened the initiative towards a long-term agenda to combat resistance through multipronged approaches.

The supply and trade of counterfeit and substandard medicines is another growing problem with international dimensions that compromises the quality of healthcare. The true scale of the problem is poorly documented, but some estimates suggest that 10–30 per cent of medicines on sale in developing countries are substandard or counterfeit (Cockburn et al. 2005). All countries are affected, as most recently demonstrated by tainted steroids in the United States that caused several deaths and placed 13,000 people at risk (Centers for Disease Control and Prevention 2012). The consequences can be severe. In Pakistan, more than 100 patients died following administration of contaminated cardiovascular medication (WHO 2012f). Countries that lack strong drug regulatory authorities and quality control laboratories are at particular risk. Substandard medical products may arise from unintentional lapses in good manufacturing practices. Other medical products of concern may enter the market from unknown or unlicensed producers and thus prove very difficult to trace. A known or licensed producer may intentionally distribute a substandard product as, for example, a product with a falsified expiration date or statement of active ingredients. Still other medical products may be deliberately and deceptively formulated and packaged to imitate another product often in very sophisticated ways. Drugs falsified in this way are copyright infringements and violations of intellectual property rights. While such instances are criminal activities to be addressed in appropriate courts of law, public health must be concerned whenever substandard or dangerous medicines enter the supply chain, regardless of whether the cause reflects deliberate deception, negligence, or weak capacity for quality assurance and regulatory control.

The drugs most commonly falsified include antimicrobials, hormones, and steroids. A study of malaria medicines sampled from several countries in South East Asia and sub-Saharan Africa found that 35 per cent of the samples from both regions failed chemical analysis; 46 per cent failed packaging analysis and 36 per cent were classified as falsified in South East Asia; and 35 per cent failed packaging analysis and 20 per cent were classified as falsified in sub-Saharan Africa (Nayyar et al. 2012). More recently, sophisticated and deceptive practices have included the falsification of anticancer and antiviral drugs, including those used to treat AIDS. To combat these problems, much more needs to be done to strengthen national drug regulatory authorities and quality assurance laboratories. The WHO estimates that only around 20 per cent of countries have well-developed systems for regulating medical products—of the remaining countries, around 50 per cent implement drug regulation at varying levels of effectiveness, and the remaining 30 per cent have either no drug regulation in place or a very limited capacity that barely functions. The increasing sale of medicine via the Internet further complicates efforts to protect consumers from substandard or falsified medical products (WHO n.d. b).

Past efforts to address the problem of counterfeit and substandard medicines have been hampered by the confusion of public health issues with issues of intellectual property rights and copyright infringements, and high-profile trade incidents in which legitimate generic medicines were seized, in transit, as counterfeits. In many countries, the only legal instrument available to address the public health problems caused by counterfeit and substandard medicines is legislation related to intellectual property rights, which further fuels the confusion (Attaran et al. 2012).

A changing climate

Climate change—possibly the defining issue of the twenty-first century—poses a significant addition to the spectrum of environmental hazards that threaten health. The contribution of human activities to changes in the climate system is irrefutable. The consequences of increases in global average air and ocean temperatures, widespread melting of snow and ice, and rising average sea levels are already being felt (WHO 2008b). Climate change will affect, in profoundly adverse ways, the most basic determinants of health: air, water, food, shelter, and freedom from disease. While the warming of the planet is expected to be gradual, the effects of extreme weather events—more storms, floods, heat waves, cold waves and droughts—will be abrupt and acutely felt. Such events are expected to increase in both frequency and intensity. While climate change is a global phenomenon, scientists predict that developing countries, including those that have contributed least to greenhouse gas emissions, will experience the earliest and most severe consequences, also for health (Postigo et al. 2007).

Specific effects of climate change on health include: (1) increases in malnutrition (associated with declining food production and security, especially in areas dependent on rain-fed agriculture) and related increases in the severity of childhood infectious diseases; (2) increases in death, disease, and injury due to extreme weather events; (3) increases in the number of displaced populations and the corresponding problem of 'environmental refugees'; (4) increases in episodes of diarrhoeal disease; (5) increases in outbreaks, especially of cholera due to unsafe water and flooding; (6) increases in the frequency of cardiorespiratory diseases associated with heat waves; and (7) altered distribution of vectors responsible for infectious diseases, most notably malaria and dengue (WHO 2008b).

In our interdependent world, the effects of a changing climate can have widespread consequences. Recent droughts in the Russian Federation and the United States significantly reduced world grain supplies. Whether these events are direct expressions of a changing climate is still being debated, but their contribution to record-breaking world food prices has been well documented, offering evidence of what lies ahead: more global crises caused by rising food prices (Food and Agriculture Organization of the United Nations 2012). The same is true for the two mega-disasters of 2010, the floods in Pakistan and the earthquake in Haiti, which outstripped the capacity of the international humanitarian community to respond. The disproportionate impact of climate change on the developing world will almost certainly further widen the unacceptably large gaps in health outcomes. Some have suggested that climate change could undo the progress made towards reaching the health-related MDGs. Unfortunately, these effects on health have been largely neglected in debates about climate change and the justifications for urgent action either to mitigate the causes or adapt to the consequences. Humanity, not only an endangered species like the polar bear, and human health should be the face of climate change.

The proliferation of global health initiatives

About 100 global health initiatives now exist—far more than in any other sector contributing to development. Most of these target health interventions for single infectious diseases or related groups of these diseases. A few, including the Global Fund to Fight AIDS, Tuberculosis and Malaria, the GAVI Alliance, the US President's Emergency Plan For AIDS Relief (PEPFAR), and the World Bank Multi-Country AIDS Program (MAP), contribute substantially to the funding for health provided by international donors (World Health Organization Maximizing Positive

Synergies Group 2009). In addition, an increasing number of non-governmental, faith-based, and private sector organizations are delivering health programmes in countries. New philanthropies, including the Bill & Melinda Gates Foundation, have become a potent financial force supporting the quest for new medical products for diseases of the poor and the delivery of pro-poor health interventions within countries.

Some experts in development aid view this rapid proliferation of initiatives as creating a public health landscape that is overcrowded and competitive. Problems identified include fragmentation and duplication of efforts, high transaction and operational costs, and the burden on recipient countries of multiple separate demands for monitoring and reporting. For example, in 2009, Vietnam dealt with more than 400 donor missions to review health projects or the health sector. Rwanda must report annually to various donors on 890 health indicators, with nearly 600 relating to HIV and malaria alone. Although increases in funding for health development are a welcome trend, recipient countries must digest such assistance with an extraordinary mobilization of their own very limited health resources.

In parallel, efforts to scale up the delivery of interventions have brought renewed attention to pervasive weaknesses in health systems as one of the most important barriers to programme success. Single-disease initiatives depend on a well-functioning health system to achieve their objectives yet rarely make the strengthening of health systems an explicit goal. Under the pressure of scaled-up efforts to deliver interventions, long-standing weaknesses became more visible: severe staff shortages; inefficient procurement and supply chains; frequent stock-outs; little capacity to regulate the quality and availability of medicines in either the public or private sectors; weak laboratory support; a concentration of clinical services in urban areas; a reliance on user fees to finance healthcare; little or no support from social protection or insurance schemes; crumbling government-funded services that forced reliance on more expensive private providers, even for routine care; and a glaring absence of fundamental health data for setting priorities, measuring results, monitoring progress, and adjusting priorities and strategies accordingly.

The debate about whether global health initiatives strengthen or weaken health systems and distort national priorities has been intense. It rekindles a decades-old controversy over horizontal versus vertical approaches to health development, but in a more nuanced guise, as most health services now combine vertical and integrated elements, with varying degrees of balance between them (Atun et al. 2008). Some critics argue that single-disease initiatives have deepened inequalities in health services, reduced the quality of services because of pressures to meet targets, and created expensive parallel systems for the management of programme delivery, bypassing rather than strengthening existing national systems (The Lancet 2009). Other studies suggest that single-disease initiatives make an important contribution to improved health outcomes by delivering preventive or treatment interventions for high-mortality diseases, especially when health systems are weak, a rapid response is needed, and economies of scale can reduce procurement costs and further extend coverage (Atun et al. 2008).

Evidence for the benefits of single-disease initiatives is too limited to support firm conclusions about their broad effects on health systems. Some criticisms lose their relevance as programmes successfully reduce the disease burden and graduate to a more integrated approach. For example, the adoption of a new global health sector strategy on HIV/AIDS, 2011–2015 (WHO 2011b), stressing integration with existing health services, is regarded by many as marking a formal end to AIDS exceptionalism. Similarly, the Onchocerciasis Control Programme (WHO n.d. c) in West Africa, which began as a strictly vertical programme, with helicopters applying insecticides to fast-flowing rivers, eventually evolved to a primary healthcare approach that relies on community-directed distribution of ivermectin together with other essential interventions, including bednets, vitamin A supplements, and deworming tablets. Moreover, for AIDS, tuberculosis, and malaria, it is generally agreed that single-disease initiatives upgraded the quality of clinical care by introducing standardized treatment protocols and delivering quality-assured interventions.

Concern about the growth of uncoordinated aid and its adverse consequences has been addressed by international instruments such as the Paris Declaration on Aid Effectiveness of 2005 and the Accra Agenda for Action of 2008 (OECD 2005, 2008). These set out principles for improving the quality of aid and making development assistance more effective, with clear responsibilities for donors as well as recipient countries. A growing number of partnerships are implementing these principles in a spirit of mutual accountability and with an emphasis on delivering measurable results. In 2011, a meeting in Busan, Republic of Korea, took these commitments a step further with the concept of domestic accountability, in which country ownership matures to the point that governments are ultimately held accountable, by citizens and civil society organizations, for safeguarding public health (OECD 2011b).

In 2007, the International Health Partnership and Related Initiatives, known as IHP+, was established to accelerate better health results in low- and middle-income countries by applying principles of aid effectiveness, giving particular attention to aligning contributions from donors and implementing agencies with a country's own definition of its needs and capacities (IHP+ n.d.). The initiative has grown from 27 to 56 signatories to the IHP+ Global Compact, including 25 countries in Africa. IHP+ has developed and refined tools for improving the quality of national health strategies and plans and for conducting joint assessments of these. It has also helped bring civil society into these processes at country level, giving them a greater voice in policy formulation.

Work on harmonization and simplification of financial management has accelerated through collaboration between the World Bank, the GAVI Alliance, and the Global Fund. Other development partners are also becoming involved. Through IHP+, a single monitoring and evaluation framework with a limited number of indicators was developed, based on consultations with countries and development partners. Supported in part by the achievements of the Commission on Information and Accountability for Women's and Children's Health (WHO n.d. d), the framework is being used by a growing number of countries as the basis for strengthening their health information platforms.

The 2008 global financial crisis has changed the operating environment for IHP+. Growth in development assistance for health slowed, with data for 2011 showing a 3 per cent real decline in aid as a whole (IHP+ 2012). The number of aid providers, however, has continued to increase, increasing the risk of fragmentation. There has also been less political willingness to take risks and an increased focus on value for money. These trends reinforce the need for the WHO and other agencies to continue to play an active role in initiatives that aim to improve aid effectiveness.

Recent experiences show the value of harmonizing and aligning development assistance, especially when country ambitions are pragmatic and show vision. For example, Nepal introduced free maternal healthcare in a few districts in 2009, and announced its plans to extend this throughout the country's 76 districts. Donors united behind this visionary plan, and the goal was achieved in 2011. In the Democratic Republic of Congo, a single-donor coordination arrangement, introduced by the Ministry of Health, reduced the management costs of donor funds from 28 per cent to 9 per cent. The funds saved were invested to expand coverage with insecticide-treated bednets.

Questions about the sustainability of funding for health development continue to be raised, and particularly in the current era of austerity. The domestic pressure on donors to demonstrate results for investments in health development may skew investments to areas that can yield rapid measurable results. In such calculations, childhood immunization, for example, wins out over the purchase of antiretroviral medication, creating fears that the expansion of coverage with antiretroviral therapy may lose momentum.

Strategies for maintaining momentum in an era of austerity

Despite the financial crisis that began in 2008, the international community has not backed away from its commitment to better health, especially for the poor. Instead, the focus has been on using new instruments and political agreements to better utilize existing resources, reduce waste and inefficiency, demonstrate the value of investments by tracing resources and measuring results, and to use legislation and regulatory control to reduce threats to health at their source. New solutions that work well for one problem are being adapted to address others. Mechanisms for ensuring that developing countries reap the benefits of research and development for new medical products are also being negotiated. Many of these instruments and political agreements operate at the international level, reflecting solidarity in the desire for greater healthcare equity and the transnational nature of many health threats. As such, they are building a framework for global health governance.

New instruments for accountability

Instruments and frameworks for accountability aim to ensure that resources for health are responsibly used and are fully accountable, that results are measured and transparently reported, and that strategies are adjusted when expected results fail to materialize. Two of these instruments are described in the following subsections: the Independent Monitoring Board of the Global Polio Eradication Initiative and an accountability framework and independent monitoring body established by the Commission on Information and Accountability for Women's and Children's Health. Independent accountability is a compelling new concept in public health and holds promise as a way of spending resources more wisely, improving outcomes and maintaining the confidence of donors and the support of ministries of finance.

Accountability for polio eradication

In 2008, there were heightened concerns that the hitherto successful global polio eradication programme would be derailed.

A devastating setback in Nigeria 5 years earlier resulted in a surge of cases in northern Nigeria, after bans on vaccination issued by religious leaders and supported by politicians. This seeded outbreaks in many countries that had previously been polio-free, necessitating intensive containment campaigns. Some of these campaigns were unsuccessful, leading to the re-establishment of transmission in new areas. Experts previously argued that polio could never be eradicated, that the goal was unrealistic, and that it was time to give up and move the programme from eradication to control (Arita et al. 2006).

By 2008, donors were fatigued, field staff were tired and discouraged, and commitment in many countries with indigenous wild poliovirus or with re-established transmission was wavering. Reassuring statements that the eradication effort was in the 'home stretch' had been repeatedly issued for nearly a decade and were losing credibility, and the programme faced a funding gap of $575 million for 2007–2008.

In 2008, the World Health Assembly responded to this alarming situation by asking the WHO to develop a new strategy to reinvigorate the drive to eradicate polio. As some delegates had noted, the strategy that had worked so well to reduce the worldwide number of cases by 99 per cent since 1988 was inadequate for the challenge of eliminating the remaining 1 per cent of cases. In an unusual step, the WHO established an Independent Monitoring Board (IMB) to monitor the implementation and impact of the new strategic plan and its milestones, covering the 2010–2012 timeframe (The Global Polio Eradication Initiative n.d.). The IMB uses data generated by the eradication initiative but independently develops its own analyses and presentations and does not share drafts of its assessments before they are finalized. Its reports have been frank in their analyses and criticisms of dysfunctions and missed opportunities at every level of programme performance, from local staff, to national strategic plans, to the administration and culture of the global programme. As an instrument for accountability, the value of the IMB has been enforced by its insistence that its recommendations are heeded.

The results have been impressive, showing a substantial impact on programme performance but also on the prospects of success.

At the start of 2012, India, arguably the most challenging of all the remaining sanctuaries of poliovirus, had been polio-free for a year. The worldwide number of new cases was at the lowest level since records began. In May 2012, the WHO, acting on a recommendation of the IMB, declared the completion of poliovirus eradication a programmatic emergency for global public health, requiring the institution of strong national oversight and accountability mechanisms for all affected areas. The programme was restructured on an emergency footing. Thousands of additional staff were recruited, and national emergency plans were launched in Afghanistan, Pakistan, and Nigeria, the three remaining countries with indigenous poliovirus. India sent its experienced staff to share best practices with other countries. More children were reached, for the first time, in high-risk areas. The IMB final report for 2012 revised downwards the percentage of cases yet to be eradicated to 0.1 per cent and concluded that the prospects for success were more positive than ever (Independent Monitoring Board of the Global Polio Eradication Initiative 2012).

Accountability for women's and children's health
The UN's Global Strategy for Women's and Children's Health, also known as Every Woman, Every Child, was launched in 2010

as the first major health initiative since the 2008 financial crisis (Every Woman, Every Child n.d.). It responded to stalled progress in reaching the MDGs for reducing child and maternal mortality. Donors initially pledged $40 billion to support the strategy, and that amount has since increased. The strategy targets 75 countries where 98 per cent of all maternal, neonatal, and child deaths occur and includes the delivery, on a large scale, of low-cost but high-impact interventions with a proven capacity to save lives.

Every Woman, Every Child has several unique features. First, it was almost immediately followed by the establishment of a Commission on Information and Accountability for Women's and Children's Health, jointly supported by the WHO and the International Telecommunication Union. The Commission set out a framework for accountability that includes a small but balanced set of core indicators for measuring progress, supported by a tracer set of eight coverage indicators that can monitor almost real-time changes in coverage. Second, the development of systems for reliable civil registration and vital statistics was a built-in component of the framework. Finally, an independent Expert Review Group was rapidly established to provide oversight, including the identification of best value-for-money approaches.

The Expert Review Group operates with full independence. Its first report expressed serious concerns about the failure of some promised resources to materialize, the continuing absence in 64 of the 75 countries of reliable data on the key indicators established by the Commission, and insufficient progress overall (Independent Expert Review Group on Information and Accountability for Women's and Children's Health 2012). The report made six recommendations for improving the effectiveness of the accountability framework. Predictably, the report found that 53 of the 75 priority countries suffer a severe shortage of health workers, and recommended that the strengthening of human resources for women's and children's health be addressed as a matter of immense urgency. The accountability framework for Every Woman, Every Child has proved broadly useful for other health initiatives, including the International Health Partnership and Related Health Initiatives. The framework's country monitoring and evaluation platform is used by the Global Fund and the GAVI Alliance and has influenced the framework for the global monitoring of chronic NCDs.

New instruments for global health governance
Since the start of this century, the international health community has agreed on an unprecedented number of treaties, regulations, and codes of practice aimed at improving the global governance of public health by introducing systems of rules-based obligations. Some are legally binding 'hard law' instruments. Others are voluntary 'soft law' agreements. All respond to challenges that have international dimensions and depend on broad collaboration for an effective response. Some of these are described in the following subsections.

Framework Convention on Tobacco Control
The Framework Convention on Tobacco Control (FCTC), which came into force in 2005, is the first treaty negotiated under the auspices of the WHO and one of the most rapidly ratified treaties in the history of the UN (WHO Framework Convention on Tobacco Control 2012). The legally binding treaty now has 171 signatories representing nearly 90 per cent of the world's population.

Provisions in the treaty provide rules governing the production, sale, distribution, advertisement, and taxation of tobacco products as minimum requirements for tobacco control. The FCTC and a related treaty that followed, the Protocol on the Elimination of Illicit Trade in Tobacco Products (WHO Framework Convention on Tobacco Control 2013), demonstrate what can be achieved when multiple sectors, including trade, finance, agriculture, education, labour, the environment, law enforcement, and the judicial system, collaborate in the name of health.

International Health Regulations

The revised International Health Regulations (IHR) came into force in 2007 (WHO 2008c). Administered by the WHO, the Regulations bring an orderly, rules-based structure to the detection, reporting, and containment of public health emergencies of international concern. They also provide a centralized, coordinated mechanism for sharing information and keeping the world informed. The current, revised version of the IHR was strongly influenced by experiences during the SARS outbreak of 2003, which underscored the need for better disease intelligence and more stringent requirements for reporting. Adoption of the revised Regulations moved the response to health emergencies from a passive, reactive effort to prevent spread across national borders to a proactive effort that aims to stop an outbreak before it has a chance to spread internationally

Recommendations on the marketing of unhealthy food and beverages

The marketing of unhealthy foods and beverages to children is a growing problem. Advertising and other forms of food marketing to children are widespread across the world (Hastings et al. 2003; McGinnis et al. 2006; Cairns et al. 2009). Most of this marketing is for foods high in saturated fats, trans fatty acids, sugar, and salt. There is evidence that television advertising, including transboundary advertising, influences children's food preferences, requests, and consumption patterns. In addition, studies have shown compelling evidence of an association between the consumption of sugary beverages and the prevalence of obesity and overweight in children and adolescents (De Ruyter et al. 2012; Ebbeling et al. 2012; Qibin et al. 2012). In 2010, with more than 43 million pre-school-aged children estimated to be overweight or obese, the World Health Assembly adopted recommendations aimed at fostering more responsible marketing practices in the food and beverage industries. Although some countries have introduced legislation or established national policies aimed at curtailing the marketing of unhealthy foods and beverages to children, the global recommendations depend on voluntary changes on the part of the food and beverage industries.

Some experts and civil society organizations believe that the recommendations do not go far enough, that industry self-regulation is unlikely to be effective, and that a legally binding international treaty or convention is needed. As support for their arguments, they cite repeated industry violations of the 1981 International Code of Marketing of Breast-milk Substitutes (International Baby Food Action Network 2010). Support for stronger measures also comes from studies comparing the behaviour of the food industry with that of the tobacco industry in the second half of the previous century. While there are many differences between these industries, such comparisons reveal the use of broadly similar tactics: making pledges of self-regulation, lobbying with massive resources to stifle government action, introducing 'safer' products, and paying scientists to instil doubts about the conclusiveness of evidence (Brownell and Warner 2009). If the food industry does not change pre-emptively, public opinion may turn against it, as it did with the tobacco industry. At present, public health might best contribute to the debate by continuing to document the prevalence of overweight and obesity in children, to demonstrate the multiple risks and consequences for health, and to estimate the costs.

Voluntary code of practice on healthcare worker migration

The migration of health workers from the countries that invested in their training is another critical problem that requires an international solution. A global code of practice for the international recruitment of health personnel, adopted in 2010 (WHO 2010c), establishes voluntary principles, standards, and practices for the ethical international recruitment of health personnel in order to achieve a balance, in line with the principle of mutuality of benefits, between the rights, obligations, and expectations of source countries, destination countries, and migrant health personnel. Compliance with the code's voluntary principles remains to be determined.

Pandemic Influenza Preparedness Framework

In 2011, after nearly 6 years of intense negotiations, the World Health Assembly approved the Pandemic Influenza Preparedness Framework, which breaks new ground in preparing the world to respond to future influenza pandemics in more equitable ways (WHO 2011c). The framework sets out obligations for the sharing of information and materials relating to influenza viruses of pandemic potential, and of the resulting benefits, including medicines and vaccines, once a pandemic is underway. The Framework stipulates obligations for the WHO, its Member States, and WHO-appointed influenza laboratories, but also for the pharmaceutical industry, which eventually profits from the sharing of viruses when it manufactures influenza vaccines and antiviral medicines. For example, pharmaceutical companies contributed around $28 million in 2012 to support implementation of the Framework in areas such as improving laboratory and surveillance capacities and the acquisition of medical products. Industry will make additional contributions yearly. Implementation of the Framework is overseen by an independent group of experts, continuing the trend of independent monitoring as a new norm for international public health. Although negotiations were especially tense and difficult, the resulting instrument marks an important step forward in ensuring the more equitable distribution of medical products during international public health emergencies and finding a fair way to secure a new source of funding for building capacity in the developing world.

Prospects for additional treaties

Calls for additional treaties and conventions have been made for additional transnational threats to health and other urgent problems that depend on broad-based collaboration for their solution. In 2012, two intergovernmental processes were established to consider proposals for treaties aimed at protecting countries from trade in substandard and counterfeit medicines and generating financial support for research and development in new medical products for the neglected diseases of the poor. The results of initial meetings suggest reluctance by many countries to commit to the protracted and costly negotiations needed to reach agreement on treaties. The options do, however, remain open.

Essential medicines: strategies for improving access and innovation

The need to ensure access to safe, effective, quality-assured, and affordable medicines is a long-standing concern. The first Model List of Essential Medicines was issued in 1977 as a groundbreaking way to support countries in their efforts to rationalize procurement and prescribing practices and to focus limited purchasing power on medicines that meet the priority health needs of populations (WHO 2013b). The lists, which are updated every 2 years, are widely used in the developing world and also in some wealthy countries as the basis for insurance reimbursement schemes. Concern about equitable access peaked with the spread of AIDS—when effective antiretroviral treatments became available, and survival for many millions of patients often depended on their ability to pay. AIDS made inequitable access to medicines both highly visible and ethically unacceptable. The AIDS epidemic further demonstrated that price reductions were a feasible objective; the price of antiretroviral therapy dropped by nearly 99 per cent in less than a decade.

Better access to medical products, especially for the poor, is currently being pursued on two main fronts: reducing prices for existing products and developing new products for markets with limited purchasing power where there are few incentives for industry research and development. Financial support for the development of new medicines is largely generated by intellectual property rights and the patent regime, which protects high prices for originator products and delays the market entry of less expensive generics. Generic medicines, which do not need to recoup the considerable investments needed for drug discovery, development, and marketing approval, are sold at prices closer to the costs of manufacturing, offering a significant means to reduce healthcare costs in all countries. Policies that rationalize the purchasing and prescribing of medicines can be a major source of savings in any country. In many countries, a national policy that encourages the use of generic medicines can save an estimated 60 per cent of the costs of medicines (WHO 2010a).

The WHO Prequalification Programme also operates to improve access to quality, affordable medical products. It stimulates the supply of quality-assured medicines, including generics, and encourages fair competition (WHO 2013c). The Programme was established in 2001 and initially served as a mechanism to ensure that UN agencies, the GAVI Alliance, and the Global Fund get the best quality products at the best prices for use in health campaigns. The Programme has expanded from this initial purpose and now operates in ways that allow manufacturers from developing and emerging economies to enter the market and, when strict quality and safety standards are met, to compete with established manufacturers on an equal footing. This has resulted in more abundant and reliable supplies, better forecasting, and often substantial price reductions driven by added competition, changing the dynamics of the market for medicines and public health vaccines (WHO 2012g). The programme also contributes to globally harmonized quality standards and reduces the supply of substandard products. The strengthening of capacities, including the hands-on training of drug regulators, is a central component of the programme. Strong compliance mechanisms are in place and on-site inspections to ensure adherence to good manufacturing practices are repeated at regular intervals. Products can, and frequently do, get de-listed if quality is not maintained; the prospect of de-listing has proven to be a powerful incentive to maintain standards.

Another concern about the current patent regime is its bias towards commercially profitable products and its neglect of diseases that predominantly affect the poor. International efforts to correct the current incentive scheme that drives research and development, or at least compensate for its bias towards commercially lucrative products, have been underway for more than a decade, and featured strongly in the negotiations that eventually led to adoption of the Global Strategy and Plan of Action for Public Health, Innovation and Intellectual Property (WHO 2011d).

Public–private partnerships have emerged as a promising way to compensate for the bias inherent in the patent system. In the past, the quest for new products for neglected diseases has usually been opportunistic. Existing products, often developed for veterinary purposes, were screened for their potential efficacy in treating human diseases. More recently, this process has become strategic. An unmet health need is identified, an ideal product is defined, and a public–private partnership is formed to develop the product. These projects usually bring together expertise from academia, industry, and public health, with funding from philanthropic sources. Recent examples include the Medicines for Malaria Venture, the International AIDS Vaccine Initiative, the Global Alliance for TB Drug Development, the Drugs for Neglected Diseases Initiative, and funding from the Bill and Melinda Gates Foundation to develop a malaria vaccine.

This positive trend continues to evolve. For example, the Meningitis Vaccine Project illustrates the many ancillary benefits that can accrue when a product is designed with the needs of very poor countries in mind (Meningitis Vaccine Project n.d.). African ministers of health asked for a new vaccine that could prevent almost yearly epidemics in the 26 countries that form Africa's Meningitis Belt, and defined its ideal characteristics, including a price they could afford to pay. The project required collaboration with several commercial companies, and broke new ground in the management of intellectual property rights. The technology for producing a conjugate vaccine was transferred from the United States and the Netherlands to the Serum Institute of India, which agreed to manufacture the vaccine at the target price of 50 cents per dose. In less than a decade, the new vaccine was developed by a consortium of scientists, licensed with support from Canada's regulatory authority, and prequalified by the WHO. The vaccine protects very young children, confers immunity that may last a decade, and contributes to herd immunity. The first campaigns using the new vaccine began in late 2011; more than 100 million doses had been administered by the end of 2012. Following these campaigns, some hyperendemic countries have recorded their lowest level of meningitis cases in more than a decade. The economic benefits are expected to be significant. A single case of meningitis can cost a household the equivalent of 3–4 months of income. Mounting a reactive emergency response to epidemics can absorb more than 5 per cent of a country's entire health budget. The project is groundbreaking in another sense. African countries usually have to wait years, if not decades, for new medical technologies to trickle into their health systems. In this case,

Africa was first to receive the best technology that the world, working together, could offer.

The most ambitious initiative thus far to promote innovation for neglected diseases followed the 2012 publication of a report, commissioned by WHO Member States, which proposed mechanisms for research and development (R&D) financing and coordination that could provide a sustainable solution (WHO 2012h). An intergovernmental process was established to take forward the report's recommendations and proposals in the three broad areas of monitoring R&D flows, the coordination of R&D, and finding new, innovative, and sustainable sources of funding. The substance and form of an international agreement is currently being debated. Proposals include establishing an R&D observatory, setting up a funding instrument that pools funds at the international level, and starting negotiations on an international treaty that would commit governments to spend at least 0.01 per cent of GDP on R&D to develop new products for diseases that mainly affect developing countries.

Universal health coverage

One of the strongest signs of continuing commitment to better health comes from the number of countries that are adopting policies to extend health coverage to all their citizens. Following the publication of the World Health Report 2010, *Health Systems Financing: The Path to Universal Health Coverage* (WHO 2010a), more than 70 low- and middle-income countries have requested the WHO's technical assistance in planning strategies to move towards universal coverage. Universal health coverage is arguably the single most powerful concept that public health has to offer. It is an effective social equalizer, the ultimate expression of fairness, and one of the best ways to cement the remarkable gains made during the first decade of the twenty-first century. Universal health coverage is also a unifying concept that draws together the many factors, from access to essential medicines and social protection schemes, to preventive as well as curative care, that together ultimately influence health outcomes. As studies show, universal coverage improves the efficiency of service delivery, leads to better health outcomes, and has been effectively supported by a range of health financing reforms in several lower income countries. When countries move towards universal coverage, the benefits of interventions, when taken to scale, are value-added. They not only protect health or prevent a disease, but also bring down the risks for entire populations. In addition, economists point to considerable economies of scale in service provision when interventions reach a large proportion of the population (Sachs 2012).

Universal health coverage does, however, carry some risks. One important caveat is that there is no 'one-size-fits-all' solution. No single mix of policy options is right for every country; any effective strategy must be home-grown.

Further, when public services are free, overconsumption of healthcare is possible, especially by the rich, even though their needs may be less than those of the poor. And although removing financial barriers does help the poor obtain care, it does not guarantee it. Financial barriers, such as those incurred by transportation and accommodation costs to obtain treatment, may still exist.

Finally, improving efficiency is imperative to avoid incurring unsustainable costs. The main sources of inefficiency lie in the areas of medicines (costs, inappropriate and ineffective use, underuse of generics, use of substandard and counterfeit medicines, etc.);

healthcare products and services; human resources (inappropriate or costly mix of staff, problems with recruitment, inadequate salaries); hospitals (inappropriate admissions and length of stay, too many or too few hospitals and inpatient beds); medical errors; waste, corruption, and fraud; and inappropriate balance between levels of care or between prevention, promotion, and treatment. Sustaining universal coverage requires finding the most efficient ways to meet demands for health services (WHO 2010a).

Some commentators have described the growing prominence in health policies of universal coverage as the third great transition in health, following the demographic transition that began in the late eighteenth century and the epidemiological transition that began in the twentieth century. Many argue that universal coverage should be included as a goal in the post-2015 development agenda.

Conclusion

The landscape of public health in the twenty-first century is complex, challenging, and overcrowded. Some problems arise from the explosive growth of assistance for health development that followed commitment to the health-related MDGs. Others arise from universal trends generated by the world's radically increased interdependence. All around the world, health is being shaped by the same powerful forces, blurring the distinctions between wealthy and developing countries. Solutions need to be found that work internationally as well as within countries or regional groups of countries. Inequality is growing, resulting in demands that equity be included as an explicit objective in the policies of health and other sectors. Foremost among the new challenges to health is the growing prevalence of chronic NCDs, which have overtaken infectious diseases as the leading cause of mortality worldwide. Responding to these diseases will require transformational changes in the way public health is conceived and delivered. It will also require new strategies for addressing risk factors that reside in sectors beyond the purview of health officials. Developments in tobacco legislation reveal the promise of regulatory solutions, especially for transnational threats to health; they also show that collaboration, in the name of health, among multiple sectors is entirely feasible.

Although worldwide financial uncertainty may appear to put at risk the future of financing for health development, several recent initiatives suggest that the momentum for better health has not faltered and that innovative ways will be found to reach more people with better services at lower costs. The prominence of universal health coverage in policy debates demonstrates the priority being given to fairness, as do efforts to find financing to develop new medicines for diseases of the poor. Recent agreement on several instruments for global health governance, also in areas where public health concerns cross purposes with powerful economic interests, further signals a continuing high-level commitment to health. The establishment of independent mechanisms for ensuring accountability can potentially increase confidence that money is being spent wisely and with good effect.

Public health alone cannot fundamentally change the way the world works. But public health can and should continue to be a powerful driver of positive change that dramatically improves the health and lives of populations across the planet. The WHO takes the firm view that the best days for public health do not lie in the past, but in the future.

References

Anand, S. and Barnighausen, T. (2004). Human resources and health outcomes: cross-country econometric study. *The Lancet*, 364(9445), 1603–9.

Anand, S. and Barnighausen, T. (2007). Health workers and vaccination coverage in developing countries: an econometric analysis. *The Lancet*, 369(9569), 1277–85.

Arita, I., Nakane, M., and Fenner, F. (2006). Is polio eradication realistic? *Science*, 312(5775), 852–4.

Attaran, A., Barry, D., Basheer, S., et al. (2012). How to achieve international action on falsified and substandard medicines. *BMJ*, 345, e7381.

Atun, F.A., Bennet, S., and Duran, A. (2008). *When do Vertical (Stand-Alone) Programmes Have a Place in Health Systems?* Copenhagen: WHO Regional Office for Europe. Available at: http://www.who.int/management/district/services/WhenDo VerticalProgrammesPlaceHealthSystems.pdf.

Barceló, A., Aedo, C., Rajpathak, S., et al. (2003). The cost of diabetes in Latin America and the Caribbean. *Bulletin of the World Health Organization*, 81(1), 19–27.

Bermingham, A., Chand, M.A., Brown, C.S., et al. (2012). Severe respiratory illness caused by a novel coronavirus, in a patient transferred to the United Kingdom from the Middle East, September 2012. *Euro Surveillance*, 17(40), 20290.

Blas, E. and Sivasankara Kurup, A. (2010). *Equity, Social Determinants and Public Health Programmes*. Geneva: WHO. Available at: http://whqlib-doc.who.int/publications/2010/9789241563970_eng.pdf.

Boekelheide, K., Blumberg, B., Chapin, R.E., et al. (2012). Predicting later-life outcomes of early-life exposures. *Environmental Health Perspectives*, 120(10), 1353–61.

Brownell, K.D. and Warner, K.E. (2009). The perils of ignoring history: Big Tobacco played dirty and millions died. How similar is Big Food? *Milbank Quarterly*, 87(1), 259–94.

Cairns, G., Angus, K., and Hastings, G. (2009). *The Extent, Nature and Effects of Food Promotion to Children: A Review of the Evidence to December 2008*. Geneva: WHO. Available at: http://www.who.int/diet-physicalactivity/Evidence_Update_2009.pdf.

Carrera, C., Azrack, A., Begkoyian, G., et al. (2012). The comparative cost-effectiveness of an equity-focused approach to child survival, health, and nutrition: a modelling approach. *The Lancet*, 380, 1341–51.

Centers for Disease Control and Prevention (2012). *Press Briefing Transcript. CDC, FDA, Massachusetts Department of Public Health. Joint Telebriefing Updating Investigation of Meningitis Outbreak.* [Online] Available at: http://www.cdc.gov/media/releases/2012/t1011_meningitis_outbreak.html.

Chan, M. (2008). Return to Alma-Ata. *The Lancet*, 372(9642), 866–7.

Cockburn, R., Newton, P.N., Agyarko, E.K., Akunyili, D., and White, J.H. (2005). The global threat of counterfeit drugs: why industry and governments must communicate the dangers. *PLoS Medicine*, 2(4), e100.

De Ruyter, J.C., Olthof, M.R., Seidell, J.C., and Katan, M.B. (2012). A train of sugar-free or sugar-sweetened beverages and body weight in children. *The New England Journal of Medicine*, 367(15), 1397–406.

Ebbeling, C.B., Feldman, H.A., Chomitz, V.R., et al. (2012). A randomized trial of sugar-sweetened beverages and adolescent body weight. *The New England Journal of Medicine*, 367(15), 1407–16.

Every Woman, Every Child (n.d.). Website. [Online] Available at: http://www.everywomaneverychild.org/.

Food and Agriculture Organization of the United Nations (2012). *FAO Food Price Index up 1.4 Percent in September*. [Online] Available at: http://www.fao.org/news/story/en/item/161602/icode/.

Gao, R., Cao, B., Hu, Y., et al. (2013). Human infection with a novel avian-origin influenza A (H7N9) virus. *The New England Journal of Medicine*, 368, 1888–97.

Global Health Workforce Alliance (n.d.). Website. [Online] Available at: http://www.who.int/workforcealliance/about/en/.

Gurria, A. (2011). *Remarks by OECD Secretary-General delivered at the launch of Divided we stand: why inequality keeps rising*. Paris: OECD. http://www.oecd.org/els/soc/dividedwestandwhyinequalitykeepsrising speech.htm

Hastings, G., Stead, M., McDermott, L., et al. (2003). *Review of the Research on the Effects of Food Promotion to Children*. Glasgow: University of Strathclyde, Centre for Social Marketing. Available at: http://www.food.gov.uk/news/newsarchive/2003/sep/promote.

Independent Expert Review Group on Information and Accountability for Women's and Children's Health (2012). *Every Woman, Every Child: From Commitments to Action: The First Report of the Independent Expert Review Group (iERG) on Information and Accountability for Women's and Children's Health*. Geneva: WHO. Available at: http://www.who.int/woman_child_accountability/ierg/reports/2012/IERG_report_low_resolution.pdf.

Independent Monitoring Board of the Global Polio Eradication Initiative (2012). *June 2012 Report: Every Missed Child*. [Online] Available at: http://www.polioeradication.org/Aboutus/Governance/IndependentMonitoringBoard/Reports.aspx.

Independent Monitoring Board of the Global Polio Eradication Initiative (2012). *Polio's Last Stand? Report of the Independent Monitoring Board of the Global Polio Eradication Initiative*. [Online] Available at: http://www.polioeradication.org/Portals/0/Document/Aboutus/Governance/IMB/7IMBMeeting/7IMB_Report_EN.pdf.

International Baby Food Action Network (2010). *Breaking the Rules—Stretching the Rules*. Penang: International Baby Food Action Network International Code Documentation Centre.

International Health Partnership and Related Initiatives (IHP+). (2012). *IHP+ Core Team Report May 2011–April 2012*. [Online] Available at: http://www.internationalhealthpartnership.net/fileadmin/uploads/ihp/Documents/About_IHP_/mgt_arrangemts___docs/core_team_report2011_2012WEB_EN.pdf

International Health Partnership and Related Initiatives (n.d.). Website. [Online] Available at: http://www.internationalhealthpartnership.net/en/about-ihp/.

McGinnis, J.M., Gootman, J.A., and Kraak, V.I. (eds.) (2006). *Food Marketing to Children and Youth: Threat or Opportunity?* Washington, DC: Institute of Medicine, National Academies Press. Available at: http://www.nap.edu/catalog.php?record_id=11514#toc.

Meningitis Vaccine Project (n.d.). Website. [Online] Available at: http://www.meningvax.org/.

Mullan, F., Frehzwot, S., Omaswa, F., et al. (2011). Medical schools in sub-Saharan Africa. *The Lancet*, 377, 1113–21.

Narasimhan, V., Brown, H., Pablos-Mendez, A., et al. (2004). Responding to the global human resources crisis. *The Lancet*, 363(9419), 1469–72.

Nayyar, G., Breman, J., Newton, P.N., and Herrington, J. (2012). Poor-quality antimalarial drugs in southeast Asia and sub-Saharan Africa. *The Lancet Infectious Diseases*, 12(6), 488–96.

Nordmann, P., Poirel, L., Walsh, T.R., and Livermore, D.M. (2011). The emerging NDM carbapenemases. *Trends in Microbiology*, 19, 588–95.

Ogata, S. and Sen, A. (2009) *Human Security Now. Protecting and Empowering People. United Nations Commission on Human Security, Final report*. New York: UN. Available at: http://www.unocha.org/humansecurity/human-security-now.

Ong, A.K. and Heymann, D.L. (2007). Microbes and humans: the long dance. *Bulletin of the World Health Organization*, 85, 422–3.

Organisation for Economic Co-operation and Development (2005). *Paris Declaration on Aid Effectiveness*. Paris: OECD. Available at: http://www.oecd.org/development/effectiveness/34428351.pdf.

Organisation for Economic Co-operation and Development (2008). *Accra Agenda for Action*. Paris: OECD. Available at: http://www.oecd.org/development/effectiveness/34428351.pdf.

Organisation for Economic Co-operation and Development (2011a). *Divided We Stand: Why Inequality Keeps Rising*. Paris: OECD.

Available at: http://www.oecd.org/els/soc/dividedwestandwhyine qualitykeepsrising.htm.

Organisation for Economic Co-operation and Development (2011b). *Fourth High Level Forum on Aid Effectiveness, Busan. The Busan Partnership Agreement*. Paris: OECD. Available at: http://www.oecd.org/dac/effec tiveness/49650173.pdf.

Postigo, A., Haines, A., Neira, M., and Confalonieri, U. (2007). Will increased awareness of the health impacts of climate change help in achieving international collective action? *Bulletin of the World Health Organization*, 85(11), 826–8.

Qibin, Q., Chu, A.Y., Kang, J.H., et al. (2012). Sugar-sweetened beverages and genetic risk of obesity. *The New England Journal of Medicine*, 367(15), 1387–96.

Sachs, J.D. (2012). Achieving universal health coverage in low-income settings. *The Lancet*, 380(9845), 944–7.

Sen, A. (1999). *Development as Freedom*. Oxford: Oxford University Press.

The Global Polio Eradication Initiative (n.d.). *Independent Monitoring Board*. [Online] Available at: http://www.polioeradication.org/ Aboutus/Governance/IndependentMonitoringBoard.aspx.

The Lancet (2009). Editorial: who runs global health? *The Lancet*, 373, 2083.

The Lancet (2012). *Global Burden of Disease Study 2010*. [Online] Available at: http://www.thelancet.com/themed/global-burden-of-disease.

United Nations (2000). *United Nations Millennium Declaration (United Nations General Assembly Resolution 55/2)*. New York: UN. Available at: http://www.un.org/millennium/declaration/ares552e.pdf.

United Nations (2013). *The Millennium Development Goals Report*. New York: UN. Available at: http://www.un.org/millenniumgoals/ pdf/report-2013/mdg-report-2013-english.pdf.

United Nations Children's Fund (2012). *Levels and Trends in Child Mortality. Report 2012: Estimates Developed by the UN Inter-agency Group for Child Mortality Estimation*. New York: United Nations Children's Fund. Available at: http://www.unicef.org/videoaudio/ PDFs/UNICEF_2012_child_mortality_for_web_0904.pdf.

United Nations Department of Economic and Social Affairs (2012a). *World Population Prospects: The 2012 Revision*. New York: UN. Available at: http://esa.un.org/wpp/.

United Nations Department of Economic and Social Affairs (2012b). *Probabilistic Population Projections*. New York: UN. Available at: http://esa.un.org/unpd/ppp/Figures-Output/Population/ PPP_Total-Population.htm.

United Nations Department of Economic and Social Affairs (2012c). *World Urbanization Prospects: The 2012 Revision*. New York: UN. Available at: http://esa.un.org/wpp/wpp2012/wpp2012_1.htm.

Vujicic, M., Zurn, P., Diallo, K., Adams, O., and Dal Poz, M. (2004). The role of wages in the migration of health care professionals from developing countries. *Human Resources for Health*, 2(1), 3.

WHO Framework Convention on Tobacco Control (2012). *Global Progress Report on Implementation of the WHO Framework Convention on Tobacco Control*. Geneva: WHO. Available at: http://www.who.int/ fctc/reporting/summary_analysis/en/index.html.

WHO Framework Convention on Tobacco Control (2013). *Protocol to Eliminate Illicit Trade in Tobacco Products*. Geneva: WHO. Available at: http://apps.who.int/iris/bitstream/10665/80873/1/9789241505246_ eng.pdf.

World Health Organization (2005). Constitution of the World Health Organization. Geneva: WHO. Available at: http://apps.who.int/gb/bd/ PDF/bd47/EN/constitution-en.pdf?ua=1.

World Health Organization (2006). *The World Health Report 2006: Working Together for Health*. Geneva: WHO. Available at: http://www.who.int/ whr/2006/en/.

World Health Organization (2008a). *Commission on Social Determinants of Health. Closing the Gap in a Generation: Health Equity Through Action on the Social Determinants of Health*. Geneva: WHO. Available at: http://www.who.int/social_determinants/thecommission/final-report/en/index.html.

World Health Organization (2008b). *Protecting Health from Climate Change—World Health Day 2008*. Geneva: WHO. Available at: http:// www.who.int/world-health-day/previous/2008/en/index.html.

World Health Organization (2008c). *International Health Regulations (2005)* (2nd ed.). Geneva: WHO. Available at: http://whqlibdoc.who. int/publications/2008/9789241580410_eng.pdf.

World Health Organization (2010a). *The World Health Report 2010. Health Systems Financing: The Path to Universal Coverage*. Geneva: WHO. Available at: http://www.who.int/whr/2010/en/index.html.

World Health Organization (2010b). *Hidden Cities: Unmasking and Overcoming Health Inequities in Urban Settings*. Geneva: WHO. Available at: http://www.hiddencities.org/.

World Health Organization (2010c). *Global Code of Practice on the International Recruitment of Health Personnel*. Geneva: WHO. Available at: http://www.who.int/hrh/migration/code/practice/en/.

World Health Organization (2011a). *Global Status Report on Noncommunicable Diseases 2010*. Geneva: WHO.

World Health Organization (2011b). *Global Health Sector Strategy on HIV/ AIDS 2011–2015*. Geneva: WHO. Available at: http://whqlibdoc.who. int/publications/2011/9789241501651_eng.pdf.

World Health Organization (2011c). *Pandemic Influenza Preparedness Framework for the Sharing of Influenza Viruses and Access to Vaccines and Other Benefits*. Geneva: WHO. Available at: http://www.who.int/ influenza/pip/en/.

World Health Organization (2011d). *Global Strategy and Plan of Action on Public Health, Innovation and Intellectual Property*. Geneva: WHO. Available at: http://www.who.int/phi/publications/Global_Strategy_ Plan_Action.pdf.

World Health Organization (2012a). *Monitoring the Achievement of the Health-Related Millennium Development Goals*. Executive Board document 132/11. Geneva: WHO. Available at: http://apps.who.int/ gb/e/e_eb132.html.

World Health Organization (2012b). *Trends in Maternal Mortality: 1990 to 2010. WHO, UNICEF, UNFPA and The World Bank estimates*. Available at: http://www.who.int/reproductivehealth/publications/ monitoring/9789241503631/en/index.html.

World Health Organization (2012c). *Every Woman, Every Child: from Commitments to Action. The First Report of the Independent Expert Review Group on Information and Accountability for Women's and Children's Health*. Geneva: WHO. Available at: http://www.who. int/woman_child_accountability/ierg/reports/2012/en/index. html.

World Health Organization (2012d). *World Health Day 2012: Good Health Adds Life to Years. Global Brief*. Geneva: WHO. Available at: http:// www.who.int/world-health-day/2012/en/.

World Health Organization (2012e). *Global Tuberculosis Report 2012*. Geneva: WHO. Available at: http://www.who.int/tb/publications/ global_report/en/.

World Health Organization (2012f). *Information Exchange System. Alert No. 125. Contaminated Isotab (Isosorbide Mononitrate) Incident in Lahore Pakistan*. [Online] Available at: http://www.who.int/medicines/publications/drugalerts/DrugSafetyAlert125.pdf.

World Health Organization (2012g). *The Strategic Use of Antiretrovirals to Help End the HIV Epidemic*. Geneva: WHO. http://apps.who.int/iris/ bitstream/10665/75184/1/9789241503921_eng.pdf.

World Health Organization (2012h). *Accelerating Work to Overcome the Global Impact of Neglected Tropical Diseases: A Roadmap for Implementation*. Geneva: WHO. Available at: http://www.who.int/ neglected_diseases/NTD_RoadMap_2012_Fullversion.pdf.

World Health Organization (2013a). *Noncommunicable Diseases: Fact Sheet*. [Online] Available at: http://www.who.int/mediacentre/ factsheets/fs355/en/.

World Health Organization (2013b). *WHO Model Lists of Essential Medicines*. [Online] Available at: http://www.who.int/medicines/ publications/essentialmedicines/en/index.html.

World Health Organization (2013c). *Prequalification of Medicine by WHO: Fact Sheet*. [Online] Available at: http://www.who.int/media-centre/factsheets/fs278/en/index.html.

World Health Organization (n.d. a). *Global Health Observatory*. [Online] Available at: http://www.who.int/gho/en/.

World Health Organization (n.d. b). *General Information on Counterfeit Medicines*. [Online] Available at: http://www.who.int/medicines/services/counterfeit/overview/en/index1.html.

World Health Organization (n.d. c). *Onchocerciasis Control Programme (OCP)*. [Online] Available at: http://www.who.int/blindness/partnerships/onchocerciasis_OCP/en/.

World Health Organization (n.d. d). *Accountability Commission for Health of Women and Children*. [Online] Available at: http://www.who.int/topics/millennium_development_goals/accountability_commission/en/.

World Health Organization and the World Economic Forum (2011). *From Burden to 'Best Buys': Reducing the Economic Impact of NCDs in Low- and Middle-Income Countries*. Geneva: WHO. Available at: http://www.who.int/nmh/publications/best_buys_summary/en/.

World Health Organization Centre for Health Development (n.d.). Website. [Online] Available at: http://www.who.int/kobe_centre/en/.

World Health Organization Maximizing Positive Synergies Group (2009). An assessment of interactions between global health initiatives and country health systems. *The Lancet*, 373, 2137–69.

Yoon, K.-H., Lee, J.-H., Kim, J.-W., Cho, J.H., and Choi, Y.-H. (2006). Epidemic obesity and type 2 diabetes in Asia. *The Lancet*, 368, 1681–8.

Zhang, P., Zhang, X., Brown, J., et al. (2010). Global healthcare expenditure on diabetes for 2010 and 2030. *Diabetes Research and Clinical Practice*, 87, 293–301.

Index

Page numbers in **bold** refer to main sections of the text. Page numbers in *italic* refer to figures, tables and boxes.

Since the major subject of this title is public health, entries under this keyword have been kept to a minimum, and readers are advised to seek more specific references.

Indexing style
Alphabetical order. This index is in letter-by-letter order, whereby hyphens, en-rules and spaces within index headings are ignored in the alphabetization.

Main abbreviations used
AIDS acquired immune deficiency syndrome
ANOVA analysis of variance
BMI body mass index
CJD Creutzfeldt–Jakob disease
COPD chronic obstructive pulmonary disease
HIV human immunodeficiency virus
SARS severe acute respiratory syndrome
STIs sexually transmitted infections

Other abbreviations are defined in the index
1000 Genomes Project 555